ARTHRITIS AND ALLIED CONDITIONS

A Textbook of Rheumatology

ARTHRITIS AND ALLIED CONDITIONS
A Textbook of Rheumatology

Daniel J. McCarty, M.D.

Will and Cava Ross Professor and Chairman
Department of Medicine
The Medical College of Wisconsin
Milwaukee, Wisconsin

Foreword By
Joseph Lee Hollander, M.D.

Tenth Edition

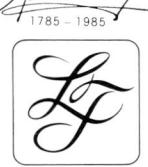

Lea & Febiger   1985   Philadelphia

Lea & Febiger
600 Washington Square
Philadelphia, Pennsylvania 19106–4198
U.S.A.
(215) 922-1330

First Edition, 1940
Second Edition, 1941
Third Edition, 1944
Fourth Edition, 1949
Fifth Edition, 1953
Sixth Edition, 1960
Seventh Edition, 1966
Eighth Edition, 1972
Ninth Edition, 1979
Tenth Edition, 1985

Library of Congress Cataloging in Publication Data

Main entry under title:

Arthritis and allied conditions.

  Includes bibliographies and index.
  1. Arthritis. 2. Rheumatism. I. McCarty, Daniel J.
[DNLM: 1. Arthritis. WE 344 A7866]
RC933.A64 1984   616.7′22   84-9748
ISBN 0-8121-0925-2

PRINTED IN THE UNITED STATES OF AMERICA

Print Number   3   2   1

Foreword

About 45 years ago my friend and former teacher, Dr. Bernard I. Comroe, started writing *Arthritis and Allied Conditions*. Realizing the need for a comprehensive textbook on rheumatic diseases, he gathered much from the literature and excerpted data from the *Rheumatism Reviews* and his own voluminous notes to produce the first edition, which appeared in 1940. The book was well received, and he produced a second and a third edition before his untimely death in 1945.

Dr. O.H. Perry Pepper, who had helped and encouraged Dr. Comroe in his efforts, convinced me that I should take on the awesome task of carrying on this project as a memorial to our mutual friend. Even in 1947, when I undertook the job, I realized that I could not keep the volume up-to-date by my own efforts, as the field was growing rapidly. A group of my colleagues in rheumatology, many of whom had worked together in the Army Arthritis Centers during World War II, were persuaded to join me in a collaborative effort, each being responsible for chapters covering portions of the field of rheumatology most familiar to him.

The fourth edition appeared in 1949, and the fifth edition in 1953, each with a Foreword by Dr. O.H. Perry Pepper. The sixth edition came out in 1960 after Dr. Pepper had died; therefore, Dr. Russell L. Cecil was kind enough to write an introductory Foreword. Regrettably, he did not survive to repeat for the seventh edition in 1966, so Dr. Robert M. Stecher did the honors, and also rewrote his introductory Foreword for the eighth edition. Bob Stecher died just before that edition came out in 1972. Then, for the ninth edition, I was asked to assume this apparently lethal task on becoming Editor Emeritus, and have survived to repeat for this tenth edition.

Editors of this textbook have come and gone, and contributors also have come and gone, but the arthritis compendium that was started by Dr. Comroe 45 years ago has continued to grow in size and in number of contributors, in complexity, and in popularity throughout the world. *Arthritis and Allied Conditions* has become accepted as the standard text in rheumatology almost everywhere. A number of other books, some of which are excellent, on clinical rheumatology or on other aspects of the field, have recently appeared. This volume, however, remains the nearest approach to an encyclopedia of rheumatology as well as the most widely sold and longest established text.

The five editions edited by me covered the major growth years of rheumatology from 1947 to 1972: from infancy to maturity. When asked why I have retired as editor, I have replied that my predecessor, Dr. Comroe, died after producing three editions. The editor of the British *Textbook of the Rheumatic Diseases,* Dr. Will Copeman, died after producing four editions of his book. After producing five editions of *Arthritis and Allied Conditions,* I felt I should quit while I was still ahead!

As it became evident to all who read the ninth edition, the new editor is extremely capable by training, research background, and editorial experience not only to carry on, but to improve the standard of excellence Dr. Comroe and I tried to achieve. Daniel J. McCarty has held the esteem of rheumatologists all over the world by his research, particularly on crystal-induced synovitis. He was editor of the journal *Arthritis & Rheumatism* for five years. He was associate editor of *Arthritis and Allied Conditions* for the eighth edition and was editor of the ninth and now this tenth edition. His clarity of thought and expression have made a book that Bernie Comroe would have been proud of, and one that is most gratifying to me. Its great success deserved repetition.

Joseph Lee Hollander, M.D.

Preface

The gold cover adorning this, the tenth edition of *Arthritis and Allied Conditions—A Textbook of Rheumatology*, symbolizes the current status of this clinical discipline. I have collected and perused its nine predecessors which faithfully record the evolution of rheumatology over the past 45 years. The enormous impact of modern science, coupled with clinical observations, controlled therapeutic trials, and epidemiologic studies, has catapulted rheumatology into a position analogous to older fields such as cardiology, gastroenterology, and infectious diseases. And just in time! The aging populations of the developed countries will need and expect the high level of care that is now available. They will also live with hope for future advances through research—a hope that we certainly share.

This book represents a synthesis of the current science and art of medicine as it exists in North America. It is an American book written entirely by scholars whose work has earned the respect of their peers. All authors are engaged in clinical and/or bench research, and patient care in our best teaching hospitals. We have not forgotten our colleagues in the developing nations. Thus, conditions such as rheumatic fever, now most unusual in the United States but still an enormous problem elsewhere in the world, are discussed fully.

The organization of this volume evolved from that used so successfully in the past. I have attempted to avoid overlap between chapters as much as possible with the idea that failure to present a comprehensive view of the field in a single volume represents editorial failure. To *edit* means to delete, not add!

Unlike the preceding nine editions, the references in this volume include titles and complete pagination to better identify the source of the author's statements, and the index has been greatly expanded. Thus, in addition to our goal of easy readability, the original literature is readily at hand for the reader who wishes to dig more deeply into a given problem.

The content of the 88 chapters that appeared in the ninth edition has been updated, and most have been completely rewritten. Sixteen new chapters have been added. That six of these are in the section on the Scientific Basis for the Study of the Rheumatic Diseases reflects the expanding role of science. New chapters relating to the biology of synoviocytes, chondrocytes, and platelets and to new knowledge of neutrophil chemotaxis, arachidonic acid metabolites, and clinical immunogenetics have been added. A chapter on computerized tomography as applied to rheumatic diseases reflects the rapid progress made in this area in recent years. The increasingly important role of nonphysician members of the health care team in caring for patients with arthritis and allied conditions has been recognized by a comprehensive chapter on the role of nurses and allied health professionals in both treatment and patient education, authored by a nurse who has been a pioneer in this area.

Newly discovered conditions such as lyme arthritis and basic calcium phosphate crystal deposition disease have been addressed in new chapters. Lastly, a chapter has been devoted to the common and vexing arthritis developing in the temporomandibular joint. It is written by dental surgeons with great personal experience in this field.

The chapter on synovial fluid analysis encompasses the many new practical techniques needed for modern differential diagnosis of arthritis. The chapter on clinical assessment of arthritis, written by a master in this field, discusses up-to-date data strategies for the conduct and assessment of the controlled drug trials so important in defining clinical treatment of the various rheumatic diseases. The chapter on radiology includes an assessment of possible uses of nuclear magnetic resonance and newer techniques for determination of bone density. The organ physiology of the joint, so vital in understanding basic treatment of arthritis with appropriate rest, exercise, and physical modalities, has been written by a clinical scholar whose concepts have revolutionized our perceptions. The new chapter on arachidonic metabolites, potent mediators of inflammation, sets the stage for the chapter on the pharmacology and practical use of the many nonsteroidal inflammatory drugs now available.

As in the ninth edition, an entire section is devoted to empirical therapy, which is still the mainstay in rheumatology. Specific therapy for gout and infectious arthritis is discussed in the chapters devoted to those diseases. An entire section comprising 16 chapters is devoted to rheumatoid arthritis, the condition that occupies fully one-half the effort of the practicing clinical rheumatologist.

I have not devoted much text to areas where real knowledge is "soft," such as the effects of weather or diet on arthritis.

The choice of topics and emphasis on each reflect the experience of your Editor, who has been involved in the direct personal care of patients with arthritis and allied conditions for the past 25 years.

I am deeply grateful to the many contributors who unselfishly devoted their time and energy to record their own experiences and to critically review the recorded experiences of others. I am also grateful to their hardworking secretaries who typed their chapters. I particularly wish to thank my own secretary, Jane Alexander, who labored long and hard in the vineyard toward the birth of this tenth edition. I am planning to completely revise this volume every six years to keep pace with the advances in the art and science of rheumatology.

Daniel J. McCarty, M.D.
Milwaukee, Wisconsin

In Memoriam
Edward C. Franklin, M.D.
Carl M. Pearson, M.D.
Gerald P. Rodnan, M.D.

Contributors

FRANK C. ARNETT, M.D.
Professor of Medicine
Head, Rheumatology Division
University of Texas School of Medicine
Houston, Texas

JOHN BAUM, M.D.
Professor of Medicine and Pediatrics
Professor of Preventive, Rehabilitation, and Family
  Medicine
University of Rochester School of Medicine and
  Dentistry
Director, Pediatric Arthritis Clinic
Strong Memorial Hospital
Director, Arthritis and Clinical Immunology Unit
Monroe Community Hospital
Rochester, New York

J. CLAUDE BENNETT, M.D.
Professor and Chairman
Department of Medicine
University of Alabama
Physician-in-Chief
University of Alabama Hospitals
Birmingham, Alabama

ROBERT M. BENNETT, M.D.
Professor of Medicine
Head, Division of Arthritis and Rheumatic Diseases
Oregon Health Sciences University
Portland, Oregon

RODNEY BLUESTONE, M.D.
Clinical Professor of Medicine
University of California
Los Angeles, California

KENNETH D. BRANDT, M.D.
Professor of Medicine
Chief, Rheumatology Division
Indiana University School of Medicine
Attending Physician
Indiana University Hospital
Indiana University Medical Center
Consulting Physician
Richard L. Roudebush Veterans Administration Medical
  Center
Indianapolis, Indiana

BRUCE J. BREWER, M.D.
Professor and Acting Chairman
Department of Orthopaedic Surgery
Medical College of Wisconsin
Senior Attending Staff
Milwaukee County Medical Complex
Milwaukee Children's Hospital
Lutheran Hospital of Milwaukee (Good Samaritan Med-
  ical Center)
Milwaukee, Wisconsin

W. WATSON BUCHANAN, M.D.
Professor of Medicine
Regional Coordinator of Rheumatology
Health Sciences Centre
McMaster University
Chedake–McMaster Hospitals
Hamilton, Ontario
Canada

ROBERT B. BUCKINGHAM, M.D.
Clinical Associate Professor of Medicine
University of Pittsburgh School of Medicine
Co-Chief, Division of Rheumatology
The Western Pennsylvania Hospital
Pittsburgh, Pennsylvania
Attending Physician
The Western Pennsylvania Hospital
Presbyterian University Hospital
St. Margarets Memorial Hospital
Pittsburgh, Pennsylvania

JOHN J. CALABRO, M.D.
Professor of Medicine and Pediatrics
University of Massachusetts Medical School
Director of Rheumatology
Saint Vincent Hospital
Worcester, Massachusetts

JUAN J. CANOSO, M.D.
Associate Professor of Medicine
Boston University School of Medicine
Chief, Rheumatology Section
Veterans Administration Medical Center
Boston, Massachusetts

GUILLERMO F. CARRERA, M.D.
Associate Professor of Radiology and Orthopaedic
  Surgery
The Medical College of Wisconsin
Chief of Diagnostic Radiology
Milwaukee Regional Medical Center
Milwaukee, Wisconsin

DENNIS A. CARSON, M.D.
Department of Basic and Clinical Research
Scripps Clinic and Research Foundation
La Jolla, California

JAMES J. CASTLES, M.D.
Professor of Internal Medicine (Rheumatology)
Associate Dean for Academic Affairs
University of California Davis Medical Center
Attending Physician
San Joaquin County General Hospital
Martinez Veterans Administration Hospital
Davis, California

C. WILLIAM CASTOR, M.D.
Professor of Internal Medicine
University of Michigan Medical School
Member, Rackham Arthritis Research Unit
Consultant, Ann Arbor Veterans Administration Hospital
Ann Arbor, Michigan

CHARLES L. CHRISTIAN, M.D.
Professor of Medicine
Cornell University Medical College
Physician-in-Chief
The Hospital for Special Surgery
Attending Physician
The New York Hospital
New York, New York

MACK L. CLAYTON, M.D.
Clinical Professor of Surgery
Associate Clinical Professor of Orthopedic Surgery
University of Colorado
Attending Orthopedic Surgeon
St. Joseph Hospital and Rose Medical Center
Denver, Colorado

ALAN S. COHEN, M.D.
Conrad Wesselhoeft Professor of Medicine
Boston University School of Medicine
Director, Arthritis Center
Boston University Medical Center
Chief of Medicine and Director
Thorndike Memorial Laboratory
Boston City Hospital
Boston, Massachusetts

DOYT L. CONN, M.D.
Professor of Medicine
Mayo Medical School
Consultant, Rheumatology and Internal Medicine
Mayo Clinic and Mayo Foundation
Rochester, Minnesota

MARY CRONIN, M.D.
Medical Staff Fellow
Arthritis and Rheumatism Branch
National Institute of Arthritis, Diabetes, Digestive and
  Kidney Diseases
Bethesda, Maryland

BRUCE N. CRONSTEIN, M.D.
Instructor in Experimental Medicine
New York University Medical Center
Clinical Assistant Attending Physician
Bellevue Hospital
Assistant in Medicine
University Hospital
New York, New York

JOHN L. DECKER, M.D.
Director, Warren Grant Magnuson Clinical Center
Associate Director for Clinical Care
National Institutes of Health
Bethesda, Maryland

JOSEPH DUFFY, M.D.
Assistant Professor of Medicine
Mayo Medical School and Mayo Clinic
Consultant, Rheumatology and Internal Medicine
Mayo Clinic and Mayo Foundation
Rochester, Minnesota

GEORGE EHRLICH, M.D.
Visiting Professor
New York University School of Medicine
New York, New York
Vice President
Ciba-Geigy Corporation
Pharmaceuticals Division
Summit, New Jersey

ANTHONY S. FAUCI, M.D.
Chief, Laboratory of Immunoregulation
National Institute of Allergy and Infectious Diseases
National Institutes of Health
Bethesda, Maryland

DOUGLAS T. FEARON, M.D.
Associate Professor of Medicine
Harvard Medical School
Rheumatologist and Immunologist
Brigham and Women's Hospital
Boston, Massachusetts

RICHARD H. FERGUSON, M.D.
Professor of Medicine
Mayo Medical School
Consultant, Rheumatology and Internal Medicine
Mayo Clinic and Mayo Foundation
Rochester, Minnesota

ADRIAN E. FLATT, M.D.
Clinical Professor of Orthopaedic Surgery
University of Texas Health Science Center at Dallas
(Southwestern Medical School)
Chief, Department of Orthopaedics
Baylor University Medical Center
Dallas, Texas

ROBERT I. FOX, M.D., Ph.D.
Department of Basic and Clinical Research
Scripps Clinic and Research Foundation
La Jolla, California

DANIEL E. FURST, M.D.
Associate Professor of Medicine and Rheumatology
University of Iowa Hospital and Clinics
Iowa City, Iowa

HARRY K. GENANT, M.D.
Professor of Radiology, Medicine, and Orthopaedic
  Surgery
Chief of Skeletal Section
Department of Radiology
University of California
San Francisco, California

MARK H. GINSBERG, M.D.
Associate Member
Department of Immunology and Division of
  Rheumatology
Scripps Clinic and Research Foundation
La Jolla, California

EDWARD J. GOETZL, M.D.
Professor of Medicine
University of California
Director, Division of Allergy and Immunology
Moffitt-Long Hospitals
University of California Medical Center
San Francisco, California

DON L. GOLDENBERG, M.D.
Associate Professor of Medicine
Clinical Program Director, Arthritis Center
Boston University School of Medicine
Associate Director, Department of Medicine
Boston City Hospital
Boston, Massachusetts

ELIOT A. GOLDINGS, M.D.
Assistant Professor of Internal Medicine
The Harold C. Simmons Arthritis Research Center
Southwestern Medical School
Attending Physician
Parkland Memorial Hospital
Dallas, Texas

IRA M. GOLDSTEIN, M.D.
Professor of Medicine
University of California
Chief, Division of Rheumatology
San Francisco General Hospital
San Francisco, California

BEVRA H. HAHN, M.D.
Professor of Medicine
Chief, Division of Rheumatology
UCLA School of Medicine
Los Angeles, California

PAUL HALVERSON, M.D.
Assistant Professor of Medicine
Medical College of Wisconsin
Attending Physician
St. Luke's Hospital
Milwaukee, Wisconsin

LOUIS A. HEALEY, M.D.
Clinical Professor of Medicine
University of Washington
Attending Physician
The Mason Clinic
Seattle, Washington

JOSEPH LEE HOLLANDER, M.D.
Emeritus Professor of Medicine
University of Pennsylvania School of Medicine
Consultant in Rheumatology
Childrens' Hospital, Pennsylvania Hospital, and
  Delaware County Memorial Hospital
Emeritus Chief, Rheumatology Section
Department of Medicine
Hospital of the University of Pennsylvania
Philadelphia, Pennsylvania

EDWARD W. HOLMES, M.D.
Professor of Medicine
Assistant Professor of Biochemistry
Chief, Division of Metabolism, Endocrinology, and
  Genetics
Duke University Medical Center
Durham, North Carolina

AUBREY J. HOUGH, JR., M.D.
Professor and Chairman
Department of Pathology
University of Arkansas for Medical Sciences
Little Rock, Arkansas

DAVID S. HOWELL, M.D.
Professor of Medicine
Director, Arthritis Division
University of Miami School of Medicine
Medical Investigator
Veterans Administration Medical Center
Miami, Florida

ALLAN E. INGLIS, M.D.
Professor of Clinical Surgery
Clinical Professor of Anatomy
Cornell University Medical College
Attending Orthopaedic Surgeon
The Hospital for Special Surgery and The New York
  Hospital
New York, New York

JOHN N. INSALL, M.D.
Professor of Orthopaedic Surgery
Cornell University Medical Center
Attending Orthopaedic Surgeon
The Hospital for Special Surgery and The New York
  Hospital
Chief of the Knee Service
The Hospital for Special Surgery
New York, New York

RUTH JACKSON, M.D.
Honorary Assistant Clinical Professor
Orthopaedic Surgery
University of Texas Health Science Center
Consultant in Orthopaedic Surgery
Baylor University Medical Center
Honorary Consultant in Orthopaedic Surgery
Parkland Memorial Hospital
Dallas, Texas

ISRAELI A. JAFFE, M.D.
Professor of Clinical Medicine
College of Physicians and Surgeons
Columbia University
Attending Physician
The Presbyterian Hospital
New York, New York

HUGO E. JASIN, M.D.
Professor of Internal Medicine
The Harold C. Simmons Arthritis Research Center
Southwestern Medical School
University of Texas Health Science Center
Senior Attending Physician
Parkland Memorial Hospital
Dallas, Texas

ROGER PAUL JOHNSON, M.D.
Professor of Orthopaedics
Medical College of Wisconsin
Senior Attending Staff
Milwaukee County Medical Complex
Froedtert Memorial Lutheran Hospital
Staff Physician
Milwaukee Children's Hospital
Elmbrook Memorial Hospital
Milwaukee, Wisconsin

JOHN PAUL JONES, JR., M.D.
Medical Research Director
Diagnostic Osteonecrosis Center and Research
  Foundation
Attending Physician
Department of Surgery
Lakeside Community Hospital
Lakeport, California

LAWRENCE J. KAGEN, M.D.
Professor of Medicine
Cornell University Medical College
Attending Physician
The Hospital for Special Surgery and The New York
  Hospital
New York, New York

ALEXANDER P. KELLY, JR., M.D.
Clinical Associate Professor of Surgery (Plastic Surgery)
University of Michigan
Associate Surgeon
Division of Plastic and Reconstructive Surgery
Ann Arbor, Michigan

FRANKLIN KOZIN, M.D.
Assistant Member
Autoimmune Disease Center
Department of Basic and Clinic Research
Department of Immunology
Division of Rheumatology
Scripps Clinic and Research Foundation
La Jolla, California

SARA B. KRAMER, M.D.
Instructor, Department of Medicine
New York University Medical Center
Clinical Assistant Attending Physician
Bellevue Hospital
Assistant in Medicine
University Hospital
New York, New York

STEPHEN M. KRANE, M.D.
Professor of Medicine
Harvard Medical School
Physician and Chief
Arthritis Unit
Massachusetts General Hospital
Boston, Massachusetts

E. CARWILE LeROY, M.D.
Professor of Medicine
Director, Division of Rheumatology and Immunology
Department of Medicine
Medical University of South Carolina
Attending Physician
Medical University Hospital
Veterans Administration Hospital
Charleston Memorial Hospital
Charleston, South Carolina

DAVID B. LEVINE, M.D.
Clinical Professor of Orthopaedic Surgery
Cornell University Medicial College
Associate Director of Orthopaedic Surgery
The Hospital for Special Surgery
Attending Orthopaedic Surgeon
The New York Hospital
New York, New York

ROBERT W. LIGHTFOOT, JR., M.D.
Associate Professor of Medicine
Chief, Rheumatology Section
Medical College of Wisconsin
Milwaukee, Wisconsin

DANIEL J. McCARTY, M.D.
Will and Cava Ross Professor and Chairman
Department of Medicine
The Medical College of Wisconsin
Milwaukee, Wisconsin

HUGH O. McDEVITT, M.D.
Professor of Medical Microbiology and Medicine
Stanford University School of Medicine
Attending Physician
Stanford University Hospital
Stanford, California

VICTOR A. McKUSICK, M.D.
William Osler Professor and Director
Department of Medicine
The Johns Hopkins University School of Medicine
Professor of Epidemiology
The Johns Hopkins University School of Hygiene and
  Public Health
Professor of Biology
The Johns Hopkins University
Physician-in-Chief
The Johns Hopkins Hospital
Baltimore, Maryland

STEPHEN E. MALAWISTA, M.D.
Professor of Medicine
Chief, Section of Rheumatology
Department of Internal Medicine
Yale University School of Medicine
Attending Physician
Yale/New Haven Hospital
New Haven, Connecticut

HENRY J. MANKIN, M.D.
Edith M. Ashley Professor of Orthopaedic Surgery
Harvard Medical School
Chief, Orthopaedic Service
Massachusetts General Hospital
Boston, Massachusetts

MART MANNIK, M.D.
Professor of Medicine
Head, Division of Rheumatology
University of Washington
Seattle, Washington

ALFONSE T. MASI, M.D.
Professor and Head, Department of Medicine
University of Illinois College of Medicine
Attending Physician
Saint Francis Medical Center and
  Methodist Medical Center of Illinois
Peoria, Illinois

THOMAS A. MEDSGER, JR., M.D.
Professor of Medicine
Chief, Division of Rheumatology and Clinical Immu-
  nology
University of Pittsburgh School of Medicine
Active Staff
Presbyterian-University Hospital
Pittsburgh, Pennsylvania

EUGENE J. MESSER, D.D.S.
Professor and Chairman
Department of Oral and Maxillofacial Surgery
Medical College of Wisconsin
Milwaukee County Medical Complex
Froedtert Memorial Lutheran Hospital
Wood Veterans Administration Medical Center
Milwaukee, Wisconsin

RONALD P. MESSNER, M.D.
Professor of Medicine
Director, Section of Rheumatology/Clinical
  Immunology
University of Minnesota School of Medicine
Mayo Memorial Building
Minneapolis, Minnesota

GLENN A. MEYER, M.D.
Professor of Neurosurgery
Medical College of Wisconsin
Attending Physician
Froedtert Memorial Lutheran Hospital
Milwaukee County General Hospital
Wood Veterans Administration Hospital
Columbia Hospital
Milwaukee, Wisconsin

ROLAND W. MOSKOWITZ, M.D.
Professor of Medicine
Case Western Reserve University
Director, Division of Rheumatic Diseases
University Hospitals
Cleveland, Ohio

HAROLD E. PAULUS, M.D.
Professor of Medicine
University of California School of Medicine
Attending Physician
University of California Medical Center
Los Angeles, California

PAUL E. PHILLIPS, M.D.
Professor of Medicine
Chief of Rheumatology
State University of New York
Upstate Medical Center
Attending Physician
University Hospital
Syracuse, New York

JANICE SMITH PIGG, B.S.N., R.N.
Nurse Consultant, Rheumatology
Rheumatic Disease Program
Columbia Hospital
Milwaukee, Wisconsin

TAINA PIHLAJANIEMI, M.D.
Research Associate
Biochemistry Department
University of Medicine and Dentistry of New Jersey
Rutgers Medical School
Piscataway, New Jersey

ROBERT S. PINALS, M.D.
Professor and Associate Chairman
Department of Medicine
University of Medicine and Dentistry of New Jersey
Rutgers Medical School
Piscataway, New Jersey
Chairman, Department of Medicine
The Medical Center at Princeton
Princeton, New Jersey

PAUL H. PLOTZ, M.D.
Clinical Professor of Medicine
National Institutes of Health
Chief, Connective Tissue Diseases Section
Arthritis and Rheumatism Branch
National Institute of Arthritis, Diabetes, and Digestive
 and Kidney Diseases
Bethesda, Maryland

THEODORE A. POTTER, M.D.
Clinical Professor of Orthopedic Surgery
Tufts University School of Medicine
Senior Staff Surgeon
New England Baptist Hospital
New England Center Hospital
Boston City Hospital
Boston, Massachusetts

DARWIN J. PROCKOP, M.D., Ph.D.
Professor and Chairman of Biochemistry
University of Medicine and Dentistry of New Jersey
Rutgers Medical School
Piscataway, New Jersey

REED E. PYERITZ, M.D., Ph.D.
Associate Professor of Medicine and Pediatrics
The Johns Hopkins University School of Medicine
Active Staff, Department of Medicine
Director of Clinical Services
Division of Medical Genetics
The Johns Hopkins Hospital
Baltimore, Maryland

ERIC RADIN, M.D.
Professor and Chairman
Department of Orthopedic Surgery
West Virginia University Medical Center
West Virginia University Hospital
Morgantown, West Virginia

MORRIS REICHLIN, M.D.
Head, Arthritis and Immunology Program
Oklahoma Medical Research Foundation
Professor and Chief
Immunology (Arthritis, Allergy) Section
Department of Medicine
University of Oklahoma Health Sciences Center
Oklahoma City, Oklahoma

GERALD P. RODNAN, M.D.*
Professor of Medicine
University of Pittsburgh
Pittsburgh, Pennsylvania

LAWRENCE ROSENBERG, M.D.
Professor, Orthopedic Surgery
Albert Einstein College of Medicine
Director, Orthopedic Research
Montefiore Medical Center
Bronx, New York

NAOMI F. ROTHFIELD, M.D.
Professor of Medicine
Chief, Division of Rheumatic Diseases
University of Connecticut Health Center
Attending Physician
Newington Veterans Administration Hospital
Dempsey Hospital
Farmington, Connecticut

DORAN E. RYAN, D.D.S.
Attending Physician
Milwaukee County Medical Complex
Froedtert Memorial Lutheran Hospital
Veterans Administration Medical Center
Associate Professor
Oral and Maxillofacial Surgery
Medical College of Wisconsin
Milwaukee, Wisconsin

LAWRENCE M. RYAN, M.D.
Associate Professor of Medicine
Medical College of Wisconsin
Attending Physician
Milwaukee County General Hospital
Senior Attending Physician
Froedtert Memorial Lutheran Hospital
Milwaukee, Wisconsin

JANE GREEN SCHALLER, M.D.
Professor and Chairman
Department of Pediatrics
Tufts University School of Medicine
Pediatrician-in-Chief
The Floating Hospital for Infants and Children
New England Medical Center
Boston, Massachusetts

FRANK R. SCHMID, M.D.
Professor of Medicine
Chief, Section of Arthritis-Connective Tissue Diseases
Attending Physician
Northwestern Memorial Hospital
Consultant, Rehabilitation Institute of Chicago and Vet-
 erans Administration Lakeside Medical Center
Chicago, Illinois

H. RALPH SCHUMACHER, M.D.
Professor of Medicine
University of Pennsylvania School of Medicine
Director, Rheumatology-Immunology Center
Veterans Administration Medical Center
Philadelphia, Pennsylvania

GORDON C. SHARP, M.D.
Professor of Medicine and Pathology
Director, Division of Immunology and Rheumatology
University of Missouri-Columbia School of Medicine
Director, University of Missouri Multipurpose Arthritis
  Center
Staff Rheumatologist and Director
Antinuclear Antibody Laboratory
University of Missouri Health Sciences Center
Columbia, Missouri

JOHN T. SHARP, M.D.
Professor, Department of Medicine
University of Colorado Health Sciences Center
Director, Joe and Betty Alpert Arthritis Center
Rose Medical Center
Denver, Colorado

JOHN W. SIGLER, M.D.
Clinical Associate Professor of Internal Medicine
University of Michigan
Division Head Emeritus
Division of Rheumatology
Ann Arbor, Michigan

PETER A. SIMKIN, M.D.
Professor of Medicine
Division of Rheumatology
Department of Medicine
University of Washington
Seattle, Washington

BERNHARD H. SINGSEN, M.D.
Associate Professor of Child Health, Internal Medicine,
  and Pathology
University of Missouri School of Medicine
Attending Physician, Pediatric Rheumatology
University of Missouri Health Sciences Center
Columbia, Missouri

JOHN L. SKOSEY, M.D., Ph.D.
Professor of Medicine and Chief
Section of Rheumatology
Department of Medicine
University of Illinois College of Medicine
Attending Physician
University of Illinois Hospital
Veterans Administration West Side Hospital
Cook County Hospital
Chicago, Illinois

HUGH A. SMYTHE, M.D.
Professor and Director of Rheumatic Diseases Unit
Wellesley Hospital
University of Toronto
Toronto, Canada

RALPH SNYDERMAN, M.D.
Frederic M. Hanes Professor of Medicine
Professor of Immunology
Chief, Division of Rheumatic and Genetic Diseases
Duke University Medical Center
Durham, North Carolina

LEON SOKOLOFF, M.D.
Professor of Pathology
Department of Pathology
Health Sciences Center
State University of New York at Stony Brook
Attending Pathologist
University Hospital
Stony Brook, New York

ISAIAS SPILBERG, M.D.
Associate Professor of Medicine
Washington University School of Medicine
Chief, Rheumatology Unit
Veterans Administration Medical Center
St. Louis, Missouri

RICHARD N. STAUFFER, M.D.
Professor of Orthopaedic Surgery
Mayo Medical School
Consultant, Mayo Clinic
Attending Physician
Rochester Methodist Hospital
St. Mary's Hospital
Rochester, Minnesota

ALLEN C. STEERE, M.D.
Associate Professor of Medicine
Yale University School of Medicine
Attending Physician
Yale/New Haven Hospital
New Haven, Connecticut

ALFRED D. STEINBERG, M.D.
Senior Investigator
Arthritis and Rheumatism Branch
National Institute of Arthritis, Diabetes, and Digestive
  and Kidney Diseases
National Institutes of Health
Bethesda, Maryland

JOHN D. STOBO, M.D.
Professor of Medicine
Head, Section of Rheumatology/Clinical Immunology
University of California
San Francisco, California

ROBERT L. SWEZEY, M.D.
Director, Arthritis and Back Pain Center
Clinical Professor of Medicine
University of California
Attending Physician
St. John's Hospital
Santa Monica Hospital
Santa Monica, California

NORMAN TALAL, M.D.
Professor of Medicine and Microbiology
The University of Texas Health Science Center
Chief, Section of Clinical Immunology
Audie Murphy Veterans Hospital
San Antonio, Texas

ENG M. TAN, M.D.
Director, W. M. Keck Foundation
Autoimmune Disease Center
Head, Division of Rheumatology
Scripps Clinic and Research Foundation
La Jolla, California

ANGELO TARANTA, M.D.
Professor of Medicine
Chief, Division of Rheumatology/Immunology
New York Medical College
Valhalla, New York
Director of Medicine
Cabrini Medical Center
New York, New York

ROBERT TERKELTAUB, M.D.
Research Associate
Scripps Clinic and Research Foundation
La Jolla, California
Visiting Attending Physician
Veterans Administration Medical Center
Department of Medicine
University of California School of Medicine
San Diego, California

N. NOEL TESTA, M.D.
Associate Clinical Professor of Orthopaedic Surgery
Associate Attending Orthopaedic Surgeon
New York University Medical Center
New York, New York

DAVID E. TRENTHAM, M.D.
Associate Professor of Medicine
Harvard Medical School
Assistant Physician
Department of Rheumatology/Immunology
Brigham and Women's Hospital
Boston, Massachusetts

PETER TUGWELL, M.D., M.Sc.
Chairman, Department of Clinical Epidemiology and
    Biostatistics
Professor, Department of Clinical Epidemiology and
    Biostatistics
Professor, Department of Medicine
McMaster University
Attending Physician
Division of Rheumatology
Chedake-McMaster Hospital
Hamilton, Ontario
Canada

STEVEN R. WEINER, M.D.
Assistant Professor of Medicine
University of California
Los Angeles, California
Chief of Rheumatology
Olive View Medical Center
Van Nuys, California

GERALD WEISSMANN, M.D.
Professor of Medicine
Director of Rheumatology
New York University Medical Center
Attending Physician
New York University Medical Center
Bellevue Hospital
Consulting Rheumatologist
Manhattan Veterans Administration Hospital
New York, New York

RALPH C. WILLIAMS, JR.
Professor and Chairman
Department of Medicine
University of New Mexico School of Medicine
Albuquerque, New Mexico

ROBERT L. WORTMANN, M.D.
Assistant Professor
Section of Rheumatology
Department of Internal Medicine
Medical College of Wisconsin
Staff Physician
Wood Veterans Administration Medical Center
Wood, Wisconsin
Milwaukee County General Hospital and Froedtert
    Memorial Lutheran Hospital
Milwaukee, Wisconsin

MORRIS ZIFF, M.D., Ph.D.
Ashbel Smith Professor of Internal Medicine
Morris Ziff Professor of Rheumatology
Director, Harold C. Simmons Arthritis Research Center
Attending Physician
Parkland Memorial Hospital
Dallas Veterans Administration Hospital
Dallas, Texas

NATHAN J. ZVAIFLER, M.D.
Professor of Medicine
University of California at San Diego School of Medicine
Attending Physician
University of California Medical Center
La Jolla, California

Contents

Section III—Clinical Pharmacology of the Antirheumatic Drugs

Section IV—Rheumatoid Arthritis

Section V—Other Inflammatory Arthritic Syndromes

*Deceased

Section VIII—Regional Disorders of Joints and Related Structures

Section IX—Osteoarthritis

Section X—Metabolic Bone and Joint Diseases

Section XI—Infectious Arthritis

Introduction to the Study of the Rheumatic Diseases

Chapter 1

Introduction

Joseph Lee Hollander

The term "rheumatism" is derived from the Greek word *rheumatismos,* which designated mucus (catarrh) as an evil humor believed to flow from the brain to the joints and other structures of the body, producing pain.[5] Since studies[10] over the past 35 years have shown that an alteration of an important constituent of joint mucin (the muco-polysaccharide:hyaluronic acid) actually occurs in at least some of the "rheumatic diseases," the term at long last may be somewhat appropriate. Any condition in which pain and stiffness of some portion of the musculoskeletal system are prominent may be termed a rheumatic disease. These conditions include the so-called diseases of connective tissue.

Arthritis is the general term used when the joints themselves are the major site of the rheumatic disease. *Fibrositis* denotes inflammation of connective tissue in any location, particularly near joints, in or near muscles or tendons. *Enthesopathy* is the term used to designate irritation of fibrous tissue attachments to bone. *Rheumatology* is the study of the rheumatic diseases, including arthritis, fibrositis, rheumatic fever, bursitis, neuralgia, gout, and any other conditions producing somatic pain, stiffness, or soreness.

Arthritis is one of the earliest known, yet most neglected, diseases. The first known example of multiple arthritis in a fossil vertebrate was found in the skeleton of a platycarpus (a large swimming reptile), which lived about 100,000,000 years ago. This skeleton may be seen in the Museum of Natural History of the University of Kansas.[8] Chronic arthritis of the spine was present in the Ape Man of 2,000,000 years ago as well as in the Java and Lansing men of 500,000 years ago and the Egyptian mummies dating to 8000 B.C.[9] The Romans built extensive baths throughout their empire because of the prevalence of arthritis, and warm springs have been utilized as spas ever since by those seeking relief.

Until recently there had not been available any concise yet comprehensive histories of arthritis or rheumatic disease. This deficiency has been remedied adequately, and the reader is referred to this account in the Bulletin of Rheumatic Diseases or in the new Primer on the Rheumatic Diseases.[2,12]

Pertinent historical data will be given in appropriate sections of this volume.

CLASSIFICATION OF ARTHRITIS AND RHEUMATISM

There are more than a hundred different forms of diseases affecting joints or related structures. Causative factors range from specific infectious agents, trauma, aging, metabolic derangements, immunologic abnormalities to the unknown. Arthritis is the usual term for most joint diseases, although some insist on the term "arthrosis" for those conditions without obvious inflammation. Because the "fire" of inflammation may be low-grade in some forms, especially in degenerative joint disease, this has been called osteoarthrosis or arthrosis, particularly in European countries. Since even the "fire" of rheumatoid arthritis may burn out, leaving the "ashes" of joint damage behind, the term arthritis may still be used for any joint disease in which inflammation has played a part, whether or not inflammation is still active.

Many classifications of diseases of joints and related structures have been suggested. All have certain disadvantages, and none can be accurate until the cause of each has been determined. For the sake of simplicity and unification of terminology, the classification originally accepted by the American Rheumatism Association in 1963,[3] and later modified with addition of newer entities by the Glossary Committee of the American Rheumatism Association,[12] is given in Table 1–1.

All classifications of rheumatic diseases are subject to additions and corrections. This revised and updated classification is already subject to change since the cause of Lyme arthritis (XA2 in Table 1–1) is apparently a spirochaete. If this is confirmed, Lyme arthritis will be moved to category IV. The current arrangement has been based on clinical patterns, pathologic changes induced in affected tissues, and causative agents when known. The arrangement of this textbook itself (see Table of Contents) is another attempt at classification.

A comprehensive Thesaurus of Rheumatology, which attempts to standardize the terms used in this field, was completed and published in 1964.[14] This epic work was needed for clarification since many

Table 1–1. Classification of the Rheumatic Diseases*

I. Diffuse connective tissue diseases
  A. Rheumatoid arthritis
  B. Juvenile arthritis
    1. Systemic onset
    2. Polyarticular onset
    3. Oligarticular onset
  C. Systemic lupus erythematosus
  D. Progressive systemic sclerosis
  E. Polymyositis/dermatomyositis
  F. Necrotizing vasculitis and other vasculopathies
    1. Polyarteritis nodosa group (includes hepatitis B associated arteritis and Churg-Strauss allergic granulomatosis)
    2. Hypersensitivity vasculitis (includes Schönlein-Henoch purpura and others)
    3. Wegener's granulomatosis
    4. Giant cell arteritis
      a. Temporal arteritis
      b. Takayasu's arteritis
    5. Mucocutaneous lymph node syndrome (Kawasaki's disease)
    6. Behcet's disease
  G. Sjögren's syndrome
  H. Overlap syndromes (includes mixed connective tissue disease)
  I. Others (includes polymyalgia rheumatica, panniculitis (Weber-Christian disease), erythema nodosum, relapsing polychondritis, and others)
II. Arthritis associated with spondylitis
  A. Ankylosing spondylitis
  B. Reiter's syndrome
  C. Psoriatic arthritis
  D. Arthritis associated with chronic inflammatory bowel disease
III. Degenerative joint disease (osteoarthritis, osteoarthrosis)
  A. Primary (includes erosive osteoarthritis)
  B. Secondary
IV. Arthritis, tenosynovitis, and bursitis associated with infectious agents
  A. Direct
    1. Bacterial
      a. Gram-positive cocci (staphylococcus and others)
      b. Gram-negative cocci (gonococcus and others)
      c. Gram-positive rods
      d. Mycobacteria
      e. Treponemes
      f. Others
    2. Viral
    3. Fungal
    4. Parasitic
    5. Unknown, suspected (Whipple's disease)
  B. Indirect (reactive)
    1. Bacterial (includes acute rheumatic fever, intestinal bypass, postdysenteric—shigella, yersinia, and others)
    2. Viral (hepatitis B)
V. Metabolic and endocrine diseases associated with rheumatic states
  A. Crystal-induced conditions
    1. Monosodium urate (gout)
    2. Calcium pyrophosphate dihydrate (pseudogout, chondrocalcinosis)
    3. Hydroxyapatite
  B. Biochemical abnormalities
    1. Amyloidosis
    2. Vitamin C deficiency (scurvy)
    3. Specific enzyme deficiency states (includes Fabry's, Farber's, alkaptonuria, Lesch-Nyhan, and others)
    4. Hyperlipidemias (types II, IIa, IV)
    5. Mucopolysaccharides
    6. Hemoglobinopathies (SS disease and others)
    7. True connective tissue disorders (Ehlers-Danlos, Marfan's, pseudoxanthoma elasticum, and others)
    8. Others
  C. Endocrine diseases
    1. Diabetes mellitus
    2. Acromegaly
    3. Hyperparathyroidism
    4. Thyroid disease (hyperthyroidism, hypothyroidism)
  D. Immunodeficiency diseases
  E. Other hereditary disorders
    1. Arthrogryposis multiplex congenita
    2. Hypermobility syndromes
    3. Myositis ossificans progressiva

Table 1–1. *Continued*

VI. Neoplasms
    A. Primary (e.g., synovioma, synoviosarcoma)
    B. Metastatic
VII. Neuropathic disorders
    A. Charcot joints
    B. Compression neuropathies
        1. Peripheral entrapment (carpal tunnel syndrome and others)
        2. Radiculopathy
        3. Spinal stenosis
    C Reflex sympathetic dystrophy
    D. Others
VIII. Bone and cartilage disorders associated with articular manifestations
    A. Osteoporosis
        1. Generalized
        2. Localized (regional)
    B. Osteomalacia
    C. Hypertrophic osteoarthropathy
    D. Diffuse idiopathic skeletal hyperostosis (includes ankylosing vertebral hyperostosis—Forrestier's disease)
    E. Osteitis
        1. Generalized (osteitis deformans—Paget's disease of bone)
        2. Localized (osteitis condensans ilii; osteitis pubis)
    F. Avascular necrosis
    G. Osteochondritis (osteochondritis dissecans)
    H. Congenital dysplasia of the hip
    I. Slipped capital femoral epiphysis
    J. Costochondritis (includes Tietze's syndrome)
    K. Osteolysis and chondrolysis
IX. Nonarticular rheumatism
    A. Myofascial pain syndromes
        1. Generalized (fibrositis, fibromyalgia)
        2. Regional
    B. Low back pain and intervertebral disc disorders
    C. Tendinitis (tenosynovitis) and/or bursitis
        1. Subacromial/subdeltoid bursitis
        2. Bicipital tendinitis, tenosynovitis
        3. Olecranon bursitis
        4. Epicondylitis, medial or lateral humeral
        5. DeQuervain's tenosynovitis
        6. Adhesive capsulitis of the shoulder (frozen shoulder)
        7. Trigger finger
    D. Ganglion cysts
    E. Fasciitis
    F. Chronic ligament and muscle strain
    G. Vasomotor disorders
        1. Erythromelalgia
        2. Raynaud's disease or phenomenon
    H. Miscellaneous pain syndromes (includes weather sensitivity, psychogenic rheumatism)
X. Miscellaneous disorders
    A. Disorders frequently associated with arthritis
        1. Trauma (the result of direct trauma)
        2. Lyme arthritis
        3. Pancreatic disease
        4. Sarcoidosis
        5. Palindromic rheumatism
        6. Intermittent hydrarthrosis
        7. Villonodular synovitis
        8. Hemophilia
    B. Other conditions
        1. Internal derangement of joints (includes chondromalacia of patella, loose bodies)
        2. Familial Mediterranean fever
        3. Eosinophilic fasciitis
        4. Chronic active hepatitis
        5. Other drug-induced rheumatic syndromes

*From Rodnan, G.P., et al.: Primer on the Rheumatic Diseases, 8th Ed., Atlanta, The Arthritis Foundation, 1983.

terms for the same clinical entity had been used (e.g., ankylosing spondylitis, rheumatoid spondylitis, rhizoméliqué spondylitis, Marie-Strümpell's disease, and so forth). The pattern was set for naming new entities and rare conditions usually known by the name of the early worker who described the syndrome. Further progress in this unification has been achieved by the *Primer on the Rheumatic Diseases*,[12] and by the new *Dictionary of the Rheumatic Diseases*.[6]

PREVALENCE AND PROBLEM OF RHEUMATIC DISEASE

According to the latest estimates derived from various surveys and quoted by the Arthritis Foundation in 1982,[1] there are more than 36,000,000 persons in the United States suffering from some form of arthritis or related disease. The epidemiology of rheumatic diseases is discussed in Chapter 2, but the preceding figure is quoted to underscore the magnitude of the problem of diagnosis and treatment of rheumatic diseases.

Although arthritis cripples many each year, it kills relatively few as compared with cancer and cardiovascular disease. However, *there is no other group of diseases that causes so much suffering by so many for so long*. Because of the tendency to disable and even permanently cripple without killing, arthritis and rheumatism belong at the top of the list of chronic diseases from the standpoint of social and economic importance. A review of National Health Survey figures several years ago showed that 26% of persons with rheumatic diseases were at least partially handicapped, and about 10% were grossly disabled. Arthritis and rheumatism result in at least 27,000,000 lost work days yearly.[4]

CAMPAIGN AGAINST ARTHRITIS AND RHEUMATISM

During the past 35 years rheumatology has become one of the most active and rapidly expanding fields of medicine. Original research has increased geometrically with the expansion and addition of many laboratories and clinical facilities devoted to this field of study. There has been a tremendous influx of new personnel into rheumatology, attracted and stimulated by many discoveries in this relatively virgin field of medicine over the past 35 years. In 1947 there were scarcely a dozen centers in the United States for research in rheumatic diseases, whereas in 1983 there are over 100. Arthritis treatment centers have increased more than 10-fold during this period, and the number of full-time specialists in rheumatology is now over 3500. (There were fewer than 100 when I began working in the field in 1937.)

The "Renaissance of Rheumatology" began shortly after World War II, when a number of young physicians who had worked together in Army Arthritis Centers returned to civilian practice. This was given tremendous impetus by the founding of the Arthritis and Rheumatism Foundation in 1948, the discovery of the effects of cortisone on arthritis inflammation in 1949, the meeting of the Seventh International Rheumatism Congress in New York in 1949, and the establishment of the National Institute of Arthritis and Metabolic Diseases in 1953. This same remarkable growth of interest and influx of expert personnel has also occurred in many countries throughout the world.

World, Regional, and National Organizations Against Arthritis

The first organization concerned with the problem of arthritis was *La Ligue Internationale contre le Rhumatisme* founded in 1927 as a small European medical club. At that time there was neither definition of the field nor any scientific background to rheumatology.[13] Over the next 20 years national societies were formed in a number of European countries, the United States, Canada, Argentina, Brazil, Mexico, Uruguay, and Chile. Because World War II disrupted normal communication between the American societies and those in Europe, the Pan-American League Against Rheumatism (PANLAR) was formed. By 1947 the European societies banded together as the European League Against Rheumatism (EULAR), which later included among its 31 members a few national societies from the Mideast as well. The national rheumatism societies that had sprung up in Australia, New Zealand, India, Japan, and the Philippines organized the Southeast Asia and Pacific Area League Against Rheumatism (SEAPAL) in 1963.

Each of these regional leagues conducts a scientific congress every four years, as does the parent organization, the International League Against Rheumatism (ILAR). Thus, there is an international meeting for exchange of new developments each year. The most recent congress of ILAR was held in Paris in 1981, that of PANLAR was in Washington in 1982, and that of EULAR in Moscow in 1983. SEAPAL held another congress in Bangkok in 1984, and ILAR will have its next congress in Sydney, Australia in 1985.

National rheumatism societies have been organized in nearly every important country of the world, reflecting the growing importance of rheumatology as a medical discipline. At each succeeding international congress more and more physicians and allied research and clinical personnel concerned with rheumatology participate.

The World Health Organization (WHO), a special agency of the Social and Economic Council of the United Nations, cooperates with and relies on the ILAR and its component units for technical guidance in rheumatology, and assists in research, epidemiology, and standardization of terminology and medical education.[11]

Government and Voluntary Agencies

The Arthritis and Rheumatism Council in the United Kingdom, the Canadian Arthritis Society, the Australian Rheumatism Council, and similar agencies of physicians and interested lay persons have been active and increasingly successful in raising funds for research and education programs over the past 30 years. In the United States, the Arthritis Foundation, originating as the Arthritis and Rheumatism Foundation in 1948, has flourished with 71 local chapters in nearly all the 50 states. Each year the Foundation raises over $24,000,000. Nearly $2,500,000 supports more than 50 arthritis clinical research centers, and a similar amount supports over 105 research training fellowships in rheumatic diseases. Chapter support for treatment clinics, research, and education programs constitutes the major function of this large voluntary agency.[1]

Government support of arthritis research and control programs has been, for the most part, inadequate everywhere. Whereas the National Institute of Arthritis and Metabolic Diseases, formed 30 years ago as one of the units of the National Institutes of Health, U.S. Department of Health, Education and Welfare, was a fine beginning, the subsequent progress has been disappointing. The wide range of both intramural and extramural research and training programs has been restricted by decreasing budgets. Hopes for increased emphasis on arthritis research had been raised by passage of the National Arthritis Act by Congress in 1975, creating a National Arthritis Commission that made intensive studies and published a comprehensive report on plans to attack the arthritis problem.[11] This program has never been adequately funded, however. The National Institute of Arthritis, Diabetes, and Digestive and Kidney Diseases continues its limited program, but hopes are high that the diluted attack will be again increased in years to come as more are made aware of the great need.

PUBLICATIONS IN RHEUMATOLOGY

An increasing number of medical scientific journals devoted exclusively to rheumatic diseases is further evidence of the growth and activity of rheumatologic research. The principal journals in English are the *Annals of the Rheumatic Diseases*, the journal of the Heberden Society,* published in Great Britain; *Arthritis and Rheumatism*, published in the United States by the American Rheumatism Association; and the *Journal of Rheumatology*, published in Canada. *Acta Rheumatologica Scandinavica*, now the *Scandinavian Journal of Rheumatology* publishes also in English. Newer rheumatology journals published in English include *Rheumatology International*, published in Italy; *Clinical and Experimental Rheumatology*, published in Italy; and *Rheumatology and Rehabilitation*, published in England. The *Bulletin on the Rheumatic Diseases*, published by the Arthritis Foundation in nine issues yearly since 1950, gives discussions of important topics in the field. The *Primer on Rheumatic Diseases*, an essential text for teaching rheumatology to medical students and house officers, has been prepared by committees of the American Rheumatism Association at intervals for many years. The Eighth Edition, the finest and most comprehensive yet, appeared in March 1983. It is essential for all those studying rheumatology.[12] Every year more monographs, textbooks, and periodicals in rheumatology appear, reflecting the increased interest of physicians and the growing complexity and wealth of knowledge about musculoskeletal diseases. The *Rheumatism Reviews*, originated by Hench et al. in 1935, has been augmented by numerous other efforts. The current and last *Rheumatism Review*, the twenty-fifth,[7] was published in March 1983.

TRAINING IN RHEUMATOLOGY

The current Rheumatism Review[7] discusses the status of training in this field. Most medical schools give little formal training in rheumatology. Many house officer training programs are also deficient in rheumatic disease study, but it was demonstrated that even those who took an elective in rheumatology were far ahead in knowledge of diagnosis and treatment than those only randomly exposed.

Subspecialty training in rheumatology has advanced greatly over the past 35 years, both in numbers of trainees and in the sophistication of training programs. Board Certification in Rheumatology has been available since 1972 as a subspecialty examination administered through the American Board of Internal Medicine. Despite the hundreds of qualified physicians who have been certified, there is still a shortage of rheumatologists in some areas of the United States.

REFERENCES

1. Arthritis Foundation: Annual Report. Atlanta, 1982, pp. 1–36.

---

*Since 1983, known as the British Society for Rheumatology.

2. Benedek, T.G., and Rodnan, G.P.: A brief history of the rheumatic diseases. Bull. Rheum. Dis., *32*:59–68, 1982.

3. Blumberg, B.S., et al.: Nomenclature and classification of arthritis and rheumatism. Bull. Rheum. Dis., *14*:339–340, 1964.

4. Hollander, J.L.: Report of epidemiology subcommittee. *In* Arthritis, Report of Governor's Task Force. Edited by W.R. Katz. Harrisburg, Pa. 1981.

5. Hormell, R.S.: Notes on the history of rheumatism and gout. New Eng. J. Med., *223*:754–760, 1940.

6. McShane, D.J., et al.: Dictionary of the Rheumatic Diseases, Vol. 1. Atlanta, The Arthritis Foundation, 1983, pp. 1–87.

7. Medsger, T.A., Jr., et al.: Twenty-fifth rheumatism review. Arthritis Rheum., *26*:241–456, 1983.

8. Murphy, G.E.: Antiquity and arthritis. Bull. Hist. Med., *14*:123–127, 1943.

9. Osgood, R.B.: Medical and social approach to the problem of rheumatism. Amer. J. Med. Sci., *200*:429–445, 1940.

10. Ragan, C., and Meyer, K.: The hyaluronic acid of synovial fluid in rheumatoid arthritis. J. Clin. Invest., *28*:56, 1949.

11. Report of the National Arthritis Commission: U.S. Dept. H.E.W., National Institutes of Health, #76, Paris, 1976, pp. 1150–1154.

12. Rodnan, G.P., et al.: Primer on the Rheumatic Diseases, 8th Ed. Atlanta, The Arthritis Foundation, 1983, pp. 1–238.

13. Rudd, E.: Rheumatology and international health. International relations of the American Rheumatism Association. Arthritis Rheum., *15*:417–424, 1972.

14. Ruhl, M.J., and Sokoloff, L.: A thesaurus of rheumatology. Arthritis Rheum., *8*:97–182, 1965.

Chapter 2

Epidemiology of the Rheumatic Diseases

Thomas A. Medsger, Jr. and Alfonse T. Masi

Epidemiology (*epi,* upon; *demos,* people; *logy,* science) is the study of the frequency and distribution of disease in populations and of those factors determining or associated with disease occurrence. This discipline has made significant contributions to the understanding and control of many conditions, both infectious and noncommunicable. Epidemiology has a broad mission, and its methodology interfaces with other major disciplines, including clinical studies, public health, and laboratory science.

Depending upon the level of disease understanding, epidemiologic investigations may be designed as descriptive, integrative, hypothesis-testing, experimental, or disease control studies. Although acute rheumatic fever studies have encompassed all levels, most rheumatic disease epidemiology has, thus far, focused on the more elementary descriptions of disease occurrence. The next stages are to infer concepts of disease by synthesizing such descriptive data and to generate testable etiologic hypotheses.

The descriptive epidemiology of the rheumatic diseases is voluminous, and important past contributions have been summarized in an annotated bibliography,[138] reviews,[66,157,159,161,202,210,231] and proceedings of international conferences.[37,89,186] Accordingly, we have emphasized more recent studies illustrating epidemiologic concepts and principles, and have selected the major disorders not associated with known infectious agents. Infection-related arthritis is covered in other chapters.

BASIC EPIDEMIOLOGIC CONCEPTS

Classification of Disease. Since case frequencies reported in population surveys depend directly upon disease definition, emphasis has been given to developing accurate, or at least reliable, criteria for the classification or diagnosis of rheumatic diseases, as described subsequently. No clear distinction exists between epidemiologic and clinical studies of disease classification, although the former tend to be based more upon defined populations and the latter on patient data from one or more medical care institutions.

Incidence and Prevalence. *Incidence* is the rate of occurrence of new cases of disease (or its manifestations) during a given period in a defined population.[81] It is determined by specifying the number of new cases that occur in a population over time. *Prevalence* is the percentage or proportion of cases, identified by interview or examination, in a population at a given point in time (point prevalence) or during a specified interval (interval or period prevalence). Point prevalence is determined in a single survey, whereas interval prevalence is determined in one or more surveys.

A numerical relationship exists between incidence (I) and prevalence (P); incidence times average duration of disease (D) equals prevalence ($I \times D = P$). Because disease duration, including likelihood of remission or mortality, may vary with factors such as onset age, sex, race, and socioeconomic status, prevalence reflects both the risk of acquiring a disease and those factors that influence its duration. Hence, incidence is a more sensitive and specific indicator of disease acquisition risk than is prevalence and is thus superior for inferring mechanisms of etiology or host predisposition to onset. Studies of incidence tend to be the more demanding because larger populations are required to derive a suitable number of new cases, and definition of disease at onset or first diagnosis may be difficult.

Sensitivity and Specificity. *Sensitivity* is defined as the probability that those who have a positive test or finding, or who are diagnosed as having the disease (by criteria), actually have it.[202] *Specificity* is the probability that those who have a negative test or finding, or who are diagnosed as not having the disease, actually do not have it. These relationships are shown in a two-by-two table comparing a true classification of a population with the results of a test or criterion result (Table 2–1).

Multifactorial Contributions to Etiology. Most chronic acquired diseases are now believed to result from the interaction of multiple factors related to the host, environment and, at times, infecting agents (Fig. 2–1). Multifactorial mechanisms of disease often obscure recognition of the

Table 2–1.   Sensitivity and Specificity Measures

Test or Criteria	True or Standard Classification		Total
	Yes	No	
Positive	a	b	a + b
Negative	c	d	c + d
Total	a + c	b + d	Total

Sensitivity equals a/a + c
Specificity equals d/b + d

primary determining factor(s) by virtue of complex interactions and sequences of events. Epidemiology helps develop an holistic perspective of disease and a conceptual synthesis that can clarify such interrelationships and reveal promising directions for future studies. This may be accomplished by identifying either a broader or narrower spectrum of a disease in the population or by recognizing characteristic disease course patterns that correlate closely with specific host, environmental, and other factors. Comprehensive approaches combining epidemiologic, clinical, and laboratory methods offer great promise in unraveling the currently obscure primary interactions in these complex disorders.

RHEUMATOID ARTHRITIS

The epidemiology of rheumatoid arthritis (RA), including juvenile rheumatoid arthritis,[137] and the relationship between seropositive and seronegative RA[203,205] have been reviewed recently.

Classification of Disease. Rheumatoid arthritis illustrates the dilemma that lack of accurate defi-

nition poses to investigators seeking to determine its frequency or natural course. Thus, differences in reported incidence and prevalence may result mainly from differences in definition or severity rather than actual disease occurrence. Although classic advanced RA can be more reliably diagnosed, it represents a minority segment of the total disease spectrum, and conclusions based upon such narrow subsets must be properly qualified and not overgeneralized. Unfortunately, recognition and definition of RA during its earliest stages are difficult because it may follow a variable nonspecific pattern for months or years before becoming "typical."

Criteria for Rheumatoid Arthritis. A committee of the American Rheumatism Association (ARA) proposed diagnostic criteria based on a set of 11 symptoms, signs, and laboratory features of RA as well as specific exclusions that increased the specificity[283] (Table 2–2). Five or more criteria (definite RA) yielded a sensitivity of 70% for rheumatologist-diagnosed definite rheumatoid arthritis and a specificity of 91%. Three or more criteria (probable RA) had a sensitivity of 88% and specificity of 77% for clinically probable or definite disease. Definite and probable categories were recommended for study or reporting purposes on the features, course, or treatment of RA, but not for establishing a diagnosis in an individual patient.[282] A less rigid classification of "possible" RA was also proposed to include early and atypical cases and patients with other disorders.[282,283] The duration of articular manifestations required to satisfy clinical criteria was purposely set at 6 weeks to elim-

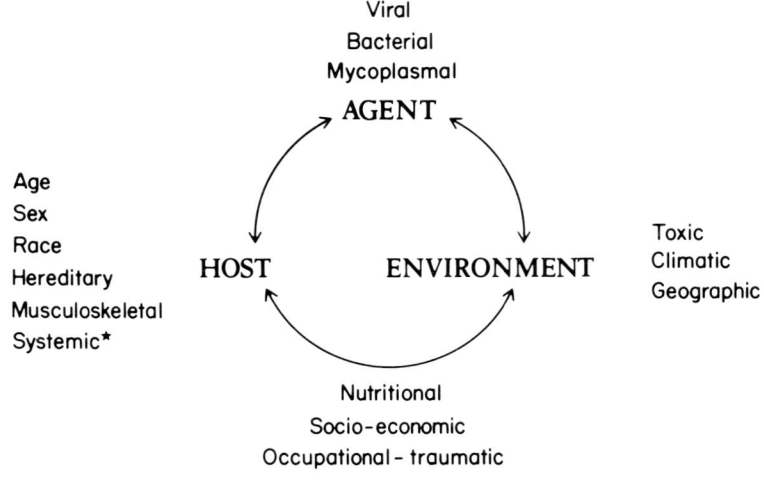

*e.g., circulatory, endocrinologic, immunologic, metabolic, neurologic, psychologic

Fig. 2–1.   Factors contributing to arthritis: holistic model of disease.

Table 2–2. Rheumatoid Arthritis Diagnostic Criteria (ARA 1958 Revision)[282,283]

1. Morning stiffness.
2. Pain on motion or tenderness in at least one joint.*
3. Swelling (soft tissue thickening or fluid, not bony overgrowth alone) in at least one joint.*
4. Swelling of at least one other joint.*†
5. Symmetrical joint swelling with simultaneous involvement of the same joint on both sides of the body.*† Terminal phalangeal joint involvement does not satisfy the criterion.
6. Subcutaneous nodules over bony prominences, on extensor surfaces or in juxta-articular regions.*
7. Roentgenographic changes typical of rheumatoid arthritis (which must include at least bony decalcification localized to or greatest around the involved joints and not just degenerative changes).†
8. Positive agglutination (antigammaglobulin) test.†
9. Poor mucin precipitate from synovial fluid (with shreds and cloudy solution).
10. Characteristic histologic changes in synovial membrane.†
11. Characteristic histologic changes in nodules.†

Categories†	Number of Criteria Required	Minimum Duration of Continuous Symptoms	Exclusions‡
Classic	7 of 11	6 weeks (nos. 1–5)	any of listed
Definite	5 of 11	6 weeks (nos. 1–5)	any of listed
Probable	3 of 11	3 weeks (one of nos. 1–5)	any of listed

*Observed by a physician.
†Refer to original reference for further specification.
‡Refer to original reference for listing of exclusions.

inate inclusion of the more acute forms of arthritis caused by infection, trauma, or rheumatic fever.

At the Second International Symposium on Population Studies in the Rheumatic Diseases held in Rome in 1961, these criteria were modified to make them more suitable for epidemiologic studies. Synovial fluid analysis, synovial histology, and microscopic confirmation of subcutaneous nodules, which could not be expected to be routinely ascertained, were eliminated.[158] Deficiencies in the criteria included the difficulty in quantitating morning stiffness and its low reliability, the low frequency of subcutaneous nodules, and marked variation in use of different serologic tests for rheumatoid factor and grading of radiographs.[137]

Another set of RA criteria proposed mainly for population studies[36] was derived from the Third International Symposium held in New York in 1966 (Table 2–3). The roentgenographic and serologic components of the Rome criteria were retained, but the New York criteria included different clinical items. They emphasized the pattern of affected joints, requiring involvement of a distal extremity joint (hand, wrist, or foot) and symmetry of an acceptable joint pair. These criteria list no exclusions or required duration of joint manifestations.

Both sets of criteria have been compared in the same populations. In the Sudbury, Massachusetts study of 4,552 adults, 118 initially met Rome criteria for probable or definite RA versus only 17 who satisfied the more selective physical examination item of the New York criteria.[260] After a 3-

Table 2–3. Rheumatoid Arthritis Population Survey Criteria (New York, 1966)*[36]

1. History, past or present, of any episode of joint pain involving three or more limb joints without stipulation as to duration. The joints on either side shall count separately, but joints that occur in groups (e.g., the PIP or MCP joints) on one side shall count only as a single joint.

2. Swelling, limitation, subluxation, or ankylosis of at least three limb joints, including one hand, wrist, or foot with symmetry of at least one joint pair. (Joints excluded from criteria are the DIP, the fifth PIP, the first carpometacarpal (CMC) joints, the hips, and the first MTP. Subluxation of the lateral MTP must be irreducible.)

3. X-ray features of grade 2 or more erosive arthritis in the hands, wrists, or feet.

4. Positive serologic reaction for rheumatoid (antigammaglobulin) factor.

*Recommendations for summation of the criteria were not made.

to 5-year follow-up, only 15% of those initially satisfying probable Rome criteria remained so classified, whereas 65% of persons initially satisfying New York criteria continued to do so. In a comparative criteria study among 1,748 Pima Indians over 14 years of age, slightly more patients satisfied New York (103) than Rome (91) criteria for probable RA.[132] Results were discordant in 64 individuals, most of whom had limitation of joint motion without swelling or subluxation, leading to the recommendation that the second New York criterion be modified to exclude limitation of motion.[132] Similarly, in population samples from England, prevalence was increased using the New York criteria compared with the ARA "definite" classification, especially among males.

Discrepancies in these results may be explained in part by the different populations studied. These data also suggest that some individuals are included who have transient, nondeforming RA. It is likely that different criteria measure different stages in the evolution of RA or identify other conditions that mimic it. For example, females with bilateral knee involvement having osteoarthritis may be included under RA by satisfying the second New York criterion.[132] Another obvious source of false positives is patients with polymyalgia rheumatica and peripheral joint involvement, who are not excluded from the Rome criteria and can easily satisfy both Rome and New York criteria.[127] Such criteria have contributed importantly to standardization of classification, but they must be reevaluated and revised periodically as knowledge of RA increases. Our enthusiasm for these criteria must also be tempered by the knowledge that clinical assessment of patients is subject to striking interobserver variation despite attempts to make clinical examination uniform.[122]

Analysis of the manner in which the eight noninvasive RA criteria classify patients at initial evaluation in a large, community-based population has shown that seven major clinical syndromes were identified frequently.[235] The natural history and long-term outcome in these RA subsets, which correspond to the most common clinical presentations, will be of great interest.

Criteria that have been developed for clinical remission in RA include: morning stiffness absent or less than 15 minutes in duration, no fatigue, no joint pain by history, no joint or tendon sheath swelling, and a normal erythrocyte sedimentation rate.[273] In the study sample of 344 RA patients, 5 or more of these criteria present in an individual patient identified clinical remission with 72% sensitivity and 100% specificity.

Age and Sex Distribution. There is general agreement that the prevalence of "definite" RA increases with age for both males and females, approaching 2% and 5%, respectively, over age 55; these studies have been comprehensively reviewed.[137] The overall sex ratio of almost three females to one male is likewise a consistent finding. However, the sex ratio is 5:1 or more with onset under age 60, but approximately 2:1 or less when onset is at an older age.[137,148,155,327] The latter ratio may be related to an abrupt increase in RA among older males.[155] Sex ratio data in younger adult RA subjects are limited, but marked female preponderance was found in some populations.[6,226] More

recently a peculiarly high younger adult female predisposition to RA was found in studies of Yakima Indians,[27] with a tendency to more progressive disease.[349] The relative infrequency of RA in younger adult males compared with other types of inflammatory arthritis has been noted also.[16]

Analysis of five-year average annual incidence rates for RA in Rochester, Minnesota showed a dramatic decrease among females from 92.3 per 100,000 from 1960 to 1964 to 39.7 per 100,000 from 1970 to 1974.[191] The authors suggested a temporal relationship between the decline in incidence and the concomitant increase in use of oral contraceptives, but their recent case-control study of the current or prior use of estrogens in women with and without RA showed no differences.[190a]

Sex-related host factors seem to play an important role in determining the onset and severity of RA. This concept is consistent with recognized pregnancy-induced remission and post-partum exacerbation or new onset of RA.[266] Males may have a protective factor that may be lost in older ages.

Decreased urinary excretion[207] and plasma levels[94] of adrenal androgens have been demonstrated in female RA patients compared with controls. Steroid sex hormones may alter either microvascular[288] or immunologic[9] function, thereby influencing predisposition to RA and related disorders.[207]

Ethnic and Geographic Distribution. All races seem capable of developing RA. Although differences in case definition make prevalence rates from various sources difficult to compare, estimates for definite RA are remarkably constant at 1.0% in Caucasian populations.[137] The prevalence of RA was similar for U.S. whites and blacks.[248] When ARA criteria for definite disease have been used, the average adult (age 15 and older) prevalence in major reported surveys has ranged from a low of 0.1% in a rural black South African community[31] to 3.0% among Finnish and rural West Caucasians.[181] The high prevalence in young adult Yakima females,[27] and Chippewa Indians,[126] may be exceptions. Climate per se does not seem to be a factor. Although most population studies of RA do not permit the calculation of incidence, estimates vary from 1 to 3/1,000 persons at risk.[137,155]

Despite their general similarity, reported population frequency differences seem real. Emphasis in future field studies should be directed at critically evaluating criteria, incidence, and course of RA in populations that offer particular logistical advantages or strongly suggest unusually high or low frequencies. Additionally, further emphasis should be placed on controlled analysis of personal, historical, and environmental factors with which the disease may be associated in order to gain clues to etiology or pathogenesis.

Environmental Factors. An increased prevalence of RA has been noted in single and divorced females,[222] as well as in association with lower income and lower educational achievement in males.[248] The contribution of personality factors to RA onset is controversial, and it is most likely that the reported associations represent the effect of the disease.[346] The marked increase in prevalence of definite RA in genetically close, related South African black urban populations, compared with rural populations, implicates sociologic and environmental factors in disease occurrence.[31,309]

Lack of association of RA in marital partners[130] and failure to demonstrate elevated antiviral antibody titers in RA,[271] do not support the usual type of infectious agent transmission. However, the association between Epstein-Barr infection and RA has been suggested by the finding of a serum antibody in RA patients reactive with an antigen in normal B lymphocytes infected with the virus.[340] Defective EBV-specific suppressor T-cell function in RA has also been described.[329] Further studies are required to elucidate this relationship (see Chap. 35).

Genetic Influences on Occurrence. Analysis of twin and family studies confined to probands with erosive seropositive arthritis showed a sixfold increase in RA prevalence among siblings or dizygotic twins versus controls.[185] In monozygotic twins, the association was over 30 times that expected among controls, and the data were most consistent with a polygenic pattern of inheritance. These results are supported by studies of HLA-DW4 and DR4 with estimated relative risk of 7 and 6, respectively.[137] DRW4 association with RA occurs irrespective of race[151] but in strong association with Felty's syndrome,[79] an unusual complication among blacks. Combined family and immunogenetic studies in RA deserve high priority.

Course of Disease. The natural history of RA is variable. Three major patterns of articular involvement have been documented in its early course in younger adults, as illustrated in Figure 2–2.[206] Most reviews of outcome in RA have dealt with patients having well-established disease and thus may be unrepresentative of the total spectrum. Essentially all studies, however, concur that serum rheumatoid factor and bony erosions indicate a poor prognosis.[137] Other early features found by multivariate analysis to be associated with worse disease on follow-up include female sex, white race, two or more swollen upper-extremity joints, Raynaud's-like phenomenon, and malaise or weakness.[95,203]

Because of the systemic nature of RA, it is not surprising that total mortality is reported to be greater than expected.[2] First evaluation findings that predict premature death include: ARA functional class, subcutaneous nodules, rheumatoid factor titer and erythrocyte sedimentation rate, bone erosions, and prednisone dosage.[234] Patients who are hospitalized prior to age 45 or 50 also have decreased survival.[146,237,336] A disproportionately frequent cause of death is infection, mainly of the respiratory tract. Cardiac deaths occur at an expected[336] or increased[237] rate, with no apparent relationship to medications used.[237] Considering the increased use of immunosuppressive drugs for severe RA, the frequency of cancer could be excessive. In one controlled study, cyclophosphamide-treated patients had a four-fold increase in occurrence of new cancers and a 15-fold increase in hematologic and lymphoreticular cancers.[19] Prolonged follow-up may be necessary before this risk is accurately determined.

As expected, disease stage and duration adversely affected work capability in this study, but social and work-related factors had the greatest influence on disability in RA.[357] Control over the pace and activities of work and self-employment status most influenced continued employment.

JUVENILE ARTHRITIS

Definition of Disease. Chronic forms of juvenile onset arthritis include juvenile rheumatoid arthritis (JRA), juvenile ankylosing spondylitis and related HLA-B27-associated disorders, numerous specific rheumatic and nonrheumatic conditions manifesting arthritis, and a residual group of unclassified arthritides. In England, the term juvenile chronic polyarthritis is often used for idiopathic, chronic juvenile onset arthritis, with "JRA" limited to the 10 to 15% of children with positive tests for serum rheumatoid factor. Although arbitrary, the upper age limit for juvenile onset is usually considered to be the sixteenth birthday.

An ARA subcommittee reviewed and validated the 1977 classification criteria for JRA using a computerized data base of 250 children with prolonged follow-up.[58] The criteria include disease manifestations present during the first six months after onset, i.e., polyarticular onset (manifestations most closely resembling those of adult seropositive RA), pauciarticular onset, and systemic onset. Rheumatoid rash was a good discriminator for the systemic onset type. In a comparison study, Soviet and American patients were remarkably similar in the frequency of subtype onset, in sex and onset age within subtype, and in the distribution by subtype after follow-up.[24] No population survey criteria for chronic juvenile onset arthritis have been proposed yet.

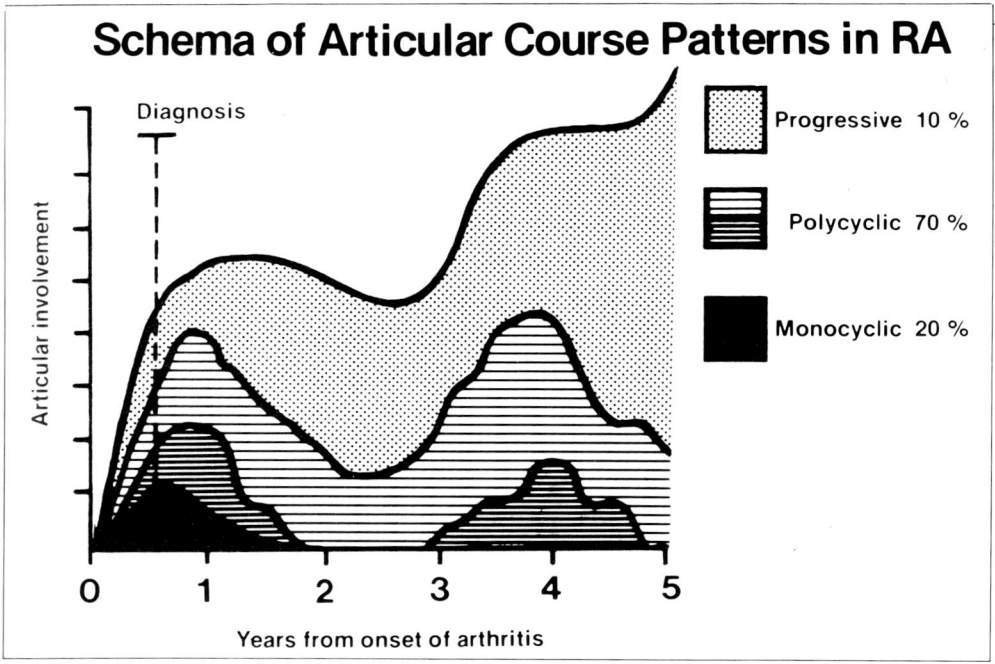

Schema of Articular Course Patterns in RA

Diagnosis

Articular involvement

Progressive 10 %

Polycyclic 70 %

Monocyclic 20 %

0   1   2   3   4   5

Years from onset of arthritis

Fig. 2–2.   Schema of articular course patterns over five years in early-diagnosed young adult rheumatoid arthritis patients.[206]

Population Frequency. Adequate data on the incidence of juvenile onset arthritis are lacking. Figures derived from referral hospitals or specialty clinics undoubtedly underestimate the occurrence and are subject to selection biases. A summary of existing prevalence estimates suggests a figure of 0.2 to 1.0 cases per 1,000 individuals.[107] One community-based epidemiologic study (Rochester, Minnesota, 1960 to 1980) has been published using 1977 ARA criteria for juvenile arthritis.[330] A comparable prevalence rate of 0.96 to 1.13 per 1,000 was reported. The overall incidence was 13.9 per 100,000 population, with patterns indicating a female predominance before age 5 (pauciarticular) and increased incidence in both sexes after age 10 (males with juvenile ankylosing spondylitis and females with JRA). A greater proportion of the patients (74%) was classified as having pauciarticular onset in this community study than in referral medical center series. Other reported juvenile arthritis incidence rates are lower, ranging from 2.2 to 9.2 per 100,000 children at risk.[134,137]

Age and Sex Distribution. Age and sex variations occur according to the previously mentioned onset patterns.[124,293] The sex ratio in the systemic onset (Still's) type is approximately equal, with the majority (over 80%) having onset under 10 years of age.[315] Numerous similar cases have been reported with onset in late adolescence and adulthood. Polyarticular onset usually begins after age

10, and females predominate,[124,315] as in young adult onset RA.

In the pauciarticular category, further subdivisions can be made. A group of young girls with serum antinuclear antibodies and chronic iridocyclitis has an average onset age of under three years.[293] Boys with HLA-B27 and one or another of the associated arthritis variants usually have onset at age 10 or older. One follow-up study showed that 15 individuals who had progressed to either clear-cut spondylitis or sacroiliitis were nearly all male and B27-positive with a mean onset age of 10.6 years.[87]

Racial and Ethnic Distributions. In a Los Angeles referral clinic and a 10-year Vancouver, Canada survey, disproportionately few children of Oriental origin were found to have arthritis.[124,134] In contrast, 16 North American Indian children with JRA were seen from a population of 22,000 in British Columbia (calculated incidence of 7.2 cases per 100,000 person-years).[134,135] Since HLA-B27 and ankylosing spondylitis are also considerably more frequent in several British Columbia Indian tribes,[113,114] it would have been helpful to know what proportion of these arthritic children were HLA-B27 positive and had spondyloarthropathy.

Familial Occurrence. Within each of three families, pairs of first-degree relatives manifested the same onset subtype and strikingly similar clinical features.[285] As anticipated, a higher than expected frequency of clinical ankylosing spondylitis and radiographic sacroiliitis has been found among male relatives, especially of those probands with sacroiliitis and HLA-B27. The presence of this antigen also identifies a group of young girls with dominant peripheral arthritis and cervical spondylitis, which may closely mimic rheumatoid arthritis.[285]

Early-onset pauciarticular arthritis with antinuclear antibody and iritis was associated with HLA-DRW5 in one study, and with HLA-DRW8 and an antigen "Tmo," related to HLA-DW7 and DW11, in others.[109,311] As in adult rheumatoid arthritis, polyarticular disease is associated with HLA-DW4. Three genetic markers, HLA-BW35, HLA-B8, and HLA-DW7, have increased frequency in systemic onset juvenile arthritis.[110,311] These studies support the clinical subgrouping and suggest genetic predisposition to their development, but a great deal of heterogeneity with respect to these markers is obvious.

Other Factors. In juvenile patients not further subclassified, those whose arthritis was preceded by an emotionally stressful event had higher antiviral antibody titers than those without such events.[279] The possible role of microbial agents in the occurrence and precipitation of chronic rheumatic disease in children has been reviewed, with emphasis on diseases that typify several different mechanisms of microbe-host interaction.[270]

Natural History. Although the prognosis in juvenile arthritis is better than in adult RA,[123,179] about one-half in one series had active disease at some time between the fifth and fifteenth years after onset, and functional class III or IV disability was present in 34 of 123 (28%).[123] Most (11 of 18) systemic-onset versus only 11 of 101 pauciarticular-onset patients had developed polyarticular involvement after 5 years.[24] Eight of nine deaths in one English series of 100 patients were in children with systemic onset.[112] In another follow-up study of 100 patients, the worst prognosis at 15 years was associated with polyarticular onset or persistent polyarthritis; all 3 deaths and 13 instances of "severe disability" derived from this group.[49] Long-term mortality ranges from 1 to 3% in U.S. series to nearly 10% in England and Europe, with differences possibly due to definition of disease and the increased frequency of secondary amyloidosis in Europe.[25] Interestingly, the sex ratio of fatal cases is equal.

Juvenile and Adult Rheumatoid Arthritis: A Continuum or Separate Diseases? Clinical and epidemiologic differences between the onset types of juvenile arthritis suggest that a variety of syndromes overlap age limits and that the age distinction between adult and juvenile cases is an artificial one. As indicated by tissue typing associations with certain juvenile onset arthritis syndromes, separate host predispositions to disease are suggested for different onset types, supporting concepts of disease not restricted to age limits.[137] Additional genetic studies are needed for more definitive conclusions.

ARTHRITIS SYNDROMES RELATED TO HLA-B27

Conceptual Developments. Over two decades ago, population and family pedigree studies indicated that ankylosing spondylitis had a strong familial predisposition, although its mode of inheritance was not defined. In addition, prior to the HLA-B27 discoveries, a genetic predisposition was suspected in several overlapping spinal and peripheral arthritis syndromes, including cases diagnosed as juvenile and adult ankylosing spondylitis, sacroiliitis, and Reiter's syndrome. These typically rheumatoid factor-negative (seronegative) conditions are now grouped into a family of spondyloarthritis syndromes,[352] and also include Yersinia-reactive arthritis, spondylitis associated with chronic inflammatory bowel disease or psoriasis, and certain forms of oligoarticular peripheral arthritis in juveniles or younger adults. It has now been clearly established that the population prevalence of these disorders varies considerably[26,65,113,114] and is highly correlated with the occurrence of B27 in the described populations.[46,65,114,351] However, these conditions may occur in the absence of B27[116,165] and appear identical in terms of clinical features and severity except for the association of acute anterior uveitis with B27 positivity.[169] In family studies, homozygosity for HLA-B27 does not seem to influence the severity or the occurrence of ankylosing spondylitis.[310] The shared B27 association of these spondyloarthritis disorders suggests a common host predisposition, conditioned perhaps by exogenous factors that may determine the clinical manifestations. HLA-D locus typing has not revealed significant associations with ankylosing spondylitis or Reiter's syndrome.[162]

Activation of ankylosing spondylitis in HLA-B27-positive persons by virtue of antigenic cross-reactivity with certain micro-organisms, specifically enteric carriage of *Klebsiella pneumoniae* has been proposed[86] but not confirmed.[344] Although various gram-negative enteric infections can precipitate Reiter's syndrome and similar reactive arthritis disorders (vide infra), no such mechanism has yet been documented for ankylosing spondylitis or psoriatic arthritis. The epidemiology of the spondyloarthritis syndromes and concepts of etiology have been reviewed.[209]

ANKYLOSING SPONDYLITIS

Ankylosing spondylitis (AS) is a chronic systemic disorder that affects primarily the axial and truncal joints with characteristic limited mobility and tendency to ankylosis, especially involving the sacroiliac joints. Because of its variable severity, the frequency of ankylosing spondylitis depends upon disease definition.[46] Prevalence varies greatly in different populations, ranging from a virtual absence in Australian aborigines[65] or black Africans[307] to a 4.2% diagnosed frequency in adult male Haida Indians.[114,135] The usual reported prevalence of "definite" AS is 1 per 1,000 population, based upon hospital or clinical survey techniques with a sex ratio of 3 males to 1 female.[200] A 20% frequency of "definite" and "possible" ankylosing spondylitis has been reported in HLA-B27-positive "healthy" males and females,[52,69] but most subjects had radiographic sacroiliitis rather than ankylosing spondylitis. A much lower prevalence of spondylitis among B27-positive individuals has been reported in other studies, including 3% in males and 0.6% in females in Hungary,[115] none in 139 persons in Australia,[61] and 1.3% in persons aged 45 or older in the Netherlands.[337] Symptomatic radiographic sacroiliitis should not be equated with clinical ankylosing spondylitis.

Criteria for Ankylosing Spondylitis. Criteria for population study of ankylosing spondylitis were proposed at the 1961 Rome symposium,[159] and a revised set was introduced in New York in 1966.[37] They are compared in Table 2–4. The Rome criteria permit diagnosis of ankylosing spondylitis without bilateral sacroiliitis on roentgenographs, whereas the New York criteria allow a "probable" diagnosis based solely upon roentgenographic evidence of sacroiliitis without clinical disease. Certainly, the latter syndrome is not synonymous with clinical AS, although both may be associated with HLA-B27 and belong to the spectrum of spondyloarthropathy. Future criteria studies should further define differences between clinically manifest ankylosing spondylitis and more limited radiographic syndromes.

Considerable variability may be expected in the determination and interpretation of symptoms of pain and stiffness in the dorsal and lumbar spine.[236] A high degree of variability has also been found in the interpretation of radiographic sacroiliitis,[137,141] especially unilateral and milder bilateral changes and in films of persons aged 50 or younger.[141] In one study, the pain item in the New York criteria had a specificity of only 4.9 percent and thus must be considered a nonspecific criterion

as it was defined.[236] However, certain manifestations of back pain may be more characteristic of spondylitis than of degenerative disease, e.g., onset before 40 years of age, insidious development, persistence longer than 3 months, morning stiffness, and relief with mild exercise.[50] In a psoriatic arthritis study, the physical findings of limited back movement in all directions and limited chest expansion had high specificity (over 95%) for roentgenographic disease, but a low sensitivity (less than 15%).[236] It has been suggested that the New York pain criterion for ankylosing spondylitis be modified by substituting the Rome pain criterion (low back pain for more than 3 months) to achieve greater specificity.[339]

Age and Sex Distribution. Ankylosing spondylitis is typically diagnosed in young adult males with the usual age of onset between 15 and 35 years. Radiographic sacroiliitis occurs in nearly equal proportions of B27-positive males and females, with[245] or without[50] peripheral arthritis, but females tend to have milder disease.[212] Ankylosing spondylitis is clinically diagnosed predominantly in males. Although marked male preponderance of about 10 to 1 was reported previously, later studies[57,209] noted a lower ratio, i.e., about 3 or 4 to 1, probably reflecting a greater proportion of women with milder disease. These findings suggest important age- and sex-related factors contributing to the disease expression.

Ethnic and Genetic Distribution. Ankylosing spondylitis is unusual in blacks.[26] Over 90% of nonrelated white males and females with ankylosing spondylitis have B27 versus only about half the blacks.[116,165] Family studies indicate that genetic susceptibility to ankylosing spondylitis closely associates with HLA-B27,[74,337] but may occur in its absence.[317] However, histocompatibility antigens B7, BW22, B40, and BW42[17] and the "public" antigen[294] have been found to associate with spondyloarthritis syndromes in B27-negative white and black Americans. These findings imply a more direct role of the B27-related antigens in pathogenesis. This concept is supported by family studies showing close segregation of AS with HLA-B27.[166,192,337] Epidemiologic data suggest the possibility of a relationship to hormonal factors as well. Diagnostically, HLA-B27 determination is most useful when the pre-test likelihood of ankylosing spondylitis or Reiter's syndrome is clinically neither low nor high, but in the middle ranges of probability where the test result can influence decision.[168]

Natural History. Prognosis of AS varies with the severity and its treatment, but it is generally favorable as the disease is often mild or self-limited. Mortality among 836 AS patients diagnosed

Table 2–4.   Ankylosing Spondylitis Population Survey Criteria

Rome, 1961[159]	*New York, 1966*[37]
CLINICAL CRITERIA	
1. Low back pain and stiffness for more than 3 months which is not relieved by rest.	Pain at the dorsolumbar junction or in the lumbar spine by history or at present.
2. Pain and stiffness in the thoracic region.	
3. Limited motion in the lumbar spine.	Limitation of motion of the lumbar spine in all three planes: anterior flexion, lateral flexion, and extension.
4. Limited chest expansion.	Limitation of chest expansion to 1 inch (2.5 cm) or less, measured at the level of the fourth intercostal space.
5. Iritis or its sequelae (history or evidence).	
RADIOLOGIC CRITERIA	
Bilateral sacroiliac changes characteristic of ankylosing spondylitis	Grade 3 to 4 bilateral sacroiliitis.
DEFINITE ANKYLOSING SPONDYLITIS	
Positive roentgenogram and 1 + clinical criteria.	Positive roentgenogram and 1 + clinical criteria.
Four of the five clinical criteria.	Grade 3 to 4 unilateral or grade 2 bilateral sacroiliitis either with limitation of back movement in all planes, or with both other clinical criteria.
PROBABLE ANKYLOSING SPONDYLITIS	
	Positive roentgenogram with no clinical criteria.

between 1935 and 1957 and not given x-ray therapy in the United Kingdom revealed an increased mortality in males only from arthritis-related causes.[275] In a U.S. clinical series of 56 AS cases (49 males) diagnosed between 1934 and 1960, reduced survival was detected only by 20 years after diagnosis or after approximately 30 years of symptomatic disease.[167] Only 4 of these individuals had received radiotherapy. A population sample of 102 AS patients from Rochester, Minnesota diagnosed from 1935 through 1973, including 73 males and 29 females, had decreased survival for the females only, beginning about 10 years after diagnosis and not attributable to irradiation, but the numbers were small.[57] The prognosis for functional capacity and occupational performance was found to be relatively good in AS after a mean duration of 38 years of disease.[55]

OTHER SERONEGATIVE SPONDYLOARTHRITIS SYNDROMES

Reiter's Disease. Reiter's disease, defined as the triad of arthritis, urethritis, and conjunctivitis, has been reported in epidemic occurrences, such as following bacillary dysentery,[251,262] and as an endemic or sporadic event following venereal urethritis.[184] An ARA subcommittee has proposed criteria for Reiter's syndrome (RS) based upon analysis of 83 RS, 53 AS, 33 seronegative RA, 53 psoriatic arthritis, and 27 gonococcal arthritis patients submitted from seven centers.[348] Clinically acceptable Reiter's syndrome consists of peripheral arthritis of more than 1 month's duration occurring in association with urethritis and/or cervicitis. These criteria had 84% sensitivity at the initial episode and 97.6% including subsequent episodes. Specificity varied among the control groups from 96 to 100%.

Although once considered to be relatively rare, Reiter's disease is now recognized commonly in young adult males and is perhaps the leading cause of noninfectious arthritis admissions to military hospitals.[16] The venereal acquisition of this disorder by women is unusual.[253] Following a bacillary dysentery epidemic in Finland in the summer of 1944, 0.2% of the enteritis victims developed Reiter's syndrome.[262] Interestingly, 10% of the enteric-acquired cases occurred in women, suggesting that Reiter's syndrome is relatively more common in women in the epidemic than endemic type.[184,253] In an epidemic in June 1962, aboard an American naval vessel, 10 of 602 (1.5%) men with

Shigella dysentery subsequently acquired Reiter's syndrome within several weeks.[251] However, in a large community outbreak of *Shigella sonnei* in Puerto Rico, no case of Reiter's syndrome was disclosed among 1,970 patients surveyed.[153] Earlier reports associated Bedsonia venereal infection with Reiter's syndrome,[292] but subsequent controlled studies have not supported such a relationship.[100] Sporadic cases of Reiter's syndrome have been reported after enteric infection with Yersinia enterocolitica, Salmonella enteritidis, and Campylobacter fetus.

A survey of Reiter's disease in venereal clinics in the United Kingdom between 1960 and 1964 yielded 1 female and 100 male cases; 35 males residing in a particular area were examined along with their relatives and spouses.[184] Radiographic evidence of sacroiliitis was found in 23% of the probands, and its frequency increased with duration of symptoms. Clinical spondylitis and radiographic changes (Rome criteria) were two to eight times as frequent among relatives as in a population control sample, and none of the spouses had spondylitis. An even wider spectrum of disease is suggested by recent studies of probands in Finland, indicating an association with acute peripheral polyarthritis among first-degree relatives.[174] The description of "incomplete" Reiter's syndrome[16] also favors a broader disease spectrum.

Following the HLA-B27 discovery, numerous clinical series of sporadic Reiter's syndrome were reported with striking B27 associations of 63 to 96% among adult Caucasian patients, highest in those individuals with clinical or roentgenographic evidence of sacroiliitis.[46,214,238] HLA-B27 shows a lower association, approximately 40%, among American black RS cases,[164] but a complementary association with B7 CREG antigens may occur.[17] Among childhood cases of RS, at least 12 of 13 reported had B27.[286] In addition, the epidemic form has been shown to be associated with B27,[51,291] with an estimated Reiter's syndrome attack frequency of one-sixth to one-third in B27-positive young adult males infected with Shigella.[51]

Reactive Arthritis. A large series of Scandinavian Reiter's disease and Yersinia reactive arthritis patients was reported with special reference to HLA-B27.[189] The male to female ratio was nearly 20:1 in RS but 1:1 in Yersinia arthritis, with a similar mean age of 30 and 31 and HLA-B27 positivity of 81 and 73%, respectively. Chronic back pain and joint symptoms were frequent in all the patient groups over the average five-year follow-up, but most patients were able to lead normal lives. In 16% of RS patients, the acute disease progressed to a chronic destructive peripheral arthritis. Follow-up of an American series of 122 RS

patients revealed that 16% had to change jobs and 11% were unemployable over a mean interval of 5.6 years of disease.[101] No specific entry factors were identified that correlated with outcome.

In addition, B27-positive individuals have been noted to be particularly prone to arthritis following gastroenteritis caused by the gram-negative organisms Yersinia enterocolitica,[189] Salmonella,[10] and Campylobacter jejuni.[32] The frequency of each was similar to that reported for Reiter's disease.

These observations suggest that a genetically susceptible host (HLA-B27-positive) may encounter an environmental inciting or infective agent that precipitates disease.

Inflammatory Bowel Disease Arthritis. Although only a small proportion of patients with ulcerative colitis or regional enteritis develop spondylitis, their risk is estimated to be 30 times greater than in the general population, and approximately 50% are HLA-B27-positive.[47] It is interesting, however, that neither asymptomatic roentgenographic sacroiliitis[144] nor peripheral arthritis alone,[46] occurring during the course of chronic inflammatory bowel disease, is associated with B27. Population frequency, family studies, and HLA-B27 associations of the arthropathy of inflammatory bowel disease have been reviewed.[209]

Psoriatic Arthritis. Spondylitis occurs in approximately 2% of individuals with psoriasis, and 35 to over 70% of these spondylitis patients are HLA-B27-positive.[209] Among patients with psoriasis and only peripheral arthritis without sacroiliitis, a slightly increased frequency of B27 has been observed in some series.[47,209] Some of these B27-positive patients may eventually develop spondylitis.

In comparison to normal subjects, patients with psoriasis and peripheral arthritis more often had HLA-BW38 (38% vs. 6%) as well as HLA-DRW4 (54% vs. 32%).[91] These and other studies[244] suggest that multiple factors, controlled by genes in the major histocompatibility complex, appear to contribute to psoriasis and psoriatic arthritis. The association of HLA-DR4 is interesting because it also associates with more advanced rheumatoid arthritis, whether seropositive or seronegative.[205] Psoriatic arthritis in childhood shows some clinical features similar to those of the adult disease.[305] A sex ratio of 17 girls to 7 boys was found in one series, consistent with the female predominance of 2:1 in childhood-onset psoriasis. Arthropathy antedated skin changes in 14 (58%) of the 24 patients, and clinical evidence of tendinitis (36%) was also more common than in the adult disease.

Peripheral arthritis is believed to occur in about 5% of psoriasis patients and presumably in higher frequency in those with more advanced skin involvement. Microvascular changes similar to those seen in RA have been identified in psoriatic synovium and implicated in pathogenesis.[91] Interestingly, autoimmunity to collagen[332] and association with HLA-DR4[91,244] are also shared features of psoriatic and rheumatoid arthritis. Furthermore, the native collagen mouse model of arthritis shows histologic and radiographic similarities to both psoriatic and rheumatoid arthritis.[331] Thus, host predisposition as evidenced by certain HLA genotypes, immunologic reactivity to collagen, and microvasculopathy may contribute to the pathogenesis of both psoriatic and rheumatoid arthritis.

HOST PREDISPOSITION TO PERIPHERAL AND SPINAL ARTHRITIS SYNDROMES

Accumulating evidence indicates significant correlations between host factors, e.g., onset age, sex, and race, with various arthritis syndromes, some having recognized genetic or immunologic markers. For example, the onset age of spondyloarthritis syndromes tends to be earlier than in RA with males greatly favored. Among newly diagnosed younger peripheral arthritis patients with clinical diagnoses of RA, unclassified arthritis, and spondyloarthritis syndromes, but without evidence of classic ankylosing spondylitis,[203] HLA-B27 correlated with maleness and younger adult onset age (15 to 29 years). In contrast, rheumatoid factor positivity was found predominantly in females with older onset age (30 to 44 years) as seen in Table 2–5. These data emphasize powerful host factor effects on the type of rheumatic disease syndrome manifested.[205] The largest group of newly diagnosed peripheral arthritis patients had neither rheumatoid factor nor B27. Their total frequency was equal in each age group studied, but a significant sex ratio reversal occurred between the juvenile and young adult ages.

Overlapping relationships among these largely undefined syndromes are schematized in Figure 2–3. Their further characterization provides an important challenge for future integrated epidemiologic, clinical, and laboratory research.[205]

CONNECTIVE TISSUE DISORDERS (ACQUIRED)

Systemic Lupus Erythematosus

A review of the epidemiology of systemic lupus erythematosus (SLE) has been published.[199]

Criteria for Classification. The use, evaluations, and criticisms of the 1971 preliminary criteria for the classification of SLE[68] were reviewed in 299 articles published in three rheumatology journals and four general medical journals.[54] The criteria were increasingly used during the eight-year study period, with 90% of authors referring to them in the last year examined, 1978. The main criticism of these criteria was the failure to incorporate new immunologic knowledge. One study suggested using two or more of serum anti-DNA antibodies, serum anti-Sm antibodies, or positive lupus band test, which were found in 80% of 50 SLE patients but in none of 77 other patients with connective tissue disease.[241] This problem was addressed in the 1982 revised criteria report with lupus and control patient data obtained from 18 institutions.[324] Criteria were developed in a "training" sample of the lupus and control patients and then tested on the remaining "test" sample to avoid the bias of testing criteria against the same patients in whom they were developed. Antinuclear, anti-DNA, and anti-Sm antibodies were added while Raynaud's phenomenon and alopecia were dropped (Table 2–6). If any 4 or more of the 11 criteria were present, serially or simultaneously, during any interval of observation, SLE could be diagnosed with 96% sensitivity and 96% specificity. The control group consisted predominantly of patients with rheumatoid arthritis. However, the revised criteria performed well in 172 SLE patients and against a combined group of 299 patients with systemic sclerosis and 119 patients with polymyositis-dermatomyositis from the Scleroderma Criteria Cooperative Study[318] (83% sensitivity, 89% specificity).[324]

Table 2–5. Distribution of Early-Diagnosed Peripheral Arthritis Patients by Onset Age, Sex, Rheumatoid Factor (RF), and HLA B27 Status*

Onset Age	RF + B27 −			RF − B27 −			RF − B27 +			Total		
	F	M	T	F	M	T	F	M	T	F	M	T
<15	1	1	2	10	20	30	2	5	7	13	26	39
15–29	9	0	9	23	12	35	4	15	19	36	27	63
30–44	15	2	17	31	8	39	4	2	6	50	12	62
<45	25	3	28	64	40	104	10	22	32	99	65	164

*Three B27 patients excluded with associated rheumatoid factor positivity. Data from the Memphis and Shelby County Arthritis Research Program.[203]

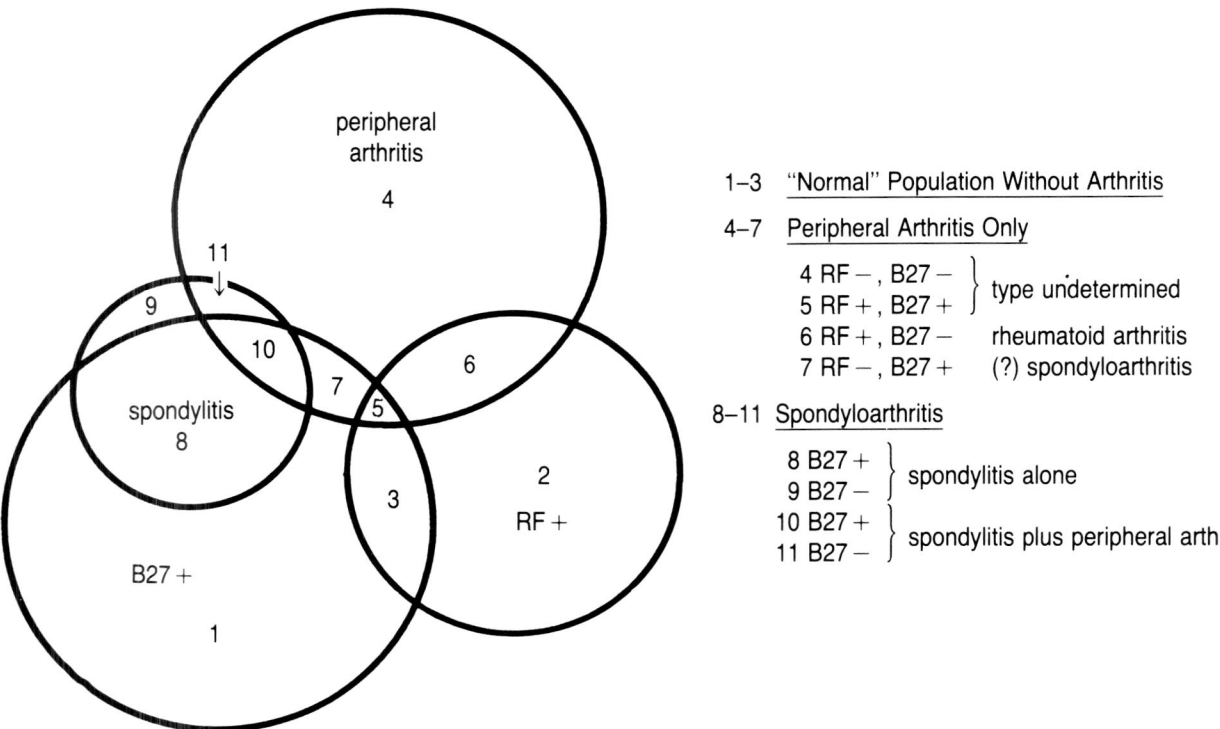

1–3 "Normal" Population Without Arthritis

4–7 Peripheral Arthritis Only

4 RF −, B27 −	type undetermined
5 RF +, B27 +	
6 RF +, B27 −	rheumatoid arthritis
7 RF −, B27 +	(?) spondyloarthritis

8–11 Spondyloarthritis

8 B27 +	spondylitis alone
9 B27 −	
10 B27 +	spondylitis plus peripheral arthr
11 B27 −	

Fig. 2–3.   Schematic relationship between spondylitis, peripheral arthritis, HLA-B27, and rheumatoid factor (RF).

Incidence and Prevalence. The occurrence of SLE in populations has been summarized (Table 2–7).[199] The first population studies were performed using mainly hospital discharge record indexes, supplemented by clinic, laboratory, or pathology records.[300,302] In New York City, the 1965 estimated annual SLE incidence was over 30 new cases per million population.[302] During 1965 to 1973, incidence was calculated as 74 per million in 120,000 San Francisco city and county residents belonging to a group health plan.[96] In the latter study, the prevalence was 1 case in 700 white women aged 15 to 64 years, and 1 in 245 black women of this age!

Reports from areas with a variety of racial types throughout the world suggest that SLE is prevalent.[199] The age-adjusted prevalence rates for Chinese, Filipinos, and Japanese living on Oahu Island, Hawaii were three to four times greater than those for whites.[295] The Crow, Arapahoe, and Sioux tribes of North American Indians had annual incidence in excess of 100 per million population, using the 1971 ARA classification criteria.[240] The estimated annual incidence of SLE was 313 per million for full-blooded Sioux, but these rates were based on relatively small numbers of cases.

It is not known whether the increasing incidence with time reflects heightened physician awareness of lupus or a true increase in frequency. The worldwide distribution of lupus suggests a multifactorial etiology and pathogenesis.

Age, Race, and Sex Distribution. Females have a striking susceptibility to SLE, particularly during the younger adult ages, as observed in virtually all epidemiologic studies reported. This dramatic incidence increases early in the second decade, peaks in the third, remains high during the childbearing years, decreases during the 45- to 64-year period, and declines further thereafter.[302] Conversely, males showed no impressive incidence variation with age in the small number of cases reported in the New York City study.[302] Over all ages, females exceed males in clinical series in a ratio of at least 5:1, and to a greater extent during the childbearing years.[93,208]

Under age 12, the female to male ratio of new SLE cases is low (2 to 3:1).[172] Similarly, this ratio approaches equality after age 65.[195,302] It may also be important that SLE may begin or exacerbate during pregnancy or the postpartum period,[83] when marked hormonal changes are occurring. The female preponderance in SLE may thus be associated more with sexual maturation or hormonal factors than with the female genotype per se.[208]

Table 2-6. 1982 Revised Criteria for the Classification of Systemic Lupus Erythematosus*[124]

Disorder	Signs
1. Malar rash	Fixed erythema, flat or raised, over the malar eminences, tending to spare the nasolabial folds.
2. Discoid rash	Erythematous raised patches with adherent keratotic scaling and follicular plugging; atrophic scarring may occur in older lesions.
3. Photosensitivity	Skin rash as a result of unusual reaction to sunlight, by patient history or physician observation.
4. Oral ulcers	Oral or nasopharyngeal ulceration, usually painless, observed by a physician.
5. Arthritis	Nonerosive arthritis involving two or more peripheral joints, characterized by tenderness, swelling, or effusion.
6. Serositis	a. Pleuritis—convincing history of pleuritic pain or rub heard by a physician or evidence of pleural effusion; OR b. Pericarditis—documented by ECG or rub or evidence of pericardial effusion.
7. Renal disorder	a. Persistent proteinuria greater than 0.5 g per day or greater than 3+ if quantitation not performed; OR b. Cellular casts—may be red cell, hemoglobin, granular, tubular, or mixed.
8. Neurologic disorder	a. Seizures—in the absence of offending drugs or known metabolic derangements, e.g., uremia, ketoacidosis, or electrolyte imbalance; OR b. Psychosis—in the absence of offending drugs or known metabolic derangements, e.g., uremia, ketoacidosis, or electrolyte imbalance.
9. Hematologic disorder	a. Hemolytic anemia—with reticulocytosis; OR b. Leukopenia—less than 4,000/mm³ total on two or more occasions; OR c. Lymphopenia—less than 1,500/mm³ on two or more occasions; OR d. Thrombocytopenia—less than 100,000/mm³ in the absence of offending drugs.
10. Immunologic disorder	a. Positive LE cell preparation: OR b. Anti-DNA: antibody to native DNA in abnormal titer; OR c. Anti-Sm: presence of antibody to Sm nuclear antigen; OR d. False positive serologic test for syphilis known to be positive for at least 6 months and confirmed by Treponema pallidum immobilization or fluorescent treponemal antibody absorption test.
11. Antinuclear antibody	An abnormal titer of antinuclear antibody by immunofluorescence or an equivalent assay at any time and in the absence of drugs known to be associated with "drug-induced lupus" syndrome.

*The proposed classification is based on 11 criteria. For the purpose of identifying patients in clinical studies, a person shall be said to have systemic lupus erythematosus if any 4 or more of the 11 criteria are present, serially or simultaneously, during any interval of observation.

Table 2–7. **Prevalence and Average Annual Incidence of SLE (Frequency per 100,000 Population)[199]**

Source	Location of Study Population	Survery Period	Type of Survey	Prevalence	Incidence
Leonhardt[199]	Scania*	1955–1961	Hospital	2.3	0.5
	Malmö	1955–1961		6.0	1.0
Siegel et al.[300,302]	New York City	1954–1956	Multi-institutional	4.0	1.5
		1960–1962		10.0	1.5
		1964–1966		15.0	3.5
		1956–1965		14.6	2.0
Kurland et al.[177]	Rochester, Minnesota	1950–1979	Multiclinic	40.0	1.8
Fessel[96]	San Francisco	1965–1973	Health plan	50.8	7.4
Serdula and Rhoads[295]	Oahu, Hawaii	1970–1975	General hospitals	5.8 (white)	
				24.1 (Chinese)	
				19.9 (Filipino)	
				20.4 (part-Hawaiian)	
				18.2 (Japanese)	
Morton et al.[240]	Crow	1971–1975	Hospital index	—	27.1
	Arapahoe			—	24.3
	Sioux			67.0†	16.6
	Other tribes			—	5.0‡
Chantler et al.[199]	Southern Nevada	15-year period	Isolated community	—	16.0

*Except Malmö.
†Period prevalence (20 cases in 30,210 population).
‡Median of other tribes.

A role for endocrine factors in the pathogenesis of systemic lupus is also suggested by its reported association with Klinefelter's syndrome[208] and metabolic data showing prolonged estrogenic stimulation in such cases.[312] Additional support comes from the protective effects of androgen (testosterone) administration in the murine lupus model.[289] Clinical and experimental data from a variety of sources suggest heightened humoral immunity and depressed cellular immunity in females compared with males; these differences appear to be mediated by sex hormones.[145]

An incidence of black versus white females of about 3:1 was first reported from New York City, based on relatively small numbers.[300] This conclusion has now been amply supported in larger case series,[96,301] and mortality analyses confirm the findings.[154] Whether the incidence is increased in black versus white males is not known because community population data are limited.

Genetic Factors. Although familial SLE has been described frequently, one cannot prove familial aggregation without a population denominator and a known frequency of disease in the population at risk.[201] However, the impressive number of reports, including males,[182] suggests a greater than chance familial occurrence.[199] Such aggregation appears to operate generally at a low level whether environmental, genetic, or infectious agent factors might be contributing.[18,43,193,228] Studies of genetically determined HLA antigens in SLE have revealed that HLA-B8 and DRW3 are partic-

ularly frequent,[59] but no clinical features or disease course correlations with these antigens have been noted.

The healthy relatives of SLE patients have increased frequency of both serum lymphocytotoxic antibodies[228] and impaired suppressor cell function,[233] but these abnormalities have not been correlated.[233] Thus, although these findings represent defects in immunoregulation, they may not necessarily lead to disease.

A newly observed association is that of congenital complete heart block with maternal SLE.[92,125] Many other cardiac abnormalities have also been noted in these infants. In at least half the cases, the women had few or no findings of lupus prior to the delivery. A striking proportion (70%) of the mothers had serum SS-A Ro antibodies in these studies.

Environmental and Socioeconomic Associations. Studies of housing quality and crowding in New York City SLE cases and controls revealed no significant associations.[304] Antinuclear antibodies have been found in the serum of consanguineous female relatives of SLE patients irrespective of household contact with the proband.[228] In addition, lymphocytotoxic antibodies have been noted in laboratory personnel who have studied lupus sera.[193] Neither SLE nor autoantibodies were more frequent in human household contacts of dogs with SLE.[64,278]

The etiologic role of type C viruses in human lupus remains controversial. In several reports, extensive studies failed to identify type C oncornavirus or its p30-related antigens.[133,171] In another report, however, immunoglobulins with specific antiviral p30 activity, distinct from antinuclear antibodies, were eluted from the glomerular immune deposits of two lupus nephritis patients previously found to have viral p30-related antigen present in the same tissue.[225] High-titer (1:20 or greater) serum antibodies to *Rickettsia haemobartonella,* an Anaplasmataceae, were found in all of 22 SLE patients compared with only 13 or 102 controls.[150] Free Haemobartonella antigen was demonstrated in the glomeruli of one of these antibody-positive patients with lupus nephritis. The specificity and primary nature of this finding are not known.

Course of Disease and Survival. Reported survival rates from the time of first diagnosis have improved over the years, from the earlier hospital-based studies indicating a four-year 51% survival,[227] to more recent clinic-based results suggesting a 10-year 70 to 90% survival.[96,108] Interpretations of such marked differences are complex and still unresolved. Clinical series have revealed a more favorable prognosis in older individuals,[78] in patients with a longer interval from onset to diagnosis, and in those without renal or central nervous system involvement[93,187] or superimposed bacterial infections.[93,108,187] In patients with lupus nephritis, a bimodal mortality pattern has been observed, with an excess of early deaths due to active lupus and sepsis and late deaths attributable to vascular events superimposed on a constant rate of death caused by renal failure.[152] It was reported earlier that juvenile-onset patients had a poorer prognosis than expected,[224] but more recent studies indicate survival is at least comparable to that in adults.[1,343] Racial differences in prognosis were not detected in the New York City study.[299]

The role of corticosteroids in survival is unclear in retrospective series, primarily because patients could not be matched for disease severity and other prognostically important organ system involvement. In one study, patients were stratified using a prognostic index that included scoring of disease severity according to clinical and laboratory evidence of intensity of involvement and number of organs affected.[11] Corticosteroid use was associated with improved survival only among high-risk patients who were identified by having at least two of the following: 4+ severity at any time, total average severity of 2+ or greater, and nephritis.

Drug-Activated SLE-Like Syndromes. The relationship of drug-induced disease to idiopathic SLE is not clear. A hospital study of 258 SLE patients revealed that 12 (4.7%) had received one or another possibly inducing drug for at least two months preceding onset.[188] During 1957 to 1966, 59 cases of drug-induced SLE were detected in a New York City hospital survey.[303] The frequency increased with age and females predominated over males, notwithstanding differences in drug exposure. No racial predisposition was observed, unlike that found in idiopathic SLE. In Rochester, Minnesota, drug-induced disease had an annual incidence of 0.8 per 100,000 compared with 1.8 for the natural disease.[230] In one series, it was reported that hydralazine-induced lupus developed only in "slow acetylators" of the drug,[265] suggesting host metabolic predisposition to this syndrome.

Systemic Sclerosis (Scleroderma)

The term scleroderma encompasses a variety of disorders associated with hardening of the skin, whereas "systemic sclerosis" implies a multisystem disorder affecting both skin and internal organs. The spectrum of systemic sclerosis ranges from classic disease with diffuse scleroderma to the CREST syndrome, in which there is prominent calcinosis, Raynaud's phenomenon, esophageal involvement, sclerodactyly, and telangiectasia.[281] Systemic sclerosis may also be encountered in the setting of "overlap" syndromes, such as "mixed connective tissue disease."[297] The coexistence of systemic sclerosis and rheumatoid arthritis was reported in five patients.[23,70] Important clinical and natural history differences between these systemic sclerosis variants suggests that they represent distinct subsets of the disease.[216] The specificity of serum anticentromere antibody for the CREST syndrome supports this concept.[325]

Classification Criteria. Criteria for classification of definite systemic sclerosis have been proposed by a subcommittee of the ARA based on a multicenter longitudinal evaluation of 264 systemic sclerosis patients and 413 patients with other connective tissue disease.[318] One major criterion (scleroderma proximal to the digits) or at least two of three minor criteria (including sclerodactyly, digital pitting scars, and bilateral basilar pulmonary fibrosis on chest roentgenogram) served to identify 256 systemic sclerosis patients (97% sensitivity) but only 10 comparison patients (98% specificity). These criteria for definite disease performed well in an external validation completed as part of the study. Assessment of the criteria made on 50 patients with systemic sclerosis and 199 patients with similar connective tissue disease from New Zealand revealed a 100% specificity and the anticipated lower sensitivity of 79%.[326] The latter is attributable to a higher proportion of patients with CREST syndrome and early, mild disease in this population-based study. Definition of early, mild, and limited scleroderma should be addressed in subsequent studies of the ARA criteria.

Age, Race, and Sex-Specific Incidence and Mortality. Three community[177,204,221] and two national[66,220] epidemiologic surveys of systemic sclerosis incidence or mortality have been performed in the United States based on hospital and/or death certificate records. The estimated annual incidence has varied, but is believed to be 5 to 10 new cases per million population at risk. An incidence of 6.3 new patients per million per year was found from 1970 to 1979 in Auckland, with no significant difference between Caucasians and Polynesians.[85] There is general agreement concerning a female to male ratio of almost 3:1, which is significantly exaggerated during the childbearing years of 15 to 44.[221] The first convincing case of systemic sclerosis in a patient with Klinefelter's syndrome was reported.[257] Childhood or adolescent onset is unusual,[334] and incidence appears to increase steadily with age, especially in females.[221] Although some excess is present in blacks, this tendency is small compared with findings in systemic lupus erythematosus.

Geographic, Occupational, and Environmental Factors. Systemic sclerosis occurs throughout the world, and in the United States, there is no recognized geographic concentration of cases.[66,220] It has been suggested that the disease is more common among underground coal and gold miners and others occupationally exposed to silica dust.[90,280] Scleroderma-like cutaneous lesions, Raynaud's phenomenon, nail fold capillary changes, and osteolysis of the distal phalanges have been described in workers exposed to vinyl chloride monomer used in the manufacture of plastics.[198] Japanese workmen exposed to the vapor of epoxy resin developed cutaneous sclerosis.[355] In Japan, silicone or paraffin implantation for breast augmentation has been followed after many years by a scleroderma-like illness.[176] An acute multisystem disease with eosinophilia, culminating in fibrosis of the skin and subcutis, reached epidemic proportions in Spain and has been attributed to the ingestion of denatured rapeseed oil.[170] Notably absent were Raynaud's phenomenon and esophageal hypomotility.

Familial Occurrence. Although reports of the familial occurrence of systemic sclerosis remain limited, there are over 10 documented instances.[219] HLA-A, B, and DR typing has been unrewarding.[194]

Natural History. The course of systemic sclerosis is variable, but survival studies, including several over nearly a decade, have revealed almost identical results.[35,217] The five-year cumulative survival rates from diagnosis ranged from 60 to 73%. Recent advances in the treatment of "scleroderma renal crisis," including renal dialysis and the use of potent antihypertensive agents, should result in improved survival during the next few years.

The coexistence of cancer and systemic sclerosis has been the subject of several reports.[84,323] They have led to speculation regarding increased frequency of cancer in systemic sclerosis patients.[41] These series have the anticipated referral biases, and no community epidemiologic study has yet been performed.

Disease Models. Several potential models of systemic sclerosis have been described. Long-term survivors of bone marrow transplantation have developed multisystem involvement resembling systemic sclerosis.[105] The chemotherapeutic agent, bleomycin, is capable of inducing scleroderma.[97] In addition, "scleroderma chicken"[106] and "tight-skinned mouse"[116a] models have been reported. Although these conditions differ in a number of ways from systemic sclerosis, they may lead to important insights into the pathogenesis of tissue fibrosis.

Polymyositis and Dermatomyositis

Polymyositis is the more inclusive term for this group of disorders characterized by chronic degenerative and inflammatory alterations of striated muscle, skin, and various internal organs. Because no clear-cut distinction exists between polymyositis and dermatomyositis, except for the characteristic skin involvement in the latter, both terms may be used interchangeably.[44,218] Polymyositis in childhood is less well recognized than the more acute dermatomyositis, but critical comparison of these two juvenile disorders has revealed similarities also favoring a common disease spectrum.[121]

Classification. Because of the variability in clinical and laboratory features, the problem of disease classification has been handled differently by various authors. One generally accepted system, that of Pearson,[264] includes adult polymyositis, adult dermatomyositis, inflammatory myositis associated with cancer, childhood myositis, and myositis associated with other connective tissue diseases (overlap syndromes).

No official criteria have as yet been proposed for either diagnosis or classification of polymyositis. However, for epidemiologic purposes, combinations of clinical and laboratory features have been suggested, with exclusion of patients having a primary diagnosis of another connective tissue disease, or other cause of primary myopathy. The classification criteria of Medsger and Masi[218] and the diagnostic criteria of Bohan and Peter[45] are most frequently used. They require various combinations of findings, including proximal muscle weakness, abnormal muscle biopsy, electromyogram, serum muscle enzymes, urine creatine excretion, and evidence of corticosteroid responsiveness (Table 2–8).

Age, Sex, and Race Incidence. A hospital-based epidemiologic survey of polymyositis (including dermatomyositis) in Memphis and Shelby County, Tennessee from 1947 to 1968 revealed an average annual incidence of 5.0 cases per million population.[218] As with scleroderma, incidence increased during the study interval, reaching 8.4 during the period from 1963 to 1968; greater awareness of diagnosis and availability of serum muscle enzyme tests were believed to explain this trend. A bimodal age distribution was found, with the first incidence peak of 4.3 in the 10 to 14 age group, a nadir of 1.0 in the 15 to 24 age group, and a second peak of 10.2 in the 45 to 64 age group. Similar results were obtained in Israel, where the overall incidence was 2.2 new cases diagnosed annually per million population from 1960 to 1976, and childhood and adult incidence peaks were also observed.[33] Such patterns contrast with SLE in females, in whom the peak incidence occurs in the 15 to 44 age group and with considerably lower incidence in the younger and older ages, especially in blacks.

In an expanded Memphis survey (1948 to 1972) of patients under age 20, the average annual incidence was 3.2 per million.[120] Under age 10, the incidence was identical in females and males (3.2F:3.1M) but, in the second decade, a significant female excess was noted (6.0F:0.7M). Thus, a female preponderance seems to emerge again in adolescence, as observed for RA, SLE, and systemic sclerosis, suggesting common factors related to sexual maturation as important in occurrence or precipitation of these conditions.

Like SLE, the incidence was four times greater in black females.[218] No overall sex difference was found in adult whites, but in blacks, females predominated twofold over males. In the Transvaal, the annual incidence of dermatomyositis among the Bantus was estimated to be not less than 2.1 cases per million, nearly 10 times that observed among whites in the same region.[98] The disease was twice as frequent as SLE in this population, it tended to occur in the "young adult" age group, and patients had some features suggesting overlap syndromes. The female to male sex ratio tends to be greater in polymyositis patients whose manifestations overlap with those of other connective tissue diseases.[44]

Genetic Factors. Familial aggregation has rarely been reported, but studies of histocompatibility antigens have shown an increased frequency of HLA-B8 and DRW3 in both children and adults.[28,103,261] DRW3 correlated with the presence of Jo-1,[15] one of several antibody systems identified in the serum of polymyositis patients.

Geographic and Socioeconomic Distribution. Polymyositis has been reported to occur in nearly all climates and geographic areas of the globe. No association with family income or household crowding and no evidence of temporal-spatial clustering of cases was found in Memphis.[218] In juveniles, a concentration of case onsets during colder months,[218] or with possible exposure to bacteriologically proved streptococcal diseases,[173] suggests the contribution of upper respiratory infection precipitating factors. High anti-Coxsackie B antibody titers have been noted in childhood polymyositis-dermatomyositis in a case-controlled study,[60] and a new experimental model of Coxsackie virus-induced myositis has been de-

Table 2–8. Diagnostic Criteria for Polymyositis-Dermatomyositis

	Manifestions
	1. Typical skin rash of dermatomyositis
	2. Symmetrical proximal muscle weakness by history and physical examination
	3. Elevation of one or more serum muscle enzymes
	4. Myopathic changes on electromyogram
	5. Typical polymyositis on muscle biopsy
	6. Elevated urine creatine excretion
	7. Objective improvement in muscle weakness on corticosteroid therapy

	Bohan and Peter[45]		*Medsger and Masi*[218]
	Dermatomyositis	*Polymyositis*	*Polymyositis*
Definite	(1) + any 3 of (2),(3),(4)or(5)	all 4 of (2),(3),(4)and(5)	(2)and(5) *or* (2),(4) and either (3)or(6)
Probable	(1) + any 2 of (2),(3),(4)or(5)	any 3 of (2),(3),(4)or(5)	(2)and(4) *or* (2) and either (3)or(6)
Possible	(1) + any 1 of (2),(3),(4)or(5)	any 2 of (2),(3),(4)or(5)	(2) and (7)

scribed in mice.[316] Complement-fixing antibodies to *Toxoplasma gondii* have been found in the serum of 7 of 20 (35%) of polymyositis patients, but rarely in individuals with dermatomyositis or in age-, race- and sex-matched controls.[272] Patients with the highest titers had disease of more recent onset (mean less than 2 years) and more frequently had anti-Toxoplasma IgM antibodies, favoring recent infection.[196] Direct immunofluorescence has identified free Toxoplasma tachyzoites in a child with dermatomyositis.[131]

Natural History. Life-table analysis of 124 patients with polymyositis[223] showed an overall 53% survival at 7 years, similar to that for systemic sclerosis. Age over 50 years, black race, and the presence of marked muscle weakness, dysphagia, and aspiration pneumonia were signs of a poor prognosis if identified at the time of first hospital diagnosis. In a series from comparable years, dysphagia and severe proximal weakness at entry also were considered signs of a poor prognosis, and the case fatality rate was 45%.[56] A lower overall fatality rate of 28%, increasing with age, was determined in 118 cases of polymyositis over a mean interval of 6 years for surviving patients.[77] The significantly increased mortality among the older patients is not explained by associated cancer alone.[77,223] Mortality data from a 1968 to 1978 United States study of nearly 2,000 deaths attributed to polymyositis or dermatomyositis showed the greatest mortality in nonwhite females.[139] It has been suggested that the prognosis in patients referred to large urban medical centers may be unrepresentative, and that milder disease with a higher remission rate is more characteristic.[140] Survival among patients with childhood polymyositis in two series is 90% or more after six years of follow-up.[223,319]

Although earlier studies suggested that many middle-aged or older adults with dermatomyositis had various associated cancers, larger more representative surveys indicate a frequency of 10% or less.[44,218] However, reliable statistical data based upon large epidemiologic surveys are not available to settle the question of magnitude or significance of association between adult dermatomyositis-polymyositis and malignant neoplasms.[22,321]

Vasculitis Syndromes

Disorders characterized by inflammation of arteries, capillaries, or veins may occur independently or in association with other rheumatic diseases. Nomenclature varies, depending upon the frame of reference, i.e., clinical, etiologic, histologic, or immunologic.[72]

Polyarteritis Nodosa. Classic polyarteritis, originally termed "periarteritis nodosa," may be the end stage of a variety of necrotizing processes affecting muscular arteries. Infectious agents have long been suspected as participants in the etiology, but have been difficult to demonstrate.

Concomitant infection with hepatitis B virus has been associated with 30 to 60% of cases of classic polyarteritis[111,333] and has been reported in circumstances hyperendemic for hepatitis B.[82,215] Immune complexes containing hepatitis B surface antigen and antibody have been demonstrated in the circulation and blood vessel walls of polyarteritis patients.[229] Use of certain intravenous drugs, particularly methamphetamines,[63] may lead to polyarteritis, presumably of toxic etiology. Other associations reported include hyposensitization treatment for allergies,[269] serous otitis media,[296] and "hairy cell" leukemia.[88] No genetic factors have yet been identified in this disorder.

The population frequency of polyarteritis is not known, but middle-aged adults are mainly affected, with a male predominance in most series.[104,242] In one series of incidence studies, based on only a few cases, the annual rate in Rochester, Minnesota was 7 to 9 per million population.[177,178] Mortality data from New York City showed 103 deaths attributed to polyarteritis nodosa from 1951 through 1959, during which time 340 deaths were attributed to SLE.[300] Similar mortality data were obtained from Baltimore[202] and a sampling of United States death certificates.[66] Unfortunately, many types of vasculitis are probably included in these reports because subclassification on the basis of pathologic features was not popular at that time.

Kawasaki Disease. Infantile polyarteritis, a rare condition with a particular affinity for involvement of the coronary arteries, affects children mainly under one year of age.[99] Kawasaki disease (mucocutaneous lymph node syndrome), presumably of infectious origin, has many similarities to infantile polyarteritis, but is a more varied systemic disorder. It has been reported in increasing, epidemic proportions in Japan,[298] but is also described worldwide. This syndrome may be a final common pathway for a variety of infectious agents. It has been reported in association with Epstein-Barr virus[21] and Pseudomonas septicemia.[163] Childhood polyarteritis is unusual. Such patients may be classified within the multiple categories that compose the broad group of necrotizing vasculitis in adults.[99] Allergic granulomatous angiitis (Churg-Strauss syndrome) usually begins with asthma, followed by fever, eosinophilia, and a systemic necrotizing granulomatous vasculitis.[62] No favored host or environmental factor has been identified, although patients often have a strong personal history of allergy.

The prognosis in polyarteritis is poor regardless

of whether it is associated with hepatitis B infection. The five-year survival in one large series was 48% for patients treated with corticosteroids and 13% for untreated patients.[104] Renal involvement and associated hypertension at initial evaluation were the features most indicative of a poor prognosis.

Hypersensitivity Vasculitis. Hypersensitivity implies an allergic or immune response to a foreign antigen and, indeed, illnesses such as serum sickness can be shown to result from the formation and tissue deposition of immune complexes containing the antigen. However, a specific offending antigen is found in only half of reported cases of small-vessel vasculitis, and thus the more uniform histologic finding of leukocytoclastic angiitis has been proposed as a better inclusive term. This pathologic change is also part of the spectrum of vessel damage seen in cases of hepatitis B infection. Henoch-Schönlein vasculitis, with skin, joint, gastrointestinal tract, and kidney target organ involvement, mainly affects children but may occur at all ages.[71] Various precipitating factors, e.g., viral or bacterial infections, drug exposures,[243] and other allergic mechanisms, have been implicated.[71]

Wegener's Granulomatosis. Wegener's granulomatosis, necrotizing granulomatous angiitis of the upper and lower respiratory tract associated with focal necrotizing glomerulonephritis, affects mainly adults of either sex with a slight (3:2) male predominance,[72] but cases have been reported in children.[256] Prognosis in this disease has been dramatically improved by the use of immunosuppressive drugs, especially cyclophosphamide.[72]

Giant Cell Arteritis. Arteritis characterized pathologically by giant cell formation may involve the aorta or any of its major branches (Takayasu's arteritis or pulseless disease), or may be relatively restricted to the cranial vessels. The syndrome of polymyalgia rheumatica (PMR) is associated with temporal arteritis in one-third of cases; the former also affects older adults, and familial aggregation is reported.[190] In both disorders, however, HLA associations have been controversial.[142,197] In contrast, Takayasu's arteritis affects mainly adolescent and younger adult females of many races,[102,345] but especially those of Oriental origin.[298] Excessive estrogen secretion has been implicated in this disorder.[252]

Epidemiology of giant cell arteritis derived from a 17-year experience in Olmstead County, Minnesota suggests steadily increasing incidence with age and an annual rate of 2.9 per 100,000 persons rising to 13 per 100,000/year in individuals over the age of 50.[143] Similar age-related incidence patterns have been reported from Sweden[34] and Scotland[147] where the overall annual incidence rates

per 100,000 persons were 6.0 and 1.3, respectively. In contrast, a United States southern urban location (Memphis and Shelby County, Tennessee) has a lower rate reported of 0.35 per 100,000.[306] Incidence was seven times higher among women than men, and among whites compared with blacks. Racial distribution does not account fully for differences between Minnesota and Tennessee. Additional studies are required to determine whether climate or other host or environmental factors are implicated. No confirmed environmental risk factors have been identified.

Criteria have been proposed for classification of PMR based on 236 unequivocal cases and 253 comparison patients from 11 rheumatic disease centers in Great Britain (Table 2–9).[40] Three or more of the seven criteria were considered to identify PMR cases. They had 92% sensitivity and 80% specificity when applied to the original study group. As expected, the criteria performed less well (80% sensitivity) in a population chosen for external validation.

Behçet's Syndrome. Behçet's syndrome is also a cause of vasculitis, especially phlebitis, and is best known for the triad of oral and genital ulceration and ocular inflammation. Several sets of diagnostic criteria have been proposed.[29,211] The disease is especially frequent in Japan and the Middle East; in the former population, its prevalence has been estimated at 1 per 10,000 population.[14] For unknown reasons, the marked male predominance (approximately 5 to 1) noted in reports from eastern Mediterranean countries is not found in smaller series from the United States.[72] Familial aggregation has been reported,[39] and increased frequency of HLA-B5 has been noted in Japan[254] and several countries in Europe.[7,287]

Conceptual Developments

The connective tissue diseases, including rheumatoid arthritis, share several features that tend to link them.

    1. Host and genetic predisposition.[42,185,311] The impressive body of epidemiologic data de-

Table 2–9. Diagnostic Criteria for Polymyalgia Rheumatica[40]

1. Age > 65 years
2. Onset of illness < 2 weeks in duration
3. Bilateral shoulder pain and/or stiffness
4. Morning stiffness duration > 1 hour
5. Depression and/or loss of weight
6. Upper arm tenderness bilaterally
7. Initial erythrocyte sedimentation rate ≥ 40 mm/hour

PMR = any three or more criteria *or* one or two criteria plus clinical or pathologic evidence of temporal arteritis.

scribed here and reports of familial occurrence indicate important underlying host predisposing factors in disease precipitation and expression. Similarities in the demographic patterns of these diseases reflect such host influences, e.g., female preponderance and increased incidence with development of sexual maturation, especially in blacks.

2. Overlapping clinical features.[44,290,297] Clinical and laboratory similarities among the diseases, and difficulty in classification of individual patients at any one time, or over a period of time, have led authors to consider them a family of "collagen vascular diseases" or "connective tissue diseases." More specifically, authors now use such terms as "sclerodermatomyositis," "lupoderma," and the "mixed connective tissue disease syndrome" (Fig. 2–4).

3. Blood vessels as an important target organ.[20,53,288,298] Vascular alterations are particularly frequent in these conditions and may affect arteries, capillaries, or veins of any size, including a spectrum of changes from noninflammatory intimal proliferative responses to acute necrotizing lesions.

4. Immunologic correlates.[38,48,111,314,347,350] Immune alterations often appear to be correlated with organ injury as a primary or secondary mechanism as indicated by the presence of circulating and tissue-localized immunoglobulins, immune complexes, complement components, and changes in cell-mediated immunity.

Clinical epidemiologic data suggest that these disorders share important pathogenetic mechanisms, but vary in manifestations, perhaps by virtue of different combinations of predisposing and precipitating factors operating on the major target tissues. Vasculature seems to be vitally involved in these diseases, with increasing recognition of the pathophysiologic contributions and interrelationships of the immune and endocrine systems.[9,145,207]

HYPERURICEMIA AND PRIMARY GOUT

Gouty arthritis, recognized since antiquity, affects mainly adult males, in contrast to RA, SLE, and most other connective tissue diseases. Gout and RA rarely coexist, but the reasons for this dissociation are unknown.[213,341]

Hyperuricemia predisposes to crystal formation, and the presence of monosodium urate crystals in intra- and peri-articular tissue spaces precipitates acute gouty inflammation. A close but not absolute correlation exists betweeen factors that influence hyperuricemia and gout.[359] The risk of developing hyperuricemia and primary gout depends on a complex interaction of multiple factors, e.g., diet, environment, age, sex, and heredity.[3,250,258,353,356]

Serum Uric Acid Values. The influence of heredity on serum uric acid (SUA) level has been debated; a polygenic hypothesis appears most ten-

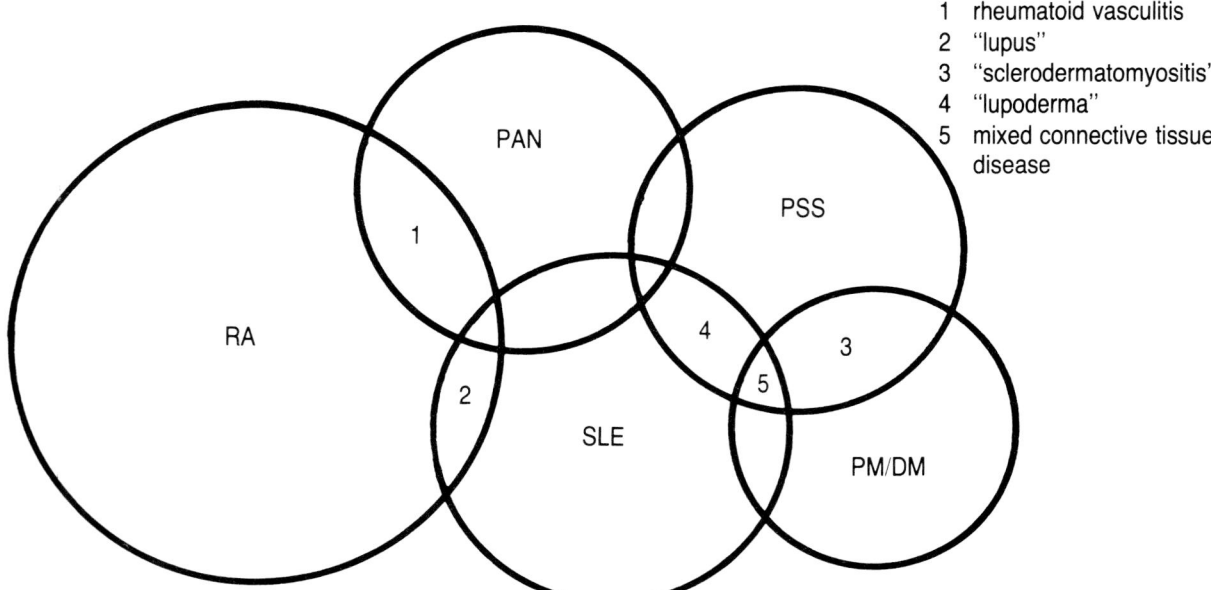

1 rheumatoid vasculitis
2 "lupus"
3 "sclerodermatomyositis"
4 "lupoderma"
5 mixed connective tissue disease

Fig. 2–4. Schematic representation of interrelationships among the connective tissue diseases. To show other recognized "overlaps" would require a three-dimensional model.

able.[239] First-degree relatives have been found to have SUA levels significantly closer to one another than do spouses, even after height and weight are considered.[8] In Japanese, black Africans, and the mixed populations of the United States and most European countries, the normal mean SUA for males is about 5 mg/dl.[80,232,255,356,359] In contrast, surveys in the South Pacific have shown populations with mean levels ranging from 6.1 to 7.3 mg/dl, all utilizing nonautoanalyzer assay methods.[128,284,353] In native Filipinos, the mean SUA was found to be normal (5.2 mg/dl) with a low frequency of gout, whereas hyperuricemia and increased frequency of gout were noted in Filipinos living in the Northeast United States, Alaska, and Hawaii.[129,328] Differences in dietary habits between the native and westernized cultures have been implicated, as well as a relatively more frequent inability in Filipinos to increase renal urate excretion to compensate for a purine load.[129]

Several population surveys in the United States have indicated that the distribution of SUA values is a continuous unimodal curve for both sexes.[80,119,232,259,356] The mean levels rise during childhood irrespective of sex, but starting at 15 to 19 years of age, the average male values are higher, with maximum difference of almost 1.5 mg/dl in the 20 to 24 age group. The mean female values gradually increase from age 40, reaching about 0.5 mg/dl of the male values after the menopause. Levels in males remain essentially constant throughout the adult ages, as do those in females from about age 50 and older.[313] These age and sex relationships suggest hormonal influences, but how such factors may be operating has not been demonstrated.[128]

Serum uric acid appears to be associated with alcohol intake[277] and with hypertension,[277,335] but not independently with ischemic heart disease[267,335] or with diabetes mellitus.[255] Cross-sectional studies have also identified correlations with physical (e.g., weight) and biochemical (e.g., hyperlipidemia) factors.[356]

Diagnostic Criteria for Gout. Criteria for population studies of gout, independent of hyperuricemia, were recommended at the 1966 New York symposium.[36] They included either: (1) the presence of monosodium urate crystals in synovial fluid or in the tissues, demonstrated by chemical or microscopic examination, or (2) the presence of two or more of the following:

a. history or observation of at least two typical gouty arthritis attacks;
b. a clear history or observation of podagra;
c. the presence of a tophus;
d. a clear history or observation of a good response to colchicine.

An ARA subcommittee proposed the following preliminary criteria for the classification of the acute arthritis of primary gout:[342]

1. the presence of characteristic urate crystals in the joint fluid, or
2. a tophus proved to contain urate crystals by chemical or polarized light microscopic means, or
3. the presence of 6 out of 12 clinical, laboratory, and radiographic features, excluding Items 1 and 2 (Table 2–10).

The combined criteria were highly sensitive (98%) and specific (98% against RA of greater than two years' duration and 89% against pseudogout and septic arthritis). This set of criteria was slightly modified for epidemiologic survey purposes. The information to be ascertained on a single patient visit, by history, or by review of clinic records had a sensitivity for gout of 85% and a specificity of 93% or greater. The reliability of these preliminary criteria must be tested against independent clinical and population samples of gout and control arthritis patients.

Age, Sex, and Race Distribution of Gout. In Great Britain, the annual incidence of diagnosis of gout was determined to be 250 to 350 new cases per million population.[73] As expected, the prevalence and incidence of gout correlate closely with levels of SUA in the population,[3,75,119,258,259,359] but gout seems to be increased also in relatives of patients, whether such individuals were initially determined to be hyperuricemic or normouricemic.[250,276] Prevalence figures as high as 15 per thousand have been estimated, with a 6:1 male to female ratio.[119,258] Family history of gouty arthritis is especially correlated with onset of gout in premenopausal women; in one study, over half of the

Table 2–10. Proposed Criteria for Acute Arthritis of Primary Gout[342]

1. More than one attack of acute arthritis
2. Maximum inflammation developed within one day
3. Monarthritis attack
4. Redness observed over joints
5. First metatarsophalangeal joint painful or swollen
6. Unilateral first metatarsophalangeal joint attack
7. Unilateral tarsal joint attack
8. Tophus (proved or suspected)
9. Hyperuricemia
10. Asymmetric swelling within a joint on x ray*
11. Subcortical cysts without erosions on x ray
12. Monosodium urate monohydrate microcrystals in joint fluid during attack
13. Joint fluid culture negative for organisms during attack

*This swelling could logically be found on examination as well as on x ray. However, the protocol did not request this information in regard to examination.

latter provided such a history.[358] The relative protection from gout in women appears to be due to their prolonged lower mean SUA levels, but other influences are possible.

Primary gout was believed to be rare among native races living in their original habitat.[30,284] However, with changing life styles at present, gout is frequently seen in Orientals, Filipinos, Polynesians, and United States blacks.[128,284,322,328] In one large study of United States blacks, the male to female ratio was only 2:1.[322]

Familial Occurrence. Gout has been recognized as a familial disorder since antiquity. The reported frequency of familial occurrence ranges from 6% to as high as 80%.[156] In 1964, the Lesch-Nyhan syndrome, a rare complete deficiency of the enzyme hypoxanthine-guanine phosphoribosyl-transferase, was reported. Patients with this x-linked condition develop severe hyperuricemia, gout, and profound neurologic complications. Since that time, a number of inborn errors of uric acid metabolism have been described,[156] some of which are associated with clinical gout and others with hypouricemia.[354,354a] Although partial enzyme deficiency states were predicted to account for a considerable portion of the hyperuricemic population, this is not the case. In fact, only rarely is an enzymatic defect in purine metabolism identified in gouty individuals.

OSTEOARTHRITIS

Osteoarthritis (OA) is considered the most frequent articular disorder among white populations. Its prevalence is based on the presence of symptomatic and nonsymptomatic roentgenographic degenerative articular changes, the latter considered to be the most reliable criterion available today.[180] Standardization of diagnostic criteria has been developed in the form of the Atlas of Standard Radiographs, which has been used in several population studies.[320] The problem of interobserver variation remains, along with its effect on cross-cultural comparisons. It has been estimated that about 30% of persons with radiographic evidence of degenerative joint changes complain of pain at such sites[67] and would thus be considered to have osteoarthritis.

At present, the factors contributing to the occurrence of OA can only be incompletely listed, with little understanding of their interaction. It is likely that each type and anatomic location of OA must be studied separately with regard to etiologic factors because cartilage degeneration may be a final common pathway of many pathophysiologic processes.[268]

Prevalence by Age, Sex, and Race. Age appears to be the most consistent factor influencing the occurrence of osteoarthritis.[268] A nationwide sample of 6,672 adults 18 to 79 years of age was studied for evidence of osteoarthritis, including radiographs of the hands and feet, in the 1960 to 1962 United States Health Examination Survey.[249] All degrees of radiographic osteoarthrosis of the extremities increased steadily with age from 4% in persons 18 to 24 years of age to 85% among individuals 75 to 79 years of age, with an average of 37% in both males and females. Males appear to be affected more commonly than females before 45 to 54 years of age, but the sex ratio is reversed thereafter.[161] Moderate or severe involvement (9% overall) was almost twice as prevalent in females (11%) as males (6%), adjusted for age.[249] No racial or urban-rural difference was found. In a study of systemic factors associated with OA, age was the most important correlate, accounting for over 40% of variance.[4]

Roentgenographic surveys of other populations have shown a number of different patterns. American Indians have a significantly increased prevalence of osteoarthrosis, with age-adjusted prevalence of all degrees of OA being 74% for males and 61% for females.[249] Moderate and severe grades of OA were highest among the Indian men, about four times the United States male prevalence. In contrast, Eskimos showed a significantly lower incidence of OA than that found in United States males and females.[13] Osteoarthrosis was less common in hands, feet, and hips of South African black women than in white English women, but hand changes were more common in black African men than in white English men.[308] Southern Chinese had a low incidence of both knee and hip osteoarthritis.[136] Several host and environmental factors, particularly those involving patterns and frequency of joint usage, have been postulated to explain these differences. Hypothesis-testing prevalence studies are needed to clarify these geographic and cultural differences.

Prevalence by Occupation and Body Measurements. Theories of the etiology of OA have included mechanical factors, e.g., ''wear and tear,'' prolonged immobilization, continuous pressure, impact loading, anatomic abnormalities, previous inflammatory joint injury, and others.[149,268] In general, epidemiologic surveys tend to confirm such associations.[161] Moderate or severe OA in men does, indeed, show significant differences by occupation and industry.[118,247,263] Clerical and sales workers had a lower than expected frequency of hand involvement, but higher than expected foot involvement.[247] The opposite was true of craftsmen, foremen, and similar workers. Finance, insurance, and real estate industry employees had significantly lower than expected hand involvement. Other studies have suggested that occupation is an important factor in determining the distribution and severity of OA,[66,160,183] but caution should be used in interpreting such data.[117] For example, competitive sports, e.g., running or football, were not found to predispose to OA of the hips or ankles, respectively.[5,274] A great deal more could be done to identify the work specifics, such as lifting, bending, twisting, and bumping, which predispose to OA in certain occupations.

A positive association has been noted between a number of body measurements and osteoarthrosis in both sexes.[246] The relationship is stronger for measurements reflecting body and limb girth and breadth rather than length. These trends are stronger in women than in men and apply to osteoarthrosis of both hands and feet, as found in other studies.[4] In one investigation of risk factors, 100 severe OA patients hospitalized for total hip replacement were compared with an age-, sex-, and race-matched control group.[175] Matched pair analysis showed osteoarthritis to be most strongly associated with increased body weight, amount of education, and a family history of arthritis, but not with tobacco or alcohol consumption or athletic activity. It should be noted, however, that cause and effect in the relationship between OA and obesity have not been clearly identified. Anthropometric comparison of 25 women with generalized OA and 27 with symptomatic osteoporosis revealed that the former were more obese and had greater muscle mass and strength despite comparable age and skeletal size.[76]

Familial Association. An influence of heredity is most conspicuous in distal interphalangeal joint involvement (Heberden's nodes), with dominant transmission in women and recessive transmission in men suspected.[268] The prevalence of radiographic evidence of generalized osteoarthrosis (involvement of three or more joint groups) is increased in families and twins of index cases, indicating an influence of genetic factors.[183] An excess of generalized osteoarthrosis has been noted in male and female siblings of affected probands, and a greater concordance has been reported in monozygotic than dizygotic twins. The increased frequencies do not fit simple mendelian inheritance patterns and may be determined by multiple genes.

PERSPECTIVES

Gout illustrates a metabolically determined form of arthritis with important interactions of genetic, dietary, other host factors, and the environment in pathogenesis. Osteoarthritis, perhaps more than other forms of arthritis, demonstrates important local and biomechanical factors influencing joint involvement, although systemic and genetic factors

also participate. To what extent degenerative and mechanical processes contribute to articular manifestations in other forms of chronic arthritis, e.g., gout and RA, is difficult to quantitate, but is nevertheless believed to be important. Similarly, the significance of genetic and other host chacteristics in many arthritis conditions is becoming increasingly recognized. Thus, a constellation of interrelated factors undoubtedly contributes to each arthritis syndrome, which may be classified by clinical, radiologic, or laboratory markers of greater or lesser accuracy. Classification of disease, identification of risk and other associated factors, and definition of its course are important challenges for future research, and especially for clinical epidemiology.

Broad perspectives of disease and of pathogenetic mechanisms can provide valuable biologic insights and new directions to profitable lines of investigation and ultimately to improved patient care. Integrated multidisciplinary studies, including longitudinal observations, are costly of time, effort, and money, but are essential to a proper understanding of these multifactorial diseases. Regrettably, support for such efforts has not kept pace with perceived needs.[12] Detailed clinical-laboratory descriptive surveys should be performed to better define the diagnostic ranges and boundaries of the major arthritis syndromes. Although advanced "typical" stages of rheumatic disorders are readily recognized, studies of the mildest or earliest detectable diseases are vital to search for factors associated with onset, predisposition, and subsequent outcome. In addition, multidisciplinary analytic studies must be designed to refine and to test specific hypotheses in populations.

REFERENCES

1. Abeles, M., et al.: Systemic lupus erythematosus in the younger patient: Survival studies. J. Rheumatol., 7:515–522, 1980.
2. Abruzzo, J.L.: Rheumatoid arthritis and mortality. Arthritis Rheum., 25:1020–1023, 1982.
3. Acheson, R.M.: Epidemiology of serum uric acid and gout: An example of the complexities of multifactorial causation. Proc. R. Soc. Med., 63:193–197, 1970.
4. Acheson, R.M., and Collart, A.B.: New Haven survey of joint diseases. XVII. Relationship between some systemic characteristics and osteoarthrosis in a general population. Ann. Rheum. Dis., 34:379–387, 1975.
5. Adams, I.D.: Osteoarthrosis and sport. J. R. Soc. Med., 72:185–187, 1979.
6. Adler, E., et al.: Rheumatoid arthritis in a Jerusalem population. 1. Epidemiology of the disease. Am. J. Epidemiol., 85:365–377, 1967.
7. Adorno, D., et al.: HLA-B5 and Behçet's disease. Tissue Antigens, 14:444–448, 1979.
8. Ahern, F.M., Johnson, R.C., and Ashton, G.C.: Family resemblances in serum uric acid level. Behav. Genet., 10:303–307, 1980.
9. Ahlqvist, J.: Endocrine influences on lymphatic organs, immune responses, inflammation and autoimmunity. Acta Endocrinol., 83(Suppl. 206):1–136, 1976.

10. Aho, K., et al.: Yersinia arthritis and related diseases: Clinical and immunogenetic implications. *In* Infection and Immunology in the Rheumatic Diseases. Edited by D.C. Dumonde. Oxford, Blackwell Scientific, 1974, pp. 341–344.

11. Albert, D.A., Hadler, N.M., and Ropes, M.W.: Does corticosteroid therapy affect the survival of patients with systemic lupus erythematosus? Arthritis Rheum., 22:945–953, 1979.

12. Allander, E., et al.: Rheumatology in perspective. The epidemiological view. Scand. J. Rheumatol., 46(Suppl.):5–49, 1982.

13. Andersen, S.: The epidemiology of primary osteoarthrosis of the knee in Greenland. Scand. J. Rheumatol., 7:109–112, 1978.

14. Aoki, K., Fujioka, K., and Katsumata, H.: Epidemiological studies in Behçet's disease in the Hokkaido district. Jpn. J. Clin. Ophthalmol., 25:2239–2243, 1971.

15. Arnett, F.C., et al.: The Jo-1 antibody system in myositis: Relationships to clinical features and HLA. J. Rheumatol., 8:925–930, 1981.

16. Arnett, F.C., et al.: Incomplete Reiter's syndrome: Discriminating features and HL-A W27 in diagnosis. Ann. Intern. Med., 84:8–12, 1976.

17. Arnett, F.C., Hochberg, M.C., and Bias, W.B.: Cross-reactive HLA antigens in B27-negative Reiter's syndrome and sacroiliitis. Johns Hopkins Med. J., 141:193–197, 1977.

18. Arnett, F.C., and Shulman, L.E.: Studies in familial systemic lupus erythematosus. Medicine, 55:313–322, 1976.

19. Baltus, J.A.M., et al.: The occurrence of malignancies in patients with rheumatoid arthritis treated with cyclophosphamide: A controlled retrospective follow-up. Ann. Rheum. Dis., 42:368–373, 1983.

20. Banker, B.Q., and Victor, M.: Dermatomyositis (systemic angiopathy) of childhood. Medicine, 45:261–289, 1966.

21. Barbour, A.G., et al.: Kawasaki-like disease in a young adult. Association with primary Epstein-Barr virus infection. J.A.M.A., 241:397–398, 1979.

22. Barnes, B.E., and Mawr, B.: Dermatomyositis and malignancy. A review of the literature. Ann. Intern. Med., 84:68–76, 1976.

23. Baron, M., et al.: The coexistence of rheumatoid arthritis and scleroderma: A case report and review of the literature. J. Rheumatol., 9:947–950, 1982.

24. Baum, J., et al.: Juvenile rheumatoid arthritis. A comparison of patients from the USSR and USA. Arthritis Rheum., 23:977–984, 1980.

25. Baum, J., and Gutowska, G.: Death in juvenile rheumatoid arthritis. Arthritis Rheum., 20:253–255, 1977.

26. Baum, J., and Ziff, M.: The rarity of ankylosing spondylitis in the black race. Arthritis Rheum., 14:12–18, 1971.

27. Beasely, R.P., Willkens, R.F., and Bennett, P.H.: High prevalence of rheumatoid arthritis in Yakima Indians. Arthritis Rheum., 16:743–748, 1973.

28. Behan, W.M.H., Behan, P.O., and Dick, H.A.: HLA-B8 in polymyositis. N. Engl. J. Med., 298:260–261, 1978.

29. Behçet's Disease Research Committee of Japan: Behçet's disease: Guide to diagnosis of Behçet's disease. Jpn. J. Ophthalmol., 18:291–294, 1974.

30. Beighton, P., et al.: Serum uric acid concentrations in an urbanized South African Negro population. Ann. Rheum. Dis., 33:442–445, 1974.

31. Beighton, P., Solomon, L., and Valkenburg, H.A.: Rheumatoid arthritis in a rural South African Negro population. Ann. Rheum. Dis., 34:136–141, 1975.

32. Bekassy, A.N., Enell, H., and Schalen, C.: Severe polyarthritis following Campylobacter enteritis in a 12-year old boy. Acta Paediatr. Scand., 69:269–271, 1980.

33. Benbassat, J., Geffel, D., and Zlotnick, A.: Epidemiology of polymyositis-dermatomyositis in Israel, 1960–1976. Isr. J. Med. Sci., 16:197–200, 1980.

34. Bengtsson, B.A., and Malmvall, B.E.: The epidemiology of giant cell arteritis including temporal arteritis and polymyalgia rheumatica: Incidences of different clinical presentations and eye complications. Arthritis Rheum., 24:899–904, 1981.

35. Bennett, R.M., Bluestone, R., and Holt, P.J.: Survival in scleroderma. Ann. Rheum. Dis., 30:581–588, 1971.

36. Bennett, P.H., and Burch, T.A.: New York symposium on population studies in the rheumatic diseases: New diagnostic criteria. Bull. Rheum. Dis., 17:458, 1967.

37. Bennett, P.H., and Wood, P.H.: Proceedings of the Third International Symposium on Population Studies of the Rheumatic Diseases. Amsterdam, Excerpta Medica Foundation, 1968.

38. Bennett, R.M., and Spargo, B.M.: Immune complex nephropathy in mixed connective tissue disease. Am. J. Med., 63:534–541, 1977.

39. Berman, L., Trappler, B., and Jenkins, T.: Behçet's syndrome: A family study and the elucidation of a genetic role. Ann. Rheum. Dis., 38:118–121, 1979.

40. Bird, H.A., et al.: An evaluation of criteria for polymyalgia rheumatica. Ann. Rheum. Dis., 38:434–439, 1979.

41. Black, K.A., et al.: Cancer in connective tissue disease. Arthritis Rheum., 25:1130–1133, 1982.

42. Block, S.R., et al.: Immunologic observations on 9 sets of twins either concordant or discordant for SLE. Arthritis Rheum., 19:545–554, 1976.

43. Block, S.R.: Studies of twins with systemic lupus erythematosus. A review of the literature and presentation of 12 additional sets. Am. J. Med., 59:533–552, 1975.

44. Bohan, A., et al.: A computer-assisted analysis of 153 patients with polymyositis and dermatomyositis. Medicine, 56:255–286, 1977.

45. Bohan, A., and Peter, J.B.: Polymyositis and dermatomyositis. N. Engl. J. Med., 292:344–347, 403–407, 1975.

46. Brewerton, D.A.: Joseph J. Bunim Memorial Lecture. HLA-B27 and the inheritance of susceptibility to rheumatic disease. Arthritis Rheum., 19:656–668, 1976.

47. Brewerton, D.A., and James, D.C.: The histocompatibility antigen (HLA 27) and disease. Semin. Arthritis Rheum., 4:191–207, 1975.

48. Brunner, C., and Davis, J.S.: Immune mechanisms in the pathogenesis of systemic lupus erythematosus. Bull. Rheum. Dis., 26:854–861, 1975.

49. Calabro, J.J., et al.: Juvenile rheumatoid arthritis: A general review and report of 100 patients observed for 15 years. Semin. Arthritis Rheum., 5:257–298, 1976.

50. Calin, A., et al.: Clinical history as a screening test for ankylosing spondylitis. J.A.M.A., 237:2613–2614, 1977.

51. Calin, A., and Fries, J.F.: An "experimental" epidemic of Reiter's syndrome revisited: Follow-up evidence on genetic and environmental factors. Ann. Intern. Med., 84:564–566, 1976.

52. Calin, A., and Fries, J.: Striking prevalence of ankylosing spondylitis in "healthy" W27 positive males and females: A controlled study. N. Engl. J. Med., 293:835–839, 1975.

53. Campbell, P.M., and LeRoy, E.C.: Pathogenesis of systemic sclerosis: A vascular hypothesis. Semin. Arthritis Rheum., 4:351–368, 1975.

54. Canoso, J.J., and Cohen, A.S.: A review of the use, evaluations, and criticisms of the preliminary criteria for the classification of systemic lupus erythematosus. Arthritis Rheum., 22:917–921, 1979.

55. Carette, S., et al.: The natural disease course of ankylosing spondylitis. Arthritis Rheum., 26:186–190, 1983.

56. Carpenter, J.R., et al.: Survival in polymyositis: Corticosteroids and risk factors. J. Rheumatol., 4:207–214, 1977.

57. Carter, E.T., et al.: Epidemiology of ankylosing spondylitis in Rochester, Minnesota: 1935–1973. Arthritis Rheum., 22:365–370, 1979.

58. Cassidy, J.T., et al.: A study of classification criteria for children with juvenile rheumatoid arthritis. Arthritis Rheum. In press, 1984.

59. Celada, A., et al.: Increased frequency of HLA-DRW3 in systemic lupus erythematosus. Tissue Antigens, 15:283–288, 1980.

60. Christensen, M.L., et al.: Antibody of Coxsackie-B virus: Increased incidence in sera from children with recently diagnosed juvenile dermatomyositis (abstract). Arthritis Rheum., 26:S24, 1983.

61. Christiansen, F.T., et al.: The prevalence of ankylosing spondylitis among B27 positive normal individuals: A reassessment. J. Rheumatol., 6:713–718, 1979.

62. Chumbley, L.C., Harrison, E.G., and DeRemee, R.A.: Allergic granulomatosis and angiitis (Churg-Strauss syndrome): Report and analysis of 30 cases. Mayo Clin. Proc., 52:477–484, 1977.

63. Citron, B.F., et al.: Necrotizing angiitis associated with drug abuse. N. Engl. J. Med., 283:1003–1011, 1970.

64. Clair, D., et al.: Autoantibodies in human contacts of SLE dogs. Arthritis Rheum., 23:251–253, 1980.

65. Cleland, L.G., Hay, J.A.R., and Milazzo, S.C.: Absence of HL-A 27 and of ankylosing spondylitis in central Australian aboriginals (abstract). Scand. J. Rheumatol., 8:30–35, 1975.

66. Cobb, S.: The Frequency of the Rheumatic Diseases. American Public Health Association Monograph. Cambridge, Harvard University Press, 1971.

67. Cobb, S., Merchant, W.R., and Rubin, T.: The relation of symptoms to osteoarthritis. J. Chronic Dis., 5:197–204, 1957.

68. Cohen, A.S., et al.: Preliminary criteria for the classification of systemic lupus erythematosus. Bull. Rheum. Dis., 21:643–648, 1971.

69. Cohen, L.M., et al.: Increased risk for spondylitis stigmata in apparently healthy HL-AW27 men. Ann. Intern. Med., 84:1–7, 1976.

70. Cohen, M.J., and Persellin, R.H.: Coexistence of rheumatoid arthritis and systemic sclerosis in four patients. Scand. J. Rheumatol., 11:241–245, 1982.

71. Cream, J.J., Gumpel, J.M., and Peachey, R.D.G.: Schonlein-Henoch purpura in the adult. A study of 77 adults with anaphylactoid or Schonlein-Henoch purpura. Q.J. Med., 39:461–484, 1970.

72. Cupps, T.R., and Fauci, A.S.: Classification of the vasculitides. Major Probl. Intern. Med., 21:1–5, 1981.

73. Currie, W.J.C.: Prevalence and incidence of the diagnosis of gout in Great Britain. Ann. Rheum. Dis., 38:101–106, 1979.

74. Daneo, V., et al.: Family studies and HLA typing in ankylosing spondylitis and sacroiliitis. J. Rheumatol., 4 (Suppl 3):5–10, 1977.

75. DeMuckadell, O.B., and Gyntelberg, G.: Occurrence of gout in Copenhagen males aged 40–59. Int. J. Epidemiol., 5:153–158, 1976.

76. Dequeker, J., Goris, P., and Uytterhoeven, R.: Osteoporosis and osteoarthritis (osteoarthrosis): Anthropometric distinction. J.A.M.A., 249:1448–1451, 1983.

77. DeVere, R., and Bradley, W.G.: Polymyositis: Its presentation, morbidity and mortality. Brain, 98:637–666, 1975.

78. Dimant, J., et al.: Systemic lupus erythematosus in the older age group: Computer analysis. J. Am. Geriatr. Soc., 27:58–61, 1979.

79. Dinant, H.J., et al.: HLA-DRW4 in Felty's syndrome (letter). Arthritis Rheum., 23:1336, 1980.

80. Dodge, H.J., and Mikkelsen, W.M.: Observations on the distribution of serum uric acid levels in participants of the Tecumseh, Michigan, community health studies. J. Chronic Dis., 23:161–172, 1970.

81. Dorn, H.F.: Methods of measuring incidence and prevalence of disease. Am. J. Public Health, 41:271–278, 1951.

82. Drueke, T., et al.: Hepatitis B antigen-associated periarteritis nodosa in patients undergoing long-term hemodialysis. Am. J. Med., 68:86–90, 1980.

83. Dubois, E.L.: The clinical picture of systemic lupus erythematosus. In Lupus Erythematosus. Los Angeles, University of Southern California Press, 1974, pp. 232–379.

84. Duncan, S.C., and Winkelmann, R.R.: Cancer and scleroderma. Arch. Dermatol., 115:950–955, 1979.

85. Eason, R.J., Tan, P.L., and Gow, P.J.: Progressive systemic sclerosis in Auckland: A ten year review with emphasis on prognostic features. Aust. N. Z. J. Med., 11:657–662, 1981.

86. Ebringer, R.W., et al.: Sequential studies in ankylosing spondylitis: Association of Klebsiella pneumoniae with active disease. Ann. Rheum. Dis., 37:146–151, 1978.

87. Edmonds, J., et al.: Follow-up study of juvenile chronic polyarthritis with particular reference to histocompatibility antigen W 27. Ann. Rheum. Dis., 33:289–292, 1974.

88. Elkon, K.B., et al.: Hairy-cell leukaemia with polyarteritis nodosa. Lancet, 2:280–282, 1979.

89. Engleman, E., Bombardier, C., and Hochberg, M.C. (Eds.): Conference on Epidemiology of Rheumatic Diseases: Specific Needs of Developing and Developed Countries. J. Rheumatol., 10:1–107, 1983.

90. Erasmus, L.D.: Scleroderma in gold-miners on the Witwatersrand with particular reference to pulmonary manifestations. S. Afr. J. Lab. Clin. Med., 3:209, 1957.

91. Espinoza, L.R., et al.: Histocompatibility typing in the seronegative spondyloarthropathies: A survey. Semin. Arthritis Rheum., 11:375–381, 1982.

92. Esscher, E., and Scott, J.S.: Congenital heart block and maternal systemic lupus erythematosus. Br. Med. J., 1:1235–1238, 1979.

93. Estes, D., and Christian, C.L.: The natural history of systemic lupus erythematosus by prospective analysis. Medicine, 50:85–95, 1971.

94. Feher, K.G., and Feher, T.: Plasma dehydroepiandrosterone, dehydroepiandrosterone sulfate and androsterone sulfate levels and their interaction with plasma proteins in rheumatoid arthritis. Exp. Clin. Endocrinol. In press, 1984.

95. Feigenbaum, S.L., Masi, A.T., and Kaplan, S.B.: Prognosis in rheumatoid arthritis. A longitudinal study of newly diagnosed younger adult patients. Am. J. Med., 66:377–384, 1979.

96. Fessel, W.J.: Systemic lupus erythematosus in the community. Incidence, prevalence, outcome, and first symptoms, the high prevalence in black women. Arch. Intern. Med., 134:1027–1035, 1974.

97. Finch, W.R., et al.: Bleomycin induced scleroderma. J. Rheumatol., 7:651–659, 1980.

98. Findlay, G.H., Whiting, D.A., and Simson, I.W.: Dermatomyositis in the Transvaal and its occurrence in the Bantu. S. Afr. Med. J., 43:694–697, 1969.

99. Fink, C.W.: Polyarteritis and other diseases with necrotizing vasculitis in childhood. Arthritis Rheum., 20:378–384, 1977.

100. Ford, D.K.: Isolation of Bedsonia agents from patients with uncomplicated non-gonococcal urethritis. Arthritis Rheum., 10:278–279, 1967.

101. Fox, R., et al.: The chronicity of symptoms and disability in Reiter's syndrome. Ann. Intern. Med., 91:190–193, 1979.

102. Fraga, A., et al.: Takayasu's arteritis: Frequency of systemic manifestations (study of 22 patients) and favorable response to maintenance steroid therapy with adrenocorticosteroids (12 patients). Arthritis Rheum., 15:617–624, 1972.

103. Friedman, J.M., et al.: Immunogenetic studies of juvenile dermatomyositis: HLA-DR antigen frequencies. Arthritis Rheum., 26:214–216, 1983.

104. Frohnert, P.P., and Sheps, S.G.: Long-term follow-up study of periarteritis nodosa. Am. J. Med., *43*:8–14, 1967.
105. Furst, D.E., et al.: A syndrome resembling progressive systemic sclerosis after bone marrow transplantation. A model for scleroderma? Arthritis Rheum., *22*:904–910, 1979.
106. Gershwin, M.E., et al.: Characterization of a spontaneous disease of White Leghorn chickens resembling progressive systemic sclerosis (scleroderma). J. Exp. Med., *153*:1640–1659, 1981.
107. Gewanter, H.L., Roghmann, K.J., and Baum, J.: The prevalence of juvenile arthritis. Arthritis Rheum., *26*:599–603, 1983.
108. Ginzler, E.M., et al.: A multicenter study of outcome in systemic lupus erythematosus. I. Entry variables as predictors of prognosis. Arthritis Rheum., *25*:601–611, 1982.
109. Glass, D., et al.: Early-onset pauciarticular juvenile rheumatoid arthritis associated with human leukocyte antigen-DRW5, iritis, and antinuclear antibody. J. Clin. Invest., *66*:426–429, 1980.
110. Glass, D.N., and Litvin, D.A.: Heterogeneity of HLA associations in systemic onset juvenile rheumatoid arthritis. Arthritis Rheum., *23*:796–799, 1980.
111. Gocke, D.J., et al.: Association between polyarteritis and Australia antigen. Lancet, 2:1149–1153, 1970.
112. Goel, K.M., and Shanks, R.A.: Follow-up study of 100 cases of juvenile rheumatoid arthritis. Ann. Rheum. Dis., *33*:25–31, 1974.
113. Gofton, J.P., et al.: Sacroiliitis and ankylosing spondylitis in North American Indians. Ann. Rheum. Dis., *31*:474–481, 1972.
114. Gofton, J.P., et al.: HL-A 27 and ankylosing spondylitis in B.C. Indians. J. Rheumatol., *2*:314–318, 1975.
115. Gomor, B., Gyodi, E., and Bakos, L.: Distribution of HLA B27 and ankylosing spondylitis in the Hungarian population. J. Rheumatol., *4*:314 (Suppl 3):33–35, 1977.
116. Good, A.E., Kawahishi, H., and Schultz, J.S.: HLA B27 in blacks with ankylosing spondylitis or Reiter's disease. N. Engl. J. Med., *94*:166–167, 1976.
116a. Green, M.C., Sweet, H.O., and Bunker, L.E.: Tight-skin, a new mutation of the mouse causing excessive growth of connective tissue and skeleton. Am. J. Pathol., *82*:493–507, 1976.
117. Hadler, N.M.: Industrial rheumatology: Clinical investigations into influence of pattern of usage on the pattern of regional musculoskeletal disease. Arthritis Rheum., *20*:1019–1025, 1977.
118. Hadler, N.M., et al.: Hand structure and function in an industrial setting. The influence of three patterns of stereotype, repetitive usage. Arthritis Rheum., *21*:210–220, 1978.
119. Hall, A.P., et al.: Epidemiology of gout and hyperuricemia. A long-term population study. Am. J. Med., *47*:27–37, 1967.
120. Hannissian, A.S., et al.: Juvenile dermatomyositis and polymyositis: An epidemiologic and clinical comparative analysis. IV. Pan American Congress on Rheumatic Diseases (Abstract.) J. Rheumatol., *1* (Suppl. 1): 119, 1974.
121. Hanissian, A.S., et al.: Comparison of childhood polymyositis and dermatomyositis: An epidemiologic and clinical comparative analysis. J. Rheumatol., *9*:390–394, 1982.
122. Hansen, T., et al.: Clinical assessment of disease activity in rheumatoid arthritis. Scand. J. Rheumatol., *8*:101–105, 1979.
123. Hanson, V., et al.: Prognosis of juvenile rheumatoid arthritis. Arthritis Rheum., *20*:279–284, 1977.
124. Hanson, V., et al.: Three subtypes of juvenile rheumatoid arthritis. Correlations of age at onset, sex, and serologic factors. Arthritis Rheum., *20*:184–186, 1977.
125. Hardy, J.D., et al.: Congenital complete heart block in the newborn associated with maternal systemic lupus erythematosus and other connective tissue disorders. Arch. Dis. Child., *54*:7–13, 1979.
126. Harvey, J., Lotze, M., and Stevens, M.B.: Rheumatoid arthritis in a Chippewa band: I. Pilot screening study of disease prevalence. Arthritis Rheum., *24*:717–721, 1981.
127. Healey, L.A.: Polymyalgia rheumatica and the American Rheumatism Association criteria for rheumatoid arthritis. Arthritis Rheum., *26*:1417–1418, 1983.
128. Healey, L.A.: Epidemiology of hyperuricemia. Arthritis Rheum., *18*:709–712, 1975.
129. Healey, L.A., and Bayani-Sioson, P.S.: A defect in the renal excretion of uric acid in Filipinos. Arthritis Rheum., *14*:721–726, 1971.
130. Hellgren, L.: Rheumatoid arthritis in both marital partners. Acta Rheum. Scand., *15*:135–138, 1969.
131. Hendricks, G.F.M., et al.: Dermatomyositis and toxoplasmosis. Ann. Neurol., *5*:393–395, 1979.
132. Henrard, J., Bennett, P.H., and Burch, T.A.: Rheumatoid arthritis in the Pima Indians of Arizona: An assessment of the clinical components of the New York criteria. Int. J. Epidemiol., *4*:119–126, 1975.
133. Hicks, J.T., et al.: Search for Epstein-Barr and type C oncornaviruses in systemic lupus erythematosus. Arthritis Rheum., *22*:845–857, 1979.
134. Hill, R.: Juvenile arthritis in various racial groups in British Columbia. Arthritis Rheum., *20*:162, 1977.
135. Hill, R.H., and Robinson, H.S.: Rheumatoid arthritis and ankylosing spondylitis in British Columbia Indians. Can. Med. Assoc. J., *100*:509–511, 1969.
136. Hoaglund, F.T., Yau, A.C.M.C., and Wong, W.L.: Osteoarthritis of the hip and other joints in Southern Chinese in Hong Kong: Incidence and related factors. J. Bone Joint Surg., *55A*:545–557, 1973.
137. Hochberg, M.C.: Adult and juvenile rheumatoid arthritis: Current epidemiologic concepts. Epidemiol. Rev., *3*:27–44, 1981.
138. Hochberg, M.C., and Lawrence, R.C.: Epidemiologic studies of the rheumatic diseases. Bibliography 1967–1980, in U.S. Department of Health and Human Services Report.
139. Hochberg, M.C., Lopez-Acuna, D., and Gittelsohn, A.M.: Mortality from polymyositis and dermatomyositis in the United States, 1968–1978. Arthritis Rheum., *26*:1465–1471, 1983.
140. Hoffman, G.S., et al.: Presentation, treatment, and prognosis of idiopathic inflammatory muscle disease in a rural hospital. Am. J. Med., *75*:433–438, 1983.
141. Hollingsworth, P.N., et al.: Observer variation in grading sacroiliac radiographs in HLA-B27 positive individuals. J. Rheumatol., *10*:247–254, 1983.
142. Hunder, G.G., et al.: HLA antigens in patients with giant cell arteritis and polymyalgia rheumatica. J. Rheumatol., *4*:321–323, 1977.
143. Huston, K.A., et al.: Temporal arteritis: A 25-year epidemiologic, clinical and pathologic study. Ann. Intern. Med., *88*:162–167, 1978.
144. Hyla, J.F., Franck, W.A., and Davis, J.S.: Lack of association of HLA B27 with radiographic sacroiliitis in inflammatory bowel disease. J. Rheumatol., *3*:196–200, 1976.
145. Inman, R.D.: Immunologic sex differences and the female predominance in systemic lupus erythematosus. Arthritis Rheum., *21*:849–852, 1978.
146. Isomaki, H.A., Mutru, O., and Koota, K.: Death rate and causes of death in patients with rheumatoid arthritis. Scand. J. Rheumatol., *4*:205–208, 1975.
147. Jonasson, F., Cullen, J.F., and Elton, R.A.: Temporal arteritis: A 14-year epidemiological, clinical and prognostic study. Scott. Med. J., *24*:111–117, 1979.
148. Josipovic, D.B., and Masi, A.T.: Marked female preponderance in rheumatoid arthritis patients with younger adult onset and positive rheumatoid factor (RF) (abstract).

Proceedings of XIV International Congress of Rheumatology, 1977, p. 249.

149. Jurmain, R.D.: Stress and the etiology of osteoarthritis. Am. J. Phys. Anthropol., 46:353–356, 1977.

150. Kallick, C.A., Thadhani, K.C., and Rice, T.W.: Identification of anaplasmataceae (Haemobartonella) antigen and antibodies in systemic lupus erythematosus. Arthritis Rheum., 23:197–205, 1980.

151. Karr, R.W., et al.: Association of HLA-DRW4 with rheumatoid arthritis in black and white patients. Arthritis Rheum., 23:1241–1245, 1980.

152. Karsh, J., et al.: Mortality in lupus nephritis. Arthritis Rheum., 22:764–769, 1979.

153. Kaslow, R.A., Ryder, R.W., and Calin, A.: Search for Reiter's syndrome after an outbreak of *Shigella sonnei* dysentery. J. Rheumatol., 6:562–566, 1979.

154. Kaslow, R.L., and Masi, A.T.: Age, sex, and race effects on mortality due to systemic lupus erythematosus in the United States. Arthritis Rheum., 21:473–479, 1978.

155. Kato, H., et al.: Rheumatoid arthritis and gout in Hiroshima and Nagasaki, Japan: A prevalence and incidence study. J. Chronic Dis., 23:659–679, 1971.

156. Kelley, W.N.: Inborn errors of purine metabolism—1977. Arthritis Rheum., 20:S221–S227, 1977.

157. Kellgren, J.H.: Epidemiology of rheumatoid arthritis. Arthritis Rheum., 9:658–674, 1966.

158. Kellgren, J.H., Jeffrey, M.R., and Ball, J.: Proposed diagnostic criteria for use of population studies: Active rheumatoid arthritis. In The Epidemiology of Chronic Rheumatism. Oxford, Blackwell Scientific Publications, 1963, p. 324.

159. Kellgren, J.H., Jeffrey, M.R., and Ball, J.: Appendix I. Proposed diagnostic criteria for use in population studies. In The Epidemiology of Chronic Rheumatism. Oxford, Blackwell Scientific Publications, 1963, pp. 324–327.

160. Kellgren, J.H., and Lawrence, J.S.: Rheumatism in miners. II. X-ray study. Br. J. Ind. Med., 9:197–207, 1952.

161. Kelsey, J.L.: Epidemiology of Musculoskeletal Diseases. New York, Oxford University Press, 1982.

162. Kemple, K., et al.: HLA-D locus typing in ankylosing spondylitis and Reiter's syndrome. Arthritis Rheum., 22:371–375, 1979.

163. Keren, G., et al.: Kawasaki's disease and infantile polyarteritis nodosa: Is Pseudomonas infection responsible? Report of a case. Isr. J. Med. Sci., 15:592–600, 1979.

164. Khan, M.A., et al.: Low association of HLA-B27 with Reiter's syndome in blacks. Ann. Intern. Med., 90:202–203, 1979.

165. Khan, M.A., et al.: HLA B27 in ankylosing spondylitis: Differences in frequency and relative risk in American blacks and Caucasians. J. Rheumatol., 4 (Suppl 3):39–43, 1977.

166. Khan, M.A., and Hammouden, M.: Genetics of HLA-associated disease: Ankylosing spondylitis and related spondyloarthropathies. Arthritis Rheum., 26:S18, 1983.

167. Khan, M.A., Khan, M.K., and Kushner, I.: Survival among patients with ankylosing spondylitis: A life table analysis. J. Rheumatol., 8:86–90, 1981.

168. Khan, M.A., and Khan, M.K.: Diagnostic value of HLA-B27 testing in ankylosing spondylitis and Reiter's syndrome. Ann. Intern. Med., 96:70–76, 1982.

169. Khan, M.A., Kushner, I., and Bran, W.E.: Comparison of clinical features in HLA-B27 positive and negative patients with ankylosing spondylitis. Arthritis Rheum., 20:909–912, 1977.

170. Kilbourne, E.M., et al.: Clinical epidemiology of toxic-oil syndrome. Manifestations of a new illness. N. Engl. J. Med., 309:1408–1414, 1983.

171. Kimura, M., Andon, T., and Kai, K.: Failure to detect type-C virus p30-related antigen in systemic lupus erythematosus: False-positive reaction due to protease activity. Arthritis Rheum., 23:111–113, 1980.

172. King, K.K., et al.: The clinical spectrum of systemic lupus erythematosus in childhood. Arthritis Rheum., 20:287–294, 1977.

173. Koch, M.J., Brody, J.A., and Gillespie, M.M.: Childhood polymyositis: A case-control study. Am. J. Epidemiol., 104:627–631, 1976.

174. Kousa, M., et al.: Family study of Reiter's disease and HLA B27 distribution. J. Rheumatol., 4:95–102, 1977.

175. Kraus, J.F., et al.: Epidemiological study of severe osteoarthritis. Orthopedics, 1:37–42, 1978.

176. Kumagai, Y., et al.: Clinical spectrum of connective tissue disease after cosmetic surgery (human adjuvant disease): Observations in eighteen patients and a review of the Japanese literature. Arthritis Rheum., 26:1–12, 1984.

177. Kurland, L.T., et al.: Epidemiologic features of diffuse connective tissue disorders in Rochester, Minnesota, 1951–1967, with special reference to systemic lupus erythematosus. Mayo Clin. Proc., 44:649–663, 1969.

178. Kurland, L.T., Chuang T-Y, and Hunder, G.G.: The epidemiology of systemic arteritis. In Epidemiology of the Rheumatic Diseases. Proceedings of the Fourth International Conference, National Institutes of Health. New York, Gower Medical Publishing, Ltd., 1984, pp. 196–205.

179. Laaksonen, A.L.: A prognostic study of rheumatoid arthritis. Acta Paediatr. Scand. (Suppl. 166): 1–79, 1966.

180. Laine, V.A.: International standardization of the diagnosis of rheumatoid arthritis and osteoarthritis, clinical aspects. Milbank Mem. Fund Q., 43:133–141, 1964.

181. Laine, V.A.I.: Rheumatic complaints in an urban population in Finland. Acta Rheum. Scand., 8:81–88, 1962.

182. Lahita, R.G., et al.: Familial systemic lupus erythematosus in males. Arthritis Rheum., 26:39–44, 1983.

183. Lawrence, J.S.: Rheumatism in Populations. London, William Heinemann Medical Books Ltd., 1977.

184. Lawrence, J.S.: Family survey of Reiter's disease. Br. J. Vener. Dis., 50:140–145, 1974.

185. Lawrence, J.S.: Heberden Oration, 1969. Rheumatoid arthritis—nature or nurture? Ann. Rheum. Dis., 29:357–379, 1970.

186. Lawrence, R.C., and Shulman, L.E. (eds.): Epidemiology of the Rheumatic Diseases. Proceedings of the Fourth International Conference. National Institutes of Health. New York, Gower Medical Publishing Ltd., 1984.

187. Lee, P., et al.: Systemic lupus erythematosus. A review of 110 cases with reference to nephritis, the nervous system, infections, aseptic necrosis and prognosis. Q. J. Med., 181:1–32, 1977.

188. Lee, S.L., Rivero, I., and Siegel, M.: Activation of systemic lupus erythematosus by drugs. Arch. Intern. Med., 117:620–626, 1966.

189. Leirisalo, M., et al.: Followup study on patients with Reiter's disease and reactive arthritis, with special reference to HLA-B27. Arthritis Rheum., 25:249–259, 1982.

190. Liang, G.C., et al.: Familial aggregation of polymyalgia rheumatica and giant cell arteritis. Arthritis Rheum., 17:19–24, 1974.

190a.Linos, A., et al.: Case-control study of rheumatoid arthritis and prior use of oral contraceptives. Lancet, 1:1299–1300, 1983.

191. Linos, A., et al.: The epidemiology of rheumatoid arthritis in Rochester, Minnesota: A study of incidence, prevalence, and mortality. Am. J. Epidemiol., 111:87–98, 1980.

192. Lockhead, J.A., et al.: HLA-B27 haplotypes in family studies of ankylosing spondylitis. Arthritis Rheum., 26:1011–1016, 1983.

193. Lowenstein, M.B., and Rothfield, N.F.: Family study of systemic lupus erythematosus: Analyses of the clinical history, skin immunofluorescence and serologic parameters. Arthritis Rheum., 20:1293–1303, 1977.

194. Lynch, C.J., et al.: Histocompatibility antigens in progressive systemic sclerosis (PSS, scleroderma). J. Clin. Immunol., 2:314–318, 1982.

195. Maddock, R.K.: Incidence of systemic lupus erythematosus by age and sex. J.A.M.A., 191:137–138, 1965.

196. Magid, S.K., and Kagen, L.J.: Serologic evidence for acute toxoplasmosis in polymyositis-dermatomyositis. Increased frequency of specific anti-Toxoplasma IgM antibodies. Am. J. Med., 75:313–320, 1983.

197. Malmvall, B-E., Bengtsson, B-A., and Rydberg, L.: HLA antigens in patients with giant cell arteritis, com-

pared with two control groups of different ages. Scand. J. Rheumatol., 9:65–68, 1980.

198. Maricq, H.R., et al.: Capillary abnormalities in polyvinyl chloride production workers. Examination by in vivo microscopy. J.A.M.A., 236:1368–1371, 1976.

199. Masi, A.T.: Clinical epidemiologic perspective of systemic lupus erythematosus. In Epidemiology of the Rheumatic Diseases. Proceedings of the Fourth International Conference. National Institutes of Health. New York, Gower Medical Publishing, Ltd., 1984, pp. 145–163.

200. Masi, A.T.: Epidemiology of B-27 associated diseases. Ann. Rheum. Dis., 38:131–134, 1979.

201. Masi, A.T.: Family, twin and genetic studies: A general review illustrated by systemic lupus erythematosus. In Population Studies in the Rheumatic Diseases. Edited by P.H. Bennett, and P.H. Wood. New York, Excerpta Medica, 1968, pp. 267–284.

202. Masi, A.T.: Population studies in rheumatic disease. Ann. Rev. Med., 18:185–206, 1967.

203. Masi, A.T., et al.: Prospective study of the early course of rheumatoid arthritis in young adults: Comparison of patients with and without rheumatoid factor positivity at entry and identification of variables correlating with outcome. Semin. Arthritis Rheum., 5:299–326, 1976.

204. Masi, A.T., and D'Angelo, W.A.: Epidemiology of fatal systemic sclerosis (diffuse scleroderma). A 15-year survey in Baltimore. Ann. Intern. Med., 66:870–883, 1967.

205. Masi, A.T., and Feigenbaum, S.: Seronegative rheumatoid arthritis: Fact or fiction? Arch. Intern. Med., 143:2167–2172, 1983.

206. Masi, A.T., Feigenbaum, S.L., and Kaplan, S.B.: Articular patterns in the early course of rheumatoid arthritis. Am. J. Med., 75 (Suppl.):16–26, 1983.

207. Masi, A.T., Josipovic, D.B., and Jefferson, W.E.: Decreased 11-deoxy-17-ketosteroid excretion in women with rheumatoid arthritis (RA): Gas liquid chromatographic (GLC) studies of RA patients and matched controls implicating a deficiency of androgenic-anabolic steroids in RA. Semin. Arthritis Rheum. In press, 1984.

208. Masi, A.T., and Kaslow, R.A.: Sex effects in systemic lupus erythematosus: A clue to pathogenesis. Arthritis Rheum., 21:480–484, 1978.

209. Masi, A.T., and Medsger, T.A.: A new look at the epidemiology of ankylosing spondylitis and related syndromes. Clin. Orthop., 143:15–29, 1979.

210. Masi, A.T., and Medsger, T.A., Jr.: Epidemiology of the rheumatic diseases. In Arthritis and Allied Conditions, 9th Ed. Edited by D.J. McCarty. Philadelphia, Lea & Febiger, 1979, pp. 11–35.

211. Mason, R.M., and Barnes, C.C.: Behçet's syndrome with arthritis. Ann. Rheum. Dis., 28:95–103, 1969.

212. McBryde, A.M., Jr., and McCollum, D.E.: Ankylosing spondylitis in women. The disease and its prognosis. N.C. Med. J., 34:34–37, 1973.

213. McCarty, D.J.: Coexistent gout and rheumatoid arthritis. J. Rheumatol., 8:253–254, 1981.

214. McKlusky, D.E., Lordon, R.E., and Arnett, F.C.: HL-A27 in Reiter's syndrome and psoriatic arthritis: A genetic factor in disease susceptibility and expression. J. Rheumatol., 1:263–268, 1974.

215. McMahon, B.J., et al.: Vasculitis in Eskimos living in an area hyperendemic for hepatitis B. J.A.M.A., 244:2180–2182, 1980.

216. Medsger, T.A., Jr.: Progressive systemic sclerosis and associated disorders. In Principles of Rheumatic Diseases. Edited by R.S. Panush. New York, John Wiley & Sons, 1981, pp. 331–350.

217. Medsger, T.A., Jr., et al.: Survival with systemic sclerosis (scleroderma). Ann. Intern. Med., 75:369–376, 1971.

218. Medsger, T.A., Jr., Dawson, W.N., Jr., and Masi, A.T.: The epidemiology of polymyositis. Am. J. Med., 48:715–723, 1970.

219. Medsger, T.A., Jr., and Masi, A.T.: Epidemiology of progressive systemic sclerosis. Clin. Rheum. Dis., 5:15–25, 1979.

220. Medsger, T.A., and Masi, A.T.: The epidemiology of systemic sclerosis (scleroderma) among male U.S. veterans. J. Chronic Dis., 31:73–85, 1978.

221. Medsger, T.A., Jr., and Masi, A.T.: Epidemiology of systemic sclerosis (scleroderma). Ann. Intern. Med., 74:714–721, 1971.

222. Medsger, A.R., and Robinson, H.: Comparative study of divorce in rheumatoid arthritis and other rheumatic diseases. J. Chronic Dis., 25:269–275, 1972.

223. Medsger, T.A., Jr., Robinson, H., and Masi, A.T.: Factors affecting survivorship in polymyositis. A life-table study of 124 patients. Arthritis Rheum., 14:249–258, 1971.

224. Meislin, A.G., and Rothfield, N.: Systemic lupus erythematosus in childhood. Analysis of 42 cases, with comparative data on 200 adult cases followed concurrently. Pediatrics, 42:37–49, 1968.

225. Mellors, R.C., and Mellors, J.W.: Type C RNA viral genome expression in systemic lupus erythematosus (SLE). The New Zealand mouse model and the human disease. Immunopathology Sixth International Convocation Immunology, 185–190, 1978.

226. Mendez-Bryan, R., Gonzalez-Alcover, R., and Roger, L.: Rheumatoid arthritis: Prevalence in a tropical area. Arthritis Rheum., 7:171–176, 1964.

227. Merrell, M., and Shulman, L.E.: Determination of prognosis in chronic disease illustrated by systemic lupus erythematosus. J. Chronic Dis., 1:12–32, 1955.

228. Messner, R.P., DeHoratius, R., and Ferrone, S.: Lymphocytotoxic antibodies in systemic lupus erythematosus patients and their relatives. Reactivity with the HLA antigenic molecular complex. Arthritis Rheum., 23:265–272, 1980.

229. Michalik, T.: Immune complexes of hepatitis B surface antigen in the pathogenesis of polyarteritis nodosa. Am. J. Pathol., 90:619–628, 1978.

230. Michet, C.J., et al.: Epidemiology of systemic lupus erythematosus and other connective tissue diseases in Rochester, Minnesota, 1950–1979. Mayo Clin. Proc. In press, 1984.

231. Mikkelsen, W.M.: In Arthritis and Allied Conditions, 8th Ed. Philadelphia, Lea & Febiger, 1972, p. 211.

232. Mikkelsen, W.M., et al.: The distribution of serum uric acid values in population unselected as to gout or hyperuricemia. Am. J. Med., 39:242–251, 1965.

233. Miller, K.B., and Schwartz, R.S.: Familial abnormalities of suppressor-cell function in systemic lupus erythematosus. N. Engl. J. Med., 301:803–809, 1979.

234. Mitchell, D.M., et al.: Predictors of mortality in rheumatoid arthritis (abstract). Arthritis Rheum., 25:S24, 1982.

235. Mitchell, D.M., and Fries, J.F.: An analysis of the American Rheumatism Association criteria for rheumatoid arthritis. Arthritis Rheum., 25:481–487, 1982.

236. Moll, J.M.B., and Wright, V.: New York clinical criteria for ankylosing spondylitis: A statistical evaluation. Ann. Rheum. Dis., 32:354–363, 1973.

237. Monson, R.R., and Hall, A.P.: Mortality among arthritics. J. Chronic Dis., 29:459–467, 1976.

238. Morris, R., et al.: HL-A W27—a clue to the diagnosis and pathogenesis of Reiter's syndrome. N. Engl. J. Med., 290:554–556, 1974.

239. Morton, N.E.: Genetics of hyperuricemia in families with gout. Am. J. Med. Genet., 4:103–106, 1979.

240. Morton, R.O., et al.: The incidence of systemic lupus erythematosus in North American Indians. J. Rheumatol., 3:186–190, 1976.

241. Moses, S., and Barland, P.: Laboratory criteria for a diagnosis of systemic lupus erythematosus. J.A.M.A., 242:1039–1043, 1979.

242. Moskowitz, R.W., Baggenstoss, A.H., and Slocumb, C.H.: Histopathologic classification of periarteritis nodosa: A study of 56 cases confirmed at necropsy. Mayo Clin. Proc., 38:345–357, 1963.

243. Mullick, F.G., et al.: Drug related vasculitis. Clinicopathologic correlations in 30 patients. Hum. Pathol., 10:313–325, 1979.

244. Murray, C., et al.: Histocompatibility alloantigens in psoriasis and psoriatic arthritis: Evidence for the influence of multiple genes in the major histocompatibility complex. J. Clin. Invest., 66:670–674, 1980.

245. Nasrallah, N.S., et al.: HLA-B27 antigen and rheumatoid factor negative (seronegative) peripheral arthritis: Studies in early-diagnosed younger patients. Am. J. Med., 63:379–386, 1977.

246. National Center for Health Statistics. PHS, Publication No. 1000, Series 11, No. 29. Washington, U.S. Government Printing Office, 1968.

247. National Center for Health Statistics. PHS, Publication No. 1000, Series 11, No. 20. Washington, U.S. Government Printing Office, 1966.

248. National Center for Health Statistics. PHS, Publication No. 1000, Series 11, No. 17, Washington, U.S. Government Printing Office, 1966.

249. National Center for Health Statistics. PHS, Publication No. 1000, Series 11, No. 15, Washington, U.S. Government Printing Office, 1966.

250. Neel, J.V., et al.: Studies of hyperuricemia. II. A reconsideration of the distribution of serum uric acid values in the families of Smyth, Cotterman, and Freyberg. Am. J. Hum. Genet., 17:14–22, 1965.

251. Noer, H.R.: An "experimental" epidemic of Reiter's syndrome. J.A.M.A., 198:693–698, 1966.

252. Numano, F., and Shimamoto, T.: Hypersecretion of estrogen in Takayasu's disease. Am. Heart J., 81:591–596, 1971.

253. Oates, J.K., and Csonka, G.W.: Reiter's disease in the female. Ann. Rheum. Dis., 18:37–44, 1959.

254. Ohno, S., et al.: Specific histocompatibility antigens associated with Behçet disease. Am. J. Ophthalmol., 80:636–641, 1975.

255. Okada, M., et al.: Factors influencing the serum uric acid level. A study based on a population survey in Hisayamatown, Kyushu, Japan. J. Chronic Dis., 33:607–612, 1980.

256. Orlowski, J.P., Clough, J.D., and Dyment, P.G.: Wegener's granulomatosis in the pediatric age group. Pediatrics, 61:83–90, 1978.

257. O'Donoghue, D.J.: Klinefelter's syndrome associated with systemic sclerosis. Postgrad. Med. J., 58:575–576, 1982.

258. O'Sullivan, J.B.: Gout in a New England town. Ann. Rheum. Dis., 31:166, 1972.

259. O'Sullivan, J.B.: The incidence of gout and related uric acid levels in Sudbury, Massachusetts. In Population Studies of the Rheumatic Diseases. Amsterdam, Excerpta Medica Foundation, 1968, pp. 371–376.

260. O'Sullivan, J.B., and Cathcart, E.S.: The prevalence of rheumatoid arthritis. Follow-up evaluation of the effect of criteria on rates in Sudbury, Massachusetts. Ann. Intern. Med., 76:573–577, 1972.

261. Pachman, L.M., Johasson, O., and Cannon, R.A.: HLA-B8 in juvenile dermatomyositis. Lancet, 2:567–568, 1977.

262. Paronen, I.: Reiter's disease: A study of 344 cases observed in Finland. Acta Med. Scand., 131 (Suppl. 212):7–114, 1948.

263. Partridge, R.E.H., and Duthie, J.J.R.: Rheumatism in dockers and civil servants: A comparison of heavy manual and sedentary workers. Ann. Rheum. Dis., 27:559–568, 1968.

264. Pearson, C.M.: Polymyositis and dermatomyositis. In Arthritis and Allied Conditions, 9th Ed. Edited by D.J. McCarty. Philadelphia, Lea & Febiger, 1979, pp. 742–743.

265. Perry, H.M., et al.: Relationship of acetyl transferase activity to antinuclear antibodies and toxic symptoms in hypertensive patients treated with hydralazine. J. Lab. Clin. Med., 76:114–125, 1970.

266. Persellin, R.H.: The effect of pregnancy on rheumatoid arthritis. Bull. Rheum. Dis., 27:922–927, 1976–1977.

267. Persky, V.M., et al.: Uric acid: A risk factor for coronary heart disease. Circulation, 59:969–977, 1979.

268. Peyron, J.G.: Epidemiologic and etiologic approach to osteoarthritis. Semin. Arthritis Rheum., 8:288–306, 1979.

269. Phanupnak, P., and Kohler, P.F.: Onset of polyarteritis nodosa during allergic hyposensitization treatment. Am. J. Med., 68:479–485, 1980.

270. Phillips, P.E.: Infection and chronic rheumatic disease in children. Semin. Arthritis Rheum., 10:92–99, 1980.

271. Phillips, P.E.: Virologic studies in rheumatoid arthritis. Rheumatology, 6:353–360, 1975.

272. Phillips, P.E., Kassan, S.S., and Kagen, L.J.: Increased toxoplasma antibodies in idiopathic inflammatory muscle disease. A case-controlled study. Arthritis Rheum., 22:209–214, 1979.

273. Pinals, R.S., Masi, A.T., and Larsen, R.A.: Preliminary criteria for clinical remission in rheumatoid arthritis. Arthritis Rheum., 24:1308–1315, 1981.

274. Puranen, J., et al.: Running and primary osteoarthritis of the hip. Br. Med. J., 2:424–425, 1975.

275. Radford, E.P., Doll, R., and Smith, P.G.: Mortality among patients with ankylosing spondylitis not given x-ray therapy. N. Engl. J. Med., 297:572–576, 1977.

276. Rakic, M.T., et al.: Observations on the natural history of hyperuricemia and gout. I. An eighteen year follow-up of nineteen gouty families. Am. J. Med., 37:862–871, 1964.

277. Ramsay, L.E.: Hyperuricaemia in hypertension: Role of alcohol. Br. Med. J., 1:653–654, 1979.

278. Reinertsen, J.L., et al.: An epidemiologic study of households exposed to canine systemic lupus erythematosus. Arthritis Rheum., 23:564–567, 1980.

279. Rimon, R., Viukari, M., and Halonen, P.: Relationship between life stress factors and viral antibody levels in patients with juvenile rheumatoid arthritis. Scand. J. Rheumatol., 8:62–64, 1979.

280. Rodnan, G.P., et al.: The association of progressive systemic sclerosis (scleroderma) with coal miners' pneumoconiosis and other forms of silicosis. Ann. Intern. Med., 66:323–334, 1967.

281. Rodnan, G.P., Jablonska, S., and Medsger, T.A., Jr.: Classification and nomenclature of progressive systemic sclerosis (scleroderma). Clin. Rheum. Dis., 5:5–13, 1979.

282. Ropes, M.W., et al.: Proposed diagnostic criteria for rheumatoid arthritis. Ann. Rheum. Dis., 16:118–125, 1957.

283. Ropes, N.W., Bennett, F.A., and Cobb, S.: 1958 revision of diagnostic criteria for rheumatoid arthritis. Arthritis Rheum., 2:16–20, 1959.

284. Rose, B.S.: Gout in Maoris. Semin. Arthritis Rheum., 5:121–145, 1975.

285. Rosenberg, A.M., and Petty, R.E.: Similar patterns of juvenile rheumatoid arthritis within families. Arthritis Rheum., 23:951–953, 1980.

286. Rosenberg, A.M., and Petty, R.E.: Reiter's disease in children. Am. J. Dis. Child., 133:394–398, 1979.

287. Rosselet, E., Saudan, Y., and Jeannet, M.: Recherche antigens HLA dans la maladie de Behçet. Ophthalmologica, 172:116–119, 1976.

288. Rothschild, B.M., and Masi, A.T.: Pathogenesis of rheumatoid arthritis: A vascular hypothesis. Semin. Arthritis Rheum., 12:11–31, 1982.

289. Roubinian, J.R., et al.: Delayed androgen treatment prolongs survival in murine lupus. J. Clin. Invest., 63:902–911, 1979.

290. Russell, A.S., et al.: Deforming arthropathy in systemic lupus erythematosus. Ann. Rheum. Dis., 33:204–209, 1974.

291. Sairanen, E., and Tillikainen, A.: HL-A 27 in Reiter's syndrome following shigellosis. Scand. J. Rheumatol., 4 (Suppl. 8):30–11, 1975.

292. Schachter, J., et al.: Isolation of Bedsoniae from the joints of patients with Reiter's syndrome. Proc. Soc. Exp. Biol. Med., 122:283–285, 1966.

293. Schaller, J.G.: Juvenile rheumatoid arthritis. Arthritis Rheum., 20:165–170, 1977.

294. Schwartz, B.D., Luehrman, L.R., and Rodey, G.E.: Public antigenic determinant on a family of HLA-B molecules: Basis for cross-reactivity and a possible link with disease predisposition. J. Clin. Invest., 64:938–947, 1979.

295. Serdula, M.K., and Rhoads, G.G.: Frequency of systemic lupus erythematosus in different ethnic groups in Hawaii. Arthritis Rheum., 2:328–333, 1979.

296. Sergent, J.S., and Christian, C.C.: Necrotizing vasculitis

after acute serous otitis media. Ann. Intern. Med., *81*:195–199, 1974.

297. Sharp, G.C., et al.: Mixed connective tissue disease—an apparently distinct rheumatic disease syndrome associated with a specific antibody to an extractable nuclear antigen (ENA). Am. J. Med., *52*:148–159, 1972.

298. Shiokawa, Y.: Vascular Lesions of Collagen Diseases and Related Conditions. Baltimore, University Park Press, 1977.

299. Siegel, M., et al.: Survivorship in systemic lupus erythematosus: Relationship to race and pregnancy. Arthritis Rheum., *12*:117–125, 1969.

300. Siegel, M., et al.: The epidemiology of systemic lupus erythematosus: Preliminary results in New York City. J. Chron. Dis., *15*:131–140, 1962.

301. Siegel, M., Holley, H.L., and Lee, S.L.: Epidemiologic studies on systemic lupus erythematosus. Comparative data for New York City and Jefferson County, Alabama, 1956–1965. Arthritis Rheum., *13*:802–811, 1970.

302. Siegel, M., and Lee, S.L.: The epidemiology of systemic lupus erythematosus. Semin. Arthritis Rheum., *3*:1–53, 1973.

303. Siegel, M., Lee, S.L., and Persee, N.S.: The epidemiology of drug-induced systemic lupus erythematosus. Arthritis Rheum., *10*:407–415, 1967.

304. Siegel, M., and Seelenfreund, M.: Racial and social factors in systemic lupus erythematosus. J.A.M.A., *191*:77–80, 1965.

305. Sills, E.M.: Psoriatic arthritis in childhood. Johns Hopkins Med. J., *146*:49–53, 1980.

306. Smith, C.A., Fidler, W.J., and Pinals, R.S.: The epidemiology of giant cell arteritis. Report of a ten-year study in Shelby County, Tennessee. Arthritis Rheum., 26:1214–1219, 1983.

307. Solomon, L., et al.: Rheumatic disorders in the South African Negro. Part I. Rheumatoid arthritis and ankylosing spondylitis. S. Afr. Med. J., *49*:1292–1296, 1975.

308. Solomon, L., Beighton, P., and Lawrence, J.S.: Rheumatic disorders in the south African Negro. Part II. Osteoarthritis. S. Afr. Med. J., *49*:1292–1296, 1975.

309. Solomon, L., Robin, G., and Valkenburg, H.A.: Rheumatoid arthritis in an urban South African Negro population. Ann. Rheum. Dis., *34*:128–135, 1975.

310. Spencer, D.G., Dick, H.M., and Dick, W.C.: Ankylosing spondylitis—the role of HLA-B27 homozygosity. Tissue Antigens, *14*:379–384, 1974.

311. Stastny, P., and Fink, C.W.: Different HLA-D associations in adult and juvenile rheumatoid arthritis. J. Clin. Invest., *63*:124–130, 1979.

312. Stern, R., et al.: Systemic lupus erythematosus associated with Klinefelter's syndrome. Arthritis Rheum., *20*:18–22, 1977.

313. Stewart, R.B., et al.: Epidemiology of hyperuricemia in an ambulatory elderly population. J. Am. Geriatr. Soc., *27*:552–554, 1979.

314. Stiller, C.R., Russell, A.S., and Dossetor, J.B.: Autoimmunity: Present concepts. Ann. Intern. Med., *82*:405–410, 1975.

315. Stillman, J.S., and Barry, P.E.: Juvenile rheumatoid arthritis: Series 2. Arthritis Rheum., *20*:171–175, 1977.

316. Strongwater, S.L., et al.: A murine model of polymyositis induced by Coxsackievirus B1 (Tucson strain). Arthritis Rheum., *27*:433–442, 1984.

317. Sturrock, R.D., et al.: Family studies in ankylosing spondylitis. Ann. Rheum. Dis., *34* (Suppl 1):39–41, 1975.

318. Subcommittee for Scleroderma Criteria of the American Rheumatism Association Diagnostic and Therapeutic Criteria Committee: Preliminary criteria for the classification of systemic sclerosis (scleroderma). Arthritis Rheum., *23*:581–590, 1980.

319. Sullivan, D.B., Cassidy, J.T., and Petty, R.E.: Dermatomyositis in the pediatric patient. Arthritis Rheum., *20*:327–331, 1977.

320. Symposium on the Epidemiology of Chronic Rheumatism, Volume II. Atlas of Standard Radiographs. Oxford, Blackwell Scientific Publications, 1963.

321. Talbott, J.H.: Acute dermatomyositis-polymyositis and malignancy. Semin. Arthritis Rheum., *6*:305–360, 1977.

322. Talbott, J.H., et al.: Gouty arthitis in the black race. Semin. Arthritis Rheum., *4*:209–239, 1975.

323. Talbott, J.H., and Barrocas, M.: Progressive systemic sclerosis (PSS) and malignancy, pulmonary and non-pulmonary. Medicine, *58*:182–207, 1979.

324. Tan, E.M., et al.: The 1982 revised criteria for the classification of systemic lupus erythematosus. Arthritis Rheum., *25*:1271–1272, 1981.

325. Tan, E.M., et al.: Diversity of antinuclear antibodies in progressive systemic sclerosis (scleroderma): Anticentromere antibody and its relationship to CREST syndrome. Arthritis Rheum., *23*:617–625, 1980.

326. Tan, P.L.J., Wigley, R.D., and Borman, C.B.: Clinical criteria for systemic sclerosis. Arthritis Rheum., *24*:1589–1590, 1981.

327. Terkeltaub, R., et al.: A clinical study of older age rheumatoid arthritis with comparison to a younger onset group. J. Rheumatol., *10*:418–424, 1983.

328. Torralba, T.P., and Bayani-Sioson, P.S.: The Filipino and gout. Semin. Arthritis Rheum., *4*:307–320, 1975.

329. Tosato, G., Steinberg, A.D., and Blaese, R.M.: Defective EBV-specific suppressor T-cell function in rheumatoid arthritis. N. Engl. J. Med., *305*:1238–1243, 1981.

330. Towner, S.R., et al.: The epidemiology of juvenile arthritis in Rochester, Minnesota 1960–1979. Arthritis Rheum., *26*:1208–1213, 1983.

331. Trentham, L.E.: Collagen arthritis as a relevant model for rheumatoid arthritis: Evidence pro and con. Arthritis Rheum., *25*:911–916, 1982.

332. Trentham, D.E., et al.: Autoimmunity to collagen: A shared feature of psoriatic and rheumatoid arthritis. Arthritis Rheum., *24*:1363–1369, 1981.

333. Trepo, C.G., et al.: The role of circulating hepatitis B antigen-antibody complexes in the pathogenesis of vascular and hepatic manifestations in polyarteritis nodosa. J. Clin. Pathol., *27*:863–868, 1974.

334. Tuffanelli, D.L., and Winkelmann, R.K.: Systemic scleroderma. A clinical study of 727 cases. Arch. Dermatol., *84*:359–371, 1961.

335. Tweeddale, M.G., and Fodor, J.G.: Elevated serum uric acid. A cardiovascular risk factor. Nephron, *23*(Suppl. 1):3–6, 1979.

336. Uddin, J., Kraus, A.S., and Kelly, H.G.: Survivorship and death in rheumatoid arthritis. Arthritis Rheum., *13*:125–130, 1970.

337. van der Linden, S.M., et al.: The risk of developing ankylosing spondylitis in HLA-B27 positive individuals: A comparison of relatives of spondylitis patients with the general population. Arthritis Rheum., *27*:241–249, 1984.

338. van der Linden, S., Valkenburg, H.A., and Cats, A.: Intra- and interobserver variation in diagnosis of sacroiliitis (abstract). Clin. Res., *31*:807A, 1983.

339. van der Linden, S., Valkenburg, H.A., and Cats, A.: Evaluation of diagnostic criteria for ankylosing spondylitis: A proposal for modification of the New York criteria. Arthritis Rheum., *27*:361–368, 1984.

340. Vaughan, J.H.: Rheumatoid arthritis, rheumatoid factor and the Epstein-Barr virus. J. Rheumatol., *6*:381–388, 1979.

341. Wallace, D.J., et al.: Coexistent gout in rheumatoid arthritis. Arthritis Rheum., *22*:81–86, 1979.

342. Wallace, S.L., et al.: Preliminary criteria for the classification of the acute arthritis of primary gout. Arthritis Rheum., *20*:895–900, 1977.

343. Walravens, P.A., and Chase, H.P.: The prognosis of childhood systemic lupus erythematosus. Am. J. Dis. Child., *130*:929–933, 1976.

344. Warren, R.E., and Brewerton, D.A.: Faecal carriage of Klebsiella by patients with ankylosing spondylitis and rheumatoid arthritis. Ann. Rheum. Dis., *39*:37–44, 1980.

345. Warshaw, J.B., and Spach, M.S.: Takayasu's disease (primary aortitis) in childhood. Case report with review of literature. Pediatrics, *35*:626–630, 1965.

346. Weiner, H.: Psychobiology and Human Disease. New York, Elsevier Scientific Publishing Co., 1977.

347. Whitaker, J.N., and Engel, W.K.: Vascular deposits of immunoglobulin and complement in idiopathic inflammatory myopathy. N. Engl. J. Med., *286*:333–338, 1972.

348. Willkens, R.F., et al.: Reiter's syndrome: Evaluation of preliminary criteria for definite disease. Arthritis Rheum., *24*:844–849, 1981.

349. Willkens, R.F., et al.: Studies of rheumatoid arthritis among a tribe of Northwest Indians. J. Rheumatol., *3*:9–14, 1976.

350. Winkelstein, A., and Rabin, B.S.: Theories of autoimmunity. Bull. Rheum. Dis., *26*:842–847, 1975.

351. Woodrow, J.C.: Histocompatibility antigens and rheumatic diseases. Semin. Arthritis Rheum., *6*:257–276, 1977.

352. Wright, V., and Moll, J.M.H.: Seronegative Polyarthritis. New York, Elsevier/North-Holland Biomedical Press, 1976.

353. Wyngaarden, J.B., and Kelley, W.N.: Epidemiology of hyperuricemia and gout. *In* Gout and Hyperuricemia. New York, Grune and Stratton, Inc., 1976, pp. 21–37.

354. Wyngaarden, J.B., and Kelley, W.N.: Hereditary xanthinuria. *In* Gout and Hyperuricemia. New York, Grune and Stratton, Inc., 1976, pp. 397–410.

354a. Wyngaarden, J.B., and Kelley, W.N.: Miscellaneous forms of hypouricemia. *In* Gout and Hyperuricemia. New York, Grune and Stratton, Inc., 1976, pp. 411–418.

355. Yamakage, A., et al.: Occupational scleroderma-like disorder occurring in men engaged in the polymerization of epoxy resins. Dermatologica, *161*:33–44, 1980.

356. Yano, K., Rhoads, G.G., and Kagan, A.: Epidemiology of serum uric acid among 8000 Japanese-American men in Hawaii. J. Chronic Dis., *30*:171–184, 1977.

357. Yelin, E., et al.: Work disability in rheumatoid arthritis: Effects of disease, social, and work factors. Ann. Intern. Med., *93*:551–556, 1980.

358. Yu, T.F.: Some unusual features of gouty arthritis in females. Semin. Arthritis Rheum., *6*:247–255, 1977.

359. Zalokar, J., et al.: Epidemiology of serum uric acid and gout in Frenchman. J. Chronic Dis., *27*:59–75, 1974.

Chapter 3

Differential Diagnosis of Arthritis; Analysis of Signs and Symptoms

Daniel J. McCarty

Rational prognosis and therapy require precise diagnosis. And diagnosis depends primarily on skillful history-taking and physical examination with subsequent help from the laboratory, the radiology department, or the surgical staff when indicated. I have assumed that the reader has acquired general clinical skills and will concentrate, therefore, on the interpretation of those aspects of the clinical history (symptoms) and the physical examination (signs) that relate to the differential diagnosis of arthritis and allied conditions (Table 3–1).

The purpose of the history and physical examination is to classify a patient's problem into one of four broad categories: inflammatory, degenerative-metabolic, functional (neurotic), or of unknown etiology. These categories represent the primary nature of the diseases listed in Table 3–2. This classification does not deny the existence of an inflammatory component in osteoarthritis, or a degenerative component of inflammatory arthritides such as RA or psoriatic arthritis. There may be an organic component even in those syndromes listed as "psychogenic," an organic peg upon which is hung a psychoneurotic hat. Conversely, there is often a functional component to most organic illnesses. The "unknown" category is important since there is a tendency by many clinicians to "force" a given patient's musculoskeletal complaints into a diagnostic pigeonhole. New syndromes and subsets of old ones are constantly being recognized. At least 10% of patients with musculoskeletal complaints that I have seen through the years cannot be given a diagnosis with certainty. In the remainder, however, a reasonable differential diagnosis can be formulated after the initial examination.

HISTORY

Chief Complaint. Patients consult physicians only for pain (or pain equivalent) or anxiety. Pain equivalents include subpainful unpleasantries such as itching, aching, stiffness, and nausea. Almost all other complaints are not presented to the doctor unless the patient, or a relative with some degree of control of the patient, is concerned (anxious) about their presence. Thus, treatment depends on relief of the pain or other unpleasant sensation, an explanation of the pertinent pathophysiology to the patient in lay terms, and a brief explanation of how the prescribed regimen is expected to correct the problem. The history should include detailed inquiry about the patient's motivation in coming to the doctor, especially in the *absence* of pain or pain equivalent. Why the anxiety? Could the notion that rheumatoid arthritis is a psychosomatic illness[5] have come from those extra office visits by anxious patients with mild disease while their stoic counterparts were at the movies? Could the patients with "fibrositis," making up 28% of new patient visits in private rheumatologic practice,[1] represent the anxious protruding tip of the mountain of individuals with tense neck and shoulder muscles? Are patients in a rheumatic disease practice more likely to come to the office with a shopping list of questions written on a slip of paper (*petit morceau de papier* syndrome)? Find out precisely why the patient consulted you, with particular attention to the reason for the anxiety underlying all chief complaints.

History of Present Illness. In general, one attempts to determine whether the patient has a systemic disease or a purely local condition. A localized condition may affect multiple sites, of course. What joints or other structures are involved?*

What was the pattern of involvement? In what order did joint involvement occur? How fast did it occur? At what time of the day did it start? If joint involvement is painful, severity can be estimated by whether it interfered with function of the affected extremity, or with sleep or work. Was involvement self-limited, migratory, or additive (progressive)? If limited, how long was the episode? *Migratory* means that the process subsided completely in an affected joint while cropping up in an erstwhile normal joint. *Progressive* or additive means that the first joint stays afflicted while

---

*"Joint" will be used hereafter, although tendon sheaths and bursae are often involved as well.

Table 3–1.   Signs and Symptoms Useful in Differential Diagnosis of Arthritis

Symptoms	Degenerative	Inflammatory	Psychogenic
Stiffness (duration)	Few minutes; ''gelling'' after prolonged rest	Hours (often); most pronounced after rest	Little or no variation in intensity with rest or activity
Pain	Follows activity; relieved by rest	Even at rest; nocturnal pain may interfere with sleep	Little or no variation in intensity with rest or activity
Weakness	Present, usually localized and not severe	Often pronounced	Often a complaint ''neurasthenia''
Fatigue	Not usual	Often severe with onset in afternoon	Often in A.M. on arising
Emotional depression and lability	Not usual	Common, coincides with fatigue; often disappears if disease remits	Often present
Signs			
Tenderness localized over afflicted joint	Usually present	Almost always; the most sensitive indication of inflammation	Tender ''all over''; ''touch me not attitude''; tend to push away or to grasp the examining hand
Swelling	Effusion common; little synovial reaction	Effusion very common; often synovial proliferation and thickening	None
Heat and erythema	Unusual but may occur	More common	None
Crepitus	Coarse to medium	Medium to fine	None, except with coexistent osteoarthritis
Bony spurs	Common	Sometimes found, usually with antecedent osteoarthritis	None, except with coexistent osteoarthritis

additional joints are involved by the pathologic process. Was treatment sought? What and how much was given and for how long? What was its effect on the disease? Side effects of therapy should be recorded.

Certain symptoms can be analyzed almost objectively, producing reliable data that deserve much weight diagnostically. The *duration of morning stiffness* is such a measurement and also serves as a convenient clinical yardstick to measure inflammatory activity (see Chap. 7). Patients are often emotional about the magnitude of morning stiffness but not about its duration. Two questions suffice: what time do you get out of bed (not awake) and about when are you as ''loose'' as you are going to get? The physician then determines the duration of stiffness by subtraction. If a single question is asked, ''How long are you stiff after getting up in the morning?'' the patient will provide an answer. This answer will nearly always be different (shorter) than that obtained with the two-question technique.

The duration of morning stiffness is directly proportional to the severity of an inflammatory process

in an extremity, whether this be arthritis, myositis, fibrositis, or sunburn. It signifies, nonspecifically, *inflammation*. Variations in its duration can be used to quantify inflammation and its response to treatment. Indeed, it is one of the best ways to follow inflammation clinically, and in this modern world of complex testing, it is both free of charge and immediately available. It is more precise than the erythrocyte sedimentation rate in following rheumatoid inflammation. True stiffness should be differentiated from the ''articular gelling'' of osteoarthritis, which lasts only for a few minutes or even seconds. The hesitant stiff first few steps of an elderly person crossing the room to switch channels on a TV set are a familiar example of the ''gelling'' phenomenon.

The sunburned limb becomes flexible sooner with each passing day, faithfully reflecting the resolution of the thermal injury and the accompanying inflammatory response. The protracted morning stiffness characteristic of polymyalgia rheumatica vanishes completely after low doses of prednisone are given. The average untreated patient with rheumatoid arthritis is stiff for about four hours after

Table 3–2. Examples of Diseases in Various Categories

Noninflammatory†	Inflammatory	Psychogenic
Erosive osteoarthritis	*Tenosynovitis { calcific (BCP) / other	*Primary fibrositis (tension rheumatism)
*Primary generalized osteoarthritis (OA)	*Rheumatoid arthritis	*Restless leg syndrome
*Isolated OA, e.g., hip, knee, first CMC	seropositive	*Hysteria
	seronegative	
*Cervical syndrome	*Systemic lupus erythematosus	
*Traumatic arthritis	Mixed connective tissue disease	
Aseptic (osteo)necrosis	Polyarteritis nodosa	
Amyloid arthropathy	Polymyositis	
*Pseudogout (some types)	Dermatomyositis	
Metabolic arthropathy	Rheumatic fever	
Hemachromatosis	*Reiter's syndrome (''reactive'' arthritis)	
Acromegaly		
Hypothyroidism	*Psoriatic arthritis	
Hyperparathyroidism	*Ankylosing spondylitis	
Ochronosis	*Juvenile rheumatoid arthritis	
Neuroarthropathy (Charcot)	Inflammatory bowel disease arthritis	
*Enthesopathy	*Crystal synovitis	
Tumors	Gout (MSU)	
Pigmented villonodular	Pseudogout (CPPD)	
Synovitis	Other (BCP, postcorticosteroid	
Synovial cell sarcoma	injection flare)	
*Mechanical abnormalities, e.g., torn menisci, tibial torsion	*Polymyalgia rheumatica	
	*Palindromic rheumatism	
*Reflex sympathetic dystrophies, e.g., shoulder-hand	Viral arthritis (e.g., rubella, mumps, hepatitis B)	
*Periarthritis of shoulder	Infectious arthritis	
*Tendonitis	Bacterial	
Blood dyscrasias, e.g., hemophilia	Tuberculous	
	Fungal	
	Immune complex arthritis, e.g., cryoglobulinemia, bacterial endocarditis, infected ventriculoatrial shunt	

*Common conditions encountered by every clinician.

†An inflammatory component may be present intermittently in some of these conditions.

arising in the morning. The mechanism of stiffness after immobilization of an inflamed part is unclear, but it may be the subjective perception of increased resistance to motion that has been measured objectively,[7] which in turn is probably related to localized tissue edema and accumulation of the metabolic products of the inflammatory process. Motion activates the milking action of the muscles on both lymphatic flow and venous return. Increased stiffness of an inflamed part occurs not only after sleeping, but after any prolonged immobility, such as watching television or movies or cat-napping.

If a structure is severely inflamed, it is *painful* on motion, just as sunburned skin over a joint is painful on motion. Overt pain at rest is found only in intense inflammation. Pain is difficult to describe, much less to quantify or localize. If trauma, including the microtrauma of motion, is pathogenetically important, then pain occurs on motion and subsides with rest. If there is no pattern of pain at all, a psychogenic factor might be involved. In patients with musculoskeletal diseases, it may arise from stimulation of synovial, capsular, periosteal, ligamentous, or tendinous nerve endings by mechanical irritation or by inflammation; from pressure on entrapped nerves, such as the median in the carpal tunnel at the wrist, the suprascapular in the shoulder, or from nerve roots in the cervical foramina; or from muscle spasm, either directly or, with increased muscle tone, on nerves coursing through the tightened muscle. It never arises from cartilage. Electromyographers report that there is little or no evidence of increased muscular contraction (spasm) about inflamed joints at rest, and to differentiate pathologically increased from normally increased electrical activity in contracting muscles is difficult. If a patient complains of parietal pain and has no increased stiffness after prolonged immobility, direct nerve irritation or a psychologic problem is immediately suspected. Elicited pain (*tenderness*) is much more important clinically and can be localized accurately.

Systemic *fatigue*, like stiffness, is a subjective phenomenon and not disease-specific. The time of onset of fatigue after arising from bed is inversely proportional to the severity of the inflammatory process. This time is determined by subtracting the point of "bone tiredness" from the time of arising. The average untreated rheumatoid patient has about 3.5 hours before fatigue sets in. The cause of such pathologic fatigue is unknown. Perhaps the products of inflammation, milked from the involved sites by muscular activity, as already outlined, produce tissue effects that subjectively represent fatigue. When asked about fatigue, patients often state that tiredness is present on arising. In the absence of insomnia, anemia, or metabolic disease, such fatigue is of neurotic origin, a desire perhaps to remain in the womb. This sensation usually disappears soon after the patient is up and about. Most of us have had this experience occasionally.

Weakness. Disuse atrophy occurs rapidly, often in a few days, in muscles that move painful joints. In the diffuse systemic rheumatic diseases, direct muscle involvement often occurs as well. With upper extremity involvement, "clumsiness" or weakness of grip may be the complaint, whereas difficulty in arising from a chair or in going up or down stairs may be experienced in lower extremity involvement. This subjective complaint can be verified and measured by measurement of grip strength or by timing a set task using lower extremity muscles.[2a]

Depression, Hysteria, and Emotional Lability. Depression may be the most common symptom of the twentieth century and is commonly seen in rheumatologic practice. It is nearly always present in patients with "fibrositis" (see Chap. 70), and, usually in reactive form, in patients with systemic rheumatic diseases including rheumatoid arthritis. In the latter group it often corresponds to the time of onset of pathologic fatigue, when emotional lability (crying, temper tantrums, or withdrawal) also occurs. These symptoms may disappear as the disease remits. Hysteria is less common and usually dramatic. A patient cannot write clearly and has pain in the fingers (writer's cramp), or cannot bend over or straighten up (camptocormia), or cannot straighten a bent extremity. *Restless legs syndrome* is fairly common and appears to be an hysterical condition or a depressive equivalent. Such patients are inordinately open to suggestion. Almost any medication that is prescribed with conviction will work miraculously, but is certain to produce unpleasant side effects, i.e., these patients are notorious "placebo-reactors" (see Chap. 70).

Systemic Review. This is part of the routine history and should be done in all cases.

Past History. A previous account of musculoskeletal or systemic disease may shed light on the current problem. Chorea or "growing pains" in childhood may aid in differentiating rheumatic fever or juvenile rheumatoid arthritis in an adult patient. A recent history of exposure to rubella or mumps may clarify an otherwise obscure arthritis. Even more important is a history of sexual deviance or promiscuity in a patient suspected of having gonorrheal arthritis or Reiter's syndrome. The personalities of patients with the latter condition are often bizarre.

Family History. A history of diabetes mellitus, hypertension, or heart disease can often be obtained accurately. Diabetes is associated with adhesive capsulitis of the shoulders, Dupuytren's contracture, and osteoarthritis. A family history of arthritis may be obtained in gout, pseudogout, ankylosing spondylitis, and rheumatoid arthritis, to name a few. I have often found it difficult to be sure of the diagnosis of arthritis from the family history, let alone what type of arthritis was actually present. This aspect of history-taking gives promise of becoming more important with recent advances in immunogenetics (see Chaps. 24, 25).

Social History. Stability of family life and the stability and type of job are important points to establish, since much of the treatment program in arthritis involves them. Avocations should also be recorded since these, too, must often be dealt with in designing a treatment program. Current drug intake should be listed here, including alcohol and tobacco. Some idea of the patient's ability to perceive reality and of emotional maturity should be obtained at this point.

PHYSICAL EXAMINATION

An "arthralgia" is often an arthritis without a physical examination.

Palpation. The rheumatologist's fingers are his stethoscope. Although various devices are useful to quantify tenderness, joint swelling, and skin temperature, none supplants the skilled examiner's fingers in the physical examination. A working knowledge of topographic anatomy is essential. The examiner must know what structure(s) lies under his hand. This is particularly true when eliciting *tenderness*, which is the most sensitive sign available, albeit not specific. The neophyte uses too little force when pressing even on superficial structures. I exert sufficient force to blanch my thumbnail,[3,4] about 74 pounds per square inch, when examining areas that are not obviously inflamed. Obviously one could reduce return office visits sharply by pressing this hard on red, swollen joints. Common sense must prevail! I use tenderness primarily to *exclude* disease. If none is present at 74 pounds per square inch, underlying inflammation, in the absence of congenital or acquired insensitivity to pain, is ruled out. If tenderness is present, then either a low pain threshold or pathologic change may be responsible. Fortunately, most tenderness due to an organic cause is accompanied by more specific findings, such as swelling, crepitus, and increased local heat. Tenderness of joints is best elicited by pressure over the areas of synovial reflexion, whereas tendons should be stretched gently and then subjected to pressure. Direct pressure should be exerted on "fibrositic" areas in every patient. These areas include the lateral neck strap muscles, the belly of the trapezius, the epicondylar area, the medial knee over the collateral ligament and anserine bursa, and the lateral thigh over the tensor fascia lata (see Chap. 70).

Areas of tenderness can be "controlled" by similar pressure over other nearby areas. A neurotic patient may be tender everywhere on the body. Such patients grasp the examiner's hand or draw the part away from the examiner's grasp—the "touch-me-not" sign. It is important to distinguish tender bones from tender soft tissues. For example, the anterior tibia is tender in most elderly subjects for reasons unknown to me. Bone tenderness is present in severe osteoporosis and other forms of systemic bone disease. In reflex sympathetic dystrophies, the entire hand (or foot) is tender. Even allowing for periarticular accentuation of tenderness, tenderness between the joints, over both bone and soft tissue, often suggests this condition rather than a true synovitis (see Chap. 85).

Deep-seated joints, such as the hips, spine, and sacroiliac joints, require even more pressure to elicit tenderness because the intervening "pad" of soft tissue attenuates the applied force. Here, I exert pressure with the weight of my body against the flat of my hand held over the hip or over my thumb in the case of spine or sacroiliac joints. It is helpful to drape the patient over the examining table with the legs hanging down and the feet touching the floor but not bearing weight (Fig. 3–1). The lumbar lordotic curve is flattened in this position. The sacroiliac joints lies between the roof of the sciatic notch and the posterior-inferior iliac spine, both of which can be identified easily. Inflammation of the sacroiliac joint is faithfully reflected by localized tenderness. Pressure can be exerted over each vertebral spine separately. The "skip areas" of spinal involvement so common in Reiter's syndrome, a septic discitis, or the precise level of lumbar degenerative disc disease, can often

be mapped out readily with this technique (see Chaps. 53, 54, 82, 101).

A skilled examiner can lay hands on every peripheral joint in the body and record the presence of tenderness on an appropriate form in about three minutes. Examination of the spine requires an additional three minutes.

Range of Motion. *Passive motion of a joint* is an ancillary method of eliciting pain and is also necessary to check for contractures or limitation of motion. When pain is present on passive motion, it is often impossible to determine its origin without further examination. For example, pain on attempting to straighten the elbow to 0° or beyond can arise from intrinsic joint disease such as synovitis, or may be due to extrinsic causes such as biceps tendonitis. Pain on motion of a hip or shoulder joint is often due to abnormalities in the joint capsule or tendons of the surrounding muscles. It is my practice to examine the anatomic structures about any joint that is painful on passive motion to determine exactly what is and what is not tender. Thus, the absence of pain on passive motion rules out pathologic abnormalities of many structures, but its presence demands further palpatory dissection of the local anatomy in search of its cause.

The *range of motion* of all joints should be determined while attempting to elicit tenderness and pain on passive motion (Fig. 3–2). Loss of normal motion can be due to articular changes such as subluxation (partial dislocation), luxation (complete dislocation), capsular contraction, intra-articular adhesions, fibrous ankylosis, a tense effusion, extremely thickened synovium, or an intra-articular loose body. Bony ankylosis occurs commonly in some conditions such as juvenile rheumatoid arthritis (JRA), ankylosing spondylitis, psoriatic arthritis, Reiter's disease and, rarely, in gout, pseudogout, rheumatoid arthritis, and osteoarthritis. Extra-articular causes such as ruptured or dislocated tendons, muscle spasm, tendon inflammation or shortening, or subchondral bony fractures are perhaps even more common causes of loss of motion.

Abnormal motion of joints should also be noted. The subchondral bony collapse of the medial tibial plateau, so common in osteoarthritis of the knee, produces a *genu varus* deformity and an abnormal lateral motion of the unstable knee owing to the slack in the medial collateral ligament. Early loss of lateral stability of the knee should be determined while the knee is flexed to about 25°. Except in carpal or tarsal joints, rheumatoid arthritis is apt to result in unstable, not-fused joints. Three common examples are the valgus and flexion deformities of laterally unstable knees, sliding atlantoaxial joints, and abnormal lateral motion of the second

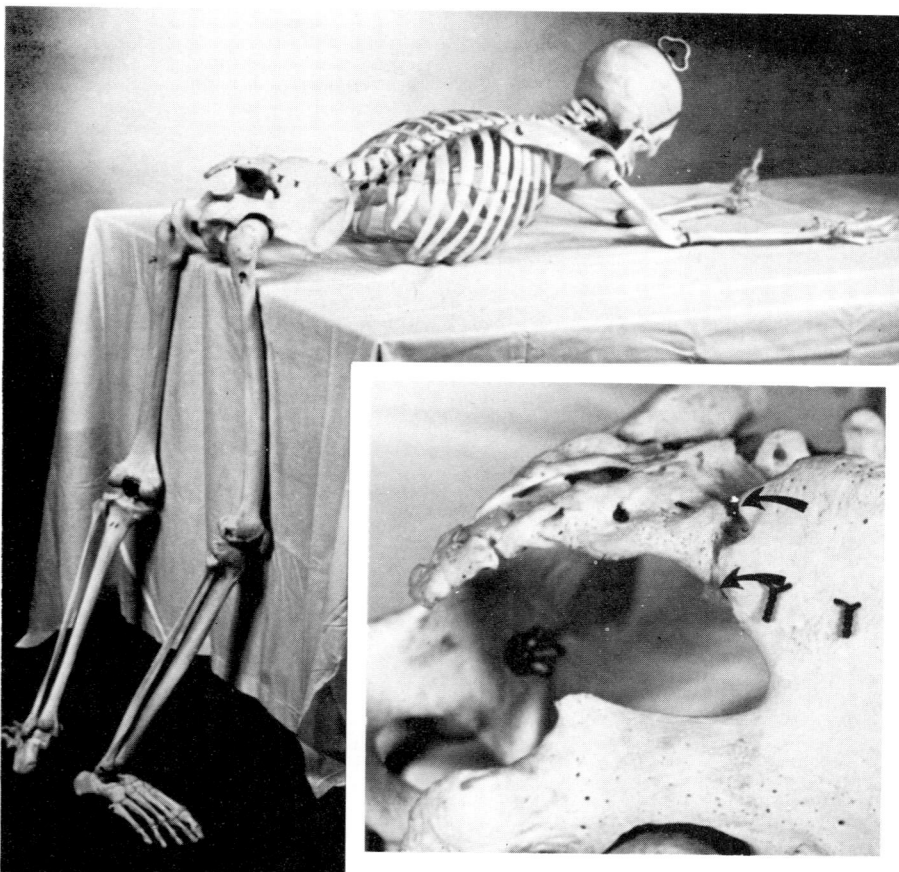

Fig. 3–1. Optimal position for examination of sacroiliac joints and lumbar spine is shown. The posterior aspect of the sacroiliac joints lies between the sciatic notch and the posterior-inferior iliac spine (insert—arrows).

MCP joint owing to erosion and rupture of its medial collateral ligament. This should be looked for with the joint flexed to 90°, which stretches the collateral ligaments to tautness. Occasionally in osteoarthritis, one knee develops a varus, and the other a valgus deformity, resulting in a "windswept" appearance and often requiring surgical correction.

Swelling. Swelling of joints, bursae, and tendons is an important sign that is always abnormal. Unlike tenderness, swelling specifically indicates organic disease. Swelling is most often due to underlying inflammation and can be due to synovial thickening, increased volume of joint fluid, or local edema. Detection of synovial thickening requires a knowledge of the anatomic synovial reflexions. Joints that lie just under the skin, such as the knee, elbow, wrist, MCP, PIP, DIP, and MTP joints, are particularly suitable. If a "pad" of thickened tissue is felt, particularly if felt in multiple areas, synovium is probably thickened owing to inflammatory proliferation, or to storage of abnormal material such as amyloid. The synovia of tendons frequently share in the proliferative process, leading to detectable swelling in the hand with bulging of palmar fat between the tendons (Fig. 3–3). Swelling of the synovium of the MTP joints leads to abnormal separation of the toes—the "window" sign (Fig. 3–4). Synovial thickening in a tendon sheath, common in Reiter's syndrome or psoriatic arthritis, produces a "sausage" finger or "sausage" toe appearance. In general, synovial swelling is most pronounced on extensor surfaces of joints where the capsule is more distensible.

Effusions are particularly common in large weight-bearing joints with distensible communicating bursae. Thus, fluid is often found in the knee, is less common in hip or ankle with their tighter joint capsules, and is much less common in upper extremity joints, where the presence of detectable fluid is related directly to joint size. Fluid is often present in rheumatoid shoulder joints, but these joints are involved in relatively few patients. The wrist has a tight capsule and fluid rarely is

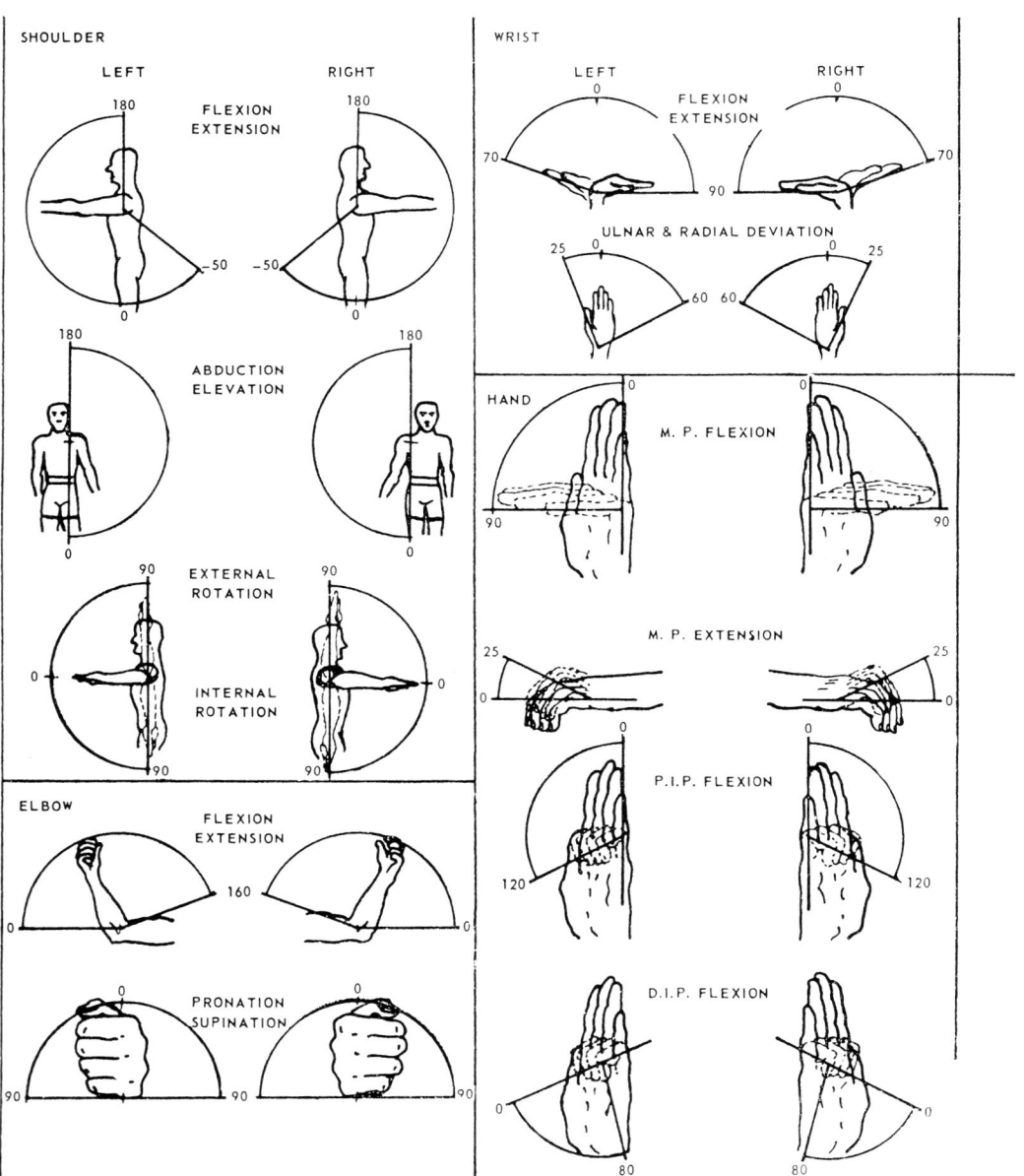

Fig. 3–2.   Normal range of motion of all joints is shown graphically. (From chart used at Children's Hospital of Buffalo.)

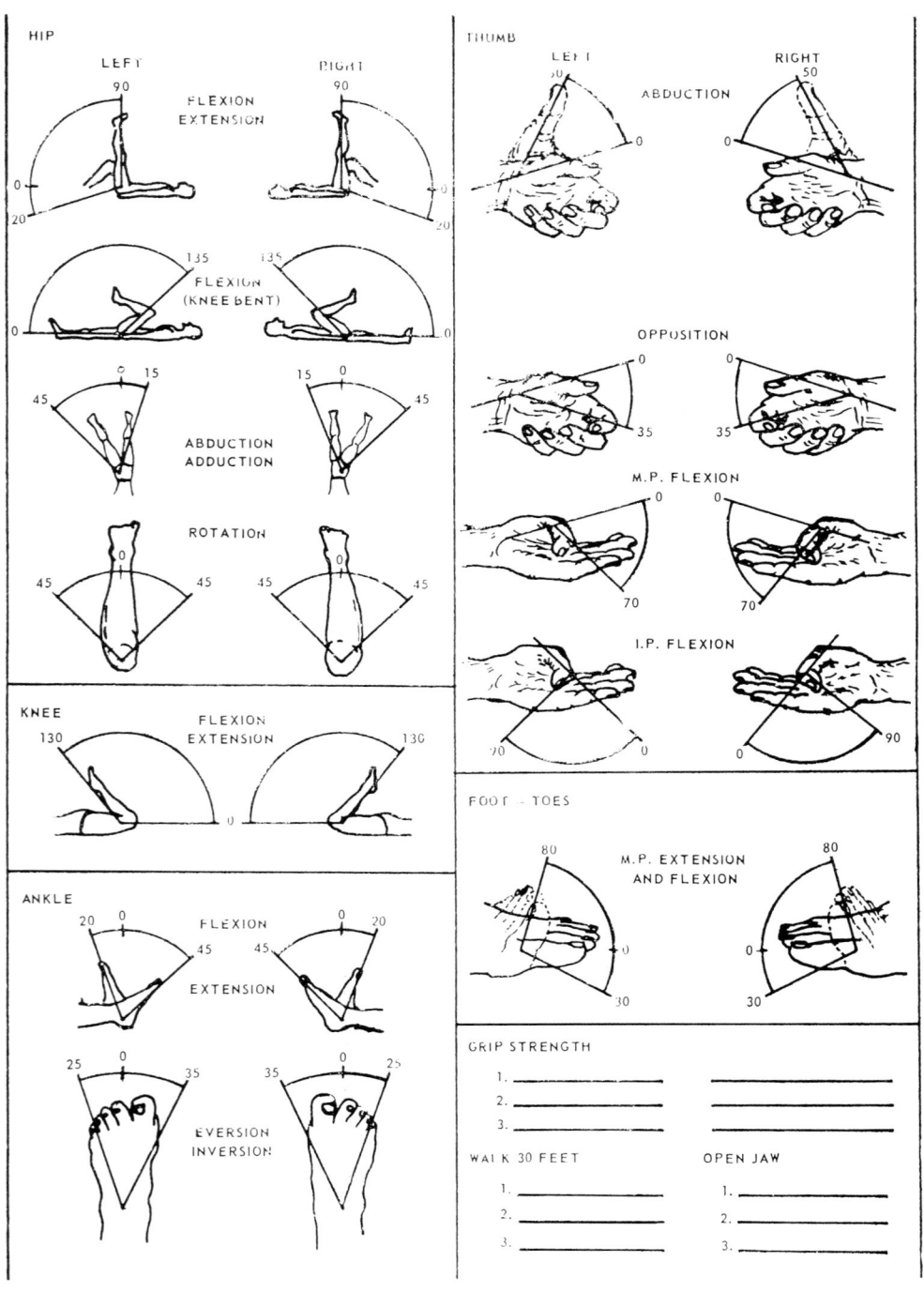

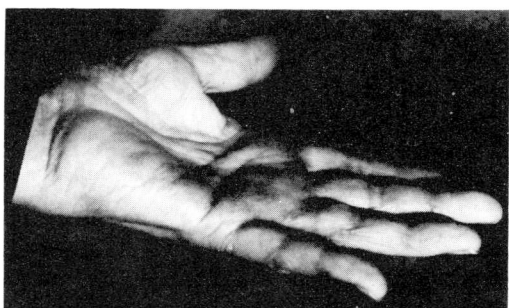

Fig. 3–3. Thickening of the synovium of the flexor digitorum tendons can be felt easily. Displaced tissues produce abnormal bulging between the tendons in the palm.

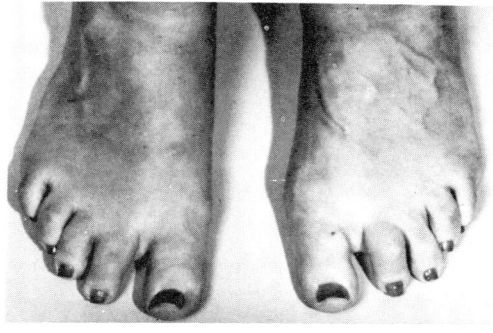

Fig. 3–4. Synovial thickening of the MTP joints spreads the forefoot, separating the toes, and producing the "window sign."

obtained unless the joint is intensely inflamed. Fluid is rarely, if ever, obtained from small hand joints. The importance of detecting fluid lies in its great diagnostic value. (See Chaps. 4 and 34 for the techniques of arthrocentesis and synovianalysis.)

Osteophytes also produce a swollen appearance and are easily palpable along the margins of joints or parts of joints that lie just under the skin, such as the MTP, knee, PIP, and DIP joints. These are hard to the touch and may be tender. They are often more striking on clinical than on radiologic examination.

Nodular swellings felt over joints or areas exposed to repeated trauma—such as the olecranon, back of the head or heel, the ischial tuberosity, the external ear, and bridge of the nose in persons wearing eyeglasses—may be due to rheumatoid nodules, gouty tophi, or (rarely) xanthomata or amyloid masses. Clinically, a nodule is only a nodule until its contents are examined microscopically. Most "nodules" over rheumatoid finger joints turn out to be synovium herniated through defects in

the joint capsule. Such herniae are usually reducible. Tendon nodules often occur in rheumatoid arthritis, systemic lupus, and rheumatic fever.

Skin Temperature. Increased warmth of skin overlying an inflamed deeper structure, sometimes accompanied by erythema in those individuals with relatively little skin pigment, is common and relatively nonspecific. Differences between the temperature of the skin over an inflamed part and the surrounding skin can be estimated to within ± 0.5° C using the *back* of the fingers. This is most helpful over large joints for obvious reasons. Unlike tenderness, which is a sensitive parameter because normal structures have none, increased warmth is inherently insensitive because normal parts are normally warm. It is more difficult to be certain of an increase of 0.5° C on a background temperature of 32° C than it is to feel secure that a PIP joint is tender when other PIP joints in the same hand are not.

Crepitus (noise). Crepitus may be heard or, more often, felt as the joints are put through a range of motion. The coarse crackle in the joints of some individuals is of no pathologic significance. This is due to tendons snapping over bony prominences or perhaps to the "cracking" phenomenon (see Chap. 9). Generally, the finer the crepitus, the more significant it is clinically. Crepitus can be felt frequently, even when no noise is heard, as a fine vibratory sensation. Crepitus can arise from the grating of roughened cartilages against one another, or from bone rubbing against bone, as in advanced osteoarthritis.

A peculiar, fine crepitus can often be felt or heard when a chronically involved rheumatoid joint is moved, especially when loaded, e.g., in knees or hips on weight-bearing. This is presumably due to friction between severely destroyed articular cartilages. It always occurs in joints showing severe generalized cartilage loss radiographically, and has been likened to the rubbing together of two sheets of old parchment. Extensive fibrin deposition in certain kinds of trauma or inflammation often gives rise to tendon crepitus. Thus, the patient with scleroderma may generate much noise while on the stairs, and the achilles tendons of the weekend golfing enthusiast may audibly rebel on Monday. Typically, the latter types of crepitus are prominent after rest and diminish with repetitive movement. They are detected easily by the first, but not the last, student to examine the patient. Some idea of the integrity of the articular cartilages can be obtained by rubbing the distal part of a joint against the firmly anchored proximal part. The patella can be rubbed up and down in its groove as the patient lies supine with the quadriceps muscle relaxed. The humeral head can be grated against the glenoid with the scapula held firmly by the examiner's other hand. The MTP, PIP, and first CMC joint surfaces can be rubbed together at the same time that stability, range of motion, and tenderness are being checked. Thus, the examiner can determine the extent of inflammation that is present and its long-term sequelae: deformity, instability, and cartilage damage.

The mechanism of knuckle cracking has been examined.[6] This phenomenon is due to mechanical subluxation of the joint, with gas formation in the joint due to the accompanying great decrease in intra-articular pressure. The subsequent vaporization of joint fluid releases enough free energy to produce an audible "crack." Once cracked, a knuckle cannot be cracked again until the gas has been absorbed and the increased space between the bone returns to normal. This takes about 30 minutes.

Weakness. Atrophy of muscle, especially the extensors, occurs rapidly about an inflamed or injured joint. Such a joint is almost always flexed to midposition, the position of maximum comfort. Muscle strength can be quantified readily by measuring grip with an appropriately rolled blood pressure cuff and by timing a repetitive action involving lower extremity muscles.[2a] It is often helpful to measure the circumference of the limb at a measured distance above or below a fixed point, such as the olecranon process or patella. Serial measurement provides a method to monitor an exercise program designed to restore missing muscle bulk (see Chap. 44).

SPECIFIC RHEUMATOLOGIC EXAMINATION

It is important that each clinician develop a standard disciplined routine examination of the musculoskeletal system just as he has for the abdominal or chest examination. The approach may differ greatly between individual physicians, but should be the same for a given clinician each time he lays hands on a patient. This routine can easily be integrated into the general examination, reference to which will be omitted for the sake of brevity in the following description. Particular attention is given to sites about which the patient specifically complains or those having abnormalities of which the patient is often unaware.

I start at the top with the temporomandibular joints, commonly involved in rheumatoid arthritis but almost never in gout. I press over the joint, which lies just below the zygomatic arch in front of the ear. The joint can also be felt by placing a finger in the external auditory canal. Ask the patient to open wide and then bite. The space between the front teeth should accommodate two to three fingers. Next the range of motion of the cervical spine is examined. Have the patient touch the chin to both shoulders (rotation). Then, with the nose kept in the midline, have him attempt to touch first one shoulder and then the other with his ear (lateral flexion). He should then place the chin to the chest, and then extend the neck as far as possible. The inion process of the occiput should come within three finger-breadths of the spinous process of C7. The usual "fibrositic" areas in the neck are pressed at the same time. Arthritic conditions generally produce limitation of rotation or lateral flexion before limitation of flexion or extension occurs. If these latter motions are disproportionately restricted, or if they are more painful than attempted lateral flexion or rotation, a lesion affecting the spinal cord itself, rather than the cervical nerve roots, should be suspected.

Next pressure is applied with the thumb over the acromioclavicular (AC) and sternoclavicular (SC) joints, which are also examined for synovial thickening. Both are commonly affected by RA, and the AC joints often develop osteoarthritic changes. The sternomanubrial cleft and the costal cartilages are next compressed, and the chest expansion measured as an index of costovertebral motion. The shoulder joints are then put through a full range of motion, always testing abduction by holding the scapula down with one hand.

The cartilages of the humeral head and glenoid are rubbed together, the fibrous capsule felt, and the supraspinatus and bicipital tendons compressed. The latter can be "twanged" like a bowstring as it lies in the bicipital groove. The extension of the elbows is next examined, and these joints are examined for synovial thickening. The olecranon and proximal ulna are palpated for bursal enlargement and for lumps that might suggest tophi, rheumatoid nodules, xanthoma, or amyloid deposits.

The wrist is put through a range of motion and examined for synovial thickening and extensor tenosynovitis or deQuervain's tenosynovitis (extensor tendons of thumb). The radiocarpal joint, the carpal joints, and the ulnar bursa (distal radioulnar joint and contiguous bursa over the distal ulna) are each pressed separately for tenderness. The integrity of the distal radioulnar joint, often eroded by RA with dorsal displacement of the ulna, is assessed. The abnormal vertical motion of the distal ulna has been likened to that of a piano key—thus the "piano key" sign. The MCP joints are pressed together laterally and then checked separately if any tenderness is elicited. Synovial thickening, range of motion, instability, and cartilage integrity are checked. Tenderness, swelling, and range of motion of all PIP and DIP joints, and of

Table 3–3. Differential Diagnosis of Inflammatory Monarthritis

A. *Crystal-induced*

  1. Gout—man, lower extremity, previous attack, nocturnal onset, precipitated by medical illness or surgical procedures, response to colchicine, hyperuricemia, sodium urate crystals in joint fluid with polymorphs predominating, and WBC 10,000 to 60,000/cmm.

  2. Pseudogout—elderly, knee or other large joint, previous attack, precipitated by medical illness or surgical procedure, flexion contractures, chondrocalcinosis on radiography, calcium pyrophosphate dihydrate crystals in joint fluid with polymorphs predominating, and WBC 5,000 to 60,000/cmm.

  3. Calcific tendonitis or equivalent—extra-articular, tendon or capsule of larger joints, previous attack same or other area, calcification on radiography, chalky or milky material aspirated from area, polymorphs with phagocytosed ovoid bodies microscopically.

B. *Palindromic rheumatism*

  Middle-aged or elderly man, very sudden onset, little systemic reaction, previous attacks, may be positive rheumatoid factors, little or no residual chronic joint inflammation, olecranon bursal enlargement.

C. *Infectious arthritis*

  1. Septic—severe inflammation, primary septic focus, drug or alcohol abuse, joint fluid with polymorphs predominating, WBC 50,000 to 300,000/cmm (pus), infectious agents identified on smear and culture, or bacterial antigens identified in joint fluid.

  2. Tubercular—primary focus elsewhere, drug or alcohol abuse, marked joint swelling for long period, joint fluid with polymorphs predominating, acid-fast organisms on smear and culture.

  3. Fungal—similar to tuberculosis.

  4. Viral—antecedent or concomitant systemic viral illness, joint fluid can be of inflammatory or noninflammatory type, either mononuclear or polymorphs may predominate.

D. *Other*

  1. Tendonitis—as in A3 but without radiologic calcification, antecedent trauma including repetitive motion.

  2. Bursitis—as above, but inflamed area is more diffuse, antecedent trauma.

  3. Juvenile rheumatoid arthritis—one or both knees swollen in pre-teen or teenager without systemic reaction, no erosions, mildly inflammatory joint fluid with some polymorphs, and no depression in synovial fluid C′H$_{50}$ levels.

the IP, MCP, and first carpometacarpal joints of the thumb are assessed. The hand is turned over and examined for palmar erythema, palmar thickening, and Dupuytren's contracture. Each tendon is compressed and felt for thickening after the finger is fully extended. The flexor carpi radialis and flexor carpi ulnaris tendons are next compressed.

The lateral motion of the spine is determined as the patient still sits. The costal cartilages are compressed and chest expansion is examined. Next, with the patient supine, each hip is flexed, abducted, and externally rotated (Patrick's maneuver). If a flexion contraction is suspected, the opposite hip is held in full flexion to flatten fully the lumbar lordosis, and the hip in question is fully extended. This maneuver prevents disguise of the flexion deformity by an increased lumbar lordosis. The hip joint is compressed from above, and then the tensor fascia lata and trochanteric bursa are compressed from the side.

The range of motion of the knee is determined. The condition of the quadriceps, presence of synovial thickening, foreign bodies, fluid, warmth, osteophytes, stability, and cartilage integrity, especially of the patellofemoral compartment, are determined. Popliteal cysts are sought, and the fat pads under the patellar tendons are compressed. The ankles and subtalar joints are examined sep-

arately, as are the posterior and anterior tibialis and peroneal tendons. Synovial thickening at the ankle is often hard to determine because there is normally some increase in the periarticular tissues here in middle age and beyond, especially in women.

The tarsal joints are compressed as a group. The MTP joints are squeezed together laterally and examined separately if any tenderness ensues. The first MTP is felt for osteophytes, range of motion, and cartilage integrity. The bunion bursa and sesamoids in the flexor hallucis tendon are examined. The latter is an extremely common site of symptomatic osteoarthritis, perhaps even more common than the patellofemoral compartment. The position of the metatarsal fat pad, nature's metatarsal support, is checked. This often slides forward under the toes in RA, leaving the swollen metatarsal heads just under the skin. The toes are next examined for ankylosis, and for "cock-up" or hammer deformities. Foot deformities such as pes cavus or pes planus are noted. The spine is examined as already described.

Each of these areas can be examined in greater detail if necessary, with abnormalities pinpointed to specific ligaments, bursae, and tendons. The interested reader is referred to the excellent monograph by Beetham and colleagues for further details on the clinical examination.[2]

Table 3–4. Differential Diagnosis of Inflammatory Polyarthritis

A. *Rheumatoid arthritis*

   1. Seropositive—woman, symmetrical joint and tendon involvement, synovial thickening, joint inflammation "in phase," nodules, weakness, systemic reaction, erosions on radiogram, rheumatoid factor present, $C'H_{50}$ level depressed in joint fluid that has 5,000 to 30,000 WBC/cmm, about 50 to 80% polymorphs. Can occur in children.

   2. Seronegative—either sex, symmetrical joint and tendon involvement, joint inflammation "in phase," little or no systemic reaction, usually no erosions radiographically, rheumatoid factor absent, $C'H_{50}$ not depressed in joint fluid that has 3,000 to 20,000 WBC/cmm, about 20 to 60% polymorphs. More asymmetrical than in seropositive cases. Some probably are adult JRA.

B. *Collagen-vascular disease*

   1. Systemic lupus—female, symmetrical joint distribution identical to RA, hair loss, mucosal lesions, rash, systemic reaction, visceral organ or brain involvement, leukopenia, positive STS, no erosions radiographically, noninflammatory joint fluid with good viscosity and mucin clot and 1,000 to 2,000 WBC/cmm, mostly small lymphocytes. Serum $C'H_{50}$ often depressed, antinuclear antibody (ANA) titer elevated, antinative human DNA antibody titer increased, anti-Sm antibody increased. Anti SSA (Ro) subset (subacute cutaneous lupus).

   2. Scleroderma—tight skin, Raynaud's, resorption of digits, dysphagia, constipation, lung, heart or kidney involvement, symmetrical tendon contractures, little or no synovial thickening, radiographic calcinosis circumscripta, positive ANA with speckled or nucleolar pattern, anti SLE_{70} (systemic) and anti-centromere antibodies (CREST syndrome).

   3. Polymyositis (dermatomyositis)—proximal muscle weakness in pelvic and pectoral girdles, tender muscles, skin changes, typical nailbed and knuckle pad erythema, symmetrical joint involvement, EMG showing combined myopathic and denervation pattern, muscle biopsy abnormal, elevated serum creatinine phosphokinase.

   4. Mixed connective tissue disease—swollen hands, Raynaud's, tight skin, symmetrical joint and tendon involvement, maybe joint erosions radiographically, positive ANA speckled pattern, anti-RNP antibody increased, good response to corticosteroid therapy in anti-inflammatory doses.

   5. Polyarteritis nodosa—symmetrical involvement, diverse clinical picture of systemic disease, histologic diagnosis.

C. *Rheumatic fever*

   Young (2 to 40 yrs), sore throat, Gp A streptococci, migratory arthritis, rash, pancarditis or pericardial involvement, elevated ASO titers, joint inflammation responds dramatically to aspirin treatment.

D. *Juvenile rheumatoid arthritis*

   Symmetrical joint involvement, rash, fever, no rheumatoid factor, radiographic periostitis, erosions late, can begin or recur in adult. ANA positive preociarticular subset may develop iridocyclitis; B27 positive boys may show bony fusion of sacroiliac and spinal joints.

E. *Psoriatic arthritis*

   Asymmetrical boggy joint and tendon swelling, skin or nail lesions may not be prominent or may follow arthritis, DIP joints may be prominently involved, radiologic periostitis or erosions, no rheumatoid factor, $C'H_{50}$ usually not depressed in inflammatory joint fluid with polymorph predominance.

F. *Reiter's syndrome*

   Male, deviant-promiscuous, urethritis, iritis, conjunctivitis, asymmetrical joints, lower extremity, nonpainful mucous membrane ulcerative lesion, balanitis circinata, keratodermia blenorrhagica, weight loss, $C'H_{50}$ increased in serum and in joint fluid with 5,000 to 30,000 leukocytes/cmm. Macrophages in joint fluid with 3 to 5 phagocytosed polymorphs ("Reiter's" cell). Can follow enteric infections or urethritis. Syndrome may be incomplete and affect females.

G. *Gonorrheal arthritis*

   Migratory arthritis or tenosynovitis finally settling in one or more joints or tendons, either sex, primary focus urethra, female GU tract, rectum or oropharynx, skin lesions, vesicles, gram-negative diplococci on smear but not on culture of vesicular fluid, positive culture at primary site, blood, or joint fluid.

H. *Polymyalgia rheumatica*

   Elderly patient (>50 yrs), symmetrical pelvic and/or pectoral girdle complaints without loss of strength, morning stiffness of long duration, fatigue prominent, weight loss, joints can be involved, especially shoulders, sternoclavicular, knees, sed rate markedly elevated, fibrinogen alpha 2 and gamma globulin elevation, anemia, complete response to low doses (10 to 20 mg) prednisone, serum CPK normal, elevated alkaline phosphatase (liver).

Table 3–4. Differential Diagnosis of Inflammatory Polyarthritis (continued)

I. *Crystal-induced*

  1. Monosodium urate (MSU) crystals: (Gout)—symmetrical arthritis, flexion contractures, prior history of acute attacks, tophi, joint inflammation out of phase, systemic corticosteroid treatment for "RA," hyperuricemia, MSU crystals in joint fluid.

  2. Calcium pyrophosphate dihydrate (CPPD) crystals: (Pseudogout)—symmetrical arthritis, flexion contractures MCP, wrist, elbow, shoulder, hips, knees, and ankles, prior acute attacks (sometimes), joint inflammation out of phase, CPPD crystals in joint fluid.

  3. Basic calcium phosphate (BCP) crystals: (Milwaukee shoulder).

J. *Other*

  Amyloid arthropathy, peripheral arthritis of inflammatory bowel disease, tuberculosis, SBE, viral arthritis.

Table 3–5. Differential Diagnosis of Inflammatory Spondyloarthropathy*

A. *Ankylosing spondylitis*—male, symmetrical sacroiliitis clinically and radiologically, limitation of spinal motion, uveitis, smooth symmetric spinal ligamentous calcification, ankylosis often complete, no skip areas, family history, HLA-B27 antigen often present, good response to phenylbutazone, indomethacin, or other NSAID.

B. *Reiter's syndrome*—promiscuous or deviant man with urethritis, skin-eye-heel, asymmetric peripheral joint involvement, sacroiliitis often asymmetrical and "skip" areas of involvement in spine, coarse asymmetrical syndesmophytes in spine, ankylosis incomplete and asymmetrical, HLA-B27 often positive, equivocal response to phenylbutazone or other NSAID.

C. *Psoriatic spondylitis*—skin and/or peripheral joints involved, asymmetric sacroiliitis, skip areas, may be ankylosing, HLA-B27 often present.

D. *Inflammatory bowel disease*—sacroiliitis, often symmetric, ankylosing, bowel disease may be silent, spinal inflammation, unlike peripheral arthritis, does not vary with and is not responsive to treatment directed at bowel inflammation, HLA-B27 often present.

E. *Other*—infection (bacterial tuberculous, fungal), osteochondritis, multiple epiphysitis in young adult.

*JRA spondyloarthropathy occurs almost entirely in HLA-B27-positive boys and is regarded as juvenile ankylosing spondylitis.

Table 3–6. Differential Diagnosis of Degenerative or Metabolic Arthropathy

A. *Primary generalized "nodal" osteoarthritis*

  Heberden's nodes DIP joints, Bouchard's nodes PIP joints, arthritis of first CMC, knee, first MTP joints, symmetric, familial, no systemic reaction, Gp 1 joint fluid.

  Variants

  1. Erosive osteoarthritis—same but with more inflammatory features. Can produce bony ankylosis.

  2. Localized osteoarthritis of DIP, first CMC, first MTP, other joints.

B. *"Non-nodal" osteoarthritis*

  1. Osteoarthritis localized to one or (usually) both knees—flexion and varus deformities in middle-aged or elderly patient, Gp 1 joint fluid, subchondral microfractures with collapse of the medial tibial plateau; medial tibiofemoral compartment predominantly involved.

  2. Primary osteoarthritis of hip—(a) unilateral—superior joint space narrowing, long leg on ipsilateral side; (b) bilateral—medial joint space narrowing with medial migration of femoral heads, equal leg lengths.

  3. Secondary osteoarthritis—any joint, due to trauma, slipped epiphysis, mechanical problem, congenital malformation, another antecedent arthritis.

  4. Osteoarthritis associated with CPPD and/or BCP crystals. Symmetric involvement, elderly patient, flexion contractures of joints listed in Table 3–4, prior acute attacks, associated metabolic diseases, familial incidence. Lateral tibiofemoral and patellofemoral compartments often predominant.

C. *Metabolic*

  Diffuse or localized musculoskeletal complaints in patient with endocrine or metabolic disease.

DATA SYNTHESIS AND DIFFERENTIAL DIAGNOSIS

The mind of the clinician stores data in much the same way as a computer. But it does more: it weights each datum and weights each datum differently in each individual. When one is writing about this process, generalizations must be made, but in full recognition of the more subtle analysis actually made in real life. The relative weights of the various signs and symptoms have been indicated in a general way in the foregoing descriptions of each.

The general category within which a patient's problem falls is usually obvious from the history and physical examination. To pinpoint the diagnosis, however, laboratory examination, including gross and microscopic joint fluid analysis as detailed in Chapter 4; radiologic work-up as described in Chapter 5 and in the various chapters dealing with specific diseases; specialized tests such as those discussed in Chapter 5; and, occasionally, biopsy for ordinary or special microscopy are indicated.

If the process is inflammatory, the diagnostic possibilities differ according to whether it is confined to one joint or is polyarticular, and whether it affects the axial (spine, shoulders, hips) or the appendicular (peripheral) joints. The differential diagnosis of some representative common inflammatory conditions is given in Table 3–3 for monarthritis, Table 3–4 for polyarthritis, Table 3–5 for inflammatory spondyloarthropathy, and Table 3–6 for degenerative arthropathy. Such brief vignettes of findings are necessarily superficial and incomplete, and are offered here with some diffidence. These may be of use to medical students and house staff in their earliest encounters with arthritic patients.

REFERENCES

1. A.R.A. Committee on Rheumatologic Practice: A description of rheumatology practice. Arthritis Rheum., 20:1278–1281, 1977.
2. Beetham, W.P., et al.: *Physical Examination of Joints,* Philadelphia, W.B. Saunders Co., 1965.
2a. Csuka, M.E., and McCarty, D.J.: A rapid method for measurement of lower extremity muscle strength. J.A.M.A. In press, 1984.
3. McCarty, D.J., Gatter, R.A., and Phelps, P.: A dolorimeter for quantification of articular tenderness. Arthritis Rheum., 8:551–559, 1965.
4. McCarty, D.J., Gatter, R.A., and Steele, A.D.: A twenty pound dolorimeter for quantification of articular tenderness. Arthritis Rheum., 11:696–698, 1968.
5. Robinson, W.D.: The etiology of rheumatoid arthritis. *In* Arthritis and Allied Conditions, 8th Ed. Edited by J.L. Hollander and D.J. McCarty. Philadelphia, Lea & Febiger, 1972, pp. 297–301.
6. Unsworth, A., Dowson, D., and Wright, V.: "Cracking joints." Ann. Rheum. Dis., 30:348–358, 1971.
7. Wright, V., and Johns, R.J.: Observations on the measurement of joint stiffness. Arthritis Rheum., 3:328–340, 1960.

Chapter 4

Synovial Fluid

Daniel J. McCarty

Paracelsus called joint fluid *synovia* (like egg).[123] "Synovial fluid" is an often used redundancy for this clear, sticky liquid that is indeed reminiscent of egg white. The reader is referred to the article by Rodnan, Benedek, and Panetta on the early history of the synovia.[123] The synovium is the tissue lining the joint space containing synovia. It terminates at the margin of the articular cartilage and is supported by the dense fibrous joint capsule, much as the pia mater and arachnoid are supported by the fibrous dura mater about the brain. It is richly supplied with both blood vessels and lymphatics. Synovia is a dialysate of blood plasma into which hyaluronate, a glycosaminoglycan of high molecular weight, is secreted by the synoviocytes (synovial lining cells). These are normally arranged in a layer only 1 to 3 cells thick, embedded in ground substance but with no basement membrane. The synovium is therefore not a true membrane, but a modified tissue space.[125]

Synovia may be obtained readily from the larger joints by needling, a procedure known as arthrocentesis, described in detail in Chapters 34 and 91.

I agree with Hollander's contention that sterile drapes and gloves are unnecessary. I have never used either in 25 years of performing arthrocentesis and have never infected a joint from the skin. The use of sterile disposable needles and syringes and thorough cleansing of the skin suffices. It is likely that some bacteria are introduced into the joint with every needle thrust through the skin. Leukocyte accumulation in canine joint fluid was greatly reduced if the skin was first cut and the needle thrust through sterile subcutaneous tissues exposed by spreading the wound.[100] Nagel and colleagues showed that a critical number of bacteria had to be inoculated before a rabbit joint could be infected experimentally.[103]

It is also impossible to thrust a needle through the vascular synovium without rupturing at least a few capillaries with subsequent micro-bleeding into the joint fluid. Thus, at least a few erythrocytes are seen in every aspirated joint fluid. Some may have entered the joint fluid by diapedesis through synovial capillaries secondary to the underlying disease, but some almost certainly are due to the needling itself. The greatest danger of joint infec-

tion from arthrocentesis lies in the inoculation of bacteria from the blood during bacteremia. I know of five examples of an arthrocentesis productive of noninflammatory sterile fluid from joints that subsequently were infected with an organism cultured from the blood at the time of the original joint aspiration.[91]

Much information about various arthritic diseases and the systemic rheumatic diseases with prominent joint involvement has been gained by gross, microscopic, and laboratory analyses of the synovia. A good deal of this information is pertinent to the contemporary practice of rheumatology and is the primary focus of this chapter. Other data, of theoretical interest only at this time, will be discussed briefly. A practical handbook of joint fluid analysis has been published recently.[40a]

Samples of the synovium may be obtained by the use of needles adapted to hollow organ biopsy, such as the Cope, or needles specifically designed for joints, such as the Parker-Pearson, the Williamson-Holt, or the Polley-Bickel. I have used all three, but the Polley-Bickel has proved most satisfactory because larger samples of tissue and a full-thickness specimen, including the articular capsule, are obtained. Synovial biopsy is of less practical value than aspiration of synovia (actually a "liquid biopsy") but is helpful in the diagnosis of the granulomatous diseases and in clinical research.

Biopsy of synovium or articular cartilage in large joints such as the knee and shoulder by direct vision through an arthroscope has been performed in many centers in recent years. Technical improvements may extend the range of this procedure to smaller joints, gradually supplanting the need for open surgical biopsy.

The structure and function of the synovium are covered in Chapters 8 and 9, and joint lubrication, including the role of the synovia, is discussed in Chapter 8.

SYNOVIANALYSIS

The term synovianalysis was coined to indicate an analogy with urinalysis.[65] Tests on synovia are at least as important in the differential diagnosis of joint disease as are those on the urine in urinary tract disease. The types of routine and special tests that may be useful are listed in Table 4–1.

Gross Analysis

The gross analysis of joint fluid is an office or bedside procedure. Its purpose is to divide a given fluid into one of five groups: normal, noninflammatory (group I of Ropes and Bauer),[125] inflammatory (group II of Ropes and Bauer), purulent, or hemorrhagic. A specific diagnosis is rarely made from gross analysis alone. Table 4–2 provides normal joint fluid values for selected items. Normal fluid is often difficult to obtain; it is scant and viscous. The normal knee joint—the body's larg-

est—contains only a few drops to a maximum of 4 ml. Although normal, postmortem, and traumatic fluids are somewhat similar, protein concentrations are sufficiently increased in the latter two that they cannot be studied as substitutes for normal fluid.[8,131] A partial list of the diseases producing fluids of the various groups is listed in Table 4–3. The noninflammatory or only mild inflammatory character of fluid from joints affected with very early rheumatoid arthritis is surprising and important.[135] Some bacterial arthritis presents group II rather than frankly purulent effusions, although I have listed them here only in the latter group. The range of values found for the various tests in each group is given in Table 4–4.

Normal fluid in increased amounts is found in the knee in myxedema, congestive heart failure, anasarca, or other conditions causing tissue edema. Fluid transudation into the joint space occurs as into any other tissue space.

Although it is often possible to obtain a large volume of joint fluid, only a few drops are needed for the most useful tests. Only one drop or less (about 0.05 ml) is needed for bacteriologic culture, for a total leukocyte count, for Wright's staining, and for a wet preparation to look for crystals and other particulates. If phase-contrast microscopy is available, the predominant type of leukocyte may be determined, their concentration and morphology estimated, and particulates studied all with one drop of fluid! Almost any joint that is severely inflamed will yield a drop of fluid after skillful puncture.

Clot Formation. Normal synovial fluid does not clot because it lacks fibrinogen as well as prothrombin, factors V and VII, tissue thromboplastin, and antithrombin.[22] Most pathologic fluids do clot, however, and the rapidity of clotting and the size of the clot are roughly proportional to the severity of inflammation present. All fluids should be transferred immediately from the syringe used for as-

Table 4–1. Synovianalysis: Types of Studies

A. *Routine*
  1. Gross analysis
    a. amount
    b. color
    c. clarity
    d. viscosity
    e. "mucin" clot
  2. Microscopic
    a. white cell concentration
    b. differential leukocyte count
    c. wet smear inspection by polarized and phase contrast microscopy
B. *Special*
  1. Microbiologic
    a. culture for bacteria, fungi, viruses, or tubercle bacilli
    b. countercurrent immunoelectrophoresis for microbial antigens
  2. Serologic
    a. hemolytic complement titration ($C'H_{50}$)
    b. complement components (C_3 and C_4) by immunodiffusion
  3. Chemical
    a. glucose
    b. protein
    c. enzymes

Table 4–2. Normal Synovial Fluid Values*

	Range	Mean	References
pH	7.3–7.43	7.38	28,46,126
WBC/cmm	13–180	63	
differential WBC (%)			
polymorphonuclear	0–25	7	
lymphocytes	0–78	24	
monocytes	0–71	48	
clasmatocytes	0–26	10	
synovial lining cells	0–12	4	
total protein g/dl	1.2–3.0	1.8	8,126,129,131,137
albumin (%)	56 –63	60	
globulin (%)	37 –44	40	
hyaluronate g/dl		0.3	53

*Values represent combined data from various reports.

Table 4–3. Examples of Diseases Producing Fluids of Different Groups

Noninflammatory (Group I)	Inflammatory† (Group II)	Purulent† (Group III)	Hemorrhagic (Group IV)
Osteoarthritis	Rheumatoid arthritis	Bacterial infections	Trauma, especially fracture
Early rheumatoid arthritis	Reiter's syndrome	Tuberculosis	Neuroarthropathy (Charcot joint)
Trauma	Crystal synovitis, acute (gout, pseudogout, other)		Blood dyscrasia (e.g., hemophilia)
Osteochondritis dissecans	Psoriatic arthritis		
Aseptic necrosis	Arthritis of inflammatory bowel disease		Tumor, especially pigmented villonodular synovitis or hemangioma
Osteochondromatosis	Viral arthritis		
Crystal synovitis; chronic or subsiding acute (gout and pseudogout)	Rheumatic fever		Chondrocalcinosis
*Systemic lupus erythematosus	Behçet's syndrome		Anticoagulant therapy
*Polyarteritis nodosa	Fat droplet synovitis		Joint prostheses
Scleroderma			Thrombocytosis
Amyloidosis (articular)			Sickle cell trait or disease
Polymyalgia rheumatica			Myeloproliferative disease
			Metal prostheses

*May occasionally be inflammatory.
†As a disease in these groups remits, the exudate (fluid) passes through a group I phase before returning to normal.

Table 4–4. Gross Analysis of Joint Fluid

Criteria	Normal	Noninflammatory (Group I)	Inflammatory (Group II)	Purulent (Group III)
1. volume (ml) (knee)	<4	often >4	often >4	often >4
2. color	clear to pale yellow	xanthochromic	xanthochromic to white	white
3. clarity	transparent	transparent	translucent to opaque	opaque
4. viscosity	very high	high	low	very low, may be high with coagulase-positive staphylococcus
5. mucin clot*	good	fair to good	fair to poor	poor
6. spontaneous clot	none	often	often	often

*Recent effusions do not give firm clot because of serum admixture.

piration into a tube containing heparin, 50 units per milliliter of joint fluids. Oxalated tubes should not be used because calcium oxalate crystals will form and, in the presence of leukocytes, will be phagocytosed, often leading to confusion.[132]

Color. Truly normal fluid is colorless, like water. It is likely that the diapedesis of red cells, accompanying even mild inflammation, and their subsequent breakdown release hemoglobin, the heme moiety of which is metabolized locally to bilirubin, giving a yellow (xanthochromic) color to the fluid. Cerebrospinal fluid becomes similarly xanthochromic after subarachnoid hemorrhage. The presence of leukocytes renders the fluid white, and the degree of whiteness is proportional to the leukocyte concentration. Pus, containing 150,000 to 300,000 leukocytes/cmm, is characteristically cream-colored, the "off-white" being due to heme pigments or to chromogen from the invading bacteria. For example, *Staphylococcus aureus* adds some golden pigment and the saprophytic *Serratia*

marcescens, a reddish hue. Gray synovial fluid containing 2,550 μg of lead/dl was obtained from a hip joint of a patient with retained bullet fragments.[122]

A grossly bloody fluid may be due to a traumatic arthrocentesis, which is usually evident during the procedure when the fluid entering the syringe may show an uneven distribution of blood. Bleeding due to trauma may decrease as aspiration continues or, more commonly, blood may appear for the first time in the syringe near the end of the procedure. A hematocrit reading should always be obtained on a truly bloody effusion to determine whether it is blood per se, or whether it is blood admixed with joint fluid. Even 5 to 10% admixture makes joint fluid look like whole blood. A truly bloody effusion, unlike that due to a "bloody tap," almost never clots.

The differential diagnosis of a bloody effusion is given in Table 4–3. If a joint swells immediately after trauma, aspiration reveals frank blood, with a hematocrit and leukocyte count approaching, or even identical to, that of whole blood from the same patient. In the absence of an underlying bleeding disorder, such as hemophilia, a fracture into the joint must be assumed to be present, and appropriate radiographic views should be obtained. Recurrent bleeding into a knee joint that appears normal on physical and radiologic examination between episodes is almost diagnostic of a hemangioma.[141]

Trauma, including neuroarthropathy, bleeding disorders, and tumors, is the most common cause of hemarthrosis, but chondrocalcinosis,[98,142] anticoagulant therapy,[74,101,152] joint prostheses,[82] thrombocytosis,[55] sickle cell trait,[18] and sickle cell disease[34a] all have been described as rarer causes. Bone marrow in joint fluid, either fat droplets or blood-forming elements, is suggestive of a fracture into the joint, although the former have been found in large number in synovial fluid leukocytes even in the absence of trauma.[49,151]

Patients with hemophilia and other coagulation defects are particularly prone to hemarthrosis (see Chap. 74), and even minor trauma may result in this condition.

Clarity. Normal joint fluids and those from joints affected with diseases that are fundamentally noninflammatory, such as osteoarthritis, are transparent. Ordinary newsprint can be read through a tube containing such fluid (Fig. 4–1A). Fluids with higher leukocyte counts from inflamed joints are opaque, and the degree of opacity is proportional to the leukocyte count.

Rarely, erythrocytes are present in sufficient number to given a cloudy, but not pink, fluid. These cells settle rapidly. Leukocytes also settle in joint fluid in vivo just as they do in a tube after aspiration.[60] Thus, both tube and joint must be inverted to mix their contents uniformly before samples are taken for counting cells. This important point has been ignored by most clinicians, and serious errors have probably occurred as a result. Fluids otherwise classified as group I may be opaque because of large numbers of monosodium urate (MSU), calcium pyrophosphate dihydrate (CPPD), or cholesterol crystals.

Viscosity. Normal and group I fluids are viscous owing to the high concentration of hyaluronate. Hyaluronate is degraded in some types of inflammatory joint disease (e.g., RA), and the viscosity is reduced appreciably. An approximation of viscosity, satisfactory for clinical purposes, can be obtained by watching the fall of a drop of fluid during transfer from aspirating syringe to glass tube. Viscous fluid "strings out" like molasses, often to a length of 10 cm or more (Fig. 4–1B). It strings out "spinbarkheit" when a drop is com-

pressed between thumb and index finger, which are then pulled apart suddenly (Fig. 4–1C). Fluids with reduced viscosity form a shorter string or even fall in discrete drops like water. More precise data can be obtained by using a viscometer[125] or by adapting an ordinary white blood cell diluting pipette,[59] but this is not necessary in everyday practice.

Mucin Clot. Although synovial fluid hyaluronic acid can be measured by several different techniques[25] the qualitative "mucin clot" test is the most practical. It estimates the degree of polymerization of hyaluronate sufficiently to classify clots as "good," "fair," or "poor." The supernatant from a centrifuged specimen is transferred to a clean glass tube. A few drops of glacial acetic acid are placed on the surface of the fluid. The heavier acid settles to the bottom of the tube, leaving a dense white precipitate of protein hyaluronate in its wake (Fig. 4–1D). This white clump remains intact even when the tube is shaken.

An alternative method of producing a mucin clot, especially useful when the amount of fluid is limited, involves the addition of one part of whole joint fluid to four parts of 2% acetic acid (usually 1 to 4 ml). "Fair" and "poor" clots are shown in Figure 4–2. Prior use of hyaluronidase prevents the formation of even a "poor" clot.

The mechanism for the failure of most fluids from inflamed joints to form good mucin clots is not well understood. The higher than normal (>2%) protein concentration in the hyaluronate, the presence in the protein-hyaluronate complex of inter-alpha trypsin inhibitor, and the lower degree of polymerization of the hyaluronate caused by its catabolism or by differences in its synthesis by the synoviocytes have all been invoked to explain it.[25]

Occasionally it is useful to reduce the viscosity of joint fluid to prepare a fluid for other tests. We have found that 1 mg (about 400 units) of testicular hyaluronidase* per milliliter of joint fluid reduces the viscosity approximately to that of serum after 30 minutes of incubation at 37°C.[52]

Analysis of Data. From the amount, color, and viscosity of the fluid and the mucin clot produced by acetic acid, a fluid can usually be classified into one of the five categories already described. No single gross measurement is of great significance or of diagnostic importance per se. Septic, normal, and hemorrhagic fluids are easily distinguished. Most confusion arises in differentiating group I from group II. We sometimes speak of "group I½." A pale yellow, clear, high viscous fluid producing a good mucin clot from a patient with sym-

---

*Worthington Biochem.

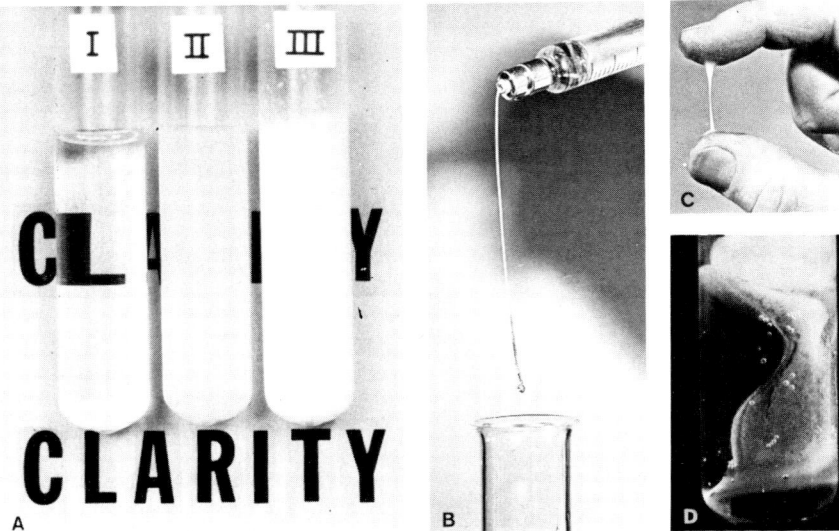

Fig. 4–1. *A,* Noninflammatory (group I), inflammatory (group II), and purulent (group III) joint fluids have been transferred to glass tubes. Group I fluids typically contain few leukocytes and are transparent, whereas fluids in groups II and III are opaque. *B,* Viscosity of a fluid can be judged by the length of "stringing" of a falling drop. This "string" is nearly 8 cm long and illustrates the relatively high viscosity of fluid from an osteoarthritic knee joint. *C,* Viscosity of joint fluid can also be tested like motor oil. The "stringing" of a drop as thumb and forefinger are separated is proportional to its viscosity. *D,* The dense white precipitate of protein hyaluronate developed after a few drops of glacial acetic acid were added to a tube containing nearly normal joint fluid. This "mucin clot" remained intact even after the tube was shaken (note bubbles), leading to its designation as "good."

metric polyarthritis is suggestive of lupus erythematosus rather than rheumatoid arthritis, for example.

Rheumatic fever is an example of a condition producing a group II fluid with good preservation of viscosity and mucin clot.[125] Group I effusions of recent onset can show reduced viscosity and mucin clot due to serum admixture. As with all tests, findings must be interpreted in light of the clinical picture.

Microscopic Synovianalysis

Microscopic synovianalysis is easily done in an office or outpatient clinic setting and requires an ordinary light microscope with oil immersion optics and a polarizing microscope equipped with a first-order red plate compensator.

Routine Cytology. A total leukocyte count is obtained on all group II or III fluids, just as for blood, except that care must be taken to thoroughly mix the contents of the tube before sampling to uniformly resuspend the cells. The cells mentioned already also sediment in vivo. This finding is particularly evident in the presence of severe inflammation when the patient is supine for an extended period because of pain. The joint contents should be mixed by barbotage before a sample is taken for analysis. Some of the unexpected divergent synovial fluid leukocyte counts that have attracted

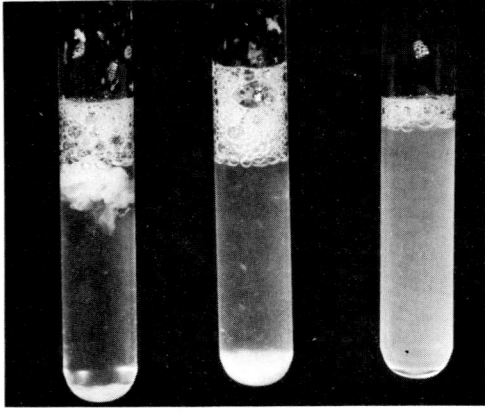

Fig. 4–2. "Mucin" clots can also be produced by adding one part of whole joint fluid to four parts of 2% acetic acid. A "fair" clot is seen on the left and a "poor" clot, composed of poorly formed shreds in a turbid solution, is in the middle. Treatment of the fluid shown in Figure 4–1D with hyaluronidase abolished mucin clot formation completely *(right).*

attention might also be due to this phenomenon.[84] Normal saline (0.9 g/dl) must be used instead of acetic acid, or the bulk of the leukocytes will be entrapped in a mini-mucin clot. Erythrocytes will be lysed preferentially if hypotonic saline (0.3 g/dl) is used as diluent. This facilitates enumeration of leukocytes, which should be done at $\times$ 400 magnification (high dry).

A thin smear for leukocyte differential counting can be prepared on either a coverslip or a glass slide. For sharp detail, as one might wish for photography, it is best to treat the fluid with hyaluronidase before making the slide. It is rarely necessary to obtain total or differential leukocyte counts on group I fluids. If these are needed, the fluid can be centrifuged and the pellet resuspended in a smaller volume before smearing. Here again, pretreatment with hyaluronidase is helpful.

A summary of the findings in normal fluids and in those of groups I, II, and III appears in Table 4–5. Although total and differential leukocyte counts are nonspecific, they are useful in differential diagnosis between groups. If a fluid is grossly opaque, yellow-white, of reduced viscosity, and gives a poor mucin clot test, generally it shows, as expected, a high total leukocyte count with polymorphonuclear cell predominance. In general, small lymphocytes, monocytes, and macrophages (or synovial lining cells) make up the remainder of the leukocytes, and some of each can be found in most joint fluids. Normal human or bovine synovial fluid contains only a few leukocytes, and polymorphonuclear cells are difficult or even impossible to find (see Table 4–2),[125,126] but normal canine fluid contains a higher leukocyte count and polymorph percentage.[100]

Occasionally, an eosinophilic predominance is found in the differential leukocyte counts.[29,58,86,102,118] The differential diagnosis of synovial fluid eosinophilia is given in Table 4–6. The association with acute or chronic urticaria is of particular interest in that Charcot-Leyden crystals have been noted,[29,102] some of which were intracellular.

Monocytosis is another peculiar and unusual finding usually occurring with acute, self-limited arthritis associated with viral disease. Chronic monocytosis has been found in a patient with ANA-negative, Ro (SSA)-positive lupus, however.[45]

Special Qualitative Cytologic Findings. Qualitatively peculiar cells that may be found in joint fluid are listed in Table 4–6. "Inclusion body cells" or "ragocytes" (raisin cells)[31] originally called "RA cells,"[64] a term implying disease specificity, which unfortunately does not exist, can be seen in many fluids of the inflammatory types (Fig. 4–3A–C). The polymorphonuclear leukocytes in rheumatoid arthritis contain much phagocytosed material, including immunoglobulins G and M,[15,111,120,149,157] rheumatoid factors,[1,111,150] fibrin,[4] antinuclear factors,[3,88] immune complexes,[54] and DNA particles.[115] The significance of these inclusions is discussed in Chapter 35. Polymorphs in inflammatory joint fluids from other diseases, however, also contain inclusion bodies with similar contents.[3,73,149,153] Inclusion bodies are best seen in a "wet" preparation of joint fluid prepared as described subsequently. They appear as vacuoles (phagosomes) by phase contrast microscopy (Fig. 4–3A,B). By ordinary light they appear as round or raisin-shaped dark granules (Fig. 4–3C), almost always located at the periphery of the phagocyte, even during locomotion (Fig. 4–4A). Such cells show vacuolization in Wright's stained smears.

Classic LE cells, usually described as an in vivo phenomenon, are seen in Wright's stained smears frequently.[66,72] These cells must be differentiated from "tart" cells, polymorphonuclear leukocytes that have phagocytosed nuclear debris. With the advent of more sophisticated immunologic tests for lupus, however, the LE cell test has become obsolete and the chance identification of LE cells in joint fluid is rarely critical or even helpful on differential diagnosis.

Dead, degranulated polymorphonuclear leukocytes may disintegrate completely or may be phagocytosed relatively intact by scavenger cells such as monocytes or macrophages. The larger macrophages can ingest 3 to 5 polymorph "cadavers" (Fig. 4–4D), whereas the smaller monocyte can never manage to ingest more than one. Macrophages with ingested polymorphs may constitute up to 2% of the entire joint fluid leukocyte population in acute Reiter's syndrome, and were originally described as the "Reiter's cell," again a misnomer implying disease specificity.[114] Such macrophages have also been described in Reiter's synovium by electron microscopy.[107] These impressive cells have been described as part of the Shwartzman reaction, a host response to bacterial

Table 4–5. Cytology of Joint Fluid

	Normal	*Gp I	Gp II	Gp III
leukocytes cmm⁻¹	<150	<3,000	3,000–50,000	50,000–300,000
polymorphonuclears (%)	<25	<25	>70	>90

*Group designations of Ropes and Bauer.[125]

Table 4–6.   Cellular Peculiarities in Synovial Fluid

I.		Quantitatively Peculiar	References
	A.	*Monocytosis*	45,148
		1. Acute, self-limited	
		Viral arthritis	
		Serum sickness	
		Idiopathic	
		2. Chronic	
		Ro (SSA) plus SLE	45
		Undifferentiated connective tissue disease	130
	B.	*Eosinophilia*	87
		1. Rheumatoid arthritis	83
		2. Rheumatic fever	83
		3. Parasitic infections	83
		4. Metastatic adenocarcinoma	83
		5. Arthropathy	83
		Air	
		Dye	58
		6. Therapeutic x-irradiation	61
		7. Urticaria	
		Acute	102
		Chronic	29,83,86
		8. Idiopathic	118
II.		*Qualitatively Peculiar*	
	A.	*Nonspecific*	
		1. Ragocytes (PMN with large peripheral granules)	1,64
		2. LE cells	66,72
		3. Reiter's cells (macrophages containing PMNs)	114
		4. Bone marrow cells	85
	B.	*Specific*	
		1. Sickled erythrocytes	18,34a
		2. Gaucher's cells	156
		3. Tumor cells	

endotoxin. Therefore, the finding in Reiter's syndrome, where an infectious etiologic trigger is often suspected,[39] is of great potential interest. Unfortunately, these cells are an inconstant feature of Reiter's syndrome, and phagocytosis of polymorphs by mononuclear cells has been found in many inflammatory joint fluids.[143] The phenomenon is particularly common in fluids from patients with juvenile rheumatoid arthritis. The finding of a single polymorph in a monocyte is common in my experience, especially in fluids from gouty joints.

Over half of all large mononuclear cells in rheumatoid synovial fluid have been found to be lymphoblasts.[147] These were almost never found in fluids from patients with septic arthritis, gout, or pseudogout. Synovial membrane type C cells[80] were identified in joint fluid by their sudanophilic property, a criterion suggesting that they are actually monocyte-derived macrophages.[147] The

lymphoblasts retained their surface markers and formed E rosettes when incubated with sheep erythrocytes (T lymphoblasts); 58 of 60 RA fluids contained these cells, suggesting disease specificity. Data showing lymphokines in rheumatoid joint fluid support this study.[79,140] Although macrophage motility inhibition factor (MIF) was detected in 16 of 22 (73%) of RA fluids, it was present also in 23% of fluids from other inflammatory arthritides and in 20% of osteoarthritis fluids. Blastogenic activity was found in 14 of 15 fluids, but in only 1 of 7 fluids from other joint diseases.[140]

Phagocytosis of hydroxyapatite crystal aggregates by polymorphonuclear leukocytes (Fig. 4–5C) has been described by wet smears, by light microscopy,[16,94] and by electron microscopy.[27,32,133] These particles, microspheroidal by scanning electron microscopy, are composed of mixtures of hydroxyapatite, largely carbonate substituted, and octacalcium phosphate or tricalcium phosphate.[99] Because these crystals are all basic calcium phosphate, the term *"BCP crystal deposition disease"* is now preferred (see Chap. 95). Cytoplasmic inclusions in joint fluid polymorphs, staining a dark purple with Wright's stain, may represent clumps of hydroxyapatite.[133] However, this finding also is nonspecific, since similar inclusions have been found in cells from effusions without demonstrable apatite crystals, and inclusions were found in only 9 of 12 fluids showing apatite crystals by electron microscopy.

Sickled erythrocytes have been found in fluid from patients with either sickle cell disease or trait.[18,34a,56] Gaucher cells and tumor cells have also been identified in synovial fluids.

There remains little doubt that platelets do gain access to joint fluid. They have been enumerated directly in RA, JRA, and OA.[34,39a,155] In studies of RA fluids, they correlated with the leukocyte count, and clumps were noted with platelets adherent to synovial fluid lymphocytes.[34] Moreover, platelet products such as beta thromboglobulin and connective tissue activity peptide III (from platelets) were detected in synovial fluids. Levels were higher in RA fluids, although polymorphonuclear leukocytes consume these proteins.

Identification of Crystals

The pathogenesis of crystal-induced inflammation is discussed in Chapter 93. Microcrystalline substances that may be found in joint fluid are listed in Table 93–1. I will focus here on the techniques useful or potentially useful in routine clinical work and in current clinical research.

"Wet Smear" Preparation. It is important that both the glass slide and coverslip are free of dust and scratches. Dust particles are positively

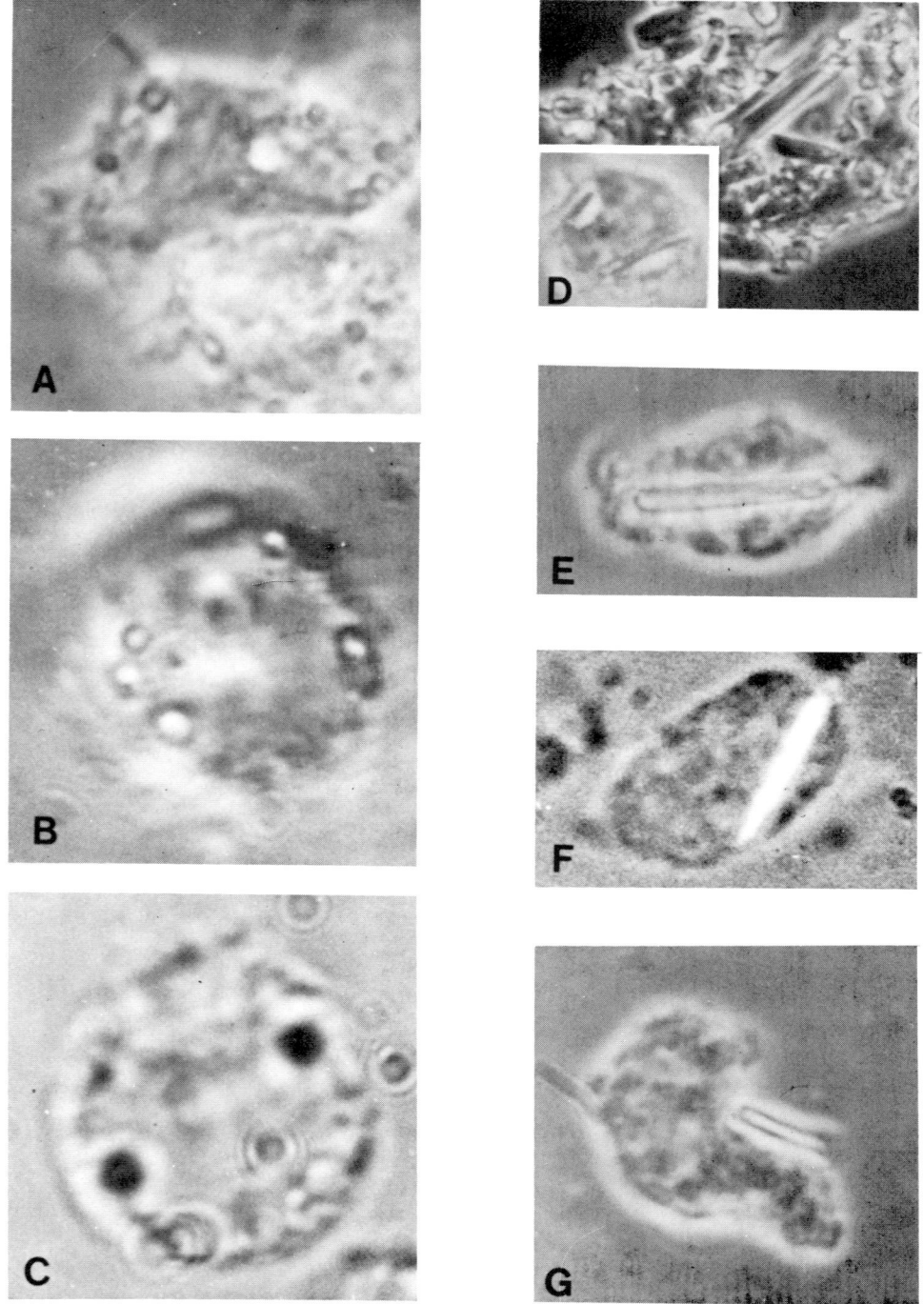

Fig. 4–3. *A*, Inclusion bodies are seen as well-defined vacuoles in a motile polymorphonuclear leukocyte (phase contrast, × 1000). *B*, The vacuoles are typically located in the periphery of the leukocyte, and often contain an eccentrically placed dark body when viewed by phase contrast microscopy under oil immersion (× 1250). *C*, By ordinary light microscopy, the inclusion bodies appear as dark, dense granules (× 1250). *D*, Crystals of triamcinolone hexacetonide, a corticosteroid ester, are similar to monosodium urate or calcium pyrophosphate crystals in size and shape (phase contrast, × 1000). These are rapidly ingested by joint fluid leukocytes and are often seen lying within phagosomes (*insert*, phase contrast, × 800, reduced by two-thirds). *E*, A large triclinic crystal of calcium pyrophosphate dihydrate within a polymorphonuclear leukocyte phagosome (phase contrast, × 1000). *F*, A phagocytosed monosodium urate crystal appears to lie free in the cytoplasm of a joint fluid polymorphonuclear leukocyte (polarized light, × 1000). *G*, A phagocyte is about to ingest a calcium pyrophosphate crystal (phase contrast, × 1000).

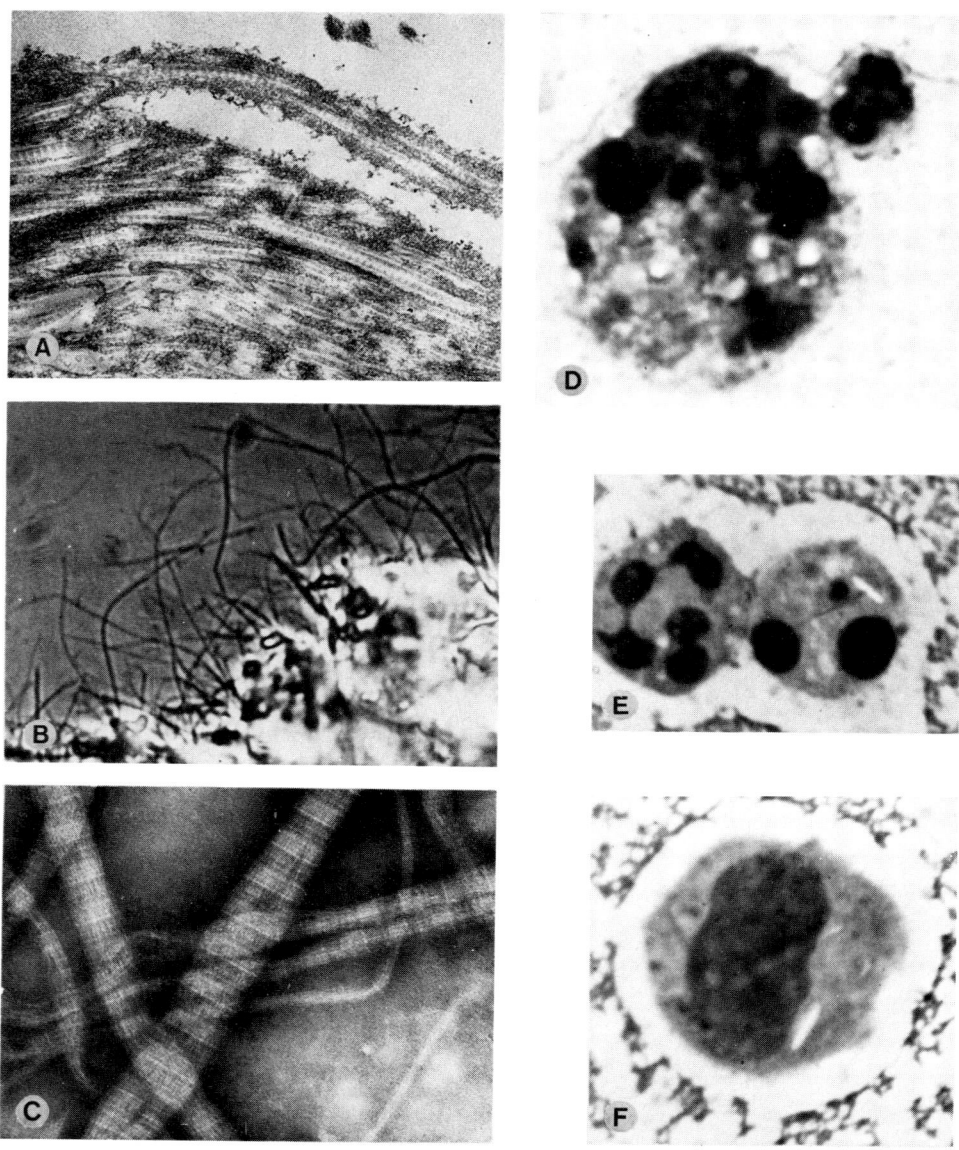

Fig. 4–4. *A,* A centrifuged pellet of fluid from an osteoarthritic knee joint showing collagen fibers (electron micrograph × 40,000). *B,* Homogenized normal cartilage produces some debris that appears fibrillar by light microscopy (phase contrast, × 1200). Other debris is birefringent and must be differentiated from microcrystals. The fibrils cannot be distinguished from fibrin by light microscopy. *C,* An electron micrograph of the fibrils shown reveals typical collagen periodicity (× 100,000). *D,* A macrophage with at least three phagocytosed polymorphonuclear leukocytes is seen in a Wright's stained smear of synovial fluid from a patient with psoriatic arthritis (× 1000 reduced by 50%). *E,* Wright's stained smear showing phagocytosed MSU crystals in a polymorphonuclear leukocyte (polarized light, × 1200). The nucleus of the cell on the right has become denser and the internuclear bridges, characteristic of the healthy polymorph, are lost. *F,* Wright's stained smear showing phagocytosis of MSU crystals by a monocyte.

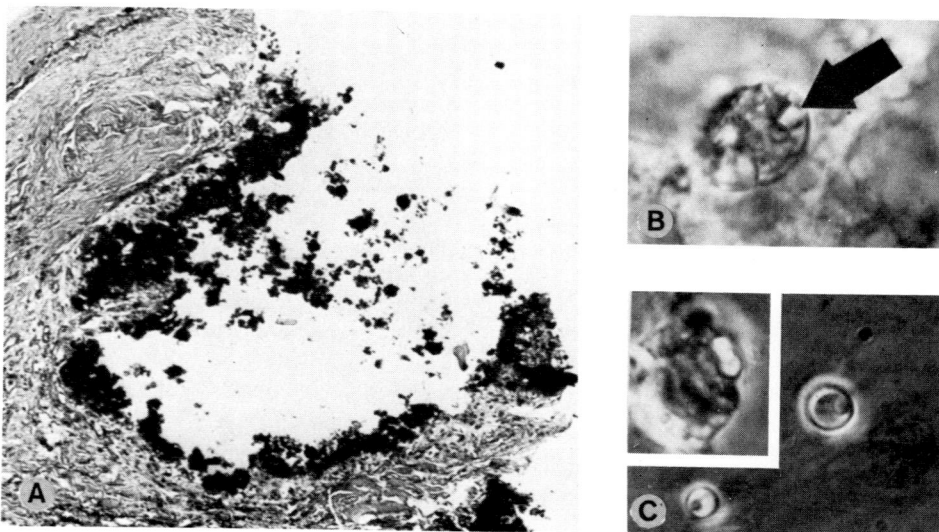

Fig. 4–5. *A,* A focus of calcification in the periarticular tissues of a knee is shown by the von Kossa's stain (× 80). The granular nature of the lesion is evident. An x-ray diffraction pattern revealed only hydroxyapatite. *B,* An inspissated chalk-like deposit removed from a shoulder joint capsule showed preservation of the sphere-like masses, some of which now contain birefringent crystals *(arrow)* (polarized light × 1250). *C,* Small spherical or disc-shaped particles containing eccentric or concentric striations were seen by phase contrast microscopy (× 1250). These were phagocytosed by polymorphonuclear leukocytes *(insert). (B* and *C* from McCarty and Gatter.[94])

birefringent. One drop (about 0.05 ml) of freshly obtained joint fluid is placed on the slide and covered with a coverslip, the edges of which are sealed immediately with clear fingernail polish. This measure retards, but does not prevent, some evaporation at the edges. Crystalline material may form at the junction of the fingernail polish and joint fluid if these touch. Such particles should be ignored. As the slides dries out, microcrystals of various types form at the edges of the fluid. These are likewise ignored. To avoid confusion, the wet preparation should be examined immediately.

Sodium heparin should be used as anticoagulant. Lithium heparin may persist in crystalline form.[144] These and calcium oxalate crystals form the use of oxalate since anticoagulant[132] can prove confounding.

Light Microscopy. Monosodium urate monohydrate (MSU) crystals are strongly birefringent and are easily seen, even by ordinary light microscopy, as needle-shaped rods.[97] MSU crystals are usually 5 to 20 µ long, but crystals as short as 1 to 2 µ may be the only ones found, especially in persistent asymptomatic effusions after an acute attack. Some patients form only small crystals, and with every acute attack, only these are found. It is important to examine a wet smear as soon as possible after aspiration, using oil immersion and, preferably, compensated polarized light microscopy. In acute gout, many intraleukocytic crystals

are found (Fig. 4–3F). They are often present for many weeks after all clinical signs of inflammation have subsided.

Fluid obtained from a hyperuricemic patient and stored in a refrigerator for some hours after aspiration may show crystals when none were present initially.[11] Such crystals are unusually long and appear to nucleate and grow in or around leukocytes. Fifty consecutive joint fluids from patients with a variety of diseases refrigerated for 24 hours failed to show crystals if none were present originally in the fresh fluid.[7] This phenomenon is rare, inconstant and, although not now interpretable, does not justify the diagnosis of gout.

MSU crystals and acute inflammation have been described in the absence of leukocytes[109] and inflammatory joint fluids have been seen from putative gout in the absence of MSU crystals.[134] In the former instance, a focus of polymorph accumulation might occur in a contiguous synovial or extrasynovial compartment, and the latter phenomenon may represent a "sympathetic" effusion in a joint near another compartment where crystal-induced inflammation is occurring. The settling phenomenon already discussed could account for some of these cases. Moreover, small MSU and CPPD crystals have been found only by electron microscopy in several instances.[9,67] The light microscopy examination also cannot definitely exclude the presence of crystals in joint fluid. Alternatively, the clinical inflammation is due to causes other than gout. In my own experience over a 25-year period, I rarely have been perplexed by either phenomenon. Repeated clinical examination during several days, as inflammation subsides and becomes more easily localized, has invariably disclosed the primary focus of inflammation.

Specific identification of MSU crystals is easiest with a quality polarizing microscope. Every arthritis center should invest in one. Some have advocated adapting an ordinary microscope with polarizing filters and a makeshift compensator using cellophane tape on a glass slide.[37,110] Although this may be better than no polarized light at all, the results using this technique or even an inexpensive polarizing microscope are inferior.

The depth of field with polarized light optics is remarkably flat, tending to minimize cellular detail, so that nonrefractile crystals and intracellular details are difficult to see. The addition of phase contrast is therefore helpful. We routinely use a polarizing microscope equipped with a rotating stage; a built-in polarizer, analyzer, and first-order red plate compensator; a phase-contrast condenser, and $\times$ 10, $\times$ 40, and $\times$ 100 phase objectives; and a $\times$ 10 or $\times$ 12.5 eyepiece.

First the wet preparation is scanned under the $\times$ 10 objective to localize suspicious objects. These objects are then observed by the use of the oil immersion objective ($\times$ 100).

The morphology of a putative microcrystal is noted, as is whether it is birefringent. The strength and sign of birefringence and the extinction angle are then noted. Thus, four different descriptive items are obtained for an observed crystal. Birefringence is a property of many substances that are ordered in three dimensions. Not all birefringent objects are truly crystalline, e.g., house dust, collagen, and pieces of cartilage. Not all crystals are birefringent, e.g., in NaCl or table salt, a cuboidal crystal, the velocity of light passing through the crystal is identical in all directions. Thus, birefringence is caused by an observable difference in the velocity of light passing through an ordered structure in different directions, analogous to the velocity of an axe being driven into a log in different directions with the same applied force. In most logs, the velocity of the axe is greatest when its blade is parallel to the grain and slowest when it is across the grain. The blade penetrates deeper in the first instance. If the difference in the depth of penetration is great, the log is said to be "grainy." If the light is passing through a "grainy" crystal, strong birefringence is seen, whereas a "nongrainy" crystal may appear weakly birefringent or even nonbirefringent (isotropic).

Another variable is the mass of ordered material being examined. That is, the amount of light being slowed up must be sufficient to be appreciated visually. If a grainy log is thin, the axe might penetrate it completely no matter what the direction of the blow, and no difference in penetrability is noted. Thus, a thin crystal or a small collagen mass may appear nonrefractile by polarized light, whereas a larger mass of the same substance shows birefringence.

MSU crystals show strong birefringence, which disappears when their long axis is parallel to that of the crossed polarizer or analyzer (Figs. 4–6A, 4–8). This is called the position of extinction and is analogous to the axe striking the log obliquely, at a 45-degree angle to the cross grain, from either side. The difference in depth of penetration is now zero. MSU crystals extinguish when their long axis is parallel to the axis of the polarizer or analyzer; this is called parallel or axial extinction. Calcium pyrophosphate dihydrate (CPPD) crystals that show any birefringence extinguish when their long axis is oblique to the axis of the polarizer or analyzer; this is called oblique or inclined extinction (Fig. 4–6B). The angle between the axis of the polarizer or analyzer and the extinct crystal is called the extinction angle; in the case of CPPD crystals, this angle is between 20 and 30 degrees.

The findings by plane-polarized light are augmented by the use of a first-order red quartz retardation plate, or "compensator." This plate slows the red component of white light by one-quarter wavelength so that the background now appears red rather than black. Now a MSU crystal appears red in the four positions of extinction shown in Figure 4–6A, and, instead of the four positions of brightness where it appeared white, it shows its optical sign of birefringence. Thus, when its long axis is perpendicular to the direction of slow vibration of the light in the compensator, it appears blue, and when its long axis is parallel to this direction, it appears yellow (Fig. 4–7A). Red is called the "sensitive tint," since it is relatively easy to shift from it to a slower (blue) or faster (yellow) wavelength of the visible spectrum, as shown in Figure 4–7B. Thus, first-order yellow and second-order blue are equidistant from first-order red. MSU crystals in blue or yellow positions of brightness or in positions of extinction are shown in Figure 4–8A.

The sign of birefringence is a characteristic of biaxial crystals like MSU and CPPD. Such crystals have two optic axes (biaxial), which means that two directions permit light to pass through the lattice without being refracted at all. Our hypothetical axe would pass through the log from one end to the other without meeting any resistance at all in two directions.

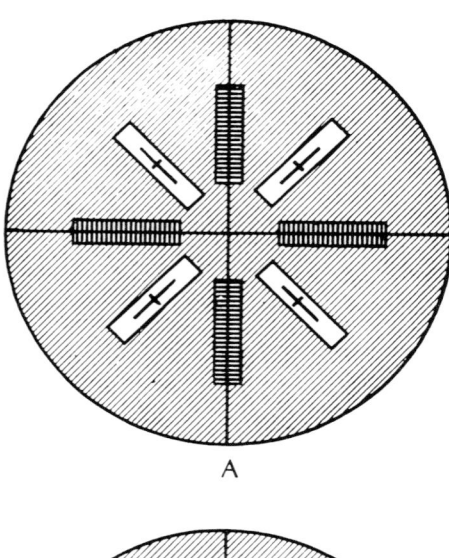

A

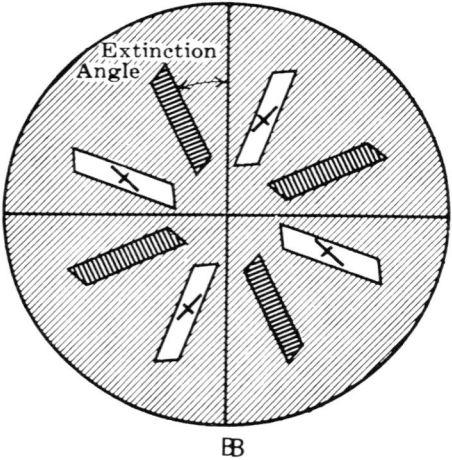

BB

Fig. 4–6. *A,* The typical properties under plane-polarized light of the strongly birefringent MSU crystal are illustrated *(top).* The crystal becomes nonrefractile when its long axis lies parallel to that of the polarizer or analyzer—the position of extinction. It is maximally bright when its long axis is in a position 45° oblique to these axes—the position of maximal brightness. This property is called axial or parallel extinction. *B,* The typical properties under plane-polarized light of the weakly birefringent CPPD crystal are illustrated *(bottom).* Here extinction occurs when the long axis of the crystal is at an oblique angle to the axis of the polarizer or analyzer. This is called oblique or inclined extinction.

The slow and fast rays of biaxial crystals bisect the angles formed by the optic axes. A crystal is optically (+) if its slow ray bisects the acute angles and optically (−) if its fast ray bisects the acute angles (Fig. 4–7C). As the fast ray of MSU crystals bisects the angle acutely in the morphologically long dimension of the crystal, it adds velocity to the light coming from the compensator and shifts

the color to a higher wavelength—second-order blue (Fig. 4–7B). In crystallographic jargon, this phenomenon is known as (−) elongation. MSU crystals are thus analogous to a "grainy" log. When the morphologically long axis of CPPD crystal is at right angles to the direction of slow vibration of light in the compensator, its slow wave bisects the acute optic axis angle, slowing the velocity of the light even further and shifting the light to first-order yellow (Fig. 4–7B). CPPD crystals are like a log, the modest grain of which lies at right angles to its long dimension.

Fiechtner and Simkin have described "sphereurates" in gouty synovial fluid[40] (Fig. 4–8B). In a few instances these were the only MSU crystalline phase present.

The use of a high-quality polarizing light microscope with a compensator provides multiple parameters, morphology, strength of birefringence, the optical sign of birefringence (elongation), and the extinction angle. Excellent descriptions of this method have been published since compensated polarized light microscopy was first used to characterize MSU[97] and CPPD[98] microcrystals, and should be consulted for further details.[40a,41,42]

Other Methods. X-ray diffraction "powder patterns" were used initially to classify pathologic calcifications in the 1960s.[43,76] Satisfactory patterns were obtained on as little as 50 μg of crystals (see Chap. 94). Specific digestion with uricase was used initially to substantiate the identity of MSU crystals,[97] but this is not necessary in routine work. The initial identification of both CPPD and dicalcium phosphate dehydrate (DCPD) was accomplished by infrared spectroscopy of crystals compressed into a sodium bromide disc.[76,95] This is a good method for identifying phosphate groups. The calcium moiety was identified in both crystals by routine chemical methods after crystal dissolution.

BCP but not CPPD or MSU crystals bind (^{14}C) diphosphonate (EHDP), and this has proved useful as a rapid, semiquantitative screening test.[52] Alizarin red staining, also used for this purpose,[113] is more sensitive but less specific. We examine the pellets of fluids that bind (^{14}C) EHDP by scanning electron microscopy (SEM).[51] Others have used rapid transmission electron microscopy (TEM), which is more sensitive and provides better definition of crystal morphology and location, e.g., intra-vs.-extracellular.[19] Particulates found can be characterized further by x-ray energy dispersive analysis.[51]

Fourier transform infrared (FTIR) spectrophotometry has been used to characterize calcium phosphate crystal aggregates.[99] These contained particulate collagen, hydroxyapatite partially substituted with carbonate and either octacalcium phosphate (OCP) or tricalcium phosphate (TCP). Chapter 95 provides more detail relative to identification of calcium-containing crystals.

Dicalcium Phosphate Dihydrate (DCPD). These orthophosphate crystals, a dimorph of brushite ($CaHPO_4 \cdot 2H_2O$), were initially identified in cadaver cartilage[92,95] by infrared spectroscopy and x-ray diffraction. They show strong (+) birefringence. They are more soluble than are CPPD crystals—K_{sp}, about 10^{-7} vs. 10^{-15}. They have been identified in articular cartilage in a patient with a destructive arthropathy.[44] Identification was made by scanning electron microscopy (see Fig. 95–3a) and by x-ray diffraction.

Basic Calcium Phosphate (BCP) Crystals. These crystals have been listed previously. The individual crystals are too small to be seen by optical microscopy. The largest are only 1 μm in one largest dimension. By TEM they appear as needles or plates. They are invariably aggregated and by phase contrast appear as ''shiny coins'' as shown in Figure 4–5B, or as microspheroidal ''snowballs'' by SEM as shown in Figure 95–3a. Particulate collagens are a constant feature of these fluids.[51,99]

Other Crystals. These crystals are listed in Table 4–7. Cholesterol crystals, usually occurring as flat rhomboid plates with notched corners, have been described in joint fluids, in inflammatory and degenerative types of joint disease, usually in longstanding effusions.[35,38,105,108,156] These crystals are usually large, often more than 100 μ in greatest dimension. They are thin plates and, although strongly birefringent, the mass refracting light in a single crystal may be insufficient to demonstrate this. When stacked like poker chips, however, their strong birefringence is evident.

Needle-shaped cholesterol crystals, as well as rhomboid plates, have been described in both joint fluid and pericardial fluid.[35,38,108] Both forms gave an identical x-ray diffraction powder pattern that resembled that of anhydrous cholesterol rather than cholesterol monohydrate.[108] Such cholesterol crystals were not pure, but contained small to moderate amounts of cholesterol ester, triglyceride, phospholipids, and small quantities of protein. These components absorbed to pure cholesterol crystals when these were added to the supernatant effusion fluid. Conversion of rhomboid cholesterol crystals to needle-shaped crystals occurred with time. These needles were large and negatively birefringent. They were readily soluble in ether, which distinguished them immediately from the smaller MSU. Small cholesterol (5- to 10-μm) crystals have been described in osteoarthritic joint fluids.[38] More importantly, cholesterol crystals are never phagocytosed. They may be sufficiently numerous to render an effusion milky, but they have no known pathogenetic or phlogistic role.

Calcium oxalate crystals form readily if joint fluid is placed in an oxalated tube. Such crystals are cuboidal or rhomboid, about 2 to 10 μ across, and are phagocytosed by viable polymorphs in the joint fluid.[132] They have been found in patients on maintenance dialysis who have hyperoxalemia.[63]

Crystals of corticosteroid esters are prepared as an injectable suspension by the drug companies by the grinding of larger crystals in a colloid mill and are often irregular in size and shape as a result. They are brightly birefringent. Most preparations are optically (+), but some are (−). They are usually 1 to 20 μ long and are avidly phagocytosed by joint fluid leukocytes.[96] They may be present in joint fluid for as long as one month after injection.[75] Storage, different crystal lots, and amount of shaking before injection may alter crystal appearance.[75]

Lithium, but not sodium, heparin anticoagulant has been reported to produce crystals in joint fluid resembling CPPD.[144] Such crystals are 2 to 5 μ long with varied shape. Calcium phosphorus mineral can precipitate from joint fluids exposed to air since the pH rises to ~8 coincident with CO_2 loss.[52] As mentioned already, birefringent fat droplets resembling a Maltese cross have been seen both free and phagocytosed, usually but not always associated with trauma.[49,50,130,151]

Aluminum phosphates have been found in French patients with renal disease who were taking aluminum-containing gels to control blood phosphorus.[104]

Fig. 4–7. *A,* The plane of slow vibration of light in the compensator is indicated here by the wedge in the diagram, inserted at a 45° angle to the crossed polarizer and analyzer. A single MSU crystal rotated under the objective now appears maximally blue (B) when its long axis is perpendicular to the plane of slow vibration of light in the compensator, and maximally yellow (Y) when it is parallel. The position of extinction (E) occurs when it lies parallel to the plane of the polarizer or analyzer. (From McCarty, D.J.[98]) *B,* First and second orders of colors produced from polarized white light are shown. (From Gatter, R.A.[42]) *C,* Optical sign determination in biaxial crystals; a crystal is (+) when the slow ray from the compensator bisects the optic axes acutely and (−) when the fast ray from the compensator bisects the optic axes acutely. (From Gatter, R.A.[42])

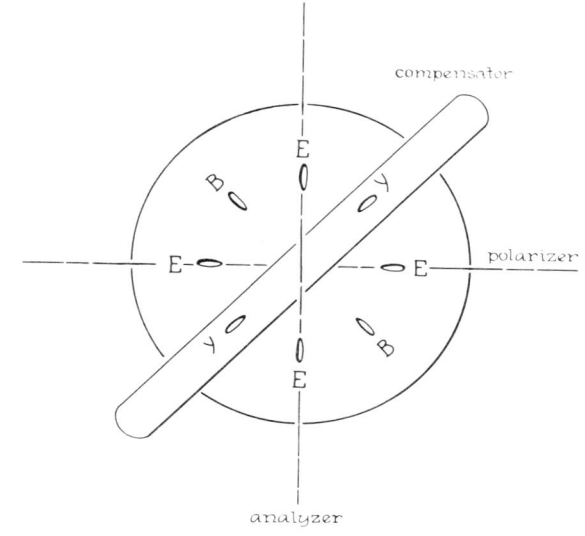

A

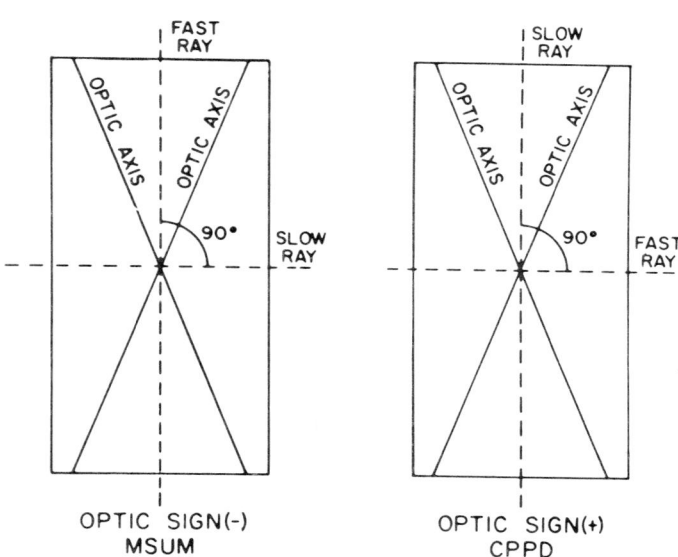

B

C

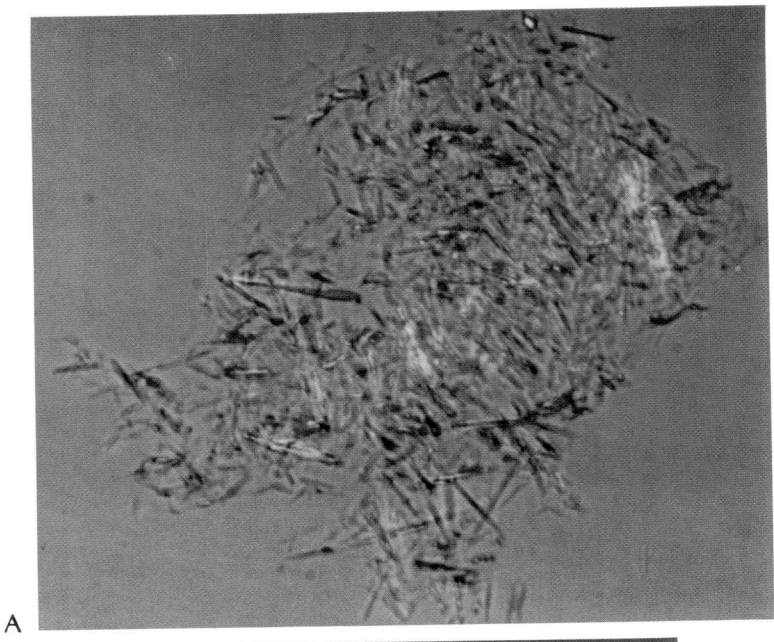

A

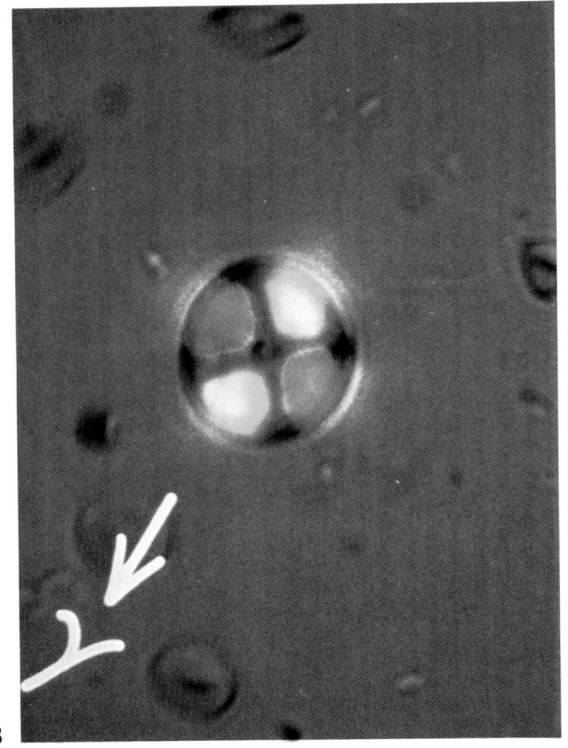

B

Fig. 4–8. *A*, MSU crystals in a drop of joint fluid from an 80-year-old dentist with chronic tophaceous gout. Viewed by compensated polarized light microscopy ($\times$ 500). *B*, Negatively birefringent spherulite in synovial fluid of a patient with gouty arthritis. These spherulites may be (rarely) present as the only MSU crystalline phase or may be accompanied by the typical needle-shaped crystals ($\times$ 1000). (From Fiechtner, J.J., and Simkin, P.A.[40])

Table 4–7. Particulate Matter of Synovial Fluid

I. Crystals
   A. Monosodium urate monohydrate (MSU)
      1. Ultramicroscopic
      2. Spherulites
   B. Calcium pyrophosphate dehydrate (CPPD)
      1. Ultramicroscopic
   C. Basic calcium phosphate (BCP)
      1. Carbonate-substituted hydroxyapatite (HA)
      2. Octacalcium phosphate (OCP)
      3. Tricalcium phosphate (TCP) (Whitlockite)
   D. Dicalcium phosphate dehydrate (DCPD) (Brushite)
   E. Calcium oxalate
   F. Cholesterol
   G. Lipid
   H. Aluminum phosphate
   I. Charcot-Leyden
   J. Artifactual—corticosteroid esters, lithium heparin, MSU, DCPD, calcium oxalate
II. Other Particulates
   A. Collagens
   B. "Wear" particles
      1. Cartilage fragments
      2. Prosthesis fragments
   C. "Rice" bodies (collagens types I, III, and V, enriched with fibrin)
   D. Fibrin
   E. Amyloid

Metal fragments have been described in joint fluid from a joint that had had a metal prosthesis inserted.[82]

Amyloid fragments have been identified in synovial fluid by polarized light microscopic examination of pellets stained with Congo red.[47]

Cartilage Fragments. Normal articular cartilage ground in a tissue homogenizer showed many nonbirefringent fibrils by ordinary light or phase contrast microscopy (Fig. 4–4B), and also birefringent chunks of cartilage.[81] The fibrils showed the typical periodicity of collagen by electron microscopy (Fig. 4–4C). Similar fibrils were seen in joint fluid pellets by both light and electron microscopy (Fig. 4–4A), and these same pellets contained hydroxyproline.[81] Collagen is a highly ordered molecule and is birefringent if enough is present to refract sufficient light. Collagen in parallel array with the highly ordered glycosaminoglycans arranged neatly between fibers is strongly (+) birefringent. Small birefringent, irregular-shaped particles are seen frequently in joint fluid and are thought to represent pieces of articular cartilage. Such fragments have been well characterized by histochemical methods in synovium, where they were thought to have become embedded after desquamation.[70]

Particulate collagens have been further identified by type.[21] Types I and III, characteristic of synovial membrane, are found in patients with RA, whereas fluids from patients with osteoarthritis contain type II, the predominant type in hyaline articular cartilage.

Wear particles have been characterized ferrographically.[36] In addition to the potential diagnostic importance of this technique, the wear particles themselves are capable of provoking collagenase and prostaglandin release from synovial cells. An excellent correlation was found between the number and microscopic features of cartilage fragments obtained by filtering synovial lavage fluid and arthroscopic appearance of the cartilaginous surface.[68] Both of these techniques have great potential for diagnosis and prognosis of selected types of arthritis.

Rice Bodies. Bits of tissue resembling polished white rice are seen in many fluids from the affected joints of patients with rheumatoid arthritis, systemic lupus, or septic arthritis. Some of these contain a core of collagen with a mantle of fibrin, whereas others contain only fibrin.[119] On analysis, it is clear that the collagen is types I, III, and V in a proportion (40-40-20) identical to that of synovial membrane.[20] Whether these rice bodies represent infarcted ischemic synovium[93] or newly synthesized collagen by synovial cells that become entwined in the particulate fibrin[119] is unclear.

Clinical Laboratory Studies

Proteins. The total protein of normal synovial fluid averages about 1.8 g/dl (see Table 4–2). In general, the smaller protein molecules such as albumin are present in greater concentration than larger molecules such as the globulins. As discussed fully in Chapter 9, the entry and egress of small molecules are explained by diffusion between synovial lining cells, whereas the factor limiting protein entry is probably the number and size of the fenestrations in subsynovial capillaries. Thus, with diseases producing inflammation and increased synovial blood flow, protein entry may often increase out of proportion to the entry of small molecules. Therefore, virtually all protein molecules found in plasma enter the joint and with increasing inflammation their concentration in synovia approaches the concentration of the patient's plasma. Protein egress from both normal and diseased joints is probably through lymphatic drainage, and there is nearly a 1:1 ratio between lymphatics and capillaries in normal synovium.

That molecular size is not the only factor limiting protein entry into normal joints is obvious from the virtual absence of prothrombin (MW 63,000)[22] and the low levels of haptoglobin (MW 85,000)[106] and fibrinogen.

Total Hemolytic Complement ($C'H_{50}$). The measurement of $C'H_{50}$, which measures the functional activity of all complement component proteins in synovial fluid, is sometimes helpful diagnostically. Normal synovial fluids show, as expected, low levels of $C'H_{50}$. Whether this is due to low levels of all or selected components is not known. In diseased synovia, the $C'H_{50}$ level is proportional to the total protein in the same fluid and to serum $C'H_{50}$, unless there is local consumption due to the nature of the inflammatory process.[22,62,77,89] Generally, synovial $C'H_{50}$ is one-third to one-half that of the patient's serum in the absence of local consumption. Table 4–8 summarizes the reported data. Thus, the serum $C'H_{50}$ is often low in systemic lupus and high in Reiter's syndrome, psoriatic arthritis, and gonococcal arthritis and correspondingly low or high in fluids obtained from joints affected with these diseases; this simply reflects the serum levels.

Marked depression of joint fluid complement occurs most predictably in seropositive rheumatoid arthritis, when sepsis and the crystal deposition diseases are excluded. Exclusion is relatively easy in both instances by the specific features of these conditions, i.e., crystals or bacteria. The depression of $C'H_{50}$ in joint fluid is a reflection of the local Arthus-like immune complex disease that is an integral feature of RA (see Chap. 35). C3 levels corrected for synovial fluid globulin levels can be substituted for $C'H_{50}$ and protein levels.[57] Activation of C3 and factor B was found in synovial fluids

from a variety of inflammatory types of arthritis but not osteoarthritis.[71] There was a correlation between the amount of conversion and the synovial fluid polymorphonuclear leukocyte count.

Other Serologic Tests. Rheumatoid factors have been measured in synovial fluid.[10,124] In most instances, their titer is identical to or slightly lower than that in the patient's serum. In a few instances they were found in the fluid and not in the serum or vice versa. Anti-gamma globulins are also found in joint fluids from other inflammatory types of arthritis and from osteoarthritic joints.[111,112] IgG and IgM rheumatoid factor titers are higher in RA fluids,[111] and their specificity is broader in RA.[112] Measurement of rheumatoid factors in synovial fluid leukocytes has been discussed in connection with inclusion bodies. Assays for rheumatoid factors in either cells or synovia have not been shown to be helpful, for either diagnosis or prognosis.

Both antinuclear antibodies[3,88] and DNA[2,69,86] have been found in synovial fluid, but no disease specificity has been found for either. The significance, if any, of antinuclear antibodies in synovia is obscure. DNA may be derived nonspecifically from the breakdown of cells during the inflammatory process.

Cryoproteins have been found in both rheumatoid and nonrheumatoid fluids.[26,89] These occurred in virtually all RA fluids and contained mixed immunoglobulins and bound complement, DNA, and rheumatoid factors. Those in non-RA fluids contained mostly fibrinogen and did not fix comple-

Table 4–8. Synovial Fluid Hemolytic Complement Levels

Disease	Serum $C'H_{50}$†	Synovial Fluid $C'H_{50}$
Rheumatoid arthritis		
seropositive*[62,116,127]	N or I	N or D (usually)
seronegative[78]	N or I	N
Juvenile RA*		N
seronegative[62,78,90]	N or I	
Systemic lupus[78,117,136,145]	N or D (usually)	N
erythematosus		
Crystal deposition disease[78,145,146]	N or I	N or D (rarely)
(gout and pseudogout)		
Reiter's syndrome[116]	N or I (usually)	N
Ankylosing spondylitis[17]	N or I	N
Psoriatic arthritis[146]	N or I	N
Septic arthritis[146]	N or I (usually)	N or D
Other diffuse connective tissue diseases		
Drug LE[145]	N	inadequate data
polyarteritis[154]	N, I, or D	inadequate data
scleroderma[145,154]	N	inadequate data
polymyositis[154]	N	inadequate data
Mixed cryoglobulinemia[121]	D	inadequate data

N = normal; I = increased; D = decreased. (N, I, or D in synovial fluid is given with respect to that predicted from serum $C'H_{50}$ and joint fluid protein.)

*Seropositive children show findings as in adult seropositive RA.

†May be decreased with systemic vasculitis, so-called hypocomplementemic RA.

ment. Fibrin and fibronectin are present in synovial fluid in both soluble and precipitated form, although levels of the latter are normal in the serum.[24]

Chemistry. Protein levels in synovia have been discussed in connection with complement proteins. In general, with increased intensity of inflammation, various proteins in synovia increase toward plasma levels. Lysosomal enzymes and other leukocyte-derived proteins, such as the antimicrobial substance lactoferrin,[5,6,30] also increase the degree of inflammation. Since lysozyme in synovia is derived from both cartilage and leukocyte lysosomes, and lactoferrin is derived from leukocyte lysosomes only, estimation of both substances simultaneously in joint fluid, with consideration of their ratio, has been advocated as diagnostically helpful in assessing the degree both of inflammation and of cartilaginous degradation.[6]

The presence of fibrin strands was alluded to in the discussion of particulate matter in synovia. Fibrin degradation products of high molecular weight, often in aggregates, quite different from those found in blood due to plasmin digestion of fibrin, have been found in inflammatory synovial fluids.[4,48] Antiplasmins were presumed to be responsible for this phenomenon. Even osteoarthritic fluids contained small amounts of these peculiar fibrin degradation products. Fibrin is chemotactic and is phagocytosed by synovial fluid leukocytes. It comprises the bulk of the ''rice body.''

Enzymes. Many studies have been performed on various enzymes in joint fluid.[25] None seems useful as a practical diagnostic tool, with the possible exception of the lysozyme-lactoferrin ratio already discussed.

Small Molecules. The synovial transport of small molecules is discussed in Chapter 9. Most small molecules diffuse into synovia from the blood; some (such as lactate, CO_2, and inorganic pyrophosphate) are produced by joint tissues and may achieve higher concentrations in synovia as compared to plasma. These molecules are discussed in Chapters 9 and 94, respectively. Antimicrobial molecules also diffuse into synovia readily, even in infected joints (see Chap. 99).

Glucose. This vital molecule enters the synovia from plasma by facilitated diffusion, and its measurement in both compartments is sometimes diagnostically helpful. True glucose (Somogyi-Nelson), not total reducing substances, must be measured. The patient must be fasting to permit measurement of a stable serum level and the attainment of equilibrium between it and the joint fluid.[125] Tense effusions may give falsely low joint fluid levels.[125] Table 4–9 summarizes the data of Cohen et al. relative to mean glucose serum-synovia differences in various joint diseases.[25] Differ-

ences greater than 40 mg/dl were seen regularly only in cases of bacterial or tubercular infection, but overlap in values between septic and nonseptic inflammatory conditions often occurred,[25,125] which limits the absolute reliability of this test.

Lipids. Normal fluid contains little lipid despite the large amount of fat in normal synovium. With inflammation, the content of lipid in synovia increases; cholesterol, phospholipids, neutral fat, and triglycerides all rise.[13,23,105,139] Cholesterol concentration may be high and, as outlined previously, cholesterol crystals may be found. Lipids of synovia may be synthesized by joint tissues[105] or may derive from the lipid-rich membrane constituents of inflammatory cells. No specific diagnostic inflammation can be obtained from lipid analysis of synovia.

In conclusion, the examination of synovia has provided an excellent rapid adjunct to the clinical examination in the differential diagnosis of arthritis. Culture for microbes and identification of crystals and other particulates provide specific clues, whereas gross parameters of analysis and selected laboratory procedures, such as total and differential leukocyte counts, total protein and hemolytic complement assay, and serum-synovial fluid differential glucose concentrations, provide ancillary data. It can be predicted that future studies of joint fluid will yield additional information of both practical and theoretic importance in the rheumatic diseases.

Microbiologic Study. Like serum, joint fluid is an excellent culture medium. Unlike serum, however, which promotes neutrophilic killing of bacteria, it inhibits the in vitro killing of *Staphylococci aureus*, the most common pathogen isolated from joints other than gonococcus, by neutrophils.[138] This effect was thought to be due to interference by osteoarthritis synovial fluid with the serum factors that promote intracellular killing. Moreover, neutrophils from rheumatoid arthritis joint fluid are relatively effete.[12] Considering the ability of the synovium to trap circulating organisms, as discussed further in Chapter 99, and the frequency of bacteremia, it is surprising a priori that septic arthritis is not more common than it is. Considering the aforementioned factors, it is easy to understand the increased incidence of joint sepsis in the presence of preexisting joint disease and in patients whose defenses are compromised by drugs or systemic diseases such as cancer or cirrhosis.

Infection must be ruled out whenever joint inflammation accompanies a septic process elsewhere in a patient (e.g., heart valve, pneumonia, urinary tract, or skin). A joint fluid leukocyte count greater than 50,000/cmm should heighten the suspicion of infection. Arthrocentesis is again indispensable, with the caveat that infectious organisms

Table 4–9.   Serum-Synovial Fluid Glucose Differences in Joint Diseases

Disease	N	OA,Tr	LE	RF	Reiter's	Gout	RA	Tb	Bact
mean Δ glucose (mg/dl)	0	5	22	6	9	11	30	70	91
number of fluids	29	79	16	12	16	86	80	27	21

From data of Cohen et al.[25]
N = normal; OA = osteoarthritis; Tr = trauma; LE = lupus erythematosus; RF = rheumatic fever; RA = rheumatoid arthritis; Tb = tuberculosis; Bact = bacterial arthritis.

may be introduced into the joint from the infected blood owing to the bleeding that almost invariably accompanies this procedure. The unsolved problem is how to make a rapid diagnosis. Antimicrobials are usually given empirically while the results of culture are awaited. Several new techniques for rapid microbiologic diagnosis have been advocated. These techniques have been reviewed elsewhere.[128]

Pneumococcal antigen has been detected in synovial fluid by counter-immunoelectrophoresis[33] and staphylococcal products by enzyme-linked immunoabsorbent (ELISA) assay in unpublished reports. Further systemic study of these promising techniques is needed.

Even more promising is the use of gas-liquid chromatographic (GLC) analysis of synovial fluid.[14] Lactic acid levels have been helpful in detecting infection, but only when above 250 mg/dl and when no antimicrobials were given previously. Succinic acid, however, separated all septic fluids due to gram-positive or gram-negative bacteria, including *N. gonorrhoeae,* in patients not given antibiotics, from fluids obtained from joints with sterile inflammatory types of arthritis. Only 5 of 39 of the latter group had detectable succinic acid levels by GLC analysis. Moreover, succinic acid was detected in joint fluids in all eight instances where antibiotics had already been given. The combination of WBC count >50,000, synovial fluid glucose <40 mg/dl, and succinic acid was nearly 100% accurate in diagnosing septic arthritis.

REFERENCES

1. Astorga, G., and Bollet, A.J.: Diagnostic specificity and possible pathogenetic significance of inclusions in synovial leukocytes. Arthritis Rheum., 8:511–523, 1965.
2. Barnett, E.V.: Detection of nuclear antigens (DNA) in normal and pathologic human fluids by quantitative complement fixation. Arthritis Rheum., 11:407–417, 1968.
3. Barnett, E.V., Bienenstock, J., and Bloch, K.J.: Antinuclear factors in synovia. J.A.M.A., 198:143–150, 1966.
4. Barnhardt, M.I., et al.: Fibrin promotion and lysis in arthritis joints. Ann. Rheum. Dis., 26:206–218, 1967.
5. Bennett, R.M., Eddie-Quartey, A.C., and Holt, P.J.L.: Lactoferrin—an iron binding protein in synovial fluid. Arthritis Rheum., 16:186–190, 1973.
6. Bennett, R.M., and Skosey, J.L.: Lactoferrin and lysozyme levels in synovial fluid. Arthritis Rheum., 20:84–90, 1977.
7. Bible, M.W., and Pinals, R.S.: Late precipitation of monosodium urate crystals. J. Rheumatol., 9:480, 1982.
8. Binette, J.P., and Schmid, K.: The proteins of synovial fluid: A study of the α1/α2 globulin ratio. Arthritis Rheum., 8:14–28, 1965.
9. Bjelle, A., Crocker, P., and Willoughby, D.: Ultramicrocrystals in pyrophosphate arthropathy. Acta. Med. Scand., 207:89–92, 1980.
10. Bland, J.H., and Clark, L.: Rheumatoid factors in serum and joint fluid. Ann. Intern. Med., 58:829–836, 1963.
11. Bluhm, G.B., Riddle, J.M., and Barnhardt, M.I.: Crystal dynamics in gout and pseudogout. Med. Times, 97:135–144, 1969.
12. Bodel, P.T., and Hollingsworth, J.W.: Comparative morphology, respiration and phagocytic function of leukocytes from blood and joint fluid in rheumatoid arthritis. J. Clin. Invest., 45:580–589, 1966.
13. Bole, G.G.: Synovial fluid lipids in normal individuals and patients with rheumatoid arthritis. Arthritis Rheum., 5:589–601, 1962.
14. Borenstein, D.G., Gibbs, C.A., and Jacobs, R.P.: Gas liquid chromatographic analysis of synovial fluid. Succinic acid and lactic acid as markers for septic arthritis. Arthritis Rheum., 25:947–953, 1982.
15. Brandt, K., Cathcart, E.S., and Cohen, A.J.: Studies of immune deposits in synovial membranes and corresponding synovial fluids. J. Lab. Clin. Med., 72:631–647, 1968.
16. Brandt, K.D., and Krey, P.R.: Chalky joint effusion. Arthritis Rheum., 20:792–796, 1977.
17. Calabro, J.J., Katz, R.M., and Maltz, B.A.: Ankylosing spondylitis. J. Pediatr., 75:912–913, 1969.
18. Casey, D.J., and Cathcart, E.S.: Hemarthrosis and sickle cell trait. Arthritis Rheum., 13:882–886, 1970.
19. Cherian, P.V., and Schumacher, H.R.: Diagnostic potential of rapid electron microscopic analysis of joint effusions. Arthritis Rheum., 25:98–100, 1982.
20. Cheung, H.S., et al.: Synovial origins of rice bodies in joint fluid. Arthritis Rheum., 23:72–76, 1980.
21. Cheung, H.S., et al.: Identification of collagen subtypes in synovial fluid from arthritis patients. Am. J. Med., 68:73–79, 1980.
22. Cho, N.H., and Neuhaus, O.W.: Absence of blood clotting substances from synovial fluid. Thrombosis et Diathesis Haemorrhagica, 5:108–111, 1960.
23. Chung, A.C., Shanahan, J.R., and Brown, E.M.: Synovial fluid lipids in rheumatoid and osteoarthritis. Arthritis Rheum., 5:176–183, 1962.
24. Clemmersen, I., Holund, B., and Andersen, R.B.: Fibrin and fibronectin in rheumatoid synovial membrane and rheumatoid synovial fluid. Arthritis Rheum., 26:479–485, 1983.
25. Cohen, A.S., Brandt, K.D., and Krey, P.R.: *In* Laboratory Diagnostic Procedures in Rheumatic Disease, 2nd Ed. Edited by A. Cohen. Boston, Little, Brown and Co., 1975.
26. Cracchiolo, A., Goldberg, L.S., and Barnett, A.V.: Studies of cryoprecipitate from synovial fluid of rheumatoid patients. Immunology, 20:1067–1077, 1971.
27. Crocker, P.R., et al.: The identification of particulate matter in biological tissues and fluids. J. Pathol., 121:37–40, 1977.
28. Cummings, N.A., and Nordby, G.L.: Measurement of synovial fluid pH in normal and arthritic knees. Arthritis Rheum., 9:47–56, 1966.
29. Dougados, M., et al.: Charcot-Leyden crystals in synovial fluid. Arthritis Rheum., 26:1416, 1983.
30. Decoteau, E.: Lactoferrin in synovial fluid of patients with

inflammatory arthritis. Arthritis Rheum., *15*:324–325, 1972.
31. Delbarre, F., Kahan, A., and Amor, B.: Le ragocyte synovial. Press Med., *72*:2129–2132, 1964.
32. Dieppe, P.A., et al.: Apatite deposition disease. Lancet, *1*:266–270, 1976.
33. Dorff, G.J., Ziolkowski, J.S., and Rytel, M.W.: Detection by counter immunoelectrophoresis of pneumococcal antigen in synovial fluid from septic arthritis. Arthritis Rheum., *18*:613–615, 1975.
34. Endresen, G.K.M.: Investigation of blood platelets in synovial fluid from patients with rheumatoid arthritis. Scand. J. Rheumatol., *10*:204–208, 1981.
34a.Espinoza, L.K., Spilberg, I., and Osterland, C.K.: Joint manifestations of sickle cell disease. Medicine, *53*:295–305, 1974.
35. Ettlinger, R.E., and Hunder, G.C.: Synovial effusions containing cholesterol crystals. Mayo Clin. Proc., *54*:366–374, 1979.
36. Evans, C.H., Mears, D.C., and McKnight, J.: A preliminary ferrographic survey of the wear particles in human synovial fluid. Arthritis Rheum., *24*:912–918, 1981.
37. Fagan, T.J., and Lidksy, M.D.: Compensated polarized light microscopy using cellophane adhesive tape. Arthritis Rheum., *17*:256–262, 1974.
38. Fam, A.G., et al.: Cholesterol crystals in osteoarthritis joint effusions. J. Rheumatol., *8*:273–280, 1981.
39. Farel, D.K., et al.: The specificity of synovial mononuclear cell response to microbiological antigens in Reiter's syndrome. J. Rheumatol., *9*:561–567, 1982.
39a.Farr, M., et al.: Platelets in the synovial fluid of patients with rheumatoid arthritis. Rheum. Internat., *4*:13–18, 1984.
40. Fiechtner, J.J., and Simkin, P.A.: Urate spherulites in gouty synovia. J.A.M.A., *245*:1533–1536, 1981.
40a.Gatter, R.A.: A Practical Handbook of Joint Fluid Analysis. Philadelphia, Lea & Febiger, 1984.
41. Gatter, R.A.: Use of the compensated polarizing microscope. Clin. Rheum. Dis., *3*:91–103, 1977.
42. Gatter, R.A.: The compensated polarized light microscope in clinical rheumatology. Arthritis Rheum., *17*:253–255, 1974.
43. Gatter, R.A., and McCarty, D.J.: Pathological tissue calcifications in man. Arch. Pathol., *84*:346–353, 1967.
44. Gaucher, A., et al.: Identification des Cristaux observes dans les arthropathies destructrices de la chondrocalcinosis. Rev. Rhum., *44*:407–414, 1977.
45. George, D., et al.: Chronic monocyte arthritis. Arthritis Rheum., *26*:674–677, 1983.
46. Goldie, I., and Nachmenson, A.: Synovial pH in rheumatoid knee joints. Acta Orthop. Scand., *40*:634–641, 1969.
47. Gordon, D.A., Pruzanski, W., and Ogryzlo, M.A.: Synovial fluid examination for the diagnosis of amyloidosis. Ann. Rheum. Dis., *32*:428–430, 1973.
48. Gormsen, J., Andersen, R.B., and Feddersen, C.: Fibrinogen-fibrin breakdown products in pathologic synovial fluids. Arthritis Rheum., *14*:503–512, 1971.
49. Graham, J., and Goldman, J.H.: Fat droplets and synovial fluid leukocytes in traumatic arthritis. Arthritis Rheum., *21*:76–80, 1978.
50. Gregg, J.R., Nixon, J.E., and Distefona, V.: Neutral fat globules in traumatized knees. Clin. Orthop., *132*:219–224, 1978.
51. Halverson, P.B., et al.: "Milwaukee shoulder": Association of microspheroids containing hydroxyapatite crystals, active collagenase and neutral protease with rotator cuff defects. II. Synovial fluid studies. Arthritis Rheum., *24*:474–483, 1981.
52. Halverson, P.B., and McCarty, D.J.: Identification of hydroxyapatite crystals in synovial fluid. Arthritis Rheum., *22*:389–395, 1979.
53. Hamerman, D., and Schuster, H.: Hyaluronate in normal human synovial fluid. J. Clin. Invest., *37*:57–64, 1958.
54. Hannestadt, K.: Rheumatoid factors reacting with autologous native G-globulin and joint fluids G aggregates. Clin. Exp. Immunol., *3*:671–690, 1968.
55. Harris, B.K., and Ross, H.A.: Hemarthrosis as the pre-

senting manifestation of myeloproliferative disease. Arthritis Rheum., *17*:969–970, 1974.
56. Hasselbacher, P.: Sickled erythrocytes in synovial fluid. Arthritis Rheum., *23*:127–128, 1980.
57. Hasselbacher, P.: Immunoelectrophoretic assay for synovial fluid C3 with correction for synovial fluid globulin. Arthritis Rheum., *22*:243–250, 1979.
58. Hasselbacher, P.: Synovial fluid eosinophilia following arthropathy. J. Rheumatol., *5*:173–176, 1978.
59. Hasselbacher, P.: Measuring synovial fluid viscosity with a white blood cell diluting pipette. Arthritis Rheum., *19*:1358–1362, 1976.
60. Hasselbacher, P., Passero, F.C., and Ludvico, C.L.: Sedimentation of leukocytes within the joint space. Pa. Med., *81*:54–55, 1978.
61. Hasselbacher, P., and Schumacher, H.R.: Bilateral protrusia acetabuli following pelvic irradiation. J. Rheumatol., *4*:189–196, 1977.
62. Hedberg, H.: The depressed synovial complement activity in adult and juvenile rheumatoid arthritis. Acta Rheum. Scand., *10*:109–127, 1964.
63. Hoffman, G.S., et al.: Calcium oxalate microcrystalline-associated arthritis in end stage renal disease. Ann. Intern. Med., *97*:36–42, 1982.
64. Hollander, J.L., et al.: Studies on the pathogenesis of rheumatoid joint inflammation. I. The "RA Cell" and a working hypothesis. Ann. Intern. Med., *62*:271–280, 1965.
65. Hollander, J.L., Jessar, R.A., and McCarty, D.J.: Synovianalysis. Bull. Rheum. Dis., *12*:263–264, 1961.
66. Hollander, J.L., Reginato, A., and Torralba, T.P.: Examination of synovial fluid as a diagnostic aid in arthritis. Med. Clin. North Am., *50*:1281–1293, 1966.
67. Honig, S., et al.: Crystal deposition disease. Am. J. Med., *63*:161–164, 1979.
68. Hotchkiss, R.N., Tew, W.P., and Hungerford, D.S.: Cartilaginous debris in the injured human knee. Clin. Orthop., *168*:144–156, 1982.
69. Hughes, G.R.V., et al.: The release of DNA into serum and synovial fluid. Arthritis Rheum., *14*:259–266, 1971.
70. Hulten, O., and Gillerstedt, N.: Uber abnutzungsproduke in Gelenken und thu resorption unter dem bilde synovits detritca. Acta Chir. Scand., *84*:1–29, 1940.
71. Hunder, G.C., McDuffie, F.C., and Mullen, B.J.: Activation of complement components C2 and B in synovial fluids. J. Lab. Clin. Med., *89*:161–171, 1977.
72. Hunder, G.C., and Pierre, R.V.: In vivo LE cell formation in synovial fluid. Arthritis Rheum., *13*:448–454, 1970.
73. Huttl, S.: Synovial effusion. A nosographic and diagnostic study. Part I. Acta Pistiniana 5, 1970.
74. Jaffer, A.M., and Schmid, F.R.: Hemarthrosis associated with sodium warfarin. J. Rheumatol., *4*:215–217, 1977.
75. Kahn, C.B., Hollander, J.L., and Schumacher, H.R.: Corticosteroid crystals in synovial fluid. J.A.M.A., *211*:807–809, 1970.
76. Kohn, N.N.: The significance of calcium phosphate crystals in the synovial fluid of arthritis patients: The "pseudogout syndrome." II. Identification of crystals. Ann. Intern. Med., *56*:738–745, 1962.
77. Kim, H.J., et al.: Clinical significance of synovial fluid total hemolytic complement activity. J. Rheumatol., *7*:143–152, 1980.
78. Kim, F.C., and Cohen, A.S.: Synovial fluid fatty acid composition in patients with rheumatoid arthritis, gout, and degenerative joint disease. Proc. Soc. Exp. Biol. Med., *123*:77–80, 1966.
79. Kinsella, T.D.: Transformation of human lymphocytes in vitro by autologous and allogenic rheumatoid synovial fluid. Ann. Rheum. Dis., *35*:8–13, 1976.
80. Kinsella, T.D., Baum, J., and Ziff, M.: Studies of isolated synovial lining cells of rheumatoid and non-rheumatoid synovial membranes. Arthritis Rheum., *13*:734–753, 1970.
81. Kitridou, R., et al.: Identification of collagen in synovial fluid. Arthritis Rheum., *12*:580–588, 1969.
82. Kitridou, R.C., et al.: Recurrent hemarthrosis after prosthetic knee arthroplasty: Identification of metal particles

in the synovial fluid. Arthritis Rheum., *12*:520–528, 1969.

83. Klofkorn, R.W., and Lehman, T.J.: Eosinophilia synovial effusions complicating chronic urticaria and angio edema. Arthritis Rheum., 25:708–709, 1982.

84. Krey, P.R., and Bailen, D.A.: Synovial fluid leukocytosis: A study of extremes. Am. J. Med., 67:436–442, 1979.

85. Lawrence, C., and Seefe, B.: Bone marrow in joint fluid: A clue to fracture. Ann. Intern. Med., 74:740–742, 1971.

86. Leon, S.A., et al.: DNA in synovial fluid and the circulation of patients with arthritis. Arthritis Rheum., 24:1142–1150, 1981.

87. Lugar, M.J., and Friedman, B.M.: Acute synovial fluid eosinophilia. J. Rheumatol., 9:961–962, 1982.

88. MacSween, R.N., Dolakos, G., and Jasani, M.K.: A clinico-immunologic study of serum and synovial fluid antinuclear factors in rheumatoid arthritis and arthritides. Clin. Exp. Immunol., 3:17–24, 1968.

89. Marcus, R.L., and Townes, A.S.: The occurrence of cryoproteins in synovial fluid; the association of a complement-fixing activity in rheumatoid synovial fluid with cold precipitable protein. J. Clin. Invest., 50:282–293, 1971.

90. Matsura, M., Ruddy, S., and Stillman, J.S.: Proceedings of the International Symposium on Rheumatoid Arthritis. Edited by W. Mullen. New York, Academic Press, 1972.

91. McCarty, D.J.: A basic guide to arthrocentesis. Hospital Med., 4:77–97, 1968.

92. McCarty, D.J., et al.: Studies on pathological calcifications in human cartilage. I. Prevalence and types of crystal deposits in the menisci of two hundred fifteen cadavera. J. Bone Joint Surg., 48:309–325, 1966.

93. McCarty, D.J., and Cheung, H.S.: Origin and significance of rice bodies in synovial fluid. Lancet, 2:715–716, 1982.

94. McCarty, D.J., and Gatter, R.A.: Recurrent acute inflammation associated with focal apatite deposition. Arthritis Rheum., 9:804–819, 1966.

95. McCarty, D.J., and Gatter, R.A.: Identification of calcium hydrogen phosphate dihydrate crystals in human fibrocartilage. Nature, 201:391–392, 1963.

96. McCarty, D.J., and Hogan, J.M.: Inflammatory reaction after intrasynovial injection of microcrystalline adrenocorticosteroid esters. Arthritis Rheum., 7:359–367, 1964.

97. McCarty, D.J., and Hollander, J.L.: Identification of urate crystals in gouty synovial fluid. Ann. Intern. Med., 54:452–460, 1961.

98. McCarty, D.J., Kohn, N.N., and Faires, J.S.: The significance of calcium phosphate crystals in the synovial fluid of arthritis patients: The "pseudogout syndrome." I. Clinical aspects. Ann Intern. Med., 56:711–737, 1962.

99. McCarty, D.J., Lehr, J.R., and Halverson, P.B.: Crystal populations in human synovial fluid. Identification of apatite, octacalcium phosphate and beta tricalcium phosphate. Arthritis Rheum., 26:1220–1224, 1983.

100. McCarty, D.J., Phelps, P., and Pyenson, P.: Crystal induced inflammation in canine joints. I. An experimental model with quantification of the host response. J. Exp. Med., 124:99–114, 1966.

101. McLaughlin, G.E., McCarty, D.J., and Seagal, B.L.: Hemarthrosis complicating anticoagulant therapy. Report of three cases. J.A.M.A., 196:1020–1021, 1966.

102. Menard, H.A., et al.: Charcot-Leyden crystals in synovial fluid (letter). Arthritis Rheum., 24:1591–1593, 1981.

103. Nagel, D.A., Albright, J.A., and Hollingsworth, J.W.: Studies on the pathophysiology and some host defense factors in staphylococcal arthritis in the rabbit and on the relationship of aseptic inflammation to infection rate. Yale J. Biol. Med., 39:119–128, 1966.

104. Netter, et al.: Inflammatory effect of aluminum phosphate. Ann. Rheum. Dis., 42:114, 1983.

105. Newcombe, D.S., and Cohen, A.S.: Chylous synovial effusion in rheumatoid arthritis. Am. J. Med., 38:156–163, 1965.

106. Niedermeier, W., Creitz, E.E., and Holley, H.L.: Trace metal composition of synovial fluid from patients with rheumatoid arthritis. Arthritis Rheum., 5:439–444, 1962.

107. Norton, W.L., Lewis, D., and Ziff, M.: Light and electron

microscopic observations on the synovitis of Reiter's disease. Arthritis Rheum., 9:747–757, 1966.

108. Nye, W.H.R., Terry, R., and Rosenbaum, D.L.: Two forms of crystalline lipid in "cholesterol" effusions. Am. J. Clin. Pathol., 49:718–728, 1968.

109. Ortel, R.W., and Newcombe, D.S.: Acute gouty arthritis and response to colchicine in the virtual absence of synovial fluid leukocytes. N. Engl. J. Med., 290:1363–1364, 1974.

110. Owen, D.S.: A cheap and useful compensated polarizing microscope. N. Engl. J. Med., 285:1152, 1971.

111. Panush, R.S., Bianco, N.E., and Schur, P.H.: Serum and synovial fluid IgG, IgA, and IgM. Antigammaglobulins in rheumatoid arthritis. Arthritis Rheum., 14:737–747, 1971.

112. Parker, L.P., Seward, C.W., and Osterland, C.K.: Occurrence of antigammaglobulins in effusion fluids of diverse aetiology. Ann. Rheum. Dis., 33:262–267, 1974.

113. Paul, H., Reginato, A.J., and Schumacher, H.R.: Alizarin red staining as a screening test to detect calcium compounds in synovial fluid. Arthritis Rheum., 26:191–200, 1983.

114. Pekin, T.J., Malinin, T.I., and Zvaifler, N.J.: Unusual synovial fluid findings in Reiter's syndrome. Ann. Intern. Med., 66:677–684, 1967.

115. Pekin, T.J., Malinin, T.I., and Zvaifler, N.J.: The clinical significance of deoxyribonucleic acid particles in synovial fluid. Ann. Intern. Med., 65:1229–1236, 1966.

116. Pekin, T.J., and Zvaifler, N.J.: Hemolytic complement in synovial fluid. J. Clin. Invest., 43:1372–1382, 1964.

117. Petz, L.D., Sharp, G.C., and Cooper, N.J.: Serum and cerebral spinal fluid complement and serum autoantibodies in systemic lupus erythematosus. Medicine, 50:259–275, 1971.

118. Podell, T.E., et al.: Synovial fluid eosinophilia. Arthritis Rheum., 23:1060–1061, 1980.

119. Popert, A.G., et al.: Frequency of occurrence mode of development and significance of rice bodies in rheumatic joints. Ann. Rheum. Dis., 41:109–117, 1982.

120. Rawson, A.J., Abelson, V.M., and Hollander, J.L.: Studies of the pathogenesis of rheumatoid joint inflammation. Ann. Intern. Med., 62:281–291, 1965.

121. Riethmuller, G., Meltzer, M., and Franklin, E.C.: Serum complement levels in patients with mixed (IgM-IgG) cryoglobulinaemia. Clin. Exp. Immunol., 1:337–339, 1966.

122. Roberts, R.D., Wong, S.W., and Thiel, G.B.: An unusual case of lead nephropathy. Arthritis Rheum., 26:1048–1051, 1983.

123. Rodnan, G.P., Benedek, T.G., and Panetta, W.C.: The early history of synovial (joint) fluid. Ann. Intern. Med., 65:821–842, 1966.

124. Rodnan, G.P., Eisenheis, C.H., and Creighton, A.S.: The occurrence of rheumatoid factor in synovial fluid. Am. J. Med., 35:182–188, 1963.

125. Ropes, M.W., and Bauer, W.: Synovial Fluid Changes in Joint Diseases. Boston, Harvard University Press, 1953.

126. Ropes, M.W., Rossmeisl, E.C., and Bauer, W.: The origin and nature of normal human synovial fluid. J. Clin. Invest., 19:795–799, 1940.

127. Ruddy, S., and Austen, K.F.: The complement system in rheumatoid synovitis. Arthritis Rheum., 13:713–723, 1970.

128. Rytel, M.W.: Rapid Diagnosis of Infectious Disease. Edited by M.W. Rytel. CRC Press, 1979, pp. 7–16.

129. Sandson, J., and Hamerman, D.: Paper electrophoresis of human synovial fluid. Proc. Soc. Exp. Biol. Med., 98:554–561, 1958.

130. Schlesigner, P.A., Stillman, M.T., and Peterson, L.: Polyarthritis with birefringent lipid within synovial fluid macrophages: Case report and ultrastructural study. Arthritis Rheum., 25:1365–1368, 1982.

131. Schmid, K., and MacNair, M.D.: Characterization of the proteins of certain postmortem human synovial fluids. J. Clin. Invest., 37:708–718, 1958.

132. Schumacher, H.R.: Intracellular crystals in synovial fluid anticoagulated with oxalate. N. Engl. J. Med., 274:1372–1373, 1966.

133. Schumacher, H.R., et al.: Arthritis associated with apatite crystals. Ann. Intern. Med., *87*:411–416, 1977.

134. Schumacher, H.R., et al.: Acute gouty arthritis without urate crystals identified on initial examination of synovial fluid. Arthritis Rheum., *18*:603–612, 1975.

135. Schumacher, H.R., and Kitridou, R.C.: Synovitis of recent onset. Arthritis Rheum., *15*:465–485, 1972.

136. Schur, P.H., and Sandson, J.: Immunologic factors and clinical activity in systemic lupus erythematosus. N. Engl. J. Med., *278*:533–540, 1968.

137. Schur, P.H., and Sandson, J.: Immunologic studies of the proteins of human synovial fluid. Arthritis Rheum., *6*:115–129, 1963.

138. Simon, G.L., Niller, H., and Borenstein, D.G.: Synovial fluid inhibits killing of Staphylococcus aureus by neutrophils. Infect. Immun., *40*:1004–1010, 1983.

139. Small, D.M., Cohen, A.S., and Schmid, K.: Lipoproteins of synovial fluid as studied by analytical ultracentrifugation. J. Clin. Invest., *43*:2070–2079, 1964.

140. Stastny, P., et al.: Lymphokines in the rheumatoid joint. Arthritis Rheum., *18*:237–243, 1975.

141. Stevens, J., et al.: Synovial hemangioma of the knee. Arthritis Rheum., *12*:647, 1969.

142. Stevens, L.W., and Spiera, H.: Hemarthrosis in chondrocalcinosis (pseudogout). Arthritis Rheum., *16*:651–653, 1972.

143. Takasugi, K., and Hollingsworth, J.W.: Morphologic studies of mononuclear cells of human synovial fluid. Arthritis Rheum., *10*:495–501, 1967.

144. Tnaphaichitr, K., Spilberg, I., and Hahn, B.: Lithium heparin crystals simulating CPPD crystals. Arthritis Rheum., *19*:966–968, 1976.

145. Townes, A.S.: Topics in clinical medicine. Johns Hopkins Med. J., *120*:337–343, 1967.

146. Townes, A.S., and Sowa, J.M.: Complement in synovial fluid. Johns Hopkins Med. J., *127*:23–37, 1970.

147. Traycoff, R.B., Pascual, E., and Schumacher, H.R.: Mononuclear cells in human synovial fluid. Arthritis Rheum., *19*:743–748, 1976.

148. Yurdakul, S., et al.: The arthritis of Behçet's disease: A prospective study. Ann. Rheum. Dis., *42*:505–515, 1983.

149. Vaughan, J.H., et al.: Intracytoplasmic inclusions of immunoglobulins in rheumatoid arthritis and other diseases. Arthritis Rheum., *11*:125–134, 1968.

150. Vaughan, J.H., Jacox, R.F., and Noell, P.: Relation of intracytoplasmic inclusions in joint fluid leukocytes to anti-G globulins. Arthritis Rheum., *11*:135–144, 1968.

151. Weinstein, J.: Synovial fluid leukocytosis associated with intracellular lipid inclusions. Arch. Intern. Med., *140*:560–561, 1980.

152. Wild, J.H., and Zvaifler, N.J.: Hemarthrosis associated with sodium warfarin therapy. Arthritis Rheum., *19*:98–102, 1976.

153. Wilkins, R.F., and Healey, L.A.: The non-specificity of synovial leukocyte inclusions. J. Lab. Clin. Med., *68*:628–635, 1966.

154. Williams, R.C., and Law, D.H.: Serum complement of connective tissue disorders. J. Lab. Clin. Med., *52*:273–281, 1958.

155. Yaron, M., and Djaldetti, M.: Platelets in synovial fluid (letter). Arthritis Rheum., *21*:607–608, 1978.

156. Zuchner, J., Uddin, J., and Gantner, G.E.: Cholesterol crystals in synovial fluid. Ann. Intern. Med., *60*:436–446, 1964.

157. Zucker-Franklin, D.: The phagosomes in rheumatoid synovial fluid leukocytes: A light, fluorescence and electron microscope study. Arthritis Rheum., *9*:24–36, 1966.

Chapter 5

Radiology of Rheumatic Diseases

Harry K. Genant

The gross pathologic processes appearing in the musculoskeletal system in rheumatic diseases are often demonstrable by radiologic examination. A specific radiologic diagnosis is sometimes possible, but more important, the detection, evaluation, and serial assessment of structural joint abnormalities can be achieved. Based on clinical, pathologic, and radiologic criteria, this chapter is organized in the following manner: imaging techniques; systemic connective tissue disorders; degenerative and ischemic disorders; crystal-induced arthropathies; infectious arthritides; and miscellaneous articular disorders. Comments are limited to musculoskeletal manifestations. Discussion of findings in other organ systems appears in specific clinical chapters of this book.

RADIOLOGIC TECHNIQUES

These techniques include magnification radiography, radionuclide joint imaging, arthrography, quantitative bone mineral analysis, and nuclear magnetic resonance. (See Chapter 6 for a discussion of computerized tomography.)

Magnification Radiography

A clear radiographic image is essential for the accurate assessment of subtle skeletal abnormalities. High-resolution magnification radiography, particularly valuable in the evaluation of arthritic and metabolic bone disorders,[17,81,97,98,113,115,117,119,120,224,244,245] is generally achieved by optical magnification of fine-grain film or direct radiographic magnification.[80,120]

The optical magnification technique consists of contact exposures obtained with conventional x-ray equipment, and nonscreen, fine-grain industrial film, such as Kodak type M or Kodak AA. The resultant image is magnified four to ten times by means of a hand lens, loupe, or projector. Clinical studies with this technique are not new. In the early 1950s, Fletcher and Rowley used fine-grain film and photographic enlargements to study peripheral arthritis.[97,98] In 1969, a monograph by Berens and Lin described radiography with industrial film and optical magnification in rheumatoid arthritis (RA).[17] More recently, Meema and Meema,[244,245] Genant and co-workers,[115,117,119,120] and Kozin et

al.[189] have reported extensive experience with this technique in various arthritic and metabolic skeletal disorders. The clinical importance of the optical magnification technique to assess selected peripheral skeletal disorders appears to be established. This technique is less feasible, however, for thicker body parts of the central skeleton because of high radiation exposure, geometric blurriness (focal-spot penumbra), and decreased contrast that results from scattered radiation.[120] For these parts, direct radiographic magnification is preferable.

Direct radiographic magnification for skeletal radiography has received increasing attention since the development and availability of x-ray tubes with small focal spots and fast rare-earth screen-film systems. The technique consists of direct geometric magnification of 2 to 4 times using a microfocus tube with a nominal focal-spot size of 100 μ.[80,120] The images are recorded with high-resolution screen-film systems. The radiographs are then processed in a standard manner and are viewed with the unaided eye. Initial clinical experience with direct radiographic magnification has been favorably reported by Doi et al.[81] and Genant et al.,[113,120] and applications for both thin and thick body parts have been established.

The images from optical and radiographic magnification are superior to those from conventional radiography; contrast is better, resolution is higher, and "noise" or quantum mottle is diminished (Figs. 5–1, 5–2). In a controlled study,[224] fine-detail radiography in patients with RA improved detection of early erosive disease. Assessment of soft tissue swelling was modestly improved in patients with early or minimal RA. These results are of particular importance in view of the prognostic significance of the presence of erosive disease in the initial examination and on short-term follow-up examinations.[330] When pronounced changes were present initially, the disease ran a rapid course; this finding indicates the need for early and aggressive therapy.

In other arthritides, too, the evaluation of subtle articular changes may be of clinical importance. For instance, the distinction between the proliferative erosions of Reiter's disease or psoriatic arthritis and the nonproliferative erosions of RA or

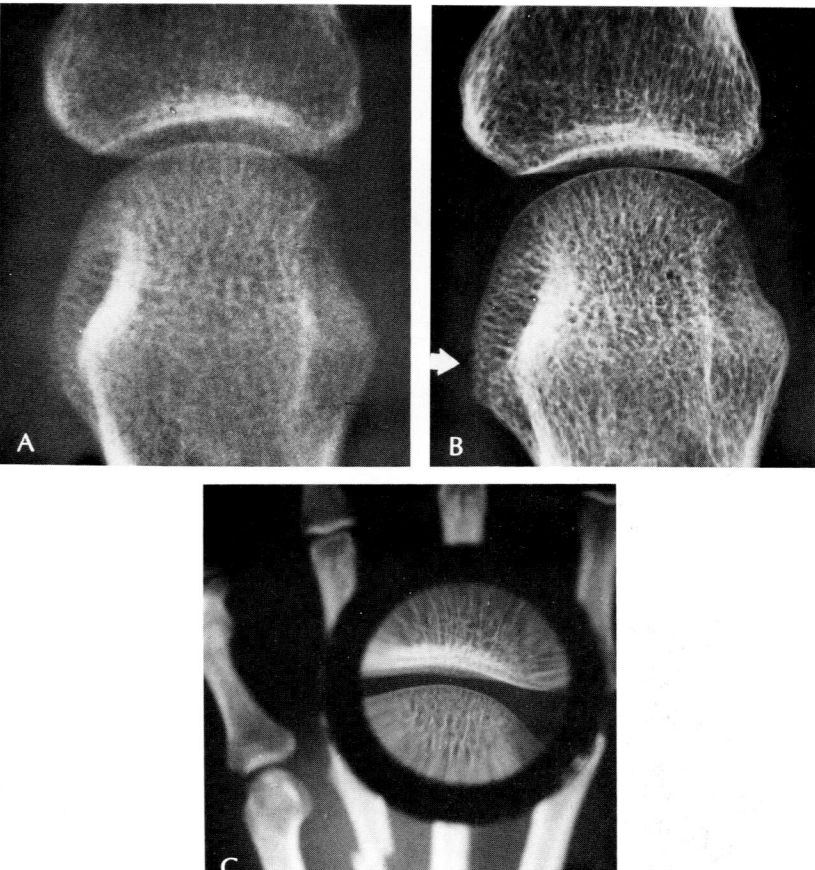

Fig. 5–1. Radiographs of a metacarpophalangeal joint in a patient with early rheumatoid arthritis obtained both by conventional screen film technique *(A)* and by industrial film technique *(B)*. Subtle surface erosion of the subchondral cortical line *(B,* arrow), characteristic of this disorder, is detected only on fine-grain film. The method of optically magnifying a radiograph with a loupe that magnifies four times is shown in *C.*

sclerodermatous arthritis is facilitated by magnification.[120] Early articular calcification in pseudogout is detected more readily with high-quality radiography.[111,272] In advanced disease with well-established structural changes, high-resolution techniques add little.

In metabolic bone disease, subtle subperiosteal resorptive changes are frequently undetected by conventional techniques, but are easily seen with magnification.[117,245] Assessment of intracortical resorption (cortical striations or "tunneling") is possible with magnification and provides an important index of bone turnover in such diseases as hyperparathyroidism, hyperthyroidism, Sudeck's atrophy, and osteomalacia.[115,117,244,245]

Radionuclide Joint Imaging

In 1965, Weiss et al. evaluated joint disease after the intravenous injection of [131]iodine (^{131}I)-labeled albumin.[376] The articular accumulation of the radionuclide was measured both by a stationary detector and by a rectilinear scanner. Tracer accumulation in affected joints was a result of several nonspecific factors, including increased synovial permeability and blood flow. The images produced with ^{131}I-labeled albumin were poor because of the physical characteristics of this nuclide.

In 1967, Alarcon-Segovia and associates first used [99m]technetium (^{99m}Tc) as the pertechnetate ([99m]TcO4), a blood pool and extracellular-fluid space tracer, for joint imaging.[3] Because of its short half-life of 6 hours, ^{99m}Tc can be used in much higher activities than can [131]I. Additionally, its 140-keV photon emission is ideally suited for use with the gamma camera (Fig. 5–3). This agent has been employed widely as a clinical investigative tool.[138,212,242,331]

Recently, bone-seeking agents have been used,

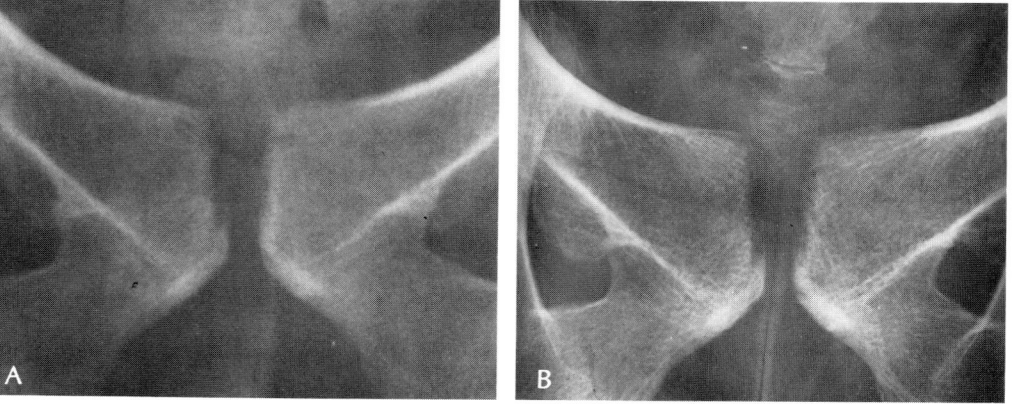

Fig. 5–2. *A,* Conventional radiograph and *B,* direct radiographic magnification view demonstrate widening of the symphysis pubis. The magnification study, reproduced photographically at the same size as the contact radiograph, demonstrates irregular destruction of the subchondral cortical line producing a ragged, lace-like appearance. These features indicate an aggressive evolving process and support the diagnosis of infectious osteitis pubis.

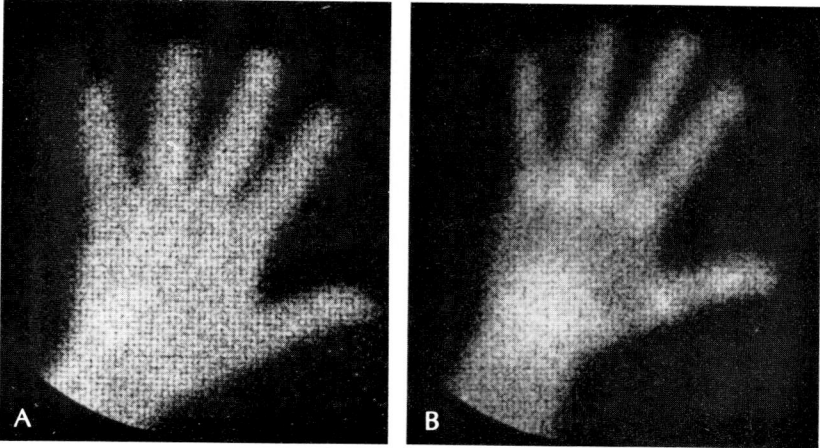

Fig. 5–3. Normal hand joints imaged with [99m]technetium (Tc)-pertechnetate *(A)* and ^{99m}Tc-EHDP *(B).* It is difficult to discern the individual joints of the hand on the pertechnetate image. The ^{99m}Tc-EHDP image demonstrates the normal pattern of decreasing activity from proximal to distal joints.

especially the ^{99m}Tc compounds (pyrophosphate, polyphosphate, or diphosphonate).[159,350] Articular disease produces early changes in the periarticular bone,[355,359] and an abnormal uptake of these radionuclides results.[12,14,77,115,141] Increased uptake of [85]strontium ([85]Sr) in the periarticular bone of diseased joints was shown in 1966.[160] This agent is not suitable for routine joint imaging because of its physical characteristics. The ^{99m}Tc-labeled bone-scanning agents are far superior,[77] with greater sensitivity than ^{99m}Tc-pertechnetate (Fig. 5–3).[14,77] Moreover, imaging with ^{99m}Tc bone-scanning agents provides a means of evaluating the central joints, that is, the hips,[74,168,315] the sacroiliac joints,[198,302] and the spine. This evaluation is not

possible with ^{99m}Tc-pertechnetate because the high activity in the surrounding soft tissue gives poor target-to-background ratios.

The ^{99m}Tc-labeled bone-scanning compounds are localized by chemabsorption onto the hydroxyapatite crystals at bone surfaces in contact with the circulating fluids.[312,357] Uptake, closely correlated to blood flow in bone,[116,269,364] is greatest in regions with high ratios of bone surface to volume and high local blood flow, such as the epiphyseal-metaphyseal cancellous bone around joints.[312] In arthritis, localization of these agents results primarily from the increased blood flow to the juxta-articular bone that accompanies synovitis and cartilage degeneration.[116,270,364] Additional contributors to increased bone localization of ^{99m}Tc-labeled phosphates include capillary permeability,[57] extraction efficiency,[55,63] and possibly binding onto organic components of bone matrix.[311]

The use of ^{99m}Tc-pertechnetate for evaluating RA has been extensively investigated. Weiss et al.,[376] Sholkoff and Glickman,[331] McCarty et al., [212,213] and Green and Hays[138] have reported diagnostic sensitivity at least equal to that of clinical evaluation and higher than that of radiographic examination. Radionuclide imaging aided assessment of early or atypical seronegative rheumatoid disease,[242,331] as well as assessment of therapeutic response. Experience with inflammatory joint disease other than RA is limited.

The sensitivity of the various examinations in early disease increases in the following sequence: conventional radiography, clinical examination, ^{99m}Tc-pertechnetate joint scan, and ^{99m}Tc-phosphate bone scan.[14] Gout (Fig. 5–4), pseudogout, Reiter's disease, psoriatic arthritis, and inflammatory osteoarthritis have all been imaged by radionuclide studies with either ^{99m}Tc-pertechnetate or bone-scanning agents.[14,77,212,242,354]

Joint-imaging techniques may establish a diagnosis in a patient with "arthralgia" when objective clinical evidence of synovitis is scant or lacking altogether (Fig. 5–5). Increased localization limited to the joints in question supports the presence of a true "arthritis," provided other causes for a positive scan, such as focal bone lesions, have been excluded. Conversely, a negative scintigram in a

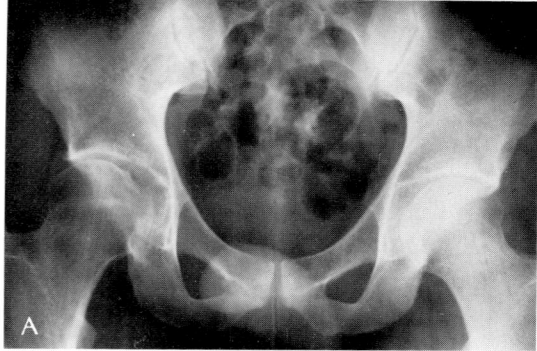

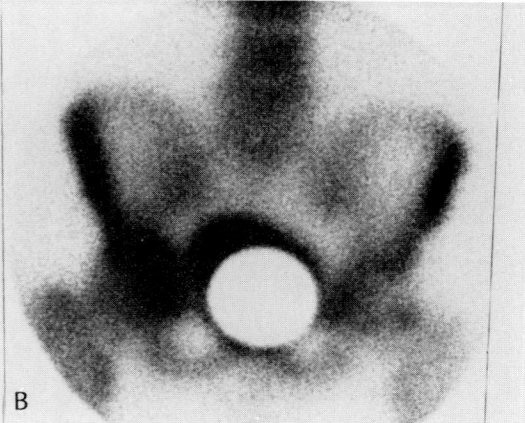

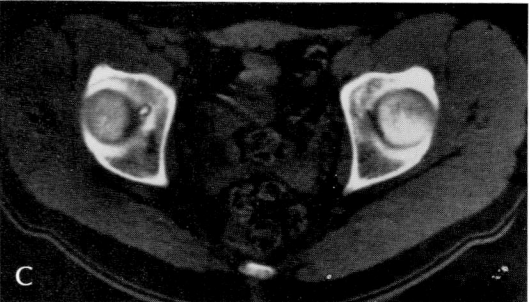

Fig. 5–5. Conventional radiograph of the pelvis *(A)* demonstrates periarticular demineralization of the right hip, but no other objective osseous or articular abnormalities. A bone scan *(B)* demonstrates a dramatic focal increased uptake in the right acetabular region that prompts an additional diagnostic study, a computed tomographic (CT) examination *(C)*, which demonstrates a focal lytic defect with a central calcified nidus diagnostic of a benign osteoid osteoma.

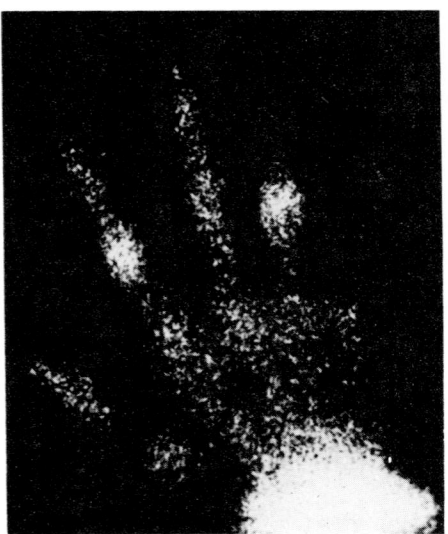

Fig. 5–4. Radionuclide image (^{99m}Tc-EHDP) of a hand with gout. Increased localization is seen in the second and fourth proximal interphalangeal joints, which are clinically involved.

patient with arthralgia militates against synovial inflammation.[159,212] The ability to "see" central joints such as hips, sacroiliac joints, and zygapophyseal joints has broadened the clinical usefulness of joint scintigraphy. This technique has been employed in a quantitative mode to detect early sacroiliitis and to distinguish this disease from other conditions, such as osteitis condensans ilii (Fig. 5–6).[127,159,198,302] The greater accuracy of computed tomography (CT) for assessing the sacroiliac joint, however, is resulting in decreased use of quantitative scintigraphy for this purpose.[189,368] Early septic arthritis of the hips, possibly a difficult clinical diagnosis, is readily detected with a bone-seeking radionuclide. A positive scintiphotograph is nonspecific; post-traumatic synovitis and rheumatoid or osteoarthritic involvement of the hip yield a similar picture.[85,122,221]

Joint imaging in the evaluation of osteoarthritis of the knee is a current orthopedic practice. Imaging with ^{99m}Tc-polyphosphate is as sensitive as arthrography in the detection of specific compartmental involvement in the knee.[355]

In aseptic necrosis of the hip resulting from fracture, corticosteroid treatment, or Legg-Perthes disease, initial radiographic findings may be subtle, absent, or confusing.[198] A characteristic anterolateral scintiphotopenic notch has been observed early in patients with aseptic necrosis. Reports of increased or decreased localization of radionuclide in adult aseptic necrosis probably reflect variables in the different agents used and in the stage of the disease at the time of study (see Chap. 86).[12,50,341]

Another important application of joint scintiphotography is in the evaluation of joint prostheses.[92,375] These devices may loosen and may produce abnormal stresses in adjacent bone. An increased uptake of radionuclide is shown in the region of abnormal stress. Pyogenic infection, another complication of joint replacement, may be detected by radionuclide scintigraphy.[381]

Radionuclide evaluation of joints has evolved slowly over the past two decades into a clinically useful method both for diagnosis and chronologic evaluation of joint disease. Many clinicians are

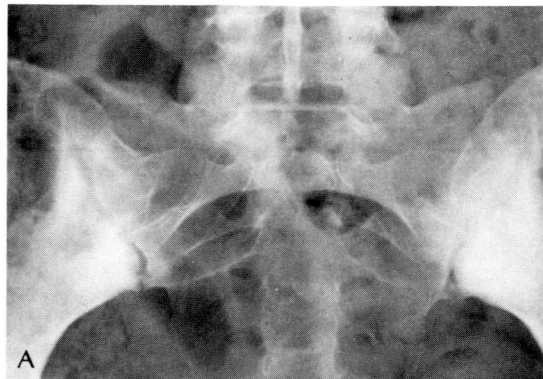

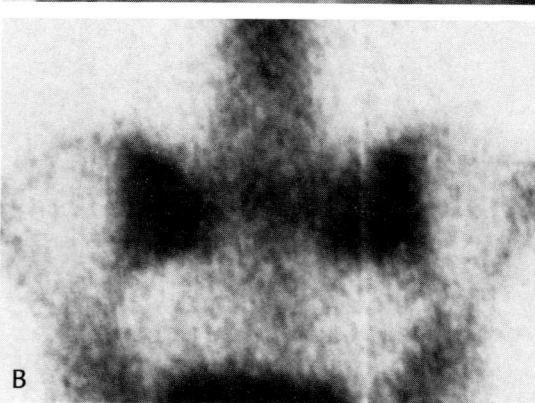

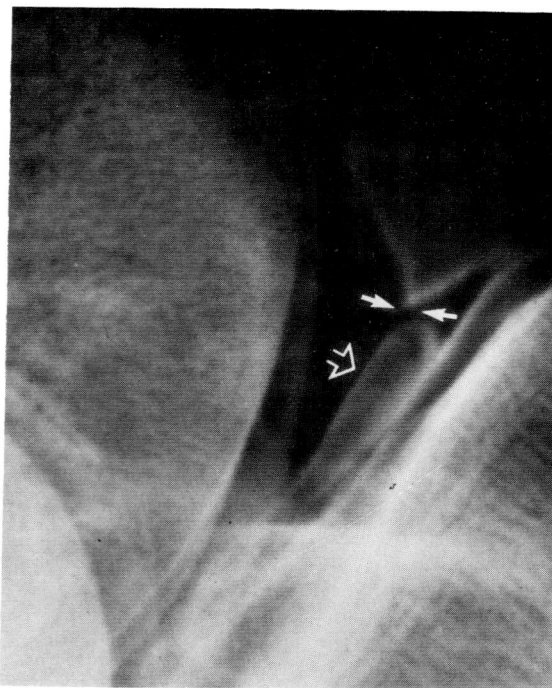

Fig. 5–6. *A*, Radiograph demonstrates sclerosis on the sacral side of the sacroiliac joints consistent with either early sacroiliitis or osteitis condensans ilii in this 27-year-old woman with low back pain. *B*, A posterior scintigram of the pelvis ([99m]Technetium-pyrophosphate) reveals symmetric, diffuse increased uptake over the sacroiliac joints. Such increased uptake is seen in early ankylosing spondylitis, but not in osteitis condensans ilii. (From Richards et al.[303])

Fig. 5–7. Spot-film taken during arthrography of the knee demonstrates a vertical tear (closed arrows) and a loose fragment (open arrow) of the posterior horn of the medial meniscus.

unaware of the progress in this field and do not avail themselves of these techniques to maximum advantage. Clinical examination is the primary method to diagnose arthritis and will probably remain so. Radionuclide imaging, although sensitive, is nonspecific. Radiography is specific, but insensitive. When used appropriately, each may help in the detection and evaluation of many forms of articular disease.[159]

Arthrography

Arthrography is used to examine the intra-articular anatomic features of a joint after injection of radiopaque material. This technique dates back to 1905,[378] but was not used clinically until 1939.[202] Technical advances in the 1960s, such as fluoroscopic guidance, smaller focal spots, stressing devices, and double-contrast techniques (air and iodinated contrast medium) simplified the procedure, which often provides useful information.[41,103,261,305,361]

The predominant application of arthrography has been assessment of internal derangements of the knee, particularly meniscal injuries, with an accuracy of 90 to 95% in the detection of tears and lacerations of the medial meniscus (Fig. 5–7).[7] Arthrography is well established in assessment of this common injury, particularly when clinical findings are equivocal or atypical.[41,103,145,261,305] Lateral meniscal injuries, far less common, may be more difficult to detect arthrographically because of the more complex anatomic structure. Most such tears, however, are detected accurately by the experienced arthrographer.[73,102,216] With a double-contrast technique, the entire lining of the joint can be opacified, and extrameniscal lesions may be assessed as well.[342] These lesions include abnormalities of the articular cartilage, such as osteochondritis dissecans, chondromalacia patellae, osteochondral fractures, and foci of cartilaginous fibrillation or ulceration in osteoarthritis.[163] Synovial abnormalities, such as the hypertrophy of RA, pigmented villonodular synovitis,[384] and synovial chondromatosis can be seen.[64] Tears of the cruciate ligaments may be visible,[201] as well as disruption of the joint capsule and collateral ligaments, as evidenced by extravasation of contrast material outside the confines of the joint. Finally, large, ruptured popliteal (Baker's) cysts are readily demarcated and are thus differentiated from lesions of acute thrombophlebitis (Fig. 5–8).[38]

Arthrography of other joints has been increasingly employed. Positive-contrast or double-contrast arthrography of the shoulders graphically demonstrates the integrity, shape, and capacity of the glenohumeral articulation.[130,187,202] This method has been used to show ruptures of the musculotendinous rotator cuff, adhesive capsulitis, and the extent of damage in recurrent dislocation and synovial masses in RA (Fig. 5–9) (see Chaps. 85 and 95).

Arthrography in congenital dislocation of the hip has been used for many years to assess the nonossified acetabular labrum and the cartilaginous capital femoral epiphysis,[249] particularly when attempts at reduction are unsuccessful. The procedure has been used to determine the state of the cartilage surface in Legg-Perthes disease[137] and has been accepted widely as a means to evaluate pain after total arthroplasty of the hip.[109,259,317] Loosening of the prosthesis or infection, or both, is detectable with a high degree of accuracy, although false-positive and false-negative results are seen.[259] Arthrography has been applied to many other articulations, generally to assess capsular integrity or the state of articular cartilage and synovial lining.[90,151,287,379] It is often essential for evaluation of the temporomandibular joint (see Chap. 81).

Quantitative Bone Mineral Analysis

The detection and serial assessment of metabolic bone disorders by noninvasive methods has been a subject of considerable interest and importance to clinicians and researchers (see also Chap. 97). Although conventional radiography offers a readily available, simple approach to this problem, it is insensitive and poorly reproducible.[105,117,309] Consequently, quantitative techniques, with variable but generally improved precision and accuracy, have been devised.

First, the *measurement of cortical thickness* is simple and easy, is reproducible, and is supported by a large body of normative data.[76,105,260,366] This technique may lack sensitivity in the assessment of many metabolic bone disorders because only endosteal bone resorption is detected. Intracortical resorption (cortical porosity or "tunneling") and trabecular bone resorption, important determinants of high bone turnover, are not measured (Fig. 5–10).[88,115,117,135,335,344]

Second, *photodensitometry*,[58,82,219,245] a technique with an x-ray source, radiographic film, and a known standard wedge, is reproducible and is possibly more sensitive than simple cortical measurement, but complicated technical requirements have limited its clinical use.

Third, an easier, more precise technique is *photon absorptiometry*, which determines the linear attenuation coefficient of bone by means of transmission scanning with a ^{125}I source interfaced to a sodium iodine scintillation detector.[49,194,335] Many different techniques have been used, but the most widely accepted is the Norland-Cameron,[48] which measures the radial shaft, although other tubular

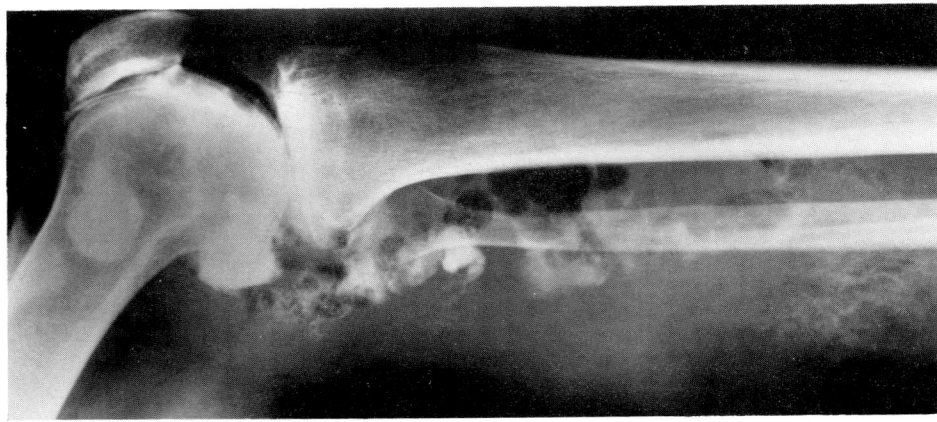

Fig. 5–8. Arthrographic demonstration of a large Baker's cyst that has ruptured, allowing contrast material and air to escape into the soft tissues of the calf.

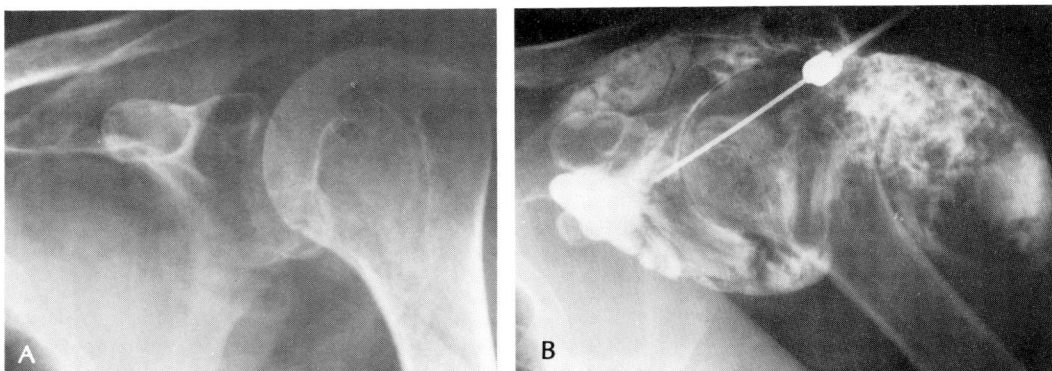

Fig. 5–9. Conventional radiograph *(A)* and shoulder arthrogram *(B)* of a patient with rheumatoid arthritis demonstrates massive synovial hypertrophy, accumulation of rice bodies, and distention and rupture of the synovial spaces into subachromial and subdeltoid bursae.

bones can be examined. Considerable normative data are available, and many clinical studies support its usefulness.[114,117,144,335] Its reproducibility is approximately 2%, with an accuracy of about 6%.[48] The measurement is primarily an integral of cortical bone because the diaphysis, generally the site measured, contains little cancellous bone. The metaphysis, containing proportionally more trabecular bone, as much as 25 to 40% of total integral bone, is more difficult to measure and is a less-precise site because of repositioning errors.[320] The impetus for measurement of cancellous bone is its surface-to-volume ratio, which is greater than that of cortical bone, and its early and dramatic alteration in many metabolic disorders.[76,135,144,344]

Methods that can measure separately cancellous bone or regions composed largely of cancellous bone have been devised for this reason. These newer methods include x-ray spectrophotometry,[71,191,281] dual photon absorptiometry,[382] total- or partial-body neutron activation analysis,[217,218,225] Compton scatter determination,[373] and more recently, CT scanning.[26,28,108,112,118,167,280,313] Of these, only dual photon absorptiometry and CT are widely available for bone mineral determination. Quantitative computed tomography (QCT) promises several advantages over other competing techniques: (1) transaxial display of data, to permit identification of anatomic features and separate determination of cortical, cancellous, or integral bone density; (2) capability of determining linear absorption coefficient for a readily defined volume of bone; (3) in the dual-energy mode, the ability to determine mineral content in the presence of variable fat and soft tissue; and (4) the nearly universal availability of the apparatus (Fig. 5–11). Studies in patients have shown a precision of 1 to 3% and an accuracy of 5 to 8%; these findings indicate that

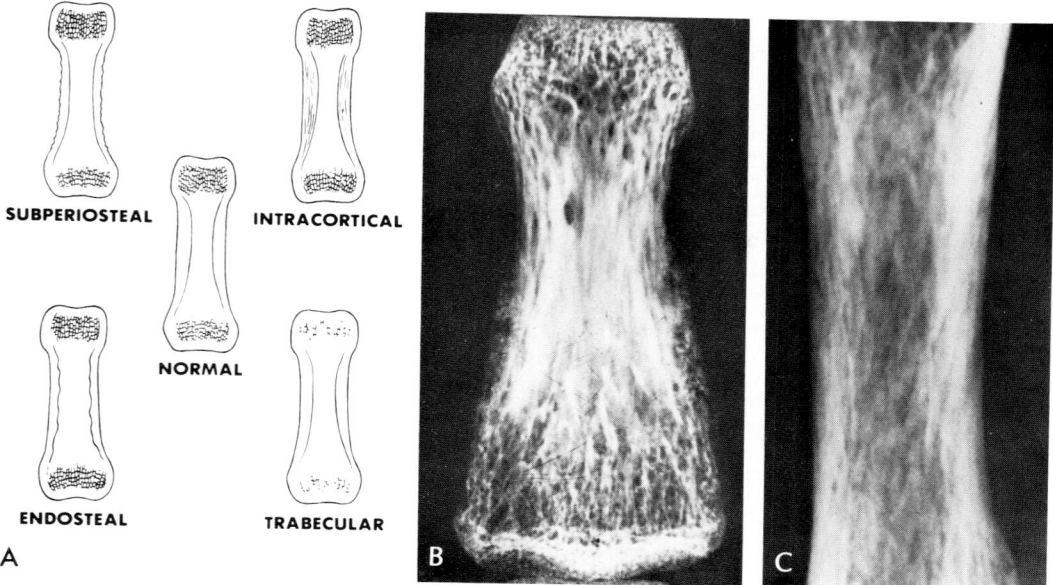

Fig. 5–10. *A,* Schematic representation of sites of bone resorption in that phalanx, that is, subperiosteal, endosteal, trabecular, and intracortical. *B,* Striking subperiosteal bone resorption is shown in a phalanx of a patient with renal osteodystrophy and secondary hyperparathyroidism. *C,* Advanced intracortical and endosteal bone resorption is shown in the metacarpal joint of patient with reflex sympathetic dystrophy syndrome.

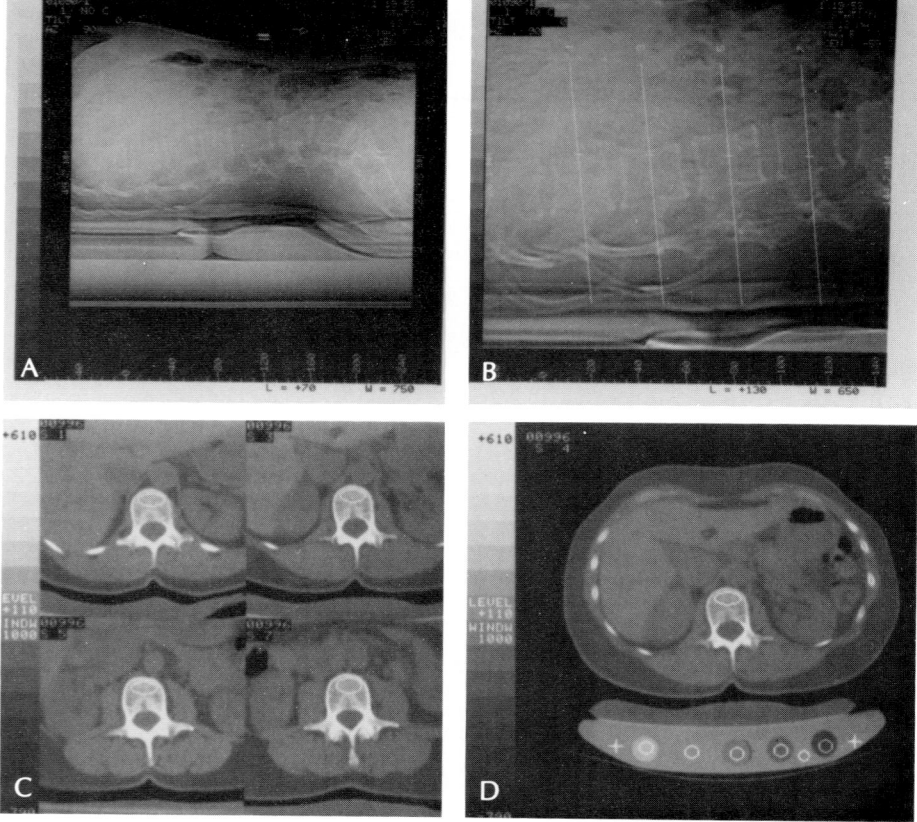

Fig. 5–11. *A to D,* A composite figure demonstrating the technique for quantitative computed tomographic vertebral mineral determination. A computed radiograph (scout view) provides localization for the midplane of four vertebral bodies. The cresent-shaped calibration standard is scanned simultaneously with the patient, and representative volumes of purely trabecular bone are quantified in the anterior portion of the vertebral body.

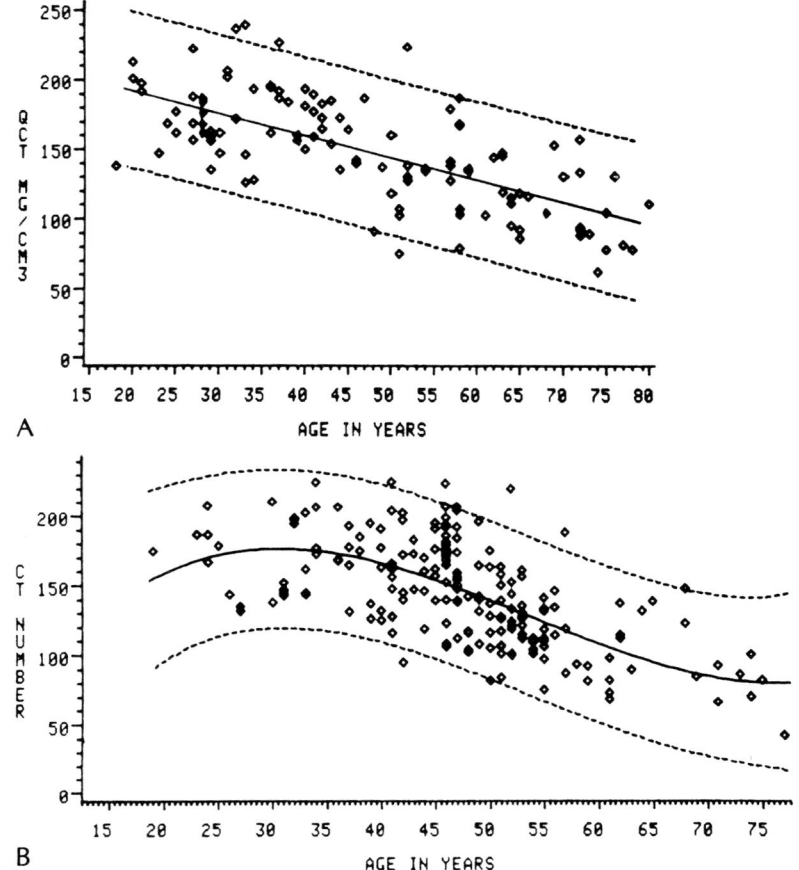

Fig. 5–12. *A,* Quantitative computed tomography (QCT) shows vertebral mineral content in relation to age in normal males; linear regression and a 95% confidence interval are also shown. *B,* QCT shows vertebral mineral content in relation to age in normal females; cubic regression and a 95% confidence interval are also present.

QCT can be used reliably to assess bone mineral content in the axial skeleton. Cross-sectional studies using QCT[108] have defined the normal age-related bone loss in men and women and have shown the capability for predicting fracture risk (Fig. 5–12). Longitudinal clinical studies[112] have shown the high shortening of spinal QCT, as compared to standard peripheral contrast measurements for assessing rates of bone loss and monitoring response to therapy (Fig. 5–13).

Nuclear Magnetic Resonance

The phenomenon of nuclear magnetic resonance (NMR) was discovered in 1946,[22,277] and since that time, NMR spectroscopy has been widely applied in chemistry and physics as an analytic tool. It was not until 1973, however, that Lauterbur proposed and demonstrated the feasibility of using NMR signals as the basis of an imaging technique.[196] Since

then, NMR imaging technology has advanced at a pace even more rapid than that of CT imaging.

The physical principles on which NMR imaging is based are completely different from those of any previous imaging technique. Because the NMR phenomenon reflects events occurring at the molecular level, NMR imaging may provide physiologic and biochemical as well as anatomic information about the tissues studied. In this sense, it appears to combine the anatomic information of CT and the physiologic information of nuclear medical studies in one technique, with the added advantage that it uses no ionizing radiation and has no known harmful biologic effects. This advantage accounts for the widespread interest in the technique.

NMR depends on the behavior of certain nuclei in a magnetic field.[226,252] Any nucleus with an odd number of protons or neutrons acts as if it has a magnetic moment, that is, a small magnetic field.

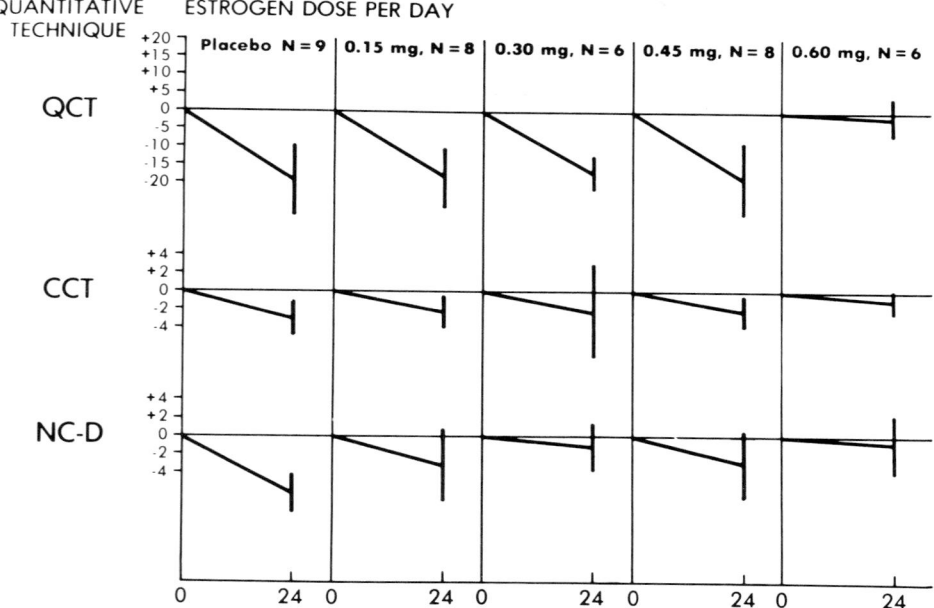

Fig. 5–13.   Bone mineral losses 24 months following oophorectomy are shown as a function of estrogen dose and quantitative bone mineral technique. Quantitative computed tomography (QCT), combined cortical thickness (CCT) of the second metacarpal joint, and Norland-Cameron photon absorptiometry (NC-D)$_2$ of the radiodiophesis are shown.

Hydrogen is the element most commonly used for NMR imaging, however, because of its relative abundance in biologic tissue and its high sensitivity to magnetic perturbation.

When the hydrogen proton is placed in a uniform magnetic field, it aligns its field in the direction of the external magnetic field. Because the proton also has spin, however, it does not align directly with the magnetic field, but precesses around the axis of the magnetic field lines in a fashion similar to a spinning top wobbling in the earth's gravitational field (Fig. 5–14). This precession or resonance occurs at a fixed frequency called the "Lamour frequency," which is directly proportional to the strength of the magnetic field. Because many protons are present in the sample and are precessing in random phase relative to one another, the net magnetic moment of all the protons in the sample are parallel to the magnetic field. Applying a radio frequency pulse at the Lamour frequency causes the net magnetic moment to tilt from its alignment with the external field. The amount of tilt depends on the strength and duration of the applied radio frequency pulse. Because the tilted protons continue to precess, the net magnetic moment also precesses. This process of precession or magnetic resonance produces the radio frequency signal, which, when detected, provides the basis for the NMR image. The intensity of the emitted NMR

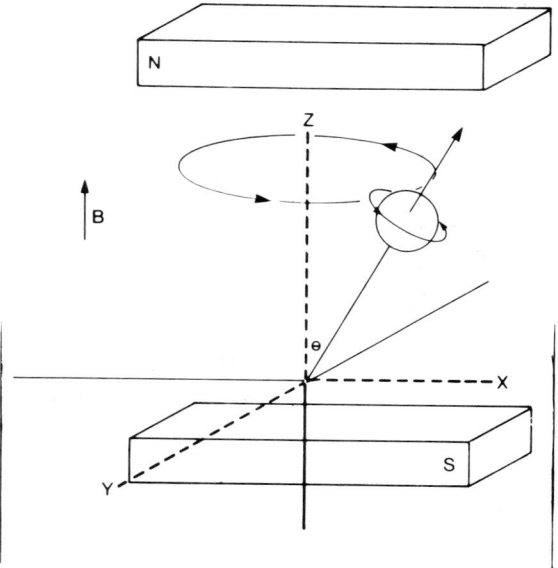

Fig. 5–14.   Schematic representation of a spinning hydrogen proton, which, when placed in a uniform magnetic field, is caused to precess or to resonate.

radio frequency signal from any given point in the patient depends on several factors, including hydrogen density and unique magnetic properties called the T1 and T2 relaxation times. The assessment of these parameters provides the potential for physiologic and biochemical information about the tissues sampled.

Recent reports have documented the ability of NMR to demonstrate normal anatomic features (Fig. 5–15) and pathologic conditions in a variety of cerebral, cardiovascular, and abdominal applications.[226] To date, however, the role of NMR in the diagnosis and assessment of musculoskeletal and articular disorders has not been extensively explored.[54,109,251,252] Preliminary indications do exist about the strengths and weaknesses of the NMR technique in this role.

A general feature of NMR imaging, which makes it well suited for a number of orthopedic and rheumatologic applications, is its superior soft tissue contrast, as compared to that of CT imaging. Muscle, cartilage, fibrous structures such as ligaments and tendons, nerves, and blood vessels each have unique NMR imaging characteristics based on differing T1 and T2 relaxation times, whereas these same tissues all have similar CT attenuation values and are principally differentiated from each other on the basis of their anatomic appearance. In addition to excellent tissue contrast, NMR has the capability of providing direct coronal, sagittal, or multiplanar imaging, as well as the routine axial imaging afforded by CT. Although the spatial resolution of NMR is approaching that of CT, the time required to obtain a single sectional image is substantially longer with NMR. To counter this disadvantage, instrumentation now provided by NMR is capable of obtaining multiple simultaneous sections. For example, 20 separate anatomic sections may be obtained in a single scanning sequence of approximately 20 minutes.

NMR is clearly an exciting and rapidly evolving diagnostic imaging technique that undoubtedly will have an impact on medical diagnostic imaging and may become a useful instrument in the assessment of a variety of musculoskeletal and articular disorders.

Areas of early and promising musculoskeletal investigation include NMR assessment of lumbar (Fig. 5–16) and cervical intervertebral disc herniation and avascular necrosis of the femoral heads (Fig. 5–17). The assessment of the articular cartilage and capsular structures of the hips and knees (Fig. 5–18) suggests a potential role in diagnosing a variety of arthropathies, whereas the capability for detecting and analyzing joint effusions raises the possibility of differentiating inflammatory from noninflammatory articular processes noninvasively.

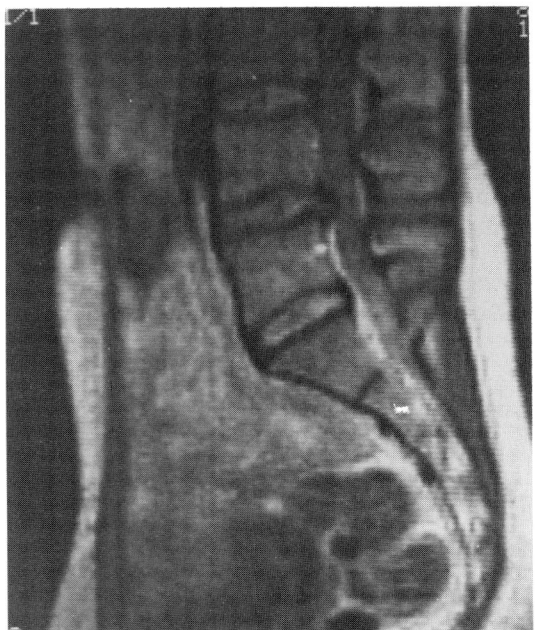

Fig. 5–15. High-resolution sagittal image of the head and upper neck demonstrating excellent visualization of the brain stem and spinal cord, as well as minute delineation of the C1 to C2 articulations.

Fig. 5–16. Sagittal image of the lower lumbar spine demonstrates a focal disc herniation at the L4 to L5 level with protrusion of the nucleus pulposus in the midline displacing the thecal sac posteriorly.

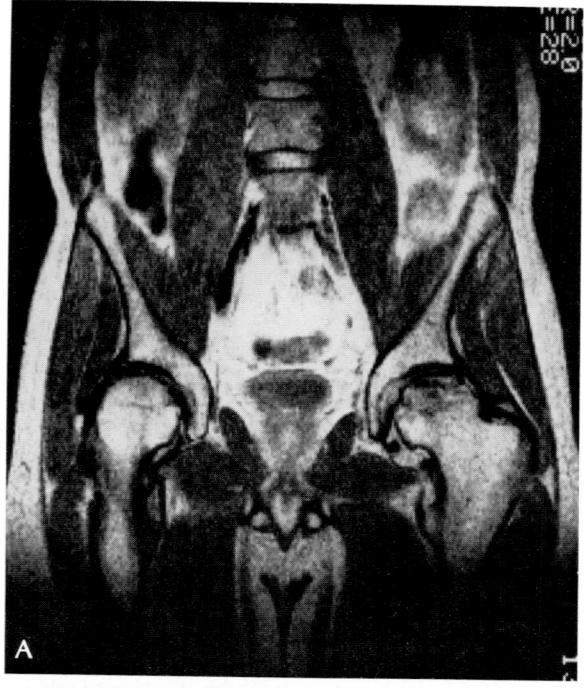

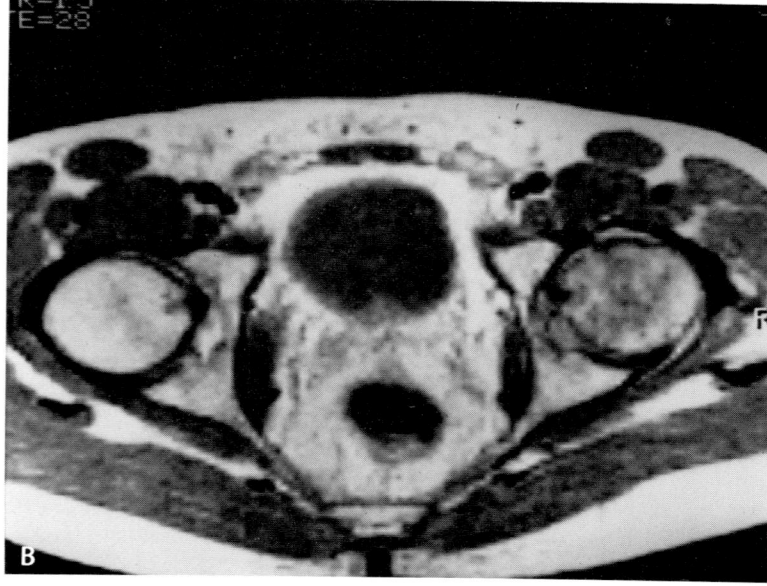

Fig. 5–17. Images produced by nuclear magnetic resonance in a patient with unilateral osteonecrosis of the femoral head. *A,* Coronal image demonstrates the loss of the normal, bright, homogeneous signal on the left side, accompanied by subchondral collapse; areas of low-intensity signal in dark indicate reactive bone formation. Capsular distention by a bright-signal joint effusion can be identified as well. *B,* An axial image demonstrates mottled, inhomogeneous loss of high-intensity signal throughout the superior aspect of the femoral head and an associated joint effusion.

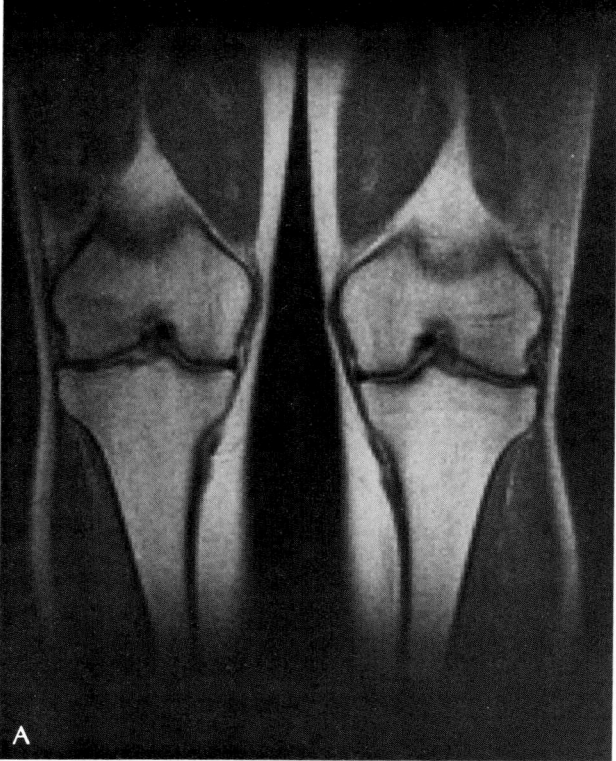
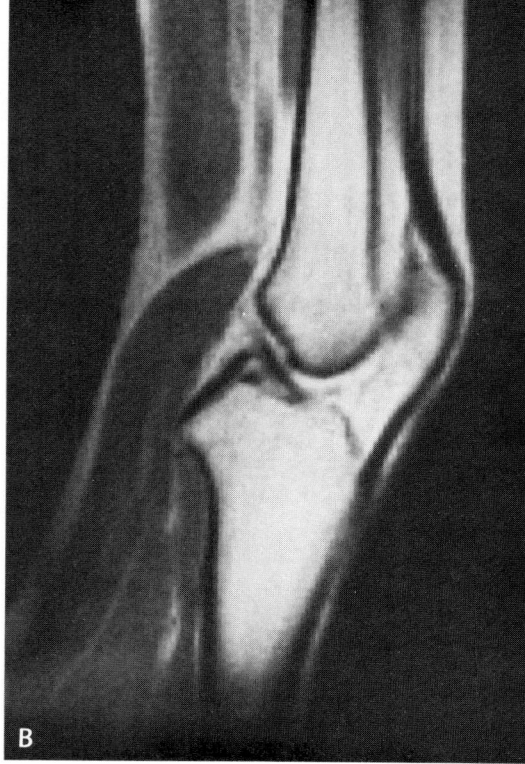

Fig. 5–18.   The osseous and articular structures of a normal knee are shown in coronal *(A)* and sagittal *(B)* planes. The hyaline and fibrocartilage of the knee can be seen on the coronal images, whereas on the sagittal image, the black anterior and posterior cruciate ligaments as well as the patellar tendon can be easily identified. Note the homogeneous, high-intensity signal of the fat-containing marrow.

SYSTEMIC CONNECTIVE TISSUE DISORDERS

Rheumatoid Arthritis

RA, a systemic connective tissue disorder of unknown origin has protean manifestations, of which destruction of the articular and periarticular structures is foremost.

Distribution

Any synovial joint of the body may be involved, but especially the knees and the small joints of the hands, wrists, and feet. The process may begin with a monoarticular, or asymmetric, pauciarticular distribution, which in time becomes polyarticular and symmetric.[16,17,101,175,228,346,347] Occasionally, advanced disease is asymmetric and nonuniform. Early in the course of disease, the dominant hand may be more affected than the nondominant;[175,268] similarly, hemiparalysis may protect the disused extremity.[385] Axial skeletal involvement in adult RA usually occurs later, is less striking than peripheral involvement, and is generally limited to the cervical spine or, less commonly, to the sacroiliac joints.[87,235,346]

General Appearance

Radiologic manifestations that reflect the gross pathologic changes of RA are seen in the periarticular soft tissue, the interosseous cartilage space, and the subchondral bone.[17,101,346,347]

Soft Tissues.   Swelling of the soft tissues is a hallmark of rheumatoid involvement of the peripheral joints; its radiologic assessment in the central skeleton is often unreliable. This swelling develops early in the disease,[43,222,339] and it invariably precedes cartilaginous and osseous changes; thus, bone changes are unlikely if periarticular soft tissues are normal, except when the disease is quiescent.[224] Swelling results from accumulation of joint fluid, synovial proliferation, and periarticular edema. Radiographically, symmetric, uniform swelling around the joints is most easily detected in the small joints of the hands and wrists. The changes in these joints are a bulbous periarticular radiodensity, displacement or obliteration of pericapsular and occasionally, subcutaneous, fat lines, and loss of normal skin folds, such as knuckle pads in the hands (Figs. 5–19, 5–20). Less commonly, asymmetric nodules or lumps appear as a result of either pronounced synovial hypertrophy or rheumatoid nodule formation.[228,346] A rare form of RA, in which the prominent feature is multiple subcutaneous and intra-articular nodules with little joint inflammation or destruction, has been called "rheumatoid nodulosis" (see Fig. 6–16).[104,123] In late stages of RA, the soft tissue swelling may subside and may result in generalized atrophy of all soft tissues, including fat and muscle. Occasionally, large periarticular soft tissue masses may result from accumulation of synovial fluid in sacs, such as the popliteal, olecranon, or iliopsoas bursae. Arthrography may be useful in the delineation of these fluid-filled structures (see Fig. 5–8).[38]

Cartilage. Narrowing of the interosseous space, reflecting cartilage loss, takes place later than the initial soft tissue swelling. Such narrowing is uniform in a given joint and perhaps reflects the greater importance of synovial fluid enzymatic degradation of cartilage than direct erosion by the granulomatous pannus (Figs. 5–19, 5–20).[149,238] This

involvement is recognized by the simple loss of distance that separates the articular ends of bone when viewed tangentially. A false interpretation of narrowing of the cartilage may result from oblique projections or when flexion contractures exist. In early disease, a comparison of the interosseous space with that of adjacent or contralateral uninvolved joints is essential. Weight-bearing views of the larger joints of the lower extremities are helpful. Occasional apparent widening of the joint may reflect capsular distention by hypertrophied synovium and excessive fluid, accompanied by joint laxity. In late disease, the interosseous space may be irregularly narrow or widened by a result of the advanced destruction and fragmentation of subchondral bone and the disruption of supporting capsular and ligamentous structures.

Osteopenia. Regional osteoporosis generally accompanies soft tissue swelling in RA. Initially, it is most apparent in the periarticular regions that contain predominantly trabecular bone, which has a high surface-to-volume ratio and resorbs rapidly with increased local blood flow.[115,135,344] This resorption of cancellous bone produces periarticular demineralization (Figs. 5–19 to 5–21). It is indi-

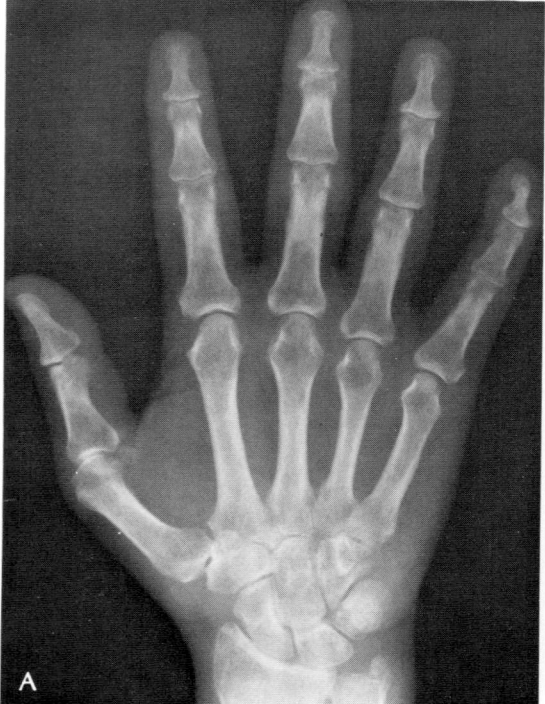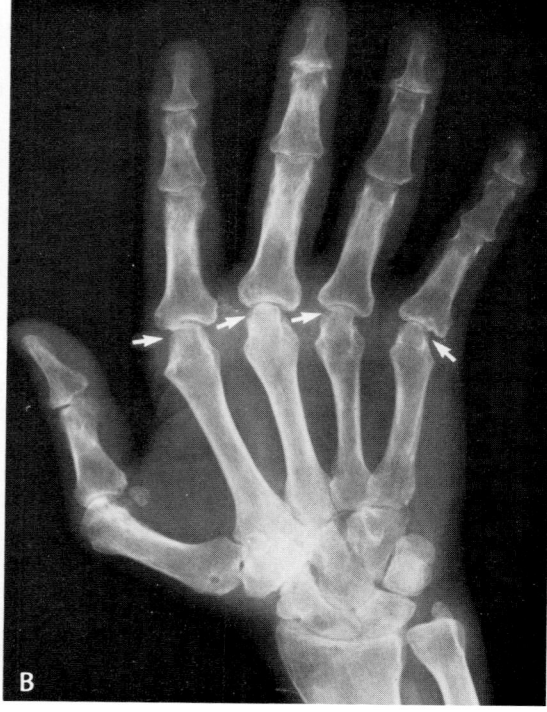

Fig. 5–19. Evolution of changes in rheumatoid arthritis. *A,* Early changes consist of mild periarticular soft tissue swelling and demineralization accompanied by minimal uniform cartilage narrowing, best seen here in the radiocarpal and third distal interphalangeal joints. *B,* Two years later, demineralization, articular destruction (arrows), and typical metacarpophalangeal and wrist deformity have occurred. Subluxation of the first metacarpophalangeal joint, an early finding, has progressed, and ulnar deviation of these joints has begun.

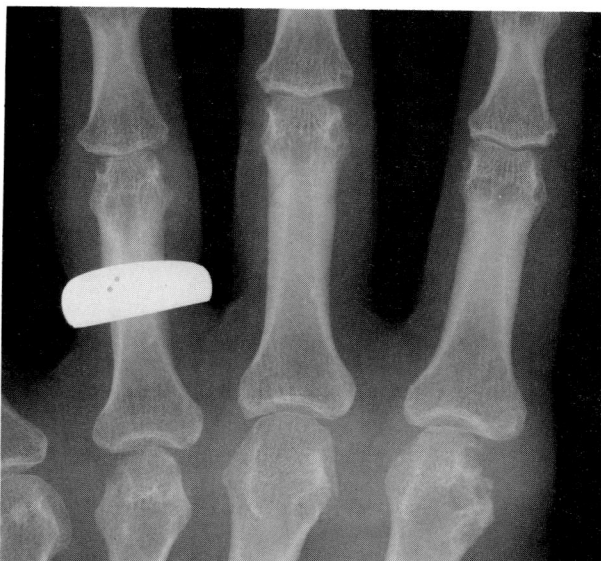

Fig. 5–20. Proximal interphalangeal and metacarpophalangeal joints in rheumatoid arthritis demonstrating typical surface and deeper pocketed erosions at the bases of the middle phalanges and over the condylar surfaces of the proximal phalanges and metacarpals. Cartilage loss is variable, and soft tissue swelling is associated with the erosive changes.

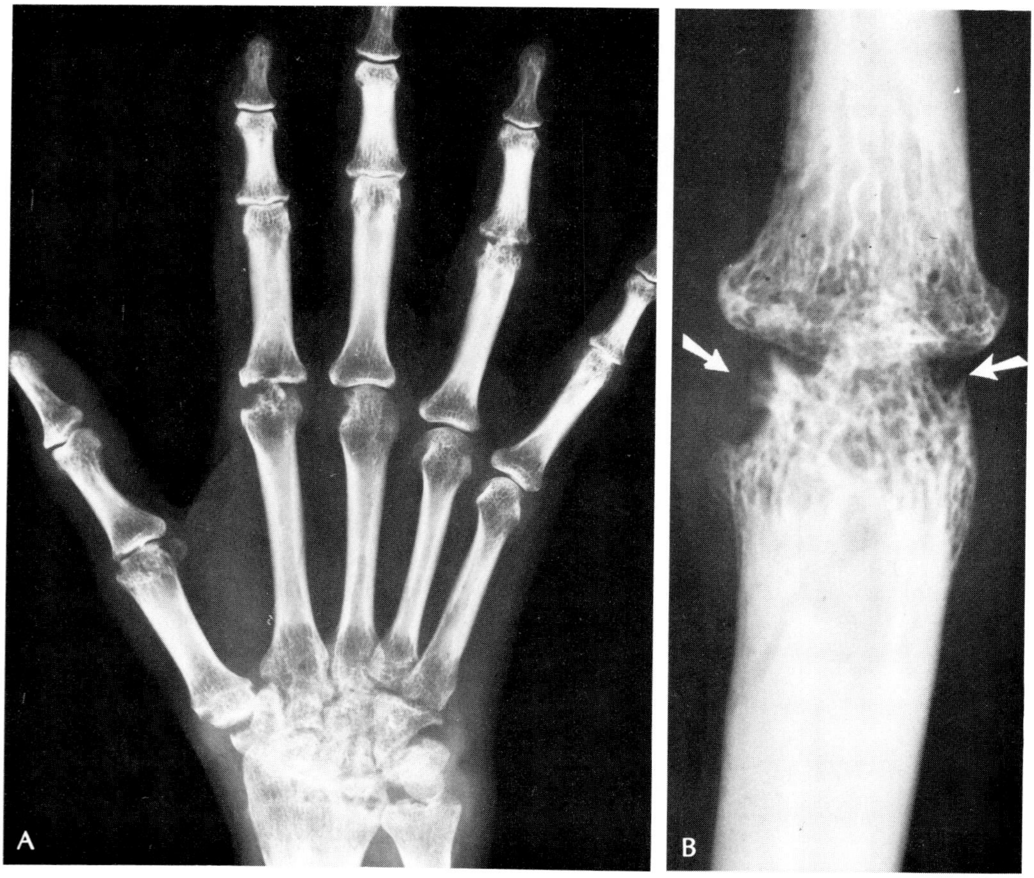

Fig. 5–21. *A*, Typical radiographic changes of moderately advanced rheumatoid arthritis with periarticular demineralization, cartilage narrowing, erosive disease showing a proximal distribution, and sparing of the distal interphalangeal joints. *B*, Magnification of the fourth proximal interphalangeal joint demonstrates fusiform soft tissue swelling and extensive erosion (arrows) of the head of the proximal phalanx.

cated by increased radiolucency and, occasionally, by a relative accentuation of the primary trabeculae as the secondary trabeculae are resorbed. Cortical bone may later be lost, as evidenced by irregular endosteal resorption that produces scalloped inner cortical surfaces and by intracortical resorption that causes linear striation or "tunneling" from widened resorptive spaces.[115,224,344] The relative importance of hyperemia, local metabolic factors, and disuse in mediating the cancellous and cortical bone loss in early and middle stages of the disease is controversial and probably multifarious. In late disease, the regional, irregular, patchy osteopenia is superseded by a more uniform demineralization that parallels the generalized atrophy of soft tissue and cartilage (see Fig. 5–26).[119,344,346] Disuse, immobilization, and, in some instances, corticosteroid therapy contribute to this generalized osteopenia.

Occasionally, a destructive arthropathy is seen in RA, but osseous mineralization, both cancellous and cortical, is well maintained. This change appears most frequently in laborers and in stoic individuals who maintain high levels of physical activity despite inflammatory joint disease (see Figs. 5–24, 5–25).[53] Conversely, occasionally severe osteopenia is seen when articular destruction is minimal, especially in patients without physical demands on their joints and with weak muscles and a low threshold of pain.

Erosion. Articular erosions, a form of bone resorption along the surface of subchondral compact bone, are the most distinctive radiologic manifestation of RA. Their radiographic appearance provides an important parameter for serial assessment of activity of disease and response to therapy.[180,224] Erosions are usually preceded by soft tissue swelling and focal osteopenia, features that are more sensitive, but less specific. The osteopenia frequently affects the joints likely to become involved in the more definitive erosive process (see Figs. 5–19 to 5–21, 5–27). Erosions generally begin at the joint margin in the region of synovial reflection where the cartilage ends and the capsule inserts (the "bare" areas of exposed bone) (see Fig. 5–25).[17,228,238] In this area, as pannus develops and erodes cartilage locally, the underlying cortical and deeper cancellous bone becomes rarefied and indistinct, and is later focally destroyed, producing the initial *surface erosion.* This process results in a characteristic "dot-dash" or serrated appearance of the cortical line (see Figs. 5–1, 5–24, 5–27).[16,41,97] The location of these early erosive changes is constant and predictable for a given joint, as dictated by its anatomic features and the radiographic projection.

As the erosive process advances, greater destruc-

tion and resorption of bone produce a whittled or, alternatively, cavitated appearance (Figs. 5–19, 5–20, 5–22, 5–23). This latter manifestation, termed "pocketed erosion," appears cystic when viewed en face, but when viewed tangentially, it has a broad, serrated interface with the joint surface (Fig. 5–24).[126,282,346] A similar cystic appearance, termed "geode" or "pseudocyst," is an uncommon complication of RA and other specific joint afflictions.[53,220,282,297] Single or multiple, variably sized, subchondral, cyst-like radiolucencies develop, particularly in weight-bearing or heavily used joints and appear completely intraosseous radiographically (Figs. 5–22, 5–25). Their pathogenesis involves penetration of subchondral cortex by proliferating pannus, usually at the joint margin, with subsequent expansion into the weak cancellous bone. The original osteum (opening into the joint space) of the geode is frequently not detected radiographically, but is usually identifiable in histologic sections.[68]

In late articular erosions of RA, extensive destruction accompanied by resorption and occasional fragmentation may be seen.[293] Bizarre osseous deformities result from the stress of altered joint mechanics and the limited shearing strength of bone tissue. The adjacent bare, unprotected articular ends of bone in these patients may become tapered or may resemble a "pencil in cup" (Fig. 5–26).[131] Rarely, if resorption is extreme, an "arthritis mutilans" picture may result, although this manifestation is more common in psoriatic arthritis. As in any process that causes loss of cartilage and weakening of the supporting structures, secondary degenerative changes consisting of reactive sclerosis or subchondral eburnation may develop, but in RA, osteophyte formation is usually minimal or absent.

Alignment. As disease progresses and capsular, ligamentous, and tendinous structures become weakened or destroyed, diastasis, subluxation, or eventual dislocation may take place (Figs. 5–19, 5–26). These changes are most common in the small peripheral joints and in the cervical spine. Altered joint mechanics and muscle imbalance contribute to this appearance, and the manner of joint deformity is determined by the specific local anatomic features. In any event, restriction of joint mobility and flexion deformity resulting from chronic inflammation and secondary fibrosis are to be expected in well-established disease.

Ankylosis. Bony ankylosis, although not prominent in adult RA, develops in approximately 10% of patients with advanced disease and involves predominantly the peripheral joints, especially the carpal and tarsal joints.[223]

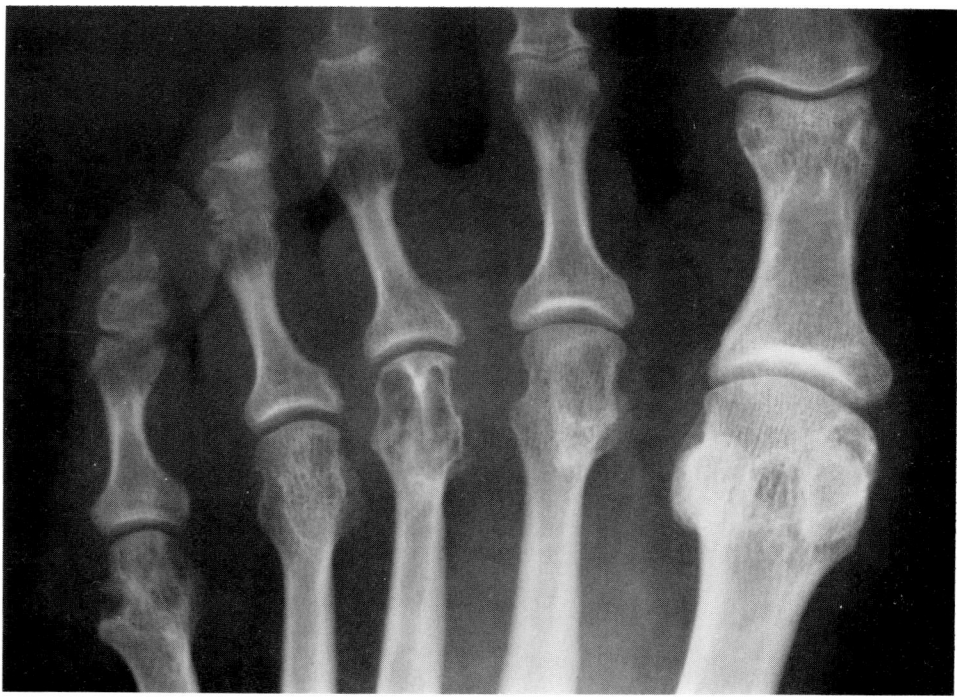

Fig. 5–22.   Foot in rheumatoid arthritis showing typical surface and deeper pocketed erosions involving the metatarsal heads as well as the interphalangeal joint of the first digit. Relative preservation of cartilage and mineralization is a common finding in the weight-bearing foot.

Findings in Specific Joints

The general radiographic findings as described apply broadly, but specific joints express disease variably and deserve further analysis.

Hands and Wrists. Clinicians and radiologists alike have focused particularly on the hands and wrists in RA because of the early involvement (Fig. 5–27), the functional importance, the characteristic appearance of the disease at these sites, and the ease with which high-quality radiographs of these thin body parts are obtained.[17,43,224,238,347]

The most common sites of early involvement include the ulnar styloid, the first through the third metacarpophalangeal joints, and the second and third proximal interphalangeal joints (Fig. 5–28). Involvement of the proximal interphalangeal joints usually is easily recognized from the fusiform soft tissue swelling, often accompanied by regional osteopenia. Uniform cartilage loss occurs early at this site, and erosion appears later. Erosive disease, which parallels the synovial and capsular anatomic features, is extensive over the proximal phalangeal condyles and is more limited over the base of the distal phalanges (see Figs. 5–20, 5–21). Flexion or extension deformities are frequent in advanced disease; bony ankylosis is rare. Erosive articular disease rarely is seen in the distal interphalangeal joints, although swelling and tenderness are common.[209,346]

Soft tissue swelling in the metacarpophalangeal joints, although clinically prominent, is more difficult to evaluate than in the proximal interphalangeal joints, but this swelling appears as discrete capsular distention in high-quality radiographs.[17,96,224] The cartilage at this site becomes narrow later, whereas erosion, particularly of the radial aspect of the metacarpal head, is an early and important sign of RA.[43,97] Small, discrete, pocketed erosions develop at the proximal phalangeal base near the capsular insertion. As the erosive process evolves, narrowing ensues, and eventually complete destruction of the joint with ''pencil in cup'' deformity is seen, accompanied by palmar subluxation and ulnar deviation (see Fig. 5–26).

In the wrist (see Fig. 5–27), soft tissue swelling is usually prominent and is easily recognized, particularly adjacent to the ulnar styloid, as a result of synovitis of the extensor carpi ulnaris tendon sheath. This involvement frequently leads to characteristic focal demineralization and surface erosion of the medial ulnar styloid. Additional erosion of the distal ulna results from synovitis of the pre-

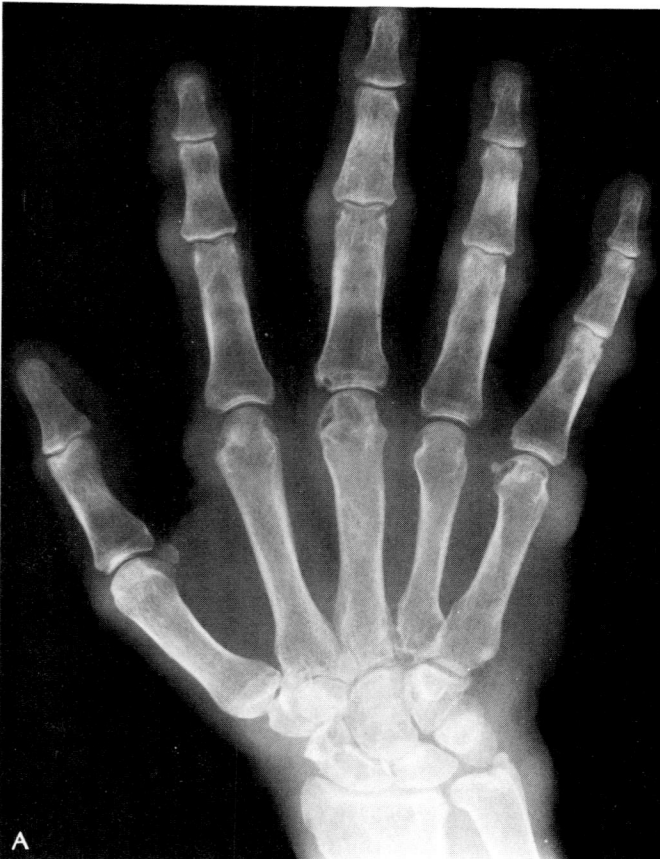

Fig. 5–23. *A*, Striking, nodular, soft tissue swelling, predominantly asymmetric and advanced, subchondral, cyst-like erosions are seen in this patient with "rheumatoid nodulosis." *B*, The left wrist of the same patient demonstrates striking geode (pseudocyst) formation with preservation of mineralization, cartilage space, and articular surfaces.

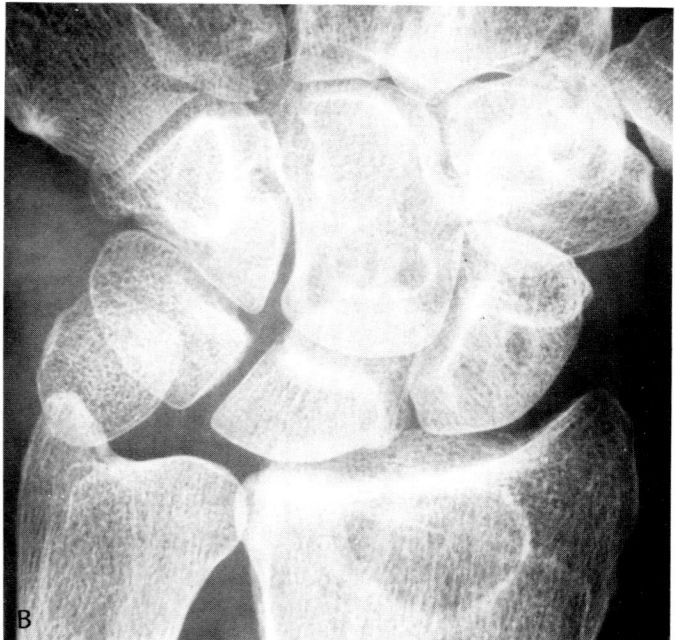

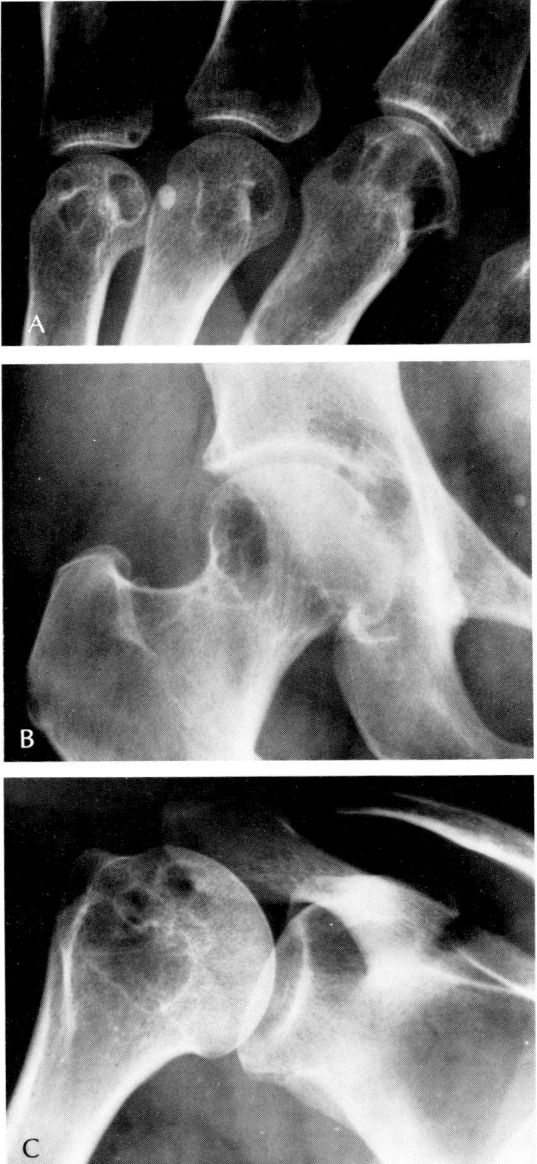

Fig. 5–24. Deep, cystic, pocketed erosions at the chondro-osseous junctions of the metacarpal heads *(A)*, the hip *(B)*, and the shoulder *(C)*. Notice the relative preservation of mineralization and cartilage space in these examples of "robust" rheumatoid arthritis.

styloid recess that erodes the tip of the styloid and from synovitis in the inferior radioulnar compartment that erodes the foveal region.[287] Other early and common sites of erosion include the waist of the navicular, the radial styloid, the pisiform and triquetrum bones, and the palmar aspect of the distal radial articular surface.[238] Cartilaginous loss occurs early at the wrist (see Fig. 5–19) and is uniform throughout the various compartments, owing to development of early, abnormal com-

munications among these separate spaces.[151] In RA, joints that communicate are involved simultaneously and uniformly.[228.238]

Anatomic alignment at the wrist generally becomes altered, with medial migration of the carpus at the radiocarpal joint,[59] which allows the navicular bone to occupy the hollow of the radius (see (Figs. 5–19, 5–25). This rotational change may result in foreshortening of the navicular and lunate bones. Frequently, a widened space is seen be-

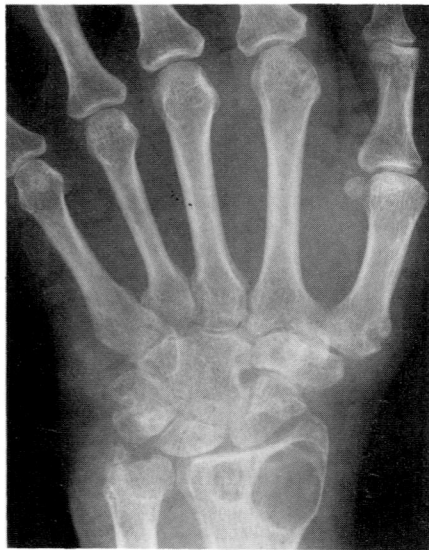

Fig. 5–25. The wrist in rheumatoid arthritis demonstrates a large subchondral cyst (geode) in the distal radius and soft tissue swelling with erosion at the ulnar styloid.

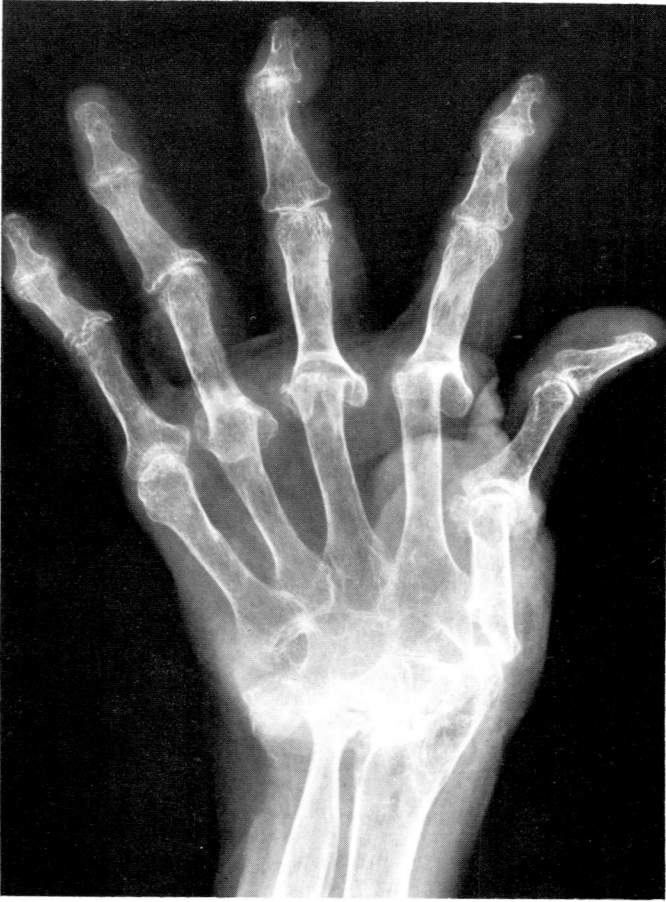

Fig. 5–26. Advanced rheumatoid arthritis showing soft tissue atrophy, severe generalized osteoporosis, resorption, and fragmentation of the metacarpophalangeal and wrist joints, accompanied by remodeling of bone.

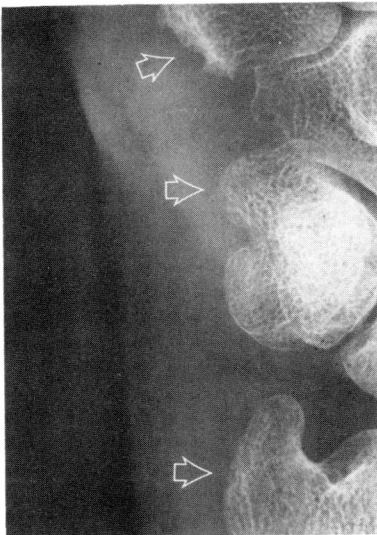

Fig. 5–27. Early changes in rheumatoid arthritis consist of soft tissue swelling adjacent to the surface erosions (arrows) at the ulnar styloid, the triquetrum, and the base of the fifth metacarpal.

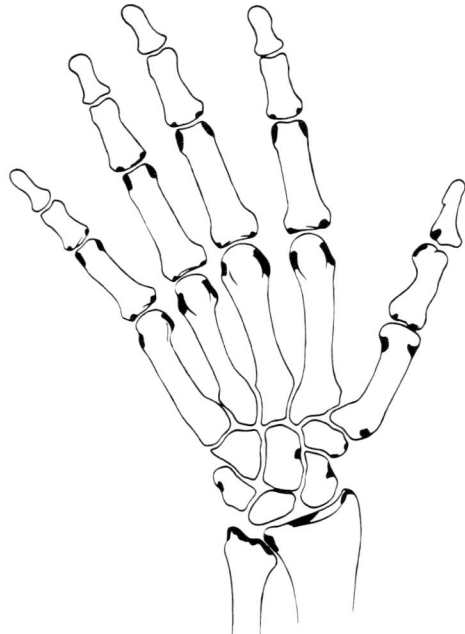

Fig. 5–28. Schematic representation of the hand demonstrating the frequent sites of early erosion in rheumatoid arthritis.

tween the navicular and capitate bones. Involvement of the inferior radioulnar compartment with destruction of the triangular cartilage results in diastasis and, occasionally, in complete dorsal dislocation of the distal ulna. In the lateral view, either dorsal or palmar subluxation and deviation of the carpus in regard to the distal radius may be seen. Bony ankylosis is more common at the carpus than at any other site. Finally, a near-total resorption or fragmentation, or both, of the carpus, penciling of the distal ulna, and cup-shape resorption of the distal radius are seen in end-stage disease (see Figs. 5–12, 5–26).[131,293]

Feet. Rheumatoid involvement of the feet (see Fig. 5–22) is as frequent as, or more frequent than, that of the hand, although unlike the hand, the feet may be abnormal radiographically while clinically silent.[36,46,356] For this reason, radiographs of the forefeet should be obtained if the diagnosis is in question, as well as to evaluate the extent of disease. Characteristically, soft tissue swelling and osteopenia are detected initially in the metatarsophalangeal joints, particularly the fourth and fifth.[47,228,346] These early, nonspecific changes are followed by surface or pocketed erosions of the metatarsal heads that eventually develop into large, cystic erosions or geodes possibly resembling gout.[282] Abnormal separation of the metatarsal heads may result from capsular distension accompanied by weakening and destruction of ligamentous structures, to produce a "spread foot" appearance.

Other characteristic deformities include hallux valgus, which may become extreme, and hammer or cocked-up toes. Cocked-up toes are caused by hyperextension at the metatarsophalangeal joints, with inferior subluxation of the proximal phalanges and hyperflexion of the proximal or distal interphalangeal joints.[47] Fibular deviation of the forefoot is frequent and may be associated with midfoot deformities, such as pes cavus from contracture of the plantar fascia or, less commonly, flatfoot. Erosive disease may develop in the interphalangeal joints, but this is difficult to detect radiographically except in the first phalangeal joint because of the accompanying deformities of the toes. Tarsal involvement simulates that seen in the carpus. Although the talonavicular joint space is frequently the first to undergo narrowing and destruction, the entire tarsal articulation is soon uniformly narrowed. Erosive disease is not always prominent, whereas bony ankylosis is common in late disease.

The heel is involved in 2.5 to 6% of patients and is characterized by swelling of the Achilles tendon and plantar aponeurosis at the insertions of these tendons into the calcaneus.[47,288] The pre-Achilles fat triangle between the tendon and the posterosuperior surface of the calcaneus becomes obliterated by synovitis and fluid in the retrocalcaneal bursa. At these sites, the calcaneus becomes demineralized focally and is then affected by loss of cortical definition and, finally, erosion. Reactive periostitis, although not as prominent as in psoriatic and Reiter's arthritis, leads to spur formation.

Large Weight-Bearing Joints of the Lower Extremities. These joints are affected by changes of a similar nature, with some distinctive features. The *knees*, for example, are early sites of clinical involvement, but erosions are late manifestations. Typically, an advanced, uniform, tricompartmental cartilage loss is noted, with or without joint effusion and soft tissue swelling (Figs. 5–29, 5–30). Osteopenia is prominent, except in the immediate subchondral bone, in which a thin zone of sclerosis appears frequently. Osteophytosis is absent or minimal, even·in advanced disease. Erosions, when present, are at the margins of the femoral condyles and at the periphery of the tibial plateau. Flexion contractures are common, but advanced deformity and destruction of the subarticular bone and joint are unusual. Posterior communication into the semimembranosus-gastrocnemius bursa is a common manifestation of recurrent joint effusions. This communication can result in a large accumulation of fluid (Baker's cyst), which occasionally may rupture into the soft tissues of the calf and may simulate thrombophlebitis (see Fig. 5–8).[38] Similarly, the joint may become de-

compressed by the development of large, subarticular geodes.

Hip involvement, although less common, is characterized by periarticular osteopenia and concentric narrowing of cartilage (Fig. 5–31). Subsequent to concentric loss of cartilage, the femoral head migrates axially, with remodeling of the weakened acetabular bone that produces the characteristic protrusio acetabuli. This deformity is particularly common in patients treated with corticosteroids.[4,346] Erosions are more common at this site than in the knee. Reactive sclerosis may develop, but osteophytosis is minor in relation to the amount of joint destruction. Rarely, cystic marginal erosions are a preliminary finding (see Fig. 5–24, *B*).

Shoulder. Rheumatoid involvement of the shoulder is characterized by synovitis of the capsular, tendinous, and bursal structures of the glenohumeral and acromioclavicular articulations (Fig. 5–32).[193] Erosions are most common at the site of insertion of the rotator cuff in the greater tuberosity (see Fig. 5–24, *C*). Destruction and attrition of the supraspinatus tendon may cause abnormal communication between the joint and the subacromial or subdeltoid bursae and may permit the humerus to migrate superiorly to pseudoarticulate with the inferior surface of the acromion. Erosion at the acromioclavicular joint is common and initially leads to widening and, occasionally, to tapering of the distal clavicle. It may be associated with erosion of the inferior aspect of the

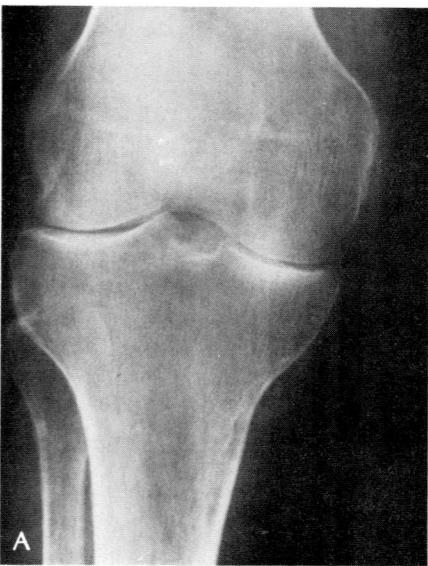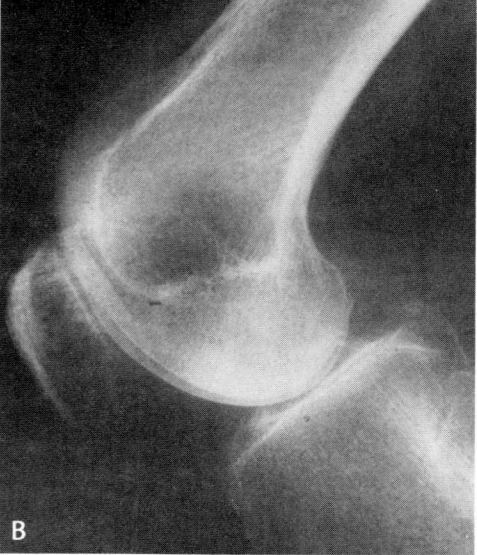

Fig. 5–29. *A,* Anteroposterior views of weight-bearing knees demonstrate bilateral uniform cartilage narrowing and minimal subarticular demineralization, but no osteophytosis. *B,* Similar uniform cartilage loss is seen on a lateral flexion view. The uniform narrowing is characteristic of rheumatoid arthritis. The process is more advanced in the left knee.

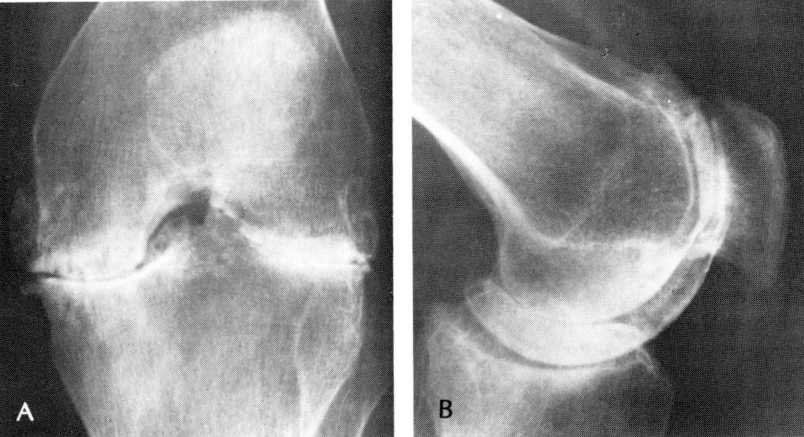

Fig. 5–30. Anteroposterior *(A)* and lateral *(B)* views of moderately advanced changes of rheumatoid arthritis in a knee with complete tricompartmental cartilage loss accompanied by subchondral sclerosis, but minimal osteophytosis.

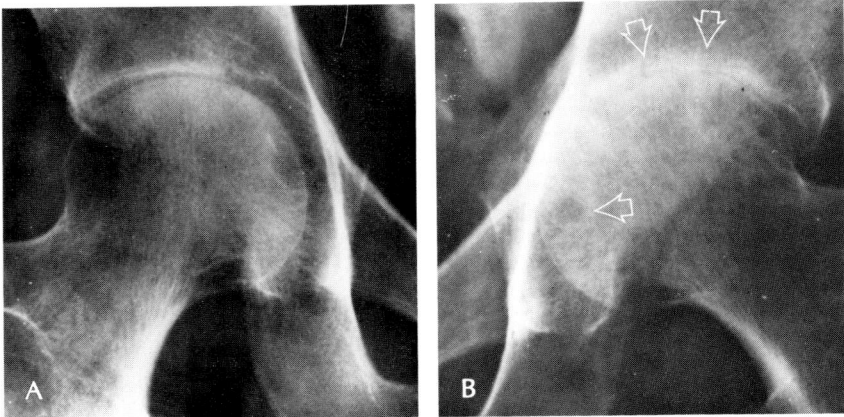

Fig. 5–31. *A,* Hips in moderately advanced rheumatoid arthritis demonstrate bilateral periarticular demineralization and concentric narrowing. *B,* Mild erosion (arrows) of the femoral head and acetabular roof with early protrusio acetabulum.

clavicle at the insertion of the coracoclavicular ligament and with erosion involving the third through seventh ribs posteriorly. Erosion of the ribs may be a pressure-related phenomenon resulting from rubbing by the scapula posteriorly. Scleroderma, poliomyelitis, hyperparathyroidism, and restrictive lung disease have all been associated with similar rib erosion.[347]

Cervical Spine. Because joint motion apparently heightens susceptibility to rheumatoid disease, the frequent affliction of the cervical spine is not surprising, especially in the upper portion, which provides flexion and rotation of the skull. Radiologic evaluation of the cervical spine is important to determine the extent, pattern, and severity of disease. Changes detected usually parallel those in the peripheral joints, although occasionally, advanced radiographic findings may be present in the absence of focal symptoms or generalized disease.[20,60,147,329,377]

The most characteristic radiographic change is subluxation at the atlantoaxial articulation (Fig. 5–33), manifested by abnormal separation between the anterior surface of the odontoid and the posteroinferior surface of the anterior mass of Cl. If this distance in the lateral flexion view exceeds 2.5 to 3 mm in adults, subluxation is established.[62,230] Such subluxation may be attributable to laxity or rupture of the transverse ligament or to erosion of the odontoid. Another indication of subluxation between C1 and C2 is a change in the vertical distance in lateral flexion and extension views, of greater

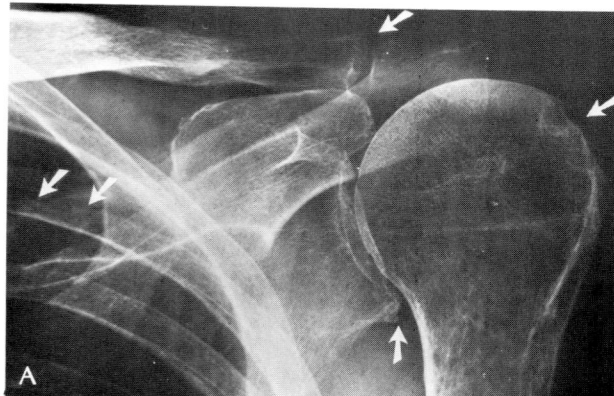

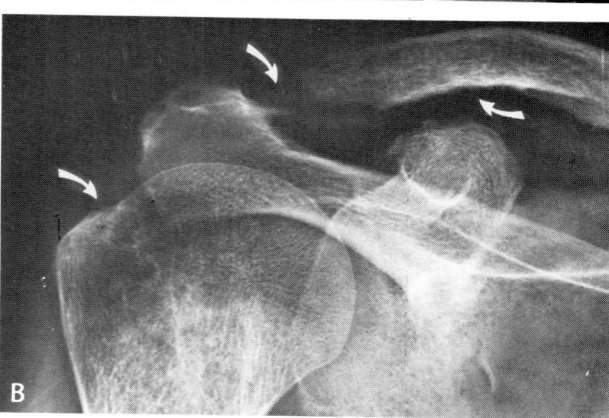

Fig. 5–32. *A,* Shoulder of a patient with rheumatoid arthritis with erosions (arrows) at the inferior glenoid, greater tuberosity, and acromioclavicular joint. The superior subluxation of the humeral head indicates attrition of the supraspinatus tendon. Note also superior rib erosion. *B,* Similar erosive articular disease can be seen in a patient with advanced hyperparathyroidism (curved arrows).

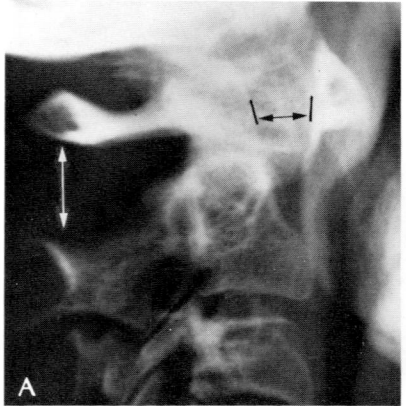
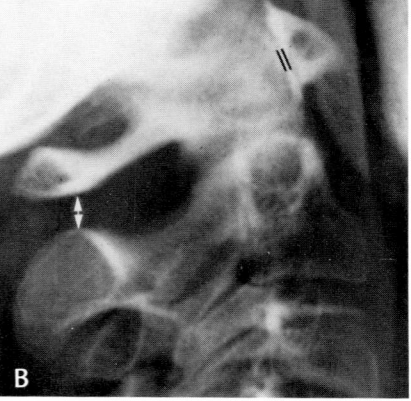

Fig. 5–33. Flexion *(A)* and extension *(B)* views of the cervical spine with C1 to C2 subluxation demonstrate increased separation between the dens (odontoid) and the anterior mass of the atlas (black arrows), as well as excessive vertical motion between the posterior arch of C1 and the spinous process of C2 (white arrows).

than 7 mm between the posterior arch of C1 and the spinous process of C2.[62] Multiple subluxations from C2 to C6 occasionally produce a "stepladder" appearance (Fig. 5–34).[60] The correlation between and radiographic detection of subluxation and neurologic deficit is poor, but prompt recognition of the underlying structural changes is important because neurologic complications are usually reversible with corrective measures.

Narrowing of the apophyseal joints and the disc space, without osteophytosis or eburnation, is common.[20,236,329] The superior cervical levels or, less commonly, the entire cervical spine may be affected. Erosion and destruction produce blurring and obliteration of the apophyseal and neurocentral joints. Similar erosive destruction takes place at the synovial joints of the lateral occipitoatlantoaxial articulations and the anterior and posterior odontoid articulations. The odontoid becomes irregular or pointed and, rarely, may be fractured or entirely resorbed.[230] Extensive erosion and softening of the basiocciput and lateral masses of C1 and C2 may cause vertical subluxation or translocation of the spine with respect to the skull. Basilar invagination or an upturning of the foramen magnum is then recognized by an extension of the tip of the odontoid greater than 4.5 mm superior to McGregor's line. This line connects the hard palate to the most caudad portion of the occipital curvature.[236]

The vertebral end plates become eroded as pannus grows from the neurocentral joints along the posterolateral aspects of the vertebral bodies (Fig. 5–34), whereas mechanical instability contributes to the destruction of the posterior vertebral margins.[227] The end-plate destruction and associated disc narrowing have been termed "rheumatoid discitis" and may simulate septic infection of the disc.[20,62] Rarely, erosions in the posterior elements cause destruction and pointing of the spinous processes, usually of the medial and inferior cervical region (Fig. 5–34). These lesions, like those in the ribs already mentioned, may represent pressure-related or mechanical resorption rather than destruction by pannus.

Generalized osteoporosis of the cervical spine is frequent in RA and may be striking, particularly in active disease.[20,62] In later phases, subchondral sclerosis and secondary degenerative changes may ensue, especially if active synovitis and concomitant hyperemia have subsided.[20] Bony ankylosis of the cervical spine occurs in adult RA much less often than in juvenile RA (JRA) and involves mostly the C2 and C3 apophyseal joints (Fig. 5–34).

The differential diagnosis of adult RA in the cervical spine includes ankylosing spondylitis, psoriatic arthritis, degenerative disc disease, and JRA, all of which are discussed in separate sections of this chapter. RA and primary degenerative disc disease (spondylosis) are usually easily distinguished. Spondylosis typically narrows a disc at one or several levels of the medial or inferior cervical spine,

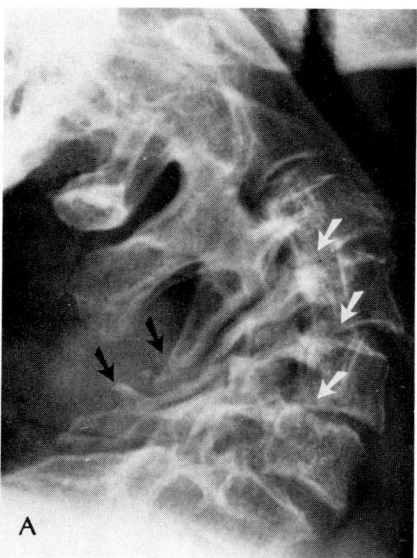 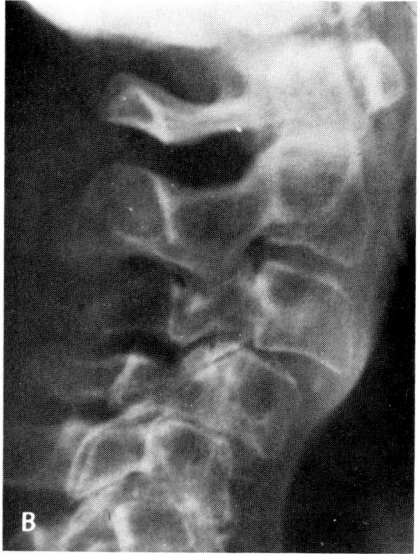

Fig. 5–34.   *A,* Advanced rheumatoid arthritis (RA) of the cervical spine consisting of resorption of the dens (odontoid) and spinous processes (black arrows), ankylosis of the C2 to C3 apophyseal joints, erosions at the joints of Luschka and adjacent end plates (white arrows), moderate disc narrowing, anterior subluxation of C6 to C7, and finally, generalized demineralization. *B,* Typical "stepladder" subluxations and disc narrowing in advanced RA.

accompanied by prominent osteophytosis and sclerosis, but with minimal or no subluxation. Occasionally, RA and degenerative disc disease occur together, resulting in a mixed radiologic appearance that is difficult to interpret.

Juvenile Rheumatoid Arthritis

JRA represents a heterogeneous group of childhood arthritides of which seronegative polyarthritis, or Still's disease, is the largest subgroup and accounts for approximately 70% of cases.[4] Other, smaller subgroups include seropositive adultpattern RA in late childhood and ankylosing spondylitis (HLA-B27-positive).[4,318] This discussion is concerned predominantly with the first subgroup, that is, Still's disease or JRA. In addition to the appreciable difference in the systemic manifestations that accompany JRA, as compared to adult RA, the specific radiographic manifestations also vary. In general, the articular manifestations of JRA are milder, are less symmetric, and are more likely to be monoarticular or pauciarticular. Involvement of the cervical spine is greater, destruction of cartilage and bone occurs later, reactive periosteal new bone is more common, and disturbance of growth and maturation is more severe.[4,142,239,347]

JRA is initially monoarticular in about one-third of patients, but it usually becomes pauciarticular or polyarticular. A few patients have polyarthritis at the onset of disease. The joints most commonly involved are the knees, ankles, wrists, hands, feet, cervical spine, and hips.[4,142,239,346]

Early changes in the knees consist of effusion of the joint and periarticular osteoporosis, followed by prominent overgrowth of the distal femoral epiphysis and, to a lesser extent, of the proximal tibia. The patella may be enlarged, and its inferior aspect may be deformed, producing concavity or squaring. The femoral and tibial shafts appear slender and have thin or atrophic cortices. Skeletal maturation is accelerated, with alterations in linear growth, which may be advanced or retarded.[31] Similar changes may be noted in hemophilia, tuberculosis, and pigmented villonodular synovitis. In time, the interosseous space becomes narrow, but erosive articular changes are uncommon. Compression fractures of the epiphyses may produce a flattened appearance.[7,239] Metaphyseal radiolucent bands may simulate those of leukemia and acute disuse osteoporosis.[239,346] Later, sclerotic growtharrest lines may be seen in the metaphyseal regions.

The wrists and hands are commonly involved in JRA, particularly the carpus, in which early loss of cartilage is accompanied by an angular appearance of the carpal bones that results from accelerated but abnormal maturation (Figs. 5–35, 5–36).[4,239,346] The disease progresses to ankylosis in approximately 10% of patients, whereas extensive carpal erosive destruction is usual.[223,243] The metacarpophalangeal and proximal interphalangeal joints are less often involved than in adult RA, but involvement of the distal interphalangeal joints is more common. Soft tissue swelling of the small joints of the hands may be present, or an associated periosteal reaction, initially near sites of capsular insertion, but later involving the entire shaft. Such periosteal reaction may be the sole osseous manifestation in JRA and, in advanced phases, may result in a peculiar rectangular shape of the tubular bones (Figs. 5–35, 5–37, 5–38).[239,346]

Overgrowth of the capital femoral epiphysis, increased obliquity of the acetabular roof, lateral subluxation, coxa valga, shortening of the femoral neck, and overgrowth of the lesser trochanter are all prominent features. Protrusio acetabuli is far less common than in adults, but is seen in children with late onset of the disease, particularly those who receive corticosteroid treatment.[346] A proliferative collar of new bone formation at the chondro-osseous junction may be seen in late stages, but is less common than in ankylosing spondylitis.[250] Bony ankylosis occurs less often than in the carpus, tarsus, or cervical spine (Fig 5–39). Rarely, late reconstitution of articular cartilage "space" is observed radiographically.[18] Involvement of the temporomandibular joint is common in well-established disease and may result in micrognathia because of retardation at the proximal endochondral growth center.[239] Frequently, with this involvement, no specific symptoms are related to the temporomandibular joint. Both the body and the ramus of the joint may be shortened, and the antagonal notch becomes prominent.

Cervical spine abnormalities in JRA are generally more frequent and more severe than in adult RA, and the pattern of disease differs.[4,142,239,346] The characteristic widespread ankylosis of apophyseal joints and subsequent hypoplasia of the vertebrae are unique to JRA (see Fig. 51–3). The early onset of osteophytosis and of eburnation is also common as a secondary degenerative process caused by destruction of cartilage. Subluxation at C1 to C2, however, is frequent in both RA and JRA. The apophyseal joints characteristically fuse early in JRA. Multiple levels are usually involved and produce a rigid cervical spine. Fusion of the vertebral bodies is less frequent and occurs generally in response to ankylosis or immobilization of the posterior elements. When the spine is fused early in childhood, abnormal growth and development of the vertebral bodies and discs result in a dwarfed appearance.[239,242] Erosion of neurocentral joints and of vertebral endplates does not take place, in con-

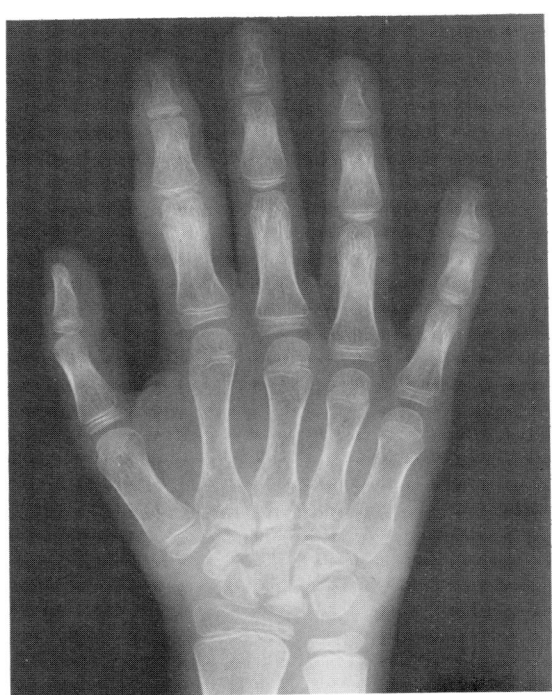

Fig. 5–35. Characteristic radiographic changes in juvenile rheumatoid arthritis consisting of prominent soft tissue swelling involving the second and fifth digits and the wrist. The most advanced change, at the carpus, consists of irregular cartilage loss and early erosive disease. The second digit demonstrates periosteal new bone or cloaking involving the proximal phalanx and resulting in a club-like enlargement, when compared with adjacent proximal phalanges.

Fig. 5–36. Radiograph of the right hand in juvenile rheumatoid arthritis demonstrating mild flexion deformities, prominent pericapsular and tendinous calcifications resulting from local corticosteroid injections, and bone infarction of the distal ulna related to systemic corticosteroid therapy.

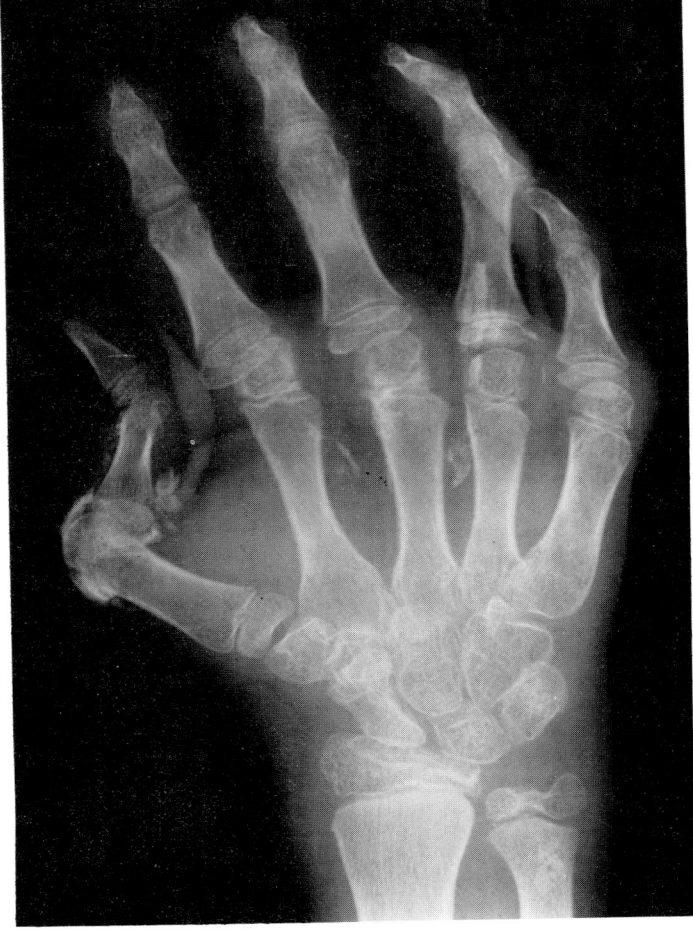

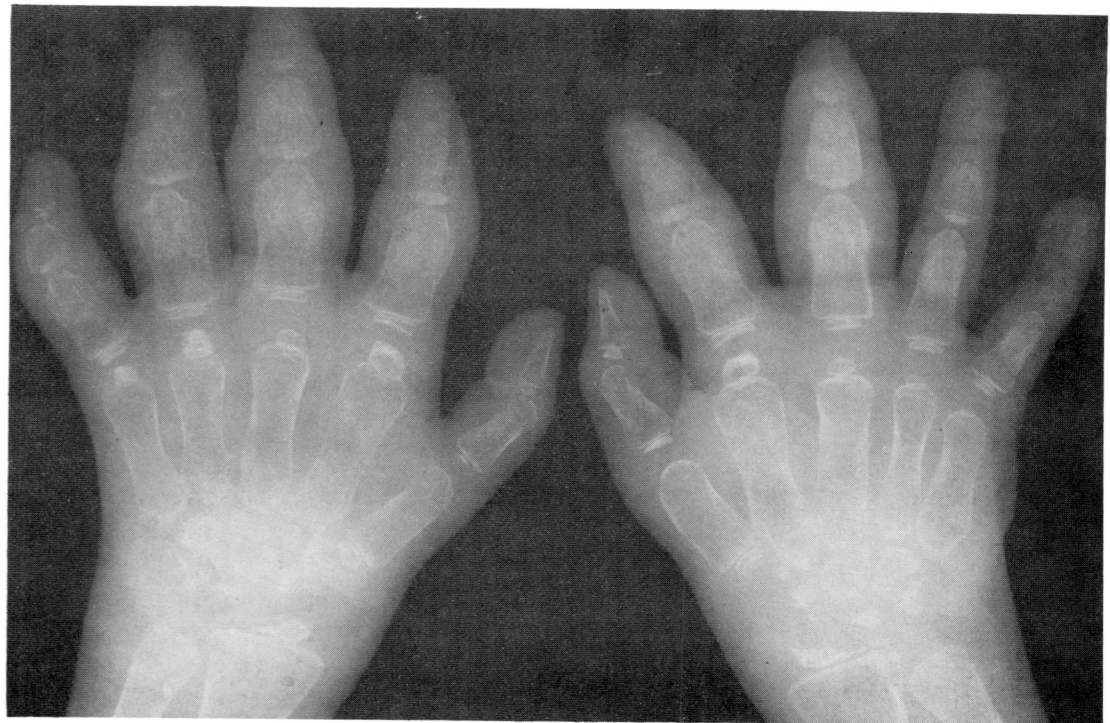

Fig. 5–37. Radiograph of hands and wrists of a patient with juvenile rheumatoid arthritis showing generalized soft tissue swelling. Periosteal new-bone formation (''cloaking'') has produced a rectangular configuration of the tubular bones. Advanced resorption, destruction, and sclerosis of the carpus have occurred.

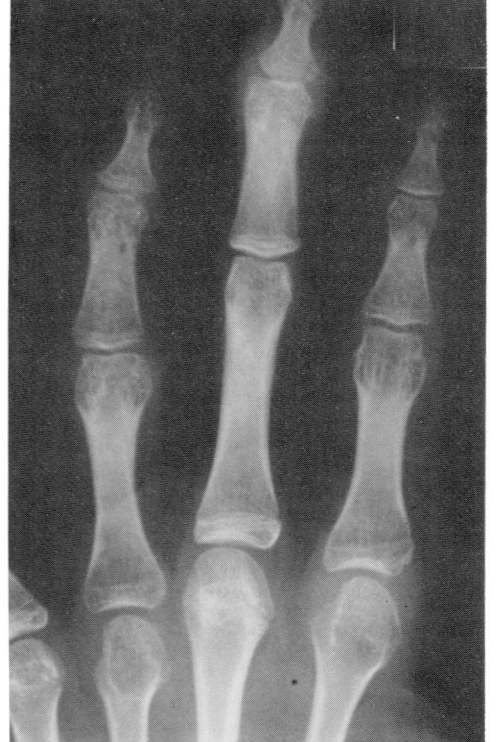

Fig. 5–38. Dramatic alteration in growth patterns in juvenile rheumatoid arthritis are demonstrated by shortening of the fourth metacarpal bone, related to premature fusion of the epiphysis, and club-like overgrowth of the second and fourth phalangeal heads and the third and fourth middle phalangeal heads.

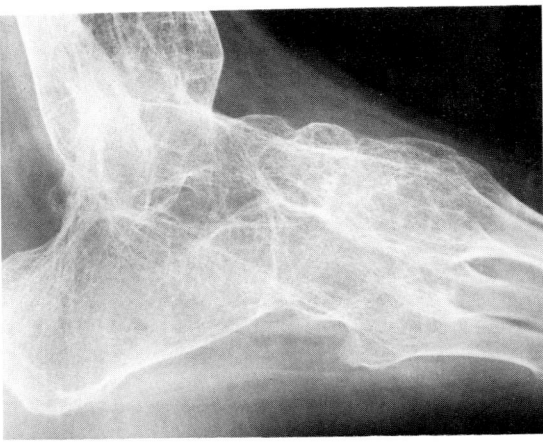

Fig. 5–39. Complete ankylosis of the hindfoot and ankle in a patient with juvenile rheumatoid arthritis. Trabeculae crossing the "joint space" are the hallmark of true bony ankylosis.

trast to adult RA. Vertebral compressive fractures are common as a consequence of the osteoporosis of the disease process and corticosteroid therapy.[4] These fractures occur predominantly in the thoracic spine and result in wedge deformity and occasionally in scoliosis. The sacroiliac joints are not usually involved, except in HLA-B27-positive boys, and are rarely symptomatic.[4,235] The radiographic manifestations consist of mild erosion with little reactive sclerosis, and only rarely ankylosis.

The radiographic differentiation between JRA and ankylosing spondylitis or psoriatic arthritis may be difficult, particularly in the cervical spine, because of the frequent ankylosis in these disorders. In JRA, however, extensive involvement of the sacral, lumbar, and thoracic joints and ossification of the paraspinal ligaments are rare and help to differentiate this condition.[9] The radiographic appearance of JRA and that of hemophiliac arthropathy may overlap, although the hemophiliac disorder has a greater tendency for pauciarticular involvement, subchondral cyst formation, and secondary reactive sclerosis (Fig. 5–40), perhaps because of the remitting nature of this disorder.

Systemic Lupus Erythematosus

Systemic lupus erythematosus (SLE) is a chronic disease with many manifestations, of which polyarthralgia and polyarthritis are the most common. Nearly 50% of patients have these symptoms initially, and in more than 90% they develop eventually. Exclusive of soft tissue swelling, radiographic changes occur in only 5 to 30% of these patients.[75,84,154] As in RA, involvement is frequently polyarticular and symmetric, with an iden-

tical pattern of joint involvement. Unlike in RA, severe progressive joint destruction is rare.[21,75,262]

In the hands, the most common finding is nonspecific soft tissue swelling, either fusiform from capsular distention or more generalized from tenosynovitis. Rarely, eccentric, lumpy, soft tissue swelling is present as a result of rheumatoid nodules.[143] The proximal interphalangeal, metacarpophalangeal, and wrist articulations are predominantly affected by these soft tissue changes. Periarticular osteoporosis is seen in approximately 20% of patients, and more generalized osteoporosis which is frequent in late disease, is often accentuated by corticosteroid therapy.[21] Mild, uniform narrowing of the cartilage is seen in a minority of patients.

The most characteristic radiographic change is pronounced joint deformity, without erosive or destructive bony alteration (Fig. 5–41). The synovitis of SLE is much milder than that of RA, without pannus and granulation tissue, and does not result in erosive disease. Rather, the periarticular, capsular, and ligamentous supporting structures are involved and account for the characteristic displacement and angular deformities.[5,21,32,190,192] Most commonly, ulnar deviation and volar subluxation of the metacarpophalangeal joints, hyperextension at the proximal interphalangeal joints, flexion of the distal interphalangeal joints, and ulnar drift of the radiocarpal mass take place. These manifestations are easily reducible, unlike those in RA, and do not produce significant disability. Occasionally, the tendons in the hands may rupture completely and may require surgical repair. The amount of deformity and malalignment appears to correlate with the chronicity of disease. The rare patient with SLE with destructive bony changes probably has concomitant RA (overlap syndrome)[21,179] or avascular necrosis.

Avascular necrosis is seen in approximately 5% of patients with SLE, usually in those taking corticosteroids.[156,188,200,363] Most commonly this disorder affects the femoral heads and is indistinguishable from other causes of avascular necrosis. Other sites include the distal femoral condyle, humeral head, talus, and carpus. Articular collapse and fragmentation accompanied by sclerosis may simulate primary destructive arthropathies.

Soft tissue calcification in the form of subcutaneous linear densities, lumps, and plaques, vascular calcification, or, less commonly, small, punctate calcifications around joints may be found in approximately 5 to 10% of patients with SLE.[39,177] These changes, most frequent in the legs, are associated with ulceration of the skin. The soft tissue calcifications in SLE are nonspecific and are found with greater frequency and severity in other con-

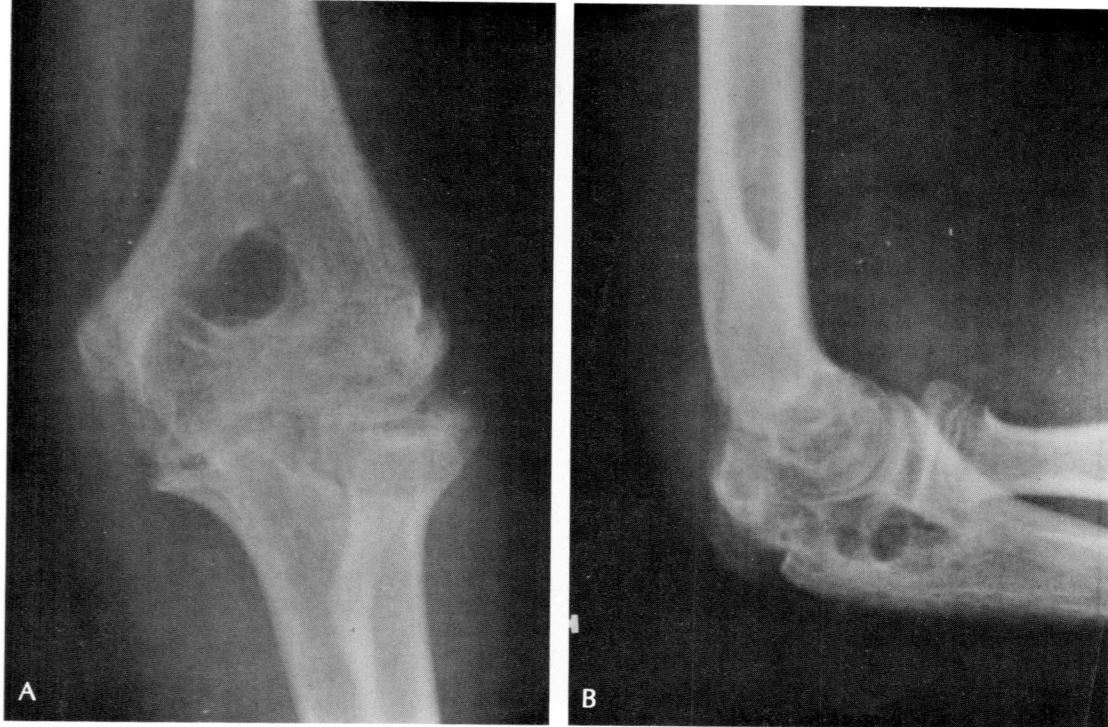

Fig. 5–40. Anteroposterior *(A)* and lateral *(B)* radiographs of the elbow with hemophiliac arthropathy. Changes consist of irregular cartilage loss, deformity of the articular surfaces, large subchondral cyst formation, and reactive sclerosis.

nective tissue disorders, particularly progressive systemic sclerosis (PSS) and dermatomyositis.

Progressive Systemic Sclerosis

PSS (scleroderma) is a generalized disorder of connective tissue characterized by inflammation, fibrosis, and degeneration.[349] The frequent clinical manifestations of Raynaud's phenomenon and arthralgia are associated with characteristic radiographic changes in about two-thirds of these patients.[11,27,204,308,360] Soft tissue atrophy, resorption of bone, flexion contracture, and subcutaneous calcification all appear at various stages of the disease. Within 6 months of the onset of PSS, radiographic changes may be seen in about one-third of patients.[386] During the early, edematous phase, soft tissue swelling in the hands is diffuse, with some periarticular accentuation. It is associated with obliteration of subcutaneous fat lines, periarticular fat, and knuckle folds. The distal pulp of the fingers is atrophied in about 40% of patients, and tapering is a characteristic feature; this radiographic change correlates closely with clinical Raynaud's phenomenon.[386]

Arteriographic study invariably shows partial or complete obliteration of the digital arteries.[338] Periarticular osteoporosis is common. Later, and independent of Raynaud's phenomenon, soft tissue calcification and bony erosion may be seen (Fig. 5–42). Calcinosis, which occurs in 7 to 10% of these patients, is generally a late manifestation and is most common in the palmar aspect of the digital pulp. Occasionally, it appears diffusely in subcutaneous or periarticular structures, such as tendons, capsules, and bursae. This calcification has been identified as hydroxyapatite,[61] which may produce lumps that break through necrotic tissue to the skin surface. Uncommonly, periarticular calcification is seen around the wrists, elbows, shoulders, hips, and knees. Calcification that is intra-articular and produces a chalky effusion is rare (Fig. 5–43).[30,290] A common subgroup of PSS is the CRST syndrome,[365,386] in which calcinosis, Raynaud's phenomenon, sclerodactyly, and telangiectasia are concomitant.

Bony erosion is of several types and is noted in 25 to 40% of patients. Typically, resorption of the distal phalangeal tufts begins in the palmar aspect, occasionally progressing proximally to involve the greater part of the phalanx.[11,319] Rarely, resorption

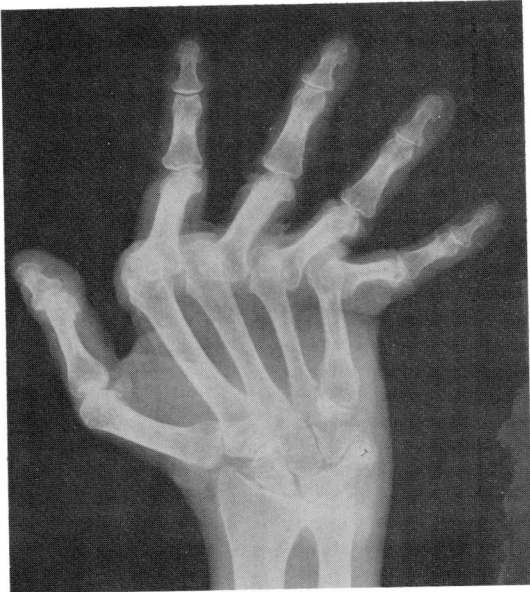

Fig. 5–41. Pronounced joint deformity in systemic lupus erythematosus is evidenced by dislocation and ulnar deviation at the metacarpophalangeal joints and ulnar drift of the carpus.

and lysis of the distal radius, ulna, and clavicle,[132] the superior ribs,[155] and the angle of the mandible[326] have been reported.

The second form of bone resorption is erosive articular disease, which simulates RA in its marginal location,[278,386] but affects distal, more than proximal, joints, and is a late manifestation of disease (Fig. 5–44). These modest erosive changes may reflect the mild, nonproliferative synovitis of PSS. In late stages, when atrophy of soft tissue is pronounced and restriction of motion is advanced, generalized osteoporosis and uniform loss of cartilage are common. Additionally, fixed flexion deformities develop, particularly in the small joints of the hands, elbows, and knees. These deformities may simulate RA, but with fewer erosions, or they may resemble SLE, but are not reducible.

Overlap Syndromes

Connectve-tissue overlap syndromes, in which features of several distinct diseases are concomitant, have been widely reported.[56,83,197,314,333] A recently recognized subgroup has been termed *mixed connective tissue disease* (MCTD) and is associated with a particular antinuclear antibody, the specificity of which is controversial[264,271,328] (see Chaps. 60 and 64).

The radiographic characteristics of MCTD have been examined systematically.[333,362] In the hand, soft tissue atrophy, osteoporosis, soft tissue cal-

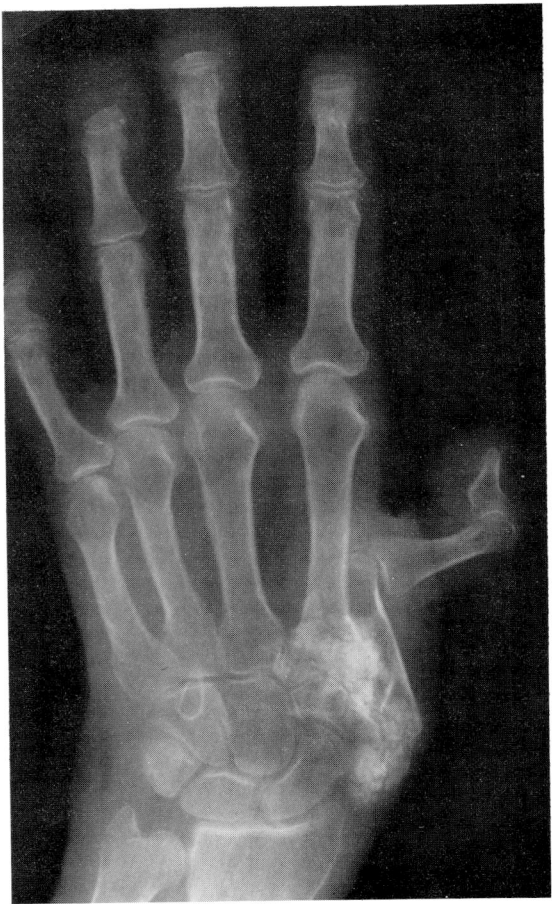

Fig. 5–42. Moderately advanced sclerodermatous changes consisting of resorption of the distal phalangeal tufts, subluxations of the thumb, and prominent periarticular soft tissue calcification near the base of the thumb.

cification, flexion deformities, cartilage narrowing, tuft resorption, and marginal joint erosion may be shown. A given patient may appear normal radiographically or may manifest any combination of these changes, paralleling the clinical diversity of the syndrome. Radiographic features of PSS (tuft resorption and distal interphalangeal erosions), RA (polyarticular erosive disease) (Fig. 5–45), and SLE (deforming, nonerosive arthritis) may be apparent. Of particular interest is the observation of bony erosions in approximately one-third of seronegative patients.

Seronegative Spondyloarthropathy

This section encompasses a group of spondylitic disorders that share many common features. These conditions include ankylosing spondylitis, colitic arthritis, psoriatic arthritis, and Reiter's syndrome. They are characterized clinically and radiographi-

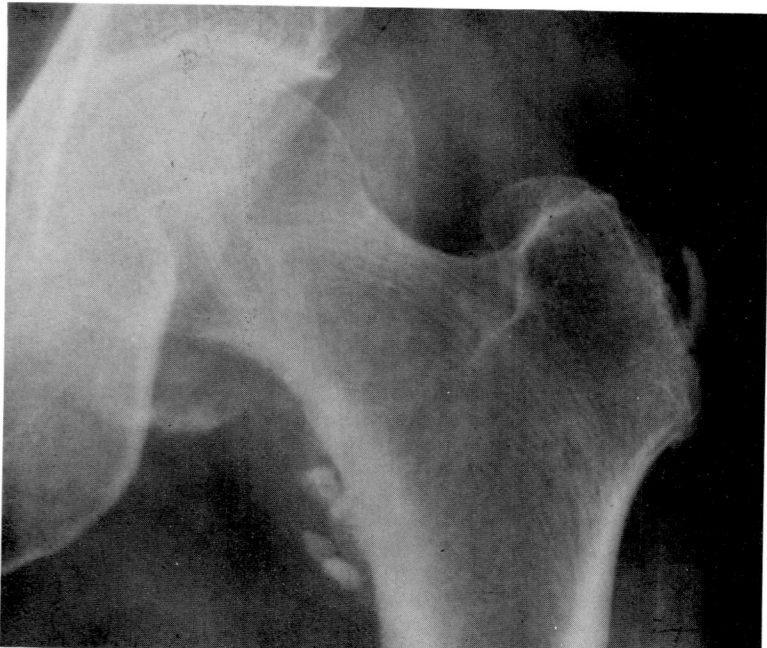

Fig. 5–43. Left hip in scleroderma demonstrating extra-articular calcifications and, in addition, homogeneous increased density representing intra-articular hydroxyapatite accumulation, rare in this disorder.

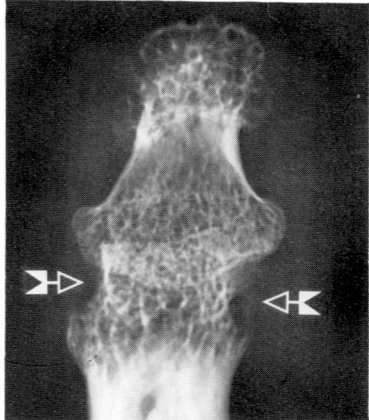

Fig. 5–44. Marginal erosions (arrows) of the distal interphalangeal joint in scleroderma.

cally by prominent axial involvement, proliferative new-bone formation, and bony anky-losis.[15,33,44,110,214,273,324,327] The pathologic changes consist of *enthesopathy*,[9,227,324] that is, inflammation and degeneration at sites of ligamentous or tendinous insertion in bone, which are called *entheses*, and prominent synovitis. These disorders are also linked to the HLA-B27 histocompatibility antigen.[35,89,321,327] Thus, the clinical, radiologic, pathologic, and immunogenetic features permit a

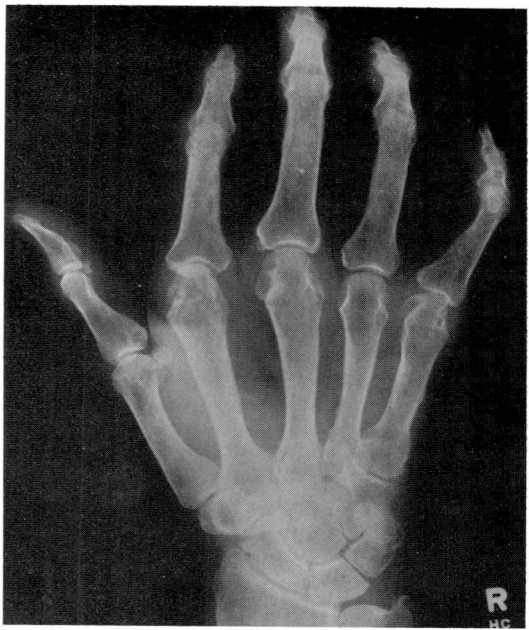

Fig. 5–45. A spectrum of radiographic findings in the hand of mixed connective tissue disease. Atrophy of distal soft tissue pulp, flexion contractures in the distal and proximal interphalangeal joints, marginal erosions at the metacarpophalangeal joints and the ulnar styloid, and ulnar drift of the carpus are all identified.

common grouping of these arthropathies, although their distinctive clinical features allow diagnostic differentiation.

Ankylosing Spondylitis

The use of CT scanning for evaluation of the sacroiliac joints is discussed in Chapter 6.

Ankylosing spondylitis (see also Chap. 53) is an inflammatory condition of unknown origin that occurs predominantly in young men.[67] The axial skeleton is most frequently and most severely involved, although nearly one-third of these patients, particularly adolescents, complain of isolated peripheral joint symptoms.[4,48] In addition to synovitis of the diarthrodial joints, less severe than in RA, these patients have prominent inflammation at ligamentous, tendinous, and capsular attachments to bone (entheses).[9,214,286,294] The most common early clinical symptom is low back pain related to sacroiliitis, which in approximately 90% of patients is noted on initial radiographic examination of this joint.[15] Abnormal sacroiliac joints may be seen radiographically even before the onset of focal symptoms.[48] Almost all male patients have radiographic changes at this site within 12 months of clinical onset of the disorder.[214] Thus, careful radiographic analysis of the sacroiliac joints is important and may require several projections because the articulations are not isoplanar.[15,298] An anteroposterior projection with 20° cephalad angulation of the beam offers an optimal view of the lower portion of the joint, and a 30° anteroposterior oblique projection defines the medial and superior articular surfaces. Alternatively, a single posteroanterior projection, with the patient prone and the beam angled 20° caudad, frequently demonstrates most aspects of the articulation and obviates the need for additional views.[15]

Early radiographic change in the sacroiliac joint consists of loss of the discrete subchondral cortical line, a result of focal absorption and erosion accompanied by reactive sclerosis in the adjacent cancellous bone (Fig. 5–46).[48,324] The iliac side of the articulation is affected first because of its thinner cartilage; the sacral side may initially appear normal.[298,345] At its inception, the process may be unilateral or asymmetric, but it soon becomes bilateral, and eventually symmetric.[15,214] With progressive erosion, joint widening becomes apparent in association with pronounced patchy sclerosis that extends some distance into the subarticular bone. The process may arrest at any phase, but characteristically it progresses to narrowing of the joint and, finally, to intracapsular and intraarticular bony ankylosis. Occasionally, part of the original joint line may persist. Once the joint has fused solidly, the sclerosis resolves gradually, and

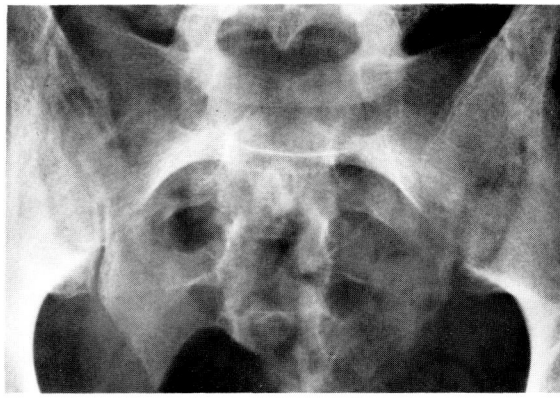

Fig. 5–46. A 20° upshot of the sacrum demonstrates to advantage the inferior aspects of the sacroiliac joints. Early septic sacroiliitis is present on the patient's left, as evidenced by the loss of a discrete subchondral cortical line and by slight joint "widening." Focal demineralization and absence of sclerosis distinguish it from early ankylosing spondylitis.

a generalized osteopenia of the pelvis develops (see Fig. 53–3, *B*).[214,345]

Pelvic Involvement

Radiographic findings in the pelvis are not limited to the sacroiliac joints. Features of generalized enthesopathy include erosion accompanied by prominent periostitis, proliferative bone formation, and reactive sclerosis, seen at the symphysis, the greater or lesser trochanters, and the margins of the ilium and ischium at the insertions of muscles and tendons (Fig. 5–47). The resultant bony spiculation and sclerosis have been termed "whiskering" and are prominent features of established disease.[15,214]

Spinal Involvement

Spinal involvement in ankylosing spondylitis invariably follows sacroiliitis by at least several months and frequently longer.[214] The changes consist of anterior vertebral squaring, syndesmophytosis, apophyseal joint ankylosis, and ligamentous ossification. The changes begin in the lumbar spine and progress predictably and uniformly to involve the thoracic and cervical spinal regions.[214,324] In women with ankylosing spondylitis, cervical involvement may occur without significant thoracic or lumbar involvement.[291] "Squaring" results from a loss of the normal concavity of the anterior surface of the vertebral body. This squaring, an important observation in lateral radiographs, may be caused by osteitis and erosion of the anterosuperior and inferior vertebral margins and may produce the so-called "shiny corners" and the squared ap-

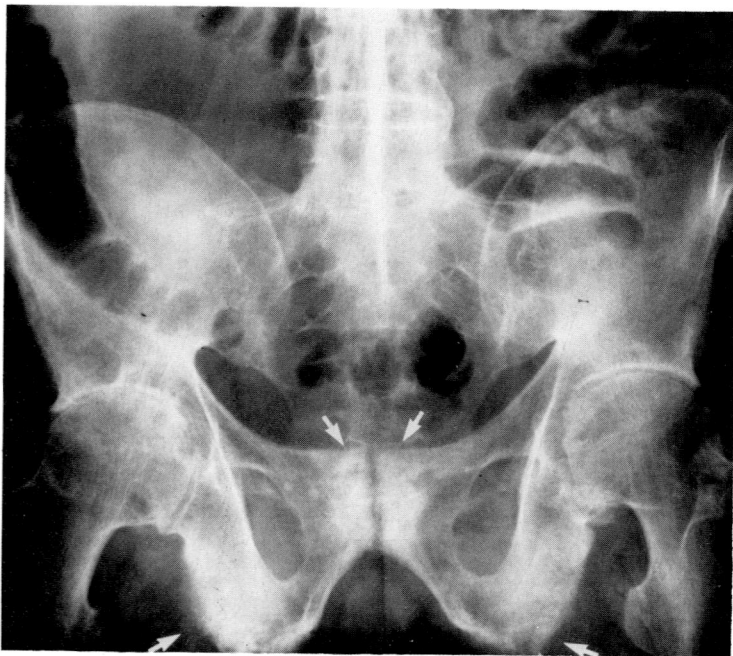

Fig. 5–47. Anteroposterior view of the pelvis in advanced ankylosing spondylitis showing fused sacroiliac joints and characteristic osteitis and periostitis (arrows) around the ischium and pubic symphysis. Concentric hip narrowing and moderate reactive sclerosis can be seen.

pearance (Fig. 5–48).[15,214] This manifestation is due to inflammation at the insertion of the outer fibers of the anulus fibrosus in the vertebral rim, with appositional new bone forming in the periosteal tissue adjacent to the vertebral body, to "fill in" the concavity of the vertebral waist (Fig. 5–49).[324] Radiographic squaring is common in early ankylosing spondylitis and is best evaluated in lateral views of the lumbar and cervical regions because the thoracic vertebrae may appear squared even in normal individuals.[214,273]

Syndesmophytes are vertically oriented paravertebral ossifications in the outer fibers of the anulus fibrosus and the adjacent connective tissues along the anterior and lateral aspects of the spine at the level of the disc interspace.[9,44,214] They differ from *osteophytes,* which originate from the cartilaginous end plate in response to degeneration of the disc and are horizontally oriented. These important radiographic signs, classified as *marginal or nonmarginal and symmetric or asymmetric,* differentiate ankylosing spondylitis from other spondylitic disorders.[44,214,273,324,345] *Marginal* syndesmophytes (Fig. 5–50) appear to arise from the edge or margin of the vertebral body and form a fine vertical bridge. The *nonmarginal* syndesmophytes, typical of psoriatic arthritis (Figs. 5–51, 5–52) and Reiter's syndrome (Fig. 5–53), arise in the adjacent connective tissue along the waist or midpor-

tion of the vertebral body and are broad and coarse.[44,214,352] In ankylosing spondylitis, syndesmophytes are typically marginal and symmetric and eventually result in the classic "bamboo spine." These syndesmophytes are detected initially in the superior or thoracolumbar regions, particularly in the anteroposterior projection.[214,324] In the cervical and thoracic regions, they are difficult to evaluate because of the superimposition of lateral masses or costovertebral junctions and because of the spinal curvatures.

Involvement of the apophyseal joints in ankylosing spondylitis may result in erosion, narrowing, and sclerosis, detectable in anteroposterior and oblique views of the lumbar spine and in lateral (Fig. 5–54) and oblique views of the cervical spine. Detection of involvement of the thoracic apophyseal joints is more difficult.[15] Paraspinal muscle spasm probably accounts for the early loss of lumbar and cervical lordosis seen in lateral radiographs.[48] Later, the apophyseal joints become ankylosed, resulting in rigid fixation of the entire spine. Occasionally, in patients with advanced disease, dense linear tracks may be seen posteriorly. These tracks result from ossification of the interspinous ligaments in the midline plane and, less commonly, of the capsules and ligaments that span the apophyseal joints in the parasagittal plane.[214] Thus, anteroposterior radiographs in the lumbar

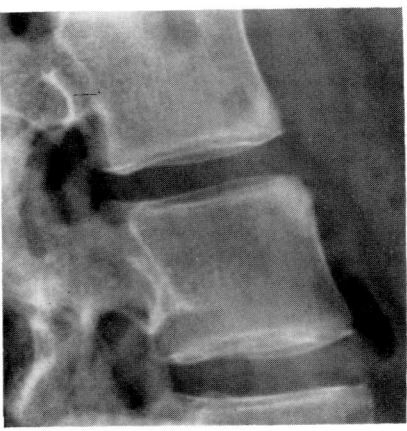

Fig. 5–48. Lateral lumbar spine in early ankylosing spondylitis shows osteitis at the site of insertion of the anulus fibrosus that produces "shiny corners" and contributes to "squaring."

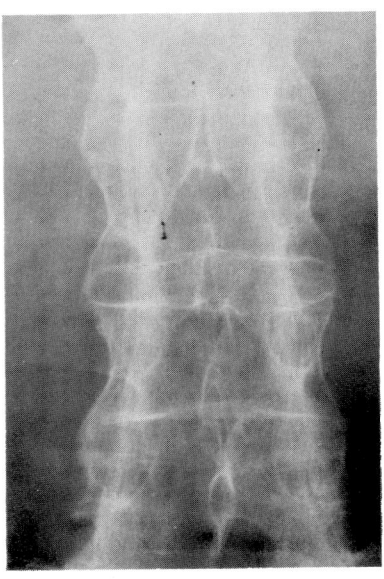

Fig. 5–50. Anteroposterior view of lumbar spine in ankylosing spondylitis showing fine, linear syndesmophytes.

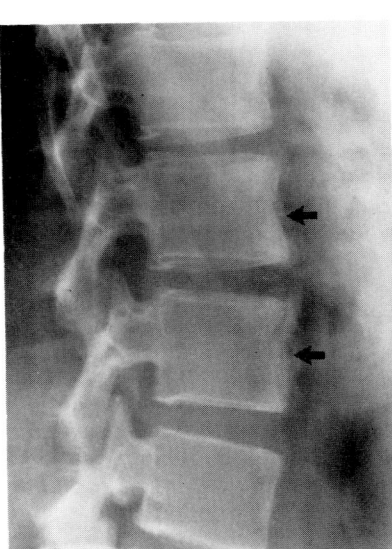

Fig. 5–49. Lateral view of the lumbar spine in ankylosing spondylitis demonstrating appositional new bone in the periosteal tissue anterior to the vertebral bodies (arrows), producing a "squared" appearance.

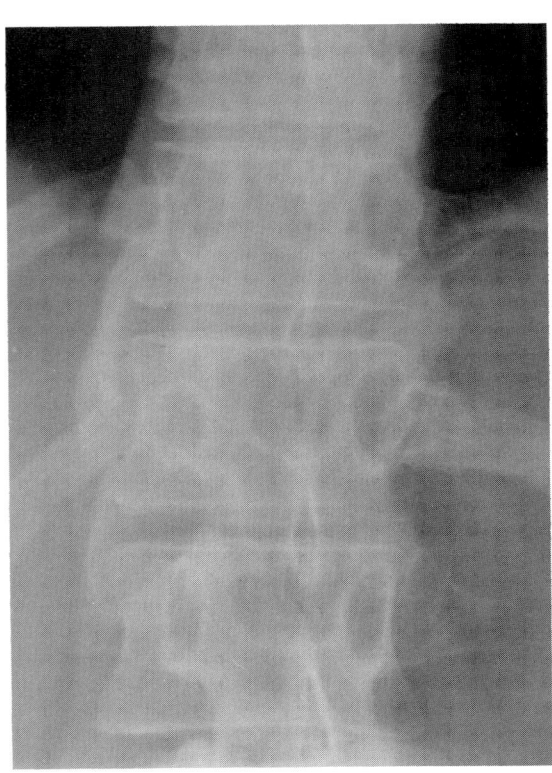

Fig. 5–51. Anteroposterior view of the lumbar spine in psoriatic spondylitis demonstrates broad, asymmetric, nonmarginal syndesmophytes characteristic of psoriatic arthritis or Reiter's syndrome.

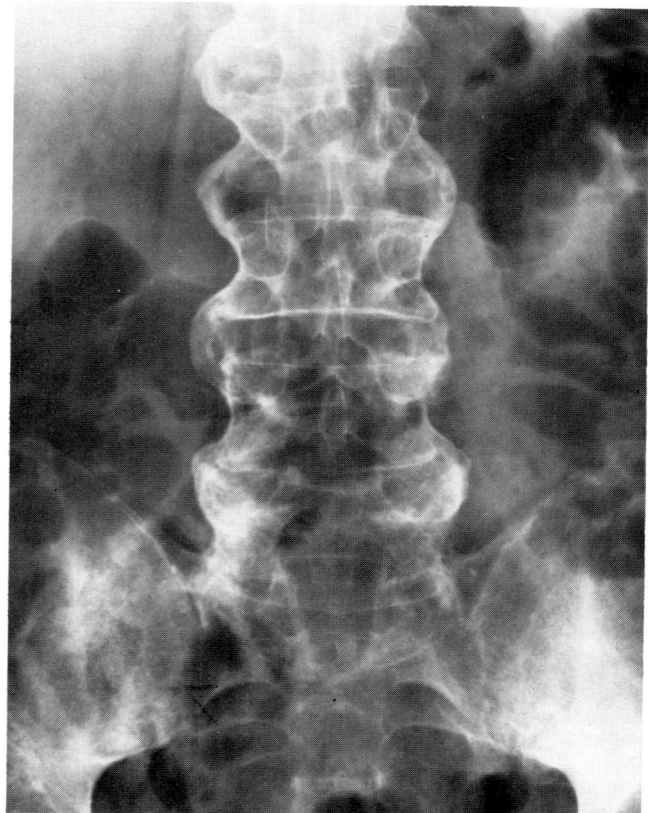

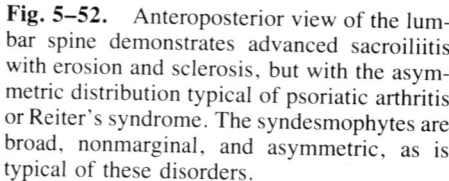

Fig. 5–52. Anteroposterior view of the lumbar spine demonstrates advanced sacroiliitis with erosion and sclerosis, but with the asymmetric distribution typical of psoriatic arthritis or Reiter's syndrome. The syndesmophytes are broad, nonmarginal, and asymmetric, as is typical of these disorders.

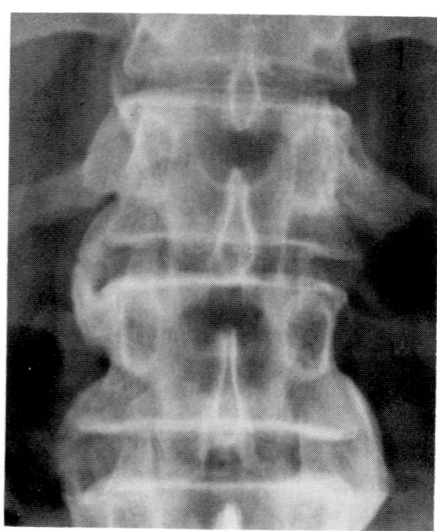

Fig. 5–53. Anteroposterior view of the thoracolumbar junction demonstrates nonmarginal, asymmetric syndesmophytes in a patient with Reiter's syndrome.

region have a distinct "triple-track" appearance. The synovial structures of the atlantoaxial joint may be involved, although less frequently and less severely than in RA. Varied degrees of subluxation may result, with erosion and pronounced reactive sclerosis of the dens.

Spinal osteoporosis is a prominent feature of ankylosing spondylitis, a result of immobilization and inflammation.[148,273] Mild, uniform narrowing of the disc and, rarely, biconcave end-plate compressions complicate the late stage of ankylosing spondylitis.[15] A frequently asymptomatic, but sometimes painful, complication in approximately 5% of patients is "spondylodiscitis" (see Fig. 53–8), consisting of fragmentation and erosion of adjacent end plates at the level of an isolated disc.[107,203,307,345] This appearance may simulate infection and most likely results from excessive motion at the involved segment, with or without fracture of the ankylosed posterior elements.

Peripheral Joint Involvement

Involvement of the appendicular skeleton, noted clinically and radiographically in most patients with ankylosing spondylitis, is usually transient and nondeforming in the peripheral joints. In the

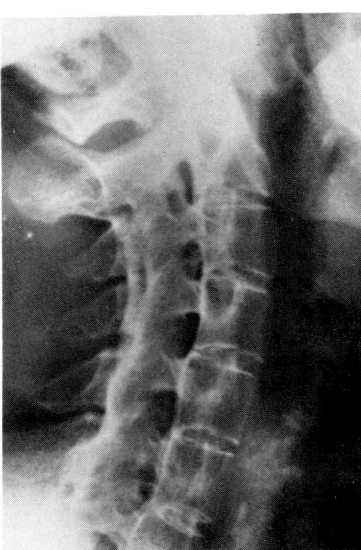

Fig. 5–54. Lateral view of the cervical spine in advanced ankylosing spondylitis demonstrates extensive ankylosis of the apophyseal joints, as well as "squaring" of the vertebral bodies, but no identifiable syndesmophytosis.

large proximal joints, however, advanced destructive arthropathy and clinical disability are common.[15,47,286,324,345] The hips are often involved early in ankylosing spondylitis, as indicated by distinct radiographic changes in nearly 50% of patients. Initially, a small focus or nub of new bone forms at the lateral junction of the head and neck. This zone of bone proliferation eventually enlarges to a ridge of exophytic overgrowth that surrounds the perimeter of the femoral head like a collar. Loss of cartilage is secondary to synovial inflammation and causes narrowing with axial migration of the femoral head, occasionally complicated by protrusio acetabuli (see Fig. 5–47).[86] Mild-to-moderate erosive disease and reactive sclerosis develop, but unlike in osteoarthritis, with little or no formation of subchondral cysts. Although hip motion is frequently limited, bony ankylosis is uncommon. Total arthroplasty of the hip is attended by an increased risk of postoperative heterotopic ossification and ankylosis.[292]

In nearly one-third of patients with chronic disease, the shoulders and knees are affected with deforming arthropathy that simulates RA, but with a proliferative bone response.[15,241,243] The small peripheral joints are commonly involved with transient soft tissue swelling, but generally appear normal radiographically.[324] About 20% of patients may have mild asymmetric erosive arthritis, distinguishable from RA by associated periostitis and lack of

osteoporosis.[286] Erosions and spurs, similar to those of psoriasis, Reiter's syndrome, or RA, but less striking, may be shown in the calcaneus.[15,288] Uncommonly, in the presence of HLA-B27 homozygosity, severe peripheral joint destruction occurs.[6] Rarely, RA coexists with ankylosing spondylitis.[205]

Arthritis of Inflammatory Bowel Disease

Arthritic manifestations develop in 5 to 20% of patients with inflammatory bowel disease (see also Chap. 56), most often secondary to ulcerative colitis, but sometimes complicating Crohn's disease.[99,214,215,254] Most commonly, a migratory transient synovitis involves the knees, ankles, or wrists with effusion and soft tissue swelling. These manifestations closely parallel the clinical activity of inflammatory bowel disease. Radiographic changes other than soft tissue swelling are rare. A second form of arthritis that accompanies inflammatory bowel disease involves the axial skeleton and runs a course independent of the clinical activity of bowel disease; it may even precede enteropathic manifestations. This process is indistinguishable from ankylosing spondylitis, except that it is usually milder.[214]

Psoriatic Arthropathy

In approximately 7% of patients with psoriasis, arthritis develops (see Figs. 55–6 to 55–8).[8,178,186,214] Axial manifestations resemble ankylosing spondylitis in many respects, whereas the peripheral manifestations may simulate RA. Manifestations of both axial and peripheral joints are nearly indistinguishable radiographically from those of Reiter's syndrome, a condition that clinically overlaps with psoriasis in many respects. The radiographic changes in the axial skeleton result from enthesopathy and synovitis.

Sacroiliitis is an early, frequent feature, but differs from that of ankylosing spondylitis in that asymmetry is seen in about 50% of patients.[214,324] The spondylitis of psoriasis is characterized by the frequent development of broad, coarse, nonmarginal, asymmetric syndesmophytes, in addition to the fine syndesmophytes of ankylosing spondylitis (see Figs. 5–51, 5–52).[44,186,214,352] Anterior squaring and apophyseal ankylosis are less common than in ankylosing spondylitis, and the distribution of spondylitis is often random and disorganized. "Skip" areas are frequent, and advanced cervical spine changes may be seen in the absence of involvement of the thoracic, lumbar, or even sacroiliac joints.[153,186] Atlantoaxial subluxation is frequent, but is generally less dramatic than in RA. In advanced instances, psoriatic spondylitis may result in extensive diffuse, anterior and posterior fusion, although far less commonly than in ankylosing spondylitis.

Peripheral psoriatic arthritis affects predominantly the small joints of the hands and feet; occasionally, destructive changes appear in the larger diarthrodial joints.[8,324,345] The spectrum of changes ranges from those characteristic of psoriatic arthropathy to those indistinguishable from RA.[178] Typically, pauciarticular or polyarticular asymmetric arthropathy affects the distal interphalangeal joints and, less severely, the proximal interphalangeal, metacarpophalangeal, metatarsophalangeal, carpal, or tarsal joints.[275,345] The posterosuperior and inferior aspects of the calcaneus are also frequent target sites (Fig. 5–55), and in about one-fourth of patients, diffuse swelling of an entire digit ("sausage finger") from tenosynovitis may be present. Osteoporosis is uncommon, but may arise during inflammatory stages of disease. Characteristic erosions which develop at articular margins and at capsular attachments (Fig. 5–56, 5–57),

consist of a combination of focal bone resorption and fluffy new-bone formation, often seen together with linear periosteal new bone.[153,324,345] The periosteal new bone is extra-articular, beginning at the capsule of inflamed joints and extending along the tubular bone shafts. In progressive disease, isolated, destroyed joints are seen, whereas other joints may be normal or only mildly affected.

Occasionally, complete erosion of the articular ends of bone, accompanied by intervening proliferation of granulation tissue, results in joints that appear widened radiographically. Although uncommon, such widening suggests psoriatic arthritis and is rare in other forms of inflammatory joint disease. In approximately 5 to 10% of patients, a rapidly progressive, destructive, peripheral arthropathy develops, leading to a resorption and telescoping of the digits termed "arthritis mutilans,"[8] (Fig. 5–58).

In 10 to 15% of patients, a proximal, symmetric arthritis in the hands develops, nearly indistin-

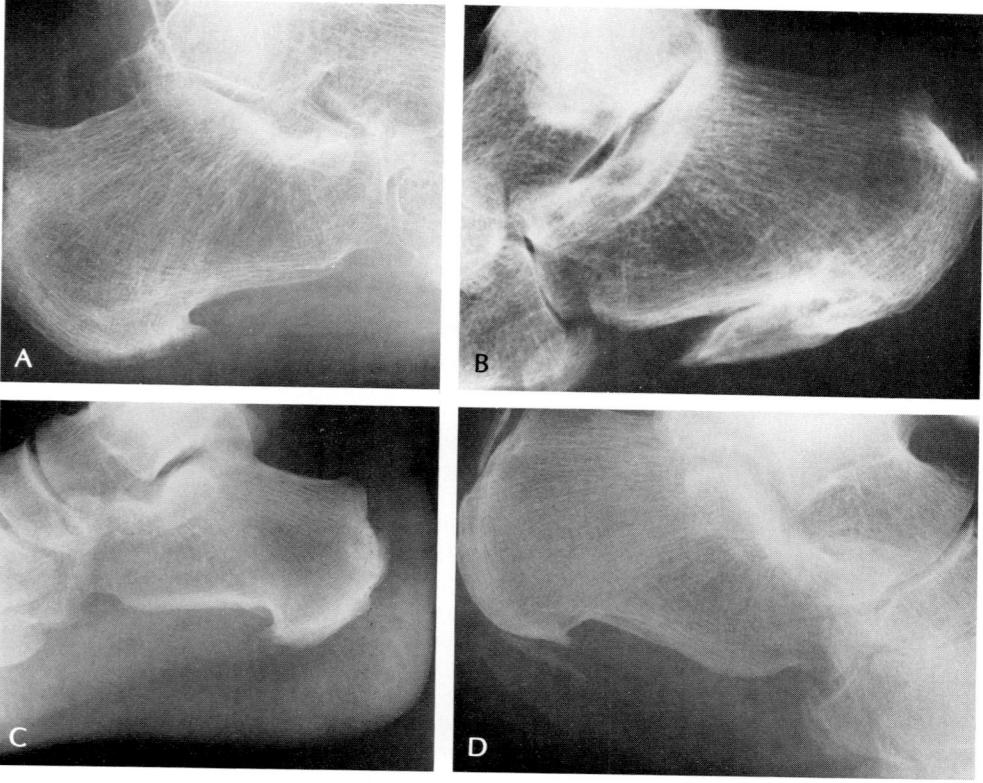

Fig. 5–55. *A,* Lateral view of the calcaneus demonstrates spurs associated with proliferative erosions owing to the evident inflammation at ligamentous and fascial insertion sites of the calcaneus. These changes are most prominent in psoriatic and Reiter's arthritis. *B,* Large posterior and inferior spurs can be seen with well-corticated margins indicating chronic, inactive disease. This nonspecific finding may be seen in any of the HLA-B27-associated arthritides during later stages. *C,* Typical, well-corticated, degenerative spurs of the calcaneus, a frequent appearance in the elderly population. *D,* Linear and punctate calcifications in the Achilles tendon and plantar aponeurosis are an occasional finding in calcium pyrophosphate dihydrate crystal deposition or pseudogout.

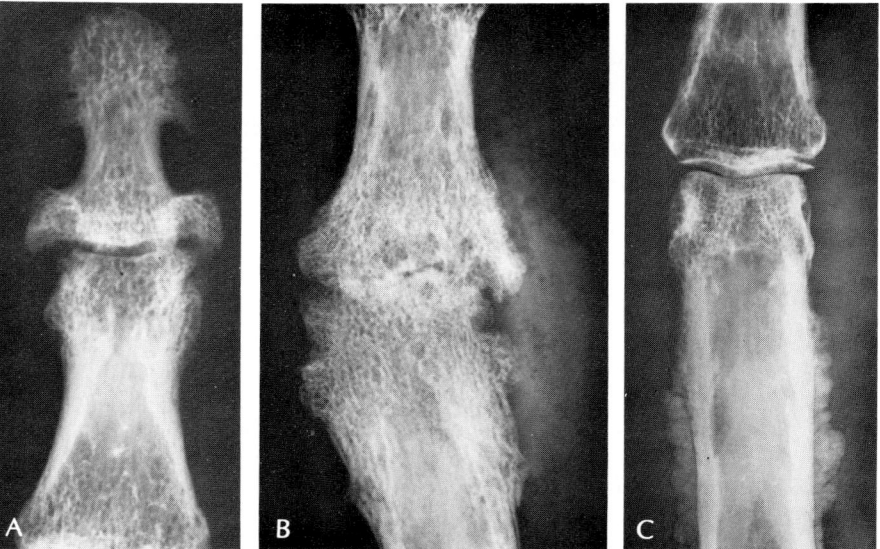

Fig. 5–56. Close-up views of psoriatic arthritis. *A,* Extensive proliferative erosion with prominent new-bone formation producing overgrowth at the base of the phalanx. *B,* Complete loss of cartilage and proliferative erosions with fluffy and linear new-bone formation. *C,* Linear and cloud-like periosteal new bone in the proximal and middle phalangeals in response to tenosynovitis.

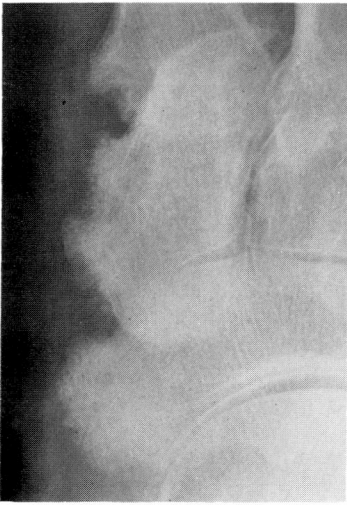

Fig. 5–57. Soft tissue swelling and irregular, fluffy periostitis, or proliferative erosion, involving the tarsus in psoriasis.

guishable from RA. This condition may represent coexistent disease because some of these patients are seropositive for RA.[8] Most, however, are seronegative, with features resembling RA proximally combined with one or more psoriatic features distally. These cases are a part of the spectrum of psoriatic arthropathy.

Over all, the radiographic features of psoriatic arthritis correlate poorly with cutaneous disease. Exceptions include advanced spondylitis and arthritis mutilans, which appear predominantly in patients with severe psoriasis;[8] another is the distal interphalangeal arthropathy that correlates with psoriatic nail changes. Recently, the association of palmoplantar pustulosis with progressive sternoclavicular hyperostosis has been observed.[91]

Reiter's Syndrome

Reiter's syndrome (see also Chap. 54) has a classic constellation of clinical manifestations including urethritis, circinate balanitis, uveitis, keratoderma blenorrhagicum, and arthritis. When the syndrome is incomplete, the diagnosis may be aided by careful radiographic assessment. Characteristically, these features of arthritis consist of asymmetric, pauciarticular involvement of the feet, knees, ankles, and lower spine. The upper extremity is generally spared, except for soft tissue swelling and, rarely, periostitis.[275,324,332,345] One or several joints of the feet, most commonly the first interphalangeal and proximal interphalangeal joints, are the sites of pronounced soft tissue swelling, moderate periarticular osteoporosis, proliferative erosion, and periosteal new-bone formation (Fig. 5–59). Advanced destruction of the joint is uncommon.[332] The peripheral manifestations simulate psoriatic arthropathy closely and may be indistinguishable clinically or radiographically. Features that may differentiate Reiter's syndrome from

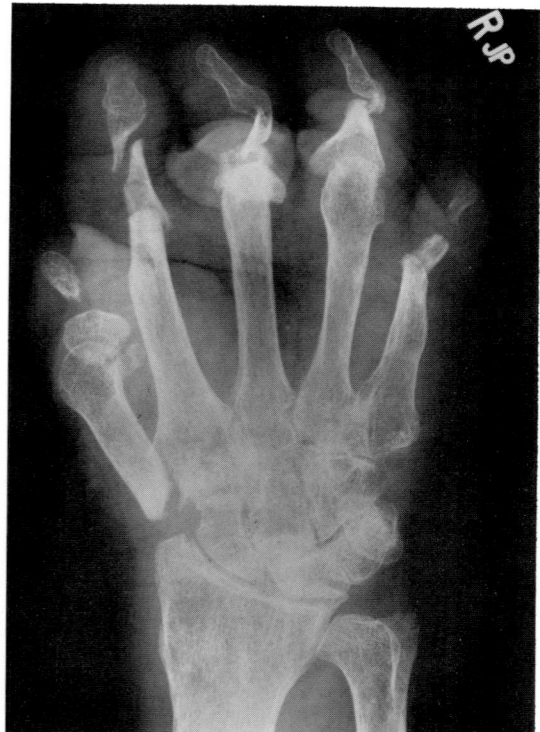

Fig. 5–58. Advanced distal articular destruction with "pencil-in-cup" configuration and telescoping of the digits in arthritis mutilans of psoriatic arthritis. Distal bony ankylosis is noted at several articulations as well.

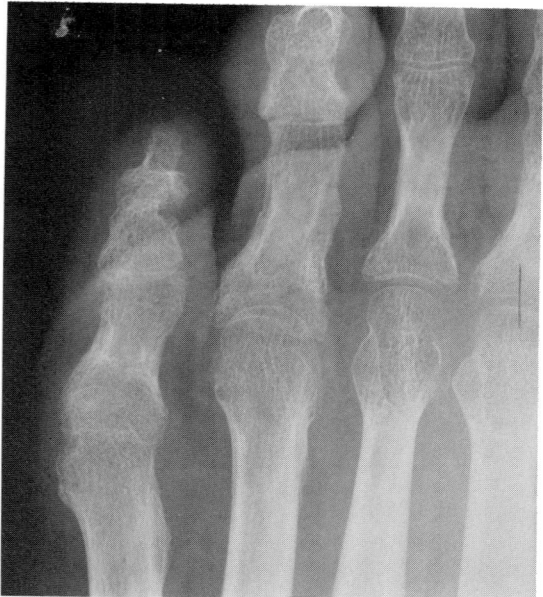

Fig. 5–59. Magnified view of proliferative erosion and formation of periosteal new bone, mild demineralization, and overlying soft tissue swelling, producing "sausage" toes in a man with Reiter's syndrome. An identical appearance can be seen in psoriatic arthritis.

psoriatic arthritis include predominant distribution in the lower extremity, involvement of fewer joints, sparing of the distal interphalangeal joints, and greater periarticular osteoporosis.[324,345] Both processes affect the calcaneus and produce erosion and spurs, as a result of plantar fasciitis, Achilles tendinitis, and retrocalcaneal bursitis.[288] Changes in the ankles and knees, although clinically disabling, are frequently unimpressive in radiographs.

Sacroiliitis, often asymmetric, is common in patients with Reiter's syndrome, whereas additional findings of spondylitis, such as nonmarginal asymmetric syndesmophytes (see Fig. 5–53), are less common than in psoriasis.[186,214,345] Anterior squaring and extensive posterior ankylosis, as seen in ankylosing spondylitis, are rare. Thus, the arthritis of Reiter's syndrome closely resembles that of psoriatic arthropathy, but the distribution and severity of involvement frequently differ.

DEGENERATIVE AND ISCHEMIC ARTHROPATHIES

Osteoarthritis

Osteoarthritis, also known as osteoarthrosis or degenerative joint disease (see also Chap. 89) is a common affliction of diarthrodial and, to some extent, amphiarthrodial joints characterized by predominantly noninflammatory deterioration and abrasion of articular cartilage accompanied by formation of new bone at joint surfaces and margins.[164,165] Osteoarthritis occurs in two major forms: primary (idiopathic) and secondary.[345] The distinction between the two is neither clear nor universally accepted.

Primary osteoarthritis develops in joints without antecedent history of insult and affects predominantly the distal and proximal interphalangeal joints, first carpometacarpal joint in the hands, the spine, and the larger weight-bearing joints, such as the hips and knees.[182,340,345] Initial involvement is commonly limited to one or several joints, but the disorder may arise simultaneously in many joints. This latter form of polyarticular disease has been termed *primary generalized osteoarthritis,*[182] and it affects predominantly the hands of middle-aged women, but frequently involves the knees, hips, and spine as well.

Secondary osteoarthritis results from alterations in metabolism or mechanics of the joint subsequent to other conditions. These conditions are infection, osteonecrosis, epiphyseal dysplasia,[376] acromegaly (Fig. 5–60), ochronosis, Wilson's disease,[95] pseudogout, neurologic deficit,[181] or simple trauma. Al-

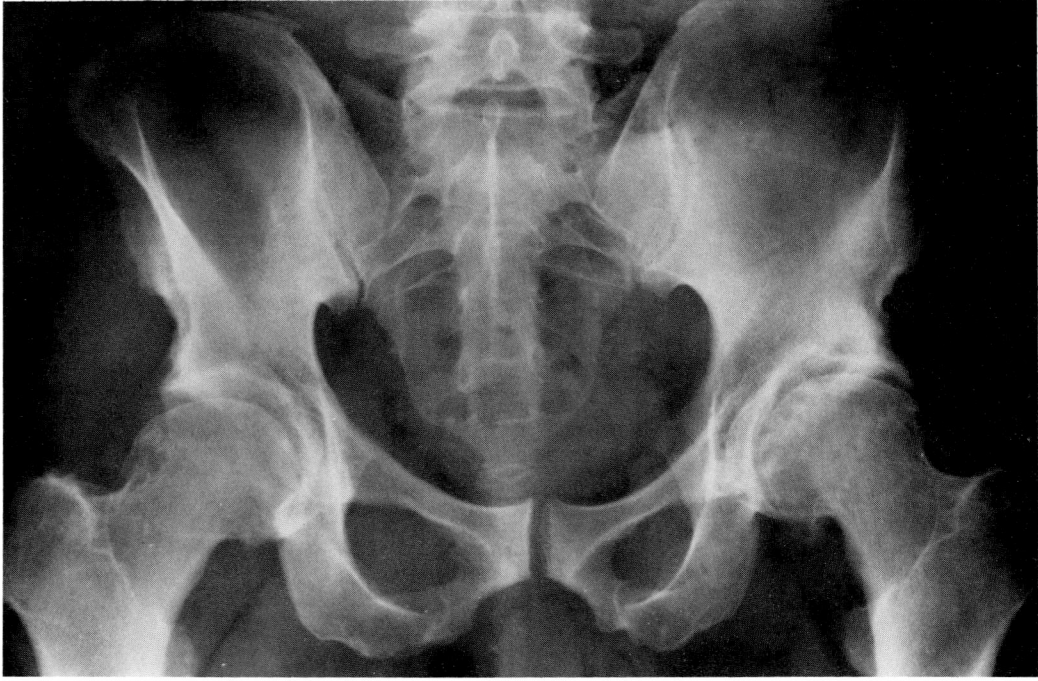

Fig. 5–60. Osteoarthritis of the hips in a patient with acromegaly demonstrate widening of the cartilage space on the right side with a collar of osteophyte at the chondro-osseous junction. The left hip demonstrates more advanced degeneration with subchondral sclerosis, pseudocyst formation, and large, marginal osteophytes. Generalized bony hypertrophy at tendon insertions is noted as well.

ternatively, secondary osteoarthritis may be super-imposed late in the course of other common primary arthritides, such a RA, JRA, and gout.[345] Unusual and destructive degenerative arthritis has been described in association with excessive trauma in vigorous sports activity.[157] Regardless of the predisposing factors, once cartilage damage begins, the characteristic sequence of pathologic events ultimately provides similar radiographic features. Thus, the late radiographic appearance of primary osteoarthritis is frequently indistinguishable from that of the secondary condition, but secondary osteoarthritis may be modified by the specific appearance and distribution of the underlying process.

Generally, the radiographic manifestations of established osteoarthritis consist of irregular narrowing of the joint, subchondral sclerosis and cyst formation, marginal osteophytosis, minimal soft tissue swelling, mild-to-moderate joint deformity, and preservation of normal mineralization. The variable expression of these components depends on the stage of the disease, the precipitating factors, and the dictates of local joint anatomy.

Findings in Specific Joints

Hips. Osteoarthritis of the hips (Figs. 5–61 to 5–63), or coxarthrosis, occurs about equally in pri-

mary and secondary forms.[340] In the latter, underlying disorders include congenital dislocation of the hip, osteonecrosis, epiphysiolysis, and trauma. In presumed primary osteoarthritis of the hip, several retrospective analyses suggest that unrecognized, subtle acetabular dysplasia or epiphysiolysis can be uncovered,[257] but others indicate that such altered anatomic features may be a result of remodeling secondary to the degenerative process rather than its cause.[150,158,285]

Radiographically, this disease presents several patterns.[158,285] Most commonly, a proximal migration of the femoral head develops with loss of the weight-bearing interosseous space superiorly (Figs. 5–61, A, 5–62). Early subchondral sclerosis is followed by flattening of the femoral head, related to microfractures and osteonecrosis and compounded by osteophytosis with remodeling at the medial and lateral aspects of the cartilaginous surfaces of the femoral head.[150,158] Similarly, the acetabular roof may remodel, with flattening and extensive marginal osteophytosis. In patients with advanced disease, cystic changes are invariable in the subchondral bone of the femoral head and adjacent acetabular roof, generally in areas of maximum stress. The pseudocysts, or geodes, are round or piriform, may be single or multiple, have

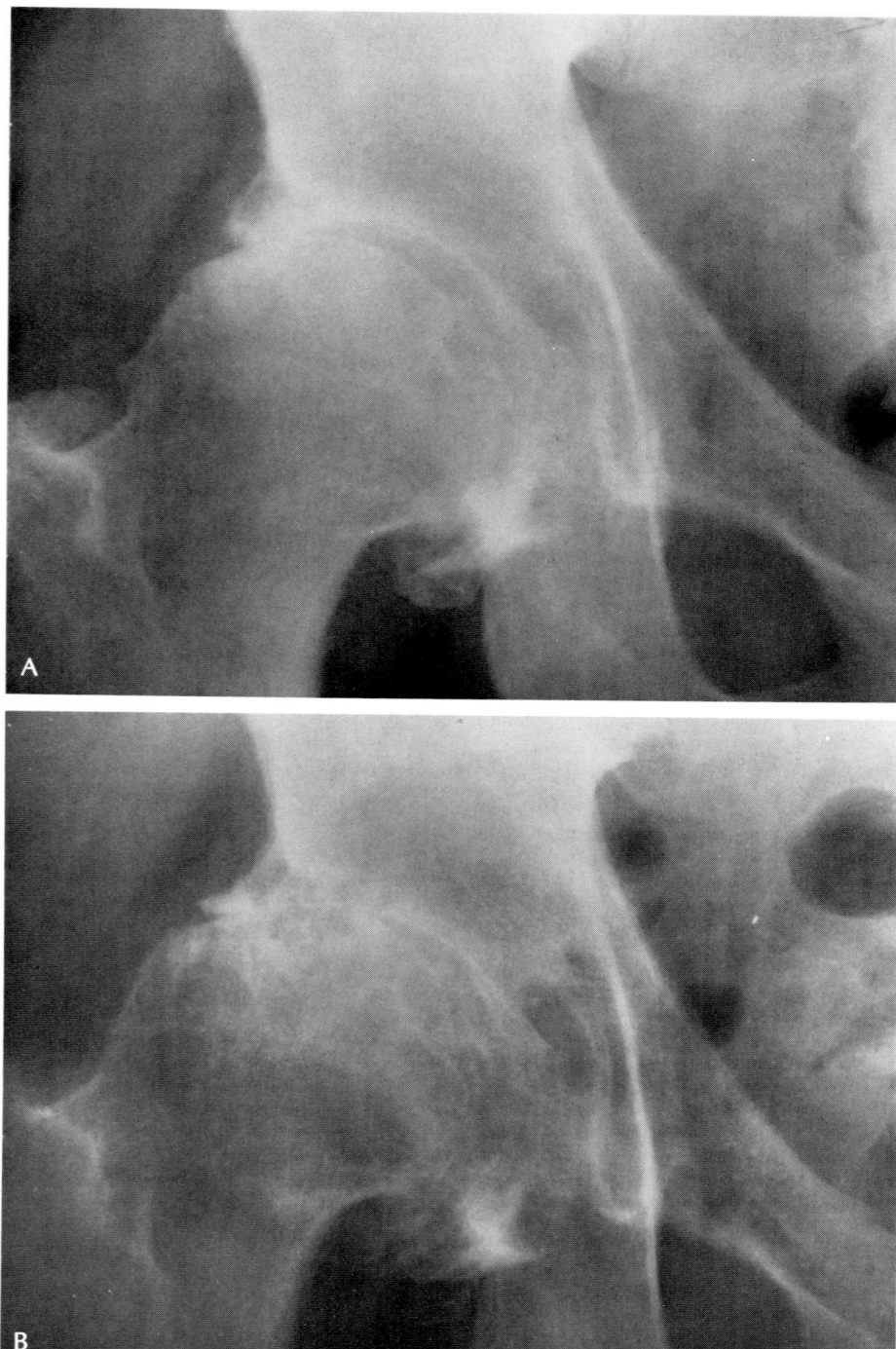

Fig. 5–61. *A*, Natural progression of osteoarthritis in the hips with asymmetric cartilage loss, principally of the weight-bearing superior cartilage, superior and lateral migration of the femoral head, and early, marginal osteophyte formation. *B*, Three years later, more advanced changes consist of subchondral cyst formation, further lateral migration, and extensive, marginal osteophyte formation.

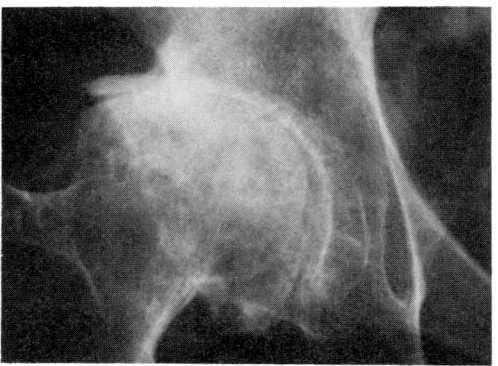

Fig. 5–62. Advanced osteoarthritis in the hip with superolateral migration, extensive marginal osteophytosis, and remodeling of the femoral head and acetabular roof.

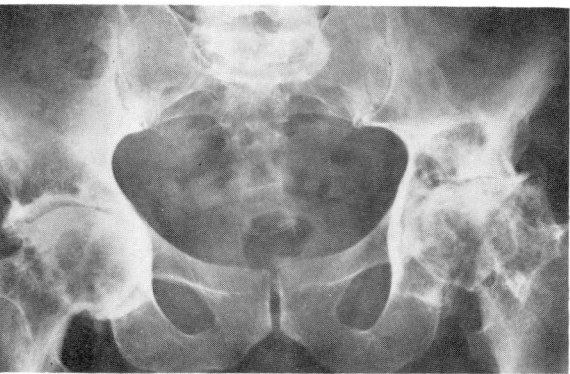

Fig. 5–63. Extensive bilateral osteoarthritis of the hips with reactive sclerosis, cartilage loss, mild protrusio acetabuli, and extensive subchondral cyst formation, particularly on the left side.

finely sclerotic margins, and may lead eventually to collapse and fragmentation of the articular surfaces. They may result from intrusion of synovial fluid and granulation tissue through weakened fibrillated cartilage or from contusion of subarticular cancellous bone with subsequent necrosis and liquefaction.[279,297] *Buttressing* results from periosteal new-bone formation along the femoral neck, predominantly on the medial aspect. With superior femoral migration, lateral displacement frequently coexists, accompanied by prominent osteophytosis filling in the foveal region of the medial acetabulum.

A second, less common pattern of migration, often bilateral and more likely to be part of primary generalized osteoarthritis, consists of a medial drift of the femoral head associated with cartilage loss and subchondral sclerosis at the abutting surfaces. In this instance, the superolateral aspect of the joint widens; this feature helps one to distinguish this pattern from the axial migration and concentric narrowing of RA (Fig. 5–63). Osteophytosis and buttressing take place with medial migration, but are generally milder than with superior migration. In late stages of medial drift, mild protrusio acetabuli may be seen as in RA, except that instead of osteoporosis, reactive bone formation is pronounced.

In an uncommon variant of degenerative hip disease, the primary manifestation is formation of a subchondral cyst in either the femoral head or the acetabular roof, or both, with preservation of cartilage and absence of subchondral sclerosis and osteophytosis.[171]

Knees. Osteoarthritis in the knees is characterized by nonuniform loss of cartilage, generally of the medial or patellar compartment alone, or a combination of the two. Narrowing of the lateral compartment may also be present, but rarely as an isolated finding. Unlike in RA, tricompartmental, uniform narrowing is rare.[1,355] Tricompartmental involvement or isolated patellofemoral disease suggests underlying calcium pyrophosphate dihydrate (CPPD) crystal deposition. In general, significant narrowing of joint space is localized to only a single compartment. Anteroposterior weight-bearing views are necessary to assess the extent of cartilage loss and corresponding degrees of varus (most common) or valgus deformity (Fig. 5–64). Focal cartilage loss is frequently accompanied by discrete, local subchondral sclerosis, most commonly of the medial tibial plateau.

Osteophyte formation, unlike loss of cartilage, is likely to be generalized, although most advanced in the narrowest compartment.[1] Osteophytosis may produce exophytic bony ridges that outline the articular margins, but, unlike this process in the hip, do not extend onto the articular surfaces. Osteophytosis, most extensive in areas of capsular recesses, is modified by mechanics of the local joint because it is horizontally oriented on the narrow, compressed side, and vertically oriented on the wide, distracted side of the joint. Subchondral cyst formation in the knee, unlike that in the hip, is rare. In the presence of severe cartilage loss, remodeling takes place and produces a beveled or scalloped appearance of the tibial plateau and a flattening of the femoral condyle. These advanced changes are frequently associated with some type of subluxation, such as joint widening, horizontal translocation, or angular deviation. Finally, pain, diminished range of motion, instability, and crepitus correlate only moderately with the extent of radiographic findings.[140,355]

Hands. Osteoarthritic involvement of the hands is common and causes much discomfort, but only moderate disability.[181,345] The distribution and appearance are radiographically characteristic and are

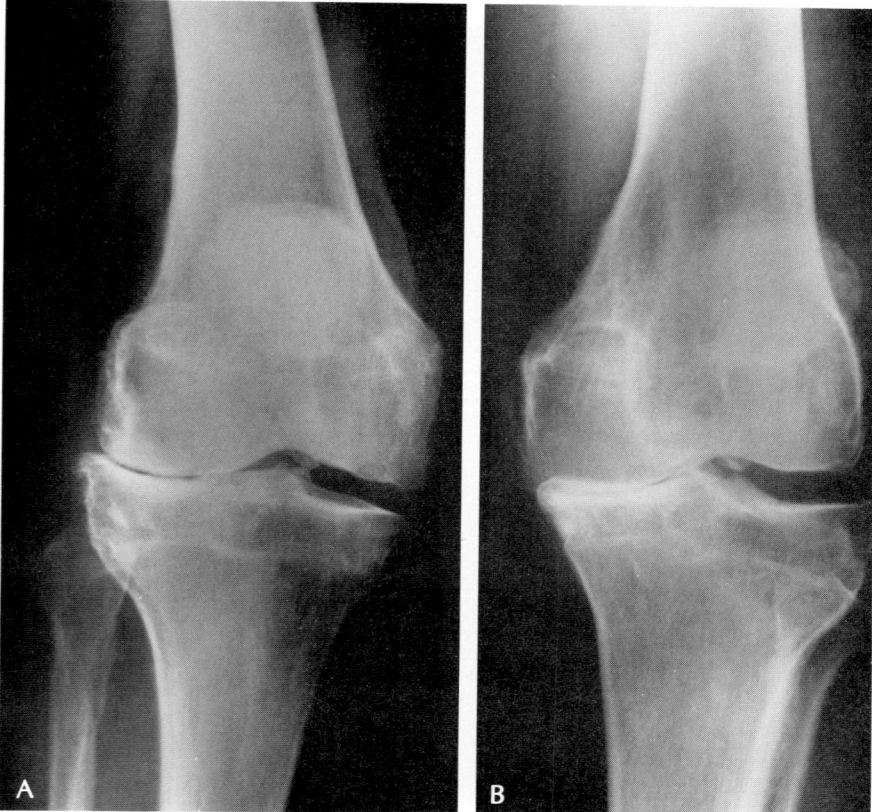

Fig. 5–64. *A* and *B*, Moderately advanced osteoarthritis of the knees is present with atypical distribution showing marked varus with total loss of medial cartilage and secondary reactive sclerosis involving the left knee *(B)*, whereas the right knee *(A)* demonstrates atypical valgus deformity with near-total loss of lateral cartilage and secondary sclerosis. This asymmetric pattern results in a "windswept" appearance.

generally differentiated easily from other common forms of arthritis. Typically, the distal interphalangeal, proximal interphalangeal, first carpometacarpal, and naviculomultangular articulations undergo irregular narrowing, subchondral sclerosis, marginal osteophytosis, and mild subluxation (Figs. 5–65, 5–66). As the process evolves, large rounded or pointed bony excrescences are associated with well-defined overgrowth of the phalangeal condyles. The articular space is completely lost, and a peculiar zig-zag appearance of the articulating surfaces results from translocation and the mechanical erosion of bone on bone. Intense eburnation and formation of subarticular cysts may accompany the process. Soft tissue swelling, although common, is localized to the immediate articular region and may appear lumpy. This feature distinguishes it from the more extensive, fusiform swelling of RA. Erosive disease is generally not a feature, although crumbling, fragmentation, and collapse of subchondral bone may simulate a truly

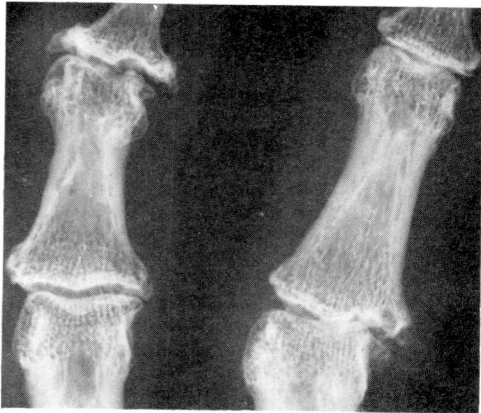

Fig. 5–65. The interphalangeal joints in osteoarthritis, showing irregular narrowing, mild subluxation, prominent osteophyte formation, and subchondral sclerosis. Cystic erosive change can be seen.

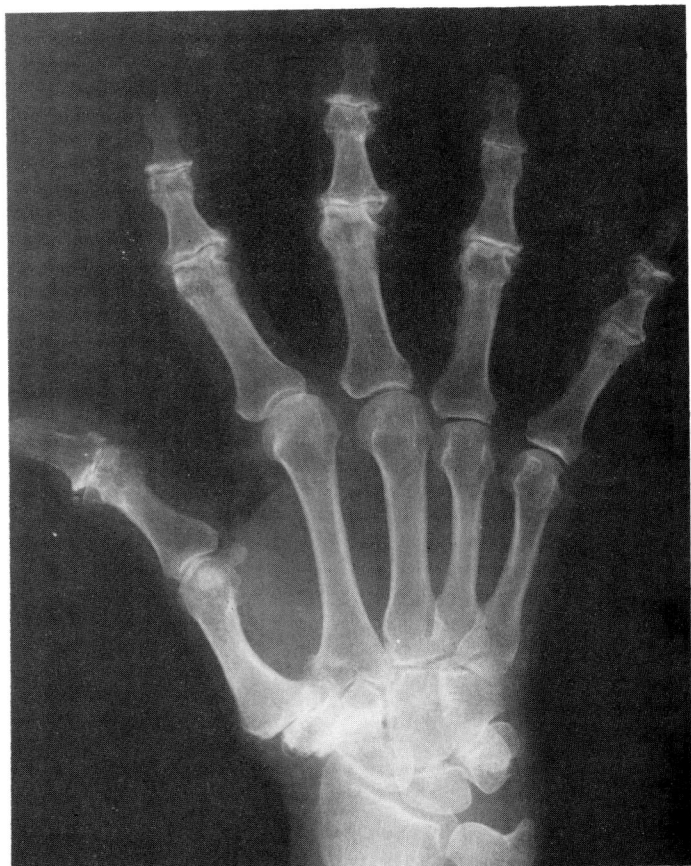

Fig. 5–66. More advanced primary, generalized osteoarthritis consisting of striking changes at the distal and proximal interphalangeal joints, as well as at the first carpometacarpal joint.

erosive process. Rarely, an interphalangeal joint becomes ankylosed.[337] The metacarpophalangeal joints uncommonly develop extensive degenerative changes, but a uniform loss of cartilage is frequently demonstrated, occasionally with "hook-like" osteophytes.[240] The proximal hand and wrist are spared, except for the first carpometacarpal and naviculomultangular joints. Narrowing of the radiocarpal joint suggests underlying CPPD crystal deposition.

The term *primary generalized osteoarthritis* is used when a polyarticular disease in the hands appears with a rapid clinical onset and development of multiple Heberden's and Bouchard's nodes. The condition may be accompanied by similar degenerative changes in the knees, hips, or apophyseal joints of the spine.[181,345] This form of osteoarthritis, which is most common in middle-aged women, particularly after menopause, generally runs its course over several years and later leaves the patient with only moderate pain and deformity. The hands are usually bilaterally involved, although sparing of the ipsilateral side in hemiparalysis has been noted.[128]

Erosive osteoarthritis, an uncommon variant limited to the hands and, rarely, to the feet, also affects predominantly middle-aged women and has the same distribution of joint involvement as primary generalized osteoarthritis.[184,274] Erosive osteoarthritis differs quantitatively in that a pronounced inflammatory component causes prominent soft tissue swelling and erosive disease, features not simply degenerative in nature (Fig. 5–67). The appearance simulates that of RA, but with a more distal distribution, with destruction of subchondral bone of the articular surfaces rather than the marginal "bare areas" and with a much greater tendency to reactive bone formation. Similarly, erosive osteoarthritis may simulate psoriatic arthritis, particularly in its distal distribution, but it lacks the fine, periosteal new-bone formation and fluffy, proliferative marginal erosions of the psoriatic disorder.[231] The precise nature of erosive osteoarthritis is unclear, but it may represent part of the spectrum of primary generalized osteoarthritis.[274] Alternatively, seronegative RA may be superimposed on a degenerative process to produce this appearance in some patients. In any event, as the process evolves, the inflammatory and erosive components subside, and the more degenerative

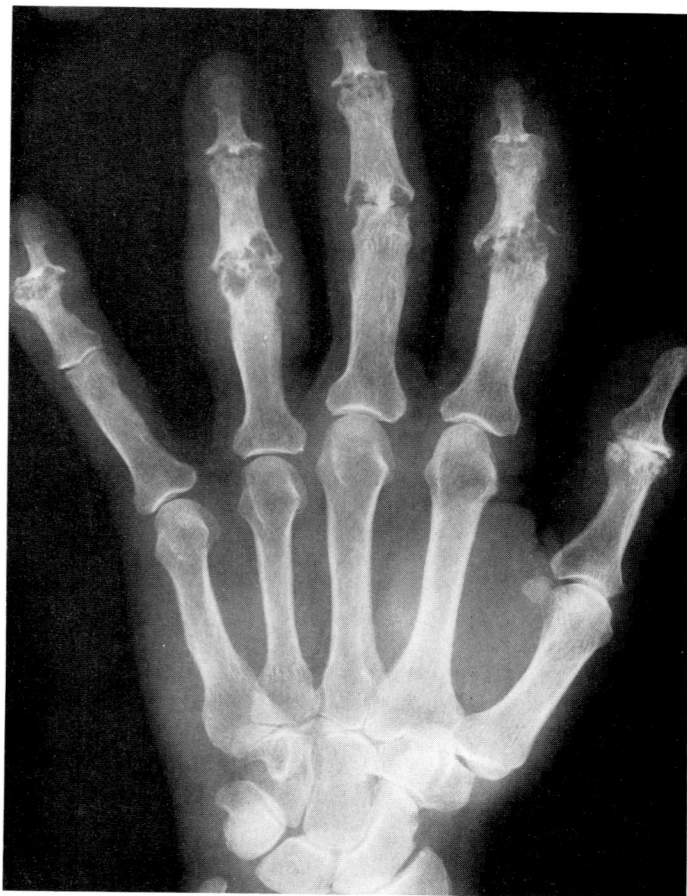

Fig. 5–67. Left hand of a patient with erosive osteoarthritis demonstrating fusiform soft tissue swelling and cystic erosions without periarticular demineralization.

features supervene, leaving an appearance identical to that of primary generalized osteoarthritis.

Spine. Degenerative disease affects all levels of the spine, but symptoms generally are greatest in the cervical and lumbar regions. Various terms have been applied to this process, depending on the location of predominant change. Therefore, *intervertebral osteochondrosis* applies to degeneration of the nucleus pulposus, *spondylosis deformans* refers to degeneration of the anulus fibrosus, and *osteoarthritis* describes degeneration of the apophyseal joints. These distinctions may be artificial because each vertebral level consists of a three-joint complex, and similar degeneration of cartilage and fibrous tissue, accompanied by mild reactive bone formation, occurs pathologically in each subgroup. The radiologic findings reflect the gross pathologic changes and are dictated by the local anatomic features and mechanics. Although the degenerative process may occur in one site independently, parallel changes are usually found in the nucleus pulposus, anulus fibrosus, and apophyseal joints.

In the cervical spine (Fig. 5–68),[37,161] degener-ation of the disc is manifested by irregular narrowing of the intervertebral space, accompanied by subchondral eburnation and osteophytic overgrowth that extends most prominently anterolaterally. The medial and inferior cervical regions are predominantly affected, in contrast to the superior cervical involvement seen in RA. Advanced narrowing of the disc with minimal osteophytosis or, conversely, advanced osteophytosis with minimal narrowing is noted. The apophyseal and neurocentral (Luschka) joints are similarly involved with narrowing, sclerosis, and osteophytosis. These osteophytes are best seen in 45° oblique views, which may reveal narrowing of the neural foramina. The correlation between the degree of radiographic change and the severity of symptoms is poor, although significant clinical manifestations are uncommon in the presence of a radiographically normal cervical spine.[37,61]

Degenerative disease of the lumbar spine, which appears similar to that of the cervical spine, is manifested by variable disc narrowing, osteophytosis, and apophyseal joint sclerosis (Fig. 5–69). The lower lumbar and first sacral levels are most

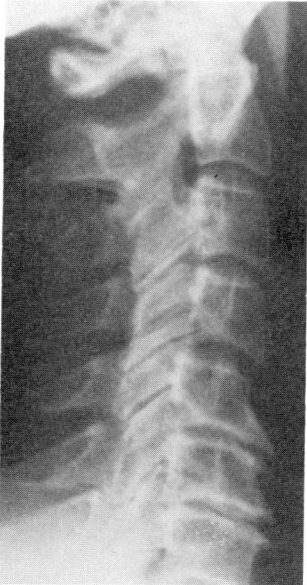

Fig. 5–68. Moderately advanced degenerative disc disease involving the medial and inferior cervical regions with narrowing, osteophytosis, and subchondral sclerosis. Minor degenerative changes are also present in inferior apophyseal joints.

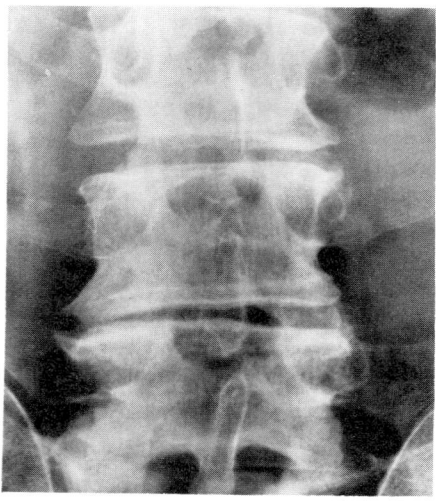

Fig. 5–69. Typical degenerative disc disease of lumbar spine consisting of irregular narrowing, subchondral sclerosis, and horizontally oriented osteophytes.

commonly involved. Occasionally, a vacuum disc results from advanced desiccation and fragmentation of the nucleus pulposus. Additionally, radiographs may show evidence of herniation of the nucleus pulposus through a weakened cartilaginous end plate into the subchondral bone, producing striking reactive sclerosis in the adjacent vertebral

body. This appearance may simulate infection or osteoblastic metastasis. It is most commonly observed at the L4 to L5 segment and is referred to as discogenic vertebral sclerosis (Fig. 5–70).[233]

Ankylosing Hyperostosis

Ankylosing hyperostosis, also called Forestier's disease[100] or diffuse idiopathic skeletal hyperostosis (DISH),[295,299] is a common condition that affects predominantly middle-aged and elderly men. It is a bone-forming diathesis[110,324,327] similar to the spondyloarthropathies, but it is primarily degenerative rather than inflammatory.[100,273,295] Ankylosing hyperostosis is frequently asymptomatic, a radiographic curiosity, but occasionally it produces limitation of motion and discomfort. It is characterized by pronounced ''flowing mantles'' of ossification in the thoracic, lumbar, and cervical spine, without accompanying narrowing of disc space, osteoporosis, or ankylosis of the posterior apophyseal joint.[295] Ossification appears earliest in the thoracic region (Fig. 5–71) along the anterior and anterolateral aspects of the spine. Radiographs of the frontal chest or abdomen reveal knobby, ossified, paraspinal masses. Even more often, this exuberant ossification is detected in a lateral radiograph of the chest, as an undulating bony mantle lying anterior to the vertebral body and deep to, or incorporated into, the anterior longitudinal ligament.[100] The left side of the thoracic spine is gen-

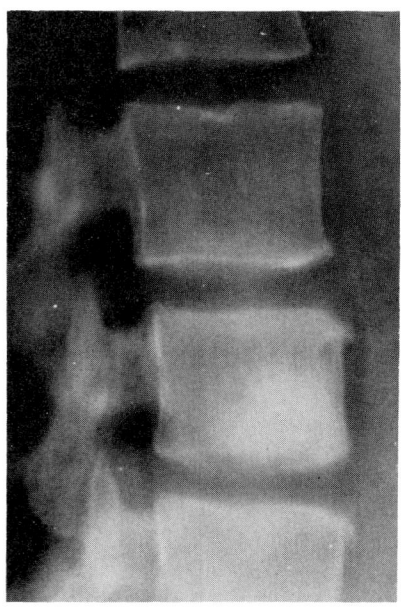

Fig. 5–70. Discogenic vertebral sclerosis at the L4 to L5 level consisting of intense reactive sclerosis extending into the anterior two-thirds of the vertebral body and accompanied by mild disc narrowing.

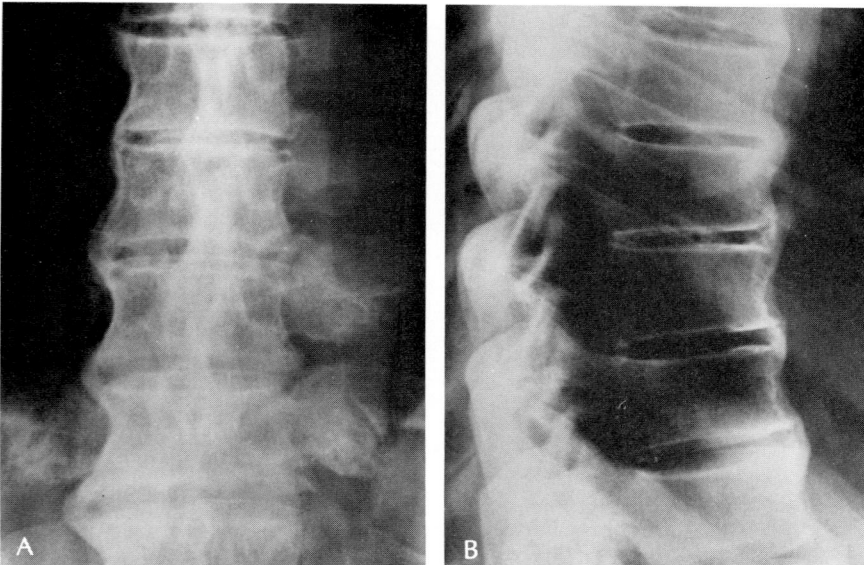

Fig. 5–71. Anteroposterior *(A)* and lateral *(B)* views of the thoracic spine demonstrating an undulating mantle of ossification with preservation of disc space and normal mineralization, characteristic of diffuse idiopathic skeletal hyperostosis.

erally spared, possibly because of aortic pulsation. Small notches or slots frequently detected anteriorly at the disc levels represent fissures or fractures and account for the preservation of motion, albeit limited in the spine (Fig. 5–72).[273]

The mantle is sometimes finer and less undulating and simulates the squaring of ankylosing spondylitis in lateral radiographs, but a faint radiolucent separation from the underlying vertebral body usually is detectable. Occasionally, the appearance is extreme (Fig. 5–73), with broad and coarse vertically oriented ossification resembling the nonmarginal asymmetric syndesmophytes of psoriasis.[324] A distinct spinal encroachment syndrome due to posterior longitudinal ligament ossification has been reported, perhaps part of the spectrum of ankylosing hyperostosis.[248,255,301]

The axial manifestations are frequently accompanied by distinct peripheral changes consisting of well-corticated exophytic overgrowth at areas of musculotendinous and capsular insertion that has led to the term diffuse idiopathic skeletal hyperostosis.[295,299] The hyperostosis, particularly of the phalangeal tufts, may simulate acromegaly, but is unassociated with soft tissue and cartilage hypertrophy.

Neuroarthropathy

The terms *Charcot* or *neuropathic* describe painless, unstable, and frequently deformed joints that accompany neurologic deficit (see also Chap. 71).

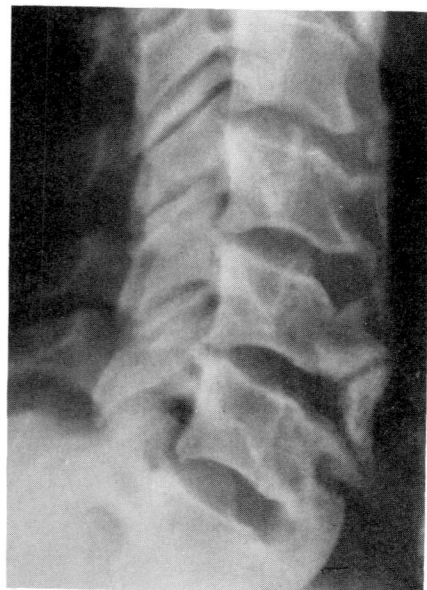

Fig. 5–72. Lateral cervical spine demonstrates extensive anterior ossification, with characteristic clefts and preservation of disc spaces in diffuse idiopathic skeletal hyperostosis.

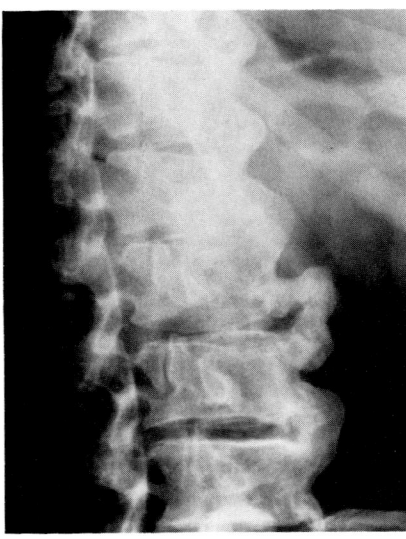

Fig. 5–73. Oblique view of the thoracolumbar spine demonstrates large osteophytes fused with a thick, undulating mantle of ossification involving the anterior longitudinal ligament, the anulus fibrosus, and the adjacent connective tissue in a patient with ankylosing hyperostosis. This appearance can mimic the large, nonmarginal, asymmetric syndesmophytes of psoriatic and Reiter's arthritis, although the distribution is generally different.

In the early phase of the process, the affected joint is not deformed or unstable and may be painful, warm, and swollen from an accompanying synovitis and microfractures.[13,129,176,181,263] The many diseases that may predispose patients to this disorder are all associated with loss of proprioception and varied degrees of hypoesthesia, especially diminished deep pain sensation, which is a sine qua non. Most common among these diseases are tabes dorsalis, diabetes mellitus, syringomyelia, and spinal cord injury or anomaly.

The radiographic features depend on the underlying disease and on the stage and rate of evolution. In established neuroarthropathy, these features consist of joint effusion, subluxation, subarticular sclerosis, fracture and fragmentation, marginal osteophytosis, and heterotopic calcification and ossification (Fig. 5–74, 5–75). Any of these features may exist separately, or they may be combined, as is common in advanced disease.[176,181,263] Although initially a single joint is usually involved, others are eventually affected.[13,51,94,176] The common sites of neuropathic involvement are the midfoot, ankle, and knee, and less commonly, the hip, spine, shoulder, and wrist, although other joints may be affected. When the condition evolves rapidly,[93,263] radiographs may show massive effusion of the joint accompanied by striking calcific detritus, which generally is intra-articular, but may

extravasate into the surrounding soft tissue planes (Fig. 5–76).[152,169] Later, both in the rapidly and slowly evolving forms of neuroarthropathy, one sees similar radiographic features of extensive subarticular bone resorption, the atrophic phase, with joint deformity and instability. This resorption is followed by intense sclerosis, prominent osteophytosis, and periarticular ossification, the hypertrophic phase. The adjacent shafts of bone may show periosteal new-bone formation, which is usually solid and well defined and thereby indicates chronicity. The late changes, which are similar to those of advanced degenerative joint disease, differ primarily in degree.

A purely atrophic form of neuroarthropathy affects the peripheral articulations of the upper extremity and the forefoot in diabetic patients.[325] Radiographically, striking resorption and tapering and frequent dislocation of the articular ends of bone are seen, but little reactive periosteal or heterotopic new-bone formation. The appearance is that of arthritis mutilans simulating psoriatic arthropathy or, less commonly, RA, Ehlers-Danlos syndrome, or leprosy.[325]

Two factors that may contribute to Charcot arthropathy are systemic or intra-articular corticosteroid therapy and CPPD crystal deposition disease. The former has been termed steroid arthropathy,[156,247,256,348] possibly beginning as osteonecrosis, but soon resulting in advanced joint destruction. Its radiographic appearance is identical to that of Charcot joints associated with a primary neurologic deficit. Generalized CPPD crystal deposition and luetic Charcot arthropathy of the knee frequently coexist.[169] A neuropathic picture of severe destructive arthropathy can be seen in the metacarpophalangeal, shoulder, hip, knee, and other joints affected by CPPD crystal deposition even in the absence of any neurologic deficit (see Chap. 94).

Osteonecrosis

Osteonecrosis includes a spectrum of conditions with similar pathologic and radiologic features (see also Chap. 86). These conditions include avascular necrosis of bone, juvenile osteochondrosis, and osteochondritis dissecans.

Avascular necrosis may affect the metadiaphyseal regions of bone and may cause characteristic, finely sclerotic, medullary bone infarcts, or it may affect the intra-articular epiphyseal region, resulting in clinical and radiologic features of secondary arthropathy.[24,233] Common subarticular sites are the femoral and humeral heads, distal femoral condyle, proximal tibial plateau, carpal navicular, and proximal talus.[370,380] The precise focus in a given joint is dictated by the vascular supply and the location

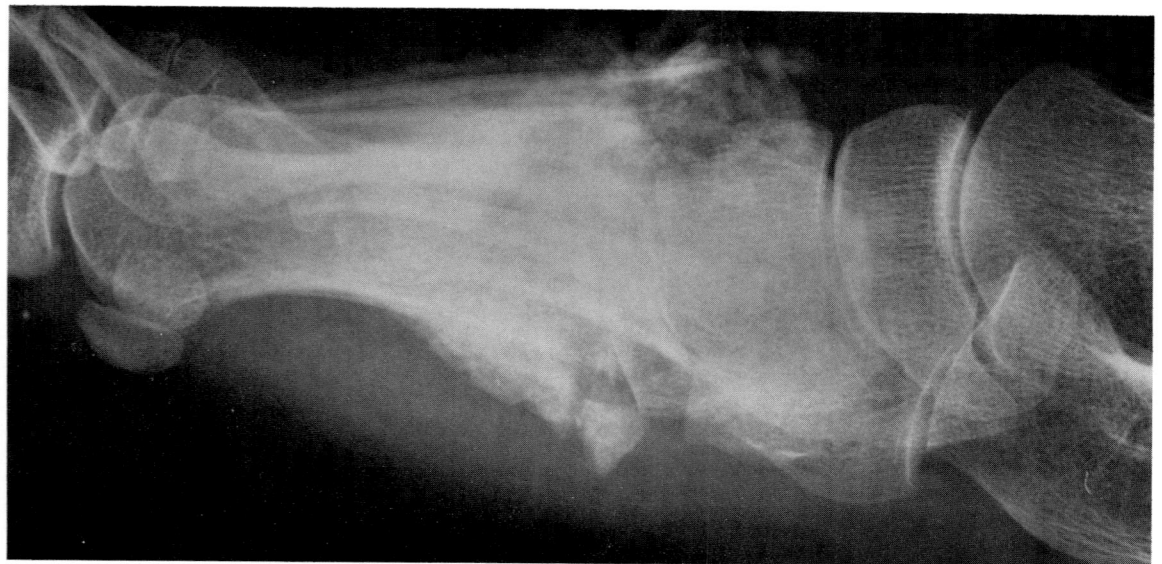

Fig. 5–74.   Advanced diabetic neuroarthropathy of the midfoot consisting of fragmentation of the metatarsal, tarsal, and intertarsal articulations, heterotopic ossification, and marked soft tissue swelling.

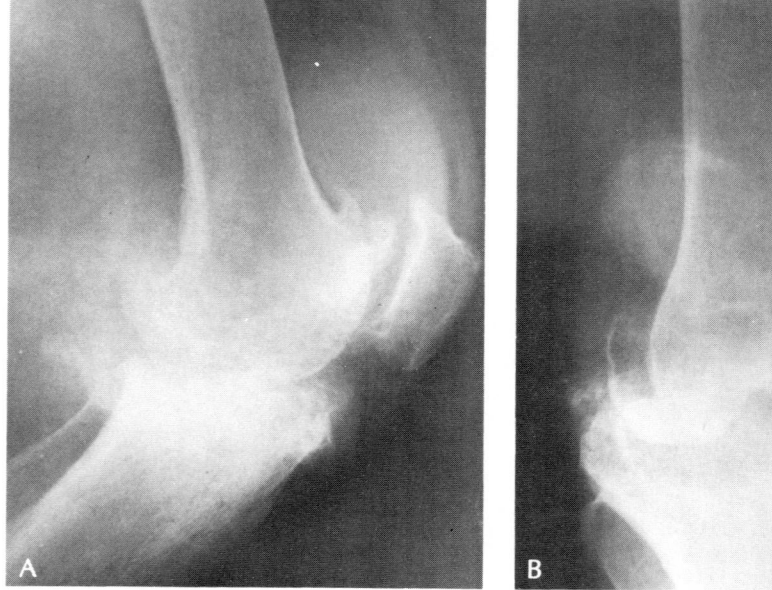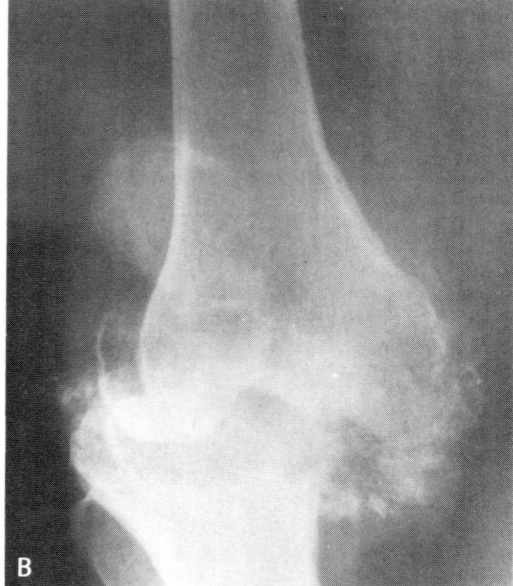

Fig. 5–75.   A and B, Extensive destructive arthropathy of a neuropathic joint in a patient with calcium pyrophosphate dihydrate crystal deposition and tabes dorsalis. Subluxations, subchondral bone resorption, and heterotopic ossification are associated with joint effusion.

of the weight-bearing surface.[233] Common predisposing factors include trauma, corticosteroid therapy, hemoglobinopathy, pancreatitis, alcoholism, renal osteodystrophy, systemic lupus erythematosus, and decompression sickness.[121,247,256,348] The femoral head is the most common site of avascular necrosis and is representative radiographically of changes in other joints.

The radiographic appearance may be normal initially, whereas a bone scan frequently demonstrates a focal, "cold," avascular area surrounded by a "hot," hyperemic zone.[74,139,159] Later, radiographic changes consist of subtle, mottled sclerosis and lysis of the superior aspect of the femoral head. A slight loss of the normal concentric shape or minimal flattening is noted, followed by the develop-

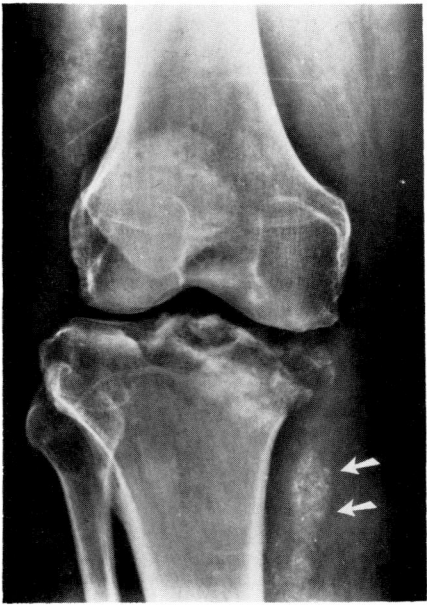

Fig. 5–76. Acute joint neuropathy in a patient with tabes dorsalis and chondrocalcinosis. The extensive destruction and fragmentation of bone evolved during a period of several days. The powdered bone provides an "autoarthrogram;" the knee, ruptured posteriorly, has spilled "contrast material" into the calf (arrows).

ment of a pathognomonic, faint, radiolucent crescent line that parallels the articular surface and represents a separation or fracture of subchondral bone (Fig. 86–2).[237] This appearance is best seen in lateral projections of the hip because the anterosuperior aspect of the femoral head is most frequently involved. That the articular space and the adjacent acetabulum are initially unaffected differentiates this process from the primary arthropathies. Subsequently, sclerosis, lysis, fragmentation, and collapse progress (see Figs. 86–3 to 86–5), with resultant compromise of the articular space and, eventually, secondary osteoarthritis. A patient in a late stage of avascular necrosis is usually distinguishable from one with primary osteoarthritis by a greater destruction of the femoral head with dissolution of the cortical outline and relative preservation of the acetabulum,[237] but this distinction is not always possible.

When osteonecrosis develops as an idiopathic process during childhood, it is frequently termed *juvenile* osteochondrosis.[269] It may represent ischemic or traumatized juxta-articular bone and may involve the hips (Legg-Calvé-Perthes's disease), the tarsal navicular (Köhler's disease), the vertebral end plates (Scheuermann's disease), and other sites.[269] The radiographic appearance, like that of

avascular necrosis, consists of sclerosis, fragmentation, and collapse. The process is clinically self-limited and radiography demonstrates progressive resolution.

Osteochondritis dissecans is a similar ischemic or traumatic subarticular process predominantly in young persons that is more focal in nature.[334] The condition is frequently monoarticular, but it may be bilateral, affecting predominantly the medial femoral condyle, capitellum (Fig. 5–77), talus, femoral head, and patella. It results in a small "button," or osteocartilaginous fragment, that separates partially from the remainder of the articular surface or breaks off completely as a loose body. Tomographic examination is frequently helpful in the delineation of this small osteochondral defect, as is arthrography in the assessment of the integrity of the overlying cartilage.

CRYSTAL DEPOSITION DISEASES

Gout

Gout is a form of crystal-induced disease caused by monosodium urate monohydrate crystal deposition that affects predominantly the small diarthrodial joints (see also Chapter 91).[29,129,284,345,346,372] The feet, hands, wrists, ankles, and elbows are most frequently involved, both clinically and radiographically. During the initial acute episodes of gout, the only radiographic manifestations are soft tissue swelling, usually related to capsular distention, and mild focal demineralization. Even in chronic gout, radiographic evaluation may fail to reveal articular abnormalities. After years of recurrent disease, characteristic asymmetric, oligoarticular involvement may appear, consisting of nodular, periarticular soft tissue swelling, absent or minimal osteoporosis, relative maintenance of articular space, and intra- and

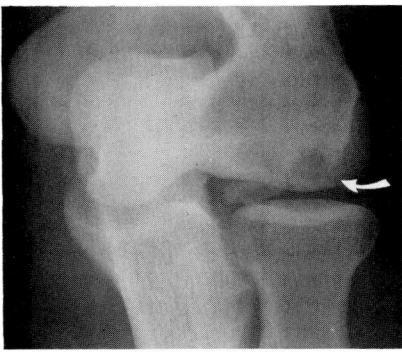

Fig. 5–77. Osteochondritis dissecans of the capitellum showing a small lytic defect (arrow) in the subarticular bone and a "button" of osteocartilaginous fragment, loose in the joint.

extra-articular bony erosions. Polyarticular involvement, uniform loss of cartilage, and pronounced articular destruction with malalignment are rare and are seen only in advanced disease, particularly since the advent of effective therapy for hyperuricemia.[266]

Tophi characteristic of gout appear radiographically as eccentric discrete foci, often with a homogeneous or mottled increased density. They arise in periarticular and, less commonly, nonarticular regions. Discrete calcification within tophi is uncommon and is seen mainly in patients with underlying renal disease and altered calcium metabolism.[345,346,374] Tophi may develop in any location, but they are particularly common over the dorsum of the foot, around the calcaneus, and in the bursae, particularly of the elbows.

Erosive disease is common in established gout and results from pressure, remodeling, and destruction secondary to tophaceous deposits in periarticular structures. Characteristically, erosions are sharply marginated with a fine, sclerotic border and may appear punched out, as opposed to the ill-defined and focally demineralized erosions of RA (Fig. 5–78).[229,369,372] In about 40% of patients with gouty erosions, a characteristic overhanging margin or lip results from displacement of cortex and apposition of new bone, with remodeling around the tophus.[229] This appearance is uncommon in other erosive articular disorders. Frequently, large cystic erosions develop, particularly in the carpal and tarsal articulations.[284,372] Less commonly, rheu-

matoid-like erosive disease seen at synovial reflections and at sites of capsular insertion may be related to urate crystal-induced proliferative synovitis.[284] Of importance in this regard is the rare coexistence of gout and RA.[174,206]

The joint space is generally well preserved in gout because destruction of cartilage is focal, rather than generalized. Characteristically, erosive disease occurs in a patient with a normal joint space, although generalized and uniform loss of cartilage may be present in late stages of gout.[284,346,372] Rarely, bony ankylosis develops, predominantly in the interphalangeal, carpal, and tarsal joints. Periosteal new-bone formation may be associated with gouty erosion by enlarging the ends and, less commonly, the shafts of involved bones and thereby causing bizarre deformities.[353] Secondary degenerative changes with typical subchondral sclerosis and osteophyte formation become manifest in advanced disease. Patients with end-stage disease may have arthritis mutilans simulating psoriatic arthritis or RA[284,353] (Fig. 5–79).

Involvement of the sacroiliac joints, spine, hips,

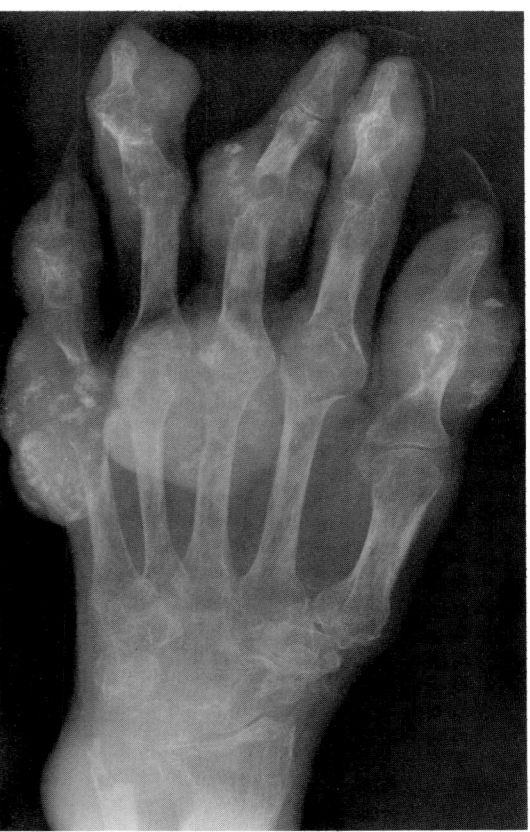

Fig. 5–79. Advanced destructive gouty arthropathy resembling arthritis mutilans.

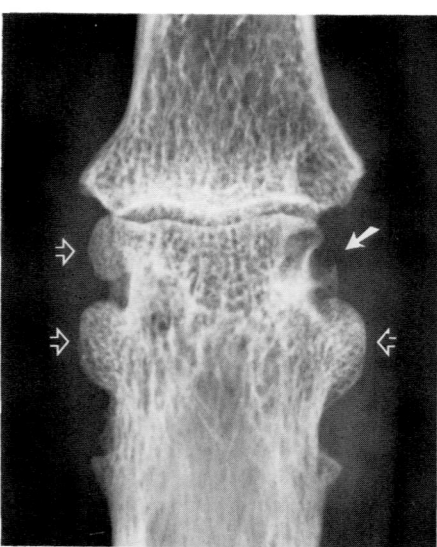

Fig. 5–78. Proximal interphalangeal joint in gout demonstrates maintenance of normal mineralization and articular space, but well-defined erosion (closed arrow) and lobulated bone response (open arrows).

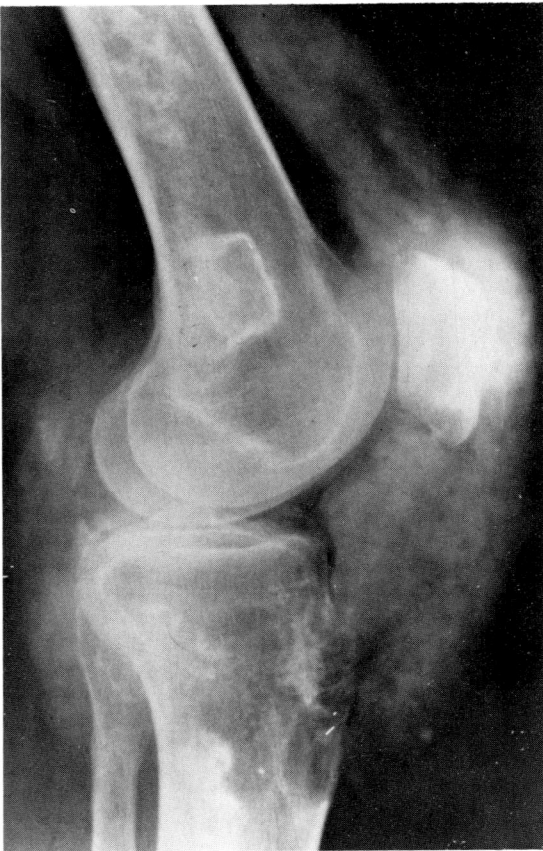

Fig. 5–80. Extensive tophaceous deposits around the knee accompanied by prominent intramedullary bone infarcts in a patient with gout.

or shoulders is uncommon, although isolated reports of involvement at these sites have appeared.[284,346] These unusual sites are affected generally in the presence of advanced, long-standing polyarticular arthropathy or, less commonly, in rapidly evolving disease of early onset.[283,284] Here the manifestations are not characteristic, but consist of bony erosion, cystic changes, variable narrowing of cartilage, and reactive sclerosis.

Uncommonly recognized in chronic gout are intramedullary bone infarction (Fig. 5–80) and avascular necrosis of subarticular regions.[52,79,345,346] These complications may result in collapse of subchondral bone and may be indistinguishable from other conditions that cause avascular necrosis of the femoral heads. The cause of ischemia in this instance is unknown, but it may be related to alterations in platelet adhesiveness or local pH.[23,284] Intra-articular calcification, occasionally noted in gout, may represent calcium urate (unproved) or CPPD crystal deposition in the fibrocartilage. This type of calcification is seen most commonly in the knees, hips, and wrists, and its appearance is similar to that of other forms of CPPD crystal deposition disease, although it may be more limited in distribution.[79,134,284,345,346] Probably, this form of chondrocalcinosis is caused by CPPD deposition because gout and pseudogout appear to coexist frequently.

Pseudogout

Articular chondrocalcinosis is the abnormal deposition of calcium salts in the hyaline and fibrocartilage of joints (see also Chaps. 94 and 95). These salts may consist of hydroxyapatite, dicalcium phosphate dihydrate, or CPPD crystals.[208] The last form, often accompanied by acute or chronic synovitis, is by far the most common and is called *pseudogout,* or *CPPD crystal deposition disease.*[211] Periarticular apatite-type calcifications have been noted radiographically to be more common (30%) in patients with CPPD type cartilaginous deposits than in controls (3%).[121a] Patients with both apatite and CPPD deposition had an increased frequency of Heberden's nodes.

Articular Calcification

The conspicuous radiographic features of pseudogout consist of linear and punctate calcifications of fibrocartilage and hyaline cartilage of multiple joints, frequently bilateral and symmetric.[111,173,210,234,289,383] Characteristically, fibrocartilage is most densely calcified in the meniscus, the articular disc of the wrist, the symphysis pubis, the glenoid and acetabular labra, and the anulus fibrosus of the intervertebral disc. Hyaline cartilage calcification differs in appearance from that of fibrocartilage; it is finer and more linear, and parallels the subchondral bone. It is situated in the midzonal layer initially and thus remains separate and distinct from the subchondral bony cortical line.[85] The synovial lining of joints may calcify, producing irregular, radiodense foci sufficient for radiographic detection. Intra-articular calcification of fragmented synovium or cartilage appears occasionally, particularly in the knees, and suggests loose bodies (Fig. 5–81),[210,264,289] or even synovial chondromatosis.[88] At times, calcification of joint capsules is predominant, as in the hips, shoulders, elbows, and small joints of the hands. Less commonly, extra-articular tendon, bursa, and soft tissue calcification takes place, as in the Achilles, triceps, quadriceps, and supraspinatus tendons and in the hip adductors.[234,289] The joint calcifications in both sporadic and familial forms of CPPD crystal deposition disease are qualitatively similar, although more widespread and extensive in the familial form.

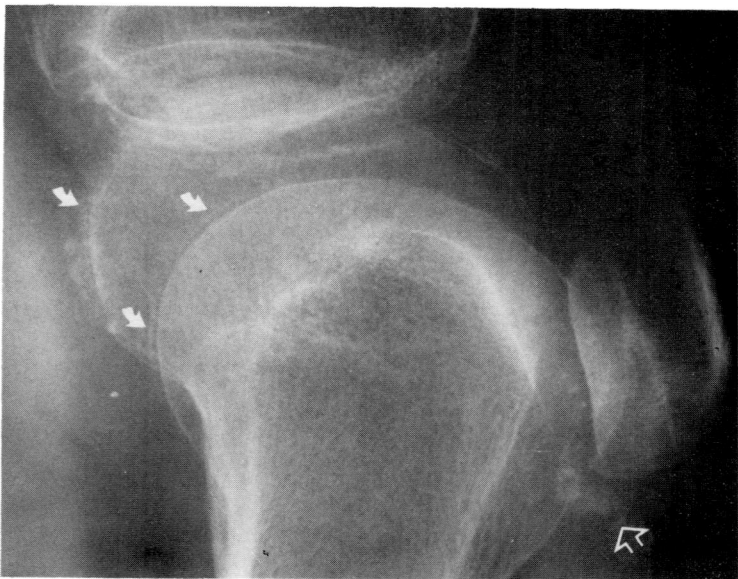

Fig. 5–81. Lateral view of the knee showing linear calcification of hyaline cartilage parallel to subchondral compact bone of the femoral condyles (small arrows). Calcification within the suprapatellar bursa simulates synovial chondromatosis (open arrow).

Arthropathy. That degenerative arthropathy accompanies articular chondrocalcinosis in pseudogout is well recognized. Martel et al.,[234] Resnick and co-workers,[289,296] and others[19,303] have emphasized the distinct features that distinguish this condition from typical primary osteoarthritis. The arthropathy consists of narrowing of the joint space, eburnation, marginal osteophytosis, and discrete subchondral cysts, all features of osteoarthritis, but differing in that cysts are more prominent and osteophytosis is variable. In pseudogout, for example, the pronounced and often isolated involvement of the patellofemoral compartment,[289] the radiocarpal joint (Fig. 5–82), and the metacarpophalangeal joints (Fig. 5–83) are distinguishing characteristics.[234,296] Severe destructive changes may evolve rapidly and may produce a Charcot-like appearance in the presence of normal[169,210,246,289,303] or minimally abnormal neurologic function (see Figs. 5–75, 5–76). The knees, shoulders, hips, and wrists are the most common joints affected by this destructive and deforming arthropathy, although other joints such as the metacarpophalangeal and elbow may also be involved (Fig. 5–84).

Abnormalities in Specific Joints. The knee is the most commonly involved joint clinically and radiographically (95% of patients). Chondrocalcinosis in the knee is identified as linear or punctate calcification in the inner two-thirds of the fibrocartilaginous meniscus (see Fig. 5–81). Its appearance ranges from fine to dense, and it produces

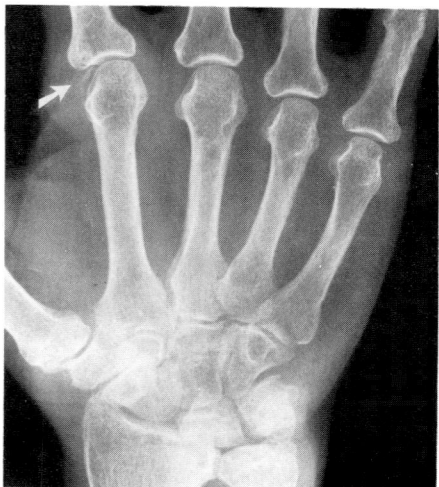

Fig. 5–82. Advanced arthropathy of the radiocarpal joint consisting of narrowing, eburnation, subchondral cyst formation, and mild fragmentation. Articular calcification of the wrist is not identified. Capsular and synovial calcification of the second metacarpophalangeal joint with mild associated subchondral radiolucency is seen (arrow). Although degenerative changes at the first carpometacarpal joint are consistent with osteoarthritis, striking radiocarpal involvement is not. The dissociation between calcification and degenerative arthropathy is also illustrated.

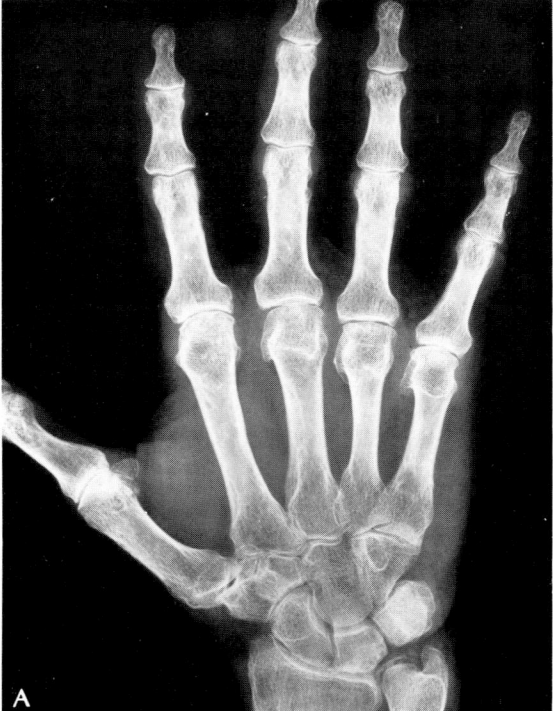

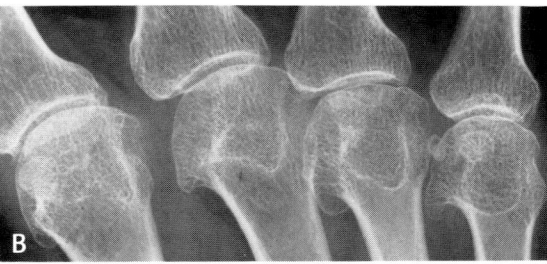

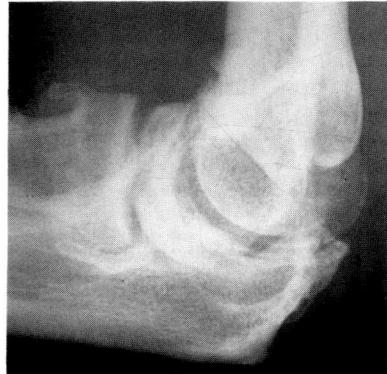

Fig. 5–84. Lateral radiograph of the elbow in patient with calcium pyrophosphate dihydrate crystal deposition disease, showing extensive arthropathy with joint narrowing, eburnation, obteophytosis, and intra-articular fragmentation of bone.

Fig. 5–83. Radiographs of the hand of a patient with hemochromatosis. *A*, Diffuse osteopenia and calcification of the articular disc of the wrist, associated with arthropathy of the radiocarpal joint. *B*, Close-up view of the metacarpophalangeal joints showing joint narrowing, subchondral collapse, and striking proliferation of bone that produces a ''squared off'' appearance.

a wedge-shaped calcification of the medial and lateral margins of the joint. The hyaline cartilage is less frequently involved and appears as a fine, linear density that parallels the subchondral bone of the tibial plateau or femoral condyles. This density is often well demonstrated in the lateral radiographs (see Fig. 5–81). Calcification of the fibrous cruciate ligaments and the quadriceps tendon is common. Synovial calcification and intra-articular calcified loose bodies are more frequent in this joint that in any other in this condition.

Changes resembling those of osteoarthritis are frequent but variable in the knee and consist of

narrowing of joint space, osteophytosis, and eburnation. As narrowing and osteophytosis become more advanced, articular chondrocalcinosis may become obscured, although CPPD crystals may still be seen in joint fluid aspirates. In some instances, knee arthropathy may be destructive, with rapid evolution of erosion, fragmentation of subchondral bone, and periarticular ossification, resulting in severe joint deformity. These Charcot-like knees (see Figs. 5–75, 5–76) may develop in patients with otherwise uncomplicated CPPD disease, or they may be associated with neurologic deficit[169,303] or hyperparathyroidism.[44]

The *wrist* and *hand* are the second most common regions involved with CPPD crystal deposition disease in most reported series.[19,210,234,289] Characteristically, the articular disc of the distal radioulnar joint, a triangular fibrocartilaginous structure, is the earliest and most frequent site of calcification (see Fig. 5–83, *A*). Fine linear calcification of the hyaline cartilage of the intracarpal and carpometacarpal joints may be an accompanying manifestation. Arthropathy at the wrist (see Fig. 5–82) is characteristic, suggesting the underlying presence of CPPD crystals even when chondrocalcinosis is absent radiographically.[234,289,296] The radiocarpal joint is predominantly affected, with narrowing of joint space, eburnation, and occasional formation of discrete subchondral bone cysts. That the first carpometacarpal joint is generally spared helps one to distinguish pseudogout from osteoarthritis, in which this joint is typically involved and the radiocarpal joint is spared. Characteristic calcification may even be seen in the metacarpophalangeal joints, with opacities in the capsular and synovial tissues, particularly of the second joint. Fine, linear hyaline cartilage calcification is less common. Narrowing of the metacarpophalangeal joints, subchondral sclerosis, and fragmentation with occasional pseudocyst formation are distinctive. Such changes are rare at this site in osteoarthritis,[234,289] but are particularly pronounced in hemochromatosis,[146,323] often with associated CPPD crystal deposition (see Fig. 5–83, A,B). Periarticular calcification of distal and proximal interphalangeal joints is seen rarely.

In the *pelvis,* calcification of the symphysis pubis is a frequent finding, particularly in familial series,[279,388] in which it is nearly invariable. This involvement consists of punctate calcifications of the fibrocartilage, that produce a vertical density in the midline of the symphysis.

Involvement of the hip and shoulder is frequent radiographically, with a reported incidence of 15 to 50%. It consists of calcification of hyaline articular cartilage that results in a curvilinear density parallel to the subchondral bony cortex and an irregular, mottled calcification of the fibrocartilage of the labrum, capsule, tendons, and bursae, with prominent amorphous periarticular deposits. Although associated degenerative arthropathy is frequent, advanced changes are only occasionally reported.[246,289,303]

In the *spine,* a frequent site of articular chondrocalcinosis, the outer fibers of the articular disc (anulus fibrosus) are the site of crystal deposition. The nucleus pulposus is not involved,[111,210] except in advanced familial cases.[279,383] Dense calcification of the entire intervertebral disc may simulate ochronosis.[265] Arthropathy consists of degeneration of the disc with narrowed interspaces and subchondral sclerosis, generally most pronounced in the lumbar and cervical regions.[234,289]

Involvement of the *elbow* may be characteristic (Fig. 5–84) because this joint is not affected by primary osteoarthritis.[234,289] Linear calcification of articular cartilage, calcification of capsule and triceps tendon, and eventual narrowing of joint space and eburnation are seen.[289] Flexion contractures of the elbow are frequent.

Less commonly affected by either calcification or associated arthropathy are the ankles, acromioclavicular and sternoclavicular joints, and the metatarsophalangeal joints (Fig. 5–85). The infrequency of disease, specifically in the first metatarsophalangeal joint, helps one to distinguish the pseudogout syndrome from true gouty arthritis.[210,234,289] Although a degenerative arthropathy of the sacroiliac joint in pseudogout is seen occasionally,[210,211] radiographically visible chondrocalcinosis is common only in severe familial cases.[383]

Differential Diagnosis. In patients with articular CPPD deposits with or without degenerative arthropathy, certain associated diseases must be considered. These include hemochromatosis,[146,272,323] Wilson's disease,[95] and primary hyperparathyroidism,[45,78,136,246] as well as the familial forms[279,304,383] (see Chap. 94). The radiographic features of *hemochromatosis* with articular chondrocalcinosis (see Fig. 5–83) may be identical to those of idiopathic CPPD crystal deposition disease, particularly in the knees, hips, and wrists. These changes are seen in 25 to 50% of affected patients. The destructive arthropathy of the metacarpophalangeal joints, with bony proliferation, collapse, fragmentation, and subchondral cyst formation, associated with generalized skletal osteopenia, may suggest the underlying disorder. *Wilson's disease* may have radiographic features similar to those in hemochromatosis, including abnormalities of the metacarpophalangeal joints, although articular chondrocalcinosis is infrequent and bone fragmentation is common.[2,95]

Articular chondrocalcinosis in *primary hyperparathyroidism* with CPPD deposition is well recognized, with a reported incidence of 10 to 18%.[78,117,136] Conversely, in several large series of CPPD crystal deposition disease, the frequency of concomitant primary hyperparathyroidism is reported to be 2 to 7%.[69,207] Many of these patients have symptomatic pseudogout. The erosive and destructive arthropathy may be aggravated by parathyroid hormone, with weakening of subchondral bone and secondary fragmentation and collapse.[45,300] Of interest is the frequent periarticular and soft tissue calcification in *secondary hyperparathyroidism* associated with renal disease. This calcification results from hydroxyapatite crystal deposition.[78] CPPD deposits are commonly associated with secondary hyperparathyroidism, but their deposition is more common in the spine (see Chap. 94).

Gout and articular calcification coincide with greater-than-chance frequency.[69,79,210,211,234,253] Calcification in these instances is generally limited to the knees and is associated with advanced tophaceous gout.[79,234] Chondrocalcinosis again involves the menisci, but is faint and asymmetric. Only rarely does calcification appear in the wrist.[79,234] The simultaneous existence of urate and calcium pyrophosphate crystals in some patients with gout is well known.[69,253]

CPPD crystal deposition disease may be coincidental to other rheumatic diseases,[42,134,253] such as RA and systemic lupus erythematosus, and has accompanied septic arthritis. In such instances, the radiographic appearance of articular calcification or the detection of CPPD crystals in joint fluid aspirates may prove a "red herring," with symp-

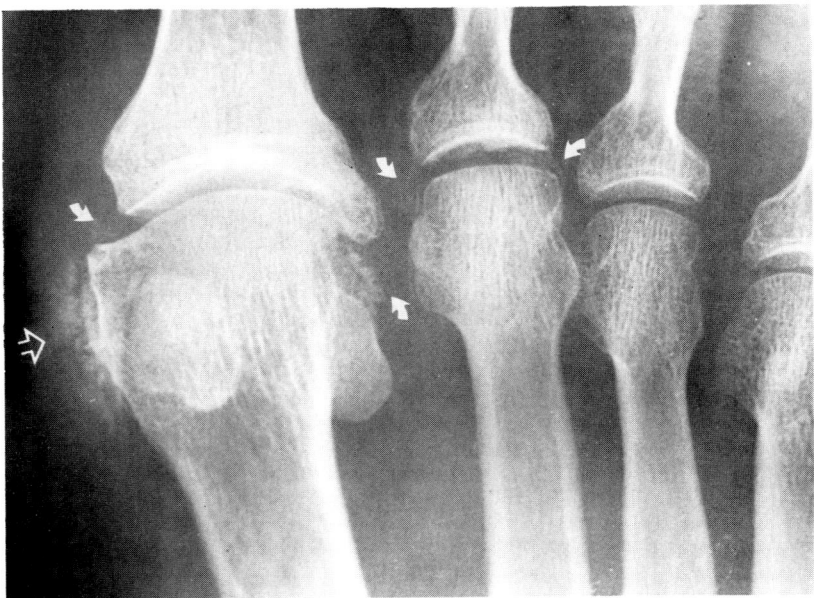

Fig. 5–85. Articular and capsular deposits (arrows) similar to those of calcium pyrophosphate dihydrate deposition disease in the metatarsophalangeal joints and calcific deposits in the bursa (open arrow) of the first metatarsophalangeal joint are seen.

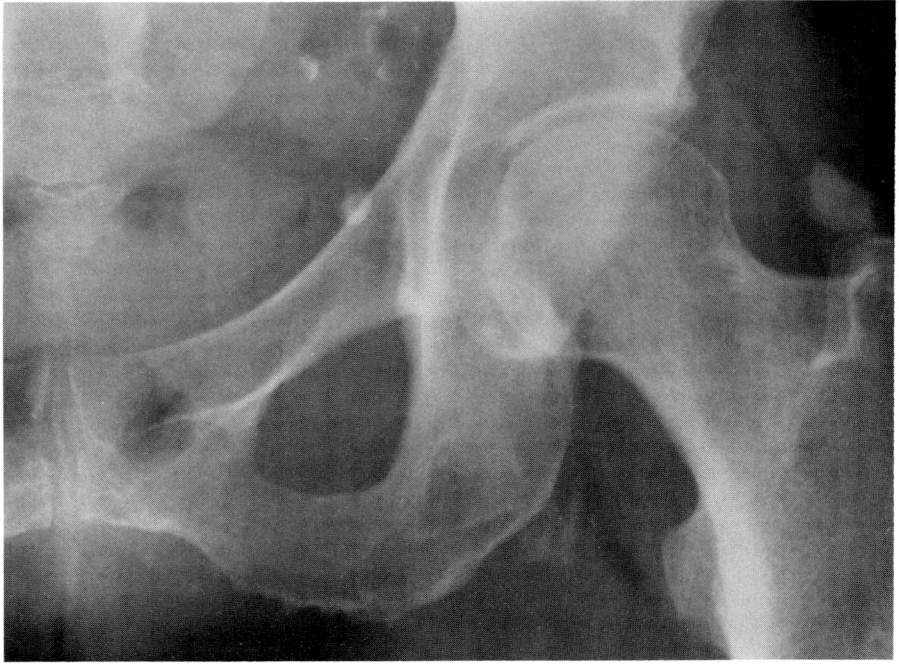

Fig. 5–86. Anteroposterior view of the pelvis demonstrates mottled, cloud-like calcification of the greater trochanteric region characteristic of basic calcium phosphate crystal deposition; fine linear and punctate calcification involving the symphysis pubis and hamstring insertions are characteristic of calcium pyrophosphate dihydrate crystal deposition disease.

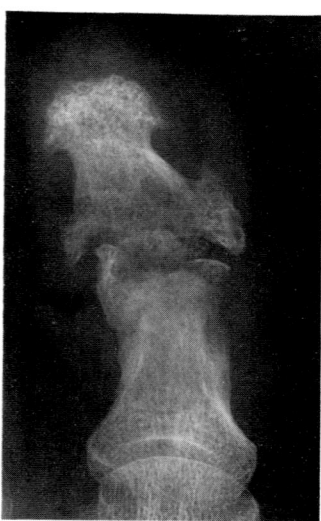

Fig. 5–87. Chronic osteomyelitis and joint infection in diabetic patient. Joint destruction and extensive sclerosis with remodeling indicate chronicity.

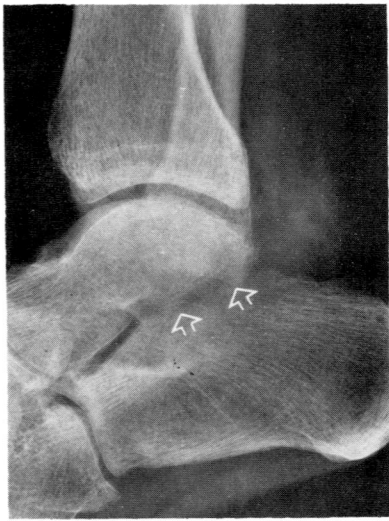

Fig. 5–88. Lateral ankle radiograph of a patient with gonoccocal arthritis showing complete dissolution of the subchondral cortical line of the subtalar joint (arrows) with adjacent focal demineralization.

toms primarily related to the noncrystal disease process (see Chaps. 4, 93, and 94).

Hydroxyapatite (Basic Calcium Phosphate) Deposition Disease

Calcific periarthritis or *peritendinitis calcarea*,[133,276] a basic calcium phosphate (BCP) crystal deposition disease affecting tendons and bursae,[25] must be considered in the differential diagnosis (Fig. 5–86) of the crystal-induced arthropathies (see also Chap. 95). Characteristically, the supraspinatus tendon and subacromial bursa of the shoulder are involved, but often several areas are affected, including the tendons and capsules of the hips, elbows, and wrists. Generally, the calcification is periarticular, a homogeneous solitary deposit not involving the articular cartilage. This feature distinguishes it from CPPD crystal deposition disease. Recent studies have shown that BCP crystals may also be deposited intra-articularly,[25,290,322] either as a primary phenomenon or secondary to another disease. A continuum of abnormalities from monoarticular periarthritis to polyarticular disease and finally joint destruction may occur. The diagnosis of BCP crystal deposition diseases is discussed in Chapters 4 and 95.

JOINT INFECTION

Septic Arthritis

Joint infection is generally diagnosed clinically, but radiographic examination is of great value in assessing the extent of joint destruction (see also Chaps. 99 to 101). It may be of little use in the early diagnosis because of the lack of both sensitivity and specificity. Specific radiographic features are a late manifestation.[72,170,343,371] Radionuclide joint scanning, although nonspecific, may be helpful early in these conditions because of its high sensitivity.

The radiographic appearance depends on the age of the patient, the mechanism of inoculation, the virulence of the organism, the stage of disease, the influence of therapy, the local anatomic features, and the presence of underlying articular disorders. Any joint may be infected, but the spine, hips, and knees are the most common, and next in order are the wrists, ankles, shoulders, and sacroiliac joints. Small peripheral joints are uncommonly involved, except for those of the feet in the presence of vascular insufficiency (Fig. 5–87).

Articular "seeding" may result from direct hematogenous spread to the synovium and, secondarily, from subarticular osteomyelitis or overlying superficial cellulitis. The first is the most common mechanism. Articular destruction complicating osteomyelitis is seen in adults and in infants in whom the subarticular blood supply is continuous with the major nutrient supply to the diaphysis and metaphysis.[358,371] In children, however, the cartilaginous epiphyseal growth plate acts as an effective barrier to the spread of pyogenic infection from its common site of origin in the metaphysis. Thus, isolated osteomyelitis without septic arthritis is more common in this age group. An exception is when the metaphysis is situated within the joint

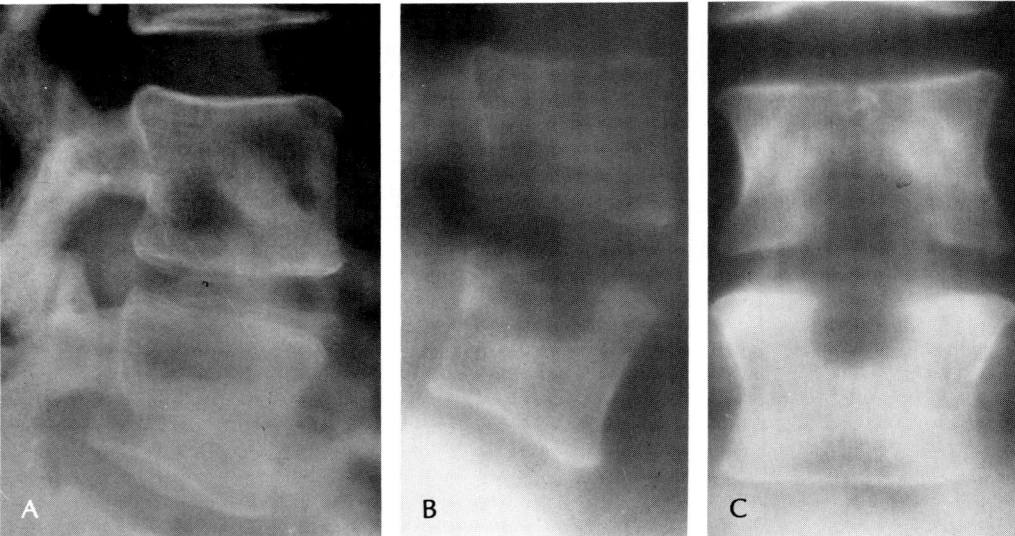

Fig. 5–89. Septic infection of the spine due to staphylococci. *A,* Conventional lateral radiograph demonstrates mild disc-space narrowing and dissolution of the vertebral end plate. The extensive destruction of the cancellous bone may only be detected tomographically, as shown in lateral *(B)* and anteroposterior *(C)* projections.

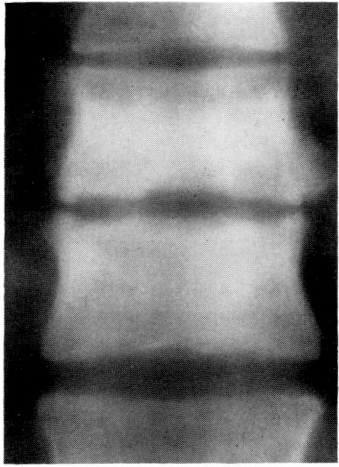

Fig. 5–90. Chronic infection of the spine has resulted in end-plate destruction, disc-space narrowing, and extensive sclerosis of the vertebral bodies. The appearance here has been modified by incomplete therapy.

capsule, such as that of the hip, in which instance osteomyelitis is frequently accompanied by septic arthritis. Another exception is osteomyelitis caused by tuberculous or fungal infection, which readily destroys and crosses the epiphyseal plate and induces secondary arthritis.[70,343]

Pyogenic infection of the diarthrodial joints may result from a variety of organisms, the most common of which are staphylococci, streptococci, pneumococci, gonococci, and in recent years, pseudomonas.[72,343] Generally the process is monarticular except in instances of underlying systemic disease, immunosuppressive therapy, or drug abuse.[72,162,185,316] Pyogenic infection is characterized radiographically by capsular distention recognizable several days after the onset of symptoms and soon followed by patchy osteoporosis related to hyperemia and disuse. The early resorption of cancellous bone is nonspecific and affects predominantly the region immediately adjacent to the subarticular cortex and the epiphyseal plate. Initially, the joint space may be widened because of effusion, but uniform loss of articular space soon appears from rapid, generalized destruction of cartilage.[40,70] Within several weeks, diffuse lysis of the subchondral cortical line is produced (Fig. 5–88), resulting in an appearance distinct from that of tuberculous arthritis or RA in which articular erosions are focal and marginal.[72] Later, complete destruction of cartilage and subchondral bone causes fragmentation, reactive sclerosis, and pronounced deformity.

Spinal Involvement

Pyogenic infection in the spine is usually less acute than that in diarthrodial joints, with slower evolution of clinical and radiographic manifestations.[72,343] The earliest radiographic changes consist of focal demineralization and loss of the distinct margin of the vertebral end plate, generally accompanied by slight narrowing of disc space (Fig.

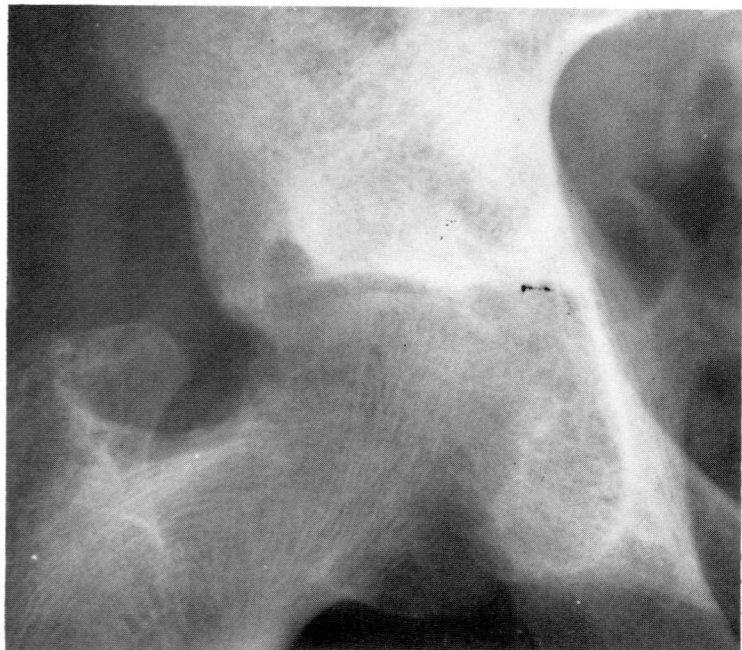

Fig. 5–91. Chronic tuberculous infection of the hip demonstrating marginal erosion, moderate cartilage loss, destruction of the medial femoral head, and reactive sclerosis in the supra-acetabular region.

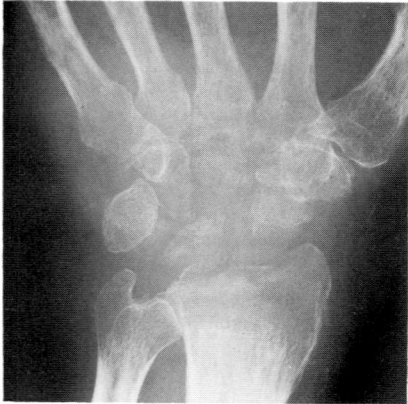

Fig. 5–92. Late tuberculous arthritis involving the wrist and carpus and resulting in destruction of cartilage and subarticular bone, accompanied by pronounced periarticular demineralization and soft tissue swelling.

5–89, A). Irregular erosion and destruction of the vertebral end plate then take place, with progressive narrowing of disc space, a result of herniation of the nucleus pulposus into the body (Fig. 5–89, B,C). Paraspinal masses representing abscesses may be seen particularly in the anteroposterior views of the thoracic spine and lateral views of the cervical spine. Later, striking reactive sclerosis, osteophytic spur formation, collapse, and occa-

sionally bony ankylosis may be seen (Figs. 5–90, 101–2).

Nonpyogenic Joint Infection

Tuberculosis is the most common cause of nonpyogenic infection.[70,318,343] Other nonsuppurative infections are uncommonly implicated, such as coccidioidomycosis, blastomycosis, actinomycosis, sporotrichosis, and brucellosis.[66,72,183] These subacute or chronic processes are more likely to result in radiographic changes when initially encountered than are pyogenic infections.[343]

Tuberculous involvement of diarthrodial joints is characterized radiographically by mild-to-moderate soft tissue swelling, marginal erosions on non-weight-bearing surfaces, and preservation of cartilage.[72,258,343] Mixed demineralization and patchy sclerosis are common (Figs. 5–91, 101–1, 102–2). In children, epiphyseal overgrowth may simulate RA as a result of the diffuse synovial involvement and chronic hyperemia.[343] The late appearance of tuberculosis may be indistinguishable from that of a chronic pyogenic infection (Figs. 5–92, 102–3). Rarely, one sees distinctive "kissing" sequestra of abutting articular surfaces.

Tuberculosis of the spine is characterized by narrowing of the disc space, end-plate destruction, and large, occasionally calcified paraspinal abscesses. Moderate reactive sclerosis may be seen. The posterior elements are generally spared, whereas ad-

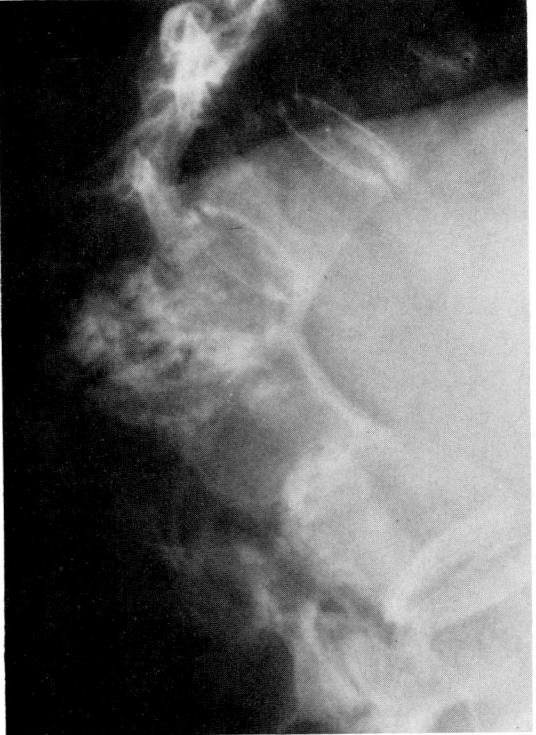

Fig. 5–93. Classic residual effect of advanced tuberculosis of the spine (Pott's disease), with calcified paraspinous abscess, gibbous deformity, and secondary bony ankylosis.

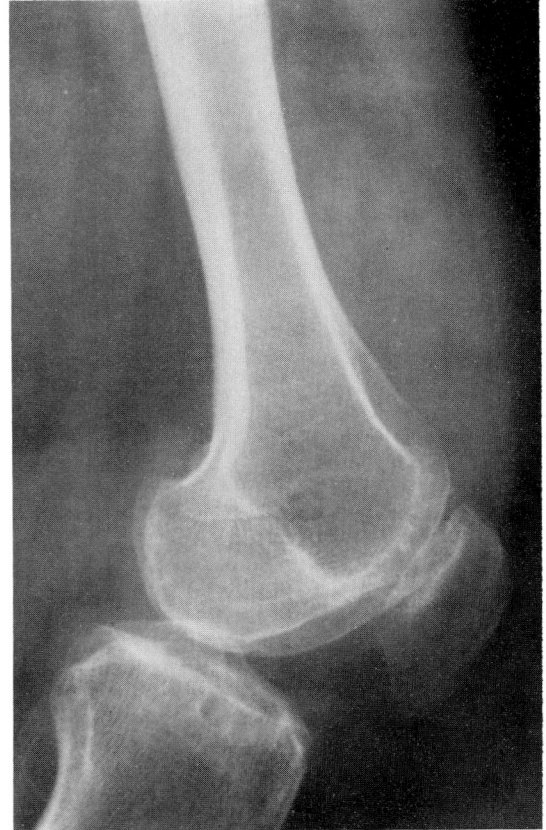

Fig. 5–94. Lateral radiograph of a young adult with long-standing joint swelling related to pigmented villonodular synovitis. The mass of mottled soft tissue in the superpatella region represents the hypertrophied synovium. One sees overgrowth of the femoral condyles, irregularity of the subarticular surface, and some loss of articular cartilage space.

jacent vertebral bodies are frequently involved at several levels. Striking anterior collapse and wedging may result in a characteristic gibbous deformity (Fig. 5–93). Occasionally, in both tuberculosis and coccidioidomycosis, isolated focal destruction of the anterior surface of the vertebral body may cause a scalloped or scooped-out erosion deep to the anterior longitudinal ligament.[72]

MISCELLANEOUS ARTICULAR DISORDERS

Neoplasia and Metaplasia (see also Chap. 84)

True primary neoplastic processes involving the articular soft tissue structures are rare, whereas benign proliferative and metaplastic alterations are common. Pigmented villonodular synovitis is included in the latter group and involves the synovium of joints, tendons, and bursae.[34,129,336] It may appear in a diffuse or nodular form[124] and as an intra- or extra-articular process. It is generally monarticular, although pauciarticular cases have been reported.[65] The most common site is the knee (Fig. 5–94); occasionally the hip, ankle, shoulder,

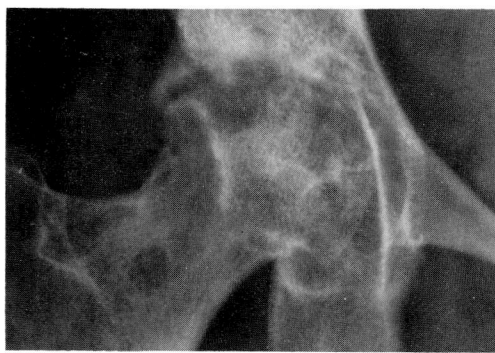

Fig. 5–95. Cartilage narrowing and cystic erosive changes in the acetabulum and femoral head and neck from pigmented villonodular synovitis.

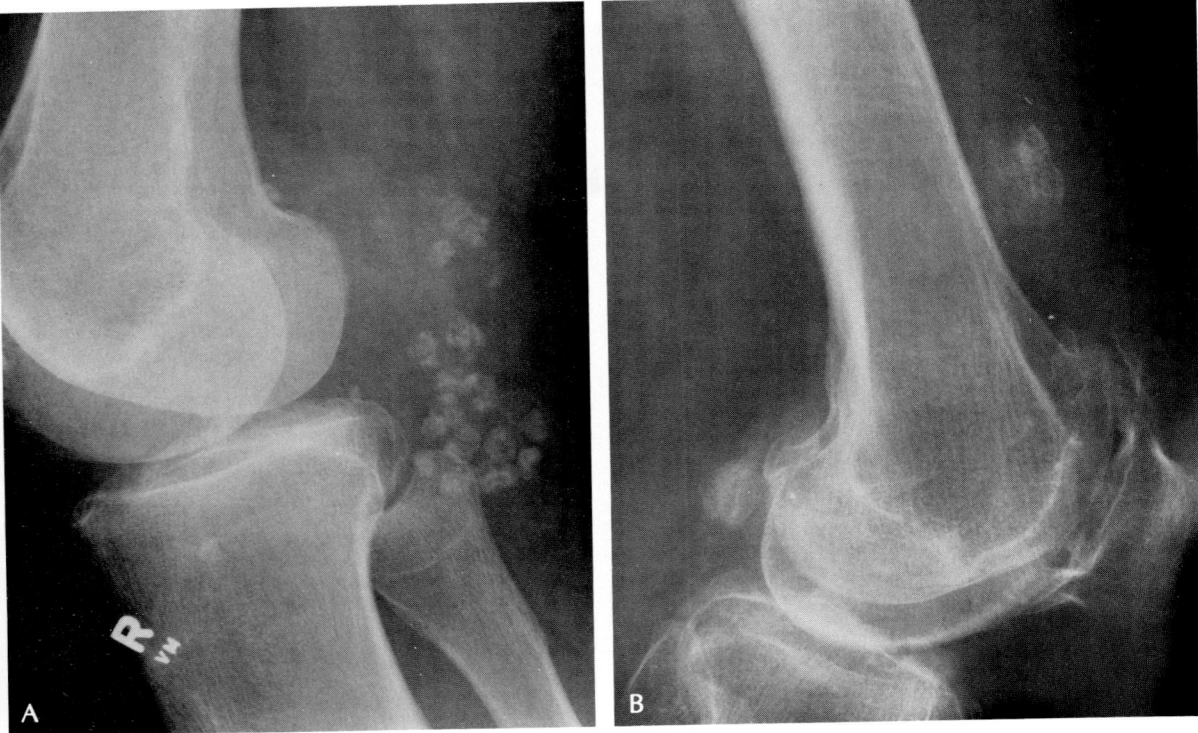

Fig. 5–96. *A,* Primary synovial osteochondromatosis with multiple loose bodies extruded into a Baker's cyst. *B,* Advanced degenerative joint disease with effusion and secondary osteochondromatosis.

and other joints may be affected.[336] In approximately two-thirds of patients, either diffuse or nodular soft tissue swelling is visible radiographically. Slight increased radiodensity may be identified, but calcification is not a feature.

Nearly half the patients have bony changes consisting of subchondral, juxta-articular cystic areas of radiolucency with finely sclerotic borders. These changes represent pressure erosions by lobulated masses. Osteoporosis is not a feature, and narrowing of cartilage is unusual and may help to differentiate pigmented villonodular synovitis from rheumatoid or tuberculous synovitis, with which it is frequently confused. Secondary osteoarthritis may be a late sequela. Because of its large and distensible synovial space, the knee is more likely to be the site of isolated soft tissue alteration, whereas in the hip, which is less capacious, isolated bony changes of sclerosis and cystic erosion develop frequently (Fig. 5–95). Extra-articular tendon sheath involvement (giant cell tumor), predominantly around the small peripheral joints, results in discrete, nodular, soft tissue swelling and focal punched-out erosions. The isolated nodular form of pigmented villonodular synovitis, when situated intra-articularly, may be best delineated arthrographically.[124]

Osteochondromatosis represents a rare, diffuse metaplasia of subsynovial fibroblasts to chondroblasts, which form multiple cartilaginous nodules.[129,387] Some of these become pinched off to form loose bodies within the joint space. The nodules may or may not calcify. This process is generally monarticular, and the knee is by far the most common site of involvement. Radiographically, many small, round, calcified, or ossified bodies are seen, some of which may be free or loose within the joint (Fig. 5–96). Secondary osteoarthritis is often superimposed. Rarely, the condition is detected by arthrography before the cartilaginous bodies are calcified.[64] The radiographic appearance of well-established osteochondromatosis is characteristic, however, and should be distinguished easily from the more common entities that give rise to only one or several intra-articular loose bodies, such as osteoarthritis, osteochondritis dissecans, or neuroarthropathy.

Other rare, benign lesions that affect soft tissues of the joint include lipoma, chondroma, and hemangioma.[172,195] Primary malignant tumors of the joint are rare. Synovioma, or synovial-cell sar-

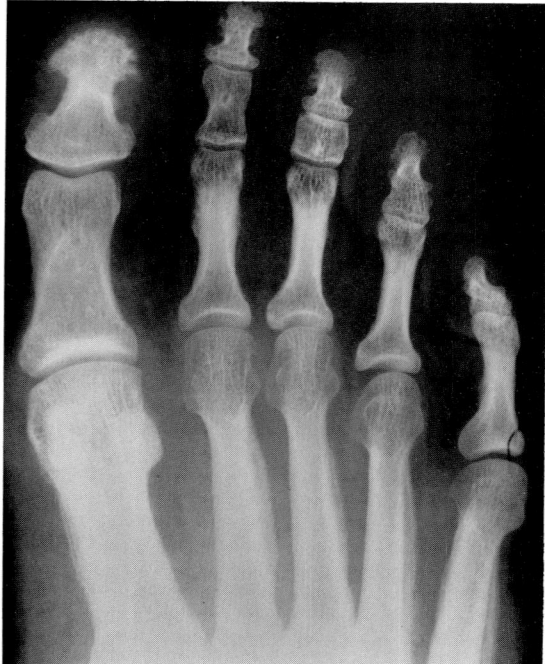

Fig. 5–97. Striking hyperostosis of the distal phalangeal tufts accompanied by marked periosteal new bone in the phalangeal and metatarsal shafts, a finding in pachydermal periostosis or pulmonary hypertrophic osteoarthropathy.

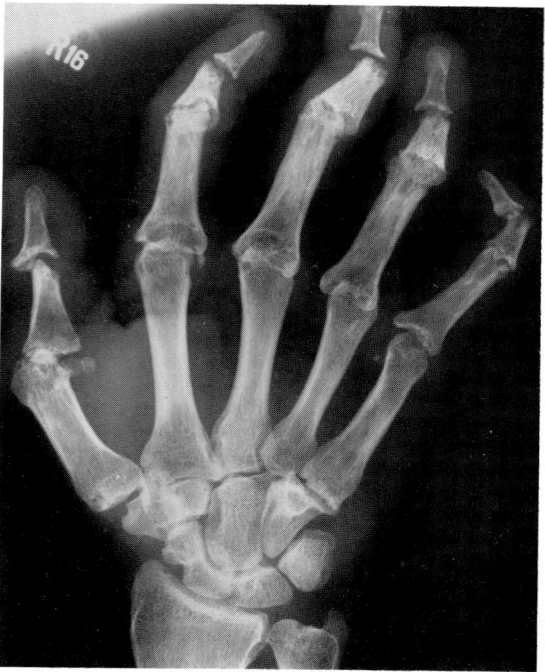

Fig. 5–98. Marked articular destruction involves the distal and proximal interphalangeal and the metacarpophalangeal articulations associated with nodular soft tissue swelling and angular deformities. Normal mineralization is preserved, and the wrist is spared. These findings are indicative of multicentric reticulohistiocytosis (lipoid dermatoarthritis).

coma, is more likely to involve the tendon sheaths of the lower extremity than the synovium of a joint.[46] This tumor results in a large, soft tissue mass frequently containing calcific deposits and occasionally eroding adjacent bone by pressure.

Although metastatic carcinoma and sarcoma frequently implant in subarticular bone, such implants in the synovial tissue are rare. Synovitis in widespread metastatic disease, particularly that with pulmonary manifestations, is more likely to be a feature of associated hypertrophic pulmonary osteoarthropathy.

Hypertrophic Osteoarthropathy

Idiopathic hypertrophic osteoarthropathy or pachydermoperiostosis[306,367] is a genetically determined autosomal dominant disorder with marked variability in expressivity and phenotypically is more severe in males (see also Chap. 76). The syndrome generally appears at puberty and progresses slowly for approximately 10 years. It is usually self-limited thereafter. The process is characterized by clubbing of the digits (Fig. 5–97), periarticular soft tissue swelling at the knees, ankles, or wrists, periosteal new-bone formation, coarsening of the facial features with thickening,

furrowing, and oiliness of the skin. The ends of the fingers and toes may become grossly enlarged and bulbous. The principal symptoms of pachydermoperiostosis are hyperhydrosis of the hands and feet, and occasionally bone and articular pain. Some patients may initially have chronic swelling of the knees due to associated synovitis and joint effusion.

These appendicular manifestations may be entirely simulated by those seen in secondary hypertrophic osteoarthropathy or Marie-Bamberger disease. In this condition, articular manifestations with joint swelling and effusion may be the initial harbingers of an underlying process such as carcinoma of the lung or may be late sequelae of chronic pulmonary, cardiac, or hepatic failure.

Lipoid Dermatoarthritis (Multicentric Reticulohistiocytosis)

This is a rare articular disorder of unknown origin. It occurs in adults and is characterized by proliferation of histiocytic nodules in the skin and mucous membranes in the presence of a severe mutilating arthritis.[125] The disease affects women

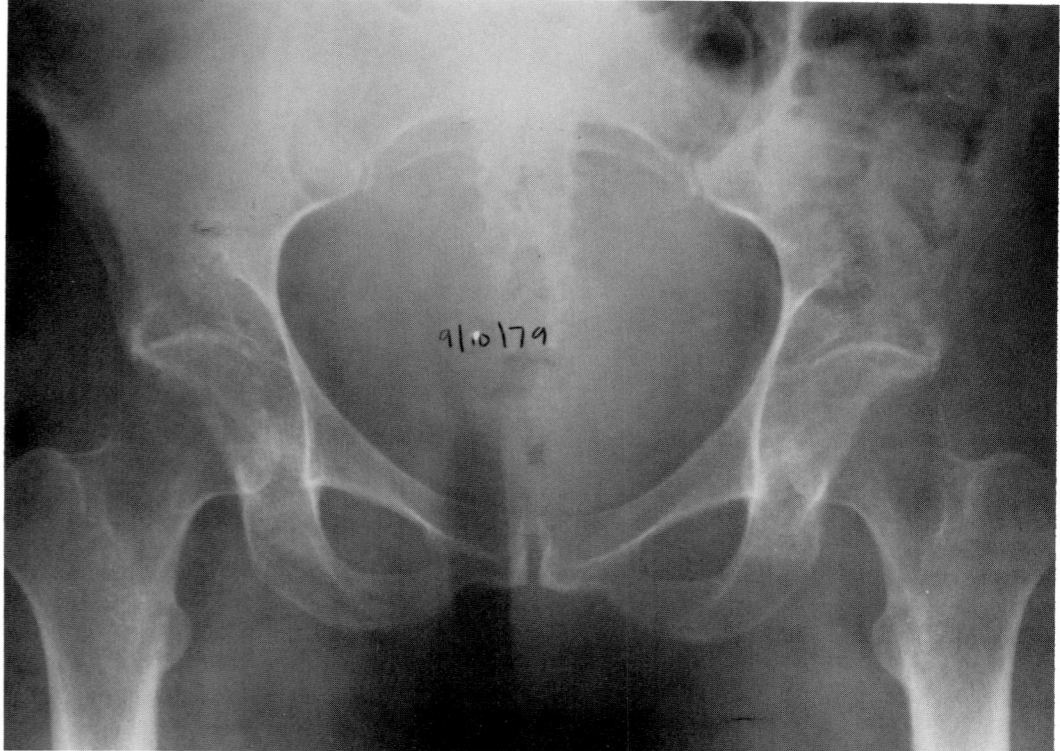

Fig. 5–99. Striking, bilateral, periarticular demineralization of the hips involves both the femoral heads and the acetabulae. This patient was in the third trimester of pregnancy when the migratory osteoporosis or transient demineralization began, a recognized association.

three times more commonly than men. Two-thirds of patients have polyarthritis followed by skin changes. The remainder have skin nodules on presentation.

The nodules in multicentric reticulohistiocytosis are pruritic, firm, and reddish brown in color. Common locations include the hands and face (seen in over 90% of patients) as well as the forearms, neck, and chest. The nodules may wax and wane. Radiographic features other than the nodules include marginal erosions with a predilection for the interphalangeal joints of the hands and feet, absence of osteoporosis, and symmetric involvement (Fig. 5–98).[10] Half these patients develop arthritis mutilans.

Migratory Osteoporosis

Migratory osteoporosis or regional transient osteoporosis is recognized as a clinical and radiologic syndrome characterized clinically by the development of severe and often incapacitating pain around a major joint, usually the ankle, the knee, or the hip (Fig. 5–99) in middle-aged and elderly adults.[166,199,310] Hematologic and biochemical stud-

ies are essentially normal. Radiologic examination initially reveals no abnormality, but one or two months after the onset of symptoms, widespread osteoporosis is demonstrated around the affected joint. The clinical symptoms resolve spontaneously within approximately four to ten months, with subsequent partial remineralization of the osteoporotic areas. In about a third to a quarter of patients, the cause is unknown (idiopathic form). In the remainder, a history of minor or major trauma, including surgery, suggests that the entity is analogous to Sudeck's atrophy.[351]

REFERENCES

1. Ahlback, S.: Osteoarthrosis of the knee. Acta Radiol. [Diagn.], *277 [Suppl.]*:7–72, 1968.
2. Aksoy, M., et al.: Osseous changes in Wilson's disease. A radiologic study of nine patients. Radiology, *102*:505–509, 1972.
3. Alarcon-Segovia, D., et al.: Scintillation scanning of joints with technetium99m. (Abstract.) Arthritis Rheum., *10*:262, 1967.
4. Ansell, B.M., and Kent, P.A.: Radiological changes in juvenile chronic polyarthritis. Skeletal Radiol., *1*:129–144, 1977.
5. Aptekar, R.G., Lawless, O.J., and Decker, J.L.: Deforming non-erosive arthritis of the hand in systemic lupus erythematosus. Clin. Orthop., *100*:120–124, 1974.

6. Arnett, F.C., Jr., et al.: Homozygosity for HLA-B27: impact on rheumatic disease expression in two families. Arthritis Rheum., 20:797–804, 1977.

7. Badley, B.W.D., and Ansell, B.M.: Fractures in Still's disease. Ann. Rheum. Dis., 19:135–142, 1960.

8. Baker, H., Golding, D.N., and Thompson, M.: Psoriasis and arthritis. Ann. Intern. Med., 58:909–925, 1963.

9. Ball, J.: Enthesopathy of rheumatoid and ankylosing spondylitis. Ann. Rheum. Dis., 30:213–222, 1971.

10. Barrow, M.V., and Holubar, K.: Multicentric reticulo-histiocytosis: a review of 33 patients. Medicine, 48:287–305, 1969.

11. Bassett, L.W., et al.: Skeletal findings in progressive systemic sclerosis (scleroderma). AJR, 136:1121, 1981.

12. Bauer, G.C.H.: The use of radionuclides in orthopaedics. IV. Radionuclide scintimetry of the skeleton. J. Bone Joint Surg., 50A:1681–1709, 1968.

13. Beetham, W.P., Jr., Kaye, R.L., and Polley, H.F.: A case of extensive polyarticular involvement, and discussion of certain clinical and pathologic features. Ann. Intern. Med., 58:1002–1012, 1963.

14. Bekerman, C., et al.: Radionuclide imaging of the bones and joints of the hand. A definition of normal and a comparison of sensitivity using 99mTc-pertechnetate and 99mTc-diphosphonate. Radiology, 118:653–659, 1976.

15. Berens, D.L.: Roentgen features of ankylosing spondylitis. Clin. Orthop., 74:20–33, 1971.

16. Berens, D.L., et al.: Roentgen changes in early rheumatoid arthritis. Radiology, 82:645–653, 1964.

17. Berens, D.L., and Lin, R.K.: Roentgen Diagnosis of Rheumatoid Arthritis. Springfield, IL, Charles C Thomas, 1969.

18. Bernstein, B., et al.: Hip joint restoration in juvenile rheumatoid arthritis. Arthritis Rheum., 20:1099–1104, 1977.

19. Bjelle, A., and Sundén, G.: Pyrophosphate arthropathy: a clinical study. J. Bone Joint Surg., 56B:246, 1974.

20. Bland, J.H.: Rheumatoid arthritis of the cervical spine. J. Rheumatol., 1:319–342, 1974.

21. Bleifeld, C.J., and Inglis, A.E.: The hand in systemic lupus erythematosus. J. Bone Joint Surg., 56A:1207–1215, 1974.

22. Bloch, F., Hansen, W.W., and Parkard, M.E.: Nuclear induction. Phys. Rev., 69:127, 1946.

23. Bluhm, G.B., and Riddle, J.M.: Platelets and vascular disease in gout. Semin. Arthritis Rheum., 2:355–366, 1973.

24. Boettcher, W.G., et al.: Non-traumatic necrosis of the femoral head. I. Relation of altered hemostasis to etiology. J. Bone Joint Surg., 52A:312–321, 1970.

25. Bonavita, J.A., Dalinka, M.K., and Schumacher, H.R., Jr.: Hydroxyapatite deposition disease. Radiology, 134:621, 1980.

26. Boyd, D.P., Genant, H.K., and Korobkin, M.T.: Improved accuracy of CT body scanning as applied to bone mineral quantification. (Abstract.) In Proceedings of the Sixty-second Annual Meeting of the Radiological Society of North America, Chicago, Illinois, November 15, 1976.

27. Boyd, J.A., Patrick, S.I., and Reeves, R.J.: Roentgen changes observed in generalized scleroderma: report of 63 cases. A.M.A. Arch. Intern. Med., 94:248, 1954.

28. Bradley, J.G., et al.: Presented at the Sixty-second Annual Meeting of the Radiological Society of North America, Chicago, Illinois, November 15, 1976.

29. Brailsford, J.F.: The radiology of gout. Br. J. Radiol., 32:472–478, 1959.

30. Brandt, K.D., and Krey, P.R.: Chalky joint effusion. The result of massive synovial deposition of calcium apatite in progressive systemic sclerosis. Arthritis Rheum., 20:792–796, 1977.

31. Brattstrom, M.: Asymmetry of ossification and rate of growth of long bones in childen with unilateral juvenile gonarthritis. Acta Rheumatol. Scand., 9:102–115, 1963.

32. Braunstein, E.M., et al.: Radiologic findings in late-onset systemic lupus erythematosus. AJR, 140:587, 1983.

33. Braunstein, E.M., Martel, W., and Moidel, R.: Ankylosing spondylitis in men and women: a clinical and radiographic comparison. Radiology, 144:91, 1982.

34. Breimer, C.W., and Freiberger, R.H.: Bone lesions associated with villonodular synovitis. Am. J. Roentgenol., 79:618–629, 1958.

35. Brewerton, D.A.: Joseph J. Bunim Memorial Lecture. HLA-B27 and the inheritance of susceptibility to rheumatic disease. Arthritis Rheum., 19:656–668, 1976.

36. Brook, A., and Corbett, M.: Radiographic changes in early rheumatoid disease. Ann. Rheum. Dis., 36:71–73, 1977.

37. Brooker, A.E.W., and Barter, R.W.: Cervical spondylosis. A clinical study with comparative radiology. Brain, 88:925–936, 1965.

38. Bryan, R.S., DiMichele, J.D., and Ford, G.I., Jr.: Popliteal cysts. Arthrography as an aid to diagnosis and treatment. Clin. Orthop., 50:203–208, 1967.

39. Budin, J.A., and Feldman, F.: Soft tissue calcifications in systemic lupus erythematosus. Am. J. Roentgenol., 124:358–364, 1975.

40. Butt, W.P.: Radiology of the infected joint. Clin. Orthop., 96:136–149, 1973.

41. Butt, W.P., and McIntyre, J.L.: Double-contrast arthrography of the knee. Radiology, 92:487–499, 1969.

42. Bywaters, E.G.L.: Calcium pyrophosphate deposits in synovial membrane. Ann. Rheum. Dis., 31:219–221, 1972.

43. Bywaters, E.G.L.: The early radiological signs of rheumatoid arthritis. Bull. Rheum. Dis., 11:231–234, 1960.

44. Bywaters, E.G.L., and Dixon, A.S.: Paravertebral ossification in psoriatic arthritis. Ann. Rheum. Dis., 24:313–331, 1965.

45. Bywaters, E.G.L., Dixon, A.S., and Scott, J.T.: Joint lesions of hyperparathyroidism. Ann. Rheum. Dis., 22:171–187, 1963.

46. Cade, S.: Synovial sarcoma. J. R. Coll. Surg. (Edinb.), 8:1–51, 1962.

47. Calabro, J.J.: A critical evaluation of the diagnostic features of the feet in rheumatoid arthritis. Arthritis Rheum., 5:19–29, 1962.

48. Calabro, J.J., and Maltz, B.A.: Current concepts: ankylosing spondylitis. N. Engl. J. Med., 282:606–610, 1970.

49. Cameron, J.R., Mazess, R.B., and Sorenson, J.S.: Precision and accuracy of bone mineral determination by direct photon absorptiometry. Invest. Radiol., 3:141–150, 1968.

50. Cameron, R.B.: Strontium-85 scintimetry in nontraumatic necrosis of the femoral head. Clin. Orthop., 65:243–261, 1969.

51. Campbell, W., and Feldman, F.: Bone and soft tissue abnormalities of the upper extremity in diabetes mellitus. Am. J. Roentgenol., 124:7–16, 1977.

52. Carrabba, M., and Cherie Ligniere, G.: Reumatismo, 21:417, 1969.

53. Castillo, B.A., El Sallab, R.A., and Scott, J.T.: Physical activity, cystic erosions and osteoporosis in rheumatoid arthritis. Ann. Rheum. Dis., 24:522, 1965.

54. Chafetz, N., et al.: Recognition of lumbar disk herniation with NMR. AJR, 141:1153–1156, 1983.

55. Charkes, N.D., Philips, C., and Malmud, L.S.: Bone tracer uptake: evaluation by a new model. (Abstract.) J. Nucl. Med., 16:519, 1975.

56. Clark, J.A., Winkelmann, R.K., and Ward, L.E.: Serologic alterations in scleroderma and sclerodermatomyositis. Mayo Clin. Proc., 46:104–107, 1971.

57. Coates, G., et al.: An analysis of factors which influence the local accumulation of bone seeking radiopharmaceuticals. (Abstract.) J. Nucl. Med., 16:520, 1975.

58. Colbert, C., Mazess, R.B., and Schmidt, P.B.: Bone mineral determination in vitro by radiographic photodensitometry and direct photon absorptiometry. Invest. Radiol., 5:336–340, 1970.

59. Collins, L.C., et al.: Malposition of carpal bones in rheumatoid arthritis. Radiology, 103:95–98, 1972.

60. Conlon, P.W., Isdale, I.C., and Rose, B.S.: Rheumatoid arthritis of the cervical spine: an analysis of 333 cases. Ann. Rheum. Dis., 25:120–126, 1966.

61. Cornbleet, T., Reed, C.I., and Reed, B.P.: X-ray dif-

fraction studies in calcinosis. J. Invest. Dermatol., 13:171–174, 1949.

62. Corrigan, A.B.: Radiological changes in rheumatoid cervical spines. Australas. Radiol., 13:370–375, 1969.
63. Costeas, A., Woodard, H.G., and Laughlin, J.A.: Depletion of 18F from blood flowing through bone. J. Nucl. Med., 11:43–45, 1970.
64. Crittenden, J.J., Jones, D.M., and Santarelli, A.G.: Knee arthrogram in synovial chondromatosis. Radiology, 94:133–134, 1970.
65. Crosby, E.B., Inglis, A., and Bullough, P.G.: Multiple joint involvement with pigmented villonodular synovitis. Radiology, 122:671–672, 1977.
66. Crout, J.E., Brewer, N.S., and Tompkins, R.B.: Sporotrichosis arthritis: clinical features in seven patients. Ann. Intern. Med., 86:294–297, 1977.
67. Cruickshank, B.: Pathology of ankylosing spondylitis. Clin. Orthop., 74:43–58, 1971.
68. Cruickshank, B., MacLeod, J.G., and Shearer, W.S.: Subarticular pseudocysts in rheumatoid arthritis. J. Fac. Radiol., 5:218–226, 1954.
69. Currey, H.L., et al.: Significance of radiological calcification of joint cartilage. Ann. Rheum. Dis., 25:295–306, 1966.
70. Curtiss, P.H.: The pathology of joint infections. Clin. Orthop., 96:129–135, 1973.
71. Dalén, N., and Jacobson, B.: Bone mineral assay: choice of measuring sites. Invest. Radiol., 9:174–185, 1974.
72. Dalinka, M.K., et al.: The radiology of osseous and articular infection (review). C.R.C. Crit. Rev. Clin. Radiol. Nucl. Med., 7:1–64, 1975.
73. Dalinka, M.K., Lally, J.F., and Gohel, V.K.: Arthrography of the lateral meniscus. Am. J. Roentgenol., 121:79–85, 1974.
74. Danigelis, J.A., et al.: 99mTc-polyphosphate bone imaging in Legg-Perthes disease. Radiology, 115:407–413, 1975.
75. Decker, J.L., et al.: Systemic lupus erythematosus. Contrasts and comparisons. Ann. Intern. Med., 82:391–404, 1975.
76. Dequeker, J.: Bone and ageing. Ann. Rheum. Dis., 34:100–115, 1975.
77. Desaulniers, M., et al.: Radiotechnetium polyphosphate joint imaging. J. Nucl. Med., 15:417–423, 1974.
78. Dodds, W.J., and Steinbach, H.L.: Primary hyperparathyroidism and articular cartilage calcification. Am. J. Roentgenol., 104:884–892, 1968.
79. Dodds, W.J., and Steinbach, H.L.: Gout associated with calcification of cartilage. N. Engl. J. Med., 275:745–749, 1966.
80. Doi, K., Genant, H.K., and Rossman, K.: Comparison of image quality obtained with optical and radiographic magnification techniques in fine-detail skeletal radiography: effect of object thickness. Radiology, 118:189–195, 1976.
81. Doi, K., Genant, H.K., and Rossman, K.: Effect of film graininess and geometric unsharpness on image quality in fine-detail skeletal radiography. Invest. Radiol., 10:35–42, 1975.
82. Doyle, F.H.: Some quantitative radiological observations in primary and secondary hyperparathyroidism. Br. J. Radiol., 39:161–167, 1966.
83. DuBois, E.L., et al.: Progressive systemic sclerosis (PSS) and localized scleroderma (morphea) with positive LE cell test and unusual systemic manifestations compatible with systemic lupus erythematosus: presentation of 14 cases including one set of identical twins, one with scleroderma and the other with SLE. Review of the literature. Medicine, 50:199–222, 1971.
84. DuBois, E.L., and Tuffanelli, D.L.: Manifestations of systemic lupus erythematosus. JAMA, 190:104–111, 1964.
85. Duszynski, D.O., et al.: Early radionuclide diagnosis of acute osteomyelitis. Radiology, 117:337–340, 1975.
86. Dwosh, I.L., Resnick, D., and Becker, M.A.: Hip involvement in ankylosing spondylitis. Arthritis Rheum., 19:683–692, 1976.
87. Elhabali, M., et al.: Tomographic examinations of sacro-

iliac joints in adult patients with rheumatoid arthritis. J. Rheumatol., 6:417–425, 1979.
88. Ellman, M.H., Krieger, M.I., and Brown, N.: Pseudogout mimicking synovial chondromatosis. J. Bone Joint Surg., 57A:863–865, 1976.
89. Esdaile, J.M., et al.: HLA B27 in rheumatoid factor-negative polyarthritis. Ann. Intern. Med., 86:699–702, 1977.
90. Eto, R.T., Anderson, P.W., and Harley, J.D.: Elbow arthrography with the application of tomography. Radiology, 115:283–288, 1975.
91. Fallet, G.H., Arroyo, J., and Vischer, T.L.: Sternocostoclavicular hyperostosis: case report with a 31-year followup. Arthritis Rheum., 26:784–790, 1983.
92. Feith, R., et al.: Strontium87 MSR bone scanning for the evaluation of total hip replacement. J. Bone Joint Surg., 58B:79–83, 1976.
93. Feldman, F., Johnson, A.M., and Walter, J.F.: Acute axial neuroarthropathy. Radiology, 111:1–16, 1974.
94. Feldman, M.J., et al.: Multiple neuropathic joints, including the wrist, in a patient with diabetes mellitus. JAMA, 209:1690–1692, 1969.
95. Finby, B., and Bearn, A.G.: Roentgenographic abnormalities of the skeletal system in Wilson's disease (hepatolenticular degeneration). Am. J. Roentgenol., 79:603–611, 1958.
96. Fischer, E.: In Entzundliche und degenerative Erkrankungen der Gelenke und der Wirbelsaule under Ausschluss der Tuberkulose. Edited by W. Dihlmann. Stuttgart, Georg Thieme, 1974.
97. Fletcher, D.E., and Rowley, K.A.: The radiological features of rheumatoid arthritis. Br. J. Radiol., 25:282–295, 1952.
98. Fletcher, D.E., and Rowley, K.A.: Radiographic enlargements in diagnostic radiology. Br. J. Radiol., 24:598–604, 1951.
99. Ford, D.K., and Vallis, D.G.: The clinical course of arthritis associated with ulcerative colitis and regional ileitis. Arthritis Rheum., 2:526–536, 1959.
100. Forestier, J., and Lagier, R.: Ankylosing hyperostosis of the spine. Clin. Orthop., 74:65–83, 1971.
101. Forrester, D.M., and Nesson, J.W.: The Radiology of Joint Disease. Philadelphia, W.B. Saunders, 1973.
102. Freiberger, R.H., and Kaye, J.J.: Arthrography. New York, Appleton-Century-Crofts, 1979.
103. Freiberger, R.H., Killoran, P.J., and Cardona, G.: Arthrography of the knee by double contrast method. Am. J. Roentgenol., 97:736–747, 1966.
104. Ganda, O.P., and Caplan, H.I.: Rheumatoid disease without joint involvement. JAMA, 228:338–339, 1974.
105. Garn, S.M., Poznanski, A.K., and Nagy, J.M.: Bone measurement in the differential diagnosis of osteopenia and osteoporosis. Radiology, 100:509–518, 1971.
106. Gelman, M.I.: Arthrography in total hip prosthesis complications. Am. J. Roentgenol., 126:743–750, 1976.
107. Gelman, M.I., and Umber, J.S.: Fractures of thoracolumbar spine in ankylosing spondylitis. Am. J. Roentgenol. 130:485–491, 1978.
108. Genant, H.K.: Osteoporosis. Part I. West. J. Med., 139:75–84, 1983.
109. Genant, H.K. (Ed.): Spine Update 1984. San Francisco, Radiology Postgraduate Education Foundation, University of California, 1983.
110. Genant, H.K.: Proceedings of the 20th Annual Postgraduate Course in Diagnostic Radiology. San Francisco, University of California, 1977.
111. Genant, H.K.: Roentgenographic aspects of calcium pyrophosphate dihydrate crystal deposition disease (pseudogout). Arthritis Rheum., 19[Suppl.]:307–328, 1976.
112. Genant, H.K., et al.: Quantitative computed tomography of vertebral spongiosa: a sensitive method for detecting early bone loss after oophorectomy. Ann. Intern. Med., 97:699–705, 1982.
113. Genant, H.K., et al.: Direct radiographic magnification for skeletal radiography: an assessment of image quality and clinical application. Radiology, 123:47–55, 1977.
114. Genant, H.K., et al.: Skeletal demineralization and

growth retardation in inflammatory bowel disease. Invest. Radiol., *11*:541–549, 1976.

115. Genant, H.K., et al.: Reflex sympathetic dystrophy syndrome: a comprehensive analysis using fine-detail radiography, photon-absorptiometry, and bone scintigraphy. Radiology, *117*:21–32, 1975.

116. Genant, H.K., et al.: Bone-seeking radionuclides: an in vivo study of factors affecting skeletal uptake. Radiology, *113*:373–382, 1974.

117. Genant, H.K., et al.: Primary hyperparathyroidism: A comprehensive study of clinical, biochemical and radiological manifestations. Radiology, *109*:513–524, 1973.

118. Genant, H.K., and Boyd, D.: Quantitative bone mineral analysis using dual energy computed tomography. Invest. Radiol., *12*:545–551, 1977.

119. Genant, H.K., Doi, K., and Mall, J.C.: Comparison of non-screen technique (medical versus industrial film) for fine-detail skeletal radiography. Invest. Radiol., *11*:486–500, 1976.

120. Genant, H.K., Doi, K., and Mall, J.C.: Optical versus radiographic magnification for fine-detail skeletal radiography. Invest. Radiol., *10*:160–172, 1975.

121. Gerle, R.D., et al.: Osseous changes in chronic pancreatitis. Radiology, *85*:330–337, 1965.

121a. Gerster, J.C., Rappoport, G., and Ginalski, J.M.: Prevalence of periarticular calcifications in pyrophosphate arthropathy and their relation to nodal osteoarthritis. Ann. Rheum. Dis., *43*:255–257, 1984.

122. Gilday, D.L., Paul, D.J., and Paterson, J.: Diagnosis of osteomyelitis in children by combined blood pool and bone imaging. Radiology, *117*:331–335, 1975.

123. Ginsberg, M.H., et al.: Rheumatoid nodulosis: an unusual variant of rheumatic disease. Arthritis Rheum., *18*:49–58, 1975.

124. Goergen, T.G., Resnick, D., and Niwayama, G.: Localized nodular synovitis of the knee: a report of two cases with abnormal arthrograms. Am. J. Roentgenol., *126*:647–50, 1976.

125. Gold, R.H., et al.: Multicentric reticulohistiocytosis (lipoid dermatoarthritis): an erosive polyarthritis with distinctive clinical, roentgenographic and pathologic features. Am. J. Roentgenol., *124*:610–624, 1975.

126. Goldberg, R.P., et al.: Femoral neck erosions: sign of hip joint synovial disease. AJR, *141*:107, 1983.

127. Goldberg, R.P., et al.: Application and limitation of quantitative sacroiliac joint scintigraphy. Radiology, *128*:683–686, 1978.

128. Goldberg, R.P., Zulman, J.I., and Genant, H.K.: Unilateral primary osteoarthritis of the hand in monoplegia. Radiology, *135*:65, 1980.

129. Goldman, A.B.: Some miscellaneous joint diseases. Semin. Roentgenol., *17*:60–80, 1982.

130. Goldman, A.B., and Ghelman, B.: The double-contrast shoulder arthrogram. Radiology, *127*:655, 1978.

131. Gondos, B.: The pointed tubular bone, its significance and pathogenesis. Radiology, *105*:541–545, 1972.

132. Gondos, B.: Roentgen manifestations in progressive systemic sclerosis (diffuse scleroderma). Am. J. Roentgenol., *84*:235–247, 1960.

133. Gondos, B.: Observations on periarthritis calcarea. Am. J. Roentgenol., *77*:93–108, 1957.

134. Good, A.E., and Rapp, R.: Chondrocalcinosis of the knee with gout and rheumatoid arthritis. N. Engl. J. Med., *277*:286–290, 1967.

135. Gordan, G.S., and Vaughan, C.: Clinical Management of the Osteoporoses. Acton, MA, Publishing Sciences Group, 1976.

136. Grahame, R., Sutor, D.J., and Mitchener, M.B.: Crystal deposition in hyperparathyroidism. Ann. Rheum. Dis., *30*:597–604, 1971.

137. Grech, P.: Video-arthrography in hip dysplasia. Clin. Radiol., *23*:202–207, 1972.

138. Green, F.A., and Hays, M.T.: The pertechnetate joint scan. II. Clinical correlations. Ann. Rheum. Dis., *31*:278–281, 1972.

139. Greiff, J.: Determination of the vitality of the femoral head with ^{99m}Tc-Sn-pyrophosphate scintigraphy. Acta Orthop. Scand., *51*:109–117, 1980.

140. Gresham, G.E., and Rathey, U.K.: Osteoarthritis in knees of aged persons. Relationship between roentgenographic and clinical manifestations. JAMA, *233*:168–170, 1975.

141. Greyson, N.D.: Radionuclide bone and joint imaging in rheumatology. Bull. Rheum. Dis., *30*:1034–1039, 1979.

142. Grokoest, A.W., Snyder, A.L., and Schlaeger, R.: Juvenile Rheumatoid Arthritis. Boston, Little, Brown, 1962.

143. Hahn, B.H., Yardley, J.H., and Stevens, M.B.: ''Rheumatoid'' nodules in systemic lupus erythematosus. Ann. Intern. Med., *72*:49–58, 1970.

144. Hahn, T.J., Boisseau, V.C., and Aviolo, L.V.: Effect of chronic corticosteroid administration on diaphyseal and metaphyseal bone mass. J. Clin. Endocrinol., *39*:274–282, 1974.

145. Hall, F.M.: Pitfalls in knee arthrography. Radiology, *118*:55–62, 1976.

146. Hamilton, E., et al.: The arthropathy of idiopathic haemochromatosis. Q. J. Med., *37*:171–182, 1968.

147. Hancock, D.O.: Cervical spine in chronic rheumatoid arthritis. Clin. Rheum. Dis., *4*:443–459, 1978.

148. Hanson, C.A., Shagrin, J.W., and Duncan, H.: Vertebral osteoporosis in ankylosing spondylitis. Clin. Orthop., *74*:59–64, 1971.

149. Harris, E.D., Jr.: Recent insights into the pathogenesis of the proliferative lesion in rheumatoid arthritis. Arthritis Rheum., *19*:68–72, 1976.

150. Harrison, M.H.M., Schajowicz, F., and Trueta, J.: Osteoarthritis of the hips: a study of the nature and evolution of the disease. J. Bone Joint Surg., *35B*:598–626, 1953.

151. Harrison, M.O., Freiberger, R.H., and Ranawat, C.S.: Arthrography of the rheumatoid wrist joint. Am. J. Roentgenol., *112*:480–486, 1971.

152. Harrison, R.B.: Charcot's joint: two new observations. Am. J. Roentgenol., *128*:807–809, 1977.

153. Harvie, J.N., Lester, R.S., and Little, A.H.: Sacroiliitis in severe psoriasis. Am. J. Roentgenol., *127*:579–584, 1976.

154. Harvey, A.M., et al.: Systemic lupus erythematosus: review of the literature and clinical analysis of 138 cases. Medicine, *33*:291–437, 1954.

155. Haverbush, T.J., et al.: Osteolysis of the ribs and cervical spine in progressive systemic sclerosis (scleroderma). A case report. J. Bone Joint Surg., *56A*:637–640, 1974.

156. Heimann, W.G., and Freiberger, R.H.: Avascular necrosis of the femoral and humeral heads after high-dosage corticosteroid therapy. N. Engl. J. Med., *263*:672–675, 1960.

157. Hellmann, D.B., Helms, C.A., and Genant, H.K.: Chronic repetitive trauma: a cause of atypical degenerative joint disease. Skeletal Radiol., *10*:236–242, 1983.

158. Hermodsson, I.: Roentgen appearance of coxarthrosis. Relation between the anatomy, pathologic changes, and roentgen appearance. Acta Orthop. Scand., *41*:169–187, 1970.

159. Hoffer, P.B., and Genant, H.K.: Use of bone scanning agents in the evaluation of arthritis. Semin. Nucl. Med., *6*:121–137, 1976.

160. Holopainen, T., and Rekonen, A.: Uptake of radioactive strontium (^{85}Sr) in joints damaged by rheumatoid arthritis measured by external counting of radiation. Acta Rheumatol. Scand., *12*:102–111, 1966.

161. Holt, S., and Yates, P.O.: Cervical spondylosis and nerve root lesions. Incidence at routine necropsy. J. Bone Joint Surg., *48B*:407–423, 1966.

162. Holzman, R.S., and Bishko, F.: Osteomyelitis in heroin addicts. Ann. Intern. Med., *75*:693–696, 1971.

163. Horns, J.W.: Single contrast knee arthrography in abnormalities of the articular cartilage. Radiology, *105*:537–540, 1972.

164. Howell, D.S.: Pemberton lecture. Degradative enzymes in osteoarthritic human articular cartilage. Arthritis Rheum., *18*:167–177, 1975.

165. Howell, D.S., et al.: A view on the pathogenesis of osteoarthritis. Bull. Rheum. Dis., *29*:996–1001, 1979.

166. Hunder, G.G., and Kelly, P.J.: Roentgenologic transient osteoporosis of the hip. A clinical syndrome? Ann. Intern. Med., *68*:539, 1968.

167. Isherwood, I., et al.: Bone-mineral estimation by computer-assisted transverse axial tomography. Lancet, 2:712–715, 1976.

168. Ishibashi, A., et al.: Early diagnosis of aseptic necrosis of the bone after renal transplantation. (Abstract) J. Nucl. Med., 16:538–539, 1975.

169. Jacobelli, S., et al.: Calcium pyrophosphate dihydrate crystal deposition in neuropathic joints: four cases of polyarticular involvement. Ann. Intern. Med., 79:340–347, 1973.

170. Jacobs, J.C.: Septic infections of bones and joints: medical management. Arthritis Rheum., 20:590, 1977.

171. Jacobs, P.: Primary cystic arthrosis of the hip. Br. J. Radiol., 36:129–134, 1963.

172. Jaffe, H.L.: Tumors and Tumorous Conditions of the Bones and Joints. Philadelphia, Lea & Febiger, 1958, pp. 577–579.

173. Jensen, P.S., and Putman, C.E.: Current concepts with respect to chondrocalcinosis and the pseudogout syndrome. Am. J. Roentgenol, 123:531–539, 1975.

174. Jessee, E.F., et al.: Coexistent rheumatoid arthritis and chronic tophaceous gout. Arthritis Rheum., 23:244–247, 1980.

175. Johnson, J.S., et al.: Rheumatoid arthritis, 1970–1972. Ann. Intern. Med., 78:937–953, 1973.

176. Johnson, J.T.H.: Neuropathic fractures and joint injuries. Pathogenesis and rationale of prevention and treatment. J. Bone Joint Surg., 49A:1–30, 1967.

177. Kabir, D.I., and Malkinson, F.D.: Lupus erythematosus and calcinosis cutis. A.M.A. Arch. Dermatol., 100:17–22, 1969.

178. Kammer, G., et al.: Psoriatic arthritis: a clinical, immunologic and HLA study of 100 patients. Semin. Arthritis Rheum., 9:75–97, 1979.

179. Kantor, G.L., Bickel, Y.B., and Barnett, E.V.: Coexistence of systemic lupus erythematosus and rheumatoid arthritis. Report of a case and review of the literature, with clinical, pathologic and serologic observations. Am. J. Med., 47:433–444, 1969.

180. Karten, I., et al.: Articular erosions in rheumatoid arthritis. J. Chronic Dis., 25:449–456, 1972.

181. Katz, I., Rabinowitz, J.G., and Dziadiw, R.: Early changes in Charcot's joints. Am. J. Roentgenol., 86:965–974, 1961.

182. Kellgren, J.H., and Moore, R.: Generalized osteoarthritis and Heberden's nodes. Br. Med. J., 1:181–187, 1952.

183. Kelly, P.J., et al.: Brucellosis of the bones and joints. Experience with 36 patients. JAMA, 174:347–353, 1960.

184. Kidd, K.L., nd Peter, J.B.: Erosive osteoarthritis. Radiology, 86:640–647, 1966.

185. Kido, D., Bryan, D., and Halpern, M.: Hematogeneous osteomyelitis in drug addicts. Am. J. Roentgenol., 118:356–363, 1973.

186. Killebrew, K., Gold, R.H., and Sholkoff, S.D.: Psoriatic spondylitis. Radiology, 108:9–16, 1973.

187. Killoran, P.J., Marcove, R.C., and Freiberger, R.H.: Shoulder arthrography. Am. J. Roentgenol., 103:658–668, 1968.

188. Klipper, A.R., et al.: Ischemic necrosis of bone in systemic lupus erythematosus. Medicine, 55:251–257, 1976.

189. Kozin, F., et al.: Computed tomography in the diagnosis of sacroiliitis. Arthritis Rheum., 24:1479–1486, 1981.

190. Kramer, L.S., et al.: Deforming, nonerosive arthritis of the hands in chronic systemic lupus erythematosus (SLE). (Abstract.) Arthritis Rheum., 13:329–330, 1970.

191. Krokowski, E.: In Proceedings of a Symposium on Bone Mineral Determinations. Studsvik, Stockholm, 1974.

192. Labowitz, R., and Schumacher, J.R., Jr.: Articular manifestations of systemic lupus erythematosus. Ann. Intern. Med., 74:911–921, 1971.

193. Laine, V.A., Vaino, K.J., and Pekanmaki, K.: Shoulder affections in rheumatoid arthritis. Ann. Rheum. Dis., 13:157–160, 1954.

194. Lanzl, L.H., and Strandjord, N.: In Proceedings of a Symposium on Low-energy X- and Gamma Sources and Applications. Chicago, Illinois Institute of Technology Research, October 20, 1964.

195. Larsen, I.J., and Landry, R.M.: Hemangioma of the synovial membrane. J. Bone Joint Surg., 51A:1210–1215, 1969.

196. Lauterbur, P.: Image formation by induced local interactions: examples employing nuclear magnetic resonance. Nature, 242:190–191, 1973.

197. Lawson, J.P.: Joint manifestations of the connective tissue diseases. Semin. Roentgenol., 17:25, 1982.

198. Lentle, B.C., et al.: The scintigraphic investigation of sacroiliac disease. J. Nucl. Med., 18:529–533, 1977.

199. Lequesne, M., et al.: Partial transient osteoporosis. Skeletal Radiol., 2:1–9, 1977.

200. Lightfoot, R.W., and Lotke, P.A.: Osteonecrosis of metacarpal heads in systemic lupus erythematosus: value of radiostrontium scintimetry in differential diagnosis. Arthritis Rheum., 15:486–492, 1972.

201. Liljedahl, S.O., Lindvall, N., and Wetterfors, J.: Roentgen diagnosis of rupture of anterior cruciate ligament. Acta Radiol. [Diagn.], 4:225–239, 1966.

202. Lindblom, K.: Arthrography roentgenography in ruptures of the tendon of the shoulder joint. Acta Radiol., 20:548–562, 1939.

203. Little, H., et al.: Asymptomatic spondylodiscitis. An unusual feature of ankylosing spondylitis. Arthritis Rheum., 17:487–493, 1974.

204. Lovell, C.R., and Jayson, M.I.V.: Joint involvement in systemic sclerosis. Scand. J. Rheumatol., 8:154–160, 1979.

205. Luthra, H.S., Ferguson, R.H., and Conn, D.L.: Coexistence of ankylosing spondylitis and rheumatoid arthritis. Arthritis Rheum., 19:111–114, 1976.

206. McCarty, D.J., Jr.: The pendulum of progress in gout: from crystals to hyperuricemia and back. Arthritis Rheum., 7:534–541, 1964.

207. McCarty, D.J., et al.: Diseases associated with calcium pyrophosphate dihydrate crystal deposition. Am. J. Med., 56:704–714, 1974.

208. McCarty, D.J., Jr., et al.: Studies on pathological calcifications in human cartilage. I. Prevalence and types of crystal deposits in the menisci of 215 cadavers. J. Bone Joint Surg., 48A:309–325, 1966.

209. McCarty, D.J., and Gatter, R.A.: A study of distal interphalangeal joint tenderness in rheumatoid arthritis. Arthritis Rheum., 9:325–336, 1966.

210. McCarty, D.J., and Haskin, M.E.: The roentgenographic aspects of pseudogout (articular chondrocalcinosis). Am. J. Roentgenol., 90:1248–1257, 1963.

211. McCarty, D.J., Jr., Kohn, N.N., and Faires, J.S.: The significance of calcium phosphate crystals in the synovial fluid of arthritic patients: the "pseudogout syndrome." I. Clinical aspects. Ann. Intern. Med., 56:711–737, 1962.

212. McCarty, D.J., Polcyn, R.E., and Collins, P.A.: 99mTechnetium scintiphotography in arthritis. II. Its nonspecificity and clinical and roentgenographic correlations in rheumatoid arthritis. II. Technic and interpretation. Arthritis Rheum., 13:21–32, 1970.

213. McCarty, D.J., Polcyn, R.E., and Collins, P.A.: I. Technic and interpretation. Arthritis Rheum., 13:11, 1970.

214. McEwen, C., et al.: Ankylosing spondylitis and spondytis accompanying ulcerative colitis, regional enteritis, psoriasis and Reiter's disease. Arthritis Rheum., 14:291–318, 1971.

215. McEwen, C., et al.: Arthritis accompanying ulcerative colitis. Am. J. Med., 33:923–941, 1962.

216. McIntyre, J.L.: Arthrography of the lateral meniscus. Radiology, 105:531–536, 1972.

217. Mack, P.B.: Radiographic Bone Densitometry. Washington, D.C., National Aeronautics and Space Administration, 1975, pp. 31–46.

218. McNeill, K.G., et al.: In vivo neutron activation analysis for calcium in man. J. Nucl. Med., 14:502–506, 1973.

219. McTammany, J.R., Moser, K.M., and Houk, V.N.: Disseminated bone tuberculosis. Review of the literature and presentation of an unusual case. Am. Rev. Respir. Dis., 87:889–895, 1963.

220. Magyar, E., et al.: The pathogenesis of the subchondral pseudocysts in rheumatoid arthritis. Clin. Orthop., 100:341–344, 1974.

221. Majd, M., and Frankel, R.S.: Radionuclide imaging in skeletal inflammatory and ischemic disease in children. Am. J. Roentgenol., *126*:832–841, 1976.

222. Makela, P., and Haatja, M.: Soft tissue radiography for evaluating clinical activity of rheumatoid arthritis. Acta Radiol. [Diagn.], *19*:389–400, 1978.

223. Maldonado-Cocco, J.A., et al.: Carpal ankylosis in juvenile rheumatoid arthritis. Arthritis Rheum., *22*:728–736, 1979.

224. Mall, J.C., et al.: The efficacy of fine-detail radiography in the evaluation of patients with rheumatoid arthritis. Radiology, *112*:37–42, 1974.

225. Manzke, E., et al.: Relationship between local and total bone mass in osteoporosis. Metabolism, *24*:605–615, 1975.

226. Margulis, A.R., et al. (Eds.): Clinical Magnetic Resonance Imaging. San Francisco, Radiology Research and Education Foundation, University of California, 1983.

227. Martel, W.: Pathogenesis of cervical discovertebral destruction in rheumatoid arthritis. Arthritis Rheum., *20*:1217–1225, 1977.

228. Martel, W.: Radiologic manifestations of rheumatoid arthritis with particular reference to the hand, wrist and foot. Med. Clin. North Am., *52*:655–665, 1968.

229. Martel, W.: The overhanging margin of bone: a roentgenologic manifestation of gout. Radiology, *91*:755–756, 1968.

230. Martel, W.: The occipito-atlanto-axial joints in rheumatoid arthritis and ankylosing spondylitis. Am. J. Roentgenol., *86*:223–240, 1961.

231. Martel, W., et al.: Erosive osteoarthritis and psoriatic arthritis: radiologic comparison in the hand, wrist, and foot. AJR, *134*:125, 1980.

232. Martel, W., et al.: Radiologic features of Reiter disease. Radiology, *132*:1, 1979.

233. Martel, W., et al.: Traumatic lesions of the discovertebral junction in the lumbar spine. Am. J. Roentgenol., *127*:457–464, 1976.

234. Martel, W., et al.: A roentgenologically distinctive arthropathy in some patients with the pseudogout syndrome. Am. J. Roentgenol., *109*:587–605, 1970.

235. Martel, W., and Duff, I.F.: Pelvo-spondylitis in rheumatoid arthritis. Radiology, *77*:744–756, 1961.

236. Martel, W., and Page, J.W.: Cervical vertebral erosions and subluxations in rheumatoid arthritis and ankylosing spondylitis. Arthritis Rheum., *3*:546–556, 1960.

237. Martel, W., and Sitterley, B.H.: Roentgenologic manifestations of osteonecrosis. Am. J. Roentgenol., *106*:509–522, 1969.

238. Martel, W., Hayes, J.T., and Duff, I.F.: The pattern of bone erosion in the hand and wrist in rheumatoid arthritis. Radiology, *84*:204–214, 1965.

239. Martel, W., Holt, J.F., and Cassidy, J.T.: Roentgenologic manifestations of juvenile rheumatoid arthritis. Am. J. Roentgenol., *88*:400–423, 1962.

240. Martel, W., Snarr, J.W., and Horn, J.R.: The metacarpophalangeal joints in interphalangeal osteoarthritis. Radiology, *108*:1–7, 1973.

241. Mason, R.M., et al.: A comparative radiological study of Reiter's disease, rheumatoid arthritis and ankylosing spondylitis. J. Bone Joint Surg., *41*:137–148, 1959.

242. Maxfield, W.S., Weiss, T.E., and Shuler, S.E.: Synovial membrane scanning in arthritic disease. Semin. Nucl. Med., *2*:50–70, 1972.

243. Medsger, T.A., Jr., and Christy, W.C.: Carpal arthritis with ankylosis in late onset Still's disease. Arthritis Rheum., *19*:232–242, 1976.

244. Meema, H.E., and Meema, S.: Improved roentgenologic diagnosis of osteomalacia by microradioscopy of hand bones. Am. J. Roentgenol., *125*:925–935, 1975.

245. Meema, H.E., and Meema, S.: Comparison of microradioscopic and morphometric findings in the hand bones with densitometric findings in the proximal radius in thyrotoxicosis and in renal osteodystrophy. Invest. Radiol., *7*:88–96, 1972.

246. Menkes, C.J., et al.: Destructive arthropathies in chondrocalcinosis. Rev. Rhum. Mal. Osteoartic., *40*:115–123, 1973.

247. Miller, W.T., and Restifo, R.A.: Steroid arthropathy. Radiology, *86*:652–657, 1966.

248. Minagi, H., and Gronner, A.T.: Calcification of the posterior longitudinal ligament: a cause of cervical myelopathy. Am. J. Roentgenol. Radium Ther. Nucl. Med., *105*:365–369, 1969.

249. Mitchell, G.P.: Arthrography in congenital displacement of the hip. J. Bone Joint Surg., *45B*:88–95, 1963.

250. Mitnick, J.S., Mitnick, H.J., and Genieser, N.B.: Proliferative changes of the hip in juvenile rheumatoid arthritis. AJR, *136*:369, 1980.

251. Modic, M.T., et al.: Nuclear magnetic resonance imaging of the spine. Radiology, *148*:757–762, 1983.

252. Moon, K.L., Jr., et al.: Nuclear magnetic resonance imaging in orthopaedics: principles and applications. J. Orthop. Res., *1*:101–114, 1983.

253. Moskowitz, R.W., and Katz, D.: Chondrocalcinosis coincidental to other rheumatic disease. Arch. Intern. Med., *115*:680–683, 1965.

254. Mueller, C.E., Seeger, J.F., and Martel, W.: Ankylosing spondylitis and regional enteritis. Radiology, *112*:579–581, 1974.

255. Murakami, J., et al.: Computed tomography of posterior longitudinal ligament ossification: its appearance and diagnostic value with special reference to thoracic lesions. JCAT, *6*:41–50, 1982.

256. Murray, R.O.: Iatrogenic lesions of the skeleton. Caldwell lecture, 1975. Am. J. Roentgenol., *126*:5–22, 1976.

257. Murray, R.O.: The aetiology of primary osteoarthritis of the hip. Br. J. Radiol., *38*:810–824, 1965.

258. Murray, R.O.: Observations on cystic tuberculosis of bone, with report on 2 cases. Proc. R. Soc. Med., *47*:133–138, 1954.

259. Murray, W.R., and Rodrigo, J.J.: Arthrography for the assessment of pain after total hip replacement. A comparison of arthrographic findings in patients with and without pain. J. Bone Joint Surg., *57A*:1060–1065, 1975.

260. Newton-John, H.F., and Morgan, D.B.: The loss of bone with age, osteoporosis, and fractures. Clin. Orthop., *71*:229–252, 1970.

261. Nicholas, J.A., Freiberger, R.H., and Killoran, P.J.: Double-contrast arthrography of the knee. Its value in the management of 225 knee derangements. J. Bone Joint Surg., *52A*:203–220, 1970.

262. Noonan, C.D., et al.: Roentgenographic manifestations of joint disease in systemic lupus erythematosus. Radiology, *80*:837–843, 1963.

263. Norman, A., Robbins, H., and Milgram, J.E.: The acute neuropathic arthropathy—a rapid, severely disorganizing form of arthritis. Radiology, *90*:1159–1164, 1968.

264. Notman, D.D., Kurata, N., and Tan, E.M.: Profiles of antinuclear antibodies in systemic rheumatic diseases. Ann. Intern. Med., *83*:464–469, 1975.

265. O'Brien, W.M., LaDu, B.H., and Bunim, J.J.: Biochemical, pathologic and clinical aspects of alcaptonuria, ochronosis and ochronotic arthropathy. Review of world literature. Am. J. Med., *34*:813–838, 1963.

266. O'Duffy, J.D., Hunder, G.G., and Kelly, P.J.: Decreasing prevalence of tophaceous gout. Mayo Clin. Proc., *50*:227–228, 1975.

267. Ondrouch, A.S.: Cyst formation in osteoarthritis. J. Bone Joint Surg., *45B*:755–760, 1963.

268. Owsianik, W.D.J., et al.: Radiological articular involvement in the dominant hand in rheumatoid arthritis. Ann. Rheum. Dis., *39*:508–510, 1980.

269. Pappas, A.M.: The osteochondroses. Pediatr. Clin. North Am., *14*:549–570, 1967.

270. Paradis, G.R., and Kelly, P.J.: Blood flow and mineral deposition in canine tibial fractures. J. Bone Joint Surg., *57A*:220–226, 1975.

271. Parker, M.D.: Ribonucleoprotein antibodies: frequency and clinical significance in systemic lupus erythematosus, scleroderma, and mixed connective tissue disease. J. Lab. Clin. Med., *82*:769–775, 1973.

272. Parlee, D.E., Freundlich, I.M., and McCarty, D.J., Jr.: A comparative study of roentgenographic techniques for detection of calcium pyrophosphate dihydrate deposits

(pseudogout) in human cartilage. Am. J. Roentgenol., 99:688–694, 1967.

273. Patton, J.T.: Differential diagnosis of inflammatory spondylitis. Skeletal Radiol., 1:77–85, 1976.

274. Peter, J.B., Pearson, C.M., and Marmor, L.: Erosive osteoarthritis of the hands. Arthritis Rheum., 9:365–388, 1966.

275. Peterson, C.C., Jr., and Silbiger, M.L.: Reiter's syndrome and psoriatic arthritis. Their roentgen spectra and some interesting similarities. Am. J. Roentgenol., 101:860–871, 1967.

276. Pinals, R.S., and Short, C.L.: Calcific periarthritis involving multiple sites. Arthritis Rheum., 9:566–574, 1966.

277. Purcell, E.M., Torrey, H.C., and Pound, R.V.: Resonance absorption by nuclear magnetic moments in solid. Physiol. Rev., 69:37, 1946.

278. Rabinowitz, J.G., Twersky, J., and Guttadauria, M.: Similar bone manifestations of scleroderma and rheumatoid arthritis. Am. J. Roentgenol, 121:35–44, 1974.

279. Reginato, A., et al.: Polyarticular and familial chondrocalcinosis. Arthritis Rheum., 13:197–213, 1970.

280. Reich, N.E., et al.: Determination of bone mineral content using CT scanning. Am. J. Roentgenol., 127:593–594, 1976.

281. Reiss, K.H., Killig, K., and Schuster, W.: Dual-photon x-ray beam applications. In Proceedings International Conference on Bone Mineral Measurement. DHEW Publication 75-863. Edited by R.B. Mazess. Washington, D.C., Department of Health, Education and Welfare, 1974, pp. 80–87.

282. Rennell, C., et al.: Subchondral pseudocysts in rheumatoid arthritis. Am. J. Roentgenol., 129:1069–1072, 1977.

283. Resnick, D.: Crystal induced arthropathy: gout and pseudogout. JAMA, 242:2440–2442, 1979.

284. Resnick, D.: The radiographic manifestations of gouty arthritis. C.R.C. Crit. Rev. Radiol., 9:265–335, 1977.

285. Resnick, D.: Patterns of migration of the femoral head in osteoarthritis of the hip. Roentgenographic-pathologic correlation and comparison with rheumatoid arthritis. Am. J. Roentgenol., 124:62–74, 1975.

286. Resnick, D.: Patterns of peripheral joint disease in ankylosing spondylitis. Radiology, 110:523–532, 1974.

287. Resnick, D.: Rheumatoid arthritis of the wrist: why the ulnar styloid? Radiology, 112:29–35, 1974.

288. Resnick, D., et al.: Calcaneal abnormalities in articular disorders. Rheumatoid arthritis, ankylosing spondylitis, psoriatic arthritis, and Reiter syndrome. Radiology, 125:355–366, 1977.

289. Resnick, D., et al.: Clinical, radiographic and pathologic abnormalities in calcium pyrophosphate dihydrate deposition disease (CPPD). Radiology, 122:1–15, 1977.

290. Resnick, D., et al.: Intra-articular calcification in scleroderma. Radiology, 124:685–688, 1977.

291. Resnick, D., et al.: Clinical and radiographic abnormalities in ankylosing spondylitis: a comparison of men and women. Radiology, 119:293–297, 1976.

292. Resnick, D., et al.: Clinical and radiographic "reankylosis" following hip surgery in ankylosing spondylitis. Am. J. Roentgenol., 126:1181–1188, 1976.

293. Resnick, D., and Gmelich, J.T.: Bone fragmentation in the rheumatoid wrist: radiographic and pathologic considerations. Radiology, 114:315–321, 1975.

294. Resnick, D., and Niwayama, G.: Entheses and enthesopathy: anatomical, pathological, and radiological correlation. Radiology, 146:1, 1983.

295. Resnick, D., and Niwayama, G.: Radiographic and pathologic features of spinal involvement in diffuse idiopathic skeletal hyperostosis. Radiology, 119:559–568, 1976.

296. Resnick, D., and Utsinger, P.D.: The wrist arthropathy of "pseudogout" occurring with and without chondrocalcinosis. Radiology, 113:633–641, 1974.

297. Resnick, D., Niwayama, G., and Coutts, R.D.: Subchondral cysts (geodes) in arthritis disorders: pathologic and radiographic appearance of the hip joint. Am. J. Roentgenol., 128:799–806, 1977.

298. Resnick, D., Niwayama, G., and Goergen, T.G.: Comparison of radiographic abnormalities of the sacroiliac joint in degenerative disease and ankylosing spondylitis. Am. J. Roentgenol., 128:189–196, 1977.

299. Resnick, D., Shaul, S.R., and Robins, J.M.: Diffuse idiopathic skeletal hyperostosis: Forestier's disease with extraspinal manifestations. Radiology, 115:513–524, 1975.

300. Resnick, D.L.: Erosive arthritis of the hand and wrist in hyperparathyroidism. Radiology, 110:263–269, 1974.

301. Resnick, D.R., et al.: Association of diffuse idiopathic skeletal hyperostosis (DISH) and calcification and ossification of the posterior longitudinal ligament. Am. J. Roentgenol., 131:1049–1053, 1978.

302. Richards, A.J., et al.: Osteitis condensans ilii. Lancet, 1:812, 1975.

303. Richards, A.J., and Hamilton, E.B.: Destructive arthropathy in chondrocalcinosis articularis. Ann. Rheum. Dis., 33:196–203, 1974.

304. Richardson, B.C., et al.: Hereditary chondrocalcinosis in a Mexican-American family. Arthritis Rheum., 26:1387–1396, 1983.

305. Ricklin, P., Ruttimann, A., and del Buono, M.S.: Meniscus Lesions: Practical Problems of Clinical Diagnosis, Arthrography and Therapy. New York, Grune & Stratton, 1971, pp. 31, 50, 105.

306. Rimoin, D.L.: Pachydermoperiostosis (idiopathic clubbing and periostosis): genetic and physiologic considerations. N. Engl. J. Med., 272:923–930, 1965.

307. Rivelis, M., and Freiberger, R.H.: Vertebral destruction at unfused segments in late ankylosing spondylitis. Radiology, 93:251–256, 1969.

308. Rodnan, G.P., and Medsger, R.A.: The rheumatic manifestations of progressive systemic sclerosis (scleroderma). (Review.) Clin. Orthop., 57:81–93, 1968.

309. Rose, G.A.: The radiologic diagnosis of osteoporosis, osteomalacia and hyperparathyroidism. Clin. Radiol., 15:75–83, 1964.

310. Rosen, R.A.: Transitory demineralization of the femoral head. Radiology, 94:509–512, 1970.

311. Rosenthall, L., and Kaye, M.: 99mTechnetium pyrophosphate kinetics and imaging in metabolic bone disease. J. Nucl. Med., 16:33–39, 1975.

312. Rowland, R.E.: Exchangeable bone calcium. Clin. Orthop., 49:233–248, 1966.

313. Ruegsegger, P., et al.: Quantification of bone mineralization using computed tomography. Radiology, 121:93–97, 1976.

314. Sack, K.E., and Genant, H.K.: Radiologist's guide to the use of the laboratory in diagnosing rheumatic diseases. Radiology, 139:585, 1981.

315. Sagar, V.V., et al.: A potential method to detect bone changes of femoral head in patients with cup-arthroplasty. (Abstract.) J. Nucl. Med., 16:564, 1975.

316. Salahuddin, N.I., et al.: Pseudomonas osteomyelitis. Radiologic features. Radiology, 109:41–47, 1973.

317. Salvati, E.A., Freiberger, R.H., and Wilson, P.D., Jr.: Arthrography for complications of total hip replacement. A review of 31 arthrograms. J. Bone Joint Surg., 53A:701–709, 1971.

318. Schaller, J.G.: The seronegative spondyloarthropathies of childhood. Clin. Orthop., 143:76–83, 1979.

319. Scharer, L., and Smith, D.W.: Resorption of the terminal phalanges in scleroderma. Arthritis Rheum., 12:51–63, 1969.

320. Schlenker, R.A., and von Seggen, W.W.: The distribution of cortical and trabecular bone mass along the lengths of the radius and ulna and the implications for in vivo bone mass measurements. Calcif. Tissue Res., 20:41–52, 1976.

321. Schlosstein, L., et al.: High association of an HL-A antigen, W27, with ankylosing spondylitis. N. Engl. J. Med., 288:704–706, 1973.

322. Schumacher, H.R., et al.: Arthritis associated with apatite crystals. Ann. Intern. Med., 87:411–416, 1977.

323. Schumacher, H.R., Jr.: Hemochromatosis and arthritis. Arthritis Rheum., 7:41–50, 1964.

324. Schumacher, T.M., et al.: HLA-B27 associated arthropathies. Radiology, 126:289–297, 1978.

325. Schwarz, G.S., Berenyi, M.R., and Siegel, M.W.: Atrophic arthropathy and diabetic neuritis. Am. J. Roentgenol., *106*:523–529, 1969.

326. Seifert, M.H., Steigerwald, J.C., and Cliff, M.M.: Bone resorption of the mandible in progressive systemic sclerosis. Arthritis Rheum., *18*:507–512, 1975.

327. Shapiro, R.F., et al.: HLA-B27 and modified bone formation. Lancet, *1*:230–231, 1976.

328. Sharp, G.C., et al.: Mixed connective tissue disease—an apparently distinct rheumatic disease syndrome associated with a specific antibody to an extractable nuclear antigen. Am. J. Med., *52*:148–159, 1972.

329. Sharp, J., Purser, D.W., and Lawrence, J.S.: Rheumatoid arthritis of the cervical spine in the adult. Ann. Rheum. Dis., *17*:303–313, 1958.

330. Sharp, J.T., et al.: Methods of scoring the progression of radiologic changes in rheumatoid arthritis. Correlation of radiologic, clinical and laboratory abnormalities. Arthritis Rheum., *14*:706–720, 1971.

331. Sholkoff, S.D., and Glickman, M.G.: Scintiphotographic evaluation of arthritis activity. Invest. Radiol., *4*:207–214, 1969.

332. Sholkoff, S.D., Glickman, M.G., and Steinbach, H.L.: Roentgenology of Reiter's syndrome. Radiology, *97*:497–503, 1970.

333. Silver, T.M., et al.: Radiological features of mixed connective tissue disease and scleroderma—systemic lupus erythematosus overlap. Radiology, *120*:269–275, 1976.

334. Smillie, I.S.: *Osteochondritis*. Edinburgh, E. & S. Livingston, 1960.

335. Smith, D.M., Johnston, C.C., Jr., and Yu, P.L.: In vivo measurement of bone mass. Its use in demineralized states such as osteoporosis. JAMA, *219*:325–329, 1972.

336. Smith, J.H., and Pugh, D.G.: Roentgenographic aspects of articular pigmented villonodular synovitis. Am. J. Roentgenol., *87*:1146–1156, 1962.

337. Smuckler, N.M., Edeiken, J., and Giuliano, V.J.: Ankylosis in osteoarthritis of the finger joints. Radiology, *100*:525–530, 1971.

338. Soila, P.: Some features of angiographic findings in rheumatoid arthritis and scleroderma. Acta Rheumatol. Scand., *10*:189–192, 1964.

339. Soila, P.: The roentgen demonstration of soft tissue change in rheumatoid arthritis. Acta Rheumatol. Scand., *3*:328–334, 1957.

340. Sokoloff, L.: The pathology of rheumatoid arthritis and allied disorders. *In* Arthritis and Allied Conditions, 8th Ed. Edited by J.L. Hollander and D.J. McCarty, Jr. Philadelphia, Lea & Febiger, 1972, pp. 309–332.

341. Stadalnik, R.C., et al.: Vascularity of the femoral head: ¹⁸fluorine scintigraphy validated with tetracycline labeling. Radiology, *114*:663–666, 1975.

342. Staple, T.W.: Extrameniscal lesions demonstrated by double-contrast arthrography of the knee. Radiology, *102*:311–319, 1972.

343. Steinbach, H.L.: Infections of bones. Semin. Roentgenol., *1*:337–369, 1966.

344. Steinbach, H.L.: The roentgen appearance of osteoporosis. Radiol. Clin. North Am., *2*:191–207, 1964.

345. Steinbach, H.L., and Jensen, P.S.: Roentgenographic changes in the arthritides (Part II). Semin. Arthritis Rheum., *5*:203–246, 1976.

346. Steinbach, H.L., and Jensen, P.S.: Roentgenographic changes in the arthritides (Part I). Semin. Arthritis Rheum., *5*:167–202, 1975.

347. Steinbach, H.L., Gold, R.H., and Preger, L.: Roentgen Appearance of the Hand in Diffuse Disease. Chicago, Year Book Medical Publishers, 1975.

348. Steinberg, C.L., Duthie, R.B., and Piva, A.E.: Charcot-like arthropathy following intra-articular hydrocortisone. JAMA, *181*:851–854, 1962.

349. Subcommittee for Scleroderma Criteria of the American Rheumatism Association Diagnostic and Therapeutic Criteria Committee: Preliminary criteria for the classification of systemic sclerosis (scleroderma). Arthritis Rheum., *23*:581–590, 1980.

350. Subramanian, G., et al.: ⁹⁹ᵐTc-labeled polyphosphate as a skeletal imaging agent. Radiology, *102*:70–74, 1972.

351. Sudeck, P.: Uber die akute entzundliche Knochenatrophie. Arch. Klin. Chir., *62*:147, 1900.

352. Sundaram, M., and Patton, J.T.: Paravertebral ossification in psoriasis and Reiter's disease. Br. J. Radiol., *48*:628–633, 1975.

353. Swezey, R.L., et al.: Resorptive arthropathy and the opera-glass hand syndrome. Semin. Arthritis Rheum., *2*:191–244, 1972–73.

354. Sy, W.M., Bay, R., and Camera, A.: Hand images: normal and abnormal. J. Nucl. Med., *18*:419–424, 1977.

355. Thomas, R.H., et al.: Compartmental evaluation of osteoarthritis of the knee. A comparative study of available diagnostic modalities. Radiology, *116*:585–594, 1975.

356. Thould, A.K., and Simon, G.: Assessment of radiological changes in the hands and feet in rheumatoid arthritis. Their correlation with prognosis. Ann. Rheum. Dis., *25*:220–228, 1966.

357. Tilden, R.L., et al.: ⁹⁹ᵐTc-polyphosphate: histological localization in human femurs by autoradiography. J. Nucl. Med., *14*:576–578, 1973.

358. Trueta, J.: The three types of acute haematogenous osteomyelitis. J. Bone Joint Surg., *41B*:671–680, 1959.

359. Trueta, J.: Osteoarthritis of hip. Ann. R. Coll. Surg., *15*:174–192, 1954.

360. Tuffanelli, D.L., and Winkelmann, R.K.: Systemic scleroderma. A clinical study of 727 cases. Arch. Dermatol., *84*:359–371, 1961.

361. Turner, A.F., and Budin, E.: Arthrography of the knee: a simplified technique. Radiology, *97*:505–508, 1970.

362. Udoff, E.J., et al.: Mixed connective tissue disease: the spectrum of radiographic manifestations. Radiology, *124*:613–618, 1977.

363. Urman, J.D., et al.: Aseptic necrosis presenting as wrist pain in SLE. Arthritis Rheum., *20*:825–828, 1977.

364. Van Dyke, D., et al.: Bone blood flow shown with F¹⁸ and the positron camera. Am. J. Physiol., *209*:65–70, 1965.

365. Velayos, E.E., et al.: The 'CREST' syndrome: comparison with systemic sclerosis (scleroderma). Arch. Intern. Med., *139*:1240–1244, 1979.

366. Virtama, P., and Helela, T.: Radiographic measurements of cortical bone. Variations in a normal population between 1 and 90 years of age. Acta Radiol. 293 *[Suppl.]*:7–268, 1969.

367. Vogl, A., and Goldfischer, S.: Pachydermoperiostosis: primary or idiopathic hypertrophic osteoarthropathy. Am. J. Med., *33*:166–187, 1962.

368. Vogler, J.B., et al.: The normal SI joint: a computed tomographic study of asymptomatic patients. Radiology, *151*:433–437, 1984.

369. Vyjnanek, L., Lavicka, J., and Blahos, J.: Roentgenological findings in gout. Radiol. Clin. (Basel), *29*:256–264, 1960.

370. Waldenstrom, J.: First stages of coxa plana. J. Bone Joint Surg., *20*:559–566, 1938.

371. Waldvogel, F.A., Medoff, G., and Swartz, M.N.: Osteomyelitis: a review of clinical features, therapeutic considerations and unusual aspects. N. Engl. J. Med., *282*:198–206, 260–266, 316–322, 1970.

372. Watt, I., and Middlemiss, H.: The radiology of gout. Clin. Radiol., *26*:27–36, 1975.

373. Webber, C.E., and Kennett, T.J.: Bone density measured by photon scattering. I. A system for clinical use. Phys. Med. Biol., *21*:760–769, 1976.

374. Weinfeld, A., Ross, M.W., and Sarasohn, S.H.: Spondylo-epiphyseal dysplasia tarda. A cause of premature osteoarthritis. Am. J. Roentgenol., *101*:851–859, 1967.

375. Weiss, P.E., et al.: ⁹⁹Tc-Methylene diphosphonate bone imaging in the evaluation of total hip prostheses. Radiology, *133*:727–729, 1979.

376. Weiss, T.E., et al.: Iodinated human serum albumin (I¹³¹) localization studies of rheumatoid arthritis joints by scintillation scanning. Arthritis Rheum., *8*:976–987, 1965.

377. Weissman, B.N.W., et al.: Prognostic features of atlantoaxial subluxation in rheumatoid arthritis patients. AJR, *144*:745, 1982.

378. Werndorff, R., and Robinsohn, L.: Kongressverhandl. Deutsch Gesellsch. Orthop., 9, 1905.
379. Weston, J.: Lymphatic filling during positive contrast arthrography in rheumatoid arthritis. Australas. Radiol., 13:368–369, 1969.
380. Williams, J.L., Cliff, M.M., and Bonakdarpour, A.: Spontaneous osteonecrosis of the knee. Radiology, 107:15–19, 1973.
381. Williamson, B.R.J., et al.: Radionuclide bone imaging as a means of differentiating loosening and infection in a patient with total hip prosthesis. Radiology, 133:723, 1979.
382. Wilson, C.R., and Madsen, M.: Dichromatic absorptiometry of vertebral bone mineral content. Invest. Radiol., 12:180–184, 1977.
383. Winterbauer, R.H.: Multiple telangiectasia, Raynaud's phenomenon, sclerodactyly, and subcutaneous calcinosis: a syndrome mimicking hereditary hemorrhagic telangiectasia. Bull. Johns Hopkins Hosp., 114:361–383, 1964.
384. Wolfe, R.D., and Giuliano, V.J.: Double-contrast arthrography in the diagnosis of pigmented villonodular synovitis of the knee. Am. J. Roentgenol., 110:793–799, 1970.
385. Yaghmai, I., Rooholamini, S.M., and Faunce, H.F.: Unilateral rheumatoid arthritis: protective effect of neurologic deficits (case report). Am. J. Roentgenol., 128:299–301, 1977.
386. Yune, H.Y., Vix, V.A., and Klatte, E.C.: Early fingertip changes in scleroderma. JAMA, 215:1113–1116, 1971.
387. Zimmerman, C., and Sayegh, V.: Roentgen manifestations of synovial osteochondromatosis. Am. J. Roentgenol., 83:680–686, 1960.
388. Zitnan, D., and Sit'aj, S.: Chondrocalcinosis articularis. Section I. Clinical and radiological study. Ann. Rheum. Dis., 22:142–168, 1963.

Chapter **6**

Computed Tomography in the Evaluation of Low Back Pain

Guillermo F. Carrera

Low back pain affects many individuals in industrialized societies, and can be an important (occasionally the primary) complaint in patients under evaluation for rheumatic disease. The lumbar spine and sacroiliac joint are affected by many conditions that can result in localized or radiating back pain, sometimes accompanied by evidence of neural dysfunction. Radiographic evaluation of the lumbar spine and sacroiliac joints is complicated by numerous factors. In the peripheral skeleton, relatively thin osteoarticular structures surrounded by uniform soft tissues are the rule. Conventional high-resolution radiography can provide exquisite demonstration of peripheral skeletal structure and abnormality. The lumbar spine and sacroiliac joints, in contrast, are anatomically complex structures. The presence of overlying abdominal visceral contents, the thickness of the trunk, and the importance of demonstrating neural structures (in the lumbar spine) render conventional radiographic techniques disappointingly insensitive in the evaluation of early or subtle abnormalities.

High-resolution computed tomography (CT) has become accepted as the best technique for evaluating the anatomy of the spine and spinal canal in the lumbar area, as well as for demonstrating the complex anatomy of the sacroiliac joints. Subtle abnormalities of the intervertebral discs, lumbar facet joints, and neural arches can now be properly evaluated using CT, and myelography avoided in most cases of mechanical backache. Radiographic findings diagnostic of sacroiliitis can be shown better in many cases using high-resolution CT than with conventional radiography. Computed tomography, therefore, offers a rapid, accurate, noninvasive technique for detecting pathologic anatomy in a wide spectrum of patients being evaluated for low back, pelvic, and radiating leg or hip pain.

CT OF THE LUMBAR SPINE

Radiographic evaluation of patients with low back and sciatic pain requires demonstration of the vertebral bodies and neural arches, and also good delineation of the soft tissue structures in the spinal canal. The diagnosis and discrimination of such

conditions as herniated nucleus pulposus, spinal canal and neural foraminal stenosis, spondylolysis, and lumbar facet arthritis comprise the most important reasons for radiographic evaluation of patients with chronic backache. Systemic disorders such as metastatic disease to the vertebral column and noninfectious spondylitis are generally diagnosed prior to detailed radiographic evaluation of the vertebral segments for low back or radiating leg pain. Computed tomography, using techniques that allow a high degree of spatial resolution and contrast resolution adequate for discriminating soft tissues in the spinal canal, can effectively diagnose most anatomically demonstrable lesions causing low back pain and can obviate the need for complex and invasive tests such as contrast myelography, gas myelography, epidural venography, and discography.[6,7,9,11,12,15,17,18]

CT TECHNIQUES

A variety of instruments for performing high-resolution CT has become available in the past several years. The techniques for obtaining adequate CT images of the lumbar spinal canal and intervertebral discs vary from instrument to instrument. The CT study of the lumbar spine as performed at the Milwaukee Regional Medical Center furnishes an example of satisfactory technique.[12]

A General Electric CT/T 8800 scanner with a tilting gantry and large patient aperture is used to examine the lumbar spine. The patients are supine to minimize motion. Factors including 25-cm field of view, 10-second scan time, 5-mm contiguous slices, 1,150 mAS, and 120 kVP allow CT imaging with contrast resolution less than 0.5%, spatial resolution of 0.75 mm, and 6-rad radiation dose to the skin per examination. A preliminary lateral localizer image (computed radiograph) is obtained prior to transaxial examination in order to select the gantry level and angle for producing optimal images in (or near) the plane of the intervertebral disc and perpendicular to the plane of the lumbar facet joints (Fig. 6–1).

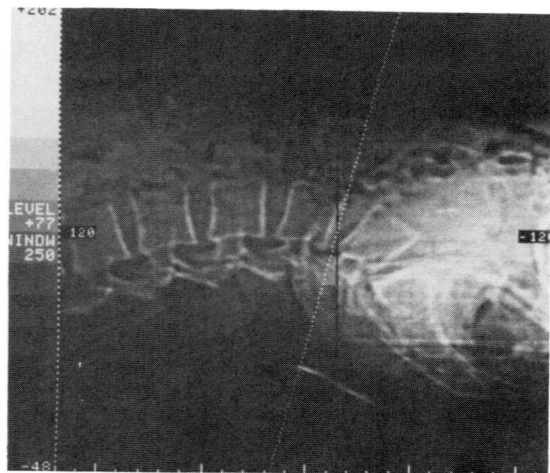

Fig. 6–1. Lateral computed radiograph shows the gantry angle and level chosen to produce an image in the mid-plane of the L4–L5 intervertebral disc and lumbar facet joints (dotted line). (From Carrera, G.F., et al.[6])

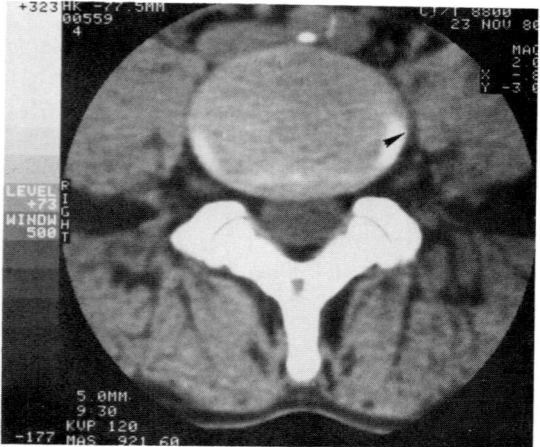

Fig. 6–2. CT image through a normal L4–L5 intervertebral disc shows a smooth, slightly convex posterior interface with the spinal canal. The disc margin is congruent with a small area of density representing vertebral end-plate (arrowhead). The spinal canal, thecal sac, nerve roots, and ligamenta flava are easily identified.

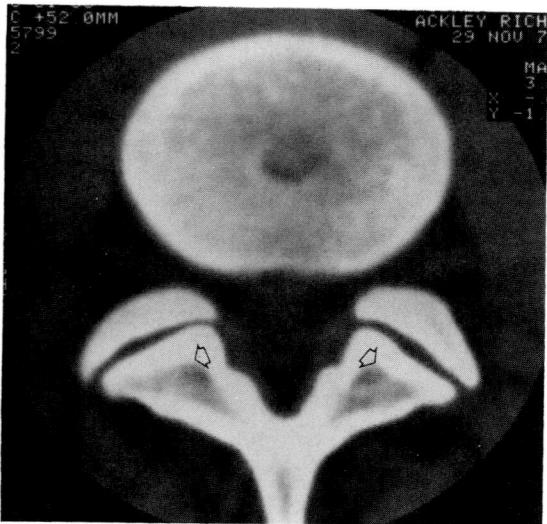

Fig. 6–3. CT scan at the L5–S1 level shows normal lumbar facet joints. The articular surfaces are straight and parallel, and normal osseous structure, including a corticomedullary discrimination (arrows), is apparent.

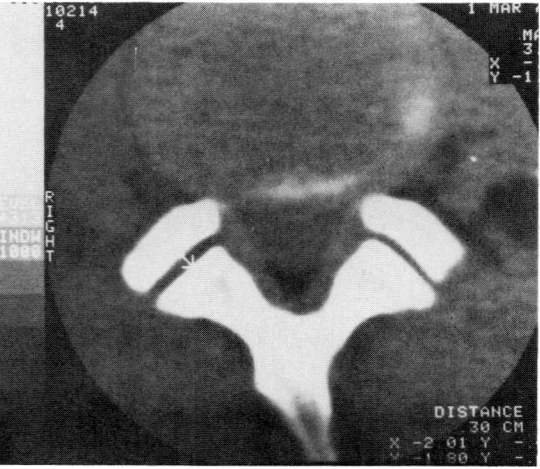

Fig. 6–4. CT scan through the L4–L5 interspace demonstrates use of a computer program to measure the right L4–L5 lumbar facet joint. In a series of normal volunteers, joint widths of 2.0 to 3.5 mm were measured. Joint narrowing should be diagnosed when a width less than 2 mm is encountered. (From Carrera, G.F., et al.[6])

NORMAL ANATOMY

CT images should be obtained at both "bone" and "soft tissue" image settings for full evaluation of the spine and spinal canal. Contiguous images covering the entire neural foramen from pedicle to pedicle allow complete assessment of the neural arch at each segment. The intervertebral discs, lumbar facet joints, bony structures of the neural arch, thecal sac, and nerve root sheaths can be clearly demonstrated. Epidural fat surrounds many important structures in the lumbar spine canal, and allows easy discrimination of thecal anatomy (Figs. 6–2, 6–3, 6–4).

HERNIATED INTERVERTEBRAL DISC

Because of the differential density of intervertebral disc material and epidural fat, the abnormal contour of a herniated intervertebral disc can be

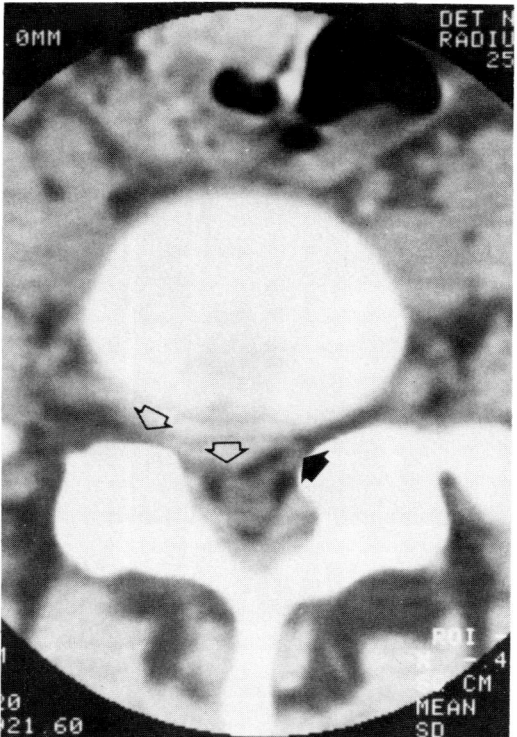

Fig. 6–5. CT image through the L5–S1 interspace shows an asymmetric posterior protrusion of intervertebral disc (open arrows). The left S1 root sheath (solid arrow) is easily identified. The right S1 root sheath has been displaced and obscured by the herniated intervertebral disc. (From Eldevik, O.P., et al.: Radiology, *145*:85, 1982.)

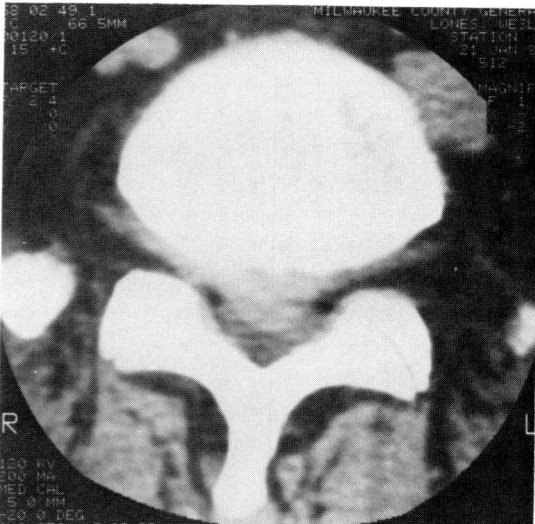

Fig. 6–6. CT image at the L5–S1 level shows a large central herniation of relatively high-density intervertebral disc. The dural sac is posteriorly compressed and deformed by this central herniated nucleus pulposus.

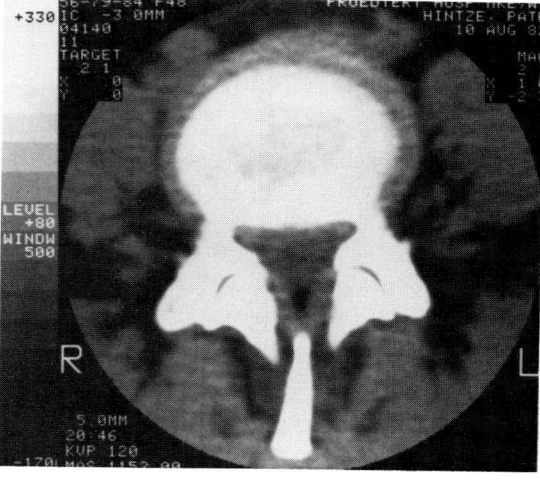

Fig. 6–7. CT image demonstrates symmetric circumferential bulge of the annulus, projecting beyond the vertebral end-plate.

clearly demonstrated using CT. Asymmetric protrusion of the intervertebral disc, either centrally or posterolaterally, can be readily appreciated, as can the effects of the intervertebral disc on adjacent nerve-root sheaths (Figs. 6–5, 6–6). Unusual lesions such as lateral disc herniations and extruded fragments can be clearly identified, often better than with myelography.[10,18]

BULGING ANNULUS

The myelographic discrimination between a diffusely bulging annulus fibrosus and a focal disc protrusion can be complex. CT can clearly demonstrate the symmetric bulge of a degenerated annulus fibrosus and allows discrimination from focal protrusion or herniation of intervertebral disc material[14] (Fig. 6–7).

LUMBAR FACET ARTHROPATHY

Subtle anatomic abnormalities of the lumbar facet joints can be easily demonstrated. Adequate CT images readily show such findings as joint space narrowing, osteophytes, reactive sclerosis, and erosions. Unusual findings, such as facet capsular calcifications, can be seen[3,6] (Figs. 6–8, 6–9, 6–10).

SPINAL STENOSIS

Spinal stenosis, either central canal stenosis or neural foraminal stenosis, remains largely a clinical diagnosis. The role of computed tomography in establishing the anatomic level of potential stenosis is still not clearly defined, but CT images dem-

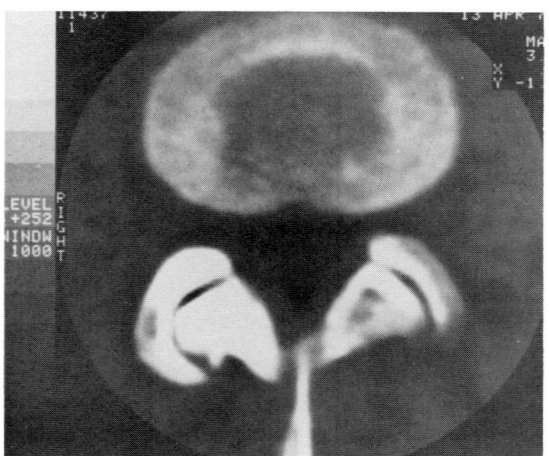

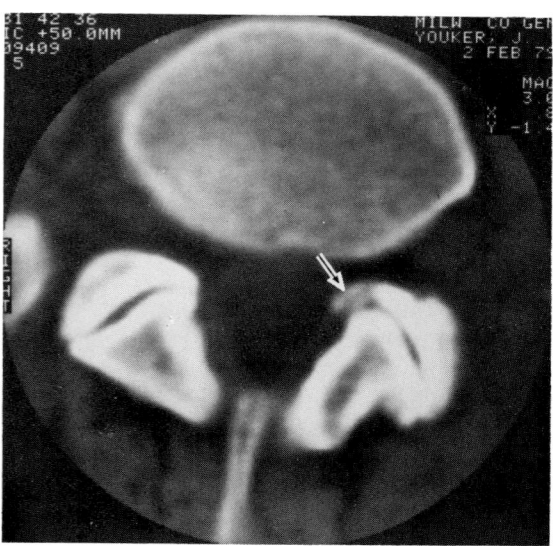

Fig. 6–8.   Extensive degenerative disease of the right L4–L5 facet joint. There is asymmetric narrowing of the joint, subchondral sclerosis involving both superior and inferior articular facets, posterior osteophyte formation, and a small amount of gas within the facet joint (vacuum phenomenon). (From Carrera, G.F., et al.[6])

Fig. 6–10.   Bilaminar calcification of the anterior capsular structures of the left L5–S1 lumbar facet joint. The innermost calcification (arrow) is in the ligamentum flavum. The calcification adjacent to the joint itself is in the anterior joint capsule. (From Carrera, G.F., et al.[6])

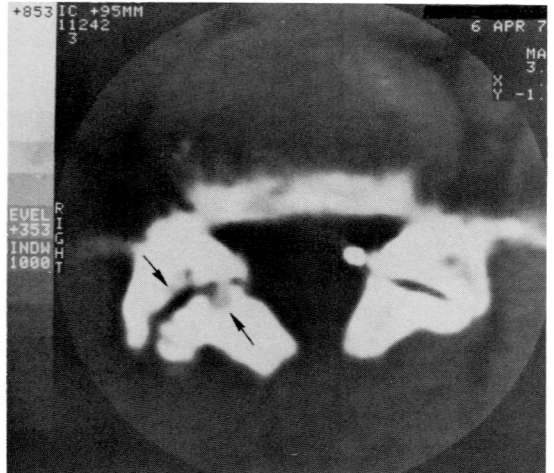

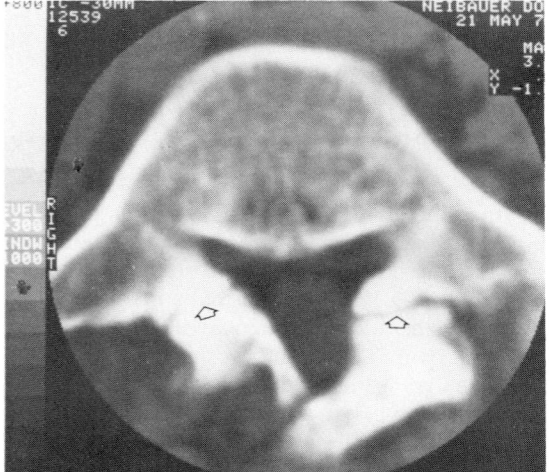

Fig. 6–9.   Extensive facet arthritis in a patient who has had a laminectomy. Prominent subchondral erosions (arrows) as well as subchondral sclerosis are present. A small drop of residual myelographic contrast material is seen adjacent to the left facet joint. (From Carrera, G.F., et al.[6])

Fig. 6–11.   CT image through the neural arch of L5 reveals irregular and sclerotic defects through the pars interarticularis (arrows). A dysmorphic pars and lamina are seen on the right. A deformed and elongated spinal canal is also apparent. These findings are characteristic of bilateral spondylolysis.

SPONDYLOLYSIS

onstrating severe constriction of the spinal canal or narrowing of the lateral recess of the neural foramen can be valuable in surgical planning for patients with the clinical diagnosis of spinal stenosis.[1,6,10,15]

Defects in the pars interarticularis can be difficult to diagnose using conventional films. If contiguous CT images are obtained from pedicle to pedicle in each vertebral segment under study, the entire neural arch is demonstrated, and defects in the pars interarticularis, degenerative changes, or evidence of maldevelopment of the pars interarticularis can be clearly seen[8] (Fig. 6–11).

IMPLICATIONS OF CT EXAMINATION OF THE LUMBAR SPINE

Conventional radiographic evaluation of the lumbar spine in patients with chronic low back and/or sciatic pain as a major or exclusive complaint is relatively insensitive for the diagnosis of herniated disc, spinal stenosis, and lumbar facet arthropathy, and these are the anatomically demonstrable, treatable causes of "mechanical" low back pain. Conventional radiographic examination of the lumbar spine is most useful in screening for a variety of focal or multifocal disorders such as metastases to the spine, infectious lesions, osteoporosis with compression fracture, trauma, and Paget's disease. High-resolution CT has been found to be more reliable than myelography in the diagnosis of intervertebral disc herniation, which is the major surgically approachable lesion in patients with chronic low back pain and sciatica.[10] CT diagnosis of lumbar facet arthropathy in patients with localized radiating back pain has proved to be an effective guide to diagnostic and therapeutic lumbar facet joint injection.[3,4]

COMPUTED TOMOGRAPHY OF SACROILIAC (SI) JOINTS

Sacroiliitis is an important feature of the seronegative spondyloarthropathies such as psoriatic arthritis, Reiter's syndrome, ankylosing spondylitis, and enteropathic spondyloarthritis. Infectious sacroiliitis is a less common but important diagnostic consideration in patients with inflammatory low back pain. Their complex anatomy and location in the pelvis, surrounded by a thick mantle of abdominal and pelvic contents, make radiographic evaluation of the SI joints using conventional techniques such as plain radiography difficult. Evidence of sacroiliitis, such as joint space narrowing, osteoporosis, subchondral sclerosis, erosion, and ankylosis, can be difficult to define.[16]

CT produces sectional images of the SI joints with high-spatial resolution, free of the confusing shadows caused by overlying soft tissue structures. The natural irregularities of these joints are easily resolved by the tomographic nature of CT images. CT has been shown to be an effective and accurate method for SI joint evaluation.[5,13] Combined with careful clinical evaluation, screening conventional radiography, and (on occasion) radioisotope studies, CT contributes greatly to the diagnosis of sacroiliac disorders.[2]

CT Technique

As in the evaluation of the lumbar spine, regardless of the CT instrument and protocol chosen, certain essential features must be addressed to produce adequate images. Essential elements of a successful CT examination include adequate spatial resolution and slice orientation in the axis of the sacrum to allow discrimination and evaluation of both ligamentous and diarthrodial compartments of the joint.

We use the General Electric CT/T 8800 scanner. A lateral localizer image is obtained first to select the best gantry level and angle for the CT cuts (Figs. 6–12, 6–13). Five-mm thick contiguous sections through the sacroiliac joints are then performed using either a small field of view or target reconstruction algorithm. The scans are displayed with a window width of 1,000 Hounsfield units (HU) and an image level of + 250 to + 350 Hounsfield units. This protocol allows discrimination of both compartments of the SI joint, and produces high-resolution, high-contrast images clearly

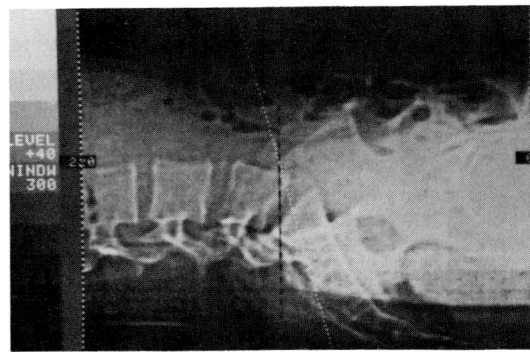

Fig. 6–12.   Lateral computed radiograph of the gantry level and angle required to produce contiguous images through the sacroiliac joint in the plane of the sacrum (dotted line).

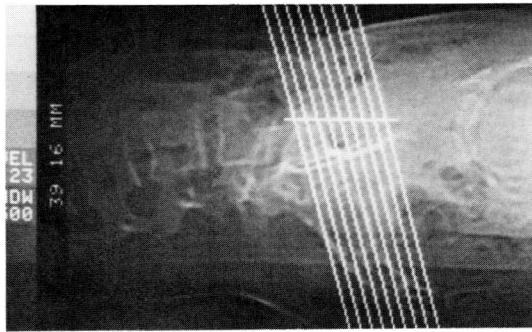

Fig. 6–13.   Lateral computed radiograph displays the CT scan sequence used to image the sacroiliac joints. (From Carrera, G.F., et al.[5])

showing the normal subchondral cortex, medullary space, and all other anatomic landmarks.[14]

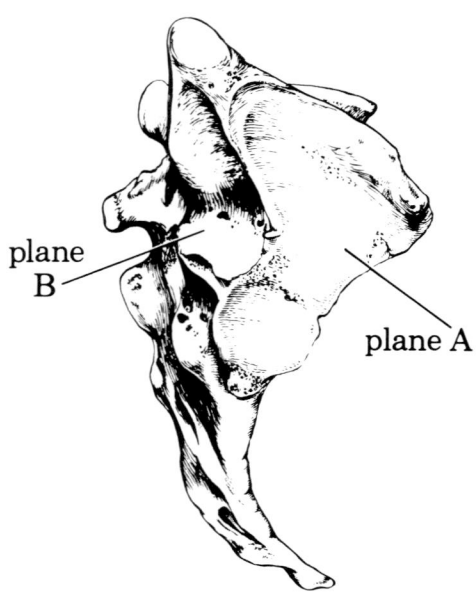

Fig. 6–14. Diagrammatic representation of a disarticulated sacroiliac joint viewed from the lateral aspect. Plane B represents the steeply oblique ligamentous portion of the joint, which lies dorsal and cephalad to the oval more sagittally oriented diarthrodial compartment of the joint (plane A). (From Carrera, G.F., et al.[5])

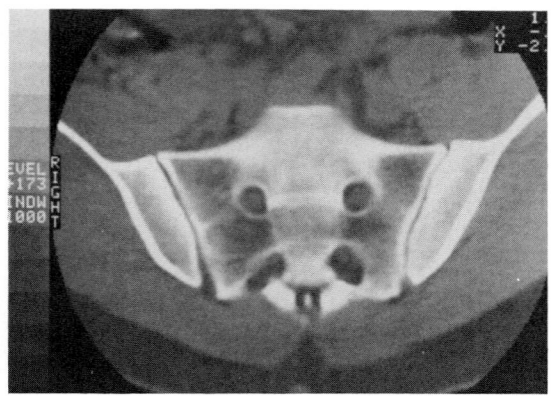

Fig. 6–15. CT scan through the diarthrodial compartment of the normal sacroiliac joints shows smooth, parallel articular surfaces. A sharp subchondral demarcation is seen on the sacral side of the joint. A somewhat broader zone of increased density is seen on the iliac side of both joints. This is a normal finding and should not be confused with subchondral reactive sclerosis. (From Carrera, G.F., et al.[5])

Normal Anatomy

The SI joint consists of two anatomic compartments. The entire dorsal surface as well as superior aspect of the joint (approximately 25 to 30% of the total craniocaudal length) is ligamentous (syndesmosis). The strong sacroiliac ligaments are surrounded by fat and traversing muscles, and insert into a series of ligamentous "pits" on the sacrum. This compartment is sharply oblique when compared to the diarthrodial (synovial) compartment. The oval-shaped diarthrodial compartment occupies the anterior and inferior portions of the sacroiliac joint and is oriented in, or near, the sagittal anatomic plane[2,14] (Figs. 6–14, 6–15).

Sacroiliitis

The findings of sacroiliitis are similar to those found on conventional films. Early synovitis and hyperemia cause osteoporosis in a juxta-articular distribution. CT shows well-defined areas of decreased absorption (decreased density of mineral) near the articular cortex, frequently separated from the subchondral bone by a band of adjacent sclerosis. As an isolated finding, this zone of decreased absorption can be difficult to interpret even on CT images. Continued inflammatory disease leads to narrowing of the articular cartilage. In a series of normal volunteers, we found the normal SI joint width to be 2.5 to 4.0 mm. We therefore diagnose narrowing when the diarthrodial compartment of the joint measures less than 2 mm by computer program. Continued inflammatory disease causes erosions of the subchondral bone, evidenced on CT by indistinct cortical margins and/or interruptions of the subchondral cortex. With progressive erosive disease, these cortical interruptions progress to frank osteodestructive lesions and deep, irregular erosions, frequently surrounded by a zone of reactive sclerosis.

Reactive sclerosis in an area of sacroiliitis is manifested by areas of increased density on CT images. Although sclerosis on both sides of the joint is frequently stated as a criterion for the reactive sclerosis of sacroiliitis, *the predominant sclerosis almost always occurs on the iliac side of the joint.* This is true even in advanced cases of sacroiliitis, and should not deter one from diagnosing reactive sclerosis due to sacroiliitis.

Ankylosis appears on CT scans, as on plain films, as mature bone bridging the sacroiliac space[2,5] (Figs. 6–16, 6–17, 6–18).

Implications of CT in Sacroiliitis

The SI joint can participate in many inflammatory and mechanical conditions, resulting in findings suggesting sacroiliitis. Indistinct articular margins, osteoporosis, and cortical erosion are

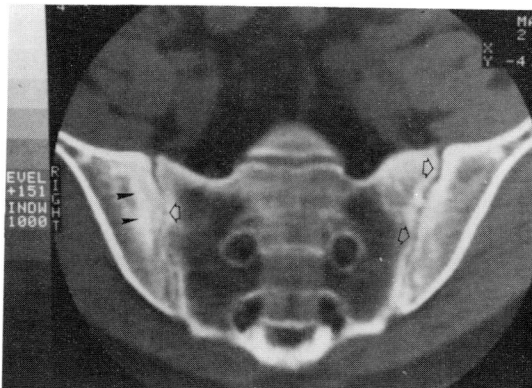

Fig. 6–16. CT scan through the diarthrodial compartment of the sacroiliac joints in a patient with ankylosing spondylitis shows advanced bilateral sacroiliitis. There is severe joint narrowing and irregularity. Small erosions (open arrows) are seen in both joints. Reactive sclerosis, present as a band of increased density separated from the subchondral plate by a lucent zone, is particularly apparent in the right joint (arrowheads). (From Carrera, G.F., et al.[5])

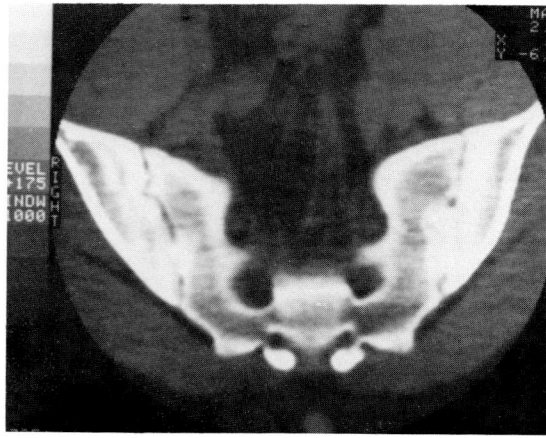

Fig. 6–18. CT scan in a patient with ankylosing spondylitis shows bilateral joint narrowing, sclerosis, and erosions. Focal ankylosis, seen as solid bars of bone traversing the joint, is present in both joints. (From Carrera, G.F., et al.[5])

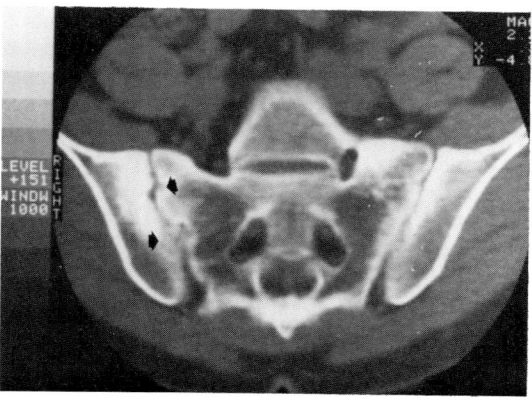

Fig. 6–17. CT scan through the diarthrodial compartment of the sacroiliac joints shows asymmetric erosive sacroiliitis. There is mild irregularity and narrowing of the left sacroiliac joint, with erosions and subchondral sclerosis. Severe subchondral sclerosis is present in the right sacroiliac joint. Large erosions (arrows) are seen in the more involved right sacroiliac joint. (From Carrera, G.F., et al.[5])

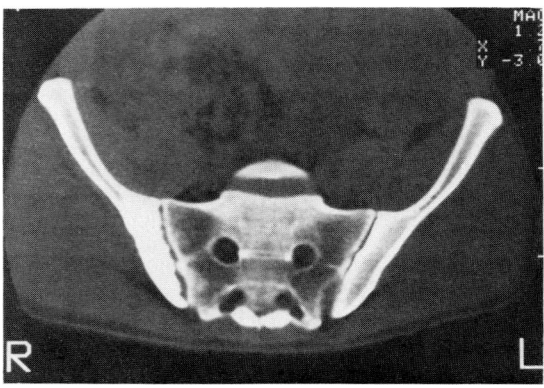

Fig. 6–19. CT scan in a patient with prostatic carcinoma shows a normal left sacroiliac joint. The right joint is irregular, but most of the irregularity is on the iliac side of the joint. A dense, sclerotic metastatic lesion is seen occupying the ilium adjacent to the right sacroiliac joint. (From Carrera, G.F.[2])

nonspecific changes that do not discriminate infectious, spondyloarthritic, or mechanical etiologies. Careful correlation of the radiographic findings (including CT) with the clinical findings is necessary to properly diagnose suspected sacroiliitis.

Bilateral sacroiliitis, particularly if spondylitis or peripheral arthritis is present, is essentially diagnostic of one of the seronegative spondyloar-

thritic syndromes. Although symmetric bilateral sacroiliitis is most characteristic of ankylosing spondylitis, and asymmetric bilateral sacroiliitis is most common in psoriatic arthritis or Reiter's syndrome, the findings in the SI joints alone frequently do not serve to discriminate these conditions. Although bilateral asymmetric sacroiliitis is somewhat more common in the latter two conditions than in ankylosing spondylitis, extensive bilateral changes are found frequently.

Pure unilateral sacroiliitis, although occasionally seen in seronegative spondyloarthritis, is more suggestive of joint infection. In the absence of strong clinical evidence for one of the seronegative spondyloarthritic syndromes, unilateral sacroiliitis suggests a presumptive diagnosis of infectious arthritis and should prompt vigorous attempts to isolate an organism.

Other etiologies for destructive SI joint disease, such as mechanical or neoplastic disorders, are generally accompanied by a history and clinical findings suggesting the primary condition. Osseous destruction on one side of the SI joint suggests metastasis, particularly if no systemic evidence of inflammatory disease is present[2] (Fig. 6–19).

CT, therefore, can play a significant role in the diagnosis and evaluation of patients with suspected sacroiliitis. When plain films are negative or equivocal, and clinical suspicion of sacroiliitis is high, CT is indicated. It is the most sensitive and accurate anatomic method now available for evaluation of the SI joints.

REFERENCES

1. Brown, H.A.: Enlargement of the ligamentum flavum—a cause of low-back pain with sciatic radiation. J. Bone Joint Surg., *20*:325, 1938.
2. Carrera, G.F.: Current concepts in the evaluation of sacroiliitis. Postgr. Rad., *3*:97, 1983.
3. Carrera, G.F.: Lumbar facet arthropathy. *In* Computed Tomography of the Spine. Edited by V. M. Haughton. New York, Churchill Livingstone, 1983.
4. Carrera, G.F.: Lumbar facet joint injection in low back pain and sciatica (I) and (II). Radiology, *136*:661–667, 1980.
5. Carrera, G.F., et al.: Computed tomography of sacroiliitis. Am. J. Roent., *136*:41–46, 1981.
6. Carrera, G.F., et al.: Computed tomography of the lumbar facet joints. Radiology, *134*:145, 1980.
7. Carrera, G.F., Williams, A.L., and Haughton, V.M.: Computed tomography in sciatica. Radiology, *137*:433, 1980.
8. Grogan, J.P., et al.: Spondylolysis studies with computed tomography. Radiology, *145*:737, 1982.
9. Hammerschlag, S.B., Wolpert, S.M., and Carter, B.L.: Computed tomography of the spinal canal. Radiology, *121*:361, 1976.
10. Haughton, V.M., et al.: A prospective comparison of computed tomography and myelography in the diagnosis of herniated lumbar disk. Radiology, *142*:103, 1982.
11. Haughton, V.M., Syvertsen, A., and Williams, A.L.: Soft tissue anatomy within the spinal canal as seen on CT. Radiology, *134*:649, 1980.
12. Haughton, V.M., and Williams, A.L.: CT anatomy of the spine. CRC Crit. Rev. Diagn. Imaging, 173, 1981.
13. Kozin, F., et al.: Computed tomography in the diagnosis of sacroiliitis. Arthritis Rheum., *24*:1479–1485, 1981.
14. Lawson, T.L., et al.: The sacroiliac joints; anatomic, plain roentgenographic, and computed tomographic analysis. J. Comput. Assist. Tomogr., *6*:307–314, 1982.
15. Lee, B.C.V., Kazam, E., and Newman, A.D.: Computed tomography of the spine and spinal cord. Radiology, *128*:95, 1978.
16. Ryan, L.M., et al.: The radiographic diagnosis of sacroiliitis: A comparison of different views with computed tomograms of the sacroiliac joint. Arthritis Rheum. In press, 1983.
17. Sheldon, J.J., Sersland, T., and LeBorgne, J.: Computed tomography of the lower lumbar vertebral column. Radiology, *124*:113, 1977.
18. Williams, A.L., Haughton, V.M., and Syvertsen, A.: Computed tomography in the diagnosis of herniated nucleus pulposus. Radiology, *135*:95, 1980.

Chapter 7

Clinical Evaluation in Rheumatic Diseases

W. Watson Buchanan and Peter Tugwell

> . . . . . . I took twelve patients in the scurvy . . . . . . Their cases were as similar as I could have made them. They lay together in one place. . . . and had one diet common to all. . . . Two of these were ordered each a quart of cyder a-day. Two others took twenty-five gutts of *elixir vitriol* three times a day. . . . . Two others took two spoonfuls of vinegar three times a day. . . . . Two of the worst patients. . . . were put on a course of sea-water. . . . Two others had each two oranges and one lemon given them every day.
>
> The consequence was, that the most sudden and visible good effects were perceived from the use of the oranges and lemons; one of those who had taken them, being at the end of six days fit for duty.
>
> James Lind, 1753

Since the dawn of time doctors have tried out their pills and potions and, even more serious, their surgery, on countless thousands of suffering patients. Conclusions as to the efficacy of treatment were often based on a single or, at most, a few observations. This method worked well and many of the major drugs in modern medicine were introduced in this way, including morphine, digitalis, penicillin, salicylates, gold, and cortisone, for which a clinical rheumatologist, the late Dr. Philip S. Hench, won a Nobel Prize in Medicine. Indeed, there are relatively few examples of great modern therapeutic advances having arisen from sheer intellectualism of the discoverer planning his research with a certain objective in view.[161] The experiments that led to the eradication of smallpox by Edward Jenner were unethical by today's standards and statistically uncontrolled.[139] James Lind is credited as the first to perform a properly controlled therapeutic trial,[179] although some 42 years were to elapse before the Lords of the Admiralty put his precepts into practice and abolished scurvy from the Royal Navy, thereby causing British seamen to be known by the sobriquet of "limeys." However, the era of controlled clinical therapeutic trials only began after the second World War, and it is gratifying that clinical rheumatologists were among the first to try out their drugs in this manner. The late Thomas N. Fraser of Glasgow, Scotland was probably the first to report a double-blind, controlled trial in rheumatic diseases when he compared injectable gold to placebo in patients with

rheumatoid arthritis.[85] In the 1950s there were several well-designed controlled trials: salicylates and corticosteroids in rheumatic fever[40] and rheumatoid arthritis,[28,79,202,203] chrysotherapy in rheumatoid arthritis,[77] and radiotherapy in ankylosing spondylitis.[56] Concurrently the statistical basis of clinical evaluation of therapeutic agents was established.[97,119–121]

With the ever-increasing number of new antirheumatic drugs being produced by the pharmaceutical industry, there is no substitute for properly designed and controlled trials to test their efficacy. Clinical impressions can be misleading: for example, two-thirds of patients with rheumatoid arthritis "improved" after tonsillectomy,[260] and even "cures" were claimed.[209] The controlled clinical trial, while being the most powerful design for assessing effectiveness of therapy,[27,30,33,146,245,248,258] needs to be critically assessed for its quality before one accepts its conclusions and needs to be placed in the appropriate clinical context.[26,81,82,89,125,126,163,228,239,253,280]

Since the quality of many clinical therapeutic trials of antirheumatic drugs leaves little ground for complacency,[224,266] an outline of the design and statistical interpretation seems appropriate.

DESIGN AND STATISTICAL INTERPRETATION

The following critical appraisal guidelines should be considered when designing or assessing clinical trials in rheumatology:[274]

1. *Appropriate unambiguous specification of*

research objective. The research objective should be clearly specified in terms of clinical significance, and should confine itself to testing one or at most two major hypotheses. The information to be tested should be judged to have an acceptably high probability of doing more good than harm on the basis of basic research, clinical pharmacokinetics, and open clinical studies.

2. *Valid trial architecture.* The design of the trial should be appropriate for the major question and should not be compromised by trying to answer too many different questions. In conditions where there is no known effective therapy, a placebo control group is appropriate, but once efficacious therapy is established it may be more reasonable to use this as the standard therapy against which subsequent therapies are compared. Randomization should be used to avoid unconscious bias—allocation procedures that allow prediction of the allocation of the individual patients entering the trial, such as alternate allocation, are still found in rheumatology journals.

Crossover and factorial designs offer statistical advantages in that fewer patients are needed, but drug interactions and carry-over effects frequently outweigh those advantages. Avoidance of the latter by a "washout" period either with placebo or no drugs can help with short-acting agents, but such a regimen is painful for the patients.

3. *Clinically sensible maneuver and minimization of the three biases of contamination, cointervention, and compliance.* It is important to use clinically sensible maneuvers. For example, the dosages used should be those recommended for clinical practice. It is no longer necessary to insist upon fixed dosage regimens. Increasing the dose in a clinically logical fashion according to the patient's response (e.g., pain relief with NSAIDs) or tolerance (e.g., gastric discomfort with aspirin) is entirely feasible in rheumatology trials.

Contamination (the administration of the intervention being tested to the control group) must be avoided in an ethical fashion by setting out clear criteria for deterioration. In this way such patients are eligible for the active agent if this occurs, yet they are analyzed as treatment failures in the placebo group (and are not included in the analysis of the active treatment group). It is unrealistic to withhold all concurrent therapy, but bias due to cointervention can be avoided by maintaining concurrent therapies in a constant fashion in all patients or, if there is clinical deterioration, by handling it in a similar way to contamination. Compliance with the protocol by both physician and patient is crucial if one is to discriminate between lack of improvement due to intrinsic lack of effect of the agent being tested and failure to comply. In trials involving oral medication, patient questionnaires are relatively inaccurate measures of compliance, and additional checks, such as surprise pill counts or the use of blood and urine markers, should be considered.[111]

4. *Appropriate patient selection.* It is more efficient (in that fewer patients are needed) to restrict entry for rheumatology trials to those with widespread evidence of active inflammation (e.g., many active joints) who comply with therapy and do not have comorbidity. These patients are most likely to respond. However, if beneficial results are obtained, it is important when generalizing the results to other patients to take into account the reduction in the magnitude of benefit in less compliant patients with milder disease and the increased risk of adverse effects in patients with comorbidity.

5. *Accurate measurement of relevant outcomes.* Appropriate outcomes should be selected that measure both the pathophysiologic effects of disease and the impact upon symptoms, signs, and disability that the therapeutic agent has the potential to improve. Important issues to be considered when selecting outcomes include their credibility to clinicians, the minimization of error, and their ability to detect the smallest clinically important improvement.

6. *Blinded assessment of outcomes.* Since a major subjective component exists in most end points used in rheumatology, major bias is likely if the assessor knows which patients are in the experimental and control groups. Whenever possible the assessor should be blinded to the allocation.

7. *Appropriate analysis.* The results should be analyzed and presented to demonstrate both their clinical and their statistical significance. Results are too often reported in a form that is appropriate for statistical analysis but that obscures the magnitude of clinical improvement in individual patients. Elaborate indices, even though they have statistical advantages, should be used only if they are interpretable by rheumatologists in terms of their clinical significance.

The analysis should be checked to ensure that all patients entered into the trial are included in the analysis. Not infrequently patients are dropped from the analysis because they "fail to improve," e.g., The Cooperating Clinics trial of gold sodium thiomalate.[43] This practice reduces the likelihood of the study demonstrating a benefit because, if the intervention is effective, a greater number of patients who failed therapy will be in the control group but who will not be analyzed.

Several different outcomes are included as major end points in many rheumatology trials. There should be evidence that the statistical significance of the results has been adjusted to avoid the increased likelihood of falsely assuming a difference. The more outcomes that are assessed, the more likely it is that one will achieve a p value of <0.05 due to chance alone (a type I error). Using multiple outcomes with statistical adjustment again penalizes the likelihood of a true difference being demonstrated. This can be avoided by classifying outcomes into major and minor and apportioning differential type I errors to them.[34]

One must include sufficient numbers of patients to minimize the risk of a true clinically important

Table 7-1. Sample Size Requirements

Rate of Events in the Control Group	Number of Trial Patients Required per Treatment Group to Show (1 sided alpha = 0.05; beta = 0.2) Clinically Significant Differences (Risk Reductions) of:	
	25%	50%
.01	17,121	3,587
.02	8,485	1,780
.03	5,606	1,178
.04	4,167	877
.05	3,304	696
.06	2,728	576
.07	2,317	490
.08	2,008	425
.09	1,768	375
.10	1,576	335
.12	1,289	274
.14	1,083	231
.16	929	199
.18	809	174
.20	713	154
.22	634	138
.24	569	124
.26	513	112
.28	466	102
.30	425	94
.35	343	76
.40	281	63
.45	233	53
.50	194	45
.55	163	39
.60	136	33
.65	114	28
.70	95	24
.75	78	21
.80	63	17
.85	50	14
.90	38	12
.95	27	9
.9999	12	5

One-tailed α = .05
β = .2

benefit not achieving statistical significance (Table 7-1). This ensures that sufficient patients are studied for the results to achieve sufficient "power," i.e., there is a measurable likelihood that the smallest clinically significant benefit would be detected. This issue is well illustrated by the current confusion over the efficacy of yttrium radiosynovectomy of the knee in rheumatoid arthritis.[23] The only double-blind controlled trial of yttrium against a placebo (saline) demonstrated a 30% (10/13 vs. 13/21) risk reduction in pain and a 33% (8/23 vs. 11/21) risk reduction in joint effusions in the patients treated with yttrium, but this clinically significant difference failed to reach conventional levels of statistical significance owing to the small sample size of 23 and 21 in the two groups. Table 7-1 shows the number of patients that need to be studied to have an 80% or greater likelihood of a risk reduction of 25% and 50% being detected.[23] If we assume that the rate of improvement in the saline placebo group found in this study is accurate, then 343 patients per group need to be studied for a 25% improvement/risk reduction (or 76 patients per group for a 50% improvement) to achieve statistical significance. Thus, this trial may have produced a false negative result. There should be evidence in the analysis that allowance was made for any differences in the baseline characteristics of the groups since randomization itself does *not* guarantee a balance of potential confounding variables. Factors that should be adjusted for in the statistical analysis if unequally distributed should include severity of symptoms or disease, duration of disease, responsiveness to previous therapy and, possibly, age and sex.

8. *Appropriate conclusions.* The results of clinical trials should be placed in the appropriate clinical context.[26,81,82,89,125,126,163,228,239,253,280] Clinicians should be cautious in generalizing to all patients in their practice who could potentially benefit, because of the frequent exclusion of the elderly and the young, the pregnant, and those with comorbid conditions.[153,160,239,253] Trials of nonsteroidal antiinflammatory analgesics are usually of short duration, and clearly the conclusions of such trials must be constrained and not extrapolated beyond the limits of the study.[166] Data obtained in open studies and in the course of normal clinical practice should not be ignored[92,125,126,253] but used in combination with results obtained in randomized controlled trials.[81,82,119,136,253]

METHODS OF ASSESSMENT

Inflammation has long been recognized as notoriously difficult to measure both in clinical practice and in the laboratory.[10] The commonly employed methods are essentially based on efforts to quantitate the cardinal features: dolor, tumor, calor, et rubor (Celsus 53BC to AD7), functio laesa (Galen c129 to c200), et rigor.[129] The methods are at best indirect, and have been aptly described by Lansbury[155] as being "analogous to estimating the size and heat of an underground fire by the amount of smoke, flame and heat detected above ground." Laboratory tests play a relatively small part in the assessment of a patient's progress, since a drug that only reduces the erythrocyte sedimentation rate but does not relieve joint pain is clearly of no interest to either patient or physician. Antirheumatic drugs available at present are relatively weak, and differences between nonsteroidal anti-inflammatory analgesics and placebo in short-term trials are relatively small[54] (Table 7–2). At present no single ideal method is capable of accurately reflecting disease activity in arthritis. Some authors have suggested aggregation of end points into a composite index.[152,154,156,173,189,201,226,255]

Composite Indexes

Such indexes have two major assets over multiple end points. First, they provide a basis for combining all the end points in order to decide on the success or failure of a therapeutic intervention where some measurements improve and others worsen. Secondly, they increase the statistical efficiency of clinical trials, allowing sample size to be reduced. Many of the indexes involve differential weighting of the individual components of the index—the appropriate basis for this differential weighting is controversial.[21] The authors prefer those that weight each component either equally or according to the relative clinical and biological importance of the components (the "clinical/biological judgmental approach"). Examples of those include the Ritchie Articular Index, which weights

each joint according to a four-point tenderness scale;[238] the Lansbury Index, which weights the joints according to size;[155] the Keitel Functional Test,[149] which weights performance of different specified exercises; and the Fellinger Rheumazahl Index,[83] which weights different signs, symptoms, and functional tests. A different, increasingly popular form of weighting is based upon the statistical properties of each component, and several techniques have been utilized that maximize the statistical significance of the results such as the pooled index-derived units of Smythe and his colleagues,[255] discriminant analysis,[201] and generalizability coefficient analysis.[74] These purely statistical weighting techniques run the risk of producing relative weights of the components that differ substantively from their relative clinical importance. For example, the sedimentation rate might make a larger contribution to the final index than the active joint count. Approaches are needed to integrate the advantages of these statistical tests with the relative clinical importance for each component.

Measurement of Error

Sir Thomas Lewis, the acknowledged father of clinical science in the United Kingdom, remarked, "It is crucial in measuring to know the error of the method; to have but an inaccurate measure may be regrettable, but to have it and not to know it is deplorable."[174] Surprisingly, few authors reporting clinical therapeutic trials of antirheumatic drugs provide any information on the error of the clinical significance of their methods.[75] This can lead to misinterpretation of the clinical significance of results. For example, the intra-observer error of digital joint circumference by the Geigy spring apparatus is approximately 2 mm.[278] In a trial of ketoprofen compared to placebo in rheumatoid ar-

Table 7–2. Mean Differences in Clinical and Laboratory Parameters Between Placebo and Salicylate, Indomethacin, Ibuprofen, and Prednisolone in 37 Patients with Rheumatoid Arthritis[54]

Clinical and Laboratory Parameters	Salicylate	Indomethacin	Ibuprofen	Prednisolone
Pain index[54]	−6	−10	−6	−7
Articular index[238]	−6	−10	−6	−7
Grip strength (mm Hg)[166]				
right	+12.3*	+14.5*	+17.5*	+16.5
left	+10.6	+11.1	+12.7	+11.3
Digital joint circumference (mm)[278]				
right	−1	−4	0	−4
left	−3	−3	−3	−1
^{99m}Tc Knee joint uptake[58]				
(percent × 10^{-2})				
right	−9.3	−12.0*	−8.3	−11.7*
left	−7.5	−10.9*	−10.9*	−12.1

Oral daily dosage: Sodium salicylate 1 g four times a day; indomethacin 25 mg four times a day; ibuprofen 400 mg three times a day; and prednisolone 5 mg three times a day. Each preparation was given in double-blind, cross-over fashion, for one week.
*Statistically significant at the 5% level.

thritis, the reported reduction in digital joint circumference using this instrument was small and less than the error of the method.[208] In addition, systematic errors not measured by the standard deviation can also occur in clinical therapeutic trials. An example of this would be assessing joint tenderness at different times of the day, which has been shown to vary.[106] Only good trial design can eliminate this type of error.[244]

Objective Versus Subjective Outcome Measures

Naturally, objective measurements are needed in clinical therapeutic trials of antirheumatoid drugs.[107] Clinical trials in rheumatology are only as good as their end points. In a comprehensive review of the literature on clinical trials of indomethacin, O'Brien showed that in those studies employing objective measurements only 25% of patients had "good" or "excellent" responses, whereas in those studies primarily based on subjective indices the average "good" or "excellent" response was 60%.[224] However, these differences might also be explained by the quality of the trial designs, since those employing objective measures were better controlled than those using patients' subjective responses. The point is not that objective measures are better than subjective, but that sensitive measures are better than insensitive.[144] The most sensitive parameter to change with antirheumatic drug therapy in rheumatoid arthritis is the patient's subjective assessment of pain relief.[54] The objective measurement of radionuclide joint uptake, on the other hand, is often unable to discriminate between active drugs and placebo.[164] It is of interest that the "softer" subjective responses ranked high in importance to a panel of clinical rheumatologists.[21]

CHOICE OF END POINTS

The choice of end points should take into account the perspectives of (1) the "doer"—researchers whose prime responsibility is to scientific rigor, and (2) the "consumer"—clinicians who will apply and integrate the results to decide whether the therapy is likely to do the patient more good than harm.

The end points in clinical trials for anti-inflammatory drugs currently recommended by the Canadian and United States governmental drug approval agencies are listed in Table 7–3.

Several advances in the measurement of patient outcomes should be considered in the selection of end points for future clinical trials. We propose a methodologic framework that addresses some of the major measurement issues relevant to the selection of end points for trials (Fig. 7–1).

Table 7–3. End Points in Clinical Trials for Anti-Inflammatory Drugs Recommended by the United States and Canadian Government Agencies Responsible for Drug Approval

All Studies	Chronic Studies
Number of painful or tender joints	ARA functional capacity
Number of swollen joints	
Duration of morning stiffness	ARA anatomic stage
Grip strength	
Time to walk 50 feet	Rheumatoid factor titer
ESR	
Clinician's opinion of patient's condition	
Patient's opinion of own condition	

(From Tugwell, P., and Bombardier, C.[274])

The end points may be divided into: (1) traditional "objective" measures of disease activity assessable by the physician or a designated independent assessor, and (2) the "subjective" outcomes based on the patient's self-report, unassessable directly by others.

The terms (jargon) published for the same measurement issues may be confusing. The terms commonly used in clinical research for the "objective" outcomes are listed at the top end of the boxes in Figure 7–1, while terms from the social sciences, such as the many types of validity, are more frequently used for "subjective" outcomes and are listed at the lower end of the boxes. We will now discuss each of the component boxes in this figure.

Comprehensiveness/Content Validity

The particular outcomes selected should include or predict all those components of health status important to the rheumatologist and the patient that are relevant to the intervention being assessed.

If the eight Ds (Table 7–4)[281] that encompass the spectrum of health status in measurable terms are considered, and matched to the end points commonly used in rheumatologic clinical trials, the "objective" outcomes cluster into the Disease Activity category (although some such as grip strength and walking time could also be classified in the Disability and Dysfunction category). The inclusion of end points that reflect the other Ds, such as those that assess pain and quality of life (physical, social, and emotional function), are increasingly popular with the development of better methods for assessing them.

It is impossible to include all aspects of the eight Ds in the end points selected for a rheumatology clinical trial. Those selected have to act as "indicators," "markers," or "proxies" for the other components not being measured directly. This is particularly pertinent to the assessment of physical and social function because so many activities

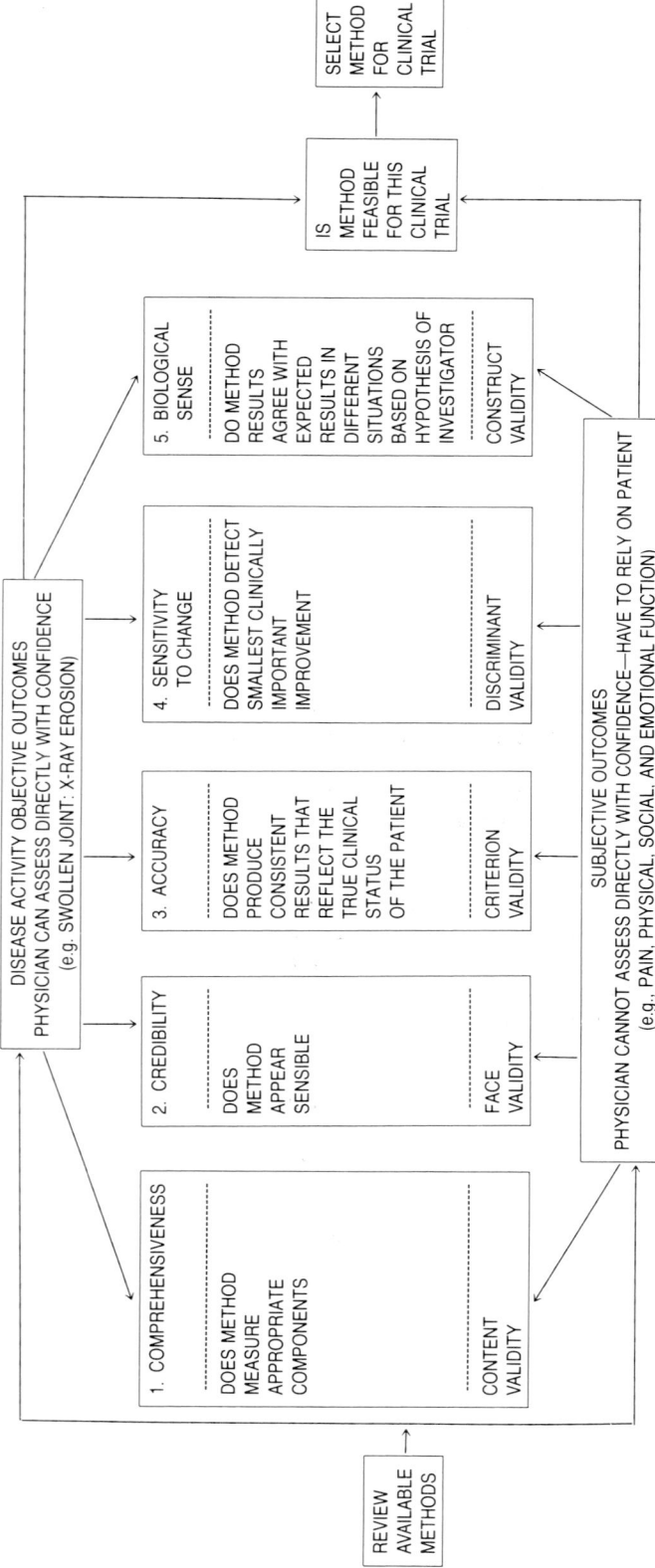

Fig. 7–1. Methodologic framework for development and selection of end points in rheumatology clinical trials. (From Tugwell, P., and Bombardier, C.[274])

Table 7–4.   Comprehensiveness—The Eight Ds

The Ds—Examples from Arthritis Studies
Disease Activity
Painful/tender/swollen joints
Grip strength
Sedimentation rate
Morning stiffness
Walking time
Radiographic erosions
Isotope uptake
*D*istress
Pain
*D*eath (infrequent)
*D*isadvantages/Drug Effects
*D*isability and *D*ysfunction
Physical function
Self care
Mobility
Physical ability
Social function
Work
Household
Emotional function
*D*isharmony (family function)
*D*issatisfaction

(Modified from White, K.L.[281])

within these categories may be affected by the arthritis.

The approaches currently used to select components or items for outcomes, where there are too many items to use them all, are extremely important because they set the terms of reference, which cannot be altered during any subsequent sophisticated testing of reliability and validity. There are major differences between the approaches currently used that will affect the credibility and interpretation of the results of the end points developed in different ways. There are two major approaches: judgmental and statistical.

Judgmental Approaches

Clinician/Investigator. Various methods can be used ranging from selection by a single investigator to use of sophisticated group consensus techniques.[114,257] These methods are guided by the following considerations: (1) The frequency of occurrence, i.e., the assessment of whether the outcome (pain, component of disease activity, or functional disability) is sufficiently common in the patients being studied that it is worthwhile including. (2) Clinical importance, i.e., the importance of the outcome in the clinical management of the patient. (3) Potential for response to intervention, i.e., the likelihood of the outcome to respond to the intervention being tested in the clinical trial.

Patient's Preference

Group Data. Patients with arthritis are polled to assess which components of the eight Ds are affected by the arthritis and the relative importance of each component. The results of the frequency and the importance are integrated in one of several ways, and the items are ranked highest in the group selected.

Individualized Goal Attainment. Each patient identifies the most important symptoms and functional disability due to the arthritis, and then improvement in these individualized outcomes is measured.

Statistical Approaches

Statistical methods are used in a variety of ways, including: (1) to identify which outcomes can be used as "markers" to represent other outcomes (e.g., agreement statistics),[35] (2) to identify which outcomes best discriminate between control and experimental patients (e.g., discriminant analysis),[221] and (3) to identify which outcomes can be fitted into a hierarchical scale (e.g., Guttman/Cumulative Scaling).[264]

Credibility/Face Validity

The method chosen to assess the outcome of interest should appear equally sensible both to the investigators and to the clinician who will be interested in applying the results in clinical practice. There are two main components to this approach:

Willingness of Investigators or Practicing Clinicians to Accept Patient's Opinion. This, of course, has a major influence upon the choice of end points for inclusion in the clinical trial. If they are not acceptable, then patient questionnaires for the assessment of pain and quality of life are not credible, and the investigator must resort to instruments, such as thumb-crushing dolorimeters, and direct observation of the patient's disabilities, which would be impractical for most studies.

Extent to which Reporting of Results of Method is Interpretable. The clinical meaning of the way in which the end points are quantified and indices are used certainly influences the confidence of those wishing to apply the results.

Accuracy/Criterion Validity

The method chosen should consistently reflect the best available estimate of the true clinical status of the patient. This is done by measuring and then minimizing the sources of error.

Types of Error. The two main types of error that should be shown to be minimal are random and systematic. The results obtained from a new end point method (clinical, laboratory, or functional status of the patient) can be conceptualized as being potentially contributed to by three components as follows:

Result = True value + Random error (Imprecision/Unreliability) + Systemic error (Bias)

An example of the difference between these two types of error is shown in Figure 7–2. It is not always appreciated that the standard deviation measures the random error but does not reflect systematic bias, the minimization of which requires good trial design and is as important as sophisticated statistics. Thus, it is important to minimize these two types of error that influence the accuracy of the end point selected.

The major sources of variability are those due to (1) patient variability caused by extraneous factors affecting the assessment, such as the variation in joint tenderness at different times of the day,[106] and the inconsistent response to questions of a patient who is distracted, tired, or has organic memory loss; (2) observer variability, such as that found when different observers use different examination techniques and/or infer different conclusions when examining for joint tenderness;[238] (3) instrument variability, such as that found with different size cuffs used for measuring grip strength.

These three sources of variability need to be considered for each end point method by repeat observations in patients whose clinical condition is unchanged until acceptable levels of agreement are achieved. Statistical approaches are used that take into account the level of agreement expected due to chance alone (such as Cohen's Kappa).[35]

Sensitivity to Change/Discriminant Validity

In view of the relatively small, although important, overall effects or differences between many drugs in arthritis, it is important to demonstrate that the end points selected can detect the smallest clinically significant change of interest to practicing physicians. This can be assessed by comparing the ability of the end point method to detect the smallest clinically important differences detected by experienced rheumatologists and the patients themselves.

Biologic Sense Construct Validity

One assesses the extent to which the results of the method match the hypothesized expectations of the investigator when compared with other indirect assessments. This approach is important when

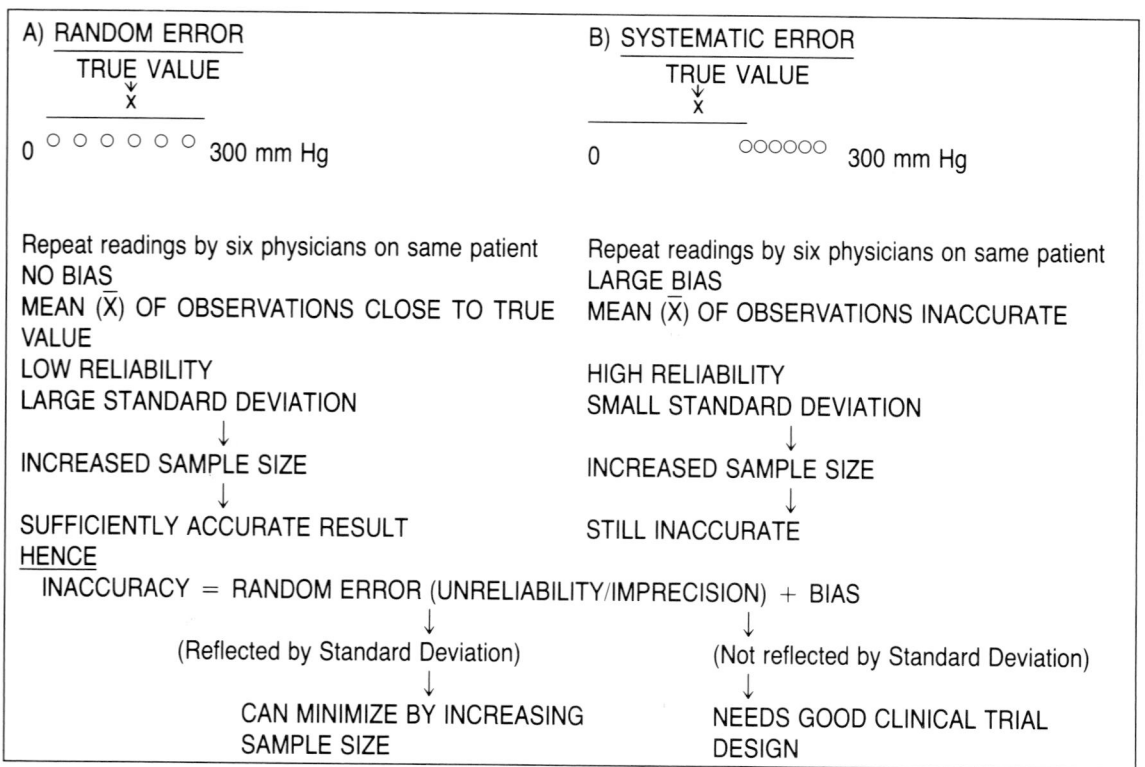

Fig. 7–2. Random error versus systematic error: an example of each using repeat readings of grip strength. (From Tugwell, P., and Bombardier, C.[274] Reproduced by courtesy of the Editor of the Journal of Rheumatology.)

there are no good direct methods for measuring the true value. There are two main types of construct validity:

Convergent Construct Validity. One assesses how well the results of the end point method being considered agree with other accepted methods. For example, a new method for assessing physical disability would be expected to agree with the results of a standard active joint count. One might hypothesize that a new isotope scan should show higher numbers of involved joints in hospitalized patients (since they are expected to have more extensive disease) than in ambulatory patients.

Divergent Construct Validity. One assesses how well the results of the new end point method being considered demonstrate differences in groups of patients who would be expected to show differences. For example, if one is testing out a new psychologic function scale, patients who have more active joints and pain could be hypothesized to be more depressed and anxious than patients with fewer active joints and less pain. Hence, a new psychologic scale should demonstrate differences between these two groups of patients.

PAIN

Since pain is the major complaint of the rheumatic sufferer, measurement of pain relief becomes extremely important in assessing clinical response to antirheumatic drug medication. "Pain is known to us by experience and described by illustrations" wrote Sir Thomas Lewis,[173] and the absence of a more precise definition highlights the difficulty in recognizing and grading the pain response. Pain is an entirely subjective phenomenon, and can only be measured by the patient who experiences it. Keele proposed a pain chart on which the patient recorded his pain on an adjectival scale: slight, moderate, severe, and agonizing.[148] In practice, few patients record their pain as agonizing; most tend to select moderate. However, on other scales the moderate score often corresponds to either slight or severe.[128] The adjectival scale is controversial because there are insufficient descriptions available to be placed regularly in the same rank order by patients.[130] Numerical values can be given to the adjectival scale as follows: 0 = no pain, 1 = slight pain, 2 = moderate pain, 3 = severe pain, and 4 = extremely severe or agonizing pain. Such a scale is capable of discriminating between nonsteroidal anti-inflammatory analgesics and placebo in short-term clinical therapeutic trials.[165]

Currently the most popular method of recording pain is by the visual analogue scale.[68,69,131,145,234,259] This is a line that is taken to represent the continuum of pain, the ends defining the extremes of the experience, i.e., "no pain" and "as severe as it could be" (Fig. 7–3). The patient marks the line at a point corresponding to his estimate of pain, and the distance from O is taken to represent the severity of pain. Scott and Huskisson have shown that the performance of a visual analogue scale is profoundly affected by its design.[249] Thus, for example, descriptions of pain at intervals along the line result in a clustering of points opposite the descriptions, converting the visual analogue scale into a graphic rating scale, which they claimed resulted in loss of sensitivity[131] (Fig. 7–4).

If, however, the descriptions are evenly spread along the line, the results are uniformly distributed, and the aforementioned problem with clustering is avoided.[250] There is excellent agreement between repeated measurements of pain using the visual analogue scale.[250,259] Some 5% of patients have difficulty in understanding the concept of a visual analogue scale, at least initially, and time taken for careful explanation before the trial commences is well spent. The line should have stops at either end to limit the distribution of results.[133] The conventional length of the line is 10 cm, and it is important to note that this will change with photocopying.[67] Normal subjects asked to remember the position of a mark on the line perform less well than patients with pain.[67] The method has, however, been found applicable to patients regardless of ethnic background and even to children under five years of age.[251]

Beecher has aptly stated that, "Pain is measured in terms of its relief."[10] Huskisson has made a plea to measure pain relief rather than pain directly.[128] Jacobsen contended that patients should not have access to previous scores when measuring subjective states like pain.[138] However, Scott and Huskisson found that the reverse was true.[249] They observed that as time goes on patients tend to overestimate pain severity, but quickly correct their scores when shown their starting point. This observation is clearly important in long-term studies, and in rheumatic disease trials it is now our practice to provide the patient with his previous scores. Pain varies at different times of the day, and it is therefore wise to standardize the timing of measurements.[128]

Other methods of measuring pain, such as assessment of pain threshold and pain tolerance[129] and measurement of catecholamine excretion rates,[130] have not found acceptance in clinical trial practice.

JOINT COUNT

Various methods have been used to evolve a scoring system of joint tenderness.[8,9,29,45–47,116,154,156,157,189,231,238] These indices are based on applying firm digital pressure to the joint margins,

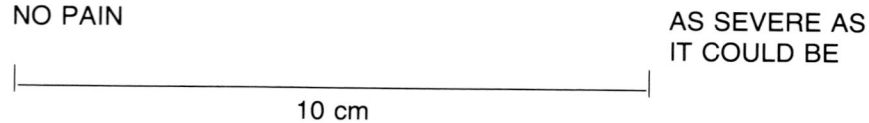

NO PAIN

AS SEVERE AS
IT COULD BE

|——————————————————————————|

10 cm

Fig. 7–3. Visual analogue pain scale. This scale may be either vertical or horizontal.[250] The ends of the line should be marked; otherwise, some patients will record their pain beyond the ends of the line.

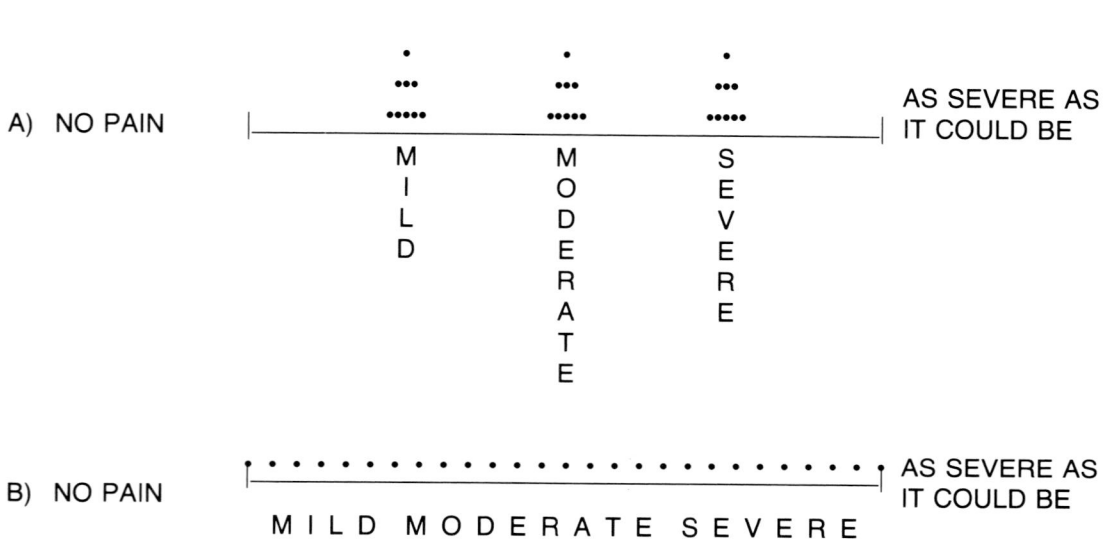

A) NO PAIN | AS SEVERE AS IT COULD BE

M M S
I O E
L D V
D E E
   R R
   A E
   T
   E

B) NO PAIN | AS SEVERE AS IT COULD BE

MILD MODERATE SEVERE

Fig. 7–4. *A,* The use of descriptive terms along a visual analogue scale converts it to a graphic rating scale so that sensitivity is lost. *B,* The scale, however, is satisfactory if the descriptive terms are spread out evenly along the line.

and grading the degree of tenderness by the patient's response. The articular index of Lansbury[154,157] was designed to provide information on the extent of articular involvement. An estimate of disease activity was based upon joint size, as determined by the area of the articular surface, but the degree of joint inflammation was not taken into account. It should be noted that there are no data on the area of the articular surface in joints of the human body. The articular index of Lansbury has a close correlation with the systemic index described by the same author,[156] and both have proved useful in charting the individual patient's progress, although most workers have found they take considerable time to perform.

The Cooperating Clinics Committee of the American Rheumatism Association employs a simple count of clinically active joints, as determined by pain on passive motion, tenderness on pressure, or inflammatory joint swelling.[45,46] This index has been widely used for the assessment of antirheumatic drugs, both in short- and long-term clinical therapeutic trials. Ward and his colleagues have provided evidence that scoring a few selected "signal" joints gives a better assessment of drug effect than a total joint count.[277] Only one trial in which

"signal" joints were used has been reported.[277] If "signal" joints become accepted, then the instruments variously described as dolorimeters* and palpameters[73,124,143,190,194,263] may come back into vogue, since at present they cannot generally be applied to all the joints.

The articular index devised by Ritchie and colleagues[238] is based on the summation of joint responses after firm digital pressure. The responses are recorded: 0 = the patient has no tenderness, +1 = the patient says it is tender, +2 = the patient says it is tender and winces, and +3 = the patient says it is tender, winces, and withdraws the limb. Tenderness of the cervical spine, hip joints, and talocalcaneal and midtarsal joints is elicited by passive movement. Some joints are treated as single units: temporomandibular, sternoclavicular, acromioclavicular, and metacarpophalangeal, metatarsophalangeal, and proximal interphalangeal joints of the hands. The total sum of the Ritchie articular index is 78, and it has been shown to reflect exacerbations of disease and improvement

---

*Ed. note: The dolorimeter was developed and standardized against the Lansbury indices with the idea of making precise serial measurements of "one slice of the inflammatory pie."[194]

induced by antirheumatic drugs. The Ritchie index correlates well (r = 0.89) with the articular index of the Cooperating Clinics Committee of the American Rheumatism Association.[238] Both indices show clear differences in short-term clinical therapeutic trials of antirheumatic drugs compared with placebo. The articular index of the Cooperating Clinics Committee of the American Rheumatism Association gives lower mean differences between active drugs and placebo, but this finding is offset by its smaller variability. Both articular indices are satisfactory for clinical trial purposes. The intraobserver error with the Ritchie index when performed within 30 minutes is highly acceptable (mean difference between 1 and 2 units). The interobserver error is high, and it has been calculated that differences less than 20 between two observers in an individual patient cannot be interpreted as significant. This finding once again emphasizes the need for a single observer to make the measurements in a clinical therapeutic trial. The Ritchie articular index of joint tenderness correlates with the patient's assessment of pain,[54] in the upper limbs with grip strength, and in the lower limbs with the time to walk 50 feet.[238] The Ritchie Articular Index of joint tenderness has the advantage that it can be performed by nonmedical personnel with an amanuensis within $2\frac{1}{2}$ minutes.[238] It is the method chosen by the European League against Rheumatism Standing Committee on International Clinical Studies.[171]

GRIP STRENGTH

Various instruments[49,53,71] have been devised to measure grip strength during the past century,[127] but they have failed to provide any advantage over the Davis bag[247] or sphygmomanometer cuff.[47,73,231] The intraobserver error with the Davis bag is up to 10 mm Hg, but twice this between different observers.[166] Day-to-day and week-to-week variations in patients with stable disease gave no greater difference than that observed in intraobserver studies.[166] A circadian rhythm has been noted in one study in normal subjects[286] and in patients with rheumatoid arthritis[152a] but not in another study.[166] It seems prudent to standardize the time of measurement of grip strength, as with other indices, in clinical therapeutic trials in patients with rheumatic disease. The determinants of grip strength are the strength of the muscles in the forearm and hand, and the pain and degree of joint destruction in the wrist, hand, and finger joints: grip strength, as previously noted, correlates with the Ritchie articular index of joint tenderness in the upper limbs, and also with a functional index[168] in the upper limbs. Grip strength is not particularly sensitive to change with antirheumatic drug ther-

apy,[54,166] and its continued use in clinical trials rests largely on its simplicity and rapidity.

Myers and colleagues have described the use of an electronic apparatus that measures pressure-time recordings as well as maximum grip.[219] This method requires more study to determine its value as an outcome measure in clinical trials. Downie et al. found a poor correlation between measured grip strength and that assessed using a visual analogue scale.[70]

DIGITAL JOINT CIRCUMFERENCE

Jeweler's rings were first used by Boardman and Hart to measure the circumference of the proximal interphalangeal joint of the thumb.[19] These measurements correlate well with those obtained with the Geigy plastic spring gauge apparatus.[19] Webb et al. found a relatively small intraobserver error with the Geigy plastic spring gauge (approximately 2 mm) but a large interobserver error (approximately 10 mm).[278] The results of digital joint circumference measurement in patients with rheumatoid arthritis are reproducible from day-to-day and week-to-week in stable disease.[278] No correlation has been found with radionuclide(^{99m}Tc) joint uptakes,[38] and Rhind et al.[236] found no correlation with other clinical measurements. A diurnal rhythm in digital joint circumference has been found by some[19,86] but not all[278] investigators. Reduction in joint circumference can only occur in patients who have soft tissue inflammatory joint swelling: in this instance, "signal" joints have proved to be of value.[278] Willkens et al. have introduced an "arthrocircameter" with a fully flexed polyethylene loop that more readily adapts to irregular shapes than the Geigy spring gauge.[283] However, there is still no proof of its superiority over the latter.

The circumference of the knee joint has been shown to decrease with nonsteroidal anti-inflammatory analgesics,[54] but has failed to gain acceptance in clinical therapeutic trials of antirheumatic drugs.

MORNING STIFFNESS, "LIMBERING-UP" TIME, TIME OF ONSET OF FATIGUE, AND SLEEP

Huskisson emphasized that rigor is an important component of joint inflammation, and few clinicians or patients would disagree.[129] The problem of measuring morning stiffness, "limbering-up" time, and time of onset of fatigue is essentially due to lack of precise definition and inadequate methods of quantitation.[129,169,261] Many patients have difficulty in separating pain from stiffness,[261] although in our experience this can be resolved with careful explanation. The duration of morning stiffness does correlate reasonably well with other clinical and laboratory parameters,[236] but appears to be due to extra-articular rather than intra-articular parameters.[288] Morning stiffness, limbering-up time, and time to onset of fatigue do improve with antirheumatic drug medication. Huskisson has pointed out that the morning stops at noon, and that assessment of morning stiffness should have an adjustment for the time of first getting out of bed.[129] Laboratory methods of quantitating joint stiffness[7,137,285] are applicable to only a few joints and have not, as yet, been used in clinical therapeutic trials.

One of the functions that is most disturbed in rheumatoid arthritis is sleep. Only one study has been reported on the effects of a nonsteroidal anti-inflammatory drug in rheumatoid arthritis.[150] It showed that somatic movements monitored overnight by a video recorder were not significantly different, but the quality of sleep was improved with the nonsteroidal anti-inflammatory drug.

RANGE OF JOINT AND SPINAL MOVEMENT

The range of motion of peripheral joints in normal subjects has been determined by the American Academy of Orthopaedic Surgeons[2] and the subject reviewed in detail by Wright.[285] Range of movement of the knee by a goniometer is highly reproducible,[141,210] but is of limited value in assessing antirheumatic drug therapy.

Much effort has been put into defining spinal movement and chest expansion in assessing progress in ankylosing spondylitis. Normal range of spinal movement for different ages in the two sexes has been established.[211] Spinal movement has been measured by several methods, including the Dunham spondylometer,[72,94,108,109,235,260] skin distraction,[187,211–213,248] an inclinometer,[180] and now abandoned radiologic procedures.[4,142,271,282] Reynolds has compared the three clinical techniques for measuring spinal mobility.[235] The spondylometer was found to be the quickest method, but applicable to certain movements only, the goniometer the most versatile and of accepted accuracy, and the skin distraction method inaccurate and complicated.

How does measurement of fingertip to floor, occiput to wall, range of spinal movement, and chest expansion perform in clinical trials? In a review of 22 reports in the literature, we found that only 8 showed differences (and these were extremely small) in spinal movement and only 6 in chest expansion as a result of nonsteroidal anti-inflammatory analgesic therapy, although other parameters suggested that the drugs were efficacious. At present we doubt the value of these time-consuming measurements in clinical therapeutic trials in ankylosing spondylitis.

FUNCTIONAL INDICES

Disability is a major feature of rheumatic disease, but its measurement has proved difficult. Nevertheless, as previously mentioned, improvement in function was the principal measurement in the first controlled clinical therapeutic trial in rheumatic diseases.[85] Early descriptive methods based on four- or five-point scales can only detect major changes in functional ability and are too insensitive to detect differences with antirheumatic drug medication.[170,262] More elaborate scoring systems in common use in rehabilitation centers employing as many as 100 or more separate "activities of daily living" have either proved too complex and time-consuming or not sufficiently sensitive to detect change with antirheumatic drug therapy.[42,115,140,166,176,177,184,188,191,199]

Timing of certain movements or set maneuvers related to "activities of daily living," such as tying knots, picking up pins, hopping on one foot, standing on toes, flailing arms, walking a certain distance, and climbing and descending stairs, are now seldom used, with the exception of "the time to walk 50 feet."[8,48,168,190,231,246,273] An unresolved problem with functional assessments, whether global or limited to a particular movement, is that they do not differentiate reversible disability due to joint inflammation from the irreversible form that is associated with joint destruction and ligamentous laxity. More elaborate questionnaires have been designed to test the quality of life as well as functional impairment in patients with rheumatoid arthritis,[11,31,87,115,147,168,175,204] but their value in short- and long-term trials still must be determined. A "signal function" approach analogous to the "signal" joint approach of Ward[277] (discussed previously in the section on joint counts), which involves the identification of "specific responsive functional disabilities" important to the patient, has the potential to detect clinically significant changes in function.[274]

THERMOGRAPHY

Increase in heat is a cardinal feature of inflammation and, in joint disease, can be measured in various ways.[9] Skin temperature, as determined by thermography, correlates with the intra-articular temperature, albeit some 4 to 5°C higher, and with synovial perfusion as determined by xenon joint clearance,[133] plethysmography, and synovial fluid cell count, protein concentration, and volume.[9] The thermographic pattern also correlates with the anatomic site of synovial hyperemia,[51] and release of cathepsin D.[229]

Most thermographic equipment is designed around an indium antimonide detector that is sensitive to infrared energy in the wavelengths of 2μ

to 5μ. Infrared quantitative thermography, when carefully conducted with attention to methodologic requirements, especially control of ambient temperature, is capable of demonstrating reproducible changes in disease activity, and shows significant changes following treatment with nonsteroidal anti-inflammatory analgesics,[8,103,132,237] intra-articular corticosteroids,[9,15,16] D-penicillamine,[25] and cyclophosphamide.[104] A thermographic index has been described and validated.[137]

Thermography provides a noninvasive and reproducible method of assessing improvement in joint inflammation. The initial cost of equipment is high, and the procedure must be carried out with strict attention to ambient temperature. As a result, thermography has not been widely used in clinical therapeutic trials of antirheumatic drugs. A study by Paterson et al. comparing clinical indices, radioisotope uptake, and thermography in assessing knee joint inflammation revealed differences in the time course of the rate of change of the various methods, emphasizing the need to interpret the results of each separately.[227] A differential thermometer may provide an alternative to thermography, but more work is needed to evaluate its usefulness.[272] Clinical evaluation of temperature changes over joints has rarely been used in clinical trials of antirheumatic drugs,[172] and changes in color have never been used, since generally only septic or acute gouty joints become red.

ROUTINE LABORATORY TESTS

Several laboratory tests reflect to some extent the severity of joint inflammation. The most frequently employed test is the erythrocyte sedimentation rate (ESR). Nonsteroidal anti-inflammatory analgesics do not reduce the ESR[45,215,287] although, peculiarly, fenclofenac does,[12] and oral corticosteroids cause only a temporary reduction lasting approximately one week. The value in determining the ESR and other acute-phase reactants, such as C-reactive protein, haptoglobin, fibrinogen, and alpha-2 macroglobulin, would appear to be in trials of slow-acting drugs such as gold, chloroquine, and D-penicillamine.[6,196–198,236,242,276] Improvement in the albumin-to-globulin ratio and level of gammaglobulin also may be used to monitor slow-acting drugs, such as oral gold.[34] Immunoglobulin concentrations fall with gold,[289] D-penicillamine,[18] cyclophosphamide,[44] and levamisole treatment.[270] Nonsteroidal anti-inflammatory drugs have no effect on the titer of IgM rheumatoid factor, which has been variously noted to fall with gold, chloroquine, D-penicillamine, and cytotoxic agents,[3,14,44,52,55,151,181,200,214,218,230] but not with low-dose oral corticosteroids. No correlation has been found between immunologic parameters and clinical effects in patients treated with azathioprine or cyclophosphamide.[1,269] Laurent and Panayi concluded that on present evidence rheumatoid factor titers are not a reliable measure of patient response to antirheumatic drug treatment.[162] Tests of lymphocyte function are relevant only to drugs that might exert their action by this means (e.g., levamisole).[207,217]

A normocytic normochromic anemia is common in rheumatoid arthritis[110,216] and responds to drugs such as gold, D-penicillamine, and orgotein,[110,205,216,218] although it correlates poorly with disease activity.[48] A low serum iron concentration,[36] eosinophilia,[284] and thrombocytosis[118,135] are found in active disease, but have not as yet been used as outcome measures.

The essential amino acid L-tryptophan is displaced from serum albumin by nonsteroidal anti-inflammatory analgesics and other drugs such as gold, D-penicillamine, and chloroquine.[5] Rheumatoid arthritis has an increase in the protein-bound fraction and a corresponding fall in free plasma tryptophan correlating with disease activity.[5,6,192] The significance, however, of these changes in tryptophan to clinical therapeutic trials remains to be determined.

Serum concentrations of sulfhydryl groups are reduced in rheumatoid arthritis[182] paralleling disease activity.[102,183] There is evidence that both nonsteroidal anti-inflammatory analgesics and drugs such as gold, D-penicillamine, and levamisole may increase sulfhydryl group reactivity,[41,68,80,90,102] but the value of this laboratory parameter in clinical therapeutic trials remains to be proved.

Serum copper concentrations are elevated in rheumatoid arthritis, and correlate with ceruloplasmin levels and disease activity.[4,280] Whether serum copper estimations would be of use in clinical trials remains to be determined.

Synovial fluid analysis is relevant only in clinical trials of intra-articular drugs,[105] and synovial biopsies are worthless because of the marked differences in synovial lesions in the same joint.[50]

RADIOLOGY

Claims for reduction in the number of fresh erosions and healing of erosions with corticosteroids,[78,79] chrysotherapy,[43,77,178,185,186,254] D-penicillamine,[91] and cyclophosphamide[44] have led to renewed interest in radiologic assessment in patients with rheumatoid arthritis.[95] Gofton[95] has pointed out that in only three long-term clinical therapeutic trials in rheumatoid arthritis did the radiologic improvement reach statistical significance.[44,202,254] Hernandez et al. have reported healing of rheumatoid juxta-articular erosions with first-line drugs.[117] Various methods have been used to score changes in radiographs of the hands and wrists.[43,96,159,206] There appears to be no advantage of the Brewerton[22] or Nørgaard[222,223] views compared to the conventional posterioanterior views in detection of erosions at the metacarpophalangeal joints.[206] Some of the radiologic methods of interpreting change in rheumatoid arthritis suffer from a lack of observer error studies.[252] With the exception of Larsen et al.,[158] all workers have found a disquieting degree of observer disagreement.[17,96,206] This is hardly surprising since observer agreement in most human endeavors has been found to be low.[88] Mewa et al.[206] concluded that an erosion index cannot reliably be used in therapeutic trials as an outcome measure unless steps are taken to overcome observer disagreement, a view also shared by Gofton.[95]

RADIONUCLIDES

Various radionuclides have been used to quantify joint inflammation.[57,66,275] These may be administered intra-articularly and the rate of clearance from the joint determined or, alternatively, they may be administered intravenously and the rate of accumulation over a joint (or joints) measured. The clearance of radioactive xenon (^{133}Xe) after intra-articular injection provides an indirect measurement of synovial blood flow[93,99] and has been used to investigate physiologic and pharmacologic control of the synovial microcirculation.[58,60,99,100,265] The ^{133}Xe clearance method correlates with clinical assessment of joint inflammation[59,61,63] but has shown poor discrimination between antirheumatic drug medication and placebo compared to standard methods in clinical therapeutic trials.[61,64]

The accumulation of radionuclide in joints after intravenous injection can be measured as a quantitative determination of peak count rate or monitored by a display scintiscan.[13,20,59,63,134,167,193,195] None of the various methods for quantifying synovitis using radionuclides has proved entirely satisfactory,[275] but measurement of the absolute uptake per unit joint area seems to give the best separation between normal joints and joints affected with rheumatoid arthritis.[240] The optimum time to scan after intravenous injection of the isotope remains undecided. Some workers find 15 minutes adequate, whereas others argue for a longer time.[20,54,112,193,195] Pertechnetate (^{99m}TcO$_4$) has been found superior to radioiodinated (I^{125}) human fibrinogen.[167] The newer technetium pyrophosphate or diphosphonate compounds absorb to juxta-articular bone and are consequently less useful than ^{99m}TcO$_4$ itself.[123,164] It should be noted that increased uptake of the former also occurs in bone in rheumatoid arthritis.[241]

Notwithstanding these problems, isotope joint uptakes have an acceptable reproducibility and correlate reasonably well with clinical assessments of joint inflammation and the rate of clearance of intra-articularly injected radioactive xenon.[59,63,101,193,195] Polyarticular isotope indices have been described.[134,167,225,232] Radionuclide joint uptakes in both large and small joints are reduced with nonsteroidal anti-inflammatory analgesics, and therapy with corticosteroids, gold, and D-penicillamine[38,54,65,232,267] and synovectomy.[62]

At a conference on outcome measures in rheumatologic clinical trials in inflammatory peripheral joint disease, a pessimistic view was expressed regarding the use of radionuclide joint scans,[164] the limiting factors being the initial capital cost of equipment, the lack of portability, and the time required for each individual measurement. Nevertheless, there is still a role for radionuclide measurements in clinical therapeutic trials of antirheumatic drugs, provided due attention is directed to methodology and interpretation, and especially since these techniques provide an objective measurement of articular inflammation.

In ankylosing spondylitis, the sacroiliac joint/sacral ratio of radionuclide uptake shows considerable overlap between patients and control, thus reducing its diagnostic value.[32,256] However, significant reduction in sacroiliac joint/sacral ratios has been reported with as little as 3 weeks of treatment with nonsteroidal anti-inflammatory drugs.[122,220,243] Further study is required to evaluate this method in clinical therapeutic trials in ankylosing spondylitis.

CONCLUSIONS

No single measure adequately reflects change in articular inflammation produced by a nonsteroidal anti-inflammatory analgesic, slow-acting drug, or any other therapeutic modality. As discussed previously, there is a reasonable correlation between subjective clinical measures and objective tests, such as radionuclide joint scanning or thermography. It is important, however, to appreciate that there are differences in the rate of change among the different outcome measurements, whether subjective or objective.[227] It is unwise to rely on a single outcome measure. The ranking of 20 measures of disease activity by experienced rheumatologists indicated preference for a "joint count," patient-rated measure of pain relief, global assessment of change in disease activity, and patient-rated measure of pain.[101] The clinical investigator, however, would be wise to choose those tests with which he is most familiar and those whose reproducibility he has documented thoroughly. A judicious combination of subjective and objective measurements is recommended. If composite indices are used, these should be first subjected to the rigor of reproducibility and sensitivity to change. The outcome methods that should be used in short- and long-term rheumatologic therapeutic trials are summarized in Table 7–3. A joint count, a measure of pain relief, and a global assessment of progress by both patient and physician should be used in short- and long-term trials. In addition to those major outcome measures, we consider it wise to employ at least four of the minor procedures. Measurement of function, other than time to walk 50 feet, and rheumatoid factor titers are probably inappropriate for short-term trials, but are desirable for long-term trials.

Finally, it is important for the clinical investigator to attempt to answer only one question at a time. If his intent is to determine whether a nonsteroidal analgesic has anti-inflammatory effect, then patients must be chosen who are capable of demonstrating such an effect, and the appropriate outcome measures must be used. Often clinical therapeutic trials fail because too many questions are asked and because too many details are required for the clinician to record at each visit. It is necessary to "prune" many of the work sheets now being produced of much unnecessary data. For instance, it is not important to record the height at each visit in a short-term trial of a nonsteroidal anti-inflammatory analgesic! The less the clinician has to record, the more reliable will be his data.

All this is common sense, but as Voltaire in his *Dictionnaire Philosophique* remarked, common sense is not common.

REFERENCES

1. Alepa, F.P., Zvaifler, N.J., and Sliwinski, A.J.: Immunologic effects of cyclophosphamide treatment in rheumatoid arthritis. Arthritis Rheum., *13*:754–760, 1970.
2. American Academy of Orthopaedic Surgeons: Joint Motion: Method of Measuring and Recording. Edinburgh, Churchill Livingstone, 1966.
3. Amor, B., and Mery, C.: Chlorambucil in rheumatoid arthritis. Clin. Rheum. Dis., *6*:567–584, 1980.
4. Anderson, J.A.D.: The thoraco-lumbar spine. In Measurement of Joint Movement. Edited by V. Wright. Clin. Rheum. Dis., *8*:631–653, 1982.
5. Aylward, M., and Maddock, J.: Total and free tryptophan concentrations in rheumatic disease. J. Pharm. Pharmacol., *25*:570–572, 1973.
6. Aylward, M., et al.: A study of the influence of various anti-rheumatic drug regimens on serum acute phase proteins, plasma tryptophan and erythrocyte sedimentation rate in rheumatoid arthritis. Rheumatol. Rehabil., *14*:101–114, 1975.
7. Backlund, L., and Tiselius, P.: Objective measurements of joint stiffness in rheumatoid arthritis. Acta Rheumatol. Scand., *13*:175–288, 1967.
8. Bacon, P.A., Collins, A.J., and Cosh, J.A.: Thermographic assessment of the anti-inflammatory effect of flurbiprofen in rheumatoid arthritis. Scand. J. Rheumatol., *4* (Suppl. 8):11–17, 1975.
9. Bacon, P.A., et al.: Thermography in the assessment of inflammatory arthritis. Clin. Rheum. Dis., *2*:51–65, 1976.
10. Beecher, H.K.: *Measurement of Subjective Responses.* Oxford, Oxford University Press, 1959.
11. Bergner, M., et al.: The sickness impact profile: Validation of a health status measure. Med. Care, *14*:57–67, 1976.
12. Berry, H., et al.: Antirheumatic activity of fenclofenac. Ann. Rheum. Dis., *39*:473–475, 1980.
13. Berry, H., et al.: Radioisotope scanning using a gamma camera. Ann. Rheum. Dis., *37*:76–77, 1978.
14. Berry, H., et al.: Azathioprine and penicillamine in treatment of rheumatoid arthritis: A controlled trial. Br. Med. J., *1*:1052–1054, 1976.
15. Bird, H.A., et al.: Comparison of intra-articular methotrexate with intra-articular triamcinolone hexacetonide by thermography. Curr. Med. Res. Opin., *5*:141–146, 1977.
16. Bird, H.A., Ring, E.F.J., and Bacon, P.A.: A thermographic and clinical comparison of the intra-articular steroid preparations in rheumatoid arthritis. Ann. Rheum. Dis., *38*:36–39, 1979.
17. Bland, J.H., et al.: A study of inter- and intra-observer error in reading plain roentgenograms of the hands. Am. J. Roentgenol., *105*:853, 1969.
18. Bluestone, R., and Goldberg, L.S.: Effects of D-penicillamine on serum immunoglobulins and rheumatoid factor. Ann. Rheum. Dis., *32*:50–52, 1973.
19. Boardman, P.L., and Hart, F.D.: Clinical measurement of the anti-inflammatory effects of salicylates in rheumatoid arthritis. Br. Med. J., *4*:264–268, 1967.
20. Boerbooms, A.M., and Buys, W.C.: Rapid assessment of ^{99m}Tc pertechnetate uptake in the knee joint as a parameter of inflammatory activity. Arthritis Rheum., *21*:348–352, 1978.
21. Bombardier, C., Tugwell, P., and Sinclair, A.: Preference for endpoint measures in clinical trials: Results of structured workshops. J. Rheumatol., *9*:797–800, 1982.
22. Brewerton, D.A.: Instrumental and technical roles. A tangential radiographic projection for demonstrating involvement of the metacarpal heads in R.A. Br. J. Radiol., *40*:233–234, 1967.
23. Bridgman, J.F., et al.: Irradiation of the synovium in the treatment of rheumatoid arthritis. Q. J. Med. New Series, *42*:357–367, 1973.
24. Brown, D.H., et al.: Serum copper and its relationship to clinical symptoms in rheumatoid arthritis. Ann. Rheum. Dis., *3*:174–176, 1979.
25. Bucknall, R.C., et al.: A thermographic assessment of the anti-inflammatory effect of D-penicillamine in rheumatoid arthritis. Scand. J. Rheum., *4*(Suppl. 8):21–29, 1975.
26. Burkhardt, R., and Kienle, G.: Controlled clinical trials and medical ethics. Lancet, *2*:1356–1359, 1978.
27. Byar, D.P., et al.: Randomized clinical trials—perspectives on some recent ideas. N. Engl. J. Med., *295*:74–80, 1976.
28. Bywaters, E.G.L., Dixon, A., St. J., and Wild, J.B.: Deoxycortone and ascorbic acid in the treatment of rheumatoid arthritis. Lancet, *1*:951–953, 1950.
29. Camp, A.V.: An articular index for the assessment of rheumatoid arthritis. Orthopedics, *4*:39–45, 1971.
30. Carbone, P.P.: The case for clinical trials. CA, *30*:53–54, 1980.
31. Chambers, L.W., et al.: The McMaster Health Index Questionnaire as a measure of quality of life for patients with rheumatoid disease. J. Rheumatol., *9*:780–784, 1982.
32. Chalmers, I.M., et al.: Sacroiliitis detected by bone scintiscanning: a clinical, radiological and scintigraphic follow-up study. Ann. Rheum. Dis., *38*:112, 1979.
33. Chalmers, T.C., Block, J.B., and Lee, S.: Controlled studies in clinical cancer research. N. Engl. J. Med., *287*:75–78, 1972.
34. Chaput de Saintonge, D.M., and Charman, V.L.: Bizepam or nitrazepam? A question of cost. Br. J. Clin. Pharmacol., *4*:422–444, 1977.
35. Cicchetti, D.V., and Fleiss, J.L.: Comparison of the null distributions of weighted kappa and the coordinal statistic. Appl. Psych. Meas., *1*:195–201, 1977.
36. Cockel, R., et al.: Serum biochemical values in rheumatoid disease. Ann. Rheum. Dis., *30*:166–170, 1971.

37. Collins, A.J., et al.: Quantitation of thermography in arthritis using multi-isothermal analysis I. Thermographic index. Ann. Rheum. Dis., 33:113–115, 1974.
38. Collins, K.E., et al.: Radioisotope study of small joint inflammation in rheumatoid arthritis. Ann. Rheum. Dis., 30:401–405, 1971.
39. Collins, K.E., et al.: Radioisotope study of small joint inflammation in rheumatoid arthritis. Radioactive technetium (^{99m}Tc) uptake in the proximal interphalangeal joints and the effects of oral corticosteroids. Ann. Rheum. Dis., 30:401–405, 1971.
40. Combined Rheumatic Fever Study Group: A comparison of prednisone and acetylsalicylic acid on the incidence of residual rheumatic heart disease. N. Engl. J. Med., 262:895–902, 1960.
41. Conference Proceedings: Do drugs alter the course of rheumatoid arthritis? Ann. Rheum. Dis., 41:549–550, 1982.
42. Convery, F.R., et al.: Polyarticular disability: A functional assessment. Arch. Phys. Med. Rehabil., 58:494–499, 1977.
43. Cooperating Clinics Committee of the American Rheumatism Association: A controlled trial of gold salt therapy in rheumatoid arthritis. Arthritis Rheum., 16:353–358, 1973.
44. Cooperating Clinics Committee of the American Rheumatism Association: Controlled trial of cyclophosphamide in rheumatoid arthritis. N. Engl. J. Med., 283:883–889, 1970.
45. Cooperating Clinics Committee of the American Rheumatism Association: A three-month trial of indomethacin in rheumatoid arthritis with special reference to analysis and inference. Clin. Pharmacol. Ther., 8:11–38, 1967.
46. Cooperating Clinics Committee of the American Rheumatism Association: A seven-day variability study of 499 patients with peripheral rheumatoid arthritis. Arthritis Rheum., 8:302–334, 1965.
47. Copeman, W.S.C., et al.: A study of cortisone and other steroids in rheumatoid arthritis. Br. Med. J., 2:849–855, 1950.
48. Reference deleted.
49. Cousins, G.R.: Effect of trained and untrained testers upon the administration of grip strength tests. Res. Q., 26:273–276, 1955.
50. Cruickshank, B.: Interpretation of multiple biopsies of synovial tissue in rheumatic diseases. Ann. Rheum. Dis., 11:137–143, 1952.
51. Davidson, J.W., and Thomson, J.G.: Thermographic survey in chronic rheumatic diseases. Medical Thermography, 1978, pp. 267–271.
52. Day, A.T.: Penicillamine in rheumatoid disease: A long term study. Br. Med. J., 1:180–183, 1974.
53. De Choisy, J.: A new method of assessing grip strength and wrist and arm movement in the arthritic patients. Rheumatol. Rehabil. (Suppl.), 12:81–84, 1973.
54. Deodhar, S.D., et al.: Measurement of clinical response to anti-inflammatory drug therapy in rheumatoid arthritis. Q. J. Med. New Series, 42:387–401, 1973.
55. De Seze, S., and Kahn, M.F.: Immunosuppressive drugs in rheumatoid arthritis: Clinical results. Adv. Clin. Pharmacol., 6:89, 1974.
56. Desmaris, M.H.L.: Radiotherapy in arthritis. Ann. Rheum. Dis., 12:25–28, 1953.
57. Dick, W.C.: The use of radioisotopes in normal and diseased joints. Semin. Arthritis Rheum., 1:301–325, 1972.
58. Dick, W.C., et al.: The effect of thymoxamine on peripheral blood vessels as monitored by the ^{133}Xe clearance technique. J. Pharm. Pharmacol., 23:204–208, 1971.
59. Dick, W.C., et al.: Isotope studies in normal and diseased knee joints: ^{99m}Tc uptake related to clinical assessment and to synovial perfusion measured by the ^{133}Xe clearance technique. Clin. Sci., 40:327–336, 1971.
60. Dick, W.C., et al.: Studies on the sympathetic control of normal and diseased synovial blood vessels: The effect of α and β receptor stimulation and inhibition, monitored by the ^{133}xenon clearance technique. Clin. Sci., 40:197–209, 1971.
61. Dick, W.C., et al.: Clinical studies on inflammation in human knee joints: Xenon (^{133}Xe) clearances correlated with clinical assessment in various arthritides and studies on the effect of intra-articularly administered hydrocortisone in rheumatoid arthritis. Clin. Sci., 38:123–133, 1970.
62. Dick, W.C., et al.: Effect of synovectomy on the clearance of radioactive xenon (^{133}Xe) from the knee joint of patients with rheumatoid arthritis. J. Bone Joint Surg., 5213:70–76, 1970.
63. Dick, W.C., et al.: Indices of inflammatory activity. Relationship between isotope studies and clinical methods. Ann. Rheum. Dis., 29:643–648, 1970.
64. Dick, W.C., et al.: Effects of anti-inflammatory drug therapy on clearance of ^{133}Xe from knee joints of patients with rheumatoid arthritis. Br. Med. J., 3:278–280, 1969.
65. Dick, W.C., Collins, K.E., and Buchanan, W.W.: Clinical studies on inflammation in small diarthroidial joints. Technetium (^{99m}Tc) percentage uptakes in various arthritides and studies on the effect of aspirin in rheumatoid arthritis. Clin. Sci., 42:383–393, 1972.
66. Dick, W.C., and Grennan, D.M.: Radioisotopes in the study of normal and inflamed joints. Clin. Rheum. Dis., 2:67–76, 1976.
67. Dickson, J.S., and Bird, H.A.: Reproducibility along a 10 cm vertical visual analogue scale. Ann. Rheum. Dis., 40:87–89, 1981.
68. Dixon, J.S., et al.: Discriminatory indices of response of patients with rheumatoid arthritis treated with D-penicillamine. Ann. Rheum. Dis., 39:301–311, 1980.
69. Downie, W.W., et al.: Studies with pain rating scales. Ann. Rheum. Dis., 37:378–381, 1978.
70. Downie, W.W., Leatham, P.A., and Rind, V.M.: The visual analogue scale in the assessment of grip strength. Ann. Rheum. Dis., 37:382–384, 1978.
71. Dresner, E., Pugh, L.G.C., and Wild, J.B.: ACTH in rheumatoid arthritis compared with intramuscular adrenaline and with deoxycortone and ascorbic acid. Lancet, 1:1149–1153, 1950.
72. Dunham, W.F.: Ankylosing spondylitis—measurement of hip and spine movement. Br. J. Phys. Med., 12:126–129, 1949.
73. Duthie, J.J.R.: Clinical trials of ACTH: Preliminary report. Edinburgh Med. J., 57:341–364, 1950.
74. Eberl, R.: Are morning stiffness and time to onset of fatigue really measurable? Is measurement of ranges of motion useful? How much change is clinically significant? In Controversies in the Clinical Evaluation of Analgesic-Anti-Inflammatory–Antirheumatic Drugs. Edited by H.E. Paulus, G.E. Ehrlich, and E. Lindenlaub. Stuttgart, Schattauer Verlag, 1981, pp. 113–117.
75. Eberl, D.R., et al.: Repeatability and objectivity of various measurements in rheumatoid arthritis. A comparative study. Arthritis Rheum., 19:1278–1286, 1976.
76. Empire Rheumatism Council: Gold therapy in rheumatoid arthritis: Final report of a multicentre controlled trial. Ann. Rheum. Dis., 20:315–334, 1961.
77. Empire Rheumatism Council: Gold therapy in rheumatoid arthritis: Report of a multicentre controlled trial. Ann. Rheum. Dis., 19:95–119, 1960.
78. Empire Rheumatism Council: Multicentre controlled trial comparing cortisone acetate and acetylsalicylic acid in the long-term treatment of rheumatoid arthritis. Ann. Rheum. Dis., 16:277–289, 1957.
79. Empire Rheumatism Council: Multicentre controlled trial comparing cortisone acetate and acetylsalicylic acid in the long-term treatment of rheumatoid arthritis. Ann. Rheum. Dis., 14:353–370, 1955.
80. Evans, P.H.: Serum sulphydryl changes in rheumatoid coal workers pneumoconiosis patients treated with D-penicillamine. Proc. R. Soc. Med., 70 (Suppl. 3):95–97, 1977.
81. Feinstein, A.R.: On steroids for publication of therapeutic research. J. Chronic Dis., 33:65–66, 1980.
82. Feinstein, A.R.: Should placebo-controlled trials be abolished? Eur. J. Clin. Pharmacol., 17:1–4, 1980.
83. Fellinger, K., et al.: Computer Dokumentation einer Rheumastation. Z. Rheumatol., 32:257–271, 1973.
84. Finkelstein, A.E., et al.: New oral gold compound for

treatment of rheumatoid arthritis. Ann. Rheum. Dis., 35:251–257, 1976.

85. Fraser, T.N.: Gold therapy in rheumatoid arthritis. Ann. Rheum. Dis., 4:71–75, 1945.

86. Fremont-Smith, F., Harter, J.G., and Halberg, F.: Circadian rhythmicity of proximal interphalangeal (PIP) joint circumference in patients with rheumatoid arthritis. Arthritis Rheum., 12:294, 1969.

87. Fries, J.F., et al.: Measurement of patient outcome in arthritis. Arthritis Rheum., 23:137–145, 1980.

88. Garland, L.H.: On the scientific evaluation of diagnostic procedures. Radiology, 3:309–327, 1949.

89. Gehan, E.A., and Freireich, E.J.: Non-randomized controls in cancer clinical trials. N. Engl. J. Med., 290:198–203, 1974.

90. Gerber, P.A., Cohen, N., and Giustra, R.: The ability of nonsteroidal anti-inflammatory compounds to accelerate a disulphide interchange reaction of serum sulphydryl groups and 5.5′-dithiobis (2-Nitrobenzoid acid). Biochem. Pharmacol., 16:115–123, 1967.

91. Gibson, T., et al.: Evidence that D-penicillamine alters the course of rheumatoid arthritis. Rheumatol. Rehabil., 15:211–215, 1976.

92. Gilbert, J.P.: Randomization of human subjects. N. Engl. J. Med., 291:1303–1306, 1974.

93. Goetzl, E.J., et al.: A physical approach to the assessment of disease activity in rheumatoid arthritis. J. Clin. Invest., 50:1167–1180, 1971.

94. Goff, B., and Rose, G.K.: The use of a modified spondylometer in the treatment of ankylosing spondylitis. Rheumatism, 20:63–66, 1964.

95. Gofton, J.P.: Problems associated with the measurement of radiological progression of disease in rheumatoid arthritis. J. Rheumatol., 10:177–179, 1983.

96. Gofton, J.P., and O'Brien, W.M.: Effects of auranofin on the radiological progression of joint erosion in rheumatoid arthritis. J. Rheumatol., 9 (Suppl. 8):169–172, 1982.

97. Greenberg, B.G.: Conduct of cooperative field and clinical trials. Am. Stat., 13:13–28, 1959.

98. Grennan, D.M., et al.: Relationship between hemoglobin and other clinical and laboratory parameters in rheumatoid arthritis. Curr. Med. Res. Opin., 3:104–108, 1975.

99. Grennan, D.M., et al.: Histamine receptors in the synovial microcirculation. Eur. J. Clin. Invest., 5:75–82, 1975

100. Grennan, D.M., Zeitlin, I.J., and Dick, W.C.: Effects of inflammatory mediators on synovial blood flow. Prostaglandins, 9:799–816, 1975.

101. Haataja, M.: Evaluation of the activity of rheumatoid arthritis. Scand. J. Rheumatol., 4 (Suppl. 7):1–54, 1975.

102. Haataja, M., Nissila, M., and Ruutsalo, H.K.: Serum sulphydryl levels in rheumatoid patients treated with gold thiomalate and penicillamine. Scand. J. Rheumatol., 7:212–214, 1978.

103. Haberman, J.A., et al.: Thermography in arthritis. Arthritis Rheum., 14:387, 1971.

104. Hall, N.D., et al.: A combined clinical and immunological assessment of four cyclophosphamide regimes in rheumatoid arthritis. Agents Actions, 9:97–102, 1979.

105. Hall, S.H., et al.: Intra-articular methotrexate clinical and laboratory study in rheumatoid and psoriatic arthritis. Ann. Rheum. Dis., 37:351–356, 1978.

106. Harkness, J.A.L., et al.: Circadian variation in disease activity in rheumatoid arthritis. Br. Med. J., 284:551–554, 1982.

107. Hart, F.D., and Huskisson, E.C.: Measurement in rheumatoid arthritis. Lancet, 1:28–30, 1972.

108. Hart, F.D., and MacLagan, N.F.: Anklylosing spondylitis: A review of 184 cases. Ann. Rheum. Dis., 14:77–89, 1955.

109. Hart, F.D., Strickland, D., and Cliffe, P.: Measurement of spinal mobility. Ann. Rheum. Dis., 33:136–139, 1974.

110. Harvey, A.R., et al.: Anemia associated with rheumatoid disease. Arthritis Rheum., 26:28–34, 1983.

111. Haynes, B., Taylor, W., and Sackett, D.L. (Eds.): Compliance in Health Care. Baltimore, Johns Hopkins University Press, 1979.

112. Hays, M.T., and Green, F.A.: The pertechnetate joint scan. Ann. Rheum. Dis., 31:272–277, 1972.

113. Hill, A.B.: The clinical trial. Br. Med. Bull., 7:278–282, 1951.

114. Health Services Research Group: Development of the index of medical underservice. University of Wisconsin. Health Serv. Res., 10:168–180, 1975.

115. Helewa, A., Goldsmith, C.H., and Smythe, H.A.: Independent measurement of functional capacity in rheumatoid arthritis. J. Rheumatol., 9:793–796, 1982.

116. Hench, P.S., et al.: Effects of cortisone acetate and pituitary ACTH on rheumatoid arthritis, rheumatic fever and certain other conditions: Study in clinical physiology. Arch. Intern. Med., 85:545–666, 1950.

117. Hernandez, L.A., et al.: Rheumatoid juxta-articular erosions: Healing with first line drugs. Rheumatology, 7:41–45, 1978.

118. Hernandez, L.A., et al.: Thrombocytosis in rheumatoid arthritis: A clinical study of 200 patients. Rhumatologie, 5:635–640, 1975.

119. Hill, A.B.: The clinical trial. Br. Med. Bull., 1:278–282, 1951.

120. Hill, A.B.: The clinical trial. N. Engl. J. Med., 247:113–119, 1952.

121. Hill, A.B.: Statistical Methods of Clinical and Preventive Medicine. New York, Oxford University Press, 1962.

122. Ho, G., Jr., et al.: Quantitative sacroiliac scintigraphy. A critical assessment. Arthritis Rheum., 22:837–844, 1979.

123. Hoffer, P.B., and Genant, H.K.: Radionuclide joint imaging. Semin. Nucl. Med., 6:168–184, 1976.

124. Hollander, J.L., and Young, D.C.: The palpameter, an instrument of quantification of joint tenderness. Arthritis Rheum., 6:277, 1963.

125. Horwitz, R.I., and Feinstein, A.R.: The application of therapeutic-trial principles to improve the design of epidemiologic research: A case-control study suggesting that anticoagulants reduce mortality in patients with myocardial infarction. J. Chronic Dis., 34:575–583, 1981.

126. Horwitz, R.I., and Feinstein, A.R.: Improved observational method for studying therapeutic efficacy. Suggestive evidence that lidocaine prophylaxis prevents death in acute myocardial infarction. J.A.M.A., 246:2455–2459, 1981.

127. Hunsicker, P.A., and Donnelly, R.V.: Instruments to measure strength. Res. Q., 26:408–419, 1955.

128. Huskisson, E.C.: Measurement of pain. J. Rheumatol., 9:768–769, 1982.

129. Huskisson, E.C.: Assessment in clinical trials. Clin. Rheum. Dis., 2:37–49, 1976.

130. Huskisson, E.C.: Catecholamine excretion and pain. Br. J. Clin. Pharmacol., 1:80–82, 1974.

131. Huskisson, E.C.: Measurement of pain. Lancet, 2:1127–1131, 1974.

132. Huskisson, E.C., et al.: Measurement of inflammation. Comparison of technetium clearance and standard thermography with standard methods in a clinical trial. Ann. Rheum. Dis., 3:99–102, 1973.

133. Huskisson, E.C., and Scott, P.J.: Flectafenine: A new analgesic for use in rheumatic diseases. Rheumatol. Rehabil., 16:54–57, 1977.

134. Huskisson, E.C., Scott, J., and Balme, H.W.: Objective measurement of R.A. using technetium index. Ann. Rheum. Dis., 35:81–82, 1976.

135. Hutchinson, R.M., Davis, P., and Jayson, M.I.V.: Thrombocytosis in rheumatoid arthritis. Ann. Rheum. Dis., 35:138–142, 1976.

136. Ingelfinger, F.J.: The randomized clinical trial. N. Engl. J. Med., 287:100–101, 1972.

137. Ingpen, M.L.: The quantitative measurement of joint changes in rheumatoid arthritis. Ann. Phys. Med., 9:322–327, 1968.

138. Jacobsen, M.: The use of rating scales in clinical research. Br. J. Psychiatry, 111:545–546, 1965.

139. Jenner, E.: An Enquiry into the Causes and Effects of The Variolae Vaccinae (1798). Denver, The Range Press, 1949.

140. Jette, A.M.: Functional capacity evaluation: An empirical approach. Arch. Phys. Med. Rehabil., 61:85–89, 1980.

141. Johnson, F.: The knee. Clin. Rheum. Dis., 8:677–702, 1982.
142. Jonck, L.M., and van Niekerk, J.M.: A roentgenological study of the motion of the lumbar spine in the Bantu. S. Afr. J. Lab. Clin. Med., 7:67–71, 1961.
143. Jonus, O.: Objective assessment in rheumatoid arthritis. Br. Med. J., 2:1244–1249, 1950.
144. Joyce, C.R.B.: Patient cooperation and the sensitivity of drug trials. J. Chronic Dis., 15:1025–1036, 1962.
145. Joyce, C.R.B., et al.: Comparison of fixed interval and visual analogue scales for rating chronic pain. Eur. J. Clin. Pharmacol., 8:415–420, 1975.
146. Juhl, E., Christensen, E., and Tygstrup, N.: The epidemiology of the gastrointestinal randomized clinical trial. N. Engl. J. Med., 296:20–22, 1977.
147. Kaplan, R.M., Bush, J.W., and Berry, C.C.: Health status: Types of validity for an index of well-being. Health Serv., 11:478–507, 1976.
148. Keele, K.D.: Pain chart. Lancet, 255:6–8, 1948.
149. Keitel, W., et al.: Ermittlung der prozentualen. Funktionsminderung der Gelenke durch einen Bewegungsfunktionstest in der Rheumatologie. Dtsch. Gesundheitwesen, 26:1901–1903, 1971.
150. Khong, T.K., et al.: Sleep disturbance due to arthritis: The efficacy of piroxicam in rheumatoid arthritis. New York, Academic Professional Information Service, 1982, pp. 55–57.
151. Klinefelter, H.F., and Achurra, A.: Effect of gold salts and antimalarials on the rheumatoid factor titre in rheumatoid arthritis. Scand. J. Rheumatol., 2:177–182, 1973.
152. Kotzin, B.L., et al.: Treatment of intractable rheumatoid arthritis with total lymphoid irradiation. N. Engl. J. Med., 305:969–976, 1981.
153. Lacher, M.J.: Physicians and patients as obstacles to a randomized trial. Clin. Res., 26:375–379, 1978.
154. Lansbury, J.: Clinical appraisal of the activity index as a measure of rheumatoid activity. Arthritis Rheum., 11:599–604, 1968.
155. Lansbury, J.: Methods for evaluating rheumatoid arthritis. In Arthritis and Allied Conditions, 6th Ed. Edited by J.L. Hollander. Philadelphia, Lea & Febiger, 1960.
156. Lansbury, J.: Report of a three-year study on the systemic and articular indexes in rheumatoid arthritis. Arthritis Rheum., 1:505–522, 1958.
157. Lansbury, J., and Haut, D.D.: Quantitation of the manifestations of rheumatoid arthritis 4. Area of joint surfaces as an index of total joint inflammation and deformity. Am. J. Med. Sci., 232:15–155, 1956.
158. Larsen, A., et al.: Interobserver variation in the evaluation of radiologic changes of rheumatoid arthritis. Scand. J. Rheumatol., 8:109–112, 1979.
159. Larsen, A., Dale, K., and Eek, M.: Radiographic evaluation of rheumatoid arthritis and related conditions by standard reference films. Acta Radiol. [Diagn] (Stockh.), 18:481–491, 1977.
160. Lasagna, L.: Placebo and controlled trials under attack. Eur. J. Clin. Pharmacol., 15:373–374, 1979.
161. Lasagna, L.: In Drugs in Our Society. Edited by P. Talalay. Baltimore, Johns Hopkins Press, 1964, p. 27.
162. Laurent, M.R., and Panayi, G.S.: Biochemical parameters in the assessment of anti-inflammatory drugs. A review. Agents Actions, 7 (Suppl.):310–317, 1980.
163. Leading article: Controlled trials: Planned deceptions? Lancet, 1:534–535, 1979.
164. Lee, P.: Isotopes in the measurement of joint inflammation. J. Rheumatol., 9:767, 1982.
165. Lee, P., et al.: Evaluation of analgesic action and efficacy of antirheumatic drugs. J. Rheumatol., 3:283–294, 1976.
166. Lee, P., et al.: An assessment of grip strength measurement in rheumatoid arthritis. Scand. J. Rheumatol., 3:17–23, 1974.
167. Lee, P., et al.: The technetium radioiodinated human fibrinogen and clinical indices in the assessment of disease activity in rheumatoid arthritis. J. Rheumatol., 1:432–440, 1974.
168. Lee, P., et al.: The evaluation of a functional index in rheumatoid arthritis. Scand. J. Rheumatol., 2:71–77, 1973.
169. Lee, P., et al.: The evaluation of antirheumatic drugs. Curr. Med. Res. Opin., 1:427–443, 1973.
170. Lee, P., and Dick, W.C.: The assessment of disease activity and drug evaluation in rheumatoid arthritis. In Recent Advances in Rheumatology I. Part 2. Edited by W.W. Buchanan, and W.C. Dick. New York, Churchill Livingstone, 1976, pp. 1–32.
171. Lequesne, M.: European guidelines for clinical trials of new antirheumatic drugs. EULAR Bull (Suppl)., 9:171–175, 1980.
172. Levinson, J.E., et al.: Comparison of tolmetin sodium and aspirin in the treatment of juvenile rheumatoid arthritis. J. Pediatr., 91:799–804, 1977.
173. Lewi, P.J., and Symeons, J.: Levamisole in rheumatoid arthritis—a multivariate analysis of a multicentre study. J. Rheumatol. (Suppl. 4), 5:17–25, 1978.
174. Lewis, T.: Pain. New York, Macmillan Publishing Co., 1942.
175. Liang, M.H., Cullen, K., and Larson, M.: In search of a more perfect mousetrap (health status or quality of life instrument). J. Rheumatol., 9:775–779, 1982.
176. Liang, M.H., and Jette, A.M.: Measuring functional ability in chronic arthritis. Arthritis Rheum., 24:80–86, 1981.
177. Liang, M., Schurman, D.J., and Fries, J.: A patient administered questionnaire for arthritis assessment. Clin. Orthop., 131:123–129, 1978.
178. Lidsky, M.D., Sharp, J.T., and Billings, S.: Double-blind study of cyclophosphamide in rheumatoid arthritis. Arthritis Rheum., 16:148–153, 1973.
179. Lind, J.: A Treatise of the Scurvy. Edinburgh, A Kincaid and A Donaldson Publishers, 1753, pp. 147–148.
180. Loebl, W.Y.: Measurement of spinal posture and range of spinal movement. Ann. Phys. Med., 9:103–110, 1967.
181. Lorber, A., et al.: Chrysotherapy: Suppression of immunoglobulin synthesis. Arthritis Rheum., 21:785–791, 1978.
182. Lorber, A., et al.: Serum sulphydryl determinations and their significance in connective tissue diseases. Ann. Intern. Med., 61:423–434, 1964.
183. Lorber, A., Bovy, R.A., and Chang, C.C.: Sulphydryl deficiency in connective tissue disorders. Correlation with disease activity and protein alterations. Metabolism, 20:446–455, 1971.
184. Lowman, E.W.: Rehabilitation of the rheumatoid cripple: A five-year study. Arthritis Rheum., 1:38–43, 1958.
185. Luukkainen, R., Isomaki, H., and Kajander, A.: Effect of gold treatment on the progression of erosions in R.A. patients. Scand. J. Rheumatol., 6:123–127, 1977.
186. Luukkainen, R., Kajander, A., and Isomaki, H.: Effect of gold in progression of erosions in rheumatoid arthritis. Better results with early treatment. Scand. J. Rheumatol., 6:189–192, 1977.
187. Macrae, J.F., and Wright, V.: Measurement of back movement. Ann. Rheum. Dis., 28:584–589, 1969.
188. Mahoney, F.I., and Barthel, D.W.: Functional evaluation: The Barthel index. MD Stat. Med. J., 14:61–65, 1965.
189. Mainland, D.: The estimation of inflammatory activity in rheumatoid arthritis. Role of composite indices. Arthritis Rheum., 10:71–77, 1967.
190. Mandel, L.: Assessment of therapeutic agents in rheumatoid arthritis. Can. Med. Assoc. J., 74:515–521, 1956.
191. Mason, R.M., et al.: Assessment of drugs in outpatients with rheumatoid arthritis. Ann. Rheum. Dis., 26:373–388, 1967.
192. McArthur, J.N., Dawkins, P.D., and Smith, M.J.H.: The displacement of L-tryptophan and dipeptides from bovine albumin in vitro and from human plasma in vivo by antirheumatic drugs. J. Pharm. Pharmacol., 23:393–398, 1971.
193. McCarty, D.J., et al.: ^{99m}technetium scintiphotography in arthritis. I. Technic and interpretation. Arthritis Rheum., 13:11–21, 1970.
194. McCarty, D.J., Gatter, R.A., and Phelps, P.: A dolorimeter for quantification of articular tenderness. Arthritis Rheum., 8:551–559, 1965.
195. McCarty, D.J., Polcyn, R.E., and Collins, P.A.: ^{99m}technetium scintiphotography in arthritis. II. Its non-specificity and clinical and roentgenographic correlations

in rheumatoid arthritis. Arthritis Rheum., *13*:21–32, 1970.

196. McConkey, B., et al.: Effects of gold, dapsone and prednisolone and C-reactive protein and serum haptoglobin and erythrocyte sedimentation rate in rheumatoid arthritis. Ann. Rheum. Dis., *38*:141–144, 1979.

197. McConkey, B., et al.: The effects of some anti-inflammatory drugs on the acute phase reactants in rheumatoid arthritis. Q. J. Med. New Series, *42*:785–791, 1973.

198. McConkey, B., Crockson, R.A., and Crockson, A.P.: The assessment of rheumatoid arthritis. A study based on measurements of serum acute phase reactants. Q. J. Med. New Series, *41*:115–125, 1972.

199. McEwan, C.: Evaluation of the patient as a whole and evaluation of the individual functional units of the musculoskeletal system. In The Surgical Management of Rheumatoid Arthritis. Edited by L. Preston, and C. McEwen. Philadelphia, W.B. Saunders Co., 1968.

200. McKenzie, A.H., and Scherbel, A.L.: Chloroquine and hydroxychloroquine in rheumatological therapy. Clin. Rheum. Dis., *6*:545–566, 1980.

201. McQuire, R.J., and Wright, V.: Statistical approach to indices of disease activity in rheumatoid arthritis. Ann. Rheum. Dis., *30*:574–580, 1971.

202. Medical Research Council: Long-term results in early cases of rheumatoid arthritis treated with either cortisone or aspirin. Br. Med. J., *1*:847–850, 1957.

203. Medical Research Council: A comparison of cortisone and aspirin in the treatment of early cases of rheumatoid arthritis. Br. Med. J., *1*:1223–1227, 1954.

204. Meenan, R.F., Gertman, P.M., and Mason, J.H.: Measuring health status in arthritis: The arthritis impact measurement scales. Arthritis Rheum., *23*:146–152, 1980.

205. Menander-Huber, K.B.: Orogotein in the treatment of rheumatoid arthritis. In International Workshop New Aspects of Therapy for Inflammation. Eur. J. Rheum. Inflamm. (Suppl.), *4*:201–211, 1981.

206. Mewa, A.A.M., et al.: Observer differences in detecting erosions in radiographs of rheumatoid arthritis. A comparison of posteroanterior, Norgaard and Brewerton views. J. Rheumatol., *12*:216–221, 1983.

207. Mille, B., et al.: Double-blind placebo controlled crossover evaluation of levamisole in rheumatoid arthritis. Arthritis Rheum., *23*:172–182, 1980.

208. Mills, S.B., Bloch, M., and Bruckner, F.E.: Double-blind crossover study of ketoprofen and ibuprofen in management of rheumatoid arthritis. Br. Med. J., *4*:82–84, 1973.

209. Miltner, L.J., and Kulowski, J.: The effect of treatment and eradication of foci and infection in chronic arthritis (focal infection). J. Bone Joint Surg., *15A*:383–393, 1973.

210. Mitchell, W.S., Miller, J., and Sturrock, R.: An evaluation of goniometry as an objective parameter for measuring joint motion. Scott. Med. J., *20*:57–59, 1975.

211. Moll, J.M.H., and Wright, V.: Normal range of spinal mobility. Ann. Rheum. Dis., *30*:381–386, 1971.

212. Moll, J.M.H., Liyanage, S.P., and Wright, V.: An objective chemical method to measure lateral spinal flexion. Rheum. Phys. Med., *11*:225, 1972.

213. Moll, J.M.H., Liyanage, S.P., and Wright, V.: An objective clinical method to measure spinal extension. Rheum. Phys. Med., *11*:293–312, 1972.

214. Mouridsen, H.T., Baerentsen, O., and Rossing, N.: Lack of effective gold therapy on abnormal IgG and IgM metabolism in rheumatoid arthritis. Arthritis Rheum., *17*:391–396, 1974.

215. Mowat, A.G.: Hematological abnormalities in rheumatoid arthritis. Semin. Arthritis Rheum., *1*:195–198, 1971.

216. Mowat, A.G., Hothersall, T.E., and Aitchison, W.R.C.: Nature of anaemia in rheumatoid arthritis. Ann. Rheum. Dis., *28*:303–309, 1969.

217. Multicentre Study Group: Levamisole in rheumatoid arthritis: A randomised double-blind study comparing two dosage regimens of levamisole with placebo. Lancet, *2*:1007–1012, 1978.

218. Multicentre Trial Group: Controlled trials of D(−) pen-

icillamine in severe rheumatoid arthritis. Lancet, *2*:75–280, 1973.

219. Myers, D.B., Grennan, D.M., and Palmer, D.G.: Hand grip function in patients with rheumatoid arthritis. Arch. Phys. Med. Rehabil., *61*:369–373, 1980.

220. Namey, T.C., McIntyre, J., and Dune, M.: Nucleoradiographic studies of axial spondyloarthropathies. Arthritis Rheum., *20*:1058, 1977.

221. Nie, N.H., et al.: SPSS Statistics Package for the Social Sciences, 2nd Ed. New York, McGraw-Hill, 1975.

222. Nørgaard, F.: Earliest roentgenological changes in polyarthritis of the rheumatoid type: Rheumatoid arthritis. Radiology, *85*:325–329, 1965.

223. Nørgaard, F.: Earliest changes in polyarthritis of the rheumatoid type. Radiology, *92*:299–303, 1969.

224. O'Brien, W.M.: Indomethacin: A survey of clinical trials. Clin. Pharmacol. Ther., *9*:94–107, 1968.

225. Oka, M., et al.: Measurement of systemic inflammatory activity in rheumatoid arthritis by the ^{99m}Tc method. Scand. J. Rheumatol., *2*:101–107, 1973.

226. Oka, M., Rekonen, A., and Ruotsi, A.: Tc^{99m} in the study of systemic inflammatory activity in rheumatoid arthritis. Acta Rheum. Scand., *17*:27–30, 1971.

227. Paterson, J., et al.: The assessment of rheumatoid inflammation in the knee. Ann. Rheum. Dis., *37*:48–52, 1978.

228. Pocock, S.J.: The combination of randomized and historical controls in clinical trials. J. Chronic Dis., *29*:175–188, 1976.

229. Poole, A.R., et al.: Extracellular release of cathepsin-D from cells in human normal and rheumatoid synovial membranes. Ann. Rheum. Dis., *33*:405–408, 1974.

230. Popert, A.J., et al.: Chloroquine diphosphate in rheumatoid arthritis. Ann. Rheum. Dis., *20*:18–33, 1961.

231. Quin, C.E., Mason, R.M., and Knoweldon, J.: Clinical assessment of rapidly acting agents in rheumatoid arthritis. Br. Med. J., *2*:810–813, 1950.

232. Rekonen, A., Juikka, J., and Oka, M.: Measurement of joint inflammation. Scand. J. Rheumatol., *3*:75–78, 1974.

233. Report by the Joint Committee of the Medical Research Council: A comparison of prednisolone with aspirin or other analgesics in the treatment of rheumatoid arthritis. Ann. Rheum. Dis., *18*:173–188, 1959.

234. Revill, S.I., et al.: The reliability of a linear analysis for evaluating pain. Anesthesia, *31*:1191–1198, 1976.

235. Reynolds, P.M.G.: Measurement of spinal mobility: A comparison of three methods. Rheumatol. Rehabil., *14*:180–185, 1975.

236. Rhind, V.M., Bird, H.A., and Wright, V.: A comparison of clinical assessments of disease activity in rheumatoid arthritis. Ann. Rheum. Dis., *39*:35–137, 1980.

237. Ring, E.F.J., et al.: Quantitation of thermography in arthritis using multi-isothermal analysis II. Effect of nonsteroidal anti-inflammatory therapy on the thermographic plus index. Ann. Rheum. Dis., *33*:353–356, 1974.

238. Ritchie, D.M., et al.: Clinical studies with an articular index for the assessment of joint tenderness in patients with rheumatoid arthritis. Q. J. Med., *37*:393–406, 1968.

239. Ritter, J.M.: Placebo-controlled, double-blind clinical trials can impede medical progress. Lancet, *1*:1126–1127, 1980.

240. Rosenspire, K.C., et al.: Comparison of four methods of analysis of ^{99}Tc pyrophosphate uptake in RA joints. J. Rheumatol., *7*:461–468, 1980.

241. Rosenspire, K.C., et al.: Investigation of the metabolic activity of bone in rheumatoid arthritis. J. Rheumatol., *7*:469–473, 1980.

242. Runge, L.A., et al.: Treatment of rheumatoid arthritis with levamisole. A controlled trial. Arthritis Rheum., *20*:1445–1448, 1977.

243. Russell, A.S., Lentle, B.C., and Percy, J.S.: Investigation of sacroiliac disease. J. Rheumatol., *2*:45–51, 1975.

244. Sackett, D.L.: Bias in analytic research. J. Chronic Dis., *32*:51–63, 1979.

245. Sartwell, P.E.: Retrospective studies—a review for the clinician. Ann. Intern Med., *81*:381–386, 1974.

246. Savage, O.: Criteria for measurement in chronic diseases.

Report on a Symposium on Clinical Trials. Pfizer, Kent, 32, 1958.

247. Savage, O.: Criteria for measurement in chronic diseases. Proc. R. Soc. Med. (Suppl. 59): 85–88, 1958.

248. Schöber, P.: Tendenwirbelsäule und Kreuzschmerzen. Munch. Med. Wschr., 84:336–338, 1937.

249. Scott, J., and Huskisson, E.C.: Accuracy of subjective measurements made with or without previous scores: An important source of error in serial measurement of subjective states. Ann. Rheum. Dis., 38:558–559, 1979.

250. Scott, J.T., and Huskisson, E.C.: Graphic representation of pain. Pain, 2:175–184, 1976.

251. Scott, P.J., Ansell, B.M., and Huskisson, E.C.: Measurement of pain in juvenile chronic polyarthritis. Rheumatol. Rehabil., 16:54–57, 1977.

252. Sharp, J.T., et al.: Methods of scoring the progression of radiological changes in rheumatoid arthritis. Arthritis Rheum., 14:706–720, 1971.

253. Sheiner, L.B.: Clinical trials and the illusion of objectivity. In Drug Therapeutics—Concepts for Physicians. Edited by K.L. Melman. New York, Elsevier-North Holland, 1979, pp. 167–182.

254. Sigler, J.W., Bluhm, G.B., and Duncan, H.: Gold salts in the treatment of RA. A double-blind study. Ann. Intern. Med., 80:21–26, 1974.

255. Smythe, H.A., Helewa, A., and Goldsmith, C.H.: "Independent assessor" and "polled index" as techniques for measuring treatment effects in rheumatoid arthritis. J. Rheumatol., 4:144–152, 1977.

256. Spencer, D.G., et al.: Scintiscanning in ankylosing spondylitis: A clinical, radiological and quantitative radioisotopic study. J. Rheumatol., 6:426–431, 1979.

257. Spiegel, A.D., and Hyman, H.H.: Basic Health Planning Methods. Germantown, Aspens Systems Corp., 1978.

258. Spodick, D.H., et al.: Letter to the editor. J. Chronic Dis., 33:127–128, 1980.

259. Sriwatanakul, K., et al.: Studies with different types of visual analog scales for measurement of pain. Clin. Pharmacol. Ther., 34:234–239, 1983.

260. Stainsby, W.J., and Nicholls, E.: Results of treatment in rheumatoid arthritis with reference to foci of infection and streptococcus vaccine. J. Lab. Clin. Med., 18:881–890, 1933.

261. Steinberg, A.D.: On morning stiffness. J. Rheumatol., 5:3–6, 1978.

262. Steinbrocker, O., Traeger, C.H., and Batterman, R.C.: Therapeutic criteria in rheumatoid arthritis. J.A.M.A., 140:659–662, 1949.

263. Steinbrocker, O.: A simple pressure gauge for measured palpation in physical diagnosis and therapy. Arch. Phys. Med., 30:289–290, 1949.

264. Stewart, A.L., Ware, J.E., and Brook, R.H.: Advances in measurement of functional status: Construction of aggregate indices. Med. Care., 19:473–488, 1981.

265. St. Onge, R.A., et al.: The effect of external heat and exercise on the [133]xenon clearance rate in normal and diseased human joints, and of injection volume, methacholine, and atropine on the [133]xenon clearance rate in the normal canine joint. Rev. Rheum., 38:87–101, 1971.

266. Sturrock, R.D., et al.: Eine Bewertung der Phenylalkanoinsaure—Derivate in der Behandlung rheumatischer Erkrankungen sowie einige Erlauterungen zur den klinischen Versuchsmethoden. Z. Rheumaforsch., 34:55–67, 1975.

267. Sturrock, R.D., Nicholson, R., and Wojtulewski, J.: Technetium counting in rheumatoid arthritis: Evaluation in the small joints of the hands. Arthritis Rheum., 17:417–420, 1974.

268. Sturrock, R.D., Wojtulewski, J., and Hart, F.D.: Spondylometry in a normal population and in ankylosing spondylitis. Rheumatol. Rehabil., 12:135–142, 1973.

269. Swanson, M.A., and Schwartz, R.S.: Immunosuppressure therapy: The relation between clinical response and immunology competence. N. Engl. J. Med., 277:163–170, 1967.

270. Szpilman, H., et al.: Levamisole, cell-mediated immunity and serum immunoglobulins in rheumatoid arthritis. Lancet, 2:208–209, 1976.

271. Tanz, S.S.: Motion of the lumbar spine: A roentgenologic study. Am. J. Roentgenol., 69:399–412, 1953.

272. Thomas, D., et al.: Knee-joint temperature measurement using a differential thermistor thermometer. Rheumatol. Rehabil., 19:8–13, 1980.

273. Tugwell, P., et al.: The ability of MACTAR Disability Questionnaire to Detect Sensitivity to Change in Rheumatoid Arthritis. Clin. Res., 31:129A, 1983.

274. Tugwell, P., and Bombardier, C.: A methodologic framework for developing and selecting endpoints in clinical trials. J. Rheumatol., 9:758–762, 1982.

275. Wallace, D.J., Brachman, M., and Klinenberg, J.R.: Joint scanning in rheumatoid arthritis. A literature review. Semin. Arthritis Rheum., 11:172–176, 1981.

276. Walsh, L., Davies, P., and McConkey, B.: Relationship between erythrocyte sedimentation rate and C-reactive protein in rheumatoid arthritis. Ann. Rheum. Dis., 38:362–363, 1979.

277. Ward, J.R., Niethammer, T.A., and Egger, M.J.: Can we just measure signal joints? Should ring size and walking time be analyzed only in selected patients? In Symposia Medica Hoechst 16 Controversies in the Clinical Evaluation of Analgesic Anti-inflammatory—Anti-rheumatic Drugs. Edited by H.E. Paulus, G.E. Ehrlich, and E. Lindenlaub. Stuttgart, Schattauer Verlag, 1981, pp. 103–112.

278. Webb, J., et al.: Evaluation of digital joint circumference measurements in rheumatoid arthritis. Scand. J. Rheumatol., 2:127–131, 1973.

279. Weinstein, M.C.: Allocation of subjects in medical experiments. N. Engl. J. Med., 291:1278–1285, 1974.

280. White, A.G., et al.: Copper—an index of erosive activity. Rheumatol. Rehab., 17:3–5, 1978.

281. White, K.L.: Improved medical care: Statistics and the health services system. Public Health Rep., 82:847–854, 1967.

282. Wiles, P.: Movements of the lumbar vertebrae during flexion and extension. Proc. R. Soc. Med., 26:647–651, 1935.

283. Willkens, R.F., Gleichert, J.E., and Gade, E.T.: Proximal interphalangeal joint measurement by arthrocircameter. Ann. Rheum. Dis., 32:585–586, 1973.

284. Winchester, R.J., et al.: Observation on the eosinophilia of certain patients with rheumatoid arthritis. Arthritis Rheum., 14:650–655, 1971.

285. Wright, V.: Measurement of Joint Movement. Philadelphia, W.B. Saunders Co., 1982.

286. Wright, V.: Some observations on diurnal variation of grip strength. Clin. Sci., 18:17–23, 1959.

287. Wright, V., et al.: Erythrocyte sedimentation rate (ESR). In Controversies in the Clinical Evaluation of Analgesic Anti-inflammatory-Anti-rheumatic Drugs. Edited by H.E. Paulus, G.E. Ehrlich, and E. Lindenlaub. Stuttgart, Schattauer Verlag, 1981, pp. 161–163.

288. Wright, V., and Johns, R.J.: Physical factors concerned with the stiffness of normal and diseased joints. Bull. Johns Hopkins Hosp., 106:215–231, 1960.

289. Zuckner, J., et al.: D-penicillamine in rheumatoid arthritis. Arthritis Rheum., 13:131–138, 1970.

Scientific Basis for the Study of the Rheumatic Diseases

Chapter **8**

Structure and Function of Joints

Henry J. Mankin and Eric Radin

The rigidity of structure and segmental stability of the human frame are provided by the bony skeleton. Interruptions in the rigid framework, the *joints*, allow controlled and almost frictionless movement. The bones and joints provide structural support and protection to vital parts, yet allow sufficient directed movement for the functions of locomotion and prehension. The purpose of this chapter is to discuss the structure and function of the joints, in detail. Although all joints will be considered, synovial joints and the intervertebral disc will be emphasized, since they constitute most joints and are most often involved by the disease processes discussed in this volume.

CLASSIFICATION OF JOINTS

Human joints are most often classified according to the type of motion that occurs. Three groups are recognized: the immovable joints (synarthroses); slightly movable joints (amphiarthroses); and movable joints (diarthroses).[44] Another less commonly used classification is based on the nature of the specialized forms of connective tissue that are present.[44] The two classifications are interrelated in that the constituent bones of the immovable joints or slightly movable joints are connected by fibrous or cartilaginous membranes (syndesmoses or synchondroses), whereas the component bony parts of the movable joints, although covered by hyaline cartilage, are completely separated and contain between them a joint cavity enclosed by a synovial membrane (synovial joints).[36,44]

Synarthroses are generally found in the skull. The contributing bony plates that comprise the joints are held firmly to each other by fibrous or cartilaginous elements. *Amphiarthroses* are characterized by the presence of broad, flattened discs of fibrocartilage connecting the articulating surfaces. The bony portions of the joint are usually covered by hyaline cartilage, and the entire structure is invested by a fibrous capsule. Such joints are those between the vertebrae, the distal tibiofibular articulation, and the pubic symphysis. *Diarthroses* include most of the joints of the extremities. The joint space, articular cartilage, and synovial membrane allow the wide ranges of motion nec-

essary for the functions of locomotion and prehension.[36,44]

SYNOVIAL JOINTS

General Structure

The synovial joints comprise most of the body's articulations and are characterized by wide ranges of almost frictionless movement. The articulating body surfaces present at their ends a thin plate of dense cortical bone, known as the articular end-plate. Beneath this lies the cancellous bone often containing red (hematopoietic) marrow. Tightly adherent to the bony end-plate are the hyaline articular cartilages, specialized connective tissue structures that are the bearing and gliding surfaces. The joint cavity is a tissue space, containing only a few milliliters of synovial fluid (Fig. 8–1).

The movement of the cartilaginous surfaces on one another provides the joint with *mobility* but, by definition, joints must also have *stability* in order to prevent movement in abnormal planes or excessive slipping under load. Stability is provided by the bony configuration of the joint, the ligamentous and capsular support systems, and the muscles controlling the joint. Each joint has a unique configuration. For example, the hip is a ball and socket; the knee is a rounded, condylar, cam-shaped, four-bar linkage that allows not only flexion and extension but rotation; the ankle is a complexly shaped mortised hinge; each intervertebral facet joint is a slightly convex-concave flat on a slightly convex flat; the shoulder is a ball on a disc, and so on. The configuration of each individual joint provides the maximum contact area for the most usual positions of loading, with a range of motion and sufficient stability to allow high-efficiency performance.[53] Each joint has somewhat different load and positional requirements, reflected appropriately in its individual design. Uniaxial, biaxial, or polyaxial motion occurs, depending on the fit of the component parts at the various ranges. Thus, the bony structure of the ankle joint (a hinge joint) is the primary factor that dictates that motion will occur mainly in the sagittal plane through an axis running transverse to the long axis of the limb through the body of the talus. The medial malleolus, anterior lip, and posterior margin of the tibia

179

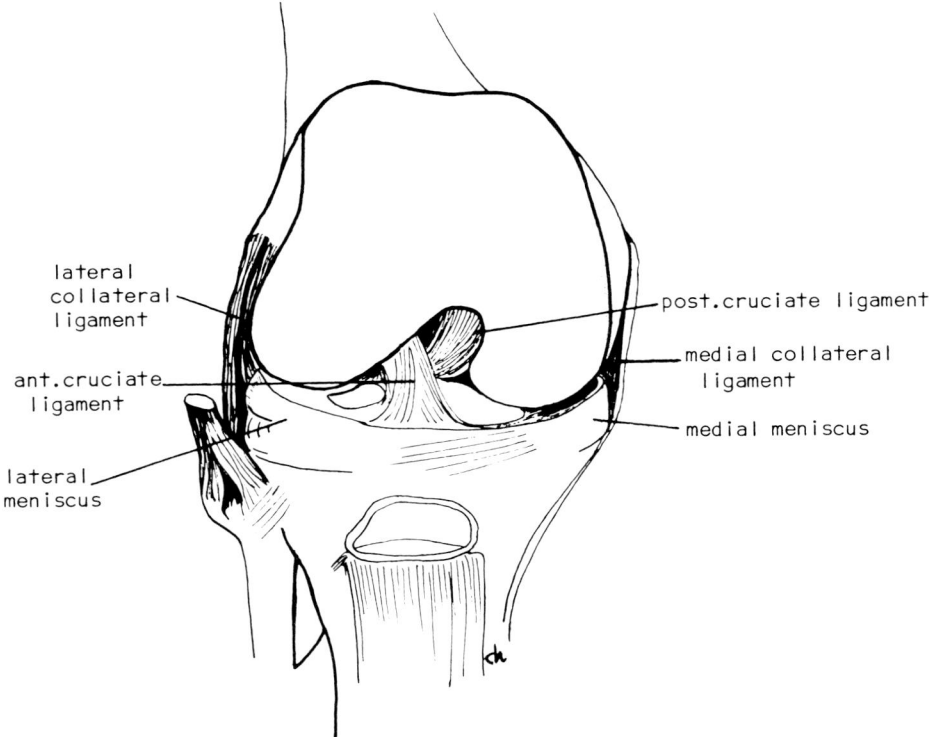

lateral
collateral
ligament

ant.cruciate
ligament

lateral
meniscus

post.cruciate ligament

medial collateral
ligament

medial meniscus

Fig. 8–1. An artist's conception of the human knee joint. The patella and capsule have been removed. Note that the distal femur and proximal tibia are covered by hyaline articular cartilage. Affixed to the surface of the tibia are the medial and lateral menisci. The medial and lateral collateral ligaments, stout collagenous bands, provide stability in the coronal plane. The cruciate ligaments control stability in the sagittal plane.

and the fibular malleolus prevent abnormal movement by their bony impingement on the talus and provide the stability necessary for normal dorsi- and plantar flexion under heavy load. On the other hand, the ball-and-shallow-socket bony configuration of the shoulder joint contributes almost nothing to its stability, which is provided almost entirely by the capsule, ligaments, and investing musculature.[110]

Accessory structures that aid in maintaining the integrity of the joint are the fibrous capsule and ligaments.[12,57,110] The fibrous capsule consists of dense connective tissue, investing the entire joint and inserting into bone, usually close to the articulating surfaces. Within the capsule are thick bands of parallel collagen fibers known as ligaments. These too insert on the bony parts and vary in their tightness from anatomic site to site, depending considerably on the position of the joint.

Within the joint capsule and defining the interarticular space is a specialized layer of connective tissue cells, the synoviocytes, which secrete the synovial fluid.[47,61] Deep to this layer are varying amounts of highly vascular adipose, fibrous or areolar tissue supporting the synoviocytes and allow-

ing the sac to be appropriately loose in certain ranges of motion, without allowing the synovial folds to become entrapped between the joint surfaces.[8,105] The synovial sac is "incomplete" in that, although it faithfully replicates the inner surface of the capsule, is reflected at the capsular insertion into the bone, and then extends along the bone to the margin of the articular cartilage, it does not cover the cartilage surfaces.[8] The synovial tissue is endowed with nerve endings[61] which, along with those in the capsule and spindles in the muscles, ligaments, and tendons, are responsible for the keen proprioceptive sense and deep pain perception that protect the joint.[15,95,103]

Certain of the body's joints have within their cavities complete or incomplete fibrocartilaginous discoid partitions known as menisci. The menisci are inconstant in some areas (e.g., acromioclavicular joint) and highly developed and well defined in others (e.g., knee, temporomandibular joint, and sternoclavicular joints).[44] Synovium does not cover the avascular, aneural fibrocartilaginous menisci, which are firmly fixed to the joint margin by attachment to bone and to ligaments or capsule, preventing abnormal movement or intra-articular displacement during joint function.[12]

Embryology and Development

Shortly after the limb buds appear in the human embryo (26 to 28 days), an axial condensation or blastema develops within them.[119] At approximately five postovulatory weeks, the blastema becomes chondrified in the region of future bones; the chondrification proceeds in a proximodistal sequence.[119] The precartilage so formed undergoes an orderly sequence of maturation that proceeds in a fashion approximating epiphyseal cartilage maturation. The bony segments differentiate and become surrounded by a two-layered perichondrium.[37,39] The joint ends of the rudimentary bones are surrounded by concentric rings of flattened cells, and the site of the future joint is the intersection (known as the interzone) of the arcs of cells from one bony rudiment with those of the adjacent one.[46]

Early development of the large joints of the limbs involves two critical phases: the formation and differentiation of the interzones, and the appearance of cavities. At first the cells of the interzone appear identical, but soon develop into three layers: a central loosely arranged layer and two denser layers on either side, which subsequently become the articular cartilages.[46,119] The mesenchyme that surrounds the joints (synovial mesenchyme) becomes vascularized, and the capsule and the peri- and intra-articular structures (ligaments, menisci, and synovial membrane) differentiate from it.[37,39] By eight postovulatory weeks, the component parts of the developing joint resemble the adult joint, except that the joint space has not yet appeared.[39,46,89]

At the end of the embryonic period or early in the fetal period (47 to 60 days), minute spaces appear in the undifferentiated interzone synovial mesenchyme of the larger joints. These spaces result from autolysis and liquefaction of the cells and are thought to be mediated by locally synthesized enzymes.[119] Lysosomal bodies are noted in embryonic cells early in their differentiation, and the enzymes contained within the sacs are believed to be released in response to an alteration in pH or oxygen tension.[120] The enzymes destroy the matrix and cells, forming minute cavities, which subsequently coalesce to form the joint cavity. The joint space is lined by articular cartilage rudiments centrally, but peripherally by a single layer of flattened cells, which becomes the synovial membrane. Early in fetal life the synovial membrane is a relatively smooth, two-cell-layered lining with a subjacent vascular network. Subsequently, convolutions and villiform irregularities appear.

In terms of congenital abnormalities of joints, there is a critical period in the life of the developing fetus when an alteration in physiologic balance resulting from a genetic error or an intrauterine insult could lead to a major disturbance in joint structure. The upper limb buds appear at 26 days and the lower at 28, and the cavitation to form the joint does not occur until approximately 60 days.[46] It is reasonable to suppose that the joints are in maximum danger of maldevelopment as a result of insult occurring between the third and sixth week after conception. Insults before this time may include joint and limb abnormalities, but will probably be considerably more extensive (somitic in distribution), and those that occur after complete development of the joint (80 days) are unlikely to have a significant effect.[119]

Structure and Chemistry of Component Parts

Ligaments and Capsule. Ligaments and capsular structures vary considerably in thickness and position, depending on the joint studied and the site within that joint.[44] Structures range from the thin, redundant articular capsule of the shoulder joint[110] to the thick, dense collagenous collateral and cruciate ligaments of the knee.[12,41] In some, the ligaments are condensations within the capsule, and in others they are discrete and separated from the capsule by an areolar layer. Capsular redundancy is an important aspect of joint function, particularly in relation to the range of motion. The inferior medial portion of the capsule of the shoulder joint is a loose, redundant sac, which does not become tense until the shoulder is fully abducted or flexed.[110] The posterior capsule of the knee is quite loose in flexion, but so tight in extension that it becomes an important stabilizer.[12]

Although there is some variation, depending on the site studied, the periarticular ligaments and capsule are fairly uniform in histologic appearance, chemical composition, and tissue organization. The structures consist principally of parallel bundles or fascicles of collagen, sparsely populated with fibrocytes.[57] Blood vessels traverse a tortuous course between the fascicles, and an occasional nerve fiber is noted, most frequently perivascular, but occasionally free in the ligament or capsule.[56] The collagen fibers range from 150 to 1500 nm in diameter, and an occasional elastic fiber is interspersed.[22,57] Together the fibrous proteins (collagen and elastin) account for over 90% of the dry weight of the tissue.[2,3,31] The collagen of ligaments and capsule is mostly type I $(2\alpha_1{}^1, 1\alpha_2)$, similar but not identical in biochemical composition, glycosylation, and cross-linking to that found in dermis and bone.[48]

Mammalian ligaments and capsule are hyperhydrated with estimates of water ranging up to approximately 70%.[2,3] Most of the remaining inorganic solids consist of collagen (and elastin), although a small but important fraction is in the form of proteoglycans.[2,3,59] The glycosaminoglycan chains associated with these macromolecules differ somewhat from those found in cartilage in that approximately 35% is in the form of hyaluronic acid, with chondroitin sulfate (40%) and dermatan sulfate (20%) comprising the remainder.[2,3]

The insertions of ligaments and capsule into the adjacent bones demonstrate a zonal organization. Parallel bundles of collagen first become invested with a fibrocartilaginous stroma and, as they near the bone, become calcified.[22] The collagen fibers, continuous with the ligament, then enter the cortical osseous tissue in a manner analogous to Sharpey's fibers[88] (Fig. 8–2). The gradual transition of ligaments to mineralized fibrocartilage and then to bone enhances the ability of the insertions to distribute forces evenly and decreases the likelihood of pull-out failure.[22]

Articular Cartilage. The articular cartilages are the principal "working" components of the diarthrodial joint and, in large measure, are responsible for the almost frictionless movement of the articulating surfaces on each other[18] (Fig. 8–3). These specialized connective tissue components are firmly attached to the underlying bones, and measure less than 5 mm in thickness in human joints,[44] with considerable variation depending on joint and site within the joint.[75,79,116] Articular cartilage is dense and white on gross inspection, but tends to become somewhat yellow with age.[126] It feels semisolid. Contrary to expectations, the surface is not smooth.[105] Studies using the scanning electron microscope have demonstrated gentle undulations and irregular depressions that appear to correspond to the location and shape of cells lying just beneath the surface. These depressions average

20 to 40 μm in diameter and occur with a frequency of 430/mm² (Fig. 8–4).[19,20]

The articular cartilages are both avascular and alymphatic. Thus, at least in adult humans, they derive their nutrition by a double diffusion system.[8,29,69] Since the blood vessels in synovium are situated along the (outer) capsular surface,[24] the articulating (inner) surface is relatively avascular, and nutrients must first diffuse across the synovial membrane into the synovial fluid and then through the dense matrix of the cartilage to reach the chondrocyte (see Chap. 9).[8,14,67] Because there are no nerves in articular cartilage, the bearing surfaces of the joint depend on nerve endings in the capsule, synovium, muscles, and subchondral bone for appreciation of pain and proprioception.[37,38,95,103]

Histologic and ultrastructural examination of the cartilage demonstrates a vast preponderance of extracellular matrix and only sparse cellularity[69,123] (see Fig. 8–3). The distribution of cells is not random, and four zones have been described:[123] a tangential or gliding zone in which the cells are elongated with their long axes parallel to surface; a transitional zone in which the cells are rounded and appear randomly distributed; a radial zone, in which the cells appear to line up in short irregular columns; and a calcified zone, the matrix and cells of which are heavily encrusted with hydroxyapatite. The calcified zone is separated from the radial zone superficial to it by a wavy, irregular bluish line (on hematoxylin and eosin staining) called the "tidemark,"[33,34] and on its deep surface merges with the end-plate of the underlying bone[45] (Fig. 8–5). The tidemark is similar in appearance and composition to the cement lines in bone and may act as a limit to calcification[45] or, as has been suggested by Redler et al.,[104] may represent a variation in the structure of the collagen fibers to increase the resistance to shearing forces.

The biochemical composition of articular carti-

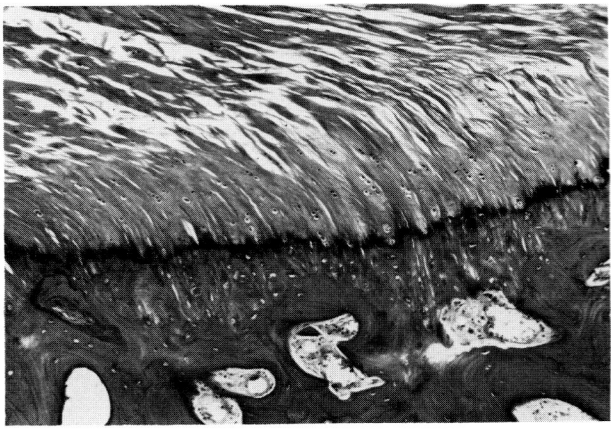

Fig. 8–2. Photomicrograph showing the insertion of a collateral ligament of an interphalangeal ligament into the cortex of the phalanx. Note the parallel bundles of collagen that comprise the ligament, becoming first fibrocartilaginous, then calcified, prior to entering the substance of the cortical bone in a fashion similar to Sharpey's fibers. (H & E, × 50)

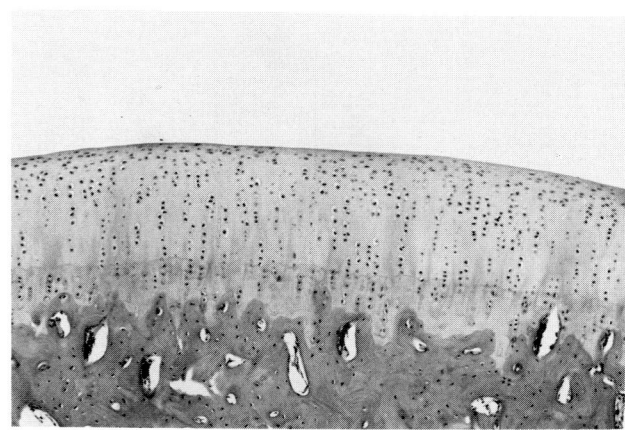

Fig. 8–3. Low-power photomicrograph of adult articular cartilage. Note the zonal distribution of the cells, the calcified layer separated from the radial zone by the "tidemark," and the cortical bone of the underlying bony end plate. Articular cartilage is sparsely cellular, and the bulk of the tissue consists of extracellular matrix. (H & E, ×40)

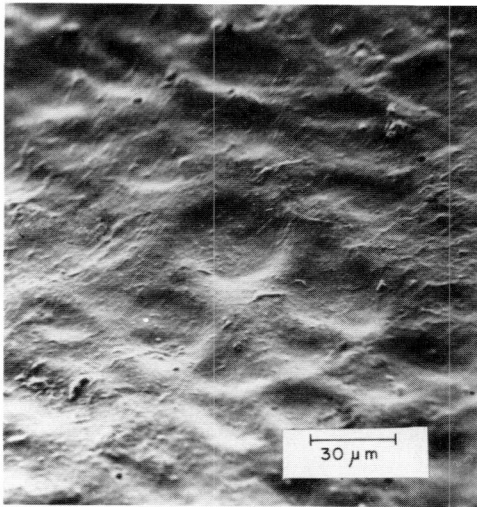

Fig. 8–4. Scanning electron micrograph of the surface of articular cartilage demonstrating irregularly placed rounded or ovoid depressions averaging 20 to 40 μm in diameter. (× 440) (Courtesy of Dr. Ian Clark.)

lage is quite different from that of other connective tissues involved in the joint. Water content ranges up to almost 80%.[72,76] The water of articular cartilage is freely exchangeable with synovial fluid and appears to be held in the form of proteoglycan-collagen gel.[72] Collagen is the most prevalent organic constituent, accounting for over 50% of the remaining material.[59,69,82] The most superficial collagen fibers are arranged in bundles and sheets parallel to the surface of the cartilage forming a "skin," but distribution is more random in the deeper layers[59,127] (Fig. 8–6). Collagen of cartilage (type II) is of a different genetic species from that of skin or bone (type I) and consists of three identical α_1^{II} chains in a helical form.[77,78] The chains differ from those of type I collagen principally in the increased quantity of hydroxylysine and excessive glycosylation (see Chap. 10).[42,52,77,78] The remainder of the organic solids are mostly proteoglycans,[69,81] macromolecules consisting in their simplest form (subunit) of a linear protein core approximately 180 to 210 nm in length, to which are attached glycosaminoglycans of three species: chondroitin 6-sulfate; chondroitin 4-sulfate; and keratan sulfate in varying numbers depending on the age of the individuals and site.[9,21,82,88] The molecular weight of the subunit is about two million Daltons, with as many as 50 glycosaminoglycan chains extended at right angles from the core protein.[108,109] Since the three polysaccharides are markedly anionic, the molecule exerts an enormous electronegative domain, causing it to remain stiffly extended in space (see Chap. 11).[81,108] This factor is probably a key one in maintenance of the resiliency of the tissue. The component glycosaminoglycans vary with age, with chondroitin 4-sulfate and chondroitin 6-sulfate being the principal constituents in immature animals, whereas in adults chondroitin 4-sulfate is diminished to less than 5% and keratan sulfate accounts for about 50%.[21,30,69,70,82] It is unlikely that the subunit exists as such in the natural state, and most of the proteoglycan is in the form of highly ordered, large aggregates.[83,108] Aggregation of the subunits has been shown to occur along a thin filament of hyaluronic acid, which accounts for less than 1% of the total glycosaminoglycan present within the tissue,[83] but is obviously of critical importance in maintenance of the physical properties.[49,108]

Articular cartilage also contains other materials in small quantities. Approximately 5 to 6% of the tissue is in the form of inorganic constituents, mostly calcium salts.[81] Lipids[11] and lysozyme[58] each account for 1% of the dry weight, and studies have suggested the presence of a glycoprotein or

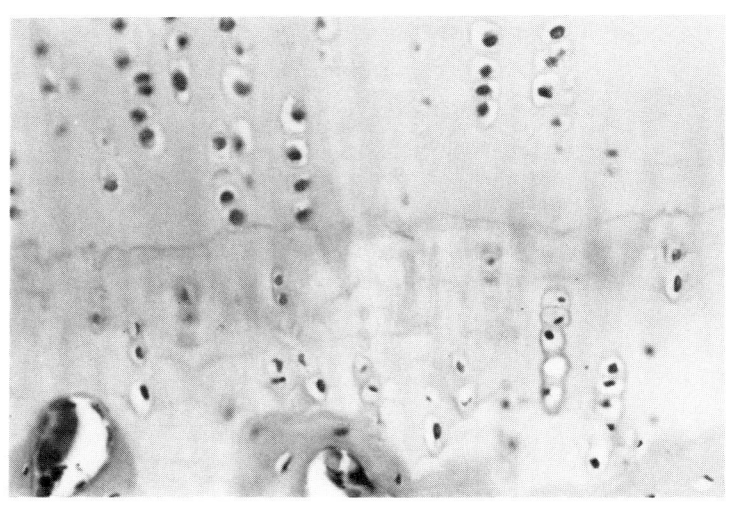

Fig. 8–5. Photomicrograph of mature articular cartilage showing the "tidemark," a wavy bluish line (or series of lines) separating the calcified zone below from the radial zone above. The matrix and cells of the calcified zone are heavily encrusted with apatitic salts. (H & E, × 250)

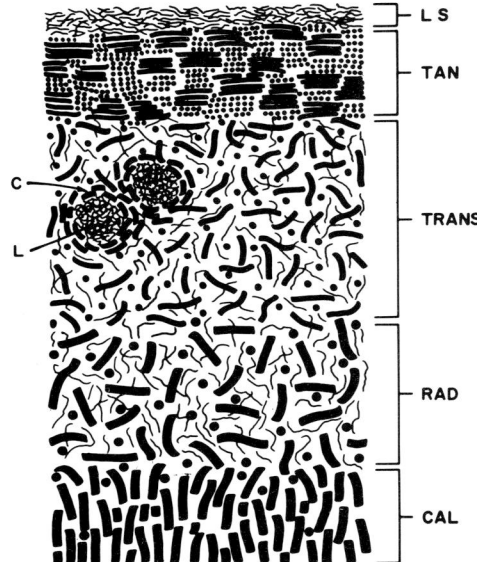

Fig. 8–6. Diagram of the fibrous architecture of human articular cartilage according to a scheme proposed by Lane and Weiss. The lamina splendens (LS) is a layer several micra deep, composed of the fine fibers that cover the articular surface. Beneath this lies the tangential zone (TAN), which consists of tightly packed bundles of individual collagen fibers arranged parallel to the articular surface, often at right angles to each other. The collagen fibers in the transitional zone (TRANS) are randomly arranged. Collagen fibers of the radial zone (RAD) are also randomly arranged, but are of larger diameter, while those of the calcified zone (CAL) are arranged perpendicular to the articular surface. (From Lane, J.M., and Weiss, C.[59])

"matrix protein," constituting up to 15% of the total dry weight.[81] In addition, a fibronectin-like material has been described.[70a]

Studies on the metabolism of articular cartilage contradict the inert appearance of the tissue, demonstrating a surprising rate of synthesis and degradation of the component matrix materials.[68] Specifically, it has been demonstrated by radiotracer studies that the articular chondrocytes are responsible for the synthesis of the proteoglycan,[68,107] and that at least a small portion of it turns over at a rapid rate.[71] Collagen is also synthesized locally by the cartilage cells, but is considerably more stable than the proteoglycan.[64,106] The rapid turnover of at least a small portion of the proteoglycan suggests the presence of an internal remodeling system, and evidence has accumulated that this is based on the release of lysosomal enzymes from the chondrocytes, which have as their principal substrate the proteoglycan.[4,111–113] Although it would seem logical that a hyaluronidase would also be involved (since it could break down both the hyaluronate backbone of the aggregate and the glycosaminoglycan chains), no evidence has been found for its presence in articular cartilage,[10] and it is more likely that the degradative activity is on the basis of cathepsin D[4,111] and neutral proteoglycanase.[80,112,113] Collagenase has been found in osteoarthritic articular cartilage, but not in normal tissues.[28,93]

Synovial Membrane and Synovial Fluid of Diarthrodial Joints. The synovial fluid and synovial membrane are discussed in Chapters 4 and 9 respectively, and hence are reviewed only briefly here. The synovial membrane is a vascular connective tissue lining the inner surface of the capsule but not covering the articular cartilage. As indicated, there is considerable anatomic difference between the lining cells (synoviocytes) and the subsynovial tissues, which consist of avascular connective tissue framework with varying amounts of fibrous, areolar, and fatty tissues with elements of the reticuloendothelial system interspersed.[5,40,47] (Fig. 8–7). The synoviocytes themselves are the unique feature of this tissue and, as will be discussed, have been divided according to ultrastructural and cytochemical characteristics into types A and B,[7] which vary in their functional activities (fibrogenesis, phagocytosis, synthesis of hyaluronate, synthesis of immune globulins).[5,40,47] Ultrastructural studies have shown that the surface or lining cells form a discontinuous layer, lacking a basement membrane, and that cell processes (which may interdigitate) project from the cells toward the surface.[5,40,61] Thin branching filaments, probably of reticular origin, appear to serve as a supportive membrane for the cells, rather than collagen fibers, which are usually absent.[61]

The synovial membrane is richly endowed with a plexus of blood vessels in the subsynovial layers, which is thought to be responsible for the transfer of blood constituents into the synovial cavity and the formation of synovial fluid.[1,24] Filtration may be variable depending on the constituent studied, and it is apparent that there is a selective element to the transudative process. There is excellent evidence to demonstrate that the synovial cells synthesize and secrete hyaluronate, an "additive" to the plasma constituents that form the synovial fluid and an important aspect in lubrication mechanisms.[1,47] Studies have also supported the concept that the synovial cells synthesize low-molecular-weight mediator substances, such as "catabolin," which may significantly affect the articular chondrocytes.[25,55]

Normal synovial fluid is clear, pale yellow, and viscous. It is normally present in very small amounts. One to four milliliters is found in the human knee, and less in smaller joints. The viscosity of the fluid is due to the presence of the hyaluronate and proteinaceous materials, which have considerable importance in lubrication.[102,124,125]

Menisci of Diarthrodial Joints. As already stated, menisci normally occur only in the knee and temporomandibular, sternoclavicular, distal radioulnar, and acromioclavicular joints. They consist of complete or incomplete flattened, triangular, or somewhat irregularly shaped fibrocartilaginous discs, firmly attached to the fibrous capsules and often to one of the adjacent bones[36,44] (Fig. 8–8A, B).

Menisci, like articular cartilages, are avascular, aneural, and alymphatic. They presumably derive their nutrition from synovial fluid, but also by diffusion from vascular plexuses, which are present in the soft tissues adjacent to their attachment to bone or fibrous capsule. Examination of the menisci of the knee under polarized or light microscopy has shown that the collagen fibers are arranged circumferentially, presumably to withstand the tension of load bearing[16] (Fig. 8–8B).

The fibrocartilage of the meniscus has a biochemical composition considerably different from that of articular cartilage.[60,94,121] The water content ranges between 70 and 78%. Inorganic ash accounts for approximately 3% of the wet weight. The remainder of the material, the inorganic solids, are principally collagen with type I $(2\alpha_1',1\alpha_2)$ predominating.[59] Collagen accounts for 60 to 90% of the organic solids.[94] Elastin is present in low concentration ($<1\%$).[94] Proteoglycans constitute less than 10% of the dry weight, and their constituent glycosaminoglycans are principally chondroitin sulfates with keratan sulfate representing a minor component.[60,121]

Subchondral Bone. Although at the ultrastructural and biochemical levels the bone making up the subchondral cortex and the cancellous bone that supports it are indistinguishable from bone from other sites, the organization of the subchondral bone is quite specific. The subchondral plate on which the calcified cartilage lies is thinner than

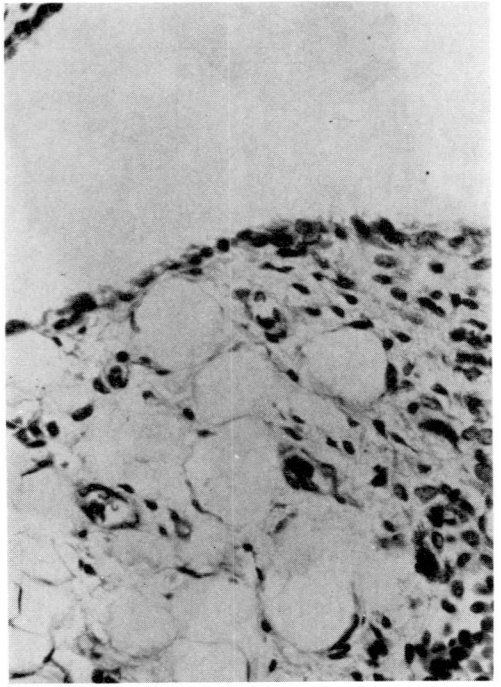

Fig. 8–7. Photomicrograph of normal synovium showing the surface layers of synovial cells and the presence of areolar and fatty synovial tissue. (H & E, × 225)

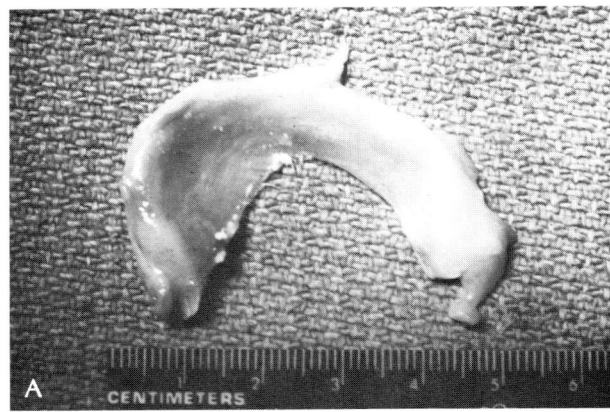

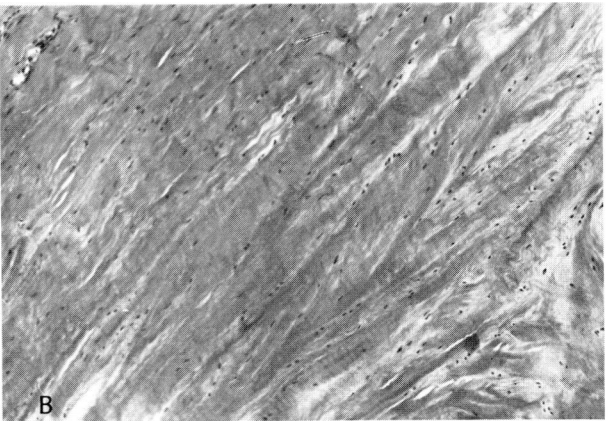

Fig. 8–8. *A,* Photograph of a normal human medial meniscus. Note the semilunar shape with a thin free edge and considerably thickened marginal attachment site. Menisci increase the stability of the joint and serve as weight-bearing structures in the knee. *B,* Low-power photomicrograph of a fibrocartilaginous human medial meniscus. Note the presence of large numbers of parallel bundles of collagen and the sparse cellularity. (H & E, × 40)

cortical bone in most areas and may contain variable numbers of mature haversian systems. The distribution of these systems has not been well established, but they appear to run parallel to the joint rather than parallel to the long axis of the bone (Fig. 8—9). The sheets and interconnecting struts of cancellous bone that support the plate and fill the epiphyseal end of the bone differ considerably from joint to joint, but are highly ordered and characteristic for any one joint. The major plates are arranged at right angles to the predominating stresses and, together with the subchondral bony end-plate, are approximately 10 times more deformable than is the cortical bony shaft.[101]

Function

The compressive stress under which diarthrodial joints function is considerably greater than that associated with support of body weight. Since muscular contraction is responsible for creating the equilibrium of moments, which provides stability to the loaded joint, the major joints of the lower extremity—the knee, the hip, and the ankle—usually function under loads approximating $2\frac{1}{2}$ to 10 times that of body weight.[54] Similar compressive stresses (about 200 to 500 pounds per square inch)

are not uncommon in the joints of the upper extremity. Further, the load on joints is not constant, since activities are intermittent and often create high peak dynamic loads.[118] Joint motion is characterized by frequent rapid starts and equally rapid stops, both of which, but especially the starts, are associated with high compressive loads. It is remarkable that under such potentially punishing mechanical conditions most joints function throughout the life of the individual without evidence of destruction of their major load-bearing areas.

Role of Ligaments, Joint Capsule, and Surrounding Muscles. The ligaments, joint capsule, and surrounding muscles provide stability to joints. The role of muscles in this regard cannot be overemphasized. Even though all periarticular structures are intact, complete paralysis of muscle abolishes the stability of a joint, and partial paralysis creates significant functional limitations. Muscles are most important in stabilizing the large proximal joints—the shoulder and the hip—which are of ball and socket design and thus have the least configurational stability. Energy conservation requires that the diameter of the extremities become smaller as one moves farther from the center of the body, so that bulky musculature can only exist close to

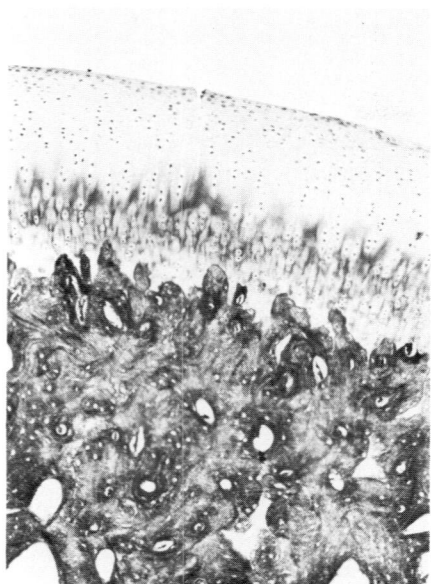

Fig. 8–9.   Photomicrograph of distal femur of an adult rabbit showing the subchondral bone. Note the relationship of the bone to the cartilage and the compact nature of the subchondral plate. The haversian canals appear to be parallel to the joint surface. (Masson trichrome, × 50)

the trunk. The wrist and foot cannot be totally surrounded by muscles as are the more centrally placed joints. Although muscles remain important in the stabilization of small joints, the configuration of the bone and the dense ligamentous interconnections of the wrist and foot play the major role in their stability.

The contribution of the joint capsule to joint stability has already been discussed. The capsular volume of joints varies considerably from joint to joint and also with position of the joint. Variations in intra-articular pressure (IAP) with joint position have been extensively studied by Eyring and Murray[32] and subsequently by Myers and Palmer.[84] The range of IAP in the knee varies from 5 cm of water at 15 to 60 degrees of flexion to 60 cm of water at full extension and full flexion. These authors have also found that there is a position for each joint where the intracapsular volume is potentially largest (for example, 30 degrees of knee flexion).[32] Joints with significant effusions are maintained in this position in order to maximize intracapsular volume and minimize IAP.

Ligamentous structures prevent the joint from subluxation or dislocation and act to constrain and guide joint motion.[12,41] Ligaments are variable in their architecture and are complicated not only in structure but in relationship to adjacent tissues. In

the fingers, ligaments are closely approximated to tendinous insertions. The collateral ligaments of the knee are constructed so that some portion of their fibers is under tension in all degrees of flexion. In combination with the cruciate ligaments, the collateral ligaments of the knee guide the complicated rolling and gliding motion of the distal femur on the proximal tibia (Fig. 8–1).[12,41]

Role of Articular Cartilage.   Articular cartilage represents the bearing surface of the joint and is structured to resist the repetitive rubbing and considerable deformation that this surface is subjected to over years. The cartilage matrix, for the most part, is composed of a systematically oriented fibrous network of collagen and highly charged proteoglycan molecules. The collagen fibers at the surface run parallel to the surface and act as a membrane holding the matrix together. The collagen fibers in the basilar region of the articular cartilage run vertically and actually connect the articular cartilage with its underlying calcified bone, preventing shear failure during joint motion. The fibers in the mid-zone of the cartilage appear to be randomly oriented, but when the cartilage is subjected to axial compression, the fibers tend to line up perpendicular to the compressive force (Fig. 8–10),[65] the most advantageous arrangement in resisting a compressive load. The lack of vessels in articular cartilage would appear to be of significant functional advantage. Under physiologic conditions, articular cartilage can be compressed to as much as 40% of its original height; if blood vessels traversed it, they would be rendered useless. On the basis of the diffusion rates in the tissue, and the metabolic requirement of the cells, Maroudas has calculated that the maximal thickness of the cartilage assuring chondrocyte viability is 6 mm.[74] Patellar cartilage, the thickest in the human body, is under 6 mm thick. Mechanical considerations clearly indicate that such thin layers have little meaningful roles as shock absorbers. The appearance of articular cartilage may belie its mechanical integrity. One must judge cartilage biochemically or mechanically in order not to be misled.[6,26]

The function of articular cartilage is that of a bearing and contact surface. If the articular cartilage is removed, the subchondral bony plates of the joint will not fit well. It is the relatively deformable articular cartilage that provides the largest possible surface contact area when force is applied to a joint.[50] Simon and colleagues have shown that cartilage thickness is related to the degree of underlying bony incongruity.[117] Cartilage thickness is maximal in joints that fit less well and thinnest in joints that are most congruous. Cartilage thickness appears to depend on physiologic and mechanical factors.[5] Articular cartilage acts to transmit load to

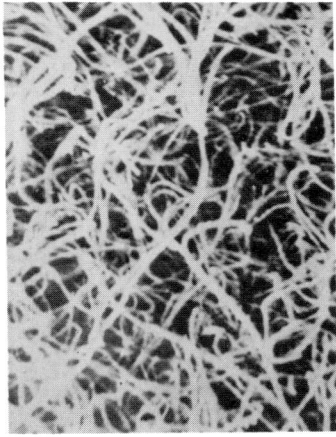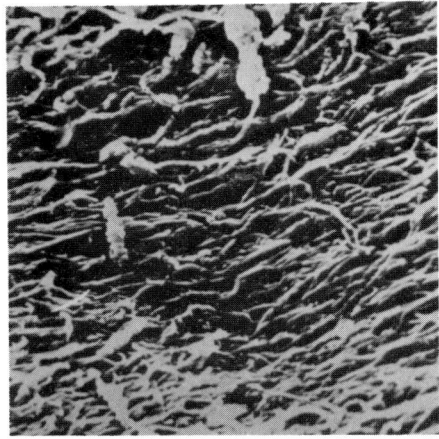

Fig. 8–10. On the left a scanning electron micrograph of the mid-zone collagen fibers of articular cartilage in the unloaded state. Note the essentially random orientation. The picture on the right is the same area of the cartilage with compressive load applied. Note how the fibers line up perpendicular to the load. (From McCall, J.[65])

the underlying bony bed, but does little to distribute that load.[100] In fact, it is the subchondral bone that deforms under physiologic load.[79] Joints must be slightly incongruous in the unloaded state[17] (Fig. 8–11), so that when they deform under load they will become congruous. Deformation of subchondral bone is important in achieving an effective

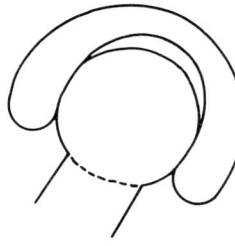

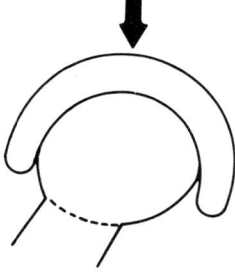

Fig. 8–11. Normally unloaded joints are not completely congruous; under load they become so. It is deformation of the articular cartilage and subchondral bone that allows maximal contact under load. The larger the contact under load the lower the force per unit area and the stress on these tissues. (From Radin, E.L., et al.[98])

distribution of stress within a joint. This deformation of the subchondral bone reults in a low-frequency, physiologically occurring, trabecular microfracture.[91] It has been suggested that microfractures of the interconnected plates of subchondral bone and the subsequent healing result in structural patterns that provide maximum strength.[96] The subchondral bone pattern accurately reflects the stress distribution within the joint. From the overall orientation of the trabecular pattern of a joint radiogram one can determine whether this pattern of stresses is normal or abnormal.[24] In cases of localization of stress, subchondral bone becomes sclerotic and dense (Fig. 8–12).

Role of Menisci. The sites of intra-articular fibrocartilages or menisci have already been mentioned. Analyses of the types of joint that contain menisci show that they are basically hinge joints that also rotate. In order to achieve this type of motion, the edges of the hinge are rounded off, and it is the menisci that fill the gap (Fig. 8–13).[97] Without these "washers," such joints would have fairly small central articular cartilage contact areas and would be less stable. The menisci bear load[33] and also act as shock absorbers by "barrelling."[115]

Joint Lubrication. The joint is lubricated by synovial fluid that contains hyaluronate, a large glycoprotein molecule whose average molecular weight is in excess of a million. It is this giant molecule that is responsible for the *"thixotropic"* flow characteristics of the synovial fluid (the more slowly it flows the more viscous it becomes). Based on the observations regarding the thixotropic character of the fluid, scientists originally concluded that joints were lubricated by a hydrodynamic system in which the fluid is held between the bearing

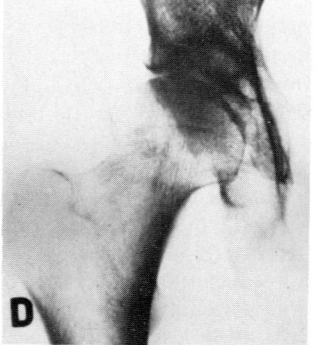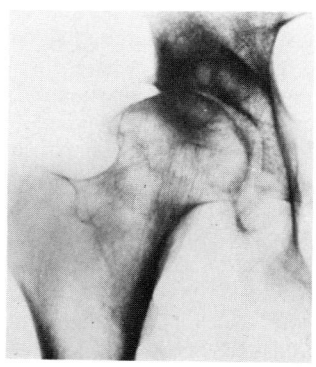

Fig. 8–12. Radiogram of an osteoarthritic hip that is beginning to sublux laterally. Note the condensation of bone at the lateral rim of the acetabulum and directly across from that area in the femoral head. Where stress is increased above normal, bone becomes sclerotic. If the stress is even greater, case cysts will form. Unloaded bone becomes relatively osteopenic.

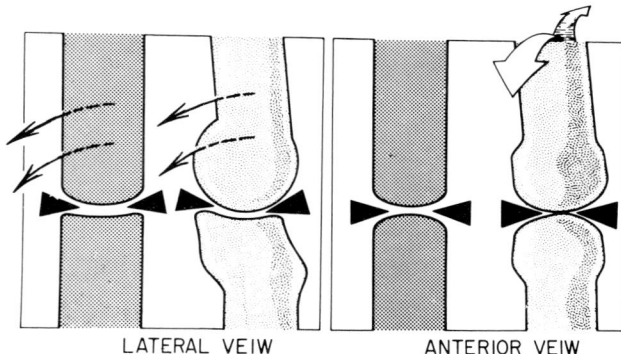

LATERAL VEIW   ANTERIOR VEIW

Fig. 8–13. The knee is a hinge with rounded off corners to allow rotation as well as flexion in extension. "Washers" are needed in such a design to maintain stability, particularly in full extension. (From Radin, E.L.[97])

surfaces by the continuing rotation of one part of the bearing. Joints are poorly suited to this form of lubrication, however, since they oscillate rather than rotate.[18] The finding that the coefficient of friction remains unchanged in joints lubricated with hyaluronidase-treated synovial fluid negated the hydrodynamic theory.[62]

The frictional resistance of animal joints lubricated with synovial fluid has been measured to be as low as .002, which is twice as low as that of rubber on steel and one-tenth that of an ice skate on ice.[99] Two hydrated cartilage surfaces under load are separated by a thin film of fluid under physiologic circumstances, and there is ample evidence that this fluid is water "squeezed" from the hyperhydrated cartilage.[66] Although the major part of water in cartilage is in the form of a proteoglycan-collagen gel,[72] it is freely exchangeable with synovial fluid, and a significant portion can be liberated by pressure on the cartilage.[27] Since in the adult there is little or no traverse of water through the subchondral plate or flow through the substance of the cartilage, the water displaced by cartilage compression is expressed onto the surface of the cartilage, preferentially peripheral to the zone of impending contact. Mow and Mansour have concluded that, under the most usual circumstances of

joint motion, water tends to be pushed out just in front of the contact area.[81] When the compression is released, the matrix within the cartilage contains enough of a fixed charge to osmotically attract the water and small solutes back into the matrix, and the cartilage regains its original height.[63] Thus the fluid film that exists between moving cartilage layers is made up of the cartilaginous interstitial fluid, which is squeezed onto the surface as the cartilage compresses the already present synovial fluid trapped in the contact zone. This mechanism of lubrication is referred to as *hydrostatic.*

The hydrostatic mechanism obviously functions best under substantial loads, since under small loads there would be little cartilage compression and little weeping of fluid onto the surface. Physiologically, however, joints frequently move under relatively light load. Under such circumstances a hydrostatic mechanism would not generate a substantial fluid film, particularly just at the moment motion begins. Thus it would be advantageous to have a second lubrication mechanism function primarily under these conditions. Such a mechanism exists, and it involves the binding of a special glycoprotein found in synovial fluid, *the lubricating glycoprotein,*[125] which is affixed to the cartilage surfaces and keeps them from touching, a mechanism referred to as *boundary lubrication*. Joints are thus lubricated by two complementary systems: a hydrostatic system, which functions primarily at high loads, and a boundary system, most effective at low loads.

Hyaluronate appears to have no place in cartilage-on-cartilage lubrication, but does play an important role as the boundary lubricant for synovial tissue.[124] Since the friction of cartilage rubbing on cartilage is so low, the preponderance of frictional resistance in joint movement is in the periarticular soft tissues, which also in most joints make up the bulk of the articulating area within the joint capsule (Fig. 8–14). Hyaluronate serves as a boundary lubricant in this system.[124]

INTERVERTEBRAL DISCS

General Structure

Intervertebral discs are fibrocartilaginous complexes that form the articulation between the bodies of two adjacent vertebrae. Motion between any two vertebral segments is limited to a few degrees in any plane by the configuration of the discal tissue and intervertebral facets, but the sum of the motion in the joints of the entire column provides the range necessary for the extraordinary mobility of the human spine. Discs from various regions of the spine (cervical, thoracic, and lumbar) vary in size and shape, but are basically identical in their organization.[19,20] Each consists of three components: the outer fibrous restraining band, the annulus fibrosus; the central semifluid mass, the nucleus pulposus; and the restraining superior and inferior sur-

faces, the vertebral cartilaginous plates (Fig. 8–15A, B).

The annulus fibrosus consists of a concentric ring of fibrous lamellae that encases the nucleus and unites the vertebral bodies by contiguity of the fibrous structure with the margin of vertebral segment and with the investing anterior and posterior longitudinal ligaments.[23,44] The fibrous layers of the annulus are approximately 20 μm thick and show an organization on polarized microscopic examination such that alternating sheets of collagen are set at an angle to each other.[48,86] Flexibility is achieved by random arrangement of the fibers (0.1 to 0.2 μm in diameter) within the substance of the plates of collagen and by a relatively high proportion of proteoglycan and interstitial fluid in the annulus as compared with the more rigid tendons or ligaments.[54] The annulus is not uniformly thick throughout the substance. The plates in the anterior third of the disc are stoutest and most distinct, whereas those in the posterior aspect are more closely packed and somewhat thinner.[90]

The second component of the disc is the nucleus pulposus, which occupies the central portion of the disc and is surrounded by the annulus. Actually, the nucleus is not centrally placed within the confines of the annulus, but usually lies closer to the posterior margin of the disc.[90] The nature of this material and its function in the joint is most evident when, on transverse or sagittal sectioning of the disc, it is found to bulge prominently beyond the plane of the section. The nucleus consists of a viscid fluid structure, which histologically is sparsely cellular and consists principally of loose delicate fibrous strands embedded in a gelatinous matrix.[12] In the central portion of the nucleus, the fibers appear randomly distributed, but as they approach the superior and inferior cartilage plates they assume an oblique angular orientation to become embedded in the cartilage at the peripheral attachment of the nucleus.[48,54,90] The structural interspace between the nucleus and the annulus is difficult to appreciate, and in many older subjects the two tissues blend imperceptibly.[23]

The disc is contained superiorly and inferiorly by cartilaginous plates, which are firmly fixed to the bony end-plates of the adjacent vertebral segments and differ little in structure from the hyaline articular cartilage seen in diarthrodial joints, except that they have no collagenous "skin," or indeed any discrete superficial surface.[23,90] Instead, the cartilage serves as an anchor for the fine filamented fibers of the nucleus pulposus in its central portion and the coarse fibrous plates of the annulus fibrosus peripherally.

JOINTS CONTAIN TWO

SYSTEMS WHICH REQUIRE

LUBRICATION

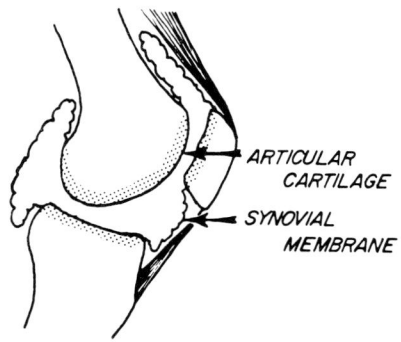

ARTICULAR CARTILAGE

SYNOVIAL MEMBRANE

Fig. 8–14. In most joints the surface area of synovium that rubs on itself and on articular cartilage is far greater than the area of the cartilage that rubs on cartilage. The synovium is redundant so that it will not interfere with joint motion.

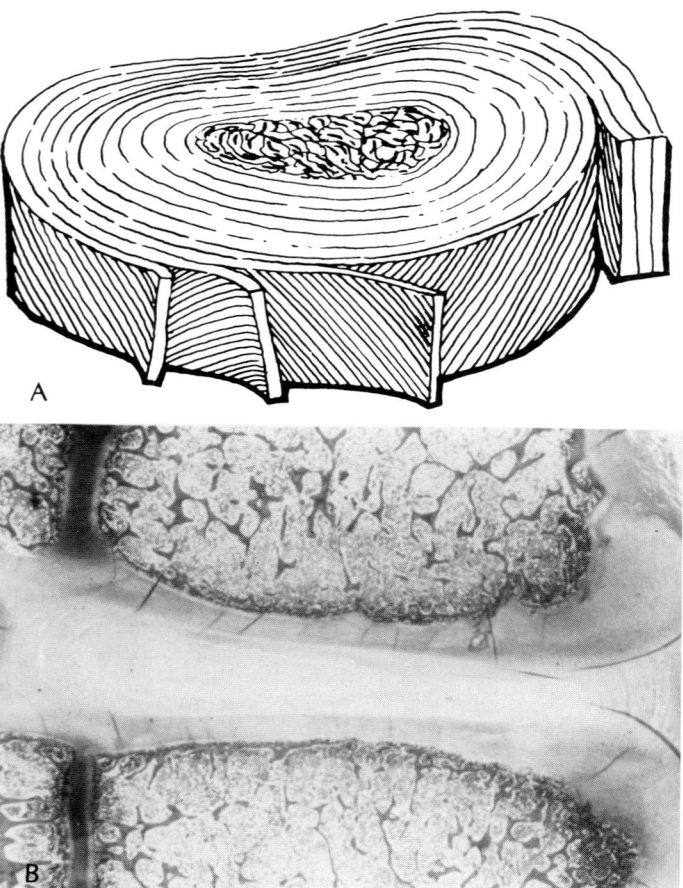

Fig. 8–15. *A,* Artist's concept of the structure of the intervertebral disc. Note that the concentric layers of the lamina fibrosa show varied orientation of collagen fibers. Centrally placed is the nucleus pulposus, a semifluid mass. *B,* Low-power photomicrograph of the intervertebral disc showing the cartilage plates covering the bony end plates of the vertebral segments. Circumferential rings of fibrous tissue comprise the lamina fibrosa, and in the center is a poorly staining material, the nucleus pulposus. (H & E, × 4)

Embryology and Development

The development of the intervertebral disc in man occurs early in fetal life. Following formation of the morula, the mass of primitive cells becomes the blastocyst, which rapidly undergoes proliferation and differentiation into ectoderm and endoderm, which in turn combine to form the embryonic disc.[114] A primitive streak develops at the caudal end of the dorsum of the embryonic disc. The groove deepens, and at the most caudal portion, the primitive node develops. At this site, cells arising from the mesoderm give rise to the notochord, which thickens and rolls up into the neural folds to form the neural tube.[129,130] The mesodermal tissues on each side of the notochord form the primitive somites, and at approximately the third week of gestation, distinct spinal segments can be iden-

tified. The central portions of the somite on either side of the notochord form the vertebral column, mesodermal cells from each side joining to form the vertebral bony elements, including not only the cartilaginous end-plates but the annulus fibrosus and the peripheral portions of the nucleus pulposus.[114] The notochord, which originally lies centrally placed in the vertebral body and disc, is compressed as chondrification of the vertebra progresses and within a short time is destroyed.[127] No notochordal remnants can be found in the vertebral body in the mature fetus or adult (except in an occasional patient who develops a chordoma). That portion of the notochord that lies in the intervertebral disc area, however, becomes the major central portion of the nucleus pulposus.[130] The annulus develops early in embryonic life from the densely aggregated cells about each pole of the somitic segment and eventually surrounds the notochord completely. Ossification begins in the vertebral body at the 50- to 60-mm stage (third month) as vessels invade the cartilaginous precursors, but the end-plates remain cartilaginous and serve as the attachment site for the adult nucleus pulposus and annulus fibrosus.[35]

Biochemistry

The annulus fibrosus is principally collagenous in structure, but is relatively hyperhydrated as compared with other fibrous tissues, with water estimates ranging between 65 and 70%.[86] Collagen accounts for approximately 50 to 55% of the dry weight. The remainder of the material consists of proteoglycan, the principal glycosaminoglycans, including chondroitin sulfate and keratan sulfate.[43] A small amount of glycoprotein is present.[92]

The nucleus has a much higher water content than the annulus, with estimates for immature animals ranging up to 88%. The value falls to about 65% in aged individuals.[86] Collagen is also present in the nucleus (mostly type II), but accounts for a considerably smaller percentage of the dry weight (20 to 30%) than in other joint connective tissues.[43,86] Most of the material within the nucleus consists of proteoglycan[43] and other as yet poorly defined proteinaceous materials.[92] The distribution of glycosaminoglycans varies considerably, depending on the age of the patient and the amount of degeneration that has occurred, but chondroitin 6-sulfate (approximately 40%), chondroitin 4-sulfate (5%), keratan sulfate (approximately 50%), and hyaluronic acid (<2%) have all been reported.[43] Pearson et al. have described the presence of other proteins, probably glycoproteins, which are believed to be important in maintaining the physical properties of the material.[92] Lysosomal enzymes have been described that presumably play a role in the normal turnover of the proteoglycans.[87] Synthetic activity takes place in the outer ring of cells of the nucleus.[122]

Function

Over the last several years, there have been several investigations by physicians and engineers in an attempt to define the functional behavior of the intervertebral disc.[51,73,85] It is evident that the unit serves as a load-bearing structure, and that the resistance to axial loading (compression) is mediated through the compressibility of the hyperhydrated nucleus which, with its surrounding envelope of annulus, resists and modifies pressures by ''barrelling'' (losing height while gaining in width).[13,51,85] The application of compressive force to the disc compresses the nucleus pulposus, which tends to push on the annulus fibrosus containing the nucleus. The annulus is designed to absorb most of the barrelling of the disc by stretching its collagen network. The disc should not be considered a separate unit, however, but an integral part of the intervertebral joint that includes the facet joints and the anterior and posterior longitudinal ligaments. All components acting together maintain the axial resistance to compression and stability of the spine.[73,128]

REFERENCES

1. Adkins, E.W.O., and Davies, D.V.: Absorption from the joint cavity. Q.J. Exp. Physiol., 30:147–154, 1940.
2. Akeson, W.H.: An experimental study of joint stiffness. J. Bone Joint Surg., 43A:1022–1034, 1961.
3. Akeson, W.H., Amiel, D., and LaViolette, D.: The connective tissue response to immobility: A study of chondroitin 4- and 6-sulfate and dermatan sulfate changes in periarticular connective tissue of control and immobilized knees of dogs. Clin. Orthop., 51:183–197, 1967.
4. Ali, S.Y., et al.: The degradation of cartilage matrix by an intracellular protease. Biochem. J., 93:611–618, 1964.
5. Armstrong, C.G., and Gardner, D.L.: Thickness and distribution of human femoral head articular cartilage. Ann. Rheum. Dis., 36:407–412, 1977.
6. Armstrong, C.B., and Mow, V.C.: Variations in the intrinsic mechanical properties of human articular cartilage with age, degeneration, and water content. J. Bone Joint Surg., 64A:88–94, 1982.
7. Barland, P., Novikoff, A.B., and Hamerman, D.: Electron microscopy of the human synovial membrane. J. Cell Biol., 14:207–220, 1962.
8. Barnett, C.H., Davies, D.V., and MacConnail, M.A.: Synovial Joints: Their Structure and Mechanics. Springfield, Illinois, Charles C Thomas, 1961.
9. Bayliss, M.T., et al.: Structure of proteoglycans from different layers of human articular cartilage. Biochem. J., 209:387–400, 1983.
10. Bollet, A.J., Bonner, W.M., and Nance, J.L.: The presence of hyaluronidase in various mammalian tissues. J. Biol. Chem., 238:3522–3527, 1963.
11. Bonner, W.M., et al.: Changes in the lipids of human articular cartilage with age. Arthritis Rheum., 18:461–473, 1975.
12. Brantigan, O.C., and Voshell, A.F.: Mechanics of ligaments and menisci of the knee joint. J. Bone Joint Surg., 23A:44–66, 1941.
13. Broberg, K.B.: On the mechanical behavior of the intervertebral discs. Spine, 8:151–165, 1983.
14. Brower, T.D., Akahoski, Y., and Orlic, P.: Diffusion of dyes through articular cartilage in vivo. J. Bone Joint Surg., 44A:456–463, 1962.
15. Browne, K., Lee, J., and Ring, P.A.: The sensation of passive movement at the metatarso-phalangeal joint of the great toe in man. J. Physiol., 126:448–458, 1954.
16. Bullough, P.G., et al.: The strength of the menisci of the knee as it relates to their fine structure. J. Bone Joint Surg., 52B:564–570, 1970.
17. Bullough, P., Goodfellow, J., and O'Connor, J.: The relationship between degenerative changes and load-bearing in the human hip. J. Bone Joint Surg., 55:746–758, 1973.
18. Charnley, J.: Symposium on Biomechanics. London, Institute of Mechanical Engineering, 1969.
19. Clark, I.C.: Human articular surface contours and related surface depression frequency studies. Ann. Rheum. Dis., 20:15–23, 1971.
20. Clark, I.C.: Surface characteristics of human articular cartilage—a scanning electron microscope study. J. Anat., 108:23–30, 1971.
21. Clemmensen, I., et al.: Demonstration of fibronectin in human articular cartilage by an indirect immunoperoxidase technique. Histochem. J., 76:51–56, 1982.
22. Cooper, R.P., and Misol, S.: Alterations during immo-

bilization and regeneration of skeletal muscle in cats. J. Bone Joint Surg., 52A:919–953, 1972.

23. Coventry, M.B.: Anatomy of the invertebral disc. Clin. Orthrop., 67:9–15, 1969.
24. Davies, D.V., and Edwards, D.A.W.: Blood supply of synovial membrane and intraarticular structures. Ann. Coll. Surg. Engl., 2:142–156, 1948.
25. Dingle, J.T.: Catabolin—a cartilage catabolic factor from synovium. Clin. Orthop., 156:219–231, 1980.
26. Donohue, J.M., et al.: The effects of indirect blunt trauma on adult canine articular cartilage. J. Bone Joint Surg., 65A:948–957, 1983.
27. Edwards, J.: Lubrication and Wear in Living and Artificial Human Joints. London, Institute of Mechanical Engineering, 1967.
28. Ehrlich, M.G., et al.: Collagenase inhibitors in osteoarthritic and normal cartilage. J. Clin. Invest., 59:226–233, 1977.
29. Ekholm, R.: Articular cartilage nutrition; how radioactive gold reaches cartilage in rabbit knee joints. Acta Anat. (Suppl. 15), 1–76, 1951.
30. Elliott, R.J., and Gardner, D.L.: Changes with age in the glycosaminoglycans of human articular cartilage. Ann. Rheum. Dis., 38:371–377, 1979.
31. Enneking, W.F., and Horowitz, M.: The intraarticular effects of immobilization on the human knee. J. Bone Joint Surg., 54A:973–985, 1972.
32. Eyring, E.J., and Murray, W.R.: The effect of joint position on the pressure of intraarticular effusion. J. Bone Joint Surg., 46A:1235–1241, 1964.
33. Fairbank, T.J.: Knee joint changes after meniscectomy. J. Bone Joint Surg., 30B:664–670, 1948.
34. Fawns, H.T., and Landells, I.W.: Histological studies of rheumatic conditions. I. Observations on the fine structure of the matrix of normal bone and cartilage. Ann. Rheum. Dis., 12:105–113, 1953.
35. Gardner, E.: The development and growth of bones. J. Bone Joint Surg., 45A:856–862, 1963.
36. Gardner, E.: The physiology of joints. J. Bone Joint Surg., 45A:1061–1066, 1963.
37. Gardner, E.: Physiology of movable joints. Physiol. Rev., 30:127–176, 1950.
38. Gardner, E.: Innervation of the knee joint. Anat. Rec., 101:109–130, 1948.
39. Gardner, E., and O'Rahilly, R.: The early development of the knee joint in staged human embryos. J. Anat., 102:289–299, 1968.
40. Ghadially, F.N., and Roy, S.: Ultrastructure of Synovial Joints in Health and Disease. London, Butterworth, 1969.
41. Girges, F.G., Marshall, J.L., and Monajem, A.: The cruciate ligaments of the knee joint. Clin. Orthop., 106:216–231, 1975.
42. Goldwasser, M., et al.: Analysis of the type of collagen present in osteoarthritic human cartilage. Clin. Orthop., 167:296–302, 1982.
43. Gower, W.E., and Pedrini, F.: Age related variations in protein polysaccharides from human nucleus pulposus, annulus fibrosus, and costal cartilage. J. Bone Joint Surg., 51A:1154–1162, 1969.
44. Gray, H.: Anatomy of the Human Body, 29th ed. Edited by C.M. Goss. Philadelphia, Lea & Febiger, 1973.
45. Green, W.T., Jr., et al.: Microradiographic study of the calcified layer of articular cartilage. Arch. Pathol., 90:151–158, 1970.
46. Haines, R.W.: The development of joints. J. Anat., 81:33–55, 1947.
47. Hamerman, D., Rosenberg, L.D., and Schubert, M.: Diarthrodial joints revisited. J. Bone Joint Surg., 52A:725–774, 1970.
48. Happey, F., et al.: Preliminary observation concerning the fine structure of the intervertebral disc. J. Bone Joint Surg., 46B:563–567, 1964.
49. Hardingham, T.E., and Muir, H.: Hyaluronic acid in cartilage. Biochem. Soc. Trans., 1:282–284, 1973.
50. Hayes, W.C., and Mockros, L.F.: Viscoelastic properties of human articular cartilage. J. Appl. Physiol., 31:462–568, 1971.
51. Hirsch, C., and Nachemson, A.: New observations on

mechanical behavior of lumbar discs. Acta Orthop. Scand., 23:254–283, 1954.
52. Hui-chou, C.S., and Lust, G.: The type of collagen made by the articular cartilage in joints of dogs with degenerative joint disease. Coll. Relat. Res., 2:245–256, 1982.
53. Inman, V.T.: Functional aspects of the abductor muscles of the hip. J. Bone Joint Surg., 29:607–619, 1947.
54. Inoue, H., and Tetsuaki, T.: Three dimensional observation of collagen framework of lumbar intervertebral discs. Acta Orthop. Scand., 46:949–956, 1975.
55. Jubb, R.W., and Fell, H.B.: The effect of synovial tissue on the synthesis of proteoglycan by the articular cartilage of young pigs. Arthritis Rheum., 23:545–555, 1980.
56. Kellgren, J.A., and Samuel, E.P.: The sensitivity and innervation of the articular capsule. J. Bone Joint Surg., 32B:84–92, 1950.
57. Kennedy, J.C., Weinberg, H.W., and Wilson, A.S.: The anatomy and function of the anterior cruciate ligament. J. Bone Joint Surg., 56A:223–235, 1974.
58. Kuettner, K.E., Eisenstein, R., and Sorgente, N.: Lysozyme in calcifying tissues. Clin. Orthop., 112:316–339, 1975.
59. Lane, J.M., and Weiss, C.: Current comment: Review of articular cartilage collagen research. Arthritis Rheum., 18:553–562, 1975.
60. Lehtonen, A., Viljanto, J., and Karkkainen, J.: The mucopolysaccharides of herniated human invertebral discs and semilunar cartilages. Acta Chir. Scand., 133:303–306, 1967.
61. Lever, J.D., and Ford, E.H.R.: Histological, histochemical and electron microscopic observations on synovial membrane. Anat. Rec., 132:525–539, 1958.
62. Linn, F.C., and Radin, E.L.: Lubrication of animal joints. III. The effect of certain chemical alterations of the cartilage and lubricant. Arthritis Rheum., 11:674–682, 1968.
63. Linn, F.C., and Sokoloff, L.: Movement and composition of interstitial fluid of cartilage. Arthritis Rheum., 8:481–493, 1965.
64. Lippiello, L., Hall, D., and Mankin, H.J.: Collagen synthesis in normal and osteoarthritic human cartilage. J. Clin. Invest., 59:593–600, 1977.
65. McCall, J.: In Lubrication and Wear in Joints. Edited by V. Wright. London, Sector Publ. Ltd., 1969.
66. McCutchen, C.W.: Mechanism of animal joints. Nature, 184:1284–1285, 1959.
67. McKibben, B., and Holdsworth, F.S.: The nutrition of immature joint cartilage in the lamb. J. Bone Joint Surg., 48B:793–803, 1966.
68. Mankin, H.J.: The metabolism of articular cartilage in health and disease. In Dynamics of Connective Tissue Macromolecules. Edited by P.M.C. Burleigh, and A.R. Poole. New York, American Elsevier Publishing Co., Inc., 1975, pp. 327–353.
69. Mankin, H.J.: The reaction of articular cartilage to injury and osteoarthritis. N. Engl. J. Med., 291:1285–1292; 1335–1340, 1974.
70. Mankin, H.J.: The reaction of articular cartilage to injury and osteoarthritis. N. Engl. J. Med., 291:1335–1340, 1974.
70a. Clemmensen, I., et al.: Demonstration of fibronectin in human articular cartilage by an indirect immunoperoxidase technique. Histochemistry, 76:51–56, 1982.
71. Mankin, H.J., and Lippiello, L.: The turnover of adult rabbit articular cartilage. J. Bone Joint Surg., 51A:1591–1600, 1969.
72. Mankin, H.J., and Thrasher, A.Z.: Water content and binding in normal and osteoarthritic human cartilage. J. Bone Joint Surg., 57A:76–80, 1975.
73. Markolf, K.L.: Deformation of the thoracolumbar intervertebral joints in response to external loads. J. Bone Joint Surg., 54A:511–533, 1972.
74. Maroudas, A.: Distribution and diffusion of solutes in articular cartilage. Biophys. J., 10:365–379, 1970.
75. Meachim, G.: Effect of age on the thickness of adult articular cartilage at the shoulder joint. Ann. Rheum. Dis., 30:43–46, 1971.
76. Miles, J.S., and Eichelberger, L.: Biochemical studies of

human cartilage during the aging process. J. Am. Geriatr. Soc., *12*:1–20, 1964.
77. Miller, E.J.: A review of biochemical studies in the genetically distinct collagens of the skeletal system. Clin. Orthop., *92*:260–280, 1973.
78. Miller, E.J., and Matukas, V.J.: Chick cartilage collagen: A new type of chain not present in bone or skin of the species. Proc. Natl. Acad. Sci. U.S.A., *64*:1264–1268, 1969.
79. Mital, M.A.: Human Hip Joints. M.S. Thesis. Glasgow University Strathclyde, 1970.
80. Morales, T.I., and Kuettner, K.: The properties of the neutral proteinase released by primary chondrocyte cultures and its action on proteoglycan aggregate. Biochim. Biophys. Acta, *705*:92–101, 1982.
81. Mow, V.C., and Mansour, J.M.: The nonlinear interaction between cartilage deformation and interstitial fluid flow. J. Biomech., *10*:31–39, 1977.
82. Muir, I.H.M.: Biochemistry. *In* Adult Articular Cartilage. Edited by M.A.R. Freeman. New York, Grune and Stratton, 1973, pp. 100–131.
83. Muir, H., and Hardingham, T.E.: Structures of proteoglycans. *In* MTP International Review of Science. Biochemistry Series One, Vol. 5: Biochemistry of Carbohydrates. Edited by W.J. Whelan. Baltimore, University Park Press, 1975, pp. 153–222.
84. Myers, D.B., and Palmer, D.G.: Capsular compliance and pressure-volume relationhips in normal and arthritic knees. J. Bone Joint Surg., *54B*:710–716, 1972.
85. Nachemson, A., and Morris, J.M.: In vivo measurements of intradiscal pressure. J. Bone Joint Surg., *46A*:1077–1092, 1964.
86. Naylor, A.: The biochemical changes in the human intervertebral disc in degeneration and nuclear prolapse. Orthop. Clin. North Am., *2*:343–358, 1971.
87. Naylor, A., et al.: Enzymatic and immunological activity in the invertebral disc. Orthop. Clin. North Am., *6*:51–58, 1975.
88. Noyes, F.R., et al.: Biomechanics of ligament failure. J. Bone Joint Surg., *56A*:1406–1418, 1974.
89. O'Rahilly, R., and Gardner, E.: The development of the knee joint of the chick and its correlation with embryonic staging. J. Morphol., *98*:49–88, 1956.
90. Parke, W.W., and Schiff, D.C.M.: The applied anatomy of the invertebral disc. Orthop. Clin. North Am., *2*:309–324, 1971.
91. Pauwels, F.: *In* Atlas of the Biomechanics of the Normal and Abnormal Hip. New York, Springer Verlag, 1976.
92. Pearson, C.H., et al.: The non-collagenous proteins of the human intervertebral disc. Gerontologie, *15*:189–202, 1969.
93. Pelletier, J.P., et al.: Collagenase and collagenolytic activity in human osteoarthritic cartilage. Arthritis Rheum., *26*:63–68, 1983.
94. Peters, T.J., and Smillie, I.S.: Studies on the chemical composition of the menisci of the knee joint with special reference to the horizontal cleavage lesion. Clin. Orthop., *86*:245–252, 1972.
95. Peterson, H.A., Winkelmann, R.K., and Coventry, M.B.: Nerve endings in the hip joint of the cat: Their morphology, distribution and density. J. Bone Joint Surg., *54A*:333–343, 1972.
96. Pugh, J.W., Rose, R.M., and Radin, E.L.: A possible mechanism of Wolff's law: Trabecular microfractures. Arch. Int. Physiol. Biochim., *81*:27–40, 1973.
97. Radin, E.L.: Biomechanics of the knee joint. Orthop. Clin. North Am., *4*:539–546, 1973.
98. Radin, E.L., et al.: The mechanics of joints as it relates to their degeneration. *In* American Academy of Orthopaedic Surgeons: Symposium on Osteoarthritis. St. Louis, The C.V. Mosby Co., 1976.
99. Radin, E.L., and Paul, I.L.: Response of joints to impact loading. I. In vitro wear. Arthritis Rheum., *14*:356–362, 1971.
100. Radin, E.L., and Paul, I.L.: Does cartilage compliance reduce skeletal impact loads? The relative force—attenuating properties of articular cartilages, synovial fluid, periarticular soft tissues and bone. Arthritis Rheum., *13*:139–144, 1970.
101. Radin, E.L., Paul, I.L., and Lowy, M.: A comparison of the dynamic force transmitting properties of subchondral bone and articular cartilage. J. Bone Joint Surg., *52A*:444–456, 1970.
102. Radin, E.L., Swann, D.A., and Weisser, P.: Separation of a hyaluronate free lubricating fraction from synovial fluid. Nature, *288*:377–378, 1970.
103. Ralston, H.J., III, Miller, M.R., and Kasahara, M.: Nerve endings in human fasciae, tendons, ligaments, periosteum, and joint synovial membrane. Anat. Rec., *136*:137–147, 1960.
104. Redler, I., et al.: The ultrastructure and biochemical significance of the tidemark of articular cartilage. Clin. Orthop., *112*:357–362, 1975.
105. Redler, I., and Zimny, M.L.: Scanning electron microscopy of normal and abnormal articular cartilage and synovium. J. Bone Joint Surg., *52A*:1395–1404, 1970.
106. Repo, R.U., and Mitchell, N.: Collagen synthesis in mature articular cartilage of the rabbit. J. Bone Joint Surg., *53B*:541–548, 1971.
107. Roden, L., and Schwartz, N.B.: Biosynthesis of connective tissue proteoglycans. *In* MTP International Review of Science, Biochemistry Series. Vol. 5: Biochemistry of Carbohydrates. Edited by W.J. Whelan. Baltimore, University Park Press, 1975, pp. 95–152.
108. Rosenberg, L.: Structure of cartilage proteoglycan. *In* Dynamics of Connective Tissue Macromolecules. Edited by P.M.C. Burleigh, and A.R. Poole. New York, American Elsevier Publishing Co., Inc., 1975, pp. 105–128.
109. Rosenberg, L., Hellman, W., and Kleinschmidt, A.K.: Electron microscopic studies of proteoglycan aggregates from bovine articular cartilage. J. Biol. Chem., *250*:1877–1883, 1975.
110. Rothman, R.H., Marvel, J.P., Jr., and Heppenstall, R.B.: Anatomic considerations in the glenohumeral joint. Orthop. Clin. North Am., *6*:341–352, 1975.
111. Sapolsky, A.I., et al.: The action of cathepsin D in human articular cartilage on proteoglycans. J. Clin. Invest., *52*:624–633, 1973.
112. Sapolsky, A.I., and Howell, D.S.: Further characterization of a neutral metalloprotease isolated from human articular cartilage. Arthritis Rheum., *25*:981–988, 1982.
113. Saposky, A.I., Howell, D.S., and Woessner, J.F., Jr.: Neutral proteinases and cathepsin D in human articular cartilage. J. Clin. Invest., *53*:1044–1053, 1974.
114. Sherk, H.H., and Nicholson, J.T.: Comparative anatomy and embryology of the cervical spine. Orthop. Clin. North Am., *2*:325–341, 1971.
115. Shrive, N.G., O'Connor, J.J., and Goodfellow, J.W.: Load-bearing in the knee joint. Clin. Orthop., *131*:279–287, 1978.
116. Simon, W.H.: Scale effects in animal joints. I. Articular cartilage thickness and compressive stress. Arthritis Rheum., *13*:244–256, 1970.
117. Simon, W.H., Friedenberg, S., and Richardson, S.: Joint congruence. A correlation of joint congruence and thickness of articular cartilage in dogs. J. Bone Joint Surg., *55A*:1614–1620, 1973.
118. Simon, S.R., et al.: Peak dynamic force in human gait. J. Biomech., *14*:817–822, 1981.
119. Sledge, C.B.: Some morphologic and experimental aspects of limb development. Clin. Orthop., *44*:241–264, 1966.
120. Sledge, C.B., and Dingle, J.T.: Activation of lysosomes by oxygen. Nature, *205*:140–141, 1965.
121. Solheim, K.: The glycosaminoglycans of human semilunar cartilage. J. Oslo City Hosp., *15*:127–132, 1965.
122. Souter, W., and Taylor, T.K.F.: Sulphated acid mucopolysaccharide metabolism in the rabbit intervertebral disc. J. Bone Joint Surg., *52B*:371–384, 1970.
123. Stockwell, R.A., and Meachim, G.: The chondrocytes. *In* Adult Articular Cartilage. Edited by M.A.R. Freeman. New York, Grune and Stratton, 1973, pp. 51–99.
124. Swann, D.A., et al.: Role of hyaluronic acid in joint lubrication. Ann. Rheum. Dis., *33*:318–326, 1974.
125. Swann, D.A., and Radin, E.L.: The molecular basis of

articular lubrication. I. Purification and properties of a lubricating fraction from bovine synovial fluid. J. Biol. Chem., *274*:8069–8083, 1972.

126. Van Der Korst, J.K., Sokoloff, L., and Miller, E.J.: Senescent pigmentation of cartilage and degenerative joint disease. Arch. Pathol., *86*:40–46, 1968.

127. Weiss, C., Rosenberg, L., and Helft, A.J.: An ultrastructural study of normal young adult human articular cartilage. J. Bone Joint Surg., *50A*:663–674, 1968.

128. White, A.A., III, and Gordon, S.L.: Synopsis: Workshop on Idiopathic Low-back Pain. Spine, *7*:141–149.

129. Willis, T.A.: The phylogeny of the intervertebral disk: A pictorial review. Clin. Orthop., *54*:215–233, 1967.

130. Wolfe, H.J., Putschar, W.G.J., and Vickery, A.L.: Role of the notochord in human intervertebral disk. I. Fetus and infant. Clin. Orthop., *39*:205–212, 1965.

Chapter 9

Synovial Physiology

Peter A. Simkin

Synovial joints are the bearings through which the human machine accomplishes its work. Surrounding tissues help to maintain, support, and renew these complex living bearings throughout the lifetime of the individual. Principal among these tissues is the synovium, which supports the normal joint in at least three important physiologic ways: it provides an unobtrusive, low-friction lining; it transports needed nutrients into the joint space while it removes metabolic wastes; and it plays an important role in maintaining joint stability. These physiologic functions in health and their alterations in disease are reviewed here. A fourth important role is to produce and to dispense the biologic lubricants discussed in Chapter 8.

SYNOVIAL LINING

Since motion is the business of joints, the synovial lining must be able to adapt to the full range of positions permitted by the surrounding tendons, ligaments, and joint capsule. As a finger flexes, for instance, the palmar synovium of each interphalangeal joint contracts while the dorsal synovium expands. As the finger re-extends, the roles are reversed (Fig. 9–1). This expansion and contraction of synovium appear more consistent with an accordion-like process of folding and unfolding than with an elastic stretching of the tissue.

Most expansion and contraction of the synovium take place over unopposed surfaces of articular cartilage. For any joint to flex or extend, there must be a disparity in the surface areas of opposing cartilages. When the joint moves, the smaller area glides across or around the larger. Cartilage not in contact with opposing cartilage is temporarily covered by synovium as, for example, are the knuckles of a clenched fist. As the cartilage surfaces move upon each other to return to their initial position, an effective lubrication system must prevent pinching of the adjacent, vascular synovial tissue. Were this system to fail, repeated hemarthroses would prove rapidly incapacitating. This lubrication problem has not received the attention devoted to that of cartilage on cartilage. Swann et al. have suggested, however, that the hyaluronate molecules that render synovial fluid viscous may find their major physiologic role in lubricating the synovium.[38]

The well-lubricated synovium must expand and contract within the confines of the joint capsule. The process is easier when the volume of synovial tissue is at a minimum and is impeded when the volume is excessive. The cellular infiltration, hyperplasia, and edema of active synovitis may thus limit joint motion when the synovium gathers as a mass lesion. This problem seems likely to be most acute in full flexion, since the capsule of "hinge" joints is normally thicker on the flexor surface, and compression of extracapsular soft tissue further compromises the available space. In addition to its effect on range of motion, this process may also contribute to the stiffness of many arthritic patients.

Studies of relaxed metacarpophalangeal joints undergoing passive manipulation have found that increased stiffness is readily demonstrable in the hands of patients with rheumatoid arthritis and that this stiffness is greater in flexion than in extension.[1,43] Stiffness in normal joints is a complex phenomenon influenced by the time of day, varying inversely with grip strength and temperature, increasing progressively with age, occurring to a greater degree in men than in women, and affected by muscles, tendons, and other periarticular structures as well as by the capsule and synovium.[37] In the more severe stiffness characteristic of rheumatoid arthritis, the typical morning pattern suggests that tissue edema develops during periods of rest and then partially resolves with activity. The sensation of stiffness presumably results when redundant, edematous tissue interferes with free use of the joint.

SYNOVIAL TRANSPORT

In their classic studies of synovial effusions, Ropes and Bauer likened the synovial fluid to a dialysate of plasma.[30] They found a wide assortment of electrolytes and small molecules in the effusions at concentrations equivalent to those of plasma. The dialysate concept adequately explained the relative exclusion of most proteins in the presence of full equilibration of smaller molecules. Only hyaluronate, which is locally synthe-

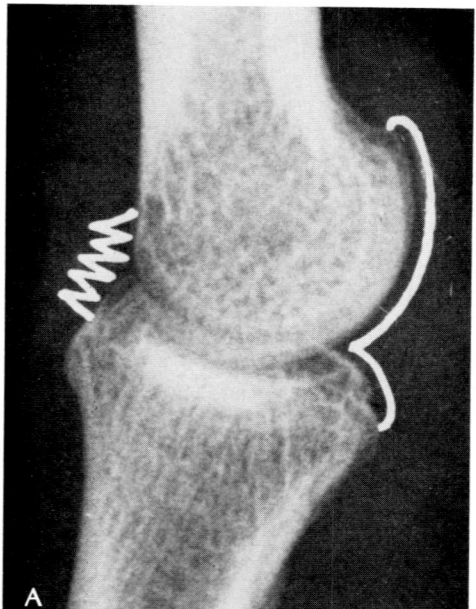

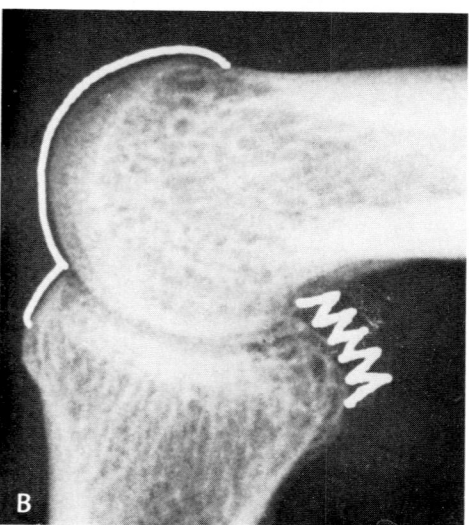

Fig. 9–1. Lateral views of an interphalangeal joint in extension (*A*) and in flexion (*B*). The greater surface area of proximal articular cartilage permits the distal bone to move around the proximal. Redundant synovium (shown schematically) gathers above the superior margin in extension and below the inferior margin during flexion.

sized by synovial cells, departed significantly from this pattern.

This model, however, is too simple to fairly reflect the problem of synovial permeability. The synovium is not a single inert membrane, but a complex living tissue (Fig. 9–2). As Bauer et al. also noted, transfer across the synovium "neces-

sitates passage through an endothelial wall as well as diffusion through the intercellular spaces of the synovial membrane."[3] They were thus well aware that synovial permeability includes and implies both of these barriers, but they were unable to dissect the individual contributions of the endothelium and the interstitium.

The importance of considering these barriers separately may be illustrated by the "increased vascular permeability," regarded as a hallmark of inflammation. In this phenomenon, the inflamed endothelium is thought to leak an excessive amount of protein into the interstitium. If this excess is not cleared by a comparable increase in the rate of lymphatic clearance, the extravascular concentration of protein will rise toward the plasma level. The necessary result will be a progressive diminution in the colloid osmotic pressure gradient between the two spaces. Since it is this pressure gradient that drives venular reabsorption of water, increased vascular permeability leads to edema in tissues and to effusions in joints. These principles reflect the Starling-Landis hypothesis of microvascular function and underscore the importance of the endothelium in retaining plasma proteins.[18]

It would be wrong, however, to infer that increased microvascular permeability to proteins necessarily means a significant increase in synovial permeability to smaller molecules as well. Small solutes normally cross the endothelium not only through the "large pores" available to proteins but also through a more abundant and highly permeable "small pore" system that excludes all large molecules. After leaving the microvessels, all molecules large and small must still traverse the synovial interstitium before they enter the synovial fluid. It is this tissue space, rather than the endothelium, which appears to be the most important limiting factor controlling the overall transynovial exchange of small molecules. This functional duality (proteins limited by endothelium-small solutes limited by interstitium) permits independent changes in synovial permeability to large and to small solutes.

Small Molecules

Small physiologic molecules (those less than 10,000 daltons in molecular weight) are usually in full equilibration between plasma and synovial fluid. To study the mechanism of their transynovial exchange, one must disturb this equilibrium and then measure and interpret the kinetics of the re-equilibration process. This may be done in a number of ways.

A series of experiments in normal human knees provided the best evidence examining the normal process of transynovial exchange and supporting the critical importance of interstitial diffusion.[35] In

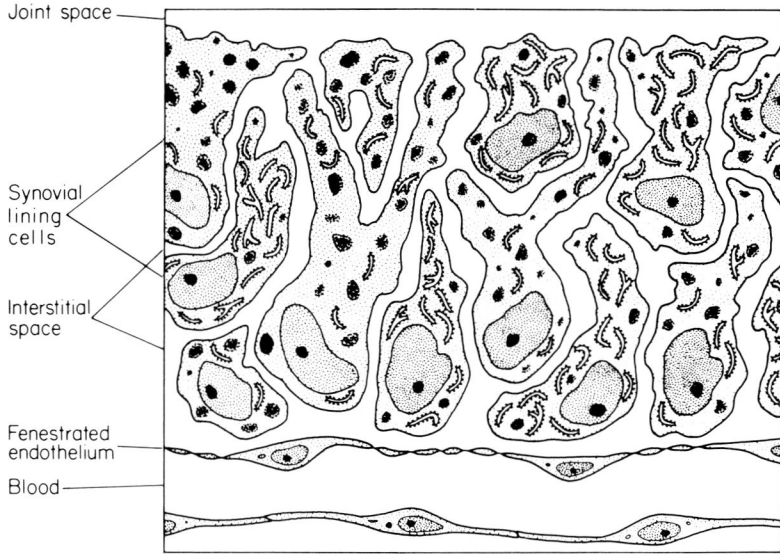

Fig. 9–2. The synovium. Molecules entering or leaving the joint space must traverse both the microvascular endothelium and the interstitial space between synovial cells. The endothelium provides the principal barrier limiting synovial permeability to proteins. The permeability of smaller molecules appears to be limited chiefly by their diffusibility across the synovial interstitium.

this model, the knee was injected with saline containing trace amounts of tritiated water, benzyl alcohol, and ^{14}C-labeled urea, urate, glucose, or sucrose. Serial samples of intrasynovial saline were then removed and assayed for those exogenous tracer compounds as well as for endogenous urea, urate, glucose, creatinine, and total protein moving from plasma into the saline. Over the course of the experiment, the concentration of endogenous molecules progressively rose toward full equilibration with plasma levels, while the concentration of exogenous molecules fell toward zero as they were cleared from the joint space. In a kinetic analysis of these data, the Fick diffusion equation permitted calculation of permeability values for each solute at the midpoint of every experiment. These experimental values, analogous to renal clearances, may be considered as the volume of intrasynovial saline equilibrating with plasma per unit time (ml/min).

For most small compounds, synovial permeability is inversely related to the dimensions of the molecule. Thus, a plot of observed synovial permeability versus diffusion coefficient (which reflects configuration as well as size) yields a rather linear function (Fig. 9–3). This proportionality suggests that most small molecules cross the synovium by a process of free diffusion. Further analysis indicates that the limiting diffusion path is relatively long and narrow. These dimensions seem most consistent with those of the narrow channels between synovial lining cells. It thus appears that synovial

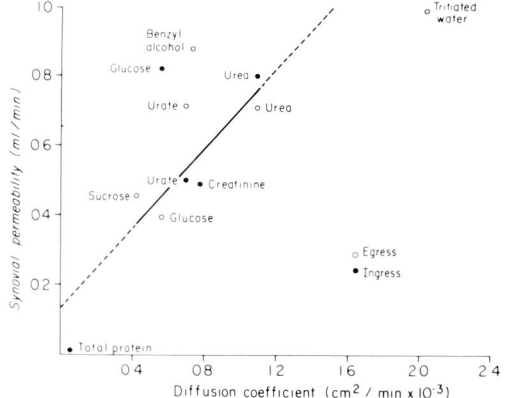

Fig. 9–3. Synovial permeability in normal, resting knees. The permeability is plotted against the diffusion coefficient. Egress and ingress are with respect to the joint space. Most data points are the mean values from 25 studies, but egress values for sucrose, glucose, urate, and urea are based on 7, 6, 6, and 6 studies, respectively. Benzyl alcohol leaving and glucose entering the joint space move rapidly because of diffusion into cells and specific transport, respectively. Protein enters slowly because of endothelial pore size limitation. Tritiated water leaves more slowly than predicted by its diffusion coefficient, probably because its egress is limited by effective synovial blood flow. All other small molecules (sucrose, urea, urate, creatinine, and glucose leaving the joint) cross the synovium at rates inversely proportional to their size as predicted by diffusion kinetics.

permeability to most small molecules is determined by a process of free diffusion, limited mainly by the intercellular spaces of the synovium (see Fig. 9–2).

Additional evidence supporting this concept has been found in a high correlation between permeability and intrasynovial volume. Distention of the joint space accelerates the transynovial exchange of all small molecules. This relationship is best explained by the probability that distention increases intercellular distances, thus facilitating the diffusion process. The positive correlation between volume and permeability provides an interesting teleologic explanation for synovial effusions since the presence of an effusion enhances the delivery of nutrients to and the removal of wastes from the perturbed joint. In addition, these observations indicate that the intrasynovial volume should be known and considered in any comparative study of synovial permeabilities.

A more recent evaluation of these and other data employed a different analysis to reach the same interpretation of the synovium as a double barrier between plasma and synovial fluid. Once again, the microvascular endothelium was believed to be most critical for proteins, and the synovial interstitium was considered to be more important in determining the exchange of small solutes.[19]

In the aforementioned studies, the bidirectional permeability of urate ions was symmetrical and consistent with simple diffusion kinetics. Dick and his associates have evidence, however, that egress of other anions from the joint space may be facilitated by a specific transport system. In their experiments, potassium perchlorate inhibited clearance of ^{99m}Tc and ^{131}I from dog stifle joints[6] and ^{99m}Tc from human knees.[15] These observations are of interest, since effective active export of halide ions would be followed passively by sodium ions and by water. Such a system would thus be a "pump" capable of moving water out of the joint space.

Several other investigators have also studied the removal of ionic sodium and iodine from human knees.[34] The radioactive ions ^{24}Na and ^{131}I emit gamma rays that readily pass through human soft tissues. A counter placed over the joint is thus able to continuously monitor the disappearance of these isotopes after their intra-articular injection. These tracings characteristically follow a simple exponential pattern, which may be usefully expressed as either a half-life value or a clearance constant. In different series of normal knees, mean clearance constants for ^{24}Na have ranged from 0.022 to 0.051 min^{-1}, while similar determinations for ^{131}I have been from 0.022 to 0.055 min^{-1}. These isotopes are thought to leave the knee by way of the blood,

an interpretation strongly supported by the work of Scholer et al.,[32] who injected knees with D_2O and either ^{22}Na or ^{24}Na, followed the appearance of these isotopes in serial samples of arterial blood, and from these data calculated clearance constants in the same range as those obtained by external counting over the joint. In addition, clearance of ^{24}Na from the knee was markedly reduced when Harris and Millard inflated a tourniquet around the thigh to 60 mm Hg, and was eliminated when they raised the pressure to 200 mm Hg.[12] These findings demonstrate that isotopic clearance depends on an effective circulation and that diffusion into adjacent tissues plays no meaningful role.

The same isotopic clearance technique has been applied to the study of patients with joint diseases. Both in degenerative joint disease and in rheumatoid arthritis there is highly variable but consistently significant (up to three-fold) increase above normal rates for the disappearance of both ^{24}Na and ^{131}I. The intrasynovial volume was not determined in these experiments, but clinical impressions suggested a positive correlation between effusion size and isotopic clearance rate. Intra-articular steroids caused a diminished clearance in a few individuals. In summary, these investigators found that isotopic clearance correlated well with clinical signs of synovial inflammation. They attributed this finding to an enhanced synovial blood flow in active synovitis.

Clinical physiologists have long been interested in accurate determinations of the synovial blood flow. The vascular supply, however, is provided by many small vessels, and is in part shared by the joint capsule, epiphyseal bone, and other perisynovial structures.[20] There is thus no possibility of directly isolating and measuring that portion of the blood supply that is specifically destined for synovium, but the synovial blood flow may be indirectly approached by examining the clearance of small marker molecules from the joint space. In the event of full equilibration between synovial fluid and perfusing plasma, the clearance of such a marker would be equal to the synovial blood flow. Because it is unlikely that such equilibration is ever complete, all experimental values must be qualified with the adjective "effective." Using tritiated water as the marker, we found a mean effective synovial blood flow of 1 ml/min in normal knees.[35] When the same test system was used in inflamed arthritic knees, many with rheumatoid arthritis had diminished effective synovial blood flow, whereas those with other forms of joint disease had a wide range of values (Fig. 9–4). Unlike the studies of free ^{24}Na and ^{131}I, these experiments were conducted with equivalent intra-articular volumes and in the presence of a mild irritant (0.9% benzyl

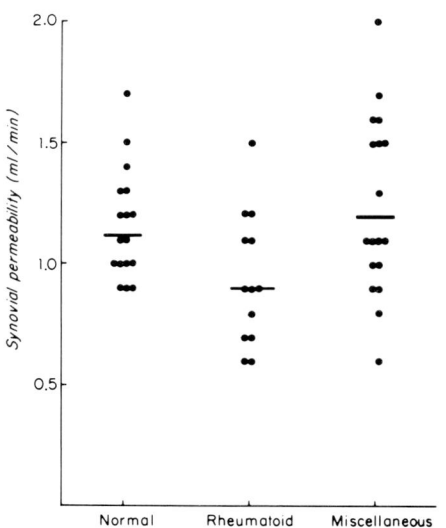

Fig. 9–4. Synovial permeability values of tritiated water from the resting knees of normal individuals, patients with rheumatoid arthritis, and subjects with other forms of arthritis. Under these experimental conditions, the effective synovial blood flow is not enhanced and may, indeed, be diminished in some of the patients with rheumatoid arthritis.

alcohol). The low rates found in many rheumatoid patients suggest that they have an impaired capacity to respond to additional stimuli, as reflected by the data in Figure 9–4.

The effective blood flow has been reexamined using a new experimental method in 11 patients with rheumatoid arthritis and 9 people with osteoarthritis.[41] In this work, trace amounts of both free ^{123}I and ^{131}I-labeled human serum albumin were injected into existing knee effusions and followed simultaneously by external counting. The apparent distribution volume was assessed by isotope dilution of the labeled albumin in a synovial fluid specimen aspirated after 24 hours. From the product of the rate constant for removal of free iodine (min^{-1}) and the volume (ml), one can determine a clearance value in ml/min (Table 9–1).

The clearance of free iodine (like that of tritiated water in the previous work) may be taken as an indicator of effective synovial blood flow. The values are comparable to those found with tritiated water but are somewhat higher, presumably because of the larger volumes that include the inter-

stitial water of the synovial tissue as well as the recoverable effusion. Once again, the mean effective blood flow was lower in the rheumatoid patients and six of the lowest seven values were found in this disease. Within the rheumatoid group, the clearance of free iodine correlated highly with synovial fluid pH (r = 0.74), lactate (r = −0.77), synovial fluid/serum ratio of glucose (r = 0.81), and temperature (r = 0.88). The high correlation between apparent blood flow and these indices of circulatory metabolic imbalance suggests that the rheumatoid synovium is often relatively hypoperfused and ischemic. Apparently, microvascular impairment may prevent an adequate circulatory response to the rheumatoid process.

The problems associated with studies of synovial blood flow must not be underestimated. Ideal conditions include equivalent intra-articular pressures and volumes, thorough and continuous mixing, measurements both in resting and in comparably active joints, and use of an injectate identical to synovial fluid in temperature and in the concentration of all major solutes, both large and small. No study has yet controlled most, let alone all, of these variables, and the problem of synovial blood flow thus remains an important area for further investigation.

Glucose

Glucose is carried in plasma, is delivered by synovial transport, and is one of the most important nutrients required by chondrocytes. Since glucose concentration is easily measured in synovial fluid and is often low with severe synovitis, physicians have long been interested in its transynovial exchange.[39] Ropes, Muller, and Bauer were the first to systematically study normal mechanisms of glucose transport into joints.[31] They found that the concentration of glucose in synovial fluid usually was close to that of plasma. Between three and four hours after meals, however, levels were regularly higher within the joint space than they were in the perfusing blood. After a series of infusion experiments in man and in cattle, they suggested that a specific transport system might facilitate the transfer of glucose from plasma to synovial fluid.

We used a different experimental approach (described previously) to confirm the presence of asymmetric glucose transport.[35] These studies used serial concentration changes within an injectate of saline to compare the egress of ^{14}C-labeled com-

Table 9–1. Joint Protein Clearance Values

	n	Vol (ml)	(min^{-1})	Clearance (ml/min)
Rheumatoid	11	106 ± 23	0.018 ± 0.007	1.92 ± 0.98
Osteoarthritis	9	109 ± 105	0.028 ± 0.017	2.40 ± 1.44

pounds with the ingress of physiologic "cold" molecules in normal human knees. Most small molecules, exemplified by urea in Figure 9–5, move freely in both directions between plasma and synovial fluid in accord with simple diffusion kinetics. In these studies, however, glucose, entered the joint space more rapidly than would be expected from its size alone, implicating a specific glucose transport system: a system that accelerates the entrance of glucose into the joint space, but does not affect its rate of return to the plasma. These studies do not establish whether the specific glucose transport occurs by active (energy requiring) transport or by facilitated diffusion, although the latter mechanism appears more likely.

The synovial fluid glucose level in inflamed joints may be significantly lower than plasma levels. Although most characteristic of sepsis, this finding is often present in rheumatoid disease (where levels may be undetectably low) and has occasionally been observed in gout, trauma, and other joint afflictions.[30] A low level thus offers no diagnostic specificity. Low glucose values may, however, offer valuable insight into the effectiveness of the synovial microcirculation. Specifically, any low value must indicate that the intrasynovial demand for glucose exceeds the supply and suggests that this circulatory-metabolic imbalance may apply for other nutrients as well. For instance, Fal-

chuk, Goetzl, and Kulka found a low glucose concentration in 3 of 15 rheumatoid synovial fluids, and all three had remarkably low PO_2, high PCO_2, high lactate, and low pH.[9] Both increased consumption and impaired delivery reasonably may be implicated in this disruption of the normal equilibration between synovial fluid and plasma.

The white blood cells of synovial fluid consume relatively little glucose in vitro and cannot be implicated as an important factor in intrasynovial hypoglycemia.[31] Additional experiments in vitro suggest that hyperplastic synovium is the major user of glucose in rheumatoid joints, and presumably active synovitis of other etiologies may be similarly implicated.[28] Clearly, synovial consumption must be an important variable. Otherwise, even a marginal microcirculation would be able to maintain equilibration between synovial fluid and plasma.

Conversely, a microcirculation of maximal effectiveness should be able to supply an increased demand for glucose. Low glucose values indicate that the demand has not been met and suggest impaired microvascular function. The overall importance of vascular impairment is strongly supported by the significant (p <0.005) correlations we found between effective synovial blood flow (^{123}I clearance) and synovial fluid pH, lactate, glucose, and temperature in 11 rheumatoid synovial effusions. Obliteration of terminal blood vessels is a well-recognized histologic manifestation of rheumatoid synovitis. This direct vascular loss could well explain local synovial ischemia. The finding that "rice bodies" in synovial fluid from rheumatoid arthritis patients contain collagen types I, III, and V in a proportion of 40/40/20, identical to that of synovial membrane, strongly suggests that such local ischemia is accompanied by microinfarction and detachment of the infarcted tissue to form the core of the "rice body."[5a] In addition, as data of Ropes and Bauer suggest,[30] the high intrasynovial pressure of some rheumatoid effusions may further compromise the synovial microvessels by tamponade. Experimental support for this concept comes from the finding that a tense effusion markedly inhibited clearance of [133]xenon from inflamed joints.[26]

In summary, a specific transport system accelerates the entrance of glucose into normal joints. Low levels of glucose often occur in the synovial effusions of intra-articular sepsis or rheumatoid arthritis. The precise mechanism of this intrasynovial hypoglycemia is unclear, but it appears to be caused both by increased local utilization and by impaired delivery of glucose into the joint space.

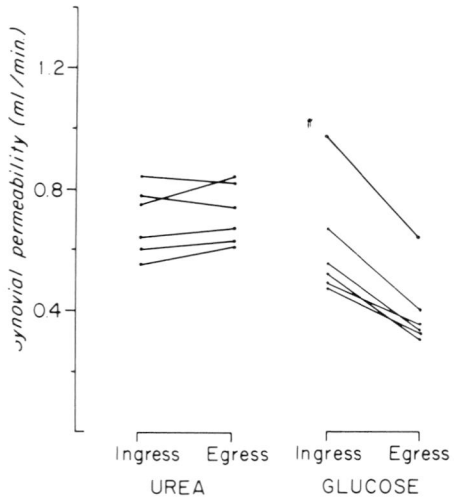

Fig. 9–5. Ingress of endogenous urea and glucose is compared with egress of the labeled molecules from resting normal knees. The synovium is symmetrically permeable to urea (mean ingress/egress = 0.97). Glucose, however, enters the joint at a rate faster than it leaves (mean ingress/egress = 1.59). These data are most consistent with a unidirectional transport system moving glucose into the joint. (From Simkin, P.A., and Pizzorni, J.E.[35])

Fat-Soluble Solutes

Since fat-soluble solutes can diffuse through, as well as between, cell membranes, they do not face the same synovial surface area restrictions as do hydrophilic molecules. The entire surface area of the synovium is available to lipophilic molecules diffusing in or out of the joint space. In our studies of normal knees,[35] this phenomenon was seen with benzyl alcohol, a fat-soluble molecule that left the joint space considerably faster than hydrophilic molecules of equivalent size.

Physiologically, the most important fat-soluble molecules are the respiratory gases: oxygen and carbon dioxide. Since 1970,[9] several investigators have studied the synovial fluid content of these crucial metabolites.[21,34] These studies show that many patients with rheumatoid arthritis (as well as a smaller number of patients with other joint diseases) have low Po_2 values and that this finding correlates highly with increased Pco_2, decreased pH, and increased lactate (Fig. 9–6). Despite the high diffusibility of oxygen, its supply is unable to meet synovial demand in such joints. The resultant hypoxia makes synovial cells utilize the metabolically expensive glycolytic pathway with a consequent increase in consumption of glucose and production of lactic acid. The latter, together with the carbonic acid produced by oxidative metabolism, leads to an intra-articular acidosis with synovial fluid pH values as low as 6.8.[10,21] All these changes reflect a severe circulatory-metabolic imbalance within the inflamed synovium, with the microvasculature being unable either to supply sufficient metabolic fuels or to adequately clear the products of their combustion. As yet, little is known about the consequences to the bearer of such compromised joints. We do not know how well the cartilage withstands local hypoxia, hypoglycemia, and acidosis. It seems likely, however, that these factors may be important in the pathogenesis of rheumatoid lesions. Circulatory-metabolic imbalance in the synovium will require more investigation before the clinician can readily recognize the problem and appropriately interpret its implications.

Lipophilic molecules (those having a high oil:water partition coefficient) pose a special problem since they accumulate in fatty tissues and are eluted slowly by the surrounding interstitial water. Recognition of this fact largely has led investigators to abandon xenon (^{133}Xe) clearance as a technique for the study of synovial blood flow. When ^{133}Xe was injected into a joint, its exponential clearance could be followed by external counting using the same techniques described for [24]Na and [131]I. For example, the clearance constant from normal knees was 0.0028,[7] an order of magnitude less than that found for sodium or iodide. Unfortunately, as Phelps, Steele, and McCarty demonstrated,[26] the recorded clearance was from perisynovial fat rather than from the joint space. The technique is therefore of little value in assessing synovial blood flow.

Drugs

Physicians treating any form of arthritis are engaged in a battle against synovial inflammation. Our principal weapons in this war are a wide variety of drugs intended to eliminate the cause or to ameliorate the effects of the inflammatory process. But

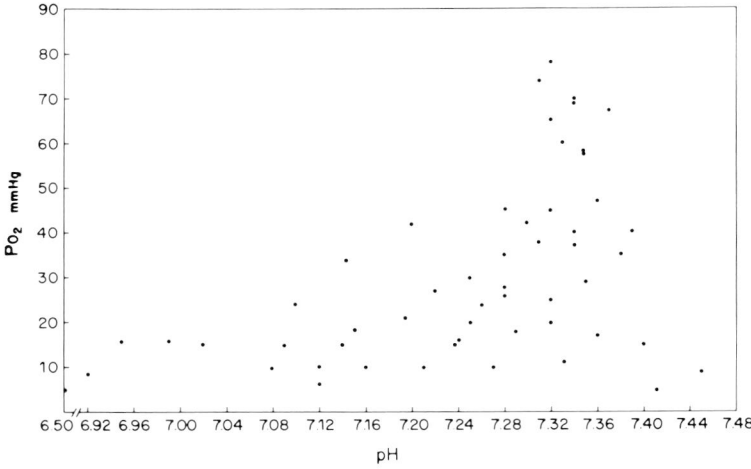

Fig. 9–6. Correlation of oxygen tension (Po_2) with pH in synovial effusion of patients with various joint diseases. The pH varies little with modest local hypoxia, but usually becomes acidotic when the Po_2 falls below 30 mm Hg. (Courtesy of Dr. D.J. McCarty.)

how well do our agents reach their target? This question has been asked primarily by examining drug levels in synovial fluid and contrasting them with concurrent concentrations in plasma. Available data, obtained under a wide variety of clinical circumstances, indicate that drugs readily cross the double barrier of microvascular endothelium and synovial interstitium to appear in the synovial fluid.

We have reviewed an expanding literature on anti-inflammatory drug levels in synovial fluids and tissue.[42] For any orally administered drug, plasma levels reflect the sequential but overlapping processes of absorption, distribution, and elimination. Peak levels are usually reached within 1 or 2 hours, and the plasma concentration subsequently falls at rates reflecting first the distribution of the drug throughout the various tissue compartments and then the metabolism and/or elimination of that specific agent. The levels in synovial fluid lag behind those of plasma, reach a later and lower peak, and then begin their own descent. At some point, the downward slopes of both curves characteristically cross, and synovial fluid levels are subsequently higher than those of plasma (Fig. 9–7). After this time, the concentration gradient leads to diffusion

of the agent from the tissues back into blood. The time required to reach this crossing or equilibration point appears to be a function primarily of the half-life of the drug. Short-lived agents such as aspirin have the earliest equilibration time, whereas long-lived drugs, i.e., phenylbutazone, have the latest with intermediate agents falling in between (Fig. 9–8). This pattern may vary somewhat with the protein content of each effusion, the degree of protein binding of the agent, and the effective blood flow. Nevertheless, the available data indicate that synovial fluid levels exceed those of plasma by a passive, nonspecific process that is most readily observed in the case of short-lived therapeutic agents. On balance, such drugs possess no apparent advantage over longer-lived agents.

Antibiotics constitute a second major class of drugs that has been studied in a similar way. Rapp et al. in patients with traumatic synovitis,[27] Nelson in children,[23] and Parker and Schmidt in adults with acute septic arthritis[25] have examined intrasynovial antibiotic concentrations. They found that such levels lag behind peak plasma concentrations, with some suggestion that the lag is greater for antibiotics of larger molecular weight, such as erythromycin. In all cases, however, effective antibiotic levels were achieved within these repeatedly aspirated joints. It remains possible, and perhaps likely, however, that antibiotic access may be limited in tense, undrained effusions. Such conditions, analogous to any other abscess, would be most likely to occur in smaller or less accessible joints

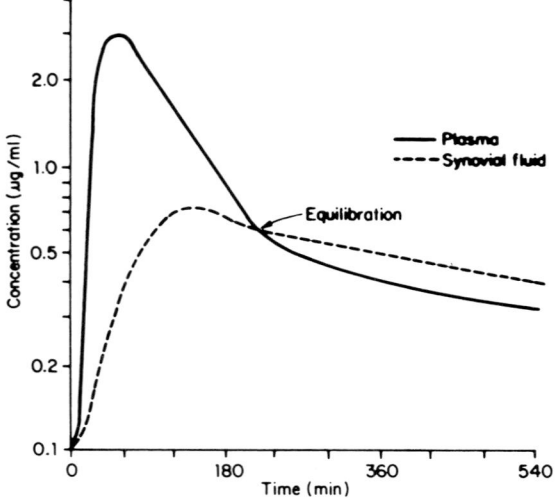

Fig. 9–7. Mean concentrations in serial samples of plasma and synovial fluid after a single oral dose of a therapeutic agent. Plasma levels rise rapidly with gastrointestinal absorption, fall somewhat as the drug is distributed throughout body compartments, and then decline steadily as a result of continuing metabolism and excretion. Synovial fluid levels initially lag behind those in plasma, but then cross over the plasma concentration (at the equilibration point) and eventually decline at a rate comparable to that in plasma. After equilibration, the drug diffuses down the concentration gradient from synovial fluid back into plasma. (Modified from indomethacin data of Emori, H.W., et al.[8])

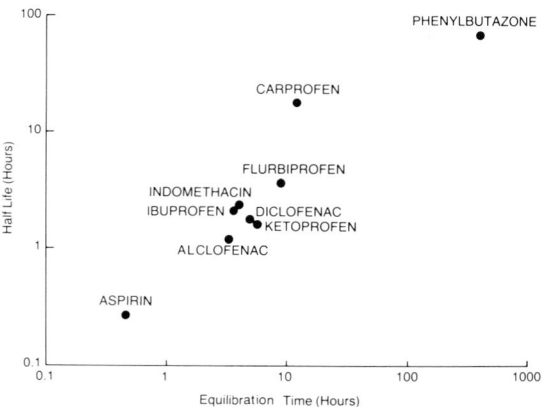

Fig. 9–8. Biological half-life vs. equilibration time for nonsteroidal anti-inflammatory drugs. The linear relationship indicates that equilibration occurs early in the case of those agents which are rapidly cleared from plasma and late in those with a long biological half-life. With usual dosage schedules, short-lived agents will often be found with synovial fluid concentrations exceeding the concurrent levels in plasma (From Wallis, W.J., and Simkin, P.A.[42])

in which high-pressure effusions may be most easily overlooked. Therefore, *it remains unwise to assume that adequate antibiotic levels are present in any septic joint unless it is regularly aspirated or surgically drained.*

Protein

The proteins of synovial fluid are qualitatively the same as those of plasma, but there are major quantitative differences.[16,30] Normal synovial fluid from the human knee contains 1.3 g of total protein per 100 ml, and most of that protein is albumin.[2] The larger molecules such as fibrinogen, large globulins, and certain complement components are largely excluded. In "noninflammatory" fluids taken primarily from the knees of edematous patients, the same relative distribution holds, but with somewhat higher total protein concentrations. Because its small volumes make it inaccessible to investigators, there are few observations of truly normal human synovial fluid and essentially none from any joint other than the knee.

With active synovitis, proteins gain more ready access to the joint space. The fluid clots after aspiration, the complement activity increases (unless ongoing consumption is present), and the concentration of each protein approaches that of plasma. The rate of total protein ingress into normal and diseased joints was examined in our studies employing serial sampling of "artificial effusions" comprised of comparable volumes of physiologic saline containing 0.9% benzyl alcohol (Table 9–2).[33] The rate of protein entry was significantly increased above normal (p <0.001) both in rheumatoid arthritis and in a diverse "miscellaneous synovitis" group including patients with osteoarthritis, septic arthritis, gout, and psoriasis. This increase in permeability to proteins was clearly not shared by smaller molecules exemplified by tritiated water $(^3H)H_2O$ in Figure 9–4. This important differential effect of inflammation is entirely consistent with the double barrier model of synovial permeability. Active synovitis lowers the endothelial barrier to proteins but does not affect, or may even increase, the interstitial barrier that is the limiting factor in transsynovial exchange of smaller molecules.

Both in normal and in diseased joints, there is continuing turnover of synovial fluid proteins. Proteins entering the joint space do so at rates inversely

proportional to their molecular size. In contrast, proteins of quite different dimensions have been found to leave the joint at essentially identical rates.[4,29] The presumed basis for this difference is that entering proteins primarily arrive by the size-selective process of diffusion, whereas all proteins leave the joint by the bulk flow of lymphatic drainage. In any stable effusion, these opposing processes are in balance, and the net flux into the joint (moles/min) is equaled by the net flux out. This net efflux of any protein may be obtained from the product of its concentration in synovial fluid (moles/ml) and the effective rate of lymphatic flow (ml/min).

We have determined the effective lymphatic flow in a series of patients with rheumatoid and osteoarthritis.[41] As in the case of effective blood flow, the lymphatic flow is assessed by the product of intracapsular volume (ml) and the rate constant for removal of a labeled marker (min^{-1}). These experiments employed ^{131}I-labeled human serum albumin as the reference protein. The clearance rate of labeled albumin (interpreted as the effective synovial lymph flow) was 0.071 ± 0.028 (SD) ml/min in 11 patients with rheumatoid arthritis and 0.039 ± 0.030 ml/min in 9 patients with osteoarthritis. The difference between the two groups was highly significant, thus providing evidence for an accelerated rate of lymphatic flow in patients with rheumatoid disease.

The principal advantage of such information is the opportunity it provides for a kinetic interpretation of synovial fluid protein concentrations. A considerable body of evidence is now on hand regarding synovial fluid levels and synovial fluid:serum (SF/S) concentration ratios of specific plasma proteins. Figure 9–9, for instance, gives Kushner and Somervilles's data on SF/S for orosomucoid, transferrin, ceruloplasmin, and α_2-macroglobulin in "normal" fluid from nonarthritic fresh cadavers and from patients with rheumatoid arthritis and osteoarthritis.[16] The SF/S of these reference proteins bears a clear inverse relationship to their molecular size consistent with passive diffusion from plasma to synovial fluid. Similar plots have been useful to these and other authors in qualitatively assessing whether immunoglobulins are locally produced in the synovium.[5] Values of SF/S above the passive regression line strongly suggest local IgG synthesis in rheumatoid synovium, for

Table 9–2.   **Synovial Permeability to Water and Protein**

	n	*THO (ml/min)*	*Protein (ml/min)*
Normal	17	1.11 ± 0.05	0.008 ± 0.001
Rheumatoid	13	0.90 ± 0.07	0.021 ± 0.002
Miscellaneous	18	1.11 ± 0.05	0.024 ± 0.003

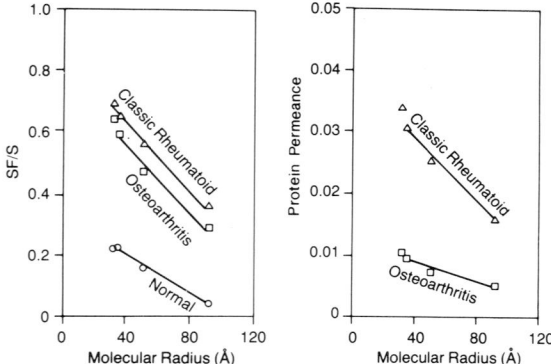

Fig. 9–9. Synovial fluid:serum ratios (SF/S) and protein permeance as function of molecular radius for four proteins (transferrin, orosomucoid, ceruloplasmin, and α_2 macroglobulin) in patients with rheumatoid arthritis and osteoarthritis. The concentration ratios differ by only a modest degree, but the permeance values illustrate the much greater microvascular permeability to protein in rheumatoid synovitis (see text).

instance, whereas an SF/S appropriate for the size of IgG makes local production unlikely in osteoarthritis. Although such assessments have been useful, these static observations provide no quantitative information regarding either synovial permeability or local production of specific proteins. In fact, SF/S reflects the point of equilibrium between the opposing rates of permeability (in) and clearance (out).[19] Without appropriate kinetic information, one cannot determine whether a high SF/S, for instance, reflects increased permeability, decreased lymphatic flow, or a combination of the two.

To illustrate these principles, we reanalyzed the data of Kushner and Somerville by making the assumption that their rheumatoid and osteoarthritic patients had effective lymphatic flow rates comparable to those measured in our patients with the same two clinical conditions.[16,41] The product of effective blood flow (ml/min) and plasma concentration (moles/ml) provides the amount of that protein (moles/min) delivered by the synovial microvasculature. The product of the effective lymph flow (ml/min) and the synovial fluid concentration (moles/ml) provides the rate (moles/min) at which the same protein enters (or leaves) a stable synovial effusion. The ratio of these entities gives the fraction of a given protein that leaves the plasma, crosses the synovium, and enters synovial fluid during each passage through the synovial microvasculature. We have termed this value the *synovial permeance* and, in Figure 9–9, have recalculated and replotted the SF/S data as permeance values. By this assessment, it becomes apparent that the

rheumatoid synovium is markedly more permeable to protein than is the synovium in osteoarthritis. This prominent difference is not apparent from examination of SF/S ratios alone. Further development of this methodology should make it possible to quantify in vivo the synovial permeability to plasma proteins in individual patients and to calculate the net intra-articular production or consumption rates for specific proteins of interest. This ability may prove valuable, for instance, in assessing net local synthesis of rheumatoid factor, consumption of complement components, and release of enzymes from leukocytes.

INTRASYNOVIAL PRESSURE

The humeral head sits snugly in the glenoid fossa, regardless of whether the arm is supported. The hip does not sublux during the swing-through phase of gait. Both at work and at rest, the opposing surfaces of articular cartilage remain in close approximation. This consistent apposition of articulating surfaces reflects a critical stabilizing capacity in normal joint function. Present data indicate that atmospheric pressure is one of the factors that sustain this apposition.

Pressures in Normal Joints

Only a film of synovial fluid separates the moving surfaces in normal joints. Unlike the distended structure so often depicted in schematic drawings, the intra-articular cavity is primarily a potential space containing so little free fluid that none can be recovered by needle aspiration. Similarly, a microscopic layer of fluid fulfills the mission of lubrication in normal bursae and tendon sheaths. Each of these spaces, then, resembles a collapsed balloon with a wet, slippery inner surface. The state of collapse is apparently maintained by a subatmospheric intracavitary pressure. This concept was introduced by Müller, who found pressures of -8, -8, and -12 cm H_2O in three human knees without effusions and values from -4 to -6 cm H_2O in four additional knees with small effusions.[22] Müller also found that intra-articular pressures were negative (subatmospheric) in anesthetized dogs and in amputated limbs. These observations have been confirmed repeatedly in the normal, resting knees of several mammalian species.[17] A pressure differential of this magnitude is sufficient to explain the close apposition of synovium on cartilage, sheath on tendon, and bursal lining on itself but how could these organs maintain such a differential without a specific pumping system and a continuous energy cost?

The exact mechanism of subatmospheric pressures remains controversial,[17] but one reasonable explanation may be drawn from animal experiments employing rigid perforated subcutaneous capsules. The pressure in such capsules is consistently subatmospheric by as much as 7 mm Hg. In this model, an equal and opposite colloid osmotic pressure may maintain the negative hydrostatic pressure within the capsule (Fig. 9–10). This balance of forces requires fixation of glycosaminoglycans in the gel-like interstitial space of surrounding tissues. The high osmotic pressure of this fixed pericapsular gel may "draw" water from the capsule with a force sufficient to generate a negative pressure within the capsule. Infusions of either hyaluronidase or collagenase through the capsules disrupt the investing interstitial gel and cause equilization of pressures without and within the capsule.[36] This model indicates, then, both that an organized matrix of relatively high colloid osmotic pressure may maintain a negative hydrostatic pressure within an enclosed tissue space and that enzymatic disruption of interstitial matrix will destroy the normal pressure relationships. Since the colloid osmotic pressure of normal, human synovial fluid approximates 10 mm Hg, that of the synovial interstitium would be predicted to be 14 mm Hg to maintain a resting intra-articular pressure at −4 mm Hg by this mechanism.

Role in Joint Stability

However achieved, a pressure differential of this magnitude may play a significant role in stabilizing joints. In concert with the action of tendons and ligaments, the "suction" of this phenomenon draws articulating surfaces into the best possible fit with each other and helps to guide the surface contacts as the joint moves through its range of motion. The magnitude of these forces was indicated by Jayson and Dixon's studies of nine normal human knees.[13] With simple isometric exercise of the quadriceps, they found the mean intra-articular pressure to be −107 mm Hg. With severe distractive forces, the baseline pressure is driven farther downward and may ultimately go so low that

dissolved gases come out of solution. This released gas appears coincident with sudden distraction of the joint surfaces and the well-known audible "knuckle crack." Both the bubble of gas and the distraction of the joint are readily demonstrated by serial radiographs.[40] This cavitation or "vacuum" phenomenon has generally been regarded as interesting, but of little practical value.

The observations are most instructive when assessed from the standpoint of joint stability, as illustrated in the finger. Normally, the extended middle finger may readily be moved throughout a lateral arc of approximately 40 degrees, thus demonstrating laxity in the collateral ligaments of the metacarpophalangeal joint. On applying progressive increments of pull to relaxed third fingers, Unsworth et al. found that a force of 10 kg was required to "crack" the average knuckle (Fig. 9–11).[40] Only at this point did significant distraction occur and did the collateral ligaments accept a significant fraction of the force operating across the joint. At this force, then, an important stabilizing factor has been overcome. A metacarpophalangeal joint surface area is too small for atmospheric pressure alone to explain this 10-kg approximating force. Surface tension is the factor most likely to provide the additional increment. In this phenomenon, the synovial fluid acts not only as a lubricant, but also as an adhesive that helps to hold the articular cartilages in close apposition.

When the metacarpophalanagel joint "cracks," the 10 kg of pull has overcome these adhesive properties. Here, as in other joints, the resultant bubble of intra-articular gas may then be used as a contrast agent for radiographic imaging of articular cartilage and other soft tissues within the joint. Radiologists have found this phenomenon to be useful in evaluating the knees, hips, and shoulders of infants and very young children, although bubbles can be induced only rarely after the age of 2. Presumably the surface area of these joints is sufficiently large in older children and adults to render

Fig. 9–10. Perforated subcutaneous capsule employed in physiologic studies of interstitial fluid. After implantation, the capsule is invested by granulation tissue. The colloid osmotic pressure of this tissue may exceed that of the fluid by an average value of 7 mm Hg, thus generating a subatmospheric pressure within the capsule. A similar discrepancy between colloid osmotic pressures of synovium and synovial fluid would explain the subatmospheric pressures reported in resting normal joints (From Guyton, A.C.[11])

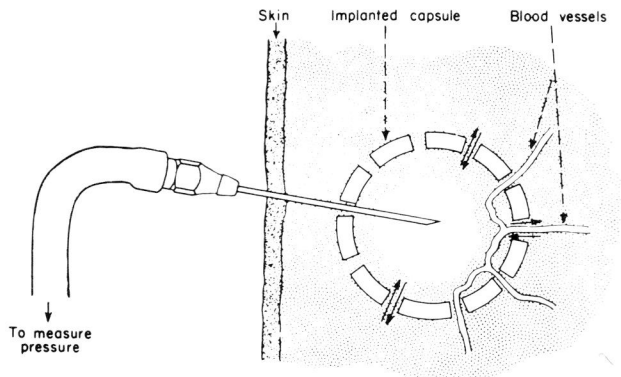

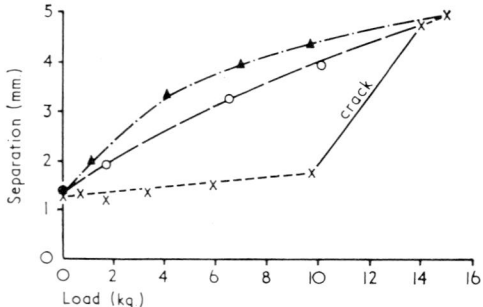

Fig. 9–11. "Cracking" of the third metacarpophalangeal joint. Despite progressive increments of pull up to 10 kg (lower curve with X's), there is little separation until the joint "cracks" with formation of a gas bubble within the joint space. When this happens, the load is no longer borne by atmospheric pressure and surface tension, but is instead transferred to the collateral ligaments of the joint. As long as the bubble remains, loading (open circles) and unloading (closed triangles) of the joint will follow the upper curves (From Unsworth, A.[40])

the average radiologist unable or unwilling to apply sufficient force to make the system fail. A simple comparison of the contact area of metacarpophalangeal joints with that of shoulders, elbows, and knees suggests that forces many times greater than 10 kg would be necessary to distract these joints. Simple atmospheric pressure, aided by adhesive properties of synovial fluid, must thus be able to contribute tremendously to the stabilization and congruent articulation of large joints. This is especially true in the polyaxial shoulder and hip joints, where ligaments can play only a limited role in maintaining joint stability.

Effect of Effusions

In the presence of effusions, the resting intra-articular pressure usually becomes positive. The degree of positivity varies widely. Pressures between 10 and 20 mm Hg are common, and values as high as 80 mm Hg have been recorded in tense rheumatoid joints.[24] Although the degree of tension is often disregarded by clinicians, the consequences of elevated intra-articular pressure may be profound. Effusions of significant volume deprive the joint of the stabilizing effects of subatmospheric pressure and substitute instead a distending force that greatly increases the stress on the ligaments and joint capsule (Fig. 9–12). In contrast to normal joints, the pressures of effusions are greatest in full flexion and full extension, with lowest intra-articular pressures occurring at 30 degrees of flexion. The thickened tissues of chronic synovitis are also less compliant than normal. This means that full flexion or extension may lead to extremely high

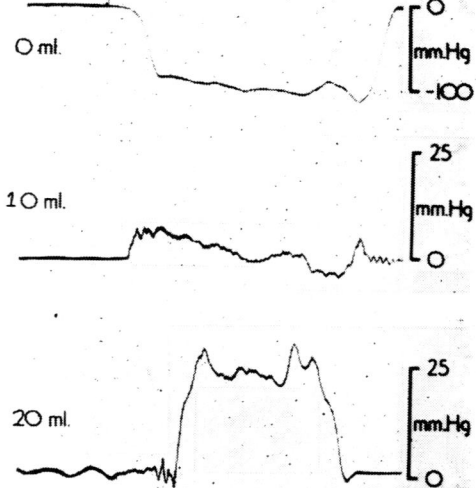

Fig. 9–12. Isometric quadriceps contraction in normal knee containing 0, 10, and 20 ml of added saline. With no injection, the intra-articular pressure is markedly subatmospheric. This is no longer seen with 10 ml of saline, and the pressure becomes significantly positive with a simulated 20-ml effusion. (From Jayson, M.I.V., and Dixon, A.[14])

pressures in many inflamed joints. With passive knee flexion, for instance, Jayson and Dixon observed a mean pressure of 802 mm Hg in three rheumatoid patients injected with 100 ml of intra-articular fluid.[13] These high pressures cause discomfort in chronically effused joints and thus limit the effective range of joint motion. They may also cause herniation through the capsule, progressive distention, or even rupture of the joint so often illustrated by "Baker's cysts" in the popliteal fossa. Such pressures also have been implicated in the pathogenesis of the subchondral cysts or "geodes" found in many kinds of joint diseases. As already mentioned, it seems likely that they may tamponade the synovial microvasculature, thus contributing to the circulatory-metabolic imbalance of severe chronic synovitis. For all of these reasons, the high pressure effusion remains an important problem for investigation and a potentially critical reason for therapeutic intervention.

OPPORTUNITIES IN SYNOVIAL PHYSIOLOGY

Rheumatologists owe a great debt to Marian Ropes and Walter Bauer. Through their own physiologic observations and their exhaustive and critical review of the work of others, Ropes and Bauer formulated most of the concepts that we still hold about how joints work in health and how they fail in disease. Despite this formidable beginning, or perhaps because it was so comprehensively done, the investigative interests of rheumatologists have largely ignored questions of articular physiology. A renewed emphasis on organ physiology of joints and on their pathophysiology seems overdue.

Accurate diagnosis and appropriate therapy lie at the heart of good clinical rheumatology. The diagnostic criteria for most rheumatic diseases are broad, resting primarily on clinical observations supported by nonspecific laboratory findings. Within any diagnostic category (as illustrated for rheumatoid arthritis by Figures 9–4 and 9–6) there is wide variation in pathophysiologic findings. As yet, however, the implications of this variation have rarely been explored. In which joints is the synovitis most likely to respond to intra-articular corticosteroids? Would the hydrostatic pressure, the pH, the oxygen tension, or some combination of physiologic parameters accurately predict joint destruction? Can such data serve as useful guides in therapeutic decision making? How well do antibiotics and other medications enter tense effusions? Does the "internal milieu" of the synovium or of cartilage predispose joints to infection by certain microorganisms? Do unique features of the synovial microvasculature lead to preferred deposition of circulating immune complexes? Are there physiologic differences between joints that would explain characteristic patterns of rheumatic diseases, such as the relative sparing by rheumatoid arthritis of the distal interphalangeal joints that are preferentially involved by osteoarthritis? Does the subchondral bone share, to some extent, the subatmospheric pressure encountered in working joints? If so, do fluctuations in intraosseous pressure contribute to the lesions of decompression sickness and of other causes of aseptic necrosis? These and many other critical questions remain virtually unexplored. Answers will come only through a new commitment to the problems of articular physiology.

REFERENCES

1. Bäcklund, L., and Tiselius, P.: Objective measurement of joint stiffness in rheumatoid arthritis. Acta Rheum. Scand., *13*:275–288, 1967.
2. Balazs, E.A., et al.: Hyaluronic acid in synovial fluid. Arthritis Rheum., *10*:357–376, 1967.
3. Bauer, W., Ropes, M.W., and Waine, H.: The physiology of articular structures. Physiol. Rev., *20*:272–312, 1940.
4. Brown, D., Cooper, A., and Bluestone, R.: Exchange of IgM and albumin between plasma and synovial fluid in rheumatoid arthritis. Ann. Rheum. Dis., *29*:644–651, 1969.
5. Cecere, F., et al.: Evidence for the local production and utilization of immune reactants in rheumatoid arthritis. Arthritis Rheum., *25*:1307–1315, 1982.
5a. Cheung, H.S., et al.: Synovial origin of rice bodies. Arthritis Rheum., *23*:72–76, 1980.
6. Deodhar, S.D., O'Boyle, P.J., and Dick, W.C.: Anion transport from the canine synovial cavity. Nature, *231*:61–63, 1971.
7. Dick, W.C., et al.: Clinical studies on inflammation in human knee joints. Clin. Sci., *38*:123–133, 1970.
8. Emori, H.W., et al.: Simultaneous pharmacokinetics of indomethacin in serum and synovial fluid. Ann. Rheum. Dis., *32*:433–435, 1973.
9. Falchuk, K.H., Goetzl, E.J., and Kulka, J.P.: Respiratory gases of synovial fluids. An approach to synovial tissue circulatory-metabolic imbalance in rheumatoid arthritis. Am. J. Med., *49*:223–231, 1970.
10. Goetzl, E.J., et al.: A physiological approach to the assessment of disease activity in rheumatoid arthritis. J. Clin. Invest., *50*:1167–1180, 1971.
11. Guyton, A.C.: A concept of negative interstitial pressure based on pressures in implanted perforated capsules. Circ. Res., *12*:399–414, 1963.
12. Harris, R., and Millard, J.B.: Clearance of radioactive sodium from knee joint. Clin. Sci. Mol. Med., *15*:9–15, 1956.
13. Jayson, M.I.V., and Dixon, A.St.J.: Intra-articular pressure in rheumatoid arthritis of the knee. Ann. Rheum. Dis., *29*:401–408, 1970.
14. Jayson, M.I.V., and Dixon, A.St.J.: Intra-articular pressure and rheumatoid geodes (bone "cysts"). Ann. Rheum. Dis., *29*:496–502, 1970.
15. Kremer, D., Deodhar, S.D., and Dick, W.C.: A function of synovial membrane of normal and diseased humans in relation to the movement of small-molecular weight ions. Clin. Sci. Mol. Med., *44*:611–615, 1973.
16. Kushner, I., and Somerville, J.A.: Permeability of human synovial membrane to plasma proteins. Relationship to molecular size and inflammation. Arthritis Rheum., *14*:560–570, 1971.
17. Levick, J.R.: Joint pressure-volume studies: Their importance, design and interpretation. J. Rheumatol., *10*:353–357, 1983.
18. Levick, J.R.: Synovial fluid dynamics: The regulation of volume and pressure. *In* Studies in Joint Disease. Vol. 2 Edited by E.J. Holborow, and A. Maroudas, New Nork, Pitman, 1983, pp. 153–240.
19. Levick, J.R.: Permeability of rheumatoid and normal human synovium to specific plasma proteins. Arthritis Rheum., *24*:1550–1560, 1981.
20. Liew, M., and Dick, W.C.: The anatomy and physiology of blood flow in a diarthrodial joint. Clin. Rheum. Dis., *7*:131–148, 1981.
21. McCarty, D.J.: Physiology of the normal synovium. *In* Joints and Synovial Fluid. Edited by L. Sokoloff. New York, Academic Press, 1980.
22. Müller, W.: Über den negativen Luftdruck im Gelenkraum. Dtsch. Z. Chir., *217*:395–401, 1929.
23. Nelson, J.D.: Antibiotic concentrations in septic joint effusions. N. Engl. J. Med., *284*:349–353, 1971.
24. Palmer, D.G., and Myers, D.B.: Some observations of joint effusions. Arthritis Rheum., *11*:745–755, 1968.
25. Parker, R.H., and Schmid, F.R.: Antibacterial activity of synovial fluid during therapy of septic arthritis. Arthritis Rheum., *14*:96–104, 1971.
26. Phelps, P., Steele, A.D., and McCarty, D.J.: Significance of Xenon-133 clearance rate from canine and human joints. Arthritis Rheum., *15*:360–369, 1977.
27. Rapp, G.F., Griffith, R.S., and Hebble, W.M.: The permeability of traumatically inflamed synovial membrane to commonly used antibiotics. J. Bone Joint Surg., *48A*:1534–1539, 1946.
28. Roberts, J.E., McLees, B.D., and Kerby, G.P.: Pathways of glucose metabolism in rheumatoid and non-rheumatoid synovial membrane. J. Lab. Clin. Med., *70*:503–511, 1967.
29. Rodnan, G.P., and MacLachlan, M.J.: The absorption of serum albumin and gamma globulin from the knee joint of man and rabbit. Arthritis Rheum., *3*:152–157, 1960.
30. Ropes, M.W., and Bauer, W.: Synovial Fluid Changes in Joint Disease. Cambridge, Harvard University Press, 1953.
31. Ropes, M.W., Muller, A.F., and Bauer, W.: The entrance of glucose and other sugars into joints. Arthritis Rheum., *3*:496–513, 1960.
32. Scholer, J.F., Lee, P.R., and Polley, H.F.: The absorption of heavy water and radioactive sodium from the knee joint of normal persons and patients with rheumatoid arthritis. Arthritis Rheum., *2*:426–432, 1959.

33. Simkin, P.A.: Synovial permeability in rheumatoid arthritis. Arthritis Rheum., 22:689–696, 1979.
34. Simkin, P.A., and Nilson, K.L.: Trans-synovial exchange of large and small molecules. Clin. Rheum. Dis., 7:99–129, 1981.
35. Simkin, P.A., and Pizzorno, J.E.: Transynovial exchange of small molecules in normal human subjects. J. Appl. Physiol., 36:581–587, 1974.
36. Stromberg, D.D., and Widerhielm, C.A.: Effects of oncotic gradients and enzymes on negative pressures in implanted capsules. Am. J. Physiol., 219:928–932, 1970.
37. Such, C.H., et al.: Quantitative study of stiffness in the knee joint. Ann. Rheum. Dis., 34:286–291, 1975.
38. Swann, D.A., et al.: Role of hyaluronic acid in joint lubrication. Ann. Rheum. Dis., 33:318–326, 1974.
39. Taylor, T.: Glucose metabolism and respiration. Clin. Rheum. Dis., 7:167–175, 1981.
40. Unsworth, A., Dowson, D., and Wright, V.: "Cracking joints": A bioengineering study of cavitation in the metacarpophalangeal joint. Ann. Rheum. Dis., 30:348–358, 1971.
41. Wallis, W.J., et al.: Unpublished.
42. Wallis, W.J., and Simkin, P.A.: Antirheumatic drug levels in human synovial fluid and synovial tissue: Observations on extravascular pharmacokinetics. Clin. Pharmacokinet., 8:496–522, 1983.
43. Wright, V., and Johns, R.J.: Quantitative and qualitative analysis of joint stiffness in normal subjects and in patients with connective tissue diseases. Ann. Rheum. Dis., 20:36–45, 1961.

Chapter 10

Collagen in Normal and Diseased Connective Tissue

Darwin J. Prockop and Taina Pihlajaniemi

Collagen is the major macromolecule of most connective tissues, and it is probably the most abundant protein in the human body. The other major macromolecules characteristic of connective tissues are elastin, a related fibrous protein, and a class of sugar-rich polymers known as proteoglycans (see Chap. 11). The amounts of collagen in tissues vary. Soft organs such as the liver contain little of the protein, whereas collagen accounts for over 70% of the dry weight of tissues such as skin and tendon (Table 10–1). Because collagen constitutes the bulk of most connective tissues, it makes a major contribution to their properties. Recent information about the biochemistry and chemistry of collagen (1) explains how the protein performs its important physiologic functions; (2) provides a molecular explanation for a number of genetic diseases of connective tissue; and (3) offers the promise of providing a basis for understanding the more common diseases of connective tissue that involve both genetic and environmental components.

FORMATION OF COLLAGEN FIBERS AND RELATED COLLAGEN STRUCTURES

Early in evolution nature had to solve the question, How can cells be held together to constitute

a multicellular organism? A major answer to this question was the formation of extracellular collagen fibrils and fibers.

Collagen fibrils have approximately the same tensile strength as steel wires, and they act in most complex organisms to hold together the cells of various tissues. The assembly of extracellular collagen fibrils is based on two relatively simple principles. The first principle is "*self-assembly*," whereby a protein monomer of relatively small size aggregates with itself in a precise manner to form a much larger biological structure.[13,77,78] In the case of collagen, large connective tissue structures, such as ligaments and tendons, are comprised of small bundles of collagen fibrils. The fibrils themselves are formed by the self-assembly of the collagen monomer (Fig. 10–1). The collagen monomer permits such self-assembly because it is relatively long and rigid, it has the correct distribution of charge and hydrophobic amino acid side chains along its surface, and it has the correct length.

The second principle in the formation of collagen fibrils is that most collagens are first synthesized as precursors known as *procollagens* (Figs. 10–1, 10–2).[4,12,13,15,77,78] The procollagens contain additional amino acid sequences at both the N- and C-terminal ends of the monomers. These additional amino acid sequences constitute as much as one-

Table 10–1. Collagen, Elastin, and Proteoglycan Contents of Some Tissues*

Tissue	Collagen† (g/100 g dry wt)	Elastin‡ (g/100 g dry wt)	Proteoglycans§ (g/100 g dry wt)
Liver	4	0.2	
Lung	10	5	
Aorta	18	30	6
Ligamentum nuchae	17	75	
Cartilage	55		29
Cornea	68		5
Skin	72	0.6	
Tendon (Achilles)	86	4	0.5
Bone (mineral-free, cortical)	88		0.8

*Values are averages from references cited by Grant and Prockop.[33]
†Values for ligamentum nuchae, cartilage, and bone from bovine tissues; remainder from human tissue.
‡Values for ligamentum nuchae and Achilles tendon from bovine tissues; values for liver and skin from rat tissues; and remainder from human tissues.
§Value for aorta from rabbit tissues; value for cornea from human tissues; and remainder from bovine tissues.

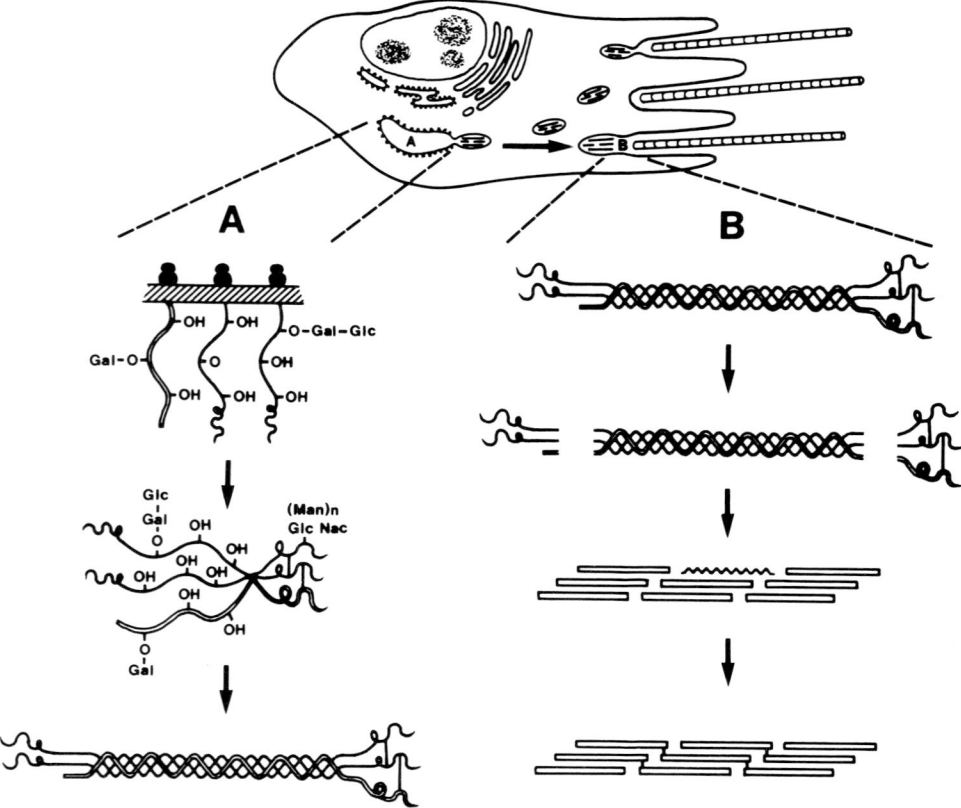

Fig. 10–1. Schematic representation of how a fibroblast assembles collagen fibrils. *A*, Intracellular post-translational modifications of proα chains, association of C-propeptide domains, and folding into triple-helical conformation. *B*, Enzymic cleavage of procollagen to collagen, self-assembly of collagen monomers into fibrils, and cross-linking of fibrils. (From Prockop, D.J., and Kivirikko, K.I.[78] Reprinted by permission of the New England Journal of Medicine.)

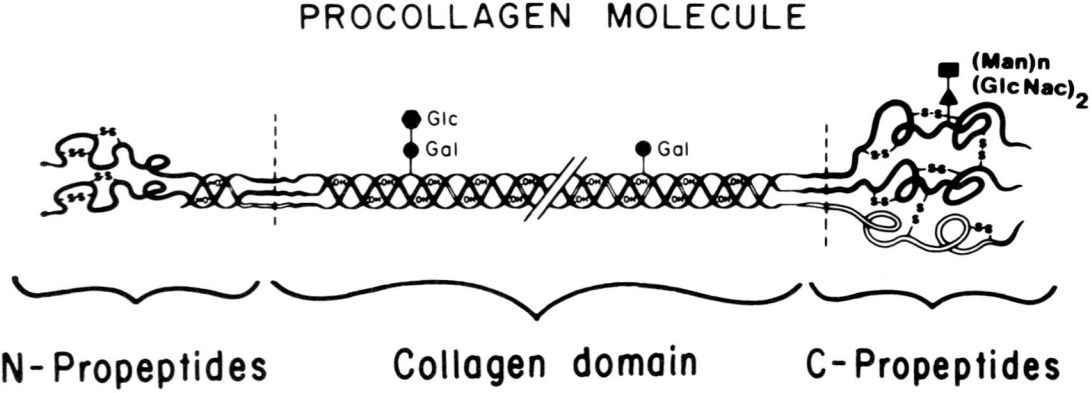

Fig. 10–2. Structure of a type I procollagen molecule. The molecule consists of two proα1(I) and one proα2(I) chains. It has the three distinct domains indicated. The C-propeptides of both kinds of proα chains contain a mannose-rich oligosaccharide. (From Prockop, D.J., and Kivirikko, K.I.[78] Reprinted by permission of the New England Journal of Medicine.)

third of the mass of the procollagens. They have several important biological functions, one of which is that they prevent the protein from self-assembling into fibrils and fibers prematurely.

At least 10 different kinds of collagen have now been identified in human connective tissues; therefore, these collagens can be considered a family of proteins (Table 10–2). The major subclassifications of the collagens is into the "fibrillar" and the "nonfibrillar" types. The fibrillar types form distinctive fibrils that are readily identified by their cross-striations, and they provide the tensile strength required to hold tissues together. The small differences in their amino acid sequences are probably a major determinant in producing the kinds of fibrils that fibrillar collagens form in vivo (Fig. 10–3). The nonfibrillar collagens form network-like structures that serve as a scaffold for the binding of epithelial and endothelial cells. They also serve as filtration barriers in tissues such as the kidney. The most important difference between nonfibrillar collagens and fibrillar collagens is that the monomers of the nonfibrillar collagens contain large globular domains in addition to collagen domains. The presence of the globular domains means that the monomers self-assemble into structures that are more complex than the orderly array of fibrils seen in the structures formed by fibrillar collagens.

Types I, II, and III collagens are the major fibrillar collagens.[13,77,78] Type I collagen is found ubiquitously in most connective tissues, including skin, bone, tendons, and ligaments. Type II collagen is the major collagen of hyaline cartilage. Type III collagen is less abundant than type I or type II collagen, but small amounts are found in most tissues that contain type I. Aorta and synovial

membranes, however, are particularly rich in type III collagen; bone contains type I without any accompanying type III collagen.

Type IV collagen is the major nonfibrillar collagen of the body and is the major constituent of most basement membranes.[13,77,78,82] Type V collagen is found in a variety of tissues, particularly in blood vessels and smooth muscle cells.[15] Type VI collagen and a family of other minor collagens are found in small amounts in various tissues.[9,15,32,56,67,82,84]

Types I and III collagens are the best studied and have been most closely linked to human diseases. This discussion will focus primarily on these types.

The monomer of type I procollagen contains two proα1(I) chains and a slightly different proα2(I) chain (see Fig. 10–2). In contrast, the monomer of type III procollagen is comprised of three identical proα1(III) chains that differ slightly in their structure from type I proα chains. Both type I and type III procollagen contain an N-propeptide domain, a collagen domain, and a C-propeptide domain.[12,13,77,78] Although the propeptides are, in general, globular structures similar to other globular proteins, the N-propeptide contains a short triple-helical subdomain similar to the collagen domain of the same protein. The C-propeptides are entirely globular, and they contain a mannose-rich oligosaccharide.

In the collagen domains of the proteins, each of the three chains is coiled into a left-handed helix with about three amino acids per turn. The three helical chains then twist around each other into a right-handed super-helix to form a rigid structure similar to a long and thin segment of rope. Each α chain contains about 1,000 amino acid residues

Table 10–2.   Structurally and Genetically Distinct Collagens*

Type	Tissue Distribution	Polypeptide Chains	Chemical Characteristics
I	Bone, tendon, skin, dentin, ligament, fascia, arteries, and uterus	$[\alpha 1(I)]_2\alpha 2$	Hybrid composed of two kinds of chains. Low content of hydroxylysine and glycosylated hydroxylysine.
II	Hyaline cartilage	$[\alpha 1(II)]_3$	Relatively high content of hydroxylsine and glycosylated hydroxylysine.
III	Skin, arteries, and uterus	$[\alpha 1(III)]_3$	High content of hydroxyproline and low hydroxylysine. Contains interchain disulfide bonds.
IV	Basement membranes	$\alpha 1(IV),\alpha 2(IV)$	High content of cystine, hydroxylysine, and glycosylated hydroxylysine. Contains large globular regions.
V	Blood vessels, other tissues	$\alpha 1(V),\alpha 2(V),\alpha 3(V)$	

*Type VI and five or more additional types have been identified, but these are less abundant and are not as well characterized as types I, II, III, IV, and V. For more complete descriptions of these collagens see Bachinger et al.,[4] Bornstein and Sage,[12] Burgeson,[15] Gibson et al.,[32] Mayne et al.,[56] Odermatt et al.,[67] Schmid and Conrad,[84] and Timpl et al.[97]

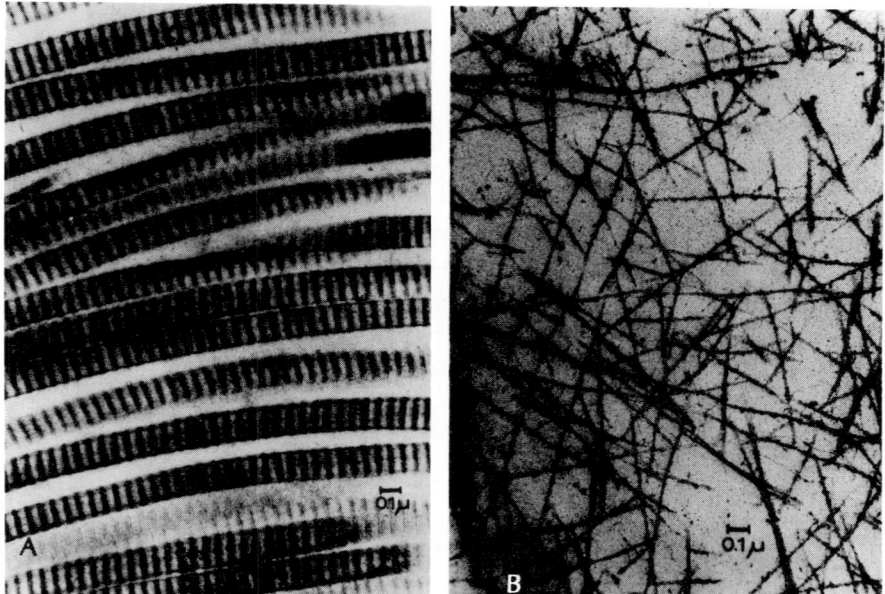

Fig. 10–3.   General scheme for the formation of type I collagen fibrils in tendon and type II collagen fibrils in hyaline cartilage. Most current evidence suggests that the differences in fibril morphology as shown here are due to small differences in the genetically determined amino acid sequences. Morphology is probably also influenced by the presence of other connective tissue components, such as proteoglycans. (From Prockop, D.J., et al.[77] Reprinted by permission of the New England Journal of Medicine.)

and, with the exception of short sequences at the ends of the chains, every third amino acid is glycine. Therefore, the molecular formula of an alpha chain can be represented as $(Gly-X-Y)_{333}$ where X and Y are amino acids other than glycine. Glycine, the smallest amino acid, must be present in every third position because the amino acid residue in this position occupies a restricted space in which the three helical chains come together in the center of the triple helix. The X and Y positions are frequently occupied by proline and 4-hydroxyproline, respectively. Because proline and hydroxyproline are ring amino acids, they provide rigidity to the structure. Other amino acids in the X and Y positions appear in clusters of charged hydrophobic amino acids whose side groups point away from the center of the triple helix. The pattern in which these clustered hydrophobic and charged amino acids appear on the surface of the monomer determines the precise manner in which the protein self-assembles (see Fig. 10–1, *B*).

The genes for type I and type III procollagen have several unusual features.[27,61,63,98,106,107] One is that the protein coding sequences, or the exons of the genes, are divided by about 50 intervening sequences (Fig. 10–4). Most of the exons coding for the α chain domains are either 54 or 108 bases in length, and each of these exons begins with the

codon for glycine and ends with the codon for a Y-position amino acid. These unexpected features of the genes have been interpreted as evidence that the procollagen gene originally arose as a 54-base primitive exon that was duplicated extensively at some stage during evolution.[27,107] However, it is also possible that the 54-base pattern of the exons arose through mechanisms designed to protect the gene from unequal crossover mutations. The exon pattern is similar in the $pro\alpha1(I)$ and the $pro\alpha2(I)$ genes, but the intervening sequences in the $pro\alpha2(I)$ genes are longer. Therefore, the $pro\alpha1(I)$ gene is 18,000 bases,[21] whereas the $pro\alpha2(I)$ gene is 38,000 bases.[63] The same exon pattern has been seen in type II procollagen genes of chick embryos[83] and in type III procollagen genes from the same species.[108] The globular C-propeptides of types I, II, and III procollagens are coded for by relatively large exons.

The gene for the $pro\alpha1(I)$ chain is on human chromosome 17,[40] whereas the gene for the $pro\alpha2(I)$ chain is on human chromosome 7.[40] A gene for type IV procollagen is also present on chromosome 17,[43] and a type I-like collagen gene, whose identity has not been fully established, has been located on chromosome 7.[91]

A variety of mRNAs of differing length for $pro\alpha1(I)$ and $pro\alpha2(I)$ chains have been found in

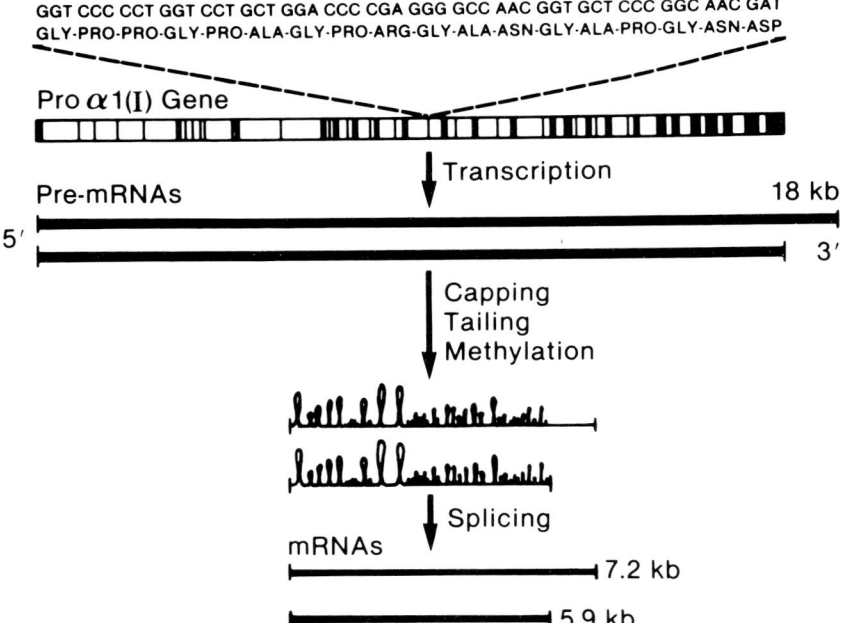

GGT CCC CCT GGT CCT GCT GGA CCC CGA GGG GCC AAC GGT GCT CCC GGC AAC GAT
GLY-PRO-PRO-GLY-PRO-ALA-GLY-PRO-ARG-GLY-ALA-ASN-GLY-ALA-PRO-GLY-ASN-ASP

Fig. 10–4. Schematic representation of the structure and of transcription of the proα1(I) gene. The top portion shows a typical 54-base pair exon encoding for a sequence of (Gly-X-Y)$_6$. The pattern of exons and introns in the proα1(I) gene is schematically represented on the basis of the similar pattern of the chick proα2(I) gene.[96,106] The gene is transcribed into two different pre-mRNAs, apparently because the first signal for termination of transcript is not entirely efficient. The initial RNA transcripts are about 18,000 bases (kilobases or kb) in length. Splicing out the intervening sequences reduces them to mRNAs of about 7.2 and 5.9 kb. The processing of the initial RNA transcripts also includes addition of a ''cap'' of the unusual base 7-methylguanylate at the 5'-end, addition of a ''tail'' of polyadenylate at the 3'-end, and methylation of a few bases. The two mRNAs with 3'-non-coding ends of different length are both used to synthesize proα1(I) chains with the same primary structure on polysomes. (From Prockop, D.J., and Kivirikko, K.I.[78] Reprinted by permission of the New England Journal of Medicine.)

fibroblasts synthesizing type I procollagen. The explanation for these mRNAs of different length is probably that the signals for the termination of transcription and for polyadenylation at the 3' end of RNA transcripts are relatively inefficient. As a result, two mRNAs of different length are synthesized from the proα1(I)[21] gene and at least three mRNAs of different size from the proα2(I) gene.[63,64] Both genes appear to be present as single copies per haploid genome.[21,25] However, the steady-state levels of the mRNA for proα1(I) and proα2(I) chains are 2:1.[29] There appear to be major differences, therefore, in the rates at which the two genes are transcribed or the initial RNA transcripts of the genes are processed. However, the two kinds of proα chains are synthesized in a ratio of 2:1. It is apparent, then, that the mRNAs for proα1(I) and proα2(I) are translated at this same rate.[29]

POST-TRANSLATIONAL MODIFICATIONS

The intracellular assembly of the procollagen molecule is a complex process that requires at least

eight specific enzymes and several nonspecific enzymes (see Fig. 10–1). In the course of the intracellular processing of the polypeptide chains, over 100 amino acids in each proα chain are modified. After the procollagen molecule is secreted, one-third of the mass is cleaved from the protein in the course of this conversion to the collagen monomer.[36,46,77]

The complex processing that occurs both co-translationally and post-translationally in fibroblasts includes the following steps (Table 10–3): (1) cleavage of ''signal'' peptides at the N-termini of the chains; (2) hydroxylation of Y-position proline and lysine residues to 4-hydroxyproline and to hydroxylysine; (3) hydroxylation of a few Y-position proline residues to 3-hydroxyproline; (4) addition of galactose or both galactose and glucose to some of the hydroxylysine residues; (5) addition of a mannose-rich oligosaccharide to the C-propeptide; (6) association of the C-terminal propeptides through a process directed by the structure of the C-terminal propeptide; and (7) formation of

Table 10–3.   **Stages in Collagen Metabolism**

Process	Biological Significance
Intracellular	
1. Transcription and translation	Determination of primary structure
2. Hydroxylation of prolyl residues	Stabilization of triple helix
3. Hydroxylation of lysyl residues	Site of attachment of galactose and glucose
	Needed for most stable cross-links
4. Galactosylation of hydroxylysyl residues	
5. Glycosylation of galactosyl-hydroxylysyl residues	
6. Glycosylation of procollagen propeptides	
7. Chain association, disulfide bonding, and helix formation	Helix required for normal rate of procollagen secretion
8. Translocation and secretion of complete procollagen molecule	
Extracellular Steps	
1. Conversion of procollagen to collagen	Fibril formation
2. Aggregation of collagen molecules	Fibril formation
3. Oxidation of lysyl and hydroxylysyl residues and subsequent cross-linking	Stabilization of fibrils
4. Degradation by collagenase(s)	Fibril turnover

both intrachain and interchain disulfide bonds in the propeptides.

After the procollagen molecules are assembled and secreted from fibroblasts, the N-propeptides are cleaved by a procollagen N-proteinase, and the C-propeptides are cleaved by separate procollagen C-proteinase.[36,46,77,100] The collagen then self-assembles into fibrils. After the fibrils are formed, a lysyl oxidase oxidizes lysine and hydroxylysine residues to aldehyde derivatives that form cross-links with similar residues in adjacent molecules (Fig. 10–1, *B*).[85]

Specific functions can be assigned to several of these enzymatic modifications.[36,47,100] The conversion of proline residues to 4-hydroxyproline is necessary for the α chain domains to fold into a triple-helical conformation at body temperature. The hydroxylation of lysine residues to hydroxylysines is required for addition of sugar residues to hydroxylysine residues. This process is also required to form the most stable kinds of cross-links found in collagen fibrils. The disulfide bonds found between C-propeptides are probably required as a first step in the formation of the triple helix. To form collagen fibrils, however, the C-propeptides must be cleaved from procollagen. Fibrils can form without cleavage of the N-propeptide, but the protein containing the N-propeptides forms fibrils that are thin and irregular in their morphology. Stabilizing the fibril structure clearly requires lysyl oxidase reaction.[85] Without the formation of cross-links initiated by lysyl oxidase, the fibrils do not achieve their maximal tensile strength.

Studies on the post-translational enzymes have demonstrated an unusual relationship between the conformation of the protein being processed and the enzymatic reactions themselves. In particular, the proα chains must be nonhelical to be substrates for some of the enzymes, but they must be triple-helical in order to be substrates for the others. Specifically, proα chains must be nonhelical in order to be substrates for 3-prolylhydroxylase, 4-prolylhydroxylase, lysylhydroxylase, and the two transferases that add sugars to hydroxylysine residues.[47,48] Modification by these enzymes ceases once the protein folds into a triple-helical conformation. In addition, extensive work has demonstrated that after the protein has folded, it is rapidly secreted from fibroblasts. Conversely, if folding of the protein is delayed by circumstances, such as agents that inhibit the hydroxylation of prolyl residues, the time required for secretion is greatly increased. In contrast to the hydroxylating and glycosylating enzymes, the enzyme procollagen N-proteinase has the striking property of requiring that the protein be triple-helical in order to be cleaved by the enzyme.[100] In addition, lysyl oxidase will not oxidize lysine or hydroxylysine residues unless the protein has self-assembled into collagen fibrils.[85]

One additional feature of interest about the post-translational modifications is that ascorbic acid is required by the prolylhydroxylases and lysylhydroxylases. Therefore, absence of ascorbic acid probably explains the failure of wounds to heal in scurvy. The hydroxylases also require oxygen, and limitations of oxygen may explain the failure of tissue repair in vascular insufficiency.[47,77]

GENETIC DISEASES SHOWN TO INVOLVE COLLAGEN

Within the past several years, definitive evidence has been developed for the involvement of collagen in a spectrum of genetic diseases (see also Chap. 75). The list of such genetic diseases of collagen now includes several specific forms of osteogenesis imperfecta (OI), the Marfan syndrome (MS), Ehlers-Danlos syndrome (EDS), and several related disorders (Table 10–4). Each of these conditions has proved to be highly heterogeneous at the molecular level. Many of them, however, can now be understood in terms of the basic information available about the biosynthesis of collagen. Although these diseases are relatively rare, they clearly provide paradigms for understanding more common diseases of connective tissue.

Molecular Defects in Osteogenesis Imperfecta

Although brittle bones are the most characteristic feature of OI, the disease is now recognized to involve most other tissues rich in type I collagen, such as ligaments, tendons, fasci, sclerae, and teeth.[11,39,57,59,72,90,104]

Several different schemes for the classification of OI have been presented, each of which has considerable merit. The most commonly referred to classification, however, is the scheme of four major types as proposed by Sillence and his associates (Table 10–5).[87,88] In this classification, the type I form of OI is characterized by mildly brittle bones, blue sclerae, and an autosomal dominant mode of inheritance. This type is further subclassified as type IA if teeth are normal and type IB if opalescent teeth are present. Type II is the most severe form. The connective tissues are so fragile that the disease is usually lethal at birth. Type III is a moderately severe form with a recessive mode of inheritance but highly variable manifestations. Type IV is also a highly variable form characterized by a dominant mode of inheritance and normal sclerae.

The current information of molecular defects in OI demonstrates that the disease is even more heterogeneous than the clinical manifestations suggest. Unfortunately, definitive data are available on only a few patients, and it is difficult to present many generalizations as to the kinds of molecular defects found in each clinical phenotype (Table 10–6). Therefore, the information is best considered on a case-by-case basis as examples of specific ''variants'' of the disease.

The Lethal Variant Proα1(I)[5]. The most thoroughly studied variant of OI occurred in a patient who died at birth with connective tissues so weak that the head separated from the trunk during delivery.[5,22,70,105] The defect in this variant has been defined at the gene level and shown to be a deletion of about 500 bases near the center of one allele for the proα1(I) gene (Fig. 10–5).[22] Because of the deletion of the gene, fibroblasts from the patient synthesized both normal-length mRNAs for proα1(I) chains and mRNAs for proα1(I) chains, which are shortened by about 250 bases. The deletion in the proα1(I) gene was ''in register'' in the sense that the coding sequences on either side of the deletion were in the correct phase to be translated into polypeptide chains. Therefore, the shortened mRNAs were translated into shortened proα1(I) chains.[5,105] Because the structure of the shortened chains was normal beyond the deletion, these chains became disulfide-linked to the normal proα1(I) and proα2(I) chains synthesized by the same fibroblast.[105] As a result, three-fourths of the procollagen trimers assembled by the fibroblasts contained either one or two shortened proα1(I) chains (Fig. 10–6). The stability of procollagen trimers is directly related to the length of the α chain domain of the protein. In the case of the proα1(I)[5] variant, the shortening in the proα1(I) chains was so great that the presence of even one shortened chain in a procollagen molecule prevented it from folding into a stable triple helix. Such molecules, therefore, were rapidly degraded either intracellularly or after secretion from the cells. As a consequence, a mutation that altered half the proα1(I) chains inactivated half the normal

Table 10–4. Genetic Diseases in which Collagen Defects have been Demonstrated

Disease	Major Manifestations	Tissues Involved in Most Variants
Osteogenesis imperfecta (OI)	Brittle bones	Bone, skin, ligaments, tendons, fasciae, sclerae, ears, teeth
Marfan syndrome (MS)	Long, thin extremities	Skeleton, eye, aorta, ligaments
Ehlers-Danlos syndrome (EDS)	Skin changes and joint laxity	Skin, ligaments, tendons, fascia, great vessels, bowel, and bones in some types
Menkes steely-hair syndrome	Cerebral degeneration	Brain, hair, arteries, bone, and bladder
Epidermolysis bullosa	Blistering of skin	Skin

Table 10–5. Classification of Osteogenesis Imperfecta (OI) based on Clinical Manifestations and Mode of Inheritance as Proposed by Sillence et al.[87,88]

	Bone Fragility	Blue Sclerae	Dentinogenesis Imperfecta	Presenile Hearing Loss	Inheritance*
I	Mild	Present	Absent in IA† Present in IB‡	Present in some	AD
II	Extreme	Present	Present in some	Unknown	AR or S
III	Severe	Bluish at birth	Present or absent	Low incidence	AR
IV	Variable	Normal	Absent in IVA† Present in IVB‡	Low incidence	AD

*AD = autosomal dominant; AR = autosomal recessive; S = sporadic.
†A = normal teeth.
‡B = opalescent teeth.

Table 10–6. Molecular Defects Identified in Osteogenesis Imperfecta (OI) and the Marfan Syndrome (MS)

Disease*	Molecular Defect†	Secondary Events
OI-I	Proα1(I)° Proα2(I)^s Other unidentified	Resistance to procollagen N-proteinase
OI-II	Proα1(I)^s	Unstable 3-helix; increased synthesis of proα1(III)
	Proα2(I)^s + Proα2(I)°	Increased synthesis of proα1(IV) and proα2(IV)
	Other unidentified	
OI-III	Proα2(I)^{cx} Proα1(I)^{cx} or Proα2(I)^{cx} Other unidentified	Synthesis of proα1(I) trimers Increased mannose in C-propeptide
MS	Proα2(I)^L Decreased cross-linking of elastin Other unidentified	

*OI-I, OI-II, and OI-III refer to the different types of OI as classified by Sillence and his associates (see Table 10–5).
†The molecular defects in most patients with OI and MS are still unknown. The statements here generally apply to single patients or to families with each type of disease in which the molecular defect has been defined.

proα1(I) and half the normal proα2(I) chains synthesized by the fibroblasts (Fig. 10–6).

This inactivation of normal proα chains by shortened proα1(I) chains can be regarded as "protein self-inactivation" or "protein suicide" by analogy with "suicide inhibitors" of enzymes that bind irreversibly and inactivate enzymes. The phenomenon may be general and may help to explain how many heterozygous gene defects, which reduce the amount of normal gene product by only one-half, can produce a dominantly inherited disease. In the case of the variant called proα1(I)^s, the phenomenon of protein inactivation (or protein suicide) reduced the biological useful procollagen synthesized by the fibroblasts in one-quarter of the normal amount. This level of synthesis of type I procollagen was apparently insufficient to produce connective tissues with adequate tensile strength. Because the parents of the proband were phenotypically normal, the deletion in the proα1(I) chain apparently was a new, sporadic mutation.

Three Variants of Proα2(I)^s. Three OI variants have been shown to synthesize shortened proα2(I) chains of type I procollagen. Two involve deletions of amino acids from the N-terminal region of the proα2(I) chain.[16,89] The third involves a similar deletion from near the middle of the proα2(I) chain.[28]

The two variants with deletions near the N-terminal region of the proα2(I) chain were similar in that 20 to 30 amino acids were missing from the chain, and the deletions were located between amino acid residue number 7 and number 347 of the α2(I) chain. In one of these variants, half the proα2(I) chains synthesized by fibroblasts are shortened, whereas the other half are normal.[89] A similar situation was apparently present in the second variant,[16] but the clinical presentations differed. In one, the disease was apparently a sporadic one produced by a new mutation.[16] The proband was a middle-aged woman with multiple fractures and blue sclerae. In the second, the proband had

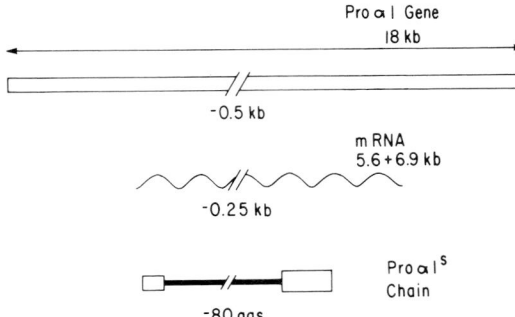

Fig. 10–5. Illustration of the molecular defect in one lethal variant of OI.[5,22,70,105] One allele for proα1(I) chains contains a deletion of about 0.5 kb in the middle of the gene. As a result, the mRNAs transcribed from the gene are shortened by 0.25 kb and about 80 amino acid residues. (From Prockop, D.J., and Kivirikko, K.I.[78] Reprinted by permission of the New England Journal of Medicine.)

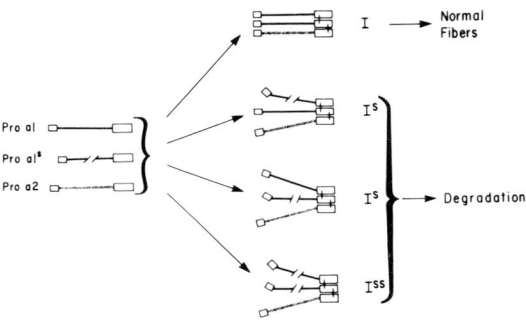

Fig. 10–6. Illustration of the phenomenon of "protein suicide" in a lethal variant of OI described in Figure 10–5. Because the deletion in the middle of the proα1(I) chain is in phase, the shortened proα1(I) chains associate with proα1(I) chains of normal length. The resulting trimers cannot fold into a stable triple-helix at body temperature and are rapidly degraded. (From Prockop, D.J., and Kivirikko, K.I.[78] Reprinted by permission of the New England Journal of Medicine.)

markedly loose joints, blue sclerae, and roentgenographic evidence of wormian bones but no fractures.[89] His mother, who had the same molecular defect, was short and had blue sclerae but no other findings. Several affected members of the same family had a history of blue sclerae and fractures. This family is probably best considered as having an atypical variant of OI with a high degree of incomplete penetrance. The major clinical manifestations in some members of the family, however, were those of EDS.

The reasons for the differences in the clinical manifestations of these two variants with similar deletions in about the same region of the proα2(I)

chains are not aparent. They may be explained by the possibility that one of the deletions is closer to the N-terminus of the proα2(I) chains and involves different amino acids.

In the second variant, the consequences of the deletion on the properties of procollagen were examined.[89] Two effects were found: (1) the deletion made procollagen molecules containing the shortened proα2(I) chain resistant to procollagen N-proteinase, apparently because the shortening altered the conformation of the cleavage site, and (2) procollagen trimers containing the shortened proα2(I) chains formed a triple-helical structure that was less stable than the triple-helical structure formed by normal type I procollagen. The data did not clearly resolve which of these two effects was the more important in vivo. The simplest explanation for the observations was that the shortening of the proα2(I) chains created a partial unfolding of the N-terminal region of the procollagen molecule. As a consequence, the N-propeptides were incompletely cleaved by procollagen N-proteinase. The persistence of the partially processed procollagen molecules in tissues probably explained the clinical manifestations of loose joints and fractures in some members of the family who inherited the defect.

The third variant that synthesized shortened proα2(I) chains was a lethal disease.[28] Two unrelated mutations were found, one in each of the two alleles for proα2(I) chains. The mutation in one allele produced a shortened chain, and the mutation in the second allele made it nonfunctional so that no mRNA was synthesized from the gene. The consequences of these two mutations were a decreased rate of synthesis of proα2(I) chains and shortening of all the proα2(I) chains synthesized by the patient's fibroblasts. The deletion of amino acids was again an "in-register" deletion so that the amino acid sequences of either side were normal. Therefore, the shortened chains were incorporated in the triple-helical trimers of procollagen. These trimers, however, apparently were not processed and assembled into normal collagen fibrils. In addition, because there was a relative overproduction of proα1(I) chains compared to proα2(I) chains, the patient's fibroblasts probably synthesized trimers of proα1(I) chains, which do not have the same functional properties as normal trimers of type I procollagen. One additional observation on this variant was of interest. The father of the proband had one normal and one nonfunctioning allele for proα2(I). However, he was phenotypically normal, an observation that demonstrated that a nonfunctioning allele for the proα2(I) chain may be of no consequence. The mother of the proband had two normal proα2(I) alleles. Apparently, the allele that the proband had inherited from his mother underwent a sporadic mutation which generated the shortened proα2(I) chains.

The Variants Proα1(I)^{cx} and Proα2(I)^{cx}. Two variants of OI have mutations that change the structure of the C-propeptides of type I procollagen.[30,30a,65,69] Both appear to have a progressively deforming disease best classified as type III (see Table 10–5). The molecular defect in one of these variants has been only partially characterized, but a more precise characterization has been obtained for the second.

In the first variant, the patient's fibroblasts synthesized and secreted a type I procollagen that was less soluble than normal.[69] Examination of the structure of the C-propeptides of the type I procollagen demonstrated that it contained increased amounts of mannose. It was not established whether the excess mannose was in the proα1(I) or the proα2(I) chain. In addition, it was not established that the defect specifically involved a change in the amino acid sequence of the C-propeptides. The most likely explanation for the data, however, is that the mutation altered the amino acid sequence of the C-propeptide of one chain and that this change in amino acid sequence decreased the solubility of the procollagen and probably produced inappropriate aggregation of the protein in tissues. The increased mannose content may have directly contributed to the altered solubility of the protein, but it may also have been a secondary and less important phenomenon.

In the second variant with altered C-propeptides, the defect was precisely located to a change in amino acid sequence of the C-propeptide of the proα2(I) chain.[30,30a,65] The dramatic finding in this patient was that none of the type I collagen in his skin, and presumably other tissues, contained any proα2(I) chains.[65,76] Since type I collagen had existed as a heterotrimer of two α1(I) and one α2(I) chains for about 800 million years of evolution,[10] it was generally assumed that the α2(I) chain is essential for life. This patient, however, had a form of OI that is only moderately debilitating. Examination of his fibroblasts demonstrated that the cells contained normal levels of mRNA for proα2(I) chains and that proα2(I) chains were synthesized by the fibroblasts.[30] However, none of the proα2(I) chains associated with proα1(I) chains. Therefore, the only procollagen trimer assembled and secreted by the fibroblasts consisted of three proα1(I) chains. Because the structure of the C-propeptide is critical for chain association, the results strongly suggested the molecular defect was an alteration of the structure of the C-propeptides of the proα2(I) chains. This suggestion has recently been confirmed by examination of both DNA and RNA from the patient's and his parents' fibroblasts.[30a] The rate of proα2(I) synthesis by the patient's fibroblasts was less than that seen in control fibroblasts, apparently as a secondary consequence of the mutation in the coding sequences for the C-propeptide.[30] A similar molecular defect was probably present in an OI variant studied earlier.[58]

Less Well-Defined Mutations in OI. An extensive study of patients with the type I form of OI demonstrated that cultured fibroblasts from three patients synthesized proα1(I) chains at a decreased rate as reflected by a decrease in the ratio of newly synthesized proα1(I) to proα2(I) chains.[6] Such defects may prove to be common in type I OI.

Fibroblasts from two patients with a lethal variant synthesized proα1(I) chains that migrated more slowly in polyacrylamide gels than normal chains.[102] The observations suggested that the fibroblasts were synthesizing lengthened proα1(I) chains, but this conclusion has not yet been definitely substantiated. In one of these variants, the ratio of mRNAs for proα1(I) to proα2(I) chains was 1:1 instead of the normal ratio of 2:1. Therefore, this patient appears to have one allele for a structurally altered proα1(I) chain and a second allele for proα1(I), which was not transcribed into mRNA.

Studies on one patient revealed that some of his proα1(I) chains contained cysteine, an amino acid not normally found in type I collagen.[76] In other variants, abnormalities in the migration of both α1(I) and α2(I) chains were found.[7,8] In still other variants, some of which may be the same as those studied by other investigators, changes in the ratio of α1(I) to α2(I) chains in pepsin digests of skin were observed.[31] The data suggested a mutation in one or more genes for type I procollagen, but the precise nature of the molecular defects is unclear.

Other Observations in OI. A frequent finding in OI is that the type I procollagen is overmodified, i.e., it has an increased content of hydroxylysine and glycosylated hydroxylysine.[44,90,99] The most probable explanation for this observation is that the proα chains have changes to their structure that delay the time at which the chains fold into the triple helix. Any condition that delays helix formation will, in itself, produce an overmodification, since folding into the triple helix normally terminates and limits the extent of the post-translational modifications.

Another common observation in OI is a decrease in the ratio of type I to type III collagen in skin extracts, or a decrease in the ratio of the amounts of type I and type III procollagen secreted by cultured fibroblasts.[70,90] Some of these observations probably reflect either a decreased rate of synthesis of type I procollagen or the synthesis of a structurally abnormal type I procollagen, which is rapidly degraded in vivo. Some patients with OI, however, have type III collagen in bone, a tissue that normally does not contain this protein.[62,73] In these variants, therefore, the decrease in the ratio may represent an increased synthesis of type III collagen because of "gene switching."

Some observations point to mutations that change the expression of genes for other components of extracellular matrix. In fibroblasts from three patients with type II OI, an increased rate of synthesis of type IV collagen was observed.[28] Fibroblasts from several patients synthesized increased amounts of hyaluronic acid.[101] These effects may or may not be secondary to mutations in genes for type I procollagen.

Molecular Defects in Marfan Syndrome

Marfan syndrome (MS) (see Table 10–4) is characterized by long, thin extremities, redundant ligaments and joint capsules, ectopia lentis, and dilation and rupture of the aorta.[11,57,66,72,79,104] As in OI, most of the affected tissues are rich in type I collagen. In addition, many of the characteristics of MS can be produced in young animals by inhibiting the cross-linking of collagen either by severe copper deficiency or by administration of nitriles, which inhibit lysyl oxidase. Therefore, several investigators have suggested that MS is produced by mutations in the synthesis or structures of type I procollagen. Evidence for this suggestion has, however, been developed in only a few patients.

The most definitive evidence for collagen defect in MS comes from studies on one patient in whom some of the proα2(I) chains had an insert of about 20 amino acids in the C-terminal third of the α chain domain (see Fig. 10–6).[17] In addition, the collagen in skin from this patient was more extractable than normal. The most likely explanation for these observations is that the inserted amino acids altered the register of the α2 chain relative to other collagen molecules in fibrils, and therefore appropriate cross-links were not formed.

A series of more indirect observations also suggests defects in collagen genes in MS. In one patient, the rate of synthesis of type I procollagen in explants of aorta was decreased.[34] In several independent studies, about one-third of the patients had increased excretion of peptide-bound hydroxyproline in the urine, an observation suggesting an increased rate of collagen turnover.[45] In some patients, skin collagen was more extractable than normal.[11,71,77] This observation and related findings suggest a defect in the cross-linking of collagen. A deficiency in stable cross-links of collagen was, in fact, observed in four patients.[14] However, extensive searches for a deficiency of lysyl oxidase, the critical enzyme for synthesis cross-links, have proved to be negative.[17,81]

Some observations suggest defects in noncollagen genes. Aortas from six patients had a decreased content of elastin.[1,35] In addition, fibroblasts from some patients showed increased synthesis of hyaluronic acid.[2]

Molecular Defects in Ehlers-Danlos Syndrome, The Menkes Steely-Hair Syndrome, and Related Diseases

EDS produces joint hypermobility and skin changes, such as thinness, extensibility, and fragility (see Table 10–4).[11,53,57,60,66,72,104] EDS has been classified into nine different types based primarily on the clinical manifestations (Table 10–7). As with OI, the precise molecular defects have been defined in only a few variants of EDS (Table 10–8), but these variants are instructive for understanding the others. Some forms are caused by mutations in genes for type I or type III procollagens, others by defects in enzymes required for the processing of type I procollagen. The defects in the processing enzymes mean that, at the molecular level, many forms of EDS resemble the Menkes syndrome and several related disorders.

Defects of Type III Procollagen in Ehlers-Danlos Syndrome Type IV. Type IV EDS is a rare but severe form of the syndrome. It frequently produces rupture of large arteries and hollow organs. All the patients apparently have a defect in type III procollagen.

One group of variants has a decreased rate of synthesis of proα1(III) chains by cultured fibroblasts.[3,20,73,74,75] In another group, proα1(III) chains are synthesized at about a normal rate, but the secretion of type III procollagen is decreased.[18,23] By analogy with the defects seen in OI (discussed previously), these variants probably involve changes in the primary structure of proα1(III) chains, which either prevent or delay folding of the chains into the triple-helix and therefore interfere with normal secretion. This conclusion is supported by the observation that fibroblasts from some patients have greatly distended cisternae of the rough endoplasmic reticulum.[20,103] In another variant, fibroblasts secrete normal amounts of type III procollagen, but the protein contains both normal proα1(III) chains and proα1(III) chains with a slower electrophoretic mobility because of an alteration of amino acid sequence in the chain.[95] The type III procollagen containing the abnormal chains is unusually sensitive to digestion by proteinases, and therefore may be rapidly degraded in vivo.

Hydroxylysine Deficiency in Ehlers-Danlos

Table 10–7.   Classification of EDS based on Clinical Manifestations and Mode of Inheritance

Type	Joint Hyper-mobility	Skin Extensibility	Fragility	Bruising	Other Manifestations	Inherit-ance
I	Marked	Marked	Marked	Marked	Hernias, premature rupture of fetal membranes	AD*
II	Moderate	Moderate	Absent	Moderate		AD
III	Marked	Minimal	Minimal	Minimal		AD
IV	Limited to small joints	Minimal	Marked	Marked	Ruptures of large arteries and bowel; thin skin with prominent venous net-work; characteristic facies in some	AD or AR
V	Minimal	Moderate	Moderate	Moderate		XR
VI	Moderate	Moderate	Mild	Moderate	Ocular rupture; blue sclerae and other ocular abnor-malities; scoliosis in some	AR
VII	Marked	Moderate	Moderate	Moderate	Multiple dislocations	AR or AD
VIII	Moderate	Moderate	Moderate	Moderate	Advanced periodontitis	AD
IX	Mild	Mild	Absent	Absent	Bladder diverticuli with spontaneous ruptures; her-nias and skeletal abnor-malities; skin laxity	XR or AR

*AD = autosomal dominant; AR = autosomal recessive; XR = X-linked recessive.

Table 10–8.   Molecular Defects Identified in Ehlers-Danlos Syndromes (EDS)

EDS-IV	Proα(III)^o	Decreased synthesis of type III procollagen
	Proα1(III)^L	Unstable 3-helix of type III procollagen
	Proα1(III)^X	Decreased secretion rate of type III procollagen
	Other unidentified	
EDS-VI	Lysyl hydroxylase deficiency	Hydroxylysine-deficient collagen and defective cross-linking
	Other unidentified	
EDS-VII	Procollagen N-proteinase deficiency	Persistence of pNcollagen
	Proα2(I)^X	Resistance to procollagen N-proteinase and persistence of pNcollagen
	Other unidentified	
EDS-IX	Defect in Cu metabolism	Lysyl oxidase deficiency and defective cross-linking

Type VI. The characteristic of the type VI form of EDS is ocular changes, which frequently pro-duce rupture of the eye. Severe skeletal deformities are also common. In the first family studied, there was both a deficiency of lysyl hydroxylase and a marked decrease in the hydroxylysine content of type I collagen in skin and other tissues.[52,71] The low hydroxylysine content probably explains the clinical symptoms because hydroxylysine is nec-essary for the synthesis of the most stable cross-links of collagen.[47,77]

Several families similar to the first have been identified,[41,51] but there are at least two other var-iants. In the second variant, assays of cultured fi-broblasts show a deficiency of lysyl hydroxylase, but the hydroxylysine content of collagen extracted from tissues is essentially normal.[41,94] The third variant has the same clinical picture, but there is no evidence of either a deficiency of lysyl hydrox-ylase or a decrease in the hydroxylysine content of collagen.[42] The molecular basis for this variant, therefore, is unclear.

Impaired Cleavage of N-Propeptides in Ehlers-Danlos Type VII. The type VII form of EDS is characterized by laxity of joints severe enough to produce dislocations of the knees and unreducible dislocations of the hips. Two variants involve impaired removal of the N-propeptides from procollagen, but they are caused by distinctly different mutations.

In the type VIIA form, the N-propeptides are incompletely removed from type I procollagen because of a deficiency of procollagen N-proteinase.[55] Partially processed proα1(I) and proα2(I) chains are found in tissue extracts, and the disease closely resembles dermatosparaxis, a recessively inherited disease found in cattle, sheep, and cats.[37,50,59,60,77] Examination of tissues from these animals, as well as studies on the self-assembly of the purified protein in vitro, has indicated that the partially processed procollagen that contains N-propeptides will form fibrils, but the fibrils are thin and irregular in outline. The failure of the fibrils to become thicker and more rounded probably explains the joint laxity in these individuals.

In the type VIIB form of EDS, the molecular defect is a structural alteration of the proα2(I) chain, which prevents cleavage by procollagen N-proteinase.[93] The consequence of the defect is again persistence of partially processed collagen containing the N-propeptide of the proα2(I) chain.

Altered Copper Metabolism and Deficient Lysyl Oxidase Activity in Ehlers-Danlos Syndrome Type IX, Menkes Syndrome, and Related Diseases. A variety of diseases of copper metabolism have been found to be associated with changes in collagen. These disorders include diseases previously classified as EDS type IX,[19,68] the Menkes syndrome,[26] and X-linked cutis laxa.[19] Because of similarities at the molecular level, it has been suggested that all these diseases be classified as EDS type IX.[24,68] Under this classification, one variant of type IX is characterized by bladder diverticula with spontaneous rupture, inguinal hernias, mild skin changes, and skeletal abnormalities. The variant previously called the Menkes syndrome includes many of these changes together with arterial disease and deterioration of the central nervous system so severe that the condition is lethal.

The variants of type IX are all characterized by low levels of copper and ceruloplasmin in serum, but high levels of copper in most cells.[26,49,54,68,80,92] The mutant cells also have increased amounts of the cation-binding protein metallothionein.[26,68] The change in metallothionein may be a primary alteration or it may be secondary to undefined alterations in copper metabolism. The low extracellular levels of copper probably decrease the cross-linking of collagen because the critical enzyme in the cross-linking of collagen (lysyl oxidase) requires copper.[85,86] Because all the disorders are X-linked, it is likely that the essential genes involved in copper metabolism are closely linked on the X-chromosome. The variability in the clinical manifes-

tations, however, suggests that several different genes are involved.

Other Observations in Ehlers-Danlos Syndrome. The type V form of EDS is a moderately severe disorder in which a deficiency of lysyl oxidase has been reported in a few patients.[77] However, other families have not revealed any deficiencies of this enzyme,[85] and the initial observations of the deficiency probably need to be confirmed.

Alterations in the morphology of collagen fibers have been observed in almost every type of EDS and in animals with related disorders, but it has not yet been possible to relate the morphologic changes to specific molecular defects.[24,38,59,60]

CONCLUSIONS

This new information about genetic diseases of collagen has important implications for a broad range of common diseases. In addition, at least three surprises have been encountered.

One of the surprises has been the phenomenon called "protein suicide" discussed previously (see Fig. 10–6). A second surprise has been the broad range of different clinical manifestations produced by different mutations that change the structure of type I procollagen. The results demonstrate that a structural change in one part of the molecule produces a disease that primarily affects skin and ligaments (Fig. 10–7), but a similar change in another part of the same protein produces a disease that primarily affects bone. In effect, these diseases demonstrate that some parts of the type I procollagen molecule are critical for normal bone formation, whereas other parts are critical for the normal function of other connective tissues. A third surprise is the apparently high frequency of mutations that shorten or lengthen proα chains. In simple bacterial genes, DNAs with repetitive nucleotide sequences have been shown to readily undergo unequal crossover mutations in which the genes become shorter and longer. Such mutations may well be common in procollagen because of the higher repetitive structure of its coding sequences (see Fig. 10–4).

The variants of OI and related diseases discussed here represent mutations in single genes of the collagen family that have overwhelming effects on the individual. The information about these diseases, however, makes it possible, perhaps for the first time, to think concretely about more common diseases that are "multifactorial" and that involve both genetic and environmental components.

There are, in fact, several reasons why mutations in collagen genes may be involved, as contributing factors, in relatively common diseases of midlife and beyond. One is a general consideration of the

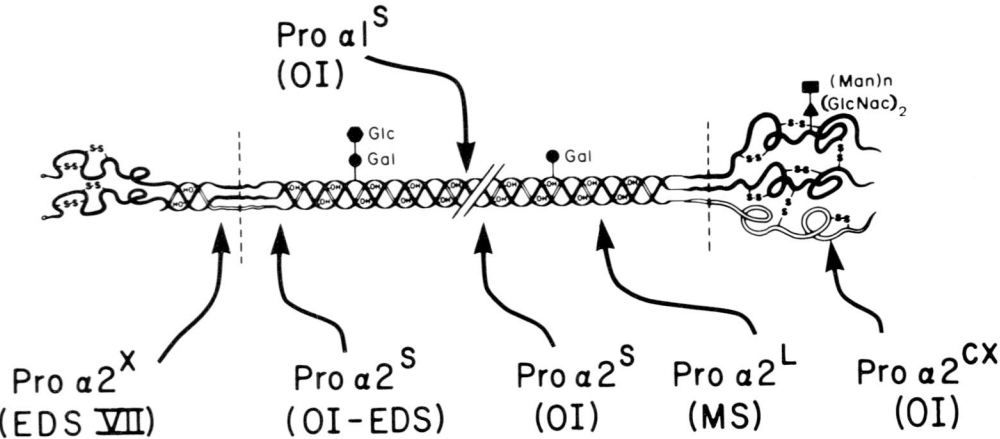

Fig. 10–7.   Approximate locations of mutations in the structure of type I procollagen. OI = osteogenesis imperfecta; EDS = Ehlers-Danlos syndrome; MS = Marfan syndrome.

kinds of mutations one can expect to find in examining human collagen genes more thoroughly than has been done to date. From the example of a few patients with lethal OI (see Figs. 10–5, 10–6, Table 10–6), it is apparent that, at one extreme, there are mutations in type I procollagen genes that are incompatible with life. At the other extreme, it is likely that a detailed examination of genes from different individuals will reveal "neutral mutations," i.e., changes in the genes that change the amino acid sequence of the protein but have no effect on its normal function. Between these two extremes, however, it is likely that mutations will be encountered that have subtle effects and require a long time to manifest themselves. Such "subtle mutations" may be particularly important in considering collagen. Collagen is a remarkably stable protein, and most of the collagen an individual acquires during the growth spurt of adolescence remains with him the rest of his life. A broad time scale must therefore be considered in examining the biological consequences of mutation in procollagen genes. One can readily imagine mutations that have no apparent consequence during childhood or early adult life. The same mutations, however, might produce changes in the size or in other features of collagen fibrils to make connective tissues less fit than normal to withstand the stresses of 30 or 40 years of confrontation with the environment. These mutations may predispose an individual to a slow manifestation of chronic diseases such as osteoporosis or osteoarthritis. The work on genetic diseases of collagen is clearly providing the experimental tools and the basic information necessary to examine such subtle mutations in collagen genes. Examining the medical consequences of the subtle mutations is likely to move the study of

genetic diseases from the special realm of rare maladies to diseases of a broader population. In effect, it may be possible in the future to provide specific, molecular definitions of what physicians have long recognized as the "genetic predisposition" of many families and individuals to a variety of common chronic diseases.

REFERENCES

1. Abraham, P.A., et al.: Marfan syndrome: Demonstration of abnormal elastin in aorta. J. Clin. Invest. 7:1245–1252, 1982.
2. Appel, A., Horwitz, A.L., and Dorfman, A.: Cell-free synthesis of hyaluronic acid in Marfan syndrome. J. Biol. Chem., 254:12199–12203, 1979.
3. Aumailley, M., et al.: Biochemical and immunological studies of fibroblasts derived from a patient with Ehlers-Danlos syndrome type IV demonstrate reduced type III collagen synthesis. Arch. Dermatol. Res., 269:169–177, 1980.
4. Bachinger, H.P., et al.: Structural implications from an electron microscopic comparison of procollagen V with procollagen I, pC-collagen I, procollagen IV, and a Drosophila procollagen. J. Biol. Chem., 257:24590–24592, 1982.
5. Barsh, G.S., and Byers, P.H.: Reduced secretion of structurally abnormal type I procollagen in a form of osteogenesis imperfecta. Proc. Natl. Acad. Sci. USA, 78:5142–5146, 1981.
6. Barsh, G.S., David, K.E., and Byers, P.H.: Type I osteogenesis imperfecta: A nonfunctional allele for proα2(I) chains of type I procollagen. Proc. Natl. Acad. Sci. USA, 79:3838–3942, 1982.
7. Bateman, J.F., et al.: Structural defects of type I procollagen in lethal perinatal osteogenesis imperfecta. Connect. Tissue Res., 9:203, 1982a.
8. Bateman, J.F., et al.: Defective type I procollagen secretion in lethal perinatal osteogenesis imperfecta. Connect. Tissue Res. 9:203, 1982b.
9. Benz, H., et al.: Isolation and partial characterization of a new human collagen with an extended triple-helical structural domain. Proc. Natl. Acad. Sci. USA, 80:3168–3172, 1983.
10. Bernard, M.P., et al.: Nucleotide sequences of cDNAs for the proα1 chain of hyman type I procollagen. Statistical evaluation of structures which are conserved during evolution. Biochemistry, 22:5213–5223, 1983.

11. Bornstein, P., and Byers, P.H.: Disorders of collagen metabolism. *In* Metabolic Control and Disease. Edited by P.K. Bondy, and L.E. Rosenberg. Philadelphia, W.B. Saunders Co., 1980, pp. 1089–1153.

12. Bornstein, P., and Sage, H.: Structurally distinct collagen types. Annu. Rev. Biochem. *49*:957–1003, 1980.

13. Bornstein, P., and Traub, W.: The chemistry and biology of collagen. *In* The Proteins. Vol. 4. Edited by H. Neurath, and R.L. Hill. New York, Academic Press, 1979, pp. 411–632.

14. Boucek, R.J., et al.: The Marfan syndrome: A deficiency in chemically stable collagen cross-links. N. Engl. J. Med. *305*:988–991, 1981.

15. Burgeson, R.E.: Genetic heterogeneity of collagens. J. Invest. Dermatol. *79*:25s–30s, 1982.

16. Byers, P.H., et al.: Abnormal α2-chain in type I collagen from a patient with a form of osteogenesis imperfecta. J. Clin. Invest., *71*:689–697, 1983.

17. Byers, P.H., et al.: Marfan syndrome: Abnormal α2-chain in type I collagen. Proc. Natl. Acad. Sci. USA, *78*:7745–7749, 1981d.

18. Byers, P.H., et al.: Altered secretion of type III procollagen in in form of type IV Ehlers-Danlos syndrome. Biochemical studies in cultured fibroblasts. Lab. Invest., *44*:336–341, 1981c.

19. Byers, P.H., et al.: X-linked cutis laxa. Defective cross-link formation in collagen due to decreased lysyl oxidase activity. N. Engl. J. Med. *303*:61–65, 1980.

20. Byers, P.H., Barsh, G.S., and Holbrook, K.A.: Molecular mechanisms of connective tissue abnormalities in the Ehlers-Danlos syndrome. Col. Rel. Res., *1*:475–489, 1981a.

21. Chu, M.-L., et al.: Characterization of the human proα1(I) collagen gene. Fed. Proc., *42*:1758, 1983a.

22. Chu, M.-L., et al.: Internal deletion in a collagen gene in a perinatal lethal form of osteogenesis imperfecta. Nature, *304*:78–80, 1983b.

23. Clark, J.G., et al.: Lung collagen in type IV Ehlers-Danlos syndrome: Ultrastructural and biochemical studies. Am. Rev. Respir. Dis., *122*:971–978, 1980.

24. Cupo, L.N., et al.: Ehlers-Danlos syndrome with abnormal collagen fibrils, sinus of valsalva aneurysms, myocardial infarction, panacinar emphysema and cerebral heterotopias. Am. J. Med., *71*:1051–1058, 1981.

25. Dagleish, R., et al.: Copy number of a human type I α2 collagen gene. J. Biol. Chem., *257*:13816–13822, 1982.

26. Danks, D.M.: Hereditary disorders of copper metabolism in Wilson's disease and Menkes' disease. *In* The Metabolic Basis of Inherited Disease, 5th ed. Edited by J.B. Stanbury, et al. New York, McGraw-Hill Book Co., 1983, pp. 1251–1268.

27. de Crombrugghe, B., and Pastan, I.: Structure and regulation of a collagen gene. Trends Biochem. Sci., 11–23, 1982.

28. de Wet, W.J., et al.: Synthesis of a shortened proα2(I) chain and decreased synthesis of proα2(I) chains in a proband with osteogenesis imperfecta. J. Biol. Chem., *258*:7721–7728, 1983a.

29. de Wet, W.J., Chu, M.-L., and Prockop, D.J.: The mRNAs for the proα1(I) and proα2(I) chains of type I procollagen are translated at the same rate in normal human fibroblasts and in fibroblasts from two variants of osteogenesis imperfecta with altered steady-state ratios of the two mRNAs. J. Biol. Chem., *258*:14385–14389, 1983b.

30. Deak, S., et al.: The molecular defect in a non-lethal variant of osteogenesis imperfecta: Synthesis of proα2(I) chains which are not incorporated into trimers of type I procollagen. J. Biol. Chem., *258*:15192–15197, 1983.

30a. Dickson, L., et al.: Nuclease S1 mapping of a homozygous mutation in the carboxy-propeptide coding region of the proα2(I) collagen gene in a patient with osteogenesis imperfecta. Proc. Natl. Acad. Sci. USA. In press, 1984.

31. Francis, M.J.O., et al.: The relative amounts of the collagen chains α1(I), α2 and α1(III) in the skin of 31 patients with osteogenesis imperfecta. Clin. Sci., *60*:617a–623, 1981.

32. Gibson, G.J., Schor, S.L., and Grant, M.E.: Effect of matrix macromolecules on chondrocyte gene expression: Synthesis of a low molecular weight collagen species by cells cultured within collagen gels. J. Cell Biol., *93*:767–774, 1982.

33. Grant, M.A., and Prockop, D.J.: The biosynthesis of collagen. N. Engl. J. Med., *286*:194, 242, 291, 1972.

34. Halbritter, R., et al.: Case report and study of collagen metabolism in Marfan's syndrome. Klin. Wochenschr., *59*:83–90, 1981.

35. Halme, T., et al.: Desmosines in aneurysms of the ascending aorta (annuloaortic ectasia). Biochim. Biophys. Acta. *717*:105–110, 1982.

36. Heathcote, J.C., and Grant, M.E.: Extracellular modification of connective tissue proteins. *In* The Enzymology of Post-translational Modifications of Proteins. Edited by R.B. Freedman, and H.C. Hawkins. London, Academic Press, 1980, PP. 457–605.

37. Holbrook, K.A., et al.: Dermatosparaxis in a Himalayan cat: II. Ultrastructural studies of dermal collagen. J. Invest. Dermatol., *74*:100–104, 1980.

38. Holbrook, K.A., and Byers, P.H.: Structural abnormalities in the dermal collagen and elastic matrix from the skin of patients with inherited connective tissue disorders. J. Invest. Dermatol., *79*:7s–16s, 1982.

39. Hollister, D.W., Byers, P.H., and Holbrook, K.A.: Genetic disorders of collagen metabolism. Adv. Hum. Genet., *12*:1–87, 1982.

40. Huerre, C., et al.: Human type I procollagen genes are located on different chromosomes. Proc. Natl. Acad. Sci. USA, *79*:6627–6630, 1982.

41. Ihme, et al.: Biochemical characterization of variants of the Ehlers-Danlos syndrome type VI.. Eur. J. Clin. Invest., *13*:357–362, 1983.

42. Judisch, F.G., Waziri, M., and Krachmer, J.H.: Ocular Ehlers-Danlos syndrome with normal lysyl hydroxylase activity. Arch. Ophthalmol., *94*:1489–1491, 1976.

43. Kefalides, N.A.: Persistence of basement membrane collagen phenotype in hybrids of human vascular endothelium and rodent fibroblasts. Fed. Proc., *38*:816–817, 1979.

44. Kirsch, E., et al.: Disorder of collagen metabolism in a patient with osteogenesis imperfecta (Lethal type): Increased degree of hydroxylation of lysine in collagen types I and III. Eur. J. Clin. Invest., *11*:30–47, 1981.

45. Kivirikko, K.I.: Urinary excretion of hydroxyproline in health and disease. Int. Rev. Connect. Tissue Res., *5*:93–163, 1970.

46. Kivirikko, K.I., and Myllyla, R.: Biosynthesis of collagens. *In* Connective Tissue Biochemistry. Edited by K.A. Piez, and A.H. Reddi. New York, Elsevier, North-Holland. In press, 1984.

47. Kivirikko, K.I., and Myllyla, R.: Post-translational modifications. *In* Collagen in Health and Disease. Edited by J.B. Weiss, and M.I.V. Jayson. New York, Churchill Livingstone, 1982a, pp. 101–120.

48. Kivirikko, K.I., and Myllyla, R.: Collagen glycosyltransferases. Int. Rev. Connect. Tissue Res., *8*:23–72, 1979.

49. Kivirikko, K.I., and Peltonen, L.: Abnormalities in copper metabolism and disturbances in the synthesis of collagen and elastin. Med. Biol. *60*:45–48, 1982b.

50. Kohn, L.D., et al.: Calf tendon procollagen peptidase. Its purification and endopeptidase mode of action. Proc. Natl. Acad. Sci. USA, *71*:40–44, 1974.

51. Krane, S.M.: Hydroxylysine-deficient collagen disease: A form of Ehlers-Danlos syndrome type VI. *In* American Academy of Orthopaedic Surgeons Symposium on Heritable Disorders of Connective Tissue. Edited by W.H. Akeson, P. Bornstein, and M.J. Glimsincher. St Louis, The C.V. Mosby Co., 1982, pp. 61–75.

52. Krane, S.M., Pinnell, S.R., and Erbe, R.W.: Lysyl-protocollagen hydrolysase deficiency in fibroblasts from siblings with hydroxylysine-deficient collagen. Proc. Natl. Acad. Sci. USA., *69*:2899–2903, 1972.

53. Krieg, T., et al.: Molecular defects of collagen metabolism In the Ehlers-Danlos syndrome. Int. J. Dermatol., *20*:415–425, 1981.

54. Kuivaniemi, H., et al.: Abnormal copper metabolism and

deficient lysyl oxidase activity in a heritable connective tissue disorder. J. Clin. Invest., *69*:730–733, 1982.

55. Lichtenstein, J.R., et al.: Defect in conversion of procollagen to collagen in a form of Ehlers-Danlos syndrome. Science, *182*:298–300, 1973.

56. Mayne, R., Reese, C.A., and Wiedemann, H.: New collagenous molecules from chicken hyaline cartilage. *In* New Trends in Basement Membrane Research. Edtied by K. Kuhn, H.-H. Schoene, and R. Timpl. New York, Raven Press, 1982, pp. 121–126.

57. McKusick, V.A.: Heritable Disorders of Connective Tissue. Saint Louis, The C.V. Mosby Co., 1972.

58. Meigel, W.N., et al.: A constitutional disorder of connective tissue suggesting a defect in collagen biosynthesis. Klin. Wochenschr., *52*:906–912, 1974.

59. Minor, R.R.: Collagen metabolism. A comparison of diseases of collagen and diseases affecting collagen. Am. J. Pathol., *98*:227–278, 1980.

60. Minor, R.R., et al.: Defects in collagen fibrillogenesis causing hyperextensible, fragile skin in dogs. J. Am. Vet. Med. Assoc. *182*:142–148, 1983.

61. Monson, J.M., and McCarthy, B.J.: Identification of a Balb/c mouse proα1(I) procollagen gene: Evidence for insertions or deletions in gene coding sequences. DNA, *1*:59–69, 1981.

62. Müller, P.K., et al.: Presence of type III collagen in bone from a patient with osteogenesis imperfecta. Eur. J. Pediatr., *125*:29–37, 1977.

63. Myers, J.C., et al.: Analysis of the 3′ end of the human proα2(I) collagen gene: Utilization of multiple polyadenylation sites in cultured fibroblasts. J. Biol. Chem., *258*:10128–10135, 1983.

64. Myers, J.C., et al.: Cloning a cDNA for the proα2 chain of human type I collagen. Proc. Natl. Acad. Sci. USA, *78*:3516–3520, 1981.

65. Nicholls, A.C., Pope, F.M., and Schloon, H.: Biochemical heterogeneity of osteogenesis imperfecta: New variant. Lancet, *1*:1193, 1979.

66. Nimmi, M.E.: Collagen: Structure, function, and metabolism in normal and fibrotic tissues. Semin. Arthritis Rheum., *13*:1–86, 1983.

67. Odermatt, E., et al.: Structural diversity and domain composition of a unique collagenous fragment (intima collagen) obtained from human placenta. Biochem. J., *211*:295–302, 1983.

68. Peltonen, L., et al.: Alterations in copper and collagen metabolism in the Menkes syndrome and a new subtype of the Ehlers-Danlos syndrome. Biochemistry. In press, 1984.

69. Peltonen, L., Palotie, A., and Prockop, D.J.: A defect in the structure of type I procollagen in a patient who had osteogenesis imperfecta: Excess mannose in the COOH-terminal propeptide. Proc. Natl. Acad. Sci. USA, *77*:6179–6183, 1980.

70. Penttinen, R.P., et al.: Abnormal collagen metabolism in cultured cells in osteogenesis imperfecta. Proc. Natl. Acad. Sci. USA, *72*:586–589, 1975.

71. Pinnell, S.R., et al.: A heritable disorder of connective tissue. Hydroxylysine-deficient collagen disease. N. Engl. J. Med., *286*:1013–1020, 1972.

72. Pinnell, S.R., and Murad, S.: Disorders of collagen. *In* The Metabolic Basis of Inherited Disease. Edited by J.B. Stanbury, et al. New York, McGraw-Hill Book Co., 1983, pp. 1425–1449.

73. Pope, F.M., et al.: Osteogenesis imperfecta (lethal) bones contain types III and V collagens. J. Clin. Pathol., *33*:53408, 1980a.

74. Pope, F.M., et al.: EDS IV (acrogeria): New autosomal dominant and recessive types. J.R. Soc. Med., *73*:180–186, 1980b.

75. Pope, F.M., et al.: Patients with Ehlers-Danlos syndrome type IV lack type III collagen. Proc. Natl. Acad. Sci. USA, *72*:1314–1316, 1975.

76. Pope, F.M., and Nicholls, A.C.: Molecular abnormalities of collagen in osteogenesis imperfecta. Mainz Symposium on Bone Dysplasias. 1982.

77. Prockop, D.J., et al.: The biosynthesis of collagen and its disorders. N. Engl. J. Med., *301*:13–23, 77–85, 1979.

78. Prockop, D.J., and Kivirikko, K.I.: Heritable disorders of collagen. The lessons of rare maladies provide a basis for understanding common diseases. N. Engl. J. Med. In press, 1984.

79. Pyeritz, R.E., and McKusick, V.A.: The Marfan syndrome: Diagnosis and management. N. Engl. J. Med., *300*:772–777, 1979.

80. Rowe, D.W., et al.: Decreased lysyl oxidase activity in the aneurysm-prone mottled mouse. J. Biol. Chem., *252*:939–942, 1977.

81. Royce, P.M., and Danks, D.M.: Normal lysyl oxidase activity in skin fibroblasts from patients with Marfan's syndrome. IRCS Med. Sci., *10*:41, 1982.

82. Sage, H.: Collagens of basement membranes. J. Invest. Dermatol., *79*:51s–59s, 1982.

83. Sandell, L.J., et al.: Identification of the gene coding for type II procollagen. J. Biol. Chem., *258*:11617–11621, 1984.

84. Schmid, T., and Conrad, H.E.: A unique low molecular weight collagen secreted by cultured chick embryo chondrocytes. J. Biol. Chem., *257*:12444–12450, 1982.

85. Siegel, R.C.: Lysyl oxidase. Int. Rev. Connect. Tissue Res., 8:73–118, 1979.

86. Siegel, R.C., Black, C.M., and Bailey, A.J.: Cross-linking of collagen in the X-linked Ehlers-Danlos type V. Biochem. Biophys. Res. Commun., *88*:281–287, 1979.

87. Sillence, D.O.: Osteogenesis imperfecta: An expanding panorama of variants. Clin. Orthop. Rel. Res., *159*:11–25, 1981.

88. Sillence, D.O., Senn, A., and Danks, D.M.: Genetic heterogeneity in osteogenesis imperfecta. J. Med. Genet. *16*:101–116, 1979.

89. Sippola, M., and Prockop, D.J.: A shortened proα2(I) chain in a mild variant of osteogenesis imperfecta. The altered structure makes type I procollagen resistant to procollagen N-proteinase. J. Cell Biol., *97*:229a, 1984.

90. Smith, R., Francis, M.J.O., and Houghton, G.R.: The Brittle Bone Syndrome. Osteogenesis Imperfecta. London, Butterworths, 1983.

91. Solomon, E., et al.: Regional localization of the human α2(I) collagen gene on chromosome 7 by molecular hybridization. Cytogenet. Cell Genet., *35*:64–66, 1983.

92. Starcher, B., et al.: Abnormal cellular copper metabolism in the blotchy mouse. J. Nutr., *108*:1229–1233, 1978.

93. Steinmann, B., et al.: Evidence for a structural mutation of procollagen type I in a patient with the Ehlers-Danlos syndrome type VII. J. Biol. Chem., *255*:8887–8893, 1980.

94. Steinmann, B., et al.: Ehlers-Danlos syndrome in two siblings with deficient lysyl hydroxylase activity in cultured skin fibroblasts but only mild hydroxylysine deficit in skin. Helv. Paediatr. Acta, 30:255–274, 1975.

95. Stolle, C.A., et al.: Synthesis of an altered type III procollagen in a patient with type IV Ehlers-Danlos syndrome. A structural change in the α1(III) chain which makes the protein more susceptible to proteinases (abstract). J. Cell Biol., 1983.

96. Tate, R., et al.: The procollagen genes: Further sequence studies and interspecies comparisons. Cold Spring Harbor Symp., *47*:1039–1049, 1982.

97. Timpl, R., et al.: A network model for the organization of type IV collagen molecules in basement membranes. Eur. J. Biochem., *120*:203–211, 1981.

98. Tolstoshev, P., and Crystal, R.: The collagen alpha-2 chain gene. J. Invest. Dermatol., *79*:60S–64S, 1982.

99. Trelstad, R.L., Rubin, D., and Gross, J.: Osteogenesis imperfecta congenita. Evidence for a generalized molecular disorder of collagen. Lab Invest., *36*:501–508, 1977.

100. Tuderman, L., and Prockop, D.J.: Procollagen N-proteinase. Properties of the enzyme purified from chick embryo tendons. Eur. J. Biochem., *125*:545–549, 1982.

101. Turakainen, H., et al.: Synthesis of hyaluronic acid and collagen in skin fibroblasts cultured from patients with osteogenesis imperfecta. Biochim. Biophys. Acta, *628*:388–397, 1980.

102. Uitto, J., et al.: Synthesis of lengthened proα1(I) chains of type I procollagen by skin fibroblasts from two patients

with lethal osteogenesis imperfecta. Clin. Res., *31*:468A, 1983.

103. Uitto, J., et al.: The Ehlers-Danlos syndrome type IV: Clinical, genetic, and biochemical studies of a family. *In* American Academy of Orthopaedic Surgeons Symposium on Heritable Disorders of Connective Tissue. Edited by W.J. Akeson, P. Bornstein, and M.J. Glimcher. Saint Louis, The C.V. Mosby Co., 1982, pp. 82–95.

104. Uitto, J., Ryhanen, L., and Tan, E.M.L.: Collagen: Its structure, function, and pathology. *In* Progress in Diseases of the Skin. Vol. 1. Edited by R. Fleischmajer. New York, Grune and Stratton, 1981, pp. 103–141.

105. Williams, C.J., and Prockop, D.J.: Synthesis and processing of a type I procollagen containing shortened proα1(I) chains by fibroblasts from a patient with osteogenesis imperfecta. J. Biol. Chem., *258*:5915–5921, 1983.

106. Wozney, J., et al.: Structure of the proα2(I) collagen gene. Nature, *294*:129–135, 1981.

107. Yamada, Y., et al.: The collagen gene: Evidence for its evolutionary assembly by amplification of a DNA segment containing an exon of 54 bp. Cell, *22*:887–892, 1980.

108. Yamada, Y., et al.: Isolation and characterization of a genomic clone encoding chick α1 and type III collagen. J. Biol. Chem., *258*:2758–2761, 1983.

Chapter 11

Structure and Function of Proteoglycans

Lawrence Rosenberg

Articular cartilage and nucleus pulposus are highly specialized connective tissues composed of relatively few cells distributed throughout an abundant extracellular matrix. The extracellular matrix gives each tissue unusual mechanical properties essential for normal joint function. Articular cartilage provides a smooth covering for the osseous components of diarthrodial joints and contributes to the almost frictionless gliding of opposing joint surfaces. Articular cartilage is a relatively hard, yet elastic tissue. Nucleus pulposus is softer, more compressible and deformable, and has the capacity to undergo substantial changes in shape and volume with motion of the intervetebral joint. Both tissues transmit load, absorb impact, and sustain shearing forces, yet resist wear to a surprising degree.

The remarkable mechanical properties of these connective tissues are directly related to the structure and properties of the extracellular matrix. The extracellular matrix is composed mainly of collagen, proteoglycans, and water. Collagen is an insoluble fibrous protein with tensile strength. Proteoglycans are elastic molecules that tend to expand in solution and resist compression into a smaller volume of solution. The mechanical properties of normal articular cartilage and nucleus pulposus result from the structure and properties of the fibrous composite formed when proteoglycans at high concentration are entangled and constrained in a dense network of collagen fibers. Our understanding of the mechanical properties of normal articular cartilage and nucleus pulposus must be based upon knowledge of the structures and physicochemical properties of proteoglycans and collagen and their interactions.

Current interest in the structure and properties of the molecular species comprising the intercellular substance of cartilage is based on other, more compelling considerations. Degradation of proteoglycans is a central event in osteoarthritis and rheumatoid arthritis, resulting in a loss of the capacity of articular cartilage to resist wear, and an acceleration of the destructive process. Each of these forms of arthritis may be viewed as a series of biochemical processes in which connective tissue macromolecules of elaborate structure are shattered in a characteristic fashion by specific enzymes. The clinical effect of the cartilage destruction is pain, limitation of motion of the affected joint, and increasing functional disability. A comprehensive view of the pathogenesis of a particular form of arthritis should include knowledge of the sequence of events at the cellular level involved in cartilage destruction, and of the biochemical mechanisms underlying each event. The first section of this chapter describes the cartilage proteoglycans that are degraded in diseases such as osteoarthritis and rheumatoid arthritis.

CARTILAGE PROTEOGLYCANS

In the formation of both collagen and proteoglycans, a basic structural unit of relatively low molecular weight is first formed. Many basic units then assemble into an ordered aggregate form of much higher molecular weight. The aggregate form exhibits the specific functional properties of the biochemical species, whereas the basic structural unit does not, at least to the same degree. Such a process is frequently encountered in biochemistry.

The basic structural unit of cartilage ground substance is the proteoglycan monomer. A diagrammatic model of the structure of a cartilage proteoglycan monomer is shown in Figure 11–1. It consists of a protein core from which arise many chondroitin sulfate and keratan sulfate side chains. Chrondroitin sulfate and keratan sulfate are covalently attached mainly to serine and threonine residues within the protein core. Proteoglycan monomers from different cartilages and nucleus pulposus vary considerably in molecular weight and chemical composition, particularly the relative amounts of chondroitin sulfate and keratan sulfate. Indeed, proteoglycan monomers from the same cartilage are polydisperse and vary in size and composition. However, an average representative proteoglycan monomer would have a protein core of approximately 200,000 in molecular weight, measuring about 300 nm long. To this protein core would be attached approximately 100 chondroitin sulfate side chains, each 20,000 to 30,000 in molecular

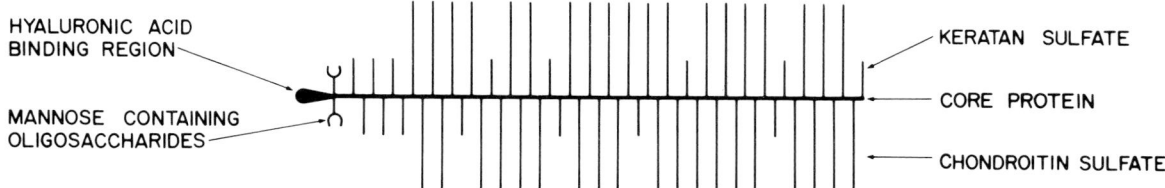

Fig. 11–1.   Diagrammatic model of the structure of the cartilage proteoglycan monomer.

weight, and approximately 50 to 60 nm long. Keratan sulfate chains, 5,000 to 10,000 in molecular weight and 10 to 20 nm in length, would also be attached to the protein core. The entire proteoglycan monomer would be approximately 2 to 3 million in molecular weight.

Chondroitin sulfate and keratan sulfate are linear polymers composed of sugar residues. They are members of the group of polysaccharides called glycosaminoglycans or mucopolysaccharides found in the ground substance of various connective tissues. The glycosaminoglycans are composed of two different sugar residues that alternate regularly in the polysaccharide chain. One sugar residue is an amino sugar, formed when the hydroxyl group of the number two carbon of glucose or galactose is replaced by an amino group, which is acetylated. Therefore, in the glycosaminoglycans, one sugar residue is the hexosamine N-acetylglycosamine or N-acetylgalactosamine. The other sugar residue is usually glucuronic acid, in which the number six carbon of glucose carries a carboxyl group. Each glycosaminoglycan is described in terms of the sugar residues that comprise its disaccharide repeating unit. The structures of the glycosaminoglycans and their linkage regions to protein core are shown in Figure 11–2.

The structure of the disaccharide repeating unit of chondroitin 6-sulfate is shown on the left of Figure 11–3. Chondroitin 6-sulfate chains are composed of approximately 40 to 60 repeating units consisting of glucuronic acid alternating with N-acetylgalactosamine. N-acetylgalactosamine carries an ester sulfate group on carbon number six. The chondroitin sulfate chains are covalently bound to serine residues within the protein core via the neutral sugar trisaccharide galactose-galactose-xylose shown on the right of Figure 11–3.[52,62,64] The structure of the keratan sulfate repeating unit is shown on the left of Figure 11–4. Keratan sulfate consists of galactose residues alternating regularly with N-acetylglucosamine residues. Keratan sulfate carries an ester sulfate group on the number six carbon of N-acetylglucosamine, and some or most of the galactose residues of keratan sulfate

may be sulfated. Keratan sulfate chains consist of approximately 10 to 20 repeating units covalently bound mainly to threonine or serine residues of the protein core via N-acetylgalactosamine. As shown on the right of Figure 11–4, N-acetylneuraminic acid (sialic acid) and galactose residues are attached to the N-acetylgalactosamine residue linking each keratan sulfate chain to protein.[48,49]

The most important feature of the chemical structure of chondroitin sulfate and keratan sulfate is that the repeating units of the glycosaminoglycans carry closely spaced negatively charged groups. Glycosaminoglycan repeating units are approximately 450 to 500 in molecular weight and 1 nm in length. Chondroitin 6-sulfate carries an ester sulfate group attached to carbon number six of N-acetylgalactosamine and the negatively charged carboxyl group of glucuronic acid. Thus, chondroitin 6-sulfate carries negatively charged groups at approximately 0.5-nm intervals. Keratan sulfate carries an ester sulfate group on carbon number six of N-acetylglucosamine, and some or most of the galactose residues may be sulfated, so that keratan sulfate carries negatively charged groups at 0.5- to 1-nm intervals. Because of the repelling forces of the closely spaced negatively charged groups, the glycosaminoglycan chains arising from proteoglycan monomer core protein are maintained in a stiffly extended conformation. The chondroitin sulfate and keratan sulfate chains stick out from core protein like the bristles on a brush, as shown in Figure 11–1. The proteoglycan monomer assumes an extended conformation and spreads out into a relatively large volume of solution. The stiffness of the glycosaminoglycan chains makes the molecule resistant to compression into a smaller volume of solution. This property is partially responsible for the elasticity of cartilage.

In addition to chondroitin sulfate and keratan sulfate, proteoglycan monomers contain two types of oligosaccharides.[16,53] The first type consists of oligosaccharides that resemble the linkage region of keratan sulfate to core protein, and that are linked via N-acetylgalactosamine by O-glycosidic

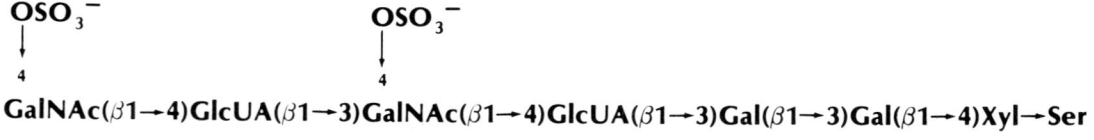

$$\overset{OSO_3^-}{\underset{4}{\downarrow}} \qquad \overset{OSO_3^-}{\underset{4}{\downarrow}}$$

GalNAc(β1→4)GlcUA(β1→3)GalNAc(β1→4)GlcUA(β1→3)Gal(β1→3)Gal(β1→4)Xyl→Ser

CHONDROITIN 4-SULFATE

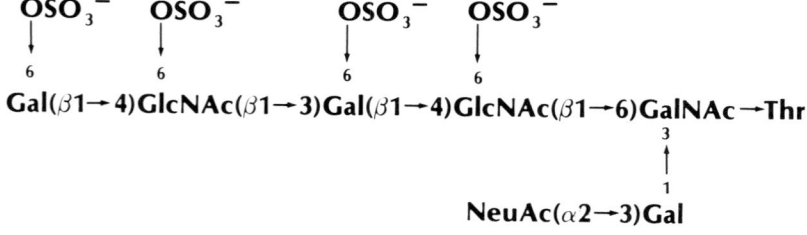

Gal(β1→4)GlcNAc(β1→3)Gal(β1→4)GlcNAc(β1→6)GalNAc→Thr

NeuAc(α2→3)Gal

KERATAN SULFATE

GlcNAc(β1→4)GlcUA(β1→3)GlcNAc(β1→4)GlcUA(β1→3)Gal(β1→3)Gal(β1→4)Xyl→Ser

HYALURONATE

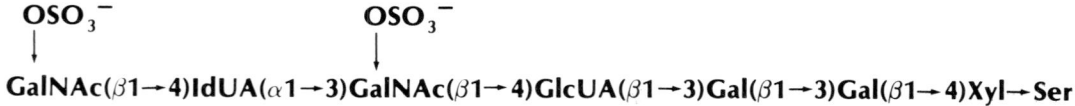

GalNAc(β1→4)IdUA(α1→3)GalNAc(β1→4)GlcUA(β1→3)Gal(β1→3)Gal(β1→4)Xyl→Ser

DERMATAN SULFATE

GlcNAc(α1→4)IdUA(α1→4)GlcNAc(α1→4)GlcUA(β1→3)Gal(β1→3)Gal(β1→4)Xyl→Ser

HEPARAN SULFATE

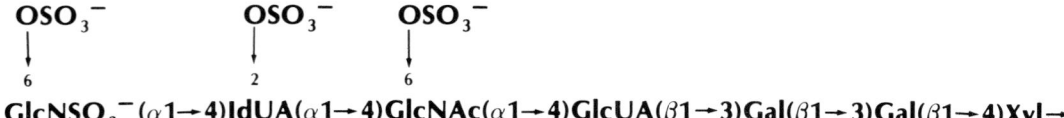

GlcNSO$_3^-$(α1→4)IdUA(α1→4)GlcNAc(α1→4)GlcUA(β1→3)Gal(β1→3)Gal(β1→4)Xyl→Ser

HEPARIN

Fig. 11–2. Structures of the glycosaminoglycans and their linkage regions to protein. GlcUA = glucuronic acid; IdUA = iduronic acid; GlcNAc = N-acetylglucosamine; GalNAc = N-acetylgalactosamine; Gal = galactose; Xyl = xylose; NeuAc = N-acetylneuraminic acid. Two disaccharide repeating units are shown to emphasize the microheterogeneity that exists in some cases. Heparan sulfate and heparin show many structural similarities. However, heparan sulfate contains more GlcNAc(α1→4)GlcUA repeating units, fewer glucosamine residues are N-sulfated, and fewer iduronic acid residues are sulfated at C2.

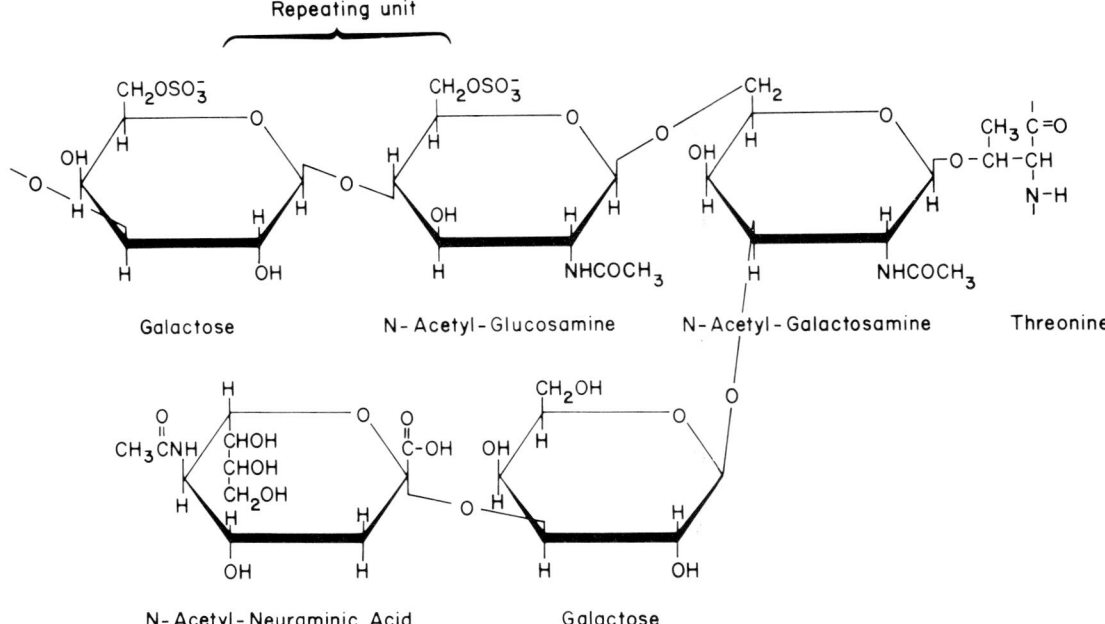

Fig. 11–3. Structure of chondroitin 6-sulfate and of its linkage region to protein. The disaccharide repeating unit of chondroitin 6-sulfate consists of glucuronic acid and N-acetylgalactosamine 6-sulfate. The chondroitin sulfate chain is covalently bound to serine via the trisaccharide containing galactose and xylose.

Fig. 11–4. Structure of keratan sulfate and its linkage region to protein. The disaccharide repeating unit of keratan sulfate consists of galactose and N-acetylglucosamine 6-sulfate. The keratan sulfate chain is covalently bound mainly to threonine via N-acetylgalactosamine.

bonds to the hydroxyl groups of threonine or serine residues of core protein:

$$NeuAc(2{\rightarrow}3)Gal(1{\rightarrow}3)GalNAc$$

$$\begin{array}{c} NeuAc \\ {\scriptstyle 2} \\ {\downarrow} \\ {\scriptstyle 6} \end{array}$$
$$NeuAc(2{\rightarrow}3)Gal(1{\rightarrow}3)GalNAc$$

$$NeuAc(2{\rightarrow}3)Gal(1{\rightarrow}4)GlcNAc$$
$$\begin{array}{c} {\downarrow} \\ {\scriptstyle 6} \end{array}$$
$$NeuAc(2{\rightarrow}3)Gal(1{\rightarrow}3)GalNAc$$

These oligosaccharides are located mainly in the chondroitin sulfate-rich region of core protein. In developing (fetal) hyaline cartilages, the proportion

of keratan sulfate linkage region-like oligosaccharides is high, and the proportion of keratan sulfate chains in the chondroitin sulfate-rich region is low. In mature hyaline cartilages, the proportion of keratan sulfate chains is high, and the proportion of keratan sulfate linkage region-like oligosaccharides is low.

The second type of oligosaccharide is mannose-containing oligosaccharide, probably linked by N-glycosylamine bonds to asparagine residues in core protein. Although the structures of the mannose–containing oligosaccharides are only now being elucidated, they are probably similar to those of the mannose-rich oligosaccharides linked by N-glycosidic bonds to asparagine. These oligosaccharides are present in many glycoproteins. In proteoglycan monomers, the mannose-containing ol-igosaccharides are located near the hyaluronic acid-binding region as shown in Figure 11–1.

STRUCTURE OF CARTILAGE PROTEOGLYCAN AGGREGATES

In native cartilage, most of the proteoglycan exists in the form of aggregates of high molecular weight.[31–46,65,68–71] The molecular architecture of a proteoglycan aggregate is shown in Figure 11–5. Hyaluronic acid forms the filamentous backbone of the aggregate.[33–36,38,69] The aggregate is formed by the noncovalent association of many proteoglycan monomers with hyaluronate. Proteoglycan monomers of varying size arise laterally at regular intervals from the opposite sides of the hyaluronic

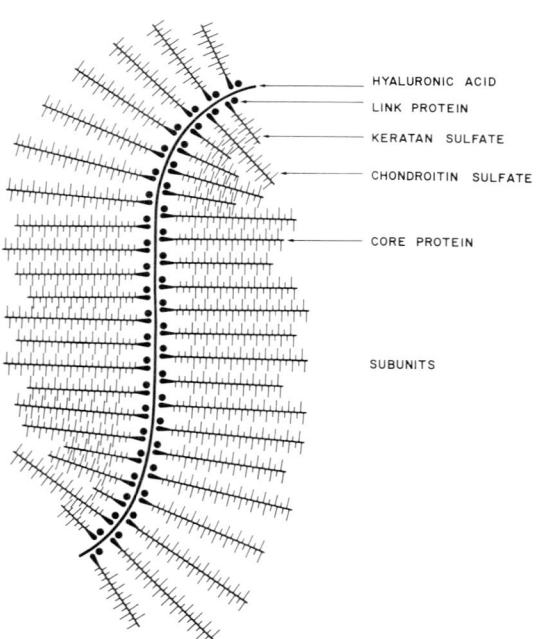

PROTEOGLYCAN   AGGREGATE

HYALURONIC ACID
LINK PROTEIN
KERATAN SULFATE
CHONDROITIN SULFATE

CORE PROTEIN

SUBUNITS

Fig. 11–5. Diagrammatic model of the cartilage proteoglycan aggregate. The filamentous backbone of the aggregate is hyaluronic acid. Proteoglycan monomers of varying size arise at regular intervals from the opposite sides of the hyaluronic acid chain. One end of the proteoglycan monomer core protein has a globular conformation and contains the hyaluronic acid binding region of the core protein. The other end of the core protein has an extended conformation and contains the attachment sites for chondroitin sulfate and keratan sulfate chains. The polydispersity in size and composition of proteoglycan monomers from mature cartilages results from the variable length of the chondroitin sulfate-rich region of proteoglycan monomer core protein. (From Rosenberg, L.[65])

acid chain. A low-molecular-weight ''link'' protein is also a component of the aggregate. Link protein appears to stabilize or to strengthen the bond between proteoglycan monomer and hyaluronate.

A closer examination of the model shown in Figure 11–5 indicates that proteoglycan monomer core protein consists of three distinct regions that differ in structure and function. One end of the proteoglycan monomer core protein contains little or no chondroitin sulfate or keratan sulfate, and consists of a region of core protein approximately 60,000 in molecular weight with a globular conformation. This region contains the hyaluronic acid binding of proteoglycan monomer core protein.[41,46,67] Extending toward the other end of the molecule is a region of the protein core to which essentially all the chondroitin sulfate chains and some of the keratan sulfate chains are attached. It is called the chondroitin sulfate-rich region. Between the hyaluronic acid binding region and the chondroitin sulfate-rich region is located a third region consisting of a short peptide to which are attached mainly keratan sulfate chains.[44,67] This region is called the keratan sulfate-rich region.[44] In the proteoglycan aggregate, the link proteins are centrally located in the region where proteoglycan monomer binds to hyaluronate. The link proteins bind simultaneously to the hyaluronic acid binding region of proteoglycan monomer core protein, and to hyaluronate, and stabilize the binding of proteoglycan monomer to hyaluronate.

Proteoglycan aggregates in different tissues vary greatly in size and composition owing to differences in hyaluronic acid chain lengths, and to differences in the size, chemical composition, and numbers of proteoglycan monomers noncovalently bound to hyaluronic acid in the proteoglycan aggregates. The mechanical properties of different tissues are related to these variations in the size and composition of proteoglycan aggregates. Even proteoglycan aggregates isolated from a particular cartilage are markedly polydisperse. They consist of a population of molecules in which individual members vary greatly in molecular weight owing mainly to differences in the length of hyaluronic acid chain that forms the filamentous backbone of the proteoglycan aggregate. However, a representative proteoglycan aggregate from articular cartilage would consist of over 100 proteoglycan monomers (each two million daltons in molecular weight) noncovalently bound together with link protein to a hyaluronic acid chain 4,000 nm in length. Such an aggregate would be over 200 million daltons in molecular weight.

Because of the repelling forces of the thousands of negatively charged groups, these huge proteoglycan aggregates spread out into an enormous domain of solution. The volume of solution occupied by proteoglycan aggregates in vitro is far greater than that available to them in native cartilage, where the aggregates expand until they are constrained by the surrounding network of collagen fibers. The aggregates in native cartilage exhibit elastic forces that are balanced by the tensile forces of collagen fibers. When articular cartilage is subjected to a compressive force, the aggregates are temporarily compressed into a smaller domain, and water is simultaneously extruded from the cartilage. When the compressive force is relieved, the aggregates expand, the articular cartilage simultaneously imbibes water, and the volume of the cartilage increases until further increases in volume are prevented by the collagen fibers. This kind of interaction is the basis for the elastic properties of articular cartilage.

The aforementioned structural concepts have been derived from studies of the chemical composition and physical properties of proteoglycan monomers and aggregates from different cartilages and from chemical binding studies between proteoglycan monomers, hyaluronate, and link protein. These studies required that proteoglycan monomers and proteoglycan aggregates first be isolated from cartilage. The procedure now generally used for the isolation of proteoglycan aggregates and monomers from cartilage involves four steps: (1) dissociative extraction; (2) reassociation; (3) equilibrium density gradient centrifugation under associative conditions; and (4) equilibrium density gradient centrifugation under dissociative conditions.

The purpose of step 1, dissociative extraction, is to bring proteoglycans into solution and to separate them from the insoluble network of collagen fibers. In native cartilage, most of the proteoglycan exists in the form of huge proteoglycan aggregates that are intricately entangled with, enmeshed in, and constrained by the dense network of collagen fibers. Little proteoglycan diffuses out of fresh, wet cartilage when it is stirred in the cold in isotonic solvents at neutral pH. The dissociative extraction method for extracting proteoglycans depends upon one of the fundamental properties of the proteoglycan aggregate.

The noncovalent bonds between proteoglycan monomers, hyaluronate, and link protein are broken in concentrated solutions of guanidine hydrochloride (GuHCl) or divalent cations.[56,68,74] When fresh, wet cartilage is slowly stirred at 4° in 4 molar GuHCl, pH 5.8 to 6.3, proteoglycan aggregates dissociate. Proteoglycan monomers, hyaluronate, and link proteins diffuse out of the insoluble collagen network at a rapid rate into the extraction

solvent. The extract is separated from the insoluble collagenous cartilage residue by filtration. The filtered extract also contains a variety of noncollagenous matrix proteins that must be separated from the proteoglycans. To accomplish this, proteoglycan monomer, hyaluronate, and link proteins are first reassembled into proteoglycan aggregates by dialyzing off the guanidine hydrochloride. This is step 2: reassociation.

In step 3, matrix proteins are separated from the proteoglycan aggregates by equilibrium density gradient centrifugation under associative conditions. Cesium chloride is added to the reassociated extract, and the solution is centrifuged to equilibrium in a preparative ultracentrifuge. A gradient is established in which the concentration of CsCl and the denstiy of the solution increase with distance from the top to the bottom of the solution. The gradient is divided into six equal fractions. The fractions from the bottom to the top of this associative gradient are called A1 through A6.[42,67] Proteoglycan aggregates are of high buoyant density and distribute in fraction A1 in the bottom one-sixth ($\rho \approx 1.6$ g/ml) of the gradient. The matrix proteins are of low buoyant density and distribute in fraction A6 ($\rho \approx 1.4$ g/ml) at the top of the gradient. Fraction A1 is the preparation used for the physical characterization of proteoglycan aggregates by sedimentation velocity experiments[68] and by electron microscopy.[69]

In step 4, equilibrium density gradient centrifugation under dissociative conditions, the proteoglycan aggregate is separated into its component species. Fraction A1 from the associative gradient, which contains proteoglycan aggregate, is dissolved in 4 mol/l GuHCl. The aggregate is dissociated into proteoglycan monomer, hyaluronate, and link protein. Cesium chloride is added. The solution is centrifuged to equilibrium in a preparative ultracentrifuge. Six fractions called A1–D1 (bottom) through A1–D6 (top) are taken from this dissociative gradient. The effects of the dissociative gradient are shown diagrammatically in Figure 11–6.[67] Link protein is separated into the top of the gradient. Hyaluronic acid distributes in the middle of the 4 mol/l GuHCl–3mol/l CsCl dissociative gradient. Proteoglycan monomers from mature hyaline cartilages distribute throughout the dissociative gradient. Individual members of the polydisperse population of proteoglycan monomers from mature hyaline cartilages band at buoyant densities determined mainly by their chondroitin sulfate and keratan sulfate to protein ratios.

Figure 11–6 also expresses diagrammatically the structural basis for the polydispersity of proteoglycan monomers from a particular mature hyaline cartilage. The polydispersity of proteoglycan

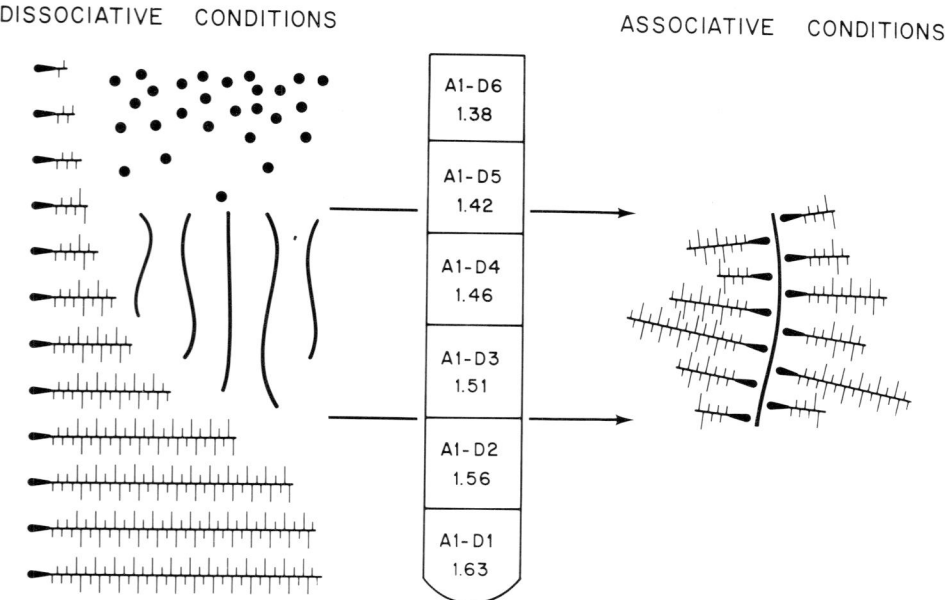

DISSOCIATIVE CONDITIONS   ASSOCIATIVE CONDITIONS

A1-D6 1.38
A1-D5 1.42
A1-D4 1.46
A1-D3 1.51
A1-D2 1.56
A1-D1 1.63

Fig. 11–6. Diagrammatic representation of the structural basis for the polydispersity of cartilage proteoglycan monomer. The polydispersity of the proteoglycan monomer is determined mainly by the variable length of the chondroitin sulfate-rich region of the protein core. The chondroitin sulfate-to-protein ratio, buoyant density, and molecular weight of an individual proteoglycan monomer molecule are directly related to the length of the chondroitin sulfate-rich region of core protein.

monomers appears to be determined mainly by the variable length of the chondroitin sulfate-rich region of proteoglycan monomer core protein. Proteoglycan monomer core protein contains a hyaluronic acid bonding region of constant size and composition, located in the region where the monomer binds to hyaluronate. Proteoglycan monomer core protein also contains a chondroitin sulfate-rich region of variable length (composed of variable numbers of possibly homologous peptides providing attachment sites for chondroitin sulfate chains), which extends toward the other terminus. The chondroitin sulfate to protein ratio, buoyant density, and molecular weight of an individual proteoglycan monomer are determined mainly by the length of the chondroitin sulfate-rich region of the core protein.

This concept for the structural basis of the polydispersity of proteoglycan monomer is based on the results of several studies. In the first series of studies, the variable length of the chondroitin sulfate-rich region has been deduced indirectly from the chemical composition and physical properties of individual members of the polydisperse population of proteoglycan monomers. For example, Table 11–1 shows the chemical composition and physical properties of eight relatively monodisperse proteoglycan monomer fractions

separated from the polydisperse population of proteoglycan monomers from bovine articular cartilage.[67] As shown in Table 11–1, the chondroitin sulfate content of each fraction, as indicated by the values for uronate or galactosamine, increases as the sedimentation coefficient of the proteoglycan monomer increases from 5.7S to 14S. These data indicate that the molecular weight of a proteoglycan monomer increases in proportion to its chondroitin sulfate content. The chondroitin sulfate to protein ratio of the fractions also increases and is largely responsible for the differences in the buoyant densities of the fractions. One possible structural basis for this pattern of polydispersity might be that all proteoglycan monomer contains the same core protein, i.e., polypeptide chains identical in molecular weight and composition in which chondroitin sulfate chains of different lengths are attached. However, the amino acid composition of proteoglycan monomers of different molecular weights is not constant. As shown in Table 11–1, the amino acid composition varies characteristically with molecular weight. The molecules of lowest weight are highest in cysteine, methionine, and aspartic acid, and lowest in serine and glycine. As the molecular weight increases, serine and glycine increase and cysteine, methionine, and aspartic acid decrease.

Table 11–1. Chemical Composition and Physical Properties of Eight Monodisperse PGS Fractions Isolated from Bovine Articular Cartilage

Column	1	2	3	4	5	6	7	8
Yield, g/g	.019	.039	.036	.045	.074	.053	.209	.451
Uronate, %	9.7	10.3	11.5	15.3	16.1	17.1	19.0	20.1
Galactosamine	6.6	8.1	12.7	14.3	15.4	14.8	17.5	18.7
Hexose	12.5	13.5	12.9	14.3	13.3	11.7	11.8	12.2
Glucosamine	10.4	11.1	10.0	9.1	8.6	5.6	6.5	6.0
Sialate	3.0	3.1	2.9	2.4	2.8	1.8	1.8	1.4
Protein	30.7	23.9	17.3	13.0	14.9	10.3	11.1	9.9
s_{20}^0, subunit	5.7	7.8	8.8	9.7	10.3	10.8	12.7	14.3
s_{20}^0, aggregate		18.8	32.1					
Amino Acid Composition Residues/1000								
Aspartic acid	96	92	71	68	70	62	65	60
Threonine	61	65	68	63	65	62	62	61
Serine	69	77	90	105	103	115	123	125
Glutamic acid	139	138	149	147	141	150	146	150
Proline	84	96	101	111	110	104	105	101
Glycine	81	87	93	102	102	117	114	118
Alanine	75	76	77	74	76	71	73	70
Half-cystine	20	21	17	14	17	12	13	12
Valine	60	56	56	59	56	59	59	57
Methionine	12	10	10	6	8	6	7	5
Isoleucine	35	34	33	32	31	32	33	40
Leucine	81	78	74	73	74	74	78	78
Tyrosine	42	27	33	29	20	27	25	24
Phenylalanine	40	45	41	43	41	39	38	38
Lysine	32	28	24	19	19	15	15	13
Histidine	14	17	12	11	11	12	13	13
Arginine	58	55	51	44	47	42	41	37

What is the structural basis for this change in amino acid composition with molecular weight? The hyaluronic acid binding region of proteoglycan monomer core protein has been isolated.[46] It is characterized by its relatively high cysteine, methionine, and aspartic acid contents, and its relatively low serine and glycine contents. The chondroitin sulfate-rich region of proteoglycan monomer core protein is composed of variable numbers of possibly homologous peptides each containing Ser-Gly within a region, with the primary structure and conformation required for the initiation of the synthesis of a chondroitin sulfate chain.[2,3] The changes in the amino acid composition of proteoglycan monomer with molecular weight reflect the changes in the proportions of these two major domains of core protein. Proteoglycan monomers of the lowest molecular weight consist mainly of the hyaluronic acid binding region. As the molecular weight of a proteoglycan monomer increases, the size of the chrodroitin sulfate-rich region increases, as indicated by the increase in serine and glycine contents. Thus, the polydispersity of proteoglycan monomers results mainly from the variable length of the chondroitin sulfate-rich region of proteoglycan monomer core protein.

Direct evidence for the variable length of the chondroitin sulfate-rich region has been presented in our electron microscopic study of the dimensions of cartilage proteoglycans.[7] A polydisperse population of proteoglycan monomers from bovine nasal cartilage was separated into a series of relatively monodisperse fractions with sedimentation coefficients ranging from 8.3 S to 21.1 S. There was no difference in the lengths of the chondroitin sulfate chains or in the spacing between chains in the different proteoglycan monomer fractions, indicating that neither increased chondroitin sulfate chain length nor decreased spacing between chains contributed to increases in monomer molecular weight. However, the length of the proteoglycan monomer core protein increased and the numbers of chondroitin sulfate chains per monomer increased as the sedimentation coefficients of the monomers increased, demonstrating that the length of the chondroitin sulfate-rich region increases as the molecular weight of the monomer increases.

Electron microscopic measurements were also made of the chondroitin sulfate-rich region in proteoglycan monomers bound to hyaluronate in proteoglycan aggregates.[7] Figure 11–7 shows the molecular architecture of a cartilage proteoglycan aggregate on nitrocellulose films. On these films, proteoglycan monomers bound to hyaluronic acid in proteoglycan aggregates consist of two distinct segments: a peripheral thick segment corresponding to the chondroitin sulfate-rich region, and a

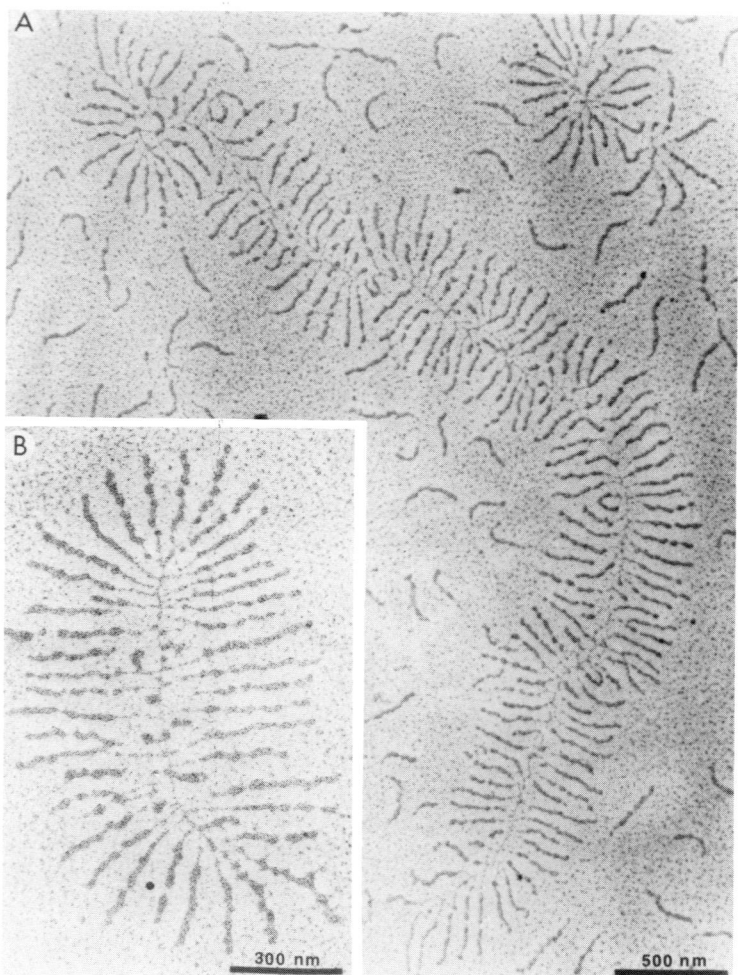

Fig. 11–7. Electron micrographs of proteoglycan aggregates from bovine fetal epiphyseal cartilage. The size of an individual proteoglycan aggregate is determined mainly by the length of the hyaluronic acid central filament. Proteoglycan aggregates isolated from a particular tissue vary in size over a broad range, owing to variations in (1) the length of the hyaluronic acid central filament; (2) the numbers of proteoglycan monomers present in individual aggregates; (3) the sapcing between monomers; and (4) the lengths of the proteoglycan monomers. On nitrocellulose films, chondroitin sulfate chains condense along the protein core, so that the chondroitin sulfate-rich region appears as a relatively homogeneous, dense widened area (thick segment). The centrally located thin segment is devoid of chondroitin sulfate chains and contains the hyaluronic acid binding region. (From Buckwalter, J.A., and Rosenberg, L.C.[6])

central thin segment that can be traced directly to the hyaluronic acid central filament. This segment contains the hyaluronic acid binding region. Direct measurements of these domains demonstrated that the size of a proteoglycan monomer is determined mainly by the length of the chondroitin sulfate-rich region. The same methods might be used to investigate the structural changes in proteoglycans that occur in osteoarthritis.

STRUCTURE AND FUNCTION OF LINK PROTEINS

Cartilage proteoglycan aggregates contain two link proteins with molecular weights of approximately 44,000 and 48,000, based on sodium dodecyl sulfate-polyacrylamide gel electrophoresis.[75] Evidence has been presented (1) that the link proteins are components of native proteoglycan aggregates in vivo and (2) that the isolation of link proteins in association with proteoglycan aggregates is not an artifact resulting from the dissociative extraction and reassociation procedures commonly used to prepare proteoglycan aggregates.[18] Link protein has been isolated to homogeneity.[75] As indicated in Figure 11–6, fractions of low buoyant density (D5, D6) from the top of dissociative density gradients contain link protein mixed with small amounts of proteoglycan monomer. Link protein has been isolated from these fractions by gel chromatography on Sephacryl S-200 in 4 mol/l GuHCl, and characterized. Baker and Caterson have separated the two forms of link protein by preparative electrophoresis.[1] The two link proteins differ in their carbohydrate composition. The link protein of higher molecular weight contains about 9% carbohydrate and more mannose and N-acetylglucosamine. The link protein of lower molecular weight contains about 3% carbohydrate. The two forms of link protein are essentially identical in amino acid composition and in their peptide maps. The studies of Baker and Caterson suggest that the two forms of link protein are identical in the primary structure of their polypeptide chains, but differ in their olgosaccharide components.[1]

In the proteoglycan aggregate, the two link proteins are centrally located in the region where proteoglycan monomer binds to hyaluronate, as indicated by the following observations (Fig. 11–8): In proteoglycan aggregates, the chondroitin sulfate-rich region of proteoglycan monomer core protein is readily cleaved by trypsin[46] or clostripain.[9] When proteoglycan aggregate is digested with tryp-

sin or clostripain, the chondroitin sulfate-rich region is shattered into small fragments. However, the central portion of the proteoglycan aggregate, which consists of link protein, the hyaluronic acid binding region of core protein, and hyaluronic acid, is relatively resistant to degradation by trypsin or clostripain. After digestion of proteoglycan aggregate with trypsin or clostripain, a complex consisting of link protein, hyaluronic acid binding region, and hyaluronate may be isolated, as shown in Figure 11–8. These observations indicate that the link proteins are centrally located in the proteoglycan aggregate in the region where proteoglycan monomer binds to hyaluronate.

Link protein stabilizes proteoglycan aggregates against dissociation, apparently in binding simultaneously to proteoglycan monomer and hyaluronic acid, as shown in Figure 11–5.[31,75] The capacity of link protein to stabilize proteoglycan aggregates against dissociation has been demonstrated in sedimentation velocity experiments in the analytical ultracentrifuge.[75] If a solution is prepared that contains proteoglycan monomer and hyaluronate, a link-free aggregate is formed that is stable at pH 7, and that can be demonstrated in the analytical ultracentrifuge (Fig. 11–9). The link-free aggregate is unstable at low pH, so that the amount of aggregate decreases at pH 5. The link-free aggregate is completely dissociated at pH 4. However, if link protein is added to the solution and a link protein-containing aggregate is formed, a greater amount of aggregate is present at pH 7, and the aggregate is stabilized against dissociation at pH 5.

Taken together, the aforementioned observations

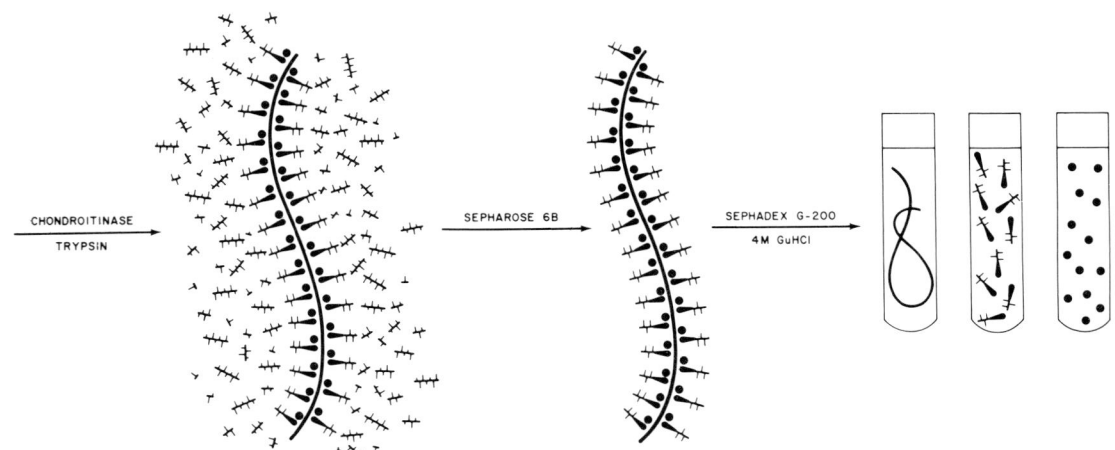

Fig. 11–8. Demonstration of the central location of link protein in proteoglycan aggregate. The chondroitin sulfate-rich region of proteoglycan monomers in aggregates is selectively cleaved by trypsin or clostripain, whereas the hyaluronic acid binding region and link protein are not. Following digestion with trypsin or clostripain, a complex that contains link protein can be isolated: the hyaluronic acid binding region and hyaluronate.

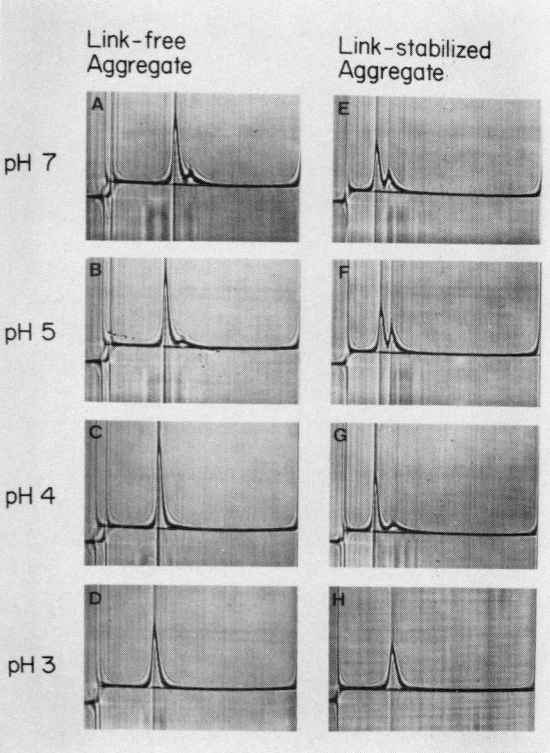

Link-free
Aggregate

Link-stabilized
Aggregate

pH 7

pH 5

pH 4

pH 3

Fig. 11–9. Demonstration of the capacity of link protein to stabilize the proteoglycan aggregates against dissociation. On the left, a link-free aggregate has been prepared by mixing proteoglycan monomer and hyaluronate. The schlieren patterns show that the link-free aggregate is relatively stable at pH 7, but largely dissociated at pH 5. On the right, a link-stabilized aggregate has been prepared by mixing proteoglycan monomer, link protein, and hyaluronate. More aggregate is present at pH 7, and the aggregate is not dissociated at pH 5. (From Tang, et al.[75])

indicate that the two forms of link protein probably represent two identical multifunctional subunits, each of which contains binding sites for both proteoglycan monomer and hyaluronate, fused into single and identical polypeptide chains. Rigorous proof of this concept requires that the two forms of link protein be separated from one another, and that the functional capacity of each form of link protein to bind to hyaluronate, to bind to proteoglycan monomer, and to stabilize proteoglycan aggregate against dissociation be examined.

DERMATAN SULFATE PROTEOGLYCANS

Dermatan sulfate proteoglycans are widely distributed in the extracellular matrix of undifferentiated mesenchymal tissue, fibrous connective tis-

sues, blood vessel wall, skin, sclera, and lung. Compared with cartilage proteoglycan monomers, dermatan sulfate proteoglycan monomers are usually much smaller, do not bind with link protein to hyaluronate to form large stable aggregates, but self-associate to form relatively small, unstable aggregates. Systematic studies of the properties of dermatan sulfate proteoglycans have been initiated only recently, and detailed information about their structure and function is only now becoming available. However, this class of proteoglycans will be important, not only in understanding the properties of tissues, such as blood vessel wall where the proteoglycan is an essential structural component of normal extracellular matrix, but also in understanding alterations in the structure and properties of articular cartilage that occur during aging and in response to injury. For example, a dermatan sulfate proteoglycan is present in the extracellular matrix of undifferentiated fetal limb bud mesenchyme, which is largely replaced by cartilage proteoglycan after the advent of chondrogenesis, but then reappears in increased concentration in some aging articular cartilages. The substitution during aging of a small dermatan sulfate proteoglycan with feeble elastic properties for the large cartilage proteoglycan aggregate with potent elastic properties may have deleterious effects on the elastic properties of articular cartilage.

The structure of the glycosaminoglycan dermatan sulfate is shown in Figure 11–10. The disaccharide repeating unit of dermatan sulfate, shown on the left of Figure 11–10, consists of L-iduronic acid and N-acetylgalactosamine. L-iduronic acid is the C-5 epimer of D-glucuronic acid, in which the carboxyl group is in an axial rather than an equatorial position. The N-acetylgalactosamine residue of the dermatan sulfate repeating unit carries an ester sulfate group usually on carbon number four, but sometimes on carbon number six.[22] As indicated in the middle of Figure 11–10, dermatan sulfate chains also contain disaccharide repeating units composed of glucuronic acid and N-acetylgalactosamine.[20–23,27,28,55] The N-acetylgalactosamine residues in these chondroitin sulfate-like repeating units may be 4- or 6-sulfated. Thus, dermatan sulfate may be considered a hybrid in which the glycosaminoglycan chain is a copolymer of dermatan sulfate and chondroitin sulfate repeating units.

Dermatan sulfate has been isolated from skin,[58] heart valves,[15] blood vessels,[5,17,50,51,60] lung,[79] kidney,[59] nucleus pulposus,[8,14,54] and umbilical cord.[23] Dermatan sulfate accounts for much of the glycosaminoglycan present in lung[79] and in the blood vessels of nonhuman primates[77,78] frequently used in the studies of the pathogenesis of vascular dis-

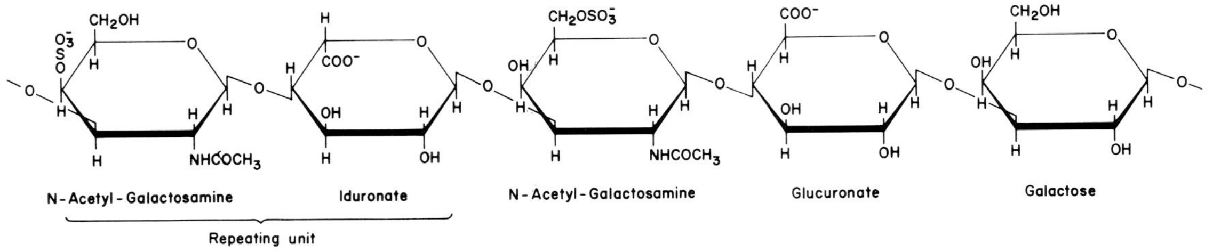

Fig. 11–10. Structure of dermatan sulfate. The repeating unit of dermatan sulfate, shown on the left, consists of L-iduronic acid and N-acetylgalactosamine 4- or 6-sulfate. Dermatan sulfate chains also contain some disaccharide-repeating units consisting of glucuronic acid and N-acetylgalactosamine 4- or 6-sulfate. Dermatan sulfate is therefore a hybrid glycosaminoglycan. Dermatan sulfate chains are covalently bound to serine via the same linkage region as chondroitin sulfate; the first galactose of this linkage region is shown on the right.

eases. In these tissues, dermatan sulfate exists covalently bound to a core protein in the form of a proteoglycan monomer. The linkage region of dermatan sulfate to protein is identical to that of chondroitin sulfate[4,20] shown in Figure 11–2.

Proteoglycans containing dermatan sulfate are distributed in the extracellular matrix where they interconnect collagen fibers, elastin, and cells. Wight and Ross studied the ultrastructural localization of proteoglycans in the intima of nonhuman primate arteries.[77,78] Numerous polygonal granules 20 to 50 nm in diameter with a marked affinity for ruthenium red were distributed throughout the extracellular matrix. The granules possessed filamentous projections 3 to 6 nm thick that appeared to interconnect adjacent granules. The granules and their filaments interconnected collagen fibers at regular intervals in register with the periodicity of the collagen fibers and elastic fibers, and appeared to form connections between the plasma membranes of smooth muscle cells and intercellular fibers. Most of the intercellular granules and filaments were removed with chondroitinase ABC. Wight and Ross also found[78] that 60 to 80% of the glycosaminoglycan synthesized and secreted into the medium by arterial smooth muscle cells in culture was dermatan sulfate, whereas only 10 to 20% was chondroitin 4- or 6-sulfate. Taken together, the results indicate that most of the extracellular matrix granules are dermatan sulfate proteoglycans. Wight and Ross suggested that the dermatan sulfate proteoglycan might function to hold collagen fibers, elastin, and cells together, and at the same time maintain tissue turgor as a result of their elastic properties. They suggested that the proteoglycans might function as a type of plastic interstitial substance, important in absorbing and/or dissipating stress. Dermatan sulfate proteoglycans in the interstitium of lung parenchyma may possess similar functions.

Bovine sclera is a rich source of dermatan sulfate proteoglycans that may be isolated in amounts suf-ficient for its detailed characterization, and for studies of its unusual properties. Dermatan sulfate proteoglycans have been extensively studied by Fransson, Coster, and their co-workers.[10–13,19,24–26] The dermatan sulfate proteoglycans were extracted from bovine sclera with 4 molar GuHCl in the presence of protease inhibitors. They were purified by ion-exchange chromatography on DEAE-cellulose in 6 molar urea, by equilibrium density gradient centrifugation, and by gel chromatography on Sepharose CL-2B in 4 molar GuHCl. Two proteoglycan monomers of different size, called proteoglycans I and II, were separated by gel chromatography on Sepharose CL-2B in 4 molar GuHCl. Under associative conditions on gel chromatography, the larger proteoglycan monomer (I) self-associated into aggregates, whereas the smaller proteoglycan monomer (II) did not. The sizes of proteoglycans I and II under associative conditions were not increased by the addition of hyaluronic acid, indicating that the dermatan sulfate proteoglycan monomers did not react with, or bind to, hyaluronate to form proteoglycan aggregates of the kind formed by cartilage proteoglycans.

The molecular weights of the scleral proteoglycan monomers were determined by sedimentation velocity, diffusion, and sedimentation equilibrium experiments in 6 mol/l GuHCl. In 6 mol/l GuHCl, the molecular weights of proteoglycan monomers I and II were 160,000 to 200,000 and 70,000 to 100,000, respectively. The molecular weight of the dermatan sulfate side chain was 24,000. Proteoglycan monomer I contained 45% protein, and proteoglycan monomer II contained 60% protein. Thus, the molecular weights of the protein cores of monomers I and II are approximately 85,000 and 46,000, respectively. This finding indicates that proteoglycan monomer II contains one or two dermatan sulfate chains bound to a core protein that is approximately 46,000 in molecular weight, whereas proteoglycan monomer I contains four or five dermatan sulfate chains bound to a core protein that is approximately 85,000 in molecular weight.

Sedimentation equilibrium and light scattering studies under associative conditions in 0.15 mol/l NaCl, pH 7.4, revealed that proteoglycan monomers I and II self-associated to form aggregates of higher molecular weight. Moreover, the propensity to form aggregates and the size of the aggregates formed varied under different conditions and were dramatically increased under the conditions prevailing in the light scattering experiments. Proteoglycan monomer I self-associated into aggregates with molecular weights of 500,000 to 800,000 in sedimentation equilibrium experiments in 0.15 mol/l NaCl, whereas proteoglycan monomer II showed little tendency to self-associate and gave molecular weights of 90,000 to 110,000. In light scattering experiments, both proteoglycan monomers I and II exhibited an enhanced propensity for self-association. Under associative conditions in 0.15 mol/l NaCl, proteoglycan monomers I and II showed molecular weights of 3.1×10^6 and 3.4×10^6, respectively. Thus, dermatan sulfate proteoglycans, even in a maximally aggregated state, have molecular weights that are approximately the same as those of cartilage proteoglycan monomers, and 20 to 100 times less than those of cartilage proteoglycan aggregates.

One of the most interesting properties of the dermatan sulfate proteoglycan is its capacity to undergo different degrees of self-association depending upon the experimental conditions. Thus, under the conditions of light scattering experiments, where the macromolecules are not subjected to shearing forces or pressure, the highest degree of self-association into aggregates of large size readily occurs. In sedimentation equilibrium experiments, where the macromolecules are subjected to pressure, the degree of self-association is somewhat less. In gel chromatography experiments, the larger dermatan sulfate proteoglycan (proteoglycan I) self-associates slightly to form small aggregates, whereas the smaller dermatan sulfate-containing proteoglycan (proteoglycan II) does not. The possibility exists that the proteoglycan aggregates formed by the self-association of dermatan sulfate proteoglycans are reversibly dissociated by shearing forces and/or pressure. Because of the small size of dermatan sulfate proteoglycan monomers, and the instability of the small aggregates formed by the self-association of these proteoglycans, the substitution of dermatan sulfate proteoglycans for cartilage proteoglycans in aging articular cartilage, or in the reparative tissue-filling cartilage defects, would have deleterious effects on the biomechanical properties of the articular cartilage.

MODULATION OF PROPORTIONS OF DERMATAN SULFATE PROTEOGLYCANS AND CARTILAGE PROTEOGLYCANS IN DEVELOPING AND AGING CARTILAGES

Prior to the advent of chondrogenesis, the developing limb bud consists of a core of mesenchyme covered by ectoderm. The mesenchymal cells are closely spaced and separated by relatively small amounts of extracellular matrix. Before chondrogenesis begins, the extracellular matrix of the mesenchyme contains mainly type I collagen and a dermatan sulfate proteoglycan, and much smaller amounts of cartilage proteoglycan. With the advent of chondrogenesis, synthesis of the cartilage proteoglycan suddenly increases, and synthesis of the dermatan sulfate proteoglycan greatly decreases. Goetinck and his co-workers have extensively studied the biosynthesis of the dermatan sulfate proteoglycan and the cartilage proteoglycan during the chondrogenesis that occurs in limb bud development.[29,30,57,61,72,73]

Heretofore, it has been assumed that the small dermatan sulfate proteoglycan that is a major component of the extracellular matrix of undifferentiated mesenchymal tissue is eventually completely replaced by cartilage proteoglycan after chondrogenesis during fetal development. However, more recent studies have shown that the dermatan sulfate proteoglycan is present in low concentrations in epiphyseal cartilage throughout fetal development.[66] Moreover, in some aging cartilages, the dermatan sulfate proteoglycan appears in increased concentration, in amounts over ten times greater than those present in fetal epiphyseal cartilages. The dermatan sulfate proteoglycan isolated from bovine fetal epiphyseal cartilage and from aging bovine articular cartilage is polydisperse. Its molecular weight ranges from 80,000 to 140,000. Antisera have been prepared against the dermatan sulfate proteoglycan monomer and against the cartilage proteoglycan monomer from the same cartilage. The antiserum to the cartilage proteoglycan monomer does not react with the dermatan sulfate proteoglycan monomer, and the antiserum to the dermatan sulfate proteoglycan monomer does not react with the cartilage monomer. Thus, the two proteoglycan monomers possess different protein cores.

The substitution of dermatan sulfate proteoglycan for cartilage proteoglycan in the articular cartilage of some aging individuals, or in the reparative tissue-filling cartilage defects, would have profound effects on the biochemical properties of the articular cartilage. Cartilage proteoglcyan aggregates, formed by the noncovalent association of proteoglycan monomers, link protein and hyaluronate and are stabilized against dissociation by link protein. There is no indication that they dissociate when subjected to shearing forces or pressure. On the other hand, aggregates formed from dermatan sulfate proteoglycans are smaller than the cartilage proteoglycan aggregates. They may dissociate into small dermatan sulfate proteoglcyan monomers when subjected to shearing forces or to pressure similar to that to which articular cartilage is exposed. The small dermatan sulfate proteoglycans would be less effectively enmeshed with and constrained by the surrounding network of collagen fibers. In the next several years, research should reveal what effects the partial substitution of dermatan sulfate proteoglycans with feeble elastic properties for cartilage-specific proteoglycans with potent elastic properties has on the biomechanical properties of articular cartilage.

REFERENCES

1. Baker, J.R, and Caterson, B.: The isolation and characterization of the link proteins from proteoglycan aggregates of bovine nasal cartilage. J. Biol. Chem., 254:2387–2393, 1979.
2. Baker, J.R., Roden, L., and Stoolmiller, A.C.: Biosynthesis of chondroitin sulfate proteoglycan. Xylosyl transfer to Smith-degraded proteoglycan and other exogenous acceptors. J. Biol. Chem., 247:3838–3847, 1972.
3. Baker, J.R., Roden, L., and Yamagata, S.: Smith-degraded cartilage proteoglycan as an acceptor for xylosyl transfer. Biochem. J., 125:93P, 1971.
4. Bella, A., Jr. and Danishefsky, I.: The dermatan sulfate-protein linkage region. J. Biol. Chem., 243:2660–2664, 1968.
5. Berenson, G.S.: A study of acid mucopolysaccharides of bovine aorta with the aid of a chromatographic procedure for separating sulfated mucopolysaccharides. Biochim. Biophys. Acta, 28:176–183, 1958.
6. Buckwalter, J.A., and Rosenberg, L.C.: Structural changes during development in bovine fetal epiphyseal cartilage. II. Electron microscopic studies of proteoglycan monomers and aggregates. Coll. Rel. Res., 3:489–504, 1983.
7. Buckwalter, J.A, and Rosenberg, L.C.: Electron microscopic studies of cartilage proteoglycans. Direct evidence for the variable length of the chondroitin sulfate-rich region of proteoglycan subunit core protein. J. Biol. Chem., 257:9830–9839, 1982.
8. Butler, W.F., and Wels, C.M.: Glycosaminoglycans of cat intervertebral disc. Biochem. J., 122:647–652, 1971.
9. Caputo, C.B., et al.: Characterization of fragments produced by clostripain digestion of proteoglycans from the Swarm rat chondrosarcoma. Arch. Biochem. Biophys., 204:220–233, 1980.
10. Carlstedt, I., Coster, L., and Malmstrom, A.: Isolation and characterization of dermatan sulphate and heparan sulphate proteoglycans from fibroblast cultures. Biochem. J., 197:217–225, 1981.
11. Coster, L., et al.: Self-association of dermatan sulphate proteoglycans from bovine sclera. Biochem. J., 197:483–490, 1981.
12. Coster, L., et al.: The co-polymeric structure of pig skin dermatan sulphate. Distribution of L-iduronic acid sulphate residues in co-polymeric chains. Biochem. J., 145:379–389, 1975.
13. Coster, L., and Fransson, L.A.: Isolation and characterization of dermatan sulphate proteoglycans from bovine sclera. Biochem. J., 193:143–153, 1981.
14. Davidson, E.A., and Woodhall, B.: Biochemical alterations in herniated intervertebral discs. J. Biol. Chem., 234:2951–2954, 1959.
15. Deiss, W.P., and Leon, A.S.: Mucopolysaccharides of heart valve; mucoprotein. J. Biol. Chem., 215:685–689, 1955.
16. De Luca, S., et al.: Proteoglycans from chick limb bud chondrocyte cultures. Keratan sulfate and oligosaccharides which contain mannose and sialic acid. J. Biol. Chem., 255:6077–6083, 1980.
17. Engel, U.R.: Glycosaminoglycans in the aorta of six animal species. A chemical and morphological comparison of their topographic distribution. Atherosclerosis, 13:45–60, 1971.
18. Faltz, L.L., et al.: Characteristics of proteoglycans extracted from the Swarm rat chondrosarcoma with associative solvents. J. Biol. Chem., 54:1375–1380, 1979.
19. Fransson, L.A.: Interaction between dermatan sulphate chains. I. Affinity chromatography of copolymeric galactosaminoglycans on dermatan sulfate substituted agarose. Biochim. Biophys. Acta, 437:106–115, 1976.
20. Fransson, L.A.: In Chemistry and Molecular Biology of the Intercellular Matrix. Edited by E.A. Balazs. New York, Academic Press, 1970, p. 823.
21. Fransson, L.A.: Structure of dermatan sulfate. 5. Hybrid structure of dermatan sulfate from hog intestinal mucosa. Arkiv. Kemi, 29:95–99, 1968.
22. Fransson, L.A.: Structure of dermatan sulfate. III. The hybrid structure of dermatan sulfate from umbilical cord. J. Biol. Chem., 243:1504–1510, 1968.
23. Fransson, L.A.: Structure of dermatan sulfate. IV. Glycopeptides from the carbohydrate-protein linkage region of pig skin dermatan sulfate. Biochim. Biophys. Acta, 156:311–316, 1968.
24. Fransson, L.A., et al.: Self-association of scleral proteodermatan sulfate. Evidence for interaction via the dermatan sulfate side chains. J. Biol. Chem., 257:6333–6338, 1982.
25. Fransson, L.A., et al.: Interactions between dermatan sulfate chains. III. Light-scattering and viscometry studies of self-association. Biochem. Biophys. Acta, 586:179–188, 1979.
26. Fransson, L.A., and Coster, L.: Interaction between dermatan sulphate chain. II. Structural studies on aggregating glycan chains and oligosaccharides with affinity for dermatan sulphate-substituted agarose. Biochim. Biophys. Acta, 582:132–144, 1979.
27. Fransson, L.A, and Roden, L.: Structure of dermatan sulfate I. Degradation by testicular hyaluronidase. J. Biol. Chem., 242:4161–4169, 1967.
28. Fransson, L.A., and Roden, L.: Structure of dermatan sulfate. II. Characterization of products obtained by hyaluronidase digestion of dermatan sulfate. J. Biol. Chem., 242:4170–4175, 1967.
29. Goetinck, P.F., and Pennypacker, J.P.: Controls in the acquisition and maintenance of chondrogenic expression. In Vertebrate Limb and Somite Morphogenesis. Edited by I.A. Ede, J.F. Hinchliffe, and M. Balls. Cambridge, Cambridge University Press, 1977.
30. Goetinck, P.F., Pennypacker, J.P., and Royal, P.D.: Proteochondroitin sulfate synthesis and chondrogenic expression. Exp. Cell Res., 87:241–248, 1974.
31. Hardingham, T.E.: The role of link-protein in the structure of cartilage proteoglycan aggregates. Biochem. J., 177:237–247, 1979.
32. Hardingham, T.E., Ewins, R.J.F., and Muir, H.: Cartilage proteoglycans. Structure and heterogeneity of the protein core and effects of specific protein modifications on the binding and hyaluronate. Biochem. J., 157:127–143, 1976.
33. Hardingham, T.E., and Muir, H.: The specific interaction of hyaluronic acid with cartilage proteoglycans. Biochim. Biophys. Acta, 279:401–405, 1972.
34. Hardingham, T.E., and Muir, H.: Hyaluronic acid in cartilage. Biochem. Soc. Trans. (Dublin), 1:282–284, 1973.
35. Hardingham, T.E., and Muir, H.: Binding of oligosaccharides of hyaluronic acid to proteoglycans. Biochem. J., 135:905–908, 1973.
36. Hardingham, T.E., and Muir, H.: Hyaluronic acid in cartilage and proteoglycan aggregation. Biochem. J., 139:905–908, 1973.
37. Hascall, V.C., and Heinegard, D.: Aggregation of cartilage

proteoglycans. I. The role of hyaluronic acid. J. Biol. Chem., *249*:4232–4241, 1974.

38. Hascall, V.C., and Heinegard, D.: Aggregation of cartilage proteoglycans. II. Oligosaccharide competitors of the proteoglycan-hyaluronic acid interaction. J. Biol. Chem., *249*:4242–4249, 1974.

39. Hascall, V.C, and Sajdera, S.W.: Physical properties and polydispersity of proteoglycan from bovine nasal cartilage. J. Biol. Chem., *245*:4920–4930, 1970.

40. Hascall, V.C., and Sajdera, S.W.: Protein polysaccharide complex from bovine nasal cartilage. The function of glycoprotein in the formation of aggregates. J. Biol. Chem., *244*:2384–2396, 1969.

41. Heinegard, D.: Polydispersity of cartilage proteoglycans. Structural variations with size and buoyant density of the molecules. J. Biol. Chem., *252*:1980–1989, 1977.

42. Heinegard, D.: Extraction, fractionation and characterization of proteoglycans from bovine tracheal cartilage. Biochim. Biophys. Acta. *285*:181–192, 1972.

43. Heinegard, D.: Hyaluronidase digestion and alkaline treatment of bovine tracheal cartilage proteoglycans. Isolation and characterization of different keratan sulfate proteins. Biochim. Biophys. Acta, *285*:193–297, 1972.

44. Heinegard, D., and Axelsson, I.: Distribution of keratan sulfate in cartilage proteoglycans. J. Biol. Chem., *252*:1971–1979, 1977.

45. Heinegard, D., and Hascall, V.C.: Characterization of chondroitin sulfate isolated from trypsin-chymotrypsin digest of cartilage proteoglycans. Arch. Biochem. Biophys., *165*:427–441, 1974.

46. Heinegard, D., and Hascall, V.C.: Aggregation of cartilage proteoglycans. III. Characteristics of the proteins isolated from trypsin digests of aggregates. J. Biol. Chem., *249*:4250–4256, 1974.

47. Hoffman, P., Linker, A., and Meyer, K.: Uronic acid of chondroitin sulfate B. Science, *124*:1252, 1956.

48. Hopwood, J.J., and Robinson, H.C.: The alkali labile linkage region between keratan sulphate and protein. Biochem. J., *141*:57–69, 1974.

49. Hopwood, J.J., and Robinson, H.C.: The structure and composition of cartilage keratan sulphate. Biochem. J., *141*:517–526, 1974.

50. Kumar, V., et al.: Acid mucopolysaccharides of human aorta. Part 1. Variations with maturation. J. Atheroscler. Res., *7*:573–581, 1967.

51. Kumar, V., et al.: Acid mucopolysaccharides of human aorta. Part 2. Variation with atherosclerotic involvement. J. Atheroscler. Res., *7*:583–590, 1967.

52. Lindahl, U., and Roden, L.: The chondroitin-4 sulfate-protein linkage. J. Biol. Chem., *241*:2113–2119, 1966.

53. Lohmander, L.S., et al.: Oligosaccharides on proteoglycans on the Swarm rat chondrosarcoma. J. Biol. Chem., *255*:6084–6091, 1980.

54. Lyons, H., et al.: Changes in the protein polysaccharide fractions of nucleus pulposus from human intervertebral disc with age and disc herniation. J. Lab. Clin. Med., *68*:930–939, 1966.

55. Malmstrom, A., et al.: The copolymeric structure of dermatan sulphate produced by cultured human fibroblasts. Different distribution of iduronic acid- and glucuronic acid-containing units in soluble and cell-associated glycans. Biochem. J., *151*:477–489, 1975.

56. Mason, R.M., and Mayes, R.W.: Extraction of cartilage protein-polysaccharides with inorganic salt solutions. Biochem. J., *131*:535–540, 1973.

57. McKeown, P.J., and Goetinck, P.F.: A comparison of the proteoglycans synthesized in Meckel's and sternal cartilage from normal and nanomelic chick embryos. Dev. Biol., *71*:203–215, 1979.

58. Meyer, K., and Chaffee, E.: Mucopolysaccharides of skin. J. Biol. Chem., *138*:491–499, 1941.

59. Murata, K.: Polydisperse distribution of acidic glycosamino-glycans in bovine kidney tissue. Connect. Tissue Res. *4*:131–140, 1976.

60. Murata, K., Nakazawa, K., and Hamai, A.: Distribution of acidic glycosaminoglycans in the intima, media and adventitia of bovine aorta and their anticoagulant properties. Atheroscler., *21*:93–103, 1975.

61. Pennypacker,: J.P., and Goetnick, P.: Biochemical and ultrastructural studies of collagen and proteoglychondroitin sulfate in normal and nanomelic cartilage. Dev. Biol., *50*:35–47, 1976.

62. Roden, L., and Armand, G.: Structure of the chondroitin 4-sulfate-protein linkage region. Isolation and characterization of the disaccharide 3-O-β-D-glucuronosyl-D-galactose. J. Biol. Chem., *241*:65–70, 1966.

63. Roden, L., and Dorfman, A.: The metabolism of mucopolysaccharides in mammalian tissues. V. The origin of L-iduronic acid. J. Biol. Chem., *233*:1030–1033, 1958.

64. Roden, L., and Smith, R.: Structure of the neutra; trisaccharide of the chondroitin-4 sulfate-protein linkage region. J. Biol. Chem., *241*:5949–5954, 1966.

65. Rosenberg, L.: Structure of cartilage proteoglycans. *In* Dynamics of Connective Tissue Macromolecules. Edited by P.M.C. Burleigh, and A.R. Poole. New York, Elsevier-North Holland Pub. Co., 1973, pp. 105–128.

66. Rosenberg, L., et al.: Isolation, characterization and immunofluorescent localization of a dermatan sulfate-containing proteoglycan from bovine fetal epiphyseal cartilage. *In* Limb Development and Regeneration, Part B. Edited by R.O. Kelley, P.F. Goetinck, and J.A. MacCabe. New York, Alan R. Liss, Inc., 1983, pp. 67–84.

67. Rosenberg, L., et al.: Proteoglycans from bovine proximal humeral articular cartilage. Structural basis for the polydispersity of proteoglycan subunit. J. Biol. Chem., *251*:6439–6444, 1976.

68. Rosenberg, L., et al.: A comparison of proteinpolysaccharides of bovine nasal cartilage isolated and fractionated by different methods. J. Biol. Chem., *245*:4112–4122, 1970.

69. Rosenberg, L., Hellman, W., and Kleinschmidt, A.: Electron microscopic studies of proteoglycan aggregates from bovine articular cartilage. J. Biol. Chem., *250*:1877–1883, 1975.

70. Rosenberg, L., Pal, S., and Beale, R.: Proteoglycans from bovine proximal humeral articular cartilage. J. Biol. Chem., *248*:3681–3690, 1973.

71. Rosenberg, L., Schubert, M., and Sandson, J.: The protein-polysaccharides of bovine nucleus pulposus. J. Biol. Chem., *242*:4691–4701, 1967.

72. Royal, P.D., and Goryinck, P.F.: *In vitro* chondrogenesis in mouse limb mesenchymal cells: Changes in ultrastructure and proteoglycan. J. Embryol. Exp. Morphol., *39*:79–95, 1977.

73. Royal, P.D., Sparks, K.J., and Goetinck, P.F.: Physical and immunochemical characterization of proteoglycans synthesized during chondrogenesis in the chick embryo. J. Biol. Chem., *255*:9870–9878, 1980.

74. Sajdera, S.W., and Hascall, V.C.: Protein polysaccharide complex from bovine nasal cartilage. A comparison of low and high shear extraction procedures. J. Biol. Chem., *244*:77–87, 1969.

75. Tang, L.H., et al.: Proteoglycans from bovine nasal cartilage. Properties of a soluble form of link protein. J. Biol. Chem., *254*:10523–10531, 1979.

76. Wasteson, A., Hook, M., and Westermark, B.: Demonstration of a platelet enzyme degrading heparan sulfate. F.E.B.S. Lett., *64*:218–221, 1976.

77. Wight, T., and Ross, R.: Proteoglycans in primate arteries. I. Ultrastructural localization and distribution in the intima. J. Cell Biol., *67*:660–674, 1975.

78. Wight, T., and Ross, R.: Proteoglycans in primate arteries. II. Synthesis and secretion of glycosaminoglycans by arterial smooth muscle cells in culture. J. Cell Biol., *67*:675–686, 1975.

79. Wusteman, F.S.: Glycosaminoglycans of bovine lung parenchyma and pleura. Experientia, *28*:887–888, 1972.

Chapter 12

Regulation of Connective Tissue Metabolism

C. William Castor

The several connective tissues of mammals comprise a large and metabolically active protion of the body mass; they are no longer considered an inert fabric serving merely to support and bind together the parenchymal and neural structures. Mesenchymal derivatives account for 75% of the human body mass, and collgen alone constitutes one-third of total body protein. The family of proteoglycans and glycosaminoglycans in the connective tissue ground substance probably amounts to less than 100g per person, emphasizing the enormous importance of these hydrophilic polyanions in regulating the movement of water and solutes in the extracellular matrix, and in influencing its mechanical and lubricating properties.

Embryonic mesodermal cells differentiate to form different connective tissues, including fibroelastic, reticular, adipose, and elastic connective tissue, as well as bone, cartilage, synovial membrane, and the vascular system. A "connective tissue" consists of cellular and intercellular (matrix) components; the latter category is subdivided into fibrillar (collagen, elastin) and ground substance materials including glycosaminoglycans, proteoglycans, glycoproteins, water, electrolytes, and other solutes. The proportion of these constituents varies with anatomic location and functional requirements. Thus, tendon and fascia have a disproportionate fibrillar component, whereas Wharton's jelly of the umbilical cord is predominantly ground substance; a greater cellular content is found in cartilage and synovial membrane. The vascular endowment of connective tissues ranges from the relative avascularity of cartilage to a profusion of interconnecting loops of fenestrated capillaries found in synovial membrane.

Mechanical support and protection are among the important functions performed by connective tissues. Bone protects viscera from mechanical injury, preserves intricate pressure relationships necessary for the life of the organism, and serves as a lever system via which tendons and fascia transmit mechanical energy derived from muscle contraction. The smooth transmission of mechanical energy to move the organism or its parts is facilitated by lubrication from ground substance components located in the gliding planes of tendon sheaths, bursae, and joints. Since connective tissue matrix is everywhere interposed between the vascular system and epithelial structures, it functions as an organ of transport, conveying nutrients to the periphery and returning metabolic wastes. Energy reserves in the form of neutral fat are stored in, and released from, adipose connective tissue in response to direct hormonal influence, but the role of other metabolically active constituents, such as the glycoproteins of the ground substance, is less obvious.

No summary of the general functions of connective tissue would be complete without mention of its reparative potential. When injury disrupts the anatomic continuity of an organism, connective tissue rapidly bridges the defect. The cellular components effectively neutralize or destroy noxious agents, remove debris, and produce a framework of fibers and ground substance that restores anatomic continuity and (usually) functional capacity to the injured part.

CONNECTIVE TISSUE METABOLISM

An analysis of connective tissue metabolism is concerned with the chemical and physical processes involved in the formation of the connective tissues and their maintenance in a functional state, as well as those processes involved in their degradation and remodeling. The anabolic aspect of connective tissue formation includes the formation of new cells, fibrillar proteins, and ground substance components; catabolic events are concerned with the degradation and removal of these materials.

A plethora of factors with potential importance for the regulation of metabolism in diverse connective tissues is now being recorded and includes an ever-growing list of autacoids ("Growth factors," protein mediators of intercellular matrix formation, complex lipids, nucleotides, peptides, and biogenic amines) in addition to hormones and vitamins. In contrast to conventional hormones, many autacoid mediators are formed within the tissue they influence and have a limited radius of action, and their operational concentrations may not be accurately reflected in the plasma.

FACTORS REGULATING CELL REPLICATION AND GLYCOSAMINOGLYCAN FORMATION

The actions of many substances with regulatory potential have been studied only in vitro, and have yet to be shown important in vivo or in man. Evaluation of signal molecules important in cell-to-cell communication continues to be fraught with difficulties. Most growth-promoting "factors" begin life as one element of a complex biologic mixture, declaring their presence via some measurable action in a bioassay system. One problem obscuring the significance of many autacoid factors is the peculiar array of assay systems that often feature the effect of a protein isolated from one species on a narrow range of biochemical functions of cells or tissues from yet another species. Fortunately, several autacoid factors have now been sufficiently purified to permit amino acid sequence and other structural studies. Availability of nearly homogeneous proteins has not only permitted structural studies and assignment of biologic activities to specific molecules, but has made possible the development of immunologic and receptor binding assays to assist in detection and measurement of these regulatory proteins. Although these techniques bring their own problems, they do offer an approach to measuring growth regulatory factors in man. Major emphasis in this section is placed on materials and mechanisms that appear to have importance in man for the regulation of connective tissue cell proliferation and the formation and breakdown of intercellular matrix materials in both basal and perturbed states. Characteristics of several mediators that stimulate connective tissue growth are recorded in Table 12–1.

Epidermal Growth Factor (Urogastrone)

Epidermal growth factor (EGF) was first described in the mouse submaxillary gland, and was later isolated from human urine as "urogastrone."[56] Excellent reviews summarize historical aspects of the discovery, isolation, and mechanism of action of EGF.[31,71] EGF isolated from mouse submaxillary gland and human urine has been sequenced and shown to be a heat-stable acidic polypeptide chain with 53 amino acid residues and 3 intramolecular disulfide bonds. Mouse EGF is synthesized and stored in the submandibular gland where it is found in granular form in convoluted tubules. The localization of EGF in human platelet alpha granules suggests that it may be synthesized by megakaryocytes.[104] In the mouse, EGF is known

to be regulated by androgens; other evidence indicates that thyroid hormones and adrenalcortical hormones also regulate EGF in this species.[57] In senescent mice, the submandibular glands contain decreased amounts of EGF.[58]

In vitro actions of EGF include stimulation of cell proliferation in epithelial and fibroblastic cells of many types. EGF induces increased synthesis of DNA, RNA, cyclic nucleotides, and enhanced transport of nutritional precursors. In the appropriate cell types, EGF stimulates synthesis and secretion of specialized proteins (such as prolactin or collagen) and complex carbohydrates (such as hyaluronic acid). EGF-stimulated prolactin synthesis in rat pituitary cells was thought to depend on an increased transcription rate of the prolactin gene.[99] Nanogram amounts of EGF cause selective dose-dependent synthesis of collagen fibers by epithelial cells derived from rat liver.[84] However, mouse EGF has little effect on collagen formation in cultures of rat liver fibroblasts,[83] and EGF actually reduces collagen synthesis in mouse osteoblastic cultures.[68] These data underline growth factor bioassay ambiguities that may arise from the species or tissue type of the target system.

In vivo, EGF stimulates cell proliferation, keratinization, and premature eruption of incisors, inhibits gastric acid secretion, and promotes healing of corneal ulcers. Intravenous infusion of EGF into merino sheep leads to temporary cessation of follicular activity and to the appearance of an abnormal wool protein.[52] A role for EGF was postulated during embryonic development when it was demonstrated that palatogenesis was controlled in part by EGF; the presumed mechanism involved increased concentration of environmental hyaluronic acid, perhaps critical for palatal shelf elevation or fusion of medial epithelium.[147]

Fibroblasts have specific receptors for EGF, and binding of the peptide is said to be nearly irreversible. The gene for the human EGF receptor is believed to reside on chromosome 7.[33] Binding sites for EGF in skin fibroblasts from patients with neurofibromatosis are markedly diminished when compared with age- and passage-matched normal strains.[161] Monoclonal antibodies against the EGF receptor induce some of the effects of EGF itself, including stimulation of thymidine incorporation into DNA. This observation supports the idea that information in the EGF-membrane receptor system resides primarily in the membrane receptor itself.[132] The binding characteristics of human placental membrane EGF receptor have been characterized;[69] studies leading to solubilization and isolation of the receptor suggest an apparent molecular weight of 160,000 to 180,000 daltons.[70] EGF binding to cellular receptors is followed by phosphorylation of

Table 12–1.   Growth Factors that Stimulate Connective Tissue Cell Replication and Extracellular Matrix Synthesis

	Source	Purification Status	Molecular Weight	Possible Clinical Significance
1. EGF	Platelets	Sequenced	6,045	Wound healing, neurofibromatosis
2. CTAP-III	Platelets	Sequenced	9,278	Inflammation, wound healing, artherosclerosis, neoplasia
3. PDGF	Platelets	Partially sequenced	31,000	Inflammation, wound healing, atherosclerosis, neoplasia
4. IGF-I	Plasma	Sequenced	7,649	Leprechaunism, mediates hGH action
5. IGF-II	Plasma	Sequenced	7,471	Mediates hGH action
6. NGF	Uncertain in man	Active subunit sequenced	13,259	Maintenance of sympathetic nervous system, neural neoplasms, Alzheimer's disease
7. CTAP-PMN	Human PMN	Highly purified, nonhomogeneous	12,000–16,000	Wound healing, inflammation
8. Interleukin-1	Human monocytes	Highly purified, nonhomogeneous	11,000–15,000	Mediates immune responses, connective tissue growth, and wound healing; an endogenous pyrogen
9. CTAP-U	Human urine	Highly purified, nonhomogeneous	25,000–35,000	Unclear

the receptors, internalization, and proteolytic processing in lysosomes. "Remodeled" receptor fragments may serve as intracellular signals for the multiple specific activities attributed to EGF.[46]

Platelet Factors

Nondialyzable factor(s) in monkey serum promote proliferation of monkey arterial muscle cells in vitro; dialyzed serum prepared from recalcified platelet-poor plasma (SDP) is much less mitogenic. Addition of platelets and calcium to platelet-poor plasma restores mitogenic activity to SDP. Furthermore, addition to SDP of a supernatant prepared from thrombin-aggregated platelets also stimulates proliferation of smooth muscle cells. These observations support the conclusion that much of the growth-promoting activity of dialyzed serum derives from platelets. This finding may be important in understanding the response of arteries to localized injury and may partially explain the source of serum factors that promote cell proliferation in vitro.[127]

It is clear that human platelets contain both cationic and anionic growth factors; one laboratory reported three different forms.[67] Current interest centers on three classes of defined entities: cationic proteins such as connective tissue activating peptide-III (CTAP-III), several molecular forms of "platelet-derived growth factors" (PDGF), and epidermal growth factor (EGF) which appears to be one of the anionic platelet-derived growth factors.

Connective Tissue Activating Peptide-III (CTAP-III), a thrombin-releasable growth-promoting factor in human platelets, has been isolated and studied in detail.[22–24] CTAP-III, isolated from fresh or outdated human platelets, is a 9,278-dalton sin-

gle-chain protein with an isoelectric point of 8.5. Amino acid sequence and immunologic studies showed CTAP-III to differ from β-thromboglobulin (β-TG) only by the addition of an amino terminal tetrapeptide.[10,26] Proteolytic removal of the amino terminal tetrapeptide degrades CTAP-III to β-TG and obliterates growth factor activity. Growth factor activity, as measured by enhanced DNA or GAG synthesis in human fibroblast cultures, also depends on the intact status of one or both of the two interchain disulfide bonds. Depending on the characteristics of the preparation, nanogram to microgram quantities of CTAP-III stimulate synthesis of DNA, hyaluronic acid, sulfated GAG chains, proteoglycan monomer, and proteoglycan core protein in human fibroblast cultures. CTAP-III also stimulates glucose transport, formation of prostaglandin E_2, hyaluronic acid synthetase activity, and the synthesis and secretion of plasminogen activator.

Isoelectric point-related microheterogeneity has been identified which modifies growth factor activity. Specific antisera directed against CTAP-III ablate its mitogenic activity. CTAP-III antigen and biologic activity have been found in platelets of growth hormone-deficient children, indicating that CTAP-III is not human growth hormone-dependent.[21] Elevated levels of pCTAP-III were found by radioimmunoassay in RA, in systemic lupus, and in other forms of vasculitis. Plasma CTAP-III levels appear to parallel clinical disease activity,[90,101] suggesting a possible pathogenetic role.

Data concerning other preparations of *platelet-derived growth factor(s) (PDGF)* have suggested a molecule with two disulfide linked chains, each with a molecular weight of 14,000 to 16,000 daltons.[76] PDGF is generally believed to exist in two forms, PDGF-I and -II, whose molecular weights are, respectively, 31,000 and 28,000 daltons.[36] Differences in glycosylation led some workers to postulate four molecular forms of PDGF.[114] Preliminary sequence studies of PDGF show little resemblance to CTAP-III.[4] Of considerable interest are two reports that suggest that a transforming protein from simian sarcoma virus and PDGF are so closely related as to suggest that they are derived from the same or closely related genes.[39,156]

PDGF has induced tyrosine-specific phosphorylation in human fibroblast membranes[43] and has stimulated synthesis of as many as five species of intracellular proteins.[108] Partially purified PDGF modified lipid metabolism by enhancing cholesterol synthesis and the number of LDL receptors in monkey aortic muscle cells.[28] The action of PDGF in promoting polyamine transport in arterial smooth muscle cells may relate to its role in cell division.[142] It now appears that PDGF is capable of stimulating cell division without the need for "progression factors" in plasma.[66] Other effects of PDGF include evidence that it is chemotactic for fibroblasts and vascular smooth muscle cells.[59] A related study has showed that three platelet alpha granule proteins, platelet factor 4, β-TG and PDGF, each exhibited chemotactic activity for human skin fibroblasts.[133]

Studies of PDGF interactions with fibroblast receptors have suggested that PDGF and EGF are not processed via a common pathway, although PDGF and its receptor also may be internalized and degraded.[14,65,72] Phylogenetic surveys utilizing a radioreceptor assay indicate that a PDGF-type protein is restricted to chordate members of the animal kingdom.[137]

EGF was designated as an anionic growth factor of platelets on the basis of radioimmunoassay and radioreceptor assay data; it is located in the platelet alpha granules and is released during blood coagulation.[104]

Insulin-Like Growth Factors (IGA I, II) and Somatomedins

Cell replication in connective tissue occurs not only in response to acute or chronic injury, but also as a maintenance process. Although it is not certain that "replacement cell replication" depends on omnipresent plasma signals, several interesting materials in plasma are known to sitmulate DNA synthesis. The advent of a radioimmunoassay that specifically recognized insulin demonstrated that only 7% of the "insulin-like activity" of serum was actually insulin (and consequently suppressible by anti-insulin serum); the remainder was originally designated as nonsuppressible insulin-like activity (NSILA). The NSILA materials are themselves growth hormone-dependent, and in turn have growth promoting activity in chick embryo fibroblast cultures and in several other systems. NSILA has now been resolved into two entities: insulin-like growth factors I and II (IGF-I, IGF-II) whose covalent structures are known.[122,123] IGF-I is a single chain containing 70 residues (7,649 daltons) with 3 disulfide bonds and marked homology with proinsulin. IGF-II is a 7,471-dalton protein with 3 interchain disulfide bonds; it shows substantial homology with IGF-I and with proinsulin. Radioimmunoassay and radioreceptor assays indicate that IGF-I closely resembles *somatomedin C*.[150] Sequence analysis now confirms their identity.[7,79,143]

Growth hormone affects cartilage by inducing the formation of secondary substances, *somatomedins* ("sulfation factors"), which in turn interact with chondrocytes to modify their metabolism. Somatomedins in serum stimulate $^{35}SO_4$ uptake by cartilage from hypophysectomized rats; serum from hypophysectomized rats is less stimulatory than that from normal rats, and administration of growth hormone restores stimulatory activity to serum of hypophysectomized animals.[130] Bioassay of somatomedins in human serum discloses high levels in acromegaly, and low levels after hypophysectomy and in patients with pituitary dwarfism. Administration of human growth hormone (hGF) to hypophysectomized patients or pituitary dwarfs restores human somatomedin levels to the normal range. At least three somatomedins (A, B, C) are present in human plamsa. Somatomedin A (SM-A) isolated from human plasma was reported to have a molecular weight of approximately 7,000 with asparagine at its N-terminus. SM-A stimulates incorporation of $^{35}SO_4$ into GAG in chick cartilage and DNA synthesis in both chick embryo and human fibroblasts.[119] Although IGF-I and -II bind to "multiplication stimulation activity" (MSA) "receptors," it is not appropriate to conclude that IGF and MSA are identical; the data may mean that there are multiple types of receptors for IGF materials.[118] One review characterizes MSA as a rat plasma "somatomedin" that shares properties with IGF-I, -II, and insulin.[117] Somatomedin B stimulates DNA synthesis in human glial cells and human embryonic lung fibroblasts; when infused into hypophysectomized rats, it markedly stimulates proline uptake in skin, tibia, liver, and kidney.[128]

IGF-I and -II are equally potent in stimulating DNA synthesis in chick embryonic tissue and $^{35}SO_4$ uptake in rat costal cartilage.[159] Both IGF species enhance mitosis in rabbit lens epithelial cells.[120] IGF stimulates 2-deoxy-glucose (2-dG) uptake in skeletal muscle, fat, and heart cells, presumably not acting through the insulin receptor. However, while IGF is 50 to 100 times more potent than insulin on growth parameters, it is only one-sixtieth as potent as insulin with respect to 2-dG uptake by fat cells.[110]

Skin fibroblasts have been shown by radioimmunoassay to secrete material resembling SM-C. Secretion is blocked by cycloheximide and stimulated by hGH, platelet-derived growth factors, and fibroblast growth factors (FGF), but not by EGF, thyroxine, or cortisol.[30]

Radioimmunoassay of IGF-I and -II shows IGF-I levels to be elevated in acromegaly and depressed in hGH deficiency. Oversecretion of IGF-II with acromegaly is not seen; however, the values are low in hGH deficiency, supporting the idea that both factors are growth hormone-dependent. Extra pancreatic tumors associated with hypoglycemia are not associated with increased levels of IGF-I and -II.[160]

Leprechaunism, a syndrome characterized by growth retardation, poor muscle development, and absence of fat, may result from deficiency of insulin-like growth factor activity. Some patients with this syndrome are reported to be deficient in cellular receptors for IGF-I.[149]

Nerve Growth Factor (NGF)

Nerve growth factor (NGF) is present in many tissues, but is found in unusually high concentrations in some snake venoms and in the male mouse submaxillary gland.[3] It elicits overgrowth of sympathetic chain ganglia in vivo, generates a halo-like outgrowth of nerve fibers from embryonic sympathetic ganglia cultured in vitro, and is believed to be important in the regulation of neural cell growth and differentiation. NGF regulates the survival of peripheral sympathetic and spinal sensory neurons.

NGF isolated from the mouse submaxillary gland is a hexameric 140,000-dalton protein complex composed of α, β and γ subunits. The α subunit subserves a regulatory function, the γ subunit is an arginine esteropeptidase, and the biologic activity resides in the β subunit.[61] The β subunit of NGF (βNGF) has been sequenced, revealing a primary peptide with a molecular weight of 13,259 daltons that associates in two subunits with a molecular weight of 26,518 daltons. βNGF has three disulfide bonds with many acidic residues present in amide form, accounting for its basic nature. The biologic acitivity of βNGF is inhibited in the hexameric complex, which in turn protects the active component from proteolysis.

Antibodies to NGF cause total destruction of the sympathetic nervous system. NGF may be viewed as a protein hormone that exerts positive pleiotropic stimulation on developing nerve tissue, being required in small amounts to maintain the mature sympathetic nervous system. NGF activity immunologically identical to that of submaxillary glands has been found in blood and other peripheral organs. Structural similarities between NGF and proinsulin lead to the suggestion that NGF is an evolutionary derivative of a primitive ancestral form of proinsulin.[47]

There is a puzzling lack of data confirming the presence of NGF in human tissues. One review emphasizes the possible role of nerve growth factor in neoplasms, including sarcoma, neuroblastoma, and gliomas.[153] Older data suggest that NGF was secreted by a human glioblastoma cell strain.[6] In addition, human melanoma cells in culture have been shown by indirect immunofluorescence to possess surface NGF; NGF receptors were thought to be present on the basis of both immunofluorescence and ^{125}I-NGF binding.[135] Highly purified receptor for NGF has also been prepared from membranes of a human melanoma cell line by affinity chromatography.[112] The similarity of the physiologic deficits in Alzheimer's disease and the functions subserved by NGF has led to speculation that Alzheimer's disease may be caused either by a deficiency of NGF or by decreased responsiveness of cholinergic neurons to NGF.[64]

Interleukin 1 (see also Chaps. 16, 17, and 37)

Interleukin 1 (IL-1), the first well-defined human "monokine," was originally known as lymphocyte activating factor (LAF). It is a potent thymocyte mitogen, and may be an important mediator of inflammation in man, even to the point of acting as an endogenous pyrogen.[50,85] Interleukin 1 is secreted by activated macrophages of both man and mouse; synthesis of IL-1 also may be initiated by a cell contact dependent process involving activated lymphocytes, and promoted by endotoxins and phagocytosis. Interleukin 1 stimulates helper T-cell release of Interleukin 2, a T-cell growth factor. IL-1 not only has a role in promoting T-cell proliferation, but it modifies in vitro immune responses and induces PGE$_2$ and collagenase synthesis and secretion by human synovial cells.[96,105,111] Both the murine and human forms of IL-1 have been purified to near homogeneity.[85,97] Human IL-1 is heat-labile and stable to acid and thiols; it appears to have a molecular weight of 11,000 to 15,000 daltons and an isoelectric point near 7.1. Recent work indicates that the IL-1 stimulates DNA synthesis in normal human connective tissue cells and promotes formation of important extracellular matrix components, including collagen and glycosaminoglycans. It is similar to, perhaps identical to, MCF (see Chap. 37).

Fibroblast Growth Factor (FGF)

Protein fractions from bovine brain and pituitary gland are "fibroblast growth factors" (FGF) in the sense that they stimulate DNA synthesis in one or more tissue culture systems, including mouse fibroblasts, chick myoblasts, and ovarian cell strains. At least one form is present as a contaminant of bovine TSH and LH preparations and stimulates DNA synthesis in rabbit chondrocytes. A potent FGF from bovine pituitary gland stimulates DNA synthesis in mouse 3T3 fibroblasts at concentrations ranging from 2×10^{-13} M to 1×10^{-10} M. It also stimulates DNA synthesis in a strain of human dermal fibroblasts. Isoelectric focusing separates FGF into basic (pI 8 to 9) and acidic (pI 4 to 5) fractions; an acidic (pI 4.7) 12,000-dalton fraction stimulates DNA synthesis in fibroblasts, adrenal, and glial cells.[49] FGF has been shown to enhance proliferation of mouse Schwann cells in vitro, an activity not shared by EGF.[81] Experiments in which FGF was used to treat the amputated limb stumps of adult frogs suggest that the peptide is active on parenchymal cells in this in vivo context.[55]

Human pituitary glands also contain a factor mitogenic for fetal rabbit chondrocytes. This material is acid-labile and heat-sensitive, and has a pI of 7.9 and a molecular weight of 40,000. It is believed to be distinct from growth hormone, prolactin, LH, FSH, vasopressin, and oxytocin, and unlike bovine brain and pituitary fibroblast growth factors.[77]

Angiogenic Factors

Regulation of angiogenesis in normal embryonic and adult tissues is a remarkably understudied subject. Information concerning the control of vascular proliferation in neoplasia indicates that a tumor angiogenesis factor (TAF) from some tumor cells diffuses over distances of 2 to 5 mm, causing migration of host capillaries to vascularize clusters of neoplastic cells. Extracts of lymph nodes and other tissues occasionally show traces of TAF activity. Preliminary purification studies suggest that the molecular weight of the angiogenesis-promoting substance is approximately 100,000.[45] Partially purified TAF bioassayed on chick chorioallantoic membrane strongly stimulates new vessel formation with minimal evidence of lymphocyte accumulation. Tumor angiogenic factor increases cell growth of capillary, but not aortic, endothelial cells grown on a collagen substrate.[78]

The inflammatory response in graft versus host reactions in mice leads to formation of new host blood vessels, the number of vessels induced in skin being a function of the number of donor lymphocytes injected.[136] Isogeneic lymphocyte injections have no effect on vascularity of the injection site. Invasion by endothelial cells during neovascularization may require production of both plasminogen activator and latent collagenase.[121] Increased amounts of these enzymes are produced by bovine capillary endothelial cells in the presence of a retinal extract, a hepatoma lysate, and adipocyte conditioned medium, all said to be "angiogenic."

An *endothelial cell growth factor* (ECGF) isolated from bovine hypothalamus stimulates proliferation of quiescent populations of human umbilical vein endothelial cells.[91] ECGF is anionic and found in high (70,000-dalton) and low (17,000- to 25,000-dalton) molecular weight forms. This material stimulates DNA synthesis in mouse fibroblasts and human umbilical vein endothelial cells at 10 and 100 ng/ml, respectively.

Tumor-induced angiogenesis can be inhibited by a diffusible factor present in cartilage.[15] Heat inactivation of cartilage destroys the antiangiogenesis activity of this notably avascular tissue. A cationic protease isolated from cartilage was believed to act by inhibiting the ability of endothelial cells to penetrate and to vascularize cartilage. Such factors might be influential in the resistance of some tissues to invasion by blood vessels, reparative processes, and neoplasms.[82]

Newly Described Factors

Transforming growth factors (TGFs) are acidic, heat-stable proteins secreted by certain human tumor cell lines in culture that confer a transformed phenotype on untransformed fibroblasts.[145] TGFs extracted with acid ethanol are low molecular weight polypeptides (6,000 to 10,000 daltons) containing essential disulfide bonds.[124] Binding assays suggest that some TGFs are related to EGF. Some are potentiated by EGF. Production of TGFs by transformed cells and the response of normal cells to TGFs raise the possibility that cells may release factors that then bind to their own cell surface, thus stimulating their own growth.[144]

Cartilage-derived growth factors[11] in bovine scapular cartilage include a cationic polypeptide with a molecular weight of 16,400, which is believed to be a matrix-associated growth factor. A second component associated with chondrocyte chromatin has a higher molecular weight (20,000 to 22,000); both materials are mitogenic for mouse fibroblasts and human chondrocytes.

Connective tissue activating peptide (CTAP-PMN) is a human granulocyte-derived factor that stimulates DNA and GAG synthesis by human fibroblasts; it is relatively heat-stable, sensitive to thiols, and has a molecular weight between 12,700 and 15,700. Such a factor might play a role in chronic proliferative synovitis or in other settings where exudative inflammation is accompanied by connective tissue growth.[100]

A protein factor in human urine that activates connective tissue cells has been identified and partially purified. It appears to be distinct from EGF. Urinary connective tissue activating factor (CTAP-U) is nondialyzable, labile to protease, stable to thiols, heat, and acid, and has an acidic isoelectric point. Purified preparations of CTAP-U have biologic activities that cause human connective tissue cells in vitro to synthesize incremental amounts of ^{14}C-hyaluronic acid, ^{35}S-proteoglycans, and ^{3}H-DNA. The cell spectrum responsive to this substance includes human synovial cells, human chondrocytes, and skin fibroblasts.[54] The site of origin and biologic significance of CTAP-U are unknown.

A factor derived from bovine retina (EDGF) is mitogenic for corneal endothelium, chondrocytes, and epidermal cells. Despite the low pI (4.5), EDGF was believed to be distinct from EGF on immunologic grounds.[109] In the bovine ocular vitreous, partially characterized factors exhibit both stimulatory and inhibitory actions when tested for proliferative effects against endothelial, smooth muscle, and fibroblastic cells in culture.[116] Stromal fibroblastic cells from rabbit cornea release a factor that stimulates DNA synthesis in corneal epithelial cells in vitro.[29]

An antibody-independent role for complement in the activation of human fibroblasts was suggested by experiments showing that fresh serum-mediated enhancement of proliferation requires binding of C1 complex to fibroblast surfaces. The C1q component presumably serves as a recognition site.[80]

FACTORS REGULATING GLYCOSAMINOGLYCAN (GAG) FORMATION

Structural characteristics of complex glycosaminoglycans are determined by the specificity of glycosyl transferases that in turn are determined by structural genes. Processes essential for synthesis of GAG include: (1) synthesis of sugar nucleotide precursors, (2) formation of sugar nucleotide transferases, and (3) synthesis of a specific protein core that can be appropriately xylosylated. Clearly, one might interfere with GAG synthesis at many levels. For example, selective inhibition of proteoglycan core protein formation with BUdR causes reduced synthesis of chondroitin sulfate.[40]

Molecular mechanisms directing the qualitative and quantitative make-up of ground substance GAG are poorly understood at best. Factors mod-

ifying the function of UDP-glucose dehydrogenase and UDP-glucose 4′-epimerase may play a significant role, since in circumstances where the dehydrogenase shows greater affinity for UDP-glucose than the competing epimerase enzyme, chondroitin sulfate synthesis would be favored over keratan sulfate.[35] Similarly, UDP-xylose, an inhibitor of UDP-glucose dehydrogenase activity, does not inhibit UDP-glucose 4′-epimerase activity; thus, the concentration of UDP-xylose could direct UDP-glucose utilization toward the synthesis of either chondroitin sulfate or keratan sulfate.

Hormones and Vitamins

Knowledge of hormonal regulation of GAG metabolism is fragmentary, but the evidence indicates that normal levels of GAG synthesis are supported by *insulin*, and depressed by *glucocorticoids*. On the other hand, excess *thyroid hormone* modifies the GAG milieu by retarding synthesis of sulfated GAGs and increasing the rate of hyaluronate degradation. *Triiodothyronine* at physiologic concentration has been shown to inhibit formation of glycosaminoglycans, primarily hyaluronic acid, by human skin fibroblasts.[139] *Parathyroid hormone* stimulates rodent bone in organ culture to form increased amounts of hyaluronate and to release calcium.[89] This effect has been seen with nanogram amounts of hormone and blocked by even smaller amounts of calcitonin. A direct relationship between the increased formation of hyaluronate and the removal of calcium during parathormone-induced bone resorption is not clearly established.

In human synovial cultures, high medium concentrations of *ascorbic acid* result in accumulation of increased amounts of hyaluronic acid.[20] Guinea pigs given large doses of ascorbic acid develop minor increases in aortic sulfated GAGs and hepatic aminotransferase activity.[51] *Retinoic acid*, a natural metabolite of vitamin A, inhibits sulfate fixation into GAG by chondrocytes in vitro at 10^{-9} M.[134] This is not a general phenomenon, however, since the relative proportion of N-sulfated GAG (heparan or heparin) increases as chondroitin-4 sulfate decreases.

Prostaglandins and Cyclic Nucleotides

Prostaglandins, particularly those of the E series, stimulate the formation of hyaluronic acid both in vitro and in vivo at pharmacologic concentrations. However, physiologic concentrations of prostaglandins potentiate GAG synthesis induced by CTAP-I and -III.[17,24] In addition, E series prostaglandins stimulate incorporation of $^{35}SO_4^=$ into GAG synthesized by human dermal fibroblasts in cell culture. *Cyclic 3′5′ adenosine monophosphate* in pharmacologic concentrations also enhances GAG synthesis, particularly hyaluronic acid, by human synovial and dermal fibroblasts; in lesser concentrations, cAMP potentiates the actions of CTAP-I and -III.[19,24] Exposure of 3T3 mouse fibroblasts and their SV40 transforms counterparts to pharmacologic concentrations of cyclic AMP modestly increases synthesis and secretion of chondroitin-4/6 sulfate as well as dermatan sulfate.[53] These actions of cyclic AMP may represent specific examples of cyclic nucleotide regulation of differentiated cell function.

Regulation by Protein Factors

Connective Tissue Activating Peptide-I (CTAP-I) from human lymphocytes is a low molecular weight protein (approximately 11,000 daltons) characterized by an essential sulfhydryl residue and low aromatic amino acid content.[18] Although CTAP-I is released by human lymphocytes in cultures, the process is not mediated by conventional lymphocyte mitogens. Major effects of CTAP-I on cultured synovial cells include: release of E series prostaglandins into the medium; delayed accumulation of intracellular cyclic AMP and, subsequently, accelerated glycolysis and GAG synthesis by activated synovial cells. Synovial cells are stimulated by CTAP-I to increase hyaluronate synthesis 4- to 50-fold; two to four times as much sulfated GAG is formed. Augmented hyaluronate synthesis by synovial cells in response to CTAP-I requires synthesis of RNA and protein, but not DNA. One can visualize how CTAP-I might enhance differentiated functions of connective tissue cells during perturbed states such as inflammation, but it is uncertain whether it has an important effect on the basal synthesis of connective tissue glycosaminoglycans. *CTAP-II* isolated from cultures of human laryngeal carcinoma cells is similar to CTAP-I in its isolation characteristics, electrophoretic mobility, and molecular weight, but is substantially different in amino acid composition.[22] This peptide also has a biologically essential sulfhydryl residue and, like CTAP-I, the tumor cell factor stimulates glycolysis and GAG synthesis by human synovial cells. CTAP-II may be an example of a tumor-related factor responsible for the generation of a connective tissue matrix suitable for an expanding tumor cell mass.

REGULATION OF COLLAGEN METABOLISM

Formation of the several known types of mature collagen fibrils is a multistep process, and many loci in the pathway are sensitive to regulatory action. Intracellular events leading to the formation of the collagen molecule include: (1) synthesis of mRNA specific for collagen; (2) formation of polyribosomal clusters; (3) association of polyribosomes and endoplasmic reticulum; (4) formation of an alignment segment of the polypeptide chains (registration peptide); (5) hydroxylation of specific proline and lysine residues; (6) glycosylation of selected hydroxylysine residues; and (7) conversion of procollagen to collagen by the action of procollagen peptidase and extrusion of tropocollagen into the extracellular milieu[102] (see Chap. 10).

Extracellular events include: (1) formation of peptide-bound aldehydes at specific lysine and hydroxylysine residues; (2) formation of intramolecular cross-links via an aldol condensation reaction; (3) formation of intermolecular cross-links peptide-bound aldehydes and unmodified amino groups of lysine or hydroxylysine residues as Schiff bases; and (4) aggregation of collagen fibers in the extracellular matrix to reflect specific structural characteristics in a given tissue.[102]

Stimulation of Collagen Formation by Low-Molecular-Weight Agents

A notable gap in our understanding of connective tissue metabolism concerns *factors responsible for initiating or terminating collagen synthesis* in response to specific biologic requirements. A useful review has covered circumstances that modulate and regulate collagen synthesis in vitro, including cell density, aging, ascorbate, cell-to-cell interaction, and serum factors.[98] Although it is well known that *molecular oxygen, ferrous iron, α ketoglutarate,* and *ascorbic acid* are required for collagen synthesis in man, there is little to suggest that these factors play a major regulatory role except in deficiency states. *Ascorbic acid* promotes aggregation of ribosomes in the endoplasmic reticulum to facilitate collagen synthesis. Hydroxylation of lysine and proline in vivo can be inhibited by ascorbic acid deficiency or by chelation of ferrous iron by agents such as α,α'-dipyridyl. Human synovial cells incubated with pharmacologic concentrations of ascorbic acid form increased amounts of both soluble and fibrillar collagen.[20] Embryonic human lung fibroblasts depend on ascorbic acid for full hydroxylation of collagen, but not for maximal rate of synthesis.[107] Excess *vitamin A* modestly stimulates collagen accumulation[41] and may reverse the retarding effect of glucocorticoids on collagen formation. Although lysosomal labilizing compounds such as vitamin A, digitonin, testosterone, and papain are reported to stimulate collagen synthesis and repair, vitamin E slightly reduces tensile strength and collagen accumulation in healing wounds and does not alter glucocorticoid inhibition of this process.[42]

Collagen synthesis is selectively increased by

bleomycin in human fetal lung fibroblast cultures; prolyhydroxylase activity is also markedly elevated, as are collagen degradation processes.[141] *Uroporphyrin I* also markedly stimulates collagen biosynthesis in human skin fibroblast cultures,[152] while modest increments of collagen are seen in sponge granulation tissue incubated with serotonin, bradykinin, histamine, and vasopressin.[1] Similarly, modest stimulation of proline and lysine hydroxylation occurs following exposure of chick embryo tissue to high concentrations of prostaglandins E_1 and $F_{1\alpha}$.[13] Collagen accumulation in female rat skin is promoted by estradiol, which apparently retards degradation rather than stimulating synthesis.[138]

Protein Factors Promoting Collagen Accumulation

Although autacoid mediators may play a role in regulating collagen metabolism, few have been described and none has been chemically characterized. "Lymphokine"-rich supernates (possibly IL-1) generated by PHA stimulation of human blood mononuclear cells modestly enhance collagen accumulation by WI-38 embryonic lung fibroblasts.[75] *Lymphokines* from human lymphocytes have been shown to stimulate synovial cell proliferation in culture as well as collagen synthesis, effects that are enhanced if the lymphocytes are lectin-activated.[106]

A *coupling factor* thought to mediate coupling of bone formation to bone resorption has been described.[44] This protein, extracted from human bone matrix, has been substantially purified and shown to stimulate bone growth by assays measuring bone cell DNA synthesis and incorporation of labeled proline into collagen. Coupling factor apparently is released during the course of bone resorption. It increases the growth rate of embryonic bone in culture, and apparently is specific for bone and cartilage but does not affect skin, kidney, muscle, or liver. Another *bone-derived growth factor* (BDGF) has been isolated from the conditioned medium used to nourish the calvariae of 21-day fetal rats. Two forms are found: one with a molecular weight of approximately 20,000 to 30,000, the other with a molecular weight between 6,000 and 13,000. Both fractions stimulate DNA, RNA, and proteoglycan synthesis in rabbit chondrocyte cultures. Others have shown that protein extracted from rat bone stimulates proliferation of both human and rat fibroblasts.[131]

Unfractionated growth factors secreted by platelets have been shown to stimulate selective synthesis of collagen by human skin fibroblasts.[140] A *basic protein* secreted by rat macrophages stimulates formation of soluble collagen by rat fibro-

blasts in a cellulose sponge granuloma, while depressing the formation of noncollagen proteins.[73] In experiments with fetal rat calvariae, *insulin* stimulates formation of type I collagen, an activity not shared with PTH, EGF, or 1,25 dihydroxyvitamin D_3.[16]

Agents Depressing Collagen Synthesis

Since collagen synthesis may require a membrane-bound mRNA-ribosome complex, it is possible that any agent that significantly modifies membrane integrity may depress collagen biosynthesis. Cutaneous application of adrenal *glucocorticoids* decreases the thickness of rat dermis and its collagen content.[25] Direct suppression of collagen accumulation by hydrocortisone has also been shown in human fibroblast cultures.[20] Pharmacologic concentrations of natural and synthetic glucocorticoids inhibit incorporation of ^{14}C-proline into nondialyzable hydroxyproline in short-term tissue slice experiments.[148] In mechanically damaged aortic tissue, prednisone markedly modifies the repair process, especially inhibiting the biosynthesis of collagen.[93] In uninjured aortic tissue, prednisone acts mainly antianabolically on the metabolism of collagen, as part of a general inhibition of protein synthesis.[92] Depression of collagen biosynthesis by adrenocortical hormones may reflect changes in the mRNA-tRNA complex, since steroids cause a reduction in the amount of particulate RNA.

Parathyroid hormone (PTH)-treated cultures of fetal rat calvaria show slow reversible inhibition of bone collagen synthesis, which is not opposed by calcitonin, an effect that may be mediated by cyclic AMP.[37] This phenomenon may be specific for bone collagen, since there is little change in noncollagen protein or cartilage collagen. Both *osteoclast-activating factor* (OAF) from human lymphocytes and PTH inhibit collagen synthesis in fetal rat calvaria at concentrations that stimulate bone resorption. It is interesting that OAF-stimulated bone resorption is effectively inhibited by cortisol.[115] Since OAF, PTH, and PGE_2 are potential mediators of neoplastic and inflammatory bone loss, their interactions have been studied. The biologic actions of these agents are additive only at low concentrations. Human peripheral blood mononuclear cells, particularly B lymphocytes, may release soluble factors that preferentially inhibit collagen synthesis by normal human dermal fibroblasts.[94]

Lysyl oxidase activity is inhibited by β-aminoproprionitrile, EDTA, isonicotinic acid hydrazide, and D-penicillamine. Low doses of penicillamine act primarily by blocking aldehyde residues; higher levels are required to affect the activity of lysyl oxidase. The consequences of acutely inhibiting lysyl oxidase in healing wounds have been noted in rats treated with β-aminopropionitrile, where transient lysyl oxidase inhibition in metabolically active wounds is associated with reduced wound strength.[5]

Chelating agents alter the incorporation and hydroxylation of proline and lysine, and the glycosylation of hydroxylysine.[12] For example, α, α'-dipyridyl and 8-hydroxyquinoline inhibit hydroxylation of proline and lysine as well as glycosylation of lysine derivatives. However, EDTA, chlorpromazine, tetracycline, hydralyzine, and procainamide inhibit hydroxylation and glycosylation in excess of their effect on the incorporation of ^{14}C-proline and ^{14}C-lysine. Penicillamine-type drugs affect incorporation of proline and lysine only at high concentrations. In a related vein, zinc deficiency may reduce collagen biosynthesis and depress the cross-linking process.[95]

PHYSICAL FACTORS REGULATING CONNECTIVE TISSUE METABOLISM

Clinicians have long known that *temperature* affects the musculoskeletal system, providing relief from pain and reducing stiffness and resistance to motion in articulations and fascial planes. Although the molecular basis for these effects is not understood, it is clear that increased temperature reduces resistance to flow of viscous hyaluronate solutions, and that collagen also undergoes temperature-related changes in physical state. Mammalian collagenase is four times as active at the higher temperatures within rheumatoid knee joints (36°C) than at normal joint temperature (33°C).[63] In a similar vein, small increases in joint temperature are associated with a marked increase in the responsiveness of synovial cells to CTAP-I-induced acceleration of glycolysis and hyaluronate formation.[27] *Shortwave diathermy*, a heat-inducing modality, increases uptake of $^{35}SO_4$ and GAG concentration in rabbit articular tissues.[151] *Ionizing radiation* directed at normal and rheumatoid synovial cells in vitro stimulates hyaluronate formation and glucose utilization, an effect that requires both RNA and protein synthesis and is inhibited by hydrocortisone.[158]

Mechanical factors may influence organization of the extracellular matrix and the metabolic activity of the resident cells. The collagen fibers themselves may act as electrochemical transducers, transmitting information (force) to initiate changes in cellular metabolism important to the maintenance of the appropriate GAG and collagen matrix. Release of the normal *distractive forces* from rabbit Achilles tendons by tenotomy has resulted in increased accumulation of a GAG thought to be hyaluronic acid. The type and proportion of proteoglycan in *tension-* and *pressure*-bearing segments of rabbit tendons relate directly to the functional needs of the tissue.[51] Tendon segments subjected to substantial tension show thick collagen fibers of high tensional strength associated with a small amount of dermatan sulfate. Pressure-bearing segments contain chondroitin-4/6 sulfate with its greater water inclusion properties. Continuous mechanical pressure applied to cartilage appears to reduce both proteoglycan synthesis and breakdown. Further evidence for the importance of the *mechanical stimulation* to cell metabolism comes from in vitro experiments in which arterial smooth muscle cells were subjected either to stretching stimuli or to agitation without stretching. Repeated stretching and relaxation of rabbit aortic medial cells markedly stimulate the synthesis of types I and III collagen, hyaluronate, and chondroitin-6 sulfate, but do not affect the rate of synthesis of chondroitin-4 sulfate or dermatan sulfate.[87]

Electrical Field Effects

Current interest in electrical field stimulation of fracture healing stems from work on piezoelectrical effects in bone.[48] The known tissue interactions with nonionizing electromagnetic fields have been carefully reviewed.[2] Methods of applying electrical current in the management of nonunited fractures include constant direct current, pulsing direct current, alternating current, and induced current; these modalities are introduced to patients by either invasive or noninvasive methods.[86] Most reports indicate that the various modes of electrical stimulation result in healing of 65 to 75% of fractures classified as nonunions.

Studies of mechanisms involved in electrical modulation of bone healing have focused attention on the idea that mechanically induced electrical polarization of biological systems, resulting from the deformation of crystalline biopolymers (as collagen), may have major physiologic importance. An important observation was the demonstration that cartilage is electrically polarized on mechanical deformation with generation of electrical potentials ranging from 0.5 to 2.0 mv. The joint face of articular cartilage becomes positively charged in a cyclical fashion in the face of intermittent loading.[9] Cells subjected to electrical fields in vitro show increased *protein synthesis* as well as *sulphate uptake* into presumptive GAGs.[146] In addition, mouse fibroblasts subjected to an interrupted DC field show modest stimulation of DNA and collagen synthesis.[8] Other studies show that DNA synthesis in cartilage cells may be stimulated by oscillating electric fields, an effect said not to occur with skin fibroblasts.[126] Verapamil or tetrodotoxin blocks this electrical field effect, supporting the hypothesis that altered Na^+ and Ca^{2+} fluxes are important in triggering DNA synthesis in these cells. Epiphyseal cartilage shows changes in cAMP produced by electrical and mechanical perturbation.[103] In an animal model of disuse osteoporosis, pulsed electromagnetic fields increased the rate of synthesis of proteoglycan and collagen and diminished bone resorption.[32] In another study, electromagnetic fields inhibited bone cell responsiveness to parathyroid hormone in vitro.[88]

The accumulated data suggest that mechanical and electrical coupling in living organisms, at least in selected tissues, results in polarization of cells and other tissue components with subsequent alterations in ion fluxes and cell membrane function. These translate into biological responses important to growth, repair, and remodeling of tissues.

FACTORS RELATED TO CONNECTIVE TISSUE MATRIX DEGRADATION

Rheumatoid synovial tissue incubated in vitro elaborates collagenase as free enzyme or trypsin-releasable proenzyme. Collagenase secreted by synovial cells may complex with native collagen fibrils at physiologic temperatures and subsequently be activated by plasmin generated from plasminogen via a plasminogen activator. Synthesis of both latent collagenase and plasminogen activator by synovial cells is inhibited by as little as 10^{-9} M dexamethasone or by larger amounts of other glucocorticoids, whereas progesterone has no inhibitory effect.[157] Indomethacin increases collagenase synthesis in cell culture while inhibiting the formation of prostaglandin E_2. Thus, it is unlikely that PGE_2 formation is a required antecedent of collagenase synthesis.[34] Collagenase production has been stimulated in macrophages by endotoxin and by lymphocyte products,[154,155] in tadpole explants by cyclic AMP, and in bone cell cultures by heparin.[62]

Since the action of mammalian collagenase on bone presupposes previous demineralization of the matrix, the action of agents promoting calcium loss is of considerable importance. Prostaglandin stimulation of bone resorption is greatest with PGE_2. Stimulation increases linearly over a range of 10^{-9} M through 10^{-3} M, when measured by release of ^{45}calcium from prelabeled fetal bone. The relatively flat dose response curve of PGE_2 differentiates it from other bone resorption agents such as PTH, vitamin D_3, and OAF, all of which show steeper dose response curves and cause more rapid bone resorption than do prostaglandins. The mechanism of action of prostaglandins in this phenomenon is not well understood.[38] There is evidence that rheumatoid synovial tissue in organ culture synthesizes primarily PGE_2 and PGF_{2a}, and it is possible that the prostaglandin E_2 produced by rheumatoid synovium may contribute to the tissue destruction of juxta-articular bone in RA.[125]

A factor produced by pig synovial membrane in organ culture induces living cartilage to resorb its own proteoglycan in vitro. This material, termed *catabolin,* has been partially purified, with a molecular weight of 17,000 and a pI of approximately 4.6.[129] Other connective tissue cells, and possibly lymphocytes, may produce similar activities. It is possible that catabolin has a physiologic function related to the induced resorption of connective tissue matrix following injury. Activated human mononuclear cells (including both T-lymphocytes and monocytes) release catabolin-like factors that mediate degradation of matrix proteoglycan and collagen in intact cartilage explants via chondrocyte activation.[74] CTAP-III, a chemically defined factor, is known to stimulate synthesis and secretion of plasminogen activator by human synovial cells in culture.[113] Factors in the medium from lectin-stimulated human monocytes also stimulate plasminogen activator synthesis and secretion by human synovial fibroblast cultures.[60]

CONCLUDING COMMENTS

The foregoing summary hardly suggests that connective tissue metabolism is regulated by a dominant central control mechanism. Rather, connective tissue cells function as a community of diverse interacting cell types exerting a high degree of mutual local control over neighboring cells. In perturbed states (as with injury), those metabolic phenomena with survival value stand out—and their major thrust is repair. Metabolic functions of cells during the repair process are genetically programmed activities largely regulated by autacoid mediators, feedback control mechanisms, and environmental factors converging on the cell to yield an appropriate metabolic response. The polypeptide effector substances of connective tissue may be analogous to peptides like the endorphins, which act in the local endocrine control of nervous system function. In the era ahead, present tentative speculations about roles of "growth factors" and their receptors in disease processes are likley to gel, become organized, and provide new avenues on which to approach refractory biologic problems, including those characterized by degenerative and inflammatory change in connective tissue, such as the various forms of arthritis.

REFERENCES

1. Aalto, M., and Kulonen, E.: Effects of serotonin, indomethacin and other antirheumatic drugs on the synthesis of collagen and other proteins in granulation tissue slices. Biochem. Pharmacol., *21*:2835–2840, 1972.

2. Adey, W.R.: Tissue interactions with nonionizing electromagnetic fields. Physiol. Rev., *62*:435–514, 1981.

3. Angeletti, R.H., and Bradshaw, R.A.: Nerve growth factor from mouse submaxillary gland: Amino acid sequence. Proc. Natl. Acad. Sci. U.S.A., *68*:2417–2420, 1971.

4. Antoniades, H.N., and Hunkapillar, M.W.: Human platelet-derived growth factor (PDGF): Amino-terminal amino acid sequence. Science, *220*:963–965, 1983.

5. Arem, A.J., et al.: Effect of lysyl oxidase inhibition on healing wounds. Surg. Forum, *26*:67–69, 1975.

6. Arnason, B.G.W., et al.: Secretion of nerve growth factor by cancer cells. J. Clin. Invest., *53*:2a, 1974.

7. Bala, R.M., and Bhaumick, B.: Purification of a basic somatomedin, from human plasma Cohn fraction IV-1, with physiochemical and radioimmuno-assay similarity to somatomedin-C and insulin-like growth factor. Can. J. Biochem., *57*:1289–1298, 1979.

8. Baserga, R., and Sasaki, T.: Protein synthesis in the prereplicative phase of isoproterenol-stimulated DNA synthesis. J. Cell Biol., *39*:9a, 1968.

9. Bassett, C.A.L., and Pawluk, R.J.: Electrical behavior of cartilage during loading. Science, *178*:982–983, 1972.

10. Begg, G.S., et al.: Complete covalent structure of human beta-thromboglobulin. Biochemistry, *17*:1739–1744, 1978.

11. Bekoff, M.C., and Klagsbrun, M.: Characterization of growth factors in human cartilage. J. Cell. Biochem., *20*:237–245, 1982.

12. Blumenkrantz, N., and Asboe-Hansen, G.: Effect of chelating agents on the biosynthesis of collagen. Acta Derm. Venereol. (Stockh.) *53*:94–98, 1973.

13. Blumenkrantz, N., and Sondergaard, J.: Effect of prostaglandin E1 and F1 on biosynthesis of collagen. Nature (New Biol.), *239*:246, 1972.

14. Bowen-Pope, D.F., and Ross, R.: Platelet-derived growth factor. Specific binding to cultured cells. J. Biol. Chem., *257*:5161–5171, 1982.

15. Brem, H., Arensman, R., and Folkman, J.: Inhibition of tumor angiogenesis by a diffusible factor from cartilage. *In* Extracellular Matrix Influences on Gene Expression. Edited by H.C. Slavkin, and R.C. Greulich. New York, Academic Press, 1975, pp. 767–772.

16. Canalis, E.: Effect of hormones and growth factors on alkaline phosphatase activity and collagen synthesis in cultured rat calvariae. Metabolism, *32*:14–20, 1983.

17. Castor, C.W.: Connective tissue activation. VII. Evidence supporting a role for prostaglandin and cyclic nucleotides. J. Lab. Clin. Med., *85*:392–404, 1975.

18. Castor, C.W.: Synovial cell activation induced by a polypeptide mediator. Ann. N.Y. Acad. Sci., *256*:304–317, 1975.

19. Castor, C.W.: Connective tissue activation. VI. The effects of cyclic nucleotides on human synovial cells *in vitro*. J. Lab. Clin. Med., *83*:46–66, 1974.

20. Castor, C.W.: Regulation of collagen and hyaluronate formation in human synovial fibroblast cultures. J. Lab. Clin. Med., *75*:798–810, 1970.

21. Castor, C.W., et al.: Connective tissue activating peptide-III. XXII. A platelet growth factor in human growth hormone deficient patients. J. Clin. Endocrinol. Metab., *52*:128–132, 1981.

22. Castor, C.W., et al.: Connective tissue activation. XIV. Composition and actions of a human platelet autacoid mediator. Arthritis Rheum., *22*:260–272, 1979.

23. Castor, C.W., et al.: Connective tissue activation. XI. Stimulation of glycosaminoglycan and DNA formation by a platelet factor. Arthritis Rheum., *20*:859–868, 1977.

24. Castor, C.W., et al.: Connective tissue activation: Stimulation of DNA and glycosaminoglycan synthesis by a platelet factor (Abstract). Arthritis Rheum., *20*:110, 1977.

25. Castor, C.W., and Baker, B.L.: The local action of adrenocortical steroids on epidermis and connective tissue of the skin. Endocrinology, *47*:234–241, 1950.

26. Castor, C.W., Miller, J.W., and Waltz, D.A.: Structural and biological characteristics of connective tissue activating peptide (CTAP-III), a major human platelet-derived growth factor. Proc. Natl. Acad. Sci. U.S.A., *80*:765–769, 1983.

27. Castor, C.W., and Yaron, M.: Connective tissue activation. VIII. The effects of temperature studies *in vitro*. Arch. Phys. Med. Rehabil., *57*:5–9, 1976.

28. Chait, A., et al.: Platelet-derived growth factor stimulates activity of low density lipoprotein receptors. Proc. Natl. Acad. Sci. U.S.A., *77*:4084–4088, 1980.

29. Chan, K.Y., and Haschke, R.H.: Epithelial-stromal interactions: Specific stimulation of corneal epithelial cell growth *in vitro* by a factor(s) from cultured stromal fibroblasts. Exp. Eye Res., *36*:231–246, 1983.

30. Clemmons, D.R., Underwood, L.E., and Van Wyk, J.J.: Hormonal control of immunoreactive somatomedin production by cultured human fibroblasts. J. Clin. Invest., *67*:10–19, 1981.

31. Cohen, S.: The epidermal growth factor (EGF). Cancer, *51*:1787–1791, 1983.

32. Cruess, R.L., Kan, K., and Bassett, C.A.L.: The effect of pulsing electromagnetic fields on bone metabolism in experimental disuse osteoporosis. Clin. Orthop., *173*:245–250, 1983.

33. Davies, R.L., et al.: Genetic analysis of epidermal growth factor action: Assignment of human epidermal growth factor receptor gene to chromosome 7. Proc. Natl. Acad. Sci., *77*:4188–4192, 1980.

34. Dayer, J-M., et al.: Production of collagenase and prostaglandins by isolated adherent rheumatoid synovial cells. Proc. Natl. Acad. Sci. U.S.A., *73*:945–949, 1976.

35. DeLuca, G., Rindi, S., and Speziale, P.: Proceedings: Regulatory mechanisms of glycosaminoglycan biosynthesis at the level of nucleotide-sugars precursors. Ital. J. Biochem., *25*:179–181, 1976.

36. Deuel, T.F., et al.: Human platelet-derived growth factor. Purification and resolution into two active protein fractions. J. Biol. Chem., *256*:8896–8899, 1981.

37. Dietrich, J.W., et al.: Hormonal control of bone collagen synthesis *in vitro*: Effects of parathyroid hormone and calcitonin. Endocrinology, *98*:943–949, 1976.

38. Dietrich, J.W., Goodson, J.M., and Raisz, L.G.: Stimulation of bone resorption by various prostaglandins in organ culture. Prostaglandins, *10*:231–240, 1975.

39. Doolittle, R.F., et al.: Simian sarcoma virus onc gene, v-sis, is derived from the gene (or genes) encoding a platelet-derived growth factor. Science, *221*:275–276, 1983.

40. Dorfman, A.: Adventures in viscous solutions. Mol. Cell Biochem., *4*:45–74, 1974.

41. Ehrlich, H.P., Tarver, H., and Hunt, T.K.: Effects of vitamin A and glucocorticoids upon inflammation and collagen synthesis. Ann. Surg. *177*:222–227, 1973.

42. Ehrlich, H.P., Tarver, H., and Hunt, T.K.: Inhibitory effects of vitamin E on collagen synthesis and wound repair. Ann. Surg., *175*:235–240, 1972.

43. Ek, B., and Heldin, C-H.: Characterization of a tyrosine-specific kinase activity in human fibroblast membranes stimulated by platelet-derived growth factor. J. Biol. Chem., *257*:10486–10492, 1982.

44. Farley, J.R., and Baylink, D.J.: Isolation and partial purification of a putative coupling factor from human bone. Trans. Assoc. Am. Physicians, *XCIV*:80–87, 1981.

45. Folkman, J., and Cotran, R.: Relation of vascular proliferation to tumor growth. Int. Rev. Exp. Pathol., *16*:207–248, 1976.

46. Fox, C.F., Linsley, P.S., and Wrann, M.: Receptor remodeling and regulation in the action of epidermal growth factor. Fed. Proc., *41*:2988–2995, 1982.

47. Frazier, W.A., Angeletti, R.H., and Bradshaw, R.A.: Nerve growth factor and insulin. Science, *176*:482–488, 1972.

48. Fukada, E., and Yasuda, I.: On the piezoeffect of bone. J. Physiol. Soc. Jpn., *12*:1158, 1957.

49. Gambarini, A.G., and Armelin, H.A.: Purification and partial characterization of an acidic fibroblast growth factor from bovine pituitry. J. Biol. Chem., *257*:9692–9697, 1982.

50. Gery, I., Gershon, R.K., and Waksman, B.H.: Potentiation of the T-lymphocyte response to mitogens. I. The responding cell. J. Exp. Med., *136*:128–142, 1972.

51. Gillard, G.C., et al.: The proteoglycan content and the

axial periodicity of collagen in tendon, Biochem. J., *163*:145–151, 1977.

52. Gillespie, J.M., et al.: Changes in the proteins of wool following treatment of sheep with epidermal growth factor. J. Invest. Dermatol., *79*:197–200, 1982.

53. Goggins, J.F., Johnson, G.S., and Pastan, I.: The effect of dibutyryl cyclic adenosine monophosphate on synthesis of sulfated acid mucopolysaccharides by transformed fibroblasts. J. Biol. Chem., *247*:5759–5764, 1972.

54. Gordon, M.A., and Castor, C.W.: Connective tissue activation: Urinary excretion of agent(s) stimulating GAG and DNA synthesis. Arthritis Rheum., *24*:S106, 1981.

55. Gospodarowicz, D., et al.: Fibroblast growth factor: Its localization, purification, mode of action, and physiological significance. *In* Advances in Metabolic Disorders. Vol. 8, Edited by R. Luft, and K. Hall. New York, Academic Press, 1975, pp. 301–335.

56. Gregory, H., and Preston, B.M.: The primary structure of human urogastrone. Int. J. Pept. Protein Res., *9*:107–118, 1977.

57. Gresik, E.W., et al.: Hormonal regulation of epidermal growth factor and protease in the submandibular gland of the adult mouse. Endocrinology, *109*:924–929, 1981.

58. Gresik, E.W., Brennan, M., and Azmitia, E.: Age-related changes in EGF and protease in submandibular glands of C57BL/6J Mice. Exp. Aging Res., *8*:87–90, 1982.

59. Grotendorst, G.R., et al.: Platelet-derived growth factor is chemoattractant for vascular smooth muscle cells. J. Cell. Physiol., *113*:261–266, 1982.

60. Hamilton, J.A., and Slywka, J.: Stimulation of human synovial fibroblast plasminogen activator production by mononuclear cell supernatants. J. Immunol., *126*:851–855, 1981.

61. Harper, G.P., and Thoenen, H.: Nerve growth factor: Biological significance, measurement, and distribution. J. Neurochem., *34*:5–16, 1980.

62. Harris, E.D., Jr.: Recent insights into the pathogenesis of the proliferative lesion in rheumatoid arthritis. Arthritis Rheum., *19*:68–72, 1976.

63. Harris, E.D., Jr., and McCroskery, P.A.: The influence of temperature and fibril stability on degradation of cartilage collagen by rheumatoid synovial collagenase. N. Engl. J. Med., *290*:1–6, 1974.

64. Hefti, F.: Is Alzheimer disease caused by lack of nerve growth factor? Ann. Neurol., *13*:109–110, 1983.

65. Heldin, C.-H., Wasteson, A., and Westermark, B.: Interaction of platelet-derived growth factor with its fibroblast receptor. J. Biol. Chem., *257*:4216–4221, 1982.

66. Heldin, C.-H., Wasteson, A., and Westermark, B.: Growth of normal human glial cells in a defined medium containing platelet-derived growth factor. Proc. Natl. Acad. Sci. U.S.A., *77*:6611–6615, 1980.

67. Heldin, C.-H., Wasteson, A., and Westermark, B.: Partial purification and characterization of platelet factors stimulating the multiplication of normal human glial cells. Exp. Cell Res., *109*:429–437, 1977.

68. Hiramatsu, M., et al.: Effect of epidermal growth factor on collagen synthesis in osteoblastic cells derived from newborn mouse calvaria. Endocrinology, *111*:1810–1816, 1982.

69. Hock, R.A., and Hollenberg, N.D.: Characterization of the receptor for epidermal growth factor-urogastrone in human placenta membranes. J. Biol. Chem., *255*:10731–10736, 1980.

70. Hock, R.A., Nexo, E., and Hollenberg, M.D.: Solubilization and isolation of the human placenta receptor for epidermal growth factor-urogastrone. J. Biol. Chem., *255*:10737–10743, 1980.

71. Hollenberg, M.D.: Epidermal growth factor-urogastrone, a polypeptide acquiring hormonal status. Vitam. Horm., *37*:69–110, 1979.

72. Huang, J.S., et al.: Platelet-derived growth factor. Specific binding to target cells. J. Biol. Chem., *257*:8130–8136, 1982.

73. Jalkanen, M., and Penttinen, R.: Enhanced fibroblast collagen production by a macrophage-derived factor (CEMF). Biochem. Biophy. Res. Commun., *108*:447–453, 1982.

74. Jasin, H.E., and Dingle, J.T.: Human mononuclear cell factors mediate cartilage matrix degradation through chondrocyte activation. J. Clin. Invest., *68*:571–581, 1981.

75. Johnson, R.L., and Ziff, M.: Lymphokine stimulation of collagen accumulation. J. Clin. Invest., *58*:240–252, 1976.

76. Johnsson, A., et al.: Platelet-derived growth factor: Identification of constituent polypeptide chains. Biochem. Biophys. Res. Commun., *104*:66–74, 1982.

77. Kaspert, S., et al.: Chondrocyte growth factor from the human pituitary gland. J. Biol. Chem., *257*:5226–5230, 1982.

78. Keegan, A., et al.: Purified tumour angiogenesis factor enhances proliferation of capillary, but not aortic, endothelial cells *in vitro*. J. Cell Sci., *55*:261–276, 1982.

79. Klapper, D.G., Svoboda, M.E., and Van Wyk, J.J.: Sequence analysis of somatomedin-C: Confirmation of identity with insulin-like growth factor I. Endocrinology, *112*:2215–2217, 1983.

80. Korotzer, T.I., et al.: Complement-dependent induction of DNA synthesis and proliferation of human diploid fibroblast. J. Cell. Physiol., *105*:503–512, 1980.

81. Krikorian, D., Manthorpe, M., and Varon, S.: Purified mouse Schwann cells: Mitogenic effects of fetal calf serum and fibroblast growth factor. Dev. Neurosci., *5*:77–91, 1982.

82. Kuettner, K.E., et al.: Regulation of epiphyseal cartilage maturation. *In* Extracellular Matrix Influences on Gene Expression. Edited by H.C. Slavkin, and R.C. Greulich. New York, Academic Press, 1975, pp. 435–440.

83. Kumegawa, M., et al.: Effect of epidermal growth factor on collagen formation in liver-derived epithelial clone cells. Endocrinology, *110*:607–612, 1982.

84. Kumegawa, M., et al.: Epidermal growth factor stimulates collagen synthesis in liver-derived epithelial clone cells. Biochim. Biophys. Acta, *675*:305–308, 1983.

85. Lachman, L.B.: Human interleukin 1: Purification and properties. Fed. Proc., *42*:121–127, 1983.

86. Lechner, F., Ascherl, R., and Uraus, W.: Treatment of pseudarthroses with electrodynamic potentials of low frequency range. Clin. Orthop., *161*:71–81, 1981.

87. Leung, D.Y., Glagov, S., and Mathews, M.B.: Cyclic stretching stimulates synthesis of matrix components by arterial smooth muscle cells *in vitro*. Science, *191*:475–477, 1976.

88. Luben, R.A., et al.: Effects of electromagnetic stimuli on bone and bone cells *in vitro:* Inhibition of responses to parathyroid hormone by low-energy low-frequency fields. Proc. Natl. Acad. Sci., U.S.A., *79*:4180–4184, 1982.

89. Luben, R.A., and Cohn, D.V.: Effects of parathormone and calcitonin on citrate and hyalurate metabolism in cultured bone. Endocrinology, *98*:413–419, 1976.

90. MacCarter, D.K., Hossler, P.A., and Castor, C.W.: Connective tissue activation. XXIII: Increased plasma levels of a platelet growth factor (CTAP-III) in patients with rheumatic diseases. Clin. Chim. Acta, *115*:125–134, 1981.

91. Maciag, T., Hoover, G.A., and Weinstein, R.: High and low molecular weight forms of endothelial cell growth factor. J. Biol. Chem., *257*:5333–5336, 1982.

92. Manthorpe, R., et al.: Effects of glucocorticoid on connective tissue of aorta and skin in rabbits. Biochemical studies on collagen, glycosaminoglycans, DNA and RNA. Acta Endocrinol., *77*:310—324, 1974.

93. Manthorpe, R., Garbasch, C., and Lorenzen, I.: Glucocorticoid effect on repair processes in vascular connective tissue. Morphological examination and biochemical studies on collagen RNA and DNA in rabbit aorta. Acta Endocrinol., *80*:380–397, 1975.

94. McArthur, W., et al.: Immune modulation of connective tissue functions: Studies on the production of collagen synthesis inhibitory factor by populations of human peripheral blood mononuclear cells. Cell. Immunol., *74*:126–139, 1982.

95. McClain, P.E., et al.: Influence of zinc deficiency on synthesis and cross-linking of rat skin collagen. Biochim. Biophys. Acta, *304*:457–465, 1973.

96. Mizel, S.B., et al.: Stimulation of rheumatoid synovial cell collagenase and prostaglandin production by partially purified lymphocyte-activating factor (interleukin 1). Proc. Natl. Acad. Sci. U.S.A., 78:2474–2477, 1981.

97. Mizel, S.B., and Mizel, D.: Purification to apparent homogeneity of murine interleukin 1. J. Immunol., 126:834–837, 1981.

98. Muller, P.K., et al.: Some aspects of the modulations and regulation of collagen synthesis in vitro. Mol. Cell. Biochem., 34:73–85, 1981.

99. Murdoch, G.H., et al.: Epidermal growth factor rapidly stimulates prolactin gene transcription. Nature, 300:192–194, 1982.

100. Myers, S.L., and Castor, C.W.: Connective tissue activation. XV: Stimulation of glycosaminoglycan and DNA synthesis by a polymorphonuclear leucocyte factor. Arthritis Rheum., 23:556–563, 1980.

101. Myers, S.L., Hossler, P.A., and Castor, C.W.: Connective tissue activation XIX: Plasma levels of the CTAP-III platelet antigen in rheumatoid arthritis. J. Rheumatol., 7:814–819, 1980.

102. Nimni, M.E.: Collagen: Its structure and function in normal and pathological connective tissues. Semin. Arthritis Rheum., 4:95–150, 1974.

103. Norton, L.A., Rodan, G.A., and Bourret, L.A.: Epiphyseal cartilage cAMP changes produced by electrical and mechanical perturbations. Clin. Orthop., 124:59–68, 1977.

104. Oka, Y., and Orth, D.N.: Human plasma epidermal growth factor/β-urogastrone is associated with blood platelets. J. Clin. Invest., 72:249–259, 1983.

105. Oppenheim, J.J., and Gery, I.: Interleukin 1 is more than an interleukin. Immunology Today, 3:113–119, 1982.

106. Parrott, D.P., et al.: The effect of lymphokines on proliferation and collagen synthesis of cultured human synovial cells. Eur. J. Clin. Invest., 12:407–415, 1982.

107. Paz, M.A., and Gallop, P.M.: Collagen synthesized and modified by aging fibroblasts in culture. In Vitro, 11:302–312, 1975.

108. Pledger, W.J., et al.: Platelet-derived growth factor-modulated proteins: Constitutive synthesis by a transformed cell line. Proc. Natl. Acad. Sci. U.S.A., 78:4358–4362, 1981.

109. Plouet, J., et al.: Eye-derived growth factor from retina and epidermal growth factor are immunologically distinct and bind to different receptors on human foreskin fibroblasts. FEBS Lett., 144:85–88, 1982.

110. Poggi, C., et al.: Effects and binding of insulin-like growth factor I in the isolated soleus muscle of lean and obese mice: Comparison with insulin. Endocrinology, 105:723–730, 1979.

111. Postlethwaite, A.E., et al.: Interleukin 1 stimulation of collagenase production by cultured fibroblasts. J. Exp. Med., 157:801–806, 1983.

112. Puma, P., et al.: Purification of the receptor for nerve growth factor from A875 melanoma cells by affinity chromatography. J. Biol. Chem., 258:3370–3375, 1983.

113. Ragsdale, C.G., et al.: Connective tissue activation: Stimulation of plasminogen activator by CTAP-III. Arthritis Rheum., 25:S100, 1982.

114. Raines, E.W., and Ross, R.: Platelet-derived growth factor. High yield purification and evidence for multiple forms. J. Biol. Chem., 257:5154–5160, 1982.

115. Raisz, L.G., et al.: Effect of osteoclast activating factor from human leukocytes on bone metabolism. J. Clin. Invest., 56:408–413, 1975.

116. Raymond, L., and Jacobson, B.: Isolation and identification of stimulatory and inhibitory cell growth factors in bovine vitreous. Exp. Eye Res., 34:267–286, 1982.

117. Rechler, M.M., et al.: Multiplication stimulating activity (MSA) from the BRL 3A rat liver cell line: Relation to human somatomedins and insulin. J. Supramol. Struct. Cell. Biochem., 15:253–286, 1981.

118. Rechler, M.M., et al.: Interactions of insulin-like growth factors I and II and multiplication-stimulating activity with receptors and serum carrier proteins. Endocrinology, 107:1451–1459, 1980.

119. Rechler, M.M., et al.: Purified human somatomedin A and rat multiplication stimulating activity. Mitogens for cultured fibroblasts that cross-react with the same growth peptide receptors. Eur. J. Biochem., 82:5–12, 1978.

120. Reddan, J.R., and Dziedzic, D.C.: Insulin-like growth factors, IGF-1, IGF-2 and somatomedin C trigger cell proliferation in mammalian epithelial cells cultured in a serum-free medium. Exp. Cell Res., 142:293–300, 1982.

121. Rifkin, D.B., et al.: The involvement of proteases and protease inhibitors in neovascularization. Acta Biol. Med. Ger., 40:1259–1263, 1981.

122. Rinderknecht, E., and Humbel, R.E.: The amino acid sequence of human insulin-like growth factor I and its structural homology with proinsulin. J. Biol. Chem., 253:2769–2776, 1978.

123. Rinderknecht, E., and Humbel, R.E.: Primary structure of human insulin-like growth factor II. FEBS Lett., 89:283–286, 1978.

124. Roberts, A.B., et al.: New class of transforming growth factors potentiated by epidermal growth factor: Isolation from non-neoplastic tissues. Proc. Natl. Acad. Sci. U.S.A., 78:5339–5343, 1981.

125. Robinson, D.R., et al.: Prostaglandin synthesis by rheumatoid synovium and its stimulation of colchicine. Prostaglandins, 10:67–85, 1975.

126. Rodan, G.A., Bourret, L.A., and Norton, L.A.: DNA synthesis in cartilage cells is stimulated by oscillating electric fields. Science, 199:690–692, 1978.

127. Ross, R., et al.: A platelet-dependent serum factor that stimulates the proliferation of arterial smooth muscle cells in vitro. Proc. Natl. Acad. Sci. U.S.A., 71:1207–1210, 1974.

128. Rudman, C.G., and Parsons, J.A.: Autoradiographic comparison of growth factors: Influence of growth hormone and somatomedin B on patterns of proline incorporation. Clin. Endocrinol., 15:319–324, 1981.

129. Saklatvala, J.: Characterization of catabolin, the major product of pig synovial tissue that induces resorption of cartilage proteoglycan in vitro. Biochem. J., 199:705–714, 1981.

130. Salmon, W.D., Jr., and Daughaday, W.H.: A hormonally controlled serum factor which stimulates sulfate incorporation by cartilage in vitro. J. Lab. Clin. Med., 49:825–836, 1957.

131. Sampath, T.K., DeSimone, D.P., and Reddi, A.H.: Extracellular bone matrix-derived growth factor. Exp. Cell Res., 142:460–464, 1982.

132. Schreiber, A.B., et al.: Monoclonal antibodies against receptor for epidermal growth factor induce early and delayed effects of epidermal growth factor. Proc. Natl. Acad. Sci. U.S.A., 78:7535–7539, 1981.

133. Senior, R.M., et al.: Chemotactic activity of platelet alpha granule proteins for fibroblasts. J. Cell Biol., 96:382–385, 1983.

134. Shapiro, S.S., and Poon, J.P.: Effect of retinoic acid on chondrocyte glycosaminoglycan biosynthesis. Arch. Biochem. Biophys., 174:74–81, 1976.

135. Sherwin, S.A., Sliski, A.H., and Todaro, G.J.: Human melanoma cells have both nerve growth factor and nerve growth factor-specific receptors on their cell surfaces. Proc. Natl. Acad. Sci. U.S.A., 76:1288–1292, 1979.

136. Sidky, Y.A., and Auerback, R.: Lymphocyte-induced angiogenesis: A quantitative and sensitive assay of the graft-vs.-host reaction. J. Exp. Med., 141:1084–1100, 1975.

137. Singh, J.P., Chaikin, M.A., and Stiles, C.D.: Phylogenetic analysis of platelet-derived growth factor by radioreceptor assay. J. Cell Biol., 95:667–671, 1982.

138. Skosey, J.L., and Damgaard, E.: Effect of estradiol benzoate on the degradation of insoluble collagen of rat skin. Endocrinology, 93:311–315, 1973.

139. Smith, T.J., et al.: Regulation of glycosaminoglycan synthesis by thyroid hormone in vitro. J. Clin. Invest., 70:1066–1073, 1982.

140. Stavenow, L., Kjellstrom, T., and Malmquist, J.: Stimulation of collagen production in growth-arrested myocytes and fibroblasts in culture by growth factor(s) from platelets. Exp. Cell Res., 136:321–325, 1981.

141. Sterling, K.M., Jr., et al.: Bleomycin-induced increase of collagen turnover in IMR-90 fibroblasts: An in vitro

model of connective tissue restructuring during lung fibrosis. Cancer Res., *42*:3502–3506, 1982.

142. Subbaiah, P.V., and Bagdale, J.D.: Polyamines and atherosclerosis. Platelet releasate and other mitogens stimulate putrescine transport in arterial smooth muscle cells. Atherosclerosis, *44*:49–60, 1982.

143. Svoboda, M.E., et al.: Purification of somatomedin-C from human plasma: Chemical and biological properties, partial sequence analysis, and relationship to other somatomedins. Biochemistry, *19*:790–797, 1980.

144. Todaro, G.J., et al.: Transforming growth factors (TGFs): Properties and possible mechanisms of action. J. Supramol. Struct., *15*:287–301, 1981.

145. Todaro, G.J., Fryling, C., and DeLarco, J.E.: Transforming growth factors produced by certain human tumor cells: Polypeptides that interact with epidermal growth factor receptors. Proc. Natl. Acad. Sci. U.S.A., *77*:5258–5262, 1980.

146. Transactions of the First Annual Meeting of the Bioelectrical Repair and Growth Society. Vol. I. Philadelphia, 1981.

147. Turley, E., and Hollenberg, M.D.: Epidermal growth factor stimulates glycosaminoglycan synthesis during palatogenesis. Pharmacologist, *22*:249, 1980.

148. Uitto, J., Teir, H., and Mustakallio, K.K.: Corticosteroid-induced inhibition of the biosynthesis of human skin collagen. Biochem. Pharmacol., *21*:2161–2167, 1972.

149. Van Obberghen-Schilling, E.E., et al.: Receptors for insulin-like growth factor I are defective in fibroblasts cultured from a patient with leprechaunism. J. Clin. Invest., *68*:1356–1365, 1981.

150. Van Wyk, J.J., Svoboda, M.E., and Underwood, L.E.: Evidence from radio-ligand assays that somtomedin-C and insulin-like growth factor-I are similar to each other or different from other somatomedins. J. Clin. Enbdocrinol. Metab., *50*:206–208, 1980.

151. Vanharanta, H., Eronen, I., and Videman, T.: Shortwave diathermy effects on ^{35}S-sulfate uptake and glycosaminoglycan concentration in rabbit knee tissue. Arch. Phys. Med. Rehabil., *63*:25–28, 1982.

152. Varigos, G., Schiltz, J.R., and Bickers, D.R.: Uroporphyrin I stimulation of collagen biosynthesis in human skin fibroblasts. J. Clin. Invest., *69*:129–135, 1982.

153. Vinores, S.A., and Perez-Polo, J.R.: Nerve growth factor and neural oncology. J. Neurosci. Res., *9*:81–100, 1983.

154. Wahl, L.M., et al.: Collagenase production by lymphokine-activated macrophages. Science, *187*:261–263, 1975.

155. Wahl, L.M., et al.: Collagenase production by endotoxin-activated macrophages. Proc. Natl. Acad. Sci. U.S.A., *71*:3598–3601, 1974.

156. Waterfield, M.D., et al.: Platelet derived growth factor is structurally related to the putative transforming protein P^{28sis} of simian sarcoma virus. Nature, *304*:35–39, 1983.

157. Werb, Z., et al.: Endogenous activation of latent collagenase by rheumatoid synovial cells. Evidence for a role of plasminogen activator. N. Engl. J. Med., *296*:1017–1023, 1977.

158. Yaron, M., et al.: Hyaluronic acid production by irradiated human synovial fibroblasts. Arthritis Rheum., *20*:702–708, 1977.

159. Zapf, J., Schoenle, E., and Froesch, E.R.: Insulin-like growth factors I and II: Some biological actions and receptor binding characteristics of two purified constituents of nonsuppressible insulin-like activity of human serum. Eur. J. Biochem., *87*:285–296, 1978.

160. Zapf, J., Walter, H., and Froesch, E.R.: Radioimmunological determination of insulin-like growth factors I and II in normal subjects and in patients with growth disorders and extrapancreatic tumor hypoglycemia. J. Clin. Invest., *68*:1321–1330, 1981.

161. Zelkowitz, M.: Neurofibromatosis fibroblasts: Abnormal growth and binding to epidermal growth factor. Adv. Neurol., *29*:173–188, 1981.

Chapter **13**

Structure and Function of Synoviocytes

Dennis A. Carson and Robert I. Fox

The synovial membrane is the thin layer of tissue that lines the inner surfaces of joints, bursae, and tendon sheaths, with the exception of hyaline cartilage. The synoviocyte layer is located between the joint cavity and underlying fibroblasts or adipose tissue that constitute the subsynovium. The synovial living cell layer is normally 1 to 3 cells thick (Fig. 13–1, A). However, in arthritic joints, the precise identification of the synovial cell layer is difficult because of the markedly increased thickness of this layer, the lack of a basement membrane demarcating it, and the often imperceptible blending of synovial cell layer into the subsynovium (see Fig. 13–1, B, C). The cellular composition of the synovial layer is heterogeneous in normal and disease states, consisting of fibroblastoid, macrophage-like, and dendritic cells.

The synovial lining fibroblasts help form and modify the synovial fluid and extracellular matrix. Compared with typical connective tissue fibroblasts, the synovial lining fibroblasts have more secretory granules, and probably synthesize more hyaluronic acid and less collagen. The synovial macrophages keep the joint fluid free of debris by phagocytosing and degrading particulate material. The synovial dendritic cells may assist in this latter function by releasing collagenase into the joint fluid. No single property distinguishes the synovial lining macrophages from other connective tissue histiocytes.[22]

Changes in the structure and function of the synovial lining cells associated with repeated trauma, infection, metabolic imbalance, or deposition of immune complexes may contribute to the development of degenerative and inflammatory joint disease. For these reasons, an adequate comprehension of the specialized properties of synoviocytes is a major goal of rheumatologic research. Unfortunately, progress in the area has been hampered by several obstacles. It is difficult to obtain a pure cell population from a heterogeneous synovial lining that is only a few cells thick. Moreover, the isolated synoviocytes seldom maintain a stable, differentiated phenotype during repeated passages in vitro. Indeed, if one accepts the hypothesis that

synoviocytes represent the reversible adaptation of connective tissue macrophages and fibroblasts to the particular environment of the joint, then the results of experiments with long-term cell lines may have limited applicability. Instead, the elucidation of the properties that truly differentiate synovial lining cells from other fibroblasts and tissue histiocytes may depend on the results of histochemical studies performed with tissue sections and on biochemical analyses conducted with short-term, nondividing explant cultures.

Wherever possible, this chapter emphasizes those aspects of cell morphology, metabolism, and function that distinguish the synovial lining cells from the cell types.

STRUCTURE OF THE NORMAL SYNOVIAL MEMBRANE

On gross inspection, the normal human synovial membrane is smooth and shiny. Its minute folds, or microvilli, can be seen easily under a light microscope. The folds permit the expansion of the synovial membrane in response to joint movement or changes in intra-articular pressure.

The actual synovial lining comprises an ill-defined layer, 1 to 3 cells deep, that overlies a subsynovial layer composed of fibroblasts, adipocytes, unclassified cells, collagen fibers, and proteoglycans.[16] No basement membrane separates the synovial intima from the underlying connective tissue. Although abundant blood vessels and lymphatics penetrate the subsynovial tissue, they do not reach the actual synovial lining.

The ultrastructure of the synovial lining reveals the presence of two morphologically distinct types of cells, originally termed "A" and "B" cells by Barland.[2] Type A synovial lining cells resemble tissue macrophages.[2,16] They possess a dense and heterochromatin-rich nucleus, abundant cytoplasmic vacuoles, and a poorly developed rough endoplasmic reticulum (Fig. 13–2). These cells possess finger-like extensions, filopodia, which protrude into and surround particles of extracellular matrix. In contrast, type B synovial cells have ultrastructural characteristics of connective tissue fi-

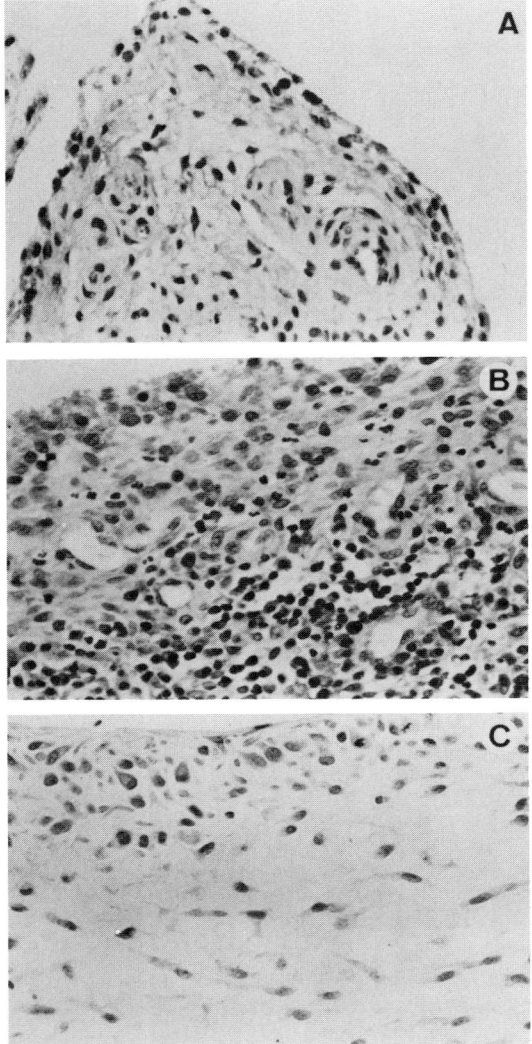

Fig. 13–1. Histology of the synovial membrane in normal and rheumatoid arthritis joints. *A,* The normal synovial lining layer is 1 to 3 cells thick. The subsynovial tissue consists of fibrocytes, blood vessels, and a few histiocytes, all between collagen bundles. *B,* A biopsy of rheumatoid arthritis synovial membrane has hyperplasia and lymphocytic infiltration. *C,* A synovial biopsy from a different rheumatoid arthritis patient shows thickening of the synovial membrane associated with fibroblastic proliferation, but with few infiltrating lymphocytes.

broblasts.[18,41] They have a pale nucleus, relatively few vacuoles and filopodia, a well-developed Golgi apparatus, and a prominent rough endoplasmic reticulum (Fig. 13–3). Approximately 70 to 80% of the normal synovial lining cells have fibroblast (type B cell) characteristics. The remaining 20 to 30% resemble macrophages (type A cells)[2,18]

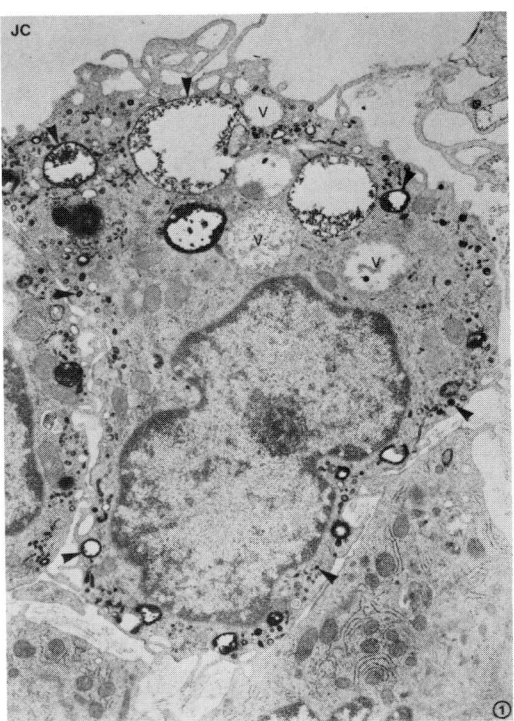

Fig. 13–2. Electron micrograph ($\times$ 14,000) of a type A rat synovial macrophage after intra-articular injection of horseradish peroxidase. Numerous small vessles and large vacuoles contain the ingested peroxidase reaction product, as indicated by the arrows. Other large vacuoles (V) are partly filled with a moderate electron-dense material. (From Graabaek, P.M.[18])

(Table 13–1). Cells with ultrastructural characteristics intermediate between fibroblasts and macrophages, the intermediate or type C cells, have also been described by several authors.[16,33]

When examined in situ, the secretory synovial fibroblasts may be oriented asymmetrically, with the nucleus at one end. At the opposite end, large cytoplasmic processes interdigitate to form the actual surface of the joint cavity. The shape of the synovial macrophages may be round or elongated, with slender cytoplasmic processes.

If synovial cells are dispersed from the surrounding matrix with trypsin and collagenase, and then are allowed to adhere to a plastic surface, the morphology of the cells may change substantially. Many of the cells assume a dendritic or stellate character with prominent, branching cytoplasmic processes[31,62] (Fig. 13–4). Cells with this morphology are not apparent on examination of serial sections of the synovial membrane. Although related to the synovial macrophages, the dendritic cells are relatively deficient in lysosomes, and lack

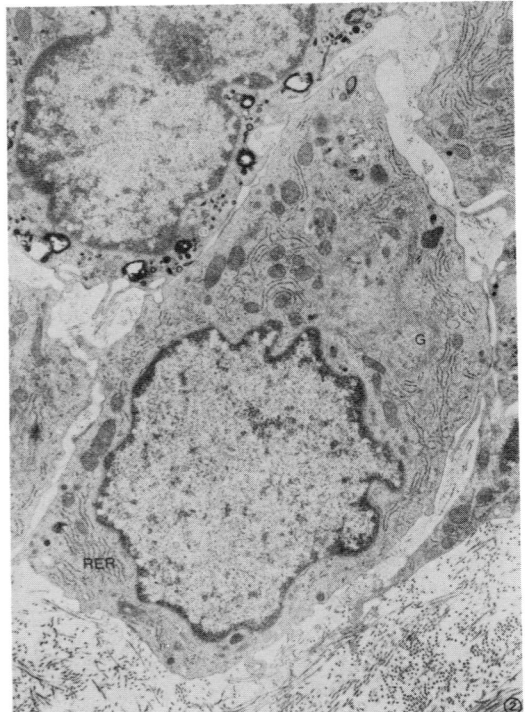

Fig. 13–3. Electron micrograph ($\times$ 14,000) of a type B rat synovial fibroblast after intra-articular injection of horseradish peroxidase. The peroxidase reaction product has not been ingested. The prominent Golgi region (G) and rough endoplasmic reticulum (RER) are visible. Note the adjacent horseradish peroxidase positive synovial cell, which is the same as that shown in Figure 13–2. (From Graabaek, P.M.[18])

significant phagocytic activity[31,45,46,57,62] (see Table 13–1).

SYNOVIAL LINING CELLS

Embryology

Certain aspects of the embryology of joints are important in understanding the structure and function of the synovial lining cells. In the fourth to sixth week of gestation, the synovial mesenchyme arises from a cellular aggregate or blastema associated with early limb-bud formation.[42] The primitive synovial mesenchyme is the progenitor of the secretory lining cells, the subsynovial fibroblasts, and the cells of the joint capsule.

The exact origin of the synovial cells has remained controversial.[9,18] Some workers feel that both type A and type B cells are derived from a unique precursor, such as the "intermediate" cell that has features of primitive fibroblasts.[22] However, experimental data now indicate that some type A synovial phagocytes arise from the circulating bone marrow-derived monocyte pool. Mac-

rophages do not appear in the developing synovial membrane until the subsynovial tissue becomes vascularized.[33] Furthermore, if adult mice of one strain are lethally irradiated and reconstituted with bone marrow from a genetically distinct strain, the synovial macrophages are gradually replaced by cells with the genetic markers of the bone marrow donor.[11,27] In contrast, the secretory synovial fibroblasts continue to display the genetic markers of the recipient strain of mice for at least 60 days following transplantation. One cannot exclude the possibility that during the period of observation the repopulation of the synovial fibroblasts had not yet occurred. Nevertheless, a reasonable interpretation of the data is that most synovial macrophages arise from bone marrow-derived precursors, whereas most synovial fibroblasts develop from the primitive mesenchyme of the limb-bud.

The origin of synovial dendritic cells is a topic of current research interest. In tissue sections, they express Ia antigens and may express ATPase.[45,46] Some of these cells have morphologic features similar to Langerhans' cells of skin and interdigitating cells of lymph node.[24,27,56] These latter cells probably arise from bone marrow-derived cells. Dendritic or stellate cells are often observed in tissue cultures derived from enzyme digests of synovial tissue.[31,62] However, the precise relationship of these cells to the type A cells in situ remains unclear.

Even though fibroblasts belong to a different cell lineage than the macrophages, they may undergo phenotypic conversion when a selective pressure is applied. In one study, murine fibroblast cells were induced in vitro to express macrophage markers such as Ia antigen, phagocytosis, lysozyme, and nonspecific esterase.[32] In another study, rabbit synoviocytes with the morphologic appearance of fibroblasts were observed to phagocytose latex particles and release collagenase after maintenance in tissue culture.[61] Perhaps a fraction of the synovial fibroblasts are primitive mesenchymal cells that can reversibly differentiate into macrophages.

The stimuli that cause connective tissue fibroblasts and macrophages to assume the structure and function of synovial lining cells have not been defined precisely. The formation of the joint cavity during embryogenesis is preceded by the appearance of small clefts in the primitive synovial mesenchyme, with accompanying cell and matrix lysis.[42,47] The clefts gradually enlarge and eventually coalesce to form the complete joint cavity, surrounded by a synovial lining. In one experimental model, injection of air into the subcutaneous tissues of rats induced the formation 10 to 14 days later of a cavity with a lining resembling synovium.[12] The lining was composed of macro-

Table 13–1. Properties of Synovial Lining Cells

	Cell Type		
	Macrophage (Type A Cell)	Fibroblast (Type B Cell)	Dendritic Cell
Cytoplasm & Organelles			
Vacuoles	+		
Filopodia	+		
Endoplasmic Reticulum		+	
Lysosomes	+		
Prostaglandins			+
Collagenase			+
Hyaluronic Acid		+	
Chondroitin Sulfate		+	
Fibronectin		+	
Mononuclear Cell Factors	+		
Plasminogen Activator		+	
Plasma Membrane			
HLA-DR	+		+
Fc Receptor	+		–
C3 Receptor	+		–
Function			
Phagocytosis	+		
Interaction with T-lymphocytes	+		+
Glycosaminoglycan and proteoglycan synthesis		+	

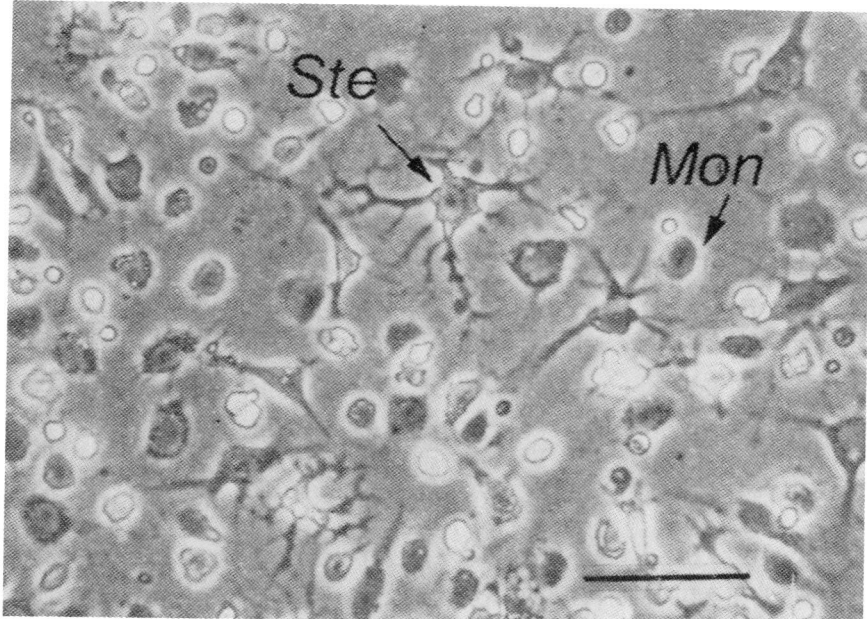

Fig. 13–4. Photomicrograph using phase contrast optics of a primary culture of rheumatoid synovium. Stellate cells (Ste) and probable monocytes (Mon) are designated by the arrows. (From Krane, S.M.[31])

phages and fibroblasts in a laminar arrangement, overlying a collagenous subintima and a zone of high vascularity. However, the composition of the fluid in the cavity was not analyzed. These results suggest, but do not prove, that tissue cavitation can stimulate fibroblasts and macrophages to develop into synovial lining cells. Apparently, the conversion is not irreversible. The morphology and biochemical properties of normal synovial fibroblasts propagated in tissue culture do not differ reproducibly from fibroblasts obtained from other anatomic sites.[20] Presumably, a continuous interaction among the synovial lining cells, the synovial fluid, and the extacellular matrix is necessary to maintain their differentiated state.

Life Span

Under physiologic conditions, synovial lining cells proliferate slowly and have a prolonged life span.[21,38,40] Fewer than 1% of normal superficial lining cells in explanted synovium incorporate tritiated thymidine into DNA during a brief incubation (Fig. 13–5). The frequency of dividing synovial cells in patients with rheumatoid arthritis is considerably higher, although never exceeding a few percent of the total.[38,40]

The slow turnover of synovial cells may partly explain the prolonged retention of foreign materials deposited on the synovial membrane.[59] In patients with rheumatoid arthritis, synovial phagocytes occasionally harbor gold particles long after chrysotherapy has been discontinued.

Despite their intrinsically slow proliferation rate in vivo, synovial fibroblasts from normal adults retain the potential for rapid cell division. Following synovectomy or joint injury, the synovial lining can regenerate completely. The fibroblasts in the new lining layer probably derive from the mitosis of residual synoviocytes as well as fibroblasts in the subsynovial tissue. The synovial macrophages and dendritic cells, like other specialized tissue histiocytes, probably have a limited capacity for cell division. Following injury or synovectomy, the synovial macrophages probably are replaced by precursor monocytes from the systemic circulation and subsynovial space rather than from direct cell division. It is conceivable that a constant migration of monocytes from the circulation is required for the persistence of chronic inflammatory synovitis. Whether synovial lining cells ever actively migrate back into the subsynovial tissue, or into the systemic circulation, is not known.

Composition and Biochemistry

Because synovial lining cells are difficult to obtain in quantity, knowledge of their composition

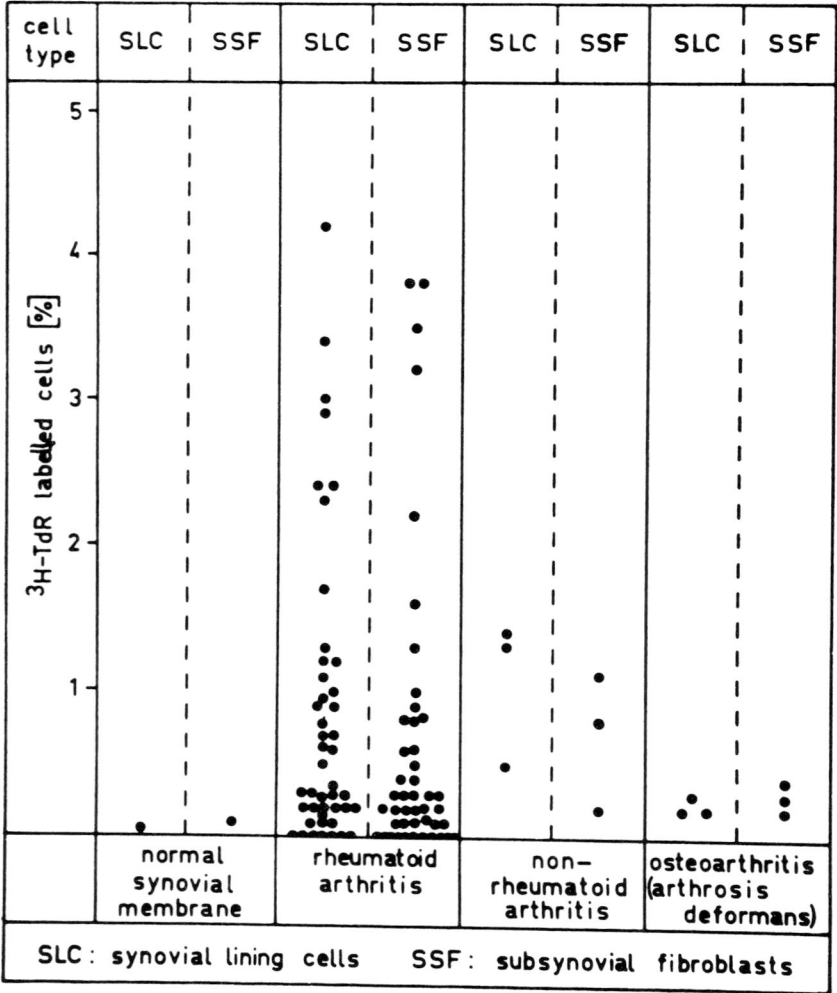

Fig. 13–5. Tritiated thymidine [³H]-TdR, labeling indices of synovial lining cells (SLC) and fibroblasts (SSF) in various conditions. (From Mohr, W., et al.[38])

and biochemistry has come partly from quantitative histochemical studies of carefully sectioned tissues,[15,16] and partly from metabolic analysis of dispersed cells maintained in short-term tissue culture.[1,19,25,26,31,54]

Nucleotide Metabolism. The DNA content of synoviocytes should be similar to that of other human diploid cells, i.e., about 8×10^{-12} g/cell. The RNA content in the secretory fibroblast is greater than in the phagocytic macrophage, reflecting the well-developed rough endoplasmic reticulum of the former cell type.[16,18,41] Explanted synovial fibroblasts synthesize RNA and DNA in medium lacking exogenous purines and pyrimidines.[38] Hence, they presumably retain the capacity for de novo purine and pyrimidine biosynthesis. Although not yet formally demonstrated, it seems likely that synovial macrophages, like other cells of the monocyte-macrophage series, should contain xanthine oxidase.

The endogenous production of pyrophosphate and hypoxanthine increases when cells proliferate. As shown in Figure 13–5, synovial cell turnover is accelerated in osteoarthritic and rheumatoid synovium. The potential contribution of endogenously generated pyrophosphate and uric acid to the pathogenesis of calcium pyrophosphate and monosodium urate deposition disease has not been fully evaluated.

Lysosomes. The abundant lysosomes of synovial lining macrophages have been studied in detail because of their potential role in the production of joint inflammation.[20,22,46,57] The organelles typically contain tartrate-inhibitable acid phosphatase(s) (Fig. 13–6), β-N-acetylglucosaminidase, cathepsin D, and nonspecific esterase. The lysosomes lack significant amounts of alkaline phosphatase, peroxidase, and chloroacetate-reactive esterase.[57]

Lysosomes are less prominent in the synovial cells that assume a stellate or dendritic appearance in tissue culture.[23,28,31,62] However, the cytoplasmic processes of the dendritic cells do have numerous granules that contain immunoreactive collagenase in a latent form.[63]

Prostaglandins. The synovial membrane contains freely available unsaturated phospholipids, as detected by the acid hematin reaction.[20] Increased amounts of unsaturated phospholipids have been observed in rheumatoid synovial cells. The elevation may be related to an accelerated rate of prostaglandin synthesis. With immunofluorescent and immuno-electron-microscopic techniques, prostaglandin E has been detected in intracytoplasmic granules, presumably lysosomes, of synovial macrophages.[53] The prostaglandins are probably synthesized endogenously, since microsomal preparations from rheumatoid synovial lining contain enzymes capable of generating PGE_2 and $PGF_2\alpha$.[3] Similarly, isolated adherent rheumatoid synovial cells produce prostaglandins in tissue culture.[4,5,36] Neither the enzymes mediating prostaglandin synthesis nor the prostaglandin molecules themselves have been detected within synovial fibroblasts. The leukotriene content and synthetic capacity of normal and rheumatoid synoviocytes are topics of current research.

Carbohydrates. Human synovial cells consume glucose and oxygen, and generate lactic acid in vivo.[17] They contain an active glycolytic pathway, tricarboxycylic acid cycle, and hexose monophosphate shunt.[20] Cytochemical assays have also yielded evidence for mitochondrial oxidative activity. The quantitative importance of nonoxidative and oxidative glucose metabolism for the generation of ATP by synovial cells under various conditions has not been determined precisely.

In chronic synovitis, synovial cells consume increased amounts of oxygen and generate more lactic acid. These changes undoubtedly reflect the enhanced proliferative and protein synthetic activity of the cells, as well as the entry into the joints of inflammatory cells from the circulation. The increased metabolic activity can cause a substantial fall in synovial fluid glucose, pH, and oxygen tension.[17] These changes may ultimately limit the energy-generating capacity of the synovial lining cells

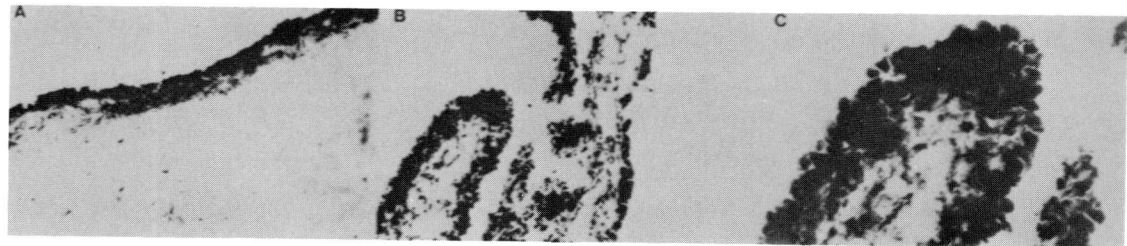

Fig. 13–6. Cryostat section of a normal *(A)* and a rheumatoid synovium *(B and C)* stained for acid phosphatase. Note the intense staining at the lining areas. (From Theofilopoulos, A.N., et al.[57])

and adjacent chondrocytes, with resultant exacerbation of joint destruction.

Glycosaminoglycans. A basic physiologic function of the synovial lining fibroblasts is the synthesis and secretion of hyaluronic acid. This acidic glycosaminoglycan is a major component of the joint fluid, and forms part of the extracellular matrix that surrounds the synovial lining cells. The hexuronic acid moiety of hyaluronic acid derives from UDP-glucuronic acid, which is formed by the action of UDP-glucose dehydrogenase.[48] Specific glycosyltransferases represent the rate-limiting step in hyaluronate formation.[3,54] Both UDP-glucose dehydrogenase and hyaluronic acid synthase activity are present in normal synovial lining fibroblasts progagated in vitro.

Human synovial lining fibroblasts incorporate radioactive sulfate into chondroitin sulfate and dermatan sulfate.[35] The two glycosaminoglycans, in association with proteoglycan core proteins, are part of the extracellular synovial lining matrix. They are also detectable in joint fluid. In accord with the necessity to modify continually the joint fluid and extracellular matrix, the synovial lining fibroblasts probably synthesize and secrete proteoglycans constitutively. However, several distinct polypeptide hormones can affect the rate of production.[1,46] When the synovium is injured, the synovial macrophages, and other inflammatory cells, release specific connective tissue activating factors that enhance proteoglycan synthesis by the adjacent fibroblasts. The newly formed extracellular matrix coats the synovial lining and protects it from further injury. The control of connective tissue activation is discussed in detail in Chapter 12.

Collagen. It is not clear to what extent the synovial fibroblasts normally produce collagen. Although significant amounts of types 1 and 3 collagen are synthesized by synovial fibroblasts in vitro, this may represent an adaptation of the cells to tissue culture. Collagen is not a significant component of the synovial fluid, and collagen fibers are notably sparse in the superficial synovial layers. In one early study, normal rabbit synovial slices incorporated less proline (a collagen precursor) than glycine, tryptophan, or histidine into protein. The results were interpreted to indicate that collagen represented only a minor fraction of synovial protein synthesis in vivo.[26]

Collagenase and Plasminogen Activator. As mentioned earlier, the nonphagocytic synovial dendritic cells contain collagenase in granules associated with the stellate processes.[63] When exposed to soluble factors produced by activated adjacent synovial macrophages, the dendritic cells release the collagenase in a latent form into the extracellular space.[60] In a parallel fashion, normal synovial fibroblasts have been reported to release the proteolytic enzyme plasminogen activator, following exposure to supernatants of mononuclear phagocytes.[31,60,61] The plasminogen activator converts the latent collagenase to an active form. It also degrades fibrinogen directly, and thereby prevents fibrin formation. The collagenase and plasminogen activator work in concert with the phagocytic mechanism to prevent the accumulation of particulate material in the joint fluid.

Fibronectin. The adhesive glycoprotein fibronectin has been detected between the intimal lining cells of both normal and rheumatoid synovial membrane with immunohistochemical techniques.[50] Fibronectin is known to interact with hyaluronic acid to form a meshwork that may influence the attachment, the spreading and, indirectly, the replication of synovial fibroblasts. The source of the fibronectin in the synovial lining is not known precisely. It may derive in part from the endothelial cells in the subsynovial tissue.

CHANGES IN SYNOVIOCYTES IN RHEUMATOID ARTHRITIS (RA)

In RA, the synovial lining becomes hyperemic and thickened with extensive growth and folding into villi.[64] The proliferation of synovial cells is an early event in pathogenesis and precedes the appearance of plasma cells.[49] The synovial layer may increase in thickness to 10 or more cells (see Fig. 13–1, *B* and *C*). In addition, individual synovial cells hypertrophy to double in size, predominantly owing to increased cytoplasm.[13] During the first months of disease, there may be significant variation in the degree of synovial hypertrophy and hyperplasia in different regions of the same joint.[7] However, significant regional variations are less frequent in cases of long duration. In some patients, synovial giant cells are present (Table 13–2); these cells have 2 to 12 nuclei and resemble hypertrophied synoviocytes. Their location and features are distinct from "foreign body" giant cells and Langerhan "giant cells."[6,13,55] However, they are not specific for RA since synovial giant cells are found in other types of arthritis (see Table 13–2).

Both macrophage (type A) and fibroblast (type B) cells are increased in number in most RA patients, although some patients have a more pronounced increase in type B and intermediate cell types.[16] At the electron microscopic level, numerous differences are apparent between the type A cells in RA patients as compared with those of normal individuals. The size and number of lysosomes are increased. The Golgi apparatus is smaller and fewer filopodia are present. The mitochondria are frequently swollen and contain fewer cristae. The type B cells show increased

Table 13–2. Percentage Incidence of Histopathologic Parameters in 10 Diagnostic Categories*

	Clinical Diagnoses (Number of Accessions in Percentages)						
	Definite or Classic Rheumatoid Arthritis (127)	Juvenile Rheumatoid Arthritis (23)	Psoriatic Arthropathy (13)	Reiter's Syndrome (9)	Ankylosing Spondylitis (17)	Enterocolitic Arthropathy (7)	Osteo-arthritis (74)
1. Hypertrophy of synoviocytes	82.7	73.9	84.6	77.8	35.3	85.7	68.9
2. Hyperplasia of synoviocytes	63.0	69.6	76.9	77.8	47.1	57.1	63.5
3. Synovial giant cells	18.1	8.7	30.8	0	17.6	0	10.8
Synovial giant cells, superficial	15.7	4.3	23.1	0	17.6	0	6.8
Synovial giant cells in subsynoviocyte tissue	7.9	4.3	15.4	0	5.9	0	5.4
4. Ulceration of synovial surface	26.0	13.0	15.4	0	11.8	0	5.4
5. Fresh fibrin on synovial surface	32.5	21.7	38.5	0	23.5	28.6	24.3
6. Organizing fibrin on synovial surface	50.4	39.1	53.8	11.1	17.6	14.3	13.5
7. Fibrin in subsynoviocyte tissue	7.1	0	0	0	0	0	1.4
8. Proliferating fibroblasts	68.5	26.1	84.6	33.3	11.8	14.3	14.9

*Data from Cooper et al.[6]

rough endoplasmic reticulum and intermediate-sized filamentous fibers of the vimentin type.[16,43] The matrix of RA joints contains periodically banded collagen fibers as well as "fibrinoid" material that does not show cross-striation.[39] The fibroblasts in the subsynovium of RA joints do not show the changes noted in type A or type B cells and appear similar to fibroblasts in skin or normal joints.[16] At the junction of pannus and articular cartilage, both fibroblasts and type A cells are present, with the type A cells forming the cells actually invading the cartilage.[51,52]

Quantitative cytochemical measurements have revealed that synoviocytes from RA patients contain higher levels of various enzymes than normal synoviocytes; examples include elevated amounts of glucose 6-phosphatase, cathepsin D, enzymes of the glycolytic pathway, and prostaglandin synthetase.[1,20] Enzymes commonly found in monocytes, such as nonspecific esterase and lysozyme, are present in most of the synovial lining cells.[28,29] The intense staining of tissue sections for acid phosphatase (see Fig. 13–6) is due to the increased

thickness of the synovium and to the increased lysozyme content per synoviocyte. Henderson has reviewed many additional studies that have been performed on tissue slices and cells eluted from synovial membrane.[21] The relationship of these activities to those expressed by synoviocytes in situ remains a topic of intense research interest.

Studies have used monoclonal antibodies to further characterize antigens expressed by synovial cells.[15,23,28,30,45,62,65] Frozen tissue sections can be stained with particular monoclonal antibodies that have been produced from mice immunized with human antigens. Synovial cells binding the monoclonal antibody are then detected with fluorescent or peroxidase conjugated anti-mouse IgG antiserum. Most rheumatoid synovial lining cells express Ia antigen, the gene product of the HLA-DR locus (Fig. 13–7, *A* and *B*). Synovial lining cells also express OKM-1 *(C)* and T200 *(D)* antigens; these markers are found on monocytes but not on fibroblasts.[34,58] These results suggest that synovial proliferation in rheumatoid arthritis is due to bone marrow-derived cells. However, it remains possi-

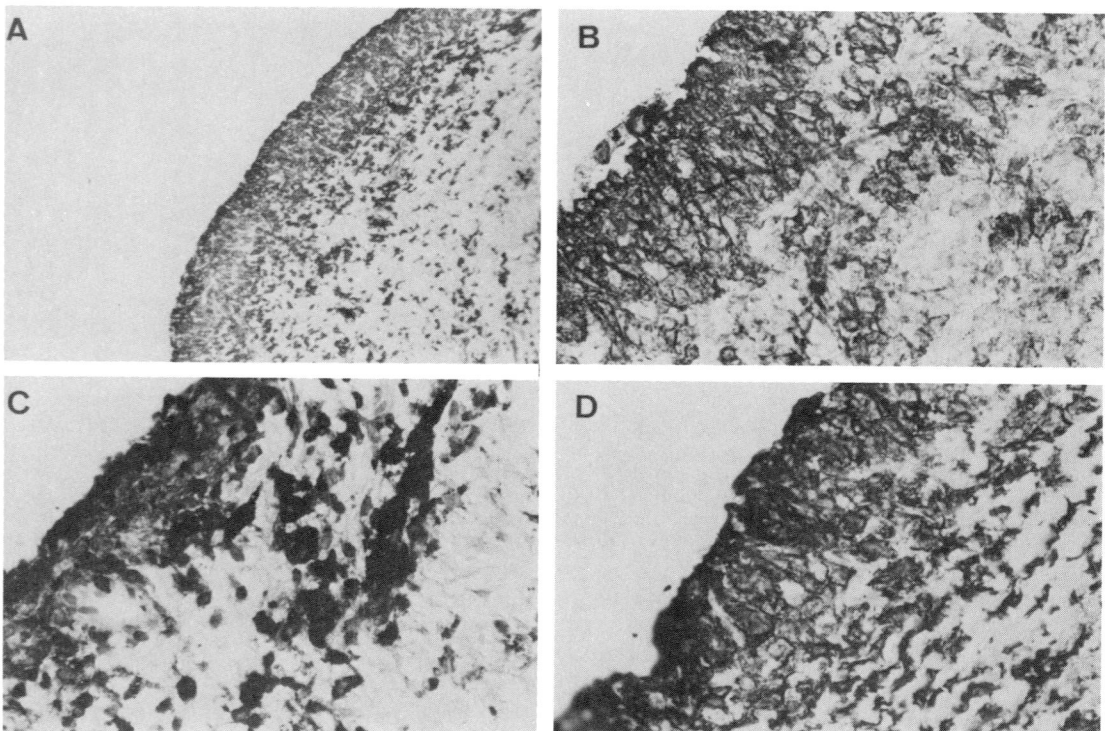

Fig. 13–7. Immunohistologic characterization of rheumatoid synovial membrane. Frozen tissue sections were reacted with monoclonal antibodies and peroxidase-coupled goat anti-mouse IgG. The presence of a positive reaction is shown by dark staining. *A,* Reaction with monoclonal anti-Ia antibody to detect the gene product of the HLA-DR gene locus. *B,* A higher magnification (× 400) demonstrates that virtually all lining cells express Ia-antigen. *C,* Staining of the synovial lining cells with antibody OKM-1 that detects an antigen on monocytes. *D,* Reaction with the T200 antigen, a marker found on hematopoietic cells but not with normal fibroblasts.

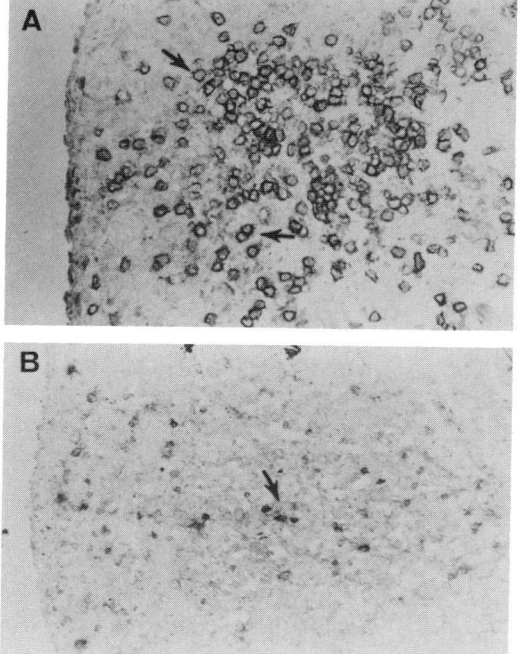

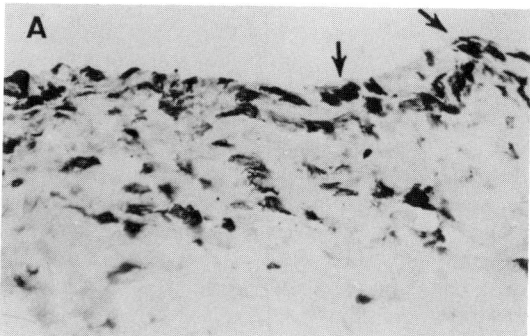

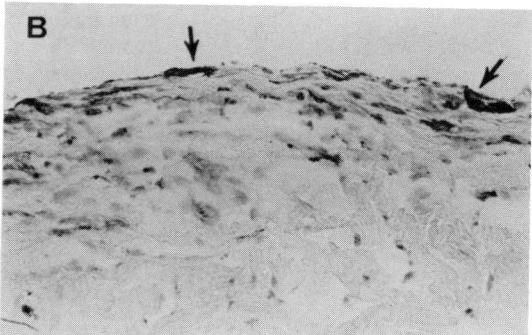

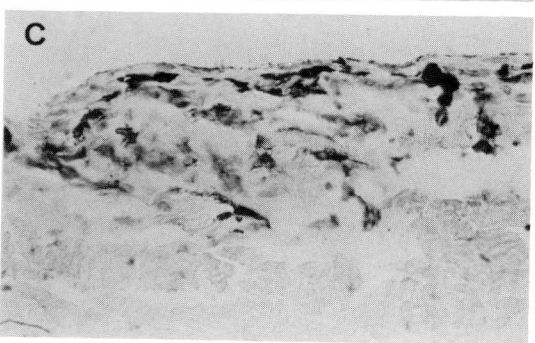

Fig. 13–8. Most mononuclear cells in the rheumatoid synovium are T cells based on staining with monoclonal antibody Leu 4 *(A)*; examples of the positively stained cell membranes are shown by arrows. Scattered B cells, detected by anti-kappa/lambda antibody *(B)*, are also present; an example of the cytoplasmic and membrane staining is shown by the arrow.

ble that primitive mesenchymal cells can be induced to express these markers. Immunohistologic techniques can also be used to demonstrate that most mononuclear cells infiltrating the rheumatoid synovium are T cells (Fig. 13–8, *A*), although some B cells *(B)* are also present. In contrast to rheumatoid synovium, normal joints have a smaller proportion of synovial cells rective with anti-Ia antibody (Fig. 13–9, *A*), OKM-1 *(B)*, and T-200 *(C)* antibodies. These results emphasize the increased number of macrophage-dendritic cells found in the rheumatoid joint.[23,45,46]

In vitro functional studies have shown that rheumatoid synovial cells can stimulate mixed lymphocyte cultures or present antigens to T cells more efficiently than synoviocytes from normal or osteoarthritic joints.[27] Synovial cells are also able to bind immune complexes, presumably through their receptors for the Fc portion of IgG or for complement components[57] (Fig. 13–10). Thus, synovial cells are able to concentrate particular antigens and present them in an immunogenic form to lymphocytes. The binding of immune complexes to synovial macrophages may release polypeptide factors

Fig. 13–9. Normal synovial membrane tissue sections stained with anti-Ia *(A)*, OKM-1 *(B)*, and T200 *(C)* monoclonal antibodies. Examples of positively stained cells are shown by the arrows.

that in turn stimulate the proliferation and metabolic activity of the adjacent connective tissue.[3,31,61] One such mononuclear cell factor is related to, or is the same as, the cytokine interleukin-1 (IL-1).[31,37] Minute amounts of IL-1 induce synovial dendritic cells and fibroblasts to release collagenase and plasminogen activator, respectively. Besides this specific effect on synovial cell function, IL-1 promotes the activation and proliferation of T-lymphocytes, and is a potent pyrogen.[37,44] Additional factors, termed connective tissue activating peptides, derived from platelets and mononuclear cells, are able to influence synovial proliferation and proteoglycan synthesis (see Chap. 12).

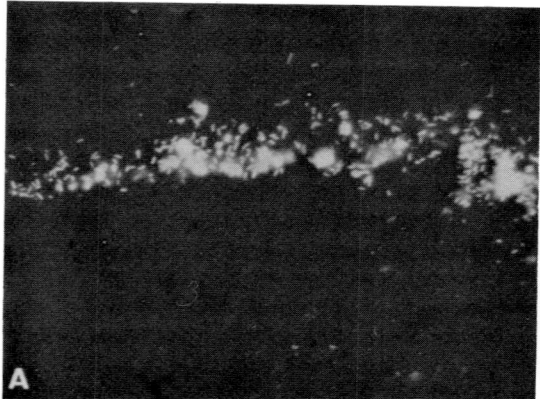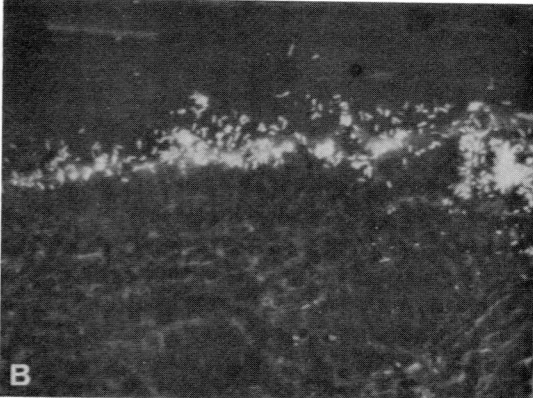

Fig. 13–10. Cryostat section of a normal synovium with attachment on the lining areas of fluorescinated gram-negative bacteria that had fixed complement as viewed by fluorescence *(A)* and phase *(B)* microscopy. (From Theofilopoulos, A.N., et al.[57])

Harris and co-workers have pointed out the similarity between the destructive process in rheumatoid synovium and localized cancer.[3] They found that suspensions of synovial cells could survive after transplantation into nude (athymic) mice. These cells become organized into a pannus-like structure with fibroblasts, multinucleated giant cells, and collagen fibers. In comparison, normal human skin fibroblasts or normal rabbit synovial cells cannot be recovered from the injection site of nude mice.

In sum, the synovial lining cells have a notable capacity to (1) bind antigen-antibody complexes, (2) present antigen to T lymphocytes, (3) produce cytokines that promote the activation and proliferation of T lymphocytes, and (4) respond to signals from mononuclear cells. Hence, it is not surprising that the persistence of antigenic material in the synovium, or the intermitent deposition of immune complexes from the circulation, induces the infiltration of lymphocytes and plasma cells, and the disruption of the normal synovial architecture. Indeed, in some patients with RA, the synovial membrane eventually transforms into a lymphoid tissue that produces abundant immunoglobulin and lymphokines in situ. This metamorphosis serves to remind us again that the specialized structure and function of the synovial lining represent an adaptation to the milieu of the joint space and adjacent subsynovial tissue. When the external environment is altered, the character of the synovial lining changes accordingly.

PHARMACOLOGIC APPROACHES TO MODIFYING THE FUNCTION OF SYNOVIOCYTES

To varying degrees, all forms of chronic inflammatory synovitis are associated with hyperplasia of synovial fibroblasts, metabolic activation of synovial macrophages and dendritic cells, infiltration of leukocytes from the subsynovial space, and matrix disorganization. Not surprisingly, therefore, pharmacologic agents that block lysosomal enzyme release, prostaglandin synthesis, free radical formation, or cellular proliferation favorably alter the course of joint inflammation.[8] If the same drugs could be administered in a form that localized preferentially to the synovial macrophages, and persisted for long periods, a more specific antiarthritic effect could be obtained. An objective for future research will be to develop anti-arthritic substances that (1) impede the homing of monocytes to the synovial membrane, (2) block the synthesis of interleukin-1 and related lymphokines, (3) impair the ability of dendritic cells to present antigen to T-lymphocytes, and (4) interfere with the binding of polypeptide growth factors to specific receptors on synovial fibroblasts and dendritic cells. Agents with these properties could stop directly the reciprocal interactions between synovial macrophages, dendritic cells, fibroblasts, and subsynovial lymphocytes that are necessary for sustained joint inflammation. The possibility also exists that pathways in intermediary metabolism of particular importance to the function of the synovial lining cells, when compared to histiocytes and fibroblasts in other tissues, will be discovered.

REFERENCES

1. Amento, E.P., et al.: Modulation of synovial cell products by a factor from a human cell line: T-lymphocyte induction of a mononuclear cell factor. Proc. Natl. Acad. Sci. U.S.A., 79:5307–5311, 1982.
2. Barland, P., Novikoff, A.B., and Hamerman, D.: Electron microscopy of the human synovial membrane. J. Cell. Biol., 14:207–214, 1962.
3. Brinkerhoff, C., and Harris, E.: Survival of rheumatoid

synovium implanted into nude mice. Am. J. Pathol., *103*:411–418, 1981.

4. Cheung, H.S., Halverson, P.D, and McCarty, D.J.: Release of collagenase, neutral protease, and prostaglandins from cultured mammalian synovial cells by hydroxyapatite and calcium pyrophosphate dihydrate crystals. Arthritis Rheum., *24*:1338–1344, 1981.

5. Collins, A.J., et al.: Prostaglandin synthetase activity in synovial tissue from patients with rheumatoid arthritis after therapy with aspirin-like drugs. *In* Prostaglandins and Inflammation. Edited by G.P. Lewis. Vienna, Hans Huber, 1976, p. 138.

6. Cooper, N., et al.: Diagnostic specificity of synovial lesions. Hum. Pathol., *12*:314–328, 1981.

7. Cruickshank, B.: Interpretation of multiple biopsies of synovial tissues in rheumatic diseases. Ann. Rheum. Dis., *11*:137–145, 1952.

8. Davies, P., et al.: The effect of anti-rheumatic agents on macrophage function. Int. J. Immunopharmacol., *4*:111–118, 1982.

9. Davies, D., and Palfray, A.: Studies on the Anatomy and Function of Bones and Joints. (Edited by F. Evans.) Berlin, Springer-Verlag, 1966, pp. 1–16.

10. Edwards, J.C.W.: The origin of type A synovial lining cells. Immunobiology, *161*:227–231, 1982.

11. Edwards, J.C.W., and Willoughby, D.A.: Demonstration of bone marrow-derived cells in synovial lining by means of giant intracellular granules as genetic markers. Ann. Rheum. Dis., *41*:177–182, 1982.

12. Edwards, J.C.W., Sedgwick, A.D., and Willoughby, D.A.: The formation of a structure with the essential features of synovial lining by subcutaneous injection of air. J. Pathol., *134*:147–156, 1981.

13. Fassbender, H.: Rheumatoid arthritis. *In* Pathology of Rheumatic Diseases. New York, Springer-Verlag, 1980.

14. fox, R., et al.: Synovial fluid lymphocytes differ from peripheral blood lymphocytes in patients with rheumatoid arthritis. J. Immunol., *128*:351–354, 1982.

15. Fox, R., and Adamson, T.: Human lymphocyte cell surface antigens defined by monoclonal antibodies. *In* New Directions in Clinical Laboratory Assays. Edited by R. Nakamura. New York, Masson Press, 1984, pp. 265–295.

16. Gadially, F.N.: Fine structure of joints. *In* The Joints and Synovial Fluid. Vol. I. Edited by L. Sokoloff. New York, Academic Press, 1978, pp. 105–177.

17. Goetzl, E.J., et al.: Physiological approach to the assessment of disease activity in rheumatoid arthritis. J. Clin. Invest., *50*:1167–1173, 1971.

18. Graabaek, P.M.: Ultrastructural evidence for two distinct types of synoviocytes in rat synovial membrane. J. Ultrastruct. Res., *78*:321–339, 1982.

19. Hamilton, J.A., et al.: Streptococcal cell walls and synovial cell activation. J. Exp. Med., *155*:1702–1717, 1982.

20. Henderson, B.: The biochemistry of the human synovial lining with special reference to alterations in metabolism in rheumatoid arthritis. Pathol. Res. Pract., *172*:1–24, 1981.

21. Henderson, B., Glynn, L.E., and Chayen, J.: Cell division in the synovial lining in experimental allergic arthritis: Proliferation of cells during the development of chronic arthritis. Ann. Rheum. Dis., *41*:275–281, 1982.

22. Hermanns, W., and Schulz, L.C.: Enzyme histochemical studies of the homogeneity of the mononuclear phagocyte system with special reference to the synovium. Agents Actions [Suppl.], *11*:117–129, 1982.

23. Janossy, G., et al.: Rheumatoid arthritis: A disease of T-lymphocytes/macrophage immunoregulation. Lancet, *2*:839–842, 1981.

24. Katz, S.I., Tamaki, K., and Sax, D.H.: Epidermal Langerhans cells are derived from cells originating in bone marrow. Nature, *282*:324–326, 1979.

25. Kinsella, T.D., Baum, J., and Ziff, M.: Studies of isolated synovial lining cells of rheumatoid and non-rheumatoid synovial membranes. Arthritis Rheum., *13*:734–735, 1971.

26. Kitlowski, N.P., et al.: Protein synthesis in articular cartilage and synovium of the rabbit. Arthritis Rheum., *8*:456–458, 1965.

27. Klareskog, L., et al.: Immune functions of human synovial cells. Arthritis Rheum., *25*:488–499, 1982.

28. Klareskog, L., et al.: Appearance of anti-HLA-DR-reactive cells in normal and rheumatoid synovial tissue. Scand. J. Immunol., *14*:183–192, 1981.

29. Klareskog, L., Forsum, U., and Wigzell, H.: Murine synovial intima contains Ia, Ie/c positive bone marrow-derived cells. Scand. J. Immunol., *15*:509–514, 1982.

30. Konttinen, Y., et al.: Characterization of the immunocompetent cells of rheumatoid synovium from tissue sections and eluates. Arthritis Rheum., *24*:71–79, 1981.

31. Krane, S.M.: Aspects of the cell biology of the rheumatoid synovial lesion. Ann. Rheum. Dis., *40*:433–448, 1981.

32. Krawisz, B., Florine, D., and Scott, R.: Differentiation of fibroblast-like cell into macrophages. Cancer Res., *41*:2891–2899, 1981.

33. Krey, P.R., et al.: The human fetal synovium. Histology, fine structure and changes in organ culture. Arthritis Rheum., *14*:319–325, 1971.

34. Kung, P.: Strategies for generating monoclonal antibodies: A review. Transplant. Proc., *12*:141–146, 1980.

35. Marsh, J.M., et al.: Synthesis of sulfated proteoglycans by rheumatoid and normal synovial tissue in culture. Ann. Rheum. Dis., *38*:166–170, 1979.

36. McGuire, M.K.B., et al.: Messenger function of prostaglandins in cell-to-cell interactions and control of proteinase activity in the rheumatoid joint. Int. J. Immunopharmacol., *4*:91–102, 1982.

37. Mizel, S.B.: Interleukin 1 and T cell activation. Immunol. Rev., *63*:51–73, 1982.

38. Mohr, W., Benecke, G., and Amohing, W.: Proliferation of synovial lining cells and fibroblsts. Ann. Rheum. Dis. *34*:219–224, 1975.

39. Norton, W., and Ziff, M.: Electron microscopic observations on rheumatoid synovial membranes. Arthritis Rheum., 9:589, 1966.

40. Nykanen, T., et al.: Characterization of the DNA-synthesizing cells in rheumatoid synovial tissue. Scand. J. Rheum., *7*:118–122, 1978.

41. Okada, Y., Nakanishi, I., and Kajikawa, K.: Ultrastructure of the mouse synovial membrane. Arthritis Rheum., *24*:835–843, 1981.

42. O'Rahilly, R., and Gardner, E.: The embryology of movable joints. *In* The Joints and Synovial Fluid. Vol. I. Edited by L. Sokoloff. New York, Academic Press, 1978, pp. 48–97.

43. Osung, O., Chandra, M., and Holborow, E.: Intermediate filaments in synovial lining cells in rheumatoid arthritis are of the vimentin type. Ann. Rheum. Dis., *41*:74–77, 1982.

44. Palacios, R.: Mechanism of T cell activation: Role and functional relationship of HLA antigens and interleukins. Immunol. Rev., *63*:73–111, 1982.

45. Poulter, L.W., et al.: Involvement of interdigitating (antigen-presenting) cells in the pathogenesis of rheumatoid arthritis. Clin. Exp. Immunol., *51*:247–254, 1983.

46. Poulter, L.W., et al.: Histochemical discrimination of HLA-DR positive cell populations in the normal and arthritic synovial lining. Clin. Exp. Immunol., *48*:381–388, 1982.

47. Rajah, K.T., and Merker, H.J.: Joint formation in culture. Arthritis Rheum., *34*:200–205, 1975.

48. Ross, G.T., Marsh, J.M., and Roback, D.W.: Uridine diphosphate glucose dehydrogenase in rheumatoid synovial cells in culture. J. Rheumatol., *8*:710–715, 1981.

49. Schumacher, H.R.: Synovial membrane and fluid morphologic alterations in early rheumatoid arthritis: Micorvascular injury and virus-like particles. Ann. N.Y. Acad. Sci., *15*:519, 1966.

50. Scott, C.L., et al.: Significance of fibronectin in rheumatoid arthritis and osteoarthrosis. Ann. Rheum. Dis., *40*:142–153, 1981.

51. Shiozawa, S., Jasin, H., and Ziff, M.: Absence of immunoglobulins in rheumatoid cartilage-pannus junctions. Arthritis Rheum., *23*:816–821, 1980.

52. Shiozawa, S., Shiozawa, K., and Fujita, T.: Morphologic observations in the early phase of the cartilage-pannus junction. Arthritis Rheum., *26*:472–477, 1983.

53. Shiozawa, S., Williams, R.C., Jr., and Ziff, M.: Immu-

noelectron/microscopic demonstration of prostaglandin E in rheumatoid synovium. Arthritis Rheum., *25*:685–693, 1982.

54. Sisson, J.C., Castor, C.W., and Klavons, J.A.: Connective tissue activation XVIII. Stimulation of hyaluronic acid synthetase activity. J. Lab. Clin. Med., *96*:189–197, 1980.
55. Soren, A., and Waugh, T.: The giant cells in synovial membrane. Ann. Rheum. Dis., *40*:496–500, 1981.
56. Steinman, R.M., et al.: Identification of a novel cell type in peripheral lymphoid organs of mice. V. Purification of spleen dendritic cells, new surface markers, and maintenance in vitro. J. Exp. Med., *149*:1–8, 1979.
57. Theofilopoulos, A.N., et al.: Evidence for the presence of receptors for C3 and IgG–Fc on human synovial cells. Arthritis Rheum., *23*:1–9, 1980.
58. Trowbridge, I., Omary, B., and Battifora, H.: Human analogue of murine T200 glycoprotein. J. Exp. Med., *152*:842, 1980.
59. Webb, F.W., Ford, P.M., and Glynn, L.E.: Persistence of antigen in rabbit synovial membrane. Br. J. Exp. Pathol., *52*:31–41, 1971.
60. Werb, Z., et al.: Endogenous activation of latent collagenase by rheumatoid synovial cells. N. Engl. J. Med., *266*:1017–1021, 1977.
61. Werb, Z., and Reynolds, J.J.: Stimulation by endocytosis of the secretion of collagenase and neutral proteinase from rabbit synovial fibroblasts. J. Exp. Med., *140*:1482–1490, 1976.
62. Winchester, R.J., and Burmester, G.J.: Demonstration of Ia antigens on certain dendritic cells and on a novel elongate cell found in human synovial tissue. Scand. J. Immunol., *14*:439–444, 1981.
63. Woolley, D.E., Harris, E.D., and Brinckerhoff, C.E.: Collagenase immunolocation in cultures of rheumatoid synovial cells. Science, *200*:773–775, 1978.
64. Wyllie, J., Haust, M., and More, R.: The fine structure of synovial lining cells in rheumatoid arthritis. Lab. Invest., *15*:519, 1966.
65. Young, C., et al.: Immunohistologic characterization of synovial membrane lymphocytes in rheumatoid arthritis. Arthritis Rheum., *27*:32–39, 1984.

Chapter 14

Chondrocyte Structure and Function

E. Carwile LeRoy

In the diarthrodial joint, articular cartilage is the single most important tissue for smooth, repetitive, pain-free movement (Fig. 14–1). The articular cartilage, itself an example of hyaline cartilage, is a highly organized, relatively acellular tissue. At its articular surface, dense arches of collagen are filled by hydrated proteoglycans under pressure with few cells. Deeper within the cartilage are gradual increases in chondrocyte density and changes in cell morphology, as well as in matrix composition, until one reaches the tidemark—the junction between noncalcified, avascular hyaline cartilage and ossified, vascularized subchondral bone.[8,21,26,28]

This chapter is concerned primarily with chondrocytes, a subject about which our understanding is meager. Nonetheless, focus on the chondrocyte is timely because an increasing number of phenomena concerning cartilage degradation are being recognized as chondrocyte-dependent.[4] The direct role of the synovium in cartilage and bone destruction, elegantly summarized in Chapter 37 and elsewhere,[14] is not discussed in detail here; rather, emphasis is placed on the emerging chondrocyte-dependent mechanisms of synovial-cartilage interaction and of cartilage metabolism. In addition, the major role of chondrocytes and cartilage in the development and differentiation of the skeleton is not treated here; it, too, is discussed extensively elsewhere.[6]

THE CHONDROCYTE

The term *chondrocyte* derives from the Greek *chondros,* meaning cartilage (itself derived from the word for grain). In fixed tissue, the cells within cartilage are easily identified (Figs. 14–2 through 14–5). When they are separated from surrounding cartilaginous matrix, however, it is remarkably difficult to define distinctive morphologic features of these cells.[11,31,32] In the absence of matrix in vitro, chondrocytes acquire fibroblast-like morphologic features, as do osteocytes.[1] Only recently have synthetic matrixes (e.g., agarose) been shown to sustain the distinctive cartilage phenotype of chondrocytes in vitro.[2]

A characteristic chondrocyte is oval and 10 to

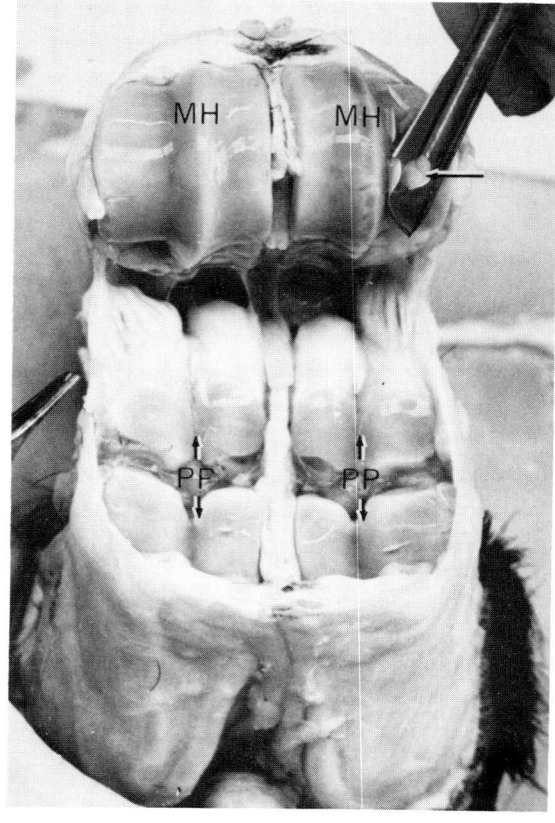

Fig. 14–1. The metacarpophalangeal joint of an 18-month-old bovine was opened from the dorsal side, and the metacarpal bone (Mc III + IV) was bent backward. The joint surfaces of the metacarpal head (MH) and the bone of the two proximal phalanges (PP) are exposed. Cartilage is shaved from the joint surfaces with a scalpel (arrow). (Reproduced from *The Journal of Cell Biology,* 1982, volume 93, page 743 by copyright permission of The Rockefeller University Press.)

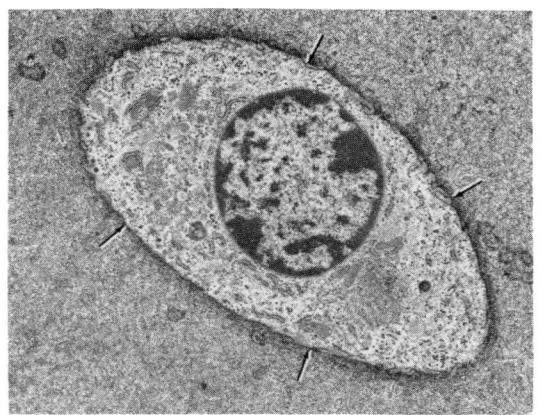

Fig. 14–2. Chondrocyte of normal articular cartilage shows prominent rough endoplasmic reticulum and numerous free ribosomes. It is surrounded by a rim of dense, finely fibrillar, RR-positive territorial matrix (arrows). The extraterritorial matrix is somewhat less dense and also stains positively with ruthenium red (RR) (× 6,100). (Reproduced from *The Journal of Cell Biology*, 1982, volume 93, page 743 by copyright permission of The Rockefeller University Press.)

structures such as basal laminae (basement membranes, absent from cartilage as befits its exclusively mesenchymal origin).[31] Chondrocytes are primarily distinguished by the unique combination of matrix molecules that they secrete, by the highly ordered arrangement of this matrix, by their role in sustaining cartilage in its pristine state with low levels of cell division, and by their large distances from nutrient-supplying microvessels (Figs. 14–6 through 14–11).[15,25]

The absence of microvessels and the low rate of cell proliferation are unique and distinguishing features of cartilage. Both may relate to the higher organization of joint structure in which nutrition comes from the vascularized synovium through synovial fluid into the cartilage, aided by the physicochemical features of synovial fluid and by the mechanical "pumping" effects of movement and weight-bearing on the "circulation" of nutrients and of waste products in and out of the cartilage. In specialized situations, nutrition may also come from the bone marrow circulation.[28]

Both chondrocytes in situ and chondrocytes grown on plastic and in close proximity suspension cultures secrete proteoglycan (ruthenium red positive) material that forms a finely granular shell around the cell made up of globules interconnected with fine fibrils. The term "territorial matrix" has been used for this structure, shown in Figure 14–2 surrounding a chondrocyte *in situ*. Its function is unknown. The territorial matrix may also contain one or more of the minor collagens of cartilage, which share structural similarities with type V collagens.[3,10,16]

30 μ in diameter, may vary from spheroidal to flattened in situ, has many projecting cell processes, has a fine plasma (cell) membrane, and shows no evidence of organelles, which in other cells permit cell-to-cell communication. The absence of morphologic evidence of intercellular communication suggests a degree of independence for each chondrocyte, influenced more by matrix signals for macromolecular synthesis and by soluble signals for matrix degradation than by signals from other chondrocytes. Theoretically, if adequately stimulated, a few chondrocytes could both synthesize and destroy large areas of cartilage. Thus, the domain of the individual chondrocyte, both for biosynthesis and for degradation, is unlimited by cell contact or by the presence of limiting

CHONDROCYTE METABOLISM

Chondrocytes have the usual array of metabolic pathways, including anaerobic and aerobic glycolysis, protein turnover, and lipid and fatty acid interchange, as well as the arachidonic acid cascade producing both prostaglandins and leukotrienes.

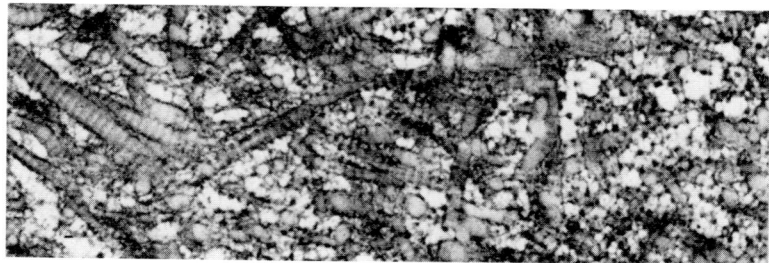

Fig. 14–3. The extraterritorial matrix typically consists of a network of tightly packed and highly cross-linked collagen fibrils. This network is embedded in a ground substance containing RR-positive proteoglycans (× 25,000). (Reproduced from *The Journal of Cell Biology*, 1982, volume 93, page 743 by copyright permission of The Rockefeller University Press.)

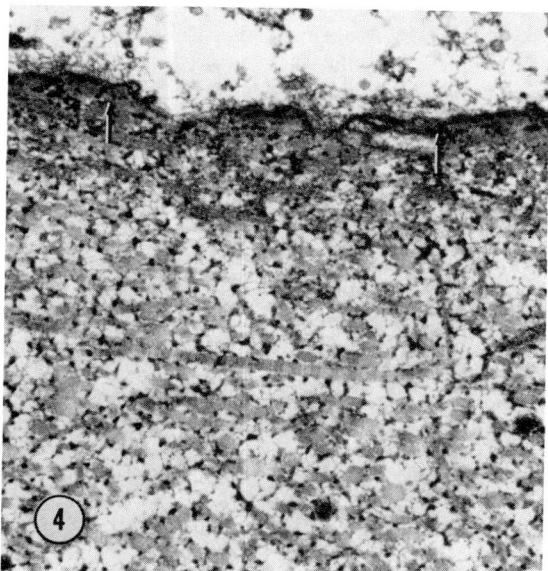

Fig. 14–4. Articular cartilage was digested for 90 minutes in 1% pronase at 37°C. Pronase removed large parts of the proteoglycan, thereby exposing collagen fibers. Under this condition, pronase does not noticeably digest the territorial matrix (arrows) (× 53,000). (Reproduced from *The Journal of Cell Biology,* 1982, volume 93, page 743 by copyright permission of The Rockefeller University Press.)

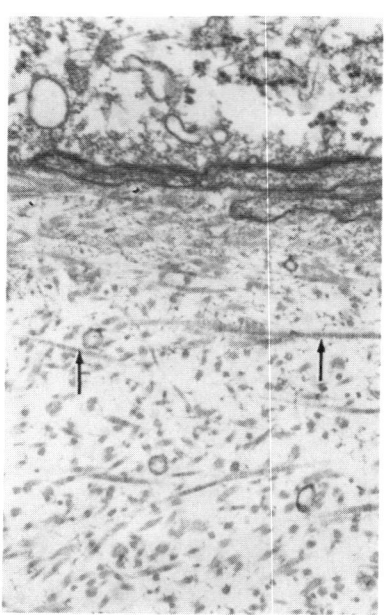

Fig. 14–5. Pronase-digested cartilage slices were exposed to 0.4% of nonpurified, bacterial collagenase for 2 hours at 37°C (total incubation period: 3 hours). This enzyme cleaves the remaining proteoglycan and starts to degrade the collagen network (arrows). The fiber diameter of collagen is reduced when compared to that in Figure 14–4 (× 37,000). (Reproduced from *The Journal of Cell Biology,* 1982, volume 93, page 743, by copyright permission of The Rockefeller University Press.)

Perhaps the most distinctive product of chondrocyte metabolism is type II collagen, found exclusively in hyaline cartilage, the nucleus pulposus, and the vitreous of the eye. The discovery of type II collagen by Miller and colleagues was the first indication that collagens were a family of proteins derived from as many as a dozen or more gene products with differing properties and distinct compositions in different tissues. The three chains of type II collagen appear to be identical: the molecules have a high concentration of hydroxylysine, and the hydroxylysine is heavily glycosylated with glucose and galactose residues, imparting to cartilage collagen a distinctive charge profile that may influence its association with cartilage proteoglycans. Among the interstitial family of collagens (types I, II, III) type II collagen is most resistant to the degradative action of mammalian collagenase, a property for which we can be thankful, considering the limited capacity of hyaline cartilage to repair itself in its own image.[3,12,19]

Type II collagen is not the only collagenous protein in articular cartilage. Although nomenclature is confusing, several laboratories agree that other collagens exist in the form of as many as seven structurally distinct collagen polypeptide chains and from the expression of as many as nine distinct collagen genes. The role of minor cartilage collagens is still unclear; there are structural homologies with the incompletely characterized pericellular type V collagen, the function of which is also unknown (see Chap. 10).[3,9]

Chondrocytes also synthesize proteoglycans which, with type II collagen, comprise the two major matrix constituents of hyaline cartilage. Cartilage proteoglycans are distinctive macromolecules that may reach 2×10^6 daltons in aggregated molecular weight (see Chap. 11). They consist of proteoglycan core proteins to which glycosaminoglycan side chains of at least two types (chondroitin and keratan sulfate) are covalently bound. Each proteoglycan is in turn bound to hyaluronic acid by the interaction of linkage proteins to form the superaggregate proteoglycan molecules, which look like fern leaves on rotary shadowed electron micrographs and which dominate large volumes of water packed under pressure in the collagen arches (more Gothic than Roman) of articular cartilage. Movement of water in and out of these proteoglycan aggregates provides the resilient elastic prop-

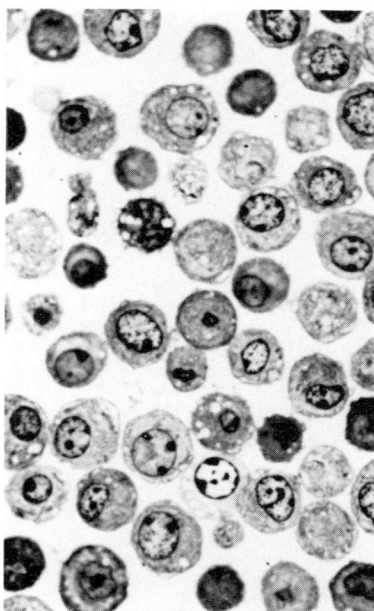

Fig. 14–6. Isolated chondrocytes were obtained after a final trypsin digestion (0.25%) and after passing the digest through a Nitex filter (90 μm). The cell viability is ~95% (× 830). (Reproduced from *The Journal of Cell Biology*, 1982, volume 93, page 743 by copyright permission of The Rockefeller University Press.)

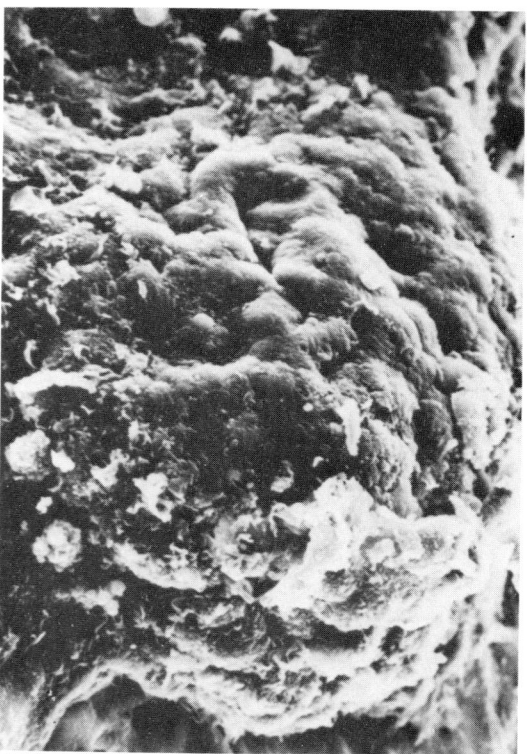

Fig. 14–7. Chondrocyte nodule consisting of an aggregation of cells and matrix is shown in a scanning electron micrograph after incubation of high-density culture for 14 days (× 600). (Reproduced from *The Journal of Cell Biology*, 1982, volume 93, page 743 by copyright permission of The Rockefeller University Press.)

erties of cartilage. The synthesis of proteoglycans by chondrocytes also provides the basis for the distinctive tinctorial property of cartilage: that of metachromasia on staining. Metachromasia is one of the first histologically recognizable features of cartilage in skeletal development, it is a constant feature of healthy articular cartilage, and its loss is one of the earliest features of damaged articular cartilage.[7,13,18,20]

The collagen scaffolding in all human tissue interacts with tissue cells via a family of attachment proteins. Cartilage is no exception. The attachment protein that binds type II collagen to chondrocytes has been identified and named chondronectin, which is distinct from the other attachment proteins and, as expected, has one or more high-avidity binding sites selective for type II collagen. Chondronectin, an attachment glycoprotein found uniquely in hyaline cartilage and in chondrocyte-conditioned medium, is a 180,000-dalton molecule composed of two 70,000-dalton subunits. It binds preferentially to type II collagen, stimulates chondrocyte attachment to type II collagen at concentrations of 5 to 10 ng/ml, and is immunologically distinct from fibronectin and from laminin. Fibronectin does not stimulate chondrocyte attachment to type II collagen, nor does chondronectin stim-

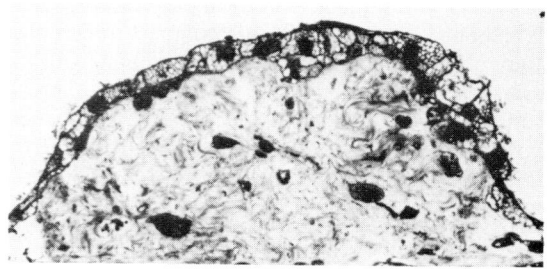

Fig. 14–8. Transverse thick section of a chondrocyte nodule shows abundant extracellular matrix and a few chondrocytes. The nodule is covered by one to three layers of flattened chondrocytes (× 300). (Reproduced from *The Journal of Cell Biology*, 1982, volume 93, page 743 by copyright permission of The Rockefeller University Press.)

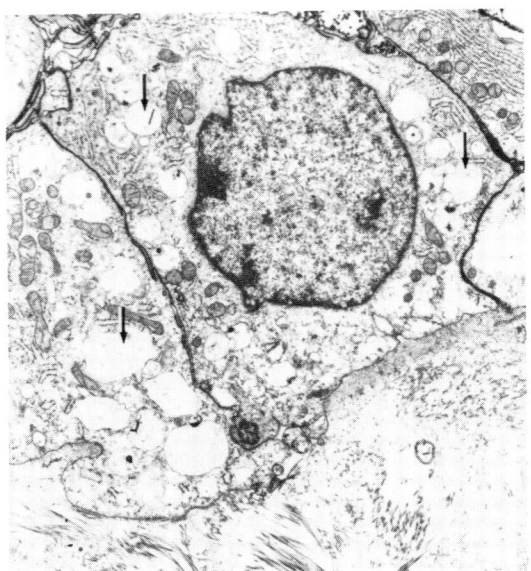

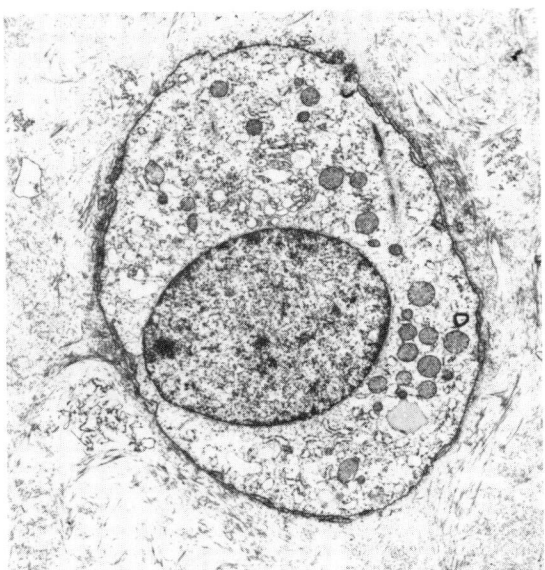

Fig. 14–9. The flattened superficial cells of chondrocyte nodules are surrounded by a prominent territorial matrix. Their cytoplasm contains well-developed rough endoplasmic reticulum and numerous empty-appearing vacuoles (arrows), ($\times$ 5,000). (Reproduced from *The Journal of Cell Biology*, 1982, volume 93, page 743 by copyright permission of The Rockefeller University Press.)

Fig. 14–10. A chondrocyte in the nodule center is surrounded by abundant extracellular matrix, which consists of a rather dense network of collagen fibers. Some collagen fibers are arranged in bundles. The chondrocyte displays a round, eccentrically located nucleus, clusters of mitochondria, rough endoplasmic reticulum, and a prominent Golgi complex ($\times$ 6,500). (Reproduced from *The Journal of Cell Biology*, 1982, volume 93, page 743 by copyright permission of The Rockefeller University Press.)

ulate fibroblast attachment to type I collagen. The kinetics of attachment suggest that other factors such as proteoglycans may be involved in the chondronectin-mediated attachment of chondrocytes to type II collagen.[9]

CHONDROCYTE GENE SWITCHING

The expanding family of collagens (up to 14 genetically distinct extracellular structural proteins) and the exquisite sensitivity of chondrocytes to respond to matrix signals combine to make the study of mass and cloned cultures of chondrocytes a fertile field for the investigation of gene expression. Two well-characterized chondrocyte phenotypes can be demonstrated. Switching from one to the other phenotype and back again can be demonstrated to involve multigene switching. The differentiated chondrocyte phenotype is expressed as type II collagen and as the characteristic cartilage proteoglycan, whereas the dedifferentiated phenotype is expressed as collagen types I, I trimer, III, V, and as less well-characterized differences in proteoglycan synthesis. The differentiated phenotype is also expressed by a characteristic cell shape (see Fig. 14–2) and a high level of connective tissue protein synthesis, whereas the dedifferentiated

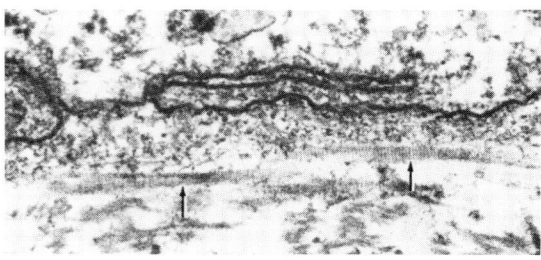

Fig. 14–11. Detail of Figure 14–10 shows chondrocyte territorial matrix and cross-banded collagen fibers of the extraterritorial matrix ($\times$ 21,500). (Reproduced from *The Journal of Cell Biology*, 1982, volume 93, page 743 by copyright permission of The Rockefeller University Press.)

chondrocyte phenotype is expressed as a sheathlike cell with low levels of collagen and proteoglycan synthesis. Thus chondrocytes can be shown to switch reversibly between two phenotypes involving distinct morphologic changes and complex gene switching of several families of connective tissue proteins. Further understanding of this intricate process should increase the ability to cope with the diseases that degrade articular cartilage.[12]

Chondrocytes in vitro show exquisite dependence on the presence of cartilage matrix to continue the synthesis and secretion of type II collagen. In the absence of cartilage matrix (presumably type II collagen and/or chondronectin), chondrocytes rapidly change morphology from rounded to sheath-like and switch from type II to type I collagen synthesis. This switch can be stimulated by the interstitial attachment protein fibronectin. Removal of fibronectin and type I collagen and reexposure to type II collagen or to cartilage direct the chondrocyte to return to type II collagen synthesis. Artificial gels such as agarose can maintain chondrocytes in their phenotypically differentiated state almost as well as can cartilage matrix. Perhaps the cell responds to the charge distribution to which it is exposed.[2]

CHONDROCYTE METABOLISM IN CARTILAGE DEGRADATION

When substantial areas of articular cartilage are removed by injury, resulting chondrocyte and inflammatory cell responses lead to the formation of fibrocartilage, a less well-organized matrix in which type I collagen is the prominent structural protein. Fibrocartilage provides a depressed surface for joint function, which is grossly less efficient than that provided by hyaline cartilage. Movement on fibrocartilage is superior to movement on bone mechanically and symptomatically, but it is distinctly inferior to normal joint function on surfaces of hyaline cartilage. Thus, repair of cartilage is functionally less desirable than is protection of the original cartilage and prevention of its degradation.

The initial response to injury by articular cartilage does not fall precisely into the classic paradigm of necrosis, inflammation, and repairs.[18] Necrotic cells can be seen, but usually, in the situation of injury confined to the articular cartilage, the first change is loss of metachromasia associated with a measurable increase in water content. This change has been interpreted as evidence of the release from chondrocytes of neutral or other proteases that cleave critical peptide bonds holding the proteoglycan aggregate together ("neutral proteoglycanase").[7] The altered proteoglycan is of smaller molecular weight, loses its metachromasia, imbibes water, and is mechanically less resilient. Associated with these early changes in the matrix are changes in the chondrocytes themselves. Nearest the injury, chondrocytes divide (mitosis) and proliferate (clusters) and show evidence of increased proteoglycan and increased collagen (type II) synthesis. This amplification and enhanced synthetic

capacity of chondrocytes may be prostaglandin-mediated since cyclo-oxygenase inhibition (aspirin) inhibits at least one aspect of this chondrocyte response, i.e., the increased proteoglycan synthesis accompanying the loss of metachromasia.

Such superficially injured cartilage remains morphologically similar to hyaline cartilage, and its chondrocytes continue to synthesize type II collagen. Conversion to fibrocartilage and type I collagen synthesis seems to require more extensive injury with the recruitment of inflammatory or blood-borne cells. In this context it is probably too simple to think of all stages of osteoarthritis (osteoarthrosis) as the conversion of hyaline cartilage to fibrocartilage via the single gene switch from type II to type I collagen synthesis.

The relationship of chondrocytes to inorganic pyrophosphate (PPi) elaboration in normal, osteoarthritic, and chondrocalcinotic cartilage is discussed in Chapter 94 and elsewhere.[13,17]

CHONDROCYTE-DEPENDENT CARTILAGE DEGRADATION

The Chondrocyte Signal. Classic approaches to understanding cartilage degeneration have emphasized two pathways: mechanical and inflammatory. It seems likely that the understanding of both these approaches deserves revision in light of recent information suggesting that cartilage degeneration, in some experimental systems at least, requires the participation of viable chondrocytes.

Explanations of the mechanisms of mechanically induced cartilage degradation have emphasized physical injury to cartilage and/or to subchondral bone as initiating the influx of synovial fluid, blood plasma-derived soluble factors, or blood- or marrow-derived cellular elements that directly perpetuate cartilage degradation enzymatically. It has long been observed that chondrocytes divide and multiply (proliferation) in and near areas of mechanical damage.[18] Most interpretations of this observation have emphasized the likelihood that proliferation represents an attempt to repair the cartilage. Studies of cell proliferation in general, and of chondrocyte proliferation in particular, suggest that proteolytic enzymes capable of digesting proteoglycans (neutral proteases and acid proteases) and possibly also cartilage collagen (elastase-like serine proteases and collagenase) are released when chondrocytes multiply. Thus, chondrocyte proliferation in response to mechanical, soluble (lymphokine/monokine/cytokine), or cellular factors may participate in cartilage destruction of a chondrocyte-dependent type.[29] (See also Chapter 88.)

The second traditional mechanism described for cartilage breakdown, the direct invasion by inflammatory cells (e.g., the rheumatoid pannus) and the release by these cells of well-characterized enzymes that degrade both proteoglycan and collagen, has been best studied and most emphasized (see Chaps. 16, 18, and 37). Inflammatory cells of all types (neutrophils, lymphocytes, monocytes, platelets) contain large quantities of enzymes capable of degrading all the matrix elements of cartilage. These enzymes have been characterized and their activities demonstrated in neutral environments (neutral proteases, such as collagenase and elastase) and in acid environments (acid proteases, such as cathepsins), suggesting that blood-borne influences can degrade cartilage under both physiologic (neutral pH) and pathologic (inflammation, acid pH, phagolysosome milieu) situations.[14] These enzymes and the processes of inflammation have heretofore been considered necessary and sufficient for cartilage destruction without any contribution from the chondrocyte. Several lines of investigation, however, now suggest that signals from other cells stimulate chondrocytes to initiate cartilage destruction.[23] Whether these signals emanate from all cells, as well as the number of signal molecules needed, has not yet been determined. Furthermore, whether such signal molecules can diffuse through healthy cartilage to reach chondrocytes is also unclear, but the participation of chondrocytes in inflammatory destruction of their own matrix, at least in some conditions, seems certain. The further study of these signal molecules as cytokines is necessary for understanding the mechanisms of cartilage destruction. Cartilage matrix could protect chondrocytes from signal recognition; the known presence of protease inhibitors in cartilage could prevent the effector arm of chondrocyte-dependent cartilage degradation. Many potential signal molecules come to mind: interleukin-1, platelet-derived growth factor, and the proliferative activity of interleukin-2. The best-described catabolic signal for cartilage breakdown has been appropriately termed "catabolin."[4,22]

This third and novel mechanism for cartilage destruction, the catabolic activation of chondrocytes by soluble informational molecules of synovial or other origin, is a recent observation that warrants further definition to determine its role in situ in joint diseases of many types. Fell and Jubb, and more recently Saklatvala and Dingle, noted that viable chondrocytes are essential for cartilage breakdown at sites distant from the contact of synovium and that the signal for cartilage breakdown is an acidic molecule or family of molecules produced and released by synovial and other soft tissue cells.[23] A mechanism of cartilage degradation distant from the synovial cell mass is appealing as an explanation for cartilage loss associated with min-

imal degrees of synovitis. Steinberg and Sledge have added another dimension to these observations.[30] They showed that viable cartilage continues to degrade proteoglycan for 8 days following only 1 day of exposure to synovium or to the supernatant of synovial tissue cultures, suggesting that once the catabolic activation of chondrocytes occurs, it continues of its own accord, at least in vitro.[30] Thus, remote stimulation of chondrocyte-dependent cartilage degeneration both in space and in time has been demonstrated in these experiments and suggests the potential for widespread and continued degradative influences of synovitis by the catabolic activation of chondrocytes.[30]

Catabolins have been defined as proteins of molecular weight 15,000 to 25,000 (porcine synovial catabolin = 17,000) daltons produced by soft connective tissues that induce cartilage resorption in vitro. It remains possible that this activity is similar to that of other cytokines such as the monocyte factor, which stimulates synovial cells to secrete collagenase, PGE_2, and collagen, and which is now thought to be similar or identical to interleukin-1 (see Chap. 37). The precise mechanism by which catabolin induces chondrocytes to resorb cartilage has not been demonstrated.[22–24]

The Chondrocyte Effector Arm. The capability of the endogenous chondrocyte to digest its components has been partially characterized (see Chap. 88). Chondrocytes have been shown to synthesize and secrete (1) collagenase, (2) another metalloproteinase of more general specificity, (3) a neutral proteinase with a particular propensity to degrade proteoglycan, and (4) one or more acid cathepsins. This full complement of proteases allows the chondrocyte to degrade cartilage without any assistance from abnormal mechanical stresses or blood or soft tissue-derived inflammatory cells.[5,13,27]

Why there is so little evidence of matrix breakdown by chondrocytes in healthy cartilage is not clear. One factor may well be that the signal for protease secretion is absent. A further protective factor may be the protease inhibitors known to be present in cartilage. These seem to be or more than one type and of broad specificity. It seems likely that these inhibitors must be overcome before matrix degradation can begin. Whatever the balance of biologic activities, the imperturbability of the chondrocyte and the imperviousness of the articular cartilage to vascular influences (angiogenesis, inflammation) are remarkably constant biologic features of articular hyaline cartilage, which effectively support the physical demands placed upon it.

REFERENCES

1. Adams, S.L., et al.: Regulation of the synthesis of extracellular matrix components in chondroblasts transformed by a temperature-sensitive mutant of Rous sarcoma virus. Cell, 30:373, 1982.
2. Benya, P.D., and Shaffer, J.D.: Dedifferentiated chondrocytes reexpress the differentiated collagen phenotype when cultured in agarose gels. Cell, 30:215, 1982.
3. Burgeson, R.E., et al.: Human cartilage collagens. Comparison of cartilage collagens with human type V collagen. J. Biol. Chem., 257:7852, 1982.
4. Dingle, J.T., et al.: A cartilage catabolic factor from synovium. Biochem. J., 184:177, 1979.
5. Ehrlich, M.G., et al.: Collagenase and collagenase inhibitors in osteoarthritic and normal human cartilage. J. Clin. Invest., 59:226, 1977.
6. Elmer, W.A.: Developmental cues in limb bud chondrogenesis. Coll. Rel. Res., 2:257, 1982.
7. Eyre, D.R., et al.: Biosynthesis of collagen and other matrix proteins by articular cartilage in experimental osteoarthrois. Biochem. J., 818:823, 1980.
8. Freeman, M.A.R.: Adult Articular Cartilage. Tunbridge Wells, Kent, England, Pitman Medical Publishing Company, 1979.
9. Furthmayr, H.: Immunochemistry of the extracellular matrix. Vol. I, Methods. Boca Raton, Florida, CRC Press, 1982.
10. Gay, S., et al.: Collagen molecules comprised of α1(V)-chains (B-chains): An apparent localization in the exocytoskeleton. Coll. Rel. Res., 1:53, 1981.
11. Ghadially, F.N.: Fine structures of joints. In The Joints and Synovial Fluid: Fine Structure of Joints. Vol. I. Edited by L. Sokoloff, New York, Academic Press, 1978.
12. Gibon, G.J., et al.: Identification and partial characterization of three low-molecular-weight collagenous polypeptides synthesized by chondrocytes cultured within collagen gels in the absence and in the presence of fibronectin. Biochem. J., 211:417, 1983.
13. Howell, D.S., and Talbott, J.H.: Osteoarthritis symposium. Semin. Arthritis Rheum., XI(Suppl.)1:1, 1981.
14. Krane, S.M., Dayer, J.M., and Goldring, S.R.: Considerations of possible cellular events in the destructive synovial factor of rheumatoid arthritis. Adv. Inflam. Res., 3:1, 1982.
15. Kuettner, K.E., et al.: Synthesis of cartilage matrix by mammalian chondrocytes in vitro. I. Isolation, culture characteristics, and morphology. J. Cell Biol., 93:743, 1982.
16. Kuettner, K.E., et al.: Synthesis of cartilage matrix by mammalian chondrocytes in vitro. II. Maintenance of collagen and proteoglycan phenotype. J. Cell Biol., 93:751, 1982.
17. McCarty, D.: Heberden oration, 1982. Crystals, joints, and consternation. Ann. Rheum Dis., 42:243, 1983.
18. Mankin, H.J.: The response of articular cartilage to mechanical injury. J. Bone Joint Surg., 64A:460, 1982.
19. Meachim, G., and Stockwell, R.A.: The matrix. In Adult Articular Cartilage. Edited by M.A.R. Freeman. Tunbridge Wells, Kent, England, Pitman Medical Publishing Company, 1979.
20. Palmoski, M.J., Colyer, R.A., and Brandt, K.D.: Marked suppression by salicylate of the augmented proteoglycan synthesis in osteoarthritis cartilage. Arthritis Rheum., 23:83, 1980.
21. Roth, V., Mow, V.C., and Grodzinsky, A.J.: Biophysical and electromechanical properties of articular cartilage: In Skeletal Research: An Experimental Approach. Edited by D.J. Simmons, and A.S. Kunin. New York, Academic Press, 1979.
22. Saklatvala, J.: Characterization of catabolin, the major product of pig synovial tissue that induces resorption of cartilage proteoglycan in vitro. Biochem. J., 199:705, 1981.
23. Saklatvala, J., and Dingle, J.T.: Identification of catabolin, a protein from synovium which induces degradation of cartilage in organ culture. Biochem. Biophys. Res. Commun., 96:1225, 1980.
24. Saklatvala, J., Sarsfield, S.J., and Pillsworth, L.M.C.: Characterization of proteins from human synovium and mononuclear leucocytes that induce resorption of cartilage proteoglycan in vitro. Biochem. J., 209:337, 1983.
25. Schwartz, E.R.: Cartilage cells and organ culture. In Skeletal Research: An Experimental Approach. Edited by D.J. Simmons, and A.S. Kunin. New York, Academic Press, 1979.
26. Serafini-Fracassini, A., and Smith, J.W.: The Structure and Biochemistry of Cartilage. Edinburgh and London, Churchill Livingstone, 1974.
27. Silverman, E., et al.: Recognition of a factor in juvenile arthritis synovial fluid which enhances cartilage degradation. Arthritis Rheum., 26:S34, 1983 (abstract).
28. Sokoloff, L.: The Joints and Synovial Fluid, Vol. I. New York, Academic Press, 1978.
29. Steinberg, J.J., Kincaid, S.B., and Sledge, C.B.: Inhibition of cartilage breakdown by hydrocortisone in a tissue culture model of rheumatoid arthritis. Ann. Rheum. Dis., 42:323, 1983.
30. Steinberg, J.J., and Sledge, C.B.: Synovial factor and chondrocyte-mediated breakdown of cartilage: Inhibition by hydrocortisone. J. Orthop. Res., 1:13, 1983.
31. Stockwell, R.A.: Biology of Cartilage Cells. Cambridge, England, Cambridge University Press, 1979.
32. Stockwell, R.A., and Meachim, G.: The chondrocytes. In Adult Articular Cartilage. Edited by M.A.R. Freeman. Tunbridge Wells, Kent, England, Pitman Medical Publishing Company, 1979.

Chapter 15

Immunoglobulins and Their Genes

J. Claude Bennett

An immunoglobulin molecule is a complex entity with two major biologic functions:

1. The recognition of foreign substances (receptor function).
2. The elimination or destruction of these foreign substances (effector function).

This requires that the immune system be designed so that it has the potential to interact with almost an infinite number of antigens. Consequently, it must generate an enormous degree of molecular diversity in order to react with these substances in highly specific ways. Among the whole family of immunoglobulin molecules, by far the most complex heterogeneity is found at the level of structural differences that relate to the specificity of an antibody (idiotype). It is clear that the specificity of all antibodies is determined by differences in the primary structure in the combining region, and this is the major factor responsible for heterogeneity of immunoglobulins. In addition, there are structural differences defining the recognized classes of immunoglobulins, whose existence has been demonstrated in all members of the species (isotype). Both serologic and amino acid sequencing studies have revealed the existence of a limited number of these classes and subclasses of antibodies, which differ from each other in specific structural ways, although they are invariably related. They also each seem to have unique biological properties. Finally, as one would expect, there are subtle yet specific genetic polymorphisms of immunoglobulins, as have been identified for many other families of protein molecules (allotype).

Several general features of the immunoglobulins deserve mention here in the context of our understanding of this system in relation to rheumatologic diseases. First, as will be described in this chapter, the various classes and subclasses of immunoglobulins seem to have special functions that relate to immunologic defense mechanisms. For example, IgA is the major class of immunoglobulin that is present in all external secretions, and is responsible for protecting the mucosal surfaces from the primary attack of exogenous substances. A second general consideration is that either as a result of cross reactivities or alteration of antigens that are presented to the immune system of the host, or

perhaps due to unique genetic rearrangements of immunoglobulin genes, certain sets of clones of cells may produce antibodies that are reactive with self-constituents. Such aberrations in the immune response are most often encountered in rheumatoid arthritis, in SLE, and in related disorders. One would assume, as is discussed in other chapters of this text, that these immunologic reactions play a significant role in the pathogenesis of some of the manifestations of these diseases.

STRUCTURE OF AN ANTIBODY MOLECULE

The basic structure of all immunoglobulins is the same. Immunoglobulins are made of two types of polypeptide chains (Fig. 15–1). The larger one is called the heavy (H) chain. The other, because it is smaller, is known as the light (L) chain. Each immunoglobulin subunit consists of two identical H and two L chains, which are generally held together by disulfide bonds, and hence the molecular formula is H_2L_2.[10–12] The disulfide bonds joining the H and L chains connect the carboxy termini of the light chains to the heavy chains. The interheavy chain disulfide bridges vary in number from 1 to 11 for the different classes and subclasses, and are generally located in the center of the H chain in a region known as the "hinge," which is unusually rich in cysteine and proline. The molecular weight of the light chain is about 25,000; that of the heavy chain varies between 55,000 and 65,000 daltons. The differences in size are related to differences in the structure of the "hinge," i.e., in the γ3 subclass of IgG, or to the presence of an extra domain in the μ and ϵ heavy chains.[31] Each polypeptide chain can be divided into a series of globular subunits or domains, each of which is about 110 residues in length and characterized by a highly conserved intrachain disulfide bridge, which spans about 60 residues and makes the domain compact.[9] The domains are separated by more extended regions known as the interdomain stretches. Based on amino acid sequence studies showing a high degree of homology between different domains, it would appear that they are the result of a series of gene duplications. In those classes, and in subclasses where functional localization of various biologic

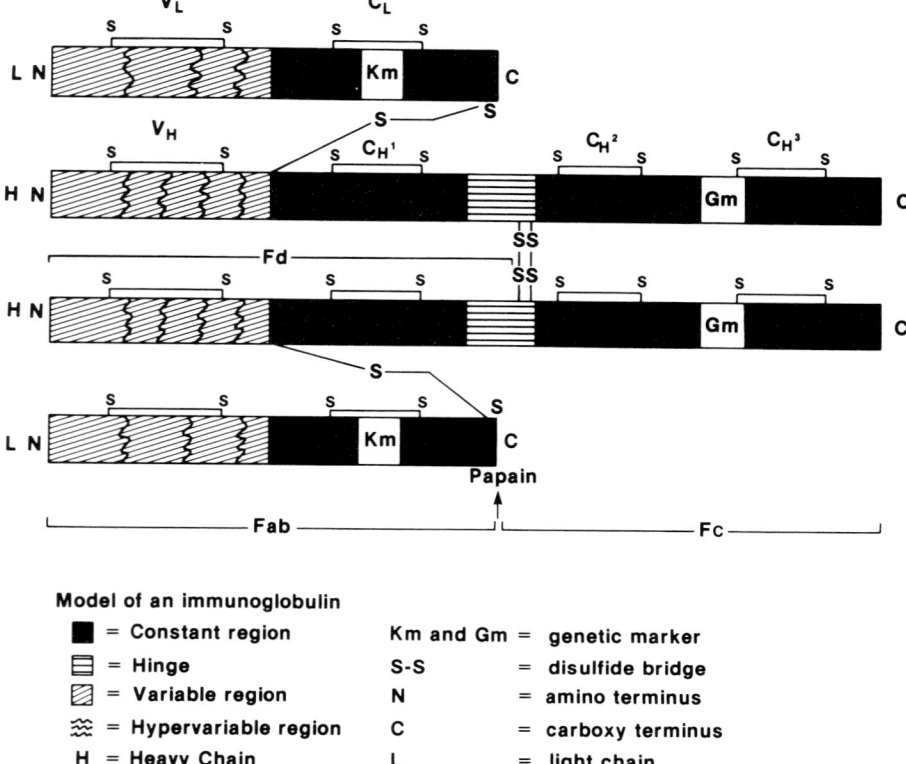

Fig. 15–1. Basic model of the immunoglobulin molecule structure. See text for description.

properties has been achieved, it seems that the different domains may have evolved to serve different biologic functions.[43]

Comparison of the amino acid sequences of a large number of homogeneous immunoglobulins has documented that each of the chains can be divided structurally and functionally into two major regions. One of these, the amino terminal 110–120 residues, is known as the variable (V) region because of the amino acid sequence variation among different myeloma proteins and antibodies belonging to a given class.[16] The remaining half of the L chain and three-quarters of the H chain are known as the constant regions (C) because their structure is virtually the same for all molecules belonging to a single immunoglobulin class or subclass.

Abundant structural, functional, and x-ray diffraction evidence now supports the concept that the variable regions are directly involved in the antigen-binding sites of the molecule and that the sites are composed of one or more "hypervariable regions," which in the three-dimensional structure of the molecules are in close proximity and thus able to react with the antigen.[6] There are three hypervariable regions in the light chains and four in the heavy chains which, though far separated in

the linear sequence, are in close proximity in the fully folded molecule. It would appear from immunologic analyses that the hypervariable regions are intimately involved in the idiotypic determinants of the antibody, and that antibodies with the same specificity commonly have similar if not identical hypervariable regions.[2] Spanning the remainder of the variable segments are the so-called framework regions, which show less variability among different molecules and contribute to the variable region subclass specificity. Numerous amino acid sequence studies of myeloma proteins and Bence Jones proteins have revealed the existence of subclasses of V regions for λ and κ chains, and at least three H chain variable region subclasses, which are found in all general classes and subclasses of heavy chains.[19] The antigen-binding sites (there is one per H-L pair) are located at the tip of the molecule and consist of both the H and L chain; however, in most antibodies studied to date, the H chain plays a greater role in determining the specificity of the antibody than does the L chain.[6]

The constant region consists of either three or four domains and, in most classes, it also contains the interdomain or hinge region in the center of the molecule. Comparison of the structure of the constant regions of different classes and subclasses of H chains shows striking homologies among many of them.[27] In the case of the four subclasses of IgG, this homology is greater than 95%. The structural features of the C regions seem to determine those biologic functions that distinguish different classes and subclasses of immunoglobulins from each other and to influence the localization and sites of action of all immunoglobulins. Thus, the C_H2 domain seems to be important in most subclasses in complement fixation and in regulating the catabolic properties of an antibody, while the C_H3 domain is important in the interaction of immunoglobulins with receptors on many cells, including monocytes, polymorphonuclears, lymphocytes, and endothelial cells. Obviously, these interactions with a variety of cells are important in initiating the process of phagocytosis, in allowing certain subclasses to traverse the placenta, and in profoundly influencing many of the biologic functions of lymphocytes, platelets, and other cells. The antigenic determinants reactive with rheumatoid factors seem to be located in more than one domain.[39]

Although the H and L chains are the true structural subunits of immunoglobulins, a simple way of obtaining biologically active fragments with differing biologic properties is by proteolytic digestion, which occurs preferentially at the hinge region.[13] The products obtained differ for different enzymes. Thus, papain yields an Fc and two Fab fragments, while pepsin degrades the Fc fragment and yields the two Fab fragments still joined by a disulfide bridge—(Fab')2. Other enzymes, or these enzymes under slightly different conditions, yield different types of fragments that have proved to be equally useful in dissecting the biologic functions of the molecule. These proteolytic fragments, which generally include one or more intact domains, have provided us with a great deal of useful biologic information, since the Fab fragments composed of the light chain and Fd fragment (see Fig. 15–1) can combine with antigen while the Fc fragment can be used to study the secondary biologic properties of immunoglobulins.

CLASSES AND SUBCLASSES

Although the basic structure of all antibody molecules is similar, there exists in all species of animals studied to date a series of immunoglobulin classes and subclasses (Fig. 15–2). They appear to have evolved from each other, but differ in the structure and, consequently, the function of the constant domains of the heavy chains. These are all under control of a series of closely linked genes, as will be discussed later. In a broad sense one can regard the classes and subclasses in a similar man-

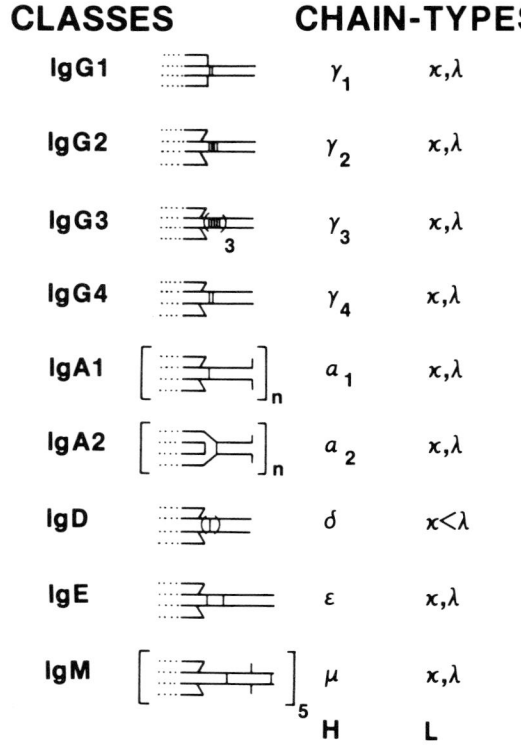

Fig. 15–2. Basic subunit diagrams of the various immunoglobulin classes depicting their disulfide bonding patterns and, in the case of IgA$_1$, IgA$_2$, and IgM, indicating that they may exist as polymeric structures. See text for further description. (Redrawn from Hilschmann, N., et al.: Naturwissenschaften, *65*:617, 1978.)

ner. For example, IgG$_{1,2,3,4}$ all have the same basic structural design differing only in the primary sequence of their constant regions and the location of their interchain disulfide bonds. The H chain in each of these subclasses is referred to as $\gamma_{1,2}$ and so forth. The L chain may be of either the κ or the λ type. IgA exists as two subclasses, with H chain designations as α_1 and α_2, respectively, and again the light chains may either be of the κ or λ type. IgD and IgE have H chains designated δ and ε, respectively, and in the case of IgM, which exists as a pentamer, the H chain is termed μ. Again, in all classes, the L chain may either be κ or λ. Furthermore, additional polypeptide chains are found in those classes in which molecules exist as polymers. One such chain, the J chain, is present in both IgAs and IgMs when they are in the polymeric state.[26] This 15,000-dalton molecule appears to be important in initiating the disulfide bonded polymer formation.[21] In the case of IgA, a 70,000-dalton secretory component binds to the molecule and is present only in the external secretions. It seems to be important in playing a receptor-like role for IgA, in allowing the secretory event to take place, and possibly in protecting the polymers against proteolysis.[40] Table 15–1 lists the five major classes of immunoglobulins in man and describes some of their physical, chemical, and biologic features. Table 15–2 treats the four subclasses of IgG and the two of IgA in a similar fashion.

IgG. IgG is the major immunoglobulin class that provides the bulk of antibody activity in response to most antigens. Most IgG molecules are avid in reacting with complement and in initiating the enzymatic cascade consequent to complement fixation. However, IgG_1 and IgG_3 are most effective. IgG_4 does not fix complement effectively in the native state, but has been reported to do so after proteolytic cleavage. Studies with various types of fragments suggest that complement fixation is a property of the C_H2 domain. There are some differences in the ability of different subclasses to interact with receptors on the surface of polymorphonuclear leukocytes, monocytes, and lymphocytes. As a consequence, IgG_1 and IgG_3 are most active in opsonization by polymorphonuclear leukocytes and monocytes and participate most effectively in the phenomenon of antibody-mediated cytotoxicity. The Fc fragments of all four subclasses of IgG can interact with rheumatoid factors. Howeve, IgG_1 and IgG_3 tend to do so more effectively. The structural and genetic studies[28] clearly indicate that the subclasses and classes of IgG are under separate genetic control.

IgM. The biologic and clinical significance of this class of immunoglobulin was initially appreciated when it was recognized that rheumatoid factors present in serum are generally macroglobulins with antibody activity to IgG. However, in the last 20 years, its significance in many other areas of the immune response has been fully established. IgM exists in two forms. One is the basic subunit, the 8S 180,000 dalton IgM with a molecular formula μ_2L_2.[32] This is a minor fraction in serum, but appears to be the major component on lymphocyte surfaces.[24] The other and major form is the 19S, 900,000-dalton pentameric IgM $(\mu_2L_2)5J$, in which five subunits are disulfide bridged and generally contain one molecule of J chain, which joins two of the subunits by a disulfide bridge.[21] IgM is the predominant immunoglobulin in many primary immune responses and can, at times, as in the case of rheumatoid factors, cold agglutinins, and isoagglutinins, remain the major or sole antibody for long periods of time.[14,42] It differs from most other immunoglobulins in having a heavy chain that is larger owing to the presence of an extra domain. IgM is avid in complement fixation, and studies suggest that this property resides in the $C\mu4$ domain.[17] As is the case for all immunoglobulins, the valence of the μ_2L_2 subunit is two. Because it consists of five subunits, IgM has ten combining sites for small antigens, but because of steric factors, half the sites appear to be blocked when IgM reacts with large protein antigens. As a consequence, the valence for large antigens is five, and rheumatoid factor exists in serum in the form of a 22S complex $(\mu_2L_2)5\text{-}(IgG)5$.[14]

IgA. Second in concentration to IgG in serum is the IgA fraction, which generally exists in the form of a monomer (α_2L_2), but on occasion, especially in patients with myeloma, as a polymer $(\alpha_2L_2)2,3\text{-}J$. Although in serum there appears to be no particular function for IgA, it plays a major role in the so-called secretory immune system.[30,37] The secretory IgA has several unique features. First, it is synthesized largely by plasma cells located in, or originating from, the lymphoid tissues in the intestinal tract. In the secretions, the molecule usually exists in the form of a polymer linked to another molecule, the 70,000-dalton secretory component (SC), which is synthesized by the epithelial cells lining the gut.[30] The function of the SC remains uncertain. On the one hand, it appears to serve as a receptor for IgA[5] and thus may play a role in attracting IgA-bearing lymphocytes to the gut and other organs of secretion, or IgA to the

Table 15–1. Selected Properties of Immunoglobulin Classes

	IgG	IgA	IgM	IgD	IgE
Molecular weight	160,000	170,000 or polymer	900,000	160,000	180,000
Sedimentation constant	7S	7S (9, 11, 13)	19S	7S	8S
Approx. concentration serum (mg%)	1000–1500	250–300	100–150	.3–30	.0015–.2
Valance	2	2 (monomer)	10	2	2
Molecular formula	γ_2L_2	$(\alpha_2L_2)_n$	$(\mu_2L_2)_5$	δ_2L_2	ϵ_2L_2
Half-life (days)	23	6	5	3	2.5
Special property	Placental passage	Secretory Ig	Primary response Lymphocyte surface	Lymphocyte surface	Reagin

Table 15–2.   Selected Biologic Properties of Classes and Subclasses of Immunoglobulins

	IgG				IgA		IgM	IgD	IgE
	1	*2*	*3*	*4*	*1*	*2*			
% of Total	65	20	10	5	90	10			
Major genetic factors	Gm a, f, z	n	b, g	4 a, b	A₁m	A₂m			
Complement fixation	+ +	+	+ +	–	–	–	+ +	–	–
Complement fixation (alternative)					+	+		±	±
Placental pasage	+	+	+	+	–	–	–	–	–
Fix to mast cells or basophils	–	–	–	–	–	–	–	–	+
Bind to:									
—Macrophages	+	±	+	±	–	–	–	–	–
—Polys	+	+	+	+	+	+	–	–	–
—Platelets	+	+	+	+	–	–	–	–	–
—Lymphocytes	+	+	+	+	–	–	+	–	–
Reaction with Staph A	+	+	–	+	–	–	–	–	–
Half-life (days)	23	23	8–9	23	6	6	5	3	2.5
Synthesis mg/kg/day	25	?	3.5	?	24	?	7	.4	.02

surface of the epithelial cells within which the molecule combines to the secretory component. A second function may be to make the secretory IgA complex more resistant to proteolytic digestion since several in vitro studies have shown that the complex is more resistant to degradation than the IgA without secretory component.[4] The observation that several bacterial enzymes digest IgA₁ and not IgA₂ in the hinge region[29] may explain why IgA₂ is relatively more abundant in external secretions than in the serum, where it makes up a minor fraction of IgA.

The importance of this immune system in the host defense cannot be overestimated. Most infectious agents enter via the gastrointestinal and respiratory tracts and initiate a local immune response involving, primarily, the IgA fraction. Consequently, as was demonstrated in the polio vaccination program, oral vaccinations in general may prove to be more effective than those by the systemic route. It seems likely that this local immune system plays a major role also in the genitourinary, lacrimal, salivary, and respiratory systems, and that it may be the primary defense against a variety of environmental pathogens, even though IgA is less able to activate the complement system or to initiate phagocytosis.

IgD. IgD is a minor immunoglobulin and, even though some serum antibodies have been identified in this class in man, it appears to serve no unusual function and is absent from the serum of mice and primates. Its primary role in man and all these species appears to be to function as one of the two major surface receptors on B lymphocytes together with monomeric IgM.[41] Although it seems likely that the interaction of these surface molecules with

antigen is necessary to trigger and perhaps also to suppress lymphoid function, there are no data available to define a distinct biologic function in this regard for either of these two surface antigen recognition units. Free IgD differs from the other immunoglobulins in being unusually susceptible to digestion by a variety of proteolytic enzymes.[35]

IgE. The distribution of IgE is largely extravascular, and its turnover is rapid with a half time of about two days. The major type of antibody associated with IgE is the reaginic antibody that plays a role in a variety of allergic conditions. Through their interaction with receptors on mast cells and basophils, the IgE reaginic antibodies, in the presence of antigens, cause the release of histamine and various other vasoactive substances, which are responsible for the clinical manifestations of various allergic states.[18] IgE antibodies may play a protective role in numerous parasitic infections, perhaps by increasing vascular permeability, thus permitting other types of antibodies to be active.

Immunoglobulin Gene Organization. As has been discussed in earlier sections of this chapter, pairs of light and heavy chains fold into discrete structural V region domains that bind the antigens. These domains consist of approximately 107 amino acids from a light chain and approximately 125 amino acids from a heavy chain. Within the V region domain three short polypeptide loops (hypervariable regions) from each of the heavy and the light chains form the antigen-binding sites. This extraordinary degree of variability defined within the V regions gives rise to the idiotypes.

Extensive amino acid sequence determination on various myeloma proteins, both from man and from mouse, led to an appreciation that the heavy chains and the two types of light chains, kappa and lambda, are each encoded by a separate multigene family. The extraordinary variability of the V region of a single immunoglobulin polypeptide chain in conjunction with a nearly invariant constant region gave rise to the concept that the functionally distinct V and C regions of these polypeptides are encoded by independent genetic elements within each gene family.[8] That is, more than one gene is required to encode a single polypeptide chain.

The development of the technology for recombinant DNA led to the ability to clone immunoglobulin genes and to develop extensive libraries of gene fragments that could be used to determine the molecular organization of immunoglobulin genes.[7,22,33,36] The initial studies of the light chains confirmed the prediction, and showed a large separation between the V and C regions.[35] As shown in Figure 15–3, embryonic DNA contained gene elements coding for the leader sequence, a V region gene separated by over 3 kilobases from a C region gene, and an interspersed J region gene, which accounted for residues 98 through 110. In the proc-

ess of message formation, the V and J regions were linked together through a deletion of the intervening sequence.[3] In the case of a myeloma cell, there was already some juxtaposition in which the V-J joining had occurred, but the C sequences were still at some distance. This was faithfully transcribed in the primary RNA, and additional splicing occurred before a mature messenger was produced. This finding agreed with the two gene/one polypeptide hypothesis, i.e., V and C sequences are encoded separately in the germ line and are rearranged to form an active V-C gene in antibody-producing cells.[8] The coding regions are referred to as *exons* and the intervening sequences as *introns*.

In the case of the V kappa sequences, which have a minimum of perhaps 300 different groups, it seems that a library of possible V kappa genes exists from which selected sequences undergo combination with one of the four J_κ regions. This would provide a mechanism for the generation of considerable diversity, since J_κ segments are not restricted to any one V_κ group. Such V-J joining might occur through a mechanism of inverted palindrome read-

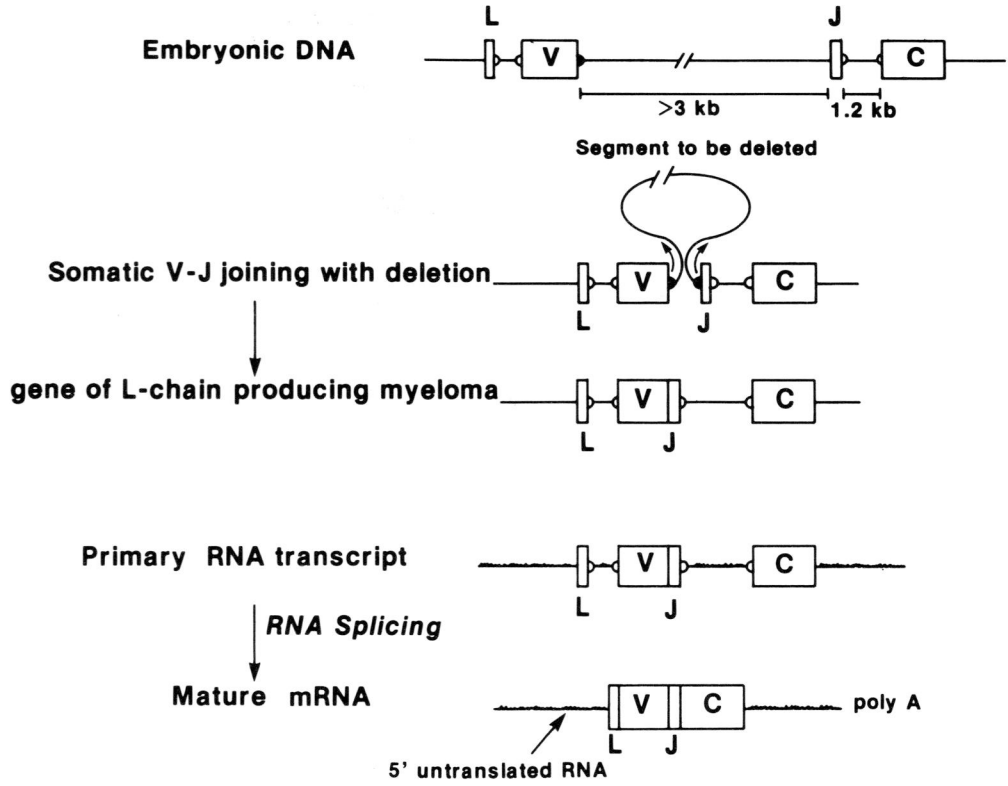

Fig. 15–3. Genetic events involved in gene segment organization and messenger RNA splicing during the development of an immunoglobulin-secreting cell line. (L = leader sequence; V = variable region; J = joining region; C = constant region of the genome.) See text for further description.

ing. It is also evident from the way in which the jointing occurs that sequence variation may be seen at the point of a junction. This would explain the exceptional variability at position 96 that has been observed in the mouse kappa chains.[23,25]

The heavy chain genes are developed in a similar way with the provisions for the immunoglobulin class switching that occurs during ontogeny.[20] In this situation, the various constant region areas related to each class or subclass can be spliced to a given V region through a switching recognition point. This event is shown in its simplest form in Figure 15–4. The actual picture, relative to the constant regions, is a bit more complex. From what we know about the globular domains of the immunoglobulin C regions, and what we have already learned about genes existing in fragments, we should not be surprised to see that the C genes exist with the CH_1 domain separated from the hinge region domain, separated from a CH_2 domain, separated from a CH_3 domain,[1] as shown in Figure 15–5. Such a separation of the domains, requiring splicing before the final message is read, explains how certain of the heavy chain diseases may develop.[15]

Furthermore, the total variable region is a bit more complex for the heavy chains, involving the splicing together of three segments (V, D, and J) rather than two as occurs in the light chain. The new area in heavy chain genes is called D because

it may be viewed as a diversity generating segment[7,33] (Fig. 15–6).

As can be seen in this joining scheme, a single V_H region is drawn from the V library, a single D is drawn from the D library, and a single J from the J library, all of which are then spliced together. Perhaps through a recognition mechanism, suggested by rather consistent intervening sequences, appropriate joining takes place. Thus, the whole pattern for differentiation of immunoglobulin heavy chains involves the joining of V, D, and J segments, plus the necessary switching of S segments that are homologous to each other and that identify recognition sets for splicing in the various C genes. If the heavy chain gene family had 200 V, 12 D, and 4 J gene segments, 9.6×10^3 V_H genes $(200 \times 12 \times 4)$ could be generated by combinatorial joining.[38] Similarly, class-specific switching may allow one V_H gene to be associated with eight different C_H genes, permitting distinct effector functions to be employed. Four sources for the generation of somatic diversity may be seen: (1) combinatorial diversity, by combining the various gene segments; (2) junctional site diversity at the V_L-J_L, V_H-D, and D-J_H junctions, due to imprecise joining; (3) junctional insertion diversity where several nucleotides are inserted without template direction; and (4) somatic mutational events, especially near the junctional areas. Obviously, mechanisms 2, 3, and 4 greatly amplify the poten-

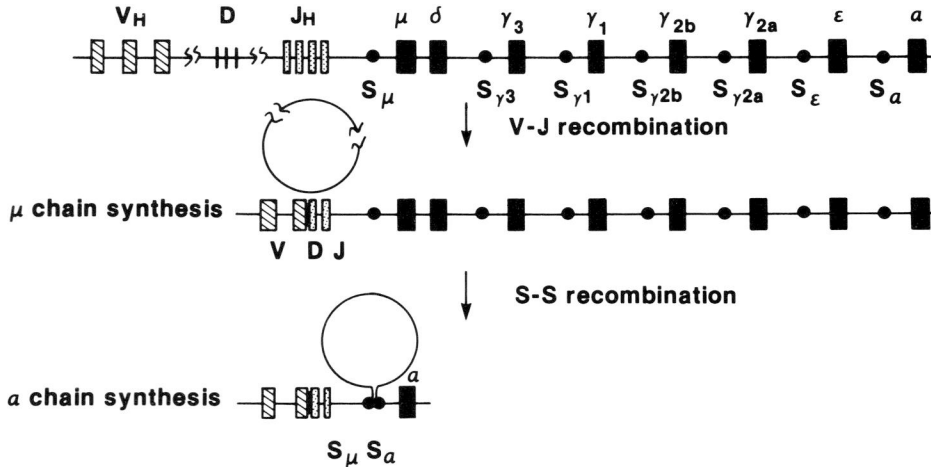

Fig. 15–4. Immunoglobulin H chain class switching in the mouse. The molecular events involved in switching from expression of one class of immunoglobulin to another are depicted, showing first the gene organization during μ chain synthesis. In the second situation is shown a switch region recombination event resulting in a deletion of all the DNA up to the α gene necessary for ultimate expression of the α polypeptide chain. (Adapted from Honjo, H.: Ann. Rev. Immunol., *1*:515, 1983.)

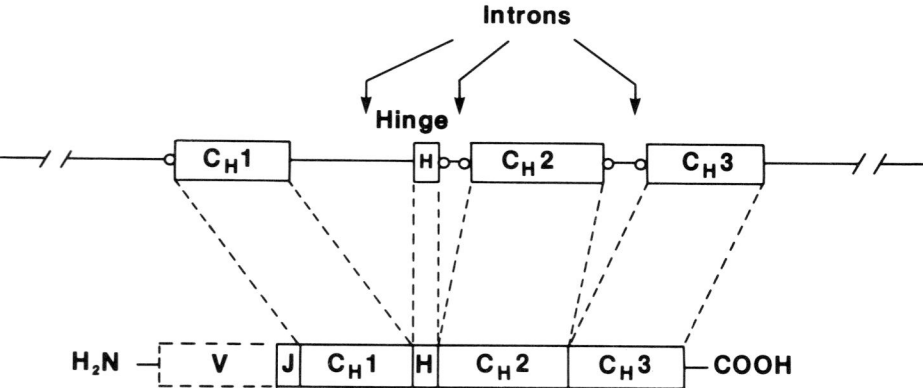

Fig. 15–5.   Molecular events involved in gene segment splicing for the constant region domains of the heavy chain. See text for further description.

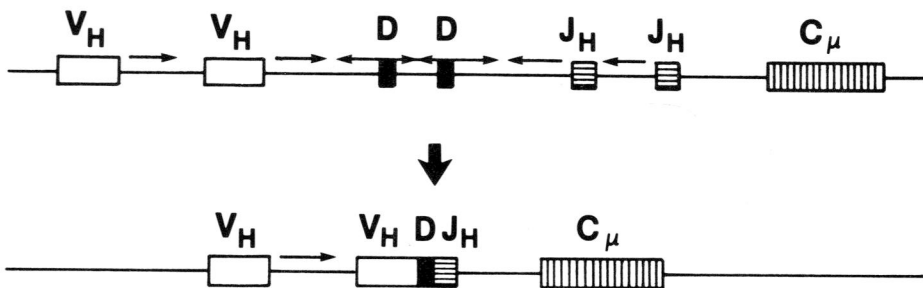

Fig. 15–6.   Gene segment joining mechanisms generate diversity within the V region of the heavy chains. Shown is a combination of events selecting out V, D, and J regions of the heavy chain.

tial diversity implied in the combinatorial calculations.

CLINICAL SIGNIFICANCE

Although one must be careful not to overutilize and overemphasize technical assays in clinical situations where they are interesting but not very useful, one must not overlook the importance of the immune system in analyzing the clinical status of the patients with rheumatic diseases. Clearly, evaluation of autoantibodies, and particularly the clonal repertoire of response in disease states, is likely to be of increasing importance at not only the fundamental level but also the applied clinical level as well. The real significance for understanding the immunoglobulins as they relate to rheumatic diseases, however, stems from the knowledge it has given us of the immune system, its regulation, its genetic organization, and the new avenues of approach it has provided us to define ways in which perturbations of this system take place. Only through these new approaches can we ever hope to modify in a predetermined and clinically effective way such perturbations. Additionally, studies of immunoglobulin genes have provided an excit-

ing new avenue for the study of somatic cell differentiation and molecular diversity in general. As we come to understand the ways in which all these mechanisms are regulated at the molecular level, only then will we be able to apply the appropriate tools to reverse an immunologic disease process and bring it under control.

REFERENCES

1. Adams, J.M., et al.: Organization and expression of murine immunoglobulin genes. Immunol. Rev., *59*:5–14, 1981.
2. Brient, B.W., and Nisonoff, A.: Quantitative investigations of idiotypic antibodies. IV. Inhibition by specific haptens of the reaction of anti-haptin antibody with its anti-idiotypic antibody. J. Exp. Med., *132*:951–962, 1970.
3. Brock, C., et al.: A complete immunoglobulin gene is created by somatic recombination. Cell, *15*:1–14, 1978.
4. Brown, W.R., Newcomb, R.W., and Ishizaka, K.: Proteolytic degradation of exocrine and serum immunoglobulins. J. Clin. Invest., *49*:1374–1380, 1970.
5. Crago, S.S., Kulhavy, R., Prince, S.J., and Mestecky, J.: Secretory component on epithelial cells is a surface receptor for polymeric immunoglobulin. J. Exp. Med., *147*:1832–1837, 1978.
6. Davie, D.R., and Metzger, H.: Structural basis of antibody function. Annu. Rev. Immunol., *1*:87–117, 1983.
7. Davis, M.M., et al.: An immunoglobulin heavy chain gene is formed by at least two recombinational events. Nature, *283*:733–739, 1980.
8. Dreyer, W.J., and Bennett, J.C.: The molecular basis of

antibody formation: A paradox. Proc. Natl. Acad. Sci. U.S.A., *54*:864–869, 1965.

9. Edelman, G.W.: The covalent structure of a human γG-immunoglobulin. XI. Functional implication. Biochemistry, *9*:3197–3205, 1970.

10. Edelman, G.M.: Antibody structure and molecular immunology. Science, *180*:830–840, 1973.

11. Feinstein, D., and Franklin, E.C.: Two antigenically distinguishable subclasses of human A myeloma proteins differing in their heavy chains. Nature, *121*:1496–1498, 1966.

12. Fleishman, J.B., Pain, R.H., and Porter, R.R.: Reduction of γ-globulins, Arch. Biochem. (Suppl.), *I*:174–180, 1962.

13. Franklin, E.C., and Frangione, B.: Structural variants of human immunoglobulin. *In* Contemporary Topics in Molecular Immunology. Edited by F.P. Inman, and W.J. Mandy. New York, Plenum Publishing Corp., 1975, pp. 89–126.

14. Franklin, E.C., et al.: An unusual protein component of high molecular weight in the serum of certain patients with rheumatoid arthritis. J. Exp. Med., *105*:425–438, 1957.

15. Franzione, B., and Franklin, E.C.: Heavy chain diseases: Clinical features and molecular significance of the disordered immunoglobulin structure. Semin. Hematol., *10*:53–64, 1973.

16. Hilschmann, N., and Craig, L.: Amino acid sequence studies with Benca-Jones proteins. Proc. Natl. Acad. Sci. U.S.A., *53*:1403–1409, 1965.

17. Hurst, M., et al.: The structural basis for binding of complement by immunoglobulin M. J. Exp. Med., *140*:1117–1121, 1974.

18. Ishizaka, K., Ishizaka, T., and Lee, E.N.: Biologic function of the Fc fragments of E myeloma protein. Immunochemistry, *7*:687–702, 1970.

19. Kabat, E.A., Wu, T.T., and Bilofsky, H.: Variable regions of immunoglobulin chains. NIH Publ. #80–2008, 1979.

20. Kataoka, T., Miyata, T., and Honjo, T.: Repetitive sequences in class-switch recombination regions of immunoglobulin heavy chain genes. Cell, *23*:357–368, 1981.

21. Koshland, M.E.: Structure and function of the J chain. *In* Advances in Immunology. Edited by F. Dixon, and H.G. Kunkel. New York, Academic Press, 1975, pp. 41–69.

22. Leder, P.: Mechanisms of gene evolution. J.A.M.A., *248*:1582–1591, 1982.

23. Leder, P.: The genetics of antibody diversity. Sci. Am., *246*:102–115, 1982.

24. Marchalonis, J.J., Cone, R.E., and Atwell, J.L.: Isolation and partial characterization of lymphocyte surface immunoglobulins. J. Exp. Med., *135*:956–971, 1972.

25. Max, E.E., Seidman, J.B., and Leder, P.: Sequences of five potential recombination sites enclosed close to an immunoglobulin κ constant region. Proc. Natl. Acad. Sci. U.S.A., *76*:3450–3454, 1979.

26. Mestecky, J., Zikan, J., and Butler, W.T.: Immunoglobulin M and secretory immunoglobulin A: Presence of a common polypeptide chain different from light chains. Science, *171*:1163–1165, 1971.

27. Milstein, C., and Pink, J.R.L.: Structure and evolution of immunoglobulins. Prog. Biophys. Mol. Biol., *21*:211–263, 1970.

28. Natvig, J.B., and Kunkel, H.G.: Human immunoglobulins: Classes, subclasses, genetic variants, and idiotypes. Adv. Immunol., *16*:1–59, 1973.

29. Plaut, A.G., et al.: Neisseria gonorrhoeae and Neisseria meningitidis: Extracellular enzyme cleaves human immunoglobulin A. Science, *190*:1103–1105, 1975.

30. Poger, M.E., and Lamm, M.E.: Localization of free and bound secretory component in human intestinal epithelial cells: A model for the assembly of secretory IgA. J. Exp. Med., *139*:629–642, 1974.

31. Putnam, F.W., et al.: Complete amino acid sequence of the Mu heavy chain of a human IgM immunoglobulin. Science, *182*:287–291, 1973.

32. Rothfield, N., Frangione, B., and Franklin, E.C.: Slowly sedimenting mercaptoethanol-resistant antinuclear factors related antigenically to M immunoglobulins (γ_{1M}-globulin) in patients with systemic lupus erythematosus. J. Clin. Invest., *44*:62–72, 1965.

33. Sabano, H., et al.: Identification and nucleotide sequence of a diversity DNA segment (D) of immunoglobulin heavy-chain genes. Nature, *290*:562–570, 1981.

34. Seidman, J.G., and Leder, P.: The arrangement and rearrangement of antibody genes. Nature, *276*:790–795, 1978.

35. Spiegelberg, H.L.: NH_2-terminal amino acid sequence of the Fc fragment of IgD resembles IgE and IgG sequences. Nature, *254*:723–725, 1975.

36. Takahashi, N., et al.: Structure of human immunoglobulin gamma genes: Implications for evolution of a gene family. Cell, *29*:671–679, 1982.

37. Tomasi, T.B., et al.: Characteristics of an immune system common to certain external secretions. J. Exp. Med., *121*:101–123, 1965.

38. Tonegawa, S.: Somatic generation of antibody diversity. Nature, *302*:575–581, 1983.

39. Turner, M.W., et al.: Genetic (Gm) antigens associated with subfragments from the Fc fragment of human immunoglobulin G. Nature, *221*:1166–1169, 1969.

40. Underdown, B.J., and Dorrington, K.J.: Studies on the structural and confirmational basis for the relative resistance of serum and secretory immunoglobulin A to proteolysis. J. Immunol., *112*:949–959, 1974.

41. Vitetta, E., and Uhr, J.: Immunoglobulin-receptors revisited. Science, *189*:964–969, 1975.

42. Williams, R.C., Kunkel, H.G., and Capra, J.D.: Antigenic specificities related to the cold agglutinin activity of gamma M globulins. Science, *161*:379–381, 1968.

43. Yasmeen, D., et al.: The structure and function of immunoglobulin domains. IV. The distribution of some effector functions among the $C_\gamma 2$ and $C_\gamma 3$ homology regions of human immunoglobulin G[1]. J. Immunol., *116*:518–526, 1976.

Chapter 16

Structure and Function of Monocytes and Macrophages

Ralph Snyderman

The human immune system has evolved the capability of performing a number of vital protective functions, including defending against microbial dissemination, resisting the development of neoplasms, and removing denatured substances and nonvital tissues. Efficiency in the elimination of substances by the immune system depends upon its ability to identify what is to be destroyed, and to rapidly eliminate the identified agent. The immune system has unique features that permit the mediation of surveillance and the removal of "unwanted" materials. In addition to fixed structures, such as the thymus, spleen, lymph nodes, and bone marrow, the immune system is comprised of motile cells that are able to localize rapidly at virtually any site within the host. For example, billions of leukocytes accumulate at sites of bacterial invasion within hours after their penetration into tissues. The immune system is also the only tissue that has the potential to destroy other components of the host. The destructive potential of the immune system is a necessary factor in its host protective function, but is also responsible for the tissue destruction common to most rheumatic disorders.

Conceptually, the immune system can be divided into three functional units that mediate recognition, recruitment (amplification), and effector functions. The interaction of foreign or denatured substances with either nonspecific or specific recognition components of the immune system results in the generation of inflammatory mediators that then recruit and activate effector cells. Amplification systems are the source mediators, termed "phlogistic" agents, which alter vascular permeability, enhance local blood flow, and stimulate the egress, chemoattratcion, and activation of effector cells that destroy the inciting agent.[198]

The macrophage is central to recognition, amplification, and effector functions of the immune system. Since the seminal observations of Eli Metchnikoff in the late nineteenth century, the phagocytic nature of macrophages has been recognized as an important component of host defense against infection.[152,204,238,240] Macrophages are wandering phagocytes that contain a broad repertoire of intracellular degradative and oxidative enzymes. Both polymorphonuclear leukocytes and macrophages have chemotactic, phagocytic, antibacterial, and secretory capabilities. Unlike the polymorphonuclear leukocytes, however, macrophages play a crucial role in immunoregulation, have the ability to further differentiate (become activated), and often are the first components of the immune system to encounter an antigen. The nature of the interaction of macrophages with an antigen may subsequently determine the immunogenicity of the antigen or its ability to induce tolerance.[180,182] Processing of antigen by macrophages is obligate for most subsequent lymphocyte responses. Lymphocytes and their secretory products, called *lymphokines,* may augment macrophage egress to inflammatory sites, enhance effector functions, or regulate macrophage functions in other ways. In turn, macrophages produce cytokines, termed *monokines,* which affect other cell types, and as part of their comprehensive secretory capabilities, may modulate their own function in inflammatory foci.

Macrophages are thus essential for the initiation and execution of nearly all immune processes. Macrophage differentiation and its roles as an effector, immune accessory, and secretory cell are reviewed here with emphasis on relevance to the rheumatic diseases.

STRUCTURE AND DEVELOPMENT OF MONONUCLEAR PHAGOCYTE SYSTEM

The mononuclear phagocyte system consists of a group of cells, located in different tissues throughout the body, which share a common stem cell origin in the bone marrow as well as certain functional and cytochemical characteristics.[239,240] In the blood, the cells are termed monocytes, whereas once they have migrated into tissues, they are called macrophages. The term mononuclear phagocyte is inclusive of all the cells in this lineage. The mononuclear phagocyte system is a vital component of the immune system in that it is the source of fixed tissue macrophages of the reticuloendothelial system as well as wandering phagocytic cells. The single most important characteristic of the mononuclear phagocyte is its ability to phagocytize and digest other substances, particularly substances coated (opsonized) by antibody. Mononuclear phagocytes are also capable of differentiating into cells with altered functional properties depending on the environmental stimuli. As such, the mononuclear phagocyte system is admirably suited to its role as the primary effector in numerous host defensive situations.

General Characteristics of the Mononuclear Phagocyte System. Cells of the mononuclear phagocyte system share several important characteristics even though the cells acquire tremendous biochemical and functional diversity depending on their tissue locus.[241,244] Morphologic features, such as low nuclear/cytoplasmic ratios, bilobed nuclei, and membrane ruffling are features evident at the light and electron microscopic level. Enzymatic features of macrophages that can be demonstrated cytochemically or enzymatically include the presence of nonspecific esterase, peroxidase, (depends on the state of differentiation), lysozyme, 5′nucleotidase, and aminopeptidase.[105,106,141] Membrane characteristics of macrophages include the presence of receptors for chemotactic factors, Fc, C3b, certain sugars, as well as a variety of macrophage-specific antigenic determinants (see section on macrophage surface antigens). The morphology of cells in the mononuclear phagocyte system is variable, and is determined by the state of maturation, degree of differentiation, or content of ingested material. All macrophages share the ability to phagocytize particles and to adhere to charged surfaces. The cytotoxic and microbicidal capacities of macrophages are highly variable and relate to their state of activation[154] (see section on macrophage activation).

In different tissues, macrophages acquire certain distinct structural and metabolic properties. For example, alveolar macrophages develop a high oxidative metabolic capacity, whereas splenic and peritoneal macrophages remain primarily dependent on anaerobic glycolysis.[21] Structurally, the macrophages that egress into tissues or into inflammatory sties as single cells may form granulomas and can develop into sheets of epithelioid cells, or they may fuse to become multinucleated giant cells, or differentiate into osteoclasts.[58] Most data regarding the development of the mononuclear phagocyte system have been derived from the study of murine, guinea pig, rat, or human species. The macrophages studied have been blood monocytes, the resident peritoneal or alveolar macrophages, or macrophages called to an inflammatory site by phlogistic agents (elicited macrophages). The development of continuous cell lines with macrophage characteristics has allowed the further study

of macrophage origins, differentiation, and functional development.[1,109,115,171,173]

Origin of Mononuclear Phagocyte System. The earliest components of the mononuclear phagocyte system can be identified in the bone marrow. Primitive stem cells are called colony-forming units (CFUs), and those committed to the granulocyte/monocyte line are termed GM-CFUs. Dividing cells resident in the bone marrow include the CFUs, GM-CFUs, monoblasts, and promonocytes, whereas monocytes, the next level of cell maturity, are generally nondividing cells that first circulate in the blood and then egress into tissues, where they are called macrophages. Once in tissue or sites of granulomatous inflammation, macrophages may be long-lived. Although monocytes are considered to be stem cells, a subpopulation appears capable of dividing at local tissue sites.[238,240] Macrophages enter various tissues and populate serous cavities (i.e., resident peritoneal macrophages), the lungs (alveolar macrophages), hepatic and splenic sinusoids (Kupffer's and sinusoidal cells), the brain (microglial elements), and bone (osteoclasts). The type A synovial lining cell is also an important part of the mononuclear phagocyte system (Fig. 16–1).

Bone Marrow Macrophage Progenitors. Progression from the multipotential stem cell to the circulating monocyte is observed as macrophages develop.[76,77,213] The GM-CFUs are the distinct progenitor cells for this lineage, and can be induced to express Fc receptors.[30] Erythrocytes and lymphocytes have separate progenitors. Human GM-CFU proliferation is regulated by several diffusible factors, as are GM-CFUs in other species. Among these are colony-stimulating factors (CSF). CSF is a term used to describe substances that stimulate individual hemapoietic precursor cells to divide and differentiate. CSF that act specifically on macrophage differentiation have been isolated.[220] CSF for GM-CFUs are contained in supernatants of certain cell cultures (conditioned medium) such as stimulated lymphocytes, fibroblasts, and cell cultures of some tumor cell lines. CSF are acidic glycoproteins with molecular weight (MW) in the range of 40,000 to 70,000 daltons.[156,219,220] CSF for macrophages bind to cells of this lineage with high affinity, suggesting the presence of specific receptors. In contrast to the stimulatory effects of CSF, the combination of prostaglandins (PGE$_1$ and PGE$_2$) and acidic isoferritin activities (AIA)[26,159] depresses macrophage differentiation. Prostaglandins apparently play a role in the regulation of monocytopoiesis via their inhibitory effects on the GM-CFU cycle, thus providing a negative feedback loop. Since macrophages can synthesize prodigious amounts of PGEs,[189,190] they may have the capacity to autoregulate their own progenitor

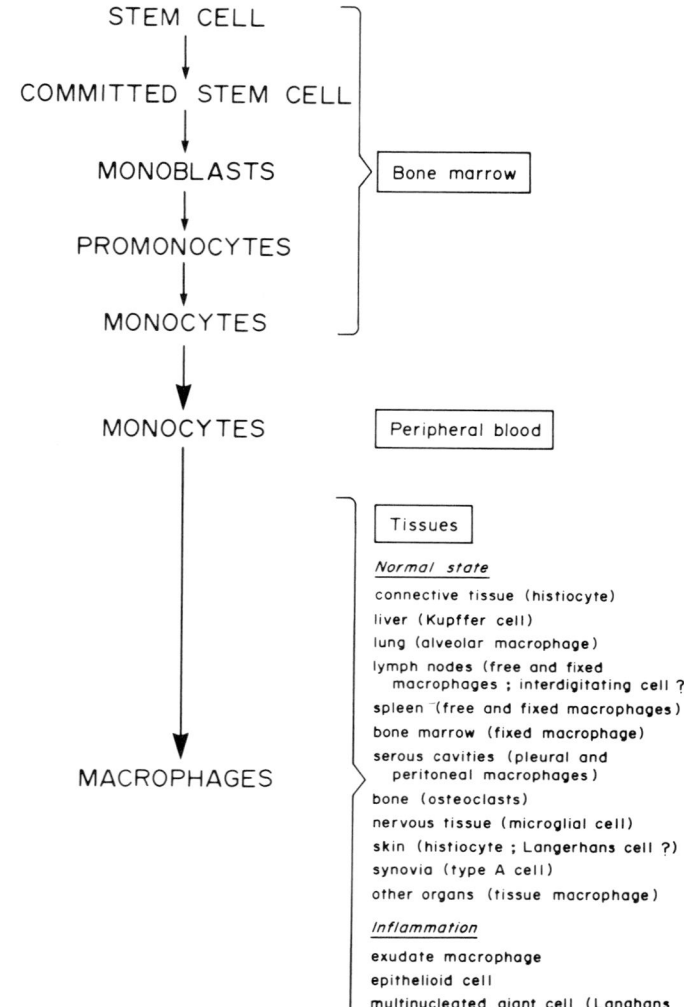

STEM CELL

↓

COMMITTED STEM CELL

↓

MONOBLASTS

↓

PROMONOCYTES

↓

MONOCYTES

Bone marrow

↓

MONOCYTES

Peripheral blood

Fig. 16–1.   Mononuclear phagocyte system.

↓

MACROPHAGES

Tissues

Normal state
connective tissue (histiocyte)
liver (Kupffer cell)
lung (alveolar macrophage)
lymph nodes (free and fixed
    macrophages ; interdigitating cell ?)
spleen (free and fixed macrophages)
bone marrow (fixed macrophage)
serous cavities (pleural and
    peritoneal macrophages)
bone (osteoclasts)
nervous tissue (microglial cell)
skin (histiocyte ; Langerhans cell ?)
synovia (type A cell)
other organs (tissue macrophage)

Inflammation
exudate macrophage
epithelioid cell
multinucleated giant cell (Langhans
    type and foreign-body type)

cells.[158] Macrophages also appear to be the source of AIA. AIAs are 21,000-dalton MW subunits of ferritin, and are major components of this protein. AIAs in conjunction with prostaglandins inhibit the stimulatory effects of CSF. Another cell-derived inhibitory factor acting on stem cells is lactoferrin.

In normal bone marrow, cells have been detected that produce a factor that suppresses the development of GM-CFUs.[214] The cells producing this factor have Fc gamma receptors and do not require activation by mitogens for the elaboration of this substance. Another factor regulating growth of macrophage precursors has been called synergistic activity (SA). When added with CSF to normal murine bone marrow cultures, SA results in the selection of a subset of macrophage progenitors that exhibit a high proliferative potential.[116] Activity such as this could induce a rapid turnover of

macrophages when needed in an inflammatory setting.

Differentiation.   The first level of differentiation from the stem cell is the monoblast, a round (ca. 12-micron cell) that can be grown in culture from murine but not yet from human bone marrow.[76,213,238–240,242,244] It is characterized by a small amount of basophilic cytoplasm, a ruffled membrane, and is esterase-positive; monoblasts also are adherent phagocytes with Fc receptors and apparently divide only once into two promonocytes. Promonocytes are larger cells with an indented nucleus and more cytoplasm than monoblasts, and are also peroxidase-positive. The cell cycle time for promonocytes is longer than that for the monoblasts (ca. 12 vs. 16 hours).[77,135] The promonocyte pool, which is twice as large as the monoblast pool, matures in the bone marrow for ca. 60 hours, then becomes part of the circulating or marginal pool for approximately 9 hours. Inflammatory stimuli result in an increased proliferation of promonocytes, and an enhanced release of immature monocytes from bone marrow, thus accelerating entry into the circulating/marginal pool.[135] Monocytes constitute a minority population (less than 8%) of nucleated circulating blood elements.[252] Yet, this pool constitutes a readily available source of tissue macrophages. Since marrow reserves of preformed monocytes are small relative to the pool of reserve polymorphonuclear leukocytes, and the proliferative capacity of monocytes is limited, the participation of macrophages in host defense depends on the continued expansion of this small pool in response to various inflammatory stimuli. In mice, the circulation half-time is approximately 22 hours and can last from 10 to over 70 hours in man.[238,241] The marginating monocyte pool is approximately four times the circulating pool. The extravascular pool, represented by the monocytes that have egressed into tissues, is large. Once out of the circulating pool, these cells, now termed macrophages, never return. The kinetics of monocyte maturation are similar in mice and in humans.

In general, there are three mechanisms whereby monocyte levels are modulated by inflammatory stimuli: (1) earlier release of premature monocytes that would normally have been retained in the marrow; (2) temporary shortening of the cell cycle time, resulting in an increased output of younger monocytes, and (3) a sustained enlargement of the precursor pool as accomplished by an increase in the proportion of promonocytes.[252] Several possibilities for the regulation of monocytopoiesis during acute inflammation have been proposed.[242,246] In the normal steady state, monoblast production is controlled by bone marrow regulators of monocytopoiesis (i.e., local production of CSF). When an inflammatory stimulus develops, however, local macrophages may, after phagocytosis of an antigen, release a substance that has been called factor-increasing monocytopoiesis (FIM). This agent circulates to the bone marrow and stimulates increased monoblast production. This factor has been characterized as a protein of 18,000 to 24,000 daltons and elicits a rapid monocytopoiesis when injected into normal mice.[246]

Tissue Macrophages. Although most tissue macrophages arise from emigration from the circulating/marginating pool, there is some mitotic potential of precursor cells at local tissue sites.[251] Data concerning the fate of macrophages that have emigrated into tissues derive primarily from studies of experimentally induced granulomatous inflammation.[12,213] A hematogenous origin is currently held for peritoneal, alveolar, hepatic, and neural

tissue macrophages, but in chronic granulomatous foci, there is evidence for local replication as well.[2,213,241,251] A small portion of circulating blood monocytes may be capable of dividing once at local tissue sites.[238] Depending on the particulate nature and digestibility of the antigenic stimulus, macrophages may become long-lived immobile nondividing cells (i.e., fuse to become giant cells that do not divide), or they may become epithelioid macrophages.

In certain tissue sites, the macrophages may dramatically affect the regulation of the local environment. Two examples of this premise are the interactions between the synovial phagocytic cell and its neighboring plasma cells and lymphoblasts in the synovial membrane, and the potential of alveolar macrophages to produce soluble factors affecting proliferation of lymphocytes to antigens and mitogens.[130]

The ability of blood monocytes to become resident cells in specific tissues is thought to be a random process, and one in which the further differentiation at the specific tissue is a consequence of local trophic influences. However, as more is learned about the development of macrophages and their heterogeneity, it would not be surprising to find that specific bone marrow precursors or subclasses of monocytes possess unique capacity for differentiation, thus eventually selecting their specific final tissue destination.

MACROPHAGES AS EFFECTOR CELLS

Mechanisms of Macrophage Accumulation. The accumulation of macrophages at local tissue sites is the result of a complex process that involves the adherence of monocytes to the vascular endothelium, their migration through gaps between the endothelial cells, penetration of the basement membrane, and then locomotion through tissue spaces to the inflammatory site. The initial binding of blood monocytes to endothelial cells is likely to involve fibronectin, a complex high-molecular-weight molecule found in plasma, which is capable of binding to monocytes as well as to endothelial cells.[40,160] The passage of monocytes through vascular basement membrane may depend on their ability to secrete collagenase.[253,268] The actual migration of the cells to the inflammatory site appears to be mediated by the chemotactic process.[205] Chemotactic factors are molecules that have the property of causing the directed migration of cells along a concentration gradient. As will be described, several different types of chemotactic factors are produced at sites of inflammatory reactions, and the type of factor produced is dependent upon the stimulus to inflammation. Monocytes and macrophages have cell surface receptors for chemotactic factors.[16,202,203,260] The binding of chemoattractants to the surface of resting blood monocytes leads to change in the shape of the round cells to their motile triangular configuration.[35] Associated with this change are several metabolic events apparently required for chemotaxis to occur (to be discussed). These processes lead to a rapid change in the cytoskeleton of the cells and allow reorientation of actin filaments to the front of the cell with rearrangement of cytoskeletal elements in a way to provide front-to-back polarization. The net effect of the interaction of chemoattractants with monocytes or macrophages is the migration of the cells along a chemotactic gradient toward the site of inflammation (Fig. 16–2). Several chemotactic factors that appear to result in macrophage accumulation in vivo have been described.

Complement-Derived Chemotactic Factors. The fifth component of complement, C5, is composed of two chains termed the α-chain and the β-chain.[93] Activation of C5 by the earlier acting

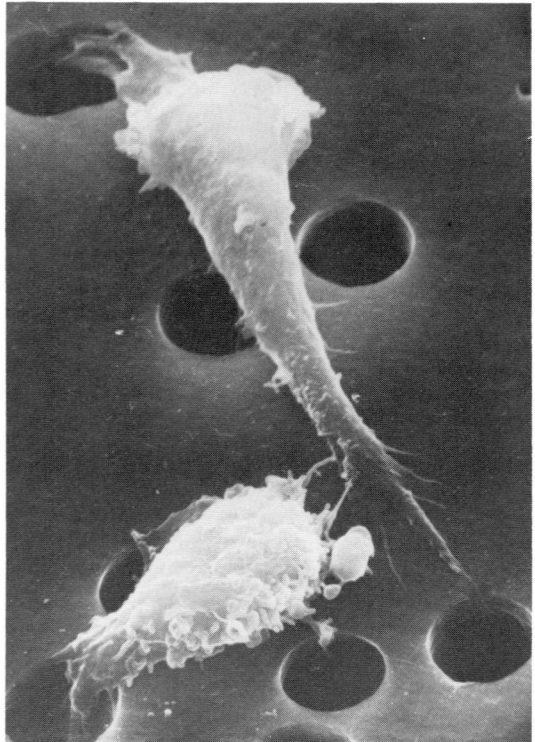

Fig. 16–2. Scanning electron micrograph of two human blood monocytes migrating through 5.0-micrometer pores of a polycarbonate filter in response to a chemotactic lymphokine (× 4,000). The cell at the top has completely emerged through a pore and has advanced diagonally across the filter's surface. On the lower left another cell has begun to emerge through the filter. (From Synderman, R., and Mergenhagen, S.E.[205])

complement components (see Chap. 21) or a cleavage of C5 by proteases leads to the release of a fragmentation product termed C5a.[98,193] C5a is a potent mediator of inflammatory reactions in that it is a chemotactic factor for both polymorphonuclear leukocytes[98,193] and monocytes-macrophages.[201,211] It also has anaphylatoxin activity in that it increases vascular permeability, contracts vascular smooth muscle, degranulates mast cells, and can cause hypotension.[98,193] C5a is a protein consisting of 74 amino acids, the carboxy-terminal constituent being arginine.[93,94] In addition to initiating monocyte-macrophage chemotaxis, C5a at higher concentrations can also lead to secretion of lysosomal enzymes by macrophages and stimulation of the respiratory burst with production of superoxide anion. C5a has been identified at inflammatory sites in vivo[206] and has also been detected in synovial effusions from patients with RA.[258] C5a in the circulation is rapidly degraded to C5a des Arg through the action of a carboxypeptidase.[93] This molecule retains chemotactic activity for mononuclear phagocytes, although it appears to be less active than C5a itself. C5a and/or C5a des Arg are important chemoattractants in inflammatory conditions initiated by immune complexes,[207] bacterial endotoxins, or nonspecific tissue trauma, which causes release of tissue proteases.[210]

Cell-Derived Chemotactic Factors. Stimulation of lymphocytes by specific antigen or mitogens results in the synthesis and release of biologically active agents termed lymphokines. One particular lymphokine, termed lymphocyte-derived chemotactic factor (LDCF) is a chemoattractant for monocyte-macrophages.[8,201] This material has a molecular weight of approximately 12,000 and has been isolated from supernatants of stimulated lymphocyte cultures as well as from delayed hypersensitivity reactions in vivo.[168]

Other Chemotactic Factors from Macrophages. Several other chemotactic factors for monocyte-macrophages have been described. One well-defined group is the synthetic N-formylated methionyl oligopeptides.[184] These synthetic peptides are thought to be analogous to chemotactic factors produced by rapidly dividing bacteria. Certain N-formyl methionyl peptides (i.e., f-met-leu-phe) are potent chemoattractants for monocytemacrophages. Indeed, monocytes and macrophages have specific membrane receptors for N-formyl methionyl peptides.[16,42,203,260] By recognizing these peptides, mononuclear phagocytes may be able to accumulate at sites of bacterial growth. Collagen (type I) as well as collagen degradation products are also chemoattractants for monocytes.[167] In addition to these chemotactic factors, kallikrein, proteins released by tumor cells, and a product released by fibroblasts have also been described as having monocyte-macrophage chemotactic activity.[66,107,134] Another potential source of chemoattractants for macrophages are the metabolites of arachidonic acid.[11,236] The interaction of certain phlogistic agents, such as C5a, with inflammatory cells activates a cellular phospholipase that cleaves arachidonic acid from membrane phospholipids.[164] Metabolism of arachidonic acid by macrophages can result in the production of leukotriene B4 (5'12 dihydroxyeicosatetraenoic acid).[31,189,190] LTB4 is a chemoattractant for neutrophils and macrophages and has been detected in rheumatoid synovial effusions.[63,69]

Mechanisms of Macrophage Chemotaxis. The precise biochemical mechanisms by which the binding of chemoattractants leads to directed migration by macrophages is not fully understood, but is an area of considerable research. N-formylmethionyl peptides, in particular N-f-met-leu-phe, have provided an important tool for the study of chemotaxis since these peptides are structurally defined and quite potent. Monocytes and macrophages have specific receptors for the N-formylated peptides.[16,203,260] The equilibrium disassociation constant (K_D) for f-met-leu-phe by human blood monocytes is 30×10^{-9}M, and there are approximately 65,000 receptors per human blood monocyte.[16] The receptor is a glycoprotein with a molecular weight of approximately 62,000 daltons.[109] The chemotactic factor receptor in macrophage membranes exists in a high and low affinity, with the two affinities being in part interconvertible and regulated by guanine di- and trinucleotides. This finding suggests that a nucleotide regulatory protein may be involved in regulating the biologic activity of the chemotactic factor receptor.[202] Similar regulation has been suggested for certain neurotransmitter receptors.[216] The binding of chemoattractants to their receptor on human monocytes leads to the activation of phospholipase C and thus degradation of phosphatidylinositol.[164] There is evidence that transmethylation reactions mediated by S-adenosyl-methionine are required for activation of the phospholipase and regulation of the affinity of the chemoattractant receptor.[163] Degradation of phosphatidylinositol leads to the formation of diacylglycerol, which is further metabolized to phosphatidic acid, arachidonate, and LTB4.[111,117,127,176] Both phosphatidic acid and LTB4 are calcium ionophores.[191] The combination of increased and intracellular calcium associated with diacylglycerol would be expected to activate a calcium-dependent protein kinase termed protein kinase C, which may be involved in triggering macrophage responses to chemoattractants.[208] Interestingly, arachidonic acid itself has been found to directly activate protein

kinase C as well as the respiratory burst enzyme in human polymorphonuclear leukocytes.[132] Thus, release of arachidonate by phospholipases activated by chemoattractants may be a second messenger involved in triggering macrophage responses.

MACROPHAGE RECEPTORS

The function of receptors is to trigger cells to respond appropriately to environmental stimuli. Considering the broad range of macrophage functions, it is not surprising that their plasma membranes should be well endowed with receptors that selectively initiate various physiologic functions.[124,263] Biochemically, receptors are discrete cellular structures that bind specific ligands with high affinity and limited capacity. Functionally, the binding of a receptor with its ligand triggers a discrete biologic response by the cell.

Fc Receptors. Clearance of immune complexes and endocytosis of opsonized particles is an important function of macrophages. These cells contain receptors for the Fc portion of immunoglobulin on their surfaces.[10,79,85,92,195,232–234] Cross-linkage of such receptors stimulates endocytosis. Fc receptors for distinct immunoglobulin subclasses are present on both human monocytes and murine macrophages. Studies in macrophages from species such as guinea pig, rat, mouse, and man have demonstrated Fc receptor specificity for individual subclasses of IgG. For example, mouse macrophages have distinct receptors for IgG2a, IgG2b/IgG1, and IgG3.[53–55,256] These receptors are termed $FcR_{\gamma 2a}$, $FcR_{\gamma 2b/\gamma 1}$, $FcR_{\gamma 3}$, respectively. Some evidence suggests that the signals generated by the binding of IgG to the different classes of Fc receptors in murine macrophages may stimulate different biologic activities (i.e., phagocytosis vs. cytotoxicity).[257] The murine Fc receptors themselves have differential susceptibility to proteases and phospholipases and cap independently.[9,234] In murine macrophages, all classes of Fc receptors appear to be single-chain glycoproteins of approximately 50,000 daltons. The mechanism by which the binding of IgG to its receptor initiates cellular function is largely unknown, but in the case of the $FcR_{\gamma 2b/\gamma 1}$ receptor, a ligand-dependent ion-channel initiating influx is operative.[278] Fc receptors appear to react differently with respect to their ability to bind monomers and aggregates of immunoglobulins. Receptors for monomeric IgG are thought to bind cytophilic antibody of the human IgG1 and IgG3 subclasses. The function of such receptors may be to couple antibody to monocytes so that the cells are better able to recognize specific antigens. Receptors for monomeric IgG are protease-sensitive and do not lead to endocytosis of antigen unless they are subsequently cross-linked by other antibodies to the antigen. There are Fc receptors that bind only aggregates of IgG or antigen-antibody complexes. This binding results in internalization of the antigens. It is estimated that macrophages contain approximately 500,000 such receptors per cell.[233] Specific Fc receptors for IgE and IgM have been reported on mononuclear phagocytes and cell lines from several species, but the functional role of these receptors is not clear.[23,62]

Complement Receptors. Monocytes and macrophages respond chemotactically to low doses of C5a, implying the presence of a specific receptor for these peptides.[211] Indeed, a common receptor for C5a and C5a des Arg has been demonstrated on human polymorphonuclear leukocytes.[32] The C5a receptor initiates lysosomal enzyme secretion and activation of the respiratory burst enzyme in mononuclear phagocytes. Macrophages also contain receptors for fragments of the fourth and third component of complement. Complement receptor 1 (CR1) binds the C3b as well as C4b.[169] Complement receptor 2 (CR2) binds C3bi, a degradation product of C3b produced by the action of C3b inactivator. The receptors for C3b and C3bi are antigenically distinct and are independently mobile in the plane of the membrane. Moreover, the C3bi receptor requires Ca^{+2} and Mg^{+2} for optimal activity, whereas the C3b receptor does not.[273] Structurally, the C3b receptor is a 205,000d single-chain membrane glycoprotein,[61] whereas the C3bi receptor is composed of two membrane glycoprotein chains of MW 180,000d and 100,000d, respectively.[272,274] Binding of antigens to macrophages via complement receptors does not appear to directly initiate endocytosis unless there is further stimulation of the macrophage by Fc receptors or other phlogistic stimuli.[18,272,274] The primary function of complement receptors appears to be the attachment of complement-bearing antigens to the surface of the macrophage. In the presence of low levels of IgG, complement receptors do enhance phagocytosis.

Receptors for Glycoproteins. Clearance of serum proteins such as enzymes, as well as bacteria, may be mediated by receptors for specific sugars or glycoproteins on macrophages. A mannosyl-glucosyl receptor on macrophages mediates clearance of mannosyl, glucosyl, and acetylglucosamine terminal glycoproteins from the circulation. The clearance of lysosomal hydrolases appears to be via the mannosyl-glucosyl receptor of Kupffer's cells[218] and alveolar macrophages.[217] A mouse macrophage recognition system involving lectin-like receptors has been described and can bind the cell wall sugars of certain microorganisms.[261] The role of receptors that bind sugars may be important in removing denatured proteins, effete

cells, or bacteria from the circulation. The terminal sugar on most glycoproteins is sialic acid. This terminal residue may be lost when cells or proteins are exposed to neuraminidase or denatured by some other means. Exposure of sugar residues other than sialic acid can then be recognized by the manosylglucosyl receptor or perhaps other sugar receptors on macrophages. This model provides an excellent example of ''nonspecific recognition'' mediated by macrophages.[110]

Receptors for Lipoproteins. Macrophages are important in the clearance of lipids from the circulation, and accumulation of fatty substances within macrophages may be involved in the pathogenesis of atherosclerosis. Human and murine macrophages have surface receptors for low-density lipoproteins that allow them to internalize and degrade modified lipoproteins.[71]

Hormone Receptors on Macrophages. Macrophages contain receptors for several hormones that are likely in the regulation of macrophage funcitons.[263] Many classes of hormone receptors have been demonstrated either indirectly or on macrophages. These include receptors for polypeptide hormones, steroid hormones, and catecholamines. Direct binding studies have shown that macrophages contain adrenergic, insulin, glucagon, thyrotropin, as well as receptors for somatomedin, prostaglandins, and dexamethasone.[263] Rheumatoid synovial adherent macrophages have a steroid receptor.[25] Indirect evidence suggests that macrophages also have receptors for histamine, serotonin, parathyroid hormone, calcitonin, vitamin D, estrogen, and progesterone. Beta-adrenergic agonists inhibit chemotaxis as well as secretion and superoxide anion production, whereas alpha adrenergic receptors, serotonin receptors, and muscarinic-cholinergic receptors appear to enhance chemoattractant-mediated functions.[65,183,222]

Other Receptors on Macrophages. Functional evidence suggests that macrophages have receptors for a wide variety of agents that may affect their biologic activity. Colony-stimulating factor (CSF) binds to monocytes and macrophages. The binding site for CSF may be involved in the differentiation of these cells.[220] α-2 Macroglobulin-protease complexes are rapidly endocytized by macrophages and may provide an important mechanism for the clearance of proteolytic enzymes. Macrophages appear to have a membrane-binding site for α-2 macroglobulin-protease complex, but not for native α-2 macroglobulins.[52] Macrophage activating factor (MAF) has been shown to be identical or closely related to γ-interferon.[146,187] The potency of this material for activating macrophages suggests a receptor for γ-interferon on the cells. Similarly, macrophage migration inhibitory factor (MIF) probably binds to a receptor on macrophages since its activity is blocked by sugars such as 1-fucose as well as by pretreating the cells with fucosidase.[86,172,178] The receptor for MIF/MAD on guinea pig macrophages has been identified as a glycolipid.[44] Clearance of iron could be mediated by a lactoferrin receptor that has been described on murine macrophages.[245] Lactoferrin release from neutrophil specific granules could be internalized by macrophages, thereby sequestering iron in the reticuloendothelial system.[245]

ENDOCYTOSIS

A central feature of macrophage function, which enables the cells to perform their many roles in host defense, is their ability to avidly ingest a wide variety of materials. Endocytosis is the generalized term for internalization of extracellular substances by invagination of the plasma membrane. Subsequent membrane fusion results in the formation of membrane-bound vesicles within the cell. The term pinocytosis is used to describe the internalization of fluids and solutes, while phagocytosis refers to the ingestion of particulate materials.

Pinocytosis. Murine macrophages internalize twice their cell surface area per hour in pinocytic vesicles that deliver their contents to secondary lysozymes.[229] Recycling of the membrane from the lysosomal compartment back to the plasma membrane is an ongoing event since the size of the vacuolar system and membrane remains relatively constant. Thus, pinocytosis is an ongoing process by macrophages and may provide a means for the rapid recycling of plasma membrane to lysosomal compartments and back.[143]

Phagocytosis. The ingestion of particles by macrophages requires two processes: the binding of the particle to the macrophage plasma membrane, and the actual ingestion of the particulate material.[194,224] Binding of particles to macrophages is enhanced by serum factors termed opsonins which, by definition, are agents that enhance phagocytosis, but the cells are capable of binding and ingesting nonposonized material as well. In this latter case, lectin-like receptors or carbohydrate receptors may be involved in stimulating the phoggocytic process. The metabolic requirements for phagocytosis of nonopsonized particles apparently differ in that the latter but not the former are blocked by 2-deoxyglucose.[136,137] Contact of macrophages with opsonized particles results in their attachment to the macrophage plasma membrane followed by the elaboration of pseudopods at the location of the particle. The responses by the macrophage to bound particles are segmental in that they occur only in the proximity of the material to be phagocytized.[81] Bystander particles, not containing opsonins, may be ignored while adjacent opsonized particles are phagocytized. The development of the pseudopodia is dependent upon the polymerization of actin filaments directly beneath the particle to be ingested,[277] and phagocytosis is blocked by cytochalasin B, an gent that inhibits actin polymerization (Fig. 16–3). Energy for the movement of the macrophage membrane around an opsonized particle is likely to derive from ATP and occurs in a "zipper"-like fashion.[80] That is, the movement of the membrane around an opsonized particle to be phagocytized proceeds sequentially by interaction of receptors on the macrophage with ligands on the particle. If macrophages confront particles that are only partially covered with opsonin, the pseudopiods advance only as far as the opsonins are present and do not form a complete phagosome. When the particle bound to the macrophage is circumferentially opsonized, the macrophage membrane covers its entire surface and fuses. At this point, the particle is inside the macrophage and is surrounded by what had been the macrophage plasma membrane. The internalized structure is termed a "phagosome." Concomitant with the formation of the phagosome is the migration of lysosomal granules toward it. The lysosomal granules fuse with the membrane of the forming phagosome and discharge their contents into it.[185] The fusion of lysosomal granules with the phagosome causes the formation of a structure called a "phagolysosome." In addition to exposing the opsonized particle to the enzyme contents of lysosomal granules, the binding process leads to activation of the "respiratory burst enzyme," NADPH oxidase, which is associated with the plasma membrane.[132] Activation of this enzyme leads to the production of superoxide anion, which is further metabolized into several toxic oxygen products, including hydrogen peroxide, hydroxyl radical, hypochlorous ion, and singlet oxygen.[100,112,145] These products are toxic to most microbial agents. The combination of toxic oxygen products with the contents of lysosomal granules makes it unlikely that all but the most resistant microorganisms will survive following phagocytosis by macrophages (see Fig. 16–3). During the process of phagocytosis, incomplete fusion of phagosomes prior to discharge of lysosomal contents, ("regurgitation while feeding") can cause the release of toxic products into the extracellular environment.

Both Fc and C3 receptors promote phagocytosis; however, there are striking differences in their ability to do so. Cross-linking of Fc receptors triggers phagocytosis whether or not the macrophages have been stimulated by inflammatory agents. In contrast, macrophages isolated from noninflammatory

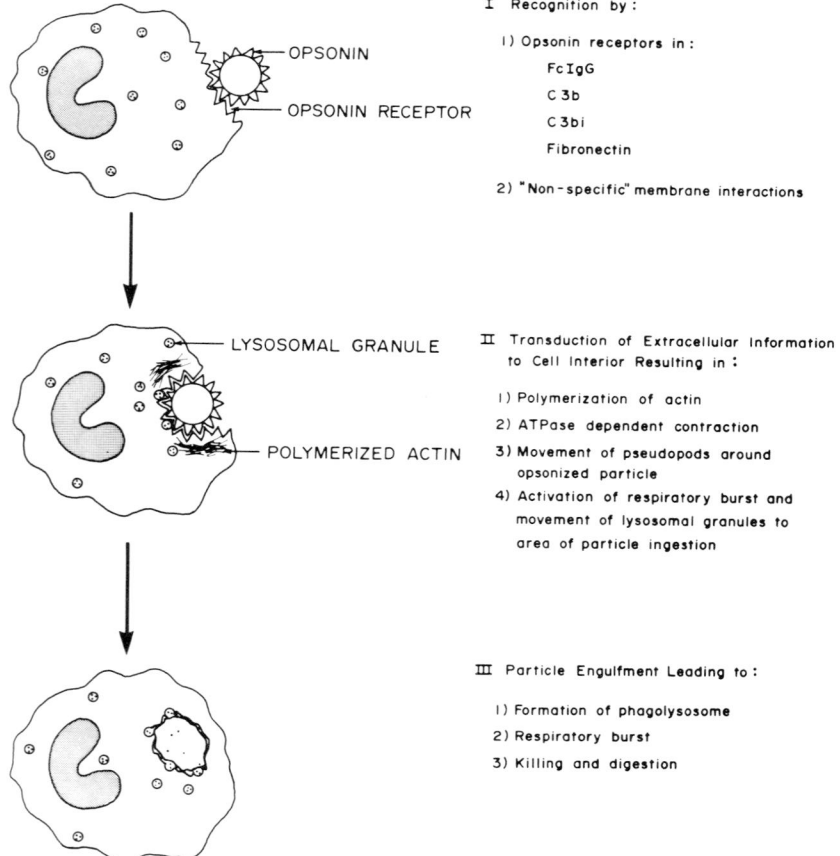

I Recognition by :

  1) Opsonin receptors in :

    FcIgG

    C 3b

    C 3bi

    Fibronectin

  2) "Non-specific" membrane interactions

II Transduction of Extracellular Information to Cell Interior Resulting in :

  1) Polymerization of actin

  2) ATPase dependent contraction

  3) Movement of pseudopods around opsonized particle

  4) Activation of respiratory burst and movement of lysosomal granules to area of particle ingestion

III Particle Engulfment Leading to :

  1) Formation of phagolysosome

  2) Respiratory burst

  3) Killing and digestion

Fig. 16–3.   Mechanisms of phagocytosis.

environments (i.e., resident peritoneal macrophages) bind but do not internalize particles coated with either C3b or C3bi alone. If the cells are stimulated with phorbol-myristate-acetate, a tumor promoter that initiates the respiratory burst as well as lysosomal enzyme secretion, the macrophages then ingest both C3b- and C3bi-coated particles.[272,274] These data indicate that for C3b or C3bi receptors to stimulate ingestion, a second signal is needed and that this can be provided by phlogistic stimuli. In addition to phagocytizing opsonized particles, macrophages readily ingest immune complexes as well as aggregated immunoglobulins. These agents, like opsonized particles, stimulate the respiratory burst and secretory events by macrophages. However, immune complexes and cryoglobulins can also interfere with the phagocytosis of particles by monocytes, perhaps by blocking Fc receptors. Although little is known about regulation of phagocytosis in rheumatic diseases, it has been postulated that immune complexes in the synovial fluid can prevent effective phagocytosis and elim-

ination of particulate antigens.[225] In patients with rheumatoid arthritis, immune clearance is decreased, perhaps owing to the saturation of reticuloendothelial clearance mechanisms by intermittent exposure to immune complexes.[118] Rheumatoid patients with vasculitis who have circulating immune complexes have defects of monocyte phagocytosis of yeast particles, which is a complement-dependent opsonic function. Patients with circulating immune complexes and cutaneous vasculitis, but without rheumatoid arthritis, also display an impairment of complement-mediated monocyte phagocytosis.[95] Stimulation of phagocytosis depends heavily on membrane phenomena in that it is decreased when macrophages are treated with antibodies to their membrane components.[89]

MACROPHAGES AS SECRETORY CELLS

Macrophages secrete numerous products that affect a wide range of host functions. The vast array of secretory products of macrophages is just now being recognized, and secretion may be as important a macrophage function as is endocytosis. Macrophages secrete products in several different patterns. Secretion can be triggered by phlogistic products such as chemoattractants or opsonized particles.[186] Other types of secretion are constitutive and do not require any known exogenous stimulation.[74] Many products of macrophage secretion are stored within the cell's lysosomal compartments; however, other products are not preformed and are synthesized as they are released.

Acid Hydrolases. Abundant amounts of acid hydrolases are present in lysosomes within macrophages.[46] Following exposure to inflammatory substances such as chemoattractants or opsonized particles, macrophages rapidly secrete these preformed products. In general, substances capable of inducing chronic inflammation in vivo induce macrophage secretion of acid hydrolases in vitro.[262] Peptidoglycans of streptococcal cell walls, potent inducers of inflammatory reactions in vivo, are also potent stimulators of acid hydrolase secretions.[7,196] The secretion of hydrolases by chemoattractants occurs at doses generally 10 times higher than those required to initiate chemotaxis, implying that secretion may not occur until macrophages reach the inflammatory site where chemoattractants are in highest concentration.[208] Acid hydrolases may contribute to tissue destruction at inflammatory sites if the pH there is sufficiently low. Hydrolases may also amplify inflammatory reactions by cleaving C5 or other proinflammatory molecules, thereby producing additional biologically active cleavage products.[210] Other substrates for acid hydrolases may be collagen, proteoglycans, and the basement membrane of blood vessels.[280]

Plasminogen Activator. Plasminogen activator is a neutral protease that converts plasminogen to plasmin.[73,235] Plasmin not only degrades fibrin but also can activate C1, cleave C3, and convert Hageman factor into prekallikrein activator.[104] Plasminogen activator is secreted at low levels by nonactivated macrophages or monocytes, but its secretion is markedly enhanced by phlogistic stimuli.[247] The secretion of plasminogen activators by monocytes or macrophages may allow them to migrate through fibrin clots to arrive at inflammatory tissue sites. The ability of plasminogen activator to cleave Hageman factor as well as to activate complement at site of inflammation may also provide additional phlogistic agents. Plasminogen activator can also activate collagenase from its proenzyme form and thereby stimulate the destruction of collagen.[59]

Collagenase. Collagenase is a neutral protease secreted in small amounts by unstimulated macrophages, but phagocytosis or endotoxin enhances secretion.[254,268] Lymphokines also induce macrophages to produce collagenase.[253] Degradation of collagen in chronic inflammatory sites, such as the rheumatoid synovium, could be caused, at least in part, by collagenases secreted by macrophages.[49] Macrophage factors (i.e., IL-1) can stimulate collagenase and prostaglandin formation from rheumatoid tissues containing stellate cells.[48]

Elastase. Elastase is a neutral protease whose secretion is stimulated by phagocytic stimuli as well as by inflammatory mediators.[267] Human monocytes secrete elastase when exposed to immune complexes.[170] Release of elastase at inflammatory sites can lead to irreversible tissue damage by destroying vascular structures.

Lysozyme. Lysozyme is an important component of macrophage secretions, which is capable of degrading the cell walls of bacteria. Lysozyme is a cationic protein that hydrolyzes n-acetyl muramic β1-4 n-acetyl glucose linkages in bacterial cell walls.[215] Lysozyme has been found in human osteoarthritic cartilage.[91] Lysozyme is considered to be a constitutive secretion product of macrophages in that it is not stimulated by phagocytosis or by phlogistic agents.[46] Lysozyme is secreted at high levels by macrophages in culture irrespective of their degree of activation.[72,185] Other enzymes secreted by macrophages are angiotensin-converting enzyme, arginase, and nonspecific esterases.[72,91]

Anti-Proteases. Regulation of proteolytic enzyme activity is important in limiting tissue destruction following the release of proteases into extracellular tissue sites. Two antiproteases are contained in macrophages: α2-macroglobulin and α1-antiprotease.[90,99] 2-Macroglobulin binds several proteases, including kallikrein, thrombin, elastase, collagenase, plasmin, and plasminogen activator. Following the binding of a protease, α2-macroglobulin itself is modified and is then internalized and destroyed by macrophages. This provides an important regulatory mechanism for inhibiting the damage due to secretion of proteases by inflammatory cells. Human monocytes secrete α2-macroglobulin in culture, but regulation of secretion has not been elucidated.[22]

α1-Antiprotease is a potent inhibitor of serine proteinases and works by forming enzyme-inhibitor complexes. Among the important proteases inhibited by α1-antiprotease is elastase. Low levels of α1-antiprotease have been associated with emphysema and with adult respiratory distress syndrome where α1-antiprotease levels in alveolar secretions are low because of the release of toxic neutrophil products.[38] Antiprotease-protease complexes are indeed taken up by synovial inflammatory macrophages.[249] Abnormalities of antiproteases in rheumatic diseases have not been extensively evaluated and should provide an important area for future research.

Pro-Coagulants. In addition to stimulating fibrinolysis by secretion of plasminogen activator, macrophages and monocytes have procoagulant activity that is stimulated by their interaction with endotoxin, immune complexes, C3b or by phagocytosis of bacteria.[67] The procoagulant activity of macrophages has similarities to tissue thromboplastin. The physiologic significance of thromboplastin generation by monocytes is speculative, but in pathologic situations may contribute to the development of intravascular clotting. A role for tissue thromboplastin-like activity released by monocytes has been suggested in the pathophysiology of allograft rejection.[237] Monocytes from patients with rheumatic disease appear to have higher thromboplastin generating activity than do monocytes from normal persons. However, when phlogistic stimuli are introduced, monocytes from the latter make more thromboplastin than do monocytes from rheumatoid patients. The development of microvascular thromboses and fibrin deposition in chronic inflammatory states could be related to the release of thromboplastins from macrophages.[125]

Complement Components. Macrophages synthesize a number of complement components.[24,57] The synthesis of complement by macrophages might provide a source for opsonins and mediators of inflammation directly at local tissue sites. C1, C4, C2, C3, C5, as well as factor B, factor D, and properdin are products of macrophages. Considering the fact that the cleavage products of C3b and factor B of the alternative pathway are potent macrophage activators,[17,75] release of complement components at sites of inflammation could play an important role in macrophage activation.[51] Monocytes from rheumatoid patients make more C2 than do those from osteoarthritis patients.[122]

Arachidonic Acid Metabolites. Stimulation of macrophages or monocytes by phlogistic agents activates cellular phospholipases, particularly phospholipase C, which degrades membrane phospholipids,[164] resulting in the release of arachidonic acid.[45,111,117,132,176] Arachidonic acid can be further metabolized into prostaglandins or leukotrienes by the action of either cyclo-oxygenase or lipoxygenase (see Chap. 22). Prostaglandin E_2 appears to be the predominant prostaglandin synthesized by macrophages.[189,190] This substance is secreted by unstimulated peritoneal macrophages, but the amount of secretion is markedly increased following exposure to phlogistic stimuli. Macrophages also synthesize leukotrines and thromboxanes. The most predominant leukotrienes are of the 12 hydroxyeicosotetraenoic acid series.[36] Leukotrienes C and D,

formerly termed slow reactive substances of anaphylaxis, are also released by stimulated macrophages. Alveolar macrophages also produce 12 HETE, LTB_4, PGF_2, thromboxane A2, and PAF.[11,31,103,129] PGE_2 stimulates the production of cAMP in cells with PGE_2 receptors including macrophages.[248] Cyclic AMP is an inhibitor of many cellular reactions including chemotaxis, phagocytosis, the respiratory burst, lymphocyte mitogenesis, and lymphocyte-mediated cytotoxicity. Prostaglandins are stimulators of osteoclast activation and enhance bone absorption.[29] Thromboxanes are vasoconstrictors, whereas leukotriene B4 is chemotactic for neutrophils and macrophages.[236] Leukotriene C and D stimulate smooth muscle contraction and bronchoconstriction. Macrophage-induced suppressor activity,[197] which has been described in numerous inflammatory conditions including RA, may be mediated by their release of prostaglandins.[16,192,255,259]

Growth-Promoting Factors Produced by Macrophages. Macrophages produce a number of products that stimulate the growth of other cells. The best defined of these is interleukin-1 (IL-1), previously termed lymphocyte-activating factor (LAF). IL-1 is a polypeptide with a molecular weight of 12,000 daltons.[138–140] IL-1 acts independently or in concert with mitogenic agents to stimulate lymphocyte proliferation. IL-1 secretion by macrophages can be stimulated by a number of phlogistic agents, including immune complexes. Interestingly, IL-1 contains several other activities in addition to its lymphocyte-activating activity. IL-1 may be identical to leukocytic pyrogen, an agent important in initiating fever following challenge with endotoxin or immune complexes. IL-1 may also be identical to mononuclear cell factor (MCF), a material that stimulates synovial stellate cells to produce collagenase.[49,138]

Macrophages also produce other less well-defined growth factors. Colony-stimulating activity, which causes hematopoietic progenitor cells to form colonies in vitro, is released following the addition of endotoxin to macrophage cultures. Macrophages also release activities that stimulate fibroblast proliferation.[20] The nature of colony-stimulating activity as well as fibroblast-stimulating activity for macrophages is still poorly defined.[269] Macrophages also synthesize low levels of type 1 interferon, while type 2 interferon may act as a differentiation signal to macrophages by enhancing their expression of surface membrane components.[177,250]

Reactive Oxygen Products. An important mechanism by which macrophages kill microbial agents and tumor cells is through the release of toxic oxygen products.[13,100] Stimulation of macrophages by phagocytosis or with phlogistic agents, such as chemoattractants, initiates a "respiratory burst." This phenomenon is associated with an increase of cellular oxygen consumption and the activation of a membrane-associated enzyme termed NADPH oxidase.[101,132] This enzyme uses NADPH as its preferred substrate and converts molecular oxygen into superoxide anion (O_2^-). Further metabolism of superoxide leads to the formation of hydrogen peroxide through the enzyme superoxide dismutase. Hydrogen peroxide plus O_2 in the presence of iron reacts to form singlet oxygen (•OH) and hydroxyl radical (OH^-). In the presence of the enzyme myeloperoxidase plus a halide such as chloride ion, singlet oxygen leads to the production of hypochlorous ion.[113] Toxic oxygen products such as hydrogen peroxide, singlet oxygen, hydroxyl radical, and hypochlorous ion are potent oxidizing agents and inactivate the sulfhydryl groups of enzymes or proteins. The release of toxic oxygen products by macrophages is markedly affected by their state of activation. Macrophages activated to kill inteacellular parasites or tumor cells are capable of secreting large amounts of hydrogen peroxide.[100,147] Resident peritoneal macrophages or inflammatory macrophages not stimulated with agents such as BCG are far less capable of producing hydrogen peroxide. An interesting activity of oxidizing agents is their ability to inactivate biologically active products such as chemoattractants or antiproteases.[37,38] The mechanism of this inactivation appears to be through oxidation of methionine residues to sulfoxides.[38] Oxidizing agents may thus play additional roles in inflammation other than through their cytotoxic activity. For example, production of superoxide anion decreases the viscosity of synovial fluid through depolymerization of hyaluronate.[131]

Fibronectin Secretion by Macrophages. Fibronectin, a macromolecular glycoprotein, mediates the adherence of cells such as fibroblasts to substrata. Activated macrophages synthesize and release fibronectin. This molecule is chemotactic for fibroblasts; activated macrophages may thus provide the stimulus for fibrogenesis at inflammatory sites.[5,166,228,275]

Release of Factors Affecting Lipid Metabolism. Apolipoprotein E is a 34,000 to 37,000-dalton glycoprotein that regulates lipoprotein and cholesterol metabolism. Peritoneal macrophages secrete large amounts of apolipoprotein E after the cells have been loaded with cholesterol.[71] Apolipoprotein E and cholesterol are released independently, but after secretion they associate with high-density lipoproteins and form particles that can deliver cholesterol to the liver.[15a] Liver cells contain receptors for apolipoprotein E, which stimulates the uptake of apolipoprotein E-associated lipids. The magnitude of apolipoprotein E secretion by cholesterol-laden macrophages suggests an important role for mononuclear phagocytes in atherogenesis.[14,15,265] The release of apolipoprotein E by macrophages is inhibited by their treatment with endotoxin, suggesting a mechanism for the hyperlipidemia associated with endotoxemia.[265] In addition, very low-density lipoproteins (VLDL) induce triglyceride synthesis by macrophages.[68] These findings suggest a potentially important role for macrophages in regulating lipid metabolism.

Other Factors. Alveolar macrophages, isolated by bronchial lavage and placed in culture, make soluble factors that suppress the proliferation of peripheral blood lymphocytes to antigens and mitogens. These factors suppress T cells to a greater extent than B cells. Thus, the alveolar macrophage, formerly thought to have only nonspecific defensive functions, may actually have the capacity to adjust its own microenvironment.[130] A nonspecific immune suppressor factor has been isolated from macrophages treated with soluble immune response suppressor factor (SIRS).[12]

MICROBICIDAL ACTIVITY OF MACROPHAGES

When phagocytized by macrophages, microbial agents are exposed to hydrolases, toxic oxygen products, lysozyme, and a number of other antibacterial proteins. The antimicrobial activity of macrophages is one of their most important functions.[179] However, a number of infectious agents may escape destruction by macrophages. These predominantly intracellular pathogens include some viruses, and mycobacterial, chlamydial, rickettsial, and listerial organisms. Parasites such as *Trypanosoma*, *Leishmania*, and *Toxoplasma* can replicate in macrophages, whereas fungal organisms, including *Cryptococcus* and *Aspergillus*, and bacteria such as *Corynebacteria*, *Salmonella*, *Brucella*, *Pasteurella*, and *Nocardia* can also survive macrophage phagocytosis. The ability of these organisms to escape destruction by macrophages is, however, far from complete. In particular, macrophages in the "activated" state kill the aforementioned organisms far more readily than do nonactivated macrophages. The concept of macrophage activation is important to its host defensive functions, particularly in regard to antimicrobial and tumoricidal activity.[39]

MACROPHAGE ACTIVATION

Macrophages and granulocytes share functions in common; however, there are some striking differences. One of the most important of these is the ability of macrophages to alter their functional activity in response to environmental stimuli. When isolated from blood or from noninflammatory tissue sites such as the peritoneal cavity, macrophages have chemotactic, phagocytic, and antimicrobial activity. All these functions, however, as well as the magnitude of the respiratory burst, are greatly enhanced during the process of activation. Exposure of macrophages to products synthesized by stimulated lymphocytes (i.e., lymphokines such as γ-interferon) as well as by small doses of endotoxins[43,126,144] leads to macrophage activation. The functional characteristics of the activated macrophage include the ability to kill intracellular parasites as well as tumor cells in the absence of antitumor antibody.[3,146] Microbicidal activity for trypanosomes can be induced in human monocyte-derived macrophages if the cells are first exposed to soluble factors produced by lymphocytes.[150,151] Soluble factors from spleen cells enhance macrophage antimicrobial functions for *Chlamydia* by enhancing hydroxyl-radical production.[28] Macrophages can also utilize peroxidase enzymes released by other cells at inflammatory sites to augment their own killing potential.[123]

Evidence suggests that macrophage activation can be divided into several distinct steps.[3,106,133] Experimentally, this can be demonstrated with murine macrophages isolated from the peritoneal cavity. Resident macrophages have the least amount of lysosomal enzymes and low microbicidal and tumoricidal activity. Macrophages elicited with nonimmune inflammatory agents (inflammatory macrophages) such as proteose peptone or thioglycollate have higher levels of intracellular lysozymes and are more phagocytic, but are still unable to kill intracellular parasites or tumor cells. Macrophages elicited from BCG-induced inflammatory sites are fully activated and readily kill intracellular organisms as well as tumor cells. Intermediate between inflammatory and activated macrophages are "primed" macrophages obtained from animals injected with the complex polysaccharide pyran. These cells can be rendered fully active in vitro following treatment with macrophage-activating factor and small doses of endotoxin.[3,181]

MACROPHAGE-MEDIATED TUMOR CYTOTOXICITY

The development of direct tumor cell cytotoxicity by macrophages is associated with their ability to selectively bind to tumor as opposed to nontumor cells (Fig. 16–4).[3,161] In addition, activated macrophages develop increased lysosomal hydrolase activity and a greater potential to produce hydrogen peroxide. In the presence of tumor cells, activated macrophages secrete a novel serine protease (M.W. approximately 40,000), not found in unactivated

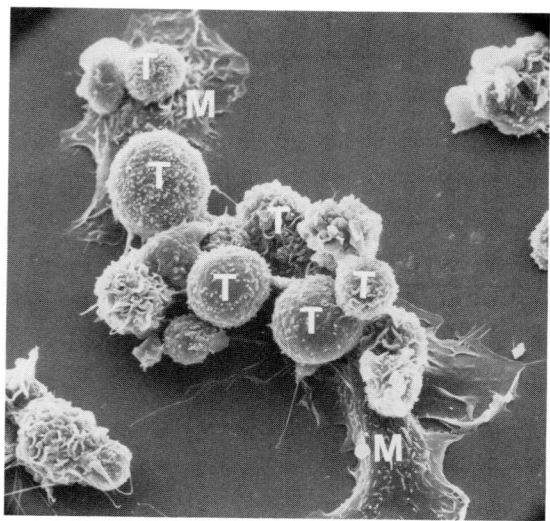

Fig. 16–4. Scanning electron micrograph of macrophages binding multiple tumor cells (× 3,800). M = macrophage; T = tumor cell. (Courtesy of Dr. Dolph O. Adams, Duke University Medical Center.)

macrophages.[2] The release of this cytolytic factor as well as the production of hydrogen peroxide by activated macrophages appears to be responsible for tumor cell killing.[148] Macrophages are also capable of killing tumor cells in the presence of antibody. This phenomenon is termed antibody-dependent cell-mediated cytotoxicity (ADCC) and does not require activated macrophages. Although the biochemical correlates of macrophage activation are not currently known, there are several functional changes including enhanced binding activity to tumor cells as well as enhanced secretion of the cytolytic protease.[102,128] Activated macrophages also have alterations in their cell surface characteristics, including a decrease of 5' nucleotidase and decreased numbers of mannose receptors.[56,96] Transmethylation reactions mediated by S-adenosyl-methionine are required for direct tumor cell lysis.[4]

How do clinically apparent tumors survive macrophage-mediated destruction? Tumors have been shown to produce factors that depress the ability of macrophages to accumulate at sites of inflammation in vivo and depress macrophage and monocyte chemotactic responsiveness in vitro.[149,153,200,209,223] Defects of monocyte chemotaxis in vitro have also been noted in humans with cancer. Interestingly, the defect is reversed by tumor removal.[199] The inhibitor of chemotaxis associated with neoplasms may be due to the synthesis by tumor cells of a protein with similarities to the P15E structural component of oncogenic retroviruses.[33,34] By releasing this immunosuppressive protein, cancer cells may protect themselves from macrophage-mediated immune destruction.

MACROPHAGES AS IMMUNOREGULATORY CELLS

The importance of macrophages as effector cells has been recognized for over a century. What is now apparent is that these cells are also essential in the afferent limb of the immune response. Macrophages are required, at some point, in almost all immunologic reactions and regulate the function of both B and T lymphocytes.[120,157,180,182] The regulatory aspect of macrophages in immune reactions begins with the antigen binding to the cell. The degree to which antigen is phagocytized and digested is of importance since this affects the quantity that will ultimately react with other immunocompetent cells. When administered in vivo, most antigen is destroyed by macrophages, with the fate of the remainder being determined in part by its site of administration. Antigen penetrating the circulation accumulates in splenic macrophages, whereas antigen administered in local tissue sites localizes in macrophages within draining lymphoid follicles.[230,231] Antigen bound to macrophages is taken up by an active metabolic process involving micropinocytosis and becomes associated with Ia gene products. Limited regions of antigen molecules act as determinants (epitopes) for the stimulation of specific clones of T cells in the generation of helper cells for antibody production. ''Antigen presentation'' is the phenomenon whereby macrophages alter antigen so that subsequent macrophage-lymphocyte interactions lead to the initiation of an immune response (see also Chap. 17). Antigen presentation by macrophages to lymphocytes occurs in the context of compatibility between these two cell types at the Ia locus.[279] Immune responses proceed only if Ia compatibility exists. A physical interaction between macrophages and lymphocytes appears to be necessary for subsequent immunologic responses to occur. There are some exceptions in the requirement of macrophages for activation of lymphocytes by antigen. Complex lipopolysaccharides and polysaccharides such as endotoxins appear to interact directly with B cells. Macrophage independent immune responses, however, appear to be the exception rather than the rule.

In addition to specific antigen presentation, macrophages also affect immune responses through the secretion of nonantigen-specific factors such as interleukin-1 (IL-1).[139,140] IL-1 is required for lymphocyte blastogenesis initiated by antigen or nonspecific mitogens. Macrophages can also inhibit immune responses by the secretion of prostaglandins.[6,108,142,259]

Role of Ia Expression. The expression of Ia antigens on macrophages is regulated via a specific soluble protein secreted by activated T-lymphocytes. This material has been termed macrophage-Ia-positive recruiting factor (MIRF). When injected intraperitoneally in mice, MIRF increases the percentage of Ia-positive macrophage from a basal level of less than 10% to up to 90%. MIRF is an immunoregulatory molecule that affects the differentiation of immature phagocytes derived from a bone marrow stem cell precursor into Ia-positive macrophages.[212] The expression of Ia on human mononuclear cells is affected by agents that change their phagocytic and secretory functions. Endotoxin and zymosan, a complex polysaccharide derived from yeast cell walls, enhance both phagocytic and secretory abilities of human monocytes, but reduce Ia positivity in macrophage preparations. This reduction in Ia expression correlates with decreased efficiency by the cells in antigen-induced regulatory functions.[276]

Other Macrophage Surface Antigens. Several other antigens on the surface of macrophages have been defined, but their function is as yet unknown. An antigen called Mac-1 is present on 90% of resident peritoneal macrophages, as well as on macrophages elicited by phlogistic stimuli. This antigen has been expressed on peritoneal macrophages, irrespective of whether they were resident cells or were elicited by either inflammatory agents or specific immune reactions. In all cases, the macrophages contained a similar amount of Mac-1 proteins of molecular weight 170,000 and 95,000 daltons. Mac-1 is thus a general marker for macrophages, and is expressed independently of Ia expression.[87] An additional series of four Mo antigens (Mo 1–4) defined by monoclonal antibodies has been described.[227]

Role of Dendritic Cells. A newly described nonlymphoid cell appears to be an important component of immune responses.[88,221] This cell has been called a dendritic cell because of its striking stellate appearance. Dendritic cells have potent antigen presentation functions and are strongly Ia-positive. They are adherent to surfaces, but do not express Fc receptors, and are nonphagocytic. The cells are thus not ''officially'' recognized as macrophages. They do function, however, in stimulating allogeneic, syngeneic, and soluble antigen responses. The dendritic cell may be equivalent to the ''interdigitating cell'' in the T-cell nodal region of the lymph node where antigen is known to localize. However, marker studies have not yet proved this conclusively.[108]

The elongated cell in human synovial tissue that

is sometimes called a dendritic cell has been isolated from synovial explants of patients with rheumatoid disease. This cell is a potent source of collagenase and should best be called a stellate cell.[50,271] These cells are Ia-positive and are not phagocytic[270] (see also Chap. 13).

EFFECT OF PHARMACOLOGIC AGENTS ON MACROPHAGE FUNCTION

Corticosteroids. Mononuclear phagocytes contain glucocorticoid receptors,[266] and glucocorticoids have a profound effect on macrophage function both in vivo and in vitro. Hydrocortisone given intravenously in humans induces a monocytopenia within four hours and is associated with depressed monocyte accumulation at inflammatory sites.[60] Alternate-day prednisone has less effect on monocyte function than does daily administration of the drug.[41] Corticosteroids also depress the release of monocytes from the bone marrow and decrease the formation of GM-GFU from bone marrow cells in vitro.[226,264] Monocytes isolated from individuals taking prednisone have depressed bactericidal activity in vitro, although chemotactic and phagocytic responsiveness is normal.[174] Treatment of human monocytes with corticosteroids in vitro, however, depresses their ability to respond to chemoattractants.[222] Similarly, incubation of monocytes with hydrocortisone depresses their ability to bind opsonized erythrocytes.[188] Other functions of monocytes depressed by glucocorticoids include the secretion of collagenase, elastase, and plasminogen activator.[82,247,264] Production of superoxide anion is also depressed by glucocorticoids,[119] as is differentiation of human monocytes to macrophages in vitro.[175] In contrast, human spontaneous monocyte-mediated cytotoxicity in vitro is enhanced by hydrocortisone treatment.[114]

Gold Compounds. Gold sodium thiomalate inhibits mixed leukocyte reactions of mononuclear cell preparations at doses of the drugs compatible with those attained by therapy in vivo.[84] Incubation of human blood monocytes with gold sodium thiomalate causes the cells to develop large intracytoplasmic vacuoles and diminishes pinocytosis and phagocytosis of IgG opsonized erythrocytes.[121] Gold depresses the phagocytic activity of macrophages isolated from rheumatoid synovium as well.[99] There may be some selectivity to the effect of gold in rheumatoid patients vis à vis normal subjects since suppression of monocyte phagocytosis is greater in the former.[47]

Cytotoxic Agents. These agents frequently decrease circulating monocyte levels, probably by affecting the development of monocytes in the bone marrow.[27,243] High doses of cyclophosphamide or methotrexate may also affect the accumulation of

macrophages at inflammatory sites.[27,64] Vincristine similarly depresses the ability of macrophages to accumulate at sites of infection.[155]

Penicillamine. In experimental animals, administration of D-penicillamine has a stimulatory effect on reticuloendothelial function. This effect is accompanied by an increased uptake of radio-labeled aggregated human gammaglobulin by rat peritoneal macrophages.[19]

Levamisole. This immunostimulatory drug was initially developed as an antiparasitic agent. It enhances monocyte chemotaxis in vitro and appears to reverse defects of monocyte function associated with certain viral infections such as influenza.[162,165]

MACROPHAGES IN RHEUMATIC DISEASES

The human immune system has evolved highly complex mechanisms designed to recognize specific epitopes on a variety of antigens. Nonetheless, the phagocytic cell is still central to the recognition and elimination of antigen, whether it be via fixed tissue macrophages as components of the reticuloendothelial system, or by wandering macrophages at tissue sites throughout the body. Macrophages participate in virtually all aspects of immunity. The properties that allow macrophages to be so efficient in destroying non-self render them capable of being major participants in the tissue destruction associated with inflammatory diseases. In RA, polymorphonuclear leukocytes are the predominant phagocytic cells in the synovial fluid, but macrophages predominate in the synovium.[78] Although the stimulus initiating the inflammatory event in RA is unknown, it is clear that synovial macrophages produce copious amounts of prostaglandins; release hydrolytic enzymes such as collagenase, elastase, and plasminogen activator; and secrete interleukin-1. The cartilage-degrading lysosomal enzymes, collagenase and elastase, are derived from macrophages in the synovial pannus that invades the surrounding hard tissues. Cartilage-specific collagen may activate macrophages and the alternative pathway of complement, thus interrelating two facets of the immunopathology of RA.[83] Proteases aid in superficial cartilage destruction by virtue of their ability to uncross-link collagen fibers, making them more susceptible to proteolytic destruction. Stellate synovial cells are stimulated by interleukin-1 to produce abundant amounts of collagenase. Early in the development of RA, cartilage loss with decreased proteoglycan content is manifested. Lysosomal proteases degrade aggregates of proteoglycans which, when released from cartilage as solubilized components, are then sensitive to further enzymatic attack. Interleukin-1 secreted by macrophages also stimulates lympho-

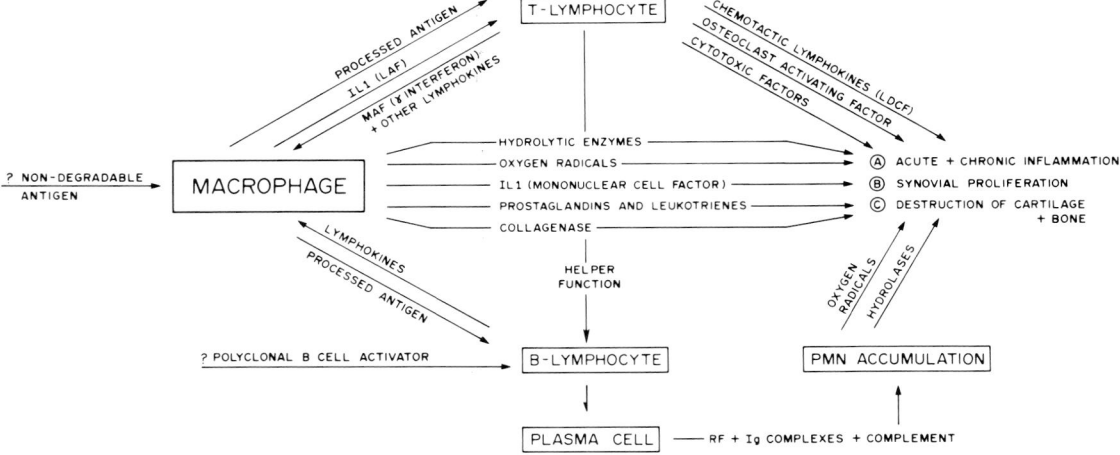

Fig. 16–5. Model for the pathogenesis of articular inflammation in rheumatoid arthritis. IL 1 = interleukin 1; LAF = lymphocyte activating factor; LDCG = lymphocyte-derived chemotactic factor; MAF = macrophage activating factor; RF = rheumatoid factor.

cytes to produce lymphokines, at least one of which, termed osteoclast-activating factor (OAF), appears to be involved in demineralization of bone. Prostaglandins, leukotrienes, and other arachidonic acid metabolites may be responsible for long-term leaching of mineral from bony matrix. The net effect of an acute and chronic inflammatory response in the synovium is continued cellular influx, proliferation, and invasion of synovium into the surrounding structures of the joint (Fig. 16–5) (see also Chaps. 35 and 37).

REFERENCES

1. Abboud, C.N., et al.: Hydrophobic adsorption chromatography of colony-stimulating activities and erythroid-enhancing activity from the human monocyte-like cell line. G.C.T. Blood, 58:1148, 1981.
2. Adams, D.O.: The granulomatous inflammatory responses. Am. J. Pathol., 84:163–191, 1976.
3. Adams, D.O., Johnson, W.J., and Marino, P.A.: Mechanisms of target recognition and destruction in macrophage-mediated tumor cytotoxicity. Fed. Proc., 41:2212, 1982.
4. Adams, D.O., Pike, M.C., and Snyderman, R.: The role of transmethylation reactions in regulating the binding of BCG-activated murine macrophages to neoplastic target cells. J. Immunol., 127:225, 1981.
5. Alitalo, K., Hovi, T., and Vaheri, A.: Fibronectin is produced by human macrophages. J. Exp. Med., 151:602, 1980.
6. Allison, A.C.: Mechanisms by which activated macrophages inhibit lymphocyte responses. In Immunological Review 40. Copenhagen, Munksgaard, 1978.
7. Allison, A.C., Cardella, D., and Davies, P.: Immune complexes and induced release of lysosomal enzymes from mononuclear phagocytes in the pathogenesis of rheumatoid arthritis. In Immunological Aspects of Rheumatoid Arthritis, Rheumatology. Vol. 6. Edited by J. Clot, and J. Sany. Basel, S. Karger, 1975.
8. Altman, L.C., et al.: A human mononuclear leukocyte chemotactic factor: Characterization, specificity, and kinetics of production by homologous leukocytes. J. Immunol., 110:801, 1973.
9. Anderson, C.L., and Grey, H.M.: Physicochemical separation of two distinct Fc receptors on murine macrophage-like cell lines. J. Immunol., 121:648, 1978.
10. Arend, W.P., and Mannik, M.: The macrophage receptor for IgG: Number and affinity of binding sites. J. Immunol., 110:1455, 1973.
11. Arnou, B., et al.: Release of platelet activating factor and arachidonic acid metabolites from alveolar macrophages. Agents Actions, 11:555, 1981.
12. Aune, T.M., and Pierce, C.W.: Identification and initial characterization of a nonspecific suppressor factor (macrophage-SF) produced by soluble immune response suppressor (SIRS)-treated macrophages. J. Immunol., 127:1828, 1981.
13. Babior, B.M.: Oxygen-dependent microbial killing by phagocytes. N. Engl. J. Med., 298:659, 1978.
14. Basu, S.K., et al.: Biochemical and genetic studies of the apoprotein E secreted by mouse macrophages and human monocytes. J. Biol. Chem., 257:9788, 1982.
15. Basu, S.K., et al.: Mouse macrophages synthesize and secrete a protein resembling apolipoprotein E. Proc. Natl. Acad. Sci. U.S.A., 78:7545, 1981.
15a. Basu, S.K., Goldstein, J.L., and Brown, M.S.: Independent pathways for secretion of cholesterol and apolipoprotein E by macrophages. Science, 219:871, 1983.
16. Benyunes, M.C., and Snyderman, R.: Characterization of an oligopeptide chemoattractant receptor on human blood monocytes using a new radioligand. Blood, 63:588, 1984.
17. Bianco, C., Eden, A., and Cohn, Z.A.: The induction of macrophage spreading: Role of coagulation factors and the complement system. J. Exp. Med., 144:1531, 1976.
18. Bianco, C., Griffin, F.M., Jr., and Silverstein, S.C.: Studies of the macrophage complement receptor. Alteration of receptor function upon macrophage activation. J. Exp. Med., 141:1278, 1975.
19. Binderup, L., Bramm, E., and Arrigoni-Martelli, E.: Effect of D-penicillamine in vitro and in vivo on macrophage phagocytosis. Biochem. Pharmacol., 29:2273, 1980.
20. Bitterman, P.B., et al.: Human alveolar macrophage growth factor for fibroblasts. Regulation and partial characterization. J. Clin. Invest., 70:806, 1982.
21. Blusse van, O., Abbas, A., and van Furth, R.: Origin, kinetics, and characteristics of pulmonary macrophages in the normal steady state. J. Exp. Med., 149:1504, 1979.
22. Boldt, D.H., Chan, S.K., and Keaton, K.: Cell surface alpha 1-protease inhibitor on human peripheral mononuclear cells in culture. J. Immunol., 129:1830, 1982.

23. Boltz-Nitulescu, G., Plummer, J.M., and Spiegelberg, H.L.: Fc receptors for IgE on mouse macrophages and macrophage-like cell lines. J. Immunol., *128*:2265, 1982.

24. Brade, V., and Bentley, C.: Synthesis and release of complement components by macrophages. *In* Mononuclear Phagocytes: Functional Aspects. Edited by R. van Furth. The Netherlands, Martinus Nijhoff, 1980.

25. Braidman, L.P., et al.: Evidence for a steroid receptor in rheumatoid synovial tissue cells. Agents Actions (Suppl.), 7:233, 1980.

26. Broxmeyer, H.E., et al.: Monocyte-macrophage-derived acidic isoferritins: Normal feedback regulators of granulocyte-macrophage progenitor cells in vitro. Blood, 60:595, 1982.

27. Buhles, W.C., Jr., and Shifrine, M.: Effects of cyclophosphamide on macrophage numbers, functions and progenitor cells. J. Reticuloendothel. Soc., 21:285, 1977.

28. Bryne, G.I., and Faubian, C.L.: Lymphokine-mediated microbiostatic mechanisms restrict *Chlamydia psittaci* growth in macrophages. J. Immunol., *128*:469, 1982.

29. Byvoet, O.L., et al.: ADP in Paget's disease of bone. Role of the Mononuclear phagocyte system. Arthritis Rheum., 23:1193, 1980.

30. Calcagno, M., et al.: Evidence of the existence of a factor that induces Fc receptors on bone marrow cells. Blood, 59:756, 1982.

31. Chang, J., Liu, M.C., and Newcombe, D.S.: Identification of two monohydroxyeicosatetraenoic acids synthesized by human pulmonary macrophages. Am. Rev. Respir. Dis., *126*:457, 1982.

32. Chenoweth, D.E., and Hugli, T.E.: Demonstration of specific C5a receptor on intact human polymorphonuclear leukocytes. Proc. Natl. Acad. Sci. U.S.A., 75:3943, 1978.

33. Cianciolo, G.J., et al.: Murine malignant cells synthesize a 19,000 dalton protein which is physiochemically and antigenically related to the immunosuppressive retroviral protein, P15E. J. Exp. Med., *158*:885, 1983.

34. Cianciolo, G.J., et al.: Inhibitors of monocyte responses to chemotaxins are present in human cancerous effusions and react with monoclonal antibodies to the P15E structural protein of retroviruses. J. Clin. Invest., 68:831, 1981.

35. Cianciolo, G.J., and Snyderman, R.: Monocyte responsiveness to chemotactic stimuli is a property of a subpopulation of cells that can respond to multiple chemoattractants. J. Clin. Invest., 67:60, 1981.

36. Claeys, M., et al.: 15-HETE formation by rabbit peritoneal tissue. Agents Actions, *11*:589, 1981.

37. Clark, R.A., and Szot, S.: Chemotactic factor inactivation by stimulated human neutrophils mediated by myeloperoxidase-catalyzed methionine oxidation. J. Immunol., *128*:1507, 1982.

38. Cochrane, C., Spragg, R., and Revak, S.: Studies on the pathogenesis of the adult respiratory distress syndrome: Evidence of oxidant activity in bronchoalveolar lavage fluid. J. Clin. Invest., 71:754, 1983.

39. Cohn, Z.A.: The activation of mononuclear phagocytes: Fact, fancy, and future. J. Immunol., *121*:813, 1978.

40. Czop, J.K., McGowan, S.E., and Center, D.M.: Opsonin-independent phagocytosis by human alveolar macrophages; augmentation by human plasma fibronectin. Am. Rev. Respir. Dis., *125*:607, 1982.

41. Dale, D.C., Fauci, A.S., and Wolff, S.M.: Alternate-day prednisone. Leukocyte kinetics and susceptibility to infections. N. Engl. J. Med., *291*:1154, 1974.

42. Daniele, R.P., Diamond, M.S., and Holian, A.: Demonstration of a formyl peptide receptor on lung macrophages; correlation of binding properties with chemotaxis and release of superoxide anion. Am. Rev. Respir. Dis., *126*:274, 1982.

43. David, J.R.: Macrophage activation by lymphocyte mediators. *In* Infection and Immunity in the Rheumatic Diseases. Edited by D.C. Dumonde. London, Blackwell Scientific, 1974.

44. David, J.R., et al.: MIF/MAF-macrophage interactions: Biochemical characterization of a putative glycolipid receptor for MIF and the existence and properties of two distinct MIFs. *In* Mononuclear Phagocytes: Functional Aspects. Edited by R. van Furth. The Hague. Martinus Nijhoff, 1980.

45. Davies, P., et al.: Synthesis of arachidonic acid oxygenation products by various mononuclear phagocyte populations. *In* Mononuclear Phagocytes: Functional Aspects. Edited by R. van Furth. The Hague. Martinus Nijhoff, 1980.

46. Davies, P., and Allison, A.C.: The macrophage as a secretory cell in chronic inflammation. Agents Actions, 6:60, 1976.

47. Davis, P., Miller, C.L., and Johnston, C.A.: Effect of gold salts on adherent mononuclear cells in tissue culture. J. Rheumatol. (Suppl.), 5:98, 1979.

48. Dayer, J.M., et al.: Purification of a factor from human blood monocyte which stimulates production of collagenase and PGG2 by cells cultured from rheumatoid synovial tissues. FEBS Lett., *124*:253, 1981.

49. Dayer, J.M.: Production of collagenase and prostaglandins by isolated adherent rheumatoid synovial cells. Proc. Natl. Acad. Sci. U.S.A., 73:945, 1976.

50. Dayer, J.M., and Krane, S.M.: The interaction of immunocompetent cells and chronic inflammation as exemplified by rheumatoid arthritis. Clin. Rheum. Dis. 4:517, 1978.

51. de Ceulaer, C., Papagoglau, S., and Whaley, K.: Increased biosynthesis of C components by cultured monocytes, synovial fluid macrophages and synovial membrane cells from plasma. J. Immunol., *41*:37, 1980.

52. Debanne, M.T., Bell, R., and Dolovich, J.: Uptake of proteinase-macroglobulin complexes by macrophages. Biochim. Biophys. Acta., *411*:295, 1975.

53. Diamond, B., Bloom, B.R., and Scharff, M.D.: The Fc receptors of primary and cultured phagocytic cells studied with homogeneous antibodies. J. Immunol., *121*:1978, 1978.

54. Diamond, B., and Scharff, M.D.: IgG1 and IgG2b share the Fc receptor on mouse macrohages. J. Immunol., *125*:631, 1980.

55. Diamond, B., and Yelton, D.E.: A new Fc receptor on mouse macrophages binding IgG3. J. Exp. Med., *153*:514, 1981.

56. Edelson, P.J.: Macrophage ecto-enzymes: Their identification, metabolism, and control. *In* Mononuclear Phagocytes: Functional Aspects. Edited by R. van Furth. The Hague, Martinus Nijhoff, 1980.

57. Einstein, L.P., Schneeberger, E.E., and Colten, H.R.: Synthesis of the second component of complement by long-term primary cultures of human monocytes. J. Exp. Med., *43*:114, 1976.

58. Ericsson, J.L.E.: Origin and structure of the osteoclast. *In* Mononuclear Phagocytes: Functional Aspects. Edited by R. van Furth. The Hague, Martinus Nijhoff, 1980.

59. Evans, C., Mgars, D., and Cosgrove, C.: Release of neutal proteinase from mononuclear phagocytes and synovial cells in response to cartilaginous wear particles in vitro. Biochim. Biophys. Acta, *677*:287, 1981.

60. Fauci, A.S., and Dale, D.C.: The effect of in vivo hydrocortisone on subpopulations of human lymphocytes. J. Clin. Invest., *52*:240, 1974.

61. Fearon, D.T.: Identification of the membrane glycoprotein that is the C3b receptor of the human erythrocyte, polymorphonuclear leukocyte, and monocyte, J. Exp. Med., *152*:20, 1980.

62. Finbloom, D.S., and Metzger, H.: Binding of immunoglobulin E to the receptor on rat peritoneal macrophages. J. Immunol., *129*:2004, 1982.

63. Ford-Hutchinson, A.W., et al.: Leukotriene B, a potent chemokinetic and aggregating substance released from polymorphonuclear leukocytes. Nature, *286*:264, 1980.

64. Gadeberg, O.V., Rhodes, J.M., and Larsen, S.: The effect of various immunosuppressive agents on mouse peritoneal macrophages and on the in vitro phagocytosis of *Escherichia coli* 05:K3:H5 and degradation of ^{125}I-labelled HSA-antibody complexes by these cells. Immunology, 28:59, 1975.

65. Gallin, J.I., et al.: Agents that increase cyclic AMP inhibit

accumulation of cGMP and depress human monocyte locomotion. J. Immunol., *120*:492, 1978.

66. Gallin, J.I., and Kaplan, A.P.: Mononuclear cell chemotactic activity of kallikrein and plasminogen activator and its inhibition by C1 inhibitor and α2-macroglobulin. J. Immunol., *113*:1928, 1974.

67. Geczy, C.L., and Meyer, P.A.: Leukocyte procoagulant activity in man: An in vitro correlate of delayed-type hypersensitivity. J. Immunol., *128*:331, 1982.

68. Gianturco, N., et al.: Hypertriglyceridemic very low density lipoproteins induce triglyceride synthesis and accumulation in mouse peritoneal macrophages. J. Clin. Invest., *70*:168, 1982.

69. Goetzl, E.J., and Pickett, W.C.: The human PMN leukocyte chemotactic activity of complex hydroxy-eicosatetraenoic acids (HETEs). J. Immunol., *125*:1789, 1980.

70. Reference deleted.

71. Goldstein, J.L., et al.: Binding site on macrophages that mediates uptake and degradation of acetylated low density lipoprotein, producing massive cholesterol deposition. Proc. Natl. Acad. Sci. U.S.A., *76*:333, 1979.

72. Gordon, S.: Lysozyme and plasminogen activator:constitutive and induced secretory products of mononuclear phagocytes. *In* Mononuclear Phagocytes: Functional Aspects. Edited by R. van Furth. The Hague, Martinus Nijhoff, 1980.

73. Gordon, S.: Macrophage neutral proteinase and chronic inflammation. Ann. N.Y. Acad. Sci., *278*:176, 1976.

74. Gordon, S., Todd, J., and Cohn, Z.A.: In vitro synthesis and secretion of lysozyme by mononuclear phagocytes. J. Exp. Med., *139*:1228, 1974.

75. Gotze, O., et al.: The stimulation of mononuclear phagocytes by components of the classical and the alternative pathways of complement activation. *In* Mononuclear Phagocytes: Functional Aspects. Edited by R. van Furth. The Hague, Martinus Nijhoff, 1980.

76. Goud, J.L.M., Schotte, C., and van Furth, R.: Identification and characterization of the monoblast in mononuclear phagocyte colonies grown in vitro. J. Exp. Med., *142*:1180, 1975.

77. Goud, J.L.M., and van Furth, R.: Proliferative characteristics of monoblasts grown in vitro. J. Exp. Med., *142*:1200, 1975.

78. Greenberg, P., and Zvaifler, N.J.: Immunobiology of rheumatoid arthritis. *In* Pathobiology Annual. Vol. 6. Edited by H. Ioachim. New York, Appleton-Century Crofts, 1976.

79. Grey, H.M., and Anderson, C.L.: Structural characteristics of Fc receptors on macrophages. *In* Mononuclear Phagocytes: Functional Aspects. Edited by R. van Furth. The Hague, Martinus Nijhoff, 1980.

80. Griffin, F.M., Jr., et al.: Studies on the Mechanism of phagocytosis. I. Requirements for circumferential attachment of particle–bound ligands to specific receptors on the macrophage plasma membrane. J. Exp. Med., *142*:1263, 1975.

81. Griffin, F.M., and Silverstein, S.: Segmental response of the macrophage plasma membrane to a phagocytic stimulus. J. Exp. Med., *139*:323, 1974.

82. Hamilton, J., Vassalli, J.D., and Reich, E.: Macrophage plasminogen activator: Induction by asbestos is blocked by anti-inflammatory steroids. J. Exp. Med., *144*:1689, 1976.

83. Hanauskeok-Abel, H.M., Pointz, B.F., and Schorlemmer, H.U.: Cartilage-specific collagen activates macrophages and the alternative pathway of C: Evidence for an immunopathogenic concept of RA. Ann. Rheum. Dis., *41*:168, 1982.

84. Harth, M., and Stiller, C.R.: Inhibitory effects of gold and other drugs on mononuclear cell responses: A comparison. J. Rheumatol. (Suppl.), *5*:112, 1979.

85. Heusser, C.H., Anderson, C.L., and Grey, H.M.: Receptors for IgG: Subclass specificity of receptors on different mouse cell types and the definition of two distinct receptors on a macrophage cell line. J. Exp. Med., *145*:131, 1977.

86. Higgins, T.J., et al.: Possible role of macrophage gly-

colipids as receptors for migration inhibitory factor (MIF). J. Immunol., *121*:880, 1978.

87. Ho, M.K., and Springer, T.A.: Mac-1 antigen: Quantitative expression in macrophage population and tissues, and immunofluorescent localization in spleen. J. Immunol., *128*:2281, 1982.

88. Hoefsand, E.C.M.: Macrophages, Langerhans' cells, interdigitating and dendrite accessory cells: A summary. Adv. Exp. Med. Biol., *155*:463, 1982.

89. Holland, P., Holland, N.H., and Cohn, Z.A.: The selective inhibition of macrophage phagocytic receptors by antimembrane antibodies. J. Exp. Med., *135*:458, 1982.

90. Hovi, T., Mosher, D., and Vaheri, A.: Cultured human monocytes synthesize and secrete α2-macroglobulin. J. Exp. Med., *145*:1580, 1978.

91. Howell, D.S., et al.: Presence and role of lysozyme in human osteoarthritic cartilage. J. Rheumatol., *1*:31, 1974.

92. Huber, H., et al.: Human monocytes: Distinct receptor sites for the third component of complement and for immunoglobulin G. Science, *162*:1281, 1968.

93. Hugli, T.E.: The structural basis for anaphylatoxin and chemotactic functions of C3a, C4a, and C5a. *In* Critical Reviews in Immunology I, 4. Boca Raton, Fl., CRC Press Review, 1981.

94. Hugli, T.E., and Muller-Eberhard, H.J.: Anaphylatoxins:C3a and C5a. Adv. Immunol., *26*:1, 1978.

95. Hurst, N.P., and Nuki, G.: Evidence for defect of C-mediated phagocytes by monocytes from patients with RA and cutaneous vasculitis. Br. Med. J., *282*:2081, 1980.

96. Imber, M.J., et al.: Selective reduction of mannose specific binding on activated vs. inflammatory macrophage monolayers. J. Biol. Chem., *257*:5129, 1982.

97. Isaacson, P., et al.: Alpha-1-antitrypsin in human macrophages. J. Clin. Pathol., *34*:982, 1981.

98. Jensen, J., Snyderman, R., and Mergenhagen, S.E.: Chemotactic activity: A property of guinea pig, C5 anaphylatoxin. *In* Cellular and Humoral Mechanisms in Anaphylaxis and Allergy. Proceedings of the Third International Congress on Allergy and Anaphylaxis. Basel, Switzerland, 1969.

99. Jessop, J.D., and Wilkins, M.: The effect of gold salts on the phagocytic activity of synovial macrophages in organ culture. J. Rheumatol. (Suppl.), *5*:137, 1979.

100. Johnston, R.B., Jr.: Oxygen metabolism and the microbicidal activity of macrophages. Fed. Proc., *39*:93, 1978.

101. Johnston, R.B., Jr., Chadwick, D.A., and Pabst, M.J.: Release of superoxide anion by macrophages: Effect of in vivo or in vitro priming. *In* Mononuclear Phagocytes: Functional Aspects. Edited by R. van Furth. The Hague, Martinus Nijhoff, 1980.

102. Johnston, W.J., Whisnant, C.C., and Adams, D.O.: The binding of BCG-activated macrophages to tumor targets stimulates secretion of cytolytic factor. J. Immunol., *127*:1787, 1981.

103. Kaltreider, H.B.: Alveolar macrophages. Enhancers or suppressors of pulmonary immune reactivity? (Editorial). Chest, *82*:261, 1982.

104. Kaplan, A.P.: The Hageman factor dependent pathways of human plasma. Microvasc. Res., *8*:92, 1974.

105. Karnovsky, M.L.: Biochemical characteristics of activated macrophages. Ann. N.Y. Acad. Sci., *256*:266, 1975.

106. Karnovsky, M.L., and Lazdins, J.K.: Biochemical criteria for activated macrophages. J. Immunol., *121*:809, 1978.

107. Katz, A.B., Papper, D.S., and Ewart, M.R.: Generation of chemotactic activity for leukocytes by the action of thrombin on human fibrinogen. Nature, *24*:56, 1973.

108. Katz, D.R., et al.: A comparative study of accessory cells derived from the peritoneum and from solid tissues. Adv. Exp. Med. Biol., *155*:421, 1982.

109. Kay, G.E., Lane, B.C., and Snyderman, R.: Induction of selective biological responses to chemoattractants in a human monocyte-like cell line. Infect. Immun., *41*:1166, 1983.

110. Kay, M.B.: Mechanism of removal of senescent cells by

human macrophages in situ. Proc. Natl. Acad. Aci. U.S.A., 72:3521, 1975.

111. Kennerly, D.A., et al.: Diacylglycerol metabolism in mast cells: A potential role in membrane fusion and arachidonic acid release. J. Exp. Med., 150:1039, 1979.
112. Klebanoff, S.J.: Oxygen intermediates and the microbicidal event. In Mononuclear Phagocytes: Functional Aspects. Edited by R. van Furth. The Hague, Martinus Nijhoff, 1980.
113. Klebanoff, S.J.: A peroxidase-mediated antimicrobial system in leukocytes. J. Clin. Invest., 46:1078, 1967.
114. Kleinerman, E.S., et al.: Pharmacology of human spontaneous monocyte-mediated cytotoxicity: I. Enhancement by salicylates and steroids. Arthritis Rheum., 24:774, 1981.
115. Koren, H.S., Handwerger, B.S., and Wunderlich, J.R.: Identification of macrophage-like characteristics in a cultured murine tumor line. J. Immunol., 114:894, 1975.
116. Kriegler, A.B., et al.: Partial purification and characterization of a growth factor for macrophage progenitor cells with high proliferative potential in mouse bone marrow. Blood, 60:503, 1982.
117. Lapetina, E.G., and Cuatrecasas, P.: Stimulation of phosphatidic acid production in platelets precedes the formation of arachidonate and parallels the release of serotonin. Biochim. Biophys. Acta, 573:394, 1979.
118. Lawley, T.J.: Immune complexes and RES function in human diseases. J. Invest Dermatol., 74:339, 1980.
119. Lehmeyer, J.E., and Johnston, R.B., Jr.: Effect of anti-inflammatory drugs and agents that elevate intracellular cyclic AMP on the release of toxic oxygen metabolites by phagocytes: Studies in a model of tissue-bound IgG. Clin. Immunol. Immunopathol., 9:482, 1978.
120. Lipsky, P.E., and Rosenthal, A.S.: Macrophage-lymphocyte interaction I. Characteristics of the antigen-independent binding of guinea pig thymocytes to syngeneic macrophages. J. Exp. Med., 138:900, 1973.
121. Lipsky, P.E., Ugai, K., and Ziff, M.: Alterations in human monocyte structure and function induced by incubation with gold sodium thiomalate. J. Rheumatol. (Suppl.), 5:130, 1979.
122. Littman, B.H., and Ruddy, S.: Accelerated synthesis of second complement component (C2) by mononuclear cells from synovial fluid. Clin. Res., 25(3):485A, 1977.
123. Lockley, R.M., Wilson, C.B., and Klebanoff, S.J.: Role of endogenous and acquired peroxidase in the toxoplasmacidal activity of murine and human mononuclear phagocytes. J. Clin. Invest., 69:1099, 1982.
124. Loor, F., and Roelants, G.E.: The dynamic state of the macrophage plasma membrane. Attachment and fate of immunoglobulin, antigen and lectins. Eur. J. Immunol., 4:649, 1974.
125. Lyberg, T., et al.: Effect of immune-complex containing sera from patients with rheumatic diseases on thromboplastin activity of monocytes. Thromb. Res., 25:193, 1982.
126. Mackaness, G.B.: Influence of immunologically committed lymphocytes on macrophage activity in vivo. J. Exp. Med., 129:973, 1969.
127. Maino, V.C., Hayman, M.J., and Crumpton, M.J.: Relationship between enhanced turnover of phosphatidylinositol and lymphocyte activation by mitogens. Biochem. J., 146:247, 1975.
128. Marino, P.A., and Adams, D.O.: Interaction of bacillus calmette-guerin-activated macrophages and neoplastic cells in vitro. Cell Immunol., 54:11, 1980.
129. Martin, T.R, et al.: Leukotriene B₄ production by the human alveolar macrophage: A potential mechanism for amplifying inflammation in the lung. Am. Rev. Respir. Dis., 129:106, 1984.
130. McCombs, C.C., et al.: Human alveolar macrophages suppress the proliferative response of peripheral blood lymphocytes. Chest, 82:266, 1982.
131. McCord, J.M.: Free radical and inflammation: Protection of synovial fluid by superoxide dismutase. Science, 185:529, 1974.
132. McPhail, L.C., and Snyderman, R.: Oxygen-dependent microbicidal activity of leukocytes. In Contemporary Top-

ics in Immunobiology. "Regulation of Leukocyte Function." Edited by Ralph Snyderman. New York, Plenum Press. In press, 1984.
133. Meltzer, M.S., et al.: Macrophage activation for tumor cytotoxicity: Analysis of intermediary reactions. J. Reticuloendoethel. Soc., 26:403, 1979.
134. Meltzer, M.S., Stevenson, M.D., and Leonard, E.J.: Characterization of macrophage chemotoxins in tumor cell cultures and comparison with lymphocyte-derived chemotactic factors. Cancer Res., 37:721, 1977.
135. Meuret, G., Batara, E., and Furste, H.O.: Monocytopoiesis in normal man: Pool size, proliferation activity and DNA synthesis time of promonocytes. Acta Haematol., 54:261, 1975.
136. Michl, J., Ohlbaum, D.J., and Silverstein, S.C.: 2-Deoxyglucose selectively inhibits Fc and complement receptor-mediated phagocytosis in mouse peritoneal macrophages. I. Description of the inhibitory effect. J. Exp. Med., 144:1465, 1976.
137. Michl, J., Ohlbaum, D.J., and Silverstein, S.C.: 2-Deoxyglucose selectively inhibits Fc and complement receptor-mediated phagocytosis in mouse peritoneal macrophages.II. Dissociation of the inhibitory effect of 2-deoxyglucose on phagocytosis and ATP generation. J. Exp. Med., 144:1484, 1976.
138. Mizel, S.B., et al.: Stimulation of rheumatoid synovial cells: Collagenase and prostaglandin production by partially purified lymphocyte activating factor (IL-1). Proc. Natl. Acad. Sci. U.S.A., 78:2474, 1981.
139. Mizel, S.B., and Mizel, D.: Purification to apparent homogeneity of murine interleukin 1. J. Immunol., 126:834, 1981.
140. Moller, G.: Interleukins and lymphocyte activation. Immunol. Rev., 63:1, 1982.
141. Monahan, R.A., Dvorak, H.F., and Dvorak, A.M.: Ultrastructural localization of nonspecific esterase activity in guinea pig and human monocytes, macrophages, and lymphocytes. Blood, 58:1089, 1981.
142. Morley, J.: Anti-inflammatory effects of prostaglandins. In Rheumatoid Arthritis. Edited by J.L. Gordon, and B. Hazelman. Amsterdam, Elsevier, 1977.
143. Muller, W.A., Steinman, R.M., and Cohn, Z.A.: Membrane flow during endocytosis. In Mononuclear Phagocytes: Functional Aspects. Edited by R. van Furth. The Hague, Martinus Nijhoff, 1980.
144. Nakagawara, A., et al.: Lymphokines enhance the capacity of human monocytes to secrete reactive oxygen intermediates. J. Clin. Invest., 70:1042, 1982.
145. Nathan, C.F.: The release of hydrogen peroxide from mononuclear phagocytes and its role in extracellular cytolysis. In Mononuclear Phagocytes: Functional Aspects. Edited by R. van Furth. The Hague, Martinus Nijhoff, 1980.
146. Nathan, C.F., et al.: Identification of interferon-γ as the lymphokine that activates human macrophage oxidative metabolism and antimicrobial activity. J. Exp. Med., 158:670, 1983.
147. Nathan, C.F., et al.: Extracellular cytolysis by activated macrophages and granulocytes. II. Hydrogen peroxide as a mediator of cytotoxicity. J. Exp. Med., 149:100, 1979.
148. Nathan, C.F., and Cohn, Z.A.: Role of oxygen dependent mechanisms in antibody-induced lysis of tumor cells by activated macrophages. J. Exp. Med., 152:198, 1980.
149. Nelson, M., and Nelson, D.S.: Macrophages and resistance to tumors. I. Inhibition of delayed-type hypersensitivity reactions by tumor cells and by soluble products affecting macrophages. Immunology, 34:277, 1978.
150. Nogueira, N., et al.: Trypanosoma cruzi: Induction of microbicidal activity in human mononuclear phagocytes. J. Immunol., 128:2142, 1982.
151. Nogueira, N., and Cohn, Z.A.: Trypanosoma cruzi: Mechanisms of entry and intracellular fate in mammalian cells. J. Exp. Med., 143:1402, 1976.
152. Normann, S.I., and Sorkin, F.: Macrophages and natural killer cells. Regulation and function. Adv. Exp. Med. Biol., 155:1, 1982.
153. Normann, S.J., and Sorkin, F.: Inhibition of macrophage

chemotaxis by neoplastic and other rapidly proliferating cells in vitro. Cancer Res., *37*:705, 1977.

154. North, R.J.: The concept of the activated macrophage. J. Immunol., *121*:806, 1978.

155. North, R.J.: Suppression of cell-mediated immunity to infection by an antimitotic drug. Further evidence that migrant macrophages express immunity. J. Exp. Med., *132*:535, 1970.

156. North, R.J., and Mackaness, G.B.: Immunological control of macrophage proliferation in vitro. Infect. Immun., *8*:68, 1973.

157. Panayi, G.S., Corregall, V., and Youlden, L.F.: Immunoregulation in the rheumatic diseases. Scand. J. Rheumatol. (Suppl.), *38*:9, 1982.

158. Pelus, L.M.: Association between CFU–GM expression of HLA-DR antigen and control for granulocyte and macrophage production. A new role for prostaglandin E1. J. Clin. Invest., *70*:568, 1982.

159. Pleus, L.M., Broxmeyer, H.G., and Moore, M.A.: Regulation of human myelopoiesis by prostaglandin E and lactoferrin. Cell Tissue Kinet., *14*:515, 1981.

160. Perri, R.T., et al.: Fibronectin enhances in vitro monocyte-macrophage-mediated tumoricidal activity. Blood, *60*:430, 1982.

161. Piessens, W.F.: Increased binding of tumor cells by macrophages activated in vitro with lymphocyte mediators. Cell. Immunol., *35*:303, 1978.

162. Pike, M.C., Daniels, C.A., and Snyderman, R.: Influenza induced depression of monocyte chemotaxis: Reversal by levamisole. Cell. Immunol., *32*:234, 1977.

163. Pike, M.C., and Snyderman, R.: Transmethylation reactions regulate affinity and functional activity of chemotactic factor receptors on macrophages. Cell, *28*:107, 1982.

164. Pike, M.C., and Snyderman, R.: Transmethylation reactions are required for initial morphologic and biochemical responses of human monocytes to chemoattractants. J. Immunol., *127*:1444, 1981.

165. Pike, M.C., and Snyderman, R.: Augmentation of human monocyte chemotaxis response by levamisole. Nature, *261*:136, 1976.

166. Postlethwaite, A.E., et al.: Induction of fibroblast chemotaxis by fibronectin: Localization of the chemotactic region to a 140k nongelatin binding fragment. J. Exp. Med., *153*:494, 1981.

167. Postlethwaite, A.E., and Kang, A.: Collagen and collagen peptide-induced chemotaxis of human monocytes. J. Exp. Med., *143*:1299, 1976.

168. Postlethwaite, A.E., and Snyderman, R.: Characterization of a cell mediated reaction in the guinea pig. J. Immunol., *114*:274, 1975.

169. Rabellino, E.M., Ross, G.D., and Polley, M.J.: Membrane receptors of mouse leukocytes. I. Two types of complement receptors for different regions of C3. J. Immunol., *120*:879, 1978.

170. Ragsdale, C.G., and Arend, W.P.: Neutral protease secretion by human monocytes. Effect of surface-bound immune complexes. J. Exp. Med., *149*:954, 1979.

171. Ralph, P.: Functions of macrophage cell lines. *In* Mononuclear Phagocytes: Functional Aspects. Edited by R. van Furth. The Hague, Martinus Nijhoff, 1980.

172. Remold, H.G.: Requirement for α-L-fucose on the macrophage membrane receptor for MIF. J. Exp. Med., *138*:1065, 1973.

173. Rhodes, J.: Altered expression of human monocyte Fc receptors in malignant disease. Nature, *265*:253, 1977.

174. Rinehart, J.J., et al.: Effects of corticosteroid therapy on human monocyte function. N. Engl. J. Med., *292*:236, 1975.

175. Rinehart, J.J., Wuest, D., and Ackerman, G.A.: Corticosteroid alteration of human monocyte to macrophage differentiation. J. Immunol., *129*:1436, 1982.

176. Rittenhouse-Simmons, S.: Production of diglyceride from phosphatidylinositol in activated human platelets. J. Clin. Invest., *63*:580, 1979.

177. Roberts, N.H., Jr., et al.: Virus-induced interferon production by human macrophages. J. Immunol., *123*:365, 1979.

178. Rocklin, R.E.: Role of monosaccharides in the interaction of two lymphocyte mediators with their target cells. J. Immunol., *116*:816, 1976.

179. Rodley, G.E., et al.: Defective bactericidal activity of monocytes in fatal granulomatous disease. Blood, *33*:813, 1969.

180. Rosenthal, A.L., and Shevach, E.M.: The function of macrophages in T-lymphocyte antigen recognition. *In* Contemporary Topics in Immunobiology. Edited by W.O. Weigle. New York, Plenum Publishing Corp., 1976.

181. Ruco, L.P., and Meltzer, M.S.: Macrophage activation for tumor cytotoxicity: Induction of tumoricidal macrophages by PPD in BCG immune mice. Cell. Immunol., *32*:203, 1977.

182. Russell, I.J., and Tomasi, T.B.: Mechanisms and abnormalities of immune regulation. *In* Pathobiology Annual. Edited by H.L. Ioachim. New York, Raven Press, 1978.

183. Sandler, J.A., et al.: The effect of serotonin (5-hydroxytryptamine) and derivatives on guanosine 3′,5′-monophosphate on human monocytes. J. Clin. Invest., *55*:431, 1975.

184. Sciffmann, E., Corcoran, B., and Wahl, S.: N-formylmethionyl peptides as chemoattractants for leukocytes. Proc. Natl. Acad. Sci. U.S.A., *72*:1059, 1975.

185. Schnyder, J., and Baggiolini, M.: Secretion of lysosomal enzymes by macrophages. *In* Mononuclear Phagocytes: Functional Aspects. Edited by R. van Furth. The Hague, Martinus Nijhoff, 1980.

186. Schnyder, J., and Baggiolini, M.: Secretion of lysosomal hydrolases by stimulated and nonstimulated macrophages. J. Exp. Med., *148*:435, 1978.

187. Schreiber, R.D., et al.: Macrophage-activating factor produced by a T cell hybridoma: Physicochemical and biosynthetic resemblance to interferon. J. Immunol., *131*:826, 1983.

188. Schreiber, A.D., et al.: Effect of corticosteroids on the human monocyte IgG and complement receptors. J. Clin. Invest., *56*:1189, 1975.

189. Scott, W.A., et al.: Regulation of arachidonic acid metabolism by macrophage activation. J. Exp. Med., *155*:1148, 1982.

190. Scott, W.A., et al.: Resting macrophages produce metabolites from exogenous arachidonic acid. J. Exp. Med., *155*:535, 1982.

191. Serhan, C.N., et al.: LTB$_4$ and phosphatidic acid are calcium ionophores. J. Biol. Chem., *257*:4746, 1982.

192. Shibata, Y., Tamura, K., and Ishida, N.: In vivo analysis of the suppressive effects of immunosuppressive acidic protein, a type of α1-acid glycoprotein, in connection with its high level in tumor-bearing mice. Cancer Res., *43*:2889, 1983.

193. Shin, H.S., et al.: Chemotactic and anaphylatoxic fragment cleaved from the fifth component of guinea pig complement. Science, *162*:136, 1968.

194. Silverstein, S.C., and Loike, J.D.: Phagocytosis. *In* Mononuclear Phagocytes: Functional Aspects. Edited by R. van Furth. The Hague, Martinus Nijhoff, 1980.

195. Silverstein, S.C., Steinman, R.M., and Cohn, Z.A.: Endocytosis. Ann. Rev. Biochem., *46*:669, 1977.

196. Smialowicz, R.J., and Schwab, J.H.: Processing of streptococcal cell walls by rat macrophages and human monocytes, in vitro. Infect. Immun., *17*:591, 1977.

197. Smolen, J.S., et al.: The human autologous mixed lymphocyte reaction. I. Suppression by macrophages and T-cells. J. Immunol., *127*:1987, 1981.

198. Snyderman, R.: Mechanisms of inflammation and tissue destruction in the rheumatic diseases. *In* Cecil Textbook of Medicine, 16th ed. Edited by L.H. Smith, and J.B. Wyngaarden. Philadelphia, W.B. Saunders Co., 1982.

199. Snyderman, R., et al.: Abnormal monocyte chemotaxis in patients with breast cancer. Evidence for a tumor-mediated effect. J. Natl. Cancer Inst., *60*:737, 1978.

200. Snyderman, R., et al.: Effects of neoplasms on inflammation: Depression of macrophage accumulation after tumor implantation. J. Immunol., *116*:585, 1976.

201. Snyderman, R., et al.: Human mononuclear leukocyte chemotaxis: A quantitative assay for mediators of humoral

and cellular chemotactic factors. J. Immunol., *108*:857, 1972.

202. Snyderman, R., et al.: A chemoattractant receptor on macrophages exists in two affinity states regulated by guanine nucleotides. J. Cell Biol., *98*:444, 1984.

203. Snyderman, R., and Fudman, E.J.: Demonstration of a chemotactic factor receptor on macrophages. J. Immunol. *124*:2754, 1980.

204. Snyderman, R., and Goetzl, E.J.: Molecular and cellular mechanisms of leukocyte chemotaxis. Science, *213*:830, 1981.

205. Snyderman, R., and Mergenhagen, S.E.: Chemotaxis of macrophages. *In* Immunobiology of the Macrophage. Edited by D.S. Nelson. New York, Academic Press, 1976.

206. Snyderman, R., Phillips, J.K., and Mergenhagen, S.E.: Biological activity of complement in vivo. Role for C5 in the accumulation of polymorphonuclear leukocytes in inflammatory exudates. J. Exp. Med., *134*:1131, 1971.

207. Snyderman, R., Phillips, J.K., and Mergenhagen, S.E.: Polymorphonuclear leukocyte chemotactic activity in rabbit serum and guinea pig serum treated with immune complexes. Evidence for C5a as the major chemotactic factor. Infect. Immun., *1*:521, 1970.

208. Snyderman, R., and Pike, M.C.: Transductional mechanisms of chemoattractant receptors on leukocytes. *In* Contemporary Topics in Immunobiology, "Regulation of Leukocyte Function." Edited by R. Snyderman. New York, Plenum Publishing Corp. In press, 1984.

209. Snyderman, R., and Pike, M.C.: An inhibition of macrophage chemotopic produced by neoplasms. Science, *192*:370, 1976.

210. Snyderman, R., Shin, H.S., and Dannenberg, A.M., Jr.: Macrophage proteinase and inflammation: The production of chemotactic activity from the fifth component of complement by macrophage proteinase. J. Immunol., *109*:896, 1972.

211. Snyderman, R., Shin, H.S., and Hausman, M.S.: A chemotactic factor for mononuclear leukocytes. Proc. Soc. Exp. Biol. Med., *138*:387, 1971.

212. Sother, M.G., Unanue, E.R., and Beller, D.I.: Regulation of macrophage populations. III. The immunologic induction of exudates rich in Ia-bearing macrophages is a radiosensitive process. J. Immunol., *128*:447, 1982.

213. Spector, W.G.: The macrophage: Its origin and role in pathology. *In* Pathobiology Annual. Vol. 4. Edited by H.L. Ioachim. New York, Raven Press, 1974.

214. Spitzer, G., and Verma, D.S.: Cells with Fc gamma receptors from normal donors suppress granulocytic macrophage colony formation. Blood, *60*:758, 1982.

215. Spitznagel, J.K.: Non-oxidative antimicrobial reactions of leukocytes. *In* Contemporary Topics in Immunobiology. "Regulation of Leukocyte Function." Edited by R. Snyderman. New York, Plenum Press. In press, 1984.

216. Stadel, J.M., DeLean, A., and Lefkowitz, R.J.: Molecular mechanisms of coupling in hormone receptor-adenylate cyclase systems. Adv. Enzymol., *53*:1, 1982.

217. Stahl, P., et al.: Evidence for receptor-mediated binding of glycoproteins, glycoconjugates, and lysosomal glycosidases by alveolar macrophages. Proc. Natl. Acad. Sci. U.S.A, *75*:1399, 1978.

218. Stahl, P., et al.: In vivo and in vitro evidence for a lysosomal enzyme uptake system in macrophages. *In* Mononuclear Phagocytes: Functional Aspects. Edited by R. van Furth. The Hague, Martinus Nijhoff, 1980.

219. Stanley, E.R., et al.: Colony stimulating factor and the regulation of granulopoiesis and macrophage production. Fed. Proc., *34*:2272, 1976.

220. Stanley, E.R., and Gilbert, L.J.: Regulation of macrophage production by a colony-stimulating factor. *In* Mononuclear Phagocytes: Functional Aspects. Edited by R. van Furth. The Hague, Martinus Nijhoff, 1980.

221. Steinman, R.M., et al.: Dendritic cells and macrophages—current knowledge of their distinctive properties and functions. *In* Mononuclear Phagocytes: Functional Aspects. Edited by R. van Furth. The Hague, Martinus Nijhoff, 1980.

222. Stephens, C.G., and Snyderman, R.: Cyclic nucleotides

223. Stevenson, M.M., and Meltzer, M.S.: Depressed chemotactic responses in vitro of peritoneal macrophages from tumor-bearing mice. J. Natl. Cancer Inst., *57*:847, 1976.

224. Stossel, T.P.: Phagocytosis: Recognition and ingestion. Semin. Hematol., *12*:83, 1975.

225. Svensson, B.O., Norberg, R., and Torshensson, R.: Effects of cytoglobulins and aggregated IgG on in vitro monocyte phagocytosis. Scand. J. Rheum. (Suppl.), *31*:57, 1980.

226. Thompson, J., and van Furth, R.: The effect of glucocorticosteroids on the proliferation and kinetics of promonocytes and monocytes of the bone marrow. J. Exp. Med., *137*:10, 1973.

227. Todd, R.F., III, and Schlossman, S.F.: Analysis of antigenic determinants on human monocytes and macrophage. Blood, *59*:775, 1982.

228. Tsukamoto, Y., Helsel, W.E., and Wahl, S.M.: Macrophage production of fibronectin, a chemoattractant for fibroblasts. J. Immunol., *127*:673, 1981.

229. Tulkens, P., Schneider, Y.J., and Trouet, A.: Membrane recycling (shuttle?) in endocytosis. *In* Mononuclear Phagocytes: Functional Aspects. Edited by R. van Furth. The Hague, Martinus Nijhoff, 1980.

230. Unanue, E.R., et al.: Regulation of immunity and inflammation by mediators from macrophages. Am. J. Pathol., *85*:465, 1976.

231. Unanue, E.R., and Calderon, J.: Evaluation of the role of macrophages in immune induction. Fed. Proc., *34*:1737, 1975.

232. Unkeless, J.C.: Fc receptors of mouse macrophages. *In* Mononuclear Phagocytes: Functional Aspects. Edited by R. van Furth. The Hague, Martinus Nijhoff, 1980.

233. Unkeless, J.C.: The presence of two Fc receptors on mouse macrophages: Evidence from a variant cell line and differential trypsin sensitivity. J. Exp. Med., *145*:931, 1977.

234. Unkeless, J.C., and Eisen, H.: Binding of monomeric immunoglobulins to Fc receptors of mouse macrophages. J. Exp. Med., *142*:1520, 1975.

235. Unkeless, J.C., Gordon, S., and Reich, E.: Secretion of plasminogen activator by stimulated macrophages. J. Exp. Med., *139*:834, 1974.

236. Valone, F.H.: Regulation of human leukocyte function by lipoxygenase products of arachidonic acid. *In* Contemporary Topics in Immunobiology. "Regulation of Leukocyte Function." Edited by R. Snyderman. New York, Plenum Publishing Corp. In press, 1984.

237. van Dingle, C.J.W., and van Agan, W.B.: Generation of tissue thromboplastin by human monocytes. *In* Mononuclear Phagocytes: Functional Aspects. Edited by R. van Furth. The Hague, Martinus Nijhoff, 1980.

238. van Furth, R.: Mononuclear Phagocytes: Functional Aspects. The Hague, Martinus Nijhoff, 1980.

239. van Furth, R.: An approach to the characterization of mononuclear phagocytes involved in pathologic processes. Agents Actions, *6*:91, 1976.

240. van Furth, R.: Origin and kinetics of mononuclear phagocytes. Ann. N.Y. Acad. Sci., *278*:161, 1976.

241. van Furth, R.: Mononuclear Phagocytes in Immunity, Infection and Pathology. Oxford, Blackwell Scientific Publications, 1975.

242. van Furth, R., et al.: The regulation of the participation of the mononuclear phagocyte system in inflammatory responses. *In* Experimental Models of Chronic Inflammatory Disease. Edited by L.E. Glynn, and H.D. Schlumberger. Va Bayer Symposium. Germany, Gross Leder, 1977.

243. van Furth, R., et al.: The effect of azathioprine (Imuran) on the cell cycle of promonocytes and the production of monocytes in the bone marrow. J. Exp. Med., *141*:531, 1975.

244. van Furth, R., et al.: The mononuclear phagocyte system: A new classification of macrophages, monocytes and their precursor cells. Bull. W.H.O., *46*:845, 1972.

245. van Snick, J.L., and Masson, P.L.: Binding of human

lactoferrin to mouse peritoneal cells. J. Exp. Med., *144*:1568, 1976.

246. van Waarde, D., Hulsing-Hessilink, E., and van Furth, R.: Properties of a factor increasing monocytopoiesis (FIM) occurring in serum during the early phase of an inflammatory reaction. Blood, *50*:727, 1977.

247. Vassalli, J.D., Hamilton, J., and Reich, E.: Macrophage plasminogen activator. Modulation of enzyme production by anti-inflammatory steroids, mitotic inhibitors and cyclic nucleotides. Cell, *8*:271, 1976.

248. Verghese, M.W., and Snyderman, R.: Hormonal activation of adenylate cyclase in macrophage membranes is regulated by guanine nucleotides. J. Immunol., *130*:869, 1983.

249. Vischer, T.L., Flory, E., and Muirden, K.: Proteinase complexes are taken up by synovial macrophages during joint inflammation. Adv. Exp. Med. Biol., *135*:635, 1982.

250. Vogel, S.N., et al.: Correction of defective macrophage differentiation in C3H/HeJ mice by an interferon-like molecule. J. Immunol., *128*:380, 1982.

251. Volkman, A.: Disparity in origin of mononuclear phagocyte populations. J. Reticuloendothel. Soc., *19*:249, 1976.

252. Volkman, A.: Monocyte kinetics and their changes in infection. *In* Immunobiology of the Macrophage. Edited by D.S. Nelson. New York, Academic Press, 1976.

253. Wahl, L.M., et al.: Collagenase production by lymphokine-activated macrophages. Science, *187*:261, 1975.

254. Wahl, L.J., et al.: Collagenase production by endotoxin activated macrophages. Proc. Natl. Acad. Sci. U.S.A., *71*:3598, 1974.

255. Walinsky, S.I., et al.: Role of prostaglandins in the development of depressed cell mediated immune response in rheumatoid arthritis. Cell Immunol. Immunopathol., *17*:3, 1980.

256. Walker, W.S.: Separate Fc receptors for immunoglobulins IgG2a and IgG2b on an established cell line of mouse macrophages. J. Immunol., *116*:911, 1976.

257. Walker, W.S.: Mediation of macrophage cytolytic and phagocytic activities by antibodies of different classes and class-specific Fc receptors. J. Immunol., *119*:367, 1977.

258. Ward, P.A., and Zvaifler, N.: Complement-derived chemotactic factors in inflammatory fluids of humans. J. Clin. Invest., *50*:606, 1971.

259. Webb, D.R., and Nowowiejski, I.: Control of suppressor cell activation via endogenous prostaglandin synthesis: The role of T cells and macrophages. Cell. Immunol., *63*:321, 1981.

260. Weinberg, J.B., Muscato, J.J., and Niedel, J.: Monocyte chemotactic peptide receptor. J. Clin. Invest., *68*:621, 1981.

261. Weir, D.M., and Ogmundsdottir, H.M.: Cellular recognition by phagocytes: Role of lectin-like receptor(s). *In* Mononuclear Phagocytes: Functional Aspects. Edited by R. van Furth. The Hague, Martinus Nijhoff, 1980.

262. Weissmann, G.: Lysosomal mechanism of tissue injury in arthritis. N. Engl. J. Med., *286*:141, 1972.

263. Werb, Z.: Hormone receptors and hormonal regulation of macrophage physiological functions. *In* Mononuclear

Phagocytes: Functional Aspects. Edited by R. van Furth. The Hague, Martinus Nijhoff, 1980.

264. Werb, Z.: Biochemical actions of glucocorticoids on macrophages in culture. Specific inhibition of elastase, collagenase, and plasminogen activator secretion and effects on other metabolic functions. J. Exp. Med., *147*:1695, 1978.

265. Werb, Z., and Chin, J.R.: Endotoxin suppresses expression of apoprotein E by mouse macrophages in vivo and in culture. J. Biol. Chem., *258*:10642, 1983.

266. Werb, Z., Foley, R., and Munck, A.: Interaction of glucocorticoids with macrophages. Identification of glucocorticoid receptors in monocytes and macrophages. J. Exp. Med., *147*:1684, 1978.

267. Werb, Z., and Gordon, S.: Elastase secretion by stimulated macrophages. J. Exp. Med., *142*:361, 1975.

268. Werb, Z., and Gordon, S.: Secretion of a specific collagenase by stimulated macrophages. J. Exp. Med., *142*:345, 1975.

269. Wharton, W., Walker, E., and Stewart, C.C.: Growth regulation by macrophages. *In* Macrophages and Natural Killer Cells: Regulation and Function. Edited by S.J. Normann and E. Sorkin. New York, Plenum Publishing Corp., 1982.

270. Winchester, R.J., and Burmester, G.R.: Demonstration of Ia antigens on certain dendrite cells and on a novel elongate cell found in human synovial tissue. Scand. J. Immunol., *14*:439, 1981.

271. Wooley, D.E., et al.: Collagenase immunolocalization in cultures of rheumatoid synovial cells. Science, *200*:773, 1978.

272. Wright, S.D., et al.: Identification of the C3bi receptor of human monocytes and macrophages with monoclonal antibodies. Proc. Natl. Acad. Sci. U.S.A., *80(18)*:5699, 1983.

273. Wright, S.D., and Silverstein, S.C.: Phagocytosin g macrophages exclude soluble macromolecules from the zone of contact with ligand-coated targets. Cell Biol., 95:433a, 1982.

274. Wright, S.D., Van Voorhis, W.C., and Silverstein, S.C.: Identification of the C3b′ receptor on human leukocytes using a monoclonal antibody. Fed. Proc., *42*:1079, 1983.

275. Wyler, D., and Postlethwaite, A.E.: Fibroblast stimulation in schistosomiasis. IV. Isolated egg granulomas elaborate a fibroblast chemoattractant in vitro. J. Immunol., *130*:1371, 1983.

276. Yem, A.W., and Parmely, M.J.: Modulation of Ia-like antigen expression and antigen-presenting activity of human monocytes by endotoxin and zymosan A. J. Immunol., *127*:2245, 1981.

277. Yin, H.L., and Stossel, T.P.: Control of cytoplasmic actin gel-sol transformation by gelsolin, a calcium-dependent regulatory protein. Nature, *281*:583, 1979.

278. Young, J.D.E., et al.: Macrophage membrane potential changes associated with $\gamma 2b/\gamma 1$ Fc receptor-ligand binding. Proc. Natl. Acad. Sci. U.S.A., *80*:1357, 1983.

279. Ziegler, K., and Unanue, E.R.: Identification of a macrophage antigen-processing agent required for I-region-restricted antigen presentation to T-lymphocytes. J. Immunol., *127*:1869, 1981.

280. Ziff, M.: Phagocytes and substrates in the joint. Scand. J. Rheum. (Suppl.), *40*:10, 1981.

Chapter 17

Lymphocytes: Structure and Function

John D. Stobo

In the six years that have elapsed since the previous writing of this chapter, there has been a tremendous increase in information concerning lymphocyte structure and function. This increase has resulted from technologic advances such as somatic cell hybridization, lymphocyte cloning, and recombinant DNA. Somatic cell hybridization has been most useful in producing monoclonal antibodies with specificity for cell surface molecules that not only mark functional subpopulations of lymphocytes, but also play a crucial role in lymphocyte function. The technique of lymphocyte cloning has enabled the establishment and maintenance of individual clones of immunocompetent cells so that their specific immune reactivities and fine specificities can be examined carefully. The technologies derived from recombinant DNA have provided approaches to examine the structure, organization, and activity of gene coding for immunologically relevant molecules such as immunoglobulin (Ig). The accumulation of knowledge concerning lymphocyte structure and function that has resulted from these advances has generated a vocabulary that often confuses and discourages the neophyte. Therefore, this chapter will first define basic terminology necessary to comprehend the discussion of lymphocyte biology and then will discuss the structure and function of specific populations of lymphocytes.

TERMINOLOGY

Interleukins

Interleukins are soluble materials released by one population of leukocytes, usually mononuclear cells, which exert a biologic effect on another population of leukocytes. Three different interleukins, abbreviated IL, have been described.

IL-1. IL-1 refers to a 12,000 to 15,000 molecular weight polypeptide synthesized by macrophages and perhaps by other cells such as granulocytes, fibroblasts, and keratinocytes.[19] The old terminology for IL-1 is leukocyte activating factor. Synthesis of IL-1 by macrophages is necessary for full T cell activation to occur.

IL-2. IL-2 refers to a 15,000 to 17,000 molecular weight polypeptide synthesized by T cells.[5] The old terminology for IL-2 is T cell growth factor (TCGF). As the term TCGF implies, IL-2 is necessary for the full activation, growth, and expansion of activated T cells. IL-2 has been used to maintain clones of activated T cells in vitro.

IL-3. IL-3 is a poorly characterized material presumably synthesized by activated T cells. The biologic effect of IL-3 was originally defined by its ability to induce the expression of the enzyme $20\text{-}\alpha\text{-hydroxysteroid}$ dehydrogenase ($20\text{-}\alpha\text{-SDA}$) among early cells of the T cell lineage.[7] The role that IL-3 plays in modulating immune reactivity is not known. Some investigators believe that IL-3 is identical to previously described colony stimulating factors.

In addition to these designated interleukins that exert an effect on T cells, there exist two soluble materials that are synthesized by T cells and have an effect on the differentiation of B cells:

B Cell Growth Factor (BCGF)

The biologic effect of BCGF may be a result of two factors of 17,000 to 20,000 and 12,000 to 13,000 molecular weight.[10] BCGF is synthesized by T cells and is required for the differentiation of a subpopulation of activated B cells.

T Cell Replacing Factor (TRF)

TRF is a factor with a relatively high molecular weight (30,000 to 50,000). It is synthesized by T cells and is required for the differentiation of B cells into plasma cells.[2]

Cell Surface Molecules

Various surface molecules play an important role in the function and differentiation of immunocompetent cells (see also Chap. 24).

Products of Genes in the Major Histocompatibility Complex (MHC). MHC genes are present on the short arm of chromosome 17 in mice and chromosome 6 in humans.[6,8] Genes in this locus code for the synthesis of transplantation antigens and can be divided into two broad groups based on differences in the structure and tissue distribution of the molecules for which they code.

Class I Molecules. These molecules have a molecular weight of 45,000 and exist as a bimolecular complex noncovalently associated with B_2 microglobulin on the surface of all nucleated cells. B_2 microglobulin has a molecular weight of 13,000 and is encoded for by genes distinct from those in the MHC. Genes in the human HLA-A and HLA-B loci code for the synthesis of class I molecules.

Class II Molecules. Class II molecules exist as a bimolecular complex of an α chain (34,000 molecular weight) and a β chain (29,000 molecular weight) expressed on the surface of only B cells and antigen presenting cells. (Both the α and β chains are coded for by MHC genes.) Class II molecules are products of immune response genes and are also referred to as immune response associated or Ia molecules.

The technique of somatic cell hybridization has allowed the production of monoclonal antibodies that have specificity for molecules useful in marking functional subpopulations of cells. The production of such monoclonal antibodies involves immunizing an animal, typically a mouse or rat, with cells followed by fusion of the immune spleen cells to a plasmacytoma. In this way, spleen cells producing antibodies are then assayed for the production of useful antibody. This results in the generation of antibody with a singular specificity from a single clone of hybrids. The monoclonal antibodies most commonly used to mark populations of human cells are listed in Table 17–1.[22] The finding that both OK* and Leu† reagents depict the same population of cells indicates that they each have specificity for the same molecule. For ex-

ample, OKT4 and Leu 3 bind to the same 57,000 molecular weight molecule.

THYMOCYTE DIFFERENTIATION

The appearance of functional peripheral T cells requires that precursor cells first undergo a series of differentiation steps within the microenvironment of the thymus. Stem cells from the bone marrow enter the thymus, migrate from the cortex to the medulla, and finally emigrate to peripheral lymphoid tissue, a process that takes approximately three days. This migration is accompanied by the acquisition of functional maturity (cortical thymocytes are the least and medullary thymocytes the most mature cells) and the differential expression of certain cell surface molecules. For example, it can be demonstrated in mice that movement of thymocytes from the cortex to the medulla is accompanied by a loss of some cell surface molecules (e.g., TL) and the acquisition of others (e.g., Lyt). A similar situation exists in humans.[23] Utilizing monoclonal antibodies with specificity for surface molecules, researchers have been able to trace the migration of thymocytes through the thymus (Fig. 17–1). The earliest lymphoid cells within the thymus, the prothymocytes, react with the monoclonal antibodies anti-T10 and anti-T9 (i.e., they are $T10^+$ and $T9^+$). As maturation proceeds and thymocytes move toward the medulla, they lose the T9 marker, maintain the T10 molecule, and become reactive with the monoclonal antibodies anti-T6, anti-T8, and anti-T4. At this point, the T8 and T4 determinants are present on the same cell. Further differentiation, occurring in the medulla, is accompanied by the development of the two distinct populations of thymocytes. Both populations react with the monoclonal antibodies anti-T10 and anti-T3. However, one population reacts with anti-T4, but not anti-T8, and the other with anti-T8, but not anti-T4. As the cells gain further maturity, they lose the T10 molecule and exit into the periphery where they can be broadly divided into two populations: $T3^+$, $T4^+$ (50 to 60% of peripheral T

---

*OK refers to monoclonal antibodies from Ortho Pharmaceuticals, Raritan, N.J.

†Leu designates monoclonal antibodies available from Becton-Dickinson, Mountain View, CA.

Table 17–1.   Monoclonal Antibodies Commonly Used to Mark Populations of Human Cells

Monoclonal Antibody*	Population Depicted
OKT3, Leu 4	10% of thymocytes, all (100%) peripheral blood T cells.
OKT4, Leu 3	75% of thymocytes, 60% of peripheral blood T cells. Includes cells that proliferate in response to soluble antigen, helper T cells, T cells that can induce the activation of suppressor T cells, and cytotoxic T cells directed against foreign class II molecules.
OKT5, OKT8, Leu 2	80% of thymocytes, 30% of peripheral blood T cells. Includes T cells that can suppress immune reactivities and effector T cells whose cytotoxicity requires recognition of class I molecules.

*OK = monoclonal antibodies from Ortho Pharmaceuticals, Raritan, N.J.
 Leu = monoclonal antibodies from Becton-Dickinson, Mountain View, CA.

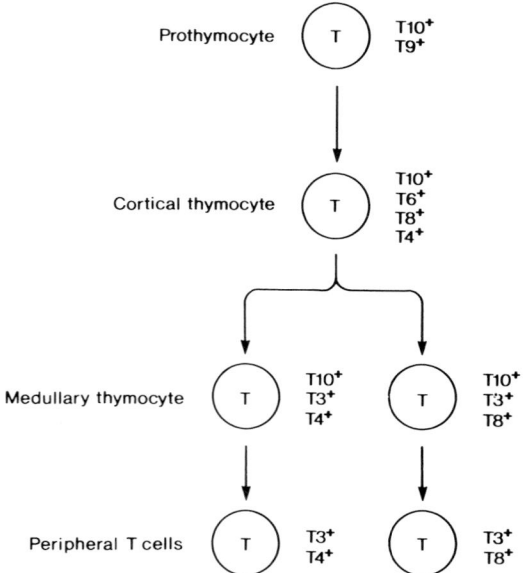

Fig. 17–1. Thymocyte differentiation as depicted by changes in the expression of cell surface markers. The designation T10⁺, T9⁺, and so forth indicates that the cell displays a cell surface molecule detectable with a specific monoclonal antibody (e.g., anti-T10, anti-T9, and so forth).

cells) and T3⁺, T8⁺ (20 to 30% of peripheral T cells).

The finding that acquisition of functional maturity among thymocytes occurs concomitant with the acquisition of certain surface molecules (i.e., T3, T4, T8) suggests that these molecules play a role in mediating the function of the cells. As will be shown subsequently, this suggestion is correct.

It can be clearly demonstrated that recognition of foreign antigens by immunocompetent, peripheral T cells requires that they not only see determinants inherent in the antigen, but also determinants inherent in self class I or class II molecules. For example, activation of virus-specific, effector, cytotoxic T cells requires that the T cell "see" virus in conjunction with class I molecules displayed by the virus-infected target cell. Activation of delayed hypersensitivity or helper T cells by foreign antigen requires that the T cell see determinants inherent in the foreign antigen in conjunction with self class II molecules displayed on the surface of antigen presenting cells. In other words, a basic requirement for the expression of T cell immunity is recognition of self class I or class II molecules. Compelling data indicate that this self-recognition is either imprinted or selected for during the differentiation of thymocytes in the thymus.³² The following illustration serves to em-

phasize this point. If animals of strain X are infected with virus Y, the cytotoxic T cells that are generated will demonstrate specificity for the X class I molecules plus Y. These cytotoxic T cells will not lyse T cells from a different animal strain (e.g., Z) infected with the same virus, Y. If, however, the thymus of strain X is removed and replaced with a thymus from strain Z animals, then virus-specific cytotoxic T cells appearing in the periphery will have specificity for Y seen in conjunction with strain Z and not X class I molecules. In other words, even though the stem cells are derived from the strain X host, the specificity to the cytotoxic T cells is determined by the thymic milieu in which they develop, i.e., the strain Z thymus.

It is not clear if this self-recognition represents a selective or inductive process. On the one hand, it is possible that the pool of prothymocytes consists of many different clones of cells, each of which is capable of recognizing a different class I or class II molecule. Only those capable of recognizing self class I or class II would be selected for during differentiation. On the other hand, expression of recognition units for self class I or class II may be induced during differentiation. Two observations indirectly support a selective process. First, only 10% of stem cells entering the thymus exit to the periphery. This could indicate that the other 90% that undergo intrathymic death do not display receptors for self class I or class II molecules, and therefore are not "selected" for exit to the periphery. Second, thymic stromal cells display high densities of class I and class II molecules. This provides a means by which thymocytes displaying receptors for self class I or class II molecules can be selected for as they migrate through the thymus.

If class I and class II molecule–bearing thymic stromal cells can "select" for T cells displaying the appropriate self-receptor, then an obvious question is, how does this occur? Although there is no clear answer, there is an interesting hypothesis that implicates four enzymes, adenosine deaminase (ADA), purine nucleoside phosphorylase (PNP), 5'nucleotidase (5'NT), and terminal deoxynucleotidyl transferase (TdT); and thymic stromal cells displaying class I and class II molecules in the selective maintenance of self-reactive thymocytes.¹² During the normal cellular metabolism of purines, ADA and PNP convert deoxyadenosine to deoxyinosine and deoxyguanosine to guanine, respectively. In the absence of these enzymes the substrates deoxyadenosine and deoxyinosine can be converted to deoxyATP (dATP) and deoxyGTP (dGTP). Both compounds are toxic to cells. High levels of both 5'NT and TdT protect against the toxic effects of dATP and dGTP. 5'NT shifts the reaction back toward synthesis of deoxyadenosine and deoxyguanosine. TdT metabolizes the toxic products. Therefore, if cells contain low levels of ADA or PNP, toxic levels of dATP and dGTP will accumulate. If levels of TdT are sufficiently high, these toxic products will be metabolized. If not, they accumulate resulting in cell death.

Although all thymocytes have some of each enzyme, the absolute amounts of each vary with thymocyte differentiation (Fig. 17–2). Prothymocytes have relatively high levels of all four enzymes. Therefore, toxic levels of dATP and dGTP do not accumulate. During late cortical development, 5'NT remains elevated, while activity of ADA, PNP, and TdT decreases. The result is an accumulation of potentially lethal levels of dATP and dGTP in the rapidly dividing cortical thymocytes. It is postulated that cortical thymocytes bearing receptors for self class I or class II molecules displayed by thymic stromal cells are brought into close contact with these cells. The thymic stromal cells then metabolize and remove the toxic dATP and dGTP. Because cortical thymocytes lacking receptors for self class I or class II molecules cannot take advantage of the same metabolic cooperation, they die. A morphologic observation provides support for this proposed selective cooperation between thymocytes and stromal cells. During the differentiation of rodent thymocytes, it can be demonstrated that thymic stromal cells are capable of engulfing as many as 50 thymocytes. The stromal cells then allow the thymocytes to proliferate, and

subsequently discharge them, unharmed, back into the thymic environment. It is presumably during this intracellular engulfment that stromal cells remove toxic deoxynucleotides from thymocytes.

In summary, the functional maturation of thymocytes proceeds in stages that correlate with their movement through the thymus and their expression of certain cell surface markers. An important consequence of this maturation is the generation of T cells capable of recognizing self class I or class II molecules. Although the exact mechanism by which this self-recognition occurs is unknown, metabolic rescue of thymocytes containing toxic levels of dATP or dGTP by class I and class II bearing thymic stromal cells may be involved.

CIRCULATION OF PERIPHERAL BLOOD LYMPHOCYTES

Movement of lymphocytes from the circulation into lymphoid organs such as peripheral lymph nodes and Peyer's patches is mediated by specific interactions between lymphocytes and endothelial cells that line post-capillary high endothelial venules (HEV). Lymphocyte binding to HEV can be demonstrated both in vivo and in vitro. Several observations indicate that interactions between HEV and lymphocytes involve cell surface recognition units that determine the homing pattern of lymphocytes.[4] If lymphocytes isolated from a peripheral lymph node are injected back into an animal from which they were removed, they preferentially localize to the peripheral lymph nodes and not to the spleen or Peyer's patches. An iden-

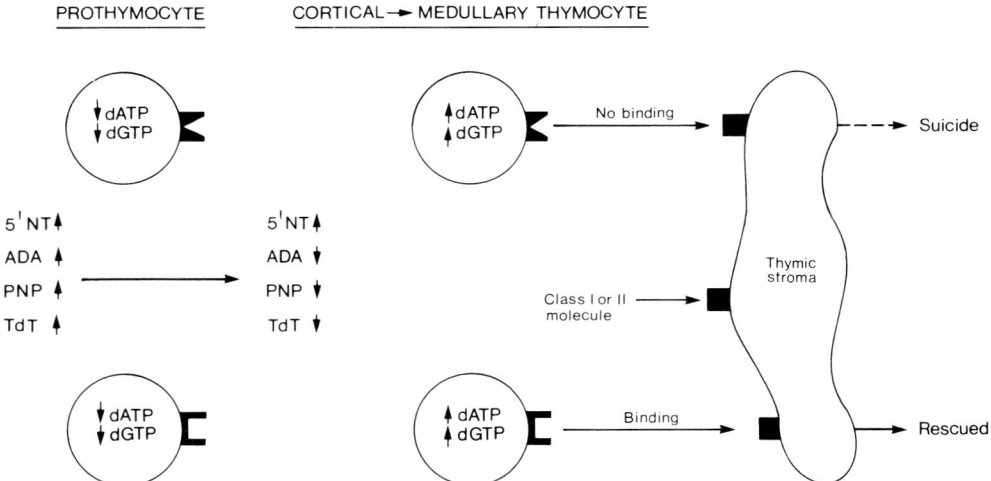

Fig. 17–2. Hypothetical scheme for the selection of thymocytes displaying receptors for self class I or class II molecules. TdT = terminal deoxynucleotidyl transferase; ADA = adenosine deaminase; PNP = purine nucleoside phosphorylase; 5'NT = 5'nucleotidase; dATP = deoxyadenosine triphosphate; dGTP = deoxyguanosine triphosphate. ↑ or ↓ indicates the relative amount of each enzyme or metabolite.[12]

tical preferential homing pattern of Peyer's patch lymphocytes to Peyer's patches and not to peripheral lymphocyte nodes can be demonstrated. Therefore, localization of lymphocytes to lymphoid tissue is directed and not random. Treatment of the lymphocytes with enzymes that digest cell surface molecules destroys their homing pattern so that it becomes random. This finding suggests that a lymphocyte surface molecule is important in determining homing patterns. Gallatin and colleagues have produced a monoclonal antibody with specificity for an 80,000 molecular weight molecule displayed on the surface of these murine lymphocytes that preferentially home to peripheral lymph nodes and not on the surface of the cells in Peyer's patches.[4] This antibody blocks binding of lymphocytes to lymph node HEV, but not to Peyer's patch HEV. Coating of lymphocytes with the antibody followed by infusion into an animal inhibits homing to and movement into peripheral lymph nodes, but not into Peyer's patches. The structure of the molecule on HEV, which interacts with the lymphocyte homing molecule, has not been determined. These observations account for the preferential localization of functional populations of lymphocytes to specific lymphoid tissues, e.g., localization of lymphocytes involved in IgA production to Peyer's patches.

PHENOTYPIC AND FUNCTIONAL HETEROGENEITY AMONG PERIPHERAL T CELLS

Immunologic reactivities that involve the participation of T cells include effector and regulatory functions such as delayed hypersensitivity and cytotoxicity, as well as regulatory functions such as help and suppression. The results of studies performed in mice clearly indicate that these different reactivities do not represent the capabilities of a single clone of pluripotential cells. Instead, discrete populations of T cells exist, each of which mediates a single or limited number of effector or regulatory functions.

Functional capabilities of discrete populations of murine T cells correlate with their expression of certain cell surface markers. For example, murine T cells participating in delayed hypersensitivity, as well as regulatory cells that help B cells differentiate into plasma cells, display a determinant Lyt 1 but lack another determinant, Lyt 2. In contrast, cytotoxic effector cells and suppressor T cells are both Lyt 1$^+$ and Lyt 2$^+$.

Based on the demonstrated correlation between function and expression of certain cell surface moleculares in mice, monoclonal antibodies capable of depicting functional subpopulations of human T cells were developed. The most commonly used

are those that depict the molecules T3, T4, and T8.[24] All peripheral T cells display T3. T3 positivity, therefore, is a marker of T cells. Approximately 50 to 60% of T3$^+$ cells are also T4$^+$, and 20 to 30% are T8$^+$. Most importantly, the effector and regulatory functions of T4$^+$ cells are different than those of T8$^+$ cells (Table 17–2). The T4$^+$ cells contain effector cells for delayed hypersensitivity reactions, as well as cells capable of inducing activation of suppressor cells. The T8$^+$ population contains cytotoxic effector and suppressor effector T cells. Therefore, the human T3$^+$, T4$^+$, T8$^-$, and T3$^+$, T4$^-$, T8$^+$ populations represent the functional equivalents of murine Lyt 1$^+$ 2$^-$ and Lyt 1$^+$ 2$^+$ populations, respectively.

Each of these major human T cell populations can be further fractionated by differences in cell surface markers that also correlate with differences in function (Fig. 17–3).[21] Approximately 80% of T4$^+$ cells display a molecule easily detectable by a circulating antibody present in the serum of some patients with active juvenile rheumatoid arthritis (i.e., they are JRA$^+$). This same population reacts with a monoclonal antibody, anti-TQ1 and, after activation with pokeweed mitogen, maintains the display of a molecule depicted by the monoclonal antibody, OKT17. The remaining 20% of T4$^+$ T cells are JRA$^-$, TQ1$^-$ and lose the OKT17 marker after activation with pokeweed mitogen. Both populations of T4$^+$ cells are required for maximal immunoglobulin (Ig) production, i.e., they are both helpers for Ig synthesis. However, only the T4$^+$, JRA$^-$, TQ1$^+$ and not the T4$^+$, JRA$^-$, TQ1$^-$ population is capable of inducing the activation of suppressor cells existing among the T8$^+$ T cells. In an analogous fashion, functional and phenotypic heterogeneity can be demonstrated among T8$^+$ T cells.[28] Cytotoxic effector cells can be induced by activation with allogeneic cells to express a differentiation antigen detectable with the monoclonal antibody, OKT20. In contrast, T8$^+$ suppressor cells remain OKT20$^-$ after activation with alloantigens.

T CELL ACTIVATION

Activation of T cells by antigen is a complex process that requires interactions between at least two distinct types of cells, T cells and accessory cells, and two soluble materials, IL-1 and IL-2 (Fig. 17–4). The role of accessory cells in T cell activation is twofold. First, they are required to process and appropriately present antigen to T cells. Second, they serve as sources of IL-1, a soluble material necessary for full T cell activation to occur.

The precise biochemical events involved in the processing of antigen by accessory cells remain to

Table 17–2.   Phenotypic and Functional Heterogeneity Among Peripheral Blood T Cells

		T Cell Phenotype*	
	Immune Function	*T3$^+$, T4$^+$, T8$^-$*	*T3$^+$, T4$^-$, T8$^+$*
A.	Proliferation in response to stimulation with:		
	Mitogens (PHA, Con A)	+	+
	Soluble antigens	+	−
	Alloantigens	+	±†
B.	Synthesis of IL-2	+	+
C.	Effectors for delayed hypersensitivity	+	−
D.	Cytotoxicity		
	Restricted by class I molecules	−	−
	Restricted by class II molecules	+	−
E.	Regulatory Function		
	Help	+	−
	Inducer of suppression	+	−
	Suppressor effector	−	+

*Te$^+$, T4$^+$, T8$^+$ indicate that the cell reacts with the monoclonal antibody OKT3, OKT4, and OKT8, respectively.
†"±" indicates some activity, but less than "+." "−" indicates no activity.

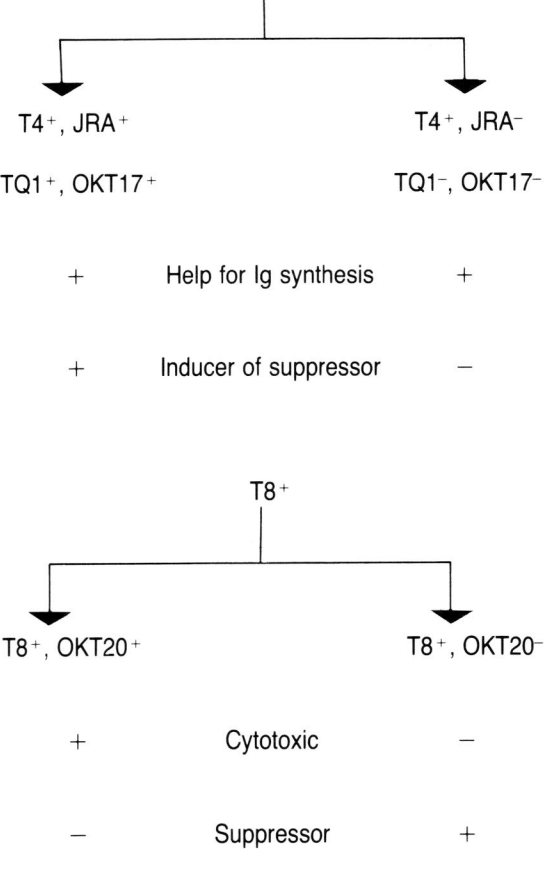

Fig. 17–3.   Phenotypic and functional heterogeneity existing within T4$^+$ and T8$^+$ cells. See text for explanation of phenotypes.

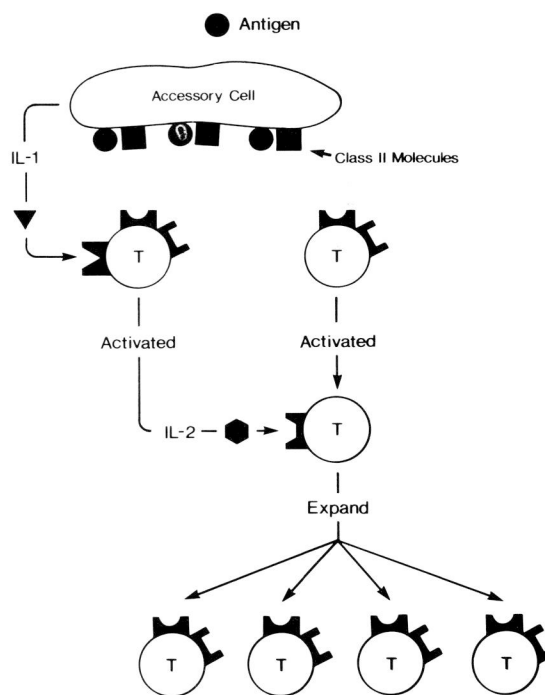

Fig. 17–4.   Events involved in T cell activation. Two signals are required to initiate T cell activation: antigen seen in conjunction with class II (Ia) molecules and IL-1. These activated T cells synthesize IL-2, which acts on a second population of T cell that has been induced to express IL-2 receptors by appropriate interactions with antigen plus class II molecules. This results in expansion of antigen reactive T cells and is an important mechanism for the development of large numbers of helper and cytotoxic T cells.

be elucidated. To date, it appears to be an energy-dependent process that does not require active phagocytosis, but may require pinocytosis of antigen.[25] Although events involved in presentation of antigen by accessory cells are equally obscure, it is clear that this process requires that the accessory cell display an appropriate density of class II molecules. Activation of T cells by antigen requires that the T cells see two sets of determinants: those inherent in antigen and those inherent in self class II molecules. Whether antigen is physically associated with or only physically proximate to class II molecules on the surface of accessory cells is not known. Nonetheless, it is clear that interactions between antigen-reactive T cells and either antigen alone or class II bearing accessory cells alone is not sufficient to induce their activation. Determinants inherent in antigen and class II molecules must be seen in association with each other. This has implications for the structure of the T cell antigen receptor as discussed subsequently.

A second crucial role for accessory cells in T cell activation is the synthesis of IL-1.[19] Human IL-1 was originally defined by its direct mitogenicity for thymocytes or its ability to enhance blastogenesis of thymocytes initiated by stimulation with suboptimal concentrations of mitogens. (Human IL-1 will work with mouse thymocytes, but mouse IL-1 will not work on human thymocytes.) Some antigens, such as endotoxin, can directly activate accessory cells to synthesize IL-1. Other antigens induce IL-1 synthesis indirectly by first stimulating T cells, which subsequently release a soluble material capable of inducing IL-1 synthesis by accessory cells. T-derived soluble materials that can induce IL-1 production by accessory cells include a factor that resembles colony stimulating factor in its biologic activity. Synthesis of IL-1 by accessory cells can be inhibited by steroids and by prostaglandins of the E series.

Although IL-1 is directly mitogenic for thymocytes, it cannot by itself induce proliferation among thymus-derived lymphocytes. Instead, IL-1 acts in concert with a second signal to enhance T cell activation and proliferation. This second signal is represented by antigen and class II molecules appropriately presented by accessory cells or by lectins that bind directly to T cell surfaces (Fig. 17–4). Either signal alone is insufficient.

IL-1 has a wide range of metabolic effects on various cells. A common denominator is the induced synthesis of other biologically active materials. For example, IL-1 can induce synthesis of fibrinogen by hepatocytes and of prostaglandins by myocytes and hypothalamic cells. In its role as a requisite signal for T cell activation, IL-1 also appears to exert its effect by inducing the synthesis

of a second biologically active material, IL-2, as well as receptors for IL-2.

Human IL-2 is synthesized by T cells that are appropriately activated by two signals, e.g., antigen seen in conjunction with class II molecules and IL-1[5]. Addition of IL-2 alone to resting T cells has no effect on their growth or metabolism, but when it is added to T cells appropriately activated by some other stimulus, the cells proliferate and grow. Indeed, repeated addition of fresh IL-2 to activated T cells can be used to perpetuate and expand their growth. The major effect of IL-2 on the immune system is to act as a growth or differentiation factor, thus expanding the number of activated T cells.

If the same T cell that synthesizes IL-2 also responded to it, then each time a cell is activated by antigen and IL-1 it would become an autonomous, malignant-like cell line. Therefore, it has been hypothesized that T cells that can be activated to synthesize IL-2 do not respond to it, a hypothesis supported by studies of IL-2 synthesis and response among cloned T cell lines. IL-2 synthesized by activated T cells acts on a different population of T cells, which do not synthesize IL-2, but which do display IL-2 receptors and, therefore, are capable of responding.

In summary, interactions between the different cells and soluble materials required for T cell activation are represented by the following scheme (see Fig. 17–4). Antigen appropriately presented by accessory cells bearing class II molecules acts in concert with IL-1 secreted by the accessory cells to activate a clone of antigen-reactive T cells. These activated cells then synthesize and secrete IL-2. IL-2 acts on another T clone of similar antigenic specificity, which has been induced by interactions with antigen to display surface IL-2 receptors. IL-2 then promotes expansion of this clone, which can manifest either effector or regulatory functions.

What type of cell serves as the physiologic accessory cell for T cell activation in vivo is controversial. Some investigators claim that only dendritic cells, and not macrophages, are important accessory cells. On the other hand, others claim that macrophages and their tissue progeny, Kupffer's cells in the liver and Langerhans' cells in the skin, can function as accessory cells. These cells contain the basic machinery for accessory cell function, i.e., they display class II molecules and synthesize IL-1. Available data support the moderate view that both macrophages or their descendants, in addition to dendritic cells, can function as accessory cells. Which cell type is most relevant to T cell activation may depend on the antigen involved and its tissue localization.

T CELL EFFECTOR FUNCTION

Delayed Hypersensitivity

Delayed hypersensitivity is the prototype of T cell effector function and is involved in host defense to viruses, fungi, and mycobacteria. Macrophages operate at both afferent and efferent limbs of this response. Activation of clones of T cells specific for the antigen requires the accessory cell-dependent pathways discussed in the previous section, antigen presentation, and synthesis of IL-1. Accessory cells mediating this function include Langerhans' cells of the skin when this is the portal of entry for the antigen, or alveolar macrophages when exposure occurs via the tracheobronchial tree. The number of T cells specific for a given antigen is relatively small (1 to 10 out of every 100,000 T cells), but once activated, this small number of T cells magnifies their reactivity through the synthesis and liberation of soluble materials termed *lymphokines,* such as *migration inhibition factor* and *macrophage activating factor.* Migration inhibition factor inhibits the random migration of macrophages as they wander through tissues. This results in the accumulation of macrophages adjacent to where T cells have been activated. Macrophage activating factor enhances the microbiocidal and tumoricidal activity of the accumulated macrophages, thus arming them for eradication of the foreign organism or cell. To date, it has not been possible to purify macrophage activating factor activity free of gamma interferon, suggesting that they may be the same molecules. The morphologic expression of delayed hypersensitivity reactions is the accumulation of mononuclear cells (lymphocytes, macrophages) and the formation of a granuloma.

In humans, the effector cells mediating delayed hypersensitivity reactions are OKT4$^+$; OKT8$^+$ cells can inhibit this reactivity. This relationship between effector and regulatory cells in the expression of delayed hypersensitivity is exemplified by the immune reactivity seen in response to infection with *Mycobacterium leprae.*[29] Patients with tuberculoid leprosy develop high levels of T cell reactivity to *M. leprae,* resulting in the killing and clearing of the organism. In contrast, patients with lepromatous leprosy exhibit specific in vivo and in vitro unresponsiveness to *M. leprae,* and the organisms multiply in the skin. It is possible that in lepromatous leprosy, T cells reactive to *M. leprae* do not exist, or the activity of potentially reactive T cells may be suppressed. Several observations suggest that the latter is true. First, in the lesions of tuberculoid leprosy, OKT4 cells predominate over OKT8$^+$ cells, whereas OKT8$^+$ cells predominate in lepromatous lesions. Second, depletion of OKT8$^+$ cells results in the appearance of in vitro reactivity to *M. leprae* in some patients with lepromatous leprosy. Third, addition of exogenous IL-2 to in vitro cultures of cells from patients with lepromatous leprosy partly restores their reactivity to *M. leprae.* Therefore, the absence of cell-mediated immunity to *M. leprae* seen in lepromatous leprosy represents suppression of potentially reactive OKT4$^+$ cells by OKT8$^+$ cells rather than an absence of reactive T cells. Furthermore, such suppression appears to involve inhibition of either IL-2 secretion or activity. This mechanism of suppression is probably not limited to leprosy, and similar interactions between effector and regulatory cells in the expression of delayed hypersensitivity must occur in other systems.

The best in vivo correlate of delayed hypersensitivity is the skin test. The best in vitro correlate measures the ability of a specific antigen to induce the synthesis of migration inhibition factor by T cells. Antigen-induced T cell proliferation is not a good in vitro correlate of in vivo delayed hypersensitivity, since T cell proliferation is not necessary for delayed hypersensitivity reactions.

Cytotoxicity

The specificity and function of cytotoxic T cells were first explored in systems that analyzed T cell reactivity to foreign transplantation antigens (i.e., alloantigens) such as occur in the rejection of an allograft or in graft vs. host reactions.[18] In vivo studies led to in vitro studies of T cell reactivity to alloantigen. These studies demonstrated that the mixing of lymphocytes from distinct animal species or from different individuals resulted in the proliferation of T cells similar to that seen when T cells were stimulated with antigen or mitogen. This proliferation, termed the *mixed lymphocyte reaction* occurs among Lyt 1$^+$, 2$^-$, 3$^-$ cells in mice or OKT4$^+$ cells in humans in reponse to recognition of foreign class II molecules. Following the proliferation, it is possible to demonstrate the existence of effector T cells that are cytotoxic for the allogeneic stimulator cells. This cytotoxic effector activity is mediated by Lyt 1$^+$, 2$^+$ cells in mice and OKT8$^+$ cells in humans, which recognize foreign class I, and not class II, molecules. The generation of cytotoxic effector cells also requires the presence of IL-2.

To summarize, generation of T cells cytotoxic to allogeneic target cells occurs in the following manner (Fig 17–5). OKT4$^+$ cells recognize foreign class II molecules, are activated, and proliferate (the mixed lymphocyte reaction). Activation results in the liberation of IL-2. (IL-2 synthesis does not require cell division.) IL-2 then stimulates the growth and expansion of OKT8$^+$ cytotoxic effector

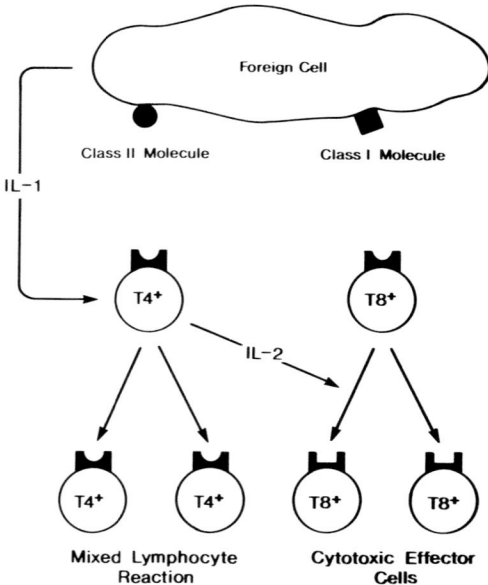

Fig. 17–5. Events involved in the generation of alloreactive T cells. Foreign class II molecules in the presence of IL-1 lead to activation and proliferation among T4+ T cells. This proliferation is termed the mixed lymphocyte reaction. As a consequence of T4 activation, IL-2 is synthesized. This IL-2 allows the expansion and growth of T8+ T cells that have specificity for foreign class I molecules.

cells, which have been activated by recognition of foreign class I molecules. IL-2 is crucial for the expansion and maintenance of cytotoxic effector cells and, once generated, cytotoxic T cells can be maintained for months in vitro provided that fresh IL-2 is added periodically.

In an experimental model, infection of mice with a virus also resulted in the generation of cytotoxic Lyt 1+, 2+ T cells. As already indicated, the activity of these effector cells requires that they see viral antigen in conjunction with self class I molecules. They will not lyse cells displaying class I molecules alone nor will they lyse virally infected cells displaying class I molecules different than self. Therefore, the specificity of these cytotoxic T cells is similar to that noted for alloreactive cytotoxic T cells in that both require recognition of class I molecules. In the one instance, however, self class I molecules are seen in association with virus, whereas in the other, foreign class I molecules are seen alone.

The following experiment was performed to determine the relationship between these two specificities.[1] A clone of T cells cytotoxic for virus plus self class I antigens was assayed for its cytotoxic activity against a panel of targets displaying dif-

ferent, foreign class I molecules in the absence of virus, and the T cell line could lyse one of the foreign targets. Reactivity to foreign class I molecules appeared to represent cross-reactivity by a cell whose original specificity was for virus seen in association with self class I molecules. The frequency of T cell clones reacting to a single foreign class I molelcule (1/100) was greater than that for T cell clones reactive to an individual virus plus self class I (1/1000). Therefore, the total reactivity to a foreign class I molecule must represent the sum of the reactivities occurring among several clones each of which has specificity for a different virus plus self class I. In teleologic terms, this makes sense. The immune system must have been designed to prevent infection rather than to frustrate transplantation surgeons. Although viruses have been used as the prototype antigen in this discussion, similar class I restricted cytotoxicity can be demonstrated for other intracellular organisms as well as for cells that have been modified by reactivity with haptens.

An analogous situation exists for the relationship between T cells with specificity for foreign class II molecules and those that view self class II molecules in conjunction with soluble antigen. A clone of T cells reactive to a single antigen seen in the context of self class II can cross-react with a single foreign class II molecule in the absence of antigen.[26] The frequency of T cell clones reactive to a foreign class II molecule (1/100) is greater than the frequency of T cell clones reactive to antigen plus self class II (1/10,000).

It has been possible to generate in humans OKT4+ T cells that are cytotoxic for cells displaying foreign class II, but not class I molecules. The biologic significance of such cells has not been established.[17]

ONTOGENY OF B CELLS

In birds, development of peripheral B cells requires that stem cells undergo differentiation in a portion of the hindgut called the bursa of Fabricius. Extirpation of this bursa results in a B cell-depleted, agammaglobulinemic bird. In mammals, there is no discrete bursal homologue. Instead, the differentiation of stem cells into B cells occurs in the liver during fetal life and in the bone marrow during adult life.

The stepwise differentiation of B cells is represented by the development of three different cell types: pre-B cell, B cell, and plasma cell. A pre-B cell contains cytoplasmic immunoglobulin, but does not express surface Ig. A B cell expresses Ig on its surface, but does not secrete large amounts of Ig. A plasma cell does not express surface Ig, but does secrete large amounts of Ig into the environment. The development of B cells through these three stages can best be presented by recounting the genetic and molecular events involved in Ig synthesis. (For a more complete discussion of Ig genes, see Chapter 15.)

Genes encoding for the synthesis of Ig heavy chains can be divided into four major domains: variable (V), diversity (D), joining (J), and constant (C).[11] Each domain consists of a variable number of genes: $v = 100$, $D = 10$, $J = 5$, $C = 5$. The production of an intact heavy chain involves two major gene rearrangements. In the first, a single V gene links with a single D gene, which in turn links with a single J gene. In the second, the VDJ complex links with a C gene that codes for the constant region of the heavy chain. (The five C region genes represent each of the five Ig classes, μ, δ, γ, ϵ, and σ, and are represented on the chromosome $5' \rightarrow 3'$ in that order.) Genes encoding for the synthesis of light chains can be divided into three domains, V-J-C, each of which is also composed of a variable number of genes. Synthesis of an intact light chain involves rearrangements among these genes that result in a single VJC complex. In cells not synthesizing immunoglobulin, e.g., a fibroblast, no rearrangement of heavy or light chain genes occurs and this is referred to as their *germ line configuration*. In cells that do synthesize Ig, the Ig genes are rearranged. Therefore, rearrangement of Ig genes can be equated with the synthesis of heavy or light chains. Each stage of B cell development can be characterized by specific patterns of Ig gene rearrangement as follows (Fig. 17–6).

Pre-B Cell

The first event in B cell differentiation is reflected by rearrangements among heavy chain genes. A VJD gene complex associates with a Cμ gene. An intact heavy chain is synthesized and appears in the cytoplasm. Next, rearrangements occur among the light chain genes in an interesting fashion. The first rearrangements occur on one allele of the κ light chain. If this results in an effective VJC complex, than an intact κ light chain is synthesized. If an effective rearrangement does not occur, then rearrangement switches to the other allele of the κ gene. If an effective VJC complex results, κ light chain synthesis ensures. If not, rearrangements switch first to one allele and, if unsuccessful, to the other allele of the λ genes. If no effective light chain gene rearrangement occurs, then normal B cell development does not proceed.

Once an effective light chain gene rearrangement ensues, light chains are synthesized, appear in the cytoplasm, and become associated with heavy chains.

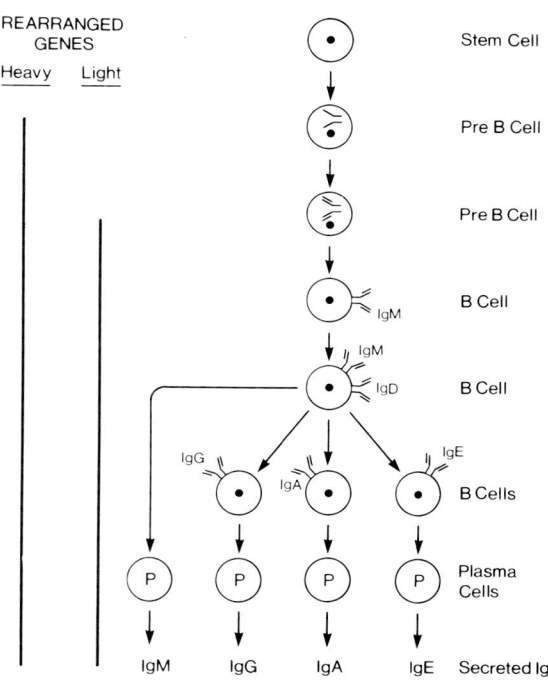

Fig. 17–6. Events involved in the differentiation of B cells. The scheme traces the differentiation of B cells. The black lines to the left indicate the presence of rearranged genes that correlate with various stages of B cell differentiation.

B Cell

The switch from the pre-B cell to B cell stage is characterized by the appearance of membrane immunoglobulin. The B cell first only expresses IgM (monomeric, 7S IgM) and next synthesizes and expresses both IgM and IgD. At the gene level this is represented by the association of a single VDJ complex with both Cμ and Cδ genes. Since VDJ genes code for the portions of Ig molecules that dictate their antigen specificity and C genes code for portions that determine immunoglobulin class, it is easy to see how a single cell can synthesize two different classes of immunglobulin each of which has the same antigenic specificity. The display of both IgM and IgD appears to be an important event in B cell activation. B cells displaying only surface IgM are difficult to activate and, in some models, appear particularly susceptible to the induction of tolerance. In contrast, the appearance of surface IgD provides a receptor that allows appropriate signals to push B differentiation forward. At the next stage of B cell development, the B cells express only IgD. From this point, they differentiate into cells that display only IgG, IgE, or IgA.

Plasma Cell

At this stage, all gene rearrangements have been completed, and the cell is engaged in secreting large amounts of immunoglobulin of a single antigenic specificity and immunoglobulin class. In general, it can be assumed that B cells displaying a specific immunoglobulin class give rise to plasma cells secreting Ig of that same class. For example, IgG-bearing B cells generate IgG-secreting plasma cells, IgA-bearing B cells give rise to IgA-secreting plasma cells, and IgE-bearing B cells generate IgE-secreting plasma cells.

This ordered sequence of immunoglobulin class expression that occurs during B cell differentiation is mirrored by the ontogeny of B cells and immunoglobulin production. In human fetuses, synthesis of IgM begins at 10 to 11 weeks of age, IgG at 12 weeks, and IgA after 30 weeks of age. Adult levels of IgM occur by one year of age, IgG by five years of age, and IgA by early teens.

REGULATION OF B CELL DIFFERENTIATION AND IG PRODUCTION

Although B cells displaying IgM can develop in the absence of T cells, the development of B cells displaying other Ig classes and the differentiation of B cells into plasma cells requires the presence of T cells. A complete picture of the T cell factors and cellular interactions involved in the B cell differentiation and immunoglobulin production requires data obtained in mice (Fig. 17–7). Mouse splenic B cells can be divided broadly into two equal populations based on their display of the differentiation marker Lyb5. (Lyb5$^+$ cells constitute 50% and Lyb5$^-$ cells 50% of the splenic B cell pool.) Both populations require T cells for their differentiation and development into plasma cells. However, in the case of the Lyb5$^+$ population, the interaction with T cells is not restricted by class II molecules. Differentiation of the Lyb5$^+$ B cell population can be mediated by T cells displaying nonhomologous class II molecules or by soluble factors obtained from these T cells. Since the events involved in triggering differentiation among the Lyb5$^+$ population have been studied in most detail, the discussion will focus on them.

Three different stimuli are required to induce proliferation among resting Lyb5$^+$ cells.: (1) a stimulus that appropriately perturbs membrane Ig receptors, (2) a T cell-derived factor designated BCGF, and (3) IL-1.

Initial events that cause physiologic activation of resting Lyb5$^+$ B cells is represented by the cross-linking of surface receptors for antigen (i.e., surface Ig) by multivalent antigens. In vitro, this initial event can be mimicked by cross-linking surface Ig

with anti-IgM. This signal initiates increased RNA synthesis and the cell moves from resting (G$_0$) into an early activation (G$_1$) phase. Interaction with the two soluble materials, BCGF and IL-1, is needed to move the cell from the G$_1$ and S phase where DNA synthesis and replication occur. Although not purified to homogeneity, human BCGF produced from mitogen-activated peripheral blood lymphocytes appears to consist of two components with molecular weights of 17,000 to 20,000 and 12,000 to 13,000. BCGF does not bind to resting B cells, but does bind to B cells activated with anti-IgM. Therefore, it appears that activation of B cells by appropriate interactions with antigen results in the expression of BCGF receptors. The third signal required to initiate DNA synthesis among Lyb5$^+$ B cells is IL-1, liberated by accessory cells such as macrophages.

The combination of these three signals, anti-IgG (or multivalent antigen), BCGF, and IL-1, is sufficient to induce B cell proliferation, but is not sufficient for development of antibody-secreting plasma cells. *This fact emphasizes that B cell proliferation cannot be equated with antibody secretion.* Development of antibody-secreting plasma cells from activated B cells requires the action of still another T cell-derived factor, TRF. This factor is poorly characterized, but in both mice and humans it appears to have a molecular weight (i.e., 30,000 to 50,000) higher than that described for IL-1, IL-2, or BCGF.

To summarize, induction of Ig synthesis among a subpopulation of murine peripheral blood B cells represented by those bearing the Lyb5 differentiation markers is initiated by appropriate interactions between surface Ig receptors for antigen and multivalent antigens and proceeds through interactions with BCGF, IL-1, and TRF (Fig. 17–7). Only the initiating event is antigen-specific. BCGF, IL-1, and TRF act in an unrestricted manner, and T cells synthesizing BCGF or TRF do not have to share the same class II molecules displayed by the B cells. None of these factors specifically binds to antigen. The specificity of their action depends on the state of activation of the B cell upon which they exert their effect.

Events involved in the activation of the other 50% of peripheral B cells (i.e., Lyb5$^-$ cells) are less clearly understood. T cells are required in conjunction with antigen to induce their activation. However, in contrast to T-B cell interactions involved in the early stages of the activation of Lyb5$^+$ cells, this interaction probably requires direct cell-to-cell contact and can occur only if the T cell and B cell bear the same class II molecules. Various soluble materials have been claimed to substitute for this T cell help. Most of them contain class II

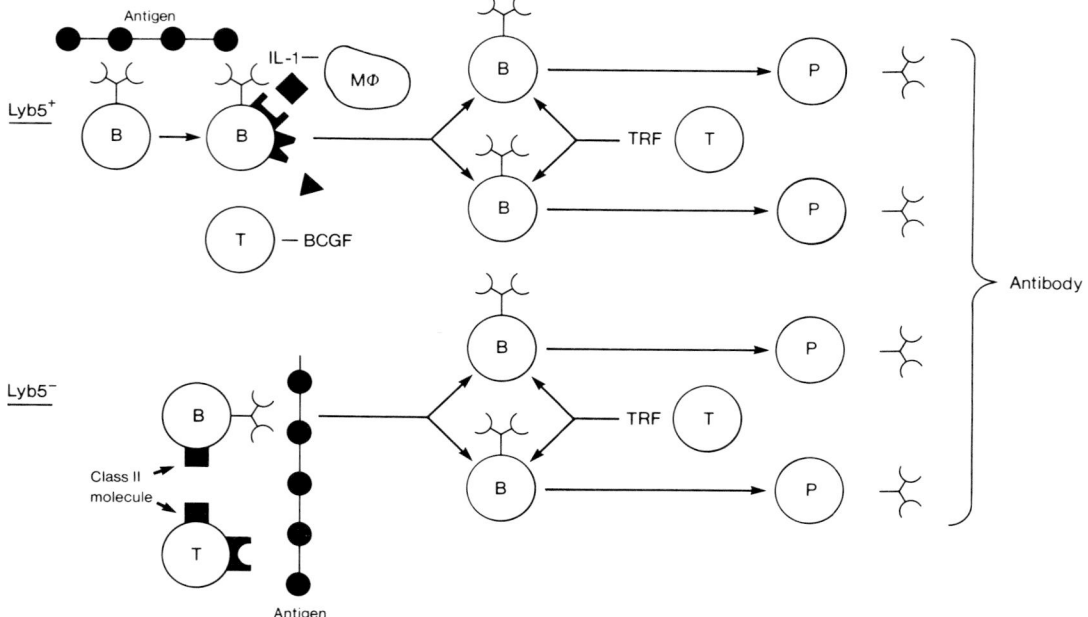

Fig. 17–7. Differentiation of Lyb5$^+$ and Lyb5$^-$ B cells into plasma cells. Differentiation of Lyb5$^+$ cells requires appropriate activation of Lyb5$^+$ B cells by antigen plus BCGF synthesized by T cells and IL-1 synthesized Mϕ (macrophages). Differentiation of Lyb5$^-$ B cells requires direct interactions with antigen and T cells displaying homologous iA molecules. In both models, TRF is required for B cells to differentiate into plasma cells.

determinants, some bind antigen, and all are poorly characterized. As indicated for differentiation of Lyb5$^+$ B cells, the generation of antibody-secreting plasma cells from Lyb5$^-$ B cells also requires a T cell-derived TRF (Fig. 17–7). Thus, although initial events involved in activating Lyb5$^+$ and Lyb5$^-$ B cells may differ, subsequent events involved in their differentiation into plasma cells may be similar. The events involved in the activation and differentiation of both Lyb5$^+$ and Lyb5$^-$ cells are summarized in Figure 17–5.

Recently, an increasing number of studies indicate that T cells also can influence the specific class of immunoglobulin produced.[9] These isotype specific helper T cells can exert their effect either by influencing the differentiation of B cells or by driving B cell development into plasma cells. For example, there appears to exist a specific population of T cells that affect the development of IgA bearing from IgM bearing B cells.[3] Another population of T cells specifically drives IgA bearing B cells into IgA-secreting plasma cells.[14] In each instance, the effect can be replaced by a soluble factor derived from the T cells. Isotypic specific helper T cells have been demonstrated thus far for IgG, IgE, and IgA production. Signals that activate these T cells may be initiated via T cell receptors capable of binding to the Fc portion of the isotype

that they regulate. T cells specifically involved in regulating the production of IgE bear receptors capable of binding to the Fc portion of IgE.[31] T cells capable of generating IgA-bearing from IgM-bearing cells preferentially home to gut associated lymphoid tissue, which may account for the relatively high levels of IgA in gastrointestinal secretions.

To attain immunologic homeostasis, perturbations initiated among the T cell pool driving B cell activation and differentiation must be accompanied by signals capable of inhibiting or halting this same process and this is accomplished by suppressor T cells. The balanced activation of suppressor T cells occurs in response to feedback signals from (1) activated B cells, and (2) activated helper T cells. Activation of a subpopulation of OKT4$^+$ helper T cells (OKT4$^+$, JRA$^+$, TQ1$^+$, OKT17$^+$) results in signals that induce the generation of suppresor effectors among OKT8$^+$ T cells.[24] Such suppressor effector cells then exert their effect on Ig production either indirectly through inactivation of helper T cells, or directly through inhibition of B cell differentiation.[30] In some cases, it has been possible to obtain soluble factors capable of mediating immunosuppression. Most of these factors have two features in common. First, they specifically bind only the antigen whose response is being suppressed. Second, they bind to I-J antisera. The J locus is thought to represent a region of the murine immune response locus that controls activation of suppressor cells. Utilizing genetic probes, researchers have demonstrated that this locus does not exist in murine I region.[8] To date, no one has isolated and fully characterized an I-J molecule. Therefore, the localization of I-J in the genome and the significance of I-J molecules in physiologic immunosuppression is uncertain.

The synthesis of immunoglobulin requires interactions among distinct populations of T cells. For control and antigen specificity, a recognition system for communication between the appropriate populations of T cells must exist. This system involves the recognition of idiotypes. Idiotypes are located in the antigen combining region of immunoglobulin molecules. Antibodies with specificity for different antigens have different amino acid sequences in the region of the molecule that binds to the antigen, and these structural differences can be recognized antigenically by the immune system. It is possible to make an antibody against idiotypic determinants (i.e., an anti-idiotype) present in an antibody of a given specificity that reacts only with that antibody and not with others. The *idiotype network* involved in regulating immune reactivity proceeds as follows. In response to an antigenic challenge, T cells and B cells bearing a receptor specific for the antigen are activated. The expansion of these cells produces an immunologic response to the idiotypes in their antigen receptors characterized by the production of anti-idiotypic antibodies. This, in turn, reults in the production of anti-anti-idiotypes. This reaction does not go on indefinitely, and the loop closes with the production of anti-anti-anti-idiotype. This is because the anti-anti-anti–idiotype contains determinants that structurally resemble antigen and, therefore, bind to the original antibody produced against the antigen.

T CELL RECEPTOR FOR ANTIGEN

The search for the T cell receptor for antigen has been challenging and elusive. As indicated previously, it is clear that activation of T cells reactive to either soluble, conventional, or viral antigens requires that they recognize determinants inherent in either the antigen or virus in conjunction with self class II or class I determinants, respectively. This has led to the development of two models concerning the general structure of the T cell receptor. The first, the "modified self model," suggests that the T cell receptor exhibits specificity for a new determinant generated by interactions between antigen or virus and self class II or class I molecules. The second, the "dual recognition model," proposes that the T cell receptor is composed of two distinct units, one that recognizes antigen and one that recognizes self class II or I molecules. Interactions with both units of the receptor are required for T cell activation to occur. There are not sufficient data to determine which of these models is correct. There is, however, evidence that clearly indicates that if the "dual recognition model" is appropriate, the two recognition units are closely linked on the T cell membrane.

To characterize the T cell receptor for antigen, several investigators have tried to show that at least a portion of the receptor consists of a molecule structurally resembling immunoglobulin, but none have been successful yet. The recent availability of probes for immunoglobulin genes provides another approach to this question. Several laboratories have examined T cell clones and T cell lines for either rearranged Ig genes indicating their activation or for Ig messenger RNA. Most studies have demonstrated that Ig genes in T cells exist in the germ line configuration and are not rearranged as they are in Ig expressing B cells. This finding indicates either that Ig genes in T cells are not active or that their activation occurs by some mechanism different from that used in B cells. Although some studies have demonstrated the existence of T cell messenger RNA, which hybridizes with Ig probes, the message is usually defective and does not translate for the synthesis of Ig molecules. Therefore, the probing of T cells with either molecular or genetic probes has failed to elucidate the structure of the T cell receptor for antigen.

Three observations have indicated that activation of T cells by antigen involves more than a single receptor.[15,16] The first is that molecules that serve to mark populations and subpopulations of T cells play an important role in their function (Table 17–3). Antibodies to T8 block the cytolytic capabilities of T8[+] cells, owing to the antibody blocking T cell recognition of class I molecules and preventing interactions between effector and target cells, and not to the inhibition of the cytolytic mechanism of the T cell. Antibodies to T4 block recognition of class II molecules by OKT4[+] T cells. Since activation of T4[+] and T8[+] cells by antigen requires associative recognition of class II and class I molecules, respectively, one might conclude that these data support the concept that the T4 and T8 molecules are actually the antigen receptor. This possibility is ruled out by the demonstration that T4 and T8 molecules isolated from clones of T cells with specificity for different antigens are structurally identical. Receptors with specificity for distinct antigens should manifest

Table 17–3.   Characteristics of T Cell Surface Molecules Important in T Cell Recognition of Antigen

T Cell Surface Molecule	Mol. Wt.	Functional Effect of Antibodies Against the Molecule
T3	20,000–23,000	1) Activates T cells 2) Inhibits proliferative responses to Ag 3) Inhibits cytotoxicity restricted by class I or class II molecules
T4	60,000	1) Inhibits proliferation to class II alloantigens 2) Inhibits cytotoxicity to class II antigens
T8	76,000*	1) Inhibits proliferation to class I alloantigens 2) Inhibits cytotoxicity restricted by class I molecules
T clonotypic (Tc)	43,000† 49,000	Inhibits reactivity of only a specific clone of T cells reactive with the antibody

*nonreducing conditions
†reducing conditions

structural differences in the antigen-combining regions.

A second important observation in delineating the nature of the T cell receptor is that it is possible to generate monoclonal antibodies that block, in an antigen-specific fashion, activation of T cell clones (see Table 17–3). For example, some monoclonal antibodies block class I or class II molecule restricted reactivity among only a single clone of T8+ or T4+ cells, respectively. Molecules reactive with these antibodies consist of a bimolecular complex (43,000 and 49,000 daltons molecular weight chains) linked together on the cell surface by disulfide bonds. These molecules do exhibit structural polymorphism in that the structure of the molecules isolated from clones reactive to distinct antigens is different. These clonotypic molecules (termed here Tc for convenience) appear to be excellent candidates for the T cell antigen receptor.

The third observation important in understanding the nature of the T cell receptor for antigen is that the T3 molecule, displayed by all T cells, plays a central role in T cell activation by antigen (see Table 17–3). Antibody-induced removal of T3 from T4 or T8 positive cells inhibits their reactivity. The re-expression of T3 coincides with recovery of activity. It can be demonstrated that antibody-induced removal of T3 also results in the co-capping of the bimolecular complex depicted by the antigen-specific, clonotypic antibodies, Tc. Moreover, immunoprecipitation of T3 from cell surfaces results in the concomitant precipitation of the clonotypic, bimolecular complex. These observations, coupled with the fact that the number of T3 molecules on the T cell surface is similar to the number of displayed Tc molecules (~30,000), suggest that T3 and Tc are physically associated on the cell surface.

Based on these three major observations, a model concerning structures involved in recognition of antigen by T cells can be constructed (Fig.

17–8).[20] Three classes of molecules appear to be involved: T4 or T8, T3, and Tc. The T4 and T8 molecules displayed by all T4+ and T8+ cells is involved in recognizing nonpolymorphic determi-

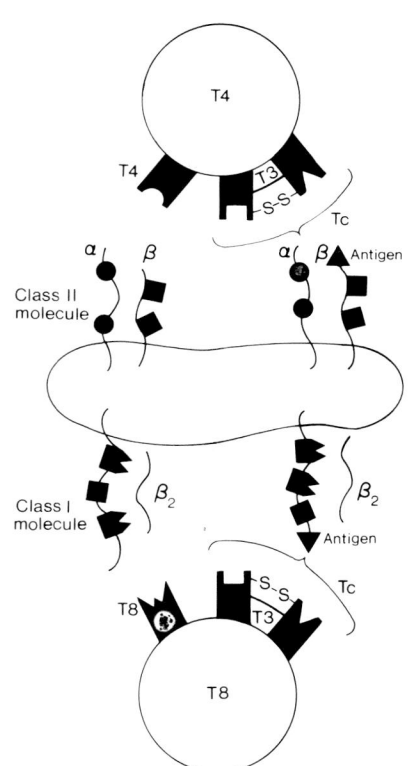

Fig. 17–8.   T cell molecules involved in the recognition of antigen. In this model, T4 and T8 recognize nonpolymorphic determinants in class II (●) and class I (X) molecules, respectively. This stabilizes binding between the T cell and the cell-associated antigen. One chain of Tc binds antigen (▲) while the other binds polymorphic class II or class I determinants (■). T3 stabilizes the Tc receptor. S-S = a disulfide bond.

nants present in class II and class I molecules, respectively. One chain of the Tc might recognize polymorphic class I or class II determinants, while the other portion of the Tc molecule might recognize antigen. T3 could be associated with one or both Tc chains and could serve to stabilize the Tc receptor.

In this model, the T4 and T8 receptors serve to stabilize interactions between unprimed T cells and cells bearing class II and class I molecules, respectively. This stabilization is necessary so that appopriate perturbation of the Tc-T3 complex can occur and thus initiate cell activation. This concept is supported by the observation that reactivity among primed T cells is not easily blocked by anti-T4 or anti-T8. The primed T cells, as opposed to non-primed cells, can generate a stable interaction between antigen and the T3-Tc complex without the need for T4 or T8.

An important issue concerns the nature of the polymorphic recognition unit represented by Tc. This complex can be found on murine T cell hybrids selected for their loss of genes coding for the synthesis of immunoglobulin light chains and MHC determinants.[13] Therefore, light chains and MHC determinants are not part of the receptor. Whether Tc is encoded for by immunoglobulin heavy chain genes and its relationship to conventional immunoglobulin molecules remains a fascinating and important question.

REFERENCES

1. Brunner, K.T., et al.: Cytolytic T lymphocyte clones recognizing murine sarcoma virus induced tumor antigens. *In* Isolation, Characterization, and Utilization of T Lymphocyte Clones. Edited by C.G. Fathman, and F.W. Fitch. New York, Academic Press, 1982, pp. 297–310.
2. Dutton, W.: Suppressor T cells. Transplant. Rev., 26:39–55, 1975.
3. Elson, C.O., Heck, J.A., and Strober, W.: T cell regulation of murine IgA synthesis. J. Exp. Med., 149:632–643, 1979.
4. Gallatin, W.M., Weissman, I.R., and Butcher, E.C.: A cell-surface molecule involved in organ-specific homing of lymphocytes. Nature, 304:30–34, 1983.
5. Gillis, S.: Interleukin 2: biology and biochemistry. J. Clin. Immunol., 3:1–13, 1983.
6. Gonwa, T.A., Peterlin, B.M., and Stobo, J.D.: Human Ir genes: Structure and function. *In* Advances in Immunology. Vol. 34. Edited by H. Kunkel, and F. Dixon. New York, Academic Press, 1983, pp. 71–93.
7. Hapel, A.J., et al.: Establishment of continuous cultures of Thy 1.2+, Lyt 1+, 2- T cells with purified interleukin 3. Cell, 25:179–186, 1981.
8. Hood, L., Steinmetz, M., and Malissen, B.: Regulation of B cell growth and differentiation by soluble factors. Ann. Rev. Immunol., 1:529, 1983.
9. Hoover, R.G., et al.: Occurrence and potential significance of increased numbers of T cells with Fc receptors in myeloma. Immunol. Rev., 56:115–139, 1981.
10. Howard, M., and Paul, W.: Regulation of B-cell growth and differentiation by soluble factors. Annu. Rev. Immunol., 1:307–334, 1983.
11. Leder, P.: Genetic control of immunoglobulin production. Hosp. Pract., 18:73–82, 1983.
12. Ma, D.D.F., et al.: The role of purine metabolic enzymes and terminal deoxynucleotidyl transferase in intrathymic T cell differentiation. Immunol. Today, 4:65–67, 1983.
13. Marrack, P., and Kappler, J.: Use of somatic cell genetics to study chromosome contributing to antigen plus I recognition by T cell hybridomas. J. Exp. Med., 157:404–418, 1983.
14. Mayer, L., Fu, S.M., and Kunkel, H.G.: Human T cell hybridomas secreting factors for IgA-specific help, polyclonal B cell activation, and B cell proliferation. J. Exp. Med., 156:1860–1871, 1982.
15. Meuer, S.C., et al.: Evidence for the T3 associated 90K heterodimer as the T-cell antigen receptor. Nature, 303:808–810, 1983.
16. Meurer, S.C., et al.: Clonotypic structures involved in antigen-specific human T cell function: Relationship to the T3 molecular complex. J. Exp. Med., 157:705–719, 1983.
17. Meuer, S.C., Schlossman, S.F., and Reinherz, E.L.: Clonal analysis of human cytotoxic T lymphocytes: T4+ and T8+ effector T cells recognize products of different major histocompatibility complex regions. Proc. Natl. Acad. Sci. U.S.A., 79:4395–4399, 1982.
18. Nabholz, M., and MacDonald, H.R.: Cytolytic T lymphocytes. Ann. Rev. Immunol., 1:273–306, 1983.
19. Oppenheim, J.J., and Gery, I.: Interleukin 1 is more than an interleukin. Immunol. Today, 3:113–119, 1982.
20. Reinherz, E.L., Meuer, S.F., and Schlossman, S.F.: The delineation of antigen receptor on human T lymphocytes. Immunol. Today, 4:5–9, 1983.
21. Reinherz, E.L., et al.: Heterogeneity of human T4+ inducer T cells defined by a monoclonal antibody that delineates two functional subpopulations. J. Immunol., 128:463–468, 1982.
22. Reinherz, E.L., and Schlossman, S.F.: The characterization and function of human immunoregulatory T lymphocyte. Immunol. Today, 2:69–75, 1981.
23. Reinherz, E.L., and Schlossman, S.F.: The differentiation and function of T lymphocytes. Cell, 19:821–827, 1980.
24. Reinherz, E.L., and Schlossman, S.F.: Regulation of immune response-inducer and suppressor T lymphocyte subsets in human beings. N. Engl. J. Med., 303:370–373, 1980.
25. Rosenthal, A.S.: Current concepts: Regulation of the immune response role of the macrophage. N. Engl. J. Med., 303:1153–1159, 1980.
26. Schwartz, R.H., and Sredni, B.: Alloreactivity of antigen specific T cell clones. *In* Isolation, Characterization and Utilization of T Lymphocyte Clones. Edited by C. G. Fathman, and R.W. Fitch. New York, Academic Press, 1982, pp. 375–382.
27. Singer, A., and Hodes, R.J.: Mechanisms of T cell-B cell interaction. Annu. Rev. Immunol., 1:211–242, 1983.
28. Thomas, Y., et al.: Further dissection of the functional heterogeneity within the OKT4+ and OKT8+ human T cell subsets. J. Clin. Immunol., 2:8S–14S, 1982.
29. Van Voorhis, W.C., et al.: The cutaneous infiltrates of leproxy: Cellular characteristics and the predominant T cell phenotypes. N. Engl. J. Med., 307:1593–1597, 1982.
30. Webb, D.R., Kapp, J.A., and Pierce, C.W.: The biochemistry of antigen specific T cell factors. Annu. Rev. Immunol., 1:423–438, 1983.
31. Yodoi, J., Hirashima, M., and Ishizaka, K.: Regulatory role of IgE-binding factors from rat T lymphocytes. V. The carbohydrate moieties in IgE-potentiating factors and IgE-suppressive factors. J. Immunol., 128:289–295, 1982.
32. Zinkernagle, R., and Doherty, P.: MHC restricted cytotoxic T cells: Studies on the biologic role of polymorphic major transplantation antigens determining T cell restriction—specificity, function and responsiveness. Adv. Immunol., 27:51–177, 1979.

Chapter **18**

Polymorphonuclear Leukocytes

Sara B. Kramer, Bruce N. Cronstein, and Gerald Weissmann

The polymorphonuclear leukocytes (PMNs) are highly specialized cells whose primary function is the phagocytosis and destruction of microorganisms and other noxious agents. In addition to their role in host defense, PMNs are commonly present at sites of immunologically mediated tissue injury. It has recently been appreciated that they mediate many of the events that occur at foci of acute inflammation.

Metchnikoff proposed, in the closing years of the nineteenth century, that leukocytes may liberate substances that are capable of damaging adjacent tissues.[83] Not until the mid-twentieth century was the crucial role of PMNs demonstrated in a variety of experimental immunologically induced inflammatory reactions. The first such lesion shown to be dependent on neutrophils was the Arthus reaction. The specific depletion of PMNs by either nitrogen mustard or heterologous antineutrophil antisera could abort or inhibit the Arthus reaction in several species. Despite deposition of antigen, antibody, and complement components in the vessels of antiserum-treated animals, no microscopic evidence of vascular injury could be found.[18,23,51,101,133] Other experimental models of immunologic injury have a similar dependence on the neutrophil for tissue damage. These models include the necrotizing arteritis of experimental serum sickness in rabbits,[67] the proteinuria associated with acute nephrotoxic vasculitis in rats and rabbits[17] and arthritis in rabbits induced by an intra-articular reversed passive Arthus reaction.[24] In the last of these experimental systems, intra-articular injections of purified suspensions of PMNs reconstituted the immunologic lesions in neutrophil-depleted rabbits.

As documented in these studies, PMNs play an important role in the mediation of immunologically induced tissue injury. PMNs accomplish this role by the generation of toxic metabolites and by the release of various inflammatory substances. In particular, PMNs actively release substances contained within their cytoplasmic granules or lysosomes. These lysosomal substances not only cause tissue damage directly but can interact with components of the complement and kinin systems to generate other mediators of inflammation and tissue damage.

GENERAL DESCRIPTION OF THE PMN

Morphology. Mature PMNs are easily distinguished from other circulating cells. They range in size from 8 to 15 μm in diameter and have a multilobed nucleus (Fig. 18–1) PMN types can be further distinguished by visualizing blood smears stained with Wright's stain. Three types of granulocytes, the neutrophils, eosinophils, and basophils, have thus been identified.

The most common type of PMN in blood and other kinds of tissues is the PMN neutrophil. This type of PMN is probably the most important for the mediation of tissue injury and for host defense. The neutrophil nucleus has 2 to 5 lobes. Cytoplasm is plentiful, and multiple granules are pink on Wright's stain. Electron microscopy demonstrates few mitochondria and sparse endoplasmic reticulum (see Fig. 18–1).

Eosinophils, which comprise 1 to 3% of the total leukocyte population in the peripheral blood, have large cytoplasmic granules that stain red. These cells appear to be involved in the host response to parasites, although their function and role in host defense and response to injury are currently being studied.

The third type of PMN is the basophil. This cell can be distinguished by the large bluish-black cytoplasmic granules seen in Wright's stained smears. These granules contain histamine and heparin. Basophils mediate immediate hypersensitivity (type I immunologic) reactions and constitute less than 1% of the leukocyte population in the peripheral blood.

Although basophils and eosinophils are involved in inflammation, the preponderant PMN cell type found in sites of inflammation, as well as in the peripheral blood, is the neutrophil. Because of this numerical preponderance and because their role in the mediation of inflammation and tissue injury in the connective tissue diseases has been more intensively studied, the discussion in the remainder of this chapter will refer exclusively to neutrophils.

PRODUCTION OF PMNS

Polymorphonuclear leukocytes have an extremely rapid rate of turnover[15] and circulate for short periods of time. The half-life of the mature neutrophil in the circulation is 6 to 7 hours. Because several days are required for the neutrophil to mature in the bone marrow, a large pool of marrow precursors is necessary for maintenance of the population of PMNs in the circulation. The factors responsible for stimulation of neutrophil production, such as granulopoietin, are now being isolated, although their source is not known.[68]

In the bone marrow, maturation of neutrophils proceeds through several histologically characteristic stages. The precursors of PMNs (myelocytes and promyelocytes) synthesize lysosomes or granules in the Golgi apparatus.[30] Two granule types are morphologically distinct. The first type of granule to appear during the maturation process is called the primary or azurophil granule (because of its staining characteristics on Wright-Giemsa stain). These granules are large and contain several hydrolytic enzymes and bactericidal materials (discussed in greater detail later). Secondary granules (also known as specific granules) appear only after the full cellular complement of primary granules has been synthesized. The secondary granules are smaller than primary granules and contain their own different group of enzymes and bactericidal materials. There are more secondary granules than primary granules in the mature neutrophil, despite the later appearance of the secondary granules during cellular maturation. Some evidence suggests other subcellular storage sites for "granular" enzymes.[89] These enzymes can be released upon appropriate stimulation.

In addition to the morphologic changes seen during maturation, the cellular metabolism also undergoes a transition. Neutrophil precursors contain many mitochondria and appear to use oxidative metabolism to fuel their protein synthesis. As the cell matures, there is a shift to anaerobic glycolysis as the primary energy source, presumably in preparation for function of hypoxic tissues.[8,117] The neutrophil precursors also acquire mobility, plasticity, and the capacity to ingest particles as they mature. Immature neutrophils that are released into the circulation prematurely have diminished bactericidal activity.[82]

PMN FUNCTION

In order to accomplish their role in host defense, PMNs ingest their targets for further intracellular digestion and destruction.

Phagocytosis. Upon exposure to suitable particles, PMNs invaginate their surface membrane at the point of contact and surround the particle. The resulting intracellular vacuole, called a phagosome or phagocytic vesicle, pinches off from the surface of the cell and becomes completely internalized within the cytoplasm of the PMN.[72,88,146] After phagocytosis, the cells are rounded and have less available surface membrane. Resting PMNs that have not been exposed to particles have a large surface area, seen in the form of surface pseudopods and blebs (Fig. 18–2). Despite the relatively large surface area, cell surface membrane is finite in extent, and limitations in availability of surface membrane may limit the number of particles that can be ingested by a single cell. Fusion of granule membranes with phagosome membranes begins the process of digestion of the phagocytosed particles. The lysosomal granules then discharge their contents into the phagosome in a process known as degranulation.[19,46,97] The phagosome, now called a phagolysosome, contains an array of microbicidal proteins and degradative enzymes.

GRANULE CONTENTS

Neutrophils are well adapted to their role as microbicidal and scavenging cells. Their granules contain an assortment of microbicidal enzymes and proteases necessary to meet the challenge of many different types of bacteria as well as to scavenge damaged tissues. Many of these granular enzymes are also capable of damaging viable host tissues. Since they are usually sequestered within the granule and phagolysosome, however, these enzymes do not usually present a threat to the host. Generally, a minimal amount of granule contents is released by the cell during the phagocytic process, but under certain pathologic conditions massive release of granule contents can promote tissue injury and lead to further inflammation. Extracellular release of granule contents can be accomplished by several mechanisms that are discussed subsequently.

The granules of neutrophils contain many different types of compounds, including microbicidal enzymes, proteases, and proteins whose microbicidal properties are nonenzymatic. Lysozyme, a bactericidal enzyme found in specific and azurophilic granules, hydrolyzes cell wall peptidoglycans of many species of bacteria.[13,130] Specific granules also contain nonenzymatic compounds, including lactoferrin,[130] a bacteriostatic protein, and vitamin B_{12} binding protein.[59] Collagenase[90] and alkaline phosphatase[14] are neutral hydrolases also found in specific granules.

Azurophil granules also contain lysozyme.[13,130] In contrast to the specific granules, however, the azurophil granules also contain myeloperoxidase, low-molecular-weight bactericidal cationic proteins,[144] chondroitin sulfate, and the neutral and acid hydrolases.[72,99,130] Myeloperoxidase, together with H_2O_2 and a halide, constitutes one of the killing mechanisms of the neutrophils.[65] The low-molecular-weight bactericidal cationic proteins are a

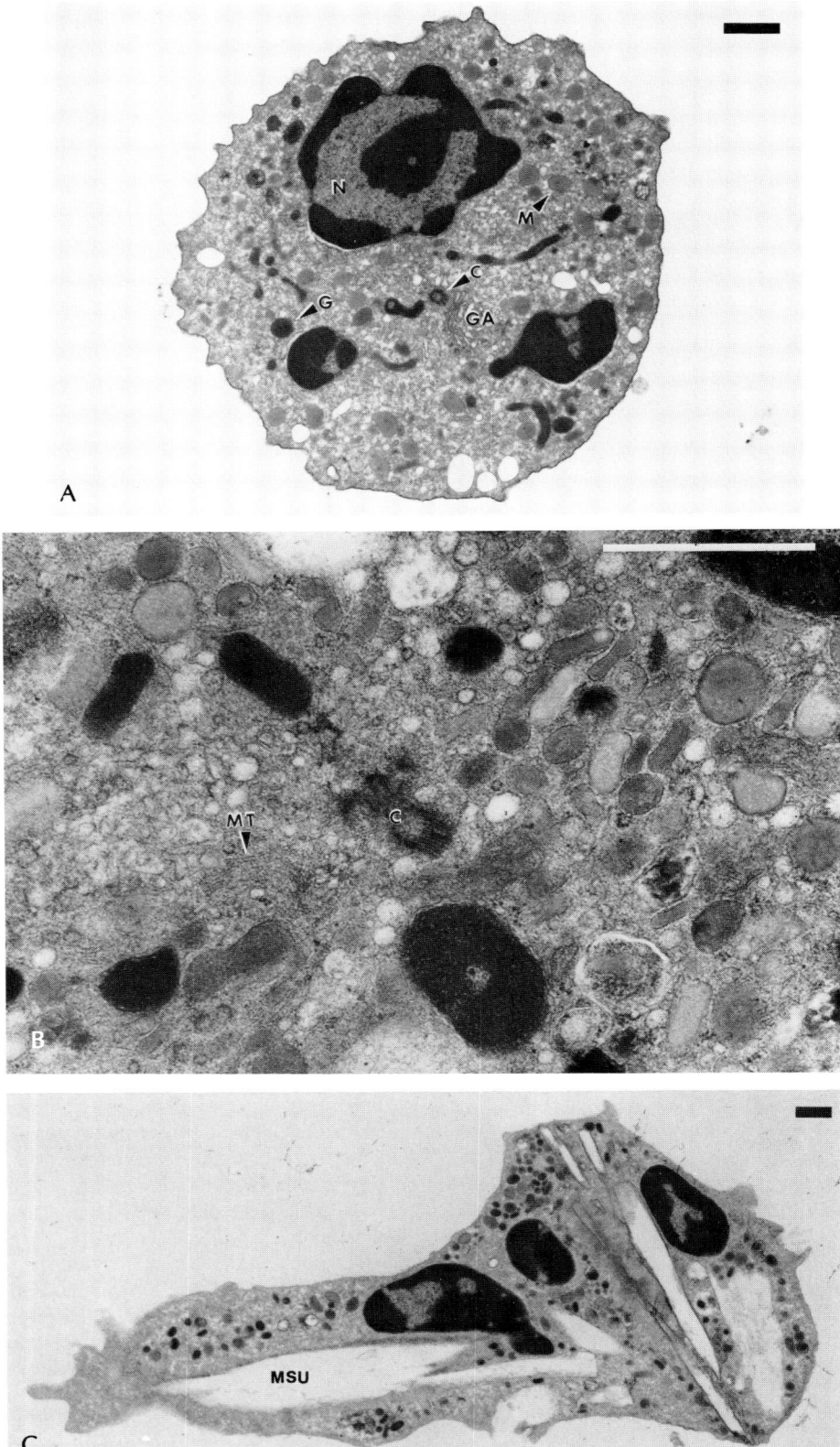

heterogeneous group of proteins most active at acid pH and with different bactericidal specificities for gram-positive and gram-negative bacteria.[145] When released into the extracellular milieu, these proteins can also cause increased vascular permeability or histamine release. The acid and neutral hydrolases have digestive or scavenging functions as well as antibacterial properties. A representative group of granule contents is listed in Table 18–1.

The proteases are the granule contents with the greatest potential for causing tissue damage. As a group, these enzymes have a broad substrate specificity. We will describe in more detail the neutral serine proteases, cathepsin G and elastase, and the metalloenzyme, collagenase. Although these are not the only proteolytic enzymes found in neutrophils, they probably account for most of the damage to extracellular structures induced by lysosomal enzymes.

Cathepsin G. Human neutrophil "chymotrypsin-like" enzyme is recognized by its ability to hydrolyze phenylalanine esters.[108,116] The enzyme has a molecular weight of 26,000 and has been localized to azurophil granules from which it can be extracted.[32] It is immunologically distinct from PMN elastase. Conditions required for isolation from granules are also different. The enzyme has a broad substrate specificity and has been reported to hydrolyze hemoglobin,[116] fibrinogen,[116] casein,[108] cryocasein,[132] insoluble collagen,[56] and cartilage proteoglycans.[132] The enzyme is inhibited by the human plasma inhibitors alpha 1-antitrypsin, by alpha 2-macroglobulin and, most effectively, by alpha 1-antichymotrypsin.

Collagenase. This neutral protease has been localized to the azurophil granule by some investigators[97] and to the specific granule by others.[90] Collagenase is a metalloenzyme with an apparent molecular weight of approximately 76,000.[74,96] Collagenase hydrolyzes solubilized native collagen, but cannot cleave collagen fibrils without the participation of an additional neutral protease.[74] The preferred substrate for this enzyme is type I collagen, the predominant collagen type of bone and tendon.[49] Like other metalloproteases, collagenase is inhibited by EDTA and cysteine, but unlike the other neutral proteases, PMN cytosol does not inhibit collagenase activity. Plasma inhibitors of collagenase include alpha 1-antitrypsin and

alpha 2-macroglobulin, which must first undergo proteolytic cleavage by collagenase as part of its mechanism of action.[96]

Elastase. Elastase is a neutral protease that has been localized to the azurophil granule.[25] The isolated enzyme is a basic glycoprotein with a molecular weight of approximately 30,000 to 34,000.[25] This protein, together with collagenase, constitutes 5% of the dry weight of the PMN. The substrate specificity of elastase is broad, and the enzyme has been reported to hydrolyze elastin from tendons, lung, basement membrane, native collagen, fibrils, proteoglycans, cryocasein, hemoglobin, fibrinogen and, in concert with collagenase, histone.[54,132] Elastase digests elastic arteries in vitro and provokes vascular injury when injected in vivo. Alpha 1-antitrypsin, alpha 2-macroglobulin, and PMN cytosol are effective inhibitors of elastase activity. Of the enzymes discussed here, elastase is probably the most important because of its abundance and broad substrate specificity.

Taken together, these enzymes have a remarkably broad substrate specificity, although of greater importance to the rheumatologist is the degradation of the two major components of articular cartilage: collagen and proteoglycans. The neutral proteases may also contribute to the inflammatory response by generating chemotactic factors from C5[137] and cleavage of plasma kininogen[84] and leukokininogen to kinins.[56] The existence of multiple plasma and cytosolic inhibitors for these proteolytic enzymes testifies to their potential for destruction when not confined to the granule.

CYTOSKELETAL STRUCTURES

Microtubules and microfilaments are the major constituents of the cytoskeletal structure of PMNs. These structures are involved in degranulation, cell motility,[1,105] and maintenance of the internal organization of neutrophils, and also may mediate a transfer of information between plasma membrane and the cell interior.

Microtubules are polymers of tubulin, a 55,000 MW protein. The centrioles, located between the Golgi apparatus and nucleus, have an electron-dense organizing center from which almost all the microtubules associated with these structures originate. The microtubules then radiate outward passing close to and appearing to graze membrane-

Fig. 18–1. *A*, A transmission electron photomicrograph of a resting neutrophil ($\times$ 11,700). N = nucleus; GA = golgi apparatus; G = granules; C = centrioles; M = mitochondrion. *B*, A higher power of this neutrophil demonstrating radiation of microtubules (MT) from centrioles (C) ($\times$ 44,100). *C*, The electron photomicrograph shows a neutrophil that has ingested monosodium urate crystals (MSU) ($\times$ 7,600). Marker indicates 1 μm. (Photomicrographs courtesy of Dr. Abby Rich.)

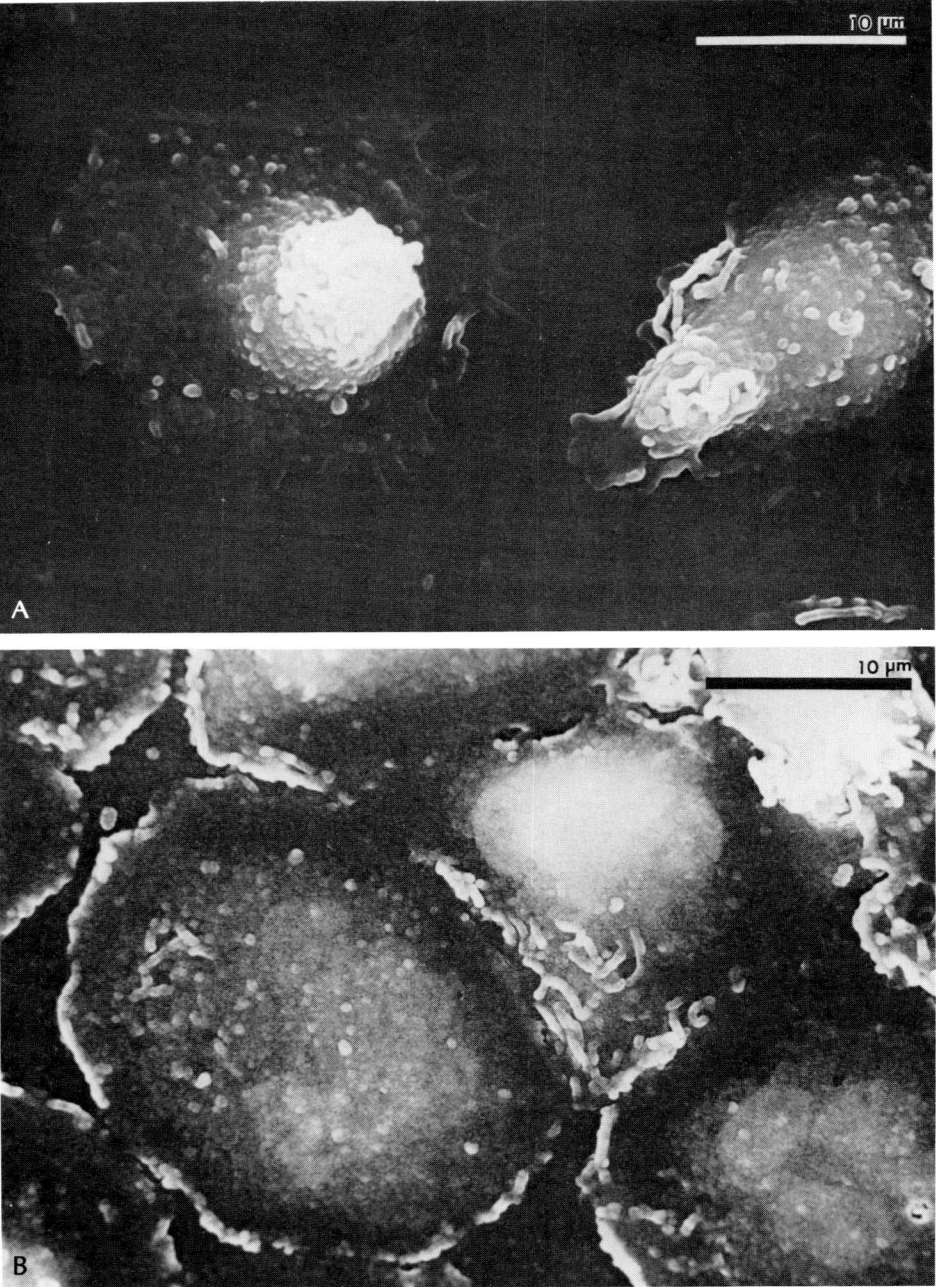

Fig. 18–2. *A*, A scanning electron micrograph of two resting neutrophils. Note the ruffled edges, irregular shape, and large number of pseudopods extending from the cell surface. *B*, Neutrophils adherent to a surface coated with IgG. Note the flattened, rounded shape and loss of pseudopods as the neutrophils spread out and attempt to ingest the antibody coated surface. (Photomicrographs courtesy of Dr. Abby Rich.)

Table 18–1. Neutrophil Granules and Their Contents

Substance	Azurophilic Granules (Primary)	Specific Granules (Secondary)
Microbicidal enzymes	Myeloperoxidase Lysozyme	Lysozyme
Neutral proteases	Elastase Cathepsin C Cathepsin G Collagenase	Alkaline phosphatase Collagenase
Acid proteases	β-glucuronidase Acid β-glycerophosphatase N-acetyl β-glucosaminidase α-mannosidase Arylsulphatase β-galactosidase α-fucosidase Cathepsin B Cathepsin D	
Nonenzymatic	Cationic proteins Chondroitin sulfate	Lactoferrin Vitamin B_{12}-binding protein

bound organelles such as granules[139] (see Fig. 18–1B).

The "assembly" and "disassembly" of microtubules are controlled in several ways both in vitro and in vivo. Calcium ions promote dissolution of polymerized tubulin, as does decreased pH or osmolality of medium.[107] Cyclic GMP and agents that elevate intracellular levels of cGMP, such as phorbol myristate acetate and carbamylcholine, promote assembly of tubulin, whereas cAMP and agents that elevate intracellular levels of cAMP, such as PGE_1 and isoproterenol, promote disassembly. The redox state of the cells may also regulate assembly of microtubule proteins.[81] Micromolar concentrations of the plant alkaloids colchicine and vinblastine induce reversible dissolution of microtubules. Studies done with the aid of these agents, especially colchicine, have made it possible to identify the function of these structures.

Microtubules are of particular importance in PMN function. Numerous studies have shown that degranulation during phagocytosis is affected by agents that influence the state of assembly of microtubules.[77,140,142,143,147] Cyclic nucleotide-modulated increments and decrements in degranulation correlate with increments and decrements in microtubule numbers.[39] Cyclic GMP can induce assembly of microtubules in the absence of a stimulus, but is itself incapable of stimulating degranulation.

The evidence at present suggests that translocation of phagosomes rather than fusion is modulated by microtubules. Correlations between tubule assembly and disassembly and the degree of de-

granulation probably reflect earlier events in the degranulation sequence.

Assembly may enhance, and disassembly diminish, the chances for contact between neutrophil granules and stimulated areas of the plasma membrane. Other structures, perhaps contractile proteins, might play a more direct role in fusion between granules and the phagosome.

Microfilaments are 6 nm in diameter and constitute the contractile system of the neutrophils. These structures, identified as actin polymers, are prominent in areas of the cell involved in adhesion and particle ingestion.[105] The neutrophil contractile system bears a striking resemblance to that of skeletal muscle. Actin, myosin (with actin-activated Mg^{2+}-ATPase activity), actin binding protein, and a cofactor that allows actin to activate the Mg^{2+}-ATPase have all been isolated from phagocytic cells.[12] During normal phagocytosis, contractions occur in two directions. Contraction occurs under the particle to form an invagination that is directed along microtubule-defined tracks toward the cytocenter. Filaments are seen associated with the phagocytic vacuole, but granules fuse with vacuoles in the cytocenter, and microfilaments are not usually seen near sites of active fusion.

The second type of movement involves a filamentous web at the cell surface containing actin and myosin. Contraction of this web, which interacts with actin-binding protein, results in a lateral movement of the plasma membrane that serves to close the phagocytic vacuole like a purse string. The microfilment system can be inhibited by interference with production of metabolic energy or by chelation of calcium, providing one possible mechanism for the modulation of degranulation by calcium. More specific disruption of the contractile system can be achieved using the fungal metabolite cytochalasin B, which interferes with the function of actin-binding protein.[134] Cytochalasin B inhibits the "purse string" contraction by either preventing the formation of actin-binding gels or by solubilizing them and thus preventing sol to gel transformation of cytoplasmic extracts.[134,138] Cytochalasin B is a powerful inhibitor of PMN migration and phagocytosis; this observation in conjunction with ultrastructure data suggests a vital role for microfilaments in these active processes.[1]

STIMULUS-RESPONSE COUPLING IN PMNS

In response to an appropriate stimulus such as bacteria, foreign peptides, or certain soluble agents, neutrophils will aggregate, migrate toward the source of chemoattractants, ingest appropriately coated particles, degranulate, and generate toxic oxygen metabolites. The nature of this interaction between stimuli and neutrophils is now becoming clearer and can serve as a paradigm of cellular activation.

OPSONINS AND THEIR RECEPTORS

The ability and speed with which PMNs ingest a particle are, at least in part, dependent upon the surface characteristics of the particle. Surface charge and hydrophobicity profoundly influence ingestion, although the optimal surface characteristics for phagocytosis are not completely understood. Certainly one explanation for the ability of some bacteria to evade phagocytic attack by PMNs is a subtle alteration of the bacterial surface that makes them less appetizing.

Humoral factors produced by the host greatly facilitate phagocytosis by neutrophils. Thus, particles exposed to fresh serum are ingested more readily than untreated particles. Humoral factors that coat peptides in preparation for ingestion by PMNs are known as opsonins, from the Greek "to prepare victuals." Opsonins have traditionally been divided into "heat-stable" and "heat-labile" factors. Immunoglobulins, in particular IgG (specifically subclasses IgG1 and IgG3), which are resistant to the effects of heating, comprise the heat-stable opsonins. The immunoglobulin molecule must be intact to promote phagocytosis. By proteolytic digestion of immunoglobulin molecules, two functional portions can be distinguished: the Fab portion of the antibody molecule, which binds to specific antigenic sites on the particle, and the Fc portion, which binds to a specific receptor on the neutrophil membrane. This membrane receptor has been isolated and partially characterized as a protein with a molecular weight of 53,000 to

66,000. By using either a specific monoclonal antibody or labeled immune complexes, workers have found that there are 112,000 to 135,000 Fc receptor sites per cell.[33]

Serum complement can also act as an opsonin and is characteristically heat-labile. The most active opsonic agent generated from serum complement is C3b. This factor is generated from the proteolytic cleavage of C3, resulting either from activation of the classical pathway of complement or from the properdin system (alternate pathway). A receptor for C3b has been isolated from human erythrocytes and was shown to be identical to that found on neutrophils. The isolated receptor has been further characterized as a protein with a molecular weight of approximately 205,000. By use of a specific labled antibody to this receptor, there are estimated to be almost 60,000 receptors per cell for C3b.[29]

Tuftsin is a tetrapeptide fragment of IgG that acts as a nonspecific stimulus for phagocytosis.[93]

THE ACTIVATION PROCESS

Once the neutrophil has engaged an appropriately opsonized particle, a number of cellular responses occur. Following binding of the stimulus to an appropriate receptor, there is a lag period before a measurable physiologic response, such as granule release or aggregation, can be demonstrated.[61,124] This lag period, which is stimulus-specific, represents the time required for transmission of an excitatory signal and translation into an appropriate cellular response.

One of the cellular alterations that is classically found as a first step in stimulus-response coupling is a change in the plasmalemmal transmembrane potential. In PMNs, where changes in transmembrane potential can only be demonstrated indirectly, rapid hyperpolarization followed by depolarization has been found after appropriate stimulation.[71]

In addition to changes in membrane potential, calcium has been proposed as a second messenger for neutrophil activation. Four criteria for second messenger status have been met for calcium: (1) Translocation of extracellular calcium by the ionophore A23187 activates PMNs, and removal of calcium from the extracellular milieu markedly reduces PMN responses to various stimuli.[36,95,129] (2) Activated PMNs take up labeled calcium from the extracellular milieu and, after a variable period, actively extrude this calcium. Free cytoplasmic calcium increases rapidly after stimulation, and this phenomenon may represent mobilization of intracellular stores of calcium.[69,92,103,120] (3) By cytochemical and ultrastructural techniques, calcium has been localized to several areas within the PMN.

There are discrete deposits along the plasmalemma in resting PMNs, in the heterochromatic region of the nucleus, in the azurophil granules, and in association with glycogen. (4) Evidence suggests that membrane-associated calcium is released soon after PMN activation, possibly giving rise to the elevation of free cytosolic calcium.[48,91,128]

Cyclic nucleotides are also classic "second messengers" in several secretory cells. Rapid transient rises in cAMP have been documented to occur after activation of PMNs with some, but not all stimuli.[44,53,126] This increase in cAMP concentration is not necessary for cellular responses of PMNs because an inhibitor of cAMP formation does not affect measured PMN responses after activation by stimuli that normally give rise to cAMP increases.[123] Agents that elevate intracellular cAMP levels, such as isoproterenol and theophylline, tend to diminish the response of PMNs to stimulation.[147] This finding suggests that cyclic nucleotides play a role as a modulator, but not as a signal for cell function.

METABOLIC RESPONSE TO ACTIVATION

Upon activation of the PMN by contact with appropriately opsonized particles, several metabolic changes take place. Among these responses are "the respiratory burst" with increased oxygen consumption,[7,115] increased hexose monophosphate shunt activity,[27] increased hydrogen peroxide[52] and superoxide anion generation,[5] increased phospholipid turnover,[63] and phosphorylation of proteins.[2]

Protein phosphorylation is involved in the regulation of intracellular activities of many cell types. Both cAMP-sensitive and phospholipid-sensitive protein kinase activities have been found in activated PMNs.[50,136] Phorbol esters, activators of PMNs, bind directly to a protein kinase C and thus are able to bypass the standard activation sequence.[94] Appropriate stimulation of human PMNs leads to enhanced phosphorylation of four protein bands and dephosphorylation of one protein band.[2]

Stimulation of PMNs leads to enhanced lipid turnover. Increased turnover of the phosphatidyl inositol/phosphatidic acid cycle may play a role in regulation of intracellular calcium levels.[122] Additionally, breakdown of phosphatidyl inositol or its di- and tri-phosphorylated derivatives by phospholipase C could lead to generation of diacyl glyceride, a known activator of protein kinase C.[122] Phospholipid turnover can also provide free arachidonic acid that can be further metabolized to prostaglandins and products of the lipoxygenase pathway as discussed later.

The rapid consumption of oxygen by stimulated PMNs leads to production of almost stoichiometric quantities of hydrogen peroxide (H_2O_2), superoxide anion radicals (O_2), singlet oxygen, and hydroxyl radicals. A critical first step in these events appears to be the reduction of molecular oxygen to superoxide anion by a plasma membrane-bound NADPH-dependent oxidase. Consumption of NADPH by this oxidase leads to enhanced glucose metabolism by the hexose monophosphate shunt. Superoxide anion is enzymatically (by superoxide dismutase) or spontaneously converted to hydrogen peroxide, which may in turn react with additional superoxide anion to form hydroxyl radicals. All these oxygen species are highly reactive and possess varying degrees of bactericidal and cytocidal activity.[28]

Evidence from granule- and nucleus-free subcellular particles derived from human neutrophils strongly suggests that superoxide anion is generated by enzymes in the plasma membrane.[70] Owing to the plasma membrane localization of the superoxide anion generating system, toxic microbicidal agents are concentrated around ingested organisms once the phagosome is formed by the cell membrane. Focusing these toxic bactericidal materials into the phagolysosome minimizes release of toxic oxygen species.

RELEASE OF PROSTAGLANDINS, THROMBOXANES, AND LEUKOTRIENES

Neutrophils release activated products of arachidonate when exposed to phagocytic stimuli. They include products of the cyclo-oxygenase pathway, prostaglandins (PGs) and thromboxanes, and products of the lipoxygenase pathways, the leukotrienes. The exact role of these compounds and their interaction with each other and with other mediators of inflammation are not completely understood. In addition, these compounds appear to have both anti- and proinflammatory effects.

Upon stimulation, arachidonic acid is released from membrane phospholipids via the enzyme phospholipase. This step is inhibited by anti-inflammatory steroids. These [20]carbon polyunsaturated fatty acids then interact with the active oxygen species generated during the respiratory burst.[102] Two enzyme systems are operative at this point: cyclo-oxygenase to produce prostaglandins and thromboxanes or the lipoxygenases to produce leukotrienes.

Cyclo-oxygenase, also called prostaglandin synthetase, is inhibited by aspirin and the other nonsteroidal anti-inflammatory drugs (NSAIDs). The fatty acid endoperoxides thus formed (the PGG and PGH series) are weak potentiators of edema caused by bradykinin and histamine,[73] but more importantly they serve as intermediates in the formation of other prostaglandins and thromboxanes via isomerization of the more stable PGs. Of these, PGE_2 and PGI_2 appear to be the primary mediators of inflammation because (1) they cause vasodilatation and inflammation when injected; (2) injection of these substances into the midbrain of experimental animals causes fever; and (3) they act synergistically with mediators, such as bradykinin and histamine, to cause edema and vasodilatation and to sensitize tissues to painful stimuli by other agents. These compounds are present in elevated concentrations in inflammatory exudates, and their synthesis is inhibited by most anti-inflammatory drugs.[109] There is also some evidence that PGs are anti-inflammatory. The PGE series can stimulate cAMP production. It can thereby suppress immediate hypersensitivity reactions and reactions associated with cellular immunity, such as lectin-induced T-cell mitogenesis[40] and degranulation by neutrophils.[126]

The products of the lipoxygenase pathway have recently been elucidated, and their role in inflammation is becoming increasingly evident. The predominating pathway of leukotriene metabolism depends on the cell type: the 12-lipoxygenase is the major enzyme in platelets, the 15-lipoxygenase is most active in T-lymphocytes, and the 5-lipoxygenase predominates in neutrophils. The scheme of arachidonic acid metabolism via the 5-lipoxygenase pathway is depicted in Figure 18–3. Lipoxygenase is not inhibited by the NSAIDs, except for benoxaprofen,[22] but is inhibited by ETYA. The lipoxygenase acts together with activated oxygen species to form 5-HETE, which is converted to the unstable epoxide LTA_4.[104] LTA_4 can then be either enzymatically hydrolyzed to LTB_4 or acted upon by glutathione-5-transferase to produce LTC_4. LTC_4 can be further modified by glutamyl transpeptidase to form LTD_4 and LTE_4.[41,42]

LTB_4, a potent inflammatory stimulus, is released upon activation of neutrophils.[58] In nanomolar or less amounts, it causes leukocyte chemotaxis[35,78,100,125] and adhesion to endothelial cells.[21] At higher concentrations, LTB_4 in the presence of PMNs elicits extravasation of plasma from vessel walls.[114] In nanomolar amounts, LTB_4 also activates neutrophils. Within seconds after addition to neutrophil suspensions, LTB_4 causes aggregation, degranulation, generation of superoxide anion, and mobilization of membrane-associated calcium.[31,121]

Monosodium urate (MSU) crystals stimulate the formation of arachidonate metabolites by neutrophils and platelets.[79] Recent work from this laboratory has shown that neutrophils exposed to nonlytic quantities of MSU generate 5-HETE, LTB_4 (and its nonenzymatically formed isomers 6-*trans*-LTB_4, 12-*epi*-6-*trans*-LTB_4) and 20-COOH-LTB_4

via the 5-lipoxygenase pathway. Neutrophils pretreated with colchicine once exposed to MSU are unable to form LTA_4 from 5-HPETE and thus do not form LTB_4 and its isomers. This shifts metabolism of arachidonate to other metabolites such as 5S, 12S-diHETE that antagonize the action of LTB_4. Thus, LTB_4 and other products of arachidonate produced by platelets appear to be important mediators of inflammation in gouty arthritis, and colchicine may specifically affect the biosynthesis of these substances[119] (see also Chap. 93).

The cysteine-containing leukotrienes (LTC_4, LTD_4, and LTE_4) produced by macrophages and basophils comprise immunologically mediated slow reactive substances (SRS-A) and hence have diverse biological effects. The discussion here is confined to the influence upon the inflammatory response. In nanomolar concentrations, SRS-A causes an intense dose-dependent contraction of arterioles most marked in the terminal arterioles. Although the vasoconstriction is short-lived, it is followed by a dose-dependent and reversible leakage of macromolecules at the postcapillary venules.[114] Thus, together with PGE_2 and PGI_2, SRS-A contributes to edema formation. These actions appear to occur via a direct action of the vessel walls since they are rapidly occurring and do not require PGs, histamine, or PMNs.

The proinflammatory effects of the various products of arachidonic acid are summarized in Table 18–2.

DEGRANULATION

Degranulation in the neutrophil normally accompanies phagocytosis. This close relationship suggests common or similar triggering mechanisms[46,80] and has been discussed earlier in the section describing stimulus-response coupling. After binding of a phagocytosable particle, a localized contraction occurs just underneath the point of contact and at right angles to the plasma membrane resulting in a cup-shaped depression into which the particle fits. The margins of the depression move inward to enclose the particles in a complete phagocytic vacuole or phagosome. This movement is inhibited by cytochalasin B, which interferes with microfilaments, and thus measurement of degranulation is possible. Azurophil and specific granules (lysosomes) join this newly formed vacuole at its internal border and discharge their contents. This process is called degranulation. The fusion of the granule and plasma membranes is inhibited by corticosteroids. Most of the time, the vacuole closes and prevents escape of the enzymes; however, if there is too much to digest, the vacuole may remain open, and some enzymes may be secreted extra-

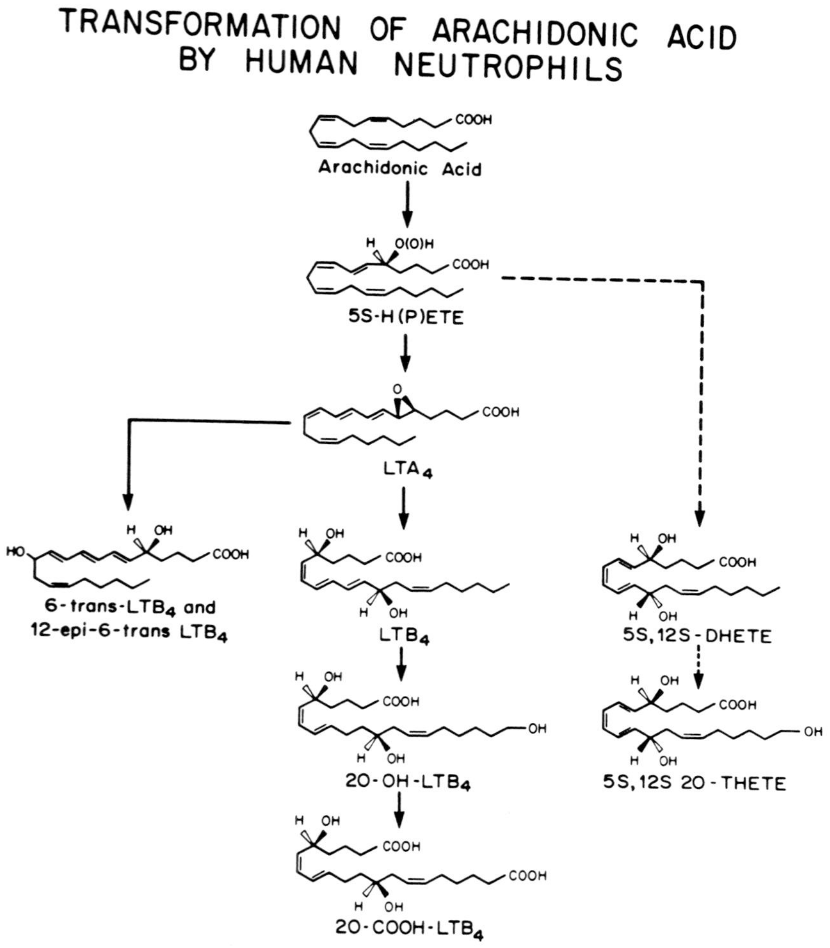

TRANSFORMATION OF ARACHIDONIC ACID
BY HUMAN NEUTROPHILS

Fig. 18–3. Scheme of arachidonic acid metabolism via 5-lipoxygenase.

Table 18–2. Inflammatory Effects of Products of Metabolites of Arachidonate

	Products of Cyclo-oxygenase	Products of Lipoxygenase
Vasodilatation	PGE_2 PGF_2	Not demonstrated
	PGE_2 PGF_2 (PGG, PGH weak with bradykinin and histamine)	LTC_4 LTD_4
Pain, hyperalgesia	PGE_2 PGI_2	Not demonstrated
Fever	PGE_2	Not demonstrated
Neutrophil migration and adhesion	PGE_2, PGF_2, PGI_2 (inhibit)	LTB_4
Released by PMN in response to monosodium urate	Not demonstrated	LTB_4 and Isomer, 5S, 12S DHETE

cellularly and may attack host tissues.[46] This mechanism of host injury will be discussed in detail.

Degranulation occurs not only during phagocytosis, but also when neutrophils are exposed to secretagogues, chemoattractants, lectins, tumor promotors, and calcium ionophores. In the laboratory, the extracellular release of granule contents can be readily induced by exposing neutrophils to secretagogues in the presence of cytochalasin B. This technique has allowed kinetic studies of the stimulus-secretion coupling response. Continuous monitoring of secretion from cytochalasin B-treated cells has revealed a distinct lag period between exposure to stimulant and lysosomal enzyme release. The lag period was stimulus-dependent, the shortest being 15 seconds for the chemotactic peptide FMLP[127] and the longest 60 seconds for calcium ionophore A23187.[141] These results were comparable to those seen for O_2 generation using the same stimuli. Further work has shown that, in general, the lag periods for specific granules are slightly less than those for azurophils.[126,127]

Several possible explanations for this lag period have been considered. Some suggest that the lag period reflects the time required to assemble or to disassemble cytoskeletal structures, to piece together a multicomponent oxidase system, or physically to transport secretory granules through the cytoplasm. The theory that has received most attention suggests that the lag period is a reflection of the amount of time required to accumulate a crucial second messenger as discussed previously.

BACTERICIDAL MECHANISMS

Neutrophils play a major role in host defense against bacteria and fungi. Destruction of invading bacteria by neutrophils is most efficiently accomplished within phagosomes where the granule contents are concentrated around the invading organism yet remain isolated from the cytoplasm and from the extracellular tissues. The phagosome is well adapted for this function with an internal milieu of pH 3.5 to 4.0, which is optimal for the acid hydrolases delivered by azurophil granules and which promotes the conversion of superoxide anion produced during the respiratory burst to hydrogen peroxide. Hydrogen peroxide has a certain amount of bactericidal effect itself, but its potency is actually augmented via the action of myeloperoxidase, an enzyme present in the azurophilic granules of neutrophils. This enzyme catalzyes the oxidation of halide ions (most likely Cl^- in vivo)[36] with resultant halogenation of bacteria.[64] Myeloperoxidase may also be able to directly degrade amino acid constituents of the bacterial wall.

The respiratory burst also gives rise to other active oxygen species with bactericidal activity, including hydroxyl radical and singlet oxygen.[4] Although it is difficult to determine which of these active oxygen species is most responsible for destruction of microbes, it is likely that some combination of the aforementioned process is responsible for destruction in vivo. The large number of killing mechanisms provides the PMN with an armory of sufficient redundancy and "overkill" to deal with a broad spectrum of microorganisms and to provide a "fail-safe" system in the event that one component of active oxygen species is inoperative.

EXTRUSION OF PMN GRANULE ENZYMES IN TISSUE INJURY

Having presented evidence that polymorphonuclear leukocytes and their lysosomal proteases have the potential to provide significant tissue injury, we will outline the mechanisms by which these proteases and other lysosomal constituents are extruded from the cell and given access to their specific substrates.

Cell Death. One mechanism is simply "cell death" (Fig. 18–4, upper left). When polymorphonuclear leukocytes are exposed to a variety of toxins (for example, phospholipases in snake venom or materials that could be encountered in some septic forms of arthritis), injury to the plasma membrane is an early consequence. All intracellular materials are released pari passu from the injuried cell, including those ordinarily sequestered within lysosomes. Biologic detergents, such as the amphipath melitti, act in this manner to cause primary lysis of the cell membrane and, only subsequently, disruption of lysosomes.[79] Under these circumstances, cytoplasmic enzymes, potassium, and other cellular constituents, in addition to lysosomal hydrolases, escape into the surrounding tissue.

Perforation from Within. Another mechanism conforms to the "suicide sac" hypothesis of deDuve. Under some circumstances, materials gain access to the interior of the vacuole system of the cells, wherein they cause membranes of lysosomes to rupture from within (see Fig. 18–4, upper right). Damage to the organelles leads to the release of lysosomal enzymes concomitantly with the release of cytoplasmic enzymes and other intracellular constituents because the cell dies by a kind of "perforation from within" of its vacuolar system. Crystalline substances, such as monosodium urate and silica, act upon phagocytic cells in this fashion.[87] Hence, this form of lysosomal enzyme release is a primary promoter of inflammation in gout.

Using neutroplasts (neutrophil fragments without granules that retain the ability to phagocytize crystals), we have demonstrated that phagocytosis alone is not sufficient for lysis-from-within.

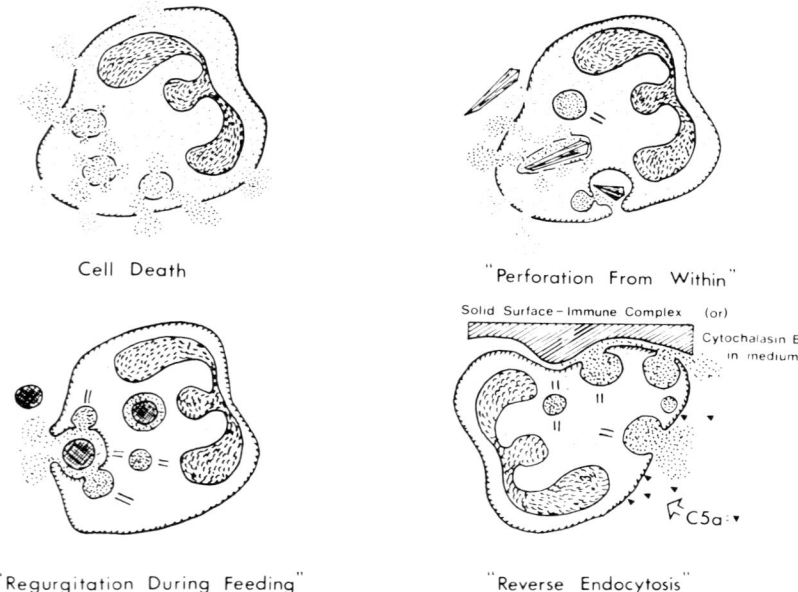

Cell Death

"Perforation From Within"

"Regurgitation During Feeding"

"Reverse Endocytosis"

Fig. 18–4. Mechanisms of lysosomal enzyme release causing tissue injury.

Rather, the release of granule contents from the phagolysosome is responsible for lysis-from-within.[106]

Whereas these first two mechanisms of lysosomal enzyme release may account for tissue injury in some instances, two additional mechanisms involving intact, viable PMNs are now recognized. Both are relevant to the pathogenesis of immune tissue injury, and often have been proved amenable to modification by a number of pharmacologic agents, particularly those that affect the state of assembly of cytoplasmic microtubules or the level within cells of cyclic nucleotides.

Regurgitation During Feeding. One mechanism of lysosomal enzyme release from intact, viable PMNs has been termed "regurgitation during feeding" (see Fig. 18–4, lower left). Under some circumstances (e.g., following the ingestion by these cells of insoluble immune complexes, as are encountered in synovial fluid during rheumatoid arthritis, or other particulates), a phagosome is formed that merges at its internal border with primary lysosomes. Because of either incomplete fusion of the vacuolar membrane or the persistence of endocytic channels, regurgitation of lysosomal hydrolases occurs, and inflammatory materials are released into the surrounding tissues without associated phagocytic cell death or release of cytoplasmic enzymes.[149] Biochemical and morphologic evidence for this mechanism, called "regurgitation during feeding," has been presented for a variety of systems involving particle ingestion by phago-

cytic cells. The cell engaging in phagocytosis remains viable, but it releases lysosomal contents that are free to act upon surrounding tissues. This is a common mechanism of tissue injury in a variety of disease states. Ohlsson has shown that the neutral proteases, elastase and collagenase, are regurgitated by this mechanism.[96]

Harlin et al., using human neutrophils activated with serum-treated zymosan, demonstrated endothelial cell detachment caused by neutral protease digestion of endothelial cell surface proteins, including fibronectin.[43]

Reverse Endocytosis. Another mechanism of selective lysosomal enzyme extrusion from PMNs has been termed "reverse endocytosis" or "frustrated phagocytosis" (see Fig. 18–4, lower right). In this process material previously stored within lysosomes is exported to the external milieu. Cells, for example, that encounter immune complexes (both soluble and insoluble) or aggregated immunoglobulins deposited upon solid surfaces, such as millipore filters or collagen membranes, adhere to these surfaces and selectively release their lysosomal constituents.[45] Enzyme release under these conditions seems to occur by a process of reverse endocytosis, during which merger of granules with the plasma membrane results in discharge of lysosomal enzymes directly to the outside of the cell as though into a phagocytic vacuole. Phagocytosis per se does not occur, and the viability of the adherent cells is not altered. This mechanism of enzyme release is probably pertinent to the pathogenesis of tissue injury in various diseases in which immune complexes are deposited upon cell surfaces or extracellular structures, such as vascular basement membranes. For example, nephritis, common in systemic lupus erythematosus, could be generated by this form of granule enzyme release, stimulated by the surface deposition of immune complexes (DNA, anti-DNA IgG, and complement components).

Recent work has led to the appreciation that PMN cell surface recognition of, and stimulation by, three distinct ligands can provoke granule translocation, membrane fusion, and selective extracellular release of granule contents. These ligands include Fc regions of IgG molecules that have undergone a conformational change either as a result of combining with antigen or as a result of heat aggregation (Fc receptor stimulus), fragments of the third component of complement (C3b receptor stimulus). and the soluble, low–molecular-weight complement component C5a. For example, immune complexes prepared by reacting heat-aggregated human IgG with rheumatoid factor or heat-aggregated IgG per se, either in suspension or deposited upon nonphagocytizable surfaces, are capable of provoking the selective discharge of lysosomal constituents from human PMNs (by "regurgitation during feeding" or "reverse endocytosis").[37,147–149] PMNs exposed to fragments of C3 fixed on nonphagocytizable surfaces respond in a similar manner (in the presence of IgG). C5a, generated by activation of either the classic or alternative complement pathways, is capable of interacting with human PMNs in the absence of particles (or immunoglobulins) to stimulate membrane fusion between lysosomal granules and between these organelles and the plasma membrane.[37] In cytochalasin B-treated PMNs[37] and in PMNs adherent to nonphagocytizable surfaces,[148] this phenomenon leads to selective extracellular release of lysosomal enzymes by the process of "reverse endocytosis."

The exocytosis, or degranulation, that follows PMN cell surface stimulation by immune reactants appears to involve both major classes of PMN granules: azurophil and specific. Consequently, acid hydrolases such as beta-glucuronidase (from azurophilic granules) as well as lysozyme (from specific granules) can be detected in the medium surrounding such stimulated cells.[37,147–149] In contrast, some nonimmune stimuli appear to provoke selective discharge (by exocytosis) of only specific granule constituents (e.g., lysozyme) from human PMNs. These stimuli include the tumor promoter, phorbol myristate acetate,[39] concanavalin A,[47] and ionized calcium,[38] in either the presence or the absence of the divalent cation ionophore A23187. These ob-

servations, together with reported sequential degranulation during phagocytosis,[6] indicate that slightly different mechanisms are responsible for discharge of the two types of granules.

Oxygen metabolites have also been implicated in extracellular cytolysis of host cells. Because the generation of oxygen metabolites occurs along with phagocytic uptake, these metabolites come in contact with surrounding tissues in one of the four methods outlined previously. It is likely that these oxygen metabolites cause the same degree of tissue damage in autoimmune disease once tissue-free radical scavengers that inhibit oxygen-metabolite-mediated cytolysis are exhausted.[112]

PHARMACOLOGIC CONTROL OF PMN FUNCTION

Because lysosomal enzyme release and generation of toxic oxygen metabolites may contribute to the pathogenesis of tissue injury during inflammation as well as to the propagation of the inflammatory reaction, it is likely that a reduction in the extracellular release of these toxic substances could be beneficial in disease states characterized by aberrant inflammation. Attention has thus been directed to the problem of pharmacologic inhibition of enzyme release and superoxide anion generation. As would be expected, no inhibitors will alter the enzyme release found after cell death or after "perforation from within" as is seen with crystal-induced enzyme release. In general, two major types of compounds have been studied for their effect on granular enzyme release: those that affect the state or formation of cytoplasmic microtubules directly and those that influence the intracellular level of cyclic nucleotides, cAMP and cGMP. Exogenous cAMP (plus theophylline) as well as agents that elevate intracellular levels of cAMP (e.g., PGE₁ or isoproterenol) reduced enzyme release.[147] Exogenous cGMP and agents that elevate levels of cGMP (e.g., serotonin, carbamylcholine) enhance lysosomal enzyme release.[147] Similarly, agents that promote disassembly of cytoplasmic microtubules (e.g., colchicine and vinblastine) reduce lysosomal enzyme release, and agents that promote microtubule assembly (e.g., deuterium oxide) enhance lysosomal enzyme release. For some of these agents, such as colchicine, that specifically inhibit leukotriene generation by neutrophils, alternative mechanisms of action may exist.[119]

The nonsteroidal anti-inflammatory agents that, as a group, share the ability to block prostaglandin synthesis appear to have a variety of effects on neutrophils. Aspirin and piroxicam inhibit neutrophil degranulation, aggregation, and superoxide anion generation. Ibuprofen inhibits only aggregation and degranulation, and indomethacin inhibits only aggregation[60] (see also Chap. 28).

Other agents also have a selective inhibitory effect on neutrophils. Adenosine, a naturally occurring purine, and some of its analogues selectively inhibit superoxide anion generation by neutrophils.[20]

Some of the anti-inflammatory effects of glucocorticosteroids can be attributed to inhibition of PMN locomotion, phagocytosis, and degranulation. One interesting explanation of this inhibition is that these drugs stabilize membranes, thus inhibiting fusion between membrane surfaces upon which both phagocytosis and degranulation depend.[26]

PMNs, through their ability to release potentially toxic enzymes and oxygen metabolites, play a crucial role in the pathology of arthritis and other inflammatory conditions. Successful therapy of these conditions may be achieved by use of drugs directed at inhibition of PMN responses to inflammatory stimuli.

HERITABLE DISORDERS

PMN function is regulated by a multitude of extrinsic and intrinsic factors, and disruption of any one of these factors can lead to PMN malfunction. To date at least 15 primary (probably inheritable) defects of neutrophil function with resultant recurrent infections have been identified, and at least twice as many conditions (including SLE and RA) secondarily resulting in decreased PMN function have also been reported.[57] The defects identified include perturbations of neutrophil interactions with external stimulatory factors, such as activated complement components, causing impaired chemotaxis and ingestion or impaired phagocytosis due to opsonin or turftsin deficiency.

Abnormalities of PMN function can be classified in terms of the major responses of neutrophils to inflammatory stimuli. Intrinsic inherited defects that are of interest here can be classified in terms of defects of chemotaxis, ingestion, degranulation, receptor coupling, adherence, or bactericidal mechanisms. Studies of these rare defects have provided insight into normal neutrophil function.

One of the most intriguing of the heritable diseases is Chédiak-Higashi syndrome, a rare autosomal recessive disorder that is characterized clinically by a propensity to skin and subcutaneous infections and partial albinism. The PMNs and monocytes from patients with this disorder contain large azurophilic granules that do not fuse with phagosomes.[111] Degranulation is delayed. The respiratory burst is normal. PMNs from these patients have been found to have increased levels of cAMP.[10] Studies have shown that the basic cause

of this syndrome is inadequate tubulin polymerization resulting in nonfunctional microtubules and impaired chemotaxis[16] and degranulation.[98] Indeed, cells from patients with this disorder exhibit functional abnormalities like those of normal cells treated with colchicine, a microtubule-disrupting drug.[34,55] Agents that increase intracellular cGMP such as carbachol and bethanechol, and ascorbic acid, which decreases cAMP, promote microtubule assembly and seem to ameliorate dysfunction in vitro.[10,98]

A neutrophil actin abnormality has been reported in a single patient whose PMNs failed to ingest particles and to respond to chemotactic stimuli resulting in recurrent infections.[11] The cytoplasm from this patient's PMNs was deficient in microfilaments. In vitro polymerization of isolated actin was poor. These neutrophils exhibited hyperactive degranulation.

A single patient with recurrent bacterial infections has been identified as having a deficiency of a granulocyte membrane glycoprotein (gp150).[3] This deficiency resulted in a defect in receptor-coupled PMN functions of superoxide anion generation and degranulation stimulated by C3 and Fc receptors. The membrane glycoprotein was distinct from the receptors themselves and was present in reduced amounts in granulocytes from each of the patient's parents, suggesting a genetic basis for this deficiency.

Lactoferrin deficiency has also been associated with altered granulocyte function in a single patient with recurrent bacterial infections.[9] His neutrophils were characterized by bilobed nuclei, a deficit of specific granules that had abnormal membranes and less than 8% of the specific granule proteins lactoferrin and vitamin B_{12} transport protein. These neutrophils also displayed impaired phagolysosome fusion, as demonstrated by the presence of an increased number of primary granules and their products. Adherence, aggregation, the ability to decrease cell surface charge in response to stimulation by FMLP (a chemoattractant), as well as hydroxyl radical production in response to phagocytosis were all impaired. Addition of lactoferrin to in vitro suspensions of these PMNs normalized adherence and aggregation. The association of lactoferrin deficiency with these abnormalities suggests that specific granule products play a part in modulating granulocyte function.

Increasing interest has focused recently upon heritable intrinsic disorders of the bactericidal respiratory burst mechanisms. The importance of the microbicidal system described by Klebanoff,[66] consisting of myeloperoxidase, hydrogen peroxide, and halide ions, is brought to light by some of these conditions. Chronic granulomatous disease

(CGD) is what now appears to be a group of inheritable disorders characterized by recurrent bacterial and fungal infections. In patients with this disease, the respiratory burst that normally accompanies phagocytosis by neutrophils and monocytes is completely defective and, hence, microbial killing is diminished.[62] In a multicenter European study, two distinct inheritance patterns for this disorder were demonstrated: the well-recognized X-linked inheritance pattern and a newly identified autosomal recessive inheritance.[118] The same study also identified two distinct abnormalities of the cellular machinery involved in the respiratory burst. In the X-linked form of the disease, cytochrome b-245 was not detected in affected males. In the autosomal recessive form of the disease, PMNs from the affected individuals had normal cytochrome b-245, but it was not reduced in response to phorbol myristate acetate. In this subset of patients, the disease seems to result from an abnormality of an activation system or an absence or malfunction of a proximal electron donor in the electron-transport chain. Another report described a patient with an X-linked disorder similar to but not as severe as CGD.[75] This patient was thought to have a defect in an oxidase enzyme activity with a decreased affinity for NADPH.

PMNs from patients with CGD can kill some bacteria, namely those that generate sufficient hydrogen peroxide to facilitate the oxidase system, thereby providing the means of their own destruction. However, some peroxide-generating bacteria produce catalase as well (e.g., *S. aureus* and *E. coli*), thus destroying those small amounts of peroxide and once again leaving the killing system without a substrate. Indeed, it is to catalase-positive aerobic bacteria that CGD patients most often succumb.

Glucose 6-phosphate dehydrogenase deficiency causes a defect in hydrogen peroxide production that is rarely of clinical significance. The defect results in inability to maintain adequate levels of NADPH. PMNs from patients with this deficiency usually have near normal or only slightly reduced bactericidal activity unless the enzyme activity is entirely absent, in which case the syndrome loosely resembles CGD.

Myeloperoxidase (an enzyme contained within azurophilic granules) deficiency also disrupts the Klebanoff system. This autosomal recessive trait is usually of no clinical consequence, and neutrophils from these patients often accumulate more hydrogen peroxide than do normal cells.[113] Some impairment of bactericidal activity has been reported for the PMNs of patients lacking lysozyme[131] and secondary granules.[135] One family has been reported with a deficiency of the enzyme

glutathione reductase, which appears to be inherited as an autosomal recessive disorder. Glutathione (GSH) protects cells against oxidative damage by the highly reactive compounds produced during the respiratory burst. In so doing, GSH is oxidized to its dimer GSSG. This enzyme catalyzes the reconversion of GSSH to GSH. The PMNs from the affected family members appear normal and function normally in the presence of small numbers of bacteria, but with greater numbers of bacteria hydrogen peroxide generation is increased with a concomitant shortening in the duration of the respiratory burst.[76,110]

Other inherited neutrophil disorders include a familial defect in chemotaxis[85] and the "lazy leukocyte syndrome."[86]

REFERENCES

1. Allison, A.C., Davies, P., and DePetris, S.: Role of contractile microfilaments in macrophage movement and endocytosis. Nature New Biol., *232*:153–155, 1971.
2. Andrews, P.C., and Babior, B.M.: Endogenous protein phosphorylation by resting and activated human neutrophils. Blood, *61*:333–340, 1983.
3. Arnaout, M.A., et al.: Deficiency of a granulocyte-membrane glycoprotein (gp 150) in a boy with recurrent bacterial infections. N. Engl. J. Med., *306*:693–699, 1982.
4. Babior, B.M.: Oxygen-dependent microbial killing by phagocytes. N. Engl. J. Med., *298*:659–668, 1978.
5. Babior, B.M., Kipnes, R.S., and Curnutte, J.T.: Biological defense mechanisms: The production by leukocytes of superoxide, a potential bacterial agent. J. Clin. Invest., *52*:741–744, 1973.
6. Bainton, D.F.: Sequential degranulation of the two types of polymorphonuclear leukocyte granules during phagocytosis of microorganisms. J. Cell Biol., *58*:249–264, 1973.
7. Baldridge, C.W., and Gerard, R.W.: The extra respiration of phagocytosis. Am. J. Physiol., *103*:235–236, 1933.
8. Beck, W.S.: The control of leukocyte glycolysis. J. Biol. Chem., *232*:251–270, 1958.
9. Boxer, L.A., et al.: Lactoferrin deficiency associated with altered granulocyte function. N. Engl. J. Med., *307*:404–410, 1982.
10. Boxer, L.A., et al.: Correction of leukocyte function in Chediak-Higashi syndrome by ascorbate. N. Engl. J. Med., *295*:1041–1045, 1976.
11. Boxer, L.A., Hedley-White, E.T., and Stossel, T.P.: Neutrophil actin dysfunction and abnormal neutrophil behavior. N. Engl. J. Med., *291*:1093–1099, 1974.
12. Boxer, L.A., and Stossel, T.P.: Interactions of actin, myosin, and an actin-binding protein of chronic myelogenous leukemia leukocytes. J. Clin. Invest., *57*:964–976, 1976.
13. Bretz, U., and Baggiolini, M.: Biochemical and morphological characterization of azurophil and specific granules of human neutrophilic polymorphonuclear leukocytes. J. Cell Biol., *63*:251–269, 1974.
14. Bretz, U., and Baggiolini, M.: Association of the alkaline phosphatase of rabbit polymorphonuclear leukocytes with the membrane of the specific granules. J. Cell Biol., *59*:696–707, 1973.
15. Cartwright, G.E., Athens, J.W., and Wintrobe, M.M.: The kinetics of granulopoiesis in normal man. Blood, *24*:780–803, 1964.
16. Clark, R.A., and Kimball, H.R.: Defective granulocyte chemotaxis in the Chediak-Higashi syndrome. J. Clin. Invest., *50*:2645–2652, 1971.
17. Cochrane, C.G., Unanue, E.R., and Dixon, F.J.: A role of polymorphonuclear leukocytes and complement in nephrotoxic nephritis. J. Exp. Med., *122*:99–116, 1965.

18. Cochrane, C.G., Weigle, W.O., and Dixon, F.J.: The role of polymorphonuclear leukocytes in the initiation and cessation of the Arthus vasculitis. J. Exp. Med., *110*:481–494, 1959.

19. Cohn, Z.A., and Hirsch, J.G.: The influence of phagocytosis on the intracellular distribution of granule-associated components of polymorphonuclear leucocytes. J. Exp. Med., *112*:1015–1022, 1960.

20. Cronstein, B.N., et al.: Adenosine: A physiological modulator of superoxide anion generation by human neutrophils. J. Exp. Med., *153*:1160–1177, 1983.

21. Dahlen, S.-E., et al.: Leukotrienes are potent constrictors of human bronchi. Nature (London), *288*:484–486, 1980.

22. Dawson, W., et al.: The pharmacology of benoxaprofen with particular reference to effects on lipoxygenase product formation. Eur. J. Rheumatol. Inflam., *5*:61–68, 1982.

23. DeShazo, C.V., et al.: The effect of complement depletion of neutrophil migration in acute immunologic arthritis. J. Immunol., *108*:1414–1419, 1972.

24. DeShazo, C.V., Henson, P.M., and Cochrane, C.G.: Acute immunologic arthritis in rabbits. J. Clin. Invest., *51*:50–57, 1972.

25. Dewald, B., et al.: Subcellular localization and heterogeneity of neutral proteases in neutrophilic polymorphonuclear leukocytes. J. Exp. Med., *141*:709–723, 1975.

26. Dunham, P., et al.: Membrane fusion: Studies with a calcium-sensitive dye, arsenazo III, in liposomes. Proc. Natl. Acad., Sci. U.S.A., *74*:1580–1584, 1977.

27. Evans, W.H., and Karnovsky, M.L.: The biochemical basis of phagocytosis. IV. Some aspects of carbohydrate metabolism during phagocytosis. Biochemistry, *1*:159–166, 1962.

28. Fantone, J.C., and Ward, P.A.: Role of oxygen-derived free radicals and metabolites in leukocyte-dependent inflammatory reactions. Am. J. Pathol., *107*:397–418, 1982.

29. Fearon, D.J.: Identification of the membrane glycoprotein that is the C3b receptor of the human erythrocyte, polymorphonuclear leukocytes, B lymphocyte, and monocyte. J. Exp. Med., *152*:20–30, 1980.

30. Fedorko, M.E., and Hirsch, J.G.: Cytoplasmic granule formation in myelocytes: An electron microscope radioautographic study on the mechanism of formation of cytoplasmic granules in rabbit heterophilic myelocytes. J. Cell Biol., *29*:307–316, 1966.

31. Feinmark, S.J., et al.: Stimulation of human leukocyte degranulation by leukotriene B4 and its omega-oxidized metabolites. FEBS Lett., *136*:141–144, 1981.

32. Feinstein, G., and Janoff, A.: A rapid method for purification of human granulocyte cationic neutral proteases: Purification and characterization of human granulocyte chymotrypsin-like enzyme. Biochim. Biophys. Acta, *403*:477–492, 1975.

33. Fleit, H.B., Wright, S.D., and Unkeless, J.C.: Human neutrophil Fc receptor distribution and structure. Proc. Natl. Acad. Sci. U.S.A., *79*:3275–3279, 1982.

34. Gallin, J.I.: Abnormal phagocyte chemotaxis: Pathophysiology, clinical manifestations, and management of patients. Rev. Infect. Dis., *3*:1196–1220, 1981.

35. Goetzl, E.J., and Pickett, W.C.: The human polymorphonuclear leukocyte chemotactic activity of complex hydroxy-eicosatetraenoic acids (HETEs) J. Immunol., *125*:1789–1791, 1980.

36. Goldstein, I.M., et al.: Calcium-induced lysozyme secretion from human polymorphonuclear leukocytes. Biochem. Biophys. Res. Commun., *60*:807–812, 1974.

37. Goldstein, I.M., et al.: Mechanisms of lysosomal enzyme release from human leukocytes: Microtubule assembly and membrane fusion induced by a component of complement. Proc. Natl. Acad. Sci. U.S.A., *70*:2916–2920, 1973.

38. Goldstein, I.M., Hoffstein, S., and Weissmann, G.: Influence of divalent cations upon complement-mediated enzyme release from human polymorphonuclear leukocytes. J. Immunol., *115*:665–670, 1975.

39. Goldstein, I.M., Hoffstein, S., and Weissmann, G.: Mechanisms of lysosomal enzyme release from human polymorphonuclear leukocytes. J. Cell Biol., *66*:647–652, 1975.

40. Goodwin, J.S., Bankhurst, A.D., and Messner, R.P.: Suppression of human T-cell mitogenesis by prostaglandin: Existence of a prostaglandin-producing suppressor cell. J. Exp. Med., *146*:1719–1734, 1977.

41. Hammarstrom, S.: Metabolism of leukotriene C3 in the guinea pig. Identification of metabolites formed by lung, liver, and kidney. J. Biol. Chem., *256*:9573–9578, 1981.

42. Hammarstrom, S., et al.: Rapid *in vivo* metabolism of leukotriene C_3 in the monkey, Macaca Irus. Biochem. Biophys. Res. Commun., *101*:1109–1115, 1981.

43. Harlin, J.M., et al.: Neutrophil-mediated endothelial injury in vitro. Mechanisms of cell detachment. J. Clin. Invest., *68*:1394–1403, 1981.

44. Henson, P.M.: Mechanisms of mediator release from inflammatory cells. *In* Mediators of Inflammation. Edited by G. Weissmann. New York, Plenum Publishing, 1974, pp. 9–50.

45. Herlin, T., Petersen, C.S., and Esmann, V.: The role of calcium and cyclic adenosine 3′,5′-monophosphate in the regulation of glycogen metabolism in phagocytozing human polymorphonuclear leukocytes. Biochim. Biophys. Acta, *542*:63–76, 1978.

46. Hirsch, J.G., and Cohn, Z.A.: Degranulation of polymorphonuclear leucocytes following phagocytosis of microorganisms. J. Exp. Med., *112*:1005–1014, 1960.

47. Hoffstein, S., et al.: Concanavalin A induces microtubule assembly and specific granule discharge in human polymorphonuclear leukocytes. J. Cell. Biol., *68*:781–787, 1976.

48. Hoffstein, S.T.: Ultrastructural demonstration of calcium loss from local regions of the plasma membrane of surface-stimulated human granulocytes. J. Immunol., *123*:1395–1402, 1979.

49. Horwitz, A.J., Hance, A.J., and Crystal, R.G.: Granulocyte collagenase: Selective digestion of type I relative to type III collagen. Proc. Natl. Acad. Sci. U.S.A., *74*:897–901, 1977.

50. Huang, C-K., et al.: Effects of chemotactic factors on the protein phosphorylation of rabbit peritoneal neutrophils. Fed. Proc., *42*:1080, 1983.

51. Humphrey, J.H.: The mechanism of Arthus reactions. I. The role of polymorphonuclear leucocytes and other factors in reversed passive Arthus reactions in rabbits. Br. J. Exp. Pathol., *36*:268–282, 1955.

52. Iyer, G.Y.N., Islam, D.F.M., and Quastel, J.H.: Biochemical aspects of phagocytosis. Nature, *192*:535–541, 1971.

53. Jackowski, S., and Sha'afi, R.I.: Response of adenosine cyclic 3′,5′-monophosphate level in rabbit neutrophils to the chemotactic peptide FMLP. Mol. Pharmacol., *16*:473–481, 1979.

54. Janoff, A., et al.: Human neutrophil elastase: In vitro effects on natural substrates suggest important physiological and pathological actions. *In* Proteases and Biological Control. Edited by E. Reich, D.B. Rifkin, and E. Shaw. New York, Cold Spring Harbor Laboratory, 1975, pp. 603–620.

55. Johnson, R.B., Jr.: Biochemical defects of polymorphonuclear and mononuclear phagocytes associated with disease. *In* The Reticuloendothelial System. Edited by A.J. Sbarra, and R.R. Strauss. New York, Plenum Publishing Corp., 1980, pp. 397–421.

56. Johnston, M., and Greenbaum, L.M.: Leukokinin-forming system in the ascitic fluid of a murine mastocytoma. Biochem. Pharmacol., *22*:1386–1389, 1973.

57. Johnston, R.B., Jr.: Defects of neutrophil function. N. Engl. J. Med., *307*:434–436, 1982.

58. Jubiz, W., et al.: A novel leukotriene produced by stimulation of leukocytes with formylmethionylleucylphenylalanine. J. Biol. Chem., *257*:6106–6110, 1982.

59. Kane, S.P., and Peters, T.J.: Analytical subcellular fractionation of human granulocytes with reference to the localization of vitamin B_{12}-binding proteins. Clin. Sci. Molec. Med., *49*:171, 1975.

60. Kaplan, H.B., et al.: Effects of non-steroidal anti-inflam-

matory agents on human neutrophil functions *in vitro* and *in vivo*. Biochem. Pharmacol., *33*:371, 1984.

61. Kaplan, H.B., et al.: The roles of degranulation and superoxide anion generation in neutrophil aggregation. Biochim. Biophys. Acta, *721*:55–63, 1982.

62. Karnovsky, M.L.: Steps toward an understanding of chronic granulomatous disease. N. Engl. J. Med., *308*:274–275, 1983.

63. Karnovsky, M.L., and Wallach, D.F.H.: The metabolic basis of phagocytosis III. Incorporation of inorganic phosphate into various classes of phosphatides during phagocytosis. J. Biol. Chem., *236*:1895–1901, 1961.

64. Klebanoff, S.J.: Iodination of bacteria: A bactericidal mechanism. J. Exp. Med., *126*:1063–1078, 1967.

65. Klebanoff, S.J.: Myeloperoxidase: Contribution to the microbicidal activity of intact leukocytes. Science, *169*:1095–1097, 1970.

66. Klebanoff, S.J., and Hamon, C.B.: Role of myeloperoxidase–mediated antimicrobial systems in intact leukocytes. J. Reticuloendothel. Soc., *12*:170–196, 1972.

67. Kniker, W.T., and Cochrane, C.G.: Pathogenic factors in vascular lesions of experimental serum sickness. J. Exp. Med., *122*:83–98, 1965.

68. Kohsaki, M., et al.: In vivo stimulation of murine granulopoiesis by human urinary extract from patients with aplastic anemia. Proc. Natl. Acad. Sci. U.S.A., *80*:3802–3806, 1983.

69. Korchak, H.M., Hoffstein, S.T., and Weissmann, G.: The neutrophil granule. *In* The Secretory Granule. Edited by A.M. Poisner, and J.M. Trifaro. New York, Elsevier Medical Press, 1982, pp. 317–356.

70. Korchak, H.M., et al.: Granulocytes without degranulation: Neutrophil function in granule-depleted cytoplasts. Proc. Natl. Acad. Sci. U.S.A., *80*:4968–4972, 1983.

71. Korchak, H.M., and Weissmann, G.: Changes in membrane potential of human granulocytes antecede the metabolic responses to surface stimulation. Proc. Natl. Acad. Sci. U.S.A., *75*:3818–3822, 1978.

72. Korn, E.D., and Weisman, R.A.: Phagocytosis of latex beads by acanthamoeba II. Electron microscopic study of the initial events. J. Cell Biol., *34*:219–227, 1969.

73. Kuehl, E.A.A., et al.: Role of prostaglandin endoperoxide PGG$_2$ in inflammatory processes. Nature, *265*:170–172, 1977.

74. Lazarus, G.S., et al.: Role of granulocyte collagenase in collagen degradation. Am. J. Pathol., *68*:565–576, 1972.

75. Lew, P.D., et al.: A variant of chronic granulomatous disease: Deficient oxidative metabolism due to a low-affinity NADPH oxidase. N. Engl. J. Med., *305*:1329–1333, 1981.

76. Loos, H., et al.: Familial deficiency of glutathione reductase in human blood cells. Blood, *48*:53–62, 1976.

77. Malawista, S.E.: Vinblastine can inhibit lysosomal degranulation without suppressing phagocytosis in human blood leukocytes. *In* Immunopathology of Inflammation. Edited by B.K. Forscher, and J.C. Houck. Amsterdam, Exerpta Medica, 1971, pp. 118–120.

78. Malmsten, C.L., et al.: Leukotriene B$_4$: A highly potent and stereospecific factor stimulating migration of polymorphonuclear leukocytes. Acta Physiol. Scand., *110*:449–451, 1980.

79. Malmsten, C., et al.: The role of prostaglandin endoperoxides and thromboxanes in platelet aggregation. *In* Advances in Prostaglandin and Thromboxane Research, Vol. 1. Edited by B. Samuelsson, and R. Paoletti. New York, Raven Press, 1976, pp. 737–746.

80. Mandell, G.L.: Intraphagosomal pH of human polymorphonuclear neutrophils. Proc. Soc. Exp. Biol. Med., *134*:447–449, 1970.

81. Mellon, M.G., and Rebhun, L.I.: Sulfhydryls and the in vitro polymerization of tubulin. J. Cell Biol., *70*:226–238, 1976.

82. Messner, R.P., et al.: A transient defect in leukocytic bactericidal capacity. Clin. Immunol. Immunopathol., *1*:523–532, 1973.

83. Metchnikoff, E.: Sur la lutte des cellules de l'organisme contre l'invasion des microbes. Ann. Inst. Pasteur, *1*:321, 1887.

84. Michell, R.H., Karnovsky, M.J., and Karnovsky, M.L.: The distribution of some granule-associated enzymes in guinea-pig polymorphonuclear leucocytes. Biochem. J., *116*:207–216, 1970.

85. Miller, M.E., et al.: A new familial defect of neutrophil movement. J. Lab. Clin. Med., *82*:1–8, 1975.

86. Miller, M.E., et al.: Lazy-leucocyte syndrome. A new disorder of neutrophil function. Lancet, *1*:665–669, 1971.

87. Movat, H.Z., Habal, F.M., and Mac Moline, D.R.L.: Neutral proteases of human PMN leukocytes with kininogenase activity. Int. Arch. Allergy Appl. Immunol., *50*:257–281, 1976.

88. Mudd, J., McCutcheon, M., and Lucke, B.: Phagocytosis. Physiol. Rev., *14*:210–275, 1934.

89. Murphy, G., et al.: The latent collagenase and gelatinase of human polymorphonuclear neutrophil leucocytes. Biochem. J., *192*:517–525, 1980.

90. Murphy, G., et al.: Collagenase is a component of the specific granules of human neutrophil leucocytes. Biochem. J., *162*:195–197, 1977.

91. Naccache, P.H., et al.: Involvement of membrane calcium in the response of rabbit neutrophils to chemotactic factors as evidenced by the fluorescence of chlorotetracycline. J. Cell Biol., *83*:179–186, 1979.

92. Naccache, P.H., et al.: Changes in ionic movements across rabbit polymorphonuclear leukocyte membranes during lysosomal enzyme release. Possible ionic basis for lysosomal enzyme release. J. Cell Biol., *75*:635–649, 1977.

93. Najjar, V.A., and Nishioka, K.: Tuftsin: A natural phagocytosis stimulating peptide. Nature, *228*:672–673, 1970.

94. Niedel, J.E., Kohn, I.J., and Vandenback, G.R.: Phorbol diester receptor copurifies with protein kinase C. Proc. Natl. Acad. Sci. U.S.A., *80*:36–40, 1983.

95. O'Flaherty, J.T., et al.: Substances which aggregate neutrophils. Am. J. Pathol., *92*:155–166, 1978.

96. Ohlsson, K.: Granulocyte collagenase and elastase and their interactions with alpha 1-antitrypsin and alpha 2-macroglobulin. *In* Proteases and Biological Control. Edited by D.B. Reich and E. Shaw. New York, Cold Spring Harbor Laboratory, 1975, p. 591.

97. Ohlsson, K., Olsson, I., and Spitznagel, J.K.: Localization of chymotrypsin-like cationic protein, collagenase, and elastase in azurophil granules of human neutrophilic polymorphonuclear leukocytes. Hoppe Seylers Z. Physiol. Chem., *358*:361–366, 1977.

98. Oliver, J.M., and Zurier, R.B.: Correction of characteristic abnormalities of microtubule function and granule morphology in Chediak-Higashi syndrome with cholinergic agonists. Studies in vitro in man and in vivo in the beige mouse. J. Clin. Invest., *57*:1239–1247, 1976.

99. Olsson, I., and Venge, P.: Cationic proteins of human granulocytes I. Isolation of the cationic proteins from the granules of leukaemic myeloid cells. Scand. J. Haematol., *9*:204–214, 1972.

100. Palmer, R.M., et al.: Chemokinetic activity of arachidonic and lipoxygenase products on leukocytes of different species. Prostaglandins, *20*:411–418, 1980.

101. Parish, W.E.: Effects of neutrophils on tissues. Experiments on the Arthus reaction, the flare phenomenon, and post-phagocytic release of lysosomal enzymes. Br. J. Dermatol., *81*:28–35, 1969.

102. Perez, H.D., Weksler, B., and Goldstein, I.: A new mechanism for the generation of biologically active products from arachidonic acid. Clin. Res., *27*:464a, 1979.

103. Pozzan, T., et al.: Monitoring cytoplasmic free calcium concentration $(Ca^{++})_i$ in living polymorphonuclear leukocytes. Clin. Res., *31*:320–329, 1983.

104. Radmark, O., et al.: Leukotriene A.: Stereochemistry and enzymatic conversion to leukotriene B. Biophys. Res. Commun., *92*:954–961, 1980.

105. Reaven, E.P., and Axline, S.G.: Subplasmalemmal microfilaments and microtubules in resting and phagocytizing cultivated macrophages. J. Cell Biol., *59*:12–27, 1976.

106. Rich, A.M., et al.: Granules are necessary for death of neutrophils after phagocytosis of crystalline monosodium urate. Submitted, 1984.

107. Rich, A.M., and Hoffstein, S.: Inverse correlation between neutrophil microtubule numbers and enhanced random migration. J. Cell Sci., 48:181–191, 1981.

108. Rindler-Ludwig, R., and Braunsteiner, H.: Cationic proteins from human neutrophil granulocytes: Evidence for their chymotrypsin-like properties. Biochim. Biophys. Acta, 379:606, 1975.

109. Robinson, D.R., Curran, D.P., and Hamer, P.J.: Prostaglandins and related compounds in inflammatory rheumatic diseases. In Advances in Inflammation Research. Edited by M. Ziff, G. Velo, and S. Gorini, 3:17–27, 1982.

110. Roos, D., et al.: Protection of phagocytic leukocytes by endogenous glutathione: Studies in a family with glutathione deficiency. Blood, 53:851–866, 1979.

111. Root, R.K., Rosenthal, A.S., and Balestra, D.J.: Abnormal bactericidal, metabolic, and lysosomal functions of Chediak-Highashi syndrome leukocytes. J. Clin. Invest., 51:649–665, 1972.

112. Sacks, T., et al.: Oxygen radicals mediate endothelial cell damage by complement-stimulated granulocytes. J. Clin. Invest., 61:1161–1167, 1978.

113. Salmon, S.E., et al.: Myeloperoxidase deficiency. Immunologic study of a genetic leukocyte defect. N. Engl. J. Med., 282:250–252, 1970.

114. Samuelsson, M.: Leukotrienes: Mediators of immediate hypersensitivity reactions and inflammation. Science, 220:568–575, 1983.

115. Sbarra, A.J., and Karnovsky, M.L.: The biochemical basis of phagocytosis I. Metabolic changes during the ingestion of particles by polymorphonuclear leukocytes. J. Biol. Chem., 234:1355–1362, 1959.

116. Schmidt, W., and Havemann, K.: Isolation of elastase-like and chymotrypsin-like neutral proteases from human granulocytes. Hoppe Seylers Z. Physiol. Chem., 355:1077–1082, 1974.

117. Scott, R.E., and Horn, R.G.: Ultrastructural aspects of neutrophil granulocyte development in humans. Lab. Invest., 23:202–215, 1970.

118. Segal, A.L., et al.: Absence of cytochrome b-245 in chronic granulomatous disease. N. Engl. J. Med., 308:245–251, 1983.

119. Serhan, C.N., et al.: Formation of leukotrienes and hydroxy acids by human neutrophils and platelets exposed to monosodium urate. Prostaglandins, 27:563–581, 1984.

120. Serhan, C.N., et al.: Changes in phosphatidylinositol and phosphatidic acid in stimulated human neutrophils. Relationship to calcium mobilization, aggregation, and superoxide radical generation. Biochim. Biophys. Acta, 762:420–428, 1983.

121. Serhan, C.N., et al.: Leukotriene B4 and phosphatidic acid are calcium ionophores: Studies employing arsenazo III in liposomes. J. Biol. Chem., 257:4746, 1982.

122. Serhan, C.N., et al.: Phosphatidate and oxidized fatty acids are calcium ionophores. Studies employing arsenazo III in liposomes. J. Biol. Chem., 256:2736–2741, 1981.

123. Simchowitz, L., Spilberg, I., and Atkinson, J.P.: Evidence that the functional responses of human neutrophils occur independently of transient elevations in cAMP levels. Fed. Proc., 42:1080, 1982.

124. Sklar, L.A., et al.: A continuous, spectroscopic analysis of the kinetics of elastase secretion by neutrophils. J. Biol. Chem., 257:5471–5475, 1982.

125. Smith, M.J., Ford-Hutchinson, A.W., and Bray, M.A.: Leukotriene B.: A potential mediator of inflammation. J. Pharmacol., 32:517–518, 1980.

126. Smolen, J.E., Korchak, N.M., and Weissmann, G.: Increased levels of cyclic adenosine-3',5'-monophosphate in human polymorphonuclear leukocytes after surface stimulation. J. Clin. Invest., 65:1077–1085, 1980.

127. Smolen, J.E., Korchak, H.M., and Weissmann, G.: Initial kinetics of lysosomal enzyme release and superoxide anion generation in human polymorphonuclear leukocytes. Inflammation, 4:145, 1980.

128. Smolen, J.E., and Weissman, G.: The fluorescence response of chlorotetracycline-loaded human polymorpho-nuclear leukocytes. I. The effect of various stimuli and calcium antagonists. Biochim. Biophys. Acta, 720:172–180, 1982.

129. Smolen, J.E., and Weissmann, G.: Stimuli which provoke secretion of azurophil enzymes from human neutrophils induced increments in adenosine cyclic 3',5'-monophosphate. Biochim. Biophys. Acta, 672:197–206, 1981.

130. Spitznagel, J.K., et al.: Character of azurophil and specific granules purified from human polymorphonuclear leukocytes. Lab. Invest., 30:774–787, 1974.

131. Spitznagel, J.K., et al.: Selective deficiency of granules associated with lysozyme and lactoferrin in human polymorphs (PMN) with reduced microbicidal capacity. J. Clin. Invest., 51:93a, 1972.

132. Starkey, P.M., and Barrett, A.J.: Neutral proteinases of human spleen. Biochem. J., 155:255–263, 1976.

133. Stetson, C.A.: Similarities in the mechanisms determining the Arthus and Shwartzman phenomena. J. Exp. Med., 94:347–358, 1951.

134. Stossel, T.P., and Hartwig, J.H.: Interactions of actin, myosin, and a new actin-binding protein of rabbit pulmonary macrophages. II. Role in cytoplasmic movement and phagocytosis. J. Cell Biol., 68:602–619, 1976.

135. Strauss, R.G., et al.: An anomaly of neutrophil morphology with impaired function. N. Engl. J. Med., 290:478–484, 1974.

136. Tsung, P.K., Sakamoto, T., and Weissmann, G.: Protein kinase and phosphatases from human polymorphonuclear leukocytes. Biochem. J., 145:437–438, 1975.

137. Ward, P.A., and Hill, J.H.: C5 chemotactic fragments produced by an enzyme in lysosomal granules of neutrophils. J. Immunol., 104:535–536, 1970.

138. Wehring, R.R.: Cytochalasin B inhibits actin-related gelation of HeLa cell extracts. J. Cell Biol., 71:303–307, 1976.

139. Weissmann, G., et al.: The secretory code of the neutrophil. In Cellular Interactions. Edited by J.T. Dingle and J.L. Gordon. New York, Elsevier North-Holland Biomedical Press, 1981, pp. 15–31.

140. Weissmann, G., et al.: A general method, employing arsenazo III in liposomes, for study of calcium ionophores: Results with A23187 and prostaglandins. Proc. Natl. Acad. Sci. U.S.A., 77:1506–1510, 1980.

141 Weissmann, G., et al.: The secretory code of the neutrophil. J. Reticuloendothal. Soc., 26:687–700, 1979.

142. Weissmann, G., Smolen, J.E., and Korchak, H.M.: Release of inflammatory mediators from stimulated neutrophils. N. Engl. J. Med., 303:27–34, 1980.

143. Wright, D.G., and Malawista, S.E.: Mobilization and extracellular release of granular enzymes from human leukocytes during phagocytosis: Inhibition by colchicine and cortisol but not by salicylate. Arthritis Rheum., 16:749–758, 1973.

144. Zeya, H.I., and Spitznagel, J.K.: Cationic protein bearing granules of polymorphonuclear leukocytes: Separation from enzyme-rich granules. Science, 163:1069–1071, 1969.

145. Zeya, H.I., and Spitznagel, J.K.: Arginine-rich proteins of polymorphonuclear leukocyte lysosomes. Antimicrobial specificity and biochemical heterogeneity. J. Exp. Med., 127:927–941, 1968.

146. Zucker-Franklin, D. and Hirsch, J.G.: Electron microscope studies on the degranulation of rabbit peritoneal leukocytes during phagocytosis. J. Exp. Med., 120:569–576, 1964.

147. Zurier, R.B., et al.: Mechanisms of lysosomal enzyme release from human leukocytes. II. Effects of cAMP and cGMP, autonomic agonists, and agents which affect microtubule function. J. Clin. Invest. 53:296–309, 1974.

148. Zurier, R.B., Hoffstein, S., and Weissmann, G.: Cytochalasin B.: Effect on lysosomal enzyme release from human leukocytes. Proc. Natl. Acad. Sci. U.S.A., 70:844–848, 1973.

149. Zurier, R.B., Hoffstein, S., and Weissmann, G.: Mechanisms of lysosomal enzyme release from human leukocytes. J. Cell Biol., 58:27–48, 1973.

Chapter **19**

Granulocyte Chemotaxis

Isaias Spilberg

The recruitment of granulocytes at the site of tissue injury is the histopathologic hallmark of acute inflammation. A vast array of information has been accumulated, which suggests that a common pathway of events is followed by the responding cells in arriving at the exact location of tissue damage, independent of whether the potentially injurious substance is a bacterium, an immune complex, or a urate crystal. The local accumulation of cells is an active phenomenon. Loss of vascular integrity is not required for the cells to leave the circulation. Microscopic studies clearly indicate that neutrophils coursing through vessels adjacent to an inflamed area are sidetracked from their normal pattern of flow. They clump together, adhere to the endothelial wall, and then actively crawl between endothelial cells, traversing the interstitial matrix to arrive at the site of tissue injury. Once there, the neutrophil in all likelihood releases additional mediators, thereby amplifying the inflammatory process. The critical role that granulocyte chemotaxis plays in normal host defense is dramatically underscored by the clinical and laboratory descriptions of several potentially lethal immunodeficiency states in which the defined alteration of host defense is depressed cellular migration. The reverse is observed in primary inflammatory disorders in which the chronic stimulation of inflammatory cells leads to organ dysfunction. In some clinical conditions, excessive chemotactic factor elaboration and depressed neutrophil function may coexist.

DEFINITION AND METHODOLOGY

Chemotaxis is the directed migration of cells along a chemical gradient. This must be distinguished from *chemokinesis* in which cells are chemically stimulated to move faster, but not necessarily along a gradient.[50] The key distinction is that during chemotaxis the cells orient and maintain the same orientation during their locomotion. The two processes can be experimentally distinguished by exposing the cells to a series of gradients obtained by varying the concentration of the test substance. Substances that are truly chemotactic give the greatest enhancement of vectorial cellular movement when they are spatially separated from

the responding cells so that a diffusion gradient results. Studies on individual cells reveal that on exposure to a chemotactic factor the initial pseudopod is extended toward the gradient peak.[48,49] The cells seem capable of sensing the strength of the gradient across their diameter. Migration following this extension is in a vector toward maximal chemical concentration. In contrast, cells responding chemokinetically show increased migration but no net vector of migration. This response can be correlated with absolute mediator concentration, as opposed to the strength of the gradient.[25] Besides being chemotactic, chemoattractants characteristically also induce chemokinesis.[4]

Current methods used to study granulocyte movement in vitro fall into two general categories: (1) observation of the motion of individual cells, and (2) measurement of the migration of a cell population. In the first method, locomotion is analyzed by time-lapse cinematography of individual cells on a warmed glass slide.[48] This technique has permitted the detailed description of the morphology of granulocytes in motion, but has been less frequently utilized to study various clinical states and drug effects. Study of the locomotion of individual cells is not clinically applicable because of problems in quantifying the cellular events, and because of technical difficulties in establishing stable concentration gradients and in surveying the effects of a large number of agents on granulocyte motion. These difficulties are partially avoided by assessing the migration of cell populations using the Boyden chamber and the "under agarose" assays.

In the Boyden chamber method,[51] granulocytes are added to the upper and the potential chemoattractant is added to the lower of two compartments that are separated by a micropore filter. After a suitable incubation period, migration is quantified microscopically by counting the stained granulocytes that have migrated through the filter, or by determining the actual distance traveled into the filter by the "leading front" of cells. Filter pore sizes utilized in these experiments have ranged from .65 to 5 μm—sizes too small to enable the cells to passively traverse the filter. The adaptation of computer-assisted image anaylyzers to the described technique has been a major advance allowing for more accurate quantitation. A modification of the Boyden chamber assay,[16] which reduces human error, utilizes two micropore filters and radiolabeled leukocytes. Migration is quantified by counting the radioactivity in cells that have passed completely through the first filter and into the second. Highly purified cell populations are required, however, in order to equate radioactivity with the migration of a given granulocyte class. The limitations of the filter technique include filter lot variability, inability to study isolated cells, and the artificial constraint imposed by inflexible pores.

The second population method, also limited by the inability to study individual cells, utilizes an agarose gel matrix to allow the cell to crawl between the underlying petri dish and the gel.[31] This technique permits a visual evaluation of the chemotactic and chemokinetic effects of an attractant, but is less sensitive than the membrane techniques. Population techniques do not allow for ready identification of neutrophil subsets with varied migratory capabilities. All methods require a control for endogenous random granulocyte motility.

In vivo assessment of neutrophil motility[28] is possible but provides information that is difficult to quantify. A superficial skin abrasion made with a sterile scapel blade, the "skin window" first described by Rebuck, is covered with a coverslip that can be removed at suitable times and stained for the cells to be counted. This in vivo assay is a useful clinical monitor of total cell migration but cannot distinguish between chemotaxis and chemokinesis.

White cell motility in vitro is influenced by the concentration of protein, partial pressure of oxygen, pH, temperature, and tonicity of the suspending medium.[49] It is unclear, however, whether the extremes necessary to alter leukocyte function in vitro apply to in vivo situations.

CHEMOTACTIC FACTORS

Substances reportedly chemotactic for granulocytes vary greatly in size and chemical composition as well as in the extent to which they have been studied. The initial interaction between cell and chemotactic factor appears to be via "factor specific" receptors. Such receptors have been described for formylated peptides on both neutrophils[2,46] and macrophages.[38,44] It may well be that these chemotactic factors, which are active at 10^{-10}M, play a key role in the attraction of neutrophils to the site of metabolically actively growing bacteria, since similar material can be isolated from the filtrates of E. coli growing in broth.[34] The ready availability of these small peptides, especially N-formyl-methionine-leucine-phenylalanine (F-met-

leu-phe), has led to study of the mechanism by which receptor binding is translated into oriented cell migration. The biological significance of receptor interaction is evidenced by a striking correlation between binding affinities and chemotactic activities of a large number of formylated peptides of varying amino acid sequence.[34,37]

The bulk of chemotactic activity of complement is due to C5a and C5a des Arg.[36] The latter is the residual C5a molecule after serum carboxypeptidase(s) cleaves the terminal arginine residue, and is probably the major circulating form of C5a. C5a des Arg differs from C5a in that it has no anaphylatoxin activity, has roughly 10% of the chemotactic activity of native C5a, and probably requires a serum protein "helper factor" to exert its activity.[32] C5a is active at a concentration of 10^{-9}M, and a specific receptor recognizing it has been demonstrated on human neutrophils.[10] The structure of the cellular receptor for C5a and other chemotactic factor receptors remains largely unknown.

The phagocytosis of urate or calcium pyrophosphate crystals by neutrophils leads to the synthesis and secretion of a glycopeptide that is chemotactically active, at concentrations of less than 10^{-7}M, for neutrophils and monocytes.[39] The production of this chemotactic factor, first described by Phelps, is exquisitely sensitive to suppression by low doses of colchichine, and this has been proposed as the primary mechanism by which the drug acts in acute gout and pseudogout.[43] Neutrophils have a distinct receptor for this chemotactic factor.[41] The intraarticular injection of the crystal-induced chemotactic factor into the joints of rabbits induces an acute synovitis without a significant increase in vascular permeability.[39]

The clinical success of nonsteroidal anti-inflammatory drugs in the rheumatic diseases has prompted an intense search among the metabolites of arachidonic acid[19] for a pivotal mediator of inflammation. The most potent chemotactic factor described to date comes from the lipoxygenase pathway[20] of neutrophils. Leukotriene B4 or 5(S), 12(R)-hydroxy-eicosa-6, 14-CIS 8, 10-transtetraneoic acid (LTB$_4$) is chemotactically active for neutrophils at concentrations less than 10^{-10}M. Human neutrophils possess a specific receptor for LTB$_4$.[20] Other derivatives are active, but less potent, chemotactic factors. Since their production is stimulated by exposure of cells to other chemotactic factors, they may well function to modulate the inflammatory process.

Type I allergic reactions are characterized by tissue infiltration with eosinophils and neutrophils and are mediated by the specific interaction of antigen with IgE on the surface of mast cells and basophils. Exposure in vitro or in vivo of sensitized mast-cell-rich tissues to a stimulating antigen results in the release of chemotactic factors for both eosinophils[24] and neutrophils.[3] The eosinophil chemotactic factor of anaphylaxis (ECF-A) is composed of at least two tetrapeptides: val-gly-ser-glu and ala-gly-ser-glu.[18] They exist preformed in granules of mast cells and basophils, and apparently their release is under the same control as histamine secretion. ECF-A exhibits peak activity at approximately $5 \times 10^{-8}M$ and is capable of inducing chemotaxis and enzyme release from eosinophils, but not from neutrophils. A specific receptor for ECF-A has been described[7] that exhibits marked conformational specificity toward related tetrapeptides. The less well-studied basophil can also respond chemotactically to C5a and to an as yet unidentified product of lymphocyte culture.[5] Several other chemotactic factors have been described,[4,15,33,34] some of which are listed in Table 19–1.

Chemotactic factors have multiple effects on granulocytes both in vitro and in vivo. Exposure of cells to high concentrations of chemotactic factors in vitro causes prompt reversible aggregation. Infusion of chemotactic factors intravenously into animals elicits a transient neutropenia and pulmonary sequestration of granulocytes, with an accompanying decrease in the PO_2 and increase in the alveolar-arterial oxygen gradient. This phenomenon may be analogous to that occurring in vivo with the initiation of hemodialysis,[12] a procedure that activated C5a. Incubation of neutrophils in vitro with most chemotactic factors induces lysosomal enzyme release and superoxide production.[4] Factors vary in their potency, and fairly stringent incubation conditions are sometimes necessary to demonstrate this activity. Although

exocytosis has been proposed as a mechanism for modulating the chemotactic response by way of chemotactic factor destruction and direct cellular effects, the in vivo significance is unclear. Neutrophil lysosomal contents are, however, capable of activating complement and the coagulation cascade, as well as degrading collagen and proteoglycans.

Incubation of cells with chemotactic factors in the absence of a gradient leads to a reversible state of chemotactic unresponsiveness (without decreased chemokinesis) termed *deactivation*. This state has been shown to be, in part, agent-nonspecific and, therefore, unlikely to occur simply as a result of receptor binding or "down regulation" of receptors.[34,40] In vivo deacativtion can be demonstrated in man[9] and may contribute to the accumulation of cells in an inflammatory focus by limiting the egress of cells attracted by a chemotactic gradient. Normal serum contains an irreversible inactivator of chemotactic peptides. This chemotactic factor inactivator can inhibit Arthus reactions and immune-complex-induced pulmonary damage.[23]

Cellular Effects of Chemotactic Factors

Leukocytes migrating in a chemotactic gradient exhibit a polarized morphology.[1,50] There is a leading pseudopod adherent to substrate, which is generally free of organelles, followed by the cell body containing the nucleus and a tail that may contain organelles. The position of the centriole is usually maintained between the leading pseudopod and the bulk of the nucleus, and this has been used as a marker for orientation. The tail is not necessarily adherent to the substratum, although at times it may have extensions (retraction fibers) that are rich in

Table 19–1.   Granulocyte Chemotactic Factors

Chemotactic Factor	Characteristics	Comments	Reference
C5a	Glycoprotein, MW 11,200	Specific receptor; formed during hemodialysis	10
C5a des Arg		Needs helper factor	32
Crystal-induced CF	Glycoprotein, MW 11,500	Specific receptor; synthesis inhibited by colchicine	41
Arachidonate metabolites	LTB$_4$ product of lipoxygenase pathway, MW 330	Specific receptor; at least as potent as C5a	20
Eosinophil chemotactic factor of anaphylaxis (ECF-A)	Val-Gly-Ser-Glu and other tetrapeptides, 300–500 MW	Specific receptor from mast cells	18
Histamine	Amine, MW 111; specific for eosinophils	From mast cells, basophils	11
Ragweed antigen-induced neutrophil chemotactic factor	Protein; MW 150,000	Probably from mast cells	3
Formylated peptides	F-Met-Leu-Phe, MW 440, and related peptides	Specific receptor on neutrophils, macrophages	2
Bacterial products	MW 150–1500	From *E. coli* culture filtrate	34
Platelet factor 4	MW 7,800	From platelets	14
Denatured proteins	Various proteins including albumin and hemoglobin	No specific receptor identified	45

microfilaments. Direct observation of migrating cells has shown that they crawl along a substrate, changing direction by a series of turns, each less than 90° from the previous direction. Actin-containing microfilaments are necessary for migration to take place, and microtubules are probably required for accurate maintenance of orientation.[1] Patients with altered granulocyte migration accompanying defects in microfilaments[8] and microtubules[15] have been described.

The biochemical steps by which receptor binding is translated into chemotaxis are still unclear. Chemotactic factor binding to neutrophils stimulates several rapid and transient metabolic events, including activation of Na^+K^+ ATPase, membrane hyperpolarization, tyrosylation of tubulin, increased glucose and oxygen consumption, and changes in cyclic nucleotide levels and arachidonic acid metabolism.[30,34]

Stimulation of metabolic processes by chemotactic factor does not necessarily indicate that the stimulation contributes directly to chemotaxis nor that the events are interdependent. For instance, chemotactic factors induce a rapid increase in neutrophil membrane potentials. Cells from patients with chronic granulomatous disease, a disorder marked by inability of neutrophils to undergo the normal respiratory burst of increased oxygen consumption and superoxide production, do not respond to chemotactic factors with membrane hyperpolarization.[35] However, their chemotactic response is still 60% of normal. Microtubule polymerization occurs during both chemotaxis and exocytosis, although the two processes can be separated by altering membrane fluidity[47] or by using the chemotactic factor gly-his-gly, an agent that polymerizes microtubules but does not stimulate exocytosis.[42]

The observation that methylation plays a necessary role in chemotaxis, coupled with studies implicating increased intracellular calcium and arachidonate metabolism as prerequisites for neutrophil chemotaxis,[21,29,33] allows for the synthesis of a possible scheme of chemotactic activation. Exposure of neutrophils to chemotactic factors leads to decreased methylation of phospholipids. This correlates with a rapid increase in the availability of arachidonate and its subsequent metabolism. The arachidonate increase is a result of cleavage of phospholipids by phospholipase A_2, an enzyme readily inhibited by high-dose glucocorticoids that induce synthesis of a specific protein that inhibits both phospholipase A_2 and chemotaxis.[21] Endogenous inhibitor activity is suppressible by the increased intracellular calcium evoked by chemotactic factors. Products of the lipoxygenase pathway increase in response to increased arachidonate mobilization. Several of these products have been shown to be chemotactic themselves, and the incorporation of LTB_4 into the plasma membrane further enhances chemotactic factor-induced calcium influx. The increased intracellular calcium is capable of activating the actin system and cell migration. The exact mechanism by which these events allow the cell to maintain orientation along a chemotactic gradient has yet to be elucidated. One possibility rests on the observation that chemotactic factors induce the tyrosylation of tubulin. This is prevented by inhibitors of phospholipase A_2 or of calcium influx.[34] Thus, chemotactic factor-receptor interaction may provoke alterations in phospholipid metabolism that in turn alter local membrane fluidity and allow for changes in calcium influx, receptor movement, cytoskeletal assembly and attachment, and membrane flow resulting in pseudopod extension. The actual migratory response may require continued increased intracellular calcium as well as the maintenance of local membrane changes in the areas of the peak chemotactic gradient. The exact role that other chemotactic factor stimulated events, such as esterase activation, play in this scheme has yet to be explored.

CHEMOTAXIS AND THE RHEUMATIC DISEASES

Studies on various rheumatic disease states have reportedly demonstrated altered chemotaxis, both reduced and enhanced.[15,26] Clear-cut distinction between chemotaxis and chemokinesis has not always been provided, and interpretation of several of these studies is therefore limited. As a rule, peripheral blood granulocytes from patients with rheumatic disorders behave in a normal fashion, but the serum from some patients may be defective in its ability to induce chemotaxis. Peripheral neutrophils of some patients with rheumatoid arthritis, Felty's syndrome, and SLE have exhibited abnormal migration in vitro with the extent of the defect correlating with disease activity. Increased chemotaxis has been reported in neutrophils from patients with Beçhet's syndrome and familial Mediterranean fever.[26] A caveat in the interpretation of these data lies in the fact that circulating neutrophils are not homogeneous.[15] Studies on peripheral blood cells may actually reflect a subpopulation of cells that are not participating in the ongoing inflammatory process, either because of intrinsic cellular properties or because of secondary extracellular factors, such as in vivo deactivation.

An inadequate capacity to generate chemotactic activity in serum has been described in some patients with SLE. The patient's sera contains an inhibitor of a factor required by C5a des Arg to be fully chemotactic.[32] A profound defect in the capacity to generate chemotactic activity from serum is frequently seen in a rheumatic disease-like syndrome associated with a genetic deficiency in early complement components.[15] Patients with Clr, C_4, or C2 deficiencies are prone to develop an SLE-like illness or, more rarely, a dermatomyositis-like syndrome or necrotizing vasculitis. Patients with C3 deficiency have a more pronounced serum chemotactic defect and are prone to recurrent infections but, as a rule, do not develop rheumatic-like syndromes.

ANTI-INFLAMMATORY AGENTS AND CHEMOTAXIS

Anti-inflammatory drugs are thought to act on the leukocyte, limiting motility and/or effector function of the cell. There is, however, a general dearth of information convincingly documenting such effects on chemotaxis. Corticosteroids are the most potent anti-inflammatory compounds available, and in vivo assays of cell motility reveal that hydrocortisone is capable of reducing neutrophil accumulation for up to 12 hours.[6] In vitro studies, however, have not fully demonstrated a primary defect on chemotaxis. A single dose of intravenous dexamethasone did not alter neutrophil migration assessed in vitro even when the cells were obtained from volunteers at near the peak of the steroid-induced granulocytosis.[17] Colchicine, a drug capable of depolymerizing microtubules, has been shown to impair chemotaxis in vitro when assessed by the filter technique, but not by the agarose method that does not require the cell to penetrate a filter with rigid channels.[13] Studies utilizing an experimental model for crystal arthritis indicated that pharmacologic doses of intravenous colchicine impaired phagocyte synthesis and secretion of the crystal-induced chemotactic factor implicated in the pathogenesis of acute gout and pseudogout. However, the peripheral blood granulocytes of the colchicine-treated rabbits retained their full ability to respond to a chemotactic challenge.[43] Normal chemotaxis has also been demonstrated testing peripheral neutrophils from colchicine-treated patients. Anecdotal reports document the clinical efficacy of colchicine in small groups of patients with the arthritis of sarcoidosis, familial Mediterranean fever, and Behçet's syndrome.[26] Any relation of this apparent beneficial effect and altered neutrophil chemotaxis has yet to be elucidated. Various drugs have been shown to alter granulocyte chemotaxis in vitro,[15,22,27] including gold compounds, levamisol, and the nonsteroidal anti-inflammatory agents. Often the drugs have been tested in vitro at greater than their pharmacologic levels, and clear-cut distinction between chemotaxis and che-

mokinesis has not always been presented. Additional studies are needed before conclusions can be drawn regarding their in vivo effect.

In summary, leukocyte chemotaxis is the result of a complex series of intracellular events that cause directional migration of potentially destructive cells into an inflamed area. Intelligent manipulation of the inflammatory response at this locus will require a greater understanding of the chemotactic process in order to suppress unwanted granulocyte-mediated tissue damage without compromising host defense to an intolerable degree.

REFERENCES

1. Allan, R.B., and Wilkinson, P.C.: A visual analysis of chemotactic locomotion of human leukocytes: Use of a new chemotactic assay with Candida albicans as a gradient source. Exp. Cell Res., *111*:191–198, 1978.
2. Aswanikumar, S., Corcoran, B., and Schiffmann, E.: Demonstration of a receptor on rabbit neutrophils for chemotactic peptides. Biochem. Biophys. Res. Commun., *74*:810–817, 1977.
3. Atkins, P.C., et al.: Further characterization and biologic activity of ragweed antigen-induced neutrophils chemotactic activity in men. J. Allergy Clin. Immunol., *64*:251–258, 1979.
4. Becker, E.L.: Chemotaxis. J. Allergy Clin. Immunol., *66*:97–105, 1980.
5. Boetcher, D.A., and Leonard, E.J.: Basophil chemotaxis: Augmentation by a factor from stimulated lymphocyte cultures. Immunol. Commun., *2*:421–428, 1973.
6. Boggs, D.R., Athens, J.W., and Cartwright, G.E.: The effect of adrenal glucocorticosteroids upon the cellular composition of inflammatory exudates. Am. J. Pathol., *44*:763–773, 1964.
7. Boswell, R.N., Austen, K.F., and Goetzl, E.L.: A chemotactic receptor for Val-Gly-Ser-Glu on human eosinophil polymorphonuclear leukocytes. Immunol. Commun., *5*:469–479, 1976.
8. Boxer, L.A., Hedley-Whyte, E.T., and Stossel, T.P.: Neutrophil actin dysfunction and abnormal neutrophil behavior. N. Engl. J. Med., *291*:1093–1099, 1974.
9. Center, D.M., et al.: Inhibition of neutrophil chemotaxis in association with experimental angioedema in patients with cold urticaria: A model of chemotactic deactivation in vivo. Clin. Exp. Immunol., *35*:112–118, 1979.
10. Chenoweth, D.E., and Hugli, T.E.: Demonstration of specific C5a receptor on intact human polymorphonuclear leukocytes. Proc. Natl. Acad. Sci. U.S.A., *75*:3943–3947, 1978.
11. Clark, R.A.F., Gallin, J.I., and Kaplan, A.P.: The selective eosinophil chemotactic activity of histamine. J. Exp. Med., *142*:1462–1476, 1975.
12. Craddock, P.R., et al.: Complement (C5a)-induced granulocyte aggregation in vitro. A possible mechanism of complement mediated leukostasis and leukopenia. J. Clin. Invest., *60*:260–264, 1977.
13. Daughaday, C.C., Bohrer, A.N., and Spilberg, I.: Lack of effect of colchicine on human neutrophils chemotaxis under agarose. Experientia, *37*:199–200, 1981.
14. Duel, T.F., et al.: Platelet factor 4 is chemotactic for neutrophils and monocytes. Proc. Natl. Acad. Sci. U.S.A., *78*:4584–4587, 1981.
15. Gallin, J.I.: Abnormal phagocyte chemotaxis: Pathophysiology, clinical manifestations, and management of patients. Rev. Infect. Dis., *3*:1196–1220, 1981.
16. Gallin, J.I., Clark, R.A., and Goetzl, E.J.: Radioassay of leukocyte locomotion: A sensitive technique for clinical studies. *In* Leukocyte Chemotaxis: Methods, Physiology and Clinical Implications. Edited by J.I. Gallin, and P.G. Quie. New York, Raven Press, 1978, pp. 79–86.
17. Glasser, L., Huestic, D.W., and Jones, J.F.: Functional capabilities f steroid recruited neutrophils harvested for

clinicl transfusion. N. Engl. J. Med., *297*:1033–1036, 1979.

18. Goetzl, E.J., and Austen, K.F.: Purification and synthesis of eosinophilic tetrapeptides of human lung tissue: Identification as eosinophil chemotactic factor of anaphylaxis. Proc. Natl. Acad. Sci. U.S.A., *72*:4123–4127, 1975.

19. Goetzl, E.J.: Oxygenation products of arachidonic acid as mediators of hypersensitivity and inflammation. Med. Clin. North Am., *65*:809–829, 1981.

20. Goldman, D.W., and Goetzl, E.J.: Specific binding of leukotrine B_4 to receptors on human polymorphonuclear leukocytes. J. Immunol., *129*:1600–1604, 1982.

21. Hirata, F., et al.: A phospholipase A_2 inhibitory protein in rabbit neutrophils induced by glucocorticoids. Proc. Natl. Acad. Sci. U.S.A., *77*:2533–2536, 1980.

22. Ho, P.P.K., Young, A.L., and Southard, G.L.: Methyl ester of N-formyl-methionyl-leucyl-phenylalanine. Chemotactic responses of human blood monocytes and inhibition of gold compounds. Arthritis Rheum., *21*:133–136, 1978.

23. Johnson, K.J., Anderson, T.P., and Ward, P.: Suppression of immune complex induced inflammation by the chemotactic factor inactivator. J. Clin. Invest., *59*:951–958, 1977.

24. Kay, A.B., Stechschulte, D.J., and Austen, K.F.: An eosinophilic chemotactic factor of anaphylaxis. J. Exp. Med., *133*:602–619, 1971.

25. Keller, H.U., et al.: A proposal for the definition of terms related to locomotion of leukocytes and other cells. Clin. Exp. Immunol., *27*:377–380, 1980.

26. Levy, M., et al.: Enhanced polymorphonuclear chemotaxis—a common feature of diseases responsive to colchicine. Med. Hypotheses, *7*:15–20, 1981.

27. Meacock, S.C.R., and Kitchen, E.A.: Some effects of nonsteroidal anti-inflammatory agents on leukocyte migration. Agents Actions, *6*:320–324, 1976.

28. Miller, M.E.: Cell movement and host defenses. Ann. Intern. Med., *78*:601–603, 1973.

29. Naccache, P.H., et al.: Pharmacological differentiation between chemotactic factor induced calcium redistribution and transmembrane flux in rabbit neutrophils. Biochem. Biophys. Res. Commun., *89*:1224–1230, 1979.

30. Nath, J., et al.: Stimulation of tubulin tyrosylation in rabbit leukocytes evoked by the chemoattractant Formyl-methionyl-leucyl-phenylalanine. J. Cell Biol., *91*:232–234, 1981.

31. Nelson, R.D., Quie, P.G., and Simmons, R.L.: Chemotaxis under agarose: A new and simple method for measuring chemotaxis and spontaneous migration of human polymorphonuclear leukocytes and monocytes. J. Immunol., *115*:1650–1656, 1975.

32. Perez, H.D., et al.: Chemotactic activity of C5a des arg: Evidence of a requirement of an aniodic peptide "helper factor" and inhibiton by a cationic protein in serum from patients with SLE. Mol. Immunol., *17*:163–169, 1980.

33. Schiffmann, E.: Leukocyte chemotaxis. Annu. Rev. Physiol., *44*:553–568, 1982.

34. Schiffmann, E., and Gallin, J.I.: Biochemistry of phagocyte chemotaxis. Curr. Top. Cell Regul., *15*:203–261, 1979.

35. Seligmann, B.E., and Gallin, J.I.: Use of lipophilic probes of membrane potentials to assess human neutrophil activation. J. Clin. Invest., *66*:493–503, 1980.

36. Shin, H.S., et al.: Chemotactic and anaphylatoxic fragment cleaved from the fifth component of guinea pig complement. Science, *162*:361–363, 1968.

37. Showell, et al.: Structure-activity relations of synthetic peptides as chemoattractants and inducers of lysosomal enzyme secretion for neutrophils. J. Exp. Med., *143*:1154–1169, 1976.

38. Snyderman, R., and Fudman, E.J.: Demonstration of a chemotactic factor receptor on macrophages. J. Immunol., *124*:2754–2757, 1980.

39. Spilberg, I., and Mandell, B.: Crystal-induced chemotactic factor. *In* Advances in Inflammation Research. Vol. 5. Edited by G. Weissmann. New York, Raven Press, 1983, pp. 57–65.

40. Spilberg, I., Mandell, B., and Hoffstein, S.: A prposed model for chemotactic factor deactivation: Evidence for microtubule modulation of polymorphonuclear leukocyte chemotaxis. J. Lab. Clin. Med., *94*:361–369, 1979.

41. Spilberg, I., and Mehta, J.: Demonstration of a specific neutrophil receptor for a cell-derived chemotactic factor. J. Clin. Invest., *63*:85–88, 1979.

42. Spilberg, I., et al.: Dissociation of the neutrophil functions of exocytosis and chemotaxis. J. Lab. Clin. Med., *92*:297–302 1978.

43. Spilberg, I., et al.: Mechanism of action of colchicine in acute urate crystal induced arthritis. J. Clin. Invest., *64*:775–780, 1979.

44. Spilberg, I., et al.: Determination of a specific receptor for formyl-methionyl-leucyl-phenylalanine on the pulmonary alveolar macrophage and its relationship to chemotaxis and superoxide production. J. Lab. Clin. Med., *97*:602–609, 1981.

45. Wilkinson, P.C., and Allen, R.B.: Binding of protein chemotactic factors to the surface of neutrophil leukocytes and its modifications with lipid bacterial toxins. Mol. Cell Biochem., *20*:25–40, 1978.

46. Williams, L.T., Snyderman, R., Pike, M.C., and Lefkowitz, R.J.: Specific receptor sites for chemotactic peptides on human polymorphonuclear leukocytes. Proc. Natl. Acad. Sci. U.S.A., *74*:1204–1206, 1977.

47. Yuli, I., Tomonaga, A., and Snyderman, R.: Chemoattractant receptor functions in human polymorphonuclear leukocytes are divergently altered by membrane fluidizers. Proc. Natl. Acad. Sci. U.S.A., *79*:5906–5910, 1982.

48. Zigmond, S.H.: Mechanisms of sensing chemical gradients by polymorphonuclear leukocytes. Nature, *249*:450–452, 1974.

49. Zigmond, S.H.: Ability of polymorphonuclear leukocytes to orient in gradients of chemotactic factors. J. Cell Biol., *75*:606–616, 1977.

50. Zigmond, S.H.: Chemotaxis of polymorphonuclear leukocytes. J. Cell Biol., *77*:269–287, 1978.

51. Zigmond, S.H., and Hirsh, J.G.: Leukocyte locomotion and chemotaxis: New methods for evaluation and demonstration of a cell derived chemotactic factor. J. Exp. Med., *137*:387–410, 1973.

Chapter 20

Platelets in Rheumatic Disease

Robert Terkeltaub and Mark H. Ginsberg

The involvement of blood platelets in inflammatory processes has become recognized as an important aspect of platelet biology.[31,32,49] In this chapter we address the structure and function of platelets as they relate to their potential role in rheumatic disease. We also review the evidence for platelet involvement in the pathogenesis of human rheumatic diseases and some clinically significant events involving platelets in certain rheumatic diseases.

Platelet Morphology and Function

Normal platelets are anucleate discoid cell fragments approximately 2 μm in diameter. They are derived from marrow megakaryocytes as fragments budding from the peripheral cytoplasm as reviewed in detail elsewhere.[52] The cell contains at least three types of storage organelles: (1) The alpha granule is a storage site of several platelet-specific proteins and adhesive glycoproteins.[37] (2) The dense body, which is less numerous than the alpha granule, is the main storage site for biogenic amines. The major biogenic amine in human platelets is serotonin, and virtually the entire blood content of serotonin is borne in platelet dense bodies. Adenine nucleotides, calcium, and pyrophosphate are also stored in the dense bodies.[11] (3) Lysosomes containing several neutral and acid hydrolases are also present.[28]

The normal platelet life span is 7 to 10 days, with circulating cells being removed either by the reticuloendothelial system when senescent or by incorporation into hemostatic plugs. The cells have little or no ability to synthesize proteins.

The main function of platelets is to initiate hemostasis by forming and helping to consolidate a cellular plug at sites of vascular injury.[7] Platelets may also contribute to atherogenesis, clearance of particulate material from the blood, wound-healing, and transplant rejection.

Four lines of evidence indicate that platelets participate in inflammation: (1) They contain and release,[63] upon stimulation, mediators of inflammation. (2) They are stimulated by phlogistic agents. (3) They participate in the pathogenesis of animal models of rheumatic disease. (4) There is evidence suggesting platelet localization and activation at sites of tissue injury in some human rheumatic diseases. Since these cells respond rapidly to stimuli, they may participate in the earliest steps of the production of inflammation. As the pharmacology of platelet inhibitors attains ever-growing sophistication, intervention in rheumatic disease at the level of the platelet may become a reality.

Platelet-Derived Mediators of Inflammation

Platelet-derived mediators of inflammation may be newly synthesized, as in the case of metabolites of arachidonic acid, or preformed and concentrated in storage organelles. The materials released from stimulated platelets may contribute to the inflammatory process by modulating vascular tone and permeability, attracting more inflammatory cells, inducing tissue damage, and initiating repair by mitogenic effects on connective tissue. Table 20–1 lists some of the platelet mediators capable of contributing to these events.

POTENTIAL ACTIVATORS OF PLATELETS IN RHEUMATIC DISEASES

A number of agents stimulate platelets, and several of these materials may be involved in the initiation or propagation of inflammatory responses. Table 20–2 lists some of these agents. They first include "traditional" hemostatic platelet activators such as thrombin, ADP, prostaglandins, and exposed subendothelial collagen known to be present at sites of vascular injury. Activation of platelets may also be affected by several different types of immunologic reactions as reviewed in detail elsewhere.[31]

Platelet Activating Factor

Platelet activating factor (PAF) is a recently characterized phospholipid mediator released from stimulated human mast cells, neutrophils, and macrophages.[65] It aggregates platelets at subnanomolar concentrations and may stimulate other cell types, including neutrophils. Injection of PAF into animals induces thrombocytopenia, leukopenia, hypotension, and platelet-dependent bronchoconstriction. PAF generation and PAF cell stimulation are not inhibited by nonsteroidal anti-inflammatory drugs (NSAID) in vitro.

Table 20–1. **Platelet-Derived Mediators of Inflammation**

Class	Mediator	Actions	References
I Cyclo-oxygenase-dependent	thromboxane A_2	vasoconstrictor, proaggregant, increases neutrophil adherence	65, 68
	thromboxane B_2	more stable thromboxane A_2 derivative	65, 68
	prostaglandins D_2, E_2, $F_2\alpha$	vasoactive, modulate hemostasis and leukocyte function	65, 68
	HHT	chemotactic	27
II Lipoxygenase-dependent	12-HPETE	vasoconstrictor, cyclo-oxygenase inhibitor, stimulates leukocyte LTB_4 synthesis	26, 43
	12-HETE	chemotactic	26, 43
III Dense body contents	serotonin	vasoconstrictor, increases vascular permeability, fibrogenic	11
IV Alpha granule contents	platelet-derived growth factor (PDGF)	connective tissue mitogen	58
	platelet factor 4 (PF4)	proaggregant, inhibits collagenase	34
V "Granule" contents	cationic permeability factor	stimulates mast cell histamine release, chemotactic	50
	serum activating enzymes	generate C5a in serum	67
	cathepsins A, C, D, E	acid proteinases	19
	elastase	neutral proteinase	33, 42
	collagenase	neutral proteinase	9
	α-1 Antitrypsin, α-2 macroglobulin	proteinase inhibitors	48
	α-2 Antiplasmin	primary plasmin inhibitor	55

Table 20–2. **Potential Activators of Platelets in Rheumatic Disease**

Types of Activation	Activator
Hemostatic activation	Thrombin
	Collagen
	ADP
	Prostaglandins, thromboxanes
Immunologic activation	Platelet activating factor (PAF)
	Immune aggregates
	Antibodies to certain drugs (e.g., quinidine)
	Antiplatelet antibodies
Nonimmunologic activation	Monosodium urate crystals
	Microorganisms
	Double-stranded DNA
Enhancers of activation	Complement
	Single-stranded DNA
	Certain bacterial lipopolysaccharides

Platelet Activation by Immune Aggregates

Human platelets possess a receptor for the Fc portion of IgG.[53] Thus, IgG-containing immune complexes, aggregated gamma globulin, and IgG-coated surfaces stimulate human platelets.[31] Certain drug-induced thrombocytopenias probably are examples of immune complex-mediated platelet sequestration and lysis. Quinidine-induced purpura is the best studied of these, and immunologically nonspecific adsorption of drug-antibody complexes to the platelet surface seems important in its pathogenesis.[61] Such binding may well be mediated by the platelet Fc receptor. Among antirheumatic drugs, aspirin, acetaminophen, phenylbutazone,[2] and gold compounds in some cases[30] have been implicated as causative agents of immunologically mediated thrombocytopenias.

Antiplatelet Antibodies

Antibodies to antigens on the platelet surface may arise in autoimmune states, e.g., in systemic lupus erythematosus (SLE) or idiopathic thrombocytopenic purpura (ITP), or as a result of iso-immunization after transfusion or pregnancy. In addition, antilymphocyte and antithymocyte globulins may also possess antiplatelet activity.[10] Antiplatelet antibodies may either stimulate platelets or inhibit platelet function, and thrombocytopenia may be produced via increased reticuloendothelial clearance.[3] In the case of alloantibodies, anti-P1A1 has been clearly shown to react with a major cell surface glycoprotein,[41] and antilymphocyte globulins react in part with beta 2-microglobulin on the cell surface.[10] In the case of autoantibodies, studies are just beginning to characterize their antigens.

Monosodium Urate Crystal-Platelet Interactions

Platelets and monosodium urate crystals, the causative agent of gout, have the potential to interact at many intravascular and extravascular sites.

The study of platelet-crystal interaction has proved useful as a model system for cellular activation in gout and other microcrystalline diseases. Monosodium urate crystals have been shown to induce a selective secretion of dense body constituents followed by platelet lysis in vitro.[22] More recent work suggests that platelet membrane glycoproteins mediate platelet stimulation by urate crystals.[35]

Complement Enhancement of Platelet Activation

In addition to complement-dependent sequelae to the binding of antiplatelet antibodies,[31] platelet participation in the activation of complement has been described.[56] This occurs by C5 cleavage by platelet-bound thrombin. Such complement activation may enhance thrombin stimulation via the cyclo-oxygenase pathway.[57]

Platelets and DNA

Free DNA has been described in serum and plasma in several conditions associated with tissue injury, including vasculitides and SLE. Single- and double-stranded (native) DNA both bind to platelets. Native DNA induces in vitro serotonin release from platelets.[14,20] Single-stranded DNA, but not native DNA, enhances the platelet release reaction induced by heat-aggregated IgG.[14]

Lipopolysaccharide Enhancement of Platelet Responses

The bacterial lipopolysaccharide (LPS) component of gram-negative bacteria may be responsible for a number of in vivo effects, including pyrogenicity, toxicity, and lethality. LPS may also have several important immunologic actions, in part mediated by effects in Fc receptor-bearing cells such as macrophages and B cells. The lipid A region of LPS is responsible for many of these effects. Isolated lipid A and lipid A-rich LPS of certain strains have been found to enhance immune-aggregate-induced platelet serotonin release approximately 50-fold[24] and to enhance secretion of other platelet constituents as well.

PLATELETS IN ANIMAL MODELS OF RHEUMATIC DISEASES

Another important aspect of platelet participation in rheumatic disease is their possible role in inducing inflammation and tissue damage. Numerous studies of animal models of human disease have assessed the effect of platelet depletion on tissue injury and have measured platelet deposition at sites of inflammatory tissue damage. Platelet deposition at sites of tissue injury has been detected quantitatively by the accumulation of ^{51}Cr-labeled platelets or by ultrastructural pathology in such animal models as sponge implantation,[6] reverse passive Arthus reaction in skin,[40] and IgE-mediated anaphylaxis.[54] Protective effects of platelet depletion have been reported in models such as IgE anaphylaxis, the Shwartzman reaction, the Arthus reaction in the joint,[45] and serum sickness nephritis,[39] where released platelet permeability factors may influence the deposition of immune complexes in blood vessel walls. In the case of the Arthus reaction and IgE-dependent skin reactions in the rabbit, platelet depletion does not prevent the lesions, but may be associated with some lessening of the intensity of the reaction. This finding exemplifies the inherent redundancy of the inflammatory response. It should be pointed out that platelet deposition is without effect in various other animal models. It is important to study platelets in human disease directly rather than with animal models because of the known functional differences between human and nonprimate platelets.

PLATELETS AS MEDIATORS IN HUMAN INFLAMMATORY DISEASE

Evidence of Platelet Localization at Sites of Human Tissue Injury

Light microscopic recognition of platelets in inflammatory lesions is difficult. Ultrastructural techniques have demonstrated platelets in synovial fluids[69] and platelet aggregation in rheumatoid synovium[59] or in glomerular capillaries.[18] More recently, the platelet-specific protein platelet factor 4 and beta thromboglobulin (β-TG) have been demonstrated in rheumatoid synovial fluids.[23,46] At present, there is suggestive evidence of platelet localization at sites of human immune injury, but newer investigation using immunolocalization techniques for platelet-specific antigens and ^{111}indium-labeled platelets with external imaging is anticipated in the next few years.

Evidence of Platelet Activation in Human Rheumatic Diseases

Measurement of platelet activation in human immunologic diseases has dual significance. First, it implicates platelets in the disease. Secondly, it may provide a means of monitoring drug effects on platelet activation in a disease and an opportunity to elucidate the relationship between disease activity and platelet activation.

Approaches to date have included measurement of platelet turnover in patients with immunologic diseases. This test is inconvenient and does not measure activation per se, but rather the increased turnover that presumably accompanies platelet activation. Assays for detection of platelet activators in blood and tissue fluids of immunologic disease patients have also been used.[25,60] Presence of these activators also represents only an indirect indication of in vivo platelet activation. The availability of assays for detection of in vivo secretion of platelet-specific proteins[38] has provided a rapid and simple approach to measure the state of platelet activation in disease. Studies of several rheumatic diseases by these methods have provided evidence of platelet activation.

Platelets in Scleroderma. Platelet interaction with small vessel subendothelium exposed by immune endothelial injury has been advanced as a possible factor in the early pathogenesis of scleroderma. This process would be followed by smooth muscle cell migration and intimal proliferation with luminal narrowing and ultimate fibrosis. Serotonin is believed to be a modulator of vasoconstriction (Raynaud's phenomenon) and fibrogenesis in this disease.[62,64] Evidence of in vivo platelet participation of scleroderma includes evidence of decreased serotonin content of platelets in affected patients[70] and the report of in vivo platelet adhesion to subendothelium in a case study.[8] Elevated levels of circulating platelet aggregates and plasma β-TG have been observed in scleroderma with significant reductions of these levels achieved in a group of patients treated with dipyridamole and aspirin.[36]

Platelets in SLE. Defective platelet aggregation independent of NSAID therapy is seen in a significant proportion of SLE patients.[15,66] Increased plasma levels of β-TG[16] and an acquired deficiency of platelet dense body contents (storage pool deficiency) have been associated with this defect and suggest in vivo platelet activation. Potential platelet activators in SLE include immune complexes, antiplatelet antibodies, exposed subendothelial collagen (vasculitis), and thrombin, via activation of the clotting cascade.[29] Increased plasma levels of free DNA are frequently observed in SLE. Single-stranded (ssDNA) and native DNA both bind to platelets, and both have been shown to modulate platelet activation in vitro. Treatment of SLE platelet-rich plasma with deoxyribonuclease has been shown to restore defective aggregation to collagen in platelets of some SLE patients with an acquired storage pool deficiency, suggesting this abnormality to be possibly mediated by DNA.[15]

Acute and chronic thrombocytopenias may be encountered in SLE. The course of chronic thrombocytopenia in SLE may be similar to that in chronic idiopathic thrombocytopenic purpura.[44] In addition to antiplatelet antibodies, it has been suggested that antibodies to platelet-bound ssDNA may play a pathogenetic role in this condition.[13]

Platelet involvement in SLE proliferative glomerulonephritis as well as other forms of glomerulonephritis is recognized and reviewed elsewhere.[51] Thrombotic thrombocytopenic purpura has been reported in association with SLE.[1]

Platelet Abnormalities in Rheumatoid Arthritis. Various studies have shown that sera and synovial fluids from rheumatoid arthritis (RA) patients can activate normal platelets.[70] Increased plasma concentrations of β-TG have been found in some RA patients.[47] The presence of increased amounts of platelet activating material in RA sera and synovia may be of particular importance because of the frequent occurrence in RA of heightened platelet production and net thrombocytosis. The degree of thrombocytosis correlated directly with parameters of active disease and inversely with the hematocrit.[5] A relationship appears to exist between thrombocytosis and extra-articular manifestations of RA, particularly cutaneous vasculitis.

Thrombocytopenia may be encountered as a complication of gold, penicillamine, or cytotoxic therapy of RA, as reviewed in Chapters 29, 31, and 33. A decreased platelet life span and thrombocytopenia may also be observed in Felty's syndrome.

Platelet Pharmacology in Rheumatic Diseases. Inhibition of platelet function is a consequence of the administration of many drugs with anti-inflammatory properties. As reviewed elsewhere,[21] therapy with aspirin (ASA) and many NSAIDs may affect certain aggregation and release reactions in the platelets. Importantly, even low doses of ASA irreversibly acetylate platelet cyclooxygenase and, thus, recovery of platelet function from ASA requires several days. In contrast, most other NSAIDs inhibit platelets only when present in blood in pharmacologic concentrations. Antimalarial agents such as chloroquine also inhibit platelet function, but this inhibition is of uncertain clinical significance.[17] Several other agents that inhibit platelets or platelet-derived mediators may potentially find therapeutic roles in rheumatic diseases. Included among these are agents that antagonize serotonin, elevate platelet cyclic AMP, stabilize the cell membrane, and block certain membrane receptors.[12] The therapy of Raynaud's phenomenon with serotonin antagonists[62] or adenylate cyclase stimulants, e.g., prostacyclin,[4] holds some promise at present.

REFERENCES

1. Amorosi, E.L., and Ultmann, J.E.: Thrombotic thrombocytopenic purpura. Medicine (Baltimore), 45:139–159, 1966.
2. Aster, R.H.: Thrombocytopenia due to enhanced platelet destruction. In Hematology. Edited by W. Williams, et al. New York, McGraw-Hill Book Co., 1977, pp. 1326–1359.
3. Aster, R.H., and Jandl, J.: Platelet sequestration in man. J. Clin. Invest., 43:856–870, 1964.

4. Belch, J.J., et al.: Successful treatment of Raynaud's syndrome with prostacyclin. Thromb. Haemost., *45*:255–256, 1981.

5. Bennett, R.M.: Hematological changes in rheumatoid disease. Clin. Rheum. Dis., *3*:433–465, 1977.

6. Bolam, J.P., and Smith, M.J.: Accumulation of platelets at acute inflammatory sites. Br. J. Pharmacol., *61*:158–159, 1977.

7. Born, G.U.: Platelets in hemostasis and thrombosis. *In* Platelets: Cellular Response Mechanisms and Their Biological Significance. Edited by A. Rotman, et al. New York, Wiley Interscience, 1980, pp. 3–17.

8. Case records of the Massachusetts General Hospital: Case 34-1978. N. Engl. J. Med., *299*:466–474, 1978.

9. Chesney, C.M., Harper, E., and Colman, R.W.: Human platelet collagenase. J. Clin. Invest., *53*:1647–1655, 1974.

10. Csako, G., Suba, E.A., and Wistar, R.: Activation of human platelets by antibodies to thymocytes and beta 2-microglobulin. Clin. Lab. Immunol., *7*:33–38, 1982.

11. Da Prada, M., Richards, J.G., and Kettler, R.: Amine storage organelles in platelets. *In* Platelets in Biology and Pathology. Vol. 2. Edited by J.L. Gordon. Amsterdam, Elsevier/North-Holland, 1981, pp. 107–146.

12. Didisheim, P., and Fuster, V.: Actions and clinical status of platelet-suppressive agents. Semin. Hematol., *15*:55–72, 1978.

13. Dorsch, C.A.: Enhancement of binding of single-strand DNA to human platelets by aggregated IgG and ADP. Arthritis Rheum., *23*:666–667, 1980.

14. Dorsch, C.A., and Killmayer, J.: The effect of native and single stranded DNA on the platelet release reaction. Arthritis Rheum., *26*:179–185, 1983.

15. Dorsch, C.A., and Meyerhoff, J.: Mechanisms of abnormal platelet aggregation in systemic lupus erythematosus. Arthritis Rheum., *25*:966–973, 1982.

16. Dorsch, C.A., and Meyerhoff, J.: Elevated plasma beta-thromboglobulin levels in systemic lupus erythematosus. Thromb. Res., *20*:617–622, 1980.

17. Dubois, E.L.: Antimalarials in the management of discoid and systemic lupus erythematosus. Semin. Arthritis Rheum., *8*:33–51, 1978.

18. Duffy, J.L., et al.: Intraglomerular fibrin, platelet aggregation, and subendothelial deposits in lipoid nephrosis. J. Clin. Invest., *49*:251–258, 1970.

19. Erlich, H.P., and Gordon, J.L.: Proteinases and platelets. *In* Platelets in Biology and Pathology. Vol. 1. Edited by J.L. Gordon. Amsterdam, Elsevier/North-Holland, 1976.

20. Fiedel, B.A., Schoenberger, J.S., and Gewurz, H.: Modulation of platelet activation by native DNA. J. Immunol., *123*:2479–2483, 1979.

21. Fuster, V., and Chesebro, J.H.: Antithrombotic therapy: Role of platelet-inhibitor drugs. Mayo Clin. Proc., *56*:102–112, 185–195, 265–273, 1981.

22. Ginsberg, M.H., et al.: Release of platelet constituents by monosodium urate crystals. J. Clin. Invest., *60*:999–1007, 1977.

23. Ginsberg, M.H., Breth, G., and Skosey, J.L.: Platelets in the synovial space. Arthritis Rheum., *21*:994, 1978.

24. Ginsberg, M.H., and Henson, P.M.: Enhancement of platelet response to immune complexes and IgG aggregates by lipid A-rich bacterial lipopolysaccharides. J. Exp. Med., *147*:207–218, 1978.

25. Ginsberg, M.H., and O'Malley, M.: Serum factors releasing serotonin from normal platelets. Ann. Intern. Med., *87*:564–567, 1977.

26. Goetzl, E.J.: Oxygenation products of arachidonic acid as mediators of hypersensitivity and inflammation. Med. Clin. North Am., *65*:809–828, 1981.

27. Goetzl, E.J., and Gorman, R.R.: Chemotactic and chemokinetic stimulation of human eosinophil and neutrophil polymorphonuclear leukocytes by HHT. J. Immunol., *120*:526–531, 1978.

28. Gordon, J.L.: Blood platelet lysosomes and their contribution to the pathophysiological role of platelets. *In* Lysosomes in Biology and Pathology. Vol. 4. Edited by J.T. Dingle, and R.T. Dean. Amsterdam, Elsevier/North-Holland, 1975, pp. 3–31.

29. Hardin, J.A., et al.: Activation of blood clotting in patients with systemic lupus erythematosus. Am. J. Med., *65*:430–436, 1978.

30. Harth, M., et al.: Gold induced thrombocytopenia. J. Rheumatol., *5*:165–172, 1978.

31. Henson, P.M., and Ginsberg, M.H.: Immunological reactions of platelets. *In* Platelets in Biology and Pathology. Vol. 2. Edited by J.L. Gordon. Amsterdam, Elsevier/North-Holland, 1981, pp. 265–308.

32. Henson, P.M., Ginsberg, M.H., and Morrison, D.C.: Mechanisms of mediator release from inflammatory cells. *In* Cell Surface Reviews V. Membrane fusion. Edited by G. Poste, et al. Amsterdam, Elsevier/North-Holland, 1978, pp. 407–462.

33. Henson, P.M., Gould, D., and Becker, E.L.: Activation of stimulus-specific serine esterases in the initiation of platelet secretion. J. Exp. Med., *144*:1657–1672, 1976.

34. Hiti-Harper, J., Wohl, H., and Harper, E.: Platelet factor 4, an inhibitor of collagenase. Science, *199*:991–992, 1978.

35. Jaques, B.C., and Ginsberg, M.H.: The role of cell surface proteins in platelet stimulation by monosodium urate crystals. Arthritis Rheum., *25*:508–521, 1982.

36. Kahaleh, M.B., Osborn, I., and Leroy, E.C.: Elevated levels of circulating platelet aggregates and beta-thromboglobulin in scleroderma. Ann. Intern. Med., *96*:610–613, 1982.

37. Kaplan, K.L.: Platelet granule proteins: Localization and secretion. *In* Platelets in Biology and Pathology. Vol. 2. Edited by J.L. Gordon. Amsterdam, Elsevier/North-Holland, 1981, p. 77–90.

38. Kaplan, K.L., and Owen, J.: Plasma levels of beta-thromboglobulin and platelet factor 4 as indices of platelet activation in vivo. Blood, *57*:199–202, 1981.

39. Kniker, W.T., and Cochrane, C.G.: The localization of circulating immune complexes in experimental serum sickness. J. Exp. Med., *127*:119–136, 1968.

40. Kravis, T.C., and Henson, P.M.: Accumulation of platelets at sites of antigen-antibody mediated injury. J. Immunol., *118*:1569–1580, 1977.

41. Kunicki, T.J., and Aster, R.H.: Isolation and immunologic characterization of the human platelet alloantigen, P1A1. Mol. Immunol., *16*:353–360, 1979.

42. Legrand, Y., Pignaud, G., and Caen, J.P.: Human blood platelet elastase and proelastase. Hemostasis, *6*:180–189, 1977.

43. Maclouf, J., de Laclos, B.F., and Borgeat, P.: Stimulation of leukotriene biosynthesis in human blood leukocytes by platelet-derived 12-HPETE. Proc. Natl. Acad. Sci. U.S.A., *79*:6042–6046, 1982.

44. McMillan, R.: Chronic idiopathic thrombocytopenic purpura. N. Engl. J. Med., *304*:1135–1147, 1981.

45. Margaretten, W., and McKay, D.G.: The requirement for platelets in the active Arthus reaction. Am. J. Pathol., *64*:257, 1971.

46. Myers, S.L., and Christine, T.A.: Measurement of beta-thromboglobulin connective tissue activating peptide-III platelet antigen concentrations in pathologic synovial fluids. J. Rheumatol., *9*:6–12, 1982.

47. Myers, S.L., Hossler, P.A., and Castor, C.W.: Connective tissue activation XIX. Plasma levels of CTAP-III platelet antigen in rheumatoid arthritis. J. Rheumatol., *7*:814–819, 1980.

48. Nachman, R.L., and Harpel, P.C.: Platelet alpha-2 macroglobulin and alpha-1 antitrypsin. J. Biol. Chem., *251*:4514–4521, 1976.

49. Nachman, R.L., and Polley, M.: The platelet as an inflammatory cell. *In* Advances in Inflammation Research. Vol. 1. Edited by G. Weissmann, et al. 1979, pp. 169–173.

50. Nachman, R.L., Weksler, B., and Ferris, B.: Characterization of human platelet vascular permeability-enhancing factor. J. Clin. Invest., *51*:549–556, 1972.

51. Parbtani, A., Frampton, G., and Cameron, J.S.: Measurement of platelet release substances in glomerulonephritis. Thromb. Res., *19*:177–189, 1980.

52. Penington, D.G.: Formation of platelets. *In* Platelets in Biology and Pathology. Vol. 2. Edited by J.L. Gordon. Amsterdam, Elsevier/North-Holland, 1981, pp. 19–42.

53. Pfueller, S.L., Jenkins, C.S., and Luscher, E.F.: A com-

parative study of the effect of modification of the surface of human platelets on the receptors for aggregated immunoglobulins. Biochim. Biophys. Acta, *465*:614–626, 1977.

54. Pinckard, R.N. et al.: Intravascular aggregation and pulmonary sequestration of platelets during IgE-induced systemic anaphylaxis in the rabbit. J. Immunol., *119*:2185–2194, 1977.

55. Plow, E.F., and Collen, D.: The presence and release of alpha 2-antiplasmin from human platelets. Blood, *58*:1069–1074, 1981.

56. Polley, M.J., and Nachman, R.L.: The human complement system in thrombin-mediated platelet function. J. Exp. Med., *147*:1713–1726, 1978.

57. Polley, M.J., and Nachman, R.L.: The human complement system in thrombin-mediated platelet function. *In* Platelets in Biology and Pathology. Vol. 2, Edited by J.L. Gordon. Amsterdam, Elsevier/North-Holland, 1981, pp. 309–319.

58. Ross, R., et al.: Cell proliferation: Platelet and macrophage derived growth factor. *In* Advances in Inflammation Research. Vol. 1. Edited by G. Weissmann, et al. New York, Raven Press, 1979, pp. 183–188.

59. Schumacher, H.R.: Synovial membrane and fluid morphologic alterations in early rheumatoid arthritis: Microvascular injury and virus-like particles. Ann. N.Y. Acad. Sci., *256*:39–64, 1975.

60. Shapleigh, C., et al.: Platelet-activating activity in synovial fluids of patients with rheumatoid arthritis, juvenile rheumatoid arthritis, gout, and noninflammatory arthropathies. Arthritis Rheum., *23*:800–807, 1980.

61. Shulman, N.R.: Immunoreactions involving platelets. J. Exp. Med., *107*:665–690, 697–710, 711–729, 1978.

62. Siebold, J.R., and Jageneau, A.H.: Ketanserin in the treatment of Raynaud's phenomenon. Arthritis Rheum., *26*:S27, 1983.

63. Skaer, R.J.: Platelet degranulation. *In* Platelets in Biology and Pathology. Vol. 2. Edited by J.L. Gordon. Amsterdam, Elsevier/North-Holland, 1981, pp. 321–348.

64. Sternberg, E., et al.: Development of a scleroderma-like illness during therapy with L-5-hydroxytryptophan and carbidopa. N. Engl. J. Med., *303*:782–787, 1980.

65. Vargaftig, B.B., et al.: Pharmacology of arachidonate metabolites and of platelet-activating factor. *In* Platelets in Biology and Pathology. Vol. 2. Edited by J.L. Gordon. Amsterdam, Elsevier/North-Holland, 1981, pp. 373–406.

66. Weiss, H.J., et al.: Acquired storage pool deficiency with increased platelet-associated IgG. Am. J. Med., *69*:711–717, 1980.

67. Weksler, B.B., and Coupal, C.E.: Platelet-dependent generation of chemotactic activity in serum. J. Exp. Med., *137*:1419–1430, 1973.

68. Weksler, B.B., and Goldstein, I.M.: Prostaglandins: Interactions with platelets and polymorphonuclear leukocytes in hemostasis and inflammation. Am. J. Med., *68*:419–428, 1980.

69. Yaron, M., and Djaldetti, M.: Platelets in synovial fluid. Arthritis Rheum., *21*:607, 1978.

70. Zeller, J., et al.: Serotonin content of platelets in inflammatory rheumatic diseases. Arthritis Rheum., *26*:532–540, 1983.

Chapter 21

Complement Mediators of Inflammation

Douglas T. Fearon

Activation of the complement system leads to the generation of mediators that can induce an acute inflammatory response. This well-characterized function of the complement system normally serves to protect the individual from microbial infection by causing the accumulation of leukocytes and by modulating their function at sites of complement activation. However, these same functions of complement may be detrimental if activation is excessive or is triggered by host rather than foreign material, as may occur in the presence of large amounts of immune complexes comprised of autoantibodies. Accordingly, several experimental models of immunologically mediated diseases have emphasized the central position of the complement system in linking the humoral immune response to the recruitment of leukocytes to sites of immune complex deposition. Observations derived from these models have led to one view of the complement system as having only deleterious effects in rheumatic diseases. However, an opposing view, which is based on the apparently frequent occurrence of autoimmune disease in individuals having inherited abnormalities of the complement system, suggests that this system may have beneficial or protective effects by regulating immune complex formation and clearance. This chapter presents the biochemistry and cell biology of the proteins and cellular receptors of the complement system from which any hypotheses concerning the role of complement in rheumatic disease must be derived.

BIOCHEMISTRY OF THE COMPLEMENT SYSTEM

The complement system consists of 18 plasma proteins (Table 21–1) whose designations conform to two conventions. The classic components, which are the plasma proteins responsible for hemolysis of antibody-sensitized erythrocytes, are symbolized with a capital C and a number designating the component, e.g., C1, C4, C2, C3, and C5 through C9. The alternative pathway factors, so-called because they were discovered after the classic components, are denoted with a capital letter, e.g., B, D, and P (properdin). A bar over a letter or number,

as in $\overline{C1s}$, indicates the enzymatically active form of the protein, and cleavage fragments are suffixed with lower-case letters, e.g., C3a and C3b. The most critical step in the elaboration of the biologic functions of the complement system is generation of the major cleavage fragment of C3, C3b; all complement proteins may be grouped into functional divisions according to their interactions with C3 (Fig. 21–1). There are two pathways for initial cleavage of C3, the classic and the alternative; a single amplification mechanism comprised of alternative pathway proteins, which augments C3 cleavage once initial C3b has been generated; and a final common effector sequence that the initiating and amplifying pathways activate after C3b has been generated (Fig. 21–1).

Classic Pathway of Activation

The classic activating pathway (Fig. 21–2) is comprised of five proteins, three of which—C1q, C1r, and C1s—are bound together in the presence of calcium to form C1, and C4 and C2. Initiation of the pathway follows binding of the C1q subcomponent of the Fc region of IgM or IgG1–3 that is present in antigen-antibody complexes. Activation of C1 requires the calcium-dependent intact C1 complex, and interaction of at least two of the six binding sites of C1q with immunoglobulin. The latter requirement has been surmised from studies showing that while a single IgM molecule with its five Fc regions will suffice for conversion of C1 to $\overline{C1}$, at least two adjacent IgG molecules are necessary for this step to occur. Interaction of two C1q binding sites is thought to induce a steric change in the proenzyme C1r, thereby permitting autocatalytic activation to $\overline{C1r}$. The serine protease-active site of $\overline{C1r}$ converts C1s to $\overline{C1s}$ by cleavage of a peptide bond to reveal its serine protease site. $\overline{C1s}$ sequentially acts on its two complement protein substrates, C4 and C2. C4 is cleaved into two fragments, the larger of which, C4b, continues the complement reaction, while the smaller fragment, C4a, has weak anaphylatoxic activity. Generation of C4b reveals a site that transiently has the capacity to bind covalently to membranes or immune

Table 21–1. **Physicochemical Characteristics of Proteins of the Complement System**

	Approximate Molecular Weight (Daltons)	Serum Concentration ($\mu g/ml$)	Cleavage Fragments
Classic pathway of activation			
C1q	400,000	100	
C1r	95,000	50	
C1s	85,000	50	
C4	209,000	430	C4a, C4b, C4c, C4d
C2	117,000	30	C2a, C2b
Alternative pathway of activation and amplification			
Factor P (properdin)	160,000	25	
Factor D	25,000	2	
Factor B	93,000	240	Bb, Ba
C3	190,000	1300	C3a, C3b, iC3b, C3c, C3d,g
Attack sequence			
C5	206,000	75	C5a, C5b
C6	128,000	60	
C7	120,000	55	
C8	153,000	80	
C9	79,000	160	
Control proteins			
C$\bar{1}$INH	105,000	180	
Factor I (C3b/C4b inactivator)	93,000	50	
Factor H (β1H)	150,000	520	
C4bp	1.2×10^6	250	

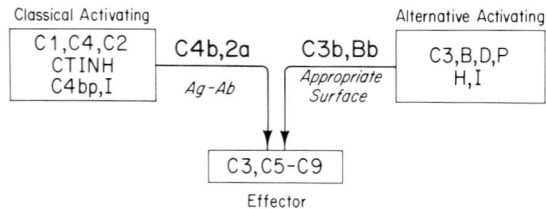

Fig. 21–1. Relation of the classic and alternative pathways of complement activation to C3 and the effector sequence of complement. Antigen-antibody complexes (Ag-Ab) initiate formation of the classic pathway C3 convertase, which can cleave C3 to generate C3b and activate C5 to C9. The alternative pathway amplification C3 convertase C3b,Bb is assembled when C3b that was initially generated by the priming C3 convertase C3,Bb or by C4b,2a is deposited on a surface with appropriate biochemical characteristics. This C3 convertase is termed "amplifying" because the product of C3 cleavage, C3b, is a subunit of the enzyme.

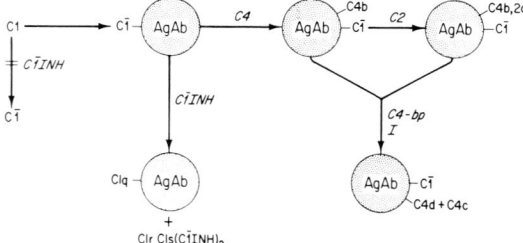

Fig. 21–2. The classic activating pathway. C$\bar{1}$, bound to and activated by antibody (Ab) within the antigen-antibody complex (AgAb), sequentially cleaves C4, whose major C4b fragment binds to AgAb and C2 to form the classic pathway C3 convertase, C4b,2a. The reaction is regulated by C$\bar{1}$INH, which binds to and inhibits C$\bar{1}$, and by the combined effects of C4-bp and I, which result in cleavage of C4b into the inactive fragments, C4c and C4d.

complexes, thereby localizing the reaction to the initiating complex containing C$\overline{\text{I}}$. This binding of C4b occurs by a transacylation reaction involving an internal thiolester present in the α-polypeptide of C4 and nucleophiles, such as amino or hydroxyl groups on the immune complex. The bound C4b then forms a reversible magnesium-dependent

complex with C2, which is cleaved into its larger C2a and smaller C2b fragments by C$\overline{\text{T}}$. The C2a cleavage fragment remains bound to C4b, and the complex is termed the classic C3 convertase because of its capacity to cleave C3. The enzymatic site for C3 cleavage resides on the C2a fragment, and irreversible decay-dissociation of C2a from C4b,2ba releases C2i and abolishes C3 convertase activity. C4b is capable of reforming the convertase upon cleavage of additional native C2 with C̄1̄.

In addition to lability of the classic C3 convertase, activation of C3 by this pathway is limited by three control proteins: C̄1̄ inhibitor (C̄1̄INH), C4 binding protein (C4bp), and C3b/C4b inactivator (I). C̄1̄INH inhibits autoactivation of C1r, C̄1̄r activation of C1s, and C̄1̄s cleavage of C4 and C2. Irreversible C̄1̄r₂–C̄1̄INH₂ and C̄1̄s₂–C̄1̄INH₂ complexes are formed, which dissociate from C1q. C̄1̄INH also functions as a control protein for the Hageman factor-initiated pathways since it inhibits the capacity of activated Hageman factor to activate prekallikrein and factor XI of the clotting system and suppresses the kinin-generation of kallikrein. Inherited deficiency of this control protein results in the disease, hereditary angioedema, and is associated with chronically depressed serum levels of C4 and C2 because of their cleavage by uninhibited C1 that is spontaneously generated.

C4bp forms complexes with C4b, thereby blocking the binding of C2 and promoting the cleavage of C4b by I into the C4c and C4d fragments. The latter fragment remains bound to immune complexes and expresses the Rogers and Chido antigen.

Alternative and Amplifying Pathways for Generation of C3b

An alternative pathway for C3 cleavage was discovered when zymosan, an insoluble polysaccharide-containing derivative of yeast cell walls, was observed to inactivate C3 in serum without apparent utilization of C1, C4, C2, or specific antibody. Various substances are now known to activate this pathway and include: microbial polysaccharides, such as endotoxin; rabbit erythrocytes and lymphocytes; some human lymphoblastic and virus-infected cell lines; and large, insoluble immune complexes. Cleavage of C3 by the alternative pathway occurs in two distinct phases: continuous, low-grade generation of C3b and subsequent amplified cleavage of C3 by an enzyme that is initially formed with C3b derived from the low-grade reaction (Fig. 21–3). This C3b-dependent C3 convertase is not only essential for expression of the alternative pathway, but it is inherently capable of amplifying C3 cleavage initiated by the classic pathway.

The constituent proteins of the amplification pathway are C3b, B, D, P, and two control proteins, I and H (see Table 21–1). Initial cleavage of C3 by the alternative pathway occurs continuously and in the absence of activators. C3 that possibly differs from the native form of the protein, in having acquired a C3b-like conformation, forms a fluid phase C3 convertase on interaction with B and D. Small amounts of C3 are cleaved by this enzyme, generating the larger C3b and smaller C3a

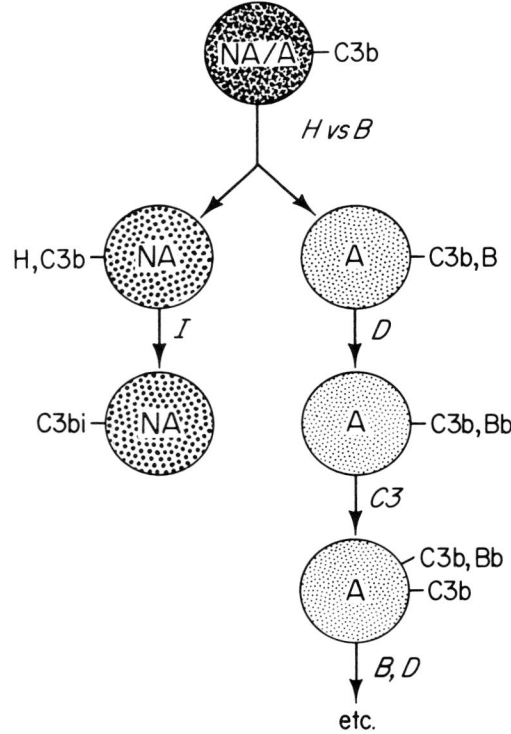

Fig. 21–3.   Competition between B and H for binding to membrane-associated C3b. C3b binds to both non-activating (NA) and activating (A) cell surfaces, and discrimination between these surfaces by the alternative pathway occurs after this step. On a nonactivating cell, certain membrane constituents, such as sialic acid, promote the binding of H, which facilitates conversion of C3b to C3bi by I. On an activating cell, these membrane constituents are diminished or absent, and binding of B leads to formation of C3b,Bb, which can catalyze deposition of more C3b. Not shown is P, which enhances activation by binding to C3b and stabilizing the C3b,Bb complex.

fragments. As occurs following cleavage of C4, a thiolester within the α-polypeptide of C3b is capable of undergoing a transacylation reaction with amino or hydroxyl groups on nearby cell surfaces, leading to covalent attachment of C3b. This attachment may take place only in the immediate vicinity of C3b because of the short half-life of the thiolester in C3b, which otherwise reacts with H_2O. The bound C3b reversibly binds B in the presence of magnesium, thereby exposing a peptide bond in B that is susceptible to cleavage by D, a serine protease. The major cleavage fragment of B, Bb, remains bound to C3b to form the labile bimolecular complex, C3b,Bb, that is the amplification C3 convertase. The proteolytic site for C3 cleavage resides on the Bb fragment and can be expressed only as long as Bb is bound to C3b. Thus, the rapid irreversible decay-release of Bb, which becomes inactive Bbi, that occurs with a half-life of 4 minutes at 30°C results in loss of C3-cleaving activity. This intrinsic control of convertase function is overcome by P, which binds to C3b and retards decay-release of Bb from the complex, extending the half-life of C3b,Bb up to 40 minutes at 30°C.

Regulation of the amplification of C3 convertase is effected by H and I. H binds reversibly to C3b, inhibiting uptake of B or displacing B or Bb, which have already complexed with C3b. In addition, binding of H apparently induces an allosteric change in C3b so that I can cleave the α-polypeptide to generate inactive iC3b. The critical roles of these regulatory proteins are apparent in patients with homozygous deficiencies of H or I who have markedly depressed serum concentrations of C3 and B secondary to their hypercatabolism.

Whether a cell or particle activates the alternative pathway is determined by the relative affinity of bound C3b for B and for H, respectively. C3b that is fixed to the surface of a nonactivator binds H with almost a 100-fold greater affinity ($K_a = 1 \times 10^7$ M^{-1}) than that with which it binds B ($K_a = 1 \times 10^5$ M^{-1}) in the presence of 0.5 mM free Mg^{2+}. Fluid phase C3b also appears to complex with H more readily than it does with B. In contrast, C3b on the surface of a cell or particle that activates the alternative pathway binds both proteins with almost equal avidity. Its association constant for H decreases while that for B remains unchanged. With nonactivating surfaces, formation of the amplification C3 convertase is impaired because H effectively blocks uptake of B by C3b and promotes irreversible cleavage-inactivation of C3b by I. With activators, B can effectively compete with H for binding to C3b, and amplification of C3 cleavage occurs.

A cell surface constituent that regulates the affinity of membrane-associated C3b for H is sialic acid, which is present in some glycoproteins and glycolipids of cells. Naturally occurring activators of the human alternative pathway, such as zymosan or rabbit erythrocytes, have absent and diminished amounts of sialic acid on their surfaces, respectively. Enzymatic removal of sialic acid from sheep erythrocytes or chemical cleavage of its polyhydroxylated side chain converts this cell from a nonactivator to an activator of the pathway by decreasing the affinity of membrane-bound C3b for H. The capacity of the alternative complement pathway to respond to cells that are relatively deficient in surface sialic acid may be relevant to its apparent role in natural resistance to infections. Most bacteria and all plants lack sialic acid. However, some bacterial species that have capsular sialic acid, such as type III, group B *Streptococcus*, groups B and C *Neisseria meningitidis*, and K1 *Escherichia coli*, are pathogenic for humans.

Specific antibody augments activation of the human alternative pathway by zymosan, rabbit erythrocytes, pneumococci, streptococci, and measles virus-infected HeLa cells, independent of any effects on the classic activating pathway. F(ab')$_2$ fragments are as active as intact IgG, Mg^{2+} but not Ca^{2+} is required, and the reactions can occur in C2-deficient human serum. Three mechanisms may account for the potentiating activity of antibody: alteration of the target cell surface by covering sialic acid residues; provision of additional binding sites for C3b, either on the antibody molecules themselves or on membrane constituents; and alterations of the spatial distribution of bound C3b to enhance formation of C5 convertase sites.

Effector Component Reactions

The C4b,2a and C3b,Bb enzymes are identical in their substrate specificities. They both cleave C3 at the Arg77-Ser78 bond of the α-polypeptide chain to generate C3a and C3b, and C5 at the Arg74-X75 bond of its α-polypeptide chain to generate C5a and C5b fragments. The C3 convertases acquire C5 convertase activity only after C3b has attached to a site on the target that is adjacent to the enzyme. This C3b may function by interacting with the substrate C5 rather than with the enzyme because it exhibits an affinity for C5 and C5b,6. The C5b fragment combines with C6 and C7, probably while it is still associated with the C5 convertase, and this trimolecular complex transfers from C3b to the membrane of the target. Uptake of C8 by membrane-associated C5b-7 apparently leads to further insertion of the complex into the bilayer, and binding of as many as five molecules of C9 to a single C5b-8 complex creates stable transmembrane channels.

The C5b-9 complex can damage membranes by two means. The first is by formation of the transmembrane channel, which appears on electron microscopy as a hollow, thin-walled cylinder of approximately 10 nm height. This structure allows the passage of salt, water, and small proteins leading to net uptake of water by a cell, with consequent swelling and gross disruption of the membrane. The second means of membrane damage involves the disorganization of the lipid bilayer that occurs when large numbers of amphiphilic C5b-9 complexes are formed in target membranes. Membrane damage by this means may be important for lysis of viruses whose envelope membranes do not function as osmotic barriers.

BIOLOGY OF COMPLEMENT

Some of the cleavage fragments of complement proteins that are produced during activation of the system serve as ligands for specific receptors on certain cells, including polymorphonuclear leukocytes, eosinophils, monocytes and macrophages, mast cells, and lymphocytes. These ligand-receptor interactions elicit the cellular responses that may culminate in an inflammatory reaction (Table 21–2).

The ligands that are generated during complement activation are of two general types: those that are bound to the target of complement activation, and those that are freely diffusible in the fluid phase. Examples of the former are C1q, C4b, and C3b, which directly promote the removal of microorganisms through endocytosis by leukocytes (opsonins). The diffusible ligands, which are low-molecular-weight cleavage peptides such as C3a and C5a, act as local hormones that cause receptor-mediated cellular responses of secretion, altered metabolism, and migration in the microenvironment. These ligand-receptor interactions indirectly promote the clearance of complement-activating material by causing the accumulation of large numbers of phagocytic cells.

Biologic Reactions Induced by Interaction of Cellular Receptors with Bound Complement Ligands

C3a has long been recognized to be capable of interacting with mast cells and basophils and has been reported also to modulate certain lymphocyte functions. Binding of C3a to specific receptors on mast cells and basophils causes the secretion of granule contents, including histamine, indicating a role for the peptide in altering vascular permeability. The demonstration that C3a suppresses the maturation of B lymphocytes, but not their purification, induced by antigen and polyclonal activators, has been attributed to inhibition of the production of T cell-derived helper factors. The cell type that C3a interacts with in this reaction is not known. Removal of the C-terminal arginine by serum carboxypeptidase to generate C3a des Arg abolishes both biologic functions of the peptide.

C3e is a peptide of 10,000 molecular weight that is thought to be derived from the C3c fragment by unknown proteolytic enzymes. This peptide causes leukocytosis when injected into rabbits, and specific binding of C3e to neutrophils has been reported.

C5a may be the most critical of the diffusible

Table 21–2. Cell Types Bearing Complement Receptors

Receptor	Cell Type	Cellular Response
C1q	Neutrophil	Respiratory burst
	Monocyte	?
	Null cell	Enhanced ADCC
	B lymphocyte	?
C4a, C3a	Mast cell	Secretion
C3b	Erythrocyte	Immune complex clearance, production of iC3b and C3d,g
	Neutrophil	Phagocytosis; adsorptive pinocytosis
	Monocyte/macrophage	Same as neutrophil
	Eosinophil	Enhanced phagocytosis
	B lymphocyte	?
	T lymphocyte	?
	Glomerular podocyte	?
CR2 (C3d)	B lymphocyte	?
CR3 (iC3b)	Neutrophil	Phagocytosis
	Monocyte	Phagocytosis
	Large granular lymphocyte	Enhanced ADCC
C3e	Neutrophil	Release from bone marrow
C5a	Mast cell	Secretion: leukotriene synthesis?
	Neutrophil	Chemotaxis; secretion; increased stickiness; increased C3b receptor expression
	Monocyte/macrophage	Chemotaxis; secretion; spreading; leukotriene synthesis?
Factor H	B lymphocyte	Secretion of factor I; mitogenesis
	Monocyte	Respiratory burst
	Neutrophil	?

cleavage fragments of complement proteins. Receptors for this peptide exist on mast cells, basophils, neutrophils, and probably on eosinophils, monocytes, and macrophages. Binding to mast cells and basophils induces secretion of histamine and other secretory granule constituents. Incubation of guinea pig lung strips with C5a causes production of slow-reacting substances of anaphylaxis, which are comprised of the C-6 sulfidopeptide leukotrienes, but the cell type responding in this reaction to C5a has not been identified. Interaction of C5a on neutrophils causes a range of cellular responses: increased ''stickiness'' that may promote adhesion to endothelial cells, chemotaxis along a concentration gradient of C5a, increased expression of C3b receptors on the plasma membrane, increased oxygen consumption and superoxide generation, and secretion of specific granules. In general, these responses of the neutrophil promote its localization to a tissue site in which complement activation is occurring, and prepare it for endocytosis of the complement-activating material. C5a is also chemotactic for monocytes and induces slow secretion of glycolytic and proteolytic enzymes by this cell type. An interesting finding indicates that C5a causes production of interleukin-1 by macrophages and augments in vitro lymphocyte responses to antigen. In contrast to the effects of carboxypeptidase H on the activity of C3a, conversion of C5a to C5a des Arg by this enzyme does not abolish the biologic activities of the peptide except, perhaps, that of inducing secretion of histamine by mast cells.

Biologic Reactions Induced by Interaction of Cellular Receptors with Bound Complement Ligands

Three complement proteins attach to the target of complement activation—C1q, C3b and its further degradation fragments, and factor H—and have the capacity to interact with specific receptors present on leukocytes and certain other cell types. Therefore, these proteins can be considered as bifunctional ligands.

The C1q subcomponent of activated $\overline{\text{C1}}$ becomes accessible for interacting with C1q receptors on leukocytes when $\overline{\text{C1}}$INH binds to the $\overline{\text{C1}}\text{r}_2$ and $\overline{\text{C1}}\text{s}_2$ subcomponents, which causes them to dissociate from C1q. C1q receptors have been found on neutrophils, monocytes, B lymphocytes, a small population of T cells, and some lymphocytes lacking B and T cell markers. These receptors probably mediate the attachment of C1q-coated particles and soluble immune complexes, but the consequences of these binding interactions by each cell type are incompletely understood. It has been shown that latex particles coated with C1q induce a respiratory

burst by neutrophils, and that antibody-dependent cellular cytotoxicity mediated by lymphocytes is enhanced by the presence of C1q on target cells.

Three different receptors for fragments of C3 that are bound to complement-activating substances are thought to exist: the C3b receptor, CR2, and CR3. The C3b receptor, which has also been termed the immune adherence receptor and CR1, binds C3b and C4b. This receptor, which is a 250,000 molecular weight glycoprotein, is found on erythrocytes, neutrophils, monocytes, macrophages, eosinophils, mast cells, all B lymphocytes, a minority of T cells, and glomerular podocytes. The function of C3b receptors on erythrocytes may be to facilitate clearance of immune complexes bearing C3b from the blood. Because of its factor H-like activity, the erythrocyte C3b receptor also promotes the cleavage by factor I of immune complex-bound C3b to iC3b, and to the fragments C3d,g and C3c. The C3b receptor on neutrophils and monocytes facilitates the phagocytosis of C3b-bearing particles and adsorptive pinocytosis of soluble C3b-bearing complexes. The functions of C3b receptors on B and T lymphocytes and glomerular podocytes are not yet understood. Although these receptors can mediate phagocytosis by mast cells of particles bearing C3b, endocytosis of particles would not seem to be a major role for this cell type.

CR2 binds iC3b, C3d,g, and C3d and has been reported to be a glycoprotein that is thought to reside only on B cells. These fragments of C3 are produced by cleavage of bound C3b with I in the presence of H or the C3b receptor, and by trypsin. The function of this receptor is incompletely understood, although studies have found that either soluble ligand or antibody to the receptor inhibits the mixed lymphocyte and some mitogen-induced proliferative response of T cells. CR2 has recently been found to be the receptor for the Epstein-Barr virus.

The C3 receptor termed CR3 appears to have specificity for iC3b. Initial studies of the cell types bearing CR3 found it to be present on B cells, monocytes, and neutrophils, although its recent identification as the membrane protein that is recognized by the monoclonal antibodies, anti-Mac-1 and OKM1, indicates that CR3 resides only on large granular lymphocytes, macrophages, and neutrophils. This receptor is involved in the phagocytosis of iC3b-coated particles by neutrophils and monocytes, and enhances ADCC reactions of large granular lymphocytes.

Receptors for factor H reside on B cells, perhaps some T cells, neutrophils, and monocytes. Factor H probably interacts with its receptors after first binding to C3b on the complement-activating target, and is therefore considered as a bound, rather than a freely diffusible, ligand. Polymerized human factor H induces proliferation of mouse B cells, and causes a chemiluminescent response of human monocytes.

INHERITED DEFICIENCIES OF COMPLEMENT PROTEINS

Inherited deficiencies of complement proteins are relatively rare, but in many instances the deficiency may be considered to have been a contributing factor to disease (Table 21–3). Individuals with an inherited deficiency of a complement component may present with a history of repeated bacterial infections, autoimmune disease, or angioedema, the syndrome being dependent on which component is absent.

Bacterial Infections

Individuals with homozygous deficiency of C3 generally suffer repeated bacterial infections, making clear the central role of C3 in maintaining normal host defenses by opsonizing foreign organisms to promote thir phagocytosis by neutrophils and macrophages. Interruption of complement activation at the C3 step also prevents the bactericidal reaction of the C5b-9 complex and the generation of C5a chemotactic factor, which would otherwise localize leukocytes to the infection site. When H or I is absent from the plasma, there is uncontrolled, spontaneous activation of the alternative pathway, hypercatabolism of C3 and B, and impaired host defense against bacterial infections.

Individuals with homozygous deficiencies of C5, C6, C7, or C8 appear to be unusually susceptible to systemic neisserial infections, suggesting that direct complement-mediated cytolysis by the C5b-9 complex may be an important factor in resistance to these organisms.

Rheumatic Diseases

Individuals having homozygous deficiencies or structural abnormalities of components of the classic pathway of complement activation, C1q, C1r, C1s, C4, and C2, appear to be predisposed to various diseases thought to have an autoimmune basis. In addition, several reports of glomerulonephritis in C3-deficient persons indicate that impaired resistance to bacterial infection may not be the only manifestations of the absence of this component. Further supporting the association of rheumatic disease with inherited abnormalities of the complement system is the finding of low numbers of erythrocyte C3b receptors in patients having systemic lupus erythematosus and their consanguineous relatives, and the absence of C3b receptors on glomerular podocytes of patients with proliferative glomerulonephritis of lupus. Several explanations may account for these associations: the null gene for the complement protein is in linkage disequilibrium with certain alleles of immune response (Ir) genes that predispose to autoimmunity; the complement deficiency causes altered processing and clearance of immune complexes; and the deficiency impairs the generation of complement-derived immunoregulatory factors.

There complement components, C4, C2, and factor B, are coded by genes within the major histocompatibility complex (MHC) between the HLA-D and HLA-B loci. The hypothesis that C4 and C2 deficiency do not themselves predispose to rheumatic disease postulates that the primary as-

Table 21–3.   Diseases Associated with Complement Component Deficiencies

Deficient Component	Associated Diseases
C1q	Lupus-like syndromes, glomerulonephritis, chronic sepsis, skin disease
C1r	Lupus-like syndromes, glomerulonephritis, chronic discoid lupus erythematosus
C1s	Systemic lupus erythematosus
C2	Systemic lupus erythematosus, chronic discoid lupus erythematosus, dermatomyositis, vasculitis and Schönlein-Henoch purpura, inflammatory bowel disease, glomerulonephritis, juvenile rheumatoid arthritis
C4	Systemic lupus erythematosus
C3	Recurrent bacterial infections, nephritis
C5	Systemic lupus erythematosus, recurrent *Neisseria* infections
C6	Recurrent *Neisseria* infections, Raynaud's phenomenon
C7	Raynaud's phenomenon with sclerodactyly, systemic lupus erythematosus, recurrent *Neisseria* infections
C8	Recurrent *Neisseria* infections, systemic lupus erythematosus, xeroderma pigmentosum
C9	None
P_	Recurrent *Neisseria* meningitis
C1INH	Hereditary angioedema, chronic discoid lupus erythematosus, systemic lupus erythematosus
I	Recurrent bacterial infections
H	Recurrent bacterial infections
C3b receptor	Partial deficiency on erythrocytes of patients with systemic lupus erythematosus

sociation is with an allele of an Ir gene that is linked to the C4 or C2 null genes. Evidence supporting this explanation is the linkage disequilibrium between the C2 null gene, which has a frequency of approximately 0.01, and HLA-DR2, and the finding that HLA-DR2 is found more frequently in patients with systemic lupus erythematosus than among normal individuals. However, genes coding for deficiencies of the complement proteins, C1q, C1r, C1s, and C3, are not located within the MHC, and this explanation cannot apply to the disease associations of these deficiencies.

The complement system can prevent the formation of large, insoluble immune complexes and can disaggregate preformed insoluble antigen-antibody complexes in vitro (see Chap. 23). The former reaction appears to be dependent primarily on the classic activating pathway, whereas the latter, which is mediated by the binding of C3b to antibody within the immune complex, is principally dependent on activation of C3 by the alternative pathway. Thus, the absence of C1, C4, C2, or C3 may permit the formation in tissues of relatively larger aggregates of antigen-antibody classes which could induce an inflammatory reaction. Similarly, deficiencies of these components, or of C3b receptors on erythrocytes, may have the common consequence of impairing the clearance from the circulation of soluble immune complexes by decreasing their opsonization and cellular uptake. These complexes possibly may then deposit in sites other than the reticuloendothelial system where they could induce tissue damage.

The third possibility by which complement deficiencies may predispose to autoimmune disease relates to the recent findings that certain cleavage fragments of C3 may have down-regulatory effects on cellular immune responses. The absence of the components of the classic activating pathway or of C3 would prevent the generation of these fragments by immune complexes, thereby blocking this putative negative feedback role of the complement system. Although it is still not possible to choose between these various explanations, it is becoming more apparent that the complement system, and in particular the classic pathway, has an essential role in the homeostasis of the immune response and should no longer be considered as having only deleterious effects in inflammatory diseases.

ACQUIRED DEFICIENCIES OF COMPLEMENT PROTEINS

An acquired deficiency of a complement protein is caused by hypercatabolism alone or in combination with hyposynthesis. Hypercatabolism reflects complement activation, usually secondary to the presence of excessive amounts of immune complexes, and often correlates with the occurrence of clinical disease. Two unusual mechanisms of acquired hypercatabolism of C3 involve *autoantibodies directed to the C3 convertase of the classic and alternative pathways*. The former has been found in some patients with systemic lupus erythematosus, and the latter, which has been termed *C3 nephritic factor*, occurs in some patients with membranoproliferative glomerulonephritis and partial lipodystrophy. These antibodies bind to and stabilize their respective C3 convertases, thereby causing augmented C3 cleavage.

Relative functional depressions of C1, C4, C2, and C3 in synovial fluid of patients with seropositive rheumatoid arthritis are taken as evidence of intra-articular activation of the classic pathway, whereas depressions of these components in plasma are generally seen only in those patients having rheumatoid vasculitis. In patients with systemic lupus erythematosus, the plasma concentrations of C3 are frequently depressed in association with active renal disease, and response to therapy can sometimes be monitored by observing a return to normal plasma levels of the component, presumably indicating lower amounts of complement-activating immune complexes. Thus, acquired deficiencies of complement proteins usually indicate activation of the system by normal mechanisms and frequently indicate the presence of an immunologically mediated pathobiologic process.

CLINICAL ASSESSMENTS OF COMPLEMENT FUNCTION

Activation of a complement protein results in loss of its precursor, native activity, and in the generation of cleavage fragments that are usually more rapidly cleared from plasma than is the native form of the protein. If hypercatabolism is not compensated for by increased synthesis, the finding of a depressed concentration of a complement protein in plasma or other body fluids is evidence for activation of the system. Complement can be measured by assaying the function of its components by hemolytic assays that detect only native, unaltered proteins, or by measuring the protein concentration of individual components and their cleavage fragments, usually by immunoprecipitation assays. The most frequently employed functional assay of complement activity is the determination of the amount of serum or other body fluid required to lyse 50% of a sample of sheep erythrocytes that have been sensitized with rabbit antibody, and is reported as CH_{50} units. The test measures the overall activity of C1–C9; is not influenced by the alternative pathway proteins B, D, or P; is relatively insensitive to a modest decrease in the activity of a single component; and requires that the sample be assayed immediately or promptly frozen at $-70°C$. The CH_{50} is useful as an initial screen to detect marked consumption of complement proteins or homozygous deficiencies of individual components. Although specific functional assays for all components of both pathways have been developed, these require specialized reagents that are not available in most clinical laboratories, and individual components are usually measured by radial immunodiffusion assays.

For the evaluation of patients found to be hypocomplementemic, determination of the C4 and C3 protein concentrations is most informative. Low concentrations of C4 indicate that classic pathway activation has occurred, since C4 is extremely sensitive to C1. Depressed levels of C3 suggest that rather intense activation of either pathway is occurring and, if found to be associated with normal levels of C4, indicate that exclusive activation of the alternative pathway is occurring. A limitation of these assays is that they do not discriminate between native C4 and C3 and their high molecular weight cleavage fragments, C4c and C3c, respectively, because most of the antigenic determinants on the native proteins are also expressed by these degradation products. In compartments that are separated from the vascular system, such as synovial and pleural spaces, clearance of degradation fragments is slow, so that measurement of the protein concentrations will underestimate the extent of complement activation. Assays for C4a des Arg and C3a des Arg that have become available may be more informative since they would provide direct evidence for complement activation. Finally, the involvement of complement in a pathologic process can be directly assessed by immunofluorescent staining of individual complement proteins in the involved tissue and by studies of the metabolism of radiolabeled complement proteins. The former is a useful diagnostic procedure, and the latter technique is useful in clinical investigative studies.

CONCLUDING COMMENTS

The complement system has two pathways for activation: the classic and alternative. The former,

through its C1 component, is especially suitable for the recognition of immune complexes, and the latter, by its capacity to interact directly with bacterial cell surfaces in the absence or presence of specific antibody, may be critical for host defense. Activation of either pathway leads to the formation of C3 and C5 convertases that generate the soluble and target-bound cleavage fragments of C3 and C5 that may interact with specific cellular receptors to mediate most of the biologic effects of the complement system. Because many of these effects promote an inflammatory response, the primary role of complement in rheumatic diseases had generally been considered to be deleterious. However, the recognition of autoimmune diseases in a large proportion of individuals having inherited deficiencies of the components of the classic pathway, C1, C4, and C2, and of the C3b receptor, suggests that the complement system may also have a critical role in modulating the immune response. Understanding the molecular and cellular bases for the apparent predisposition of these individuals to rheumatic disease is essential for the definition of the pathobiologic and homeostatic functions of the complement system.

GENERAL REFERENCES

1. Colten, H.R.: Biosynthesis of complemnt. Adv. Immunol., 22:67–118, 1976.
2. Fearon, D.T., and Austen, K.F.: The alternative pathway of complement: A system for host defense to microbial infection. N. Engl. J. Med., 303:259–263, 1980.
3. Fearon, D.T., and Wong, W.W.: Complement ligand-receptor interactions that mediate biological responses. Ann. Rev. Immunol., 1:243–271, 1983.
4. Hugli, T.E.: The structural basis for anaphylatoxin and chemotactic functions of C3a, C4a and C5a. CRC Crit. Rev. Immunol., 4:321–366, 1981.
5. Lachmann, P.J., and Peters, D.K.: Clinical Aspects of Immunology, 4th Ed. Oxford, Blackwell Scientific, 1982.
6. Lachmann, P.J., and Rosen, F.S.: Genetic defects of complement in man. Springer Semin. Immunopathol., 1:339–353, 1978.
7. Muller-Eberhard, H.J., and Schreiber, R.D.: Molecular biology and chemistry of the alternative pathway of complement. Adv. Immunol., 29:1–53, 1980.
8. Reid, K.B.M., and Porter, R.R.: The proteolytic activation systems of complement. Annu. Rev. Biochem., 50:433–464, 1981.

Chapter 22

Arachidonic Acid Metabolites

Edward J. Goetzl and Ira M. Goldstein

The important roles of products of the oxygenation of arachidonic acid and other polyunsaturated fatty acids as mediators of inflammation and hypersensitivity have been delineated more clearly over the past decade.[4,40,113] In many different types of cells, arachidonic acid is released from membrane phospholipids in response to specific stimuli. The arachidonic acid is converted by the cyclo-oxygenase pathway to diverse prostaglandins and thromboxanes and by lipoxygenase pathways to hydroxy-eicosatetraenoic acids (HETEs) and more complex polar metabolites. The cyclo-oxygenase and lipoxygenase pathways share a dependence on the availability of free arachidonic acid and oxygen and exhibit other common characteristics, such as a critical involvement of unstable epoxide and peroxide intermediates and the requirement for more than one type of cell for optimal generation of some products.

Most of the mediators derived from the oxygenation of arachidonic acid *fulfill physiologic activities in normal organ function*. For example, prostaglandins may participate in the regulation of ovulation, parturition, and vascular tone.[114] In some circumstances, deficient or excessive concentrations of the same products may initiate or modulate pathologic reactions. Such is the case for the contributions of prostaglandins to dysmenorrhea, anomalous central and peripheral vascular responses, and Bartter's syndrome.[114] The more recently characterized lipoxygenase products of arachidonic acid also appear to serve physiologic roles and have the capacity to evoke responses that are deleterious in some individuals. Lipoxygenase products are important mediators of inflammation and hypersensitivity and, in some instances, such as the constriction of pulmonary airways and stimulation of epithelial cell secretion, are 100 to 1000 times more potent than cyclo-oxygenase products.[4,41,43,113]

The purposes of this chapter are to describe the general features of the pathways of enzymatic and nonenzymatic oxygenation of arachidonic acid, the structural and biologic characteristics of the resultant mediators of inflammation, the possible roles of such mediators in rheumatic diseases, and the capacity to influence pharmacologically the generation and actions of the mediators.

MOBILIZATION AND OXYGENATION OF ARACHIDONIC ACID

The rate of metabolism of arachidonic acid by oxidative pathways in most types of cells is controlled primarily by the rate of release of arachidonic acid from phospholipids (Fig. 22–1). Although the events that initiate release of arachidonic acid are different for each type of cell, three general mechanisms have been implicated in the release process. In polymorphonuclear leukocytes and some mast cells, the primary mechanism is the degradation of phospholipids by phospholipase A_2,[64,68] which releases arachidonic acid principally from phosphatidylcholine. The second mechanism was suggested by the observations that phosphatidylinositol donates arachidonic acid at a significantly enhanced rate in stimulated leukocytes.[10,46,111,128] The action of a phosphatidylinositol-specific phospholipase C results in the generation of diacylglycerol, from which arachidonic acid is released by a diacylglycerol lipase.[111,128] A third mechanism involves the conversion of phosphatidylethanolamine by sequential methylation to a phospholipase A_2-susceptible phosphatidylcholine, which serves as the source of arachidonic acid in some leukocytes.[64,68,100] The importance of the last pathway in mononuclear leukocytes and some mast cells was implied by the similar time-course of the degradation of phosphatidylethanolamine-derived phosphatidylcholine and the release of arachidonic acid, as well as by the capacity of phospholipase inhibitors and inhibitors of phospholipid methylation to block leukocyte functional responses.[100] The fate of free arachidonic acid is either reacylation into phospholipids or oxygenation to more polar compounds.

The cyclo-oxygenation of arachidonic acid consists of a sequence of complex molecular rearrangements and oxygenations that lead to the formation of 15-hydroperoxy-9-α,11α-peroxidoprosta-5,13-dienoic acid, which is an endoperoxide designated PGG_2 (see Fig. 22–1).[113] Reduction of the C-15 hydroperoxy-group of PGG_2 generates the more polar endoperoxide, PGH_2

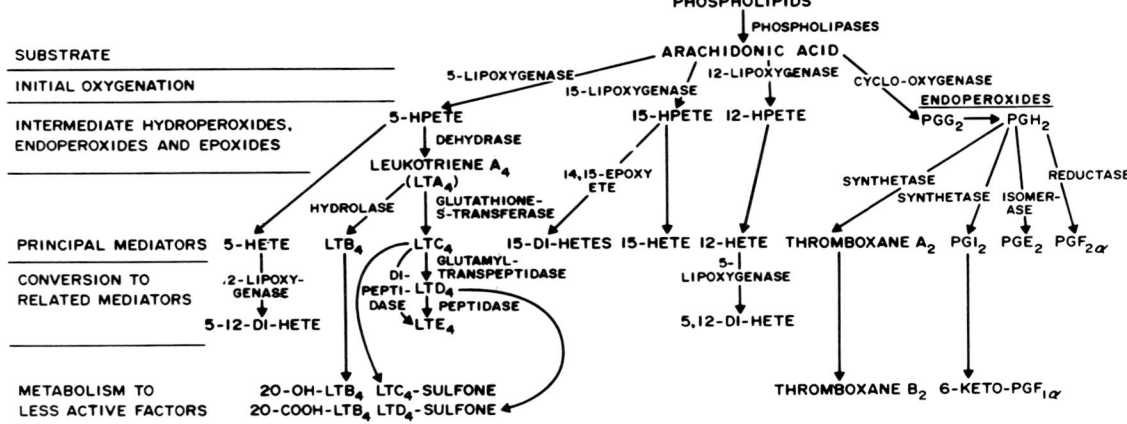

Fig. 22–1. Common characteristics of the cyclo-oxygenation and lipoxygenation of arachidonic acid. PG = prostaglandin; HETE = hydroxy-eicosatetraenoic acid; DI-HETE = dihydroxy-eicosatetraenoic acid; HPETE = hydroperoxy-eicosatetraenoic acid; LT = leukotriene.

which serves as the common precursor for prostaglandins, prostacyclin, and thromboxanes. PGH_2 is converted to PGE_2 by an isomerase and to $PGF_{2\alpha}$ by a reductase, while a distinct synthetase in the walls of blood vessels transforms PGH_2 to prostacyclin, or PGI_2.[70,90,113]

PGH_2 is converted to thromboxane A_2 in platelets and some other types of cells.[58,113] Thromboxane A_2 and each of the prostaglandins have a unique profile of actions on blood vessels, smooth muscle, platelets, and other cells (Table 22–1). PGE_2 and PGI_2 decrease tone and increase the permeability of vessels in the microcirculation.[75,91] In contrast, thromboxane A_2 and $PGF_{2\alpha}$ increase microvascular tone, and $PGF_{2\alpha}$ decreases slightly the natural permeability of microvasculature as well as the increased permeability induced by other agonists.[75,91] Although less potent than some of the lipoxygenase products of arachidonic acid, $PGF_{2\alpha}$, PGI_2, and thromboxane A_2 constrict, and PGE_2 dilates, both large and small airways of the lungs.[91] The potent bidirectional effects of thromboxane A_2 and PGI_2 on platelet aggregation and other functions are intravascular activities critical to the control of hemostasis and the development of some atherosclerotic lesions.[86] Identical bidirectional effects of thromboxane A_2 and PGI_2 are expressed in relation to the adherence of leukocytes to surfaces (see Table 22–1). Other direct and modulatory effects of prostaglandins on leukocyte functions are generally less pronounced than the corresponding activities of lipoxygenase products.[41] PGE_2 derived largely from macrophages suppresses the secretory and proliferative responses of subsets of T-lym-

phocytes to antigens and mitogenic lectins[55,129–131] which appears to account for part of the suppressive function of macrophages and perhaps some T-lymphocytes.[56]

The lipoxygenation of arachidonic acid by different pathways shares some features with the cyclo-oxygenation reactions and is equally complex (see Fig. 22–1). An unstable hydroperoxy-eicosatetraenoic acid (HPETE) is the initial metabolite of each lipoxygenase pathway. The HPETE is either reduced to the more stable corresponding HETE or is transformed to an epoxide which serves as the precursor for more highly substituted and polar products.[41,113] The HPETEs and epoxides are analogous to the endoperoxides and to thromboxane A_2, respectively, in the cyclo-oxygenase pathway. Similarly, the HETEs and related derivatives are analogous to the prostaglandins. In both types of pathways, oxidation and hydrolysis are the predominant mechanisms for either conversion to less active mediators or degradation (see Fig. 22–1). HETEs and more complex products of the lipoxygenase pathways, such as leukotrienes, have the capacity to alter microvascular and smooth muscle function and to initiate and modify leukocyte activities, but have no documented effects on platelets (see Table 22–1).[41,113]

Products of arachidonic acid are susceptible to precise quantification by both chromatographic and immunochemical techniques. The prostaglandins, HETEs, and other lipoxygenase products can be assayed directly, while thromboxane A_2 and PGI_2 are assessed in terms of their stable metabolites thromboxane B_2 and 6-keto-$PGF_{1\alpha}$, respectively.

Table 22–1. Primary Inflammatory Effects of Arachidonic Acid Products

	LTB_4	LTC_4	LTD_4	TxA_2	PGF_2	PGI_2	PGE_2
Microvasculature	Increases permeability Decreases tone; may increase tone transiently	Increases permeability Decreases tone; may increase tone transiently	Increases permeability Decreases tone; may increase tone transiently	Increases tone	Decreases permeability Increases tone	Increases permeability Decreases tone	Increases permeability Decreases tone
Pulmonary airways	Constricts small > large LTD_4 > LTC_4 >> LTB_4	Constricts small ≈ large	Constricts small ≈ large	Constricts	Constricts small ≈ large	Constricts small ≈ large	Dilates
PMN leukocytes and macrophages	Stimulates chemotaxis; other specific functions Increase adherence to surfaces	Increase adherence to surfaces	Increase adherence to surfaces	Increases adherence to surfaces		Enhances random migration Decreases adherence to surfaces Decreases some responses to other stimuli	Enhances random migration Decreases some responses to other stimuli
T-lymphocytes	Inhibits transformation and secretion; induces suppressor cells						Inhibits transformation and secretion
Platelets				Aggregates (through ADP)		Inhibits aggregation (through cAMP); elicits pain	
Other actions	Stimulates pulmonary airway secretion of mucous glycoproteins LTC_4/D_4 > LTB_4	Stimulates pulmonary airway secretion of mucous glycoproteins LTC_4/D_4 > LTB_4	Stimulates pulmonary airway secretion of mucous glycoproteins LTC_4/D_4 > LTB_4				

NONENZYMATIC PATHWAYS LEADING TO PRODUCTION OF BIOLOGICALLY ACTIVE ARACHIDONIC ACID METABOLITES

Since enzymatic conversion of arachidonic acid to biologically active hydroxy-derivatives proceeds throuh the formation of hydroperoxides, it is not surprising that similar derivatives can be generated nonenzymatically by free radical-mediated reactions. Turner et al., for example, found that exposure of arachidonic acid either to air for 24 hours or to ultraviolet irradiation resulted in the generation of oxidized lipids that were chemotactic for human polymorphonuclear leukocytes.[126,127] The products that were generated in this fashion were identified as positional isomers of hydroxy-eicosatetraenoic acids.

Perez et al. described another mechanism whereby arachidonic acid can be converted nonenzymatically to biologically active products.[98] Chemotactic activity for human polymorphonuclear leukocytes was generated upon exposure of arachidonic acid to a superoxide-generating system consisting of xanthine oxidase and acetaldehyde. Generation of chemotactic activity in this experimental system was time-dependent and could be inhibited significantly by scavengers of singlet oxygen, as well as by scavengers of superoxide, hydrogen peroxide, and hydroxyl radicals. Silica gel thin-layer radiochromatography demonstrated a product with chemotactic activity that was distinct from unaltered arachidonic acid and from 12-HETE. The isolated product was chemotactic for human polymorphonuclear leukocytes at a concentration (approximate) of 3.0 ng/ml and chemokinetic at concentrations of 0.75 to 1.5 ng/ml. Interestingly, the chemotactic lipid also influenced aggregation of human platelets. Addition of the isolated chemotactic lipid to normal platelet-rich plasma for one to two minutes did not induce any platelet shape change or aggregation. However, subsequent platelet aggregation responses to threshold concentrations of either sodium arachidonate or the endoperoxide analogue, 9,11-azo-prostanoid III,[19] were delayed or inhibited, depending upon the amount of chemotactic lipid that was added. Similarly, biphasic aggregation responses to adenosine diphosphate were delayed, and the second phase of aggregation was inhibited by prior exposure of the platelets to the chemotactic lipid. Thrombin-induced aggregation of washed platelets also was inhibited by the chemotactic lipid, with concomitant inhibition of serotonin release.

The precise identity of the chemotactic lipid formed from arachidonic acid by exposure to a superoxide-generating system was not determined. There is evidence, however, that hydroxyl radicals and singlet oxygen can convert arachidonic acid to several biologically active products. Fridovich and Porter, for example, found that exposure to xanthine oxidase and acetaldehyde converted arachidonic acid to a series of conjugated diene hydroperoxides (i.e., HPETEs).[37] The 15-hydroperoxide and 5-substituted hydroperoxide were the major products formed. Co-oxidation of arachidonic acid by the xanthine oxidase-acetaldehyde system was inhibited by either superoxide dismutase or catalase and was stimulated by the addition of ferrous salts. These findings suggested that hydroxyl radicals, or similar reactive species generated by the iron-catalyzed interaction of superoxide with hydrogen peroxide, were responsible for the formation of hydroperoxy-acids from arachidonate. Porter et al. also found that arachidonic acid could be oxidized by exposure to either air or singlet oxygen (generated by photolysis) to yield a mixture of hydroperoxides, including 5-HPETE, 12-HPETE, and 15-HPETE.[101,102]

Phagocytic leukocytes (particularly polymorphonuclear leukocytes) generate abundant amounts of oxygen-derived free radicals upon stimulation of their plasma membranes[50] and are capable of producing lipid peroxides.[125] Consequently, under conditions that exist at most foci of inflammation, it is possible that potent chemoattractants are generated from arachidonic acid by mechanisms involving free radicals. Generation of chemotactic products from arachidonic acid may be important for amplifying inflammatory responses.

Another chemoattractant formed by the action of oxygen-derived free radicals was described by Petrone et al.[99] These investigators found that potent chemotactic activity for human polymorphonuclear leukocytes could be generated in vitro by exposing normal human plasma to a source of superoxide anion radicals (i.e., xanthine oxidase and sodium xanthine). Generation of chemotactic activity in this system was inhibited by superoxide dismutase, but not by catalase. When plasma that had been exposed to superoxide anion radicals was injected intradermally into rats, large numbers of polymorphonuclear leukocytes accumulated at the injection sites. Infiltration by these cells was evident as early as 30 minutes after injection and increased with time. A similar response was observed when rats were injected intradermally with xanthine oxidase and xanthine. No leukocyte infiltration was observed, however, if superoxide dismutase was injected simultaneously with the enzyme and substrate.

The chemotactic activity that was formed by exposing plasma to superoxide was heat-labile (56°C for 30 minutes), nondialyzable, and stable to ly-ophilization. The bulk of the activity was recovered after gel filtration and ion exchange chromatography of treated plasma in fractions containing albumin. Albumin per se, however, was not chemotactic. Rather, the chemotactic factor appeared to consist of a chloroform-extractable component (i.e., lipid) that was bound to albumin. Although the nature of the lipid was not determined, it is intriguing to speculate that it may be a hydroperoxy- or hydroxy-derivative of arachidonic acid.

Based on these findings, it has been proposed that (1) superoxide anion radicals produced by stimulated leukocytes interact with a plasma precursor to form a potent chemotactic factor that propagates and amplifies inflammatory reactions, and (2) superoxide dismutase ameliorates inflammation by preventing the formation of superoxide-dependent chemotactic activity.

PROINFLAMMATORY EFFECTS OF PROSTAGLANDINS

There is ample evidence that stable prostaglandins, thromboxanes, and prostacyclin are mediators of inflammation.[4,41,76] First, these compounds are capable of provoking many of the cardinal signs of inflammation (e.g., erythema, fever, pain, edema). Second, they are synthesized by phagocytic cells and are released in large amounts during inflammatory reactions. Finally, synthesis of stable prostaglandins, thromboxanes, and prostacyclin is inhibited by many anti-inflammatory drugs. Details concerning the proinflammatory effects of prostaglandins are summarized in the sections that follow.

Erythema and Fever. It has been demonstrated conclusively that products of the cyclo-oxygenase pathway of arachidonic acid metabolism contribute to the erythema, local increases in temperature, and fever associated with many forms of acute and chronic inflammation. PGI_2, PGE_1, PGE_2, PGD_2, and PGA_2, for example, have been found capable of provoking vasodilatation.[91,135,136] The most potent of these compounds, PGI_2, markedly increases the diameter of precapillary arterioles.[62] In contrast, the cyclic endoperoxides (e.g., PGH_2) and thromboxane A_2 are potent vasoconstrictors.[91]

Prostaglandins of the E series, as well as arachidonic acid, produce fever in experimental animals when injected directly into the cerebral ventricles.[21,89] In addition, levels of prostaglandins are increased in the cerebrospinal fluid of animals rendered febrile by both endogenous and exogenous pyrogens.[24,137] These observations, together with the fact that almost all nonsteroidal anti-inflammatory agents also are antipyretic agents,[119] support the hypothesis that products of arachidonic acid

formed by the cyclo-oxygenase pathway contribute to the development of hyperpyrexia.

Pain and Edema. The roles played by stable prostaglandins in provoking the pain and edema that accompany inflammation are more complex. For example, in a number of experimental models, stable prostaglandins (e.g., PGE compounds) have been found incapable of provoking pain directly.[31,32] They do, however, produce hyperalgesia and act synergistically with other mediators (e.g., histamine, bradykinin) to augment pain.[31,33] PGE_2, for example, when injected into human skin, causes a marked potentiation of the pain produced by intradermal injections of either histamine or bradykinin.[31] PGE_2 not only enhances the intensity of the pain provoked by these mediators, but prolongs the duration as well.

As is the case with pain, prostaglandins appear to be incapable of directly causing edema, but act synergistically with other mediators. Williams and Peck, for example, showed that intradermal injections of E-type prostaglandins in rabbits produce large increases in local blood flow with little, if any, plasma exudation.[136] Bradykinin and histamine, on the other hand, increased vascular permeability (resulting in plasma exudation) for 10 to 15 minutes after injection, but were far less potent with respect to their ability to increase blood flow. Prostaglandins potentiated the vascular permeability changes provoked by histamine and bradykinin. The ability of any individual prostaglandin to potentiate plasma exudation was directly related to its ability to enhance blood flow. It appears, therefore, that the edema of acute inflammation is not due directly to products of the cyclo-oxygenase pathway of arachidonic acid metabolism, but can be modulated by inhibitors of this pathway (e.g., nonsteroidal anti-inflammatory agents).

More recent evidence suggests that products of arachidonic acid play a role in provoking changes in vascular permeability mediated by complement and polymorphonuclear leukocytes. For example, purified rabbit and human C5a des Arg (which lacks intrinsic anaphylatoxin activity) caused increased vascular permeability in rabbit skin only in the presence of added prostaglandins (e.g., PGE_1 and PGE_2) and only in animals with normal numbers of circulating polymorphonuclear leukocytes.[69,132] As indicated previously, prostaglandins probably enhance exudation of plasma across (or through) the endothelium by inducing vasodilatation and increased flow.

Other products of the cyclo-oxygenase pathway may promote vascular permeability changes. Prostacyclin (PGI_2), for example, dilates blood vessels and augments edema provoked by other mediators.[62,63] Thromboxane A_2 also may provoke some forms of vascular injury by enhancing adherence of polymorphonuclear leukocytes to endothelial surfaces.[45,121]

Tissue Injury (Resorption of Bone). Apart from their ability to influence vascular tone and permeability, prostaglandins show little evidence of directly causing tissue injury. It has been suggested, however, that at least some of the tissue damage that accompanies inflammation is produced indirectly by free radicals (e.g., hydroxyl radicals), which are generated during the enzymatic conversion of PGG_2 to PGH_2.[76] Inhibition of the formation of such free radicals or their elimination by scavengers may account for the potent anti-inflammatory effects of some drugs that do not inhibit the synthesis of stable prostaglandins.

Although prostaglandins generally are incapable of causing tissue injury, it has been demonstrated that PGE_2 stimulates bone resorption in vitro and in vivo.[73,108,117] PGE_2 produced by rheumatoid synovia promotes resorption of bone in the absence of other major products of the rheumatoid tissue.[108] In addition, rheumatoid synovial tissue in culture produces approximately 10 times more PGE_2 than normal synovial tissue. It appears likely, therefore, that prostaglandins (particularly PGE_2) produced by hypertrophic and hyperplastic synovial tissue contribute to the destruction of juxta-articular bone in rheumatoid arthritis. Since PGE compounds also inhibit collagen biosynthesis in vitro,[104] enhanced production of prostaglandins by rheumatoid synovium may lead to additional detrimental effects in adjacent connective tissue.

Generation of Prostaglandins at Sites of Inflammation. Large amounts of stable prostaglandins have been detected at foci of inflammation, and these compounds are synthesized by phagocytic cells (i.e., polymorphonuclear leukocytes, monocytes, and macrophages).[53,79,145] Human polymorphonuclear leukocytes released prostaglandins of the E and F series to the surrounding medium when these cells were exposed to suitably opsonized zymosan particles.[145] Prostaglandin E was found in the highest concentration in the medium, and the prostaglandin E to prostaglandin F ratio was approximately 3:1. Prostaglandin release was not due to contamination of the reaction mixtures with platelets and was inhibited by indomethacin and by aspirin. Stimulated human polymorphonuclear leukocytes also generated thromboxane A_2.[51,52] Finally, and perhaps most relevant to the types of inflammation observed in patients with rheumatoid disease, inflamed synovial tissue synthesized large amounts of PGE compounds.[34,71,106–108]

Inhibition of Prostaglandin Biosynthesis by Anti-Inflammatory Drugs. The most compelling evidence that stable prostaglandins are mediators of inflammation has come from studies of the effects of various drugs on the biosynthesis of these compounds. Most nonsteroidal anti-inflammatory agents and anti-inflammatory adrenal corticosteroids inhibit the biosynthesis of stable prostaglandins.

From the foregoing discussion, it might be concluded that stable prostaglandins are important mediators of inflammation and that many anti-inflammatory drugs produce their beneficial effects by inhibiting prostaglandin biosynthesis, but some observations suggest alternative conclusions.

INHIBITION OF LEUKOCYTE FUNCTIONS BY PROSTAGLANDINS

Abundant evidence has been accumulated during the past decade indicating that several functions of cells involved in acute and chronic inflammatory reactions (i.e., polymorphonuclear leukocytes, monocytes, macrophages, lymphocytes) can be modulated by cyclic nucleotides. For example, selective extracellular release of proinflammatory lysosomal constituents from stimulated human peripheral blood polymorphonuclear leukocytes in vitro, as well as release of mediators of inflammation from other cell types, can be inhibited either by cyclic 3',5'-adenosine monophosphate (cAMP) directly or by pharmacologic agents that increase levels within cells of this cyclic nucleotide.[13,133,134] Therefore, consistent with their ability to increase cellular levels of cAMP, some prostaglandins (e.g., PGE_1, PGE_2) act as "extracellular messengers" and inhibit release of mediators of inflammation from leukocytes.[138] Prostaglandins of the E series, as well as PGI_2, also inhibit leukocyte chemotaxis,[38,61] adherence to various substrates (including endothelium),[14,15] phagocytosis,[20] and generation of oxygen-derived free radicals.[82] Inhibitory effects on various functions of B- and T-lymphocytes have been reported as well. For example, PGE_1 and PGE_2 (with or without the phosphodiesterase inhibitor, theophylline) suppress proliferative responses of human lymphocytes to mitogens, lymphocyte-mediated cytotoxicity, and antibody production by B-lymphocytes.[54,56,97,123,131]

In contrast to the effects of cAMP, cyclic 3',5'-guanosine monophosphate (cGMP) and agents that elevate levels within cells of cGMP enhance some leukocyte functions. PGF_2, for example, increases levels of cGMP in polymorphonuclear leukocytes and enhances selective release from these cells of lysosomal constituents.[133,134,138] $PGF_{2\alpha}$ enhances other functions of polymorphonuclear leukocytes,[61] and augments certain functions of B- and T-lymphocytes.[54,97] It is not surprising, therefore, that considerable attention has been focused recently on the potential roles played by prostaglandins in regulating inflammatory reactions as well as both humoral and cellular immune reactions. It has been suggested, for example, that by local, preferential biosynthesis of one or another of the prostaglandins, the very cells that release mediators of inflammation provide a mechanism for modulating inflammatory responses. PGF compounds may enhance inflammation, whereas PGE compounds, by acting as feedback inhibitors, actually may provide a "shutoff" signal, and reduce inflammation.

ANTI-INFLAMMATORY EFFECTS OF PROSTAGLANDINS IN EXPERIMENTAL ANIMALS

From the foregoing discussion, it seems possible that prostaglandins that inhibit leukocyte functions in vitro also may exhibit anti-inflammatory effects in vivo. Examples of some anti-inflammatory effects of prostaglandins in various forms of experimentally induced inflammation are discussed in the following sections.

Adjuvant Arthritis. Adjuvant disease in the rat includes a severe and persistent polyarthritis that appears 10 to 14 days after a single intradermal injection of complete Freund's adjuvant.[96] PGE_2 significantly reduces tibiotarsal joint swelling in rats with adjuvant arthritis.[2] In subsequent studies,[39,142-144] it was observed that PGE_1 (500 μg administered intraperitoneally twice daily) either prevented or suppressed adjuvant arthritis, while the same treatment with PGA_2 had no effect on the disease. Arthritis was prevented when rats were treated either from the day of adjuvant injection or from day seven. When treatment was begun on day 14, the typical explosive course of the arthritis was suppressed. Established inflammation was reduced significantly even when treatment was begun on day 21. Similar results were obtained with PGE_1 and PGE_2 in adrenalectomized rats.

Whereas treatment of rats with PGE compounds did not suppress delayed hypersensitivity reactions to mycobacterial antigens, anti-sheep red blood cell antibody titers were reduced. Treatment with PGE compounds also reduced the numbers of circulating lymphocytes. Despite these and other observations relative to the effects of prostaglandins on humoral and cellular immune reactivity, the mechanism whereby PGE compounds suppress adjuvant arthritis in rats is still unknown.

Carrageenan-Induced Inflammation. PGE_1 and PGE_2 also suppressed inflammation in rats injected with carrageenan.[143] Administration of PGE compounds into subcutaneous air blebs at the time of carrageenan injection reduced the number of polymorphonuclear leukocytes that entered the focus of inflammation. PGE_1 and PGE_2 also produced concentration-dependent reductions in exudate lysosomal enzyme (i.e., beta-glucuronidase) and cytoplasmic enzyme (i.e., lactate dehydrogenase) levels. Ultrastructural studies revealed that carrageenan was ingested by invading leukocytes and enclosed within phagocytic vacuoles, the membranes of which subsequently ruptured. More lysosomes apparently remained intact after carrageenan uptake by bleb leukocytes from PGE-treated than from control rats. There also was no loss of phagosomal membrane integrity in cells from treated rats.

Another carrageenan-induced lesion has been used to evaluate the effectiveness of anti-inflammatory drugs. Carrageenan-induced edema in the rat footpad is associated with three distinct phases of mediator-induced vascular permeability changes.[25] The initial phase probably results from the release of histamine and serotonin and is inhibited by antihistamines. The second phase has been attributed to the action of bradykinin. The third phase of persistent edema has been attributed to the local production of prostaglandins (particularly PGE_2) by inflammatory cells. Interestingly, treatment of rats systemically with either PGE_1[39] or the more stable derivative, 15-(S)-15-methyl PGE_1,[27] significantly inhibits carrageenan-induced rat footpad edema. Both the acute phase of edema formation and the later phases are reduced in a dose-dependent fashion by PGE_1 and PGE_2, but not by $PGF_{2\alpha}$.

The effects of PGE compounds on carrageenan-induced rat footpad edema are in accord with the findings reported previously that PGE_1 and 15-(S)-15-methyl PGE_1 (but not PGA_2 or $PGF_{2\alpha}$) markedly reduce the increases in vascular permeability induced in rats by intradermal injections of histamine, serotonin, bradykinin, the complement-derived anaphylatoxin C3a, and compound 48/80.[28] Suppression by the PGE compounds of vascular permeability changes is associated ultrastructurally with preservation of tight junctions between endothelial cells. Interference with the local effects of vasopermeability mediators may account for the suppressive effects of PGE compounds on immune complex-induced inflammation and tissue injury in experimental animals.

Immune Complex-Induced Inflammation. Vascular permeability changes after induction of reversed passive Arthus reactions in rat skin were suppressed significantly by pretreatment with either PGE_1 or its stable derivative, 15-(S)-15-methyl PGE_1.[77] Suppression also was observed in animals treated with PGE_2 and PGD_2, but not $PGF_{2\alpha}$. Interestingly, the stable derivative of PGE_1 also was effective when administered orally. Diminished vascular permeability in treated animals was accompanied by markedly reduced exudation of poly-morphonuclear leukocytes. For the most part, leu-kocytes remained within dermal venules and capillaries despite the observations by transmission electron microscopy and/or by immunofluores-cence microscopy that immune complexes and complement were deposited in the walls of these blood vessels. Ingestion of immune complexes by leukocytes also was reduced in treated animals. Polymorphonuclear leukocytes harvested from the blood of rats treated with PGE_1 exhibited depressed chemotactic responses in vitro as well as dimin-ished lysosomal enzyme secretion after incubation with a chemotactic peptide.

Suppression of human polymorphonuclear leu-kocyte degranulation also has been observed fol-lowing intravenous infusion of PGE_1 for the treat-ment of peripheral vascular disease.[29] A detailed study of this phenomenon[30] revealed evidence that administration systemically of 15-(S)-15-methyl PGE_1 reduces the binding affinity of the receptor on rat polymorphonuclear leukocytes for the syn-thetic chemotactic peptide, N-formyl-methionyl-leucyl-phenylalanine (FMLP). Whereas the dis-sociation constant (K_D) for FMLP binding was in-creased two- to three-fold, treatment with PGE_1 did not alter the total number of receptor sites per cell. Consistent with these findings, polymorpho-nuclear leukocytes from PGE_1-treated rats exhib-ited significantly decreased responses to FMLP in vitro (i.e., degranulation and generation of super-oxide anion radicals). These studies suggest that some of the anti-inflammatory effects observed after administration of PGE compounds may be mediated by altered functional responses of poly-morphonuclear leukocytes to chemotactic peptides.

In addition to inhibiting immune complex-in-duced inflammation, 15-(S)-15-methyl PGE_1 has been found capable of suppressing inflammation caused by antitissue antibodies. The nephrotoxicity in rats caused by single intravenous injections of antibodies directed against glomerular basement membranes was suppressed significantly by treat-ment with PGE_1.[78] Treatment reduced glomerular hypercellularity and proteinuria, but did not affect binding of the antibodies to the glomerular base-ment membrane.

Murine Systemic Lupus Erythematosus. Fe-male F_1 hybrids of New Zealand black (NZB) and white (NZW) mice spontaneously develop a dis-ease that resembles systemic lupus erythemato-sus.[80] The disease is associated with the appearance of circulating autoantibodies (e.g., anti-DNA an-tibodies) and progressive, immune complex-me-diated glomerulonephritis. When female NZB/NZW F_1 hybrid mice were treated with PGE_1 (200 μg subcutaneously either once or twice daily) from 6 through 52 weeks of age, they not only were protected from the development of anemia and ne-phritis but also lived longer than untreated ani-mals.[139-141] At 52 weeks, 18 of 19 treated mice were alive versus only 2 of 19 untreated controls. Survival of NZB/NZW mice also was prolonged when treatment with PGE_1 was begun at 24 weeks, at a time when these animals begin to develop nephritis. Interestingly, although treatment with PGE_1 did not prevent development of antibodies to nuclear antigens (including anti-DNA antibodies), it did prevent deposition of immunoglobulins and complement in glomeruli as well as the develop-ment of proliferative nephritis. The milder disease observed in male NZB/NZW mice also was pre-vented by treatment with PGE_1.

In contrast to these, as yet unexplained, effects of pharmacologic amounts of PGE compounds on the course of murine lupus, evidence has appeared suggesting that inhibition of endogenous prosta-glandin biosynthesis also may suppress this dis-ease. Female NZB/NZW F_1 hybrid mice fed a diet rich in eicosapentaenoic acids (i.e., fatty acids con-taining five double-bonds) did not develop pro-teinuria and lived longer than similar mice fed a normal diet.[103] None of the animals fed the special diet died or exhibited proteinuria for the duration of the study (up to 13.5 months). Anti-double-stranded DNA antibodies also were reduced by approximately 50% in treated animals. Because eicosapentaenoic acid inhibits conversion of arach-idonic acid into thromboxanes and stable prosta-glandins, it was concluded that arachidonic acid metabolites may play a role in the pathogenesis of murine lupus. Clearly, more work will be required to elucidate the mechanisms whereby prostaglan-dins modulate immune complex-mediated inflam-mation and tissue injury.

LEUKOTRIENES AS POTENT MEDIATORS OF INFLAMMATION AND HYPERSENSITIVITY

The 5-lipoxygenation of arachidonic acid in leu-kocytes generates 5-hydroperoxy-eicosatetraenoic acid (5-HPETE), which is the precursor for the production of a family of complex 5-hydroxy-ei-cosatetraenoic acids (5-HETEs), termed leuko-trienes, that contain additional polar substituents and three conjugated double bonds (see Fig. 22–1). The highly reactive 5,6-epoxy-eicosa-7,9,11,14-tetraenoic acid (leukotriene A_4 and LTA_4, where the subscript 4 indicates the total number of double bonds in the molecule) is derived from 5-HPETE.[11] LTA_4 is hydrated enzymatically to form 5(S),12(R)-dihydroxy-eicosa-6,14,cis-8,10,trans-tetraenoic acid (LTB_4),[12] a potent stimulus of chemotaxis and other functions of leukocytes in vitro and in vivo.[36,47] LTA_4 also combines enzymatically with glutathione to yield 5-hydroxy-6-sulfido - glutathionyl - 7,9 - trans - 11,14 - cis - ETE (LTC_4), which is converted enzymatically to 5-hydroxy-6-sulfido-cysteinyl-glycine-ETE (LTD_4) and subsequently to 5-hydroxy-6 - sulfido - cysteinyl - ETE (LTE_4).[113] A γ-glutamyltranspeptidase also transforms LTE_4 to a γ-glutamyl-LTE_4 designated LTF_4.[6] LTC_4, LTD_4, and LTE_4 are potent contractile and vasoactive factors, and represent the principal constituents of the slow-reacting substance of anaphylaxis (SRS-A) generated by immunologic stimulation of human lung and other tissues.[83] The conversion of HPETE to an epoxide, which reacts with one or more polar compounds, is a fundamental mechanism observed in each of the pathways. 15-HPETE similarly is transformed to an unstable 14,15-epoxide that is convertd to two isomers of 14,15-diHETE and four of 8,15-diHETE. Although the epoxide derived from 12-HPETE has not been characterized fully, the complex metabolites identified include an 11,12-diHETE and several trihydroxy-eicosatetraenoic acids. Although the biochemical and cellular characteristics of the generation of leukotrienes by leukocytes and other cells have not been defined fully, cell-to-cell interactions appear to be important for the achievement of maximal rates of production of the mediators. The addition of platelets to polymorphonuclear (PMN) leukocytes in vitro enhances the rate of generation of isomers of LTB_4.

Fluid and tissue concentrations of the lipoxygenase products are regulated predominantly by the activities of the pathways of generation, as has been demonstrated by the greater than 80% suppression of the levels achieved with different classes of lipoxygenase inhibitors. In addition, further metabolism of leukotrienes may convert the primary principles either to mediators with different activities or to inactive products (see Fig. 22–1). The transformation of LTB_4 to 20-hydroxyl-LTB_4 and 20-carboxyl-LTB_4 reduces both the polymorphonuclear leukocyte chemotactic and aggregating potency and the smooth muscle contractile and microvascular activities in several in vitro systems.[60] The peroxidation of LTC_4 in human eosinophils rapidly yields sulfoxides and a sulfone of LTC_4, the latter of which retains smooth muscle and microvascular activities, and two 6-trans isomers of LTB_4, which exhibit leukocyte chemotactic activity that is not expressed by LTC_4.[44] The SRS-A activities of LTD_4 are diminished substantially by peptidolytic conversion to LTE_4,[81] and the activities of LTC_4, LTD_4, and LTE_4 are eliminated by 15-hydroxylation.[4,92] The quantitative importance and biological significance of the secondary pathways of metabolism of the leukotrienes have not been established in vivo. The bulk of the radioactivity of [³H]-LTC_4 given systemically to rats accumulates in the liver and kidneys, which both degrade and excrete the mediator in the bile and urine, respectively.[1,93] Other pathways for the metabolic inactivation of leukotrienes in distinct tissue compartments may contribute to their elimination after local reactions.

Although some of the smooth muscle and microvascular effects of LTB_4 may be attributable to stimulation by LTB_4 of the generation of thromboxanes and prostaglandins,[120] the activation of PMN leukocytes is initiated by the occupancy of receptors on the cell surface that selectively recognize LTB_4 as compared to other chemotactic factors. The dependence of the PMN leukocyte chemotactic activity on the structural integrity of several relatively polar domains of LTB_4 and the capacity of chemotactically less active derivatives and analogues of LTB_4 to inhibit the responses to LTB_4, but not to peptide chemotactic factors,[48] suggested that a subset of receptors was dedicated to LTB_4 and did not bind functionally similar stimuli of different structures. The application of direct binding assays has confirmed the presence on PMN leukocytes of a distinct subset of stereospecific receptors with a high affinity for LTB_4.[49] Similarly, specific receptors for LTC_4 and LTD_4 have been found in lung tissues, but have not been characterized with isolated smooth muscle cells.

The first functional classification of leukotrienes was based on the observations that the contractile and vasoactive factors, LTC_4 and LTD_4, lacked the capabilities of LTB_4 to stimulate leukocyte chemotaxis and other functions.[40,113] However, 3.0 to 300 nM LTC_4 and LTD_4 enhanced the adherence of PMN leukocytes to surfaces to the same extent as LTB_4 and peptide chemotactic factors.[45] Indomethacin inhibited the increase in PMN leukocyte adherence evoked by LTC_4 and LTD_4 and the concurrent elevation in the concentration of endogenous thromboxane B_2, suggesting that the adherence-enhancing activity of the C-6 peptide leukotrienes was mediated by PMN leukocyte-derived thromboxane A_2.[45] Similar studies of the effects of indomethacin on the constriction of pulmonary airways by LTB_4 in animal models indicate that cyclo-oxygenase products of arachidonic acid are generated by the action of LTB_4 on lung tissues and contribute significantly to the physical outcome observed.[120] Thus, the involvement of cyclo-oxygenase metabolites in the biologic effects of lipoxygenase mediators may be a more general phenomenon.

Diverse metabolites of the 15-lipoxygenation and 5-lipoxygenation of arachidonic acid, including LTB[4], are generated in substantial quantities by human and murine T-lymphocytes.[5,42,72] 15-HETE, at concentrations attained in suspensions of stimulated lymphocytes, inhibits murine lymphocyte transformation[5] and human T-lymphocyte migration.[94] In contrast, LTB[4] and, to a lesser extent, 5-HETE enhance the migration of human T-lymphocytes in vitro.[94] A broader analysis of the direct effects of leukotrienes on other functions of purified human T-lymphocytes demonstrated that 10^{-8}M–10^{-6}M LTB[4], but not LTC[4], LTD[4], or LTE[4], inhibits significantly both proliferative and synthetic responses to mitogens[95] and antigens. In more complex interactions, LTB[4] also induced T-lymphocyte suppressor and cytotoxic activities. Enhancement by LTB[4] of T-lymphocyte cytotoxic activity required endogenous thromboxane production, while both adherent mononuclear leukocytes and endogenous prostaglandin production were essential for the suppressor activity exhibited by LTB[4]-stimulated T-lymphocytes.[109,110]

The results of the earliest comprehensive assays of arachidonic acid metabolites in human disease demonstrated highly significant increases in the concentrations of PGE[2], PGF[2α], free arachidonic acid, and HETEs in psoriatic lesions as compared to uninvolved skin of the same patients.[59] Concurrent studies indicated that synovial fluid of patients with rheumatoid arthritis contains higher concentrations of PGE[2] and, to a lesser extent, PGF[2α] and thromboxane B[2], than synovial fluid of subjects with noninflammatory arthropathies.[106,107] In addition, explants of synovial tissue and cultures of adherent synovial cells from patients with rheumatoid arthritis produced greater quantities of PGE[2] and some other cyclo-oxygenase products in vitro than did tissue from subjects with nonrheumatoid arthropathies.[9,34,71,108] The finding of significantly increased levels of LTB[4] in synovial fluid of patients with rheumatoid arthritis or spondyloarthritis and of 5-HETE in rheumatoid synovial tissue was the first documentation of abnormal activity of the lipoxygenase pathway in human arthritis.[74] Interest in the pathophysiologic significance of the metabolism of arachidonic acid in human inflammatory states was enhanced by the detection of heightened tissue sensitivity to lipoxygenase products in psoriasis. The activity of soluble guanylate cyclase from psoriatic lesions and uninvolved skin of psoriasis patients was stimulated two- to three-fold by arachidonic acid or 12-L-HETE, whereas that from normal subjects was not altered, although baseline levels were substantially lower than those of patient samples.[16] Although available data do not permit a meaningful integration of the abnormalities of arachidonic acid metabolism and of other systems in human inflammatory disease, a tentative model may be provided for rheumatoid arthritis. Macrophages and polymorphonuclear leukocytes that infiltrate the synovium in large numbers contribute to the elevated levels of PGE[2], thromboxanes, 5-HETE, and LTB[4]. Synoviocytes also generate cyclo-oxygenase products, LTB[4], and 5-HETE. These products, along with complement-derived molecules, such as C5a, stimulate the local influx of more leukocytes. Other leukotrienes and, with a lower potency, LTB[4], might increase the permeability of regional microcirculatory beds.

ANTI-INFLAMMATORY ACTIONS OF DRUGS THAT INHIBIT OXYGENATION OF ARACHIDONIC ACID

The pharmacologic characteristics of inhibitors of the oxygenation of arachidonic acid[87] and their uses clinically as anti-inflammatory drugs[119] have been reviewed comprehensively. Here we describe the properties of clinically relevant inhibitors of generation and antagonists of biologically active metabolites of arachidonic acid in relation to their mechanism of action and the consequent effect on inflammation (Table 22-2). Although numerous difficulties limit the applicability of information gained from in vitro analyses and studies of animal models, such information will be utilized to reinforce points that are not clearly established by clinical data.

Some of the inhibitors, most notably corticosteroids, suppress the release of arachidonic acid by phospholipases and thus effectively inhibit the cyclo-oxygenase and lipoxygenase pathways. Other agents exhibit selectivity either for or within one of the major pathways. For example, therapeutic doses of most nonsteroidal anti-inflammatory drugs inhibit cyclo-oxygenation, while sparing lipoxygenase activities. Phenylbutazone inhibits preferentially the formation of PGE[2], whereas gold has a similar effect on PGF[2α] synthesis without influencing that of PGE[2].[124] Most commonly, the antirheumatic drugs have more than one type of effect on the reactions of oxygenation of arachidonic acid. Most nonsteroidal anti-inflammatory drugs and corticosteroids have other suppressive effects on inflammation, such as scavenging oxygen radicals, altering cyclic nucleotide metabolism, influencing the activities of various enzymes or transport systems, or blocking unrelated receptors. The capacity of the cyclo-oxygenase and lipoxygenase inhibitor eicosatetraynoic acid (ETYA) to suppress neutrophil chemotaxis to the synthetic peptide, N-formyl-methionyl-leucyl-phenylalanine (FMLP), for example, is attributable in part to inhibition of the binding of FMLP to chemotactic receptors.[3] Indomethacin inhibits

Table 22–2. Inhibitors of Generation or Effects of Metabolites of Arachidonic Acid

Class	Agent	Action
Inhibitors of synthesis	Corticosteroids	Inhibit release of arachidonic acid
	Gold compounds	Block production of $PGF_2\alpha$
	Nonsteroidal anti-inflammatory drugs	Suppress generation of prostaglandins; retard conversion of HPETEs to HETEs
	Phenylbutazone	Blocks production of PGE_2
	Salicylazosulfapyridine	Inhibits lipoxygenase activity, with less effect on cyclo-oxygenase activity
	Tocopherols	Inhibit cyclo-oxygenase and lipoxygenase activities
	Ascorbic acid	Inhibits thromboxane synthesis, stimulates release of arachidonic acid; variable effect on prostaglandin synthesis
Inhibitors of effect	Colchicine, chloroquine, probenecid, methylxanthines, some nonsteroidal anti-inflammatory drugs	Suppress transport of prostaglandins into cells and/or the actions of prostaglandins

cyclic nucleotide phosphodiesterase activity, leading to elevated intracellular levels of cAMP, at concentrations that suppress cyclo-oxygenase activity.[122] Some actions of inhibitors of the oxygenation of arachidonic acid may attenuate their anti-inflammatory effects. Indomethacin and salicylates up-regulate some cellular receptors for prostaglandins,[88,105] which may augment or unmask the proinflammatory activities of prostaglandins.

Adrenal Corticosteroids

Since 1950, a staggering number of publications have appeared attesting to the ability of adrenal corticosteroids to suppress undesirable immune and inflammatory reactions (see also Chap. 32). Despite this, we still know relatively little about the precise mechanisms by which the anti-immunologic and anti-inflammatory benefits of these compounds are achieved. Evidence has appeared suggesting that adrenal corticosteroids may act to ameliorate inflammation by interfering with the metabolism of arachidonic acid. Several investigators, for example, have documented that corticosteroids inhibit production of PGE_2 and $PGF_{2\alpha}$ by inflamed synovial tissue.[34,71] In addition, it has been documented that corticosteroids inhibit production by stimulated leukocytes of thromboxane A_2 and stable prostaglandins, and that this inhibitory effect could be overcome by supplying the cells with exogenous arachidonic acid.[26,51] Several observations suggest that corticosteroids inhibit prostaglandin biosynthesis by binding to specific glucocorticoid receptors and by inducing synthesis and release of one or more cellular proteins that inhibit phospholipase activity.

Macrocortin. Three groups of investigators independently observed that inhibition by cortico-

steroids of prostaglandin production by rat renal papillae,[22] perfused guinea pig lungs,[35] and rat peritoneal leukocytes (a mixture of macrophages and polymorphonuclear leukocytes)[18,26] required prolonged incubations and could be prevented with agents that inhibit either DNA-directed RNA synthesis (e.g., actinomycin D) or protein synthesis (e.g., puromycin, cycloheximide). Incubation of rat peritoneal leukocytes with hydrocortisone for 90 minutes resulted in release into the medium surrounding these cells of a nondialyzable "factor" that inhibited production of prostaglandins by fresh leukocytes.[18] The steroid-induced inhibitor of prostaglandin biosynthesis was identified subsequently as a polypeptide, termed "macrocortin."[7] Studies in vitro established that at least some macrocortin is stored in leukocytes (the location was not determined) and that treatment with hydrocortisone for 150 minutes reduces intracellular macrocortin levels by 90%.[17] This phenomenon was confirmed in vivo. One hour after rats were injected with dexamethasone, macrocortin was undetectable in peritoneal leukocytes. After two hours, the macrocortin content of these cells returned to control levels. Markedly increased levels (two to three times control) were detected three to four hours after treatment. Steroids, therefore, appear to stimulate both release and synthesis of macrocortin by rat leukocytes. Interestingly, both effects are inhibited by actinomycin D and cycloheximide. Macrocortin was partially purified from steroid-stimulated guinea pig lungs and rat peritoneal leukocytes, and was found to have an apparent molecular weight of 15,000 (determined by chromatography on Sephadex G-50). The activity of the partially purified material resisted heating at 70°C and acidification to pH 2.0, but was diminished significantly by boiling and by treatment with either trypsin or papain. More recently, the same group of investigators identified a 40,000 dalton substance that exhibited similar biologic activity.[8]

Lipomodulin. Preincubation of rabbit peritoneal leukocytes with adrenal corticosteroids for 16 hours resulted in inhibition of phospholipase A_2 activity in situ, measured by chemotactic factor-induced release of [^{14}C]-arachidonic acid previously incorporated into membrane phospholipids.[65] The inhibitory potency of various corticosteroids correlated well with their anti-inflammatory activity and with their ability to bind to glucocorticoid receptors. Evidence was presented that corticosteroids induced the synthesis of a 40,000-molecular-weight protein ("lipomodulin"), which is expressed on the leukocyte cell surface (i.e., susceptible to digestion with pronase), and which directly inhibited the activity of porcine pancreatic phospholipase A_2. When human fibroblasts were stimulated with bradykinin in the presence of a monoclonal antibody directed against lipomodulin, the cells responded by releasing greater than normal amounts of previously incorporated [^{14}C]-arachidonic acid.[66] This apparent enhancement of phospholipase activity was blocked by adding an excess of lipomodulin (partially purified from supernatants of rabbit polymorphonuclear leukocytes incubated for 16 hours with 1.0 μm fluocinolone acetonide). The activity of partially purified lipomodulin was decreased markedly after treatment with sera from patients with systemic lupus erythematosus, rheumatoid arthritis, and dermatomyositis, as well as with sera from NZB/NZW and MRL/1 mice. The decrease in phospholipase A_2-inhibitory activity paralleled the amount of [^{35}S]-methionine-labeled lipomodulin that was precipitated by these sera. *Sera from patients with various rheumatic diseases apparently contain "autoantibodies" directed against lipomodulin.* It was suggested that such "autoantibodies" facilitate activation of phospholipase A_2 in vivo and play a role in the pathogenesis of immunologically-induced inflammation and tissue injury.

Despite a report suggesting that macrocortin and lipomodulin share similar immunologic properties,[67] it is not entirely clear that they are identical. It also is unclear whether similar proteins are synthesized by corticosteroid-treated human leukocytes.

Whereas most nonsteroidal anti-inflammatory agents effectively inhibit production by leukocytes of prostaglandins by inhibiting cyclo-oxygenase activity, these agents do not influence the formation of lipoxygenase products (e.g., hydroxy-acids, leukotrienes). Anti-inflammatory corticosteroids, on the other hand, may act more "proximally" to

suppress phospholipase activity, thereby reducing the availability of arachidonic acid as a substrate and thus limiting production of inflammatory mediators by both the cyclo-oxygenase and lipoxygenase pathways.

Nonsteroidal Anti-Inflammatory Drugs

The ability of most drugs to inhibit the generation of prostaglandins, thromboxanes, or HETEs has been assessed principally in vitro or in animal models (see also Chap. 28). However, indomethacin and related agents block the production of prostaglandins by human synovial and cutaneous tissues and cells[23,108] and in human subjects[57,112] at clinically relevant concentrations. The specificity of drug action has not been established in most instances. This will be an important goal for future clinical trials in view of the observations that some nonsteroidal agents inhibit the conversion of HPETEs to HETEs.[118] Because HPETEs are potent inhibitors of some steps in the cyclo-oxygenation and further metabolism of arachidonic acid, the HPETEs that accumulate may contribute to the suppression of prostaglandin and thromboxane synthesis by some nonsteroidal agents.

Pronounced inhibition of the effects of prostaglandins on vascular tissue or smooth muscle and of their proinflammatory activities has suggested that some drugs block the transport and/or actions of prostaglandins (see Table 22–2). The competitive inhibition of the effects of prostaglandins was assessed in dog lung or rat intestinal blood vessels for chloroquine and methylxanthines; in uterine or intestinal muscle for indomethacin, naproxen, and cyproheptadine; and in a model of inflammation for colchicine.[84,85,115,116] Antagonism of the effects of an exogenous prostaglandin would seem to be an operationally specific test of mechanism. Few studies, however, have established direct antagonism by receptor analyses or have ruled out an involvement of secondary mediators that might have been the target of the inhibitors. For the lipoxygenase pathways, neither selective inhibitors of generation nor antagonists of the mediators have been assessed in models of inflammation or in clinical states.

REFERENCES

1. Appelgren, L.E., and Hammarstrom, S.: Distribution and metabolism of [^{3}H]-labeled leukotriene C_4 in the mouse. J. Biol. Chem., *257*:531–535, 1982.
2. Aspinall, R.L., and Cammarata, P.S.: Effect of prostaglandin E_2 on adjuvant arthritis. Nature (London), *224*:1320–1321, 1969.
3. Atkinson, J.P., et al.: 5,8,11,14-eicosatetraynoic acid (ETYA) inhibits binding of N-formyl-methionyl-leucylphenylalanine (FMLP) to its receptor on human granulocytes. Immunopharmacology, *4*:1–9, 1982.

4. Bach, M.K.: Mediators of anaphylaxis and inflammation. Annu. Rev. Microbiol., *36*:371–413, 1982.
5. Bailey, J.M., et al.: Regulation of T-lymphocyte mitogenesis by the leukocyte product 15-hydroxy-eicosatetraenoic acid (15-HETE). Cell. Immunol., *67*:112–120, 1982.
6. Bernström, K., and Hammarstrom, S.A.: A novel leukotriene formed by transpeptidation of leukotriene E. Biochem. Biophys. Res. Commun., *109*:800–804, 1982.
7. Blackwell, G.J., et al.: Macrocortin: A polypeptide causing the antiphospholipase effect of glucocorticoids. Nature (London), *287*:147–149, 1980.
8. Blackwell, G.J., et al.: Glucocorticoids induce the formation and release of anti-inflammatory and anti-phospholipase proteins into the peritoneal cavity of the rat. Br. J. Pharmacol., *76*:185–194, 1982.
9. Blotman, R., et al.: PGE_2, $PGF_{2\alpha}$, and TXB_2 biosynthesis by human rheumatoid synovia. *In* Advances in Prostaglandin and Thromboxane Research. Vol. 8. Edited by B. Samuelsson, P.W. Ramwell, and R. Paoletti. New York, Raven Press, 1980.
10. Bonser, R.W., et al.: Esterification of an endogenously synthesized lipoxygenase product into granulocyte cellular lipids. Biochemistry, *20*:5297–5301, 1981.
11. Borgeat, P., and Samuelsson, B.: Arachidonic acid metabolism in polymorphonuclear leukocytes: Unstable intermediate in formation of dihydroxy acids. Proc. Natl. Acad. Sci. U.S.A., *76*:3213–3217, 1979.
12. Borgeat, P., and Samuelsson, B.: Metabolism of arachidonic acid in polymorphonuclear leukocytes. Structural analysis of novel hydroxylated compounds. J. Biol. Chem., *254*:7865–7869, 1979.
13. Bourne, H.R., et al.: Modulation of inflammation and immunity by cyclic AMP. Receptors for vasoactive hormones and mediators of inflammation regulate many leukocyte functions. Science, *184*:19–28, 1974.
14. Boxer, L.A., et al.: Inhibition of polymorphonuclear leukocyte adhesion by prostacyclin. J. Lab. Clin. Med., *95*:672–678, 1980.
15. Bryant, R.E., and Sutcliffe, M.C.: The effect of 3′,5′-adenosine monophosphate on granulocyte adhesion. J. Clin. Invest., *54*:1241–1244, 1974.
16. Cantieri, J.S., Graff, G., and Goldberg, N.D.: Cyclic GMP metabolism in psoriasis: Activation of soluble epidermal guanylate cyclase by arachidonic acid and 12-hydroxy-5,8,10,14-eicosatetraenoic acid. J. Invest. Dermatol., *74*:234–237, 1980.
17. Carnuccio, R., et al.: The inhibition by hydrocortisone of prostaglandin biosynthesis in rat peritoneal leukocytes is correlated with intracellular macrocortin levels. Br. J. Pharmacol.,*74*:322–324, 1981.
18. Carnuccio, R., DiRosa, M., and Persico, P.: Hydrocortisone-induced inhibitor of prostaglandin biosynthesis in rat leukocytes. Br. J. Pharmacol., *68*:14–16, 1980.
19. Corey, E.J., et al.: Synthesis and biological properties of a 9,11-azoprostanoid: Highly active biochemical mimic of prostaglandin endoperoxides. Proc. Natl. Acad. Sci. U.S.A., *73*:3355–3358, 1975.
20. Cox, J.P., and Karnovsky, M.L.: The depression of phagocytosis by exogenous cyclic nucleotides, prostaglandins and theophylline. J. Cell Biol., *59*:480–490, 1973.
21. Cranston, W.I.: Central mechanisms of fever. Fed. Proc., *38*:49–51, 1979.
22. Danon, A., and Assouline, G.: Inhibition of prostaglandin biosynthesis by corticosteroids requires RNA and protein synthesis. Nature (London), *273*:552–554, 1978.
23. Dayer, J.-M., Robinson, D.R., and Krane, S.M.: Prostaglandin production by rheumatoid synovial cells. J. Exp. Med., *145*:1399–1404, 1977.
24. Dey, P.K., et al.: Further studies on the role of prostaglandin in fever. J. Physiol., *241*:629–646, 1974.
25. DiRosa, M., Giroud, J.P., and Willoughby, D.A.: Studies of the mediators of the acute inflammatory response induced in rats in different sites by carrageenan and turpentine. J. Pathol., *104*:15–29, 1971.
26. DiRosa, M., and Persico, P.: Mechanism of inhibition of prostaglandin biosynthesis by hydrocortisone in rat leukocytes. Br. J. Pharmacol., *66*:161–163, 1979.

27. Fantone, J.C., Kunkel, S.L., and Weingarten, B.: Inhibition of carrageenan-induced rat footpad edema by systemic treatment with prostaglandins of the E series. Biochem. Pharmacol., *31*:3126–3128, 1982.
28. Fantone, J.C., Kunkel, S.L., Ward, P.A., and Zurier, R.B.: Suppression by prostaglandin E_1 of vascular permeability induced by vasoactive inflammatory mediators. J. Immunol., *125*:2591–2596, 1980.
29. Fantone, J.C., Kunkel, S.L., and Ward, P.A.: Suppression of human polymorphonuclear function after intravenous infusion of prostaglandin E_1. Prostaglandins Med., *7*:195–198, 1981.
30. Fantone, J.C., et al.: Anti-inflammatory effects of prostaglandin E_1: *In vivo* modulation of the formyl peptide chemotactic receptor on the rat neutrophil. J. Immunol., *130*:1495–1497, 1983.
31. Ferreira, S.H.: Prostaglandins, aspirin-like drugs and analgesia. Nature New Biol., *240*:200–203, 1972.
32. Ferreira, S.H., and Vane, J.R.: New aspects of the mode of action of nonsteroid anti-inflammatory drugs. Annu. Rev. Pharmacol., *14*:57–73, 1974.
33. Ferreira, S.H., Nakamura, M., and Castro, M.S.A.: The hyperalgesic effects of prostacyclin and prostaglandin E_2. Prostaglandins, *16*:31–37, 1978.
34. Floman, Y., Floman, N., and Zor, U.: Inhibition of prostaglandin E release by anti-inflammatory steroids. Prostaglandins, *11*:591–594, 1976.
35. Flower, R.J., and Blackwell, G.J.: Anti-inflammatory steroids induce biosynthesis of a phospholipase A_2 inhibitor which prevents prostaglandin generation. Nature (London), *278*:456–459, 1979.
36. Ford-Hutchinson, A.W., et al.: Leukotriene B_4, a potent chemotactic and aggregating substance released from polymorphonuclear leukocytes. Nature (London), *286*:264–265, 1980.
37. Fridovich, S.E., and Porter, N.A.: Oxidation of arachidonic acid in micelles by superoxide and hydrogen peroxide. J. Biol. Chem., *256*:260–265, 1981.
38. Gallin, J.I., et al.: Agents that increase cyclic AMP inhibit accumulation of cGMP and depress human monocyte locomotion. J. Immunol., *120*:492–496, 1978.
39. Glenn, E.M., and Rohloff, N.: Anti-arthritic and anti-inflammatory effects of certain prostaglandins. Proc. Soc. Exp. Biol. Med., *139*:290–294, 1971.
40. Goetzl, E.J.: Mediators of immediate hypersensitivity derived from arachidonic acid. N. Engl. J. Med., *303*:822–825, 1980.
41. Goetzl, E.J.: Oxygenation products of arachidonic acid as mediators of hypersensitivity and inflammation. Med. Clin. North Am., *65*:809–828, 1981.
42. Goetzl, E.J.: Selective feed-back inhibition of the 5-lipoxygenation of arachidonic acid in human T-lymphocytes. Biochem. Biophys. Res. Commun., *101*:344–350, 1981.
43. Goetzl, E.J.: Leukocyte recognition and metabolism of leukotrienes. Fed. Proc., *42*:3128–3131, 1983.
44. Goetzl, E.J.: The conversion of leukotriene C_4 to isomers of leukotriene B_4 by human eosinophil peroxidase. Biochem. Biophys. Res. Commun., *106*:270–275, 1982.
45. Goetzl, E.J., Brindley, L.L., and Goldman, D.W.: Enhancement of human neutrophil adherence by synthetic leukotriene constituents of the slow-reacting substance of anaphylaxis. Immunology, *50*:35–41, 1983.
46. Goetzl, E.J., Goldman, D.W., and Valone, F.H.: Lipid mediators of leukocyte function in immediate-type hypersensitivity reactions. *In* Biochemistry of the Acute Allergic Reaction. Fourth International Symposium. Edited by E.L. Becker, A.S. Simon, and K.F. Austen. New York, Alan R. Liss, 1981.
47. Goetzl, E.J., and Pickett, W.C.: The human PMN leukocyte chemotactic activity of complex hydroxy-eicosatetraenoic acids (HETEs). J. Immunol., *125*:1789–1791, 1980.
48. Goetzl, E.J., and Pickett, W.C.: Novel structural determinants of the human neutrophil chemotactic activity of leukotriene B. J. Exp. Med., *153*:482–487, 1981.
49. Goldman, D.W., and Goetzl, E.J.: Specific binding of

leukotriene B_4 to receptors on human polymorphonuclear leukocytes. J. Immunol., *129*:1600–1604, 1982.

50. Goldstein, I.M., et al.: Complement and immunoglobulins stimulate superoxide production by human leukocytes independently of phagocytosis. J. Clin. Invest., *56*:1155–1163, 1975.

51. Goldstein, I.M., et al.: Prostaglandins, thromboxanes, and polymorphonuclear leukocytes. Mediation and modulation of inflammation. Inflammation, *2*:309–317, 1977.

52. Goldstein, I.M., et al.: Thromboxane generation by human peripheral blood polymorphonuclear leukocytes. J. Exp. Med., *148*:787–792, 1978.

53. Goldyne, M.E., and Stobo, J.D.: Synthesis of prostaglandins by subpopulations of human peripheral blood monocytes. Prostaglandins, *18*:687–694, 1979.

54. Goldyne, M.E., and Stobo, J.D.: Immunoregulatory role of prostaglandins and related lipids. Crit. Rev. Immunol., *2*:189–223, 1981.

55. Goodwin, J.S., Kaszubowski, P.A., and Williams, R.C., Jr.: Cyclic AMP response to prostaglandin E on subpopulations of human lymphocytes. J. Exp. Med., *150*:1260–1264, 1979.

56. Goodwin, J.S., and Webb, D.R.: Regulation of the immune response by prostaglandins. Clin. Immunol. Immunopathol., *15*:106–122, 1980.

57. Granström, E., and Kindahl, H.: Radioimmunoassay for urinary metabolites of prostaglandin $F_{2\alpha}$. Prostaglandins, *12*:759–783, 1976.

58. Hamberg, M., Svensson, J., and Samuelsson, B.: Thromboxanes: A new group of biologically active compounds derived from prostaglandin endoperoxides. Proc. Natl. Acad. Sci. U.S.A., *72*:2994–2998, 1975.

59. Hammarstrom, S., et al.: Increased concentrations of nonesterified arachidonic acid, 12 *L*-hydroxy-5,8,10,14-eicosatetraenoic acid, prostaglandin E, and prostaglandin $F_{2\alpha}$ in epidermis of psoriasis. Proc. Natl. Acad. Sci. U.S.A., *72*:5130–5134, 1975.

60. Hansson, G., et al.: Identification and biological activity of novel ω-oxidized metabolites of leukotriene B_4 from human leukocytes. FEBS Lett., *130*:107–112, 1981.

61. Hatch, G.E., Nichols, W.K., and Hill, H.R.: Cyclic nucleotide changes in human neutrophils induced by chemoattractants and chemotactic modulators. J. Immunol., *119*:450–456, 1977.

62. Higgs, G.A., et al.: Microcirculatory effects of prostacyclin (PGI_2) in the hamster cheek pouch. Microvasc. Res., *18*:245–254, 1979.

63. Higgs, E.A., Moncada, S., and Vane, J.R.: Inflammatory effects of prostacyclin (PGI_2) and 6-oxo-$PGF_{2\alpha}$ in the rat paw. Prostaglandins, *16*:153–162, 1978.

64. Hirata, F., et al.: Chemoattractants stimulate degradation of methylated phospholipids and release of arachidonic acid in rabbit leukocytes. Proc. Natl. Acad. Sci. U.S.A., *76*:2640–2643, 1979.

65. Hirata, F., et al.: A phospholipase A_2 inhibitory protein in rabbit neutrophils induced by glucocorticoids. Proc. Natl. Acad. Sci. U.S.A., *77*:2533–2536, 1980.

66. Hirata, F.: Presence of autoantibody for phospholipase inhibitory protein, lipomodulin, in patients with rheumatic diseases. Proc. Natl. Acad. Sci. U.S.A., *78*:3190–3194, 1981.

67. Hirata, F., et al.: Identification of several species of phospholipase inhibitory protein(s) by radioimmunoassay for lipomodulin. Biochem. Biophys. Res. Commun., *109*:223–230, 1982.

68. Hirata, F., and Axelrod, J.: Phospholipid methylation and biological signal transmission. Science, *209*:1082–1090, 1980.

69. Issekutz, A.C., and Movat, H.Z.: The effect of vasodilator prostaglandins on polymorphonuclear leukocyte infiltration and vascular injury. Am. J. Pathol., *107*:300–309, 1982.

70. Johnson, R.A., et al.: The chemical structure of prostaglandin X (prostacyclin). Prostaglandins, *12*:915–928, 1976.

71. Kantrowitz, F., et al.: Corticosteroids inhibit prostaglandin production by rheumatoid synovia. Nature (London), *258*:737–739, 1975.

72. Kelly, J.P., and Parker, C.W.: Effects of arachidonic acid and other unsaturated fatty acids on mitogenesis in human lymphocytes. J. Immunol., *122*:1556–1562, 1979.

73. Klein, D.C., and Raisz, L.G.: Prostaglandins: Stimulation of bone resorption in tissue culture. Endocrinology, *86*:1436–1440, 1970.

74. Klickstein, L.B., Shapleigh, C., and Goetzl, E.J.: Lipoxygenation of arachidonic acid as a source of polymorphonuclear leukocyte chemotactic factors in synovial fluid and tissue in rheumatoid arthritis and spondyloarthritis. J. Clin. Invest., *66*:1166–1170, 1980.

75. Kuehl, F.A., Jr.: Role of prostaglandin endoperoxide PGG_2 in inflammatory processes. Nature (London), *265*:170–173, 1977.

76. Kuehl, F.A., Jr., and Egan, R.W.: Prostaglandins, arachidonic acid, and inflammation. Science, *210*:978–984, 1980.

77. Kunkel, S.L., et al.: Suppression of immune complex vasculitis in rats by prostaglandin. J. Clin. Invest., *64*:1525–1529, 1979.

78. Kunkel, S.L., Zanetti, M., and Sapin, C.: Suppression of nephrotoxic serum nephritis in rats by prostaglandin E_1. Am. J. Pathol., *108*:240–245, 1982.

79. Kurland, J.I., and Bockman, R.J.: Prostaglandin E production by human blood monocytes and mouse peritoneal macrophages. J. Exp. Med., *147*:952–957, 1978.

80. Lambert, P.H., and Dixon, F.J.: Pathogenesis of the glomerulonephritis of NZB/W mice. J. Exp. Med., *127*:507–521, 1968.

81. Lee, C.W., et al.: Metabolism of leukotriene D by human polymorphonuclear leukocytes. Fed. Proc., *41*:487, 1982.

82. Lehmeyer, J.E., and Johnston, R.B.: Effect of anti-inflammatory drugs and agents that elevate intracellular levels of cyclic AMP on the release of toxic oxygen metabolites by phagocytes: Studies in a model of tissue-bound IgG. Clin. Immunol. Immunopathol., *9*:482–490, 1978.

83. Lewis, R.A., et al.: Slow reacting substances of anaphylaxis: Identification of leukotrienes C-1 and D from human and rat sources. Proc. Natl. Acad. Sci. U.S.A., *77*:3710–3714, 1979.

84. Manku, M.S., and Horribin, D.F.: Chloroquine, quinine, procaine, quinidine and clomipramine are prostaglandin agonists and antagonists. Prostaglandins, *12*:789–801, 1976.

85. Manku, M.S., and Horribin, D.F.: Chloroquine, quinine, procaine, quinidine, tricyclic antidepressants, and methylxanthines as prostaglandin agonists and antagonists. Lancet, *2*:1115–1117, 1976.

86. Marcus, A.J.: The role of prostaglandins in platelet function. *In* Progress in Hematology, Vol. 11. Edited by E.B. Brown. New York, Grune & Stratton, 1979.

87. Metz, S.A.: Anti-inflammatory agents as inhibitors of prostaglandin synthesis in man. Med. Clin. North Am., *65*:713–757, 1981.

88. Metz, S.A., Robertson, R.P., and Fujimoto, W.Y.: Inhibition of prostaglandin E synthesis in cultured pancreas augments glucose-induced insulin secretion. Diabetes, *30*:551–557, 1981.

89. Milton, A.S., and Wendlandt, S.: A possible role for prostaglandin E_1 as a modulator for temperature regulation in the central nervous system of the cat. J. Physiol. (London), *207*:76P–77P, 1970.

90. Moncada, S., et al.: An enzyme isolated from arteries transforms prostaglandin endoperoxides to an unstable substance that inhibits platelet aggregation. Nature (London), *263*:663–665, 1976.

91. Moncada, S., and Vane, J.R.: Pharmacology and endogenous roles of prostaglandin endoperoxides, thromboxane A_2 and prostacyclin. Pharmacol. Rev., *30*:293–331, 1979.

92. Morris, H.R., et al.: Slow reacting substances (SRSs). The structure identification of SRSs from rat basophil leukaemia (RBL-1) cells. Prostaglandins, *19*:185–201, 1980.

93. Ormstad, K., et al.: Uptake and metabolism of leukotriene C4 by isolated rat organs and cells. Biochem. Biophys. Res. Commun., *104*:1434–1440, 1982.

94. Payan, D.G., and Goetzl, E.J.: The dependence of human

T-lymphocyte migration on the 5-lipoxygenation of endogenous arachidonic acid. J. Clin. Immunol., *1*:266–270, 1981.

95. Payan, D.G., and Goetzl, E.J.: Specific suppression of human T-lymphocyte function by leukotriene B$_4$. J. Immunol., *131*:551–553, 1983.

96. Pearson, C.M., and Wood, F.D.: Studies of polyarthritis and other lesions induced in rats by injection of mycobacterial adjuvant. I. General clinical and pathological characteristics and some modifying factors. Arthritis Rheum., *2*:440–459, 1959.

97. Pelus, L.M., and Strausser, H.R.: Prostaglandins and the immune response. Life Sci., *20*:903–914, 1977.

98. Perez, H.D., Weksler, B.B., and Goldstein, I.M.: Generation of a chemotactic lipid from arachidonic acid by exposure to a superoxide-generating system. Inflammation, *4*:313–328, 1980.

99. Petrone, W.F., et al.: Free radicals and inflammation: Superoxide-dependent activation of a neutrophil chemotactic factor in plasma. Proc. Natl. Acad. Sci. U.S.A., *77*:1159–1163, 1980.

100. Pike, M.C., Kredich, N.M., and Snyderman, R.: Phospholipid methylation in macrophages is inhibited by chemotactic factors. Proc. Natl. Acad. Sci. U.S.A., *76*:2922–2926, 1979.

101. Porter, N.A., et al.: The autoxidation of arachidonic acid: Formation of the proposed SRS-A intermediate. Biochem. Biophys. Res. Commun., *89*:1058–1064, 1979.

102. Porter, N.A., Logan, J., and Kontoyiannidou, V.: Preparation and purification of arachidonic acid hydroperoxides of biological importance. J. Org. Chem., *44*:3177–3181, 1979.

103. Prickett, J.D., Robinson, D.R., and Steinberg, A.D.: Dietary enrichment with the polyunsaturated fatty acid eicosapentaenoic acid prevents proteinuria and prolongs survival in NZB X NZW F$_1$ mice. J. Clin. Invest., *68*:556–559, 1981.

104. Raisz, L.G., and Koolemans-Beynen, A.R.: Inhibition of bone collagen synthesis by prostaglandin E$_2$ in organ culture. Prostaglandins, *8*:377–385, 1974.

105. Rice, M.G., McRae, J.R., and Robertson, R.P.: The prostaglandin E receptor: Induction of density changes in rat liver plasma membrane. Clin. Res., *28*:522A, 1980.

106. Robinson, D.R., Dayer, J.-M., and Krane, S.M.: Prostaglandins and their regulation in rheumatoid arthritis. Ann. N.Y. Acad. Sci., *332*:279–294, 1979.

107. Robinson, D.R., McGuire, M.B., and Levine, L.: Prostaglandins in rheumatic diseases. Ann. N.Y. Acad. Sci., *256*:318–329, 1975.

108. Robinson, D.R., Tashjian, A.H., Jr., and Levine, L.: Prostaglandin-stimulated bone resorption by rheumatoid synovia. J. Clin. Invest., *56*:1181–1188, 1975.

109. Rola-Pleszczynski, M., Borgeat, P., and Sirois, P.: Leukotriene B$_4$ induces human suppressor lymphocytes. Biochem. Biophys. Res. Commun., *108*:1531–1537, 1982.

110. Rola-Pleszczynski, M., Gagnon, L., and Sirois, P.: Leukotrine B$_4$ augments human natural cytotoxic cell activity. Biochem. Biophys. Res. Commun. In press, 1983.

111. Rubin, R.P., Sink, L.E., and Freer, R.J.: Activation of (arachidonyl) phosphatidylinositol turnover in rabbit neutrophils by the calcium ionophore A23187. Biochem. J., *194*:497–505, 1981.

112. Samuelsson, B.: Quantitative aspects of prostaglandin synthesis in man. Adv. Biosci., *9*:7–12, 1973.

113. Samuelsson, B.: Prostaglandins, thromboxanes, and leukotrienes: Formation and biological roles. The Harvey Lectures. Series 75. New York, Academic Press, 1981.

114. Samuelsson, B., Ramwell, P.W., and Paoletti, R. (eds.): Advances in Prostaglandin and Thromboxane Research, Vols. 6–8. New York, Raven Press, 1980.

115. Sanner, J.H.: Substances that inhibit the actions of prostaglandins. Arch. Intern. Med., *133*:133–146, 1974.

116. Sanner, J.H., and Eakins, K.E.: Prostaglandin antagonists. *In* Prostaglandins. Chemical and Biochemical Aspects. Edited by S.M.M. Karim. Baltimore, University Park Press, 1976.

117. Seyberth, H.W., et al.: Prostaglandins as mediators of

hypercalcemia associated with certain types of cancer. N. Engl. J. Med., *293*:1278–1283, 1975.

118. Siegel, M.I., et al.: Arachidonate metabolism via lipoxygenase and 12L-hydroperoxy-5,8,10,14-icosatetraenoic acid peroxidase sensitive to anti-inflammatory drugs. Proc. Natl. Acad. Sci. U.S.A., *77*:308–312, 1980.

119. Simon, L.S., and Mills, J.A.: Drug therapy: Nonsteroidal anti-inflammatory drugs (two parts). N. Engl. J. Med., *302*:1179–1185; 1237–1243, 1980.

120. Sirois, P., et al.: *In vivo* effects of leukotriene B$_4$, C$_4$, and D$_4$. Evidence that changes in blood pressure are mediated by prostaglandins. Prostaglandins Med., *7*:363–373, 1981.

121. Spagnuolo, P.J., Ellner, J.J., Hassid, A., and Dunn, M.J.: Thromboxane A$_2$ mediates augmented polymorphonuclear leukocyte adhesiveness. J. Clin. Invest., *66*:406–414, 1980.

122. Stefanovich, V.: Inhibition of 3',5' cyclic AMP phosphodiesterase with anti-inflammatory drugs. Res. Commun. Chem. Pathol. Pharmacol., *7*:573–582, 1974.

123. Stobo, J.D., Kennedy, M.S., and Goldyne, M.E.: Prostaglandin E modulation of the mitogenic response of human T cells: Differential response of T cell subpopulations. J. Clin. Invest., *64*:1188–1195, 1979.

124. Stone, K.J., Mather, S.J., and Gibson, P.P.: Selective inhibition of prostaglandin biosynthesis by gold salts and phenylbutazone. Prostaglandins, *10*:241–251, 1975.

125. Stossel, T.P., Mason, R.J., and Smith, A.L.: Lipid peroxidation by human blood phagocytes. J. Clin. Invest., *54*:638–645, 1974.

126. Turner, S.R., Campbell, J.A., and Lynn, W.S.: Polymorphonuclear leukocyte chemotaxis toward oxidized lipid components of cell membranes. J. Exp. Med., *141*:1437–1441, 1975.

127. Turner, S.R., Tainer, J.A., and Lynn, W.S.: Biogenesis of chemotactic molecules by the arachidonate lipoxygenase system of platelets. Nature (London), *257*:680–681, 1975.

128. Walsh, C.E., et al.: Effect of phagocytosis and ionophores on release and metabolism of arachidonic acid from human neutrophils. Lipids, *16*:120–124, 1981.

129. Webb, D.R., and Nowowiejski, I.: Mitogen-induced changes in lymphocyte prostaglandin levels: A signal for the induction of suppressor cell activity. Cell. Immunol., *41*:72–85, 1978.

130. Webb, D.R., and Osheroff, P.L.: Antigen stimulation of prostaglandin synthesis and control of immune responses. Proc. Natl. Acad. Sci. U.S.A., *73*:1300–1304, 1976.

131. Webb, D.R., Rogers, T.J., and Nowowiejski, I.: Endogenous prostaglandin synthesis and the control of lymphocyte function. Ann. N.Y. Acad. Sci., *332*:262–270, 1980.

132. Wedmore, C.V., and Williams, T.J.: Control of vascular permeability by polymorphonuclear leukocytes in inflammation. Nature (London), *289*:646–650, 1981.

133. Weissmann, G., et al.: Yin-yang modulation of lysosomal enzyme release from polymorphonuclear leukocytes by cyclic nucleotides. Ann. N.Y. Acad. Sci., *256*:222–231, 1975.

134. Weissmann, G., et al.: Reciprocal effects of cAMP and cGMP on microtubule-dependent release of lysosomal enzymes. Ann. N.Y. Acad. Sci., *253*:750–762, 1975.

135. Williams, T.J.: Prostaglandin E$_2$, prostaglandin I$_2$, and the vascular changes of inflammation. Br. J. Pharmacol., *65*:517–524, 1979.

136. Williams, T.J., and Peck, M.J.: Role of prostaglandin-mediated vasodilation in inflammation. Nature (London), *270*:530–532, 1977.

137. Ziel, R., and Krupp, P.: Influence of endogenous pyrogen on cerebral prostaglandin-synthetase system. Experientia, *32*:1451–1453, 1976.

138. Zurier, R.B., et al.: Mechanisms of lysosomal enzyme release from human leukocytes. II. Effects of cAMP and cGMP, autonomic agonists, and agents which affect microtubule function. J. Clin. Invest., *53*:297–309, 1974.

139. Zurier, R.B., et al.: Prostaglandin E$_1$ treatment of NZB/NZW F$_1$ hybrid mice. II. Prevention of glomerulonephritis. Arthritis Rheum., *20*:1449–1456, 1977.

140. Zurier, R.B., et al.: Prostaglandin E$_1$ treatment of NZB/

NZW mice. I. Prolonged survival of female mice. Arthritis Rheum., *20*:723–728, 1977.

141. Zurier, R.B., et al.: Prostaglandin E treatment prevents progression of nephritis in murine lupus erythematosus. J. Clin. Lab. Immunol., *1*:95–98, 1978.

142. Zurier, R.B., and Ballas, M.: Prostaglandin E_1 (PGE_1) suppression of adjuvant arthritis. Histopathology. Arthritis Rheum., *16*:251–258, 1973.

143. Zurier, R.B., Hoffstein, S., and Weissmann, G.: Suppression of acute and chronic inflammation in adrenalectomized rats by pharmacologic amounts of prostaglandins. Arthritis Rheum., *16*:606–618, 1973.

144. Zurier, R.B., and Quagliata, F.: Effect of prostaglandin E_1 on adjuvant arthritis. Nature (London), *234*:304–305, 1971.

145. Zurier, R.B., and Sayadoff, D.M.: Release of prostaglandins from human polymorphonuclear leukocytes. Inflammation, *1*:93–101, 1975.

Chapter **23**

Characteristics of Immune Complexes and Principles of Immune Complex Diseases

Mart Mannik

Immunologic mechanisms of tissue injury include: (1) IgE-mediated anaphylaxis; (2) complement-induced cell lysis; (3) immune complex mediated injury; (4) cell-mediated immune injury involving specifically sensitized lymphocytes or antibody-dependent cellular cytotoxity; and (5) antibody-mediated neutralization of biologically active molecules. In a given disease more than one mechanism may be operative to cause the clinical manifestations. This chapter will focus on injury mediated by immune complexes.

Tissue injury in immune complex mediated diseases results from the presence of antigen-antibody complexes in tissues. The basement membranes of blood vessels, glomeruli, choroid plexus, and other organs are common locations for deposits of immune complexes. The antigen-antibody deposits may arise from deposition in tissues of circulating immune complexes or from local formation. The diseases mediated by immune complexes share common pathogenic mechanisms, but the underlying causes vary owing to the different origins of the antigens in immune complexes. Since the immune complex diseases have common pathologic mechanisms, their clinical manifestations include common features such as glomerulonephritis, vasculitis, arthritis, skin eruptions, pleuritis, and pericarditis. Such multiple organ involvement is frequent in disorders that result from deposition of immune complexes from circulation. Diseases resulting from local immune complex formation, on the other hand, usually are associated with involvement of a single organ such as the kidney or thyroid gland. In disorders associated with circulating immune complexes, considerable variations occur in the extent of the manifestations among patients and even in a given patient during the course of the disease. The reasons for such variations are still not known. Differences in the nature of the immune complexes, differences in the involved antigens, or alterations in the mechanisms for disposal of

circulating immune complexes may account for variations in the disease expression.

A disease can be categorized as an immune complex disease with certainty when the specific antibodies and antigens that participate in the disease process are identified. Specific antibodies and antigens have been identified in some of the currently established immune complex disorders by elution from one or more target organs, followed by immunochemical identification of the recovered materials. In other disorders the specific antigens in the lesions have been identified by immunofluorescence microscopy, using specific antibodies to the suspected antigens. The currently known human immune complex diseases can be categorized according to the source of antigen, i.e., administered antigens, antigens released from microorganisms, antigens originating from endogenous tissues, and antigens released from tumors. The chronicity of many immune complex diseases results from the continued or recurrent presence of the antigen. Table 23–1 provides several examples of established human immune complex diseases. The list of suspected immune complex diseases is long, and appropriate reviews should be consulted for further detail.[21,41,44] The clinical manifestations of these "suspected" disorders resemble the findings in established immune complex diseases. Immunoglobulins and complement components exist in glomeruli, blood vessels, and other organs characteristic of immune complex diseases, but the specific antigens and antibodies are still not identified.

NATURE OF IMMUNE COMPLEXES

The essential constituents of all antigen-antibody complexes are antigens and antibodies. In any given immune complex, the number of antigen and antibody molecules may vary, depending on the characteristics of each of the reactants and the features of the antigen-antibody union. The biological properties of immune complexes are related to the nature of the molecules forming the complexes, as well as the number of reactants in each complex.

Table 23–1. Examples of Established Human Immune Complex Diseases*†

1. *Due to administered antigens*
   Serum sickness (animal antitoxins and antiserums, other animal proteins and hormones, drugs)
2. *Due to microbial antigens*
   Post-Streptococcal glomerulonephritis (plasma membrane antigens of beta-hemolytic Streptococci)
   Glomerulonephritis of bacterial endocarditis (bacterial antigens)
   Glomerulonephritis of infected ventriculoatrial shunts (*Staphylococcus epidermidis* antigen)
   Glomerulonephritis of syphilis (treponemal antigen)
   Glomerulonephritis of typhoid fever (*Salmonella* Vi antigen)
   Immune complex disease of hepatitis B infection (hepatitis B antigen)
   Glomerulonephritis of toxoplasmosis (*Toxoplasma* antigen)
   Glomerulonephritis of quartan malaria (*Plasmodium malariae* antigen)
   Glomerulonephritis of schistosomiasis (*Schistosoma mansoni* antigen)
3. *Due to autologous antigens*
   Systemic lupus erythematosus (DNA, nucleoprotein)
   Rheumatoid arthritis (IgG as antigen for rheumatoid factors)
   Mixed cryoglobulinemia (IgG as antigen)
   Glomerulonephritis due to renal tubular antigen (renal tubular antigen)
   Thyroiditis with thyroid carcinoma (thyroglobulin)
   Nephropathy of autoerythrocyte-sensitization (red cell stroma)
4. *Due to tumor antigen*
   Colonic carcinoma with nephritis (specific tumor antigen, carcinoembryonic antigen)
   Bronchogenic carcinoma with nephritis (specific tumor antigen)
   Clear cell renal carcinoma with nephritis (proximal tubule brush border antigen)

*The identified antigens are indicated in parentheses.
†Selected references identifying the involved antigens were provided in a previous edition.[30]

Antigens

Antigens are defined as substances that interact specifically with available antibodies or sensitized lymphocytes. The term *immunogen* is reserved for a substance that upon administration to a suitable host will elicit an immune response. This distinction is made because all substances that react with antibodies or with sensitized lymphocytes do not necessarily induce an immune response. Antigens may be proteins, polysaccharides, nucleic acids, lipoproteins, or other chemicals. The actual portion of an antigen molecule that interacts with the antibody-combining site or with a specific receptor of a sensitized lymphocyte is defined as an *antigenic determinant*. The number of antigenic de-

terminants on a molecule defines its valence for the interaction with specific antibodies. Five to six amino acids or six to seven monosaccharide units form the optimal size of an antigenic determinant for the interaction with a specific antibody-combining site. Small molecules with a single antigenic determinant are called haptens. Macromolecules, on the other hand, may be multivalent with several distinct antigenic determinants. Most macromolecular proteins fall into the latter category of antigenic molecules, whereas molecules like DNA with a repeating sequence are more likely to have repeating single antigenic determinants. The number of antigenic determinants of a molecule profoundly influences the kinds of antigen-antibody complexes that may form with the specific antibodies. Clearly, the molecular complexity of antigens increases as one considers microorganisms, cells, or tissues as antigens. For detailed discussions of antigens and antigenic determinants, the reader should consult immunochemical texts.[12]

Chemical features of the antigen may influence the biological properties of immune complexes. A few examples serve to emphasize this point. For instance, exposed galactose residues in a glycoprotein may hasten the removal from circulation of small-latticed immune complexes by interaction with galactose receptors on hepatocytes.[16] Large molecular weight DNA is removed quickly from circulation by the liver and, as a consequence, immune complexes containing such DNA are also quickly removed from circulation.[15] Furthermore, highly anionic (negatively charged) molecules may contribute to complement activation by immune complexes. Finally, cationic (positively charged) antigens can interact with fixed negative charges in tissues and then contribute to local immune complex formation, including the kidney, as will be emphasized later.

Antibodies

Antibodies are the other essential constituents of antigen-antibody complexes; they may belong to the IgG, IgA, IgM, IgD, or IgE classes of immunoglobulins (for detailed discussion of antibody structure see Chapter 15). IgG, monomeric IgA, IgD, and IgE have a valence of two. Dimeric IgA and trimeric IgA molecules have a valence of four and six respectively. IgM molecules exhibit a valence of ten or five, depending on the nature of the antigen. Interestingly, when bivalent IgG molecules interact with a polyvalent antigen with appropriately spaced repeating antigenic determinants, then both antibody-binding sites preferentially react with the same antigenic molecule, giving an apparent valence of one to the antibody molecule. This type of reaction is termed a monogamous bivalent reaction and does not favor the formation of immune complexes with many antigen and many antibody molecules.[23] Antibodies to DNA, for example, may bind with monogamous bivalent interactions to DNA of sufficient size and, in this interaction, cross-linking of DNA strands by antibodies is not favored.[35]

Lattice of Immune Complexes

When antigen-antibody union takes place, various immune complexes may form, ranging from a union of one antigen molecule and one antibody molecule to unions of many molecules of each reactant. The *lattice of immune complexes* is defined as the number of antigen molecules and the number of antibody molecules in a given immune complex. Examples of various lattice formations are schematically depicted in Figure 23–1.

The lattice formation of immune complexes influences their biological properties. Several variables alter the lattice formation of immune complexes. The valence of most antibody molecules is two, as pointed out previously. Polymeric IgA molecules and IgM molecules might form different lattice structures. The valence of antigen molecules profoundly alters the lattice of formed complexes. A monovalent antigen can only form Ag_2Ab_1 complexes; larger lattices and immune precipitates can-

not be formed. Bivalent antigens, depending on the distance between the antigenic determinants, may form Ag_1Ab_1, Ag_2Ab_2, circular Ag_3Ab_3, or larger open or closed complexes. Only multivalent antigens form immune complexes with high degrees of lattice and undergo immune precipitation.

The molar ratio of antigen to antibody influences the degree of lattice formation, as illustrated by the classic precipitation curves. When an increasing amount of antigen is added to a constant amount of antibody, then an increasing amount of precipitate is formed in the antibody excess zone. At the point of equivalence, maximum amount of precipitate is formed, and free antigen and free antibody are not detectable in the supernatant. Addition of antigen beyond the point of equivalence results in soluble immune complexes, and the amount of formed precipitate decreases. With increasing antigen excess, the lattice formation of soluble immune complexes decreases. When a large excess of antigen is used, small soluble immune complexes are formed, consisting of Ag_1Ab_1, Ag_2Ab_2, or Ag_2Ab_1 complexes. In addition, the absolute concentrations of antigen and antibody influence the lattice formation independent of the antigen-antibody molar ratio. At a given degree of antigen excess, more small-latticed immune complexes (Ag_1Ab_1 and Ag_2Ab_2) are formed at microgram

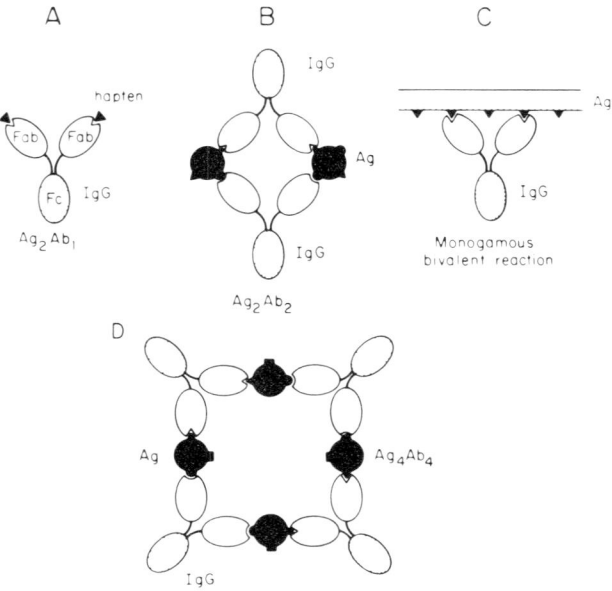

Fig. 23–1. Schematic representation of immune complexes (AgAb) with varying degrees of lattice formation. In *A* the interaction of two small monovalent antigen molecules (haptens) with one antibody molecule is depicted. Diagram *B* shows a small-latticed (Ag_2Ab_2) immune complex formed by multivalent antigen and IgG molecules. Diagram *C* depicts the monogamous bivalent interaction formed by an antigenic molecule with repeating antigenic determinants. A large-latticed (Ag_4Ab_4) immune complex is depicted in *D*, formed with antibodies of two different specificities and an antigen with two different antigenic determinants.

concentrations of reactants than at the same antigen-antibody ratio at milligram concentrations.

The association constant between the antigen and antibody influences the lattice formation of immune complexes. Low-affinity antibodies form smaller immune complexes than high-affinity antibodies with all other variables constant. The principles of determining association constants for monovalent antigens are well established. The principles and methods of measuring association constants for large, multivalent antigens and antibodies are complicated and may lead to errors, depending on the assumed simplifications. The reader interested in further study of the association constants and their measurement should consult texts on immunochemistry.[12]

The characteristics of immune complexes in human diseases have not yet been examined in sufficient detail to relate their features to the disease processes and disease outcome. The concepts established in experimental animals, however, have pointed to the need to develop this information.

BIOLOGICAL PROPERTIES OF IMMUNE COMPLEXES

The key properties of antigen-antibody complexes with respect to immune complex diseases are activation of the complement systems, interaction with cell receptors, and deposition in tissues. These functions depend on the nature of antibodies in the complexes and the degree of lattice formation of the complexes. Other biological properties of immune complexes, such as the influence on the immune response and alteration of the functions of lymphocytes, are less well understood at this time, but have been reviewed elsewhere.[21] Polyclonal B cell activation by immune complexes, however, is a biological property of immune complexes that may have considerable importance in the concepts of autoimmune disorders. Studies in experimental animals have demonstrated that antigen-antibody complexes can lead to antigen independent B cell proliferation and to synthesis of specific antibodies not related to the constituents of immune complexes.[33]

Complement Fixation by Immune Complexes

Complement fixation by immune complexes may proceed through the classic or the alternative pathways of complement activation (see Chap. 21 for discussion of the complement system).

Antibodies of the IgG and IgM class activate the complement system through the classic pathway, provided sufficient lattice formation is present. Among the IgG class of antibodies, IgG1, IgG2, and IgG3 subclasses ae efficient in complement

activation, and the IgG4 subclass is inefficient. The initial step of complement activation through the classic pathway occurs by binding of Clq to the immune complexes. The available evidence indicates that the complexes form a multivalent ligand to bind Clq, thereby activating the complement system, rather than by conformational changes induced by the antigen-antibody interaction. This view is consistent with the observations that even monomeric IgG molecules bind weakly to isolated Clq as examined by analytical ultracentrifugation, including all subclasses of IgG. With multiple IgG molecules, immune complexes are expected to form even firmer bonds with Clq, thus leading to complement activation. As a generalization, with increasing number of IgG molecules, immune complexes become increasingly more effective in binding to Clq and in activation of the complement system. Similarly, with heat-aggregated IgG, effective complement activation is achieved. The number of IgM molecules required in soluble immune complexes has not been carefully delineated, but on cell surface one IgM antibody molecule may suffice to activate the complement system. The other classes of antibodies in immune complexes do not fix complement.

The alternative complement pathway is activated by all immune complexes that activate the classic complement pathway by generating C3b and thereby activating the C3b-dependent loop of the alternative pathway.

Another potentially important activity of the complement system on biological properties of immune complexes is the ability of the complement system to solubilize immune precipitates. When immune precipitates are formed between antigen and antibody at equivalence, and fresh serum is added as a source of complement, then the immune precipitates are converted to soluble, large-latticed immune complexes that contain covalently bound products of C3.[40] This binding of C3 breakdown products to antibody molecules is essential for dispersion of the immune precipitates and for the prevention of reformation of immune precipitates. These solubilized complexes are large. For example, when the system of bovine serum albumin and antibodies to bovine serum albumin is employed, the solubilized complexes have sedimentation constants of 25 to 30 Svedberg units. It is an attractive possibility that complement may prevent the formation of immune precipitates in vivo by a similar mechanism. In patients with systemic lupus erythematosus, the ability of serum to solubilize immune precipitates is decreased,[4] presumably because of lowered complement levels.

Interaction of Immune Complexes with Cell Surface Receptors

The primary interaction of immune complexes with cells occurs through the Fc receptors on neutrophils, monocytes (including tissue macrophages throughout the body, as well as Kupffer's cells in the liver), platelets, and certain lymphocyte populations. These receptors are specific for IgG and do not interact with other classes of immunoglobulins. The carboxy terminal end of the $C\gamma3$ domain (third constant homology region) of the IgG molecules reacts with the Fc receptor of the listed cells. In addition to the Fc receptors, phagocytic cells and some lymphocytes also possess complement receptors. (For detailed discussion of receptors on lymphocytes, monocytes, and neutrophils, see Chaps. 16, 17, and 18, respectively.)

The lattice structure of immune complexes influences significantly their interaction with the Fc receptors. Monomeric IgG molecules bind to these cell surface receptors weakly, but do not trigger the interiorization or engulfment of the attached molecules by the cell. Attachment of complexes with sufficient lattice, on the other hand, results in phagocytosis of the complexes. Small-latticed immune complexes, such as those prepared with divalent and monovalent antigens or prepared by high degrees of polyvalent antigen excess, are not phagocytized by neutrophils or by monocytes. Large-latticed immune complexes, defined as containing more than two antibody molecules, are attached to the Fc receptors and then apparently undergo further condensation or rearrangement to even larger lattices prior to phagocytosis.[14] This condensation to larger lattices was thought to result from the increased local concentration of the soluble immune complexes by interaction with Fc receptors on the monocyte surface. Monomeric IgG1 and IgG3 are effective in inhibiting the attachment of immune complexes to the Fc receptors of neutrophils and monocytes, but IgG2 and IgG4 are ineffective.

The interaction of immune complexes with monocyte receptors occurs via the Fc receptors and can lead to phagocytosis and degradation of the ingested immune complexes. If the immune complexes have reached a sufficient lattice to activate complement, then the C3b bound to immune complexes can facilitate their binding to and phagocytosis by monocytes through the interaction with C3b receptors on these cells. For example, if heat-aggregated IgG, as a surrogate for immune complexes, contains more than 16 IgG molecules, it is effective in complement activation, and phagocytosis of these large aggregates by monocytes is facilitated by presence of complement.[26]

The principles of interactions of monocytes and immune complexes also apply to tissue macrophages, including Kupffer's cells in the liver. The interaction of immune complexes with Kupffer's cells is the basis for their removal from circulation.

As discussed in Chapter 18, during phagocytosis of large-latticed immune complexes, particularly when these materials are attached to a nonphagocytizable surface, lysosomal enzymes spill to the surrounding medium. This event is thought to be highly important in mediating tissue damage during immune complex deposition.

Human platelets interact with immune complexes without the presence of complement components, leading to platelet aggregation and release of platelet constituents that activate the clotting system (see Chap. 20). Platelet aggregation and release of platelet constituents require large-latticed immune complexes. During this release platelets are not lysed. Thus, through interactions with platelets, immune complexes can activate the clotting system, which then may contribute to the final pathways of tissue injury.

Human erythrocytes possess a receptor for C3b that mediates the binding of immune complexes to the red cells. Erythrocytes from patients with active SLE have a decrease in these receptors.[24] In one study, even the relatives of patients with SLE had decreased C3b receptors on erythrocytes, suggesting an inherited defect.[45] The role of this inherited defect in red cell receptors for C3b in pathogenesis of SLE remains to be determined. Furthermore, studies in monkeys have suggested that the C3b receptors on red cells contribute to the removal from circulation of very large immune complexes.[9]

Fate of Circulating Immune Complexes

Once immune complexes are formed in circulation, their subsequent fate and tissue deposition depend on several variables, including the lattice of immune complexes, the status of the mononuclear phagocyte system, the nature of antibodies in the complexes, and the nature of antigen molecules in the complexes. The principles involved in the removal of immune complexes from circulation have been studied in experimental animals.

When immune complexes with known degrees of lattice formation are injected into mice, rabbits, or monkeys, large-latticed immune complexes, composed of lattices larger than Ag_2Ab_2, are rapidly removed from the circulation by the mononuclear phagocyte system, predominantly by the Kupffer's cells of the liver. Small-latticed complexes, composed of Ag_2Ab_2 and Ag_1Ab_1 complexes, persist longer in circulation but are removed more quickly than the antibodies alone. Complement components are not required in this rapid uptake of large-latticed complexes since the depletion of complement with cobra venom factor or with aggregated IgG does not alter the kinetics or quantity of immune complexes cleared by the mononuclear phagocyte system.[31] The mechanism of immune clearance by Kupffer's cells depends on Fc receptors of these cells. Furthermore, Kupffer's cells in hepatic sinusoids are not covered by endothelial cells and are thus directly exposed to the circulating complexes.

The mononuclear phagocyte system in the liver, previously called the reticuloendothelial system, is saturable with carbon particles or with other substances. Competitive uptake, and the inhibition of uptake of one substance by another, is an established phenomenon. The saturation of the mononuclear phagocyte system by large-latticed immune complexes was established by injecting increasing doses of immune complexes.[31] Saturation of this system leads to prolonged circulation of large-latticed immune complexes and thereby to increased risk of tissue deposition. This saturation was detected by using aggregated IgG as a probe for Kupffer's cell function in experimental animals as a surrogate of immune complexes. Small-latticed immune complexes in experimental animals do not alter the clearance kinetics or hepatic uptake of this probe.[25] Patients with systemic lupus erythematosus or other immune complex disease have decreased clearance of antibody-coated red cells in comparison to normal persons.[28] Normal persons with certain histocompatibility antigens (HLA-DR2 and MT-1), however, also have a similar defect.[27] The antibody-coated red cells measure principally uptake by the spleen. Nevertheless, the clearance of these coated cells indicates a malfunction in patients with active systemic lupus erythematosus.

As pointed out, the class and subclass of antibody molecules influence the efficacy of their interactions with monocyte receptors in vitro. These observations suggest that large-latticed immune complexes, containing antibodies that are ineffective in interacting with monocyte receptors, would circulate longer than complexes containing antibodies that interact effectively with these receptors. For example, when the interchain disulfide bonds of the IgG class of antibodies are cleaved by reduction and alkylation, immune complexes made with such antibodies interact ineffectively with monocyte receptors in vitro. The clearance kinetics of such complexes are altered. The large-latticed complexes are removed slowly from circulation of rabbits, monkeys, and mice owing to decreased hepatic uptake. Because of the prolonged circulation of these large-latticed immune complexes, deposition in renal glomeruli is enhanced.[31]

In experimental animals, immune complexes containing IgA class of antibodies are taken up rapidly by the liver when eight or more IgA antibodies are present in the immune complexes.[38] The critical number of eight antibody molecules is achieved either by eight monomeric IgA molecules or by four dimeric IgA molecules. The uptake of these large IgA complexes occurs by nonparenchymal cells and is not blocked by IgG aggregates, indicating that the Fc (IgG) receptors on Kupffer's cells are not involved in removal of these complexes from circulation of mice.

The nature of antigens in immune complexes can alter the fate of circulating immune complexes. For example, certain antigens are rapidly removed from circulation by the mononuclear phagocyte system without the presence of antibodies. Small-latticed immune complexes prepared with such antigens are also quickly removed from circulation. Specific examples of the role of antigens on the fate of immune complexes were already cited in the section on the nature of immune complexes.

Tissue Deposition of Immune Complexes

As already pointed out, the presence of immune complexes in a variety of organs is associated with inflammation and tissue damage. Glomeruli, renal peritubular capillaries, renal tubular basement membranes, small and medium blood vessels in many organs, dermal-epidermal junction, choroid plexus, the basement membrane of thyroid follicles, interstitial spaces in synovial tissue, and articular cartilage are examples of the many sites where immune complexes have been identified. The presence of immune complexes at various sites may arise from deposition of circulating immune complexes or from local formation of antigen-antibody complexes at the site of their presence. The local formation of immune complexes can arise from interaction of antibodies with structural components of the tissue or from selective deposition or presence of an antigen at a given location, followed by specific immune complex formation. A clinical example of local immune complex formation with structural antigens in tissues occurs in Goodpasture's syndrome. Here, antibodies develop to the glomerular basement membrane antigens that also react with the alveolar basement membrane, leading to presence of antibodies uniformly deposited along the glomerular and alveolar basement membranes.

The Arthus reaction is the basic model of local immune complex disease, induced in actively or passively immunized animals by local injection of the antigen. Vasculitis at the site of antigen injection is caused by immune complexes in small vessels, leading to complement fixation and influx of polymorphonuclear leukocytes and later mononuclear cells.[11] Antigen-induced local immune complex disease can be generated experimentally in specific organs, such as joints, pleural cavity, and lungs. Antigen-induced synovitis is an example of local antigen-induced disease, and the formation of immune complexes plays a significant part in the inflammatory process. In these experiments, the injected antigen in the form of immune complexes remains bound to the superficial layers of cartilage and ligaments for prolonged periods, thus prolonging the inflammation. As another example, once tolerance to an endogenous substance is broken, then the autologous tissues can serve as a continued source of antigen to maintain a chronic local inflammatory process. A well-studied example is the thyroiditis induced by injection of heterologous thyroglobulin. Tolerance is broken to thyroglobulin, antibodies are synthesized to thyroglobulin, and immune complexes form at the follicular basement membrane of thyroid follicles.[7] The key point in this disease model is that the follicular basement membrane is the site where the antigen and antibody union occurs, and the formed complexes remain largely localized in this area.

Information is not available to distinguish in human diseases the immune complexes that have arisen at a given location by deposition from circulation from those developed by local formation. The presence of circulating immune complexes in association with tissue deposition should not be considered as unequivocal evidence that the circulating immune complexes were deposited in the tissues. In recent years considerable progress has been made in understanding the development of immune complexes in glomeruli. Therefore, special emphasis will be given to the concepts that have evolved from studies in experimental animals.

In human glomerulonephritis, including the nephritis of systemic lupus erythematosus, and in experimental models of glomerulonephritis, immune deposits are found in three locations. These locations are the mesangium, the subendothelial area, and the subepithelial area (Fig. 23–2). The glomerular mesangium, consisting of matrix and resident mesangial cells, is considered as glomerular interstitial tissue, surrounded by the glomerular capillary loops that are confined by the Bowman's capsule. The glomerular capillary wall is both a size and a charge barrier to macromolecules in circulation. Fixed negative charges are present in the glomerular basement membrane, both in the lamina rara interna (subendothelial area) and the lamina rara externa (subepithelial area). These fixed negative charges in the glomerular capillary wall significantly contribute to the mechanisms of immune complex formation and deposition in glomeruli.

Experimental evidence indicates that some immune deposits in glomeruli arise from deposition of immune complexes from circulation and that other immune deposits in glomeruli develop by local formation of antigen-antibody complexes.

In chronic serum sickness models in experimental animals, the renal lesions contained mesangial, subendothelial, and subepithelial immune deposits. Initially, all these deposits were thought to arise from deposition of circulating immune complexes. Experiments with injection of preformed immune complexes into unimmunized animals, however, showed that complexes in circulation deposit in the subendothelial area and in the mesangium. No deposits were found in the subepithelial area, using rabbit IgG antibodies to human serum albumin, bovine serum albumin, or to the dinitrophenyl antigenic determinants on bovine serum albumin.[31] Several lines of evidence indicate that the lattice of circulating immune complexes is highly important to their deposition in glomeruli. First, when mixtures of large-latticed (greater than Ag_2Ab_2) and small-latticed (Ag_2Ab_2 and Ag_1Ab_1) immune complexes in antigen excess are injected into mice, glomerular deposition of complexes progresses only while the large-latticed complexes remain in circulation. Second, the injection of small-latticed (Ab_2Ab_2, Ag_1Ab_1) immune complexes into mice causes no glomerular immune deposits. Third, when large-latticed immune complexes are deposited in glomeruli, the injection of a large excess of antigen results in complete removal of extracellular glomerular immune deposits, presumably by conversion of the immune deposits to small-latticed immune complexes.[31] Finally, immune complexes deposited from circulation into the subendothelial or mesangial areas must undergo condensation or rearrangement into even larger complexes or small precipitates to persist in glomeruli and to become visible as electron-dense deposits. Proof for this concept was obtained by injecting into mice large-latticed immune complexes that were covalently cross-linked so that these complexes could not rearrange or condense into precipitates. These complexes were only transiently deposited in glomeruli and did not evolve into electron-dense deposits. In contrast, when similar complexes without covalent bonds were administered to mice, the deposits that evolved then persisted and became visible as electron-dense deposits.[32]

These observations collectively indicate that large-latticed immune complexes, containing more than two antibody molecules, become locally concentrated in glomeruli, possibly as a result of transient interactions with glomerular structures. Then, as a consequence of this increased local concentration, they condense into even larger deposits,

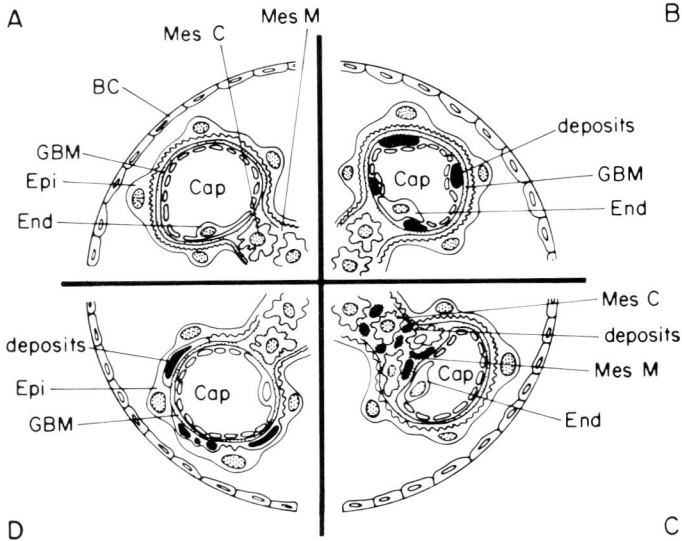

Fig. 23–2. Schematic representation of different localization of immune complexes within the glomerular capillaries. *A*, Normal capillary loop; *B*, pattern of subendothelial deposits; *C*, pattern of mesangial deposits; *D*, pattern of subepithelial deposits. BC = Bowman's capsule; US = urinary space; GBM = glomerular basement membrane; Cap = capillary lumen; Epi = epithelial cells with foot processes; End = endothelial cells with fenestrated cytoplasmic extensions covering the basement membrane; Mes C = mesangial cells; Mes M = mesangial matrix.

comparable to immune precipitates, that become visible as electron-dense deposits in the subendothelial or mesangial areas of the glomeruli. Immune deposits that do not undergo such rearrangement, such as nonprecipitating antigen-antibody systems, persist in glomeruli only a relatively short time.

Electrostatic interactions constitute one mechanism for local increase in concentration of immune complexes in glomeruli. When chemically modified, cationic (positively charged) antibodies were used to prepare soluble immune complexes, the injection of these complexes caused extensive subendothelial deposits that persisted in this location much longer than complexes prepared with unaltered antibodies.[18] The lattice of the injected complexes is still important in that large-latticed complexes (containing more than two antibody molecules) result in deposits that persist for several days, whereas cationized antibodies or small-latticed immune complexes are present by immunofluorescence microscopy only for a few hours, owing to the interaction with the fixed negative charges in glomerular capillary walls. Since the glomerular capillary wall is partially permeable to cationic molecules of even 400,000 molecular weight, but not to cationic molecules of about 1 × 10⁶ molecular weight,[42] the large-latticed complexes with more than two antibody molecules attach to the fixed negative charges in the lamina rara

interna, achieve increased local concentration, and then condense to even larger deposits that persist and become visible as electron-dense deposits. Similar deposits also evolve in the mesangial matrix. Other mechanisms must be involved in the retention and condensation of immune complexes in the mesangial matrix since even highly anionic (negatively charged) antibodies in large-latticed immune complexes result in mesangial deposits.[19]

Several experimental models exist for local immune complex formation in glomeruli due to antigens that become attached or planted in glomeruli. Intravenously injected aggregated IgG or aggregated albumin becomes entrapped in the mesangial matrix, and when antibodies to these aggregated proteins are administered, immune deposits form and an acute inflammatory response ensues in the mesangial area of the glomeruli. Concanavalin A binds to the glomerular basement membrane, and when antibodies to Concanavalin A are administered, lumpy-bumpy immune deposits evolve.[10]

Considerable evidence indicates that the subepithelial immune deposits, as seen in membranous glomerulonephritis, are locally formed rather than deposited from circulation.[10] Evidence for this was marshalled in rats with the Fx1A antigen, derived from the brush border of proximal tubules, and with repeated perfusion of rat kidneys with bovine serum albumin and antibodies to bovine serum albumin. In these experiments the possible formation of immune complexes in the perfusate was excluded. In the first example, the Fx1A antigen is located in the subepithelial area, and the perfused antibodies combine with the antigen to form subepithelial immune deposits. In the second example, some of the perfused bovine serum albumin reaches the subepithelial area and is followed by antibody to form subepithelial immune complexes. The role of the charge on antigens has been extensively studied on glomerular localization. For example, cationized (positively charged) human IgG localizes in rat kidneys and persists there with a half-life of 4.2 hours due to interaction with the fixed negative charges in the glomeruli. When antibodies to IgG are injected after the antigen, then subepithelial immune deposits form, and the antigen persists with a half-life of 21 days in rat glomeruli.[34] Furthermore, the chronic administration of cationic antigens results in extensive membranous glomerulonephritis with subepithelial deposits to a greater extent than achieved with neutral or anionic antigens.[5,17] For the persistence of immune deposits in the subepithelial area and the formation of electron-dense deposits, precipitating antigen-antibody systems are required. Nonprecipitating antigen-antibody systems form only transient deposits that do not become visible as electron-dense deposits.[2] It is also possible that positively charged antibodies become planted in the glomeruli first, followed by antigen, to form immune deposits in glomeruli.[3] Obviously, much work is required to identify and characterize the antigens involved in human glomerulonephritis, but the studies in experimental models have established principles that can be useful in this needed work.

When subepithelial deposits have formed, the glomerulus does not become hypercellular and monocytes do not accumulate; yet, proteinuria becomes prominent. The injury that leads to proteinuria is largely mediated by complement since extensive proteinuria did not evolve in C3-depleted rats with subepithelial deposits.[39]

EXPERIMENTAL MODELS OF IMMUNE COMPLEX DISEASES

The study of immune complex diseases in experimental animal models was first to establish many principles involved in these disorders. The experimental models can be classified as spontaneous disease models, diseases induced by administration of antigen (serum sickness), and abnormalities induced by injection of preformed immune complexes. Furthermore, the serum sickness models can be considered as acute or chronic abnormalities, depending on a single or multiple administration of antigen.

The best known example of spontaneous immune complex disease is murine lupus in the New Zealand and other strains of mice (see Chap. 26).

Acute Immune Complex Diseases

The study of acute immune complex disease or serum sickness in rabbits provided perhaps the greatest initial insight into the pathologic events in immune complex diseases. In this system, large quantities of an antigen are required for intravenous injection in unimmunized rabbits to produce significant disease. For example, 500 mg of bovine serum albumin (BSA) is used for a 2-kg rabbit.[13] When radiolabeled antigen is employed, the events of antigen disappearance can be easily followed (Fig. 23–3). Initially, the concentration of the injected antigen decreases rapidly as a result of intra- and extravascular equilibration. Thereafter, the concentration of the antigen declines gradually as a result of catabolism. When the immune response to the BSA develops after about eight days, then the concentration of the antigen drops rapidly because of antigen-antibody complex formation, resulting in immune clearance of the foreign material. During the immune clearance phase and just prior to this event, circulating immune complexes are easily identified by the presence of a radiolabel on the injected BSA. At the time of immune clearance, the rabbit serum complement level decreases.

Coincident with the immune clearance of the injected BSA, resulting from the formation of large-latticed immune complexes, the rabbits develop glomerulonephritis, vasculitis of many organs, and synovitis. The injected antigen, rabbit IgG, and complement components are present in the glomerular and vascular lesions. This model does not distinguish whether the tissue deposits result from deposition of circulating complexes or from local formation. Vasculitis can be abrogated in this model when complement components (C3) are depleted with cobra venom factor prior to the onset of the immune clearance phase of the disease, thus preventing the development of complement-derived chemotactic factors. The vascular damage is also abrogated by neutropenia induced by nitrogen mustard.[8] Thus, the vascular damage is not caused per se by the deposition of immune complexes, but requires an influx of neutrophils. The development of glomerular lesions is more complex, since the depletion of complement components or neutrophils does not abrogate histologic lesions. On the other hand, a decrease in circulating monocytes decreases proteinuria, indicating that monocytes are involved in mediating the renal damage in this model.[22] The natural course of this acute illness in rabbits is self-limited and abates with return of complement to normal levels and

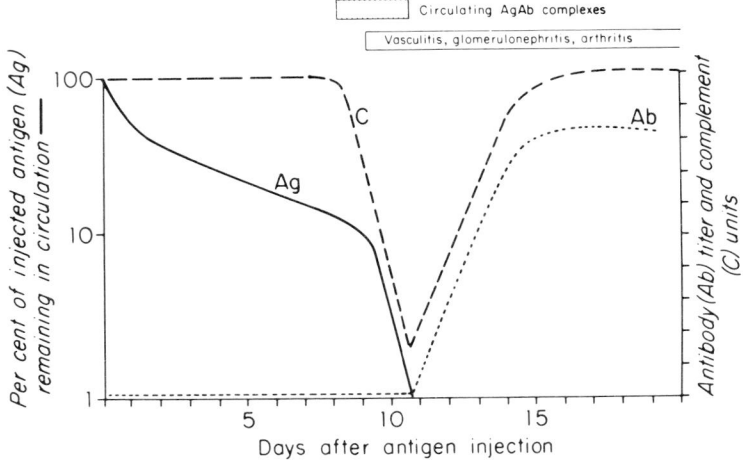

Fig. 23–3. Schematic representation of events in acute serum sickness. The percentage of injected antigen (Ag) in circulation initially declines rapidly as a result of intra- and extravascular equilibration, then decreases as a result of catabolism, and about nine days after injection undergoes immune clearance as a result of antibody synthesis. At the time of immune clearance, circulating immune complexes are detectable and complement (C) is consumed. Vasculitis, glomerulonephritis, and arthritis develop because of immune complex deposition. With the clearance of immune complexes by the mononuclear phagocyte system, the pathogenic process ceases, free antibody (Ab) becomes detectable, and the inflammatory lesions gradually subside.

gradual disappearance of the inflammatory lesions. The immune response in rabbits to BSA persists, but the pathogenic process ceases when the antigen is removed. Similarly, in human diseases when the presence of antigens ceases, the immune complex manifestations abate. The self-limited course of serum sickness from an injected foreign protein and the cessation of glomerulonephritis by appropriate antimicrobial treatment of infective endocarditis serve as excellent examples.

Chronic Immune Complex Disease

The acute serum sickness in rabbits is easily converted to a chronic disease model by injecting repeated doses of the same antigen. If the injected dose of BSA is varied according to the immune response in each rabbit, providing an antigen excess relative to the total amount of antibody, then the disease progresses, invariably leading to a chronic glomerulonephritis and renal failure. On the other hand, if a fixed dose of antigen is given (e.g., 12.5 mg of BSA per injection), then the progression of disease varies according to the immune response of the rabbit.[20] Rabbits that mount a vigorous immune response develop no progressive disease, presumably owing to formation of large-latticed immune complexes that are effectively and promptly removed from the circulation. Rabbits that mount a relatively low immune response have demonstrable immune complexes in circulation, ranging from 500,000 to 700,000 daltons by sucrose density gradient ultracentrifuga-

tion; these persist in circulation up to 24 hours. These animals develop diffuse proliferative glomerulonephritis with deposits of immune complexes in capillary loops in the subepithelial area. As discussed previously under tissue deposition of immune complexes, current evidence indicates that these deposits may have arisen by the alternating presence of antigen and antibody. Rabbits that develop a moderate immune response have circulating complexes of about one million daltons that persist in circulation only for a few hours. These animals develop hypercellularity in glomeruli and mesangial deposits of immune complexes. In addition to glomerular pathology, chronic and frequent antigen administration to immunized animals also causes immune complex mediated interstitial renal lesions.[6]

Disease Induced by Preformed Immune Complexes

Vasculitis and glomerulonephritis are readily induced in mice by injecting large doses or repeated doses of soluble preformed immune complexes. Similar experiments have not succeeded in rabbits, but this may have resulted from inadequate doses of injected complexes as compared to the doses required in mice.[21] Nevertheless, the observation that injected, preformed immune complexes can cause vasculitis and glomerulonephritis confirmed that circulating immune complexes cause lesions, and opened the way for further study of the physiology of circulating immune complexes and elucidation of mechanisms for their deposition in tissues as described previously. Glomerular deposition of preformed immune complexes has already been discussed in detail.

TESTS FOR DETECTION OF IMMUNE COMPLEXES AND CLINICAL APPLICATION OF THESE TESTS

The preceding sections pointed out the relevance of circulating immune complexes to the persistence and chronicity of immune complex mediated disease processes in experimental animals. Therefore, it seems desirable to quantify and to characterize the immune complexes in human diseases to predict disease outcome or even to identify the origin of involved antigens. Many methods have been proposed for the estimation of circulating immune complexes in human diseases. The presence of immune complexes has been demonstrated and claimed in many disorders.[1,41,44,46] No single assay, however, provides an accurate measure of all immune complexes. The most frequently used assays for immune complexes are listed in Table 23–2.

The physical methods for detection of immune complexes depend on separation of these materials from other serum components. Size separations by ultracentrifugation or gel filtration are insensitive and laborious. In addition, small complexes are difficult to distinguish from normal serum macromolecules. These methods alone or in combination with biological methods remain tools for research laboratories. Addition to serum of low concentrations of polyethylene glycol can precipitate immune complexes, but some normal serum proteins are also precipitated with this quick technique. Cryoprecipitation is a property of some but not all immune complexes; furthermore, certain myeloma proteins and Waldenström macroglobulins have the same property.

The biological methods for detection of immune complexes have been extensively employed. All these methods depend on one or the other biological properties of immune complexes already discussed earlier in this chapter. As pointed out, many of these properties depend on the lattice of immune complexes and on the class or subclass of antibodies in the complexes and even on properties of the antigens. Therefore, these biological tests detect various immune complexes with variable efficiency. Another problem is the lack of an ideal standard for the biological assays for immune complexes. Aggregated human IgG is most commonly used as a surrogate standard for immune complexes, but the degree of aggregation is often not adequately standardized. The results are usually expressed as equivalents of μg or ng of aggregated human IgG. Some investigators prefer to express the results as standard deviations above the normal range, established with serums from normal persons.

Table 23–2.   Selected Examples of Methods for Detection of Immune Complexes

Methods	Comments
1. *Physical methods*	
Analytical ultracentrifugation	Relatively insensitive
Sucrose density gradient ultracentrifugation and gel filtration	Can be combined with biological assays to relate activity and size of complexes
Precipitation with polyethylene glycol	Immune complexes are less soluble in polyethylene glycol than other serum proteins
Cryoprecipitation	Some immune complexes, but also other proteins, are insoluble at 4°C
2. *Interaction with Clq*	
Precipitation of radiolabeled Clq with complexes in polyethylene glycol	Extensively used method, able to detect as little as 10 μg of aggregated IgG
Clq-coated polystyrene tubes	Clq-coated tubes bind complexes, detected with radiolabeled antibodies to IgG
3. *Interactions with rheumatoid factors (RF)*	
Solid-phase radioimmunoassay, RF bound to cellulose	Complexes inhibit binding of ^{125}I aggregated IgG by RF
Solid-phase radioimmunoassay aggregated IgG bound to agarose	Complexes inhibit binding of RF to aggregated IgG conjugated to agarose
4. *Interactions with bovine conglutinin*	
Conglutinin-coated tubes	Coated tubes bind immune complexes that contain C3bi, detected with ^{125}I-antihuman-IgG
5. *Interaction with Fc and complement receptors on cells*	
Raji cell assay	C3b and other complement receptors bind immune complexes, detected with ^{125}I-antihuman IgG
Interaction with macrophage receptors	Immune complexes inhibit uptake of aggregated IgG by macrophages

The assays using Clq detect immune complexes that can bind this complement protein. A fluid-phase or a solid-phase assay is used. These methods detect immune complexes containing IgM or IgG that can interact with Clq. As a generalization, immune complexes with large lattices are detected more effectively than immune complexes with small lattices.[43] Thus, the same degree of positivity can arise from the presence of a relatively small amount of large-latticed immune complexes or a relatively large amount of small-latticed immune complexes. Monomeric IgG can interfere to some degree with these tests. Some patients have in serum materials sedimenting with normal IgG (6.6 Svedberg units) that bind to Clq, but the nature of these IgG molecules has not been elucidated. Furthermore, anionic molecules, including DNA, endotoxin, and heparin, can bind to Clq molecules and render the Clq insoluble in polyethylene glycol. On the other hand, in a solid-phase Clq assay, these substances do not interfere with the test results, since binding to Clq is detected by antibodies to IgG or to IgM.

Rheumatoid factors bind to the Fc fragment of IgG and with higher efficiency when the IgG molecules are polymerized in immune complexes or nonspecifically aggregated. Thus, these assays only detect immune complexes containing IgG, and the presence of complement components is not required. Polyclonal rheumatoid factors from patients with rheumatoid arthritis or monoclonal rheumatoid factors from patients with B-cell malignant tumors may be employed for these assays. Again, the assays with rheumatoid factors detect larger complexes more effectively than small complexes. In addition, high concentrations of monomeric IgG can cause false positive tests.

The conglutinin assay detects only immune complexes that have activated complement and contain C3bi. If C3b is present prior to inactivation by the C3b inactivator, the complexes are not detected. Once C3bi is cleaved into C3d and C3c, the immune complexes are no longer effectively detected by this assay. Other systems have taken advantage of specific antibodies to C3b or C3d, adsorbed on the surface of plastic tubes. The binding to the test tube of immune complexes with these complement components is then detected by antibodies to specific immunoglobulins. These systems also detect material in the size range of norml IgG that can arise from solubilization of immune precipitates by complement, consisting of C3d bound to IgG without the presence of antigen molecules.[36]

The most commonly used assay employing cell receptors is the Raji cell assay. The Raji cells are lymphoblastoid B cells derived from a patient with Burkitt's lymphoma. These cells lack surface immunoglobulins, have low-affinity receptors for IgG and high-affinity receptors for activated complement components. Hence, this assay detects immune complexes that have C3b and other complement components bound to them. The binding of immune complexes to the cells is detected with antibodies to IgG or other immunoglobulins. Therefore, the presence of lymphocytotoxic antibodies can lead to false positive results. Even antibodies to nuclear antigens may give false positive tests since these cells extrude or bind DNA at times.

Because all the assays for immune complexes mentioned are not antigen specific, these tests are not specific to a given disease and provide no assistance in reaching a specific diagnosis. The development of assays that identify specific antigens in systemic lupus erythematosus and other disorders may become useful in the future.[29] Several studies have been reported with rheumatic diseases and other disorders, relating the concentration of circulating immune complexes to the severity of the disease. Positive correlations have been reported in patients with SLE, rheumatoid arthritis, certain leukemias, other cancers, Lyme arthritis, and other diseases.[1,41,46] Prospective studies demonstrating the usefulness of one or more tests for immune complexes in decisions of clinical management of rheumatic or other diseases, however, have been lacking or inconclusive. Therefore, some groups have recommended only sparing and judicious use of tests for immune complexes in clinical diagnosis and management[37] until more data become available from researchers. A clinician thoroughly familiar with the interpretation of these tests may find the assays for immune complexes useful as an adjunct with other tests or in place of other tests, such as complement or complement component levels, in guiding therapeutic interventions. The indiscriminate use of these tests, however, should be discouraged.

REFERENCES

1. Agnello, V.: Immune complex assays in rheumatic diseases. Hum. Pathol., 14:343–349, 1983.
2. Agodoa, L.Y.C., Gauthier, V.J., and Mannik, M.: Precipitating antigen-antibody systems are required for the formation of subepithelial electron dense immune deposits in rat glomeruli. J. Exp. Med., 158:1259–1271, 1983.
3. Agodoa, L.Y.C., Gauthier, V.J., and Mannik, M.: Antibody localization in glomerular basement membrane (GBM) may precede in situ immune deposit formation. Arthritis Rheum., 26:S74, 1983.
4. Aguado, M.T., et al.: Decreased capacity to solubilize immune complexes in serum from systemic lupus erythematosus patients. Arthritis Rheum., 24:1225–1229, 1981.
5. Border, W.A., et al.: Induction of membranous nephropathy in rabbits by administration of an exogenous cationic antigen: Demonstration of a pathogenic role for electrical charge. J. Clin. Invest., 69:451–461, 1982.
6. Brentjens, J.R., et al.: Extra-glomerular lesions associated with deposition of circulating antigen-antibody complexes in kidneys of rabbits with chronic serum sickness. Clin. Immunol. Immunopathol., 3:112–126, 1974.

7. Claggett, J.A., Wilson, C.B., and Weigle, W.O.: Interstitial immune complex thyroiditis in mice. The role of autoantibody to thyroglobulin. J. Exp. Med., *140*:1439–1456, 1974.
8. Cochrane, C.G.: Mediation of immunologic glomerular injury. Transplant. Proc., *1*:949–958, 1969.
9. Cornacoff, J.B., et al.: Primate erythrocyte-immune complex-clearing mechanism. J. Clin. Invest., *71*:236–247, 1983.
10. Couser, W.G., and Salant, D.J.: In situ immune complex formation and glomerular injury. Kidney Int., *17*:1–13, 1980.
11. Crawford, J.P., Movat, H.Z., Ranadive, N.S., and Hay, J.B.: Pathways to inflammation induced by immune complexes: Development of the Arthus reaction. Fed. Proc., *41*:2583–2587, 1982.
12. Day, E.D.: Advanced Immunochemistry. Baltimore, Williams & Wilkins, 1972.
13. Dixon, F.J., et al.: Pathogenesis of serum sickness. A.M.A. Arch. Pathol., *65*:18–28, 1958.
14. Dower, S.K., et al.: Mechanism of binding of multivalent immune complexes to Fc receptors. 1. Equilibrium binding. Biochemistry, *20*:6326–6334, 1981.
15. Emlen, W., and Mannik, M.: Clearance of circulating DNA-antiDNA immune complexes in mice. J. Exp. Med., *155*:1210–1215, 1982.
16. Finbloom, D.S., et al.: The influence of antigen on immune complex behavior in mice. J. Clin. Invest., *68*:214–224, 1981.
17. Gallo, G.R., et al.: Nephritogenicity and differential distribution of glomerular immune complexes related to immunogen charge. Lab. Invest., *48*:353–362, 1983.
18. Gauthier, V.J., Mannik, M., and Striker, G.E.: Effect of cationized antibodies in preformed immune complexes on deposition and persistence in renal glomeruli. J. Exp. Med., *156*:766–777, 1982.
19. Gauthier, V.J., Striker, G.E., and Mannik, M.: Glomerular localization of immune complexes prepared with anionic antibodies or with cationic antigens. Lab. Invest. In press, 1984.
20. Germuth, F.G. Jr., and Rodriguez, E.: Immunopathology of the Renal Glomerulus. Boston, Little, Brown and Co., 1973.
21. Haakenstad, A.O., and Mannik, M.: The biology of immune complexes. *In* Autoimmunity. Edited by N. Talal. New York, Academic Press, 1977, pp. 277–360.
22. Holdsworth, S.R., Neale, T.J., and Wilson, C.B.: Abrogation of macrophage-dependent injury in experimental glomerulonephritis in the rabbit. Use of an antimacrophage serum. J. Clin. Invest., *68*:686–698, 1981.
23. Hornick, C.J., and Karush, F.: Antibody affinity. III. The role of multivalence. Immunochemistry, *9*:325–340, 1972.
24. Iida, K., Mornaghi, R., and Nussenzweig, V.: Complement receptor (CR₁) deficiency in erythrocytes from patients with systemic lupus erythematosus. J. Exp. Med., *155*:1427–1438, 1982.
25. Jimenez, R.A.H., Haakenstad, A.O., and Mannik, M.: Hepatic uptake of small-latticed immune complexes does not alter mononuclear phagocyte system function. Immunology, *48*:205–210, 1983.
26. Kijlstra, A., van Es, L.A., and Daha, M.R.: The role of complement in the binding and degradation of immunoglobulin aggregates by macrophages. J. Immunol., *123*:2488–2493, 1979.
27. Kimberly, R.P., et al.: Impaired Fc-mediated mononuclear phagocyte system clearance in HLA-DR2 and MR1-positive healthy young adults. J. Exp. Med., *157*:1698–1703, 1983.
28. Kimberly, R.P., and Ralph, R.: Endocytosis by the mononuclear phagocyte system and autoimmune disease. Am. J. Med., *74*:481–483, 1983.
29. Maire, M.A., et al.: Identification of components of IC purified from human sera. I. Immune complexes purified from sera of patients with SLE. Clin. Exp. Immunol., *51*:215–224, 1983.
30. Mannik, M.: Characteristics of immune complexes and principles of immune complex diseases. *In* Arthritis and Allied Conditions, 9th Ed. Edited by D.J. McCarty. Philadelphia, Lea & Febiger, 1979, pp. 256–267.
31. Mannik, M.: Pathophysiology of circulating immune complexes. Arthritis Rheum., *25*:783–787, 1982.
32. Mannik, M., Agodoa, L.Y.C., and David, K.A.: Rearrangement of immune complexes in glomeruli leads to persistence and development of electron dense deposits. J. Exp. Med., *157*:1516–1528, 1983.
33. Morgan, E.L., and Weigle, W.O.: Polyclonal activation of murine B lymphocytes by immune complexes. J. Immunol., *130*:1066–1070, 1983.
34. Oite, T., et al.: Quantitative studies of in situ immune complex glomerulonephritis in the rat induced by planted, cationized antigen. J. Exp. Med., *155*:460–474, 1982.
35. Papalian, M., et al.: Reaction of systemic lupus erythematosus antinative DNA antibodies with native DNA fragments from 20 to 1200 base pairs. J. Clin. Invest., *65*:469–477, 1980.
36. Pereira, A.B., Theofilopoulos, A.N., and Dixon, F.J.: Detection and partial characterization of circulating immune complexes with solid-phase anti-C3. J. Immunol., *125*:763–770, 1980.
37. Report of IUIS/WHO Working Group: Use and abuse of laboratory tests in clinical immunology: Critical considerations of eight widely used diagnostic procedures. Clin. Exp. Immunol., *46*:662–674, 1981.
38. Rifai, A., and Mannik, M.: Clearance kinetics and fate of mouse IgA immune complexes prepared with monomeric or dimeric IgA. J. Immunol., *130*:1826–1832, 1983.
39. Salant, D.J., et al.: A new role for complement in experimental membranous nephropathy in rats. J. Clin. Invest., *66*:1339–1350, 1980.
40. Takahashi, M., et al.: Mechanism of solubilization of immune aggregates by complement. Implication for immunopathology. Transplant Rev., *32*:121–139, 1976.
41. Theofilopoulos, A.N., and Dixon, F.J.: The biology and detection of immune complexes. Adv. Immunol., *28*:89–220, 1979.
42. Vogt, A., et al.: Interaction of cationized antigen with rat glomerular basement membrane: In situ immune complex formation. Kidney Int., *22*:27–35, 1982.
43. Wener, M.H., and Mannik, M.: Influence of immune complex lattice on the Clq solid phase assay as determined with covalently cross-linked immune complexes. Clin. Exp. Immunol., *52*:543–550, 1983.
44. Williams, R.C., Jr.: Immune Complexes in Clinical and Experimental Medicine. Cambridge, Harvard University Press, 1980.
45. Wilson, J.G., et al.: Mode of inheritance of decreased C3b receptors on erythrocytes of patients with systemic lupus erythematosus. N. Engl. J. Med., *307*:981–986, 1982.
46. Zubler, R.H., and Lambert, P.H.: Detection of immune complexes in human diseases. Prog. Allergy, *24*:1–48, 1978.

Chapter 24

Genetic Structure and Functions of the Major Histocompatibility Complex

Hugh O. McDevitt

The mammalian major histocompatibility complex (MHC) is defined as the genetic region that determines the structure of those cell surface molecules that elicit the strongest transplantation rejection reaction. Historically, the MHC was characterized in just this fashion. In recent years, it has become apparent that the major transplantation antigens are the gene products of a complex genetic system intimately related to the development of immune responsiveness at several levels. Possibly because of this role in regulating immune responsiveness, the major histocompatibility antigens also show a striking relationship with a number of human diseases, as well as animal disease models. Ankylosing spondylitis, a number of diseases related to ankylosing spondylitis such as Reiter's disease, rheumatoid arthritis (RA), and psoriasis are all associated with the major transplantation antigen system in man, as discussed in Chapter 25. Knowledge of the genetic structure of the MHC and of the defined functions of these genes is important in understanding these associations and, possibly, the pathogenesis of these diseases.

The genetic structure of the MHC in mouse and man, the biochemistry of the identifiable gene products, and the function of these genes and gene products in relation to regulation of the immune response and disease susceptibility are described in this chapter. Although these genes may have other, as yet undiscovered, functions, it is already clear that they play a major role in regulating immune responsiveness.

GENETIC STRUCTURE AND BIOCHEMISTRY

Our understanding of the MHC is most advanced in the mouse and in man. The genes, gene products, and functions of this system in both species appear to be similar in most respects. The genetic organization of the MHC varies in the two species, however, and the nomenclature differs radically. The genetic analysis of the murine MHC is more advanced. For this reason, the genetic structure of

the murine MHC is presented first, followed by a discussion of the homologous genes in the human MHC.

The MHC was the second histocompatibility-determining locus described in the mouse and therefore is designated H-2. The MHC includes three major classes of genes and gene products.

Definitions

Class I Molecules

These cell surface glycoproteins are found on all nucleated cells and platelets. These molecules were originally detected by isoimmunization to produce isoantisera. The presence or absence of H-2 incompatibility in a donor-recipient pair is correlated with rapid, as opposed to subacute or slow, graft rejection. Isolation of cDNA clones encoding some of the Class I MHC proteins has revealed, in both mouse and man, a large number of Class I MHC genes. The mouse has 30 to 40 Class I MHC genes, and man has at least 20 Class I genes.

Class I genes fall into two subclasses. The first comprises the typical or "classic" major histocompatibility antigens, which, as noted previously, are expressed on all nucleated cells and platelets and exhibit a high degree of genetic polymorphism. In the mouse, these genes are designated H-2K, H-2D, H-2L, and H-2R. The second subclass of Class I MHC genes differs from the foregoing in that this subclass has a restricted tissue distribution and a minimal degree of genetic polymorphism. These gene products are expressed on thymocytes, on subsets of peripheral thymus-derived lymphocytes, and on thymus-derived leukemias. The known genes of this type are *Tla* (thymus leukemia antigen) and Qa-1, Qa-2, and Qa-3, which are expressed on functionally distinct peripheral T-cell subpopulations. Some of the Class I genes in the Qa-Tla region are pseudogenes, with stop codons that lead to failure of expression. Some of them are probably expressed, although their gene products have not yet been detected biochemically or serologically and their functions have not yet been characterized.

Class II Genes and Gene Products

These entities are the products of the murine I region. The I region was originally identified because immune response (Ir) genes, which determined the ability of a particular inbred strain of mouse to respond to synthetic polypeptide antigens, were localized to the chromosomal segment to the right of the *H2-K* locus. Subsequently, a number of other immunologic functions were localized to this chromosomal segment, and a new set of cell surface alloantigens, originally designated as the *I*-region *associated*, or *Ia* antigens, were also mapped to this same chromosomal segment. The Ia antigens are the Class II MHC gene products, and their structure and function are described in detail later in this chapter.

S Region Genes

These S region genes are the structural genes for several of the complement components in the classic and alternate pathways of complement activation, including C2, C4, and properdin factor B.

Characteristics and Structure

These three classes of gene products are found in both the murine and the human MHC. Each set of gene products is involved in or regulates one or more aspects of the immune response. The functional characteristics of each of the three classes of genes are discussed following a brief description of the genetic fine structure of the murine MHC and the biochemical characteristics of each of the three sets of gene products.

Class I

Figure 24–1 (top) is a schematic diagram of the linkage map of the seventeenth mouse chromosome. The histocompatibility-2 (H-2) region is a small chromosomal area approximately 15 centimorgans to the right of the centromere.*

The H-2 region, a small portion of the seventeenth mouse chromosome, covers a genetic distance of 1.0 centimorgan. Although this distance is small in terms of the size of the seventeenth chromosome, it is sufficient to encode as many as 200 polypeptides of approximately 20,000 daltons. The exact number of genes in the H-2 complex is still not known, but it is likely to be less than 200.

As discussed later, at least 40 to 50 genes have been identified in the H-2 complex. The true number of genes is probably somewhere between 50 and 200, most likely in the low hundreds.

Figure 24-1 (center) is a schematic diagram of the genetic fine structure of the H-2 region itself. The left-hand and right-hand limits of the H-2 region are given by the H-2K and H-2D loci. These loci determine the structure of the classic, serologically detected major transplantation antigens found on the surface of all nucleated cells as well as on platelets and red cells. The H-2K and H-2D,L,R gene products are 44,000-M.W. glycoproteins located in the cell membrane as a 2-chain molecule in which each H-2K or H-2D,L,R polypeptide chain is tightly bound to a 12,000-M.W. polypeptide known as β_2-microglobulin. The molecular weight of the 2-chain molecule is 56,000. The H-2K and H-2D,L and R genes code for the 44,000 M.W. glycoprotein of the H-2 molecule on the cell surface. The β_2-microglobulin molecule is under the control of a structural gene on a separate chromosome. This arrangement of a heavy and a light chain is reminiscent of immunoglobulin structure, a similarity strengthened by the marked amino acid sequence homology between β_2-microglobulin and a portion of the constant region of the IgG immunoglobulin heavy chain. This finding has led to speculation that immunoglobulins may have evolved from a primitive recognition system represented by the transplantation antigen system.

Support for this hypothesis comes from extensive amino acid sequence data, as well as from nucleotide sequencing of cDNA clones of Class I MHC gene products. Class I MHC molecules, as well as Class II MHC molecules, show extensive amino acid sequence homology with the amino acid sequences of the constant regions of immunoglobulin heavy-chain polypeptides. Thus, Class I and Class II MHC molecules, β_2-microglobulin, and immunoglobulin molecules all share marked, definite amino acid sequence homology that indicates a common ancestral gene, which evolved by a process of tandem gene duplication into many Class I and Class II MHC genes, the β_2-microglobulin gene, and many constant and variable-region genes for both heavy and light immunoglobulin chains.

The structure of Class I and Class II MHC molecules is shown in Figures 24–2 and 24–3. The Class I MHC molecule is composed of the MHC-encoded heavy chain, which is organized into three folded globular domains and associates with the β_2-microglobulin single globular domain to form a four-domain molecule with a two-fold axis of symmetry, as indicated in Figure 24–2. Most of the alloantigenic sites for Class I molecules are located

---

*Genetic distances are expressed as cross-over frequencies. Thus, 2 loci on the same chromosome that show genetic recombination or crossing over 15 times in 100 potentially informative matings are said to be 15 map units, or cross-over units, or centimorgans, apart.

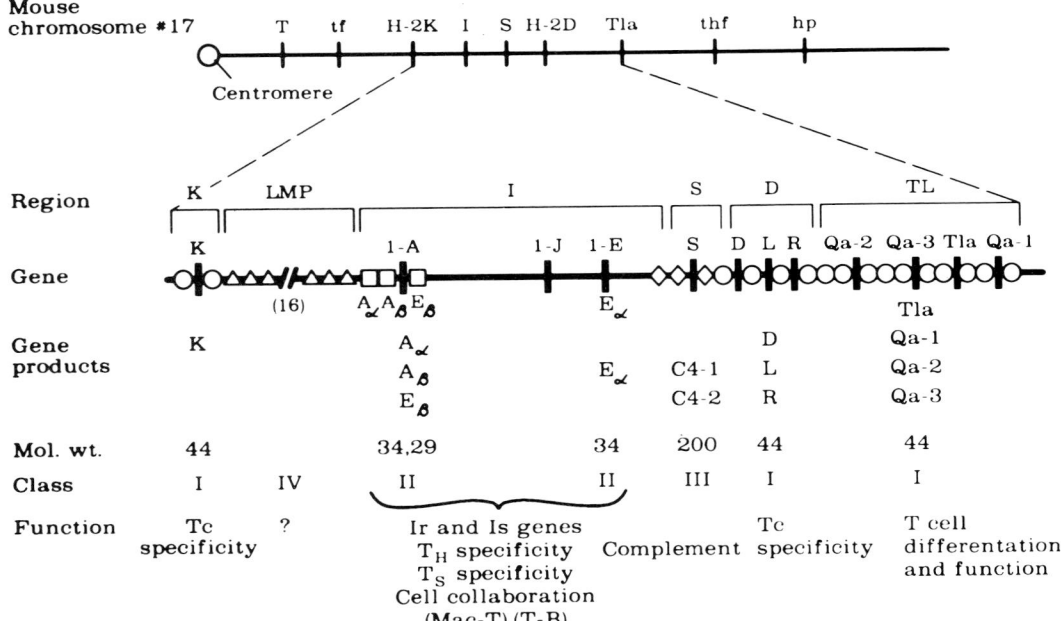

Fig. 24–1. A schematic diagram of the genes of the murine major histocompatibility system. These genes in the mouse are located on the seventeenth chromosome, shown at the top of the diagram. The major histocompatibility system is shown in an expanded version in the second tier of the diagram, in which it is broken up into subregions. Class I major histocompatibility genes are found in the K, D, and TL regions, whereas Class II major histocompatibility genes (defined in the text) are found in the I region. Class III genes encoding several of the components of the complement system are found in the S region, and 16 polypeptides are encoded by genes in the LMP region. The function of Class I and Class II genes is described in the text, and the function of Class IV genes is unknown.

in the first and second domains, and the third domain has the most marked amino acid sequence homology with immunoglobulin-constant region domains and is probably closely associated with the β_2-microglobulin molecule. When visualized in this manner, a striking similarity exists between the (hypothetic) spatial organization of the Class I MHC molecules and that of the Class II MHC molecules, which are seen in Figure 24–3. Both are similar to the Fab fragment of an IgG immunoglobulin molecule.

Class II

Class II MHC molecules also have four domains, but in this case, two of the domains are in a 34,000-M.W. heavy chain, designated the α chain, whereas the other domains are in a 29,000-M.W. light chain, designated the β chain of the Class II molecule. Once again, the α chain and the β chain have two domains. The second domain of the α chain and the first and second domains of the β chain have approximately 100 amino acid residues each, with an intrachain disulfide loop with a spacing of approximately 60 amino acid residues and definite immunoglobulin amino acid sequence ho-

mology around the cysteine residues. All these characteristics indicate definite structural homology with immunoglobulin molecules. Analysis of predicted (from cDNA clones) amino acid sequence of multiple alleles of the α and β chains of murine Class II molecules indicates that most of the alloantigenic sites, that is, the sites of variation among different genetic forms or alleles of the gene product, are clustered in the first domains of the α and β chains. In addition, in both the α and β chains, the sites of allelic variation cluster into 3 regions around residues 5 to 15, 45 to 60, and 70 to 85, with slight differences between α and β chains; these are the regions of "allelic hypervariability."

These allelic hypervariable regions, their localization, and their spacing are reminiscent of the location and spacing of hypervariable regions in immunoglobulin molecules. This analogy suggests that the first and second domains of the α and β chains are folded in the "classic immunoglobulin fold" in a series of antiparallel sheets, so the allelic hypervariable regions are all located at one end of the molecule. Depending on the three-dimensional position of the first domain of the α and β chains,

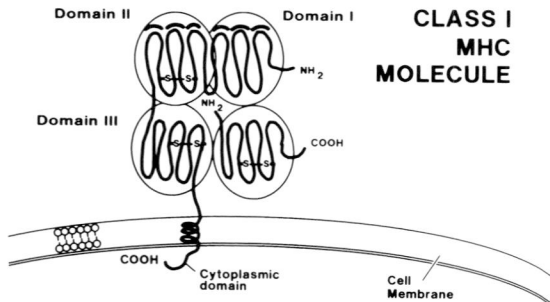

CLASS I MHC MOLECULE

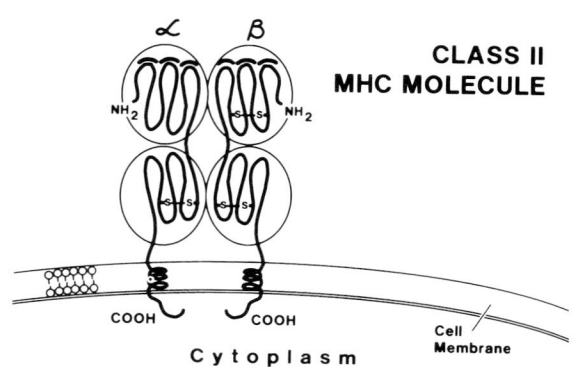

CLASS II MHC MOLECULE

Fig. 24–2. A schematic diagram of a Class I major histocompatibility (MHC) protein. The heavy chain (molecular weight 44,000) is organized into three globular protein domains labeled I, II and III, a transmembrane domain, and a short cytoplasmic domain. Domains I, II, and III of the heavy chain and the β_2-microglobulin domain unite to form a protein composed of four globular domains arranged as indicated in the diagram with a twofold access of symmetry. This arrangement is derived from preliminary analysis of crystals of a human Class I MHC protein. Analysis of Class I mutants in the mouse has suggested that most of the variation in amino acid sequence, which affects immunologic recognition, occurs in the first and second domains of the heavy chain of the Class I MHC protein. The sites of these variations are indicated as arcs, but their true position is unknown.

it is possible that a single alloantigenic site could be generated, with at least six "allelic hypervariable" regions. These sites of allelic variation, presumably all clustered at one end of the molecule, are probably responsible for the differences in immune responsiveness among various inbred strains of mice.

Figure 24–2 illustrates the similarity of Class I molecules in spatial organization to the Class II molecule. In addition, the knowledge that the major alloantigenic sites occur in the first and second domains of the Class I molecules suggests that the Class I molecules may have a similar "active" site at one end of the molecule, notably, the end projecting from the cell membrane's surface. Despite the similar spatial organization, a sharp division in function exists between the Class I and Class II MHC molecules, as discussed later.

The major histocompatibility antigens are unusual among mammalian isoantigenic systems in their high degree of stable, balanced polymorphism. A polymorphism is said to exist in a population when two or more different forms of the same gene and gene product are found in the population, both of which are present in more than 1% of individuals. One of the most striking characteristics of the MHC in both mouse and man is that the Class I transplantation antigens show an enormous degree of genetic polymorphism. In the

Fig. 24–3. A schematic diagram of a Class II major histocompatibility (MHC) protein. This protein is composed of two polypeptide chains, an α chain of 34,000 M.W. and a β chain of 29,000 M.W. As indicated in the diagram, three of these domains have intrachain disulfide loops with spacing reminiscent of immunoglobulin domains. Analyses of nucleotide sequence of complementary DNA clones of several different genetic forms (alleles) of the Aα chain and the Aβ chains have shown that the major sequence differences between different alleles of the α and β chains occur in the first domain, and within the first domain, they occur in three "allelic hypervariable" regions positioned similarly to the hypervariable regions in immunoglobulin molecules. The position of these allelic hypervariable regions in space is still unknown. In the diagram, they are depicted at the end of the molecule (indicated by arcs) that is open to the aqueous environment in a manner similar to that seen in the three-dimensional folding of the antibody molecule.

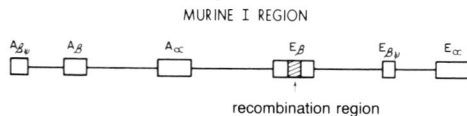

Fig. 24–4. A schematic diagram of the genetic organization of the murine I region.

mouse, continued sampling of new wild mouse isolates from different geographic regions has shown that each new population tested has at least one or two new and previously undetected antigenic specificities. Given the worldwide distribution of *Mus musculus,* the polymorphism at these loci is enormous. In man, a high degree of polymorphism for the homologous loci is also seen.

The genetic fine structure of the murine *I* response region, as determined by serologic and biochemical methods, is shown in Figure 24–1. The genetic organization of this region as shown by recombinant DNA techniques is shown in Figure 24–4. It is now apparent that the I-A subregion encodes two genes for the A$_\beta$ polypeptide chain, of which one is expressed, and one expressed gene for the A_α polypeptide chain. In addition, the I-A subregion encodes a part of the E_β polypeptide chain. The remainder of the I-E molecule falls into the I-E subregion, which encodes the $E\alpha$ polypeptide chain. To date, it has not been possible to identify a gene responsible for the antigenic determinants mapped to the I-J subregion. This subregion was originally defined as encoding antigenic determinants selectively expressed on antigen specific suppressor T cells. Although monoclonal antibodies already isolated can detect an antigenic determinant on suppressor T cells and suppressor-T-cell factors, none of the methods of molecular biology have yet succeeded in the search for a gene to encode these I-J antigenic determinants. It is possible that these determinants arise from differential processing of messenger RNA from genes in the I region, or multiple cross-overs have given rise to a false map position for the I-J gene. The existence of distinct antigenic determinants on suppressor T cells seems to be beyond doubt, but the gene encoding these determinants, their nature, and their location remains to be determined.

The subject, of course, is important because of the possibility of using antisera to T-suppressor-cell antigenic determinants for a variety of types of immunotherapy.

Class III

The murine S region includes genes encoding the second and fourth components of complement, C2 and C4, and properdin factor B, the analogue of C2 in the alternate pathway of complement activation. Recent evidence in man indicates that the corresponding genes in man show not only duplication, at least of the gene for C4, but also a much higher degree of genetic polymorphism than originally suspected. Thus, the S region, like the other regions of the MHC, includes multiple copies of closely related genes showing an unusually high degree of genetic polymorphism.

No amino acid sequence homology exists between the Class III MHC genes and the Class I and Class II genes; however, the close functional interactions between antibody molecules and components of the complement system, the regulation of antibody production by the Class II MHC molecules, and the possibility that complement molecules may also be involved in activation of cells in the immune system suggest that Class III MHC molecules may be functionally related to the Class I and Class II MHC molecules. This interrelationship has considerable clinical as well as biologic significance. Evidence now indicates that C2 genes are associated with unusual susceptibility to certain rheumatic diseases, particularly a syndrome resembling systemic lupus erythematosus. The mechanism for this association must await further characterization of the C2, C4, and properdin factor B gene products, their genetic polymorphism, and the association of particular forms of C2, C4, and Bf with particular diseases.

FUNCTION OF MHC GENES

A major function of the Class I and Class II MHC molecules is to influence the manner in which foreign antigens are seen by the immune receptors on thymus-derived lymphocytes.

Thymus-Derived Lymphocytes

Peripheral, functionally mature thymus-derived lymphocytes are divided into several distinct subcategories (see also Chap. 17).

Cytotoxic or Killer T-Lymphocytes

These lymphocytes are responsible for direct cell-mediated cytotoxicity, independent of immunoglobulin molecules, and for a variety of types of cellular immunity, including graft rejection. These cells are called cytotoxic T cells, or T_c cells.

Helper T Cells

These T cells interact with antigen on the surface of antigen-presenting macrophages and B cells and also interact with other T-cell subsets. Thus, helper T cells, when presented with antigen on the surface of antigen-presenting macrophages or B cells, stimulate B cells to proliferate and to produce antibody. Helper T cells can interact with precursors of cytotoxic T cells and precursors of suppressor T cells to stimulate the production of suppressor or cytotoxic T cells.

Suppressor T Cells

Suppressor T cells interact directly with other T-cell subsets, presumably in the presence of antigen, to suppress the action and proliferation of helper T cells and to suppress the production of cytotoxic T cells from cytotoxic-T-cell precursors. They may also act directly on B cells.

Cell Surface Antigens

During the past several years, it has become apparent that cytotoxic T cells and helper T cells can be distinguished on the basis of the presence on the surface of these cells of distinct cell surface antigens. Thus, in the mouse, helper T cells express a large amount of a cell surface antigen designated Lyt-1 and no Lyt-2,3, whereas cytotoxic T cells express little Lyt-1 and large amounts of Lyt-2,3.

Class I and Class II MHC molecules appear to influence the manner in which these cells recognize foreign antigen. As an oversimplification, it appears that cytotoxic T cells see antigen *in the context* of Class I MHC molecules, whereas helper T cells see antigens *in the context* of Class II MHC molecules.

The key words in this description are "seen in the context of." The experimental phenomenon is as follows: After immunization with cells bearing viruses, minor histocompatibility antigens, or haptens complexed to cell surface antigens, the cytotoxic T cells that develop are capable of killing target cells *only* when the target cell has on its surface both the foreign antigenic determinant, such as the virus, minor histocompatibility antigen, or hapten, and the *same* Class I MHC gene product, H-2K,D,L, or R, present on the immunizing cells used to elicit the cytotoxic T cells. Similarly, following injection of soluble protein antigens, the helper cells (T_H) that develop are capable of recognizing antigen, of proliferating in response to that antigen, and of giving helper signals *only* if they are presented with antigen on the surface of antigen-presenting macrophages that express Class II MHC molecules of the *same* genotype present on the antigen-presenting macrophages in the initial immunization process.

In both cases, cytotoxic and helper T cells can "see" antigen only if it is present on the cell surface in association with the particular genotype of the Class I or Class II MHC molecule active in the initial immunization. This phenomenon, designated "MHC restriction," is a major determinant of the specificity and degree of immune responsiveness mediated by cytotoxic and helper T cells on exposure to many foreign antigens.

Because most associations between the human MHC, that is, the *human leukocyte antigen* or HLA complex, and susceptibility to a variety of autoimmune diseases are apparently functions of the human Class II MHC molecules, the way in which the Class II MHC genotype influences immune responsiveness is described in greater detail.

First, it is now clear that the macrophage, or adherent or accessory cell, population is composed of a variety of distinct cell types. The only cell type capable of "presenting" antigen to T cells in such a way as to stimulate them to proliferate and to differentiate are those adherent, accessory, or macrophage populations that express Class II MHC molecules. Moreover, studies during the past 15 years have shown that Class II MHC genotype influences whether or not a particular antigen elicits an immune response in an inbred strain of a particular genotype, and it also affects the specificity of the antibody produced. Thus, for simple polypeptide antigens with few antigenic determinants, Class II MHC genotype determines whether an immune response develops or whether active immu-

nosuppression is the result of the immunizing event. For more complex protein antigens, Class II MHC genotype influences the specificity of the cellular and humoral immune response to that antigen.

One of the best examples of this phenomenon comes from an analysis of the immune response of inbred guinea pigs to bovine insulin. One inbred strain of guinea pigs, designated strain 2, responds primarily to antigenic determinants on the A chain of bovine insulin. A different strain of inbred guinea pigs, strain 13, fails to recognize antigenic differences in the A chain of beef, sheep, and horse insulin, but recognizes antigenic differences between any of these insulins and the guinea pig insulin B chain. Thus, both strains are capable of responding to bovine insulin, but strain 2 guinea pigs respond to antigenic determinants on the insulin A chain, and strain 13 guinea pigs respond to antigenic determinants on the insulin B chain. These differences are due to differences in Class II MHC genes.

More complex experiments, using strain (2 by 13) F_1 guinea pigs, show that this difference in responsiveness is expressed in the antigen-presenting macrophage. The results show that strain 2 macrophages are capable of "presenting" only the insulin A chain antigenic determinants, whereas strain 13 macrophages are capable of "presenting" only the insulin B chain antigenic determinants.

Numerous other examples of this sort have been described in mice and in the human; localization is to the I-A, or I-E, Class II MHC molecule in the mouse and to corresponding molecules in the human.

The critical question raised by these phenomena is, how do the Class II MHC molecules influence the manner in which T cells see foreign antigens? One hypothesis suggests a close molecular association between Class II MHC molecules and the foreign antigen on the surface of the antigen-presenting macrophage, and this complex is seen by the T-cell antigen receptor. In this view, the genotype of Class II molecule on the antigen-presenting macrophage in some manner determines which antigenic determinants on the foreign antigen are recognized by the T cell. This concept is the "determinant selection" hypothesis, shown schematically in Figure 24–5. An alternate hypothesis postulates that combinations of a variety of self-molecules with self-Class II MHC molecules induce neonatal tolerance to cross-reacting antigenic figurations generated by molecular association of foreign antigenic determinants with self-Class II MHC molecules. This tolerance is then expressed as a defect in the repertoire of T-cell receptors in the helper-T-cell population. At present, abundant

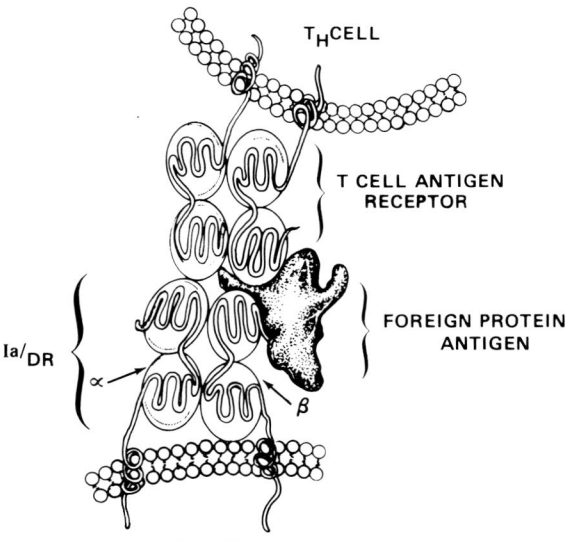

Fig. 24–5. A schematic diagram of the interaction between the T-helper (T_H) lymphocyte (which is responsible for triggering proliferation and differentiation of B-lymphocytes to produce antibody), and the foreign antigen on the surface of an antigen-presenting adherent cell or macrophage. The T-lymphocyte is "restricted" in its ability to recognize a foreign antigen on the surface of the antigen-presenting cell by the genotype of the Class II histocompatibility protein on the antigen-presenting cell. The T-helper lymphocyte can recognize foreign antigen only if it is in association with a Class II molecule of the same genotype as found on the initial-antigen presenting cell that induced the initial proliferation and differentiation of the T-helper lymphocyte.

evidence indicates that both antigen and Class II MHC molecules must be present on the surface of antigen-presenting macrophages to induce a T-cell response.

Although as yet no direct evidence suggests that foreign antigens and Class II MHC molecules *associate* on the surface of the antigen-presenting macrophage, much indirect evidence of this association exists. It is also possible, however, that deletions in the T-cell-receptor repertoire could be induced by neonatal tolerance to self-antigens and self-Class II MHC molecules. It is therefore likely that both these mechanisms are active, and Class II MHC genotype can influence immune responsiveness and the specificity of immune responses by both mechanisms.

Class II MHC genotype in the mouse also determines the development of specific immune suppression. Thus, for some antigens in some MHC genotypes, the antigen may fail to elicit any helper T cells. The result may be nonresponsiveness, or one may see suppressor T cells and active

immune suppression of the immune response to the antigen in question. This effect is due to Class II MHC genotype, and the suppressor T cells in this case are restricted to the H2-I region and are antigen specific. This point is of critical importance because it shows that Class II MHC genotype can lead to the development of active suppression of the immune response to a particular foreign antigen, as well as to the development of T helper cells that actively stimulate the response to a particular foreign antigen.

One other point on the function of Class II MHC molecules in regulating the immune response is important in considering the way in which these genes regulate susceptibility to disease. In the mouse, immune response to some synthetic polypeptide antigens requires "hybrid" Class II MHC molecules. Thus, an animal of the H-$2^{k/k}$ genotype expresses A_α, A_β, E_α, and E_β polypeptides only of the k genotype. Such an animal is a nonresponder to a given polypeptide antigen. Animals of the H-$2^{b/b}$ genotype are also nonresponders to this antigen. The F_1 offspring of a cross between H-$2^{k/k}$ and H-$2^{b/b}$ parents are capable of responding to this antigen, however. In several cases, this capability is due to the presence in the F_1 hybrid of Ia molecules of the composition $E_\alpha{}^k:E_\beta{}^b$. Many biochemical, serologic, and genetic studies have shown that in F_1 heterozygotes, A_α and A_β chains of different genotypes form all possible molecular combinations, and the same occurs with E_α and E_β chains. This form of gene interaction, or gene complementation, has been amply documented in the mouse and is an important potential source for generating diversity in the regulation of immune responsiveness. The point is described in detail because it is possible, if not likely, that genetic control of human susceptibility to a variety of autoimmune diseases may be mediated by a similar type of gene interaction among different alleles of α and β chains of Class II MHC molecules.

HUMAN MAJOR HISTOCOMPATIBILITY COMPLEX

The human MHC has been designated the *h*uman *l*eukocyte *a*ntigen or HLA system. The HLA system is found on the short arm of human chromosome 6 and spans a genetic distance of approximately 2.0 centimorgans. A schematic diagram of the HLA system is presented in Figure 24–6.

Class I HLA Antigens

Amino acid sequence studies clearly show that the HLA-A and HLA-B gene products are homologous with the H-2K and D gene products. The HLA-C gene product appears to be a tandem duplication of the HLA-B gene product. All these

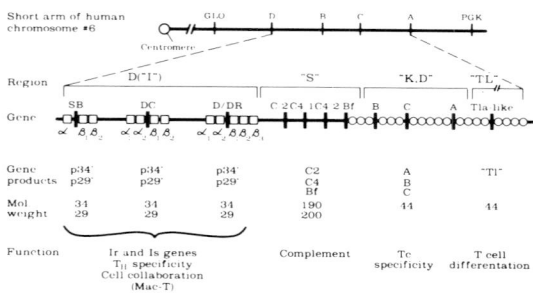

Fig. 24–6. A schematic diagram of the genes of the human major histocompatibility system. These genes are located in man on the sixth chromosome, shown at the top of the diagram. The major histocompatibility system is shown in an expanded version in the second tier of the diagram in which it is divided into subregions. Class I major histocompatibility genes are found in the "K," "D," and "TL" regions, whereas Class II major histocompatibility genes (defined in the text) are found in the "D" (or "I") region. Class III genes encoding several of the components of the complement system are found in the "S" region. The function of Class I and Class II genes is described in the text.

Class I MHC molecules are 44,000-M.W. cell surface glycoproteins, found on the surface of all nucleated cells in association with a 12,000-M.W. β_2-microglobulin chain, as with the murine Class I MHC molecules.

Current evidence from recombinant DNA studies indicates the presence of 15 to 30 Class I MHC genes in the human. The major categories expressed on all nucleated cells are the HLA-A, HLA-B, and HLA-C molecules. In addition, many Tla-like genes are present in the human and are presumably similar to the Tla and Qa subset of nonpolymorphic Class I MHC antigens in the mouse. These genes and their products have not yet been fully characterized.

HLA-A, HLA-B, and HLA-C antigens are routinely typed by using maternal isoantisera. During the course of pregnancy, leakage of fetal lymphocytes into the maternal circulation is sufficient to enable approximately 30% of women to develop a significant titer of anti-HLA antibodies in the immediate weeks following delivery. These maternal isoantibodies are directed against specific antigenic determinants on the HLA-A, HLA-B, HLA-C, and HLA-D isoantigens. Thus, any particular maternal isoantiserum contains a number of antibodies directed against these gene products and, in addition, appears to have several different antibodies specific for any single gene product, such as HLA-A. Maternal isoantiserum from a primipara reacts with the offspring's lymphocytes and with the lymphocytes of the father, as well as with those of anyone

else in the population who shares any of the alleles of the HLA-A, HLA-B, and HLA-C loci with the father and the offspring. The maternal isoantiserum can thus be used to define the presence of these antigens in other members of the population.

By using a varied sampling of maternal sera and a large panel of normal donor lymphocytes, combined with computer analysis of paired associations of reactions of sera with particular lymphocytes, it has been possible to define many allelic antigenic specificities at the HLA-A, HLA-B, and HLA-C loci. Approximately 20 different allelic antigenic specificities are present at the HLA-A locus, nearly 40 allelic antigenic specificities are found at the HLA-B locus, and 8 distinct antigenic specificities occur at the HLA-C locus. These allelic antigenic specificities have been assigned numbers; for example, HLA-A1, A2, and A3, HLA-B12, B15, B16, B17, and B27, and HLA-C1, C2, and C3 (Table 24–1).

Table 24–1. Alleles of the Human Class II Major Histocompatibility Proteins*

HLA-Dw	HLA-DR
Dw1	DR1
Dw2	DR2
Dw3	DR3
Dw4	DR4
Dw5	DR5
Dw6	DR6
Dw7	DRw7
Dw8	DRw8
Dw9	DRw9
Dw10	DRw10
Dw11	
Dw12	

*The alleles of the HLA-D region are given two designations, depending on the method of genotyping. HLA-Dw genotyping is done by mixing lymphocytes from unrelated individuals and measuring the resulting proliferation if they differ at the HLA-D region. This method of genotyping detects differences not only in HLA-DR molecules, but also in HLA-DC and HLA-SB molecules, although the latter probably are minor components of the mixed lymphocyte reaction. Isoantisera in some mothers react selectively with the HLA class II histocompatibility proteins, primarily the HLA-DR molecules. When genotyping is done by this serologic method, the genotype is designated HLA-DR. The two methods do not always detect the same antigenic differences among individuals. For example, HLA-DR4 can be subdivided into HLA-Dw4, HLA-Dw10, and several other as yet unclassified HLA-Dw types including those designated LD40 and DYT. In another example, the HLA-DR2 serologic designation includes HLA-Dw2 and HLA-Dw12, the latter found primarily in Japanese populations. Both genotyping methods are inadequate and do not precisely identify allelic variations in the HLA-DR, HLA-DC, and HLA-SB molecules. The number of alleles of the HLA-DR system is much larger than this list indicates.

Class II Molecules

As Figure 24-6 indicates, several striking differences exist between the genetic regions encoding Class II MHC molecules in mouse and in man. The first of these differences is that the Class II MHC genes in man lie outside the genetic region encoding the Class I antigens, namely, to the left of the HLA-B locus and apparently to the left of all the Class I MHC genes. In contrast, in the mouse, the I region genes map between the H2-K and D regions.

The other major such difference between mouse and man is that in the human, more Class II genes and gene products exist compared to the mouse. Current evidence from recombinant DNA studies analyzing both cDNA and genomic DNA clones, combined with evidence from serologic and biochemical studies, indicates three sets of human Class II MHC genes, now designated HLA-DR, HLA-DC, and HLA-SB. One DR-α chain gene, DR-β chain genes, two DC-α chain genes, at least two DC-β chain genes, and one to two SB-2 and four SB-β chain genes are known to exist. Thus, at least four to five α chain genes and six to eight β chain genes are found in man. At least three α chain genes and six to eight β chain genes are expressed at the cell surface, so the expressed complexity of the Class II MHC molecules in man is greater than in the mouse. The reasons for this striking difference in complexity of Class II MHC gene products is not immediately apparent, but it may be related to the range of ecologic environments inhabited by man or to the difference in life span of the two species.

Methods for determining genotype of the HLA-DR, HLA-DC, and HLA-SB molecules are currently complicated, expensive, and time consuming and are undergoing rapid development. The genes of the HLA-DR region are typed either by their abilities to stimulate the mixed lymphocyte culture reaction, in which case the gene product is designated the Dw allele, or by maternal isoantisera specific for the HLA-DR gene products, in which case the genotype is designated the HLA-DR allele. Methods for genotyping HLA-DC and HLA-SB gene products are even more complex and at present can only be considered as research methods.

Preliminary studies in a number of laboratories have shown that the DNA sequences flanking the various HLA Class II MHC α and β chain genes can be used to develop a method of molecular genotyping. Different alleles of these genes have different DNA sequences in the flanking regions of the gene that lead to variations in the size of the fragments produced when the genomic DNA is cut with restriction endonuclease enzymes. Initial studies have shown that restriction fragment size for HLA-DR-β and HLA-DC-β cDNA probes correlates with genotype, as determined by isoantisera identifying gene products of the HLA-DR region. The use of probes for the DR, DC, and SB α and β chain genes, combined with several restriction enzymes, should permit precise genotyping through the use of this restriction fragment length polymorphism. It is also apparent from these early studies that particular combinations of restriction fragments remain together as sets on a given chromosome, so particular chromosomal, or haplotypic, combinations of HLA-DR, HLA-DC, and HLA-SB genotypes can be readily identified through the analysis of restriction fragment length polymorphism.

As Table 24-1 shows, ten HLA-DR alleles are currently identified by maternal isoantisera. Recent studies from a number of laboratories have shown that these DR alleles are actually broad inclusion groups, which can be subdivided either by typing by the mixed lymphocyte reaction or biochemically by immunoprecipitation and analysis with two-dimensional gel protein electrophoresis. Thus, the HLA-DR4 allele actually includes five different Dw types, as determined by mixed lymphocyte reaction typing using homozygous typing cells, and most of these five subtypes of HLA-DR4 have biochemically distinct HLA-DR4-β chains.

These findings indicate that the actual number of HLA-DR alleles is much greater than Table 24-1 indicates, and they raise the possibility that particular HLA-DR4 subtypes may be associated with susceptibility to particular diseases. Preliminary studies from one laboratory have already indicated that such is the case with respect to inherited susceptibility to juvenile rheumatoid arthritis (JRA).

As in the mouse, the Class II MHC antigens in man are expressed primarily on B-lymphocytes, antigen-presenting macrophages, and on antigen- or mitogen-activated T-lymphocytes. Amino acid sequence studies show clearly that the HLA-DR molecules are the human analogue of the murine I-E molecules, whereas the HLA-DC molecules are the human analogue of the I-A molecules in the mouse. The HLA-SB molecules, by predicted amino acid sequence based on cDNA sequences, appear to have amino acid sequences homologous to both HLA-DR and HLA-DC sequences and show the same degree of homology (approximately 75%) to HLA-DR and HLA-DC amino acid sequences.

Much experimental evidence indicates that the HLA-D region gene products are the molecules that elicit the mixed lymphocyte culture reaction, are the antigenic determinants that elicit HLA-DR isoantisera in maternal sera, and have essentially the same functions as the Class II MHC gene products in the mouse. Thus, these molecules probably regulate the immune response to specific antigens, and particular antigenic determinants in man, in the same fashion as in the mouse.

Recent studies have indicated that the immune response to streptococcal cell-wall antigens, to cedar pollen allergens, and to ragweed pollen allergens is under the control of genes linked to the HLA complex. Sufficient evidence, now available, indicates that the ability of antigen-presenting accessory cells to present antigen to T cells is closely related to HLA-D region gene products in man in the same manner as with the corresponding molecules in the mouse. Thus, these genes probably regulate the immune response in man and may play a major role in resistance to environmental pathogens and in the development of autoimmunity. In a similar manner, much experimental evidence indicates that Class I MHC antigens in man have a major influence on the specificity of cytotoxic T cells, as well as on the specificity and degree of cytotoxic cell-mediated immunity for environmental pathogens, such as the influenza virus.

HLA-Linked Complement Genes

As indicated in Figure 24–6, genes determining the structure of several of the components of the classic and alternate pathways of complement activation are encoded in the HLA system. Included are the structural gene for the second component of complement, two structural genes for the fourth component of complement, and the structural gene for properdin factor B, which is the initial component in the alternate pathway of complement activation.

The complement genes have an unusually high degree of polymorphism, comparable to that of the other gene products of the HLA system. Thus, 4 alleles of the C2 gene, 13 alleles of the C4A gene, 22 alleles of the C4B gene, and 11 alleles of the properdin factor B gene are known.

The complement components are activated by aggregation of antigen antibody complexes, are thereby related to the immune response, and are involved in the effector arm of this response. Abundant evidence suggests the existence of particular chromosomal or haplotypic combinations of HLA-A, HLA-B, HLA-C, and HLA-D regions and complement alleles on a particular chromosome. These chromosomal combinations or haplotypes occur more frequently than would be predicted by chance alone and therefore presumably have some functional survival value, which has not yet been detected. Thus, the HLA-A10, B18, DR2, C2 deficiency haplotype occurs more frequently than would be expected by chance. Other combinations

of particlar alleles of C4, or properdin factor B with particular alleles of HLA-A, HLA-B, and HLA-D region genes have also been documented. Some of these combinations appear to play a role in disease susceptibility and thus raise the question of a possible functional interaction between these complement components and Class I and Class II MHC gene products in the induction or the regulation of the immune response. These functional roles are not yet understood.

Population Genetics and Disease Associations

Specific combinations of particular alleles at the HLA-A, HLA-B, HLA-C, and HLA-D loci occur together on the same chromosome in a particular population more often than would be expected by chance. This phenomenon, known as *linkage disequilibrium,* is the opposite of linkage equilibrium. Equilibrium can be said to exist when any given allele of one gene is found on the same chromosome in combination with any specified allele of a second linked gene in a frequency determined by the product of the gene frequencies of the two specified alleles at the two loci. This linkage equilibrium develops because genetic crossing over occurs between the two loci and scrambles any particular combination of particular alleles at these loci. For a newly introduced (mutant) allele of one of the two genes, genetic equilibrium develops more rapidly for genes that are farther apart, but even for closely linked genes, genetic equilibrium ultimately develops, given sufficient numbers of generations and a random choice of breeding partner.

The HLA system constitutes one of the most remarkable examples of linkage disequilibrium in the human genome. Several chromosomal combinations or haplotypes, which are sets of particular alleles of linked genes on one chromosome, the haploid number, occur in a particular population at a much higher frequency than would be predicted by chance. Thus, in Caucasians, the HLA-A1, B8, Dw3 combination occurs more frequently than would be predicted by the product of the gene frequencies of these three alleles in the population. The same is true for the HLA-A3, B7, Dw2 haplotype, among others. These alleles are thus said to be in linkage disequilibrium.

Although the occurrence of linkage disequilibrium could be due to suppression of crossing over between the linked genes, no evidence indicates significant suppression in this system. In the absence of any special genetic mechanism, therefore, geneticists have concluded that linkage disequilibrium reflects a selective survival advantage of a particular combination of alleles at linked loci. In most systems including the HLA system, the precise mechanism of selective survival advantage is unclear. The clear evidence in mice that HLA-A and HLA-B can influence cytotoxic-T-cell specificity, and presumably responsiveness, and the knowledge that two or more genes in the I region may be required to develop a specific immune response to a particular antigen suggest at least one mechanism, however. Particular combinations of HLA-A, HLA-B, and HLA-D alleles might confer a strong selective survival advantage to a population that is exposed to a particular selective force such as a viral or bacterial infection. This advantage would presumably vary with climate and other environmental factors, and similar variation in the occurrence of linkage disequilibrium has also been observed. Thus, for example, the HLA-A3, B7, Dw2 haplotype is much more prevalent in Scandinavian countries and in temperate European areas than in Mediterranean countries and in countries closer to the equator. This comparison in all cases is among Caucasian populations of European origin.

In Caucasians, the HLA-A1, B8, Dw3 haplotype is associated with a number of autoimmune diseases, including myasthenia gravis, thyrotoxicosis, Addison's disease, juvenile-onset diabetes mellitus, Sjögren's syndrome, and chronic active hepatitis. The HLA-A3, B7, Dw2 haplotype is associated with susceptibility to multiple sclerosis. A particularly intriguing example of this type is the frequent occurrence of the HLA-A10, B18, Dw2 haplotype with a deficiency in the structural gene for the second component of complement. Most cases of absolute deficiency of the second component of complement, a recessive defect, carry at least one dose of this haplotype. In addition, the HLA-A10, B18, Dw2 C2 deficiency haplotype in a heterozygote appears to be associated with an increased incidence of autoimmune syndromes resembling systemic lupus erythematosus (see Chap. 61).

POSSIBLE MECHANISMS FOR THE RELATION TO DISEASE SUSCEPTIBILITY

Animal Models

In some animal models, H-2 genotype has a marked effect on susceptibility or resistance to a particular disease. Susceptibility or resistance to Gross virus-induced leukemogenesis in the mouse is a definite function of H-2 type. $H-2^k$ mice are much more susceptible to leukemogenesis, whereas $H-2^b$ mice are resistant. Friend virus leukemogenesis is also associated with H-2 genotype. Susceptibility to Gross virus leukemogenesis appears to be a function of a gene locus in the left-hand part of the H-2 system, but it has not yet been possible to determine whether this susceptibility is an I-region gene function or a function of $H-2K^k$ or a gene to the left of H-2K. On the other hand, susceptibility or resistance to Friend virus leukemogenesis appears to be a function of the H-2D locus. The same is true for susceptibility or resistance to the induction of thymic leukemia by the radiation leukemia virus (RadLV). Resistance is mediated by the $H-2D^d$ allele. Although it seems likely that some of these forms of resistance or susceptibility are due to the effect of specific immune response genes, and others to the effect of H-2K or H-2D on the development of cytotoxic immune responsiveness, experimental proof for this hypothesis is lacking.

A number of other traits are under the influence of H-2 genotype. Thus, in mice of identical genetic background, H-2 genotype has an influence on intracellular cyclic adenosine monophosphate levels in the liver. The mechanisms of these associations are not known, but some of them appear to be caused by the effect of genes *within* the H-2 system. These effects may be indirectly due to the interaction between molecules coded by the H-2 system and receptors for hormones on the cell surface. Proof for this speculation is still lacking, but H-2K, H-2D, and I region antigens are distributed on many cell types and may have pleomorphic effects in addition to regulating immune responsiveness. This factor is of particular interest when we attempt to understand the association with the HLA system of diseases, such as hemochromatosis, that appear to have no immunologic basis.

HLA and Disease

More than 40 diseases are associated with the HLA system. It is beyond the scope of this discussion to review all these associations and to treat them in detail. Those related to the rheumatic diseases are summarized in Table 24–2 and are discussed more fully in Chapter 25. Several generalizations are pertinent, however.

First, association of a particular allele of a particular HLA gene with susceptibility to a disease is dominant because the affected individual is usually heterozygous; homozygosity in the HLA system is uncommon. Second, although up to 80%, or even more, of individuals with a given disease may possess a particular allele of an HLA gene, such as the more than 95% of patients with ankylosing spondylitis who carry HLA-B27, the majority of individuals with this allele do *not* have one of the HLA-associated diseases. Thus, only 20% of HLA-B27-positive individuals in the population have any manifestations of ankylosing spondylitis or sacroiliitis, and only a tiny fraction

Table 24–2. Associations between HLA Genes and Susceptibility to Some Diseases*

Disease	HLA Gene	Patients (%)	Normal Subjects (%)	Relative Risk (expressed in terms of frequency)
Ankylosing spondylitis	B27	90	9	87
Reiter's disease	B27	79	9	37
Gluten-sensitive enteropathy (celiac disease)	DR3	80	26	11
Addison's disease	DR3	70	26	6
Hyperthyroidism	DR3	56	26	4
Juvenile-onset (insulin-dependent) diabetes mellitus	DR3	56	28	3
Juvenile-onset (insulin-dependent) diabetes mellitus	DR4	75	32	6
Myasthenia gravis	DR3	50	28	2.5
Systemic lupus erythematosus	DR3	70	28	6
Multiple sclerosis	DR2	60	26	4
Rheumatoid arthritis	DR4	50	20	4

*Associations between a particular allele of a particular HLA gene locus and susceptibility to a disease are given in terms of the frequency of an allele in patients and in a normal control population. Relative risk is a mathematic expression of the relative frequency of a disease in individuals carrying a particular allele versus the frequency of the disease in individuals not carrying that allele. The minority of individuals who have HLA-B27 develop ankylosing spondylitis, but their risk of developing the disease is still 87 times greater than that of HLA-B27-negative individuals. Most other HLA disease associations are with the HLA-DR region, and most of these are with HLA-DR2, 3, and 4. A striking number of diseases are associated with HLA-DR3. Susceptibility to insulin-dependent diabetes mellitus is mediated by both the DR3 and DR4 alleles. Family studies in these patients have shown that most are HLA-DR3,3 homozygotes, HLA-DR4,4 homozygotes, or HLA-DR3,4 heterozygotes. The relative risk is much higher for DR3/4 heterozygotes (approximately 30) than for either for DR3 or DR4 homozygotes. This is an exception to the general rule that susceptibility to disease mediated by HLA genes is dominant. Insulin-dependent diabetes is also of interest because the HLA-DR2 allele confers resistance to the disease and therefore has a protective effect. The data in this table are incomplete and list only 10 of the more than 40 diseases in which susceptibility is in part mediated by genes of the HLA system.

of HLA-Dw2-positive individuals develop multiple sclerosis.

Third, good reason exists to suspect that most of the HLA-associated diseases involve not only the susceptible genotype in the HLA system, but also susceptibility at other genetic loci, as well as the probable additional interaction of an environmental factor.

Fourth, with a few exceptions, almost every disease associated with an allele of an HLA gene shows the strongest association with an allele of the HLA-D locus. The most notable exceptions are ankylosing spondylitis and Reiter's disease, which are associated with HLA-B27, and idiopathic hemachromatosis, which is associated most strongly with HLA-A3. These few exceptions aside, almost all other diseases associated with the HLA system show the strongest association with the HLA-D locus. Thus, the initial discovery that multiple sclerosis was associated with HLA-A3, B7 was followed by the clear demonstration that this association was really due to a much stronger association with HLA-Dw2. The apparent association with HLA-A3, B7 can now be attributed to the linkage disequilibrium among these three alleles. HLA-Dw2 occurs in 50 to 60% of patients with multiple sclerosis, whereas HLA-B7 is found in only 36%.

These foregoing generalizations, and especially the fourth, have a major bearing on our attempts to understand the mechanism underlying the association between the HLA system and susceptibility to disease. Because the origin and pathogenesis of these diseases are, for the most part, still a mystery, any attempt to explain the mechanism of association with HLA must be speculative. Thus, the association of ankylosing spondylitis and Reiter's disease with HLA-B27 might be due to a direct effect of the B27 allele on the development of cytotoxic-T-cell responsiveness to an exogenous antigen that triggers an immune response to a cross-reacting self-antigen. Alternatively, the association could reflect the effect of a gene closely linked to HLA-B27 and in strong linkage disequilibrium with it. Definitive family studies have not yet been conducted.

Similarly, the association of many autoimmune diseases, including RA, with the HLA-D locus raises the speculation that either a hyper- or a hyponormal immune response to an exogenous antigen or to a self-antigen is an underlying factor. For example, the association of Graves' disease and myasthenia gravis with HLA-Dw3 might be due to a hypernormal immune response to an environmental agent that cross-reacts with either the thyrotropin receptor or the acetylcholine receptor, or alternatively, it might be due to a deficit in suppressor T cells that maintain the suppression of what might otherwise be a damaging autoimmune response to the thyrotropin or acetylcholine receptor. Some of these possibilities are susceptible to experimental testing, but evidence is still lacking.

The existence of linkage disequilibrium within the HLA system, already discussed, means that it is possible that none of the measured genes are responsible for the association; rather, the association may be due to a linked gene in linkage disequilibrium with the measured genes. For example, the association of Graves' disease and juvenile-onset diabetes mellitus, as well as a number of other autoimmune diseases in Caucasians, with HLA-Dw3 might be caused by a strong linkage disequilibrium between HLA-Dw3 and the genes predisposing persons to these diseases. In this view, HLA-A, HLA-B, HLA-C, and HLA-D are not true disease-susceptibility genes. That such might be the case is indicated by recent studies in the Japanese population showing that Graves' disease and juvenile-onset diabetes mellitus are indeed associated to the same extent with a particular HLA-D locus type, but the D locus type is different from that found in the Caucasian population.

This finding raises the possibility that the predisposing gene is the same in the two populations and that it is in linkage disequilibrium with different HLA-D types in the two populations. In this regard, the multiplicity of loci in the I region of the mouse is pertinent. The HLA-D region is subdivided into several loci: HLA-DR, HLA-DC, and HLA-SB. Some of these HLA-D associated loci might be of major importance in determining disease susceptibility.

A summary of the reported associations between the major histocompatibility antigens and various rheumatic and other diseases is provided in Table 24–2. Our understanding of the molecular mechanisms by which genes in the HLA system and the H-2 system regulate immune responsiveness is still rudimentary, and our knowledge of many of the gene products of the HLA system, particularly of the HLA-D region, is equally incomplete. Recent progress in both areas makes it likely that the next 10 years will see major advances in our understanding of the relationship between this complex genetic system and susceptibility to rheumatic diseases.

REFERENCES

1. Hood, L., Steinmetz, M., and Malissen, B.: Genes of the Major Histocompatibility Complex. Annu. Rev. Immunol. *1*:529–568, 1983.
2. Kaufman, J.A., et al.: The class II molecules of the human and murine major histocompatibility complex. Cell, *36*:1–13, 1984.
3. Klein, J.: The major histocompatibility complex. *In* Immunology: The Science Of Self-Non Self Discrimination. New York, John Wiley and Sons, 1982.
4. Ryder, L.P., Svejgaard, A., and Dausset, J.: Genetics of HLA disease association. Annu. Rev. Genet., *15*:169–188, 1981.

Chapter 25

Immunogenetics and Arthritis

Frank C. Arnett

A multitude of rheumatic diseases, particularly those believed to arise from disordered immuno-regulation, have recently been associated with HLA antigens encoded by genes from within the major histocompatibility complex (MHC). Noso-logic concepts of disease entities and clusters, pre-viously justified on clinical and serologic grounds, have been strengthened by commonalities and dif-ferences in HLA correlations. Equally important are the clues of pathogenesis underlying these rap-idly evolving observations. Precise localization of the responsible genes and determination of their biologic functions in health and disease are cur-rently areas of intense and potentially fruitful in-vestigation (see Chap. 24).

HLA AND THE SPONDYLITIC DISORDERS

Genetic predisposition to this family of diseases clusters around HLA-B, especially with the B27 antigen marker (Fig. 25–1). Each clinical disorder, however, demonstrates unique HLA correlations.

Ankylosing Spondylitis (AS). About 90% of Caucasian patients possess HLA-B27 compared to 6 to 8% of the general population in the United States and Europe (relative risk = 100 to 150).[15,23,74] American blacks, whose B27 frequency is lower at 2 to 4%, develop the disease less often and also show a weaker B27 association of only 48 to 60%.[34] The prevalence of AS generally par-allels the B27 antigen frequency in different pop-

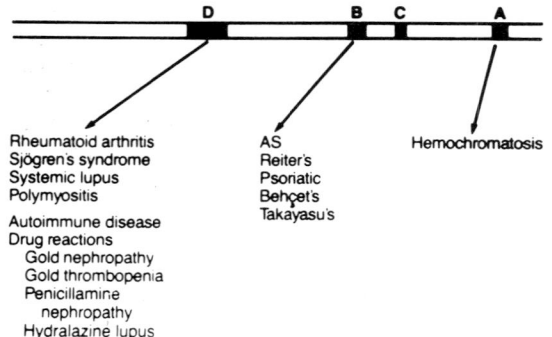

Rheumatoid arthritis
Sjögren's syndrome
Systemic lupus
Polymyositis

Autoimmune disease
Drug reactions
  Gold nephropathy
  Gold thrombopenia
  Penicillamine
    nephropathy
  Hydralazine lupus

AS
Reiter's
Psoriatic
Behçet's
Takayasu's

Hemochromatosis

Fig. 25–1. HLA chromosomal region disease associ-ations.

ulations, both being notably low in African blacks and Japanese and high in certain American Indians, especially the Haida, Pima, and Chippewa.[41,74] Ap-proximately 20% of B27-positive individuals have clinical and/or radiographic evidence of spondyli-tis.[17]

Multiple cases in families almost invariably seg-regate with B27 unless there are members with psoriatic arthritis or inflammatory bowel dis-ease.[32,74] Homozygosity for the antigen may pro-mote more severe disease in terms of peripheral arthritis and uveitis.[7] HLA-B27-negative patients rarely have uveitis or cardiac involvement,[15,35] and B27 is less frequent (50 to 70%) in isolated sac-roiliitis, perhaps a milder form of disease.[9,43] An excess of B7 cross-reacting antigens (the B7-Creg)[9] and the psoriatic-associated specificities, Bw38 and Bw39, occur in B27-negative patients[35] (Table 25–1).

Reiter's Syndrome. HLA-B27 is found in 63 to 76% of patients with either postdysenteric or postvenereal Reiter's syndrome.[16,39] *Forme frustes,* such as incomplete Reiter's syndrome, isolated cir-cinate balanitis, uveitis, keratodermia (pustular psoriasis), and dactylitis have also been associated with this antigen.[53] B27-negative patients rarely develop sacroiliitis or uveitis and generally pursue a milder course.[16,39,53]

A 20% disease risk for reactive arthritis has been calculated for B27-positive individuals who ac-quire one of the inciting enteric pathogens *(Shi-gella, Salmonella,* or *Yersinia)* or nongonococcal urethritis.[41,53,74] Family studies show that 10 to 12% of patients' relatives will also have arthritis, usually peripheral, which segregates with B27.[32,74] In fact, Reiter's syndrome and AS each tend to ''breed true'' within families and certain populations.[32,41] A particularly high prevalence has been found in Navaho Indians who live in areas where shigellosis is endemic.[45]

Psoriatic Arthritis. Neither psoriasis vulgaris nor peripheral psoriatic arthritis is associated with HLA-B27.[41,74] Instead, psoriasis shows an excess of HLA-B17, B13, B37, Cw6, and DR7.[47] Pso-riatic arthritis, moreover, is associated with addi-tional HLA types, including Bw38 and Bw39 (both formerly Bw16) and possibly DR4.[12,23,47] Disease

Table 25–1. HLA and the Spondyloarthropathies

	Frequency of HLA-B27	Other Associated HLA Antigens
Ankylosing spondylitis	85–90%	B7-Creg*; Bw16 (38 and 39)
with uveitis or carditis	95–100%	—
Acute anterior uveitis	50–56%	—
Reiter's syndrome	63–76%	B7-Creg*
with sacroiliitis, uveitis, carditis	90–100%	—
Inflammatory bowel diseases	Not increased	None
peripheral arthritis	Not increased	None
spondylitis	30–50%	None
Psoriasis vulgaris	Not increased	B13, B17, B37, Cw6, DR7
peripheral arthritis	Not increased	Bw38, Bw39, ?DR4
spondylitis	40–50%	Bw38, Bw39, ?DR4
Normal Caucasians	6–10%	—

*Includes B7, Bw22, B40, Bw42 in addition to B27.

susceptibility appears to lie closer to HLA-B or -C loci than to DR. HLA-B27 is increased only in psoriatic spondylitis occurring in 40 to 50%.[12,23,41,47] HLA-Bw38 and Bw39 may also promote axial involvement.

Enteropathic Arthritis. The inflammatory bowel diseases (IBD), ulcerative colitis, and Crohn's disease, as well as their complicating peripheral arthritides, show no HLA correlations.[44] Enteropathic spondylitis, however, is associated with HLA-B27 in 30 to 50% of cases.[22,41,44] Family studies suggest that non-HLA linked genes that predispose to IBD may also confer susceptibility to axial arthropathy even in the absence of expression of the bowel lesion.[22]

HLA-B27: Primary or Linked Gene

It is unknown whether B27 is itself the disease-conferring gene (or product), or only a marker for another closely linked immune response or disease-susceptibility locus. Evidence favoring a direct role for the HLA-B locus includes the following: (1) HLA-B27 is the strongest HLA-disease association. Recombinational events between B27 and another linked gene occurring over eons should have weakened the association unless linkage was extraordinarily tight.[74] (2) The B27-disease link transcends geographic and ethnic barriers.[41] (3) No stronger correlations exist at HLA-A, -C or -D loci.[74] (4) Most patients with B27-negative disease have another cross-reactive B locus antigen, either B7, Bw22, B40, or Bw42 (the B7-Creg).[9] A "public" specificity or polypeptide epitope termed "X" has been discovered on the molecules of each of these "private" B7-Creg specificities,[59] thus providing indirect evidence that HLA-B is the primary locus. (5) Environmental agents as triggers or perpetuators for AS are strongly suspected and are already known for Reiter's disease. Interactions

between infectious agents and B27 molecules would provide compelling evidence for direct participation by the B locus. Reports have described antibodies to certain *Klebsiella* strains that were cytotoxic for B27-positive lymphocytes from AS patients.[66] Evidence has been presented for a *Klebsiella* cell wall component that alters the cell surface B27 molecule and makes the lymphocyte susceptible to lysis by *Klebsiella* antibody.[66] Other investigators have been unable to reproduce these findings.[36] Similarly, preliminary data suggest that a pathogenic *Yersinia* from Europe selectively stimulates T cells from American patients with Reiter's syndrome and adheres to these cells at HLA receptor sites.[14]

The clinical differences between AS and Reiter's syndrome and their tendency to "breed true" suggest either structural diversity in B27 molecules or a separate B27-linked gene for each. Structural differences in B27 molecules have been demonstrated, but whether these segregate into disease patterns is unclear.[29]

HLA-B27: Clinical Uses

Diagnosis of a spondyloarthropathy depends on careful clinical and radiographic assessment. Occasionally, testing for B27 may provide useful additional information. The following are examples of such situations. (1) A patient, usually young, whose chronic low back pain is inflammatory in character, may have sacroiliac roentgenograms that are normal or equivocal. A positive B27 does not establish a diagnosis of spondylitis, but it is supportive. The likelihood of a false-positive is only 8% (the normal population frequency), and a negative test makes spondylitis improbable since 90% of patients are positive. (2) Patients with incompletely expressed Reiter's syndrome and postvenereal or postdysenteric reactive arthritis are often diagnostic problems. A positive B27 test along with careful bacteriologic exclusion may prove useful. (3) Finally, B27 positivity may help properly classify the child with seronegative juvenile arthritis. Although not absolutely predictive, it provides a high likelihood for a future spondylitic course.

RHEUMATOID ARTHRITIS

Rheumatoid arthritis, a disorder clinically, radiographically, and serologically distinctive from the spondyloarthropathies, shows important genetic differences as well. Susceptibility does not appear to arise from HLA-A, -B, or -C loci, but rather from the HLA-D region (see Fig. 25–1). Stastny first demonstrated a frequently occurring mixed lymphocyte response (MLR) in patients with rheumatoid arthritis, later defined by homozygous typing cells as HLA-Dw4.[63] This specificity occurred in 54% of Caucasian seropositive rheumatoids, but in only 16% of normal controls. With the advent of serologic typing for D-related (DR) B cell alloantigens, HLA-DR4 was found to occur in even higher frequency in seropositive patients, 70% as compared to 25 to 28% of normal individuals (relative risk = 6).[27,63] Again, only rheumatoid factor-positive patients showed this association, and the frequency of DR4 was further increased in those with the highest serologic titers.[62] In fact, seronegative rheumatoid arthritis demonstrated no excess of DR4 or any other HLA antigen, suggesting that it develops on a different genetic background or is a separate disorder.[62] Healthy women who were rheumatoid factor-positive also showed no excess of Dw4.[21] The DR4 association with seropositive rheumatoid arthritis is equally distributed between males and females and does not relate to age of disease onset.[62] On the other hand, although DR4 maintains a statistically significant correlation with the disease in most ethnic groups, including Japanese, Latin Americans, and Europeans, its frequency is highly variable.[62] Only 36 to 46% of American blacks with rheumatoid arthritis have the antigen, and its frequency is lower (10 to 14%) in normal blacks.[3,33,62] Studies in Ashkenazi Jews and Asian Indians show no association of disease with DR4, but rather an excess of HLA-DR1 in the former.[57] Two American Indian tribes, each with a high frequency of seropositive disease, show striking HLA contrasts. The Mille Lacs Chippewas show a high population frequency of DR4 (68%), which has been uniformly found in those with rheumatoid arthritis.[30] The Yakimas, however, in whom DR4 normally occurs in 38%, show no DR or Dw associations with disease.[70]

Family studies also support a strong predisposition to rheumatoid arthritis carried on DR4-bearing haplotypes.[62] Multiple affected members usually share the same DR4 haplotype, but not uniformly. Furthermore, all DR4-positive family members do not express disease. Thus, a simple Mendelian dominant model with incomplete penetrance cannot be proposed currently for all families. In addition, it is unclear whether homozygosity for DR4 increases disease risk or severity, although several studies imply an effect, especially on aggressive articular destruction and Felty's syndrome. In fact, DR4 itself has been associated with radiographic erosions.[27a]

The genetic susceptibility conferred by the HLA-D region appears to be more intimately related to serologically definable factors rather than to mixed lymphocyte determinants. Parallelism between Dw4 and DR4 in Caucasians is lost when other ethnic groups, such as Japanese, blacks, and American Indians, are studied, and Dw4 shows no association with rheumatoid arthritis in these populations, in sharp contrast to DR4.[30,62] More recent studies suggest that newer B cell alloantigen systems determined by the D region but distinct from DR may correlate more strongly with rheumatoid arthritis. MT3, which is in tight linkage disequilibrium with DR4, 7, 9 and possibly w10, and MB3, which associates with DR4, 5, and 9, may be more strongly associated.[64]

IMMUNE RESPONSE TO COLLAGEN

A definite role for collagen autoimmunity in the initiation or perpetuation of rheumatoid arthritis has not yet been shown. Nevertheless, evidence from animal models and from in vitro human studies suggests that immune responses to collagen subtypes are controlled by the MHC and may be relevant to human disease. The induction of type II collagen arthritis in both rat and mouse models requires certain MHC-linked alleles.[28,75] Specifically, I region genes, the murine counterparts of HLA-D, are necessary for disease expression in mouse strains.[75] Both cell-mediated and humoral mechanisms are operative in producing the inflammatory articular lesions. In humans, T-cell-dependent responses to denatured collagen as measured by leukocyte inhibitory factor release were correlated with DR4-positivity in both rheumatoid patients and in normal individuals.[60] Furthermore, this "hyper-responsiveness" of the DR4-positive cell was related to an inherent lack of suppressor influence.[60]

SUSCEPTIBILITY TO DRUG TOXICITY

The risk of developing certain immunologically mediated adverse reactions to drugs used in the treatment of rheumatoid arthritis is increased in patients possessing certain HLA antigens. Gold-induced proteinuria/nephrotic syndrome, an immune complex nephropathy, occurs most commonly in DR3-positive individuals.[76] Of 24 rheumatoid patients who developed proteinuria on sodium aurothiomalate, 19 (80%) possessed DR3 (relative risk = 32). Similarly, 69% of patients developing penicillamine-induced nephropathy had DR3.[76] Thus, a similar renal lesion induced by two different drugs has been associated with the same genetic marker, a phenomenon solidifying clinical observations that penicillamine proteinuria is more likely in patients having previous gold nephropathy. Gold-induced thrombocytopenia, an immune-mediated peripheral destruction of platelets, also correlates with DR3 positivity.[18] Of 15 patients studied, 12 (80%) were positive for this tissue antigen (relative risk = 8.9). Notably, penicillamine-induced myasthenia appears to be more common (62%) in DR1-positive patients.[19a] Additional HLA associations with adverse effects or favorable responses (DR3 reported for aurothioglucose)[67a] from these and other therapeutic agents require further attention. Furthermore, it may soon become practical to determine DR status prior to initiation of drug therapy, with exclusion or more careful monitoring of patients at highest risk. The expected frequency of DR3 in a rheumatoid population, especially when DR4 is the dominant antigen, is approximately 10%.

JUVENILE CHRONIC ARTHRITIS (JCA)

Juvenile-onset chronic arthritis (JCA), often termed juvenile rheumatoid arthritis (JRA), is a heterogeneous group of rheumatic diseases beginning in childhood and often persisting into adult-

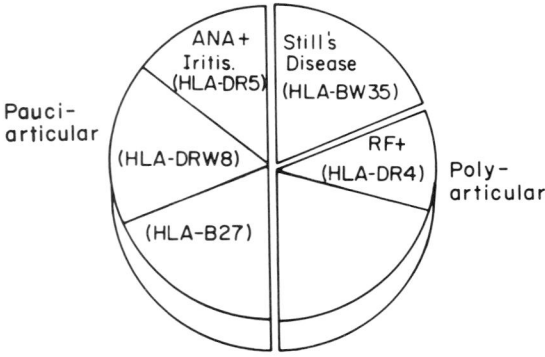

Fig. 25–2. Clinical/serologic subsets of juvenile arthritis and their HLA antigen associations. (Courtesy of The Johns Hopkins University Press.)

hood. Clinical subgroups have been established based on modes of presentation, numbers of affected joints, ocular disease, and serologic markers such as rheumatoid factor and antinuclear antibodies (ANA).[56] The application of HLA antigens has confirmed the rationale for establishing these subgroups and has provided impetus to more guided investigations into pathogenesis (Fig. 25–2).

Juvenile Spondylitis. Following the discovery of the strong association of HLA-B27 with ankylosing spondylitis and Reiter's disease, this antigen was also found in 26 to 42% of patients with juvenile chronic arthritis.[42,56] The majority are boys with late-onset pauciarticular involvement, usually affecting lower-extremity joints, who may later develop more typical symptoms and signs of spondylitis.[56] Others, however, persist with a dominant peripheral arthritis. Girls may also be affected, and a deforming polyarthritis continuing into adulthood may ensue.[8] Cervical spine involvement with apophyseal joint fusion is a predominant finding in this unique B27-subset.[8]

Seropositive Polyarticular Onset. Only 10 to 15% of children with JCA have demonstrable IgM rheumatoid factor. This subset, in particular, clinically resembles adult rheumatoid disease because of the chronicity and severity of joint disease and the frequent appearance of subcutaneous nodules. HLA-DR4, as in adult-onset rheumatoid disease, is significantly increased in such patients. Neither DR4 nor any other HLA antigen has been found in excess in seronegative patients with polyarticular onset.[42]

Pauciarticular Onset. This mode of onset, particularly at a young age in girls, is often accompanied by ANA positivity, which correlates strongly with the development of chronic iridocyclitis. HLA-Dw5 and DR5 correlate with ANA and the ocular lesion. HLA-Dw8 and DRw8 also associate with pauciarticular disease and may overlap with Dw5/DR5 in predisposing to eye disease. LD-TMo is a still ill-defined MLC specificity cross reacting with Dw7 and Dw11, which has been found in 20% of pauciarticular patients and 1% of normals.[42]

Acute Febrile Onset (Still's Disease). There may be an association of Still's disease with HLA-Bw35, but no HLA-D correlations have been detected.[42]

SYSTEMIC LUPUS ERYTHEMATOSUS (SLE)

Systemic lupus erythematosus (SLE) is a multisystem inflammatory disorder characterized by multiple autoantibodies to plasma and cellular constituents and by immune complex formation resulting in immune-mediated tissue injury. Under-lying genetic influences on its development and expression have long been suspected because of familial clustering of cases (10 to 12% of patients have another affected relative) and the 71% concordance of disease in monozygotic twins.[73] It is now clear that MHC-linked genes are exerting a profound effect on disease expression, and are probably acting in concert with one or more non-HLA linked loci. Several B cell alloantigens coded by the HLA-D region, as well as hereditary deletions of nearby structural genes for the complement components C2 and C4, all show significant associations with SLE.[58,73]

Early studies of HLA-A and -B loci antigens in SLE patients suggested a weak link to B8 and, in retrospect, probably reflected linkage disequilibrium between B8 and DR3. It has now been well established that HLA-DR2 and HLA-DR3 occur in significantly increased frequencies in white patients (relative risk 2 to 3 for each).[27,52] Reports from different centers and geographic locations show great variability as to which DR specificity is more common, with some showing only an excess of DR2 and others DR3.[2,11,13,24] In most studies, DR2 and DR3 each occur in 40 to 60% of patients, with 75% possessing one or the other antigen. Both antigens are also common in normal Caucasians (DR2 in 22% and DR3 in 25%). Investigations in other racial groups are limited, but it appears that DR2 and DR3 may be increased in black Americans.[2,3] The combination of DR2 and DR3 in the same individual does not appear to increase susceptibility to disease, and any impact of homozygosity for either is still unknown.

The more recently recognized B cell alloantigens MB1/MT1 and possibly MT2 are also increased in SLE patients. MB1/MT1, previously defined by serum Ia-715, is in tight linkage disequilibrium with DR1, 2, and w6 and occurs in approximately 85% of white SLE patients as compared to 46% of normals (relative risk 2 to 3).[2,52] MT2, previously defined by serum Ia-172 and a dominant antigen in Sjögren's syndrome,[46,72] is strongly affiliated with DR3, 5, w6, and w8 and occurs in mild excess in some SLE series.[5] It remains unclear whether DR or MT are the primary loci for disease predisposition.

Families containing more than one relative with SLE frequently have additional members with other immunologic disorders (e.g., thyroid disease, autoimmune hemolytic anemia, thrombocytopenic purpura) or serologic abnormalities (e.g., ANA, anti-ssDNA, false-positive tests for syphilis).[9a,38,54] Studies of HLA haplotypes in such families show that neither affected SLE members nor relatives with other immune disorders or abnormal serolo-

gies share HLA haplotypes any more often than would be expected by chance alone.[9a] In fact, formal genetic analyses using these disease/serologic abnormalities as "traits" show a Mendelian-dominant segregation pattern with no linkage to HLA. On the other hand, the SLE relatives appear to have randomly inherited DR2- or DR3-bearing haplotypes, whereas their relatives with other diseases and serologic reactions have not. These observations raise the possibility that HLA may be acting only in a modifying role since certain of its alleles are randomly superimposed on another dominant immunoregulatory gene common to many autoimmune disorders. Theoretically, such HLA effects should be manifested as clinical or serologic phenomena highly characteristic for SLE.

Certain autoantibody responses, some distinc-

HLA AND SEROLOGIC ASSOCIATIONS IN SYSTEMIC LUPUS ERYTHEMATOSUS

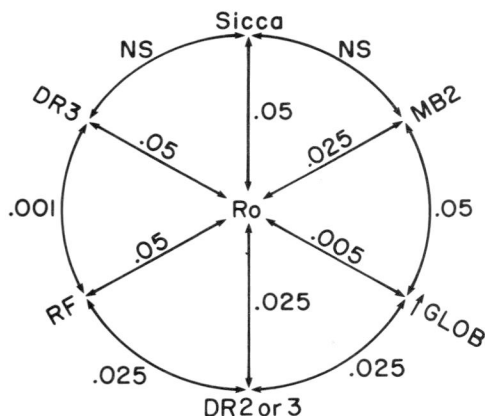

Fig. 25–3. Schematic representation of significant clinical, serologic, and HLA associations of the anti-Ro (SSA) antibody in 70 patients with SLE. (From Ahearn, J.M., et al.[2])

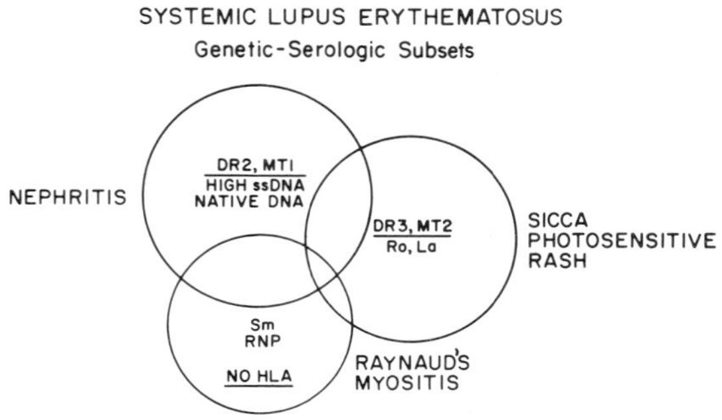

SYSTEMIC LUPUS ERYTHEMATOSUS
Genetic-Serologic Subsets

Fig. 25–4. Circles represent major autoantibody systems in SLE and their respective HLA associations. Adjacent clinical features have been correlated with these antibodies. (From Alvarellos, A., et al.[5])

tive of SLE, show strong associations with DR antigens. Anti-nDNA measured by a *Crithidia luciliae* assay and high titers of anti-ssDNA show significant correlations with DR2.[2,5] The anti-Ro(SS-A)/anti-La(SS-B) antibody system, found in 25% of lupus patients, associates strongly with DR3 and, to a lesser degree, with DR2.[2,5,13] Hyperglobulinemia and rheumatoid factor also show intimate clustering with anti-Ro(SS-A), DR3, and DR2. Clinically evident sicca complex is often present in such SLE patients (Fig. 25–3). Anti-Sm and anti-RNP show no positive HLA relationships.[2,5] Interestingly, several of these autoantibodies correlate with disease features in SLE; however, their direct participation in producing the lesions of SLE has not been proved, except for anti-nDNA in the renal lesion (Fig. 25–4).

CLINICAL-SEROLOGIC-GENETIC LUPUS SUBSETS

Several newly recognized lupus subsets further support the role of HLA antigens in predisposing to autoantibody production, which in turn may prove to be pathogenic. An intimate link between Ro antibody, HLA-DR3, DR2, and cutaneous disease seems likely in these disorders.

Subacute Cutaneous Lupus Erythematosus (SCLE). A predominantly cutaneous disease, SCLE is marked by nonscarring, often photosensitive, annular, and/or papulosquamous lesions.[61] Serious systemic manifestations such as nephritis and nervous system involvement are unusual, and such patients are frequently ANA- and anti-DNA negative. Anti-Ro(SS-A) has been found in 63% and anti-La(SS-B) in 25% of these patients. HLA-DR3 is strongly associated with SCLE, occurring in 77% of patients.[61]

Neonatal Lupus. Neonatal lupus is a syndrome characterized by photosensitive annular skin lesions and/or serious congenital heart block appearing shortly after birth.[25] Placentally transferred anti-Ro(SS-A) antibodies are uniformly found in these infants, and their anti-Ro positive mothers are often asymptomatic. HLA-DR3 has been found in most mothers studied; however, the affected infants do not necessarily inherit DR3.[37] Thus, tissue injury in the neonate, whether by anti-Ro or other factors, does not require the presence of DR3.

Lupus-Like Disease in Hereditary Complement Deficiencies. This disease has been recorded for nearly all components of the cascade.[58] Heterozygous C2 deficiency, the most common defect, occurs in 1 in 300 normal individuals, and the homozygous state in approximately 1 in 10,000.[58] A lupus-like syndrome characterized by prominent cutaneous disease, including annular lesions, mild systemic features, and a paucity of ANA and anti-

DNA, occurs in approximately one-third of homozygous C2 deficients.[1] Again, the anti-Ro(SS-A) antibody has been found to occur in 70% of such patients.[51] The "null" gene for C2 deficiency is linked to an A25,B18,Dw2/DR2-bearing haplotype. The prevalence of SLE in heterozygotes for C2 deficiency is unknown; however, the partially deficient C2 state has been found in approximately 6% of unselected SLE patients.[58]

Two structural genes for C4 (C4A and C4B) also map between the HLA-B and -D loci.[55] Homozygous C4 deficiency, requiring gene deletions of both C4A and C4B on both homologous chromosomes, is exceedingly rare but has been reported in a few patients with SLE.[67] Partial deficiency, however, resulting from "null" alleles at C4A or C4B, are relatively common (11% for C4A and 13.5% for C4B). In fact, a C4A silent allele is in strong linkage disequilibrium with the HLA-A1,B8,Cw7 and DR3 haplotype, a gene cluster strongly associated with diseases of autoimmunity. One study recorded one or more C4 "null" alleles in 79% of 29 patients with SLE compared to 43% of normal controls.[24] It remains unclear whether the partial complement deficiency or its linked D region genes, or both, are contributing to disease susceptibility.

A genetically determined partial deficiency of C3b receptors has been reported in SLE.[71] The structural genes for both C3b and C3b receptors have been tentatively mapped to HLA.[19]

DRUG-INDUCED LUPUS

Hydralazine-induced lupus provides a model in which several genes are necessary after exposure to a sufficient quantity of drug.[11] The syndrome occurs primarily in slow acetylators of the drug. Female sex, another heritable factor, increases predisposition. Finally, HLA-DR4 has been found in 73% of such patients, occurring in 54% of affected females and 100% of males. Thus, it appears that hydralazine does not promote the expression of a "lupus diathesis," since neither DR2 nor DR3 is the predisposing HLA type. Similarly, penicillamine-induced lupus in rheumatoid patients has been reported in a small series where the majority had A11, B15, DR4, and DRW8.[17a]

SJÖGREN'S SYNDROME

Sjögren's syndrome (the sicca complex) is an autoimmune exocrinopathy characterized by unbridled B cell proliferation, lymphocytic infiltration of multiple glandular and extraglandular organs, and a myriad of autoantibodies.[65] The disorder may occur alone (primary Sjögren's syndrome) or secondarily in the settings of rheumatoid

arthritis, systemic lupus, and other connective tissue diseases.

Genetic predisposition to primary Sjögren's syndrome has been linked to HLA-B8 and more strongly to HLA-DR3.[46] In addition, early studies of B cell reactivity to serum Ia-172, now known to be an MT2 defining reagent, demonstrated that most primary and rheumatoid-associated Sjögren's patients were positive.[46] It now appears likely that MT2, a B cell alloantigen in linkage with DR3,5,w6, and w8, is the major HLA specificity conferring susceptibility to both primary and secondary forms of this disorder.[72] MT2 is positive in approximately 90% of patients with primary Sjögren's syndrome, and is usually carried on B8,DR3 haplotypes. MT2 is also significantly associated with rheumatoid-Sjögren's and SLE-Sjögren's, as compared to both normal controls and rheumatoid and lupus controls without the sicca complex (Fig. 25–5). In these instances, MT2 may be carried with DR3 but is more often allied with DR5, DRw6, or DRw8. Furthermore, since MT2 is not linked to DR4 or DR2, the primary HLA associations for RA and SLE, respectively, this sicca-promoting factor is usually inherited on the alternate HLA haplotype.[72]

Similar to the situation in SLE, the expression of the anti-Ro(SS-A)/anti-La(SS-B) antibody system appears to be intimately related to DR3 and DR2.[72] In addition, anti-Ro associates strongly with hyperglobulinemia, rheumatoid factor, leukopenia, and vasculitis.[4] Thus, although susceptibility to disease seems intimately related to the MT system, the production of certain autoantibodies appears more closely allied to the DR specificities, suggesting close interaction between MHC linked genes.

POLYMYOSITIS/DERMATOMYOSITIS

Adult polymyositis in whites has been associated with HLA-DR3, whereas disease in blacks correlates with HLA-DRw6.[31] Supporting the possibility that dermatomyositis might be an immunogenetically different disorder, no HLA excesses have been found. Furthermore, a negative association of HLA-DR4 with all forms of myositis has been found, a phenomenon that suggests that DR4 may afford protection against the acquisition of inflammatory muscle disease. Childhood dermatomyositis also shows a significant association with HLA-B8 and, more strongly, HLA-DR3.[26] The saline extractable precipitating antibody Jo-1, which is highly specific for polymyositis, has also been noted to correlate with HLA-DR3 and DRw6.[6]

PROGRESSIVE SYSTEMIC SCLEROSIS (SCLERODERMA)

Although progressive systemic sclerosis (PSS) shares many overlapping clinical and immunologic features with SLE and Sjögren's syndrome, evidence suggesting MHC influences on pathogenesis is weak.[69] An increased frequency of DR5 has been reported, as well as an excess of DR3, especially in the CREST variant. The B8/DR3 haplotype was also increased in a series of European patients and correlated with impaired cellular immunity. More recently, DR1 was found in 27.5% of 68 patients with diffuse scleroderma and 19.5% with CREST compared to 11.5% in normals.[69] Possibly of note was a significant correlation of DR1 (46%) with anticentromere antibodies.

OTHER AUTOIMMUNE DISORDERS

Multiple diseases resulting from aberrations in immune function have been associated with specific HLA types, the majority coded by the HLA-D region.[40] It is not uncommon to find many of these disorders occurring in patients with HLA-D-related rheumatic disorders or in their family members.[38,54] In addition, several defects and disorders not believed to be of immune origin have also been linked to the MHC. A listing of these illnesses and HLA antigen correlations appears in Table 25–2.

BEHÇET'S DISEASE

Behçet's disease is strongly affiliated with HLA-B5 in Japanese, Turkish, Tunisian, Israeli, Greek, Italian, French, and possibly Swiss and British patients.[50] For unclear reasons, no HLA-A or -B an-

SJÖGREN'S SYNDROME(SS)

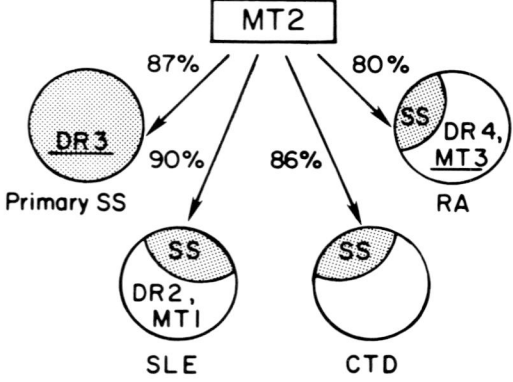

* MT2 occurs in 46% of normal Caucasians

Fig. 25–5. Schematic representation of data presented in Wilson, R.W., et al.[72] showing the MT2 specificity predisposing to Sjögren's syndrome in its primary and secondary settings. (From Wilson, R.W., et al.[72])

Table 25–2. HLA and Nonrheumatic Diseases

Immunologic Disorders	HLA Associations
Graves' disease	B8, Dw3, DR3
Hashimoto's thyroiditis	Dw3
Addison's disease	B8, Dw3, DR3
Chronic active hepatitis	B8, Dw3, DR3
Celiac disease	B8, Dw3, DR3
Dermatitis herpetiformis	B8, Dw3, DR3
Myasthenia gravis	B8, Dw3, DR3
Juvenile diabetes	B8, Dw3, DR3 and B15, DR4
Multiple sclerosis	B7, Dw2, DR2
Optic neuritis	B7, Dw2
Goodpasture's syndrome	DR2
Pernicious anemia	B7, Dw2
Ragweed allergy (Ra 5)	B7, Dw2
Ragweed allergy (Rye I & II)	B8, Dw3
IgA deficiency	B8, DR3
Defective Fc receptors	B8, Dw3
Nonimmunologic Disorders	
21-hydroxylase deficiency	HLA-linked (Bw47)
Hemochromatosis	HLA-linked (A3)
Atrial septal defect (secundum)	HLA-linked
Spinocerebellar ataxia	HLA-linked
Depressive disorders	HLA-linked
Longevity (>90 years in males)	A1, Cw7, B8, DR3

tigens, including B5, are increased in Americans with the disease. In Japan, HLA-Bw51, a "split" of B5, appears to be the primary antigen occurring in 62% of patients and 21% of normals (relative risk = 6). Other antigens that may be implicated include Aw31, DR5, DR7, and MT2.[49]

TAKAYASU'S ARTERITIS

Takayasu's arteritis (aortic arch syndrome, pulseless disease of young women) has been strongly associated with HLA-B5 in Japanese patients.[48] More recently, Bw52, a "split" of B5, has been demonstrated to be the major specificity.[48] A weaker link exists for Dw12, an antigen in linkage with Bw52. No HLA-DR, MB, or MT antigens have been implicated in Japanese. On the other hand, ten affected Americans showed no B locus association but, instead, high frequencies of HLA-DR4 (70%) and MB3 (100%).[68]

OTHER VASCULITIDES

Giant cell arteritis and polymyalgia rheumatica have been weakly correlated with HLA-DR4 in French and American patients.[10] Similarly, an excess of HLA-DR2 was found in Wegener's granulomatosis, but no HLA-A,B,C, or DR associations have been found for polyarteritis or Churg-Strauss vasculitis.[20]

REFERENCES

1. Agnello, V.: Complement deficiency states. Medicine (Baltimore), 57:1–23, 1978.
2. Ahearn, J.M., et al.: Interrelationships of HLA-DR, MB, and MT phenotypes, autoantibody expression, and clinical features in systemic lupus erythematosus. Arthritis Rheum., 25:1031–1040, 1982.
3. Alarif, L.I., et al.: HLA-DR antigens in blacks with rheumatoid arthritis and systemic lupus erythematosus. J. Rheumatol., 10:297–300, 1983.
4. Alexander, E.L., et al.: Sjögren's syndrome: Association of anti-Ro (SS-A) antibodies with vasculitis, hematologic abnormalities, and serologic reactivity. Ann. Intern. Med., 98:155–159, 1983.
5. Alvarellos, A., et al.: Relationships of HLA-DR and MT antigens to autoantibody expression in SLE. Arthritis Rheum., 26:1533–1535, 1983.
6. Arnett, F.C., et al.: The Jo-1 antibody system in myositis: Relationships to clinical features and HLA. J. Rheumatol., 8:925–930, 1981.
7. Arnett, F.C., et al.: Homozygosity for HLA-B27. Impact on rheumatic disease expression in two families. Arthritis Rheum., 20:797–804, 1977.
8. Arnett, F.C., Bias, W.B., and Stevens, M.B.: Juvenile-onset chronic arthritis. Clinical and roentgenographic features of a unique HLA-B27 subset. Am. J. Med., 69:369–376, 1980.
9. Arnett, F.C., Hochberg, M.C., and Bias, W.B.: Cross-reactive HLA antigens in B27-negative Reiter's syndrome and sacroiliitis. Johns Hopkins Med. J., 141:193–197, 1977.
9a. Arnett, F.C., et al.: Systemic lupus erythematosus. Current state of the genetic hypothesis. Semin Arthritis Rheum., In press, 1984.
10. Barrier, J., et al.: Increased prevalence of HLA-DR4 in giant cell arteritis. (Letter.) N. Engl. J. Med., 305:104–105, 1981.
11. Batchelor, J.R., et al.: Hydralazine-induced systemic lupus erythematosus: Influence of HLA-DR and sex on susceptibility. Lancet, 2:1107–1109, 1980.
12. Beaulieu, A.D., et al.: Reappraisal of HLA antigen frequencies in psoriasis and psoriatic arthritis. Arthritis Rheum. (Suppl.), 25:S133, 1982.
13. Bell, D.A., and Maddison, P.J.: Serologic subsets in systemic lupus erythematosus: An examination of autoantibodies in relationship to clinical features of disease and HLA antigens. Arthritis Rheum., 23:1268–1273, 1980.
14. Brenner, M.B., et al.: A new experimental approach to Reiter's disease. Arthritis Rheum. (Suppl.), 25:S63, 1982.
15. Brewerton, D.A., et al.: Ankylosing spondylitis and HL-A27. Lancet, 1:904–907, 1973.
16. Brewerton, D.A., et al.: Reiter's disease and HL-A27. Lancet, 2:996–998, 1973.
17. Calin, A., and Fries, J.F.: The striking prevalence of ankylosing spondylitis in "healthy" w27 positive males and females: A controlled study. N. Engl. J. Med., 293:835–839, 1975.
17a. Chalmers, A., et al.: Systemic lupus erythematosus during penicillamine therapy for rheumatoid arthritis. Ann. Intern. Med., 97:659–663, 1982.
18. Coblyn, J.S., et al.: Gold-induced thrombocytopenia: A clinical and immunogenetic study of twenty-three patients. Ann. Intern. Med., 95:178–181, 1981.
19. Curry, R.A., et al.: Evidence for linkage between HLA antigens and receptors for complement components C3b and C3d in human-mouse hybrids. Immunogenetics, 3:465–471, 1976.
19a. Delamere, J.P. et al.: Penicillamine induced myasthenia in rheumatoid arthritis: Its clinical and genetic features. Ann. Rheum. Dis., 42:500–504, 1983.
20. Elkton, K.B., et al.: HLA antigen frequencies in systemic vasculitis: Increase in HLA-DR2 in Wegener's granulomatosis. Arthritis Rheum., 26:102–105, 1983.
21. Engleman, E.G., et al.: Mixed lymphocyte reaction in healthy women with rheumatoid factor. Lack of association with Dw4. Arthritis Rheum., 21:690–693, 1978.
22. Enlow, R.W., Bias, W.B., and Arnett, F.C.: The spondylitis of inflammatory bowel diseases. Evidence for a non-HLA linked axial arthropathy. Arthritis Rheum., 23:1359–1365, 1980.
23. Espinoza, L.R., et al.: Histocompatibility typing in the

seronegative spondyloarthropathies. Semin. Arthritis Rheum., *11*:375–381, 1982.

24. Fielder, A.H.L., et al.: Family study of the major histocompatibility complex in patients with systemic lupus erythematosus: Importance of null genes of C4A and C4B in determining disease susceptibility. Br. Med. J., *286*:425–428, 1983.

25. Franco, H.L., et al.: Autoantibodies directed against sicca syndrome antigens in the neonatal lupus syndrome. J. Am. Acad. Dermatol., *4*:67–72, 1981.

26. Friedman, J.M., et al.: Immunogenetic studies of juvenile dermatomyositis: HLA-DR antigen frequencies. Arthritis Rheum., *26*:214–216, 1983.

27. Gibofsky, A., et al.: Contrasting patterns of newer histocompatibility determinants in patients with rheumatoid arthritis and systemic lupus erythematosus. Arthritis Rheum. (Suppl.), *21*:S134–138, 1978.

27a. Gran, J.T., Husby, G., and Thorsby, E.: HLA antigens in palindromic rheumatism, nonerosive rheumatoid arthritis and classical rheumatoid arthritis. J. Rheumatol., *11*:136–140, 1984.

28. Griffiths, M.M., et al.: Immunogenetic control of experimental type II collagen-induced arthritis. I. Susceptibility and resistance among inbred strains of rats. Arthritis Rheum., *24*:781–789, 1981.

29. Grumet, F.C., et al.: Monoclonal antibody (B27M2) subdividing HLA-B27. Hum. Immunol., *5*:61–72, 1982.

30. Harvey, J., et al.: Heterogeneity of HLA-DR4 in the rheumatoid arthritis of a Chippewa band. J. Rheumatol., *8*:797–803, 1981.

31. Hirsch, T.J., et al.: HLA-D related (DR) antigens in various kinds of myositis. Hum. Immunol., *3*:181–186, 1981.

32. Hochberg, M.C., Bias, W.B., and Arnett, F.C.: Family studies of HLA-B27 associated arthritis. Medicine (Baltimore), *57*:463–475, 1978.

33. Karr, R.W., et al.: Association of HLA-DRw4 with rheumatoid arthritis in black and white patients. Arthritis Rheum., *23*:1241–1245, 1980.

34. Khan, M.A., et al.: HLA-B27 in ankylosing spondylitis: Differences in frequency and relative risk in American Blacks and Caucasians. J. Rheumatol., (Suppl. 3), *4*:39–43, 1977.

35. Khan, M.A., Kushner, I., and Braun, W.E.: Genetic heterogeneity in primary ankylosing spondylitis. J. Rheumatol., *7*:383–386, 1980.

36. Kinsella, T.D., Fritzler, M.J., and McNeil, D.J.: Ankylosing spondylitis. A disease in search of microbes. J. Rheumatol., *10*:2–4, 1983.

37. Lee, L., et al.: Immunogenetics of the neonatal lupus syndrome. (Abstract.) Arthritis Rheum., (Suppl.), *26*:S71, 1983.

38. Lippman, S.M., et al.: Genetic factors predisposing to autoimmune diseases. Autoimmune hemolytic anemia, chronic thrombocytopenic purpura and systemic lupus erythematosus. Am. J. Med., *73*:827–840, 1982.

39. McClusky, O.E., Lordon, R.E., and Arnett, F.C.: A genetic factor in disease susceptibility and expression. J. Rheumatol., *1*:263–268, 1974.

40. Mann, D.L., and Murray, C.: HLA alloantigens: Disease association and biologic significance. Semin. Hematol., *16*:293–308, 1979.

41. Masi, A.T., and Medsger, T.A., Jr.: A new look at the epidemiology of ankylosing spondylitis and related syndromes. Clin. Orthop. Rel. Res., *143*:15–29, 1979.

42. Miller, M.L., and Glass, D.N.: The major histocompatibility complex antigens in rheumatoid arthritis and juvenile arthritis. Bull. Rheum. Dis., *31*:21–25, 1981.

43. Möller, E., and Olhagen, B.: Studies on the major histocompatibility system in patients with ankylosing spondylitis. Tissue Antigens, *6*:237–246, 1975.

44. Morris, R.I., et al.: HLA w27—a useful discriminator in the arthropathies of inflammatory bowel disease. N. Engl. J. Med., *290*:1117–1119, 1974.

45. Morse, H.G., et al.: High frequency of HLA-B27 and Reiter's syndrome in Navajo Indians. J. Rheumatol., *7*:900–902, 1980.

46. Moutsopoulos, H.M., et al.: Genetic differences between

47. Murry, C., et al.: Histocompatibility alloantigens in psoriasis and psoriatic arthritis. J. Clin. Invest., *66*:670–675, 1980.

48. Numano, F., et al.: HLA-DR, MT and MB antigens in Takayasu disease. Tissue Antigens, *21*:208–212, 1983.

49. O'Duffy, J.D., Lehner, T., and Barnes, C.G.: Summary of the Third International Conference on Behçet's Disease. J. Rheumatol., *10*:154–158, 1983.

50. Ohno, S., et al.: Close association of HLA-Bw51 with Behçet's disease. Arch. Ophthalmol., *100*:1455–1458, 1982.

51. Provost, T.T., Arnett, F.C., and Reichlin, M.: C2 deficiency, lupus erythematosus and anticytoplasmic Ro(SS-A) antibodies. Arthritis Rheum., *26*:1279–1282, 1983.

52. Reinertsen, J.L., et al.: B lymphocyte alloantigens associated with systemic lupus erythematous. N. Engl. J. Med., *299*:515–518, 1978.

53. Renlund, D.G., Kim, W.S., and Arnett, F.C.: Reiter's syndrome. Johns Hopkins Med. J., *150*:39–44, 1982.

54. Reveille, J.D., et al.: Familial systemic lupus erythematosus: Immunogenetic studies in eight families. Medicine (Baltimore), *62*:21–35, 1983.

55. Rittner, C., and Bertrams, J.: On the significance of C2, C4 and factor B polymorphisms in disease. Hum. Genet., *56*:235–247, 1981.

56. Schaller, J.G.: Juvenile rheumatoid arthritis—series 1. Arthritis Rheum. (Suppl. 2), *20*:165–170, 1977.

57. Schiff, B., et al.: Association of Aw31 and HLA-DR1 with adult rheumatoid arthritis. Ann. Rheum. Dis., *41*:403–404, 1982.

58. Schur, P.H.: Complement and lupus erythematosus. Arthritis Rheum., *25*:793–798, 1982.

59. Schwartz, B.D., Luehrman, L.K., and Rodey, G.E.: Public antigenic determinant on a family of HLA-B molecules. Basis for cross-reactivity and a possible link with disease predisposition. J. Clin. Invest., *64*:938–947, 1979.

60. Solinger, A.M., and Stobo, J.D.: Immune response gene control of collagen reactivity in man: Collagen unresponsiveness in HLA-DR4 negative nonresponders is due to the presence of T-dependent suppressive influences. J. Immunol., *129*:1916–1920, 1982.

61. Sontheimer, R.D., et al.: Serologic and HLA associations in subacute cutaneous lupus erythematosus. Ann. Intern. Med., *97*:664–671, 1982.

62. Stastny, P.: Joint report: Rheumatoid arthritis. *In* Histocompatibility Testing 1980. Edited by P.I. Terasaki. Los Angeles, UCLA Tissue Typing Laboratory Press, 1980, pp. 681–686.

63. Stastny, P.: Association of the B-cell alloantigen DRw4 with rheumatoid arthritis. N. Engl. J. Med., *298*:869–871, 1978.

64. Stobo, J.D.: Personal communication.

65. Strand, V., and Talal, N.: Advances in the diagnosis and concept of Sjögren's syndrome (autoimmune exocrinopathy). Bull. Rheum. Dis., *30*:1046–1052, 1980.

66. Sullivan, J.S., Prendergast, J.K., and Gezy, A.F.: Hypothesis: The etiology of ankylosing spondylitis: Does a plasmid trigger the disease in genetically susceptible individuals? Hum. Immunol., *6*:185–187, 1983.

67. Toppeiner, G., et al.: Systemic lupus erythematosus in hereditary deficiency of the fourth component of complement. J. Am. Acad. Dermatol., *7*:66–79, 1982.

67a. van Riel, P.L.C.M., et al.: Association of HLA antigens, toxic reactions and therapeutic response to auranofin and aurothioglucose in patients with rheumatoid arthritis. Tissue Antigens, *22*:194–199, 1983.

68. Volkman, D.J., Mann, D.L., and Fauci, A.: Association between Takayasu's arteritis and a B-cell alloantigen in North Americans. N. Engl. J. Med., *306*:464–465, 1982.

69. Whiteside, T.L., Medsger, T.A., Jr., and Rodnan, G.P.: HLA-DR antigens in progressive systemic sclerosis (scleroderma). J. Rheumatol., *10*:128–131, 1983.

70. Willkens, R.F., et al.: HLA antigens in Yakima Indians with rheumatoid arthritis. Lack of association with HLA-Dw4 and HLA-DR4. Arthritis Rheum., *25*:1435–1439, 1982.

71. Wilson, J.G., et al.: Mode of inheritance of decreased C3b receptors on erythrocytes of patients with systemic lupus erythematosus. N. Engl. J. Med., *307*:981–986, 1982.

72. Wilson, R.W., et al.: Sjögren's syndrome: Influence of multiple HLA-D region specificities on clinical and serologic expression. Arthritis Rheum. In press, 1984.

73. Winchester, R.J., and Nunez-Roldan, A.: Some genetic aspects of systemic lupus erythematosus. Arthritis Rheum., *25*:833–837, 1982.

74. Woodrow, J.C.: Histocompatibility antigens and rheumatic diseases. Semin. Arthritis Rheum., *6*:257–276, 1977.

75. Wooley, P.H., et al.: Type II collagen-induced arthritis in mice: I. MHC (I region) linkage and antibody correlates. J. Exp. Med., *154*:668–700, 1981.

76. Wooley, P.H., et al.: HLA-DR antigens and toxic reaction to sodium aurothiomalate and d-penicillamine in patients with rheumatoid arthritis. N. Engl. J. Med., *303*:300–302, 1980.

Chapter 26

Arthritis and Autoimmunity in Animals

Eliot A. Goldings and Hugo E. Jasin

Spontaneously occurring and experimental animal models of disease have traditionally provided important insights into mechanisms of human disease and have allowed for the development of effective therapeutic agents in many areas of human pathology. In the case of human rheumatoid arthritis (RA) and other autoimmune diseases, the sketchy knowledge available regarding causative factors and pathogenic mechanisms makes the task of selection of a pertinent animal model for any particular research endeavor extremely difficult. This difficulty is compounded by the absence of animal models that imitate closely the human diseases, and by the realization that more than one pathogenic mechanism may induce identical clinical and pathologic manifestations.

In most models of chronic arthritis, regardless of the inducing mechanisms employed, the synovial inflammatory reaction tends to show a monotonous picture of lining cell layer hyperplasia, infiltration of the subsynovium with macrophages, lymphocytes, and plasma cells and, in severe cases, the development of invasive pannus and cartilage destructive changes. The expression of autoimmunity may result from widely different genetic and regulatory abnormalities in mice depending on the strain under study. Thus, the studies carried out with animal models usually yield results and conclusions with limited applicability to the human counterpart. The fruitful transfer of knowledge derived from studies on animal models to human disease should be the result of a careful consideration of the common features in both species. Overinterpretation of data on the part of the investigator should be avoided.

The list of animal models of arthritis and autoimmunity is long. An exhaustive description of all experimental and spontaneous models is clearly impossible. Models expressing a significant number of clinical, pathologic, and pathophysiologic features in common with human natural counterparts have been selected for discussion here. A considerable amount of information is available on these models since they have attracted investigators pre-cisely because of the features they share with human diseases.

ANIMAL MODELS OF ARTHRITIS

Experimental Models with Immune Pathogenesis

Adjuvant Arthritis of Rats. Polyarthritis induced by a single injection of Freund's adjuvant containing bacterial components has been studied extensively. Its induction and severity are fairly predictable, leading to its widespread use by pharmacologists to study the potential value of immunosuppressive and anti-inflammatory drugs in the treatment of human chronic inflammatory arthritides. It is species-specific and can be produced only in rats. The development of adjuvant arthritis was first described by Stoerk et al.[114] in 1954 in rats injected with complete Freund's adjuvant (containing heat-killed acid-fast bacilli) and spleen homogenate. In 1956, Pearson[85] made similar observations using muscle homogenate instead of spleen cells, and showed that polyarthritis also followed use of complete Freund's adjuvant only, without addition of any tissue homogenate. Numerous studies have since dealt with multiple aspects of this model.[142]

Adjuvant arthritis is induced by intradermal injection of complete Freund's adjuvant into the back, tail, or foot pad, or directly into a lymph node. Not all breeds are equally susceptible to the disease. Rat strains such as Lewis and Sprague-Dawley develop arthritis with an incidence of over 90%, whereas the AVN, Buffalo, and other strains demonstrate significant resistance with an incidence of less than 10%. It has been shown that susceptibility to adjuvant arthritis is controlled in part by genes in or close to the rat major histocompatibility complex.[4]

After adjuvant injection, there is a latent period of about 10 to 12 days prior to the appearance of polyarthritis, which consists of the abrupt onset of acute or subacute inflammation affecting the ankles, wrists, and tarsal and interphalangeal joints. Spine and tail structures are involved often concomitantly with the appearance of the peripheral arthritis. Extra-articular manifestations such as tendonitis, keratitis, iridocyclitis, nodular lesions on exposed surfaces, skin rashes, urethritis, and diarrhea are common. The arthritis is usually self-limited. It increases in severity to a peak at 20 to 25 days after the adjuvant injection, then it involutes slowly. In some animals, there is a tendency to spontaneous recurrences of a cyclic nature, usually at about 60 and 100 days postinoculation. As a result of the acute process, in over 50% of the animals, the arthritis progresses to irreversible joint destruction and ankylosis.

The early synovial lesion consists of a perivascular mononuclear cell infiltrate and edema. Burstein and Waksman[10] showed that the earliest cells appearing in the affected tissues were proliferating mononuclear cells, probably macrophages derived from rapidly dividing bone marrow precursors. Thus, the synovial lesions mimic in many ways the cellular events occurring at the site of a delayed hypersensitivity reaction in the skin. Soon after the onset of the synovial lesions, the inflammatory process becomes more intense. In addition to the increased cellular infiltration, there is fibrin deposition, joint effusion, and a concomitant proliferative response of fibroblasts and osteoblasts. Pannus invades the subchondral bone and occasionally the surface of the articular cartilage, leading to widespread joint destruction with fibrous and bony ankylosis.

The pathologic appearance of the extra-articular lesions has been well described by Pearson et al.[86] In general, they resemble the synovial inflammatory changes described previously. The nodular lesions in the skin, eye, tendons, and genitalia are characterized by perivascular accumulation of mononuclear cells, predominantly histiocytic in appearance. There may be focal areas of fibrin deposition and occasional foci of necrosis. The proliferative aspects of the inflammatory synovitis are also seen in the extra-articular lesions with intense proliferative response of fibroblasts and osteoblasts. In the affected tendons, the fibroblast response leads to pannus formation contributing to fibrous ankylosis and further restriction of joint motion.

Several features strongly suggest that adjuvant disease is induced by a delayed hypersensitivity reaction to a disseminated antigen, i.e., the histologic picture described, the induction of the disease by complete Freund's adjuvant, the latent period between inoculation and clinical expression of the inflammatory response, and the experimental studies to be described. The nature of the antigen(s) is not now known, but there are compelling reasons suggesting that affected rats may develop an aberrant immune response to ubiquitous autoantigen(s). The early studies on the pathogenesis of this model disease addressed the possibility that a latent infection was being activated as a result of the administration of adjuvant. However, multiple studies failed to uncover an infectious agent, and the disease could not be transferred by contact or by infusion of serum or joint tissue into an unaffected rat.[86] A viral etiology is still not ruled out since antiviral agents, including one that does not induce interferon synthesis, can ameliorate the expression of disease.[71] That adjuvant arthritis is due to a delayed hypersensitivity reaction to an unknown antigen was strongly suggested by passive transfer of sensitized T lymphocytes to naive recipients who then developed the disease.[122]

Although the nature of the sensitizing antigen(s) has not yet been elucidated, the finding that the arthritis can still be induced after replacing the mycobacterium in the Freund's adjuvant by apparently nonimmunogenic small molecular weight adjuvants[12] suggests that the antigen(s) involved may be endogenous. Indeed, Trentham et al. showed that rats with classic adjuvant arthritis develop both cell-mediated and humoral immunity to type II collagen.[125] However, the importance of this autoimmune reaction to collagen in the development of tissue injury is not yet completely understood.

There are many reasons why rat adjuvant arthritis has been one of the most frequently used experimental models of inflammatory arthritis to study the mechanisms of action and therapeutic effects of various anti-inflammatory and immunomodulatory agents.[94,119] The most attractive features of this model include: (1) similarities of its clinical and histopathologic picture to human RA and Reiter's syndrome; (2) the immunologic nature of the pathogenic mechanisms involved in the induction of the disease, (3) the ease and reproducibility of induction and clinical course in susceptible rat strains, and (4) the availability of reproducible objective quantitation of the severity of inflammatory joint involvement. Less attractive is its species specificity, and the tendency for bony proliferation and bony ankylosis, both found in Reiter's syndrome but almost never in RA.

Type II Collagen-Induced Arthritis. The arthritis induced in rats by immunization with homologous or heterologous type II collagen was first described by Trentham et al. in 1977.[127] This model is of particular interest since both cell-mediated and humoral immune responses to collagen have been described in patients with RA,[111,116] systemic lupus erythematosus,[47] progressive systemic sclerosis,[117] relapsing polychondritis,[41] and other inflammatory conditions.[116] The arthritis is induced in rats[127] or mice[23,141] by injection of native type II collagen in complete or incomplete Freund's adjuvant. The absolute requirement of homologous or heterologous *native* collagen type II as the inducing antigen is of great interest. Immunization of rats or mice with denatured collagen type II, with peptide fragments, or with collagen types I or III has been unsuccessful in generating arthritis. The ability of both incomplete and complete Freund's adjuvant to induce the arthritis is also significant. Because the disease has many clinical and histopathologic similarities to adjuvant arthritis, collagen type II theoretically could act as an adjuvant in lieu of mycobacterium and give rise to adjuvant disease. However, studies have failed to show any evidence that collagen type II behaves as an adjuvant.[26] Although animals with either adjuvant disease or collagen type II-induced arthritis develop cell-mediated and humoral immunity to collagen,[125] several features suggest that the two experimental models may have a different pathogenesis.[61]

In Wistar, Lewis, or Sprague-Dawley rats the incidence of clinically apparent arthritis is about 40 to 80%.[127] The onset of polyarthritis is usually abrupt, occurring 14 to 60 days after immunization, with peak onset at 20 days. Although the joints of the hindlimbs usually become involved, forepaw inflammation occurs only in about 10% of those developing arthritis. Involvement is predominantly distal, with ankles and tarsal and interphalangeal joints most commonly affected. Inflammation reaches maximum severity within 4 or 5 days, and swelling usually persists for 5 to 8 weeks. The involved joints usually develop permanent deformity. In contrast to adjuvant arthritis, the spine is not involved and no extra-articular manifestations are observed. However, about 10% of the animals develop erythema and nodular or diffuse induration of the ears, lesions clinically and histologically different from the ear lesions associated with adjuvant disease.

The disease in mice is induced by intradermal immunization of type II collagen in adjuvant followed by an intraperitoneal booster injection of collagen 21 days later. The onset of collagen-induced arthritis in mice is extremely variable, occurring 19 to 112 days after the initial immunizing injection, with a mean of 47 days. The incidence of arthritis is also variable, depending on the genetic susceptibility of the inbred strains used. In susceptible strains, the ankle joints are most often involved. Swelling and redness usually involve the entire foot, doubling the size of the dorsum of the foot and intermalleolar thicknesses. Spine involvement or extra-articular manifestations do not develop in mice either.

The earliest alterations include profuse fibrin deposition over the synovial and articular cartilage surfaces. Subsequently, the synovial lining cells become hyperplastic; the cells appear round with increased number of filopodia. Fibrin deposition and hyperplasia may be seen in joints that do not go on to develop cellular infiltrates. As arthritis progresses in about 20% of the animals, the subsynovium becomes infiltrated with mononuclear cells and polymorphonuclear leukocytes. The latter disappear about 6 or 7 weeks postimmunization. The synovial proliferative changes lead to the formation of villi and of invasive pannus covering the articular surface of the cartilage. In the later stages, the synovium is hypertrophied and fibrotic. The articular cartilage and the subchondral bone covered by pannus show widespread erosive changes and periosteal new bone formation leading to joint ankylosis.[11,127] In mice, the histologic changes are similar.[23,141]

The histologic appearance of the auricular chondritis that develops in about 10% of the immunized rats is of interest since it is similar to the picture seen in patients with relapsing polychondritis (see Chap. 69). The involved ears show focal cellular perichondrial infiltrates. The early lesions consist of polymorphonuclear leukocytes scattered over a mononuclear cell background with necrosis of chondrocytes and matrix loss adjacent to the cell infiltrates. In later stages, the cartilage is surrounded by multinucleated giant cells and histiocytes. Occasionally, the inflammatory process leads to complete destruction of the normal auricular cartilage. The costal cartilages, tracheae, major bronchi, and aortic valves of the affected rats show no evidence of inflammation.[25,127]

There is compelling evidence that the inflammatory arthritis in this model is mediated by a specific immune response to homologous or heterologous native type II collagen. The disease can be transferred passively with spleen and lymph node cells obtained from sensitized donor animals.[126] However, the exact pathogenetic mechanisms responsible for the induction and maintenance of the chronic arthritis are not completely understood, since the disease is associated with the development of high levels of both cell-mediated and humoral immunity. Studies indicate that antibodies with specificity for the helical structure of collagen type II may be important in the induction of arthritis. Clague et al.[14] found a correlation between antibody titers and the development of arthritis in different strains of rats.

It is possible to passively transfer the disease in rats with serum containing anticollagen type II antibodies.[115] Immunogenetic studies using inbred mice also have emphasized the importance of humoral immunity in the induction of arthritis. Immunization of mice with collagen type II induces equally good skin test reactivity to both native and denatured collagen, but humoral antibodies are more specific for the helical conformation of native collagen.[118,141] The antibody responses to collagen are under genetic control. Mice with H-2^b and H-2^s genotypes are high responders to collagen type I, whereas the H-2^q determines high responses to collagen type II. With few exceptions, the mouse strains susceptible to the development of arthritis are also high responders to collagen II. Although arthritis does not develop in the absence of an antibody response to collagen II, the reverse is not always true. B10.S and B10.D2 mice are not susceptible to the development of arthritis, but their antibody responses to collagen type II reach high values. It has been argued that overt arthritis may depend on the development of a critical level of an antibody specific for a particular epitope on native type II collagen.[118] In B10 mice, the antibodies may have a different specificity, akin to those (directed primarily against covalent structural determinants) appearing after immunization with denatured collagens, although these may cross-react with the native molecule. The role of immunity to collagen in the pathogenesis of RA or other connective tissue diseases has not yet been established. It is likely that additional studies with this experimental model may contribute to a better delineation of the role of this autoimmune mechanism in human disease.

Antigen-Induced Arthritis. One of the major distinctive clinical features of RA is its chronic, relentless course. Both experimental arthritis models described previously may resemble the human disease in their histologic picture, but both have a relatively short clinical course. It has been suggested that chronicity of RA may be due to a local immune response directed against a self-replicating infectious agent or to renewable autoantigen (see Chap. 35). For these reasons, chronic infectious arthritis models or chronic arthritis induced by intra-articular injection of antigen into previously immunized animals may be better suited to study mechanisms involved in the long-term maintenance of chronic joint inflammation.

Experimental arthritis produced by intra-articular injection of antigen was first described over 70 years ago,[43] but this model attracted widespread attention only after Dumonde and Glynn[36] produced chronic arthritis in rabbits sensitized to autologous or heterologous fibrin and subsequently injected intra-articularly with the insoluble antigen. The chronic synovitis was postulated to be caused by a local delayed hypersensitivity reaction. Other soluble antigens, such as ovalbumin,[19,22] bovine serum albumin,[22] ferritin,[121] or horseradish peroxidase[52] injected intra-articularly in rabbits

previously immunized to the antigen in complete Freund's adjuvant, also gave rise to a long-standing arthritis, lasting in some cases over 6 months. A chronic arthritis with the same features has been described in mice[9] or rabbits immunized with antigen in complete Freund's adjuvant. Several authors have emphasized the use of complete adjuvant since chronic arthritis does not develop in animals immunized with incomplete Freund's adjuvant, indicating the need for a vigorous immune response to the injected antigen.

A few hours after the antigen injection, acute joint inflammation associated with severe swelling and exudation develops. Swelling decreases slowly over 2 weeks to a variable plateau. About one-third of the animals show a thickened synovium for 8 to 24 weeks. Inflammatory synovial fluid is obtained from the joint cavity in the first week following injection; thereafter, the chronic synovitis is not associated with free exudate. Invasive pannus and cartilage erosions develop 4 to 6 weeks after intra-articular injection, but the affected animals may not show any visible functional impairment.

Severe acute synovitis developing within a few hours after the intra-articular injection of antigen represents an Arthus reaction in animals with high titers of precipitating IgG antibodies.[35] Microscopically, 2 to 12 hours postinjection, there is widespread engorgement of many large and small vessels throughout the synovium. Tissue infiltration, with large numbers of polymorphonuclear leukocytes, hemorrhagic changes, vascular thrombosis, and tissue necrosis are seen in most specimens. In the initial 2 to 4 days the joint cavity is filled with an exudate loaded with erythrocytes and polymorphonuclear leukocytes. The synovial membrane and cartilage are often covered by a thick coat of fibrin. The articular cartilage shows widespread necrosis of the superficial chondrocytes and depletion of intercellular matrix. Three to six days postinjection, the acute phase of the synovitis begins to subside. The polymorphonuclear leukocyte infiltrate becomes less prominent, and mononuclear cells with the appearance of tissue macrophages and histiocytes appear in the subsynovium. The lining layer shows active proliferation reaching a thickness of 6 to 8 cell layers in many areas. The fibrinous exudate becomes infiltrated with round cells and fibroblasts and shows early evidence of organization. At this stage, the subsynovial cellular infiltrate is composed of heterophiles and large mononuclear cells, but few lymphocytes and plasma cells.

By 3 to 4 weeks, there is diffuse proliferation of synovial lining cells, scattered areas of fibrosis in the deeper layers, and lymphocytes and plasma cells infiltrating the subsynovium. Moreover, at this stage of chronic synovitis, there is a tendency to form collections of lymphocytes, resembling lymphoid follicles, similar to those seen in established rheumatoid synovitis. The articular cartilage shows small scattered erosions and, in some areas, early invasive pannus extends onto the articular surface. In later stages, 4 to 6 months postinjection, about 30% of the animals show evidence of active progressive chronic synovitis. Synovial proliferation and subsynovial infiltration with clumps of lymphocytes and plasma cells are still prominent. The articular cartilage shows progressive damage with widespread erosions and replacement by fibrous tissue. In many areas, the chondrocytes appear dead and the remaining matrix is disrupted by amorphous deposits and fibrin. Electron microscopic studies confirm the light microscopic appearance, and the superficial layer of residual cartilage contains amorphous electron-dense deposits, identified as immune complexes.[21,128] The collagen fiber meshwork is disorganized and, in many areas, the fibers lose their typical banding.

An acute Arthus reaction[35] in the injected joints is not surprising, since its prerequisite high titers of precipitating IgG antigen-specific antibody are certainly present in most rabbits. However, the mechanism maintaining long-term chronic synovitis in this model is a matter of debate. Dumonde and Glynn emphasized the use of complete adjuvant to establish a strong delayed hypersensitivity reaction to the antigen as a requirement for the development of the chronic stage of the disease.[36] Support for this hypothesis was adduced as the development of chronic synovitis correlated better with the magnitude of cell-mediated immunity than with antibody titers in individual rabbits.[42,78] Alternatively, studies by Cooke et al. suggested that humoral mechanisms may play an important part in the development of chronic synovitis in this model.[22] The inflamed synovial membranes synthesize immunoglobulins in vitro to the same extent as spleen or lymph node tissues. Moreover, 30 to 40% of these immunoglobulins represent specific antibody to the antigen injected up to 8 weeks previously suggesting that a sustained local antibody response is maintained by persisting antigen. Further study shows that the injected antigen is selectively retained in the joints of previously immunized animals and is released slowly.[21] The major portion of the retained antigen is localized to avascular collagenous tissues in the joint, i.e., articular cartilage, menisci, and intra-articular ligaments, and is associated with specific antibody and complement components. Antigen retained in the form of immune complexes may serve as the stimulus for prolonged local antibody synthesis in the synovium, providing a source of complement-fixing

antigen-antibody complexes provoking a sustained inflammatory response. Local trapping of antigen depends on the presence of antibody in the extravascular compartment, since immune complex formation probably occurs within the articular collagen fiber meshwork.[58,67] The exact role of the trapped immune complexes remains to be established, but when menisci containing immune complexes are surgically inserted into the suprapatellar pouches of previously immunized animals, a chronic inflammatory capsule develops around the donor tissue, reminiscent of the inflammatory pannus seen in rheumatoid cartilage.[69]

The chronic nature of this experimental immune synovitis probably depends both on the presence of a critical number of circulating lymphocytes specific for the antigen injected and on enough circulating antibody to retain sufficient antigen to establish a sustained local chronic inflammatory process. Local antibody synthesis may help maintain the sequestered complexes in antibody excess, ensuring their insolubility and slow release. The relevance of this model with regard to pathogenic mechanisms in RA is strengthened by the observation that most pannus-free rheumatoid articular cartilage and meniscus specimens contain trapped immune complexes with the same localization shown for the rabbit model.[20]

Chronic arthritis might be due to the long-term retention of local antigen in the affected joints because antigen has been detectable for many weeks after injection, but the arthritis may last more than 6 months in some animals. Although the number of retained molecules needed to provoke arthritis is extremely small,[137] an inflammatory process of long duration may be due to the development of an immune reaction to an autoantigen, probably a product of the inflammatory process itself.[89]

Streptococcal Cell Wall-Induced Arthritis. Attempts to induce chronic experimental arthritis with streptococcal cell wall preparations arose from the observation that a single intradermal injection of sonically disrupted group A streptococci provokes a prolonged intermittent inflammatory lesion in rabbit skin.[29] This was related to the long-term persistence of the cell-wall material in macrophages.[83] Further work by the same group led to the development of interesting models of chronic arthritis in rabbits[99] and rats[27] and a carditis resembling rheumatic fever in mice.[28]

In rabbits, a single intra-articular injection of isolated fragments of group A streptococcal cell walls induces acute synovitis with maximal swelling 2 days after injection and subsidence in 4 to 5 days. Subsequent chronic synovitis may not be severe enough to be detectable clinically. A single intraperitoneal injection of large amounts of cell-wall sonicate induces acute polyarthritis in 100% of susceptible rat strains. By day 2 after injection, most animals show from 2 to 35 acutely inflamed joints, usually involving ankles, wrists, and interphalangeal, tarsophalangeal, carpophalangeal, tarsal, and carpal joints. About 50% of these animals have findings lasting 10 to 12 weeks that are characterized by exacerbations and partial remissions. Many chronically involved joints show gross deformities or ankylosis. The course of polyarthritis is marked by at least two cycles of exacerbations and complete remissions in 40% of rats peaking on weeks 5 and 10 after injection. Rats exhibiting this intermittent pattern of polyarthritis sometimes also have chronic deformities and ankylosis. This peculiar clinical course and the observation that the susceptibility to polyarthritis varies from strain to strain[27] suggest that this model may share pathogenic mechanisms with adjuvant-induced arthritis.

The early microscopic changes in the rabbit model consist of accumulation of a fibrinopurulent exudate, focal synovial necrosis, and intense infiltration with polymorphonuclear leukocytes. Two to three weeks after the intra-articular injection, the exudative process is slowly replaced by hypertrophy of synovial villi, hyperplasia of the lining layer, and diffuse infiltration of the subsynovium by macrophages and giant cells. The macrophages are mostly replaced by focal accumulations of lymphocytes 4 to 6 weeks after injection. At the end of 9 weeks, inflammatory changes are minimal.

In susceptible rat strains, such as outbred Sprague-Dawleys, polyarthritis can be severely erosive. The initial acute inflammatory synovitis may be detected as early as 5 hours postinjection and is monotonously similar in all of the models discussed here. Acutely, synovitis is characterized by congestion, edema, profuse deposition of fibrin, lining cell layer hyperplasia, and intense infiltration with leukocytes and macrophages. The joint capsules and periarticular and subcutaneous tissues are also involved acutely. This acute process is slowly replaced by a chronic erosive arthritis, with proliferative synovitis and intense subsynovial infiltration with macrophages and lymphocytes. In severely involved joints, pannus invades cartilage and subchondral bone, replacing these tissues by vascular granulation tissue and disrupting their normal architecture. Chronic synovitis may subside without causing irreversible destructive changes in other joints. In most animals, synovitis is observed microscopically for 10 weeks after injection. Between 11 and 30 weeks only one-third of the rats still show active lesions.

The peptidoglycan portion of the streptococcal cell walls has been implicated in the genesis of the inflammatory changes. This macromolecule con-

sists of a backbone of alternating N-acetylglucosamine and N-acetyl-muramic acid units linked by β-1,4 bonds. In the streptococcus, the acetyl muramic acid residues are covalently linked to pentapeptide side-chains composed of L-alanine, D-glutamine, L-lysine, and two D-alanine residues. The carbohydrate backbone is also linked to group-specific polysaccharide chains. The peptidoglycan moiety may be responsible for the toxic effects on the tissues while the polysaccharide side-chains protect the mucopeptide from digestion by intracellular lysozymes.[100] Such resistance to biodegradation leading to long-term persistence within macrophages correlates with prolonged inflammatory reactions.[99] In the rabbit arthritis model, the peptidoglycan persists in synovial macrophages for at least 5 weeks, and its presence within the joint correlates with the evolution of the inflammatory process.[99] Peptidoglycan could be detected within mononuclear cells up to 63 days after injection, and in spleen and liver throughout the 180 days of the study.[30]

Although the peptide and polysaccharide moieties of the cell wall fragments are both antigenic, specific immune mechanisms may play a secondary role in the development of arthritis. First, the acute inflammatory synovitis may be detected as early as 5 hours after the intraperitoneal injection. Moreover, although many animals develop humoral[53] and cell-mediated immune responses[59] to the bacterial antigen, there is little or no correlation between the immune responses and the development or severity of arthritis. Since bacterial peptidoglycans are potent macrophage activators, the inflammatory reaction may be the result of this process. The undigestible peptidoglycan-polysaccharide complexes may persist in macrophages that release peptide mediators of inflammation and lysosomal proteases with the subsequent tissue injury and repair.

The pathogenic background of these four chronic arthritis models resides in the concept that an inflammatory process develops as a result of an immune response against a locally persisting foreign antigen or autoantigen. Undigestible bacterial products persisting within cells may generate tissue injury through the same final common inflammatory pathway.

Experimental Production of Rheumatoid Factors. In human diseases characterized by intense and sustained antigenic stimulation, a significant proportion of patients develops positive tests for rheumatoid factor (see Chap. 41). Stimulation of autoantibody may be the result of nonspecific polyclonal activation of B lymphocytes containing a subpopulation of precursor cells programmed for rheumatoid factor synthesis. The experimental counterpart of this clinical finding has been reproduced in rabbits hyperimmunized with bacterial vaccines.[13] Repeated injections of streptococcal vaccines in susceptible rabbits induce the synthesis of large amounts of IgM and IgG rheumatoid factors,[8] which in some animals appear homogenous with common idiotypic determinants.[7] Rheumatoid factor production following hyperimmunization appears to be under genetic control since large quantitative differences have been observed between rabbit families. The development of rheumatoid factors due to inordinate B-lymphocyte activation after hyperimmunization with foreign antigens may share common mechanisms with chronic graft vs. host reactions in mice.

Infectious Arthritis

Mycoplasma Arthritis. Mycoplasmas are small bacteria with fastidious growth requirements, but without rigid cell walls, and are found in latent form in almost all species of laboratory animals. Many strains of these microorganisms are arthritogenic, producing chronic arthritis spontaneously or under experimental conditions. In swine, cattle, and rats, both epizootic and sporadic infections with *Mycoplasma hyorhinis* and *M. arthritidis* have been reported. In addition, experimental arthritis has been described in pigs, rats, and rabbits.[16,18,108,133]

The clinical course of arthritis produced by *M. arthritidis* in rats or mice is somewhat different. In rats, the site of injection develops a well-capsulated abscess that soon resolves. Arthritis onset is relatively acute, developing a few days after injection and peaking 7 to 14 days later. It rapidly subsides 2 to 3 weeks later.[132] In mice, the injection with viable organisms commonly produces severe and extensive abscesses. However, arthritis is less severe than in the rat, and is characterized by gradual progression for as long as 9 months with periods of remission and exacerbation.[16]

The acute suppurative synovitis in the rat frequently leads to irreversible severe joint destruction. In mice, the synovium shows an initial acute phase with polymorphonuclear leukocyte infiltration and mild proliferative changes; the chronic phase is characterized by massive synovial proliferation, mononuclear cell infiltration, articular cartilage and juxta-articular bone erosions, and pannus formation.

Mycoplasmas can be recovered from the affected joints at all stages of the disease, although the number of microorganisms tends to be lower during the chronic inflammatory phase. The mechanisms of arthritogenesis of mycoplasma are not well understood, but several biologic characteristics may account for its ability to maintain chronic inflammation. Mycoplasmas can attach to and modify host cell membranes, mediate T- and B-lymphocyte activation, induce lymphocyte cytotoxicity, stimulate interferon production, and activate complement.[17] The role of the immune response to the injected agents in the development and maintenance of the synovitis has not been defined. Partial protection against the development of arthritis develops in animals previously injected or in mice injected with formalin-killed *M. arthritidis*.[18]

The rabbit model of mycoplasma arthritis developed at the University of Utah is of particular interest since it may represent an example of chronic "infectious" arthritis persisting in the apparent absence of the etiologic agents.[133] Following intra-articular injection of viable *M. arthritidis* or *M. pulmonis*, an acute and chronic inflammatory reaction develops that may persist at least one year. The disease is characterized by an initial acute synovitis with heterophile infiltration during the first week, followed by a proliferative synovitis and subsynovial infiltration with lymphocytes and plasma cells often organized around blood vessels and mimicking lymphoid follicles. Invasive pannus and articular cartilage erosions may develop in two-thirds of the rabbits injected with *M. arthritidis*.

Despite the sustained synovitis persisting for many months, viable mycoplasmas or mycoplasma antigens cannot be found in joint tissues 7 weeks after injection. However, high antibody titers in synovial fluids persist for many weeks, suggesting a local immune response to the mycoplasma. Granular deposits containing IgG and complement in synovium and cartilage are detectable after the local disappearance of mycoplasma antigens.[135] Other studies indicate that it is possible to induce a chronic monoarthritis by intra-articular injection of nonviable mycoplasma in rabbits previously exposed to live *M. arthritidis*.[134] Here there is strong correlation between synovial fluid antibody levels and the severity of the synovitis. In addition, immune complexes in cartilage and menisci are detected 7 weeks after the intra-articular injection. These observations suggest that immune mechanisms similar to those operative in antigen-induced arthritis may also play an important role both in this model and in the arthritis generated with live organisms. Alternatively, the failure to detect antigenic material in synovium or cartilage also suggests that the late chronic synovitis could be maintained by the development of immunity against an autoantigen present within the joint.

Erysipelothrix Insidiosa Arthritis. Spontaneous or experimental *E. insidiosa* (previously called *E. rhusiopathiae*) arthritis has been reported in swine, dogs, and rabbits.[3,102,103] This model has some features in common with mycoplasma arthritis. *E. insidiosa* arthritis is also characterized by an early acute stage followed by a prolonged chronic synovitis that may last several years and lead to severe destructive changes. The histologic changes are similar to the chronic synovitis induced by mycoplasma. The synovium shows hypertrophy and perivascular infiltration with lymphocytes, plasma cells, and macrophages. In severe cases, pannus formation and cartilage erosive changes are common.

This model also shares other interesting characteristics, not only with mycoplasma arthritis but also with RA itself. Viable organisms can be recovered from the affected joints only in the early stages of the disease. Using a technique based on RNA-DNA hybridization capable of detecting one organism per 50 mammalian cells, Steinman and Hsu were unable to demonstrate the presence of *E. insidiosa* in synovial specimens from miniature pigs with chronic arthritis produced by intravenous injection of the organism.[113] However, other studies suggest that bacterial products may play a role in the induction of arthritis. White et al. showed that arthritis can be reproduced in rabbits by multiple intravenous injection of a cell-free extract of *Erysipelothrix*.[138] Bacterial products labeled with fluorescein localize in the inflamed synovium. In rabbits and dogs with experimental *E. insidiosa* arthritis,[3,102] serum rheumatoid factors can be readily detected. Moreover, rheumatoid factor-like material has been found in leukocyte inclusions obtained from rabbits with *Erysipelothrix* arthritis.[3]

The mechanisms responsible for chronicity in these infectious arthritis models have not been elucidated. Failure to detect bacterial products within the joint does not eliminate the possibility that these may still be directly or indirectly responsible for the maintenance of chronic inflammation. However, the alternative hypothesis that a second independent pathophysiologic process initiated by the infection may take over as the chronic stimulus is attractive, particularly in view of the current ideas on the pathogenetic mechanisms operative in RA (see Chap. 35).

Viral Arthritis. A spontaneous chronic viral arthritis in goats has been described.[24] A retrovirus with antigenic similarities to the visna virus has been shown to be responsible for the production of chronic progressive arthritis, tendonitis, and bursitis in adult animals and a demyelinating encephalomyelitis in kids. The arthritis is characterized by progressive mononuclear cell infiltration and lining cell hyperplasia, hypertrophy, and necrosis. Viral particles are present in lining layer cells up to 45 days after inoculation, and live virus has been isolated from inoculated goats up to 79 days after infection.

Two spontaneous forms of feline chronic progressive arthritis have been described. One is characterized by prominent periosteal bone formation around affected joints. The other resembles RA and is associated with the development of subchondral marginal erosions and joint deformity. A feline syncytium-forming virus has been either isolated or detected serologically in all cats tested.[87]

A self-limiting chronic experimental arthritis has been induced in both inoculated and contralateral rabbit knees by injection of herpes virus of the hominis strain.[136] The arthritis persists for 3 months, at which time no evidence of live virus can be detected. Histologically, subsynovial vessel formation, lymphocyte infiltration, and lining cell layer hyperplasia are seen. Some animals develop cartilage erosions and reactive periostitis.

ANIMAL MODELS OF AUTOIMMUNITY

Several well-characterized murine models for human systemic lupus erythematosus (SLE) are discussed in this chapter. Because the genetic background remains constant among different members of an inbred mouse strain, the sequence and spectrum of disease expression are rather homogenous within that strain. The reproducibility of disease features within strains has permitted investigations of both the immunopathogenesis and therapy of SLE. For example, modification of the environment, diet, hormonal status, or the administration of either drugs or certain forms of irradiation to mice of a given strain each has profoundly altered the expression of the autoimmune syndrome characteristic of that strain. Several strains in addition to New Zealand mice have been developed that express SLE-like autoimmunity. The clinical and immunopathologic manifestations of their illness have been described in detail.[2] It has become painfully clear that pathogenic mechanisms or therapeutic success in one strain may not operate and fail in the others.[124] In recent years, therefore, investigators have performed experiments in several autoimmunity-prone strains before arriving at universal conclusions. Since the clinical manifestations of SLE in man also exhibit considerable heterogeneity, this comparative approach in murine lupus research is more likely to yield information regarding basic common mechanisms relevant to our understanding and treatment of lupus in man.

New Zealand Mice

The prototype murine model of spontaneous autoimmunity is the New Zealand Black (NZB) mouse. The immunopathology of this strain has been reviewed.[79] Virtually all NZB mice, male and female, develop a severe autoimmune hemolytic anemia associated with reticulocytosis and hepatosplenomegaly by one year of age. An indolent membranous glomerulonephritis often develops that terminally can acquire proliferative features. Approximately 12 to 20% of NZB mice develop a lymphoid cancer in their second year of life. Overall, untreated NZB mice live a life span equivalent to "middle age" in man.

The immunologic abnormalities present in NZB mice are manifold, and their cellular basis is complex. Although the disease can be transferred with bone marrow cells,[80] defects of mature B- and T-lymphocytes and of macrophages have been documented in various experimental systems.[112,124] Consequently, considerable debate exists regarding the mechanism by which the activation of autoantibody-producing B cells occurs. It is clear that the immunopathology is a consequence of the overproduction of antibodies directed toward self-determinants. For example, accelerated maturation from the pre-B cell to the mature B cell occurs in the bone marrow of NZB mice at an early age.[70] Moreover, unusual Ly-1 positive B cells present in the spleens[57] can account for the spontaneous, well-documented, polyclonal production of IgM in NZB mice.[77,81] Whether microenvironmental factors such as those exerted by cells of a monocyte/macrophage lineage, either in the bone marrow or spleen, might play a role in driving the differentiation of these B cells is not clear.[70] Functionally, the abnormality appears to reside within the B cells assayed in various systems, such as cloning in soft agar[70] or susceptibility to tolerance induction.[50,51] Theoretically, accelerated maturation of B cells could arise from defective thymic-derived lymphocyte regulation. Defects in T cells include abnormal responses to mitogens and in the autologous mixed lymphocyte reaction,[49] production of interleukin-2,[32] cytotoxic and suppressor T cell generation, and susceptibility to tolerance induction.[44,76,109,112] Moreover, a defect in the generation of auto-anti-idiotypic antibodies to control the development of Coombs antibodies in NZB mice has been suggested.[15]

When NZB mice are mated with New Zealand White (NZW) mice, the F_1 offspring manifest an autoimmune syndrome distinct from that found in the parental NZB strain. NZB/W female mice develop an extensive membranoproliferative glomerulonephritis leading to death between 8 and 10 months of age. Congenitally athymic (nude) female NZB/W mice similarly develop fatal glomerulonephritis during the first year of life, indicating that autoimmune disease in this strain is T cell independent.[45] Male survival into the second year of life has been related to hormonal differences.[97] The glomerular lesions are associated with the deposition of DNA anti-DNA immune complexes and complement.[74] Murine retroviral glycoprotein antigen, GP-70, and its specific antibody also have been eluted from glomerular lesions in NZB/W mice.[62,65] The relative nephritogenicity of these two antigen:antibody systems in murine lupus is still unclear.

NZB/W mice may be a model for human Sjögren's syndrome because of mononuclear cell infiltration of lacrimal and salivary glands, and renal interstitium. NZB/W mice also develop lymphoid cancer, but to a lesser degree than in the NZB parent strain.[79,120] The Coombs positive hemolytic anemia so characteristic of NZB mice is not clinically significant in the NZB/W F_1 hybrid. Similarly, overt central nervous system and skin disease are not apparent, but immune complex deposition in the choroid plexus[75] and at the dermal-epidermal junction[46] has been detected.

Because of the prominence of glomerulonephritis in the female NZB/W mice, this model has been touted as the experimental analogue of lupus nephritis in man. The role of various drugs as well as diet and hormonal manipulations have been studied in these mice. Treatment with either corticosteroids or cyclophosphamide prolongs life, but greatly increases the incidence of neoplasm.[130,31] Prolonged survival also follows treatment with prostaglandin E1,[64,143] essential fatty acid deprivation,[60] low-calorie diet,[63] zinc deprivation,[5] or total lymphoid irradiation.[73,104]

The genetics of autoimmunity expressed in New Zealand mice has been studied in detail and reviewed.[101] Sophisticated studies using recombinant inbred lines derived from F_2 generation matings between NZB and nonautoimmune mice have showed independent segregation of genes determining the various autoantibodies (anti-erythrocyte, natural thymocytotoxic, and anti-single stranded DNA autoantibodies), those determining polyclonal B cell activation, and those determining the expression of retroviruses.[31,92] Similarly, each of these genes segregates independently from other immunologic markers such as immunoglobulin heavy chain allotypes and the major histocompatibility locus. Therefore, multiple genes are involved in the autoimmune disease of NZB mice. Moreover, interactions occur among various genes within the NZB mouse as well as with NZW genes in the NZB/W F_1 mouse hybrid.[101] In addition, environmental factors impinging on this complex genetic background have been observed in a strain of NZB mice that expresses an X-linked immunodeficiency, primarily involving the lack of a B cell population, designated Lyb5. Such congeneic NZB.CBA/N mice ordinarily do not manifest polyclonal B cell activation or develop significant autoimmunity, but do acquire the latter if continually stimulated by various polyclonal activators.[105] The NZB model of autoimmunity demonstrates well the complex interaction between multiple genes whose expression may be further modified by the unpredictable external environment.

MRL Mice

As noted previously, genetic analyses of New Zealand mice rule out the concept of a single "autoimmunity" gene. In the late 1970s, additional models were developed in the Jackson Laboratory by Murphy and Roths. The MRL/Mp-*lpr/lpr*, also known as MRL/1, is a model for an accelerated membranoproliferative glomerulonephritis associated with anti-DNA production.[2] Both male and female members of this strain die between 5 and 7 months of age. A congeneic strain designated MRL/Mp⁻⁺/⁺, also known as MRL/n, develops a low-grade autoimmune syndrome, dying midway in the second year of life. This latter mouse develops antibody to the Sm antigen,[39] a specific marker for SLE in man, but does not develop the impressive lymphoproliferative disorder present in the *lpr/lpr* counterpart. The MRL/Mp-*lpr/lpr* mouse is the only strain that develops a detectable synovitis in up to 75% of individuals in addition to immune complex glomerulonephritis.[2,56] A high correlation between serum IgM rheumatoid factor and the development of erosive arthritis has been recorded.[56] This feature has been used to promote the MRL/Mp-*lpr/lpr* mouse as a natural occurring model of RA. This strain may also develop a necrotizing polyarteritis with dense infiltration by polymorphonuclear leukocytes and fibrinoid necrosis of medium-size arterial walls of kidneys, genital organs, and heart in 75% of individuals.[2,6]

The advantage of the MRL/Mp-*lpr/lpr* strain for drug and diet studies relates to the rapid pace of the autoimmune syndrome and the death of the mouse, both of which are markedly accelerated compared to the NZB/W female. The therapeutic efficacy of PGE1,[64] total lymphoid irradiation,[123] and cyclophosphamide[106] have been clearly shown in this model in addition to their previously noted beneficial effect in NZB/W mice. The therapeutic effect of PGE1 administration as well as low-calorie diet was more closely linked to the inhibition of formation of circulating endogenous retroviral envelope glycoprotein GP-70-anti-GP-70 immune complexes than to the inhibition of anti-native DNA autoantibodies.[63,64] The deposition of retroviral immune complexes in glomeruli may be highly pathogenic in MRL/Mp-*lpr/lpr* and NZB/W mice and critically important for the development of vasculitis in the former strain.[6]

The genetics of this model appears simpler than in the NZB mouse. The *lpr* gene is a single locus

autosomal recessive gene that merely functions as an accelerating factor interacting with MRL background genes present in the MRL/Mp⁻⁺/⁺ mouse. The effect of the *lpr* gene by itself can be more clearly appreciated by the successful transfer of this gene to mice with no known autoimmune potential. Thus, C57BL/6-*lpr/lpr* and C3H/HeJ-*lpr/lpr* mice develop substantial lymphoadenopathy, anti-DNA antibody,[88] and immune complex glomerulonephritis leading to death at approximately one year of age.[95]

Clues to the mode of action of the *lpr* gene have been detected. In contrast to the NZB, NZB/W, and BXSB/Mp strains where neonatal thymectomy will dramatically accelerate the development of autoimmunity, such a maneuver will abolish its development in the MRL/Mp-*lpr/lpr* mouse.[124,139] The T cell dependence of MRL disease is further supported by the observation of massive proliferation of T cells in the spleen and lymph nodes of the *lpr* mouse[124] that have been shown further to be rich in helper cell activity with respect to antibody formation.[124] More recently, T cell-derived lymphokines, designated B cell differentiation factors, have been detected in the supernatants of cultured lymphoid cells from *lpr* mice whether on the MRL or C57BL/6 backgrounds.[91] It is probable that these factors play an important role in the activation and maturation of nearby B cells and in their secretion of IgG autoantibodies. Mice with the *lpr* gene also have been shown to exhibit defects in the production of interleukin-2 (T cell growth factor) as well as in the production of receptors for interleukin-2.[1,140] The presence of such defects in all murine SLE strains suggests that these are not the primary expression of the *lpr* gene.[32] Similarly, increased Ia-positive peritoneal macrophages have been detected in MRL/Mp-*lpr/lpr* and NZB mice in association with autoantibody formation, but their absence in *lpr* mice with the C57BL/6 and C3H/HeJ backgrounds indicates that this feature is not tightly linked to the expression of the *lpr* gene.[72]

BXSB Mice

Another strain developed by Murphy and Roths, the BXSB/Mp mouse, is unusual in that males develop autoimmunity quite early, dying at 5 to 7 months of age, whereas the female BXSB/Mp mice develop an indolent autoimmune syndrome that does not lead to death until well into the second year of life. The BXSB/Mp male mice develop a Coombs positive hemolytic anemia and, more importantly, a rapidly progressive immune complex membranoproliferative glomerulonephritis.[2] In addition, a degenerative vascular disease involving the coronary arteries is noted in some mice of this strain,[2,6] but is far more striking in the male offspring of the mating between BXSB/Mp males and NZW females.[55] Coronary disease is observed in 100% of the (NZWxBXSB)F$_1$ males and is responsible for death at approximately 5 months of age. The pathology reveals a paucity of cellular infiltrate in the coronary vessels. The pathogenesis of this lesion has been linked to sustained low levels of circulating immune complexes in contrast to the necrotizing polyarteritis of MRL/Mp-*lpr/lpr* mice, which is associated with high levels of circulating immune complexes that trigger an inflammatory reaction once deposited.[6] It is conceivable that vasospastic compounds such as thromboxanes may play a significant role in the pathogenesis of this lesion (see Chap. 22). Thus, this model may be ideally suited to examine the effect of thromboxane inhibitors, prostaglandin E1, as well as diet modification, particularly with regard to lipid content on the development of degenerative coronary vascular disease. As with MRL/Mp-*lpr/lpr* mice, the BXSB male and the (NZWxBXSB)F$_1$ male are ideal models for study of drug, diet, and other therapeutic modalities since their life span is markedly shortened and each has distinctive immunopathology.

Immunologic and genetic pathogenetic factors in the SLE syndrome in BXSB/Mp male mice involve a Y chromosome-linked factor that is not mediated via male hormones.[38,82] An abnormal B cell function of BXSB/Mp male mice may be augmented by thymectomy.[107] An enhanced response to normal T cell-derived lymphokines by BXSB/Mp- and NZB-derived B cells, activated by either lipopolysaccharide or anti-immunoglobulin, has been demonstrated.[90] This observation, together with a defined defect in tolerance induction at the B cell level,[54] indicates that the disease in the BXSB/Mp male, like that in the NZB mouse, involves an inherent B cell abnormality in its pathogenesis.

Parent to F$_1$-Induced Graft Versus Host Reactions

A model has been developed by Gleichmann and coworkers.[40,48] Essentially, a chronic graft-versus-host reaction (GVHR) is achieved by the transfer of parental helper T cell-enriched, suppressor T cell-depleted, spleen cells into nonirradiated F$_1$ hosts. Similarly, a chronic GVHR is achieved with certain strain combinations favoring the generation of T cell help even with the transfer of unfractionated spleen cells [e.g., DBA/2→(C57BL/10xDBA/2) F$_1$, or combinations differing only at the I region locus]. In both cases, the chronic GVHR triggers an SLE-like syndrome. Precedent for SLE-like autoimmunity and the development of scleroderma-like skin disease ensuing from a

GVHR was first reported in rats[110] and later in mice.[66] The donor T cells recognize allogeneic F$_1$ major histocompatibility antigens, resulting in chronically augmented nonspecific T cell helper function. These mice develop a whole series of autoantibodies characteristic of SLE,[48] including antinuclear antibodies, Coombs antibody, natural thymocytotoxic autoantibody, and anti-DNA antibody, with immunopathologic consequences such as the development of immune complex glomerulonephritis.[93]

This murine model of SLE is created rather than inherited, offering the advantage of careful experimental manipulation and analysis. Gleichmann has proposed that F$_1$ host B cells are primed in vivo by autoantigens with multiple repeating antigenic determinants, rendering them responsive to abnormal T cell help that is neither major histocompatibility complex restricted nor specific for the same autoantigens to which the B cells are committed. Such a novel mechanism could account for the development of the various autoantibodies observed in human and murine SLE. Thus, helper T cell activation generated by the acquisition of mutant major histocompatibility complex determinants (particularly of the I region in mice and D region in man) or the modification of I- or D-region antigens by viruses or drugs might trigger the onset of autoimmunity and the lupus syndrome. This process may ensue from appropriate T cell recognition of autoantigens in the context of "new" I- or D-region antigens present on macrophages rather than from the generation of nonspecific T cell help.[37] Pharmacologic, dietary, or other therapeutic approaches to the modification of the autoimmune disease produced in this model have not yet been reported.

CONCLUDING COMMENTS

All models discussed here, in addition to SLE-prone inbred Palmerston North mice,[1,33,129] moth-eaten mice,[34,98] and the most recently described C3H/HeJ-*gld/gld* mice,[95] have in common the production of characteristic autoantibodies leading to immune complex mediated injury. The immunopathologic features of these various models are summarized in Table 26–1. None develops significant neurologic disorders, serositis, or skin involvement. Nevertheless, they provide models of glomerulonephritis, vasculitis, and synovitis that resemble the analogous manifestations of human SLE.

The immunoregulatory disorders associated with such pathology are varied. In certain instances, the induction of excess helper T lymphocyte activity, as in the cases of the chronic GVHR mice and the *lpr* mice, may in fact be the dominant mechanism. In the BXSB/Mp male and in the New Zealand

Table 26–1. Mouse Models of Systemic Lupus Erythematosus

Model	Immunopathology	Accelerating Factor	Mean Mortality Male; Female (months)	T Cell Dependence	Primary B Cell Abnormality	Autoantibodies
NZB	Autoimmune hemolytic anemia; membranous glomerulonephritis; lymphoid hyperplasia and cancer	Environment	15½; 14	No	Yes	Antierythrocyte Anti-single stranded DNA NTA*
(NZBxNZW)F₁	Membranoproliferative glomerulonephritis; Sjögren's syndrome	Estrogens	15; 9	No	Yes	Antinative DNA Anti GP-70
MRL/Mp-lpr/lpr	Membranoproliferative glomerulonephritis; polyarteritis; erosive arthritis; lymphadenopathy	Autosomal recessive lpr gene	6; 5	Yes	No	Antinative DNA Anti-Sm Rheumatoid factor Anti GP-70
BXSB/Mp	Proliferative glomerulonephritis; degenerative coronary disease	Y chromosome (not hormonal)	5; 20	No	Yes	Antinative DNA Antierythrocyte
Chronic GVHR†	Glomerulonephritis; arthritis; Sjögren's syndrome	—	>12	Yes	No	Anti-DNA Antierythrocyte NTA

*NTA: Natural thymocytotoxic autoantibody
†GVHR: Graft-versus-host reaction

mice, tissue injury may result from intrinsic abnormalities of B lymphocytes, although defective suppressor T cell and excessively active monocyte/macrophage mechanisms may be operative as well. Cognizance of these heterogenous models of SLE in mice should stimulate further clinical investigation of SLE and lead to a better understanding of the pathogenic mechanisms and to the development of more effective therapies.

REFERENCES

1. Altman, A., et al.: Analysis of T cell function in autoimmune murine strains. J. Exp. Med., *154*:791, 1981.
2. Andrews, B.A., et al.: Spontaneous murine lupus-like syndromes: Clinical and immunopathological manifestations in several strains. J. Exp. Med., *148*:1198, 1978.
3. Astorga, G.P.: Immunologic studies of an experimental chronic arthritis resembling rheumatoid arthritis. Arthritis Rheum., *12*:589, 1969.
4. Battisto, J.R., et al.: Susceptibility to adjuvant arthritis in DA and F344 rats. A dominant trait controlled by an autosomal gene locus linked to the major histocompatibility complex. Arthritis Rheum., *25*:1194, 1982.
5. Beach, R.S., Gershwin, M.E., and Hurley, L.S.: Nutritional factors and autoimmunity: II. Prolongation of survival in zinc-deprived NZB/W mice. J. Immunol., *128*:308, 1982.
6. Berden, J.J.M., Hang, L., McConahey, P.J., and Dixon, F.J.: Analysis of vascular lesions in murine SLE. I. Association with serologic abnormalities. J. Immunol., *130*:1699, 1983.
7. Bokisch, V.A., et al.: Isolation and immunochemical characterization of rabbit 7S anti-IgG with restricted heterogeneity. J. Exp. Med., *137*:1354, 1973.
8. Bokisch, V.A., Bernstein, D., and Krause, R.M.: Occurrence of 19S and 7S anti-IgG's during hyperimmunization of rabbits with streptococci. J. Exp. Med., *136*:799, 1972.
9. Brackertz, D., Mitchell, G.F., and Mackay, I.R.: Antigen-induced arthritis in mice. I. Induction of arthritis in various strains of mice. Arthritis Rheum., *20*:841, 1977.
10. Burstein, N.A., and Waksman, B.H.: The pathogenesis of adjuvant disease in the rat. II. A radioautographic study of early lesions with the use of H³-thymidine. Yale J. Biol. Med., *37*:195, 1964.
11. Caulfield, J.P., et al.: Morphologic demonstration of two stages in the development of type II collagen-induced arthritis. Lab. Invest., *46*:321, 1982.
12. Chang, Y-H, Pearson, C.M., and Chedid, L.: Adjuvant polyarthritis. V. Induction by N-acetylmuramyl L-alanyl-D-isoglutamine, the smallest peptide subunit of bacterial peptidoglycan. J. Exp. Med., *153*:1021, 1981.
13. Christian, C.L.: Rheumatoid factor properties of hyperimmune rabbit sera. J. Exp. Med., *118*:827, 1963.
14. Clague, R.B., et al.: Native type II collagen-induced arthritis in the rat. 2. Relationship between the humoral immune response to native type II collagen and arthritis. J. Rheumatol., *7*:775, 1980.
15. Cohen, P.L., and Eisenberg, R.A.: Anti-idiotypic antibodies to the Coombs antibody in NZB F₁ mice. J. Exp. Med., *156*:173, 1982.
16. Cole, B.C., et al.: Chronic proliferative arthritis of mice induced by Mycoplasma arthritidis. I. Induction of disease and histopathological characteristics. Infect. Immun., *4*:344, 1971.
17. Cole, B.C., et al.: Chronic proliferative arthritis of mice induced by Mycoplasma arthritidis. II. Serological responses of the host and effect of vaccines. Infect. Immun., *4*:431, 1971.
18. Cole, B.C., and Cassell, G.H.: Mycoplasma infections as models of chronic joint inflammation. Arthritis Rheum., *22*:1375, 1979.
19. Consden, R., et al.: Production of a chronic arthritis with
20. Cooke, T.D., et al.: Identification of immunoglobulins and complement in rheumatoid collagenous tissues. Arthritis Rheum., *18*:544, 1975.
21. Cooke, T.D., et al.: The pathogenesis of chronic inflammation in experimental antigen-induced arthritis. II. Preferential localization of antigen-antibody complexes to collagenous tissues. J. Exp. Med., *135*:323, 1972.
22. Cooke, T.D., and Jasin, H.E.: The pathogenesis of chronic inflammation in experimental antigen-induced arthritis. I. The role of antigen on the local immune response. Arthritis Rheum., *15*:327, 1972.
23. Courtenay, J.S., et al.: Immunization against heterologous type II collagen induces arthritis in mice. Nature, *283*:666, 1980.
24. Crawford, T.B., Adams, D.S., and Cheevers, W.P.: Chronic arthritis in goats caused by a retrovirus. Science, *207*:997, 1980.
25. Cremer, M.A., et al.: Auricular chondritis in rats. An experimental model of relapsing polychondritis induced with type II collagen. J. Exp. Med., *154*:535, 1981.
26. Cremer, M.A., Stuart, J.M., and Townes, A.H.: A study of native type II collagen for adjuvant activity. J. Immunol., *124*:2912, 1980.
27. Cromartie, W.J., et al.: Arthritis in rats after systemic injection of streptococcal cells or cell walls. J. Exp. Med., *146*:1585, 1977.
28. Cromartie, W.J., and Craddock, J.G.: Rheumatic-like cardiac lesions in mice. Science, *154*:285, 1966.
29. Cromartie, W.J., Schwab, J.H., and Craddock, J.G.: The effect of a toxic cellular component of group A streptococci on connective tissue. Am. J. Pathol., *37*:79, 1960.
30. Dalldorf, F.G., et al.: The relation of experimental arthritis to the distribution of streptococcal cell wall fragments. Am. J. Pathol., *100*:383, 1980.
31. Datta, S.K., et al.: Analysis of recombinant inbred lines derived from "autoimmune" (NZB) and "high leukemia" (C58) strains: Independent multigenic systems control B cell hyperactivity, retrovirus expression, and autoimmunity. J. Immunol., *129*:1539, 1982.
32. Dauphinee, M.J., et al.: Interleukin 2 deficiency is a common feature of autoimmune mice. J. Immunol., *127*:2483, 1981.
33. Davidson, W.F.: Immunologic abnormalities of the autoimmune mouse, Palmerston North. J. Immunol., *129*:751, 1982.
34. Davidson, W.F., et al.: Phenotypic and functional effects of the motheaten gene on murine T and B lymphocytes. J. Immunol., *122*:884, 1978.
35. DeShazo, C.V., Henson, P., and Cochrane, C.G.: Acute immunologic arthritis in rabbits. J. Clin. Invest., *51*:50, 1972.
36. Dumonde, D.C., and Glynn, L.E.: The production of arthritis in rabbits by an immunological reaction to fibrin. Br. J. Exp. Pathol., *43*:373, 1962.
37. Eisenberg, R.A., and Cohen, P.L.: Class II major histocompatibility antigens and the etiology of systemic lupus erythematosus. Clin. Immunol. Immunopathol., *29*:1, 1983.
38. Eisenberg, R.A., and Dixon, F.J.: Effect of castration on male-determined acceleration of autoimmune disease in BXSB mice. J. Immunol., *125*:1959, 1980.
39. Eisenberg, R.A., Tan, E.M., and Dixon, F.J.: Presence of anti-Sm reactivity in autoimmune mouse strains. J. Exp. Med., *147*:582, 1978.
40. Elson, C.J.: Autoantibodies typical of SLE and graft-vs-host reactions. Immunol. Today, *3*:181, 1982.
41. Foidart, J.M., et al.: Antibodies to type II collagen in relapsing polychondritis. N. Engl. J. Med., *299*:1203, 1978.
42. Fox, A., and Glynn, L.E.: Persistence of antigen in non-arthritic joints. Ann. Rheum. Dis., *34*:431, 1975.
43. Gardner, D.L.: The experimental production of arthritis. Ann. Rheum. Dis., *19*:297, 1960.
44. Gerber, N.L., et al.: Loss with age in NZB/W mice of thymic suppressor cells in the graft-vs-host reaction. J. Immunol., *113*:1618, 1974.

45. Gershwin, M.E., et al.: Studies of congenital immunologic mutant New Zealand mice. IV: Development of autoimmunity in congenitally athymic (nude) New Zealand black x white F_1 hybrid mice. J. Immunol., 125:1189, 1980.
46. Gilliam, J.N., Hurd, E.R., and Ziff, M.: Subepidermal deposition of immunoglobulin in NZB/NZW F_1 hybrid mice. J. Immunol., 114:133, 1975.
47. Gioud, M., et al.: Antibodies to native type I and II collagens detected by an enzyme linked immunosorbent assay (ELISA) in rheumatoid arthritis and systemic lupus erythematosus. Collagen Rel. Res., 2:557, 1982.
48. Gleichmann, E., Van Elven, E.H., and VandenVeen, J.P.W.: A systemic lupus erythematosus (SLE)-like disease in mice induced by abnormal T-B cell cooperation. Preferential formation of autoantibodies characteristic of SLE. Eur. J. Immunol., 12:152, 1982.
49. Glimcher, L.H., et al.: The autologous mixed lymphocyte reaction in strains of mice with autoimmune disease. J. Immunol., 125:1832, 1980.
50. Goldings, E.A.: Defective B cell tolerance induction in New Zealand Black mice. I. Macrophage independence and comparison with other autoimmune strains. J. Immunol., 131:2630, 1983.
51. Goldings, E.A., et al.: Defective B cell tolerance in adult (NZBxNZW)F_1 mice. J. Exp. Med., 152:730, 1980.
52. Graham, R.C., and Shannon, S.L.: Peroxidase arthritis. I. An immunologically mediated response with ultrastructural cytochemical localization of antigen and specific antibody. Am. J. Pathol., 67:69, 1972.
53. Greenblatt, J.J., Hunter, N., and Schwab, J.H.: Antibody response to streptococcal cell wall antigens associated with experimental arthritis in rats. Clin. Exp. Immunol., 42:450, 1980.
54. Hang, L., et al.: The cellular basis for resistance to induction of tolerance in BXSB systemic lupus erythematosus male mice. J. Immunol., 129:787, 1982.
55. Hang, L.M., Izui, S., and Dixon, F.J.: (NZW x BXSB) F_1 hybrid, a model of acute lupus and coronary vascular disease with myocardial infarction. J. Exp. Med., 154:216, 1981.
56. Hang, L., Theofilopoulos, A.N., and Dixon, F.J.: A spontaneous rheumatoid arthritis-like disease in MRL/1 mice. J. Exp. Med., 155:1690, 1982.
57. Hayakawa, K., et al.: The "Ly-1 B" cell subpopulation in normal, immunodefective and autoimmune mice. J. Exp. Med., 157:202, 1983.
58. Hollister, J.R., and Mannik, M.: Antigen retention in joint tissues in antigen-induced synovitis. Clin. Exp. Immunol., 16:615, 1974.
59. Hunter, N., et al.: Cell-mediated immune response during experimental arthritis induced in rats with streptococcal cell walls. Clin. Exp. Immunol., 42:441, 1980.
60. Hurd, E.R., et al.: Prevention of glomerulonephritis and prolonged survival in New Zealand black/New Zealand white F_1 hybrid mice fed an essential fatty acid-deficient diet. J. Clin. Invest., 67:476, 1981.
61. Iizuka, Y., and Chang, Y-H.: Adjuvant polyarthritis. VII. The role of type II collagen in pathogenesis. Arthritis Rheum., 25:1325, 1982.
62. Izui, S., et al.: Retroviral gp70 immune complexes in NZB x NZW F_2 mice with murine lupus nephritis. J. Exp. Med., 154:517, 1981.
63. Izui, S., et al.: Low-calorie diet selectively reduces expression of retroviral envelope glycoprotein gp70 in sera of NZBxNZW F_1 hybrid mice. J. Exp. Med., 154:1116, 1981.
64. Izui, S., et al.: Selective suppression of retroviral gp70-anti-gp70 immune complex formation by prostaglandin E_1 in murine systemic lupus erythematosus. J. Exp. Med., 152:1645, 1980.
65. Izui, S., et al.: Association of circulating retroviral gp70-anti-gp70 immune complexes with murine systemic lupus erythematosus. J. Exp. Med., 149:1099, 1979.
66. Jaffee, B.D., and Claman, H.H.: Chronic graft-versus-host disease (GVHD) as a model for scleroderma: 1. Description of model systems. Cell. Immunol., 77:1, 1983.
67. Jasin, H.E.: Mechanism of trapping of immune complexes

68. Jasin, H.E., et al.: Immunologic models used for the study of rheumatoid arthritis. Fed. Proc., 32:147, 1973.
69. Jasin, H.E., and Cooke, T.D.: The inflammatory role of immune complexes trapped in joint collagenous tissues. Clin. Exp. Immunol., 33:416, 1978.
70. Jyonouchi, H., et al.: Age-dependent deficiency of B lymphocyte lineage precursors in NZB mice. J. Exp. Med., 155:1665, 1982.
71. Kapusta, M.A., Young-Rodenchuk, M., and Kourounakis, L.: Restoration of diminished splenic responses to phytohemagglutinin and concanavalin A in adjuvant-induced disease by irrazole: Possible role of a virus and suppressor cells. J. Rheumatol., 6:507, 1979.
72. Kelley, V.E., and Roths, J.B.: Increase in macrophage Ia expression in autoimmune mice: Role of the Lpr gene. J. Immunol., 129:923, 1982.
73. Kotzin, B.L., and Strober, S.: Reversal of NZB/NZW disease with total lymphoid irradiation. J. Exp. Med., 150:371, 1979.
74. Lambert, P.H., and Dixon, F.J.: Pathogenesis of glomerulonephritis of NZB/W mice. J. Exp. Med., 127:507, 1968.
75. Lambert, P., and Oldstone, M.: Host IgG and complement deposits in choroid plexus during spontaneous immune complex diseases. Science, 180:408, 1973.
76. Laskin, C.A., et al.: Studies of defective tolerance induction in NZB mice. Evidence for a marrow pre-T cell defect. J. Exp. Med., 155:1025, 1982.
77. Manny, N., Datta, S.K., and Schwartz, R.S.: Synthesis of IgM by cells of NZB and SWR mice and their crosses. J. Immunol., 111:1220, 1979.
78. Menard, H.A., and Denners, J-C.: Use of a hapten-carrier system in experimental immune arthritis in the rabbit. Arthritis Rheum., 20:1402, 1977.
79. Milich, D.R., and Gershwin, M.E.: The pathogenesis of autoimmunity in New Zealand mice. Semin. Arthritis Rheum., 10:111, 1980.
80. Morton, J.B., and Siegel, B.V.: Transplantation of autoimmune potential. I. Development of antinuclear antibodies in H-2 compatible recipients of NZB bone marrow. Proc. Natl. Acad. Sci. U.S.A., 71:2162, 1974.
81. Moutsopoulos, H.M., et al.: Demonstration of activation of B lymphocytes in New Zealand mice at birth by an immunoradiometric assay for murine IgM. J. Immunol., 119:1639, 1977.
82. Murphy, E., and Roths, J.B.: A Y chromosome associated factor in strain BXSB producing accelerated autoimmunity and lymphoproliferation. Arthritis Rheum., 22:1188, 1979.
83. Ohanian, S.H., and Schwab, J.H.: Persistence of group A streptococcal cell walls related to chronic inflammation of rabbit dermal connective tissue. J. Exp. Med., 125:1137, 1967.
84. Pearson, C.M.: Arthritis in animals. In Arthritis and Allied Conditions, 9th Ed. Edited by D.J. McCarty. Philadelphia, Lea & Febiger, 1979.
85. Pearson, C.M.: Development of arthritis, periarthritis and periostitis in rats given adjuvants. Proc. Soc. Exp. Biol. Med., 91:95, 1956.
86. Pearson, C.M., Waksman, B.H., and Sharp, J.T.: Studies of arthritis and other lesions induced in rats by injection of mycobacterial adjuvant. V. Changes affecting the skin and mucous membranes. Comparison of the experimental process with human disease. J. Exp. Med., 113:485, 1961.
87. Pedersen, N.C., Pool, R.R., and O'Brien, T.: Feline chronic progressive polyarthritis. Am. J. Vet. Res., 41:522, 1980.
88. Pisetsky, D.S., et al.: lpr gene control of the anti-DNA antibody response. J. Immunol., 128:2322, 1982.
89. Phillips, J.M., Kaklamanis, P., and Glynn, L.E.: Experimental arthritis associated with autoimmunization to inflammatory exudates. Ann. Rheum. Dis., 25:165, 1966.
90. Prud'homme, G.J., et al.: B cell dependence on and response to accessory signals in murine lupus strain. J. Exp. Med., 157:1815, 1983.

in joint collagenous tissues. Clin. Exp. Immunol., 22:473, 1975.

91. Prud'homme, G.J., et al.: Identification of a B cell differentiation factor(s) spontaneously produced by proliferating T cells in murine lupus strains of the lpr/lpr genotype. J. Exp. Med., *157*:730, 1983.

92. Raveche, E.S., et al.: Genetic studies in NZB mice: V. Recombinant inbred lines demonstrate that separate genes control autoimmune phenotype. J. Exp. Med., *153*:1187, 1981.

93. Rolink, A.G., Gleichmann, H., and Gleichmann, E.: Diseases caused by reactions to T lymphocytes to incompatible structures of the major histocompatibility complex. VII. Immune-complex glomerulonephritis. J. Immunol., *130*:209, 1983.

94. Rosenthale, M.E., and Nagra, C.L.: Comparative effects of some immunosuppressive and antiinflammatory drugs on allergic encephalomyelitis and adjuvant arthritis. Proc. Soc. Exp. Biol. Med., *125*:149, 1967.

95. Roths, J.B., et al.: Modification of expression of *lpr* by background genome. Fed. Proc., *42*:1075, 1983.

96. Roths, J.B., Murphy, E.D., and Eicher, E.M.: A new mutation, *gld*, that produces lymphoproliferation and autoimmunity in C3H/HeJ mice. J. Exp. Med., *159*:1, 1984.

97. Roubinian, J.R., Papoian, R., and Talal, N.: Androgenic hormones modulate autoantibody responses and improve survival in murine lupus. J. Clin. Invest., *59*:1066, 1977.

98. Schultz, L.D., and Green, M.C.: Motheaten, an immunodeficient mutant of the mouse. II. Depressed immune competence and elevated serum immunoglobulins. J. Immunol., *116*:936, 1976.

99. Schwab, J.H., et al.: Association of experimental chronic arthritis with the persistence of group A streptococcal cell walls in the articular tissue. J. Bacteriol., *94*:1728, 1967.

100. Schwab, J.H., and Ohanian, S.H.: Degradation of streptococcal cell wall antigens in vivo. J. Bacteriol., *94*:1346, 1967.

101. Shirai, T.: The genetic basis of autoimmunity in murine lupus. Immunol. Today, *3*:187, 1982.

102. Sikes, D., et al.: Electrophoretic and serologic changes of blood serum of arthritic (rheumatoid) dogs infected with *Erysipelothrix insidiosa*. Am. J. Vet. Res., *32*:1083, 1971.

103. Sikes, D., Crimmins, L.T., and Fletcher, O.J.: Rheumatoid arthritis of swine: A comparative pathologic study of clinical spontaneous remissions and exacerbations. Am. J. Vet. Res., *30*:753, 1969.

104. Slavin, S.: Successful treatment of autoimmune disease in (NZB/NZW)F₁ female mice by using fractionated total lymphoid irradiation. Proc. Natl. Acad. Sci. U.S.A., *76*:5274, 1979.

105. Smathers, P.A., et al.: Effects of polyclonal immune stimulators upon NZB.*xid* congenic mice. J. Immunol., *128*:1414, 1982.

106. Smith, H.R., et al.: Cyclophosphamide induced changes in the MRL-*lpr/lpr* mouse: Effects upon cellular composition, immune function, and disease. Arthritis Rheum., *26*:S76, 1983.

107. Smith, H.R., et al.: Evidence for thymic regulation of autoimmunity in BXSB mice: Acceleration of disease by neonatal thymectomy. J. Immunol., *130*:1200, 1983.

108. Sokoloff, L.: Animal model of human disease. Rheumatoid arthritis. Am. J. Pathol., *73*:261, 1973.

109. Staples, P.J., and Talal, N.: Relative inability to induce tolerance in adult NZB and NZB/NZW F₁ mice. J. Exp. Med., *129*:123, 1969.

110. Stastny, P., Stembridge, V.A., and Ziff, M.: Homologous disease in the adult rat, a model for autoimmune disease. I. General features and cutaneous lesions. J. Exp. Med., *118*:635, 1963.

111. Steffen, C.: Collagen as an autoantigen in rheumatoid arthritis. *In* Advances in Joint Diseases. Edited by A. Maroudas, and E.J. Holborow. Marshfield, Massachusetts, Pitman Publishing, 1981.

112. Steinberg, A.D., et al.: The cellular and genetic basis of murine lupus. Immunol. Rev., *55*:121, 1981.

113. Steinman, C.R., and Hsu, K.: Specific detection and semiquantitation of microorganisms in tissue by nucleic acid hybridization. II. Investigation of synovia from pigs

with chronic *Erysipelothrix* arthritis, Arthritis Rheum., *19*:38, 1976.

114. Stoerk, H.C., Bielinski, T.C., and Budzilovich, T.: Chronic polyarthritis in rats injected with spleen in adjuvants. (Abstract.) Am. J. Pathol., *30*:616, 1954.

115. Stuart, J.M., et al.: Type II collagen-induced arthritis in rats. Passive transfer with serum and evidence that IgG anti-collagen antibodies can cause arthritis. J. Exp. Med., *155*:1, 1982.

116. Stuart, J.M., et al.: Incidence and specificity of antibodies to types I, II, III, IV and V collagen in rheumatoid arthritis and other rheumatic diseases as measured by I¹²⁵-radioimmunoassay. Arthritis Rheum., *26*:832, 1983.

117. Stuart, J.M., Postlethwaite, A.E., and Kang, A.H.: Evidence for cell-mediated immunity to collagen in progressive systemic sclerosis. J. Lab. Clin. Med., *88*:601, 1976.

118. Stuart, J.M., Townes, A.S., and Kang, A.H.: Nature and specificity of the immune response to collagen in type II collagen-induced arthritis in mice. J. Clin. Invest., *69*:673, 1982.

119. Swingle, K.F.: Evaluation of anti-inflammatory activity. *In* Anti-inflammatory Agents. Edited by R.A. Scherrer, and M.W. Whitehouse. New York, Academic Press, 1974.

120. Talal, N., and Steinberg, A.D.: The pathogenesis of autoimmunity in NZB mice. *In* Current Topics in Microbiology and Immunology. Edited by W. Arber, et al. New York, Springer-Verlag, 1974, pp. 64–79.

121. Tateishi, H., Jasin, H.E., and Ziff, M.: Electron microscopic study of synovial membrane and cartilage in a ferritin-induced arthritis. Arthritis Rheum., *16*:133, 1973.

122. Taurog, J.D., Sandberg, G.P., and Mahowald, M.L.: The cellular basis of adjuvant arthritis. I. Enhancement of cell-mediated passive transfer by concanavalin A and by immunosuppressive pretreatment of the recipient. Cell. Immunol., *75*:271, 1983.

123. Theofilopoulos, A.N., et al.: Inhibition of T cell proliferation and SLE-like syndrome of MRL/1 mice by whole body or total lymphoid irradiation. J. Immunol., *125*:2137, 1980.

124. Theofilopoulos, A.N., and Dixon, F.J.: Etiopathogenesis of murine SLE. Immunol. Rev., *55*:179, 1981.

125. Trentham, D.E., et al.: Autoimmunity to collagen in adjuvant arthritis of rats. J. Clin. Invest., *66*:1109, 1980.

126. Trentham, D.E., et al.: Passive transfer of cells of type II collagen-induced arthritis in rats. J. Clin. Invest., *62*:359, 1978.

127. Trentham, D.E., Townes, A.S., and Kang, A.H.: Autoimmunity to type II collagen: An experimental model of arthritis. J. Exp. Med., *146*:857, 1977.

128. Ugai, K., Ziff, M., and Jasin, H.E.: Interaction of polymorphonuclear leukocytes with immune complexes trapped in joint collagenous tissues. Arthritis Rheum., *22*:353, 1979.

129. Walker, S.E., et al.: Palmerston-North mice, a new animal model for systemic lupus erythematosus. J. Lab. Clin. Med., *92*:945, 1978.

130. Walker, S.E., et al.: Prolonged lifespan and high incidence of neoplasms in NZB/NZW mice treated with hydrocortisone sodium succinate. Kidney Int., *14*:151, 1978.

131. Walker, S.E., and Bole, G.G., Jr.: Augmented incidence of neoplasia in NZB/NZW mice treated with long-term cyclophosphamide. J. Lab. Clin. Med., *82*:619, 1973.

132. Ward, J.R., and Jones, R.S.: The pathogenesis of mycoplasmal (PPLO) arthritis in rats. Arthritis Rheum., *5*:163, 1962.

133. Washburn, L.R., et al.: Chronic arthritis of rabbits induced by mycoplasmas. I. Clinical, microbiologic and histologic features. Arthritis Rheum., *23*:825, 1980.

134. Washburn, L.R., Cole, B.C., and Ward, J.R.: Chronic arthritis of rabbits induced by mycoplasmas. III. Induction with nonviable *Mycoplasma arthritidis* antigens. Arthritis Rheum., *25*:937, 1982.

135. Washburn, L.R., Cole, B.C., and Ward, J.R.: Chronic arthritis of rabbits induced by mycoplasmas. II. Antibody

response and the deposition of immune complexes. Arthritis Rheum., *23*:837, 1980.

136. Webb, F.W., et al.: Experimental viral arthritis induced with herpes simplex. Arthritis Rheum., *16*:241, 1973.

137. Webb, F.W., Ford, P.M., and Glynn, L.E.: Persistence of antigen in rabbit synovial membrane. Br. J. Exp. Pathol., *52*:31, 1971.

138. White, T.G., Puls, J.L., and Mirikitani, F.K.: Rabbit arthritis induced by cell-free extracts of *Erysipelothrix*. Infect. Immun., *3*:715, 1971.

139. Wofsy, D., et al.: Thymic influences on autoimmunity in MRL/lpr mice. Scand. J. Immunol., *16*:51, 1982.

140. Wofsy, D., et al.: Deficient interleukin 2 activity in MRL/Mp and C57BL/6J mice bearing the lpr gene. J. Exp. Med., *154*:1671, 1981.

141. Wooley, P.H., et al.: Type II collagen-induced arthritis in mice. I. Major histocompatibility complex (I region) linkage and antibody correlates. J. Exp. Med., *154*:688, 1981.

142. Zahiri, H., et al.: Adjuvant experimental polyarthritis. Can. Med. Assoc. J., *101*:269, 1969.

143. Zurier, R.B., et al.: Prostaglandin E treatment prevents progression of nephritis in murine lupus erythematosus. J. Clin. Lab. Immunol., *1*:95, 1978.

Chapter 27

Infectious Agents in Chronic Rheumatic Disease

Paul E. Phillips and Charles L. Christian

Genetic factors, immune responses, and inflammation are clearly involved in the pathogenesis of the systemic connective tissue diseases (CTD). Histocompatibility antigen gene associations with specific CTD have been increasingly defined; these genes probably affect immunoregulation, which seems to be deranged in most CTD. Humoral and cellular immune responses to various antigens, many of self-origin, apparently result in inflammation in various tissues.

The role of chronic infection in pathogenesis is less clear. Hypotheses are based on both animal models of disease and human arthritides in which the etiologic roles of microbial agents are explicit. The striking clinical and pathologic similarities between certain naturally occurring infectious diseases in animals and human diseases, such as rheumatoid arthritis (RA), systemic lupus erythematosus (SLE), and vasculitis, have stimulated a search for microbial etiologies of the human syndromes. With a few exceptions, such as hepatitis B-associated vasculitis and, more recently, Lyme disease, these efforts have been unsuccessful. However, as the few successes demonstrate so well, this generally negative experience is not definitive. For instance, successful microbial rescue may require as yet unrecognized experimental conditions: some clearly infectious agents, such as those in Whipple's disease and, until recently, Lyme disease, cannot be propagated in the laboratory under any known conditions. Furthermore, chronic arthritis in experimental animals that is initiated by infection may progress even when the microbial agent is no longer demonstrable. Even after a specific microorganism has been identified, the problem is to define what role it plays: is it a nonspecific, perhaps even trivial, trigger, or is its persistence in some form essential to the recurring and chronic patterns of the CTD?

This chapter focuses on microbes as inciting or perpetuating factors in the pathogenesis of CTD. The role of chronic infection in animal models is discussed. Known infections causing rheumatic disease in man illustrate the various microbe-host interactions that could lead to CTD and, lastly, evidence for specific microbial involvement in each CTD is reviewed with emphasis on recent studies and controversial areas.

MICROBE-HOST INTERACTION

It is difficult to test hypotheses for microbial roles in the CTD experimentally because the three principal factors in microbe-host interactions—host susceptibility, tropism of the microbe, and the host response—vary greatly. The first two determine whether infection actually occurs. Host susceptibility may involve genetic factors, for instance, determining presence of specific microbial receptors on cells. It is also affected by preexisting immunity, including cross-reactivity toward other antigenically related microbes, and by the size and route of the microbial inoculum. Susceptibility may also influence the course and outcome of infection, but here microbial tropism and the host immune response are more important. Tropism refers not only to the species, but also to the cell type and tissues preferentially infected, and to whether infection is local or systemic. Local or distant damage may be caused by microbial replication or release of toxins. In the nonimmune host, the initial response may include interferon production, complement activation, local inflammation, and pyrogen or toxin release. Thereafter, the host develops specific immunity, and additional mechanisms for cell and tissue damage become operative. The importance of each immune mechanism in eliminating infection varies with the specific microbe, but systemic spread is generally reduced or terminated by development of circulating antibody. However, circulating or in situ immune complexes with microbial antigens may be formed and may result in inflammation. Specific cellular immunity destroys intact bacteria and virus-infected cells. Residual or released microbes and their components are further degraded and eliminated by specific humoral and cellular recognition. The successful conclusion of these events is termination of infection and its symptoms, but if the microbe or its antigens persist, or if reinfection occurs, recurrent or chronic inflammatory disease may result. This can also happen if the host responds immunologically to self-antigens, whether altered by inflammation or cross-reacting with microbial antigens. Rheumatic disease results if any of these mechanisms involve joint or other connective tissues and, depending on the specific microbe-host interaction, can vary in both severity and duration.

MODELS FOR INFECTION IN THE CONNECTIVE TISSUE DISEASES

Animal Models: Articular CTD

How the various microbes, from bacteria to viruses, cause arthritis in these animal models is often unclear (see also Chap. 26). Synovial membranes appear to be effective localizers of several microbial forms that are capable of inducing systemic infection. Whether this tropism is related to efficient removal of organisms by phagocytic mechanisms or by some other aspect of joint milieu is moot.

Bacteria. A chronic proliferative synovitis that occurs naturally in swine is caused by *Erysipelothrix insidiosa* infection.[191] The initial phase of infection is characterized by systemic sepsis, including involvement of the joints from which the bacteria can be recovered, but the later chronic phase that resembles RA may persist and progress in the absence of demonstrable microorganisms. Even serologic evidence of *E. insidiosa* infection may decline while the proliferative synovitis progresses. Whether the disease is maintained by persistence of latent infection or by some independent process has not been determined. Studies employing the technique of nucleic acid hybridization have not detected microbe-related DNA in synovial tissue of animals with the chronic phase of disease, although this may reflect the sensitivity of the method.[202] Alternatively, it has been postulated that the central event in bacteria-induced chronic synovitis may be the persistence of nonbiodegradable microbial cell wall components.[84] Interperitoneal injection of cell walls of group A streptococci in rats or guinea pigs induces a biphasic, first acute and then chronic, arthritis. Soluble peptidoglycan-polysaccharide polymers of varying sizes from streptococci have different biologic properties; the most severe chronic synovitis, resembling RA, is obtained with polymers of intermediate size (estimated 50×10^6 daltons).[38,70] Radioimmunoassays specific for cell wall antigens demonstrate maximal antigen concentration in liver and spleen after a single interperitoneal injection; the development of arthritis correlates with the degree of cell wall deposited in and persisting in joints.[58] Studies of streptococcal cell wall-induced arthritis in 16 inbred rat strains demonstrate evidence of two or

more genetic loci influencing susceptibility to disease and suggest that the host mechanism predisposing to arthritis is a failure to limit dissemination of poorly degradable cell wall material.[223]

Mycoplasma. Infection of swine with *Mycoplasma hyorhinis* and infection of mice and rats with *M. arthritidis* and *M. pulmonis* can, after an acute septic phase, produce a chronic proliferative synovitis that clinically and histologically resembles human RA.[42] Arthritis produced by mycoplasma species also occurs in cattle, goats, sheep, cats, chickens, and turkeys. A model of central nervous system necrotizing vasculitis is induced in turkeys by *M. gallisepticum*.[208] The acute phase of *M. hyorhinis* arthritis in swine lasts for approximately 3 weeks and is followed by a chronic villous synovitis that may persist for months.[16] As with *E. insidiosa* arthritis, microorganisms are infrequently recovered from the joints after the first few weeks of disease. In one study, mycoplasma antigens, in the absence of demonstrable organisms, were found in synovial tissue by immunofluorescence.[63] A possible explanation for the persistence of chronic synovitis in mice infected with *M. pulmonis* or *M. arthritidis* was suggested by the demonstration of shared antigens between mycoplasma and synovial tissue.[30,89] Intra-articular injection of nonviable *M. arthritidis* into preimmunized rabbits resulted in a chronic inflammatory response.[222] Animals with chronic erosive synovitis induced by infectious *M. arthritidis* had immune deposits of immunoglobulin and complement in deep layers of articular cartilage. However, proof that mycoplasmal antigens persist in synovial tissue during the chronic phase of disease is still lacking. Several mycoplasma species are mitogenic for lymphocytes of unsensitized animals. The degree of transformation is different in various inbred strains of mice. This variability has been shown to be under Ir gene control.[39,41]

Chlamydia. Infection with this class of microorganism, which includes the agents responsible for trachoma, psittacosis, and lymphogranuloma venereum, induces chronic polyarthritis in sheep.[44] Lambs less than 4 months of age are most frequently affected. The majority recover from an acute illness that is characterized by polyarthritis, but a minority of animals manifest a chronic villous synovitis that resembles RA. The acute phase of disease is effectively treated with various antibiotics but, like the models of arthritis resulting from *Erysipelothrix* and mycoplasma infection, the chronic synovitis is not influenced by therapy.

Viruses. A reovirus has been isolated from chickens with arthritis and is capable of inducing joint and tendon synovitis experimentally in this species.[219] A mild chronic synovitis has been induced in rabbits and guinea pigs by intra-articular injection of herpes simplex virus.[15] Neither intact virions nor viral antigens have been detected in synovial tissue at intervals beginning one month after inoculation.

A type E retrovirus, the caprine arthritis-encephalitis virus, is associated with demyelinating leukoencephalopathy in 2- to 4-month old goats and with a chronic progressive synovitis affecting joints, bursa, and tendons in adult animals.[25,43] More detailed characterization of this model of disease has potential relevance to human disease for several reasons: (1) it is the only model of virus-induced chronic arthritis in mammals; (2) its gross and microscopic pathology closely resembles that of RA; (3) the virus appears to have a degree of tropism for synovial tissue in vitro; and (4) it affords an opportunity to explore the mechanisms involved in the persistence and pathogenicity of retroviruses.

A dramatic model of viral-induced autoimmunity results from the inoculation of mice with reovirus type 1. Polyendocrinopathy is associated with the development of autoantibodies reactive with multiple endocrine organs; monoclonal antibodies derived from spleen cell hybridomas have varied specificities for tissue and hormonal determinants.[92]

Animal Models: Systemic CTD

Several laboratory models are induced by chronic viral infection and exhibit features of SLE or necrotizing vasculitis. In all these experimental conditions, disease is mediated by immune complexes formed by reaction of host antibody with tissue or blood-borne virus and/or viral antigens. The most extensively studied experimental models are the chronic diseases associated with persistent lymphocytic choriomeningitis viral infection, Aleutian mink disease, and equine viral arteritis.

Chronic Lymphocytic Choriomeningitis. Mice inoculated with virus shortly after birth, or infected transplacentally in utero, exhibit high titers of virus in blood and organs. They develop widespread necrotizing vascular lesions that are immunologically mediated by antiviral antibody.[156] The susceptibility to chronic disease correlates with H-2 histocompatibility antigens in various mouse strains. Immune complex nephritis similar to that found in chronic lymphocytic choriomeningitis is associated with other persistent viral infections: lactic dehydrogenase virus, Gross murine leukemia virus, and mouse mammary tumor virus.[29]

Aleutian Disease of Mink. A viral agent, first characterized in the Aleutian strain of mink, produces a chronic infection and an illness characterized by proliferation of lymphoid cells, plasma-

cytosis, marked hypergammaglobulinemia, glomerulitis, hepatitis, and arteritis.[102] The injury to several organ systems results from immune complexes formed by host antiviral antibodies and persisting virus. Immunity to the virus, either actively or passively acquired, enhances disease rather than offering protection. The disease progresses slowly for months after infection. The virus is transmitted both vertically and horizontally.

Equine Viral Arteritis. The viral agent responsible for this naturally occurring syndrome can be propagated in cultured cells. When inoculated into horses, it produces a widespread necrosis of small muscular arteries in 5 to 10 days. The character and distribution of lesions are similar to those of human polyarteritis. Although immunologic mechanisms may play a role in pathogenesis, the occurrence of lesions as early as 5 days after inoculation suggests that direct injury of arteries by virus may be involved.[64]

SLE-Like Disease in Inbred Strains of Mice. Spontaneous disease in the New Zealand black (NZB) mouse strain, and in its F_1 hybrid with the New Zealand white strain, presents a spectrum of autoimmune phenomena and disease manifestations that resemble human SLE. Other murine strains exhibiting features of SLE have been identified, including BXSB, MRL, and Palmerston North mice. In spite of the similar immunopathologic expressions, these multiple strains differ regarding the influence of sex status, hormonal manipulations, thymectomy, diet, and PGE_1 therapy.[59,206] In addition to obvious genetic factors in these inbred mouse strains, and the evidence that immunologic processes mediate the murine disease, it has been postulated that type C retroviruses might have etiopathogenetic roles.[227] Attention has focused on an endogenous type C virus that is transmitted vertically from parent to progeny and is xenotropic, i.e., can only be propagated in cells foreign to the species of origin. The major envelope component of this class of viruses is a 70,000-MW glycoprotein (gp70). In some lupus strains, this is present in high concentration in blood and spleen, is complexed with antibody in serum, and is deposited in renal glomeruli in an immune complex pattern.[227] The relative importance of gp70 compared to nucleic acids and other autologous substances as antigens for formation of pathogenic complexes is not certain. In the sense that type C viral antigens can be integral components of cells, the development of host immunity to them may be only another manifestation of the autoimmunity so abundantly expressed in lupus strains.

Some questions regarding the importance of type C viruses in the pathogenesis of NZB disease have been raised. Chronic infection with polyoma virus, lymphocytic choriomeningitis, or an infectious retrovirus enhances the SLE-like expression of NZB disease,[206] and some inbred strains of mice exhibit disease similar to that of NZB mice with lesser expression of type C viruses. In studies of F_1 hybrids and back-crosses between NZB and SWR mice (a negative or low-virus expression strain), autoimmunity and disease manifestations were dissociated from the recovery of xenotropic virus.[45] Nor was disease in these genetic hybrids associated with subvirion type C expression.[46]

Canine SLE. A sporadic disease in dogs resembles human SLE. Manifestations include autoimmune hemolytic anemia, polyarthritis, thrombocytopenia, glomerulonephritis, arteritis, positive LE cell tests, and antinuclear antibodies. Cell-free filtrates prepared from spleens of these animals, when administered to newborn random-bred puppies, induce antinuclear antibodies within 12 months of inoculation, but disease manifestations are absent.[129] Mice injected neonatally with dog spleen extracts also exhibit antinuclear antibodies, and some develop lymphomas from which murine type C viruses can be isolated. These studies are compatible with the concept of viral transmission of canine SLE, but they did not lead to characterization of an agent.

Human Models: Articular CTD

The acute and subacute rheumatic symptoms occurring during certain recognized infections in man are potential models for the pathogenesis of CTD primarily affecting joints, such as RA.[161] The pathogenesis of these models is also not entirely clear, but a general classification can be made based on the relative importance of (1) presence of the microbe or its antigens in the local tissue, (2) the host immune response to the microbe, and (3) local presence of a host antigen cross-reactive with the microbe (Table 27–1). The causative microbes in most of these models are also candidate etiologic agents in the CTD themselves.

The arthritis occurring (rarely) after smallpox vaccination is an example of rheumatic disease resulting primarily from local presence of the microbe in the joint. The virus replicates there, causing cell necrosis and inflammation, perhaps via viral stimulation of synovial prostaglandin synthesis,[226] resulting in a monarthritis lasting several

weeks. The virus is then eliminated by the host immune response, inflammation resolves, and the arthritis does not recur. Arthritis thus results primarily from direct virus-induced cell damage; the major contribution of the immune response is to eliminate the virus. Unless a local host antigen were altered by the inflammation to become a perpetuating stimulus, this is an unlikely model for articular CTD.

The arthritis occurring with acute hepatitis B (HB) virus infection is an example of rheumatic disease resulting from the immune response to the microbe or its antigens present elsewhere than the joint. Polyarthralgias, arthritis, and urticaria occur early, with hypocomplementemia and HB antigenemia. The symptoms resolve with appearance of HB antibody and clinical hepatitis, disappearance of HB antigen, and normalization of serum complement. This serum sickness-like illness results from formation and deposition of circulating HB antigen-antibody immune complexes. Without any perpetuating antigen, this is also an unlikely model; the role of persistent HB infection in various immunologically mediated diseases is discussed subsequently.

Rubella, acquired either naturally or by immunization, is an example of rheumatic disease resulting from the immune response to the microbe or its antigens present locally. Polyarthralgias and, less often, arthritis occur following viremia, coincident with or after antibody appearance. Virus has been found in the joint early in infection and possibly as late as 4 months after vaccination. Thus, although rubella replication generally does not destroy cells, it might cause joint disease directly early in infection. Most rheumatic symptoms occur later, probably from the immune response to virus or its antigens persisting locally for some weeks or months in joint tissues, before being eliminated. An inflammation-altered host antigen might also contribute to perpetuation.

Rarely, rubella arthritis becomes chronic.[168] Studies on whether virus persistence is necessary for chronicity had generally been negative, but recently the virus was isolated from peripheral blood lymphocytes of 6 patients with chronic rubella arthritis 1 to 6 years after infection.[35] This is somewhat surprising considering the difficulty of isolation even during the acute period. That previous

Table 27–1. Models for CTD Primarily Involving Joints: Human Arthritis with Known Infections

	Vaccinia Arthritis	Acute Hepatitis B Arthritis	Rubella Arthritis	Rheumatic Fever with Carditis
Local infection	+	0	+	0
Host immune response	0	+	+	+
Local cross-reactive host antigen	0	0	0	+

failures may have been due to insensitive methods was illustrated, however, by virus isolations from acute rubella arthritis synovial fluid requiring up to 11 blind cell culture passages in vitro, 3 being the routine.[72] In the chronic rubella arthritis study, serum antibody levels were normal, but lymphocyte proliferation in response to rubella antigen was increased compared to controls.[35] These studies suggest that the virus may persist in chronic rubella arthritis, stimulating the cellular immune response. In animals, the pathogenesis of antigen- and mycoplasma-induced arthritis is probably similar to that of rubella arthritis. This model is applicable to articular CTD and has been a favorite hypothesis for several decades, but little direct evidence supports either the model or rubella as a candidate agent in CTD.

Rheumatic fever, with carditis as the local target, is the best model for rheumatic disease due to a cross-reactive immune response to a local host antigen and to a component of a microbial agent; local presence of the microbe is not necessary. Following a distant streptococcal infection in the pharynx, the host antibody response to a streptococcal antigen cross-reacts with a host antigen present in the heart, resulting in local inflammation. The cycle is repeated or intensified with recurrent infections. Although the cross-reactive host antigen has been demonstrated, its pathogenic role is less certain since it is not present in other affected tissues such as synovium. Thus, although the explanation outlined here seems best, others are possible. This model, postulating a host antigen in tissues cross-reactive with a microbial antigen, is also an attractive hypothesis for articular CTD. Again, direct evidence is lacking both for the model and for streptococcal infection as a candidate agent for CTD.

The rubella and rheumatic fever models can be combined to form a plausible general hypothesis for microbial involvement in the articular CTD. All three factors could be important: local presence

Table 27–2. Current Hypothesis for a Microbial Role in Articular CTD

Sequence
Microbial replication (? locally)
Immune response
Local microbial/cross-reactive/altered host antigen(s)
Local inflammation
Perpetuating host/microbial antigen(s) persistence
Recurrent/chronic local inflammation

Alternative Sequence
Endogenous bacterial antigens (? cross-reactive)
Rheumatoid factors
Local (and systemic) immune complexes

of microbial and/or cross-reactive host antigens, and the immune response (Table 27–2). A microbial infection, possibly in joint tissues, could induce an immune response resulting in local inflammation due to local presence of the microbial antigen, an inflammation-altered host antigen, and/or a cross-reactive host antigen. Local persistence of one or more of these antigens then provides the perpetuating stimulus for recurrent or chronic arthritis, perhaps with microbial reinfections as an additional stimulus for exacerbations.

Many variations of this basic theme can be constructed to account for specific features of particular diseases. One is the bacterial debris hypothesis (see Table 27–2), in which endogenous gut bacteria provide microbial host antigen, and various immune complexes are then formed by specific antibody, alteration of host IgG, and the induction of rheumatoid factors.[23] Formation of such complexes locally in joints results in articular CTD, whereas circulating complexes lead to systemic CTD. This mechanism could account for rheumatic disease after intestinal bypass surgery[220] or inflammatory bowel disease. Alternatively, endogenous or exogenous microbial antigens may cross-react with host antigens, perhaps HLA-determined.[228]

Human Models: Systemic CTD

Except for the bacterial debris hypothesis, the articular models are not readily applicable to the systemic CTD. The association of necrotizing vasculitis with hepatitis B (HB) virus infection was the first example of a CTD caused by chronic virus infection.[76] It is an excellent model for other systemic CTD, like SLE.

Although there may be some geographic variation, 30 to 50% of American and European patients with systemic vasculitis have evidence of chronic HB infection.[186,210] The clinical presentation of HB-positive patients may differ somewhat from the HB-negative group, but they are otherwise similar in the profound severity of their illness, their articular, central nervous system, renal and other system involvement, their often poor response to treatment, and generally poor prognosis.[103]

HB surface antigen (HBsAg) is usually found in the blood using immunologic or ultrastructural methods. It is also present in vasculitic lesions by immunofluorescence, along with IgM and C3. The frequency of vasculitis is low in chronic HBsAg carriers, about 1% in a hemodialysis group.[53] Infection can be acquired parenterally or by contact, with vasculitis beginning 1.5 to 18 months later.[138] Clinical hepatitis occurs, if at all, 3 to 4 months before the vasculitis.[103] The later appearance of specific antibody correlates with the recovery from acute illness. Antibody to core antigen is present in most patients, even those with persisting HBsAg.[210]

There is considerable evidence for a circulating immune complex pathogenesis of HB vasculitis. This includes the aggregated electron microscopic appearance of HB viral components from serum suggesting they are complexed with antibody, the immunoreactants found in the lesions, the hypocomplementemia usually found during active disease, and the occasional presence of HBsAg and specific antibody simultaneously in blood.[76,79,141,186,210] However, direct demonstration of immune complexes has been difficult, with some types of tests negative and others positive, and the presence of complexes often does not correlate with clinical activity. In fact, both direct and indirect evidence of immune complexes is often present in other HB-associated diseases and even in asymptomatic carriers.[104,120,127,207] In addition, the demonstration of specific antibody together with antigen in the vascular lesions has been difficult,[103,141] although this was recently accomplished in serum.[104]

Thus, vasculitis probably results from the immune response to persistent systemic virus replication, with circulating immune complex formation and deposition. The clearance of such complexes may be impaired by defective Kupffer's cell function due to viral damage and/or overload. Composition, size, complement fixing ability, and timing of the complexes are factors affecting potential pathogenicity. In situ immune complex formation may also occur, and factors in addition to the humoral immune response are probably involved. For instance, at the subcellular level, host genetic control of virus and virus component production apparently leads to the vast excess of circulating HBsAg. Still unrecognized virus strain variations or an abnormal cellular immune response might also be involved. Thus, HB infection can be viewed as the cause of a subset of necrotizing vasculitis, but only in concert with other equally critical host factors. An extraordinarily broad spectrum of immunopathology can occur during HB infections, ranging from the often fatal vasculitis or the acute arthritis discussed here to both acute and chronic asymptomatic infections.[54,103] HB may also play role in glomerulonephritis and essential mixed cryoglobulinemia.

A general hypothesis for microbial involvement in the systemic CTD can be constructed using the HB vasculitis model (Table 27–3). This hypothesis differs from that for articular CTD in the systemic distribution both of the microbial and/or host antigens, and of the immune interactions with them. Antigenic debris from endogenous gut bacteria or cross-reactive host antigens could also be involved here. Both hypotheses include various alternatives

Table 27–3.   Current Hypothesis for a Microbial Role in Systemic CTD

Sequence
Microbial replication systemically (? endogenous bacteria)
Immune response (? rheumatoid factors)
? Cross-reactive host antigen
Immune complexes, systemic/? local
Inflammation
Microbial/host antigen persistence
Recurrent/chronic inflammation

to account for the uncertain role of genetic factors, and the uncertain nature and location of the inciting and perpetuating microbial or host antigens. Other environmental agents, e.g., drugs or sunlight, may either mimic a microbial effect or unbalance a precarious host-microbial relationship in favor of disease. The microbe then may not be the immediate cause, but rather part of a multifactorial etiology and pathogenesis. These broad hypotheses provide a framework for future experimentation, e.g., identification of an immune response to the antigens, whatever their origin, which should be present in joint tissues of at least some articular CTD patients.

EVIDENCE IMPLICATING INFECTIOUS AGENTS IN THE CTD

Many attempts at implicating different microorganisms in most rheumatic syndromes have been made over the last 50 years. With the exception of HB vasculitis and Lyme disease, promising early findings have generally proved fruitless. Earlier enthusiasms, including references, were discussed in the previous edition[162] and in several more recent reviews.[48,139,160] Subsequent efforts are reviewed here.

Articular CTD

Rheumatoid Arthritis. In part because of the availability of specimens from this common disease, extensive microbial isolation studies with an imposing array of methods have been done.[135,160] Attempts at isolating bacteria have not yielded consistent or reproducible results.[19] Nevertheless, interest in the possible role of bacteria or their fragments has increased, largely because of their obvious role in reactive and enteropathic arthritis, and their possible role in ankylosing spondylitis.[23] Immunologic evidence has been found for the presence of bacterial antigens in rheumatoid synovial fluids,[18] but a mass spectrometric study of synovial fluids and tissues was negative.[172] Specific immunity to bacteria has not been extensively studied, but the prevalence of antibodies to streptococcal mucopeptide was similar in RA and controls.[170]

The situation is similar for mycoplasma: interest

in their possible role persists, mainly because of mycoplasma-induced chronic arthritis in animals, but numerous earlier attempts to detect either the microorganisms or specific immunity to them have been generally negative.[31,40,205] Neither the presence of an incompletely characterized transmissible agent in rheumatoid synovium nor the role of amebic infection in RA has been confirmed.

The enthusiasm for studying particular classes of microbes has been generated largely by available methodology: thus the sequence from bacteria to mycoplasma and, during the last 15 years, to viruses. Earlier studies, both published and unpublished, were predominantly negative, as were more recent attempts at detecting both DNA and RNA viruses in RA tissues.[87,88,151,152] Occasionally, viruses have been detected, as with the isolation of a cytomegalovirus[85] or the virus-like particles found by electron microscopy.[197] Although the viruses are apparently transmissible in mice, they are still poorly characterized.[193a] Cytomegalovirus antibodies were not increased generally in RA,[34] but were elevated in some patients with early disease.[133] Such data, as have many earlier studies, suggest a possible etiologic role for the virus, but can also represent isolation of an innocent passenger in vivo, or acquisition of a laboratory contaminant in vitro.

Increased prevalence or titer of virus antibodies in RA sera has been sought as indirect evidence for a viral role. Recent interest has centered on Epstein-Barr virus (EBV).[50,66,215] The initial observation was that most RA, but not normal, sera reacted by immunodiffusion with a nuclear antigen from a B-lymphoblastoid (EBV-infected) cell line.[8] Subsequent studies focused on determining whether this RA-nuclear antigen (RANA) was an EBV antigen. Serologic studies, generally using the more sensitive indirect immunofluorescent assay, confirmed that anti-RANA was found in 70 to 95% of RA patients compared to generally less than 20% of various control groups,[6,34,65] with one exception.[216] Antibodies to two other EBV components, the capsid and early antigens, and sometimes the EBV-associated nuclear antigen (EBNA), were also increased in RA sera and generally correlated with anti-RANA titers both in RA and the various control groups and in normal subjects.[5,34,65,216] Normal subjects with infectious mononucleosis, the disease caused by initial EBV infection, also developed anti-RANA during later convalescence, generally in concert with anti-EBNA.[32]

No correlations were found between anti-RANA and the clinical features of RA in most of these studies, including those done in early disease,[133,192] nor was any correlation found with the genetic marker for RA, HLA-DRw4, in either patients or controls.[33,184] There was a clear relationship between anti-RANA and the presence of rheumatoid factor in RA,[5,148] but in vitro absorption of rheumatoid factor, which causes false-positive and false-negative tests in some systems,[9,190] did not affect anti-RANA or anti-EBNA titers.[34] That RANA and EBNA may be distinct antigens, although closely related, was shown by their expression during different phases of the cell cycle in vitro, and by their independent segregation in somatic cell hybrids.[195,196] However, the two antibodies may recognize different epitopes on the same molecule.[215] These studies, although differing in some details, show that RANA results from EBV infection in vitro, that anti-RANA is found in vivo only after EBV infection, and that the prevalence and titers of anti-RANA and other EBV antibodies are generally increased in RA.

The second line of evidence stemmed from the observation that RA peripheral blood lymphocytes behave differently in vitro after exposure to EBV. RA lymphocytes make more rheumatoid factor in vitro than controls, and spontaneous transformation (i.e., without added EBV) into lymphoblastoid cell lines also occurs more frequently.[194] RA lymphocytes transform more rapidly following EBV inoculation, owing to defective EBV-specific suppressor T cell function,[17,209] and not to deficient natural killer activity.[98] The actual defect may be the failure of RA T cells to produce gamma interferon, owing to their enhanced sensitivity to the suppressive action of prostaglandins produced by the adherent cell population.[90,91]

Several studies found that the defective cellular regulation of EBV in vitro is not reflected by increased viral release or antigen expression in vivo. Oropharyngeal virus excretion was similar in RA and controls.[1,51] EBV antibody levels in RA synovial fluids were similar to those in sera, suggesting that local synthesis, in response to possibly locally enhanced virus expression, was not occurring.[5] Neither RANA nor other EBV antigens nor EBV genomes were found in RA tissues, including synovium.[7]

Taken together, the studies suggest that the increased antibody response to EBV antigens in RA could be caused by increased viral expression in B cells in vivo. These studies also suggest that the abnormal behavior of RA lymphocytes in vitro may be caused by deficient production of gamma interferon by T cells that are hypersensitive to the suppressive effect of prostaglandins produced by the macrophage-monocyte population. The cause of the T cell abnormality is unknown, but is probably not EBV infection, which thus seems unlikely to be a prime cause of RA. Further studies will be needed to determine whether the increased expression of EBV in B cells, its effect on their function, or the immune response to it may have a role in perpetuation of the disease.

Rubella has been a perennial etiologic candidate in RA, but recent studies, like earlier ones, have yielded conflicting results. Repeated virus isolation was reported over a 2-year period from 6 patients with varying types of chronic arthritis including RA, but the specific identification of the isolates as rubella was not detailed.[80] Apparently rubella-specific immune responses have also been found; B cells secreting antibody to rubella, but only rarely to other viruses, were found in both peripheral blood and synovium of 7 RA patients.[36] When indirect leukocyte migration inhibition was used, the cellular response of both rheumatoid synovial and blood lymphocytes to rubella antigen was somewhat more depressed than to other virus antigens,[37] but when lymphocyte proliferation was used, blood lymphocytes were generally hyporesponsive to virus antigens, including rubella.[224] In another study, the synovial lymphocytes of 1 of 10 RA patients proliferated specifically in response to rubella, and virus was isolated from the same joint.[69] However, two careful studies using sophisticated methodology failed to detect any evidence of rubella in RA joint or other tissues.[88,152] Further studies on the possible role of rubella in RA need more rigorous classification of patients, better controls, and specific identification of any virus isolates.

Both humoral and cellular immune responses to still other viruses have been examined in RA. Antibodies in serum and synovial fluid to the other herpesviruses (simplex, varicella-zoster, and cytomegalovirus) and measles were generally normal.[5,34,133] B cells secreting antibody to measles, mumps, respiratory syncytial, and various herpesviruses were rarely found in blood and never in synovial tissue.[36] Measles antibodies were elevated in RA sera using immunofluorescence,[190] but neither this nor elevation of any other virus antibody has been found generally. The cellular response of blood lymphocytes to measles and several parainfluenza viruses, but not to several herpesviruses, was decreased.[224] Although RA synovial fluid lymphocytes responded normally to mumps antigen,[69] they differed from blood lymphocytes in being unable to support herpes simplex virus replication. This was apparently mediated by a cell-to-cell interaction, perhaps by interferon.[10]

With these largely negative attempts at implicating specific viruses by various methods, there has been growing interest in detecting an antigen, microbial or not, unique to rheumatoid synovial cells. Cultured RA synovial cells, usually fibroblasts, have been the target, either alive or as extracts, in most studies. They are then reacted with sera or blood lymphocytes from both RA and controls to detect the "specific" immune response.[82,83,147,179] A more complex approach involves injecting RA or control synovial cells into rabbit joints, and subsequent autologous immunization with their own cultured joint cells.[198] None of these approaches has yet led to demonstration of a unique antigen in RA joint tissues.

In juvenile RA (JRA), models for microbial involvement are similar to those in the adult disease, and earlier attempts at implicating specific agents both in JRA and in the other childhood rheumatic diseases have generally been negative.[161] In more recent studies, rubella was isolated from the joint of one JRA patient,[80] and JRA blood lymphocytes were also somewhat hyporesponsive to viral antigens, including rubella.[37] Antibodies to streptococcal mucopeptide were not strikingly increased.[170] In contrast to adult RA, both blood and joint lymphocytes from JRA supported herpes simplex viral growth normally.[99]

Thus, at present, there is little firm evidence to implicate microbial agents in either RA or JRA. The abnormalities observed with EBV most likely reflect an underlying immunoregulatory disturbance, the cause of which is still undetermined. The studies directly or indirectly implicating other viruses require confirmation.

The Seronegative Spondyloarthropathies. These rheumatic syndromes share many clinical features, such as spondylitis and peripheral arthritis, the absence of rheumatoid factor, and a high prevalence of the histocompatibility antigen gene HLA-B27 (Table 27–4). This gene strongly predisposes toward illness in most Caucasian populations, and is also associated with increased severity. Those lacking B27 may have immuno-

Table 27–4.   Microorganisms Implicated in the Seronegative Spondyloarthropathies

Reactive arthritis
Enteric infection
Reiter's: *Shigella, Salmonella*
Reactive: *Yersinia, Campylobacter, Brucella*
Venereal infection
Reiter's: *Chlamydia*; ? mycoplasma,
Neisseria
Enteropathic arthritis
Inflammatory bowel disease: ? enteric flora
Whipple's: Whipple's bacterium
Intestinal-bypass: *E. coli, B. fragilis*
"Dermatopathic" arthritis
Hidradenitis suppurativa/acne conglobata
?? Psoriatic
Ankylosing spondylitis: ? *Klebsiella*

logically cross-reactive antigens in the B7 group, but predisposing genes in other populations, particularly nonCaucasian, have not been identified.[2,13,124] Many of these syndromes are also associated with infections, mainly by enteric bacteria.[139,160]

There is considerable clinical overlap among the various spondyloarthropathies, but particularly between Reiter's disease and reactive arthritis. When their distinctive extra-articular features are lacking, they are difficult to distinguish from seronegative RA, which has led to proposals that enteric infection is a major factor in RA,[23] and even in other CTD.[121] Clinically and pathogenetically, Reiter's disease can be considered a form of reactive arthritis.[124] Both can follow enteric infection. In post-dysenteric Reiter's disease, *Shigella flexneri* subtypes 1b and 2a have been positively incriminated, but *S. sonnei* has not.[193] Reactive arthritis has been principally observed in Scandinavia following *Yersinia entercolitica* bowel infections, but also after *Salmonella,* and more recently *Campylobacter jejuni* and brucellosis.[2,118,213] The arthritis following *Yersinia* occurs almost exclusively following infection with serotypes 0:3 and 0:9, which are prevalent in both Europe and Japan. Plasmids seem to determine enteropathogenicity,[94] but whether they are necessary for arthritogenicity is unknown.

Reactive arthritis patients with B27 not only usually have more severe disease, but also show several immunologic abnormalities. T-lymphocytopenia has been found, along with decreased suppression of immunoglobulin synthesis in vitro.[77] *Yersinia* antibody titers are usually elevated, IgA antibodies being particularly associated with the arthritis.[81] The specific cellular response to *Yersinia* is higher than in seronegative RA patients lacking B27,[77] but is lower than in patients with *Yersinia* infection without arthritis. The latter study also found a depressed response to *E. coli,* suggesting that the enterobacterial common antigen is involved in pathogenesis of the arthritis.[123] Formation of circulating immune complexes, possibly with bacterial antigens, may be responsible for the rheumatic symptoms.[134] Measures of leukocyte chemotaxis and chemokinesis are higher in B27-positive subjects with or without *Yersinia* arthritis; thus, B27 may predispose to more severe and prolonged symptoms via an enhanced inflammatory response.[125,175]

Reiter's syndrome more commonly follows venereal infection, but the responsible organisms continue to be debated. Candidates include *Chlamydia trachomatis,* various mycoplasma, and *Neisseria gonorrhoeae.*[78,119] Earlier studies on the role of chlamydia in sexually acquired reactive arthritis, including Reiter's syndrome, have been inconclu-

sive.[119] Recent studies have again implicated these intracellular microorganisms in adults by both higher urethral isolation rates and increased antibody levels,[114] and perhaps in children as well.[180] Arthritis occurred more often in patients with B27, or with high IgG antibody to chlamydia.[114] Chlamydia were isolated from the joint in one case, and infection was definitely implicated even in B27-negative cases.[217] A clear pattern of specific cellular responses has not been reported, but more sensitive assays may yield definitive information.[27] The exact chlamydial antigen involved is also unknown, but its major glycolipid shares both immunologic and physical characteristics with lipopolysaccharide from enteric bacteria.[153] The synovial lymphocyte response in Reiter's syndrome to venereal (chlamydia, ureaplasma) or enteric antigens (*Salmonella, Shigella, Yersinia, Campylobacter*) is often increased and can distinguish between the venereal and enteric forms. It also helps to classify "idiopathic" knee arthritis in the same manner. The synovial lymphocyte response to the particular microbial antigen is far greater than the blood lymphocyte responses in virtually all cases.[68] Except for the synovial response to ureaplasma, earlier enthusiasm for mycoplasma in Reiter's has waned. However, these agents are definitely involved in nongonococcal urethritis, and new species continue to be isolated using more sensitive methods.[211] They continue, therefore, to be candidate agents. Virologic studies have been generally negative. One study has suggested the cellular response to *N. gonorrhoeae* is increased in Reiter's disease.[181]

The emerging picture is that multiple microorganisms, both enteric and venereally transmitted, can trigger Reiter's syndrome and reactive arthritis. Recognized agents are *Yersinia,* certain species of *Shigella* and *Salmonella, Campylobacter,* probably *Chlamydia,* and possibly *Mycoplasma* (see Chap. 54).

In enteropathic arthritis (see Table 27-4), both spondylitis and peripheral arthritis occur, but only the former is associated with B27. In inflammatory bowel disease, a previously reported transmissible agent has not been confirmed. Whipple's disease is caused by an unculturable bacterium, which may invade joint tissues to cause symptoms. After intestinal bypass for morbid obesity, marked overgrowth of *E. coli* and *Bacteroides fragilis* can occur in the resulting blind loop. Circulating immune complexes containing antibodies to these bacteria may then cause arthritis, which disappears when the bypass is taken down.[122,220] "Dermatopathic" arthritis may also occur; severe chronic skin infections are associated with a reactive arthritis-like picture.[182] In psoriatic arthritis, high anti-DNAase B levels seem to implicate strepto-cocci, but the specificity of the antibody has not been shown.[214]

In ankylosing spondylitis (AS), where B27 is nearly always present, microbes had not been implicated at all until recent studies of enteric bacteria.[74,116,160] Initially, antigenic cross-reactivity was found between *Klebsiella pneumoniae* (formerly *Aerobacter aerogenes*) and the B27 antigen, and *Klebsiella* bowel infection was more prevalent in active AS.[56,228] Although the latter finding has not been confirmed,[55,221] Australian workers have presented considerable additional evidence for a cross-reactive antigen.[74] Lymphocytes from B27-positive AS proliferated less in response to *Klebsiella* antigens than did those from B27-negative AS or B27-positive or -negative normal controls. In addition, antisera to certain *Klebsiella* strains were cytotoxic to lymphocytes from 80% of B27-positive AS, 60% of B27-positive Reiter's, and 20% of B27-positive uveitis patients, but not from B27-negative patients or B27-positive or -negative healthy controls.[74,185] Other workers have failed to confirm these findings, particularly the cytotoxicity.[12,20,62,189]

The Australian group also found that B27-positive but not B27-negative normal lymphocytes were lysed by the antisera after incubation either with a culture filtrate of the particular *Klebsiella* strains[75] or, more recently, with a factor from lymphoblastoid cell lines from B27-positive AS patients.[157] The modifying factor in the culture filtrate was a 26,000 to 30,000-dalton bacterial outer membrane component. Approximately 8% of random *Klebsiella* isolates had this cross-reactive antigen; they did not share particular capsular serotypes, bacteriophage types, or cultural characteristics.[74,159] Both T- and B-lymphocytes, platelets, fibroblasts, and lymphoblastoid cell lines, but not spermatozoa or erythrocytes, from B27-positive AS patients carried this cross-reacting antigen. It persisted for many generations in cultured cells, but lymphocytes from HLA identical normal siblings of B27-positive AS patients did not carry it.

This work was interpreted as showing that a membrane antigen from particular *Klebsiella* strains cross-reacts with a cell surface antigen determined by HLA-B27, or a closely associated gene, in AS and a few other spondyloarthropathies. After in vitro exposure to the *Klebsiella* or to B27-positive AS cell lines, normal B27-positive lymphocytes acquire the antigen. Thus, in vivo the cellular antigen seems to be acquired with disease and is not transmitted genetically, whereas in vitro it is transmissible both horizontally and vertically. One possible explanation might be a bacterial plasmid that can also infect human cells.[74] However, with the lack of confirmation from other laboratories, this interesting hypothesis is encountering increasing criticism, particularly directed at the appropriateness of control groups, at the possible in vitro effects of in vivo drug treatment, and at technical variables.[116]

In other attempts at implicating microbes in the spondyloarthropathies, various candidates, including bacteria, chlamydia, mycoplasma, and viruses, were similarly cytotoxic for B27-positive and B-27-negative fibroblasts.[52] Serum antibodies to chlamydia and to measles were not increased in AS.[3,109] Another finding indirectly suggesting a role for infection in B27-associated disease was the temporary T-lymphopenia found in both patients with acute uveitis and their household contacts, and in quiescent AS, but not their contacts. This result suggested horizontal transmission of an infective agent during attacks of uveitis.[28]

Although not classified as a spondyloarthropathy, Lyme disease does share some clinical features, and now has a proven infectious cause. It is characterized by a sometimes recurrent pauciarthritis occurring after a characteristic rash, usually in children, and often with multisystem involvement.[201] The B cell alloantigen DR2 predisposes to neurologic and joint involvement. From the beginning there was strong circumstantial evidence for a tick-transmitted infectious agent, but it was isolated only recently: the *Ixodes dammini* spirochete.[199] Specific IgM antibody is high during the acute phase, whereas specific IgG antibody is high in patients with later complications such as arthritis. The symptoms of Lyme disease, both systemic and articular, appear to be immune complex mediated.[86] Early treatment with tetracycline seems to prevent the major late complications, including arthritis. The spirochete has been more readily recovered from the ticks than from patient specimens and still has not been identified in joints.[199,200] Thus, the pathogenesis of chronic arthritis in Lyme disease remains unclear; with the etiologic agent now isolated, it should be possible to demonstrate whether local persistence of the spirochete is necessary. Although this spirochete is probably not a common cause of chronic arthritis, other fastidious microorganisms, such as the mycoplasma isolated earlier during the Lyme search,[212] could well be involved. The evolving story of Lyme disease is fascinating because it clarifies the role of a microbe in a chronic inflammatory disease.

The clinical similarities of the spondyloarthropathies and their frequent association with both HLA-B27 and microbial infection suggest common pathogenetic mechanisms. The latter may include deposition of immune complexes containing bacterial antigens, or cross-reactivity of such antigens with host target tissue or responding cell antigens. Particular problems in implicating enteric bacteria are the many different species present in the bowel, which change with time, and the lack of adequate bacteriologic typing facilities, including plasmid analysis, in most centers. The possible roles of chlamydia and mycoplasma need to be examined using the most sensitive isolation and serologic methods. Problems in implicating any of these three classes of microorganisms are: (1) they are often found as normal flora, although only genetically susceptible individuals may acquire disease; and (2) many patients have been treated with antibiotics before they can be studied. Nonetheless, a role for endogenous bacteria in some of the seronegative spondyloarthropathies seems certain and should stimulate interest in their possible role in other chronic arthritides.[23]

Systemic CTD

Systemic Lupus Erythematosus. Interest in the role of microbes, and particularly viruses, has declined both because of their secondary role in New Zealand mouse disease and because of the many negative studies over the past 15 years.[160,162,165] Regarding bacteria, the prevalence and titer of serum antibodies to a hemotropic rickettsia in the Anaplasmataceae family were higher in SLE.[108] Earlier the same workers identified *Anaplasma*-like structures on SLE erythrocytes, and subsequently a related microorganism apparently caused a febrile multisystem illness.[11] Further confirmation hinges on isolation but, like the recently isolated microorganisms *Legionella* and the Lyme spirochete, *Anaplasma* are difficult to cultivate.[178] Earlier mycoplasma isolations from SLE patients and other transmissible effects have not been confirmed.

Regarding viruses, the tubuloreticular structures found by electron microscopy in many SLE patients are thought to be not viral but a secondary manifestation of cellular injury. In vitro, they could be induced by interferon, levels of which are higher in SLE sera.[177] Various other inclusions have been seen in SLE tissues, but none are convincingly viral.

During the mid-1970s, interest turned to type C or oncornaviruses, now called retroviruses. These RNA viruses have a unique enzyme (RNA-dependent DNA polymerase) and a characteristic electron-microscopic appearance. They are found in many subhuman species and are sometimes oncogenic, but the first human retrovirus, the human T cell leukemia virus, was isolated only recently.[167] They were initially implicated in New Zealand mouse disease, but it now appears that any viral pathogenetic role is secondary.[165]

Initial studies, principally using immunofluorescence and radioimmunoassays with antiviral antisera, suggested that type C virus expression was enhanced in SLE. However, specificity was difficult to prove, especially since these viruses acquire envelopes as they bud from host cells, incorporating and adsorbing components from both the cell and the culture medium. Thus, the antiviral antisera invariably contained nonviral reactivities that often persisted even after extensive absorption.[165] Nevertheless, subsequent studies from two groups tended to confirm their original immunofluorescence findings of type C virus-related antigens present in renal glomeruli.[140,176] In the latter study, immunoglobulin was eluted from SLE kidneys and reacted with type C antigens when immunoprecipitation was used. Although various controls were included, the use of serum IgG would have been desirable to control for the large number of nonviral specificities usually present in SLE. The positive findings in SLE kidneys have not yet been independently confirmed.

Many studies failing to show enhanced type C viral expression in SLE have accumulated.[162] Some, including the type C-like particles in placentas and serum antibodies to type C viruses using cytotoxicity or viral enzyme inhibition, showed equal "expression" in SLE and normals.[21,87] Most studies, however, showed no viral expression at all. These studies included attempts at detection of viral antigens in SLE tissues by radioimmunoassay, as in one of the original positive studies, but employing improved techniques,[115] studies using nucleic acid hybridization, and extensive attempts at viral isolation.[14,96,164] Thus, a pathogenetic role for any of the subhuman-type C viruses studied in the past seems unlikely. However, retroviruses remain candidate agents because of the recent isolation of a bona fide human virus, the human T cell leukemia virus.[167] With its T cell tropism, this virus certainly could cause immunoregulatory disturbances.[110] Furthermore, a related type E retrovirus, which is tropic for macrophages and can also cause immunoregulatory disturbances, has been implicated in an RA-like disease of goats.[146]

Other viruses, viral antigens, or viral genomes that have not been found more frequently, or at all, in SLE tissues, include myxoviruses such as measles and influenza, hepatitis B, and papovaviruses.[162,218] Measuring specific antibody levels has not provided any clues either. Serum antibody levels, particularly against measles and rubella, are often increased in SLE compared to controls, but this seems to be part of the general overproduction of antibodies so characteristic of SLE.[160] Furthermore, the viral antibody tests may also measure antibodies to nonviral antigens (medium, cellular components) that may also be increased in SLE.[166] In contrast, the response to immunization with both bacterial and viral antigens often seems to be blunted in SLE both in vivo and in vitro.[105,143,149] The nature of the defect is not clear, but theoretically might reflect prior commitment to other antigens.

A recent finding is that the La and Sm autoantibodies found frequently in SLE recognize intracellular ribonucleoprotein particles (small nuclear RNAs complexed with protein). EBV and adenovirus can code for these small RNAs, and the autoantibodies recognize a binding site on the RNA.[71,126] In another study, antibodies to native DNA in SLE sera inhibited adenovirus DNA synthesis in vitro.[101] These autoantibodies react, probably primarily, with nonviral antigens, so whether adenovirus or EBV is involved in their induction in vivo is unknown. Nevertheless, these studies provide an example of how a virus could, via a cross-reacting antigen, trigger autoimmune abnormalities.

Cellular reactivity to viral antigens is generally reduced in SLE, probably owing to a generalized functional lymphocyte defect rather than to a failure of specific immune recognition.[169,225] Inferferon levels are frequently high in sera from patients with active SLE, which initially suggested an antiviral response.[100] Elevated levels have also been found in other CTD[144] and, more recently, antibodies to interferon have also been found in SLE.[203] Interferons are a heterogeneous group of substances, including various kinds of viral- and immune-induced compounds, which can alter many cellular, including lymphocyte, functions. It is not clear whether the elevated levels in CTD are a cause or a result of lymphocyte dysfunction,[144] but it seems more likely that they are a direct result of lymphocyte activation than of viral infection.

Studies of antilymphocyte and other autoantibodies in family members of SLE patients, human contacts of canine SLE, and canine contacts of human SLE suggested the possibility of horizontal transmission of an infectious agent.[4,67] More recent studies failed to support this possibility, particularly between humans and dogs.[174] These autoantibodies are also heterogeneous, and although they may result from an occult viral infection, they may simply reflect disordered immunoregulation.

In spite of the lack of evidence implicating a specific infectious agent, it is still likely that SLE requires an initiating event, probably environmental and possibly infectious. In the setting of genetically determined perturbations of the immune system, an infectious trigger could be a trivial event clinically, and such a trigger could be different in different patients. Once triggered, the immuno-

logic abnormalities might be self-perpetuating so that the persistent infection and foreign antigens as found in HB vasculitis might not be needed. Current evidence has not implicated any specific microbial agents, with the possible exception of *Anaplasma* in some patients.

Polymyositis and Dermatomyositis. The possible roles of *Toxoplasma* and picornaviruses continue to be investigated.[106,107,160] Approximately 15% of polymyositis patients have high serum *Toxoplasma* antibody levels, many with specific IgM antibody suggesting current or recent infection. However, isolation attempts have been negative, and the clinical response to specific antimicrobial treatment has been equivocal.[106,132,163] The microorganism has been demonstrated in the muscle of several patients using immunofluorescence.[95,173] The etiologic role of toxoplasmosis remains to be established, since latent infection is common and could be secondarily activated by the myositis.

Various possible viral inclusions have been found in myositis using the electron microscope; the most convincing were the crystalline picornavirus-like arrays. However, one study found these inclusions could be digested with amylase, suggesting they were in fact glycogen.[112] Virus isolation attempts and virus antibody studies have generally not been revealing, but in some patients have implicated coxsackieviruses, which belong to the picornavirus family, and rarely, hepatitis B and BCG vaccination.[111] The myositis-specific Jo-1 antibody was found to inhibit histidyl-tRNA synthetase, a cellular enzyme that may be involved in the replication of RNA viruses such as picornaviruses.[137] This work is analogous to that showing autoantibodies in SLE recognize cellular nucleic acids that may also be involved in viral replication.[71,101,126]

Influenza occasionally causes a severe acute myositis, but may also cause a syndrome called benign acute childhood myositis, which may be a mild form of polymyositis.[183] Viruses have also been implicated occasionally in other forms of inflammatory muscle disease.[142] That such a variety of infectious agents has been implicated, but so rarely and in such a variety of myopathies, suggests again that infectious triggers can be different in different patients. The underlying mechanisms are probably also different, varying from direct invasion of muscle to various immunoregulatory disturbances. In summary, *Toxoplasma* has been implicated in some cases of chronic myositis; the role of picornaviruses is less certain.

Miscellaneous CTD

Necrotizing vasculitis without evidence of HB infection presumably has other causes, possibly also infectious.[160] Some adults have presented with serous otitis media and episcleritis, a distinctive clinical picture suggesting infection, but virus antibody levels in these patients did not implicate a specific agent.[187] Streptococcal infection, rubella vaccination, cytomegalovirus, and trichinosis have all been implicated rarely in systemic vasculitis, but in most non-HB cases no agent can be implicated.[73] Herpes simplex and the human T cell leukemia virus have been implicated in cutaneous vasculitis, as has varicella zoster in CNS vasculitis.[93,113,131]

Infantile polyarteritis is the most severe form of Kawasaki disease, also called the mucocutaneous lymph node syndrome. Many cases seem to be linked to previous respiratory illnesses, but no specific agents have been identified.[22,47] A pathogenetic role for rickettsia[204] has not been confirmed. Another study implicated rug shampoo exposure believed to mobilize house dust mites.[158] In Henoch-Schönlein vasculitis, preceding upper respiratory infections were observed in most cases, but specific agents were not implicated.[61]

An infectious cause, particularly viral, has long been suspected in Behçet's disease. Most studies have been negative,[136,154] but several have suggested a possible viral role. As in RA synovial lymphocytes, herpes simplex virus replication was impaired in blood lymphocytes from patients with Behçet's disease and, in addition, chromosomal abnormalities were frequent.[49] Nucleic acid hybridization suggested the herpes genome persists in lymphocytes.[57] As in SLE, interferon levels were also increased in Behçet's sera.[155]

In polymyalgia rheumatica and giant cell arteritis, no evidence has been found to implicate HB infection,[26,60] but a possible example of horizontal transmission between spouses has been reported.[97] The rarity of these vasculitis syndromes continues to be a major impediment to investigating their possible infectious etiologies.

Goodpasture's syndrome may follow influenza rarely. Virus-like structures have been found with the electron microscope, but there has been no further evidence for an infectious etiology. In children, a variety of antigens may be involved in glomerulonephritis.[117] Streptococcal infection has long been recognized as one of these, although the exact mechanism is still obscure.[150] Although an earlier study was negative, elevated cytomegalovirus antibodies, including IgM antibodies suggesting active infection, were recently found in Sjögren's syndrome.[188] Cytomegalovirus, as well as other viruses, has rarely been associated with both autoimmune hemolytic anemia and idiopathic thrombocytopenia. In the latter, another study reported finding HB and other viral antigens frequently, but appropriate controls were lacking.[130] Herpesviruses were implicated in a syndrome consisting of arthralgias with acute urinary retention.[145]

Other Hepatitis B Syndromes

The spectrum of immunologic responses to HB infection is broad, ranging from the asymptomatic persistent virus carrier, through the acute arthritis-hepatitis syndrome, to fatal necrotizing vasculitis. Two other immunologically mediated diseases have been associated with HB infection: membranous glomerulonephritis and essential mixed cryoglobulinemia.[103] The former has been associated with HB infection predominantly in childhood, where it appears to be the single most common cause.[117] Hepatitis is often present, but may be subclinical or overshadowed by the renal disease. Considerable evidence has been found for an immune complex pathogenesis, but the viral antigen involved is still unclear.

The association of essential mixed cryoglobulinemia with HB infection is more controversial. Initially, most patients were reported to have HB infection,[128] but this finding was not confirmed subsequently.[24,171] This was in part owing to differences in the numbers of patients with chronic liver disease who had a higher HB prevalence and whom many would term secondary rather than essential cryoglobulinemia.[171] Nevertheless, it seems clear that HB infection, chronic liver disease, and cryoglobulinemia are associated, and that many of the clinical manifestations of the latter are due to immune complex mediated vasculitis. HB infection in man continues to be unique because of the wide spectrum of associated immunologic disease. Much is yet to be learned about both the viral and host factors involved in pathogenesis.

Problems and Prospects

There are many potential problems in studies of the role of infectious agents in rheumatic disease.[162] Proper design can avoid many of these, but others will be recognized only by experimentation. Proper selection of patients, controls, and specimens is critical. Sensitivity of detection methods is also important, but must be balanced with the need for specificity. Culture procedures should allow early recognition of contaminants. Antisera with cross-reactivities to culture components present on the microbial envelopes are particularly troublesome, a situation that monoclonal antibodies should help clarify.

Multiple factors, host and environmental, are probably involved in the pathogenesis of the CTD. In addition, each of these diseases is a syndrome, with different factors, and perhaps different environmental agents, involved in different subsets.

Recognizable subsets include necrotizing vasculitis with hepatitis B infection, and possibly polymyositis with *Toxoplasma* infection, and various enteric bacteria in the spondyloarthropathies. Further investigation of these should be fruitful, but identification of other research areas of high potential is more difficult. As in the past, much may depend on serendipitous observations. Serum antibody levels or lymphocyte responses to newly discovered agents, such as the Lyme spirochete or the human T cell leukemia virus, or in strictly defined populations, e.g., by a genetic factor such as HLA-B27, may be helpful. Determination of the specificities of the local, as opposed to the systemic, immune response in chronic arthritis, and identification of the antigen and antibodies involved in immune complexes in blood, synovial fluid, and tissues are more direct approaches. Specifically directed microbial isolation and antigen detection studies should use the most sensitive methods available. Longitudinal epidemiologic studies to elucidate transmission by contact or other vectors may also be worthwhile.

Perhaps the most immediately rewarding area will be further definition of the genetic loci involved in the CTD and their mechanisms of action. Genetically determined cell surface components probably act in combination with microbial antigens to allow immunologic recognition of the microbe as foreign. Any microbial antigen cross-reacting with cell surface components could then affect immune responses to other antigens, regulating them either up or down. Initially the disturbed response might involve only the microbial agent or a host antigen, but with time, hyperresponsiveness to host antigens becomes established in most CTD. Identifying specific responses, particularly locally in the tissues where they occur, and the antigens involved, may clarify perpetuating mechanisms. Correlation of such responses with predisposing genetic factors might then allow prospective study of high-risk subjects so that a microbial triggering event can be identified. Thus, it may be more useful for now to focus on disease-perpetuating mechanisms in the host rather than on the inciting event and microbial candidates. The application of monoclonal antibodies, both reagents prepared in animals and reagents derived from CTD patients themselves, combined with the techniques of molecular biology should eventually allow precise dissection of the roles of genetic and microbial factors and of disordered immunoregulation in the pathogenesis of the CTD.

REFERENCES

1. Aitcheson, C.T., et al.: Frequency of transforming Epstein-Barr virus in oropharyngeal secretions of rheumatoid arthritis patients. Intervirology, *19*:135–143, 1983.

2. Alarcon, G.S., et al.: Reactive arthritis associated with brucellosis: HLA studies. J. Rheumatol., *8*:621–625, 1981.

3. Alcalay, M., et al.: Ankylosing spondylitis and chlamydial infection in apparently healthy HLA B27 blood donors. J. Rheumatol., *6*:439–446, 1979.

4. Allen, J.I., et al.: Antilymphocyte antibodies in systemic lupus erythematosus patients and their relatives: Reactivity with nonhuman lymphocytes. Clin. Immunol. Immunopathol., *9*:371–378, 1978.

5. Alspaugh, M.A., et al.: Elevated levels of antibodies to Epstein-Barr virus antigens in sera and synovial fluids of patients with rheumatoid arthritis. J. Clin. Invest., *67*:1134–1140, 1981.

6. Alspaugh, M.A., et al.: Lymphocytes transformed by EBV: Induction of nuclear antigen reactive with antibody in RA. J. Exp. Med., *147*:1018–1027, 1978.

7. Alspaugh, M.A., Shoji, H., and Nonoyama, M.: A search for rheumatoid arthritis-associated nuclear antigen and Epstein-Barr virus specific antigens or genomes in tissues and cells from patients with rheumatoid arthritis. Arthritis Rheum., *26*:712–720, 1983.

8. Alspaugh, M.A., and Tan, E.M.: Serum antibody in RA reactive with a cell-associated antigen. Arthritis Rheum., *19*:711–719, 1976.

9. Anderson-Visoná, K., and Villarejos, V.M.: Identity of antibody to hepatitis B e/I antigen as an atypical rheumatoid factor. J. Infect. Dis., *141*:603–608, 1980.

10. Appleford, D.J.A., and Denman, A.M.: Fate of herpes simplex virus in lymphocytes from inflammatory joint effusions. I. Failure of the virus to grow in cultured lymphocytes. II. Mechanisms of non-permissiveness. Ann. Rheum. Dis., *38*:443–455, 1979.

11. Archer, G.L., et al.: Human infection from an unidentified erythrocyte-associated bacterium. N. Engl. J. Med., *301*:897–900, 1979.

12. Archer, J.R.: Search for cross-reactivity between HLA-B27 and *Klebsiella pneumoniae*. Ann. Rheum. Dis., *40*:400–403, 1981.

13. Arnett, F.C., Hochberg, M.C., and Bias, W.B.: Cross-reactive HLA antigens in B27-negative Reiter's syndrome and sacroiliitis. Johns Hopkins Med. J., *141*:193–197, 1977.

14. Aulakh, G.S., et al.: Search for type C oncornavirus-related genetic information in tissues from patients with systemic lupus erythematosus. Arthritis Rheum., *21*:880–884, 1978.

15. Bacon, P.A., et al.: Experimental herpes virus arthritis: Factors in chronicity. Ann. Rheum. Dis., *33*:413–421, 1974.

16. Barden, J.A., and Decker, J.L.: *Mycoplasma hyorhinis* swine arthritis. I. Clinical and microbiologic features. Arthritis Rheum., *14*:193–201, 1971.

17. Bardwick, P.A., et al.: Altered regulation of EBV-induced lymphoblast proliferation in RA lymphoid cells. Arthritis Rheum., *23*:626–632, 1980.

18. Bartholomew, L.E., and Bartholomew, F.N.: Antigenic bacterial polysaccharide in rheumatoid synovial effusions. Arthritis Rheum., *22*:969–977, 1979.

19. Bartlett, R., and Bisset, K.A.: Isolation of *Bacillus licheniformis* var. Endoparasiticus from the blood of rheumatoid arthritis patients and normal subjects. J. Med. Microbiol., *14*:97–105, 1981.

20. Beaulieu, A.D., et al.: Klebsiella related antigens in ankylosing spondylitis. J. Rheumatol., *10*:102–105, 1983.

21. Belkin, R.N., Anderson, K., and Phillips, P.E.: Lack of type C virus antibodies in systemic lupus erythematosus. J. Rheumatol., *9*:613–616, 1982.

22. Bell, D.M., et al.: Kawasaki syndrome: Description of two outbreaks in the United States. N. Engl. J. Med., *304*:1568–1575, 1981.

23. Bennett, J.C.: The infectious etiology of RA: New considerations. Arthritis Rheum., *21*:531–538, 1978.

24. Bombardieri, S., et al.: Liver involvement in essential mixed cryoglobulinemia. La Ricerca in Clinica e in Laboratorio, *9*:361–368, 1979.

25. Brassfield, A.L., et al.: Ultrastructure of arthritis induced

by a caprine retrovirus. Arthritis Rheum., *25*:930–936, 1982.

26. Bridgeford, P.H., et al.: Polymyalgia rheumatica and giant cell arteritis: Histocompatibility typing and HB infection studies. Arthritis Rheum., *23*:516–518, 1980.

27. Brunham, R.C., et al.: Cellular immune response during uncomplicated genital infection with *Chlamydia trachomatis* in humans. Infect. Immun., *34*:98–104, 1981.

28. Byrom, N.A., et al.: T and B lymphocytes in patients with acute anterior uveitis and AS, and in their household contacts. Lancet, *2*:601–603, 1979.

29. Cafruny, W.A., and Plageman, P.G.W.: Immune response to lactate dehydrogenase-elevating virus: Isolation of infectious virus-immunoglobulin G complexes and quantitation of specific antiviral immunoglobulin G response in wild-type and nude mice. Infect. Immun., *37*:1001–1006, 1982.

30. Cahill, J.R., et al.: Role of biological mimicry in the pathogenesis of rat arthritis induced by *Mycoplasma arthritidis*. Infect. Immun., *3*:24–35, 1971.

31. Cassell, G.H., et al.: Arthritis of rats and mice: Implications for man. Isr. J. Med. Sci., *17*:608–615, 1981.

32. Catalano, M.A., et al.: Antibody to the RA nuclear antigen: Its relatioshp to in vivo EBV infection. J. Clin. Invest., *65*:1238–1242, 1980.

33. Catalano, M.A., et al.: Correlation between anti-RANA and anti-EBNA titers in normal subjects with and without HLA-DRw4. Arthritis Rheum., *23*:1049–1052, 1980.

34. Catalano, M.A., et al.: Antibodies to EBV-determined antigens in normal subjects and in patients with seropositive RA. Proc. Natl. Acad. Sci. U.S.A., *76*:5825–5828, 1979.

35. Chantler, J.A., Ford, D.K., and Tingle, A.J.: Persistent rubella infection and rubella-associated arthritis. Lancet, *1*:1323–1325, 1982.

36. Chattopadhyay, H., et al.: Demonstration of anti-rubella antibody secreting cells in RA patients. Scand. J. Immunol., *10*:47–54, 1979.

37. Chattopadhyay, H., Chattopadhyay, C., and Natvig, J.B.: Hyporesponsiveness to virus antigens of rheumatoid synovial and blood lymphocytes using the indirect leucocyte migration inhibition test. Scand. J. Immunol., *10*:585–592, 1979.

38. Chetty, C., Klapper, D.G., and Schwab, J.H.: Soluble peptidoglycan-polysaccharide fragments of the bacterial cell wall induce acute inflammation. Infect. Immun., *38*:1010–1019, 1982.

39. Cole, B.C., et al.: Specificity of a mycoplasma mitogen for lymphocytes from human and various animal hosts. Infect. Immun., *36*:662–666, 1982.

40. Cole, B.C., and Cassell, G.H.: Mycoplasma infections as models of chronic joint inflammation. Arthritis Rheum., *22*:1375–1381, 1979.

41. Cole, B.C., Daynes, R.A., and Ward, J.R.: Stimulation of mouse lymphocytes by a mitogen derived from *Mycoplasma arthritidis*. III. Ir gene control of lymphocyte transformation correlates with binding of the mitogen to specific Ia-bearing cells. J. Immunol., *129*:1352–1359, 1982.

42. Cole, B.C., and Ward, J.R.: Mycoplasma as arthritogenic agents. *In* The Mycoplasmas, Vol. II. Edited by J.G. Tully, and J.R. Whitcomb. New York, Academic Press, 1979, pp. 367–398.

43. Crawford, T.B., Adams, D.S., and Cheevers, W.P.: Chronic arthritis in goats caused by a retrovirus. Science, *207*:997–999, 1980.

44. Cutlip, R.C., Smith, P.C., and Page, L.A.: Ovine chlamydial polyarthritis: Sequential development of articular lesions in lambs after intraarticular exposure. Am. J. Vet. Res., *34*:71–75, 1973.

45. Datta, S.K., et al.: Genetic studies of autoimmunity and retrovirus expression in crosses of New Zealand black mice. I. Xenotropic virus. J. Exp. Med., *147*:854–871, 1978.

46. Datta, S.K., et al.: Genetic studies of autoimmunity and retrovirus expression in crosses of New Zealand black mice. II. The viral envelope glycoprotein gp70. J. Exp. Med., *147*:872–881, 1978.

47. Dean, A.G., et al.: An epidemic of Kawasaki syndrome in Hawaii. J. Pediatr., *100*:552–557, 1982.

48. Denman, A.M., et al.: Virus infections and chronic rheumatic disorders. Eur. J. Rheumatol. Inflam., *5*:425–431, 1982.

49. Denman, A.M., et al.: Lymphocyte abnormalities in Behçet's syndrome. Clin. Exp. Immunol., *42*:175–185, 1980.

50. Depper, J.M., and Zvaifler, N.J.: Epstein-Barr virus. Its relationship to the pathogenesis of rheumatoid arthritis. Arthritis Rheum., *24*:755–761, 1981.

51. Depper, J.M., Zvaifler, N.J., and Bluestein, H.G.: Oropharyngeal Epstein-Barr virus excretion in rheumatoid arthritis. Arthritis Rheum., *25*:427–431, 1982.

52. Dilley, D., Fan, P.G., and Bluestone, R.: Absence of cytotoxic effect of selected pathogens on HLA B27 positive fibroblasts. Proc. Soc. Exp. Biol. Med., *159*:184–186, 1978.

53. Drueke, T., et al.: Hepatitis B antigen-associated periarteritis nodosa in patients undergoing long-term hemodialysis. Am. J. Med., *68*:86–90, 1980.

54. Duffy, J., et al.: Polyarthritis, polyarteritis and hepatitis B. Medicine, *55*:19–37, 1976.

55. Eastmond, C.J., et al.: A sequential study of the relationship between faecal *Klebsiella aerogenes* and the common clinical manifestations of ankylosing spondylitis. Ann. Rheum. Dis., *41*:15–20, 1982.

56. Ebringer, R.W., et al.: Sequential studies in ankylosing spondylitis: Association of *Klebsiella pneumoniae* with active disease. Ann. Rheum. Dis., *37*:146–151, 1978.

57. Eglin, R.P., Lehner, T., and Subak-Sharpe, J.H.: Detection of RNA complementary to herpes-simplex virus in mononuclear cells from patients with Behçet's syndrome and recurrent oral ulcers. Lancet, *2*:1356–1361, 1982.

58. Eisenberg, R., et al.: Measurement of bacterial cell wall in tissues by solid-phase radioimmunoassay: Correlation of distribution and persistence with experimental arthritis in rats. Infect. Immun., *38*:127–135, 1982.

59. Eisenberg, R.A., et al.: Male determined accelerated autoimmune disease in BXSB mice: Transfer by bone marrow and spleen cells. J. Immunol., *125*:1032–1036, 1980.

60. Elling, H., Skinhoj, P., and Elling, P.: Hepatitis B virus and polymyalgia rheumatica: A search for HBsAg, HBsAb, HBcAB, HBeAg, and HBeAb. Ann. Rheum. Dis., *39*:511–513, 1980.

61. Emery, H., Larter, W., and Schaller, J.G.: Henoch-Schonlein vasculitis. Arthritis Rheum., *20*:385–388, 1977.

62. Enlow, R.W., et al.: Human lymphocyte response to selected infectious agents in Reiter's syndrome and ankylosing spondylitis. Rheumatol. Int., *1*:171–175, 1982.

63. Ennis, R.S., et al.: *Mycoplasma hyorhinis* swine arthritis. II. Morphologic features. Arthritis Rheum., *14*:202–211, 1971.

64. Estes, P.C., and Cheville, N.F.: The ultrastructure of vascular lesions in equine viral arteritis. Am. J. Pathol., *58*:235–253, 1970.

65. Ferrell, P.B., et al.: Seroepidemiological study of relationships between Epstein-Barr virus and rheumatoid arthritis. J. Clin. Invest., *67*:681–687, 1981.

66. Ferrell, P.B., and Tan, E.M.: Epstein-Barr (EB) virus antibodies in rheumatoid arthritis. Springer Semin. Immunopathol., *4*:181–191, 1981.

67. Folomeeva, O., et al.: Comparative studies in antilymphocyte, antipolynucleotide, and antiviral antibodies among families of patients with systemic lupus erythematosus. Arthritis Rheum., *21*:23–27, 1978.

68. Ford, D.K.: Infectious agents in Reiter's syndrome. Clin. Exp. Rheum., *1*:273–277, 1983.

69. Ford, D.K., et al.: Synovial mononuclear cell responses to rubella antigen in rheumatoid arthritis and unexplained persistent knee arthritis. J. Rheumatol., *9*:420–423, 1982.

70. Fox, A., et al.: Arthropathic properties related to the molecular weight of peptidoglycan-polysaccharide polymers of streptococcal cell walls. Infect. Immun., *35*:1003–1010, 1982.

71. Francoeur, A.M., and Mathews, M.B.: Interaction be-

tween VA RNA and the lupus antigen La: Formation of a ribonucleo-protein particle in vitro. Proc. Natl. Acad. Sci. U.S.A., *79*:6772–6776, 1982.

72. Fraser, J.R.E., et al.: Rubella arthritis in adults. Isolation of virus, cytology and other aspects of the synovial reaction. Clin. Exp. Rheum., *1*:287–294, 1983.

73. Frayha, R.A.: Trichinosis-related polyarteritis nodosa. Am. J. Med., *71*:307–312, 1981.

74. Geczy, A.F., et al.: HLA-B27, *Klebsiella* and ankylosing spondylitis: Biological and chemical studies. Immunol. Rev., *70*:23–50, 1983.

75. Geczy, A.F., et al.: Characterization of a factor(s) present in *Klebsiella* culture filtrates that specifically modifies an HLA-B27-associated cell-surface component. J. Exp. Med., *152*:331s–340s, 1980.

76. Gocke, D.J., et al.: Association between polyarteritis and Australia antigen. Lancet, *2*:1149–1153, 1970.

77. Goebel, K.-M., Goebel, F.-D., and Baier, R.: Impaired cell-mediated immunity among HLA-B27 related rheumatoid variants responding to Yersinia antigen. J. Clin. Lab. Immunol., *8*:75–81, 1982.

78. Goldenberg, D.L.: "Postinfectious" arthritis. New look at an old concept with particular attention to disseminated gonococcal infection. Am. J. Med., *74*:925–928, 1983.

79. Gower, R.G., et al.: Small vessel vasculitis caused by hepatitis B virus immune complexes. J. Allergy Clin. Immunol., *62*:222–228, 1978.

80. Grahame, R., et al.: Chronic arthritis associated with the presence of intrasynovial rubella virus. Ann. Rheum. Dis., *42*:2–13, 1983.

81. Granfors, K., et al.: Persistence of IgM, IgG, and IgA antibodies to yersinia in yersinia arthritis. J. Infect. Dis., *141*:424–429, 1980.

82. Griffiths, M.M., Smith, C.B., and Maryon, E.B.: Lack of antibody in rheumatoid sera to autologous synovial macrophages and dendritic cells by antibody-dependent cellular cytotoxicity assays (ADCC). J. Rheumatol., *8*:647–652, 1981.

83. Gruhn, W.B., and McDuffie, F.C.: Studies of serum Ig binding to synovial fibroblast cell cultures from patients with RA. Arthritis Rheum., *23*:10–16, 1980.

84. Hadler, N.M., and Granovetter, D.A.: Phlogistic properties of bacterial debris. Semin. Arthritis Rheum., *8*:1–16, 1978.

85. Hamerman, D., Gresser, I., and Smith, C.: Isolation of cytomegalovirus from synovial cells of a patient with rheumatoid arthritis. J. Rheumatol., *9*:658–664, 1982.

86. Hardin, J.A., Steere, A.C., and Malawista, S.E.: Immune complexes and the evolution of Lyme arthritis. Dissemination and localization of abnormal C1q binding activity. N. Engl. J. Med., *301*:1358–1363, 1979.

87. Hart, H., McCormick, J.N., and Marmion, B.P.: Viruses and lymphocytes in RA. II. Examination of lymphocytes and sera from patients with RA for evidence of retrovirus infection. Ann. Rheum. Dis., *38*:514–525, 1979.

88. Hart, H., and Norval, M.: Search for viruses in rheumatoid macrophage-rich synovial cell populations. Ann. Rheum. Dis., *39*:159–163, 1980.

89. Harwick, H.J., et al.: Arthritis in mice due to infection with *Mycoplasma pulmonis.* II. Serological and histological features. J. Infect. Dis., *133*:103–112, 1976.

90. Hasler, F., et al.: Analysis of the defects responsible for the impaired regulation of Epstein-Barr virus-induced B cell proliferation by rheumatoid arthritis lymphocytes. I. Diminished gamma interferon production in response to autologous stimulation. J. Exp. Med., *157*:173–188, 1983.

91. Hasler, F., et al.: Analysis of the defects responsible for the impaired regulation of EBV-induced B cell proliferation by rheumatoid arthritis lymphocytes. II. Role of monocytes and the increased sensitivity of rheumatoid arthritis lymphocytes to prostaglandin E. J. Immunol., *131*:768–772, 1983.

92. Haspel, M.V., et al.: Virus-induced autoimmunity: Monoclonal antibodies that react with endocrine tissues. Science, *220*:304–306, 1983.

93. Haynes, B.F., et al.: Identification of human T cell leukemia virus in a Japanese patient with adult T cell leukemia and cutaneous lymphomatous vasculitis. Proc. Natl. Acad. Sci. U.S.A., *80*:2054–2058, 1983.

94. Heesemann, J., et al.: Plasmids of human strains of *Yersinia enterocolitica:* Molecular relatedness and possible importance for pathogenesis. J. Infect. Dis., *147*:107–115, 1983.

95. Hendrickx, G.F.M., et al.: Dermatomyositis and toxoplasmosis. Ann. Neurol., *5*:393–395, 1978.

96. Hicks, J.T., et al.: Search for Epstein-Barr and type C oncornaviruses in SLE. Arthritis Rheum., *22*:845–857, 1979.

97. Hickstein, D.D., Gravelyn, T.R., and Wharton, M.: Giant cell arteritis and polymyalgia rheumatica in a conjugal pair. Arthritis Rheum., *24*:1448–1450, 1981.

98. Highton, J., and Panayi, G.S.: Spontaneous cytotoxicity of rheumatoid and normal peripheral blood mononuclear cells against 4 human lymphoblastoid cell lines. Ann. Rheum. Dis., *39*:559–562, 1980.

99. Hollingworth, P., et al.: Fate of herpes simplex virus in lymphocytes from blood and joint effusions of systemic and pauciarticular juvenile chronic arthritis. Ann. Rheum. Dis., *42*:14–16, 1983.

100. Hooks, J.J., et al.: Immune interferon in the circulation of patients with autoimmune disease. N. Engl. J. Med., *301*:5–8, 1979.

101. Horwitz, M.S., Friefeld, B.R., and Keiser, H.D.: Inhibition of adenovirus DNA synthesis in vitro by sera from patients with systemic lupus erythematosus. Mol. Cell. Biol., *2*:1492–1500, 1982.

102. Ingram, D.G., and Cho, H.J.: Aleutian disease in mink: Virology, immunology and pathogenesis. J. Rheumatol., *1*:74–92, 1974.

103. Inman, R.D.: Rheumatic manifestations of hepatitis B virus infection. Semin. Arthritis Rheum., *11*:406–420, 1982.

104. Inman, R.D., et al.: Isolation and characterization of circulating immune complexes in patients with hepatitis B systemic vasculitis. Clin. Immunol. Immunopathol., *21*:364–374, 1981.

105. Jarrett, M.P., et al.: Impaired response to pneumococcal vaccine in systemic lupus erythematosus. Arthritis Rheum., *23*:1287–1293, 1980.

106. Kagen, L.J.: Polymyositis and dermatomyositis. *In* Modern Topics in Rheumatology. Edited by G.R.V. Hughes. London, Heinemann, 1976, pp. 135–143.

107. Kallen, P.S., et al.: Infectious myositis and related syndromes. Semin. Arthritis Rheum., *11*:421–439, 1982.

108. Kallick, C.A., Thadhani, K.C., and Rice, T.W.: Identification of *Anaplasmataceae* (haemobartonella) antigen and antibodies in SLE. Arthritis Rheum., *23*:197–205, 1980.

109. Kalliomäki, J.L., et al.: Antibodies to measles virus in ankylosing spondylitis. Scand. J. Rheumatol., *12*:29–31, 1983.

110. Kapusta, M.A.: The virus-activated suppressor cell hypothesis in experimental and human rheumatic diseases. J. Rheumatol., *7*:309–315, 1980.

111. Kass, E., et al.: Dermatomyositis associated with BCG vaccination. Scand. J. Rheumatol., *8*:187–191, 1979.

112. Katsuragi, S., Miyayama, H., and Takeuchi, T.: Picornavirus-like inclusions in polymyositis-aggregation of glycogen particles of the same size. Neurology, *31*:1476–1480, 1981.

113. Kazmierowski, J.A., Peizner, D.S., and Wuepper, K.D.: Herpes simplex antigen in immune complexes of patients with erythema multiforme. J.A.M.A., *247*:2547–2550, 1982.

114. Keat, A.C., et al.: Evidence of *Chlamydia trachomatis* infection in sexually acquired reactive arthritis. Ann. Rheum. Dis., *39*:431–437, 1980.

115. Kimura, M., Andoh, T., and Kai, K.: Failure to detect type C virus p30-related antigen in SLE: False positive reaction due to protease reactivity. Arthritis Rheum., *23*:111–113, 1980.

116. Kinsella, T.D., Fritzler, M.J., and McNeil, D.J.: Ankylosing spondylitis. A disease in search of microbes. J. Rheumatol., *10*:2–4, 1983.

117. Kleinknecht, C., et al.: Membranous glomerulonephritis

with extra-renal disorders in children. Medicine, 58:219–229, 1979.

118. Kosunen, T.U., et al.: Arthritis associated with *Campylobacter jejuni* enteritis. Scand. J. Rheumatol., 10:77–80, 1981.

119. Kousa, M.: Evidence of chlamydial involvement in the development of arthritis. Scand. J. Infect. Dis., 32(Suppl.):116–121, 1982.

120. Lambert, P.H., et al.: Quantitation of immunoglobulin-associated HBs antigen in patients with acute and chronic hepatitis, in healthy carriers and in polyarteritis nodosa. J. Clin. Lab. Immunol., 3:1–8, 1980.

121. Larsen, J.H.: *Yersinia enterocolitica* infections and rheumatic disease. Scand. J. Rheumatol., 9:129–137, 1980.

122. Leff, R.D., Aldo-Benson, M.A., and Madura, J.A.: The effect of revision of the intestinal bypass on post intestinal bypass arthritis. Arthritis Rheum., 26:678–681, 1983.

123. Leino, R., et al.: Depressed lymphocyte transformation by yersinia and *Escherichia coli* in yersinia arthritis. Ann. Rheum. Dis., 42:176–181, 1983.

124. Leirisalo, M., et al.: Followup study on patients with Reiter's disease and reactive arthritis, with special reference to HLA-B27. Arthritis Rheum., 25:249–259, 1982.

125. Leirisalo, M., et al.: Chemotaxis in Yersinia arthritis. Arthritis Rheum., 23:1036–1044, 1980.

126. Lerner, M.R., et al.: Two small RNAs encoded by Epstein-Barr virus and complexed with protein are precipitated by antibodies from patients with systemic lupus erythematosus. Proc. Natl. Acad. Sci. U.S.A., 78:805–809, 1981.

127. Levo, Y., et al.: Laboratory stigmata of connective tissue disorders in asymptomatic carriers of hepatitis B virus. Am. J. Med. Sci., 282:116–119, 1981.

128. Levo, Y., et al.: Association between hepatitis B virus and essential mixed cryoglobulinemia. N. Engl. J. Med., 296:1501–1504, 1977.

129. Lewis, R.M., et al.: Canine systemic lupus erythematosus. Transmission of serological abnormalities by cell-free filtrates. J. Clin. Invest., 52:1893–1907, 1973.

130. Lurhuma, A.Z., Riccomi, H., and Masson, P.L.: The occurrence of circulating immune complexes and viral antigens in idiopathic thrombocytopenic purpura. Clin. Exp. Immunol., 28:49–55, 1977.

131. MacKenzie, R.A., Forbes, G.S., and Karnes, W.E.: Angiographic findings in herpes zoster arteritis. Ann. Neurol., 10:458–464, 1981.

132. Magid, S.K., and Kagen, L.J.: Serologic evidence for acute toxoplasmosis in polymyositis-dermatomyositis. Increased frequency of specific anti-toxoplasma IgM antibodies. Am. J. Med., 75:313–320, 1983.

133. Male, D., et al.: Antibodies to EB virus- and cytomegalovirus-induced antigens in early rheumatoid disease. Clin. Exp. Immunol., 50:341–346, 1982.

134. Manicourt, D.H., and Orloff, S.: Immune complexes in polyarthritis after Salmonella gastroenteritis. J. Rheumatol., 8:613–620, 1981.

135. Marmion, B.P.: Infection, autoimmunity and RA. Clin. Rheum. Dis., 4:565–586, 1978.

136. Martin, D.K., et al.: Lymphoproliferative responses induced by streptococcal antigens in recurrent aphthous stomatitis and Behçet's syndrome. Clin. Immunol. Immunopathol., 13:146–155, 1979.

137. Mathews, M.B., and Bernstein, R.M.: Myositis autoantibody inhibits histidyl-tRNA synthetase: A model for autoimmunity. Nature, 304:177–179, 1983.

138. McMahon, B.J., et al.: Vasculitis in Eskimos living in an area hyperendemic for hepatitis B. J.A.M.A., 244:2180–2182, 1980.

139. Medsger, T.A. (ed.): Twenty-fifth rheumatism review. Arthritis Rheum., 26(3), 1983.

140. Mellors, R.C., and Mellors, J.W.: Type C RNA virus-specific antibody in human SLE demonstrated by enzymoimmunoassay. Proc. Natl. Acad. Sci. U.S.A., 75:2463–2467, 1978.

141. Michalak, T.: Immune complexes of hepatitis B surface antigen in the pathogenesis of periarteritis nodosa. Am. J. Pathol., 90:619–628, 1978.

142. Mikol, J., et al.: Inclusion-body myositis: Clinicopathological studies and isolation of an adenovirus type 2 from muscle biopsy specimen. Ann. Neurol., 11:576–581, 1981.

143. Mitchell, D.M., et al.: Kinetics of specific anti-influenza antibody production by cultured lymphocytes from patients with systemic lupus erythematosus following influenza immunization. Clin. Exp. Immunol., 49:290–296, 1982.

144. Moutsopoulos, H.M., and Hooks, J.J.: Interferon and autoimmunity. Clin. Exp. Rheum., 1:81–84, 1983.

145. Murphy, T.F., Senterfit, L.B., and Christian, C.L.: Arthralgia associated with acute urinary retention. A syndrome of probable viral etiology. Am. J. Med., 68:386–388, 1980.

146. Narayan, O., et al.: Activation of caprine arthritis-encephalitis virus expression during maturation of monocytes to macrophages. Infect. Immun., 41:67–73, 1983.

147. Neill, W.A.: Cell-mediated cytotoxicity for cultured autologous rheumatoid synovial membrane cells. Ann. Rheum. Dis., 39:570–575, 1980.

148. Ng, K.C., et al.: Anti-RANA antibody: A marker for seronegative and seropositive RA. Lancet, 1:447–449, 1980.

149. Nies, K., et al.: Antitetanus toxoid antibody synthesis after booster immunization in systemic lupus erythematosus. Arthritis Rheum., 23:1343–1350, 1980.

150. Nissenson, A.R. (moderator): Poststreptococcal acute glomerulonephritis: Fact and controversy. Ann. Intern. Med., 91:76–86, 1979.

151. Norval, M., Hart, H., and Marmion, B.P.: Viruses and lymphocytes in RA. I. Studies on cultured rheumatoid lymphocytes. Ann. Rheum. Dis., 38:507–513, 1979.

152. Norval, M., and Smith, C.: Search for viral nucleic acid sequences in rheumatoid cells. Ann. Rheum. Dis., 38:456–462, 1979.

153. Nurminen, M., et al.: The genus-specific antigen of *Chlamydia*: Resemblance to the lipopolysaccharide of enteric bacteria. Science, 220:1279–1281, 1983.

154. O'Duffy, J.D., Lehner, T., and Barnes, C.G.: Summary of the Third International Conference on Behçet's disease. J. Rheumatol., 10:154–158, 1983.

155. Ohno, S., et al.: Detection of gamma interferon in the sera of patients with Behçet's disease. Infect. Immun., 36:202–208, 1982.

156. Oldstone, M.B.A., and Dixon, F.J.: Pathogenesis of chronic disease associated with persistent lymphocytic choriomeningitis virus infection. I. Relationship of antibody production to disease in neonatally infected mice. J. Exp. Med., 129:483–499, 1969.

157. Orban, P., et al.: A factor shed by lymphoblastoid cell lines of HLA-B27 positive patients with ankylosing spondylitis specifically modifies the cells of HLA-B27 positive normal individuals. Clin. Exp. Immunol., 53:10–16, 1983.

158. Patriarca, P.A., et al.: Kawasaki syndrome: Association with the application of rug shampoo. Lancet, 2:578–580, 1982.

159. Pease, P.E., et al.: An investigation into the properties of klebsiella strains isolated from ankylosing spondylitis patients. J. Hyg. (Camb.), 89:119–123, 1982.

160. Phillips, P.E.: Infection and the pathogenesis of CTD. *In* Scientific Basis of Rheumatology. Edited by G.S. Panayi. London, Churchill-Livingstone, 1982, pp. 1–21.

161. Phillips, P.E.: Infection and chronic rheumatic disease in children. Semin. Arthritis Rheum., 10:92–99, 1980.

162. Phillips, P.E., and Christian, C.L.: Infectious agents in chronic rheumatic diseases. *In* Arthritis and Allied Conditions, 9th Ed. Edited by D.J. McCarty. Philadelphia, Lea & Febiger, 1979, pp. 320–328.

163. Phillips, P.E., Kassan, S.S., and Kagen, L.J.: Increased toxoplasma antibodies in idiopathic inflammatory muscle disease: A case-control study. Arthritis Rheum., 22:209–214, 1979.

164. Phillips, P.E., Sellers, S.A., and Cotronei, S.L.: Type C oncornavirus isolation studies in systemic lupus erythematosus. III. Isolation of a putative retrovirus by triple cell fusion. Ann. Rheum. Dis., 37:234–237, 1978.

165. Pincus, T.: Studies regarding a possible function for viruses in the pathogenesis of systemic lupus erythematosus. Arthritis Rheum., 25:847–856, 1982.

166. Pincus, T., et al.: Reactivities of SLE sera with cellular and virus antigen preparations. Arthritis Rheum., 21:873–879, 1978.

167. Poiesz, B.J., et al.: Detection and isolation of type C retrovirus particles from fresh and cultured lymphocytes of a patient with cutaneous T cell lymphoma. Proc. Natl. Acad. Sci. U.S.A., 77:7415–7419, 1980.

168. Polk, B.F., et al.: A controlled comparison of joint reactions among women receiving one of two rubella vaccines. Am. J. Epidemiol., 115:19–25, 1982.

169. Pons, V.G., et al.: Decreased cell-mediated cytotoxicity against virus-infected cells in SLE. J. Med. Virol., 4:15–23, 1979.

170. Pope, R.M., Rutstein, J.E., and Straus, D.C.: Detection of antibodies to streptococcal mucopeptide in patients with rheumatic disorders and normal controls. Int. Arch. Allergy Appl. Immunol., 67:267–274, 1982.

171. Popp, J.W., et al.: Essential mixed cryoglobulinemia without evidence for hepatitis B virus infection. Ann. Intern. Med., 92:379–383, 1980.

172. Pritchard, D.G., Settine, R.L., and Bennett, J.C.: Sensitive mass spectrometric procedure for the detection of bacterial cell wall components in rheumatoid joints. Arthritis Rheum., 23:608–610, 1980.

173. Quilis, M.R., and Damjanov, I.: Dermatomyositis as an immunologic complication of toxoplasmosis. Acta Neuropathol. (Berl.), 58:183–186, 1982.

174. Reinertsen, J.L., et al.: An epidemiologic study of households exposed to canine SLE. Arthritis Rheum., 23:564–568, 1980.

175. Repo, H., et al.: Chemotaxis in yersinia arthritis. In vitro stimulation of neutrophil migration by HLA-B27 positive and negative sera. Arthritis Rheum., 25:655–661, 1982.

176. Reynolds, J.T., and Panem, S.: Characterization of antibody to C-type virus antigens isolated from immune complexes in kidneys of patients with systemic lupus erythematosus. Lab. Invest., 44:410–419, 1981.

177. Rich, S.A.: Human lupus inclusions and interferon. Science, 213:772–775, 1981.

178. Ristic, M., and Kreier, J.P.: Hemotropic bacteria. N. Engl. J. Med., 301:937–939, 1979.

179. Robinson, A.D., and Muirden, K.D.: Cellular immunity to possible synovial antigens in rheumatoid arthritis. Ann. Rheum. Dis., 39:539–544, 1980.

180. Rosenberg, A.M., and Petty, R.E.: Reiter's disease in children. Am. J. Dis. Child., 133:394–398, 1979.

181. Rosenthal, L., and Danielsson, D.: Induction of DNA synthesis in lymphocytes in vitro by various bacteria, with special reference to Neisseria gonorrhoeae, in patients with uro-arthritis (Reiter's disease). Scand. J. Rheumatol., 7:101–108, 1978.

182. Rosner, I.A., et al.: Spondyloarthropathy associated with hidradenitis suppurativa and acne conglobata. Ann. Intern. Med., 97:520–525, 1982.

183. Ruff, R.L., and Secrist, D.: Viral studies in benign acute childhood myositis. Arch. Neurol., 39:261–263, 1982.

184. Schweiger, F., Bell, D.A., and Little, A.H.: Coexistence of rheumatoid arthritis in married couples: A search for etiological factors. J. Rheumatol., 8:416–422, 1981.

185. Seager, K., et al.: Evidence for a specific B27-associated cell surface marker on lymphocytes of patients with ankylosing spondylitis. Nature, 277:68–70, 1979.

186. Sergent, J.S., et al.: Vasculitis with hepatitis B antigenemia: Long term observations in nine patients. Medicine, 55:1–18, 1976.

187. Sergent, J.S., and Christian, C.L.: Necrotizing vasculitis after acute serous otitis media. Ann. Intern. Med., 81:195–199, 1974.

188. Shillitoe, E.J., et al.: Antibody to cytomegalovirus in patients with Sjögren's syndrome. As determined by an enzyme-linked immunosorbent assay. Arthritis Rheum., 25:260–265, 1982.

189. Shinebaum, R., et al.: Effect of Klebsiella capsular antisera on lymphocytes from patients with ankylosing spondylitis. J. Med. Microbiol., 14:451–456, 1981.

190. Shirodaria, P.V., et al.: Measles virus-specific antibodies and immunoglobulin M antiglobulin in sera from multiple sclerosis and rheumatoid arthritis patients. Infection. Immun., 25:408–416, 1979.

191. Sikes, D., Crimmins, L.T., and Fletcher, O.J.: Rheumatoid arthritis of swine. A comparative pathologic study of clinical spontaneous remissions and exacerbations. Am. J. Vet. Res., 30:753–769, 1969.

192. Silverman, S.L., and Schumacher, H.R.: Antibodies to Epstein-Barr viral antigens in early rheumatoid arthritis. Arthritis Rheum., 24:1465–1468, 1981.

193. Simon, D.G., et al.: Reiter's syndrome following epidemic shigellosis. J. Rheumatol., 8:969–973, 1981.

193a.Simpson, R.W., et al.: Association of parvoviruses with rheumatoid arthritis of humans. Science, 223:1425–1428, 1984.

194. Slaughter, L., et al.: In vitro effects of EBV on peripheral blood monocytes from patients with rheumatoid arthritis and normal subjects. J. Exp. Med., 148:1429–1434, 1978.

195. Slovin, S.F., et al.: Discordant expression of 2 Epstein-Barr virus-associated antigens, EBNA and RANA, in man-rodent somatic cell hybrids. J. Immunol., 127:585–590, 1981.

196. Slovin, S.F., Vaughan, J.H., and Carson, D.A.: Changes in the expression of two EBV-associated antigens EBNA and RANA, during the cell cycle of transformed human B lymphoblasts. Int. J. Cancer, 26:9–12, 1980.

197. Smith, C.A.: On a possible viral etiology of rheumatoid arthritis. J. Rheumatol., 6:113–116, 1979.

198. Smith, C., Habermann, E., and Hamerman, D.: A technique for investigating the antigenicity of cultured rheumatoid synovial cells. J. Rheumatol., 6:147–155, 1979.

199. Steere, A.C., et al.: The spirochetal etiology of Lyme disease. N. Engl. J. Med., 308:733–740, 1983.

200. Steere, A.C., et al.: Elevated levels of collagenase and prostaglandin E2 from synovium associated with erosion of cartilage and bone in a patient with chronic Lyme arthritis. Arthritis Rheum., 23:591–599, 1980.

201. Steere, A.C., et al.: Lyme arthritis: An epidemic of oligoarticular arthritis in children and adults in 3 Connecticut communities. Arthritis Rheum., 20:7–17, 1977.

202. Steinman, C.R., and Hsu, K.: Specific detection and semiquantitation of microorganisms in tissue by nucleic acid hybridization. II. Investigation of synovia from pigs with chronic erysipelothrix arthritis. Arthritis Rheum., 19:38–42, 1976.

203. Suit, B.E., et al.: Detection of anti-interferon antibodies in systemic lupus erythematosus. Clin. Exp. Rheum., 1:133–135, 1983.

204. Tasaka, K., and Hamashima, Y.: Studies on rickettsialike body in Kawasaki disease. Acta Pathol. Jpn., 28:235–245, 1978.

205. Taylor-Robinson, D.: Mycoplasmal arthritis in man. Isr. J. Med. Sci., 17:616–621, 1981.

206. Theofilopoulos, A.N., and Dixon, F.J.: Autoimmune diseases. Immunopathology and etiopathogenesis. Am. J. Pathol., 108:321–365, 1982.

207. Thomas, H.C., et al.: Metabolism of the third component of complement in acute type B hepatitis, HBs antigen positive glomerulonephritis, polyarteritis nodosum, and HBs antigen positive and negative chronic active liver disease. Gastroenterology, 76:673–679, 1979.

208. Thomas, L., Davidson, M., and McCluskey, R.T.: Studies of PPLO infection. I. The production of cerebral polyartheritis by Mycoplasma gallisepticum in turkeys; the neurotoxic properties of the mycoplasma. J. Exp. Med., 123:897–912, 1966.

209. Tosato, G., Steinberg, A.D., and Blaese, R.M.: Defective EBV-specific suppressor T-cell function in rheumatoid arthritis. N. Engl. J. Med., 305:1238–1243, 1981.

210. Trepo, C.G., et al.: The role of circulating hepatitis B antigen/antibody immune complexes in the pathogenesis of vascular and hepatic manifestations in polyarteritis. J. Clin. Pathol., 27:863–868, 1974.

211. Tully, J.G., et al.: A newly discovered mycoplasma in the human urogenital tract. Lancet, 1:1288–1291, 1981.

212. Tully, J.G., et al.: Helical mycoplasmas (spiroplasmas) from *Ixodes* ticks. Science, *212*:1043–1045, 1981.
213. van de Putte, L.B.A., et al.: Reactive arthritis after *Campylobacter jejuni* enteritis. J. Rheumatol., *7*:531–535, 1980.
214. Vasey, F.B., et al.: Possible involvement of group A streptococci in the pathogenesis of psoriatic arthritis. J. Rheumatol., *9*:719–722, 1982.
215. Vaughan, J.H., Carson, D.A., and Fox, R.I.: The Epstein-Barr virus and RA. Clin. Exp. Rheum., *1*:265–272, 1983.
216. Venables, P.J.W., et al.: Titers of antibodies to RANA in rheumatoid arthritis and normal sera. Arthritis Rheum., *24*:1459–1464, 1981.
217. Vilppula, A.H., et al.: Chlamydial isolations and serology in Reiter's syndrome. Scand. J. Rheumatol., *10*:181–185, 1981.
218. Viola, M.V., et al.: Absence of measles proviral DNA in systemic lupus erythematosus. Nature, *275*:667–669, 1978.
219. Walker, E.R., et al.: Ultrastructural study of avian synovium infected with an arthrotropic reovirus. Arthritis Rheum., *20*:1269–1277, 1977.
220. Wands, J.R., et al.: Arthritis associated with intestinal-bypass procedure for morbid obesity. N. Engl. J. Med., *294*:121–124, 1976.
221. Warren, R.E., and Brewerton, D.A.: Faecal carriage of klebsiella by patients with ankylosing spondylitis and rheumatoid arthritis. Ann. Rheum. Dis., *39*:37–44, 1980.
222. Washburn, L.R., Cole, B.C., and Ward, J.R.: Chronic arthritis of rabbits induced by mycoplasmas. III. Induction with nonviable *Mycoplasma arthritidis* antigens. Arthritis Rheum., *25*:937–946, 1982.
223. Wilder, R.L., et al.: Strain and sex variation in the susceptibility to streptococcal cell wall-induced polyarthritis in the rat. Arthritis Rheum., *25*:1064–1072, 1982.
224. Wolf, R.E.: Hyporesponsiveness of lymphocytes to virus antigens in RA. Arthritis Rheum., *21*:238–242, 1978.
225. Wolf, R.E., and Ziff, M.: Lymphocyte response to virus antigens in SLE. Arthritis Rheum., *19*:1271–1277, 1976.
226. Yaron, M., et al.: RNA and DNA viral stimulation of prostaglandin E production by human synovial fibroblasts. Arthritis Rheum., *24*:1582–1586, 1981.
227. Yoshiki, T., et al.: The viral envelope glycoprotein of murine leukemia virus and the pathogenesis of immune complex glomerulonephritis in New Zealand mice. J. Exp. Med., *140*:1011–1027, 1974.
228. Young, C.R., Ebringer, A., and Archer, J.R.: Immune response inversion after hyperimmunization: Possible mechanism in the pathogenesis of HLA-linked diseases. Ann. Rheum. Dis., *37*:152–158, 1978.

Clinical Pharmacology of the Antirheumatic Drugs

Chapter 28

Aspirin and other Nonsteroidal Anti-Inflammatory Drugs

Harold E. Paulus and Daniel E. Furst

Many arthritic diseases are characterized by inflammation, causing tissue injury and loss of function. Therapy is therefore directed toward limiting the inflammatory process and its consequences. The several major categories of antirheumatic drugs differ substantially in their characteristics, mode of action, and clinical effects.

The nonsteroidal anti-inflammatory drugs (NSAID) are agents that reduce the signs and symptoms of established inflammation within the first few days of administration. Examples include aspirin, indomethacin, ibuprofen, fenoprofen, naproxen, tolmetin, sulindac, meclofenamate, diflunisal, and piroxicam. They seem effective only while blood levels of drug are sustained; withdrawal of an NSAID is soon followed by recurrence of the signs and symptoms of inflammation. Although moderated, chronic inflammatory arthritis is often not completely suppressed by NSAID, and damage to joints continues to occur during the administration of such a drug.

Slowly acting antirheumatic drugs (SAARD), also called remission-inducing drugs (RID) or disease-modifying antirheumatic drugs (DMARD), are a diverse group of compounds that share a common pattern of clinical response. Administration of one of these drugs has no immediate therapeutic benefit, but after weeks or months, the onset of clinical improvement may be detected. With continued administration, some or all disease manifestations may eventually be completely suppressed. If drug administration is discontinued, however, the manifestations of disease gradually recur. During a remission induced by SAARD, damage to joints and other tissues probably stops, although it resumes when the drug is discontinued. Examples of SAARD include the organic gold compounds, antimalarial drugs, antimetabolites, alkylating agents, d-penicillamine, and levamisole. All were developed for other indications and were then applied to the treatment of rheumatic diseases as an afterthought. Some SAARD suppress immune responses; levamisole normalizes subnormal immune responses, but other such agents have no generally accepted effect on the immune system.

The corticosteroids themselves share some characteristics with NSAID in that they rapidly moderate established inflammation and probably do not prevent the progression of joint damage. On the other hand, high doses of prednisone have prolonged effects on immunoglobulin synthesis, and the appearance of some drug effects may be delayed, as in treatment of vasculitis or nephritis.

The NSAID are discussed here. Although knowledge of their cellular and molecular effects on various aspects of the inflammatory process is increasing, the use of these drugs in rheumatic diseases remains empiric.

GENERAL CONSIDERATIONS

Chemistry

Although they appear different from one another, the NSAID can be grouped by chemical structural similarities (Fig. 28–1).

A limited correlation exists between the pKa* of a drug and both its plasma half-life† and its anti-inflammatory activity. Thus, as the pKa decreases, the plasma half-life decreases, probably owing to more rapid renal tubular excretion of the drug. A pKa of less than 3 diminishes anti-inflammatory activity and increases uricosuric activity.[250] Most NSAID have a pKa in the range of 3.5 to 5 and are not usually uricosuric.[250]

Pharmacologic Activities

All NSAID have antipyretic and analgesic activities in animal models and anti-inflammatory activity in various in vitro and in vivo tests. Because NSAID moderate established inflammation, they might be anticipated to affect numerous inflammatory processes.

---

*pKa = pH at which a salt is half-ionized.
†Plasma half-life (t 1/2) = the time necessary for the plasma concentration to decrease by half.

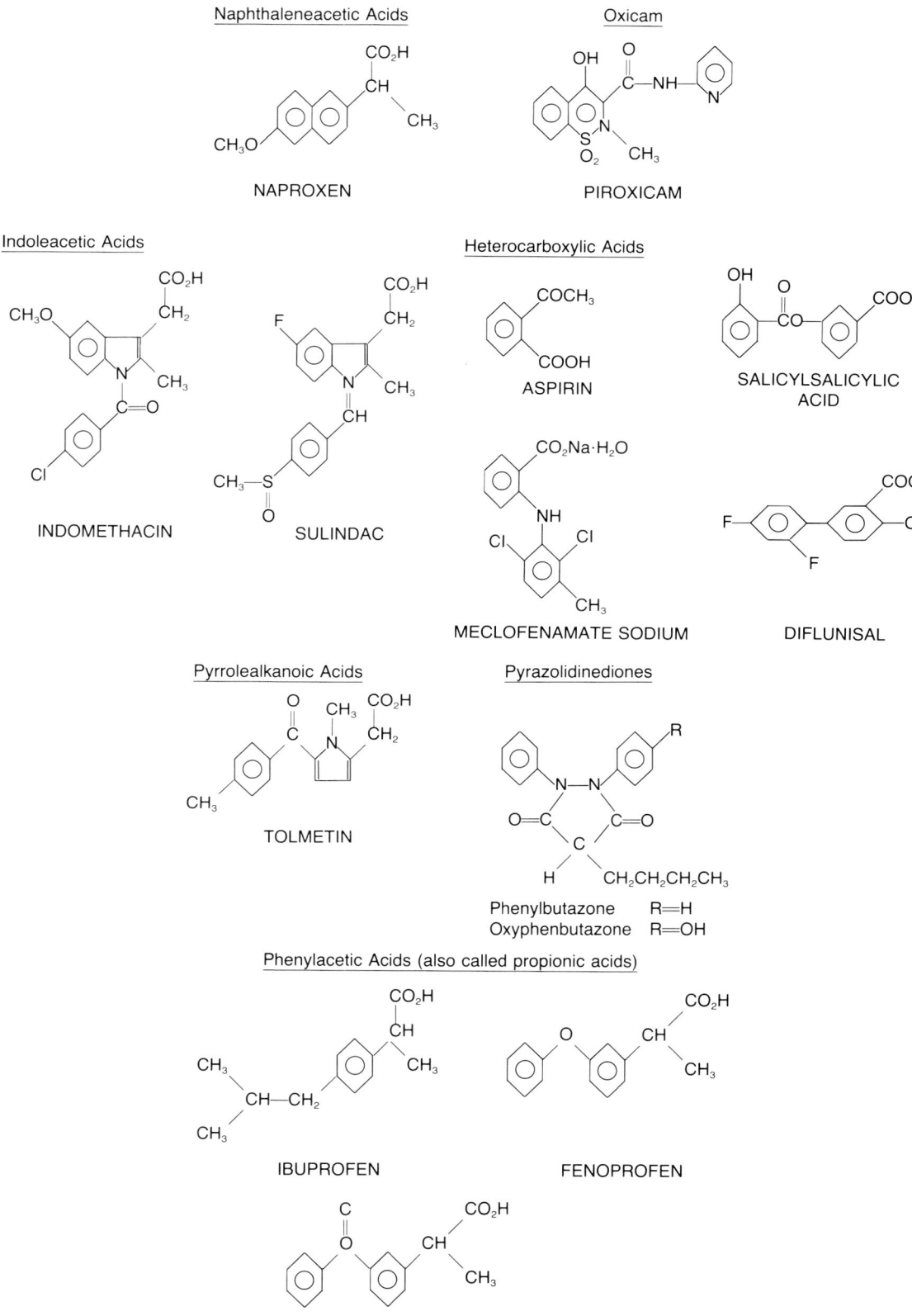

Fig. 28–1. Chemical structures of some nonsteroidal anti-inflammatory drugs.

Effects on Arachidonic Acid Metabolites

Arachidonic acid is a constituent of cell membrane phospholipids. This fatty acid is produced in response to inflammatory stimuli, and its synthesis is inhibited by glucocorticosteroids. Arachidonic acid is metabolized to form a remarkable array of biologically active substances (Fig. 28–2). The characterization and identification of these metabolites has focused attention on the mechanisms of acute and chronic inflammation (see Chap. 22). Chemotactic lipids may be produced by nonenzymatic oxidation of arachidonic acid, and various products result from its oxidation with the enzymes cyclo-oxygenase or lipoxygenase. NSAID block the conversion of arachidonic acid to the endoperoxides prostaglandins G_2 (PGG_2) and H_2 (PGH_2) by inhibiting the membrane-bound enzyme, cyclo-oxygenase (Fig. 28–2). In platelets, these endoperoxides are transformed into thromboxane A_2, whereas in inflamed tissue, PGE_2 is formed. The inhibition of endoperoxide formation by NSAID blocks the synthesis of both prostaglandins and thromboxanes.[298]

Vane has postulated that the antipyretic, anti-inflammatory, and analgesic properties of aspirin-like drugs are accounted for by their effect on prostaglandin synthetase (cyclo-oxygenase).[289] Prostaglandins have been demonstrated to cause inflammation in various experimental situations. PGE_1 is a potent pyrogen in animals,[186] and $PGF_2\alpha$ has caused fever in patients when given systemically to stimulate uterine contraction.[289] Edema, erythema, and some of the histologic changes of inflammation have been associated with prostaglandin administration to animals. Further, a variety of free radicals derived from molecular oxygen, including superoxide, hydroxyl, and perhydroxyl radicals, are involved in the biosynthesis of prostaglandins and can provoke cell injury themselves. These free radicals are produced by activated neutrophils, and probably by other elements of the inflammatory reaction. Many NSAID may act as free radical scavengers (antioxidants), in addition to inhibiting the formation of free radicals in the arachidonic acid pathway.

Thromboxane A_2 stimulates aggregation of platelets. In the gastric mucosa, prostaglandins decrease acid production and increase gastric mucin secretion and gastroesophageal sphincter tone. In the kidney, vasodilatory prostaglandins help to regulate renal blood flow, glomerular filtration rate, and sodium and water excretion. Other specific effects of prostaglandins in various tissues include dilatation of the ductus arteriosus and contraction of uterine muscle fibers.

The inhibition of arachidonic acid metabolism by systemic administration of drugs has a variety of effects. Generally, NSAID inhibit cyclo-oxygenase; aspirin does so in an irreversible fashion, and the others reversibly in a concentration-related manner. Pain associated with arachidonic acid metabolites is reduced. Fever is moderated and platelet aggregation is decreased. Gastric acid production increases, gastric mucin production decreases, and gastroesophageal sphincter tone may decrease, producing dyspepsia. Under certain circumstances, renal blood flow may decrease, causing a rise in creatinine levels, edema, hyperkalemia, and sometimes renal papillary necrosis. Uterine cramps may be suppressed, and a patent ductus arteriosus may be closed.

The order of potency* of cyclo-oxygenase inhibition by various NSAID correlates well with their potency in the carrageenan rat paw edema model of inflammation. Cyclo-oxygenases obtained from different tissues have different sensitivities to inhibition by NSAID, however, and the relative potencies of these drugs vary according to the tissue preparations used to test them. For example, acetaminophen is reported to be as effective as aspirin in inhibition of cyclo-oxygenase obtained from the brain, but it has much less activity than aspirin on the enzyme obtained from the spleen; this finding may help to explain the effective antipyretic and analgesic activities of acetaminophen, but its lack of anti-inflammatory properties.[91] Aspirin, a potent inhibitor of cyclo-oxygenase, acts by acetylating the enzyme. The relative lack of activity of nonacetylated salicylate in cyclo-oxygenase inhibition assays is anomalous in that salicylate derived from nonacetylated sources suppresses inflammation as effectively as equivalent doses of aspirin in the treatment of patients with rheumatoid arthritis (RA).[21]

Additional evidence that suppression of cyclo-oxygenase activity does not completely explain the anti-inflammatory effects of NSAID is found in experiments with rats whose tissues have been made deficient in arachidonic acid by a diet deficient in a fatty acid essential to its production. When these rats that are deficient in arachidonic acid are injected with carrageenan, the expected paw edema is produced, but to a lesser degree than in normal rats. This finding suggests that the inability to produce metabolites of arachidonic acid indeed decreases the inflammatory response. When rats deficient in arachidonic acid with paw edema were given aspirin, however, paw edema further

---

*Potency = the relative quantity of drug required to produce a particular effect. Thus, one drug is more potent than another if less is required to produce a certain effect.

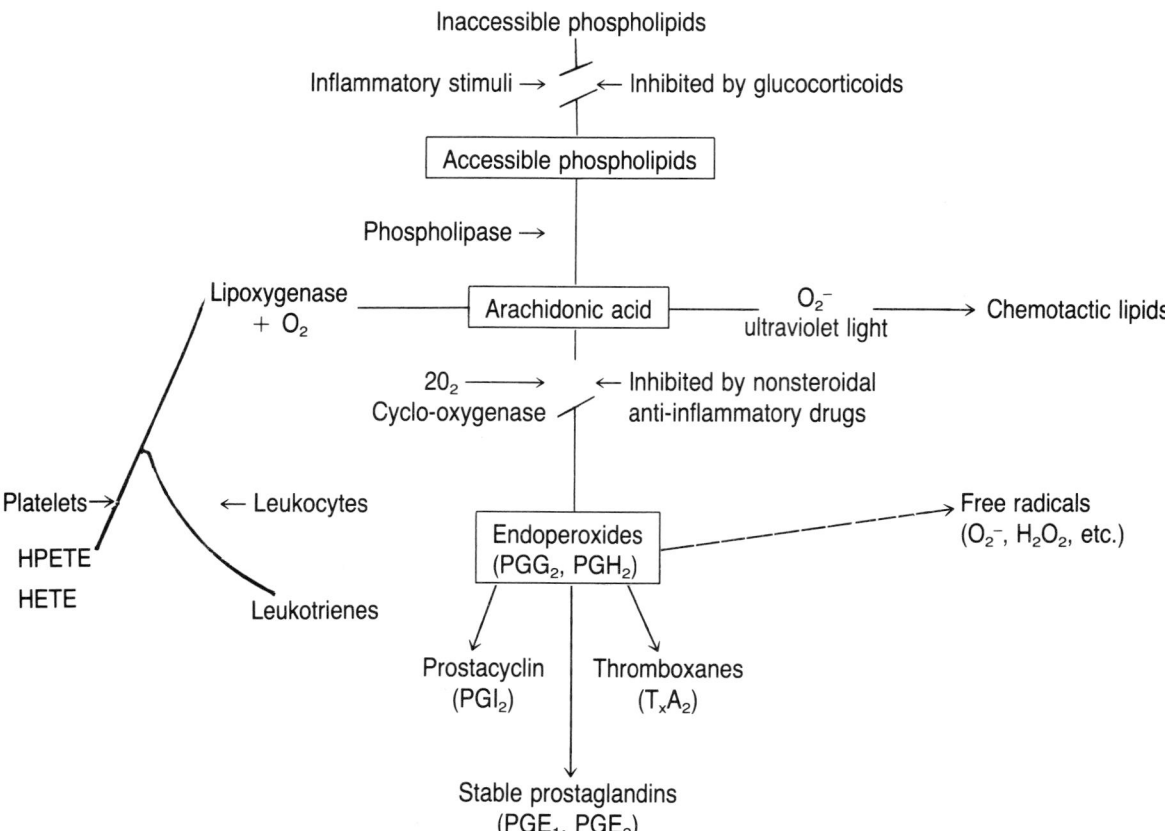

Fig. 28–2.   Arachidonic acid metabolism.

decreased. Quantitatively, this aspirin-induced decrease in paw edema was similar to that produced by aspirin in the nondeficient rats. This evidence suggests that the anti-inflammatory effects of NSAID are not completely explained by the suppression of cyclo-oxygenase.[75]

The foregoing observations have encouraged interest in the lipoxygenase pathway of arachidonic acid metabolism (Fig. 28–2). This pathway has been demonstrated to be active in rabbit and in human polymorphonuclear leukocytes.[298] Leukotriene B_4 (LTB_4) induces polymorphonuclear leukocyte aggregation, O_2^- generation, and degranulation.[221] It causes neutrophils to accumulate at local sites of inflammation by stimulating chemotaxis and enhancing leukocyte adherence to and diapedesis across postcapillary venule walls, and it also stimulates the production of guanylate and adenylate cyclase.[246] Piroxicam was reported by Abramson et al. to inhibit LTB_4-induced leukocyte aggregation,[1] but ibuprofen had no effect. Benoxaprofen was reported to be only a weak inhibitor of cyclo-oxygenase, but a more effective inhibitor of lipoxygenase, whereas indomethacin was a good inhibitor of cyclo-oxygenase and a poor inhibitor of lipoxygenase; ketoprofen was an effective inhibitor of both.[60] Perhaps differing effects on various aspects of arachidonic acid metabolism may be responsible for differences in clinical responses to specific NSAID, although such differences have not yet been clearly defined.

Effects on Other Soluble Factors

Bradykinin generation increases capillary permeability. Several NSAID inhibit bradykinin-induced edema at concentrations at the upper end of pharmacologic dosing regimens,[180] and these agents also inhibit serotonin release and the action of catecholamines in studies of platelet function in vitro and in turpentine-induced pleurisy. Yet the high concentrations needed make it unlikely that inhibition of kinin or amine release is a major mechanism of the clinical effect of NSAID. Enzymes involved in oxidative phosphorylation, transferases, RNA synthetases, and polymerases have been proposed as possible sites of action of NSAID, but effects on these enzyme systems are seen in isolated, unphysiologic preparations.[265]

In concentrations within the therapeutic range, aspirin is an effective uncoupler of oxidative phosphorylation only in tissue isolates.[264,265] Further, some effective uncouplers of oxidative phosphorylation such as 2′, 4-dinitrophenol are devoid of anti-inflammatory activity.[263] Rat fetal tissue histidine decarboxylase, needed for histamine formation, is inhibited by 1 mM aspirin, and 4 g aspirin daily reduce histamine excretion by half in man.[164]

Effects on Cellular Elements

Granulocyte and monocyte migration and phagocytosis can be inhibited in vitro by aspirin, phenylbutazone, indomethacin, and several other NSAID,[46,72] but the high concentrations required may produce general depression of cellular mechanisms. Lymphocyte transformation and DNA synthesis are suppressed by aspirin, phenylbutazone, oxyphenbutazone, indomethacin, and flufenamic acid.[64,301] Indomethacin, 10^{-1} and $10^{-5}M$, inhibits prostaglandin dehydrogenase and potentiates PGE_1-mediated cyclic adenosine monophosphate (cAMP) generation in human synoviocytes.[50] The actions of NSAID on cAMP phosphodiesterase are of particular interest because increased cAMP levels are associated with decreased lymphocyte and leukocyte responsiveness.[297] Caution must be exercised in interpreting these results because many factors may cause a rise or fall in cAMP, and the foregoing changes may have little to do with lymphocyte activity. Inhibition of neutrophil activation and lymphocyte immunoglobulin formation have been documented with therapeutic concentrations of indomethacin (1.5 to 10 μg/ml).[1,109]

Analgesia

Clinically, aspirin and other NSAID are effective analgesics. Based on cross-perfusion studies, the analgesic action of salicylates is generally considered to be peripheral,[264] in contrast to the central action of narcotics. When an isolated organ with nerves intact to the whole animal A, but with its circulation from animal B, is injected with minute amounts of bradykinin, pain is induced in animal A. Aspirin injected into the circulation of animal B blocks the bradykinin-invoked pain response in animal A; and aspirin injected into the circulation of animal A, in which it perfuses not the isolated organ, but the central nervous system of that animal, does not block the bradykinin-induced pain. Thus, salicylates and other NSAID can suppress chemically induced peripheral pain, but they do not block the transmission or perception of painful stimuli.[166]

Antipyresis

NSAID are effective antipyretics in man, generally in short-term, placebo-controlled studies of patients with fevers of various causes. Little evidence suggests that any one drug has a better therapeutic ratio* than another.

---

*Therapeutic ratio = beneficial effects/toxic effects.

Antirheumatic and Anti-inflammatory Effects

The anti-inflammatory effects of the NSAID were noted centuries ago, with the use of salicylates by Pliny for gout.[232] It was not until 1964, however, that aspirin was shown conclusively to be effective in rheumatoid arthritis (RA). Fremont-Smith and Bayles showed decreased ring size, increased range of motion, and increased grip strength in most of the 11 patients with RA whom they treated.[94] Their findings were confirmed and were extended by placebo-controlled studies using aspirin in doses of at least 4.0 g/day.[23]

NSAID have been compared with placebo, with aspirin, and often with each other in the treatment of RA. The more recent, controlled studies have been double-blind, randomized trials with well-defined criteria for evaluation of rheumatoid activity. Most trials of the newer NSAID suggest that these drugs are comparable, in anti-inflammatory doses, to aspirin with respect to efficacy, but these NSAID are somewhat less toxic.

The anti-inflammatory effects of NSAID have been documented best in RA, but such effects in other rheumatic diseases have been explored to some extent. Aspirin is probably efficacious against rheumatic fever. In juvenile RA (JRA), it is definitely the drug of first choice, presumably because of its combined analgesic, antipyretic, and anti-inflammatory activities.[247] Studies in Reiter's syndrome and psoriatic arthritis have been uncontrolled, but NSAID are widely used in these illnesses. A number of NSAID are superior to placebo in treating ankylosing spondylitis, whereas aspirin is effective only occasionally.[104,106,124] Although aspirin is both anti-inflammatory and uricosuric in high doses, it is rarely used to treat gout.[312] Other NSAID are more effective than aspirin; indomethacin is one of the drugs of choice in the treatment of acute gout.[99,268,308] The use of aspirin and aspirin-like drugs in the treatment of osteoarthritis is appropriate and is nearly universal,[127] although it is not clear whether they are acting as analgesic or anti-inflammatory drugs in this situation.

Effects on Platelet Function

Most NSAID decrease platelet aggregation induced by adenosine diphosphate, collagen, or epinephrine by inhibiting platelet cyclo-oxygenase.[195] For most NSAID, this effect is reversible and depends on the presence of adequate drug concentrations in the platelet, but aspirin irreversibly acetylates this enzyme.[146] Because platelets lack mitochondria and are unable to synthesize additional cyclo-oxygenase, this effect persists until the acetylated platelets are replaced by newly formed platelets from the bone marrow. As little as 300 mg aspirin may produce an antiaggregation effect that is still detectable 4 to 6 days later. Nonacetylated salicylates, which have minimal effect on prostaglandin synthesis, also have little or no effect on platelet aggregation and are a better choice for patients undergoing surgical procedures or at increased risk of bleeding.[75,314]

The antiplatelet aggregation effect of NSAID has been used in studies of aspirin for the prevention of cerebral and coronary artery occlusive events. It is thought that the production of thromboxane A_2 by platelets must be inhibited, whereas that of prostacyclin (PGI_2) by vascular endothelium must be maintained for most effective anticoagulation by aspirin.[182] Thromboxane A_2 promotes platelet aggregation, but PGI_2 prevents this aggregation and is also vasodilatory. Both thromboxane A_2 and PGI_2 are products of the cyclo-oxygenase pathway, however; aspirin should inhibit the production of both substances. Several approaches have been used to produce differential inhibition of thromboxane A_2 in platelets without inhibiting PGI_2 in vascular endothelium. Because platelets are unable to produce new cyclo-oxygenase to replace that which has been acetylated by aspirin, whereas nucleated endothelial cells can replace the acetylated enzyme when the brief exposure to aspirin ceases, the use of infrequent (once daily), low doses of aspirin should cause continual suppression of platelet cyclo-oxygenase, but only transient suppression of PGI_2 production by endothelial cells.[299] Another approach involves the use of slow-release aspirin or enteric-coated aspirin, which does not produce measurable aspirin concentrations in the systemic circulation, presumably because of complete metabolism of the slowly absorbed aspirin on its first pass through the liver. In this situation, platelet cyclo-oxygenases are irreversibly acetylated during their brief exposure to aspirin in the portal circulation, but PGI_2 production is normal because the endothelial cells of the systemic circulation are not exposed to aspirin.[262]

Other Effects

Induction of uterine muscle contraction was one of the earliest observed effects of prostaglandins. This effect can be suppressed by NSAID, and several of these agents have been recommended for treatment of menstrual cramps.[118] Indomethacin, used to assist in the closure of patent ductus arteriosus in infants, frequently averts the need for surgical intervention.[177]

Some Pharmacokinetic Definitions

One-Compartment Open Model

This term is defined as the representation of the body as a single homogeneous unit. It assumes that a dose of drug is instantaneously mixed throughout the body, that plasma level changes reflect changes occurring at the tissue level, and that elimination from the body occurs in an exponential fashion. The word "open" refers to the presence of a way into and out of the body; that is, it is not a closed system (Fig. 28–3).

Two-Compartment Open Model

This term is defined as the representation of the body as two compartments. These compartments do not reflect specific anatomic or physiologic areas. They are generally viewed as a "central" compartment, representing highly perfused tissues, and a "peripheral" compartment, representing poorly perfused tissues. Any representation of the body as a two-compartment model results in a biexponential decline in plasma levels as a function of time after intravenous injection (Fig. 28–4).

Absorption Half-Life

This is the time required after administration of a drug for its concentration in blood or plasma to increase from a given level to twice that level.

Distribution Half-Life (t 1/2 α)

In a two-compartment open model, during the initial (distribution) phase of the biexponential curve, this half-life is the time required for the plasma drug level to decrease by half, after administration of an intravenous bolus. Conceptually, this term reflects the change in plasma drug level as the drug distributes from the central compartment into the peripheral compartment (Fig. 28–5).

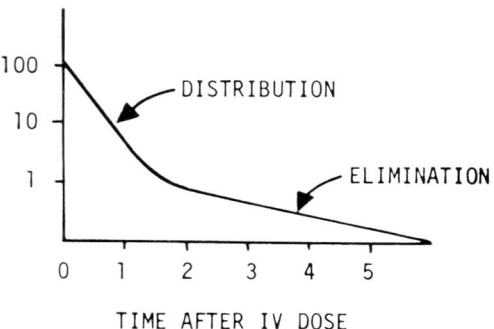

Fig. 28–4. Plasma level versus time curve for a two-compartment open model. IV = intravenous.

Elimination Half-Life, (Beta Half-life, t 1/2 β)

In a two-compartment open model, during the final (elimination) phase of the biexponential curve, this half-life is the time required for the plasma drug level to decrease by half, after an intravenous bolus. Conceptually, this term reflects the change in plasma drug level in the central compartment, once distribution is complete, as the drug leaves the body (Fig. 28–5).

Area Under the Log Serum Concentration Versus Time Curve (AUC)

This area is the calculated area under the graphic representation of drug levels using a semilogarithmic plot of plasma drug level versus time. It is considered to represent the amount of drug that actually reaches the circulation (Fig. 28–5).

Interactions

Drug-Drug Interactions

Most NSAID are acidic compounds that bind tightly to serum albumin and therefore may displace, or may be displaced by, one another or by other drugs. NSAID may displace sulfonylurea oral hypoglycemic agents from albumin and may cause transient hypoglycemia.[121] In a patient treated with warfarin, phenylbutazone increased the prothrombin time by 85%.[3]

Drug-Patient Interactions

Cirrhosis may prolong phenylbutazone half-life.[156] Acute renal failure decreased renal drug excretion and also decreased protein binding of salicylate (40 mg/100 ml) and of phenylbutazone (50 mg/100 ml) by 26% and 20%, respectively.[6] Borga et al. showed a decrease in the binding constants for salicylate in uremic patients.[25] Thus, uremia

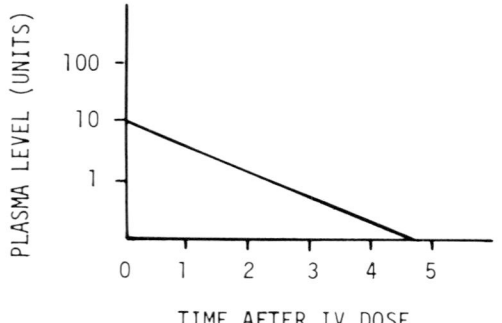

Fig. 28–3. Plasma level versus time curve for a one-compartment open model. IV = intravenous.

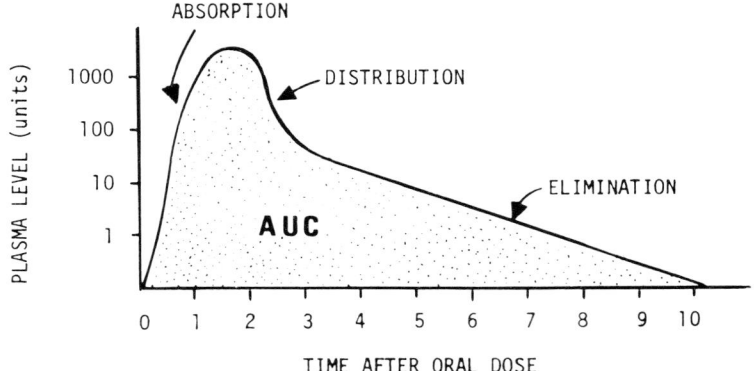

Fig. 28–5.   Plasma level versus time curve for a two-compartment open model, following an oral dose. Absorption, distribution, and elimination phases and the area under the curve (AUC) are demonstrated.

caused an increased unbound fraction* of salicylate, probably by decreasing the binding affinity of albumin. These effects may be true for other NSAID and must be considered in patients with renal impairment.

In 1982, benoxaprofen was withdrawn because of a number of deaths associated with its use. Most deaths were of elderly patients who developed hepatic or renal failure after weeks to months of therapy with benoxaprofen, probably associated with marked increases in drug concentration. The usual plasma half-life of benoxaprofen in persons with normal renal function is about 30 hours, but in persons with decreased creatinine clearance, the half-life may approach 150 hours, leading to excessive accumulation of the drug.[117]

Effect of Aging.   The age of the patient may affect NSAID metabolism. The serum half-life of phenylbutazone is often longer in elderly patients than in young adults (mean: 104.6 versus 81.2 hours)[204] and shorter in children (40.3 versus 75.8 hours).[4] For indomethacin, elderly and younger patients have equal serum half-lives and AUC, despite much lower renal clearance of the drug in older patients. Some workers postulate that a greater gastrointestinal elimination in the older group accounts for the lack of accumulation of drug.[280] Care must be taken when treating elderly patients with NSAID because toxicity may be increased by age-related aberrations in drug distribution, metabolism, or excretion.

Various physiologic, pharmacokinetic, and pharmacodynamic changes may occur with increased age. Cardiac output decreases; flow to the heart, brain, and muscles is preserved, but flow to the liver and kidneys decreases by about 1 to 2% per year.[18] Hepatic synthetic reactions such as conjugation and glucuronidation are probably less affected than preparative reactions such as oxidation and hydrolysis;[112] creatinine clearance and tubular maxima decrease. Little overall change occurs in drug absorption, although isolated examples exist of selective decreases in drug bioavailability in elderly patients; an example is acetaminophen.[73,112]

With increased age, serum albumin concentration decreased from a mean of 3.9 to 3.0 g/dl.[123] Salicylate binding decreased from 92% in the young to 79% in the elderly, at total salicylate concentrations of 140 mg/l.[154] Thus, an increased unbound salicylate fraction can result in increased toxicity in the elderly. Changes in drug receptors may occur with aging. Elderly rats have fewer glucocorticoid binding sites per mole of fat cells than young rats, whereas binding affinity is comparable in all age groups.[234] Isoproterenol-stimulated, intracellular cAMP production is decreased in the lymphocytes of the elderly, as compared to young, normal, human volunteers; this finding suggests that a postreceptor defect may occur with age.[71]

The net result is an increase in the incidence of adverse reactions with age. For NSAID, the most dramatic example is the occurrence of hepatorenal failure in elderly patients treated with benoxaprofen. Similarly, although no increase in efficacy was found when comparing treatment with d-penicillamine in young (mean age 41 years) RA patients with that in elderly patients (mean age 65 years) with RA, the incidence of severe toxicity was approximately twice as great in the elderly as in the young patients (53 versus 27%, respectively).[142]

Genetics.   The metabolism of phenylbutazone and aspirin is under genetic control. Such control

---

*Unbound fraction = that fraction of drug in blood or plasma that is not bound to plasma protein or cells.

is polygenic for phenylbutazone and is also affected by environmental factors.[97,291]

Adverse Effects

The side effects of NSAID are qualitatively similar, although the frequency of particular side effects varies with the compound. Table 28–1 lists some of NSAID and the reported incidence and occurrence of side effects. Because true incidence figures are not available and because definitions of severity of side effects vary from study to study, the table gives an admittedly incomplete overview of toxic effects.

Gastrointestinal Effects

These side effects are common to all NSAID and may be considered a characteristic of this class of drugs. These effects may be related to common mechanisms of action. For example, PGE_1, PGE_2, and PGA inhibit gastric acid secretion in animals and man. PGF_2 increases cardiac sphincter tone in man, and PGE_1 and PGE_2 prevent ulcers.[83,230] Inhibition of these putative protective functions of prostaglandins by NSAID may explain some gastrointestinal toxicity. In addition, phenylbutazone, oxyphenbutazone, and indomethacin decrease gastric mucus production and increase shedding of cells from the gastric mucosa in animals and man.[184] A number of NSAID increase acid secretion, cause local congestion and hemorrhage, and have other local effects such as precipitation of protective glycoprotein.[151,167] Some of these drugs have extensive enterohepatic recirculation.[76,77,105,238] Such recirculation through the bowel correlates with the gastrointestinal toxicity of indomethacin and may be responsible for the similar toxicity of other NSAID.[77] Microscopic bleeding is usually less severe with most other NSAID than with aspirin.[173,251]

Hepatic Effects

Reversible hepatocellular toxicity with aspirin has been reported by a number of authors in patients with JRA and systemic lupus erythematosus and has also been seen with other NSAID. In some cases, abnormal liver function tests return to normal even though the drug is continued, although in other cases, hepatic dysfunction may be severe enough to prolong prothrombin times.[10,220,255] A United States Food and Drug Administration (FDA) conference concluded that hepatic toxicity should be considered a class characteristic of these agents. During prospective clinical trials reported to the FDA, 67 of 1,252 patients (5.4%) with RA treated with aspirin developed persistent elevations of one or more liver function tests such as serum glutamic-oxaloacetic transaminase (SGOT), serum glutamic-pyruvic transaminase (SGPT), lactic dehydrogenase (LDH), alkaline phosphatase, and total bilirubin. Elevation of SGOT or SGPT levels appears to be a reversible early warning, and it may be prudent to monitor these tests monthly during the first year of treatment with NSAID. Advanced age, decreased renal function, multiple drug use, higher drug doses, increased duration of therapy, JRA, and systemic lupus erythematosus are likely to increase the risk of liver toxicity with NSAID.[210] Although the chemical structural characteristics associated with hepatotoxicity have not been clearly defined, some drugs, such as benoxaprofen, appear to present a greater-than-average risk.

Renal Effects

NSAID may temporarily decrease creatinine clearance and may increase serum creatinine concentrations in patients predisposed by hypovolemia or impaired renal function, probably by impairing the vasodilatory function of renal prostaglandins. These changes often disappear spontaneously, even with continued use of the drug.[145,155] NSAID should be used with caution in patients with congestive heart failure, liver disease associated with ascites, hypertension, excessive diuresis, minimal renal arterial insufficiency, mild impairment of glomerular filtration, or multiple drug use. Rarer renal complications include the following: acute renal failure with marked proteinuria and minimal change glomerulopathy, as reported with fenoprofen;[270] acute interstitial nephritis sometimes associated with eosinophilia or other signs of a hypersensitivity reaction;[141] and papillary necrosis.[200,259] Renal toxicity is rare in prospective trials of NSAID in which carefully selected and closely monitored patients are studied, however, and a review of 46 patients treated with aspirin for an average of more than 20 years did not find any serious renal disease.[87] Nonetheless, older patients with borderline renal function may develop serious toxicity.[90a]

SPECIFIC AGENTS

These include aspirin and other salicylate compounds, as well as other NSAID.

Aspirin and Other Salicylate Preparations

We use here the generic term, salicylates, to include all salicylates, including aspirin, but not diflunisal (see the appropriate section later in this chapter) and use the term aspirin only with reference to acetylsalicylic acid.

Pharmacologic Properties

Absorption. Salicylate absorption is thought to be a passive process proportional to the concentra-

Table 28–1. Adverse Effects of Nonsteroidal Anti-Inflammatory Drugs

Drug	Gastro-intestinal Bleeding	Peptic Ulcer	Abdominal Pain, Heartburn, Dyspepsia	Rash	Headache	Tinnitus	Renal Failure	Blood Dyscrasia	Other
Placebo			+++		+				1, 3
Aspirin	+	++	++++	+++	++	++++	+		4(?), 5
Azapropazone	?	+	+++	+++				?	
Carprofen	?	+	+++	+++					5
Diflunisal (Dolobid)	+	+	+++	+++	+++	++			2(+++), 4
Fenoprofen (Nalfon)	+	+	+++	++		++	+	+	2(++), 3(++) 4(?)
Flurbiprofen	?		++++	?		?			
Ibuprofen (Motrin)	+	+	+++	+++		++	+	+	2(++),3(+++),5
Indomethacin (Indocin)	+	+	++++	+	++++	++		+	2(++),3(++++), 5
Ketoprofen	+	+	++++	+++	+++	++			2(+++)
Meclofenamate (Meclomen)	+	++	+++	+++	+++	++	+	+	2(++++), 3(+++), 4
Naproxen (Naprosyn)	+	+	+++	+++	+++	+++	+	+	3(+++)
Phenylbutazone (Butazolidin) (and oxyphenbutazone) (Tandearil)	+	+	+++	++	+	+	+	+	4 . 5
Piroxicam (Feldene)	+	+	+++	++	++	++		+	3(++)
Salicylate (nonacetylated)	?	?	+++	?		++++			
Sulindac (Clinoril)	+	+	+++	+++	+++	++		+	2(+++), 3(+++), 5
Tolmetin (Tolectin)	+	++	+++	+	+++	++	+	+	3(+++)

? = insufficient data; incidence: + = <1%; ++ = 3%; +++ = 3%–9%; ++++ = > 10%; □ denotes important side effects; 1 = drowsiness; 2 = diarrhea; 3 = dizziness; 4 = interaction with warfarin; 5 = hepatic toxicity.

tion of the drug in the bowel, that is, a first-order process. The usual preparations of salicylates and aspirin are completely absorbed, with a peak plasma salicylate level occurring within 2 hours after a 975-mg dose.[159] Aspirin's plasma half-life is only 15 minutes because it is rapidly deacetylated to form salicylate; thus, little aspirin (acetylsalicylic acid) is found in the circulation.[236] Its metabolite, salicylic acid, is the substance usually measured.

Distribution. Salicylate is bound to albumin at 2 sites, and this binding varies nonlinearly with increasing concentrations of drug. Thus, at serum concentrations below 100 mg/l (10 mg/dl), it is approximately 92% bound, but at 300 mg/l, it is only 80% bound.[25] As higher concentrations of the drug are reached, more is unbound and thus is available to distribute into tissues.[98] Acid-base status also affects salicylate distribution because non-ionized drug diffuses through cell membranes more easily than ionized drug. Because salicylate has a pKa of 3.0, most of it is in an ionized form at pH 7.4; a decrease in pH increases the proportion of nonionized drug. In rats, when arterial pH changes from 7.4 to 7.2, the amount of nonionized salicylate doubles, albeit only from .004 to .008%. This change is reflected by much wider tissue distribution of the drug, as demonstrated by autoradiography of ^{14}carbon (^{14}C)-labeled salicylic acid.[125] Thus, in severe salicylate poisoning, an early, rapid decrease in serum salicylate concentration may reflect increased distribution of salicylate into tissues because of acidosis and may indicate that both the clinical situation and the acidosis are growing worse, rather than better.

Metabolism and Elimination. Once aspirin is deacetylated, its metabolism is the same as all other salicylates. Five metabolites formed in the liver, and salicylic acid itself, are excreted in the urine.[161] Four of these metabolites, salicylic acid, gentisic acid, gentisuric acid, and salicylacylglucuronide, are eliminated by first-order kinetics*; as the plasma concentration of salicylic acid increases, the excretion rates of these compounds increase proportionately. Two, salicylurate and salicylphenylglucuronide, are eliminated by capacity-limited

(Michaelis-Menton) kinetics* because the enzymes that catalyze their formation become saturated. Thus, with salicylate concentrations greater than approximately 50 mg/l, salicylurate and salicylphenylglucuronide are formed at their maximum rates and, no matter how much the serum concentration of salicylic acid increases, their rate of production remains approximately the same.[161] At low doses, the predominant excretory form is salicylurate and the drug is eliminated rapidly, but as the dose increases, serum concentrations may build up more rapidly than expected. For example, with daily doses of 1 g aspirin, the body contains approximately 0.5 g salicylate when steady state† has been reached, but with 4 g daily, it contains about 5.6 g salicylate. The ratio is thereby changed from 0.5 to 1.4. With a single 650-mg dose of aspirin, the serum salicylate half-life is 3.5 to 4.5 hours; when given at a dose of 4.5 g daily, the average half-life is 15 to 20 hours.[161] Serum half-life correlates more closely with serum salicylate concentration than with dose and increases as serum concentrations increase.[75] At higher doses, it takes much longer to reach steady state and to excrete the drug. Thus, salicylates are eliminated by parallel first-order and capacity-limited kinetics. Over the range of 100 to 300 mg/l, compensating mechanisms may render the relationship between dose and blood level more proportional.[98]

Salicylic acid excretion varies with urine pH. In 4 normal subjects, increasing the urine pH from 5.8 to 6.6, by administering sodium bicarbonate orally, decreased steady-state salicylate serum levels from 270 ± 79 mg/l to 150 ± 46 mg/l, by increasing salicylic acid excretion.[160]

Metabolism of salicylates may be induced by aspirin.[97,191]‡

Variability of Dose Response. Equal doses in different individuals may elicit variable responses[211] (Fig. 28–6). *No evidence establishing a relationship between a given serum salicylate level and clinical efficacy has been published.* Salicylate metabolism in man has a genetic influence.[97]

In summary, the handling of salicylate by the body is complicated by the effects of systemic pH

---

*First-order kinetics = a process in which the amount of drug eliminated per unit of time is directly proportional to the amount of drug in the body at that time. Zero-order kinetics = a process in which the amount of drug eliminated per unit of time is independent of the amount of drug in the body; that is, despite increasing amounts of drug in the body, the amount eliminated per unit of time remains constant.

*Capacity-limited (Michaelis-Menton) kinetics = a combination of first-order and zero-order kinetics. When the body contains a small amount of drug, elimination approximates first order. When the amount in the body exceeds a threshold, it approaches zero order because of saturation of capacity-limited metabolic processes.

†Steady state = that point during long-term drug therapy at which the rate of absorption of drug, usually equated with its rate of administration, equals its rate of elimination. During steady state, the amount of drug in the body remains the same.

‡Induction of metabolism = an increased rate of drug metabolism, owing to an increase in the activity or amount of an enzyme that metabolizes it.

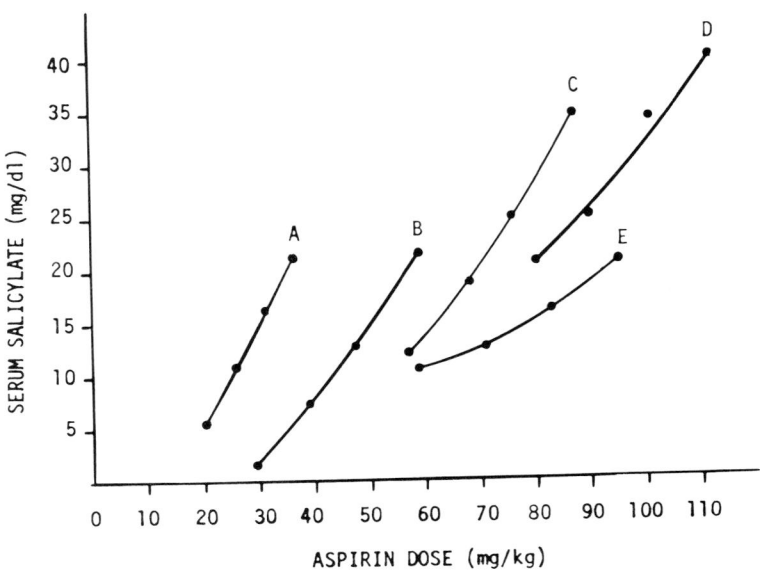

Fig. 28–6.   Relationships of aspirin doses and serum salicylate concentrations in five patients (A, B, C, D, and E) with rheumatoid arthritis. Note the striking differences in serum levels attained by different patients taking similar aspirin doses.

and nonlinear protein binding on distribution, by the effects of parallel first-order and capacity-limited metabolism, by the induction of salicylurate and salicylphenylglucuronide metabolism, and by the effects of urinary pH on excretion.

Acetylated Versus Nonacetylated Salicylates

Salicylates exist in many dosage forms. All the formulations, once metabolized to salicylate, are further metabolized and eliminated in a similar fashion. They may differ in their rates of disintegration, dissolution, and absorption, however.[75] Aspirin is a much more potent cyclo-oxygenase inhibitor in vitro than nonacetylated salicylates, although the efficacy of the two drugs is comparable in in vivo models of inflammation such as carrageenan-induced edema,[89] as well as in RA.[21]

In vitro tests of platelet aggregation and adhesiveness, and the availability of platelet factor 4, are inhibited for 72 hours after a single 300-mg aspirin dose, probably because of irreversible acetylation of platelet membranes. Nonacetylated salicylates, on the other hand, do not affect these in vitro tests of platelet aggregation.[314] This difference in the prevention of platelet aggregation is important because it dictates different uses of acetylated and nonacetylated salicylates in circumstances in which one does, or does not, wish to influence platelet aggregation. Further, a relationship appears to exist between in vitro cyclo-oxygenase inhibition and the bronchospasm associated with

the use of various NSAID.[75] Thus, aspirin-sensitive asthmatic patients may still be able to use a nonacetylated salicylate for anti-inflammatory therapy. Finally, prostaglandins increase renal blood flow, and it would theoretically be advantageous to use an anti-inflammatory drug that does not affect prostaglandin synthesis in patients with borderline or poor renal function.

Aspirin Formulations

Many tablet and capsule forms of aspirin are available. The most desirable formulation is one that has rapid tablet disintegration, rapid dissolution and small particle size, to enhance rapid absorption, decreased contact time with the gastrointestinal mucosa, and less direct gastrointestinal irritation.[75] "Buffered" tablets are formulated with calcium and magnesium antacids that increase the pH in the microenvironment of the tablet and allow rapid dissolution of aspirin in the high-pH dissolution layer; after diffusion into the acidic gastric juice, the aspirin probably reprecipitates as fine granules, allowing rapid absorption and less gastrointestinal irritation. Tablets containing sufficient antacid to raise the gastric pH above 5 may increase salicylate excretion by raising the urinary pH.[314]

Enteric dosage forms are designed to be insoluble below pH 3 and soluble above pH 5. Unfortunately, erratic, delayed, or even incomplete absorption may occur with some preparations or in patients with rapid gastrointestinal transit.[29] In addition, if gastric emptying is abnormal, large numbers of undissolved tablets may accumulate in the stomach, with the potential to cause serious toxicity when they advance into the intestine.[116] In general, enteric-coated tablets result in later and lower peak concentrations, but in overall bioequivalence if disintegration and dissolution occur completely.[206]

Time-release preparations of aspirin use microencapsulated aspirin particles. The matrices in these tablets consist of waxes, resins, plastics, or polymers with different disintegration rates. This formulation results in different and delayed absorption rates with flattened plasma salicylate concentration versus time curves.[75] The advantage of these slow-releasing preparations is that the drug may be given less frequently; their disadvantage is the potential for incomplete absorption.

Rectal suppositories have been used in attempts to circumvent gastrointestinal irritation. The absorption half-life of suppositories is much longer (3 hours) than the absorption half-life of oral preparations (15 to 30 minutes), and the bioavailability of suppositories depends on retention time. For example, only 20 to 40% of the dose was absorbed in under 2 hours, whereas 60% was absorbed in 4 to 5 hours.[75] Generally, salicylate bioavailability from suppositories is less than that of oral salicylate preparations.[75]

Nonacetylated Salicylates

Sodium Salicylate. This compound is rapidly absorbed, and although it is a less-potent analgesic than aspirin, it does appear to be an effective anti-inflammatory agent that causes less gastrointestinal bleeding.[75,153]

Choline Salicylate. This strongly basic choline ion of salicylic acid is hygroscopic and was initially marketed in liquid form. Although it provided a well-absorbed alternative to tablets, patients frequently developed a dislike for its taste during long-term administration.[198]

Choline Magnesium Trisalicylate. This compound provides 500 mg salicylic acid for each ''500 mg'' choline magnesium trisalicylate. It has been used to treat RA and osteoarthritis and it appears to cause less gastrointestinal blood loss than aspirin and to have fewer adverse gastrointestinal effects in general.[75,108]

Salicylsalicylic Acid. Although practically insoluble in the stomach, salicylsalicylic acid is soluble in the near-neutral pH of the small intestine. A 500-mg dose is equivalent to 698 mg salicylic acid. Only 77% of the possible salicylate in salicylsalicylic acid is found in the blood as salicylic acid, however, possibly because part of the salicylsalicylic acid is metabolized to its glucuronide and is excreted before it can be broken down to salicylate.[75] Like aspirin, this agent appears effective in the treatment of both osteoarthritis and RA.[168] It also causes less gastrointestinal blood loss than aspirin.[62,151]

Adverse Effects

Hypersensitivity to aspirin is estimated to occur in 0.2% of patients. The symptoms may be anaphylaxis with shock, asthma, urticaria, or angioedema. In a survey of 284 aspirin-intolerant individuals, 85% developed respiratory symptoms such as wheezing and asthma, 9.5% had urticaria or angioedema, and 6% had both skin and respiratory symptoms.[245] A triad of nasal polyposis, asthma, and aspirin sensitivity is influenced by both genetic and environmental factors.[245] It is due to an altered pharmacologic response, rather than to allergy to the drug. In sensitive individuals, bronchial asthma has also been associated with ingestion of indomethacin, ibuprofen, and fenoprofen,[275] as well as with tartrazine, a common yellow food dye that is structurally similar to indomethacin.[245]

Hepatotoxicity. As discussed earlier, abnormal liver function tests have been reported in patients taking aspirin, particularly those with active systemic lupus erythematosus, RA, or JRA.[10,255]

Nephrotoxicity. The nephrotoxic potential of NSAID described earlier in this chapter is shared by aspirin.[145] Renal papillary necrosis has been reported in patients taking aspirin alone, as well as in patients taking aspirin-containing analgesic mixtures.[197] A survey of 908 patients in New Zealand, however, showed no association between aspirin ingestion and renal disease, even when large quantities of aspirin were ingested.[200]

Gastrointestinal Toxicity. Gastrointestinal irritation, with dyspepsia, nausea, and vomiting, is a common side effect of aspirin, but usually is not serious and is relieved if the drug is withheld. Gastrointestinal blood loss due to aspirin is well documented by studies using ^{51}chromium (^{51}Cr)-labeled red blood cells to monitor fecal blood loss.[126,227] In one study, during control periods, average blood loss was 0.5 ± 0.5 ml/day (SD), whereas after 2.6 g aspirin daily for 4 days, average blood loss was 3.0 ± 2.2 ml/day. No correlation was found between symptoms of gastric distress and occult gastrointestinal bleeding.[126] The clinical significance of this occult bleeding is uncertain; during 67 months of aspirin therapy, only 1.6% of 244 patients had a drop in hemoglobin greater than 20%.[14] Aspirin damages the gastric mucosa, probably at the tight junctions of the mucosal cells; thereafter, gastric acid passes through the damaged mucosa and injures capillaries and venules.[56] Thus, achlorhydria helps to prevent aspirin induced occult gastrointestinal blood loss.[130]

It is not clear whether aspirin induces peptic ulcers or major gastrointestinal bleeding. In 15,000 patients without a predisposing cause, occasional aspirin use did not increase the incidence of major gastrointestinal bleeding, but use of aspirin for 4 or more days per week for at least 12 weeks was associated with diagnoses of benign gastric ulcers.[162]

In addition to the direct effects of aspirin on the gastric mucosa, its effects on platelets, bleeding time, and prothrombin time may place patients with pre-existing peptic ulcers or coagulation difficulties at a greater risk of major gastrointestinal bleeding. In such patients, aspirin should be avoided, or used with great caution if absolutely necessary. Non-acetylated salicylates, which do not affect the foregoing coagulation parameters, may be used, although caution must still be exercised.

Salicylate Intoxication

Aspirin toxicity is less frequent with the widespread use of "child-proof" caps. Further, the recent controversy as to the possible pathogenetic role of aspirin in Reye's syndrome will probably lead to decreased use of aspirin in infants and small children.[208] Nevertheless, aspirin is still a frequent cause of toxicity in children and adults.

General Metabolic Effects. Oxygen consumption increases rapidly after salicylate administration in either animals or man.[263] An associated increase in PCO_2 helps to produce metabolic acidosis in infants and young children, but is overcompensated by hyperventilation in adults.[263] Particularly in children, high fevers may be encountered; marked sweating accompanies the fever, and serious dehydration can result.[263] Clinically important hyper- and hypoglycemia have been observed during aspirin intoxication.[263]

Central Nervous System Effects. Reversible concentration-related tinnitus and hearing loss occur. Although most patients notice the onset of tinnitus at levels between 200 and 300 mg/l, it is not an accurate guide to dosage in patients with pre-existing hearing loss.[196]

The sensitivity of the respiratory center to changes in PCO_2 and pH is increased by aspirin. In dogs, the injection of low concentrations of salicylate into the cisterna magna caused a prompt increase in ventilatory volume and frequency, minutes before any changes occurred in PCO_2.[277] At high serum salicylate concentrations, respiratory depression occurs.[263]

Vomiting is thought to have both central and peripheral causes. Both intravenous and rectal salicylate doses cause vomiting, despite negligible gastric salicylate concentrations. A local effect is also considered likely because vomiting occurs at lower serum concentrations after oral than after intravenous salicylates (282 versus 392 mg/l) and because both vagal and spinal afferent pathways must be interrupted to afford complete protection against vomiting caused by oral salicylate.[263]

Other reported neurologic effects of aspirin toxicity include headache, hyperkineticity, excitement, hallucinations, delirium, convulsions, stupor, coma, and absent Babinski and deep-tendon reflexes.[263]

Acid-Base Disturbances. Acid-base changes during salicylate intoxication are related to the following: respiratory alkalosis due to stimulation of the respiratory center; loss of acids, salts, and fluids due to vomiting; fluid and salt losses due to profuse sweating; and metabolic acidosis due to uncoupling of oxidative phosphorylation and accumulation of organic acids. Children and infants are much more susceptible to metabolic acidosis than adults because the ability of children to increase alveolar ventilation is quickly overcome by accumulated acids.[185,263]

The combination of dehydration, salt and sodium losses caused by sweating, vomiting, and respiratory alkalosis can result in profound potassium depletion.[185] In this situation, respiratory alkalosis and urinary acidosis may coexist. Potassium and bicarbonate must be replaced, in addition to fluids and sodium. The net result of salicylate toxicity on the acid-base status of an individual patient depends on the relative contribution of each of the foregoing actions.

Treatment. Correlation of serum salicylate values with the severity of symptoms is difficult. Acidosis decreases salicylate ionization and increases membrane permeability, and the fraction of unbound salicylate increases with the total drug concentration. These effects increase diffusion of salicylates from blood into the tissues and lead to severe symptoms in the face of "relatively low" serum salicylate levels. Thus, in judging the severity of an overdose, the patient's history and symptoms, arterial blood pH, serum albumin concentration, and serum salicylate level all must be considered.

When a patient with a known aspirin overdose is first seen, induction of vomiting or gastric lavage should *always* be done because aspirin delays gastric emptying. One report states that 20.3 g salicylate were recovered by gastric lavage 9 hours after ingestion. If the patient is conscious, induced vomiting may empty the stomach more efficiently and more completely than lavage.[183,185]

Fluid and electrolyte therapy, with potassium supplements, replaces losses and induces diuresis. When potassium therapy is begun, alkalinization of the urine is recommended to increase the excretion of salicylates. Too-rapid alkalinization may be dangerous.[185] Careful monitoring of fluid and electrolyte balance is necessary to prevent overhydration, especially in the elderly.

Respiratory depression, convulsions, and hyperpyrexia must be treated if they occur. If a patient has significant hemorrhage, an unusual complication of salicylate overdose, vitamin K should be administered, and routine treatment of gastrointestinal bleeding should be undertaken.[185,263]

More severe salicylate intoxication may be treated by peritoneal dialysis or hemodialysis. Hemodialysis is a rapid and efficient method for removing salicylates.[185,263] Schreiner and Teehan recommend consideration of hemodialysis with known acute absorption of 0.5 g/kg or blood levels above 800 mg/l.[253] Clinical judgment, however, rather than a single serum salicylate value, must guide one in deciding whether to undertake dialysis.

Dosage

Tablets containing 300 or 600 mg are available, as are enteric-coated tablets containing 300 to 1200 mg.

The dose of aspirin depends on the therapeutic goals. For anti-inflammatory effects, blood levels between 200 and 300 mg/l (20 and 30 mg/100 ml) are usually desired, requiring doses between 2 and 6 g daily. Because the doses needed to achieve therapeutic concentrations vary widely, the appropriate dose *must be individualized*. The maximum tolerated dose should be approached slowly because it may take as long as a week after each dosage change to achieve a new steady-state level.

For analgesia, doses in the range of 1.8 g daily usually suffice: the dosage may be increased to tolerance or effect, before changing to other analgesics.

Phenylbutazone

Pharmacology and Pharmacokinetics

Phenylbutazone (Butazolidin) has been available as an analgesic, antipyretic, and anti-inflammatory drug for more than 30 years. Its major active metabolite, oxyphenbutazone, has been marketed as a separate preparation (Tandearil). Its absorption may vary from less than 70 to 90%.[309]

The serum elimination half-life of this drug is age dependent, from 40 hours in children to 80 hours in adults.[4,69] It is protein bound (94 to 99%), highly metabolized, and slowly excreted; only 88% of a dose is recovered.[69] Long-term dosing (5 days in man) results in enzyme induction in rats and shortened antipyrine half-life in man.[49] Phenylbutazone and oxyphenbutazone increase renal tubular sodium reabsorption and also affect the renal excretion of some other drugs.[90,218] These drugs are

aldosterone agonists and occupy the same renal tubular binding sites.

Renal failure increases free phenylbutazone serum concentrations by approximately 500%, decreases serum half-life, and decreases total serum concentration. These effects were postulated to be due to decreases both in albumin concentration and in binding affinity for phenylbutazone.[6] Because phenylbutazone is extensively protein bound and affects both drug metabolism and excretion, the results of interactions with other drugs are difficult to predict. Pretreatment of normal albumin with aspirin increases the affinity of the albumin for phenylbutazone.[48] Sulfa drugs are displaced from albumin by phenylbutazone, but the effect is transient and does not change the active, that is, unbound, concentration of drug after re-equilibration to steady state.[176]

Phenylbutazone potentiates the effects of tolbutamide by decreasing its renal excretion.[202] A marked increase in prothrombin time was documented when phenylbutazone was given to a patient receiving warfarin.[3]

Uses

Although effective against RA, gout, ankylosing spondylitis, osteoarthritis, miscellaneous nonarticular syndromes, and other diseases, phenylbutazone should *not* be used in doses greater than 400 mg daily because the incidence of side effects rises sharply without increased therapeutic effects. Further, with the advent of other NSAID and the adverse effects outlined in the next section, phenylbutazone cannot be considered a drug of first choice in any disease.

In RA, phenylbutazone or oxyphenbutazone is approximately as effective as anti-inflammatory doses of aspirin.[267] One study showed a trend toward a dose-response relationship with doses up to 300 mg daily; another study showed statistical differences between 50- and 300-mg daily doses in 29 patients with RA.[37,205] Phenylbutazone and indomethacin are equally effective in acute gout,[268] as well as in ankylosing spondylitis.[106] It is marginally more effective than 3.9 g aspirin daily in the treatment of patients with osteoarthritis.[235] Phenylbutazone and oxyphenbutazone have also been used in nonarticular syndromes and miscellaneous other diseases.[286]

Adverse Effects

Table 28–1 outlines the general adverse effects of phenylbutazone. Gastrointestinal side effects include nausea and vomiting in approximately 4% of patients, ulcers in 1 to 2%, and significant bleeding in 1 patient for each 330,000 prescriptions filled.[52,54] Phenylbutazone decreased gastric mucus production in dogs and increased cellular shedding without a rise in growth of new gastric mucosal cells.[184]

Aplastic anemia, leukemia, agranulocytosis, and thrombocytopenia have been reported.[54] Probably, no relationship exists between phenylbutazone and leukemia.[152] Aplastic anemia, pancytopenia, granulocytopenia, or thrombocytopenia occurs approximately 2 to 10 times for each million prescriptions filled, for both oxyphenbutazone and phenylbutazone.[54]

Phenylbutazone-induced renal tubular reabsorption of sodium can cause significant edema or hypertension. This antidiuretic effect of phenylbutazone is said to disappear in 6 to 10 days of treatment, despite continued use of the drug.[274] Nevertheless, sodium retention caused by phenylbutazone may precipitate congestive heart failure or pulmonary edema in patients with borderline cardiovascular status.[199] Like other NSAID, phenylbutazone is an aldosterone agonist.

Other reported side effects include rashes, myocarditis, hepatitis, induction of anti-native-DNA antibodies, sialadenitis, sweating, vertigo, and anaphylaxis.[51,93,111,274,282]

Overall, undesirable side effects, not all requiring discontinuance of the drug, occur in approximately 28% of patients taking phenylbutazone at a dose of 400 mg daily or less for up to 5 years.[267]

Dosage

The drug is supplied in 100-mg tablets.

Because phenylbutazone has a long serum half-life of 70 to 80 hours, dosing once a day is theoretically possible. Two or 3 doses per day are common, however. Doses greater than 400 mg/day are not recommended for long-term therapy; higher doses are associated with an increased incidence of serious side effects.

Significant drug interactions may occur when phenylbutazone is used with sulfa drugs and their derivatives, some anticoagulants, and other drugs easily displaced from albumin. The toxicity and usefulness of phenylbutazone may be affected by liver disease, renal disease, and age; in these instances, lower doses than usual may be necessary.

Indomethacin

Indomethacin (Indocin) is an indole-acetic acid with anti-inflammatory, analgesic, and antipyretic properties.[250] Its potent inhibition of cyclo-oxygenase has resulted in its use in several unexpected areas of medicine.

Pharmacology and Pharmacokinetics

Indomethacin is completely and rapidly absorbed, reaching peak plasma levels 1 to 3 hours after oral dosing and slightly later after administration of rectal suppositories. The plasma disappearance curve of indomethacin is biphasic, indicating that the kinetics fit a 2-compartment model, with an elimination half-life of 2.2 to 11.2 hours in adults. Kinetic analysis indicates the presence of a nonsamplable "hypothetic organ" that causes a slower elimination of drug from the circulation than expected.[149] Completeness of absorption in man has been shown. Only 2% of a 25-mg oral dose is excreted in the feces as unchanged indomethacin.[77] Both intravenous and oral indomethacin are about 65% excreted in the urine and 35% excreted in the feces, however, a finding that suggests biliary excretion of metabolized drug.[77] Whereas 16% of a dose appears as unchanged drug in the urine, the rest is inactive metabolites. Gastrointestinal toxicity was related to the amounts of indomethacin and its metabolites excreted in the bile in 5 animal species.[77] Because between 27 and 43% of the drug is excreted in the bile in man, and much is reabsorbed, it is not surprising that indomethacin has significant gastrointestinal toxicity. Indomethacin is 98 to 99% bound to albumin, with between 8 and 15 binding sites.[181]

A slow-release preparation (75-mg capsule) of indomethacin has been marketed recently; its bioavailability and efficacy appear to be the same as formulations already available, but it may be taken twice a day.[293]

Indomethacin's elimination seems to be age dependent to some extent. The mean half-life in newborn infants whose mothers were taking indomethacin was 14.7 hours, although the half-life of the drug in the mothers was 2.2 hours.[281] Seven elderly patients (mean age 75.8 years) cleared 13% of a dose of indomethacin through their kidneys, whereas 7 younger patients (mean age 33 years) cleared 30% by this route. Despite these findings, the serum half-lives and AUC were the same for both groups.[280] Thus, although renal elimination was decreased in the elderly, total elimination was the same, perhaps because of compensatory increased gastrointestinal elimination. Because of this characteristic, one would expect greater gastrointestinal toxicity from indomethacin in the elderly.

Although single doses of indomethacin may affect renal function, 2 weeks of treatment with indomethacin, 150 mg daily, did not decrease renal function as measured by creatinine clearance, fractional sodium or potassium excretion, and free water reabsorption, in 6 normal subjects or in patients with previously normal renal function. Peripheral renin activity was decreased in all patients.[304] Life-threatening hyperkalemia has been reported, mostly in elderly patients receiving large doses for gouty arthritis.[90a]

The interaction between aspirin and indomethacin is complex; the decreased indomethacin AUC after long-term administration of both drugs is due to a combination of reduced indomethacin absorption, increased biliary clearance, and decreased renal clearance.[148] Clinically, no difference in response was noted between aspirin and indomethacin given alone or in combination, although the incidence of side effects increased when the drugs were given together.[36]

Indomethacin causes sodium retention and decreases the natriuretic effect of furosemide, but this effect is easily overcome by increasing the dose of the diuretic.[209] Probenecid interferes with the excretion of indomethacin, probably by competing for a common tubular secretion mechanism.[12] The marked increase in indomethacin serum levels during concurrent probenecid administration was reported to increase the effect of indomethacin in 28 patients with RA who were given both drugs at bedtime;[38] this finding may be important when the drugs are used together to treat gout. Diflunisal caused a 210% increase in indomethacin AUC, from 0 to 12 hours, when the 2 drugs were given concomitantly.[279] Moreover, indomethacin increased lithium carbonate levels by 42% in 7 subjects, probably because of decreased renal lithium clearance.[119] In normal subjects, indomethacin did not change the anticoagulant effect induced by warfarin.[292]

Uses

Despite some initial controversy, it is generally agreed that indomethacin is approximately as effective as aspirin in RA.[203,310] It may be more effective than aspirin in some patients and is a reasonable alternative in patients who are intolerant to aspirin.

Indomethacin is effective in acute gouty arthritis. Doses as high as 600 mg have been used for the first day, following by 150 to 200 mg daily, continuing until 3 to 4 days after all pain has disappeared.[268] A daily dose of 100 mg is effective in patients with ankylosing spondylitis.[19] Its effect on osteoarthritis is documented in several short-term studies in which indomethacin, in doses of 75 to 225 mg/day, was compared with placebo,[295] as well a with other NSAID.[63] Doses greater than 100 mg daily are rarely indicated in this older population, however. Indomethacin has also been used in the following conditions: psoriatic arthritis, with about a 50% response rate; rheumatic fever, with an effectiveness equal to that of aspirin; Reiter's syndrome, with about a 75% response rate; and JRA, in which 12 of 13 children studied responded. Con-

trolled trials are not available in any of these conditions.[203]

Indomethacin has also been used in other diseases as an anti-inflammatory drug or for its potent effect on prostaglandin synthesis. It has been reported to be effective in the nephrotic syndrome,[9] pericarditis,[193] pleuritic pain,[244] pancreatic cholera,[131] hypercalcemia related to some neoplasms,[129] premature labor,[315] treatment of patent ductus arteriosus in infants,[177] leprosy,[140] dysmenorrhea,[150] and uveitis.[213] These usages of indomethacin are investigative, with a few patients treated for only a short time.*

Adverse Effects

In 1968, O'Brien reviewed published reports of toxicity to indomethacin.[203] In 15 studies, some undesirable reaction was reported in 35.6% of patients. Gastrointestinal side effects occurred in 12.5 to 44% of patients, and 2 to 5% developed ulcers with bleeding. Such ulcers may be gastric, duodenal, or jejunal and may be silent.[203,269] Gastrointestinal toxicity may be related to the amount of drug excreted in the bile. Local effects on gastric mucosa include inhibition of mucin secretion, increased acid secretion, and local congestion.[167]

Central nervous system effects, reported in 10 to 25% of patients,[203] include characteristic morning frontal headache, vertigo, feelings of dissociation or unreality, depression, and rarely, hallucinations or psychosis. In a retrospective study, the occurrence of retinal abnormalities was the same in an indomethacin-treated group as in control subjects. Both groups showed changes consistent with age and arteriosclerosis.[44]

Other rarely reported toxicities include hepatitis, acute renal failure, angina pectoris, induction of antiplatelet antibodies, asthma, arthropathy of the hips, peripheral neuropathy, rashes, and two cases of pulmonary hypertension in infants of mothers given indomethacin to inhibit premature labor, perhaps related to early closure of the ductus arteriosus in utero.[54,57,79,143,179,203] Through secretion into breast milk, the drug may have caused convulsions in a six-day-old breast-fed infant.[84] Despite reports that indomethacin is a coronary vasoconstrictor in patients with coronary artery disease, no decrease in exercise tolerance was found in patients with stable angina pectoris.[278†]

Schaller reviewed the serious adverse experi-

---

*Editors' note: We have been impressed with the effects of indomethacin's in treating the pleural and pericardial involvement in systemic lupus erythematosus.

†Editors' note: The sodium-retaining effects of indomethacin are weak, but we have noted recurrent edema in a patient with Addison's disease.

ences reported in children taking indomethacin and concluded that the drug should be given to children under age 14 only if lack of efficacy or toxicity associated with other NSAID warranted the risk; selected patients with JRA or juvenile ankylosing spondylitis may be treated with indomethacin for short periods, but the drug is not recommended for long-term use.[248]

Dosage

Capsules containing 25 or 50 mg are available, as well as 75-mg timed release capsules.

Indomethacin has a much shorter plasma elimination half-life than phenylbutazone; steady-state levels are reached within 1 to 2 days; dosing (25 mg) may be necessary every 4 or every 8 hours, depending on the half-life of the drug in individual patients. The slow-release (75-mg capsules) preparation may be used twice daily.

New uses for indomethacin and NSAID may arise from their potent effects on prostaglandin synthesis. Gastrointestinal and central nervous system effects may be troublesome, and their incidence may increase with age.

Ibuprofen

Ibuprofen (Motrin, Rufen, Advil, Nuprin), a propionic acid with a pka of 4.4 was first marketed in 1969 in Great Britain and in 1974 in the United States. Ibuprofen is more than 90% absorbed, and peak levels occur 45 to 90 minutes after tablet ingestion. Food delays absorption. The plasma-time concentration curves of the drug can be satisfactorily described by a single-compartment open model, with a half-life of approximately 2 hours. Increasing the dose linearly increases the AUC of unbound drug.[169] Despite its short half-life, pharmacologic effects continue for much longer.[58] In a small pilot study, a fixed daily dose of ibuprofen was as effective when given every 12 hours as when given every 6 hours.[40] It is 98% protein bound and is cleared predominantly by the liver.[58] All metabolites are inactive, and induction of metabolism does not occur. In 13 subjects, most of the drug was either hydroxylated or carboxylated; only 12% was excreted by the kidney as the glucuronide, and only 1% appeared unchanged in the urine.[58] Despite strong protein binding, significant interaction between warfarin and ibuprofen does not occur in normal subjects.[212] Ibuprofen causes transient inhibition of platelet aggregation of shorter duration than that caused by aspirin. It also prolongs the prothrombin time slightly after 3 weeks of use.[58]

Double-blind trials of ibuprofen (up to 1,200 mg/day) versus placebo, aspirin (2.3 to 4.8 g/day), or other NSAID yielded equivocal results in RA, with definite analgesia, but questionable anti-inflammatory activity.[58] At higher doses of 2,100 to 2,400 mg/day, the anti-inflammatory effect was more evident.[107] One study comparing doses of 2,400 mg to 3,200 mg ibuprofen daily in 61 patients with RA showed no difference between these dosing regimens.[194] Although side effects were less frequent at lower doses, they were equal to the side effects of aspirin at the higher doses.[107,163]

Ibuprofen, at a daily dose of 1,200 mg, is reported to be an effective analgesic in osteoarthritis.[58] At 1,800 mg daily, ibuprofen was as effective as 3.6 g aspirin in 437 osteoarthritis patients.[103] Success has also been shown in JRA, in comparison to aspirin;[27] in alkylosing spondylitis, although indomethacin on phenylbutazone is usually preferred;[139] and in gout.[139] In nonarticular rheumatism, indomethacin and ibuprofen are equally effective, although ibuprofen causes fewer side effects.[287] In addition, ibuprofen has been used successfully to inhibit uterine contraction and to treat dysmenorrhea.[45] Animal experiments indicate that ibuprofen limits the size of infarctions when given intravenously immediately after coronary artery occlusion. The mechanism of this effect is unknown.[137]

Adverse Reactions

Dyspepsia occurred in 9 to 17% of cases, and clinically significant gastrointestinal bleeding has been reported in 4 cases per million filled prescriptions.[107] Although ibuprofen, like other NSAID, reversibly affects platelet aggregation, it has been given to hemophiliac patients with no greater effect than in normal subjects.[174] The incidence of occult gastrointestinal blood loss was less with ibuprofen than with aspirin (1.5 versus 3.3 ml/day).[251] Headaches, drowsiness, tinnitus, vertigo, and rash occur, but are uncommon.[54] An unusual, idiosyncratic aseptic meningitis has been reported following ibuprofen administration in a few patients with systemic lupus erythematosus or mixed connective tissue disease.[303] As with other NSAID, ibuprofen has been associated with edema and precipitation of congestive heart failure in susceptible individuals, probably because of the effects of these drugs on renal homeostasis by cyclo-oxygenase inhibition. Ibuprofen has also been implicated in papillary necrosis,[259] as well as in acute renal failure.[144] Other, rare, adverse reactions include asthma, agranulocytosis, and hepatic dysfunction.[114,273,275]

Doses are given every 6 or 8 hours because of the short serum half-life of this drug, although one study compared 6- and 12-hour dosing intervals.[40] Because so little of it is cleared unchanged by the kidneys, the dose does not need to be modified in patients with renal failure. Although ibuprofen is predominantly cleared by the liver, alcoholic liver disease does not alter its kinetics.[138] Ibuprofen is tightly bound to albumin; nonetheless, no drug interactions of consequence have been reported.[58] This lack of interaction may be a significant advantage for patients taking warfarin anticoagulants. Because ibuprofen is principally metabolized by oxidation, probenecid, which inhibits glucuronidation, does not raise ibuprofen serum concentrations.[110]

Overdose. Ibuprofen was released in 1984 for nonprescription sale to the general public as 200-mg tablets for use as an analgesic, with a maximum daily dose of 1,200 mg. Increased availability as an alternative to aspirin and acetaminophen will increase the potential for accidental or deliberate overdoses. Ibuprofen overdose has been rare, despite its extensive use as an NSAID. Only 75 cases of ibuprofen overdose were noted among 58,000 overdoses recorded in a 2-year survey by the British National Poisons Information Service.[53] Alleged overdoses ranged from 200 mg to 40 g; plasma concentrations as high as 704 mg/l were measured in asymptomatic patients. One 78-year-old man had increased plama creatinine levels after taking between 9.6 and 16 g ibuprofen, with an increased plasma concentration of 360 mg/l, but he recovered. Only a single death was recorded. A 67-year-old woman died following vomiting, deafness, confusion, hyperventilation, coma, hypotension, and cardiac arrest after an overdose of both ibuprofen and salicylate.[53]

Symptoms of abdominal pain, nausea, vomiting, drowsiness, sweating, nystagmus, diplopia, headache, and tinnitus were reported in some patients who recovered from overdoses of ibuprofen alone. Treatment generally included an emetic or gastric lavage, observation, and administration of fluids.[53]

Dosage

The drug is available as 200-, 300-, 400-, or 600-mg tablets.

Because of its short plasma half-life, ibuprofen is usually given 4 times a day; 1,200 to 1,600 mg daily are adequate for analgesia, but 3,000 to 3,600 mg daily may be needed for an anti-inflammatory effect in RA. These higher doses are more likely to be associated with gastrointestinal side effects.

Naproxen

Naproxen (Naprosyn) is completely absorbed from tablet, capsule, or aqueous suspension. The absorption rate is increased by bicarbonate, is decreased by other antacids, and is slightly decreased by food. A linear relationship exists between dose and serum concentration for doses up to 500 mg, but the relationship becomes nonlinear thereafter. A 50% increase of dose to 750 mg results in only a 25% increase in the AUC. This phenomenon is associated with increases in unbound fraction and renal excretion, and indicates that protein-binding sites may be saturated at that level.[34,241] The drug is 97.6 to 99.5% protein bound at doses below 500 mg.[34] The plasma levels of naproxen fit a 2-compartment open model with an elimination half-life of 12 to 15 hours. No difference is noted in half-life between adults and children.[34,241] From 77 to 100% is recovered in the urine, as conjugated drug (50 to 60%) or as metabolites (27 to 46%); only 0.5 to 2.5% appears in the feces.[34,241] In a study of patients taking 250 mg naproxen twice daily, mean synovial fluid concentrations were 50% of serum concentrations 3 to 4 hours after a dose and 74% of serum concentrations after 15 hours.[133]

The addition of aspirin decreased naproxen blood levels and decreased the AUC by 15%; however, when naproxen was given to subjects taking salicylates, the AUC of salicylate was decreased by only 2%.[34,256] An 8-week crossover study showed that a regimen of naproxen, 500 mg daily, added to aspirin, 1.3 to 5 g daily, was better than aspirin alone, with respect to patient preference, walking time, grip strength, and morning stiffness, but not with respect to inflamed joint count or joint swelling.[307] No kinetic interactions have been found between naproxen and diflunisal,[74] but concomitant probenecid administration has increased steady-state naproxen concentrations by 50% and has increased plasma half-lives from 14 to 37 hours.[240]

Naproxen displaces warfarin from human serum albumin in vitro: a 14 to 17% increase in free warfarin concentration was found when therapeutic concentrations of naproxen were added.[311] In vivo studies show an increase in free warfarin concentrations in some subjects when these two drugs are used together, so patients treated with both warfarin and naproxen should be observed closely on initiation or change in therapy.[132] Unbound serum naproxen concentrations are increased in patients with renal insufficiency, but the half-life of the drug is unaltered.[8]

In patients with RA, naproxen, at a dose of 400 to 750 mg daily, was more effective than placebo and was as effective as aspirin;[34] it was also roughly comparable to 150 mg indomethacin or to 2.4 g fenoprofen daily. Naproxen was also more effective than 2,400 mg ibuprofen or 1,500 mg flufenamic acid, although statistically significant differences were not found.[34] A dose-related increase in efficacy has been shown in 50 patients with RA treated with up to 1,000 mg naproxen daily,[171] and a relationship of serum level to efficacy response was shown in 24 patients with RA given up to 1,500 mg naproxen daily for 2 weeks.[61] In this study, trough naproxen concentrations, measured just before a dose, below 18 μg/ml were associated with no response, whereas 76% of patients with trough concentrations above 50 μg/ml responded.

Naproxen, 250 mg/day, was as effective as aspirin, 60 to 80 mg/kg/day, in patients with JRA, although bleeding time was prolonged in some patients.[178] Naproxen, 250 mg twice daily, was more effective than placebo and was equal to indomethacin in osteoarthritis of large joints.[16,34] Many trials, using naproxen 500 to 750 mg versus other NSAID, such as proquazone, diclofenac, indomethacin, and flurbiprofen, did not show major differences between drugs in treating osteoarthritis.[34] Small numbers of patients with ankylosing spondylitis, acute gout, and "nonarticular rheumatism" have also been treated successfully with daily doses of 500 to 1,000 mg naproxen.[34,124,308]

Side effects are similar to those of indomethacin and aspirin, but they are less frequent[16,34] (see Table 28–1).

Dosage

Tablets containing 250, 375, or 500 mg are available. Because naproxen has a long elimination half-life, it can be given twice a day. Naproxen protein-binding sites become saturated at doses greater than 500 to 750 mg a day, and at higher doses, renal clearance increases. Despite this effect, increasing doses raise serum concentrations, and doses as high as 1,500 mg daily have been used. Unchanged drug may be cleared to a modest extent, so some drug may accumulate in patients with renal impairment. Naproxen is tightly and extensively bound to serum protein, making drug-drug interactions more likely. In RA, the relationship between serum concentration and efficacy suggests that serum levels may be useful to adjust doses.

Sulindac

Sulindac (Clinoril), a sulfoxide, is a prodrug because its sulfide metabolite is much more active than the parent drug in in vitro tests of anti-inflammatory activity and in animal studies of inflammation. For example, the sulfide is 500 times as active as the sulfoxide as a prostaglandin synthesis inhibitor. Sulindac is reversibly metabolized to the sulfide and is irreversibly metabolized to an inactive sulfone. In animal studies, the drug is transformed to the sulfide in all tissues, although the major sites of transformation are the kidney and liver. Except in lung and plasma, more sulfide is present than sulfoxide.[78] All forms of this drug undergo enterohepatic recirculation, with 5 to 30 times more sulindac than sulfide excreted in the bile. Sulindac is more than 88% bioavailable, although some may already be in the inactive sulfone form when absorbed. Peak plasma levels are achieved within an hour in fasted humans. The plasma half-life of sulindac itself is 7.8 hours, but the more active sulfide metabolite has a half-life of 16 to 18 hours. A large proportion of the drug is retained in the body after a 400-mg dose; the reason for this unexpected retention is unknown. Both the sulfoxide and sulfide are tightly protein bound (93 to 98%); 45 to 50% of a single dose is excreted in the urine, whereas 25 to 30% is found in the feces. Although over 90% of the drug is recovered in the urine and feces, only 10% is recovered as sulfide, all in the feces.[76]

Two-hour postprandial blood glucose levels did not change when sulindac was given with tolbutamide for 7 days, although the fasting blood sugar levels of these patients did decrease from 120.5 to 112.9 mg/100 ml.[243] Sulindac had little effect on prothrombin time in volunteers taking warfarin, although those given warfarin without sulindac had a faster return of prothrombin times to normal than those taking warfarin and sulindac combined. This effect may indicate some inhibition of the excretion or metabolism of warfarin by sulindac; 4 patients developed hypothrombinemia in response to sulindac.[120] Aspirin did not change the peak plasma concentrations or AUC of sulindac, but it did decrease these parameters for the sulfide by 20 to 25%.[188] Unlike other NSAID, sulindac does not inhibit cyclo-oxygenase in the kidney because that organ can reoxidize the sulfide back to the inactive prodrug sulfoxide form, thus protecting itself.[192a]

Doses of 150 to 200 mg sulindac twice a day are more effective than placebo and are equivalent to 3.6 to 4.8 g aspirin in the treatment of both RA and osteoarthritis of the large joints.[32,68] Sulindac is more effective than ibuprofen, 1,200 mg daily, in osteoarthritis of the hip.[32] A 1-year double-blind study of 387 patients with osteoarthritis compared 100 to 400 mg sulindac to 1.6 to 4.8 g aspirin daily; about 80% in both groups had an excellent or satisfactory response.[5] Sulindac, at a dose of 100 to 200 mg twice a day, may be as effective as indomethacin or phenylbutazone in ankylosing spondylitis, nonarticular shoulder pain, and gout.[32,65,102,165]

Adverse effects are less common with sulindac than with equieffective doses of aspirin. Of 864 patients with osteoarthritis or RA enrolled in controlled trials of sulindac versus aspirin, 10.4% of sulindac-treated patients discontinued the drug because of adverse effects, as compared to 17.3% of aspirin-treated patients.[5,188] As with other NSAID, gastrointestinal side effects were most common. In osteoarthritis patients, 1 ulcer was found in 387 patients; overall, the incidence of ulcer was 0.4%

in 1,865 patients.[5] Gastrointestinal blood loss while taking sulindac for a week was 2 ml daily, whereas blood loss while taking aspirin was 15 ml daily.[224]

Sulindac has the usual range of NSAID side effects, including rare reactions such as bone marrow aplasia, Stevens-Johnson syndrome, congestive heart failure, acute renal failure, aseptic meningitis, and severe hepatitis.[13,88,158,192,207]

Dosage

Tablets containing 150 or 200 mg are available. Sulindac is given twice daily in doses of 300 to 400 mg/day. Gastrointestinal side effects may be decreased because the sulfide, which may be the active irritant, does not build up rapidly in the gastrointestinal tract. Because sulindac is tightly protein bound, drug-drug interactions are possible. May have advantages in patients with renal insufficiency.

Tolmetin

Tolmetin (Tolectin), a pyrrole derivative, is not chemically related to any of the previously described NSAID, although it shares their probable mechanism(s) of action and animal pharmacology.[33] Tolmetin is absorbed rapidly, with peak plasma concentrations in about 30 to 45 minutes. Plasma disposition curves have been fitted to 1- and 2-compartment open models, with elimination half-lives between 2.1 and 6.8 hours.[11,96,257] The longer half-life relates to the drug's elimination phase and makes up only a small portion of the drug's AUC; 99% of the drug is excreted in the urine. All metabolites are inactive; 10 to 17% unchanged tolmetin is recovered in urine, but may be an artifact because the glucuronide metabolite may spontaneously dissociate to tolmetin in the urine. Animal studies indicate that tolmetin does not have a significant enterohepatic circulation.[122]

Tolmetin is 99% protein bound,[96] but it did not influence warfarin-induced prolonged prothrombin times when added to an anticoagulant regimen for 3 weeks.[302] Magnesium-aluminum hydroxide (Maalox) did not decrease tolmetin's AUC.[11] In vitro, aspirin and salicylic acid substantially decreased tolmetin binding to albumin.[258] Tolmetin added to established aspirin therapy in RA patients for 10 weeks did not have any additional clinical effect.[231] The combined administration of tolmetin and aspirin for 18 days resulted in a fourfold increase in free tolmetin (from 1% to 3.8%), a 16% decrease in tolmetin AUC, and a 17% increase in tolmetin clearance.[217,257]

Tolmetin, at a dose of 1,200 to 1,500 mg daily, is better than placebo and is probably equal to 3.9 to 4.5 g aspirin, 100 to 150 mg indomethacin, 2,400 mg ibuprofen, or 400 mg phenylbutazone

per day in the treatment of RA.[33] In 107 children with JRA, tolmetin was equal to aspirin in effectiveness.[157] In 10 gouty patients, it neither decreased serum uric acid levels nor suppressed acute gouty arthritis.[135] In an open study of 30 patients with ankylosing spondylitis, 90% had a satisfactory response.[249]

Gastrointestinal side effects severe enough to discontinue medication included ulcers in 3.6% of 420 patients; gastrointestinal bleeding occurred in 1% of 420 patients, and occasional nausea, pain, or diarrhea was noted.[41,85] The rare side effects of other NSAID can also occur in tolmetin-treated patients, despite the unique chemical structure of this agent. Thus, acute renal failure and interstitial nephritis, aseptic meningitis, anaphylactic reactions, and IgM-related allergic thrombocytopenic purpura have been documented.[141,223,242,272] An artifactual "pseudoproteinuria" may occur in patients taking tolmetin. When the sulfosalicylic acid test for urine protein is used, the acid precipitates the major metabolite of tolmetin, with an appearance resembling that of proteinuria. Use of tetrabromphenol blue (Albustix) or similar nonacidic or specific methods circumvents this laboratory artifact.[86]

Dosage

Tolmetin is given in doses of 600 to 1800 mg daily, divided into 3 or 4 doses; 200- and 400-mg tablets are available. Up to 2,000 mg daily in RA and up to 1,600 mg daily in osteoarthritis have been prescribed. Most of the drug is metabolized and then excreted in the urine. Because enterohepatic recirculation appears to be minimal, this drug is theoretically more useful in the elderly. No advantage exists to the simultaneous use of tolmetin and aspirin in RA. Tolmetin does not appear to be of use in gout, but it is an alternative to aspirin in the treatment of JRA.

Fenoprofen

Fenoprofen (Nalfon) is an arylpropionic acid with a pKa of 4.5. Unlike ibuprofen, both isomers of fenoprofen are equally active anti-inflammatory agents and are not interconverted in vivo.[201] Fenoprofen is 80% bioavailable, its disposition is well described by a 2-compartment open model, and it has an enterohepatic circulation in humans. The elimination half-life of the drug is short (70 to 160 minutes); 90% of a single dose is excreted in the urine as glucuronides, and only 1 to 3% is eliminated as unchanged fenoprofen. The drug is 99% bound to serum proteins.[113,237,238]

Aspirin, at a daily dose of 3.9 g, decreased the area under the log plasma concentration-time curve of fenoprofen by 25 to 50% and decreased its serum half-life by 39% after multiple dosing in normal subjects. The mechanism of this effect was not clear because aspirin and fenoprofen bind at different sites on albumin, so drug displacement is not likely. It was postulated that aspirin might have induced increased metabolism of fenoprofen.[237] Absorption of fenoprofen is decreased by food, with a 20% decrease in AUC, as compared to the fasting state.[47] On the other hand, magnesium-aluminum hydroxide does not decrease absorption. No other significant drug-drug interactions with fenoprofen appear to exist, despite its high protein binding, although probenecid would be expected to increase fenoprofen serum concentrations.

Fenoprofen, at 1.2 to 3.2 g a day, is better than placebo and is generally comparable to a daily dose of aspirin of 3.6 g or more in the treatment of RA.[115] Similarly, fenoprofen, at 1.8 to 2.4 a day, is effective in osteoarthritis.[35] It appeared to be effective in treating acute gout when a daily dose of 3.2 g was used in an open trial of 27 patients.[294] In a 2-week, double-blind, cross-over study of 19 patients with ankylosing spondylitis, 1,800 mg fenoprofen daily was as effective as 150 mg indomethacin.[261]

Occult blood loss from the gatrointestinal tract in man is less with short-term fenoprofen administration than with aspirin (2.25 versus 5 ml/day).[170] In a study of patients with RA, fewer gastrointestinal side effects and less tinnitus were noted with fenoprofen than with aspirin.[115] Like other NSAID, fenoprofen has been associated with rare hepatic dysfunction, agranulocytosis, and thrombocytopenia, as well as uncommon rashes, headaches, and drowsiness.[300] Of more concern is fenoprofen-induced renal failure, documented in at least 15 patients.[270] Although oliguria may or may not be present, and the association with nephrotic syndrome is variable, interstitial nephritis and minimal-change glomerulonephritis are characteristic. Eosinophilia is seen in 30% of patients, and T-cell predominance and IgE-bearing B cells have been documented in renal tissue.[270]

Dosage

The drug is available as a 200- or 300-mg capsule or a 600-mg tablet.

Fenoprofen should be given 4 times a day. It is an effective drug, but thus far accounts for a majority of NSAID-induced nephropathy, so it should be used cautiously.

Meclofenamate Sodium

Meclofenamate sodium (Meclomen) is the third generation of the fenamates. Flufenamic acid and mefenamic acid have also been marketed, but are used infrequently and are not discussed here. Me-

clofenamate sodium is a cyclo-oxygenase inhibitor that may inhibit phospholipase A_2 and may also impair prostaglandin activity at its receptor site.[175]

Meclofenamate is rapidly absorbed, with peak concentrations in 1 to 2 hours.[105] It is highly metabolized, and one of its metabolites, hydroxymethyl meclofenamic acid, has anti-inflammatory activity.[105] From 50 to 70% of the drug is excreted in the urine, and 25 to 30% appears in the feces.[105] It probably undergoes enterohepatic recirculation. The elimination half-life of meclofenamic acid is 3.3 hours; no information is available on the half-life of the active metabolite.[105,266] Meclofenamic acid is 99.8% albumin bound, but is displaced from albumin by salicylate.[266]

After a 3-week regimen of 3.6 g aspirin or 400 mg sodium meclofenamate daily, occult gastrointestinal blood loss averaged 11 and 7 ml per day, respectively.[266] Neither food nor magnesium-aluminum hydroxide (Maalox) affected its bioavailability, but sodium bicarbonate resulted in more rapid absorption and higher peak plasma levels.[266] Concomitant aspirin therapy decreased plasma meclofenamate concentrations; the AUC was 10% less when meclofenamate was given with aspirin.[15] Warfarin requirements were decreased by an average of 16% (range 0 to 25%) when given with meclofenamate sodium, but no interaction with proproxyphene or sulfinpyrazone appeared to be clinically significant.[15]

Meclofenamate sodium is effective in treating RA.[214] In 6- to 8-week trials, regimens of 200 mg and 300 mg daily were better than placebo; a daily dose of 300 mg was equivalent to 3.6 g aspirin or 150 mg indomethacin. In patients with osteoarthritis, 300 mg daily was better than placebo and was equivalent to phenylbutazone and naproxen regimens. With meclofenamate sodium, 76% of patients studied, versus 42% receiving placebo, felt overall improvement.[215] Meclofenamate appeared to be as effective as indomethacin in the treatment of ankylosing spondylitis or extra-articular conditions such as painful shoulder syndrome.[24,59,82] High doses, such as 800 mg the first day, followed by 300 mg/day for 6 days, were equivalent to 150 mg indomethacin daily in the treatment of acute gout.[81] A 4-week, open, uncontrolled study of 39 patients with JRA indicated that the drug was effective at daily doses of 3 to 7.5 mg/kg.[28] The 18% dropout rate in this study was higher than in previous similar studies of other NSAID by the same group (0 to 3%), however, and thus the usefulness of meclofenamate may be limited in children.[28]

Adverse Experiences

The types of adverse reactions with meclofenamate sodium are similar to those with other

NSAID, but gastrointestinal problems seem to be more common. Among 2,500 patients in controlled studies, diarrhea, the most common side effect, occurred in 11%, as compared to 2% of aspirin-treated patients.[219] Abdominal pain occurred in 7%, versus 1% with aspirin. Withdrawal of the drug for diarrhea occurred in only 2.2% of meclofenamate sodium-treated patients, however, as opposed to 1.8% of aspirin-treated patients.[219] The diarrhea was of small-bowel origin.[219] In long-term studies of 109 patients with RA in which 60% completed a year of treatment and 17% completed 2 years of treatment, gastrointestinal side effects were even more common and occurred in 30.6 to 43.3% of patients.[80] Therapy was discontinued in 29% because of these effects, which included abdominal pain in 8%, diarrhea in 7%, and peptic ulcers in 2.8%.[80] One of every 6 patients receiving meclofenamate sodium had a decrease in hemoglobin or hematocrit level, although no evidence of increased blood loss, bone marrow suppression, or hemolysis was found. Patients with osteoarthritis appeared to have fewer side effects than those with RA.[80,219]

Dosage
The drug is available in 50- and 100-mg capsules. The daily dosing regimen recommended for meclofenamate sodium is 200 to 400 mg, given in 4 divided doses. Although effective, it may have greater incidence of gastrointestinal side effects than other NSAID.

Piroxicam

Piroxicam (Feldene), a carboxamide, was marketed in the United States in 1982. It is 1 of only 3 NSAID with a high pKa, of 6.32; phenylbutazone and oxyphenbutazone are the others.[55] In most other ways, piroxicam is similar to other NSAID. Thus, it is antipyretic, variably analgesic, and anti-inflammatory, and it reversibly inhibits platelet aggregation. Its principal mechanism of action is probably cyclo-oxygenase inhibition, but at high concentrations it also inhibits neutrophil migration, phagocytosis, and lysozymal enzyme release.[55] Piroxicam's long elimination half-life (mean 38 hours; range 14 to 158 hours) makes it suitable for administration once a day.[55] It is well absorbed, highly metabolized, and renally excreted, although only 10% of a dose is excreted unchanged into the urine.[55] Its metabolites are clinically inactive.[55] The accumulation of this drug is linear, and it is 99% protein bound at a concentration between 5 and 50 µg/ml.[55] Synovial fluid concentrations are approximately 50% of serum concentrations.[55] Unlike many other NSAID, piroxicam is not displaced from albumin by aspirin, and drug-drug interactions are often insignificant; for example, no in-

teraction was found with several antacids or digoxin.[55] Partial thromboplastin times, however, were prolonged when this drug was given with acenocoumarol.[55]

Piroxicam has been studied in patients with RA, osteoarthritis, gout, ankylosing spondylitis, and acute musculoskeletal disorders.[55] In a 4-week, double-blind cross-over study of 22 patients with RA, 20 mg piroxicam daily was better than placebo with respect to joint tenderness, joint swelling, morning stiffness and global assessment. Seventy-nine patients with RA underwent a 12-week, parallel, double-blind comparison of aspirin, 3 g or more, and piroxicam, 20 mg daily. Stable prednisone and gold therapy were allowed. Patients in both drug groups improved equally with respect to pain, stiffness, joint pain and swelling, 50-foot walking time, and visual analogue scales. Grip strength improved more in patients taking aspirin, as did erythrocyte sedimentation rates.[306]

Piroxicam, at 20 mg daily, was comparable in efficacy to 100 to 200 mg indomethacin daily in 32 patients with RA. In osteoarthritis, piroxicam, 20 mg/day, was comparable to a daily dose of 2.6 to 3.9 g aspirin and was statistically superior in reducing the number of painful joints and in increasing lower-extremity range of motion.[2] In a 6-week, double-blind, randomized, parallel study of 30 patients with osteoarthritis given 20 mg piroxicam or 75 mg indomethacin daily, both drugs produced similar results. For gout (40 mg/day piroxicam for 1 to 5 days) and ankylosing spondylitis (10 to 30 mg/day), only "positive-control" (versus indomethacin) or uncontrolled trials were done, but results indicated efficacy.[22,233]

Adverse Effects

Based on studies of over 3,500 patients who have used the drug, the incidence and type of side effects from piroxicam are similar to those of other NSAID.[216] Gastrointestinal side effects occurred in 19% of patients studied and required discontinuance of the drug in 3.5%. One percent developed ulcers, as compared to 2.9% of those taking aspirin. Other gastrointestinal symptoms included dyspepsia, nausea, diarrhea, and cramping pain. Daily doses of piroxicam of 30 to 40 mg were associated with a higher incidence of ulcers than doses of 20 mg daily (up to 29% versus 1%). In one study, 4 of 10 patients taking 40 mg/day piroxicam and concurrent aspirin developed peptic ulcers.[19] Headaches and dizziness were unusual and occurred in about 3% of patients, as compared to 11 to 22% of those taking indomethacin. Other unusual side effects included rashes, liver dysfunction, allergic reactions, edema, and hematologic manifestations (0.9 to 2.4%).[19,216] Tinnitus occurred in 0.6% of patients.

Dosage

The drug is available as 10- and 20-mg capsules. Piroxicam has a half-life of 38 hours, so once-daily administration is sufficient. On the other hand, the drug has a narrow therapeutic range; 20 mg daily is the dose most frequently prescribed, a 10-mg dose is often ineffective, and a dose of 30 mg or more appears to be more toxic than the standard dose.

Diflunisal

Diflunisal (Dolobid) is difluorophenyl salicylic acid.[59] It is not broken down into salicylic acid, although its metabolism is similar to that of salicylates. Like most NSAID, its principal mechanism of action is probably cyclo-oxygenase inhibition.[59] Diflunisal may bind cyclo-oxygenase at a site close to, but not identical to, the aspirin and indomethacin binding site, however; it is also an effective free radical scavenger. Thus, the mechanism of action of this drug may differ from that of aspirin in some details.[59] Diflunisal was marketed in Great Britain in 1977 and in the United States in 1982.[70]

Diflunisal is well absorbed. Like salicylates, it is subject to capacity-limited metabolism. Ninety percent is metabolized to 2 glucuronides, acyl and phenyl, that are excreted in the urine; 5% of a dose is excreted unchanged in the urine.[59] Protein binding is greater than 98%. Because the drug exhibits capacity-limited kinetics, plasma disappearance half-times increase with larger doses (8 to 10 hours with 500 mg daily; 15 hours with 1,000 mg daily). With creatinine clearance of less than 30 ml/min, its half-life increases markedly; total body clearance decreases, but less than expected; raised biliary clearance probably compensates for the lowered renal clearance.[59]

Concurrent naproxen and diflunisal administration decreases urinary naproxen excretion, but plasma naproxen profiles do not change; this finding implies compensatory biliary naproxen clearance. Diflunisal has decreased the renal clearance and increased plasma concentrations of indomethacin after their coadministration, however.[59] In one study, free warfarin concentrations increased minimally when diflunisal was given; similarly, diflunisal increased plasma concentrations of hydrochlorothiazide and acetaminophen. No interactions were detected when diflunisal was given with tolbutamide, furosemide, or magnesium hydroxide; however, aluminum hydroxide decreased diflunisal absorption by 40%.[59]

Published clinical studies with diflunisal to date have been limited to single-dose studies for pain and longer-term studies in patients with osteoarthritis. For postoperative oral surgical pain, 500- and 1,000-mg doses of diflunisal were superior to placebo, and the effect generally lasted 12 hours. For peak analgesia, diflunisal doses of 500 and 1,000 mg, were equivalent to each other, equal to 600 mg acetaminophen with 60 mg codeine, and better than 650 mg aspirin, 600 mg acetaminophen, 100 mg acetaminophen with 100 mg propoxyphene, and 100 mg proproxyphene napsylate. For overall analgesia, measured as pain intensity differences, 1,000 mg diflunisal appeared superior to the comparison drugs at both 4 and 12 hours, whereas a 500-mg dose was superior only at 12 hours.[17]

In the treatment of osteoarthritis of the hips and knees, 5 studies included 1,218 patients, of whom 657 were receiving diflunisal.[283] Daily doses of 500, 750 and 1,000 mg were statistically better than placebo in all 10 disease activity criteria. When 791 patients were given aspirin, in daily doses of 2,000 to 3,000 mg, or diflunisal, in daily doses of 500 to 750 mg, in a 12-week, double-blind, parallel study, diflunisal was better than aspirin at 8 and 12 weeks for night pain, weight-bearing pain, stiffness, functional activity, and global response. Diflunisal, at 500 to 750 mg/day, was also better than 800- to 1,200-mg doses of ibuprofen.[283]

Adverse Effects

As expected for an NSAID, 25% of 657 patients had gastrointestinal effects: 0.5% had ulcers or hemorrhage; 17% had dyspepsia, pain, or cramps; and 9% had diarrhea or nausea. In addition, 0 to 5% had rashes, dizziness, or drowsiness. In these studies, diflunisal was associated with fewer gastrointestinal effects than aspirin (47% for aspirin versus 25% for diflunisal), and tinnitus occurred in only 1%. Diflunisal caused less microscopic gas-

---

Dosage

The drug is supplied as 250- and 500-mg tablets.

Although it is a molecular modification of salicylic acid, diflunisal is not metabolized to salicylate and is not equivalent to the nonacetylated salicylates or aspirin in dose or mode of action.

Diflunisal has capacity-limited metabolism, and consequently, serum half-lives are raised by increasing doses. When one is using the usually recommended daily dose of 1,000 mg, half-lives are about 12 hours and allow twice-daily administration. Although a dose of 1,000 mg a day has no antiplatelet effects, a dose of 1,500 mg daily reversibly inhibits platelet aggregation. Diflunisal is currently recommended only for osteoarthritis or as an analgesic.

---

trointestinal bleeding than aspirin, as measured with ^{51}chromium (^{51}Cr)-labeled red cells; after 2 weeks, 8.8 ml/24 hours with aspirin, as compared with 2.1 ml/24 hours with diflunisal and 1.6 ml/24 hours with placebo.[225]

Other Nonsteroidal Anti-Inflammatory Drugs

An efficient system has been developed for detecting chemicals with NSAID properties. Many such agents are being developed. Many await approval for marketing, and some have already been marketed in various parts of the world. Only a few examples are given here.

Azapropazone

Azapropazone, a pyrazole derivative, is similar in many ways to phenylbutazone, but thus far does not appear to cause agranulocytosis. It inhibits prostaglandin synthesis and is active in most animal models of inflammation.[136] After 600-mg oral doses, it reaches a peak level in 4.4 hours. The drug has an absolute bioavailability of 83 ± 19% (SD) and an excretion half-life in normal subjects of 14.3 ± 2.8 hours. Most of the drug is excreted in the urine, 60% as unchanged azapropazone. It has a prolonged terminal half-life of 31 hours in elderly patients (mean age 85 years), primarily associated with decreased renal function.[229] Severe renal or hepatic disease decreases clearance of the drug, but moderate hepatic disease has only a minimal effect.[26] Albumin binding is greater than 99.5% in normal subjects. Drug interactions include the following: (1) displacement of albumin-bound warfarin by azapropazone; (2) increase in phenytoin plasma levels; and (3) induction of hypoglycemia by the interaction between azapropazone and tolbutamide.[7,290]

Azapropazone, at 1,200 mg/day, was more effective in controlled trials in patients with RA than placebo, 3.9 g aspirin, 100 mg indomethacin, or 600 mg phenylbutazone daily;[39] in patients with osteoarthritis, it was more effective than 2.25 g aspirin or 1,600 mg ibuprofen daily.[39] Azapropazone has been studied in patients with psoriatic arthritis and Reiter's disease,[39] and it has been effective in the treatment of acute and chronic gout.[67] As with phenylbutazone, another pyrazole derivative, azapropazone is also uricosuric.[67] In 63 patients with osteoarthritis and in 73 with RA, no clear difference was found between 600 mg azapropazone twice daily and 300 mg 4 times daily.[276]

Because daily doses of 1,800 mg azapropazone are associated with an increased incidence of gastrointestinal side effects, doses of 1,200 mg/day are prescribed in most clinical studies of rheumatic

diseases. In our tabulation of approximately 300 patients, in some of the published studies, 13% of patients had side effects: 0.9% developed peptic ulcers, 3% has nausea or dyspepsia, and 3% had rashes. Other side effects usually seen with NSAID were also reported. No significant laboratory abnormalities were noted, but much more experience will be needed before potential hematologic adverse reactions can be excluded.

Carprofen

Carprofen is a carbazole derivative. In animal and in vitro studies, it is a cyclo-oxygenase inhibitor, has an enterohepatic circulation, is highly metabolized, and inhibits in vitro tests of platelet aggregation.[101,239] In man, the relative bioavailability of carprofen is 88%; 75% of a usual dose appears in the urine, and 25% appears in the feces.[222] From 3 to 5% of urinary excretion and 7% of fecal excretion are unchanged drug.[222] The elimination half-life of the drug is 13 to 27 hours.[222] Aspirin decreases carprofen's AUC by 37%, and probenecid decreases urinary excretion of the drug by more than 50% in the first 24 hours after a single dose.[252,313]

Although few large clinical trials have been published, a daily dose of 600 mg carprofen appears to be more effective than placebo in RA and approximately as effective as 100 to 150 mg indomethacin and 2.4 to 3.6 g aspirin.[134,172] A crossover study in 14 patients with osteoarthritis indicated that a dose of 300 mg carprofen was approximately equivalent to 100 mg indomethacin.[66] Similarly, an open trial showed that carprofen was effective against gout.[313]

Published data suggest that carprofen has the same type and frequency of side effects as other NSAID, with gastrointestinal adverse effects the most common.[66,134,172] Rashes are slightly more frequent than with other NSAID, but they do not usually require discontinuance of the drug.[66,134,172] Liver function tests are occasionally abnormal, but acute renal failure has not yet been documented in the literature.[134]

Flurbiprofen

Flurbiprofen, a phenylalkanoic acid derivative and a cyclo-oxygenase inhibitor, has anti-inflammatory effects in various animal models.[30] Flurbiprofen is rapidly absorbed, with peak concentrations in 1.5 to 3 hours and an elimination half-life of 3 to 4 hours.[30] It is more than 99% albumin bound at therapeutic concentrations; it is present in higher concentrations in synovial fluid than in serum after 9 hours.[30,228] Flurbiprofen is extensively metabolized and is principally excreted through the kidneys, although it may have an enterohepatic recirculation.[30] In clinical trials in patients with RA and ankylosing spondylitis, flurbiprofen, at doses of 150 to 300 mg per day, was comparable to aspirin, indomethacin, ibuprofen, sulindac, or mefenamic acid.[30] A 100-mg dose of flurbiprofen twice daily may be more effective than a 50-mg dose 4 times a day.[147] In studies in patients with osteoarthritis, daily doses of 150 to 300 mg were as effective as ibuprofen or naproxen.[30] The drug was also reported to be effective in ankylosing spondylitis when comparisons were made with placebo, and with daily doses of naproxen, 750 mg, ibuprofen, 1,600 mg, indomethacin, 75 to 100 mg, and phenylbutazone, 300 to 400 mg.[30,187]

Brogden et al., in their compendium of the studies on flurbiprofen, indicated that gastrointestinal effects occur in 15 to 20% of patients.[30] Gastrointestinal adverse effects were more frequent with flurbiprofen than with low doses of ibuprofen or with 750 mg naproxen daily. Dyspepsia, epigastric pain, and other gastrointestinal side effects occurred in 15 to 25% more patients taking flurbiprofen than taking aspirin, but the withdrawal rate was the same for both drugs. Headaches, loss of hearing, and tinnitus were less frequent than with moderate doses of aspirin or indomethacin.[30] In long-term, open studies in 1,220 patients, the incidence of adverse reactions was 52.5%, but no age-related increase in these reactions was noted.[260]

Ketoprofen

Ketoprofen is a propionic acid derivative that has been marketed in Europe since 1973. It inhibits both the cyclo-oxygenase and lipoxygenase pathways of arachidonic acid metabolism.[60] Following a single oral dose, the drug is rapidly and completely absorbed, with peak plasma levels 1 to 2 hours after the dose. Disappearance from plasma is rapid because the drug's half-life is 1.5 hours and is entirely due to hepatic hydroxylation and glucuronidation of the parent compound; no unchanged ketoprofen is excreted in the urine.[284] Because its plasma clearance depends on hepatic metabolism, renal insufficiency has only a modest effect on its half-life and does not cause significant accumulation of ketoprofen or require dose adjustment.[271] Food decreases the rate, but not the completeness, of ketoprofen absorption. Ketoprofen is about 99% bound to plasma proteins, but treatment with this drug does not affect the activity of digoxin or warfarin. Aspirin displaces ketoprofen from its albumin-binding sites, increases plasma clearance of unbound drug, and thus decreases total plasma ketoprofen concentrations; however, unbound concentrations do not change, and ketoprofen efficacy is probably unaffected.[305] Probenecid raises both total and unbound ketopro-

fen plasma levels, prolongs the plasma half-life, decreases protein binding of ketoprofen, and lowers the rate of hepatic conjugation, by competitive inhibition.[285]

Daily doses of ketoprofen range from 50 to 400 mg, although 150 to 200 mg are usually prescribed in 3 doses. The drug, in clinical studies, was superior to placebo in patients with RA.[92] Ketoprofen, 150 to 200 mg a day, was equivalent to 3.6 to 4.0 g aspirin, 100 to 150 mg indomethacin, 300 to 400 mg phenylbutazone, 2.6 g fenoprofen, or 500 mg naproxen daily in treating RA.[92,128] Ketoprofen is effective in JRA, but perhaps less so than indomethacin.[20] Patients with osteoarthritis responded to ketoprofen as well as to aspirin or phenylbutazone, although indomethacin was slightly more effective.[92] In daily doses of 100 to 150 mg, ketoprofen was effective in a few patients with ankylosing spondylitis or gout.[92]

Gastrointestinal and central nervous system side effects predominate. Studies of gastrointestinal blood loss with ^{51}Cr-labeled red blood cells showed that 4.3 ml/day were lost when 200 mg ketoprofen were administered daily for a week. This finding compared to 10.1 ml/day with 3.6 g aspirin/day and 1.2 ml/day with placebo.[173]

CHOICE AND USE OF NONSTEROIDAL ANTI-INFLAMMATORY DRUGS

Of prime importance is the need to individualize dosage. In all kinetic studies of NSAID, one of the most striking findings is the great range of serum concentrations in individual patients. Such variability is best documented with aspirin, with which three- or fourfold differences in steady-state serum salicylate levels occur in small groups of patients taking the same weight-adjusted doses. Although the range of individual responses is obscured in many of the kinetic studies summarized here because mean values are used for clarity of presentation, substantial individual variability is actually present with respect to the pharmacology of these drugs.[95] Therefore, in treating any patient, it is essential to adjust the therapy to the patient's response, rather than to assume the appropriateness of an average recommended dose or dosage interval.

For aspirin and the nonacetylated salicylates, dosage can be most effectively individualized by monitoring serum salicylate concentrations; we aim for values between 10 and 30 mg/100 ml (100 to 300 μg/ml or 100 to 300 mg/l). These values overlap those at which symptoms of mild salicylism are seen. Thus, the development of tinnitus can be used as a general guide to adequate salicylate levels, although this observation is inconstant and is not valid in patients with pre-existing hearing loss.

A relationship between naproxen serum levels and efficacy has been proposed;[61] if confirmed, recommendations for "therapeutic" naproxen serum levels may be useful as a guide for adjusting the dosage of this drug. Although easily measured, serum concentrations are not readily available for most NSAID. We recommend starting with the average recommended dose and then cautiously increasing stepwise to the maximum recommended dose until optimal therapeutic effects or minimal side effects develop. For some patients, the optimal dose may be low, whereas others may not achieve a satisfactory response even with the maximum recommended doses. With increasing clinical experience, the maximum doses of many of the newer NSAID have been raised.

Because aspirin has a long tradition in rheumatology, it has been customary to give it to nearly everyone and to add other medications to baseline aspirin therapy. With the proliferation of NSAID, it is now possible to give a single patient many NSAID simultaneously. We do not think that the data justify this practice. Studies in rat paw edema have not demonstrated additive anti-inflammatory effects with coadministration of more than one NSAID,[189] and rat adjuvant arthritis studies have shown decreased anti-inflammatory effect when a second drug was added to a background NSAID.[288] In one study, no increase in anti-inflammatory effect in RA patients was achieved by a combination of 100 mg indomethacin and 4 g aspirin daily, as compared to each drug given alone, and the toxicity of the combination was greater.[36] Similarly, when tolmetin was added to a background of aspirin therapy, no additive clinical effect was found.[231]

The addition of aspirin has been demonstrated to decrease plasma levels of several NSAID,[190] and it may increase the risk of gastrointestinal bleeding with piroxicam.[19] The addition of 500 mg naproxen daily to aspirin, 1.3 to 5.2 g daily, however, was more effective than aspirin alone in RA,[307] but the patients receiving the larger aspirin doses showed the least improvement. This finding suggests that the combination was more effective only if the baseline therapy was suboptimal. The patients in this study may have been receiving all their benefit from the naproxen alone. A study of only 10 RA patients concluded that the combination of 3.9 g aspirin and 600 mg benoxaprofen daily was more effective than either drug alone; the additive effect was postulated to be due to the addition of lipoxygenase inhibition by benoxaprofen to the cyclooxygenase inhibition by aspirin.[226] Unless new data supporting specific combinations of NSAID become available, *we do not recommend concurrent administration of more than one NSAID.* Efficacy

is unlikely to be increased, and toxicity may well be additive.

How should one choose an NSAID for a particular patient? Factors to consider include complicating illnesses and other drug intake. For example, if a patient is taking warfarin or has an ulcer, the effects of NSAID on coagulation must be weighed. If a patient is taking a sulfonylurea hypoglycemic agent, treatment with phenylbutazone may require a change in its dose. In addition to individually variable dose-response relationships, some patients probably respond much better to one NSAID than they do to another, although the reasons for this phenomenon are unknown. In a number of well-designed cross-over studies, 4 or more NSAID were compared; the number of subjects per study ranged from 32 to 141.[42,43,100,128,254,296] In general, the preferences of the patient and the physician were the only measures useful in ranking the drugs. In 5 studies in RA, no first choice was noted in 2, whereas naproxen ranked first in 2 and indomethacin first in 1 study. Indomethacin and naproxen were the most frequently preferred among 6 NSAID studied in ankylosing spondylitis,[296] and tolmetin was the first choice among 4 NSAID studied in osteoarthritis.[42] No study demonstrated an overwhelming preference for any single drug, however; each drug was strongly preferred by some patients. In all these comparative studies, aspirin was preferred by fewer patients, usually because it caused more side effects. It also appeared to be less effective against symptoms of ankylosing spondylitis.[106,296]

Because one cannot predict which NSAID will be most effective for an individual patient, treatment should be initiated with one drug, and the dose should be increased gradually until the optimal or maximum tolerated dose is reached. That dose should be continued for several weeks. If the patient has an inadequate therapeutic response, the first drug should be replaced with a second NSAID, and the process should be repeated. These individual therapeutic trials can be repeated with new drugs; one should persist for at least two weeks at the optimal tolerated dose, until the most effective drug for that particular patient has been found. Our prejudice against pyramiding NSAID does not apply to the appropriate addition of a slowly acting antirheumatic agent, such as a gold compound or d-penicillamine, to initial therapy with an NSAID.

REFERENCES

1. Abramson, S., et al.: The neutrophil in rheumatoid arthritis: its role and the inhibition of its activation by nonsteroidal anti-inflammatory drugs. Semin. Arthritis Rheum., *13(Suppl. 1)*:148–153, 1983.
2. Abruzzo, J.L., Gordan, G.V., and Meyers, D.R.: Double-blind study comparing piroxicam and aspirin in the treat-

ment of osteoarthritis. Am. J. Med., *72(Suppl. 2A)*:45–49, 1982.

3. Aggeler, P.M., et al.: Potentiation of anticoagulant effect of warfarin by phenylbutazone. N. Engl. J. Med., *276*:496–501, 1967.

4. Alvares, A.P., et al.: Drug metabolism in normal children, lead poisoned children, and normal adults. Clin. Pharmacol. Ther., *17*:179–183, 1975.

5. Andelman, S.Y.: Long-term double blind comparison of sulindac and aspirin in the treatment of osteoarthritis. Postgrad. Med. Comm., *Special Report*:21–32, 1979.

6. Andreasen, F.: Protein binding of drugs in plasma from patients with acute renal failure. Acta Pharmacol. Toxicol., *32*:417–429, 1973.

7. Andreasen, P.B., et al.: Hypoglycemia induced by azapropazone-tolbutamide interaction. Br. J. Clin. Pharmacol., *12*:581–583, 1981.

8. Antilla, M., Haataja, M., and Kasanen, A.: Pharmacokinetics of naproxen in subjects with normal and impaired renal function. Eur. J. Clin. Pharmacol., *11*:263–268, 1980.

9. Arisz, L., et al.: The effect of indomethacin on proteinuria and kidney function in the nephrotic syndrome. Acta Med. Scand., *199*:121–125, 1976.

10. Athreya, B.H., et al.: Aspirin-induced hepatotoxicity in JRA. Arthritis Rheum., *18*:347–352, 1975.

11. Ayres, J.R., et al.: Linear and non-linear assessment of tolmetin pharmacokinetics. Res. Commun. Chem. Pathol. Pharmacol., *17*:583–593, 1977.

12. Baber, N., et al.: The interaction between indomethacin and probenecid. Clin. Pharmacol. Ther., *24*:298–306, 1978.

13. Ballas, Z.K., and Donta, S.T.: Sulindac induced aseptic meningitis. Arch. Intern. Med., *142*:165–166, 1982.

14. Barager, F.D., and Duthie, J.J.R.: Importance of aspirin as a cause of anemia and peptic ulcer in rheumatoid arthritis. Br. Med. J., *1*:1106–1108, 1960.

15. Barager, F.D., and Smith, T.C.: Drug interaction studies with sodium meclofenamate (Meclomen). Curr. Ther. Res., *23(Suppl.)*:51–59, 1978.

16. Barnes, C.G., et al.: A double blind comparison of naproxen with indomethacin in osteoarthritis. J. Clin. Pharmacol., *15*:347–354, 1975.

17. Beaver, W.T., Forbes, J.A., and Shackleford, R.W.: A method for the 12 hour evaluation of analgesic efficacy in outpatients with postoperative oral surgery pain. Pharmacotherapy, *3*:23S–37S, 1983.

18. Bender, A.D.: The effect of increasing age on the distribution of peripheral blood flow in man. J. Am. Geriatr. Soc., *13*:192–198, 1965.

19. Benoxaprofen and piroxicam: two new drugs for arthritis. Med. Lett. Drugs Ther., *24*:63–66, 1982.

20. Bhettay, E., and Tomson, A.J.G.: Double-blind study of ketoprofen and indomethacin in juvenile chronic arthritis. S. Afr. Med. J., *54*:276–282, 1978.

21. Blechman, W.J., and Lechner, B.L.: Clinical comparative evaluation of choline magnesium trisalicylate and acetylsalicylic acid in rheumatoid arthritis. Rheumatol. Rehabil., *18*:119–124, 1979.

22. Bluestone, R.: Safety and efficacy of piroxicam in the treatment of gout. Am. J. Med., *72 (Suppl. 2A)*:66–69, 1982.

23. Boardman, P.L., and Hart, F.D.: Clinical measurement of the anti-inflammatory effect of salicylates in rheumatoid arthritis. Br. Med. J., *4*:264–268, 1967.

24. Bonssina, I., Gunthner, W., and Marti' Masso', R.: Double-blind multicenter study comparing meclofenamate sodium with indomethacin and placebo in the treatment of extra-articular rheumatic disease. Arzneim. Forsch., *33*:649–652, 1983.

25. Borga, O., et al.: Protein binding of salicylate in uremic and normal plasma. Clin. Pharmacol. Ther., *20*:464–475, 1976.

26. Breuing, K.H., et al.: Disposition of azapropazone in chronic renal and hepatic failure. Eur. J. Clin. Pharmacol., *20*:147–155, 1981.

27. Brewer, E.J.: Non-steroidal anti-inflammatory agents. Arthritis Rheum., *20*:513–516, 1977.

28. Brewer, E.J., et al.: Sodium meclofenemate (Meclomen) in the treatment of juvenile rheumatoid arthritis. J. Rheumatol., *9*:129–134, 1982.

29. Briggs, D.F., Couts, R.T., and Walter, L.J.: A note on the bioavailability of five Canadian brands of acetylsalicylic acid tablets. Can. J. Pharm. Sci., *12*:23–25, 1977.

30. Brogden, R.N., et al.: Flurbiprofen: a review of its pharmacological properties and therapeutic use in rheumatic diseases. Drugs, *18*:417–438, 1979.

31. Brogden, R.N., et al.: Naproxen up to date: a review of its pharmacological properties and therapeutic efficacy and use in rheumatic diseases and pain states. Drugs, *18*:241–277, 1979.

32. Brogden, R.N., et al.: Sulindac: a review of its pharmacological properties and therapeutic efficacy in rheumatic diseases. Drugs, *16*:97–114, 1978.

33. Brogden, R.N., et al.: Tolmetin: a review of its pharmacological properties and therapeutic efficacy in rheumatic diseases. Drugs, *15*:429–450, 1978.

34. Brogden, R.N., et al.: Naproxen: a review of its pharmacological properties and therapeutic efficacy and use. Drugs, *9*:326–363, 1975.

35. Brooke, J.W.: Fenoprofen therapy in large joint osteoarthritis: double blind comparison with aspirin and long-term experience. J. Rheumatol., *3(Suppl. 2)*:71–75, 1976.

36. Brooks, P.M., et al.: Indomethacin-aspirin interaction: a clinical appraisal. Br. Med. J., *3*:69–71, 1975.

37. Brooks, P.M., et al.: Phenylbutazone. A clinico-pharmacological study in rheumatoid arthritis. Br. J. Clin. Pharmacol., *2*:437–442, 1975.

38. Brooks, P.M., et al.: The clinical significance of indomethacin-probenecid interactions. Br. J. Clin. Pharmacol., *1*:287–290, 1974.

39. Brooks, P.M., and Buchanan, W.W.: Azapropazone: its place in the management of rheumatoid conditions. Curr. Med. Res. Opin., *4*:94–99, 1976.

40. Brugueras, N.E., LeZotte, L.A., and Moxley, T.E.: Ibuprofen: a double-blind comparison of twice-a-day therapy with four-times-a-day therapy. Clin. Ther., *2*:13–21, 1978.

41. Caldwell, J., et al.: Double blind comparison of the efficacy and side-effect liability of tolmetin and indomethacin. *In* Tolmetin. Edited by J.R. Ward. Princeton, Excerpta Medica, 1975, pp. 71–84.

42. Caldwell, J.R., et al.: Four-way, multicenter, cross over trial of ibuprofen, fenoprofen calcium, naproxen and tolmetin sodium in osteoarthritis. South. Med. J., *76*:706–711, 1983.

43. Capell, H.A., et al.: Patient compliance: a novel method of testing nonsteroidal anti-inflammatory analgesics in rheumatoid arthritis. J. Rheumatol., *6*:584–593, 1979.

44. Carr, R.E., and Siegel, I.M.: Retinal function in patients treated with indomethacin. Am. J. Ophthalmol., *75*:302–306, 1973.

45. Chan, W.Y., and Daword, M.Y.: Prostaglandins in primary dysmenorrhea: comparison of prophylactic and non-prophylactic treatment with ibuprofen and use of oral contraceptives. Am. J. Med., *70*:535–541, 1981.

46. Chang, Y.-H.: Studies on phagocytosis II. The effect of NSAID on phagocytosis and on urate crystal-induced joint inflammation. J. Pharmacol. Exp. Ther., *183*:235–244, 1972.

47. Chernish, S.M., et al.: The physiological disposition of fenoprofen in man. IV. J. Med. (Basel), *83*:249–257, 1972.

48. Chignell, C.F., and Starkweather, D.K.: Optical studies of drug protein complexes. Mol. Pharmacol., *7*:229–237, 1971.

49. Cho, A.K., Hodshon, B.J., and Brodie, B.B.: Effect of phenylbutazone on liver microsomal demethylase. Biochem. Pharmacol., *19*:1817–1823, 1970.

50. Ciosek, C.P., Jr., et al.: Indomethacin potentiates PGE-stimulated C-AMP accumulation in human synoviocytes. Nature, *251*:145–150, 1974.

51. Cohen, L., and Banks, P.: Salivary gland enlargement in phenylbutazone. Br. Med. J., *1*:1420, 1966.

52. Cooke, A.R.: Drugs and gastric damage. Drugs, *11*:36–44, 1976.

53. Court, H., Streete, P., and Volans, G.: Acute poisoning with ibuprofen. Hum. Toxicol., *2*:381–384, 1983.

54. Cuthbert, M.F.: Adverse reactions to nonsteroidal anti-inflammatory drugs. Curr. Med. Res. Opin., *2*:600–610, 1974.

55. Dahl, S.L., and Ward, J.R.: Pharmacology, clinical efficacy and adverse effects of piroxicam, a new nonsteroidal anti-inflammatory agent. Pharmacotherapy, *2*:80–90, 1982.

56. Davenport, H.W.: Salicylate damage to the gastric mucosa barrier. N. Engl. J. Med., *276*:1307–1312, 1967.

57. Davidson, C., and Manohitharajah, S.M.: Drug-induced antiplatelet antibodies. Br. Med. J., *3*:545, 1973.

58. Davies, E.F., and Avery, G.S.: Ibuprofen: a review of its pharmacological properties and therapeutic efficacy in rheumatic disorders. Drugs, *2*:416–446, 1971.

59. Davies, R.O.: Review of the animal and clinical pharmacology of diflunisal. Pharmacotherapy, *3*:23S–37S, 1983.

60. Dawson, W., et al.: The pharmacology of benoxaprofen with reference to effects on lipoxygenase product formation. Eur. J. Rheumatol. Inflammation, *5*:61–68, 1982.

61. Day, R.O., et al.: Relationship of serum naproxen concentration to efficacy in rheumatoid arthritis. Clin. Pharmacol. Ther., *31*:733–740, 1982.

62. Deodhar, S.D., et al.: A short-term comparative trial of salsalate and indomethacin in rheumatoid arthritis. Curr. Med. Res., *5*:185–188, 1977.

63. Desproges-Gotteron, R., Comte, B., and Leroy, V.: A double blind comparison of alclofenac and indomethacin in osteoarthritis of the hip. Curr. Ther. Res., *13*:393–397, 1971.

64. Dewse, C.D.: Inhibition of DNA synthesis in cultured human lymphocytes by phenylbutazone and oxyphenbutazone. J. Pharm. Pharmacol., *28*:596–598, 1976.

65. Diamond, H.S., and Bankhurst, A.D.: Double blind comparison of sulindac and phenylbutazone in acute gouty arthritis. Postgrad. Med. Comm., *Special Report*:75–80, 1979.

66. Dickey, R.A., et al.: Double-blind cross-over trial of carprofen in osteoarthritis. (Abstract.) *In* Proceedings of the International Meeting on Inflammation, Verona, September 24 to 27, 1979, p. 75.

67. Dieppe, P.A., et al.: The treatment of gout with azapropazone: clinical and experimental studies. Eur. J. Rheumatol. Inflammation, *3*:392–400, 1981.

68. Dieppe, P.A., et al.: Sulindac and osteoarthritis of the hip. Rheumatol. Rehabil., *15*:112–115, 1976.

69. Dieterle, W., et al.: Metabolism of phenylbutazone in man. Arzneim. Forsch., *26*:572–577, 1976.

70. Diflunisal. Med. Lett. Drugs Ther., *24*:76–78, 1982.

71. Dillon, N., et al.: Age and beta-adrenoceptor-mediated function. Clin. Pharmacol. Ther., *27*:769–772, 1980.

72. DiRosa, M., Papadimitrion, J.M., and Willoughby, D.A.: A histopathological and pharmacological analysis of the mode of action of NSAID. J. Pathol., *105*:239–256, 1971.

73. Divoll, M., et al.: Effect of food on acetaminophen absorption in young and elderly subjects. J. Clin. Pharmacol., *22*:571–576, 1982.

74. Dresse, A., et al.: Effect of diflunisal on the human plasma levels and on the urinary excretion of naproxen. Arch. Int. Pharmacodyn. Ther., *236*:276–284, 1978.

75. Dromgoole, S.H., Furst, D.E., and Paulus, H.E.: Rational approaches to the use of salicylates in the treatment of rheumatoid arthritis. Semin. Arthritis Rheum., *11*:257–283, 1982.

76. Duggan, D.E., et al.: Disposition of sulindac. Clin. Pharmacol. Ther., *21*:326–335, 1977.

77. Duggan, D.E., et al.: Enterohepatic circulation of indomethacin and intestinal irritation. Biochem. Pharmacol., *24*:1749–1754, 1975.

78. Duggan, D.E., Hooke, K.F., and Hwang, S.S.: Kinetics of the tissue distribution of sulindac and metabolites. Drug Metab. Dispos., *8*:241–246, 1980.

79. Eade, O.E., et al.: Peripheral neuropathy and indomethacin. Br. Med. J., *2*:66–67, 1975.

80. Eberl, R.: Long-term experience with meclofenamate sodium. Arzneim. Forsch., *33(Suppl. 4a)*:667–678, 1983.

81. Eberl, R., and Dunky, A.: Meclofenamate sodium in the treatment of acute gout. Arzneim. Forsch., *33(Suppl. 4a)*:641–643, 1983.

82. Ebner, W., Ballarin, J.M.P., and Bonssina, I.: Meclofenamate sodium in the treatment of ankylosing spondylitis. Arzneim. Forsch., *33(Suppl. 4a)*:660–663, 1983.

83. Editorial. Lancet, *2*:961–962, 1975.

84. Eeg-Olofsson, O., et al.: Convulsions in a breast fed infant after maternal indomethacin. Lancet, *2*:215, 1978.

85. Ehrlich, G.E., et al.: Long-term therapy with rheumatoid arthritis. *In* Tolmetin. Edited by J. R. Ward. Princeton, Excerpta Medica, 1975, pp. 85–101.

86. Ehrlich, G.E., and Wortham, G.F.: Pseudo-proteinuria in tolmetin-treated patients. Clin. Pharmacol. Ther., *17*:467–468, 1975.

87. Emkey, R.D., and Mills, J.A.: Aspirin and analgesic nephropathy. JAMA, *247*:55–57, 1982.

88. FDA Drug Bulletin. November, 1979.

89. Ferriera, S.H.: Prostaglandins and nonsteroidal anti-inflammatory drugs. *In* Prostaglandins and Thromboxanes. Edited by F. Berti, B. Samuelson, and G. P. Velvo. New York, Plenum Press, 1976, pp. 353–360.

90. Field, J.B.: Effect of phenylbutazone on renal excretion. N. Engl. J. Med., *278*:218, 1968.

90a. Findling, J.W., et al.: Indomethacin-induced hyperkalemia in three patients with gouty arthritis. JAMA, *244*:1127–1128, 1980.

91. Flower, R.J., Vane, J.R.: Inhibition of prostaglandin synthetase in brain explains the antipyretic activity of paracetamol (4 acetamidophenol). Nature, *240*:410–411, 1972.

92. Fossgreen, J.: Ketoprofen, a survey of current publications. Scand. J. Rheumatol., *5 (Suppl. 14)*:7–32, 1976.

93. Fowler, P.D., Woolf, D., and Alexander, S.: Phenylbutazone and hepatitis. Rheumatol. Rehabil., *14*:71–75, 1975.

94. Fremont-Smith, K., and Bayles, T.B.: Salicylate therapy in rheumatoid arthritis. JAMA, *192*:1133–1136, 1965.

95. Fries, J.F., and Britton, M.C.: Fenoprofen calcium in rheumatoid arthritis. Arthritis Rheum., *16*:629–634, 1973.

96. Furst, D.E., et al.: Comparison of tolmetin kinetics in rheumatoid arthritis and matched healthy controls. J. Clin. Pharmacol., *23*:329–335, 1983.

97. Furst, D.E., Gupta, N., and Paulus, H.E.: Salicylate metabolism in twins. J. Clin. Invest., *60*:32–38, 1977.

98. Furst, D.E., Tozer, T.N., and Melmon, K.L.: Salicylate clearance, the resultant of protein binding and metabolism. Clin. Pharmacol. Ther., *26*:380–389, 1979.

99. Gall, E.P.: Hyperuricemia and gout: a modern approach to diagnosis and treatment. Postgrad. Med., *65*:163–171, 1979.

100. Gall, E.P., et al.: Clinical comparison of ibuprofen, fenoprofen calcium, naproxen, and tolmetin sodium in rheumatoid arthritis. J. Rheumatol., *9*:402–407, 1982.

101. Gaut, Z.N., et al.: Stereoisomeric relationships among anti-inflammatory activity, inhibition of platelet aggregation and inhibition of prostaglandin synthetase. Prostaglandins, *10*:59–66, 1975.

102. Gengos, D., Pingeon, R.A., and Andrew, A.: Double blind evaluation of sulindac and oxyphenbutazone in the treatment of acute pain of the shoulder. Postgrad. Med. Comm., *Special Report*:69–74, 1979.

103. Giansiracusa, J.E., et al.: Ibuprofen in osteoarthritis. South. Med. J., *70*:49–52, 1977.

104. Gibson, T., and Laurent, R.: Sulindac and indomethacin in treatment of ankylosing spondylitis: A double-blind crossover study. Rheumatol. Rehabil., *19*:189–192, 1980.

105. Glazko, A.J., et al.: Metabolic disposition of meclofenamic acid (Meclomen) in laboratory animals and in man. Curr. Ther. Res., *23(Suppl.)*:22–41, 1978.

106. Godfrey, R.G., et al.: A double-blind crossover trial of

aspirin, indomethacin and phenylbutazone in ankylosing spondylitis. Arthritis Rheum., *15*:110–111, 1972.

107. Godfrey, R.G., and de la Cruz, S.: Effect of ibuprofen dosage on patient response in rheumatoid arthritis. Arthritis Rheum., *18*:135–137, 1975.

108. Goldenberg, A., Rudnicki, R.D., and Koonce, M.L.: Clinical comparison of efficacy and safety of choline magnesium trisalicylate and indomethacin in treating osteoarthritis. Curr. Ther. Res., *24*:245–260, 1978.

109. Goodwin, J.S., and Ceuppens, J.L.: Effect of nonsteroidal anti-inflammatory drugs on immune function. Semin. Arthritis Rheum., *13(Suppl. 1)*:134–143, 1983.

110. Graham, G.G., et al.: The pharmacokinetics of ibuprofen in healthy subjects and patients with rheumatoid arthritis. Personal Communication, 1982.

111. Grayson, M.F., Martin, V.N., and Markham, R.L.: Antinative DNA antibodies as a reaction to pyrazole. Ann. Rheum. Dis., *34*:373–375, 1975.

112. Greenblatt, D.J., Sellers, E.M., and Shader, R.I.: Drug disposition in old age. N. Engl. J. Med., *306*:1081–1088, 1982.

113. Gruber, C.M., Jr.: Clinical pharmacology of fenoprofen: a review. J. Rheumatol., *3(Suppl. 2)*:8–17, 1976.

114. Gryffe, C.I., and Rubenzahl, S.: Agranulocytosis and aplastic anemia possibly due to ibuprofen. Can. Med. Assoc. J., *114*:877–880, 1976.

115. Gum, O.B.: Fenoprofen in rheumatoid arthritis: a controlled multicentered study. J. Rheumatol., 3(Suppl. 2):26–31, 1976.

116. Halla, J.T., Fallahi, S., and Hardin, J.G.: Acute and chronic salicylate intoxication in a patient with gastric outlet obstruction. Arthritis Rheum., *24*:1205–1207, 1981.

117. Hamdy, R.C., et al.: The pharmacokinetics of benoxaprofen in elderly subjects. Eur. J. Rheumatol. Rehabil., *5*:69–75, 1982.

118. Hanson, F.W.: Naproxen sodium, ibuprofen and placebo in dysmenorrhea. J. Reprod. Med., *27*:423–427, 1982.

119. Hansten, P.D. (Ed.): Lithium and indomethacin. Drug Interaction Newsl., *1*:47–48, 1981.

120. Hansten, P.D. (Ed.): Sulindac and warfarin. Drug Interaction Newsl., *1*:26, 1981.

121. Hansten, P.D.: Drugs which may enhance the effects of diphenylhydantoin. *In* Drug Interactions. Philadelphia, Lea & Febiger, 1973, pp. 54–69.

121a. Hansten, P.D.: Effects of monoamine oxidase inhibitors (MAOI) on the actions of other drugs, and combined toxicity with other drugs. *In* Drug Interactions. Philadelphia, Lea & Febiger, 1973, pp. 185–198.

122. Hashimoto, M., et al.: Studies on disposition and metabolism of tolmetin, a new anti-inflammatory agent, in rats and mice. I and II. Drug Metab. Dispos., *7*:14–23, 1979.

123. Hayes, M.J., Langman, M.J.S., and Short, A.H.: Changes in drug metabolism with increasing age: warfarin binding and plasma proteins. Br. J. Clin. Pharmacol., *2*:69–72, 1975.

124. Hill, H.F.H., and Hill, A.G.S.: Ankylosing spondylitis: open long-term and double-blind cross over studies with naproxen. J. Clin. Pharmacol., *15*:355–362, 1975.

125. Hill, J.B.: Salicylate intoxication. N. Engl. J. Med., *288*:1110–1113, 1973.

126. Holt, P.R.: Measurement of gastrointestinal blood loss in subjects taking aspirin. J. Lab. Clin. Invest., *56*:717–729, 1960.

127. Howell, D.S.: Osteoarthritis—etiology and pathogenesis. *In* Symposium on Osteoarthritis. St. Louis, C.V. Mosby, 1976, pp. 80–85.

128. Huskisson, E.C., et al.: Four new anti-inflammatory drugs: responses and variations. Br. Med. J., *1*:1048–1049, 1976.

129. Ito, H., et al.: Indomethacin responsive hypercalcemia. N. Engl. J. Med., *293*:558–559, 1975.

130. Jabbari, M., and Vallberg, L.S.: Role of acid secretion in aspirin-induced gastric mucosal injury. Can. Med. Assoc. J., *102*:178–182, 1970.

131. Jaffe, B.N., et al.: Indomethacin responsive pancreatic cholera. N. Engl. J. Med., *97*:817–820, 1977.

132. Jain, A., et al.: Effect of naproxen on the steady state

serum concentration and anticoagulant activity of warfarin. Clin. Pharmacol. Ther., *25*:61–66, 1979.

133. Jalava, S., et al.: Naproxen concentrations in serum, synovial fluid and synovium. Scand. J. Rheumatol., *6*:155–157, 1977.

134. Jensen, E.M., et al.: Treatment of rheumatoid arthritis with carprofen (Imadyl) or indomethacin: a randomized multicenter trial. Curr. Ther. Res., *28*:882–887, 1980.

135. Jentsch, D.D.: Tolectin treatment for rheumatoid arthritis and gout. *In* Thirteenth International Congress of Rheumatology. Princeton, Excerpta Medica, 1975, p. 114.

136. Jones, C.J.: The pharmacology and pharmacokinetics of azapropazone—a review. Curr. Med. Res. Opin., *4*:3–16, 1976.

137. Jugdutt, B.I., et al.: Salvage of ischemic myocardium by ibuprofen during infarction in the conscious dog. Am. J. Cardiol., *46*:74–82, 1980.

138. Juhl, R.P., et al.: Ibuprofen and sulindac kinetics in alcoholic liver disease. Clin. Pharmacol. Ther., *34*:104–109, 1983.

139. Kantor, T.G.: Ibuprofen. Ann. Intern. Med., *91*:877–882, 1979.

140. Karat, A.B., Thomas, G., and Rao, P.S.: Indomethacin in the management of erythema nodosum leprosum: a double blind controlled trial. Lepr. Rev., *40*:153–158, 1969.

141. Katz, S.N., et al.: Tolmetin association with reversible renal failure and acute interstitial nephritis. JAMA, *246*:243–245, 1981.

142. Kean, W.F., et al.: Efficacy and toxicity of d-penicillamine for rheumatoid disease in the elderly. J. Am. Geriatr. Soc., *30*:94–100, 1982.

143. Kelsey, W.M., and Scharyj, M.: Fatal hepatitis probably due to indomethacin. JAMA, *199*:586–587, 1967.

144. Kimberly, R.P., et al.: Apparent acute renal failure associated with therapeutic aspirin and ibuprofen administration. Arthritis Rheum., *22*:281–285, 1979.

145. Kimberly, R.P., and Plotz, P.H.: Aspirin induced depression of renal function. N. Engl. J. Med., *296*:418–423, 1977.

146. Kocsis, J.J., et al.: Duration of inhibition of platelet prostaglandin aggregation by ingested aspirin or indomethacin. Prostaglandins, *3*:141–144, 1973.

147. Kowanko, J.C., et al.: Circadian variations in the signs and symptoms of rheumatoid arthritis and in the therapeutic effectiveness of flurbiprofen at different times of the day. Br. J. Clin. Pharmacol., *11*:477–484, 1981.

148. Kwan, K.C., et al.: Effect of concommitant aspirin administration on the pharmacokinetics of indomethacin in man. J. Pharmacokinet. Biopharm., *6*:451–475, 1978.

149. Kwan, K.C., et al.: Kinetics of indomethacin absorption, elimination and enterohepatic circulation in man. J. Pharmacokinet. Biopharm., *4*:255–280, 1976.

150. Ladipo, O.A.: Primary dysmenorrhea treated with indomethacin. Int. J. Gynecol. Obstet., *15*:221–222, 1977.

151. Lanza, F.L., et al.: A comparative endoscopic evaluation of the damaging effects of nonsteroidal anti-inflammatory agents in the gastric and duodenal mucosa. Am. J. Gastroenterol., *75*:17–21, 1981.

152. Leavesley, G.M., et al.: Phenylbutazone and leukemia. Is there a relationship? Med. J. Aust., *2*:963–965, 1969.

153. Leonards, J.R., and Levy, G.: Gastrointestinal blood loss from aspirin and sodium salicylate tablets in man. Clin. Pharmacol. Ther., *14*:62–66, 1973.

154. Lesko, L.J., et al.: Salicylate protein binding in young and elderly serum as measured by diafiltration. (Abstract.) Clin. Pharmacol. Ther., *33*:257, 1983.

155. Levenson, D.J., Simmons, C.E., and Brenner, B.M.: Arachidonic acid metabolism, prostaglandins and kidney. Am. J. Med., *72*:354–374, 1982.

156. Levi, A.J., Sherlock, S., and Walker, D.: Phenylbutazone and isoniazid metabolism in patients with liver disease in relation to previous drug therapy. Lancet, *1*:1275–1279, 1968.

157. Levinson, J.E., et al.: Comparison of tolmetin sodium and aspirin in the treatment of juvenile rheumatoid arthritis. J. Pediatr., *91*:799–804, 1977.

158. Levitt, L., and Pearson, R.W.: Sulindac-induced Ste-

ven's-Johnson toxic epidermal necrolysis syndrome. JAMA, *243*:1262–1263, 1980.

159. Levy, G., and Hollister, L.E.: Inter- and intrasubject variations in drug absorption kinetics. J. Pharm. Sci., *53*:1446–1452, 1964.
160. Levy, G., and Leonards, J.R.: Urine pH and salicylate therapy. JAMA, *217*:81, 1971.
161. Levy, G., Tsuchiya, T.: Salicylate accumulation kinetics in man. N. Engl. J. Med., *287*:430–432, 1972.
162. Levy, M.: Aspirin use in patients with major upper GI bleeding and peptic ulcer disease. N. Engl. J. Med., *290*:1157–1162, 1974.
163. Lewis, J.R.: Evaluation of ibuprofen (Motrin). A new antirheumatic agent. JAMA, *233*:365–366, 1975.
164. Liakakos, D., Vlachos, P., and Anoussakis, L.: Effect of acetylsalicylic acid (aspirin) on bone collagen in children. Clin. Chim. Acta, *44*:427–429, 1973.
165. Liebling, M.R.: Multi-clinic double blind trial of sulindac in ankylosing spondylitis. Postgrad. Med. Comm., *Special Report*:61–68, 1979.
166. Lim, R.K.S.: Analgesia. *In* The Salicylates. Edited by M.J.H. Smith and P.K. Smith. New York, John Wiley and Sons, 1966, pp. 155–202.
167. Lin, T.M., et al.: Action of the anti-inflammatory agents, acetylsalicylic acid, indomethacin and fenoprofen on gastric mucosa of dogs. Res. Commun. Chem. Pathol. Pharmacol., *11*:1–14, 1975.
168. Liyange, S.P., and Tambar, P.K.: Comparative study of salsalate and aspirin in osteoarthrosis of the hip or knee. Curr. Med. Res. Opin., *5*:450–453, 1978.
169. Lockwood, G.F., et al.: Pharmacokinetics of ibuprofen in man. I. Free and total area/dose relationships. Clin. Pharmacol. Ther., *34*:97–103, 1983.
170. Loebl, D.H.T., et al.: Gastrointestinal blood loss. Effect of aspirin, fenoprofen, and acetaminophen in rheumatoid arthritis as determined by sequential gastroscopy and radioactive fecal markers. JAMA, *237*:976–979, 1977.
171. Luftschein, S., et al.: Increasing doses of naproxen in rheumatoid arthritis: use with and without costicosteroids. J. Rheumatol., *6*:397–404, 1979.
172. Lussier, A., et al.: Comparative evaluation of carprofen and indomethacin in rheumatoid arthritis. Int. J. Clin. Pharmacol., *18*:482–487, 1980.
173. Lussier, A., and Arsenault, A.: Gastrointestinal blood loss induced by ketoprofen, aspirin and placebo. Scand. J. Rheumatol., *5 (Suppl. 14)*:73–76, 1976.
174. McIntyre, B.A., Philip, R.B., and Inwood, M.J.: Effect of ibuprofen on platelet function in normal subjects and hemophiliac patients. Clin. Pharmacol. Ther., *24*:616–621, 1978.
175. McLean, J.R., and Gluckman, M.I.: On the mechanism of the pharmacologic activity of meclofenamate sodium. Arzneim. Forsch., *33*:627–630, 1983.
176. McQueen, E.G., and Wardell, W.M.: Drug displacement from protein binding: isolation of a redistributional drug interaction *in vivo*. Br. J. Pharmacol., *43*:312–324, 1971.
177. Mahoney, L., et al.: Prophylactic indomethacin for patent ductus arteriosus. N. Engl. J. Med., *306*:506–510, 1982.
178. Makela, A.: Naproxen in the treatment of juvenile rheumatoid arthritis. Scand. J. Rheumatol., *6*:193–205, 1977.
179. Manchester, D., Margolis, H.S., and Sheldon, R.E.: Possible association between maternal indomethacin and primary pulmonary hypertension of the newborn. Am. J. Obstet. Gynecol., *126*:467–469, 1976.
180. Martelli, E.A.: Antagonism of inflammatory drugs on bradykinin-induced increase of capillary permeability. J. Pharm. Pharmacol., *19*:617–620, 1967.
181. Mason, R.W., and McQueen, E.G.: Protein binding of indomethacin: Binding of indomethacin to human plasma albumin and its displacement from binding by ibuprofen, phenylbutazone and salicylate, *in vitro*. Pharmacology, *12*:12–19, 1974.
182. Massotti, G., et al.: Differential inhibition of prostaglandin production and platelet aggregation by aspirin. Lancet, *2*:1213–1217, 1979.
183. Matthew, H., et al.: Gastric aspiration and lavage in acute poisoning. Br. Med. J., *1*:1333–1337, 1966.
184. Max, M., and Menguy, R.: Influence of aspirin and phen-

ylbutazone on the rate of turnover of gastric mucosal cells. Digestion, *2*:67–72, 1969.
185. Melmon, K.L., Rowland, M., and Morreli, H.: The clinical pharmacology of salicylates. Calif. Med., *110*:410–422, 1969.
186. Melton, A.S., and Wendland, T.S.: A possible role for PGE, as a modulator for temperature regulation in the CNS of the cat. J. Physiol., *207*:76–77, 1970.
187. Mena, H.R., and Willkens, R.F.: Treatment of ankylosing spondylitis with flurbiprofen or phenylbutazone. Eur. J. Clin. Pharmacol., *11*:263–266, 1977.
188. Merck, Sharpe and Dohme. FDA presentation. May, 1977.
189. Mielens, Z.E., et al.: Interactions of aspirin with nonsteroidal anti-inflammatory drugs in rats. J. Pharm. Pharmacol., *20*:567–569, 1968.
190. Miller, D.R.: Combination use of nonsteroidal anti-inflammatory drugs. Drug. Intell. Clin. Pharm., *15*:3–7, 1981.
191. Miller, F.U., Hundt., H.K.L., and deKock, A.C.: Decreased steady-state salicylic acid plasma levels associated with chronic aspirin ingestion. Curr. Med. Res. Opin., *3*:417–422, 1975.
192. Miller, J.L.: Marrow aplasia and sulindac. (Letter.) Ann. Intern. Med., *92*:129, 1979.
192a.Miller, M.J.S., Bednar, M.M., and McGiff, J.C.: Renal metabolism of sulindac, a novel non-steroidal anti-inflammatory agent. Adv. Prostaglandin Thromboxane Leukotriene Res., *11*:487–491, 1983.
193. Minuth, A.N., et al.: Indomethacin treatment of pericarditis in chronic hemodialysis patients. Arch. Intern. Med., *135*:807–810, 1975.
194. Molnar, J.P., and Moxley, T.E.: Ibuprofen, a double-blind comparison of two dosages, 2400 mg and 3200 mg daily, for treating rheumatoid arthritis. Curr. Ther. Res., *26*:581–591, 1979.
195. Moncada, S., and Vane, J.R.: Pharmacology and endogenous roles of prostaglandin endoperoxides, thromboxane A_2, and prostacyclin. Pharmacol. Rev., *30*:293–331, 1979.
196. Mongan, E., et al.: Tinnitus as an indication of therapeutic serum salicylate levels. JAMA, *226*:142–145, 1973.
197. Murray, T., and Goldberg, M.: Analgesic abuse and renal disease. Annu. Rev. Med., *26*:537–550, 1975.
198. Nevinny, D., and Gowans, J.C.D.: Observations on the usefulness of a new liquid salicylate in arthritis. Int. Rec. Med., *173*:242–247, 1960.
199. Nevins, M., et al.: Phenylbutazone and pulmonary oedema. Lancet, *2*:1358, 1969.
200. New Zealand Rheumatism Association Study: Aspirin and the kidney. Br. Med. J., *1*:593–596, 1974.
201. Nickander, R.C., Kraay, R.J., and Marshall, W.S.: Anti-inflammatory and analgesic effects of fenoprofen. Fed. Proc., *30*:563, 1971.
202. Ober, K.F.: Mechanisms of interaction of tolbutamide and phenylbutazone in diabetic patients. Eur. J. Clin. Pharmacol., *7*:291–294, 1974.
203. O'Brien, W.M.: Indomethacin: a survey of clinical trials. Clin. Pharmacol. Ther., *9*:94–106, 1968.
204. O'Malley, K., et al.: Effect of age and sex on human drug metabolism. Br. Med. J., *3*:607–609, 1971.
205. Orme, M., et al.: Plasma concentration of phenylbutazone and its therapeutic effect—studies in patients with rheumatoid arthritis. Br. J. Clin. Pharmacol., *3*:186–191, 1976.
206. Orozco-Alcola, J.J., and Baum, J.: Regular and enteric coated aspirin: a re-evaluation. Arthritis Rheum., *22*:1034–1037, 1979.
207. Park, G.D., et al.: Serious adverse reactions associated with sulindac. Arch. Intern. Med., *142*:1292–1294, 1982.
208. Partin, J.S., et al.: Serum salicylate concentrations in Reye's disease. Lancet, *1*:191–194, 1982.
209. Patak, R.V., et al.: Antagonism of the effects of furosimide by indomethacin in normal and hypertensive man. Prostaglandins, *10*:649–659, 1975.
210. Paulus, H.E.: Government affairs: FDA Arthritis Advi-

sory Committee meeting. Arthritis Rheum., *25*:1124, 1982.

211. Paulus, H.E., et al.: Variations of serum concentrations and 'half-life' of salicylate in patients with rheumatoid arthritis. Arthritis Rheum., *14*:527–532, 1971.

212. Penner, J.A., and Albrecht, P.H.: Lack of interaction between ibuprofen and warfarin. Curr. Ther. Res., *18*:862–871, 1975.

213. Perkins, E.S., and MacFaul, P.A.: Indomethacin in the treatment of uveitis: a double blind trial. Trans. Ophthalmol. Soc. U.K., *85*:53–58, 1965.

214. Petrick, T.J., and Black, M.E.: Double-blind multicenter studies with meclofenamate sodium in the treatment of rheumatoid arthritis in the United States and Canada. Arzneim. Forsch., *33*:631–635, 1983.

215. Petrick, T.J., and Bovenkerk, W.E.: Multicenter studies in the United States and Canada of meclofenamate sodium in osteoarthritis of the hip and knee. Arzneim. Forsch., *33*:644–648, 1983.

216. Pitts, N.E.: Efficacy and safety of piroxicam. Am. J. Med., *72(Suppl. 2A)*:77–87, 1982.

217. Plostnicks, J., et al.: Human metabolism of tolmetin. *In* Tolmetin. Edited by J. H. Ward. Princeton, Excerpta Medica, 1975, pp. 23–33.

218. Pond, S.M., Birkett, D.J., and Wade, D.N.: Mechanisms of inhibition of tolbutamide metabolism: phenylbutazone, oxyphenbutazone, and sulfaphenazole. Clin. Pharmacol. Ther., *22*:573–579, 1977.

219. Preston, S.N.: Safety of meclofenamate sodium. Curr. Ther. Res., *23(Suppl.)*:107–112, 1978.

220. Rachelefsky, G.S., et al.: Serum enzyme abnormalities in juvenile rheumatoid arthritis. Pediatrics, *48*:730–736, 1976.

221. Radin, A., et al.: Leukotriene B$_4$ (LTB$_4$) as a mediator of inflammation: human neutrophil (PMN) activation and calcium (Ca) ionophoresis. Arthritis Rheum., *25 (Suppl.)*:S-8, 1982.

222. Ray, J.E., and Wade, D.N.: The pharmacokinetics and metabolism of ^{14}C-carprofen in man. Biopharm. Drug Dispos., *3*:29–38, 1982.

223. Restivo, C., and Paulus, H.E.: Anaphylaxis from tolmetin. JAMA, *240*:246, 1978.

224. Richter, J.A., and Swader, J.: Comparison of fecal blood loss after use of aspirin and sulindac. Postgrad. Med. Comm., *Special Report*:81–85, 1979.

225. Rider, J.A.: Comparison of fecal blood loss after use of aspirin and diflunisal. Pharmacotherapy, *3*:61S–64S, 1983.

226. Ridolfo, A.S., et al.: A double blind study comparing benoxaprofen, aspirin, and benoxaprofen plus aspirin in patients with rheumatoid arthritis. Eur. J. Rheumatol. Inflammation, *5*:239–245, 1982.

227. Ridolfo, A.S., et al.: Effect of fenoprofen and aspirin on gastrointestinal microbleeding in man. Clin. Pharmacol. Ther., *14*:226–230, 1973.

228. Risdall, P.C., et al.: The disposition and metabolism of flurbiprofen in several species including man. Xenobiotica, *8*:691–704, 1978.

229. Ritch, A.E.S., Perera, W.N.R., and Jones, C.J.: Pharmacokinetics of azapropazone in the elderly. Br. J. Clin. Pharmacol., *14*:116–119, 1982.

230. Roberts, A., et al.: Gastric antisecretory and antiulcer properties of PGE$_2$, 15-Methyl PGE$_2$, and 16, 16-Dimethyl PGE$_2$. Gastroenterology, *70*:359–370, 1976.

231. Robinson, H., et al.: Concomitant tolmetin and aspirin therapy in rheumatoid arthritis. *In* Tolmetin. Edited by J. H. Ward. Princeton, Excerpta Medica, 1975, pp. 102–111.

232. Rodnan, G.P., and Benedek, T.G.: The early history of anti-rheumatic drugs. Arthritis Rheum., *13*:145–165, 1970.

233. Romberg, O.: Comparison of piroxicam with indomethacin in ankylosing spondylitis. A double-blind cross over trial. Am. J. Med., *72(Suppl. 2A)*:58–62, 1982.

234. Roth, G.S., and Livingston, J.N.: Reductions in glucocorticoid inhibition of glucose oxidation and presumptive glucocorticoid receptor content in rat adipocytes during aging. Endocrinology, *99*:831–839, 1976.

235. Rotstein, J.: Phenylbutazone and aspirin in osteoarthritis, a controlled study. Curr. Ther. Res., *17*:444–451, 1975.

236. Rowland, M., and Riegelman, S.: Absorption kinetics of aspirin in man following oral administration of an aqueous solution. J. Pharm. Sci., *61*:379–395, 1972.

237. Rubin, A., et al.: Interactions of aspirin with non-steroidal anti-inflammatory drugs in man. Arthritis Rheum., *16*:635–645, 1973.

238. Rubin, A., et al.: Physiological disposition of fenoprofen in man. J. Pharm. Sci., *61*:739–745, 1972.

239. Rubio, F., et al.: Metabolism of carprofen in rats, dogs, and human. J. Pharm. Sci., *69*:1245–1253, 1980.

240. Runkel, R., et al.: Naproxen-probenecid interaction. Clin. Pharmacol. Ther., *24*:706–713, 1978.

241. Runkel, R., et al.: Pharmacokinetics of naproxen overdoses. Clin. Pharmacol. Ther., *20*:269–277, 1976.

242. Ruppert, G.B., and Barth, W.F.: Tolmetin-induced aseptic meningitis. JAMA, *245*:67–68, 1981.

243. Ryan, J.R., et al.: On the question of an interaction between sulindac and tolbutamide in the control of diabetes. Clin. Pharmacol. Ther., *21*:231–233, 1977.

244. Sacks, P.V., and Kanarek, D.: Treatment of acute pleuritic pain. Comparison between indomethacin and a placebo. Am. Rev. Respir. Dis., *108*:666–669, 1973.

245. Samter, M.: Intolerance to aspirin. Hosp. Pract., *8*:85–90, 1973.

246. Samuelsson, B.: Leukotrienes: a new class of mediators of immediate hypersensitivity reactions and inflammation. Adv. Prostaglandin Thromboxane Leukotriene Res., *11*:1–13, 1983.

247. Schaller, J.G.: Treatment of juvenile rheumatoid arthritis. *In* Arthritis and Allied Conditions. 9th Ed. Edited by D. J. McCarty. Philadelphia, Lea & Febiger, 1979, pp. 602–609.

248. Schaller, J.G.: Report to the FDA Arthritis Advisory Committee, May 19–20, 1977.

249. Schattenkirchner, M., Schattenkirchner, U., and Muller-Fassbender, H.: Klinische erfahrungen mit Tolectin in der Langzeitbehandlung der Spondylitis ankylosans. Therapiewoche, *27*:2298–2306, 1977.

250. Scherrer, R.A.: Aryl- and hetero-arylcarboxylic acids. *In* Antiinflammatory Agents. Vol. 1. Edited by R. A. Scherrer and M. W. Whitehouse. New York, Academic Press, 1974, pp. 45–89.

251. Schmid, F.R., and Culic, D.D.: Anti-inflammatory drugs and gastrointestinal bleeding: comparison of aspirin and ibuprofen. J. Clin. Pharmacol., *16*:418–425, 1976.

252. Schneck, D.W., et al.: The effect of aspirin on the disposition of carprofen in humans. Pharmacology, *21*:166, 1979.

253. Schreiner, G.E., and Teehan, B.P.: Dialysis of poisons and drugs. Trans. Am. Soc. Artif. Intern. Organs, *18*:563–599, 1972.

254. Scott, D.L., et al.: Variations in responses to nonsteroidal anti-inflammatory drugs. Br. J. Clin. Pharmacol., *14*:691–694, 1982.

255. Seaman, W.E., and Plotz, P.H.: Effect of aspirin on liver tests in patients with RA or SLE and in normal volunteers. Arthritis Rheum., *19*:155–160, 1976.

256. Segre, E.J., et al.: Naproxen-aspirin interactions in man. Clin. Pharmacol. Ther., *15*:374–379, 1974.

257. Selley, M.L., et al.: Pharmacokinetic studies of tolmetin in man. Clin. Pharmacol. Ther., *17*:599–605, 1975.

258. Selley, M.L., Madsen, B.W., and Thomas, J.: Protein binding of tolmetin. Clin. Pharmacol. Ther., *24*:694–705, 1978.

259. Shah, G.M., Muhalwas, K., and Winer, R.L.: Renal papillary necrosis due to ibuprofen. Arthritis Rheum., *24*:1208–1210, 1981.

260. Sheldrake, F.E., Webber, J.M., and March, B.D.: A long-term assessment of flurbiprofen. Curr. Med. Res. Opin., *5*:106–114, 1977.

261. Shipley, M., Berry, H., and Bloom, B.: A double blind cross over trial of indomethacin, fenoprofen and placebo in ankylosing spondylitis, with comments on patient assessment. Rheumatol. Rehabil., *19*:122–125, 1980.

262. Siebert, D.J., et al.: Aspirin kinetics and platelet aggregation in man. Clin. Pharmacol. Ther., *33*:367–374, 1983.

263. Smith, M.J.H.: The metabolic basis of the major symptoms in acute salicylate intoxication. Clin. Toxicol., *1*:387–407, 1968.

264. Smith, M.J.H.: Toxicology. *In* The Salicylates. Edited by M.J.H. Smith and P.K. Smith. New York, John Wiley and Sons, 1966, pp. 233–306.

265. Smith, M.J.H., and Dawkins, P.D.: Salicylates and enzymes. J. Pharm. Pharmacol., *23*:729–744, 1971.

266. Smith, T.C.: Clinical pharmacology studies of sodium meclofenamate (Meclomen). Curr. Ther. Res., *23(Suppl.)*:42–50, 1978.

267. Smyth, C.J., and Clark, G.M.: Phenylbutazone in rheumatoid arthritis. J. Chronic Dis., *5*:734–750, 1957.

268. Smyth, C.J., and Percy, J.S.: Comparison of indomethacin and phenylbutazone in acute gout. Ann. Rheum. Dis., *32*:351–353, 1973.

269. Somogyi, A., Kovacs, K., and Selye, H.: Jejunal ulcers produced by indomethacin. J. Pharm. Pharmacol., *21*:122–123, 1969.

270. Stachura, I., Jayakumar, S., and Bourke, E.: T and B lymphocyte subsets in fenoprofen nephropathy. Am. J. Med., *75*:9–16, 1983.

271. Stafanger, G., et al.: Pharmacokinetics of ketoprofen in patients with renal impairment. *In* Ketoprofen Symposium. Paris, Rhone-Poulenc Sante, 1980, pp. 21–26.

272. Stefanini, M., and Nassif, R.I.: Acute thrombocytopenic purpura traced to tolmetin related antibody. Va. Med., *109*:171–175, 1982.

273. Stempel, D.A., and Miller, J.J., III.: Lymphopenia and hepatic toxicity with ibuprofen. J. Pediatr., *90*:657–658, 1977.

274. Strandberg, B.: Phenylbutazone in the treatment of rheumatic diseases. Acta Rheumatol. Scand., *(Suppl. 10)*:5–50, 1965.

275. Szczeklik, A.: Analgesics, allergy and asthma. Br. J. Clin. Pharmacol., *10*:4015–4019, 1980.

276. Templeton, J.S.: Azapropazone twice or four times daily? Eur. J. Rheumatol. Inflammation, *3*:401–407, 1981.

277. Tenney, S.M., and Miller, R.M.: The respiratory and circulatory actions of salicylates. Am. J. Med., *19*:498–503, 1955.

278. Thadani, U., et al.: Effect of indomethacin on hemodynamics and exercise tolerance in angina pectoris. (Abstract B-23.) *In* Proceedings of the Conference of the American Society of Clinical Pharmacology and Therapeutics. San Diego, March, 1983.

279. Tjandramaga, T.B., et al.: Interaction of diflunisal with indomethacin. *In* World Conference on Clinical Pharmacology and Therapeutics. (Abstract 658.) London, August 3 to 9, 1980.

280. Traeger, A., et al.: Pharmacokinetics of indomethacin in the aged. A. Alternesforsch., *27*:151–155, 1973.

281. Traeger, A., Noschel, H., and Zaumseil, J.: Pharmacokinetics of indomethacin in pregnant and parturient women and in their newborn infants. Zentralbl. Gynaekol., *95*:635–641, 1973.

282. Trimble, G.X.: Phenylbutazone-induced pericarditis. Br. Med. J., *2*:1184, 1965.

283. Umbenhauer, E.R.: Diflunisal in the treatment of pain in osteoarthritis. Pharmacotherapy, *3*:55S–60S, 1983.

284. Upton, R.A., et al.: Ketoprofen pharmacokinetics and bioavailability based on an improved sensitive and specific assay. Eur. J. Clin. Pharmacol., *20*:127–133, 1981.

285. Upton, R.A., et al.: Ketoprofen-probenecid interaction in man. (Abstract 102.) *In* World Conference on Clinical Pharmacology and Therapeutics. London, August 3 to 9, 1980.

286. Valtonen, E.J.: Phenylbutazone in the treatment of Tietze's syndrome. Ann. Rheum. Dis., *26*:133–135, 1967.

287. Valtonen, E.J., and Busson, M.: A comparative study of ibuprofen and indomethacin in nonarticular rheumatism. Scand. J. Rheumatol., *7*:183–188, 1978.

288. Van Armen, C.G., Nuss, G.W., and Risley, E.A.: Interactions of aspirin, indomethacin, and other drugs in adjuvant-induced arthritis in the rat. J. Pharmacol. Exp. Ther., *187*:400–414, 1973.

289. Vane, J.R.: Inhibition of prostaglandin biosynthesis as the mechanism of action of aspirin-like drugs. *In* International Congress on Prostaglandins. Edited by S. Bergstrom and S. Bernhard. Oxford, Pergamon Press, 1973, pp. 395–411.

290. Verbeeck, R.K., Blackburn, J.L., and Loewen, G.R.: Clinical pharmacokinetics of nonsteroidal anti-inflammatory drugs. Clin. Pharmacokinet., *8*:297–331, 1983.

291. Vessell, E.S., and Page, J.G.: Genetic control of drug levels in man: phenylbutazone. Science, *159*:1479–1480, 1968.

292. Vessell, E.S., Passananti, G.T., and Johnson, A.O.: Failure of indomethacin and warfarin to interact in normal human volunteers. J. Clin. Pharmacol., *15*:486–495, 1975.

293. Vignon, E., and Chapuy, M.C.: Bioavailability of indomethacin: study of sustained release preparation. Rev. Rhum. Mal. Osteo-Artic., *46*:505–508, 1979.

294. Wanasukapunt, S., Lertratanakul, Y., and Rubinstein, H.M.: Effect of fenoprofen calcium on acute gouty arthritis. Arthritis Rheum., *19*:933–935, 1976.

295. Wanka, J., and Dixon, A.S.J.: Treatment of osteoarthritis of the hip with indomethacin, a controlled clinical trial. Ann. Rheum. Dis., *23*:288–294, 1964.

296. Wasner, C., et al.: Nonsteroidal anti-inflammatory agents in rheumatoid arthritis and ankylosing spondylitis. JAMA, *246*:2168–2172, 1981.

297. Weissmann, G.: Pathways of arachidonate oxidation to prostaglandins and leukotrienes. Semin. Arthritis Rheum., *13(Suppl. 1)*:123–129, 1983.

298. Weissmann, G.: Prostaglandins in acute inflammation. *In* Current Concepts. Kalamazoo, MI, Upjohn, 1980, pp. 1–32.

299. Weksler, B.B., et al.: Differential inhibition by aspirin of vascular and platelet prostaglandin synthesis in atherosclerotic patients. N. Engl. J. Med., *308*:800–805, 1983.

300. Wendland, M.L., Wagoner, R.D., and Holley, K.E.: Renal failure associated with fenoprofen. Mayo Clin. Proc., *56*:103–107, 1980.

301. Whitehouse, M.W.: Evaluation of potential antirheumatic drugs *in vitro* using lymphocytes and epithelial cells. The selective action of indoxole, methyl glyoxal and chloroquine. J. Pharm. Pharmacol., *19*:590–595, 1967.

302. Whitsett, T.L., et al.: Tolmetin and warfarin: a clinical investigation to determine if an interaction exists. *In* Tolmetin. Edited by J.H. Ward. Princeton, Excerpta Medica, 1975, pp. 160–167.

303. Widener, H.L., and Littman, D.H.: Ibuprofen induced meningitis in systemic lupus erythematosus. JAMA, *239*:1062–1064, 1978.

304. Williams, R.L., et al.: Effects of indomethacin and carprofen on renal homeostasis in rheumatoid arthritis patients and in healthy individuals. J. Clin. Pharmacol., *21*:493–500, 1981.

305. Williams, R.L., et al.: Ketoprofen-aspirin interactions. Clin. Pharmacol. Ther., *30*:226–231, 1981.

306. Willkens, R.F., et al.: Double-blind study comparing piroxicam and aspirin in the treatment of rheumatoid arthritis. Am. J. Med., *72(Suppl. 2A)*:23–26, 1982.

307. Willkens, R.F., and Segre, E.J.: Combination therapy with naproxen and aspirin in rheumatoid arthritis. Arthritis Rheum., *19*:677–682, 1976.

308. Willkens, R.F., Case, J.B., and Huix, F.J.: The treatment of acute gout with naproxen. J. Clin. Pharmacol., *15*:363–366, 1975.

309. Withey, R.J., et al.: Physiological availability of solid dosage forms of phenylbutazone. J. Clin. Pharmacol., *11*:187–196, 1971.

310. Wright, V., Walker, W.C., and McGuire, R.J.: Indomethacin in the treatment of rheumatoid arthritis. Ann. Rheum. Dis., *28*:157–162, 1969.

311. Yacobi, A., and Levy, G.: Effect of naproxen on protein binding of warfarin. Res. Commun. Chem. Pathol. Pharmacol., *15*:369–372, 1976.

312. Yu, T.F., and Gutman, A.B.: Study of the paradoxical effects of salicylates in low, intermediate and high dosage on the renal mechanism for excretion of urate in man. J. Clin. Invest., *38*:1298–1315, 1959.

313. Yu, T.F. and Perel, J.: Pharmacokinetic and clinical studies of carprofen in gout. J. Clin. Pharmacol., *20*:347–351, 1980.

314. Zucker, M.B., and Rothwell, K.G.: Differential influences of salicylate compounds on platelet aggregation and serotonin release. Curr. Ther. Res., *23*:194–199, 1978.

315. Zuckerman, H., Reiss, U., and Rubinstein, I.: Inhibition of human premature labor by indomethacin. Obstet. Gynecol., *44*:787–792, 1974.

Chapter 29

Gold Compounds

John L. Skosey

Gold compounds have been used in therapeutics since medieval times. In the late nineteenth and early twentieth centuries, they were used primarily for the treatment of tuberculosis and other infections with an enthusiasm not warranted by their effectiveness.[25] Forestier is credited with having pioneered the use of these compounds in the treatment of rheumatoid arthritis (RA).[14] The first use of gold in RA, as Solganal, was recorded by Lande in 1927.[25a] Because of excessive toxicity associated with the large doses initially used, the popularity of these agents declined. In recent times, however, gold compounds have found a major place in the treatment of RA and certain related conditions. Table 29–1 lists currently available gold compounds.

CHEMISTRY

Elemental gold was used in ancient times to treat pruritus of the palms. Gold leaf has been used as an adjunct in the therapy of cutaneous ulcers. Radioactive gold (^{198}Au) in colloidal form has been used to treat malignant pleural and peritoneal effusions and has been injected intra-articularly in patients with RA. With these minor exceptions, gold is used in compounds in which the metal in the monovalent aurous form (Au$^+$) is stabilized by attachment to a sulfur-containing ligand.[40] The gold preparations used in the United States include aurothioglucose (Solganal) and sodium aurothiomalate (Myochrysine). Each of these compounds is approximately 50% gold by weight. Sodium aurothiosulfate (Sanochrysine), aurothioglycoanilide (Boron), and sodium aurothiopropanol sulfonate (Allochrysine) are available in other parts of the world. Each of these preparations is administered by intramuscular injection. Triethylphosphine gold thioglucosetetra-acetate (Auranofin), which is absorbed after oral ingestion, has been widely studied, but has not yet been released for use in the United States.[18]

PHARMACOLOGIC ACTIONS

Gold compounds exhibit a number of actions that may be of pharmacologic interest. The origin of RA and the related diseases for which these drugs are widely used is not known, and the relative importance of many putative pathogenic influences remains uncertain. Similarly, the importance of the multiple pharmacologic effects of gold compounds in the treatment of RA is unclear.

Antimicrobial Effects

Koch demonstrated that potassium aurocyanide [KAu(CN)$_2$] arrested the growth of *Mycobacterium tuberculosis*, in vitro. Subsequently, gold compounds have been shown to arrest or inhibit growth of, or to kill, various strains of bacteria, mycoplasma, and protozoa, in vitro, and to protect against the effects of these micro-organisms in vivo.[27] These compounds are regularly ineffective, however, in protecting against viral infections. The early observations of the effects of gold compounds on tubercle bacilli led to their use in RA, a chronic disease considered to have characteristics in common with tuberculosis.[14]

A number of arguments have challenged the thesis that antimicrobial effects represent an important therapeutic action of gold compounds in RA. First, in spite of great interest in a possible infectious cause of RA, no infectious agent has been identified

Table 29–1. Gold Compounds

Generic Name	Trade Name
Gold sodium thiomalate	Myochrysine
Aurothioglucose	Solganal
Gold thioglycoanilid	Lauron
Gold sodium thiosulfate (IV)	Sanochrysine, Crisalbine
Colloidal gold sulfide (oral, IV)	Aurol-sulfide
Calcium aurothioglycolate	Myoral
Sodium aurothiobenzimidazole carboxylic acid (IV)	Triphal
Methylglucamide of aurothiodiglycollic acid	Parmanil
Sodium auroallylthiourea benzoate (IV)	Lopion
Sodium aurothiopropanol sulfonate	Allochrysine
Sulfhydryl gold naphthyl trisulfocarbonium	Aurocein
Triethylphosphine gold thioglucosetetra-acetate (oral)	Auranofin

IV = Intravenous.

(Adapted from Gottlieb and Gray.[18])

consistently in this disease (see Chaps. 27 and 35). If an infectious agent were involved in the pathogenesis of RA, a virus would be most likely, and gold compounds do not affect viral growth. Moreover, no evidence suggests that treatment with gold compounds reduces the incidence of specific infectious diseases in patients with RA. Finally, unlike in experimental models of infectious arthritis in which gold compounds must be administered early in the disease to be effective, these preparations are often beneficial in RA even when administered months or years after onset of the disease.[27]

Alteration of Immune Function

Immunologic considerations include experimental disease and the effects of gold compounds on lymphocytes, monocytes and macrophages, and immune complexes.

Experimental Immunologically Mediated Disease

Gold compounds have an inconsistent effect on adjuvant arthritis in rats.[27] In allergic encephalomyelitis, the onset of clinical signs of disease is delayed by treatment with gold compounds given in doses 50 times greater, on the basis of weight, than those used in human disease. Lymph node cells from animals treated with gold compounds are capable of transferring the disease; this finding suggests that the drug inhibits inflammation itself, rather than acting on a more basic immune process.

Lymphocytes

Lymphocytes tested in vitro from patients with RA exhibit a decreased response to mitogens, in comparison with cells from control subjects. Responses of lymphocytes obtained from these patients after treatment with sodium aurothiomalate approach a normal range.[21] Lymphocytes from patients treated with oral gold compounds exhibit a further decrease in mitogen response, however.[30] These differences in the effects of sodium aurothiomalate and oral preparations may reflect differences in the distribution of elemental gold because a greater amount is found in cells after administration of the oral preparation. Serum from patients with active RA suppresses lymphocyte responses to mitogens, an effect probably due to its content of immune complexes. Following treatment with sodium aurothiomalate, immune complex levels fall, and the inhibitory effects of serum are diminished.[26] Both oral and injectable gold compounds added in vitro suppress lymphocyte responses to mitogens.[30] Given the conflicting effects of gold compounds on lymphocyte mitogenic responses, it is difficult to conclude that the major

therapeutic effect of these drugs is mediated through alteration of lymphocyte function. Treatment with gold compounds interferes with immunoglobulin synthesizing cells, as indicated by decreases in the serum levels of rheumatoid factor and other immunoglobulins and, as noted previously, immune complexes in patients treated with these drugs.[21]

Monocytes and Macrophages

Gold compounds variably affect the function of monocytes and macrophages. Aurosomes develop in phagocytic cells of various tissues of patients treated with gold compounds.[15] These structures are described as lysosomal bodies with myelinoid membranes enclosing rod-like inclusions, presumably derived from the membranes, and electron-dense deposits of gold. Aurosomes are formed following administration to experimental animals of a variety of soluble gold salts, including the therapeutically inactive form, sodium chloroaurate ($NaAuCl_4$). Sodium thiomalate treatment induces the formation of a structure that lacks the characteristic dense (gold) deposit, but possesses the myelinoid membrane with rod-like inclusions. As already noted, sodium aurothiomalate inhibits the proliferative responses of lymphocytes to mitogens, in vitro. Similar effects are observed with the auric compound, $NaAuCl_4$.[28,29] This inhibition is probably secondary to suppression of monocyte factors required for lymphocyte responses because it can be overcome by the addition of fresh monocytes not previously exposed to gold compounds. On the other hand, the response of splenic lymphocytes from rats with adjuvant arthritis is inhibited by adherent spleen cells, and this inhibition is overcome by treatment of the animals with gold sodium thiomalate.[4] It is not clear whether the enhancement by sodium aurothiomalate of mitogen responses of peripheral blood lymphocytes from patients with RA is similarly mediated through suppression of monocyte-macrophages. Thus, although it is difficult to reconcile the in vitro and in vivo effects of gold compounds on lymphocyte proliferation, it appears that, in each case, these effects are mediated through actions on cells of the monocyte-macrophage system.

Treatment of mice with large doses of sodium aurothiomalate increases the susceptibility of these animals to infection with a usually avirulent strain of Semliki forest virus. This increased susceptibility has been attributed to impairment of phagocytosis and degradation of virus by the mouse macrophages.[35] Increased phagocytosis of carbon particles by macrophages of patients with RA is also decreased and approaches normal levels with chrysotherapy. Gold compounds, in vitro and in vivo, inhibit chemotaxis by macrophages.[47] Thus, ample opportunity exists for the effects of gold compounds in RA to be mediated through alteration of macrophage function. Definition of the importance of these effects awaits clarification of the role of the monocyte-macrophage system in the pathogenesis of RA and related conditions.

Immune Complexes

Circulating immune complexes measured by C1q binding activity are often elevated in patients with RA and consist largely of IgM rheumatoid factor complexes to IgG. During treatment with gold compounds, immune complex levels often fall, but only when evidence of decreased joint inflammation is already present. This process suggests that the effect on immune complexes reflects suppression of inflammation, rather than an effect on a primary pathogenetic process.[26]

Anti-Inflammatory Effects

These effects include actions on acute phase proteins and oxygen-derived free radicals.

Acute Phase Proteins

Serum levels of acute phase proteins such as C-reactive protein (CRP), fibrinogen, haptoglobin, ceruloplasmin, α_1-antitrypsin, and α_1-acid glycoprotein rise nonspecifically in response to inflammation. High levels of CRP may correlate with severe arthritis and the development of erosive disease. Although evidence suggests a role for some of these proteins in the pathogenesis of inflammation, the significance of these observations is not yet clear. Treatment with gold results in a fall in the serum level of acute phase proteins, paralleling clinical improvement.[26,47]

Oxygen-Derived Free Radicals

Inflammatory mediator cells such as neutrophils and macrophages, when stimulated, produce metabolites of oxygen that possess a high degree of chemical reactivity. These metabolites, which include superoxide anion, hydrogen peroxide, hydroxyl radical, singlet oxygen, and hypochlorous acid, are, for convenience, referred to collectively as oxygen-derived free radicals, even though they do not all have the unpaired electron characteristic of free radicals. Gold compounds may protect against the oxidant properties of these free radicals. Levels of natural scavengers of free radicals, such as reduced glutathione in erythrocytes[34] and serum free sulfhydryl moieties and ceruloplasmin,[26] are diminished in active RA, possibly as a result of the action of free radicals produced during the inflammatory process. These natural scavengers return to normal levels during treatment with gold

compounds. In vitro, both sodium aurothiomalate and triethylphosphine gold thioglucosetetra-acetate inhibit leukocyte iodination, a function that requires free radical action.[46] Free radicals inactivate α_1-proteinase inhibitor, which can protect against damage due to lysosomal enzymes released by inflammatory mediator cells. Gold compounds protect α_1-proteinase inhibitor from oxidative damage resulting from the action of free radicals in vitro. That this effect of the drugs is shared by their thiol ligands, thiomalate, thioglucose, and thioglucosetetra-acetate, emphasizes the potential role of the sulfhydryl moieties of these drugs in their biologic effects.[44,45]

Enzyme Inhibition

Gold compounds directly inhibit a number of enzymes. This property probably resides in the ability of the elemental gold cation to bind to sulfhydryl groups at critical sites of the enzyme.

A potential site of action of gold compounds in the treatment of erosive synovitis is their inhibition of enzymes such as elastase, collagenase, and hyaluronidase, which are capable of degrading connective tissue components.[27,47] As previously noted, gold compounds and their sulfhydryl ligands may inhibit enzymes indirectly by protecting α_1-proteinase inhibitor from oxidative damage, and gold is concentrated within lysosomes, where it can combine with enzymes. The activity of lysosomal enzymes extracted from cells exposed to gold compounds, or from animals treated with gold compounds, is diminished. Gold is also capable of inhibiting metabolic enzymes involved in such functions as macromolecular synthesis and oxidative phosphorylation.[27] The gold moiety of sodium aurothiomalate or of triethylphosphine gold thioglucosetetra-acetate inhibits a trypsin-like neutral protease on the surface of Ehrlich ascites tumor cells.[43] This enzyme is responsible for the activation of procollagenase, which is believed to be an important requirement for tumor invasiveness through connective tissue. A similar mechanism may contribute to the invasiveness of synovial pannus. Sodium aurothiomalate inhibits proliferation of, and collagen synthesis by, cultured human synovial cells.[17]

Other Pharmacologic Effects

The amino acid tryptophan has been postulated to have anti-inflammatory effects, and its plasma level increases when it is displaced from protein-binding sites by gold compounds.[27,47] Other amino acids or oligopeptides with putative anti-inflammatory effects might be similarly displaced. Gold binds with and irreversibly inactivates the first component of complement. That the treatment of rats with gold sodium thiosulfate alters the electron-microscopic morphologic features of tail tendon collagen and changes the physicochemical measurements suggests increased intermolecular cross-linking. Gold compounds protect albumin and gamma globulin from the effects of a number of denaturing agents.

PHARMACOKINETICS

When patients are given weekly injections of 50 mg gold sodium thiomalate, the concentration of elemental gold in serum reaches a peak of approximately 700 μg/dl about 2 hours after injection. The level then declines to half this value over the next 7 days. Gold thioglucose, supplied in a sesame oil vehicle, is absorbed more slowly and produces a lower peak gold level. Serum levels a week after injection are comparable to those attained when gold sodium thiomalate is used, however. After 6 to 8 weeks of weekly injections, the serum gold level stabilizes at 300 to 400 μg/dl. Maintenance gold therapy of 50 mg every 3 to 4 weeks results in a steady-state serum gold level of 75 to 125 μg/ dl. A small amount of injected gold is first found in the erythrocytes several days after administration and reaches a peak in these cells at about 7 days. It is bound primarily to hemoglobin and replaces hydrogen in the sulfhydryl groups. The finding that gold is not present in erythrocytes for several days after injection suggests that it is incorporated into bone marrow precursors.[18]

Erythrocytes of smokers contain a much higher fraction of total blood gold than erythrocytes of nonsmokers, 18%, as opposed to 3%. This difference has been attributed to the raised levels of cyanide and thiocyanate in the blood of smokers. These compounds can form complexes with gold that are then able to enter erythrocytes.[19] Ninety-two percent of intravascular gold is bound to serum proteins, mostly albumin, with smaller amounts bound to complement and immunoglobulins. With higher doses and, consequently, higher blood levels of gold, albumin-binding sites become saturated, and the percentage bound to other serum proteins increases.[18]

Approximately 40% of the gold in sodium aurothiomalate given weekly is excreted. Of the excreted gold, approximately 70% is found in urine and 30% in feces.[18] The concentration in breast milk is low, but the serum gold level in newborns of mothers receiving chrysotherapy is over half that in the maternal circulation.[8]

About 25% of gold from the oral gold preparation, triethylphosphine gold thioglucosetetra-acetate, is absorbed. The blood gold level achieved is proportional to the dose of ingested gold, but it is lower than that with injectable gold. A whole blood gold level of approximately 125 μg/dl is achieved after continuous therapy with 9 mg per day, the highest dose thus far tested. In contrast to the findings with injectable gold preparations, 25 to 50% of whole blood gold is in the cellular fraction. In the serum fraction, 82% is bound to albumin, and the remainder is bound primarily to globulins. The excretion of the aforementioned oral gold preparation is much more complete than that of injectable gold preparations; 95% is recovered in feces and 5% in urine. The greater fecal excretion probably reflects the incomplete absorption of the oral preparation.[18]

The amount of gold retained depends on the compound, the dose, and the frequency and route of administration. In patients receiving weekly injections, approximately 60% of gold is retained, whereas only 20% is retained when injections are given monthly. Less (30%) is retained from triethylphosphine gold thioglucosetetra-acetate. None is retained when a dose of 2 mg is given daily for a similar period. Gold is stored in highest concentration in organs with the highest content of reticuloendothelial tissue: lymph nodes, adrenal glands, liver, kidney, bone marrow, and spleen. Equilibrium is achieved rapidly between blood and synovial fluid, where the gold concentration is about half that of blood. Gold accumulates in synovial macrophages, more rapidly in inflamed than in noninflamed synovium. Low concentrations of gold are detected in skin and its appendages and in the cornea and lens of the eye.[18]

Interest has been increasing in the potential therapeutic role of the sulfhydryl ligands of the gold compounds, but few data are available on the pharmacokinetics of these moieties. When patients receive weekly injections of sodium aurothiomalate, the thiomalate part of the drug disappears rapidly from plasma; about 60% is recovered in urine by the end of the first day after injection. In mice, thiomalate is retained primarily in the kidney, liver, spleen, lung, muscle, and skin.[23]

THERAPEUTIC USES

Gold compounds are used most commonly for the treatment of RA,[10,12,13] although they have been used in the therapy of other inflammatory diseases as well. The mode of administration has been dictated primarily by tradition. A small initial dose of 10 mg sodium aurothiomalate or aurothioglucose, designed to identify idiosyncratic reactions, is given intramuscularly. This dose is followed in a week by an injection of 25 or 50 mg; 50 mg is then given weekly until a total of 1 g drug (500 mg elemental gold) has been administered. It is customary then to continue "maintenance" therapy, 50 mg every 2 weeks for 4 to 8 injections, then every 3 weeks for 4 to 6 injections, then monthly. The frequency and dosage of maintenance therapy are altered according to the clinician's perception of therapeutic and toxic responses. Other regimens in which the dosage or frequency of injection is either increased or decreased have produced variable results, which are sometimes better and sometimes worse, than the traditional regimen, and the value of maintenance therapy has been questioned. Nonetheless, most practitioners currently follow the traditional method of administrating gold compounds.

Triethylphosphine gold thioglucosetetra-acetate, which is 29% elemental gold by weight, is administered orally, at a dose of 6 to 9 mg daily.

Gold compounds are seldom used in the treatment of RA before the patient has had an adequate trial of aspirin or another nonsteroidal anti-inflammatory drug. If the response to these drugs is insufficient, a gold compound may be added to the treatment regimen. The disease should probably be present for at least 1 year, to ensure that chrysotherapy is not given unnecessarily to a patient who could possibly have a spontaneous remission of disease. Exceptions exist, however. For example, the development of juxta-articular erosions or persistent inflammation unresponsive to first-line drugs would dictate earlier institution of therapy with gold compounds. Results of chrysotherapy are best when it is initiated earlier, rather than later, in the natural history of the disease, particularly, as would be expected, to retard joint erosion.[32,42]

The contraindications for therapy with gold compounds are relative, rather than absolute. They include pre-existing proteinuria and dermatitis, which would be difficult to distinguish from toxic effects of the drug. Anemia or leukopenia are not contraindications and may, when they are the result of the underlying disease process such as anemia of chronic inflammation or Felty's syndrome, improve the treatment. As noted previously, gold crosses the placenta and can be recovered in the fetal concentration in significant quantities, but children born to mothers treated with gold compounds throughout pregnancy do not have abnormalities attributable to therapy.[8]

Forestier, in an early report of his experience with the use of gold compounds in the treatment of RA and related diseases, stated that toxicity would require discontinuing the drug in 25% of patients, and 60% would be "greatly benefited."[14] Although individual reports vary widely in the relative frequencies of therapeutic success and toxicity, these figures are within the generally accepted range. It is often stated that beneficial effects are not observed for weeks or months after the institution of therapy, but some studies demonstrate gradual improvement in morning stiffness, pain, systemic symptoms, and other measures of inflammation, which by extrapolation, seem to have begun soon after the institution of therapy.[41] The effect on sedimentation rate and on other laboratory correlates of inflammation lags behind the clinical findings. Although the beneficial effect of gold compounds on the clinical manifestations of inflammation is important, the ability of these agents to retard the progression of articular damage is of even more significance. A number of studies have demonstrated that treatment of patients with RA with gold compounds retards cartilage loss and the development of cysts and erosions and, in some cases, even improves mineralization, as assessed by serial radiographs.[22]

Gold compounds are effective in patients with psoriatic arthritis with a rheumatoid pattern of involvement and in the treatment of peripheral arthritis in patients with spondylitis. Similar toxicity is also observed, but contrary to earlier teachings, cutaneous toxicity does not appear to be excessively severe or frequent when gold compounds are used in psoriatic arthritis, nor does chrysotherapy appear to benefit the skin of psoriatic patients.[39]

Gold compounds have been used in the treatment of juvenile RA (JRA) with success. The dose must be adjusted for the age and size of the child.

Chrysotherapy has been used for the treatment of palindromic rheumatism and of intermittent hydrarthrosis (see Chap. 58). It is said to be ineffective in the treatment of ankylosing spondylitis. Reports exist of its successful use in the treatment of nonrheumatic disorders such as pemphigus and asthma.[36]

TOXICITY

Unfortunately, the incidence of toxicity is high and frequently necessitates cessation of therapy (Fig. 29–1). During a standard course (20 injections of 50 mg) of therapy with gold compounds, approximately 35% of patients experience toxic side effects, and these effects are severe enough to require discontinuance of the drug in about 14% (Table 29–2). With continued maintenance therapy, the incidence of toxicity and treatment termination increases, so that by 4 to 5 years, only 16 to 50% of patients still receive treatment (Fig. 29–1).[38] Dermatitis is by far the most common side effect; proteinuria, neutropenia, and thrombocytopenia occur much less frequently. Uncommon side effects include the nitritoid reaction consisting of a cutaneous flush soon after injection, postinjection flares of inflammation, and gastrointestinal, pulmonary, and neurologic effects. The incidence of toxic effects is similar with both sodium aurothiomalate and aurothioglucose, but nitritoid re-

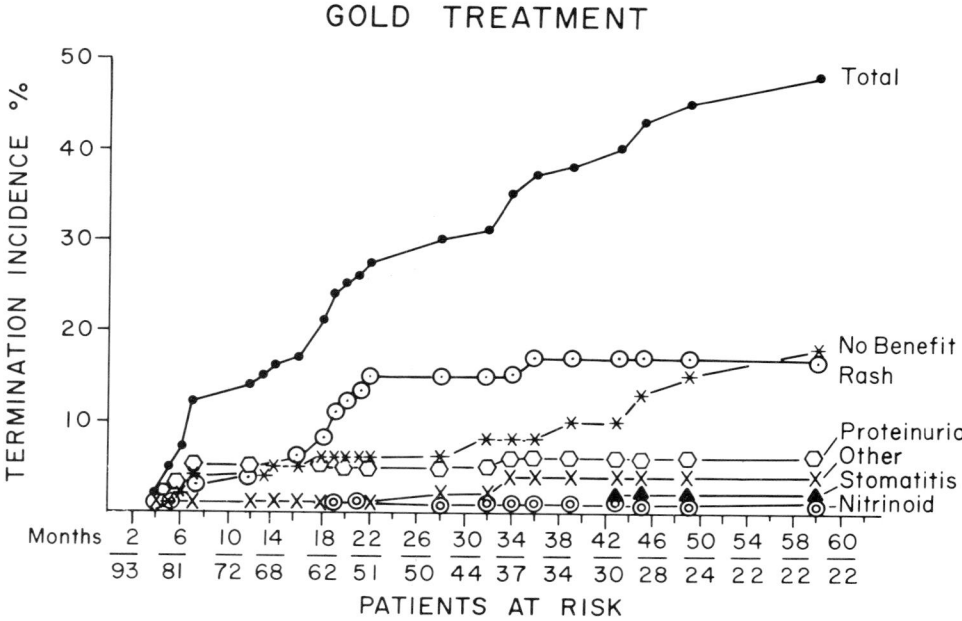

Fig. 29–1. Termination incidence for rash, for lack of benefit, for proteinuria, for other reasons, and for total causes during gold therapy. (From Richter, J.A., et al.[38])

Table 29–2. **Toxicity of Gold Compounds**

Mucocutaneous Effects
  Pruritus
  Rash
  Mucous membrane ulcers
Bone Marrow Effects
  Leukopenia
  Thrombocytopenia
Renal Effects
  Proteinuria
  Acute renal failure (hypersensitivity reaction)
Gastrointestinal Effects
  Diarrhea
  Enterocolitis
  Hepatocellular damage
Pulmonary Effects
  Reduced pulmonary function
Neurologic Effects
  Polyneuropathy
Chrysiasis
Nitritoid reaction
Postinjection inflammation flare

actions and postinjection flares are practically limited to patients receiving the former compound. The incidence of toxicity with the oral preparation is similar to that of the injectable compounds, but diarrhea is the most common side effect, and rash is less frequent. Early results suggest that the overall toxicity of oral gold preparations may be less than that of parenteral gold compounds.[11] Concomitant administration of glucocorticoids does not alter the incidence or severity of toxic reactions to gold compounds.

Toxicity to gold may be mediated by immune mechanisms under genetic control. Antibodies of the IgE class directed toward sodium aurothiomalate have been associated with toxic reactions.[6] Eosinophilia often accompanies gold toxicity. An increased incidence of toxicity, especially proteinuria, to gold compounds is seen in patients with HLA antigen haplotypes A1, B8, Cw7, and Dr3.[2] This and other findings suggest that immunologically mediated drug toxicity may be influenced by histocompatibility genes, which, in turn, may control cells concerned with immune responses.

Mucocutaneous Effects

Rash, pruritus, and mucous membrane ulcers are among the most common side effects in patients treated with gold compounds. The rash is invariably pruritic, although pruritus can occur without the rash. The rash is often similar to lichen planus or, less commonly, pityriasis rosea. It is often located in cutaneous folds, such as around the neck, the armpits, the groin, or under the breasts. Usually, however, it has no distinguishing characteristics. Eosinophilia variably accompanies rash and, when present, may precede or appear simultaneously with it. Severe reactions such as exfoliative dermatitis or toxic epidermal necrolysis occur rarely. Although mucocutaneous reactions represent the side effects most commonly associated with therapy with gold compounds, they also occur frequently in control populations. The reported incidence of toxic reactions in control populations may be spuriously high, however, because in some studies, the control injection consisted of small doses of gold compound. These small doses, although ineffective therapeutically, may well have been capable of inducing hypersensitivity reactions.

Bone Marrow Suppression

Although rare, the complication of bone marrow suppression is serious. Approximately 5% of patients develop some degree of leukopenia or thrombocytopenia. Usually, these disorders are minor and are not associated with increased risk of infection, bleeding, or other serious complications. Aplastic anemia has occurred, however, and it can be life-threatening in patients treated with gold compounds.

Renal Effects

Proteinuria is second only to rash as a manifestation of toxicity and occurs in up to 10% of patients treated with gold compounds. Proteinuria as the result of therapy with gold must be differentiated from that occurring as the result of renal amyloidosis, a complication of RA still common in many parts of the world.[5] The renal damage is usually mild, especially if recognized early and if treated by drug withdrawal. Nephrotic syndrome and renal failure have occurred, however. Immune complexes have been demonstrated in glomerular basement membrane. The nature of the antigen has not been determined. Early studies suggested that the immune complexes contained elemental gold, but later studies have not borne out this hypothesis. The findings of aurosomes in proximal and distal renal tubule cells and increased urinary excretion of urinary lysosomal enzymes as an early manifestation of nephrotoxicity have led to the suggestion that the initial injury is to renal tubules. Released antigens then complex with autoantibodies and give rise to autoimmune membranous nephropathy.[1] Rarely, acute renal failure may develop as a hypersensitivity reaction.

Other Toxic Reactions

Less common toxic reactions in patients treated with gold compounds involve the gastrointestinal tract, the lung, and the nervous system. As noted previously, mild diarrhea is the most common side effect of treatment with the oral gold preparation. Life-threatening enterocolitis has been reported as a complication of parenteral therapy.[33] The gastrointestinal tract may be affected throughout its length, and a clinical picture similar to toxic megacolon may develop. Histologic examination of biopsies reveals ulceration, edema, hemorrhage, and dense mononuclear cell infiltration. *Reversible liver damage* has been reported, associated with various histologic abnormalities and sometimes with lymphadenopathy, pulmonary infiltrates, and rash.[31]

Acute pulmonary damage, characterized by symptoms of rapidly progressing dyspnea, cough, occasionally with sputum production, pleuritic chest pain, fever, and rash, has been reported. Roentgenograms demonstrate diffuse infiltrates with patchy consolidation involving both lungs ("gold lung") (Fig. 29–2). Pulmonary function tests demonstrate a restrictive lung defect, reduced lung volume, and marked reduction in diffusing capacity. Histologic examination of lung biopsies demonstrates edema, interstitial fibrosis, and alveolar wall thickening with marked lymphocytic and plasma cell infiltration.[9] *Polyneuropathy* occurs uncommonly following therapy with gold compounds. Either a *mixed sensory and motor neuropathy,* which is predominantly distal, or an *acute polyneuropathy* of the Guillain-Barré type is seen. Axonal degeneration and segmental demyelination is seen in histological examination of sural nerve biopsies.[24]

Corneal chrysiasis, or deposition of elemental gold in the cornea, detected by slit-lamp examination, occurs in up to 87% of patients who have received as much as 1,500 mg sodium aurothiomalate. It is of no clinical significance. More extensive deposition of elemental gold in skin occurs rarely and may be mistaken for cyanosis.[3] Gold compounds may cause reactions similar to those caused by nitrites. These *nitritoid reactions* consist of facial flushing, nausea, dizziness, and sometimes, hypotension. *Postinjection reactions* of transient stiffness, arthralgia, myalgia, and constitutional symptoms account for only a few withdrawals from therapy in large control series. They occur, however, in as many as 15% of patients and may result in unnecessary and premature cessation of therapy.[20] Both nitritoid and postinjection reactions are more common in patients receiving sodium aurothiomalate than in those treated with aurothioglucose. These reactions usually cease when the latter drug is substituted.

Management of Toxic Reactions

Most toxic side effects of therapy with gold compounds, if detected early, can be managed simply by discontinuing the drug. Nitritoid and postinjection reactions respond to a change in gold compound. More severe toxicity, such as nephrosis with significant proteinuria, exfoliative dermatitis, or other severe skin toxicity, or marked leukopenia

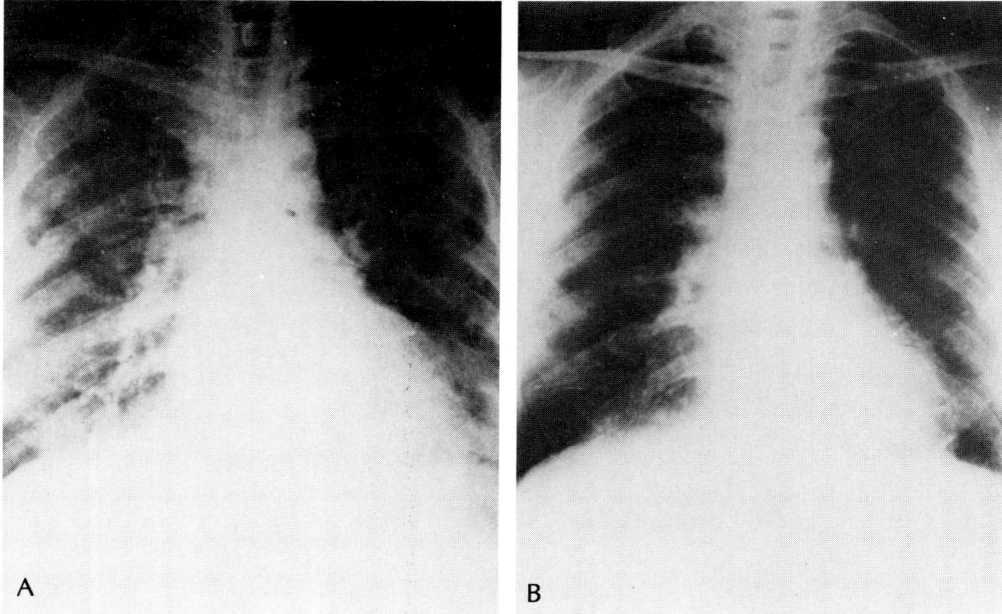

Fig. 29–2.   Posteroanterior chest radiographs of a patient with "gold lung." *A,* On hospital admission, and *B,* three months later, after successful treatment. (From Cooke, N., and Bamji, A.[9])

or thrombocytopenia, requires the use of glucocorticoids,[7] the equivalent of 40 to 60 mg prednisone daily, in divided doses. A combination of glucocorticoids and agents capable of chelating gold, such as British anti-Lewisite (BAL), has sometimes been used with apparent success. No clear-cut evidence suggests that chelating agents provide additional benefit, however. N-acetylcysteine (Mucomyst), which binds but does not chelate monovalent gold, has been used alone in doses of 2 to 9 g infused intravenously over 2 to 6 hours to treat hematologic reactions to gold. This agent lacks the toxicity of BAL and is apparently effective.*[16] Enterocolitis, when associated with eosinophilia, has been reported to respond to cromolyn sodium, 20 mg q.i.d.[33].

Monitoring Toxicity during Therapy

Prior to each injection, the patient should be questioned regarding symptoms of toxicity. Pruritus usually precedes other manifestations of rash. Traditionally, also prior to each injection, patients have a complete blood count, including a differential white count and either a platelet count or examination of the peripheral smear for platelet adequacy, and a urinalysis, particularly assessing proteinuria. Excessive reliance should not be placed on these laboratory tests to exclude toxic reactions. Leukopenia or thrombocytopenia can occur precipitously. The patient should be advised to contact the physician should fever, oral ulceration, purpura or other bleeding, or other sign of bone marrow suppression develop. Usually, however, a gradual decline in peripheral blood elements is observed and allows for reduction in dosage or cessation of treatment. Hematuria is an unlikely result of treatment with gold compounds. If it occurs, another cause should be sought.

Reinstitution of Therapy after Toxic Reactions

Following severe reactions, such as marked thrombocytopenia or leukopenia, exfoliative dermatitis, nephrotic syndrome, colitis, or pulmonary reaction, therapy with gold compounds should not be reinstituted. After mild toxic reactions, however, it is often possible to resume therapy with gold compounds at a lower dose or at decreased frequency. Should a toxic reaction recur, another second-line drug, such as penicillamine or azathioprine, may be given. Most studies have shown that toxicity to gold compounds is not predictive of the probability or the type of potential toxic reaction to one of the other drugs.

---

*Editor's note: We have successfully treated a patient with severe aplastic anemia with 10 g n-acetylcysteine given every 24 hours through a Hickman catheter and using an infusion pump. Treatment for 4 months was necessary to reverse gold toxicity and to stabilize the bone marrow output at normal levels.

REFERENCES

1. Ainsworth, S.K., et al.: Gold nephropathy: ultrastructural, fluorescent, and energy-dispersive x-ray microanalysis study. Arch. Pathol. Lab. Med., *105*:373–378, 1981.
2. Bardin, T., et al.: HLA system and side effects of gold salts and D-penicillamine treatment of rheumatoid arthritis. Ann. Rheum. Dis., *41*:599–601, 1982.
3. Beckett, V.L., et al.: Chrysiasis resulting from gold therapy in rheumatoid arthritis: Identification of gold by x-ray microanalysis. Mayo Clin. Proc., *57*:773–777, 1982.
4. Binderup, L., Bramm, E., and Arrigoni-Martelli, E.: The effect of some antirheumatic drugs *in vivo* on the response of spleen cells to concanavalin A in rats with chronic inflammation. Int. J. Immunopharmacol., *4*:57–66, 1982.
5. Bourke, B.E., Woodrow, D.F., and Scott, J.T.: Proteinuria in rheumatoid arthritis—drug-induced or amyloid? Ann. Rheum. Dis., *40*:240–244, 1981.
6. Bretza, J., Wells, I., and Novey, H.S.: Association of IgE antibodies to sodium aurothiomalate and adverse reactions to chrysotherapy for rheumatoid arthritis. Am. J. Med., *74*:945–950, 1983.
7. Coblyn, J.S., et al.: Gold-induced thrombocytopenia. Ann. Intern. Med., *95*:178–181, 1981.
8. Cohen, D.L., Orzel, J., and Taylor, A.: Infants of mothers receiving gold therapy. (Letter.) Arthritis Rheum., *24*:104–105, 1981.
9. Cooke, N., and Bamji, A.: Gold lung. Rheumatol. Rehabil., *20*:129–135, 1981.
10. Cooperating Clinics Committee of the American Rheumatism Association: A controlled trial of gold salt therapy in rheumatoid arthritis. Arthritis Rheum., *16*:353–358, 1973.
11. Davis, P., and Harth, M. (Eds.): Proceedings—Therapeutic innovation in rheumatoid arthritis: worldwide auranofin symposium. J. Rheumatol., *9 (Suppl. 8)*:1–209, 1982.
12. Empire Rheumatism Council: Gold therapy in rheumatoid arthritis. Final report of a multicentre controlled trial. Ann. Rheum. Dis., *20*:315–352, 1961.
13. Empire Rheumatism Council: Gold therapy in rheumatoid arthritis. Report of a multi-centre controlled trial. Ann. Rheum. Dis., *19*:95–119, 1960.
14. Forestier, J.: Rheumatoid arthritis and its treatment by gold salts. J. Lab. Clin. Med., *20*:827–840, 1935.
15. Ghadially, F.N., et al.: The morphology and atomic composition of aurosomes produced by sodium aurothiomalate in human monocytes. Ann. Pathol., *2*:117–125, 1982.
16. Godfrey, N.F., et al.: IV N-acetyl-cysteine treatment of hematologic reactions to chrysotherapy. J. Rheumatol., *9*:519–526, 1982.
17. Goldberg, R.L., et al.: A mechanism of action of gold sodium thiomalate in diseases characterized by a proliferative synovitis: reversible changes in collagen production in cultured human synovial cells. J. Pharmacol. Exp. Ther., *218*:395–403, 1981.
18. Gottlieb, N.L., and Gray, R.G.: Pharmacokinetics of gold in rheumatoid arthritis. Agents Actions, *8 [Suppl.]*:529–538, 1981.
19. Graham, G.G., et al.: The effect of smoking on the distribution of gold in blood. J. Rheumatol., *9*:527–531, 1982.
20. Halla, J.T., Harden, J.G., and Linn, J.E.: Postinjection nonvasomotor reactions during chrysotherapy. Arthritis Rheum., *20*:1188–1191, 1977.
21. Highton, J., et al.: Changes in immune function in patients with rheumatoid arthritis following treatment with sodium aurothiomalate. Ann. Rheum. Dis., *40*:254–262, 1981.
22. Iannuzzi, L., et al.: Does drug therapy slow radiographic deterioration in rheumatoid arthritis? N. Engl. J. Med., *309*:1023–1028, 1983.
23. Jellum, E., and Munthe, E.: Fate of the thiomalate part after intramuscular administration of aurothiomalate in rheumatoid arthritis. Ann. Rheum. Dis., *41*:431–432, 1982.
24. Katrak, S.M., et al.: Clinical and morphological features of gold neuropathy. Brain, *103*:671–693, 1980.
25. Keers, R.Y.: The gold rush 1925–35. Thorax, *35*:884–889, 1980.
25a. Lande, K.: Die gunstique Baunflussung Schleichender Dauerinfekte durch Solganal. MMW, *74*:1132–1134, 1927.
26. Laurent, M.R., and Panayi, G.S.: Biochemical parameters in the assessment of anti-inflammatory drugs—a review. Agents Actions, *7 [Suppl]*:310–317, 1977.
27. Leibfarth, J.H., and Persellin, R.H.: Mechanisms of action of gold. Agents Actions, *11*:458–472, 1981.
28. Lipsky, P.E., and Ziff, M.: The mechanisms of action of gold and D-penicillamine in rheumatoid arthritis. *In* Advances in Inflammation Research. Vol. III: Rheumatoid Arthritis. Edited by M. Ziff, G.P. Velo, and S. Gorini. New York, Raven Press, 1982, pp. 219–235.
29. Lipsky, P.E., and Ziff, M.: Inhibition of antigen- and mitogen-induced human lymphocyte proliferation by gold compounds. J. Clin. Invest., *59*:455–466, 1977.
30. Lorber, A., Jackson, W.H., and Simon, T.M.: Assessment of immune response during chrysotherapy. Comparison of gold sodium thiomalate vs. auranofin. Scand. J. Rheumatol., *10*:129–137, 1981.
31. Lowthian, P.J., Cleland, L.G., and Vernon-Roberts, B.: Hepatotoxicity with aurothioglucose therapy. Arthritis Rheum., *27*:230–232, 1984.
32. Luukkainen, R.: Chrysotherapy in rheumatoid arthritis: with particular emphasis on the effect of chrysotherapy on radiographical changes and on the optimal time of initiation of therapy. Scand. J. Rheumatol., *34 [Suppl.]*:1–56, 1980.
33. Martin, D.M., et al.: Gold-induced eosinophilic enterocolitis: response to oral cromolyn sodium. Gastroenterology, *80*:1567–1570, 1981.
34. Munthe, E., Kass, E., and Jellum, E.: Evidence for enhanced radical scavenging prior to drug response in rheumatoid arthritis. *In* Advances in Inflammation Research. Vol. III: Rheumatoid Arthritis. Edited by M. Ziff, G.P. Velo, and S. Gorini. New York, Raven Press, 1982, pp. 211–218.
35. Oaten, S.W., Jagelman, S., and Webb, H.E.: Further studies of macrophages in relationship to avirulent Semliki forest virus infections. Br. J. Exp. Pathol., *61*:150–155, 1980.
36. Okatani, Y.: A few clinical statistical observations on the use of Solganal-B-oleosum in bronchial asthma. J. Asthma Res., *17*:165–173, 1980.
37. Rainsford, K.D., Brune, K., and Whitehouse, M.W. (Eds.): Trace elements in the pathogenesis and treatment of inflammation. Agents Actions Supplements, *8*:1–617, 1981.
38. Richter, J.A., et al.: Analysis of treatment terminations with gold and antimalarial compounds in rheumatoid arthritis. J. Rheumatol., *7*:153–159, 1980.
39. Richter, M.B., Kinsella, P., and Corbett, M.: Gold in psoriatic arthropathy. Ann. Rheum. Dis., *39*:279–280, 1980.
40. Sadler, P.J.: The biological chemistry of gold: a metallodrug and heavy-atom label with variable valency. Struct. Bond., *29*:171–214, 1976.
41. Schattenkirchner, M., et al.: Auranofin and sodium aurothiomalate in the treatment of rheumatoid arthritis. J. Rheumatol., *9 (Suppl. 8)*:184–189, 1982.
42. Sharp, J.T., Lidsky, M.D., and Duffy, J.: Clinical responses during gold therapy for rheumatoid arthritis: changes in synovitis, radiologically detectable erosive lesions, serum proteins, and serologic abnormalities. Arthritis Rheum., *25*:540–549, 1982.
43. Short, A.K., et al.: β-Naphthylamidase activity of the cell surface of Ehrlich ascites cells. Reversible control of enzyme activity by metal ions and thiols. Br. J. Cancer, *44*:709–716, 1981.
44. Skosey, J.L., et al.: Drug interference with inactivation of

serum alpha-1-proteinase inhibitor by oxygen radicals. *In* Oxy Radicals and Their Scavenger Systems. Vol. II: Cellular and Medical Aspects. Edited by R.A. Greenwald and G. Cohen. New York, Elsevier Biomedical, 1983, pp. 264–267.

45. Skosey, J.L., and Chow, D.C.: Inactivation of serum elastase inhibitory capacity by products of stimulated neutrophils: protection by gold salts and D-penicillamine. *In* Advances in Inflammation Research. Vol. III: Rheumatoid

Arthritis. Edited by M. Ziff, G.P. Velo, and S. Gorini. New York, Raven Press, 1982, pp. 245–253.

46. Sliwinski, A.J., and Guertin, M.A.: Gold suppression of human neutrophil function *in vitro*. Biochem. Pharmacol., *31*:671–676, 1982.

47. Vernon-Roberts, B.: Action of gold salts on the inflammatory response and inflammatory cell function. J. Rheumatol., *6 (Suppl. 5)*:120–129, 1979.

Chapter 30

Antimalarials

Nathan J. Zvaifler

Enthusiasm for the use of antimalarial drugs to treat rheumatic diseases has waxed or waned over the past quarter century. The original enthusiasm for these compounds related to their therapeutic efficacy and seemingly mild side effects, but the eventual recognition of serious and sometimes progressive retinal damage curtailed their use. There has been recent rebirth of interest in these compounds because of an appreciation that ocular toxicity is infrequent and can be minimized by careful attention to safe drug doses.[38]

THERAPEUTIC EFFICACY

Antimalarial treatment of inflammatory arthritis began in 1951. Quinacrine was used in the initial study by Page.[35] Subsequently, other synthetic antimalarial compounds were tried, but most were eliminated because of toxicity. Two of the 4-aminoquinolines, however, are still regularly employed: chloroquine phosphate, currently favored in Europe, and hydroxychloroquine sulfate, the only FDA-approved agent of this class readily available in the United States. Both of these demonstrated efficacy in controlled double-blind studies of patients with adult rheumatoid arthritis (RA). Three have evaluated chloroquine[11,17,37] and two hydroxychloroquine.[20,27] Although not exactly alike in design, they are remarkably similar in the clinical parameters assessed. Chloroquine in an 11-week study[11] and hydroxychloroquine in a 12-week study[20] showed drug-placebo differences all favoring drug, but none reached statistical significance. As the duration of studies increased to 6 months or longer, more impressive drug-placebo differences emerged.[17,27,37] For instance, in 1960 Friedman and Steinberg studied 107 RA patients who took chloroquine for one year.[17] Statistically significant improvement in grip strength, joint tenderness, walking time, and erythrocyte sedimentation rate was found in the treated patients as compared to those given placebo. The chloroquine group also appeared to show less progression of radiographic changes. Chloroquine treatment compared favorably with gold or azathioprine in a group of patients with RA of less than five years in duration.[14] A retrospective life-table analysis was performed on RA patients receiving either gold, penicillamine, levamisole, or hydroxychloroquine for 12 to 22 months. Therapeutic benefits were comparable with each drug, but terminations because of complications were lowest in the hydroxychloroquine group, and approximately 50% of those taking hydroxychloroquine at 400 mg per day were satisfied with the results of their treatment.[38] Other long-term assessments of antimalarials attest to their efficacy and mild toxicity in the treatment of RA.[5] In the most recent report of the long-term (uncontrolled) use of hydroxychloroquine, 12% of 108 patients with RA treated at least 6 months achieved a complete remission, and another 14% showed a 75% reduction in active joint count. Overall, 63% of the group had some improvement.[1] Patients with early disease appeared to be more responsive, as has been noted by others, but chronic RA does not preclude a good response to antimalarial treatment.

DRUG METABOLISM

Chloroquine phosphate and hydroxychloroquine sulfate are similar 4-aminoquinoline compounds differing only in a single hydroxyl group at the end of the side chain. Both are rapidly and completely absorbed when given by mouth, and their subsequent metabolism is about the same, except that chloroquine is excreted primarily in the urine, whereas fecal excretion of hydroxychloroquine is greater.[3,7,29,30] Fifty percent of the administered drug can be recovered; the remainder is eliminated as metabolites.[7] Plasma levels reflect a direct dose-response relationship, and the concentrations attained during conventional long-term therapy range between 200 and 400 μg/l for chloroquine and slightly higher for hydroxychloroquine.[3,29,47] The serum concentration does not distinguish responders from nonresponders, but there is direct correlation between the frequency of side effects and serum-drug concentration. Approximately 80% of chloroquine-treated patients develop significant complications when their serum concentrations exceed 800 μg/l of chloroquine. The amount of drug that accumulates in various tissues is independent of the plasma level. Fat, bone, tendon, and brain, for example, have only small amounts of the 4-aminoquinolines, whereas organs such as the bone marrow, kidney, lungs, and liver contain concentrations several hundred times greater than those found in serum or plasma. The most dramatic accumulation is in the melanin-containing ocular tissues.[9,29] Chronic oral feeding of chloroquine to pigmented rats results in a drug concentration in the iris, choroid, and pigment epithelium of the retina that is 40 to 80 times higher than in the liver.[9] Moreover, there is a nonlinear (geometric) accumulation of the drug in the eyes of experimental animals given amounts of chloroquine simulating human doses of 250 mg, 500 mg, and 750 mg daily.[36]

PHARMACOLOGIC EFFECTS

Although the 4-aminoquinoline compounds have multiple pharmacologic actions, most are only observed at concentrations far exceeding the plasma levels obtained with conventional doses. The significance of plasma levels to mechanism of action of the drug is probably irrelevant since concentrations many times greater are achieved intracellularly, particularly in cell nuclei and in lysosomes.[2,12,28,44] Several properties of the chloroquines might be relevant to their antirheumatic action. The lysosomal accumulation may interfere with endocytosis and vesical fusion, decreasing the digestive efficiency of phagolysosomes, and may inhibit the recycling of cell surface receptors.[26,44] Chloroquine in basic form diffuses freely across membranes, including those of lysosomes. Inside this organelle the pH is 4 to 5 maintained by an ATP-driven proton pump, and the drug is protonated. The protonated drug is trapped inside the lysosome, and the pH rises away from the pH optimum of the lysosomal enzymes. Whether these acute effects, demonstrated in tissue-cultured macrophages, relate to the long-term effects of the drug is unknown.[33,46] Theoretically, they could modulate the release of deleterious enzymes in local inflammatory environments, such as the joint. In several experimental studies, the antimalarial drugs have been shown to reduce inflammation. They can trap free radicals, impair chemotaxis, and suppress prostaglandin production.[4,10,36,43] These anti-inflammatory properties would obviously be of advantage in the treatment of RA, but they are usually observed only at concentrations unlikely to occur in the tissues of treated patients. In addition, antimalarials have more in common with the slow-acting, remission-inducing drugs than they do with nonsteroidal anti-inflammatory agents. The former, including gold, penicillamine, and levamisole, appear to provide the therapeutic benefits through their effects on the immune system.[48] The demonstration that chloroquine can interfere with the generation of immu-noglobulin-secreting cells by selectively inhibiting the release of interleukin-1 from monocytes at concentrations as low as 0.8 μg/ml is, therefore, of great interest.[39]

CHLOROQUINE RETINAL TOXICITY

The earliest lesion of the retinopathy caused by the 4-aminoquinolines occurs in the macular areas of the fundus.[8,42] Granularity and edema are the initial findings followed by bilateral, symmetric pigmentary changes ranging from subtle stippling to the typical "bull's-eye" or "doughnut" appearance of advanced chloroquine macular retinopathy.[19,23,34] Classically, the lesion consists of central macular hyperpigmentation surrounded by a clear ring of depigmentation and then an outer ring of pigment (hence the bull's-eye). Only after extensive retinal damage are there changes in other parts of the fundus, pallor of the optic disk, arteriolar attenuation of segmental constriction, or loss of peripheral vision. Bernstein has described an early "premaculopathy" with fine pigmentary stippling of the macula and loss of the foveal light reflex.[8] Unlike "true retinopathy," it is asymptomatic, never affects visual acuity, and is almost always reversible following drug discontinuation.

Pathologic changes in chloroquine and hydroxychloroquine-induced retinopathy are seen mainly as a migration of the retinal pigment epithelial cells into the adjacent retinal layer and a loss of rods and cones.[13,16,31,42,45] The actual pathogenesis is not known, but probably is a direct result of the drug's interaction with the retinal pigmented epithelium,[9,30] whose primary function is to phagocytize and digest photoreceptor membranes shed from the tips of rods and cones. Photoreceptor shedding occurs regularly when the retina is exposed to light, and the 4-aminoquinolines appear to interfere with the efficient elimination of the cellular debris.[26] Several factors have been reported to influence retinal toxicity, including duration of treatment, total drug dose, plasma level, and the antimalarial drug studied.[8] Chloroquine, for instance, seems to be more toxic than hydroxychloroquine.[38,41] However, the most important determinant is the daily dose administered.[15,18,36] The relationship of drug dose to retinal injury is supported by nonlinear deposition of chloroquine into the pigmented ocular tissues of experimental animals.[36]

The incidence of chloroquine retinopathy has been variously reported from 1 in 1000 to 15% of those taking the drug.[22,42] A more reasonable estimate of the frequency of true retinopathy is probably a few percent,[8] but several studies have shown no significant retinal changes in patients taking 250 mg of chloroquine daily for long periods when compared with patients with the same diseases not receiving the drug.[24,40] In a risk/benefit analysis of hydroxychloroquine, only 4 of 99 patients taking 400 mg daily for more than one year developed an early maculopathy that caused no visual loss and reversed completely when the drug was discontinued.[38] Reasons for discrepancy in reporting include a lack of agreement about what constitutes chloroquine retinopathy, absence of correlation between observed retinal change and the degree of visual impairment, and an impression that the connective tissue disorders themselves can produce similar retinal abnormalities.[40]

Several techniques are available for detecting early retinal change. The most useful are ophthalmoscopic and photographic observations of the macular area to document change in pigmentation, combined with sensitive central visual field testing.[8] Electroretinograms, electro-oculograms, dark adaptation, retinal threshold profiles, and color vision are all ancillary techniques that are seldom required. An Amsler grid is provided each patient to permit self-testing at home (Fig. 30–1).

The development of clear-cut retinopathy demands immediate discontinuation of the offending drug. It is not clear whether it is necessary to stop with premaculopathy, but given the current availability of alternative treatments, this is advisable. Enhanced excretion of the 4-aminoquinolines by acidification of blood and urine or the use of chelating agents are theoretical possibilities that have never been tested.[9] Discontinuation of the drug at the first sign of retinopathy usually halts and occasionally reverses the progression of the pigmentary lesion.[22,32]

TREATMENT OF RHEUMATOID ARTHRITIS WITH ANTIMALARIALS

Chloroquine and hydroxychloroquine are used in the treatment of RA.* Chloroquine is taken in a single dose of 250 mg, usually before retiring, and hydroxychloroquine is administered in a 200-mg dose twice a day. Side effects consist of nausea, diarrhea, skin rash, ototoxicity, hemolytic anemia and rarely, neuromyopathy. In addition, chloroquine may deposit in the corneal epithelium where it can be detected by slit-lamp examination. Visual symptoms are often absent, but patients may complain of seeing halos about street lights or lamps. These deposits disappear with reduction in dose or withdrawal of the medication, leave no residual abnormalities, and have no known association with the development of retinopathy.[8] An uncommon

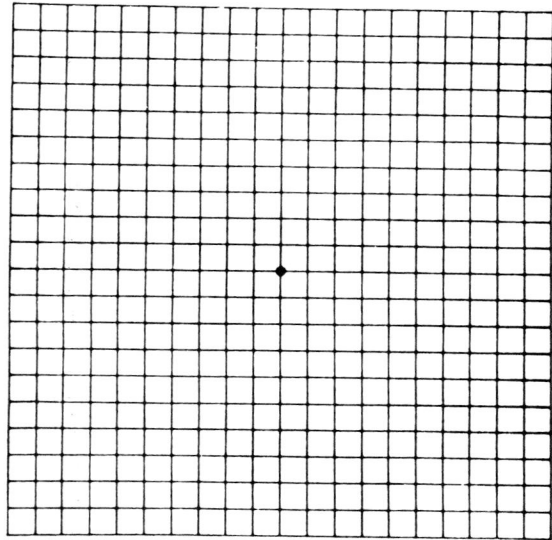

Fig. 30–1. Amsler grid. The following instructions are given to patients:

Proper use of the Amsler grid will enable you to detect subtle changes in your vision due to even a small amount of fluid from under your retina.

To perform the test, wear the glasses that you normally use while reading. If you wear bifocals, use the bottom portion or reading portion of the glass. Attach the grid to a wall at eye level and stand 12 to 14 inches away from it. Cover one eye. With the other eye, look at the center dot.

While you are looking at the center dot, you should be able to see the four corners of the square. You should also be able to see that the large square is composed of many smaller squares.

The first day you observe the grid, mark with a pencil any areas of distortion, any gray or blurry spots, or any blank spots. This is your baseline pattern.

Each Monday morning thereafter, look at the center dot of the grid. If you notice new areas of distortion, wavy instead of straight lines, or enlargement of the blank spot, especially toward the center, please call me promptly.

dose-related problem is impairment in accommodation. This direct toxicity to the ciliary body is immediately reversible upon dose reduction or discontinuation. Skin rashes are usually macular or maculopapular, occasionally urticarial; individuals sensitive to one agent may tolerate the other. An unusual patchy increase in skin pigment and blanching of the hair and the eyebrows are occasionally seen and may be a harbinger of retinopathy. Sunburn is accentuated and even occurs in persons who normally tan.

Antimalarials are seldom prescribed as the only antirheumatic medication, but are usually given in combination with salicylates or small doses of corticosteroids. Clinical improvement occurs slowly,

---

*Chloroquine diphosphate, originally available as Aralen, can now be obtained only in the generic form as a 125- or 250-mg tablet. Hydroxychloroquine sulfate (Plaquenil) is available as a 100- or 200-mg tablet.

seldom before 4 weeks; usually 3 to 6 months of drug administration are required before significant benefits are observed. It is neither necessary nor desirable to exceed 250 mg of chloroquine or 400 mg of hydroxychloroquine a day. The results of therapy should be critically appraised after 3 or 4 months; if improvement has occurred, the drug is continued, but with the provision that a funduscopic examination will be performed soon thereafter and then at 6-month intervals by an ophthalmologist acquainted with the drug's ocular toxicity. This program is associated with a low incidence of true retinopathy.[40] Others suggest a baseline assessment before starting treatment,[8] and the manufacturer of hydroxychloroquine sulfate (Plaquenil) recommends three monthly ophthalmologic examinations. Ophthalmologic examination should include color vision and two-point discrimination with a red target. We give all patients an Amsler grid (see Fig. 30–1) and instruct them to test themselves weekly. This may detect retinal macular edema, the earliest sign of toxicity.

After 6 months, if improvement has been sustained, a trial at a lesser dose is indicated. Chloroquine can be taken at 125 mg daily or 250 mg every other day; hydroxychloroquine is usually reduced to 200 mg (one tablet) daily. Withdrawal symptoms do not result from discontinuing the drug.

Laaksonen and his associates advise using serum drug concentration to monitor therapy in juvenile RA.[25] They consider 250 to 280 μg/l to be the maximum safe concentration for serum chloroquine and 370 to 470 μg/ml for hydroxychloroquine. These levels are usually attained by treatment with chloroquine diphosphate at 4 mg/kg/day and hydroxychloroquine sulfate at 5 to 7 mg/kg/day, but significant individual variations have been noted.[25]

Antimalarials have been recommended for treatment of Sjögren's syndrome (keratoconjunctivitis)[21] and psoriasis, but this may be hazardous because of the development of exfoliative dermatitis.[6] Their role in the therapy of systemic lupus erythematosus is discussed in Chapter 61.

REFERENCES

1. Adams, E.M., Yocum, D.E., and Bell, C.L.: Hydroxychloroquine in the treatment of rheumatoid arthritis. Am. J. Med., 75:321–326, 1983.
2. Allison, A.C., and Young, M.R.: Uptake of dyes and drugs by living cells in culture. Life Sci., 3:1407–1414, 1964.
3. Alving, A.S., et al.: Studies on the chronic toxicity of chloroquine. J. Clin. Invest., 27:60–65, 1948.
4. Authi, K.S., and Traynor, J.R.: Effects of antimalarial drugs on phospholipase A₂. Br. J. Pharmacol., 66:496, 1979.
5. Bagnall, A.W.: The value of chloroquine in rheumatoid disease. Can. Med. Assoc. J., 77:182–194, 1957.
6. Baker, H.: The influence of chloroquine and related drugs on psoriasis and keratodermia blenorrhagicum. Br. J. Dermatol., 78:161–166, 1966.
7. Berliner, R.W., et al.: Studies on the chemotherapy of human malarias. II. The physiologic deposition, anti-malarial activity and toxicity of several derivations of 4 aminoquinolene. J. Clin. Invest., 27:98–107, 1948.
8. Bernstein, H.N.: Ophthalmologic considerations and testing in patients receiving long-term antimalarial therapy. In A Reassessment of Plaquenil in the Treatment of Rheumatoid Arthritis (Symposium). Am. J. Med., 75:25–34, 1983.
9. Bernstein, H.N., et al.: The ocular deposition of chloroquine. Invest. Ophthalmol., 2:384–394, 1963.
10. Blackwell, G.J., et al.: Phospholipase A₂ activity of guinea pig isolated perfused lungs: Stimulation and inhibition by anti-inflammatory steroids. Br. J. Pharmacol., 62:79–89, 1978.
11. Cohen, A.S., and Calkins, E.: A controlled study of chloroquine as an antirheumatic agent. Arthritis Rheum., 1:297–312, 1958.
12. Cohen, S.N., and Yielding, K.L.: Spectrophotometric studies on the interaction of chloroquine with dioxyribonucleic acid. J. Biol. Chem., 240:3123–3131, 1965.
13. Dale, A.J., Parkhill, E.M., and Layton, D.O.: Studies on chloroquine retinopathy in rabbits. J.A.M.A., 193:241–243, 1965.
14. Dwosh, I.L., et al.: Azathioprine in early rheumatoid arthritis. Comparison with gold and chloroquine. Arthritis Rheum., 20:685–692, 1977.
15. Elman, A., et al.: Chloroquine retinopathy in patients with rheumatoid arthritis. Scand. J. Rheumatol., 5:161–166, 1976.
16. Francois, J., and Maudgal, M.C.: Experimental chloroquine retinopathy. Ophthalmologica (Basel), 148:442–452, 1964.
17. Friedman, A., and Steinberg, V.L.: Chloroquine in rheumatoid arthritis. A double blindfold trial of treatment for one year. Ann. Rheum. Dis., 19:243–250, 1960.
18. Frisk-Holmberg, M., et al.: Chloroquine serum concentrations and side effects: Evidence for dose dependent kinetics. Clin. Pharmacol. Ther., 25:345–350, 1979.
19. Giles, C.L., Henderson, J.W.: The ocular toxicity of chloroquine therapy. Am. J. Med. Sci., 249:230–235, 1965.
20. Hamilton, E.B.D., and Scott, J.T.: Hydroxychloroquine sulfate (Plaquenil) in treatment of rheumatoid arthritis. Arthritis Rheum., 5:502–512, 1962.
21. Heaton, J.M.: The treatment of Sjögren's syndrome with hydroxychloroquine. Am. J. Ophthalmol., 55:983–986, 1963.
22. Henkind, P., and Rothfield, N.E.: Ocular abnormalities in patients treated with synthetic anti-malarial drugs. N. Engl. J. Med., 269:243–249, 1963.
23. Hobbs, H.E., Sorsby, A., and Freedman, A.: Retinopathy following chloroquine therapy. Lancet, 2:478–480, 1959.
24. Knox, J.M., and Freeman, R.G.: Prophylactic use of chloroquine to prevent skin cancer. Arch. Dermatol., 87:315–322, 1963.
25. Laaksonen, A.L., Kosklahde, V., and Juva, K.: Dosage of antimalarial drugs for children with juvenile rheumatoid arthritis and systemic lupus erythematosus. Scand. J. Rheumatol., 3:103–108, 1974.
26. Mackenzie, A.H.: Pharmacologic actions of 4-aminoquinoline compounds. In A Reassessment of Plaquenil in the Treatment of Rheumatoid Arthritis (Symposium). Am. J. Med., 75:5–10, 1983.
27. Mainland, D., and Sutcliffe, M.I.: Hydroxychloroquine sulfate in rheumatoid arthritis: A six month double blind trial. Bull. Rheum. Dis., 17:287–290, 1962.
28. Marquez, V.E., et al.: Binding to deoxyribosenucleic acid and inhibition of ribonucleic acid polymerase by analogs of chloroquine. J. Med. Chem., 17:856–862, 1974.
29. McChesney, E.W., et al.: Studies of the metabolism of some compounds of the 4 amino-7-chloroquine series. J. Pharmacol. Exp. Ther., 151:482–493, 1966.
30. McChesney, E.W., Banks, W.F., Jr., and McAuliff, J.P.: Laboratory studies of the 4-aminoquinoline antimalarials: II. Plasma levels of chloroquine and hydroxychloroquine

in man after various oral regimens. Antibiot. Chemother., *12*:583–594, 1962.

31. Meier-Ruge, W.: Experimental investigation of the morphogenesis of chloroquine retinopathy. Arch. Ophthalmol., *73*:540–544, 1965.

32. Nocik, R.A., Weinstock, F.J., and Vignos, P.S.: Ocular complications of chloroquine. Am. J. Ophthalmol., *58*:774–778, 1964.

33. Ohkuma, S., and Poole, B.: Fluorescence probe measurement of the intralysosomal pH in living cells and the perturbation of pH by various agents. Proc. Natl. Acad. Sci. U.S.A., *75*:3327, 1978.

34. Okun, E., et al.: Chloroquine retinopathy: A report of 8 cases with ERG and dark adaptation finding. Arch Ophthalmol., *58*:774–778, 1964.

35. Page, F.: Treatment of lupus erythematosus with mepacrine. Lancet, *2*:755–758, 1951.

36. Perez, R., et al.: Chloroquine binding to melanin characteristics and significance. Arthritis Rheum., *7*:337–338, 1964.

37. Popert, A.J., et al.: Chloroquine diphosphate in rheumatoid arthritis: A controlled trial. Ann. Rheum. Dis., *20*:18–35, 1961.

38. Runge, L.A.: Risk/benefit analysis of hydroxychloroquine sulfate treatment in rheumatoid arthritis. *In* A Reassessment of Plaquenil in the Treatment of Rheumatoid Arthritis (Symposium). Am. J. Med., *75*:52–56, 1983.

39. Salmeron, G., and Lipsky, P.E.: Immunosuppressive po-

tential of antimalarials. *In* A Reassessment of Plaquenil in the Treatment of Rheumatoid Arthritis (Symposium). Am. J. Med., *75*:19–24, 1983.

40. Scherbel, A.L., et al.: Ocular lesions in rheumatoid arthritis and related disorders with particular reference to retinopathy. N. Engl. J. Med., *273*:360–366, 1965.

41. Toben, D., Krohel, G., and Rynes, R.: Hydroxychloroquine, a seven year experience. Arch. Ophthalmol., *100*:81–83, 1982.

42. Von Sallmann, L., and Bernstein, N.H.: Adverse effects of chloroquine and related antimalarial drugs on ocular structure. Bull. Rheum. Dis., *14*:327–330, 1963.

43. Ward, P.A.: The chemosuppression of chemotaxis. J. Exp. Med., *124*:209–225, 1966.

44. Weissmann, G.: Labilization and stabilization of lysosomes. Fed. Proc., *23*:1038–1044, 1964.

45. Wetterholm, D.H., and Winter, F.C.: Histopathology of chloroquine retinal toxicity. Arch. Ophthalmol. (Chicago), *71*:82–87, 1964.

46. Wibo, M., and Poole, B.: Protein degradation in cultured cells. J. Cell Biol., *63*:430, 1974.

47. Wollheim, F.A., Hanson, A., and Laurell, C.B.: Chloroquine treatment in rheumatoid arthritis. Scand. J. Rheumatol., *7*:171–176, 1978.

48. Zvaifler, N.J.: Immunopathology of inflammatory diseases: Rheumatoid arthritis as an example. Therapeutic control of inflammatory diseases. *In* Advances in Inflammation Research. Vol. 7. Edited by I. Otterness, R. Capitola, and S. Wong. New York, Raven Press, 1984, pp. 1–12.

Chapter 31

Penicillamine

Israeli A. Jaffe

Penicillamine is a 5-carbon amino acid that is a structural analogue of cysteine, in which (CH_3) groups replace (H) at the beta-carbon position (Fig. 31–1). It is a component of penicillin, and may be prepared from it by acid hydrolysis. However, most of the penicillamine currently employed in clinical medicine is prepared synthetically. D-penicillamine (DPA) is the only isomeric form available for therapeutic use. Its chemical structure was first elucidated by Abraham and Chain,[1] and it was first demonstrated in vivo by Walshe, who identified it chromatographically in urine obtained from cirrhotic patients receiving penicillin for intercurrent infections.[83] In clinical medicine, DPA is employed as a chelating agent in treatment of Wilson's disease, where it promotes the renal excretion of the excessive tissue copper stores. It is also used in certain forms of heavy metal intoxication such a lead poisoning; however, it is not of value in the treatment of toxicity from intramuscular gold therapy in rheumatoid arthritis (RA). It is given to patients with cystinuria because it forms a soluble mixed disulfide with cystine, thereby inhibiting cystine calculus formation and subsequent pyelonephritis.

Its widest application is in the treatment of RA, where it is classified as a slow-acting (disease-modifying) agent. Anecdotal evidence supporting its use in the treatment of systemic sclerosis has appeared,[47,76] but its efficacy in this disorder has not yet been substantiated by controlled clinical trials (see Chap. 66).

METABOLISM, PHARMACOKINETICS, AND BIOCHEMICAL PHARMACOLOGY

An understanding of the metabolism and pharmacokinetics of DPA has only recently been appreciated because of the technical difficulty of measuring drug concentrations in blood and in urine. The application of high-performance liquid chromatography (HPLC)[71,73] and radioactive tracer studies in man[64] gave almost identical results in independent studies.[49,65,87] Orally administered DPA is rapidly absorbed, possibly by a specific amino acid carrier system.[84] It is found in the plasma within 20 minutes after ingestion,[87] and its absorption is reduced by as much as 50% if it is given postprandially.[65,75] This may be due to oxidation to the disulfide by certain dietary components, or to chelation by divalent cations in food. Oral iron, for example, reduces absorption by as much as 25%.[32]

There is a double peak in the plasma concentration of the drug with time after either oral or intravenous administration, suggesting a two-compartment model. The first plasma peak occurs 60 to 80 minutes after oral administration, and the second at 110 to 140 minutes. Plasma concentrations of 0.9 µg are achieved after 2 hours. Most of the drug measurable in the plasma is in the form of the mixed disulfide, penicillamine-cysteine, or the internal disulfide, penicillamine-penicillamine. In plasma from RA patients taking 750 mg/day, 11 µ mol/l was free DPA and 23 µ mol/l (68%) was disulfide. Thus, most of the DPA circulates as disulfide. Distribution studies show that radiolabeled DPA is rapidly lost from liver and kidney, but only slowly from collagen and elastin-rich tissues such as bone and skin.[70]

In the urine, only small amounts of free DPA are found, most of it existing in three biotransformed fractions, and one metabolically transformed form. The biotransformed products are the two mixed disulfides found in the plasma and homocysteine-penicillamine-disulfide.[65] The metabolically transformed metabolite is S-methyl-D-penicillamine.[66] The same urinary products, in approximately the same concentrations, are found in patients with either RA, Wilson's disease, or cystinuria, after oral administration of the drug. As indicated, radiolabeled DPA is rapidly cleared by the kidney and, within 10 hours after dosing, 80% of the final amount that will ultimately be recovered from the urine is already present.[64] The remainder

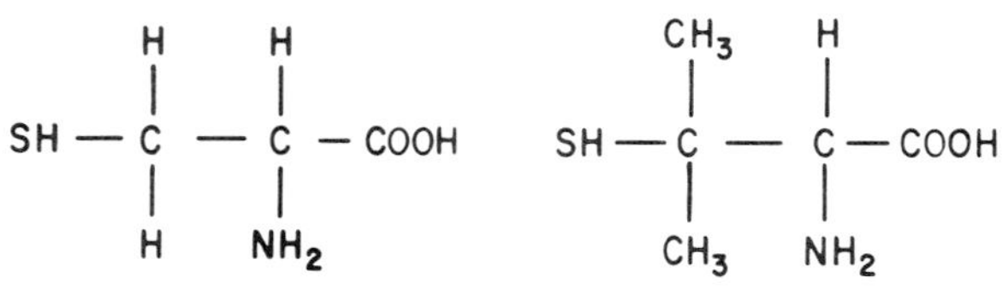

Fig. 31–1. Penicillamine *(right)* is an analogue of cysteine *(left)* in which hydrogen atoms are replaced by methyl groups in the β-carbon position.

is excreted slowly, with another 5% recovered after 1 to 4 days. Penicillamine-cysteine mixed disulfide has been detected in the urine 3 months after discontinuation of DPA,[86] suggesting a "depot" or tissue-bound compartment, possibly in the skin.[70] This may, in part, explain the persistence of both clinical improvement and some adverse reactions long after the drug has been stopped.

Between 16 and 30% of an orally administered dose can be recovered from the feces, as the two mixed disulfides. About half of an orally administered dose cannot be accounted for either in the urine or in feces, presumably that portion bound to plasma and tissue proteins. The measurement of plasma levels of DPA by HPLC is not generally available and is an investigative tool. In addition, the reported studies were for the most part acute, with values obtained after a single oral or intravenous dose of DPA. Similar measurements in RA patients in a steady state on long-term therapy have not been performed in a systematic, prospective fashion. Without such information, no correlations can be made between blood levels, clinical response, secondary failures, and the appearance of certain adverse effects.

Three major *biochemical* properties of DPA occur in man.

1. *Chelation* of copper and other divalent cations is the basis for the application of the drug in Wilson's disease and heavy metal poisoning. The elevated serum copper levels found in RA have led to a suggestion that the beneficial effects of DPA in RA are due to its copper chelating property. Most of the elevated serum copper in RA patients is ceruloplasmin copper, not free copper. It is now generally accepted that changes toward normal in ceruloplasmin levels represent a reflection of clinical improvement rather than its cause, since ceruloplasmin is an acute phase protein.

2. *Thiazolidine bindings* by DPA occurs in two important areas. A thiazolidine between DPA and pyridoxal phosphate results in vitamin B_6 antagonism in man.[45] Vitamin B_6 is necessary to maintain the integrity of the immune response, and this has been considered as a possible means by which DPA might exert an immunosuppressive effect. However, attempts to reverse the effectiveness of DPA in RA by the administration of large amounts of vitamin B_6 have been without effect, and other nonsulfhydryl drugs with antivitamin B_6 properties, such as isoniazid, are ineffective in RA.[41] The second important area is the binding of DPA with the aldehyde groups of collagen, thereby inhibiting collagen cross-linking and collagen biosynthesis.[62] This property, called dermolathyrism, has led to the trial of DPA in systemic sclerosis, particularly for the sclerodermatous features (see Chap. 66).

The alterations in dermal collagen by DPA with the dosages now used are of no clinical significance. However, with high doses given for prolonged periods, hemorrhagic bullae over pressure points have been encountered. As shown by a controlled trial, as well as clinical experience, DPA *does not* interfere with wound healing. It may be safely given until the time of surgery, and then resumed when oral feeding is reinstituted.[4]

3. The *interchange* reaction between sulfhydryl (SH) and disulfide (S-S) groups, as exemplified by mixed disulfide formation, was the biochemical rationale for the initial use of DPA in RA. The drug was used against IgM rheumatoid factor (RF). IgM-RF is a polymer of monomeric subunits, linked by S-S bonds (see Chap. 15). In vitro, DPA and other SH compounds reduce and disrupt these S-S bonds with irreversible loss of serologic reactivity against IgG.[34] DPA was given in an attempt to produce this phenomenon in vivo in RA patients,[43] but it soon became apparent that while the RF titer usually did decrease, a direct effect of DPA on RF was not the explanation.[46] The SH-SS interchange reaction is nonetheless important in understanding the metabolism of the drug, particularly its affinity for proteins in plasma and tissues.

PENICILLAMINE IN RHEUMATOID ARTHRITIS

Although DPA was first given to RA patients to study its possible effect on IgM-RF, it was soon observed that, in addition to the titer changes, there was a favorable effect on the clinical and laboratory indices of disease activity.[41] Anecdotal studies supported these initial observations, but it was the successful completion of the United Kingdom multi-center double-blind clinical trial in 1973 that firmly established the efficacy of the drug in RA.[61] Shortly thereafter, it was registered for that indication by the Committee on Safety of Medicines in Great Britain, and in 1978 was similarly approved by the United States Food and Drug Administration. Subsequent controlled clinical trials have shown that it is at least as effective as injectable gold[37] and azathioprine.[9] A daily dose of 600 mg is statistically the equal of a daily dose of 1,200 mg at the end of one year, with a notable decrease in adverse reactions, according to a well-executed trial.[20] DPA is not of value in ankylosing spondylitis nor in any of the HLA B27-associated spondyloarthropathies.[11,51]

Indications and Contraindications. DPA is *indicated* for the treatment of RA, seropositive and seronegative, and has been shown to be of value in palindromic rheumatism.[35] It has been used successfully in treatment of chronic polyarthritis in children of the non-HLA B27 type, with results similar to those obtained with injectable gold.[3] DPA has been reported to be of particular value in patients with extra-articular manifestations of RA, such as vasculitis,[42] rheumatoid lung disease,[53] Felty's syndrome,[12] amyloidosis,[50] and rheumatoid nodulosis.[30] DPA is *contraindicated* if the patient is receiving gold, cytotoxic drugs, or phenylbutazone. It should be used with extreme caution in the presence of renal insufficiency, which should be regarded as a relative contraindication. DPA should not be continued if a patient becomes pregnant, although abortion is not indicated. Although there are reports of successful pregnancies in patients with Wilson's disease treated with DPA throughout gestation,[74] other reports suggest that the drug may have been responsible for fetal abnormalities.[60] Hence, patients contemplating pregnancy should not be started on DPA treatment. DPA may safely be administered to patients with a history of hypersensitivity to penicillin.[8] Although RA patients who are HLA-DRw3-positive may be at somewhat greater risk for the development of penicillamine nephrotoxicity,[89] this HLA type is not a contraindication to the use of the drug.

The *positioning* of DPA in the overall therapeutic strategy in RA is similar to that for injectable gold: rheumatoid disease that is sustained, progressive, and inadequately responsive to the conventional symptomatic therapies. Gold and DPA are classified as disease modifying, antirheumatic drugs (DMARDS), and should be considered *before* systemic corticosteroids are instituted. Whether DPA is selected before or after a trial of injectable gold is of little consequence, for the physician will generally use that agent with which he is most familiar, initially. All studies have shown that a prior *failure of response*, or the development of an *untoward reaction* to either one of these drugs, does not preclude a favorable outcome with the other.[31,48,78,85] A serious adverse reaction to gold indicates a greater likelihood for development of a major toxicity with DPA, but this is not invariable, and often a toxicity, should it occur, involves a different organ system. No time interval is required in switching from injectable gold to DPA (or the reverse), provided that there is no residual evidence of toxicity to the drug used first.

MODE OF ADMINISTRATION

As indicated earlier, all preparations of DPA currently available for clinical use are the pure (D-)isomer. The (DL) form is no longer available for pharmaceutical use. In the United States, DPA is prepared as gelatin-filled capsules of 125 mg or 250 mg, or a scored tablet of 250 mg. A 50-mg tablet is made in Great Britain.

A single daily oral dose of 250 mg is given with water in the postabsorptive state. The most effective blood level is achieved when it is given 1 to 2 hours before breakfast. When divided doses are employed, the second dose is given 2 to 3 hours after the evening meal. As indicated earlier, food markedly impairs absorption and decreases bioavailability.[65,75] DPA should be given after meals only if the before-meal dosage results in anorexia, nausea, or vomiting. After 8 weeks at 250 mg/day, the dose is usually doubled, for 8 weeks is the average time required for any change in dosage to be reflected clinically. Further increments are made in a similar manner, as symptoms warrant and tolerance permits. The use of 125-mg daily increments is recommended, particularly if anorexia, nausea, or pruritus is encountered during the induction phase. When the daily dose is greater than 1.0 g/day, A b.i.d. regimen should be employed.

At the end of 2 years, most patients require 750 to 1,000 mg daily, and some require 750 mg twice daily. The dosage of DPA is not fixed, but must be adjusted upward or downward as the clinical picture evolves. Although the lower dosages of 500 mg/day are somewhat safer, some investigators believe that although disease activity may be reduced at these doses, disease modification as evidenced by radiographic assessment requires 1.0 g/day or more. Usually, the dosage must be increased with time, for reasons that are not understood. Although DPA is not approved for JRA in the United States, the European experience suggests that 300 to 500 mg/day is effective.[3] Supplements of vitamin B_6, 50 to 100 mg/day, and trace metals, in the form of commercially available vitamin-mineral preparations, are recommended for children and adults whose nutritional status is impaired. These supplements should always be given as far apart from the DPA dosage as feasible. Clinical evidence of a vitamin B_6 deficiency produced by the drug is extremely unusual, but peripheral neuropathy has been reported, which was reversed only after vitamin B_6 administration.[68]

Interactions between DPA and other drugs are likely because of the highly reactive nature of the molecule. Other antirheumatic drugs, analgesics, antibiotics, and vitamins should not be taken at the same time as the DPA, and ideally at least 2 hours should be allowed between DPA and any other drug. Since it is administered once or twice daily, this is easily achieved. As discussed earlier, there is a specific interaction with oral iron, which was first demonstrated by a marked decrease in DPA-induced cupruresis in the presence of oral iron.[55] Furthermore, when oral iron is taken concomitantly with DPA, and is withdrawn while DPA is being continued, an excessive incidence of toxicity, particularly nephropathy, has been observed.[33] When

DPA and hydroxychloroquine are given simultaneously, there is a decrease in both the efficacy and toxicity of the DPA, suggesting the possibility of drug interaction. Although this has not been confirmed in other studies, it seems prudent not to combine these two slow-acting drugs until more data are available.[14] Large doses of ascorbic acid are thought to inactivate DPA and should be avoided. There is no interaction between DPA and the nonsteroidal drugs or aspirin.

PATTERN OF CLINICAL RESPONSE

As with all the slow-acting drugs, up to 16 weeks may be required after the start of treatment before there is evidence of a clinical response. All symptomatic therapies must therefore be continued as required until well into the course of DPA. In particular, corticosteroids should be maintained in constant dosage, and 1 to 2 years may be required before gradual withdrawal is attempted. When improvement begins, the favorable clinical signs are similar to those of a true natural remission, or a remission induced by a successful course of gold. Patients first notice a decrease in the intensity and duration of morning stiffness. Later, as pain subsides, there is often objective evidence of a reduction in synovitis, although synovial thickening present for a long period usually remains unaltered. The quality and duration of uninterrupted sleep improve, and the easy fatigability decreases. Improvement in the laboratory parameters of disease activity, such as a decrease in the Westergren ESR, C-reactive protein, thrombocytosis, and a rise in hemoglobin, is usually seen by 6 to 9 months.[41] After 1 year, the titer of RF falls, as measured by the latex fixation and sensitized sheep cell tests. With lower doses, these changes are less dramatic. Two or more years of therapy are required before there is radiologic evidence of healing of osseous lesions[29] (Fig. 31–2).

The response pattern is nonlinear, and is usually characterized by periods of exacerbation despite continuance of the drug. These tend to be self-limited, but often require an increase in the daily maintenance dose, or conversion to a twice daily regimen, in an attempt to regain control. Usually, these flares gradually decrease in frequency and, after several years, the improvement becomes more sustained. Rarely, a worsening of the arthritis represents a manifestation of penicillamine-induced lupus (see the section on autoimmune syndromes). This condition responds only to withdrawal of the drug and can be determined only by such a trial, for a positive test for antinuclear antibody (ANA) is not diagnostic. ANA may appear, disappear, or remain unaltered during treatment with DPA.

After maximum clinical benefit has been achieved, there is conflicting opinion regarding the optimum total duration of therapy before the DPA should be gradually withdrawn. Some studies indicate that if the disease appears to be well controlled and the drug well tolerated, it should be continued indefinitely. I have studied patients on continuous maintenance therapy for 18 to 22 years, and every attempt at even a modest reduction by 125 mg/day at 3-month intervals has resulted in exacerbation. In a prospective study, 38 RA patients judged to be in remission for more than 12 months were randomly divided into two groups: one to remain on the same dosage and the other to have the drug withdrawn by 125 mg/day at monthly intervals. Of the 19 patients continuing with the previous dosage, 17 remained in remission during a 9- to 12-month follow-up period. Of the 19 whose dosage was reduced, 15 experienced an exacerbation within 2 to 7 months. This represents an 80% flare rate in those in whom withdrawal was attempted.[2]

ADVERSE EFFECTS AND TOXICITY

The numerous and varied side effects that may accompany DPA therapy represent the major factor limiting its use.[77,79,88] Some of these are *dose-related*, and can often be successfully managed by brief interruptions of therapy or alterations in dosage. Others are *idiosyncratic*, independent of dose or duration of treatment. The latter usually preclude any attempt at reinstitution of the DPA, as the same untoward reaction will almost always recur. Because compliance and follow-up examinations are essential to prevent the more serious complications, prescriptions for DPA should be clearly marked *nonrefillable*, and the amount of drug dispensed should not exceed that required for the interval between scheduled visits. Safety monitoring requires visits to the physician at 2-week intervals for the first 6 months, and monthly thereafter. A complete blood count, including a direct platelet count and a urinalysis, is performed each time, with additional laboratory tests if clinically indicated (see the section on hematologic effects).

Skin and Mucous Membranes. The most frequently encountered side effects involve the skin in the form of pruritus or various rashes. Pruritus can often be controlled with a modest reduction in dosage or the addition of an antihistaminic drug such as hydroxyzine (Atarax) or cyproheptadine (Periactin). Rashes appearing early in therapy can usually be treated either by the aforementioned measures or by temporary drug withdrawal. These rashes appearing after 1 year of therapy are more recalcitrant and often require discontinuance of DPA. Oral ulcers may appear within the first 6 months; these clear when the drug is stopped, and

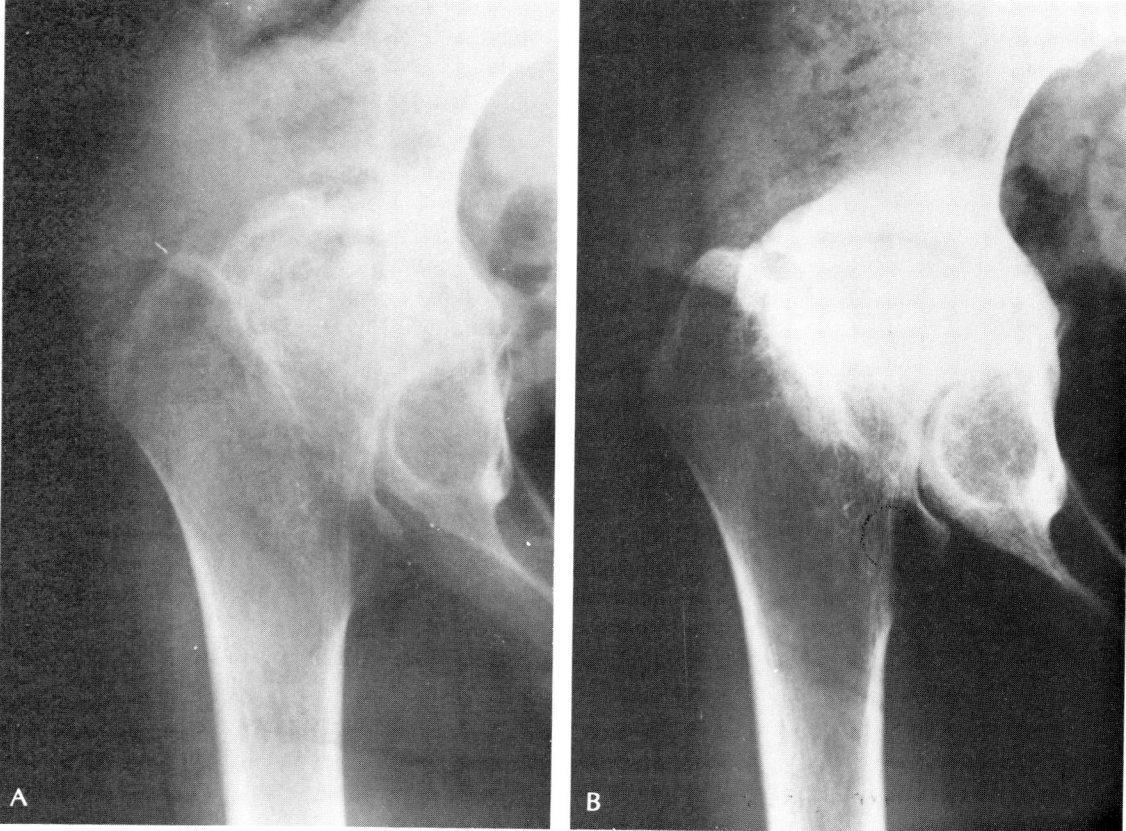

Fig. 31–2. The radiographic changes in the right hip joint of a 31-year-old woman with rheumatoid arthritis. *A,* The pretreatment radiogram shows considerable osteoporosis and bone destruction, with protrusio acetabuli. *B,* After 3 years of D-penicillamine treatment, which had resulted in clinical and laboratory evidence of remission, the osseous lesion has largely remineralized, with healing of the protrusio. Identical changes were noted in the left hip joint.

recur in about half the cases upon rechallenge, even with very low doses. At least one attempt at retreatment is warranted if the arthritis is responding.

More serious is the development of a bullous eruption, clinically indistinguishable from pemphigus, except for the rarity of involvement of the oral mucosa. As in pemphigus, there is intraepidermal acantholysis, epidermal intercellular deposition of immunoglobulin, and circulating antibody to the intercellular region of the epidermis. Nevertheless, other histologic and immunohistologic features differ from those seen in the spontaneously occurring disease.[82] *The appearance of any bullous dermatoses during DPA treatment mandates immediate discontinuation of DPA without rechallenge.* This toxicity is usually seen during the second year of treatment, but has occurred after only 2 months. Resolution generally occurs within 2 to 4 weeks after termination of drug but, in some cases, corticosteroids and immunosuppressive agents have been required.

Gastrointestinal Tract. Anorexia, nausea, and vomiting occur infrequently with the graduated dosage regimens now used. Hypoguesia or dysguesia, a blunting, distortion, or complete loss of taste perception, is often seen. It is benign, self-limited, and not dose related, with taste normalizing within 2 to 3 months regardless of whether the DPA has been stopped. Patients should be reassured, and treatment continued. Some authors recommend the addition of copper or zinc salts to accelerate the return of taste, but their efficacy is not proved, and decreasing the bioavailability of the DPA is possible. Hepatotoxicity and cholestasis have been reported rarely.[58,69] In both Wilson's disease and primary biliary cirrhosis, improvement in liver function has been found with DPA therapy. Diarrhea and peptic ulcer disease have not been associated with the drug.

Hematologic Effects. Marrow depression may be abrupt and may occur at any time during the course of therapy. This is the most serious toxicity and is potentially life-threatening, reinforcing the necessity for strict safety monitoring. If the white blood cell count falls below 3,000/mm³ or the platelet counts falls below 100,000/mm³, the drug should be stopped. Some of the pure thrombocytopenias and neutropenias are *dose-related*, and DPA can be resumed with careful titration of the dose. This is not the case in drug-induced aplastic anemia. This condition is *idiosyncratic* and may occur at any time, even at the lowest doses. Differentiation can usually be made by bone marrow examination, which is characterized by marked hypocellularity in the complete aplasias. Because thrombocytopenia, agranulocytosis, and/or aplastic anemia may develop in the *interval* between routine laboratory tests, patients must be instructed that in the event of abnormal bleeding, menorrhagia, high fever, sore throat, or a flu-like syndrome, the drug should be temporarily discontinued, the physician contacted, and supplementary tests obtained.

The effect of penicillamine is cumulative, and patients should be told that brief interruptions of DPA do not compromise the final therapeutic result, but do provide an added measure of safety. The dose-related depressions in the white blood cell and platelet count begin to rise in about a week, but the aplasias persist for weeks to months. There is disagreement as to whether antimicrobial drugs and antifungal agents should be administered prophylactically during this period, or whether reverse-isolation alone with careful monitoring for development of infection will suffice.[25] Corticosteroids do not hasten recovery and impair host resistance to infection. Blood and platelet transfusions are given as required. There may be a place for cytotoxic drugs in resistant cases of aplastic anemia.[25] Several cases of pure red-cell aplasia have been caused by the drug, one of which responded to cyclophosphamide. Thrombotic thrombocytopenic purpura has been reported in an RA patient during DPA treatment.[81] Bone marrow grafts have not been successful in DPA-associated aplastic anemia.

Renal Toxicity. Proteinuria occurs in 15 to 20% of RA patients given DPA, owing to an immune complex mediated membranous nephropathy. The causative antigen has not been identified.[6] In the absence of nephrotic syndrome, the degree of urinary protein excretion may be titrated against the maintenance dose; often a modest reduction in dose reduces proteinuria. In general, the drug may be continued as long as the protein excretion does not exceed 2 g/24 hours. If the serum albumin falls or nephrotic syndrome appears, the drug must be stopped. Sometimes nephropathy presents as nephrotic syndrome. Proteinuria may persist for up to one year after stopping the drug, but the lesion

is ultimately reversible. Rechallenge has been attempted in patients after clearing of proteinuria with variable results. Some patients can tolerate the drug without recurrence of nephropathy.

Microscopic hematuria had been considered a serious event, but incorrectly so in most instances. It is usually benign and clears despite continued DPA therapy.[7] Its cause is not known. Increasing microscopic hematuria or the appearance of gross hematuria both require that treatment be stopped, for they may portend the development of crescentic glomerulonephritis or Goodpasture's syndrome.[6] In DPA-induced Goodpasture's syndrome, staining of the glomerular basement membrane is granular, not linear as in the natural disease, and antiglomerular basement membrane antibody is not detected in the serum. Some authors therefore classify this lesion as immune complex nephritis with lung hemorrhage.[54] Clinically it is indistinguishable from Goodpasture's syndrome. Plasmapheresis and intensive immunosuppressive therapy may be required to restore renal function.[28]

Pulmonary Effects. The appearance of hemoptysis during DPA treatment should suggest the possibility of drug-induced Goodpasture's syndrome. Hematuria is present, and characteristic infiltrates are seen on chest radiogram. Another entity, fibrosing alveolitis, has been associated rarely with DPA administration. Basilar rales, a typical radiographic appearance, and rapid improvement after withdrawal of the DPA are characteristic.[22]

Bronchiolitis obliterans has been observed in some patients, but a causative role for the drug has not been established.[23] Obliterative bronchiolitis is *not* reversible upon stopping DPA, has been described in other connective tissue diseases, and is considered to be part of the spectrum of rheumatoid lung disease.[15] Patients with RA most likely to develop extra-articular features are also most likely to be treated with DPA. Bronchiolitis obliterans has not occurred in patients with Wilson's disease given DPA, where *all* of its other adverse effects have appeared. Thus, obliterative bronchiolitis during treatment with DPA is considered a chance association and not an adverse reaction to the drug.

Neuromuscular System. Myasthenia gravis (MG) may be induced by DPA in patients with Wilson's disease[57] and RA,[13] and it is most likely to develop during the second year of treatment, similar to the time of appearance of pemphigus. Antibodies to acetylcholine receptors (AChR) are found frequently, and disappear along with clinical resolution of the MG after drug withdrawal.[72] An anticholinesterase drug is often needed since months may elapse before the MG reverses. Corticosteroids and plasmapheresis have been needed rarely because of respiratory muscle weakness. Unusual muscular weakness and fatigue on repetitive acts, diplopia, and dysphagia in RA patients receiving DPA should suggest drug-induced MG. An EMG, tests for serum AChR antibody, and a Tensilon test should be performed. The DPA must be stopped because MG will recur on rechallenge. In DPA-induced MG, the AChR antibody reacts with human motor end-plate preparations, and does not have the species heterogeneity characteristic of the antibody in spontaneously developing MG.[26] A negative test result must be interpreted with caution since there is no standard end-plate preparation and many are obtained from animal muscle.

Drug-induced MG is associated with BW35, DR1, and the combination of BW35 and DR1. In spontaneous MG, B8 and DR3 predominate,[27] whereas in RA without MG, DR4 is often found. The differences in the specificity of the antibody and in the genetic associations may relate to the pathogenesis of DPA autoimmunity.

Polymyositis or dermatomyositis are well-recognized toxicities of DPA.[67] The proximal myopathy and rash are indistinguishable from the spontaneous disease. Prompt recognition is important so that the drug may be discontinued and a fatal outcome avoided.[21]

A reversible peripheral neuropathy responsive to vitamin B_6 has been alluded to previously,[68] but this is extremely rare, and if neuropathy develops in DPA treatment of RA, other causes such as vasculitis should be entertained.

THE AUTOIMMUNE SYNDROMES

DPA induces a wide spectrum of syndromes closely simulating spontaneously occurring autoimmune diseases. Many of these have already been discussed, and they may occur in Wilson's disease and cystinuria as well as in RA. Thus, this is a property of DPA and not the abnormal immune system that might be found in RA patients.[38] In addition to those entities already reviewed, DPA may induce a lupus-like syndrome similar to that induced by other drugs, except that antibodies directed toward native, double-stranded DNA develop.[18] In the usual drug-induced SLE, the antibody is to single-stranded (denatured) DNA (see Chaps. 61 and 62). Patients develop myalgias, pleurisy, and joint pain, difficult to differentiate from an exacerbation of the underlying RA. Renal disease, however, occurs rarely.[17]

Sjögren's syndrome and chronic thyroiditis have been encountered, but may have been associated with the underlying RA. The rare occurrence of breast gigantism, sometimes with galactorrhea, has been considered to be immune-mediated when secondary to DPA; however, it responds to danazol.[80] The effectiveness of DPA in ameliorating the clin-

ical and laboratory features of RA, while at the same time having the potential to induce autoimmunity, has raised the issue of whether these two properties might be linked, perhaps at the level of immune regulation.[19,24] Alternatively, the SH group of DPA may interact with the S-S bonds of proteins on cell surfaces (receptors) via the SH-SS interchange mechanisms, rendering them antigenic. DPA-induced MG, pemphigus, and Goodpasture's syndrome may mimic *clinically* the naturally occurring disease, but there are subtle differences in histology, immunohistology, and immunology.

MECHANISM OF ACTION OF DPA IN RA

The mechanism by which DPA suppresses RA is not known. In the laboratory, DPA is neither cytotoxic, anti-inflammatory, nor immunosuppressive. It does not suppress adjuvant arthritis in rats. Because it is useful only in RA, there is a connotation of disease "specificity," compared to other slow-acting agents. Marked reductions in immune complex levels in serum and synovial fluid and in both IgM *and* IgG RF levels are usually found with DPA (Figs. 31–3, 31–4), suggesting that the drug may be working at a fundamental level.[40] Other SH compounds with a DPA-like action in RA have been examined in the laboratory.[39] Neither chelation, antivitamin B_6 effects, induction of the collagen defect (dermolathyrism), nor mixed disulfide formation was a property of any of the other clinically useful SH drugs. Hence none of these properties of DPA seems relevant to its mode of action in RA.[39] In vitro studies of the effect of DPA on the responsiveness of lymphocytes to mitogenic stimulation and on lymphocyte-macrophage interaction have produced results that are conflicting and difficult to interpret.[10] One in vitro study showed that DPA in the presence of copper produced a selective inhibition of human helper T-cell function; T-suppressor cells and B-lymphocytes were not affected.[52] This could explain immunosuppression, but fails to account for the apparent "specificity" of DPA for RA. It is not possible to synthesize all the extensive laboratory observations into a unified hypothesis to explain mechanism. Further studies may resolve the question.

OTHER SH COMPOUNDS WITH A DPA-LIKE ACTION IN RA

Other SH compounds have been used in treatment of RA patients in an effort to find one with a more favorable therapeutic ratio.[39] In 1963 researchers showed that 5-thiopyridoxine produces clinical and serologic changes similar to DPA,[44] findings that were recently confirmed.[36] The di-

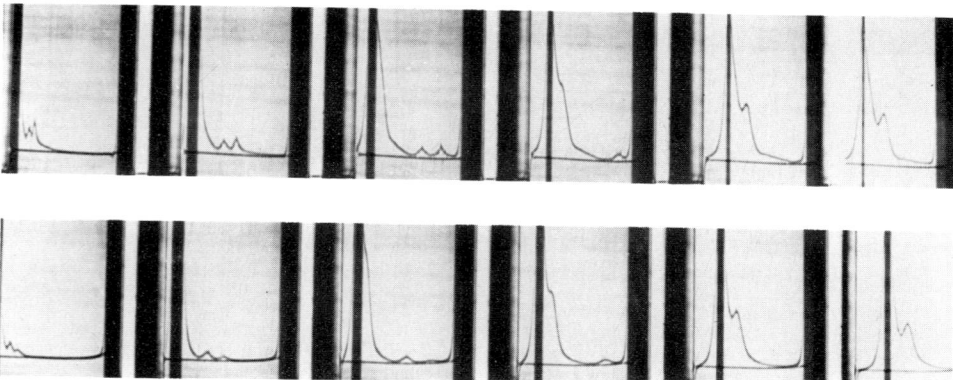

Fig. 31–3. Ultracentrifugal pattern of serum proteins before treatment *(top)* and after the patient had been taking penicillamine for 13 weeks *(bottom)*. The serum was diluted 1:1 with saline. Centrifugation was at 52,640 rpm and proceeds from left to right. Photographs were obtained at 16, 32, 48, 64, 80, and 90 minutes. The post-treatment pattern exhibits a reduction in the 22S complex, 19S macroglobulin, and in the intermediate γ-globulin complexes. (Courtesy Dr. H. Kunkel.)

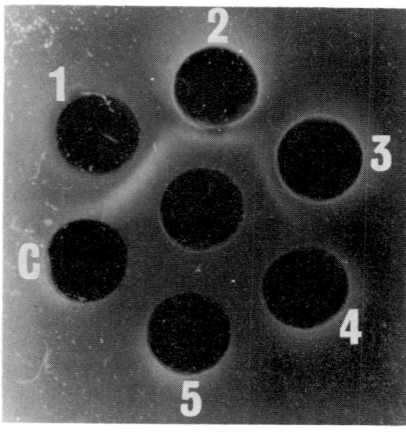

Fig. 31–4. Effect of penicillamine therapy on complexes, a measured by precipitation with purified IgM rheumatoid factor. Well 1 contains synovial fluid, and well 2 contains serum from the same patient before penicillamine therapy. Well 3 shows a decrease in the amount of complex after 6 weeks of penicillamine therapy. Wells 4 and 5 reveal the absence of demonstrable serum complexes at 3 and 6 months, respectively, after initiation of penicillamine therapy. Well C is a normal serum control. There is no post-treatment specimen of synovial fluid, because the synovial effusion had completely reabsorbed. (Courtesy Dr. R. Winchester.)

sulfide of this compound, pyrithioxine, is readily dissociated to the SH form and is also effective.[16] Thiopronine was comparable in efficacy to DPA in a controlled trial.[63] Another SH compound found to be effective in RA is the antihypertensive drug, captopril.[56,59] Its molecular structure suggested that it might have DPA-like activity in RA. In the early studies of captopril in hypertension, when excessively high doses (by present standards) were given, a toxicity profile emerged similar to that of DPA. There was a high incidence of rash, proteinuria due to immune-complex nephritis, taste disturbances, oral ulcers, neutropenia, and pemphigus.[5] The incidence of these adverse reactions was low compared to DPA, and even lower with the dosages of captopril now used to treat hypertension and refractory heart failure, but the qualitative similarity of these untoward reactions led to a trial of captopril in RA.[56,59] No controlled studies have yet been performed, but the preliminary data are encouraging. In doses of 100 to 200 mg/day in normotensive RA patients, no postural hypotension was encountered, provided that diuretics and vasodilator drugs were not given simultaneously.

In all these studies with the other SH drugs, two facts emerge. First, patients with RA could respond to one of these other SH compounds, having previously failed to respond to DPA or having "escaped" from the effects of DPA. Second, all these drugs had adverse effects similar to those of DPA, including the induction of autoimmunity,[38] but the same toxicity was not necessarily replicated in the same patient, nor would there necessarily be any toxicity in a particular patient to the newer drug. These findings are identical to those noted with DPA and injectable gold. Thus, an RA patient with DPA-induced proteinuria might respond well to pyrithioxine or captopril, with no proteinuria, perhaps with a rash, or possibly with no adverse effect at all. The availability of a family of these SH drugs would vastly enhance the therapeutic measures against RA.

REFERENCES

1. Abraham, E.P., et al.: Penicillamine: A characteristic degradation product of penicillin. Nature, *152*:107, 1943.

2. Ahern, M., Hall, N., and Maddison, P.: D-penicillamine (DPA) withdrawal in rheumatoid arthritis (RA). Ann. Rheum. Dis., *43*:213–217, 1984.

3. Ansell, B.M., and Hall, M.A.: Penicillamine in chronic arthritis of childhood. J. Rheum., *8* (Suppl. 7):112–115, 1981.

4. Ansell, B.M., Moran, H., and Arden, G.P.: Penicillamine and wound healing in rheumatoid arthritis. Proc. R. Soc. Med., *70* (Suppl. 3):75–77, 1977.

5. Atkinson, A., and Robertson, J.: Captopril in the treatment of clinical hypertension and of cardiac failure. Lancet, 2:836–839, 1979.

6. Bacon, P.A., et al.: Penicillamine nephropathy in rheumatoid arthritis. Q. J. Med., *45*:661–684, 1976.

7. Barraclough, D., Cunningham, T.J., and Muirden, K.D.: Microscopic hematuria in patients with rheumatoid arthritis on D-penicillamine. Aust. N.Z. J. Med., *11*:706–708, 1981.

8. Bell, C.L., and Graziano, F.M.: The safety of administration of penicillamine to penicillin sensitive individuals. Arthritis Rheum., *26*:801–803, 1983.

9. Berry, H. et al.: Trial comparing azathioprine and penicillamine in rheumatoid arthritis. Ann. Rheum. Dis., *35*:542–543, 1976.

10. Binderup, L., Bramm, E., and Arrigoni-Martelli, E.: D-penicillamine in vivo enhances lymphocyte DNA synthesis: Role of macrophages. Scand. J. Immunol., *11*:23–28, 1980.

11. Bird, H.A., and Dixon, A. St.J.: Failure of D-penicillamine to affect peripheral joint involvement in ankylosing spondylitis or HLA B27 associated arthropathy. Ann. Rheum. Dis., *36*:289, 1977.

12. Blau, S., and Meiselas, L.: Regression of splenomegaly with hematologic recovery in Felty's syndrome due to D-penicillamine. A case report. Meadowbrook Hosp. J., *5*:16, 1971–1972.

13. Bucknall, R.C., Dixon, A. St.J., and Glick, E.N.: Myasthenia gravis associated with penicillamine treatment for rheumatoid arthritis. Br. Med. J., *1*:600–602, 1975.

14. Bunch, T.W., et al.: Controlled trial of hydroxychloroquine and d-penicillamine singly and in combination in the treatment of rheumatoid arthritis. Arthritis Rheum., *27*:267–276, 1984.

15. Case Records of the Massachusetts General Hospital, Case 3-1982.: N. Engl. J. Med., *306*:157–165, 1982.

16. Camus, J.P., et al.: Etude d'une serie de 70 polyarthritis rhumatoides traitees par la pyrithioxine avec un recul de un an. Revue de Rhum., *45*:487–490, 1978.

17. Chalmers, A., et al.: Systemic lupus erythematosus during penicillamine therapy for rheumatoid arthritis. Ann. Intern. Med., *97*:659–663, 1982.

18. Crouzet, J., et al.: Lupus induit par la D-penicillamine au cours du traitement de la polyarthrite rheumatoid—Deux observations et Étude immunologique systematique au cours de ce traitement. Ann. Med. Interne., *125*:71–79, 1974.

19. Dawkins, R.L., and Zilco, P.J.: Penicillamine: friend and foe? Aust. N.Z. J. Med., *9*:493–494, 1979.

20. Dixon, A. St.J., et al.: Synthetic D(—) penicillamine in rheumatoid arthritis. Double-blind controlled study of a high and low dose regimen. Ann. Rheum. Dis., *34*:416–421, 1975.

21. Doyle, D.R., McCurley, T.L., and Sergent, J.S.: Fatal polymyositis in D-penicillamine-treated rheumatoid arthritis. Ann. Intern. Med., *98*:327–330, 1983.

22. Eastmond, C.J.: Diffuse alveolitis as a complication of penicillamine treatment for rheumatoid arthritis. Br. Med. J., *1*:1506, 1976.

23. Editorial: Obliterative bronchiolitis. Lancet, *1*:603–604, 1982.

24. Editorial: Penicillamine—the therapeutic paradox. Lancet, 2:1209–1210, 1981.

25. Gale, R.P., et al.: Aplastic anemia: biology and treatment. Ann. Intern. Med., *95*:477–494, 1981.

26. Garlepp, M., et al.: Heterogeneity of the acetylcholine receptor autoantigen. Muscle Nerve, *4*:282–288, 1981.

27. Garlepp, M.J., Christiansen, F.T., and Dawkins, R.L.: Myasthenia gravis induced by penicillamine. *In* Immuno-genetics in Rheumatology. Edited by R.L. Dawkins, F.T. Christiansen, and P.J. Zilco. Amsterdam. Excerpta Medica, 1982.

28. Gavaghan, T.E., et al.: Penicillamine-induced "Goodpasture's syndrome": Successful treatment of a fulminant case. Aust. N.Z. J. Med., *11*:261–265, 1981.

29. Gibson, T., et al.: Evidence that D-penicillamine alters the course of rheumatoid arthritis. Rheumatol. Rehabil., *15*:211–215, 1976.

30. Ginsberg, M.H., et al.: Rheumatoid nodulosis. An unusual variant of rheumatoid disease. Arthritis Rheum., *18*:49–58, 1975.

31. Hala, J.T., Cassidy, J., and Hardin, J.G.: Sequential gold and penicillamine therapy in rheumatoid arthritis. Am. J. Med., *72*:423–426, 1982.

32. Hall, N.D., et al.: Serum SH reactivity: A simple assessment of D-penicillamine absorption. Rheumatol. Int., *1*:39–41, 1981.

33. Harkness, J.A.L., and Blake, D.R.: Penicillamine nephrophathy and iron. Lancet, 2:1368–1369, 1982.

34. Heimer, R., and Federico, M.: Depolymerization of the 19S antibodies and the 22S rheumatoid factor. Clin. Chim. Acta, *25*:41–43, 1958.

35. Huskisson, E.C.: Treatment of palindromic rheumatism with D-penicillamine. Br. Med. J., *II*:979–980, 1976.

36. Huskisson, E.C., et al.: 5-thiopyridoxine in rheumatoid arthritis: Clinical and experimental studies. Arthritis Rheum., *23*:106–110, 1980.

37. Huskisson, E.C., et al.: Trial comparing penicillamine and gold in rheumatoid arthritis. Ann. Rheum. Dis., *33*:532–535, 1974.

38. Jaffe, I.A.: Induction of auto-immune syndromes by penicillamine therapy in rheumatoid arthritis and other diseases. Springer Semin. Immunopathol., *4*:193–207, 1981.

39. Jaffe, I.A.: Thiol compounds with penicillamine-like activity and possible mode of action in rheumatoid arthritis. Clin. Rheum. Dis., *6*:633–645, 1980.

40. Jaffe, I.A.: Penicillamine treatment of rheumatoid arthritis: Effect on immune complexes. Ann. N.Y. Acad. Sci., *256*:330–337, 1975.

41. Jaffe, I.A.: The effect of penicillamine on the laboratory parameters in rheumatoid arthritis. Arthritis Rheum., *8*:1064–1079, 1965.

42. Jaffe, I.A.: Rheumatoid arthritis with arteritis. Report of a case treated with penicillamine. Ann. Intern. Med., *61*:556–563, 1964.

43. Jaffe, I.A.: Comparison of the effect of plasmapheresis and penicillamine on the level of circulating rheumatoid factor. Ann. Rheum. Dis., *22*:71–76, 1963.

44. Jaffe, I.A.: The effect of penicillamine and mercaptopyridoxine in rheumatoid arthritis. Abst. 243: Fifth European Congress of Rheumatic Disease. Stockholm, 1963.

45. Jaffe, I.A., Altman, K., and Merryman, P.: The anti-pyridoxine effect of penicillamine in man. J. Clin. Invest., *43*:1869–1873, 1964.

46. Jaffe, I.A., and Merryman, P.: Effect of increased serum sulfhydryl content on titre of rheumatoid factor. Ann. Rheum. Dis., *27*:14–18, 1968.

47. Kang, B., et al.: Successful treatment of far-advanced progressive systemic sclerosis by D-penicillamine. J. Allergy Clin. Immunol., *69*:297–305, 1982.

48. Kean, W.F., et al.: Prior gold therapy does not influence the adverse effects of D-penicillamine in rheumatoid arthritis. Arthritis Rheum., *25*:917–922, 1982.

49. Kukovetz, W.R., et al.: Bioavailability and pharmacokinetics of D-penicillamine. J. Rheumatol., *10*:90–94, 1983.

50. Lake, B., and Andrews, G.: Rheumatoid arthritis with secondary amyloidosis and malabsorption syndrome. Effect of D-penicillamine. Am. J. Med., *44*:105–115, 1968.

51. Leca, A.P., and Camus, J.P.: Ankylosing spondylitis: Treatment failures with D-penicillamine. Nouv. Presse Med., *4*:112, 1975.

52. Lipsky, P.E., and Ziff, M.: Inhibition of human helper T-cell function in vitro by D-penicillamine and $CuSO_4$. J. Clin. Invest., *65*:1069–1076, 1980.

53. Lorber, A.: Penicillamine therapy for rheumatoid lung dis-

ease: Effects of protein sulfhydryl groups. Nature, 210:1235–1237, 1966.

54. Loughlin, G.M., et al.: Immune-complex mediated glomerulonephritis and pulmonary hemorrhage simulating Goodpasture's syndrome. J. Pediatr., 93:181–184, 1978.

55. Lyle, W.H., Pearcy, D.F., and Hui, M.: Inhibition of penicillamine-induced cupruresis by oral iron. Proc. R. Soc. Med., 70 (Suppl. 3):48–49, 1977.

56. Martin, M.F.R., et al.: Captopril: A new long-term agent for treating rheumatoid arthritis. Ann. Rheum. Dis., 42:231, 1983.

57. Masters, C.L., Dawkins, R.L., and Zilco, P.J.: Penicillamine associated myasthenia gravis, anti-acetylcholine receptor and anti-striational antibodies. Am. J. Med., 63:689–694, 1977.

58. McLeod, B.D., and Kinsella, T.D.: Cholestasis associated with D-penicillamine therapy for rheumatoid arthritis. Can. Med. Assoc. J., 120:965–966, 1979.

59. Merlet, C.L., et al.: Captopril in rheumatoid arthritis. Abstract 1389: Fifteenth International Congress of Rheumatology, Paris, 1981.

60. Mjölnerod, O.K., et al.: Congenital connective tissue defect probably due to D-penicillamine treatment in pregnancy. Lancet, 1:673–675, 1971.

61. Multi-Centre Trial Group: Controlled trial of D(—)penicillamine in severe rheumatoid arthritis. Lancet, 1:275–280, 1973.

62. Nimni, M.E., and Bavetta, L.A.: Collagen defect induced by penicillamine. Science, 150:905–907, 1965.

63. Pasero, G., et al.: Controlled multicenter trial of thiopronin and D-penicillamine for rheumatoid arthritis. Arthritis Rheum., 25:923–929, 1982.

64. Patzschke, K., et al.: Pharmakokinetische untersuchungen nach oraler applikation von radioaktiv markiertem D-penicillamin an probanden. Z. Rheumatol., 36:96–105, 1977.

65. Perett, D.: The metabolism and pharmacology of D-penicillamine in man. J. Rheumatol. (Suppl. 7), 8:41–50, 1981.

66. Perett, D., Sneddon, W., and Stephens, A.D.: Studies on D-penicillamine metabolism in cystinuria and rheumatoid arthritis: Isolation of S-methyl-D-penicillamine. Biochem. Pharmacol., 25:259–264, 1976.

67. Petersen, J., et al.: Penicillamine induced polymyositis-dermatomyositis. Scand. J. Rheumatol., 7:113–117, 1978.

68. Pool, K.D., Feit, H., and Kirkpatrick, J.: Penicillamine-induced neuropathy in rheumatoid arthritis. Ann. Intern. Med., 95:457–458, 1981.

69. Rosenbaum, J., Katz, W.A., amd Schumacher, H.R.: Hepatotoxicity associated with use of D-penicillamine in rheumatoid arthritis. Ann. Rheum. Dis., 39:152–154, 1980.

70. Ruocco, V., et al.: Specific incorporation of penicillamine into the epidermis of mice: An autoradiographic study. Br. J. Dermatol., 108:441–444, 1983.

71. Russell, A., et al.: A rapid, sensitive technique to assay penicillamine levels in blood and urine. J. Rheumatol., 6:15–19, 1979.

72. Russell, A.S., and Lindstrom, J.M.: Penicillamine induced myasthenia gravis associated with antibodies to acetylcholine receptor. Neurology, 28:847–852, 1978.

73. Saetre, R., and Rabenstein, D.L.: Determination of penicillamine in blood and urine by high performance liquid chromatography. Anal. Chem., 50:276–280, 1978.

74. Scheinberg, I.H., and Sternlieb, I.: Pregnancy in penicillamine-treated patients with Wilson's disease. N. Engl. J. Med., 293:1300–1303, 1975.

75. Schuana, A., et al.: Influence of food on the bioavailability of penicillamine. J. Rheumatol., 10:95–97, 1983.

76. Steen, V.D., Medsger, T.A., and Rodnan, G.P.: D-penicillamine therapy in progresive systemic sclerosis (scleroderma). Ann. Intern. Med., 97:652–659, 1982.

77. Stein, H.B., et al.: Adverse effects of D-penicillamine in rheumatoid arthritis. Ann. Intern. Med., 92:24–29, 1980.

78. Steven, M.M., et al.: Does the order of second-line treatment in rheumatoid arthritis matter? Br. Med. J., 1:79–81, 1982.

79. Stockman, A., et al.: Difficulties in the use of D-penicillamine in the treatment of rheumatoid arthritis. Aust. N.Z. J. Med., 9:495–503, 1979.

80. Taylor, P.J., Cumming, D.C., and Corenblum, B.: Successful treatment of D-penicillamine-induced breast gigantism with danazol. Br. Med. J., 1:362–363, 1981.

81. Trice, J.M., Pinals, R.S., and Pitman, G.I.: Thrombotic thrombocytopenic purpura during penicillamine therapy in rheumatoid arthritis. Arch. Intern. Med., 143:1487–1488, 1983.

82. Troy, J.L., et al.: Penicillamine-associated pemphigus: Is it really pemphigus? J. Am. Acad. Dermatol., 4:547–555, 1981.

83. Walshe, J.M.: Wilson's disease: New oral therapy. Lancet, 1:25–26, 1956.

84. Wass, M., and Evered, D.F.: Transport of penicillamine across mucosa of the rat small intestine in vitro. Biochem. Pharmacol., 19:1287–1295, 1970.

85. Webley, M., and Coomes, E.: An assessment of penicillamine therapy in rheumatoid arthritis and the influence of previous gold therapy. J. Rheumatol., 6:20–24, 1979.

86. Wei, P., and Sass-Kortsak, A.: Urinary excretion and renal clearance of D-penicillamine in humans and the dog. Gastroenterology, 58:288, 1970.

87. Weisner, R.H., et al.: The pharamcokinetics of D-penicillamine in man. J. Rheumatol. (Suppl. 7), 8:51–55, 1981.

88. Weiss, A., et al.: Toxicity of D-penicillamine in rheumatoid arthritis. Am. J. Med., 64:114–120, 1978.

89. Wooley, P.H., et al.: HLA-DR antigens and toxic reaction to sodium aurothiomalate and D-penicillamine in patients with rheumatoid arthritis. N. Engl. J. Med., 303:300–302, 1980.

Chapter 32

Glucocorticoids

James J. Castles

Glucocorticoids are a class of naturally occurring adrenal hormones with characteristic effects on the intermediary metabolism of glucose. In clinical therapeutics, these steroids are used because of their potent anti-inflammatory properties. In 1949, Hench and associates reported therapeutic benefits of a glucocorticoid (cortisone) in patients with rheumatoid arthritis.[43] This accomplishment was rewarded with the Nobel Prize in Medicine just one year later and led to the use of glucocorticoids for the treatment of a variety of inflammatory disorders, including most of the rheumatic diseases. Shortly after the introduction of glucocorticoids, it became apparent that their administration could also result in numerous serious side effects. As a consequence, the clinical use of glucocorticoids requires sober assessment of the benefits to be gained versus the risks involved.

The biochemical, physiologic, and pharmacologic effects of glucocorticoids in man are reviewed here. Some general guidelines for the use of these agents are summarized, as are some of their side effects. Glucocorticoids produce useful anti-inflammatory and/or immunosuppressive effects in many rheumatic diseases, and discussion of their specific applications is found in the chapters dealing with these conditions.

CHEMISTRY OF GLUCOCORTICOIDS AND STRUCTURE-FUNCTION RELATIONSHIPS

Endogenous Glucocorticoids. Cortisol (hydrocortisone) is the predominant glucocorticoid secreted by the human adrenal (Fig. 32–1) constituting 90% of the total hormonal output of the adrenal cortex.[71] Interestingly, cortisone itself, the first corticoid to be isolated[53] and used clinically,[43] is not secreted to any significant extent.

Cortisol synthesis by the adrenal cortex is regulated directly by the anterior pituitary hormone, adrenocorticotropic hormone (ACTH), which in turn is under the control of a neuroendocrine peptide, corticotropin releasing factor (CRF), produced by the hypothalamus.[76] Under normal situations, a human adult produces 16 mg of cortisol per day (range 12 to 29 mg/day).[79] In parallel with the normal diurnal rhythm of ACTH release,

plasma concentrations of cortisol are higher in the early morning hours (16 μg/100 ml at 8:00 am) than later in the day (4 μg/100 ml at 4:00 pm).[42] Various stressful stimuli can augment the release of CRF from the hypothalamus, and this leads to discharge of ACTH from the pituitary and stimulation of cortisol production. This sequence is subject to negative feedback inhibition with increasing plasma levels of cortisol causing a decrease in further ACTH production.[54] Exogenous synthetic glucocorticoids are also effective feedback inhibitors. Stressful stimuli can overcome the normal negative feedback control mechanisms.

Synthetic Glucocorticoids. After it became apparent that the natural glucocorticoids produce undesirable side effects when used in the pharmacologic doses required to control inflammatory disorders, the chemical structure of cortisol was modified in attempts to dissociate the anti-inflammatory actions of glucocorticoids from the catabolic "side effects." These actions are merely an exaggerated response to nonphysiologic concentrations of these hormones. Unfortunately, the analogues developed still do not dissociate the anti-inflammatory from the catabolic actions, although some do have less sodium-retaining capacity (mineralocorticoid effect) than does cortisol. Because of the inability to chemically synthesize a glucocorticoid with a dissociation of the effects on inflammation from those on organic metabolism, both responses may be due to hormonal effects on the same basic process. The relative potency of some commonly used glucocorticoid preparations on inflammation, on carbohydrate metabolism, and on sodium excretion is listed in Table 32–1.[5,42,50]

Studies of synthetic glucocorticoid derivatives indicate that certain features of the structure of glucocorticoids are essential for biological activity. The areas circled on the cortisol structure depicted in Figure 32–1 cannot be altered without complete loss of glucocorticoid activity.[23] Note that a hydroxyl group is required at carbon number 11. Consequently, cortisone and prednisone, which are 11-keto compounds, lack glucocorticoid activity until converted to cortisol and prednisolone by the liver.[67] Therefore, the glucocorticoid preparations marketed for topical or local use are 11-β hydroxyl

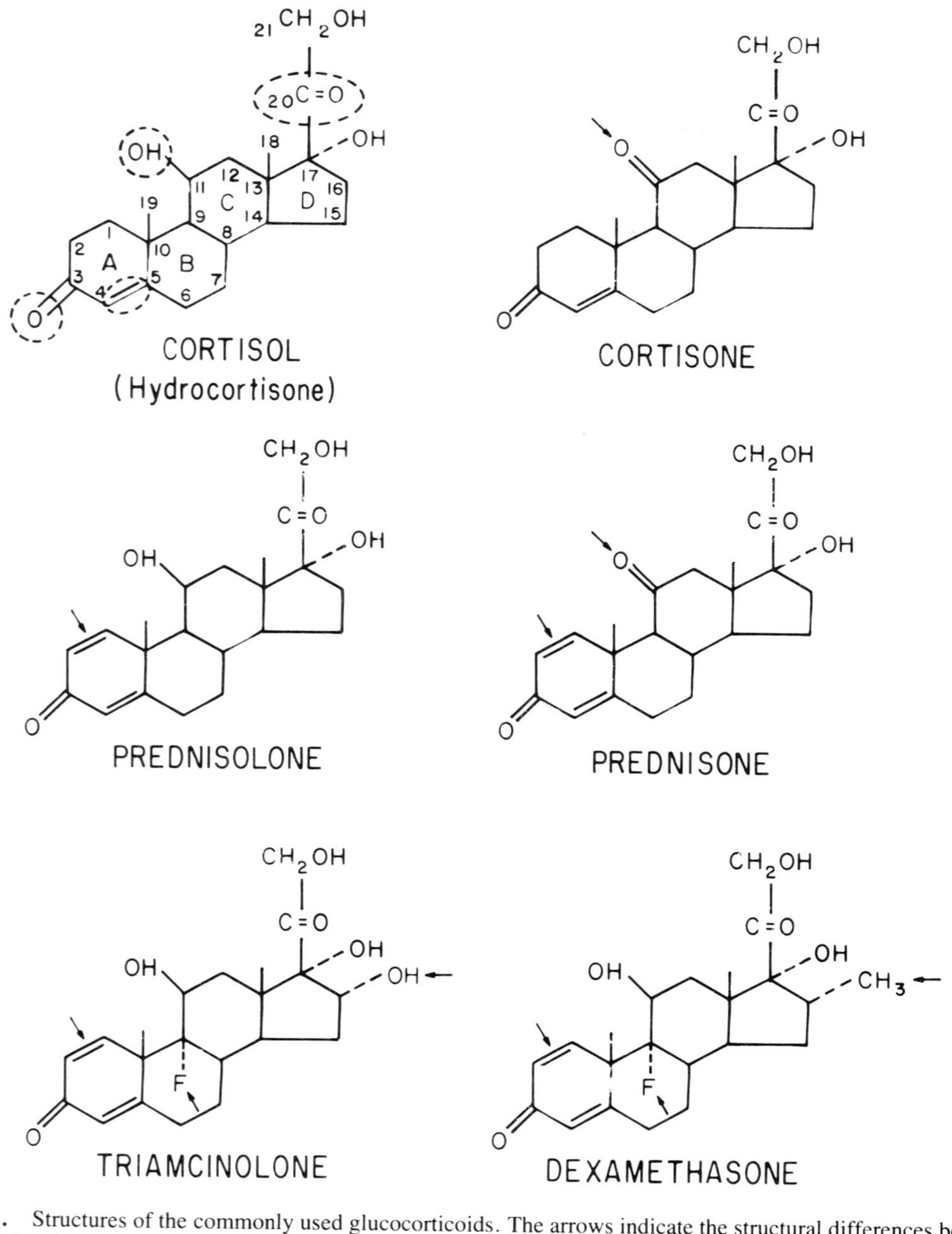

Fig. 32–1. Structures of the commonly used glucocorticoids. The arrows indicate the structural differences between cortisol and each of the other compounds.

compounds and do not require enzymatic conversion for biological activity. Because this conversion may be erratic in patients with liver disease, some practitioners advise the use of prednisolone (or cortisol) rather than prednisone (or cortisone) for systemic steroid therapy in such patients.[5] The introduction of a 1,2 double bond into the cortisol structure (prednisolone and prednisone) enhances the catabolic and anti-inflammatory potency relative to the sodium-retaining properties. Fluorina-

tion of cortisol in the 9 α position (9 α-fluorocortisol) increases all biologic activities, but most markedly the sodium-retaining potency, and the addition of a 9 α-fluoride to prednisolone coupled with a 16 α-hydroxyl group (triamcinolone) or 16 α-methyl group (dexamethasone) results in agents with significant enhancement of anti-inflammatory and catabolic properties, but virtually no mineralocorticoid effects.[42] Indeed, triamcinolone use may be accompanied by sodium loss. Dexameth-

Table 32–1. Biologic Activity of Commonly Used Glucocorticoids*

	Equivalent Dose (mg)	Anti-Inflammatory Potency	Carbohydrate Effect	Mineralocorticoid Potency
Cortisol	20	1.0	1.0	1.0
Cortisone	25	0.8	0.8	0.8
Prednisolone	5	4.0	4.0	0.8
Prednisone	5	4.0	4.0	0.8
Triamcinolone	4	5.0	5.0	0
Dexamethasone	0.75	30.0	30.0	0

*Modified from Axelrod, L.,[5] Haynes, R.C., Jr. and Murad, F.,[42] and Jasani, M.K.[50]

asone use results in euphoria and appetite stimulation, whereas its fluorinated isomer triamcinolone depresses both mood and appetite.

ABSORPTION AND METABOLISM OF GLUCOCORTICOIDS

Cortisol and its numerous synthetic analogues are efficiently absorbed from the gastrointestinal tract. Parenteral administration of glucocorticoids requires the use of water-soluble esters of which hydrocortisone sodium succinate and dexamethasone sodium phosphate are examples. Glucocorticoids are erratically absorbed from sites of local application such as the skin and joint spaces. When topical glucocorticoids are used chronically or over large areas of the skin, absorption from this site may result in systemic effects, including suppression of the hypothalamic-pituitary-adrenal (HPA) axis.

Normally, most (70 to 80%) of the cortisol in plasma is reversibly bound to a carrier glycoprotein, corticosteroid-binding globulin (CBG, transcortin), and most of the remaining fraction is bound to albumin. CBG has a high affinity for the binding of cortisol, but low total binding capacity, and the affinity for synthetic glucocorticoids is lower than it is for cortisol. The glucocorticoids bound to CBG or albumin are not biologically active, and dissociation from these carrier proteins must occur before the free glucocorticoid can exert its biologic effect. When the concentration of plasma glucocorticoids is increased above the physiologic range, concentrations of both free and albumin-bound steroids increase but, because of the limited binding capacity of CBG, there is little change in the concentration bound to this carrier. Therefore, hypoalbuminemic patients who require glucocorticoid therapy should receive lower doses of these agents in order to minimize side effects while still retaining the desired pharmacologic result.[58]

Glucocorticoids are rapidly metabolized to inactive steroids by the liver with reduction of the 4,5 double bond and the ketone group on carbon 3. These "tetrahydro" derivatives are subsequently conjugated with glucuronic acid or sulfate

and excreted by the kidneys; less than 1% of administered glucocorticoids are excreted unaltered.[32,42] Drugs that induce hepatic microsomal enzymes, such as diphenylhydantoin, phenobarbital, and rifampin, accelerate the metabolism of glucocorticoids. Therefore, concomitant administration of these agents in patients receiving steroids should be avoided, if possible, or the steroid dose should be increased appropriately.[10] Concurrent administration of a glucocorticoid and a salicylate may result in a blood salicylate concentration that is lower than expected because of increased renal clearance of salicylates; therefore, *reduction of the dose of steroids in a patient receiving a fixed dose of salicylate may increase blood salicylate concentration possibly to a toxic level.*[56]

The circulating plasma half-life of a glucocorticoid does not strictly correlate with its biologic potency or duration of action. In general, compounds with the longer plasma half-lives tend to have longer durations of action and are biologically more potent. However, since the duration of action of most glucocorticoids is many hours longer than their survival times in plasma, other factors such as distribution in body fluids, cell permeability, and affinity to binding proteins probably play a role in determining biologic potency and duration of action of the various steroids. Additionally, duration of action of any of the glucocorticoids is directly related to the dose administered. However, even when equipotent doses of glucocorticoids are administered, the absolute duration of action of any glucocorticoid preparation is variable according to the particular physiologic/pharmacologic effect being measured. Perhaps the most useful categorization of the duration of action of various glucocorticoids has been provided by Harter, who measured the length of time that equipotent anti-inflammatory doses of various glucocorticoids suppressed ACTH secretion.[39] From this study, glucocorticoids have been classified as: short-acting (cortisol, cortisone, prednisone, and prednisolone); intermediate-acting (triamcinolone); and long-acting (dexamethasone).[39] As a consequence of these differences in duration of action, pharmacologic doses of dexamethasone are more likely to produce undesirable side effects than are equipotent doses of cortisol or prednisone.[23]

BIOCHEMICAL AND METABOLIC EFFECTS OF GLUCOCORTICOIDS

Glucocorticoids, like other hormones, do not induce cells to function in a manner in which they are otherwise incapable, but rather they influence the rates at which ordinary processes occur. In addition, glucocorticoids often regulate cellular metabolism through complex interactions with the effects of other hormones; this has been termed the "permissive" role of steroids by Ingle.[48] In the following sections, the effects of glucocorticoids on certain metabolic processes are reviewed.

Carbohydrate Metabolism. The name "glucocorticoid" derives from the action of the adrenocorticosteroids on the intermediary metabolism of glucose. Glucocorticoids have a sparing effect on the utilization of glucose by peripheral tissues, and they increase hepatic gluconeogenesis. In diabetic subjects, glucocorticoids cause a marked increase in blood glucose concentration.[12] In normal subjects, the glucocorticoid-induced rise in blood glucose is only temporary and returns to normal because of a compensatory increase in insulin secretion.[65]

Hyperglycemia is the aggregate result of different glucocorticoid effects on different tissues. These hormones inhibit glucose uptake by adipose tissues, skin, fibroblasts, and lymphoid tissues.[63] In muscle, glucocorticoids induce a relative resistance to the usual insulin stimulation of glucose transport.[12,63] In addition to inhibiting glucose utilization by peripheral tissues, glucocorticoids accelerate protein catabolism, especially in muscle.[63] Enhanced protein catabolism results in the egress of amino acids into the circulation, and these amino acids become substrates for hepatic gluconeogenesis, which quantitatively is probably the most significant contributor to hyperglycemia.[6]

Glucose production by the liver is increased by direct stimulation by glucocorticoids of the rate-limiting steps in gluconeogenesis and, as just mentioned, by an increase in substrate supply (amino acids) to the liver from protein breakdown in other tissues.[6] The enhanced activity of the enzymes involved in gluconeogenesis is the combined result of induction of de novo enzyme synthesis and direct stimulation of enzyme activity.[2] Glycogen deposition in the liver is also increased by glucocorticoids by activation of glycogen synthetase and as a secondary response to hyperglycemia.[6]

In normal subjects, impaired glucose tolerance is not a persistent feature of steroid administration because of a compensatory increase in insulin production,[65] but prolonged administration may exhaust the pancreatic beta cells and result in steroid diabetes. Unlike diabetes mellitus, steroid diabetes is usually mild, not prone to ketoacidosis, readily controlled by diet and/or insulin, and usually reversible upon cessation of steroid therapy.[31]

Protein Metabolism. In numerous tissues (including muscle, bone, skin, and lymphoid, adipose, and connective tissues), glucocorticoids cause decreased synthesis and increased degradation of total proteins.[6] The diminished protein synthesis in lymphoid cells is thought to result from a decreased intracellular energy supply secondary to glucocorticoid-induced inhibition of glucose transport.[63] The basis of decreased protein synthesis in the other tissues is uncertain; there is some evidence that this results from inhibition of amino acid transport or from decreased synthesis of messenger RNA.[82] On the other hand, total protein synthesis in the liver is enhanced.[6,11] Production of specific enzymes may be increased or decreased in a tissue irrespective of the effect of glucocorticoids on total protein production by that tissue.[86]

The myopathy, osteoporosis, cutaneous and subcutaneous atrophy, and delayed wound healing seen in patients receiving prolonged pharmacologic doses of glucocorticoids are at least partially explicable on the basis of the negative protein balance induced by these hormones.

Lipid Metabolism. In adipose tissue, glucocorticoids alone have little direct effect on lipid metabolism. However, these hormones are necessary ("permissive") for the usual lipolytic effects of catecholamines.[74] Therefore, in concert with catecholamines, glucocorticoids stimulate lipolysis resulting in the release of free fatty acids and glycerol. The latter provides an additional substrate for hepatic gluconeogenesis.[6] Because glucocorticoids also inhibit glucose uptake in fat cells, resulting in decreased production of glycerol phosphate and free fatty acids, lipogenesis is also inhibited.[63]

In the intact animal, the stimulation of lipolysis and inhibition of lipogenesis induced by the combination of glucocorticoids and catecholamines is countered by insulin, which inhibits lipolysis and stimulates lipogenesis. As a consequence, most patients have no consistent alteration in serum lipid pattern or concentration during glucocorticoid administration.[74]

Nucleic Acid Metabolism. In liver, glucocorticoids exert a significant stimulatory effect on RNA metabolism, including stimulation of uptake of purine and pyrimidine precursors; increased synthesis of nucleotide precursors; increased synthesis of all types of RNA, including transfer RNA, ribosomal RNA, and messenger RNA; and increased activity of DNA-dependent RNA polymerase.[28] Stimulation of RNA synthesis is a prerequisite for the glucocorticoid-induced increase in hepatic protein production and for the induction of certain enzymes. In other steroid-sensitive tissues, bulk RNA synthesis is generally inhibited,[86] and the characteristic effects of glucocorticoids appear to require the synthesis of a specific messenger RNA, which then directs the synthesis of specific proteins that probably mediate the response(s).[63]

In contrast to a stimulatory effect on RNA synthesis, glucocorticoids inhibit DNA synthesis in liver, muscle, and kidney.[59] (DNA synthesis is also inhibited in lymphocytes, adipocytes, and fibroblasts, but this is probably secondary to glucocorticoid-induced inhibition of glucose uptake by these cells.[63]) Other tissues, such as gastrointestinal mucosa, testis, and bone marrow, are resistant to glucocorticoid effects on DNA metabolism. The inhibition of DNA synthesis in certain tissues may account for the growth suppression seen in children receiving pharmacologic doses of glucocorticoids for prolonged periods.[59] In addition, this growth suppression may also result from glucocorticoid suppression of growth hormone secretion,[30] although growth hormone replacement in steroid-treated children has failed to overcome growth arrest.[61] Glucocorticoid inhibition of somatic growth is generally reversible, and most children undergo compensatory growth spurts when steroid therapy is discontinued.[59]

Electrolyte and Water Metabolism. Although the mineralocorticoids, of which aldosterone is the predominant species secreted by the human adrenal, are the major adrenal corticosteroids involved in the regulation of electrolyte metabolism, the glucocorticoids also have some mineralocorticoid effects, but of much lower potency. In general, glucocorticoids enhance renal tubular reabsorption of sodium and promote potassium excretion,[62] but the net effect of these hormones on sodium and potassium balance in the intact animal is influenced by a plethora of other factors.[34] In addition to demonstrating renal action, corticosteroids also enhance sodium retention and promote potassium loss by salivary glands, sweat glands, and intestinal mucosa.

Besides effects on monovalent cation transport, corticosteroids, mainly glucocorticoids, may enhance free water clearance,[34] although the precise mechanism of this effect is uncertain.

In clinical use, administration of glucocorticoids, especially the synthetic analogues, does not usually result in significant and/or prolonged abnormalities in electrolyte or water metabolism in an otherwise normal subject. Occasionally, hypokalemic alkalosis occurs, but this is easily treated

with potassium chloride supplementation. In those rare instances where sodium retention results in edema formation, administration of a low-sodium diet and diuretics allows continuation of steroid therapy.[42]

MOLECULAR BASIS OF GLUCOCORTICOID ACTION

Over the past 15 years, the accumulated experimental data suggest that the molecular basis of action of glucocorticoids may coincide with a general pattern that applies to all steroid hormones.[13] The subcellular processes involved (Fig. 32–2) include: (1) interaction of the steroid with a specific hormone receptor in the cytoplasm of the responsive cell; (2) activation of the steroid-receptor complex; (3) transport into the nucleus of the active steroid-receptor complex; (4) interaction of the active steroid-receptor complex with nuclear chromatin, resulting in modulation of transcription of specific messenger RNAs that are translated in the cytoplasm into specific proteins; and (5) mediation of physiologic effects by the specific proteins.[29,51]

Cytoplasmic glucocorticoid receptors have been identified as proteins with a high affinity and stereospecificity.[7] In the absence of an appropriate glucocorticoid, the cytoplasmic receptor exists in an inactive (''aporeceptor'') form. In the presence of a glucocorticoid, such as cortisol or dexamethasone, the aporeceptor and steroid interact noncovalently to form a complex in which the conformational state of the protein receptor is changed to an active form.[77] Some steroids (for example, 11-deoxycortisol) bind to the aporeceptor, but are inefficient in inducing the conformational change required for an active complex; as a consequence, these steroids are relatively less potent as glucocorticoids. Other steroids (testosterone and estradiol-17β) bind to the aporeceptor, but maintain its conformation in the inactive state; these hormones are capable of blocking the cellular effects of glucocorticoids in vitro.[73,75] These correlations between binding of steroid to a receptor protein and biologic activity imply that these receptors have an obligatory role in glucocorticoid action. Further support for this concept is provided by the observation that some mouse cell lymphomas are resistant to glucocorticoid-induced cytolysis, and this resistance correlates with the absence of cytoplasmic receptors for glucocorticoids.[72]

Transfer of the active steroid-receptor complex from the cytoplasm to the nucleus generates a steroid-receptor complex of lower sedimentation coefficient; the nature of the change in the receptor protein from cytoplasm to nucleus is uncertain.[7,77] In the nucleus, the active steroid-receptor complex interacts with chromatin and, perhaps by reversibly

GLUCOCORTICOID RESPONSIVE CELL

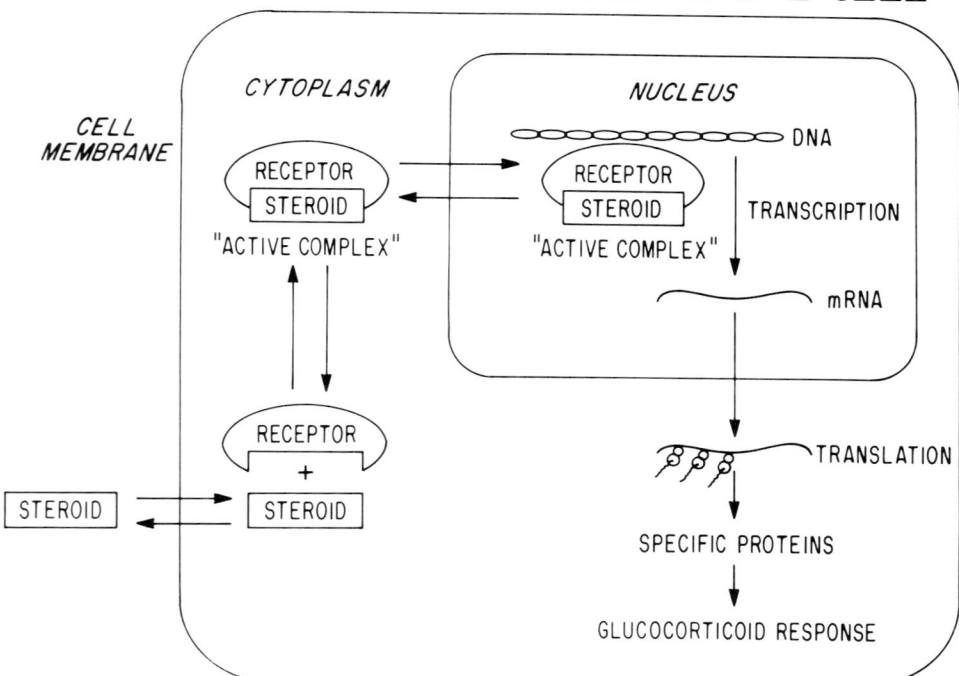

Fig. 32–2. Model for the molecular basis of glucocorticoid action. See text for details.

modifying chromosomal proteins, increases or decreases selectively the de novo synthesis of specific messenger RNAs that direct the synthesis of specific proteins.[29,51]

Correlation between the actions of the specific proteins modulated by glucocorticoids and the physiologic response of the cell or tissue has not been clearly ascertained in most instances. In liver, certain of the rate-limiting enzymes of gluconeogenesis are induced by glucocorticoids and this, in part, explains the accelerated hepatic synthesis of glucose.[2] In lymphoid tissue, it has been proposed that glucocorticoids induce the synthesis of a protein that ultimately inhibits glucose uptake; the physiologic response of this cell results from glucose starvation.[63] In neutrophils, glucocorticoids induce the synthesis of a phospholipase A$_2$ inhibitory protein (lipomodulin), which results in a decrease in the phospholipase A$_2$ catalyzed release of the prostaglandin intermediate, arachidonic acid, from cellular phospholipids.[45] In other glucocorticoid-responsive tissues, the specific protein(s) mediating the observed physiologic response(s) are unknown.

PHYSIOLOGIC EFFECTS OF GLUCOCORTICOIDS

Some of the physiologic effects of glucocorticoids on various organ systems have already been mentioned. In addition, these hormones have characteristic effects on the cardiovascular system, the central nervous system, and the skeletal muscle, which are discussed in detail in excellent reviews by Lefer,[57] Henkin,[44] and Ramey,[69] respectively. Because the clinical rationale for the use of glucocorticoids is based on their effects on the inflammatory process and the immune system, the following discussion is limited to these topics.

Effects on Inflammation. Glucocorticoids suppress the classic clinical features of inflammation, i.e., heat, swelling, and pain, by a presumed effect on the usual capillary bed response of vascular dilatation, increased permeability, and cellular migration.[3] The migration of polymorphonuclear leukocytes from the vascular space toward an inflammatory stimulus is suppressed. This may result from an effect of glucocorticoids on the granulocyte surface, since these steroids reduce the ability of granulocytes to adhere to vascular endothelium[24,60] and to aggregate[80] in the area of an injury. Glucocorticoids decrease the total number of granulocytes present in an inflammatory focus even though these hormones produce a neutrophilic leukocytosis in peripheral blood by accelerating the release of neutrophils from the bone marrow, increasing their circulating half-life, and reducing their egress from the blood.[9,64]

Numerous in vitro studies suggest that glucocorticoids also suppress neutrophil phagocytosis and bactericidal capacity; however, the drug concentrations used in these studies are rarely achieved in vivo.[27] A more accurate assessment of the effects of glucocorticoids on granulocyte function may be found in those studies that have used neutrophils from patients treated with steroids. In these instances, all granulocyte functions are normal,[27] except for a decreased ability to reduce nitroblue tetrazolium.[14]

As certain glucocorticoid hormones stabilize the membranes of liver lysosomes, thus decreasing the capacity of these organelles to release their enzymes,[89] and as lysosomal enzymes are involved in the inflammatory process, it has been proposed that this effect of glucocorticoids is a significant factor in their anti-inflammatory activity. However, this hypothesis has been challenged by the observation that glucocorticoids do not enhance the stability of granulocyte lysosomal membranes.[66,92]

In addition to suppressing the neutrophil response to an inflammatory focus, glucocorticoids also inhibit monocyte accumulation.[1] This reaction is perhaps secondary to the monocytopenia induced by these drugs,[26] which results from delayed release of mature monocytes from the bone marrow.[83] Monocytes/macrophages exposed to glucocorticoids are impaired in random motility, chemotaxis, and bactericidal activity.[64,70] In addition, chronic steroid therapy depresses macrophage-mediated antibody-dependent cell killing, probably by interfering with the ability of the macrophage to bind to the antibody-coated target cell.[64]

Glucocorticoids have been found to affect certain of the noncellular components of the inflammatory response, but the precise significance of these in the overall anti-inflammatory effect is uncertain. In some species, glucocorticoids depress complement components but, in man, there is no consistent effect on complement metabolism.[64] There are conflicting reports on the effects of glucocorticoids on kinin activation.[64] Collagenases, which are produced by numerous cell types, including neutrophils, macrophages, and synovial cells, have been postulated to have a major role in the degradation of articular cartilage and other joint structures as seen in rheumatoid arthritis; interestingly, glucocorticoids inhibit the production of collagenase by isolated rheumatoid synovial cells.[21] Additionally, glucocorticoids block the production of plasminogen activator by human neutrophils[64] and rheumatoid synovial cells.[90] The resultant decrease in the generation of plasmin inhibits the activation of collagenase from its latent form.[90] Perhaps the most significant glucocorticoid effect on a noncellular component of the inflammatory response is

on prostaglandin metabolism. Glucocorticoids inhibit prostaglandin production by rheumatoid synovia[52] and neutrophils[45] by inhibiting arachidonic acid release from phospholipids.[46] This inhibition is mediated by glucocorticoid induction of a phospholipase A_2 inhibitory protein.[45] Such inhibition also effectively prevents the synthesis of leukotrienes via the lipoxygenase pathway. Glucocorticoid inhibition of prostaglandin synthesis is different from the inhibition of prostaglandin production mediated by the nonsteroidal anti-inflammatory agents. These agents inhibit the cyclooxygenase enzyme that converts arachidonic acid to the cyclic endoperoxide intermediate in the prostaglandin synthetic pathway.

Effects on Wound Healing. Consistent with their general catabolic effects, glucocorticoids suppress wound healing.[47] These steroids inhibit the usual proliferation of fibroblasts associated with scar formation.[41] In addition, de novo synthesis of collagen by fibroblasts is also suppressed.[87] In clinical practice, glucocorticoid suppression of wound healing results in scar tissue of decreased tensile strength with a wound that is in constant danger of dehiscence.[37]

Effects on the Immune System. Glucocorticoids are among the group of pharmacologic agents used for immunosuppression, and their effects on the immune response result from effects on several interrelated processes.

It has long been known that glucocorticoids cause involution of lymphoid tissues in certain animal species, resulting in lymphocytopenia and atrophy of lymph nodes, spleen, and thymus;[49] this results from death of lymphocytes.[27] Lymphocytopenia also occurs after glucocorticoid administration in man; however, this condition is not a result of lymphocytolysis since the human lymphocytes, as well as those of the monkey and guinea pig, are relatively resistant to this effect of corticosteroids in comparison to mouse, rat, and rabbit lymphocytes.[15] Glucocorticoid-induced lymphocytopenia in man involves all subpopulations of lymphocytes, but T-lymphocytes are decreased proportionately more than B-lymphocytes.[25,93] The differing sensitivities of T- and B-lymphocytes may result from the ability of B cells to metabolize cortisol more rapidly than T cells.[55] Within the total T-lymphocyte population, T cells with Fc receptors for IgM and IgE are depleted to a greater degree than are T cells with Fc receptors for IgG.[17] Since the lymphocytopenia is not due to lymphocytolysis, it probably results from redistribution of lymphocytes from the recirculating portion of the intravascular lymphocyte pool to the extravascular recirculating lymphocyte pool, probably the bone marrow.[17] It has been proposed that this redistribution is caused by an effect of glucocorticoids on the lymphocyte surface.[17]

An effect of glucocorticoids on humoral immunity has not been clearly defined and has not been reproducible. A five-day course of high-dose methylprednisolone can decrease serum immunoglobulin levels in humans,[11] but there is no clearly predictable effect of glucocorticoids on the specific antibody response to an antigen. In some instances, glucocorticoids suppress a specific antibody response, but this is generally more predictable during a primary reponse to an antigen than during an anamnestic response.[33] The mechanism of a glucocorticoid effect on antibody production is probably operative at various levels. The redistribution of B-lymphocytes into the extravascular recirculating lymphocyte pool can account for a decreased antibody response.[27] In addition, the ability of glucocorticoids to diminish monocyte and macrophage access to sites of antigen deposition[84] and to inhibit some functions of these cell types[70,88] may interfere with the antigen processing necessary for a humoral immune response.[16] On the other hand, it remains unclear whether glucocorticoids can directly modulate immunoglobulin biosynthesis by B cells.[17]

The ability of glucocorticoids to suppress cutaneous delayed hypersensitivity, a local manifestation of the cell-mediated immune response, is a well-known clinical phenomenon.[33] Glucocorticoids are potent inhibitors of various cell-mediated immune responses, and it is this property that makes them valuable immunosuppressive agents in transplant recipients.[33] Information from numerous in vivo and in vitro studies of cell-mediated immunity suggests that glucocorticoids do not disturb most functions of the effector lymphocyte in this response, the T-lymphocyte, and that some of the alterations observed in T-lymphocyte functions are explicable on the basis of glucocorticoid-induced changes in the distribution of circulating lymphocytes.[27] Most of the suppression of cellular immunity results from effects of glucocorticoids on monocytes/macrophages, which are required for expression of a cell-mediated immune response. As the number of circulating monocytes/macrophages is decreased, their access to local sites of potential immunologic reactions[1,26,91] is inhibited, and their response to several of the soluble products released by activated T-lymphocytes (lymphokines) is depressed.[27] With regard to direct effects on the lymphocytic component of the cell-mediated immune response, glucocorticoids have been shown to suppress the lymphocyte blastogenic response to various mitogens,[64] to decrease T cell-mediated cytotoxic reactions,[81] and to inhibit interleukin-2 production by T cells.[17]

In addition to their effects on the humoral and cell-mediated immune responses, corticosteroids may in some instances have an effect on the products of an abnormal immune response. For example, glucocorticoids interfere with the passage of immune complexes across vascular basement membranes[35] and inhibit the immune clearance of sensitized erythrocytes.[4]

From the preceding discussion, it is clear that glucocorticoids may be beneficial in purely inflammatory diseases solely because of their effects on the inflammatory process. In immunologically mediated disease, glucocorticoids can be therapeutic as a result of both their anti-inflammatory and immunosuppressive effects; however, the relative contributions of these effects to the therapeutic responses in human immunologic diseases have not been ascertained.[27]

It is also clear that the administration of glucocorticoids can result in a compromised host. Because of altered defense mechanisms against infectious agents, patients on chronic high-dose glucocorticoid regimens have a heightened risk of infection. This risk results mainly from the effects of glucocorticoids on leukocytes rather than from their effects on the immune system.[19] This increased susceptibility to infection of any variety should always be kept in mind both prior to use of glucocorticoids and any time a patient receiving these agents develops a fever. Because of the lowered host resistance to infection, including tuberculosis, the Center for Disease Control recommends the prophylactic administration of isoniazid (INH) to patients with positive tuberculin reactivity who are to be treated with glucocorticoids for prolonged periods.[18] However, some investigators have questioned this routine practice because of the risk of liver disease due to INH.[78]

COMPLICATIONS AND SIDE EFFECTS OF GLUCOCORTICOID THERAPY

The side effects of glucocorticoids are the anticipated catabolic actions of supraphysiologic concentrations of these hormones. They can occur in any patient receiving more than 20 to 30 mg daily of cortisone or its equivalent. In general, the incidence and severity of side effects parallel increasing doses and duration of treatment. The potential occurrence of side effects should impose restraint and judicious evaluation on any physician considering the use of glucocorticoids in any clinical situation.

Specific details concerning the potential side effects are not reviewed here. A synopsis of the complications that can occur is found in Table 32–2. For details, the reader is referred to the excellent review by David et al.[20] Most of the side effects, with the notable exceptions of osteoporosis and

Table 32–2. Side Effects of Glucocorticoid Therapy

1. CUTANEOUS
  Thin, fragile skin
  Acne
  Hirsutism
  Striae
  Purpura
  Plethora
  Panniculitis
  Impaired wound healing
2. MUSCULOSKELETAL
  Myopathy
  Osteoporosis
  Aseptic necrosis of bone
3. GASTROINTESTINAL
  *Peptic ulceration (often gastric)
  Gastric hemorrhage
  Intestinal perforation
  Pancreatitis
4. CARDIOVASCULAR AND RENAL
  Hypertension
  Edema secondary to sodium and water retention
  Hypokalemic alkalosis
5. CENTRAL NERVOUS SYSTEM
  Psychiatric disorders
  Benign intracranial hypertension
	6. OCULAR
	  Posterior subcapsular cataracts
	  Glaucoma
	  Ocular infections
	7. ENDOCRINE
	  Growth arrest
	  Secondary amenorrhea
	  Impotence
	  Suppression of hypothalamic-pituitary-adrenal axis
	8. METABOLIC
	  Glucose intolerance
	  Hyperosmolar nonketotic coma
	  Hyperlipidemia
	  Obesity (centripetal)
	9. VASCULAR
	  *Vasculitis
	  *Thromboembolism
	  *Accelerated arteriosclerosis
	10. HOST DEFENSE SYSTEM
	  Increased risk of infection
	11. PREGNANCY
	  *Increased fetal wastage

*The relationship of these "side effects" to glucocorticoids is subject to debate at present.

aseptic necrosis of bone, tend to be reversible after discontinuing or tapering glucocorticoids; however, the time course and extent of reversibility are frequently unpredictable. Since osteoporosis and the resultant fractures, usually involving the axial skeleton, can be a bothersome side effect of chronic glucocorticoid therapy, some have advocated the use of vitamin D and calcium for prophylaxis,[8,38] but the long-term utility of this approach is uncertain.

The one side effect that is certain to occur in virtually every patient receiving more than one week of supraphysiologic doses of glucocorticoids is suppression of the hypothalamic-pituitary-adrenal (HPA) axis. HPA suppression can result in symptoms of acute adrenal insufficiency (fever, tachycardia, hypotension, and vascular collapse), especially during periods of stress, unless replacement doses of glucocorticoids are given. Since it is virtually impossible to predict the severity or duration of HPA suppression after a patient has received glucocorticoids, Axelrod recommends that any patient who has received a glucocorticoid in doses equivalent to 20 to 30 mg of prednisone per day for more than a week should be considered to have HPA suppression for as long as one year after termination of therapy.[5] As a consequence, these patients should receive steroid replacement during surgery or other metabolically stressful events.[5] Numerous regimens have been described

for administration of replacement steroids to patients who are or who may be HPA-suppressed and are to be subjected to a stressful procedure such as a surgical operation. I have used the regimen described by Plumpton,[68] which is summarized in Table 32–3.

GENERAL GUIDELINES FOR THE USE OF GLUCOCORTICOIDS

The specific rationale, indications, and dosage of glucocorticoids for treatment of various rheumatic diseases are discussed in the chapters dealing with disease entities. In view of the hazards of glucocorticoids, especially when administered in high doses for prolonged periods, Thorn recommends that the following questions be addressed prior to initiating steroid therapy.[85] Answers to these questions will permit the physician to weigh the potential risks versus the benefits of therapy.

Table 32–3. Glucocorticoid Replacement Regimen for Patients With Suppressed HPA Undergoing a Surgical Procedure*

Day of operation: hydrocortisone hemisuccinate 100 mg IM every 6 hours plus maintenance dose of steroid, if any. First to third postoperative day: same as #1. Fourth postoperative day: discontinue hydrocortisone, but continue maintenance dose of steroid, if any.

*Data from Plumpton, et al.[68]

1. How Severe is the Underlying Disorder?

The more severe the underlying disorder, the easier it is to justify the use of glucocorticoids. For example, the use of these agents for the treatment of life-threatening illnesses, such as status asthmaticus or severe polymyositis, can easily be defended. However, in diseases that do not usually threaten survival, such as rheumatoid arthritis or bronchial asthma, it would be more sensible to utilize more conservative therapy rather than risk the development of steroid side effects.

2. What is the Anticipated Duration and Effective Dosage of Steroid that Will be Required?

Because the occurrence of side effects from glucocorticoids is related to dosage and duration of administration, the smallest possible dose should be used for the shortest possible period of time. A 1- to 2-week course of steroids for the treatment of a contact dermatitis is not likely to be associated with serious complications. However, more prolonged periods of therapy are increasingly more fraught with hazard.

3. Is There Any Predisposition to Steroid Complications?

Although there are no absolute contraindications to glucocorticoid therapy, should the severity of the underlying disease warrant their use, the presence of any of the following should be deterrents to the use of steroids: diabetes mellitus, osteoporosis, peptic ulcer disease or gastritis, tuberculosis or other chronic infections, hypertension or other cardiovascular disease, psychiatric illnesses, and age, especially in women.

4. What Glucocorticoid Preparation Should be Used?

Whenever possible, a local steroid preparation should be used if it will provide the required therapeutic result: for example, the use of intra-articular microcrystalline glucocorticoid ester to treat an inflammatory monoarthritis. If systemic therapy is required, agents with minimal salt-retaining effects should be used. If only a brief course is warranted or if an alternate-day regimen is used, then a short-acting agent such as prednisone is preferred to minimize HPA suppression.

5. Can Other Modes of Therapy be Used Concomitantly to Minimize the Dose of Glucocorticoid Required?

The use of other therapeutic agents along with glucocorticoids may decrease the amount of steroid required to control the underlying disease. For example, the concomitant administration of certain nonsteroidal anti-inflammatory agents may have a steroid-sparing effect in a patient with a rheumatic disease.

6. What Type of Regimen Should be Used for Administering Glucocorticoids?

Because of the unavailability of effective anti-inflammatory glucocorticoids that do not also have the potential of causing side effects, numerous schedules for the administration of glucocorticoids have been developed with the aim of optimizing therapeutic response and minimizing the side effects. It is now clear that a single alternate-day dosage[40] significantly decreases the incidence of side effects with little or no suppression of the HPA axis.[5] In some clinical situations, an alternate-day regimen does not control disease activity for the full 48-hour period. The administration of supplemental nonsteroidal anti-inflammatory agents during the "breakthrough" periods may suffice to control the disease. On the other hand, the administration of alternate-day glucocorticoids may fail to significantly alter the prolonged inflammatory and/or immunologic events for which they are being administered. In these cases, glucocorticoids may be administered in divided daily doses or as a single daily dose. The latter is preferred since a single daily dose of glucocorticoids *in the morning* is less likely to produce HPA suppression than administration of the same amount of steroid in divided doses throughout the day.[5]

Once the disease under treatment is in adequate control, the potential of developing side effects dictates that the glucocorticoid dosage be decreased to the lowest level that will sustain the desired effect. If daily administration has been required to induce such response, the first step in dose reduction should be conversion to an alternate-day regimen; this conversion can be achieved as outlined in Table 32–4. Even in clinical situations in which alternate-day administration of glucocorticoids fails to induce a clinical remission, once a remission is achieved, then an alternate-day regimen usually maintains it.[27]

Titrating the minimum dosage of glucocorticoid required to control disease activity is frequently difficult and time-consuming. Any time the drug

Table 32–4. Protocol for Changing from a Single Daily Dose Regimen to a Single Alternate-Day Regimen*‡

Day	Prednisone (mg)
1–7	60
8	60
9	40
10	70
11	30
12	80
13	20
14	90
15	10
16	95
17	5
18	95
†19	5

*All doses taken on awakening in the morning.
†The dosage on the high-dose day can be reduced at 5- to 7-day intervals.
‡Modified from Dluhy, et al.[23]

is reduced, the disease may relapse, occasionally with symptoms even worse than before treatment. This type of response may require a return to higher steroid dosages. Tapering should be attempted again once symptoms are controlled.

As the dosage of exogenous corticoids is decreased toward physiologic ranges, true adrenal insufficiency may occur, especially during physiologically stressful events. It is important to recognize the signs of addisonian crisis, which often begins with nausea and vomiting and progresses to include hypotension, tachycardia, and hyperthermia, and the associated metabolic abnormalities, including hypoglycemia, hyperkalemia, hyponatremia, and hypochloremia. Intravenous administration of glucocorticoids is needed to reverse this serious medical emergency.

During glucocorticoid dose reduction, occasional patients develop a syndrome that cannot be clearly related to a relapse of their basic disease or to true adrenal insufficiency.[22,36] This symptom complex has been referred to as *steroid pseudorheumatism* and includes complaints of excessive fatigability, weakness, diffuse aching in muscles, bones, and joints, and emotional lability. The pathogenesis of pseudorheumatism is unknown, but its occurrence often requires a temporary increase in steroid dosage.

7. Is the Patient Reliable? All patients who are to receive glucocorticoids must be reliable and cooperative. Because of the hazards of side effects, each patient must be educated about the dangers of increasing dosage at their own discretion, and must be warned of the hazards of abruptly discontinuing therapy, especially in the event of severe physical stress, such as infection or surgery. It is advisable that all patients receiving glucocorticoids carry identifying information.

REFERENCES

1. Allison, F., Smith, M.R., and Wood, W.B.: Studies on the pathogenesis of acute inflammation. II. The action of cortisone in inflammatory response to thermal injury. J. Exp. Med., *102*:669–676, 1955.
2. Ashmore, J., and Weber, G.: Hormonal control of carbohydrate metabolism in liver. *In* Carbohydrate Metabolism and Its Disorders, Vol. I. Edited by F. Dickens, P.J. Randle, and W.J. Whelan. New York, Academic Press, 1968, pp. 335–374.
3. Ashton, N., and Cooke, C.: *In vivo* observations of the effects of cortisone upon the blood vessels in rabbit ear chambers. Br. J. Exp. Pathol., *33*:445–450, 1952.
4. Atkinson, J.P., and Frank, M.M.: Cortisone inhibition of complement independent erythrocyte clearance. Blood, *44*:629–637, 1974.
5. Axelrod, L.: Glucocorticoid therapy. Medicine, *55*:39–65, 1976.
6. Baxter, J.D., and Forsham, P.H.: Tissue effects of glucocorticoids. Am. J. Med., *53*:573–589, 1972.
7. Baxter, J.D., and Funder, J.W.: Hormone receptors. N. Engl. J. Med., *301*:1149–1161, 1979.
8. Baylink, D.J.: Glucocorticoid-induced osteoporosis. N. Engl. J. Med., *309*:306–308, 1983.
9. Bishop, C.W., et al.: Leukokinetic studies: XIII. A non-steady-state kinetic evaluation of the mechanism of cortisone-induced granulocytosis. J. Clin. Invest., *47*:249–260, 1968.
10. Brooks, P.M., et al.: Effects of enzyme induction on metabolism of prednisolone. Clinical and laboratory study. Ann. Rheum. Dis., *35*:339–343, 1976.
11. Butler, W.T., and Rossen, R.D.: Effect of corticosteroids on immunity in man. I. Decreased serum IgG concentration caused by 3 or 5 days of high doses of methylprednisolone. J. Clin. Invest., *52*:2629–2640, 1973.
12. Cahill, G.F.: Action of adrenal cortical steroids on carbohydrate metabolism. *In* The Human Adrenal Cortex. Edited by N.P. Christy. New York, Harper & Row Publishers, Inc., 1971, pp. 205–239.
13. Chan, L., and O'Malley, B.W.: Steroid hormone action: Recent advances. Ann. Intern. Med., *89*:694–701, 1978.
14. Chretien, J.H., and Garagusi, V.F.: Suppressed reduction of nitroblue tetrazolium by polymorphonuclear neutrophils from patients receiving steroids. Experientia, *27*:1343, 1971.
15. Claman, H.N.: Corticosteroids and lymphoid cells. N. Engl. J. Med., *287*:388–397, 1972.
16. Craddock, C.G., Winkelstein, A., and Matsuyuki, Y.: The immune response to foreign red blood cells and the participation of short-lived lymphocytes. J. Exp. Med., *125*:1149–1172, 1967.
17. Cupps, T.R., and Fauci, A.S.: Corticosteroid-mediated immunoregulation in man. Immunol. Rev., *65*:133–155, 1982.
18. Current trends: Preventive therapy of tuberculosis infection. Morbid. Mortal. Week. Rep., *24*:71–78, 1975.
19. Dale, D.C., and Petersdorf, R.G.: Corticosteroids and infectious diseases. Med. Clin. North Am., *57*:1277–1287, 1973.
20. David, D.S., Grieco, M.H., and Cushman, P., Jr.: Adrenal glucocorticoids after twenty years. A review of their clinically relevant consequences. J. Chronic Dis., *22*:637–711, 1970.
21. Dayer, J.M., et al.: Production of collagenase and prostaglandins by isolated adherent rheumatoid synovial cells. Proc. Natl. Acad. Sci. U.S.A., *73*:945–949, 1976.
22. Dixon, R.B., and Christy, N.P.: On the various forms of corticosteroid withdrawal syndrome. Am. J. Med., *68*:224–230, 1980.
23. Dluhy, R.G., Lauler, D.P., and Thorn, G.W.: Pharmacology and chemistry of adrenal glucocorticoids. Med. Clin. North Am., *57*:1155–1165, 1973.
24. Ebert, R.H., and Barclay, W.J.: Changes in connective tissue reaction induced by cortisone. Ann. Intern. Med., *37*:506–518, 1952.
25. Fauci, A.S., and Dale, D.C.: Alternate-day prednisone therapy and human lymphocyte subpopulations. J. Clin. Invest., *55*:22–32, 1975.
26. Fauci, A.S., and Dale, D.C.: The effect of *in vivo* hydrocortisone on subpopulations of human lymphocytes. J. Clin. Invest., *53*:240–246, 1974.
27. Fauci, A.S., Dale, D.C., and Balow, J.E.: Glucocorticoid therapy: Mechanisms of action and clinical considerations. Ann. Intern. Med., *84*:304–315, 1976.
28. Feigelson, P., Yu, F.L., and Henousee, J.: Effect of glucocorticoids on hepatic enzyme induction and purine nucleotide and RNA metabolism. *In* The Human Adrenal Cortex. Edited by N.P. Christy. New York, Harper & Row Publishers, Inc., 1971, pp. 257–272.
29. Feldman, D., Funder, J.W., and Edelman, I.S.: Subcellular mechanisms of action of adrenal steroids. Am. J. Med., *53*:545–560, 1972.
30. Frantz, A.G., and Rabkin, M.T.: Human growth hormone: Clinical measurement, response to hypoglycemia and suppression by corticosteroids. N. Engl. J. Med., *271*:1375–1381, 1964.
31. Frawley, T.F., Kistler, H., and Shally, T.: Effects of anti-inflammatory steroids on carbohydrate metabolism, with emphasis on hypoglycemic and diabetic states. Ann. N.Y. Acad. Sci., *82*:868–885, 1959.
32. Fukushima, D.K., et al.: Metabolic transformation of hy-

drocortisol-4-C¹⁴ in normal men. J. Biol. Chem., *235*:2246–2252, 1960.

33. Gabrielsen, A.E., and Good, R.A.: Chemical suppression of adaptive immunity. Adv. Immunol., *6*:91–229, 1967.
34. Gaunt, R.: Action of adrenal cortical steroids in electrolyte and water metabolism. *In* The Human Adrenal Cortex. Edited by N.P. Christy. New York, Harper & Row Publishers, Inc., 1971, pp. 273–301.
35. Germuth, F.G., Valdes, A.J., and Senterfit, L.B.: A unique influence of cortisone on transit of specific macromolecules across vascular walls in immune complex disease. Johns Hopkins Med. J., *122*:137–153, 1968.
36. Good, T.A., Benton, J.W., and Kelley, V.C.: Symptomatology resulting from withdrawal of steroid hormone therapy. Arthritis Rheum., *2*:299–321, 1959.
37. Green, J.P.: Steroid therapy and wound healing in surgical patients. Br. J. Surg., *52*:523–525, 1965.
38. Hahn, T.J., et al.: Altered mineral metabolism in glucocorticoid-induced osteopenia. J. Clin. Invest., *64*:655–665, 1979.
39. Harter, J.G.: Corticosteroids: Their physiologic use in allergic disease. N.Y. State J. Med., *66*:827–840, 1966.
40. Harter, J.G., Reddy, W.J., and Thorn, G.W.: Studies on an intermittent corticosteroid dosage regimen. N. Engl. J. Med., *269*:591–596, 1963.
41. Harvey, W., Graham, R., and Ranayi, G.S.: Effects of steroid hormones on human fibroblasts *in vitro*. I. Glucocorticoid action on cell growth and collagen synthesis. Ann. Rheum. Dis., *33*:437–441, 1974.
42. Haynes, R.C., Jr., and Murad, F.: Adrenocorticotrophic hormone; Adrenocortical steroids and their synthetic analogs; inhibitors of adrenocortical steroids biosynthesis. *In* The Pharmacological Basis of Therapeutics, 6th Ed. Edited by A.G. Gilman, L.S. Goodman, and A. Gilman. New York, Macmillan Publishing Co., 1980, pp. 1466–1496.
43. Hench, P.S., et al.: The effect of a hormone of the adrenal cortex (17-hydroxy-11-dehydrocorticosterone; compound E) and of pituitary adrenocorticotrophic hormone on rheumatoid arthritis. Mayo Clin. Proc., *24*:181–197, 1949.
44. Henkin, R.I.: The role of adrenal corticosteroids in sensory processes. *In* Handbook of Physiology, Section 7: Endocrinology. Volume VI. Adrenal Glands. Edited by H. Blaschko, G. Sayer, and A.D. Smith. Washington, D.C., American Physiological Society, 1975, pp. 209–230.
45. Hirata, F., et al.: A phospholipase A₂ inhibitory protein in rabbit neutrophils induced by glucocorticoids. Proc. Natl. Acad. Sci. U.S.A., *77*:2533–2536, 1980.
46. Hong, S.L., and Levine, L.: Inhibition of arachidonic acid release from cells as the biochemical action of anti-inflammatory corticosteroids. Proc. Natl. Acad. Sci. U.S.A., *73*:1730–1734, 1976.
47. Howes, E.L., et al.: Retardation of wound healing by cortisone. Surgery, *28*:177–181, 1950.
48. Ingle, D.J.: Permissive action of hormones. J. Clin. Endocrinol. Metab., *14*:1272–1274, 1954.
49. Ingle, D.J.: Atrophy of the thymus in normal and hypophysectomized rats following the administration of cortin. Proc. Soc. Exp. Biol. Med., *38*:443–444, 1938.
50. Jasani, M.K.: The importance of ACTH and glucocorticoids in rheumatoid arthritis. Clin. Rheumat. Dis., *1*:335–365, 1975.
51. Johnson, L.K., et al.: Studies on the mechanism of glucocorticoid hormone action. *In* Gene Regulation by Steroid Hormones. Edited by A.K. Roy, and J.H. Clark. New York, Springer-Verlag, 1980, pp. 153–187.
52. Kantrowitz, F., et al.: Corticosteroids inhibit prostaglandin production by rheumatoid synovia. Nature, *258*:737–739, 1975.
53. Kendall, E.C., et al.: Isolation in crystalline form of hormone essential to life from suppressed cortex: Its chemical nature and physiologic properties. Trans. Assoc. Am. Physicians, *49*:147–152, 1934.
54. Kendall, J.W.: Feedback control of adrenocorticotrophic hormone secretion. *In* Frontiers of Neuroendocrinology. Edited by L. Martini, and W.F. Ganong. New York, Oxford University Press, 1971, pp. 177–207.
55. Klein, A., et al.: A difference between human B and T

lymphocytes regarding their capacity to metabolize cortisol. J. Steroid Biochem., *13*:517–520, 1980.
56. Klinenberg, J.R., and Miller, F.: Effect of corticosteroids on blood salicylate concentration. J.A.M.A., *194*:601–604, 1965.
57. Lefer, A.M.: Corticosteroids and circulatory function. *In* Handbook of Physiology, Section 7: Endocrinology. Volume VI. Adrenal Glands. Edited by H. Blaschko, G. Sayers, and A.D. Smith. Washington, D.C., American Physiological Society, 1975, pp. 191–207.
58. Lewis, G.P., et al.: Prednisone side-effects and serum-protein levels, a collaborative study. Lancet, *2*:778–780, 1971.
59. Loeb, J.N.: Corticosteroids and growth. N. Engl. J. Med., *295*:547–552, 1976.
60. MacGregor, R.R., Spagnuolo, P.J., and Lentnek, A.L.: Inhibition of granulocyte adherence by ethanol, prednisone and aspirin measured with an assay system. N. Engl. J. Med., *291*:642–646, 1974.
61. Morris, H.G., Jorgensen, J.R., and Elrich, H.: Metabolic effects of human growth hormone in corticosteroid-treated children. J. Clin. Invest., *47*:436–451, 1968.
62. Mulrow, P.J., and Forman, B.H.: The tissue effects of mineralocorticoids. Am. J. Med., *53*:561–572, 1972.
63. Munck, A.: Glucocorticoid inhibition of glucose uptake by peripheral tissues: Old and new evidence, molecular mechanism, and physiological significance. Perspect. Biol. Med., *14*:265–289, 1971.
64. Parillo, J.E., and Fauci, A.S.: Mechanisms of glucocorticoid action on immune processes. Annu. Rev. Pharmacol. Toxicol., *19*:179–201, 1979.
65. Perley, M., and Kipnis, D.M.: Effect of glucocorticoids on plasma insulin. N. Engl. J. Med., *274*:1237–1241, 1966.
66. Persellin, R.H., and Ku, L.C.: Effects of steroid hormones on human polymorphonuclear leukocyte lysosomes. J. Clin. Invest., *54*:919–925, 1974.
67. Peterson, R.E., et al.: The physiological deposition and metabolic fate of cortisone in man. J. Clin. Invest., *36*:1301–1312, 1957.
68. Plumpton, F.S., Besser, G.M., and Cole, P.V.: Corticosteroid treatment and surgery. II. The management of steroid cover. Anaesthesia, *24*:12–18, 1969.
69. Ramey, E.R.: Corticosteroids and skeletal muscle. *In* Handbook of Physiology, Section 7: Endocrinology, Volume VI. Adrenal Glands. Edited by H. Blaschko, G. Sayers, and A.D. Smith. Washington, D.C., American Physiological Society, 1975, pp. 245–261.
70. Rinehart, J.J., et al.: Effects of corticosteroids on human monocyte function. J. Clin. Invest., *54*:1337–1343, 1974.
71. Romanoff, E.B., Hudson, P., and Pincus, G.: Isolation of hydrocortisone and corticosterone from human adrenal vein blood. J. Clin. Endocrinol. Metab., *13*:1546–1548, 1953.
72. Rosenau, W., et al.: Mechanism of resistance to steroids: Glucocorticoid receptor defect in lymphoma cells. Nature New Biol., *237*:20–24, 1972.
73. Rousseau, G.G., Baxter, J.D., and Tomkins, G.M.: Glucocorticoid receptors: Relation between steroid binding and biological effects. J. Mol. Biol., *67*:99–115, 1972.
74. Rudman, D., and DiGirolamo, M.: Effect of adrenal steroids on lipid metabolism. *In* The Human Adrenal Cortex. Edited by N.P. Christy. New York, Harper & Row Publishers Inc., 1971, pp. 241–255.
75. Samuels, H.H., and Tomkins, G.M.: Relation of steroid structure to enzyme induction in hepatoma tissue culture. J. Mol. Biol., *52*:57–74, 1970.
76. Sayers, G., and Portanova, P.: Regulation of the secretory activity of the adrenal cortex: Cortisol and corticosterone. *In* Handbook of Physiology, Section 7: Endocrinology. Volume VI. Adrenal Glands. Edited by H. Blaschko, G. Sayers, and A.D. Smith. Washington, D.C., American Physiological Society, 1975, pp. 41–53.
77. Schmidt, T.J., and Litwack, G.: Activation of the glucocorticoid-receptor complex. Physiol. Rev., *62*:1131–1192, 1982.
78. Schotz, M., et al.: The prevalence of tuberculosis and positive tuberculin skin tests in a steroid-treated asthmatic population. Ann. Intern. Med., *84*:261–265, 1976.

79. Siiteri, P.K.: Qualitative and quantitative aspects of adrenal secretion of steroids. *In* The Human Adrenal Cortex. Edited by N.P. Christy. New York, Harper & Row Publishers, Inc., 1971, pp. 1–39.

80. Skubitz, K.M., et al.: Corticosteroids block binding of chemotactic peptide to its receptor on granulocytes and cause disaggregation of granulocyte aggregates *in vitro*. J. Clin. Invest.,*68*:13–20, 1981.

81. Stavy, L., Cohen, I.R., and Feldman, M.: The effect of hydrocortisone on lymphocyte-mediated cytolysis. Cell. Immunol., *7*:302–312, 1973.

82. Steele, R.: Influence of corticosteroids on protein and carbohydrate metabolism. *In* Handbook of Physiology, Section 7: Endocrinology. Volume VI. Adrenal Glands. Edited by H. Blaschko, G. Sayers, and A.D. Smith. Washington, D.C., American Physiological Society, 1975, pp. 135–167.

83. Thompson, J., and Van Furth, R.: The effect of glucocorticoids on the proliferation and kinetics of promonocytes and monocytes of the bone marrow. J. Exp. Med., *137*:10–21, 1973.

84. Thompson, J., and Van Furth, R.: The effect of glucocorticosteroids on the kinetics of mononuclear phagocytes. J. Exp. Med., *131*:429–442, 1970.

85. Thorn, G.W.: Clinical considerations in the use of corticosteroids. N. Engl. J. Med., *274*:775–781, 1966.

86. Tomkins, G.M., and Martin, D.W., Jr.: Hormones and gene expression. Annu. Rev. Genet., *4*:91–106, 1970.

87. Uitto, J., Teir, H., and Mustakallio, K.K.: Corticosteroid-induced inhibition of the biosynthesis of human skin collagen. Biochem. Pharmacol., *21*:2161–2167, 1972.

88. Vernon-Roberts, B.: *The Macrophage*. Cambridge University Press, 1972, pp. 92–119.

89. Weissmann, G., and Thomas, L.: Studies on lyosomes. II. The effect of cortisone on the release of acid hydrolases from a large granule fraction of rabbit liver induced by an excess of vitamin A. J. Clin. Invest., *42*:661–669, 1963.

90. Werb, Z., et al.: Endogenous activation of latent collagenase by rheumatoid synovial cells. N. Engl. J. Med., *296*:1017–1023, 1977.

91. Weston, W.L., Mandel, M.J., and Yeckley, J.A.: Mechanism of cortisol inhibition of adaptive transfer of tuberculin sensitivity. J. Lab. Clin. Med., *82*:366–371, 1973.

92. Wiener, S.L., et al.: The mechanism of action of a single dose of methylprednisolone on acute inflammation *in vivo*. J. Clin. Invest., *56*:679–689, 1975.

93. Yu, D.T.Y., et al.: Human lymphocyte subpopulations: Effect of corticosteroids. J. Clin. Invest., *53*:565–571, 1974.

Chapter **33**

Immunoregulatory Drugs

John L. Decker and Alfred D. Steinberg

Immunoregulatory agents are now in widespread use in clinical medicine. Rheumatic disorders with immune concomitants have been treated with immunosuppressive drugs for three decades. Initially, it had been perceived that the immune hyperactivity associated with such diseases as rheumatoid arthritis (RA) and systemic lupus erythematosus (SLE) might be reduced by such therapy and that clinical improvement might result. In earlier years, the drugs were given without an appreciation of the complexity of the immune system, a complexity now apparent but incompletely understood. We are at the threshold of an era of potentially more specific therapies; however, current practice is still largely empiric. We review in this chapter the immunoregulatory drugs now in use and suggest future applications of modern technology.

CONCEPT OF IMMUNE REGULATION

The cellular basis for immune responsiveness and the regulation of antibody production and cell-mediated immunity are becoming better understood. B cells and their progeny make antibody, the magnitude of which is determined by such factors as: (1) prior exposure to antigen and the generation of memory B cells; (2) the amount of help from T cells; (3) the magnitude of T-cell suppression; and (4) anti-idiotype- and antibody-mediated effects, which may be indirect. If an antigen is presented in association with an immune enhancer, the response may be augmented. On the other hand, a more tolerogenic form of the antigen may specifically impair antibody production to that antigen. For most antigens, antigen-presenting cells are necessary, as is the elaboration of interleukin 1 (IL-1), an important signal for subsequent lymphocyte activation. T cells produce factors that regulate the differentiation and proliferation of both B and T cells. An immune circuit has been constructed in which promoting and inhibiting cells and their products interact to determine the ultimate magnitude of the antibody response.[111] A similar circuit operates in cell-mediated immunity (see Chaps. 15, 16, 17 and 23).

As a result of the network of immune responses, different immunoregulatory agents theoretically could be used to interfere selectively with individual portions of the network. This possibility is tempered by the recognition that perturbation of a network at one point may produce an effect at a distance. Such distant effects might operate to keep the system in balance and might negate the specific immunoregulatory interference. Thus, an "immunosuppressive" drug might actually increase the immune response if suppressor functions are inhibited to a greater extent than are helper functions.[5] Similarly, an "immune enhancer" might actually enhance suppressor circuits and might impair the primary immune responses.[14,36,90,126,128] The recognition of the complexity of the immune system forces us to view immunoregulatory agents not only with regard to an effect on a specific pathway, but also with regard to the overall effect on an immune response or the immune system as a whole. Because the immune system consists of a number of subpopulations of cells that interact with one another in a complex manner, and because both positive and negative feedback inhibition occur, interference with a given cell population may have widespread effects that might not be predicted from the properties of the administered agent. Furthermore, the timing of such interference is important. An agent given in one schedule may be an immune enhancer and may suppress tumor growth, but the same agent may enhance suppressor cell function and may encourage tumor growth when given in another schedule.[36] Thus, drugs may enhance or suppress different immune responses, depending on: (1) the cell population with which they directly interact; and (2) the cells that are indirectly affected by virtue of disruption or augmentation of normal feedback control mechanisms.

GENERAL PRINCIPLES OF PHARMACOLOGIC IMMUNOREGULATION

Many drugs have immunoregulatory properties. These include drugs specifically given for such properties as well as others with secondary immunoregulatory effects, such as antihistaminics, polypeptide hormones, cardioactive glycosides, foods and food additives, anticonvulsants, antiarrhythmics, and a host of other drugs. Many immunoregulatory drugs were initially developed for the chemotherapy of malignant diseases and were subsequently tried in patients with nonmalignant diseases (Table 33–1). Many of these drugs were originally tested in rodents, and the observed effects are not directly applicable to humans. Nevertheless, comparisons can be made because many of the drugs are metabolized on the basis of body surface area, which allows for rough interspecies approximations.[35] Thus, a dose in mg/kg for a full-grown mouse may be divided by 12 to give an approximate dose for adult humans in mg/kg (surface area:body weight ratio of mouse to man). The factor is 6 for rat-human comparisons, and may be as high as 2 or more for human infants, as compared with adults.

Most of the control of immune reactions involves control of lymphocyte proliferation and differentiation. Table 33–2 gives the essential features of the cell cycle. The transition from G_0 to G_1 represents activation of the cell. RNA and new protein synthesis occur, and receptors for further steps toward either proliferation or differentiation are formed at the cell membrane. The interactions of these receptors with their ligands determine whether the cell will proceed toward proliferation $(S + G_2 + M)$ or differentiation (for example, immunoglobulin secretion for a B cell). Cytotoxic and cytostatic drugs interfere with events in cellular proliferation, but most of these drugs were developed as antineoplastic agents and are not specific for the receptors in triggering cells to differentiate or proliferate. The antineoplastic drugs either kill cells or prevent their subsequent division (see Table 33–2). Future attempts at immunoregulation could take advantage of the receptors specific for the stages in G_1. Drugs primarily active during S phase kill rapidly dividing cells, but have minimal effects on resting cells. Other drugs act throughout the cell cycle and kill resting as well as proliferating cells. A drug that induces nonlethal chromosomal damage in a resting cell prevents the cell from dividing and therefore appears to have a greater effect on proliferating cells.

Most purine and pyrimidine analogues are given in repeated, small doses because such a schedule allows continued access to cells in all phases of the cell cycle. On the other hand, methotrexate and certain alkylating agents, as well as irradiation, may be more effective when given in large doses intermittently. Unfortunately, these various antiproliferative agents all kill nonlymphoid cell populations along with the cells involved in immunity. Therefore, the usefulness of a particular therapeutic regimen depends on the relative sensitivities of the different tissues as well as the regenerative capacities of the affected cell populations. Although these parameters are difficult to estimate, the principles and hypothetic equations for them have been outlined.[8]

In the study of immunoregulatory drugs in patients, it is often difficult to know whether observed changes should be ascribed to a direct effect of the therapeutic agent on lymphoid cells or to other effects on the underlying disease process. Peripheral blood cellular changes may reflect recirculation patterns rather than total body alterations and may give one little insight into the composition and function of lymph nodes, spleen, and thymus. Another problem is the circadian rhythms of endocrine, metabolic, renal, and immune functions.[79] The great variability in drug toxicity and effectiveness may reflect such circadian patterns.[79]

Another problem in evaluating the effects of immunosuppressive drugs in rheumatic diseases derives from their common use in low daily doses. Animals with autoimmune diseases respond best to immunosuppressive therapy given early and in large doses.[115] It is possible that a re-evaluation of the timing (early rather than late) and method of administration (large boluses of one drug intermittently and perhaps another in between) may improve the effectiveness of such drugs.[28,38,39,51,134]

More recently, greater emphasis has been placed on immune deficits in certain rheumatic diseases. Patients with SLE have impaired T-cell function extending to both effector and regulatory types.[105] Some suggest that a T-cell stimulant might improve these functions and might help to control the disease. In practice, empiric data still dictate therapy, but as immunologic tools become more precise, immunoregulatory intervention may come to rest on a better theoretic footing.

Immunosuppression

The many processes in an immune response allow for suppression at several points; this suppression may be either antigen-specific or nonspecific. Antigen-specific suppression of immunity may be achieved through the use of specific antigen or specific antibody. Antigen-nonspecific immunosuppression has been studied after a variety of treatments. Surgical ablation of lymphoid tissues, for example, splenectomy, or removal of lymphoid cells through thoracic duct drainage or leukapheresis may result in antigen-nonspecific immunosuppression.

Physical (such as with irradiation), chemical (a variety of drugs; see Table 33–1), biologic (such as antibodies), and living agents (such as bacille Calmette Guerin [BCG]) may bring about antigen-specific or antigen-nonspecific immunosuppression, depending on whether they are given in relation to a specific antigen or have unique specificities. For example, if a large dose of cyclo-

Table 33–1. Immunosuppressive, Cytostatic, and Cytotoxic Drugs

Mechanism of Action	Examples	
	Generic Name	Brand Name
Alkylating Agents		
Chemical reactivity with nucleophilic centers of cellular DNA, RNA, and proteins.	Nitrogen mustard	Mustargen
	Cyclophosphamide	Cytoxan
	Chlorambucil	Leukeran
	Busulphan	Myleran
	L-phenylalanine mustard	Alkeran
	Triethylenemelamine	TEM
	Triethylene thiophosphoramide	Thiotepa
Purine Analogs		
Incorporation into DNA as the deoxyribotide and into RNA as the ribotide. Interference with nucleic acid synthesis through feedback inhibition of purine synthesis by inhibition of the formation of phosphoribosylamine from glutamine and phosphoribosyl pyrophosphate (and the incorporation of purines into purine nucleosides).	Azathioprine	Imuran
	6-Mercaptopurine	Purinethol
	6-Thioguanine	Thioguanine
Pyrimidine Analogs		
Inhibition of enzymes in the synthetic pathways for ribonucleotides and/or deoxyribonucleotides, including thymidylate synthetase, orotic acid decarboxylase, aspartate carbamyltransferase, and dihydro-orotase.	5-Fluorouracil	Fluorouracil
	6-Azauridine	—
	5-Fluoro-2-deoxyuridine (FUDR)	—
	Cytarabine (ARA-C; cytosine arabinoside)	Cytosar
Folic Acid Antagonists		
Binding to dihydrofolate reductase, preventing conversion of dihydrofolic acid to tetrahydrofolic acid, thereby interfering with transport of one-carbon fragments for purine and protein biosynthesis as well as methylation of deoxyuridylic acid to thymidylic acid (necessary for DNA synthesis).	Methotrexate	Methotrexate
Antibiotics		
1. Inhibition of DNA-dependent RNA polymerase by binding to guanine-rich DNA.	1. Mithramycin	Mithracin
2. Alkylating-agent-type action.	2. Mitomycin-C	—
3. Binding to DNA, thereby inhibiting DNA synthesis.	3. Daunorubicin; Actinomycin D	Daunomycin Cosmegen
Enzymes		
Hydrolysis of L-asparagine to L-aspartate and ammonia; also catalysis of the metabolism of L-glutamine at a slower rate.	L-Asparaginase	—
Alkaloids		
Interference with assembly of protein subunits of the mitotic spindle, thereby causing metaphase arrest in dividing cells. Inhibition of RNA and protein synthesis.	Vinblastine	Velban
	Vincristine	Oncovin
Methylhydrazines		
Formation of hydroxyl radicals causing changes in DNA similar to ionizing radiation (small DNA breaks) and unifunctional alkylating agents.	Procarbazine	Matulane
Hydroxyureas		
Killing cells engaged in DNA synthesis and prevention of others from entering the S phase.	Hydroxyurea	Hydrea

Table 33–2. Cell Cycle and Immune Regulation

Phase of Cell Cycle	Cellular Events	Drugs Acting Largely on this Phase
G_0	Interphase	Prednisone (in doses <50 mg/m²/d)
	Resting cell	Many cell-cycle-nonspecific agents*
G_1	RNA synthesis	Vinblastine (interference with cell membrane
	Receptor formation	amino acid transport kills cells in late G_1)
		Inhibitors of protein and RNA synthesis, as well
		as specific probes for activation antigens and re-
		ceptors found on activated cells.
S	DNA synthesis	Cytosine arabinoside
		Methotrexate
		Hydroxyurea
		Thioguanine
		Cyclophosphamide (although it acts throughout the
		cell cycle)
G_2	Postsynthetic rest	Daunorubicin
M	Mitosis	Vincristine and vinblastine (cell must be exposed
		to each during S phase, even though the drugs' ef-
		fect is not expressed until M)

*Cell-cycle-nonspecific agents: alkylating drugs; 6-mercaptopurine; azathioprine; L-asparginase; azaserine, mithramycin; procarbazine; prednisone >100 mg/m²/d.

phosphamide is given with an antigen, the subsequent antibody response to that antigen is suppressed to a greater extent than is an antibody response to an unrelated antigen. The precise timing of administration of these agents in relation to antigen exposure determines the degree, duration, and relative specificity of the immunosuppressed state.

Several agents, given together, may produce varied results. Thus, drug A may have no effect on the results of treatment with drug B, drug A may reduce those results, or drug A may increase those results. With regard to immunoregulatory drugs, simultaneous treatment with two, three, or more drugs may give a greater result than would be expected by the summing of the expected results of treatment with the individual drugs separately.[69] It is even possible for two or three drugs to produce results greater than their additional individual effects. This phenomenon is termed "drug synergy."[8,34] This type of drug interaction has been documented with regard to such phenomena as primary immune responses,[34] tolerance,[51] and treatment of autoimmune disease.[38,115]

Immunosuppressive and anti-inflammatory effects may be difficult to separate. In fact, "inflammation" may be an important effector mechanism of the immune system. Such is especially true of the cell-mediated immune system, but also of certain antibody-mediated reactions. Thus, anti-inflammatory action and immunosuppressive actions may be inextricably intertwined. Similarly, immune stimulation may be difficult to separate from stimulation of inflammation.

Nonspecific Suppression

Immune responses can be reduced or eliminated by many antigen nonspecific mechanisms. The most drastic are mechanisms that eliminate much of the body's immune function, such as total body irradiation and large doses of cyclophosphamide used prior to bone marrow transplantation. Nonspecific suppression, which might be useful in the treatment of patients with nonmalignant inflammatory diseases, is based on a balance in the reduction in certain immune functions, without eliminating the body's ability to defend itself against infectious agents. Thus, one attempts to maintain adequate granulocyte and phagocytic function while reducing the capacity to produce antibody or to mount cell-mediated immune reactions. Physical removal of part of the immune system is one approach. The spleen is an important contributor to immune function in humans; its removal leads to reduced autoantibody production in many patients with SLE, idiopathic thrombocytopenic purpura, autoimmune hemolytic anemia, and other antibody-mediated diseases. *Splenectomy* also reduces removal of antibody-coated cells by the reticuloendothelial system. These benefits are obtained with little impairment of granulocyte function. Patients do lose the capacity to eliminate antibody-coated bacteria easily, however, and as a result, the predisposition to certain infections, such as pneumococcal septicemia, is enhanced. Appropriate immunization, such as with pneumococcal vaccines, may reduce many of the risks that follow splenectomy.

Removal of lymphocytes is accomplished by

thoracic duct drainage. Almost all the cells in the lymph are lymphocytes, and most are T cells. Therefore, thoracic duct drainage could be effective in T-cell-mediated disorders, as has already been shown for RA.[73] The risk of infection and the relative difficulty of long-term drainage has led to *leukapheresis* as an alternative.[57] By appropriately gating cells, a population enriched in lymphocytes and monocytes may be removed from peripheral veins, and the desirable granulocytes, erythrocytes, platelets, and plasma may be returned to the body. This procedure is not as simple as taking a few pills, but could be used in many patients if it were effective and long-lasting treatment. An approach that combines some of the benefits of both splenectomy and thoracic duct drainage is *total lymphoid irradiation.*[60,125] Initially designed for the treatment of lymphoid malignant disorders, this treatment has been employed in patients with RA and SLE. It involves the administration of small dosages of irradiation to the spleen and most of the lymph nodes while shielding much of the mediastinum and spine. Certain chemicals that preferentially eliminate lymphoid cell function are also able to bring about antigen-nonspecific suppression.

Because suppressor cells suppress immune response and autoimmune disease,[80,111] drugs preferentially augmenting suppressor cells may prove useful. In addition, the soluble products of suppressor cells are capable of inducing suppression.[111,114,133] Suppressor factors now can be isolated and produced in large quantities. These factors may allow in vivo natural immunosuppression without some of the drawbacks of drugs.

Nonspecific Immune Enhancement

Responses to a variety of antigens can be augmented by administration of an immune adjuvant with the antigen, and adjuvant is commonly used in the course of human immunizations. In addition to substances enhancing responses to antigens, there are substances called polyclonal B-cell activators. These activators stimulate cells to produce antibodies of many specificities. Such activators include naturally occurring materials such as oligonucleotides, bacterial endotoxin, and certain viruses. Synthetic polynucleotides and certain drugs also nonspecifically stimulate B cells. T cells may also be stimulated by both naturally occurring and synthetic immune stimulants. Therefore, one can stimulate B-cell or T-cell function or both. Feedback mechanisms that may be activated may counteract the stimulation, however.

Freund's adjuvant is most widely used and consists of a combination of killed mycobacteria, paraffin oil, and an emulsifying agent. A synthetic drug, N-acetyl muramyl-L-alanyl-D-isoglutamine (muramyl dipeptide), mimics Freund's adjuvant and is even effective orally.[19] Water-soluble preparations of a peptidoglycan isolated from Freund's adjuvant can stimulate delayed hypersensitivity. The effects of such stimulation in human rheumatic disorders remain to be determined.

IMMUNOREGULATORY AGENTS IN CURRENT USE

6-Mercaptopurine and Azathioprine

6-Mercaptopurine (6MP) is an analogue of hypoxanthine in which the hydroxyl group on the sixth carbon atom is replaced by a thiol group. Azathioprine is 6MP with an imidazole group attached to the sulfur atom. Although azathioprine is broken down in the body to produce 6MP, some differences between the two drugs may be important. For example, the imidazole group of azathioprine gives it different rates of: (1) passage through cell membranes; and (2) conversion to active products. The imidazole moiety split off from azathioprine causes a reduction in the immunosuppressive effects of concomitantly administered 6MP.[109] Azathioprine and 6MP also differ in predilection for various tissues.

Both azathioprine and 6MP are absorbed after oral administration. Typical oral doses give peak blood levels of 0.1 to 2.0 μg/ml; however, large intravenous doses may yield levels as high as 25 μg/ml.[20,30,67] The plasma half-life of 6MP is less than 90 minutes in adults and is even shorter in children. Both drugs are metabolized and excreted by degradation after tissue uptake and urinary excretion. Most of the 6MP given orally is oxidized to nontoxic thiouric acid by xanthine oxidases.[20,67] Because the major catabolism of 6MP involves xanthine oxidase, allopurinol, a xanthine oxidase inhibitor, cannot be given with 6MP or azathioprine without reducing the dose of the antimetabolite by about 75%.

Small quantities of 6MP are converted to the ribonucleotides of 6MP, 6-methylmercaptopurine, and 6-thioguanine (6TG) by the enzymes of the purine metabolic pathways. These ribonucleotides inhibit DNA synthesis by several processes. For example, 6MP ribonucleotide (thioinosinic acid) competitively inhibits the enzymes that convert: (1) inosinic acid to xanthylic and adenylosuccinic acids; and (2) adenylosuccinic acid to adenylic acid. In addition, 6-methylmercaptopurine ribonucleotide causes feedback inhibition of the formation of 5-phosphoribosylamine which inhibits renewed purine synthesis. 6TG is incorporated into DNA as an abnormal base leading to errors in transcription and replication.

In humans, azathioprine and 6MP suppressed

both antibody production and cell-mediated immunity when given after antigen; no immunosuppression occurred when the drugs were given before antigen.[1,46] Induction of specific tolerance with regard to antibody production to subsequent immunization was achieved by treatment with antigen and 6MP, followed by antigen challenge the day after 6MP was stopped.[64]

In vitro responses to mitogens and antigens are little reduced by standard oral doses of azathioprine. In general, modest doses of 6MP or azathioprine have no effect on delayed skin hypersensitivity if prior sensitization has occurred. In contrast, induction of primary sensitization is inhibited in some patients. Survival of organ grafts, such as kidney, is prolonged by either 6MP or azathioprine.

Azathioprine or 6MP is usually given 2 to 5 mg/kg/day orally. The primary toxicity of both drugs is to the bone marrow. Leukopenia is more common than thrombocytopenia or major anemia. A rapid fall in white blood cell count with marrow maturation arrest resembling an idiosyncratic reaction has occurred in some patients within a week of initiation of therapy. The maximum bone marrow suppressive effect of the usual doses takes about 2 weeks to occur. Occasionally, red blood cell aplasia results from long-term azathioprine use; this disorder may respond to cyclophosphamide therapy.[83] In some patients, 6MP and azathioprine administration have been associated with allergic hepatitis (Table 33–3). Some patients develop an influenza-like illness with fever, diffuse achiness, and malaise. This reaction is idiosyncratic, and such individuals cannot take even small doses of these drugs. Lymphoreticular malignant diseases, especially intracerebral lymphomas, are increased in kidney transplant recipients receiving purine an-

alogue immunosuppression.[49] The incidence of epithelial tumors, especially of the skin and uterine cervix, is also increased. The relative risk of malignant disease in other situations has not been accurately determined; however, leukemia and intracerebral reticulum cell sarcoma have been reported in patients with RA and SLE who have received azathioprine.

Infections caused by common microbes or by more exotic organisms such as *Pneumocystis carinii* and *Candida* are enhanced. Such infections suggest an abnormality in T-cell-macrophage defenses, especially because polymorphonuclear leukocyte function is normal in patients receiving azathioprine.[68]

Deoxycoformycin, an analogue of deoxyadenosine, is a potent inhibitor of adenosine deaminase. Severe alterations in T-cell function and mild abnormalities of B-cell function occur in the genetically determined deficiency of adenosine deaminase in man. Studies are now being conducted with inhibitors of adenosine deaminase as potential immunosuppressive agents, with deoxycoformycin as the prototype.[106]

Alkylating Agents

Alkylating drugs contain an alkyl radical substituted with one or more reactive end groups, usually chlorine atoms. Each of these reactive end groups in the alkylating compound can react with another molecule to which it becomes covalently bound. If an alkylating agent has two or more reactive groups, then two or more molecules can be bound covalently to the alkylating agent and thereby linked to each other (cross-linked). The cross-linking of DNA leads to impaired cellular division because the strands cannot be replicated.[39] Alkylating agents also alter the function of impor-

Table 33–3.   Toxic Effects of Immunosuppressive Drugs

Drug Effect (Typical Adult Doses)	Azathioprine (50–150 mg/day)	Cyclophosphamide (25–100 mg/day) (0.5–1.0 g/m² IV)*	Chlorambucil (4–12 mg/day)	Methotrexate (7.5–35 mg/week)†
Lethal bone marrow damage	+	+	+ +	+
Liver damage	+	0	+	+ +
Azoospermia	0	+ +	+ +	0
Anovulation	0	+ +	+ +	0
Clastogenicity	+	+ +	+ +?	+
Carcinogenicity	+ +	+ +	+ +	0
Teratogenicity	0	+	+	+ +
Special	Idiosyncratic: acute agranulocytosis Allergic hepatitis	Bladder toxicity: Cystitis Fibrosis Cancer Alopecia		Ulcerations of gastrointestinal tract mucosa Many other effects

*Administered at intervals of 3 weeks to 3 months. Severe toxicity occurs if given more frequently than every 3 weeks, especially at high doses.
†Divided into 3 doses, each separated by 12 hours.

tant cellular proteins and ribonucleic acids. These drugs appear to predispose to the development of leukemia and other lymphoreticular malignant diseases.[16,39,91,112]

A follow-up study of 81 patients treated with cyclophosphamide showed a 4-fold increase in malignant disease, compared to age and sex matched with RA. Lymphoreticular malignant disease occurred in 4 patients, a 15-fold increase over that expected in the general population.[7]

Nitrogen Mustard

Nitrogen mustard (mechlorethamine, HN2) is a bifunctional alkylating agent that acts through the cell cycle. After intravenous administration, clearance from the blood is rapid; 90% is cleared within the first minute. Nitrogen mustard is detoxified in the body and is cleared by the urine. Typical doses are 0.4 to 0.6 mg/kg intravenously every 3 to 4 weeks. Nausea and vomiting may be reduced by premedication. Thrombosis or phlebitis may occur if the drug comes in direct contact with the intima of the injected vein. Leukopenia and thrombocytopenia are common within a few days and may last as long as 3 weeks after a single dose. The therapeutic index of nitrogen mustard in experimental animals with regard to immunosuppressive effects is much lower than that of cyclophosphamide.

Cyclophosphamide

Cyclophosphamide is a cyclic phosphamide mustard. The ring structure reduces the reactivity of the terminal chlorine atoms. The drug is metabolized primarily by liver microsomal enzymes to a number of alkylating metabolites. Phosphorylation also occurs, separating cyclophosphamide from other alkylating agents.

The serum half-life of cyclophosphamide in adult man is about 5 hours. Because cyclophosphamide and its metabolites are excreted by the kidney, the clearance of active metabolites is reduced in patients with renal insufficiency, and toxicity is increased unless dosages are reduced. The metabolism of cyclophosphamide is also influenced by a number of drugs that affect the hepatic mixed-function oxidases that metabolize cyclophosphamide, including corticosteroids and phenobarbital.[39]

Cyclophosphamide acts primarily during the S phase of the cell cycle, thereby inactivating rapidly proliferating cells. It is also able to alter nonproliferating cells that may undergo some repair, but often are sufficiently injured so that subsequent reproduction is impaired. The drug reduces antibody production. Large intravenous doses of cyclophosphamide have been used to prepare patients for bone marrow grafting.[17] Smaller doses, which may be given orally or intravenously, have been used successfully in kidney transplantation and in a variety of inflammatory diseases. In addition to its ability to suppress both cell-mediated and humoral immunity, cyclophosphamide has some anti-inflammatory properties.[118]

The toxicity of cyclophosphamide (Table 33–3) includes features shared with other cytotoxic agents such as bone marrow depression and predisposition to infection. Bone marrow depression is primarily manifested by leukopenia. This side effect is dose related; however, a previously tolerated dose may lead to marked leukopenia a year or two into treatment. Leukopenia may persist for many months after drug withdrawal. Alopecia, expected at high doses, is rarely a problem at low doses. On reducing or stopping the drug, hair growth generally returns to normal. Damage to the urinary collecting system is the major preventable toxicity of cyclophosphamide. The metabolites of cyclophosphamide damage transitional epithelium, a process enhanced by high concentrations of metabolites in contact with the bladder for long periods of time. Bladder fibrosis, intractable hemorrhage, cystitis, and bladder carcinoma may result.[4,39,49] Prophylactic administration of large volumes of fluid and frequent emptying of the bladder are effective deterrents. Acetylcysteine appears to prevent bladder complications. Other forms of malignant disease, especially lymphoma and leukemia, may result from cyclophosphamide treatment.[7,91]

Cyclophosphamide and the other alkylating agents damage the germinal epithelium of either sex. Treatment of adult males with high doses usually leads to permanent azoospermia within a year. Libido and potency remain normal, and both Leydig and Sertoli cells appear to be spared. Prepubertal testes have a better chance of a return to normal spermatogenesis after drug withdrawal. In the ovary, proliferation of thecal cells necessary for the formation of the follicle is inhibited; the drug also has a direct effect on ova. Amenorrhea often occurs in premenopausal women within a year or two of initiation of therapy; the older the woman, the faster the onset. Estrogen levels are reduced. Thus, cyclophosphamide may give rise to secondary immunoregulatory effects mediated by sex hormone changes.

Large doses of cyclophosphamide can produce myocardial or pulmonary toxicity. The drug also has a rare antidiuretic-hormone (ADH)-like effect,[24] requiring the administration of saline solution in addition to glucose solutions, to prevent hyponatremia. Prophylactic treatment with antiemetics can reduce by several hours the nausea and vomiting that often follow large doses.

Chlorambucil

Chlorambucil is a bifunctional alkylating agent, structurally related to nitrogen mustard. It is metabolized to 2(4-N,N bis 2-chloroethylamino-phenyl) acetic acid by beta oxidation of the butyric acid. This primary metabolite is responsible for most of the cytotoxic activity of chlorambucil.[71]

At low doses, chlorambucil appears to affect lymphopoiesis to a greater extent than granulo-poiesis.[119] Higher doses suppress all hematopoietic stem cells. Chlorambucil in combination with low doses of other drugs produced a synergistic effect on lymphopoiesis without altering granulocyto-poiesis.[119] The effectiveness of chlorambucil has been enhanced without increasing toxicity by giving the drug attached to anti-T-lymphocyte globulin (ATG). Chlorambucil bound to antibody can be specifically directed to a target organ without reducing the alkylating activity of the drug.[40]

The usual dosage of chlorambucil in humans is 0.05 to 0.20 mg/kg/day orally. Either leukopenia or thrombocytopenia may occur during the course of chlorambucil therapy. Although these effects usually are rapidly reversible on early withdrawal of drug, occasional patients have failed to recover bone marrow function, including several patients with connective tissue diseases.[96] Additional problems include nausea, vomiting, hepatitis (perhaps a hypersensitivity reaction), infertility in both sexes (as in cyclophosphamide therapy), and mutagen-icity (see Table 33–3). Chlorambucil seems to be particularly associated with various types of acute leukemia,[16] especially if treatment is extended beyond 3 years.

Methotrexate

Methotrexate is a folic acid analogue that binds to the enzyme folic reductase with an affinity 10^5 times that of the natural substrate, dihydrofolic acid. This binding prevents the conversion of dihydrofolic acid to tetrahydrofolic acid and subsequently N^5N^{10}-methylenetetrahydrofolic acid, the one carbon transfer necessary for thymidine synthesis and, ultimately, for DNA synthesis and cellular proliferation. Thus, methotrexate kills proliferating cells. Administration of folinic acid (N^5-formyltetrahydrofolic acid) can overcome the methotrexate-induced block, thereby "rescuing" cells that have not been irreversibly damaged.

Methotrexate can be administered orally or parenterally. The absorption after oral administration is only 60%. Half the methotrexate in the circulation is bound to serum proteins. This protein-bound drug is displaceable by other drugs, such as salicylates and sulfonamides, which bind to the same serum proteins. The plasma half-life of methotrexate is about 2 hours.[45] Because little deg-radation occurs, the majority of the drug is excreted in the urine unchanged within 24 hours. Despite substantial biliary excretion, little fecal excretion of the drug occurs because of nearly complete intestinal reabsorption.

Methotrexate-induced immunosuppression depends on drug dosage and schedule. Weekly administration is much less effective in inhibiting antibody production than daily administration.[46,101,120]

Toxic effects of methotrexate include stomatitis, nausea, vomiting, diarrhea, leukopenia, and thrombocytopenia (see Table 33–3). Folinic acid can reduce the toxic effects of methotrexate.[41,78] Long-term daily treatment or treatment in patients with underlying liver diseases may lead to cirrhosis. Intermittent administration is less toxic than daily doses. Adult doses range from 5 to 40 mg/week. The drug may be given parenterally once a week or orally in 3 divided doses separated by 8 to 12 hours each weekend. Use of methotrexate in the first 3 months of pregnancy is associated with a high risk of teratogenesis. For patients with impaired renal function, toxicities may be reduced by decreasing the drug dose. An increased risk of malignant disease has not been associated with methotrexate use.

5-Fluorouracil

5-Fluorouracil is a pyrimidine analogue that competes with uracil, but cannot be converted to thymidine. The fluorodeoxyuridine that is formed inhibits the enzyme thymidylate synthetase, a rate-limiting enzyme for DNA synthesis. The drug works throughout the cell cycle. It is almost completely catabolized by the liver; small quantities are excreted by the kidneys. Daily administration is associated with more severe side effects than intermittent therapy. Mucocutaneous erythema often precedes toxic ulcerative stomatitis and gastrointestinal ulcerations. Other side effects include nausea and vomiting, thrombocytopenia, granulocytopenia, alopecia, erythematous dermatitis, and cerebellar ataxia.

Hydroxyurea

Hydroxyurea kills selectively proliferating cells and prevents other cells from entering S phase. Peak blood levels are found between 1 and $2\frac{1}{2}$ hours after oral administration. More than half the drug is excreted by the kidney in the first 8 hours. A rapid fall in leukocyte and platelet counts is observed in the first 48 hours, followed by a recovery within a week. Side effects include oral and gastrointestinal ulcerations, nausea and vomiting, and a maculopapular rash.

Vincristine

Vincristine, an alkaloid extracted from the periwinkle plant, *Vinca rosea*, interferes with the assembly of the protein subunits (tubulin) of the mitotic spindle. The drug is considered an M (mitosis) phase cell-cycle-specific agent; however, the expression in M phase requires exposure to the drug during earlier phases of the cell cycle.

After intravenous injection, most of the drug is cleared from the blood within 30 minutes. It is excreted almost entirely into the bile. The bone marrow is affected 12 to 18 hours after injection, with a return to normal by about 36 hours. Mild leukopenia or thrombocytopenia may occur at high doses or after prolonged therapy. Otherwise, thrombocytosis may be observed. The major side effect is neurotoxicity: peripheral neuropathy, vocal cord paralysis, cranial nerve palsies (bilateral ptosis, diplopia), cerebellar signs, convulsions, coma, and depression. Many patients develop severe constipation culminating in paralytic ileus. It is necessary to hydrate adequately every patient receiving vincristine and to administer prophylactic stool softeners or laxatives. Other side effects include bladder atony, alopecia, patchy liver necrosis, oral and gastrointestinal ulcerations, rash, nausea and vomiting, mutagenicity, orthostatic hypotension, and inappropriate secretion of ADH. Severe inflammatory reactions occur if the drug extravasates; these painful reactions may lead to phlebitis and cellulitis. Because the drug is handled by the hepatobiliary system, neurotoxicity is increased in the presence of hepatic damage or biliary obstruction.

Vinblastine

Vinblastine, a related alkaloid, has more reversible binding to the mitotic spindle. It is not as neurotoxic as vincristine and is less likely to produce severe paralytic ileus. A novel approach to directed immunosuppression is treatment of idiopathic thrombocytopenia with drug-loaded platelets to kill the cells that are destroying the platelets.[2]

Levamisole

This 3-ringed antihelminthic drug is stable in aqueous solutions in acid, but is hydrolyzed in alkaline aqueous solutions. It is readily absorbed from the gastrointestinal tract and has a plasma half-life of about 4 hours in man. After an oral dose of 150 mg, peak blood levels of 0.5 μg/ml are achieved at 2 hours.[121] In addition to gastrointestinal absorption, levamisole is rapidly absorbed from tissue sites. It is metabolized by the liver, and the metabolites are excreted in the urine and to a lesser degree in the feces. Small amounts of unmetabolized levamisole may be found in urine, milk, tears, and respiratory secretions.

Levamisole augments nonspecific inflammatory functions by increasing chemotaxis of polymorphonuclear leukocytes and monocytes and their phagocytic functions.[107] These effects can be dramatic when these functions are impaired, but the drug has little effect on normal responses. Although the drug may favorably alter immune effector functions in disease states, it may have no favorable effect on clinical infections.[47,126] In general, the drug increases resistance to secondary infections to a much greater extent than to primary infections.

In addition to its effects on effector-cell functions, the drug also has a more direct action on earlier stages of T-cell function. Helper, amplifier, cytotoxic, and suppressor T-cell functions are augmented by levamisole.[100] Patients with impaired delayed hypersensitivity showed restoration of skin reactivity after levamisole therapy. Again, the drug appears to increase subnormal responses, but not normal responses.

Levamisole increased the numbers of circulating T cells in patients with subnormal values, usually at the expense of non-T, non-B cells; this finding suggests maturation of pre-T cells to T cells.[94] The drug may have an indirect stimulatory effect on antibody production.[75] The multiple actions of levamisole may explain its contradictory effects in experimental autoimmune diseases; the drug improves some and worsens others. Levamisole may be more effective if combined with appropriate lymphocyte-depleting agents.[134]

Levamisole has been used in patients with malignant diseases, aphthous stomatitis, herpes labialis, Crohn's disease, RA, and SLE.[65,76,97,121] Unfortunately, side effects are frequent and toxic. Granulocytopenia is the most dangerous and seems especially frequent in patients with rheumatic diseases,[76,121] perhaps owing to the induction of leukoagglutinins demonstrable only after drug withdrawal. Agranulocytosis may be especially common in patients with HLA-B27.[102] It has been suggested that corticosteroids might protect against the levamisole-induced granulocytopenia; however, several deaths from granulocytopenia occurred in patients receiving both drugs. Other side effects of levamisole are nausea and vomiting, fatigue and drowsiness, urticarial skin rash, and drug fever. The drug stimulates the sympathetic and paraasympathetic nervous systems, has positive chronotropic and inotropic effects on the heart, and inhibits alkaline phosphatases. Thus, despite some favorable effects in patients with RA, the side effects probably outweigh the benefits.

BIOLOGIC IMMUNOREGULATORY AGENTS AND FUTURISTIC IMMUNE REGULATION

With the advent of modern molecular biology and cloning techniques, it is possible to produce large amounts of a given antibody molecule or a particular factor in intercellular communication. Such materials may revolutionize approaches to immunoregulation. Many of the naturally occurring biologic materials have been or will be synthesized chemically, so the division between chemical and biologic is arbitrary. Nevertheless, the substances discussed here are those that can be produced by living cells.

Many different biologic materials are capable of modifying immune responsiveness.[129] These materials include antibodies, interferons, interleukins (IL), chalones, hormones, and activating and suppressing factors. Transfer factor is capable of imparting antigen-specific delayed hypersensitivity from one person to another. Further studies may lead to clinically useful agents. Grafts of lymphoid organs such as thymus or thymic epithelium have been used in immune deficiency states. Bone marrow reconstitution has been employed in several diseases. Thymic hormones or synthetic materials with similar action on the adenyl cyclase-cyclic adenosine monophosphate (cAMP) system have the potential to modulate immunity; these materials have been tried in humans with uncertain outcome because of the lack of randomized trials. Living agents such as BCG have been used in man. The capacity for viruses to alter immunity leaves open the future possibility of purposeful infection with particular viruses. Finally, toxins have been coupled to antibodies or other materials with specificity so that they can be delivered to the desired sites.

Two types of agents stand out for possible future use: factors and antibodies.

Factors

Macrophages are induced to produce IL-1 by a T-cell product (one of the colony-stimulating factors). IL-1 is necessary for T cells maximally to produce the following factors: IL-2 (T-cell proliferation factor), T-cell differentiation factor, B-cell proliferation factor, B-cell differentiation factor, immune interferon, colony-stimulating factor, IL-3, and a variety of suppressor factors. The administration of one of these factors could have a profound influence on many immune responses. The same is true of agents that increase or decrease the production of or responses to such factors. Because these factors act on specific cell membrane receptors, antibodies to the receptors could increase or decrease the effects of the factors as well as analogues. One such factor, interleukin 2, the T-cell-derived factor that induces T-cell proliferations, is currently given to patients with acquired immune deficiency syndrome. Interferon has been used to treat both malignant diseases and viral infections. Because many interferons exist (19 at last count), with differing immune and antiviral activities, studies of specific interferons are necessary to determine the potential for such agents in various diseases. The possible benefit to patients of the potential for interfering with the immune system by means of immunoregulatory factors remains uncertain.

Antibodies

Monoclonal antibodies are being made all over the world against many antigenic determinants. In theory, if sufficient reason exists to make a particular antibody that can be made by a single cell, only time and energy (adequate screening) are required to produce large amounts of that antibody. Cell-cell fusion and selection by which hybridoma antibodies are produced have suggested the possibility of specifically altering the immune system.[59] Thus, a patient with a tumor with unique antigenic determinants may be treated with custom-made antibodies that will react specifically with the tumor and not with other cells.[75,77,93] Eventually, a bank of such antibodies may be available. In addition, antibodies to subpopulations of human lymphocytes exist. It is possible to treat patients with antibodies to T cells to diminish graft rejection and to treat donor bone marrow, to prevent graft-versus-host disease.[33,88,92] Soon it may be possible to modulate subpopulations of B cells, T cells, and monocytes selectively. This advance is a giant step beyond the antilymphocyte serum or anti-T-cell globulin already in use.[9,44,103,124] The latter eliminate T cells in cell-mediated immunity to a greater extent than those involved in antibody production, and toxicities have been reported, such as serum sickness and local tumor. Whether or not monoclonal antibodies are superior to polyclonal heterologous antibodies remains to be determined. An untapped source of antibodies is spontaneous antibody production by humans with diseases such as SLE and RA. Such antibody-producing cells could be cloned, and human antibodies specific for lymphocyte subpopulations could be obtained for use in other individuals. Studies have shown that anti-Ia- and anti-T-cell antibodies can effectively treat murine lupus erythematosus (see Chap. 24).

Steroid Hormones

These agents have achieved immunoregulatory status. Androgens are able to suppress numerous immune responses in experimental animals[29,111,113] and can modulate spontaneously occurring autoimmune disease[95,112,113] by multiple mechanisms still not completely understood. Androgens can affect gene expression at the level of DNA hypothalamic imprinting, thymocyte maturation, stem cell maturation or migration, and immune complex clearance. The net result is mild-to-impressive immunosuppression. The androgen has its greatest effect on autoimmune disease when the hormone(s) is present from early in life. It is not clear whether androgens may be helpful in patients with autoimmune disorders. Although effective in hereditary angioneurotic edema,[23,108] the toxicities of these agents are almost prohibitive, although the impeded androgen danazol is effective and only minimally toxic.[37]

Corticosteroids suppress the induction phase of both cellular and humoral immune responses. Once the immune response is initiated, corticosteroids are less effective. Great differences may exist, however, between the moderately high doses given in the past and the large intermittent doses of 1 g or more of methylprednisolone.

Cyclosporin A

Cyclosporin A, developed as an antifungal agent, is much more useful as an immunoregulatory drug. The drug is a cyclic peptide with N-methylated amino acids that render it resistant to the low gastric pH and to intestinal proteolytic enzymes.[12] The drug is active without further metabolism, but its poor solubility in water must be considered in parenteral use.

Cyclosporin is especially effective in reducing T-cell function without important bone marrow suppression and is therefore useful in preventing allograft rejection. This drug has been used in many patients who have received renal or other organ allografts.[87,110,131] It appears to be ushering in an era of increased boldness in nonrenal organ transplantation.[131]

The mechanism of action of cyclosporin is under investigation. The drug appears to interfere with the early stages of T-cell activation dependent on interleukin 2.[63,84,131] This effect interferes with help for both T cells and B cells and, in addition to reducing T-cell function, reduction of helper-T-cell-dependent B-cell function has been reported.[18] Cyclosporin might also have a direct effect on a subset of B cells.[62] The net effect of cyclosporin therapy in humans is increased, not decreased, serum IgG concentrations.[131]

Cyclosporin also has provided a giant leap forward in confronting the problem of graft-versus-host disease in bone marrow transplantation.[86] The problem was the prevention of graft-versus-host disease without killing important elements in the transplanted bone marrow. Cyclosporin, which impairs T-cell-mediated graft-versus-host disease without injuring the rapidly dividing transplanted stem cells, allows a much greater margin of safety. The utility of cyclosporin A in rheumatic diseases is not yet known.

Nephrotoxicity is a serious side effect, especially in patients receiving renal allografts. Immunosuppressive side effects of the drug include activation of Epstein-Barr virus and lymphoma development. Other side effects include gum hypertrophy, transient hirsutism, and liver function test abnormalities. Bacterial infections have not been troublesome in recipients of this drug.

4,4′ Diaminodiphenylsulfone (Dapsone)

This sulfone has long been used in the treatment of leprosy. It is also effective in the treatment of bullous skin diseases, especially those characterized by granulocyte infiltration, especially in dermatitis herpetiformis, erythema elevatum diutinum, and the uncommon bullous eruptions of patients with SLE.[43,58] Dapsone is absorbed well after oral administration, and its plasma half-life is approximately 1 day. The drug is acetylated in the liver, and 75% of the administered drug is excreted by the kidney.

Dapsone therapy is begun at doses of 50 mg to 100 mg/day and increased gradually to 200 to 400 mg/day. Hemolysis and methemoglobinemia often occur, but the degree of these side effects is dose related and often tolerable. Other side effects include gastrointestinal intolerance, peripheral neuropathy, nervousness, insomnia, and headache.

Ionizing Radiation

X-rays and gamma rays interact with atoms in living tissues. This interaction results in ejection of electrons and ionization of the affected atoms. When the irradiation is of high energy, the ejected electron may have enough energy subsequently to ionize several more atoms. The result of ionization is the formation of reactive free radicals within cells that vigorously interact with and damage biologically important macromolecules, especially DNA. The effects on nuclear DNA frequently impair cellular reproduction. Thus, rapidly dividing cells such as those of the immune system, bone marrow, and intestinal epithelium are preferentially affected. Lymphocytes are susceptible to death from irradiation without having to undergo subsequent division (interphase death), whereas most other cells die only after one or two postirradiation mitoses (mitotic death). Low doses of irradiation may selectively kill certain subpopulations of T and B cells. In general, precursor cells are particularly sensitive to X-irradiation because they have to undergo the most division.[3]

Many human suppressor T-cell precursor subpopulations are particularly radiosensitive, and B cells prior to terminal clonal proliferation are more sensitive to irradiation than are helper T cells because they must divide more times for full expression of activity. Thus, one subpopulation of T cells is more radiosensitive than most B cells, whereas another subpopulation of T cells is more radio-resistant than most B cells. Among the B cells, surface immunoglobulin-bearing B cells appear to be more radiosensitive than are complement receptor-bearing B cells; and ultraviolet irradiation is more damaging to T than to B cells.[50] That the effect of irradiation on the host's immune response is dose dependent reflects the differential sensitivity of lymphocyte subpopulations[72] and feedback effects. Immune responses may be increased at low doses and are usually decreased at high doses. Results of a single dose of irradiation may be different from those of smaller intermittent doses. Lymphocyte populations may be altered selectively by varying dosage schedules, by virtue of differences in ability to repair irradiation-induced damage.

Total body irradiation leads to profound immunosuppression; however, the side effects are equally profound and are acceptable only prior to bone marrow transplantation.[3] More localized delivery of irradiation, such as to selected lymph nodes, may be suppressive with reduced toxic effects on rapidly dividing cells of other organs as well as nondividing cells.

A modification of total body irradiation has been used for some time in the treatment of lymphoid malignant diseases. This procedure, called total lymphoid irradiation (TLI) attempts to irradiate the majority of the lymph nodes and spleen while shielding nonlymphoid tissues as fully as possible. Thus, the heart and spine are largely shielded. The lungs are not completely shielded, so that at high doses of irradiation, pneumonitis may be a complication. Such treatment may benefit patients with intractable RA.[60,125] Preliminary studies in mice with lupus erythematosus and in a few patients with SLE have also suggested benefit. TLI is accompanied by tolerable but substantial morbidity. Several serious infections, including two deaths, have occurred in a series of patients with RA treated with TLI. As a result, this procedure should be viewed as both experimental and potentially life-threatening unless administered at lower doses or by the most experienced radiotherapists. *Because suppressor cells are induced by TLI, and a major mechanism of action of this procedure may be the induction of suppressor cells,* it is possible that much lower doses of irradiation than used heretofore may be effective.

Ultraviolet (UV) Light

We often find that patients with RA fare better in warm, sunny climates. This benefit has been attributed to the warmth, but studies in experimental animals exposed to UV light suggest that the sun is not without effect. UV light interferes with macrophage antigen presentation, at least in part by reducing the numbers of Ia^+ macrophages. Because the development of Ia^+ by resting macrophages is critical to disease perpetuation, controlled exposure to the sun or to UV light *might* be of benefit to patients with RA. Adverse effects of UV light, such as burns and cancer, must be appreciated. In addition, UV light may induce skin cells to produce IL-1, which induces immune responsiveness in T cells. The effect of UV exposure on human disease is still unexplored.

Other Drugs

Colchicine and indomethacin, vitamins, and even heavy metals may modulate immune responses by a variety of mechanisms.[6] Agents that alter the production of certain mediators can be incorporated into the diet.[89,135] Moreover, many cytotoxic or cytostatic drugs used in cancer chemotherapy have been omitted from this chapter because they have not been evaluated in patients with rheumatic disease.

Physical Removal of Cells or Soluble Plasma Substances

The removal of unwanted antibody is well-established in the treatment of hyperviscosity syndrome or Waldenström's macroglobulinemia, either as an adjunct to immunosuppressive drug therapy or as sole treatment.[11] This removal is done by plasma exchange by a continuous-flow centrifugation.[98] Large quantities of pathogenic autoantibodies can be removed, and this technique has been reported to benefit patients with autoimmune thrombocytopenia, SLE, autoimmune hemolytic anemia, myasthenia gravis, Goodpasture's syndrome, and severe rhesus disease.[13,22,42,55] Such treatment suffers from the theoretic disadvantage of "rebound," that is, the production of pathogenic antibodies at higher pretreatment levels as a result of removal of suppressive antibodies. This problem is more common with primary than with secondary responses.[13] Adjunctive therapy with immunosuppressive drugs may prevent such a rebound. Under certain circumstances, plasma exchange can be accompanied by specific removal of specific antibodies or other substances.[123]

IMMUNOREGULATORY DRUGS IN INDIVIDUAL DISEASES

The use of a particular immunoregulatory agent in individual human disorders depends on its ability

Table 33–4. Selected Immunoregulatory Therapies of Selected Nonmalignant Disorders

Disorder	Therapy
Rheumatoid arthritis	Cyclophosphamide[21]
	Chlorambucil[56]
	Azathioprine[127]
	Methotrexate[132]
	Total lymphoid irradiation[60,125]
	Leukapheresis[57]
	Thoracic duct drainage[85]
	Levamisole[81]
Systemic lupus erythematosus	Cyclophosphamide[26]
	Chlorambucil[54]
	Azathioprine[122]
	Total lymphoid irradiation[32]
	Splenectomy[48]
	Plasmapheresis[130]
	Nitrogen mustard[25]
Polymyositis-dermatomyositis	Methotrexate[74]
	Cyclophosphamide[82]
	Azathioprine[15]
Psoriasis and psoriatic arthritis	Methotrexate[10]
	Azathioprine[66]
Wegener's granulomatosis	Cyclophosphamide[31]
	Azathioprine[53]
	Chlorambucil[70]
Paget's disease of bone	Mithramycin[99]

Table 33–5. The Ten Commandments: Guidelines for the Use of Immunosuppressive Drugs in Inflammatory Diseases of Unknown Origin

I. Severely debilitating or life-threatening disease shall be present.
II. Reversible abnormalities shall be present.
III. Conventional therapy shall be inadequate or intolerable.
IV. Full evaluation of physical, psychologic, moral, and family situation shall be done.
V. A meticulous follow-up shall be done, with periodic re-evaluation of doses and goals.
VI. Objective evaluation shall be done before and during treatment.
VII. Protocol shall be approved by peer review.
VIII. Informed consent shall be obtained.
IX. No relative or absolute contraindications, such as infection or pregnancy, shall be present.
X. Due consideration of drug interactions shall be given (for example, as between allopurinol and azathioprine).

to ameliorate the disease without undue immediate or long-term toxicity. This benefit-to-risk ratio should be greater than that of other available approaches to management. Because the manifestations of a given syndrome vary, it is reasonable that therapy should also vary. As a result of this heterogeneity, it is not possible to outline the uses of immunoregulatory agents in particular disorders without qualifying each with regard to individual involvement, severity, reversibility, and a host of

other factors. As discussed previously, rapid progress is being made in the whole field of immunoregulation; newer approaches may be just around the corner. Nevertheless, it is useful to illustrate some of the uses of some of these drugs by listing disease states in which evidence suggests that these drugs are effective (Table 33–4). Two general methods exist by which utility of a drug can be established: (1) provision of therapy that is nontoxic and successful; and (2) demonstration of greater benefit than "standard therapy" by a randomized trial. These stringent requirements are not met by most drugs used now. Certain therapies are probably effective, but have not yet been established on scientific grounds. These regimens include daily cyclophosphamide administration in patients with severe Wegener's granulomatosis and intermittent intravenous boluses of cyclophosphamide in patients with life-threatening active SLE. Cyclophosphamide has toxicities, however, and less toxic treatments for these disorders are still needed.

Table 33–4 is neither exhaustive nor a recommendation for such therapy. The extent to which cancer drugs have dominated our efforts is clear. Future studies should be directed to additional therapies, such as discussed earlier in the "futuristic" section of this chapter. For the present, however, we must rely on the drugs currently available. The guidelines set forth in Table 33–5 provide a basis for deciding whether a given patient is a candidate for such extraordinary therapy. New drugs for a given disorder are best studied in the context of a randomized trial against "standard therapy." Failure to follow this practice has left us without accurate data on the use of most immunoregulatory drugs in most of the disorders in which they are now used. Our legacy to future generations of physicians can be improved by both better drugs and better studies. A recent review suggested that gold and cyclophosphamide probably retard radiographic deterioration in RA.[52] Too few adequate studies were found to permit even tentative conclusions regarding other drugs.

REFERENCES

1. Abdou, N.I., Zweiman, B., and Casella, S.R.: Effects of azathioprine therapy on bone marrow-dependent and thymus-dependent cells in man. Clin. Exp. Immunol., *13*:55, 1973.
2. Ahn, Y.S., et al.: The treatment of idiopathic thrombocytopenia with vinblastine-loaded platelets. N. Engl. J. Med., *298*:1101, 1978.
3. Anderson, R.E., and Warner, N.L.: Ionizing radiation and the immune response. Adv. Immunol., *24*:215, 1976.
4. Ansell, I.D., and Castro, J.E.: Carcinoma of the bladder complicating cyclophosphamide therapy. Br. J. Urol., *47*:413, 1975.
5. Askenase, P.W., Hayden, B.J., and Gershon, R.K.: Augmentation of delayed-type hypersensitivity by doses of cyclophosphamide which do not affect antibody responses. J. Exp. Med., *141*:697, 1975.
6. Azar, M.M., and Good, R.A.: The inhibitory effect of vitamin A on complement levels and tolerance production. J. Immunol., *106*:241, 1971.
7. Baltus, J.A.M., et al.: The occurrence of malignancies in patients with rheumatoid arthritis treated with cyclophosphamide: a controlled retrospective follow up. Ann. Rheumat. Dis., *42*:368, 1983.
8. Berenbaum, M.C.: Suppression of specific immunity by non-specific agents. *In* Immunological Diseases. Edited by M. Samter. Boston, Little, Brown, 1971, p. 131.
9. Bishop, G., et al.: Effect of immunosuppressive therapy for renal allografts on the number of circulating sheep red blood cell rosetting cells. Transplantation, *20*:123, 1975.
10. Black, R.L., et al.: Methotrexate therapy in psoriatic arthritis. JAMA, *189*:743, 1964.
11. Bloch, K.J., and Maki, D.G.: Hyperviscosity syndromes associated with immunoglobulin abnormalities. Semin. Hematol., *10*:113, 1973.
12. Borel, J.F., et al.: Biological effects of cyclosporin A: a new antilymphocytic agent. Agents Actions, *6*:468, 1976.
13. Branda, R.F., et al.: Plasma exchange in the treatment of immune disease. Transfusion, *15*:570, 1975.
14. Brodeur, B.R., and Merigan, T.C.: Mechanism of the suppressive effect of interferon on antibody synthesis *in vivo*. J. Immunol., *114*:1323, 1975.
15. Bunch, T.W.: Prednisone and azathioprine for polymyositis. Long-term follow-up. Arthritis Rheum., *24*:45, 1981.
16. Cameron, S.: Chlorambucil and leukemia. N. Engl. J. Med., *296*:1065, 1977.
17. Camitta, B.M., Thomas, E.D., and Nathan, D.G.: Severe aplastic anemia: a prospective study of the effect of early marrow transplantation on acute mortality. Blood, *48*:63, 1976.
18. Cammisuli, S.: Inhibition of a secondary humoral immune response by cyclosporin A. Transplant. Clin. Immunol., *13*:15, 1981.
19. Chedid, L., et al.: Modulation of the immune response by a synthetic adjuvant and analogs. Proc. Natl. Acad. Sci. USA, *73*:2472, 1976.
20. Coffey, J.J., et al.: Effect of allopurinol on the pharma-

cokinetics of 6-mercaptopurine (NCS-755) in cancer patients. Cancer Res., *32*:1283, 1972.
21. Cooperating Clinics Committee of the American Rheumatism Association: A controlled trial of cyclophosphamide in rheumatoid arthritis. N. Engl. J. Med., *283*:883, 1970.
22. Dau, P.C., et al.: Plasmapheresis and immunosuppressive drug therapy in myasthenia gravis. N. Engl. J. Med., *297*:1134, 1977.
23. Davis, P.J., Davis, F.B., and Charache, P.: Long-term therapy of hereditary angioedema (HAE). Johns Hopkins Med. J., *135*:391, 1974.
24. DeFronzo, R.A., et al.: Water intoxication in man after cyclophosphamide therapy. Time course and relation to drug activation. Ann. Intern. Med., *78*:861, 1973.
25. Dillard, M.G., et al.: The effect of treatment with prednisone and nitrogen mustard on the renal lesions and life span of patients with lupus glomerulonephritis. Nephron, *10*:273, 1973.
26. Dinant, H.J., et al.: Alternative modes of cyclophosphamide and azathioprine therapy in lupus nephritis. Ann. Intern. Med., *96*:728, 1982.
27. Donabedian, H., Alling, D.W., and Gallin, J.I.: Levamisole is inferior to placebo in the hyperimmunoglobulin E recurrent-infection (Job's) syndrome. N. Engl. J. Med., *307*:290, 1982.
28. Ducker, P., and Dietrich, F.M.: Prevention of cyclosphosphamide-induced tolerance to erythrocytes by pretreatment with cortisone. Proc. Soc. Expl. Biol. Med., *133*:280, 1970.
29. Eidinger, D., and Garrett, T.J.: Studies of the regulatory effects of sex hormones on antibody formation and stem cell differentiation. J. Exp. Med., *136*:1098, 1972.
30. Elion, G.B.: Significance of azathioprine metabolites. Proc. R. Soc. Med., *65*:257, 1972.
31. Fauci. A.S., et al.: Wegener's granulomatosis: prospective clinical and therapeutic experience with 85 patients for 21 years. Ann. Intern. Med., *98*:76, 1983.
32. Field, E., et al.: Total lymphoid irradiation for treatment of intractable lupus nephritis. Arthritis Rheum., *26*:569, 1983.
33. Filopovich, A.H. et al.: Pretreatment of donor bone marrow with monoclonal antibody OKT3 for prevention of acute graft-versus-host disease in allogenic histocompatible bone marrow transplantation. Lancet, *1*:1266, 1982.
34. Friedman, E.A., Gelfand, M.C., and Bernheimer, H.P.: Synergism in immunosuppression. I. Effect of combination immunosuppressive drugs on tetanus antitoxin production in the mouse. Transplantation, *11*:479, 1971.
35. Freireich, E.J., Gehan, E.A., and Rall, D.P.: Quantitative comparison of toxicity. Cancer Chemother. Rep., *50*:219–243, 1966.
36. Gazdar, A.F., et al.: Enhancement and suppression of murine sarcoma virus induced tumors by polyriboinosinic polyribocytidylic acid. Proc. Soc. Exp. Biol. Med., *139*:279–287, 1972.
37. Gelfand, J.A., et al.: Treatment of hereditary angioedema with danazole. Reversal of clinical and biochemical abnormalities. N. Engl. J. Med., *295*:1444, 1976.
38. Gelfand, M.C., et al.: Therapeutic studies in NZB/W mice. I. Synergy of azathioprine, cyclophosphamide and methylprednisolone in combination. Arthritis Rheum., *15*:239, 1972.
39. Gershwin, M.E., Goetzl, E.J., and Steinberg, A.D.: Cyclophosphamide: use in clinical practice. Ann. Intern. Med., *80*:513, 1974.
40. Ghose, T., et al.: Immunochemotherapy of malignant melanoma with chlorambucil-bound antimelanoma globulins: preliminary results in patients with disseminated disease. J. Natl. Cancer Inst., *58*:845, 1977.
41. Gorgun, B., and Watne, A.L.: Skin homograft survival in cancer chemotherapy patients. Cancer, *19*:1316, 1966.
42. Graham-Pole, J., Barr, W., and Willoughby, M.L.N.: Continuous-flow plasmapheresis in management of severe rhesus disease. Br. Med. J., *1*:1185, 1977.
43. Hall, R.P., et al.: Bullous eruption of systemic lupus erythematosus. Ann. Intern. Med., *97*:165, 1982.
44. Harris, N.S., Merino, G., and Najarian, J.S.: Mode of

action of antilymphocyte sera (ALS). Transplant. Proc., 3:797, 1971.

45. Henderson, F.S., Adamson, R.H., and Oliverio, V.T.: The metabolic rate of tritiated methotrexate. II. Absorption and excretion in man. Cancer Res., 25:1018, 1965.

46. Hersh, E.M., Carbone, P.O., and Freireich, E.J.: Recovery of immune responsiveness after drug suppression in man. J. Lab. Clin. Med., 67:566, 1966.

47. Hogan, N.A., and Hill, H.R.: Enhancement of neutrophil chemotaxis and alteration of levels of cellular cyclic nucleotides by levamisole. J. Infect. Dis., 138:437, 1978.

48. Homan, W.P., and Dineen, P.: Role of splenectomy in the treatment of thrombocytopenic purpura due to systemic lupus erythematosus. Ann. Surg., 187:52, 1978.

49. Hoover, R., and Fraumeni, J.F., Jr.: Risk of cancer in renal-transplant recipients. Lancet, 2:55, 1973.

50. Horowitz, S., Cripps, D., and Hong, R.: Selective T cell killing of human lymphocytes by ultraviolet radiation. Cell. Immunol., 14:80, 1974.

51. Hyman, L.R., Kovacs, K., and Steinberg, A.D.: Drug-induced tolerance: selective induction with immunosuppressive drugs and their synergistic interaction. Int. Arch. Allergy Appl. Immunol., 48:248, 1975.

52. Iannuzzi, L., et al.: Does drug therapy slow radiologic deterioration in rheumatoid arthritis? N. Engl. J. Med., 309:1023, 1983.

53. Israil, H.L., and Patchefsky, A.S.: Wegener's granulomatosis of lung: diagnosis and treatment, Ann. Intern. Med., 74:881, 1971.

54. Ivanova, M.M., et al.: Controlled trial of cyclophosphamide, azathioprine and chlorambucil in lupus nephritis (a double-blind trial). (In Russian) Vopr. Revm., NS (2):11, 1981.

55. Jones, J.V., Cumming, R.H., and Bucknall, R.C.: Plasmapheresis in the management of acute systemic lupus erythematosus. Lancet, 1:709, 1976.

56. Kahn, M.F., et al.: Chlorambucil in rheumatoid arthritis. (In French) Rev. Rheum., 38:741, 1971.

57. Karsh, J., et al.: Lymphapheresis in rheumatoid arthritis. A randomized trial. Arthritis Rheum., 24:867, 1981.

58. Katz, S.I., et al.: Erythema elevatum diutinum: Skin and systemic manifestations, immunologic studies and successful treatment with dapsone. Medicine, 56:443, 1977.

59. Kohler, G., and Milstein, C.: Continuous cultures of fused cells secreting antibody of predefined specificity. Nature, 256:495, 1975.

60. Kotzin, B.L., et al.: Treatment of intractable rheumatoid arthritis with total lymphoid irradiation. N. Engl. J. Med., 305:969, 1981.

61. Kovacs, K., and Steinberg, A.D.: Cyclophosphamide-drug interaction and bone marrow transplantation. Transplantation, 13:316, 1972.

62. Kunkel, A., and Klaus, G.G.B.: Selective effects of cyclosporin A on functional B cell subsets in the mouse. J. Immunol., 125:2526, 1980.

63. Larsson, E.L.: Cyclosporin A and dexamethasone suppress T cell responses by selectively acting at distant sites of the triggering process. J. Immunol., 124:2828, 1980.

64. Levin, R.H., Landy, M., and Frei, E.: The effect of 6-mercaptopurine on immune response in man. N. Engl. J. Med., 271:16, 1964.

65. Lehner, T., Wilton, J.M.A., and Ivanyi, L.: Double blind crossover trial of levamisole in recurrent aphthous ulceration. Lancet, 2:926, 1976.

66. Levy, J., et al.: Double-blind controlled evaluation of azathioprine treatment in rheumatoid arthritis and psoriatic arthritis. Arthritis Rheum., 15:116, 1972.

67. Loo, T.L., et al.: Clinical pharmacologic observations on 6-mercaptopurine. Clin. Pharmacol. Ther., 9:180, 1968.

68. Losito, A., Williams, D.G., and Harris, L.: The effects on polymorphonuclear leukocyte function of prednisolone and azathioprine in vivo and prednisolone, azathioprine and 6-mercaptopurine in vitro. Clin. Exp. Immunol., 32:423, 1978.

69. McCarty, D.J., and Carrera, G.F.: Treatment of intractable rheumatoid arthritis with combined cyclophosphamide, azathioprine and hydroxychloroquine. JAMA, 248:1718, 1982.

70. McIlvonie, S.K.: Wegener's granulomatosis; successful treatment with chlorambucil. JAMA, 197:90, 1966.

71. McLean, A., Newell, D., and Baker, G.: The metabolism of chlorambucil. Biochem. Pharmacol., 25:2331, 1976.

72. Macario, A.J.L., and Conway de Macario, E.: Enhancement and inhibition of immunological mechanisms by immunosuppressive agents. I. Dose effect on priming and generation of memory to a bacterial antigen. Clin. Exp. Immunol., 31:281, 1978.

73. Machleder, H.I., and Paulus, H.: Clinical and immunological alterations observed in patients undergoing long-term thoracic duct drainage. Surgery, 84:157, 1978.

74. Metzger, A.L., et al.: Polymyositis and dermatomyositis; combined methotrexate and corticosteroid therapy. Ann. Intern. Med., 81:182, 1974.

75. Miller, R.A., et al.: Treatment of B-cell lymphoma with monoclonal anti-idiotype antibody. N. Engl. J. Med., 306:517, 1982.

76. Miller, B., et al.: Double-blind placebo controlled crossover evaluation of levamisole in rheumatoid arthritis. Arthritis Rheum., 23:172, 1980.

77. Miller, R.A., and Levy, R.: Response of cutaneous T cell lymphoma to therapy with hybridoma monoclonal antibody. Lancet, 2:226, 1981.

78. Mitchell, M.S., et al.: Immunosuppressive effects of cytosine arabinoside and methotrexate in man. Ann. Intern. Med., 70:535, 1969.

79. Moore-Ede, M.C., Czeisler, C.A., and Richardson, G.S.: Circadian timekeeping in health and disease. II. Clinical implications of circadian rhythmicity. N. Engl. J. Med., 309:530, 1983.

80. Morton, R.O., et al.: Suppression of autoimmunity and lymphoid proliferation in NZB mice with steroid-sensitive X-irradiation sensitive syngeneic young thymocytes. Arthritis Rheum., 19:1347, 1976.

81. Multicentre Study Group: Levamisole in rheumatoid arthritis: A randomised double-blind study comparing two dosage regimens of levamisole with placebo. Lancet, 2:1007, 1978.

82. Niakan, E., et al.: Immunosuppressive agents in corticosteroid-refractory childhood dermatomyositis. Neurology, 30:286, 1980.

83. Old, C.W., et al.: Azathioprine-induced pure red blood cell aplasia. JAMA, 240:552, 1978.

84. Palacios, R.: Cyclosporin A inhibits the proliferative response and the generation of helper, suppressor and cytotoxic T cell functions in the autologous mixed lymphocyte reaction. Cell Immunol., 61:453, 1981.

85. Paulus, N.E., et al.: Lymphocyte involvement in rheumatoid arthritis: studies during thoracic-duct drainage. Arthritis Rheum., 20:1249–1262, 1977.

86. Powles, R.L., et al.: Cyclosporin A to prevent graft-versus-host disease in man after allogeneic bone-marrow transplantation. Lancet, 1:327, 1980.

87. Preliminary results of a European trial: cyclosporin A as a sole immunosuppressive agent in recipients of kidney allografts from cadaver donors. Lancet, 2:57, 1982.

88. Prentice, H.B., et al.: Use of anti-T cell monoclonal antibody OKT3 to prevent acute graft-versus-host disease in allogeneic bone-marrow transplantation for acute leukemia. Lancet, 1:700, 1982.

89. Prickett, J.D., Robinson, D.R., and Steinberg, A.D.: Dietary enrichment with the polyunsaturated fatty acid eicosapentaenoic acid prevents proteinuria and prolongs survival in NZB X NZW F_1 mice. J. Clin. Invest., 68:556, 1981.

90. Pross, H.F., and Eidinger, D.: Antigenic competition: a review of nonspecific antigen induced suppression. Adv. Immunol., 18:133, 1974.

91. Puri, H.C., and Campbell, R.A.: Cyclophosphamide and malignancy. Lancet, 1:1306, 1977.

92. Reinherz, E., et al.: Reconstitution after transplantation with T-lymphocyte-depleted HLA haplotype-mismatched bone marrow for severe combined immunodeficiency. Proc. Natl. Acad. Sci. USA, 79:6047, 1982.

93. Ritz, J., et al.: Autologous bone-marrow transplantation in CALL-positive acute lymphoblastic leukemia after in

vitro treatment with J5 monoclonal antibody and complement. Lancet, 2:60, 1982.

94. Rosenthal, M., Trabert, U., and Mueller, W.: The effect of levamisole on peripheral blood lymphocyte subpopulations in patients with rheumatoid arthritis and ankylosing spondylitis. Clin. Exp. Immunol., 25:493, 1976.

95. Roubinian, J.R., Papoian, R., and Talal, N.: Androgenic hormones modulate autoantibody responses and improve survival in murine lupus. J. Clin. Invest., 59:1066, 1977.

96. Rudd, P., Fried, J.F., and Epstein, W.V.: Irreversible bone marrow failure with chlorambucil. J. Rheumatol., 2:421, 1975.

97. Runge, L.A., et al.: Treatment of rheumatoid arthritis with levamisole. A controlled trial. Arthritis Rheum., 20:1445, 1977.

98. Russell, J.A., Toy, J.L., and Powles, R.L.: Plasma exchange in malignant paraproteinanemias. Exp. Hematol., 5 (Suppl. 1):105, 1977.

99. Ryan, W.G., and Schwartz, T.B.: Mithramycin treatment of Paget's disease of bone: exploration of combined mithramycin-EHDP therapy. Arthritis Rheum., 23:1155, 1980.

100. Sampson, D., and Lui, A.: The effect of levamisole on cell-mediated immunity and suppressor-cell function. Cancer Res., 36:952, 1976.

101. Santos, G.W., Owens, A.H., and Sensenbrenner, L.L.: Effects of selected cytotoxic agents on antibody production in man. Ann. N.Y. Acad. Sci., 114:404, 1964.

102. Schmidt, K.L., and Mueller-Eckhardt, C.: Agranulocytosis, levamisole, and HLA-B27. Lancet, 2:85, 1977.

103. Sheil, A.G.R., et al.: Controlled clinical trial of antilymphocyte globulin in patients with renal allografts from cadaver donors. Lancet, 1:359, 1971.

104. Smith, H.R., et al.: Induction of autoimmunity in normal mice by thymectomy and administration of polyclonal B cell activators: association with contrasuppressor function. Clin. Exp. Immunol., 51:579, 1983.

105. Smith, H.R., and Steinberg, A.D.: Autoimmunity—a perspective. Annu. Rev. Immunol., 1:175, 1983.

106. Smyth, J.: Treatment of lymphoid malignancy with adenosine deaminase inhibitors. Ciba Found. Symp., 68:263, 1979.

107. Snyderman, R., and Pike, M.C.: Pathophysiologic aspects of leukocyte chemotaxis: identification of a specific chemotactic factor binding site on human granulocytes and defects of macrophage function associated with neoplasia. In Leukocyte Chemotaxis: Methods, Physiology, and Clinical Implications. Edited by J.I. Gallin, and P.Q. Quie. New York, Raven Press, 1978.

108. Spaulding, W.B.: Methyltestosterone therapy for hereditary episodic edema (hereditary angioneurotic edema). Ann. Intern. Med., 53:739, 1960.

109. Spreafico, F., et al.: Immunodepressant activity and 6-mercaptopurine levels after administration of 6-mercaptopurine and azathioprine. Transplantation, 16:269, 1973.

110. Starzl, T.E., et al.: Cyclosporin A and steroid therapy in sixty-six cadaver kidney recipients. Surg. Gynecol. Obstet., 153:486, 1981.

111. Steinberg, A.D., et al.: Genetic, environmental and cellular factors to the pathogenesis of SLE. Arthritis Rheum., 25:734, 1982.

112. Steinberg, A.D., et al.: Effects of thymectomy or androgen administration upon the autoimmune disease of MRL/Mp-*lpr/lpr* mice. J. Immunol., 125:871, 1980.

113. Steinberg, A.D., et al.: Approach to the study of the role of sex hormones in autoimmunity. Arthritis Rheum., 22:1170, 1979.

114. Steinberg, A.D., et al.: Therapeutic studies in NZB/NZW mice. VI. Age-dependent effects of concanavalin A stim-

ulated spleen cell supernate. Arthritis Rheum., 21:204, 1978.

115. Steinberg, A.D., et al.: Therapeutic studies in NZB/W mice. III. Relationship between renal status and efficacy of immunosuppressive drug therapy. Arthritis Rheum., 18:9, 1975.

116. Steinberg, A.D., and Klassen, L.W.: Role of suppressor T cells in lymphopoietic disorders. Clin. Haematol., 6:439, 1979.

117. Steinberg, A.D., and Steinberg, S.C.: Autoimmune disease and the clinical consequences of prolonged immunosuppression. In Proceedings of Symposium on Immunosuppression, 1978. Edited by G. Asher. Washington, D.C., Food and Drug Administration, 1979–1980.

118. Stevens, J.E., and Willoughby, D.A.: The anti-inflammatory effect of some immunosuppressive agents. J. Pathol., 2:367, 1969.

119. Stukov, A.N.: Experimental study of the combined effect of Leukeran, Degranol and prednisolone. Neoplasma, 22:181, 1976.

120. Swanson, M.A., and Schwartz, R.S.: Immunosuppressive therapy. The relations between clinical response and immunologic competence. N. Engl. J. Med., 277:163, 1967.

121. Symoens, J., and Rosenthal, M.: Levamisole in the modulation of the immune response: the current experimental and clinical state. J. Reticuloendothel. Soc., 21:175, 1977.

122. Szteinbok, M., et al.: Azathioprine in the treatment of systemic lupus erythematosus: a controlled study. Arthritis Rheum., 14:639, 1971.

123. Terman, D.S., Petty, D., and Harbeck, R.: Specific removal of DNA antibody *in vivo* by extracorporeal circulation over DNA immobilized in collodion charcoal. Clin. Immunol. Immunopathol., 8:90, 1977.

124. Thomas, F., et al.: Effect of antilymphocyte-globulin potency on survival of cadaver renal transplants. Prospective randomized double-blind trial. Lancet, 2:671, 1977.

125. Trentham, D.E., et al.: Clinical and immunologic effects of fractionated total lymphoid irradiation in refractory rheumatoid arthritis. N. Engl. J. Med., 305:976, 1981.

126. Tripodi, D., Parks, L.C., and Brugmans, J.: Drug-induced restoration of cutaneous delayed hypersensitivity in anergic patients with cancer. N. Engl. J. Med., 289:354, 1973.

127. Urowitz, M.B., et al.: Azathioprine in rheumatoid arthritis: a double-blind, cross-over study. Arthritis Rheum., 16:411–418, 1973.

128. Vladutiu, A.O.: Autoimmune thyroiditis: Conversion of low-responder mice to high-responders by cyclophosphamide. Clin. Exp. Immunol., 47:683, 1982.

129. Waksman, B.H., and Namba, Y.: Commentary on soluble mediators of immunologic regulation. Cell. Immunol., 21:161, 1976.

130. Wei, N., et al.: A randomized trial of plasma exchange in mild systemic lupus erythematosus. Lancet, 1:17, 1983.

131. White, D.J.G., and Calne, R.Y.: The use of cyclosporin A immunosuppression in organ grafting. Immunol. Rev., 65:115, 1982.

132. Wilkins, R.F., Watson, M.A., and Paxon, C.S.: Low dose pulse methotrexate therapy in rheumatoid arthritis. J. Rheumatol., 7:501, 1980.

133. Zembala, M., and Asherson, G.L.: T cell suppression of contact sensitivity in the mouse. II. The role of soluble suppressor factor and its interaction with macrophages. Eur. J. Immunol., 4:799, 1974.

134. Zulman, J., et al.: Levamisole maintains cyclophosphamide-induced remission in murine lupus erythematosus. Clin. Exp. Immunol., 31:321, 1978.

135. Zurier, R.B., et al.: Prostaglandin E$_1$ treatment of NZB/NZW F mice. II. Prevention of glomerulonephritis. Arthritis Rheum., 20:1449, 1977.

Chapter 34

Arthrocentesis Technique and Intrasynovial Therapy

Joseph Lee Hollander

Aspiration of joint fluid is of primary importance in the differential diagnosis of arthritis (see Chap. 4). Injection of arthritic joints provides a means of effective local treatment. Intra-articular corticosteroid therapy, used since 1951,[22] remains the most dependable method available for obtaining local relief from pain and swelling.[16] The purpose of this chapter is to describe techniques for joint aspiration and injection of medication into joints, bursal sacs, or tendon sheaths. In addition, the indications, contraindications, limitations, and precautions for both arthrocentesis and intrasynovial therapy are discussed.

EVOLUTION OF INTRASYNOVIAL THERAPY

Aspiration of joints has been performed for diagnostic reasons for many years, always with caution because of possible infection resulting from the procedure. Arthrocentesis for relief of pressure in distended joints is a time-honored orthopedic procedure to prevent stretching of capsule and ligaments and to relieve pain, but prompt reaccumulation of fluid and the danger of infection from repeated aspiration have limited its usefulness.

Injection of sterile liquid petrolatum into the joint space in an effort "to provide better lubrication" was tried many years ago, but failed because the oil was not miscible with joint fluid and was soon sequestered in one or more pouches of the synovial sac. Lipiodol, a contrast medium, injected originally for radiologic visualization of the synovial sac (arthrogram), was later tried for treatment of arthritis. This method failed, too. This medium also was localized in synovial pouches, often walled off by fibrin and the pannus of the rheumatoid inflammatory reaction.

Intra-articular injections of lactic acid had been recommended to stimulate natural local tissue reactions and evoke processes of repair in damaged joints, particularly after trauma. but this procedure was not accepted and fell into disuse.

Solutions of procaine hydrochloride or similar compounds have been injected frequently into joints, particularly after trauma. Such injections are palliative for a few hours.

Penicillin and many other antibiotics have been injected into septic joints, but the rationale for such local use has been destroyed by proof that systemically administered antibiotics attain therapeutic levels in septic joint fluid, and the chemical synovitis from their local use is often marked. Repeated aspiration of septic joints to drain accumulated debris and to decrease pressure is still of value (see Chap. 99).

In 1950, after noting the striking anti-inflammatory effect of cortisone used topically in eye inflammations, we injected cortisone suspension into 25 knee joints inflamed by rheumatoid arthritis. The effect was transitory and often minimal, however, usually without any drop in the elevated intra-articular temperature.[19] Other workers also found the local effect of cortisone in joints to be disappointing.[13]

Evidence that *hydrocortisone*, rather than cortisone, was the active anti-inflammatory hormone at the tissue level suggested that the local effect of the 17-hydroxysteroid would be greater. Hydrocortisone acetate crystal suspension became available for clinical trial in January 1951. Injection of 25 mg into an inflamed rheumatoid knee almost invariably reduced joint temperature to normal and reduced tenderness, pain, and swelling within 24 hours.[22] This consistent anti-inflammatory effect persisted from a few days to several weeks, when the effect could then be reduplicated by reinjection.[19] Other investigators soon confirmed these findings,[37,41] and the way was opened for extensive clinical studies on intrasynovial steroid therapy using many different preparations.[20,30]

In 1954, my colleagues and I showed that hydrocortisone esterified with a branched chain compound (hydrocortisone tertiary butyl acetate) was less rapidly hydrolyzed by joint enzymes, and thus one could double the duration of the local anti-inflammatory effect.[21] Relatively insoluble microcrystalline suspensions of hydrocortisone esters had always had longer effectiveness than their solutions, which were rapidly absorbed into the systemic circulation. The crystalline suspensions were apparently taken up by synovial lining cells, thus becoming a depot or repository of medication. Within a few hours after injection, soluble hormone in the synovial fluid was inactivated by hydrolysis.[39]

Suspensions of newer corticosteroid esters were assayed for local effect in joints as they became available. The analogues of *hydrocortisone* (prednisolone, methylprednisolone, triamcinolone, and dexamethasone, for example) all had local inflammatory potency greater than the original corticosteroid, but had *longer duration* of local anti-inflammatory effect only if injected as crystalline compounds.[20,21]

In 1961, I demonstrated that the much less soluble triamcinolone acetonide tertiary butyl acetate crystals, later generically designated triamcinolone hexacetonide, produced the most potent *and* longest-lasting anti-inflammatory effect of any intra-articular steroid preparation that we had assayed. After 23 years of experience with this preparation, I am still convinced of its superiority.[17]

As a result of the consistent, although temporary, palliative effect of intra-articular steroid therapy, numerous other drugs have been injected into arthritic joints. Attempts to inject salicylates into the joints were aborted by local irritation. Local injection of phenylbutazone into arthritic joints by Steinbrocker decreased inflammation, but only after a severe initial reaction.[36] Local suppression of rheumatoid inflammation by intra-articular gold compounds was reported by Lewis and Ziff, but usually a painful initial reaction from local irritation was noted.[26] Recently, orgotein, superoxide dismutase, has been reported helpful in suppressing rheumatoid inflammation when repeatedly injected into joints.[15]

Chemical Synovectomy

Cytotoxic drugs have been injected intra-articularly with the hope of suppressing synovial inflammation in rheumatoid arthritic joints. In 1957, Scherbel et al. reported "medical synovectomy" in rheumatoid knees after injection of nitrogen mustard. If the mustard was injected in combination with corticosteroid, the local reaction to the mustard was reduced, and the anti-inflammatory effect lasted from six months to two years.[34]

Extensive clinical studies with intra-articular triethylene thiophosphoramide (Thiotepa) into arthritic joints showed it to produce less initial irritation, with evidence of lasting suppression of inflammation.[9] In a long-term follow-up study of 123 cases, only 20% showed an objective improvement, with reactivation and progression of the disease in most.[11]

"Chemical synovectomy" using osmic acid was first suggested by VonReis and Swensson in 1947, and results were reported by Berglöf in 1959.[4] These workers thought osmic acid suitable for intra-articular therapy because it did not produce a violent irritation of the joint and deposited mainly in the inflamed synovium. By 1969, Laine had injected osmic acid into over 700 arthritic knees and had relieved pain and effusion in 50% for as long as a year.[24] Later reports, using osmium tetroxide, confirmed long-lasting suppression of synovial inflammation in a significant proportion of cases, but side effects included chills, fever, and evidence of liver damage.[8] When osmic acid was added to triamcinolone hexacetonide, and the combination was compared with triamcinolone hexacetonide alone, however, the osmic acid combination produced little advantage.[1]

These methods of "chemical synovectomy" have largely fallen into disuse in recent years. This may be because the results were neither as consistent nor as permanent as hoped, the reaction after injection was frequently severe and painful, and the best results followed *combinations* of the putatively suppressive agent with corticosteroid.[1,30]

Radiation Synovectomy

Radioactive colloidal gold has been injected into joints for "radiation synovectomy" since 1963, particularly for severe and chronic knee synovitis. Results have been encouraging, with frequent suppression of pain and effusion lasting up to a year.[38] Radioactive yttrium, because its beta rays penetrate deeper into the thickened synovium than radiogold, is preferred by some workers for "radiation synovectomy."[32] Local results from such therapy are impressive, but not permanent. Disturbing reports of "leakage" from the injected joint, danger of malignant disease from this treatment,[5,25] and other problems incidental to the use of radioisotopes suggest that this method should be reserved for refractory cases only, and its administration must be supervised by experts.[30]

Considerable additional promise has been given radiation synovectomy by the work of Sledge and his colleagues.[35,35a] They treated synovitis in 53 knees by injection of dysprosium-165 ferric hydroxide macroaggregates. This radionuclide is almost a pure beta emitter, has greater soft tissue penetration, and has a much shorter physical half-life (2.3 hours) than radioactive yttrium or radioactive gold, both of which have a half-life of about 64 hours. This newer radiocolloid shows little "leakage," less than 1%, as compared with about 10% for the older radiocolloids.

Results from use of the dysprosium-165 colloid about 3 months after injection showed definite clinical improvement in 79% and this improvement continued at the same level a year later, with diminished effusions and decreased synovial hypertrophy and an obvious decrease in symptoms and external signs of inflammation. Clinical improvement was not inversely proportional to roentgenographic evidence of cartilage and bone destruction, but best results were noted in joints with little radiologic change. Sledge concludes: "These encouraging results suggest that this short-lived radiocolloid has a role in the treatment of knee synovitis resistant to conventional medical therapy."

At this time, it appears that corticosteroids are still the agents of choice of most clinicians for intraarticular anti-inflammatory therapy. Detailed descriptions of indications, contraindications, side effects, and techniques for intrasynovial steroid therapy follow.

SPECIAL CONSIDERATIONS REGARDING INTRASYNOVIAL CORTICOSTEROID THERAPY

Injection of corticosteroid into a joint is neither specific treatment nor a cure for joint inflammation. After more than 32 years of experience with more than 400,000 injections into joints, tendon sheaths, or bursae in over 12,000 patients, I conclude that *no other form of treatment for arthritis has given such consistent local symptomatic relief to so many for so long with so few harmful effects.*

Relief from pain, and, more important to the physician, suppression of inflammation, can be obtained within 24 hours of treatment and may last for weeks or even months. Reinjection is done as rarely as possible, seldom more often than at least 6 weeks, and the same joint should not be reinjected more than 8 times yearly to avoid damage to the joint. Often, little difference exists among steroid preparations injected from the standpoint of duration of effectiveness, but I have found that tertiary butyl acetate esters have an increased duration of effect in most joints.[17,18] Suppression of inflammation often lasting for 6 weeks or more from triamcinolone hexacetonide injection is usual.[17] Because of the long biologic half-life of this latter agent in the joint, extra precautions must be taken to avoid overdosage or too frequent a reinjection. A maximum of 20 mg into largest joints (knee or hip), repeated no more often than every 6 weeks or *longer*, is my limit. Problems caused by overdosage are discussed later in this chapter.

Adverse Reactions

Long-term follow-up of the more than 12,000 patients treated with intrasynovial steroids has been impossible, but representative samples have been analyzed and are reported elsewhere.[17,18] I have

been concerned with possible harmful effects from this potent form of local therapy from several standpoints: (1) side effects and dangers from the injection itself; (2) acute steroid effects locally and systemically; and (3) long-term effects on the joint tissues and disease process.

Within the past few years, comprehensive and critical evaluations of intra-articular steroid therapy, including its dangers, have been published.[10,12,16] Additional illustrations of technique appear in Dixon and Graber,[10] Steinbrocker,[36] and the recent primer.[33]

Infection has occurred a total of 19 times in our total series. This low overall incidence has been made possible by the exclusive use of disposable sterile needles and syringes over the past 20 years; the incidence of infection with boiled or autoclaved equipment used earlier was definitely higher.[6,20]

A much more common, less-serious sequel of joint injection has been *postinjection flare*. This reaction is characterized by an increase in joint pain occurring after about 1 to 2% of steroid injections into joints or bursae, usually with heat, swelling, and tenderness persisting for a few hours or even for a few days. McCarty and Hogan demonstrated that this reaction is crystal-induced synovitis before the anti-inflammatory effect of the injected crystalline steroid suspension takes over.[28] Local applications of ice packs often shorten or even abort this painful reaction. *Fluid should be aspirated and cultured if this reaction persists for more than 24 hours.*

Systemic absorption of locally instilled corticosteroid always occurs to some degree. Multiple injections are avoided in patients with diabetes mellitus or with infections. Use of the least-soluble steroid esters also reduces the amount of systemic absorption.

Transitory weakness of the injected extremity has been noted,[6] and a few cases of thrombophlebitis in the injected leg had been noted in our early experience,[22] but have not been seen for many years.

The most serious complication of repeated corticosteroid injections is the development of joint instability, apparently from development of osteonecrosis of juxta-articular bone and weakened capsular ligaments. Although the incidence of this complication is less than 1% in my series, it probably would have been much greater had I not been aware of the potential problem early.[18]

Whether the osteonecrosis and ligamentous attenuation are caused by the steroid or by the overuse of a damaged joint permitted by relief of pain is not clear. Although instability usually develops in weight-bearing joints such as the knee or hip, it may also occur in the elbow or shoulder or other joint if large doses of steroid have been injected frequently. For this reason, I recommend minimally effective doses of steroid and reinjection at infrequent intervals (*at least* 6 weeks apart). I do not inject *any* joints showing appreciable instability.

McCarty has sought to prevent this problem by injecting a single larger dose of triamcinolone hexacetonide into each treated joint as a "medical synovectomy," then splinting the joint for 3 weeks or preventing weight bearing for 8 weeks.[27]* After an average of 22 months of follow-up, 88% of treated hand joints still had decreased swelling, tenderness, and synovial thickening, as compared with the inflamed joints in the opposite hand, observed as untreated control. Soft tissue atrophy near the finger and wrist joints, and capsular calcification (hydroxyapatite), which occurred frequently, seemed to result from leakage of steroid along the injection track from the large volume of steroid-local anesthetic suspension forced into these small joints. I have confirmed the value of single injections of triamcinolone hexacetonide into a joint followed by marked restriction of activity for some weeks in prolonging the period of anti-inflammatory effect. I do not try to force large volumes into small joint spaces and have not seen the atrophic changes of overlying skin and connective tissues, except in rare instances. The degree and duration of effect from such "medical synovectomy" is often greater than from alkylating agents or radiocolloids and is worthy of trial before resorting to more drastic measures.[27]

The disease process in the joint is rarely "cured" by corticosteroid injection, even though it may be suppressed to a major degree. Increased radiologic changes in treated joints have been noted after years of such therapy, but seldom more than, and usually less than, in untreated joints in the same patient.

The danger of developing a "Charcot joint" had been pointed out by Chandler et al. in 1958.[7,40] Such destruction of joints had followed frequent reinjection of large doses of steroid into a knee or hip, perhaps by allowing excessive use of a severely damaged joint. No loss of deep pain sensation or interference with the nerve supply to the joint was shown. In similar cases I have seen, patients had aseptic necrosis of subchondral bone.

Repeated injections of large doses of steroid into rabbit joints have produced marked cartilage deterioration,[3,29,31] but studies with frequent injections of large steroid doses into monkey joints did *not* show such deleterious effect on the cartilage.[14]

CLINICAL INDICATIONS FOR INTRA-ARTICULAR CORTICOSTEROID INJECTION

After years of study, I have concluded that intra-articular corticosteroid is clinically useful for local palliative therapy under the following conditions:

When one or few peripheral joints are inflamed or painful from rheumatoid arthritis, osteoarthritis, traumatic arthritis, acute or chronic gouty arthritis, or intermittent hydrarthrosis, intra-articular corticosteroid may provide palliation. This therapy may also be used with benefit in acute inflammation of the subdeltoid bursa, by injection directly into the bursal sac, but is rarely helpful in chronic or adhesive bursitis of the shoulder. Corticosteroids should never be injected into a joint in the presence of *infection and must not be injected into a joint until a diagnosis has been established* and infectious arthritis has been ruled out.

For sterile inflammation particularly active in a few peripheral joints, even in the presence of more widespread low-grade joint involvement, intra-articular therapy may help.

This therapy may be indicated in rheumatoid arthritis, to suppress activity in the most severely involved joints until the beneficial effects of gold therapy or other systemic measures become established.

In patients with rheumatoid arthritis in whom gold, corticosteroid, or other therapy is contraindicated because of cardiac failure, renal impairment, hypertension, diabetes, or some other condition, intra-articular injection may be beneficial.

When systemic therapy controls rheumatoid arthritic activity in all but a few "resistant" joints, local therapy may provide palliation.

If deformity is beginning to develop in an actively involved rheumatoid arthritic joint, corticosteroid injections together with proper physical therapy can prevent the deformity and may speed the return of normal function.

Indications for Intra-articular Corticosteroid Injection
1. When one or only a few peripheral joints are inflamed, provided infection has been excluded as the cause.
2. In a few actively inflamed joints even in the presence of more generalized low-grade involvement.
3. In rheumatoid arthritis as an adjunct to systemic drug therapy.
4. When systemic therapy is contraindicated.
5. As an adjunct to systemic therapy for control of "resistant" joints.
6. To assist in rehabilitation and to prevent joint deformity.

Editor's note: Upper extremity joints were splinted routinely for 3 weeks after injection; all injections into lower extremity joints were followed by 8 weeks of avoidance of weight bearing.

CONTRAINDICATIONS TO INTRA-ARTICULAR CORTICOSTEROID THERAPY

It cannot be stressed too often that *intra-articular corticosteroid injection is a palliative, local, and temporary treatment,* even though it can be repeated apparently indefinitely.* As a result of "trial and error" clinical use for many years, I conclude that the following either contraindicate the use of this method or render its use impractical:

The prime contraindication to local use of corticosteroid is the presence of infection in or about the joint. It is reasonable to avoid injection of a hormone known to reduce resistance to the spread of infection into the site of such an infection. Infection is more likely when arthrocentesis is performed in patients with bacteremia. Mechanical disruption of even a few capillaries with a needle may inoculate the joint fluid with organisms. The danger from infected blood is at least as great and probably greater than that from infected overlying skin.

When rheumatoid arthritis involves *many* joints actively, the injection of hydrocortisone into one or two joints is irrational.

When severe or late osteoarthritis is secondary to a static deformity or has itself produced severe instability, the injection of corticosteroid can accomplish little, unless preceded by adequate corrective measures. Similarly, in joints deformed by rheumatoid arthritis, intra-articular corticosteroids are of limited help.

In ankylosing spondylitis or osteoarthritis of spinal joints, the joints of the spine may be injected under radiologic control using image intensification. This technique requires the expert assistance of a skeletal radiologist.

In arthritis in joints with no synovial space. Only the diarthroses, the joints with synovial sacs, can be successfully treated by this method.

When injections of corticosteroid into a joint produce only minimal or transient benefit, the method should be abandoned. This lack of substantial benefit occurs in about 15% of patients.

ADMINISTRATION AND DOSAGE

Techniques for injection are described subsequently. The plan of treatment should be arranged so that no more than two or three joints are injected at one visit, to avoid absorption of large amounts of the hormone at one time, with resultant systemic effects. Subsequent injections into a given joint are

---

Contraindications to Intra-articular Corticosteroid Injection:
1. Presence of infection in or near the joint or bacteremia.
2. Multiplicity of severe joint inflammation in rheumatoid arthritis.
3. Severe joint destruction, or uncorrected static deformity.
4. Arthritis in spinal joints.
5. Arthritis in other than true diarthrodial (synovial) joints.
6. When trial injections have produced little or no benefit.

usually spaced according to the time of recurrence of symptoms in that joint. In most patients, succeeding injections duplicate the degree and duration of relief afforded by the first injection, but in some, succeeding injections have had an increasingly beneficial effect.

In some patients, a *decreasing* response has been noted, requiring a larger dose to suppress inflammation. With hydrocortisone acetate crystalline suspension, rheumatoid inflammation is suppressed completely for about 12 days, and osteoarthritic joints are symptomatically better for 2 to 3 weeks, whereas self-limiting conditions may resolve permanently. Less-soluble corticosteroid ester crystals produce correspondingly longer periods of symptomatic relief. The dose for individual joints is given with the description of technique for injection. If the suggested dose is inadequate, a larger dose may be tried. The response is not necessarily in proportion to the amount used, and larger doses than needed may actually decrease the benefit. Other steroids may be substituted for hydrocortisone if not effective. Prednisolone t-butyl acetate, 20 to 30 mg, has proved consistently effective, but triamcinolone hexacetonide, 20 mg (for knee or hip) nearly always has a *longer* local anti-inflammatory effect and is the drug of choice.[17]

TECHNIQUE FOR ARTHROCENTESIS AND INTRA-ARTICULAR INJECTION

Any peripheral joint may be injected, as may the temporomandibular, acromioclavicular, and sternoclavicular joints. The anatomic structure and depth of the spinal joints make local attempts to treat such articulations impractical, except under radiologic control.

An anatomic atlas and radiographs of the joint being aspirated should be before the physician when he attempts to inject any joint for the first time. No apparent harm is done when hydrocortisone is injected outside the joint space, but no anti-inflammatory effect is noted either. Less-soluble crystals, such as triamcinolone hexacetonide,

---

Editor's note: Tachyphylaxis (decreased response to repeated use) has been noted in some joints treated in this manner.

have been associated with marked *atrophy* of skin and subcutaneous tissue. *I do not advocate their use for soft tissue injections.*

The technique for arthrocentesis is simple. The *object* is to puncture the synovial sac, to aspirate excess fluid, and to inject the hormone with as little pain as possible, with minimal trauma to the joint and adjacent structures and without introducing infection into the joint cavity.

The *optimal site for injection* is usually on the extensor surface, where the synovial pouch is closest to the skin, and as remote as possible from major nerves, arteries, or veins.

Materials Needed

A small tray with detergent, skin antiseptic, alcohol sponges, 1% procaine solution, a corticosteroid suspension, 2 24-gauge sterile needles 3-cm long, 2 20-gauge sterile needles 5-cm long, a sterile 5-ml syringe for injecting procaine, a sterile 20-ml syringe for aspirating joint fluid, 1 or 2 sterile 2-ml syringes for injecting corticosteroid, a few gauze pads, and prepared small patch dressings (e.g., Band-Aids) constitute the equipment needed. Culture tubes and a graduated glass cylinder for measuring synovial fluid may also be included. No sterile drapes or rubber gloves are necessary.

A hypospray jet injector may be used instead of syringes and needles, particularly when multiple small joints are to be treated.[2]

Method

Once the optimal site for insertion of the aspirating needle has been chosen, the skin is cleansed twice with detergent, with antiseptic solution, and then with alcohol. If effusion is marked, it will seldom be necessary to infiltrate the tissues with procaine because the introduction of the needle will be quick and easy. In some individuals, a brief spraying of the area with ethyl chloride solution gives sufficient anesthesia for insertion of the aspirating needle. If 1% procaine infiltration is deemed advisable, a skin wheal should be made, and the subcutaneous tissue and joint capsule should be infiltrated with about 2 to 4 ml of the solution.

The aspirating needle seldom need be larger than 20 gauge. The needle is quickly inserted through skin, subcutaneous tissue, capsule, and synovial membrane. The tip of the needle is freely movable when the joint space is entered; it may even grate over the cartilage without causing pain. Any excess fluid present may then be aspirated. "Rice bodies" free in the joint may act as a flap-valve and may prevent aspiration of fluid even when a large effusion is present. These bodies often make complete aspiration of fluid impossible.

Entrance into a distended synovial sac is as easy as puncturing an inflated balloon, but entrance into a sac not distended may be as difficult as puncturing a deflated balloon. Folds of synovium or cellular debris may act as a flap-valve on the end of the needle and may prevent easy withdrawal of fluid. When this is suspected, the needle should be moved about gently, and a little of the fluid already withdrawn should be reinjected to clear the tip of the needle. Gentle aspiration is often more successful than the generation of extreme negative pressure in the syringe.

Aspiration may be facilitated by wrapping the joint, except for the site of paracentesis, with an elastic bandage to compress the free fluid into that portion of the sac being punctured. It is well to aspirate all readily accessible fluid at the time of paracentesis.[37]

The aspirating syringe is then detached, to allow the needle to remain in place in the joint. The desired amount of corticosteroid suspension, usually about 1 ml, is drawn into a small syringe. This syringe is then attached to the aspirating needle, still in situ. *If more than gentle pressure on the plunger is required to inject the solution, the needle is probably not free in the joint space, and its position should be readjusted.* Even if no fluid has been obtained, the easy movability of the needle tip and the easy introduction of the hormone suspension can give assurance that the tip is in the joint cavity. If fluid is present, the suspension may be mixed with the synovial fluid by barbitage (repeated withdrawal and reinjection).

The needle is then withdrawn, and the puncture site is covered with a sterile dressing. If much fluid has been aspirated from a weight-bearing joint, it is often advisable to apply an elastic bandage. The potentiating effect of joint immobilization has been already mentioned. This effect is particularly evident when the longer-acting, less-soluble crystals are injected.*

ASPIRATION OF SPECIFIC JOINTS AND SUGGESTED STEROID DOSAGE

Because the technique for paracentesis of individual joints has received little attention and includes many specific problems, a description for each of the joints frequently injected is given here. Additional descriptions and illustrations of technique are also available elsewhere.[10,33,36]

Editor's note: Although a controlled trial was done only on hand joints, the results in knee joints are striking. Complete suppression of inflammation for many years is often achieved in patients with rheumatoid arthritis.

Knee

The largest synovial cavity in the body and a weight-bearing structure, the knee is also one of the most frequent sites of synovial inflammation. It is the easiest joint to aspirate and to inject. A tightly distended knee joint can be aspirated from almost any angle without difficulty, but the following technique is useful for ready entrance into this joint space even if little or no excess fluid is present.

The patient lies supine with the knee fully extended. The site for puncture is on the anteromedial surface, 1 or 2 cm medial to the inner border of the patella. The needle is inserted in a lateral and slightly posterior direction between the posterior surface of the patella and the patellar groove of the femur. The needle tip may crepitate on the undersurface of the patella, demonstrating entrance into the joint space even though no fluid can be withdrawn. Figure 34–1 shows the position of the needle. Seldom are folds of synovial membrane or pannus under the patella to block ready aspiration, the feel of the needle tip against cartilage is distinctive, and the medial bony margin of the patellar groove of the femur is not as prominent as the lateral margin.

If the patella is ankylosed, or if marked flexion deformity of the knee is present, aspiration may be accomplished by puncture anteroposteriorly beside the inferior patellar tendon, through the fat pad into the knee joint space between the condyles of the femur. Puncture of the knee through the popliteal space is not advisable because of the large popliteal vessels. A Baker's cyst (popliteal cyst, a distention of the normal semimembranosus bursa) may be aspirated directly, however, if it is superficial and distended. Twenty-five to 37.5 mg hydrocortisone suspension, 30 mg of prednisolone t-butyl acetate, or 20 mg triamcinolone hexacetonide are the usual doses for injection into a knee.

A one-way valve has been demonstrated between the knee joint and the cyst to permit fluid to pass from the former to the latter, but not vice versa. Cysts are best treated therefore by injection of the knee itself.

Ankle

As shown in Figure 34–2, an anteromedial approach is usual. Prior procaine infiltration is often advisable. The needle is aimed at the tibioastragalar articulation from a point 1 cm superior and 1 cm lateral to the internal malleolus, just medial to the extensor pollicis tendon. The needle tip must penetrate about 3 cm inward and slightly laterally through the ligaments of the ankle joint capsule, and then it is more freely movable between the cartilaginous surfaces of the joint. Excess fluid an then be aspirated. If more than gentle pressure on the plunger of the syringe is needed for injection, the needle tip is probably in ligament or cartilage. The usual doses used for ankle injection are 25 mg hydrocortisone, 20 mg prednisolone t-butyl acetate, or 12.5 mg triamcinolone hexacetonide.

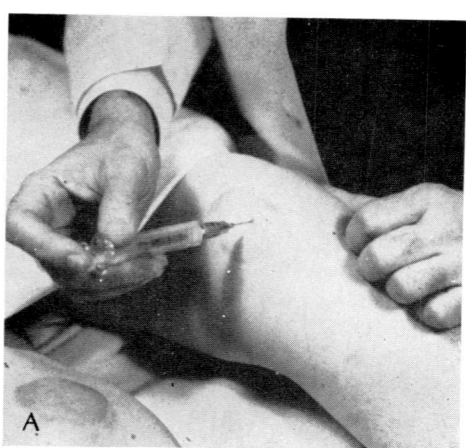
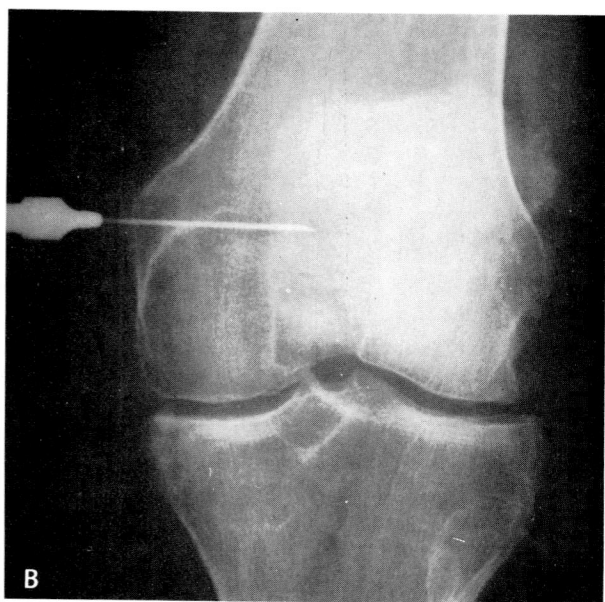

Fig. 34–1. *A,* Injection into the knee. *B,* Roentgenogram showing needle in place under medial side of patella.

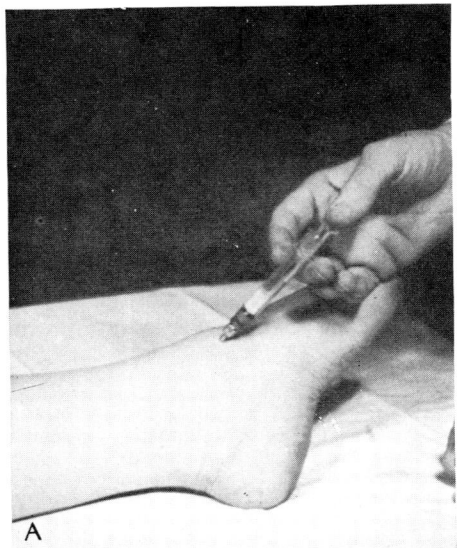

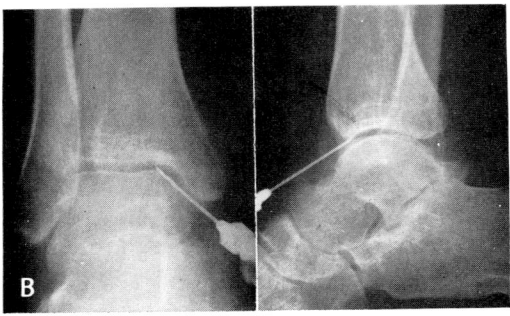

Fig. 34–2. *A*, Injection into left ankle—anteromedial approach. *B*, Roentgenogram showing anteroposterior view of needle in place in right ankle. *C*, Roentgenogram showing lateral view of needle in right ankle.

Tarsal and Tarsometatarsal Joints

A roentgenogram of the area helps to orient the operator in the location best suited for entrance into a specific space. A 22-gauge needle may be used, and procaine anesthesia is usually necessary. Because of the superficial location of the joints on the dorsum of the foot, this site is preferable to the plantar surface. The needle may have to be "teased" down between the cartilages; free fluid can only rarely be aspirated. Here the freely movable needle tip, the depth of penetration, and the lack of force needed to inject the hormone suspension ensure that the joint space has been entered. *Fluoroscopic guidance is helpful when small joints are injected.* From 10 to 15 mg hydrocortisone or prednisolone t.b.a. or 5 to 7.5 mg triamcinolone hexacetonide are usual doses for such joints.

Toes

After procaine infiltration, a 24-gauge needle is inserted from the dorsal surface, either medially or

laterally, sliding beneath the extensor tendons and between the cartilaginous surfaces, in the anatomic plane of the joint. Traction on the toe may facilitate entrance by separating the articulation. A 5-mg dose of a corticosteroid crystal suspension is usually adequate.

Hip

This joint is difficult to aspirate and inject, mainly because of the amount of soft tissue overlying it in all directions. In many cases of osteoarthritis of the hip, it has been impossible to enter the joint space with certainty, even under fluoroscopic guidance, because of the gross distortion of the normal anatomy. Occasionally, even in osteoarthritis, fluid may be aspirated from the hip joint, however, ensuring penetration to the joint space.

The patient lies with the hip in maximal extension and internal rotation. Procaine infiltration is seldom necessary. A 20-gauge needle, 5 to 6 cm long, is employed for the anterior (usual) approach, 7 to 8 cm or longer for the lateral approach. The site for puncture in the anterior approach is about 2 to 3 cm inferior to the anterior superior spine of the ilium and 2 to 3 cm lateral to the femoral pulse, depending on the size of the patient (Fig. 34–3). The needle is inserted at an angle of 60° with the skin, pointing posteromedially, through the capsular ligaments, which are tough and thick, until bone is reached. The tip is then slightly withdrawn. Fluid occasionally can be aspirated, but in any case injection meets little resistance if the tip is in the joint space. The usual dose of hydrocortisone for the hip is 37.5 mg, 30 mg prednisolone t.b.a., or 20 mg triamcinolone hexacetonide.

The lateral approach to the hip joint is also difficult, but has the advantage that the needle "follows the bone" to the hip joint. A lumbar puncture needle is inserted just anterior to the greater trochanter, in a sagittal direction, pointed toward the middle of Poupart's ligament. The needle tip slides in anterior to the periosteum of the neck of the femur and enters the joint space anteriorly and near the upper reflection of the synovial sac (see Fig. 34–3*B*).

Shoulder

Aspiration of the shoulder is easily accomplished by anterior puncture, inserting the needle just medial to the head of the humerus and inferior to the tip of the coracoid process (Fig. 34–4). A lateral insertion may also be used, particularly for injection of the subdeltoid bursa. Effusion of the shoulder joint, though rare, nearly always bulges anteriorly. Twenty-five milligrams hydrocortisone or prednisolone t-butyl acetate or 20 mg triamcinolone

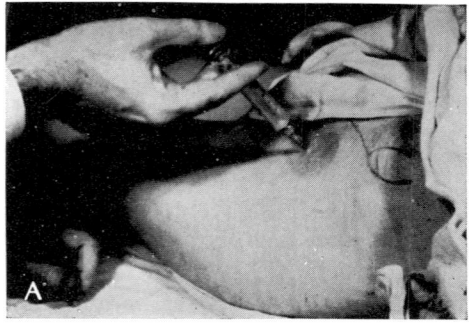

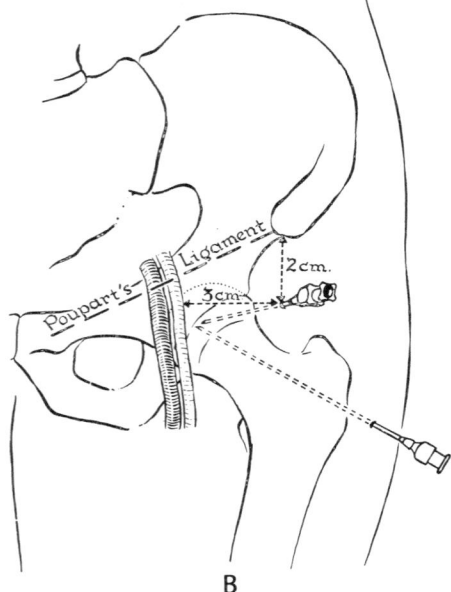

Fig. 34–3. *A*, Injection of left hip. Crescent shows location of anterosuperior spine of ilium; line is over Poupart's ligament. *B*, Diagram shows location of structures about left hip and two directions of approach for injection.

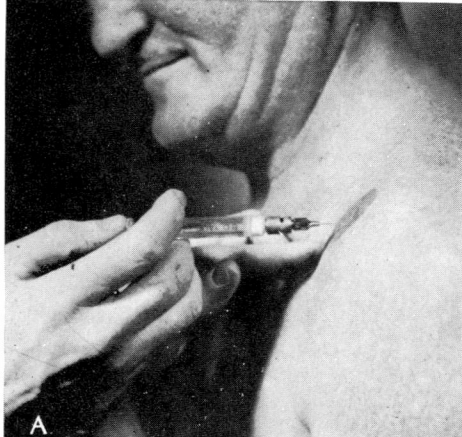

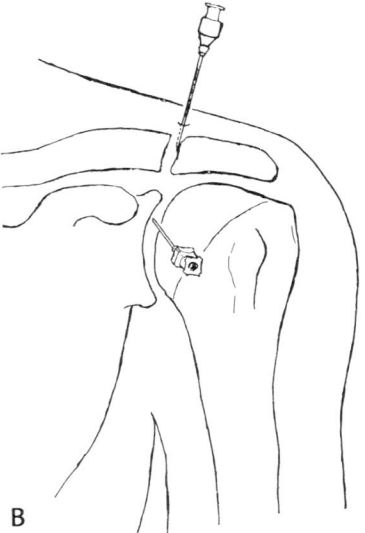

Fig. 34–4. *A*, Injection of the left shoulder joint. *B*, Diagram showing position of needle for injection of shoulder and acromioclavicular joints.

hexacetonide are the usual dose for shoulder injection.

Acromioclavicular Joint

The plane of the joint can most easily be determined by palpation. The 22-gauge needle is inserted from a superior position and slightly anteriorly until it is felt to slide between the joint surfaces (see Fig. 34–4*B*). Fifteen milligrams hydrocortisone or prednisolone or 5 to 10 mg triamcinolone acetonide are usually sufficient. Prior local use of 1% procaine is advisable.

Sternoclavicular Joint

The sternoclavicular joint is most easily entered from a point directly anterior to the joint. Because

of the fibrocartilaginous articular disc, it is a difficult joint to inject. Fifteen mg hydrocortisone or 7.5 mg triamcinolone hexacetonide are the usual injection dose.

Elbow

The elbow may either be held at 90° or be fully extended. Full extension distends the capsule as tightly as possible. The bulge of synovium, when effusion is present, is noted on the extensor surface, lateral to the olecranon process of the ulna. The aspirating needle should be inserted distally just lateral to the olecranon and just inferior to the lateral epicondyle of the humerus (Fig. 34–5). Often, particularly for injecting "tennis elbow," the lateral approach directly into the radiohumeral articulation

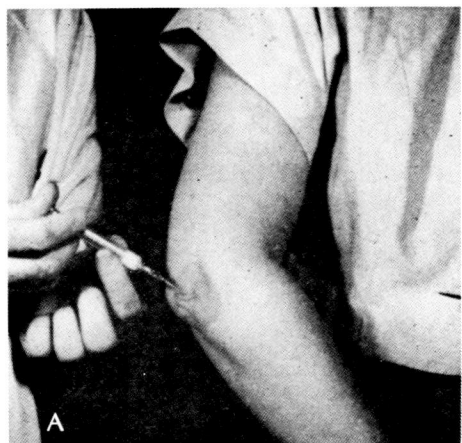

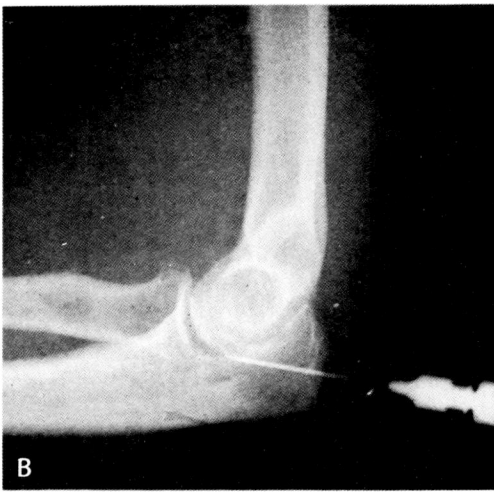

Fig. 34–5. *A*, Injection of right elbow in the position of maximum extension. *B*, Roentgenogram of left elbow showing the needle in place with the elbow at 90°. The needle is inserted *lateral* to the olecranon process of the ulna.

is desirable. The needle is inserted in a medial direction at a point just distal to the lateral epicondyle (capitulum of the humerus), and just proximal to the head of the radius, to a depth of about 2 cm, when the point of the needle feels free in the joint. Aspiration of fluid from the elbow is more difficult with this latter approach. Paracentesis medial to the olecranon is inadvisable because of proximity to the ulnar nerve. The usual hydrocortisone dose in the elbow is 20 to 25 mg and of triamcinolone hexacetonide 12.5 mg.

Wrist

This complex joint is most safely and easily aspirated dorsally (Fig. 34–6). The needle is inserted perpendicularly with the skin at a point just distal

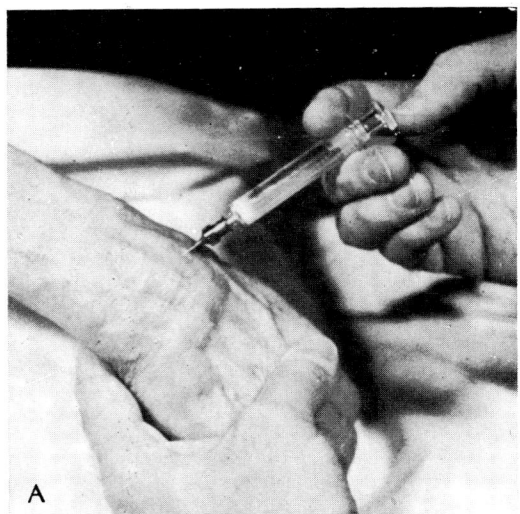

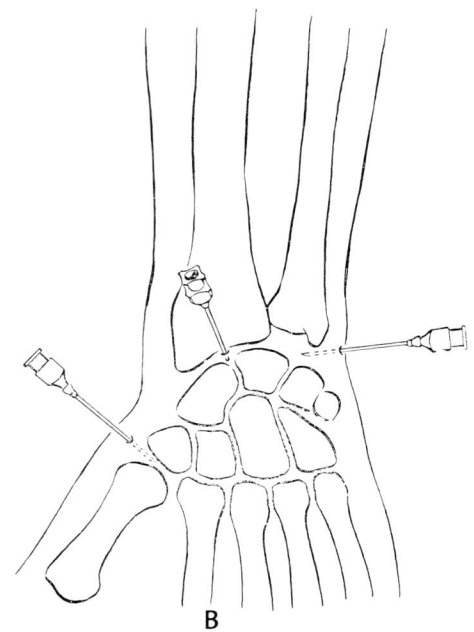

Fig. 34–6. *A*, Injection into the wrist. *B*, Diagram showing location of the needle for the dorsal approach, for injection of the ulnar bursa, and for injection into the carpometacarpal joint of the thumb.

to the radius and just ulnar to the "anatomic snuff box." If the needle can be easily inserted to a depth of 1 to 2 cm and feels free, it is probably in the correct position. Most of the small intercarpal joints have connecting synovial spaces. If marked synovial bulging is noted on the ulnar surface of the wrist, the joint may be entered by inserting the needle just distal to the ulnar styloid process and dorsal to the pisiform bone (see Fig. 34–6*B*). Fifteen to 25 mg hydrocortisone or prednisolone t.b.a. or 7.5 to 10 mg triamcinolone hexacetonide are usually an effective dose.

Carpometacarpal Joint of the Thumb

This small joint is frequently troublesome in osteoarthritis and does not communicate with the other joint spaces of the wrist. It may be entered dorsally from the radial side of the hand, as shown in Figure 34–6*B*. Five to 10 mg hydrocortisone are usually an adequate dose.

Metacarpophalangeal and Interphalangeal Joints

These joints are easily punctured from the lateral or medial approach on the *dorsal surface* (Fig. 34–7). A small needle is desirable for such injection (24 gauge) to avoid undue trauma. It is frequently necessary to "tease" the needle between the cartilages, at the same time making traction on the finger to pull the joint cartilage apart. Five to 10 mg hydrocortisone or 2.5 to 5 mg triamcinolone hexacetonide are adequate for injection into such small joints.

Temporomandibular Joint

It is sometimes desirable to inject corticosteroid into this joint for rheumatoid arthritic involvement. A roentgenogram of the area is helpful for reference. The needle should be small (24 or 25 gauge). It is inserted at a point just inferior to the zygomatic arch, about 1.3 cm (or half an inch) anterior to the tragus of the ear, and carried inward, slightly backward, and upward until it has penetrated to a depth

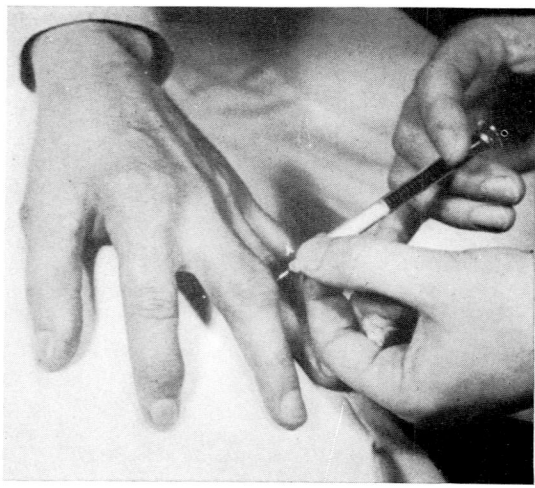

Fig. 34–7. Injection into a proximal interphalangeal joint of the finger.

of about 1.5 cm and feels free in the joint (Fig. 34–8). Since a fibrocartilaginous articular disc is present in the joint, it is often difficult to be sure that the needle is properly placed. The needle is inserted well anterior to the superficial temporal artery. Ten milligrams hydrocortisone or prednisolone t.b.a. have usually proved an adequate dose. The joint space may often be more readily entered by the needle if the patient opens his mouth wide before the puncture is made.

Usual Effective Dose of Hydrocortisone Acetate* per Joint Injection:			
Joint	*Dose (mg)*	*Joint*	*Dose (mg)*
Knee	25–37.5	Shoulder	25
Ankle	20–25	Elbow	20–25
Tarsal	10–15	Wrist	15–25
	10	Metacarpophalangeal	5–10
Interphalangeal (toes)	5	Interphalangeal (fingers)	5–10
Hip	37.5	Acromioclavicular	15
Temporomandibular	10–15	Sternoclavicular	15

*Equivalent amounts of other steroid preparations;
Hydrocortisone t-butyl acetate, same shown.
Prednisolone t-butyl acetate, 75% of doses shown.
Methylprednisolone, or triamcinolone, 75% of doses shown.
Dexamethasone t-butyl acetate, 10% of doses shown.
Triamcinolone hexacetonide, 50% of doses shown.

Bursae and Tendon Sheaths

Aspiration and injection of bursae require a knowledge of the locations of such structures, and the physician will do well to consult an anatomic atlas before attempting the procedure.[10,33,36] Unless calcific deposits are present, radiographs will be of little help. Local tenderness is often marked over any inflamed bursa, and such synovial spaces may be aspirated when distended with effusion. For the *subdeltoid bursa or supraspinatus tendinitis*, 1 ml steroid is injected after insertion of the 22-gauge needle from a lateral approach inferior to the acromion. *Bicipital tendinitis* is similarly injected from an anterolateral approach pointing up to the bicipital groove of the humerus. *Olecranon bursitis* is readily aspirated at the point of the elbow, and 0.5 ml steroid suspension may be injected without pressure. *Extensor tenosynovitis at the wrist*, which "bunches up" as the fingers are extended, can also be injected with up to 0.5 ml steroid. *Flexor tenosynovitis* at the wrist, or *carpal tunnel syndrome*, is amenable to injection using a 23-gauge needle, with 0.5 ml steroid. The needle is inserted distally from a point on the volar surface of the wrist just to the ulnar side of the palmaris flexor tendon. As the needle is inserted, the patient should hold the fist clenched, releasing it as the needle comes to rest in the ulnar bursa, so any tendon it may have impinged on will be "unhooked" before injection

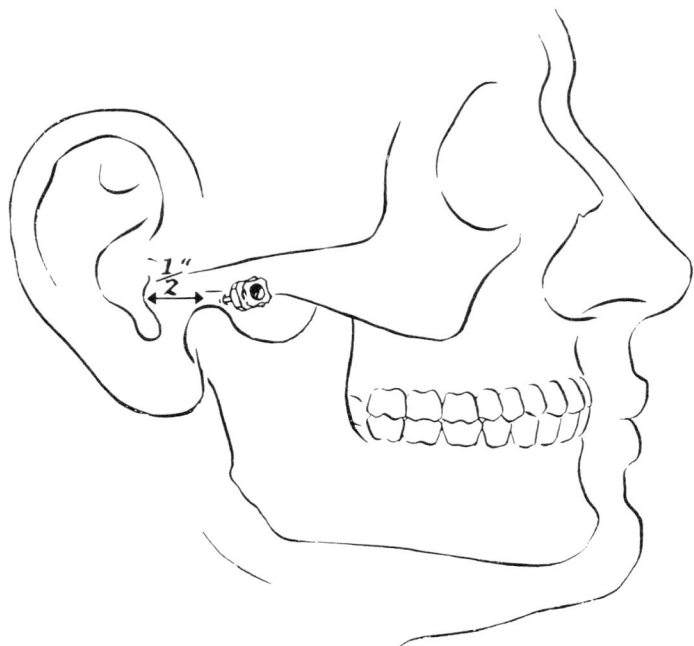

Fig. 34–8. Diagram showing location of the needle for injection of the temporomandibular joint.

is made. *Trigger finger (flexor tenosynovitis)* may be injected with 0.25 ml steroid. A 25-gauge needle is inserted at the base of the finger on the volar surface until gentle active movement of the finger by the patient makes a crepitant sensation against the needle tip. *Snapping thumb* is managed similarly.

Trochanteric bursitis of the hip can be localized by identification of the point of maximum tenderness posterior and superior to the greater trochanter. The length of the 22-gauge needle must be 4–5 cm or more. As much as 1 ml steroid suspension is injected when the needle (without procaine) strikes the tender and inflamed bursal sac. If tenderness is not pronounced, the needle is in the wrong place and should be moved.

Relief of symptoms occurs immediately when a few ml of 1% procaine are admixed with steroid if the site of injection has "hit the mark."

Numerous bursae are present at the knee, any of which may become inflamed. Direct injection into the appropriate bursa, after aspiration, may bring prompt and lasting relief. The same holds true for other bursae, including even a bunion on the inner surface of the great toe, or calcaneal bursitis of the heel, achilles tendon bursitis, or tenosynovitis.[10,33,36]

In conclusion, skill in aspiration of joints can be obtained only by study and practice, just as for any other special technique in medicine. My colleagues and I have shown over the past 32 years that this method of diagnosis and treatment of joint and bursal inflammation is effective and safe as long as careful aseptic technique is observed. Over the years, it has been confirmed that intrasynovial corticosteroid injection can give long-lasting palliation from many rheumatic inflammatory conditions.[16] Minimal effective doses of steroid should not be exceeded, and reinjection should be kept at a minimum. Patients with chronic conditions can be reinjected for many years without harm, provided that these are made no more often than every 6 weeks. The treated joint should be rested after injection, and abuse must be avoided. Other medications such as cytotoxic agents, radiogold, and radioyttrium, and osmic acid for intra-articular use are still experimental. Colloidal radioactive dysprosium has recently shown promising results.[35] One hopes that new and more effective anti-inflammatory agents will become available for intra-articular use.

REFERENCES

1. Anttinen, J., and Oka, M.: Intraarticular triamcinolone hexacetonide and osmic acid in knees. Scand. J. Rheumatol., *4*:125, 1975.
2. Baum, J., and Ziff, M.: Use of hypospray jet injector for intra-articular injections of corticosteroids. Ann. Rheum. Dis., *26*:148, 1967.
3. Behrens, F., Shepard, N., and Mitchell, N.: Alteration of rabbit articular cartilage by intraarticular injection of glucocorticoids. J. Bone Joint Surg., *58-A*:1157, 1976.
4. Berglöf, F.E.: Osmic acid in arthritis therapy. Acta Rheumatol. Scand., *5*:70, 1959.
5. Bridgman, J.F., Bruckner, F., and Bleehan, N.M.: Radioactive yttrium in the treatment of rheumatoid knee effusions. Ann. Rheum. Dis., *30*:180, 1971.

6. Brown, E.M., et al.: Locally administered hydrocortisone in rheumatic diseases. Am. J. Med., *15*:656, 1953.
7. Chandler, G.N., and Wright, V.: Deleterious effects of intra-articular hydrocortisone. Lancet, *2*:661, 1958.
8. Collan, Y., Servo, C., and Winblad, I.: An acute immune response to intraarticular injection of osmium tetroxide. Acta Rheumatol. Scand., *17*:236, 1971.
9. Currey, H.L.F.: Intraarticular thiotepa in rheumatoid arthritis. Ann. Rheum. Dis., *24*:382, 1965.
10. Dixon, A.S., and Graber, J.: Local Injection Therapy in Rheumatic Diseases. Edited by T. Dürrigl. Basel, Eular Publishers, 1983.
11. Ellison, M.R., and Flatt, A.E.: Intraarticular thiotepa in rheumatoid disease. A clinical analysis of 123 injected MP and PIP joints. Arthritis Rheum., *14*:212, 1971.
12. Eymontt, M.J., et al.: Effects on synovial permeability and synovial fluid leukocyte counts in symptomatic osteoarthritis after intraarticular corticosteroid administration. J. Rheumatol., *9*:198, 1982.
13. Freyberg, R.H., et al.: Practical considerations in the use of cortisone and ACTH in rheumatoid arthritis. Ann. Rheum. Dis., *10*:1, 1951.
14. Gibson, T., et al.: Effect of intraarticular corticosteroid injections on primate cartilage. Ann. Rheum. Dis., *36*:74, 1977.
15. Goebel, K.M., and Storck, U.: Effect of intraarticular orgotein versus a corticosteroid on rheumatoid arthritis of the knees. Am. J. Med., *74*:124, 1983.
16. Gray, R.G., Tenenbaum, J., and Gottlieb, N.L.: Local corticosteroid injection treatment in rheumatic disorders. Semin. Arthritis Rheum., *10*:231–254, 1981.
17. Hollander, J.L.: The place of intrasynovial corticosteroid therapy. Guidelines from 27 years experience. *In* 1978 Symposium on Intrasynovial Therapy of Rheumatic Diseases. XVII Nordic Congress of Rheumatology. Elsinore, Lederle, 1978.
18. Hollander, J.L.: Intrasynovial corticosteroid therapy in arthritis. Maryland State Med. J., *19*:62, 1970.
19. Hollander, J.L.: Local effects of compound F (hydrocortisone) injected into joints. Bull. Rheum. Dis., *2*:3, 1951.
20. Hollander, J.L., et al.: Nine years of experience with intrasynovial steroid therapy. Arch. Interam. Rheum., *3*:171, 1960.
21. Hollander, J.L., et al.: Local antirheumatic effectiveness of higher esters and analogues of hydrocortisone. Ann. Rheum. Dis., *13*:297, 1954.
22. Hollander, J.L., et al.: Hydrocortisone and cortisone injected into arthritic joints. JAMA, *147*:1629, 1951.
23. Hollander, J.L., Jessar, R.A., and Brown, E.M.: Intrasynovial corticosteroid therapy: a decade of use. Bull. Rheum. Dis., *11*:239, 1961.
24. Laine, V.: Osmic acid injected intra-articularly in rheumatoid arthritic knees. *In* Early Synovectomy in R.A. Edited by W. Hijmans, et al. Amsterdam, Excerpta Medica, 1969, p. 142.
25. Lee, P.: The efficacy and safety of radiosynovectomy. J. Rheumatol., *9*:165, 1982.
26. Lewis, D.C., and Ziff, M.: Intraarticular administration of gold salts. Arthritis Rheum., *9*:682, 1966.
27. McCarty, D.J.: Treatment of rheumatoid joint inflammation with triamcinolone hexacetonide. Arthritis Rheum., *15*:157, 1972.
28. McCarty, D.J., and Hogan, J.M.: Inflammatory reaction after intrasynovial injection of microcrystalline adrenocorticosteroid esters. Arthritis Rheum., *7*:359, 1964.
29. Mankin, H.J., and Conger, K.A.: Acute effects of intraarticular hydrocortisone on articular cartilage in rabbits. J. Bone Joint Surg., *48-A*:1383, 1966.
30. Medsger, T.A., et al. (Eds.): Twenty-fifth rheumatism review. Arthritis Rheum., *26*:300, 1983.
31. Moskowitz, R.W., et al.: Experimentally induced corticosteroid arthropathy. Arthritis Rheum., *13*:236, 1970.
32. Pritchard, H., Bridgman, J., and Bleehan, N.: An investigation of radioactive yttrium (90y) for the treatment of chronic knee effusions. Br. J. Radiol., *43*:466, 1970.
33. Rodnan, G.P., Schumacher, H.R., and Zvaifler, N.J. (Eds.): Primer on the Rheumatic Diseases. 8th Ed. Atlanta, Arthritis Foundation, 1983, pp. 197–199.
34. Scherbel, A.L., Schuchter, S.C., and Weyman, S.J.: Intraarticular administration of nitrogen mustard alone and combined with corticosteroid. Cleve. Clin. Qt., *24*:78, 1957.
35. Sledge, C.B., et al.: Experimental radiation synovectomy by dysprosium-165 ferric hydroxide macroaggregate. Arthritis Rheum., *20*:1339, 1977.
35a. Sledge, C.B., et al.: Therapy of chronic knee synovitis with Dy-165. In press, 1984.
36. Steinbrocker, O., and Neustadt, D.H.: Aspiration and Injection Therapy in Arthritis and Musculoskeletal Diseases. Hagerstown, MD, Harper and Row, 1972.
37. Stevenson, C.R., Zuckner, J., and Freyberg, R.H.: Intraarticular hydrocortisone acetate: a preliminary report. Ann. Rheum. Dis., *11*:112, 1952.
38. Topp, J., and Cross, E.: Treatment of persistent knee effusions with intraarticular radioactive gold. Preliminary report. Can. Med. Assoc. J., *102*:711, 1970.
39. Wilson, H., et al.: Rate of disappearance and metabolism of hydrocortisone and cortisone in the synovial cavity in rheumatoid arthritis. Proc. Soc. Exp. Biol. Med., *83*:648, 1953.
40. Wright, V., et al.: Intraarticular therapy in osteoarthritis: comparison of hydrocortisone acetate and t-butyl acetate. Ann. Rheum. Dis., *19*:257, 1960.
41. Ziff, M., et al.: Effects in rheumatoid arthritis of hydrocortisone and cortisone injected intraarticularly. Arch. Intern. Med., *90*:774, 1952.

Rheumatoid Arthritis

Chapter 35

Etiology and Pathogenesis of Rheumatoid Arthritis

Nathan J. Zvaifler

The cause of rheumatoid arthritis (RA) has eluded detection, despite a great expenditure of resources and energies. One impediment is that RA appears to be a uniquely human disease, and although experimental forms of arthritis exist, they are not entirely satisfactory models for the disorder.[106] Another problem is that most observations about RA have been made in patients with established disease. Thus, it is difficult to decide whether the abnormalities found are the cause or the result of the rheumatoid process. For instance, the characteristic physiologic changes within the joint are those of anaerobic (glycolytic) metabolism, namely, lowered synovial fluid oxygen tension, carbon dioxide accumulation, reduced pH, and increased lactic acid concentrations. These abnormalities appear to derive from an articular blood supply that, although increased over normal, is still inadequate to meet the metabolic demands of the inflamed joint.[33] Vascular lesions are well recognized in established rheumatoid synovitis and are seen at the inception of the disease,[105] but a similar state of anaerobic metabolism is likely to be found in any site of chronic inflammation.

ETIOLOGY

The products of molecular oxygen, that is, free radicals, superoxide anions, and hydroxyl molecules, which are derived at least in part from polymorphonuclear leukocytes, are important mediators of both acute and chronic inflammation.[74] The intracellular levels of the substrates and enzymes that control these deleterious substances, such as superoxide dismutase (SOD), glutathione, and glutathione peroxidase, have been observed to fall during acute rheumatoid inflammation, and it is claimed that SOD is deficient in the polymorphonuclear cells of patients with RA.[82,99] Furthermore, from in vitro studies, it appears that a reduction of intracellular SOD activity can produce abnormalities in the regulation of immunoglobulin production by B cells and lymphokine production from T-lymphocytes.[67] Although these findings are interesting and may be significant in the perpetuation of the chronic inflammatory state characteristic of

RA, it seems unlikely that they represent a true metabolic predisposition to the disease.

As noted in Chapters 24 and 25, genetic factors exist. An association of RA with a particular HLA-D locus haplotype is an intriguing and important observation, but it appears that the relevant genes may be regulators of the intensity of the host's response, particularly in the immune system, rather than a direct cause of RA.[27,114]

Therefore, considering all currently available information, it still appears that although the pathology of RA is undoubtedly related to an inflammatory response involving the immune system, the initiating event that triggers this response is most likely a specific etiologic agent.

Infectious Agents

Bacteria

Evidence implicating a specific infectious pathogen in RA is still lacking, despite more than 50 years of intensive study. The initial investigations involved bacteria, in part because of the confusion between RA and rheumatic fever. Indeed, not too long ago, treatment of RA included the eradication of foci of infection, particularly those containing streptococci. The streptococcal origin of rheumatic fever is unquestionable, but no evidence suggests that human RA is initiated by this micro-organism. Interest then shifted to diphtheroids as etiologic agents when it appeared that these organisms were present in synovial membranes and fluids.[119] Diphtheroids, however, found as normal skin flora, were subsequently discredited as contaminants. More recently, claims have been made for the isolation of diphtheroid-like organisms, such as Corynebacterium, now called Proprionibacterium, from rheumatoid synovium[93] and the demonstration of a polysaccharide antigen similar to that from Proprionibacterium acnes in phenol water extracts of synovial fluids and leukocytes.[7] Unfortunately, in both studies, similar organisms or antigens were found in nonrheumatoid tissues in sufficient numbers to question their etiologic significance in RA.

The fascination with mycoplasma as a cause of

RA is long-standing because these organisms can also produce experimental arthritis.[17] From time to time, reports have appeared of mycoplasma isolated from synovial fluid and membrane, but most studies, using a variety of sensitive detection methods, have failed to isolate these organisms. Even in experimental mycoplasma infections, however, the organisms can only be isolated from the joint tissues for a short time after the inception of the inflammatory synovitis; subsequently, they become undetectable, although the process continues as a chronic destructive arthropathy.[23] This fact makes the data obtained from human RA joints difficult to interpret.

Patients with RA have large amounts of *Clostridium perfringens* in their feces. Most normal individuals have only small numbers of these organisms, and they are limited to the colon, whereas *C. perfringens* can be demonstrated in the small intestine of about two-thirds of RA patients.[76] By modifying the diet of pigs, Mansson and his associates induced clostridial overgrowth and concomitantly observed the development of a rheumatoid-like arthritis in this animal.[77] Unfortunately, clostridial overgrowth can also be documented in other chronic inflammatory rheumatic diseases and in many individuals who have a larger-than-normal reservoir of enteric bacteria, but are without rheumatic complaints.[127]

Because of the failure to isolate live organisms, the emphasis has switched to the demonstration of bacterial antigens within articular tissues that are derived from the cell wall of organisms originating in the gastrointestinal tract. The idea that bacterial debris can be phagocytized by macrophages and synovial lining cells, but cannot be degraded, and thus persists as a chronic irritant has been championed both by Bennett[8] and by Hadler.[50] This notion of nonbiodegradable antigens gains credibility from animal models in which the systemic administration of bacterial peptidoglycans (cell wall constituents) is followed by a chronic destructive inflammatory synovitis. Attempts to detect components of bacterial cell walls in biopsies of rheumatoid synovial membranes have been unsuccessful, however, even using the unusually sensitive procedure of mass spectrometry.[97]

Viruses

The possible viral origin of RA has been vigorously pursued.[30,92] Direct viral identification, either through isolation or visualization by electron microscopy, was unrewarding.[138] As each new viral detection technique appeared, it was used to search for the putative initiating agent of RA. Sensitive methods capable of demonstrating slow viruses, noncytopathic viruses, or latent viruses, and virus rescue by co-cultivation or DNA and RNA hybridization have all been unrewarding.[78] The limited evidence that rheumatoid synovial cells might have increased activity of RNA-primed, DNA-directed DNA polymerase was best attributed to stimulated normal human lymphocyte in the tissues,[85,115] and searching joint tissues for viral nucleic acid sequences has so far proved unproductive.[86] Equally unrewarding has been the use of immunologic techniques to identify viral antigens,[42,47,48,90,94] virus-induced neoantigens,[112] or unique viral antibodies secreted by altered synovial B cells.[14,89,121] A difference was noted in the ability to infect rheumatoid synovial cells in culture with certain viruses.[45,113] This finding was suggestive of a viral interference phenomenon, but it was subsequently shown that these differences could be related to the secretion of hyaluronic acid by the synovial cells, which prevented viral attachment to the cell.[16,91] Despite these disappointments, the quest continues.

Given the complex biology of viruses, it is likely that almost any species could produce arthritis. On the other hand, only a limited number of mechanisms can explain a chronic inflammatory synovial disease such as RA. A few relevant pathogenetic models and the viruses that might be responsible are worth considering. In the first model, sequestration of an arthrotropic agent in articular cartilage or other joint structures could lead to arthritis, either directly or by invoking a localized immune response. The most likely pathogen in this model is rubella virus, which has a propensity for localization in cartilage when injected systemically.[71] Moreover, in humans, an inflammatory polyarthritis may follow both natural rubella infection and immunization with rubella vaccine.[63,88] Rubella virus has been recovered from peripheral blood lymphocytes and synovial tissues of several of these patients,[12,13,57,88,132] and in addition, Grahame and his associates have reported multiple unequivocal isolates of live rubella virus from synovial effusions of 5 adults and 1 child with chronic inflammatory, seronegative, oligoarthritis and polyarthritis who had no previous history of rubella infection.[44] With the exception of a 46-year-old man with chronic arthritis, rheumatoid factor, and nodules, however, rubella virus has not been isolated from the blood cells or synovial cells of patients with unequivocal RA.[101] Although it appears clear that rubella virus can elicit a broad spectrum of articular responses, evidence that this virus can induce or propagate RA is still insufficient.

Immune complexes accompany most, if not all, viral infections in which both continuous viral replication and a continuous host response are seen. Acute synovitis often results from circulating immune complexes, and occasionally they invoke a chronic arthritis. Hepatitis B infection is complicated by arthritis in 10 to 30% of cases, usually occurring as a prodrome of recognizable liver disease.[29,60] This form of arthritis is similar to RA in that both the small joints of the hands and the larger articulations can be affected, and women have symptoms more often than men. Hepatitis B surface antigen (HBsAg) has been demonstrated by immunofluorescence in the synovium, and Dane particles can be recognized by electron microscopy, but the virus has not been propagated in tissue culture. During the prodrome, the presence of hepatitis antigen, hypocomplementemia, and cryoprecipitates containing HBsAg, anti-HB immunoglobulins, and complement components suggests that the arthritis results from immune complexes.[130] As in other viral diseases, rheumatoid factor is often present in hepatitis B infection.[4] Sometimes, hepatitis B arthritis is complicated by persistent synovitis,[29] but in only a single reported case has the subsequent development of classic RA been documented.[81] Given the relative frequency of both diseases, this association probably occurred by chance.

A third possible way in which a virus could cause a disease such as RA is viral alteration of the immune system such that potentially harmful autoantibodies, such as rheumatoid factors, are produced. This hypothesis is currently popular. The prototype here is the Epstein-Barr virus (EBV), which is lymphotrophic. B-lymphocytes have a membrane receptor for EBV, and this virus can both infect and trigger B-lymphocytes to proliferate indefinitely and to secrete antibodies.[46,141] No antigen is required, and EBV is considered a polyclonal B-cell activator that stimulates cells to produce their genetically preprogrammed immunoglobulins. One consequence of EBV infection is autoantibody production; for instance, heterophile antibodies, cold agglutinins, hemolysins, antinuclear antibodies, and rheumatoid factors are often associated with acute infectious mononucleosis, a known EBV-induced disease in man.[15] Arthralgias have been noted in up to 10% of patients with infectious mononucleosis, but until recently, arthritis was considered to be a rare complication of heterophile-positive mononucleosis. In the dozen or so cases reported with EBV arthritis, radiologic findings have been limited to soft tissue swelling. The sedimentation rate in these patients was mildly elevated, but rheumatoid factors and antinuclear antibodies were consistently absent, and all joint complaints resolved by 30 days.[1,3,96,103,126,133] An exception is a 19-year-old woman, followed for more than 2 years, who has a persistent symmetric polyarthritis involving the small joints of the hands,

wrists, knees, and metatarsophalangeal and interphalangeal joints of the feet. This patient has remained rheumatoid-factor negative.[133]

Several other reasons for interest in the EBV are: (1) when compared with normal individuals, patients with RA have greater amounts of an unusual EBV-related antibody, that is, the rheumatoid arthritis precipitin or anti-RANA, in their serum;[10,110] (2) these patients may also have higher titers of antibodies to more conventional EBV-related antigens, although epidemiologic studies show that about 20% of RA patients have never been exposed to the virus, and similar increases in EBV antibody titers are found in patients with other chronic inflammatory connective tissue diseases;[2,36,107,128] and (3) RA patients appear to be defective in their ability to regulate EBV infections.[24,108,120]

When peripheral blood mononuclear (PBM) cells from normal subjects are exposed to EBV in vitro, they develop lymphoblastoid colonies, the precursors of established cell lines, in about 3 weeks. Rheumatoid PBM cells transform faster, in approximately 10 days. T-cell depletion reduces the time to outgrowth in the B cells of normal persons, but only a small further reduction occurs in the time needed for rheumatoid transformation.[5] RA patients also appear to lack a suppressor cell for EBV-stimulated immunoglobulin production.[124] Additional evidence of a regulatory defect is the finding that in vitro spontaneous transformation, that is, outgrowth in the absence of added EBV, occurs more often in rheumatoid non-T cells than in normal cells: approximately 40% spontaneous transformation in RA B cells versus 15% in normal B cells. Analysis of the controlling events is complicated, but it appears that several populations of E-rosetting mononuclear cells must interact to regulate the in vitro EBV infection of B-lymphocytes, and their effects are accomplished through the release of soluble mediators, including prostaglandins and interferons.[54,55]

It might be anticipated that if RA patients had a defect in their ability to regulate an EBV infection, they would harbor greater amounts of the virus than normal individuals. The more frequent "spontaneous transformation" of their B cells supports this hypothesis, but does not prove it. After infection, the EBV persists for life in a latent or sequestered form within the host's salivary epithelial cells and B-lymphocytes. A comparison of the excretion of EBV virus in the saliva of normal individuals, in RA patients, and in subjects with other rheumatic diseases taking the same medications showed no significant differences.[25] By means of a limiting dilution type of analysis, however, it has been claimed that 5 times more EBV is found in rheumatoid B cells than in normal human lympho-cytes.[123] Perhaps related to this observation is the finding that 40% of the B cells in rheumatoid joint effusions contain live virus, determined as spon-taneous transformation, whereas fewer than 10% of the B cells in synovial fluids obtained from pa-tients with other forms of inflammatory arthritis are so infected. Because the non-T cell populations of the peripheral blood of both groups of patients in this study had similar rates of spontaneous trans-formation, the implication is that the joint in RA may provide a permissive environment for the EBV.[73] Moreover, this finding clearly demonstrates that EBV can reach the joint as a passenger in trafficking B cells.

Our current understanding of EBV and RA can be summarized as follows: EBV infection, sero-logically defined, is not necessarily present at the outset or during the course of the disease in all RA patients. EBV arthritis does exist, but it is rare and is not identical to RA. The lymphocytes of RA patients are defective in their ability to regulate an in vitro EBV infection of B cells, and this defect may explain the difference reported in the expres-sion of antibodies to various EBV antigens in in-dividuals with RA. The relevance of the immuno-regulatory defect of RA patients for EBV is not proved, but the defect may have a role in the prop-agation of the disease process.

Although many facts are now available about the possible causes, epidemiology, and pathology of RA, their relationship to one another and to the disease is not clear. We shall probably not be able to understand these data until the etiologic agent responsible for the illness has been identified, but the eventual answer should explain the reason that the disease is so common (affecting approximately 1% of all adults), ubiquitous (present in almost all populations), persistent (lasting years to decades), and intimately associated with a unique antibody (rheumatoid factor) and a particular genetic con-stitution (a locus related to HLA-DR4). Our future understanding should also explain the foremost question; namely, why is RA a chronic inflam-matory disease of joints?

Articular Inflammation

The inflammatory response is usually considered a biologic adaptation to protect the host from a hostile environment. A prerequisite is that this re-sponse occurs without significant injury to the host's own tissues. Thus, the inflammation in RA must be considered inappropriate. How this comes about is not known, but a number of factors pre-dispose joints to injury and inflammation. Being moving, superficial structures, joints are subject to microtrauma almost constantly. Because the joint

lining is comprised, at least in part, of active phag-ocytic cells, it is likely that small numbers of mi-croorganisms are regularly extracted from the blood as it courses through the subsynovial ves-sels.[52] Alternatively, because the synovial lining cells are replenished by macrophage precursors in the bone marrow, organisms acquired at a distant site may be continuously transported into the joints. Equally important is the unexplained retention of immunoglobulins or antigen-antibody complexes by the macromolecules of fibrous and hyaline car-tilage.[19] In most instances, articular inflammation or synovitis is self-limited. After a variable period, the joint returns to its premorbid state, but occa-sionally, the process persists and chronic inflam-mation and eventual tissue damage ensue.

A number of reasons can be proposed to account for the chronicity of articular inflammation. The first and most obvious is persistence of the initiating event or an incomplete degradation of the primary stimulus. Chronic infection with organisms such as mycobacteria or fungi are examples in humans. In some experimental forms of chronic arthritis, such as in adjuvant arthritis and the streptococcal-cell-wall model, it appears that certain arthritogenic substances, such as peptidoglycans, are incrimi-nated.[8,50] Although injected at a distant site, these substances accumulate in the joint, and because of their unique property of being biologically non-degradable, they persist as an irritative focus. A second reason for unresolved inflammation is the development of a cross-reacting immune response between the primary stimulus and antigens peculiar to one of the articular structures. Antibody made systemically might be retained in the joint. Ex-amples include the shared antigens of streptococcal cell wall and human cartilage proteoglycan, or the chronic arthritis that develops in animals immu-nized against heterologous type II collagen.[125]

The most compelling argument, as in some other forms of chronic inflammation, is that a local im-mune reaction is responsible. In RA, this reaction could be an appropriate response to the putative causative agent sequestered in the articular cavity. Alternatively, it might represent autosensitization to a self-antigen rendered immunogenic within the joint. In RA, IgG is the obvious candidate. Perhaps in the course of a nonspecific synovitis, IgG is partially degraded by enzymes generated by the inflammatory process. Most individuals would not recognize the neoantigens produced, but those ge-netically predisposed respond with local anti-IgG production. The ensuing local antigen-antibody complex formation would beget more inflamma-tion, resulting in further alteration of immuno-globulin and a perpetuation of the inflammatory process. The association of seropositive, but not seronegative, RA with the HLA-DR4 haplotype supports this concept. A similar model could be developed using collagen as the autoantigen. Finally, the rheumatoid process might reflect a disturbance in the normal circulation of immunocompetent cells between intra- and extravascular compartments. Perhaps as a result of prior "activation," lymphocytes traffic into the joint in an unregulated manner or persist long after the provocative stimulus has gone. For whatever reason, the cells and products of the immune system, although probably not primarily involved in the initiation of RA, are certainly largely responsible for the perpetuation of the inflammatory response.

PATHOGENESIS

Rheumatoid synovitis, according to present concepts, is characterized by two discrete phases: (1) an exudative phase involving the microcirculation and lining cells of the synovium that allows an influx of plasma proteins and cellular elements into the joint; and (2) a chronic inflammatory phase occurring in the subsynovium and characterized by mononuclear cell infiltration. In well-established disease, both phases are present and are probably interrelated, but to simplify analysis, they are examined in sequence, beginning with the limited information on the initiating events, the subsequent immunologic factors that perpetuate the primary inflammatory reaction, and finally the transition of the chronic inflammatory allergic reaction in the synovium to a proliferative destructive process.

Initiation of Synovitis

The earliest events in RA are difficult to document, but the available evidence suggests that microvascular injury and mild synovial cell proliferation are the first lesions. Synovial biopsies from patients seen during the initial weeks of an arthritis that could subsequently be classified as definite or classic RA showed only mild proliferation of synovial lining cells and perivascular lymphocytes.[69,104] Polymorphonuclear leukocytes, when present, were seen in the superficial synovium; plasma cells were noted rarely. The small blood vessels were abnormal; they were obliterated by inflammatory cells and organized thrombi. Electron-microscopic examination disclosed gaps between vascular endothelial cells and endothelial cell injury. Evidence suggests the occurrence of phagocytosis by proliferating synoviocytes and in large mononuclear cells. Unfortunately, none of these findings are unique to RA and all are found at the inception of other acute inflammatory joint conditions. The microvascular changes, however, suggest that the etiologic factor is carried to the joint by the circulation.

Inflammatory Response

In contrast to the early lesions, many excellent descriptions of the histopathologic features of established RA and the immunologic events that perpetuate the primary synovial inflammatory reaction exist[34,40,53,142] (see Chap. 36.). Grossly, the synovium appears edematous and protrudes into the joint cavity as slender villous projections. Light-microscopic examination discloses a characteristic, but not pathognomonic, constellation of histologic changes. Synovial lining cells are hyperplastic and are layered to a depth of six to ten cells, in contrast to the normal thickness of one to three cell layers. Focal or segmental vascular changes are a regular feature of rheumatoid synovitis. Venous distention results from swollen endothelial cells, capillary obstruction is common, the walls of venules and arterioles are infiltrated with neutrophils, and areas of thrombosis and perivascular hemorrhage are seen. The connective tissue stroma of the normal synovial villi has few cells, but in established RA, it is usually filled with mononuclear cells. Polymorphonuclear leukocytes, common in the early lesions, are seen only occasionally. In some places, particularly around small blood vessels, lymphocytes and dendritic-appearing cells predominate; in others, plasma cells are the major type. Transitional areas have also been identified and show an intermingling of macrophages, lymphocytes, and plasma cells.[61]

Staining of the cells in situ with fluoresceinated monoclonal antibodies shows that the majority are T-lymphocytes; many have the Ia antigen, a measure of "activation," on their surface membranes.[9,37] Controversy exists over the proportion of the T cells that display helper-inducer or suppressor-cytotoxic phenotypes. The confusion relates, in part, to the region examined, because sampling in perivascular areas shows predominantly OKT4+ helper cells, whereas at a distance, the OKT8+ suppressor cells may be in the majority.[68] In some biopsies, only macrophage-mononuclear cells with large amounts of Ia on their surface membrane can be seen. A simple enumeration of the cells released from enzyme digested synovial tissues shows greater-than-expected T-cell populations with a modest increase in OKT8+ cells, as compared to companion blood samples. Although plasma cells and B-lymphocytes seem under-represented,[9,68] the rheumatoid synovium makes and contains large amounts of immunoglobulin, a finding that strongly suggests the presence of large numbers of these cells.

Immunofluorescent analysis of the plasma cells located in the subsynovium shows IgG to be the predominant class of cytoplasmic immunoglobulin because it is found in 30 to 60% of cells; IgM, occurring in 10 to 30% of cells, is less common. Most of the IgM is rheumatoid factor, but only a minority of the cytoplasmic IgG has anti-IgG activity when tested with fluorescein-labeled aggregated IgG. After pepsin treatment of the tissue, however, the number of cells staining for rheumatoid factor increases. This finding suggests that many of the plasma cells in the rheumatoid synovium make an IgG rheumatoid factor that combines in the cytoplasm with similar IgG molecules (self-associating IgG) (see Chap. 41). Surprisingly, pepsin-digested tissues from seronegative patients also show IgG-anti-Ig activity.[83,84]

Additional evidence that the B cells in the synovium of patients with RA can make immunoglobulins includes the demonstration of de novo immunoglobulin production by rheumatoid synovial explants or continuous cultures of lymphocytes released from synovium.[111] In vivo measurements of IgG synthesis show that about 20% of the IgG detected in synovial fluid is made in the synovial membrane,[109] and much of it has anti-IgG activity.[11]

Excessive synovial immunoglobulin production might come about in several ways. The fault could reside in B-cell hyperactivity caused, for instance, by a polyclonal B-cell activator. As discussed previously, the EBV is such an activator. An alternate explanation might be that B cells are driven by unrestrained T helper-inducer cells. This notion is supported by two observations: first, that the macrophage-like synovial lining cells have abundant surface Ia-like (DR) molecules and can efficiently present antigen and serve as stimulators in the mixed leukocyte reaction;[65] and second, that in certain areas of the subsynovium, T4+ helper-inducer cells are in intimate contact with dendritic-appearing cells bearing large amounts of DR antigen.[62] Such conditions are ideal for the generation of factors that support immunoglobulin production. A lack of suppressor T8+ cells, either because of an absolute reduction in their numbers or because of compartmentalization at a distance from the helper-inducer cells, could account for unbridled antibody production.[41]

The cytology of a typical rheumatoid joint effusion differs from that of the synovial membrane. Total leukocyte counts range from a few thousand to tens of thousands. Mononuclear cells, although present and with surface characteristics similar to their counterparts in the synovium, are in the minority. Neutrophils usually constitute 75 to 85% of the total. All forms are represented: early, multilobed polymorphonuclear leukocytes are admixed with effete white cells containing disintegrating nuclei and large cytoplasmic vacuoles. These vacu-

oles, when appropriately stained, can be shown to contain immunoglobulins, complement components, and antiglobulins. Similar immunoreactants are demonstrable within the cytoplasm of type A (phagocytic) synovial lining cells and in the matrix of articular cartilage.[142] Rheumatoid synovial fluids have less hemolytic complement than serum from the same patients and show evidence of activation of both the classic and alternate pathways. Complement components and biologically active fragments of the complement sequence, anaphylatoxins and chemotactic factors, have been identified in RA effusions,[131] and their presence correlates with synovial fluid immune complex levels, especially with those containing rheumatoid factors of the IgG class. Immune complexes have been isolated from rheumatoid joint effusions, and their constituent parts have been analyzed (see Chaps. 40 and 41). The dominant complexes contain anti-IgGs of both the IgM (conventional rheumatoid factor) and IgG class. This second type of complex seems particularly important in the pathogenesis of local inflammation because they self-associate to form intermediate-sized complexes that activate complement.[139] Further stabilization of complexes probably occurs by interaction with conventional IgM rheumatoid factor and enhances inflammatory properties. Other relevant antibodies, many of which are directed against by-products of the inflammatory response, include antinuclear antibodies, anti-Fab$_2$, anti-C3, and antifibrinogen, and possibly, collagen-anticollagen complexes.[125]

Electron-microscopic examination of the rheumatoid synovium shows that the hyperplasia of synoviocytes is the result of an increase in type-A (macrophage-like), type-B (secretory), and type-C (undifferentiated) cells. Superficially, the synoviocytes appear to form an uninterrupted layer, but no true basement membrane separates them from the underlying connective tissue. Capillaries are particularly abundant beneath the synovial lining, and many have large fenestrations similar to those seen in the vessels of the glomerulus, choroid plexus, and endocrine tissues.[52] Thus, material traversing these capillaries has only hyaluronate and interstitial fluid hampering its diffusion throughout the entire joint cavity.

Based on the foregoing observations, it has been suggested that the as yet unidentified cause of RA gains access to the joint and initiates an inflammatory response. Small blood vessels are injured, and mononuclear cells accumulate in the pericapillary areas. Macrophages process the pathogenic materials and present them to lymphocytes. Local antibody production ensues. The antigens and antibodies interact in synovial tissues, fluid, and cartilage and give rise to an extravascular immune complex disease (Fig. 35–1). These complexes activate the complement cascade and generate a number of biologically active materials from the complement proteins. Some, such as C3a and C5a, increase vascular permeability and allow an influx of serum proteins and cellular blood elements into the site where the complexes reside (exudation phase). Polymorphonuclear leukocytes in juxtaposition to the cartilage surface or free in the joint fluid retain the complexes with cell surface receptors for IgG and C3b. Subsequent phagocytosis stimulates: (1) the release of lysosomal proteinases, which have the potential to digest collagen, cartilage matrix, elastic tissues, and activate other biologically active mediators; (2) oxygen-free radicals, which directly produce cellular injury; and (3) oxidation of arachidonic acid that leads to the generation of proinflammatory by-products of the cyclo-oxygenase and lipoxygenase pathways (see Chaps. 18, 21, and 22).

Chronic Rheumatoid Granulomatous Response (Pannus)

Either simultaneously or in tandem, the proliferative and destructive stages of RA proceeds (see also Chap. 37). Synovial lining cells are stimulated to replicate, either by mediators generated in the inflammatory response or by lymphokines. The accumulation of lymphocytes in the rheumatoid synovium is reminiscent of a delayed-type hypersensitivity reaction. The identification of a large percentage of these lymphocytes as T cells and the finding of soluble factors derived from T cells in synovial effusions support this view. For instance, rheumatoid joint fluids inhibit the migration of guinea pig macrophages. Similar migration inhibition factor (MIF)-like material is found in supernatants from cultures of rheumatoid synovial explants.[118] Introduction of mitogen-derived lymphokines into the joints of experimental animals produces an acute and subsequently chronic inflammatory process. Further support for the role of lymphocytes is the observation that treatments such as thoracic duct drainage, lymphophoresis, and total lymph node irradiation may ameliorate rheumatoid joint inflammation and may decrease the hyperplasia of synovial lining cells.

Chronic RA is characterized by destruction of articular cartilage, ligaments, tendons, and bone.

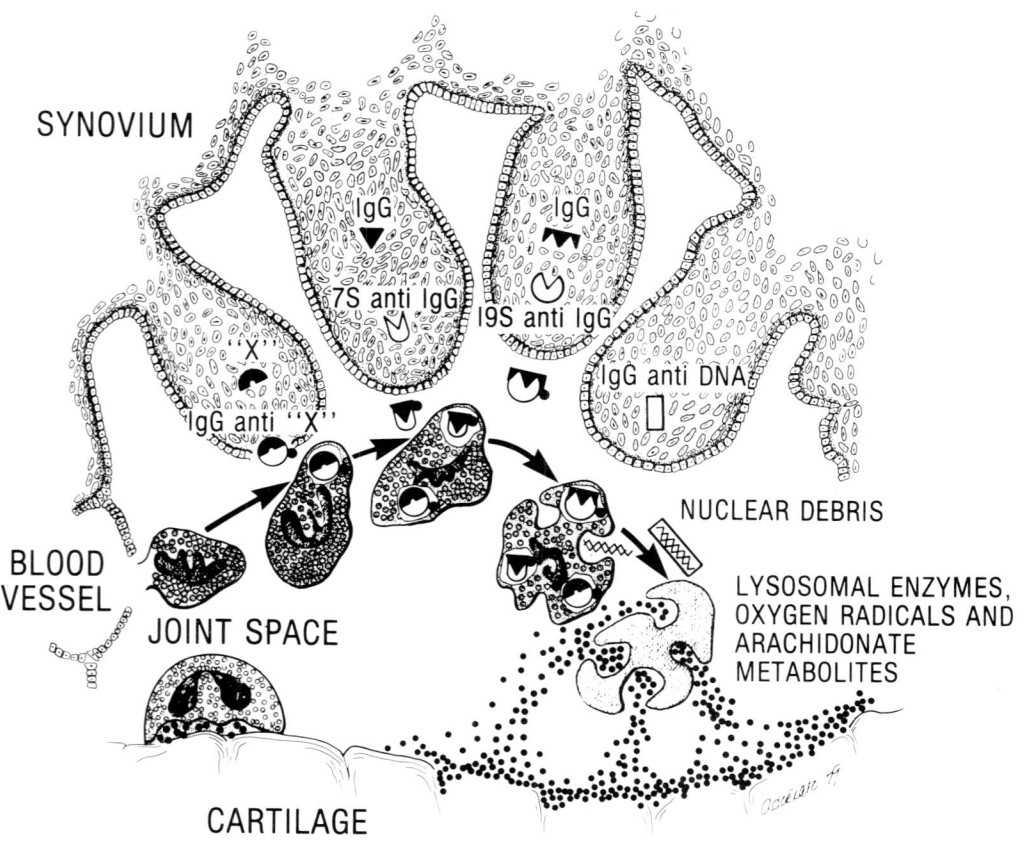

Fig. 35–1. Schematic illustration of immune complex interaction in structures involved by rheumatoid arthritis.

The damage results from a dual attack: from without, by enzymes in the synovial fluid, and from above and below, by granulation tissue.

Cartilage and other articular connective tissues are comprised primarily of proteoglycans and collagen. Proteoglycans consist of repeating disaccharide subunits linked covalently to a protein core. The earliest evidence of cartilage injury is a loss of metachromatic staining due to a leaching out of the proteoglycans. Cartilage that has lost ground substance has a diminished capacity to resist deformation and may be at risk for permanent damage through mechanical disruption. Proteoglycan loss is reversible, and complete recovery is possible, but once collagen, which forms the structural skeleton, is lost, cartilage disintegration becomes irreversible.[53]

Many potentially damaging enzymes released from phagocytic synoviocytes and polymorphonuclear leukocytes have been found in the fluid that continually bathes the cartilage surfaces. These enzymes include acid and neutral proteases that can split proteoglycan from its protein matrix.[6] Collagen, in its native triple-helical configuration, is resistant to degradation by these nonspecific proteases; however, collagenases derived from polymorphonuclear leukocytes, macrophages, and rheumatoid synovial cells can cleave (denature) the collagen polypeptide chains specifically into two fragments, which are then rapidly degraded further by proteolytic enzymes.[53] The observation of proteoglycan depletion and collagen degradation at sites distant from the advancing margin of the proliferating synovial membrane argues for the importance of synovial fluid enzymes in articular damage.[34,52]

The articular destruction in RA, however, begins at the periphery of the cartilage and in the "bare areas" of bone exposed to joint fluid but not covered by cartilage. It has been claimed that the earliest injury, which precedes the formation of recognizable pannus, is brought about by immature synovial cells arising from the recesses at the margin of the joint and creeping across the surface of cartilage. Similar cells can be seen to insert themselves between the collagen fibers when the proteoglycan has been enzymatically removed. Subsequent cartilage destruction is accomplished by the release of collagenolytic enzymes.[34] These aggressive events are short-lived, occur in waves, likely in association with the exudative (inflammatory) process, and are followed by a maturation of the granulomatous response with an ingress of proliferating fibroblasts, small blood vessels, and inflammatory cells.[34]

Several different kinds of pannus have been described. The first type, which is analogous to the "activated" synovial membrane previously described, seems to destroy cartilage by enzymatic digestion. The second, "cellular" form of pannus probably operates the same way, but its similarity to granulation tissue seen at other sites of injury suggests that the cellular and fibrous infiltrate may be the result of cartilage injury, rather than the cause of it. A third type of dense fibrous, avascular, acellular pannus may act as a mantle interfering with cartilage nutrition. Although all three types of pannus can be found simultaneously in the same joint, it is not clear whether they represent a sequential phenomenon or whether each develops independently.[66]

A better understanding of the chronic synovitis of RA has developed from in vitro studies of the effects of lymphocytes, macrophages, and their products on target cells in the synovium, cartilage, and bone. Cultured explants of rheumatoid synovial fragments produce large quantities of collagenase and prostaglandins. The responsible cells are large, measuring 20 to 30 μm in diameter or greater, and have an abundant cytoplasm, a large nucleus, and dendritic processes that give them a stellate appearance. They are not monocytes because they do not produce lysozyme, and most lack the conventional surface markers of macrophages. When placed in continuous culture, the synoviocytes initially make and secrete both collagenase and prostaglandin (PGE_2), but the production of these molecules decreases after trypsinization and serial passage of the cells.[20] Collagenase release is stimulated in such cultures by conditioned media from peripheral blood mononuclear cells.[22] Plant lectins, collagen, the Fc portion of IgG, and aggregated IgG can all further increase the amount of this stimulating factor.[21] Cellular fractionation studies have shown that monocytes or macrophages are responsible for the stimulating factor, which is called mononuclear cell factor (MCF). T cells ordinarily produce little stimulation, but when they are cultured with mononuclear cells and lectin, a marked increase in collagenase production by the adherent stellate synovial cells occurs.[20] MCF is probably identical to interleukin-1 (IL-1), a molecule whose release from macrophages is modulated by T-cell lymphokines (see Chap. 17). A much more detailed discussion of the mechanisms of hard tissue destruction in RA is given in Chapter 37.

Another important mechanism may be the destruction of cartilage brought about by the chondrocytes themselves. As noted earlier, proteoglycan loss can be observed in the absence of either pannus overgrowth or high polymorphonuclear leukocyte counts in synovial fluid,[52] particularly early in the disease. Histopathologic study of cartilage at this time reveals enlarged lacunae around the chondrocytes and some evidence of chondrocyte proliferation. These findings suggest that tissue degradation may result from factors released from chondrocytes. Synovium can elaborate a factor called *catabolin* that stimulates chondrocytes to secrete matrix-degrading enzymes.[26] Moreover, the addition of media from cultures of normal or rheumatoid synovial explants or MCF (IL-1) itself to chondrocytes stimulated the release of plasminogen activator, prostaglandin E, and collagenase.[79,98]

The inciting factors in RA remain undefined, but our understanding of the cellular and molecular mechanisms leading to chronic joint inflammation and to local tissue destruction has increased in the past few years. As seen in Figure 35–2, the central axis is the interaction between macrophage-type cells and T-lymphocytes. These cells, in concert with B cells, cause local production of antibody. Immune complexes formed locally within the joint activate complement and are phagocytized by polymorphonuclear leukocytes and the macrophage-like moiety of synovial lining cells. Accompanying this ingestion, a variety of mediators are released, giving rise to the signs and symptoms of inflammation. Leukocytes adherent to cartilage can degrade proteoglycan, and perhaps collagen, in their attempts to eliminate the sequestered immune complexes. Simultaneously, the macrophages and T cells communicate through soluble substances with the dendritic cells in the synovial lining and stimulate the release of molecules capable of causing bone and cartilage erosion, which eventuates in characteristic rheumatoid deformities and attendant functional disability.

The same complex interaction of cells and mediators is probably involved in connective tissue turnover during repair, growth, and differentiation. As in all biologic systems, control mechanisms limit the response. Thus, antibody production and lymphokine release are modulated by suppressor cells, idiotype networks, and peptides derived from IgG degradation; corticosteroids and prostaglandins modify the response to mediators and the release of degradative enzymes; and inhibitors are present in plasma and articular tissues that bind and neutralize metalloproteinases. Indeed, it is possible that an essential defect in RA is a failure in one or more of these normal regulatory systems.[75]

EXTRA-ARTICULAR MANIFESTATIONS

Although characteristically a joint disease, RA can affect a number of other tissues.[58] These extra-articular manifestations probably occur with considerable frequency, but are usually subclinical. The extra-articular events may, however, dominate the clinical picture. Terms such as "rheumatoid disease" and "malignant rheumatoid arthritis" have been used to describe this form of the disease (see also Chap. 39).

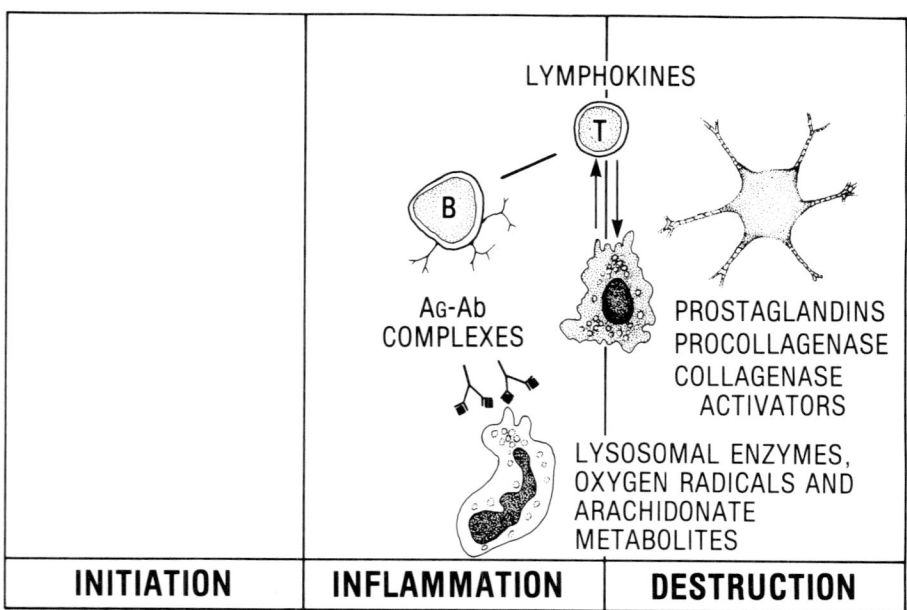

Fig. 35–2. Schematic representation of the etiology and of the cellular and immune interactions responsible for joint inflammation and destruction in rheumatoid arthritis.

Vasculitis

The spectrum of vascular lesions that accompanies RA is detailed in Chapters 39 and 63. The cause of the various vascular lesions and their relationship to one another has not been defined, but a number of observations suggest that they result from injury induced by immune complexes, especially those containing antibodies to IgG. These include: (1) the generally held view that patients with high levels of serum IgM rheumatoid factor have more systemic manifestations of the disease;[31,43,80] (2) a correlation of depressed serum complement activity, decreased concentration of C2 and C4, and hypercatabolism of C3 with the clinical signs of vasculitis;[38,80,134] (3) immunofluorescent detection of deposits of IgG, IgM, and complement (C3) in the vasa nervorum of patients with rheumatoid neuropathy, and immunoglobulins and rheumatoid factor in vessel walls of vasculitis patients;[18] and an association between vasculitis and increased levels of circulating immune complexes.[49,51,56]

As early as 1957, Kunkel and his associates identified high-molecular-weight (22S) immune complexes in the serum of RA patients. Chemical dissociation of this material revealed 7S and 19S components, the latter with anti-Ig activity.[39] Subsequently, large amounts of unusual gamma globulin complexes with sedimentation rates ranging from 9 to 17S were found in serum from patients with advanced RA.[70] These complexes, which are readily dissociated to 7S units, have been designated "intermediate complexes." Monoclonal IgM rheumatoid factors were then used to demonstrate small complexes or aggregates of IgG in the serum of approximately 50% of patients with RA.[140] This method detects aggregates that fail to precipitate with polyclonal rheumatoid factors or Clq. A later radioimmunoassay was based on the ability of test samples to inhibit the interaction of iodinated aggregated IgG with monoclonal rheumatoid factor and detected immune complex-like material in the serum of 12 of 51 (27%) RA patients examined. The presence of this material was associated with more severe disease, greater functional impairment, and more advanced joint destruction. The amount of inhibiting material was inversely related to serum C4 levels, but not to rheumatoid factor titers. Three-fourths of the patients had extra-articular manifestations including Sjögren's syndrome, leg ulcers, Felty's syndrome, neuropathy, and pulmonary fibrosis.[72] These findings have been subsequently confirmed and extended by others,[43] using a variety of immune complex assays including: Clq binding;[49,51,56,87] Raji cells;[49,51] monoclonal rheumatoid factor.[49,51]

Approximately 30% of an unselected group of patients with RA had significant amounts of cryoglobulins. Two-thirds of the cryoprecipitable protein was polyclonal IgG and IgM, with a higher IgM-to-IgG ratio than found in the whole serum from which they precipitated.[135] Systemic vasculitis, present in 3 of the original 38 patients, was associated with the largest amount of cryoglobulin. Subsequently, 5 more patients with vasculitis were studied, all of whom had detectable cryoglobulins. The cryoglobulin antiglobulin (rheumatoid factor) activity was mainly by IgM. Serial studies performed on vasculitis patients treated with cyclophosphamide disclosed a close relationship between the clinical evidence of vasculitis and the presence of cryoglobulins.[135] These findings were interpreted as evidence that the widespread vascular complications of RA are mediated, at least in part, by circulating immune complexes.

Other forms of rheumatoid factor have been described in rheumatoid vasculitis. Theofilopoulos and his associates detected IgG rheumatoid factor in 10 of 15 (67%) patients with rheumatoid vasculitis, but in only 3 of 33 without vasculitis.[122] Eighty percent of the patients with vasculitis, but only 18% of those without, had 7S IgM in their serum, a finding since confirmed by others.[116]

In summary, most patients with RA have circulating soluble materials with the characteristics of immune complexes. Antigamma globulins of the IgG and IgM classes and IgG itself are integral parts of these soluble complexes, although the clinical usefulness of their measurement is questionable.[95] Finally, whether they are responsible for vasculitis, or for the other extra-articular features, or are merely markers for severe disease remains a moot question.

Felty's Syndrome

In 1924, Felty described a symptom complex of chronic RA associated with splenomegaly and leukopenia.[35] Subsequently, additional features have been recognized, including skin hyperpigmentation, leg ulcers, generalized lymphadenopathy, anemia, and thrombocytopenia. Commonly, such patients have high titers of rheumatoid factor and antinuclear antibodies, subcutaneous nodules, and manifestations of systemic rheumatoid disease or the sicca complex (Sjögren's syndrome).[58,102]

No single explanation for the granulocytopenia that characterizes Felty's syndrome is satisfactory. Early speculations implicated hypersplenism or splenic sequestration of neutrophils. An inability to demonstrate trapping of radiolabeled cells in the spleen and the frequent failure of splenectomy to correct the leukopenia diminished the considered importance of this organ in Felty's syndrome.[129]

Consistent evidence of impaired production of granulocytes is lacking, and the bone marrow is typically hyperplastic. This finding makes the observation that serum or lymphocytes from patients with Felty's syndrome can inhibit the growth of bone marrow cells in culture less interesting.[28,117] Indeed, although neutropenia is considered the hallmark of Felty's syndrome, leukokinetic studies show that two-thirds of these patients have a normal total blood neutrophil pool. Thus, their neutropenia appears to be due to an excessive margination of neutrophils, presumably into extravascular locations.[129]

A number of observations suggest that circulating factors, particularly antibodies, play a pathogenetic role in patients with Felty's syndrome. For instance, etiocholanolone normally mobilizes granulocytes from the bone marrow. Patients with Felty's syndrome do not respond to etiocholanolone and, in one instance, infusion of plasma from a patient blocked the granulocyte-mobilizing effect of this agent.[64] Circulating IgG antibodies against neutrophils are detected in the majority of patients with Felty's syndrome.[100] Some antinuclear antibodies react only with polymorphonuclear cell nuclei. Such granulocyte reactive antinuclear factors are said to be found in virtually all patients with Felty's syndrome, in 75% of patients with RA, and in 30% of patients with systemic lupus erythematosus. These granulocyte reactive antibodies fix human complement, unlike the conventional organ-nonspecific antinuclear factors.[32,137]

Immune complexes containing IgG and IgM antibodies are demonstrable in the cytoplasm of circulating white blood cells and in the serum of the majority of patients with Felty's syndrome. Similar inclusions are formed when normal neutrophils are incubated with serum from patients with this condition.[59] Most such patients have significant amounts of serum cryoglobulins containing IgG, IgM, complement components, and antinuclear and antigamma globulin antibodies. Granulocyte-reactive antinuclear antibody was selectively concentrated in some of the cryoglobulins.[136]

Undoubtedly, multiple factors, including antibodies, immune complexes, complement activation, which influences granulocyte margination, and cellular immune reactions, either singly or in combination, are responsible for the granulocytopenia that characterizes Felty's syndrome, and it is likely that different factors or combinations of factors are operative in each patient.

REFERENCES

1. Adebonojo, F.O.: Monarticular arthritis: An unusual manifestation of mononucleosis. Clin. Pediatr., *11*:549–550, 1972.
2. Alspaugh, M.A., et al.: Elevated levels of antibodies to Epstein-Barr virus antigens in sera and synovial fluids of patients with rheumatoid arthritis. J. Clin. Invest., *67*:1134–1140, 1981.
3. Ansell, B.M.: Infective arthritis. *In* Copeman's Textbook of the Rheumatic Diseases. Edited by T. Scott. Edinburgh, Churchill-Livingstone, 1978, p. 821.
4. Atwater, E.C., and Jacox, R.F.: The latex fixation test in patients with liver disease. Ann. Intern. Med., *58*:419–425, 1963.
5. Bardwick, P.A., et al.: Altered regulation of Epstein-Barr virus induced lymphoblast proliferation in rheumatoid arthritis lymphoid cells. Arthritis Rheum., *23*:626–632, 1980.
6. Barrett, A.J.: The possible role of neutrophil proteinases in damage to articular cartilage. Agents Actions, *8*:11–18, 1978.
7. Bartholomew, L.E., and Bartholomew, F.N.: Antigenic bacterial polysaccharide in rheumatoid synovial effusions. Arthritis Rheum., *22*:969–977, 1979.
8. Bennett, J.C.: The infectious etiology of rheumatoid arthritis: New considerations. Arthritis Rheum., *21*:531–538, 1978.
9. Burmester, G.R., et al.: Ia⁺ T cells in synovial fluid and tissues of patients with rheumatoid arthritis. Arthritis Rheum., *24*:1370–1376, 1981.
10. Catalano, M.A., et al.: Antibody to the rheumatoid arthritis nuclear antigen: Its relationship to in vivo Epstein-Barr virus infection. J. Clin. Invest., *65*:1238–1242, 1980.
11. Cecere, F., et al.: Evidence for the local production and utilization of immunoreactants in rheumatoid arthritis. Arthritis Rheum., *25*:1307–1315, 1982.
12. Chantler, J.K., Ford, D.K., and Tingle, A.J.: Persistent rubella infection and rubella associated arthritis. Lancet, *1*:1323–1325, 1982.
13. Chantler, J.K., Ford, D.K., and Tingle, A.J.: Rubella associated arthritis: Rescue of rubella virus from peripheral blood lymphocytes two years post vaccination. Infect. Immun., *32*:1274–1280, 1981.
14. Chattopadhyay, H., et al.: Rheumatoid synovial lymphocytes lack concanavalin A activated suppressor cell activity. Scand. J. Immunol., *10*:479–486, 1979.
15. Chervenick, P.A.: Infectious mononucleosis. DM, December: 5–56, 1974.
16. Clarris, B.J., Fraser, J.R.E., and Rodda, S.J.: Effect of cell bound hyaluronic acid on infectivity of Newcastle disease virus for human synovial cells in vitro. Ann. Rheum. Dis., *33*:240–242, 1974.
17. Cole, B.C., et al.: New models of chronic synovitis in rabbits induced by mycoplasma: Microbiological, histopathological, immunological observations in rabbits infected with Mycoplasma arthritides and Mycoplasma pulmonis. Infect. Immun., *16*:382–396, 1977.
18. Conn, D.L., McDuffie, F.C., and Dyck, P.J.: Immunopathologic study of sural nerves in rheumatoid arthritis. Arthritis Rheum., *15*:135–143, 1972.
19. Cooke, T.D., and Jasin, H.E.: The pathogenesis of chronic inflammation in experimental antigen-induced arthritis: I. The role of antigen on the local immune response. Arthritis Rheum., *15*:327–337, 1972.
20. Dayer, J.M., et al.: Interactions among rheumatoid synovial cells and monocyte-macrophages: Production of collagenase stimulating factor by human monocytes exposed to concanavalin, A or immunoglobulin Fc fragment. J. Immunol., *124*:1712–1720, 1980.
21. Dayer, J.M., Robinson, D.R., and Krane, S.M.: Prostaglandin production by rheumatoid synovial cells: Stimulation by a factor from human mononuclear cells. J. Exp. Med., *145*:1399–1404, 1977.
22. Dayer, J.M., et al.: Production of collagenase and prostaglandins by isolated adherent rheumatoid synovial cells. Proc. Natl. Acad. Sci., USA, *73*:945–949, 1976.
23. Decker, J.L., and Barden, J.A.: *In* Infection and Immunology in the Rheumatic Diseases. Edited by D.C. Dumonde. Oxford, Blackwell Scientific Publishing, 1976.
24. Depper, J.M., Bluestein, H.G., and Zvaifler, N.J.: Impaired regulation of Epstein-Barr virus induced outgrowth

in rheumatoid arthritis is due to a T cell defect. J. Immunol., *127*:1899–1902, 1981.

25. Depper, J.M., Zvaifler, N.J., and Bluestein, H.G.: Oropharyngeal Epstein-Barr virus excretion in rheumatoid arthritis. Arthritis Rheum., *25*:427–431, 1982.

26. Dingle, J.T., et al.: A cartilage catabolic factor from synovium. Biochem. J., *184*:177–180, 1979.

27. Doherty, P.C., and Zinkernagel, R.M.: T cell mediated immunopathology in viral infections. Transplant. Rev., *19*:89–120, 1974.

28. Duckham, D.J., et al.: Retardation of colony growth of an in vitro bone marrow culture using sera from patients with Felty's syndrome, SLE, RA, and other disease states. Arthritis Rheum., *18*:323–333, 1975.

29. Duffy, J., Lidsky, M.D., and Sharp, J.T.: Polyarthritis, polyarteritis and hepatitis B. Medicine, *55*:19–37, 1976.

30. Dumonde, D.C. (Ed.): Infection and Immunology in the Rheumatic Diseases. Oxford, Blackwell Scientific Publishing, 1976.

31. Epstein, W.V., and Engleman, E.P.: The relationship of the rheumatoid factor content of serum to clinical neurovascular manifestations of rheumatoid arthritis. Arthritis Rheum., *2*:250–258, 1959.

32. Faber, V., and Elling, P.: Leukocyte specific antinuclear factors in patients with Felty's syndrome, rheumatoid arthritis, systemic lupus erythematosus, and other diseases. Acta Med. Scand., *179*:257–267, 1966.

33. Falchuk, K.H., Goetzl, E.J., and Kulka, J.P.: Respiratory gases of synovial fluids. An approach to synovial tissue circulatory-metabolic imbalance in rheumatoid arthritis. Am. J. Med., *49*:223–231, 1970.

34. Fassbender, H.G.: Potential aggressiveness of the synovial tissue in rheumatoid arthritis. *In* Articular Synovium. Edited by P. Franchimont. Basel, S. Karger, 1982, pp. 34–44.

35. Felty, A.R.: Chronic arthritis in the adult, associated with splenomegaly and leucopenia. Report of 5 cases of an unusual clinical syndrome. Bull. Johns Hopkins Hosp., *35*:16–20, 1924.

36. Ferrell, P.B., et al.: Antibodies to Epstein-Barr virus related antigens in the serum of patients with rheumatoid arthritis. J. Clin. Invest., *67*:681–687, 1981.

37. Fox, R.I., et al.: Synovial fluid lymphocytes differ from peripheral blood lymphocytes in patients with rheumatoid arthritis. J. Immunol., *128*:351–354, 1982.

38. Franco, A.E., and Schur, P.H.: Hypocomplementemia in rheumatoid arthritis. Arthritis Rheum., *14*:231–238, 1971.

39. Franklin, E.C., et al.: An unusual protein component of high molecular weight in the serum of patients with rheumatoid arthritis. J. Exp. Med., *105*:425–438, 1975.

40. Gardner, D.L.: The Pathology of Rheumatoid Arthritis. London, Arnold, 1972.

41. Gatenby, P.A., and Engelman, E.G.: Immunoregulation in the synovium of rheumatoid arthritis. Lancet, 2:1348, 1981.

42. Ghose, T., Woodbury, J.F., and Hansell, M.M.: Interaction in vitro between synovial cells and autologous lymphocytes and sera from arthritis patients. J. Clin. Pathol., *28*:550–558, 1975.

43. Gordon, D.A., Stein, J.L., and Broder, I.: The extraarticular features of rheumatoid arthritis. A systematic analysis of 127 cases. Am. J. Med., *54*:445–452, 1973.

44. Grahame, R., et al.: Chronic arthritis associated with the presence of intrasynovial rubella virus. Ann. Rheum. Dis., *42*:2–13, 1983.

45. Grayzel, A.I., and Beck, C.: Rubella infection of synovial cells and resistance of cells derived from patients with rheumatoid arthritis. J. Exp. Med., *131*:367–373, 1970.

46. Greaves, M.F., Brown, G., and Rickinson, A.B.: Epstein-Barr virus binding sites on lymphocyte subpopulations and the origin of lymphoblasts in cultured lymphoid cell lines and in blood of patients with infectious mononucleosis. Clin. Immunol. Immunopathol., *3*:514–524, 1975.

47. Griffiths, M.M., Smith, C.B., and Pepper, B.J.: Susceptibility of rheumatoid and nonrheumatoid synovial cells

to antibody dependent cell mediated cytotoxicity. Arthritis Rheum., *21*:97–104, 1978.

48. Gruhn, W.B., and McDuffie, F.C.: Studies of serum immunoglobulin binding to synovial fibroblast cultures from patients with rheumatoid arthritis. Arthritis Rheum., *23*:10–16, 1980.

49. Gupta, R.C., et al.: Comparison of three immuno-assays for immune complexes in rheumatoid arthritis. Arthritis Rheum., *22*:433–439, 1979.

50. Hadler, M.M.: A pathogenetic model for erosive synovitis: Lessons from animal arthritides. Arthritis Rheum., *19*:256–266, 1976.

51. Halla, J.T., Volanakis, J.E., and Schrohenloher, R.E.: Immune complexes in rheumatoid arthritis sera and synovial fluids: A comparison of 3 methods. Arthritis Rheum., *22*:440–448, 1979.

52. Hamerman, D., Barland, P., and Janis, R.: The structure and chemistry of the synovial membrane in health and disease. *In* The Biological Basis of Medicine. Vol. III. Edited by E.E. Bittar and N. Bittar. Philadelphia, W.B. Saunders, 1969, pp. 269–309.

53. Harris, E.D., Jr.: Pathogenesis of rheumatoid arthritis. *In* Textbook of Rheumatology. Edited by W.N. Kelley, et al. Philadelphia, W.B. Saunders, 1981, pp. 896–927.

54. Hasler, F., et al.: Analysis of the defects responsible for the impaired regulation of Epstein-Barr virus-induced B cell proliferation by rheumatoid arthritis lymphocytes. I. Diminished gamma interferon production in response to autologous stimulation. J. Exp. Med., *157*:173–188, 1983.

55. Hasler, F., et al.: Analysis of the defects responsible for the impaired regulation of Epstein-Barr virus-induced B cell proliferation by rheumatoid arthritis lymphocytes. II. Role of monocytes and the increased sensitivity of rheumatoid arthritis lymphocytes to prostaglandin E. J. Immunol., *131*:768–772, 1983.

56. Hay, F.C., Nineham, J.L., and Peumal, R.: Intra-articular and circulating immune complexes and antiglobulins (IgG and IgM). Ann. Rheum. Dis., *38*:1–7, 1979.

57. Hilderbrandt, H.M., and Maassab, H.F.: Rubella synovitis in a one-year-old patient. N. Engl. J. Med., *274*:1428–1430, 1966.

58. Hurd, E.R.: Extra-articular manifestations of rheumatoid arthritis. Semin. Arthritis Rheum., 8:151–176, 1979.

59. Hurd, E.R., Andreis, M., and Ziff, M.: Phagocytosis of immune complexes by polymorphonuclear leukocytes in patients with Felty's syndrome. Clin. Exp. Immunol., *28*:413–425, 1977.

60. Inman, R.D.: Rheumatic manifestations of hepatitis virus B infection. Semin. Arthritis Rheum., *11*:406–420, 1982.

61. Ishikawa, H., and Ziff, M.: Electron microscopic observations of immunoreactive cells in the rheumatoid synovial membrane. Arthritis Rheum., *19*:1–14, 1976.

62. Janossy, G., et al.: Rheumatoid arthritis: A disease of T lymphocyte-macrophage immunoregulation. Lancet, *2*:839–842, 1981.

63. Johnson, R.E., and Hall, A.P.: Rubella arthritis. N. Engl. J. Med., *258*:743–745, 1958.

64. Kimball, H.R., et al.: Marrow granulocyte reserves in the rheumatic diseases. Arthritis Rheum., *16*:345–352, 1973.

65. Klareskog, L., et al.: Immune functions of human synovial cells. Phenotypic and T cell regulatory properties of macrophage-like cells that express HLA-DR. Arthritis Rheum., *25*:488–501, 1982.

66. Kobayashi, I., and Ziff, M.: Electron microscopic studies of the cartilage pannus function in rheumatoid arthritis. Arthritis Rheum., *18*:475–483, 1975.

67. Kobayashi, Y., et al.: Superoxide dismutase activity of T lymphocytes and non-T lymphocytes. FEBS Lett., *98*:391–393, 1979.

68. Konttinen, Y.J., et al.: Characterization of the immunocompetence of rheumatoid synovium from tissue sections and eluates. Arthritis Rheum., *24*:71–79, 1981.

69. Kulka, J.P., et al.: Early joint lesions of rheumatoid arthritis. Arch. Pathol., *59*:129–150, 1955.

70. Kunkel, H.G., Franklin, E.C., and Muller-Eberhard, H.J.: Studies on the isolation and characterization of the "rheumatoid factor." J. Clin. Invest., *38*:424–434, 1959.

71. London, W.T., et al.: Concentration of rubella virus antigen in chondrocytes of congenitally infected rabbits. Nature, 226:172–173, 1970.

72. Luthra, H.S., et al.: Immune complexes in sera and synovial fluids of patients with rheumatoid arthritis. J. Clin Invest., 56:458–466, 1975.

73. McClurg, M., Bluestein, H.G., and Zvaifler, N.J.: Epstein-Barr virus infected lymphocytes are in rheumatoid arthritis synovial fluids. Arthritis Rheum., 26:S53, 1983.

74. McCord, J.M., Stokes, S.H., and Wong, K.: Superoxide radical as a phagocyte produced chemical mediator of inflammation. In Advances in Inflammation Research. Edited by G. Weissmann. New York, Raven Press, 1979, pp. 273–280.

75. McGuire, M.K.B., et al.: Factors influencing production of enzymes by human synovium in vitro. In Articular Synovium. Edited by P. Franchimont. Basel, S. Karger, 1982, pp. 75–94.

76. Mansson, I., and Olhagen, B.: Fecal Clostridium perfringens and rheumatoid arthritis. J. Infect. Dis., 130:444–445, 1974.

77. Mansson, I., Norberg, R., and Olhagen, B.: Arthritis in pigs induced by dietary factors: Microbiologic, clinical and histological studies. Clin. Exp. Immunol., 9:677–693, 1971.

78. Marmion, B.P.: Infection, autoimmunity and rheumatoid arthritis. Clin. Rheum. Dis., 4:565–586, 1978.

79. Meats, J.E., McGuire, M.K., and Russell, R.G.: Human synovium releases a factor which stimulates chondrocyte production of PGE and plasminogen activator. Nature, 286:891–892, 1980.

80. Mongan, E.S., et al.: A study of the relationship of seronegative and seropositive rheumatoid arthritis to each other and to necrotizing vasculitis. Am. J. Med., 47:23–35, 1969.

81. Morris, E.L., and Stevens, M.B.: Rheumatoid arthritis—a sequel to HBsAg hepatitis. Am. J. Med., 64:859–862, 1978.

82. Munthe, E., Guldal, G., and Jellum, E.: Increased intracellular glutathione during penicillamine treatment for rheumatoid arthritis. Lancet, 2:1126–1127, 1979.

83. Munthe, F., and Natvig, J.B.: Immunoglobulin classes, subclasses, and complexes of IgG rheumatoid factor in rheumatoid synovial cells. Clin. Exp. Immunol., 12:55–70, 1972.

84. Natvig, J.B., and Munthe, E.: Self associating IgG rheumatoid factor represents a major response of plasma cells in rheumatoid inflammatory tissue. Ann. N.Y. Acad. Sci., 256:88, 1975.

85. Norval, M., Ogilvie, M.M., and Marion, B.P.: DNA polymerase activity in rheumatoid synovial membranes. Ann. Rheum. Dis., 34:205–212, 1975.

86. Norval, M., and Smith, C.: Search for viral nucleic acid sequences in rheumatoid cells. Ann. Rheum. Dis., 38:456–462, 1979.

87. Nydegger, U.E., et al.: Circulating complement breakdown products in patients with rheumatoid arthritis. Correlation between plasma C3d, circulating immune complexes and clinical activity. J. Clin. Invest., 59:862–868, 1977.

88. Ogra, P.L., and Herd, J.K.: Arthritis associated with induced rubella infection. J. Immunol., 107:810–813, 1971.

89. Paget, S.A., et al.: Studies of lymphoblastoid cell lines derived from rheumatoid arthritis synovial membrane lymphocytes: tissue reactivity of secreted immunoglobulin. (Abstract.) Arthritis Rheum., 23:728, 1980.

90. Paget, S.A., Anderson, K., and Phillips, P.E.: Absence of complement dependent cytotoxicity of rheumatoid sera for rheumatoid synovial cell cultures. Arthritis Rheum., 21:249–254, 1978.

91. Patterson, R.L., et al.: Rubella and rheumatoid arthritis: Hyaluronic acid and susceptibility of cultured rheumatoid synovial cells to viruses. Proc. Soc. Exp. Biol. Med., 149:594–598, 1975.

92. Person, D.A., and Sharp, J.T.: The etiology of rheumatoid arthritis. Bull. Rheum. Dis., 27:888–893, 1976.

93. Phillips, P.E.: Infection and the pathogenesis of the connective tissue diseases. In Scientific Basis of Rheumatology. Edited by G.S. Panayi. Edinburgh, Churchill-Livingstone, 1982, pp. 1–21.

94. Phillips, P.E., Anderson, K., and Paget, S.A.: Lack of antibody in rheumatoid arthritis to cultured synovial cells using adherotoxicity. (Abstract.) Arthritis Rheum., 23:732, 1980.

95. Plotz, P.: Studies of immune complexes. Arthritis Rheum., 25:1151–1155, 1982.

96. Pollack, S., Enat, R., and Barzilai, D.: Monarthritis with heterophile negative infectious mononucleosis. Arch. Intern. Med., 140:1109–1111, 1980.

97. Pritchard, D.G., Settine, R.L., and Bennett, J.C.: Sensitive mass spectrometric procedures for the detection of bacterial cell wall components in rheumatoid joints. Arthritis Rheum., 23:608, 1980.

98. Ridge, S.C., Oronsky, A.L., and Kerwar, S.S.: Induction of the synthesis of latent collagenase and latent neutral protease in chondrocytes by a factor synthesized by activated macrophages. Arthritis Rheum., 23:448–453, 1980.

99. Rister, M., et al.: Superoxide dismutase deficiency in rheumatoid arthritis. Lancet, 1:1094, 1978.

100. Rosenthal, F.D., et al.: White cell antibodies and the aetiology of Felty's syndrome. Q. J. Med., 43:187–203, 1974.

101. Rubella Surveillance Summary, 13:40, 1964.

102. Ruderman, M., Miller, L.M., and Pinals, R.S.: Clinical and serologic observations on 27 patients with Felty's syndrome. Arthritis Rheum., 11:377–384, 1968.

103. Sauter, S.V.H., and Utsinger, P.D.: Viral arthritis. Clin. Rheum. Dis., 4:225–240, 1978.

104. Schumacher, H.R.: Synovial membrane and fluid morphologic alterations in early rheumatoid arthritis. Microvascular injury and virus-like particles. Ann. N.Y. Acad. Sci., 256:39–64, 1975.

105. Schumacher, H.R., and Kitridou, R.C.: Synovitis of recent onset. A clinicopathologic study during the first month of disease. Arthritis Rheum., 15:465–485, 1974.

106. Silver, R.M., and Zvaifler, N.J.: Immunopathogenesis of rheumatoid arthritis. In Rheumatoid Arthritis. Edited by P.D. Utsinger, N.J. Zvaifler, and G.E. Ehrlich. Philadelphia, J.B. Lippincott, 1984.

107. Silverman, S.L., and Schumacher, H.R.: Antibodies to Epstein-Barr viral antigens in early rheumatoid arthritis. Arthritis Rheum., 24:1465–1468, 1981.

108. Slaughter, L., et al.: In vitro effects of Epstein-Barr virus on peripheral mononuclear cells from patients with rheumatoid arthritis and normal controls. J. Exp. Med., 148:1429–1434, 1978.

109. Sliwinski, A.J., and Zvaifler, N.J.: In vivo synthesis of IgG by rheumatoid synovium. J. Lab. Clin. Med., 76:304–310, 1970.

110. Slovin, S.F., et al.: The rheumatoid arthritis precipitin: a misnomer. (Abstract.) Arthritis Rheum., 24:S110, 1981.

111. Smiley, J.D., Sachs, C., and Ziff, M.: In vitro synthesis of immunoglobulin by rheumatoid synovial membrane. J. Clin. Invest., 47:624–632, 1968.

112. Smith, C., Habermann, E., and Hamerman, D.: A technique for investigating the antigenicity of cultured rheumatoid synovial cells. J. Rheumatol., 6:147–155, 1979.

113. Smith, C., and Hamerman, D.: Significance of persistent differences between normal and rheumatoid synovial membrane cells in culture. Arthritis Rheum., 12:639–645, 1969.

114. Snell, G.D.: T cells, T cell recognition structures and the major histocompatibility complex. Immunol. Rev., 38:3, 1978.

115. Spruance, S.L., et al.: DNA polymerase activity of cultured rheumatoid synovial cells. Arthritis Rheum., 18:229–235, 1975.

116. Stage, D.E., and Mannik, M.: 7S γ M-globulin in rheumatoid arthritis. Arthritis Rheum., 14:440–450, 1971.

117. Starkebaum, G., Singer, J.W., and Arend, W.P.: Humoral and cellular immune mechanisms of neutropenia in patients with Felty's syndrome. Clin. Exp. Immunol., 39:307–314, 1979.

118. Stastny, P., et al.: Lymphokines in rheumatoid synovitis. Ann. N.Y. Acad. Sci., *256*:117–131, 1975.
119. Stewart, S.M., Alexander, W.R.M., and Duthie, J.J.R.: Isolation of diphtheroid bacilli from synovial membrane and fluid in rheumatoid arthritis. Ann. Rheum. Dis., *28*:477–487, 1969.
120. Stierle, H.E., et al.: Increased responsiveness of rheumatoid B lymphocytes to stimulation by Epstein-Barr virus. Rheumat. Int., *3*:7–11, 1983.
121. Taylor-Upsahl, M.M., Abrahamsen, T.G., and Natvig, J.B.: Rheumatoid factor plaque-forming cells in rheumatoid synovial tissue. Clin. Exp. Immunol., *28*:197–203, 1977.
122. Theofilopoulos, A.N., et al.: IgG rheumatoid factor and low molecular weight IgM. Arthritis Rheum., *17*:272–284, 1974.
123. Tosato, G., et al.: Elevated Epstein-Barr virus infected B cells in the blood of patients with rheumatoid arthritis. Clin. Res., *31*:522A, 1983.
124. Tosato, G., Steinberg, A.D., and Blaese, R.M.: Defective EBV-specific suppressor T cell function in rheumatoid arthritis. N. Engl. J. Med., *305*:1238–1243, 1981.
125. Trentham, D.E.: Collagen arthritis as a relevant model for rheumatoid arthritis: Evidence pro and con. Arthritis Rheum., *25*:911–916, 1982.
126. Urman, J.D., and Bobrove, A.M.: Acute polyarthritis and infectious mononucleosis. West. J. Med., *136*:151–153, 1982.
127. Utsinger, P.D.: Enteropathic arthritis. *In* Textbook of Rheumatology. Edited by W.N. Kelley, et al. Philadelphia, W.B. Saunders, 1984.
128. Venables, P.J.W., et al.: Titers of antibody to RANA in rheumatoid arthritis and normal sera. Arthritis Rheum., *24*:1459–1464, 1981.
129. Vincent, P.C., Levi, J.A., and Macqueen, A.: The mechanism of neutropenia in Felty's syndrome. Br. J. Haematol., *27*:463–475, 1974.
130. Wands, J.R., et al.: The pathogenesis of arthritis associated with acute hepatitis B surface antigen positive hepatitis. J. Clin. Invest., *55*:930–936, 1975.
131. Ward, P.A., and Zvaifler, N.J.: Complement derived leukotactic factors in inflammatory synovial fluids of humans. J. Clin. Invest., *50*:606–616, 1971.
132. Weibel, R.E., et al.: Rubella vaccination in adult females. N. Engl. J. Med., *280*:682–685, 1969.
133. Weiner, S.R., and Utsinger, P.D.: Viral arthritis: A review of the literature and report of 15 new cases. Semin. Arthritis Rheum. In press, 1984.
134. Weinstein, A., et al.: Metabolism of the third component of complement (C3) in patients with rheumatoid arthritis. Arthritis Rheum., *15*:49–56, 1972.
135. Weisman, M.H., and Zvaifler, N.J.: Cryoglobulinemia in rheumatoid arthritis. J. Clin. Invest., *56*:725–730, 1975.
136. Weisman, M.H., and Zvaifler, N.J.: Cryoimmunoglobulinemia in Felty's syndrome. Arthritis Rheum., *19*:103–110, 1975.
137. Wiik, A., and Munthe, E.: Complement fixing granulocyte specific antinuclear factors in neutropenic cases of rheumatoid arthritis. Immunology, *26*:1127–1134, 1974.
138. Wilkes, P.H., et al.: Virologic studies on rheumatoid arthritis. Arthritis Rheum., *16*:446–454, 1973.
139. Winchester, R.J.: Characterization of IgG complexes in patients with rheumatoid arthritis. Ann. N.Y. Acad. Sci., *256*:73–81, 1975.
140. Winchester, R.J., Agnello, V., and Kunkel, H.G.: Gamma globulin complexes in synovial fluids in patients with rheumatoid arthritis: Partial characterization and relationship to lowered complement levels. Clin. Exp. Immunol., *6*:689–706, 1970.
141. Yefenof, E., Klein, G., and Kvarnunzk, J.: Relationship between complement activation, complement binding, and EBV absorption by human hematopoietic cell lines. Cell. Immunol., *31*:225–233, 1977.
142. Zvaifler, N.J.: The immunopathology of joint inflammation in rheumatoid arthritis. Adv. Immunol., *16*:265–337, 1973.

Chapter 36

Pathology of Rheumatoid Arthritis and Allied Disorders

Leon Sokoloff and Aubrey J. Hough, Jr.

The principal lesions of rheumatoid arthritis (RA) are found in the diarthrodial joints and, to a lesser extent, in the related tissues—tendons and their sheaths, bursae, and periarticular subcutaneous tissue. The systemic manifestations, the subject of much study during the past three decades, suggest use of the term "rheumatoid disease." Although extra-articular lesions undoubtedly occur, their incidence should not be exaggerated; they are far less frequent and severe than lesions in the joints.

Excellent descriptions of the long-standing joint changes have been published.[41] Knowledge of the morbid anatomy of RA is limited by a number of factors. The chronicity of the disease often makes tissue available for study only in its late stages. The lesions often lack histologic specificity and vary from site to site within the joints.[27] The structures principally affected are frequently not accessible to the pathologist. For these reasons, light and immunomicroscopic study of biopsy material obtained early in the course of the illness has provided insights into the histogenesis of the lesions that have not been possible on postmortem examination.[77]

ARTICULAR LESIONS

All evidence indicates that the joint changes have their inception in the synovial tissue. Despite similarities in the character of the synovitis to that of infectious conditions and despite the prominent subchondral involvement of the bone in RA, no basis exists for believing that the synovial inflammation follows an initial seeding of the adjacent bone marrow, as it commonly does in hematogenous, infectious arthritis (Fig. 36–1).

Synovitis

The microscopic appearance of the synovial tissues is variable.[26] Three pathologic elements, although integrally related and continuous, should be distinguished: (1) exudation; (2) cellular infiltration; and (3) granulation tissue development. See also Chapter 13.

Exudation

Congestion and the edema are most marked at the internal surface of the synovium, particularly close to margins of the articular cartilage (circulus vasculosus), and have their counterpart in effusion into the joint space. In focal areas of desquamation of synovial lining cells and of necrosis of the superficial synovial tissue, compact fibrin exudes onto the surface and, to some extent, into the swollen tissues (see Chap. 9 for evidence of synovial ischemia in RA).

Cellular Infiltration

Small numbers of polymorphonuclear leukocytes emigrate with edema fluid. Foci of necrosis and purulent exudation are seen at times in older lesions, and the concept of secondary infection need not be invoked on this score.

The principal infiltrating cell, particularly in early lesions, is a small lymphocyte. It is distributed in two patterns in the superficial positions of the synovium: diffusely and in small, nodular aggregates. These cells may or may not be arranged about small blood vessels. The nodular aggregates, sometimes called *Allison-Ghormley nodules*, characteristically lack the reticular framework of lymphoid nodules. In long-standing lesions, true lymphoid follicles with germinal centers are not rare (Fig. 36–2). Close cell-to-cell contacts between lymphocytes and plasma cells have been seen with electron microscopy.[92] Many of the lymphocytes in the synovial infiltrates are T cells.[129] Recently, OKT4 and OKT8 antibodies have distinguished two categories of T cells, helper-inducer and suppressor-cytotoxic, in the synovium.[31,73] The proportion of OKT8 cells is reduced in early perivenular lesions and is increased in late areas, in which macrophage-like cells are increased in numbers and lymphocyte transformation takes place. Natural killer (NK) activity is lower in RA synovial and synovial fluid lymphocytes than in peripheral blood, where NK cell levels are normal.[29a]

In late cases, a large proportion or even a majority of the infiltrating cells are immunoglobulin-producing plasma cells.[102] When the synovium is

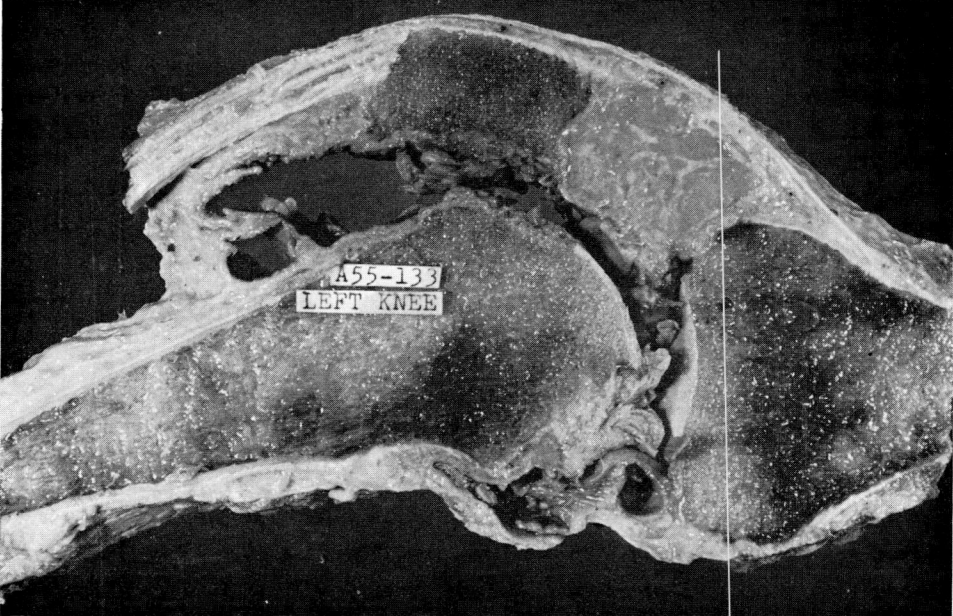

Fig. 36–1. Sagittal section of the knee in a patient with RA. Thickened, villous synovial tissue is seen in the suprapatellar pouch. A small Baker's cyst protrudes from the popliteal surface. A papillary pannus has completely replaced the articular cartilage of the patella and smaller segments on the femur and tibia. The dark portions of the marrow of the femur and tibia are areas of congestion and osteitis.

stained with labeled aggregated IgG, fluorescein, or ferritin tagging in electron micrographs, is found principally in the cytoplasm of the plasma cell, demonstrating a local synthesis of rheumatoid factors.[95] Areas of old hemorrhage are common, as evidenced by deposition of hemosiderin[97] and, sometimes, by the presence of foam cells.

Multinucleated giant cells are not common, but two types may be seen.[49] One is an ovoid pleomorphic cell, close to the synovial lining. It has three to eight peripheral nuclei (Fig. 36–3) and a basophilic cytoplasm similar to those of synovial lining cells. The other type of multinucleated cell is a foreign body phagocyte related to bone and cartilage detritus.

Granulation Tissue

As a result of these processes, the synovial tissue becomes grossly thickened. Proliferation of blood vessels and of synovial fibroblasts is most marked in areas of cellular infiltration and is accompanied by multiplication and enlargement of synovial lining cells. The lining cells become elongated in places and are oriented in a closely arranged palisade perpendicular to the surface. The hypertrophy has a villous character most marked near the joint cartilages. The papillary fronds may reach 2.5 cm in height and are approximately 1 to 2 mm in diameter (see Fig. 36–1). They may or may not ad-

here to each other. The oxygen uptake, glucose use, and lactate production of the tissue are increased as a result of both proliferation of granulation tissue and the infiltration of inflammatory cells.[29] Lining cells are stained heavily by several histochemical diaphorase procedures and have a prominent endoplasmic reticulum,[42] evidence of high metabolic and secretory activity. They also contain many lysosomes[49] and immune complex components.[145] Variable, sometimes extensive, ulceration of the synovial lining is a common feature of active RA. Necrotic fronds of the villous tissue are infiltrated with fibrin or fibrin-like protein. When sloughed into the synovial cavity, they constitute rice bodies.[4] The collagen types and proportions of rice bodies are identical to those in RA synovium.[18,75] Immunohistochemical demonstration[105] of fibrin and fibronectin[115] in loose-textured rice bodies documents organization of exudate as a feature of their development. Only in this sense is fibrin the defining feature of an "early" rice body and is collagen formation the defining feature of a late one. The initial source of the collagen is synovium and its granulation tissue that have undergone necrosis and ulceration.

Although these changes are typically present in RA, they lack histologic specificity. Statistical analysis has shown a correspondence between histologic features and clinical diagnosis in only 54

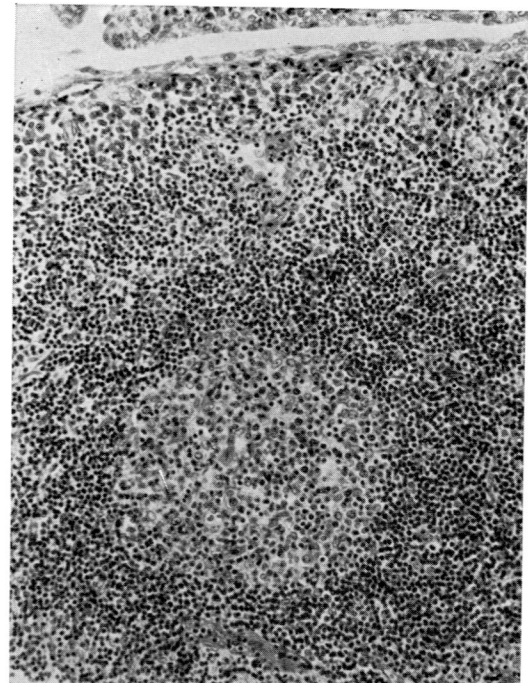

Fig. 36–2. Chronic synovitis in long-standing RA. In addition to the usual diffuse infiltration of chronic inflammatory cells into the synovial tissue, a true lymphoid follicle with a germinal center is present. The larger cells, subjacent to the swollen synovial lining, are plasma cells. (H & E, × 182.)

to 78% of chronic arthritic disorders.[26,111] Indistinguishable changes may be seen in unrelated disorders in man[46] and in other species.[122]

Subchondral Bone Lesions

An inflammatory reaction commonly occurs in the epiphyseal bone. Its histologic character is similar to that of synovial tissue, although numbers of osteoclasts are also present. The subchondral granulation tissue is continuous with that in the synovium, through defects in the cortex of the bone near the joint. These defects are presumed originally to have been normal vascular foramina, enlarged by osteitis. Grossly, the bone marrow appears congested in these areas. The bone undergoes irregular osteolysis, which accounts for the loss of radiopacity in the para-articular tissues. In juvenile patients, the osteitis may extend into the epiphyseal plate; in such instances, bone growth is retarded, and rheumatic dwarfism results. Sizable cyst-like areas of bone destruction may be present (Fig. 36–4). Bony erosion occurs preferentially in areas not covered by articular cartilage, the so-called "bare areas." The articular cortex also is involved by the osteolysis. Side by side with the osteolysis,

new bone formation occurs, and remodeling of the bone progresses under the direction of mechanical forces acting on the joint. In phalanges, "periosteitis" is frequently described as part of RA, but is not accurate, strictly speaking. The synovial recesses in the phalanges are frequently large and extend for a long distance proximally on the bone shafts. In such instances, the synovitis may evoke new bone formation in the immediately adjacent cortex. Nevertheless, periosteitis, unrelated to synovitis, is not characteristic of RA; this feature distinguishes RA from Reiter's disease and from infectious arthritis. Osteoporosis often persists in burned-out, deformed specimens and may be attributed to disuse atrophy. At times, severe and widespread osteoporosis, for which no immediate explanation can be offered, is encountered.*

Lesions of Articular Cartilage

The articular cartilage is resistant to inflammatory lysis. Its surface is involved by extension of the inflammatory process from the adjacent synovium; the granulation tissue that forms a covering mantle is known as a *pannus* (see Fig. 36–1). In contemporary specimens, the pannus is usually inconspicuous, unlike that illustrated in Figure 36–1 and in classic accounts. Perhaps this change is the result of active use associated with present-day physiatric measures or better medical therapy. The destructive changes in the cartilage are most conspicuous at the junction with the synovium; in the femoral head, this means the perifoveal as well as the peripheral margin. The eroded areas have an irregular, "chewed-out" configuration, but are sharply defined. They thus differ both in quality and in location from the cartilaginous lesions of osteoarthritis.

Like hypertrophic synovitis,[26,46] pannus formation is not a specific feature of RA. Concurrent with the ingrowth of the pannus and the subchondral granulation tissue,[71,117] the articular cartilage disappears. A possible mechanism for this process is provided in Chapter 37. Immediately adjacent chondrocytes are often necrotic. The fine structure of the surface is often disturbed, even when the cartilage appears normal grossly.[68] Whether granulations themselves destroy the cartilage or whether they represent a concomitant to an exudative, chondrolytic inflammation is unknown. Numerous explanations for the cartilage destruction accompanying pannus formation are supported by experimental and pathologic observations. Vas-

---

Editor's note: Osteoclastic activation, even at sites remote from the inflamed joints,[66] has led to speculation that lymphokines, such as osteoclast-activating factor (OAF) are responsible.

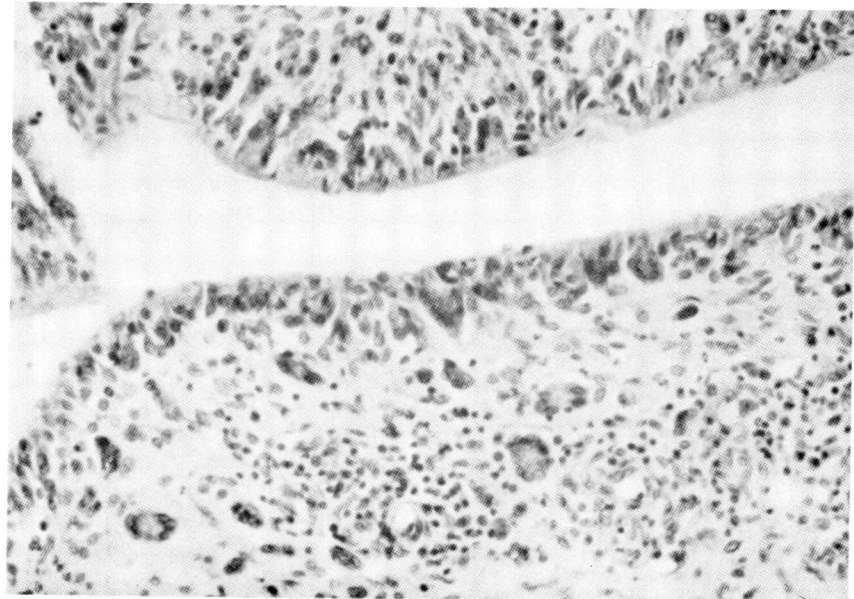

Fig. 36–3.   Synovitis in RA. Synovial lining cells are elongated and are arranged in a palisade radial to the surface. Some of the lining cells appear multinucleated, and similar giant cells are located at a slight distance from them. (H & E, × 234.)

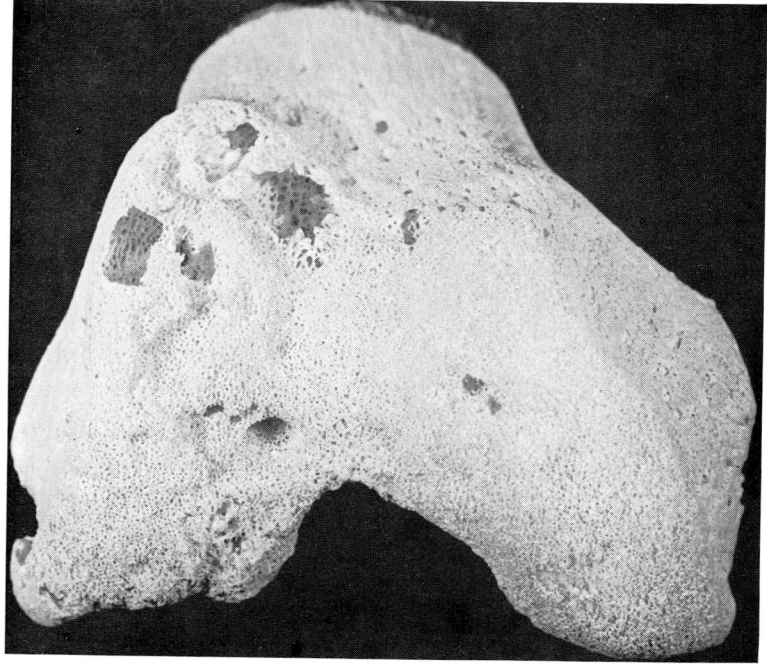

Fig. 36–4.   Advanced destruction of the articular cortex of the distal femur in RA. What appear to be cystic spaces and pores in this macerated preparation are occupied in vivo by granulation tissue in the subchondral marrow and adhesions in the joint cavity.

cularity may allow leaching out of cartilage matrix, which normally retains its integrity by being avascular.[85] Other views are that the pannus may impede the normal, nourishing percolation of interstitial fluid through the cartilage. Several different enzymatic mechanisms have been proposed for chondrolysis. These enzymes include collagenase and neutral proteases derived from polymorphonuclear leukocytes,[83,86] catheptic enzymes originating in synovial lining cells, and collagenase from the synovial granulation tissue.[50,141] Cells elaborating collagenase have been characterized by a dendritic appearance in monolayer cultures of synovium.[140] Collagen fibrils have been observed in the cytoplasm of pannus cells.[51] Recently, macrophages have been shown to elaborate catabolin-like substances that stimulate chondrocytes to resorb matrix,[61] and macrophage-like cells synthesizing prostaglandin E have been identified in RA.[117] Polymorphonuclear neutrophils are not readily apparent at the joint surface in conventional sections; however, they have been found in special concentrations at the pannus-cartilage interface by histochemical staining for polymorphonuclear elastase[83] and by electron microscopy.[86] The role of direct immune attack on articular cartilage in RA has been summarized by Cooke.[25] Using immunofluorescent staining, he found intense granular deposits of IgG and C3 in the cartilage of 85 to 92% of subjects with classic RA. Less consistent or intense amounts of IgA and IgM were present. The deposits were confined to the most superficial 0.3 mm or so of the surface. The degraded appearance of the surface was comparable to that seen in experimentally induced enzymic digestion.

Late changes may include a dense fibrous connective tissue replacing the hyaline cartilage and penetrating the subchondral bone. This process may or may not be associated with ankylosis. Secondary osteoarthritic changes are also common in long-standing lesions.

Ankylosis

The granulation tissue may form adhesions and may undergo cicatrization. The newly formed articular connective tissue has a pluripotential capacity for maturation. It may variously undergo metaplasia into synovial tissue, fibrous or hyaline cartilage, or bone; the adhesive bands may thereby cause fibrous, cartilaginous, or, rarely, bony ankylosis (Fig. 36–5).

Joint Deformities

Several factors contribute to the deformities of RA. Most important of these is the inflammatory destruction and remodeling of the articulating surfaces under the influence of the mechanical forces

of muscle pull. These changes may lead to subluxation (Fig. 36–6). Weakening of capsular and ligamentous supports by the inflammation may be of considerable importance, particularly in small joints, where these tissues are in close proximity to the synovium. Tendon contractures and ruptures also are an important element in finger and toe deformities (Fig. 36–7). Secondary osteoarthritic changes are common in long-standing lesions, but the degree of bony proliferation is ordinarily less than that seen in primary or mechanically derived degenerative joint disease.[58]

VERTEBRAL LESIONS

In RA, the cervical spine is often affected.[6] Both the diarthrodial (apophyseal) joints and the intervertebral discs may be involved.[1] Sometimes, extensive destruction of spinal ligaments occurs as well. Ball observed the destruction of the anulus fibrosus to proceed with formation of granulation tissue from synovitis of the neurocentral (Luschka) joints in 17 of 18 unselected cases. The interspinous bursae were affected in 2 of 9 subjects studied at necropsy by Bywaters.[11] Instances of cervical spine RA with little or no peripheral joint involvement have been reported. The inflammatory changes are like those described later in this chapter with regard to the tendons and ligaments of the peripheral joints. These changes cause subluxation at times and may lead to neurologic defects or, occasionally, sudden death. Destructive lesions of lumbar vertebral bodies by rheumatoid nodules have been described on several occasions.[121] Apophyseal joint involvement in this region has also been described radiologically,[12] but it is less frequent and less severe than in the cervical region.[1]

SUBCUTANEOUS NODULES

In approximately one of five patients with peripheral RA, chronic inflammatory nodules develop in para-articular subcutaneous tissue. These nodules are most common over the olecranon process of the ulna. Less frequently, they are found on the extensor aspects of the finger joints, in the achilles tendon ("pump bumps"), or in the occiput in bedridden patients. Any subcutaneous tissue subject to mechanical pressure may be involved, and individual patients show great variation in nodule development in response to pressure.

Subcutaneous nodules in RA are usually larger than those of rheumatic fever and may reach a diameter of several centimeters. Large nodules are tough, lobulated, and multicentric. They are not encapsulated and cannot be sharply dissected from underlying articular tissue, bursae, or periosteum. Geographic areas of necrosis are recognized by their yellow color because lipochrome pigments

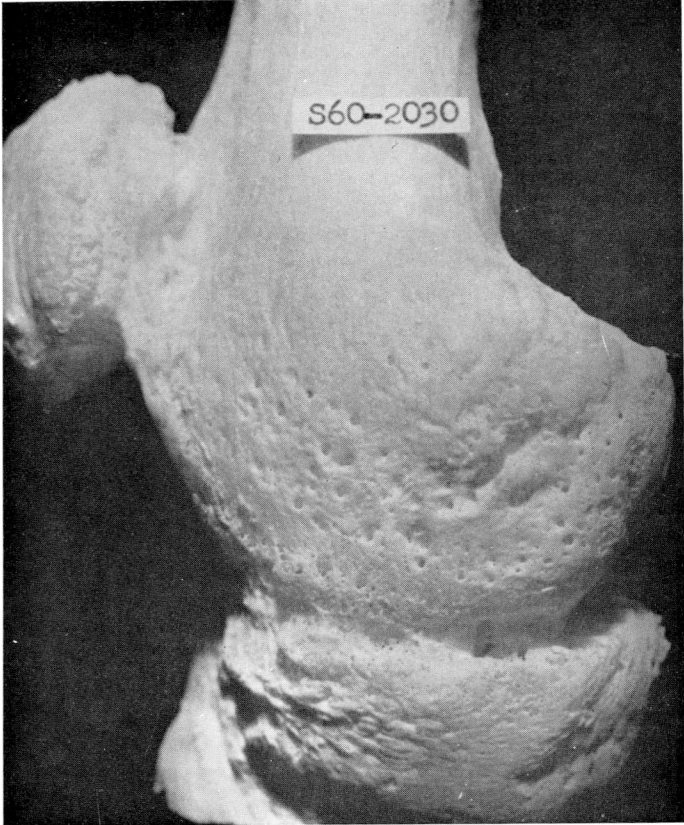

Fig. 36–5. Bony ankylosis of the knee in RA. A bridge of bone unites the patella of the femur and the condyles of the femur and tibial plateau to each other.

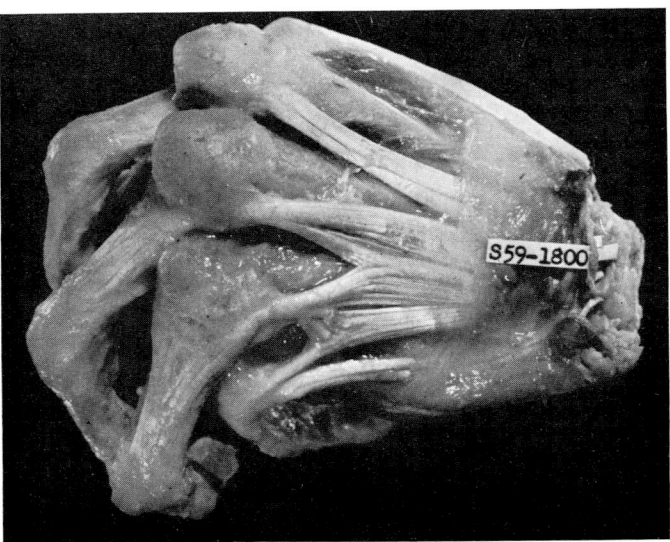

Fig. 36–6. Characteristic knuckle deformities in RA. The proximal phalanges are subluxated beneath the metacarpal heads. The tendons are displaced from their normal position over the center of the joint in association with the ulnar deviation of the fingers. No gross inflammatory change is present in the tendons, however, unlike in Figure 36–7.

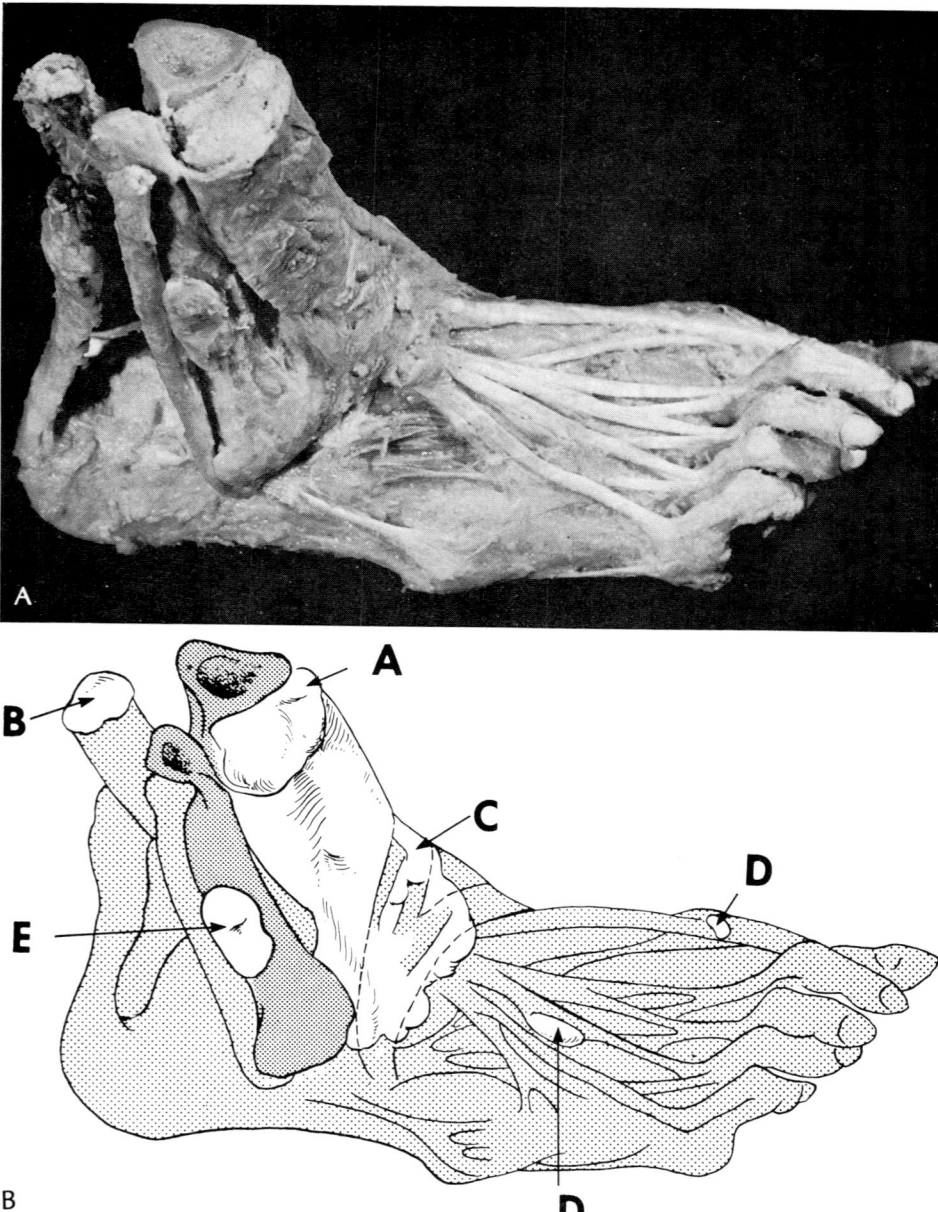

Fig. 36–7. *A* and *B*, Tendon and tendon sheath involvement in RA. *B*, White grumous exudate occupies the substance and sheaths of the anterior tibial and extensor digitorum tendons (A), and the Achilles tendon (B). The inferior extensor retinaculum (C) is irregularly infiltrated, and nodules are also present in the extensor tendons of the foot (D). The surface of the tendons is irregular and dull because of inflammatory adhesions. The changes are responsible for the cock-up deformities of the toes. A subcutaneous nodule (E) adheres to the periosteum of the fibula immediately anterior to the peroneus longus tendon.

accompany the large amounts of lipid, in the form of neutral fat, cholesterol, and phospholipids, deposited in the necrotic material.

The histologic appearance of a well-developed subcutaneous rheumatoid nodule is characteristic. It resembles many infectious or foreign body granulomas in that it has three distinct zones: (1) a central area of necrosis of subcutaneous fibrous and granulation tissue; (2) a palisade of elongated, connective tissue cells arranged radially in a corona about the necrotic zone; and (3) an enveloping granulation tissue in which chronic inflammatory cells are distributed (Fig. 36–8).

In long-standing lesions, the palisade is less apparent, and acellular fibrous tissue predominates; however, recrudescent activity may produce newer inflammatory foci adjacent to older, ''mature'' foci.

The necrotic centers have, to a varying extent, a ''fibrinoid'' appearance. This term should not be used to indicate a specific compound, a single pathogenetic significance, or identity with pathologic materials in other rheumatic or nonrheumatic disorders. It is a histologic term and simply describes the necrotic material as being oxyphilic and refractive and reacting to certain stains in the manner of fibrin rather than of collagen. The composition of the necrotic material in the rheumatoid nodule varies as the lesion progresses or ''burns out.'' It contains collagen, lipids, nucleoproteins, acid mucopolysaccharides, serum proteins, including immunoglobulins,[40,96] and, in certain active states,

material that probably is fibrin. The fibrin-like component is most prominent in active or new lesions. The lipid material may persist in an otherwise semifluid center of the nodule and may convert the nodule to a bursa-like or cystic structure. Unlike many types of persistent, lipid-rich necrotic debris, calcification of rheumatoid nodules is rare. Erosion of bone by nodules has been reported,[30] but is also a rarity.

The precise nature of the cells in the marginal palisade has not been established.[21] Although the cells to a certain degree resemble and sometimes are called epithelioid cells, as in tuberculoid granulomas, they also have fibroblastic characteristics. By electron microscopy, macrophage-like cells have been identified in the palisade zone and in the proliferating granulation tissue surrounding active nodules.[21,44] Acid phosphatase activity, indicative of a histiocytic nature, is present in these cells. Cytoplasmic fat droplets may abound in the palisaded cells and may also be present in the adjacent necrotic tissue. Whether the droplets reflect the phagocytosis of lipid, derived from the blood or from ground substance, or whether they are products of the cells has not been established. Multinucleated giant cells, occasionally seen in such areas, however, are usually of the Touton type and presumably are lipophages. The cells assume their radial arrangement because their axes are oriented against the fibers entering the zones of necrosis. The enveloping granulation tissue, vascular in its early stages,[40] ultimately cicatrizes. Lymphocytes

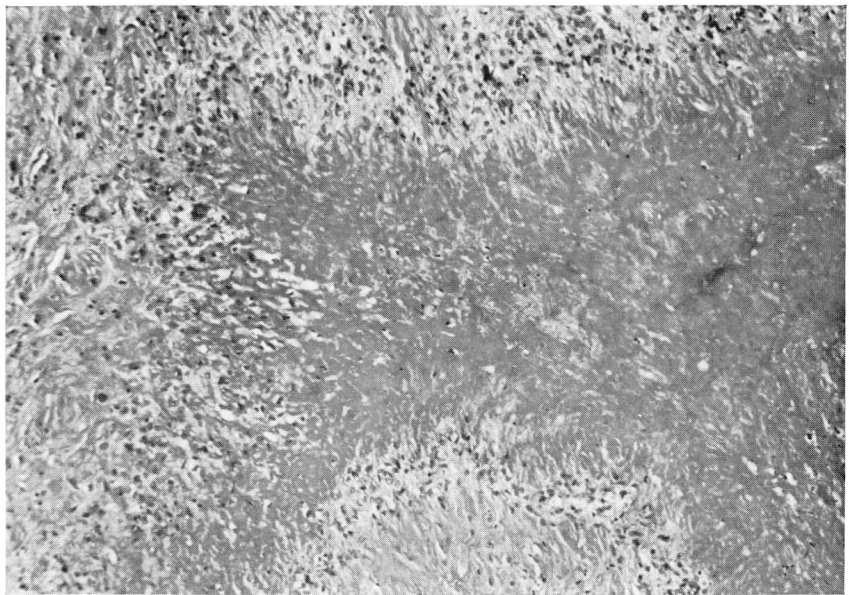

Fig. 36–8. Subcutaneous nodule of RA. Although this is a long-standing lesion, the presence of nuclear fragments in the ''fibrinoid'' central zone is presumptive evidence of recent necrosis. (H & E, × 95.)

and smaller numbers of plasma cells are disposed about some of the peripheral venules. In the proliferating areas of vascularity, the perivascular cells are primarily plump fibroblasts and mononuclear cells. Scattered eosinophils may be present in the earliest lesions.

This granuloma-like appearance of the subcutaneous nodule of RA is different from that usually found in the joints. A variant of RA has been described wherein synovitis is inconspicuous but many subcutaneous nodules are present.[45] Nodules can at times be confused diagnostically with tuberculous and other lesions such as necrobiosis lipoidica and granuloma annulare (Table 36–1). Granted that nodules may appear in advance of articular manifestations, para-articular lesions of this sort also occur in individuals who have no evidence of any rheumatic disease. These idiopathic subcutaneous nodules present a spectrum of appearances; they may resemble lesions of rheumatic fever, rheumatoid arthritis, and granuloma annulare.[84,135] The appearance of the early subcutaneous nodule is different from that of the older lesion, as discussed previously.

LESIONS OF TENDONS AND LIGAMENTS

The tendons and articular ligaments are involved pathologically with considerable, though undetermined, frequency. The inflammatory process is usually nonspecific; lymphocytes, mononuclear cells, and a few plasma cells infiltrate the bundles of collagen. In severe instances, focal areas of "fibrinoid" necrosis develop, and the lesion may be identical to a subcutaneous nodule. The nodular areas are at times palpable grossly (see Fig. 36–7). Ruptures may take place in such areas of necrosis.[33] Where the tendons lie in sheaths, tendinitis is accompanied by tenosynovitis. The ruptures and adhesions of the tendons to each other and to adjacent tissue are an integral part of the development of joint deformities in many instances.

STRIATED MUSCLE LESIONS

The skeletal muscle in severe cases of RA frequently has the histologic appearance of disuse atrophy.[76] The type 2 myofibers are affected primarily, as is usual in disuse and most other types of atrophy. An irregular diminution in the circumference of the fibers is seen, with a corresponding condensation of sarcolemmal nuclei. Immunoglobulin is localized to arteriolar walls and perimysial connective tissue in RA and in other immunologically mediated connective tissue diseases.[67,99]

In approximately 2 of every 3 patients with RA, scattered focal compact aggregates of chronic inflammatory cells, principally lymphocytes, are

Table 36–1.   Differential Pathologic Diagnosis of Subcutaneous Nodules

Lesion	Depth	Common Site	Histopathologic Characteristics*
Rheumatoid nodule	Subcutaneous	Pressure points (e.g., olecranon)	Multicentric fibrinoid necrosis; palisading
Rheumatic fever nodule	Subcutaneous	Pressure points	Fibrinoid edema; some palisading; smaller than preceding
Granuloma annulare	Dermal	Dorsum of hands and feet	Mucoid edema; palisading
Pseudorheumatoid nodule ("deep granuloma annulare")	Subcutaneous	Anterior tibial tubercle, Achilles tendon	Similar to preceding; more nonspecific granulation tissue
Necrobiosis lipoidica	Subcutaneous	Anterior thigh, leg	Necrosis of fat and collagenous tissue; foam cell reaction and variable palisading
Erythema nodosum	Subcutaneous	Anterior leg	Chronic inflammation, often granulomatous, in veins and interlobular septa
Tophus	Subcutaneous	Olecranon, dorsum of hands	Urate crystals in amorphous matrix, with foreign body reaction
Tuberculous granuloma	Subcutaneous	Olecranon bursa	Caseous necrosis; epithelioid and Langhans cells
Epidermoid cyst	Subcutaneous	Olecranon	Keratotic material within epidermoid lining
Fibrous histiocytoma (tendon sheath xanthoma)	Subcutaneous	Flexor aspect of finger	Hemosiderin-laden mononuclear and foam cells; may coexist with rheumatoid nodules
Xanthoma tuberosum	Subcutaneous	Dorsum of fingers, olecranon, Achilles tendon	Foam cells; cholesterol crystal granuloma

*A palisade is regarded in this context as a layer of elongated connective tissue cells oriented along the axis of collagenous fibers entering the zone of edema or necrosis.

seen about venules in endomysium or perimysium. The lesion is lacking in diagnostic specificity, but is more common in RA and its variants than in nonrheumatic disorders. Unlike dermatomyositis, necrosis and regenerative activity are not conspicuous features.

PERIPHERAL NERVE INVOLVEMENT

Perivascular aggregates of lymphocytes and mononuclear cells, comparable to those of striated muscle, are also present in the endoneurium and perineurium of peripheral nerves in patients with RA. Myelin and axon changes are not present unless arterial disease is a complication. Entrapment of nerves by thickened inflammatory tissue is by far the most frequent cause of neuropathy in RA.[67,91] The carpal tunnel is the most common location, but other sites are also affected. The changes in the nerves result from compression rather than from intrinsic inflammation. Other than minute perivascular cellular infiltrates, lesions have not been seen in conventional sections of the sympathetic ganglia.

LESIONS OF ARTERIES

Arterial lesions of varying severity and character have been recognized in numerous studies of RA; no unanimity exists as to their significance.[123] Several anatomic facts appear reasonably certain: (1) the arteritis affects principally small segments of terminal arteries, 250 to 400 μm in external diameter; (2) the lesions are chronic and lack distinctive histologic characteristics; and (3) although these lesions may occur in many areas, the principal sites of involvement are the peripheral nerves and skeletal muscle. At one end of the spectrum of vascular lesions is the non-necrotizing, segmental arteritis of striated muscle that can be detected only when extensive serial sections have been made. This form of arteritis has been demonstrated in approximately 10% of unselected cases. At the other end of the clinical spectrum is a fulminant systemic disease that is difficult to distinguish from polyarteritis nodosa (PAN), either on clinical or on anatomic grounds. This fulminant disease is far less common than the non-necrotizing disorder.

Among the hypotheses on the nature of the arteritis is that it results from treatment of RA with corticosteroid hormones. Corticosteroid therapy of other than rheumatic disorders has, on rare occasions, also been reported as complicated by necrotizing arteritis. Nonetheless, arteritis unquestionably may be seen in patients with RA who have not received such compounds. A widespread belief that this sort of therapy has increased the incidence of vasculitis has received no support.[107]

Another view is that the arteritis is a form of

PAN that reflects humoral hypersensitivity, sometimes postulated to underlie the development of RA. Several important differences between the usual vascular lesions of RA and those of PAN exist, however.[35] In RA, the lesions are usually mild, few, and affecting minute vessels. In PAN, the arteritis is widespread and involves medium-sized, rather than small, arteries. Obliteration of the lumen or ectasia and rupture are characteristic of PAN. The prognosis of PAN is often ominous, whereas the vascular lesions of RA have been known to exist for many years without causing detectable symptoms. In PAN, cutaneous gangrene of the extremities is most unusual, whereas it is frequent in RA when corticosteroid therapy has been administered. The nosologic status of PAN itself is also uncertain (see Chap. 63).

It seems likely that the vasculitis is a specific manifestation of RA that shares etiologic or pathogenetic factors with the joint disease and mediates the development of that disease. This view is based on the observation that vasculitis is an intrinsic part of the development of the granulomatous subcutaneous nodules.[40] In the early nodule, the important histologic processes are exudation of fibrin-rich edema fluid into subcutaneous fibrous tissue, formation of vascular granulation tissue,[44,123] proliferation of plump fibroblasts, and apparently also of macrophages, and necrosis of small arteries and more minute blood vessels.[21] The exudation and necrosis proceed centrifugally about the nodular buds of granulation tissue. These foci eventually coalesce to form the characteristic necrotic centers of the mature nodules. Some researchers emphasize the venular rather than terminal arterial disturbances in the genesis of these lesions. This process is histologically distinct from the superficial dermal necrosis of the legs occasionally resulting from RA. Another variant, leukocytoclastic vasculitis, is a feature of a variety of rheumatic disorders, but is infrequent in RA.[116]

Clinically manifest arteritis is frequently associated with high titers of rheumatoid factor, particularly of low-molecular-weight species,[88,127] as well as with the presence of subcutaneous nodules. The arteritis in peripheral nerves is one cause of the peripheral neuropathy that sometimes complicates RA (see Chap. 39).[32]

IMMUNOPATHOLOGY

Granular deposits of IgG, IgM, anti-IgG, C3, C4, and fibrinogen or fibrin, but not of albumin, are commonly found by immunofluorescent staining in the lining cells, matrix, and blood vessels of the synovium.[145] Their frequency is greater in seropositive than in seronegative patients and still more so than in noninflammatory joint diseases.

The occurrence of immunoglobulins in subcutaneous nodules has already been noted.

In overt, untreated arteritis, immunohistochemical studies have disclosed immune complex components.[43] In lesions from patients treated with corticosteroids, a proliferative endarteritis devoid of immune complex deposits has been found. Our own experience coincides with that of others that such complexes may be present at the inception of the lesion and may then be removed by leukocytes as the cellular infiltrate evolves. In other circumstances, arterioles in muscle and minute vessels in skin contain components of immune complexes,[23,24] but they are not associated with leukocytic infiltration. It is not known why such immune deposits elicit an inflammatory response in some instances and not in others.

The electron microscopic appearance of the infiltrate is consistent with an interaction among immunologic cell types involving both cellular and humoral responses.[144] A further discussion of the role of immunity in RA is found in Chapter 35.

CARDIAC LESIONS

In the past, most clinical studies found cardiac abnormalities to be uncommon; anatomic investigations, by contrast, demonstrated frequent lesions of several sorts. The disparity has been reduced by sensitive echocardiographic techniques[55] that yield clinical data[70,93,119,128] more in accord with pathologic findings.[62,108,109]

Rheumatic Heart Disease

Although rheumatic heart disease was reported in many older postmortem studies in 21 to 66% of patients, most recent papers have placed the figure, exclusive of calcareous aortic stenosis, at 6 to 10%. Several reasons exist for this lack of consistency and partly account for the high frequency of rheumatic heart disease sometimes reported in studies of RA.

Idiopathic Pericarditis

Virtually all necropsy studies have demonstrated remote or active pericarditis in approximately 40% of cases of RA. Usually, this disorder is manifested by fibrous obliteration of the pericardial cavity. Infrequently, the lesion has a granuloma-like character resembling that of the rheumatoid nodule or synovial lesion.[62] It is only the frequent association with arthritis that supports the rheumatoid nature of the process. Significant clinical consequences, recognized infrequently,[69] include pericardial constriction necessitating pericardiotomy, fatal hemopericardium, and pericardial effusion with tamponade.

Interstitial Myocarditis

In addition to occasional granuloma-like rheumatoid nodules in the myocardium, small infarcts secondary to coronary arteritis have been observed rarely, some surrounded by a palisade of elongated cells and some not. More often, however, focal idiopathic, nonspecific interstitial myocarditis is seen. In some instances, the leukocytic infiltrate includes many eosinophils. Whether allergic or other drug toxicity or viral infection complicating therapy, and not the rheumatoid disease, may be the etiologic basis of some of the myocarditis cannot be ascertained in the absence of appropriate differential diagnostic tests.

Coronary Arteritis

Coronary arteritis, affecting scattered small vessels, is an occasional finding. It has been associated with disseminated arteritis in other sites, both splanchnic and in the extremities. Myocardial infarction and aortitis[108] may be associated with coronary involvement. As in the case of peripheral arteritis, some of the variation in the frequency of coronary involvement in different laboratory studies may be influenced by selection factors. The anatomic criteria for the differential diagnosis of rheumatic heart disease are imprecise.

Calcareous Aortic Stenosis

Whether all instances of this condition are due to rheumatic inflammation is unresolved. As in the acceptable rheumatic valvular lesions, the frequency of this abnormality also was greater in several studies of patients with RA than in controls.

Rheumatoid Heart Disease

Lesions resembling the granuloma-like subcutaneous nodules occur at times in the valve leaflets, valve rings, myocardium, or epicardium in patients with peripheral RA. Although considerable histologic variation exists, the active lesions differ from those of infectious or rheumatic carditis. Their frequency is difficult to estimate, but has been reported in various series as 2 of 19, 7 of 36, 5 of 100, and 10 of 43 necropsies. The order of frequency of involvement of the valves is as follows: (1) mitral; (2) aortic; (3) tricuspid; and (4) pulmonic. The valvular lesions differ from those of rheumatic carditis in that they are neither diffuse nor verrucous.[109] As in other viscera, the histologic appearance of cardiac rheumatoid nodules is often atypical. Clinically, some have been silent; others have produced valvular insufficiency, heart block, Adams-Stokes syndrome, and an electrocardiogram resembling that of infarction.[70]

The granuloma-like lesions may co-exist with pericarditis, coronary arteritis, and interstitial myocarditis, three other frequent findings, each of which are morphologically nonspecific but lack other explanations than the rheumatoid disease. In the pathologic diagnosis of any given case, co-existing systemic lupus erythematosus (SLE) may be a possibility. The end result of burned-out lesions may be similar to those of rheumatic heart disease and may account for some reports of increased frequency of rheumatic fever in RA patients.

Aortic Insufficiency

In ankylosing spondylitis, an apparently specific form of aortic valve insufficiency has been recorded.[10] These lesions are grossly similar to those of syphilis in that the principal changes relate to the gross destruction of the elastic tissue of the root of the aorta and the adjacent valve ring, but they differ from syphilitic aortitis in that they are confined to the root and do not affect the ascending aorta. The commissures of the valve are separated, and the edges of the leaflets are rolled toward the ventricular cavity as a result of regurgitation. This lesion does not occur in peripheral RA, although rheumatoid valvulitis may occasionally involve the aortic valve and may render it incompetent.

Miscellaneous Lesions

Postmortem findings support the long-standing impression that hypertension and myocardial infarction occur infrequently in RA. Coronary atherosclerosis was no less frequent or severe than in control subjects, but the infarctive consequences were reduced,[28] perhaps because of the hematologic effects of aspirin therapy. Even so, atherosclerotic heart disease probably accounts for most clinical cardiac dysfunction encountered in patients with RA.[7] Secondary amyloidosis, a rare complication of RA, infrequently affects the myocardium. Aortic insufficiency has been reported as an occasional finding in spondyloarthropathy-associated psoriasis and Reiter's disease. A chronic form of rheumatic fever may lead to deformities (*Jaccoud's arthritis*) of the joints as well as of the heart valves. The existence of this condition has not been completely accepted by American rheumatologists. Takayasu's disease is not generally regarded as a rheumatic condition, but isolated instances of aortic arch syndrome have been associated with RA.[34]

PULMONARY LESIONS

Three patterns of chronic pulmonary disease have been proposed as occasional manifestations of RA: (1) Caplan's syndrome; (2) granulomatous lesions; and (3) idiopathic interstitial pneumonia or diffuse interstitial fibrosis.

Caplan's Syndrome

This term refers to unusually large, silicotic nodule formation seen in anthracite coal miners afflicted with RA. Histologically, these lesions do not resemble rheumatoid nodules. In addition to a silica, they contain much amorphous material. It has been suggested that the exuberant character of these nodules is due to an altered tissue reactivity to the silica particles; however, the condition has also been described in several other pneumoconioses.[56] Although the lesion appears frequently in Great Britain, it is not common in the United States.[3]

Granulomatous Lesions

These lesions, resembling rheumatoid subcutaneous nodules, are infrequent findings in patients with RA. It may be difficult to distinguish them from infectious granulomas. Rarely, accompanying vasculitis suggests Wegener's granulomatosis. Extension of the nodules to the visceral pleura is characteristic of pulmonary rheumatoid nodules, as opposed to variants of Wegener's granulomatosis.[63]

Idiopathic Interstitial Pneumonia or Diffuse Interstitial Fibrosis

Whether idiopathic interstitial pneumonia or diffuse interstitial fibrosis of the lungs is a fortuitous finding or a true manifestation of RA has been debated. The recorded lesions do not have anatomic characteristics distinguishing them from the pulmonary fibrosis observed in systemic scleroderma or the Hamman-Rich syndrome.[64] Although the histologic changes are nonspecific, IgM has been demonstrated in alveolar septa and capillary walls.[17] Idiopathic interstitial pneumonia or diffuse interstitial fibrosis is seen in approximately 2% of patients with RA. Abnormalities in pulmonary function are more common.[37] Biopsies also have been cited to support this entity.[106] The interpretation of these data is clouded by the effects of smoking.[22] Another possible factor is drug therapy; some drugs are known to produce interstitial pulmonary fibrosis in other circumstances. Transient interstitial infiltration of the lung has been described in occasional patients receiving gold (gold lung),[139] but long-term pulmonary effects from this agent have not been noted. Extensive pleural adhesions and fibrinous pleurisy are sometimes associated with pericardial disease in RA.

SPLEEN, LYMPHOID TISSUE, AND BONE MARROW LESIONS

Enlargement of the regional lymph nodes draining affected joints is common in RA. Although some reports to the contrary exist, generalized lymphadenopathy involving the deeper lymph chains is infrequent. Such enlargement is caused by a nonspecific hyperplasia associated with formation of prominent germinal centers. Plasma cells are usually few, but rheumatoid factor has been demonstrated in them.[81] Numerous reticulum cells may be found in the sinuses. The hypertrophy of the lymph nodes at times reaches dimensions sufficient to raise a suspicion of malignant lymphoma, and the histologic picture has all too often been confused with nodular lymphoma.[94] The pattern of immunoglobulin staining, however, is distinct from that of malignant lymphoma.[137]

Distinctive changes are not present in the spleen in RA. In the splenomegaly of Felty's syndrome, the most consistent finding is proliferation of reticuloendothelial cells in the sinusoids. The extent of this change is in proportion to the erythrophagocytosis.[2] Although hyperplasia of the white pulp has been described, the lymphoid tissue most often is atrophic. The relation of splenic immunopathology to the circulating antinuclear antibody directed against granulocytes in this syndrome[133] is unclear. Thymic hypertrophy is not characteristically present. The bone marrow may show a variety of nonspecific changes, including increased numbers of plasma cells and ineffective erythropoiesis with excessive iron.[136] In some instances, increased numbers of lymphoid nodules are present in bone marrow particle sections. Although uncommon, bone marrow aplasia, with or without subsequent acute leukemia, has developed after prolonged therapy with alkylating agents.

ENDOCRINE LESIONS

Because of the dramatic and rapid clinical response of RA to the administration of corticotropin and adrenocortical steroids, the adrenal cortex and the pituitary gland have been studied; neither shows morphologic changes different from those found in nonrheumatic diseases.

Lymphocytic thyroiditis, sometimes sufficiently severe as to resemble Hashimoto's struma, has been reported in some studies in as many as 17% of patients with RA.[9] Others, however, have not found it to be more frequent than in a control population.[82]

OCULAR LESIONS

The episcleritis sometimes seen in RA has its inception in focal, chronic inflammatory cell infiltration and necrosis of the sclera. When these foci become larger and chronic, they may resemble the subcutaneous nodules of RA. When the scleral necrosis is sufficient to soften the wall of the eye, uveal tissue may herniate through the scleral defect, a condition known as scleromalacia perforans.[131] This condition sometimes occurs in patients with no evidence of RA.[130]

The uveitis (iridocyclitis) of juvenile RA[20] and ankylosing spondylitis does not have distinctive properties. Band keratopathy, a characteristic equatorial corneal opacity due to deposition of calcium beneath the corneal epithelium,[54] is a sequela of the iridocyclitis, and in children it is most often, if not always, associated with the arthritic condition.

Posterior subcapsular cataracts have been observed in as many as 42% of patients with RA and other rheumatic diseases during the course of corticosteroid therapy. Little is known of their pathologic anatomy. In one well-studied, early (nine months' duration) case, preservation of lens epithelium and the architecture of the lens bow distinguished the lesion from that of the usual senile cataract. Another surgically removed lens, however, had changes indistinguishable from the senile lesion.[98]

Keratoconjunctivitis sicca, associated with diminished lacrimation, is discussed more fully elsewhere (see Chaps. 39 and 67).

SJÖGREN'S SYNDROME

Although its cardinal symptoms are referable to diminished secretion by the lacrimal and salivary glands, this condition is frequently associated with various rheumatic diseases and with serologic abnormalities (see Chap. 67). Classic peripheral RA is present in approximately one-third of cases, and almost all have rheumatoid factor. The classification of Sjögren's syndrome into primary, without associated connective tissue disease, and secondary, with connective tissue disease, types has been further enhanced by the discovery of serum antibodies against extractable nuclear antigens such as SS-B and RA precipitin[81] specific for the two types. Differences in histocompatibility antigens between the two types have been elucidated.[19]

Individuals with primary Sjögren's syndrome often demonstrate more widespread clinical disease, involving not only lacrimal and salivary glands, but also exocrine glands of the respiratory tract, gastrointestinal tract, skin, and pancreas. By light microscopy, differences in the salivary gland involvement between primary and secondary types relate to the amount of lymphoid infiltrate and the severity of glandular effacement rather than to the character of the infiltrate.

A considerable variation is found in the salivary lesions. Four principal patterns are seen. First, the predominant finding is most often like that described in Mikulicz's disease. Two different histologic elements are distinguished.[126] The first is a peculiar metaplastic change in the epithelium of the striated ducts. The columnar cells proliferate and assume a stratified, polymorphous appearance. Their cytoplasm loses its normal oxyphilia. Because of the resemblance of the cells to the myoepithelial cells that normally lie subjacent to the duct epithelium, the ducts showing solid, heaped-up cells of this sort have been referred to as "epimyoepithelial" islands. Duct-like metaplasia of acini, with irregular ectasia and attenuation, also occurs, and the acini undergo variable degrees of atrophy. The second principal component in these lesions is infiltration of lymphocytes about the intralobular ducts. At times, germinal centers appear in the lymphoid aggregates, and acini may be obliterated by the infiltrate. Nevertheless, the lobular limits are characteristically respected by the infiltrate.

The second pattern occurs in a few instances. A localized area of lymphoid infiltration associated with duct metaplasia of the sort just noted reaches tumor-like proportions. This lesion is termed benign *lymphoepithelial lesion of Godwin*. Histologically, the differential diagnosis from malignant lymphomas of the salivary glands may be difficult. Third, the cellular infiltration may be so mild and the duct so little changed that the appearance cannot be distinguished from a control population. The fourth pattern may emerge after many years. The parenchymal lobules show extreme atrophy and replacement by adipose tissue, even though lymphocytic infiltration and duct metaplasia are no longer present.

Minor salivary and labial glands are also often infiltrated with lymphocytes and may thus be suitable for biopsy. Such studies have shown a high correlation of histologic abnormality with the presence of antibodies against certain extractable nuclear antigens.[90] Myoepithelial islands, however, are infrequently seen. Labial glands of individuals with primary Sjögren's syndrome consistently have more severe histologic changes than in patients with the secondary type of the syndrome.[48] This finding correlates with clinical observations of milder disease in those individuals with Sjögren's syndrome accompanying RA.[90] Intralobular aggregates of lymphocytes are also seen in the lacrimal glands, but they are smaller than in the salivary glands and are only rarely accompanied by epimyoepithelial islands.[38] Other glandular tissues, including the pancreas, fail to disclose a comparable pattern.

The pathologic ramifications of Sjögren's syndrome are more complicated than this account suggests. Localized tumor-like nodules of infiltrating lymphoid tissue ("pseudolymphoma") have been observed in lymph nodes and lung,[125] more commonly in primary Sjögren's syndrome. Indeed, in rare instances, unequivocal malignant lymphomas, principally diffuse histiocytic lymphomas, have developed. This complication is seen in both primary and secondary types of Sjögren's syndrome, at about 40 times the expected rate for healthy individuals.[90] Isolated instances of Waldenström's macroglobulinemia, small cell lymphosarcoma, and Hodgkin's disease have also been observed. Tissue lymphoid infiltrates in primary Sjögren's syndrome, as in RA, are primarily T-lymphocytes. The numbers of OKT4 (helper-inducer) cells are increased, whereas OKT8 (suppressor) cells are decreased.[39] Thus, the polyclonal-B-cell hyperactivity, which sometimes progresses to monoclonal pseudolymphomas or lymphoma, may reflect disordered immunoregulation.

RENAL LESIONS

Although older accounts to the contrary exist, the general experience is that glomerulitis and glomerulonephritis are infrequent in uncomplicated RA.[103,134] Membranous glomerulonephritis sometimes complicates systemic gold therapy for RA.[113] The status of analgesic nephropathy is unclear.[65] Although aspirin alone in moderation seems to cause little harm, a combination of aspirin and phenacetin is particularly likely to produce the renal papillary necrosis characteristic of this syndrome.

STILL'S DISEASE

This disorder has traditionally been considered the juvenile form of RA. It differs in several respects from the adult counterpart: (1) uncommon occurrence of circulating rheumatoid factors; (2) more frequent picture of ankylosing spondylitis; (3) greater frequency of iritis and band keratopathy; (4) lesser frequency of subcutaneous nodules; (5) frequent association with an erythematous skin eruption (see Chap. 51); and (6) lower NK cell activity of peripheral blood lymphocytes.[29a] Currently, a number of distinct subsets of Still's disease are thought to exist[15] (see Chaps. 51 and 52).

Clinical Manifestations
Articular Lesions

In the systemic form of the disease, with rash and high fever, variable articular manifestations occur. The involved joints can show only a mild, nonspecific inflammation or, more rarely, a florid destructive inflammatory pannus similar to adult RA.[143] This destructive pannus, however, is more characteristic of the polyarticular form of the disease associated with rheumatoid factors and subcutaneous nodules. These patients probably have juvenile presentations of adult RA. The pauciarticular form of the disease contains a distinct subset of HLA-B27-positive male children in whom the articular inflammation and pannus are mild and are often replaced by bony ankylosis, especially in the sacroiliac and spinal joints, but frequently in the limb girdle joints as well. These patients may be victims of juvenile-onset ankylosing spondylitis; however, bony and fibrous ankylosis occurs in the polyarticular variant as well. A second subset of B27-positive girls develops spondylitis and iridocyclitis, but not sacroiliac involvement.

An additional feature of articular disease not seen in the adult RA is that the subchondral inflammatory process may arrest or distort epiphyseal bone growth and may thereby lead to so-called rheumatic dwarfism. The mandible is particularly likely to be compromised in temporomandibular arthritis because growth normally takes place in its articular condyle rather than in an epiphyseal plate. This process is the basis of the micrognathos (underslung jaw). Monarticular involvement is seen more frequently in the juvenile disorder than in the adult disease.

Subcutaneous Nodules

Subcutaneous nodules occur infrequently in all forms of Still's disease, but they are most common in the polyarticular variant.[120] The histologic appearance differs both from that of the adult rheumatoid nodule and from the nodule of rheumatic fever.[13] In material available to us, the nodules consist largely of fibrous tissue containing irregularly disposed aggregates of proliferating fibroblasts in small numbers and irregular areas of fibrinous exudation. Neither geographic areas of necrosis nor palisade formation are evident. One early lesion had proliferation of blood vessels and focal vasculitis.

Other Lesions

Ocular Changes. Iridocyclitis and subsequent band-shaped keratopathy are far more frequent in Still's disease[20] than in adult RA. Macular atrophy from secondary glaucoma may result. Ocular changes occur most frequently in the pauciarticular variant of the disease.

Spondylitis. The spinal changes resemble those of ankylosing spondylitis.

Cardiac Lesions. Pericardial involvement occurs in the juvenile form[8] approximately as frequently as in adult RA,[74] although it may be detected clinically with greater frequency.[5]

Skin Eruption. The erythema is transient. Histologically, only mild perivascular aggregation of mononuclear cells in the superficial dermis has been observed.[59]

ETIOLOGY AND PATHOGENESIS

The following considerations are oriented toward the pathologic findings in RA. A systematic treatment appears in Chapter 35.

In the past, the histologic appearance of the articular tissues has suggested that rheumatoid arthritis is an infectious disease. Many types of spontaneous or induced infectious polyarthritis in species other than man have similar histologic appearances. Arthritis caused by the enteric erysipeloid organism *Erysipelothrix rhusiopathiae* in swine, for example, is one of the leading causes of pork condemnation in federally inspected meat plants in the United States, and it closely resembles RA histologically. Similar, but generally less chronic, synovitides occur in poultry and in pigs with species-specific types of *Mycoplasma* infection.[122] These minute, filtrable bacteria were formerly called pleuropneumonia-like organisms or PPLO.[122] Another type of filtrable agent causing disease in ovine species is *Chlamydia*. Subcutaneous nodules of the sort seen in RA have not been found in these infectious diseases, however, and serologic tests for rheumatoid factor are generally negative. The affinity for joints and the frequency of arthritis in bacteremias due to these organisms have prompted many microbiologic studies in RA, but most of these have failed to disclose infectious agents, as have virologic studies.[101]

Morphologic findings in RA that might relate to hypersensitivity mechanisms include the lymphoid character of the infiltrate, the absence of demonstrable organisms, the local synthesis of rheumatoid factors, the similarities of the "fibrinoid" necrotic material in the subcutaneous nodules and synovial surface to those of acute allergic inflammation,[104] and the resemblance of certain of the vascular lesions to those of polyarteritis nodosa and experimental serum sickness. The morphologic features of the previously described cellular infiltrate allow one to reconstruct sequence of events in accord with what is known of other chronic inflammatory processes.[60]

Both T- and B-lymphocytes enter the synovium through venules and are concentrated in compact perivascular infiltrates. Variable mobility and variable recirculation of the several cell types account for large disparities in the proportions of lymphocyte populations in synovium, synovial fluid, and peripheral blood.[72,73,102] T-lymphocytes, in particular, emigrate to adjacent portions of synovium and into synovial fluid. The migrating T cells are challenged by a currently unidentified antigen(s) in the synovium and undergo blast transformation. The uncommon T-lymphoblasts accordingly are located at a distance from the perivascular infiltrates where they synthesize and release mediators of local cellular immunity. These lymphoblasts immobilize macrophages locally and also damage adjacent fibroblasts. Plasma cells and plasmablasts are immobile and often persist in the perivascular location. The OKT8 cells are retained or proliferate in areas of increased immunologic activity. This idealized schema oversimplifies the histologic features because the cell types are distributed in a variable fashion in synovium in almost pure culture in some foci. In other places, cells are dispersed singly or in small clusters at random in the superficial or deeper portions of the synovium.

The recognition of the association between HLA-B27 and ankylosing spondylitis and DW4 and RA has led to renewed interest in genetic predisposition to rheumatic syndromes. Conceivably, microbial or other antigens lodged in the joints of genetically susceptible individuals might persist or evoke chronic inflammatory responses not shown by other animals or persons. Suitable animal models that totally recapitulate human RA are not available.[122]

Certain speculations may be offered concerning histogenesis. One of the peculiarities of the morbid anatomy of the disease is that the synovial lesions are morphologically nonspecific, whereas the subcutaneous nodules are relatively specific. If no common histogenetic sequence of events occurred in the nodules and the joints, it would be difficult to understand how a common pathogenetic mechanism would produce both lesions. The following hypothesis is offered to account for this phenomenon: that the nodular type of reaction does at times occur in joints, particularly in the compact fibrous parts. The necrosis noted in superficial portions of the synovial tissue may be compared to the central zones in the nodules. At the base of the nodules, an ingrowth of fibroblasts and palisades of synovial lining or elongated cells also closely resembles those of subcutaneous nodules that have undergone central softening with formation of bursa-like cavities or pseudosynovial spaces. The simplest explanation for the differences between such synovial foci and the subcutaneous nodules is that the necrotic material in subcutaneous nodules is circumscribed by firm cicatrix, whereas in the synovial location, the necrotic debris is cast off into the joint space and appears as a rice body. In the joint, the inflammation thus diffuses into the articular cavity. In the synovium, the nonspecific components of the granulation tissue reaction seen about the nodules persist.

In the earliest days or weeks of their development, the subcutaneous nodules consist largely of vascular granulation tissue, in which the processes of necrosis and exudation proceed centrifugally about inflamed small arteries or islands of newly formed capillary or sinusoidal vessels.[44,123] Only later is coalescence of the areas of necrosis followed by the granuloma-like appearance that characterizes the mature nodule. Aside from this intrinsic association between the inflammatory process and the vasculitis, a principal reason for believing that blood vessels play a role in the development of the nodules is that, in these same patients, arteritis is frequent in other tissues as well. Accordingly, it may be proposed that disseminated arteritis is an integral manifestation of RA and that the development of the nodular and synovial lesions is in some manner mediated through the affected arteries to the terminal vascular bed of the target tissues. This hypothesis does not have universal acceptance,[107a] but it is based on unique specimen material and provides a unitary concept of the histogenesis of the disorder.[123]

ANKYLOSING SPONDYLITIS

This disorder is an entity different from RA (see Chap. 53), as gauged by genetic, immunologic, epidemiologic, and pathologic features. In the diarthrodial joints of the spine, the sacroiliac joint, and the peripheral joints, the pathologic processes are like those of peripheral RA, except bony ankylosis is more prominent.[12,100] The initial histologic events in the intervertebral discs have not been well documented. By roentgenographic studies, osteolytic resorption of the margins of the vertebral bodies, to which the anulus fibrosus is attached, occurs early.[12,100] Whether an inflammatory infiltrate is present in the bone or disc tissue at this time is not known. A metaplastic ossification of the anulus fibrosus does occur, however, and penetrates from the margin of the vertebral bodies into the anulus. At times, enchondral ossification of the anulus fibrosus may occur without inflammation.[36] Although this process is commonly referred to as ossification of the spinal ligaments, the principal changes do not affect the ligaments so much as they do the anulus fibrosus (Fig. 36–9). The ankylotic bridges are located, in anteroposterior roentgenographic projections, on the lateral aspects of the vertebral bodies. The longitudinal spinal ligaments are anterolateral and posterior, but not lateral. When extensive, the bony bridges replace not only the anulus fibrosus, but also parts of the nucleus pulposus. The ossific tissue in time is remodeled to form a continuous structure. Another feature characteristic of ankylosing spondylitis, when present, is enthesopathy, that is, inflammation and eventual ossification of tendinous attachments to the pelvis and other bones at some distance from the joints.[1]

Although this picture is not observed character-

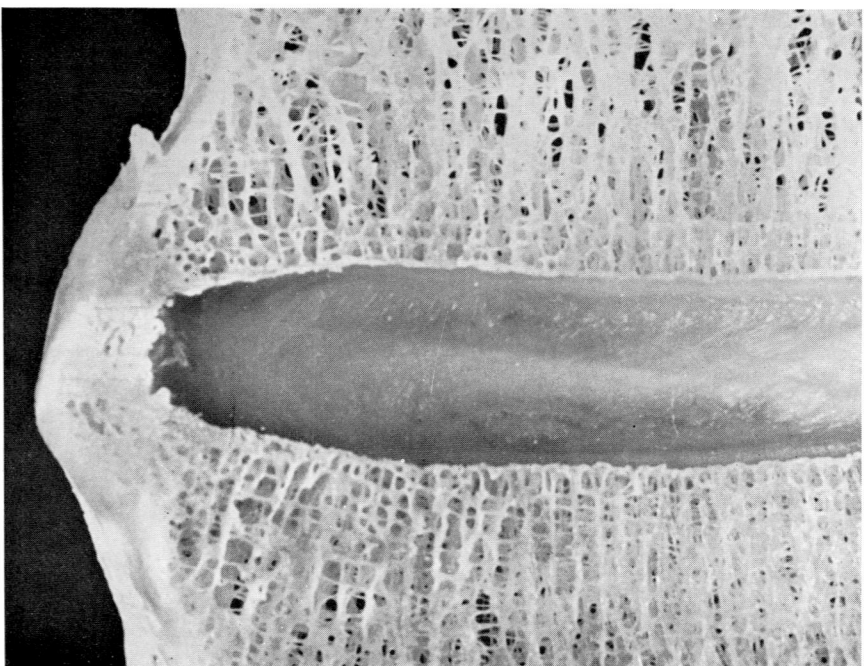

Fig. 36–9. Ankylosing spondylitis. Trabecular and cortical bone occupy the position of the anulus fibrosus. (Courtesy of Dr. Roger Terry.)

istically in the vertebral involvement of RA, similar patterns may be found in patients with Still's disease, psoriatic arthritis, and Reiter's disease, but unlike in RA, subcutaneous nodules and vascular lesions are rare. Another departure from classic RA is the prevalence of histocompatibility antigen HLA-B27.[14,114] Cardiac involvement is described previously in this chapter, as well as in Chapter 53. The ocular lesions are also described previously.

PSORIATIC ARTHRITIS

The histologic changes in the joints in this condition (see also Chap. 55) are similar to those of RA, but differ in two respects: (1) the structures affected are principally the most distal rather than proximal joints (Fig. 36–10); and (2) more extensive destruction occurs in articular and adjacent bones.[87] The osteolysis is effected by a granulation tissue in which osteoclasts are present. As a result of this resorption, the bone may "telescope" within the skin of the extremity and may give rise to the so-called opera-glass hand deformity. Aside from these changes, a bulbous swelling of the periarticular soft tissue may result from proliferation of fibrous tissue in which thick-walled blood vessels are present.

The changes in the skin in psoriasis are characteristic. The papillary element of the epidermis is hypertrophied and forms coarse, club-shaped appendages, whereas the nonpapillary portion is attenuated. This nonpapillary portion, however, is covered by a thick parakeratotic and keratotic scale. The superficial portions of the subjacent dermis are chronically inflamed and are infiltrated with large numbers of lymphocytes. A direct continuity between the dermal inflammation and the periarthritis or arthritis in psoriasis has not been established.

REITER'S DISEASE

The synovitis seen in this syndrome is similar to that seen in RA, although in the early phases of the disease, it has a more purulent character.[132] The long-standing changes also are similar, but periosteal involvement, with new bone formation in attached tendons and ligaments, is much more characteristic of Reiter's disease than of RA. In this respect, the joint lesions are reminiscent of infectious arthritis. A strong association with HLA-B27 is present.[89]

The cutaneous lesions are histologically indistinguishable from those of pustular psoriasis. Such lesions are similar to those already described, except the focal purulent infiltration of the epidermis is present (see Chap. 54).

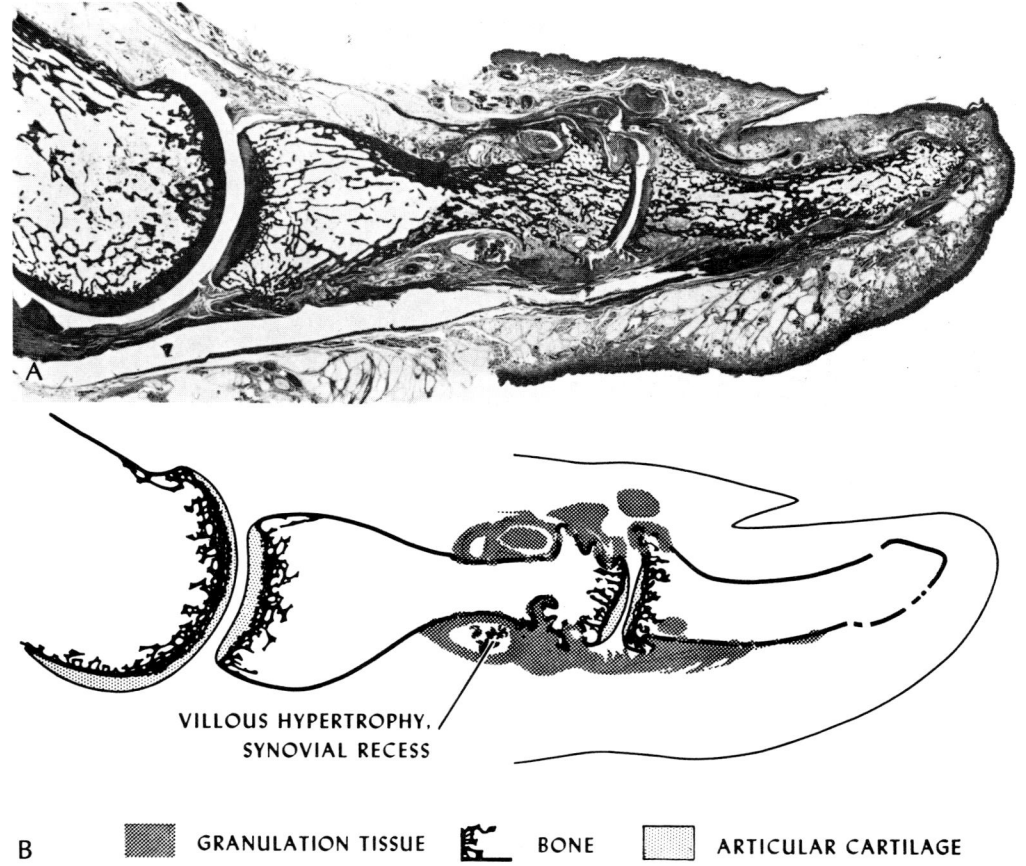

VILLOUS HYPERTROPHY,
SYNOVIAL RECESS

B   ░░░ GRANULATION TISSUE   ▓ BONE   ░ ARTICULAR CARTILAGE

Fig. 36–10.   Psoriatic arthritis of the great toe. The extensive periarticular inflammation and destruction of bone about the distal interphalangeal joint are characteristic of this disorder. The metatarsophalangeal joint is spared. (Masson's trichrome, × 2.5.)

ARTHRITIS ASSOCIATED WITH WHIPPLE'S DISEASE, REGIONAL ENTERITIS, AND ULCERATIVE COLITIS

A relationship between chronic enteritic disorders and deforming arthritis exists, not only in Reiter's disease, which may be initiated by episodes of dysentery at times, but also in other entities (see also Chap. 56).[52,75] The synovium, in the arthritis accompanying ulcerative colitis[82] and regional enteritis, shows nonspecific inflammatory changes.[77,124,142] In the arthritis accompanying Whipple's disease,[16] the rod-like inclusions characteristic of intestinal lesions have been identified by electron microscopy in the synovium.[55]

ARTHRITIS ASSOCIATED WITH AGAMMAGLOBULINEMIA

Rheumatic symptoms develop in approximately 25% of patients with congenital or acquired agammaglobulinemia or hypogammaglobulinemia. Most conspicuous among these symptoms is chronic synovitis, which resembles RA in several respects. Usually, however, fewer joints are affected, and the small joints are spared more often. Histologically, the pattern of synovitis is nonspecific and resembles that of RA, except plasma cells are generally absent.[112] Plasmacytes, however, have been seen in rare instances of arthritis associated with a deficiency of an isolated Ig type.[47]

Subcutaneous nodules, reported on several occasions in such patients, have a less characteristic appearance than the subcutaneous nodules of RA. Lobulated areas of proliferating fibroblasts and ill-defined palisades suggest the subcutaneous nodules seen in Still's disease. Vascular lesions of several types have also been described in rare instances.

AMYLOIDOSIS

In the past, secondary amyloidosis complicated RA, Still's disease, and ankylosing spondylitis in approximately 20% of severe cases. In the United States today, this complication is rare. This form of the disorder is indistinguishable from amyloidosis complicating other chronic inflammatory diseases. The principal subcomponent of amyloid in RA is the nonimmunoglobulin AA.[57] Amyloid infiltration represents the principal cause of renal dysfunction in RA, except when the joint disease coexists with SLE[103] (see Chap. 72).

BIOPSY AS A DIAGNOSTIC AID

Joint Tissues

Synovial biopsy has no place in the differential diagnosis of the several conditions discussed in this chapter. It may, however, be useful in distinguishing RA from gout and from infectious arthritides.[46] Closed and open biopsy techniques are available. Punch biopsy needles have been specifically designed for this purpose. Open biopsy, carried out under local anesthesia, is often preferable because it provides more adequate samples of tissue and causes no more discomfort to the patient. This procedure is mandatory in joints that cannot easily undergo needle biopsy with the large bone instruments. Arthroscopy is used increasingly for this purpose in large joints. In distinguishing arthritis from gout, precautions should be taken to preserve any urate crystals present by fixation of the specimen in absolute alcohol rather than in aqueous fixatives. When infection is suspected, synovial fluid and tissue should be subjected to prompt microbiologic study.

Skeletal Muscle

The principal indication for muscle biopsy in this group of disorders is the demonstration of arteritis. Because of the focal nature of this lesion, it is necessary to examine adequate amounts of tissue. The surgeon must ensure that the specimen be of sufficient size; $2 \times 1 \times 1$ cm are realistic dimensions. Disposable isometric clamps for this purpose are available commercially. Fixation should be delayed for half an hour or so after excision. Bouin's solution is a useful fixative for this tissue. In most cases, serial sections are necessary. Making 100 sections, each fifth slide stained, as routine procedure, has yielded 4 times as many positive diagnoses of arteritis as have isolated, random sections. Enzyme and immunohistochemical examinations have less diagnostic value in rheumatic diseases than do the foregoing procedures. Should these examinations be desired, the tissue should be submitted unfixed to the pathologist. Immunoglobulins usually survive at least several hours' immersion in chilled saline solution, but enzyme preparations require that the specimen be quenched immediately in low-temperature isopentane.

Peripheral Nerves

Biopsy of peripheral nerves is not often indicated in RA, but when it is, the sural nerve is the site of choice.[23]

Subcutaneous Nodules

In the differential diagnosis of a tophus, fixation of the nodule in absolute alcohol may serve the same useful purpose suggested in synovial biopsy. Epidermoid cysts in the olecranon region occasionally simulate rheumatoid nodules, and diagnostic biopsy may be indicated.[138]

Lymph Nodes

The principal indications for lymph node biopsy are: (1) the differential diagnosis of specific infectious arthritides, in which case the tissue should also be cultured; and (2) the differential diagnosis of the malignant lymphomas.

Amyloidosis

Needle punch biopsies of liver, spleen, and kidney offer no difficulties to the pathologist, but have occasionally resulted in serious visceral hemorrhages. Gingival, buccal, or rectal mucosal biopsies have at times established the presence of amyloid deposits in the walls of minute blood vessels in RA, as in other types of secondary amyloidosis. In each of these procedures, the diagnosis is valid only when positive and is not excluded when negative for amyloid material. Specific immunofluorescent staining for amyloid has not yet achieved general usefulness for several reasons.[57] Reliance must still be placed on properly controlled Congo red or similar preparations.

In summary, each of the deforming arthritides discussed in this chapter has certain similarities and common pathologic features. The inflammatory reactions in the joints, although inherently indistinguishable from each other, are nonspecific. The overlapping serologic reactions in the diffuse "collagen diseases," the histologic similarities in the subcutaneous nodules, the common patterns of vertebral bridges in spondyloarthropathy, the similarity of cutaneous lesions in Reiter's disease and pustular psoriasis, and the joint disease complicating the several sorts of chronic enteritis all defy a rigid nosologic concept. Whether they are truly "variants" of RA as was once thought, or independent diseases, as most now think, or nonspecific reaction patterns, as they appear to the pathologist, awaits more specific knowledge of their etiology and pathogenesis.

REFERENCES

1. Ball, J.: Articular pathology of ankylosing spondylitis. Clin. Orthop., *143*:30–37, 1979.

2. Barnes, C.G., Turnbull, A.L., and Vernon-Roberts, B.: Felty's syndrome—A clinical and pathological survey of two patients and their response to therapy. Ann. Rheum. Dis., *30*:359–374, 1971.

3. Benedek, G.: Rheumatoid pneumoconiosis: documentation of onset and pathogenetic considerations. Am. J. Med., *55*:515–524, 1973.

4. Berg, E., et al.: On the nature of rheumatoid rice bodies: an immunological, histochemical and electronmicroscopic study. Arthritis Rheum., *20*:1343–1349, 1977.

5. Bernstein, B., Takahashi, M., and Hanson, V.: Noninvasive techniques in the study of cardiac involvement in juvenile rheumatoid arthritis. Arthritis Rheum., *16*:535–536, 1973.

6. Bland, J.H.: Rheumatoid arthritis of the cervical spine. J. Rheumatol., *1*:319–342, 1974.

7. Bonfiglio, T., and Atwater, E.C.: Heart disease in patients with seropositive rheumatoid arthritis: a controlled autopsy study and review. Arch. Intern. Med., *124*:714–719, 1969.

8. Brewer, E., Jr.: Juvenile rheumatoid arthritis—cardiac involvement. Arthritis Rheum., *20*:231–236, 1977.

9. Buchanan, W.W., et al.: Association of Hashimoto's thyroiditis and rheumatoid arthritis. Lancet, *1*:245–253, 1961.

10. Bulkley, B.H., and Roberts, W.C.: Ankylosing spondylitis and aortic regurgitation: description of the characteristic cardiovascular lesion from study of eight necropsy patients. Circulation, *48*:1014–1027, 1973.

11. Bywaters, E.G.L.: Rheumatoid and other disease of the cervical interspinous bursae, and changes in the spinous processes. Ann. Rheum. Dis., *41*:360–370, 1982.

12. Bywaters, E.G.L.: The pathology of the spine. *In* The Joints and Synovial Fluid. Vol. II. Edited by L. Sokoloff. New York, Academic Press, 1980, pp. 427–547.

13. Bywaters, E.G.L., Glynn, L.E., and Seldis, A.: Subcutaneous nodules of Still's disease. Ann. Rheum. Dis., *17*:278–285, 1958.

14. Caffrey, M.F.P., and James, D.C.O.: Human lymphocyte association in ankylosing spondylitis. Nature, *242*:121–123, 1973.

15. Calabro, J.J., et al.: Juvenile rheumatoid arthritis: a general review and report of 100 patients observed for 15 years. Semin. Arthritis Rheum., *5*:257–298, 1976.

16. Caughey, D.E., and Bywaters, E.G.L.: The arthritis of Whipple's syndrome. Ann. Rheum. Dis., *22*:327–335, 1963.

17. Cervantes-Perez, P., Toro-Perez, A.H., and Rodriquez-Jurado, P.: Pulmonary involvement in rheumatoid arthritis. JAMA, *243*:1715–1719, 1980.

18. Cheung, H.S., et al.: Synovial origins of rice bodies in joint fluid. Arthritis Rheum., *23*:72–76, 1980.

19. Chused, T.M., et al.: Sjögren's syndrome associated with HLA-DW3. N. Engl. J. Med., *296*:895–897, 1977.

20. Chylack, L.T., Jr.: The ocular manifestations of juvenile rheumatoid arthritis. Arthritis Rheum., *20*:217–233, 1977.

21. Cochrane, W., et al.: Ultramicroscopic structure of rheumatoid nodules. Ann. Rheum. Dis., *23*:345–363, 1964.

22. Collins, R.L., et al.: Obstructive pulmonary disease in rheumatoid arthritis. Arthritis Rheum., *19*:623–628, 1976.

23. Conn, D.L., McDuffie, F.C., and Dyck, P.J.: Immunopathologic study of sural nerves in rheumatoid arthritis. Arthritis Rheum., *15*:135–143, 1972.

24. Conn, D.L., Schroeter, A.L., and McDuffie, F.C.: Cutaneous vessel immune deposits in rheumatoid arthritis. Arthritis Rheum., *19*:15–20, 1976.

25. Cooke, T.D.V.: The interactions and local disease manifestations of immune complexes in articular collagenous tissues. *In* Studies in Joint Disease. Vol. I. Edited by A. Maroudas and E.J. Holborow. London, Pittman, 1980, pp. 158–200.

26. Cooper, N.S., et al.: Diagnostic specificity of synovial lesions. Hum. Pathol., *12*:314–328, 1981.

27. Cruickshank, B.: Interpretation of multiple biopsies of synovial tissue in rheumatic diseases. Ann. Rheum. Dis., *11*:137–145, 1952.

28. Davis, R.F., and Engleman, E.C.: Incidence of myocardial infarction in patients with rheumatoid arthritis. Arthritis Rheum., *17*:527–533, 1974.

29. Dingle, J.T.: Lysosomal enzymes and the degradation of cartilage matrix. Etiological factors in the collagen diseases. Proc. R. Soc. Med., *55*:109–111, 1962.

29a. Dobloug, J.H., et al.: Natural killer (NK) cell activity of peripheral blood, synovial fluid, and synovial tissue lymphocytes from patients with rheumatoid arthritis and juvenile rheumatoid arthritis. Ann. Rheum. Dis., *41*:490–495, 1982.

30. Dorfman, H.D., Norman, A., and Smith, R.J.: Bone erosion in relation to subcutaneous rheumatoid nodules. Arthritis Rheum., *13*:69–73, 1970.

31. Duke, O., et al.: An immunohistochemical analysis of lymphatic subpopulations and their microenvironment in the synovial membrane of patients with rheumatoid arthritis using monoclonal antibodies. Clin. Exp. Immunol., *49*:22–30, 1982.

32. Dyck, P.J., Conn, D.L., and Okazaki, H.: Necrotizing angiopathic neuropathy. Mayo Clin. Proc., *47*:461–475, 1972.

33. Ehrlich, G.E., et al.: Pathogenesis of rupture of extensor tendons at the wrist in rheumatoid arthritis. Arthritis Rheum., *2*:332–346, 1959.

34. Falicov, R., and Cooney, D.F.: Takayasu's arteritis and rheumatoid arthritis: a case report. Arch. Intern. Med., *114*:594–600, 1964.

35. Fernandez-Diez, J.: General pathology of necrotizing vasculitis. Clin. Rheum. Dis., *6*:279–295, 1980.

36. François, R.J.: Le rachis dans la spondyloarthrite ankylosante. Brussels, Editions Arscia, 1975.

37. Frank, S.T., et al.: Pulmonary dysfunction in rheumatoid disease. Chest, *63*:27–34, 1973.

38. Font, R.L., Yanoff, M., and Zimmerman, L.E.: Benign lymphoepithelial lesion of the lacrimal gland and its relationship to Sjögren's syndrome. Am. J. Clin. Pathol., *48*:365–376, 1967.

39. Fox, R.I., et al.: Use of monoclonal antibodies to analyze peripheral blood and salivary gland lymphocyte subsets in Sjögren's syndrome. Arthritis Rheum., *25*:419–426, 1982.

40. Fukase, M., Koizumi, F., and Wakaki, K.: Histopathologic analysis of sixteen subcutaneous nodules. Acta Pathol. Jpn., *30*:871–882, 1980.

41. Gardner, D.L.: The Pathology of Rheumatoid Arthritis. Baltimore, Williams & Wilkins, 1972.

42. Ghadially, F.N., and Roy, S.: Ultrastructure of Synovial Joints in Health and Disease. London, Butterworths, 1969.

43. Ghose, T., et al.: Immunopathological changes in rheumatoid arthritis and other joint diseases. J. Clin. Pathol., *28*:109–117, 1975.

44. Gieseking, R., Baumer, A., and Backmann, L.: Electronenoptische Untersuchungen an Granulomen des Rheumatismus Nodosus. Z. Rheumaforsch., *28*:163–175, 1969.

45. Ginsberg, M.H., et al.: Rheumatoid nodulosis. An unusual variant of rheumatoid disease. Arthritis Rheum., *18*:49–58, 1975.

46. Goldenberg, D.L., and Cohen, A.S.: Synovial membrane histopathology in the differential diagnosis of rheumatoid arthritis, gout, pseudogout, systemic lupus erythematosus, infectious arthritis and degenerative joint disease. Medicine, *57*:239–252, 1978.

47. Grayzel, A.I., et al.: Chronic polyarthritis associated with hypogammaglobulinemia. A study of two patients. Arthritis Rheum., *20*:887–894, 1977.

48. Greenspan, J.S., et al.: The histopathology of Sjögren's syndrome in labial salivary gland biopsies. Oral Surg., *37*:217–229, 1974.

49. Grimley, P.M., and Sokoloff, L.: Synovial giant cells in rheumatoid arthritis. Am. J. Pathol., *49*:931–954, 1966.

50. Harris, E.D., Jr.: Role of collagenases in joint destruction. *In* The Joints and Synovial Fluid. Vol. I. Edited by L. Sokoloff. New York, Academic Press, 1978, pp. 243–272.

51. Harris, E.D., Jr.: Intracellular collagen fibers at the pan-

nus-cartilage junction in rheumatoid arthritis. Arthritis Rheum., 20:657–665, 1977.

52. Haslock, I.: Enteropathic arthritis. In Copeman's Textbook of the Rheumatic Diseases. 5th Ed. Edited by J.T. Scott. Edinburgh, Churchill-Livingstone, 1978, pp. 567–577.

53. Hawkins, C.F., et al.: Detection by electron microscope of rod-shaped organisms in synovial membrane from a patient with the arthritis of Whipple's disease. Ann. Rheum. Dis., 35:502–509, 1976.

54. Henkind, P., and Gold, D.H.: Ocular manifestations of rheumatic disorders. Rheumatology, 4:13–59, 1973.

55. Hernandez-Lopez, E., et al.: Echocardiographic study of the cardiac involvement in rheumatoid arthritis. Chest, 72:52–55, 1977.

56. Hunninghake, G., and Fauci, A.: Pulmonary involvement in collagen vascular diseases. Am. Rev. Respir. Dis., 199:471–503, 1979.

57. Husby, G.: Amyloidosis in rheumatoid arthritis. Ann. Clin. Res., 7:154–167, 1975.

58. Ilardi, C.F., and Sokoloff, L.: The pathology of osteoarthritis: ten strategic questions for pharmacologic management. Semin. Arthritis Rheum., 2 (Suppl. 1):3–7, 1981.

59. Isdale, I.C., and Bywaters, E.G.L.: The rash of rheumatoid arthritis and Still's disease. Q. J. Med., 25:377–387, 1956.

60. Ishikawa, H., and Ziff, M.: Electron-microscopic observations of immunoreactive cells in the rheumatoid synovial membrane. Arthritis Rheum., 19:1–14, 1976.

61. Jasin, H.E., and Dingle, J.T.: Human mononuclear cell factors mediate cartilage matrix degradation through chondrocyte activation. J. Clin. Invest., 68:571–581, 1981.

62. John, J.T., Hough, A.J., and Sergent, J.S.: Pericardial disease in rheumatoid arthritis. Am. J. Med., 66:385–390, 1979.

63. Katzenstein, A.A.: The histologic spectrum and differential diagnosis of necrotizing granulomatous inflammation in the lungs. In Progress in Surgical Pathology. Vol. II. Edited by C. Fenoglio and M. Wolff. New York, Masson, 1980.

64. Katzenstein, A.A., and Askin, F.B.: Surgical pathology of non-neoplastic lung disease. In Major Problems in Pathology. Vol. 13. Edited by J.L. Bennington. Philadelphia, W.B. Saunders Co., 1982.

65. Kennedy, A.: Analgesic nephropathy. J. Clin. Pathol., 28 (Suppl. 9):14, 1975.

66. Kennedy, A.C., et al.: Bone-resorbing activity in the sera of patients with rheumatoid arthritis. Clin. Sci. Mol. Med., 51:205–207, 1976.

67. Kim, R.C., and Collins, G.H.: The neuropathology of rheumatoid disease. Hum. Pathol., 12:5–15, 1981.

68. Kimura, H., Tateishi, H., and Ziff, M.: Surface ultrastructure of rheumatoid articular cartilage. Arthritis Rheum., 20:1085–1098, 1977.

69. Kirk, J.T., and Cosh, L.: The pericarditis of rheumatoid arthritis. Q. J. Med., 38:397–423, 1969.

70. Klein, G., and Rainer, F.: Herzmanifestationen bei rheumatischen Erkrankungen. Wien Med. Wochenschr., 4:132–135, 1977.

71. Kobayashi, I., and Ziff, M.: Electron microscopic studies of the cartilage-pannus junction in rheumatoid arthritis. Arthritis Rheum., 18:475–483, 1975.

72. Konttinen, Y.T., Reitamo, S., and Ranki, A.: Characterization of the immunocompetent cells of rheumatoid synovium from tissue sections and eluates. Arthritis Rheum., 24:71–79, 1981.

73. Kurosaka, M., and Ziff, M.: Immunoelectron microscopic study of distribution of T cell subsets in rheumatoid synovium. J. Exp. Med., 158:1191–1210, 1983.

74. Leitman, P.S., and Bywaters, E.G.L.: Pericarditis in juvenile rheumatoid arthritis. Pediatrics, 32:855–860, 1963.

75. Macrae, I., and Wright, V.: A family study of ulcerative colitis with particular reference to ankylosing spondylitis and sacroiliitis. Ann. Rheum. Dis., 32:16–20, 1973.

76. Magyar, E., et al.: Muscle changes in rheumatoid arthritis. A review of the literature with a study of 100 cases. Virchows Arch. (Pathol. Anat.), 373(A):267–278, 1977.

77. Malcolm, A.J.: Diagnostic pathology in rheumatology. Clin. Rheum. Dis., 9:27–29, 1983.

78. Martinez-Lavin, M., Vaughn, J.H., and Tan, E.M.: Autoantibodies and the spectrum of Sjögren's syndrome. Ann. Intern. Med., 91:185–226, 1979.

79. Masi, A.T., et al.: Hashimoto's disease: a clinicopathological study with matched controls. Lancet, 1:123–126, 1965.

80. McCarty, D.J., and Cheung, H.S.: Origin and significance of rice bodies in synovial fluid. Lancet, 2:715, 1982.

81. McCormick, J.N.: An immunofluorescence study of rheumatoid factors. Ann. Rheum. Dis., 22:1–10, 1963.

82. McEwen, C., et al.: Arthritis accompanying ulcerative colitis. Am. J. Med., 33:923–941, 1962.

83. Menninger, H., et al.: Granulocyte elastase at the site of cartilage erosion by rheumatoid synovial tissue. Z. Rheumatol., 39:145–156, 1980.

84. Mesara, B.W., Brody, G.L., and Oberman, H.A.: "Pseudorheumatoid" subcutaneous nodules. Am. J. Clin. Pathol., 45:684–691, 1966.

85. Meyers, D.B., and Brown, N.D.: Morphological and biomechanical studies of rheumatoid pannus and cartilage. J. Rheumatol., 9:502–513, 1982.

86. Mohr, W., Westerhellwig, H., and Wessinghage, D.: Polymorphonuclear granulocytes in rheumatic tissue destruction. III. An electronmicroscopic study of PMNs at the pannus cartilage junction in rheumatoid arthritis. Ann. Rheum. Dis., 40:396–399, 1981.

87. Moll, J.M.H., and Wright, V.: Psoriatic arthritis. Semin. Arthritis Rheum., 3:55–78, 1973.

88. Mongan, E.S., et al.: A study of the relation of seronegative and seropositive rheumatoid arthritis to each other and to necrotizing vasculitis. Am. J. Med., 47:23–25, 1969.

89. Morris, R., et al.: Medical intelligence. HL-A-W27—A useful discriminator in the arthropathies of inflammatory bowel disease. N. Engl. J. Med., 290:1117–1119, 1974.

90. Moutsopoulos, H.M., et al.: Sjögren's syndrome (sicca syndrome): Current issues. Ann. Intern. Med., 92:212–226, 1980.

91. Nakano, K.K.: The entrapment neuropathies of rheumatoid arthritis. Orthop. Clin. North Am., 6:837–860, 1975.

92. Neumark, T.: Cell-to-cell contacts between lymphoreticular cells in rheumatoid synovial membrane. Acta Morphol. Acad. Sci. Hung., 25:121–135, 1977.

93. Nomeir, A.M., et al.: Cardiac involvement in rheumatoid arthritis. Ann. Intern. Med., 79:800–806, 1973.

94. Nosanchuk, J.S., and Shnitzer, B.: Follicular hyperplasia in lymph nodes from patients with rheumatoid arthritis. Cancer, 24:343–354, 1969.

95. Nowoslawski, A., and Brzosko, W.J.: Immunopathology of rheumatoid arthritis. I. The rheumatoid synovitis. Path. Europ., 2:198–219, 1967.

96. Nowoslawski, A., and Brzosko, W.J.: Immunopathology of rheumatoid arthritis. II. The rheumatoid nodule (the rheumatoid granuloma). Path. Europ., 2:302–321, 1967.

97. Ogilvie-Harris, D.J., and Fornasier, V.L.: Synovial iron deposition in osteoarthritis. J. Rheumatol., 7:30–36, 1980.

98. Oglesby, R.B., et al.: Cataracts in patients with rheumatic diseases treated with corticosteroids. Arch. Ophthalmol., 66:625–630, 1961.

99. Oxenhandler, R., Adelstein, E.H., and Hart, M.N.: Immunopathology of skeletal muscle. The value of direct immunofluorescence in the diagnosis of connective tissue disorder. Hum. Pathol., 8:321–328, 1977.

100. Pasion, E.G., and Goodfellow, J.W.: Preankylosing spondylitis. Ann. Rheum. Dis., 34:92–97, 1975.

101. Phillips, P.E.: Virologic studies in rheumatoid arthritis. Rheumatology, 6:353–360, 1975.

102. Piatier, D., et al.: Immunofluorescence of synovial membrane. Multifactorial analysis of the results. Biomedicine, 24:359–366, 1976.

103. Pollak, V.E., Pirani, C.L., and Kark, R.M.: The kidney

in rheumatoid arthritis: studies by renal biopsy. Arthritis Rheum., *5*:1–9, 1962.

104. Poole, A.R., and Coombs, R.R.A.: Rheumatoid-like joint lesions in rabbits injected intravenously with bovine serum. Int. Arch. Allergy Appl. Immunol., *54*:97–113, 1977.

105. Popert, A.J., et al.: Frequency of occurrence, mode of development, and significance of rice bodies in rheumatoid joints. Ann. Rheum. Dis., *41*:109–117, 1982.

106. Popper, M.S., Bogdonoff, M.L., and Hughes, R.L.: Interstitial rheumatoid lung disease: a reassessment and review of the literature. Chest, *62*:243–250, 1972.

107. Prillamin, W.W., et al.: Intestinal complications in rheumatoid arthritis and their relationship to corticosteroid therapy. J. Chronic Dis., *27*:475–481, 1974.

107a.Rasker, J.J., and Kuipers, F.C.: Are rheumatoid nodules caused by vasculitis? A study of 13 early cases. Ann. Rheum. Dis., *42*:384–388, 1983.

108. Reimer, K.A., Rodgers, R.F., and Oyasu, R.: Rheumatoid arthritis with rheumatoid heart disease and granulomatous aortitis. JAMA, *235*:2510–2512, 1977.

109. Roberts, W.C., et al.: Cardiac valvular lesions in rheumatoid arthritis. Arch. Intern. Med., *122*:141–146, 1968.

110. Romanus, P., and Yden, S.: Pelvo-Spondylitis Ossificans. Copenhagen, Munksgaard, 1955.

111. Rosenberger, J.L., et al.: A statistical approach to the histopathologic diagnosis of synovitis. Hum. Pathol., *12*:329–337, 1981.

112. Rötstein, J., and Good, R.A.: Significance of the simultaneous occurrence of connective tissue disease and agammaglobulinemia. Ann. Rheum. Dis., *21*:202–206, 1962.

113. Samuels, B., et al.: Membranous glomerulonephritis in patients with rheumatoid arthritis: relationship to gold therapy. Medicine, *57*:319–327, 1978.

114. Schlosstein, L., et al.: High association of HL-A antigen W-27 with ankylosing spondylitis. N. Engl. J. Med., *288*:704–706, 1973.

115. Scott, D.L., et al.: Significance of fibronectin in rheumatoid arthritis and osteoarthrosis. Ann. Rheum. Dis., *40*:142–153, 1981.

116. Scott, D.G.I., Bacon, P.A., and Tribe, C.R.: Systemic rheumatoid vasculitis: A clinical and laboratory study of 50 cases. Medicine, *60*:288–297, 1981.

117. Shiozawa, S., Shiozawa, K., and Fujita, T.: Morphologic observations in the early phase of the cartilage-pannus junction. Arthritis Rheum., *26*:472–478, 1983.

118. Shiozawa, A., Williams, R.C., Jr., and Ziff, M.: Immunoelectron microscopic demonstration of prostaglandin E in rheumatoid synovium. Arthritis Rheum., *25*:685–693, 1982.

119. Siegmeth, W., and Eberl, R.: Gelenksfernemanifestationen der chronischen Polyarthritis. Wien Klin. Wochenschr., *88*:81–84, 1976.

120. Simon, F.E.R., and Schaller, J.G.: Benign rheumatoid nodules. Pediatrics, *56*:29–33, 1975.

121. Sims-Williams, H., Jayson, M.I.V., and Baddeley, H.: Rheumatoid involvement of the lumbar spine. Ann. Rheum. Dis., *36*:524–531, 1977.

122. Sokoloff, L.: Animal models of rheumatoid arthritis. Int. Rev. Exp. Pathol., *26*:107–145, 1984.

123. Sokoloff, L.: The pathophysiology of peripheral blood vessels in collagen diseases. *In* International Academy of Pathology, Monograph No. 4, 1963, pp. 297–325.

124. Soren, A.: Joint affections in regional ileitis. Arch. Intern. Med., *117*:78–83, 1966.

125. Talal, N., Sokoloff, L., and Barth, W.: Extra-salivary lymphoid abnormalities in Sjögren's syndrome (reticulum-cell sarcoma, "pseudolymphoma," macroglobulinemia). Am. J. Med., *43*:50–65, 1967.

126. Thackray, A.C., and Lucas, R.B.: Tumors of the Major Salivary Glands. Washington, D.C., Armed Forces Institute of Pathology, 1974, p. 127.

127. Theofilopoulos, A.N., et al.: IgM rheumatoid factor and low molecular weight of IgM. An association with vasculitis. Arthritis Rheum., *17*:272–284, 1974.

128. Turner, R., Collins, R., and Nomeir, A.M.: Extra-articular manifestations of rheumatoid arthritis. Bull. Rheum. Dis., *29*:986–990, 1979.

129. Van Boxel, J.A., and Paget, S.A.: Predominantly T-cell infiltrate in rheumatoid synovial membranes. N. Engl. J. Med., *293*:517–520, 1975.

130. Walter, J.R., and Boldt, H.A.: Scleromalacia perforans associated with a cotton wool spot of the retina in an otherwise healthy patient. Am. J. Ophthal., *55*:922–930, 1963.

131. Watson, P.G., and Hayreh, S.S.: Scleritis and episcleritis. Br. J. Ophthalmol., *60*:163–191, 1976.

132. Weinberger, H.W., et al.: Reiter's syndrome, clinical and pathological observations. A long-term study of 16 cases. Medicine, *41*:35–91, 1962.

133. Weisman, M., and Zvaifler, N.J.: Cryoimmunoglobulinemia in Felty's syndome. Arthritis Rheum., *19*:103–110, 1976.

134. Whaley, K., and Webb, J.: Liver and kidney disease in rheumatoid arthritis. Clin. Rheum. Dis., *3*:527–547, 1977.

135. Williams, J.H., et al.: Isolated subcutaneous nodules (pseudorheumatoid). J. Bone Joint Surg., *59A*:73–76, 1977.

136. Williams, R.A., et al.: *In vitro* studies of ineffective erythropoiesis in rheumatoid arthritis. Ann. Rheum. Dis., *41*:502–507, 1982.

137. Willkens, F.R., et al.: Immunopathological studies in lymph nodes in rheumatoid arthritis and malignant lymphomas. Ann. Rheum. Dis., *39*:147–151, 1980.

138. Wilson, J.T., and Sokoloff, L.: Epidermoid cysts stimulating rheumatoid nodules in the olecranon region. JAMA, *214*:593–595, 1970.

139. Winterbauer, R.H., Wilske, K.R., and Wheelis, R.F.: Diffuse pulmonary injury associated with gold therapy. N. Engl. J. Med., *294*:919–921, 1976.

140. Wooley, D.E., et al.: Collagenase production by rheumatoid synovial cells: morphological and immunohistochemical studies of the dendritic cell. Ann. Rheum. Dis., *38*:262–270, 1979.

141. Wooley, D.E., Crossley, J.J., and Evanson, J.M.: Collagenase at sites of cartilage erosion in the rheumatoid joint. Arthritis Rheum., *20*:1231–1239, 1977.

142. Wright, V.: A unifying concept for the spondyloarthropathies. Clin. Orthop., *143*:8–14, 1979.

143. Wynn-Roberts, C.R., et al.: Light and electron-microscopic findings of juvenile rheumatoid arthritis synovium: comparison with normal juvenile synovium. Semin. Arthritis Rheum., *7*:287–302, 1978.

144. Ziff, M.: Relation of cellular infiltration of rheumatoid synovial membrane to its immune response. Arthritis Rheum., *17*:313–319, 1974.

145. Zvaifler, N.J.: The immunopathology of joint inflammation in rheumatoid arthritis. Adv. Immunol., *16*:265–336, 1973.

Chapter 37

Mechanisms of Tissue Destruction in Rheumatoid Arthritis

Stephen M. Krane

In many patients with unremitting chronic rheumatoid arthritis (RA), as well as in others with nonrheumatoid chronic synovitis, disruption of the normal structure and function of the joint is a prominent feature. Indeed, much of the disability of rheumatoid disease is due to joint damage itself. Weakening of the joint capsule and ligaments, erosion of cartilage and bone, rupture of tendons, and decrease in viscosity and other alterations of the synovial fluid may be found. Under certain circumstances, when remission of the inflammatory process occurs, the resorptive processes may diminish, and some of the connective tissue components are renewed, although much of the damage is irreversible. Some of the pathogenetic mechanisms of joint destruction are discussed in this chapter.

The mechanical functions of the normal joint are determined by its structure. The usefulness of the joint as a bearing depends on the integrity of the opposing surfaces of the articular cartilage, the thickness and pattern of the subchondral bone, and the interaction of the cartilage with water, proteins, hyaluronic acid, and other components of the synovial fluid. The surfaces must be properly aligned, and their position must be maintained by the integrity of the joint capsule, ligaments, tendons, and muscles. The functional characteristics of each of these connective tissues are, in turn, determined by their chemical composition. Connective tissues in general are characterized by specialized component cells and by the type and abundance of extracellular material. This extracellular material may be considered in several subclasses. The first of these are the fibrillar components, of which collagen and elastin are the most abundant. Then are found the components of the ground substance, of which the proteoglycans make up the greatest proportion, in addition to proteins such as glycoproteins, some of which, for example, fibronectin and laminin, are involved in adherence of cells to the extracellular matrix.[68] Bone contains a calcium-phosphate mineral phase that accounts for approximately two-thirds of its weight.[40,41] The remainder of bone matrix is predominantly collagen, although

it also contains unique noncollagenous proteins such as a γ-carboxyglutamic acid-containing protein (bone GLA protein or osteocalcin), a glycoprotein called osteonectin, and a proteoglycan with a specific core protein structure.[36]

Little elastin is present in the joint structures; collagen is the major fibrillar component. The interstitial collagens of joint connective tissues are all basically composed of molecules aligned in the particular array characteristic of collagens in general.[8,40,97,116,136] The pattern is that of an approximately one-quarter stagger of the length of the molecule, with an overlap and hole zones (see Chap. 10). The collagens of several of the joint structures differ from each other in terms of primary structure, as well as in certain post-translational modifications.[38] Types I, II, and III collagen all are composed of three polypeptide chains, which are arrayed in an ordered, helical configuration. This helical configuration and the formation of the collagen fibril confer certain functional properties onto these tissues, as well as a characteristic resistance to attack by proteolytic enzymes.[43,51] The further interactions of the collagen with other components of the particular connective tissue, in turn, determine the mechanical properties of these tissues and the rate at which they are degraded.

It is possible that the earliest lesion in RA is a proliferation of the lining layer of the synovium in the presence of inflammatory cells.[16,77] The collection of inflammatory cells that usually begins in the recesses of the joint at the sites of reflection of the synovium may progress over the surface of the articular cartilage (pannus) or may burrow into the subchondral bone (Figs. 37–1 and 37–2); in other areas where tendon sheaths are involved, the inflammatory mass may burrow through the surface of the tendons. If the process continues unabated, the connective tissue structures of the joint tendons are eroded, and normal function is interrupted. The extremes of such connective tissue destruction are seen in the rupture of extensor tendons, in the loss of entire articular cartilage down to subchondral bone, and in erosions of bone that may, on rare occasion, proceed to the resorption of entire sub-

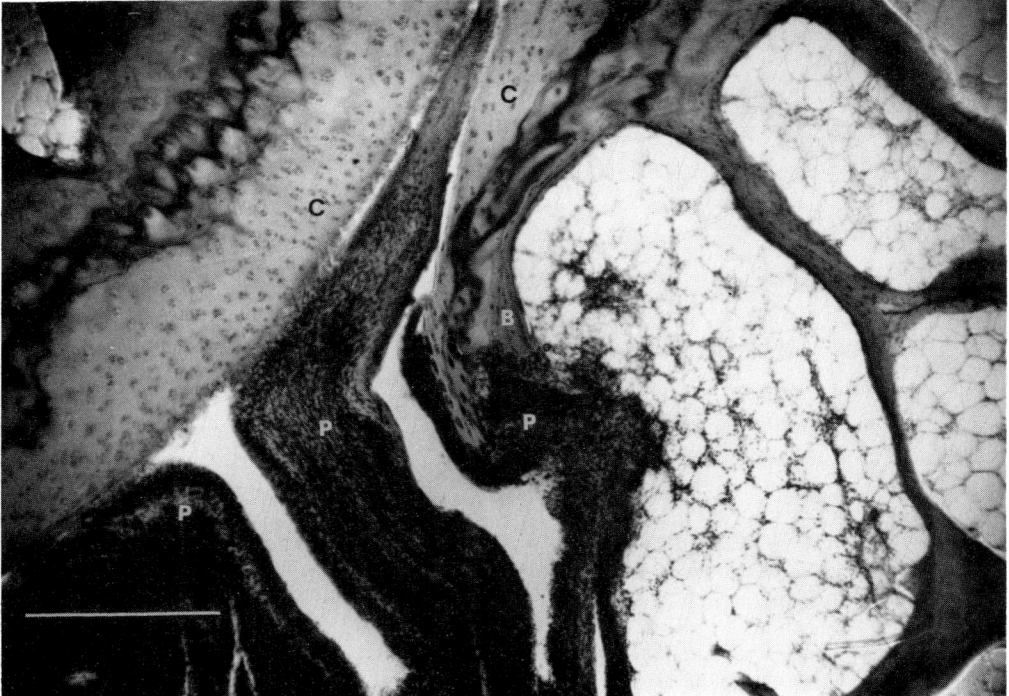

Fig. 37–1. Low-power view of typical rheumatoid arthritis of a metacarpophalangeal joint. The pannus (P) covers the surfaces of the articular cartilage (C) and in other areas has burrowed through subchondral bone (B). Bar = 400 μm.

articular regions. For the most part, the connective tissue destruction occurs predominantly in areas adjacent to the margin of the invading pannus. This process has been demonstrated by a variety of techniques including electron microscopy.[49,50] The thickness of the cartilage usually remains intact in areas not immediately adjacent to the proliferating cellular granulations, but proteoglycans may be lost in areas remote from the margin of these granulations, even in early synovitis.[60]

The type of cell or cells responsible for the destructive aspects of chronic RA has not yet been clarified. The pannus (Fig. 37–3) contains a heterogeneous population of cells.[16] In the past, identification of these cells was based almost exclusively on morphologic criteria.[16,35] In addition to chronic inflammatory cells, it was thought that the pannus contained the same cell types found in the normal synovial lining, that is, phagocytic type A cells, secretory type B cells, and type C cells with features of both type A and type B cells, which was especially characteristic of RA. Both T- and B-lymphocytes and plasma cells are present to a variable extent.[69,131] T-lymphocytes predominate and are considered to be "activated." An even higher percentage (~ 90%) of these synovial T-lymphocytes have the OKT4 surface antigen

(helper, inducer-type) than peripheral blood (~ 67%), and these are distributed differently from the OKT8 + cells.[62] Attempts have also been made to characterize the pannus cells based on certain functions in cell culture and according to the expression of surface antigens detected by other monoclonal antibodies. The most abundant adherent cell present in primary cultures of rheumatoid synovium is a large, stellate cell frequently containing long dendritic processes.[22] These *synovial stellate cells* stain by indirect immunofluoresence using antibodies to synovial collagenase,[146] but do not have Fc receptors for immunoglobulins.[22] They are probably related to fibroblasts[72,75] and are distinct from the strongly Ia-positive, Fc-negative, so-called *dendritic* or *accessory cells*.

It has been proposed that the lining cells are divisible into three populations according to the distribution of surface antigens.[10] The first is an Ia-positive, Fc-positive, phagocytic cell of the monocyte-macrophage lineage. The second is a nonphagocytic, intensely Ia-positive cell that lacks Fc receptors and other monocyte-lineage antigens and is not a B- or T-lymphocyte. This is the stellate cell particularly abundant in rheumatoid synovium. The third is Ia negative and Fc negative and is probably related to fibroblasts. This third group of

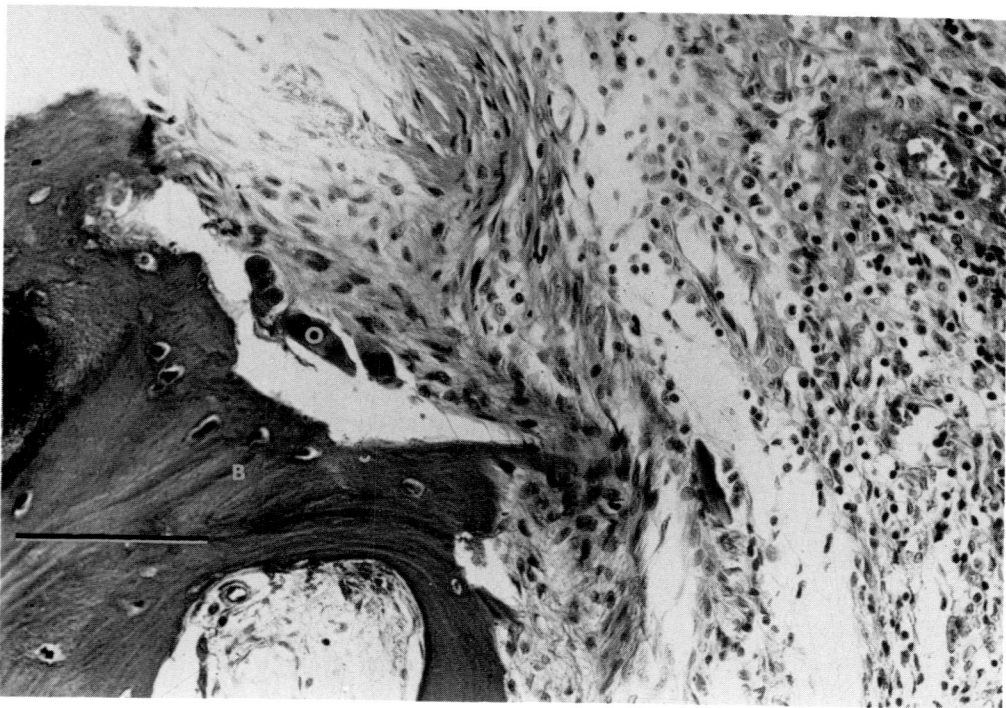

Fig. 37–2. Higher-power view of an area of rheumatoid bone erosion. Cells resembling osteoclasts (O) (artefactually pulled away from bone [B] surface) merge with other inflammatory cells. Bar = 80 μm.

cells may assume a stellate shape after exposure to prostaglandin E_2 and activation of adenylate cyclase.[4] It should be possible in the future to correlate structure and function with specific cell markers, to determine the interrelationship of these different cells.

The predominant cells in rheumatoid synovial fluids are polymorphonuclear leukocytes, which are uncommon in the pannus itself,[16] although they have been found in some instances at the cartilage-pannus junction.[96] The other cells found in the pannus may also be present in synovial fluid, however. Some of the interactions among the inflammatory cells that might be important in determining the characteristics, intensity, and direction of the destructive process are considered subsequently.

COLLAGEN DEGRADATION

In its native helical form, collagen is refractory to degradation by common proteolytic enzymes such as trypsin, chymotrypsin, and pepsin.[43,51] Although the nonhelical region at the ends of the molecule may be attacked by these proteases, the helical portion is less susceptible to attack. A possible exception to this generalization is type III collagen, which is cleaved at a specific site near the collagenase-cleavage site by enzymes such as neutrophil elastase.[37] Moreover, the fibril is even

more resistant to proteolysis than the component molecules, presumably owing to intermolecular interactions that further stabilize its structure. When collagen is denatured, that is, when the helical structure is uncoiled, proteolytic enzymes can attack peptide bonds in the polypeptide chain at many different locations. No evidence suggests, however, that collagen is denatured in vivo, even in inflammatory lesions. It had been known for years that enzymes present in bacteria such as *Clostridium histolyticum* could attack native collagen, even the helical portion, at many different loci; however, convincing demonstration of enzymes from animal tissues that could specifically carry out such an attack was lacking until Gross and Lapiere reported their observations.[45] These workers found that certain tadpole tissues in culture produced specific enzymes that attacked helical collagen molecules in solution, as well as in fibril form, in a characteristic manner. Shortly thereafter, Evanson et al. demonstrated that rheumatoid synovial tissue in culture produced enzyme(s) that degraded native collagen.[32,33] This process was accomplished by implanting fragments of synovium, obtained at the time of synovectomy, directly onto reconstituted collagen gels, resulting in lysis of the gels. Furthermore, the culture media contained soluble col-

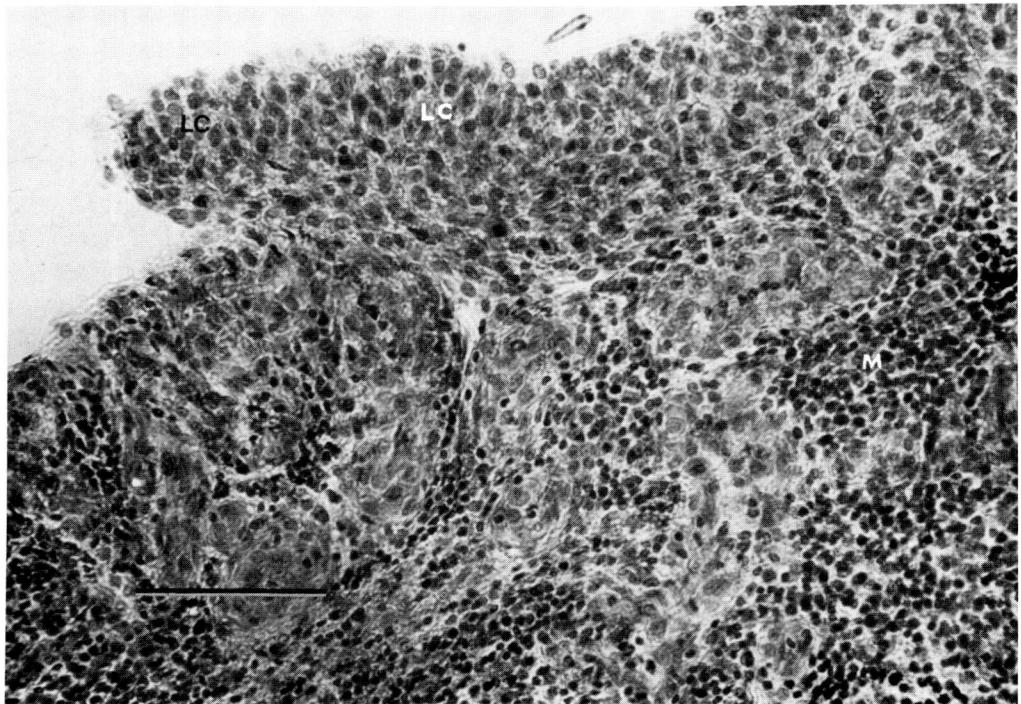

Fig. 37–3. Section of the surface of rheumatoid synovitis showing the heterogeneous population of cells. Lining cells (LC) and lymphocytes and other mononuclear cells (LM) can be seen. Bar = 80 μm.

lagenase, which could be assayed against either collagen molecules in solution or insoluble collagen fibrils.

Collagenase from rheumatoid synovial tissue culture, like that from the tadpole and other animal tissues, cleaves the collagen molecule across all three chains at a position three-quarters the distance from the amino terminal end. At 37° C, fragments cleaved from the fibril become more soluble and are then denatured. Further digestion of the solubilized fragments to smaller peptides is then accomplished, probably by neutral proteases other than collagenase. Data obtained by many investigators, using collagenases of different sources and with types I, II, and III collagens as substrates, show that the peptide bands cleaved are between specific glycyl-isoleucyl residues.[43,44] Sufficient information has been accumulated to establish criteria for determining the role of collagenase in the destruction of connective tissues in inflammatory arthritis.[74] These criteria are as follows:

Collagen degradation in RA is predominantly extracellular; this finding is consistent with evidence in vitro that collagenase is released from cultured tissues and is present in low concentrations in tissue homogenates. Under some circumstances, phagocytosis of collagen fibrils has been observed.[50] Collagenolysis in vitro is also proportional to the collagenase activity released into the culture media, and a collagenase similar to that produced by cultured synovium is found in vivo, particularly in synovial fluids.[48,76] Some of the enzyme in rheumatoid synovial fluids is probably derived from the polymorphonuclear leukocytes.[48,49] In a minority of rheumatoid fluids, collagenase activity is present without proteolytic activation,[48] but treatment (activation) with trypsin reveals activity in almost all fluids. Products similar to the specific reaction products of synovial collagenase acting on collagen in vitro have been demonstrated in vivo.[108] The pattern of inhibition of collagenase in vitro has been correlated with the pattern of collagen degradation in the rheumatoid joint; most of the collagen destruction takes place adjacent to the pannus, whereas collagen is usually preserved in regions not in contact with the pannus. Macromolecular inhibitors of collagenase are present in serum and synovial fluid and consist mainly of α2-macroglobulin as well as lower-molecular-weight inhibitors.[148] Finally, the putative collagen substrates degraded in the course of rheumatoid synovitis are indeed substrates for collagenase in vitro.[51,53,147]

Most collagenases, including the rheumatoid

synovial enzyme, cleave the interstitial collagens (types I, II, and III), but do not degrade type IV collagen, found in basement membranes, or type V collagen, found in pericellular regions. Types IV and V collagens are attacked, however, by several other neutral proteases such as elastases.[80,89] The rate at which cartilage type II collagen is attacked is slower than the rate for types I and III collagens.[51,53,139] Nevertheless, both crude and purified cartilage collagens are degraded by the rheumatoid synovial collagenase. Whether proteoglycans alter the rate or extent of collagenolysis is not certain because the proteoglycan component is usually already degraded before the collagen is attacked.

Bone erosion is a characteristic accompaniment of chronic persistent RA,[16,98] but mineralized bone collagen cannot be attacked by collagenases of any source, even from bacteria.[111,127] The presence of the calcium-phosphate mineral phase also protects the bone collagen from thermal denaturation.[7,73] Once the calcium-phosphate phase is removed, for example, by means of chelating agents or cold dilute acid, the collagen becomes susceptible to collagenolytic cleavage. The mechanisms by which the mineral is removed in vivo is not certain. Possibilities include local decreases in pH, production of a biologic chelator such as citrate, or operation of a cellular calcium or phosphate ion pump that effectively reduces local concentration of these ions and favors dissolution of the solid phase.[73] Some cellular mechanism is probably required for removal of this mineral phase. It is not certain, however, which cells are necessary for bone resorption. For example, osteoclasts normally present on endosteal surfaces could be activated through some interactions with pannus cells, or their differentiation could be induced from the hematopoietic precursor cells.[123] Alternatively, cells derived from the inflammatory tissue itself could differentiate into osteoclasts or could be involved directly in resorbing bone, without mediation by differentiated bone cells. For example, monocyte-macrophages bind to mineralized bone matrix and have some capacity to resorb dead bone.[64,102] Activation of bone cells may take place through the production of soluble mediators by pannus cells.

Robinson et al. have shown that prostaglandins, particularly PGE_2, are produced in large amounts by rheumatoid synovium in culture.[121,122] Such culture media have bone-resorbing activity toward mouse calvaria in vitro, accounted for by the PGE_2 present. The bone-resorbing activity in these studies is extractable into ether at low pH and is inhibited by indomethacin, as is the PGE_2 production. Bone-resorbing substances other than prostaglandins are also produced by rheumatoid

synovial culture media.[73] It is possible that these are accounted for in part by lymphocyte-derived osteoclast-activating factors (OAF)[58,103–105,149,150] or by monocyte-derived factors of the interleukin 1 (IL-1) type. These monocyte-derived factors are considered subsequently in further detail.

Collagenase, a typical neutral metalloprotease, is secreted from cells in a latent form. The latent collagenase can be activated by limited proteolysis, as was first demonstrated by Vaes.[130] Activation in some systems can also be accomplished by organic mercurial compounds apparently incapable of cleaving peptide bonds.[134,141] In rheumatoid synovial organ cultures, the collagenase is secreted in an active form,[32,33] whereas in cultures of rheumatoid synovial cells, collagenase is secreted in a latent form that can be activated by trypsin.[22] The occurrence of latent collagenase in rheumatoid synovial fluids has been discussed. The presence of this latent collagenase is consistent with at least two major possibilities. The first is that the cells release a procollagenase, a true zymogen, activated by cleaving off a covalently attached portion of the molecule. This process is analogous to the production of active trypsin from trypsinogen. Another possibility is that the cell producing an active collagenase also produces an inhibitor. The collagenase-inhibitor complex would thus be the latent collagenase, and its interaction with proteases would then produce active enzyme.[22,47,143]

Inhibitors of the metalloproteases have been identified.[106,107,125,133,140] More recently, however, it has been demonstrated that collagenase proteins are secreted from cultured rabbit synovial cells in the form of zymogens with M_r (molecular weight) of 55,000 and 60,000.[109] The higher-molecular-weight species is a glycosylated form of the lower-molecular-weight protein. Further evidence that the collagenase is secreted as a zymogen was obtained by translating messenger RNA (mRNA) from these cells in a cell-free translation system and by showing that the preprocollagenase was processed cotranslationally within microsomal membranes to a proenzyme of M_r indistinguishable from that of forms found in cell culture medium. Similar forms of procollagenase protein complexes detected by specific antibody are secreted by adherent rheumatoid synovial cells. These observations are most consistent with the hypothesis that the procollagenase is synthesized as a single polypeptide zymogen.

Activation of the procollagenase zymogen can also be accomplished through the action of proteases such as trypsin. Some other protease system would be required for activation of the procollagenase by neutral proteases in the synovium, such as plasmin, through a plasminogen-activator attack on plasminogen, or trypsin-like proteases secreted by cells such as mast cells. Mast cells are present in the rheumatoid synovium.[9,17] Based on observations in rabbit synovial cells, likely applicable to the inflammatory human synovium, activation of procollagenase does not take place directly, through the action of these proteases, but rather indirectly, through the action of an activator protein.[135] This activator has a molecular weight similar to the procollagenase and also exists as a zymogen. Enzymes such as plasmin may therefore activate latent collagenase by cleaving and activating the proactivator.

PROTEOGLYCAN DEGRADATION

The proteoglycans are important structural constituents of connective tissue, particularly of cartilage. Enzymatic removal of the proteoglycans in vitro diminishes the capacity of cartilage to resist deformation under a mechanical load.[54,67] On the other hand, collagen is responsible for the static form of cartilage, that is, its thickness.[54] The mechanical properties of cartilage thus depend on both the collagen and the proteoglycan components. During the process of RA, loss of proteoglycan is prominent. Even in early disease, depletion of proteoglycan may be seen in areas remote from the pannus.[60,78] Although such regions retain their form and thickness for considerable periods if the collagen network is preserved, alteration of mechanical properties is a consequence of the loss of the proteoglycans.[54]

Proteoglycan loss from articular cartilage in inflammatory joint disease probably involves cleavage of the core protein of the proteoglycan subunit. Although carbohydrases such as hyaluronidase can attack the chondroitin sulfate moiety of the proteoglycan, evidence of the presence of significant hyaluronidase activity in normal or inflamed synovial tissue is insufficient.[117] Superoxide free radical produced by polymorphonuclear leukocytes might also be involved in proteoglycan degradation, analogous to the effects of superoxide on hyaluronic acid.[92] The proteoglycan core protein is cleaved by different proteases to yield proteoglycan subunit molecules approximately the same size as the native proteoglycan subunit molecule.[5] These fragments, however, lack the capacity to bind hyaluronic acid and diffuse out of the cartilage. Which protease is responsible for this effect in inflammatory joint disease?

It had been proposed that the lysosomal acid protease, cathepsin D, was the critical enzyme.[30,36,114,115,144,145] Cathepsin D at low pH can attack proteoglycan core protein. This enzyme has been found in human and other cartilage extracts and has been demonstrated extracellularly in rheu-

matoid synovial tissue by immunofluorescence.[115] Cathepsin D or B is unlikely to play any important role in extracellular digestion, however, because the purified enzymes have no significant activity against proteoglycan substrates at pH > 6.0.[114,115] The pH in inflammatory synovial fluids is less than that in noninflammatory fluids, but not < 6.8.[34] Furthermore, inhibitors of cathepsin B and D have little effect on cartilage matrix depletion in model systems.[5]

Some of the neutral proteases described are probably responsible for degradation of proteoglycans in vivo.[5] Human granulocytes contain two different enzymes that can attack proteoglycans in solution as well as in cartilage slices. These enzymes have been characterized as an elastase and a chymotrypsin-like enzyme.[61,66,113] The elastase produces smaller fragments of the proteoglycan core than does the chymotrypsin-like enzyme. Other proteases active on proteoglycans at neutral pH have been described in human cartilage and fibroblasts.[5,124] Polymorphonuclear leukocytes are probably responsible for at least part of the proteoglycan-degrading activity in RA. Because these enzymes are inhibited by proteins found in inflammatory synovial fluids, such as α_1-antitrypsin and α_2-macroglobulin, uncontrolled degradation of tissue constituents probably does not occur.

Although the capacity of cartilage to reconstitute itself with type II collagen is limited, cartilage has a considerable capacity to restore proteoglycan.[91] This capacity has been shown particularly in experimental carrageenin-induced arthritis in the rabbit.[39,85,86] Early in the lesion, proteoglycan is lost, a loss ascribable to proteolytic activity, as well as to depression of proteoglycan biosynthesis. With recovery from inflammation, proteoglycan synthesis recovers and may exceed that found in an uninvolved joint. Inhibition of proteoglycan biosynthesis might be related to soluble factors present in the inflammatory exudate, such as prostaglandins and other soluble products of lymphocytes and monocytes,[3,31,56,90] and restoration of synthesis as inflammation subsides may occur when the concentration of these factors decreases. The "overshoot" in synthetic activity might be due to a feedback control secondary to a decrease in cartilage proteoglycan concentration.

CONTROL OF TISSUE DEGRADATION

The destruction of the joint appears to be explained by the production and release of degradative enzymes. The magnitude and duration of the synovial lesion are determined by several factors, including the relative proportion and number of each cell type in the pannus, the adjacent bone marrow and synovial fluid, the activity of the responsible cells, and the interaction of these cells with the environment, mediated either by direct cell-cell contact or by release of soluble products.

Although it has been shown that the polymorphonuclear leukocyte contains and releases neutral proteases capable of degrading proteoglycans, the origin of the collagenase-producing cell in the inflammatory synovium is uncertain. Polymorphonuclear leukocytes contain a collagenase in granular form,[79,87,88] and it is possible that some of the activity demonstrated in inflammatory synovial fluids comes from this source.[48,49] As mentioned previously, however, polymorphonuclear leukocytes are scarce in the pannus. Cells similar to fibroblasts, derived from human and rodent synovia by the common explant technique, produce collagenase through multiple passages, but most human synovial fibroblasts produce only small amounts of enzyme unless exposed to agents such as cytochalasin B.[44,55,142,143] In contrast, when rheumatoid synovial lining is dispersed with proteases, both primary cultures of the adherent cells and cells taken through several passages release large amounts of collagenase and prostaglandin (PGE_2) into the medium. Most of the collagenase secreted by these cells is in a latent form, most likely the procollagenase zymogen previously discussed.

Collagenolytic activity can be detected after proteolytic activation, even in the presence of 10% serum. Cultures in which large amounts of collagenase are secreted contain many Fc-negative stellate cells.[22,72,75] These cells are positive by indirect immunofluorescence using antibodies to rheumatoid synovial collagenase.[146] Cells that retain the capacity to synthesize and to secrete collagenase persist in culture when all monocyte-macrophages are no longer detectable and when the levels of lysozyme, an enzyme marker for monocyte-macrophages, are also undetectable. Although rodent macrophages produce collagenase when stimulated, for example, with endotoxin,[137,138] macrophages derived from human peripheral blood monocytes produce low levels of this enzyme even when stimulated.[72,75] The cells in the rheumatoid synovium that produce the collagenase are thus likely to be related to fibroblasts, rather than to macrophages. Such cells could be the nonmacrophage lining cells (synovial type B cells). The stellate morphology can be accounted for, at least in part, by the high ambient levels of PGE_2, since this appearance can be induced by stimulating endogenous PGE_2 production or by the addition of exogenous PGE_2, with subsequent activation of adenylate cyclase.[4] Even if PGE_2 production is inhibited, however, with indomethacin, and the stellate morphologic characteristics disappear, collagenase production persists. This finding indicates

that the stellate shape is not essential for the expression of collagenase synthesis.

Although the term "proliferative" is frequently applied to the rheumatoid synovial lesion, it is not yet known whether the lining cells or other cells in the heterogeneous population that comprise the lesion proliferate in situ or are derived from circulating cells. Thus, attraction of a specific cell or its precursor to the lesion by chemotaxis or the enhancement of local replication of these cells would be an important control. The role of complement components and of lymphocyte factors in the inflammatory lesion is discussed in detail elsewhere (see Chaps. 17, 21), but some comment concerning control of collagenase production is in order.

We have come to understand possible cellular interactions controlling collagenase production using these synovial cell cultures.[18,72,75] Although levels of collagenase and prostaglandins are high in primary cultures, these levels decrease when the cells are maintained in culture for several weeks or after passage of the cells by trypsinization. During this period, the small cells with macrophage markers also decrease in number. It was therefore reasoned that if macrophages were added back to synovial cells in later culture, the levels of collagenase and PGE_2 could be restored. Indeed, when peripheral blood mononuclear cells or enriched populations of monocytes were co-cultivated with synovial cells, the synovial cells were stimulated to increase synthesis of collagenase, with a dose-related increase in synthesis of PGE_2.[18,24,26,72,75] Because conditioned medium from the macrophages can produce the same effects, cell-cell contact is not essential for this stimulation. The substance responsible for this effect has been termed mononuclear cell factor (MCF). MCF, a protein with an apparent M_r of 14,000 to 25,000, has homologies with IL-1, as determined by lymphocyte activating factor (LAF) activity.[21,99] Human MCF activity co-purifies with LAF and is inactivated under conditions that inactivate LAF. Highly purified human and mouse IL-1 has MCF activity. Whether or not these biologic activities are present in identical polypeptides has yet to be determined, however.

MCF, a product of the monocyte, is released even in the absence of added stimulants in purified populations.[19] In unfractionated mononuclear cell populations, the amount of MCF is increased after incubation with lectins, such as pokeweed mitogen, which have no effects on the purified cells. When purified T-lymphocytes, which make little or no MCF by themselves, are coincubated with monocytes in the presence of lectin, MCF production is stimulated. Evidence that a soluble product of the

T-lymphocytes is responsible for this effect has been obtained using a human monocyte cell line, U937. These cells have no detectable MCF or LAF activity, but are induced to produce MCF when incubated with medium conditioned by lectin-treated T-lymphocytes.[2]

Other factors influence the production of MCF by monocyte-macrophages. The addition of aggregated immunoglobulins that increase synthesis of PGE_2 by monocyte-macrophages augments the production of MCF, assayed by measuring the ability of monocyte-macrophage-conditioned medium to increase PGE_2 and collagenase levels in synovial cell cultures.[23] This effect resides in the Fc region of the immunoglobulin molecule. Observations that self-associating rheumatoid factors are also capable of this stimulation suggest an additional role for rheumatoid factors in the pathogenesis of synovitis.[110]

The possibility that interactions of monocyte-macrophages with the extracellular matrix could also regulate MCF production is suggested by studies showing that types II and III collagens increase production of MCF by peripheral blood mononuclear cells.[27] Components of the extracellular matrix have profound effects on cell functions such as adherence and spreading, replication, and differentiation.[68] In animal models, polyarthritis has also been induced with type II collagen in incomplete Freund's adjuvant.[129] Furthermore, patients with RA have evidence of cellular immunity to several different collagens, depending on the assay systems utilized.[128] These immune effects are mediated predominantly by T-lymphocytes, whereas the effects of type II and III collagen on stimulating MCF production are observed in adherent mononuclear cells, enriched in monocytes and depleted of T-lymphocytes. Synovial fibroblast-like cells and lymphocytes are not the only targets of molecules of the IL-1 class. For example, chondrocytes also increase the production of collagenase and other proteases capable of degrading cartilage proteoglycans when exposed to factors, released from monocytes, possibly related to IL-1.[28,29,46,59,63,71,95,118,126] A substance released by synovial tissue and detected by its ability to deplete cartilage of proteoglycan, termed "catabolin," may also be a member of this family of molecules.[29] The possibility thus exists that chondrocytes may contribute to the degradation as well as to the synthesis of their own matrix under the influence of products of inflammatory synovial fluid or pannus cells.

The PGE_2 released by the synovial cells and macrophages can interact through specific receptors with these same cells, as well as with other cells in the environment, and can modulate their rate of replication, their morphology, and other functions. These functions include alteration in synthesis of matrix proteins, such as collagens by fibroblasts and chondrocytes, and proteases such as plasminogen activator and collagenase, and the release of acid hydrolases.[4,15,70,75]

Connective tissue cells in the inflammatory joint lesion are also under the influence of circulating hormones and many growth factors present in serum. Receptors for parathyroid hormone are present on synovial cells, and parathyroid hormone may have a permissive role in induction of osteoclastic bone resorption near the joint.[1,42,72] Similarly 1,25-dihydroxy-vitamin D_3 may also function in inflammation through its effects on monocyte function and maturation.[1] Substances such as platelet-derived growth factor and epidermal growth factor affect replication and function of fibroblasts and synovial cells. Castor and co-workers have described a group of factors called connective tissue activating peptides (CTAP)[11-14] (see Chap. 12). CTAP-I is derived from lymphocytes, and CTAP-III and CTAP-P2 are derived from platelets. CTAP-III has been purified, and its amino acid sequence is known. It has homologies with β-thromboglobulin. CTAP stimulate glycolysis by target cells and increase the synthesis of hyaluronic acid and proteoglycans. These peptides also potentiate prostaglandin effects on cells, as does IL-1 and may well interact with other products of mononuclear cells to affect not only the rate of cell replication and degradation of the extracellular matrix, but also repair.

The emphasis in this discussion has been on the stable prostaglandins, particularly PGE_2, because they are the most abundant products of arachidonic acid metabolism in synovial tissues. The leukotrienes, which could have several roles in synovial inflammation, such as chemotaxis, have not yet been shown to affect soft tissue matrix degradation or bone resorption.

The problem of repair is critical to the whole issue of the mechanisms of tissue destruction. The limited capacity of chondrocytes to resynthesize the appropriate (type II) collagen matrix results in an irreversible loss of cartilage thickness once the collagen has been resorbed. Even when other joint structures are destroyed and inflammation subsides, repair may be inadequate in type. For example, bone may be replaced by fibrous tissue rather than by new bone.

EFFECTS OF DRUGS

Although many features of the processes in degradation of joint structures have been defined, enormous gaps in our knowledge still exist. It is not yet possible to localize all effects of the drugs currently used to treat RA. The ultimate course of this disease and the natural history of a specific localized joint lesion in any individual patient are not predictable. Methods of following and interpreting biologic changes in a particular lesion, short of repeated biopsies, are inadequate. Drugs such as aspirin and the nonsteroidal anti-inflammatory compounds have multiple effects, but a major action is the inhibition of the cyclo-oxygenase reaction in prostaglandin biosynthesis.[100,119,121] This inhibition should lessen several deleterious effects attributed to prostaglandins, such as vasodilatation, edema, and pain. Because the prostaglandins can accelerate bone resorption as well, inhibition of their production would also be considered beneficial.[122] Under many conditions of cell and tissue culture, however, drugs such as indomethacin do not inhibit collagenase production,[75] but interfere with some anti-inflammatory effects of the prostaglandins.[101] Exposure of cells to cyclo-oxygenase inhibitors also has the paradoxic effect of sensitizing cells to the actions of prostaglandins.[20,75,112] If the suppression of ambient PGE_2 levels is proportional to the increase in cellular sensitivity, the overall effects of the drugs would be minimal. No data exist on the long-term effects on inhibition of prostaglandin synthesis on the progression of bone erosions or on the juxta-articular osteopenia of RA.

The glucocorticoids, on the other hand, have potent effects on many of the cellular functions and interactions previously described. Glucocorticoids, at levels approximating those achieved therapeutically, inhibit production of collagenase in synovial tissue and in synovial and chondrocyte culture.[25,94] These steroids also suppress levels of proteases such as plasminogen activator.[94] These effects, as well as those on collagenase, could be explained in part by specific stimulation of synthesis and release of proteins inhibitory for metalloproteases or serine proteases. Prostaglandin synthesis in synovial cells and tissue is also inhibited by glucocorticoids.[65,120,132] One mechanism for this inhibition involves the glucocorticoid-induced synthesis of an inhibitor of phospholipase A_2; this inhibitor is termed macrocortin[6] or lipomodulin.[57] Evidence also suggests that glucocorticoids inhibit prostaglandin synthesis at the level of cyclo-oxygenase in synovial tissue[120] (see Chap. 32).

The problem with the use of glucocorticoids is that anabolic processes, such as synthesis of collagen and proteoglycans, are also inhibited. Furthermore, effective local concentrations of glucocorticoids may not be obtainable without systemic toxicity. Thus, that long-term use of systemic glucocorticoids decreases the rate of joint destruction has not been convincingly demonstrated, even allowing for inhibition of repair.

Less is known of the antirheumatic effects of drugs such as gold compounds or penicillamine and of the way in which they might modulate the degradative phenomena described in this chapter. Evidence suggests that these compounds function as immunosuppressive agents. Gold compounds act, at least in part, by depression of macrophage functions, whereas penicillamine inhibits several functions of T-lymphocytes.[81-84] Thus, interaction of macrophages and T-lymphocytes, important in generating products affecting the function of other cells, would be expected to be modulated by these drugs.

REFERENCES

1. Amento, E.P., Goldring, S.R., and Kurnick, J.T.: Osteoclasts and arthritis. Adv. Immunopharmacol., 2:731–736, 1983.
2. Amento, E.P., Kurnick, J.T., and Epstein, A.: Modulation of synovial cell products by a factor from a human cell line. Lymphocyte induction of a mononuclear cell factor. Proc. Natl. Acad. Sci. U.S.A., 79:5307–5311, 1982.
3. Anastassiades, T.P., and Wood, A.: Effect of soluble products from lectin-stimulated lymphocytes on the growth, adhesiveness and glycosaminoglycan synthesis of cultured synovial fibroblastic cells. J. Clin. Invest., 68:792–802, 1981.
4. Baker, D.G., Dayer, J.-M., and Roelke, M.: Rheumatoid synovial cell morphologic changes induced by a mononuclear cell factor in culture. Arthritis Rheum., 26:8–14, 1983.
5. Barrett, A.J.: Which proteinases degrade cartilage matrix? Semin. Arthritis Rheum., 11:52–56, 1981.
6. Blackwell, G.J., Carnuccio, R., and DiRossa, M.: Macrocortin: a polypeptide causing anti-phospholipase effects of glucocorticoids. Nature, 287:147–149, 1980.
7. Bonar, L.C., and Glimcher, M.J.: Thermal denaturalization of mineralized and demineralized bone collagens. J. Ultrastruct. Res., 32:545–555, 1970.
8. Bornstein, P., and Sage, H.: Structurally distinct collagen types. Annu. Rev. Biochem., 49:957–1003, 1980.
9. Bromley, M., Fisher, W.D., and Woolley, D.E.: Mast cells at sites of cartilage erosion in the rheumatoid joint. Ann. Rheum. Dis., 43:76–79, 1984.
10. Burmester, G.R., Dimitriu-Bona, A., and Waters, S.J.: Identification of three major synovial lining cell populations by monoclonal antibodies directed to Ia antigen and antigens associated with monocytes/macrophages and fibroblasts. Scand. J. Immunol., 17:69–82, 1983.
11. Castor, C.W.: Synovial cell activation induced by a polypeptide mediator. Ann. N.Y. Acad. Sci., 256:304–317, 1975.
12. Castor, C.W., Fremuth, T.D., and Roberts, D.J.: Regulation of articular cell metabolism by CTAP mediators. Semin. Arthritis Rheum., 11:95–96, 1981.
13. Castor, C.W., Ritchie, J.C., and Scott, M.E.: Connective tissue activation-stimulation of glycosaminoglycan and DNA formation by a platelet factor. Arthritis Rheum., 20:859–867, 1977.
14. Castor, C.W., Ritchie, J.C., and William, C.H.: Connective tissue activation. Arthritis Rheum., 22:260–272, 1979.
15. Clarris, B.J., and Malcolm, L.P.: Effects of prostaglandins E_1, E_2, and $F_{2\alpha}$ on N-acetyl-β-glucosaminidase activities of human synovial cells in culture. Ann. Rheum. Dis., 42:187–191, 1983.
16. Collins, D.H.: The Pathology of Articular and Spinal Disease. London, Edward Arnold, 1955.
17. Crisp, A., Chapman, C.M., and Kirkham, S.E.: Synovial mastocytosis in adult rheumatoid arthritis. Arthritis Rheum., 26:S52, 1982.
18. Dayer, J.-M., and Krane, S.M.: The interaction of im-

munocompetent cells and chronic inflammation as exemplified by rheumatoid arthritis. Clin. Rheum. Dis., 4:517–538, 1978.

19. Dayer, J.-M., Breard, J., and Chess, L.: Participation of monocytes-macrophages and lymphocytes in the production of a factor that stimulates collagenase and prostaglandin release by rheumatoid synovial cells. J. Clin. Invest., 64:1386–1392, 1979.

20. Dayer, J.-M., Goldring, S.R., and Robinson, D.R.: Effects of human mononuclear cell factor on cultured rheumatoid synovial cells. Biochim. Biophys. Acta, 586:87–105, 1979.

21. Dayer, J.-M., Krane, S.M., and Goldring, S.R.: Cellular and humoral factors modulate connective disease destruction and repair in arthritic diseases. Semin. Arthritis Rheum., 11:77–81, 1981.

22. Dayer, J.-M., Krane, S.M., and Russell, R.G.G.: Production of collagenase and prostaglandins by isolated adherent rheumatoid synovial cells. Proc. Natl. Acad. Sci. U.S.A., 73:945–949, 1976.

23. Dayer, J.-M., Passwell, J.H., and Schneeberger, E.E.: Interactions among rheumatoid synovial cells and monocyte-macrophages: production of collagenase stimulating factor by human monocytes exposed to concanavalin A or immunoglobulin Fc fragments. J. Immunol., 124:1712–1720, 1980.

24. Dayer, J.-M., Robinson, D.R., and Krane, S.M.: Prostaglandin production by rheumatoid synovial cells. Stimulation by a factor from human mononuclear cells. J. Exp. Med., 145:1399–1404, 1977.

25. Dayer, J.-M., Robinson, D.R., and Krane, S.M.: Action of anti-inflammatory drugs on synovium. In Rheumatoid Arthritis: Cellular Pathology and Pharmacology. Edited by J.L. Gordon and B.H.L. Hazleman. Amsterdam, North Holland, 1977.

26. Dayer, J.-M., Russell, R.G.G., and Krane, S.M.: Collagenase production by rheumatoid synovial cells: stimulation by a human lymphocytic factor. Science, 195:181–182, 1977.

27. Dayer, J.-M., Trentham, D.E., and Krane, S.M.: Collagens act as ligands to stimulate monocytes to produce mononuclear cell factor (MCF) and prostaglandins (PGE₂). Collagen Rel. Res., 2:523–540, 1982.

28. Deshmukh-Pahdke, K., Nanda, S., and Lee, K.: Macrophage factor that induces neutral protease secretion by normal rabbit chondrocytes. Eur. J. Biochem., 104:175–180, 1980.

29. Dingle, J.T.: The role of catabolins in synovia-chondrocyte interactions. Adv. Immunopharmacol., 2:725–729, 1983.

30. Dingle, J.T., Barrett, A.J., and Weston, P.D.: Cathepsin D. Characteristics of immunoinhibition and the confirmation of a role in cartilage breakdown. Biochem. J., 123:1–13, 1971.

31. Eisenbarth, G.S., Beuttel, S.C., and Lebovitz, H.E.: Inhibition of cartilage macromolecular synthesis by prostaglandin A₁. J. Pharmacol. Exp. Ther., 189:213–220, 1974.

32. Evanson, J.M., Jeffrey, J.J., and Krane, S.M.: Studies on collagenase from rheumatoid synovium in tissue culture. J. Clin. Invest., 47:2639–2651, 1968.

33. Evanson, J.M., Jeffrey, J.J., and Krane, S.M.: Human collagenase: identification and characterization of an enzyme from rheumatoid synovium in culture. Science, 158:499–504, 1967.

34. Falchuk, K.H., Goetzl, E.J., and Kulka, J.P.: Respiratory gases of synovial fluids. Am. J. Med., 49:223–231, 1970.

35. Fassbender, H.G.: Histomorphological basis of articular cartilage destruction in rheumatoid arthritis. Collagen Rel. Res., 3:141–155, 1983.

36. Fell, H.B., and Dingle, J.T.: Studies on the mode of action of excess of vitamin A. Biochem. J., 87:403–408, 1963.

37. Gadek, J.E., Fells, G.A., and Wright, D.K.: Human neutrophil elastase functions as a type III collagen "collagenase." Biochem. Biophys. Res. Commun., 95:1815–1822, 1980.

38. Gay, S., Gay, R.E., and Miller, E.J.: The collagens of the joint. Arthritis Rheum., 23:937–941, 1980.

39. Gillard, G.D., and Lowther, D.A.: Carrageenin-induced arthritis II. Effect of intra-articular injection of carrageenin on the synthesis of proteoglycan in articular cartilage. Arthritis Rheum. 19:918–922, 1976.

40. Glimcher, M.J.: Handbook of Physiology. Section 7. Volume VIII. Washington, D.C., American Physiology Society, 1976.

41. Glimcher, M.J., Bonar, L.C., and Grynpas, M.D.: Recent studies of bone mineral: is the amorphous calcium phosphate theory valid? J. Crystal Growth, 53:100–119, 1981.

42. Goldring, S.R., Dayer, J.M., and Krane, S.M.: Rheumatoid synovial cell hormone responses modulated by cell-cell interactions. Inflammation, 8:107–121, 1984.

43. Gross, J.: Collagen biology: structure degradation and disease. Harvey Lect., 68:351–432, 1974.

44. Gross, J., Highberger, J.H., and Johnson-Wint, B.: Mode of action and regulation of tissue collagenases. In Collagenase in Normal and Pathological Connective Tissues. Edited by D.E. Woolley and J.M. Evanson. Chichester, John Wiley & Sons, 1980.

45. Gross, J., and Lapiere, C.M.: Collagenolytic activity in amphibian tissues: a tissue culture assay. Proc. Natl. Acad. Sci. U.S.A., 48:1014–1022, 1962.

46. Hamilton, J.A., and Slywka, J.: Stimulation of human synovial plasminogen activator production by mononuclear cell supernatants. J. Immunol., 126:851–855, 1981.

47. Harris, E.D., Jr.: Recent insights into the pathogenesis of the proliferative lesion in rheumatoid arthritis. Arthritis Rheum., 19:68–72, 1976.

48. Harris, E.D., DiBona, D.R., and Krane, S.M.: Collagenase in human synovial fluid. J. Clin. Invest., 48:2104–2113, 1969.

49. Harris, E.D., and Dimmig, T.A.: Collagenolytic enzymes in septic arthritis: potential significance for joint destruction. Arthritis Rheum., 17:498, 1974.

50. Harris, E.D., Glauert, A.M., and Murley, A.H.G.: Intracellular collagen fibers at the pannus-cartilage junction in rheumatoid arthritis. Arthritis Rheum., 20:657–665, 1977.

51. Harris, E.D., and Krane, S.M.: Cartilage collagen substrate in soluble and fibrillar form for rheumatoid collagenase. Trans. Assoc. Am. Phys., 86:82–94, 1983.

52. Harris, E.D., and Krane, S.M.: Collagenases. N. Engl. J. Med., 291:557–563, 605–609, 652–661, 1974.

53. Harris, E.D., and McCroskery, P.A.: The influence of temperature and fibril stability on degradation of cartilage collagen by rheumatoid synovial collagenase. N. Engl. J. Med., 290:1–8, 1974.

54. Harris, E.D., Parker, H.G., and Radin, E.L.: Effects of proteolytic enzymes on structural and mechanical properties of cartilage. Arthritis Rheum., 15:497–503, 1982.

55. Harris, E.D., Reynolds, J.J., and Werb, Z.: Cytochalasin B increases collagenase production by cells in vitro. Nature, 257:243–244, 1975.

56. Herman, J.H., Nutman, T.B., and Nozoe, M.: Lymphokine mediated suppression of chondrocyte glycosaminoglycan and protein synthesis. Arthritis Rheum., 24:824–834, 1981.

57. Hirata, F., Schiffman, F., and Ventasubramanian, K.: A phospholipase A₂ inhibitory protein in rabbit neutrophils induced by glucocorticoids. Proc. Natl. Acad. Sci. U.S.A., 77:2533–2536, 1980.

58. Horton, J.E., Raisz, L.G., and Simmons, H.A.: Bone resorbing activity on supernatant fluid from cultured human peripheral blood leukocytes. Science, 177:793–794, 1972.

59. Hubrechts-Godin, G., Hauser, P., and Vaes, G.: Macrophage-fibroblast interactions in collagenase production and cartilage degradation. Biochem. J., 184:643–650, 1979.

60. Janis, R., and Hamerman, D.: Articular cartilage in early arthritis. Bull. Hosp. Joint Dis., 30:136–152, 1969.

61. Janoff, A.: At least three human neutrophil lysosomal

proteases are capable of degrading joint connective tissues. Ann. N.Y. Acad. Sci., 265:402–408, 1975.
62. Janossy, G., Panayi, G., and Duke, P.: Rheumatoid arthritis: a disease of T-lymphocytes/macrophage immunoregulation. Lancet, 2:839–842, 1981.
63. Jasin, H.E., and Dingle, J.T.: Human mononuclear cell factors mediate cartilage matrix degradation through chondrocyte activation. J. Clin. Invest., 68:571–581, 1981.
64. Kahn, A.J., Stewart, C.C., and Teitelbaum, S.L.: Contact mediated bone resorption by human monocytes in vitro. Science, 199:988–989, 1978.
65. Kantrowitz, F., Robinson, D.R., and McGuire, M.B.: Corticosteroids inhibit prostaglandin production by rheumatoid synovia. Nature, 258:737–739, 1975.
66. Keiser, H., Greenwald, R.A., and Feinstein, G.: Degradation of cartilage proteoglycan by human leukocyte granule neutral proteases—a model of joint injury. J. Clin. Invest., 57:625–632, 1976.
67. Kempson, G.E.: The effects of proteoglycan and collagen degradation on the mechanical properties of adult human articular cartilage. In Dynamics of Connective Tissue Macromolecules. Edited by P.M.C. Burleigh and A.R. Poole. Amsterdam, North Holland, 1975.
68. Kleinman, H.K., Lkebe, R.J., and Martin, G.R.: Role of collagenous matrices in the adhesion and growth of cells. J. Cell Biol., 88:473–485, 1981.
69. Kobayashi, I., and Ziff, M.: Electron microscopic studies of the cartilage pannus junction in rheumatoid arthritis. Arthritis Rheum., 18:475–483, 1975.
70. Korn, J.H., Halushka, P.V., and LeRoy, E.C.: Mononuclear cell modulation of connective tissue function. J. Clin. Invest., 65:543–554, 1980.
71. Korn, J.H., Torres, D., and Downie, E.: Fibroblast prostaglandin E2 synthesis. Persistence of an abnormal phenotype after short term exposure to mononuclear cell products. J. Clin. Invest., 71:1240–1247, 1983.
72. Krane, S.M.: Aspects of cell biology of the rheumatoid synovial lesion. Ann. Rheum. Dis., 40:433–448, 1981.
73. Krane, S.M.: Degradation of collagen in connective tissue diseases. Rheumatoid arthritis. In Dynamics of Connective Tissue Macromolecules. Edited by P.M.C. Burleigh and A.R. Poole. Amsterdam, North Holland, 1975.
74. Krane, S.M.: Collagenase production by human synovial tissues. Ann. N.Y. Acad. Sci., 256:289–303, 1975.
75. Krane, S.M., Goldring, S.R., and Dayer, J.M.: Interactions among lymphocytes, monocytes and other synovial cells in the rheumatoid synovium. Lymphokines, 7:75–136, 1982.
76. Kruze, E., and Wojtecka, E.: Activation of leukocyte collagenase proenzyme by rheumatoid synovial fluid. Biochim. Biophys. Acta, 285:436–446, 1972.
77. Kulka, J.P., Bocking, E., and Ropes, M.W.: Early joint lesions of rheumatoid arthritis. Arch. Pathol., 59:129–150, 1955.
78. Lagier, R., and Taillard, W.: Softening of the cartilage and arthritis of the rheumatoid type. Acta Orthop. Scand., 40:300–316, 1969.
79. Lazarus, G.S., Daniels, J.R., and Lian, J.: Role of granulocyte collagenase in collagen degradation. Am. J. Pathol., 68:565–578, 1972.
80. Liotta, L.A., Abe, S., and Robey, P.G.: Preferential digestion of basement membrane collagen by an enzyme derived from a metastatic murine tumor. Proc. Natl. Acad. Sci. U.S.A., 76:2268–2272, 1979.
81. Lipsky, P.E.: Immunopharmacology of remission-inducing drugs in rheumatoid arthritis. Adv. Immunopharmacol., 2:345–350, 1983.
82. Lipsky, P.E., and Ziff, M.: Inhibition of human helper T cell function in vitro by D-penicillamine and CuSO4. J. Clin. Invest., 65:1069–1076, 1980.
83. Lipsky, P.E., and Ziff, M.: The effect of D-penicillamine on mitogen induced human lymphocyte proliferation synergistic inhibition by D-penicillamine and copper salts. J. Immunol., 120:1006–1013, 1978.
84. Lipsky, P.E., and Ziff, M.: Inhibition of antigen and mitogen induced human lymphocyte proliferation by gold compounds. J. Clin. Invest., 59:455–466, 1977.

85. Lowther, D.A., and Gillard, G.C.: Carrageenin-induced arthritis. I. The effect of intra-articular carrageenin on chemical composition of articular cartilage. Arthritis Rheum., 19:769–776, 1976.
86. Lowther, D.A., Gillard, G.C., and Bacter, E.: Carrageenin-induced arthritis. III. Proteolytic enzymes present in rabbit knee joints after a single intra-articular injection of carrageenin. Arthritis Rheum., 19:1287–1294, 1976.
87. Macartney, H.W., and Tschesche, H.: Latent and active human polymorphonuclear leukocyte collagenase. Eur. J. Biochem., 130:71–78, 1983.
88. Macartney, H.W., and Tschesche, H.: The collagenase inhibitor from human polymorphonuclear leukocytes. Eur. J. Biochem., 130:79–83, 1983.
89. Mainardi, C.L., Dixit, S.N., and Kang, A.H.: Degradation of type IV basement membrane, collagen by a proteinase isolated from human polymorphonuclear leukocyte. J. Biol. Chem., 255:5435–5441, 1980.
90. Malemud, C.J., and Sokoloff, L.: The effect of prostaglandins on cultured lapine articular chondrocytes. Prostaglandins, 13:845–860, 1977.
91. Mankin, H.J.: The metabolism of articular cartilage in health and disease. In Dynamics of Connective Tissue Macromolecules. Edited by P.M.C. Burleigh and A.R. Poole. Amsterdam, North Holland, 1975.
92. McCord, J.M.: Free radicals and inflammation: protection of synovial fluid by superoxide dismutase. Science, 185:529–531, 1974.
93. McCroskery, P.A., Amento, E.P., and Krane, S.M.: Mononuclear cell factor (MCF) increases procollagenase in human rheumatoid cells. Clin. Res., 31:521A, 1983.
94. McGuire, M.B., Murphy, G., and Reynolds, J.J.: Production of collaganese and inhibition (TIMP) by normal rheumatoid and osteoarthritic synovium in vitro: effects of hydrocortisone and indomethacin. Clin. Sci., 61:703–708, 1981.
95. Meats, J.E., McGuire, M.B., and Russell, R.G.G.: Human synovium releases a factor which stimulates chondrocyte production of PGE1 and plasminogen activator. Nature, 286:891–892, 1980.
96. Menninger, H., Putzier, R., and Mohr, W.: Granulocyte elastase at the site of cartilage erosion to rheumatoid synovial tissue. Z. Rheumatol., 39:145–156, 1980.
97. Miller, E.J.: The structure of collagen. In Connective Tissues Diseases. Edited by B.M. Wagner, R. Fleischmajer, and N. Kaufman. Baltimore, Williams & Wilkins, 1983.
98. Mills, K.: Pathology of the knee joints in rheumatoid arthritis. J. Bone Joint Surg., 52B:746–756, 1970.
99. Mizel, S.B., Dayer, J.-M., and Krane, S.M.: Stimulation of rheumatoid synovial cell collagenase and prostaglandin production by partially purified lymphocyte activating factor (interleukin 1). Proc. Natl. Acad. Sci. U.S.A., 78:2474–2477, 1981.
100. Moncada, S., and Vane, J.R.: Mode of action of aspirin-like drugs. Adv. Intern. Med., 24:1–22, 1979.
101. Morley, J.: Anti-inflammatory effects of prostaglandins. In Rheumatoid Arthritis: Cellular Pathology and Pharmacology. Edited by J.L. Gordon and B.L. Hazleman. Amsterdam, North Holland, 1977.
102. Mundy, G.R., Altman, A.A., and Gondek, M.D.: Director resorption of bone by human monocytes. Science, 196:1109–1111, 1977.
103. Mundy, G.R., Luben, R.A., and Raisz, L.G.: Bone resorbing activity in supernatants from lymphoid cell lines. N. Engl. J. Med., 290:867–871, 1974.
104. Mundy, G.R., Raisz, L.G., and Cooper, R.A.: Evidence for the secretion of an osteoclast stimulating factor in myeloma. N. Engl. J. Med., 291:1041–1046, 1974.
105. Mundy, G.R., Raisz, L.G., and Shapiro, J.L.: Big and little forms of osteoclast activating factor. J. Clin. Invest., 60:122–128, 1977.
106. Murphy, G., McGuire, M.B., and Russell, R.G.G.: Characterization of collagenase, other metallo-proteinases and an inhibitor (TIMP) produced by human synovium and cartilage in culture. Clin. Sci., 61:711–722, 1981.
107. Murphy, G., and Sellers, A.: The extracellular regulation of collagenase activity. In Collagenase in Normal and

Pathological Connective Tissues. Edited by D.E. Woolley and J.M. Evanson. Chichester, John Wiley & Sons, 1980.

108. Nagai, Y.: Vertebrate collagenase: further characterization and the significance of its latent form in vivo. Mol. Cell. Biochem., *1*:137–142, 1973.

109. Nagase, H., Jackson, R.C., and Brinckerhoff, C.E.: A precursor form of latent collagenase produced in a cell-free system with m-RNA from rabbit synovial cells. J. Biol. Chem., *256*:11951–11954, 1981.

110. Nardella, F., Dayer, J.-M., and Roelke, M.: Self-associating IgG rheumatoid factors stimulate monocytes to release prostaglandins and mononuclear cell factor that stimulates collagenase and prostaglandin production by synovial cells. Rheumatol. Int., *3*:183–186, 1983.

111. Newman, W.F., Mulryan, B.J., and Martin, G.R.: A chemical view of osteoclasis based on studies with yttrium. Clin. Orthop., *17*:124–133, 1960.

112. Newcombe, D.S., Ciosek, C.P., Ishikawa, Y.: Human synoviocytes: activation and desensitization by prostaglandins and 1-epinephrine. Proc. Natl. Acad. Sci. U.S.A., *72*:3124–3128, 1975.

113. Oronsky, A.L., and Perper, R.J.: Connective tissue-degrading enzymes of human leukocytes. Ann. N.Y. Acad. Sci., *265*:233–253, 1975.

114. Poole, A.R., Hembry, R.M., and Dingle, J.T.: Secretion and localization of cathepsin D in synovial tissues removed from rheumatoid and traumatized joints. Arthritis Rheum., *19*:1295–1307, 1976.

115. Poole, A.R., Hembry,. R.M., and Dingle, J.T.: Cathepsin D in cartilage. The immunohistochemical demonstration of extracellular enzyme in normal and pathological conditions. J. Cell. Sci., *14*:139–161, 1974.

116. Prockop, D.J., Kivirikko, K.I., and Tuderman, L.: Biosynthesis of collagen and its disorders. N. Engl. J. Med., *301*:13–23, 1979.

117. Pryce-Jones, R.H., Saklatvala, J., and Wood, G.C.: Neutral protease from the polymorphonuclear leukocytes of human rheumatoid synovial fluid. Clin. Sci. Mol. Med., *47*:403–414, 1974.

118. Robinson, D.R., Bastian, D., and Hamer, P.J.: Mechanism of stimulation of prostaglandin synthesis by a factor from rheumatoid tissue. Proc. Natl. Acad. Sci. U.S.A., *78*:5160–5164, 1981.

119. Robinson, D.R., Dayer, J.-M., and Krane, S.M.: Prostaglandins and their regulation in rheumatoid inflammation. Ann. N.Y. Acad. Sci., *332*:279–294, 1979.

120. Robinson, D.R., McGuire, M.B., and Bastian, D.: The effect of anti-inflammatory drugs on prostaglandin production by rheumatoid synovial tissue. Prostaglandins Med., *1*:461–477, 1979.

121. Robinson, D.R., McGuire, M.B., and Levine, L.: Prostaglandins in the rheumatic diseases. Ann. N.Y. Acad. Sci., *256*:318–329, 1975.

122. Robinson, D.R., Tashjian, A.H., and Levine, L.: Prostaglandin-stimulated bone resorption by rheumatoid synovia. J. Clin. Invest., *56*:1181–1188, 1975.

123. Rodan, G.A., and Martin, T.J.: Role of osteoblasts in hormonal control of bone resorption—a hypothesis. Calcif. Tissue Int., *33*:349–351, 1981.

124. Sapolsky, A.I., Keiser, H., and Howell, D.S.: The action of cathepsin D in human articular cartilage on proteoglycans. J. Clin. Invest., *52*:624–633, 1973.

125. Sellers, A., and Reynolds, J.J.: Identification and partial characterization of an inhibitor of collagenase from rabbit bone. Biochem. J., *167*:353–360, 1977.

126. Steinberg, J., Sledge, C.B., and Noble, J.: A tissue culture model of cartilage breakdown in rheumatoid arthritis. Biochem. J., *180*:403–412, 1979.

127. Stern, B., Golub, L., and Goldhaber, P.: Effects of demineralization and parathyroid hormone on the availability of bone collagen to degradation by collagenase. J. Periodont. Res., *5*:116–121, 1970.

128. Trentham, D.E., Dynesius, R.A., and Rocklin, R.E.: Cellular sensitivity to collagen in rheumatoid arthritis. N. Engl. J. Med., *299*:327–332, 1978.

129. Trentham, D.E., Townes, A.S., and Kang, A.H.: Autoimmunity to type II collagen: an experimental mode of arthritis. J. Exp. Med., *146*:857–863, 1977.

130. Vaes, G.: The release of collagenase as an inactive proenzyme by bone explants in culture. Biochem. J., *126*:275–289, 1972.

131. van Boxel, J.A., and Paget, S.A.: Predominantly T-cell infiltrate in rheumatoid synovial membranes. N. Engl. J. Med., *293*:517–520, 1975.

132. Vane, J.R., Flower, R.J., and Salmon, J.A.: Inhibitors of arachidonic acid metabolism, with especial reference to the aspirin-like drugs. *In* Prostaglandins and Cancer: First International Conference. Vol. 2. Edited by T.J. Powles, et al. New York, Alan R. Liss, 1982.

133. Vater, C.A., Marnardi, C.L., and Harris, E.D.: Inhibitor of human collagenase from cultures of human tendon. J. Biol. Chem., *254*:3045–3053, 1979.

134. Vater, C.A., Marnardi, C.L., and Harris, E.D.: Activation in vitro of rheumatoid synovial collagenase from cell cultures. J. Clin. Invest., *62*:987–992, 1978.

135. Vater, C.A., Nagase, H., and Harris, E.D.: Purification of an endogenous activator of procollagenase from rabbit synovial fibroblast culture medium. J. Biol. Chem., *258*:9374–9382, 1983.

136. Veis, A.: The Chemistry and Biology of Mineralized Connective Tissues. New York, Elsevier-North Holland, 1981.

137. Wahl, L.M., Wahl, S.M., and Martin, G.R.: Collagenase production by lymphokine-activated macrophages. Science, *187*:261–263, 1975.

138. Wahl, L.M., Wahl, S.M., and Mergenhagen, S.E.: Collagenase production by endotoxin activated macrophage. Proc. Natl. Acad. Sci. U.S.A., *71*:3598–3601, 1974.

139. Welgus, H.G., Jeffrey, J.J., and Eisen, A.Z.: The collagen substrate specificity of human skin fibroblast collagenase. J. Biol. Chem., *256*:9511–9515, 1981.

140. Welgus, H.G., Stricklin, G.P., and Eisen, A.Z.: A specific inhibitor of vertebrate collagenase produced by human skin fibroblasts. J. Biol. Chem., *254*:1938–1943, 1979.

141. Werb, Z., and Burleigh, M.C.: Collagenase from rabbit fibroblasts in monolayer culture. Biochem. J., *137*:373–385, 1974.

142. Werb, Z., and Reynolds, J.J.: Stimulation by endocytosis of the secretion of collagenase and neutral proteinase from rabbit synovial fibroblasts. J. Exp. Med., *140*:1482–1497, 1974.

143. Werb, Z., Mainardi, C.L., and Vater, C.A.: Endogenous activation of latent collagenase by rheumatoid synovial cells. N. Engl. J. Med., *296*:1017–1023, 1977.

144. Woessner, J.F.: Purification of cathepsin D from cartilage and uterus and its action on the protein-polysaccharide complex of cartilage. J. Biol. Chem., *248*:1634–1642, 1974.

145. Woessner, J.F.: Cartilage cathepsin D and its action on matrix components. Fed. Proc., *32*:1485–1488, 1973.

146. Woolley, D.E., Brinckerhoff, C.E., and Marnardi, C.L.: Collagenase production by rheumatoid synovial cells: morphological and immunohistochemical studies of the dendritic cell. Ann. Rheum. Dis., *38*:262–270, 1979.

147. Woolley, D.E., Glanville, R.W., and Lindberg, K.A.: Action of human skin collagenase on cartilage collagen. FEBS Lett., *34*:267–269, 1973.

148. Woolley, D.E., Roberts, D.R., and Evanson, J.M.: Small molecular-weight β_1 serum protein which specifically inhibits human collagenases. Nature, *261*:325–327, 1976.

149. Yoneda, T., and Mundy, G.R.: Monocytes regulate osteoclast activating factor production by releasing prostaglandins. J. Exp. Med., *150*:338–342, 1979.

150. Yoneda, T., and Mundy, G.R.: Prostaglandins are necessary for osteoclast-activating factor production by activated peripheral blood leukocytes. J. Exp. Med., *149*:279–283, 1979.

Chapter **38**

Clinical Picture of Rheumatoid Arthritis

Ralph C. Williams, Jr. and Daniel J. McCarty

The term "rheumatoid arthritis" (RA) was coined by Sir Alfred Baring Garrod in 1876.[36] The first convincing clear description of the disease is that of Landre-Beauvais in 1800.[63] Garrod, Charcot, and Adams each wrote extensive clinical and anatomic descriptions of the disease;[35] all three classified Heberden's nodes and primary osteoarthritis of the hip (malum coxae senilis) as variants of RA, thereby presaging the current debate on the role of inflammation in osteoarthritis.

ANTIQUITY OF THE DISEASE

Because of the lack of evidence of RA in Egyptian mummies and other skeletal remains, despite firm evidence of gout, ankylosing spondylitis, ochronosis, and infectious arthritis, including tuberculosis, Boyle and Buchanan postulated that RA is a disease of the modern era.[13] This challenge spawned a number of publications advancing evidence to the contrary. The Emperor Constantine IX (circa 980 to 1055) suffered from a rheumatoid-like polyarthritis,[18] and the Flemish painters,[22] including Rubens,[3] appear to have recorded typical rheumatoid hand deformities. Suggestive descriptive evidence for the occurrence of RA in India in the second century A.D. has been uncovered.[81] Moreover, a brief report of possible RA in an Egyptian mummy as well as in American Indian skeletons has appeared.[23] Buchanan and Murdoch have speculated further, based on observations that rheumatoid factor and antinuclear antibody positivity are under environmental rather than genetic control, that the modern epidemic of RA will spontaneously subside and perhaps will disappear.[15]

Taken together, the evidence for the existence of RA before 1500 is certainly sparse and unconvincing. Because the prevalence of RA is now about 1% of the adult population of the world (adjusted for age), and because the populations of the world were linked by roving navigators only after A.D. 1500, the original thesis of Boyle and Buchanan appears to be holding up well. Despite sanguine speculation about its future,[15,76] however, the disease remains a scourge and occupies about half the professional effort of practicing rheumatologists.[5]

CLASSIFICATION

The definition of the clinical syndrome is still a subject of some controversy, especially with respect to seronegative disease. Lawrence accepts only seropositivity and radiologic evidence of erosions as bona fide RA from an epidemiologic standpoint.[48] His data on populations and in the European twin registry only make sense if these criteria are used. Most studies use the ARA revised criteria established in 1958.[71] A tentative classification for the purposes of this discussion is given in Table 38–1.

Rheumatoid nodulosis is an uncommon variant that is usually, but not invariably, seropositive.[4,11,14,39] Such patients have little, if any, systemic reaction and often complain that they cannot grip a tennis racket or a golf club because of the interference by multiple nodules. Radiologists often diagnose gout because of the punched-out bony lesions and soft tissue nodularity. Palindromic rheumatism is much more common. Attacks are often periarticular, and few joint fluids or synovial membranes have been examined.[74] This condition is discussed in detail in Chapter 58.

Seronegative RA has various manifestations. Some patients, especially those with low titers of rheumatoid factor, convert from negative to posi-

Table 38–1.   Classification of Rheumatoid Arthritis

A. Seropositive*
1. Erosive
a. Bilateral, symmetric
b. Unilateral (rare)
2. Nonerosive
a. Bilateral, symmetric
b. Unilateral
B. Seronegative
1. Erosive
2. Nonerosive
C. Rheumatoid nodulosis
D. Palindromic rheumatism

*For IgM rheumatoid factor

tive over time; others convert, either spontaneously or while receiving remittive agents, from positive to negative. Some seronegative patients clearly have the clinical features of juvenile RA, including rash and fever,[4,31] whereas others have the characteristic involvement of larger joints such as the shoulder and knee, with lesser involvement of small hand joints and the forefoot.[55] Involvement is also often more asymmetric than in adult seropositive disease. The recognized association of spondylopathic diseases with HLA-B27 has intensified interest in the residue of patients with symmetric polyarthritis associated with persistent seronegativity.

Comparison of serologically well-characterized cases by histocompatibility typing showed the expected increase in HLA-DRW4 only in seropositive disease.[2] Vasculitis, seen in 6%, and nodules, seen in 37%, were noted only in seropositive patients, who also had greater anatomic and functional abnormalities. Destruction of joints was accelerated in 8 patients who were HLA-DRW4 positive. Another study found that seropositive patients had more severe arthritis, often with nodules, but the researchers could not otherwise separate the 2 groups on clinical or radiologic grounds.[27] Although these findings are of theoretical interest, little practical reason to consider RA subgroups appears to exist because treatment is similarly empiric in both groups.

HEREDITY

A genetic predisposition is now strongly suspected because certain histocompatibility markers, possibly related to immune-response genes, appear to be linked to the expression of RA[6,79,80] (see Chap. 25 for fuller discussion of the immunogenetics of RA). In most populations of seropositive rheumatoid patients, the frequency of HLA-DRW4 is about twice that of the general population to which these patients belong, and DR3 and DR7 are decreased. Jewish and Asian patients with RA show an association not with DRW4, but with DR1.[41] Furthermore, studies of identical fraternal twins, concordant or discordant for RA, clearly demonstrate a strong hereditary influence for seropositive erosive disease. Lawrence and Kellgren can account for about 80% of seropositive erosive RA through polygenic inheritance[49] (see Chap. 2).

GEOGRAPHIC DISTRIBUTION

A wide clinical spectrum is recognized. Thus, patients preselected by referral or by the interests of a particular clinic may not represent a true cross-section of disease presentation or clinical profile. Demographic and epidemiologic data suggest that many patients with typical disease do not ever seek medical attention.[49] In addition, environmental, social, genetic, and economic factors may play a role in the expression of the disease. Thus, the pattern of illness may appear particularly severe in homogeneous, isolated populations such as the Northwest Indians.[11]

Information about the worldwide prevalence of RA is incomplete. Because the disease occurs with high frequency after the age of 50, studies of populations in which the life expectancy is reduced, as in the era before the industrial revolution or even in the third world countries of today, provide a false impression of lowered prevalence. The prevalence of seropositive erosive RA appears to be similar all over the world, when data are corrected for the age of the population (see Chap. 2).

CLIMATE

Previous studies have reported an adverse effect of climatic changes on arthritis. Many such reports have been based on anecdotal notations by individual patients moving from one climate to another, such as from New York to New Mexico or Arizona. Careful "blind" observations by Hollander and associates, using a controlled climate chamber (climatron),[42] indicated that arthritis often worsened within a few hours of the onset of a combined rise in humidity and fall in barometric pressure. Such patients appear to be "weather sensitive." No pathogenetic mechanism has been uncovered to explain this phenomenon. In other patients, little relationship was noted between the climates and the activity of their disease. We do not recommend a change in location as part of the treatment of RA.

SPECIFIC CLINICAL FEATURES

RA is clearly a systemic disease. Its onset is frequently heralded by fatigue, diffuse myalgia, fever, loss of appetite, and vague malaise. Data collected in clinics indicate that onset of the disease occurs most often between the ages of 20 and 60, with peaks at 35 and 45 years. The disorder may begin at any time from the first few weeks of life to the ninth decade, however. Women are affected more frequently than men, in a ratio of 2 or 3 to 1, although epidemiologic studies of entire populations show a nearly equal sex ratio in patients with classic disease.[49] No clear explanation for the apparent female preponderance is available. Some women appear to develop the disease at menopause, and it is well known that onset or severe exacerbation of the disease may occur soon after termination of pregnancy. Oral contraceptives may exert a protective effect.[89]

Predominance in women parallels the effect of hormones on the immune system.[16,84] The ability of females in many mammalian species, including the human, to surpass males in both humoral and cellular immune response is well documented. Thus, if RA is somehow linked to an abnormal or harmful immune response, the result may be accentuated in females.

The influence of age on onset and expression of the disease is still not clear. Compared with control subjects, the recorded frequency of women who experienced the onset of RA between 50 and 55 years of age was higher than expected. At present, a body of evidence indicates that aging may have an interesting diversity of effects on the immune response. The incidence of autoantibodies, such as rheumatoid factors or antinuclear antibodies, increases with age.[91] This increment may be related to a decrease in number or functional activity of suppressor T cells capable of modulating and controlling the response of the immune system.[8,20]

It is often difficult to pinpoint a precipitating event in an individual patient with RA. Such events represent a variety of life stresses, including physical, psychic, infectious, or occasionally traumatic. In most patients, the disease starts gradually and insidiously, but in a few, the onset is acute, occurring within 24 to 48 hours. Prodromal symptoms of fatigue, myalgias, and malaise may be present for weeks or months before the onset of joint symptoms, but in most cases, joint pain, stiffness and swelling arise early in the disease. At times, initial joint involvement may be spotty, but a symmetric pattern of polyarthritis almost always evolves over weeks or months.[17] In one study, a tendency for the acute pattern of onset to occur before age 40 was noted, as well as an association with fever and the presence of subcutaneous nodules.[77]

Another study of the onset of RA in 102 patients showed that in 2 of 3 patients, the disease began in the winter.[34] About 10% of patients showed an acute polyarticular onset that could be pinpointed to the day; 18% could identify the week of onset, whereas the remainder could isolate the onset only to the nearest month. The male-to-female ratio was about 3:4, as in population studies. Older patients fared worst during the mean 4- to 5-year follow-up. An insidious onset and early progression to symmetric involvement carried a poor prognosis. More severe disease eventually developed when the large joints were also involved initially, or when metatarsophalangeal (MTP) joints 1 and 3 were involved early. MTP joint involvement at onset also correlated with the early occurrence of erosions.[33] More recent studies, however, showed no difference in clinical progression of the disease with respect to rapidity or age of onset.[51,83]

As the disease progresses, patients complain of joint pain at rest and on movement. Swelling of involved joints is prominent, and as the disorder persists, limitation of motion, accompanied by a diffuse wasting of adjacent muscles, is noted.

Symptoms

Systemic complaints of weakness and fatigue and localized symptoms of pain, stiffness, weakness, and paresthesias are discussed extensively in Chapter 7, which deals with the evaluation of the disease. The reader is referred to this discussion and to the summary in Table 38–2. Pain and stiffness have a circadian rhythm and are more pronounced in the morning. Both symptoms correlate with objective measurements of decreased grip strength and increased joint swelling.[46] Rarely, visceral manifestations of the disease, such as pulmonary rheumatoid nodules, antedate joint complaints.

Signs

Upper Extremity (see also Chaps. 45 and 46)

Initial swelling is due to synovitis and occurs along the lines of synovial reflection, usually most marked over the extensor surfaces, where the articular capsule is more distensible. Involved distal interphalangeal (DIP) joints show dorsal bulging, and the extensor tendon may be eroded, to produce a permanently flexed DIP joint. An extensive quantitative analysis of tenderness of the small joints of the hand showed that the DIP joints in most patients with RA were involved and that tenderness in them varied synchronously with that in the proximal small hand joints.[56] About 20% of RA patients never showed DIP joint tenderness no matter how tender the other hand joints became. The proximal interphalangeal (PIP) joints showed a symmetric, spindle-shaped swelling[62] (Fig. 38–1). These joints may develop flexion deformities in time, particularly when flexor tenosynovitis leads to subsequent tendon contracture. The PIP joints may also become hyperextended, owing to contracture of the intrinsic muscle tendons (interosseous and lumbrical), so these muscles become extensors of the joint, rather than flexors. This change leads to the ''intrinsicoid deflection'' sometimes called the ''grasshopper'' deformity when associated with simultaneous DIP joint flexion.

PIP joints in flexion deformity may suffer rupture of the central slip of the extensor digitorum tendon. When this rupture occurs, little impedes the dorsal migration of the joint through the lateral slips, through the ''buttonhole.'' This so-called ''boutonniere'' deformity is difficult to repair and is disabling. It is our practice to have this deformity repaired by a plastic or orthopedic hand surgeon as soon as possible. Results have been gratifying.

Table 38–2. Signs and Symptoms of Rheumatoid Arthritis

Sex Incidence—clinic population: 2 to 3 females to 1 male. Total population studies: equal distribution in classic disease.
Race—no particular predisposition.
Geography—more reported from temperate zones but data incomplete.
Climate—inadequate data.
Season—onset probably more frequent in the winter.
Anthropomorphic type—no definite type.
Personality pattern—no particular one.
Age of onset—any age, peaks at thirty-five and forty-five.
Prodromes—fatigue, malaise occasionally; frequently none.
Onset—usually insidious, but may be sudden or episodic.
Frequency of joint involvement—proximal interphalangeal, metacarpophalangeal, toes, wrist, knee, elbow, ankle, shoulder, temporomandibular joint.
Joint swelling—fusiform, spindle-shaped, symmetrical.
Stiffness—common after inactivity; its duration in morning used as index of activity.
Fever—usually negligible except during steroid withdrawal.
Tachycardia—may be present.
Loss of weight—may be present.
Subcutaneous nodules—in 20 to 25% of classic rheumatoid arthritis at some time during the disease.
Muscular atrophy—marked and out of proportion to the activity of disease.
Anemia—normocytic, normochromic with an element of aplasia or hemolysis, or both. Fails to respond to iron.
Skin changes—atrophy, bronzing, "liver palms" cold, moist extremities.

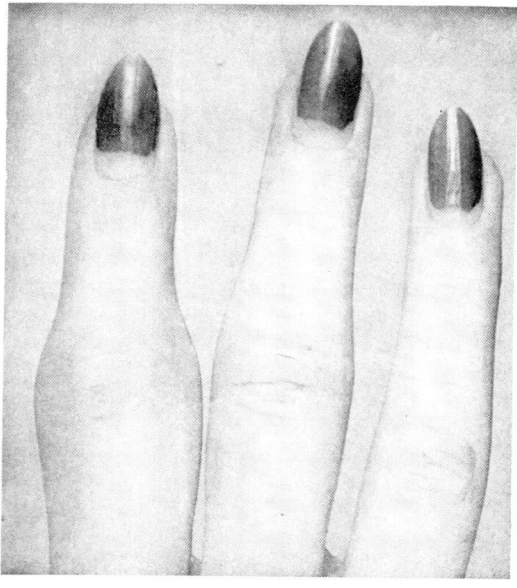

Fig. 38–1. Second, third, and fourth fingers in a young woman with rheumatoid arthritis. This figure illustrates the marked fusiform (spindle-shaped) swelling that often occurs in the proximal interphalangeal joints. It is seen best in the finger on the extreme left.

The buttonhole deformity can occur acutely and is a distressing, although uncommon, complication of local corticosteroid injection.[54]

The metacarpophalangeal (MCP) joints swell dorsally. The collateral ligaments become stretched, and the volar fibrocartilaginous plate to which they are attached and on which the base of the proximal phalanx rests drops palmward. The strong flexor muscles then pull the base of the proximal phalanx also palmward, leading to the characteristic volar subluxation (Fig. 38–2). The medial collateral ligament to the second MCP joint is often the first to be disrupted by the contiguous synovitis. The integrity of this ligament can easily be checked by flexing the second MCP joint and rocking the proximal phalanx from side to side while holding the second metacarpal firmly. Normally, the collateral ligaments are maximally tight in this position, and no side-to-side motion is possible.

With volar subluxation of the MCP joints, the extensor tendons are stretched. The pull of the forearm muscles to the ulnar side is accentuated in the presence of radial migration of the carpus. The fingers become fixed in ulnar deviation when the extensor tendons slide laterally into the groove or the ulnar side of the joint (see Fig. 38–2). The entire head of the metacarpal may now be felt just beneath the skin. Volar subluxation of the first MCP joint occurs early in the disease and is often the first evidence of deformity in the hand. Rupture of its medial collateral ligament produces the "gamekeeper's thumb" deformity, so called because it can develop in nonrheumatoid persons engaged in the wholesale slaughter of birds; the thumb of the hand used to hold the birds' necks has the deformity.

RA rarely produces bony ankylosis, except in the carpal and tarsal joints, in contradistinction to ankylosing spondylitis, psoriasis, Reiter's syndrome, and juvenile RA, all of which are associated with more bony proliferation. Osteophyte forma-

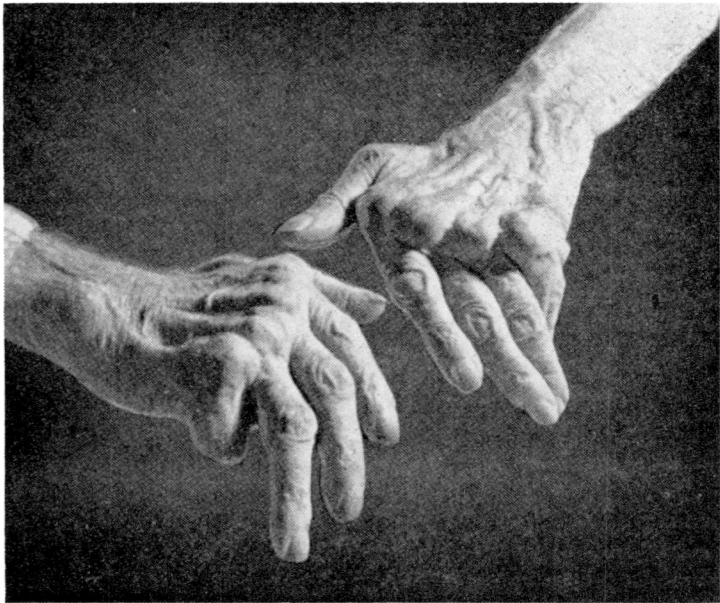

Fig. 38–2. Extreme ulnar deviation and deformity in far-advanced rheumatoid arthritis.

tion, even in severely destroyed rheumatoid joints with so-called "secondary" osteoarthritis, is almost invariably modest or absent. The only exceptions are in patients with primary osteoarthritis that antedates the onset of RA.

Flexor tenosynovitis is common in RA, and swelling can easily be felt, and often seen, as a linear tumefaction in the palm. The soft tissues of the palm typically bulge between the swollen tendons (see Fig. 3–3). These tendons may rupture, especially if rheumatoid nodules have formed within them. Such rupture occurs generally at the level of the MCP joint at which they enter the flexor sheath.[82] Flexor tenosynovitis occurred in 55 of 100 patients with RA observed for 5 years.[40] An average of 3.1 tendons were involved per patient, with the third most commonly inflamed, followed by the second, fourth, fifth, and first, in that order. In contrast, tenosynovitis in nonrheumatoid patients involved fewer tendons, and the first (thumb) tendon was most commonly involved.

Inflammation of the extensor digitorum tendons is also common and leads to swelling over the wrist and metacarpals. This occurrence is particularly troublesome in the presence of the caput ulnae syndrome, and tendon rupture, usually acute, is common.[29] Rupture of extensor tendons occurs at the wrist; the fifth tendon usually ruptures first, followed by the fourth, third, and second, in that order. Again, prompt plastic repair often gives good results (see Chap. 45). Acute ulnar deviation of the MCP joint has been described after rapid

reversal of MCP joint swelling following intra-articular corticosteroid administration.[54] This disconcerting result is presumed to be due to a stretching of the extensor tendons over the swollen joint, an adaptation that proves disastrous with rapid reduction of the swelling.

The carpus is often involved and always as a unit because its joint spaces intercommunicate. The radiocarpal joint is also a common site of RA, as are the flexor carpi radialis, flexor carpi ulnaris, and flexor digitorum tendon sheaths at the wrist.[66] The favorite site of RA in this area is the ulnar bursa, which lies in the recess of the distal ulna and is continuous with the synovial cavity of the distal radioulnar joint. The fibrous ligament holding this joint together is weakened and destroyed by synovitis, thereby allowing the ulna to migrate dorsally so that it overrides the radius (caput ulnae syndrome).[29] Early in the disorder, the ulna can be manually depressed by the examiner in much the same way as a piano key yields to pressure, the so-called "piano-key sign."

The ulnar styloid and distal ulna are often covered with inflammatory rheumatoid granulation tissue that serrates the local bony cortex. That rupture of the long extensors does not occur more often as a result of this double threat to their integrity, mechanical and chemical-inflammatory, is probably a result of lessened demands on the inflamed wrist because of pain and weakness. Resnick has shown that the rheumatoid erosions of the ulnar styloid come from synovitis in the prestyloid recess of the radiocarpal joint, which attacks its tip, from the radioulnar synovitis that attacks it inferiorly, and from extensor carpi ulnaris tenosynovitis, which attacks it dorsilaterally.[69]

The wrist joint rapidly loses its full extension when inflamed. Rest splints to preserve 30° or more of extension are commonly used, with care taken to prevent fibrous ankylosis in extension. A neutral or even a slightly flexed position is least disabling in a wrist in which all hope is lost.

Treatment consists of prophylactic excision of the distal ulna together with the surrounding inflammatory tissue. This procedure, with certain warnings (see Chap. 45), should nearly always be done at the time of repair of a ruptured extensor tendon.

Both the radiohumeral and ulnohumeral joints of the elbow are often involved in RA. The elbow rapidly develops a flexion contracture. Fortunately, the shoulder is less commonly involved in RA and, like the elbow, is easily treated by local corticosteroid injection. The acromioclavicular joint is often involved and is the chief cause of complaints of pain in the shoulder area because it hurts when the patient lies on his side during sleep. The sternoclavicular and temporomandibular joints are also more commonly involved than the shoulder. The biceps tendon may be inflamed, either at its origin or at its insertion.

An exhaustive survey of conditions that might produce hand deformities resembling those of RA has been published.[25] These include deformities due to other joint diseases such as systemic lupus erythematosus (SLE) and chronic rheumatoid fever (Jaccoud's arthritis), as well as those produced by neurologic conditions, such as reflex sympathetic dystrophy, Parkinson's disease, Wilson's disease, and others. The general pattern of joint involvement in RA is similar to that in SLE, and the two diseases cannot be distinguished on this basis.[55]

Lower Extremity (see also Chaps. 48 through 50)

The joints of the forefoot are commonly involved in RA. The metatarsophalangeal (MTP) joints are nearly always affected and are often the first to show erosive disease. We routinely obtain fine-detail radiographs of the MTP joints as well as the hands and wrists when searching for evidence of erosive disease as a clue to early aggressive treatment.[59]

Typically, in RA, the transverse (metatarsal) arch of the foot collapses, so weight bearing occurs on MTP heads 2, 3, and 4, rather than on 1 and 5 as in a normal foot (Fig. 38–3). The plantar fascia contracts, leading to a pes cavus deformity. The

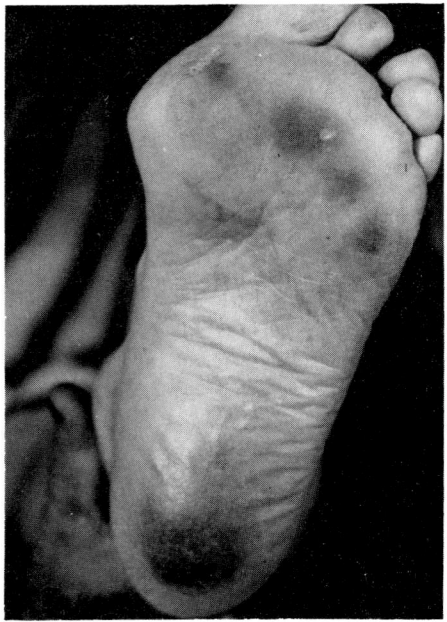

Fig. 38–3. Forefoot involvement is clearly present in this man with rheumatoid arthritis who stood on a surface lightly dusted with graphite. The weight-bearing pattern on metatarsophalangeal joints 2, 3, and 4 is abnormal. The hallux valgus, prominent bunion, high longitudinal arch, and "cocked up," overlapping toes are all typical findings in this disease.

toes become "cocked-up" and do not fit easily into a normal shoe.

The first MTP joint undergoes a progressive valgus deformity, and a bunion develops over its medial surface. A "bunionette" may develop over the lateral surface of the fifth MTP joint. The hindfoot becomes everted. One systematic study showed that 46 of 50 hospitalized patients with RA had foot joint involvement; 42 of these showed forefoot arthritis, 68% had midfoot involvement, but only 16% showed ankle joint inflammation.[58] Another study emphasized the importance of proper shoes.[90]

The ankle and subtalar joints are sometimes troublesome, but are easily injected, and once swelling subsides can be immobilized in a walking cast for eight weeks for maximal anti-inflammatory effect. Tenosynovitis of the tendons about the ankle is also common, especially of the posterior tibial tendon as it loops under the medial malleolus, and the peroneal as it passes under the lateral malleolus. The Achilles tenosynovium may become inflamed and can become eroded at its insertion on the calcaneus.

The knee joints and proximal tibiofibular joints are also commonly involved in RA. Characteristically, the inflamed knee develops a flexion contracture and a progressive valgus deformity that can become so severe that the patient can hardly move one knee past the other when walking. Uniform tricompartmental narrowing (patellofemoral, medial, and lateral tibiofemoral) of the joint space is visible radiologically. Ligamentous laxity often develops as in other rheumatoid joints, especially laxity of the medial collateral ligament and the cruciate ligaments. Synovial thickening is easily felt, and effusions are the rule (Fig. 38–4). The fat pad below the patellar tendon may become enlarged;[93] this finding is especially pronounced after systemic corticosteroid treatment because the fat pad shares in the fat redistribution process that produces moon facies. An enlarged fat pad may be mistaken for an effusion. A popliteal (Baker's) cyst may become prominent (see Fig. 38–9,A). Quadriceps muscle atrophy occurs rapidly.

Hip joint involvement in RA is fortunately uncommon. Joint space narrowing is accompanied by central migration of the femoral head.

Axial Skeleton

Sacroiliac joints are occasionally tender in seropositive erosive RA, with one side more tender than the other. These patients are often HLA-B27 positive.

Involvement of the cervical spine is more common than generally recognized.[44,52,53,92] The most frequent clinical manifestation of cervical spine involvement is painful limitation of neck motion. Radiologic evidence of cervical spine involvement consists of intervertebral disc narrowing without much in the way of osteophytes. Narrowing, erosion, or ankylosis of zygapophyseal joints may occur. Recognition of cervical spine involvement may be important in a patient with atlantoaxial joint subluxation and compression of the cervical spinal cord, owing largely to odontoid erosion from rheumatoid involvement of the bursae in front of and behind the odontoid. Such instances may represent a neurosurgical emergency,[44,53] possibly followed by signs of long-tract compression or respiratory arrest. Ligamentous distention leads to "step-ladder" subluxations.[52] Subluxation of the atlantoaxial joint is usually anterior, with more than 2.5 mm between the anterior aspect of the odontoid and the posterior aspect of the atlas ring, but it can be lateral or posterior. An analysis of 194 patients with atlantoaxial subluxation or atlantoaxial imposition (upward migration of the odontoid toward or even into the foramen magnum) showed that 20 developed spinal cord compressions. This serious complication, which occurred exclusively in seropositive disease, was more likely to occur: (1) in men; (2) when subluxation exceeded 8 mm; (3) in the presence of atlantoaxial imposition; and (4) probably, when lateral subluxation is present. Men

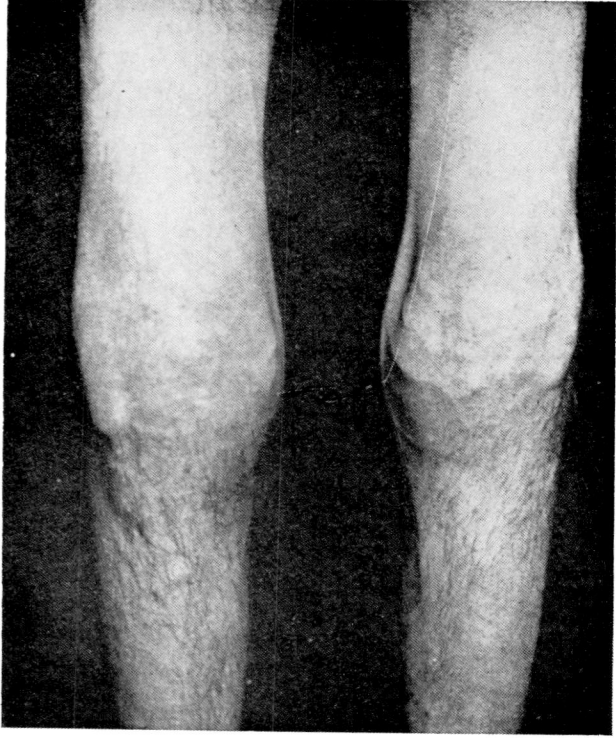

Fig. 38–4. Rheumatoid arthritis of the knees in a middle-aged man.

had a 24% chance of developing spinal cord compression, as opposed to only a 7.5% chance among the women who comprised 83% of the series. Only 2% of those with less than 9 mm of subluxation developed neurologic symptoms. Atlantoaxial impaction tripled the chance of spinal cord compression.

The sternomanubrial joints and the costal cartilages are tender in some patients, usually intermittently. The cricoarytenoid joints may also be involved, producing hoarseness. Rarely, respiration is compromised, and a tracheostomy becomes a lifesaving procedure.

Other Features

During the evolution of the disease, patients have little evidence of systemic reaction, except for occasional low-grade fever, slight tachycardia, anorexia, and weight loss. An occasional patient has an acute, fulminating course characterized by marked systemic reaction, elevated temperature, and warm, red, swollen joints. Such a picture can also be noted after abrupt withdrawal of corticosteroids as a ''rebound phenomenon.'' This manifestation of RA is accompanied by extensive fibrin deposition and is rapidly reversed by a short course of systemic corticosteroids in modest (20 to 30 mg) daily doses.

A striking aspect of the general clinical picture of the disease is noted in the degree and rapidity of accompanying muscular atrophy (see Figs. 38–2 and 38–4). The rapidity of development of muscular atrophy is not only due to disuse, but often to an active inflammatory process in the muscles as well.

Subcutaneous nodules occur over traumatized areas such as elbows, extensor surfaces of the arms, knees, knuckles, occiput, buttocks, and medial scapular areas. About 20 to 25% of all patients with RA manifest such nodules eventually. At times, these nodules can be difficult to differentiate from gouty tophi (Fig. 38–5), and similar nodules can occur in both rheumatic fever and SLE. Histologic confirmation of typical rheumatoid nodule architecture may be diagnostically helpful. A nodule is not to be considered a nodule until it has been histologically confirmed. The histologic differential diagnosis of nodules is given in Chapter 36 (see Table 36–1).

Rheumatoid nodules most often develop over the forearm, distal to the olecranon process, traumatized as the patient uses the forearms as levers to arise from a chair (Fig. 38–6). The back of the head and ears may develop nodules owing to pressure on the bed (see Fig. 38–5), the back of the heels are traumatized by shoes (''pump bumps''), the bridge of the nose by eyeglasses, and the backs

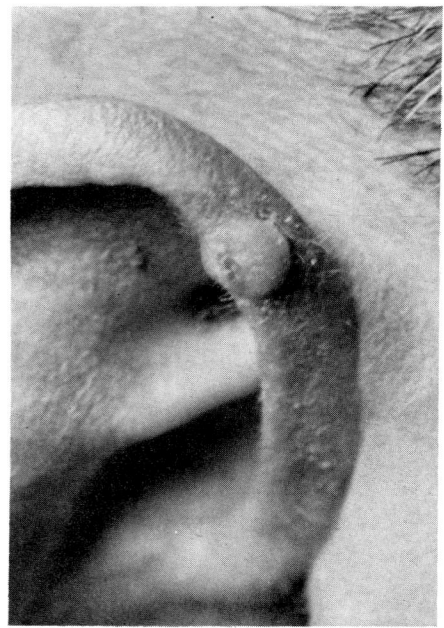

Fig. 38–5.   An ulcerating rheumatoid nodule is seen on the ear of a man with severe, deforming rheumatoid arthritis.

of the knuckles by everyday trauma. Nodules develop in the pulps of the fingers in patients who use tools and over the ischial tuberosities in patients who sit for prolonged periods on hard surfaces. Nodules may ulcerate or may become gangrenous as part of the picture of rheumatoid vasculitis. They rarely erode bone,[24] but they do not calcify. These nodules may also develop in tendons or in visceral organs, such as the meninges, cerebellum, cerebral cortex,[55] pleura, lung, pericardium, heart muscle, or cardiac valves. In the lung, the nodules may simulate carcinoma or, if they perforate and drain into a bronchus, an abscess. Nodules perforating the pleural space may cause pneumothorax or a bronchopleural fistula. Rarely, nodules form in the sclera, from a focus of scleritis, and perforate the anterior chamber, a condition called scleromalacia perforans (Fig. 38–7).

A variant of RA, rheumatoid nodulosis (Fig. 38–8) usually occurs in middle-aged men, some of whom are diabetic.[39] Few systemic features exist, and little or no joint destruction takes place. The patient retains good grip strength and feels generally well. Some of these patients have acute attacks of palindromic rheumatism. The combination of multiple nodules and acute intermittent arthritis is often mistaken for acute and tophaceous gout.

Rheumatoid nodules are thought to form around an area of vasculitis, and Sokoloff has demon-

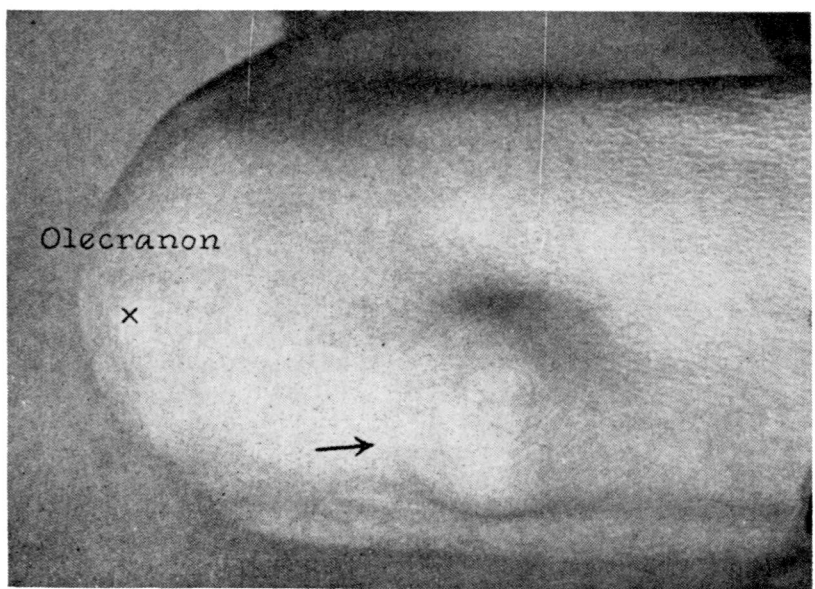

Fig. 38–6. Subcutaneous nodule on the extensor surface of the forearm distal to the elbow joint.

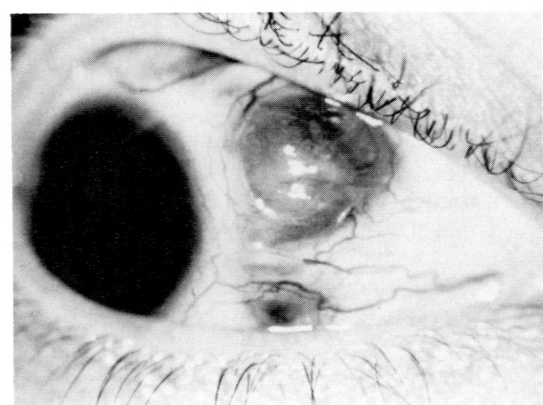

Fig. 38–7. A rheumatoid nodule is shown perforating the ocular sclera—scleromalacia perforans.

strated arterial remnants in their center by serial sectioning. As mentioned previously, these nodules can become necrotic and may ulcerate. If this happens in a nodule near a joint that lies close to the skin, a draining fistula may develop from the synovium, so-called "fistulous rheumatism." Of eight seropositive patients with this complication, seven had nodules; the fistulas were attributed to nodule necrosis in three instances, whereas four had joint sepsis and later developed fistulas and one had developed a fistula from a synovial cyst.[75]

Synovial Cysts and Synovial Hernias

The increased intra-articular pressure that occurs in rheumatoid joints tightly packed with hyper-

trophic, inflamed synovium or with a tense effusion is increased even further by active joint motion (see Chap. 9). As inflammatory damage occurs to cartilage and subchondral bone, especially at the "bare" areas of the synovial-bone contact, and to the articular capsule, focal areas of mechanical weakness develop. Such areas are particularly prominent in patients treated with corticosteroids. Increased intra-articular pressure may then force joint contents through the weakened spots to form cysts. Such nodular diverticula, about 5 mm in diameter, are commonly seen bulging from the dorsolateral surfaces of the PIP or MCP joints. These cysts contain diseased synovium that can be pushed back into the joint through the defect in the articular capsules, just as an inguinal hernia can be reduced through the inguinal ring. Cysts develop commonly from knee, wrist, carpal, PIP, MCP, and elbow joints[38] and rarely from ankle, shoulder, or hip joints (Fig. 38–9). In the hip, these cysts have been confused with inguinal hernias.[72] Plantar synovial cysts also occur,[12] as do cysts containing inflamed tenosynovium herniated through defects in tendon sheaths.

The knee joint normally communicates posteriorly with the gastrocnemius-semimembranous bursa. Increased pressure in the knee forces fluid into this structure. In fully 40% of those affected, the communicating channel between cyst and knee joint is long, tortuous, and acts as a one-way valve, so cyst contents cannot return to the joint. Bony destruction is less apparent in knees with large cysts

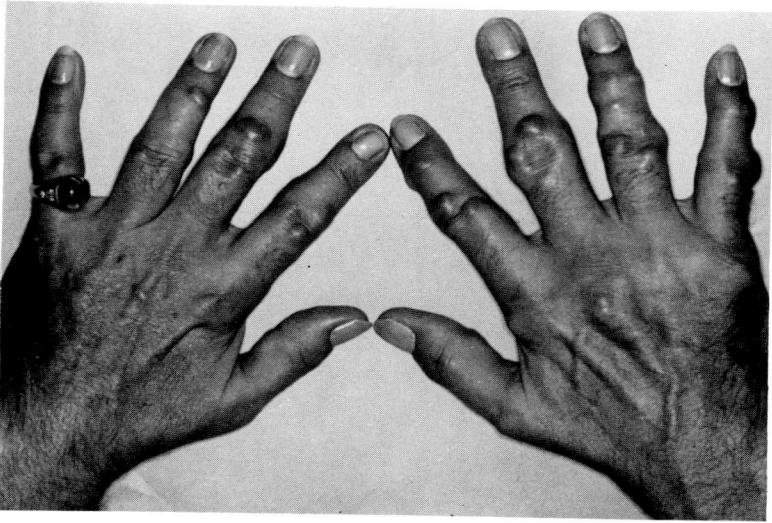

Fig. 38–8. Rheumatoid nodulosis. These multiple rheumatoid nodules and palindromic rheumatism in a diabetic man were thought at first to be gouty arthritis. A diabetologist thought the nodules were xanthomata. The patient's grip strength was nearly normal and he felt generally well.

because of the decompression of the joint that these cysts afford.[37]

Acute arthritis in a previously normal joint is often accompanied by a large effusion and a nearly normal, but less compliant, fibrous articular capsule. Measurement of intra-articular pressure may reach hundreds of millimeters of mercury, even with gentle knee flexion in bed. Rupture of the joint posteriorly may result. Joint fluid leaks into the calf and simulates acute thrombophlebitis. A positive Homans sign, calf tenderness, redness, and swelling with pitting edema may be present.[73] Such leakage may occur on a long-term basis and may lead to chronic edema of the leg; with wrist or elbow joint rupture, chronic edema of the forearm or the dorsum of the hand may result.[38]

Valvular mechanisms have been implicated in the pathogenesis of antecubital cysts and in cysts arising from other joints.[28,38] In chronic arthritis, joint rupture is unusual because the joint capsule becomes adapted by stretching. A popliteal cyst can gradually enlarge, however, dissecting distally until it nearly reaches the ankle (see Fig. 38–9,A). Cysts occurring about multiple joints and tendon sheaths, as in the patient shown in Figure 38–9, might suggest the term "rheumatoid cystoids." Such enlargement can cause entrapment neuropathy and footdrop.[61]

Popliteal cysts and lateral joint instability, indicative of capsular laxity, probably protect patients with RA against the development of pseudocysts ("geodes") of subchondral bone.[37] These latter structures also connect with the joint space

through tiny openings and are "pseudo" in that they have no synovial lining, as do the aforementioned cysts.

Pseudocysts are also thought to result from transmission of intra-articular pressure through weakened areas. Thus, cartilage and bone are spared in patients able to adapt to increased pressure by capsular laxity or by a popliteal cyst connected by a one-way valve.

Another factor of possible importance in the extreme rises of intra-articular pressure that may accompany acute inflammation is decreased articular capsular compliance.[38] Thus, the stiffer the capsule, the greater the pressure rise from an equivalent increase in synovial fluid.

Swelling in or near joints in a patient with RA is usually due to synovitis of joint, bursa, tendon sheath, to synovial cysts derived from these structures, or to rheumatoid nodules. Rarer causes include giant cell tumors[68] and intrasynovial fatty masses.[93] Four of five giant cell tumors in one report were derived from finger tendon sheaths.[68]

Nerve Entrapment Syndromes

Because RA is a proliferative disease of joint and tendon synovium, frequent entrapment of peripheral nerves by these enlarging structures might be predicted. Nerve entrapment is indeed common in RA and is important to recognize because of its treatability, but it is not found in every case, perhaps because the ligamentous destruction caused by the disease process itself releases or prevents pressure on the nerves at risk.

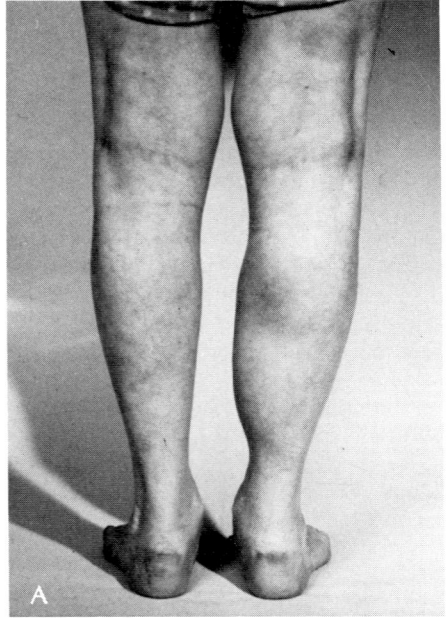

Fig. 38–9. *A,* A popliteal cyst has dissected nearly to the ankle in this woman with rheumatoid arthritis. *B,* A cyst protrudes from the ankle joint of the same patient. *C,* Cysts have developed from synovium herniated from extensor tendons at both wrists of this patient who had received corticosteroids for many years, perhaps leading to weakness of fibrous tissues.

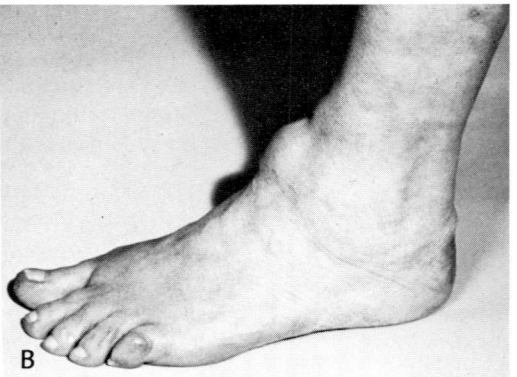

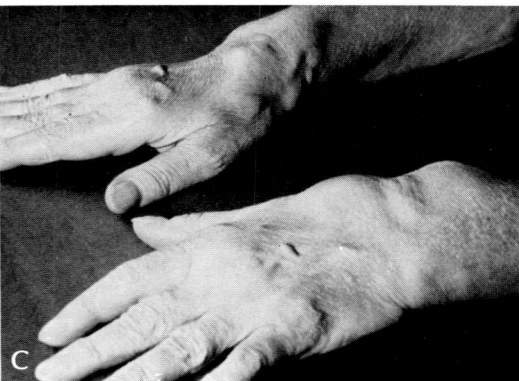

Entrapment of the median nerve at the wrist (carpal tunnel syndrome) is perhaps most common, although entrapment of the ulnar nerve at the wrist or elbow, the posterior interosseous nerve just distal to the elbow,[19] the sural nerve in the leg,[61] and one or more of the common digital nerves in the foot all occur occasionally. Involvement of the posterior interosseous nerve, a branch of the radial nerve, causes extensor paralysis of all five digits, whereas pressure on the sural nerve may cause footdrop. Such involvement must be differentiated from the neuropathy caused by rheumatoid vasculitis.

Treatment of nerve entrapment may consist of local injection of a corticosteroid suspension into the area of entrapment. If this therapy fails to provide sustained symptomatic relief and functional recovery, prompt surgical attention must be obtained. The anatomic considerations of peripheral nerves at risk from entrapment are well described and should be familiar to all those treating RA and other musculoskeletal diseases.[45,86]

Miscellaneous Findings

In some patients, generalized lymphadenopathy is present, and splenomegaly is present in about 15%. In some individuals, the palpably enlarged nodes may suggest a lymphoma. Peripheral vascular vasomotor instability is sometimes a prominent feature of the disease and is characterized by cold, clammy hands and feet with increased sweating. At times, Raynaud's phenomena may accompany or may precede initial joint manifestations, but more often these manifestations are seen in association with scleroderma, mixed connective tissue disease, or SLE. Palmar erythema, particularly over the thenar and hypothenar areas and also associated with Laennec's cirrhosis or pregnancy, is common and is often accentuated during treatment with corticosteroids. At times, patients may show pronounced atrophy of the skin with increased pigmentation and bronzing. The cutaneous manifestations have been reviewed and include those shown in Table 38–3.[78] The arthritis associated with pyoderma gangrenosum is often seronegative.[43] Leg ulceration was twice as common in patients with RA as in those with osteoarthritis in the same clinic.[87]

Disease Course

Most of the clinical progression of the disease itself can be understood as a natural consequence of the inflammatory process within the involved areas of synovium. Proliferating synovial pannus and organized chronic inflammatory tissue lead to erosion of bone and adjacent tendons. Pain and disability in such joints reduce full range of motion, and the end result is often flexion contracture, subluxation, and instability. Flexion deformities occur because the flexor muscle group is the stronger in most diarthrodial joints. Initially, the flexion contracture is maintained by flexor muscle and tendon pull, but ultimately, scarring results in actual fibrous ankylosis. When flexion contractures develop in large, weight-bearing joints such as knees or hips, persistence can lead to great functional difficulty and impairment. Thus, flexion contractures should be avoided, if possible, by proper and early use of anti-inflammatory drugs, by active exercise, and in selected patients by appropriate splinting (see Chap. 44). If flexion contractures develop in joints other than those directly involved in weight bearing, less functional impairment occurs. For instance, an elbow with a flexion contracture is more useful than one with reduced flexion.

Laboratory findings characteristic of RA include elevated acute phase reactants such as the erythrocyte sedimentation rate. Anemia, generally microcytic and normochromic, is often unresponsive

to iron therapy and may closely reflect disease activity. Laboratory and radiographic features of rheumatoid disease are discussed in Chapters 5 and 40, respectively, and rheumatoid factors are discussed in Chapter 41.

Patients with an acute onset were once thought to fare better than those with an insidious onset,[34] but this hypothesis has not stood more careful scrutiny. Although RA is usually chronic and progressive, numerous instances of prolonged or repeated periods of remission have been reported.[64,74] These periods almost always occur within a year of onset of the disease. In many instances, RA actually begins as a series of episodes, later to become sustained or unremitting. About one-quarter of patients have an intermittent or episodic course, whereas just fewer than three-quarters have a progressive, sustained, essentially lifelong illness.[65,77] A few patients, perhaps 5 to 10%, have 1 or 2 brief episodes and then appear to have prolonged, even permanent, remissions.

Exacerbations are frequently noted during the colder months of the year. Onset of disease is most common in the month of March,[77] certainly in the colder weather.[34] The relation of exacerbations to physical or emotional stress or to infection seems clearcut in a few patients. Psychometric testing or personality analysis has failed to provide a uniform character profile typical for RA.

An episode of RA may be present for a few weeks or months, or it may last for years. During active periods of disease, a certain measure of irreparable damage usually occurs. Thus, the amount of joint destruction and deformity is related to the duration of active disease periods. Control of disease activity probably reduces the degree of joint destruction. It is virtually impossible in individual instances to predict in advance the duration of disease activity or its ultimate severity, although a few clues such as elevated C-reactive protein (CRP) levels and rheumatoid factor positivity (see Chap. 40) have been described. No single clinical feature allows an accurate prediction of the subsequent course of RA, but in the presence of positive tests for rheumatoid factor, the disease often runs a sustained rather than an episodic course.[26,65] Some believe that seropositive disease starting early in childhood may have a poorer prognosis because it is present for a longer time.[65] Many studies show that high titers of rheumatoid factor are associated with more severe disease,[30,60] as well as with a higher incidence of vasculitis, nodules, and visceral manifestations.

Associated Diseases

Patients with high fever, leukocytosis, polyarthritis, rash, and a hectic course of illness are now

Table 38–3.   Cutaneous Lesions of Rheumatoid Arthritis

Nodules	Other
Typical	Lipoid nodules
Linear	Pemphigoid
	Bullous
Vasculitis	Cicatricial
Ulcers (legs, elsewhere)	Dermatitis herpetiformis
Gangrene	Granuloma annulare
Nailfold thrombi	Liver palms
Purpura	Amyloidosis
Livido reticularis	
Urticaria	
Hemorrhagia bullae	
Pyoderma gangrenosum	

From Sibbitt, W.L., and Williams, R.C.[78]

recognized as having adult Still's disease (juvenile RA).[4,31] These patients appear to represent a clinical entity distinct from adult RA.

Some patients with RA also have features of SLE.[32] The identical pattern of symmetric joint involvement in these two syndromes has already been mentioned.[55] The rarity of coexistent RA and gout still prompts isolated case reports.[7,70] Most patients with crystals and chronic synovitis turn out to have only gout.[88]* RA is associated with CPPD crystal deposition in about 1% of cases of this condition. The association with autoimmune thyroid disease[41] and with myasthenia gravis seems clear.

Prognosis

Chronic progressive RA is a debilitating disease and has long been felt to be associated with a reduced life expectancy. Debility and increased susceptibility to infection probably play some role.

In general, mortality statistics in population studies in patients with RA show no lethal effects of the disease.[1] In studies of clinic populations, a select group as previously discussed, increased mortality rates are associated with severe disease.[50,67] In a group of 100 patients with definite or classic RA followed up to 15 years, RA itself was implicated as the cause of death in 9 and as a contributor to death in 7 patients. Ischemic heart disease was the main cause of death in 11 of the 27 patients whose death was not related directly to RA. Those who died and those who survived were younger, both at age of onset and at age of death, than the whole group.[67] Men died disproportionally, and the cause of death from RA was vasculitis, infection, and amyloidosis. Another group of 311 patients with definite or classic RA followed for 11 years showed 46 deaths; 203 of these patients had been treated with large doses of azathioprine for a mean of 2.5 years; 52 of these patients had also received alkylating agents.[50] Death occurred in 46 patients with ischemic heart disease,[24] and neoplasia headed the list. Again, the death rate was higher than expected (40 versus 28) in the group aged 45 to 64 years. Death was from the usual causes occurring earlier than usual. Of note was the observation that neoplasia was not more common in patients who had received azathioprine. No leukemia was found. In this context, however, the occurrence of malignant disease in patients with RA treated with cyclophosphamide was 4 times that of a matched group of RA patients,[9] and lymphoreticular malignant disease was increased by a factor of 15.

Increasing attention has been paid to the development of a necrotizing arteritis as a final episode in the course of RA (see Chap. 63). Fortunately, this complication is rare. The clinical picture is one of multiple-system involvement, including renal, serosal, pulmonary, myocardial, or neurologic symptoms and signs. Some of these patients are difficult to distinguish from those with superimposed SLE, but the findings of peripheral neuritis, including both sensory and motor manifestations, leg ulcers, bowel infarctions, and digital gangrene or nail bed or nailfold infarcts (Fig. 38–10) have clinically often been closely associated with necrotizing vasculitis. Whether this disorder is related to corticosteroid therapy is a matter of some debate. It is generally believed that this complication has been observed more frequently since the advent of steroids, and its incidence seems to have decreased as corticosteroid treatment has fallen into disfavor. The precise pathogenesis of necrotizing vasculitis superimposed on RA is still unclear, although vasculitis in clinically normal skin of patients with RA is often present by immunofluorescence. This finding has correlated well with skin lesions and with circulating immune complexes as measured by the C1q or monoclonal rheumatoid factor methods.[47] Several experimental models in animals suggest a phlogistic or accentuating role for rheumatoid factors.[10,21,57] Other workers have found large amounts of circulating immune complexes in these patients.[85]

Few practical rules relating to prognosis can be applied to individual patients. High titers of rheumatoid factors early in the disease, an active proliferative synovitis unresponsive to anti-inflammatory agents, gold, or corticosteroids, progressive erosive disease on roentgenographic examination, and the continued progression of myopathy

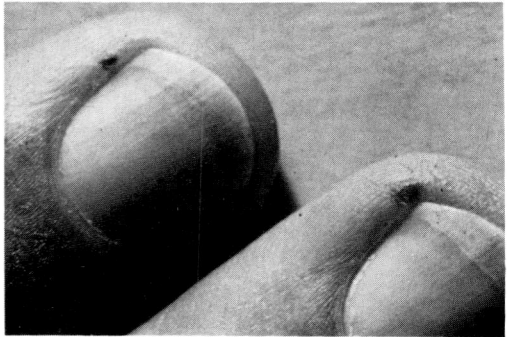

Fig. 38–10. Nailfold thrombi in a patient with rheumatoid arthritis. These or splinter hemorrhages do not always herald severe life-threatening vasculitis, but are clearly more common in patients with systemic signs and symptoms. These thrombi represent areas of infarction due to intimal proliferation in small vessels.

Editor's note: After 25 years of careful searching, I have never seen RA in a case of crystal-proved gouty arthritis.

or new crops of rheumatoid nodules generally are correlated with an unfavorable course. Regardless of the therapy or the management offered when individuals with RA are followed as a group, the number doing poorly increases with the length of observation. The chance of a complete, spontaneous remission appears to be small after one year of sustained, unremitting disease activity.[65,77] Preliminary criteria for a definition of clinical remission in RA have been published by an ARA committee charged with this task.[64] Patients who live within the limitations of their disease and who persist in active range-of-motion exercises along with a positive attitude appear to do better than those who refuse to help themselves. The effects of the disease on life expectancy have already been discussed.

REFERENCES

1. Abruzzo, J.L.: Rheumatoid arthritis and mortality. Arthritis Rheum., 25:1020–1023, 1982.
2. Alarcion, G.S., et al.: Seronegative rheumatoid arthritis. A distinct immunogenetic disease? Arthritis Rheum., 25:502–507, 1982.
3. Appleboom, T., et al.: Rubens and the question of antiquity of rheumatoid arthritis. JAMA, 245:483–486, 1981.
4. Aptekar, R.G., et al.: Adult onset of juvenile rheumatoid arthritis. Arthritis Rheum., 16:715–718, 1973.
5. ARA Committee in Rheumatology Practice: A description of rheumatology practice. Arthritis Rheum., 20:1278–1281, 1977.
6. Astorga, G.P., and Williams, R.C., Jr.: Altered reactivity in mixed lymphocytic culture from patients with rheumatoid arthritis. Arthritis Rheum., 12:547–554, 1969.
7. Atbjian, M., and Fernandez-Madrid, F.: Coexistence of chronic tophaceous gout and rheumatoid arthritis. J. Rheumatol., 8:989–992, 1981.
8. Baker, P.J., et al.: Enhancement of the antibody response to type III pneumonococcal polysaccharide in mice treated with antilymphocyte serum. J. Immunol., 104:1313–1315, 1970.
9. Baltus, J.A.M., et al.: The occurrence of malignancies in patients with rheumatoid arthritis treated with cyclophosphamide. Ann. Rheum. Dis., 42:368, 1983.
10. Baum, J., Stastny, P., and Ziff, M.: Effects of the rheumatoid factor and antigen-antibody complexes on the vessels of the rat mesentery. J. Immunol., 43:985–992, 1966.
11. Beasley, R.P., Willkins, R.F., and Bennett, P.H.: High prevalence of rheumatoid arthritis in Yakima Indians. Arthritis Rheum., 16:743–748, 1973.
12. Bienenstock, H.: Rheumatoid plantar synovial cysts. Ann. Rheum. Dis., 34:98–99, 1971.
13. Boyle, J.A., and Buchanan, W.W.: Clinical Rheumatology. Oxford, Blackwell Scientific Publications, 1971, p. 74.
14. Brower, A.C., et al.: Rheumatoid nodulosis: another cause of juxta-articular nodules. Radiology, 125:669–670, 1977.
15. Buchanan, W.W., and Murdoch, R.A.: Hypothesis: that rheumatoid arthritis will disappear. J. Rheumatol., 6:324–329, 1979.
16. Butterworth, M., McClellan, B., and Allansmith, M.: Influence of sex on immunoglobulin levels. Nature, 214:1224–1225, 1967.
17. Bywaters, E.G.L.: Symmetrical joint involvement. Ann. Rheum. Dis., 34:376, 1975.
18. Caughey, D.E.: The arthritis of Constantine IX. Ann. Rheum. Dis., 33:77–80, 1974.
19. Chang, L.W., et al.: Entrapment neuropathy of the posterior interosseous nerve. Arthritis Rheum., 15:350–352, 1972.
20. Chused, T.M., Steinberg, A.D., and Parker, L.M.: Enhanced antibody response of mice to polyinosinic poly-

21. cytidylic acid by antithymocyte serum and its age-dependent loss in NZB/W mice. J. Immunol., 111:52–57, 1973.
21. DeHoratius, R.J., and Williams, R.C., Jr.: Rheumatoid factor accentuation of pulmonary lesions associated with experimental diffuse proliferative lung disease. Arthritis Rheum., 15:293–301, 1972.
22. Dequeken, J.: Arthritis in Flemish paintings (1499–1700). Br. Med. J., 1:1203–1205, 1977.
23. Doman, R.E.: Paleopathologic evidence of rheumatoid arthritis. JAMA, 246:1899, 1981.
24. Dorfman, H.D., Norman, A., and Smith, R.J.: Bone erosion in relation to subcutaneous rheumatoid nodules. Arthritis Rheum., 13:69–73, 1970.
25. Dorwart, B.B., and Schumacher, H.R.: Hand deformities resembling rheumatoid arthritis. Semin. Arthritis Rheum., 4:53–71, 1974.
26. Duthie, J.J.R., et al.: Course and prognosis in rheumatoid arthritis. Ann. Rheum. Dis., 16:411–424, 1958.
27. Edelman, J., and Russell, A.S.: A comparison of patients with seropositive and seronegative rheumatoid arthritis. Rheumatol. Int., 3:47–48, 1983.
28. Ehrlich, G.E., and Guttmann, G.G.: Valvular mechanism in anticubital cysts of rheumatoid arthritis. Arthritis Rheum., 16:259–264, 1973.
29. Ehrlich, G.E.: Pathogenesis of rupture of extensor tendons at the wrist in rheumatoid arthritis. Arthritis Rheum., 2:332–346, 1959.
30. Epstein, W.V., and Engelman, E.P.: The relation of the rheumatoid factor content of serum to clinical neurovascular manifestations of rheumatoid arthritis. Arthritis Rheum., 2:250–258, 1959.
31. Fabricant, M.S., Chandor, S.B., and Friou, G.J.: Still's disease in adults. JAMA, 225:273–276, 1973.
32. Fischman, A.S., et al.: The coexistence of rheumatoid arthritis and systemic lupus erythematosus: a case report and review of the literature. J. Rheumatol., 8:405–415, 1981.
33. Fleming, A., et al.: Early rheumatoid disease. II. Patterns of joint involvement. Ann. Rheum. Dis., 35:361–364, 1976.
34. Fleming, A., Crown, J.M., and Corbett, M.: Early rheumatoid disease. I. Onset. Ann. Rheum. Dis., 35:357–360, 1976.
35. Garrod, A.B.: A Treatise on Gout and Rheumatic Gout (Rheumatoid Arthritis). 3rd Ed. London, Longman, Green, 1876.
36. Garrod, A.B.: A Treatise on Gout and Rheumatic Gout. London, Walton and Maberly, 1859.
37. Genovese, G.R., Jayson, M.I.V., and Dixon, A.ST.J.: Protective valve of synovial cysts in rheumatoid knees. Ann. Rheum. Dis., 31:179–182, 1972.
38. Gerber, N.J., and Dixon, A.ST.J.: Synovial cysts and juxta-articular bone cysts. Semin. Arthritis Rheum., 3:323–348, 1974.
39. Ginsberg, M.H., et al.: Rheumatoid nodulosis. Arthritis Rheum., 18:49–58, 1975.
40. Givy, R.G., and Gottlieb, N.L.: Hand flexor tenosynovitis in rheumatoid arthritis. Arthritis Rheum., 20:1003–1008, 1977.
41. Grennan, D.M., et al.: Family studies in rheumatoid arthritis—the importance of H2ADR4 and of genes for autoimmune thyroid disease. J. Rheumatol., 10:584–589, 1983.
42. Hollander, J.L.: The controlled-climate chamber for the study of the effects of meteorological changes in human diseases. Trans. N.Y. Acad. Sci., 24:167–172, 1961.
43. Holt, P.J.L., et al.: Pyoderma gangrenosum: Clinical laboratory findings in 15 patients with special reference to polyarthritis. Medicine, 59:114, 1980.
44. Isdale, I.C., and Corrigan, A.: Backward luxation of the atlas. Ann. Rheum. Dis., 29:6–9, 1970.
45. Kopell, H.P., and Thompson, W.A.L.: Peripheral entrapment neuropathies of the lower extremity. N. Engl. J. Med., 262:56–60, 1960.
46. Kowanko, I.L., et al.: Domiciliary self-measurement in rheumatoid arthritis and the demonstration of circadian rhythmicity. Ann. Rheum. Dis., 41:453–454, 1982.
47. Kozin, F., et al.: Immunoglobulin (IgG) and complement

(C') deposits in blood vessels in patients with rheumatoid arthritis. Clinical correlations. Clin. Res., 26:503A, 1978.

48. Lawrence, J.C.: Personal communication.

49. Lawrence, J.C., and Kellgren, J.H. (Eds.): Population Studies in Rheumatoid Arthritis. New York, Arthritis Foundation and National Institute of Arthritis and Metabolic Disease, United States Public Health Service, 1958, p. 13.

50. Lewis, P., et al.: Cause of death in patients with rheumatoid arthritis with particular reference to azathioprine. Ann. Rheum. Dis., 39:457–461, 1980.

51. Luukkainen, R., Isoinaki, H., and Kajander, A.: Prognostic value of the type of onset of rheumatoid arthritis. Ann. Rheum. Dis., 42:274–275, 1983.

52. Martel, W.: Pathogenesis of cervical discovertebral destruction in rheumatoid arthritis. Arthritis Rheum., 20:1217–1225, 1977.

53. Mathews, J.A.: Atlanto-axial subluxation in rheumatoid arthritis. Ann. Rheum. Dis., 28:260–266, 1969.

54. McCarty, D.J.: Treatment of rheumatoid joint inflammation with triamcinolone hexacetonide. Arthritis Rheum., 15:157–173, 1972.

55. McCarty, D.J.: Unpublished observations.

56. McCarty, D.J., and Gatter, R.A.: A study of distal interphalangeal joint tenderness in rheumatoid arthritis. Arthritis Rheum., 9:325–336, 1966.

57. McCormick, J.N., et al.: The potentiating effect of rheumatoid arthritis serum in the immediate phase of nephrotoxic nephritis. Clin. Exp. Immunol., 4:17–25, 1969.

58. Minaker, K., and Little, H.: Painful feet in rheumatoid arthritis. Can. Med. Assoc. J., 109:724–730, 1973.

59. Moberg, E., Edeland, H.G., and Wikland, L.B.: Prognostic evaluation of finger joint bony lesions in rheumatoid arthritis. Scand. J. Rheumatol., 2:139–141, 1973.

60. Mongan, E.S., Cass, R.M., and Jacox, R.F.: A study of the relation of seronegative and seropositive rheumatoid arthritis to each other and necrotizing vasculitis. Am. J. Med., 47:23–36, 1969.

61. Nakano, K.K.: Entrapment neuropathy from Baker's cysts. JAMA, 239:135, 1978.

62. Nichols, E.H., and Richardson, F.L.: Arthritis deformans. J. Med. Res., 21:149–221, 1909.

63. Parish, L.C.: An historical approach to the nomenclature of rheumatoid arthritis. Arthritis Rheum., 6:138–158, 1963.

64. Pinals, R.S., et al.: Preliminary criteria for clinical remission in rheumatoid arthritis. Bull. Rheum. Dis., 32:7–10, 1982.

65. Ragan, C., and Farrington, E.: The clinical features of rheumatoid arthritis. JAMA, 181:663–667, 1967.

66. Ranawat, C.S., and Straub, L.R.: Volar tenosynovitis of wrist in rheumatoid arthritis. Arthritis Rheum., 13:112–117, 1970.

67. Rasker, J.J., and Cosh, J.A.: Cause and age of death in a prospective study of 100 patients with rheumatoid arthritis. Ann. Rheum. Dis., 40:115–120, 1981.

68. Reginato, A.J., Martinez, V., and Schumacher, H.R.: Giant cell tumor associated with rheumatoid arthritis. Ann. Rheum. Dis., 33:333–341, 1974.

69. Resnick, D.: Rheumatoid arthritis of wrist: why the ulnar styloid? Radiology, 112:29, 1974.

70. Rizzoli, A.J., Trujeque, L., and Bankhurst, A.D.: The coexistence of gout and rheumatoid arthritis: case report and a review of the literature. J. Rheumatol., 7:316–324, 1980.

71. Ropes, M.W., et al.: 1958 revision of diagnostic criteria for rheumatoid arthritis. Bull. Rheum. Dis., 9:175–176, 1958.

72. Samuelson, C., Ward, J.R., and Albo, D.: Rheumatoid synovial cyst of the hip. Arthritis Rheum., 14:105–108, 1971.

73. Schmidt, M.F., Workman, J.B., and Barth, W.F.: Dissection or rupture of a popliteal cyst. Arch. Intern. Med., 134:694–698, 1974.

74. Schumacher, H.R.: Palindromic onset of rheumatoid arthritis. Clinical, synovial fluid, and biopsy studies. Arthritis Rheum., 25:361–369, 1982.

75. Shapiro, R.F., et al.: Fistulization of rheumatoid joints. Ann. Rheum. Dis., 34:489–498, 1974.

76. Short, C.L.: The antiquity of rheumatoid arthritis. Arthritis Rheum., 17:193–205, 1974.

77. Short, C.L., Bauer, W., and Reynolds, W.E.: Rheumatoid Arthritis. Cambridge, Harvard University Press, 1957.

78. Sibbitt, W.L., and Williams, R.C.: Cutaneous manifestations of rheumatoid arthritis. Int. J. Dermatol., 21:563–572, 1982.

79. Stastny, P.: Mixed lymphocyte cultures in rheumatoid arthritis. J. Clin. Invest., 57:1148–1157, 1976.

80. Stastny, P.: Mixed lymphocyte culture typing cells from patients with rheumatoid arthritis. Tissue Antigens, 4:571–579, 1974.

81. Sturrock, R.D., Sharma, J.N., and Buchanan, W.W.: Evidence of rheumatoid arthritis in ancient India. Arthritis Rheum., 20:42–43, 1977.

82. Tarrik, H.: Spontaneous rupture of tendons in rheumatoid arthritis. N.Z. Med. J., 79:651–653, 1976.

83. Terkeltaub, R., et al.: A clinical study of older age rheumatoid arthritis with comparison to a younger onset group. J. Rheumatol., 10:418–424, 1983.

84. Terres, A., Morrison, S.L., and Habicht, G.S.: A quantitative difference in the immune response between male or female mice. Proc. Soc. Exp. Biol. Med., 127:664–673, 1968.

85. Theofilopoulos, A.N., Wilson, C.B., and Dixon, F.J.: The Rajii cell radioimmune assay for detecting immune complexes in human sera. J. Clin. Invest., 57:169–182, 1976.

86. Thompson, W.A.L., and Kopell, H.P.: Peripheral entrapment neuropathies of the upper extremity. N. Engl. J. Med., 260:1261–1265, 1959.

87. Thurtle, O.A., and Cawley, M.D.: The frequency of ulceration in rheumatoid arthritis. A survey. J. Rheumatol., 10:507–509, 1983.

88. Trentham, D.E., and Masi, A.T.: Chronic synovitis in gout simulating rheumatoid arthritis. JAMA, 235:1358–1360, 1976.

89. Vandenbrocke, J.P., et al.: Oral contraceptives and rheumatoid arthritis: further evidence for a preventive effect. Lancet, 2:839–842, 1982.

90. Vidigal, E., et al.: The foot in chronic rheumatoid arthritis. Ann. Rheum. Dis., 34:292–297, 1975.

91. Waller, M., Toone, E.C., and Vaughan, J.E.: Study of rheumatoid factor in a normal population. Arthritis Rheum., 7:513–520, 1966.

92. Weissman, B.N., et al.: Prognostic features of atlanta-axial subluxation in rheumatoid arthritis. Radiology, 144:745–751, 1982.

93. Weston, W.J.: The intra-synovial fatty masses in chronic rheumatoid arthritis. Br. J. Rheumatol., 46:213–219, 1973.

94. Wisniewski, J.J., and Askari, A.D.: Rheumatoid nodulosis. A relatively benign rheumatoid variant. Arch. Intern. Med., 141:615–619, 1981.

Chapter **39**

Extra-Articular Rheumatoid Disease

John L. Decker and Paul H. Plotz

"Rheumatoid disease" is often suggested as a name to be preferred over "rheumatoid arthritis (RA)." The extraordinary range of manifestations and features, regarded as part and parcel of the disease, but without apparent direct relationship to its synovitis, is cited as justifying such a preference. The disease is, of course, primarily a chronic polyarthritis, and most of the ill health suffered is due to joint inflammation and dysfunction. Nevertheless, systemic manifestations, visceral features, and extra-articular findings are common.[93,226] The extra-articular manifestations are not usually overwhelming and commonly contribute only to the backdrop, whereas joint inflammation is at center stage. On other occasions, however, the threat of death due to rheumatoid arteritis or of blindness due to scleromalacia perforans can dominate the clinical foreground. Death due solely to RA is rare indeed and is due to extra-articular manifestations of the disease.

It is inappropriate to regard such findings as pleural effusions, splenomegaly, or sensory neuropathy as complications; rather, they are part of the disease. Two major disease patterns, Sjögren's syndrome and amyloidosis, are regularly associated with RA and should be regarded as concomitants. These are described in detail in Chapters 67 and 72, but they need consideration when one is evaluating such findings as purpura, neuropathy, or pulmonary infiltrates. Most extensive descriptions of the extra-articular manifestations of RA neither exclude nor specify patients with Sjögren's syndrome. In view of the prevalence of this syndrome, the inclusion of such individuals may well bias data on RA per se. Complications include such events as fractures of osteopenic bone after minimal trauma, or pyogenic infections of joints already damaged by RA.

The notable effects of various drugs are not discussed here. Nevertheless, neuromyopathy and retinal degeneration due to antimalarial agents, rashes and bone marrow effects of gold administration, major problems of peptic ulceration associated with many drugs, and posterior subcapsular cataracts and purpura due to adrenal corticosteroids are examples of drug-related phenomena that must be remembered and considered in the management of patients with RA.

Extra-articular rheumatic disease is particularly important in differential diagnosis because it presents more variety than does the joint disease. This chapter deals only with adult, usually seropositive, RA. The extra-articular manifestations of juvenile RA, ankylosing spondylitis, and other inflammatory arthropathies are often different in kind, prevalence, and implication. It is unfortunate that in many otherwise sound studies of, for example, ocular disease in arthritis, the distinctions among arthritic syndromes are not made, and thus the exact pertinence of the findings to the several confusable entities often remain unclear.

Most of the extra-articular manifestations of adult RA can be ascribed to vasculitis, to rheumatoid nodules, themselves probably the outcome of vascular inflammation, or to serositis, possibly induced by the same mechanisms as the synovitis. These manifestations are usually: (1) more frequent as the prevalence of seropositivity increases in a group of patients; and (2) more frequent in patients with higher titers of rheumatoid factor.

ANEMIA

Moderate, normocytic, normochromic anemia is the most common extra-articular manifestation of RA and is probably present at times in all patients with the disease. In women, a tendency to hypochromia and microcytosis exists. The degree of anemia is clearly related to disease activity and recedes as the disease is brought under control.[207] It is not usually sufficiently profound to cause symptoms, except in patients who have suffered major, acute hemorrhages.

The mechanisms resulting in the anemia have engaged the attention of numerous investigators over many years,[152,153,155] and many facts are clear. Chronic blood loss, due perhaps primarily to salicylates, does not seem to be a major factor,[10] because the anemia is not that of iron deficiency. Serum iron levels are low, but the serum iron-binding globulin is also low or normal rather than elevated, as is the case in iron deficiency. The gastrointestinal uptake of iron is mildly reduced to levels lower than in comparable anemia due to iron deficiency. Increased destruction of red cells due to extracorpuscular factors does occur in Felty's syndrome, and cell life spans are shortened to some degree in most patients with active RA. Nevertheless, the six- to eight-fold increase in erythrocyte production of which the normal bone marrow is capable should easily compensate for the shortened half-life in most patients. Expanded plasma volume with secondary hemodilution may play a small role.

In the normal state, the iron used in hematopoiesis is derived primarily from the breakdown of senescent red cells; the release of this iron may be diminished in RA.[161] Intravenously administered iron is rapidly cleared from the plasma, and the low baseline levels are re-established. When an iron chelating agent, desferrioxamine B, is given to rheumatoid patients, greater iron excretion occurs, suggesting that the stores of iron of these patients are increased above normal. Taken together, these studies suggest that the major defect rests in an increased uptake or diminished release of iron from a site where it is unavailable for erythropoiesis. The avidity of the site for iron appears to be directly related to disease activity. With acute suppression induced by ACTH, iron clearance returns to normal,[154] and even in the absence of iron supplements, serum and bone marrow iron levels rise dramatically, followed by a rising hemoglobin concentration. Evidence also suggests that ineffective erythropoiesis may contribute to the anemia.[37,55]

Current evidence suggests that lymph nodes[154] and synovial tissues[156] contribute to the iron sequestration. Erythrophagocytosis has been observed in both sites and, in the synovium at least, the iron is deposited only when it has been incorporated into red blood cells.[15] That the anemia of RA is best relieved not by hematinics, but by bringing the disease activity under control, fits this hypothesis.

RHEUMATOID NODULES

These familiar lesions, typically subcutaneous, are the hallmark of seropositive RA and, especially when multiple, indicate a more guarded prognosis for joint function and a greater chance for the patient to develop systemic features.

The superficial lesions are rare in the epidermis, common in the deep subcutaneous tissue, and may involve all manner of deeper connective tissue structures such as bursae, periosteum, tendon sheaths, and tendons. They vary in size from millet seed-like lesions to enormous, confluent masses of nodular tissue overlying the olecranon process or the sacrum. The lesions are usually asymptomatic and are likely to cause only cosmetic complaints. They appear insidiously and are often first noted by the physician. Usually seen in association with increasing symptoms of synovitis, the nodules are notably capricious in time of onset. They may increase in size over one or several months and may gradually shrink or disappear in a similar time period, or they may persist indefinitely. A new nodule may develop at a time when the patient feels well and is thought to be in remission. These nodules are clearly more likely to appear in areas subjected to repeated microtrauma, such as over the olecranon, over the ischial tuberosity, over the Achilles tendon at the point at which ill-fitting shoes impinge, or on the bridge of the nose where spectacles are supported. The nodules also appear in areas where no trauma is recognized, such as overlying the helix of the ear in patients who are ambulatory. In hemiplegic individuals, only the nonparalyzed limbs develop nodules.[20]

By far the most important complication is breakdown of the overlying skin and discharge of the necrobiotic central core of the granuloma. Such lesions are painful, heal poorly, and almost invariably become infected. They present a particularly difficult problem over the sacrum or over the ischial tuberosity in a bedridden patient. When the inflamed synovium dissects to the skin and discharges synovial contents and debris to the outside, the condition is termed *fistulous rheumatism*.[28,191] Excision is the only useful treatment and is usually at least temporarily successful for the uncomplicated nodule; recurrences are common, often in the original wound scar. When spontaneous drainage has occurred, wide excision is sometimes successful; skin grafting may be required when adequate closure cannot be achieved.

Other nodular lesions that can be mistaken on clinical examination for a rheumatoid nodule include gouty tophi, sebaceous cysts, basal cell carcinoma, ganglions of the hand or wrist, xanthomata, and the nodules of multicentric reticulohistiocytosis. In most patients with seropositive polyarthritis, unfortunately, little doubt exists as to the nature of the lesion. Nevertheless, excision biopsy should be performed if unusual or suspicious features are noted. Bearing the gouty tophus in mind, a portion of the nodular tissue removed should always be placed in a nonaqueous fixative. Differential diagnosis of subcutaneous nodules histologically is given in Chapter 36.

Rarely, rheumatoid nodules appear either as the predominant or only clinical manifestation of rheumatoid disease or long before the development of arthritis. Positive rheumatoid factor tests support the relationship to RA. This curious entity, sometimes called *rheumatoid nodulosis,* occurs mostly in men, though we have observed an example in a woman.[6,36,73,76,229]

Rarely, a visceral rheumatoid nodule causes a clinically important complication. Isolated examples in the aorta,[192] kidney,[232] and retroperitoneum[2] have been reported. Lung, meningeal, and choroid plexus nodules are discussed later in this chapter.

LYMPHADENOPATHY

Lymph node enlargement is common in RA. The definition of adenopathy varies widely, however, as illustrated by comparing 2 studies, one reporting nodal enlargement in 29% of patients and in 9% of control subjects, the other reporting it in 82% of patients and in 52% of control subjects.[175,193] Men showed the higher prevalence among both patients and controls. Nodal enlargement is more common in rheumatoid factor-positive patients and in those with active disease.

Clinical examination and lymphangiography both indicate that the lymph nodes immediately proximal to joints exhibiting synovitis are more likely to be enlarged than are more remote lymph nodes, although this finding is not invariable. The lymph nodes are not tender or inflamed, show no tendency to mat, and feel firm and rubbery.

In dealing with suspicious or unexpected lymphadenopathy, temporization is probably justified. The probability that the nodal enlargement will recede is high. Lymphangiograms, particularly in Sjögren's syndrome, may even mimic malignant lymphadenopathy, but enthusiasm for diagnostic biopsy must be restrained because virtually all series of lymph node biopsies in RA include patients who received radiation or cancer chemotherapy because the lesion appeared to be malignant, a treatment not justified by the subsequent course.[48,151,160]

OCULAR MANIFESTATIONS

Historically, RA was regarded as causing inflammation of two portions of the eye, the sclera and the anterior uveal tract, composed of the iris and the ciliary body. The many terms used to describe disorders of the anterior uveal tract refer to the area of most intense involvement: *iritis; iridocyclitis,* when ciliary involvement is prominent; and *anterior uveitis,* when all the structures are involved but the choroid, which constitutes the posterior uveal tract. The process is said to be *nongranulomatous* when diffuse exudative phenomena are seen rather than dense, nodular infiltrates. Such nodular infiltrates, a cardinal feature of granulomatous iridocyclitis, are typical of sarcoidosis and of chronic infections such as tuberculosis or

brucellosis. More recently, it has become apparent that anterior uveitis is no more common in RA than in the general population, corneal and conjunctival manifestations of the sicca syndrome are the most common ophthalmologic feature of RA, disease of the sclera is rare but characteristic, and many of the drugs used in RA may affect the eye.[198] Such drug-related disorders include gold deposition in the cornea, posterior subcapsular cataracts due to adrenal corticosteroids, and corneal and retinal changes related to antimalarial agents. Nongranulomatous anterior uveitis, a typical feature of both ankylosing spondylitis and juvenile RA, helps to distinguish these diseases from RA.[118,183,213] Eye involvement in these diseases is discussed in detail in Chapters 51 and 53.

The sclera, an opaque, avascular, acellular tunic of collagen, envelops the eye in continuity with the transparent cornea. Superficial to the sclera and loosely connected to Tenon's capsule and the conjunctiva lies the episclera, an ill-defined layer of vascular, loosely organized connective tissue. Rheumatoid disease affects both the episclera and the sclera.

Episcleritis appears over the anterior sclera anywhere from the extraocular muscle insertions to the cornea, but it is most frequent within a few millimeters of the limbus. It may be localized (nodular) or more diffuse.[135] Typically, episcleritis appears suddenly as a raised lesion a few millimeters in diameter, cream-colored to violaceous, and surrounded by an intense hyperemia of the deeper vessels that appears dark purple, when compared to the bright red of conjunctival hyperemia. Discomfort is common, but pain is not. The lesions may be transient, but often persist for weeks or months despite the use of topical corticosteroids. These lesions rarely ulcerate and usually remain superficial. Transient lesions heal without residua, but in the more chronic form, the conjunctiva becomes bound in a slate-colored scar. The lesions may involve one or both eyes, are sometimes multiple, and seem to be more prevalent in women. They are common in patients with rheumatoid arteritis. The specificity of the lesion is established by its histopathologic features, typical of a rheumatoid nodule.[67]

Scleritis, a rarer, more serious problem, may be manifested as a painful, inflammatory condition with widespread necrosis (necrotizing nodular sclerosis) (Fig. 39–1,*A*). More commonly, an indolent, slowly progressive, asymptomatic nodular destruction of the sclera takes place[103] (scleromalacia perforans). The incidence is greatest 10 to 15 years after the onset of RA and usually appears in patients more than 50 years of age. Reported cases include twice as many women as men and thus correspond to the sex prevalence of the underlying process.[190] Other evidence of vasculitis is usually present when scleritis develops.[103]

The lesions are most likely to appear superiorly in the sclera of the anterior eye as raised, yellow nodules with hyperemia proportional to their acuteness. The sclera may become thinned and transparent, revealing the dark blue of the underlying choroid, or the nodule may slough, leaving patches of choroid exposed (Fig. 39–1,*B*). The distinction between episcleritis and scleritis may be difficult, but ultimately it depends on thinning of the sclera. In contrast to those of episcleritis, the complications of scleritis are common and threatening to vision. They include uveitis, including choroiditis with retinal detachment, sclerosing keratitis or extension to the cornea, cataracts, secondary glaucoma, and perforation.

Treatment is not satisfactory. Topical steroids reduce the acute inflammation and may prevent some necrosis, but they do not effect closure of the scleral holes. These lesions have occasionally been successfully treated by grafting.

Less well recognized ocular complications of rheumatoid disease include Brown's syndrome, which is diplopia on upward-inward gaze, probably due to tenovaginitis of the superior oblique tendon,[113] and a distinctive peripheral corneal opacity resembling a contact lens.[129,134] Cotton-wool exudates have appeared in the course of a vasculitic flare of seropositive nodular RA.[144]

LARYNGEAL MANIFESTATIONS

Most authors ascribe laryngeal manifestations to typical rheumatoid synovitis in the diarthrodial cricoarytenoid joints, and this hypothesis has been well documented by careful postmortem dissec-tion.[25] Some feel that the symptoms are due to arteritis of the vasa nervorum of the laryngeal nerves with abductor paralysis.[230] Laryngeal disorder is included here because the larynx is omitted from the typical joint examination. This condition is potentially reversible and can be swiftly lethal.

Cricoarytenoid joint disease is found at autopsy in RA in nearly half the cases.[17,83] Detailed assessment of patients with generalized rheumatoid disease suggests that symptoms or findings are found in about 25%,[130] but clinically manifest problems are rare. Both short- and long-term symptoms are described. Pain, dysphagia, fullness or tension in the throat, hoarseness, dyspnea on exertion, and stridor may be acute. With the exception of pain, such symptoms may persist over extended periods. The number of patients with laryngeal disease but without hoarseness or voice change is remarkable. In some instances, dyspnea and stridor are believed to be absent simply because advanced arthritis limits exertion. The laryngeal symptoms may be so mild as to be overlooked without specific questioning. On occasion, they have been regarded as hysterical.

Indirect laryngoscopic examination may show acute redness and swelling overlying the arytenoid joints, but immobilized cricoarytenoid joints, with one or both vocal processes and cords adducted to the midline, are more common (Fig. 39–2). If such adduction is symmetric, the airway may be reduced to a chink. Joint pain can often be demonstrated by an attempt to move the arytenoid cartilage with a spatula. In chronic fixation in adduction, superimposed respiratory infection of any kind can put the patient at substantial risk because of laryngeal and vocal cord edema. Emergency tracheotomy may be required.[170] After control of infection, ar-

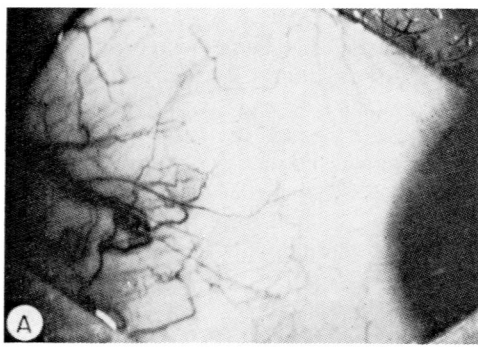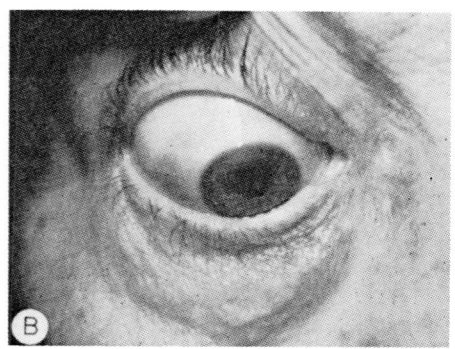

Fig. 39–1. *A*, Medial sclera showing vascularity overlying nodular scleritis in a 52-year-old woman with 18 years of seropositive RA. Subcutaneous nodules had first appeared 5 years before, and scleromalacia perforans had developed in the opposite eye 2 years earlier. (Courtesy of Dr. Vernon Wong.) *B*, This patient was 67 years old; RA had been apparent since about age 35. The darkening of the lateral sclera had the distinctly bluish hue of choroidal pigmentation, seen because of scleral thinning from previous scleritis. The destruction had occurred in 3 episodes over a year's time, the last ending a year earlier. (Courtesy of Dr. Werner Barth.)

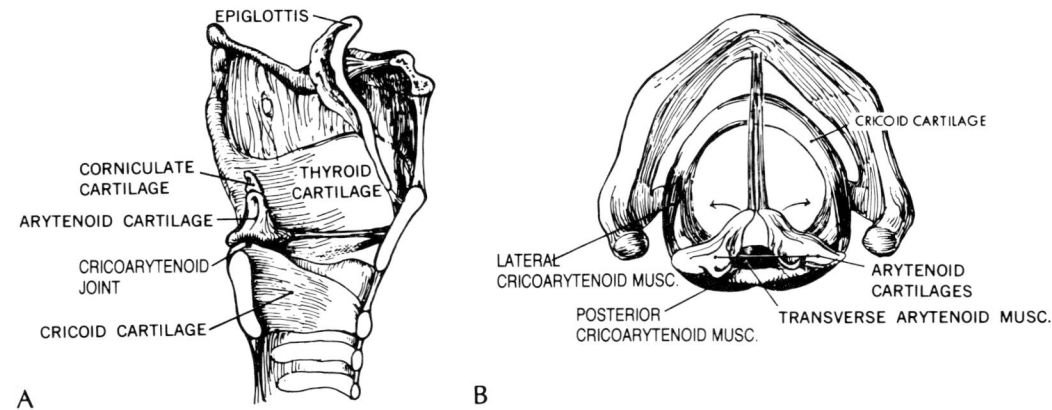

Fig. 39–2.   The cartilaginous skeleton of the larynx in lateral section *(A)* and from superiorly *(B)*. The cords and vocal processes are shown adducted by the action of the lateral cricoarytenoids. The arrows point toward abduction, the position produced by the action of the posterior cricoarytenoid muscle.

ytenoidectomy is usually preferred to permanent tracheostomy. Surgical intervention often is not needed if the joint fixation on either side is in a position other than adduction. The possible presence of compromised cricoarytenoid motion should be borne in mind whenever intubation is needed in a patient with RA.

PLEUROPULMONARY MANIFESTATIONS

The pleuropulmonary lesions of RA are diverse and uncommon. At the bedside or in the office, one is much more likely to find pulmonary symptoms or findings that can be ascribed to common causes rather than to any of the processes related to RA. Lesions such as apical scarring, bronchitis, and bronchiectasis are more prevalent than in age- and sex-matched hospitalized patients without RA.[5,216] Nevertheless pleural, nodular, pneumoconiotic, and diffuse interstitial fibrotic processes are found in association with RA or with serum rheumatoid factors in the absence of arthritis. Furthermore, the pulmonary complications of a number of antirheumatic drugs, particularly gold, D-penicillamine, and methotrexate (discussed elsewhere in this volume) have been increasingly recognized.

Pleural Manifestations

Rheumatoid pleural disease is most likely to present as an asymptomatic effusion, as basilar thickening by radiography,[194] or as widespread, prominent adhesions at autopsy.[195] Symptomatic pleurisy in brief episodes, usually in association with an increase in disease activity, but sometimes before the diagnosis of RA is apparent, does occur at a rate approximately double that seen in non-

rheumatoid patients. The incidence is higher in men than in women.[219]

Pleural effusions usually appear painlessly and may be an incidental finding, although in some instances, the collections can become massive enough to impair respiratory exchange. Effusions, like symptomatic pleurisy, may substantially antedate or herald the onset of RA and are more common in men.[125] Effusions frequently accompany rheumatoid pericarditis. The fluid is a typical serous exudate, often green or yellow-green and turbid, with either mononuclear or polymorphonuclear cells predominating. Protein content exceeds 3 g/dl, whereas the glucose content is often, but not invariably,[218] extraordinarily reduced, to levels of less than 15 mg/dl.[9,33] Rheumatoid factor titers may exceed those found in simultaneous serum samples, and complement values, especially of C4,[179] may be low, but these findings are not diagnostic of rheumatoid effusion.

Such effusions are usually chronic and often last more than a year. Extensive reactive fibrosis may appear in the persistent case and may even produce restrictive ventilatory defects requiring decortication. Pleural biopsies usually fail to recover tissue that can be definitely regarded as of rheumatoid origin; chronic, low-grade inflammation with fibrosis is the usual finding.[24] Biopsies do, of course, help to exclude other diagnoses such as tuberculosis, and because the diagnosis of rheumatoid pleurisy is essentially one of exclusion, the procedure is useful. Tumor and tuberculosis, each of which may cause an effusion with low glucose and high protein levels, need to be considered. Empyema may also be of concern, either as the entire explanation for an effusion or as a superimposed infection of a previously diseased space, as seen with the rheumatoid joint.

Although the exact role of rheumatoid disease in the aforementioned forms of nonspecific pleural disease may be debated, some patients have histologically defined rheumatoid nodules in the lungs. These nodules are often subpleural plaque-like structures that may also be found in the parietal pleura. The nodules may ulcerate from either location into the pleural space, causing pleural effusions or, more rarely, pneumothorax. Under these circumstances, the nature of the pleural fluid exactly parallels that which appears without nodules. This finding suggests that both processes are part of rheumatoid disease.

Nodular Pulmonary Disease

Although rheumatoid nodules of the lungs are often so peripheral as to involve the visceral pleura, they may develop singly or multiply, within the parenchyma itself. They appear as asymptomatic, round shadows, 0.5 to 3 cm in size, usually in a man with seropositive RA. The lesions are less common in women. Like the subcutaneous nodule, the pulmonary nodule appears and disappears without a close relationship to synovial disease activity. It may persist for years without change, or it may slowly enlarge to an enormous size. Nodular parenchymal disease in the absence of pleural findings is rare, and a thorough study is justified to exclude other causes. Such is particularly true of single "coin" lesions. Spontaneous cavitation with little pericavitary inflammation has been reported;[165] indeed, in some patients, the cavity is the first sign and only subsequently do they develop other nodules. Rarely, single or multiple pulmonary rheumatoid nodules precede the development of polyarthritis by many years.[63,95,106]

Rheumatoid Pneumoconiosis

Rheumatoid pneumoconiosis or Caplan's syndrome was described in Welsh miners with RA who, when exposed primarily to soft coal dust, showed chest roentgenographic patterns different from those of ordinary pneumoconiosis.[31] About 35% of miners with rheumatoid disease showed this peculiar condition.[146] In some instances, the pattern appeared years before the development of overt RA. The "classic" roentgenogram shows multiple, well-defined, round opacities greater than 1 cm in diameter distributed through all lung fields, especially peripherally (Fig. 39–3). Cavitation is often a feature. More commonly, patients show discrete nodular shadows varying from 0.3 to 1 cm in diameter. These smaller nodules may be few and confined to the upper zones, or they may present a "snowstorm" appearance widely distributed

throughout the chest. Other patients show scattered irregular opacities, often with evidence of cavitation, but with little simple pneumoconiosis in the background.[80] Two-thirds of patients with the "classic" picture have definite RA. Rheumatoid factor activity has been found in the serum of more than 80% of the miners with these roentgenographic changes.[32]

The syndrome has also been identified in workers with asbestos, abrasives, and silica, although some of these cases are not radiographically identical to those in miners. Pneumoconiosis is not more common among miners with RA than among those without it, nor is RA more common among miners than in the general population, as shown by studies among soft-coal miners in Pennsylvania.[13,14] Pneumoconiosis in miners with rheumatoid disease usually resembles pneumoconiosis in other miners, and only rarely does the radiologic picture of Caplan's syndrome develop. Furthermore, immunoglobulins and rheumatoid factors are not much different among miners with RA, miners with RA and pneumoconiosis, and persons other than miners with RA.

Diffuse Lung Disease

The term "rheumatoid disease" was coined in 1948 in a report describing the first recognized association of diffuse interstitial fibrosis and RA.[59] Since then, scattered descriptions of the pulmonary lesion have appeared under several names, including chronic pulmonary fibrosis, fibrosing pneumonitis, and fibrosing alveolitis.

In an extensive radiologic survey of 309 rheumatoid patients and an equal number of age- and sex-matched control subjects in which the films were read blindly, a pattern of diffuse reticulonodular fibrosis was found in 4.5% of the RA patients and in 0.3% of the control subjects. By contrast, diffuse fibrosis was roughly equal in the 2 groups, 6.8 and 5.2% respectively, and correlated with age and smoking. In the patients with RA, effusion was noted in 0.6%, and nodules were in 0.3% of the RA patients surveyed.[108] Apical fibrobullous disease has now been seen in seropositive RA, as well as in ankylosing spondylitis.[168,208]

In surveys of lung function in patients with RA, abnormalities in the diffusion capacity[70,92,162,171,181,184] have been found, as well as evidence of obstructive lung disease manifested by decreased flow rates.[41,51,75] Cigarette smoking certainly contributes to these abnormalities, although the degree of impairment exceeds that found in patients with osteoarthritis and equivalent smoking histories.[41,51] Both functional and histopathologic studies suggest that vascular changes that reduce the pulmonary capillary bed are responsible for the

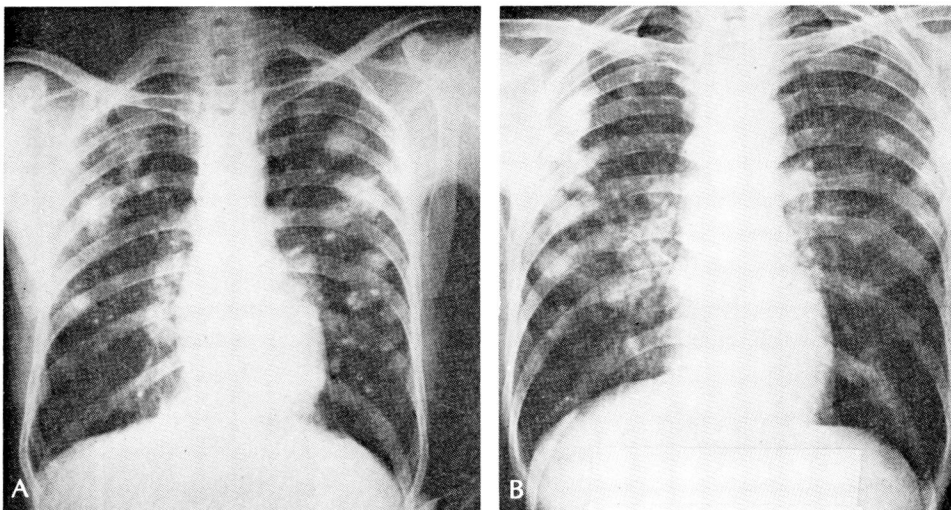

Fig. 39–3. *A* and *B*, Two examples of rheumatoid pneumoconiosis in the classic form. (Courtesy of Dr. A. Caplan.)

abnormalities in diffusion capacity.[38] If one considers patients with definite or classic disease, a substantial proportion have diffuse lung disease on the basis of mild radiographic abnormality or pulmonary dysfunction. Diffuse lung disease is most common in patients with an elevated rheumatoid factor. Muscular weakness and general debility may possibly contribute to the disease process and, at the same time, may inhibit its symptomatic expression.

Dyspnea on exertion, cough with scanty sputum, and clubbing are typical manifestations of the clinical syndrome. Diffuse or, more often, basilar crepitant rales are found. Early disease may appear radiographically as soft, fluffy patches or fine reticulonodular shadowing, almost always most prominent at the bases. Subsequently, diffuse mottling and "harder" pulmonary fibrosis gradually appear. Cysts and fibrotic "honeycombing" are typical of end-stage disease. This whole picture can evolve within a year, but a five- to ten-year course is more common. The essential histopathologic features are thickening of the alveolar walls with cells and fibrosis and the presence of large mononuclear cells, presumably of alveolar origin, within the alveolar spaces. Neither radiologic nor histologic examination provides an unequivocal link to RA because both are nonspecific. In most patients, RA precedes pulmonary fibrosis by years, but the pulmonary process can begin first.

Approximately 100 cases of RA and diffuse interstitial fibrosis have been reported, the majority in men. Many sizable groups of patients with RA have been surveyed without detection of even a single case of clinically evident diffuse interstitial fibrosis; 8 cases were identified in a study of 516 patients with RA.[217] From the chest physician's point of view, however, a substantial proportion of patients with diffuse interstitial fibrosis have RA or another connective tissue disease. Furthermore, even in those without identifiable connective tissue disease, rheumatoid factors or other abnormal antibodies are often found, suggesting common pathogenetic pathways.[50,167,211,212]

A newly recognized pulmonary manifestation of RA is bronchiolitis leading to airway obliteration.[44,74,91,102] This lesion first manifests as breathlessness of rapid onset, often in the face of a normal roentgenogram. Minimal rales may be present, and a midinspiratory squeak may be heard over the anterior chest during quiet breathing. Pulmonary functional tests show an obstructive pattern. The lung at biopsy or autopsy shows an acute inflammation of bronchiolar walls early, and later, fibrous obliteration of bronchioles. The syndrome may be rapidly fatal. Although several of these patients had been receiving D-penicillamine, others had not.

In summary, clinically evident specific pulmonary disease associated with RA is rare, whereas non-life-threatening pleural disease is common. Curiously, all the pleuropulmonary processes are more common in men and correlate with the presence of rheumatoid factor. Two patterns, rheumatoid nodules of the lung and rheumatoid pleural effusion, are clearly part of rheumatoid disease, whereas diffuse interstitial fibrosis bears a less certain relationship to the underlying disease. "Rheumatoid" pneumoconiosis is even more doubtful. The diversity of the processes discussed does not encourage the use of the loose phrase "rheumatoid lung."

CARDIAC MANIFESTATIONS

The variety and extent of cardiac lesions described in postmortem studies of RA never cease to amaze clinicians, who are usually able to recall only a handful of patients with cardiac findings that they considered to be related to RA. The autopsy findings should, however, spur these physicians to more careful and frequent evaluation of the heart, because such efforts do reveal unexpected changes.[119] Nevertheless, physicians at the bedside are probably correct in believing that most such autopsy findings are not clinically manifest, some are detectable but are not of importance to their patients and a few are the cause of significant functional impairment of the heart.

Pericarditis

Pericardial involvement in RA is common at autopsy.[22,34] Echocardiographic study indeed confirms that half the patients with definite or classic disease have small posterior pericardial effusions in life; these findings surely reflect the disease process.[8,159,172] Because most of these effusions are found in patients who have not had clinically manifested pericarditis, and who almost certainly will not have it, the existence of these effusions is no cause for changing one's therapeutic approach to the disease.

Subtle clinical pericarditis has, in fact, been identified in 10 of 100 consecutive patients with RA of sufficient severity to require hospitalization for articular problems. All patients and an equal number of age- and sex-matched control subjects were examined on at least three occasions, and all had chest roentgenograms and electrocardiograms. Pericardial friction rubs were detected in all 10 patients; only 1 had chest pain, 7 were entirely asymptomatic, and pericarditis was identified in a single control subject.[119] Women were affected more often than men, and the process was generally benign and self-limited, rarely causing symptoms or requiring therapy.

More serious, and fortunately rarer, is severe pericarditis manifested by chest pain, a large heart, heart failure, or a friction rub.[68] This disease is as common in men as in women and frequently accompanies other extra-articular disease. Rheumatoid factor is almost uniformly present. The pericardial fluid often has a low or even absent glucose level and an elevated protein level. The pathologic findings on biopsy are nonspecific and usually show fibrinous pericarditis when the process is acute or fibrosis when it is chronic. This syndrome may have severe consequences, such as tamponade or chronic constriction, despite medical therapy and pericardial taps.[78,104,127,140,176] Calcific pericarditis and cholesterol pericarditis may be late consequences. Because some patients do respond, corticosteroids in substantial doses may be tried for as long as four weeks, but many such patients are relieved only by pericardectomy.[68]

Myocardial and Coronary Artery Disease

Myocardial insufficiency and death due to congestive heart failure are frequent in RA, but how often are these cardiac effects due to RA? Probably not often. A patient with a severe debilitating disorder such as rheumatoid disease dies, as it were, by inches. Cardiac deaths are common in any group of patients who are so ill. Substantial pathologic evidence must therefore be found at necropsy before the diagnosis of rheumatoid heart disease is justified.[87] Thus, the role of interstitial foci of mononuclear cells found in the myocardium is of uncertain significance,[200] although its appearance and severity may match that of Fiedler's myocarditis. Diffuse myocarditis with frank necrosis of muscle is also seen.[123]

When disease of the coronary arteries occurs in RA, it is almost always due to arteriosclerosis. Rheumatoid arteritis, which rarely seems to involve the larger vessels supplying the heart to produce ischemia and infarction,[110] should be invoked as a cause of clinical ischemia with the greatest caution, particularly because the therapeutic implications are so different from those of arteriosclerosis. Small-vessel coronary arterial inflammation does occur in RA,[47] but is probably not a major cause of clinical heart disease unless widespread arteritis is present.

It is unclear whether the apparently increased incidence of clinical coronary artery disease in RA[34,215] can be reconciled with an apparently decreased mortality rate from myocardial infarction.[53] Further contributing to the confusion are the theoretic possibilities that corticosteroids accelerate and aspirin decelerates the course of coronary artery disease.

Endocardial Disease

Clinically apparent valvular disease that can safely be ascribed to the rheumatoid process is rare.[23,124,158] Echocardiographic examination does reveal a movement disorder of the mitral valve in up to 25% of patients, but this finding is not accompanied by any physical signs of valvular disease.[8,159,172]

The granulomas typical of rheumatoid disease, found in 5 to 10% of all seropositive patients at autopsy,[47] are responsible for the rare clinical valvular disease and conduction defects;[72,81,86] occasionally, frank aortic incompetence may result.[100,192] The pathologic process at the root of the aorta in ankylosing spondylitis may have the same clinical effects in terms of conduction difficulties and aortic insufficiency, but the process shows patchy destruction of the media of the aortic root and intimal fibrosis of regional arterioles, a different histopathologic pattern.

NEUROMUSCULAR MANIFESTATIONS

The evaluation of neuromuscular features of RA is a time-consuming and difficult task. Patients with pain, stiffness, and weakness associated with active polyarthritis may not mention symptoms that would suggest neuropathy to the examiner. The physician recognizes myasthenia, but is usually unable to exclude arthritic disease as its primary cause. Nevertheless, one often sees patients who report that "something fresh, new, and unpleasant has happened to their feet, which feel different and are painful in a different way."[88] Similarly, one cannot mistake the abrupt onset of footdrop in the ambulatory patient. These problems and others, all manifestations of RA, occur in about 10% of patients with the disease and deserve careful evaluation because of therapeutic and prognostic implications.

The classification of the neurologic lesions of RA varies widely. Diffuse distal neuropathy is considered first, and then a few specific lesions, both central and peripheral, which may have neurologic manifestations. Finally, some of the features of myopathy are mentioned. The neuropathology of rheumatoid disease has been extensively reviewed.[115]

Neuropathy

The diffuse distal neuropathy, in its most common form, is characterized by numbness of the feet, usually symmetric and stocking-like in distribution. Hyperesthesia, electric shock sensations, and burning pain occur. Examination reveals a loss of vibration sensation in most, together with loss of appreciation of light touch and pinprick. Position sense is usually retained. The findings may not exactly correspond to the symptomatic areas. Neither the symptoms nor the findings usually correspond to the distribution of a major nerve. In some patients, minor motor changes are also detectable, with muscle wasting. The Achilles reflex, particularly, may be lost. Electrophysiologic studies may be normal, but gross slowing of motor conduction in the affected limb is also observed.[39] Similar lesions are seen in the hands, and clumsiness may be a complaint. In most of those with involved hands, foot symptoms are also present. Careful assessment of the fingers has been particularly fruitful in bringing out numbness of the tips or hyperthesia along one side of a digit.[60] These patterns are typically seen in older seropositive patients with disease of 10 to 15 years' duration, and the sex distribution matches that of the disease itself. Subcutaneous nodules have been found in about half the cases. The prognosis is generally good, with partial or complete recovery in most. In some, the findings remain static, whereas progression over weeks or months can lead to more widespread findings in a few. A more subtle abnormality, impaired cardiac response to the Valsalva maneuver or to standing, has been found in patients both with and without other evidence of peripheral neuropathy.[57]

Patients with severe motor impairment based on peripheral nerve disease have a different pattern and seem to be, in large part, a separate group.[39] Although they may, either at onset or in course, have sensory deficits, the usual picture is one of rapid change in, and progressive deterioration of, motor function. At first, the abruptly developing foot- or wristdrops often represent a mononeuritis multiplex, which is motor and sensory impairment in the distribution of two or more peripheral nerves; this disorder evolves into a severe sensorimotor neuropathy with complete paralysis of several extremities and dense sensory loss.[39,164]

The prognosis for life is poor, and the more widespread the neuropathy, the worse it becomes.[65] Many of these patients die, and virtually all have arteritis, in many instances involving the vasa nervorum. This swift pattern occurs most commonly in men, invariably with nodules and high titers of rheumatoid factor (see Chap. 63).

Whether arteritis should be regarded as the cause of all diffuse neuropathy is unclear. The mechanisms for the two types of neuropathy may well be different. In the acute motor variety that accompanies widespread arteritis, vessel walls of the vasa nervorum may show signs of an immunologic process with the deposition of immunoglobulin and complement.[43] Extensive demyelination of both large and small fibers occurs.[223] By contrast, although some large-fiber demyelination and axonal degeneration occur in the more chronically affected patient with distal sensory neuropathy, the vasa nervorum show only a proliferative endarteritis.[157] Whether that finding, so common in other locations in the diffuse connective tissue diseases, is indeed the late stage of a resolving immunologic insult or represents a primary event remains unknown.

The recognized neuromuscular specific lesions of RA are all associated with pressure on neural tissue and include pressure on the spinal cord as a manifestation of cervical subluxations, the several syndromes of peripheral nerve entrapment, and manifestations resulting from rheumatoid nodules impinging on the central nervous system.

Cervical Myelopathy

Neurologic manifestations of cervical spine disease are recognized with only modest frequency when one considers the prevalence of radiographic abnormalities in the area. In a study of 333 patients requiring hospitalization for active physiotherapy and rehabilitation, a single lateral view of the cervical spine in *full flexion* was made. Atlantoaxial subluxation, defined as a distance greater than 2.5 mm in women and 3.0 mm in men between the posterior aspect of the anterior arch of the atlas and the anterior surface of the odontoid process, was found in 84 patients, and serial subluxation of other cervical vertebrae was seen in 23.[42] Other radiographic evidence of rheumatoid involvement of the cervical spine includes erosion of the apophyseal joints, of the vertebral bodies, and of the odontoid itself, which leads to a small, pointed odontoid.[18] If all radiographic abnormalities of the cervical spine are included, evidence of involvement may rise to over 80% of patients with definite or classic disease.[19] Destruction of the transverse ligament of the atlas and the anterior atlantoaxial ligament by RA permits the dens to move posteriorly into the spinal canal. Spinal cord compression is uncommon, however, perhaps primarily because of the generous size of the spinal canal at this level (Fig. 39–4,A). Cervical spinal pain is more frequent and compression findings are less frequent with atlantoaxial disease than with subluxation of lower cervical vertebrae, most common at C3 to C4, where pain is often absent and the signs of spinal cord compression may be overwhelming. At the inferior level, the spinal canal is less capacious (Fig. 39–4,B). Most often, radiographically apparent disease, even with dramatic changes, does not progress with conservative management.[199] Fewer than 10% of patients with major radiographic changes of luxation ultimately develop neurologic symptoms due to spinal cord compression or vertebral ischemia.

Cervical cord compression is most likely to develop in patients in whom it is most difficult to detect, that is, in those with long-standing, seropositive, deforming RA and extensive erosive disease, much joint instability, and tendon rupture.[42,143,163] Occasionally, pain in the cervical spine is entirely absent. The radiographic finding of atlantoaxial subluxation can be supplemented by actual palpation of the joint through the posterior pharyngeal wall. Upper motor neuron signs, such as weakness, unexplained "giving way" of the knee, flexor spasm, a positive Babinski sign, and increased deep tendon reflexes, may be identified.

Bowel and bladder dysfunction may occur. In view of the many musculoskeletal problems in the typical patient, sensory examination is important, especially because sensory changes are frequently the presenting problem.[139] Position sense and two-point discrimination are lost early. The findings range from barely detectable to full-blown tetraplegia, as in spinal cord transection. Death has resulted not only from cord compression, but also from vertebral artery thrombosis induced by kinking secondary to excessive motion of the axis.[141,220,224] Trauma is dangerous for these patients, but most particularly, care must be taken with the neck manipulation during endotracheal intubation and anesthesia induction.

Gentle collar immobilization in midposition is the best choice for conservative management. A rigid "Philadelphia" collar may be needed to control pain. Unless this therapy promptly reverses any neurologic manifestations, operative intervention should be considered. A variety of surgical procedures are available and offer some chance for a return to active life, but they should be reserved for severe cases with definite neurologic signs.[45,46]

Pressure Neuropathy

The entrapment or pressure neuropathies in RA are caused by inflammation or edema at a point, usually juxta-articular, at which nondistensible structures restrain the affected peripheral nerve. The symptoms usually subside if the local inflammation recedes consequent to rest, local corticosteroid injection, or adequate systemic therapy. Surgical intervention is dramatically successful. Compression neuropathies may occur at any stage of the disease and, in a number of instances, appear to have been the first detectable manifestations of RA.

Median nerve compression in the carpal tunnel is by far the most common pressure neuropathy, and RA is its most common systemic cause.[231] The onset is insidious, and the early changes are largely sensory. The *ulnar nerve* can be affected at elbow or wrist. The *radial or posterior interosseous nerve* is less often involved at the elbow as it passes anterior to the lateral epicondyle.[66,147] The onset is usually the abrupt loss of finger extension, with preserved wrist extension and intact extensor tendons demonstrated on extreme wrist flexion, thus distinguishing it from extensor tendon rupture. *Anterior tibial nerve* palsy with footdrop can be associated with popliteal space compression or with the external compression of braces or casts as the nerve rounds the fibular head. The *posterior tibial nerve* can be compressed in the *tarsal tunnel* beneath the flexor retinaculum distal to the medial malleolus; it is there accompanied by the tendons

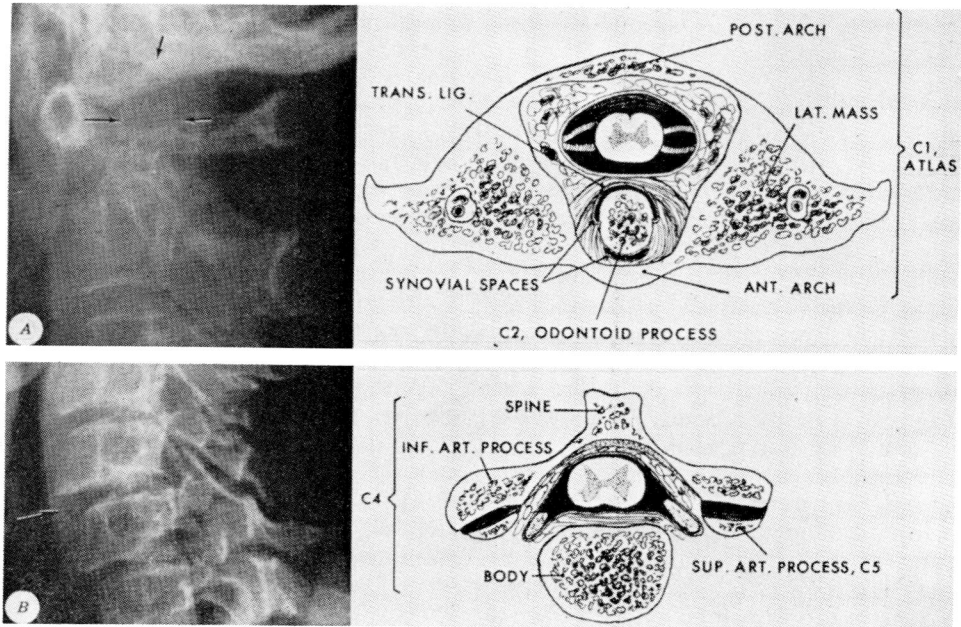

Fig. 39–4. *A,* Flexion films of the upper cervical spine with the odontoid process of C2 outlined by arrows. The dislocation measured 7 mm. The patient, a 59-year-old woman, had had seropositive RA with nodules for 17 years. She had severe deformities with finger extensor tendon destruction. She had had posterior cervical pain, but neither symptoms nor findings of neural compression. *B,* Mild subluxation of C4 on C5 in long-standing RA. This less-common change can be, but here was not, accompanied by findings of spinal cord compression. (Courtesy of Dr. John Bland.)

of the long flexors and their sheaths.[40,128] The clinical syndrome is one of burning pain and paresthesias.[82]

Rheumatoid Nodules

Only scattered case reports exist of rheumatoid nodules impinging on the central nervous system. Over the cranium, these have been found to involve primarily the dura mater or the leptomeninges.[60,138,182,203,205] The choroid plexus is rarely found to contain rheumatoid nodules at postmortem examination.[114,116] The neural tissue is uninvolved, save for occasional vasculitis.* The lesions have not been clearly related to symptoms, although one patient had "what appeared to be Jacksonian fits."[60] Extradural rheumatoid nodules involve the spinal canal and occasionally produce nerve root compression,[71,126] or even spinal cord compression.[90]

Muscle Disorder

Weakness and atrophy of skeletal muscle constitute one of the earliest and most pervasive manifestations of RA. They are evident virtually throughout the disease course and contribute to total disability. These changes affect small muscles as well as large. Muscle pain and stiffness are common symptoms. The weakness and wasting can, of course, be a sequel to neurologic dysfunction, described earlier, but more frequently they appear in the absence of discernible neurologic impairment. Although perhaps more common in muscles across painful and damaged joints, this condition appears in areas remote from synovial inflammation. The course of muscle disorder is irregular in that dramatic muscle weakness may occur over a period of three to six months, whereas for extended periods, both before and after the episode, weakness may not be prominent. Occasionally, corticosteroid therapy seems to be a major causative factor.

In essence, however, the weakness is unexplained. Striking elevations of muscle-related enzymes are not observed,[136,221] but serum creatine-creatinine ratios are increased, consistent with diminished muscle mass.[221] Electromyographic analysis has found "myositis" with "myopathy," as variously defined, to be present, but the findings are poorly related to clinically observed weakness and wasting and to neighboring joint activity.[136,204]

---

*Editor's note: I have seen one case with nodules in the substance of both the cerebrum and the cerebellum in association with rheumatoid meningitis.

Myositis, characterized by nodular or diffuse infiltrates of lymphocytes and plasma cells with muscle necrosis, and muscle cachexia, characterized by a reduction in muscle-cell bulk with both diminution in caliber and an accumulation of nuclei, are the dominant findings on biopsy. Neither change is specific for RA.[89,109] Histochemical studies demonstrate predominant atrophy of the so-called type II fibers.[58] This atrophy, also seen in other conditions, has been ascribed to limitation of muscle activity.[26]

RHEUMATOID ARTERITIS

Histopathologic terms such as "arteritis" or "vasculitis" are often used in describing the appearance of vascular lesions found in the tissues of patients with RA. Experience has shown that the presence of such lesions does not connote a single, easily distinguishable clinical syndrome, but rather reflects a pathogenetic mechanism responsible for a host of clinical manifestations of the disease. Indeed, inflammatory change in arterioles and venules has been reported to be the earliest detectable change in the two cardinal lesions, synovitis and subcutaneous nodules.[120,201] Good reason exists to believe that arterial inflammation is detectable in more than one-fourth of RA patients coming to autopsy, and the prevalence is proportional to the diligence of the search and the exact morphologic criteria used.

In recent years, however, the contributions of many students of the disease have built a *clinical picture* properly called "rheumatoid arteritis."[3,62,105,111,149] An extensive series from England has recently been reported.[186] It is characterized primarily by polyneuropathy, skin infarction and ulceration, digital gangrene, and evidence of visceral ischemia most notable in the form of intestinal infarction. The prognosis for life is poor when advanced neuropathic findings[65,164] and digital gangrene occur, and the term "malignant RA"[16] has been applied by some when such manifestations are present.

This rare clinical syndrome of rheumatoid arteritis appears in far less than 1% of patients who seek medical advice for RA. Although debatable, it seems likely that the syndrome was more prevalent in the early steroid era, from 1950 to 1960. With the smaller and more carefully regulated adrenal steroid dosage in general use today, the syndrome is again becoming less frequent.[87]

The severe form of the process seems to be more common in men than in women. It may appear abruptly after years of seropositive, erosive RA with subcutaneous nodules. Most patients who have been treated with corticosteroids show cushingoid changes and give a history of erratic, widely varying doses in the recent past. Synovitis is not usually prominent. At its worst, peripheral neuropathy may involve three or four limbs, with foot- and wristdrop often the most obvious changes (Fig. 39–5). Then fingers or toes turn blue and may later develop frank dry gangrene with autoamputation (Fig. 39–6). Malleolar or tibial skin necrosis is common, and ulcerations may become extensive, creating serious problems.

The patient is commonly febrile, with temperatures mounting to 104°F or more. Polymorphonuclear leukocytosis is frequent. Episcleritis, pleuritis, pericarditis, and myocarditis are often detected, or these may antedate the onset of neural and cutaneous changes. At times, but not frequently, central nervous system involvement and renal disease contribute to the downhill course. The blood pressure is usually consistent with iatrogenic Cushing's disease, and malignant hypertension is uncommon. The complex terminal picture may include infection, malnutrition, gastrointestinal bleeding, and congestive heart failure. In this setting, mesenteric thrombosis with bowel gangrene may constitute the final insult.

Such a pattern usually evolves over a period of three to six months, but each event may appear singly over a period of years and at widely scattered intervals. Pathologic examination shows widespread, severe necrotizing arteritis of large vessels morphologically indistinguishable from polyarteritis nodosa, save for certain variances. For example, the digital arteries usually show a bland, concentric intimal thickening and fibrosis with a generally intact elastic lamina, that is, obliterative endarteritis. In the visceral vasculature, this bland intimal fibrosis may be present in some vessels, whereas in the same area or organ, other arteries show fibrinoid necrosis of the entire wall, complete thrombosis, and intense polymorphonuclear response.[187] Arteritis may be present on a rectal biopsy in patients with the clinical syndrome and is associated with a bleak prognosis.[186]

Two features of the arterial lesions are clinically pertinent. The lesion is "nodose" in that the severe inflammation may be localized to short segments of an artery, extending for less than 100 μm, with both proximal and distal segments of the vessel anatomically undisturbed. Thus, assessment of serial sections is important in the study of biopsy material. Second, at autopsy, the overall picture is usually notably asynchronous, with healing and recanalization apparent in one section and fresh, severe arteritis in another. The healed lesions imply that the acute process is, in some measure, reversible, and thus compound the prognostic uncertainties.

The pathogenesis of the clinical syndrome of

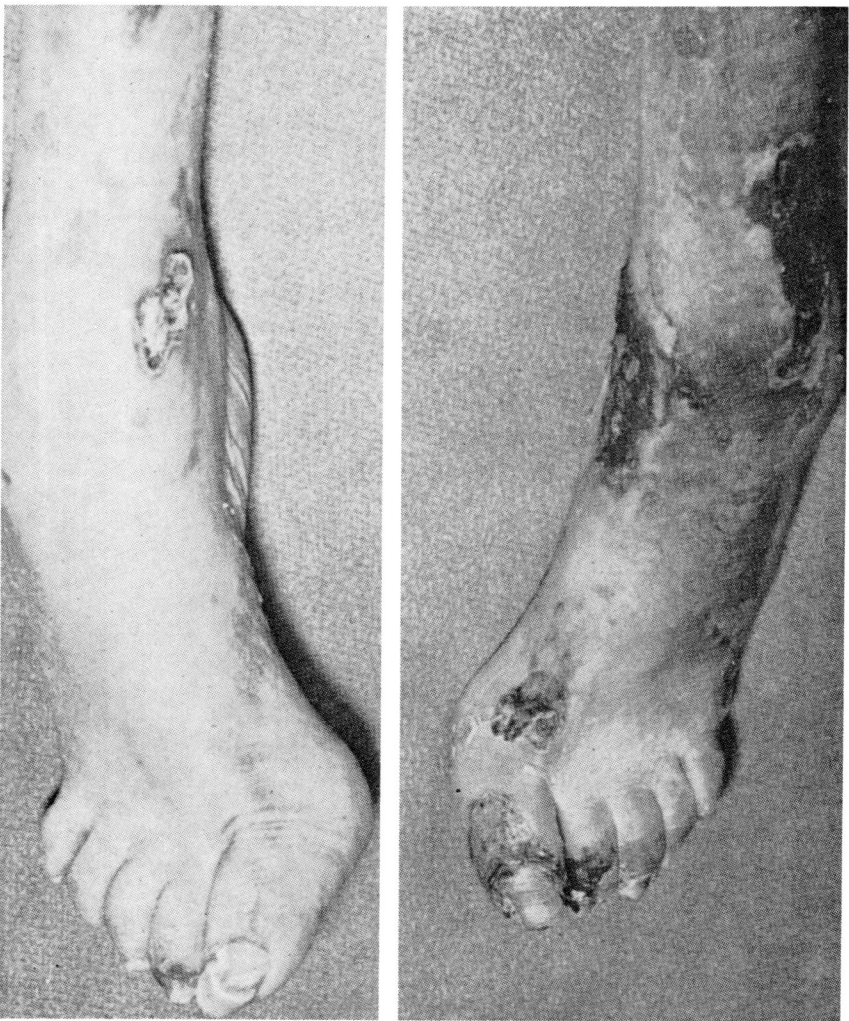

Fig. 39–5.   The feet of a 69-year-old woman who had had RA for 10 years and had been treated with large amounts of steroids. She had high titers of rheumatoid factor, abundant joint erosion visible radiographically, and biopsy-demonstrated active and healed arteritis with arterial wall necrosis. The ankle inversion of bilateral foot drop, extensive necrotic skin ulceration about the left ankle, and multiple cyanotic or gangrenous toe tips are all features of rheumatoid arteritis.

rheumatoid arteritis is unclear. It is usually considered to be a phase of RA, fortunately rare. Excellent grounds exist for believing it to be more common in the steroid-treated patient. It is virtually confined to patients with high titers of rheumatoid factor, especially IgG rheumatoid factor. In addition, LE cell preparations may be positive,[185] and antinuclear factor is usually demonstrable by fluorescence methods. No adequate explanation of the origin of the vascular necrosis exists, however. In contrast to "regular" RA, serum complement levels, especially of C4, may be reduced in the patient exhibiting manifestations of arteritis.[69] Because the progression of the syndrome is usually sufficiently

slow to permit the hope of therapeutic reversal, the mechanisms producing the lesions are of crucial importance in selecting appropriate therapy.

The management of these rare cases has not been studied systematically and has varied widely. Despite the role that corticosteroids are believed to play in inducing the process, they should not be withdrawn in a febrile phase with evolving neuropathy or progressive cutaneous lesions. If manifestations of life-threatening arteritis appear in a patient not receiving corticosteroids, the medication should be begun. Often, however, neither increasing nor beginning treatment with corticosteroids has a substantial effect on the process. In

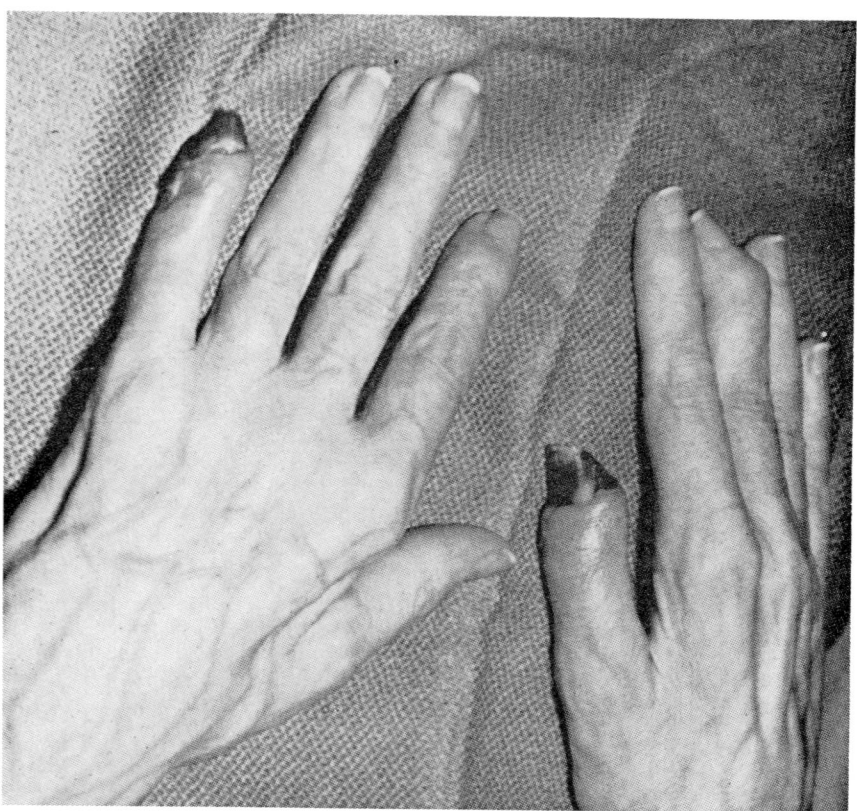

Fig. 39–6. Gangrenous fingertips of the same patient as in Figure 39–5. The necrotic fingers showed their first cyanosis five weeks earlier.

view of the reported benefits in this and other conditions, cyclophosphamide, given either orally or intravenously, should be tried in life-threatening cases.

Various forms of cytotoxic therapy with purine analogues, such as azathioprine, or with alkylating agents, such as chlorambucil or cyclophosphamide, have been used. Penicillamine treatment appears to have reversed several cases.[101] Anticoagulation has been suggested, despite the obvious attendant risks. In the full-blown clinical picture, the prognosis is sufficiently grave to warrant exceptional measures, but because of the irregular progression of the syndrome, the same cannot be said for the management of isolated lesions such as episcleritis, chronic leg ulcers, or the identification of arteritis by muscle biopsy, which may or may not herald the full syndrome.

Such is especially true of the minor digital skin lesions that often precede clinical rheumatoid arteritis, but are also seen in patients who have little or no other evidence of vascular inflammation (Fig. 39–7). These include small, often tender, nodules of the volar pads, especially over the terminal pha-

langes. These nodules may heal, leaving a transient brown scar or, in other instances, a depressed lesion with tissue loss. Infarction of the nail edges quickly results in a sharply localized black lesion, usually asymptomatic. Within weeks, the black scale flakes off and leaves unscarred, normal nail edges. These lesions are said to appear in as many as 8% of hospitalized patients with RA. They are more common in men, twice as prevalent in those receiving corticosteroid therapy,[54] and are usually accompanied by rheumatoid and antinuclear factor in the serum.[35] Gangrenous change may involve entire digits, or indeed a whole hand, but is more common in only one or two terminal phalangeal areas. Raynaud's phenomenon is by no means a prerequisite. Arteriographic studies in life and at autopsy have revealed extensive insufficiency of digital arteries, both in the presence and in the absence of overt clinical findings.[188]

The degree to which these findings are likely to be accompanied or followed by polyneuropathy or the full picture of rheumatoid arteritis with visceral infarction is not clear. Bywaters and Scott noted

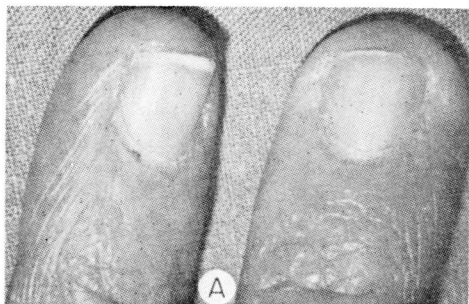
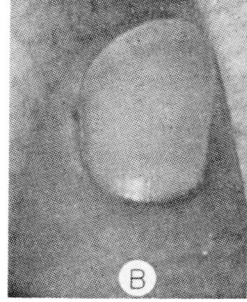
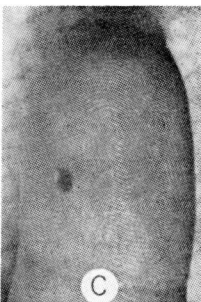

Fig. 39–7. *A*, Prominent nail fold arterioles. *B*, Nail edge infarction. *C*, Volar finger pulp brown spot. All these patients had RA.

such lesions in 34 patients; 10 deaths occurred in the group, 4 of them due to visceral infarction.[29]

FELTY'S SYNDROME

Felty observed and reported 5 middle-aged patients with deforming RA who showed weight loss, pigmentation of exposed skin surfaces, splenomegaly, and leukopenia. The white cell counts ranged from 1,000 to 4,200/mm². Differential counts in 2 cases showed fewer than 50% polymorphonuclear leukocytes.[64] The syndrome is now recognized as a variant of RA, although it appears in fewer than 5% of cases coming to medical attention.[218] The basic disease is usually deforming in nature, is accompanied by subcutaneous nodules, and is characterized by the presence of rheumatoid factor in the serum at higher titers than in patients without splenomegaly. The arthritis has its onset many years before the detection of the splenomegaly, which usually occurs in patients between 45 and 65 years of age. The patients are often severely crippled, but may have only modestly active joint disease.

The spleen ranges from barely palpable to large and is not usually tender, although splenic infarcts and traumatic rupture do occur. Slowly progressive changes in size, either an increase or a decrease, may be detected as the patient is followed. Other manifestations of systemic rheumatoid disease such as pericarditis, episcleritis, and peripheral neuropathy are often present. It almost never occurs in blacks.[209]

In the presence of splenomegaly, total white blood cell counts vary, but most patients show regular counts below 4,500 cells/mm², and counts as low as 500 have been observed. The greatest part of the reduction is in the neutrophilic leukocytes, which rarely constitute more than 40% of the cells and have been totally absent in a few patients. The number of lymphocytes is also often reduced, but to a lesser degree. Monocytes and eosinophils are not reduced, and one does occasionally see a rel-

ative eosinophilia. Bone marrow varies from hypoplastic to hyperplastic, although it is usually normal, save for a deficiency of mature neutrophils, termed "maturation arrest."[107] The anemia is hypochromic, as is usual in RA, but in addition, red cell destruction may be accelerated. After administration of chromium-labeled cells, spleen-liver uptake ratios suggested that the anemia would be alleviated by splenectomy, and such proved to be the case.[96] Increased platelet destruction has also been observed, but rarely produces purpuric manifestations.

Studies of the mechanisms of the leukopenia have revealed a number of interesting abnormalities, no one of which clearly explains the pathogenesis of the disease. Antibodies to the surface of white cells have been described,[132,178] as well as antinuclear factors specific for granulocyte nuclei.[177,222,225] The granulocytes appear to have increased immunoglobulin on their surface, and following splenectomy, the amount returns to normal.[131] Granulocytes also have large inclusions suspected to be ingested immune complexes, which, it is speculated, interfere with normal function.[97] Infused labeled white cells rapidly disappear, but those labeled cells remaining in the circulation seem thereafter to survive normally.[214] White cell production appears normal in the majority of patients, but reduced in some.[214] Not only may the infusion of Felty's plasma into a normal subject cause a transient leukopenia (though not specifically granulocytopenia),[30] but also autologous presplenectomy plasma from a patient with Felty's syndrome that is reinfused after the operation may cause the return of a defect in the bone marrow's ability to release granulocytes following an injection of the steroid, etiocholanalone.[117] A factor that can stimulate the in vitro growth of (mouse) marrow cells is diminished in the urine and serum of patients with Felty's syndrome.[56,85] Furthermore, mononuclear and T cells from Felty's syndrome patients, but not from patients with non-neutropenic RA or drug-induced neutropenia, suppressed the granulocyte colony-forming activity of normal bone marrow cells.[1] Finally, in vitro neutrophil function is normal in some respects and abnormal in others.[77,94,233] How these diverse findings relate to the development of Felty's syndrome and its response to therapy must await further investigation.

Whether the eponym should be applied to patients with splenomegaly without leukopenia or to those who have only leukopenia is uncertain. Nonpalpable splenomegaly is apparently common in RA in the absence of leukopenia.[99] Suffice it that the degree of both splenic enlargement and white count reduction can vary from month to month without apparent relationship to each other. Leukopenia and neutropenia often recur after splenectomy.

Two notable features seem to be related to the neutropenia or to the splenomegaly: chronic leg ulcers and an increase in bacterial infections. These were reported in 41 and 52%, respectively, of 27 patients.[180] Indolent ulcerations overlying the tibia or the ankles have frequently been described in patients with Felty's syndrome. The lesions are usually deep, painful, and chronically infected, with a mixed flora typical of uninvolved skin surfaces. They may be extensive, covering saucer-sized areas, or they may be only 2 to 4 cm in diameter. It is common for fresh ulcers to develop in the scars left by earlier lesions (Fig. 39–8). Some patients have had arterial and others venous insufficiency of the lower extremity, but neither loss of pulses nor marked edema is usual. Draining rheumatoid nodules can appear. Pyoderma gangrenosum, usually associated with chronic ulcerative colitis, should be excluded. After all the known causes of such lesions are considered, a group of elderly patients with leukopenia, deforming RA, and chronic leg ulcers remains. The ulcers begin as a hemorrhagic papule surrounded by a pale zone. The central area forms an eschar and eventually sloughs, leaving an ulcer that slowly spreads. Regional biopsies have shown arteritis with fibrinoid necrosis and low-grade inflammation sufficient to occlude small vessels.[121] Thus, both clinical and biopsy findings are consistent with ischemic disease in an area of poor collateral circulation.

In one study, 6 of 8 patients with this type of ulceration had either splenomegaly or leukopenia or both.[227] In one instance, leg ulcers first appeared with the leukopenia, which had developed progressively after an initially successful splenectomy. On comparison of small groups of patients, 1 with leg ulcers and 1 without, but both showing splenomegaly and leukopenia, those with leg ulcers

had disease of longer duration, smaller spleens by palpation, and a higher prevalence of positive direct LE cell preparations. Rheumatoid factor titers were high, and antinuclear factors, usually including those of IgM type, were invariably present. Conversely, when 50 LE cell-positive patients with RA were compared to 100 consecutive cases of LE cell-negative rheumatoid arthritis, spenomegaly was present in 6 of the former and in 1 of the latter.[112] Some have ascribed the condition to systemic lupus erythematosus (SLE),[4] whereas others speak of the two diseases as "overlapping." In view of the widespread and often severe erosive joint changes, the high titers, and not just the presence, of rheumatoid factors, and the almost complete freedom from central nervous system and renal disease, it seems best to classify these patients under the heading of RA and the variant, Felty's syndrome.

Chronic, recurrent, often severe bacterial infections of various sorts are seen, although one is also impressed with patients who have striking neutropenia for years, but no apparent tendency to bacterial complications. Ruderman et al. divided their series into those with more or less than 500 granulocytes mm^3; the frequency of infection was identical in both groups.[180] The infections seen included furunculosis, recurrent pulmonary disease, and urinary tract infections with typical bacterial pathogens. Patients usually respond to acute infections with some increase in granulocytes, but rarely manage a leukocytosis. Infections are a common cause of death, even in the antibiotic era, and secondary infections, resistant to antibiotics, are regularly seen.

Liver disease, even cirrhosis with portal hypertension, may occur in Felty's syndrome. A curious pathologic appearance of the liver in noncirrhotic cases, termed *nodular regenerative hyperplasia*, is distinctive.[21]

Adrenal corticosteroid therapy at tolerable dose levels does not alleviate the leukopenia and is a poor approach to the infection problem, although some have found a favorable effect on the indolent ulcers. Most physicians consider the indication for splenectomy to be limited to patients with recurrent infections. The effect of splenectomy on ulcers is irregular at best. The procedure does not have any recognized long-lasting effects on the polyarthritis and is rarely justified by the low grades of hemolytic anemia seen.

The results of splenectomy are difficult to assess because of the tendency to report favorable results and because the follow-up period is often short, although several recent longer-term follow-up reports exist.[122,210] A prompt and major granulocytosis is usually observed, and current acute infec-

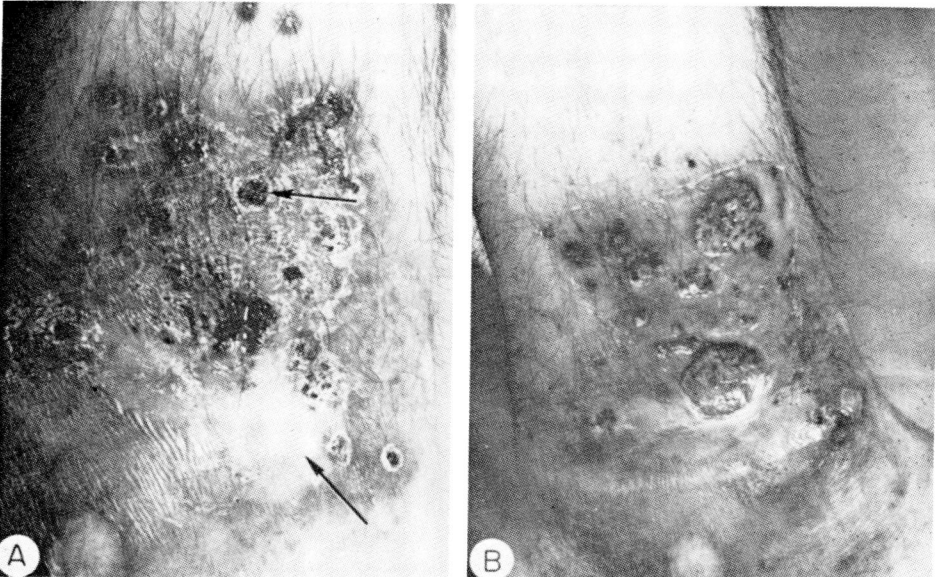

Fig. 39–8.   Proximal to the right lateral malleolus in a young man with Felty's syndrome and recurrent leg ulcers. *A*, Here abundant scar tissue (lower arrow) of earlier ulcers abruptly developed dark red and later black spots (upper arrow). *B*, Two weeks later the sharply marginated multiple ulcers exactly reflect the points of earlier infarction. (Courtesy of Dr. Robert Willkens.)

tions usually improve or disappear, but this latter outcome is by no means assured.[150] Recurrent infections may persist in those who had exhibited the problem preoperatively,[11,180] and those patients initially free of infections continue free postoperatively. What factors determine the success or failure of splenectomy in relieving granulocytopenia remain unknown, although presplenectomy bone marrow lymphocytosis may herald failure.[150] Because the pathogenesis of the disease appears not to be uniform, it is reasonable to hope that prediction of the success of splenectomy will one day be possible. It is clear that approximately one-third of patients undergoing splenectomy suffer a gradual reappearance of their neutropenia, so that within two or three years of operation, they are back to preoperative values again. In some cases, accessory splenic tissues have been identified and removed with a good response. Occasionally, the disease remits spontaneously.[11,133] On balance, splenectomy is justified for recurrent or chronic infections of significance, but one cannot make such a decision with any feeling of certainty.

The leukopenic patient alway presents a problem when chrysotherapy or cytotoxic therapy seems to be indicated by the polyarthritis. The potential role of splenectomy in permitting such therapy is dubious indeed. Chrysotherapy may be permissible if administered under strict control. Cytotoxic

agents that may produce leukopenia should not, in the current stage of knowledge, be used.

MISCELLANEOUS MANIFESTATIONS

Mention should be made of a few other common extrasynovial features of RA, the problem of peptic disease, and several organ systems involved in rare cases. Each of these aspects deserves more detailed analysis than can be presented here.

Common Features

Low-grade fever is often noted, and night sweating can be a problem. Shaking chills are unusual but do occur, accompanied by high fever, in the arteritic. Raynaud's phenomenon precedes or accompanies the disease in perhaps 10% of cases[193] and sweaty, soft palms, thenar and hypothenar erythema, and atrophic skin are cited as the result of vasomotor instability.

The psychiatric manifestations of RA have been extensively studied.[174] The key questions concern the premorbid personality and premorbid psychotrauma, in an effort to understand why one person develops the disease while another does not.[145] Whatever the findings before disease onset, however, the impact of the disease on the emotional life of the patient can be devastating and constitutes, beyond question, its most important extra-articular manifestation in terms of the *quality* of life with the disease.

Osteoporosis, regularly juxta-articular in location, but often much more widespread, is presumed to have a number of causes, including locally increased blood flow, disuse, postmenopausal status, and, commonly, the therapeutic use of adrenal corticosteroids. Fracture, resulting from the most minor trauma, is often the final, painful straw that reduces the patient to permanent bed rest. No prophylactic program is of demonstrated value, but osteopenia constitutes a compelling argument for trying to keep the patient up and moving.

Both eosinophilia[166,228] and thrombocytosis[98,189] are common, particularly in active or severe disease.

Doubtful Features

Because virtually all drugs administered to patients with RA, including aspirin, often used before the first visit to a physician, are considered by most to be "ulcerogenic," it has not been possible to establish beyond reasonable doubt that peptic ulcer is more prevalent in RA patients because they have the disease. The pathologic tissue does not usually demonstrate a rheumatoid lesion, although it is clear that rheumatoid arteritis may involve any part of the enteric vasculature.

The important practical point remains, however, that patients with treated RA manifest a high incidence of peptic ulcers and are subject to the usual complications.[7] Gross bleeding and perforation are more common than are obstructive symptoms, perhaps because gastric ulcers are more frequent in RA than in patients with uncomplicated peptic ulcer.

The therapeutic problem is most difficult. Some of the most severely crippled patients are those from whom aspirin and corticosteroids have been abruptly withdrawn for the good reason that hematemesis or perforation supervened while the patients were taking those drugs. On the other hand, healing of peptic ulceration can be seen radiologically when the patient is on a tightly defined antacid program while continuing the ulcerogenic medication. Some variation of the latter course, recognizing the risks, is to be preferred to the mandatory exclusion of medications on which virtually every articular movement may depend.

Other gastrointestinal pathologic abnormalities have been described in RA, but they are clinically irrelevant.[137]

Uncommon Features

No regularly recognized manifestations of the disease involve the endocrine or reproductive systems, except for a doubtful relationship to chronic thyroiditis.[142]

Specific rheumatoid lesions are not identified in renal tissue. Although glomerular filtration is frequently reduced,[27] owing perhaps to the effects of anti-inflammatory therapy, clinically significant renal disease is not common; most of it can probably be accounted for by amyloidosis, gold nephropathy, or chronic pyelonephritis.[202] The rare cases of glomerulopathy associated with RA have most often occurred in patients with evidence of SLE as well.[52,197]

Renal failure is not more common in patients with RA than in others.[173] Analgesic-induced nephropathy appears to be of negligible importance as a cause of renal insufficiency in the United States today,[156a] and aspirin therapy for arthritis has been explicitly exonerated as a cause of renal insufficiency.[61,169]

It is interesting that the central nervous system is spared in a disorder as widespread as rheumatoid disease. Confusion, sometimes accompanied by other central neurologic signs, has been described in elderly women withdrawn from corticosteroids and is responsive to the readministration of these drugs.[84,196] Such confusion may be caused by ignition of a cerebral vascular inflammation, or it may have an unrecognized metabolic origin.

Several surveys have shown hearing loss, usually of the sensorineural type. It is unlikely that synovial disease of the middle ear joints accounts for the deficits measured, and indeed, a handful of autopsies have shown normal ossicles.[79]

Rarely, the manifestations of the hyperviscosity syndrome dominate the clinical picture. The mechanism involves the formation of large aggregates of IgG or IgM rheumatoid factor with other immunoglobulins or with itself.

It is difficult to be sure of a general predisposition to infection because it is difficult to know what population is a suitable control.[12] Nevertheless, infection is not rare; certainly, joint infection is likely to occur in joints already damaged by the rheumatoid process and may prove fatal when it is recognized late.[148]

REFERENCES

1. Abdou, N.I., et al.: Suppressor cell-mediated neutropenia in Felty's syndrome. J. Clin. Invest., *61*:738–743, 1978.
2. Adelson, G.L., Saypol, D.C., and Walker, A.N.: Ureteral stenosis secondary to retroperitoneal rheumatoid nodules. J. Urol., *127*:124–125, 1982.
3. Adler, R.H., Norcross, B.M., and Lockie, L.M.: Arteritis and infarction of intestine in rheumatoid arthritis. JAMA, *180*:922–926, 1962.
4. Allison, J.H., and Bettley, F.R.: Rheumatoid arthritis with chronic leg ulceration. Lancet, *1*:288–290, 1957.
5. Aronoff, A., Bywaters, E.G.L., and Fearnley, G.R.: Lung lesions in rheumatoid arthritis. Br. Med. J., *2*:228–232, 1955.
6. Askari, A., Moscowitz, R.W., and Goldberg, V.M.: Subcutaneous rheumatoid nodules and serum rheumatoid factor without arthritis. JAMA, *229*:319–320, 1974.
7. Atwater, E.C., et al.: Peptic ulcer and rheumatoid ar-

thritis; a prospective study. Arch. Intern. Med., *115*:184–189, 1965.

8. Bacon, P.A., and Gibson, D.G.: Cardiac involvement in rheumatoid arthritis. Ann. Rheum. Dis., *33*:20–24, 1974.

9. Bankhurst, A.D., and Rowe, T.: Rheumatoid pleural effusions: the case for a primary glucose transport defect. J. Rheumatol., *7*:110–111, 1980.

10. Barager, F.D., and Duthie, J.J.R.: Importance of aspirin as a cause of anemia and peptic ulcer in rheumatoid arthritis. Br. Med. J., *1*:1106–1108, 1960.

11. Barnes, C.G., Turnbull, A.L., and Vernar-Roberts, B.: Felty's syndrome. Ann. Rheum. Dis., *30*:359–374, 1971.

12. Baum, J.: Infection in rheumatoid arthritis. Arthritis Rheum., *14*:135–137, 1971.

13. Benedek, T.G.: Rheumatoid pneumoconiosis. Documentation of onset and pathogenic considerations. Am. J. Med., *55*:515–524, 1973.

14. Benedek, T., Zawadzki, Z.A., and Medsger, T.A.: Serum immunoglobulins, rheumatoid factor, and pneumoconiosis in coal miners with rheumatoid arthritis. Arthritis Rheum., *19*:731–736, 1976.

15. Bennett, R.M., et al.: Synovial iron deposition in rheumatoid arthritis. Arthritis Rheum., *16*:298–304, 1973.

16. Bevans, M., et al.: The systemic lesions of malignant rheumatoid arthritis. Am. J. Med., *16*:197–211, 1954.

17. Bienenstock, H., Ehrlich, G.E., and Freyberg, R.H.: Rheumatoid arthritis of the cricoarytenoid joint: a clinopathologic study. Arthritis Rheum., *6*:48–63, 1963.

18. Bland, J.H.: Rheumatoid arthritis of the cervical spine. J. Rheum., *1*:319–342, 1974.

19. Bland, J.H., et al.: Rheumatoid arthritis of the cervical spine. Arch. Intern. Med., *112*:892–893, 1963.

20. Bland, J.H., and Eddy, W.M.: Hemiplegia and rheumatoid hemiarthritis. Arthritis Rheum., *11*:72–80, 1968.

21. Blendis, L.M., et al.: Nodular regenerative hyperplasia of the liver in Felty's syndrome. Q. J. Med., *43*:25–32, 1974.

22. Bonfiglio, T., and Atwater, E.C.: Heart disease in patients with sero-positive rheumatoid arthritis; a controlled autopsy study and review. Arch. Intern. Med., *124*:714–719, 1969.

23. Bortolotti, U., et al.: Mitral and aortic valve replacement in valvular rheumatoid heart disease. Chest, *73*:427–429, 1978.

24. Brennan, S.R., and Daly, J.J.: Large pleural effusions in rheumatoid arthritis. Br. J. Dis. Chest, *73*:133–140, 1979.

25. Bridger, M.W., Jahn, A.F., and van Nostrand, A.W.: Laryngeal rheumatoid arthritis. Laryngoscope, *90*:296–303, 1980.

26. Brooke, M.H., and Engel, W.K.: The histographic analysis of human muscle biopsies with regard to fibre types. Neurology, *19*:469–477, 1969.

27. Burry, H.C.: Reduced glomerular function in rheumatoid arthritis. Ann. Rheum. Dis., *31*:65–68, 1972.

28. Bywaters, E.G.L.: Fistulous rheumatism, a manifestation of rheumatoid arthritis. Ann. Rheum. Dis., *12*:114–121, 1953.

29. Bywaters, E.G.L., and Scott, J.T.: The natural history of vascular lesions in rheumatoid arthritis. J. Chronic Dis., *16*:905–914, 1963.

30. Calabresi, P., Edwards, E.A., and Schilling, R.F.: Fluorescent antiglobulin studies in leukopenic and related disorders. J. Clin. Invest., *38*:2091–2100, 1959.

31. Caplan, A.: Certain unusual radiological appearances in the chest of coal-miners suffering from rheumatoid arthritis. Thorax, *8*:29–37, 1953.

32. Caplan, A., Payne, R.B., and Withey, J.L.: A broader concept of Caplan's syndrome related to rheumatoid factors. Thorax, *17*:205–212, 1962.

33. Carr, D.T., and Mayne, J.G.: Pleurisy with effusion in rheumatoid arthritis, with reference to the low concentration of glucose in pleural fluid. Am. Rev. Respir. Dis., *85*:345–350, 1962.

34. Cathcart, E.S., and Spodick, D.H.: Rheumatoid heart disease; a study of the incidence and nature of cardiac lesions in rheumatoid arthritis. N. Engl. J. Med., *266*:959–964, 1962.

35. Cats, A., and Pit, A.A.: Clinical significance of rheu-

matoid vasculitis and the incidence of digital vascular lesions. Folia Med. Neerl., *12*:159–165, 1969.

36. Causey, J.Q.: Isolated subcutaneous rheumatic-like nodules in an adult. South Med. J., *65*:633–634, 1972.

37. Cavill, I., and Bentley, D.P.: Erythropoiesis in the anaemia of rheumatoid arthritis. Br. J. Haematol., *50*:583–590, 1982.

38. Cervantes-Perez, P., et al.: Pulmonary involvement in rheumatoid arthritis. JAMA, *243*:1715–1719, 1980.

39. Chamberlain, M.A., and Bruckner, F.E.: Rheumatoid neuropathy: clinical and electrophysiological features. Ann. Rheum. Dis., *29*:609–616, 1970.

40. Chater, E.H., and Wilson, A.L.: Tarsal tunnel syndrome. J. Irish Med. Assoc., *61*:326–328, 1968.

41. Collins, R.L., et al.: Obstructive pulmonary disease in rheumatoid arthritis. Arthritis Rheum., *19*:623–628, 1976.

42. Conlon, P.W., Isdale, I.C., and Rose, B.S.: Rheumatoid arthritis of the cervical spine: an analysis of 333 cases. Ann. Rheum. Dis., *25*:120–126, 1966.

43. Conn, D.L., McDuffie, F.E., and Dyck, P.J.: Immunopathologic study of sural nerves in rheumatoid arthritis. Arthritis Rheum., *15*:135–142, 1972.

44. Cooney, T.P.: Interrelationship of chronic eosinophilic pneumonia, bronchiolitis obliterans, and rheumatoid disease: a hypothesis. J. Clin. Pathol., *34*:129–137, 1981.

45. Cregan, J.C.F.: Internal fixation of the unstable rheumatoid spine. Ann. Rheum. Dis., *25*:242, 1966.

46. Crellin, R.Q., MacCabe, J.J., and Hamilton, E.B.D.: Severe subluxation of the cervical spine in rheumatoid arthritis. J. Bone Joint Surg., *52B*:244–251, 1970.

47. Cruickshank, B.: Heart lesions in rheumatoid disease. J. Pathol. Bacteriol., *76*:223–240, 1958.

48. Cruickshank, B.: Lesions of lymph nodes in rheumatoid disease and in disseminated lupus erythematosus. Scott. Med. J., *3*:110–119, 1958.

49. Cruickshank, B.: The arteritis of rheumatoid arthritis. Ann. Rheum. Dis., *13*:136–146, 1954.

50. Crystal, R.G., et al.: Idiopathic pulmonary fibrosis; clinical, histologic, radiographic, physiologic, scintigraphic, cytologic, and biochemical aspects. Ann. Intern. Med., *85*:769–788, 1976.

51. Davidson, C., Brooks, A.G.F., and Bacon, P.A.: Lung function in rheumatoid arthritis. A clinical survey. Ann. Rheum. Dis., *33*:293–297, 1974.

52. Davis, J.A., et al.: Glomerulonephritis in rheumatoid arthritis. Arthritis Rheum., *22*:1018–1023, 1979.

53. Davis, R.F., and Engleman, E.G.: Incidence of myocardial infarction in patients with rheumatoid arthritis. Arthritis Rheum., *17*:527–533, 1974.

54. Dequeker, J., and Rosberg, G.: Digital capillaritis in rheumatoid arthritis. Acta Rheumatol. Scand., *13*:299–307, 1967.

55. Dinant, H.J., and de Maat, C.E.: Erythropoiesis and mean red-cell lifespan in normal subjects and in patients with the anaemia of active rheumatoid arthritis. Br. J. Haematol., *39*:437–444, 1978. .

56. Duckham, D.J., et al.: Retardation of colony growth of in vitro bone marrow culture using sera from patients with Felty's syndrome, disseminated lupus erythematosus (SLE), rheumatoid arthritis, and other disease states. Arthritis Rheum., *18*:323–333, 1975.

57. Edmonds, M.E., et al.: Autonomic neuropathy in rheumatoid arthritis. Br. Med. J., *2*:173–175, 1979.

58. Edstrom, L., and Nordemar, R.: Differential changes in type I and type II muscle fibres in rheumatoid arthritis. Scand. J. Rheumatol., *3*:155–160, 1974.

59. Ellman, P., and Ball, R.E.: "Rheumatoid disease" with joints and pulmonary manifestations. Br. Med. J., *2*:816–820, 1948.

60. Ellman, P., Cudkowicz, L., and Elwood, J.S.: Widespread serous membrane involvement by rheumatoid nodules. J. Clin. Pathol., *7*:239–244, 1954.

61. Emkey, R.D., and Mills, J.D.: Aspirin and analgesic nephropathy. JAMA, *247*:55–57, 1982.

62. Epstein, W.V., and Engleman, E.P.: The relation of the rheumatoid factor content of serum to clinical neurovas-

cular manifestations of rheumatoid arthritis. Arthritis Rheum., 2:250–258, 1959.

63. Eraut, D., Evans, J., and Caplin, M.: Pulmonary necrobiotic nodules without rheumatoid arthritis. Br. J. Dis. Chest, 72:288–300, 1978.
64. Felty, A.R.: Chronic arthritis in the adult, associated with splenomegaly and leukopenia; a report of five cases of an unusual clinical syndrome. Bull. Johns Hopkins Hosp., 35:16–20, 1924.
65. Ferguson, R.H., and Slocumb, C.H.: Peripheral neuropathy in rheumatoid arthritis. Bull. Rheum. Dis., 11:251, 1961.
66. Fernandes, L., Goodwill, C.J., and Srivatsa, S.R.: Synovial rupture of rheumatoid elbow causing radial nerve compression. Br. Med. J., 2:17–18, 1979.
67. Ferry, A.P.: The histopathology of rheumatoid episcleral nodules; an extraarticular manifestation of rheumatoid arthritis. Arch. Ophthalmol., 82:77–78, 1969.
68. Franco, A.E., Levine, H., and Hall, A.P.: Rheumatoid pericarditis: report of seventeen cases diagnosed clinically. Ann. Intern. Med., 77:837–844, 1972.
69. Franco, A.E., and Schur, P.H.: Hypocomplementemia in rheumatoid arthritis. Arthritis Rheum., 14:231–238, 1971.
70. Frank, S.T., et al.: Pulmonary dysfunction in rheumatoid disease. Chest, 63:27–34, 1973.
71. Friedman, H.: Intraspinal rheumatoid nodule causing nerve root compression; case report. J. Neurosurg., 32:689–691, 1970.
72. Gallagher, P.J., and Gresham, G.A.: Heart block with infected cardiac rheumatoid granulomas. Br. Heart J., 35:110–112, 1973.
73. Ganda, O.P., and Caplan, H.I.: Rheumatoid disease without joint involvement. JAMA, 228:338–339, 1974.
74. Geddes, D.M., et al.: Progressive airway obliteration in adults and its association with rheumatoid disease. Q.J. Med., 184:427–443, 1977.
75. Geddes, D.M., Webley, M., and Emerson, P.A.: Airways obstruction in rheumatoid arthritis. Ann. Rheum. Dis., 38:222–225, 1979.
76. Ginsberg, M.H., et al.: Rheumatoid nodulosis, an unusual variant of rheumatoid disease. Arthritis Rheum., 18:49–58, 1975.
77. Goetzl, E.J.: Defective responsiveness to ascorbic acid of neutrophil random and chemotactic migration in Felty's syndrome and systemic lupus erythematosus. Ann. Rheum. Dis., 35:510–515, 1976.
78. Goldman, S., Gall, E.P., and Hager, W.D.: Rheumatoid pericarditis presenting as a mass lesion. Chest, 73:550–552, 1978.
79. Goodwill, C.J., Lord, I.J., and Knill Jones, R.P.: Hearing in rheumatoid arthritis. A clinical and audiometric survey. Ann. Rheum. Dis., 31:170–173, 1972.
80. Gough, J., Rivers, D., and Seal, R.M.E.: Pathological studies of modified pneumoconiosis in coal-miners with rheumatoid arthritis (Caplan's syndrome). Thorax, 10:9–18, 1955.
81. Gowans, J.D.C.: Complete heart block with Stokes-Adams syndrome due to rheumatoid heart disease; report of a case with autopsy findings. N. Engl. J. Med., 262:1012–1014, 1960.
82. Grabois, M., Puentes, J., and Lidsky, M.: Tarsal tunnel syndrome in rheumatoid arthritis. Arch. Phys. Med. Rehabil., 62:401–403, 1981.
83. Grossman, A., Martin, J.R., and Root, H.S.: Rheumatoid arthritis of cricoarytenoid joint. Laryngoscope, 71:530–544, 1961.
84. Gupta, V.P., and Ehrlich, G.E.: Organic brain syndrome in rheumatoid arthritis following steroid withdrawal. Arthritis Rheum., 19:1333–1338, 1976.
85. Gupta, R., Robinson, W.A., and Albrecht, D.: Granulopoietic activity in Felty's syndrome. Ann. Rheum. Dis., 34:156–161, 1975.
86. Handforth, C.P., and Woodbury, J.F.L.: Cardiovascular manifestations of rheumatoid arthritis. Can. Med. Assoc. J., 80:86–90, 1959.
87. Hart, F.D.: Rheumatoid arthritis: extra-articular manifestations. Br. Med. J., 3:131–136, 1969.

88. Hart, F.D., and Golding, J.R.: Rheumatoid neuropathy. Br. Med. J., 1:1594–1600, 1960.
89. Haslock, D.I., Wright, V., and Harriman, D.G.F.: Neuromuscular disorders in rheumatoid arthritis; a motorpoint muscle biopsy study. Q. J. Med., 39:335–358, 1970.
90. Hauge, T., et al.: Treatment of rheumatoid pachymeningitis involving the entire thoracic region. Scand. J. Rheumatol., 7:209–211, 1978.
91. Herzog, C.A., Miller, R.R., and Hoidal, J.R.: Bronchiolitis and rheumatoid arthritis. Am. Rev. Respir. Dis., 124:636–639, 1981.
92. Hills, E.A., and Geary, M.: Membrane diffusing capacity and pulmonary capillary volume in rheumatoid disease. Thorax, 35:851–855, 1980.
93. Hollingsworth, J.W.: Local and Systemic Complications of Rheumatoid Arthritis. Philadelphia, W.B. Saunders, 1968.
94. Howe, G.B., et al.: Polymorphonuclear cell function in rheumatoid arthritis and in Felty's syndrome. Ann. Rheum. Dis., 40:370–375, 1981.
95. Hull, S., and Mathews, J.A.: Pulmonary necrobiotic nodules as a presenting feature of rheumatoid arthritis. Ann. Rheum. Dis., 41:15–20, 1982.
96. Hume, R., et al.: Anemia of Felty's syndrome. Ann. Rheum. Dis., 23:267–271, 1964.
97. Hurd, E.R., LoSpalluto, J., and Ziff, M.: The role of immune complexes in the production of the neutropenia of Felty's syndrome. J. Rheumatol., 1 (Suppl.):105, 1974.
98. Hutchinson, R.M., Davis, P., and Jayson, M.I.V.: Thrombocytosis in rheumatoid arthritis. Ann. Rheum. Dis., 35:138–142, 1976.
99. Isomaki, H., Koivisto, O., and Kiviniity, K.: Splenomegaly in rheumatoid arthritis. Acta Rheumatol. Scand., 17:23–26, 1971.
100. Iveson, J.M.I., et al.: Aortic valve incompetence and replacement in rheumatoid arthritis. Ann. Rheum. Dis., 34:312–320, 1975.
101. Jaffe, I.A., and Smith, R.W.: Rheumatoid vasculitis—report of a second case treated with penicillamine. Arthritis Rheum., 11:585–592, 1968.
102. Jansen, H.M., et al.: Progressive obliterative bronchiolitis in a patient with rheumatoid arthritis. Eur. J. Respir. Dis., 121 (Suppl.):43–52, 1982.
103. Jayson, M.I.V., and Jones, D.E.P.: Scleritis and rheumatoid arthritis. Ann. Rheum. Dis., 30:343–347, 1976.
104. John, J.T., Jr., Hough, A., and Sergent, J.S.: Pericardial disease in rheumatoid arthritis. Am. J. Med., 66:385–390, 1979.
105. Johnson, R.L., et al.: Steroid therapy and vascular lesions in rheumatoid arthritis. Arthritis Rheum., 2:224–249, 1959.
106. Johnson, T.S., et al.: Endobronchial necrobiotic nodule antedating rheumatoid arthritis. Chest, 82:199–200, 1982.
107. Joyce, R.A., et al.: Neutrophil kinetics in Felty's syndrome. Am. J. Med., 69:695–702, 1980.
108. Jurik, A.G., Davidsen, D., and Grandal, H.: Prevalence of pulmonary involvement in rheumatoid arthritis and its relationship to some characteristics of the patients. A radiological and clinical study. Scand. J. Rheumatol., 11:217–224, 1982.
109. Kaplan, H., and Brooke, M.H.: Histochemical study of muscle in rheumatic disease. Arthritis Rheum., 14:168, 1971.
110. Karten, I.: Arteritis, myocardial infarction, and rheumatoid arthritis. JAMA, 210:1717–1720, 1969.
111. Kemper, J.W., Baggenstoss, A.H., and Slocumb, C.H.: The relationship of therapy with cortisone to the incidence of vascular lesions in rheumatoid arthritis. Ann. Intern. Med., 46:831–851, 1957.
112. Kievits, J.H., et al.: Rheumatoid arthritis and the positive LE cell phenomenon. Ann. Rheum. Dis., 15:211, 1956.
113. Killian, P.J., McLain, B., and Lawless, O.J.: Brown's syndrome; an unusual manifestation of rheumatoid arthritis. Arthritis Rheum., 20:1080–1084, 1977.

114. Kim, R.C.: Rheumatoid disease with encephalopathy. Ann. Neurol., 7:86–91, 1980.

115. Kim, R.C., and Collins, G.H.: The neuropathology of rheumatoid disease. Hum. Pathol., 12:5–15, 1981.

116. Kim, R.C., Collins, G.H., and Parisi, J.E.: Rheumatoid nodule formation within the choroid plexus. Report of a second case. Arch. Pathol. Lab. Med., 106:83–84, 1982.

117. Kimball, H.R., et al.: Marrow granulocyte reserves in the rheumatic diseases. Arthritis Rheum., 16:345–352, 1973.

118. Kimura, S.J., et al.: Uveitis and joint diseases; clinical findings in 191 cases. Arch. Ophthalmol., 77:309–316, 1967.

119. Kirk, J., and Cosh, J.: Pericarditis of rheumatoid arthritis. Q. J. Med., 38:397–423, 1969.

120. Kulka, J.P.: The vascular lesions associated with rheumatoid disease. Bull. Rheum. Dis., 10:201, 1959.

121. Laine, V.A.I., and Vainio, K.J.: Ulceration of the skin in rheumatoid arthritis. Acta Rheumatol. Scand., 1:113–118, 1955.

122. Laszlo, J., et al.: Splenectomy for Felty's syndrome. Clinico-pathological study of 27 patients. Arch. Intern. Med., 138:597–602, 1978.

123. Lebowitz, W.B.: The heart in rheumatoid arthritis (rheumatoid disease). A clinical and pathological study of 62 cases. Ann. Intern. Med., 58:102–123, 1963.

124. Liew, M., et al.: Successful valve replacement for aortic incompetence in rheumatoid arthritis with vasculitis. Ann. Rheum. Dis., 38:483–484, 1979.

125. Lillington, G.A., Carr, D.T., and Mayne, J.G.: Rheumatoid pleurisy with effusion. Arch. Intern. Med., 128:764–769, 1971.

126. Linquist, P.R., and McDonnell, D.E.: Rheumatoid cyst causing extradural compression: a case report. J. Bone Joint Surg., 52A:1235–1240, 1970.

127. Liss, J.P., and Bachman, W.T.: Rheumatoid constrictive pericarditis, treated by pericardiectomy; report of a case and review of the literature. Arthritis Rheum., 13:869–874, 1970.

128. Lloyd, K., and Agarwal, A.: Tarsal-tunnel syndrome, a presenting feature of rheumatoid arthritis. Br. Med. J., 3:32, 1970.

129. Lloyd-Jones, D., and Hembry, R.M.: Destructive corneal disease in the connective tissue disorders. Comparison with experimental animal model. Trans. Ophthalmol. Soc. U.K., 98:383–389, 1978.

130. Lofgren, R.H., and Montgomery, W.W.: Incidence of laryngeal involvement in rheumatoid arthritis. N. Engl. J. Med., 267:193–195, 1962.

131. Logue, G.: Felty's syndrome: granulocyte-bound immunoglobulin G and splenectomy. Ann. Intern. Med., 85:437–442, 1976.

132. Logue, G.L., and Silberman, H.R.: Felty's syndrome without splenomegaly. Am. J. Med., 66:703–706, 1979.

133. Luthra, H.S., and Hunder, G.G.: Spontaneous remission of Felty's syndrome. Arthritis Rheum., 18:515–517, 1975.

134. Lyne, A.J.: "Contact lens" cornea in rheumatoid arthritis. Br. J. Ophthalmol., 54:410–415, 1970.

135. Lyne, A.J., and Pitkeathley, D.A.: Episcleritis and scleritis; association with connective tissue disease. Arch. Ophthalmol., 80:171–176, 1968.

136. Magora, A., Wolf, E., and Gonen, B.: Electrodiagnostic investigation of the neuromuscular lesions in rheumatoid arthritis. Acta Rheumatol. Scand., 16:280–292, 1970.

137. Marcolongo, R., Bayeli, P.F., and Montagnani, M.: Gastrointestinal involvement in rheumatoid arthritis: a biopsy study. J. Rheumatol., 6:163–173, 1979.

138. Markenson, J.A., et al.: Rheumatoid meningitis: a localized immune process. Ann. Intern. Med., 90:786–790, 1979.

139. Marks, J.S., and Sharp, J.: Rheumatoid cervical myelopathy. Q. J. Med., 50:307–319, 1981.

140. Marshall, A.J., Brownlee, W.C., and Keen, G.: Constrictive pericarditis, pyopericardium and tamponade with rheumatoid arthritis. Ann. Rheum. Dis., 38:387–389, 1979.

141. Martel, W., and Abell, M.R.: Fatal atlanto-axial sublux-

ation in rheumatoid arthritis. Arthritis Rheum., 6:224–231, 1963.

142. Masi, A.T., et al.: Hashimoto's disease. Lancet, 1:123–126, 1965.

143. Matthews, J.A.: Atlanto-axial subluxation in rheumatoid arthrits. Ann. Rheum. Dis., 28:260–266, 1969.

144. Meyer, E., et al.: Fundus lesions in rheumatoid arthritis. Ann. Ophthalmol., 10:1583–1584, 1978.

145. Meyerowitz, S., Jacox, R.F., and Hess, D.W.: Monozygotic twins discordant for rheumatoid arthrits. Arthritis Rheum., 11:1–21, 1968.

146. Miall, W.E.: Rheumatoid arthritis in males: an epidemiological study of a Welsh mining community. Ann. Rheum. Dis., 14:150–158, 1955.

147. Millender, L.H., Nalebuff, E.A., and Holdsworth, D.E.: Posterior interosseus nerve syndrome secondary to rheumatoid synovitis. J. Bone Joint Surg., 55A:753–757, 1973.

148. Mitchell, W.S., et al.: Septic arthritis in patients with rheumatoid disease: a still underdiagnosed complication. J. Rheumatol., 3:124–133, 1976.

149. Mongan, E., et al.: A study of the relation of seronegative and seropositive rheumatoid arthritis to each other and to necrotizing vasculitis. Am. J. Med., 47:23–35, 1969.

150. Moore, R.A., et al.: Felty's syndrome: long-term follow-up after splenectomy. Ann. Intern. Med., 75:381–386, 1971.

151. Motulsky, A.G., et al.: Lymph nodes in rheumatoid arthritis. Arch. Intern. Med., 90:660–676, 1952.

152. Mowat, A.G.: Hematologic abnormalities in rheumatoid arthritis. Semin. Arthritis Rheum., 1:195–216, 1972.

153. Mowat, A.G., and Hothersall, T.E.: Nature of anemia in rheumatoid arthritis. VIII. Iron content of synovial tissue in patients with rheumatoid arthritis and in normal individuals. Ann. Rheum. Dis., 27:345–351, 1968.

154. Mowat, A.G., Hothersall, T.E., and Aitchison, W.R.C.: Nature of anaemia in rheumatoid arthritis. XI. Changes in iron metabolism induced by the administration of corticotrophin. Ann. Rheum. Dis., 28:303–309, 1969.

155. Muirden, K.D.: The anaemia of rheumatoid arthritis: the significance of iron deposits in the synovial membrane. Aust. Ann. Med., 2:97–104, 1970.

156. Muirden, K.D.: Lymph node iron in rheumatoid arthritis; histology, ultrastructure and chemical concentration. Ann. Rheum. Dis., 29:81–88, 1970.

156a. Murray, T.G., et al.: Epidemiologic study of regular analgesic use and end-stage renal disease. Arch. Intern. Med., 143:1687–1693, 1983.

157. Neumark, T., Dombay, M., and G'asp'ardy, G.: Ultrastructural studies in rheumatoid polyneuropathy. Acta Morphol. Acad. Sci. Hung., 27:205–220, 1979.

158. Newman, J.H., and Cooney, L.M., Jr.: Cardiac abnormalities associated with rheumatoid arthritis: aortic insufficiency requiring valve replacement. J. Rheumatol., 7:375–378, 1980.

159. Nomeir, A-M., Turner, R., and Watts, E.: Cardiac involvement in rheumatoid arthritis. Ann. Intern. Med., 79:800–806, 1973.

160. Nosanchuk, J.S., and Schnitzer, B.: Follicular hyperplasia in lymph nodes from patients with rheumatoid arthritis; a clinicopathologic study. Cancer, 24:343–354, 1969.

161. Owen, E.T., and Lawson, A.A.H.: Nature of anaemia in rheumatoid arthritis. VI. Metabolism of endogenous iron. Ann. Rheum. Dis., 25:547–552, 1966.

162. Oxholm, P., et al.: Pulmonary function in patients with rheumatoid arthritis. Scand. J. Rheumatol., 11:109–112, 1982.

163. Page, J.W.: Spontaneous tendon rupture and cervical vertebral subluxation in patients with rheumatoid arthritis. J. Mich. State Med. Soc., 60:888–892, 1961.

164. Pallis, C.A., and Scott, J.T.: Peripheral neuropathy in rheumatoid arthritis. Br. Med. J., 1:1141–1147, 1965.

165. Panettiere, F., Chandler, B.F., and Libcke, J.H.: Pulmonary cavitation in rheumatoid disease. Review of the literature and an additional case. Am. Rev. Respir. Dis., 97:89–95, 1968.

166. Panush, R.S., Franco, A.E., and Schur, P.H.: Rheu-

matoid arthritis associated with eosinophilia. Ann. Intern. Med., *75*:199–206, 1971.

167. Pearsall, H.R., et al.: Disseminated pulmonary infiltrates associated with protein abnormalities. II. Pulmonary findings in patients with an elevated serum rheumatoid factor titer. Bull. Mason Clin., *21*:151–155, 1967.

168. Petrie, G.R., et al.: Upper lobe fibrosis and cavitation in rheumatoid disease. Br. J. Dis. Chest, *74*:263–267, 1980.

169. Plotz, P.H.: Analgesic nephropathy: for this time and for this place. Arch. Intern. Med., *143*:1676–1677, 1983.

170. Polisar, I.A., et al.: Bilateral midline fixation of cricoarytenoid joints as a serious medical emergency. JAMA, *172*:901–906, 1960.

171. Popper, M.S., Bogdonoff, M.L., and Hughes, R.L.: Interstitial rheumatoid lung disease. Chest, *62*:243–249, 1972.

172. Prakash, R., et al.: Pericardial and mitral-valve involvement in rheumatoid arthritis without cardiac symptoms. N. Engl. J. Med., *289*:597–600, 1973.

173. Ramirez, G., Lambert, R., and Bloomer, H.A.: Renal pathology in patients with rheumatoid arthritis. Nephron, *28*:124–126, 1981.

174. Rimon, R.: A psychosomatic approach to rheumatoid arthritis; a clinical study of 100 female patients. Acta Rheumatol. Scand., *13 (Suppl.)*:1–154, 1969.

175. Robertson, M.D.J., et al.: Rheumatoid lymphadenopathy. Ann. Rheum. Dis., *27*:253–260, 1968.

176. Romanoff, H., Rozin, R., and Zlotnick, A.: Cardiac tamponade in rheumatoid arthritis: a case report and review of the literature. Arthritis Rheum., *13*:426–435, 1970.

177. Rosenberg, J.N., et al.: Eosinophil-specific and other granulocyte-specific antinuclear antibodies in juvenile chronic polyarthritis and adult rheumatoid arthritis. Ann. Rheum. Dis., *34*:350–353, 1975.

178. Rosenthal, R.D., et al.: White cell antibodies and the aetiology of Felty's syndrome. Q. J. Med., *43*:187–203, 1974.

179. Rothwell, R.S., and Davis, P.: Relationship between serum ferritin, anemia, and disease activity in acute and chronic rheumatoid arthritis. Rheumatol. Int., *1*:65–67, 1981.

180. Ruderman, M., Miller, L.M., and Pinals, R.S.: Clinical and serological observations on 27 patients with Felty's syndrome. Arthritis Rheum., *11*:377–384, 1968.

181. Scaddling, J.G.: The lungs in rheumatoid arthritis. Proc. R. Soc. Med., *62*:227–238, 1969.

182. Schachenmayr, W., and Friede, R.L.: Dural involvement in rheumatoid arthritis. Acta Neuropathol., *42*:65–66, 1978.

183. Schaller, J.G., et al.: The association of anti-nuclear antibodies with the chronic iridocyclitis of juvenile rheumatoid disease (Still's disease). Arthritis Rheum., *17*:409–416, 1974.

184. Schernthaner, G., et al.: Seropositive rheumatoid arthritis associated with decreased diffusion capacity of the lung. Ann. Rheum. Dis., *35*:258–262, 1976.

185. Schmid, F.R., et al.: Arteritis in rheumatoid arthritis. Am. J. Med., *30*:56–83, 1961.

186. Scott, D.G.I., Bacon, P.A., and Tribe, C.R.: Systemic rheumatoid vasculitis: a clinical and laboratory study of 50 cases. Medicine, *60*:288–296, 1981.

187. Scott, J.T., et al.: Digital arteritis in rheumatoid disease. Ann. Rheum. Dis., *20*:224–234, 1961.

188. Scott, J.T., El Sallab, R.A., and Laws, J.W.: The digital artery design in rheumatoid arthritis—further observations. Br. J. Radiol., *40*:748–754, 1967.

189. Selroos, O.: Thrombocytosis in rheumatoid arthritis. Scand. J. Rheumatol., *1*:136–140, 1972.

190. Sevel, D.: Rheumatoid nodule of the sclera (a type of necrogranulomatous scleritis). Trans. Ophthalmol. Soc. U.K., *85*:357–367, 1965.

191. Shapiro, R.F., Resnick, D., and Castles, J.: Fistulization of rheumatoid joints. Ann. Rheum. Dis., *34*:489–498, 1975.

192. Shearn, D.L.: Aneurysm of the sinus of valsalva secondary to rheumatoid nodulosis. Arthritis Rheum., *24*:978, 1981.

193. Short, C.L., Bauer, W., and Reynolds, W.E.: Rheumatoid Arthritis. Cambridge, MA, Harvard University Press, 1957.

194. Sievers, K., et al.: Studies of rheumatoid pulmonary disease; a comparison of roentgenological findings among patients with high rheumatoid factor titers and with completely negative reactions. Acta Tuberc. Scand., *45*:21–34, 1964.

195. Sinclair, R.J.G., and Cruickshank, B.: A clinical and pathological study of sixteen cases of rheumatoid arthritis with extensive visceral involvement ("rheumatoid disease"). Q. J. Med., *25*:313–332, 1956.

196. Skowronski, T., and Gatter, R.A.: Cerebral vasculitis associated with rheumatoid disease—a case report. J. Rheumatol., *1*:473–475, 1974.

197. Skrifvars, B.: Immunofluorescence study of renal biopsies in chronic rheumatoid arthritis. Scand. J. Rheumatol., *8*:234–240, 1979.

198. Smiley, W.K.: The eye in arthritis. Ann. Phys. Med., *10*:157–162, 1969.

199. Smith, P.H., Benn, R.T., and Sharp, J.: Natural history of rheumatoid cervical luxations. Ann. Rheum. Dis., *31*:431–439, 1972.

200. Sokoloff, L.: Cardiac involvement in rheumatoid arthritis and allied disorders: current concepts. Mod. Concepts Cardiovasc. Dis., 1964.

201. Sokoloff, L., McCluskey, R.T., and Bunim, J.J.: Vascularity of the early nodule of rheumatoid arthritis. A.M.A. Arch. Pathol., *55*:475–495, 1953.

202. Sorensen, A.W.S.: The Kidney in Rheumatoid Arthritis and the Effect of Drugs on Renal Function. Copenhagen, Munksgaard, 1966.

203. Spurlock, R.G., and Richman, A.V.: Rheumatoid meningitis. A case report and review of the literature. Arch. Pathol. Lab. Med., *107*:129–131, 1983.

204. Steinberg, V.L., and Parry, C.B.: Electromyographic changes in rheumatoid arthritis. Br. Med. J., *1*:630–632, 1961.

205. Steiner, J.W., and Gelbloom, A.J.: Intracranial manifestations in two cases of systemic rheumatoid disease. Arthritis Rheum., *2*:537–545, 1959.

206. Reference deleted.

207. Strandberg, O.: Anemia in rheumatoid arthritis. Acta Med. Scand., *180 (Suppl. 454)*:1–153, 1966.

208. Strohl, K.P., Feldman, N.T., and Ingram, R.H., Jr.: Apical fibrobullous disease with rheumatoid arthritis. Chest, *75*:739–741, 1979.

209. Termini, T.E., Biundo, J.J., Jr., and Ziff, M.: The rarity of Felty's syndrome in blacks. Arthritis Rheum., *22*:999–1005, 1979.

210. Thorne, C., and Urowitz, M.B.: Long-term outcome in Felty's syndrome. Ann. Rheum. Dis., *41*:486–489, 1982.

211. Tomasi, T.B., Jr., Fudenberg, H.H., and Finby, N.: Possible relationship of rheumatoid factors and pulmonary disease. Am. J. Med., *33*:243–248, 1962.

212. Turner-Warwick, M., and Doniach, D.: Autoantibody studies in interstitial pulmonary fibrosis. Br. Med. J., *1*:886–891, 1965.

213. Van Metre, T.D., et al.: The relationship between nongranulomatous uveitis and arthritis. J. Allergy, *36*:158–174, 1965.

214. Vincent, P.C., Levi, J.A., and Macqueen, A.: The mechanism of neutropenia in Felty's syndrome. Br. J. Haematol., *27*:463–475, 1974.

215. Voyles, W.F., Searles, R.P., and Bankhurst, A.D.: Myocardial infarction caused by rheumatoid vasculitis. Arthritis Rheum., *23*:850–855, 1980.

216. Walker, W.C.: Pulmonary infections and rheumatoid arthritis. Q. J. Med., *36*:239–251, 1967.

217. Walker, W.C., and Wright, V.: Diffuse interstitial pulmonary fibrosis and rheumatoid arthritis. Ann. Rheum. Dis., *28*:252–259, 1969.

218. Walker, W.C., and Wright, V.: Pulmonary lesions and rheumatoid arthritis. Medicine, *47*:501–520, 1968.

219. Walker, W.C., and Wright, V.: Rheumatoid pleuritis. Ann. Rheum. Dis., *26*:467–474, 1967.

220. Webb, F.W.S., Hickman, J.A., and Brew, D. St. J.:

Death from vertebral artery thrombosis in rheumatoid arthritis. Br. Med. J., 2:537–538, 1968.

221. Wegelius, O., Pasternack, A., and Kuhlback, B.: Muscular involvement in rheumatoid arthritis. Acta Rheumatol. Scand., 15:257–261, 1969.

222. Weisman, M., and Zvaifler, N.J.: Cryoimmunoglobulinemia in Felty's syndrome. Arthritis Rheum., 19:103–110, 1976.

223. Weller, R., Bruckner, F., and Chamberlain, M.: Rheumatoid neuropathy: a histological and electrophysiological study. J. Neurol. Neurosurg. Psychiatry, 33:593–604, 1970.

224. Whaley, K., and Dick, W.C.: Fatal subaxial dislocation of cervical spine in rheumatoid arthritis. Br. Med. J., 2:31, 1968.

225. Wiik, A., and Munthe, E.: Complement-fixing granulocyte-specific antinuclear factors in neutropenic cases of rheumatoid arthritis. Immunology, 26:1127–1134, 1974.

226. Williams, R.C.: Rheumatoid Arthritis as a Systemic Disease. Philadelphia, W.B. Saunders, 1974.

227. Willkens, R.F., and Decker, J.L.: Rheumatoid arthritis with serological evidence of systemic lupus erythematosus. Arthritis Rheum., 6:720–735, 1963.

228. Winchester, R.J., et al.: Observations on the eosinophilia of certain patients with rheumatoid arthritis. Arthritis Rheum., 14:650–655, 1971.

229. Wisnieski, J.J., and Askari, A.D.: Rheumatoid nodulosis. A relatively benign rheumatoid variant. Arch. Intern. Med., 141:615–619, 1981.

230. Wolman, L., Darke, C.S., and Young, A.: The larynx in rheumatoid arthritis. J. Laryngol., 79:403–434, 1965.

231. Yamaguchi, D.M., Lipscomb, P.R., and Soule, E.H.: Carpal tunnel syndrome. Minn. Med., 48:22–33, 1965.

232. Ziegler, P., and Albukerk, J.: Rheumatoid granuloma of kidney. Urology, 12:84–86, 1978.

233. Zivkovic, M., and Baum, J.: Chemotaxis of polymorphonuclear leukocytes from patients with systemic lupus erythematosus and Felty's syndrome. Immunol. Commun., 1:39–49, 1972.

Chapter 40

Laboratory Findings in Rheumatoid Arthritis

John Baum and Morris Ziff

The laboratory findings in rheumatoid arthritis (RA) are those of a chronic inflammatory disease. No specific laboratory test exists for this condition, yet a constellation of laboratory findings can aid the experienced clinician in arriving at a diagnosis and in management. The knowledge that some laboratory tests can be abnormal in this disease can often save a patient more detailed study (Table 40–1). This chapter represents a detailed survey of the incidence and frequency of abnormal laboratory tests in RA.

HEMATOLOGIC STUDIES

Erythrocytes

A recalcitrant normochromic or hypochromic normocytic anemia, usually moderate in degree, is common in RA.[191] Among Danish women with active disease, 22.7% had fewer than 10 g/dl hemoglobin; among men, 11.5% had fewer than 11 g/dl. In children, anemia is usually present,[130,259] especially in the systemic or Still's form of disease. In the series of Toumbis and co-workers,[259] 64% of children with JRA had under 10 g/dl hemoglobin.

The anemia of RA is the type seen in chronic inflammation and has been intensively studied in relation to possible contributory factors. The influence of hemolysis has been examined in detail. Early studies, using the Ashby selective agglutination technique,[5,85,86,168] indicated a reduction in the survival of erythrocytes transfused from normal donors to patients with RA. More recent investigations have used chromium-51 to label the patient's own erythrocytes for similar studies. Although Ebaugh and co-workers[70] and Weinstein[276] found evidence of some degree of hemolysis, its magnitude could not account for the development of anemia in the presence of adequate bone marrow compensation. Three studies also using chromium-51 have confirmed these earlier reports and have disclosed only a mild hemolytic tendency of an extracorpuscular type, insufficient to explain the associated anemia.[149,213,215] In contrast to iron-deficiency anemia in which excretion of porphobilinogen and aminolevulinic acid is increased, porphobilinogen excretion is increased in RA.[129]

The plasma volume in patients with RA is greater than normal.[66,126,131,216] The basis for this increase is not well understood. A compensatory increase in plasma volume for a reduced corpuscular volume is probably one factor,[95,126] and another is that a larger percentage of the body weight of patients with RA is due to lean body mass than in control subjects. This phenomenon may lead to spuriously high values for the plasma volume calculated as a percentage of body weight.

Serum iron levels are sometimes decreased.[38,70,85,125,187,215] Results using intravenously injected tracer doses of iron for hemoglobin synthesis have been normal.[85] Although the total iron binding capacity is usually higher than normal in simple iron-deficiency anemia, it is much lower in RA.[129] Although Roberts and co-workers noted a reduced capacity to absorb iron in patients with active RA and mild anemia,[215] other studies found this function to be normal in most patients.[276]

Bone marrow iron stores are absent or decreased in at least one-third of patients,[167,214] but no correlation has been demonstrated between the amount of iron in the bone marrow and the hemoglobin level or erythrocyte count. The refractoriness of the anemia in most patients to oral iron therapy is in accord with this observation because absorption of iron is usually normal.

To explain the low plasma iron level, the most constant characteristic of the anemia of inflammation, an impairment of release of iron from the reticuloendothelial tissues has been proposed.[85] In the presence of normal use of transferrin-bound iron, such impairment would account for the low iron concentration in the plasma. This suggestion is based on the observations that: (1) amounts of iron that exceed the plasma-binding capacity are deposited in the tissues and are, therefore, poorly used in patients with inflammation;[80] (2) iron injected intravenously into animals with an inflammatory reaction is diverted from normal hemoglobin formation and is deposited in storage sites;[47] and (3) the reuse of iron from senescent cells is reduced in animals with an inflammatory reaction. Insufficient release from the reticuloendothelial

Table 40–1.   Laboratory Findings in Rheumatoid Arthritis

Test	Characteristic Results
Blood Elements	
Erythrocytes	Moderate normochromic or hypochromic, normocytic anemia; low plasma iron; moderately decreased bone marrow iron stores; normal use of plasma iron; slightly decreased survival time; inadequate release of iron from tissue stores; normal transferrin levels; decreased total iron binding capacity; increased plasma volume
Leukocytes	Normal or slightly elevated polymorphonuclear leukocytes; leukocytosis possible in severe disease; leukopenia rare (Felty's syndrome); eosinophilia with severe disease and systemic complications; thrombocytosis during active disease; normal nitroblue tetrazolium test results; reduced chemotaxis; lymphocytes—normal B, T, and null cell distribution; decreased blastogenic transformation
Acute-Phase Reactants and Immuno-globulins	
Erythrocyte Sedimentation Rate (ESR)	Increased
C-Reactive Protein (CRP)	Usually positive
Serum Amyloid Protein (SAP)	Slightly elevated
Serum Proteins	Alpha-2, fibrinogen, and gamma globulins increased; albumin decreased
Immunoglobulins	IgG increased (seropositive patients mostly); IgA and IgM increased; IgD normal or low
Cryoglobulins	Rare
Urinary Gamma Globulin	Increased IgG, IgA, and free light chains
Ceruloplasmin	Elevated
Fibronectin	Normal serum levels
Immune Factors	
LE Factor	Present in 10% of patients
Antinuclear Antibody	Present in 15%; associated with more severe disease and rheumatoid-factor positivity
Rheumatoid Factor	Usually present in adults
Biologic False-Positive Serologic Test for Syphilis	Present in 5 to 10% of patients
Complement	Normal or slightly elevated levels; hypocomplementemia rare and associated with vasculitis and severe disease.

system would result in the low plasma iron concentration presumably responsible for the impaired capacity of the bone marrow to produce erythrocytes. This subject has been reviewed.[46] Intra-articular hemorrhage increases the iron content of synovial tissue in patients with RA,[29,182,184] and the retained iron could contribute to the low serum iron level and to the anemia of active RA. Another site of increased iron deposition in RA is striated muscle, in which mean iron levels twice those of normal muscles have been found.[102]

Although single measurements of serum ferritin levels have often failed to correlate with a number of clinical and laboratory parameters of joint activity, a longitudinal study found that serum ferritin levels rose during active synovitis and fell during remission. The highest levels were found in patients with systemic complications.[32] Thus, the clear correlation between serum ferritin and iron stores found in normal persons does not exist in patients with chronic inflammatory conditions such as RA.

Most patients with RA receive salicylate therapy. Occult blood in the feces has been observed in many who receive this drug.[67,197] This blood loss, although probably of minor importance, may contribute to iron deficiency, and the anemia in such patients may partially respond to iron therapy. Another factor in the anemia may be erythropoietin deficiency because serum levels in RA patients are lower than in patients with comparable degrees of iron-deficiency anemia.[272]

Leukocytes

Although white blood cell counts are usually in the normal range or are only slightly elevated, Short, Bauer, and Reynolds observed that about 25% of their patients had counts above 10,000/mm³.[234] Leukocytosis was noted in patients who had an acute and severe disease onset and acute exacerbations. In another study,[138] the white blood cell count was much higher in patients with severe RA. Although counts in the 12,000-to-20,000 range are sometimes observed without other cause,[59] this finding suggests the presence of factors other than RA. Prednisone increases the absolute number of mature granulocytes in the circulation because of an increased inflow of cells from the bone marrow, decreased margination in the capillary blood, and a decreased emigration from the circulation.[31] Leukocytosis is common in juvenile RA.[130,152,227,259]

Leukopenia is rare in RA.[234] When present, it is more likely to be observed in the chronic state of the disease. The leukopenia and splenomegaly of Felty's syndrome[79] may reflect the uptake of immune complexes by circulating polymorphonuclear cells and the subsequent removal of these cells by the spleen.[122] Neutropenia in RA has been divided into two types, one associated with splenomegaly (Felty's syndrome) and another without splenomegaly but with an increased frequency of circulating immune complexes (68 versus 31%).[41] Another possible cause of the leukopenia is the uptake and destruction of polymorphonuclear leukocytes with attached complement-fixing antineutrophil antibodies.[284]

The differential white blood cell count is usually within normal limits, but polymorphonuclear leukocytes may be increased in more acute cases.[59] Eosinophilia is not uncommon in RA. When patients in a study were selected for severity of disease or elevated rheumatoid factor titers, eosinophilia of more than 5% was found in 40% of these patients. A correlation also appeared to exist with the presence of vasculitis, pleuropericarditis, pulmonary fibrosis, and subcutaneous nodules.[254,287] Exudative fluids in pleura or pericardium often contain eosinophils.

Correlations among thrombocytosis and disease activity, anemia, sideropenia, leukocytosis, and rheumatoid factor titer have been noted.[233] Platelets from patients with RA show lower-than-normal levels of connective-tissue-activating factor.[239]

The chromosomal complement of the leukocytes of the blood in RA is normal.[25] The nitroblue tetrazolium (NBT) dye reduction test in peripheral blood leukocytes is also normal.[279] Chemotaxis of the polymorphonuclear leukocytes is diminished, possibly because of prior immune complex ingestion.[180]

Lymphocytes

In recent years, many have been interested in the function of the subpopulations of lymphocytes in various diseases. For the most part, the percentages of B, T, and null cells in the blood in RA have been in the normal range.[185,220,255,263] One group found no significant difference between the percentage and the absolute number of peripheral

blood T suppressor cells in RA and in control subjects.[163] In some patients, the number of OKT8+ (suppressor) cells/mm³ was decreased in relation to OKT4+ (helper) cells, whereas in other patients, an elevated ratio of OKT4+ to OKT8+ cells was due to a higher percentage of OKT4+ cells and a lower percentage of OKT8+ cells.[269] In another study of T-lymphocyte subpopulations in active RA, decreased Tμ (helper) cells, greatly increased T null cells, and slightly increased Fc receptor-bearing lymphocytes were found.[174]

The function of the circulating lymphocytes has also been studied. Spontaneous lymphocyte transformation was normal in patients with RA,[194] but a decreased response to concanavalin A was observed.[144,154,208,236] In early RA of under 3 months' duration, the defect was due to a decreased generation of suppressor T cells accompanied by a decrease in the B-cell response. In a study of patients with disease activity of more than 12 months' duration, the T-cell response was normal, but the B-cell response continued to be deficient.[221] The response to phytohemagglutinin (PHA) was also depressed,[144,154,236,237,239] although in several reports the decrease was not significant.[208,219] Responsiveness of peripheral blood mononuclear cells to purified streptokinase-streptodornase (SK-SD) was not much depressed, nor did hyporesponsiveness predict disease activity or prognosis.[219]

Depression of the PHA response was associated with the presence of antinuclear antibodies in 16 patients, whereas 14 patients who did not have antinuclear antibodies had normal responses.[175] A decreased response to pokeweed mitogen has also been reported,[154] but two other groups did not find the decrease to be statistically significant.[144,236] Suppressor-T-cell hypofunction was found in early active RA of under 3 months' duration, but not in late RA of more than 6 months' duration or in inactive RA.[2] Overall, mitogenic transformation of RA lymphocytes appears to be decreased.

One study of antibody-mediated lymphocyte toxicity found these antibodies to be present fivefold as frequently in RA as in normal controls,[247] but another study found no such difference.[64] Impaired monocyte "natural" killer activity has been reported in patients with active RA, and the impairment correlated with disease activity.[22]

ACUTE-PHASE REACTANTS

These substances found in blood reflect the presence and degree of inflammation. Although nonspecifically induced, they may aid in the diagnosis of RA in patients with vague symptoms. Because their serum concentration reflects the activity of the disease, they are useful in therapeutic management. A discrepancy often exists, however, between the clinical disease severity and the magnitude of the acute-phase response. For this reason, a change in the level of an acute-phase reactant is often of greater significance in guiding therapy than the actual level itself.

Erythrocyte Sedimentation Rate

The erythrocyte sedimentation rate (ESR) is the single most important laboratory test of inflammatory activity. Although the increased rate of settling of erythrocytes in the blood of patients with inflammatory diseases was known for many years, it was first measured by Fahraeus in 1918. In seeking an early test for pregnancy, Fahraeus noted that the speed of sedimentation was increased not only in pregnancy, but also in many other conditions.[74,75] Measurement of the ESR was first applied to the study of acute and chronic rheumatism by Hermann in 1924.[118]

Nature of the Sedimentation Phenomenon

ESR is related to red cell rouleaux formation and increases in proportion to the size of the erythrocyte aggregates.[120] The size of the aggregates, in turn, depends on the properties of the blood plasma rather than of the cells themselves. Cellular rouleaux formation is enhanced by adsorbed, large, asymmetric molecules. The plasma components that influence the ESR most are fibrinogen and alpha and gamma globulin.

Plasma fibrinogen increases as a result of increased synthesis by the liver in the presence of inflammation elsewhere in the body. The elevation is rapid, usually detectable 48 hours after the onset of inflammation. It usually subsides within 10 days of cessation of the inflammatory process.[99]

Early observation that the plasma fibrinogen was increased when the ESR was high led to the assumption that the two were related.[96] Moreover, a linear correlation exists between the ESR and the fibrinogen level when patients with serum globulin levels over 2.5 g/dl are excluded, the coefficient of correlation being 0.90.[81] In patients in whom the serum globulin is over 2.5 g/dl, however, the correlation is only 0.60. Under circumstances in which plasma fibrinogen is low, as in liver disease, close correlation between plasma globulin concentration and the ESR has been observed.

The addition of serum fractions to defibrinated blood has confirmed that the ESR almost entirely depends on the concentration of asymmetric molecules such as fibrinogen and alpha-2 and gamma globulins.[116] The relative effect on the ESR of these proteins, when added in equal concentration, is in the ratio 10:5:2. Detailed studies show that the closest correlation with the ESR is found when the

serum concentrations of fibrinogen, alpha-2 macroglobulin, and IgM are summed.[226]

Another factor influencing the ESR is the sialic acid residue on the erythrocyte membrane. The sialic-acid-bearing glycoproteins contribute to the forces repelling and aggregating the red blood cells. Both red cell membrane and serum sialic acid levels are higher when the ESR is elevated, although the correlation is not quantitative.[148]

A new method, called the zeta sedimentation ratio (ZSR),[178,206] requires a special centrifuge and routine control measurements. It correlates well with the Westergren method for ESR and shows less variance. It requires less blood and is faster. A microsedimentation rate using capillary tubes has been proposed for use in newborn infants.[73]

Westergren Method

The Westergren method is the most dependable of those currently used.[280] International standards have recently been developed.[124] The Westergren ESR should be performed by the classic dilution technique with citrate, or by the newer, modified technique, using ethylenediaminotetra-acetate (EDTA) and saline diluent. Use of undiluted whole blood has less reproducibility.[28] The upper limit of normal rises with age. A study of many normal individuals has shown the following normal limits, in millimeters/hour:[34] below age 50, 15 for men and 25 for women; above age 50, 20 for men and 30 for women. The reason for this increase with age has not been determined.[84] Higher normal levels are found in some populations.[83]

Wintrobe Method

The method of Wintrobe uses less than 1 ml blood for the measurement.[289] Correction for anemia is no longer recommended.[288] An advantage is that the hematocrit is measured on the same blood sample. Normal values range from 0 to 6.5 mm/hr in healthy young males and from 0 to 16 mm/hr in healthy young females. The Wintrobe method may fail to reflect the presence of active disease under circumstances in which the Westergren ESR is elevated.[91,100] Parallel determinations with the Westergren method frequently produce widely divergent results. In such a case, the ESR is usually elevated by the Westergren method and in the normal range by the Wintrobe method. When a high Westergren and a low Wintrobe ESR occur together, the clinical evidence suggests that the Wintrobe ESR is in error.

Disease Correlation

Rheumatoid Arthritis. The ESR usually is elevated and parallels the activity of the disease.[138,235] Increased values have been found in 85% of patients with RA of mild severity, and in 95% of those with moderate to severe involvement.[234] Exacerbations are usually accompanied by an increase and remissions by a decrease in the ESR. In complete remission, the values usually become normal. Nevertheless, the continuously elevated values observable in some patients with decreased joint inflammation presumably reflect the continued elevation of the serum acute phase proteins. In such circumstances, frequently repeated measurement of the ESR is unrewarding. Conversely, patients with clinically active RA may have normal sedimentation rates. This phenomenon occurred in 7.3% in one series[59] and in 5% in another.[211] In still another study, a significant correlation existed between the ESR and the plasma protein concentration and serum viscosity.[56] When a number of acute phase reactants were measured serially, the C-reactive protein and haptoglobin were more accurate than the ESR in measuring the activity of RA.[166]

Other Diseases. The ESR in primary osteoarthritis is usually normal. Nevertheless, values above 30 mm/hr were noted in 9.6% of patients by Dawson and co-workers.[59] Mild elevation of the Westergren ESR in middle-aged women with osteoarthritis is not uncommon. Thus, if the clinical findings are consistent, the diagnosis of osteoarthritis should not be excluded on the basis of a slight elevation of the ESR.

Polymyalgia rheumatica, a syndrome of pain and stiffness of the muscles of the shoulders and hip girdle appearing in the middle-aged and elderly, may be confused with RA. This disorder is characterized by high levels of the ESR. Because the symptoms usually improve before the ESR drops, sedimentation values cannot be used as a guide to management. A rapid fall in ESR with low-dose (~10 mg daily) corticosteroid treatment is diagnostically helpful, however.

Measurement of the ESR is useful in distinguishing fibrositis from RA because sedimentation values are normal in fibrositis.[60]

Congestive Heart Failure. Congestive heart failure is believed to lower the ESR, especially in young individuals with rheumatic carditis,[193,228,291] as a result of a decrease in the synthesis of fibrinogen in the passively congested liver. This widely accepted tenet has been denied on the basis of an extensive analysis of the ESR in patients with rheumatic heart disease and congestive failure.[245] Numerous exceptions are also found in the data of Saghvi,[223] who noted elevation rather than depression of the ESR in patients with heart failure as a result of rheumatic activity, respiratory infection, or myocardial damage usually associated with heart failure. Nevertheless, the available evidence suggests that the effect of hepatic congestion in congestive heart failure is to retard the ESR,[193,228,291] although the net effect of all factors may lead to elevated values.

Unexplained Elevations. In some individuals, the ESR may be persistently elevated without obvious cause. In a group of 35 patients, 14 were eventually demonstrated to have one of the following: asymptomatic pulmonary tuberculosis, macroglobulinemia of Waldenström, hepatic cirrhosis, multiple myeloma, and systemic lupus erythematosus (SLE).[151,190] The remaining 21 patients, however, continued to have persistently elevated ESR for 3 to 20 years with an otherwise benign course. Nine of these patients also had an increased gamma globulin level. The rest had unexplained elevations of either the beta lipoprotein of fibrinogen, or had paraproteins of the myeloma type on serum protein electrophoresis.

Serious illness was found on follow-up in 20 of 31 patients with unexplained elevation of the ESR.[16] Thus, an elevated ESR as an isolated abnormality should lead to careful investigation of the patient, although it may not necessarily be associated with active disease. The ESR is elevated in the majority of patients with malignant disease.[172] In 30 of 51 elderly patients who were thought to have a known cause for a high ESR, a further possible cause was found at autopsy. Cancer was found most often,[94] and extreme ESR elevation in patients with malignant disease has been associated with skeletal metastases.[196] An elevated ESR in RA of 100 mm/hr or more, however, was associated most frequently with infection (35%), and malignant disease was found in only 15%.[293] Marked elevation of the ESR occurs in multiple myeloma because of the high concentration of paraprotein in the blood.[69]

Unexplained elevated levels have also been found in a hospitalized elderly population.[35] The ESR in the aged and elderly should be viewed with special precaution. In a study of almost 500 people over age 62, the ESR was found to be greater than 20 mm/hr in 20% of men and 24% of women, without apparent cause.[176] The ESR may be elevated in women taking oral contraceptives.[43]

C-Reactive Protein and Other Tests

In RA, C-reactive protein (CRP) is present in practically all patients with clinical evidence of disease[170] and usually parallels the ESR closely. Treatment of RA with nonsteroidal anti-inflammatory drugs produced no significant change in the ESR or the CRP after 12 weeks of therapy.[11]

Unlike in rheumatic fever, salicylate and corticosteroids do not readily depress the CRP or the ESR in patients with RA. Comparison of the ESR and the CRP in 241 patients with RA showed a positive linear correlation between the measurements with a high degree of variability. The CRP was found to be a more sensitive test because gold, penicillamine, and prednisone had a greater effect on the CRP than on the ESR.[271] Corticosteroids, even in small doses, suppress the CRP. Nusinow and Arnold reported that the CRP, measured nephelometrically, correlated with erosive disease in 37 patients with RA who never received corticosteroids, not even as joint injections. These researchers believe that CRP levels above 5 mg/dl (normal <0.6 mg/dl) predict erosions, and they regard the test as an indication to begin remittive therapy early in the course of the disease.[189a]

Urinary excretion of sialylated low-molecular-weight saccharides increases in inflammatory disease and correlates closely with serum amyloid A protein and CRP levels in RA.[164] The serum amyloid P-component is slightly elevated in seropositive RA. In this case, this component appears to act as an acute-phase reactant.[249]

Plasma viscosity (PV) as an index of disease activity in RA is as reliable as the ESR or the CRP.[198] The normal range for PV is independent of age and sex, and the technique is rapid and simple, with a low incidence of false-positive and false-negative results.[198] A new acute-phase protein, vho, has been reported in high titer in RA. Titers are higher in active and seropositive patients. Serial studies, however, did not correlate titers with disease activity.[231]

Serum Proteins

Electrophoretic Studies

Increases in alpha-2 globulin and fibrinogen occur nonspecifically in the presence of inflammation. A rise in the gamma globulin level in inflammatory disease is presumptive evidence of a response to antigenic stimulation, even though the identity of the antigen is often unknown. The electrophoretic pattern changes in RA are not specific and are often within normal limits. The albumin peak is frequently low. Serum beta-2 glycoprotein 1, a protein isolated from the beta globulin fraction of serum, was reduced in RA.[140] The electrophoretic pattern in SLE resembles that seen in RA, although the gamma globulin elevation is usually more pronounced. Changes seen in the other connective tissue diseases are similar, but usually less marked.

The mechanism of the hypoalbuminemia in RA was studied,[128] using [129]I-labeled albumin for determination of pool sizes and breakdown rates in seven patients.[286] Increased albumin breakdown, a part of a general hypermetabolic state, was pro-portional to the activity of the RA. Other studies of albumin metabolism in RA showed that intravascular, extravascular, and total body albumin levels were lower in patients than in healthy control subjects.[20]

When a correction was made for hypoalbuminemia, 46% of studied patients with definite or classic RA had hypercalcemia.[137] One study found that total body calcium levels were reduced in 5.3% of men and in 6.8% of women with RA; it was further reduced in patients taking low doses of corticosteroids.[209] A study of serum carrier proteins and acute-phase proteins showed an 8 to 12% decrease in transferrin, an 18 to 28% increase in ceruloplasmin, a 70 to 80% increase in alpha-1 acid glycoprotein, and a 29% increase in alpha-1-antitrypsin.[62] Anti-chymotrypsin was elevated.[37,141,253]

Immunoglobulin levels determined by the radial diffusion technique in RA vary. Several studies have shown increased levels of IgM and IgA.[23,210] Little apparent correlation exists between the elevation of immunoglobulin levels and the duration of disease activity or rheumatoid factor titers. Seropositive patients have also shown increased levels of IgG.[268] In another study, IgA levels were also more likely to be increased in patients with seropositive RA.[256] In a detailed study of many patients, a significant increase in IgG was observed in 15% and an increase in IgA was noted in 20%. IgM was rarely increased; IgD levels were normal or low; and IgA was also decreased in 19%.[205]

Although serum levels of free light chains of immunoglobulin in RA were not much different from normal, higher levels, found in some seropositive patients, were related to a number of factors reflecting disease activity.[241]

Serum Cryoglobulins and Immune Complexes

In cryoglobulinemia, environmental cooling of blood before measuring the ESR may cause erroneous values because of the formation of microaggregates of cryoglobulin and fibrinogen.[112] A few patients with RA have significant amounts of mixed cryoglobulins.[158] The types found are IgM (K)/IgG, IgA (K)/IgG, and IgG/IgG. These cryoglobulins show rheumatoid factor activity. Cold insoluble globulin, a normal glycoprotein of human plasma, although found in increased amounts in SLE and secondary amyloidosis, is present in normal amounts in RA.[90]

A correlation of the concentration of immune complexes in serum with the presence of extra-articular manifestations of RA was shown in a study using C1q binding.[297] Researchers found circulating immune complexes determined by the C1q binding assay in 81% of RA patients with IgM rheumatoid factor.[204] Measurement of circulating immune complexes in RA by 5 different assays has shown that sensitivity, specificity, and predictive value are not sufficient to warrant their use in the management of the disease.[169]

Urinary Gamma Globulin

The quantity of urinary gamma globulins excreted was higher in RA than in control subjects.[103] These substances were composed of L chains, 7S gamma globulin, and traces of gamma A globulin. In RA the urinary excretion of IgG, IgA, and free light chains was more than three times control levels in one study.[153] The mechanism for this increased excretion is unknown.

Serologic Reactions and Complement Studies

Nonspecific Serologic Reactions

Biologic false-positive Wassermann reactions have been reported in 6.3 to 11.6% of patients with RA.[136,270] Properdin assays by the zymosan technique in 24 patients with RA gave low values in 8 and showed prozone phenomena in 5.[145] Plasma fibronectin was within the normal range in RA patients (335 μg/ml).[264]

LE Cells and Antinuclear Factors

LE cells have been found in 8 to 27% of patients with RA.[87,101,136] Gamma globulins reacting with nuclear constituents (antinuclear factors) are usually demonstrated by the fluorescent antibody technique, although other methods have been used.[260] Antinuclear antibodies occur most commonly in patients with SLE, but they may be seen with varying frequency in the other connective tissue diseases, including RA. In 710 RA patients collected from the literature by Pollak,[201] 24% had positive antinuclear antibody tests. In another series, only 3% had positive LE tests, but antinuclear antibodies were found in 14%.[277] Antinuclear factors were present mainly as macroglobulin (IgM) in rheumatoid sera, but mainly as a 7S (IgG) immunoglobulin in SLE sera.[27] Antinuclear antibodies were increased in 60% of patients with RA, but in only 13% of control subjects.[4] These antinuclear antibodies were classified as follows: IgM, 41%; IgG, 40%; and IgA, 33%. Reaction with a histone nuclear antigen was found in 24%.[4] Antiperinuclear factor, an antibody reacting with cytoplasmic granules in human cheek epithelial cells, was found in 79% of patients with RA, but only in 4% of normal subjects.[238]

Studies on the significance of positive antinuclear antibody tests in patients with RA were carried out by two groups.[52,199] Both groups concluded that these patients had more severe disease. Although one study showed a higher frequency of vasculitis associated with the antinuclear antibodies,[199] this finding was not confirmed.[52] Antinuclear antibodies were more frequent in patients who were rheumatoid-factor positive. Patients with Sjögren's syndrome had a higher prevalence of antinuclear antibodies than patients with RA alone. This finding reflects a general increase of autoantibodies in Sjögren's syndrome.[274] Half of the RA patients with granulocyte-specific antinuclear factors had protein in their urine (>150 mg/24 hours).[283] Anti-Sm and anti-RNP antibodies, characteristic markers for SLE and mixed connective tissue disease, respectively, were not found in patients with RA.[114]

Antinuclear antibodies of the IgE class in patients with RA showed a frequency of 60% with neutropenia, but only 16% without neutropenia.[195] In another series, neutropenic patients with RA were characterized by a higher frequency of IgD granulocyte-specific antinuclear antibodies, compared to RA patients without neutropenia (67 vs. 18%).[285] Antiribosomal antibodies were found in 36% of RA patients, but only in 2% of control subjects.[104] Antibody against double-stranded RNA was elevated in 33% of RA patients and was below the normal range in 11%. The lower levels were attributed to an enzyme that degraded double-stranded RNA.[133]

The occurrence in rheumatoid serum of the abnormal factors previously discussed is presumably secondary to a more fundamental process responsible for the initiation of the disease. Rheumatoid factors, antinuclear factors, and biologic false-Wassermann antibody have all been found in other conditions associated with chronic inflammation. Experimentally, prolonged hyperimmunization of rabbits with killed bacteria has resulted in the development of "rheumatoid-like" factors,[3] and even anti-DNA factors;[50] these findings suggest the relation of these antibodies to prolonged antigenic stimulation (see also Chap. 41).

Blood Groups and Histocompatibility Antigens

Low isohemagglutinins have been found in RA.[139,207] No correlation was found with the antigens of the ABO, C, or E blood groups,[51,290] nor has a significant association of HLA-A or HLA-B antigens been found in RA.[36,150,232] The presence of HLA-B27 in RA was not associated with any specific clinical or radiographic observations.[76] Stastny, however, has found a significant increase of the HLA-DRW4 antigen in patients with RA.[246] The level of HLA-DRW4 is elevated in 55% of patients with classic or definite disease, as opposed to 23% of control subjects[225] (see Chap. 25).

Other Antibodies

Antibody titers to various autoantigens and to viruses have been examined in RA. Antibody to an RA-associated nuclear antigen (RANA) was found in 90% of patients with seropositive RA.[7] Researchers also noted an increased frequency and increased levels of other antibodies to Epstein-Barr virus.[7] In another study, however, Epstein-Barr virus and cytomegalovirus antibodies were not more frequent in patients with RA than in controls.[197] Rubella antibody titers were found in 100% of 80 patients with RA and in 86.5% of matched control subjects.[61] Sera from patients with seropositive RA showed positive precipitin reactions to streptococcal mucopeptide in 73% versus 22% in normal control sera. These reactions were due, at least in part, to precipitation enhancement by rheumatoid factor. Increases in levels of antibodies to other antigens in seropositive RA patients should be suspect unless this factor has been excluded.[203] Cathepsin D agglutinators, natural antibodies to proteolytically released IgG determinants, are normally found in low titers. Levels of these substances are elevated in seropositive RA as compared to normal controls and patients with seronegative RA.[17] Anti-beta-2 microglobulin antibody was found more frequently in RA and in higher titer than in normal control subjects. The high titers were more commonly associated with pleuropulmonary lesions and nodules.[77] Factor VIII antibody, as noted clinically by reduced or absent coagulant activity, has been reported occasionally in RA.[107] Smooth muscle antibodies were found more frequently in RA than in control subjects (15.3 vs. 7.6%).[12]

Antibodies to native and denatured collagen have been found in high frequency and titer in patients with RA.[15,261] Antibodies to type I were present in 13.6%, whereas antibodies to type II were found in 14.6%.[173] Antikeratin antibodies were found in 58% of patients with classic or definite RA, but not in sera from healthy people. Thus, the finding of this antibody was specific.[295] Moreover, antibody titers to the carcinoembryonic antigen (CEA) were higher in patients with seropositive RA than in a control group.[262] Negative results were found when hepatitis-associated antigen (HAA) and anti-HAA antibodies were sought.[161] A polyclonal B-cell activator has been described in rheumatoid patients, as well as in patients with other connective tissue diseases.[71a]

Delayed hypersensitivity has also been investigated. One group using 5 antigens found decreased skin reactivity in RA patients.[197] In another investigation, 20% of patients with RA were found to be anergic. The magnitude of skin reactions and the incidence of positive reactions to multiple antigens decreased. The depression was related to age, but not to sex, duration of disease, or disease activity.[14]

Serum Complement

Serum complement levels in RA are usually either normal or elevated.[72,265] In contrast, the level of complement is reduced in most patients with active SLE.[72] Hypocomplementemia does occur in RA, and was observed in 11 of 250 patients studied.[84] This finding is associated with severe RA and a high frequency of bacterial infection.[121] Other researchers found that serum complement activity was reduced in patients with vasculitis, and the complement levels of seropositive patients were lower than those of seronegative patients.[177] Complement is found in the dermal vessels of 60% of RA patients.[230]

An inherited deficiency of complement components is associated with connective tissue disease. When the inherited deficiency of the second component of complement (C2) was investigated, 1.4% of 134 patients who were homozygous or heterozygous for the deficiency state were found to have RA.[97] The frequency of C3 deficiency is higher in patients with RA, and especially in seropositive patients, than in the general population.[40]

Elevated levels of C3b inactivator were found in patients with seropositive RA, when compared to controls.[281] Levels of immunoconglutinin, believed to be an autoantibody to complement, are also increased in RA,[48,53] but this finding is not specific because immunoconglutinin levels are also elevated in other rheumatic diseases.

LIVER AND GASTROINTESTINAL STUDIES

Mild-to-moderate abnormalities of liver function have been reported in RA, but these have been confined mainly to tests of liver function that reflect serum protein synthesis.[57,146] Histologic changes, found in up to 25% of biopsies, have been minimal.[146,179] These changes consist of slight-to-moderate fatty infiltration, slight evidence of fibrosis, and rarely, infiltration of portal areas with a few mononuclear cells. When liver biopsies were performed in 26 consecutive patients with RA, 1 showed cirrhosis, 1 fatty change, 1 hemosiderosis, 5 passive congestion, and 2 nonspecific changes. No correlation was found with any facet of the disease or activity, and the majority of the changes were nonspecific.[65] Alteration in liver size has been investigated by scintigraphy. In 7 of 32 patients with RA, a correlation was found between liver enlargement and the presence of rheumatoid factor, although results of the liver function tests in these patients were normal.[257] Clinical or biochemical evidence of liver disease was found only in 0.7% of 997 patients with RA.[281]

Serum alkaline phosphatase, serum glutamic-oxalacetic transaminase (SGOT),[24] and serum glutamic-pyruvic transaminase (SGPT)[160] levels were normal, although 15% of patients showed an elevation of serum ornithine-carbamoyl transferase.[160] Gamma glutamyl transpeptidase (GGTP) levels, considered a sensitive indicator of liver damage, were higher in RA than in degenerative joint disease (77 versus 33%) and correlated with an improvement in disease activity after penicillamine therapy.[157] Measurements of serum bilirubin and urine urobilinogen levels were within normal limits, but urine coproporphyrin excretion was elevated.[57] Measurement of the genetic types of alpha-1 antitrypsin (Pi types) showed significant increases of Pi types MZ and SZ in patients with RA,[55] although another study found no significant increase in non-MM phenotypes.[134] A significant increase, 9.2% in patients, as opposed to 3.5% in control subjects, in heterozygosity for the deficiency Z allele (Pi types MZ and SZ) was found in patients with severe, destructive RA.[54] Decreased bromsulphalein excretion was found in from 23%[57] to more than 90% of patients.[49] Serum phosphatase elevation, abnormal bromsulfalein excretion, hepatomegaly, splenomegaly, and smooth muscle antibody were observed more frequently in patients with RA than in a control group with osteoarthritis,[274] but SGPT and bilirubin levels were not different from the controls, nor was the frequency of mitochondral antibody any greater.

RA patients have a decreased amplitude of peristaltic contraction in the lower two-thirds of the esophagus.[252] The lower esophageal intrasphincteric pressure is also decreased. These findings do not seem to relate to the duration or stage of the disease. Basal and maximum acid output is subnormal in RA patients.[63] Hypergastrinemia is also a feature of RA. In one study, normal mean fasting gastrin in patients with RA was three times higher than in control subjects.[217] Examination of the intestinal mucosa of patients with RA showed that histidine-methyl-esterase activity in the intestinal mucosa biopsies was increased. Other intestinal enzymes studied did not show any significant difference from normal values.[30]

Urinary excretion of glycosaminoglycans (GAG) and of hydroxyproline was higher in patients with RA than in control subjects. Patients with active disease had the highest levels.[165] Patients with RA had higher-than-normal urinary excretion levels of hydroxyproline and zinc.[9] Free GAG levels in plasma were elevated in active RA, although total GAG levels were similar to those of controls.[88] The serum levels of an intracellular enzyme of collagen biosynthesis, prolyl hydroxylase, were elevated in RA. That raised values correlated with the level of the ESR indicates that the concentration of the enzyme reflected the degree of inflammatory activity.[142] The autoantibodies to cartilage found in a few cases of RA (1.5%) were apparently related to severe erosive disease.[71]

STUDIES OF RENAL FUNCTION AND ELECTROLYTES

Urinary abnormalities are uncommon in RA. More than a faint trace of albumin was found in the urine of only 7.2% of patients in one series.[235] Urinary tract infections were not more common in RA patients than in general,[181] although patients treated with corticosteroids had an increased incidence of bacteriuria.[42] Persistent proteinuria occurred in 24 of 183 of patients in another series.[78] When 20 patients were examined further, the proteinuria was explainable on the basis of unrelated renal disease in 12; in the remaining 8 patients, evidence of amyloidosis was present. Renal biopsy in 13 RA patients with persistent proteinuria disclosed normal kidneys in 3, arteriosclerosis or nephrosclerosis in 4, lupus nephritis in 2, and amyloidosis in 4.[202]

Scandinavian studies have reported a small-to-moderate decrease in the creatinine clearance in rheumatoid patients.[6,242–244] The average reduction was 36%.[242] Serum creatinine concentration in RA, whether measured in patients with normal or impaired renal function, was lower than in matched controls, probably because of the smaller muscle mass of RA patients.[188] Impairment of glomerular filtration was related to the stage and duration of the disease and to the presence of rheumatoid factor, but was unrelated to past history of drug intake, including phenacetin. Renal biopsies in 18 patients with classic RA but with minimal or moderate urine abnormalities showed only minimal mesangial changes in 7. Immunofluorescence studies were negative in all cases.[222] Thus, although the occurrence of occasional proteinuria and the reduction of the creatinine clearance in some patients may suggest renal abnormality in RA, histologic studies, except for those in older reports,[18] have not disclosed evidence of a specific renal abnormality other than the uncommon complication of amyloidosis.

Ammonium chloride loading experiments show normal urinary acidification in RA patients.[192] The sweat ratio of sodium to potassium increased in about half the patients in one series,[108] although information about corticosteroid therapy was not given. Increased serum copper levels have been reported,[127] but increased copper levels, associated with elevated alpha-2 globulin (ceruloplasmin) levels, are a nonspecific feature of inflammatory diseases. The increased levels were correlated with the ESR and with disease activity,[297] but not with the presence of rheumatoid factor or with the stage of disease.[159] The possible role of estrogen therapy has been discussed.[19] The urinary excretion of copper is higher in RA than in healthy subjects.[1] Although zinc levels in several studies were normal,[1,200] mean plasma zinc levels of 11.74 mol/L, versus 15.1 mol/L in controls, were decreased in the most recent study, particularly if the patients were treated only with nonsteroidal anti-inflammatory drugs.[21] A significant inverse relationship to the ESR was observed. In a study of serum trace-metal concentrations, the concentrations of copper, barium, cesium, tin, and molybdenum were elevated in RA.[186] Lower values of aluminum, nickel, strontium, chromium, cadmium,[186] and selenium were found.[1] Although plasma magnesium levels in RA are not much different from those in control subjects, the magnesium content of red blood cells is higher in these patients.[117]

ADRENAL FUNCTION TESTING

Adrenal cortical function has been evaluated on the basis of the excretion of 17-OH corticosteroids, 17-ketosteroids,[119] and other adrenal corticol metabolites.[250] Except for a decrease in excretion of 17-hydroxycorticosteroids in the early morning hours, the adrenal corticosteroid excretion pattern in RA is similar to that in other chronic diseases. Normal secretion rates of cortisol have been found.[191] Adrenal medullary function, as measured by the urinary excretion of epinephrine and norepinephrine, is within normal limits.[89,240]

MISCELLANEOUS LABORATORY STUDIES

Uric Acid Levels

Occasional studies have reported elevated levels of serum uric acid in patients with arthritides other than gout. Grayzel et al.,[106] who found elevated levels in 10 of 57 males with RA, ascribed this finding to the effect of low doses of salicylate. In other studies,[235,273] the levels of uric acid in RA were in the normal range.

Serum Cholesterol and Plasma Lipid Levels

In RA, as in other inflammatory arthritides, the total cholesterol level is reduced.[155] The mean reduction in rheumatoid-factor-positive patients was 53.7% in one series. The decrease was related to the severity and activity of the disease and was not affected by corticosteroid therapy. Plasma lipid levels have been reported to be within normal limits.[33,135] The difference in serum fatty acid concentration between RA patients and control subjects was not significant.[111] Oleic acid levels were elevated in patients with RA, whereas linolenic and arachidonic acid levels were decreased.[113]

Serum sulfhydryl levels have been reported to be low in RA, especially in the presence of vasculitis.[110,156] Ceruloplasmin levels have increased nonspecifically, a reflection of inflammatory activity.[1,212,251] Gerber found increased amounts of copper-binding substances in half of his rheumatoid patients.[93] The exact nature of these substances has not been determined. Patients with RA had low values of free serum histidine.[92] Adenosine triphosphatase (ATP)[109] and total serum lactic dehydrogenase[267] activities were within normal limits. Serum cholinesterase levels were variable.[115] Kininogen plasma levels and erythrocyte kininase levels were normal, but plasma kininase levels were decreased.[39] Serum plasmin activity correlated with the activity of the disease.[13] In a biopsy study of muscle ATP content, lower levels of muscle ATP were found in RA than in control subjects. No other muscle enzymes or metabolites studied were abnormal. The lowered levels of ATP were related to the duration of disease, and possibly to its severity.[189]

One study found increased capillary permeability in patients with RA. This finding was suggested as a possible cause of the occasional transient edema seen in these patients.[162]

Vitamin Levels

Blood levels of vitamins are commonly decreased in patients with RA. Blood concentrations of ascorbic acid are usually low.[82] Although plasma ascorbic acid levels are low in RA, low platelet levels of ascorbic acid are found only in patients taking high doses of aspirin. The platelet ascorbic acid level is a better reflection of tissue levels, whereas serum levels are a better reflection of recent intake and are susceptible to factors that affect metabolism or excretion.[218] The levels of plasma retinol-binding protein, a specific transport protein whose plasma levels reflect the availability of vitamin A and probably of zinc, were lower in patients with RA than in matched control patients with degenerative joint disease.[258] The level of blood pantothenic acid is decreased. The amount of decrease has been correlated with the activity of the disease[26] and with an increased excretion of this vitamin.[132] Riboflavin, thiamine, and occasionally nicotinic acid levels may be diminished;[132] however, folate levels are not much different from normal.[45] In one series, a low serum folate level was found in 71% of RA patients, although the authors felt that this finding might be due to aspirin-induced alterations of folic acid binding.[8] Pyridoxin excretion has been found to be depressed.[171] Fasting serum pyridoxal levels were below normal in 86% of RA patients, and serum folate levels were low. Vitamin B_{12} levels were higher in RA patients (916 pg/ml) than in patients with degenerative joint disease (624 pg/ml) and in normal controls (440 pg/ml). The vitamin B_{12} levels increased linearly with the stage of the disease and were related more closely to the hemoglobin concentration than to the erythrocyte count.[123]

Electromyography

Electromyographic findings in RA are not specific, but the frequency of abnormal findings is increased. Polyphasic potentials of short and long duration are often seen.[58,105,248] Fibrillation potentials have been reported by some authors,[58,105,292] but not by others.[10,183,248,294] Daughety and co-workers noted the presence of complicating factors such as polyneuropathy, terminal bronchopulmonary disease, and recent operation in all their patients who had fibrillation potentials.[58] Results of electrophysiologic studies of nerve conduction time in rheumatoid patients have been normal.[278]

Electrocardiography

Electrocardiographic changes were studied in a large group of patients with connective tissue diseases. Changes were found in all groups including those with RA. These changes included abnormal Q-QS, ST-segment, and T-wave patterns.[143]

Pleural Fluid Studies

A distinctive finding in RA is a low glucose concentration of pleural effusions. Glucose levels ranged from less than 5 mg/dl to 17 mg/dl in 10 of 11 effusions in one series;[44] values of 3, 0, and 0 mg/dl, respectively, were found in three effusions proved by pleural biopsy to be of rheumatoid origin.[229] The cause of this low glucose concentration is not known. Oral[47] or intravenous[68] administration of glucose failed to raise the glucose level in the effusions. A marked diminution of CH_{50}, C1, C1 inhibitor, and C2 was noted in the pleural fluid of rheumatoid-factor-positive RA.[98]

Electrodiagnostic Studies

On serial electrodiagnostic study, 20% of a series of patients with RA had evidence of carpal tunnel syndrome.[266]

REFERENCES

1. Aaseth, J., et al.: Trace elements in serum and urine of patients with rheumatoid arthritis. Scand. J. Rheumatol., 7:237–240, 1978.
2. Abdou, N.I., et al.: Suppressor T cell dysfunction and anti-suppressor cell antibody in active early rheumatoid arthritis. J. Rheumatol., 8:9–18, 1981.
3. Abruzzo, J.L., and Christian, C.L.: The induction of a rheumatoid factor-like substance in rabbits. J. Exp. Med., 114:791–806, 1961.
4. Aitcheson, C.T., et al.: Characteristics of antinuclear antibodies in rheumatoid arthritis. Arthritis Rheum., 23:528–538, 1980.
5. Alexander, W.R.M., et al.: Nature of anaemia in rheumatoid arthritis. II. Survival of transfused erythrocytes in patients with rheumatoid arthritis. Ann. Rheum. Dis., 15:12–20, 1956.
6. Allander, E., et al.: Renal function in rheumatoid arthritis. Acta Rheumatol. Scand., 9:116–121, 1963.
7. Alspaugh, M.A., et al.: Elevated levels of antibodies to Epstein-Barr virus antigens in sera and synovial fluid of patients with rheumatoid arthritis. J. Clin. Invest., 67:1134–1140, 1981.
8. Alter, H.J., Zvaifler, N.J., and Rath, C.E.: Interrelationship of rheumatoid arthritis, folic acid, and aspirin. Blood, 38:405–416, 1971.
9. Ambanelli, U., et al.: Relation between urine zinc and hydroxyproline in rheumatoid arthritis and bone diseases. J. Rheumatol., 5:477–479, 1978.
10. Amick, L.D.: Muscle atrophy in rheumatoid arthritis: an electrodiagnostic study. Arthritis Rheum., 3:54–63, 1960.
11. Amos, R.S., et al.: Rheumatoid arthritis: C-reactive protein and erythrocyte sedimentation during initial treatment. Br. Med. J., 1:1386–1387, 1978.
12. Anderson, I., Anderson, P., and Graudel, H.: Smooth muscle antibodies in RA. Acta Pathol. Microbiol. Scand., [C]88:131–135, 1980.
13. Anderson, R.B., and Winther, O.: Blood-fibrinolysis and activity of rheumatoid arthritis. Acta Rheumatol. Scand., 15:178–184, 1969.
14. Andrianakos, A.A., et al.: Cell-mediated immunity in rheumatoid arthritis. Ann. Rheum. Dis., 36:13–20, 1977.
15. Andriopoulos, N.A., et al.: Antibodies in native and denatured collagens in sera of patients with rheumatoid arthritis. Arthritis Rheum., 19:613–617, 1976.
16. Ansell, B., and Bywaters, E.G.L.: The "unexplained" high erythrocyte sedimentation rate. Br. Med. J., 1:372–374, 1958.
17. Artmann, G., Fehr, K., and Boni, A.: Cathepsin D agglutinators in rheumatoid arthritis. Arthritis Rheum., 20:1105–1113, 1977.
18. Baggenstoss, A.H., and Rosenberg, E.F.: Visceral lesions associated with chronic infectious (rheumatoid) arthritis. Arch. Pathol., 35:503–516, 1943.
19. Bajpayee, D.P.: Significance of plasma copper and caeruloplasmin concentrations in rheumatoid arthritis. Ann. Rheum. Dis., 34:162–165, 1975.
20. Ballantyne, F.C., Fleck, A., and Dick, W.C.: Albumin metabolism in rheumatoid arthritis. Ann. Rheum. Dis., 30:265–270, 1971.
21. Balogh, Z., et al.: Plasma zinc and its relationship to clinical symptoms and drug treatment in rheumatoid arthritis. Ann. Rheum. Dis., 38:329–332, 1980.
22. Barada, F.A., O'Brien, W., and Horwitz, D.A.: Defective monocyte cytotoxicity in rheumatoid arthritis. Arthritis Rheum., 25:10–16, 1982.
23. Barden, J., Mullinax, F., and Waller, M.: Immunoglobulin levels in rheumatoid arthritis: Comparison with rheumatoid factor titers, clinical stage and disease duration. Arthritis Rheum., 10:228–234, 1967.
24. Barr, J.H., Jr., et al.: Serum glutamic oxalacetic transaminase in rheumatoid arthritis and certain rheumatoid musculoskeletal disorders. Arthritis Rheum., 1:147–150, 1958.
25. Bartfeld, H.: The chromosomal complement in rheumatoid arthritis. N. Engl. J. Med., 267:551–553, 1962.
26. Barton-Wright, E.C., and Elliot, W.A.: The pathogenic acid metabolism of rheumatoid arthritis. Lancet, 2:862–863, 1963.
27. Baum, J., and Ziff, M.: 7S and macroglobulin antinuclear fluorescence factors in systemic lupus erythematosus and rheumatoid arthritis. Arthritis Rheum., 5:636–637, 1962.
28. Belin, D.C., Morse, E., and Weinstein, A.: Whither Wes-

tergren—the sedimentation rate reevaluated. J. Rheumatol., 8:331–335, 1981.

29. Bennett, R.M., et al.: Synovial iron deposition in rheumatoid arthritis. Arthritis Rheum., 16:298–304, 1973.

30. Bergstrom, K., and Havermark, G.: Enzymes in intestinal mucosa from patients with rheumatoid diseases. Scand. J. Rheumatol., 5:29–32, 1976.

31. Bishop, C.R., et al.: Leukokinetic studies. XIII. A nonsteady-state kinetic evaluation of the mechanism of cortisone-induced granulocytosis. J. Clin. Invest., 47:249–260, 1968.

32. Blake, D.R., and Bacon, P.A.: Serum ferritin and rheumatoid disease. Br. Med. J., 282:1273–1274, 1981.

33. Block, W.D., Buchanan, O.H., and Freyberg, R.H.: Serum lipids in patients with rheumatoid arthritis and in patients with obstructive jaundice. Arch. Intern. Med., 68:18–24, 1941.

34. Bottiger, L.E., and Svedberg, C.A.: Normal erythrocyte sedimentation rate and age. Br. Med. J., 2:85–87, 1967.

35. Boyd, R.V., and Hoffbrand, B.I.: Erythrocyte sedimentation rate in elderly hospital in-patients. Br. Med. J., 1:901–902, 1966.

36. Brackertz, D., et al.: Histocompatibility antigens of patients with rheumatoid arthritis. Z. Immunitaetsforsch., 146:108–113, 1973.

37. Brackertz, D., Hagmann, J., and Kueppers, F.: Proteinase inhibitors in rheumatoid arthritis. Ann. Rheum. Dis., 34:225–230, 1975.

38. Brendstrup, P.: Serum copper, serum iron and total iron-binding capacity of serum in patients with chronic rheumatoid arthritis. Acta Med. Scand., 146:384–392, 1953.

39. Briseid, K., Dyrud, O., and Rinvik, S.: Determination of plasma kininogen plasma kininase and erythocyte kininase in men with rheumatoid arthritis. Acta Pharmacol., 24:179–182, 1966.

40. Brönnestam, R.: Studies of the C3 polymorphism. Relationship between C3 phenotypes and rheumatoid arthritis. Hum. Hered., 23:206–213, 1973.

41. Bucknall, R.C., et al.: Neutropenia in rheumatoid arthritis: studies on possible contributing factors. Ann. Rheum. Dis., 41:242–247, 1982.

42. Burry, H.C.: Bacteriuria in rheumatoid arthritis. Ann. Rheum. Dis., 32:208–211, 1973.

43. Burton, J.L.: Effect of oral contraceptives on erythrocyte sedimentation rate in healthy young women. Br. Med. J., 3:214–215, 1967.

44. Carr, D.T., and Mayne, J.G.: Pleurisy with effusion in rheumatoid arthritis, with reference to the low concentration of glucose in pleural fluid. Am. Rev. Respir. Dis., 85:345–350, 1962.

45. Carr, D.T., and McGuckin, W.F.: Pleural fluid glucose. Serial observation of its concentration following oral administration of glucose to patients with rheumatoid pleural effusions and malignant effusions. Am. Rev. Respir. Dis., 97:302–305, 1968.

46. Cartwright, G.E.: The anemia of chronic disorders. Semin. Hematol., 3:351–375, 1966.

47. Cartwright, G.E., and Wintrobe, M.M.: Modern Trends in Blood Diseases. New York, Paul B. Hoeber, 1955.

48. Caspary, E.A., and Ball, E.J.: Serum immuno conglutinin in multiple sclerosis, Hashimoto's diseases, and rheumatoid arthritis. Br. Med. J., 2:1514–1515, 1962.

49. Castenfors, H., Hultman, E., and Lövgren, O.: The bromosulphthalein-test (BSP) as a measure of rheumatoid arthritis activity. Acta Rheumatol. Scand., 10:128–132, 1964.

50. Christian, C.L., DeSimone, A.R., and Abruzzo, J.L.: Anti-DNA antibodies in hyperimmunized rabbits. Arthritis Rheum., 6:766, 1963.

51. Cohen, A.S., et al.: Correlation between rheumatic diseases and Rh blood groups. Nature, 200:1214–1215, 1963.

52. Condemi, J.J.: The significance of antinuclear factors in rheumatoid arthritis. Arthritis Rheum., 8:1080–1093, 1965.

53. Coombs, R.R.A., Coombs, A.M., and Ingram, D.G.: Formation of immunoconglutinin during disease in man. In The Serology of Conglutination. Edited by R.A. Coombs, A.M. Coombs and D.G. Ingram. Springfield, IL, Charles C Thomas, 1961, p. 128–137.

54. Cox, D.W., and Huber, O.: Association of severe rheumatoid arthritis with heterozygosity for α_1-antitrypsin deficiency. Clin. Genet., 17:153–160, 1980.

55. Cox, D.W., and Huber, O.: Rheumatoid arthritis and alpha-1-antitrypsin. Lancet, 1:1216–1217, 1976.

56. Crockson, R.A., and Crockson, A.P.: Relationship of the erythrocyte sedimentation rate to viscosity and plasma proteins in rheumatoid arthritis. Ann. Rheum. Dis., 33:53–56, 1974.

57. Darby, P.W.: Liver function tests in rheumatoid arthritis. J. Clin. Pathol., 6:331, 1953.

58. Daughety, J.S., Baum, J., and Krusen, U.: Electromyography in the connective tissue diseases: preliminary report. Arch. Phys. Med. Rehabil., 45:224–230, 1964.

59. Dawson, M.H., Sia, R.H.P., and Boots, R.H.: The differential diagnosis of rheumatoid and osteoarthritis: The sedimentation reaction and its value. J. Lab. Clin. Med., 15:1065–1092, 1930.

60. Decker, J.L., et al.: Primer on the rheumatic diseases, Part III. JAMA, 190:509–530, 1964.

61. Deinard, A.S., et al.: Rubella-antibody titres in rheumatoid arthritis. Lancet, 1:526–528, 1974.

62. Denko, C.W., and Gabriel, P.: Serum proteins—transferrin, ceruloplasmin, albumin, α_1-acid and glycoprotein, α_1-antitrypsin—in rheumatic disorders. J. Rheumatol., 6:664–672, 1979.

63. DeWitte, T.J., et al.: Hypochlorhydria and hypergastrinaemia in rheumatoid arthritis. Ann. Rheum. Dis., 38:14–17, 1979.

64. Diaz-Jouanen, E., Bankhurst, A.D., and Williams, R.C., Jr.: Antibody-mediated lymphocytotoxicity in rheumatoid arthritis and systemic lupus erythematosus. Arthritis Rheum., 19:133–141, 1976.

65. Dietrichson, O., et al.: Morphological changes in liver biopsies from patients with rheumatoid arthritis. Scand. J. Rheumatol., 5:65–69, 1976.

66. Dixon, A. St.J., Ramcharan, S., and Ropes, M.W.: Rheumatoid arthritis: Dye retention studies and comparison of dye and radioactively labelled red cell methods for measurement of blood volume. Ann. Rheum. Dis., 14:51–62, 1955.

67. Dixon, A. St.J., Scott, J.T., and Harvey-Smith, E.A.: Aspirin and the anaemia of arthritis. Br. Med. J., 1:1425–1426, 1960.

68. Dodson, W.H., and Hollingsworth, J.W.: Pleural effusion in rheumatoid arthritis. Impaired transport of glucose. N. Engl. J. Med., 275:1337–1342, 1966.

69. Drivsholm, A.: Myelomatosis. Acta Med. Scand., 176:509–524, 1964.

70. Ebaugh, F.G., et al.: The anemia of rheumatoid arthritis. Med. Clin. North Am., 39:489–498, 1955.

71. Ebringer, R., et al.: Autoantibodies to cartilage and type II collagen in relapsing polychondritis and other rheumatic diseases. Ann. Rheum. Dis., 40:473–479, 1981.

71a. Eisenberg, G.M., et al.: Polyclonal B cell activator (PBA) in rheumatic diseases. Arthritis Rheum., 25:S6, 1982.

72. Ellis, H.A., and Felix-Davies, D.: Serum complement, rheumatoid factor, and other serum proteins in rheumatoid disease and systemic lupus erythematosus. Ann. Rheum. Dis., 18:215–224, 1959.

73. Evans, H.E., Glass, L., and Mercado, C.: The microerythrocyte sedimentation rate in newborn infants. J. Pediatr., 76:448–451, 1970.

74. Fåhraeus, R.: The suspension stability of the blood. Physiol. Rev., 9:241–274, 1929.

75. Fåhraeus, R.: The suspension-stability of the blood. Acta Med. Scand., 55:1–228, 1921.

76. Fallahi, S., Halla, J.T., and Hardin, J.G., Jr.: The influence of B27 antigen on the clinical and radiographic picture of definite or classical rheumatoid arthritis. J. Rheumatol., 9:13–17, 1982.

77. Falus, A., Meretey, K., and Bozsoky, S.: Prevalence of anti-beta-2-microglobulin autoantibodies in sera of rheumatoid arthritis patients with extraarticular manifestations. Ann. Rheum. Dis., 40:409–413, 1981.

78. Fearnley, G.S., and Lackner, R.: Amyloidosis in rheu-

matoid arthritis, and significance of "unexplained" albuminuria. Br. Med. J., *1*:1129–1132, 1955.

79. Felty, A.R.: Chronic arthritis in the adult, associated with splenomegaly and leukopenia: a report of 5 cases of an unusual clinical syndrome. Bull. Johns Hopkins Hosp., *35*:16–20, 1924.

80. Finch, C.A., et al.: Iron metabolism utilization of intravenous radioactive iron. Blood, *4*:905–927, 1949.

81. Fletcher, A.A., Dauphinee, J.A., and Orgyzlo, M.A.: Plasma fibrinogen and the sedimentation rate in rheumatoid arthritis and their response to the administration of cortisone and adrenocorticotropic hormone. J. Clin. Invest., *31*:561–571, 1952.

82. Forster, J.E., and Engleman, E.P.: The effect of adrenal corticosteroid therapy on blood ascorbic acid levels in rheumatoid arthritis. Arthritis Rheum., *4*:418, 1961.

83. Francis, T.I., Odusote, K., and Osuntokun, B.O.: The erythrocyte sedimentation rate in Nigerians. West Afr. Med. J., *20*:250–252, 1971.

84. Franco, A.E., and Schur, P.H.: Hypocomplementemia in rheumatoid arthritis. Arthritis Rheum., *14*:231–238, 1971.

85. Freireich, E.J., et al.: Radioactive iron metabolism and erythrocyte survival studies of the mechanism of the anemia associated with rheumatoid arthritis. J. Clin. Invest., *36*:1043–1058, 1957.

86. Freireich, E.J., et al.: Mechanism of anaemia associated with rheumatoid arthritis. Ann. Rheum. Dis., *13*:365–366, 1954.

87. Friedman, I.A., et al.: The L.E. phenomenon in rheumatoid arthritis. Ann. Intern. Med., *46*:1113–1136, 1957.

88. Friman, C., Juvani, M., and Skrifvars, B.: Acid glycosaminoglycans in plasma. Scand. J. Rheumatol., *6*:177–182, 1977.

89. Fruehan, A.E., and Frawley, T.F.: Adrenal medullary function in the connective tissue disorders. Arthritis Rheum., *6*:698–710, 1963.

90. Fyrand, O., Munthe, E., and Solum, N.O.: Studies on cold insoluble globulin. Ann. Rheum. Dis., *37*:347–350, 1978.

91. Gilmour, D. and Sykes, A.J.: Westergren and Wintrobe methods of estimating E.S.R. compared. Br. Med. J., *2*:1496–1497, 1951.

92. Gerber, D.A.: Low free serum histidine concentration in rheumatoid arthritis. A measure of disease activity. J. Clin. Invest., *55*:1164–1173, 1975.

93. Gerber, D.A.: Increased copper ligand reactivity in the urine of patients with rheumatoid arthritis. Arthritis Rheum., *9*:795–803, 1966.

94. Gibson, I.I.J.M.: The value of the erythrocyte sedimentation rate in the aged. Gerontol. Clin., *14*:185–190, 1972.

95. Gibson, J.G., Harris, A.W., and Swigert, V.W.: Clinical studies of the blood volume. VIII. Macrocytic and hypochromic anemias due to chronic blood loss, hemolysis, and miscellaneous causes, and polycythemia vera. J. Clin. Invest., *18*:621–632, 1939.

96. Gilligan, D.R., and Ernstene, A.C.: The relationship between the erythrocyte sedimentation rate and the fibrinogen content of plasma. Am. J. Med. Sci., *187*:552–556, 1934.

97. Glass, D., et al.: Inherited deficiency of the second component of complement. Rheumatic disease associations. J. Clin. Invest., *58*:853–861, 1976.

98. Glovsky, M.M., et al.: Reduction of pleural fluid complement activity in patients with systemic lupus erythematosus and rheumatoid arthritis. Clin. Immunol. Immunopathol., *6*:31–41, 1976.

99. Glynn, L.E.: Symposium on inflammation and role of fibrin in the rheumatic diseases. Bull. Rheum. Dis., *14*:323–326, 1963.

100. Goldberg, A., and Conway, H.: Observations on methods of measuring the erythrocyte sedimentation rate. Br. Med. J., *2*:315–317, 1952.

101. Goldfine, L.J., et al.: Clinical significance of the LE-cell phenomenon in rheumatoid arthritis. Ann. Rheum. Dis., *24*:153–160, 1965.

102. Goldie, I.F., et al.: A comparison of the content of iron

in normal and rheumatoid striated muscle. Scand. J. Rheumatol., *5*:205–208, 1976.

103. Gordon, D.A., Eisen, A.Z., and Vaughan, J.: Studies on urinary γ-globulins in patients with rheumatoid arthritis. Arthritis Rheum., *9*:575–588, 1966.

104. Gordon, J., Towbin, H., and Rosenthal, M.: Antibodies directed against ribosomal protein determinants in the sera of patients with connective tissue diseases. J. Rheumatol., *9*:247–252, 1982.

105. Graudal, H., and Hvid, N.: An electromyographic study on patients with arthritis. Acta Rheumatol. Scand., *5*:34–41, 1959.

106. Grayzel, A.I., Liddle, L. and Seegmiller, J.E.: Diagnostic significance of hyperuricemia in arthritis. N. Engl. J. Med., *265*:763–768, 1961.

107. Green, D., Schuette, R.T., and Wallace, W.H.: Factor VIII antibodies in rheumatoid arthritis. Arch. Intern. Med., *140*:1232–1235, 1980.

108. Gronbaek, P.: The sodium/potassium ratio in thermal sweat in patients with rheumatoid arthritis. Acta Rheumatol. Scand., *6*:102–110, 1960.

109. Györki, J., and Sandell, B.-M.: Adenosine triphosphatase activity in blood in rheumatoid arthritis. Acta Rheumatol. Scand., *7*:127–130, 1961.

110. Haataja, M.: Evaluation of the activity of rheumatoid arthritis. A comparative study on clinical symptoms and laboratory tests with special reference to serum sulfhydryl groups. Scand. J. Rheumatol., *7(Suppl.)*:1975.

111. Haataja, M., et al.: Prostaglandin precursors in rheumatoid arthritis. J. Rheumatol., *9*:91–93, 1982.

112. Haeney, M.R.: Erroneous values for the total white cell count and ESR in patients with cryoglobulinaemia. J. Clin. Pathol., *29*:894–897, 1976.

113. Hagenfeldt, L., and Wennmalm, A.: Turnover of a prostaglandin precursor, arachidonic acid, in rheumatoid arthritis. Eur. J. Clin. Invest., *5*:235–239, 1975.

114. Hamburger, M., Hodes, S., and Barland, P.: The incidence and clinical significance of antibodies to extractable nuclear antigens. Am. J. Med. Sci., *273*:21–28, 1977.

115. Hammarsten, G., et al.: Choline esterase activity in rheumatoid arthritis. Acta Rheumatol. Scand., *5*:42–48, 1959.

116. Hardwicke, H., and Squire, J.R.: The basis of the erythrocyte sedimentation rate. Clin. Sci., *11*:333–355, 1952.

117. Henrotte, J.G., et al.: Modification des taux du fer sérique et du magnésium érythrocytaire au cours des rhumatismes inflammatoires chroniques. Life Sci., *9*:609–612, 1970.

118. Hermann, H.: Die Blutkörperchensenkungsgeschwindigkeit bei arthritiden und rheumateschen Affektionen der Muskulatur. Munchen. Med. Wochenschr., *71*:1714–1716, 1924.

119. Hill, S.R., Jr., et al.: Studies on adrenal cortical activity in patients with rheumatoid arthritis: the diurnal pattern and twenty-four hour levels of urinary total 17-hydroxycorticosteroids and 17-ketosteroids. Arthritis Rheum., *2*:114–126, 1959.

120. Hollinger, N.F., and Robinson, S.J.: A study of the erythrocyte sedimentation rate for well children. J. Pediatr., *42*:304–319, 1953.

121. Hunder, G.G., and McDuffie, F.C.: Hypocomplementemia in rheumatoid arthritis. Am. J. Med., *54*:461–472, 1972.

122. Hurd, E.R., and Cheatum, D.E.: Decreased spleen size and increased neutrophils in patients with Felty syndrome. Effects of gold sodium thiomalate therapy. JAMA, *235*:2215–2217, 1976.

123. Igarai, T., et al.: Serum vitamin B_{12} levels of patients with rheumatoid arthritis. Tohoku J. Exp. Med., *125*:287–301, 1978.

124. International Committee for Standardization in Hematology: Recommendation for measurement of erythrocyte sedimentation rate of human blood. Am. J. Clin. Pathol., *68*:505–507, 1977.

125. Jeffrey, J.R.: Some observations on anemia in rheumatoid arthritis. Blood, *8*:502–518, 1953.

126. Jeffrey, M.R.: Haemodilution in rheumatoid disease. Ann. Rheum. Dis., *15*:151–159, 1956.

127. Jeffrey, M.R., and Watson, D.: Free erythrocyte por-

phyrin and plasma copper in rheumatoid disease. Acta Haematol., *12*:169–176, 1954.

128. Jeremy, R., and Wilkinson, P.: The mechanism of hypoalbuminemia in rheumatoid arthritis. Arthritis Rheum., *7*:740–741, 1964.

129. Johansson, S.V., and Strandberg, P.O.: Haem biosynthesis studied in patients with rheumatoid arthritis. J. Clin. Pathol., *25*:159–162, 1972.

130. Johnson, N.J., and Dodd, K.: Juvenile rheumatoid arthritis. Med. Clin. North Am., *39*:459–487, 1955.

131. Kalliomaki, J.L., et al.: Extracellular fluid phase in rheumatoid arthritis. Acta Rheumatol. Scand., *4*:79–85, 1958.

132. Kalliomaki, J.L., Laine, V.A., and Markkanen, T.K.: Urinary excretion of thiamine, riboflavin, nicotinic acid, and pantothenic acid in patients with rheumatoid arthritis. Acta Med. Scand., *166*:275–279, 1960.

133. Kalmakoff, J., et al.: Antibodies against double-stranded RNA in patients with rheumatoid arthritis, osteoarthritis and Paget's disease of bone. Aust. N.Z. J. Med., *11*:173–178, 1981.

134. Karsh, J., Vergalla, J., and Joines, E.A.: Alpha-1-antitrypsin phenotypes in rheumatoid arthritis and systemic lupus erythematosus. Arthritis Rheum., *22*:111–113, 1979.

135. Kelly, H.G., Hill, J.G., and Boyd, E.M.: The absence of effect of cortisone therapy upon plasma lipid levels in patients with rheumatoid arthritis. Can. Med. Assoc. J., *70*:660–662, 1954.

136. Kievits, J.H., et al.: Rheumatoid arthritis and the positive L.E.-cell phenomenon. Ann. Rheum. Dis., *15*:211–216, 1956.

137. Kennedy, A.C., et al.: Hypercalcaemia in rheumatoid arthritis. Ann. Rheum. Dis., *38*:401–412, 1979.

138. Komatsubara, Y., et al.: Multi-variate analysis of serum protein rheumatoid arthritis. Scand. J. Rheumatol., *5*:97–102, 1976.

139. Kornstad, L., Guldberg, D., and Kornstad, A.M.G.: Isohaemagglutinins anti-A and anti-B in rheumatoid arthritis and ankylosing spondylitis. Ann. Rheum. Dis., *29*:421–426, 1970.

140. Kosaka, S.: β$_2$-Glycoprotein I in rheumatoid arthritis. Tohoku J. Exp. Med., *122*:223–228, 1977.

141. Kosaka, S., and Tazawa, M.: Alpha-1-antichymotrypsin in rheumatoid arthritis. Tohoku J. Exp. Med., *119*:369–375, 1976.

142. Kuutti-Savolainen, E.-R., Kivirikko, K.I., and Laitinin, O.: Serum immunoreactive prolyl hydroxylase in inflammatory rheumatic diseases. Ann. Rheum. Dis., *39*:217–221, 1980.

143. Laitinin, O., Kentala, E., and Leirisalo, M.: Electrocardiographic findings in patients with connective tissue disease. Scand. J. Rheumatol., *7*:193–198, 1978.

144. Lance, E.M., and Knight, S.C.: Immunologic reactivity in rheumatoid arthritis. Response to mitogens. Arthritis Rheum., *17*:513–520, 1974.

145. Laurell, A.-B., and Grubb, R.: Complement, complement components, properdin and agglutination promoting factors in rheumatoid arthritis. Acta Pathol. Microbiol. Scand., *43*:310–320, 1958.

146. Lefkovits, A.M., and Farrow, I.J.: The liver in rheumatoid arthritis. Ann. Rheum. Dis., *14*:162–169, 1955.

147. Lehman, M.A., Kream, J., and Brugua, D.: Acid and alkaline phosphatase activity in the serum and synovial fluid of patients with arthritis. J. Bone Joint Surg., *46A*:1732–1738, 1964.

148. Levinsky, H., et al.: Red blood cell membrane and serum sialic acid in relation to erythrocyte sedimentation rate. Acta Haematol., *64*:276–280, 1980.

149. Lewis, S.M., and Porter, I.H.: Erythrocyte survival in rheumatoid arthritis. Ann. Rheum. Dis., *19*:54–58, 1960.

150. Lies, R.B., Messner, R.P., and Troup, G.M.: Histocompatibility antigens and rheumatoid arthritis. Arthritis Rheum., *15*:524–529, 1972.

151. Liljestrand, A., and Olhagen, B.: I. Persistently high erythrocyte sedimentation rate. Acta Med. Scand., *151*:425–439, 1955.

152. Lindjberg, I.F.: Juvenile rheumatoid arthritis. A follow-up of 75 cases. Arch. Dis. Child., *39*:576–583, 1964.

153. Lindström, F.D.: Urinary immunoglobulins in rheumatoid arthritis and other connective tissue diseases. Ann. Clin. Res., *3*:39–45, 1971.

154. Lockshin, M.D., et al.: Cell-mediated immunity in rheumatic diseases. II. Mitogen responses in RA, SLE, and other illnesses: correlation with T- and B-lymphocyte populations. Arthritis Rheum., *18*:245–250, 1975.

155. London, M.G., Muirden, K.D., and Hewitt, J.V.: Serum cholesterol in rheumatic diseases. Br. Med. J., *1*:1380–1383, 1963.

156. Lorber, A., et al.: Serum sulfhydryl determinations and significance in connective tissue diseases. Ann. Intern. Med., *61*:423–434, 1964.

157. Lowe, J.R., et al.: Gamma glutamyl transpeptidase levels in arthritis. Ann. Rheum. Dis., *37*:428–431, 1978.

158. Mackechnie, H.L., Ogryzlo, M.A., and Pruzanski, W.: Heterogeneity of IgM/IgG cryocomplexes: Immunological-clinical correlation. J. Rheumatol., *2*:225–240, 1975.

159. Makisara, P., et al.: Serum copper in rheumatoid arthritis and ankylosing spondylitis. Ann. Med. Exp. Biol. Fenn., *46*:177–178, 1968.

160. Malmquist, E., and Reichard, H.: Serum ornithine carbamoyl transferase and transaminase activity in rheumatic disease. Acta Rheumatol. Scand., *8*:170–182, 1962.

161. Marcolongo, R., and Debolini, A.: Incidence of hepatitis associated antigen HAA and homologous antibody in patients with rheumatoid arthritis. Vox Sang., *28*:9–18, 1975.

162. Marks, J., Birkett, D.A., and Shuster, S.: "Capillary permeability" in patients with collagen vascular disease. Br. Med. J., *1*:782–784, 1972.

163. Mathieu, M., Mereu, M.C., and Pisano, L.: Tγ lymphocytes of peripheral blood and synovial fluid in rheumatoid arthritis. Arthritis Rheum., *24*:658–661, 1981.

164. Maury, C.P.J., Teppo, A.-M., and Wegelius, O.: Relationship between urinary sialylated saccharides, serum amyloid A protein, and C-reactive protein in rheumatoid arthritis and systemic lupus erythematosus. Ann. Rheum. Dis., *41*:268–271, 1982.

165. Mbuyi, J.-M., et al.: Relevance of urinary excretion of alcian blue-glycosaminoglycans complexes and hydroxyproline to disease activity in rheumatoid arthritis. J. Rheumatol., *9*:579–583, 1982.

166. McConkey, B., Crockson, R.A., and Crockson, A.P.: The assessment of rheumatoid arthritis: a study based on measurements of the serum acute-phase reactants. Q. J. Med., *162*:115–125, 1972.

167. McCrea, P.C.: Marrow iron examination in the diagnosis of iron deficiency in rheumatoid arthritis. Ann. Rheum. Dis., *17*:89–96, 1958.

168. McCrea, P.C.: Latent haemolysis in rheumatoid arthritis. Lancet, *1*:402–405, 1957.

169. McDougal, J.G., et al.: Comparison of five assays for immune complexes in the rheumatic diseases. Arthritis Rheum., *25*:1156–1166, 1982.

170. McEwen, C., and Ziff, M.: Basic sciences in relation to rheumatic diseases. Med. Clin. North Am., *39*:765–782, 1955.

171. McKusick, A.B., et al.: Urinary excretion of pyridoxine and 4-pyridoxic acid in rheumatoid arthritis. Arthritis Rheum., *7*:636–653, 1964.

172. Mead, J., and Larson, D.L.: The erythrocyte sedimentation rate and other blood tests in terminal cancer. J. Am. Geriatr. Soc., *18*:489–490, 1970.

173. Meghlaoui, A., et al.: Mise au point d'une technique immunoenzymatique (ELISA) pour la détection des anticorps anti-collagéne de type I et II. Ann. Immunol. (Paris), *132C*:287–305, 1981.

174. Meijer, C.J.L.M., et al.: T lymphocyte subpopulations in rheumatoid arthritis. J. Rheumatol., *9*:18–24, 1982.

175. Menard, H.A., Dioni, J., and Richard, C.: Antinuclear antibody: predictive of lymphocyte response in rheumatoid arthritis. J. Rheumatol., *4*:21–26, 1977.

176. Milne, J.S., and Williamson, J.: The ESR in older people. Gerontol. Clin., *14*:36–42, 1972.

177. Mongan, E.S., et al.: A study of the relation of sero-

negative and seropositive rheumatoid arthritis to each other and to necrotizing vasculitis. Am. J. Med., 47:23–35, 1969.

178. Morris, M.W., Skrodzki, Z., and Nelson, D.A.: Zeta sedimentation ratio (ZSR), a replacement for the erythrocyte sedimentation rate (ESR). Am. J. Clin. Pathol., 64:254–256, 1975.

179. Movitt, E.R., and Davis, A.E.: Liver biopsy in rheumatoid arthritis. Am. J. Med. Sci., 226:516–520, 1953.

180. Mowat, A.G., and Baum, J.: Chemotaxis of polymorphonuclear leucocytes from patients with rheumatoid arthritis. J. Clin. Invest., 50:2541–2549, 1971.

181. Mowat, A.G., and Camp, A.V.: Polymyalgia rheumatica, J. Bone Joint Surg., 53B:701–710, 1971.

182. Mowat, A.G., and Hothersall, T.E.: Nature of anaemia in rheumatoid arthritis: 8. Iron content of synovial tissue in patients with rheumatoid arthritis and in normal individuals. Ann. Rheum. Dis., 27:345–351, 1968.

183. Mueller, E.E., and Mead, S.: The electromyogram in rheumatoid arthritis. Am. J. Phys. Med., 31:67–73, 1952.

184. Muirden, K.D.: The anaemia of rheumatoid arthritis: the significance of iron deposits in the synovial membrane. Aust. Ann. Med., 19:97–104, 1970.

185. Natvig, J.B., et al.: Different lymphocyte populations in rheumatoid arthritis and their relationship to anti-Ig activities. Ann. Clin. Res., 7:146–153, 1975.

186. Niedermeier, W., and Griggs, J.H.: Trace metal composition of synovial fluid and blood serum of patients with rheumatoid arthritis. J. Chronic Dis., 23:527–536, 1971.

187. Nilsson, F.: Anemia problems in rheumatoid arthritis. Acta Med. Scand., 210(Suppl.):1–193, 1948.

188. Nived, O., et al.: Is serum creatinine concentration a reliable index of renal function in rheumatic diseases? Br. Med. J., 286:684–685, 1983.

189. Nordemar, R., et al.: Muscle ATP content in rheumatoid arthritis—a biopsy study. Scand. J. Clin. Lab. Invest., 34:185–191, 1974.

189a. Nussinow, S., and Arnold, W.J.: Prognostic value of C-reactive protein (CRP) levels in rheumatoid arthritis. Arthritis Rheum., 25:524, 1982.

190. Olhagen, B., and Liljestrand, A.: II. Persistently elevated erythrocyte sedimentation rate with good prognosis. Acta Med. Scand., 151:441–449, 1955.

191. Pal. S.B.: The secretion rate of cortisol in patients with rheumatoid arthritis. Clin. Chim. Acta, 29:129–137, 1970.

192. Pasternack, A., et al.: Renal acidification and hypergammaglobulinaemia. A study of rheumatoid arthritis. Acta Med. Scand., 187:123–127, 1970.

193. Payne, W.W., and Schlesinger, B.: A study of the sedimentation rate in juvenile rheumatism. Arch. Dis. Child., 10:403–414, 1935.

194. Percy, J.S., et al.: A longitudinal study of in vitro tests for lymphocyte function in rheumatoid arthritis. Ann. Rheum. Dis., 37:416–420, 1978.

195. Permin, H., and Wiik, A.: The prevalence of IgE antinuclear antibodies in rheumatoid arthritis and systemic lupus erythematosus. Acta Pathol. Microbiol. Scand., [C] 86:245–249, 1978.

196. Peyman, M.A.: The effect of malignant disease on the erythrocyte sedimentation rate. Br. J. Cancer, 16:56–71, 1962.

197. Phillips, P.E., et al.: Virus antibody levels and delayed hypersensitivity in rheumatoid arthritis. Ann. Rheum. Dis., 35:152–154, 1976.

198. Pickup, M.E., et al.: Plasma viscosity—a new appraisal of its use as an index of disease activity in rheumatoid arthritis. Ann. Rheum. Dis., 40:272–275, 1981.

199. Pitkeathly, D.A., and Taylor, G.: Antinuclear factor in rheumatoid arthritis and related diseases. Ann. Rheum. Dis., 26:1–9, 1967.

200. Plantin, L.O., and Strandberg, P.O.: Whole-blood concentrations of copper and zinc in rheumatoid arthritis studied by activation analysis. Acta Rheumatol. Scand., 11:30–34, 1965.

201. Pollak, V.E.: Antinuclear antibodies in families of patients

with systemic lupus erythematosus. N. Engl. J. Med., 271:165–171, 1964.

202. Pollak, V.E., et al.: The kidney in rheumatoid arthritis: studies by renal biopsy. Arthritis Rheum., 5:1–9, 1962.

203. Pope, R.M., Rutstein, J.E., and Straus, D.C.: Detection of antibodies to streptococcal mucopeptide in patients with rheumatic disorders and normal controls. Int. Arch. Allergy Appl. Immunol., 67:267–274, 1982.

204. Pope, R.M., Yoshinoya, S., and McDuffy, S.J.: Detection of immune complexes and their relationship to rheumatoid factor in a variety of autoimmune disorders. Clin. Exp. Immunol., 46:259–267, 1981.

205. Pruzanski, W., et al.: Serum and synovial fluid proteins in rheumatoid arthritis and degenerative joint diseases. Am. J. Med. Sci., 265:483–490, 1973.

206. Raich, P.C., and Temperly, N.: Comparison of the Wintrobe erythrocyte sedimentation rate with the Zeta sedimentation ratio. Am. J. Clin. Pathol., 65:690–693, 1976.

207. Rawson, A.J., and Abelson, N.M.: An isohemagglutinin deficiency in relatives of rheumatoid patients. Arthritis Rheum., 7:391–397, 1964.

208. Rawson, A.J., and Huang, T.C.: Lymphocyte populations in rheumatoid arthritis. Arthritis Rheum., 19:720–724, 1976.

209. Reid, D.M., et al.: Total body calcium in rheumatoid arthritis. Br. Med. J., 285:330–332, 1982.

210. Rhodes, K., et al.: Immunological sex differences: a study of patients with rheumatoid arthritis, their relatives and controls. Ann. Rheum. Dis., 28:104–120, 1969.

211. Richardson, A.T.: Routine clinical pathology in rheumatoid arthritis. Proc. R. Soc. Med., 50:466–469, 1957.

212. Rice, E.W.: Evaluation of the role of ceruloplasmin as an acute-phase reactant. Clin. Chim. Acta, 6:652–655, 1961.

213. Richmond, J., et al.: The nature of anaemia in rheumatoid arthritis. V. Red cell survival measured by radioactive chromium. Ann. Rheum. Dis., 20:133–137, 1961.

214. Richmond, J., et al.: Nature of anaemia in rheumatoid arthritis. III. Changes in the bone marrow and their relation to other features of the disease. Ann. Rheum. Dis., 15:217–226, 1956.

215. Roberts, F.D., et al.: Evaluation of the anemia of rheumatoid arthritis. Blood, 21:470–478, 1963.

216. Robinson, G.L.: A study of liver function and plasma volume in chronic rheumatism by means of phenol-tetrabrom-phthalein sodium sulphonate. Ann. Rheum. Dis., 3:207–221, 1943.

217. Rooney, P.J., et al.: Hypergastrinaemia in rheumatoid arthritis: disease or iatrogenesis. Br. Med. J., 2:752–753, 1973.

218. Rosenthal, M., and Muller, W.: Lymphocyte subpopulations in normals and patients with rheumatoid arthritis and ankylosing spondylitis. J. Rheumatol., 2:355–358, 1975.

219. Runge, L.A.: In vitro lymphocyte response in early RA. J. Rheumatol., 8:468–476, 1981.

220. Sahud, M.A., and Cohen, R.J.: Effect of aspirin ingestion on ascorbic-acid levels in rheumatoid arthritis. Lancet, 1:937–938, 1971.

221. Sakane, T., et al.: Analysis of suppressor T cell function in patients with rheumatoid arthritis. J. Immunol., 129:1972–1977, 1982.

222. Salomon, M.I., et al.: The kidney in rheumatoid arthritis. A study based on renal biopsies. Nephron, 12:297–310, 1974.

223. Saghvi, L.M.: Sedimentation rate in heart disease. Geriatrics, 18:382–392, 1963.

224. Sanderson, C.R., Davis, R.E., and Bayliss, C.E.: Serum pyridoxal in patients with rheumatoid arthritis. Ann. Rheum. Dis., 35:177–180, 1976.

225. Scherak, O., Smolen, J.S., and Mayr, W.R.: Rheumatoid arthritis and B lymphocyte alloantigen HLA-DRw4. J. Rheumatol., 7:9–12, 1980.

226. Scherer, R., Morarescu, A., and Ruhenstroth-Bauer, G.: Die spezifische Wirkung der Plasmaproteine bei der Blutkörperchensenkung. Eine Analyse der Korrelationskoeffizienten von Blutkorperchensen—Kungsgeschwindigkeit und den Konzentrationen von zwanzig Plasmaproteinen

bei Gesunden und Kranken, insbesondere nach Herzinfarkt. Klin. Wochenschr., *53*:265–273, 1975.

227. Schlesinger, B.E.: The blood sedimentation rate in rheumatic fever. Practitioner, *157*:38–44, 1946.

228. Schlesinger, B.E., et al.: Observations on the clinical course and treatment of one hundred cases of Still's disease. Arch. Dis. Child., *36*:65–76, 1961.

229. Schools, G.S., and Mikkelsen, W.M.: Rheumatoid pleuritis. Arthritis Rheum., *5*:369–377, 1962.

230. Schroeter, A.L., Conn, D.L., and Jordon, R.E.: Immunoglobulin and complement deposition in skin of rheumatoid arthritis and systemic lupus erythematosus patients. Ann. Rheum. Dis., *35*:321–326, 1976.

231. Schwartz, M.L., et al.: The behavior of a newly described acute-phase protein in inflammatory joint disease. Inflammation, *1*:297–303, 1976.

232. Seignalet, J., et al.: HL-A antigens in rheumatoid arthritis. Vox Sang., *23*:468–471, 1972.

233. Selroos, O.: Thrombocytosis in rheumatoid arthritis. Scand. J. Rheumatol., *1*:136–140, 1972.

234. Short, C.L., Bauer, W., and Reynolds, W.E.: Red-cell, white-cell, and differential counts. *In* Rheumatoid Arthritis. Edited by C.L. Short, W. Bauer, and W.E. Reynolds. Cambridge, MA, Harvard University Press, 1957, pp. 349–356.

235. Short, C.L., Dienes, L., and Bauer, W.: Rheumatoid arthritis: a comparative evaluation of the commonly employed diagnostic tests. JAMA, *108*:2087–2091, 1937.

236. Silverman, H.A., et al.: Altered lymphocyte reactivity in rheumatoid arthritis. Arthritis Rheum., *19*:509–515, 1976.

237. Slavin, S., and Strober, S.: In vitro T cell mediated function in patients with active rheumatoid arthritis. Ann. Rheum. Dis., *40*:60–63, 1981.

238. Smit, J.W., et al.: The antiperinuclear factor: II. A light microscopical and immunofluorescence study on the antigenic substrate. Ann. Rheum. Dis., *39*:381–386, 1980.

239. Smith, A.F., and Castor, C.W.: Connective tissue activation. XII. Platelet abnormalities in patients with rheumatoid arthritis. J. Rheumatol., *5*:177–183, 1978.

240. Smyth, C.J., and Staub, A.: Catecholamine excretion in patients with rheumatoid arthritis. Arthritis Rheum., *7*:687–692, 1964.

241. Sølling, K., Sølling, J., and Rømer, F.K.: Free light chains of immunoglobulins in serum from patients with rheumatoid arthritis, sarcoidosis, chronic infectious and pulmonary cancer. Acta Med. Scand., *209*:473–477, 1981.

242. Sørensen, A.W.S.: Investigations of the kidney function in rheumatoid arthritis. II. Acta Rheumatol. Scand., *7*:138–144, 1961.

243. Sørensen, A.W.S.: The Waaler-Rose test in patients suffering from rheumatoid arthritis in relationship to 24-hour endogenous creatinine clearance. Acta Rheumatol. Scand., *7*:304–314, 1961.

244. Sørensen, A.W.S.: Investigation of the kidney function in rheumatoid arthritis. I. Acta Rheumatol. Scand., *6*:115–126, 1960.

245. Spagnuolo, M., and Feinstein, A.R.: Congestive heart failure and rheumatic activity in young patients with rheumatic heart disease. Pediatrics, *33*:653–660, 1964.

246. Stastny, P.: Mixed lymphocyte cultures in rheumatoid arthritis. J. Clin. Invest., *57*:1148–1157, 1976.

247. Steffen, C., et al.: Demonstration of lymphocytotoxins in rheumatoid arthritis in comparison with clinical course and other antibody activities. Z. Immunitaetsforsch., *145*:303–311, 1973.

248. Steinberg, V.L., and Wynn Parry, C.B.: Electromyographic changes in rheumatoid arthritis. Br. Med. J., *1*:630–632, 1961.

249. Strachan, A.F., and Johnson, P.M.: Protein SAP (serum amyloid P-component) in Waldenstrom's macroglobulinaemia, multiple myeloma and rheumatic disease. J. Clin. Lab. Immunol., *8*:153–156, 1982.

250. Stuart, F.S., et al.: Steroid biosynthetic and catabolic pathways in rheumatoid and non-rheumatoid chronic disease states. Clin. Res., *10*:237, 1962.

251. Sullivan, J.F., and Hart, K.T.: Serum benzidine oxidase. J. Lab. Clin. Med., *55*:260–267, 1960.

252. Sun, D.C.H., et al.: Upper gastrointestinal disease in rheumatoid arthritis. Am. J. Dig. Dis., *19*:405–410, 1974.

253. Swedlund, H.A., Hunder, G.G., and Gleich, G.H.: Alpha-1-antitrypsin in serum and synovial fluid in rheumatoid arthritis. Ann. Rheum. Dis., *33*:162–164, 1974.

254. Sylvester, R.A., and Pinals, R.S.: Eosinophilia in rheumatoid arthritis. Ann. Allergy, *28*:565–568, 1970.

255. Tannenbaum, H., and Schur, P.: The role of lymphocytes in rheumatic diseases. J. Rheumatol., *1*:392–412, 1974.

256. Thompson, R.A., and Asquith, P.: Quantitation of exocrine IgA in human serum in health and disease. Clin. Exp. Immunol., *7*:491–500, 1970.

257. Tiger, L.H., et al.: Liver enlargement demonstrated by scintigraphy in rheumatoid arthritis. J. Rheumatol., *3*:15–20, 1976.

258. Todesco, S.: Retinol-binding protein in rheumatoid arthritis. Arthritis Rheum., *24*:105–106, 1981.

259. Toumbis, A., et al.: Clinical and serological observations in patients with juvenile rheumatoid arthritis and their relatives. J. Pediatr., *62*:463–473, 1963.

260. Townes, A.S., Stewart, C.R., and Osler, A.G.: Immunologic studies in systemic lupus erythematosus. *In* Mechanisms of Cell and Tissue Damage Produced by Immune Reactions. Edited by Pierre Grabar and Peter Miescher. Basel, Benno Schwabe, 1961, pp. 315–325.

261. Trentham, D.E., et al.: Cellular sensitivity to collagen in rheumatoid arthritis. N. Engl. J. Med., *299*:327–332, 1978.

262. Unger, A., Panayi, G.S., and Lessof, M.H.: Carcinoembryonic antigen in rheumatoid arthritis. Lancet, *1*:781–783, 1974.

263. Van de Putte, L.B.A., et al.: Lymphocytes in rheumatoid and nonrheumatoid synovial fluids. Nonspecificity of high T cell and low B cell percentages. Ann. Rheum. Dis., *35*:451–455, 1976.

264. Vartio, T., et al.: Fibronectin in synovial fluid and tissue in rheumatoid arthritis. Eur. J. Clin. Invest., *11*:207–212, 1981.

265. Vaughan, J.H., Bayles, T.B., and Favour, C.B.: Serum complement in rheumatoid arthritis. Am. J. Med. Sci., *222*:186–192, 1951.

266. Vemireddi, N.K., Redford, J.B., and PombeJara, C.N.: Serial nerve conduction studies in carpal tunnel syndrome secondary to rheumatoid arthritis: preliminary study. Arch. Phys. Med. Rehabil., *60*:393–396, 1979.

267. Vesell, E.S., et al.: Isozymes of lactic dehydrogenase; their alterations in arthritic synovial fluid and sera. J. Clin. Invest., *41*:2012–2019, 1962.

268. Veys, E.M., and Claessens, H.E.: Serum levels of IgG, IgM and IgA in rheumatoid arthritis. Ann. Rheum. Dis., *27*:431–440, 1968.

269. Veys, E.M., et al.: Evaluation of T cell subsets with monoclonal antibodies in patients with rheumatoid arthritis. J. Rheumatol., *9*:25–29, 1982.

270. Waldenström, J., and Winblad, S.: Some observations on the relationship of certain serological reactions in various diseases with hypergammaglobulinemia. Acta Rheumatol. Scand., *4*:3–9, 1958.

271. Walsh, L., Davis, P., and McConkey, B.: Relationship between erythrocyte sedimentation rate and serum C-reactive protein in rheumatoid arthritis. Ann. Rheum. Dis., *38*:362–363, 1979.

272. Ward, H.P., Gordon, B., and Pickett, J.C.: Serum levels of erythropoietin in rheumatoid arthritis. J. Lab. Clin. Med., *74*:93–97, 1969.

273. Weaver, W.F., and Smyth, C.J.: Serum urate in degenerative joint disease and rheumatoid arthritis. Arthritis Rheum., *6*:372–376, 1963.

274. Webb, J., et al.: Liver disease in rheumatoid arthritis and Sjögren's syndrome: prospective study using biochemical and serological markers of hepatic dysfunction. Ann. Rheum. Dis., *34*:70–81, 1975.

275. Wedgewood, R.J.P., and Janeway, C.A.: Serum complement in children with "collagen diseases." Pediatrics, *11*:569–581, 1953.

276. Weinstein, I.M.: A correlative study of the erythrokinetics and disturbances in iron metabolism associated with the anemia of rheumatoid arthritis. Blood, *14*:950–966, 1959.

277. Weir, D.M., Holborow, E.J., and Johnson, G.D.: A clinical study of serum antinuclear factor. Br. Med. J., *1*:933–937, 1961.

278. Wells, R.M., and Johnson, E.W.: Study of conduction delay in median nerve of patients with rheumatoid arthritis. Arch. Phys. Med., *43*:244–248, 1962.

279. Wenger, M.E., and Bole, G.G.: Nitroblue tetrazolium dye reduction by peripheral leukocytes from rheumatoid arthritis and systemic lupus erythematosus patients measured by a histochemical and spectrophotometric method. J. Lab. Clin. Med., *82*:513–521, 1973.

280. Westergren, A.: Studies of the suspension stability of the blood in pulmonary tuberculosis. Acta Med. Scand., *54*:247–282, 1920.

281. Whaley, K., et al.: Liver disease in Sjögren's syndrome and rheumatoid arthritis. Lancet, *1*:861–863, 1970.

282. Whaley, K., Schur, P.H., and Ruddy, S.: C3b inactivator in the rheumatic diseases. Measurement by radial immunodiffusion and by inhibition formation of properdin pathway C3 convertase. J. Clin. Invest., *57*:1554–1563, 1976.

283. Wiik, A., Henriksen, K., and Faber, V.: Urinary excretion of granulocyte-specific antinuclear factors in rheumatoid arthritis. Acta Pathol. Microbiol. Scand. [C], *83*:273–279, 1975.

284. Wiik, A., and Munthe, E.: Complement-fixing granulocyte-specific antinuclear factors in neutropenic cases of rheumatoid arthritis. Immunol., *26*:1127–1134, 1974.

285. Wiik, A., and Permin, H.: The prevalence and possible significance of IgD granulocyte-specific antinuclear antibodies in neutropenic and non-neutropenic cases of rheumatoid arthritis. Acta Pathol. Microbiol. Scand. [C], *86*:19–22, 1978.

286. Wilkinson, P., et al.: The mechanism of hypoalbuminemia in rheumatoid arthritis. Ann. Intern. Med., *63*:109–114, 1965.

287. Winchester, R.J., et al.: Observations on the eosinophilia of certain patients with rheumatoid arthritis. Arthritis Rheum., *14*:650–665, 1971.

288. Wintrobe, M.M.: Clinical Hematology. 8th Ed. Philadelphia, Lea & Febiger, 1981, p. 331.

289. Wintrobe, M.M., and Landsberg, J.W.: A standardized technique for the blood sedimentation test. Am. J. Med. Sci., *189*:102–115, 1935.

290. Wood, J.W., et al.: Rheumatoid arthritis in Hiroshima and Nagasaki, Japan: Prevalence, incidence, and clinical characteristics. Arthritis Rheum., *10*:21–31, 1967.

291. Wood, P.: The erythrocyte sedimentation rate in diseases of the heart. Q. J. Med., *5*:1–19, 1936.

292. Wramner, T.: Electromyographic studies on the effect of neostigmine in rheumatoid arthritis. Acta Med. Scand., *242 (Suppl.)*:18–23, 1950.

293. Wyler, D.J.: Diagnostic implications of markedly elevated erythrocyte sedimentation rate: a reevaluation. South. Med. J., *70*:1428–1430, 1977.

294. Yates, D.A.H.: Muscular changes in rheumatoid arthritis. Ann. Rheum. Dis., *22*:342–347, 1963.

295. Young, B.J.J., et al.: Anti-keratin antibodies in rheumatoid arthritis. Br. Med. J., *2*:97–99, 1979.

296. Youssef, A.A.R., Wood, B., and Baron, D.N.: Serum copper: a marker of disease activity in rheumatoid arthritis. J. Clin. Pathol., *36*:14–17, 1983.

297. Zubler, R.H., et al.: Circulating and intra-articular immune complexes in patients with rheumatoid arthritis. Correlation of ^{125}I-C1q binding activity with clinical and biological features of the disease. J. Clin. Invest., *57*:1308–1319, 1976.

Chapter 41

Rheumatoid Factors

Mart Mannik

The term rheumatoid factor evolved from the observations of Waaler and Rose, who noted that a high proportion of serums from patients with rheumatoid arthritis (RA) agglutinated sheep erythrocytes sensitized with rabbit antibodies to erythrocytes.[12] Since then, the antibody nature of these factors has been proved, but the term "rheumatoid factors" has been retained. *Rheumatoid factors are now defined as antibodies specific to antigenic determinants on the Fc fragments of human or animal immunoglobulin G.* A number of antibodies to other antigenic determinants on immunoglobulins are known and are collectively referred to as the family of antiglobulins. These antiglobulins include antibodies specific to IgG digested by pepsin or by other enzymes, antibodies to light chains, and antibodies to IgA, IgM, and IgE. These antiglobulins are not considered rheumatoid factors because they are not directed to antigenic determinants on the Fc fragments of IgG.

Rheumatoid factors commonly exist in the three major classes of immunoglobulins and possess specificities to several antigenic determinants. The general concepts of antibody structure and function (see Chap. 15) apply to rheumatoid factors and therefore are not considered in this chapter. Seropositivity of patients with RA or with other diseases is usually defined by the latex fixation test or the red cell agglutination tests. These assays primarily reflect the presence of IgM-rheumatoid factors (IgM-RFs). The presence of rheumatoid factors is not unique to RA, and a positive test for these antibodies should not be used as the sole criterion for the diagnosis of RA.

SPECIFICITY OF RHEUMATOID FACTORS

Like any other antibodies, rheumatoid factors have specificity to defined antigenic determinants, some of which are identified on human and animal IgG molecules. Serologic and biochemical studies on human IgG have identified several antigenic determinants for IgM-RFs. These determinants may be either genetic or nongenetic. The genetic determinants on Fc fragments are the Gm antigens of IgG or closely related antigens. The nongenetic determinants exist on certain subclasses of IgG in

all persons. Thus, in a given patient, IgM-RFs may react with autologous IgG on the basis of genetic or nongenetic antigenic determinants. In some patients, the specificity is directed to genetic determinants on homologous (other human) IgG, to heterologous (animal) IgG, or to both human and animal IgG. Finally, specificity of IgM-RFs to denatured or aggregated IgG has been considered, but the issue remains controversial.

In patients with RA, IgM-RFs exist with specificity to Gm(a), also called Gm1, and to a number of other Gm antigenic determinants. The specificities of other IgM-RFs are defined to the so-called "nonmarkers," which are antigenic determinants absent from IgG molecules with a given Gm antigen, but present in other IgG molecules of the same subclass of IgG, as well as in some of the other subclasses of IgG. For example, the antigenic determinant "non-a" is absent from Gm(a)-positive IgG1 molecules, but present on IgG1 molecules positive for Gm(f), also called Gm4, as well as on IgG2 and IgG3 molecules.[31] Furthermore, some rheumatoid factors are specific to antigens common to several subclasses of IgG, regardless of genetic types. One particular antigenic determinant of this type is called the Ga antigen,[5] which constitutes a frequent antigenic determinant for IgM-RFs.

Hemagglutination inhibition experiments on IgM-RFs with carefully defined specificities have permitted localization of the various antigenic determinants on the regions of the Fc fragments of IgG subclasses,[30] as depicted schematically in Figure 41–1. The isolation of the Cγ3 domain facilitated these studies in that this IgG fragment inhibited agglutinations of known specificities. Because the Cγ2 domain was not available as an isolated preparation, but only on intact Fc fragments, the direct localization of antigenic determinants on this domain was not achieved and must remain as a deduction.

The IgM-RFs react with several different antigenic determinants on each of the subclasses of IgG, some of which determinants are found on the third (Cγ3) region of constant homology of the heavy chains of these molecules, whereas other antigenic determinants may be found on the second

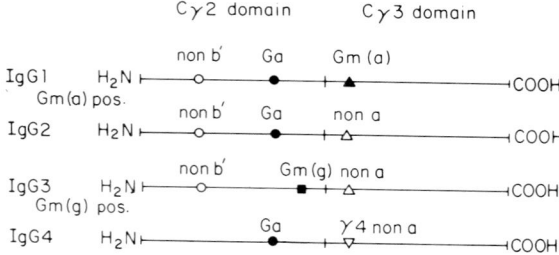

Fig. 41–1. Schematic representation of the antigenic determinants for IgM rheumatoid factors (IgM-RFs) on the second (Cγ2) and third (Cγ3) homology regions of the four subclasses of IgG. The second and third homology regions constitute the Fc fragment of an IgG molecule, as schematically depicted. The Gm(a) or Gm1-positive IgG1 molecules do not possess the "non-a" antigenic determinant, whereas the Gm(f)- or Gm4-positive IgG1 molecules have the "non-a" antigenic determinant. The Gm(g)- or Gm21-positive IgG3 molecules have the "non-b'''" antigenic determinant, whereas the Gm(b')- or Gm21-positive IgG3 molecules lack the "non-b'''" antigenic determinant. (Modified from Natvig, J.B., et al.[30])

(Cγ2) region of constant homology or may require the intact Fc fragments for their expression. A given patient may have several IgM-RFs directed to different antigenic determinants. At this time, no information is available on the way in which IgM-RFs with different specificities relate to the disease processes or to outcome.

Because IgM-RFs react better with aggregated IgG or with immune complexes than with monomeric IgG in agglutinating or precipitating test systems, the question of unique antigenic determinants on aggregated IgG or on immune complexes containing IgG has been raised. Monomeric IgG molecules with appropriate antigenic determinants react with IgM-RFs, but with low association constants. The best explanation for the increased reactivity of aggregated IgG or of immune complexes containing IgG is the polyvalency of the molecular aggregates with respect to IgM-RFs.

IgM-RFs may react with IgG from heterologous sources. For example, some IgM-RFs are specific for rabbit IgG and fail to react with human IgG, whereas others react with both.[12]

The possible heterogeneity of rheumatoid factors of the immunoglobulin G class (IgG-RFs) has not been fully examined. These antibodies react with the Fc fragments of IgG, as do all other rheumatoid factors. In one system, the antigenic determinants for the IgG-RF are present on the intact human or rabbit Fc fragments of IgG, but not on the fragments (pFc′ and Fc′) that represent the Cγ3 domain.[28] Furthermore, available evidence indicates that these antigenic determinants are located in the

area between the Cγ2 and Cγ3 domains,[27] that is, the same region of the IgG molecule that interacts effectively with the staphylococcal protein A.

The specificity of one rheumatoid factor of the immunoglobulin A class (IgA-RF) from a patient with hypergammaglobulinemic purpura is well known.[1] Because this monoclonal IgA-RF reacts with the IgG1, IgG2, and IgG4 subclasses, the antigenic determinant may well be the Ga antigen. Some rheumatoid factors that clearly react with the Fc fragments of human IgG also cross-react with DNA-histone.[2] The immunochemical basis of this cross-reactivity remains to be determined.

INTERACTIONS BETWEEN RHEUMATOID FACTORS AND THEIR ANTIGENS

On a structural basis, the valence of IgM-RFs for IgG molecules should be ten because each of the five subunits of IgM molecules possesses two binding sites (two pairs of one μ and one light chain). On analytic ultracentrifugation, however, the valence of IgM-RFs for interaction with IgG is five, and the valence of each IgM subunit is one. On the other hand, the Fab fragments obtained from purified IgM-RFs have antibody activity and a valence of one.[10,41] Therefore, in each of the five subunits of these molecules, one antibody-combining site must be sterically hindered from combining with an IgG molecule. The reasons for this phenomenon are not known. The functional antigenic valence of IgG molecules for examined interaction with IgM-RF is one, even though two gamma chains are present in each IgG molecule and the valence in respect to each antigenic determinant should be two.

The association constants for the interaction of IgM-RFs and monomeric IgG are around 10^5 L/mol.[33] Similar values exist for the interaction of IgM-RFs with specificities to known antigenic determinants on the Cγ3 domain (see Fig. 41–1), when examined with the isolated portions of IgG molecules.[40] Furthermore, the interactions of IgG myeloma proteins of several subclasses with IgM-RFs show comparable association constants for IgG1, IgG2, and IgG4, but no reaction occurs with IgG3 myeloma proteins,[34] suggesting the specificity of the used RFs is to the Ga antigen (see Fig. 41–1). The interactions of IgM-RFs with the antigenic determinants on Fc fragments of IgG are therefore weak antigen-antibody bonds.

A series of experiments has elucidated the reasons for enhanced agglutination and precipitation of IgM-RFs with aggregated IgG. First, the Fab fragments derived from IgM-RFs bind to monomeric and to heat-aggregated IgG with comparable association constants; this finding indicates that the aggregated IgG does not contain "new and better" antigenic determinants. Second, the intact IgM-RFs bind to aggregated IgG about 10^6 times more effectively than the Fab fragments from IgM-RFs.[13] These findings support the concept that the enhanced agglutination and precipitation of IgM-RFs with aggregated or polymerized IgG is due to the polyvalency of the IgG and not to the generation of new antigenic determinants on aggregated IgG molecules.

Because patients with RA may have abundant IgM-RFs reactive with autologous IgG, they may have demonstrable antigen-antibody complexes formed by these reactants.[15] These complexes sediment on analytical ultracentrifugation with 22 Svedberg units and are termed *"22S" complexes* (Figs. 41–2 and 41–3). In this interaction, each IgM-RF molecule has a valence of 5, and IgG has a valence of 1. Therefore, each IgM-RF molecule can maximally bind five IgG molecules. In serum of patients with RA, however, the 22S complex may not contain five IgG molecules because, with the binding of 5 IgG molecules to 1 IgM-RF, the sedimentation constant would be much higher.[29] The 22S complexes usually occur in patients with high titers of IgM-RFs, but a pathogenic role for these complexes is not established.

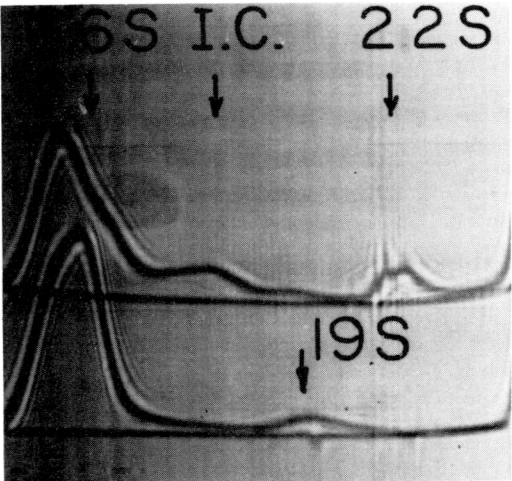

Fig. 41–2. Schlieren optical patterns of serum from a patient with rheumatoid arthritis on sedimentation velocity ultracentrifugation, illustrating the 22S and intermediate complexes. The serum was diluted 1:3 in top pattern at neutral pH (0.05 *M* phosphate, 0.15 *M* NaCl, pH 7.3) and 1:3 in bottom pattern at acid pH (0.05 *M* acetate, 0.15 *M* NaCl, pH 3.5). The photographs were taken 24 minutes after reaching 52,000 rpm. At neutral pH in the top pattern, 22S complexes and intermediate complexes (I.C.) are present. At acid pH in the bottom pattern, both immune complexes are dissociated, and the 19 and 6.6S peaks have increased.

The valence of IgG-RFs is 2 for interaction with normal IgG molecules.[37] On analytic ultracentrifugation, the serum of some patients with RA shows detectable quantities of the so-called *intermediate complexes* (see Fig. 41–2), sedimenting between 7 and 19S components of normal serum, as first demonstrated by Kunkel et al.[20] These immune complexes contain IgG-RFs. Comparable and larger immune complexes exist in the synovial fluids of patients with RA. The isolated IgG-RFs self-associate and form stable dimers of two IgG-RF, provided the antibody specificity of these molecules is directed to antigenic determinants present on the same molecules.[36,37] In this dimer formation, the antibody-combining sites of each IgG-RF molecule react with the Fc fragment of the other IgG-RF molecule, thus forming two antigen-antibody bonds per dimer (Fig. 41–4). At the same time, two antibody-combining sites remain free, and antigenic determinants must be available in each dimer to allow the observed, further-concentration-dependent aggregation of the dimers, forming tetramers, octamers, and higher polymers (see Fig. 41–4) of the IgG-RFs.[36,37]

The valence of normal IgG for interaction with IgG-RF is one, even though the valence of the Fc fragments from normal IgG or from IgG-RF is two, as expected from the presence of two polypeptide chains. Therefore, the second antigenic determinant in intact normal IgG is not available for interaction with IgG-RF, presumably because of distortion of the molecule caused by the interaction with IgG-RF.[28] In the *self-association* of IgG-RFs, the antigenic valence of the molecules has not been examined directly, but it must be two because the self-association would otherwise terminate at dimer formation and would not proceed to the formation of higher polymers.

The association constant for the interaction of IgG-RFs with normal IgG, with normal Fc fragments, and with Fc fragments derived from IgG-RF is about 10^5 L/mol.[28,36] The association constant for dimer formation of self-associating IgG-RF has not been measured directly, but by calculation it is 10^{10} L/mol.[37] This value is probably too high because energy is lost in the ring closure of dimer formation. The observed stability of the dimers is based on this high association constant because, as stated previously, unique antigenic determinants do not exist on the Fc fragments of IgG-RF. The observed association constant for further polymer formation from the IgG-RF dimers is about 10^5 L/mol.[36] The self-associating IgG-RFs thus constitute unique antibodies in that immune complexes are formed without a separate antigen molecule because these antibodies fulfill the functions both of an antibody and of an antigen.

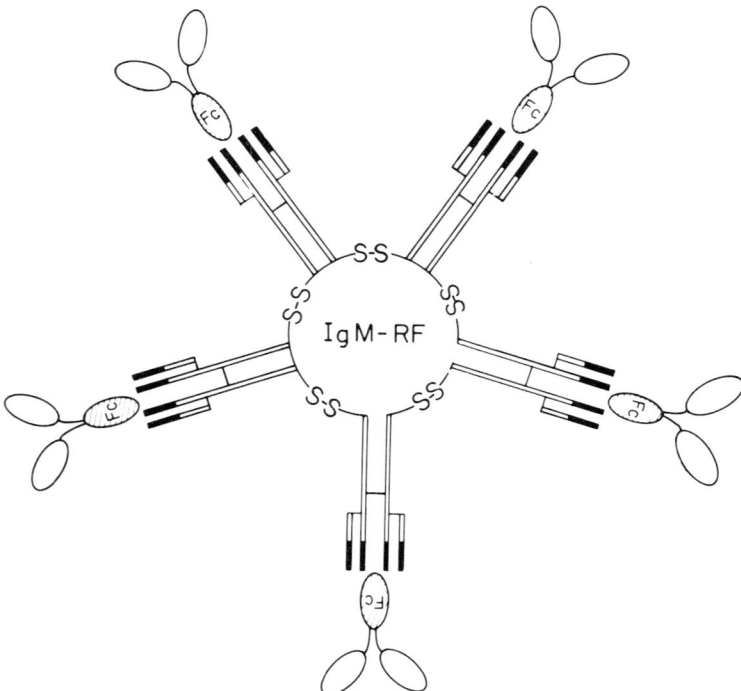

Fig. 41–3. Schematic representation of the 22S immune complex between an IgM-rheumatoid factor (IgM-RF) molecule and IgG molecules. Each IgM-RF reacts maximally with five IgG molecules, as depicted. The complexes that exist in serum most likely contain fewer than five IgG molecules.

As already discussed, the antigenic valence of normal IgG is one for the interaction with IgG-RFs. Therefore, the presence of large amounts of normal IgG in serum would terminate further polymer formation of self-associating IgG-RFs. In this termination, two normal IgG-RF molecules maximally interact with one IgG-RF dimer (see Fig. 41–4,B). This reaction is consistent with the finding of intermediate complexes in serum (see Fig. 41–2). In synovial fluids of patients with RA, larger complexes exist.[17,46] Furthermore, plasma cells in synovial tissue synthesize IgG-RFs,[14,32] and in the immediate vicinity of these cells, the concentration of IgG-RFs may be even higher than in synovial fluid. Isolated IgG-RFs precipitate from solution when concentrated at neutral pH beyond about 1.0 to 1.5 mg/ml.[9,37] Finally, the self-association of IgG-RFs occurs in the plasma cells in synovial tissues because the cytoplasm of these plasma cells binds human complement components.[32]

IgG-RFs are synthesized in the synovial tissue of patients with RA,[14] and no exogenous antigens can be identified in the immune complexes in synovial fluids of patients with this disease.[21,45,46] Thus, the self-associated IgG-RFs may contribute to the synovitis of RA (see Chap. 35). The MRL/1 mice that develop a synovitis similar to that of RA

also have self-associating IgG-RFs in their circulation[25] (see Chap. 24).

The interactions of IgA-RFs with IgG have not been examined extensively, but detailed studies of a monoclonal IgA-RF show an association constant of 1.6×10^6 L/mol.[1]

BIOLOGIC PROPERTIES OF RHEUMATOID FACTORS

The high prevalence of rheumatoid factors in many chronic infections and in aging normal persons raises the question of the central role of these antibodies. Answers to this question have been sought by studies on activation of complement systems, generation of chemotaxis, promotion of phagocytosis, and interaction with cell receptors by rheumatoid factors.

The evaluation of biologic properties of IgM-RFs has been difficult because IgG, as antigen for these antibodies, possesses its own biologic properties, particularly when aggregated nonspecifically or when complexed with antigen to serve as a polyvalent antigen for IgM-RFs. Experiments have shown, however, that IgM-RFs activate complement. Heat-aggregated human IgG, prepared from reduced and alkylated preparations, does not fix human complement, but is an effective polyvalent antigen for IgM-RFs. When IgM-RFs are

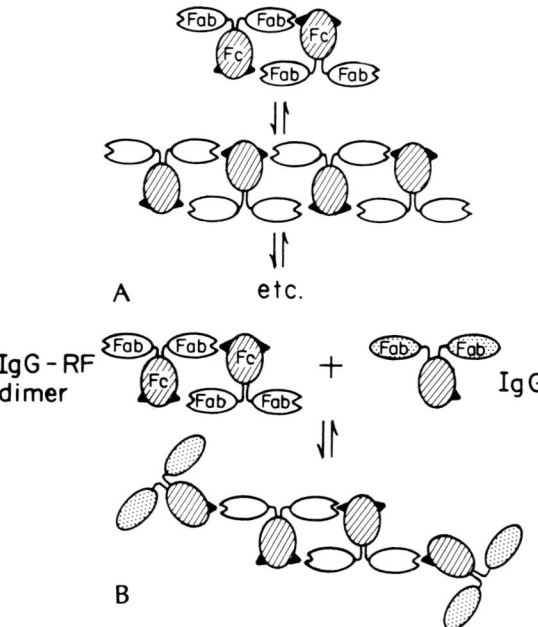

Fig. 41–4. Schematic representation of the self-association and further polymerization of IgG rheumatoid factors (IgG-RF). *A*, The formation of IgG-RF dimers is depicted. These dimers undergo concentration-dependent polymerization to tetramers, octamers, and higher polymers, owing to free antigenic determinants and free antibody-combining sites. *B*, the possible interaction of normal IgG molecules with the self-associated IgG-RF dimers is depicted. The dimers are stable in presence of excess normal IgG because two antigen-antibody bonds are formed in dimerization. Because the association constants for further polymerization are comparable to the association constant for normal IgG binding to one antibody-combining site, the presence of excess normal IgG terminates the further polymerization of the dimers, particularly because normal IgG is monovalent for interaction with IgG-RFs.

added to these aggregates, human complement is then consumed. The addition of IgM-RFs to sheep erythrocytes, sparsely sensitized with rabbit IgG antibodies, enhances complement fixation and cell lysis. Furthermore, the addition of IgM-RFs to soluble immune complexes containing IgG enhances complement fixation by these materials. Finally, red blood cells coated with aggregated human IgG, prepared from reduced and alkylated IgG or sensitized with reduced and alkylated rabbit antibodies, are lysed by the addition of IgM-RFs and human complement.[42] All these studies indicate that IgM-RFs can activate the classic complement pathway. Complement activation, in turn, explains the enhanced chemotaxis when IgM-RFs are added

to aggregated IgG or to antigen-antibody complexes.

On interaction with antigen on the surface of erythrocytes, IgG-RFs activate human complement, but less efficiently than IgM-RFs in a similar system.[38] In addition, self-associating IgG-RFs in fluid phase also activate human complement, but less efficiently than other immune complexes.[7] IgG-RF-containing immune complexes from the synovial fluid of patients bind C1q and activate complement.[45] Thus, the available evidence indicates that IgG-RFs and self-associating IgG-RFs can activate complement and may thus contribute to the synovitis of RA.

The binding of IgM-RFs to immune complexes containing IgG molecules may diminish the interaction of these complexes with Fc receptors on phagocytic cells. Similarly, the binding of IgM-RFs to cells sensitized with IgG molecules may decrease the binding of these cells to phagocytes because phagocytes do not possess IgM receptors. For example, the addition of IgM-RFs to bacteria coated with an IgG class of antibodies decreases phagocytosis of these bacteria by polymorphonuclear leukocytes in the absence of complement.[23] By a comparable mechanism, IgM-RFs have blocked the killing of target cells sensitized with IgG class of antibodies by antibody-dependent, cell-mediated cytotoxicity (ADCC). In this study, the IgM-RFs bound to the IgG molecules on target cells abrogated the reaction of IgG molecules with the Fc receptor on the killer cells.[11]

The pathophysiologic significance of some of these reactions remains uncertain. The inhibition of phagocytosis of antibody-coated bacteria by IgM-RFs may predispose patients to bacterial infections. On the other hand, the addition of IgM-RFs to antibody-coated viral particles in the presence of complement enhances the neutralization of viruses.[35]

The self-associated IgG-RFs interact with human monocytes and enhance the release of prostaglandins and a mononuclear cell factor (see Chap. 37). This factor, thought to be identical to interleukin-1, in turn acts on synovial cells in culture to increase the release of prostaglandins and collagenase.[24] Thus, these unique antibodies can contribute to the inflammatory and destructive events in synovitis. This process is likely to occur in the synovial tissue in which these antibodies are released from plasma cells and self-associate into large polymers or precipitates because of the low ambient concentration of normal IgG. In contrast, the self-association of IgG-RFs may be harmless in the plasma because the formation of high polymers is terminated by normal IgG, as explained in the preceding section. Finally, the self-associated IgG-RFs may serve as a polyvalent ligand for IgM-RFs and may thus contribute further to the inflammatory process in rheumatoid synovitis.

DETECTION OF RHEUMATOID FACTORS

Many methods have been proposed for the detection of rheumatoid factors, but few are widely employed. The purpose of this section is to consider the general principles of these methods and to discuss the nature of the rheumatoid factors detected by some of the available techniques. The details of the various methods can be found in the original articles or in works concerned with the conduct of these tests.[12,16]

The most widely used methods for detection of rheumatoid factors rely on agglutination or flocculation of IgG-coated cells or particles as the end point of the test procedure. Owing to the polyvalence of IgM-RFs, these tests emphasize the presence of IgM-RFs.

The latex test is the most common method for detection of rheumatoid factors. The bentonite flocculation test, the sensitized sheep-cell test, and the sensitized human-D-cell agglutination test have been popular in certain centers. The latex test and the bentonite flocculation test use human IgG for sensitization of the test particles. For optimal results, the IgG preparations, usually Cohn fraction II, must contain some aggregated material. The coated test particles are then agglutinated or flocculated when they are linked together by IgM-RFs. The positivity of the result is expressed as a titer, following twofold serial dilution of the tested serum. As with any agglutination test, the end point can be only approximated reliably within a dilution above or below the observed end point. Therefore, these tests are not truly quantitative. Because of the use of pooled IgG, IgM-RFs of many specificities are measured. Furthermore, these tests are not standardized from laboratory to laboratory, even though the possibilities of standardization have been debated.[18,39] Variations in the size and characteristics of latex particles cause the test results to vary. Another variable in the test system is the degree of aggregation of IgG among Cohn Fraction II preparations. Low titers of false positivity result if the tested serum is not heat inactivated because C1q may cause agglutination of sensitized or unsensitized particles.

The sensitized sheep cell agglutination test for rheumatoid factors is based on the interaction of rheumatoid factors with rabbit IgG on the red blood cell. The erythrocytes are sensitized with subagglutinating doses of the rabbit antiserum to sheep erythrocytes. Heterophile antibodies must be removed from the test serum prior to testing for rheumatoid factors. This test is less sensitive than the latex and bentonite flocculation tests for rheumatoid factors but it is more specific for RA. This test detects primarily IgM-RF, for reasons already mentioned, and does not detect rheumatoid factors specific only to antigenic determinants of human IgG.

The sensitized human-D-cell agglutination test requires human red cells, preferably homozygous D cells, and carefully selected human antibodies to D cells. This test detects IgM-RFs that react with human IgG. The selection of the human serum with antibodies to D cells is critical. When antibodies to D cells are limited to a subclass of IgG (see Fig. 41–1), rheumatoid factors with limited specificity may be detected by this method.

None of the foregoing tests for rheumatoid factors are standardized among clinical laboratories. Many additional variations and modifications of these tests have been proposed. The reader interested in these tests should consult the section on rheumatoid factors in the "Rheumatism Reviews," published every two years in the journal *Arthritis and Rheumatism*.

In some patients with RA, the routine agglutination tests for rheumatoid factors are negative because of firm binding of autologous IgG to the IgM-RFs. When such serum is submitted to gel filtration under mildly acidic conditions (pH 4.0) to dissociate the IgM-RFs from IgG, rheumatoid factor activity is found in the IgM-containing fractions.[5] Because rheumatoid factor is not detected in unseparated serum, the term *"hidden rheumatoid factor"* was coined. IgM-RFs are thus detected in some seronegative adults with RA and in some seronegative children with juvenile RA.

IgM-RFs can also be detected and quantified by nephelometric methods. The real advantages are that quantitative information is obtained and the assay is quickly completed and can be automated. This approach, however, has not replaced the inaccurate agglutination tests.

To detect and to quantify rheumatoid factors in the major classes of immunoglobulins, that is, IgG-RFs, IgM-RFs, and IgA-RFs, several solid-phase assays have been developed and tried. The basic principles of all these methods are comparable. IgG of human or animal origin is adsorbed to a test tube, is covalently linked to a solid matrix, or is solidified by chemical cross-linking. The adsorption to test tubes or microtiter plates is most frequently employed. Once the solid-phase IgG is prepared and washed, test serum is incubated with it to allow binding of all rheumatoid factors. Thereafter, the solid-phase test system is washed to remove all unbound serum proteins. The bound rheumatoid factors are then quantified by the addition of specific antiserums to IgG, IgM, or IgA, to measure the presence of IgG-RFs, IgM-RFs, or IgA-RFs, respectively. The quantitation can be accomplished by several approaches, such as by employing radiolabeled specific antibodies (radioimmunoassay) or by using enzyme-linked specific antibodies (ELISA assay). Another approach is to elute the bound rheumatoid factors, followed by quantitation of the recovered materials. This approach, however, has been fraught with problems and has been replaced by ELISA or radioimmunoassay.

Several problems are inherent in the techniques used for quantitifying rheumatoid factors with solid-phase methods. The IgG bound to solid phase is prone to nonspecific adsorption of other IgG molecules and immune aggregates.[26] In addition, the washing steps used to remove the unbound serum proteins may well dissociate and discard rheumatoid factors with low association constants that were bound to the solidified IgG. As described previously, all rheumatoid factors have low association constants to monomeric IgG, and only IgM-RFs bind with strong affinity to aggregated IgG. As a consequence, only a small fraction of IgG-RFs and a higher proportion of IgM-RFs remain bound to the solid-phase IgG. This problem can be overcome in part by employing isolated IgG-RF, IgM-RF, and IgA-RF as standards, thus calculating from the bound rheumatoid factors the actual amount of rheumatoid factors present in the tested specimen. This approach assumes that all rheumatoid factors in the test serum bind to the solid-phase IgG in a manner comparable to that of the employed standard preparation. In spite of the various problems, the solid-phase assays do provide quantitative measurements.

The quantitation of rheumatoid factors by these solid-phase assays has yielded new information and should provide even more insights. A few examples from the literature are illustrative: The serum of patients with RA who were categorized as seropositive or seronegative by the routine agglutination tests contained IgM-RFs, but the concentrations in the seropositive group were higher than in the seronegative group, and both groups had significantly higher levels of IgM-RFs than the control group.[19] The level of IgG-RFs was higher than the level of IgM-RFs, expressed in mg/ml.[44] The presence of high levels of IgG-RFs was associated with active disease in patients with RA.[4] In patients with RA treated with d-penicillamine, the IgM-RF concentration declined, whereas the concentration of IgG-RF did not change.[43] Obviously, such quantitative studies of the concentrations of rheumatoid factors during the course of the disease and during therapeutic interventions might provide additional useful insights.

These quantitative studies are also useful for the study of production of IgM-RFs on a cellular level. For example, B cells from the blood of patients with rheumatoid factors synthesize IgM-RFs. B cells from these patients can be further stimulated with pokeweed mitogen to synthesize even more IgM-RFs per cell.[3,9]

Rheumatoid factors in low titers are found in small percentages of young adults, but the prevalence of positive tests for rheumatoid factors increases with age. A high prevalence of rheumatoid factors is also found in persons with certain infections, such as infective endocarditis, syphilis, schistosomiasis, tuberculosis, and leprosy, and transiently in persons following extensive immunizations. These observations have suggested that extensive or persistent exposure to antigens and immune-complex formation induces the synthesis of rheumatoid factors. In several lung diseases, including idiopathic fibrosis, silicosis, and asbestosis, the prevalence of rheumatoid factors is also increased. The prevalence of rheumatoid factors in various disorders was reviewed by Bartfeld in 1969.[6] IgM-RFs constitute an essential ingredient of mixed cryoglobulins, and their presence is related to the pathogenesis of the disease.[22] Furthermore, IgG-RFs are an essential component in the serum protein abnormalities of hypergammaglobulinemic purpura[8] (see Chap. 67). *Thus, a positive test for rheumatoid factors should not be used as the sole criterion for the diagnosis of RA.*

Many questions remain to be answered about the significance of rheumatoid factors in apparently normal persons and in patients with diverse disorders. Above all, we still do not know why patients with RA develop these antibodies. Hypotheses for the development of rheumatoid factors include the stimulation of synthesis by immune complexes, polyclonal B-cell activation, and infection of B cells by the Epstein-Barr virus.[9] Evidence for the role of rheumatoid factors in maintaining the chronicity of the disease, however, is mounting.

REFERENCES

1. Abraham, G.N., Clark, R.A., and Vaughan, J.H.: Characterization of an IgA rheumatoid factor: binding properties and reactivity with the subclasses of human γG globulin. Immunochemistry, 9:301–315, 1972.
2. Agnello, V., et al.: Evidence for a subset of rheumatoid factors that cross-react with DNA-histone and have a distinct cross-idiotype. J. Exp. Med., *151*:1514–1527, 1980.
3. Alarcón, G.S., Koopman, W.J., and Schrohenloher, R.E.: Differential patterns of in vitro IgM rheumatoid factor synthesis in seronegative and seropositive rheumatoid arthritis. Arthritis Rheum., 25:150–155, 1982.
4. Allen, C., et al.: IgG antiglobulins in rheumatoid arthritis and other arthritides: relationship with clinical features and other parameters. Ann. Rheum. Dis., 40:127–131, 1981.
5. Allen, J.C., and Kunkel, H.G.: Hidden rheumatoid factors with specificity for native γ globulins. Arthritis Rheum., 9:758–768, 1966.

6. Bartfeld, H.: Distribution of rheumatoid factor activity in non-rheumatoid states. Ann. N.Y. Acad. Sci., *168*:30–38, 1969.

7. Brown, P.B., Nardella, F.A., and Mannik, M.: Human complement activation by self-associated IgG rheumatoid factors. Arthritis Rheum., *25*:1101–1107, 1982.

8. Capra, J.D., Winchester, R.J., and Kunkel, H.G.: Hypergammaglobulinemic purpura. Studies on the unusual anti-γ-globulins characteristic of the sera of these patients. Medicine, *50*:125–138, 1971.

9. Carson, D.A., et al.: Physiology and pathology of rheumatoid factors. Springer Semin. Immunopathol., *4*:161–179, 1981.

10. Chavin, S.I., and Franklin, E.C.: Studies on antigen-binding activity of macroglobulin antibody subunits and their enzymatic fragments. J. Biol. Chem., *244*:1345–1352, 1969.

11. Diaz-Jouanen, E., et al.: Serum and synovial fluid inhibitors of antibody-mediated lymphocytotoxicity in rheumatoid arthritis and systemic lupus erythematosus. Arthritis Rheum., *19*:142–149, 1976.

12. Egeland, T., and Munthe, E.: Rheumatoid factors. Clin. Rheum. Dis., *9*:135–160, 1983.

13. Eisenberg, R.: The specificity and polyvalency of binding of a monoclonal rheumatoid factor. Immunochemistry, *13*:355–359, 1976.

14. Fehr, K., et al.: Production of agglutinators and rheumatoid factors in plasma cells of rheumatoid and nonrheumatoid synovial tissues. Arthritis Rheum., *24*:510–519, 1981.

15. Franklin, E.C., et al.: An unusual protein component of high molecular weight in the serum of certain patients with rheumatoid arthritis. J. Exp. Med., *105*:425–438, 1957.

16. Froelich, C.J., and Williams, R.C., Jr.: Tests for detection of rheumatoid factors. *In* Manual of Clinical Immunology. 2nd Ed. Edited by N.R. Rose and H. Friedman. Washington, D.C., American Society of Microbiology, 1980.

17. Halla, J.T., Volanakis, J.E., and Schrohenloher, R.E.: Immune complexes in rheumatoid arthritis sera and synovial fluids. Arthritis Rheum., *22*:440–448, 1979.

18. Klein, F., Valkenburg, H.A., and Cats, A.: On standardization of the latex fixation test. Bull. Rheum. Dis., *26*:866–868, 1976.

19. Koopman, W.J., and Schrohenloher, R.E.: A sensitive radioimmunoassay for quantitation of IgM rheumatoid factor. Arthritis Rheum., *23*:302–308, 1980.

20. Kunkel, H.G., et al.: Gamma globulin complexes in rheumatoid arthritis and certain other conditions. J. Clin. Invest., *40*:117–129, 1961.

21. Male, D., Roitt, I.M., and Hay, F.C.: Analysis of immune complexes in synovial effusions of patients with rheumatoid arthritis. Clin. Exp. Immunol., *39*:297–306, 1980.

22. Meltzer, M., et al.: Cryoglobulinemia—a clinical and laboratory study. II. Cryoglobulins with rheumatoid factor activity. Am. J. Med., *40*:837–856, 1966.

23. Messner, R.P., et al.: Serum opsonin, bacteria, and polymorphonuclear leukocyte interactions in subacute bacterial endocarditis. Anti-γ-globulin factors and their interaction with specific opsonins. J. Clin. Invest., *47*:1109–1120, 1968.

24. Nardella, F.A., et al.: Self-associating IgG rheumatoid factors stimulate monocytes to release prostaglandins and mononuclear cell factor that stimulates collagenase and prostaglandin production by synovial cells. Rheumatol. Int., *3*:183–186, 1983.

25. Nardella, F.A., et al.: Self-associating IgG-rheumatoid factors in MRL/1 autoimmune mice. Arthritis Rheum. In press, 1984.

26. Nardella, F.A., and Mannik, M.: Nonimmunospecific protein-protein interactions of IgG: studies of the binding of

27. Nardella, F.A., Teller, D.C., and Mannik, M.: Histidine involvement in the antigenic site for self-association of IgG-rheumatoid factor. (Abstract.) Arthritis Rheum., *25*:S60, 1982.

28. Nardella, F.A., Teller, D.C., and Mannik, M.: Studies on the antigenic determinants in the self-association of IgG rheumatoid factor. J. Exp. Med., *154*:112–125, 1981.

29. Nardella, F.A., Teller, D.C., and Mannik, M.: Interaction of IgM rheumatoid factor (IgM-RF) with normal IgG (IgG) and IgG-rheumatoid factor (IgG-RF). (Abstract.) Fourth Int. Congress Immunol., *18*:5–13, 1980.

30. Natvig, J.B., Gaarder, P.J., and Turner, M.W.: IgG antigens of the Cγ2 and Cγ3 homology regions interacting with rheumatoid factors. Clin. Exp. Immunol., *12*;177–184, 1972.

31. Natvig, J.B., and Kunkel, H.G.: Human immunoglobulins: classes, subclasses, genetic variants, and idiotypes. Adv. Immunol., *16*:1–59, 1973.

32. Natvig, J.B., and Munthe, E.: Self-associating IgG rheumatoid factor represents a major response of plasma cells in rheumatoid inflammatory tissue. Ann. N.Y. Acad. Sci., *256*:88–95, 1975.

33. Normansell, D.E.: Anti-γ-globulins in rheumatoid arthritis sera. I. Studies on the 22S complex. Immunochemistry, *1*:787–797, 1970.

34. Normansell, D.E., and Young, C.W., Jr.: The IgG subclass specificity of antiIgG immunoglobulin rheumatoid factors. Immunochemistry, *12*:187–188, 1975.

35. Notkins, A.L.: Infectious virus-antibody complexes: interaction with anti-immunoglobulins, complement and rheumatoid factor. J. Exp. Med., *134*:41S-51S, 1971.

36. Pope, R.M., Teller, D.C., and Mannik, M.: The molecular basis of self-association of IgG-rheumatoid factors. J. Immunol., *115*:365–373, 1975.

37. Pope, R.M., Teller, D.C., and Mannik, M.: The molecular basis of self-association of antibodies to IgG (rheumatoid factors) in rheumatoid arthritis. Proc. Natl. Acad. Sci. U.S.A., *71*:517-521, 1974.

38. Sabharwal, U.K., et al.: Activation of the classical pathway of complement by rheumatoid factors. Assessment by radioimmunoassay for C4. Arthritis Rheum., *25*:161–167, 1982.

39. Singer, J.M.: Standardization of the latex test for rheumatoid arthritis serology. Bull. Rheum. Dis., *24*:762–769, 1974.

40. Steward, M.W., Turner, M.W., and Natvig, J.B.: The binding affinities of rheumatoid factors interacting with the Cγ3 homology region of human IgG. Clin. Exp. Immunol., *15*:145–152, 1973.

41. Stone, J.M., and Metzger, H.: Binding properties of a Waldenström macroglobulin antibody. J. Biol. Chem., *243*:5977–5984, 1968.

42. Tanimoto, K., et al.: Complement fixation by rheumatoid factor. J. Clin. Invest., *55*:437–445, 1975.

43. Wernick, R., et al.: IgG and IgM rheumatoid factors in rheumatoid arthritis. Quantitative response to penicillamine therapy and relationship to disease activity. Arthritis Rheum., *26*:593–598, 1983.

44. Wernick, R., et al.: Serum IgG and IgM rheumatoid factors by solid phase radioimmunoassay. Arthritis Rheum., *24*:1501–1511, 1981.

45. Winchester, R.J.: Characterization of IgG complexes in patients with rheumatoid arthritis. Ann. N.Y. Acad. Sci., *256*:73–81, 1975.

46. Winchester, R.J., Agnello, V., and Kunkel, H.G.: Gamma globulin complexes in synovial fluids of patients with rheumatoid arthritis. Clin. Exp. Immunol., *6*:689–706, 1970.

IgG to IgG immunoadsorbents. J. Immunol., *120*:739–744, 1978.

Chapter 42

Treatment of Rheumatoid Arthritis

Robert W. Lightfoot, Jr.

Specific information about the individual physical, medical, and surgical techniques for treating rheumatoid arthritis (RA) is given elsewhere in this book. This chapter describes an overall approach to the combined use of these therapies in the RA patient and provides a strategy for determining the appropriate treatment program in the individual patient.

The pyramid shown in Figure 42–1 schematically relates therapeutic regimens that may be used in the management of RA. The pyramid is interpreted as follows: (1) the lower items are often continued as higher elements are instituted and thus constitute a true "base" of the pyramid; (2) the elements toward the bottom of the pyramid are generally less toxic than those toward the top, and their usefulness has been established over many years; and (3) the elements toward the bottom are more generically applicable to the treatment of RA; they are used in virtually all patients, whereas those ranked higher are relevant only in certain patients. Although the pyramid in Figure 42–1 implies a fixed relationship of these regimens to one another, treatment must be designed to meet the needs of each individual patient.

As with any standard, deviation from the ideal does occur. For example, although corticosteroids generally are not considered part of the initial conservative management of an uncomplicated case of RA, their use may be warranted under certain circumstances. Similarly, although joint reconstruction generally is considered later and in chronic, recalcitrant disease, occasional patients with "early," that is, pre-erosive, disease in many joints may nonetheless benefit from surgical reconstruction of a single joint with more erosive involvement.

Several aspects of RA confound the decision-making abilities of even the best clinician. Therapy is easy to evaluate when use of a specific drug is followed by a prompt, objectively quantifiable response. Examples are the treatment of pernicious anemia with vitamin B_{12}, the treatment of diabetic ketoacidosis with insulin, and the resolution of pneumococcal pneumonia after penicillin therapy. Unlike these disorders, RA is a chronic disease without specific therapy. Its natural history may span decades, the results of therapy are usually not immediately apparent, and its course may fluctuate spontaneously. These factors often impair one's ability to determine the efficacy of treatment regimens. Furthermore, no universally accepted parameters permit specific measurement of the disease. Any attempt at therapy must take the foregoing variables into account.

GOALS OF THERAPY

Treatment of RA is directed toward: (1) alleviation of the signs and symptoms of active inflammation, both local and general; (2) prevention of tissue destruction: (3) prevention of deformity and preservation of function; and (4) reversal of phenomena threatening organ function, such as mononeuritis, myopericarditis, and lung fibrosis. Each of the elements in the therapeutic pyramid is directed toward one or more of these goals. The specific goals of a given therapy may differ among patients and with time in the same patient.

TYPES OF THERAPY

Education of the Patient

Without question, the single most important element in the management of rheumatoid disease is education of the patient. Most patients have only a vague notion of what RA is and how it differs from other forms of arthritis. Many believe, erroneously, that all patients with RA are destined to become crippled. They are often unaware that the symptoms of RA may partially remit and exacerbate spontaneously, sometimes from day to day. Intense anxiety and depression, common

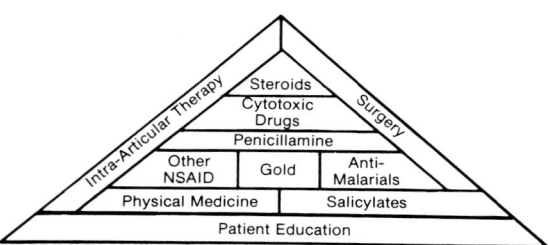

Fig. 42–1. The therapeutic pyramid. See text for details.

among these patients, result from fear and ignorance of what the future may hold and the inability to judge from day to day whether the disease is improving or worsening. Because these patients are unfamiliar with the concept of a chronic disease and do not know what to expect from its treatment, they often become discouraged if the initial steps taken by the physician are not immediately beneficial. The average patient is often unaware of the critical role he himself must play in disease management, especially with respect to ensuring an appropriate program of rest and physical therapy.

The patient should be told that RA is a chronic, lifelong disease for which no cure exists, but that a variety of measures, in the aggregate, can lead to significant improvement, that is, to "control" of the disease. *Relief of symptoms, preservation of joint function, and a reasonable life style* are three realistic goals. Patients must understand that the medications used in treatment generally do not provide overnight relief of symptoms, and they must be instructed to disregard the day-to-day variations and to think in terms of weeks or months in looking for evidence of improvement. If this concept is not emphasized, initial disappointment with the therapy may cause the patient to switch physicians often or even to seek a "cure" through quackery.

In addition to familiarizing patients with the concept of chronic disease and its management, specific points must be stressed with respect to individual therapeutic regimens.

Systemic Rest

The fever, weight loss, anemia, lymphadenopathy, and visceral involvement that may accompany RA attest to the systemic nature of the disease. A largely empiric body of evidence suggests that physical rest can rapidly ameliorate an acute exacerbation of rheumatoid disease. The optimal amount of rest varies from patient to patient. Some previously active patients have exaggerated fears of ultimately becoming crippled and may develop extreme anxiety if advised to quit work temporarily and take to bed. A modified rest program compatible with the patient's personality is appropriate in such an instance. Conversely, a systemically ill patient with multiple joint involvement and visceral disease may, of necessity, require nearly complete bed rest. Thus, the degree of physical rest prescribed varies from little to complete, depending on the individual circumstances. According to one study, complete bed rest is rarely indicated.[14]

In general, for patients with mild disease, a period of two to four hours in the afternoon at the time of onset of fatigue provides sufficient daily rest without interfering unduly with vocational responsibilities. The stiffness that follows periods of immobility should not dissuade patients from resting, and this phenomenon must be explained to the patient. As remission ensues, stiffness becomes less severe.

The ability to engage in periods of physical rest implies the ability to withdraw momentarily from psychosocial stress as well. The typical patient's fear about what to expect from this disease, the fear of possible loss of customary social and occupational roles in the family, and personal reaction to illness often cause a major psychologic stress reaction early in the disease. A rest program that does not permit respite from emotional stress is suboptimal.

In general, for patients with persistently active disease of recent onset or with "uncontrolled" inflammation at any point, a two- to three-week period of inpatient hospitalization is desirable. Physiologic studies of inflamed joints in RA (see Chap. 9) indicate that effective synovial blood flow is reduced. Because of this relative ischemia, the increased metabolic demand during joint use may cause microinfarction of synovial villi, which are the source of rice bodies found in severely involved joints.[3] Rest not only diminishes systemic stress, but probably also decreases local oxygen demand in these ischemic joints. In the study of Lee et al., hospitalized patients fared much better than those managed as outpatients.[12] Hospitalization permits definitive isolation from both physical and emotional stress. It allows time for the physician and other health professionals to educate the patient fully about the nature of the illness and the programs to be used in its treatment. Hospitalization also ensures early establishment of an optimal daily medical and physical therapeutic program.

A comprehensive treatment program requires a team of diverse health care professions including nursing, occupational and physical therapy, physiatry, orthopedic surgery, and rheumatology, as discussed in Chapters 43 and 44. The members of this team can be most effectively coordinated in the initiation of treatment if the new patient is hospitalized. In addition, questions about whether the patient is taking proper doses of medication or receiving adequate physical therapy and rest are obviated. The majority of patients experience a gratifying improvement in symptoms during this period.[12,16] If improvement does not occur, the next level on the treatment pyramid (see Fig. 42–1) can be entered without questioning whether therapy at the preceding level has failed because of noncompliance.

Physical Therapy

Rheumatoid synovitis is a chronic, inflammatory, destructive process that, if unchecked, proceeds to fibrosis of periarticular soft tissue with limitation of motion and contracture and to destruction of articular structures with ultimate subluxation, malalignment, and loss of function. The goals of physical therapy are to: (1) maintain range of motion; (2) prevent disuse atrophy of muscle; (3) minimize deformity; (4) provide adequate systemic rest; and (5) minimize excessive articular trauma, that is, provide local rest. Although the specifics of a comprehensive physical therapy program can be obtained through consultation with an appropriate specialist (see Chap. 44), the more important elements of such a program should be initiated as soon as the diagnosis is made and should be monitored by the patient's primary physician.

The patients must be convinced that the physical therapy program, including systemic rest, is as important a part of their treatment as any medication, and that, to succeed, the program must be followed on a daily basis, so it becomes as habitual as brushing teeth, combing hair, or bathing.

Preservation of Range of Motion

The initial period of conservative management of RA must include a balanced program of adequate rest to decrease inflammation and appropriate therapeutic exercise to maintain range of motion, and this program should be maintained for the duration of the disease. Patients must be educated regarding the tendency to joint contractures, and they should be instructed to move all joints gently through a full range of motion once daily. This exercise is most easily accomplished after initial morning stiffness has subsided or during or shortly after a hot bath or shower. Instruction in proper positioning of joints during rest or sleep is equally important in preventing contracture. Placing pillows under a painful knee is a major contributing factor to the development of contractures and must be actively discouraged. The patient should attempt to sleep in a position as near as possible to the anatomic, that is, with knees and elbows fully extended and with the neck and wrists in a near-neutral position.

Any exercise prescribed to maintain muscle strength and range of motion should minimize stress to the affected joints because such stress aggravates the inflammatory process.[16] Gentle isotonic or isometric exercises are preferable. Vigorous exercises such as jogging, bicycling, or calisthenics should be prohibited; they both worsen synovial hypoxia and increase direct joint trauma.[2] Any exercise that causes discomfort persisting for more than an hour or two should be decreased in amount. As the disease remits and physical tolerance increases, the exercise program can be escalated to include progressive resistive exercises.

Aerobic conditioning using a stationary exercise bicycle is of great value once control of synovitis in knees and hips has been achieved.

Splints

Joint trauma can also be minimized by the use of splints. These appliances are especially valuable in the acutely inflamed joint, in which they relieve pain, prevent deformity, and minimize the likelihood of synovial ischemic necrosis. The elegant study of Gault and Spyker has established objectively the benefits of joint immobilization in minimizing inflammation.[8] Splints should be removed at least once daily to permit range-of-motion exercises. Splints with which the physician should be familiar are volar wrist splints, used especially during sleep, and leg splints made of plaster or molded plastic, usually applied to the posterior aspect of the leg and foot by means of an elastic bandage to prevent knee flexion contractures.

Heat and Cold Application

The application of heat or cold to involved areas is often helpful in relieving pain and muscle spasm. Moist heat seems to be preferred by most patients and has the added advantage of relieving the "gel phenomenon," preparing the joint for subsequent range-of-motion exercises. Heat can be applied to painful areas in a variety of ways (see Chap. 44).

Cold applications are preferred if the inflammation is intense, as local hyperemia is already maximal.

Foot Support

RA is chiefly a disease of the small joints of the hands and feet (see Chap. 38). Typically, the metatarsophalangeal (MTP) joints are the worst affected in the foot, and patients often aptly describe a feeling of having stones under the forefoot when walking barefoot. The transverse arch collapses, and the forefoot spreads. The MTP joints are swollen and lie just under the skin, with weight borne chiefly by MTP joints 2, 3, and 4 instead of 1 and 5, as in a normal, healthy forefoot. The great toe develops a valgus position, and a bunion becomes prominent. The toes become "cocked-up" and do not fit easily into a shoe. The plantar fascia may contract and may lead to a pes cavus deformity. Involvement of the ankle and subtalar joints leads to eversion of the hindfoot.

It is important to provide proper support for the rheumatoid foot. The physician can prescribe orthopedic (modified-last) oxfords with a heel height that is comfortable for the patient, usually 1.5 to 2 inches. A medial wedge of about one-eighth inch corrects the tendency to eversion, and metatarsal bars, affixed to the leather sole of the shoe, shift the weight bearing to the midfoot and thereby relieve the constant pressure on the inflamed MTP joints. Composition soles that incorporate a metatarsal bar are now available. If the hallux valgus is severe, the shoes can be stretched to provide a "bunion pocket." Shoes with a double toe-box provide adequate space for the patient with severe toe deformities. Overweight patients may benefit from a Thomas heel.

Axial Skeletal Support

RA often involves the cervical spine, the most mobile part of the axial skeleton. It often helps to prescribe a soft cervical collar with Velcro straps to hold the neck in midposition. This collar can be worn at night as well as during the day and acts as a splint for the neck by resting the inflamed lateral interbody joints and zygapophyseal joints.

Canes or Crutches

Canes or crutches are often helpful orthotic appliances in treating RA, despite the reluctance of many American patients to accept them. Crutches are symbolic of the cripple, just what the average RA patient fears the most. Their use must be "sold" to the patient. It is best to prescribe crutches for a short while only, to prevent weight bearing in an extremity that contains a joint recently injected with corticosteroid, especially when triamcinolone hexacetonide has been administered in an effort to produce a "medical synovectomy." In such a case, maximal therapeutic benefit can be attained by avoiding weight bearing for about eight weeks (see Chap. 34).

The chief disadvantage of crutches is the stress they place on inflamed upper-extremity joints. This stress can be minimized by the use of platform crutches, with which weight is borne by the forearms. Aluminum crutches of the Canadian type are preferable because they have a metal band that uses the upper arm rather than the axilla as a fulcrum. Axillary crutches are dangerous because they predispose patients to brachial plexus stretching and injury.

A properly prescribed crutch should touch the floor about 3 inches in front of the foot when the patient is standing with arms straightened. A properly prescribed cane, so helpful in unloading the hip joint, should touch the floor similarly and should be carried in the hand contralateral to the affected extremity.

Crutches are much more effective than canes in unloading the lower extremities. The patient must be trained to use them; three- or four-point gaits are available options and are not always easy to learn, especially for the elderly. Sometimes a walker is a better option in such patients, and this simple orthotic device may permit standing or walking for periods sufficient to allow the patient independence in self-care activities, such as cooking or getting to the bathroom.

Other Appliances

The severely handicapped patient can often be helped by simple devices such as raised toilet seats and hand rails in the bathtub and kitchen. Consultation with a physiatrist who has a special interest in arthritis can help such patients achieve or maintain independence in their usual activities of daily living (see Chap. 44).

Medical Therapy

All therapy with drugs, used singly or in combination to treat RA, is empirical.

Salicylates and other NSAIDs

Salicylates, preferably as aspirin, are the cornerstone of drug treatment in RA. Their chief advantage is rapidity of therapeutic effect. A general principle of aspirin therapy is a gradual increase in the dose to produce mild toxicity, then a decrease to more tolerable doses. A usual starting dose is 0.9 g aspirin four times daily. (Details of pharmacokinetics appear in Chapter 28.) The most common cause of failure of aspirin therapy is reluctance of the patient to take the drug as directed. The average patient thinks of aspirin as little more than a headache remedy. To prescribe aspirin in large doses to such a patient without explaining the rationale behind its use is to invite noncompliance. The patient must be informed that salicylates in larger doses are anti-inflammatory and are not just analgesic. Patients should be advised that a regular daily dose must be taken for at least two weeks to maintain a blood level of between 20 and 35 mg/dl, before deciding on efficacy. Without this caution, patients often vary the dose from day to day, depending on symptoms, and thereby fail to achieve a therapeutic blood level.

The likelihood of benefit from salicylates can be maximized by hospitalization to control other variables of treatment. In the alert adult, symptoms of mild toxicity, such as tinnitus or dyspepsia, precede those of serious toxicity. Serum salicylate levels are generally determined only in outpatients with persistent synovitis despite aspirin therapy, to see whether therapeutic levels have been achieved. Aspirin is not an easy drug to use, and the average physician uses it poorly. The dose must be tailored to each patient, based on the drug kinetics discussed in Chapter 28. We routinely determine the most appropriate dose for a given patient by serial determination of serum salicylate levels drawn in the morning before the first daily dose is given.

The most common side effects of aspirin therapy

are tinnitus and gastrointestinal distress. Tinnitus responds to lowering of the dose. Ordinary aspirin should always be taken with food. It is simplest to prescribe four doses daily with meals and a bedtime snack. The dietary habits of each patient should be known. If necessary, food must be prescribed, especially breakfast. The aspirin should be taken during the meal, between bites—not before and not after, but during the meal. If these measures are not successful, alternate salicylate preparations, for example, aspirin mixed with an antacid, enteric-coated aspirin, or sodium salicylate, may be used. Patients intolerant of regular aspirin often have no gastrointestinal symptoms when taking other salicylate preparations. The newer enteric-coated preparations are well absorbed and can be substituted, if necessary, tablet for tablet, for ordinary aspirin. So effective are salicylates in the management of RA that all aforementioned agents should be tried before the physician concludes that the patient is unable to take any salicylate preparation.

Many patients experience sufficient improvement in symptoms at subtoxic doses of aspirin that additional therapies may not be required. If, after a two- to four-week trial of salicylates in therapeutic doses in an optimal setting, improvement is insufficient, or if salicylates are not tolerated, another nonsteroidal anti-inflammatory drug (NSAID) should be tried (see Chap. 28). The physician should be aware that salicylates may interfere with the absorption of some NSAID and vice versa. In deciding whether to continue salicylates during the period of NSAID administration, one must weigh the benefit obtained from salicylates at that point against this possible drug-drug interference. Although most of these drugs can cause gastrointestinal irritation, no absolute contraindication exists to using two of them concomitantly. Because no advantage has been documented, we do not endorse this practice. In a mild case of RA, six or more months of salicylates and the basic program may be in order. In more severe cases, it may be clear after three weeks of salicylate administration that additional drug therapy is needed. If the disease has been present for more than one year, or if erosive disease is already present, it is unlikely that therapy with aspirin or other NSAIDs used alone will produce satisfactory suppression of joint inflammation. We routinely begin treatment with disease-remitting agents without wasting weeks of valuable time.

Salicylates exert an analgesic effect as well. If additional analgesia is needed, acetaminophen, newer non-narcotic analgesics, and propoxyphene compounds or pentazocine, alone or in combination, may be added. Propoxyphene and pentazocine should be used cautiously because they may lead to drug dependency. Narcotic-containing analgesics should be used with extreme caution, if at all, in a chronic illness such as RA. Analgesic drugs should be considered as supplemental to the more important treatment regimens discussed here.

Second-Line Drugs

If an adequate trial of aspirin or other NSAID provides insufficient relief, if well-established RA has been present for more than one year, or if erosions have already occurred, it is necessary to begin gold or antimalarial drug therapy. As mentioned previously, the precise time at which this level of the treatment pyramid (see Fig. 42–1) should be entered varies. Gold is preferred because of the more substantial documentation of its efficacy.[1,11,20] Recent data suggest that retinal toxicity from antimalarial agents is minimal.[13] Chloroquine can be given safely for many years in doses not exceeding 4 mg/kg lean body weight daily. Hydroxychloroquine also can be given in doses lower than 6 mg/kg/day. Both antimalarial agents have equal therapeutic and toxic effects at these doses. Light exposure accelerates ocular toxicity, and patients should be advised to wear sunglasses when in bright sunlight, to minimize this effect. Patients should be advised that improvement with gold or antimalarial treatment may not be apparent for several months. Salicylate or other NSAID should be continued in full dosage throughout the period of gold or antimalarial administration.

All drug therapy of RA is empiric. Most patients require combined-drug treatment, not unlike the empiric drug regimens used in cancer chemotherapy. Thus, antimalarial drugs and gold are often used together in patients with uncontrolled inflammation, especially in those with erosions. Fine-detail roentgenograms (see Chap. 5) enable us to identify erosions early in the disease, often only a few months after onset. Most patients with erosions have positive rheumatoid factor tests.

Many rheumatologists now use penicillamine (see Chap. 31) as the next drug of choice in patients unresponsive to treatment with aspirin, gold, and/or antimalarial agents. Some even prefer penicillamine to gold, but the toxicity is often serious, even fatal. Moreover, the effect of penicillamine is inapparent for several months, and it is usual to discontinue gold therapy, but to continue the other drugs, during the period of penicillamine treatment, because gold may neutralize penicillamine by chelation. The toxicities of gold and of penicillamine are similar and have been linked to the presence of the HLA-DR3 antigen. Antimalarial agents should not be given in combination with D-penicillamine because they may interfere with its adsorption. A controlled trial using both drugs found the combination inferior to either drug used alone.[1a]

Patients with active disease despite the use of the aforementioned drugs are candidates for immunoregulatory drug therapy. Considerable evidence suggests that the immunosuppressive drugs, especially cyclophosphamide and azathioprine, are effective in controlling rheumatoid disease.[4,5] Cyclophosphamide has prevented the development of joint erosions.[4] In recently reported uncontrolled trials, methotrexate therapy led to encouraging improvement of symptoms in patients with otherwise recalcitrant disease. The rationale behind the use of these drugs is discussed in Chapter 33. All use of such toxic compounds should be supervised by a rheumatologist. Low doses of cyclophosphamide, azathioprine, and hydroxychloroquine, used in combination, have been reported to allow erosions to heal in one preliminary uncontrolled study. Immunosuppression by lymphophoresis, plasmapheresis, or total lymph-node irradiation is expensive and may have serious, as yet unrecognized, toxicity. The duration of benefits gained is yet to be defined. Both these and combined immunosuppressive drug regimens should be considered as experimental, to be used only in cases recalcitrant to all conventional therapy, and preferably administered only as part of an approved scientific protocol.

Each of the alternate drugs already mentioned has its own set of toxic effects. In some instances, evidence of drug toxicity may be delayed for months or years. The responsible clinician must be familiar with all the toxic effects of each drug and must be prepared to monitor both short- and long-term toxicity, with proper monitoring to permit the earliest possible detection of such side effects.

Corticosteroids

As indicated in Figure 42–1, the intra-articular injection of corticosteroids can play a major adjunctive role in controlling rheumatoid synovitis at all levels in the treatment pyramid. Details regarding the dosage, techniques for administration, frequency of injection, and contraindications are discussed in Chapter 34.

Systemic corticosteroid therapy is intentionally placed last in the treatment pyramid shown in Figure 42–1. Oral or intramuscular corticosteroids should be used only after a critical consideration of alternate modes of treatment and with the long-term side effects of these agents kept in mind because these drugs are much easier to start than to stop in a patient with RA. Several studies have suggested that a major subset of rheumatoid patients are prone to a dependency on corticosteroids that prevents the discontinuance of these drugs,[10,15]

and the immediate improvement that often occurs may dissuade both patient and doctor from using a better-tolerated and more effective drug regimen.

Corticosteroids may be indicated in a patient who is the family breadwinner and who must continue working. Although flares severe enough to necessitate hospitalization may be rapidly controlled with a 15-mg, single daily dose of prednisone, the physician should attempt to taper this dose to no more than a 7.5-mg dose of prednisone or equivalent corticosteroid per day, and then only as a single morning dose on arising. Because the half-life of prednisone is only about eight hours, the suppressive effect on the hypothalamic-pituitary axis is minimized, and the small dose given may be additive to the patient's endogenous corticosteroid secretion. No dose of corticosteroid is safe; even 5 mg prednisone daily can produce osteopenia (see Chap. 97).

No rationale exists for treatment with corticotropin (ACTH), and fluorinated corticosteroids, such as dexamethasone or triamcinolone, are to be avoided because they have long biologic half-lives and are likely to suppress the patient's endogenous corticosteroid output.

Specific indications for corticosteroid use therefore include life-threatening visceral disease, acute flares, and persistent, disabling symptoms in a breadwinner who must return to work. Additional indications and cautionary comments are detailed in Chapter 32.

TREATMENT STRATEGIES

A strategy cognizant of the five guidelines discussed in this section provides considerable assistance to the physician managing patients with RA.

Treatment of Specific Manifestations

One must determine which aspects of the disease process require treatment at a given time. RA can have protean manifestations involving many organ systems, and the preponderant manifestation may differ with time in the same patient. Figure 42–2 depicts the manifestations in two patients. Patient A was seen for the first time with moderate synovitis, accompanied by moderate numbers of subcutaneous nodules over the ulna and small joints of the hands. When patient B was first seen in 1969, severe incapacitating synovitis limited all activities of daily living, but more systemic features were minimal. Fifteen years later, synovitis was minimal, and the main expression of RA was severe neutropenia and digital gangrene secondary to rheumatoid vasculitis. This figure illustrates three distinct clinical presentations in two patients. It is, therefore, important to determine in advance of

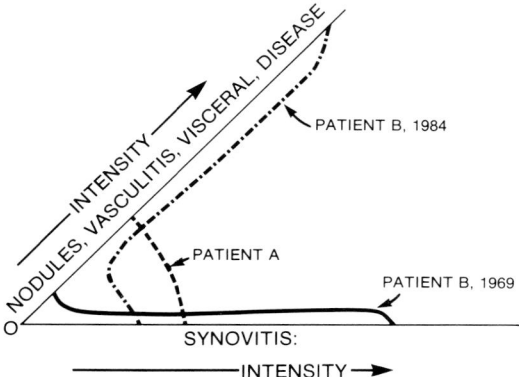

Fig. 42–2. Depiction of intra- and interpatient variability of disease expression in rheumatoid arthritis (RA). Intensity of joint inflammation and systemic involvement are represented along the lower and upper axes, respectively. Patient A had moderate synovitis and subcutaneous nodules at the time shown. Patient B had little more than synovitis when first seen in 1969. After many years and several regimens, his disease manifested as severe Felty's syndrome and vasculitis, with minimal synovitis. This figure illustrates the inter- and intrapatient variability in clinical course and manifestations seen in RA.

therapy which manifestations of RA mandate treatment. The manifestations of RA can be generally grouped as (1) signs and symptoms of joint inflammation; (2) destruction of bone and connective tissue; (3) visceral or systemic involvement; and (4) results of prior bone and soft tissue destruction.

Signs and Symptoms of Inflammation

Those signs and symptoms include joint pain, heat, and swelling. Systems designed to quantify these are discussed in Chapter 7.

Destruction of Bone and Connective Tissue

Although patients with sustained inflammatory symptoms usually also experience progressive joint destruction, progressive destructive disease need not always be accompanied by pain or other subjective symptoms. Rheumatoid scleritis, sometimes painless and noticed more by others than by the patient, may nevertheless cause erosion through the sclera. Patients with diffuse rheumatoid nodulosis,[9] who often have few or no joint complaints, may exhibit progressive, severely erosive disease in joints that have not been the seat of pain. It is of practical value therefore to consider progressive erosion and acute inflammatory signs as two possibly distinct clinical problems, one quantifiable clinically, the other often requiring roentgenographic measurement.

Manifestations of Visceral or Systemic Involvement

These manifestations include vasculitis, lung fibrosis, mononeuritis, and Felty's syndrome and are discussed at length in Chapters 39 and 63.

Results of Prior Bone and Soft Tissue Destruction

Such destruction includes subluxations, contractures, secondary degenerative changes, and (rarely) ankylosis.

Therapy should be tailored to the manifestation causing the symptoms. Gold therapy does not alleviate pain resulting from prior joint destruction, nor is surgical treatment appropriate for polyarticular inflammatory pain.

Measurement of Response to Therapy

When initiating a given therapy, one must decide how the response will ultimately be measured. Methods of clinical measurement in rheumatology are discussed in Chapter 7. Parameters such as joint count, ring size, grip strength, dolorimetry, articular index, duration of morning stiffness, erythrocyte sedimentation rate, walking time, and functional status questionnaires have all been used.[17] None of these is ideal, and it is customary to assess several parameters at the initiation of a new therapeutic regimen. In a multicenter study of criteria for remission in RA, duration of morning stiffness proved to be a far more reliable measure than other parameters.[17] Pain was less reliable, presumably because it partly reflects secondary degenerative disease in some patients with chronic RA. Clearly, if morning stiffness or grip weakness is absent at the initiation of a new regimen, this parameter will be a poor measure of response to treatment. In some patients with chronic RA, in whom it is difficult to separate symptoms due to prior joint destruction from those of active progressive rheumatoid synovitis, serial roentgenograms may be the only reliable objective parameter. This concept is discussed further later in this chapter.

Timing of Effectiveness of Therapy

One must determine in advance how long the regimen initiated generally takes before becoming effective. NSAID have a maximal effect within weeks. Gold, on the other hand, may not work until nearly the full 1000-mg induction regimen has been given, about 20 weeks. Obviously, one would not necessarily expect a measurable improvement after several weeks of gold therapy. Conversely, it would be unlikely to see additional improvement from adequate levels of NSAID after 6 or 8 weeks.

Evaluation of Regimen

Having selected parameters to be measured prior to and after initiation of therapy, one must decide, preferably in advance, what degree of change in measurements will be considered sufficient to constitute an "adequate" therapeutic response. This criterion may determine whether the regimen ultimately will be judged sufficiently successful to be continued at a maintenance level, or whether more aggressive therapy is warranted.

Combination of Therapies

One must decide whether the current regimen will be continued as the next is started. This decision is more often dictated by whether their toxicities are similar, and therefore difficult to ascribe, and whether one is rapid in onset of action while the other is slow. For example, aspirin is usually continued during gold administration because the two have different rapidity of action and toxicity. Gold is not continued when penicillamine is started because their toxicities are nearly identical. Although gold and antimalarial agents are usually initiated in sequence, the first used is often continued as the other is initiated because both are slow-acting agents, and their more serious toxicities are generally distinct and are therefore easily ascribable. On the other hand, gold is usually discontinued when immunosuppressive agents are initiated because both can cause serious bone marrow depression.

Use of the foregoing guidelines minimizes the indefinite continuance of marginal therapy, a common problem in managing any chronic, complicated, multisystem disease. It also discourages the haphazard switching of drugs in an attempt to hurry a response. As an example of this reasoning, when aspirin or other NSAID alone have failed, gold therapy is generally started to control signs of acute inflammation and to deter joint erosion in a patient in whom salicylates are inadequate. Gold would not be given to control symptoms deemed due to irreversible secondary degenerative change or to control rheumatoid vasculitis. Appropriate parameters in such a patient might be duration of morning stiffness, grip strength, and number of swollen joints, and these parameters might not be expected to change drastically for as long as 20 weeks.

A major problem is the patient with low-grade synovitis superimposed on long-term, antecedent, destructive RA. It does little good to administer gold therapy in a patient with erosive disease and metacarpalphalangeal joint subluxation whose only current symptom is mild day-long pain without soft tissue swelling, because this symptom is unlikely to reflect active inflammation, and the subluxations will not improve with gold therapy. Such patients may have the "ashes" of prior inflammatory destruction, superimposed on which is the "fire" of persistently active joint inflammation. It is often difficult to determine whether symptoms are primarily those of secondary degenerative disease, treatable only by NSAID or surgical intervention, or whether they reflect active synovitis, perhaps treatable with disease modifying agents. In these patients, already functionally compromised by the abnormal joint mechanics resulting from prior subluxation and contracture and the discomfort of destroyed joint surfaces, even minimal worsening of joint integrity can severely threaten their ability to function independently. These patients present a formidable challenge to the clinician. In many, serial roentgenograms of the involved joints at approximately yearly intervals may be the only objective parameter.

RESULTS OF THERAPY

Several studies involving many patients suggest that 50 to 70% experience significant improvement with a regimen of salicylates, rest, and physical therapy.[6,18,19] A similar percentage of response is found in controlled trials of gold therapy.[7,20] Thus, the majority of patients can control RA satisfactorily with well-accepted, conservative regimens. The role of aggressive therapy, such as penicillamine and immunoregulatory drugs, in early or mild disease is not known. Although it has not been established scientifically that conservative management or any other therapy actually alters the course of RA, gold and cyclophosphamide, at least, have been shown to alter the rate of radiologically defined deterioration.[4,20] Difficulties in diagnosing early disease, especially in initially seronegative patients, may delay the prescription of an optimal treatment regimen. The notorious spontaneous variations in disease activity make evaluation of any therapy difficult. The use of an appropriate control group is essential. Rational therapy requires that the physician use the foregoing management principles.

Use of these treatment rationales in a typical patient over time is represented in Figure 42–3. In phase I, the patient had primarily synovitis with some subcutaneous nodules, and responded gradually to NSAID. When the response is unacceptable, gold and, later, antimalarial agents were added, with better control of synovitis. When these agents became minimally effective, they were discontinued. Such "secondary failure" is common in RA patients. In phase III, when synovitis was minimal in this particular patient, nodulosis and vasculitis occurred. Later, synovitis recurred. Immunosuppressive agents were then added and even-

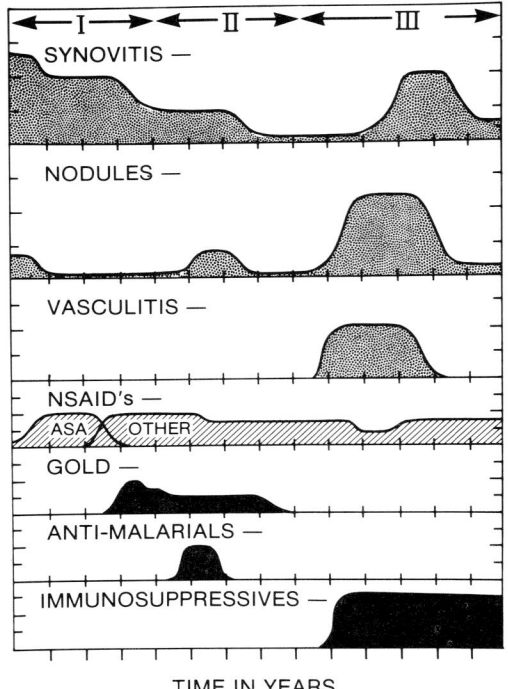

Fig. 42–3. Management choices in a hypothetical patient over several years.

tually controlled the manifestations for which they were prescribed.

In conclusion, the regimens discussed in this chapter, including rest, exercise, orthopedic shoes, splints, salicylates, NSAID, gold, antimalarial agent, penicillamine, local and systemic corticosteroids, and immunosuppresive drugs, are all beneficial in RA. They are stratified in the treatment pyramid (see Fig. 42–1) roughly in the order that benefit exceeds risk. In the case of the newer regimens now shown in the upper strata of the pyramid, future data may redefine the risk-to-benefit ratio, thus shifting their relative positions. Ultimately, protocols using combined-drug therapy may establish the effectiveness of such regimens, as in the lymphomas and leukemias. Both physician and patient must see the need to try the less toxic, better-established regimens first, rather than opting for the expedient of dramatic early response at the price of serious or long-term toxicity. In the properly educated patient, the physician's attitude, more than any other factor, inspires cooperation. A positive approach to treatment may be the single

most important factor in the successful management of RA.

REFERENCES

1. Brooks, P.M., and Buchanan, W.W.: Current management of rheumatoid arthritis. *In* Recent Advances in Rheumatology. Edited by W.W. Buchanan and W.C. Dick. New York, Churchill-Livingstone, 1976.
1a. Bunch, T.W., et al.: Controlled trial of hydroxychloroquine and D-penicillamine singly and in combination in the treatment of rheumatoid arthritis. Arthritis Rheum., 27:267–276, 1984.
2. Castillo, B.A., El Sallab, R.A., and Scott, J.T.: Physical activity, cystic erosions, and osteoporosis in rheumatoid arthritis. Ann. Rheum. Dis., 29:522–527, 1965.
3. Cheung, H.S., et al.: Synovial origins of rice bodies in joint fluid. Arthritis Rheum., 23:72–76, 1980.
4. Cooperating Clinics Committee of the American Rheumatism Association: A controlled trial of cyclophosphamide in rheumatoid arthritis. N. Engl. J. Med., 283:883–889, 1970.
5. Currey, H.L.F., et al.: Comparison of azathioprine, cyclophosphamide, and gold in treatment of rheumatoid arthritis. Br. Med. J., 3:763–766, 1974.
6. Duthie, J.J.R., et al.: Medical and social aspects of the treatment of rheumatoid arthritis, with special reference to factors affecting prognosis. Ann. Rheum. Dis., 14:133–149, 1955.
7. Empire Rheumatism Council Research Sub-Committee Report: Gold therapy in rheumatoid arthritis. Final report of a multicentre controlled trial. Ann. Rheum. Dis., 20:315–334, 1955.
8. Gault, S.J., and Spyker, J.M.: Beneficial effect of immobilization of joints in rheumatoid arthritis: a splint study using sequential analysis. Arthritis Rheum., 17:34–44, 1969.
9. Ginsberg, M.H., et al.: Rheumatoid nodulosis. An unusual variant of rheumatoid disease. Arthritis Rheum., 18:49–58, 1975.
10. Glass, D., et al.: Possible unnecessary prolongation of corticosteroid therapy in rheumatoid arthritis. Lancet, 2:334–337, 1971.
11. Ianuzzi, L., et al.: Does drug therapy slow radiographic deterioration in rheumatoid arthritis? N. Engl. J. Med., 309:1023–1028, 1983.
12. Lee, P., et al.: Benefits of hospitalization in rheumatoid arthritis. Q. J. Med., 43:205–214, 1974.
13. Mackenzie, A.H.: Dose refinements in long-term therapy of rheumatoid arthritis with antimalarials. Am. J. Med., 75:40–45, 1983.
14. Mills, J.A., et al.: Value of bed rest in patients with rheumatoid arthritis. N. Engl. J. Med., 284:453–458, 1971.
15. Moldofsky, H., and Rothman, A.I.: Personality, disease parameters and medication in rheumatoid arthritis. J. Chronic Dis., 24:363–372, 1971.
16. Partridge, R.E.H., and Duthie, J.J.R.: Controlled trial of the effects of complete immobilization of the joints in rheumatoid arthritis. Ann. Rheum. Dis., 22:91–99, 1963.
17. Pinals, R.S., Masi, A.T., and Larsen, R.A.: Preliminary criteria for clinical remission in rheumatoid arthritis. Arthritis Rheum., 24:1308–1315, 1981.
18. Ragan, C.: The general management of rheumatoid arthritis. JAMA, 141:174–177, 1949.
19. Short, C.L., and Bauer, W.: The course of rheumatoid arthritis in patients receiving simple medical and orthopedic measures. N. Engl. J. Med., 238:142–148, 1948.
20. Sigler, J.W., et al.: Gold salts in the treatment of rheumatoid arthritis. A double-blind study. Ann. Intern. Med., 80:21–26, 1974.

Chapter 43

Role of Nursing and Allied Health Professions in Treatment of Arthritis

Janice Smith Pigg

HISTORICAL PERSPECTIVE

Patients with arthritis can also benefit from the expertise and skills of professionals other than physicians. Nurses, physical therapists, occupational therapists, social workers, psychologists, and others can help patients to understand and to carry out a therapeutic program.[49] The growth of rheumatology as a subspecialty of internal medicine has been paralleled by a delayed but increasing interest on the part of such professionals in the care of patients with rheumatic diseases.[9,82]

The development of rheumatology nursing specialists, and of special interest in arthritis and allied disorders by workers in other professional disciplines, has been influenced by two factors: (1) the development of a common identity through the Arthritis Health Professions Association (AHPA), which is, like the American Rheumatism Association (ARA), a professional section of the Arthritis Foundation; and (2) the availability of grant support from federal, and to a lesser extent, state, sources.

In 1952, the Arthritis Foundation's *Manual for Arthritis Clinics* stated that "the role, necessity and value of the various paramedical personnel in the clinic is [sic] by and large self-evident. . . ."[3] The only specific role for nurses and allied health professionals noted at that time was the "unique position" of the clinic staff, identified as nurse, social worker, physical therapist, and podiatrist, in the education of the patient.

In 1965, a "Paramedical Section" of the Arthritis Foundation was formed with 40 members, primarily with the help and support of a few physicians who were ARA members.[31] Individual rheumatologists continue to exert a major influence on the recruitment and development of nurses and other health professionals who care for patients with rheumatic diseases. The "Paramedical Section" became known as the *Allied Health Professions Section* in 1968, and in 1980 became the *Arthritis Health Professions Association* to reflect both the growing numbers of physicians who were

members and the traditional distinction between nursing and the allied health professions. The word "Association" was chosen over "Section" to reflect the evolving professionalism and to parallel the name of the ARA.[94] With nearly 2,000 members as of 1983, the AHPA is the fastest-growing section of Arthritis Foundation. Although some members of AHPA are active in research, most care for patients. Nursing and physical therapy are the best-represented disciplines. Occupational therapy is a close third, and social work is a distant fourth (Table 43–1). Other professionals represented in AHPA include physicians, laboratory technologists, pharmacists, nutritionists and dietitians, podiatrists, health educators, psychologists, counselors, and others.

AHPA's growth has coincided with federal funding of arthritis-related activities that use the skills and knowledge of professionals other than physicians. The first of these activities was the Regional Medical Programs in 1974, followed by the establishment of the Multipurpose Arthritis Centers in 1977, which were developed as a part of the recommendations of the National Arthritis Act of 1974.

Most patients with arthritis are treated by general physicians, not by rheumatologists. Similarly, most professional treatment of arthritis by nonphy-

Table 43–1. Arthritis Health Professions Association (AHPA) Membership by Discipline

Members, by Discipline	Percentage of Total Membership (%)
Nurses	29
Physical therapists	28
Occupational therapists	22
Social workers	6
Physicians	5
Others	10

(Adapted from 1982–83 Membership Directory, American Rheumatism Association, Arthritis Health Professions Association, Atlanta.)

sicians is carried out by generalists. Expectations of nursing and allied health rheumatology specialists and of their nonspecialized generalist colleagues should not be the same.[115] Specialists should serve as role models, identify standards of care, provide basic and continuing professional education in their respective areas, and conduct research.[4]

In the care of patients with rheumatic diseases, the roles of nurses and allied health professionals are determined by their educational preparation, by their skills, by their rheumatologic knowledge, and by each individual's perception of the specific practice setting. Individual experiences and attitude about chronicity, deformity, and dependence are also influential.

ROLE OF ARTHRITIS HEALTH PROFESSIONALS

Most discussions of the roles of nurses and allied health professionals are expressed in generalities[23,46] or are limited to one disease condition, usually rheumatoid arthritis or osteoarthritis. Despite titles purporting to delineate roles, such literature often describes the more common rheumatic diseases and their diagnoses, addresses treatment, or broadly identifies goals in the care of patients.[75] Little is said of the specific contribution of the various disciplines in reaching these goals, nor is the responsibility of the individual discipline defined.

Beyond the traditional discipline-specific activities, roles of nurses and allied health professionals in rheumatology have been only partially described. Few standards have been defined. Process is more clearly identified but still lacks specificity, both with regard to discipline and with regard to disease treatment. Outcomes are only globally defined and rarely in measurable terms. This unsatisfactory state of affairs may reflect the newness of the field of rheumatology and the difficulty in describing roles influenced by the following: (1) the variability (stage and severity of disease) of the various rheumatic diseases; (2) the variety of practice settings; (3) the experience and preparation of the individual practitioner; (4) the availability of resources, such as time and materials; and (5) the accountability and relationships with other providers of care.

ACADEMIC PREPARATION

The preparation of nurses and allied health professionals affects their roles in caring for patients with rheumatic diseases. Most health-related disciplines require baccalaureate degrees, although the amount of preparation at entry level for registered nurses still varies from a 2-year associate

degree to a 4-year bachelor of science in nursing. A survey of rheumatology laboratory personnel revealed that 65% had bachelor's degrees, 15% had master's degrees, 12% had doctorates of philosophy, and 8% had no degrees at all.[1] Some members of health-related disciplines are registered or licensed, but such requirements vary from state to state.

A survey of the AHPA's membership showed a wide variation in academic background (Table 43–2). Detailed instruction in care of patients with arthritis is not routinely offered as a part of the basic curriculum in any of the various health disciplines. A survey of schools of occupational and physical therapy and nursing in the United States and Canada in 1979 showed that most curricula exposed students to minimal information about the rheumatic diseases.[50] Many programs no longer base their teaching on diseases or body systems, but focus on problems or processes. This change of focus may mean that a nurse or allied health professional has some knowledge, but may lack the ability to apply it to a specific arthritis patient. A survey of occupational and physical therapists in Arizona found that approximately half considered their academic background in arthritis poor to fair.[123] This finding contradicted an earlier study,[50] which found that most training program directors believed their programs were adequate in this area.

Few opportunities exist for nurses or allied health professionals to specialize in rheumatology on a graduate level.[108] Expertise in nonrheumatologic areas is often applicable to rheumatology, however, and increasing numbers of nurses and allied health professionals have advanced degrees (Table 43–3). That nurses and allied health professionals treating arthritis patients desire additional arthritis-related training after going into practice indicates the need for continuing professional education.[123] Skills and knowledge can be usefully upgraded and updated through short-term learning experiences.[1] Pre-, post-, and delayed post-testing

Table 43–2. Academic Degrees Held by the Members of the Arthritis Health Professions Association (AHPA)

Degree	Percentage of Total Membership (%)
Registered Nurse	12
Baccalaureate	57
Master's	21
Doctorate (Philosophy)	2
Doctorate (Medicine)	5
Other	3

(Adapted from 1982–83 Membership Directory, American Rheumatism Association, Arthritis Health Professions Association, Atlanta.)

Table 43–3. Academic Degree by Discipline Among Members of the Arthritis Health Professions Association (AHPA)

Discipline	Percentage of Total Membership (%)
Nursing	
Licensed Practical Nurse	3
Registered Nurse	43
Baccalaureate	30
Master's	23
Doctorate	1
Physical Therapy	
Licensed Physical Therapy	
Assistant	less than 1
Baccalaureate	84
Master's	14
Doctorate	1
Occupational Therapy	
Certified Occupational	
Therapy Assistant	2
Baccalaureate	82
Master's	15
Doctorate	less than 1

(Adapted from 1982–83 Membership Directory, American Rheumatism Association, Arthritis Health Professions Association, Atlanta.)

of participants in a multidisciplinary continuing education seminar showed that although nurses knew the most, the entire group was weak in knowledge of disease characteristics, medical management, and pharmacology.[42] This finding is predictable, however, because such care providers seldom are responsible for diagnosis or for prescribing drugs or other treatments. The traditional didactic lecture without reinforcement is ineffective. As a result, continuing education based on what the various care providers can do, rather than emphasis on the differential diagnosis and clinical effects of rheumatic disease, has been urged.[53]

Written materials[18,19,64,82,83,86,93,119,125,126] and audiovisual resources[4,45,87] are other ways to provide continuing education. Standards of care in rheumatology developed and disseminated nationally within a discipline's professional organization are one way to provide wide exposure of information to nonspecialists, as well as a way to affect roles.[82] The AHPA has produced a slide collection and instructional guide for teachers of allied health professionals to aid in providing relevant content.[4]

PRACTICE SETTINGS

Care providers other than physicians work in a variety of settings and can offer the patient a large amount of less costly time. In the hospital, the patient with arthritis is most often cared for in a general medical or surgical unit. Specialized rheu-matic disease care is most often offered in a rehabilitative, orthopedic, or rheumatic disease unit.[9,81]

The specialized staff of a categoric treatment unit can provide comprehensive care. These professionals may become particularly skillful in recognizing and reporting details that may lead the attending rheumatologist to adjust the patient's therapy. Comprehensive care includes diagnosis, application of accepted therapeutic procedures, and rehabilitation. Nursing and allied health professionals are particularly involved in the last two areas. The general activity pattern and pace of rehabilitation in the rheumatic diseases is different from those of many other disorders.[77] The energy and mobility limitations of many patients with rheumatic diseases, combined with affective learning needs, emphasis on independent function, rest and pacing requirements, and fluctuating disease activity, require a different ratio of personnel to patients than in the general hospital population.[81] A specialized rheumatology unit is best able to meet the rheumatic disease patient's unique needs for the same reason that other specialized units, such as intensive care and burn units, have been organized.

The staff members, usually nurses, therapists, and sometimes social workers, of community agencies have access to the patient at home, where many long-term aspects of management take place. Interactions with families occur more readily at home.[61] Nurses and therapists working with juvenile patients provide treatment and also serve as intermediaries among the young patients, their families, and school staff. For instance, long-range planning, including vocational rehabilitation, can be most effective when the nurse or therapist has the flexibility to move freely between the school, the home, and medical settings.[34]

Nurses and allied health professionals often provide care in the physician's office or outpatient clinic,[57] as well as in nursing homes or other extended-care facilities. The services provided by nurses and allied health professionals in these varied settings include the following: (1) physical care such as application of clinical therapeutic techniques, including those that enhance function and protect joints, relieve pain, and maintain or restore mobility and strength; (2) assessment and evaluation; (3) instruction and education; (4) psychosocial counseling and referral; and (5) support and encouragment.

Expectations must be realistic and must relate to the practice environment or to the health care delivery system. The office nurse who is expected to make appointments, handle phone calls, prepare patients for examinations, keep records, and give injections, may not also have adequate time to devote to educating patients. The educational function can sometimes be incorporated into many of these activities, however. For example, when a nurse gives a gold injection, instruction regarding side effects and essential follow-up directions should be given. Other times must also be set aside for the nurse to educate patients, however, if this is deemed to be important.

PATIENT-CARE TEAM

It is widely accepted, although still unproved, that the combined expertise of various disciplines with differing skills is needed to achieve optimal comprehensive management of an arthritis patient.[23,38,52,81,87,98,118,131] This concept is evident in the Multipurpose Arthritis Centers and in other specialized rheumatic disease units where innovative techniques in arthritis management have been and are being developed and evaluated. The problems of arthritis are diverse, and the arthritis health care team must be equally diverse to meet the needs of individual patients.

An interdisciplinary group working toward a common goal hopes for a therapeutic outcome that is better than when each discipline functions separately.[23,38,67,77] The key to success lies in the coordination of efforts and in the communication among the professionals and with the patient. The professionals' interactions are as important as the team structure itself. Any one individual or discipline cannot be given priority, or the interdisciplinary nature of the group is lost.[115] Numerous descriptions of the components of a team reflect, not surprisingly, the originator's experience, bias, and discipline.[4,9,12,19,23,38,52,53,77,81,83,93,114,115,131]

The roles of team members typically represent a distribution of responsibilities specific to a discipline by tradition or by licensure restriction. Considerable overlapping or sharing of activities is desirable when members of more than one discipline are qualified to perform a task.[38] A patient's problems often dictate the need for the intervention of the appropriate discipline, but role clarification and areas of primary responsibility must be determined.[38] In almost all multidisciplinary settings, the patient's physician is the designated leader of the team, although the role of coordinator may fall to any member.[9,23]

Within the team, however, goals and role expectations are frequently unclear.[131] The *Outcome Standards for Rheumatology Nursing Practice* point out that the identified outcomes in patients may not be affected exclusively by nurses, and collaboration with other disciplines may be required.[82] Although it is essential for those in different disciplines working together in one setting

to understand each other's roles to best effect the treatment plan, it is not yet possible to define these roles generically.

Individuals representing various disciplines can reinforce each other's instructions and can provide feedback regarding the perceptions of the patient. A Delphi study showed that, in most cases, one discipline could be designated as primary.[23] In this study, certain broad activities were not considered specific to any one discipline, and each participated according to his expertise, as well as according to the needs and resources of the setting. Because all members of the team are not always available, another member can at least partially fill the gap.[93] All patients may not need the services of all team members.

Comprehensive treatment must consist of more than a series of referrals; it must also be coordinated into interactions to use the specialized knowledge, as well as the experience and judgment of the respective disciplines, effectively.[18,115] *Such coordination should be based on the patient's needs rather than on those of the care system.* What follows are brief descriptions of the roles of specific disciplines in rheumatic disease care as I perceive them after 15 years of experience with contributions from nursing and allied health colleagues and references to the literature that can be consulted for more detail. A brief summary of the roles of the disciplines reflecting my practice setting can be found in Table 43–4.

Nurse

The nurse has sometimes been called the generalist among specialists.[2] This statement is particularly true in rheumatology in which, depending on the availability of other disciplines, the nurse's role expands to fill the needs because of broad, rather than specific, expertise. Nursing is the discipline most apt to be found in all settings, and hence it is often overlooked. Although nurses have long cared for patients with rheumatic diseases, rheumatologic nursing has only recently emerged as a specialty.[20,109,111,121,127] Most nurses caring for patients with arthritis are generalists.

Hospitalization has been advocated to provide physical rest for the patient and isolation from emotional stress during times of uncontrolled exacerbation of inflammatory disease.[42] Nursing care is therefore a major reason for hospitalization.[85]

The role of the nurse varies with the setting and with density and mix of the population of patients. The nurse has knowledge related to human responses and identification of the needs of patients and nursing skills in providing physical care and comfort, in observing and assessing physical signs, symptoms, and behavior, and in administering

Table 43–4. Primary Areas of Practice Accountability

PHYSICIAN AND/OR RHEUMATOLOGIST
  Diagnosis
  Prescription of treatment (drugs, therapy, life style)
  Management (adjustment of therapeutic regimen)
PHYSIATRIST
  Consultant to medical staff
  Therapeutic recommendations
  Determination of impairment and disability
PSYCHIATRIST
  Consultant regarding patients' emotional problems
  Recommendations of psychologic management
  Diagnosis and treatment of psychiatric disorders
NURSE
  Assessment of and interventions in patients' problems
  Coordination based on patients' needs for consistency and
    continuity of care
  Physical care, safety, and comfort
  Emotional support
  Education of patients and families (self-management of
    medications, life style, comfort measures)
  Observations and reporting
  Patients' advocate and liaison
  Reinforcement of other disciplines and instructions
  Medication administration and monitoring
PHYSICAL THERAPIST [per physician's order]
  Evaluation of joint range of motion, muscle strength,
    endurance, sensation and perception, mobility, and
    gait
  Assessment of footwear needs
  Instruction in individualized exercise program, body me-
    chanics, and transfer skills
  Selection of assistive ambulation devices
  Application of heat, cold, electrical, or other therapies
OCCUPATIONAL THERAPIST [per physician's order]
  Evaluation of functional ability
  Instruction in joint protection, energy conservation and
    work simplification, and individualized exercise pro-
    gram
  Fabrication of splints
  Assist patients in planning life style modification
  Work evaluation
SOCIAL WORKER [by referral]
  Counseling (social and emotional)
  Assist patients in development of coping skills
  Location and referral of patients to community resources
    (vocational, financial)
  Identification of patients' emotional stage
  Liaison to patients and families
PHARMACIST
  Distribution of medications
  Consultant regarding medication information
  Medication instruction
DIETITIAN
  Dietary assessment
  Monitoring of pertinent laboratory values
  Instruction to patients regarding special diet (per physi-
    cian's order) and proper nutrition
  Recommendation of nutritional supplements
HOME CARE COORDINATOR
  Coordination with community care agencies
  Provision of information on community resources
  Liaison with community agencies

(Reprinted by permission from Rheumatic Disease Program, Columbia
Hospital, Milwaukee.)

drugs. Nurses have the closest and most prolonged contact with the patient and are therefore in an excellent position to teach, to counsel, to monitor for therapeutic compliance, to coordinate continuity of care, and to communicate with the attending physicians.[8,47,98,101]

The American Nurses' Association and AHPA *Outcome Standards for Rheumatology Nursing Practice,* which relate to problems encountered by patients and their families,[82] are in accord with the definition of nursing as "the diagnosis and treatment of human responses to actual or potential health problems."[80] The rheumatologic practice standards for which the nurse is accountable include management of pain, stiffness, fatigue, self-care, self-concept, and ineffective coping, as well as knowledge of the patient relating to mobility and self-management decisions.

The nursing care of the patient with a rheumatologic condition differs not so much by medical diagnosis but according to the individual patient's needs. For example, a rheumatic disease patient with life-threatening visceral organ involvement requires a different type and amount of nursing intervention than a patient with exacerbating and remitting chronic, multiple-joint involvement, or a newly diagnosed patient, or a patient with severe and late-stage crippling disease, or a patient with a temporary and localized problem, or one with a known cause and specific treatment; yet, the medical diagnosis may be the same for each of these nursing classifications.[86]

Care also varies with the specialized role of the nurse. A staff nurse has physical, psychologic, educational, and coordinating functions.[121] These functions may be specialized for certain parts of a patient's treatment, such as surgical procedures.[11,63] A community-based public health or visiting nurse is aware of helpful community resources, can monitor the implementation of the prescribed program, can enlist family involvement, and can provide valuable feedback information concerning the home environment.[28] The functions of a nurse practitioner, certified by the American Nurses' Association, may include detailed physical examination, evaluation of the patient's response to the medical program and management, referral to others for special needs, coordination of all care-providers' needs, and continuing or follow-up care.[13,69,87,91,121] Successful nurse-managed programs have been reported for patients receiving special drugs, such as gold, penicillamine, and methotrexate, and in specific conditions, such as degenerative joint disease and gout.[109,113,120] Nurse "metrologists" are now assisting in drug studies.[10,58,59] When waiting lists for "new" patients must be established by priority, an office nurse with expertise in rheumatology can accurately assess the urgency of a patient's need for an appointment.[109,110,112]

A survey of primary care physicians in an area with an incidence of arthritis that is higher than the national average revealed that some physicians did not feel that they knew how best to incorporate the nurse's capabilities,[32] but felt that some of the nurses did not work to their capacity. Many of the physicians surveyed thought that nurses needed more education about arthritis. Most of the physicians recognized nurses as specialists in education of patients. They wanted nurses that were better able to help patients to establish treatment plans in the home and to report on progress in coping with the arthritis. This goal was felt to be impractical because of the cost, however. The frequent lack of communication between physician and nurse was recognized, as well as the expense of employing a nurse.

By the application of *nursing process* (problem solving), including *nursing diagnosis* (identification of patients' problems that lend themselves to nursing intervention), the potential role of the nurse in the care of patients with rheumatic diseases is gradually becoming more clearly delineated.[86]

Physical Therapist

Arthritis commonly requires treatment by a physical therapist (see also Chap. 44).[62] Although physical therapy is an essential part of treatment of many rheumatic diseases,[35,74,75,81,99,102,117] it is often neglected.[117] Scandinavian studies have demonstrated that patients with classic or definite rheumatoid arthritis in functional classes I, II, or III have a better disease prognosis when undergoing long-term physical therapy, including active physical conditioning training, than their counterparts receiving identical medical management, but without physical therapy.[78,79]

Physical therapy is defined as the application of physical agents, including force, and therapists are trained to evaluate a patient's musculoskeletal system by assessing joint range of motion, muscle strength, endurance, sensation and perception, gait, mobility, coordination development, respiratory pattern, functional ability, and the need for special footwear and mobility aids.

Physical therapists apply or instruct patients in an individualized therapeutic exercise program directed at correcting an impairment and at improving musculoskeletal or cardiovascular function. Therapeutic exercises are often directed toward two components of function: range of joint motion and muscle strength. Range-of-motion exercises maintain the anatomic movement of a joint. Strengthening exercises improve the muscles' ability to

work. In inflammatory joint disease, isometric exercises, which involve contraction of muscle without changing its overall length, are emphasized because of the minimal stress on the joint's supporting structures. Passive exercises can improve mobility when patients are unable to exercise independently. Active assistive exercises and active exercises increase strength, coordination, and function. Some exercises or activities aid endurance or posture. The physical therapist can advise the physician in selecting the appropriate type and intensity of exercise.

The physical therapist provides instruction in gait, body mechanics, and transfer skills. Properly selected canes, crutches, walkers, or wheelchairs often enhance a patient's mobility. Equipment must be chosen with careful consideration of all involved joints, energy conservation, convenience, and practicality. For example, painful hands or wrists may not be able to bear the load transmitted through the handle of a cane, so weight distribution through a forearm trough, or platform crutches, may be better. Aids or techniques that help in transferring may increase mobility, whereas proper use of body mechanics may increase function and may conserve limited energy. Shoe modifications may help with painful feet that limit ambulation, and shoe orthoses may prevent or correct early deformity.

The physical therapist understands the various combinations of heat, cold,[6] water, and electricity that can be applied in different forms, to relieve muscle spasm, to increase local circulation, or to relieve pain. Supervised water movement is especially valuable in treatment of arthritis, allowing exercising while using the buoyancy of water.[24,25,27,35,62,70,74,76,87,117,122]

The physical therapist plays a major part in pre- and postoperative treatment to restore optimum comfort and function and instructs patients in a home exercise program.[27,63,73] One study indicated that physicians believed that physical therapists were not sufficiently informed regarding the arthritis patient, but these physicians also recognized that they themselves were not sure how to instruct physical therapists.[32]

Occupational Therapist

Occupational therapy for rheumatic disease patients consists of a medically prescribed evaluation and treatment directed toward improving or restoring lost functions. The reference to "occupation" may be misleading unless thought of as the goal-directed use of purposeful activity. The occupational therapist aids the patient in achieving optimal function by developing new adaptive skills or by improving existing performance capacity.[106]

The work of the occupational therapist falls into the categories of assessment and therapy.[54]

Patients are appropriately referred to the occupational therapist for evaluation of performance and for help in gaining functional independence. The goals include education of the patient, physical comfort, psychosocial adjustment, and postoperative rehabilitation. To assess function, an occupational therapist evaluates motor skills, range of motion, strength, endurance, and skills of daily living, and also documents deformity.[65]

The occupational therapist can assist the patient in gaining or in maintaining functional independence at home, at work, and at school through adaptations in activities of daily living or by the provision of assistive or adaptive equipment.[103] This goal may include physical modifications of the home, work, and school environment. In addition to vocational counseling, leisure activities and play are also analyzed. Through task analysis, occupational therapists assess the work setting and activity for incorporation of disease-management principles and exploration of alternate worksites.[106]

Educating patients to prevent disability is part of the role of the occupational therapist.[124] This work includes instruction in energy conservation, by elimination of wasted body motion, work simplification, by means of streamlining of tasks to maximize efficiency, body mechanics, which are a component of energy conservation and joint protection concerned with posture during movement, joint protection to avoid postures or stress that cause deformities, the effect of disease on life style,[40] and adjustment to disease or disability.[43] The patient may also be instructed in relaxation techniques and in measures to handle emotional stress.

The occupational therapist also addresses the psychosocial components of performance, including social interaction, self-management, decision-making and problem-solving, and adjustment to disability. Orthotic devices may be fabricated by the occupational therapist and may be fitted for comfort to increase function and to prevent deformity.[41] Postoperative rehabilitation, particularly of the hand and wrist, is undertaken by the occupational therapist.[5,39,104]

A study of primary care physicians' perceptions of arthritis health professionals demonstrated confusion in understanding the difference between the physical and occupational therapist's roles, as well as misconceptions regarding the functions of the occupational therapists.[32] Although many of their functions do overlap,[5,14,15,17,55,64,66,71,87,96,105,106,128] the roles of the physical and of the occupational therapist are determined by staffing patterns, departmental philosophies, and practices, as well as

by an individual therapist's skills and interests. Broadly, the physical therapist restores the function of the muscles, whereas the occupational therapist translates that function into relevant activity.[106] The best way to differentiate their roles in each setting is to ask them.

The primary goals of occupational therapy and the ways in which they are accomplished include the following: (1) the reduction of pain and inflammation through splinting or instructing the patient in positioning to rest involved joints and the protection of joints during use; (2) maintenance of motion and joint integrity by gentle passive or active range of motion, proper positioning for lying or sitting, and use of resting splints; and (3) maintenance of function by instruction in pacing, work simplification, energy conservation measures, and alternate methods of performing activities of daily living. A major role of the occupational therapist is in helping the patient to modify his life style to reach these goals.

Social Worker

The skills of a social worker should be used in comprehensive management of patients with chronic rheumatic disease, in direct intervention with the patient and family and in helping other care providers to recognize the patient's emotional reactions. Through psychosocial assessment, the social worker can identify the patient's current stage of emotional response to the illness; that is, denial, anger, depression, or acceptance, as well as to identify his past and present ability to cope with stress and the extent of family support. The social worker's interventions with the patient and family include counseling on social and emotional concerns, development of coping skills, and location and referral to available community resources such as housing agencies, transportation resources, vocational rehabilitation programs, and financial assistance sources.

The social worker often acts as a liaison, aiding communication between care providers and patients and guiding the other care providers to appropriate responses.[9,21,56,87–89,115]

Other Disciplines

Other disciplines may be involved in the comprehensive care of the arthritis patient. The *pharmacist* not only dispenses drugs but also may assist the physician in their selection and in considerations of dosage, optimal timing, toxicity, and interactions. Education of the staff regarding medications is yet another role of the pharmacist. The pharmacist can identify patients taking over-the-counter remedies who may need medical supervision, as well as patients who have forgotten or have neglected refills. The pharmacist can also suggest ways of reducing drug costs, and when more than one physician is prescribing, may identify potential drug interactions or prescription duplications.[30,84,87,92]

The *dietitian* assesses nutritional status through diet history, monitoring of pertinent laboratory values, and appropriate anthropometrics. Acutely ill patients with increased metabolic needs, increased pain, decreased appetite, and decreased ability to eat or to swallow may require nutritional supplements to ensure adequate intake. Overweight patients require individualized meal plans, education, and counseling to maximize weight loss and weight maintenance. In addition, the dietitian provides guidance through the maze of fad diets and nutritional misinformation.

Laboratory personnel contribute their efforts toward proper diagnosis and management.[1]

Psychologists and *counselors* help to identify and to manage associated emotional problems and evaluate problems that affect the rehabilitation program. These professionals are involved in counseling and adaptation activities, including relaxation measures, and must be aware of the psychologic disorders associated with the various rheumatic diseases as well as drug-induced psychologic problems.[19,53,95,115,129,130]

The vocational rehabilitation of a person with rheumatic disease is much more complicated than that of some other physically disabled clients with more static disabilities.[53,100] Arthritis is often a progressive disability that may vary from day to day, and the same type of arthritis varies in severity from person to person. Arthritis can directly affect work competence and may have a significant psychologic impact.[115] The *vocational or rehabilitation counselor* evaluates the work abilities of the patient, offers vocational counseling and guidance, and helps the individual to retrain for specific vocational skills.[108,116]

The *podiatrist* provides routine toenail and foot care, particularly for patients with skin difficulties and deformities of the foot. In addition, the podiatrist educates patients about foot problems, including the selection of proper footwear with internal and external modifications to relieve stress areas.[97,107] The *orthotic specialist* makes and modifies prescribed appliances such as braces, splints, foot supports, and special shoes for each patient's particular needs.

Health educators and *biomedical engineers* are the newest professional groups in rheumatology. Although all disciplines are involved in educating the patient and his family, the health educator has the primary role and may be responsible for development and coordination of the education program. Biomedical engineers have become increasingly involved in research on prostheses.

FUNCTIONS

The basic treatment goals addressed in the management of arthritis are: (1) relief of pain; (2) prevention of deformity; and (3) maintenance of function. The roles of nurses and allied health professionals stem directly from these goals. Although the physician prescribes the components of the treatment program, thereby designating participation of others, not all these functions are dependent. Each discipline also has independent problem-solving activities that are usually discipline-specific. *To achieve these goals most effectively, activities should be interdependent and synergistic, so the whole is at least equal to or greater than the sum of the parts.*[9,23]

Independent Functions

Independent functions of nursing and allied health professionals include activities that are either discipline-specific, are individualized to the patient, or require that a decision be made. A discipline-specific function is physical care. A nurse does not see a physician's order to "care for the patient." Yet nurses independently see to it that the patient has physical space of his own, a bed to sleep in, food to eat, and arrangements for hygiene and personal care. Although this function is often taken for granted, it can be of vital importance to the arthritis patient who is physically dependent on others.

As a basis not only for their independent functions, but also for individualized aspects of dependent and interdependent functions, all disciplines incorporate some sort of assessment or evaluation into their programs. This individualized information is the basis of their decisions and is one of the criteria for the definition of a profession. The focus of the assessment or evaluation differs from one discipline to another. Whereas the physician structures history-taking and physical examination to elicit data on which diagnosis or management can be based, nursing and the allied health professions are oriented toward the problems of patients, such as difficulty in walking or refusal to eat. These assessments or evaluations, in addition to health, physical and functional status, include home environment and personal life style, as well as learning ability, financial resources, and emotional and social status.[33] These independent assessments can be valuable because they form a more complete picture of the patient and his needs. Such combined assessments, then, cover not only signs and symptoms and other condition-specific information, but also the patient's ability to follow a therapeutic regimen and to adapt it to his home environment and life style.

Although specific interventions are at least partly dependent functions requiring a medical order, the way in which those interventions are performed is likely to be an independent function. As an example, pain management is a frequent problem of patients with arthritis. The physician may order an analgesic to be given when needed, but whether or not to give the medication, and when to give it, is the nurse's decision based on an assessment of the specific situation. In addition to, or in place of, the drug, the nurse may decide to apply heat or cold or to try a relaxation or distraction technique.

Education of the patient, because of its inherent individualization, is another area of independent function. The following are some examples. The nurse may teach the patient pharmacologic self-management techniques based on his unique situation for a successful follow-up when the patient is on his own.

The occupational therapist, although often requiring a physician's order to teach, individualizes concepts and principles of work simplification, energy conservation, joint protection, and body mechanics. The occupational therapist takes into account the disease's systemic features, the general state of deconditioning, and the total needs of the patient in regard to psychosocial, recreational, and vocational demands, to determine an appropriately individualized institutional program.[105] Instruction in joint protection varies for different diseases. Increased joint activity may be helpful in some diseases, but harmful in others. Adjoining joints operate interdependently, so what may be protective to one joint may redirect the forces to another in a stressful manner. Although the physician orders instructions in joint protection, the occupational therapist determines the appropriate measures.

The physical therapist individualizes instruction in a home exercise program based on the patient's needs. Each discipline determines the best teaching opportunity, based on the patient's readiness to learn and the appropriate instructional technique.

Symptoms bring the patient into the health care system. If the symptoms are not relieved, the patient may leave the system to seek help elsewhere. Sometimes, the symptoms cannot be totally eliminated, so the patient's understanding of and belief in the treatment become the key to satisfaction and compliance. Reaching this understanding can be time consuming and can also require special skills in relationships. Not to merely impart knowledge, but to teach skills, including problem solving, adaptation, and coping, and to facilitate the "educational process" wherein the patient does what is

recommended and is reasonably satisfied, may be a major contribution of nurses and allied health professionals to care of the patient. The required individualization of these activities is also an independent function.

Another activity of nurses and allied health professionals may be the organization of groups of patients for the purposes of education, support, or socializing.[51,60,87] These activities, previously thought to enhance communication, to improve compliance with medical regimens, and to promote a sense of well-being, have more recently been shown to increase patients' knowledge about their disease and to improve some patients' perception of the adequacy of their families' attitudes and behavior[37,90] Use of accepted educational and counseling strategies to change behavior can assist patients to assume more responsibility for their own care. This aspect is crucial because care providers have no control over therapeutic activities performed away from direct supervision.

As the need arises, nurses and allied health professionals are involved with the family. Roles may have changed within the family, and the patient may no longer be the family's financial supporter or may no longer be able to care for the home. Like the patient, family members may be passing through similar stages of adjustment and may gain insight into management of their own emotional reactions by understanding those of the patient.[36] Both planned and informal opportunities enable the nurse and allied health professional to assume this independent role in assisting the family.

The areas of adaptation and coping with the problems arising from a chronic rheumatic disease are addressed by most care providers in an independent way. As an example, problems relating to sexuality may involve the physical therapist if the sexual dysfunction is due to limited range of motion or to weakness, the social worker in issues of emotions, personality, body image, or interpersonal relationships, the occupational therapist in applying concepts of pacing and energy conservation to overcome fatigue, and the nurse to help the patient understand the relationship of disease or medications to sexual functioning.[26]

Dependent Functions

Physicians write orders that are carried out by nursing and allied health personnel. Some activities that cannot be undertaken without a medical order are the following: (1) the administration of medications by the nurse, although timing may be left to the nurse's discretion; (2) laboratory testing, although predetermined protocol may prevail; (3) pre- and postoperative instructions and splinting although the occupational therapist or orthotist selects the splinting materials;[104] and (4) exercise programs for a specific purpose. The prescription for exercise must be individualized and may be determined by the physician or occupational therapist because the concept of the "arthritis routine" of exercises is fallacious.

Interdependent Functions

The role of any discipline, including medicine, is not carried out in a vacuum. A given discipline does not depend on the others, except within legal guidelines, to perform discipline-specific activities. Most functions, however, are best carried out interdependently with other care providers.[85] Nurses and allied health professionals independently assess the patient with regard to problems, they design and implement plans to address the identified problems, and then they evaluate the results interdependently. For example, the physician notes that a patient is not responding to treatment as expected. The nurse contributes the information that the patient is not taking the medication as directed, but is taking it only as he feels the need. The social worker indicates that the patient is on a fixed income and feels that he cannot afford the medication. As a result, instructions are clarified, medication times are adapted to the patient's home schedule, and the social worker aids in seeking financial assistance. Together, the actions of the physician, the nurse and the social worker interdependently affect the outcome. The roles complement each other while approaching the patient from each discipline's unique perspective.

In Chapter 42, education of the patient is identified as an important element in management. Education of the patient, as an independent function of nurses and allied health professionals, has been addressed earlier, but it also must be interdependent. Such interdependence provides consistency, reinforcement, and multiple and varied approaches to gain the patient's cooperation with the therapeutic regimen.[38,49]

Education of the patient and his family is also interdisciplinary. Each discipline has areas of primary accountability, but most areas overlap disciplines (Table 43–5). An example is joint protection. Although the occupational therapist is most likely to teach concepts and principles, other disciplines, usually nursing or physical therapy, provide reinforcement and instruct the patient in their application.

Education of the patient involves much more than merely providing the patient with information about disease. The information must be consistent from one professional to another. This instruction should be based on the beliefs, needs, and concerns

Table 43–5. Patient Education: Content Areas of Primary Responsibility by Discipline

NURSING
  Medications
  Pacing and rest
  Posture and positioning
  Responsibility of the patient
  Comfort measures for pain and stiffness
  Coping and adaptation
  Unproved methods of treatment
  Compliance

OCCUPATIONAL THERAPY
  Joint protection
  Energy conservation
  Use of adaptive equipment
  Relaxation
  Pacing and rest
  Exercise programs
  Posture and positioning

SOCIAL SERVICE
  Community resources
  Coping and adaptation

PHYSICAL THERAPY
  Range of motion
  Use of heat and cold therapy
  Relaxation
  Footwear
  Posture and positioning
  Exercise

MEDICINE
  Diagnosis
  Disease process
  Prognosis
  Medications

PHARMACY
  Medications
  Compliance

DIETETICS
  Nutrition
  Special diets

(Reprinted by permission from Rheumatic Disease Program, Columbia Hospital, Milwaukee.)

of the patient and should include educational activities aimed at assisting patients in changing their health behavior voluntarily.[60] This goal requires close communication and sharing of information among the various team members. Using needs assessment and measuring motivation, an educational program can improve cognitive knowledge and may motivate behavioral changes.[57]

An informed patient is more likely to comply with the prescribed therapeutic regimen and usually reports more reliably the effects, good or bad, of that regimen.[29] Failure to cooperate implies that the patient has not received full benefit from the health care provider's expertise. Failure to take the prescribed medication may exacerbate the disease. When it is assumed that the patient is taking the prescribed amount of medication without the desired results and dosage is increased, overdosage may result. Undetected failure to cooperate can lead to an incorrect evaluation of efficacy of a particular treatment regimen.[49] Regimens must be tailored to the individual characteristics of each patient and should be adjusted only when the patient is compliant. Some investigators suggest that the results of clinical trials should not be published unless they include an adequate assessment of "compliance."[48] It often takes the skills and insights of a variety of professionals to understand the reasons behind a patient's failure to comply and to then be able to help the patient.[44]

Physicians' estimate of compliance of patients are often inaccurate; nursing and allied health professionals can help to identify barriers to compliance. Patients fail to adhere to therapeutic recommendations for many reasons. *Denying* patients may not believe their illness warrants extensive care. *Angry* patients may refuse to comply as a way of punishing families or the health care provider. *Depressed* patients perceive compliance as pointless.[36] Finances, time schedules, unrealistic family expectations, and different opinions as to an adequate therapeutic trial are other possible barriers.[16,22] The problems of noncompliance often require interdisciplinary assessment and correction.

Other good examples of interdependent practice exist, such as the liaison role of the nurse.[33] The physician's referral of patients to professionals in other disciplines requires recognition of the need and reflects the quality of the interdisciplinary component of a rheumatic disease practice. Discharge planning is a cooperative effort of all disciplines with emphasis on the strengths, limitations, and goals of the individual patient. When continuing care is indicated, the decision is often shared. Interdisciplinary consultation and communication demonstrate responsibility to other professionals as well as to patients.

Administrative and Research Functions

Nurses and allied health professionals may become chiefs of departments of therapy or head nurses. Some also hold management positions in specialized rheumatic disease programs.

Some allied health professionals and nurses are also involved in independent research as principal investigators in areas such as the content and methods of programs to educate patients and families, treatment techniques, validation of measurement tools, psychosocial issues, and health status.[68] Others assist or coordinate research protocols under the direction of a physician.

The AHPA Fellowship Program was established in 1972 to develop research training opportunities and to grant support for professionals other than physicians engaged in the delivery of health care. This program mirrored the organization's shift in emphasis from its original purpose of providing a home for the allied health worker interested in arthritis to a more mission-oriented goal. The AHPA now emphasizes research and professional education in health care delivery and the effective use of clinical techniques. This emphasis complements the basic biomedical research done by the members of the ARA.[31]

FACTORS INFLUENCING EFFECTIVENESS

Recommendations made by all team members must be followed to be effective. A study of recommendations made by a rheumatologist, a physical therapist, and a psychologist to the patient's primary care physician and to the patient showed that of 58 medical recommendations, 28 were acted on by the physician and 11 by the patient.[131] Only 7 of the 45 physical therapists' suggestions were acted on by the physician, but the patients followed 26. None of the counseling or psychosocial suggestions made by the team were followed by physicians, but 35 were followed by the patients. The study recommended that patients receive written copies of the suggestions and evaluations made by the allied health professionals, to encourage patient-physician dialog regarding the suggestions.[32]

The effectiveness of the nurse or allied health professional varies with individual, environmental, organizational, financial, and interpersonal factors. Entry-level preparation, practice experience in the discipline, as well as rheumatologic skills and expertise, and individual attitudes about chronicity, deformity, and dependency all influence the care of patients with arthritis. The practice setting is another factor influencing effectiveness. When nurses, for example, care for patients other than those with arthritis, the physical care and needs of these patients may take precedence over the psychosocial and educational needs of the arthritic patient.

Support by specific departments, by hospital administrators, and by physicians is necessary for optimal function. The roles of nurses and allied health professionals in the care of patients with arthritis are often not fully understood nor are their services effectively utilized. The rheumatologist is in a position to speak to the departmental chairman or hospital administrator to request high-quality service.

The expense of employing a nurse in the office practice or concern about cost in referring the patient to a therapist may deprive the patient of needed services.[93] The recent changes in reimbursement patterns compound this problem.

The relationship between patients and nurses or allied health professionals differs from the patient-physician relationship. For various reasons, which may include physical proximity (not only the increased amount of contact time, but the intimacy of assistance provided in such tasks as bathing and toileting) and a feeling of more-equal standing, patients often confide in the nurse or allied health professional attitudes relating to compliance, financial restrictions, family relationships, and other items they did not mention to their physician. Such information is often medically relevant when conveyed to the physician.[38]

Many of these influences on effectiveness were demonstrated in a study of primary care physicians' perceptions of nurses and allied health professionals. This study revealed a lack of understanding of roles, a concern with cost, problems in communication, lack of accessibility or availability in practice, a feeling of threat to the physician's authority, and the need for flexibility of charges.[93]

In summary, the roles and functions of nurses and allied health professionals have been defined in terms of goals, problems and interventions used to solve them, organizational structure, and the perspectives of the individual disciplines. The knowledge explosion and the demand for a "holistic" approach by patients will lead to everchanging, flexible descriptions of the functions of nurses and allied health professionals. This change may lead to a more appropriate and effective use of their services.[72] Rapid translation of new information into effective disease management is a challenge to the many disciplines in the health sciences.

Roles of nurses and allied health professionals are best described by standards and expressed through the individual disciplines' practice. An understanding of these roles is necessary for the most effective utilization of expertise and skills of all disciplines involved in comprehensive care of the rheumatic disease patient.

REFERENCES

1. Adams, L.E., and Hess, E.V.: Editorial: continuing medical education in rheumatology of arthritis health professional laboratory personnel. J. Rheumatol., 7:1–4, 1980.
2. Allen, K.E., Holm, V.A., and Schiefelbusch, R.L.: Early Intervention—A Team Approach. Baltimore, University Park Press, 1978.
3. ARA Subcommittee: Manual for Arthritis Clinics. Atlanta, Arthritis and Rheumatism Foundation, 1952. (Revised 1964.)
4. Arthritis Health Professions Section: Arthritis Teaching Slide Collection for Teachers of Allied Health Professionals. Atlanta, Arthritis Foundation, 1980.
5. Artzberger, S., and Mathiewitz, V.: Splinting. In Arthritis—A Modular Curriculum for Occupational Therapy. Edited by L. Kautzmann. Milwaukee, School of Allied Health Professions, University of Wisconsin–Milwaukee, 1981.
6. Banwell, B.F.: Therapeutic heat and cold. In Rheumatic Diseases: Rehabilitation and Management. Edited by G.K. Riggs and E.P. Gall. Woburn, MA, Butterworth Publishers, 1984.
7. Baum, J., and Figley, B.A.: Psychological and sexual health in rheumatic diseases. In Textbook of Rheumatology. Vol. 1. Edited by W.N. Kelley, et al. Philadelphia, W.B. Saunders, 1981.
8. Beardsley, J., and Rowlands, D.: Nursing the rheumatic patient. In Essential Rheumatology for Nurses and Therapists. Edited by G.S. Panayi. London, Bailliere Tindall, 1980.
9. Bernhard, G.C.: Development of a rheumatology consulting practice program. In Arthritis and Allied Conditions. 9th Ed. Edited by D.J. McCarty. Philadelphia, Lea & Febiger, 1979.
10. Bird, M.: Clinical metrology. Nurs. Times, 77, 1926.
11. Brassell, M.P.: Rehabilitation nursing and the surgical patient. In Rehabilitation Management of Rheumatic Conditions. Edited by G.E. Ehrlich. Baltimore, Williams & Wilkins, 1980.
12. Brattstrom, M.D.: Teamwork in the rehabilitation of patients with chronic rheumatic disease. Ann. Clin. Res., 7:230–236, 1975.
13. Brown-Skeers, V.: How the nurse practitioner manages the rheumatoid arthritis patient. Nurs. '79, 9:26–34, 1979.
14. Chamberlain, M.A.: Occupational therapy. In Rehabilitation in the rheumatic diseases. Clin. Rheum. Dis., 7:365–375, 1981.
15. Cordery, J.C.: Joint protection—responsibility of the occupational therapist. Am. J. Occup. Ther., 19:285–291, 1965.
16. Deyo, R.A.: Compliance with therapeutic regimens in arthritis: issues, current status, and a future agenda. Semin. Arthritis Rheum., 12:233–244, 1982.
17. Douglas, J.: Occupational therapy—rehabilitation and resettlement. In Essential Rheumatology for Nurses and Therapists. Edited by G.S. Panayi. London, Bailliere Tindall, 1980.
18. Ehrlich, G.E. (Ed.): Rehabilitation Management of Rheumatic Conditions. Baltimore, Williams & Wilkins, 1980.
19. Ehrlich, G.E. (Ed.): Total Management of the Arthritis Patient. Philadelphia, J.B. Lippincott, 1973.
20. Elliott, M.: Nursing Rheumatic Disease. New York, Churchill Livingstone, 1979.
21. Erfling, J.L.: The role of the social worker in the rehabilitation of rheumatic disease patients. In Rehabilitation Management of Rheumatic Conditions. Edited by G.E. Ehrlich. Baltimore, Williams & Wilkins, 1980.
22. Ferguson, K., and Bole, G.G.: Family support, health belief, and therapeutic compliance in patients with rheumatoid arthritis. Patient Counsel. Health Educ., 1:101–105, 1979.
23. Figley, B.A.: The roles of health professionals in management of arthritis. Clin. Rheumatol. Pract., 1:43–46, 1983.
24. Figley, B.A.: Maintaining joint mobility. In Arthritis—A Modular Curriculum for Occupational Therapy. Edited by L. Kautzmann. Milwaukee, School of Allied Health Professions, University of Wisconsin–Milwaukee, 1981.
25. Figley, B.A.: Physical modalities in the management of arthritis. In Arthritis—A Modular Curriculum for Occupational Therapy. Edited by L. Kautzmann. Milwaukee, School of Allied Health Professions, University of Wisconsin–Milwaukee, 1981.
26. Figley, B.A., et al.: Comprehensive approach to sexual health in rheumatic disease. Top. Clin. Nurs., 1:69–74, 1980.
27. Figley, B.A., and Denek, C.J.: Physical Therapy in Arthritis. Ann Arbor, University of Michigan Arthritis Center, F4416 Mott, 1978.
28. Fligg, H., and Wright, V.: The community and hospital nurse in relation to arthritis. In Rehabilitation in the rheumatic diseases. Clin. Rheum. Dis., 7:321–336, 1981.
29. Fries, J.F.: General approach to the rheumatic disease

patient. *In* Textbook of Rheumatology. Vol. I. Edited by W.N. Kelley, et al. Philadelphia, W.B. Saunders, 1981.

30. Fritz, W.L.: The pharmacist's contribution to patient care. *In* Rheumatic Diseases: Rehabilitation and Management. Edited by G.K. Riggs and E.P. Gall. Woburn, MA, Butterworth Publishers, 1984.

31. Gall, E.P.: Health care research for the patient. Clin. Rheumatol. Pract., *1*:41–42, 1983.

32. Gall, E.P.: Professionalism, research and directions—the AHPA in 1983. Clin. Rheumatol. Pract., *1*:179–182, 1983.

33. Gall, E.P., and Johnson, S.A.: Arthritis: altered levels of mobility. *In* Chronic Health Problems—Concepts and Applications. Edited by S. VanDam Anderson and E.E. Bauwens. St. Louis, C.V. Mosby, 1981.

34. Giesecke, L.: School outreach is possible. Arthritis Health Professions Newslett., *13*:1–3, 1979.

35. Gross, D.: The role of physiotherapy in the overall treatment program for rheumatoid arthritis. *In* Chronic Forms of Polyarthritis. Edited by F.J. Wagenhauser. Baltimore, Williams & Wilkins, 1976.

36. Gross, M.: Psychosocial aspects of osteoarthritis—helping patients cope. Health Soc. Work, *65*:40–46, 1981.

37. Gross, M., and Brandt, K.D.: Educational support groups for patients with ankylosing spondylitis: a preliminary report. Patient Counsel. Health Educ., *3*:6–12, 1981.

38. Gross, M., et al.: Team care for patients with chronic rheumatic disease. J. Allied Health, *11*:239–247, 1982.

39. Gruen, H.: Splinting in the rheumatic diseases. *In* Rehabilitation Management of Rheumatic Conditions. Edited by G.E. Ehrlich. Baltimore, Williams & Wilkins, 1980.

40. Handley, R.K.: The occupational therapist's role in sexual adjustment to disability. Allied Health Professions Sect. Newslett., *10*:8–9, 1977.

41. Hanten, D.W.: The splinting controversy in RA physical disabilities. Am. J. Occup. Ther. (Special Interest Newslett.), *5*:1–24, 1981.

42. Haralson, K., et al.: Value of Arthritis Educational Seminars for Allied Health Professionals. (Abstract.) Denver, Arthritis Health Professions Section Meeting, 1979.

43. Harlowe, D.: Coping with change—the crisis intervention frame of reference. *In* Arthritis—A Modular Curriculum for Occupational Therapy. Edited by L. Kautzmann. Milwaukee, School of Allied Health Professions, University of Wisconsin–Milwaukee, 1981.

44. Harlowe, D.: Patient compliance: a holistic approach. *In* Arthritis—A Modular Curriculum for Occupational Therapy. Edited by L. Kautzmann. Milwaukee, School of Allied Health Professions, University of Wisconsin–Milwaukee, 1981.

45. Heiss, M.L., et al.: Patients with Rheumatic Diseases. Chicago, Educational Services Division, American Journal of Nursing, 1981.

46. Hess, E.V.: Collagen diseases. *In* Rheumatic Diseases: Rehabilitation and Management. Edited by G.K. Riggs and E.P. Gall. Woburn, MA, Butterworth Publishers, 1984.

47. Horton, J.: Rheumatology nursing. Nurs. Mirror, *155*:76, 1982.

48. Jette, A.M.: Understanding and enhancing patient cooperation with arthritis treatments. *In* Rheumatic Diseases: Rehabilitation and Management. Edited by G.K. Riggs and E.P. Gall. Woburn, MA, Butterworth Publishers, 1984.

49. Jette, A.M.: Improving patient cooperation with arthritis treatment regimens. Arthritis Rheum., *25*:447–453, 1982.

50. Jette, A.M., and Becker, M.C.: Nursing, occupational therapy, and physical therapy preparation in rheumatology in the United States and Canada. J. Allied Health, *9*:268–275, 1980.

51. Kaplan, S., and Kozin, F.: A controlled study of group counseling in rheumatoid arthritis. J. Rheumatol., *8*:91–99, 1981.

52. Katz, S., et al.: Comprehensive outpatient care in rheumatoid arthritis. JAMA, *206*:1249–1254, 1968.

53. Katz, W.A. (Ed.): Rheumatic Disease: Diagnosis and Management. Philadelphia, J.B. Lippincott, 1977.

54. Kautzmann, L. (Ed.): Arthritis—A Modular Curriculum for Occupational Therapy. Milwaukee, School of Allied Health Professions, University of Wisconsin–Milwaukee, 1981.

55. Kautzmann, L.: Joint protection in rheumatoid arthritis and degenerative joint disease. *In* Arthritis—A Modular Curriculum for Occupational Therapy. Edited by L. Kautzmann. Milwaukee, School of Allied Health Professions, University of Wisconsin–Milwaukee, 1981.

56. Kliman, C.: Role of social worker. *In* Arthritis—A Modular Curriculum for Occupational Therapy. Edited by L. Kautzmann. Milwaukee, School of Allied Health Professions, University of Wisconsin–Milwaukee, 1981.

57. Knudson, K.G., Spiegel, T.M., and Furst, D.E.: Outpatient educational program for rheumatoid arthritis patients. Patient Counsel. Health Educ., *3*:77–82, 1981.

58. Leatham, P.: An extended nursing role in the arthritis care team. Nurs. Times, *77*:1926–1927, 1981.

59. LeGallez, P.: So what's a metrologist? Nurs. Times, *77*:1926–1927, 1981.

60. Lorig, K.: Arthritis patient education. *In* Rheumatic Diseases: Rehabilitation and Management. Edited by G.K. Riggs and E.P. Gall. Woburn, MA, Butterworth Publishers, 1984.

61. Maclean, M.T.: The role of the allied health professional in an outreach rheumatology program. (Abstract.) *In* Proceedings of Allied Health Professions Section Meeting, Chicago, 1976.

62. Maloney, P.: Physiotherapy for the rheumatic patient. *In* Essential Rheumatology for Nurses and Therapists. Edited by G.S. Panayi. London, Bailliere Tindall, 1980.

63. McCann, V.H., Philips, C.A., and Quigley, T.R.: Preoperative and postoperative management—the role of allied health professionals. Orthop. Clin. North Am., *61*:379–380, 1975.

64. Melvin, Jeanne L.: Rheumatic Disease: Occupational Therapy and Rehabilitation. 2nd Ed. Philadelphia, F.A. Davis, 1982.

65. Melvin, Jeanne L.: Occupational therapy assessment. *In* Arthritis—A Modular Curriculum for Occupational Therapy. Edited by L. Kautzmann. Milwaukee, School of Allied Health Professions, University of Wisconsin–Milwaukee, 1981.

66. Melvin, Jeanne L.: Therapeutic exercises for arthritis. *In* Arthritis—A Modular Curriculum for Occupational Therapy. Edited by L. Kautzmann. Milwaukee, School of Allied Health Professions, University of Wisconsin–Milwaukee, 1981.

67. Melvin, John L.: Interdisciplinary and multidisciplinary activities and the ACRM. Arch. Phys. Med. Rehab., *61*:379–380, 1980.

68. Membership Directory 1982–83. American Rheumatism Association and Arthritis Health Professions Association, Atlanta, Sections of the Arthritis Foundation, 1983.

69. Miller, C.C.: The rheumatic disease nurse practitioner. *In* Rehabilitation Management of Rheumatic Conditions. Edited by G.E. Ehrlich, Baltimore, Williams & Wilkins, 1980.

70. Mollinger, L.: Assistive devices to improve and maintain functional ambulation. *In* Arthritis—Modular Curriculum for Occupational Therapy. Edited by L. Kautzmann. Milwaukee, School of Allied Health Professions. University of Wisconsin–Milwaukee, 1981.

71. Moyes, B., and Haslock, I.: Occupational therapy in rheumatic diseases. Rep. Rheum. Dis., *77*, 1981.

72. National Commission on Arthritis and Related Musculoskeletal Diseases: Report to the Congress of the United States. Vol. 1: The Arthritis Plan, April 1976. DHEW Publication No. (NIH)76-1150. Washington, D.C., U.S. Department of Health, Education and Welfare, 1976.

73. Navarro, A.H.: The role of the physical therapist. *In* Rheumatic Diseases: Rehabilitation and Management. Edited by G. Riggs and E. Gall. Woburn, MA, Butterworth Publishers, 1984.

74. Navarro, A.H.: Physical therapy in the management of rheumatoid arthritis. Clin. Rheumatol. Pract., *1*:125–130, 1983.

75. Navarro, A.H., and Sutton, J.D.: Rheumatoid arthritis.

VIII: The approach of the allied health professional. Md. State Med. J., *31*:27–28, 1982.

76. Neubauer, P.: The role of the physiotherapist in a multidisciplinary arthritis program. *In* Rehabilitation Management of Rheumatic Conditions. Edited by G.E. Ehrlich. Baltimore, Williams & Wilkins, 1980.

77. Nichols, P.J.R.: Rehabilitation. *In* Copeman's Textbook of the Rheumatic Diseases. Edited by J.T. Scott. New York, Churchill Livingstone, 1978.

78. Nordemar, R.: Physical training in rheumatoid arthritis: a controlled long-term study. II. Functional capacity and general attitudes. Scand. J. Rheumatol., *10*:25–30, 1981.

79. Nordemar, R., et al.: Physical training in rheumatoid arthritis: a controlled long-term study. Scand. J. Rheumatol., *10*:17–23, 1981.

80. Nursing—A Social Policy Statement. Kansas City, American Nurses' Association, 1980.

81. Ogryzlo, M.A., Gordon, D.A., and Smythe, H.A.: The rheumatic disease unit (RDU) concept. Arthritis Rheum., *105*:479–485, 1967.

82. Outcome Standards for Rheumatology Nursing Practice. Kansas City, American Nurses' Association, 1983.

83. Panayi, G.S. (Ed.): Essential Rheumatology for Nurses and Therapists. London, Bailliere Tindall, 1980.

84. Parry, D.: The pharmacist's role in the rheumatology total health care team. (Abstract.) *In* Proceedings of the Arthritis Health Professions Association Meeting, San Antonio, 1983.

85. Pigg, J.S.: Nursing care of the hospitalized patient with rheumatic disease. *In* Rehabilitation Management of Rheumatic Conditions. Edited by G.E. Ehrlich. Baltimore, Williams & Wilkins, 1980.

86. Pigg, J.S., Driscoll, P.W., and Caniff, R.: Rheumatology Nursing: A Problem Oriented Approach. New York, John Wiley and Sons. In press.

87. Pigg, J.S., and Gall, E.P.: Arthritis health professionals family tree: combined care for rheumatic disease. Arthritis Health Professions Assoc. Newslett., *3*:6,7,11, 1983.

88. Potts, M.: The role of the social worker in the management of patients with rheumatic disease. Clin. Rheumatol. Pract., *1*:77–80, 1983.

89. Potts, M.G.: The role of the social worker. *In* Rheumatic Diseases: Rehabilitation and Management. Edited by G. Riggs and E. Gall. Woburn, MA, Butterworth Publishers, 1984.

90. Potts, M.G., and Brandt, K.D.: Analysis of education support groups for patients with rheumatoid arthritis. Patient Counsel. Health Educ., *4*:161–166, 1983.

91. Raish, P.: How the rheumatology nurse practitioner improves the quality of care for the arthritis patient. (Abstract.) *In* Proceedings of the Arthritis Health Professions Section Meeting, New York, 1978.

92. Rice, M.S.: Role of the pharmacist. *In* Arthritis—A Modular Curriculum for Occupational Therapy. Edited by L. Kautzmann. Milwaukee, School of Allied Health Professions, University of Wisconsin–Milwaukee, 1981.

93. Riggs, G.K.: Philosophy of rehabilitation. *In* Rheumatic Diseases: Rehabilitation and Management. Edited by G.K. Riggs and E.P. Gall. Woburn, MA, Butterworth Publishers, 1984.

94. Riggs, G.E.: AHPA: Past, present, future. Arthritis Rheum., *256*:704–705, 1982.

95. Rogal, R.A.: Psychological considerations in the management of arthritic patients. *In* Rheumatology. Edited by R. Bluestone. Boston, Houghton Mifflin Professional Publishers, 1980.

96. Rossky, E.: Joint conservation and protection. *In* Rehabilitation Management of Rheumatic Conditions. Edited by G.E. Ehrlich. Baltimore, Williams & Wilkins, 1980.

97. Roth, R.D.: The role of the podiatrist in the rheumatology team approach. *In* Rehabilitation Management of Rheumatic Conditions. Edited by G.E. Ehrlich. Baltimore, Williams & Wilkins, 1980.

98. Roxborough, S.: Rheumatic diseases: an integrated approach to total patient care. EULAR Bull., *12*:29–30, 1983.

99. Sack, K.E.: Osteoarthritis: cause and long-term management. Compr. Ther., *84*:46–51, 1982.

100. Sales, A.P.: The role of the vocational counselor. *In* Rheumatic Diseases: Rehabilitation and Management. Edited by G.K. Riggs and E.P. Gall. Woburn, MA, Butterworth Publishers, 1984.

101. Schroeder, P.: The role of the nurse in the arthritis care team. *In* Arthritis—A Modular Curriculum for Occupational Therapy. Edited by L. Kautzmann. Milwaukee, School of Allied Health Professions, University of Wisconsin–Milwaukee, 1981.

102. Schutt, A.H.: Physical medicine and rehabilitation in the elderly arthritic patient. J. Am. Geriatr. Soc., *25*:76–82, 1977.

103. Schweidler, H.: Assistive devices, aids to daily living. *In* Rheumatic Diseases: Rehabilitation and Management. Edited by G.K. Riggs and E.P. Gall. Woburn, MA, Butterworth Publishers, 1984.

104. Seeger, M.: Splints. Braces and casts. *In* Rheumatic Diseases: Rehabilitation and Management. Edited by G.K. Riggs and E.P. Gall. Woburn, MA, Butterworth Publishers, 1984.

105. Shapiro-Slonaker, D.M.: Joint protection and energy conservation. *In* Rheumatic Diseases: Rehabilitation and Management. Edited by G.K. Riggs and E.P. Gall. Woburn, MA, Butterworth Publishers, 1984.

106. Sliwa, J.L., and Edwards, N.L.: Occupational Therapy in Arthritis. Ann Arbor, University of Michigan Arthritis Center, F4416 Mott, 1980.

107. Snyder, M.: The role of the podiatrist, prosthetist, and orthotist. *In* Rheumatic Diseases: Rehabilitation and Management. Edited by G.K. Riggs and E.P. Gall. Woburn, MA, Butterworth Publishers, 1984.

108. Spergel, P.: Vocational assessment, counseling and training. *In* Rehabilitation Management of Rheumatic Conditions. Edited by G.E. Ehrlich. Baltimore, Williams & Wilkins, 1980.

109. Sutton, J.D.: The role of the rheumatology nurse. *In* Rheumatic Diseases: Rehabilitation and Management. Edited by G.K. Riggs and E.P. Gall. Woburn, MA, Butterworth Publishers, 1984.

110. Sutton, J.D.: Patient screening for clinical priority. Arthritis Health Professions Sect. Newslett., *11,12*:1–5, 1978.

111. Sutton, J.D.: Rheumatic disease nursing: a new role. Allied Health Professions Sect. Newslett., *10*:9–11, 1977.

112. Sutton, J.D., et al.: Program entry priorities—An AHP judgement. (Abstract.) *In* Proceedings of the Arthritis Health Professions Association Meeting, Boston, 1981.

113. Sutton, J.D., et al.: Nursing intervention in degenerative joint disease. (Abstract.) *In* Proceedings of the Allied Health Professions Section Meeting, New York, 1978.

114. Swezey, R.L.: Arthritis rehabilitation: staff, facilities and evaluation. *In* Rehabilitation Management of Rheumatic Conditions. Edited by G.E. Ehrlich. Baltimore, Williams & Wilkins, 1980.

115. Swezey, R.L.: Arthritis: Rational Therapy and Rehabilitation. Philadelphia, W.B. Saunders, 1978.

116. Tesch, M.J., and Sauerberg, V.: The role of the rehabilitation counselor in the arthritis care team. *In* Arthritis—A Modular Curriculum for Occupational Therapy. Edited by L. Kautzmann. Milwaukee, School of Allied Health Professions, University of Wisconsin–Milwaukee, 1981.

117. Vignos, P.J.: Physiotherapy in rheumatoid arthritis. J. Rheumatol., *73*:269–271, 1980.

118. Vignos, P.J. Jr., et al.: Comprehensive care and psychosocial factors in rehabilitation in chronic rheumatoid arthritis: a controlled study. J. Chronic Dis., *25*:457–467, 1972.

119. Wallace, R., Heiss, M.L., and Bautch, J.C.: Staff Manual for Teaching Patients About Rheumatoid Arthritis. Revised Ed. Chicago, American Hospital Association, 1982.

120. White, B.S., et al.: Patient-oriented, nurse-supervised gold clinic. (Abstract.) *In* Proceedings of the Arthritis Health Professions Section Meeting, New York, 1978.

121. White, J.F., et al.: Rheumatology nursing: a specialty you can tailor to your talents. Nurs. '79, 9:108–110, 1979.

122. Wickersham, B.A.: Hydrotherapy. *In* Rheumatic Diseases: Rehabilitation and Management. Edited by G. K.

Riggs and E. P. Gall. Woburn, MA, Butterworth Publishers, 1984.
123. Wickersham, E.A., et al.: Arthritis: preferred learning methods among Arizona therapists. Am. J. Occup. Ther., 36:509–514, 1982.
124. Wilder, S.: Patient education. In Arthritis—A Modular Curriculum for Occupational Therapy. Edited by L. Kautzmann. Milwaukee, School of Allied Health Professions, University of Wisconsin–Milwaukee, 1981.
125. Woolf, D. (Ed.): Rehabilitation in the rheumatic diseases. Clin. Rheum. Dis., 7, 1981.
126. Wright, V., and Haslock, I.: Rheumatism for Nurses and Remedial Therapists. London, William Heinemann Medical Books, 1977.
127. Wulf, V.C.: Utilization of nurse-specialists in arthritis care. Allied Health Professions Sect. Newslett., 10:15–19, 1976.
128. Yerxa, E.J.: The role of the occupational therapist. In Rheumatic Diseases: Rehabilitation and Management. Edited by G.K. Riggs and E.P. Gall. Woburn, MA, Butterworth Publishers, 1984.
129. Ziebel, B.: The role of the counselor. In Rheumatic Diseases: Rehabilitation and Management. Edited by G.K. Riggs and E.P. Gall. Woburn, MA, Butterworth Publishers, 1984.
130. Ziebel, B.: Family dynamics. In Arthritis—A Modular Curriculum for Occupational Therapy. Edited by L. Kautzmann. Milwaukee, Allied Health Professions, University of Wisconsin–Milwaukee, 1981.
131. Ziebel, B., Wickersham, E., and Boyer, J.A.: Team arthritis consultation. Phys. Ther., 61:519–522, 1981.

Chapter 44

Rehabilitation Medicine and Arthritis

Robert L. Swezey and Steven R. Weiner

Any procedure used in the management of patients is a part of the rehabilitation process. The scientific foundations of rehabilitation medicine, as well as descriptions of the rehabilitative maneuvers customarily used by rheumatologists, physiatrists, and orthopedists in the comprehensive management of arthritis and allied disorders, are emphasized here.

The distinctions among the terms impairment, handicap, and disability must be clear to anyone treating patients with chronic diseases. An *impairment* is a damaged organ or extremity; a *handicap* is the disadvantaged function caused by impairment; a *disability* is the inability to function effectively as a consequence of the handicap that results from an impairment. Those of us who treat arthritic patients are challenged to minimize impairment, to lessen the burden of handicap, and to prevent disability.

The specialty of physical medicine and rehabilitation emphasizes comprehensive and multidisciplinary team care in the prevention and management of disability. Physical medicine uses various forms of physical energy such as light, heat, electricity, and exercise therapy to accomplish this end. Rehabilitation in the rheumatic diseases integrates physical medicine with surgery and medicine, occupational therapy, and new techniques for education and social, vocational, or psychologic counseling of patients. The goal of this multidisciplinary approach is to help patients to attain their maximum physical, psychologic, social and vocational potential for normal living, that is, rehabilitation. Successful rehabilitation depends on the efforts of qualified physicians, allied health professionals specifically trained in the management of the diseases they treat, and most important, a physician coordinator responsible for all the professional services rendered.

The objectives of comprehensive care for arthritic patients are restoration of the highest possible levels of function and independence and the attainment of optimal satisfaction and usefulness in terms of the patients themselves, their families, and their community.[140] For the patient with arthritis, this means amelioration of symptoms, restoration of mobility and strength, and above all, the development of a sense of self-worth.[275]

SOCIAL AND ECONOMIC FACTORS IN REHABILITATION

The year 1981 was designated "International Year of Disabled Persons." The International League Against Rheumatism, with its member societies in over 60 countries, was an active participant in the goals of recognition of and attention to the special needs of the disabled.[247]

Examples of the economic devastation caused by rheumatic diseases are easy to cite. Arthritis is the second leading cause of chronic disability in the United States.[49] Approximately two-thirds of the 4 million adult Americans with rheumatoid arthritis (RA) between the ages of 35 and 50 have significant impairment; 20% of the 0.06% of children under age 15 who develop juvenile RA suffer significant crippling into adult life; approximately a million men and women over age 16 in Great Britain are disabled primarily as a consequence of rheumatic diseases; the loss of nearly one-sixth of the workdays in the industrial population of England and Wales has been attributed to rheumatic complaints.[218,310] During the 1970s, approximately $426.9 million per annum were spent by the United States Veterans Administration as compensation for arthritis-related disability.[9] Also during the early 1970s, $1 billion annually was spent on disability insurance payments and aid to the permanently and totally disabled, as well as $1.4 billion on "lost" homemakers' services and $4.8 billion on lost wages. Lost federal, state, and local income taxes amounted to $955 million annually.[9] The total cost of arthritis-related disability exceeds $14 billion, and several billion dollars more will be spent in the 1980s on arthritis care and rehabilitation or on quackery.

In Sweden, rheumatic conditions represent 10% of all conditions seen by primary-care physicians, comprise 15% of the country's total health expenditures, and are the cause of one-third of all new disability pensions.[3] In the United States, over

30 million working days a year are lost to rheumatic diseases. The direct medical costs for a year in the population of patients with Stage III RA are 3 times the national average, and only 58% of these expenses are covered by insurance.[186] Indirect costs due to lost income were threefold greater than direct costs, and only 42% of these losses were recoverable.[186] The psychosocial losses associated with the economic burden and the loss of job-related identity are immeasurable. The stress of unemployment is sufficient to cause physical and mental illness even in many healthy persons; unemployment should be actively avoided in those afflicted with rheumatic diseases.[26]

Economic analyses of arthritis treatment reflect the extreme difficulty of determining cost effectiveness because of the impact of many variables on estimated and actual costs.[3,70,186] It is equally difficult to determine the effectiveness of components of rehabilitation therapy, including exercise, rest, splinting, occupational therapy, vocational counseling, psychologic and social counseling, community support, various medical and surgical therapies, and hospitalization.[131] Despite the qualifications, the assumptions, and the resistance by industry to hiring people with physical handicaps, even during periods of high employment, the most critical analyses show that rehabilitation services for arthritic disorders are cost effective and that high-quality programs are likely to be accompanied not only by increased socioeconomic benefits, but also by relief of symptoms and improved psychosocial function.[26,131,186]

Many patients with severe arthritis are capable of full or part-time work, but others need adaptive equipment, modification of work methods, and ready access to a work setting for successful employment.[241,256] Prejudice of industry, labor unions, and insurance companies toward the handicapped still often restricts opportunities for employment. Initial steps taken to eliminate restrictive underwriting provisions could increase opportunities for the handicapped worker.[9,241]

Although work for compensation is an obvious goal for the handicapped, the role of homemaker is of equal importance.[309] A legitimate goal of vocational rehabilitation and Social Security is to raise the level of function of a disabled person so that even if work in the traditional "marketplace" is not possible, independence in homemaking activities can be achieved.

COMPONENTS OF THE REHABILITATION PROCESS

These components include medical and professional personnel as well as therapeutic facilities.

Rehabilitation Therapeutic Team

The severely arthritic patient may require the diversified skills of family physicians, rheumatologists, physiatrists, and orthopedists, as well as those of the allied health care specialties (see Chap. 43). The physical, psychologic, and social derangements accompanying serious rheumatic diseases are best treated by those allied health professionals who have been specially trained in their management, but few persons possess these skills. One cannot assume that referral to a rehabilitation center that is staffed by members of all appropriate health professions will result in expert management of a patient with rheumatic disease. The Council on Rehabilitative Rheumatology of the American Rheumatism Association (ARA) and the Arthritis Health Professional Association of the Arthritis Foundation are attempting to develop arthritis rehabilitation specialists among physicians and allied health professionals, but much remains to be done.

Allied Health Professional Team

Most patients with arthritis benefit from some aspects of physical and occupational therapy; however, patients may benefit more from the combined, coordinated efforts of the health care team rather than from the individual efforts of the team professionals. The roles of the various health professionals, as described, represent a customary delineation of their responsibilities, but the boundaries blur and often overlap.

The nurse in a clinic, office, hospital, or visiting capacity must be conversant with the various arthritic diseases, therapeutic regimens, and common drug reactions.[77] The nurse must have the skills required to provide instruction, to monitor compliance in the prescribed therapeutic programs, and to give support to the arthritis patient and his family.[205]

The occupational therapist is concerned first with the patient's ability to function independently, with a minimum of fatigue and stress to the involved joints, and second with the provision or fabrication of adaptive equipment and splinting, to allow function that is otherwise difficult or impossible.[187] The occupational therapist teaches the patient to perform upper-extremity functional activities in ways that minimize joint inflammation or deformity. This therapist may play a key role in assisting the surgeon in the postoperative management of patients who have undergone upper-extremity operations. The occupational therapist can provide patients with activities that provide appropriate exercise for a variety of musculoskeletal problems, particularly when standard exercise therapy becomes boring and may result in compliance failure. The occupational therapist evaluates patients' life styles to help minimize their frustrations, and screens them for their work potential or ability to be trained in more appropriate occupations.

The physical therapist is responsible for teaching the patient therapeutic exercises, transfer skills, and ambulation methods.[127] The physical therapist also administers and instructs patients in the use of various therapeutic techniques including heat and cold application, diathermy, electrical stimulation, and traction.

The psychologist or psychiatrist is often needed to assist in the management of the psychologic problems that accompany pain and loss of function. Psychologists should be well acquainted with the rheumatic diseases and must be aware of the various organic psychologic disorders associated with them, as well as drug-induced psychologic disturbances.[242]

The social worker assists in the management of the psychologic problems and the socioeconomic stresses on families that compound the devastating effects of severe rheumatic diseases.

A vocational counselor who understands the potential for recovery and rehabilitation of the various rheumatic diseases can mobilize community and agency resources essential to restore the patient to a role of active economic participation.[182]

Patient educators provide instructional materials and structure education programs relating to the arthritic diseases and their treatments for the patients and their families. The role of the family in the rehabilitation process is crucial.[293] The family's response to the illness may be a major factor in a patient's motivation to proceed with rehabilitation, in his ability to accept losses, and in his strength to undergo changes in life style. In addition to the patient's own family, arthritis community groups can provide an extended ''family'' for emotional support, dissemination of information, and implementation of programs such as exercise classes in heated pools.

Rehabilitation counselors can work with the social worker and the vocational counselor to coordinate the patient's rehabilitation process before a formal vocational rehabilitation program begins. Counseling must also be available to deal with a patient's sexual difficulties, premarital concerns such as genetics, homemaking, and interpersonal relationships, and approach to motherhood.[10,19,40,97,293]

The most important member of the arthritis health care ''team'' is the patient himself. Patients and their families must be given every opportunity to participate in the team and its decisions.[296] The ''team'' is complex because it involves many disciplines, persons, and personalities. The sophisticated health care team is also expensive and so

must be monitored carefully to ensure that each team member functions with optimal effectiveness.[28]

Facility Considerations

The environment in which the rehabilitation process takes place varies. The most important environment is the patient's home, but the places of work, worship, educational and recreational facilities, in addition to the physician's office, clinic, hospital or rehabilitation facility, all determine limits and provide opportunities for restoration to independence.[142,153] The patient confined to a wheelchair is confronted with multiple everyday impediments: curbs, stairs, narrow doorways, insufficient space in lavatories, drinking fountains too high or too low, inaccessibility to public transportation, public telephones with coin slots out of reach, and parking spaces under 12 feet wide or located at long distances from buildings.[25,142,153] The patient who is weak, uses canes, or who walks with painful joints must be concerned with the problems of uneven terrain, ice, mud, heavy doors, resistant door knobs, lack of railings, and waiting room seats that are too low, too soft, or lack arms needed to facilitate standing and to relieve joint stress while sitting.[142,153,301]

The actual therapeutic facilities include the gymnasium, hydrotherapy area, and the area devoted to activities of daily living (ADL). Ideally, these facilities should be adjacent, interrelated, and close to psychologic, social, and vocational counseling services.[149,275] The hospital rehabilitation area should be used by both inpatients and outpatients in the same location, for continuity of care.

A small hospital requires a therapeutic gymnasium of at least 35 square meters. It should include an exercise mat, an exercise table, parallel bars and corner stairs for gait training, a full-length mirror, and areas for cervical traction, paraffin application, diathermy, ultrasound, electrical stimulation, and manual therapies. A shoulder wheel, a finger ladder, and reciprocal pulleys are desirable. A Hubbard tank, ideally a therapeutic pool, and a whirlpool are essential. A hydraulic lift is needed for transferring patients. A heavy-duty overhead wire grid accommodating a variety of pulley attachments provides flexibility when traction, reciprocal pulleys, or supporting slings are needed. More elaborate equipment, such as a standing tilt table for postural training and gravity-assisted stretching or a padded, adjustable exercise table containing cables to which graded increments of weights can be attached or isokinetic exercise equipment facilitates a variety of stretching or strengthening exercises (often prescribed postoperatively)[9] (see the section of this chapter on strengthening exercises).

Finally, space is needed for dressing rooms, lavatories, storage, and for cleaning and sterilization facilities.[24]

The occupational therapy area should provide space for evaluation of ADL.[276] Much ADL evaluation, such as bathroom and chair transfers, feeding, toileting, and personal grooming, can be performed at the patient's bedside or in a hospital bed in an outpatient facility. Although specific activities, such as preparation of food and performance of household tasks, can be simulated, it is preferable to provide actual household equipment and facilities to permit adequate training of patients in joint conservation and to illustrate home adaptations. A table for therapeutic exercise evaluations should be accessible to wheelchairs and should have an adjustable height capability; a drafting table works well. An area is needed to make and to test splints and adaptive equipment. Office space for the therapists and assistants and space for privacy for individual ADL evaluation, counseling, and training should be provided. Provisions for vocational assessment such as simulated factory, office, or outdoor physical labor or driving are useful extensions of occupational therapy functions, but more applicable to major rehabilitation facilities.

Socialization areas are desirable for group dining, visiting with families, education of patient and family, and for recreation.

DISABILITY AND MANAGEMENT

A disability may be defined as the inability of an individual to meet the sum or any part of his life's physical, psychologic, environmental, or socioeconomic demands. Legal definitions of disability focus on a person's inability to participate in gainful employment for a predetermined period.[184] Lawmakers recognize the difficulty in proving or disproving true disability in a court of law and instead rely on the diagnosis of a specific rheumatic disorder, presuming that the diagnosis itself will embrace a disorder of sufficient severity to justify the existence of a functional deficit.[184] The Arthritis Foundation has made legal determinations easier by forming a uniform database consisting of precise definitions of disorders and their respective signs and symptoms.[118] Under any nosologic classification, however, the range of functional impairment and disability is still wide.

Outcome measures of comprehensive health status examine factors such as death, discomfort, disability, therapeutic drug toxicity, and dollar cost.[86,87,165] To the arthritis patient, disability is the most important issue after control of pain. Outcome measurement in any chronic disorder needs to incorporate parameters of social, physical, and mental function.[86] Older instruments to measure outcome emphasized process rather than outcome; newer ones are more sensitive to ultimate outcome.[219] Any physician wishing to measure outcome of a rheumatologic rehabilitation patient must be aware that no one instrument is perfect although many exist. All costs and benefits cannot be measured, functional capacity is neither absolute nor constant, and undue emphasis on measurement may distract one from other critically important issues of concern to the patient.[166]

The Arthritic Impact Measurement Scale (AIMS), a brief paper and pencil test, is an example of a newer instrument to measure outcome.[183] AIMS has a high level of validity and reliability.[185]

Functional assessment is important for all physicians involved in rehabilitation. A proper functional assessment plans therapeutic intervention, defines roles in caring for the patient, and designs a rehabilitation program.[113,271]

The first instrument for functional assessment of arthritis patients consisted of four gradations; slight, moderate, severe, and extreme functional impairment.[281] In 1949, Steinbrocker's Committee for Therapeutic Criteria of the New York Rheumatism Association published a functional classification of arthritis patients not dependent on pathophysiologic parameters.[270] These early crude measures of function have been used to evaluate and to justify special rehabilitation units, to help formulate function-related goals of therapy, and to highlight the crucial point that function does not always equate with the severity of disorder.[50] The functional evaluation schemes of the 1950s and 1960s were generally lengthy, complex, and unreliable, particularly when applied to rheumatic diseases. Refinements have created instruments that are easy to record, quantifiable, and capable of reflecting more subtle changes in function. The prototype is the ADL Scale.[137] Consideration is given to a patient's ability to bathe, feed, dress, use a toilet, and to transfer from bed to chair and from chair to toilet independently.[137] Newer ADL scales given additional emphasis to a variety of psychosexual, social, vocational, and transportation functions.[141]

One must also analyze individual components of disability.[138,302] The reason for a disability is as important to the physician as its existence. Because function and disability measures are established for many reasons,[113] one method may necessarily be better to predict outcome,[271] another to measure pain[125] or pain threshold,[219] and still another to assess patients with mild impairments such as seen in a family physician's office.[253]

It is important to quantify function as a measure of the effectiveness of therapy.[56] Improvement of

Table 44–1. **Functional Criteria of the American Rheumatism Association**

1. Patient performs all usual activities without handicaps.
2. Patient performs normal activities adequately, despite occasional discomfort in one or more joints.
3. Patient is limited to few or no activities, usual occupation, or self-care.
4. Patient is largely or wholly incapacitated, is bedridden, or is confined to a wheelchair and has little or no self-care.

(From Steinbrocker, O.[270])

function is the major goal of the physician concerned with patients' rehabilitation. Therefore, the expense, time, and effort required to improve range of motion in any given joint should be justified by a concomitant improvement in function.[126]

A functional evaluation of arthritis or a related musculoskeletal condition should be brief, reproducible, quantifiable, and reasonably objective and should distinguish between upper- and lower-extremity dysfunctions. Although the evaluation is affected by the patient's pain and by psychologic factors, it should not directly measure them. A functional test is not a substitute for precise descriptions of mobility, strength, anatomic or radiographic features, or psychologic status, nor for attempts to quantify pain. Such a test should be designed to detect a functional deficit by the patient's failure to perform a specific task. Inability to pick up a key (a function test) may reflect a loss of sensation, a loss of index finger or thumb function in one or several joints, or muscular weakness of relevant muscles, but only the functional deficit would be noted. Further evaluation would be needed to determine the basis for the functional

Table 44–2. **Rheumatic Disease Self-Assessment of Function**

Dear (PATIENT'S NAME): In order to help us learn whether you need therapy, in addition to the medicine prescribed for you, please fill out this form.

DIAGNOSIS	PRESENT VOCATION (Housewife, carpenter, etc.)		
Please check (✔) the best answer for you			
HOW MUCH PAIN OR DIFFICULTY DO YOU HAVE WITH THE FOLLOWING ACTIVITIES:	AMOUNT OF DIFFICULTY		
	NONE	SOME	GREAT
EATING:			
Cutting meat, drinking from a cup, etc.			
DRESSING:			
Arms and upper part of body			
Legs and lower part of body			
Fastening buttons, zippers, or snaps			
GENERAL HAND ACTIVITIES:			
Using key, writing, dialing phone			
Opening jars, drawers or doors			
PERSONAL HYGIENE:			
Brushing teeth, combing hair, shaving			
Toileting			
MOBILITY:			
Getting on or off toilet			
Getting into or out of			
chair			
bed			
car			
tub			
shower			
Walking inside home			
outside home			
up or down stairs			
HOME ACTIVITIES:			
Gardening			
Cleaning			
Cooking			
Laundry			
Shopping			
OTHER ACTIVITIES?			

Table 44–2. Rheumatic Disease Self-Assessment of Function (Continued)

How *TIRED* are you after an average day's activity?   Slightly_____   Moderately_____
                                                       Extremely_____   Not at all_____

	YES	NO

Have you ever been treated by an occupational therapist?
  If *YES*, were you last treated:
    Less than 1 year ago?_____
    More than 1 year ago?_____		

Do you perform any home exercise program? If *YES*. was it prescribed by a doctor or a therapist?		
Do you currently use splints		
canes or crutches		
wheelchair		
other aids		

What is your *usual* means of *TRANSPORTATION?*
  Driven by family or friend _____drive self _____
  Public transportation (taxi or bus) _____other _____

COMMENTS: _____

_____

loss. Treatment of the basis for disability such as carpal tunnel release, splinting of the thumb, or exercise of intrinsic muscles, would be reflected by improved function if the patient could then pick up the key.

Scaling of levels of function is arbitrary, and the varieties of scoring systems developed are eloquent testimony to that difficulty. Redundancies in testing may be avoided by the use of one task to measure a number of related functions. For example, picking up a key requires finger tip sensation and co-ordination of the thumb to the index finger tip. The lack of tip pinch may not prevent one from picking up a key if the patient learns to compensate by sliding the key across and off the table top into his hand. It is pertinent, then, that the evaluative measures defined in the ARA Standard Data Base for Rheumatic Disease originally included only the Steinbrocker classification, grip strength, 50-foot walking time, and a description of gait as functional measures, but now include descriptors of compliance with therapeutic regimen, sexual functions, and upper- and lower-extremity activities, as well as self-care.[118]

Finally, what one can measure as "function" with a given instrument may not reflect a lack of the patient's functional performance in reality.[126] A patient may, while being tested, actually accomplish a given task that could not or would not normally be done as part of daily activity. For example, patients may be able to comb their hair laboriously, but may choose to arrange for others to do it on a regular basis.

Table 44–1 shows the most widely used brief functional evaluation for rheumatic disease, the Steinbrocker classification.[270] This classification does not distinguish upper- from lower-extremity problems and is insensitive to modest but useful gains in function.[275] Table 44–2 is a questionnaire detailing the patient's own assessment of function in rheumatic disease.

Recent reviews of newer instruments by which to assess function have found none to be ideal.[56,87,165,166] New measures of function, disability, and outcome are proposed at an alarming rate, far faster than the necessary follow-up studies of validity and reliability. All physicians should acquaint themselves with one or several measures that apply to their needs, yet may be reproduced by other physicians with minimal interobserver discrepancy. The peculiarities of "legal" methods for determining disability are also important for any physician treating arthritis patients and have been reviewed.[113]

Last, as emphasized in a recent survey of a large population of medical students of whom 69.1% had 1 to 7 separate musculoskeletal abnormalities,[232] proper physical examination is important, but function is multifaceted, dynamic, and not necessarily equivalent to the sum of the physical findings.

PHYSICAL THERAPY

Physical therapists and physiatrists have an extensive array of therapeutic techniques from which to choose, including exercise therapy, electrotherapeutics, hydrotherapy, therapeutic applications of heat and cold, manipulation, traction, and ambulation assisting devices.[12,260] Many of these therapies have their origins in antiquity and have developed their own folklore and mythology. No claim of cure or dramatic, significant improvement of a chronic rheumatic disorder by a physical therapeutic technique has ever been proved. Many current therapies have a reasonable scientific basis, however, and well-controlled statistical evaluations are under way to determine the relevance, role, and value of most interventions.[194,294] Despite the need for scientific validation of the worth of any given intervention, one should not overlook the value of the physical therapist as a rehabilitation team member who spends considerable time with the patient, lays hands on and physically interacts with the patient, and approaches fundamental problems with interventions to which patients relate much more avidly than they do to complicated drug regimens. The interpersonal contact between physical therapists and patient may be a significant factor in the overall outcome of the rehabilitation program.

Exercise Therapy

Exercise therapy is prescribed for patients with rheumatic diseases to preserve muscle strength and joint mobility, to improve functional capability, to relieve pain and stiffness, to prevent further deformities, to improve overall physical and cardiovascular conditioning, to re-establish neuromuscular coordination, to mobilize stiff or contracted joints, and to prepare for functional activity and follow-through after surgery.[11,260,282,294] Improvement of function and pain relief are the ultimate goals.

The physiatrist and the physical therapist are cognizant of the equal roles of rest and muscular relaxation and exercise. Selective rest, or immobilization of affected joints and adequate general rest, can reduce the severity of inflammatory joint disease.[155,265,266] Fatigue, a frequent constitutional complaint in inflammatory disorders, may be used as a guide to define "sufficient rest," that is, a patient is resting enough when fatigue disappears.[266] Immobilization of RA joints for as long as four weeks reduces inflammation without significant loss of mobility, although muscle strength diminishes.[108,202,222,264,266] Because of the mechan-

ical stress imposed on abnormal joints by faulty posture (body alignment), a rest position in bed that prevents hip flexion contractures, or "relative" rest in the form of modification of activities that protect a painful back or joint from stress, for example, is of major importance.[129]

Proper rest and good posture require muscle relaxation. Inadequate rest or poor posture can predispose patients to muscle aches, fibromyalgia, joint contractures, and excessive fatigue.[203] Muscle relaxation is necessary before commencing stretching exercises, and techniques such as hot packs, massage, Jacuzzi whirlpools, and ultrasound are used to relax tense patients to prepare them for stretching exercises and postural training.[110,134] Brief contraction of agonist muscles to induce relaxation of antagonists (contract-relax or rhythmic stabilization) is another technique that can augment assisted stretching exercises by relaxing muscles.[134,275]

Exercise therapy is designed to achieve specific therapeutic goals over and above the psychosocial and physiologic benefits of recreational exercise activity. Exercise during an acute arthritic flare is primarily to preserve joint range of motion and muscle strength. During the subacute stages, restoration of active joint motion is an additional goal. Exercise in the patient with chronic inflammation is designed to meet specific functional goals. Therefore, the rationale for therapeutic exercise is based on functional considerations, within the limitations imposed by the disease.

Stretching Methods

Stretching exercises are used to prevent contracture or to increase range of motion in patients who already have contractures.[275] Subluxations and other deformities associated with overstretched ligaments cannot be reversed by stretching or strengthening exercises. Contractures, however, may be slowly reversed at a rate of approximately one degree per day if the stretching is effective. First, the underlying factors predisposing a patient to contractures must be corrected. For example, the patient who places a pillow under an arthritic knee for comfort risks knee, hip, and ankle flexion contractures.[59] In addition to posture instruction and such measures as prone positioning for the patient at risk of developing hip flexion contractures, seating adjustments and supportive splinting or bracing may be required as preventive postural measures. Posture correction without the addition of range-of-motion exercise or activity may result in contractures, but such correction helps to preserve the position of useful function. Table 44–3 lists the optimal position for function in joints in which contracture cannot be avoided. *It is essential*

Table 44–3. Functional Positions for Ankylosed Joints

Joints	Function	Position	Reference
Fingers			
Metacarpophalangeal and proximal interphalangeal	Grasping	35° flexion	85
Thumb			
Interphalangeal	Pinching	Straight	85
Metacarpophalangeal	Pinching	20° flexion	
Carpometacarpal	Apposition	50° abduction	
		20° internal rotation	
Wrist			
Unilateral	Ease in toileting	Straight	79,85
Bilateral		One straight	
		One in 5° flexion	
Elbow			
Unilateral	Feeding and grooming	70° flexion	33
Bilateral	Feeding and grooming	One in 70° flexion	
	Reaching	One in 150° extension	
Shoulder	Feeding and grooming	20° flexion	33
	Dressing	45° abduction	
		20° internal rotation	
Hip*	Smooth gait	25° flexion	85
		5° abduction	
		5° external rotation	
Knee†	Smooth gait	15° flexion	35
Ankle	10° plantar flexion for high heels	Neutral	35

*Condition of opposite hip, knees, and back, and ability to sit and walk, as well as problems of daily activity must be evaluated to determine the position.
†Full extension for stability in the knee is the goal when only limited motion can be preserved.

to put all joints through a range of motion at least once daily to maintain mobility. The stretching techniques chosen to maintain motion must not aggravate joint pain and inflammation.

To understand the rationale for stretching exercises, one must recognize that contractures involve the joint capsule, the synovium, and the adjacent muscles and their fasciae.[51,145,230,305] Joint capsules vary in the looseness and irregularity of the weave of their collagen fibers. In ligaments and capsules, the collagen fibers are oriented variously to permit predetermined degrees of movement, whereas in tendons, the fibers are arranged in parallel fashion. Ligamentous and capsular structures are normally "prestressed" and shorten when normal tension or stretching forces are interrupted.[283,307] Thus, a proximal interphalangeal joint undergoing hyperextension deformity (swan neck) develops a tightening of its dorsal capsular fibers.[277,278]

In the arthritic patient, contractures typically occur in an effort to avoid pain associated with active joint disease; this avoidance response results in limitation of motion.[277,278] Contractures may also secondarily affect uninvolved joints, or they may be primarily effected by poor posture.[277] An important additional mechanism for the genesis of

joint contractures is the presence of synovial effusions. A mild or moderate effusion may have little effect on the mobility of the joint in a patient whose capsular structures are lax, although stretching of the capsule may lead to instability of the joint. In a patient whose capsular structures are less yielding, however, the synovial fluid may form a mechanical block to motion. Efforts to eliminate effusions and to minimize their recurrence are important if contractures are to be avoided.

Capsular structures and muscles undergo adaptive shortening with immobilization even in the absence of an inflammatory process.[305] When inflammation occurs, connective tissue breakdown is accelerated. Connective tissue turnover and remodeling are increased, whereas edema and pain restrict joint movement and predispose patients to joint contracture.[305]

The pathogenesis of contracture formation may be multifactorial. Although most contractures have some etiologic component of trauma, pain, internal derangement, inflammation, or immobilization, additional consideration must be given to neuropathy, including neurodystrophy, psychogenic factors, and genetic predisposition.[32,239]

Several points are relevant. First, if a progressive

load is applied gradually, connective tissue will slowly stretch, ultimately to the point of rupture, whereas an abrupt application of a lesser load will cause tearing without significant stretching.[4,282,283,292,307] Second, collagen is more susceptible to collagenase activity when stretched or when heated.[106,116,216,238] Third, repetitive movement aggravates the inflammatory and, ultimately, destructive process in an inflamed joint.[66,145,193,216]

Methods. Serial casting or splinting techniques induce gentle prolonged stretching forces. These are best applied, after relieving joint effusions, in patients with moderate and long-standing contractures. When serial or wedged cases are applied, care must be taken to prevent subluxing stresses. About five degrees of contracture can be overcome weekly with effective serial casting for knee contractures, and this schedule may be accelerated with traction.[6,145,269] Dynamic splinting, in which constant low-grade tension creates a corrective force, can be used in selective therapies and is particularly applicable in postoperative management. Examples of dynamic splinting are the use of spring and rubber-band tension-activated splint devices, or webbed belts wound to create a low-grade dynamic tension to correct contracture deformities of a finger or elbow.[2,6,136,145,227,237,269]

Range-of-Motion Exercises. Exercise to increase joint mobility should be modified according to the degree of inflammation present and, particularly, within pain tolerance.[260] To minimize exacerbations of arthritis, exercises should be performed so that any pain incurred will subside within two hours; any delayed or prolonged exacerbation of pain should largely be gone by the following day. Exercises should be selected to cause the least possible stress with the fewest possible movements, done in the least stressful manner consistent with the goal of stretching. Patients usually require "warm-up" movements before an optimal stretch can be made, but once the joint has been taken through its maximal range of motion during an exercise session (anywhere from three to ten repetitions of the movement), then the single exercise session is usually sufficient to maintain joint mobility for that day.[64,72,144,279] When increased joint mobility is the goal, the same precautions apply, but the exercise can be repeated more often, such as three to ten exercise sessions per day.

Stretching exercises are best performed when stiffness is least. This recommendation does not preclude a "loosening up" routine on arising, but it does mean that the major exercise effort for both stretching and strengthening should be done when the patient is best able to perform. Hot applications, a warm bath or shower, and anti-inflammatory and analgesic medication can be administered to be maximally effective at the time of the exercise session. Exercises can be categorized as *passive, active-assisted, active,* and *resistive.*[12] Purely passive exercise is necessary for a paralyzed limb or when pain precludes any active motion. For most arthritic patients, active-assisted exercises are used, because the patient's participation gives some control over pain, whereas the manual or mechanical assistance encourages maximal stretching. Active stretching exercises are particularly useful to preserve range of motion, and active-resistive exercises are used to maintain or to increase muscle strength.

Passive or active-assisted range-of-motion exercises may require the assistance of another person.[85] As inflammation subsides, simple assistive devices such as a cane or "wand" can be used by the patient without requiring another person. The "good" arm can push up on one end of the wand, which is grasped above by the hand ipsilateral to a contracted shoulder, to stretch upward into forward flexion[215] (Fig. 44–1). Proper positioning of the patient ensures that movement takes place in a horizontal plane, eliminating gravity. A "powdered board" or wheels on a "skate board" to minimize friction facilitates stretching exercise in the horizontal plane. In the "Codman" shoulder exercises, the patient leans forward with the shoulder and arm hanging so that gravity actually assists

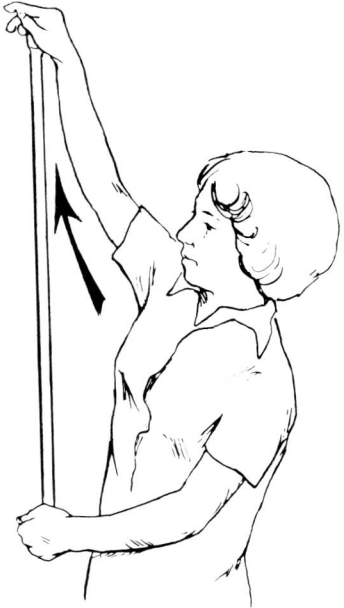

Fig. 44–1. Shoulder flexion ("wand" exercise). A stick is held with both hands approximately a shoulder's width apart. The "good" arm through the stick or wand assists the stiff shoulder in stretching. This exercise is used for subacute or chronic shoulder contractures.

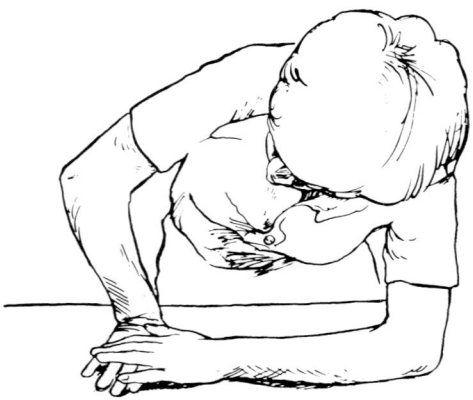

Fig. 44-2. Wrist extension (dorsiflexion). The hand is placed flat on a table. The wrist is extended by leaning the body over the table.

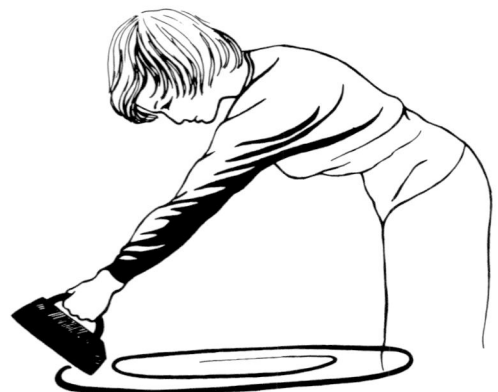

Fig. 44–3. Shoulder circumduction (Codman). A pendulum rotary motion is assisted by gravity and by holding a one-kilogram weight. If the wrist or fingers are involved, a one-kilogram wrist strap is substituted. This exercise for acute or severe restriction of shoulder motion can also be performed when the patient is lying prone, extending the arm over the side of the bed.

the pendulum-like rotary movements of the shoulder.[35] Figure 44–2 shows assisted (body weight) dorsiflexion of the wrist, and Figure 44–3 shows gravity-assisted circumduction of the shoulder. The warmth and buoyancy of water, particularly in a pool, can be employed effectively to facilitate stretching regimens[312] (Tables 44–4 and 44–5). Active exercises are best employed in late convalescence and to maintain joint mobility.

Strengthening Exercise

Strength may be required to lift a load (isotonic or dynamic strength) or to hold or resist a load in a fixed position (isometric or static strength). An isotonic stress modulated to keep the resistance throughout the range of movement constant (as the leverage changes, the load is increased or lessened to maintain a constant torque) is called an *isokinetic stress*. For example, a Nautilus machine simulates isotonic stress.

Endurance is a measure of the time that a stress can be sustained, and the duration of muscle performance may be contracted to a percentage of the level of maximum performance or to a functional assessment.[245] Static endurance is the time that a given load can be held or resisted in a fixed position (isometric contraction). Dynamic endurance is the length of time that a repetitive isotonic task can be performed and is a function of the rate of repetition, the load, and the extent to which the load is moved. Dynamic endurance is related to, but distinguishable from, power, which is the rate at which work (force $\times$ distance) is performed.

Maximal strength and endurance depend on multiple factors, including overall physical condition, muscle fiber type, motivation, pain and sensory inputs, training, learning ability, and coordination.[244] Although strength and endurance are interrelated, the requirements for sustaining a large weight are only minimally transferable to a low-resistance, repetitive task such as typing, and vice versa.

Muscle Fiber Morphology and Physiology. Skeletal muscle contains muscle fibers that are different anatomically, physiologically, histochemically, and biochemically.[69,117,121,244] The several classification systems of muscle fibers have proved confusing when attempts were made to correlate the classifications or to account for interspecies differences.[121] The oldest system divided muscle fibers by color into red, either slow or fast twitch, and white.[121] Peter's classification system used whole muscle and divided fibers, based on contraction time and enzyme capacity, into: (1) fast-twitch glycolytic; (2) fast-twitch, oxidative, glycolytic; (3) fast-twitch, fatigue-resistant; and (4) slow-twitch, fatigue-resistant.[69,121,244] The currently accepted system, an outgrowth of a Brooke and Kaiser classification,[69,117,121,244] is as follows:

Type I Fibers. These fibers are red, slow-twitch and have the highest capacity for aerobic metabolism, with a high respiratory capacity and myoglobin content, but with a low glycogenolytic capacity and low actin-myosin adenosine triphosphatase (ATPase). These fibers can do prolonged work of moderate intensity in which ATP use matches oxidative phosphorylation.

Type IIB Fibers. These white, fast-twitch, fatigable fibers have a low respiratory capacity, a high glycogenolytic capacity, a low myoglobin content, and a high actin-myosin ATPase activity.

REHABILITATION MEDICINE AND ARTHRITIS

Table 44–4. Therapeutic Considerations in Exercises for Joint Diseases

	ACUTE/SEVERE		SUBACUTE/MODERATE		CHRONIC/MILD	
	Motion	*Strength*	*Motion*	*Strength*	*Motion*	*Strength*
Goal	To maintain	To defer until pain relief permits	To maintain or increase	To maintain or increase	To maintain or increase	To maintain or increase
Method	Passive or gentle	See Subacute/Moderate	Active-assisted	Isometric	Active or active-assisted	Isometric or isotonic*
Position	To preserve function, for comfort		To preserve function, for comfort	For comfort	For comfort	Antigravity acceptable if tolerated
Repetitions	1–3/session 1–2/session/day		3–10/session 1–2/session/day	6 sec/muscle 1–2/session/day	5–10/session 1/session/day to maintain or 3–5/day to increase	6 sec/muscle 1 week to maintain; 1/day to increase strength
Time	When rested, and pain and stiffness are least		When rested, and pain and stiffness are least		When rested, and pain and stiffness are least	
Preparation	Analgesics, cold, heat, hydrotherapy as needed prior to exercise		Analgesics, heat, cold, hydrotherapy as needed prior to exercise		Analgesics, heat, hydrotherapy, cold as needed; occasionally, diathermy prior to exercise	
Precautions	Reduce intensity of exercise if postexercise pain persists over 2 hours or if pain or swelling increases the following day		See Acute/Severe. Avoid fatigue; use prescribed working splints during activity except when exercising†		See Subacute/Moderate	

*Isotonic, low-resistance, repetitive exercises to the point of fatigue for dynamic endurance.
†Compromise between the ideal and the possible may demand selective emphasis on problem joints for maximum compliance with exercises.

Table 44–5. Range-of-Motion Exercises for Specific Joints

Upper Extremity

	Proximal interphalangeal, metacarpophalangeal	Wrist	Elbow	Shoulder
Problem	Swan neck; Tight intrinsic muscles; Swelling; Restriction of motion	Supination loss; Subluxation	Flexion of at least 70° must be preserved for useful function	Rapid loss of motion, particularly flexion, abduction, and internal rotation
Method	Manually assisted, Bunnell block	Active-assisted; Use stick or door knob to assist pronation and supination; lean over hand on table top for extension*	Active, flexion-extension; best performed in horizontal plane	Gravity-assisted "Codman"† early; Active-assisted pulleys, "wall walking" later; Active and "wand"‡ when chronic
Comment	Forced grasp or ball-squeezing predisposes patients to joint derangement		Forceful stretching can exacerbate the disorder	Early institution of exercise prevents "frozen" shoulder
References and description	21,85,127,275,284	52,85,275	227,275,284	35,227,275,284

Lower Extremity

	Hip	Knee	Ankle
Problem	Flexion contracture; Loss of abduction; Motion restricted by swelling	Maintenance of extension	Tight Achilles tendon
Method	Active; Horizontal plane, side lying for extension; Supine for abduction	Active; Stretch on floor on mat	Active-assisted; Stand with palms on wall; Lean into wall to stretch heel cord of extended leg
Comment	Pool, tank or "powder board" facilitate	Pool or tub useful in acute cases	Achilles contracture requires vigorous stretching
References and description	85,227,275,284	85,227,275,284	24,85,227,275,284

*See Fig. 44–1
†See Fig. 44–2
‡See Fig. 44–3

These fibers have a capacity for short bursts of intense work, but rapidly fatigue, accumulate lactate, and require long recovery intervals.

Type IIA Fibers. These fibers are red, fast-twitch, and fatigue-resistant, with a high respiratory capacity, a high glycolytic capacity, a high myoglobin content, and a high actin-myosin ATPase activity. These fibers, intermediate between type I and type IIB, have a potential for rapid regeneration of ATP by anaerobic or aerobic metabolism.

The actual proportions of each fiber in the skeleton are fixed, and in man, approximately half are type I and half are type II.[121] Athletes often have a predominance of a single fiber type, and this factor may contribute to performance in a sport.[244] That training in man may change muscle fiber type I to type II or vice versa remains to be proved.[244]

Strength training results in: (1) an increase in type II fiber area with heavy resistance training; (2) correlation of type II fiber area with maximal isometric strength; (3) no discernible metabolic changes characteristic of low-resistance endurance training; and (4) myofibrillar protein increases resulting in enlarged or hypertrophied muscle fibers.[244]

Diseases often affect one muscle fiber type more than another; thus a basis is provided for rational exercise treatment.[243] Type II fibers have a peculiar propensity to change in size, and atrophy may occur in patients receiving corticosteroid therapy, in patients with connective tissue disease with associated myopathy, and in cancer patients.[243,245] Prolonged cast immobilization does not change the proportion of muscle fiber types, but produces greater atrophy in type I fibers, unless severe joint pain has been present, as in RA.[243–245]

Muscle is in a constant state of simultaneous degradation and synthesis.[245] The two processes are normally balanced, but this balance may be disrupted by a number of factors.[245] With inactivity, muscle strength decreases from 1.5 to 5% per day.[184] With maximal exercise, an increase of 12% per week of muscle strength may be obtained, up to 75% of maximum, when the rate of increase declines.[198] Müller has demonstrated that, in normal human subjects, even a single contraction, for a second's duration done once a day, at half maximal strength, limits the loss of muscle strength.[198]

The effect of a muscle contraction is produced by the interaction of mechanical factors, such as fiber direction, locus of insertion, joint position, and muscle length.[267] Excessive elongation, particularly at high velocities, can produce injuries ranging from minor strain to muscle rupture.[267] Muscle rupture is more common than tendon rupture in a 2:1 ratio, and most strains and ruptures occur in muscles that cross over and interact with more than one joint, such as hamstrings and rectus femoris muscle. Care must be taken with immobilization because changes in musculotendinous lengths limit range of motion. Immobilization also results in muscle atrophy[267] (see Table 44–3).

Dynamic endurance training improves the oxidative (aerobic) capacity of muscle[244] by inducing adaptive increases in mitochondrial content, in respiratory capacity, in myoglobin concentration, and in capillary number.[121] Another important biochemical change with endurance training is an increased ability to oxidize fat, carbohydrate, and ketones.[121]

Most functional activities such as grooming, dressing, feeding, light housekeeping, and walking are low-resistance, repetitive tasks. Fatigue occurs more rapidly in repetitious tasks requiring more than 10% of the maximal available static strength. Fatigue eventually occurs even if the task can be performed with only 5% of the maximal available static strength.[102,206] To lift and to maintain a load, such as holding a glass of water, a pot of tea, or a package of groceries, requires static strength and endurance sufficient to perform these tasks. The static endurance during grasp has been shown to be a function of the percentage of the total available grasp (static) strength used.[102,206] Repetitive, low-resistance activities, such as jogging or sawing, require additional dynamic endurance training for optimum function, if such training can be done without aggravating the joint disorder.

Methods. Two common methods for strengthening muscles are based on the concept that a stress sufficient to cause a muscle to fatigue stimulates the muscle to adapt by increasing in strength and endurance.[58,103] The DeLorme regimen uses a sequential, 10-step, graded reduction of isotonic stresses beginning with 10 repetitions of the greatest load that can be lifted. The "over-load principle" of Hellebrandt requires that the maximum isotonic load be lifted repeatedly in a paced exercise to the point of fatigue.[58,103] The muscle-fatigue stimulus can also be used advantageously in weakened patients because low-resistance activity (greater than 30% of maximum capability) also stimulates strengthening if carried to the point of fatigue.[103,198,244,267] These exercises are regularly prescribed in patients after trauma, joint operations, or when little joint inflammation exists.[58,103]

These fatiguing, strengthening methods contrast sharply with the brief, isometric contraction exercises. Daily isometric contractions at two-thirds maximum capability held for at least one second, and preferably for six seconds, are an optimal physiologic stimulus for static strengthening in healthy adults.[65] Only a slight increase in the rate of gain in strength was observed when the exercise was performed three times daily in normal subjects. In all these techniques, the stimulus must be increased proportionately to strength increase, to be maximally effective. The use of a maximal contraction at each exercise session obviates this problem. Once maximal static strength is achieved, it can be maintained by one exercise session per week.[198]

Specific Considerations in Rheumatic Disease. RA patients as a group have lower-than-expected aerobic capacity and physical performance, and their overall muscle strength is 60% below that of age-matched control subjects.[16,67] Such patients, however, tolerate well-tailored strengthening and endurance programs, with gains in physical performance levels in as brief a time as 6 weeks.[16,214] Long-term exercise regimens in RA patients over many years have also been well tolerated, with resultant improvement in functional and other outcome measures.[213,215] A lessening of discomfort and a better overall emotional attitude accompany such exercise.[213] In healthy adults, exercise increases plasma levels of beta endorphins and beta lipotropin, and continued training augments this effect.[38] Whether this effect occurs in the less-demanding exercises of arthritic patients remains to be determined. Additionally, regular exercise training may help to relieve depression.[100]

Exercise may increase inflammation in joints, and therefore must be designed to avoid such exacerbation.[120,206] Isometric exercises are effective in increasing strength and are well tolerated by many arthritic patients.[171] In the rabbit model of acute monosodium urate arthritis, passive range-of-motion exercise exacerbated inflammation, but isometric exercise did not.[193]

Isometrics make profound cardiovascular demands, however,[93] demands great enough to compromise patients with organic heart disease. Caution should be exercised.[93] New rehabilitation techniques of "perceived exertion" allow patients with heart disease to exercise within cardiovascular restraints and still make progress.[93]

Isometric exercises should be performed with the joint positioned for comfort, to avoid pain and to maximize the force of the muscle contraction. Pain may be reduced further by administering analgesics and by warm or cold applications before exercise. Resistance for isometric exercise can be provided by walls, floors, table tops, opposite extremities, therapists, or gymnasium equipment. A simple technique, particularly suitable for a home regimen, is the use of a minimally yielding rubber or elastic belt looped around the extremity and fixed to the opposite extremity, bed, doorknob, or chair leg (Fig. 44–4).[174] Alternatively, one can use a partially inflated beach ball, which is light, adapts comfortably to painful structures, and, like the elastic belt, moves minimally yet offers increasing

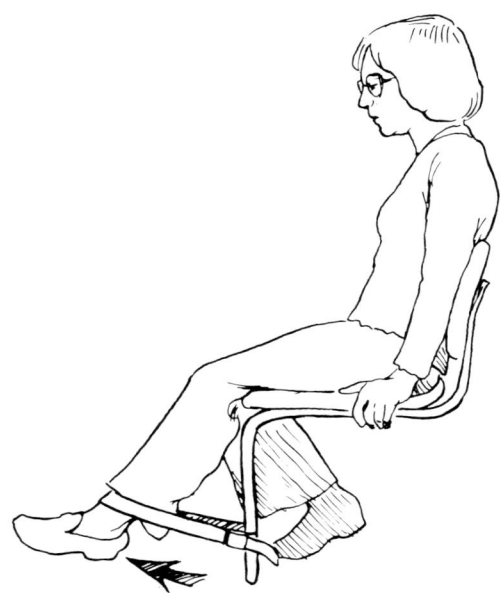

Fig. 44–4. Seated quadriceps isometric strengthening (elastic belt) exercise. An elastic belt is looped around the chair leg and the patient's ankle. The patient attempts to extend the partially flexed leg as forcibly as possible for six seconds (exhaling or counting to avoid increased intrathoracic pressure). The elastic belt yields minimally while providing "feedback" as it resists extension of the leg.

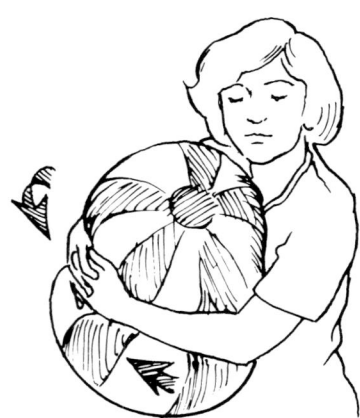

Fig. 44–5. Biceps isometric strengthening (beach ball) exercise. A partially inflated beach ball is compressed as forcibly as possible for six seconds. The beach ball is lightweight, conforms to bony contours, and offers increasing resistance during compression. Counting to ensure exhalation prevents increased intrathoracic pressure.

resistance as force is applied and thereby reinforces the proprioceptive inputs essential for a maximum contraction[275] (Fig. 44–5). Although a maximal six-second daily isometric exercise is an optimal strengthening stimulus, twice-daily exercise sessions are recommended when the patient's ability to contract maximally is uncertain (see Table 44–4).

Specific exercise techniques are beyond the scope of this chapter, but the principles and positions used by Hines in manual muscle testing, modified for joint comfort, are readily adapted for isometric exercise, and many practical exercises for arthritic patients have been described in detail.[275]

Specific Considerations in Muscle Disease. Physical therapy has been reported to be valuable in the management of patients with polymyositis, in the prevention of contractures and stiffness, in the rehabilitation of patients recovering from acute or relapsing disease, and in the treatment of muscular soreness.[274] No controlled trials substantiate this finding or support the traditional belief that resistive exercises should not be done until the serum muscle enzymes are at or near normal, however. Exercise mildly elevates levels of muscle enzymes for several hours.

Electrotherapy

Electrotherapeutics have been an integral component of physical medicine and rehabilitation therapies since 1931, when the Royal Society of Medicine combined their Section of Electrotherapeutics and the Section of Balneology and Climatology to form the specialty of "Physical Medicine."[211]

The first use of electrotherapy has been attributed to the Romans, who decapitated torpedo fish and used the natural electric charge to treat various maladies including gout.[254] Erb, in 1883, wrote that "among articular affections these constitute the real field for electricity; other methods of treatment are much more often useless."[71] By the turn of the century, use of galvanic, faradic, and static currents to treat arthritis was almost as popular as treatment at spas and natural baths.[204] Notably, no proof exists that electric current may cure any rheumatic disorder, nor have controlled experiments shown that the direct application of electric current in inflammatory arthritic disorders has any effect other than that of a counterirritant.

Iontophoresis, an early addition to electrotherapy,[146] theoretically uses a direct (galvanic) current to enhance and intensify the movement of ions from drugs that may be ionized past a biologic membrane for therapeutic purposes.[107,146,229,303] Anecdotal claims of the benefits of iontophoresis in treating most forms of arthritis have appeared.[107,168,303] Scientific evaluation of iontophoresis has been attempted, to determine its use in applying corticosteroid preparations to a small, anatomically defined area such as a joint or bursae.[20,106]

Electric and magnetic fields are now used by physicians and physical therapists for pain control, promotion of bone growth, stimulation of muscle groups, restoration of lost neuromuscular function, and movement retraining.[34,122,233,303] Further research is needed to determine what, if any, role electricity will play in the rheumatic diseases.

In 1965, Melzack and Wall proposed their gate theory of pain.[190] They suggested that intense sensory input along large-diameter nerve fibers would "close the gate" to pain sensations carried by smaller fibers. The required sensory input to the sensory mechanoreceptors could be electrical stimulation, pressure, or vibration.[94,190] The gate theory, which provided a theoretic basis for counterirritation and related pain "displacing" phenomena, has spawned a number of electrotherapeutic techniques designed to obscure pain perception by electric stimulation of cutaneous receptors, dorsal column, spinal cord, peripheral nerve, and brain.[233,303] Implantable devices, such as dorsal column and thalamic stimulators, were first used, but have largely been abandoned because of complications. The complication-free, easily applied, external transcutaneous electric nerve stimulators (TENS) and electroacupuncture[233,235] are now widely used as electrical stimulation for pain relief.[235] Transcutaneous nerve stimulation is done with an apparatus consisting of skin electrodes and a battery-powered, portable pulse generator.[235] Placement of electrodes is empiric, although guidelines suggest placement at trigger points or acupuncture points, which Melzack has found to be closely correlated.[191] The explanation for the analgesic action of TENS units was initially thought to be related to "gate control," but recent work suggests that endorphins may be released.[94,178,225,235] TENS has been used to treat many musculoskeletal conditions with varying success.[188] TENS primarily blocks C-fiber-mediated pain and, to a lesser extent, the acute pain mediated by A-delta fibers. That the periosteum, synovium, and capsule of a joint are supplied by nonmyelinated (C-fiber) sensory fibers may explain the success of TENS in reducing joint pain and in supplementing anti-inflammatory drugs during controlled trials in patients with RA, herpes zoster, and discogenic radiculopathy, and as an adjunct to the management of frozen shoulder and reflex sympathetic dystrophy.[150,178] Complications, such as interference with demand pacemakers, may occur with TENS units.

Electrical stimulation has been used to treat nonunion fractures of bone with fair success and, more germane to the arthritis patient, to treat failed arthrodesis.[14,147,204,255]

Electrical stimulation of muscle activity can retard denervation atrophy of type I fibers and, to a lesser extent, type II fibers.[221] The contraction of denervated muscle by electrical stimulation prevents the loss of oxidative enzymes and the associated atrophy,[209] although no concomitant increase in muscle strength occurs.[207] Electrical stimulation of motor nerves (faradic) to induce involuntary muscle contractions is also used as a massage technique for relief of painful muscle spasm, but no controlled trials have proved its efficacy.[270] Electrical stimulation of muscle can increase strength in normal subjects.[52]

Electroneuroprosthesis is a term describing electrical devices that stimulate the nervous system to restore lost function.[233] Such devices have been used with good results to treat foot drop, to obtain grasp in C5 fractures, to treat scoliosis, and to stimulate bowel, bladder, and diaphragmatic functions.[34,233]

Electrical stimulation has been used to facilitate muscle retraining after tendon transplants or trauma and in neurologic disorders. It is therefore a forerunner of modern biofeedback techniques.[168] Biofeedback is an outgrowth of experiments with operant conditioning done by Neal Miller showing that the effects of the autonomic nervous system are subject to training.[199] A signal, usually visual or acoustic, reflecting a physiologic "involuntary" event, is used to help the patient to gain voluntary control.[13] Electromyographic biofeedback is now used to treat upper-motor-neuron lesions, muscle tension headache, and neck and back pain and, particularly, to retrain muscles and to induce relaxation in spastic muscles of stroke patients.[13] The mechanism may be an enhancement of awareness of small muscle contractions.[195]

Biofeedback control of skin temperature in the fingers is a new technique in the treatment of Raynaud's phenomenon.[68] Biofeedback training to relieve joint or back pain has been less successful, perhaps no better than a placebo.[189] Biofeedback techniques are now widely used for pain control and relief of muscle spasm in the treatment of muscle tension headache, migraine headache, "stress," and chronic neck and temporomandibular joint syndrome, although well-controlled trials are lacking.

Hydrotherapy

Hydrotherapy combined with heat is among the oldest rehabilitative treatments for arthritis.[110,285] Hydrotherapy provides both heat and buoyancy.[275] Arm and leg basins for single joints with or without water agitators (whirlpools) and various size tubs are used.[275] Hubbard tanks or heated swimming pools are used for patients with multiple joint problems.[110] The larger tanks permit total body immersion, heat transference, therapeutic exer-

cise, swimming for conditioning, ambulatory training, and a popular spa technique, "Bad Ragaz."[110,260,275]

Contrast baths are used to treat small joints by producing hyperemia.[160] This cumbersome method has no known advantage over warm soaks or moist heat application.

Hydrotherapy has not been subject to controlled trials.[110,260,275] It is contraindicated in patients with cardiovascular disease, because of peripheral vasodilation accompanying total immersion in water at 34° C, and in patients with infections or certain inflammatory skin diseases.[110,260,275] The larger pools are also expensive to maintain and to operate, and time in them should be used judiciously.[110,275] The feeling of freedom, relaxation, and pain relief provided by pool therapy does have important psychologic value to the arthritis patient. Arthritis clubs and YMCAs with organized exercise programs at local pools can provide recreation for arthritis patients at a much more modest cost.

Therapeutic Heat and Cold

Superficial heating can be accomplished by conduction (direct contact with a warmed substance) or by convection (heat transferred by liquid- or gas-heated particles in motion). Deeper heating may be instituted by conversion, in which a nonthermal form of energy, such as sound waves, penetrates tissue, where the energy is converted to heat by absorption. How hot a tissue actually gets is a product of several factors, including the thermal properties of the tissues heated, the thermal conductivity, the pattern of relative heating, and neurovascular factors that locally regulate body temperature control.

Superficial heating may be done by direct contact with warmed substances such as sand, oil, wax (paraffin), mud, thermal springs, vapor bath, steam in a steam room, moist air in a moist air cabinet, hot water in a tub, hot packs, heating pad, and hydrocolator (silicate gel), or by the friction of rubbing with massage.[260,275] Regardless of source, the energy only penetrates a few millimeters through the epidermis, and thus intra-articular heating is minimal.[161] Although moist heat raises subcutaneous temperatures more than dry heat, this information does not influence any selection of a heating technique.[1]

Heat purportedly increases collagen extensibility in tendons,[91,139,299] decreases joint stiffness,[30,130,308] relieves pain,[106,161,226] elevates pain threshold,[18] relieves muscle spasm,[61,226,300] and affects intra-articular circulation in RA.[107a] The effect on intra-articular circulation occurs whether the heat is superficial or is applied deep to the joint, however. Heat may also increase both inflammation and pain.[62] A controlled trial of a popular superficial heating technique, paraffin baths, in RA showed no clinical benefit.[109] The benefits of heating in the treatment of rheumatic disease patients have simply not been established.[176]

Heating of skin to temperatures greater than 109° F (43° C) causes pain, and higher temperatures may cause wheal and flare reactions. Caution must be exercised when using heat in patients with sensory neuropathies, an abnormal mental state, or cardiovascular disorders. Total immersion of women during the first trimester of pregnancy in water heated to temperatures higher than 38.9° C is contraindicated, and patients with systemic lupus erythematosus, malignant diseases, infections, and open wounds have had reported adverse reactions with heating. Table 44–6 contains a summary of precautions.[157,159]

Diathermy and Ultrasound

Deep heat penetration of tissue sufficient to cause direct joint heating can be achieved with diathermy.[156,157,251] Diathermy, which literally means "heating through," consists of electromagnetic irradiation administered as shortwaves (11.0 M at 27.33 MHz) or as microwaves (12.2 cm at 2456 MHz).[156,251] Shortwave administration requires a direct applicator or a coil, and microwave administration uses an antenna. Ultrasound is a deep-heating method that uses the energy of rapidly oscillating sound waves (1.0 MHz).[156,251] It provides the deepest tissue penetration, and it is the only heating technique that raises the temperature in the adult hip.[156,162,163,251] This deep penetration can be a disadvantage when ultrasound is used over the spinal cord after laminectomy.[272] Ultrasound is reflected from metal surfaces, rather than conducted as with diathermy, and thus is safe to use in the presence of metal implants or plates.[90,164,262] No information exists on the safety of ultrasound in the presence of methyl methacrylate, used to hold joint prostheses.

Electromagnetic waves may cause burns if focused by metal or by fluid-filled spaces, such as moisture on the skin, the eye, and in bone.[76,156,159,251,272] Testicular and lenticular damage from diathermy has been reported.[252,272] The use of either shortwave or microwave diathermy in patients with cardiac pacemakers is contraindicated.[197] Precautions for use of deep heat also include those for superficial heat. In addition to causing circulatory changes and increasing the threshold for pain, diathermy can alter the viscoelastic properties of collagen.[156,272,299] This heat-related effect has been the basis for advocacy of diathermy in conjunction with prolonged stretching to overcome contracture, but the relative merits of

diathermy's effect on collagen over those of superficial heat to reduce pain and muscle spasm, and thus to facilitate stretching, have not been adequately studied.[156,226] Diathermy or ultrasound has no proved advantage over superficial heating techniques for pain relief or improvement of articular disorders.[18,44,74] Indeed, evidence that heat increases collagenase activity in rheumatoid synovia raises further doubts about the use of diathermy in inflammatory joint disease.[106]

In addition to the recommendations for prescribing heat and cold therapeutic methods in Tables 44–6 and 44–7, empiric indications exist for the use of ultrasound. Local painful areas such as fibrositic nodules, chronic ligamentous strains, neuromas, "trigger" areas in muscle, and localized tendinitis are particularly suited anatomically for focused ultrasound energy. Again, anecdotal reports of the value of treating these conditions with ultrasound abound, but controlled studies are lacking. The special therapeutic advantage of ultrasound attributable to the specific physical effects of sound waves has not been substantiated.[272]

Cold decreases electrical activity of the muscle spindle.[61,192,226] The stimulus threshold for firing is raised, thus decreasing the afferent firing rate.[226] Cold may also reduce nerve condition velocity. Cold may be better than heat for reducing pain[18,44] and muscle spasm[44,226] and, in combination with stretching, for muscle relaxation.[226] Cold causes superficial vasoconstriction, but deep vasodilation.[140] Pain relief due to cold may be due to counterirritant effects or to endorphin release.[18,140,196,223,226] Additional suggested benefits of cold include reduction of edema formation, metabolic rate, joint stiffness, muscle spasm, and joint inflammation, and enhancement of mobility.[18,61,62,123,140,196,223,226,250,304] Cold may be administered by immersion in cold water, by application of ice or cold packs, by ice massage, or by inflatable cold splints or vapocoolant sprays.[18,57,61,62,96,140,173,196,223,226,250,288] Cold is contraindicated in patients with cold allergy, Raynaud's syndrome, paroxysmal nocturnal hemoglobinuria, and cryoglobulinemia and should be used cautiously in the presence of cardiovascular insufficiency.[275]

The choice of heating or cooling for symptomatic relief is empiric. Cold seems preferable in the treatment of acute inflammatory processes or injuries, whereas traditionally heat has been used to treat subacute or chronic inflammation or injury (see Table 44–7).[88,96,152]

Traction, Massage, and Manipulation

These three physiotherapeutic techniques have been widely used in the treatment of rheumatic disease.

Table 44–6. Therapy Prescription Precautions

Therapeutic Method	Impaired sensation	Circulatory deficiency	Metal implant or contact	Pacemaker	Cardiac, respiratory, or cerebral insufficiency	Acute trauma or inflammation	Infection	Tumor	Osteoporosis	Weakness or low endurance	Weight bearing	Instability or paralysis	Psychologic factors	Intellectual factors	Economic factors
Local superficial heat or cold*	R	R				R[h]								R	
Ultrasound*	R	R	R			C	C	C							
Diathermy*	R	R	C	C		C	C	C							
Hydrotherapy with heat*	R	R			R			R		R		R		R	
Generalized (total body) heat*	R	R			R		R	R		R		R		R	
Traction	R						R	C	R			R			
Splint or Brace	R	R				R	R	C					R		R
Gait Training	R	R	R		R	R	R	R	R	R	R[d]	R		R	
Exercise (passive, active, range-of-motion, strength)		R	R		R	R	R		R	R		R			
Massage or manipulation					C[c]	C	C	C	R						
Transcutaneous nerve stimulation				C										R	R

h = Heat; c = cervical spine; d = right or left; C = contraindication or special consideration; R = relative contraindication.

*Specific operating instructions including dosage, exposure to moisture, duration of therapy, distance of energy source, and temperature of water must be followed exactly.

Table 44–7. Selection Factors in Techniques for Pain Relief

Severity of Pain	Technique	Localization of Pain	Comments
↑ Acute	Ice pack, cold compress, ice massage	↑ Focal*	Contraindicated in patients with cold intolerance or Raynaud's phenomenon
	Warm moist compress		Well tolerated, easy to apply
	Hydrotherapy: whirlpool, tub, tank, pool		Warmth and buoyancy assist in stretching exercises
	Dry heat: infrared bulb, heating pad	General	Inexpensive for home use, portable; danger of short circuit
	Paraffin, mud, sand		Provides palliation in PSS and rheumatoid arthritis
	Diathermy: microwave, short-wave, ultrasound		Pacemaker and metal implants contraindicate use
Chronic ↓		Focal* ↓	

*Transcutaneous nerve stimulation can relieve focal or regional pain

Traction

Traction, a basic component of orthopedic therapy, has an established place in the treatment of contractures occurring in the arthritic hip and knee.[136,269,280] Traction with modifications of Perry and Nickel's "halo" device is used in the treatment of spinal deformities, often in conjunction with surgical procedures.[154]

Traction in normal subjects can open posterior spinal articulations, disengage facet surfaces, widen intervertebral foramina, and elongate posterior muscles and ligaments.[36,280,306] Reduction of bulging discs in pathologic conditions has not been proved, however.[36,129,280] Pain is relieved by traction, especially in the treatment of cervical radiculopathy.[27,37,228,291] Detractors point out that cervical traction may incite cervical radiculopathy as well as temporomandibular joint symptoms.[257] The few controlled trials reported failed to show any influence on the rate of recovery,[27] and results were not much better than with other treatments with the patient at bed rest.[27,181]

No agreement exists on the method, amount of weight, duration, or frequency of cervical traction.[36] In fact, only positioning the neck in moderate flexion is widely accepted. In healthy men, 25 pounds of traction straightens the cervical lordosis;[133] 30 pounds for 7 seconds achieves posterior vertebral separation.[306] Maximal foraminal opening occurs at 24° of cervical flexion.[48] Vertebral separation is not essential for benefit in many cases and may even do harm.[27] Because traction for no more than 20 minutes daily is the rule, it is difficult to believe that relief of nerve root pressure for so short a time is the cause of any therapeutic success,

although it has been argued that facet malalignment or irritating disc fragments are occasionally reduced after distraction.[73] Traction does provide periods of supported longitudinal neck muscle stretching. The chronic state of protective muscle spasm may be overcome by traction, and this effect may explain the symptomatic relief claimed for the method. A simple method for cervical traction at home can be used for 5 minutes once or twice daily in patients with chronic cervical syndromes.[298]

The benefit of traction on the lumbar spine is equally unclear.[158,181] To separate normal lumbar vertebrae of a subject in bed, at least 25% of the body weight must be used for traction, and in lumbar disc disease, forces as high as 220 pounds for 30 minutes are frequently ineffective.[132,158,169] Vertebral separation has been demonstrated only with a split table designed to overcome friction of the body in bed. Variable subjective relief has been reported in patients with lumbar discogenic disease and with acute disc syndromes,[95] but treatment failures and increased root pain have been reported as well.[43] Pelvic traction, as usually applied in a hospital bed, is insufficient to cause vertebral separation, but may reinforce a regimen of bed rest in a noncompliant patient.[275] Until lumbar traction is more adequately studied, it is reasonable to use a split-table method, which requires only moderate weights in the range of 25 to 50% of body weight to relieve pain. Spinal traction is generally unsatisfactory in the presence of inflammation and is best avoided in patients with hemorrhagic states or malignant diseases.[275,280] Traction has been used in children for pain relief in both acute inflammatory joint disease and in septic arthritis of the hip.

Massage

Massage is an ancient method for relieving musculoskeletal tension and pain and for inducing general relaxation. Therapeutic massage techniques include stroking (effleurage) for soothing effects and deep stroking for muscle relaxation; compression (pétrissage) as a means of kneading tissues to relax muscles, to stretch adhesions, and to mobilize edema; and percussion (tapotement) to create a stimulating vibration or a more vigorous percussive counterirritant effect.[167,280] A variety of exotic massage methods are currently used in nonmedical settings. Massage is useful to relieve muscle spasm and to facilitate therapeutic exercise in selected patients when less-expensive and less time-consuming techniques prove ineffective.[36,280] Special techniques such as Cyriax friction massage, acupressure, and Shiatsu may yet find a place in the treatment of soft tissue disorders.

Manipulation

Joint manipulation, with and without anesthesia, is accepted in the management of postsurgical or post-traumatic contractures, for mobilization of a "frozen" shoulder, and, to a lesser extent, for treatment of lateral epicondylitis.[175,192]

Chiropractic cervical manipulation has resulted in transient ischemia, nonfatal brainstem infarctions, and several reported cases of stroke.[148,200,240] The exact incidence of these complications is unknown, but with an estimated quarter of a million patients per year treated by manipulation, these findings are probably rare. No mortality has been attributed to lumbar manipulation[200] or to nonspinal manipulation. Manipulation technique uses careful positioning of the patient to achieve muscle relaxation and muscle mechanical disadvantage, so an abrupt additional manipulating stretch, "thrust," stretches tight muscles and distracts joints. This distraction is often associated with an audible "cracking" sound, thought by some to be due to reduction of facet "subluxations" or to realignment of displaced fibrocartilaginous disc material.[53,167,175,192] It is uncertain whether spinal manipulation depends on joint distraction, on muscle stretching, or on actual joint or disc realignment for pain control.

Controlled trials of manipulation in acute low-back pain showed a trend to shortened duration of pain,[95] but did not alter outcome,[261] and showed no advantage over common medical therapy[8] or other physiotherapeutic techniques.[119] Manipulation therapy is contraindicated in the presence of severe osteoporosis, bone tumor, bleeding diathesis, or sepsis.[280]

Mobilization therapies such as traction, massage, and manipulation include oscillations and joint vibrations designed to relieve muscle tension, to free minor adhesions, to increase joint and muscle motion and to relieve pain.[275] Such "mobilizations" do not use the "thrust"; examples are Cyriax, Maitland, and Mennel methods.[280] They may play an adjunctive role in the management of articular and periarticular disorders.[280] Mobilization therapies may stimulate proprioceptive pathways and possibly more complex reflexes and may thereby diminish pain.[280] Additional effects may result from the impact of these techniques on pathologic tissues. They are generally safe if done by trained physicians or other health professionals. Various forms of mobilization are commonly and arbitrarily used by practitioners of "alternative" forms of therapy. Research is needed to define the possible role of these methods in the treatment of rheumatic diseases.

Vapocoolant Spray and Local Anesthetic Injections

Tonic focal areas of palpable, tender contracted muscle, so-called "trigger areas," are commonly observed in association with painful musculoskeletal disorders.[258,259,286,289] They appear to be reflex in origin, occur in predictable locations, correlate with many acupuncture points, may themselves be a source of referred pain, and often respond promptly to local measures, such as massage, cold application, cold spray, and local anesthetic injections.[191,258,259,286,289] The use of vapocoolant sprays in the local treatment of painful musculoskeletal disorders, or as a topical anesthetic prior to injections, is an outgrowth of the use of cold compresses as counterirritants.[275] (Fluorimethane is nonflammable and is therefore preferred over ethyl chloride.) The use of local anesthetic trigger-area injections historically preceded that of vapocoolant sprays.[28,289] Clinically, these injections should be tried when sprays, or spray and stretch techniques, have failed. Vapocoolant sprays have the additional advantage over local injections of suitability for home use.

In contrast to the established place of local microcrystalline adrenocorticosteroid ester injections in the treatment of articular and periarticular inflammatory or traumatic disorders, the addition of such agents to local anesthetics for trigger-area injection is unnecessary and may cause local tissue reactions.[220]

MOBILITY

A fundamental component of independent functioning for the arthritis patient is the ability to perform transfers. Modifications of bed, bath, chair, toilet, and wheelchair may be needed for the arthritic to transfer satisfactorily.[25,75,151,170,180] Patients unable to transfer independently depend for optimal mobility on the assistance of others. Instruction in specific techniques for the safe transfer of the patient from bed or chair to ambulatory-assist device to toilet, bath, or car must be provided to whomever is to be responsible for this activity.[75,92,114,170,180] Several excellent references provide details of transfer training.[114,151,170,180,234,287]

Gait

Normal gait is an efficient, energy-conserving means of locomotion.[46,60,84,128,231] Muscle weakness, joint disease and its associated pain, swelling, instability, contracture, or deformity, leg-length discrepancy, and postural deformities may lead to awkward, inefficient gait patterns that impose excessive strains on joints and on the cardiovascular system.[60,128,179,231,249] Training in gait and in the use of properly fitted canes, crutches, walkers, and braces requires supervision by a skilled therapist. Selection of a crutch, cane, or walker that minimizes hand stress (enlarged hand grip) or wrist and elbow strain (platform crutch), or one that can be used in spite of generalized weakness (a lightweight walker), can be crucial in determining the ambulatory function of an arthritic patient.[22,143,180]

The most common ambulation-assistive device is a cane. Resistance to its use can be overcome by persuasion and demonstration of its benefits.[21] A properly fitted cane or crutch (barring modifications) when multiple joints are affected, should reach 8 inches lateral to the front of the foot when the patient is standing comfortably and holding the cane or crutch handle with the elbow flexed 15 to 30°.[275] This position permits stability on standing and an easy reach to the ground ahead during walking. The cane, grasp and arm function permitting, should be held in the hand opposite to the lower-extremity joint involved by arthritis. A lightweight walking aid is particularly useful to many arthritic or elderly patients. Specific methods for gait training, including training in the use of canes and crutches, are recorded.[21,63,115,248,268]

Wheelchairs, Driving, and Public Transportation

When ambulation is impractical or impossible, a wheelchair must be prescribed. A variety of wheelchair options must be considered to ensure fit that provides support and function for painful or deformed joint structures.[22,23,25,92,212,297] Accessibility to bathrooms, clearance under tables and desks, ease of entry and exits for transferring, durability, powered versus nonpowered models, and cost are some of the factors that require analysis when recommending purchase of a wheelchair.[22,23,25] Wheelchair manufacturers or their rep-resentatives often provide important information. However, it is advisable first to consult an experienced physical or occupational therapist. Driving an automobile is often difficult, but even a patient confined to a wheelchair may be able to drive if special provisions are made. Special instructions for the handicapped arthritic driver, automobile or van modifications, and provision of suitable parking and accessibility to home, work, and recreation make mobility independence a practical goal.[29,41,83,92,143]

When driving is not a practical option, public transportation is all too often inaccessible to handicapped people.[41,83,142] In some communities, special vehicles are available to meet this need.[41,80,153] Airline travel poses many problems, although many airlines have developed special policies to assist the handicapped.

Architectural barriers that often confront the handicapped or wheelchair traveler at hotels, schools, restaurants, parks, zoos, and theatres may be avoided in part by selecting places and facilities where special access for the handicapped is provided.[29,83,128,142,170]

OCCUPATIONAL THERAPY

The occupational therapist's first concern is with the patient's ability to function independently. The second concern is to provide adaptive equipment to allow function that is otherwise difficult or impossible. This goal often requires the fabrication of splints.[17,39,187,210,275] Central to the occupational therapist's evaluation of an arthritis patient is a review of the activities of daily living (ADL) (see Table 44–2).[39,42,47,275] The occupational therapist provides an arthritic patient with concepts and techniques of joint protection, energy conservation, and function-assisted methods and devices to meet needs as determined by the ADL assessment.[39,41,42,47,187,275] Several excellent reviews on assistive devices, energy-saving techniques, and protection of arthritic joints are available.[17,29,114,143,151,170,180,208,210,275,290]

The physician should reinforce the concepts taught by the therapist, specifically: (1) joint protection, including joint ''rest'' with proper positioning to avoid deformity; (2) transferring skills to enable the patient to change position without stressing joints; (3) preferential use of the strongest (largest) joints for any given activity; and (4) conservation of energy by planning tasks to use involved joints to their greatest mechanical advantage.[39,42,47,187,208,275]

Collars and Corsets

Collars are not indicated for all neck pain, nor are corsets recommended for all back pain.[22] With the exception of the few braces that stabilize the cervical spine, collars are primarily worn for pain relief, for relief for neck muscles in spasm, and as a reminder to avoid certain movements that may exacerbate the underlying problem.[22,275] Studies on the immobilization efficiency of various cervical collars and braces have been performed on normal subjects. The lack of studies on patients with inflammatory disease of the cervical spine makes decisions regarding type of collar, duration of use, and indication for use difficult. Common practice is based on extrapolation from studies of normal subjects and from clinical experience.[22,78,112,275] Most commonly used collars do not restrict movement at the atlantoaxial joint,[5] with the exceptions of scalp fixation in a halo cast[154] or Crutchfeld tongs with longitudinal pull.[105] Stabilization of the lower cervical spine, but not of the upper cervical spine, may be obtained with a rigid cervical collar (Philadelphia collar).[275] Although controlled studies are inadequate, soft cervical collars have been found not to affect outcome as regards episodes of acute neck pain,[27] nor have they arrested the progress of subluxation in patients with RA.[263] When a cervical collar or brace is prescribed, isometric neck exercises should also be prescribed to minimize disuse atrophy.

Corsets or spinal braces are commonly used to relieve low back discomfort and to prevent exacerbation of radiculopathy.[275] Many types of corsets and braces are available, and guidelines for individual prescriptions are described in detail elsewhere.[275] Studies of corsets show only subjective relief of pain,[201] and no available brace can effectively immobilize the lumbosacral region.[217] Pain relief with a corset may be related to an increase in abdominal pressure that relieves extensor force on the spine with an overall decrease in intradiscal pressure.[99] The indications for, and instruction in the use of, neck braces are controversial.[224] The prolonged use of these braces has resulted in loss of spinal mobility and weakness of paraspinal muscles.

Splints and Braces

Splints (Table 44–8) are used to relieve pain, to improve function, to prevent trauma to unstable joints, and to prevent, contain, or correct arthritic deformities.[17,54,66,127,187,222,275,290] Although deceptively simple in appearance, their proper design and appropriate application require great sophistication.

Splints can be and have been made of cloth and metal, plaster, heat-moldable plastics, and more recently, new Fiberglas polymers, polyethylene, polypropylene, and air-pressure apparatus.[54,172,187] Splints should be light, durable, nonirritating, cosmetically appealing, and affordable.[6,26,66,127,187,275] The wearer should easily be able to apply, adjust, and remove the splint or brace without assistance. Splints are designed either for rest or for controlled motion of a given joint.[22] A properly designed splint should not unintentionally affect function, such as a wrist splint that prevents finger function, nor should stress be transferred to other joints (Fig. 44–6).[6,22,39,66,101,124,127,187,275] Research on splint use demonstrates better compliance if strength is enhanced more than dexterity.[210] Considerable education and encouragement are needed to convince patients to use splints during rest or relative inactivity.[210] Splint therapy of rheumatic disease patients requires frequent follow-up and splint adjustments.

Proved or even well-established indications for splints and braces in arthritis are few. Guidelines for postoperative splinting to maintain joint alignment and to prevent or to correct contractures, particularly in the knee and fingers, are well established.[227] Permanent reversal of joint malalignments, such as swan neck, boutonnière, or ulnar deviation, by splinting has not been demonstrated.[45] With the exceptions of contracture corrections and postoperative splinting, the indications for splints and braces should be confined to relief of pain and improvement of function (see Table 44–6).[54,89,222,246,275]

Splinting and casting can reduce joint inflammation and pain without risk of contractures if immobilization is not prolonged beyond 4 weeks.[89,222,246,275] Serial casting by a variety of techniques is an acceptable method of prevention and treatment of flexion contractures of the knee.[108,227,236] The rationale for serial or wedged casting is based on the effect of joint support on pain relief and relaxation of muscle spasm, to allow a gradual stretch of contracted connective tissue. Each cast change, which takes place every 5 to 7 days, allows for additional stretching, as well as an opportunity for range-of-motion exercise. A bivalved cast can be removed daily for observation and exercise of the extremity. Knee contractures greater than 45° usually require traction for correction. Properly applied traction has the additional advantage of minimizing impingement and compression of a subluxed tibia on the femur.[227] When the maximum possible correction is reached, as defined by the lack of increase in motion for 2 consecutive weeks, splinting may replace serial casting to maintain range of motion.

SEXUAL, SOCIAL, AND PSYCHOLOGIC CONSIDERATIONS IN REHABILITATION

Sexual problems are common among arthritic patients.[15] Chronic pain and inflammation, stiffness

Table 44–8. Useful Splints and Braces*

Region	Indication	Purpose	Type	Reference
Hand	Acute inflammation	To stabilize for pain relief	Volar resting splint†	177,187,246
		To preserve position for function		
Thumb	Carpometacarpal and metacarpophalangeal joint arthritis	To stabilize for pain relief and to permit function	Thumb post with wrist strap	177,187
	De Quervain's tenosynovitis	To relieve pain	Thumb post with wrist strap	
	Interphalangeal joint pain or instability	To improve function and relieve pain	Thumb, interphalangeal "sleeve" or "double ring"	
Wrist	Active inflammation	To improve function and relieve pain	Static "working" wrist splint‡	187
	Instability	To improve function and relieve pain	Static "working" wrist splint‡	
	Carpel tunnel syndrome	To prevent hyperflexion and nerve compression	Static "working" wrist splint‡	
Knee	Pain, instability	To relieve pain	Molded plastic hinged knee	38a,55,158,187
		To maintain position	Long leg, hinged knee with lock	
Ankle, hindfoot	Pain on weight bearing	To support foot and relieve weight-bearing stress	Cushion heel, rocker sole, below-knee weight-bearing brace	187,275
Forefoot	Pain on weight bearing	To support foot and relieve weight-bearing stress	Metatarsal pad or bar with cushion insole	51a,55

*Postoperative splints not included.
†*Resting splints maximally support affected joints, usually by sacrificing function.
‡Static working splints stabilize affected joints, but permit maximum function (see Fig. 42–6). Dynamic splints provide wire or elastic tension for traction or to assist weak muscles. Various dynamic splints, such as wire or rubber-band-assisted traction devices, are employed to maintain postoperative corrections. The Bunnell "knuckle bender" splints are occasionally helpful in treating an isolated finger contracture when inflammation is minimal. Splints for thumb interphalangeal stabilization, to correct swan neck, boutonnière, or ulnar deviation deformities, are available, but their efficacy is unproved.[33]

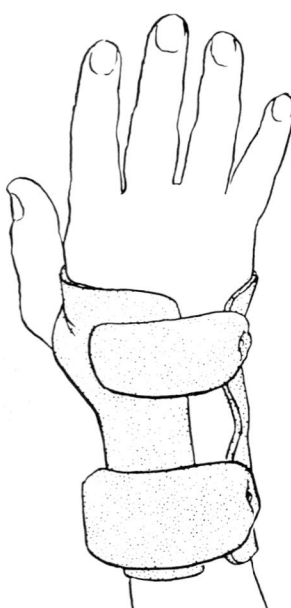

Fig. 44–6. Static "working" wrist splint. This heat-molded plastic splint with Velcro closures is designed to stabilize a painful or inflamed wrist in a neutral position (zero degrees of extension) while permitting free finger and thumb function. This splint is also useful for patients with the carpal tunnel syndrome.

or immobility especially involving the hips, neck, hands, and knees, fatigue, malaise, and medication-related and emotional disturbances all contribute.[98,104,311] A recent study showed that patients preferred a physician to a psychologist or social worker for discussion of sexual concerns[81] so it is important that the physician be attuned to the sexual problems of the arthritis patient. Problems of sexual image as a consequence of perceived disfigurement, loss of sexual drive or libido due to medication or disease-related factors, physical expression of sexuality limited by pain, stiffness, and deformity, and impotence that may be due to drug effects, pain, or psychologic factors must all be addressed.[104]

The physician can advise the patient about drugs, such as the peak levels of analgesics and anti-inflammatory agents, or surgical procedures to increase mobility, to relieve pain, and to improve appearance. The physician may also supervise the physical therapist's teaching of massage and hydrotherapy techniques as a prelude to sex, and the occupational therapist's use of splints for particularly painful extremities and demonstration of appropriate positions.[104,311] Alternate sexual positioning, depending on which joints are involved, and alternate forms of sexual expression may be needed.[98,104,311] Referral to trained sex counselors for refractory sexual dysfunction may also be indicated. Counseling regarding forms and use of contraceptive methods is often helpful.

Premarital counseling is best done with the physician and the couple together.[19] Religious, cultural, social, and disease-related histories are needed from both patient and intended spouse. Information on the specific type of arthritis, its natural course, prognosis, and how it will affect various daily activities can then be provided along with advice relative to sex.[19,104] Counseling of married couples often involves a discussion of childbirth.[104,311] Genetic counseling and concerns about the effects of the disease and medications on the bearing, nurturing, and nursing of an infant should be addressed in conjunction with the obstetrician and pediatrician.[10] The goal is an educated, confident mother and a healthy child.[10] Women afflicted with RA need help to cope with their own, often unvoiced, fears about the disease.[309] How to manage a home and how to handle a spouse's anxiety? Recent studies have debunked the myth that a disability in a parent influences a child's psychologic adjustment. Psychologic development in such children is no different from that of peers with "well" parents.[31]

Attention to psychosocial factors does not alter rheumatic disease activity, but it does affect the functional results of rehabilitation.[295] A team approach helps most in social adjustment. Educational and financial background are strong "motivational" variables that influence outcome more than the team approach itself.[295]

Psychologic problems in patients with chronic arthritis include loss of independence and self-esteem, loss of relationships with family, friends, and lovers, loss of employment, and the stress of coping with pain and disability.[242,293] The classic sequence of adaptive psychologic responses to chronic disease, that is, shock, anger, denial, resignation, and acceptance, are often altered in the arthritis patient and fluctuate with the course of the disease.[242] The approach to rehabilitation of the arthritis patient is case-specific, but must consider family dynamics and stress.[15,293] Technologic solutions to personal and social problems or reluctance to accept patients as partners in their own rehabilitation may result in poor compliance to therapeutic regimens and poorer functional outcome.[15,242,295,313]

Newer programs to supplement an arthritis rehabilitation team's efforts to deal with all facets of the patient's life and disease include the following: (1) group counseling and educational programs;[135] (2) participation of voluntary organizations that disseminate information, aid with disability-related problems such as transportation or meal preparation, and provide group psychosocial support;[7] (3) multidisciplinary pain centers in which many psychologic, physical medicine, and drug-control approaches can be used alone or together for pain management;[82,273] and (4) recreation therapy and recreational opportunities designed for the disabled.[111]

REFERENCES

1. Abramsen, D.I., et al.: Methods in training the conscious control of motor units. Arch. Phys. Med. Rehabil., 48:12–19, 1967.
2. Adamson, J.E.: Treatment of the stiff hand. Orthop. Clin. North Am., 1:467–479, 1970.
3. Alexander, R. McN., and Bennet-Clark, H.C.: Storage of elastic strain energy in muscle and other tissues. Nature, 265:114–117, 1977.
4. Allander, E., et al.: Rheumatology in perspective: the epidemiological view. Scand. J. Rheumatol., 46 (Suppl.):11–19, 1982.
5. Althoff, B., and Goldie, I.F.: Cervical collars in rheumatoid atlanto-axial subluxations: a radiographic comparison. Ann. Rheum, Dis., 39:485–489, 1980.
6. American Rheumatism Association, Arthritis Foundation and National Institute of Arthritis and Metabolic Diseases: Evaluation of splinting. Criteria for and evaluation of orthopedic measures in the management of deformities of rheumatoid arthritis. Arthritis Rheum., 7:585–600, 1964.
7. Andrews, M.C.G., and Woodford, W.F.S.: The voluntary organizations. In Rehabilitation in the Rheumatic Diseases. Edited by Douglas Woolf. Philadelphia, W.B. Saunders, 1981.
8. Aoral, D.M.L., and Navell, D.J.: Manipulation in the treatment of low back pain: a multicenter study. Br. Med. J., 2:161–164, 1975.
9. Arthritis Foundation: The Arthritis 1975 Annual Report. New York, Arthritis Foundation, 1975.
10. Asrael, W.: An approach to motherhood for disabled women. Rehabil. Lit., 43:214–218, 1982.
11. Baker, G.H.B.: Psychological management in rehabilitation. In Rehabilitation in the Rheumatic Diseases. Edited by Douglas Woolf. Philadelphia, W.B. Saunders, 1981.
12. Bardwick, P.A., and Swezey, R.L.: Physical therapy in arthritis. Postgrad. Med., 72:223–234, 1982.
13. Basmajian, J.V.: Biofeedback in rehabilitation: a review of principles and practices. Arch. Phys. Med. Rehabil., 62:469–475, 1981.
14. Bassett, C.A.L., Mitchell, S.N., and Gaston, S.R.: Pulsing electromagnetic field treatment in ununited fractures and failed arthroses. JAMA, 247:623–628, 1982.
15. Baum, J.: A review of the psychological aspects of rheumatic diseases. Semin. Arthritis Rheum., 11:352–361, 1982.
16. Beals, C.: A case for aerobic conditioning exercise in rheumatoid arthritis. (Abstract.) Clin. Res., 29:780A, 1981.
17. Bennett, R.L.: Orthotic devices to prevent deformities of the hand in rheumatoid arthritis. Arthritis Rheum., 8:1006–1018, 1965.
18. Benson, T.B., and Copp, E.P.: The effects of therapeutic forms of heat and ice on the pain threshold of the normal shoulder. Rheumatol. Rehabil., 13:101–104, 1974.
19. Bernardo, M.D.: Premarital counseling and the couple with disabilities: a review and recommendations. Rehabil. Lit., 42:213–217, 1981.
20. Bertolucci, L.C.: Introduction of antiinflammatory drugs by iontophoresis: double blind study. J. Orthop. Sports. Phys. Ther., 4:103–108, 1982.
21. Blount, W.P.: Don't throw away the cane. J. Bone. Joint. Surg., 38A:695–708, 1958.
22. Bossingham, D.H.: Wheelchairs and appliances. Clin. Rheum. Dis., 7:395–415, 1981.

23. Bossingham, D.H., and Russell, P.: The usefulness of powered wheelchairs in advanced inflammatory polyarthritis. Rheumatol. Rehabil., 19:131–135, 1980.
24. Boyle, R.W.: The Therapeutic Gymnasium. In Therapeutic Exercises. Edited by S. Licht. New Haven, Waverly Press, 1965.
25. Brattstrom, M., et al.: The rheumatoid patient in need of a wheelchair. Scand. J. Rehabil. Med., 13:39–43, 1981.
26. Brenner, M.H.: Health costs and benefits of economic policy. Int. J. Health Serv., 7:581–623, 1977.
27. British Association of Physical Medicine: Pain in the neck and arm: a multicenter trial of the effects of physiotherapy. Br. Med. J., 1:253–258, 1966.
28. Brooks, R.G., et al.: Costs of managing patients at a Canadian rheumatic disease unit. J. Rheumatol., 8:937–948, 1981.
29. Buchanan, J.M., and Symons, J.: Housing and the environment for people with arthritis. Clin. Rheum. Dis., 7:417–436, 1981.
30. Bucklund, L., and Tiselius, P.: Objective measurement of joint stiffness in rheumatoid arthritis. Acta Rheumatol. Scand., 13:275–288, 1967.
31. Bucks, F.M., and Hohmann, G.W.: Child adjustment as related to severity of paternal disability. Arch. Phys. Med. Rehabil., 63:249–253, 1982.
32. Bulgen, D.Y., Hazleman, B.L., and Voak, D.: HLA-B27 and frozen shoulder. Lancet, 1:1042–1044, 1976.
33. Bunnell, S.: Surgery of the Hand. 5th Ed. Revised by J.H. Bozes. Philadelphia, J.B. Lippincott, 1970.
34. Burgess, E.M.: Some applications of electrical energy for neuromuscular rehabilitation. Orthop. Digest., 4:14–19, 1976.
35. Cailliet, R.: Shoulder Pain. 2nd Ed. Philadelphia, F.A. Davis, 1981.
36. Cailliet, R.: Neck and Arm Pain. 2nd Ed. Philadelphia, F.A. Davis, 1981.
37. Caldwell, J.W., and Krusen, E.M.: Effectiveness of cervical traction in treatment of neck problems: Evaluation of various methods. Arch. Phys. Med. Rehabil., 43:214–221, 1962.
38. Carr, D.B., et al.: Physical conditioning facilitates the exercise-induced secretion of beta endorphin and beta-lipoprotein in women. N. Engl. J. Med., 305:560–566, 1981.
38a. Cassvan, A., Wonder, K.E., and Fultonberg, D.M.: Orthotic management of the unstable knee. Arch. Phys. Med. Rehabil., 58:487–491, 1977.
39. Chamberlain, M.A.: Occupational therapy. Clin. Rheum. Dis., 7:365–376, 1981.
40. Chamberlain, M.A.: Rehabilitation: social implications of rheumatoid arthritis to young mothers. Rheumatol. Rehabil., 16 (Suppl.):70–73, 1979.
41. Chamberlain, M.A., Buchanan, J.M., and Hanks, H.: The arthritic in the urban environment. Ann. Rheum. Dis., 38:51–56, 1979.
42. Chamberlain, M.A., Thornely, G., and Wright, V.: Evaluation of bathing and toilet aids. Rheumatol. Rehabil., 17:187–194, 1978.
43. Chrisman, O.D., Mittnacht, A., and Snook, G.A.: A study of the results following rotary manipulation in the lumbar intervertebral disc syndrome. J. Bone Joint Surg., 46A:517–524, 1964.
44. Clark, G.R., et al.: Evaluation of physiotherapy in the treatment of osteoarthrosis of the knee. Rheumatol. Rehabil., 13:190–197, 1974.
45. Convery, F.R., Conaty, J.P., and Nickel, V.L.: Dynamic splinting of rheumatoid arthritis. Orthot. Prosthet., 21:249–254, 1967.
46. Corcoran, P.J.: Energy expenditure during ambulation. In Physiological Basis of Rehabilitation Medicine. Edited by J.A. Downey and R.C. Darling. Philadelphia, W.B. Saunders, 1971.
47. Cordery, J.C.: Joint protection: a responsibility of the occupational therapist. Am. J. Occup. Ther., 19:285–294, 1965.
48. Colachis, S.C., and Strohm, B.R.: A study of tractive forces and angle of pull on vertebral interspaces in the

cervical spine. Arch. Phys. Med. Rehabil., *46*:820–830, 1965.

49. Colvez, A., and Blanchet, M.: Disability trends in the United States population 1966–1976: analysis of reported causes. Am. J. Public Health, *71*:464–471, 1981.
50. Conaty, J.P., and Nickel, V.L.: Functional incapacitation in rheumatoid arthritis: a rehabilitation challenge: a correlative study of function before and after hospital treatment. J. Bone Joint Surg., *53A*:624–637, 1971.
51. Cooke, A.F., Dawson, D., and Wright, F.: Lubrication of synovial membrane. Ann. Rheum. Dis., *35*:56–59, 1976.
51a. Cracchiolo, A., III: The use of shoes to treat foot disorders. Orthoped. Rev., *8*:73–83, 1979.
52. Currier, D.P., and Mann, R.: Muscular strength developed by electrical stimulation in healthy individuals. Phys. Ther., *63*:915–921, 1983.
53. Cyriax, J.: Textbook of Orthopedic Medicine. 7th Ed. London, Harper & Ross, 1965.
54. Davis, J., and Janecki, C.J.: Rehabilitation of the rheumatoid upper limb. Orthop. Clin. North Am., *9*:559–568, 1978.
55. Deaver, G.G.: Lower limb bracing. *In* Orthotics Etcetera. Edited by S. Licht and H. Kamenetz. New Haven, Waverly Press, 1966.
56. Decker, J.L.: Conference on outcome measures in rheumatological clinical trials: summary. J. Rheumatol., *9*:802–806, 1982.
57. DeJong, R., Hershey, W., and Wagman, I.: Nerve and conduction velocity during hypothermia in man. Anesthesiology, *27*:805–810, 1966.
58. DeLateur, B.J., Lehmann, J.F., and Fordyce, W.E.: A test of the DeLorme axiom. Arch. Phys. Med. Rehabil., *49*:245–248, 1968.
59. De Palma, A.F.: Diseases of The Knee. Philadelphia, J.B. Lippincott, 1954.
60. Dimonte, P.C., and Light, H.: Patho-mechanics, gait deviations and treatment of the rheumatoid foot. Phys. Ther., *62*:1148–1156, 1982.
61. Don Figny, R., and Sheldon, K.: Simultaneous use of heat and cold in treatment of muscle spasm. Arch. Phys. Med. Rehabil., *43*:235–237, 1962.
62. Dorwart, B.B., Hansell, J.R., and Schumacher, H.R., Jr.: Effects of cold and heat on urate crystal-induced synovitis in the dog. Arthritis Rheum., *17*:563–571, 1974.
63. Downis, E., et al.: A comparison of efficiency of three types of crutches using oxygen consumption. Rheumatol. Rehabil., *19*:252–255, 1982.
64. Edington, D.W., and Edgerton, V.R.: The Biology of Physical Activity. Boston, Houghton Mifflin, 1976.
65. Edstrom, L.: Selective changes in sizes of red and white muscle fibers in upper motor lesions and parkinsonism. J. Neurol. Sci., *11*:537–550, 1970.
66. Ehrlich, G.E.: Rest and splinting. *In* Total Management of the Arthritis Patient. Edited by G.E. Ehrlich. Philadelphia, J.B. Lippincott, 1973.
67. Ekblom, B., et al.: Physical performance in patients with rheumatoid arthritis. Scand. J. Rheumatol., *3*:121–125, 1974.
68. Emery, H., Schaller, J.G., and Fowler, R.S., Jr.: Biofeedback in the management of primary and secondary Raynaud's phenomenon. (Abstract.) Arthritis Rheum., *19*:795, 1976.
69. English, A.W.M., and Wolf, S.L.: The motor unit: anatomy and physiology. Phys. Ther., *62*:10–15, 1982.
70. Epstein, W.V.: Health services research in rheumatology. Bull. Rheum. Dis., *31*:15–19, 1981.
71. Erb, W.: Handbook of Electro-therapeutics. New York, William Wood & Company, 1883.
72. Eysenck, H.J.: A new theory of post-rest upswing on "warm-up" in motor learning. Percept. Motor Skills, *28*:992–994, 1969.
73. Farfan, A.F.: Mechanical Disorders of the Low Back. Philadelphia, Lea & Febiger, 1973.
74. Feibel, A., and Fast, A.: Deep heating of joints: a reconsideration. Arch. Phys. Med. Rehabil., *57*:513–514, 1976.

75. Ferderber, M.B.: Long-term illness: management of the chronically ill patient. Pa. Med. J., *63*:390–394, 1960.
76. Ferris, B.G., Jr.: Environmental hazards: electromagnetic radiation. N. Engl. J. Med., *275*:1100–1105, 1966.
77. Findlay, J.: Moving forward in rheumatology nursing: a report from the rheumatology nursing forum. (Editorial.) Br. J. Rheumatol., *22*:56, 1983.
78. Fisher, S.V., et al.: Cervical orthosis effect on cervical spine motion: roentgenographic and goniometric method of study. Arch. Phys. Med. Rehabil., *58*:109–115, 1977.
79. Flatt, A.E.: The Care of the Rheumatoid Hand. 3rd Ed. St. Louis, C.V. Mosby, 1974.
80. Fligg, H., and Wright, V.: The community and hospital nurse in relation to arthritis. Clin. Rheum. Dis., *7*:321–336, 1981.
81. Florian, V.: Sex counseling: comparison of attitudes of disabled and nondisabled subjects. Arch. Phys. Med. Rehabil., *64*:81–84, 1983.
82. Fordyce, W.E., et al.: Operant conditioning in the treatment of chronic pain. Arch. Phys. Med., *54*:399–408, 1973.
83. Francis, R.A.: The development of federal accessibility law. J. Rehabil., *49*:29–33, 1983.
84. Frankel, V.H., and Burstein, A.H.: Orthopedic Biomechanics. Philadelphia, Lea & Febiger, 1970.
85. Fried, D.M.: Rest versus activity. *In* Arthritis and Physical Medicine. Edited by S. Licht. New Haven, Waverly Press, 1969.
86. Fries, J.F.: Toward an understanding of patient outcome measurement. Arthritis Rheum., *26*:697–704, 1983.
87. Fries, J.F., et al.: Measurement of patient outcome in arthritis. Arthritis Rheum., *23*:137–145, 1980.
88. Gacker, T.: Heat and cold in orthopedics. *In* Therapeutic Heat and Cold. Edited by S. Licht. New Haven, E. Licht, 1965.
89. Gault, S.J., and Spyker, J.M.: Beneficial effects of immobilization of joints in rheumatoid and related arthritides: a splint study using sequential analysis. Arthritis Rheum., *12*:34–44, 1969.
90. Gersten, J.W.: Effect of metallic objects on temperature rises produced in tissue by ultrasound. Am. J. Phys. Med., *37*:75–82, 1958.
91. Gersten, J.W.: Effect of ultrasound on tendon extensibility. Am. J. Phys. Med., *34*:362–369, 1955.
92. Gibson, T., and Grahame, R.: Rehabilitation of the elderly arthritic patient. Clin. Rheum. Dis., *7*:485–496, 1981.
93. Goldberg, L.I., White, D.J., and Pandolf, K.B.: Cardiovascular and perceptual responses to isometric exercise. Arch. Phys. Med. Rehabil., *63*:211–216, 1982.
94. Goodman, C.E.: Pathophysiology of pain. Arch. Intern. Med., *143*:527–530, 1983.
95. Grahame, R.: Clinical trials in low back pain. Clin. Rheum. Dis., *6*:143–157, 1980.
96. Grant, A.E.: Massage with ice (cryokinetics) in the treatment of painful conditions of the musculoskeletal system. Arch. Phys. Med. Rehabil., *45*:233–238, 1964.
97. Greengross, W.: Rehabilitation: sex and arthritis. Rheumatol. Rehabil., *16(Suppl.)*:68–96, 1979.
98. Greengross, W.: Sex and arthritis. Rheumatol. Rehabil., *16 (Suppl.)*:68–70, 1979.
99. Grew, N.D.: Intra-abdominal pressure responds to loads applied to the torso in normal subjects. Spine, *5*:149–154, 1980.
100. Guest, J.H., et al.: Running as a treatment for depression. Compr. Psychiatry, *20*:41–54, 1979.
101. Gumpel, J.M., and Cannon, S.: A cross-over comparison of ready-made fabric wrist-splints in rheumatoid arthritis. Rheumatol. Rehabil., *20*:113–115, 1981.
102. Guniby, G., et al.: Muscle strength and endurance after training with repeated maximal isometric contractions. Scand. J. Rehabil. Med., *5*:118–123, 1973.
103. Hallebrandt, F.A.: Special review; application of the overload principle to muscle training in man. Am. J. Phys. Med., *37*:278–283, 1958.
104. Hamilton, A.: Sexual problems of the disabled. *In* Rehabilitation Medicine. 2nd Ed. Edited by P.J.R. Nichols. Baltimore, Waverly Press, 1980.

105. Hancock, D.O.: The cervical spine in rheumatoid arthritis. Clin. Rheum. Dis., *4*:443–459, 1978.
106. Harris, E., Jr., and McCroskery, P.A.: The influence of temperature and fibril stability on degradation of cartilage collagen by rheumatoid synovial collagenase. N. Engl. J. Med., *290*:1–6, 1974.
107. Harris, P.R.: Iontophoresis: clinical research in musculoskeletal inflammatory conditions. J. Orthop. Sports Phys. Ther., *4*:109–112, 1982.
107a. Harris, R.: The effect of various forms of physical therapy on radiosodium clearance from the arthritic knee joint. Ann. Phys. Med., *7*:1–17, 1963.
108. Harris, R., and Copp, E.P.: Immobilization of the knee joint in rheumatoid arthritis. Ann. Rheum. Dis., *21*:353–359, 1962.
109. Harris, R., and Millard, J.B.: Paraffin-wax baths in the treatment of rheumatoid arthritis. Ann. Rheum. Dis., *14*:278–282, 1955.
110. Harrison, R.A.: Hydrotherapy in rheumatic conditions. *In* Physiotherapy in Rheumatology. Edited by S.A. Hyde. Oxford, Blackwell Scientific Publications, 1980.
111. Harsanyi, S.L.: Toward equal opportunities in recreation for the disabled. Arch. Phys. Med. Rehabil., *56*:135–137, 1975.
112. Hartman, J.T., Palumbo, R., and Hill, B.J.: Cineradiography of the braced normal cervical spine. A comparative study of five commonly used cervical orthoses. J. Bone Joint Surg., *59A*:332–339, 1979.
113. Harvey, R.F., and Jellinek, H.M.: Functional performance assessment: a program approach. Arch. Phys. Med. Rehabil., *62*:456–461, 1981.
114. Haworth, R.J., and Nichols, P.J.R.: Hoists in the home: their recommendation and use. Rheumatol. Rehabil., *19*:42–51, 1980.
115. Haworth, R.J., Dunscombe, S., and Nichols, P.J.R.: Mobile arm supports: an evaluation. Rheumatol. Rehabil., *17*:240–244, 1978.
116. Heffman, M., and Bibby, B.G.: Effect of tension on lysis of collagen. Soc. Exp. Biol. Med. Proc., *126*:561–562, 1967.
117. Herbison, G.J., Jaweed, M.M., and Ditunno, J.F.: Muscle fiber types. Arch. Phys. Med. Rehabil., *63*:227–230, 1982.
118. Hess, E.V.: A uniform data base on rheumatic diseases. Arthritis Rheum., *19*:645–648, 1978.
119. Hoehler, F.K., Tobis, J.S., and Buerger, A.A.: Spinal manipulation for low back pain. JAMA, *245*:1835–1838, 1981.
120. Hollander, J.L., and Horvath, S.M.: The influence of physical therapy procedures on the intra-articular temperature of normal and arthritis subjects. Am. J. Med. Sci., *218*:543–548, 1949.
121. Holloszy, J.O.: Muscle metabolism during exercise. Arch. Phys. Med. Rehabil., *63*:231–234, 1982.
122. Hong, C., et al.: Magnetic necklace: its therapeutic effectiveness on neck and shoulder pain. Arch. Phys. Med. Rehabil., *63*:462–466, 1982.
123. Horvath, S.M., and Hollander, J.L.: Intra-articular temperature as measures of joint reaction. J. Clin. Invest., *28*:469–473, 1949.
124. Houston, M.E., and Goemans, P.H.: Leg muscle performance of athletes with and without knee support braces. Arch. Phys. Med. Rehabil., *63*:431–432, 1982.
125. Huskisson, E.C.: Measurement of pain. J. Rheumatol., *9*:768–769, 1982.
126. Huskisson, E.C.: Measurement in rehabilitation. (Editorial.) Rheum. Rehabil., *15*:132, 1976.
127. Hyde, S.A.: Physiotherapy in Rheumatology. Oxford, Blackwell Scientific Publications, 1980.
128. Inman, V.T., Ralston, H.J., and Todd, F.: Human Walking. Baltimore, Williams & Wilkins, 1980.
129. Jayson, M.I.V.: Back pain, spondylosis and disc disorders. *In* Copeman's Textbook of Rheumatic Diseases. Edited by J.T. Scott. London, Livingstone, 1978.
130. Johns, R.J., and Wright, V.: Relative importance of various tissues in joint stiffness. J. Appl. Physiol., *17*:824–831, 1962.
131. Johnston, M.V., and Keith, R.A.: Cost-benefits of medical rehabilitation. Arch. Phys. Med. Rehabil., *64*:147–154, 1983.
132. Judovich, B.D., and Nobel, G.R.: Traction therapy, a study of resistance forces. Am. J. Surg., *93*:108–114, 1957.
133. Judovich, B.D.: Herniated cervical disc: a new form of traction. Am. J. Surg., *84*:645–656, 1952.
134. Kabat, H.: Proprioceptive facilitation. *In* Therapeutic Exercise. 2nd Ed. Edited by S. Licht. Baltimore, Waverly Press, 1965.
135. Kaplan, S., and Kozin, F.: A controlled study of group counseling in rheumatoid arthritis. J. Rheumatol., *8*:91–99, 1981.
136. Karten, I., Koatz, A.O., and McEwen, C.: Treatment of contractures of the knee in rheumatoid arthritis. N.Y. Acad. Med. Bull., *44*:763–773, 1968.
137. Katz, S., et al.: Studies of illness in the aged. JAMA, *185*:914–919, 1963.
138. Kaufert, J.M.: Functional ability indices: measurement problems in assessing their validity. Arch. Phys. Med. Rehabil., *64*:260–267, 1983.
139. Kennedy, A.C.: Joint temperature. Clin. Rheum. Dis., *7*:177–188, 1981.
140. Kirk, J.A., and Kersely, G.D.: Heat and cold in the physical treatment of rheumatoid arthritis of the knee. Ann. Phys. Med., *9*:270–274, 1968.
141. Klein, R.M., and Bell, B.: Self-care skills: behavioral measurements with Klein-Bell ADL Scale. Arch. Phys. Med. Rehabil., *63*:335–338, 1982.
142. Kliment, S.A.: Into the Mainstream—A Syllabus for Barrier-free Environment. Washington, D.C., Rehabilitation Services Administration, U.S. Department of Health, Education and Welfare, and American Institute of Architects, Social and Rehabilitation Services, 1975.
143. Klinger, J.L.: Self Help Manual for Patients with Arthritis. Arthritis Foundation, Arthritis Health Professions Section, 1980.
144. Kottke, F.J.: Therapeutic exercise. *In* Handbook of Physical Medicine and Rehabilitation, 2nd Ed. Edited by F.H. Krusen, F.J. Kottke, and P.M. Ellwood. Philadelphia, W.B. Saunders, 1971.
145. Kottke, F.J., Pauley, D.L., and Ptak, R.A.: The rationale for prolonged stretching for correction of shortening of connective tissues. Arch. Phys. Med. Rehabil., *47*:345–352, 1966.
146. Kovacs, R.: Electrotherapy and Light Therapy. 2nd Ed. Philadelphia, Lea & Febiger, 1935.
147. Krempen, J.F., and Silver, R.A.: External electromagnetic fields in the treatment of nonunion of bones: a three-year experience in private practice. Orthop. Rev., *10*:33–39, 1981.
148. Krueger, B.R., and Okazaki, H.: Basilar infarction following chiropractic cervical manipulation. Mayo Clin. Proc., *55*:322–332, 1980.
149. Krusen, F.H., Kottke, F.J., and Ellwood, P.M.: Handbook of Physical Medicine and Rehabilitation. Philadelphia, W.B. Saunders, 1965.
150. Kumar, V.N., and Redford, J.B.: Transcutaneous nerve stimulation in rheumatoid arthritis. Arch. Phys. Med. Rehabil., *63*:595–596, 1982.
151. Laging, B.: Furniture design for the elderly. Rehabil. Lit., *27*:130–140, 1966.
152. Landen, R.R.: Heat or cold for relief of low back pain? Phys. Ther., *47*:1126–1128, 1967.
153. Lauri, G.: Housing and Home Services for the Disabled: Guidelines and Experiences in Independent Living. Hagerstown, MD, Harper & Row, 1977.
154. Lawhon, S.M., and Crawford, A.H.: Traction in the treatment of spinal deformity. Orthopedics, *6*:447–458, 1983.
155. Lee, P., et al.: Benefits of hospitalization in rheumatoid arthritis. Q. J. Med., *43*:205–214, 1974.
156. Lehmann, J.F.: Diathermy. *In* Handbook of Physical Medicine and Rehabilitation, 2nd Ed. Edited by F.H. Krusen, F. Kottke, and P.M. Ellwood. 2nd Ed. Philadelphia, W.B. Saunders, 1971.
157. Lehmann, J.F.: Diathermy. *In* Therapeutic Heat. Edited by S. Licht, Baltimore, Waverly Press, 1958.
158. Lehmann, J.F., and Brunner, G.D.: A device for the

application of heavy lumbar traction: its mechanical effects. Arch. Phys. Med. Rehabil., 39:696–700, 1958.

159. Lehmann, J.F., and Krusen, F.H.: Biophysical effects of ultrasonic energy on carcinoma and their possible significance. Arch. Phys. Med. Rehabil., 36:452–459, 1955.

160. Lehmann, J.F., and DeLateur, B.J.: Cryotherapy. In Therapeutic Heat and Cold. Edited by F. Lehmann. Baltimore, Williams & Wilkins, 1965.

161. Lehmann, J.F., Brunner, G.D., and Stow, R.W.: Pain threshold measurements after therapeutic application of ultrasound, microwave and infrared. Arch. Phys. Med. Rehabil., 39:560–565, 1958.

162. Lehmann, J.F., et al.: Heating of joint structures by ultrasound. Arch. Phys. Med. Rehabil., 49:28–30, 1968.

163. Lehmann, J.F., et al.: Comparative study of the efficiency of short-wave, microwave, and ultrasonic diathermy in heating the hip joint. Arch. Phys. Med. Rehabil., 40:510–512, 1959.

164. Lehmann, J.F., et al.: Ultrasonic effects as demonstrated in live pigs with surgical metal implants. Arch. Phys. Med. Rehabil., 40:483–488, 1959.

165. Liang, M.H., and Jette, A.M.: Measuring functional ability in chronic arthritis: a critical review. Arthritis Rheum., 24:80–86, 1981.

166. Liang, M.H., Cullen, K., and Larson, M.: In search of a more perfect mousetrap (health status or quality of life instrument). J. Rheumatol., 9:775–779, 1982.

167. Licht, S.: Massage, Manipulation and Traction. New Haven, Elizabeth Licht, 1980.

168. Licht, S.: History of electricity. In Therapeutic Electricity and Ultraviolet Radiation. Vol. 4. Edited by S. Licht. Baltimore, Waverly Press, 1969.

169. Lidsbrom, A., and Zachrisson, M.: Physical therapy on low back pain and sciatica. Scand. J. Rehabil. Med., 2:37–43, 1970.

170. Lowman, E.W., and Klinger, J.L.: Aids to Independent Living: Self-Help for the Handicapped. New York, McGraw-Hill, 1969.

171. Machover, S., and Sapecky, A.J.: Effect of isometric exercise on the quadriceps muscle in patients with rheumatoid arthritis. Arch. Phys. Med. Rehabil., 47:737–741, 1966.

172. McKnight, P.T., and Schomburg, F.L.: Air pressure splint effects on hand symptoms of patients with rheumatoid arthritis. Arch. Phys. Med. Rehabil., 63:560–564, 1982.

173. McMaster, W.G., Liddle, S., and Waugh, T.R.: Lab evaluation of various cold therapy modalities. Am. J. Sports Med., 6:291–294, 1978.

174. Magness, J.L., et al.: Isometric shortening of hip muscles using a belt. Arch. Phys. Med. Rehabil., 52:158–162, 1971.

175. Maigne, R.: Orthopedic Medicine. Springfield, IL, Charles C Thomas, 1972.

176. Mainardi, C.L., et al.: Rheumatoid arthritis: failure of daily heat therapy to affect its progression. Arch. Phys. Med. Rehabil., 60:390–393, 1979.

177. Malick, M.H.: Manual on Static Hand Splinting. Vol. 1. Pittsburgh, Harmarville Rehabilitation Center, 1972.

178. Mannheimer, C., and Carlsson, C.: The analgesic effect of transcutaneous electrical nerve stimulation (TNS) in patients with rheumatoid arthritis: a comparative study of different pulse patterns. Pain, 6:329–334, 1979.

179. Marshall, R.N., Myers, D.B., and Palmer, D.G.: Disturbance of gait due to rheumatoid disease. J. Rheumatol., 7:617–623, 1980.

180. May, E.E., Waggoner, N.R., and Hotte, E.B.: Independent Living for the Handicapped and the Elderly. Boston, Houghton Mifflin, 1974.

181. Medical Letter Staff: Traction for neck and low back disorders. Med. Lett. Drug Ther., 17:16, 1975.

182. Meenan, R.F.: The impact of chronic disease: a sociomedical profile of rheumatoid arthritis. Arthritis Rheum., 24:544–549, 1981.

183. Meenan, R.F.: The AIMS approach to health status measurement. Conceptual background and measurement properties. J. Rheumatol., 9:785–788, 1980.

184. Meenan, R.F., Liang, M.H., and Hadler, N.M.: Social

security disability and the arthritis patient. Bull. Rheum. Dis., 33:1–7, 1983.

185. Meenan, R.F., et al.: The Arthritis Impact Measurement Scales: further investigations of health status measure. Arthritis Rheum., 25:1048–1053, 1982.

186. Meenan, R.F., et al.: The costs of rheumatoid arthritis: a patient oriented study of chronic disease costs. Arthritis Rheum., 21:827–833, 1978.

187. Melvin, J.L.: Rheumatic Disease: Occupational Therapy and Rehabilitation. 2nd Ed. Philadelphia, F.A. Davis, 1982.

188. Melzack, R.: Prolonged relief of pain by brief, intense transcutaneous somatic stimulation. Pain, 1:357–373, 1975.

189. Melzack, R., and Perry, C.: Self regulation of pain. Exp. Neurol., 46:452–469, 1975.

190. Melzack, R., and Wall, P.D.: Pain mechanisms: a new theory. Science, 150:971–979, 1965.

191. Melzack, R., Stillwell, D.M., and Fox, E.J.: Trigger points and acupuncture points for pains: correlations and implications. Pain, 3:3–23, 1977.

192. Mennell, J.J.: Back Pain: Diagnosis and Treatment Using Manipulative Techniques. Boston, Little, Brown, 1960.

193. Merritt, J.L., and Hunder, G.G.: Passive range of motion, not isometric exercise, amplifies acute urate synovitis. Arch. Phys. Med. Rehabil., 64:130–131, 1983.

194. Michels, E.: Measurement in physical therapy. Phys. Ther., 63:209–215, 1983.

195. Middaugh, S.J., et al.: Electromyographic feedback: effects on voluntary muscle contraction in normal subjects. Arch. Phys. Med. Rehabil., 63:254–259, 1982.

196. Miglietta, O.: Electromyographic characteristics of clonus and the influence of cold. Arch. Phys. Med. Rehabil., 45:508–512, 1964.

197. Mikulic, M.A., Griffith, E.R., and Jebsen, R.H.: Clinical applications of standardized mobility tests. Arch. Phys. Med. Rehabil., 57:143–146, 1976.

198. Müller, E.A.: Influence of training and of inactivity on muscle strength. Arch. Phys. Med. Rehabil., 51:449–462, 1970.

199. Miller, N.E., and Banuagizi, A.: Instrumental learning by curarized rats of specific visceral response, intestinal or cardiac. J. Comp. Physiol. Psychol., 65:1–7, 1968.

200. Miller, R.G., and Burton, R.: Stroke following chiropractic manipulation of the spine. JAMA, 229:189–190, 1974.

201. Million, R., et al.: Evaluation of low back pain and assessment of lumbar corsets with and without back supports. Ann. Rheum. Dis., 40:449–454, 1981.

202. Mills, J.A., et al.: Value of bed rest in patients with rheumatoid arthritis. N. Engl. J. Med., 284:453–458, 1971.

203. Moldofsky, H., and Scarisbrick, P.: Induction of neurasthenic musculoskeletal pain syndrome by selective sleep stage deprivation. Psychosom. Med., 38:35–44, 1976.

204. Monell, S.H.: The Treatment of Disease by Electric Currents. 2nd Ed. New York, E.R. Pelton, 1900.

205. Mooney, N.E.: Coping with chronic pain in rheumatoid arthritis: patient behaviors and nursing interventions. Rehabil. Nurs., 8:20–25, 1983.

206. Mundale, M.O.: The relationship of intermittent isometric exercise to fatigue of hand grip. Arch. Phys. Med., 51:532–539, 1970.

207. Munsat, T.L., McNeal, D., and Walters, R.: Effects of nerve stimulation on human muscle. Arch. Neurol., 33:608–617, 1976.

208. Munton, J.S., et al.: An investigation into the problems of easy chairs used by the arthritic and the elderly. Rheumatol. Rehabil., 20:164–173, 1981.

209. Nemeth, P.M.: Electrical stimulation of denervated muscle prevents decreases in oxidative enzymes. Muscle Neurol., 5:134–139, 1982.

210. Nicholas, J.H., et al.: Splinting in rheumatoid arthritis: I. Factors affecting patient compliance. Arch. Phys. Med. Rehabil., 63:92–94, 1982.

211. Nichols, P.J.R.: Rehabilitation Medicine: The Management of Physical Disabilities. 2nd Ed. Butterworth, London, 1981.

212. Nichols, P.J.R., Ennis, J.A., and Norman, P.A.: Wheelchair users shoulder? Scand. J. Med. Rehabil., *11*:29–34, 1979.
213. Nordemar, R.: Physical training in rheumatoid arthritis: a controlled long-term study. II. Functional capacity and general attitudes. Scand. J. Rheumatol., *10*:25–30, 1981.
214. Nordemar, R., Edstrom, L., and Ekblom, B.: Changes in muscle fiber size and physical performance in patients with rheumatoid arthritis after short term physical training. Scand. J. Rheumatol., *5*:70–76, 1976.
215. Nordemar, R., et al.: Physical training in rheumatoid arthritis: a controlled long-term study. I. Scand. J. Rheumatol., *10*:17–23, 1981.
216. Nordschow, C.D.: Aspects of aging in human collagen: an exploratory thermoelastic study. Exp. Mol. Pathol., *5*:350–373, 1966.
217. Norton, P.L., and Brown, T.: The immobilizing efficiency of back braces. J. Bone. Joint. Surg., *39A*:111–139, 1957.
218. Nuki, G., Brooks, R., and Buchanan, W.W.: The economics of arthritis. Bull. Rheum. Dis., *23*:726–733, 1972–1973.
219. O'Driscoll, S.L., and Jayson, M.I.V.: The clinical significance of pain threshold measurements. Rheumatol. Rehabil., *21*:31–35, 1982.
220. Pace, J.B., and Nagle, D.: Piriform syndrome. West. J. Med., *124*:435–439, 1976.
221. Pachter, B.R., Eberstein, A., and Goodgold, J.: Electrical stimulation effect on denervation skeletal myofibers in rats: a light and electron microscopic study. Arch. Phys. Med. Rehabil., *63*:427–430, 1982.
222. Partridge, R.E.H., and Duthie, J.J.R.: Controlled trial of the effects of complete immobilization of the joint in rheumatoid arthritis. Ann. Rheum. Dis., *22*:91–99, 1963.
223. Pegg, S.M.H., Litter, T.R., and Littler, E.N.: A trial of ice therapy and exercise in chronic arthritis. Physiotherapy, *55*:51–56, 1969.
224. Perry, J.: The use of external support in the treatment of low-back pain. J. Bone Joint. Surg., *43*:327–351, 1961.
225. Pertovaara, A., and Hamalainen, M.A.: Vibrotactile threshold elevation produced by high-frequency transcutaneous electrical nerve stimulation. Arch. Phys. Med. Rehabil., *63*:597–600, 1982.
226. Prentice, W.E.: An electromyographic analysis of the effectiveness of heat or cold and stretching for inducing relaxation in injured muscle. J. Orthop. Sports Phys. Ther., *3*:133–140, 1982.
227. Preston, R.A.: The Surgical Management of Rheumatoid Arthritis. Philadelphia, W.B. Saunders, 1968.
228. Puri, K., and Honet, J.C.: Cervical radiculitis: methods and results of treatment in 82 patients. (Abstract.) Arch. Phys. Med. Rehabil., *55*:585, 1974.
229. Puttemans, F.J.M., et al.: Iontophoresis: mechanism of action studied by potentiometry and x-ray fluorescence. Arch. Phys. Med. Rehabil., *63*:176–179, 1982.
230. Radin, E.L., and Paul, I.L.: Joint function. Arthritis Rheum., *13*:276–279, 1970.
231. Ralston, H.J.: Energy-speed relation and optimal speed during level walking. Int. Z. Agnew Physiol., *17*:177–183, 1958.
232. Raskin, R.J., and Lawless, O.J.: Articular and soft tissue abnormalities in a "normal" population. J. Rheumatol., *9*:284–288, 1982.
233. Ray, C.D.: Electrical stimulation: new methods for therapy and rehabilitation. Scand. J. Rehabil. Med., *10*:65–74, 1978.
234. Rehabilitative Nursing Techniques—1: Bed Positioning and Transfer Procedures for the Hemiplegic. Minneapolis, Kenny Rehabilitation Institute, 1964.
235. Reuler, J.B., Girard, D.E., and Nardone, D.A.: The chronic pain syndrome: misconceptions and management, Ann. Intern. Med., *93*:588–596, 1980.
236. Rhinelander, F.W.: The effectiveness of splinting and bracing in rheumatoid arthritis. Arthritis Rheum., *2*:270–277, 1959.
237. Rhinelander, F.W., and Ropes, M.W.: Adjustable casts in the treatment of joint deformity. J. Bone Joint. Surg., *27*:311–316, 1945.
238. Rigby, B.J.: Thermal transition in the collagenous tissue of poikilothermic animals. J. Therm. Biol., *2*:80–95, 1977.
239. Risk, T.E., and Pinals, R.S.: Frozen shoulder. Semin. Arthritis Rheum., *11*:440–451, 1982.
240. Robertson, J.T.: Neck manipulation as a cause of stroke. (Editorial.) Stroke, *10*:1, 1981.
241. Robinson, H.S.: Functional and social deficits—consequences of time and disease. *In* Total Management of the Arthritis Patient. Edited by G.E. Ehrlich. Philadelphia, J.B. Lippincott, 1973.
242. Rogers, M.P., Liang, M.H., and Partridge, A.J.: Psychological care of adults with rheumatoid arthritis. Ann. Intern. Med., *96*:344–348, 1982.
243. Rose, S.J., and Rothstein, J.M.: Muscle biology and physical therapy: a historical perspective. Phys. Ther., *62*:1754–1756, 1982.
244. Rose, S.J., and Rothstein, J.M.: Muscle mutability: Part 1. General concepts and adaptation to altered patterns of use. Phys. Ther., *62*:1773–1786, 1982.
245. Rothstein, J.M.: Muscle biology: clinical considerations. Phys. Ther., *62*:1823–1830, 1982.
246. Rothstein, J.M.: Use of splints in conservative management of acutely inflamed joints in rheumatoid arthritis. Arch. Phys. Med. Rehabil., *46*:198–199, 1965.
247. Rudd, E.: International year of disabled persons, 1981. Arthritis Rheum., *24*:108–109, 1981.
248. Sankarankutty, S.M., and Rose, G.K.: A comparison of axillary, elbow and Canadian crutches. Rheumatol. Rehabil., *17*:237–239, 1978.
249. Saunders, J.B., Inman, V.T., and Eberhart, H.D.: The major determinants in normal and pathologic gait. J. Bone Joint Surg., *35A*:543–558, 1953.
250. Schmidt, K.L., et al.: Heat, cold and inflammation. J. Rheumatol., *38*:391–404, 1979.
251. Schwan, H.P., and Piersol, G.M.: The absorption of electromagnetic energy in body tissues: review and critical analysis: physiological and clinical aspects. Am. J. Phys. Med., *34*:425–448, 1955.
252. Scott, B.O.: Shortwave diathermy. *In* Therapeutic Heat and Cold. 2nd Ed. Edited by S. Licht. New Haven, Waverly Press, 1965.
253. Seltzer, G.B., Granger, C.V., and Wineberg, B.A.: Functional assessment: Bridge between family and rehabilitation medicine within an ambulatory practice. Arch. Phys. Med. Rehabil., *63*:453–457, 1982.
254. Seribonius Largus: De compisitione medicamentorum liber (translated by P. Kallaway.): the part played by electric fish in early history of bioelectricity and electrotherapy. Bull. Hist. Med., *20*:112–137, 1946.
255. Sharrard, W.J.W., et al.: The treatment of fibrous nonunion of fractures by pulsing electromagnetic stimulation. J. Bone Joint Surg., *64B*:189–193, 1982.
256. Shelkh, K., Meade, T.W., and Mattingly, S.: Unemployment and the disabled. Rheum. Rehabil., *19*:233–238, 1980.
257. Shore, N.A.: Iatrogenic temporomandibular joint difficulty: cervical traction may be the etiology. J. Prosthet. Dent., *41*:541–542, 1979.
258. Simons, D.G.: Muscle pain syndromes—Part 2. Am. J. Phys. Med., *55*:15–42, 1976.
259. Simons, D.G.: Muscle pain syndromes—Part 1. Am. J. Phys. Med., *54*:289–311, 1975.
260. Simon, L., and Blotman, F.: Exercise therapy and hydrotherapy in the treatment of the rheumatic disease. Clin. Rheum. Dis., *7*:337–347, 1981.
261. Sims-Williams, H., et al.: Controlled trial of mobilization and manipulation for back pain: hospital patients. Br. Med. J., *2*:1318–1320, 1979.
262. Skoubo-Kristensen, E., and Sommer, J.: Ultrasound influence on internal fixation with a rigid plate in dogs. Arch. Phys. Med. Rehabil., *63*:371–373, 1982.
263. Smith, P.H., Sharp, J., and Kellgren, J.A.: Natural history of rheumatoid cervical subluxations. Ann. Rheum. Dis., *31*:222–223, 1972.
264. Smith, R.D.: Bed rest at home for rheumatoid arthritis. Arthritis Rheum., *23*:263–264, 1980.

265. Smith, R.D.: Effect of hemiparesis on rheumatoid arthritis. Arthritis Rheum., 22:1419–1420, 1979.
266. Smith, R.D., and Polley, H.F.: Rest therapy for rheumatoid arthritis. Mayo Clin. Proc., 53:141–145, 1978.
267. Soderberg, G.L.: Muscle mechanics and pathomechanics: their clinical relevance. Phys. Ther., 63:216–220, 1983.
268. Sorenson, L., and Ulrich, P.G.: Ambulation Manual for Nurses. Minneapolis, American Rehabilitation Foundation, 1966.
269. Stein, H., and Dickson, R.A.: Reversed dynamic slings for knee-flexion contractures in the hemophiliac. J. Bone Joint Surg., 57A:282–283, 1975.
270. Steinbrocker, O., Traeger, C.H., and Batterman, R.C.: Therapeutic criteria in rheumatoid arthritis. JAMA, 140:659–662, 1949.
271. Stewart, C.P.U.: A prediction score for geriatric rehabilitation prospects. Rheumatol. Rehabil., 19:239–245, 1980.
272. Stoner, E.K.: Luminous and infrared heating. In Therapeutic Heat. Edited by S. Licht. New Haven, Waverly Press, 1958.
273. Swanson, D.W., et al.: Program for managing chronic pain. Mayo Clin. Proc., 51:401–408, 1976.
274. Swash, M., and Schwartz, M.S.: Neuromuscular Diseases: A Practical Approach to Diagnosis and Management. Berlin, Springer-Verlag, 1981.
275. Swezey, R.L.: Arthritis: Rational Therapy and Rehabilitation. Philadelphia, W.B. Saunders, 1978.
276. Swezey, R.L.: Arthritis rehabilitation: staff, facilities, and evaluation. In Rehabilitation of Rheumatic Conditions. Edited by G.E. Ehrlich. Baltimore, Williams & Wilkins, 1980.
277. Swezey, R.L.: Dynamic factors in deformity of the rheumatoid arthritic hand. Bull. Rheum. Dis., 22:649–656, 1971–1972.
278. Swezey, R.L., and Fiegenberg, D.S.: Inappropriate intrinsic muscle action in the rheumatoid hand. Ann. Rheum. Dis., 30:619–625, 1971.
279. Swezey, R.L.: Essentials of physical management and rehabilitation in arthritis. Semin. Arthritis. Rheum., 3:349–368, 1971.
280. Swezey, R.L.: The modern thrust of manipulation and traction therapy. Semin. Arthritis. Rheum., 12:322–331, 1983.
281. Taylor, D.: A table to indicate the degree of improvement in chronic arthritis. Can. Med. Assoc. J., 36:608–610, 1937.
282. Tipton, C.M., et al.: The influence of physical activity on ligaments and tendons. Med. Sci. Sports, 7:165–175, 1975.
283. Tkaczuk, H.: Study of tensile properties of human lumbar longitudinal ligaments. Acta Orthop. Scand., 115:54–69, 1968.
284. Toohezu, P., and Larson, C.W.: Range of Motion Exercise: Key to Joint Mobility. Rehabilitation Publication No. 703. Minneapolis, Sister Kenney Institute, 1968.
285. Trall, R.T.: The Hydropathic Encyclopedia: A System of Hydrotherapy and Hygiene. New York, Fowlers and Wells, 1853.
286. Travell, J.: Myofascial trigger points: clinical view. In Advances in Pain Research Therapy. Vol. I. Edited by J.J. Bonieg and D. Albe-Fessurd. New York, Raven Press, 1976.
287. Travell, J.: Ladies and gentleman be seated—properly. House Beautiful, July:159, 1961.
288. Travell, J.: Ethyl chloride spray for painful muscle spasm. Arch. Phys. Med. Rehabil., 33:291–298, 1952.
289. Travell, J., and Simons, D.G.: Myofascial Pain and Dysfunction: The Trigger Point Manual. Baltimore, Williams & Wilkins, 1983.

290. Tsuyuguchi, Y., Tada, K., and Kawaii, H.: Splint therapy for trigger finger in children. Arch. Phys. Med. Rehabil., 65:75–76, 1983.
291. Valtown, E.J., and Kiuro, E.: Cervical traction as a therapeutic tool. Scand. J. Rehabil. Med., 2:29–36, 1970.
292. VanBrocklin, J.D., and Ellis, D.G.: A study of the mechanical behavior of toe extensor tendons under applied stress. Arch. Phys. Med. Rehabil., 47:369–373, 1965.
293. Vershys, H.P.: Physical rehabilitation and family dynamics. Rehabil. Lit., 41:58–65, 1980.
294. Vignos, P.J.: Physiotherapy in rheumatoid arthritis. J. Rheumatol, 7:269–271, 1980.
295. Vignos, P.J., Jr., et al.: Comprehensive care and psychosocial factors in rehabilitation in chronic rheumatoid arthritis: a controlled study. J. Chronic Dis., 4:457–467, 1972.
296. Vineberg, S.E.: Psychologists in rehabilitation—manpower and training. In Rehabilitation Psychology. Edited by W.S. Neff. Washington, D.C., American Psychiatric Association, 1971.
297. Warren, C.G., et al.: Reducing back displacement in the powered reclining wheelchair. Arch. Phys. Med. Rehabil., 63:447–449, 1982.
298. Waylonis, G.W., et al.: Home cervical traction: evaluation of alternative equipment. Arch. Phys. Med. Rehabil., 63:388–391, 1982.
299. Waylonis, G.W., et al.: Home cervical traction: evaluation using rat tail tendon. Arch. Phys. Med. Rehabil., 57:122–126, 1976.
300. Weidenbacker, R.A., and Smith, C.: Does heat cause relaxation? Phys. Ther. Rev., 40:261–265, 1960.
301. Wild, D., Nayak, U.S.L., and Isaacs, B.: Description, classification and prevention of falls in old people at home. Rheum. Rehabil., 20:153–159, 1981.
302. Williams, M.E., and Hadler, N.M.: Musculoskeletal components of decrepitude. Semin. Arthritis Rheum., 11:284–287, 1981.
303. Wolf, S.L. (Ed.): Electrotherapy: Clinics in Physical Therapy. New York, Churchill Livingstone, 1981.
304. Wong, K.C.: Physiology and pharmacology of hypothermia. West. J. Med., 138:227–232, 1983.
305. Woo, S.L., Mathews, J.V., and Akisen, W.H.: Connective tissue response to immobility. Correlative study of biomechanical and biochemical measurements of normal and immobilized rabbit knees. Arthritis Rheum., 18:257–264, 1975.
306. Worden, R.E., and Humphrey, T.L.: Effect of spinal traction on the length of the body. Arch. Phys. Med. Rehabil., 45:318–320, 1964.
307. Wright, D.G., and Rennels, D.G.: A study of the elastic properties of plantar fascia. J. Bone Joint Surg., 46A:482–492, 1964.
308. Wright, V., and Johns, R.J.: Physical factors concerned with the stiffness of normal and diseased joints. Bull. Johns Hopkins Hosp., 106:215–231, 1960.
309. Wright, V., and Owen, S.: The effect of rheumatoid arthritis on the social situation of housewives. Rheum. Rehabil., 15:156–160, 1976.
310. Yelin, E., Meenan, R., Nevitt, M., and Epstein, W.: Work disability in rheumatoid arthritis: Effects of disease, social, and work factors. Ann. Intern. Med., 93:551–556, 1980.
311. Yoshimo, S., and Uchida, S.: Sexual problems of women with rheumatoid arthritis. Arch. Phys. Med. Rehabil., 62:122–123, 1981.
312. Zislis, J.M.: Hydrotherapy. In Handbook of Physical Medicine. Edited by F.H. Krusen, F.K. Kottke, and P.M. Ellwood. 2nd Ed. Philadelphia, W.B. Saunders, 1971.
313. Zola, I.K.: Socia and cultural disincentives to independent living. Arch. Phys. Med. Rehabil., 63:394–397, 1982.

Chapter 45

Correction of Arthritic Deformities of the Hand

Adrian E. Flatt

Surgical procedures are now firmly established as an important part of the rehabilitation of the arthritic patient. The hand surgeon's role in the care of arthritic deformities of the wrist and hand involves membership in a treatment team that should integrate the total care of the patient[9] (see Chaps. 43 and 44).

Because most forms of arthritis are progressive, retention of function at a satisfactory level is the goal of therapy. The progress and severity of disease vary among individual patients, and the hand surgeon must define in each patient the type of deformity and the rate of its progression, to plan maintenance of a functional hand by suitable therapeutic means. *Prevention of deformity* is the key. The earlier the patient is seen in the disease process, the easier it is to assess the rate of functional deterioration.

Surgical treatment includes the use of various forms of dynamic splinting, hand therapy, and strategically timed operative intervention. Restoration of function in a severely debilitated hand is usually more difficult and is less successful than a preventive surgical procedure early in the disease. Appearance is by far a secondary consideration because a cosmetically acceptable hand is not necessarily functional.

Arthritic hand deformity follows a spectrum of disease, with rheumatoid arthritis (RA) at one end and osteoarthritis at the other. In between are a variety of conditions such as gout, psoriatic arthritis, scleroderma, mixed connective tissue disease, and hemachromatosis. Each has its own pattern of involvement. In this chapter, I concentrate on the two main entities, RA and osteoarthritis, with only a brief discussion of the others.

RHEUMATOID DISEASE

Within the hand and wrist, the tissue primarily affected is synovium.[6] Only later are articular cartilage and subchondral bone destroyed by pannus. The intra-articular swelling of the synovium stretches and weakens the joint capsule and ligaments. This interference with joint integrity allows an imbalance of forces to occur over the joint and can eventually produce grotesque deformities.

In the past, it was said that a surgical procedure must be delayed until the disease is "burned out." This statement is not true. Although it would clearly be foolish to operate during a generalized acute "flare" of disease, active local disease or a raised sedimentation rate is not a contraindication to surgical treatment.[11] Synovectomy of an acutely inflamed joint often leads to a marked postoperative improvement in the general state of the patient. In the upper limb, almost all operations can be performed under axillary block anesthesia. It is routine for these patients to be ambulatory the day after the operation.

Operations on the wrist or hand are performed with a pneumatic tourniquet applied to the arm. The combination of local axillary anesthetic block and tourniquet control of bleeding produces no significant shock. Glucocorticoid therapy is not a contraindication to surgical treatment and does not produce any adverse general effects on the patients or delay local wound healing. Preoperatively, corticosteroids are reduced to the minimum maintenance dose. Once this dose has been established, I make no effort to increase it as a precaution against the slight operative and postoperative stress in operations on the upper limb. I do not believe that this view applies to the more massive lower-limb operations. The usual dosage is continued throughout the operative and postoperative periods. In a personal series of many hundreds of upper-limb operations, I have followed this routine with excellent results.

In three distinct phases of the disease, operative treatment can be of value to the wrist and hand. It is used: (1) prophylactically, to prevent further destruction of joint surfaces when drug therapy is unable to control synovitis; (2) late in the disease, to salvage function from grossly involved tendons and joints; and (3) in the stage of adaptation (middle phase) of disease, in which it can be of value, but is not as common as in the other two phases.

Operations can restore potential range of motion and can relieve pain, but it is fruitless to operate in the face of apathy, self-pity, or the general aura of despair so frequently associated with rheumatoid disease. Surgeons share a common responsibility with physicians in other disciplines to treat the disease, and the patient, as a whole.

The patient himself must request the operation. To try to "sell" a patient an operation is a disservice, and it is my policy to try to introduce potential candidates to others who have had the proposed operation. A short, private discussion between the two patients usually answers all potential questions rapidly and allows a decision to be made without external pressures.

Nonoperative Treatments

The classic treatments of rest, splinting, judicious exercise, and corticosteroid injections are of value throughout the course of the disease, and their use should not be restricted to early management.[14] Inflamed, painful, swollen joints benefit from rest, but as the inflammation subsides, exercise must be introduced to prevent joint stiffness and to maintain muscle strength. Short, intermittent periods of exercise are far more beneficial than prolonged vigorous workouts that can aggravate synovitis. Local injection of corticosteroids can diminish synovial reaction in both joints and around tendons; however, persistent use of long-acting corticosteroids in the same areas leads to local tissue reactions that can cause arthropathies and tendon ruptures. I believe that this form of treatment can become counterproductive, and I agree with others that three injections in one year at the same site should be the absolute maximum.[14]

Splinting is of limited value in the care of rheumatoid disease of the hands. Three major types of splints are available: passive immobilization, remedial, and assistive splints.[7] Passive immobilization splints provide rest during the acute phase of disease, remedial splints can help to overcome contractures, and assistive splints help to compensate for joint distortions and muscle weakness.

Effective splinting of the hand is an art. Much harm can be done by ill-designed or ill-fitting splints. Stiffness of the hand is inevitable if an ill-designed splint forces the fingers into a nonfunctional position, or if they are held for long periods in positions that strain the joint capsules. There is virtue in simplicity. Many ingeniously designed complex apparatus lie neglected in closets because the demands on the patient's tolerance were too great.

Wrist

The wrist is a key joint in so many functions of the hand that its impairment influences function to a far greater degree than by merely limiting motion of the joint itself. Three joints combine to produce wrist motion: the distal radioulnar joint, the intercarpal area, and the radiocarpal joint. Rheumatoid disease frequently attacks the distal radioulnar joint, and because the joint shares a common synovial cavity with the radiocarpal joint, both are frequently involved in synovitis.

Splinting

During an acute phase of arthritis, continuous passive immobilization may be necessary. As soon as symptoms begin to subside, intermittent, properly controlled muscle-building exercises are added. Many materials are now available for making splints, none completely superior to any other. A gutter-type flexor-surface splint should be made with the wrist in a maximum of 20° of extension, with the fingers in their normal functional arches and the palm and thumb abducted at least 20°.[7] Pressure is usually more evenly distributed throughout the forearm when the splint is held in place by a bandage wrap instead of by individual straps.

Remedial splinting is infinitely more satisfactory than manipulation of contractures within the hand. The gradual pull of dynamic traction creates a gentle, persistent force to which contracted tissue yields; manipulation frequently tears tissues and causes bleeding and adhesion formation. The disorders that respond best to remedial splinting are adduction contractures of the thumb, flexion contractures of the digital joints, and stiffness of the interphalangeal joints.

Assistive and prophylactic splinting techniques are still occasionally used in the treatment of varying degrees of ulnar drift. Most patients cannot tolerate the indefinite use of these splints, and in most, hand surgeons prefer to correct the internal dynamic imbalance surgically rather than impose an external corrective framework on the hand. Dynamic splinting is of great value after such reconstructive operations, particularly when it is combined with the replacement of destroyed metacarpophalangeal joints.

Surgical Treatment

As the synovial disease progresses, it destroys the ligaments supporting the radioulnar articulation and allows dorsal dislocation of the ulna in relation to the distal end of the radius. This dislocation not only restricts pronation and supination, but also creates a hazard for the long extrinsic extensor tendons. These tendons become tightly stretched against the radial side of the distal end of the ulna. Whenever the fingers are moved, the tendons rub against the irregular surface of the bone, and attrition ruptures may occur.

Excision of the spurs on the distal end of the ulna removes an actual or potential hazard to the tendons. Excision of the distal ulna itself also increases the range of pronation and supination. *Care must be taken in advising this operation.* It is best performed when no signs of disease or instability of the radiocarpal joint are present. If extensive destruction of the joint has occurred, the distal end of the ulna may be a useful prop in stabilizing the wrist; its excision may so tip the balance that the wrist may be completely dislocated. The excision of bone must be conservative and should maintain the capsular attachments and the ulnar collateral ligament of the wrist joint. Silastic replacements for excision of the distal ulna are available, but they must be used selectively. If the supporting soft tissue structures in the area are not properly reconstituted, instability and dislocation will occur.

After the operation, therapy is directed more toward restoration of pronation and supination than to restoration of wrist motion in flexion and extension. Some discomfort can be expected at the elbow as increasing movement develops around the head of the radius, but it should not be allowed to stop treatment.

In early disease of the radiocarpal joint, the radioscaphoid-lunate ligament, or Testut's ligament, serves as a conduit for synovial invasion of the radius. Gradual dissolution of the carpal insertion of the ligament leads to the classic Terry Thomas sign* of scapholunate dissociation (Fig. 45–1).

Subsequent laxity of the intercarpal joints or the radiocarpal joint from synovial disease can often be stabilized, and pain can be diminished, by the use of a molded leather wristlet held in place by lacing or by Velcro strapping. Cock-up splints made of plastic, metal, or plaster are also useful in immobilizing the wrist and in restoring some degree of function.

Tenosynovitis and Tenosynovectomy

Tenosynovitis on both palmar and dorsal surfaces of the wrist is common and, if neglected, can lead to tendon rupture. Early synovitis may be treated by splinting of the wrist, injection of corticosteroids, and general medical management. Tenosynovectomy is the proper treatment for patients who do not respond rapidly to conservative measures. The operation is effective, has a low morbidity rate, and requires only about 72 hours of hospitalization. Synovectomy of the flexor compartment effectively decompresses the median nerve and allows a surgical toilet of any spurs on

the carpal bones on the floor of the canal. Rupture of the flexor pollicis longus and of the flexors of the index finger is caused by spurs arising on the palmar aspect of the scaphoid bone.[15]

Extensor tendons rupture following infiltrative and nodular disease or as a result of attrition rupture on bony spurs at Lister's tubercle or the distal ulna. Commonly, the fifth digit loses extensor function first, followed by the fourth and then the third digit (Fig. 45–2). The extensor pollicis longus tendon also frequently ruptures. Eventually, even wrist extensor tendons can rupture and may produce a marked flexion deformity of the wrist.

Persistent dorsal synovitis or a single tendon rupture associated with synovitis should be considered an absolute indication for tenosynovectomy. During surgical exploration, any bony spurs are removed, and any intratendinous nodules are excised. Such excision may leave a ragged-looking tendon, but follow-up has shown that the area repairs well and tendon function is maintained. When one or two tendon ruptures have occurred, side-to-side junction or the transfer of the extensor indicis tendon is the usual treatment. Multiple ruptures need more complicated repairs, often involving the transfer of a flexor digitorum superficialis tendon through the interosseous membrane onto the dorsum of the hand. Some have criticized such tendon repairs by implying that the ability to make a fist after such an operation is restricted. If the procedure is properly done, however, the results are excellent (Fig. 45–2).

Early movement is the treatment of choice after synovectomy of flexor or extensor tendons. The patient should be encouraged to begin moving the wrist and fingers 24 hours after the operation, and a full range should be possible when the sutures are removed 12 to 14 days later.

Synovectomy of the true wrist joint is usually performed at the same time as tenosynovectomy of the extensor tendons. The operation usually increases the stability and motion of the joint and secondarily increases digital function by relieving wrist pain. Technically, it is difficult to effect complete clearance of the wrist joint synovium from the dorsal approach, and occasionally, the floor of the carpal tunnel has to be opened as well. I have not been impressed by the results of my attempts, or those of others, to perform intercarpal synovectomies. Theoretically, it is an admirable procedure; in practice, it is both destructive and unproductive.

Arthroplasty and Fusion

Painful or unstable wrists can be treated by arthroplasty or fusion. Retention of motion with stability is always desirable and has prompted the

---

*Mr. Terry Thomas, a British comedian with upper central dental diastema. See Clin. Orthop., *129*:321–322, 1977.

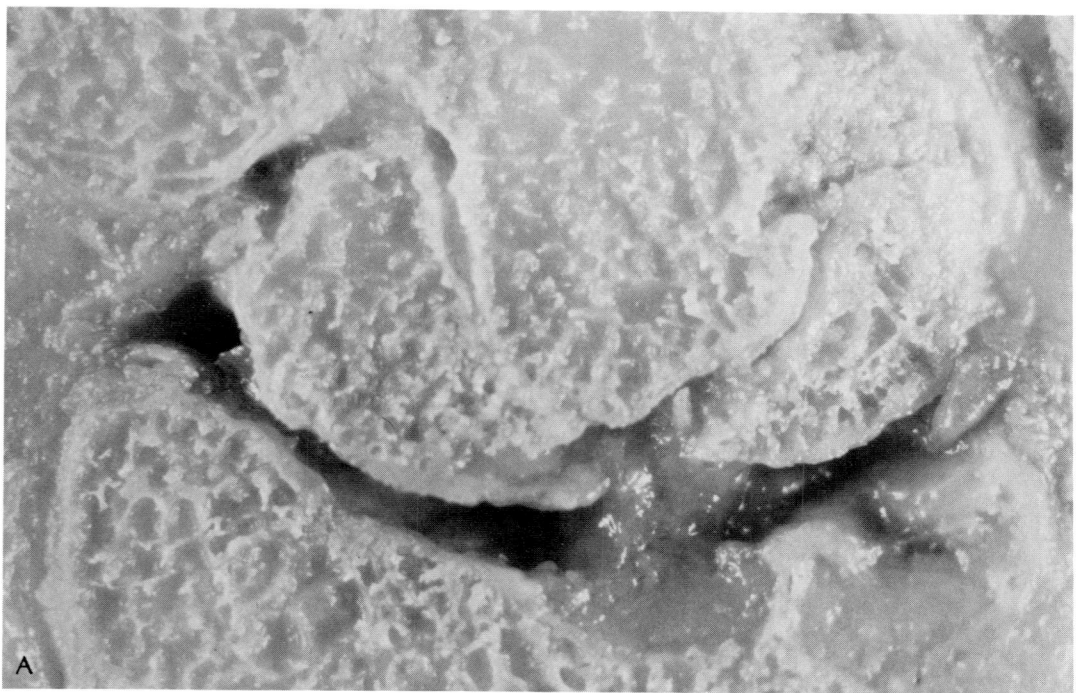

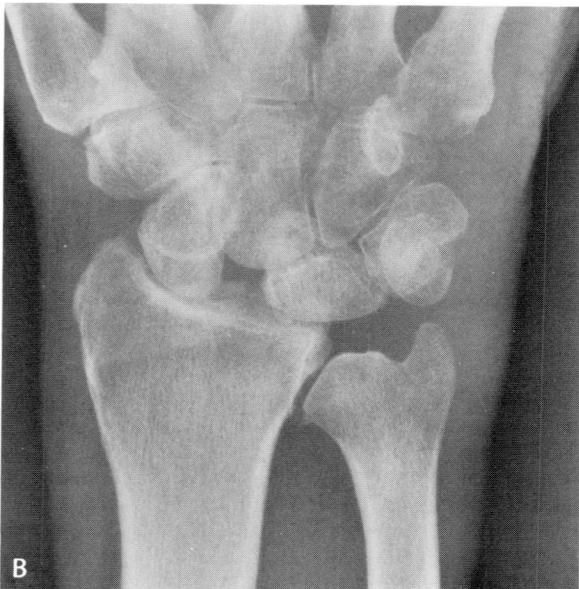

Fig. 45–1. Testut's ligament and the Terry Thomas sign. *A,* Coronal section of a rheumatoid wrist. The radius shows cavitation of its articular surface at the site of origin of Testut's ligament. The scaphoid and lunate bones are separate. *B,* The Terry Thomas sign of scapholunate dissociation. Because the lunate bone is dorsiflexed, it is superimposed on the capitate bone. (From Flatt, A.E.[7])

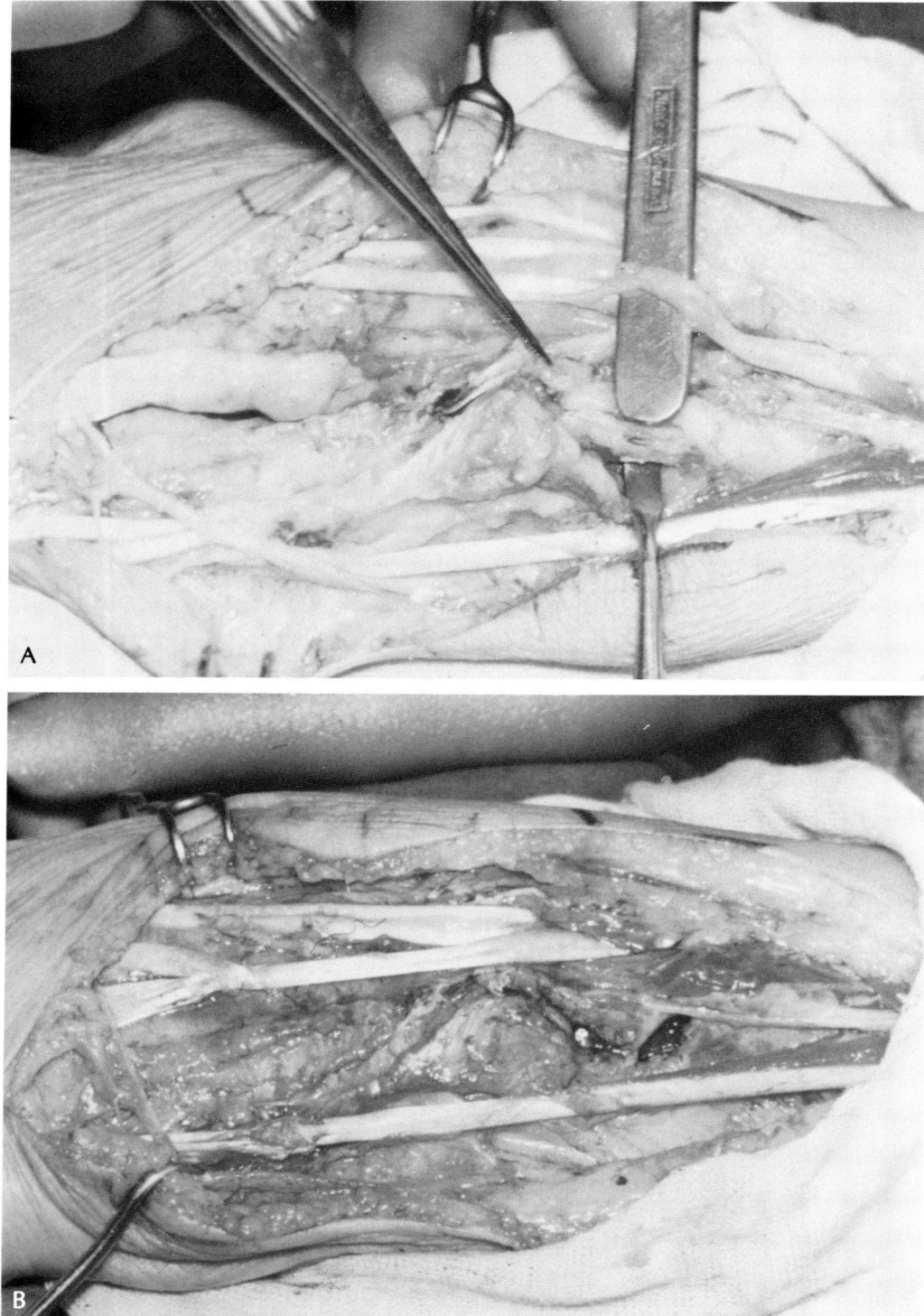

Fig. 45–2. Multiple tendon rupture. *A,* State of disease over the dorsum of the wrist. The proximal end of the extensor tendon to the ring finger lies on the scalpel blade, and the forceps hold the diseased synovium over the distal end of the ulna. *B,* In the repair, the extensor carpi ulnaris is used as an independent extensor for the small finger, and the intact long finger tendon is used to form a Y junction with the distal end of the ring finger tendon.

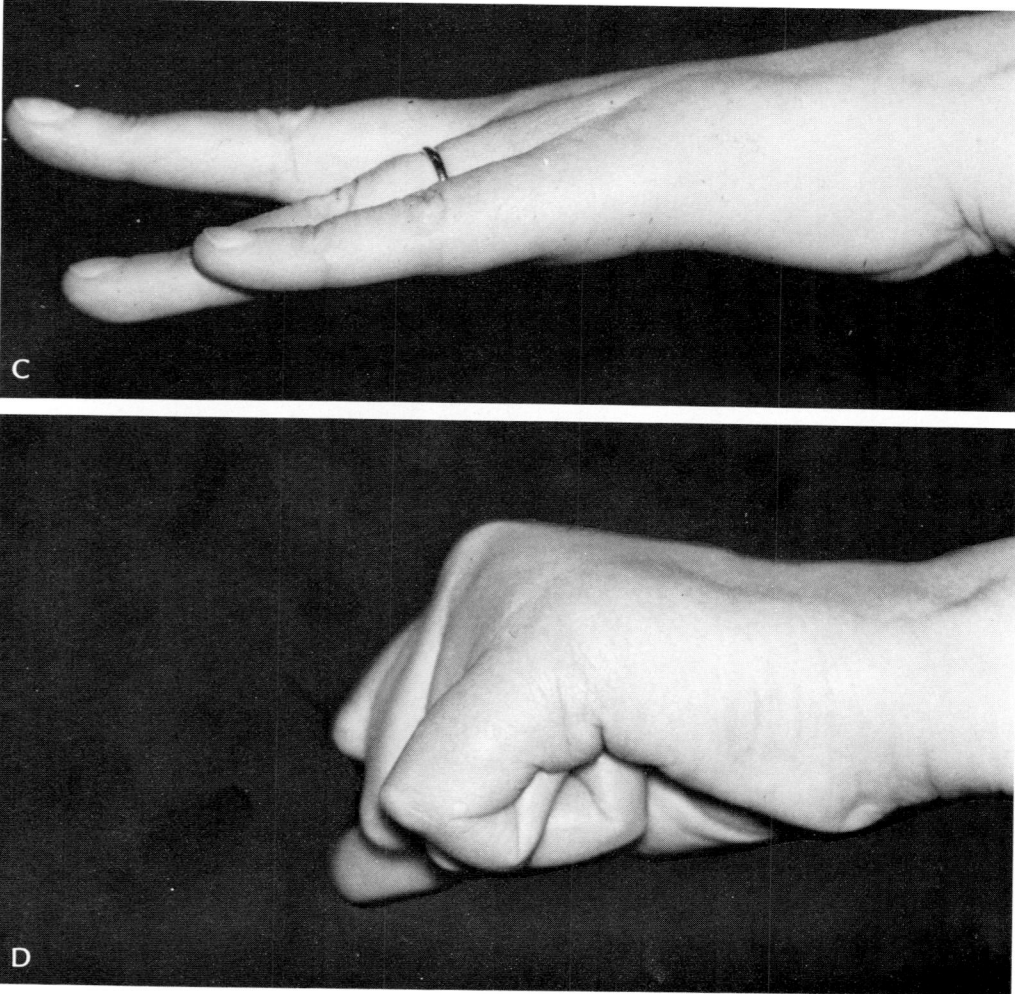

Fig. 45–2. *(Cont'd)* *C* and *D*, Two months postoperatively, a slight extensor lag exists, but the patient is able to make a good fist. (From Flatt, A.E.[7])

production of a variety of total wrist prostheses. The early results seemed encouraging, but reported problems of balancing tendon power are significant. If the device has too much mobility, the hand will assume an ''end'' position, usually dorsoradial or palmoulnar (Fig. 45–3). Currently, the results of total wrist replacement are not predictable, and no device is as generally suitable as, say, the total hip. A Silastic spacer is available, but it is not a true joint substitute. No matter what device is used, most of the proximal carpal row is removed together with the end of the radius. Follow-up studies show that an acceptable range of motion can be obtained with a Silastic spacer, despite an apparently unsatisfactory roentgenographic appearance (Fig. 45–4)

Fusion of the wrist still has its place in the treatment of rheumatoid and degenerative disease when the patient's pain is crippling, when the wrist has stiffened in a nonfunctional position, or when the joint is completely unstable. The position of fusion is of vital importance in the planes of ulnoradial deviation and in flexion and extension. Radial inclination of metacarpal bones induces ulnar deviation of the fingers.[16] To perpetuate this zigzag deformity by fusing the wrist in radial deviation dooms any metacarpophalangeal reconstruction for ulnar drift to failure (Fig. 45–5). The third metacarpal bone must be parallel to the long line of the radius if this deformity is to be avoided.[17]

In flexion and extension, the so-called ''functional'' position usually recommended is about 30° of extension. This position is that of the wrist in an otherwise normal limb. The limb of a patient with RA is usually far from normal, however, and the flexion deformity of the wrist occurs in part

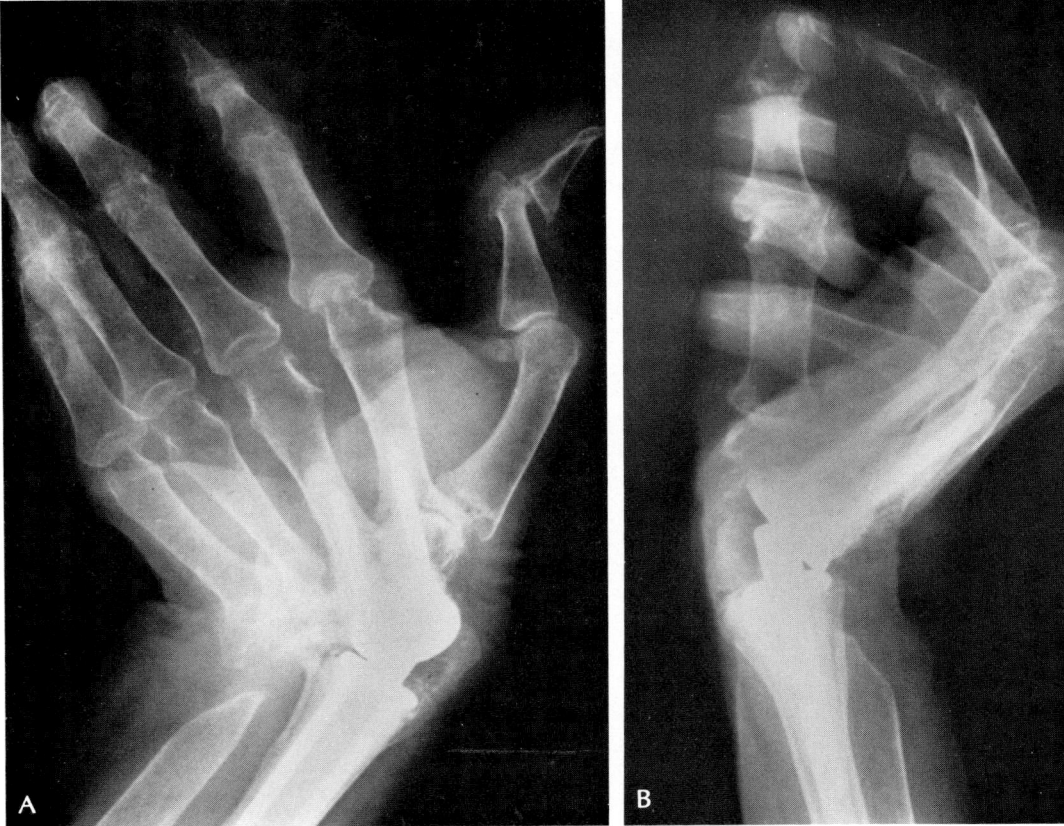

Fig. 45–3. *A* and *B,* Total wrist arthroplasty. Any unconstrained total wrist substitute must have its axes correctly placed to obtain a proper balance among the 22 extrinsic tendons crossing the wrist. This patient's wrist is locked into an end position. (From Flatt, A.E.[7])

because this is the functional position for many of the most vital uses of the hand. During feeding or dressing, the wrists are almost always flexed, and perineal toilet is impossible with the wrists held in the so-called functional position.

The wrist should be fused in a neutral position and, on some occasions, in slight flexion (Fig. 45–6). The patient is usually in a below-elbow cast for about three months, but during this time, finger movement exercises should be practiced constantly. Once the fusion is solid, exercises are done to improve pronation and supination and the strength of grip. The fusion stabilizes the carpus on the radius and frequently adds power to the grip by allowing the extrinsic flexor and extensor tendons to act solely on the fingers, instead of wasting their power on an unstable wrist.[4]

Digits

Tenosynovitis within the palm and fingers causes pain, swelling, stiffness, and occasional "triggering." Surgical synovectomy yields good results,

but in early disease, injection of corticosteroids into the tendon sheath can be helpful. Synovectomy within the flexor sheath is not difficult and is performed by a palmar approach (Fig. 45–7). Preservation and reconstruction of the pulleys retaining the flexor tendons against the phalanges are vital.

Localized nodular disease of the tendon may produce a "trigger" finger. Because nodules can occur on the flexor tendons from the level of the distal palmar crease to the middle of the proximal phalanx, *it is necessary to palpate the area with three fingers* (Fig. 45–8). To use the customary single finger over the entrance to the digital sheath would miss a nodule triggering in the decussation of the flexor digitorum superficialis tendon. In the thumb, the common level is the flexor crease over the metacarpophalangeal joint. Surgical treatment is frequently indicated, but a preliminary trial injection of a corticosteroid suspension intrasynovially is justified.

The operation is usually performed through a small incision under local anesthesia. The flexor

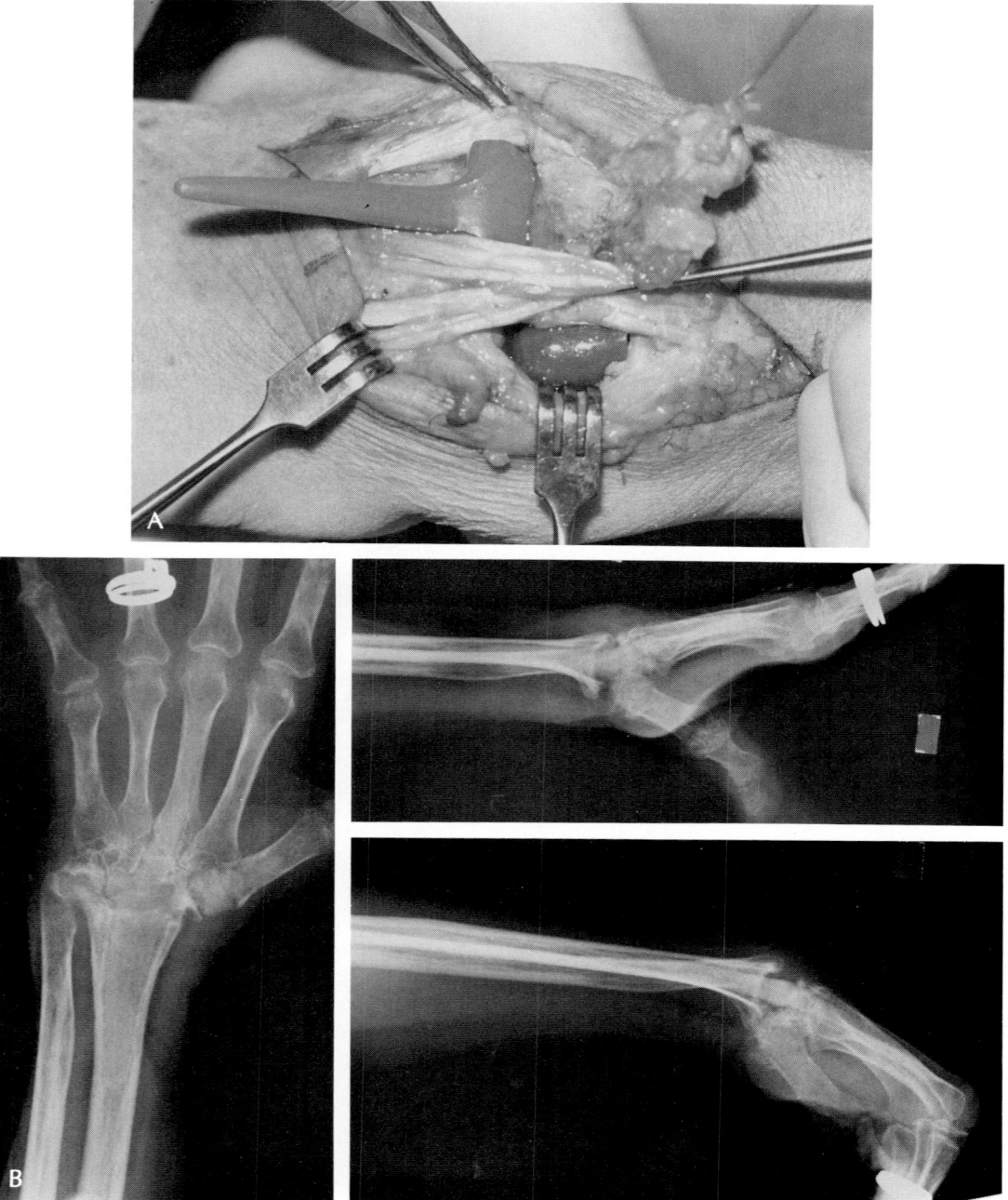

Fig. 45–4. *A*, Wrist implant resection arthroplasty. In this patient, an ulnar head replacement is judged necessary. Note the relative level of the end of the ulna implant and the crossbar of the radial component. *B*, Wrist implant follow-up. These roentgenograms are taken three years after a wrist implant; an ulnar head replacement is not judged necessary. Fifty degrees of painless motion is possible. A trapezial implant has also been used. (From Flatt, A.E.[7])

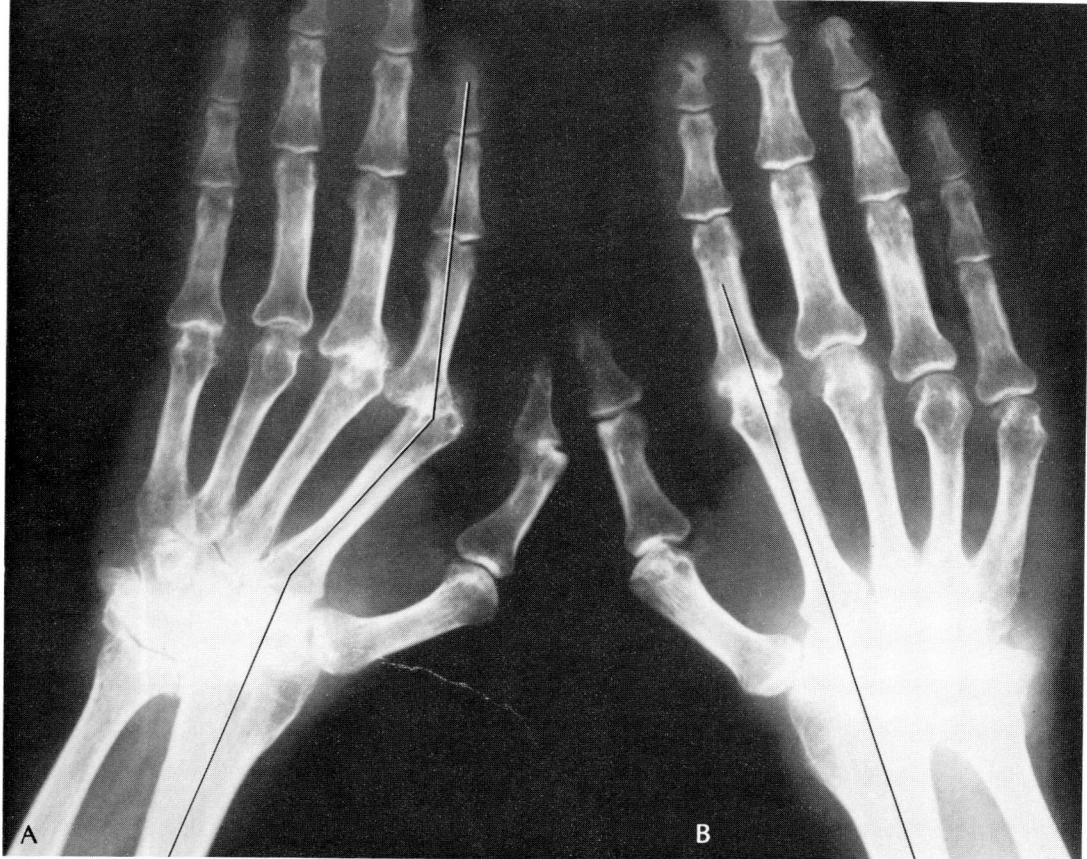

Fig. 45–5. The wrist and ulnar drift. *A,* With radial carpal collapse, the unbalanced tendon forces produce the zigzag deformity of ulnar drift. *B,* If the carpal disease is even, tendon equilibrium is not disturbed, and ulnar shift does not occur. (From Flatt, A.E.[7]).

tendon sheath is incised longitudinally for a sufficient length to allow free travel to the tendons. The patient can use the hand immediately after the operation.

Rheumatoid involvement of the extensor mechanism of the fingers produces two common types of deformity, both secondary to synovial disease. The normal restraints of joint motion and intrinsic muscle balance are destroyed, thereby causing deformity. In *boutonnière (buttonhole) deformity,* the central extensor mechanism over the proximal interphalangeal joint is eroded, and the lateral bands fall to the palmar side of the axis of the joint, with a subsequent loss of ability to extend the joint. *Swan neck deformity* results from the dorsal bowstringing of tight lateral bands, caused either by synovial attrition of the palmar plate or intrinsic muscle tendon contracture.

Intrinsic Muscle Disease

In the early stages of rheumatoid involvement of the intrinsic muscles, the average patient is not likely to notice any functional disturbance. Clinical detection of early disease is easy, however, using the intrinsic tightness test (Fig. 45–9). The test for this condition is conducted in two stages. The first stage applies passive flexion to all three digital joints. If flexion is possible, it establishes that motion is not restricted by pathologic conditions of the extrinsic extensor tendon or the digital joints. In the second stage of the test, the intrinsic muscles are tensed by pushing the metacarpophalangeal joint into full extension and then by applying dorsal pressure to the tip of the finger, in an attempt to produce passive flexion. In the normal hand, passive flexion is still possible in this position. If rheumatoid disease is affecting the intrinsic muscles, the degree of resistance to passive flexion is directly proportional to the severity of the disease.

This test is simple, yields valuable information, and should be routine in the examination of all patients with RA. Demonstration of the differential tightness of the ulnar intrinsic muscles, as opposed

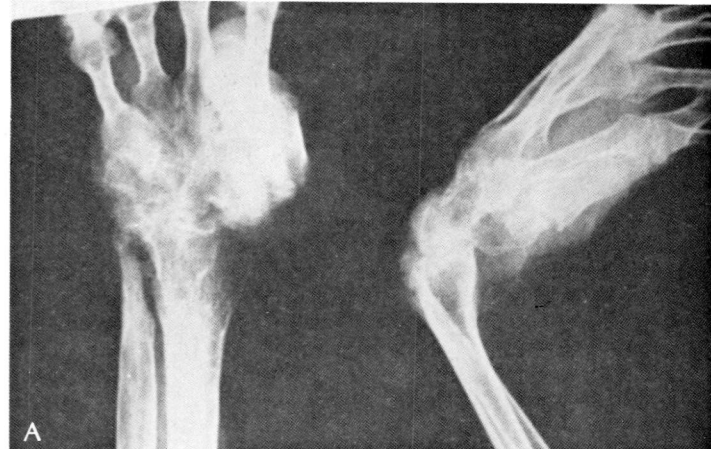

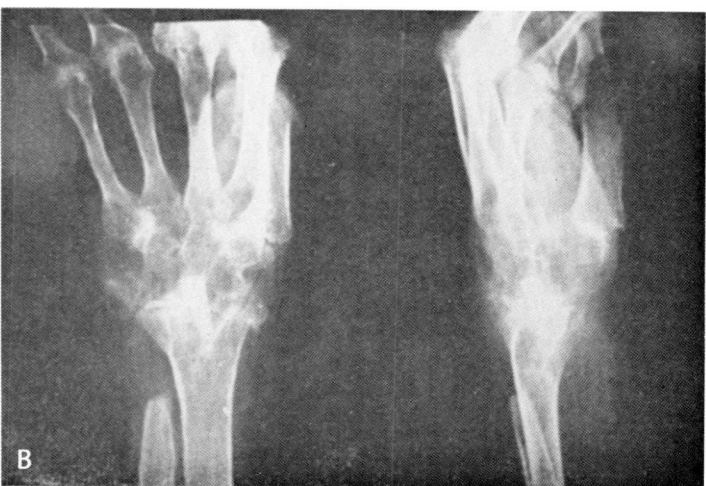

Fig. 45–6. Wrist fusion. Stabilization of the wrist is a valuable procedure, but the angle of fusion should be chosen with great care. It is not advisable to fuse the wrist in dorsiflexion because of the limitation in function imposed by such a position. *A*, Preoperative malposition in palmar flexion. *B*, Postoperative fusion in neutral position allowing improved function of the hand. (From Flatt, A.E.[7])

to the radial intrinsic muscles, can be done by fixing the metacarpophalangeal joint in extension and passively flexing the proximal interphalangeal joint, with the digit first in radial deviation and then in ulnar deviation. Tightness present in radial deviation implicates the ulnar intrinsic muscles, and vice versa.

The excess tension in the intrinsic muscles can be relieved by the *Littler release operation.* The triangular hood is excised from either side of the finger, and the pull of the intrinsic muscles on the central extensor tendon is thereby abolished. After the operation, great care must be taken to prevent the proximal interphalangeal joints from returning to their previous, hyperextended condition. Many weeks of active flexion exercises are usually needed to obtain maximum improvement. The muscles of the thumb are subject to the same disturbance, and the metacarpophalangeal joint is held in flexion, with the interphalangeal joint in hyperextension. A similar operation at the level of its metacarpophalangeal joint improves function.

In early ulnar drift, the intrinsic muscle tightness is released, but is used to correct digital deviation by *crossed intrinsic transfer.* The tighter ulnar intrinsic muscles are transferred to the radial side of the next adjacent ulnar digit (Fig. 45–10). This operation of crossed intrinsic muscle transfer transforms a dynamic deforming factor into a corrective force.

Synovectomy

Synovectomy of the digital joints is a valuable operation. It is designed to relieve symptoms and to delay subsequent destruction of articular surfaces. The operation is performed most frequently at the metacarpophalangeal joints, often at the proximal interphalangeal joints, and only rarely at the distal interphalangeal joints. The operation is properly indicated in the patient whose metacarpophalangeal joints continue to develop recurrent synovitis despite medical treatment and occasional corticosteroid injections. At the proximal interphalangeal joint, the need for synovectomy is more

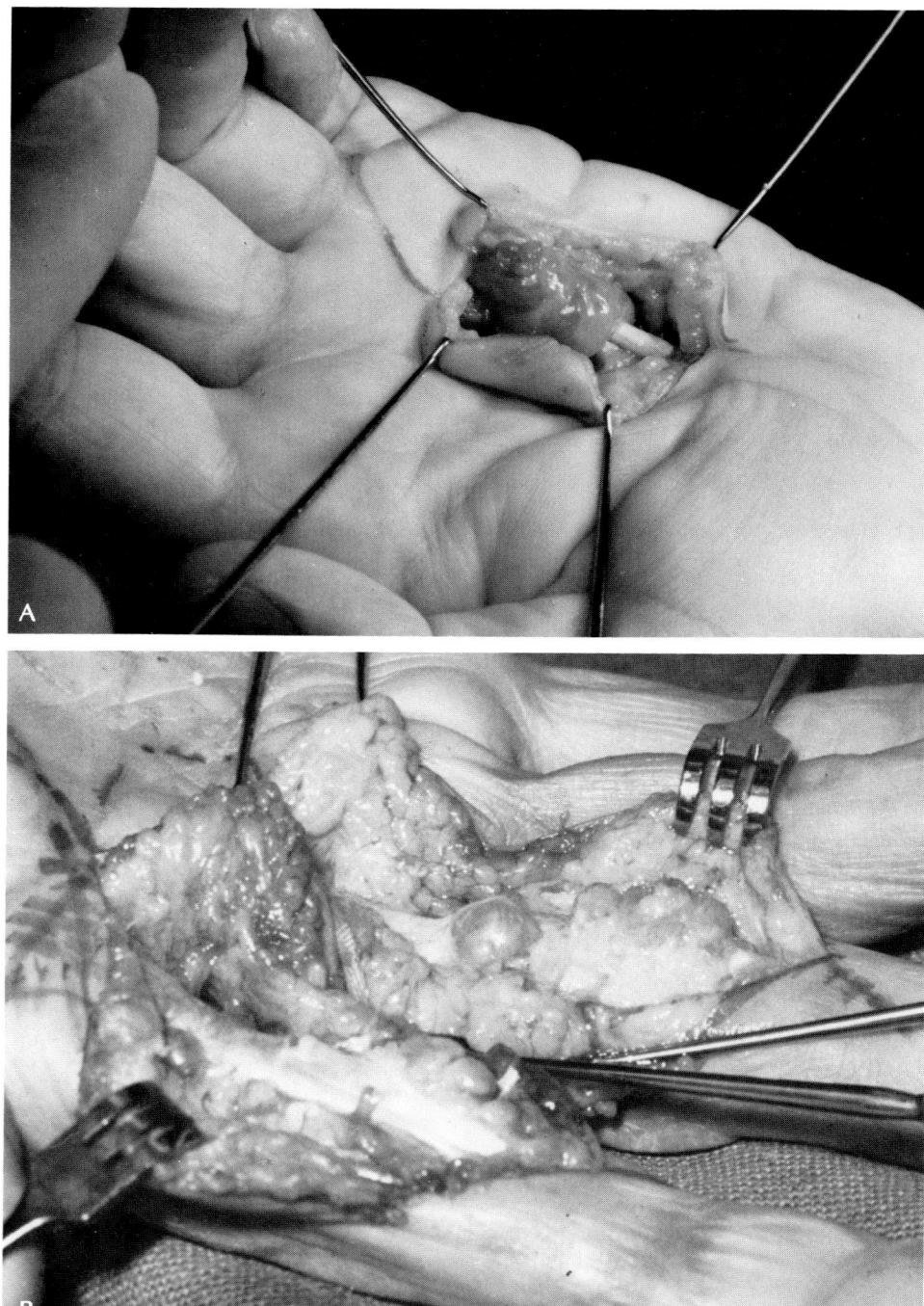

Fig. 45–7. Digital flexor tendon synovectomy. *A*, In the palm, the synovitis often bulges out as a palpable lump. *B*, The finger should be approached through a zigzag Bruner incision, which allows wide exposure. The index finger at the bottom of this illustration has been cleared of synovitis. The long finger shows the bulging synovitis prior to removal. (From Flatt, A.E.[7])

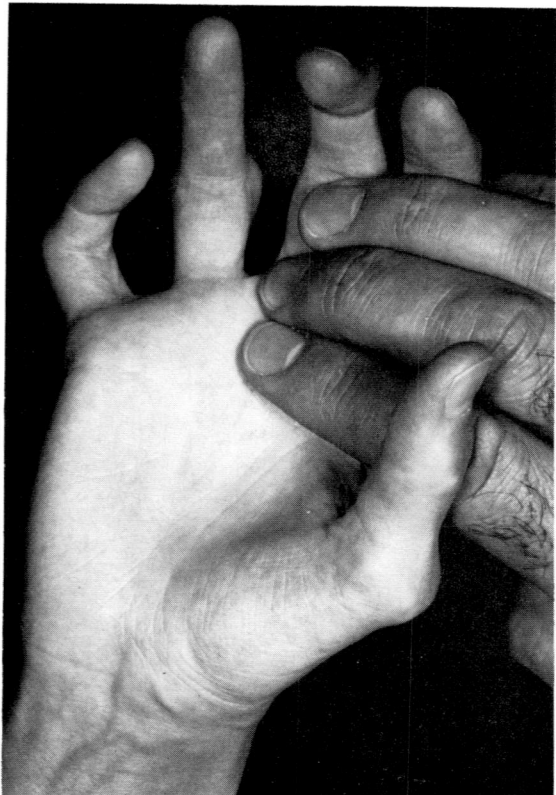

Fig. 45–8. Flexor tendon nodular disease. When a finger is "triggering," three fingers must be used to palpate a sufficient length of tendon to identify whether the nodule lies in the palm or in the area of the shaft of the proximal phalanx where the superficialis tendon decussates. (From Flatt, A.E.[7])

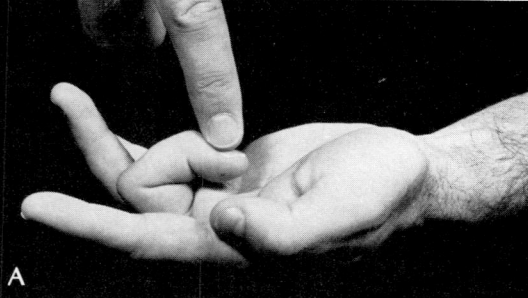

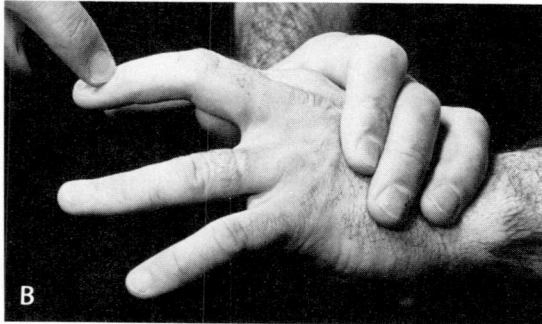

Fig. 45–9. Test for swan neck deformity. *A,* First stage of the test applies passive flexion to all three digital joints to exclude pathologic conditions of the extrinsic extensor tendon or the digital joints. *B,* Second stage of the test tenses the intrinsic muscles by holding the metacarpophalangeal joint in full extension and applying dorsal pressure to the tip of the finger. In patients with rheumatoid disease, the degree of resistance to passive flexion is directly proportional to the severity of the disease. (From Flatt, A.E.[7])

urgent because boutonnière deformity caused by the expanding synovium is difficult to treat, even in its early stages.[7]

Precise, long-term follow-up studies of surgical synovectomy are profoundly lacking. This gap in our knowledge is responsible for the greatest controversy in the care of the rheumatoid hand. Some workers challenge the use of the term "prophylactic" when applied to early synovectomy, and others counter that they have yet to see a sufficient number of patients early enough to test a prophylactic procedure adequately. I have no doubt that the operation gives symptomatic relief, but I believe that only in the earliest disease can one prevent irreversible joint changes. My own follow-up studies[5] and others in the literature[3,20] show a significant percentage of "recurrence" of rheumatoid synovitis, with higher rates in those patients suffering from more severe disease.

The operation is performed through an incision directly over the joint, and the synovium is re-

moved when the tendons on the dorsum of the joint have been retracted laterally. The technical problem is to remove all the synovium of the joint; it is particularly important to remove completely the tongue of synovium that lies between the collateral ligaments and the neck of the proximal bone of the joint. This tongue is largely responsible for the detachment of the collateral ligament from the bone and for the destruction of the subchondral cortical bone.

Synovectomy of a digital joint is commonly combined with other procedures, but when the operation is performed by itself, the usual postoperative treatment is early active motion. Passive motion should be avoided, and the patient should be advised to exercise to the limits of discomfort. If true pain is produced, the exercise program must be reduced.

Arthroplasty

Restoration of function to digital joints destroyed by rheumatoid disease is usually provided by ar-

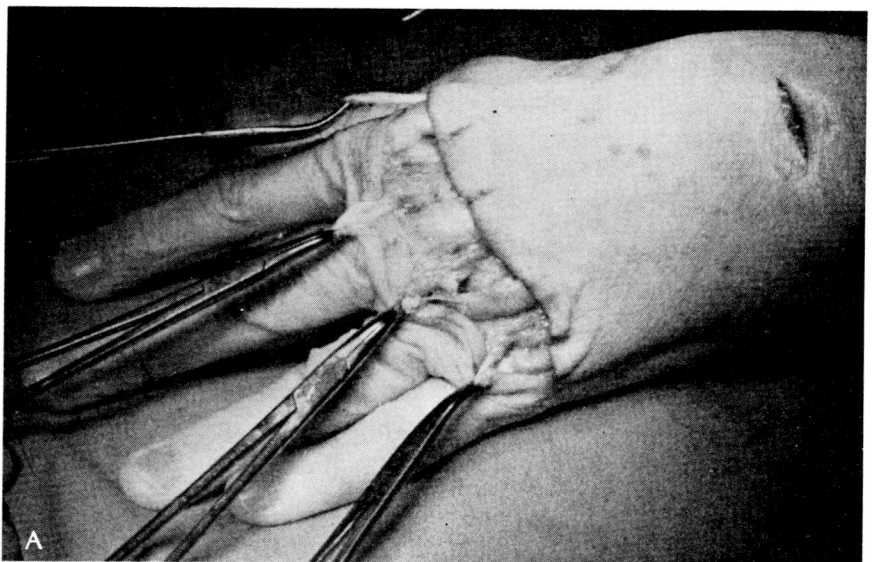

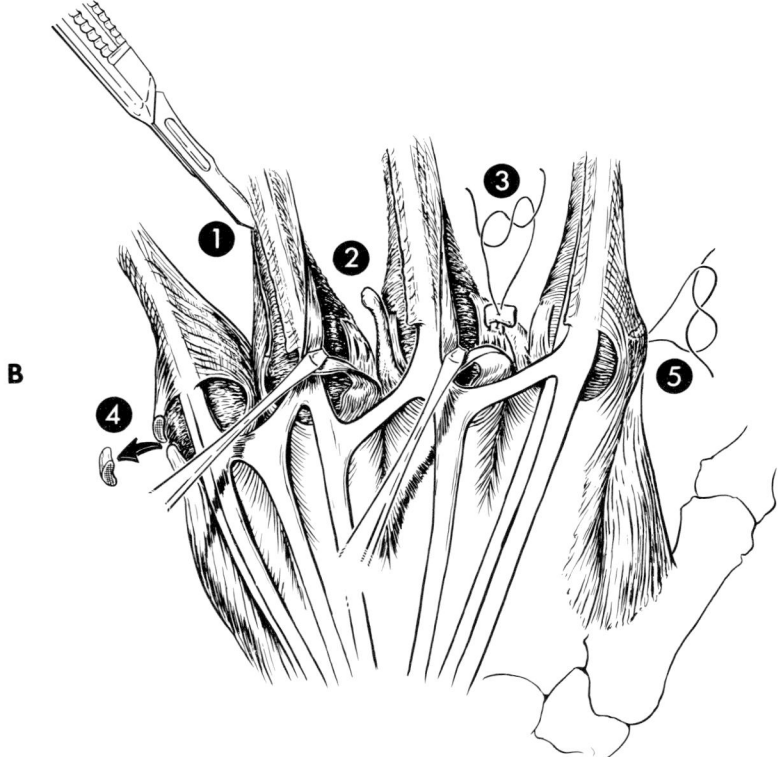

Fig. 45–10.   Crossed intrinsic transfer. *A,* The detached wing of the interosseous tendon must be dissected back proximally enough to allow free excursion. Three hemostats are on the freed-up ulnar intrinsic tendons; at the top of the figure, the extensor indicis tendon is shown in a hemostat for those who wish to continue to use this transfer. *B,* Crossed intrinsic transfer. *1,* Release of the ulnar intrinsic tendon. *2,* Its mobilization to the musculotendinous junction and the slit in the radial collateral ligament of the adjacent finger through which the transfer should be passed. *3,* The sewing in of the transfer. *4,* Abductor digiti minimi release. *5,* Repositioning of the first dorsal interosseous tendon. (From Flatt, A.E.[7])

throplasty. Fusion of these joints is of value in extreme cases, but is not generally employed because it may impair necessary hand function. Arthroplasty or prosthetic replacement cannot be done unless the patient has adequate and balanced muscle control of flexion and extension of the involved joint. The extrinsic flexor muscles are frequently stronger than the extensor mechanism, and patients may need a preoperative period of strengthening exercises for the extensor muscles.

At the metacarpophalangeal joint, excisional arthroplasty is now rare because the motion and digital alignment supplied by prosthetic substitutes are superior to those provided by arthroplasty. Three generations of implants have been tried: the original metallic implants that I used in the 1950s, the silicone rubber devices introduced by Swanson[19] and Niebauer[16] in the 1960s. and more recently, the third generation of "total" joints devised by a number of surgeons (Fig. 45–11). I no longer use the original metal implants and believe that the results achieved by the Swanson design are the standards against which other devices should be judged. I have used many of the third-generation joints and agree with Nalebuff that they are more difficult to insert, have many potential complications, and do not provide better motion or alignment than the Swanson design.[7]

The Swanson implants are not a true prosthesis, but rather are cruciform silicone rubber devices that keep the raw bone apart during the healing and scar encapsulation process. A properly performed operation with the correct postoperative therapy should relieve the pain, line up the digits, and provide an average of 60° of motion.

Complications such as infection, fracture of the implant, and recurrence of the ulnar drift do occur.[13] Infection is rare, and fracture probably occurs in about 5% of patients with implants. Such fractures are held together by the periarticular scarring, are usually asymptomatic, and are only detected radiographically. The ulnar drift may recur because of inadequate release of the shortened ulnar structures or inadequate repair on the radial sides. More frequently, it is caused by the uncorrected recurrence of the radial tilt of the carpometacarpal unit at the wrist joint (see Fig. 45–5).

Normal motion at the proximal interphalangeal joints is over 100°, and its retention is of more functional importance in the ulnar two grasping digits than in the index and long fingers, which are used more in extension for precise activities. I am willing to fuse the index finger's proximal interphalangeal joint for stability in pinch, but I strive to maintain mobility in fourth and fifth finger joints. Often, the choice is dictated by the state of the extensor mechanism. Long-standing synovial dis-

ease and flexion contractures impair the extensor mechanism to such a degree that extension against gravity is impossible. In such circumstances, fusion is necessary because it is useless to supply the motion provided by an implant if the balance between extensor and flexor power is absent.

At the distal interphalangeal joint, the preferred salvage operation is fusion in a neutral position or in about 5 to 10° flexion. Some attempt to use implant arthroplasty in this joint, but the technical difficulties are significant, and I believe that fusion gives better and more predictable functional results.

Prosthetic replacement and other salvage procedures do not, and cannot, restore normal hand function. The greatest benefit from surgical treatment is seen in properly selected patients with early disease. Early synovectomy must still be considered a particularly valuable procedure, and its judicious use may eventually abolish the need for many current salvage procedures.

OSTEOARTHRITIS

In contrast to RA, osteoarthritis of the hand primarily involves joint cartilage and bone. Soft tissue constraints are generally normal. Involvement is usually proportional to the amount of abuse of the joints. Symptoms usually do not occur until the fifth decade and are precipitated commonly by a sprain or transmission of an unusual force through the joint. Once these symptoms occur, they are unlikely to disappear completely. The most important joint affected is the carpometacarpal joint of the thumb because the thumb carries a high proportion of the work load of the hand. In prehensile activities, the thumb is half the hand, and arthritis at its base interferes with all its functions. Conservative treatment, analgesics, and splinting are all helpful, but the symptoms are frequently so disabling that operation must be considered. Two operations are possible, fusion or arthroplasty. Neither operation is ideal; each has its advocates, and both require several months of treatment before postoperative recovery is complete.

In the younger patient, fusion is preferable because the small loss of mobility of the thumb is well compensated by painless stability. The operation consists of excision of the contiguous arthritic joint surfaces, impaction of the two raw bone ends, and their immobilization by a bone graft driven into both bones. The graft is commonly taken from the tibia or, occasionally, the ilium. Immobilization in a cast that includes the thumb is necessary for three to four months after operation.

Arthroplasty is achieved by excision of the trapezium bone. The resulting space can be filled with local tissue such as a strip of rolled up tendon. It

A   FIRST GENERATION

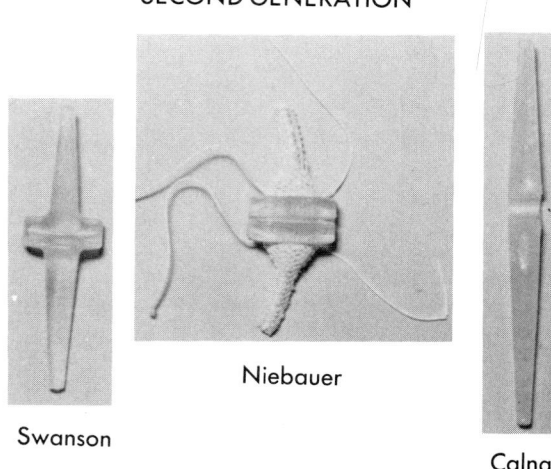

Brannon   Flatt

B   SECOND GENERATION

Fig. 45–11. The three generations of prostheses. The first generation *(A)* were made of SS 316, the second *(B)* of silicone rubber, and the third *(C)* of a variety of metals and plastics. (From Flatt, A.E.[7])

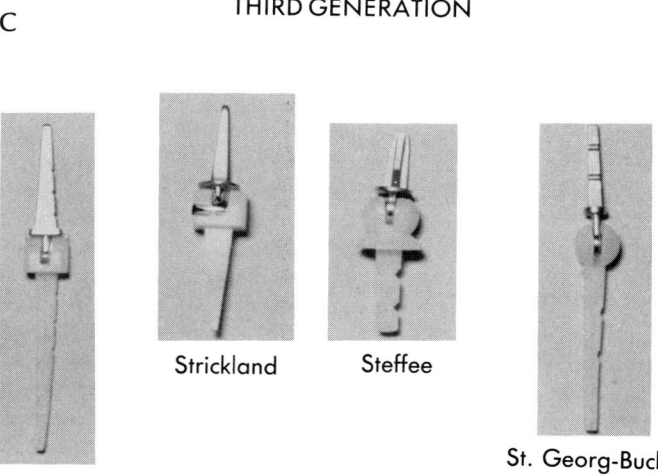

Niebauer

Swanson

Calnan

C   THIRD GENERATION

Strickland   Steffee

St. Georg-Buchholz

Schultz

can also be allowed to fill with scar, or a foreign substitute made of Silastic, metal, or high-density polyethylene can be used (see Fig. 45–4). No single replacement arthroplasty is superior to all others, and the best results probably are the result of superior surgical technique rather than choice of implant.[1]

The middle and distal joints of the thumb may also become osteoarthritic, and either the metacarpophalangeal or the interphalangeal joint can be fused with little functional loss. In multiple joint disease, however, the problem is more difficult, and treatment must be individualized by the hand surgeon because multiple-joint fusions are detrimental to hand function.

Osteoarthritis of the finger joints frequently follows trauma, usually associated with extensive soft tissue damage (Fig. 45–12). The scarring produced by the soft tissue trauma is often of greater functional importance than the changes in the joint surfaces.

Distal joint involvement is common in osteoarthritis, and radiographs show narrowing of the joint space, subchondral sclerosis, and osteophyte formation. These osteophytes are recognized clinically as Heberden's nodes. Mucous cyst formation is commonly associated with these spurs. These cysts arise from the joint synovium beneath the dorsal skin between the joint and the eponychial

fold. As the cyst increases in size, it presses on the area of the nail root and distorts the growing nail. Simple excision of the cyst is inadequate. The inciting osteophyte must also be removed[6] (Fig. 45–13). Surgical intervention at the joint is justified in the presence of severe deformity, unrelenting pain, or instability. Cosmetic excision of Heberden's nodes is poor practice, but fusion a few degrees short of full extension is common. Silastic replacement of this joint is still on trial. The condition must be distinguished from erosive osteoarthritis, in which the greater degree of destruction renders the results of surgical treatment less satisfactory.

OTHER ARTHRITIC CONDITIONS

Gouty Arthritis

The synovial response to urate crystals is similar to that seen in rheumatoid disease of the small joints of the hand and wrist. The treatment for gouty arthritis is medical, and only rarely is operation indicated. I agree with Straub and co-workers in their view that indications for surgical intervention are few and are largely restricted to the excision of gouty tophi[18] (Fig. 45–14). Although increasing evidence suggests that these tophi recede with medical treatment, I believe that they should be excised if they present a mechanical block to joint motion.

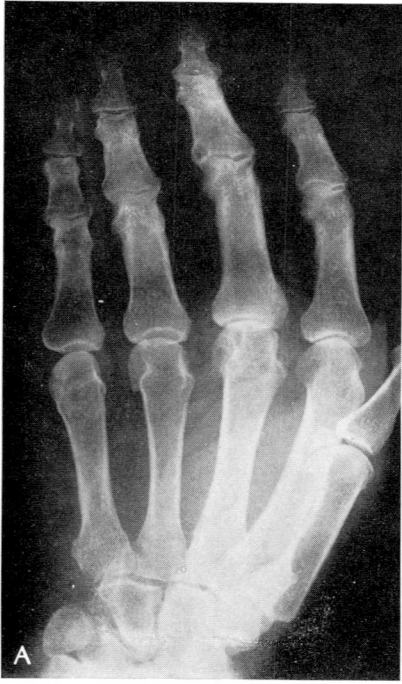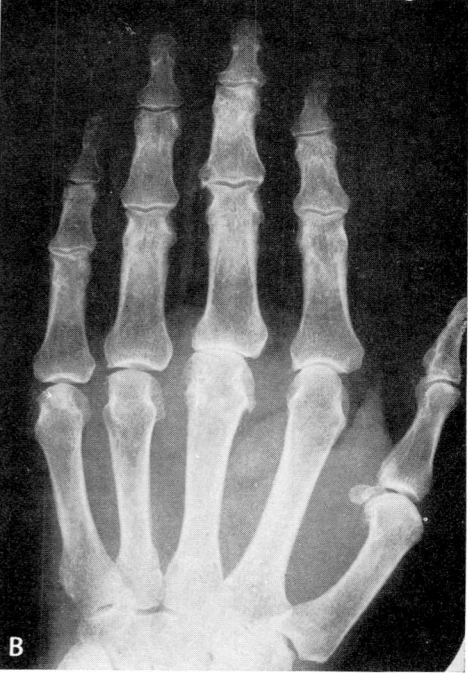

Fig. 45–12. *A* and *B*, Degenerative arthritis of fingers. This hand of a professional wrestler shows the results of repeated traumatic insults to the digital joints. (From Flatt, A.E.[7])

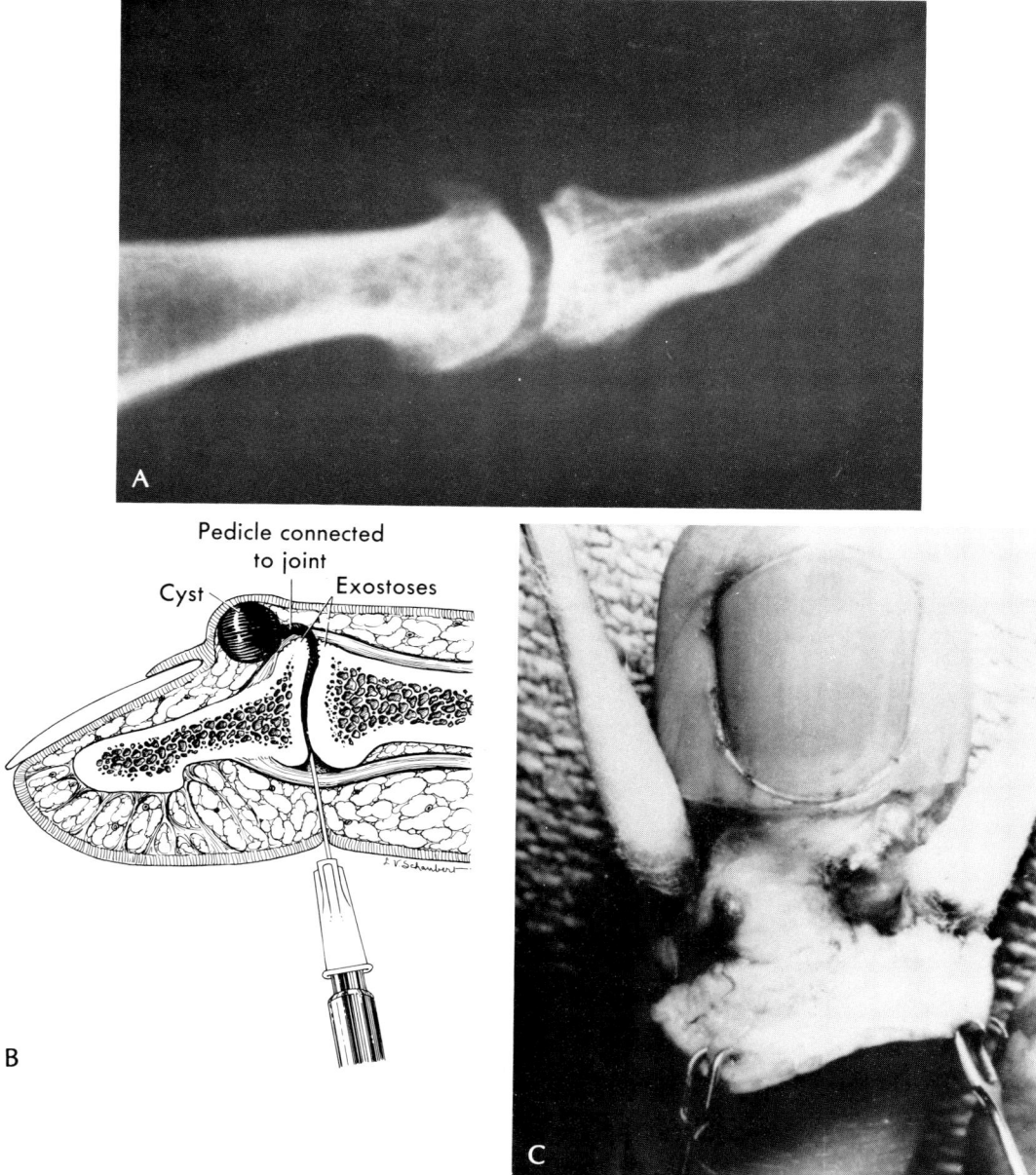

Fig. 45–13. Mucous cyst. *A,* The dorsal osteoarthritic spur frequently associated with a mucous cyst. *B,* Injection of methylene blue into the joint to fill the dorsal cyst or cysts. *C,* Dissection showing a large cyst and the presence of a small, hidden, and undiagnosed smaller cyst. (*A* and *C* Courtesy of Eugene Kilgore, II, M.D.; *B* From Flatt, A.E.[7])

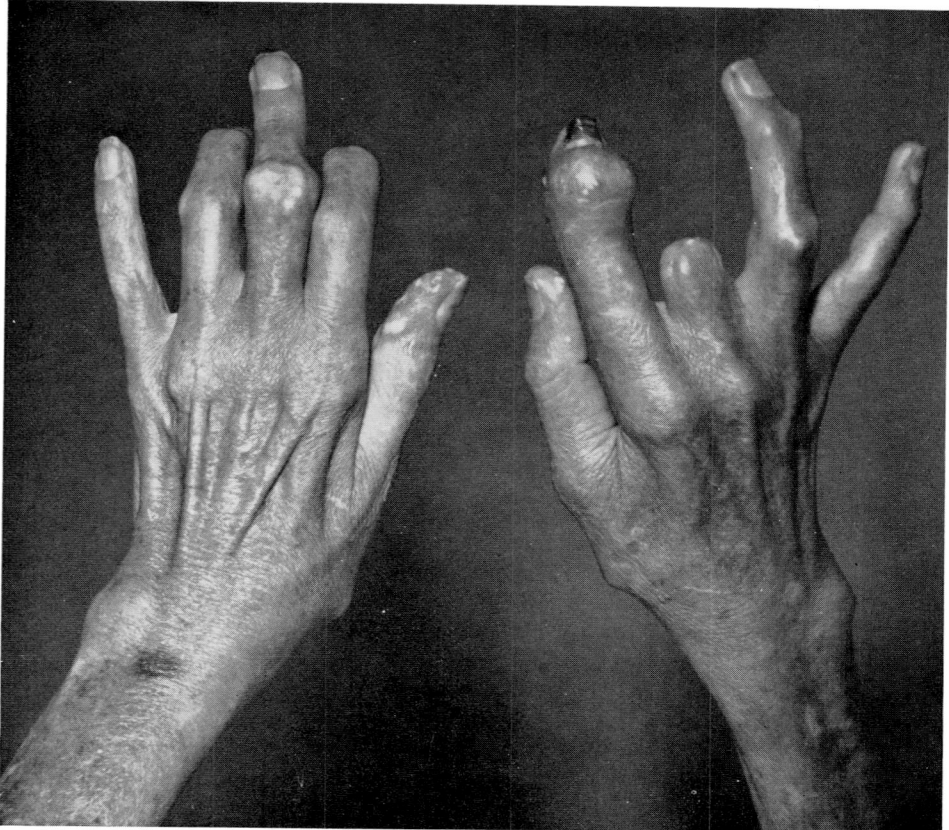

Fig. 45–14.   Gout of the hand. These hands of a 53-year-old woman illustrate the classic problems encountered in the hands of both sexes. Selective amputation has already been necessary in several digits. (From Converse, J.: Reconstructive Plastic Surgery. Philadelphia, W.B. Saunders, 1977.)

Draining sinuses and their causative tophi should be excised. Certainly, tophi causing nerve entrapment, as in the carpal tunnel syndrome, should be excised.

Occasionally, bony destruction or urate deposits are so massive that amputation of part or all of a finger may be required. Degenerative changes at the interphalangeal joint level may be great enough to warrant fusion in a functional position. No published reports exist of attempts at prosthetic replacement in gouty finger joints. Resorption of urate deposits, remodeling, and repair of damaged bones are often gratifying with proper medical treatment.

Psoriasis

No definition of psoriatic arthritis is entirely satisfactory, and the true association of psoriasis and arthritis of the hand is difficult to establish. It is known that 5 to 10% of patients with rheumatoid disease have psoriasis. Moreover, radiologic changes typically seen in psoriatic arthritis precede skin lesions in 10% of patients who eventually develop psoriasis.

Clinically, excessive fibrous tissue is present around the joints, and the metacarpophalangeal joints of the hand are stiff and flexed. Severe overriding of the bones may occur, and the medullary canals of the metacarpal bones are small in diameter. The distal interphalangeal joints often stiffen in a useful position, but the proximal interphalangeal joints frequently develop boutonnière deformities. Synovial proliferation is less pronounced than in rheumatoid disease, but destruction of articular cartilage and subchondral bone does occur. Radiologically, psoriatic arthritis is characteristically asymmetric and often unilateral. It can also involve only the bones of a single digital ray. Malalignments of the digital joints are common, and subluxation occurs.

Surgical treatment of the psoriatic arthritic hand is frustrating because it is nearly impossible to provide long-term improvement of motion. Arthroplasties do not generally improve function, and fusion prevents further deformity at the expense of motion. The results of soft tissue operations and joint replacements are less satisfactory than in rheumatoid disease.

Scleroderma

The soft tissue atrophy of the fingertips that occurs in scleroderma is usually associated with Raynaud's phenomenon. Calcification of the fingertip pulp is common in scleroderma. When calcinosis occurs, about half the cases are associated with scleroderma or some other collagen disease and with Raynaud's phenomenon. Absorption of the distal tufts of the terminal phalanges is the most common bony abnormality seen radiographically. Articular bone or cartilage destruction is seen occasionally, with absorption of bone usually involving the middle and proximal phalanges.

Surgical interventions have little to offer the victims of scleroderma. Stiffness develops in the joints of the hand, and splinting to maintain functional positions can be helpful. Assistive aids may have to be constructed for the patient. I have been able to show that digital artery sympathectomy relieves pain and aids in the healing of ulcerations.[8] I have also found that intrinsic muscle release and excision of symptomatic calcifications improve hand function.

Systemic Lupus Erythematosus

Systemic lupus erythematosus commonly involves the hand. The skin tightens, and yet deformities develop from laxity of the supporting soft tissue structures.[2] The articular cartilage is not directly involved, but it may show secondary degenerative changes following ligamentous laxity. Raynaud's phenomenon occurs in about half the patients and is the primary cause of disability, rather than the deformities caused by ligamentous laxity. Thumb carpometacarpal joint involvement is common, and replacement arthroplasty is the treatment of choice at this level. The usual treatment in recent years for metacarpophalangeal joint involvement has been Silastic arthroplasties. My results have not been as good as in rheumatoid hands because of the relentless stiffening.

Better overall results are achieved if any proximal interphalangeal joint deformities are corrected at the time of the metacarpophalangeal arthroplasties. Simple swan neck deformities are corrected by tenodesis of the superficialis tendon, and fixed deformities are treated either by arthroplasty or fusion. Boutonnière deformities can be repaired and lateral deviations can be stabilized by collateral ligament repair.

Mixed Connective Tissue Disease

The hands of these patients differ from the hands of individuals with systemic lupus erythematosus, rheumatoid disease, or scleroderma.[12] The characteristic finding is a tightness in the flexor muscles unassociated with skin or joint tightness. Occasionally, tightness of the intrinsic muscles occurs. Corticosteroid injections may be helpful, and surgical treatment may be needed to release adhesions, which occur in a high percentage of cases between the superficialis and profundus tendons. Tendon lengthening procedures are also sometimes of value.

Hemochromatosis

A rare form of arthritis is that associated with hemochromatosis. Half these patients have arthralgia and arthritis, characteristically in their hands.[10] The proximal interphalangeal, metacarpophalangeal, and radiocarpal joints are all involved, and the triangular cartilage at the wrist may be calcified. Symptoms usually begin in the metacarpophalan-

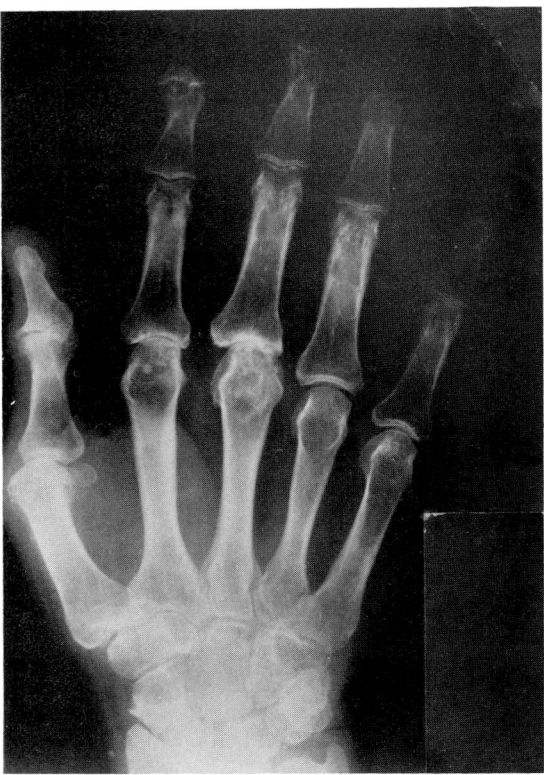

Fig. 45–15. Hemochromatosis. This surgeon's right hand has significant functional impairment because of multiple joint involvement, particularly of the metacarpophalangeal joints of the second and third digits. (From Flatt, A.E.[7])

geal joints, spread through the hand, and rapidly cause significant loss of function. I have seen few cases, but, to my chagrin, have been sensitized to the diagnosis by missing it in the hands of a surgical colleague (Fig. 45–15).

REFERENCES

1. Amadio, P.C., Millender, L.H., and Smith, R.J.: Silicone spacer or tendon spacer for trapezium resection arthroplasty—comparison of results. J. Hand Surg., 7:237–244, 1982.
2. Bleifield, C.J., and Inglis, A.E.: The hand in systemic lupus erythematosus. J. Bone Joint Surg., 56A:1207–1215, 1974.
3. Brown, P.W.: Early recurrence of rheumatoid synovium after early synovectomy in the hand and wrist. In Early Synovectomy in Rheumatoid Arthritis. Edited by W. Hijmans, W.D. Paul, and H. Herschel. Amsterdam, Excerpta Medica, 1969, pp. 201–206.
4. Clayton, M.L.: Surgical treatment at the wrist in rheumatoid arthritis. A review of 37 patients. J. Bone Joint Surg., 47A:741–750, 1965.
5. Ellison, M.R., Kelly, K.H., and Flatt, A.E.: The results of surgical synovectomy of the digital joints in rheumatoid disease. J. Bone Joint Surg., 53A:1041–1060, 1971.
6. Ellison, M.R., Kelly, K.H., and Flatt, A.E.: Ulnar drift of the fingers in rheumatoid disease. J. Bone Joint Surg., 53A:1061–1082, 1971.
7. Flatt, A.E.: Care of the Arthritic Hand. St. Louis, C.V. Mosby, 1983.
8. Flatt, A.E.: Digital artery sympathectomy. J. Hand Surg., 5:550–556, 1980.
9. Flatt, A.E., Larson, C.B., and Cooper, R.R.: Surgery for the arthritic patient. J. Am. Phys. Ther. Assoc., 44:604–619, 1964.
10. Jensen, P.S.: Hemochromatosis: a disease often silent but not invisible. Am. J. Roentgenol., 126:343–351, 1976.
11. Laine, V., and Vainio, K.: Orthopedic surgery and rheumatoid arthritis. Bull. Rheum. Dis., 15:360–361, 1964.
12. Lewis, R.A., et al.: The hand in mixed connective tissue disease. J. Hand Surg., 3:217–222, 1978.
13. Millender, L.H., et al.: Injection after silicone arthroplasty in the hand. J. Bone Joint Surg., 57A:825–829, 1975.
14. Millender, L.H., and Nalebuff, E.A.: Evaluation and treatment of early hand involvement. Orthop. Clin. North Am., 6:697–708, 1975.
15. Millender, L.H., and Nalebuff, E.A.: Preventive surgery—tenosynovectomy and synovectomy. Orthop. Clin. North Am., 6:765–792, 1975.
16. Niebauer, J.J.: Dacron-silicone prosthesis for the metacarpophalangeal and interphalangeal joints. In Symposium on the Hand. Vol. 3. Edited by L.H. Cramer and R.A. Chase. St. Louis, C.V. Mosby, 1971, pp. 91–105.
17. Pahle, J.A., and Raunio, P.: The influence of wrist position on finger deviation in the rheumatoid hand. A clinical and radiological study. J. Bone Joint Surg., 51B:664–676, 1969.
18. Straub, L.R., et al.: Surgery of gout in the upper extremity. J. Bone Joint Surg., 43A:731–752, 1961.
19. Swanson, A.B.: Flexible implant arthroplasty for arthritic finger joints. J. Bone Joint Surg., 54A:435–455, 1972.
20. Vainio, K.: Synovectomies of the hand and wrist in rheumatoid arthritis. In La Main rheumatoide. Paris, Expansion Scientifique Francaise, 1969, pp. 111–115.

Chapter 46

Correction of Arthritic Deformities of the Shoulder and Elbow

Allan E. Inglis

Functionally, the shoulder and elbow serve to position the hand in space. Limitations of function in these two articulations therefore limit the function of the hand. The shoulder, or more broadly speaking, the pectoral girdle, serves as the basal or pivotal articulation of the upper extremity. The elbow joint allows the hand to be extended away from the body for work, and equally important, to be brought toward the body for self-care. Therefore, it is essential that these joints function smoothly and painlessly in the activities of daily life.

ANATOMIC CONSIDERATIONS

Through its design characteristics, the shoulder achieves a remarkable range of motion. Six different modalities, including combinations of motions, are achieved by the glenohumeral joint. Additional shoulder flexibility is achieved through scapulothoracic motion. A high level of stability is achieved despite this high degree of flexibility. The clavicle serves to stabilize the scapula on the thoracic wall, while at the same time permitting high levels of scapular motion. The pectoral girdle is first stabilized against the thoracic wall by the muscles passing from the spine and trunk to the scapula. Further stability is achieved from those muscles passing from the trunk to the proximal humerus. Interstabilization of the glenohumeral joint is achieved by those muscles passing from the scapula to the humerus. Disorders of these stabilizing muscles, whether simple tendinitis or a small rotator cuff tear, substantially reduce the overall coordinated movements of this joint. Further stability of the shoulder is achieved through the ligaments. The ligaments between the scapula and the clavicle, those between the coracoid process of the scapula and the humerus, as well as the glenohumeral ligaments serve to stabilize the glenohumeral joint. The ligaments act to guide the joint through a range of motion and to provide stability at the extremes of motion. The intermediate stability is achieved through the coordinated action of the surrounding muscles. Biomechanically, the forces across the shoulder joint at times are extremely high, and may equal those occurring across the joints of the lower extremity.

Four types of motion are achieved in the elbow joint: flexion, extension, pronation, and supination of the forearm. Extension of the elbow permits the hand to be used at varying distances from the trunk. Chao and associates have demonstrated that if the elbow can be extended to 35°, 90% of the activities of daily living can be accomplished.[9] Rotation of the forearm is allowed through the proximal and distal radioulnar joint. Normally, about 80° of pronation and 80° of supination are permitted by these articulations. When this range of motion is reduced, the shoulder compensates by abducting for pronation and adducting for supination. This "body English" may be embarrassing to the individual with limited pronation or supination.

Normally, there is no medial-lateral movement in the elbow. The stability of the elbow joint is achieved principally by the design of the articulating surfaces and the ligamentous support. The articulating surfaces between the semilunar notch of the ulna and the trochlea of the humerus are ridged and high-walled and are aligned perfectly. The articulation between the radius and the capitellum of the humerus allows for a small amount of laxity, enough so that the radiocapitellar joint is not constantly loaded during hand function. Force transmitted through the hand and wrist is mostly transmitted from the radius to the ulna through the interosseous membrane and thence, to the humerus, scapula and, ultimately, to the spine.[13] The important function of the radiocapitellar joint, therefore, is to provide rotation of the forearm and stability to the proximal radius.

A third articulation is also important. The proximal radioulnar joint stabilizes the proximal portions of these two bones. The annular ligament passes around the neck of the radius, securing it to the ulna. The medial-lateral stability of the elbow joint is achieved through the anterior medial ligament that passes from the humerus to the sublime tubercle of the ulna.[8] Lateral stability is largely achieved by the brachioradialis muscle, extensor muscles of the wrist and, to a lesser extent, by the lateral collateral ligament. The forces across the elbow joint are almost entirely compressional. This compression loading system occurs because many of the wrist and finger flexors and extensors originate from the humeral epicondyles. Whenever the wrist is stabilized, whether it be in grasp, or release, the wrist extensors contract, thereby compressing the elbow joint. Carrying a suitcase weighing 40 pounds produces a commensurate compression force across the elbow joint rather than a distraction force.

Reduced function of the shoulder and elbow occurs in a variety of situations, including pain, weakness or paralysis, instability, or stiffness. By far, the most important of these is pain, and therapeutic measures must always place pain relief as the highest priority. The pain may be produced either by an inflammatory reaction, such as in RA or osteoarthritis or septic synovitis (fire), or by the anatomic destruction of the joint by these diseases (ashes). Such joint destruction produces painful instability. Stiffening of the joint, such as seen in degenerative or traumatic arthritis, may also produce pain. Whether the pain is due to an inflammatory reaction, instability, or stiffening, it is still the primary consideration in surgical therapy of the shoulder and elbow. The pain may be ameliorated by systemic medications or at times by intra-articular corticosteroid injections. For the stiff shoulder, an exercise program to increase range of motion and strength may be of benefit. The most difficult and therapeutically demanding pathologic processes are those that produce a combination of inflammation, joint destruction, and stiffness. In this situation, all three must be corrected simultaneously.

SURGICAL THERAPY

Arthritic Shoulder. Surgical therapy for the arthritic shoulder should never be instituted until conservative measures have been exhausted. These measures should always include the use of salicylates or other nonsteroidal anti-inflammatory drugs, a period of rest and, frequently, intra-articular injection of corticosteroid. The patient may be referred to a therapist for range of motion and strengthening exercises. These conservative measures, individually or in concert, frequently reduce symptoms to acceptable levels.

Surgical therapy for the shoulder includes synovectomy and debridement, hemiarthroplasty, arthrodesis, and total shoulder arthroplasty. Synovectomy of the shoulder is sometimes needed in rheumatoid arthritis or other primary diseases of the synovium. Synovectomy is often unsuccessful, however, and has been abandoned in most centers. The major reason for its failure is the lack of surgical accessibility of the synovium. It is extremely difficult to reach the infraglenoid recess, the subscapularis pouch, and the posterior aspect of the joint arthroscopically, or even through an anterior surgical approach. Therefore, for rheumatoid arthritis, other measures must be employed.

Debridement of the acromioclavicular joint, with acromioplasty and ligament decompression, is useful in impingement syndromes of the shoulder.[11] The glenohumeral joint is *not* opened. Surgery is directed to the area beneath the acromion process. The coracoacromial ligament is incised. The acromioclavicular joint is debrided, including osteophyte removal, and a portion of the undersurface of the acromion process is removed to provide adequate space for the greater tuberosity of the humerus to move within the space between the acromion process and the remaining humerus (Fig. 46–1). At times, it is also necessary to repair a small defect in the external rotator cuff. This operation requires prolonged convalescence during which intensive physical therapy is prescribed to achieve a functional range of motion with strength. This operation is successful in the hands of experienced surgeons. Patients can usually return to racquet sports, swimming, and other activities requiring high levels of shoulder mobility.[11]

Hemiarthroplasty of the shoulder is useful, particularly in traumatic arthritis and osteonecrosis, or when disease is confined principally to the head of the humerus and there is an intact, functioning, rotator cuff with good preservation of glenoid surface.[10] It is not necessary to cement the humeral component. Hemiarthroplasty sometimes can be used as a "salvage" procedure even when the bony glenoid process is completely destroyed. In this situation, the prosthesis articulates with the remaining glenoid labrum and remaining neck of the glenoid (Fig. 46–2). Again, intensive physical therapy is required to restore shoulder function. In a hemiarthroplasty, it is essential that a secure, functioning, external rotator cuff be established. Any tears must be repaired at the time of operation. When rotator cuff repair is necessary, an even more protracted period of convalescence and physical therapy is required. The results from hemiarthroplasty are salutary.[10] Full flexion, full abduction, full internal rotation, and external rotation to at least 45° are expected. Even if these results are achieved, however, return to racquet sports or other activities where the shoulder joint experiences high loading or force should not be expected.

Arthrodesis (fusion) is useful if obliteration of glenohumeral motion is desirable, as after severe recalcitrant infections where there has been complete loss of all the rotator muscles about the shoulder or gross destruction of both the humeral head

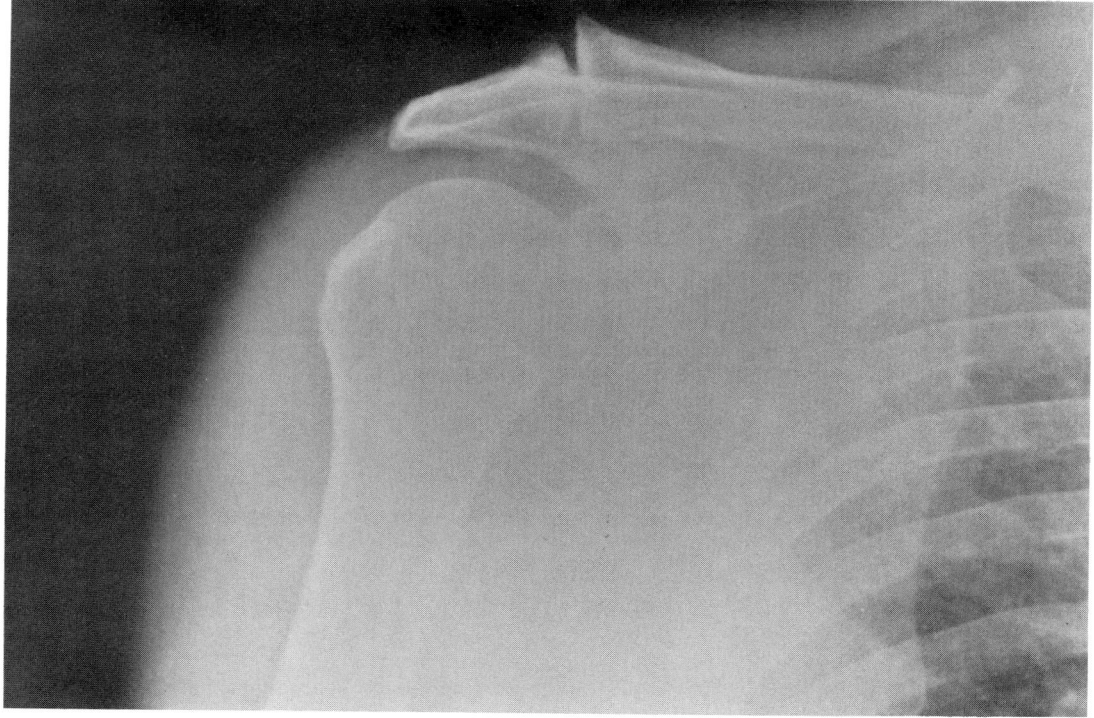

Fig. 46–1.   Osteoarthritis of the acromioclavicular joint. Note the thickening and hypertrophy of both the acromion and the end of the clavicle. Such hypertrophy irritates the subacromial bursa and injures the underlying supraspinous muscle.

and the glenoid process. This procedure is usually reserved for patients with extremely painful shoulders that do not permit use of the elbow or hand in the activities of daily living. Its major drawbacks are the long period of immobilization in a cast or splint and the occasional failure of fusion with development of a painful pseudarthrosis. A successful arthrodesis of the shoulder relieves pain but leaves limited motion. Such patients can move their hand to their face and ear, but probably not to the back of the head. The buttock area can be reached, but not the middle of the back. Forward flexion to 70° is expected. All activities that occur at a *bench* level should be possible.[1]

Total shoulder arthroplasty is useful when there is destruction of both the humeral head and the glenoid. The humeral head and the glenoid are replaced, the former with a stemmed, metallic prosthesis and the latter with a high-molecular-weight polyethylene implant. Both components are cemented in place with polymethylmethacrylate. There are two types of prostheses: constrained and nonconstrained. A constrained prosthesis is a single unit containing glenoid and humeral components. These components are attached to one another

while still allowing a high level of motion. The components of nonconstrained prostheses are not mechanically connected to one another. Stability is achieved through the newly restored capsule and the surrounding muscles. The constrained prosthesis is most useful in patients with severe irreparably damaged external rotator cuff muscles.

The constrained design produces greater stresses on the cement bone bonds. The nonconstrained shoulder joint replacement achieves greater motion, but it is important that stability be maintained through repair of the external rotator cuff. The capsule of the joint must be sufficiently intact to achieve a strong repair. Stress is less at the cement bone bond. The rehabilitative program must be intensive after either type of prosthesis has been inserted. Usually, because of pain relief, good patient cooperation is achieved during the rehabilitation period. Two levels of restored function can be observed. In patients with total shoulder arthroplasty, 80 to 90% restoration of function can be expected if the external rotator cuff was intact to begin with or was surgically restored (Fig. 46–3). Relief of pain with "Bench level" function is expected in joints in which the external rotator cuff has been

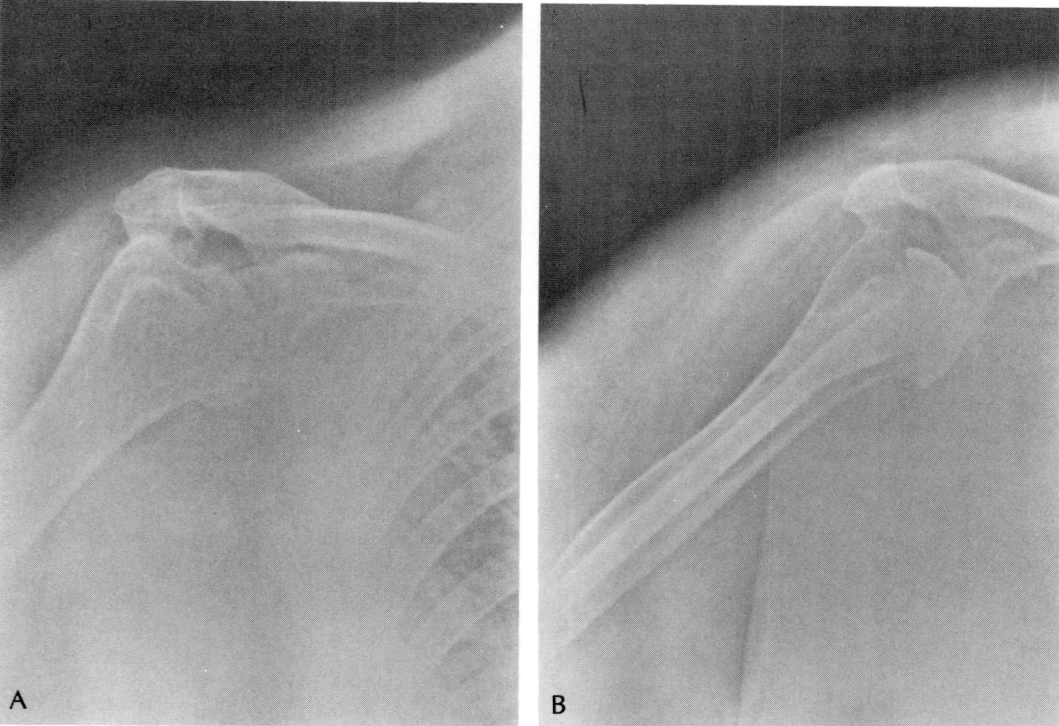

Fig. 46–2. *A*, Severe rheumatoid arthritis of the glenohumeral joint associated with complete destruction of the glenoid process. At surgery only a bony button of the remaining neck of the glenoid was evident; this structure was surrounded by remnants of the labrum and capsular fibrous tissue. *B*, After hemiarthroplasty, pain was completely relieved. Although the range of motion was "bench level," the shoulder joint was functional and the patient could reach her face and back.

partially restored or in cases where there are other residual problems in the shoulder, such as arthritis of the acromioclavicular joint or severe muscle atrophy. Total arthroplasty is being performed with increasing frequency by surgeons experienced in reconstructive shoulder surgery.[12,14] The relief of pain and restoration of function have been gratifying to most patients.

Arthritic Elbow Joint. Conservative measures should always be attempted first. These measures include the use of salicylates and other nonsteroidal, anti-inflammatory drugs. Intra-articular injections of corticosteroids and/or rest are beneficial in rheumatoid synovitis for relief of pain. Posterior splints, secured with Velcro straps, are easily prepared by occupational therapists (Fig. 46–4). Exercises, except for gentle stretching to prevent contractures, may worsen the condition because of the anatomic complexities of the elbow joint.

Surgical therapy includes: synovectomy and debridement with radial head resection, replacement arthroplasty, fascial arthroplasty, and arthrodesis.

Synovectomy and joint debridement with radial head resection are highly successful procedures in those patients with a primary disease of the synovium that has failed to respond to conservative measures.[3,7] It is particularly useful when there has been preservation of the articular surfaces of the humerus and the semilunar notch of the ulna (Fig. 46–5*A,B*). The synovium is excised and the joint edges are carefully debrided and restored to their normal anatomic state (Fig. 46–6*A,B*). The radial head is always removed to allow for normal rotation of the forearm. Ninety percent good to excellent results are expected if the appropriate indications are followed and the patient complies with the rehabilitation program. Pain and restricted motion due to degenerative arthritis can also be treated by joint debridement with radial head resection with restoration of satisfactory painless function, but the results are not as predictable as in rheumatoid arthritis. Pain relief is often complete, but it may not be accompanied by a noticeable increased range of motion. To prevent disappointments in patients with degenerative arthritis of the elbow, the goals should be carefully established before the operation.

Replacement arthroplasty of the elbow is becom-

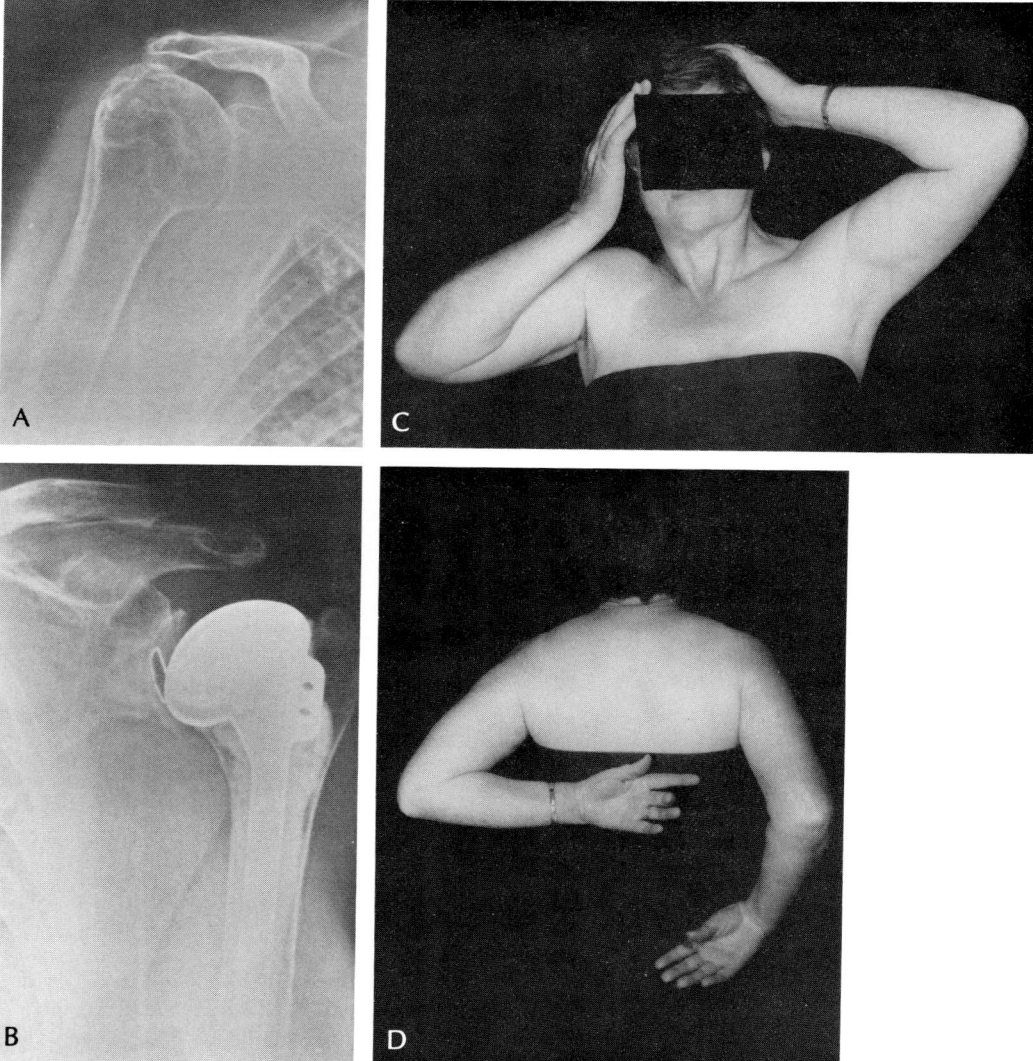

Fig. 46–3. *A,* Severe degenerative arthritis of the left shoulder with loss of cartilage from both the glenoid process and the humeral head. The patient had severe pain unrelieved by either medication or corticosteroid injections. (Radiograph negative reversed when printed.) *B,* Radiograph following total shoulder arthroplasty. Both glenoid and humeral components are secure with no evidence of loosening. *C,* Photograph obtained when the patient entered the hospital for total shoulder arthroplasty on the opposite shoulder. The left shoulder now has sufficient external rotation and abduction to permit her to reach the back of her head. *D,* Adduction and internal rotation were sufficient to enable the patient to reach the middle of her back.

ing more popular. The results over an 8- to 10-year period show that such arthroplasty is lasting and useful, particularly in patients with rheumatoid arthritis.[2,4–6] Replacement arthroplasty of the elbow may be considered in those patients who are refractory to medical management and have joint destruction. The indications for surgery in patients with traumatic arthritis and degenerative arthritis are still unclear. Certainly, a youthful patient with traumatic arthritis is not a candidate for replace-

ment arthroplasty because of his high physical demands and expectations. The stiuation is not unlike that seen in youthful patients with traumatic arthritis of the hip or knee.

There are two types of replacement arthroplasties available. *A nonconstrained elbow replacement* achieves stability through the design of the implant surfaces and adjacent ligaments and muscles. *Semiconstrained implants* with medial and lateral movement of the prosthesis allow a reduction in the

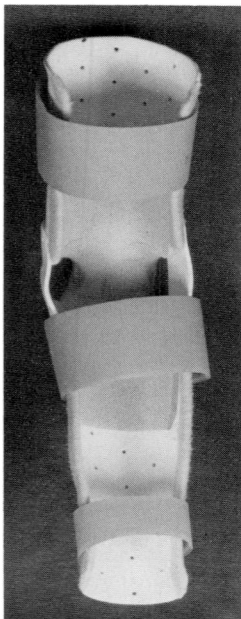

Fig. 46–4. Simple, fabricated resting splint. These splints are usually made with the elbow at 90° flexion. They are well padded with moleskin and secured with Velcro straps.

torque forces across the cement bone bond during motion, including internal and external rotation of the arm (Fig. 46–7). Such semiconstrained implants allow full flexion and extension together

with a small amount of medial-lateral laxity. Improvements in surgical technique have reduced the complication rate in both these arthroplasties to the levels expected in total hip or total knee replacement (Fig. 46–8). Rapid advancement through a therapy program can be achieved with early restoration of elbow function. Such rapid recovery is possible because of immediate intraoperative restoration of joint stability and of triceps extensor function, with retention of elbow flexion. It is expected that these patients will achieve 130° of elbow flexion and extension to 25° to 30°. Many patients achieve both full flexion and full extension.[2,5]

Complications in the shoulder and elbow are similar to those seen in implant arthroplasties of the lower extremity. The infection rate following total shoulder replacement is less than 1%, and the infection rate following total elbow arthroplasty is 3%. Nonconstrained implant loosening in total shoulder arthroplasty is less than 4% after 5 years. Our experience with semiconstrained, total elbow arthroplasty revealed that only 1 of 95 implants loosened during a 9-year period. Dislocation or separation of the components of the implant, whether it be in the shoulder or in the elbow, occurs in about 5% of cases.

We expect a 90% return of function after total shoulder arthroplasty in patients with an intact rotator cuff, and a 90% return of function after total elbow arthroplasty. These results may be compromised by arthritic disorders in adjacent articulations

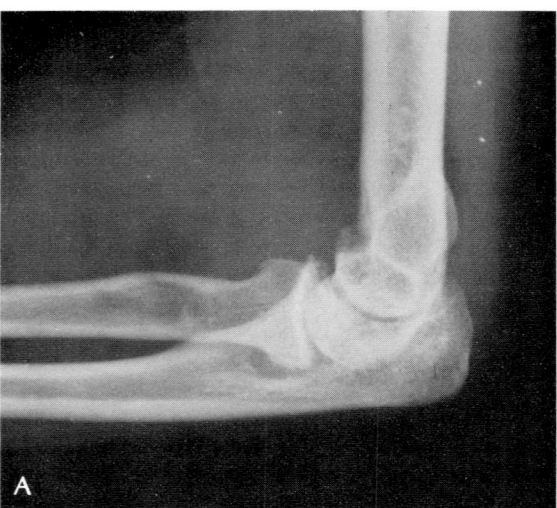
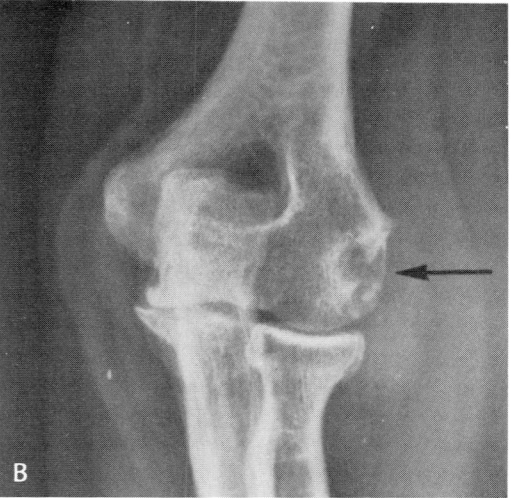

Fig. 46–5.   Radiographs of a patient with uncontrolled rheumatoid synovitis of the elbow. *A,* Note preservation of joint surfaces and minimal joint margin osteophyte formation. *B,* Anterior-posterior view. The arrow points to a 1- × 1.5-cm cystic defect in the lateral epicondyle. This defect was beneath the lateral collateral ligament and was filled with rheumatoid granulation tissue. Elbow synovectomy, debridement, and evacuation of the cystic defect were performed. Postoperatively, the patient had complete relief of pain with flexion to 125° and extension to 15°.

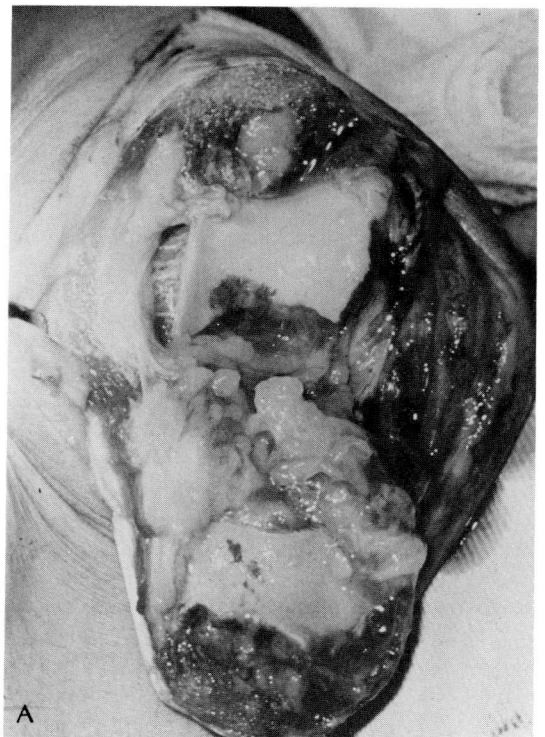

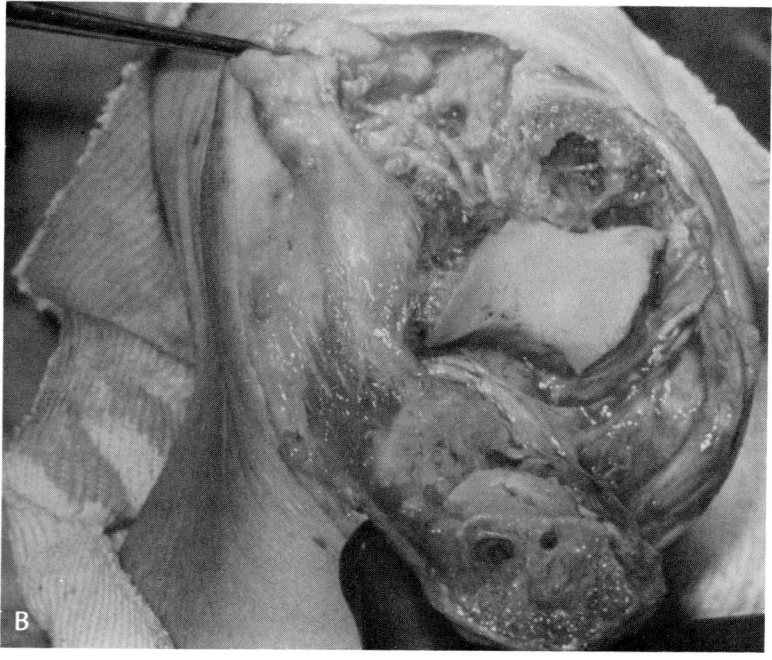

Fig. 46–6. Synovectomy and debridement of the elbow through the transolecranon approach. *A,* The osteotomized tip of the olecranon is in the foreground. Note the large rheumatoid cystic erosion in the remaining olecranon process of the ulna above. Proliferative synovitis occurs in the posterior aspect of the joint in the center of the illustration. Note the pannus formation on the surface of the trochlea of the humerus. *B,* Appearance of the joint following synovectomy and debridement. The pannus has been removed, and the joint margins debrided of all osteophytes and synovium. The radial head has been excised, followed by a complete synovectomy of the anterior compartment of the joint.

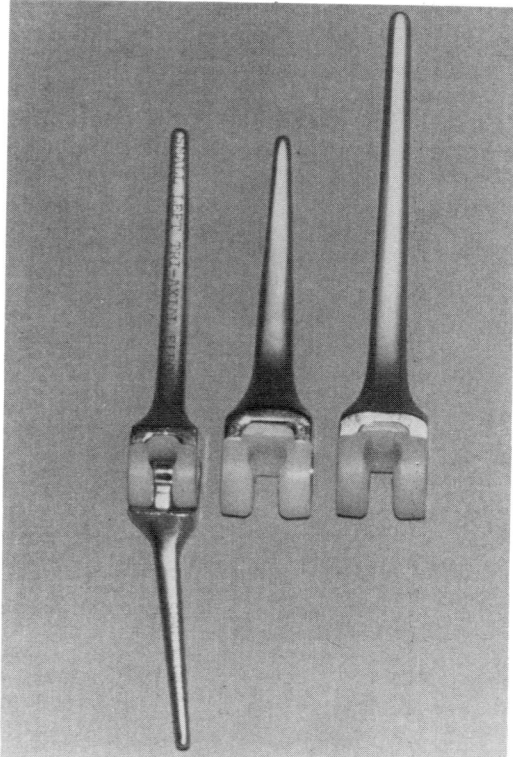

Fig. 46–7. The semiconstrained triaxial total elbow implant. The load across the implant is transmitted through the high-molecular-weight polyethylene plastic bearing. Torsional forces between the cement and the bone are reduced by the laxity in the ulnar component and the plastic bearing. This laxity reduces the potential for loosening.

such as the neck, wrist, and/or hand. The restoration of a painless, stable shoulder or a painless, flexible elbow is often of real value to patients in their activities of daily living.

Surgical therapy can be considered in patients whose pain and loss of function cannot be managed through rest, medications, and a controlled exercise program. The gain versus complications ratio is now sufficiently high that surgical therapy can be safely recommended in patients with disabling arthritis of the shoulder and elbow. The durability of these surgical procedures has been good with improvement in function and quality of life.

REFERENCES

1. Cofield, R.H., and Briggs, B.T.: Glenohumeral arthrodesis. Operative and long term functional results. J. Bone Joint Surg., *61A*:668–677, 1979.
2. Coonrad, R.W.: Seven year follow-up of Coonrad total elbow replacement. *In* Symposium on Total Joint Replacement of the Upper Extremity. Edited by A.E. Inglis. St. Louis, The C.V. Mosby Co., 1982, p. 91.
3. Eichenblat, M., Hass, A., and Kessler, I.: Synovectomy

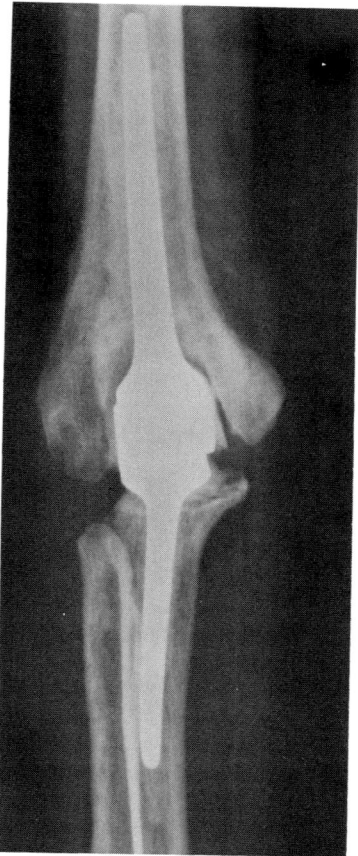

Fig. 46–8. Radiograph showing total elbow arthroplasty. This joint is pain-free with flexion to 130° and extension to 5°. This patient also has an elbow replacement on the opposite side, bilateral total hip and knee replacements, and an ankle replacement. She feels that her elbows are her "most dependable joints."

of the elbow in rheumatoid arthritis. J. Bone Joint Surg., *64A*:1074–1078, 1982.
4. Ewald, F.C., et al.: Capitellocondylar total elbow arthroplasty. J. Bone Joint Surg., *62A*:1259–1263, 1980.
5. Inglis, A.E.: Triaxial total elbow replacement: Indications, surgical technique and results. *In* Symposium on Total Joint Replacement of the Upper Extremity. Edited by A.E. Inglis. St. Louis, The C.V. Mosby Co., 1982, pp. 100–111.
6. Inglis, A.E., and Pellicci, P.M.: Total elbow replacement. J. Bone Joint Surg., *62A*:1252–1258, 1980.
7. Inglis, A.E., Ranawat, C.S., and Straub, L.R.: Synovectomy and debridement of the elbow in rheumatoid arthritis. J. Bone Joint Surg., *53A*:652–662, 1971.
8. Last, R.J.: Anatomy. Regional and Applied, 6th ed. Boston, Little, Brown and Co., 1966, p. 111.
9. Morrey, B.F., Askew, L.J., and Chao, E.Y.: A biomechanical study of normal functional elbow motion. J. Bone Joint Surg., *63A*:872–877, 1981.
10. Neer, C.S.: Replacement arthroplasty for glenohumeral osteoarthritis. J. Bone Joint Surg., *56A*:1–16, 1974.
11. Neer, C.S.: Anterior acromioplasty for the chronic impingement syndromes of the shoulder. A Preliminary Report. J. Bone Joint Surg., *54A*:41–50, 1972.
12. Neer, C.S., Watson, K.C., and Stanton, F.K.: Recent ex-

periences in total shoulder replacement. J. Bone Joint Surg., *64A*:319–337, 1982.

13. Von Langer, T., and Waschsmuth, W.: Praktische Anatomie. Berlin, Verlag von Julius Springer, 1935, p. 157.

14. Warren, R.F., Ranawat, C.S., and Inglis, A.E.: Total shoulder replacement indications and results of the Neer non-constrained prosthesis. *In* Symposium on Total Joint Replacement of the Upper Extremity. Edited by A.E. Inglis. St. Louis, The C.V. Mosby Co., 1982, pp. 56–68.

Chapter 47

Correction of Arthritic Deformities of the Spine

Glenn A. Meyer

The commonly encountered arthritic deformities of the spine are discussed here with emphasis on those that are amenable to surgical correction. The goal is to provide medically oriented physicians with information on when and how surgical treatment may be helpful to their patients. Surgical principles are emphasized with discussions of cases in which clinical, radiologic, and electrophysiologic abnormalities indicate the need for surgical consultation.

The chapter is organized by anatomic regions starting at the C1 to C2 junction and proceeding caudally. A brief description of the commonly performed operations follows.

REGIONAL DISORDERS

C1–C2 Junction

Rheumatoid arthritis is second only to trauma as the most common cause of atlantoaxial instability. Mild degrees of instability as demonstrated by lateral radiographs of the upper cervical spine in the flexed and extended positions are extremely common. Movement of up to 5 mm is rarely of concern and, if necessary, can be treated with a cervical collar. However, if serial films demonstrate a progressive instability, a stabilization procedure (fusion) is inevitable and should be performed before myelopathic symptoms ensue. Symptoms of particular concern are progressive lancinating pain in the C2 distribution of the occiput, Lhermitte's phenomenon (electric shock-like sensations radiating caudally along the spine or distally in the extremities) and, rarely, evidence of intermittent vascular insufficiency in the posterior cerebral circulation caused by impingement on the vertebral arteries. Patients with instability commonly complain of a feeling of movement and/or clicking in the upper neck as they change position. This sensation may awaken the patient and may become so severe that the patient voluntarily supports his head in his hands when changing position. Generally, any movement at the C1 to C2 interspace of more than 10 mm is an absolute indication for fusion. Disabling symptoms as described or progressive instability in the 5- to 10-mm range are relative indications for fusion. Myelopathy with a spastic quadriparesis is usually only incompletely reversible once established.[4]

In the rheumatoid patient, a pannus of inflammatory tissue or rheumatoid nodules may additionally compromise the intraspinal space. CT scanning is effective in visualizing such lesions. Less commonly, polytomography in the sagittal and parasagittal planes with or without gas myelography may provide a better visualization of the relationship among the neural structures within the bony elements because of the multisegmental view. The same view can be provided by sagittal reconstruction of axial CT scan images, but this technique usually provides less precise anatomic detail.[7,10]

Attention to technical detail is critical in establishing a solid C1 to C2 fusion. I prefer a halo vest immobilization applied a day or two prior to operation to ensure that the vest does not compromise the patient's respiratory status. If the rheumatic process has sufficiently softened or eroded the arch of C1 so that it will not hold a stabilizing wire, the occiput should be included in the fusion. Despite meticulous attention to surgical detail in performing the fusion, the rheumatoid process may involve the fusion mass and over several years destabilize a previously adequate fusion. Therefore, close clinical and radiologic follow-up of C1 to C2 instability is required of all patients with active disease before and after fusion. It is important to emphasize to these patients that they should not induce pain in attempts to maintain range of motion of the cervical spine. They may require additional training in the use of mirrors in driving their automobiles or in performing other daily tasks. Generally, methyl methacrylate fusions are not recommended for rheumatoid arthritic patients.

Infrequently, bone softening may be sufficient to allow protrusion of the cervical spine, particularly the odontoid process upward into the skull (basilar impression) with subsequent compression of the cervical medullary junction. This condition is easily demonstrated with routine radiography.

Surgical decompression usually must be done via an anterior approach.[11,12,20]

C3-T1 Segment

Similar progressive deformity, instability, and subluxation may involve any mobile segment of the cervical spine. These processes are accelerated by rheumatoid involvement and by prior laminectomy. An occasional rheumatoid arthritis patient may require fusion from the occiput to the thorax. Serial radiographs of the cervical spine are just as important as they are at the atlantoaxial junction. Most problems requiring surgery below C1 to C2 are due to degenerative disc disease and/or osteoarthritis.

The neurologic examination of patients with extreme arthritic deformity of upper extremity joints can be challenging. Joint replacement commonly interferes with the afferent side of the deep tendon reflex arc. Frequent serial examination of strength, reflex, and sensory functions of the upper extremity by the primary physician or rheumatologist provides the most reliable information. Often, additional useful information can be provided by electrodiagnostic study of muscle and nerve function. If impairment of the posterior columns of the spinal cord is suspected, useful data can be obtained from somatosensory evoked potential studies performed before and after the patient is placed in the symptom-inducing position. Serial comparison of the latencies, as well as comparisons of the data obtained on the right vs. the left side in both arm and leg, is most reliable. Most patients with advanced diseases who develop neurologic rheumatic dysfunction of the arms have a combination of nerve root compression at or near the intervertebral foramen and spinal cord compression.

Deformity of the spinal canal and intervertebral spaces may compromise circulation to the spinal cord with neurologic deficit of a seemingly radicular nature extending one or two segments above and/or below a mass lesion. Such intraspinal mass lesions are usually the result of a combination of osteophyte formation, disc bulging, and hypertrophy and bulging of ligamentous structures (induced by collapse of the intervertebral disc and concomitant shortening and thickening of elastic ligaments). Offending osteophytes most commonly originate from the specialized portion of the lateral area of the cervical vertebral body termed the uncovertebral joint (joint of Luschka).[6] Less frequently, osteophytes may form from the anterior aspect of the facet joint causing further nerve root compression located posteriorly and slightly more distally along the nerve root. Both may co-exist in the same patient causing particularly severe signs of radiculopathy and segmental muscular atrophy (Fig. 47–1).

Another condition that can produce myelopathy is *posterior longitudinal ligament ossification* (PLLO).[14] Its prevalence in Caucasians is about 0.2%, but in Japanese and certain other Orientals it is 1 to 3%. Its etiopathogenesis is obscure, although it may be associated with an equally obscure lesion, namely diffuse idiopathic skeletal hyperostosis.[15] The ossified ligament can occupy more than 50% of the spinal canal, leading to severe myelopathic signs and symptoms. The same process can occur in the *anterior longitudinal ligament* (ALLO). Treatment consists of surgical excision of the ossified ligament, usually from the entire cervical spine. After decompression, the myelopathy does not usually reverse, but further progression is prevented.

Pain alone is infrequently an indication for surgical intervention, particularly if the patient can adjust to the pain and carry on with normal activities. However, disabling sensory loss with lack of proprioceptive feedback and muscular weakness, especially with atrophy, is of great concern. Neurologic deficit of this degree is rarely completely reversible, and surgical consultation should be obtained promptly when functional deficits are first noted.

Occasionally, interspace collapse and osteophyte formation may lead to a hypomobile or completely fused vertebral segmental level. This occurrence predisposes to instability and subluxation at the next mobile level above and/or below the relatively fixed segment. Therefore, flexion/extension lateral radiograms of the cervical spine should be performed in all patients for whom operative intervention is being considered.

Occasionally, patients with a severe degree of osteoarthritis may have remodeling of the vertebral bodies with anterior wedging. When progressive and multisegmental, this condition may lead to reversal of the cervical lordosis and the ''swan neck'' deformity. This deformity may accelerate cervical myelopathy and may be the cause for severe neck pain. Swan neck deformity can be corrected by diskectomy of the intervertebral disc and by placement of multiple grafts to reestablish the anterior height of the vertebral canal. Figure 47–2 shows the pre- and postoperative roentgenograms of a patient successfully treated with a three-disc level technique. Generally, however, anterior diskectomy and fusion of more than two cervical levels is not recommended because of the greater surgical morbidity rate, including nonfusion and pseudoarthrosis formation.

Fusion of the cervical spine by the anterior or posterior technique is satisfactory, depending on

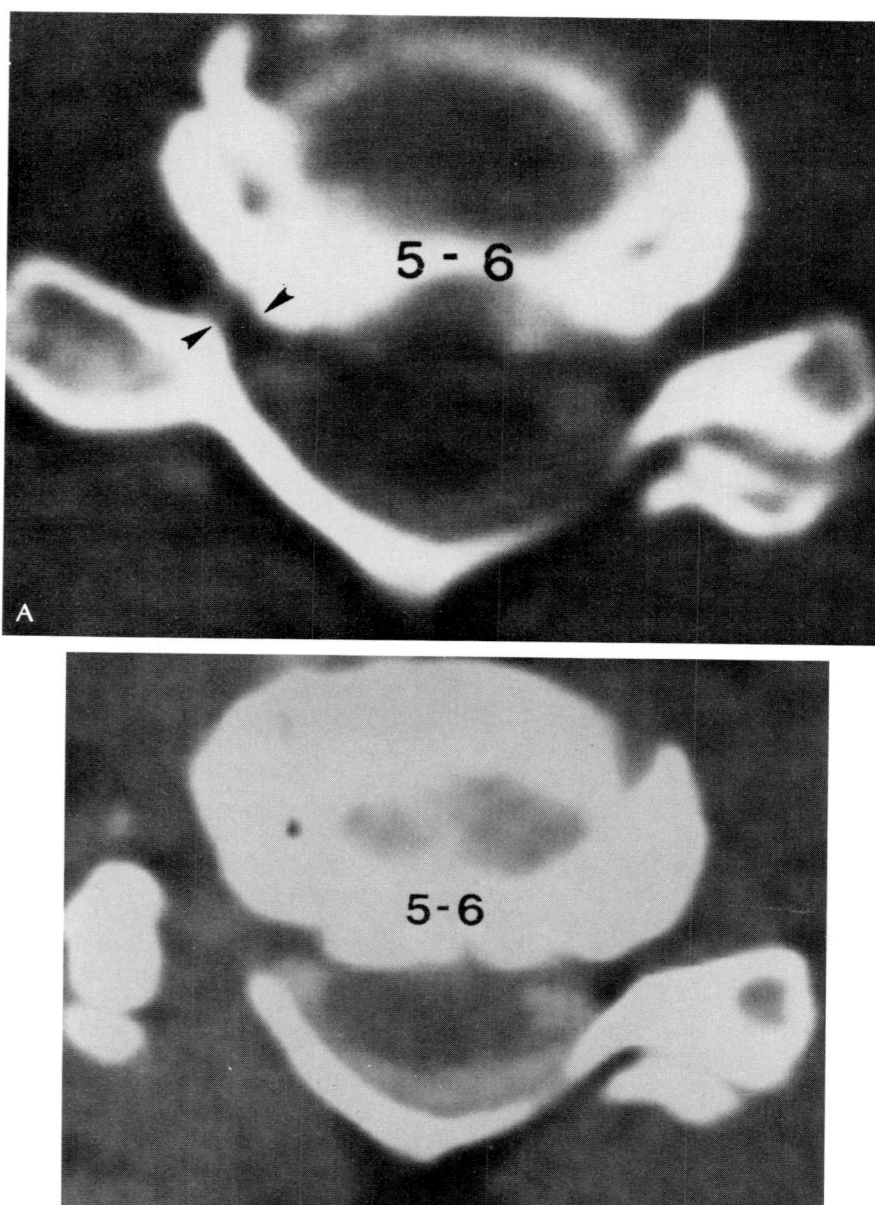

Fig. 47–1. *A*, CT scan through the intervertebral foramen of a patient with marked C6 radiculopathy secondary to an osteophyte from the left uncovertebral joint (joint of Luschka) between the arrow points. *B*, CT appearance following a high-speed air drill medial facetectomy and partial resection of the offending osteophyte with a diamond bur and curette. The intervertebral foramen can be seen now widely patent. The patient's symptoms were relieved.

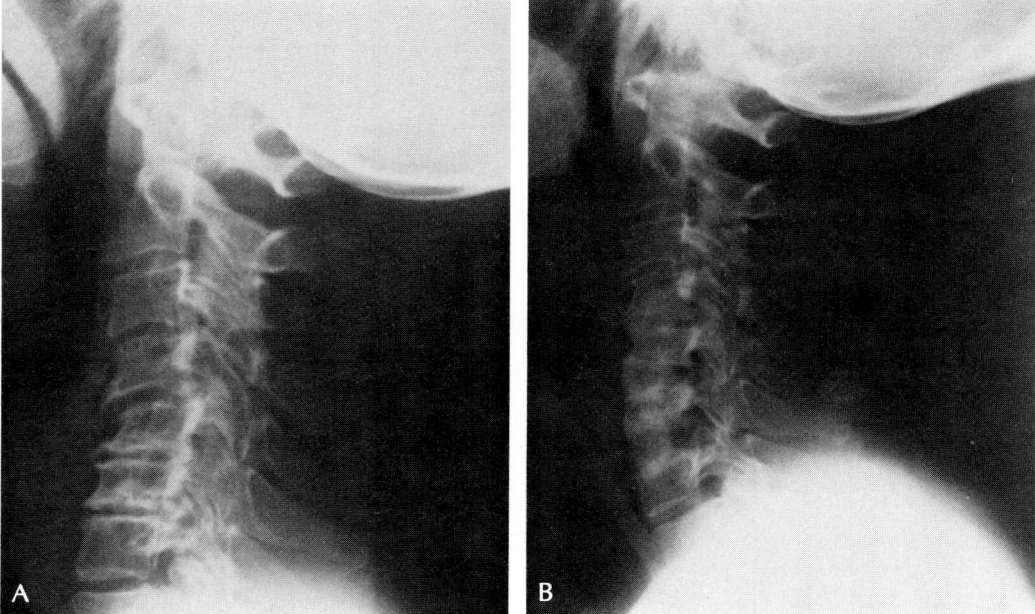

Fig. 47–2. *A,* Preoperative roentgenograms of a 64-year-old woman with severe osteoporosis and degenerative osteoarthritis. She had progressive neck pain, mild myelopathy, and cervical radiculopathy. Progressive reversal of the cervical lordosis was demonstrated on serial films. *B,* The appearance following anterior diskectomy with anterior distraction of the interspace by placement of autogenous iliac bone grafts after operation at three intervertebral levels (C4 to C5 through C6 to C7 inclusive). The cervical lordosis was partially reestablished, and symptoms were completely relieved.

the clinical situation.[1] Generally, anterior diskectomy and fusion in a stenotic cervical canal should not be performed as a primary procedure because of the risk of additional spinal cord damage and disastrous postoperative quadriplegia.

Dorsal Spine

The marked degree of structural support of the thoracic spine by the rib cage makes arthritic deformity of the thoracic spine, which requires surgical correction, a rare condition. An increase in upper thoracic kyphosis commonly develops when osteoarthritis and osteoporosis coexist. Lesser increases in the thoracic kyphosis are occasionally seen with ankylosing spondylitis and may contribute to the fixed forward flexion of the thoracolumbar spine. Fortunately, more effective medical treatment during the active phase of this disease has made this complication infrequent. Several series of osteotomy, usually performed at the thoracolumbar junction, have been reported with reasonably good results in most cases. The surgical correction of any major deformity of the thoracic spine or thoracolumbar junction is a formidable surgical undertaking with significant risk of neurologic impairment.[9,19] In my opinion, the oste-

otomy should be performed via the bilateral posterolateral extracavitary approaches to the spine with intraoperative monitoring by means of either somatosensory evoked potential or interoperative awakening of the patient to evaluate movement and sensation. The relatively new technique of motor-evoked potentials, that is, evaluation of descending pathways, holds promise, but is more difficult technically. It has the advantage of monitoring the function of the anterior aspect of the spinal cord that is usually more vulnerable during the surgical correction. Correction of thoracolumbar spine angulation is a major and hazardous surgical undertaking that should be performed in larger medical centers having specialists in spine surgery.

Lesser degrees of deformity of the thoracic spine causing nerve root compression at the foramen level are rare. In the older patient especially, neoplasia is a more common cause for localized spine pain and radiculopathy. Thoracic disc herniations with cord compression and myelopathy do occur, usually as sporadic cases not associated with arthritic conditions. The signs and symptoms of thoracic disc herniations are highly variable, and diagnosis is often delayed. Usually, the most efficient way to screen the many segments of the thoracic spine for significant deformity causing neural compression is with polytomographic gas myelography. Although effective, this procedure is technically demanding, especially in patients having scoliotic or otherwise deformed spines.

Lumbosacral Spine

During the past 15 years, arthritic deformity of the lumbar spine has been well described clinically and radiologically. Consequently, effective treatment, usually by means of surgical decompression, has become commonly available. Simple uncomplicated lumbar disc ruptures are infrequent in individuals who are over 40 (see Fig. 6–5).[13] The progressive collapse of disc height inevitably leads to facet joint overriding and subsequent arthritis, shortening and thickening of the elastic ligamentum flavum, and osteophyte formation from the joint margins (see Fig. 6–8). The clinical syndrome of neurogenic claudication of the legs secondary to *lumbar spinal stenosis* became commonly recognized in the early 1970s. Diagnostic radiologists then began to use pleuridirectional tomographic scanning in defining the size and shape of the lumbar spinal canal in axial cross section.[18] In the late 1970s, use of high-resolution CT scanning to the lumbar spine rendered tomographic equipment obsolete and made precise diagnosis routinely available.[10] The syndrome of neurogenic claudication with position (extension) or exercise-induced radiculopathy is effectively treated by lumbar laminectomy with removal of the medial portions of the facet joints and attendant hypertrophied ligaments and osteophytes. Several techniques have been described to accomplish this decompression of the nerve roots of the cauda equina.[5] The lumbar spine need not be destabilized, however, by complete removal of facet joints. Surgical undercutting, often aided by the use of high-speed drills, provides neural decompression. This procedure is just as adequate as more radical surgery and allows continued structural support from the lateral and posterior aspects of the facet joints. On rare occasions, the facet joints may be congenitally located so far medially that they must be destabilized. In a few individuals, fusion may be required of either the lateral processes bilaterally[17] or the vertebral bodies utilizing the posterior lumbar interbody fusion or PLIF technique as described by Cloward and others.[2] Generally, the results of correction of osteophytic deformity of the lumbar spine are satisfactory.

Occasionally, patients have an abrupt increase in their physical activity causing poorly tolerated stresses on other bodily systems, most commonly the cardiovascular. A few patients aged 30 to 50 may present with mild disc degenerative and ar-

thritic changes superimposed on a congenitally small spinal canal. Some of these patients have severe degeneration and bulging of all the lumbar discs, requiring extensive laminectomy, sometimes of the entire lumbar spine. However, most surgical patients are in the older age groups, and neoplasia must often be considered in the differential diagnosis. Radionuclide bone scanning, in addition to a detailed general history and physical examination, is routinely performed in the patient over 50.

SURGICAL PROCEDURES[3,16]

Laminectomy

In general, extensive laminectomies are well tolerated provided the facet joints remain to provide stability and support. Reversal of the cervical lordosis or swan-neck deformity has been described. However, with only rare exceptions, these extensive operations are performed in cases of intramedullary tumor where denervation of paraspinous musculature coexists. Nevertheless, any individual in the younger age group, particularly children and adolescents, should have serial cervical spine roentgenograms taken at increasing intervals for several years to ensure that progressive deformity is not developing.

The most frequent complication of laminectomy in the older individual is disruption of the dural membrane with the risk of persistent CSF fistula, pseudomeningocele, and/or infection. The dural sac becomes ectatic with age and must be clearly identified, covered with protective sponges, and gently retracted during decompressive techniques directed to the lateral portions of the spinal canal and the intervertebral foramina. If the dura is torn, one should attempt to repair it with fine nonabsorbable suture material. A few of the patients requiring cervical decompressive laminectomy for stenosis may need further decompression. The dural sac is then opened and the dentate ligaments are sectioned. The intradural contents should be protected by suturing a patch graft of fascia to the entire circumference of the dural defect. There are several descriptions of reconstruction techniques of the laminal arch following intraspinal operative manipulations. These techniques have little if any clinical applicability.

Fusion

Anterior cervical fusion using the technique described by Cloward and others is satisfactory at all cervical levels from C2 to C3 to C7 to T1.[1] The use of dowel grafts in round drill holes as described by Cloward is mechanically unsound, however, and a better fusion can be performed by surgical evacuation of the interspace. This procedure is aided by interspace-spreading retractors to facilitate removal of the entire cartilaginous end-plate. Bone and osteophyte are then removed as necessary to provide adequate neural decompression. Finally, an autogenous bone graft is placed by cross-sectioning the iliac crest. In the thoracic and upper lumbar areas, the fusion is best performed via a posterior-lateral exposure of the vertebral column.[8] In rare cases, a bilateral exposure is required, followed by fixation instrumentation. Direct anterior approaches to the thoracic spine require displacement of viscera and, at the thoracolumbar level, incision and reconstruction of the diaphragm. Increased morbidity accompanies these extensive intracavitary approaches to the spine and they are rarely necessary.

At lower lumbar levels and the lumbosacral level, the posterior lumbar interbody fusion (PLIF procedure) has proved satisfactory.[2] It does require removal of large portions of the facet joint or (occasionally) the entire joint and entails forceful dural sac and nerve root retraction. With anomalous conjoined lumbosacral nerve roots, the high risk of permanent nerve root damage may make this operation infeasible.

Fusions that rely on methyl methacrylate for their structural stability are rarely if ever indicated in nonmalignant disease. Acrylic, even when pins or wires are used, can and frequently does loosen with time. The risk of infection is also increased.

REFERENCES

1. Cloward, R.B.: Anterior approach for removal of ruptured cervical discs. J. Neurosurg., *15*:602–614, 1958.
2. Cloward, R.B.: The treatment of ruptured lumbar intervertebral discs by vertebral body fusion. J. Neurosurg., *10*:154, 1953.
3. Davis, C.H., Jr.: Extradural spinal cord and nerve root compression from benign lesions of the lumbar area. *In* Neurological Surgery. Vol. 4. Edited by J.R. Youmans. Philadelphia, W.B. Saunders Co., 1982, pp. 2533–2655.
4. Dirheimer, Y.: The Cranio-Vertebral Region in Chronic Inflammatory Rheumatic Diseases. New York, Springer-Verlag, 1977.
5. Ehni, G.: Significance of the small lumbar spinal canal: Cauda equina compression syndromes due to spondylosis. I. Introduction. J. Neurosurg., *31*:490–494, 1969.
6. Hall, M.C.: Luschka's Joint. Springfield, Illinois, Charles C Thomas, 1965.
7. Haughton, V., and Williams, A.: Computed Tomography of the Spine. St. Louis, The C.V. Mosby Co., 1982.
8. Larson, S.J.: The lateral extrapleural and extraperitoneal approaches to the thoracic and lumbar spine. *In* Spinal Disorders: Diagnosis and Treatment. Edited by D. Ruge and L.L. Wiltse. Philadelphia, Lea & Febiger, 1977, pp. 137–142.
9. Law, W.A.: Lumbar spinal osteotomy. J. Bone Joint Surg., *41B*:270–278, 1959.
10. Lee, B.C.P., Kaza, E., and Newman, A.D.: Computed tomography of the spine and spinal cord. Radiology, *128*:95–102, 1978.
11. Menezes, A.H., et al.: Craniocervical abnormalities. A comprehensive surgical approach. J. Neurosurg., *53*:444–455, 1980.
12. Menezes, A.H., Graf, J., and Hibri, N.: Abnormalities of the cranio-vertebral junction with cervicomedullary compression. Childs Brain, 7:15–30, 1980.
13. Meyer, G.A., Haughton, V.M., and Williams, A.L.: Diagnosis of herniated lumbar disk with computed tomography. N. Engl. J. Med., *306*:1166–1167, 1979.
14. Murakami, J., et al.: Computed tomography of posterior longitudinal ligament ossification: Its appearance and diagnostic value with special reference to thoracic lesions. J. Comput. Assist. Tomogr., *6*:41–50, 1982.
15. Resnick, D.R., et al.: Association of diffuse idiopathic skeletal hyperostosis (DISH) and calcification and ossifications of the posterior longitudinal ligament. Am. J. Roentgenol., *131*:1049–1053, 1978.
16. Rothman, R.H., and Simeone, F.A. (eds.): The Spine. Vols. 1 and 2. Philadelphia, W.B. Saunders Co., 1975.
17. Schwab, J.P., and Meyer, G.A.: Lumbar fusion. Wis. Med. J., *78*:40–42, 1979.
18. Sheldon, J.J., Russin, L.A., and Gargano, F.P.: Lumbar spinal stenosis. Radiographic diagnosis with special reference to transverse axial tomography. Clin. Orthop., *115*:53, 1976.
19. Smith-Peterson, M.N., Larson, C.B., and Aufranc, O.E.: Osteotomy of the spine for correction of flexion deformity in rheumatoid arthritis. J. Bone Joint Surg., *27A*:1–11, 1945.
20. VanGilder, J.C., and Menezes, A.H.: Craniovertebral junction abnormalities. Clin. Neurosurg., *30*:514–530, 1982.
21. Verbeist, H.: A radicular syndrome from developmental narrowing of the lumbar vertebral canal. J. Bone Joint Surg., *36B*:230, 1954.

Chapter 48

Correction of Arthritic Deformities of the Hip

Richard N. Stauffer

Deformity of the hip joint occurs as a result of a wide variety of arthritic conditions, including degenerative, inflammatory, and infectious diseases. Degenerative disease (osteoarthritis OA) is certainly the most common cause of hip joint disability. This category includes "primary" OA affecting older people, in which no predisposing causative factors can be identified, and "secondary" OA resulting from altered joint mechanics due to previous trauma, osteonecrosis of the femoral head, or various other congenital or developmental conditions of the hip (e.g., congenital hip dysplasia, slipped capital femoral epiphysis, Legg-Calvé-Perthes disease). Because of the broad spectrum of these disease categories, disability due to "arthritis" of the hip may afflict virtually all age groups, though it is most common in persons aged 60 years or over.

On the basis of epidemiologic studies, we estimate that over 100,000 people undergo reconstructive surgery for hip disease in the United States each year. The surgical procedures described for correction of hip deformities can be combined and classified as joint excision, realignment (osteotomy), arthrodesis, or prosthetic arthroplasty.

Historically, reconstructions of the hip were first attempted chiefly for tuberculosis and consisted of various types of joint excision and arthrodesis. In the 1930s, there was great interest in interposition arthroplasty. Various materials (e.g., skin, fascia, Bakelite) were interposed between the acetabulum and femoral head in an attempt to produce a smooth, congruent articulation—without notable success. The development of the mold arthroplasty by Smith Peterson (in which a Vitallium cup was interposed in the joint and provided a "mold" or scaffold for regeneration of fibrocartilage on both acetabular and femoral articular surfaces) represented a major breakthrough in reconstructive hip surgery. This procedure relieved pain, restored joint motion, and maintained stability in a *reasonably* predictable fashion, and became the standard against which other procedures were measured for over 30 years.

Osteotomy of the proximal femur was popular-

ized by Pauwels, and others, as a treatment for some forms of arthritic hip disorders. This technique, which redistributes the mechanical forces acting across the hip joint, has recently gained renewed interest for use in younger individuals.

Prosthetic replacement of the arthritic hip joint began with the use of a Vitallium femoral head prosthesis in 1942. This procedure gained popularity during the 1950s, in spite of two commonly recognized problems: loosening of the prosthetic shaft within the intramedullary canal of the femur, and erosion of the articular surface of the acetabulum by the prosthesis. These problems were addressed by the "landmark" work of Charnley and others in the late 1950s. The problem of prosthetic loosening was combated by the introduction of a self-curing acrylic cement, polymethylmethacrylate, a grouting agent designed to improve fixation between prosthetic component and bone. A prosthetic acetabular component made of high-density polyethylene was added to form a "low-friction" total hip replacement, providing a dramatic breakthrough in improved function and pain relief for individuals disabled by hip diseases. The rate of successful results from prosthetic hip replacement increased from 60 to 70% to over 90%. Clinical and basic investigations in recent years have further refined the design, mechanical function, and materials of prostheses with further improvement in clinical outcome.

The reconstructive surgical procedures currently utilized to treat hip disease are discussed in the following sections.

OSTEOTOMY

Osteotomy is aimed primarily at relieving pain and only secondarily at improving motion. This procedure involves cutting the bone of the proximal femur and realigning the fragments to alter the distribution of forces acting across the hip, or to improve the congruency of the joint. Proximal femoral osteotomies can be grouped into two general categories, angulatory and rotational, which differ somewhat as to rationale and indication.

Angulatory Osteotomy

This procedure consists or removal of a medially or laterally based wedge of bone from the intertrochanteric region of the proximal femur, to produce either a varus or valgus angulation of the femoral neck and head (Figs. 48–1, 48–2). Careful preoperative planning is required to determine the mode (and precise degree) of angulation and to produce the maximum congruency of the arthritic femoral head within the acetabulum. After the osteotomy, the bony fragments are held with some form of internal fixation, either a fixed-angle osteotomy blade plate or a compression screw plate. Partial and progressive weight-bearing with crutches is allowed. Bony union is consistently obtained within 12 weeks.

The rationale for this procedure is that the resulting, improved congruency of the joint alters the distribution of load acting across the hip. Reducing the peak pressures that exist in the arthritic joint may allow for some biologic repair of the articular cartilage (Fig. 48–3). Purely mathematical analysis has indicated that a valgus osteotomy may decrease the magnitude and direction of the compressive load across the hip (see Fig. 48–2). An unusual case in which the primary aim of the procedure was to change the direction of the resultant hip load is shown in Figure 48–4. The pain relief from this procedure has been postulated to be due

to decompression of the increased intraosseous venous pressure noted in osteoarthritis or to an interosseous neurectomy.

Angulatory osteotomy of the proximal femur was a popular form of treatment for the arthritic hip before the advent of total hip replacement. Because recent long-term follow-up studies have aroused grave concern regarding the durability of prosthetic hips, particularly in young people, osteotomy is again becoming more prevalent. Osteotomy has several definite advantages. There is a high incidence of pain relief.[6,7] It is a "conservative" procedure. All bony stock is preserved, making it possible to carry out subsequent surgery (including prosthetic hip replacement or arthrodesis) if necessary. No foreign material is placed in the hip joint. Postoperative disability is minimal, and formal rehabilitation is unnecessary. Its chief disadvantages are inconsistency of pain relief and pain relief of relatively short duration (three to five years) with gradual deterioration of the clinical result until further surgery is required.

The chief indication for angulatory osteotomy of the proximal femur is OA, particularly in a younger (under 50 years) individual. Success depends upon the presence of adequate hip motion (at least 20 degrees of coronal plane motion) and the probability that changing the angular relationship of the femoral head and acetabulum will result in better joint congruency.

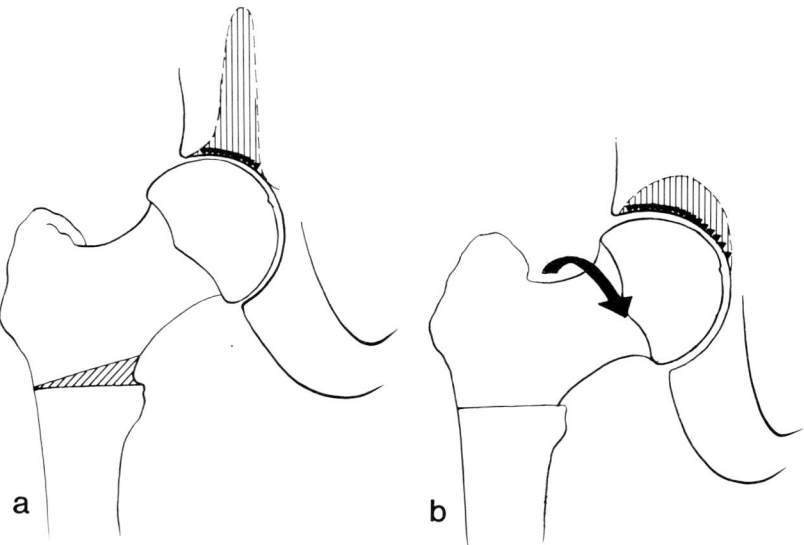

a   b

Fig. 48–1.   Schematic representation of varus osteotomy of the proximal femur. *a*, Shaded area indicates the medially based wedge of bone to be removed from the intertrochanteric area. Degenerative changes in the joint have resulted in a small area of surface contact and high compressive stress levels. *b*, Medial displacement of the femoral shaft and medial (varus) rotation of the femoral head and neck have improved congruency of the articulating surfaces, increased the load-bearing area of the joint, and reduced compression stresses.

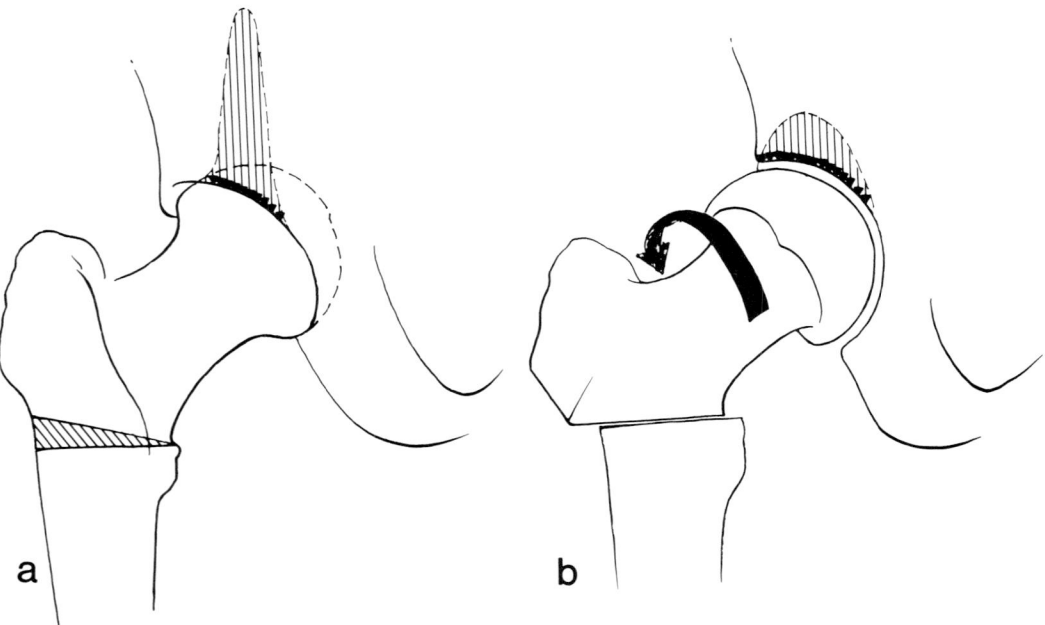

Fig. 48–2. Schematic representation of valgus osteotomy of the proximal femur. *a*, Shaded area indicates the laterally based wedge of bone to be removed from the intertrochanteric area. *b*, Lateral (valgus) rotation of the femoral head and neck. The increased congruity and enlarged surface contact area have reduced the compression stresses across the joint.

Results are difficult to evaluate objectively because the chief aim is to relieve pain—a subjective parameter. Of 103 hips followed for more than one year after varus or valgus osteotomy, 83 had satisfactory pain relief, and 20 had fair or poor results.[14] In another study of 59 consecutive osteotomies, followed for an average of 2½ years, in which clinical evaluation criteria included improved range of hip motion, need for assistive gait devices, resolution of degenerative changes on roentgenograms, and pain relief, 47 (80%) were satisfactory and 12 (20%) proved unsatisfactory.[19] Pain relief closely paralleled the roentgenographic findings of increased joint space, and resolution of body sclerosis, marginal osteophytes, and subchondral cysts.

Bombelli has been largely responsible for the increased interest in angulatory osteotomy for osteoarthritis of the hip.[6,7] Of 170 osteotomies followed for over 10 years, 76% had good or excellent long-term pain relief and function. Improved range of hip motion was inconsistent. Several authors have noted a gradual deterioration of the pain relief obtained by this procedure. In one report, 74% of patients were pain-free at one year postoperatively, but only 45% at 5 years.[13] In another series, only 25% of patients still had pain relief after 10 years.[40]

Complications include problems encountered with any major hip surgical procedure, i.e., cardiopulmonary disorders, thromboembolic disease, urinary retention, infection, delayed wound healing, hematoma, as well as two unique complications. Nonunion of the osteotomy site has been reported to range from 0 to 18%. An internal fixation device allowing compression of the osteotomy site greatly reduces the incidence of nonunion. The fixation device itself, however, often leads to another problem: irritation of the soft tissues and bursal formation in the trochanteric area. In one series, 17% of patients required eventual removal of the compression device because of localized lateral hip discomfort.[40] Because the angulatory osteotomy is performed in the intertrochanteric area, there is little danger of compromise of the extraosseous arterial blood supply to the femoral head, and avascular necrosis has not been reported as a complication.

Rotational Osteotomy

The search continues for a satisfactory surgical treatment for (avascular) osteonecrosis of the femoral head, which so frequently affects young individuals. Osteonecrosis arises as a result of compromise of the intraosseous blood supply of the femoral head from various causes (see Table 86–1). Treatment by angulatory osteotomy has been dis-

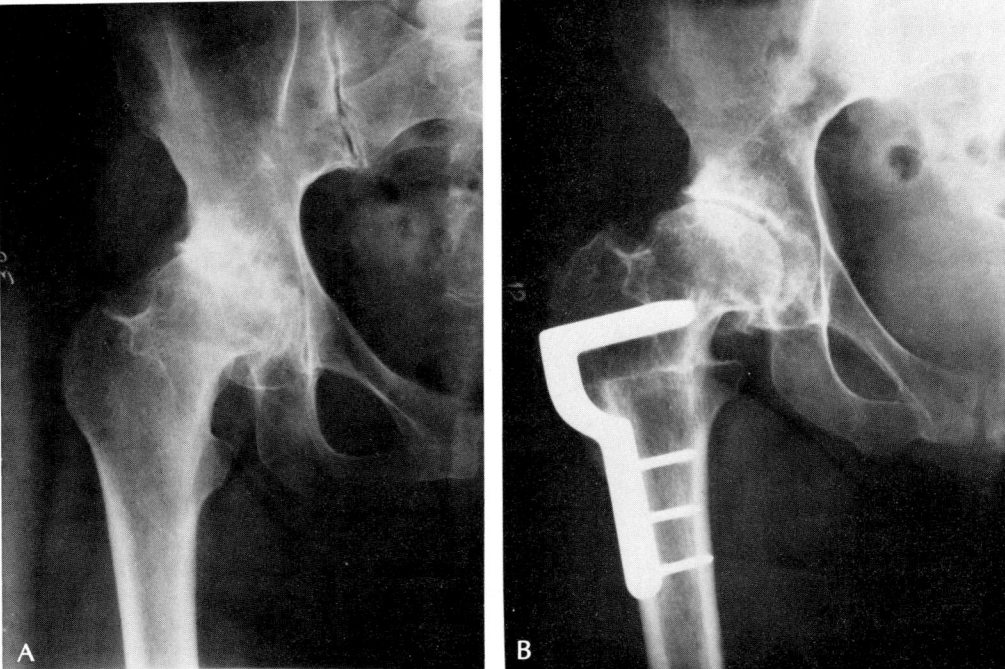

Fig. 48–3.   Roentgenographic appearance of a degenerative hip joint before and after angulatory (varus) osteotomy of the proximal femur. *A*, Degenerative arthritis of the hip in a 61-year-old man. *B*, Two and one-half years after varus osteotomy. Note the definite "widening" of the joint space, and some resolution of the degenerative sclerosis and cysts. The patient had excellent relief of hip pain.

appointing.[18] Sugioka has popularized a rotational osteotomy of the femoral head and neck.[37,38] In this procedure, the avascular segment of the femoral head, most commonly the anterior-superior portion, is rotated anteriorly, away from the area of maximum compressive loading of the joint, preventing further collapse of the segment and allowing revascularization and repair of the necrotic bone.

This procedure is technically demanding. The osteotomy is performed through the intertrochanteric area, distal to the base of the femoral neck (Fig. 48–5). Complete or circumferential division of the joint capsule is necessary. Great care is required to avoid damage to the ascending branch of the medial circumflex artery, inferiorly and posteriorly. The femoral head and neck are rotated anteriorly 50 to 70 degrees while the necrotic portion of the head is placed anterior to the weight-bearing area of the joint. Internal fixation may be achieved by various devices, most commonly a sliding compression screw plate (Fig. 48–6). Postoperatively, active range of motion exercises are started within 10 days, and non-weight-bearing ambulation with crutches is maintained for 8 to 12 weeks, followed by graduation to full weight-bearing by 6 months.

Approximately 80% relief of pain and prevention of collapse of the necrotic segment was found in one series of 100 hips followed for 2 to 7 years postoperatively.[37] The best results were obtained in those hips operated upon in the early stages of the disease process. Fully 91% excellent results occurred in hips graded state I or II (see Chap. 86), before marked collapse of the femoral head or narrowing of the joint space occurred. Hips with an extensive area of necrotic involvement showed a higher failure rate; if over two-thirds of the femoral heads were involved, 46% failed. Bilateral hip involvement showed a high failure rate (43%) also. The poor results with bilateral hip involvement can perhaps be explained by the difficulty in maintaining postoperative non-weight-bearing with crutches after both hips have undergone osteotomy.

The indication for rotational osteotomy of the femoral head and neck is avascular necrosis in a relatively young individual. Contraindications are end-stage disease with collapse of the head and degenerative changes in the acetabulum (Ficat grades III and IV),[23] more than two-thirds avascular involvement of the femoral head, and bilateral hip disease.

Still unpublished reports of experience with rotational osteotomy do not support the initial enthu-

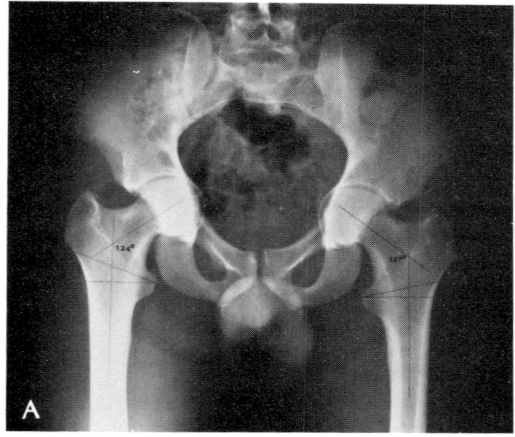

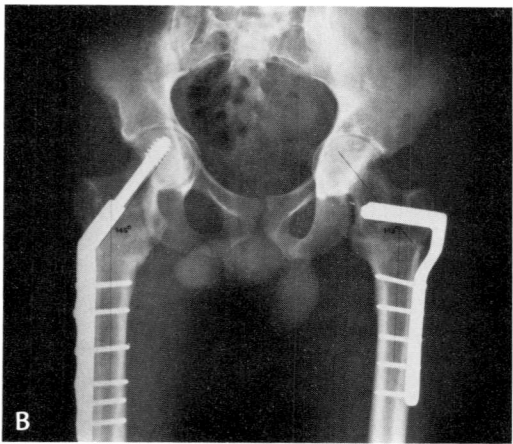

Fig. 48–4. Roentgenographic appearance of bilateral valgus osteotomies performed for protrusio acetabuli. *A*, Preoperative hip roentgenogram of a 21-year-old man with bilateral hip pain. No metabolic cause for the unusual and severe protrusion of the acetabula could be determined. The only structural abnormality was the decreased neck-shaft angle (normal is 135 degrees). This condition is presumably the result of a developmental anomaly (coxa vara) of the hips, which resulted in an increased horizontal inclination of the resultant load acting on the hip, and gradual medial protrusion of the acetabula caused by bone remodeling. *B*, Postoperative hip roentgenograms one year after bilateral valgus osteotomies. The patient's hip pain was dramatically reduced. Careful long-term follow-up will be necessary, however, to evaluate remodeling of the acetabula and possible improvement of the protrusion.

siasm. Gartland et al. reported successful results in about two-thirds of cases at one to two years, but in 12 patients followed for over three years, deterioration was progressive, and only four cases were still rated as satisfactory.[25] Most of the unsatisfactory results after three years were in patients with corticosteroid-related avascular necrosis. Ca-

banela followed 17 hips in 16 patients for 6 to 24 months.[10] Eight hips showed a good clinical result judged by pain relief, range of motion, and ability to perform daily activities; results were fair in three hips and poor in six. Radionuclide scintigrams of the femoral heads still showed complete avascularity after the osteotomy, with no improvement with time in most cases.

Complications encountered after rotational osteotomy include those general and local problems attendant to any major hip surgical procedure. Occasional delayed unions of the osteotomy site, but no nonunion, have been reported. The procedure is technically difficult, controversial, and still in the evaluation stage. Other treatment modalities currently in clinical trial for the troublesome problem of avascular necrosis of the femoral head in young people are drilling and decompression of the avascular segment, and electrical stimulation by various techniques (see Chap. 86).

ARTHRODESIS

Arthrodesis of the hip was reportedly first performed by Albert in 1885. Over the past century, this procedure has been used primarily for hip joints destroyed by sepsis. However, for the past several decades, it has been employed more commonly to treat disability caused by post-traumatic degenerative disease in the young individual. With the realization that prosthetic arthroplasty has a limited durability with unacceptable long-term results in youthful, active individuals, hip arthrodesis has enjoyed increasing popularity. Although the idea of arthrodesis or "permanent stiffening" of the hip joint, is often difficult for a patient to accept, it is often the best treatment alternative available, particularly in the young, male laborer with disabling, unilateral post-traumatic hip disease.

Many techniques for hip arthrodesis have been described. These include various intra-articular, extra-articular, and combined methods, with and without internal fixation, and with and without adjunctive bone grafts. The reported pseudarthrosis rate for all these procedures was about 25%. The most common technique now employed is an intra-articular arthrodesis using a "cobra-head" compression plate (Fig. 48–7). This device provides rigid fixation across the joint, and pseudarthrosis rates approach zero.[3] Although this plate is somewhat malleable and can be conformed to the bony contours across the hip, some form of medial displacement of the femoral head is generally necessary. This can be accomplished by medial displacement innominate osteotomy, displacement of the femoral head through the medial wall of the acetabulum, or extensive reaming of the femoral head.

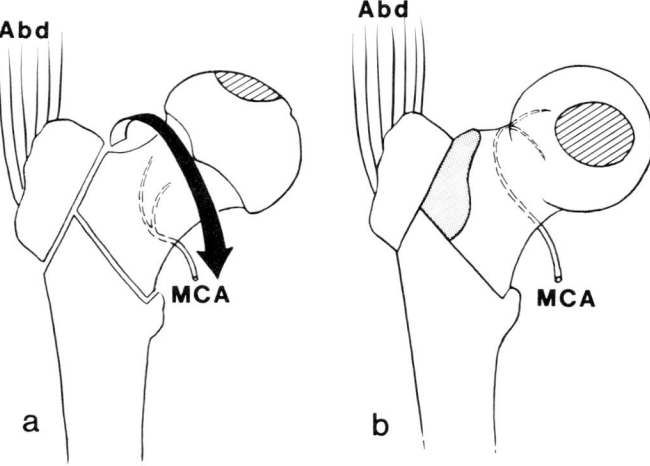

Fig. 48–5. Schematic technique of rotational osteotomy of the femoral head and neck for avascular necrosis.[37,38] *a,* The greater trochanter is osteotomized and retracted in a cephalad direction with the abductor musculature (Abd) attached. The ascending branch of the medial femoral circumflex artery (MCA) is carefully dissected and protected. The joint capsule is incised circumferentially near its distal attachment to the base of the femoral neck. The osteotomy is performed through the intertrochanteric area, perpendicular to the axis of the femoral neck. The shaded portion represents the area of avascular necrosis, which is generally in the superior and slightly anterior portion of the femoral head. *b,* After osteotomy, the femoral head and neck are rotated 50 to 70 degrees anteriorly (along with the principal blood supply to the femoral head—the MCA), thus delivering the necrotic portions well anterior to the area of maximum compression loading of the hip.

Although some degree of shortening of the extremity is inevitable with hip arthrodesis, it should be kept to a minimum, no more than 1 to 2 cm, if possible. The recommended position of fusion is 30 degrees of flexion, neutral abd-adduction, and 5 to 10 degrees of external rotation. Postoperative immobilization in a plaster spica body cast, incorporating the trunk and the operated thigh, for 8 to 12 weeks is recommended, but may not be necessary with a cooperative patient. Partial weight-bearing with crutches is started at about 2 weeks postoperatively, with full weight-bearing allowed at 10 to 12 weeks.

The primary indications for hip arthrodesis are destruction of the joint by sepsis (pyogenic or tuberculous infection), Charcot arthropathy, or disabling unilateral degenerative disease, particularly in the youthful, active male laborer. The procedure is less desirable in the young female patient because of imposed functional difficulties associated with sexual intercourse and child-bearing. Avascular necrosis of the femoral head is a relative contraindication, especially if there is extensive involvement of the head with necrotic, nonviable bone, because the disease process is frequently bilateral. D'Aubigne reported a 50% pseudarthrosis rate for hip arthrodesis performed for this condition.[18] Arthrodesis of the rheumatoid hip should be avoided,

because of the accompanying disease of the opposite hip and other lower extremity joints.

The long-term results reported with hip arthrodesis depend largely on achievement of ideal position of fusion and the integrity of other lower extremity joints. One report of 23 patients with unilateral hip fusion, followed for 10 to 30 years, showed that 21 were working regularly and leading active, vigorous lives.[11] Most were entirely satisfied with the long-term results of surgery, although over half experienced a discernible limp, and one-third had difficulty sitting. Nearly half reported difficulties with low back pain, and a few patients had pain in the ipsilateral knee or contralateral hip.

Gore et al. studied the gait mechanics of men with unilateral hip fusions.[27] Their gait was slower than normal, asymmetrical, and arrhythmic, as might be expected. Several compensatory gait mechanisms were adopted by these patients, including increased rotation and flexion of the pelvis (i.e., increased motion of the lumbar spine), increased motion of the contralateral hip, and increased flexion of the ipsilateral knee during stance phase. Because all these compensatory gait alterations impose increased stresses on the low back and other lower extremity joints, they are likely responsible for an increased rate of degenerative change in these areas over the years.

Operative complications, in addition to those

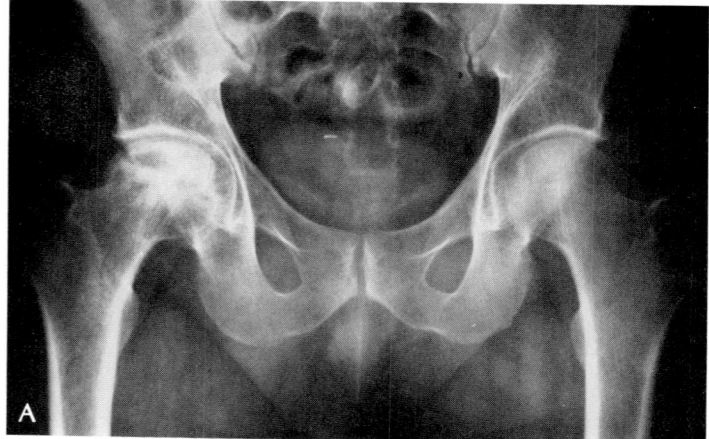

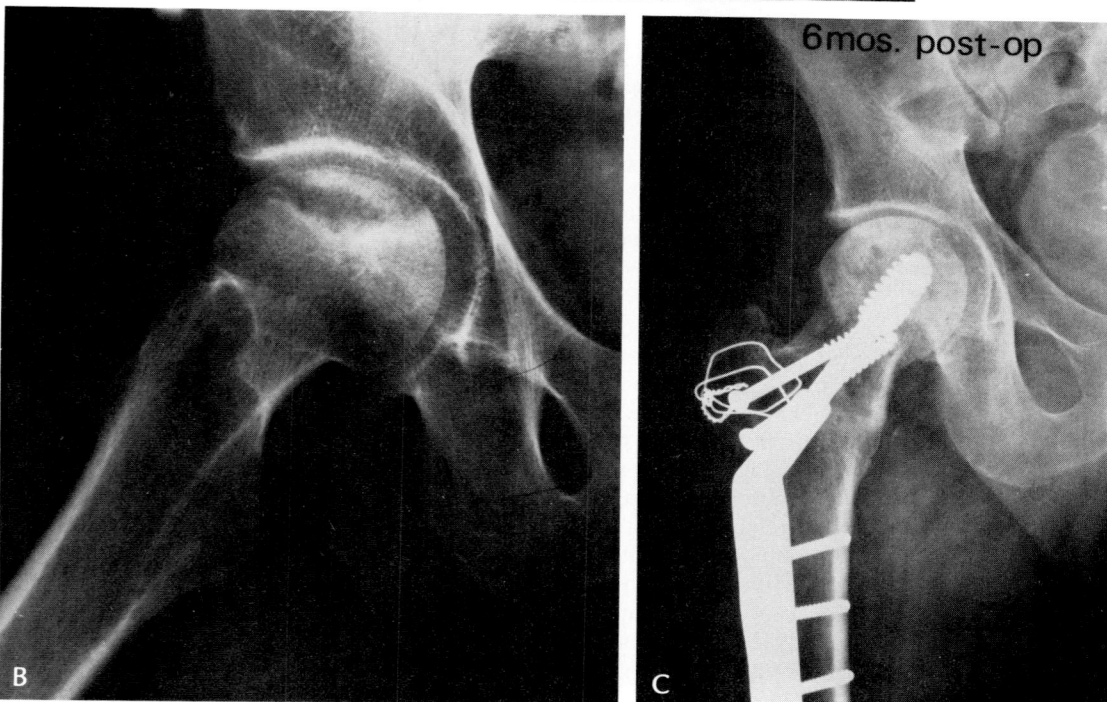

Fig. 48–6. Roentgenograms of a 36-year-old man with avascular necrosis of the right femoral head, before and after rotational osteotomy. *A*, Preoperative anteroposterior roentgenogram. Necrotic area occupies about one-third of the femoral head. There has been a slight collapse of the necrotic segment, but good preservation of the articular cartilage (normal joint "space"). *B*, Lateral preoperative roentgenogram. The necrotic segment is superior and slightly anterior. *C*, Postoperative (six months) anteroposterior roentgenogram showing bony union of the osteotomy. Fixation was achieved with a compression screw plate and two ancillary screws (to prevent rotation of the head-neck segment). The trochanteric fragment was held in place with a wire.

common to all major hip surgery procedures, include long-term degenerative disease of other joints and fracture of the femur; this latter complication has been reported in several series. Arthrodesis of the hip creates a long-rigid body segment from the lumbosacral joint to the knee. Because torsional or bending loads cannot be absorbed by the hip joint,

fracture of the femur is therefore more likely to result from a fall or twisting injury. Most series of hip fusions have a 10 to 20% incidence of pseudarthrosis, but use of newer techniques, such as medial displacement of the femoral head, and the cobra-head plate for internal fixation, have significantly reduced this complication. No nonunions

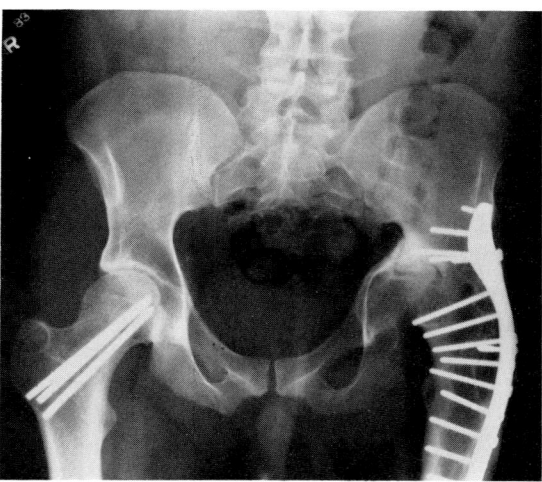

Fig. 48–7. Anteroposterior roentgenogram of a 35-year-old man three years after a compression arthrodesis of the left hip for degenerative disease secondary to slipped capital femoral epiphysis (note previous pin fixation for a similar, but less severe problem in right hip). The hip arthrodesis is solid, but the discerning observer will note an unusual serpentine stress fracture through the medial acetabular portion of the hip. The patient is currently under treatment with spica cast immobilization and an external induction-type electrical stimulator.

occurred in a series of 16 patients treated with these newer techniques.[3]

Conversion of a failed total hip arthroplasty to arthrodesis is possible when remaining bone stock is insufficient to permit reinsertion of prosthetic components, or when leaving a young patient with an unstable girdle stone-type hip is undesirable.[32] This procedure is technically difficult and requires adjunctive bone grafting and a cobra-head plate for firm fixation. It also generally results in considerable shortening of the extremity.

Conversely, conversion of an arthrodesed hip to a total arthroplasty is also possible.[8] This procedure is not particularly difficult, but depends upon the integrity of the abductor musculature and the absence of active sepsis. Conversion of an arthrodesed hip is most often indicated because of long-standing low back or ipsilateral knee pain, which occurs particularly with a malpositioned hip fusion. Rehabilitation is often prolonged compared to other total hip patients. Generally, crutch walking is necessary for six months until the abductor muscles are strong enough to prevent a limp. Satisfactory results with an average range of hip flexion of 76 degrees were found in 31 of 33 patients whose arthrodesed hips were converted to total hip arthroplasties.

PROSTHETIC HIP REPLACEMENT

A variety of prosthetic devices are currently used to replace arthritic hips. These devices are discussed here with those procedures that replace only the femoral side of the joint with no surgical alteration of the acetabulum (hemiarthroplasty) and those that involve replacement of both sides of the hip (total hip replacement).

Hemiarthroplasty

There are two generic types of prosthetic replacement of only the femoral side of the joint. The first, in use for over 40 years, involves implantation of a metallic prosthesis that replaces the head and neck of the femur with fixation by a stem that fits into the medullary canal. In the past 15 years, however, the prosthesis stem has been fixed in the medullary canal with methylmethacrylate to combat loosening (Fig. 48–8). Whether this "cement" fixation is necessary or improves the result is still being debated. The acetabulum is not surgically altered with this type of prosthesis, but careful "sizing" of the prosthesis is necessary to provide a congruent fit. A poorly fitting prosthetic femoral head may result in joint instability and

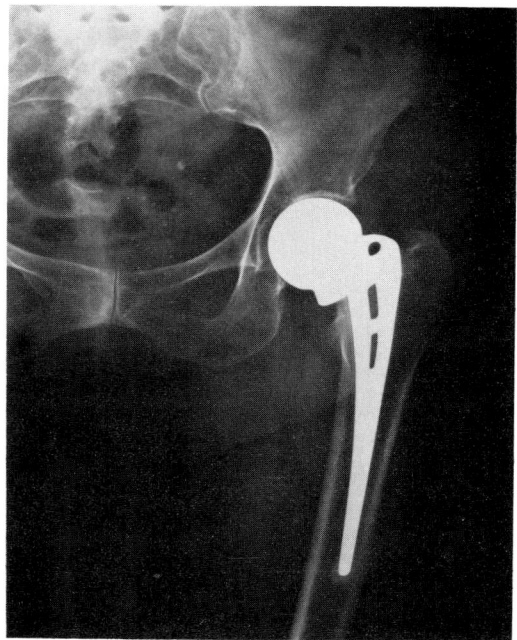

Fig. 48–8. Anteroposterior roentgenogram of a 78-year-old woman who had a femoral head prosthesis (Austin-Moore type) inserted two years previously for a displaced femoral neck fracture. Narrowing of the joint "space" superomedially indicates erosion of the prosthesis through the articular cartilage. The patient was experiencing progressive hip pain.

''point contact'' with increased localized loading and subsequent erosion of the articular cartilage of the acetabulum.[20]

The bipolar type of prosthesis consists of a metallic femoral component, generally fixed into the medullary canal with methylmethacrylate, which is ''snap fitted'' into a high-density polyethylene socket, surrounded by a metallic shell (Fig. 48–9). The rationale behind this design is that it permits motion at both the femoral head polyethylene bearing and the interface between the metal shell and the articular cartilage of the acetabulum, but both clinical and basic laboratory studies have shown that little motion actually occurs within the acetabulum because of the larger frictional properties of that interface.[33] The other theoretical advantage of this design is that later conversion into a total hip replacement is possible. Should the patient develop pain because of erosion of acetabular cartilage, the acetabular component may be replaced by one that is compatible with the femoral component and that is then cemented into the pelvis.

A prospective comparison of these two types of hip hemiarthroplasty has not yet been done, and both have their proponents. However, the indications for both types appear to be the same, namely, avascular necrosis of the femoral head, or displaced (Garden type III or IV) fracture of the femoral neck,

nonunion of femoral neck fractures, or certain arthritic diseases of the hip joint in which the acetabular cartilage has been relatively spared. Both procedures can be performed with minimal operating/anesthesia time because reaming, preparation, and cementing of the acetabulum, as in total hip replacement, are unnecessary. In addition, time is often an important factor with hip surgery in frail, elderly patients.

Disadvantages include significant problems with residual hip pain, acetabular erosion, or protrusion, and femoral stem loosening.[5,17,41] The causes of these problems include the high frictional torque between the acetabular cartilage and the large, metallic head, excessive shear forces acting across the articular cartilage with joint motion, decreased damping of high-frequency vibration (loss of shock absorption) across the joint, and uneven loading patterns due to mismatching of the radius of curvature of the acetabulum and femoral head.

The bipolar hip replacement prosthesis was developed in the early 1970s in an attempt to obviate at least some of these problems.[4,26] It was thought that the use of a small head size (22 mm) and a metal to polyethylene bearing surface, and the provision of compound motion between the inner and outer bearing surfaces, would decrease the frictional torque and high shear stress on the acetabular

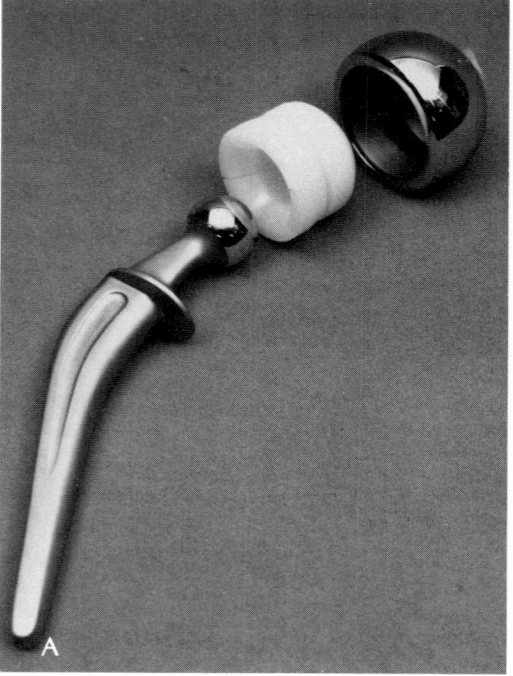
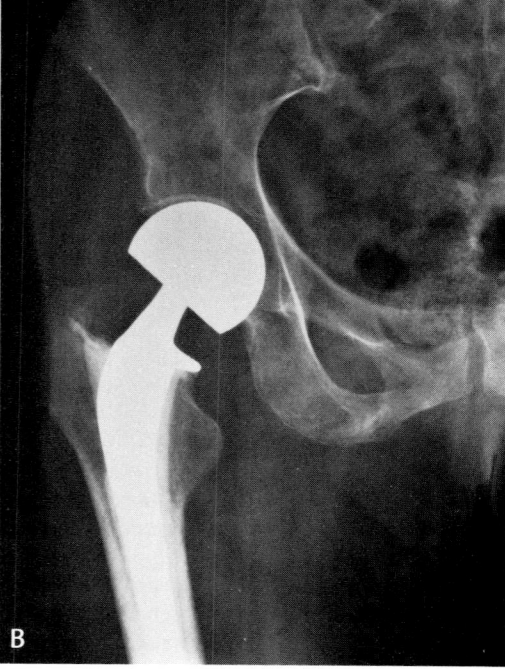

Fig. 48–9. Appearance of the bipolar hip prosthesis. *A,* Photograph of disarticular components of bipolar hip prosthesis. *B,* Roentgenographic appearance of bipolar hip prosthesis. The femoral component is cemented in place. The acetabular component is free to rotate within the pelvis.

cartilage and increase the damping characteristics of the joint, and that cementing of the femoral component would decrease the loosening problem.

Unfortunately, several other problems inherent in the design features of the bipolar device have come to light, including both outer and inner bearing separation and dislocation, and fracture of the polyethylene bearing.[22] In addition, acetabular erosion and wear, while less common with the bipolar prosthesis, have also been reported. The older designs showed a marked tendency for the acetabular component to drift into a varus position, thereby increasing the risk of dislocation or component fracture. More recent designs have largely eliminated these problems by provision of an eccentric offset between the center of the inner head and outer component.[2] This "positive eccentricity" causes the acetabular component to assume a valgus position with vertical loading of the hip.

Because of differences in patient age, preoperative diagnosis, and length of follow-up, it is difficult to compare the reported clinical results with these two types of hip hemiarthroplasty. They appear to be similar. Both offer good pain relief for the minimally ambulatory, relatively inactive, elderly individual with an acute or ununited femoral neck fracture. Results are considerably poorer for those with osteonecrosis of the femoral head or osteoarthritis, or for relatively youthful, active individuals.[5,9] Persistent hip pain and revision to total hip arthroplasty are common among these patients.

Total Hip Replacement

This procedure involves prosthetic substitution for both the femoral (metallic component) and acetabular (high-density polyethylene component) joints, producing a "low-friction" arthroplasty. Although a large number of prosthetic types are currently used (that differ to some degree in design and materials), there are two basic generic types that differ in principle. The *"conventional" total hip replacement* (THR) employs a femoral component with a stem that is fixed into the medullary canal of the femur (Fig. 48–10). The *surface replacement* type employs a metal "cap," which is fixed onto the femoral head (Fig. 48–11).

The latter type was originally developed in an attempt to obviate the problem of loosening of the "conventional" type of femoral component stem. Its proponents believed it might be useful for the younger individual with disabling disease of the hip because such patients had a high incidence of component loosening. They reasoned that if the surface type device should fail for any reason other than sepsis, adequate femoral bone stock remained to allow revision to a conventional type THR.

The surface replacement total hip enjoyed pop-

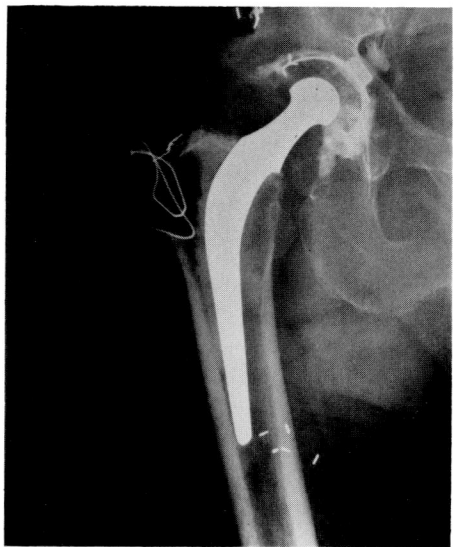

Fig. 48–10. Anteroposterior roentgenogram of basic Charnley total hip replacement five years postoperatively. Note the slight varus position of the femoral component, the poor cement filling along the medial-distal aspect of the femoral stem, and the large intramedullary canal of the femur, which is poorly "filled" by the thin stem of the femoral component. All these factors are associated with a high rate of component loosening. The 1-mm "line" between the proximal-lateral aspect of the femoral component and the prosthesis indicates some loosening of the prosthesis in the cement. This patient, however, was completely pain-free.

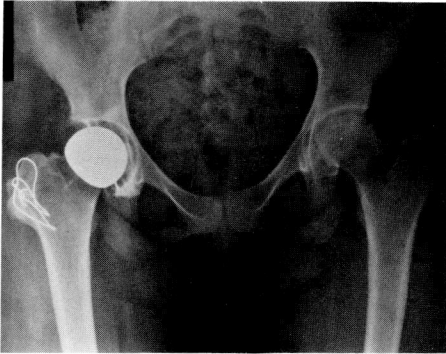

Fig. 48–11. Anteroposterior roentgenogram of a surface replacement type of THR. This patient was a 21-year-old girl with degenerative hip disease secondary to epiphyseal dysplasia. She has no signs of prosthetic loosening at five years after the operation.

ularity for several years, starting in the late 1970s. Hip function and pain relief were excellent and equivalent to conventional THR, but several reports indicating major problems with component loosening have led to its virtual abandonment.[24,29,30] Failure rates have been reported of up to 34%, even over the short term (two years), owing to loosening of the femoral component with or without avascular necrosis of the underlying femoral head, fracture of the femoral neck distal to the margin of the cup, and loosening of the acetabular component. The latter appears to be caused by the large frictional torque transmitted to the thin-walled acetabular component by the femoral component of necessarily large diameter.[34] Revision to a conventional THR has often proved difficult because of the enormous amount of bone stock lost as a result of loosening of the large acetabular component. Failure rates have been higher in osteonecrosis, in inflammatory arthritis, and in younger patients.[1] Design and materials modifications may possibly reduce or eliminate component loosening, but for the present this technique has little to recommend it.

Conventional total hip replacement (THR) provided a major "breakthrough" in reconstructive hip surgery. Patients may expect greater than a 90% chance of virtually complete relief of pain and restoration of near normal hip function. As already indicated, approximately 100,000 THRs per year are performed in the United States. The cost/benefit ratio has been found to be about 2.7 to 1.0 (6 to 1 under age 59 years, and 2.1 to 1 from 60 to 69 years).[31] No monetary benefits are estimated in patients over 70 years of age, but improvement in the *quality* of life for these elderly, retired people is undeniable and cannot be measured in monetary terms.

THR was instituted in the United States in the late 1960s, utilizing the basic principles developed by the late Sir John Charnley (see Fig. 48–10). Since then, clinical and laboratory investigations have led to a gradual evolution in design and materials of the prosthetic devices and to improvements in surgical techniques. Currently, most THR devices include a femoral component with a stem of large cross-sectional area, a collar (to provide contact and stress transmission to the calcar femorale), a neck-shaft angle of about 130 degrees, and a head diameter varying from 22 to 32 mm (see Fig. 48–12). Materials most currently used include Vitallium and titanium alloys. The acetabular component is of high-density polyethylene with an outside diameter varying from 44 to 52 mm. A metal shell or "backing" of the acetabular component has been advocated.[28] "Stiffening" of the acetabular component by addition of the metallic shell may reduce the stress transmitted to the

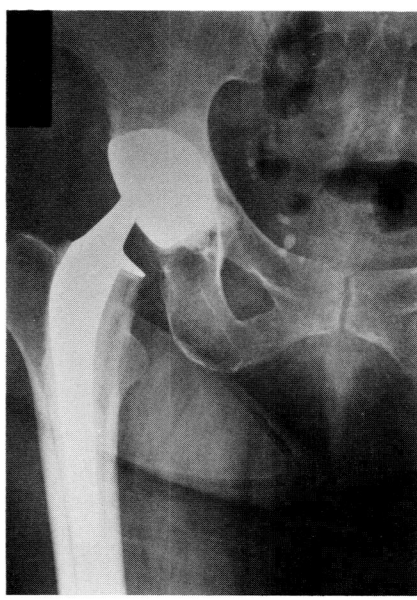

Fig. 48–12. Anteroposterior roentgenogram of a total hip replacement typical of current design and surgical technique. In comparison to Figure 48–10, note the larger stem and supporting "collar" of the femoral component, better filling (due to "pressurization and plugging") of the intramedullary canal with cement, and the metal-backed acetabular component. Osteotomy of the greater trochanter was not performed.

bone and may decrease the incidence of component loosening, but this possibility remains to be proved by long-term clinical experience.

An anterolateral hip incision and exposure without removing the greater trochanter are usual. Meticulous preparation of bony surfaces, including pressurized lavage ("water-picking") to remove blood and debris, followed by thorough drying, and pressurization of cement (i.e., polymethylmethacrylate) all improve the fixation characteristics of the bone-cement interface. Pressurization is accomplished by plugging the medullary canal of the femur, thus creating a closed space, and using a cement "syringe" to deliver the cement in a low-viscosity state.

Current postoperative management consists of bedrest for four days, followed by gait-training and partial, progressive weight-bearing with crutches for two to three months. The average hospitalization is about 12 days. Broad-spectrum antibiotic coverage, instituted during surgery and continued for 48 hours postoperatively, has been shown to significantly reduce the infection rate. Prophylactic anticoagulation (using aspirin, sodium warfarin or low-dose heparin), begun either before or shortly after surgery, greatly reduces the risk of thromboembolic complications.

Indications for THR include degenerative (either primary or secondary) or rheumatoid arthritis and avascular necrosis of the femoral head if there is complete collapse of the head and acetabular involvement. Contraindications include active sepsis, inadequate bony "stock" of either the pelvis or femur, and neuromuscular disease with imbalance of muscular forces acting across the hip (especially weakness of the abductor muscles, which might result in prosthetic dislocation). Young, active patients with a normal life expectancy also constitute a relative contraindication because of the certainty of eventual prosthetic loosening.[12,21]

Complications occur in more than 30% of patients undergoing total hip replacement.[15] The more serious of these complications and their approximate incidence, as gathered from the literature, are listed in Table 48–1. In-hospital mortality is most often due to fatal pulmonary embolism, myocardial infarction, or cardiac failure. Deep infections occur as an early complication in only 0.1 to 0.3%, but many cases of deep infection, generally due to anaerobic or other organisms of low virulence, only become clinically obvious one to three years postoperatively. A few cases of infection occurring five years postoperatively have been reported. These complications are presumably caused by hematogenous "seeding" of the hip from a distant focus. Perioperative antibiotics have been shown conclusively to lower the incidence of deep infection. Modification of the operating room environment with, for example, horizontal laminar air flow, helmet-aspirator surgical attire, and ultraviolet radiation may also reduce infection rates.

The incidence of thromboembolic disease following THR depends upon the sophistication of diagnostic techniques used. Clinically obvious thrombophlebitis occurs in fewer than 5% of patients, but when venograms or radioisotope techniques are employed, this complication may be detected in over 50% of patients. Pulmonary emboli occur clinically in about 2% but when pulmonary arteriography or lung ventilation-perfusion scans are performed, they are found in 6 to 8%. Most of these patients are asymptomatic.

Dislocation of the prosthetic components is a complication that is, to a large extent, under the control of the surgeon. Posterior dislocation of the femoral head is the most common and is generally due to malpositioning (i.e., excessive retroversion) of the acetabular component. Other causes include weakness or detachment of the abductor musculature. A lower incidence of dislocation has been found with the anterolateral approach, as opposed to the posterior or lateral transtrochanteric surgical approaches.[42] Closed reduction, followed by maintenance of an abducted position of the hip in bed for 10 to 14 days with an abductor orthosis for ambulation for 8 to 12 weeks, is often successful in preventing redislocation. When revision surgery is necessary, repeated or chronic dislocation occurs in about one-third of cases.

Heterotopic bone, which may form in response to soft tissue injury, tends to be a frequent occurrence in some individuals. Heterotopic bone formation is found, to some degree, in about 30% of THR patients, but it is severe, limiting range of hip motion, and compromising the functional result, in only 3 to 5%. It occurs more frequently in ankylosing spondylitis, in Paget's disease, and in men with the hypertrophic type of osteoarthritis. It is recommended that these high-risk patients be treated prophylactically, either with low-dose irradiation[16] (2,000 rads administered in 10 divided doses beginning four to five days postoperatively), or with diphosphonates (given orally for three months postoperatively). The former therapy is effective in preventing the formation of bone matrix (i.e., osteoid) in soft tissues about the hip; the latter prevents mineralization of any matrix that has formed.

Early concerns regarding wear of the polyethylene acetabular component have proved unfounded. Long-term follow-up studies have demonstrated wear rates of only about 0.07 mm per year. Significant wear (greater than 2 mm) detected on roentgenograms is present in fewer than .05% of cases 10 years postoperatively.[36] The apparent "wear" observed actually represents plastic deformation (creep or cold flow) of the polyethylene in most cases.

The primary long-term complication of THR, and a matter of great concern, is loosening of the prosthetic components within the bone. Loosening appears to be due to the inability of the polymethylmethacrylate (cement), a brittle material, to withstand the repetitive loading imposed by functional use of the joint over a long period. Although bone

Table 48–1. Early Complications of Total Hip Replacement

Complication	Reported Incidence (%)
Mortality	0.4
Infection	1.0
Thrombophlebitis	3.4
Pulmonary embolism	2.2
Nerve palsy	<1.0
Arterial injury	0.2
Prosthetic dislocation	3.0
Severe heterotopic bone formation	<5.0

cement at first appeared ideal in providing rigid fixation of the prosthetic components, it now seems the obvious "weak link" leading to long-term failure. Ten-year follow-up studies show loosening of the femoral component in 30 to 50% of cases.[35,36,39] Factors associated with high rates of femoral loosening include: heavy patients who are active, male sex, large-diameter femoral canal, varus positioning of the component, cross-sectional characteristics of the component stem (e.g., thin stem, sharp corners), and poor cement technique. Most instances of femoral component loosening occur by five years postoperatively, with some "equilibration" thereafter (i.e., few cases of femoral loosening appear between five and ten years postoperatively).

Acetabular component loosening is found in 10 to 20% of patients by ten years,[35,36,39] most often in younger patients (under 60 years) and in those with rheumatoid arthritis and protrusio acetabuli. This complication is associated with thin-walled polyethylene components and large-diameter prosthetic femoral heads, both of which increase the frictional torque transmitted to the bone-cement interface of the acetabulum. The rate of acetabular loosening appears to be linear with time, doubling between five and ten years postoperatively. This complication may well prove to be the most common cause of THR failure 12 to 15 years after operation.

Revision of THR surgery is most often required because of component loosening. Two reports employing standard actuarial methods of statistical analysis indicate that the probability of the Charnley THR components "surviving" 10 years without requiring revision is 88 and 94%.[36,39]

The improved component designs and materials and the surgical techniques that have evolved over the past decade should provide evidence of lower loosening rates in the future. Further refinements now under investigation include the use of more flexible stems on the femoral component, and elimination of cement used for component fixation by providing porous coatings that allow for direct bony ingrowth. The bone ingrowth/prosthesis interface should provide stable long-term fixation for the lifetime of the patient.

REFERENCES

1. Amstutz, J.C., et al.: Surface replacement of the hip with the Tharies system. J. Bone Joint Surg., 63A:1069, 1981.
2. Averill, R.: New concept in femoral head replacement: Mechanics of the device. Bull. Hosp. Joint Dis., 38:1, 1977.
3. Barmada, R., Abraham, E., and Ray, R.D.: Hip fusion utilizing the cobra head plate. J. Bone Joint Surg., 58A:541, 1976.
4. Bateman, J.E.: Experience with a multi-bearing implant in reconstruction for hip deformities. Orthop. Trans., 1:242, 1977.
5. Beckenbaugh, R.D., Tressler, H.A., and Johnson, E.W., Jr.: Results after hemiarthroplasty of the hip using a cemented femoral prosthesis. Mayo Clin. Proc., 52:349, 1977.
6. Bombelli, R.: Osteoarthritis of the Hip, 2nd Ed. New York, Springer-Verlag, 1983.
7. Bombelli, R., Arsizio, B., and Santore, R.F.: Ten year results of intertrochanteric osteotomy for osteoarthritis of the hip. Presented at 50th meeting of the American Academy of Orthopaedic Surgeons, Anaheim, California, 1983.
8. Brewster, R.C., Coventry, M.B., and Johnson, E.W., Jr.: Conversion of the arthrodesed hip to a total hip arthroplasty. J. Bone Joint Surg., 57A:27, 1975.
9. Cabanela, M.E.: Experience with bipolar femoral head replacement. Unpublished data.
10. Cabanela, M.E.: Experience with Sugioka rotational osteotomy for treatment of avascular necrosis. Unpublished data.
11. Carnesale, P.G.: Arthrodesis of the hip—long term study. J. Bone Joint Surg., 58A:735, 1976.
12. Chandler, H.P., et al.: Total hip replacement in patients younger than thirty years old. A five-year follow-up study. J. Bone Joint Surg., 63A:1426, 1981.
13. Collert, S., and Gillstrom, P.: Osteotomy in osteoarthritis of the hip. Acta Orthop. Scand., 50:555, 1979.
14. Coventry, M.B.: Osteotomy of the hip for degenerative arthritis. Mayo Clin. Proc., 44:505, 1969.
15. Coventry, M.B., et al.: 2012 Total hip arthroplasties: A study of postoperative course and early complications. J. Bone Joint Surg., 56A:273, 1974.
16. Coventry, M.B., and Scanlon, P.W.: The use of radiation to discourage ectopic bone. J. Bone Joint Surg., 63A:201, 1981.
17. D'Arcy, J., and Devas, M.: Treatment of fractures of the femoral neck by replacement with the Thompson prosthesis. J. Bone Joint Surg., 58B:279, 1976.
18. D'Aubigne, R.M., et al.: Idiopathic necrosis of the femoral head in adults. J. Bone Joint Surg., 47B:612, 1965.
19. Detenbeck, L.C., Coventry, M.B., and Kelly, P.J.: Intertrochanteric osteotomy for degenerative arthritis of the hip. Clin. Orthop., 86:73, 1972.
20. Devas, M.: Aetiology of acetabular erosion of the Thompson replacement for fractured necks of femur (abstract). J. Bone Joint Surg., 59B:128, 1977.
21. Dorr, L.D., Takei, G.K., and Conaty, J.P.: Total hip arthroplasties in patients less than forty-five years old. J. Bone Joint Surg., 65A:474, 1983.
22. Drinker, H., and Murray, W.R.: The universal proximal femoral endoprosthesis: A short-term comparison with conventional hemiarthroplasty. J. Bone Joint Surg., 61A:1167, 1979.
23. Ficat, P., et al.: Resultats therapeutique de forage-biopsie dans les osteonecroses femorocapitales primitives (100 cases). Rev. Rhumat., 38:269, 1971.
24. Freeman, M.A.R., and Bradley, G.W.: ICLH surface replacement of the hip. An analysis of the first 10 years. J. Bone Joint Surg., 65B:405, 1983.
25. Gartland, J.J., and Dethoff, J.C.: Sugioka osteotomy for avascular necrosis: Results in 12 patients with over three year follow-up. Presented at 96th annual meeting of American Orthopaedics Association, Hot Springs, Virginia, 1983.
26. Gilberty, R.P.: Low-friction bipolar hip endoprosthesis. Int. Surg., 62:38, 1977.
27. Gore, D.R., et al.: Walking patterns of men with unilateral hip fusion. J. Bone Joint Surg., 57A:759, 1975.
28. Harris, W.H., and White, R.E., Jr.: Socket fixation using a metal-backed acetabular component for total hip replacement. J. Bone Joint Surg., 64A:745, 1982.
29. Head, W.C.: Wagner surface replacement arthroplasty of the hip. Analysis of fourteen failures in forty-one hips. J. Bone Joint Surg., 63A:420, 1981.
30. Jolley, M.N., Salvatti, E.A., and Brown, G.C.: Early results and complications of surface replacement of the hip. J. Bone Joint Surg., 64A:366, 1982.
31. Kelsey, J.: Total hip replacement in the United States. (NIH Consensus Conference Program, 1982). J.A.M.A., 248:1817, 1982.

32. Kostuik, J., and Alexander, D.: Arthrodesis for failed replacement arthroplasty of the hip. Presented at 96th annual meeting of American Orthopaedics Association, Hot Springs, Virginia, 1983.
33. Krein, S.W., and Chao, E.Y.S.: A biomechanical analysis of bipolar proximal femoral endoprostheses. Unpublished data.
34. Ma, S.M., Kabo, J.M., and Amstutz, H.C.: Frictional torque in surface and conventional hip replacement. J. Bone Joint Surg., *65A*:366, 1983.
35. Salvatti, E.A., et al.: A ten-year follow-up study of our first one hundred consecutive Charnley total hip replacements. J. Bone Joint Surg., *63A*:753, 1981.
36. Stauffer, R.N.: Ten-year follow-up study of total hip replacement. J. Bone Joint Surg., *64A*:983, 1982.
37. Sugioka, Y.: Transtrochanteric rotational osteotomy of the femoral head. Proc. Hip Soc., *8*:3, 1980.
38. Sugioka, Y.: Transtrochanteric rotational osteotomy of the femoral head in the treatment of osteonecrosis affecting the hip. Clin. Orthop. *130*:191, 1978.
39. Sutherland, C.J., et al.: A ten-year follow-up of 100 consecutive Mueller curved stem total hip replacement arthroplasties. J. Bone Joint Surg., *64A*:970, 1982.
40. Weisel, H.: Intertrochanteric osteotomy for osteoarthritis: A long-term follow-up. J. Bone Joint Surg., *62B*:37, 1980.
41. Whittaker, R.P., et al.: Fifteen years' experience with metallic endoprosthetic replacement of the femoral head for femoral neck fractures. J. Trauma, *12*:799, 1972.
42. Woo, R.Y.G., and Morrey, B.F.: Dislocations after total hip arthroplasty. J. Bone Joint Surg., *64A*:1295, 1982.

Chapter 49

Correction of Arthritic Deformities of the Knee

John N. Insall

The knee is the largest joint in the body. It is essentially a hinge with an asymmetrical arc of motion such that the tibia rotates counter-clockwise (home) on the femur as the joint is extended. The joint is divided into three compartments (medial, lateral tibiofemoral, and patellofemoral) of the knee.

DEFORMITY

Most arthritic knees demonstrate some degree of instability, deformity, contracture, or a combination of these elements.

Instability initially develops because of loss of cartilage and bone, which is more or less symmetrical in rheumatoid arthritis (RA) and usually asymmetrical in osteoarthritis (OA). Thus, early in the course of RA, a symmetrical instability develops, whereas in OA knees, an angular deformity soon becomes evident (Fig. 49–1). In advanced arthritis of both types, adaptive changes take place in the ligaments.

Varus Deformity. This deformity is most commonly found in OA (Fig. 49–2). The initial disorder is loss of articular cartilage from the medial compartment. The diagnosis of OA may not be made unless a weight-bearing radiograph is obtained. Unfortunately, this important examination is often omitted (Fig. 49–3A,B). As varus deformity progresses, contracture of the medial ligament produces a fixed deformity. Adaptive changes occur in the lateral ligament and capsule, which are stretched by the stresses of walking on a knee that is now in fixed varus position. Thus, an "asymmetric instability" is now present. Extreme varus angulation may occur as a late result of Blount's disease (Fig. 49–4).

Valgus Deformity. The situation is the reverse in valgus deformity (Fig. 49–5), with contracture of the lateral capsule and iliotibial band and stretching of the medial collateral ligament. Especially in RA, there is often an associated fixed external rotation deformity of the tibia, due presumably to contracture of the iliotibial band (analogous to the similar contracture seen in poliomyelitis).

Flexion Contractures. Flexion contractures

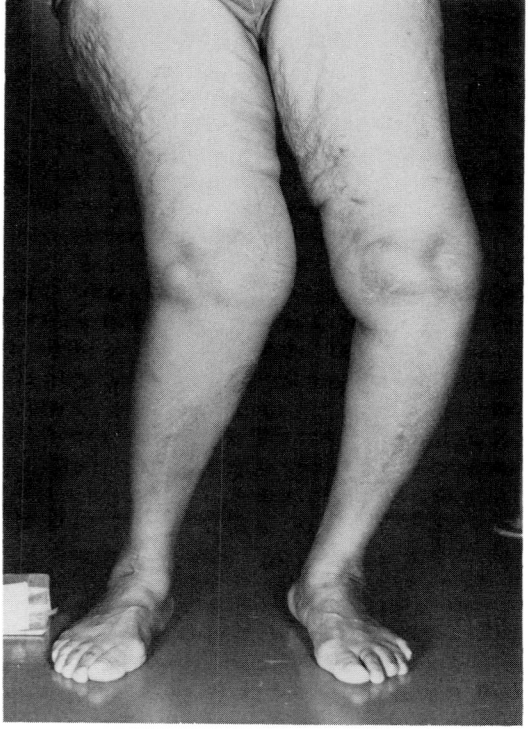

Fig. 49–1. Either varus or valgus angulation may occur in osteoarthritic knees. Both deformities have occurred in this patient, producing a "wind-swept" appearance.

are not usually pronounced in OA; in RA the more extreme degrees are seen. In patients who have not walked for years and have spent most of their time in a wheelchair, fixed flexion deformity of 90 degrees and more can occur. The contracture is caused by shortening of the posterior capsule with secondary contracture of the hamstring muscles.

Flexion Instability. Seen only in RA, flexion instability paradoxically is usually associated with flexion contracture. It is caused by bone loss from the posterior femoral condyles. When viewed on lateral radiographs, the lower femur looks like a drumstick or "chicken leg."

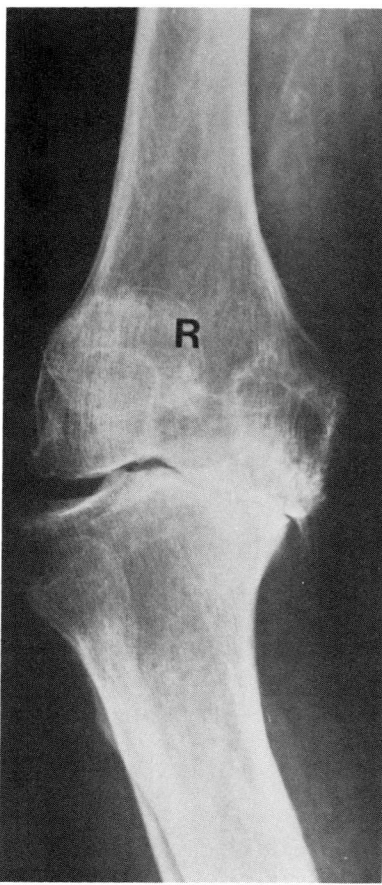

Fig. 49–2. Typical radiograph of advanced medial compartment gonarthrosis. This deformity is partially fixed by contracture of the medial soft tissues, whereas the lateral capsule is stretched.

Stiff Knee. The stiff knee (extension or quadriceps contracture) usually begins by intra-articular adhesions that bind the patella to the femur. Inevitably, a secondary quadriceps shortening occurs.

In primary OA and in osteonecrosis of the medial femoral condyle, varus deformity is the most frequent (Fig. 49–6A,B), flexion contracture is mild, and the range of motion is usually well preserved. In secondary or post-traumatic arthritis, any of the deformities may be found and the knee may be stiff. In RA, lupus erythematosus, and hemophilia, flexion contracture is common, valgus deformity is frequent, and there may be varying degrees of loss of motion. External rotation deformities of the tibia are confined to this group. Loss of motion in association with deformity is seen, particularly in juvenile rheumatoid arthritis and hemophiliac arthropathy.

CONSERVATIVE TREATMENT

To some extent, the natural history of arthritic deformity can be modified.

Active exercises that maintain strength in the quadriceps and the muscles attached to the iliotibial tract minimize the development of flexion contracture and varus deformity. *Passive exercises* and *stretching* prevent the extremes of flexion contracture that are usually seen only in those patients who "give in" to their condition.

Long leg braces are needed to control angular deformity but, because of their cumbersome nature, are seldom applicable. *Elastic supports* and knee cages (short knee braces) provide only a feeling of security and will not prevent deformity.

SURGICAL CORRECTION

Osteotomy

High tibial osteotomy is used to correct varus deformities secondary to OA or osteonecrosis. The operation is usually performed through the cancellous bone of the upper tibia proximal to the tibial tubercle. By removal of an appropriately sized wedge, the limb is corrected into approximately 10 degrees of valgus.[2,25,27,29,32] Postoperative fixation may be accomplished by either of two methods: (1) The patient may be fitted with a cast that extends from the upper thigh to above the ankle. This method requires an accurately molded cast but otherwise is simple and virtually free of complications. The foot is exposed, and the patient can wear a shoe and bear weight as tolerated. Because the cast must remain in place for at least two months, however, troublesome stiffness in the knee may develop, and the recovery period is prolonged. (2) Internal fixation[6] by a plate and screws (Fig. 49–7) avoids the need for a cast and allows early motion. However, the operation becomes more extensive, the risk of infection is greater, and the plate interferes with an arthroplasty if this procedure is required later.

High tibial osteotomy is most suitable for knees with less than 10 degrees of varus deformity, a well-preserved lateral compartment, and nearly normal ligamentous stability. It is mostly indicated for younger, active individuals, particularly those who wish to continue playing sports. Sedentary and overweight patients are better treated by an arthroplasty.

Supracondylar Femoral Osteotomy. For the treatment of valgus deformity in OA, supracondylar femoral osteotomy is used because the bone loss is predominantly femoral, and correction by tibial osteotomy produces an obliquity of the joint axis.[36] Femoral osteotomies are always fixed with a plate and screws so that early motion may begin.

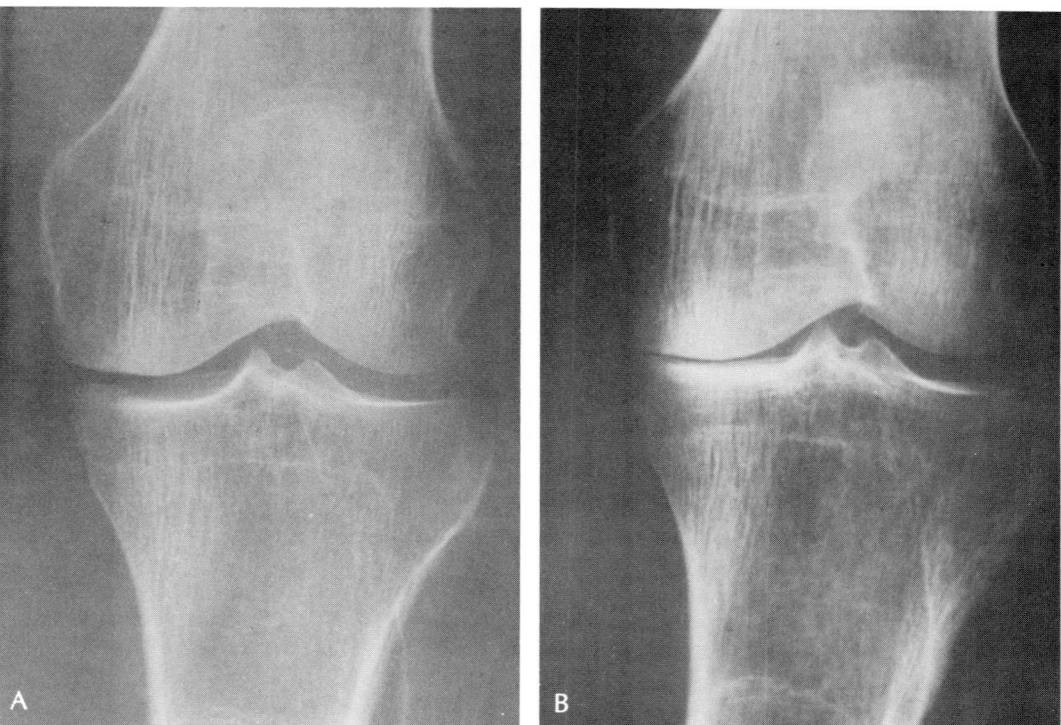

Fig. 49–3.   Weight-bearing radiographs are critical in making the diagnosis of osteoarthritis. *A*, A radiograph of a knee in the supine position. No abnormality is detectable. *B*, A radiograph of the same knee under weight-bearing conditions showing advanced narrowing of the medial compartment.

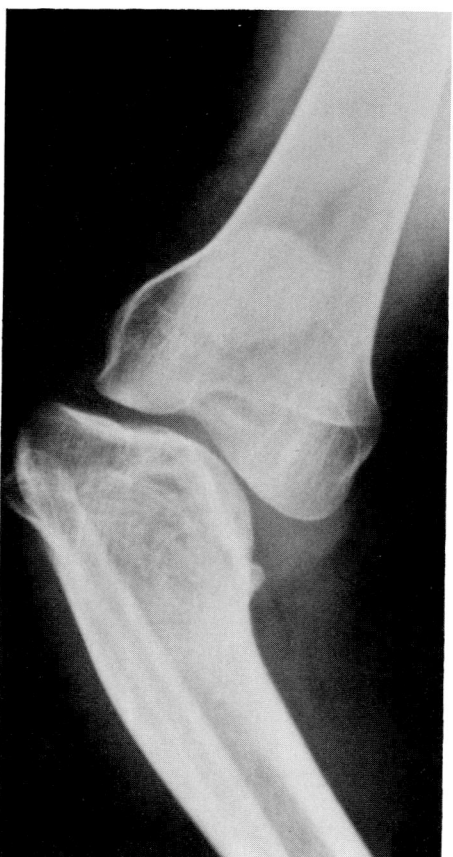

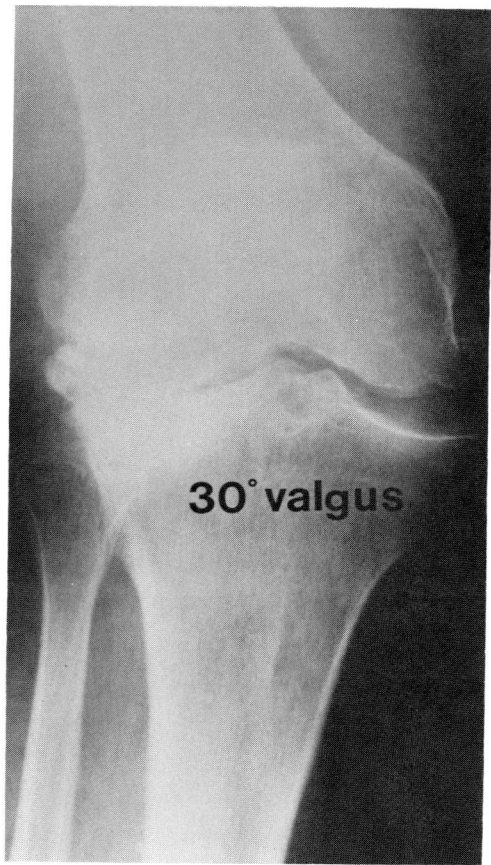

Fig. 49–4. Extreme angular deformities in Blount's disease (infantile tibia vara).

Fig. 49–5. In valgus gonarthrosis, the principal bone loss occurs from the lateral femoral condyle, whereas in varus gonarthrosis the bone loss is mostly from the tibia.

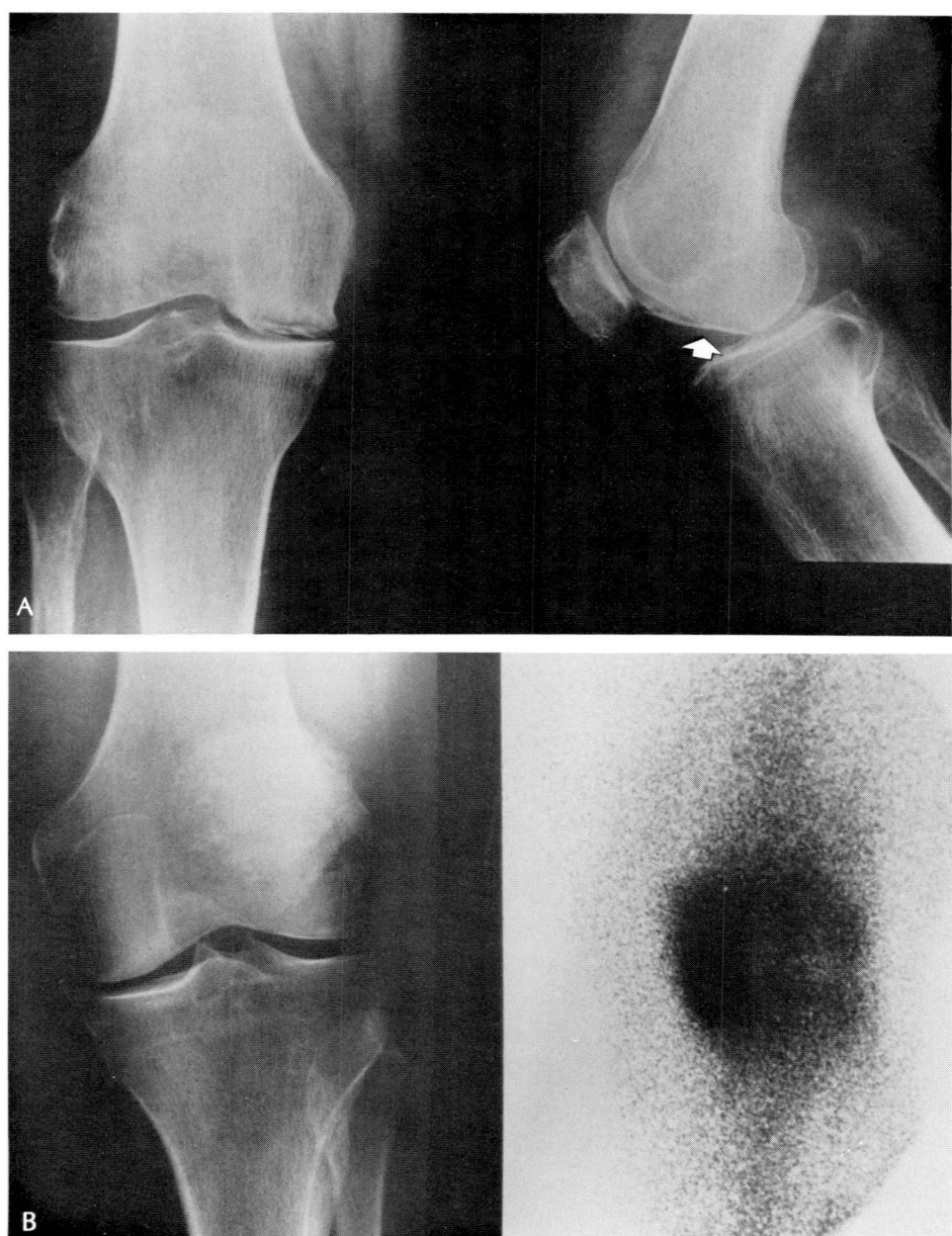

Fig. 49–6. Osteonecrosis of the medial femoral condyle (arrow). *A*, Radiograph showing well-established osteonecrosis involving most of the weight-bearing surface of the medial femoral condyle and a calcified loose fragment. Osteonecrosis differs from osteochondritis dissecans in the location of the lesion and the age group involved. *B*, Osteonecrosis often presents acutely with severe pain and swelling in the knee. In the early stages, the radiographs are negative, but the condition can be diagnosed by ^{99m}Tc diphosphonate scintigraphy.

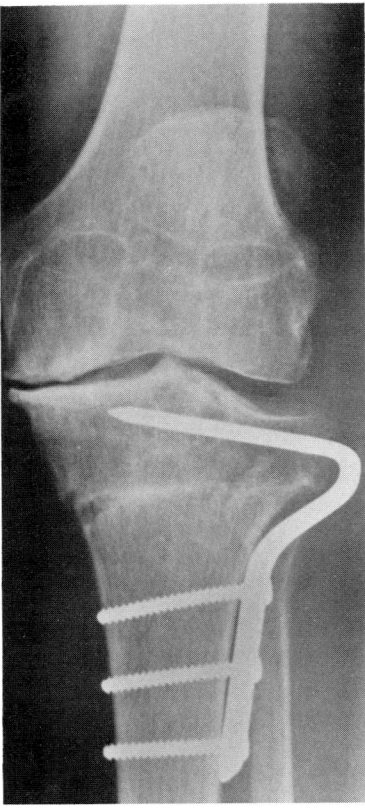

Fig. 49–7. Tibial osteotomy to correct varus angulation is a satisfactory method of surgical treatment and is the method of choice in younger, active patients. The osteotomy may be fixed with a cast or, as shown in this radiograph, by a blade plate.

Crutches are required until the osteotomy is healed (approximately two months). The indications for femoral osteotomy are approximately the same as those for tibial osteotomy.

KNEE ARTHROPLASTY

To warrant knee joint replacement, the patient's symptoms and disability must be severe, although it is no longer true that the patient should first consent to an arthrodesis. A frank discussion with the patient concerning the consequences of failure is essential, and alternative techniques, such as tibial or femoral osteotomy, should be selected when feasible. There are four contraindications to knee replacement:

1. A sound, painless arthrodesis. The prospects of a successful arthroplasty are poor.
2. Genu recurvatum associated with muscular weakness.
3. Gross quadriceps weakness.
4. Active sepsis.

Total knee arthroplasty is indicated in the following circumstances:

1. *Rheumatoid arthritis* and *juvenile rheumatoid arthritis,* regardless of age.
2. *Osteoarthritis.* The age of the patient, occupation, level of activity, sex, and weight are all factors. In general, arthroplasty should be avoided in patients under 60 years of age, manual laborers, athletes, and those grossly overweight. Men tend to abuse the arthroplasty more than women do.
3. *Post-traumatic osteoarthritis.* Knee replacement may be rarely indicated in the younger patient following intra-articular fracture or other traumatic injuries to the joint.
4. *Failure of high tibial osteotomy.* No adverse effects due to the osteotomy have been observed with regard to fixation of the tibial component of the prosthesis.
5. *Patellofemoral arthritis.* Occasionally an elderly patient presents with severe isolated patellofemoral arthritis without significant femorotibial narrowing. Although this condition is rare, such patients fare better with total joint replacement than with any other procedure.
6. *Neuropathic joint.* Joint replacement in neuropathic states is controversial but is feasible using a surface replacement, provided the joint is thoroughly debrided (Fig. 49–8*A,B*).

Various prostheses used in the knee are classified in Table 49–1. Examples are shown in Figures 49–9 and 49–10. It is generally agreed that for most knees, a bicondylar surface design is most applicable. The need to preserve cruciate ligaments is debatable.[11] The place of unicompartmental replacement is controversial, and most knees suitable for unicondylar replacement are also suitable for osteotomy.

Constrained designs are needed in a small proportion of knees and particularly in revision cases. The exact percentage of knees for which this type of design is used depends upon the experience of the surgeon and may range from 1 to 10%.

Bicondylar Prosthesis

Although coined as the name of a specific prosthesis, "total condylar" has been given a generic meaning to describe the whole range of prostheses that share general characteristics (see Fig. 49–10).

1. The femoral component has a grooved anterior flange, separating posteriorly into condylar runners.
2. The tibial component is made of one piece of high-density polyethylene containing two separate tibial plateaus that are biconcave and are sep-

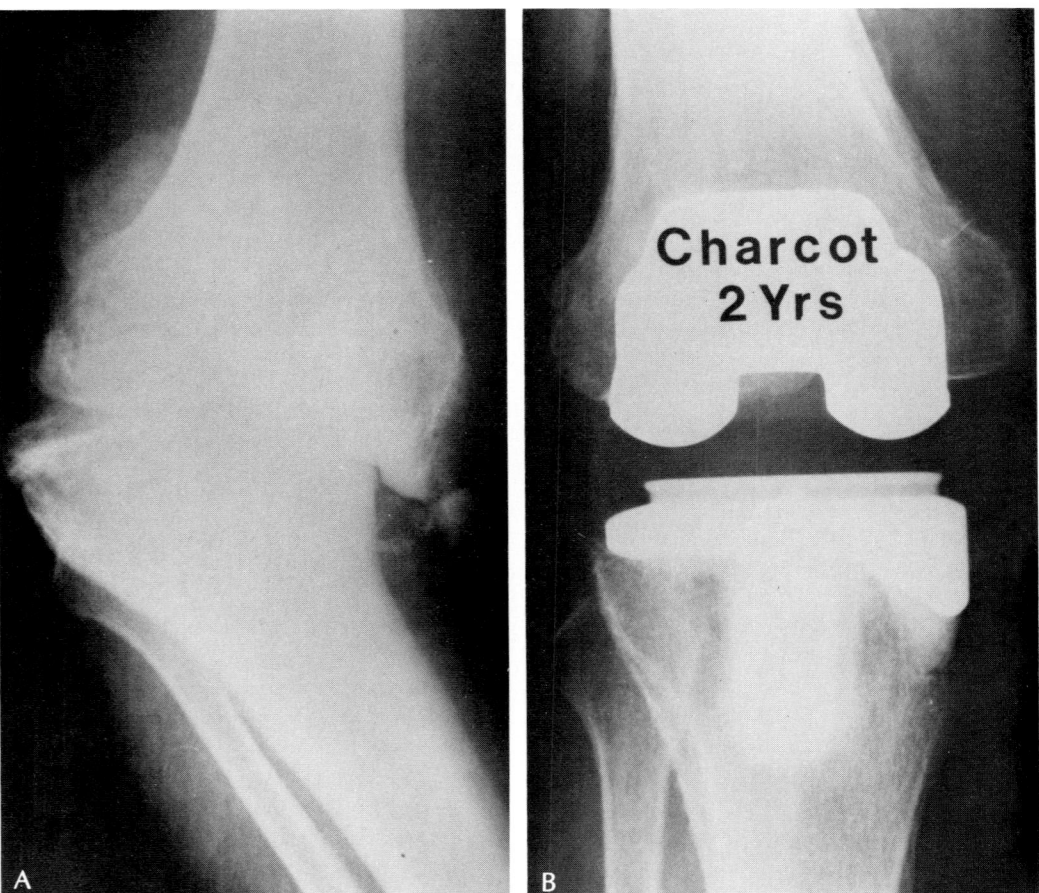

Fig. 49–8. *A,* Radiograph of neuropathic joint in a patient with tabes dorsalis. Charcot joints were once thought unsuitable for joint replacement. However, provided that a complete synovectomy and debridement are performed and the joint is correctly aligned postoperatively, successful results can be obtained. *B,* Radiograph two years after total condylar replacement. Note that the medial defect in the tibia has been filled with a wedge-shaped custom component.

Table 49–1.   Classification of Knee Prostheses*

I. SURFACE REPLACEMENTS
  A. Unicondylar
  B. Bicondylar
    1. Cruciate retaining
    2. Cruciate excising
    3. Cruciate substituting
II. CONSTRAINED PROSTHESES
  A. Loose in that some rotation and varus/valgus movement are permitted
  B. Rigid, fixed axis hinges

*See also Figures 49–9 and 49–10.

arated by an intercondylar eminence to prevent translocation. There may be a posterior cutout for the posterior cruciate ligament, and most current designs have metallic backing or an "endo skeleton." For fixation, there is either a central stem or multiple posts.

3. The polyethylene patellar component may be (1) dome-shaped, or (2) anatomic with medial and lateral facets.

Surgical Technique

Component placement, overall alignment or "axis" and, above all, soft tissue balance are critically important in determining the success of the arthroplasty.

For undeformed knees, the principle is to resect the joint and reshape the bone ends so that they may be "capped" by the components to restore the original ligamentous tension. As the components themselves are almost anatomic in size and shape, subsequent function is similar to normal, although generally the range of motion is less.

In deformed and contracted knees, a surface bicondylar prosthesis may also be used if the deformity is first corrected by "soft-tissue release." This technique allows the contracted soft tissues on the concave side of deformity to be progressively released so that the limb may be stretched into correct alignment. A resurfacing prosthesis is then inserted as would be done in an undeformed knee.

Because the technique of soft tissue release is difficult and requires experience, use of a constrained prosthesis to restore alignment and to provide stability has its attractions. Although the operation is relatively simple, unfortunately constrained prostheses are larger, invade the bone to a greater degree, and are more prone to loosening, breakage, and infection. In the event of failure, salvage is more formidable than it is for the surface replacements.

Aftercare

Intravenous antibiotics (usually oxacillin or cephalosporin) are administered preoperatively and

for 48 hours postoperatively. Thromboembolism is not considered a major threat after knee arthroplasty, although fatal pulmonary emboli have been reported. Most surgeons rely on early ambulation and muscle activity with perhaps the use of low doses of aspirin. Routine postoperative venography is practiced in some centers,[37] and intermittent compression stockings may also prove valuable. Patients with total knee replacement are allowed to walk on the third or fourth postoperative day using a walker or crutches with weight-bearing as tolerated. Range of motion is begun about the fourth day when wound healing permits. Manipulation under anesthesia may be necessary two to three weeks after surgery. Continuous passive motion machines now becoming available greatly ease the rehabilitation phase.

Complications.   Urinary retention and urinary tract infections are the most frequent general complications.

The local complications include:

1. Delayed wound healing and wound drainage.
2. Vascular complications. These complications are rare, and the absence of peripheral pulses is not necessarily a contraindication to surgery.
3. Nerve palsy, usually of the peroneal nerve.[34] This condition may follow correction of severe valgus and flexion deformities. If it is recognized early, removal of the dressing and flexion of the knee may hasten recovery.
4. Stress fractures. The patella,[38] femur, and tibia are the sites of stress fractures. Usually conservative management with a cast or traction proves satisfactory, unless the components have been loosened.
5. Component breakage. This problem is rare and usually is restricted to hinges and linked prosthetic designs.[7]
6. Component wear. Retrieval analysis of removed total joint implants has consistently revealed polyethylene particles in the synovium. Inspection of removed components often shows imbedded cement particles with scratching, pitting, and burnishing of the articular surfaces.[14] However, clinically significant wear has not yet been demonstrated with current resurfacing designs.
7. Instability, subluxation, and dislocation. Instability after surface replacement is usually due to faulty technique, which should be recognized and corrected in the operating room.
8. Component loosening. Component loosening is now mostly a problem with constrained designs. Most currently used surface replacements have acceptably low loosening rates,

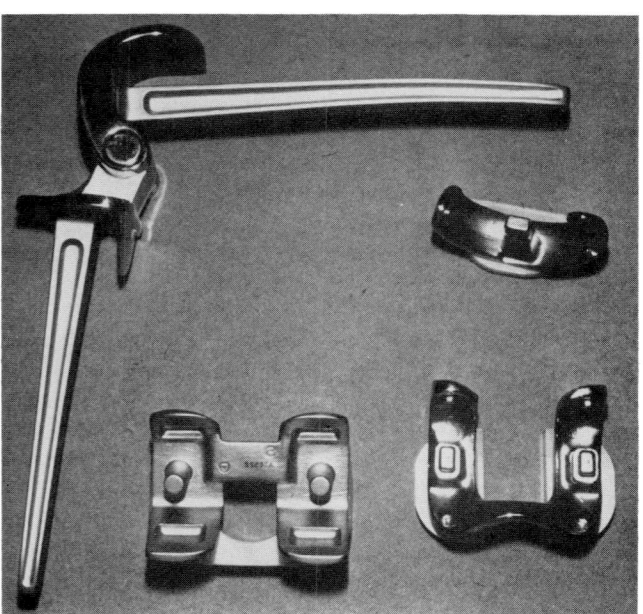

Fig. 49–9. Four of the early designs used for knee replacement. In a clockwise direction these designs are: a Guepar hinge, a unicondylar prosthesis, a duocondylar prosthesis, and a geometric prosthesis. A Guepar hinge was used for the most severely deformed knees and the unicondylar design for the least deformed, with the two bicondylar models occupying an intermediate position. The results obtained with these prostheses were unreliable, and there were many cases of component loosening. The operation of knee arthroplasty received a bad reputation based upon the early results of designs such as these.

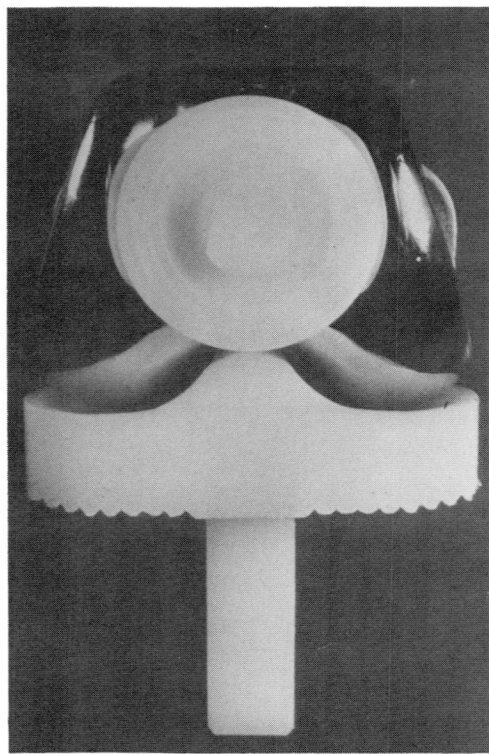

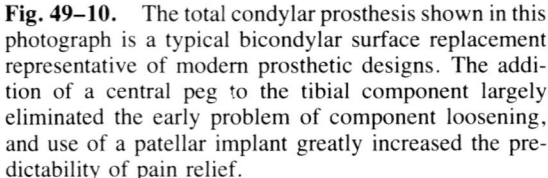

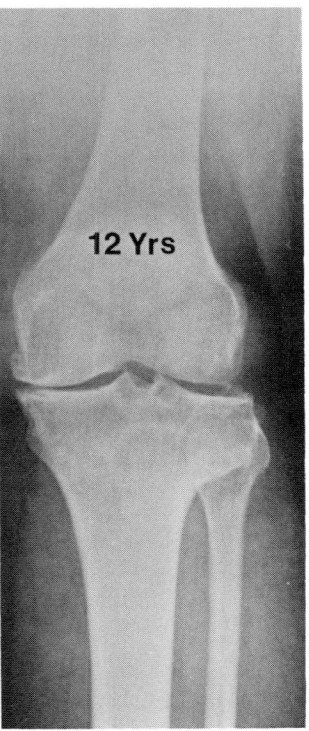

Fig. 49–10. The total condylar prosthesis shown in this photograph is a typical bicondylar surface replacement representative of modern prosthetic designs. The addition of a central peg to the tibial component largely eliminated the early problem of component loosening, and use of a patellar implant greatly increased the predictability of pain relief.

Fig. 49–11. This radiograph was taken 12 years after high tibial osteotomy in a 65-year-old woman. This knee has remained painless. Osteotomy relieves pain in most knees for about five years, but an increasing number of patients have recurrent pain after that time.

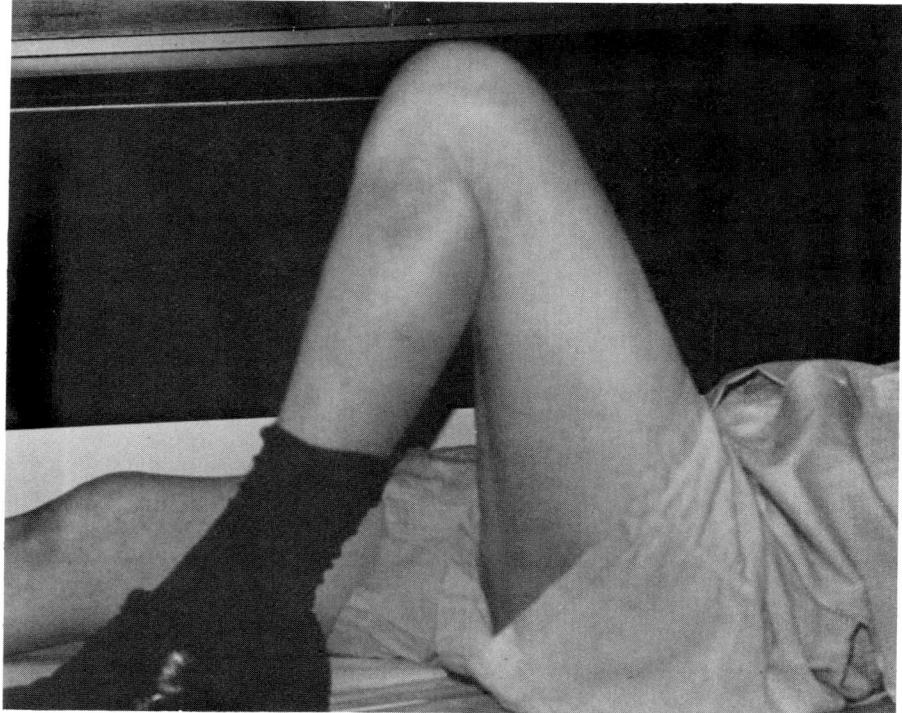

Fig. 49–12.　Current designs of knee arthroplasty allow an almost normal range of motion. This photograph shows the flexion angle obtained with a posterior stabilized condylar prosthesis.

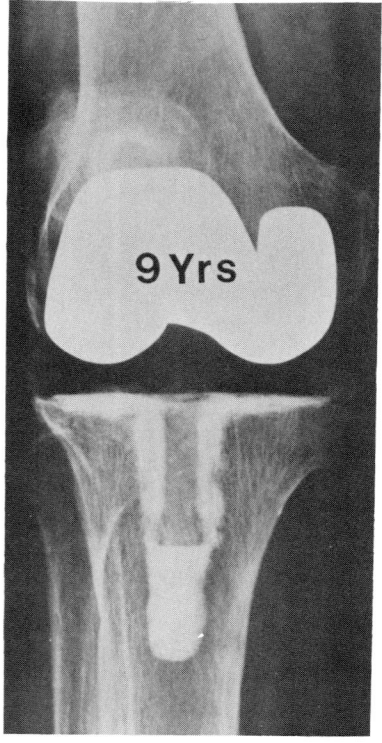

Fig. 49–13.　Continuing follow-up of total condylar prostheses suggests that these models are durable. There is little evidence to suggest that late loosening or polyethylene wear will be a significant problem. This radiograph shows the characteristic appearance of a total condylar prosthesis nine years after implantation. There is no evidence of component loosening.

and recent modifications, such as metal backing of polyethylene components and improved cementing techniques, should further reduce the loosening rate. Malalignment of the arthroplasty due to technical error predisposes to loosening.

9. Infection. Persistent symptoms following total knee replacement in the absence of a clear mechanical explanation should suggest the possibility of infection. Infection is more common in RA and when metal-on-metal constrained hinged prostheses are selected.[26] Late infections are more common than early ones. The diagnosis is usually straightforward unless antibiotics have been given previously. Antibiotic therapy should therefore be withheld in cases of suspected infection until after diagnostic aspiration of the joint. Proven or strongly suspected late deep infection is treated by surgical removal of the prosthetic components and debridement of the involved tissues. Appropriate antibiotic therapy is then given intravenously.

After completion of approximately six weeks of antibiotic therapy, the following courses are open:

1. Prolonged immobilization in a supportive brace allowing a fibrous ankylosis to develop.
2. Formal arthrodesis.[13]
3. Reimplantation of another prosthesis. This alternative can be considered in certain cases if the wound is completely benign.[22] Usually only infections due to gram-positive organisms can be managed in this manner.

RESULTS

High Tibial Osteotomy.[3,4,21,23,24,29,32] Evidence is ample that high tibial osteotomy provides a successful result in 80 to 90% of properly selected cases, for five years (Fig. 49–11). Beyond this time, however, a significant deterioration occurs. Coventry found that 62% of the patients rated themselves as having less pain even after 10 years from the time of operation.[2] Vainionpää et al. found that 26 of 103 knees deteriorated after an initial good result.[39] Joseph et al. examined 95 knees with an average follow-up of 8.5 years; 83% were excellent or good at 5 years, deteriorating to 63% in these categories at the time of last follow-up.[27] These authors also found that patients who were under 60 at the time of osteotomy did much better than those patients over the age of 60.

Femoral Osteotomy. There is a paucity of information concerning the results. At our hospital, 12 of 15 cases were satisfactory after a follow-up of 1 to 10 years.

Knee Arthroplasty. Results of early attempts at knee arthroplasty were poor, and unfortunately the operation still suffers from the bad reputation earned during these early years. With the early model prostheses, there were four major problems:[17]

Component Loosening. For both surface replacements and constrained designs, the incidence of loosening, usually of the tibial component, was unacceptably high.[8,9]

Patellofemoral Pain. None of the early designs allowed for patellofemoral replacement or resurfacing.

Infection. A major complication of metallic hinged designs was infection.

Surgical Technique. The surgical procedure was extremely difficult for early surface replacements, and the instrumentation was poor. Consequently, many prostheses were poorly inserted and often malaligned. These mistakes often led to failure.[15,31]

Current resurfacing designs[10,12,20] can now be used for most arthroplasties, and metal hinges are obsolete. Alterations to the tibial component have reduced tibial loosening to a low level. Recent designs, such as the posterior stabilized condylar knee, permit flexion to 120° or more (Fig. 49–12). Patellofemoral resurfacing is performed routinely. Instrumentation and surgical technique have been greatly improved.[16] Consequently, the results of knee arthroplasty are now as good as those for total hip replacement, and promise to be even more durable. For example, in my experience, a 5- to 9-year follow-up[17] (average 6.6 years) of the total condylar prosthesis showed 91% excellent and good results in a series of 100 consecutive replacements. Moreover, the late radiographic appearance of most of these cases remained unchanged throughout the period of follow-up, suggesting that component loosening will continue to be a minor problem (Fig. 49–13). In fact, only 2% showed a complete radiolucency around any of the three components compared with 25 to 50% of total hip prostheses followed for a similar time.

The place of unicondylar replacement is controversial (Fig. 49–14A,B). Scott and Santore studied 100 knees followed for 2 to 6 years and found satisfactory pain relief in 92.[35] However, Insall and Aglietti reported on 22 unicondylar knee replacements of similar design with a 5- to 7-year follow-up and found that only 36% remained satisfactory and 28% had been revised (Fig. 49–15).[19] Laskin,[30] using the somewhat different Marmor modular prosthesis,[33] found the results inferior to those for biocompartmental replacement.

The spherocentric prosthesis is probably the most frequently used constrained design. Kaufer

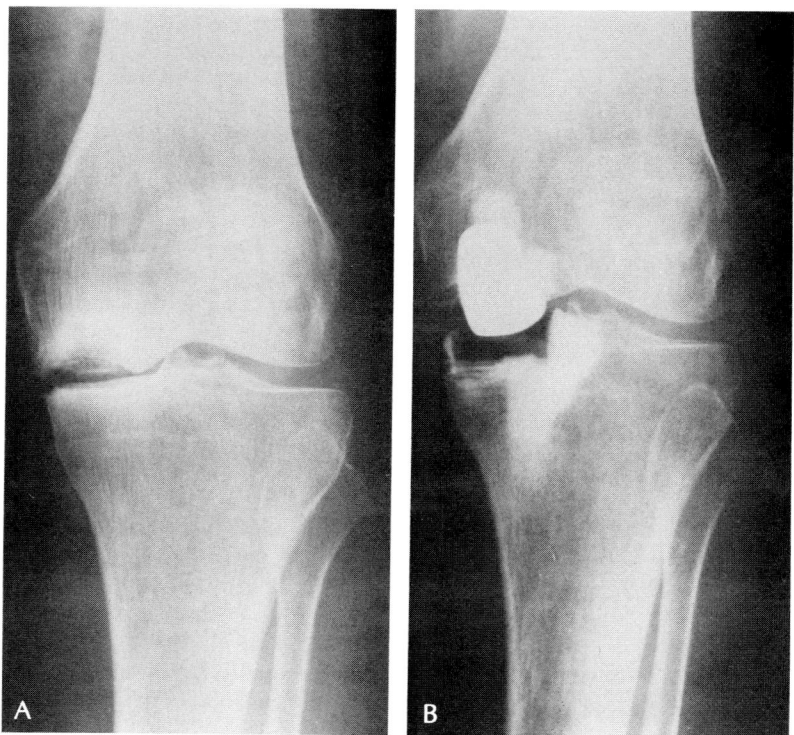

Fig. 49–14. *A,B,* Although partial or unicondylar replacement is a controversial operation, an ideal indication would be an osteonecrosis of the medial-femoral condyle in an otherwise normal knee joint as shown here.

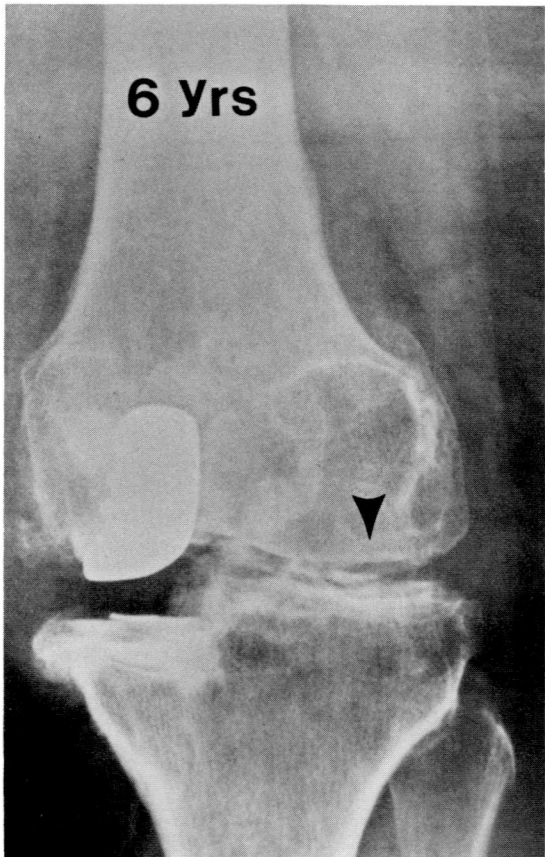

Fig. 49–15. Although unicompartmental replacement is often successful for a few years, late follow-up reveals an increasing incidence of progressive arthritis in other compartments of the joint (arrow). This complication is partly due to the abrasive effect of polyethylene and acrylic debris.

and Matthews reviewed 82 consecutive spherocentric arthroplasties with an average follow-up of 4 years.[28] There was a 10% incidence of a septic loosening and 4% infection rate. Convery et al. reported 8 cases of confirmed or suspected loosening in 36 spherocentric arthroplasties followed for an average of 3 years.[5] These results suggest that the spherocentric prosthesis, although an improvement over hinged designs, still loosens more frequently than do resurfacing models.

REFERENCES

1. Bauer, G.H., Insall, J., and Koshino, T.: Tibial osteotomy in gonarthrosis (osteo-arthritis of the knee). J. Bone Joint Surg., *51A*:1545, 1969.
2. Coventry, M.B.: Upper tibial osteotomy for gonarthrosis. Orthop. Clin. North Am., *10*:191, 1979.
3. Coventry, M.B.: Osteotomy about the knee for degenerative and rheumatoid arthritis. Indications, operative technique, and results. J. Bone Joint Surg., *55A*:23, 1973.
4. Coventry, M.B.: Osteotomy of the upper portion of the tibia for degenerative arthritis of the knee. A preliminary report. J. Bone Joint Surg., *47A*:984, 1965.
5. Convery, F.R., Minteer-Convery, M., and Malcom, L.L.: The spherocentric knee: A re-evaluation and modification. J. Bone Joint Surg., *62A*:320, 1980.
6. d'Aubigne, R.M.: Joint realignment in the management of osteoarthritis. *In* Clinical Trends in Orthopaedics. Edited by L.R. Straub, and P.D. Wilson, Jr. New York, Thieme-Stratton, Inc., 1982.
7. DeBurge, A., and GUEPAR: GUEPAR hinge prosthesis. Complications and results with two years follow-up. Clin. Orthop., *120*:47, 1976.
8. Ducheyne, P., Kagan, A., II, and Lacey, J.A.: Failure of total knee arthroplasty due to loosening and deformation of the tibial component. J. Bone Joint Surg., *60A*:384, 1978.
9. Evanski, P.M., et al.: UCI knee replacement. Clin. Orthop., *120*:33, 1976.
10. Ewald, F.C., et al.: Duo-patella total knee arthroplasty in rheumatoid arthritis. Orthop. Trans., 2:202, 1978.
11/ Freeman, M.A.R., et al.: Excision of the cruciate ligaments in total knee replacement. Clin. Orthop., *126*:209, 1977.
12. Freeman, M.A.R., and Insall, J.: Tibio-femoral replacement using two unlinked components and cruciate resection. (The ICLH and total condylar prostheses.) *In* Clinical Features and Surgical Management. Edited by M.A.R. Freeman. New York, Springer-Verlag, 1980.
13. Hagemann, W.F., Wood, G.W., and Tullos, H.S.: Arthrodesis in failed total knee replacement. J. Bone Joint Surg., *60A*:790, 1978.
14. Hood, R.W., et al.: Retrieval analysis of 70 total condylar knee prostheses. Orthop. Trans., 5:319, 1981.
15. Hood, R.W., Vanni, M., and Insall, J.N.: The correction of knee alignment in 225 consecutive total condylar knee replacements. Clin. Orthop., *160*:94, 1981.
16. Insall, J.N.: Technique of total knee replacement. *In* Instructional Course Lectures, The American Academy of Orthopaedic Surgeons, Vol. 30. St. Louis, C.V. Mosby Co., 1981.
17. Insall, J.N., et al.: The total condylar knee prosthesis in gonarthrosis: A five to nine year follow-up of the first one hundred consecutive replacements. J. Bone Joint Surg., *65A*:619–628, 1983.
18. Insall, J.N., et al.: A comparison of four models of total knee replacement prostheses. J. Bone Joint Surg., *58A*:754, 1976.
19. Insall, J.N., and Aglietti, P.: A five- to seven-year follow-up of unicondylar arthroplasty. J. Bone Joint Surg., *62A*:1329, 1980.
20. Insall, J.N., Scott, W.N., and Ranawat, C.S.: The total condylar knee prosthesis. A report of two hundred and twenty cases. J. Bone Joint Surg., *61A*:173, 1979.
21. Insall, J.N., Shoji, H., and Mayer, V.: High tibial osteotomy. J. Bone Joint Surg., *65A*:1397, 1974.
22. Insall, J.N., Thompson, F.M., and Brause, B.D.: Two-stage reimplantation for the salvage of infected total knee arthroplasty. Orthop. Trans., 6:369, 1982.
23. Jackson, J.P., and Waugh, W.: Tibial osteotomy for osteoarthritis of the knee. J. Bone Joint Surg., *43B*:746, 1961.
24. Jackson, J.P., Waugh, W., and Green, J.P.: High tibial osteotomy for osteoarthritis of the knee. J. Bone Joint Surg., *51B*:88, 1969.
25. Johnson, F., Leitl, S., and Waugh, W.: The distribution of load across the knee. J. Bone Joint Surg., *62B*:346, 1980.
26. Jones, E.C., et al.: GUEPAR knee arthroplasty results and late complications of upper tibial osteotomy. Clin. Orthop., *140*:145, 1979.
27. Joseph, D.M., Insall, J., and Msika, C.: High tibial osteotomy. A long term clinical review. Presented at the Annual Meeting of the American Academy of Orthopaedic Surgeons, Anaheim, California, 1983.
28. Kaufer, H., and Matthews, L.S.: Spherocentric arthroplasty of the knee. J. Bone Joint Surg., *63A*:545, 1981.
29. Kettelkamp, D.B., et al.: Results of proximal tibial osteotomy. The effects of tibio-femoral angle, stance-phase flexion-extension, and medial-plateau force. J. Bone Joint Surg., *58A*:952, 1976.

30. Laskin, R.S.: Unicompartmental tibiofemoral resurfacing arthroplasty. J. Bone Joint Surg., *60A*:182, 1978.
31. Lotke, P.A., and Ecker, M.L.: Influence of positioning of prosthesis in total knee replacement. J. Bone Joint Surg., *59A*:77, 1977.
32. Maquet, P.: Valgus osteotomy or osteoarthritis of the knee. Clin. Orthop., *120*:143, 1976.
33. Marmor, L.: Results of single compartment arthroplasty with acrylic cement fixation. A minimum follow-up of two years. Clin. Orthop., *122*:181, 1977.
34. Rose, H.A., et al.: Peroneal-nerve palsy following total knee arthroplasty. A review of the Hospital for Special Surgery experience. J. Bone Joint Surg., *64A*:347, 1982.
35. Scott, R.D., and Santore, R.F.: Unicompartmental replace-ment for osteoarthritis of the knee. J. Bone Joint Surg., *63A*:536, 1981.
36. Shoji, H., and Insall, J.: High tibial osteotomy for osteoarthritis of the knee with valgus deformity. J. Bone Joint Surg., *55A*:963, 1973.
37. Stulberg, B., et al.: Deep vein thrombosis following total knee replacement: An analysis of 643 arthroplasties. Presented at the Annual Meeting of the American Academy of Orthopaedic Surgeons, Anaheim, California, 1983.
38. Thompson, F.M., Hood, R.W., and Insall, J.: Patellar fractures in total knee arthroplasty. Orthop. Trans., *5*:490, 1981.
39. Vainionpää, S., et al.: Tibial osteotomy for osteoarthritis of the knee. A five- to ten-year follow-up study. J. Bone Joint Surg., *63A*:938, 1981.

Chapter 50

Correction of Arthritic Deformities of the Foot and Ankle

Mack L. Clayton

Both rheumatoid arthritis (RA) and osteoarthritis (OA) are discussed in this chapter. Because the latter process tends to be more localized in a single joint and is, therefore, a less severe problem than the generalized changes found in the RA patient, more text is allotted to RA.

GENERAL CONSIDERATIONS

Seventy-five percent of patients with RA are women, and they more often have aggressive disease. In 16% of cases of RA, the process presents in the feet and in 4% in the ankle.[16] In the later stages of the disease, however, almost all patients have some complaints related to foot involvement. In one large series of patients, metatarsophalangeal joints were involved in 46%, tarsals in 46%, toes in 23%, ankle in 68%, knees in 78%, and metacarpophalangeal joints in 71%.

Smyth and I working at the University of Colorado have noted two definite clinical subtypes of chronic RA.[7] In one group, the joints tend to stiffen with gradual loss of motion and even progress to ankylosis. The stiff type of joint involvement predominates. Soft tissue and bursal involvement predominate in the second group and cause secondary deformity. Joint destruction is slow and does not usually lead to ankylosis. The loose type tends to have gradual destruction of the joint with developing instability. This type predominates in patients with hand and foot involvement and may be accentuated by corticosteroid treatment.

These two "subtypes" may account for the marked difference in the results obtained with reconstructive surgical procedures in RA. In the first, ankylosis prone-type arthrodesis (fusion) is easy to obtain, but mobility may be difficult to regain after arthroplasty. In the loose type, arthrodesis is more difficult to obtain.

The statement in the older literature that "surgery should not be performed until the arthritis is 'burned out' or quiescent" has been shown to be false. Three main clinical forms of RA exist with regard to progression. The first group of patients has a single inflammatory cycle lasting for a number of months and then subsiding with no further attacks of arthritis. Such patients are not considered for surgery. The second group shows periods of heightened inflammatory activity followed by partial or complete remission, and then more activity and remission, with a gradual heightening of the activity. The third group of patients has steadily progressive, active inflammation. Destructive joint changes with instability and/or stiffness develop at various rates in the latter two groups.

Most patients with chronic RA seen for consideration of surgical treatment have experienced such progressive deformity and disability. Inflammation continues indefinitely. Surgery can be performed at any time, provided the patient is not in an acute condition and provided there is no general medical contraindication. This concept is not new. Smith-Petersen, Aufranc, and Larson recommended surgery when the disease is still active even in 1943.[17]

Surgery for arthritic feet is usually performed under general anesthesia, although regional anesthesia has been used successfully. If a patient has recently received corticosteroids, he will require supplementary steroids (see Chap. 32). The rate of wound healing is slowed, but the final result is unchanged. The tissues in such patients are often more fragile and must be handled atraumatically. I use perioperative intravenous antibiotics, usually an intravenous cephalosporin, on the day of the operation and for up to 24 hours afterward.

While the patient is in the hospital recovering from surgery, other involved joints are treated. Medical treatment using the team approach is carried out so that no time is wasted (see Chap. 43). The necessary period of rest after operation often decreases inflammation in other joints.

Upper-extremity procedures can be performed at the same time as foot surgery by using teams.

EVALUATION

In early RA, diagnosis may be difficult. The patient, usually female, presents with pain in the forefoot, which is usually swollen and tender. There may be mild heat and redness and local increased sweatiness. Lateral compression of the metatarsal heads increases pain. Tenderness between metatarsal heads indicates involvement of the periarticular non-weight-bearing structures, involved in RA but not in mechanical types of metatarsophalangeal disease. An exception, of course, is plantar neuroma with its characteristic findings (see Chap. 79). (Plantar neuroma also may be due to RA.) As a result of swelling of the metatarsophalangeal (MTP) joints, the toes assume a "cocked-up" position. Active and passive flexion is limited at the MTP joints. Roentgenograms may reveal only osteoporosis with soft tissue swelling (Fig. 50–1), but surface erosions of the metatarsal heads soon develop in most cases[19] (see Chaps. 5 and 38).

In early disease, proper shoes and supports with a graduated exercise regimen are helpful, and some of the deformities can be prevented. Rest may be indicated in early acute exacerbations (see Chap. 42).

Despite conservative measures, some cases progress to severely painful disabling forefoot deformities. Deformity of the knees often accentuates foot deformity. The most common deformities are hallux valgus and bunions, a spread forefoot, depressed metatarsal heads, and varying degrees of "cock-up" of the toes. This last deformity often becomes so pronounced that the toes no longer contact the floor at all when the patient stands barefoot. The proximal phalanx is dorsally subluxed on the metatarsal heads. This deformity is made

even worse as the fat pad under the transverse metatarsal arch slips anteriorly and lies under the cocked-up toes. Some toes remain slightly flexible while others are rigid with dorsal subluxation or complete dislocation of the proximal phalanges on the metatarsal heads. This condition increases the height of the forefoot and makes it difficult for the patient to wear shoes. Painful corns develop over the dorsum of the middle toe joints, and calluses develop beneath the depressed, prominent, metatarsal heads on the sole of the foot that now lies under the skin (Fig. 50–2). A painful swollen bursa often develops over the lateral aspect of the fifth MTP joint where it is known as a "bunionette."

With walking, pain arises from abnormal pressure beneath the metatarsal heads on the sole or against the shoe on the dorsum of the toes. Attempts to support the metatarsal area often produce increased pressure on the dorsum of the toes owing to their inflexibility. There is contracture of the soft tissues, including muscles, tendons, fascia, and skin, often leading to fibrous ankylosis. *However, spontaneous bony ankylosis of the metatarsophalangeal joints is rare* (about 1%). As synovitis continues, the intrinsic muscles are overpulled by the long extensors and flexors, and the cock-up deformity of the toes becomes similar to that often seen with paralysis of the intrinsic muscles of the foot. The flexor tendons subluxate laterally and migrate in a dorsal direction until they no longer flex the proximal phalanx, again increasing the

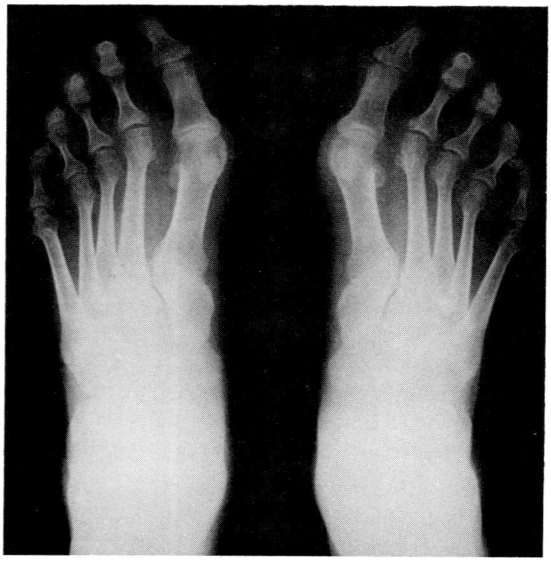

Fig. 50–1. Early rheumatoid arthritic changes with soft tissue swelling. Note erosion of bone at the metatarsophalangeal joints, particularly erosion of the metatarsal heads. Also note the interphalangeal joint of the great toes. Joint spaces are well preserved.

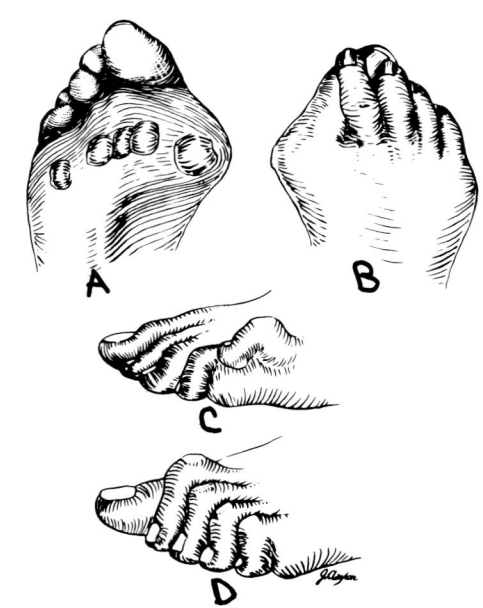

Fig. 50–2. Typical late severe deformities include hallux valgus (A), bunions (B), depressed metatarsal heads (C), and cock-up (hammer) toes (D).

cock-up deformity. This defect does not resemble the "intrinsic plus" deformity commonly seen in rheumatoid arthritis of the hand (see Chap. 45). Many variations of pathology in the involved tissues give rise to other deformities, but most patients have the basic pattern as described.

Roentgenograms help analyze the deformities. Erosion of the metatarsal heads or bases of the proximal phalanges is nearly always greater than suspected on clinical evaluation. Joint spaces are often narrowed, and subluxation or actual dislocation of the MTP joints is often seen on anteroposterior films as the proximal phalanx overlaps the metatarsal head. When the proximal phalanx is located in marked dorsal dislocation at almost 90 degrees to the metatarsal (Fig. 50–3), the "gun barrel" sign is seen. This sign is simply an axial view of the proximal phalanx in which the bony cortex appears as if one were peering straight down a gun barrel. Varying degrees of osteoporosis are present.

Several patients have had complete spontaneous dislocation at the first metatarsophalangeal joints (Fig. 50–4) as a result of rheumatoid synovial involvement of the capsule and the abductor hallucis tendon. This dislocation increases the deformity of the forefoot and increases the pressure of the bunion of the first metatarsal head. I have seen three

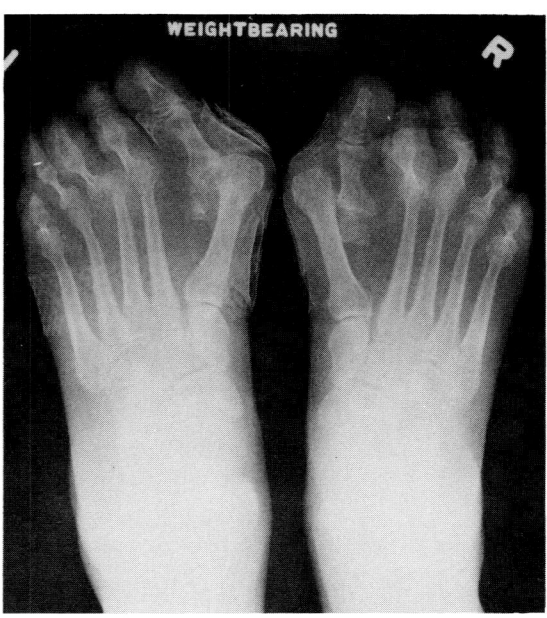

Fig. 50–4. Forefoot with dislocation of metatarsophalangeal joint of the great toe and several smaller toes. Dislocation of the first metatarsophalangeal joint without a history of trauma is pathognomonic of rheumatoid arthritis.

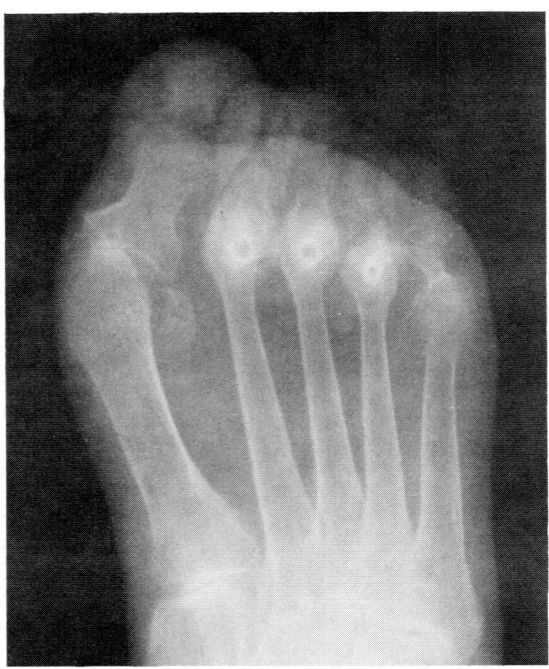

Fig. 50–3. Late deformity with multiple metatarsophalangeal dislocations. (Note "gun barrel" sign indicating 90-degree dislocation of proximal phalanges over metatarsal heads.)

feet with a spontaneous hallux varus. This unusual deformity was due to a rupture of the adductor hallucis tendon and related joint capsule by synovitis. Similar tendon ruptures in the hand are well known.

The hindfoot usually shows a progressive valgus deformity (loose type) with changes first in the talonavicular or subtalar joints and later in the midtarsals. In other cases such deformity is minimal, but there is limited motion with pain in the hindfoot due to arthritic joint changes (stiff type). Cavovarus deformity is also seen most commonly in juvenile RA, but this condition is often not symptomatic until adult life. The medial longitudinal arch becomes accentuated with the development of a pes cavus deformity.

Bursitis (or tenosynovitis) may develop around the calcaneal tendon. I have seen two cases of rupture of the Achilles tendon. Tenosynovitis also may occur near the plantar fascia insertion.

Tenosynovitis may develop in any of the tendon sheaths at the ankle level, as in the hand and wrist, and may occasionally cause tendon rupture. A ruptured posterior tibial tendon may cause rapid severe valgus of the hindfoot. Nodules often develop on the weight-bearing aspect of the os calcis and may even erode the adjacent bone.

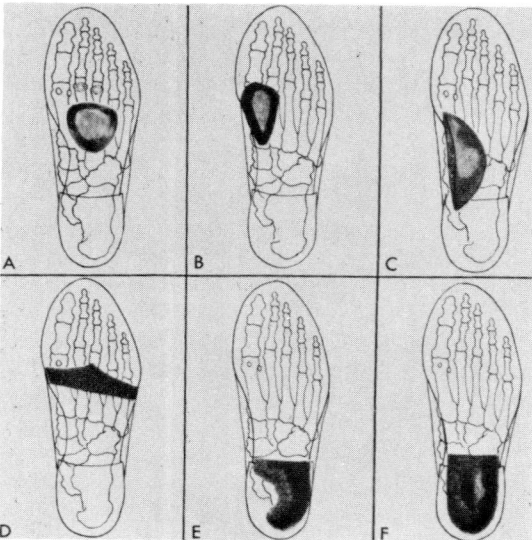

Fig. 50–5. Types of arch supports that have been helpful. The object of their use is relief of pain through mechanical realignment and pressure relief. These pads do not differ much from those used for other basic orthopedic problems, but the patient with rheumatoid arthritis requires more adjustment and ''custom fitting'' of the supports.

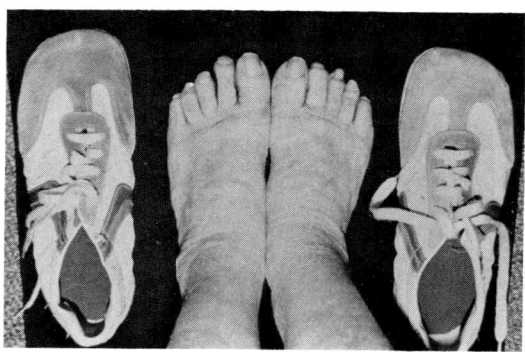

Fig. 50–6. Running shoes are useful for many patients pre- and/or postoperatively. They can be padded for pressure relief as necessary. These feet were reconstructed 6 months earlier. Fortunately, these shoes are in style, and many patients prefer them to corrective shoes.

CONSERVATIVE TREATMENT OF RHEUMATOID FOOT

Proper shoes with simple ordinary orthopedic supports should be used in the early stages coupled with an exercise regimen designed to keep the toes flexible. Simple, low- to medium-heel, basic oxford shoes with closed toes and heels are recommended. Metatarsal pads, long arch pads, or heel wedges are added if needed (Fig. 50–5). Arch sup-

ports are usually made of firm rubber and covered with leather. Steel or hard plastic alone is usually too rigid for the rheumatoid foot. The supports must be custom-made for each patient and frequently require secondary alterations. Plaster impressions of the feet are often helpful to fit the arch supports precisely. Extra-depth shoes (double-toe box) are also commercially available, and special inserts of plastizoate in combination with these have been most helpful. Running shoes are useful as a pre- or postoperative walking shoe (Fig. 50–6).

Berg, utilizing the pressure-distributing footwear that Brand developed successfully for insensitive neurotrophic feet, has treated many rheumatoid feet without surgery.[2] An extra-depth shoe with a plastizoate liner is useful in milder cases, but severely deformed feet require a sandal with special plastizoate inserts. The most severe deformities require a custom-made shoe with inserts. The principle in all cases is relief of abnormal areas of pressure, which cause the pain in long-standing deformities after the most active inflammatory synovitis has passed. Success requires constant supervision of the shoe correction and close cooperation with a knowledgeable pedorthist (shoe expert). Even after proper shoeing, a number of patients may desire an operation so that they can wear more reasonable shoes. One of the rheumatoid patient's many problems is to remain in the realm of social acceptance.

The same care must be used, however, in postoperative supports, which are necessary in practically all cases. Usually only simple metatarsal pads with or without longitudinal pads are needed. These measures are the same basic orthopedic supports used for mechanical foot deformity of any cause (see Fig. 50–5), such as marked pronation with symptoms or osteoarthritis, marked bunions, or hammertoes.

A brace may occasionally be helpful for severe valgus deformity of the hindfoot, but usually provides only temporary relief. Surgical stabilization may be necessary. A simple, outside iron, short-leg brace with an inner ''T'' strap is prescribed when the ankle joint is not particularly painful. If the ankle is painful, a double upright brace permitting only limited ankle motion may be used. Osteoarthritis of the foot most commonly involves the MTP joints of the great toes, but it can involve any other joints.

For additional discussion of conservative treatment of the rheumatoid foot, see Chapters 42 and 79.

INDICATIONS FOR SURGERY

Surgery is indicated when there is increasing deformity of the foot and/or continued pain upon weight-bearing in spite of conservative measures. In such cases, relief of the abnormal weight-bearing pressure can be obtained by surgery; the joints are extensively damaged and the feet are already "weak." The toes have lost their usual function. These patients lack the normal "takeoff" to their gait and even avoid pressure on the forefoot. Operation does not weaken the foot or impair gait further. An improved gait may decrease pain in involved knees and hips.

EVOLUTION OF SURGERY OF THE RHEUMATOID FOOT

A report called "An Operation for Severe Grades of Contracted or Clawed Toes" appeared in 1912.[12] This is still an excellent paper with many valid principles. Several of the reported patients had "infectious arthritis" (now called RA). A suitable case was described as follows:

> The toes are strongly dorsiflexed at the metatarsophalangeal joints and plantar flexed at their interphalangeal ones and are retained in this position by shortening through adaptation of tendons, ligaments and other soft structures and by bone changes due to long-continued new relationship of articular surfaces.

Operation consisted of excision of the heads and, if necessary, parts of the necks of the metatarsal bones of all the affected toes through a transverse curved plantar incision just behind the web of the toes. In the closing discussion, it was stated that:

> The operation is simply to get rid of the metatarsal heads because they make the patient's life miserable. Every step he takes hurts him so, he is afraid to get up from his chair. Mild grades of contracted toes should not be operated upon in this way.

Most of these patients had cavus feet. This finding is probably why only the metatarsal heads were resected, although a considerable amount of bone was removed well back into the neck, allowing the toes to straighten and relieving the cavus deformity.

A series of patients with chronic rheumatoid arthritic feet was presented at the Boston Orthopaedic Club in 1949.[1] Surgery had been performed with varying degrees of metatarsophalangeal joint resections through multiple dorsal incisions.

Excisional surgery has been the basic type of procedure for years, but many variations have been described. The same excisional surgery is applicable to similar painful deformities in an osteoarthritic forefoot joint.

In 1970, Raunio and Laine reviewed metatarsophalangeal joint synovectomies in 28 rheumatoid patients in many of whom the basic disease activity was judged mild.[15] With a follow-up period averaging 15 months, good results were found clinically and roentgenographically in up to two-thirds

of the cases. Overall disease activity did affect their results.

HISTORY OF HINDFOOT SURGERY IN RHEUMATOID ARTHRITIS

When the subtalar joints become inflamed, when swelling and pain occur on weight-bearing, and when planovalgus occurs, such deformity usually develops within 3 years of the onset of signs and symptoms. The most severe radiologic changes occur in the talonavicular joint, except for osteoporosis, which is most severe in the calcaneocuboid joint.

Vahvanen published a report of a controlled series of triple arthrodeses with an average follow-up of 3.7 years.[18] The symptoms of subtalar joint inflammation were usually completely resolved, and the deformity was often corrected. Slight to moderate valgus deformity (10 to 15 degrees) commonly remained but did not cause discomfort with walking. Union usually occurred with the procedure. Nonunion occurred (9.3%) most often in the talonavicular joint. Autogenous bone grafting was recommended in the most severe cases. The use of bone graft and staples helped in the hindfoot reconstruction but did not prevent the calcaneus from slipping into a valgus position if weight-bearing was permitted sooner than 6 to 8 weeks. Triple arthrodesis did not adversely affect the stability of the ankle joint, nor did it increase progression of disease in that joint. It was recommended that the operation be performed before the hindfoot deformity became fixed. This usually occurred within 3 years of the development of progressive symptoms in the hindfoot.

The talonavicular joint is often the earliest hindfoot joint to demonstrate involvement with RA.[8,14] Associated peroneal muscle spasm might be the initial result, creating eversion deformity of the hindfoot. In a patient unresponsive to conservative measures but in whom the hindfoot is still flexible, talonavicular fusion relieves pain and corrects deformity. Progression of the deformity does not occur, and the hindfoot is stabilized in neutral position (slight valgus) by the fusion of this single joint.

In the hindfoot, the basic procedure is stabilization by arthrodesis. Osteoarthritic involvement of the hindfoot is treated in the same manner if supports fail to give relief, which they usually do.

SURGERY OF THE FOREFOOT

The marked contracture of soft tissues accompanying rheumatoid deformities demands adequate bony resection for cosmetic correction and pain relief. The MTP joints are resected with excision of enough bone to correct the deformity. In severely

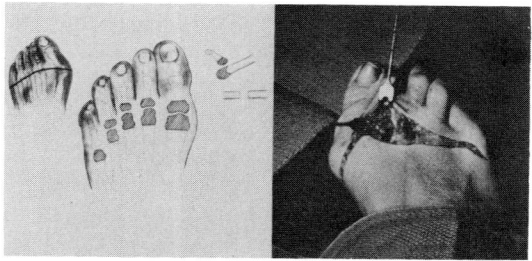

Fig. 50–7. Transverse incision beginning at the dorsal aspect of the fifth metatarsophalangeal joint and extending to the medial aspect of the first metatarsal head. The shaded areas of bone were excised.

involved cases, I generally resect all the metatarsal heads and a portion of the necks. The proximal

portion of each of the proximal phalanges is also removed as indicated. The toes are manipulated straight to correct the cock-up deformities, but formal fusion of the distal joints of the small toes is not performed.

All ten toes are corrected in one operation in most patients. Occasionally, in spite of the lack of underlying skin changes, such as a callus, a metatarsal head is resected because it would otherwise remain too prominent after removal of an offending adjacent head. The surgical procedure is always tailored to the individual patient. In many cases, it is preferable to operate through a transverse dorsal incision at the base of the toes (Fig. 50–7).[7] Exposure is easier than through multiple dorsal incisions. If there is a borderline circulation, however, multiple dorsal incisions are preferred. There

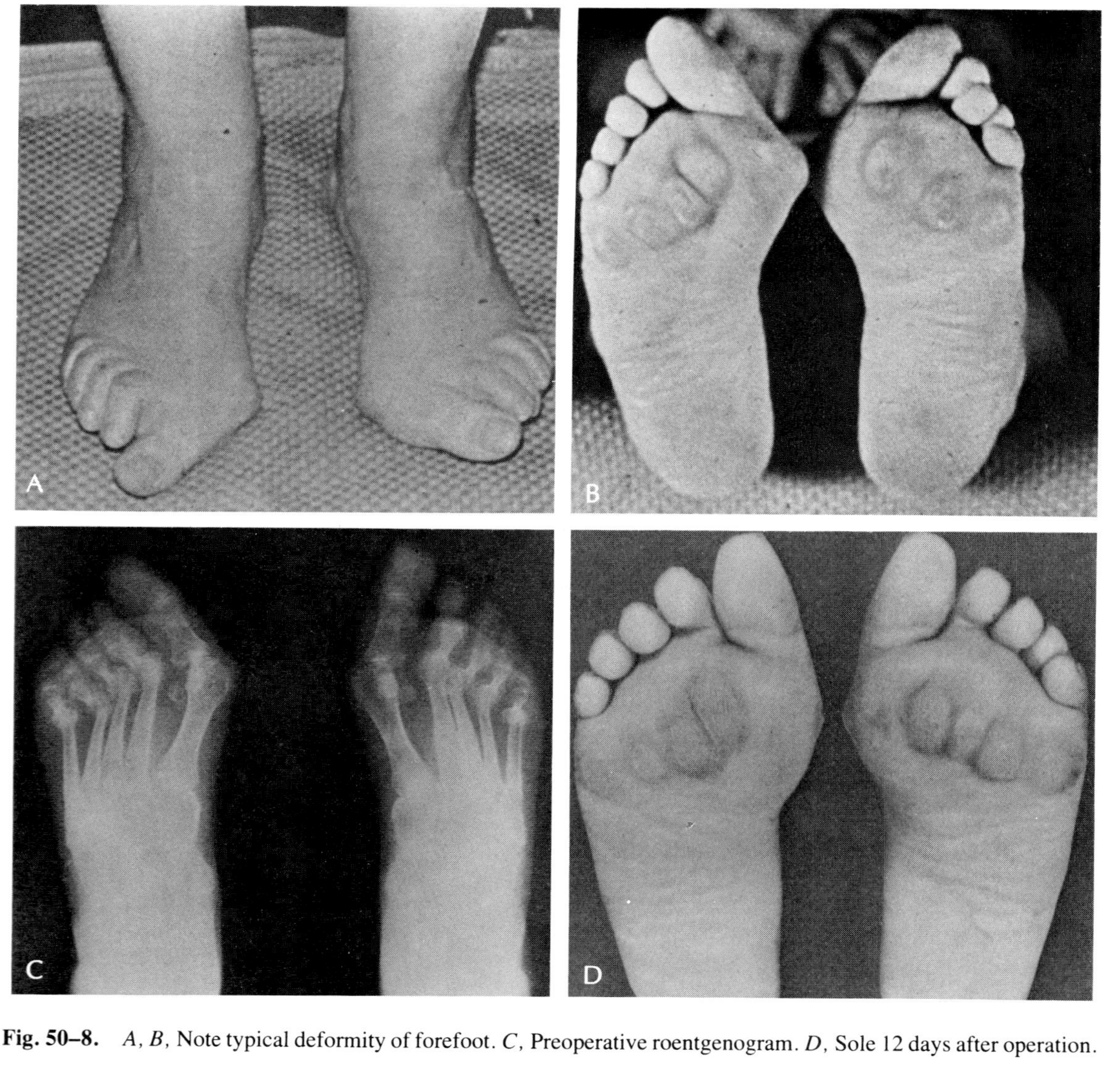

Fig. 50–8. *A, B,* Note typical deformity of forefoot. *C,* Preoperative roentgenogram. *D,* Sole 12 days after operation.

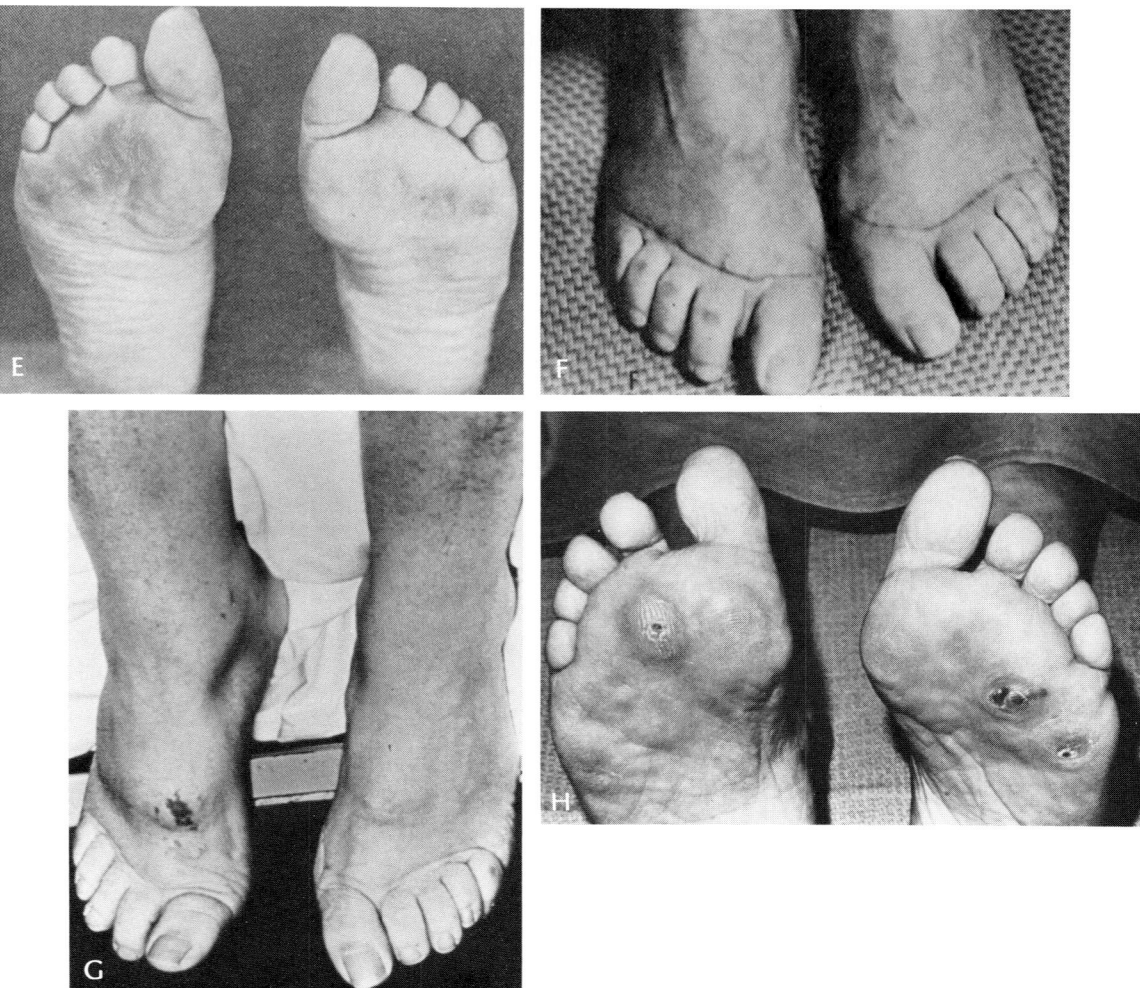

Fig. 50–8. *Continued*   *E, F,* Three months after operation. *G, H,* Thirteen years after operation. Recurrent pressure problems were partially relieved by supports. Osteotomy of the second metatarsal on the right foot was performed at the time of other surgery, and symptoms were relieved.

are also indications for a plantar incision and, in general, the incision used is that with which the surgeon is most comfortable. A tourniquet, either an Esmarch bandage at the level of the ankle or a pneumatic thigh tourniquet, is generally utilized, but the operation can be performed without a tourniquet if necessary.

After resection of the metatarsal heads and (usually) a portion of the proximal phalanges, the plantar aspect of each metatarsal is beveled to give a smooth weight-bearing surface. Ideally, the first and second metatarsal stumps should be approximately the same length with gradual tapering evenly across the third, fourth, and fifth. The more deformity, the more bone that is resected. The extensor tendons are usually divided except for that to the great toe, and the interphalangeal joints of

the lesser toes are gently manipulated straight. The tourniquet is then released, bleeding is controlled, and drains are placed as indicated. The skin is carefully closed with fine interrupted sutures or small staples. The less trauma to these tissues, the better and more rapid the healing. Application of a large conforming dressing to hold the toes exactly in the desired position is important. The patients are permitted to take a few steps in approximately 5 days. Sutures are removed after 2 to 3 weeks.

Ambulation is started with a wooden-soled, laced-top convalescent shoe, and the patients are discharged after 1 to 2 weeks. A convalescent type split shoe is fitted between 3 and 4 weeks with the patient gradually being weaned into simple medium-heel oxford shoes. Patients not needing crutches for other disability do not require crutches after forefoot surgery. A metatarsal pad, approximately three-sixteenths inch to one-quarter inch in height, is generally used postoperatively because of the altered configuration of the distal metatarsals. In some patients, a three-sixteenth inch metatarsal bar may also be added. As a rule, no attempt is made to resect corns, calluses, or thickened bursae between the metatarsal heads at the time of surgery (Fig. 50–8A to H) because relief of abnormal pressure allows these to gradually disappear.

Patients should be told that 2 to 3 months are needed for maximum recovery from bilateral forefoot surgery, although they are usually ambulatory in 1 to 2 weeks.

The operation described previously provided good results in 85% of patients after at least 3 years of follow-up.[3-6] About 10% required additional surgery, usually only minor procedures. These results have been reproduced by others.[9-11,13] Cosmesis was not considered in reporting these results.

Other procedures used in the forefoot with less severe deformity utilize the same basic principles of adequate bony resection, e.g., the Keller procedure (resection of bunion and base of proximal phalanx) for hallux valgus and bunion (Fig. 50–9) and joint excision for hammertoe with or without pinning (Fig. 50–10). The basic principle of adequate bony resection holds true. However, in a rheumatoid patient, if more than two metatarsal heads require surgery, it is preferable to perform the entire forefoot resection so that one may achieve a new weight-bearing alignment across the entire metatarsophalangeal region. Further decompression is obtained by resecting the base of the phalanges for proper realignment without unnecessarily shortening the metatarsals.

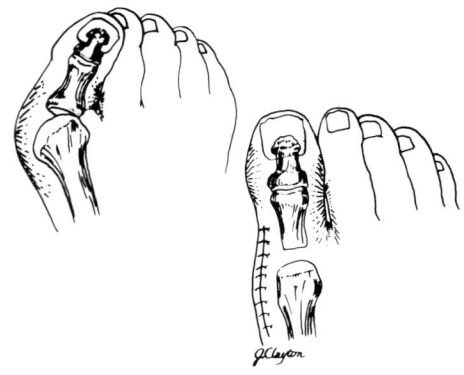

Fig. 50–9. Keller procedure, excision of bunion and osteophytes of the metatarsal head, and excision of proximal portion of the proximal phalanx. In addition, a silicone implant may be used, particularly for cosmesis in women.

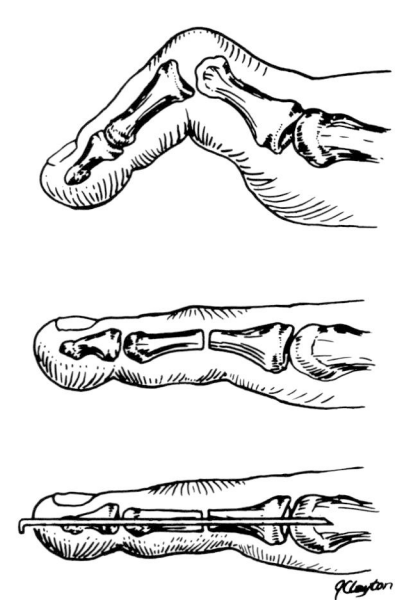

Fig. 50–10. Middle joint resection for hammertoe (ankylosis of toes is neither necessary or desirable). Pin should not cross the metatarsophalangeal joint unless necessary to maintain correction. Pin is usually left in place for 3 to 4 weeks.

I have used a number of silicone hinge great toe implants (Swanson). Cosmetically, they are helpful and the patients like them. Over 90% of my RA patients are women for whom cosmesis is important (Fig. 50–11).

The first MTP is the most common joint affected in the foot by osteoarthritis, which often produces pain and hallux rigidus due to loss of dorsiflexion, a motion that is necessary in the stance phase of normal gait. A resection arthroplasty (Keller procedure) is most commonly done (see Fig. 50–9); in selected cases, a silicone implant may be utilized (Fig. 50–12). In a few early cases simple spur removal is indicated.

Intramedullary Kirschner wires are often used to stabilize the lesser metatarsophalangeal joint resection. A plantar plate may be used to cover the weight-bearing area of the metatarsal head, providing an interposition arthroplasty (Fig. 50–13). Centralization of the flexor tendons beneath the resected end of the metatarsal and use of a Kirschner wire promote fibrosis in the area that prevents later subluxation. However, convalescence is slower with the use of a silicone implant or intramedullary wire fixation.

After 3 years of follow-up, the cosmetic results obtained from either Silastic prostheses or plantar plate arthroplasty have been good in my experience. The functional results are similar to those

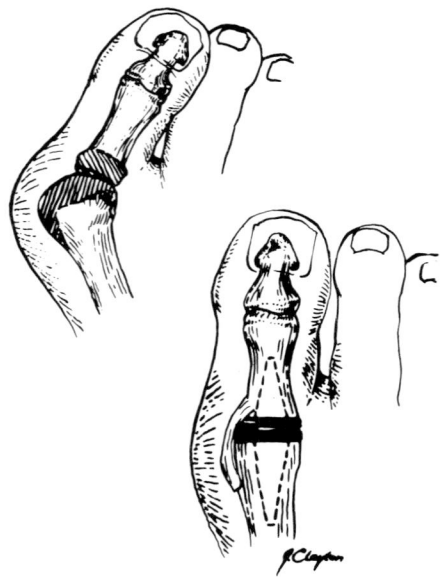

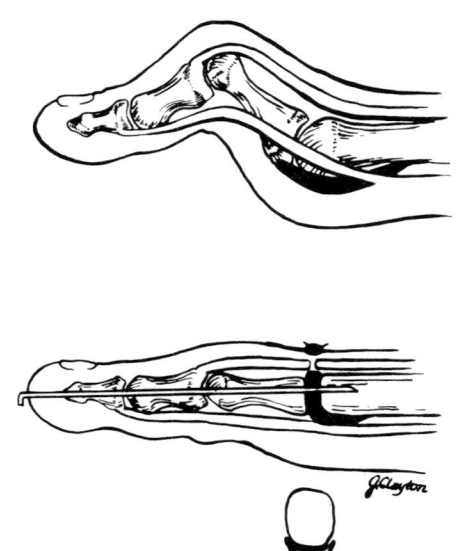

Fig. 50–11. Silicone hinge (Swanson) prosthesis for selected rheumatoid forefoot arthroplasty. Its use requires the same precise rebalancing of the soft tissues around the implant as it does in the hand.

Fig. 50–13. Plantar plate arthroplasty. After double resection at the metatarsophalangeal joint, the plantar plate is freed from the flexor tendon and brought up across the end of the resected metatarsal and impaled by the Kirschner wire. To provide a pad beneath the metatarsal head and to keep the important flexor tendons centralized, the extensor tendon is not sutured.

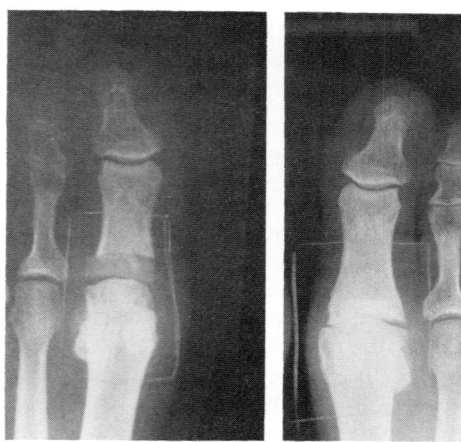

Fig. 50–12. *Right,* Active, tennis-playing, 54-year-old woman with pain and limited dorsiflexion of right great toe. Note marked narrowing, sclerosis, and mild osteophytes in right first metatarsophalangeal joint. Diagnosis is osteoarthritis (hallux rigidus). *Left,* Postoperative Keller procedure with silicone implant (film reversed). Patient had excellent cosmetic and functional result. She has no complaints and still is playing tennis three years later. In a few cases where there has been a reaction, it has been necessary to remove the silicone implant, but these toes still functioned well because of the encapsulation that had occurred around the implant.

found after resections. (However, past experience shows that procedures that remove less bone have had more recurrences.) In general, the more cosmetic procedures are reserved for younger patients. In an older patient in whom early resumption of activities is so important, simple excisional forefoot arthroplasty without any additional fixation provides both early mobilization and pain relief (Fig. 50–14).

SURGERY OF THE HINDFOOT

The valgus deformity of the hind part of the rheumatoid foot with its insidious progression often resembles a paralytic valgus deformity. Arthrodesis, the surgery of choice in the hindfoot, is indicated when pain and deformity persist despite conservative measures. Osteoarthritis of the hindfoot is usually post-traumatic and much rarer than RA. The indications for operation are the same.

If the deformity is not passively correctable, triple arthrodesis (subtalar, talonavicular, and calcaneocuboid) with joint excision to correct the deformity is utilized. Internal fixation is usually used and, in very unstable cases, cast immobilization is necessary without weight-bearing for 6 to 8 weeks, followed by use of a walking cast for another month. If the hindfoot is quite stable, weight can be borne sooner. It takes 4 to 6 months for complete recovery.

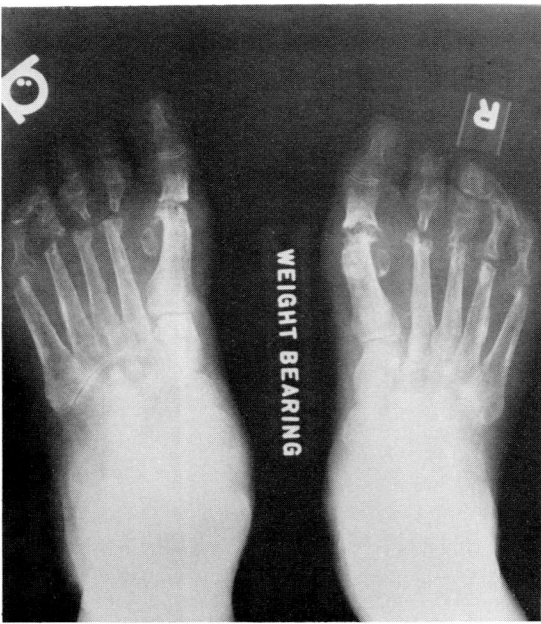

Fig. 50–14. Sixty-six-year-old woman with general-ized RA three years after bilateral forefoot reconstruc-tions. She had no complaints referable to her feet. These feet illustrate the old catch phrase, "it is a good thing the patient doesn't walk on the x-rays." Note the good overall soft tissue contour of the feet as well as the relative length of the metatarsals.

If the talonavicular joint is the most involved, and if the foot is in a reasonable position, fusion of this joint alone suffices to stabilize the hindfoot. Hindfoot arthrodesis gives good results in about 85% of cases, with relief of pain at the expense of motion.

Rheumatoid nodules may require excision, but recurrence is common unless recurrent pressure is prevented. Tenosynovitis appears around the foot and ankle and may require tenosynovectomy if other measures, such as injection of corticosteroids into the tendon sheath, fail.

CARE OF THE RHEUMATOID ANKLE

Ankle involvement of a disabling degree is un-usual in RA. The patient often complains of "a painful ankle" for any pain in the hindfoot, and hindfoot deformity may increase ankle pain.

Proper shoes and supports for foot deformity are utilized. If no relief is obtained, a short leg double upright brace, without a joint, may be added to the shoe. Such braces may be masked by wearing boots. If relief is not obtained, surgery should be considered.

Synovectomy may help in patients with pain and marked synovial proliferation before cartilage de-struction or loss of motion has occurred, but such cases are rare.

Arthrodesis of the ankle relieves pain arising from the joint, but because it often increases symp-toms in the other joints of the hindfoot, it is not often indicated in RA. Rarely, if triple arthrodesis increases ankle deformity and pain, arthrodesis of the ankle is indicated.

Total ankle arthroplasty is useful in RA because of the almost uniform involvement of other joints of the hindfoot. In general, if hindfoot arthrodesis is indicated, it should be performed first and an ankle arthroplasty performed 6 weeks or more after wound healing (Fig. 50–15). Total ankle replace-ment is usually performed through an anterior in-cision utilizing a metal-plastic articulation and methylmethacrylate (bone cement). A cast is uti-lized for a few weeks or early motion is prescribed according to the circumstances. Protected weight-bearing is usually necessary for about 3 months.

In a good result about 20 to 30 degrees of motion are obtained. Pain relief is not as predictable as with hip or knee replacement and may be due to the proximity of other involved joints in the hind-foot. I have obtained only about 70% totally sat-isfactory results. The forces on the ankle are great (up to eight times body weight); extreme osteo-porosis is a contraindication. Some of my best re-sults have been in patients in whom a triple ar-throdesis was followed by an ankle replacement.

Fusion of the ankle and hindfoot (plantar ar-throdesis) leaves a stiff foot but relieves pain; in severe cases it is a helpful salvage procedure.

CARE OF THE OSTEOARTHRITIC ANKLE

In osteoarthritis (usually post-traumatic) in some early cases, debridement of anterior osteophytes is helpful because symptoms are often caused by im-pingement rather than generalized ankle osteoar-thritis. In more severe cases, ankle arthrodesis is an excellent procedure that is preferable to total ankle replacement. With a normal hindfoot (triple joints), an ankle fusion in neutral position (90 de-grees angle between the foot and the tibia) still permits about 25 degrees of plantar flexion from neutral. This result allows a normal gait with an ordinary heel or with a one-inch dress heel for women. If the hindfoot joints are also damaged, the motion is less. Ankle arthrodesis may be per-formed by various approaches with or without sup-plementary bone grafts (Fig. 50–16). Immobili-zation usually lasts between 3 and 4 months with 6 to 8 weeks of non-weight-bearing. Approxi-mately 6 months are needed for maximum recovery.

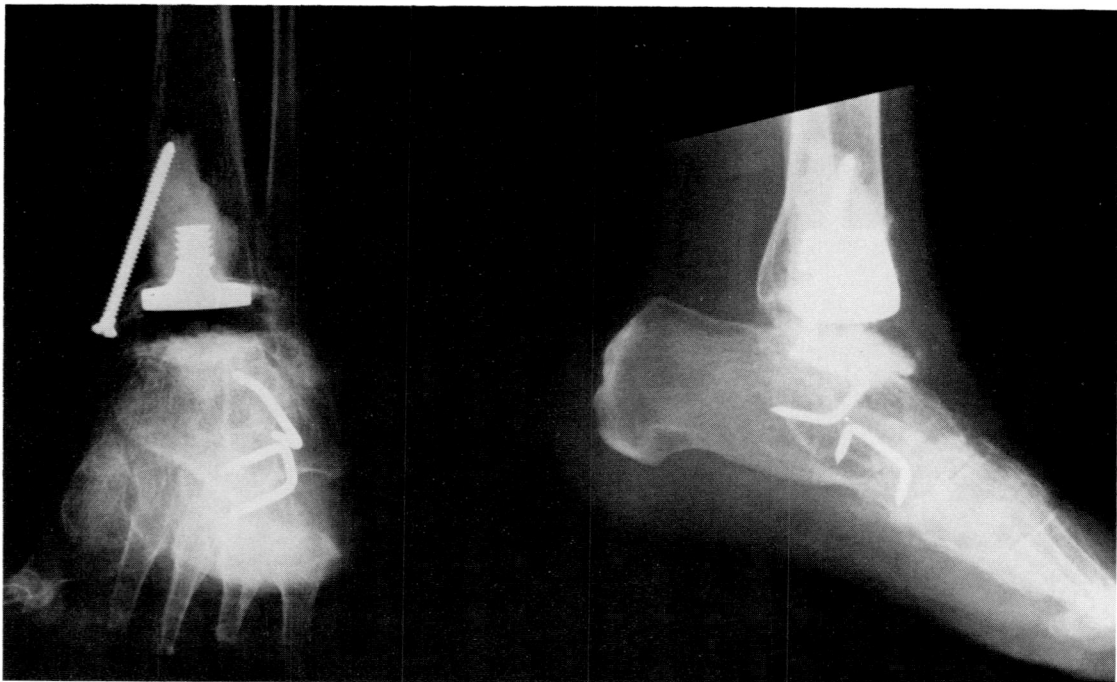

Fig. 50–15. Total ankle arthroplasty performed 3 months after a triple arthrodesis. Note staples across subtalar and calcaneocuboid joint with fusion of these joints and the talonavicular bone. Overall alignment of the foot is good. The screw in the medial malleolus was inserted for a fracture at the time of surgery and has healed in normal alignment. The patient was immobilized for 6 weeks after the ankle surgery and has 30 degrees of painless motion in her ankle.

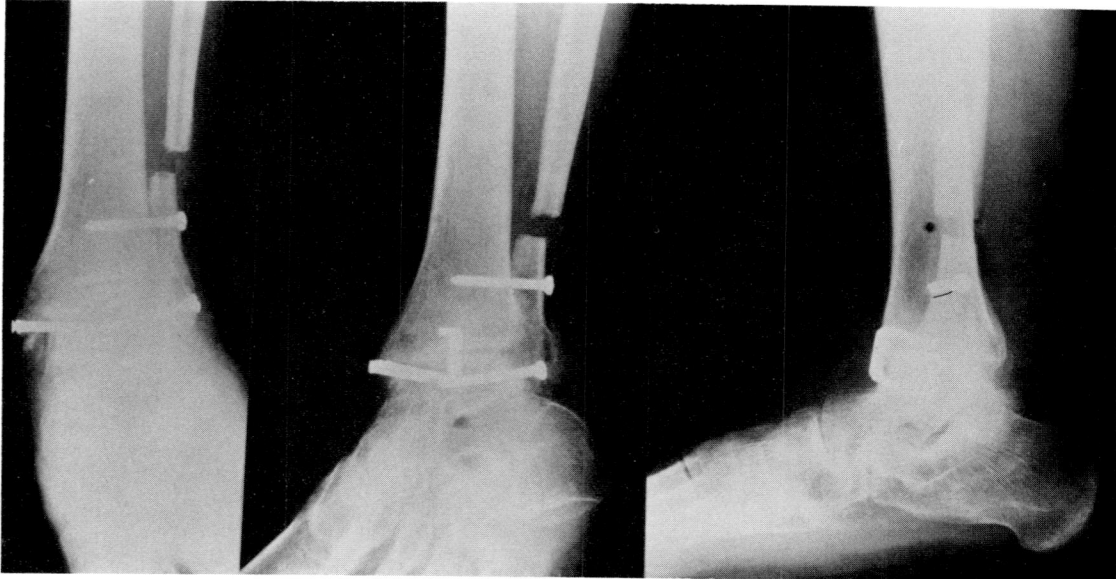

Fig. 50–16. Postoperative ankle fusion for old fracture-dislocation of ankle resulting in traumatic osteoarthritis with severe pain. Ankle fusion has been performed with a lateral approach using a living fibular graft and supplementary staple fixation. The ankle is fused in a neutral position on the lateral film. Note the normal joints in the hindfoot that allow 20 to 25 degrees of plantar flexion and dorsiflexion and a normal gait.

REFERENCES

1. Aufranc, O., and Larson, C.B.: Personal communication.
2. Berg, E., et al.: Non-operative care of the painful rheumatoid foot. American Academy of Orthopaedic Surgeons, Exhibit, 1978.
3. Clayton, M.L.: Results of surgery in rheumatoid feet. Excerpta Medica Intl. Congress Series No. 165, October, 1967.
4. Clayton, M.L.: Surgery of the lower extremity in rheumatoid arthritis. J. Bone Joint Surg., 45A:1517, 1963.
5. Clayton, M.L.: Surgery of the forefoot in rheumatoid arthritis. Clin. Orthop., 16:136, 1960.
6. Clayton, M.L.: Surgery of the forefoot in rheumatoid arthritis. Arthritis Rheum., 2:84–85, 1959.
7. Clayton, M.L., Leidholt, J.D., and Smyth, C.J.: Surgery of the forefoot in rheumatoid arthritis. Motion picture available through the American Academy of Orthopaedic Surgeons, Chicago, Illinois.
8. Elabor, J.E., Thomas, W.H., Weinfeld, M.S., and Potter, T.: Talonavicular arthrodesis for rheumatoid arthritis of the hindfoot. Orthop. Clin. North Am., 7:821, 1976.
9. Funk, F.J., Jr.: Surgery of the foot in rheumatoid arthritis. Semin. Arthritis Rheum., 1:25, 1971.
10. Funk, F.J., Jr.: Surgery of the foot in rheumatoid arthritis. J. Med. Assoc. Ga., 58:8, 1959.
11. Gschwend, N.: Surgical Treatment of Rheumatoid Arthritis. Stuttgart, New York, Georg Thieme Verlag, 1980.
12. Hoffman, P.: An operation for severe grades of contracted or clawed toes. Am. J. Orthop. Surg., 9:441, 1912.
13. Marmor, L.: Rheumatoid deformity of the foot. Arthritis Rheum., 6:749, 1963.
14. Potter, T.A.: Rheumatoid arthritis of the foot. Exhibit American Medical Association Meeting, Denver, November, 1961.
15. Raunio, P., and Laine, H.: Synovectomy of the metatarsophalangeal joints in rheumatoid arthritis. Acta Rheumatol. Scand., 16:12, 1970.
16. Short, C.L., Bauer, W., and Reynolds, W.F.: Rheumatoid Arthritis. Cambridge, Harvard University Press, 1957.
17. Smith-Petersen, M.N., Aufranc, O.E., and Larson, C.B.: Useful surgical procedures for rheumatoid arthritis involving joints of the upper extremity. Arch. Surg., 46:764, 1943.
18. Vahvanen, V.: Rheumatoid arthritis in the pantalar joints. Acta Orthop. Scand. Suppl. 107, Helsinki, 1967.
19. Vainio, K.: The rheumatoid foot. A clinical study with pathological and roentgenological comment. Ann. Chir. Gynaecol. Fenn., 45:Suppl. 1, 1956.

Other Inflammatory Arthritic Syndromes

Chapter 51

Juvenile Rheumatoid Arthritis

John J. Calabro

Juvenile rheumatoid arthritis (JRA) is a heterogeneous condition that continues to pose considerable diagnostic challenges. This situation is not surprising in a disorder as protean as JRA, with its variable modes of onset and myriad signs, symptoms, and manifestations. The historical background and classification of this major chronic rheumatic disorder of childhood are briefly reviewed.

HISTORICAL BACKGROUND, CLASSIFICATION, AND NOMENCLATURE

Historical Background

Since childhood inflammatory arthritis was first cited in 1864 by Cornil,[43] much of the literature has been directed at clinical descriptions and efforts to classify various ''subgroups.'' As early as 1890, Diamentberger reported on the predominant involvement of large joints, the flares and remissions that characterize the course of disease, the frequent disturbances of growth, and the generally favorable prognosis.[45]

A report of 22 cases by George Frederick Still in 1897 has become the classic early description of JRA,[83] an extraordinary example of exceptional clinical observation. Moreover, Still was the first to document that joint disease could be accompanied by prominent systemic manifestations, such as high spiking fever, lymphadenopathy, splenomegaly, hepatomegaly, pleuritis, and pericarditis. In fact, the term *Still's disease* is sometimes used to describe a systemic onset, one of the major presentations of JRA. Systemic onset may also occur in adults with RA, although less frequently. Known in the past as the *Still-Chauffard syndrome,* it has gained recent recognition as ''Still's disease in the adult''[17] and ''adult-onset JRA.''[5]

Classification and Nomenclature

The classification of chronic inflammatory arthritis beginning in childhood is currently undergoing widespread revision. Although JRA is the preferred term, it is commonly employed by European and British authors to describe a subgroup of children, predominantly teenage girls with a polyarticular onset, who have IgM rheumatoid factors.[40] Chronic inflammatory arthritis of childhood is also referred to as juvenile polyarthritis, juvenile chronic polyarthritis, juvenile arthritis, or juvenile chronic arthritis. The last classification, however, coined by British and European investigators, embodies several categories, including juvenile ankylosing spondylitis, psoriatic arthritis, and other childhood spondyloarthropathies, as well as the polyarthropathies associated with systemic lupus erythematosus (SLE) and other childhood connective tissue disorders.[3]

As a childhood disorder with radically different kinds of onset, JRA will most certainly pose difficulties in early diagnosis. In fact, two recent surveys disclose that errors in diagnosis occur in close to half of all children referred to specialists.[26,47] In an effort to simplify the problem, a plethora of diagnostic criteria for JRA has emerged.[26,40] Those criteria designated for adult RA,[70] even when modified,[64] are difficult to apply to children because JRA differs from adult RA in several major ways (Table 51–1).[26,86] As a result, separate criteria for JRA

Table 51–1. Major Differences Between 100 Children and 100 Adults with Rheumatoid Arthritis: Consecutive Referrals to an Arthritis Clinic

	Frequency (%)	
	Children	Adults
Type of Onset		
Systemic	20	3
Pauciarticular*	32	6
Polyarticular	48	91
Characteristics		
High fever	20	3
Rheumatoid rash	40	2
Generalized lymphadenopathy	43	21
Splenomegaly	33	7
Chronic iridocyclitis	9	0
Subcutaneous nodules	8	20
Leukocytosis†	56	23
Rheumatoid factors‡	19	76

*Pauciarticular onset associated with chronic iridocyclitis and antinuclear antibodies has not been reported in adults.

†Leukocytosis is not only more frequent in children, but the level of the white cell count is also higher, usually from 15,000 to 30,000.

‡By the latex-fixation test, titer of 1:160 or greater.

have been adopted by the American Rheumatism Association.[14] Diagnosis requires not only disease of more than six weeks' duration, but also exclusion of other disorders sharing similar clinical manifestations such as arthritis, fever, and rash.

PREVALENCE AND ETIOLOGY

JRA is arbitrarily confined to disease beginning before age 16. It is rare before the age of 6 months, and 2 onset peaks are generally observed, between ages of 1 and 3 and 8 and 12. Girls are afflicted almost twice as frequently as boys.

In an English survey, 1 case of JRA was noted for every 1,500 school children.[18] No comparable survey has been conducted in the United States, where there may be as many as 200,000 cases. This rough estimate is based on 5% of adults with RA, however.[8] Despite such prevalence, the cause of JRA is yet to be clarified.[26] The roles of possible contributing factors are critically reviewed.

Infection, Trauma, and Stress

In the search for the origin of JRA, a variety of micro-organisms have been indicted, but none has been confirmed as a cause. Suspicion of a streptococcal origin is based on elevated antistreptolysin-O (ASO) titers, found in as many as 30% of patients with JRA.[23,80] These titers now appear to be nonspecific, also observed in other childhood disorders.[32] Failure to suppress these elevated titers in JRA patients with monthly intramuscular injections of benzathine penicillin appears to bear out their nonspecific nature.[32] Rubella was also suspected when rubella antibody levels were found to be higher in patients with JRA than in control subjects.[62] The subsequent disclosure of elevations of multiple viral antibodies, including rubella, and their direct correlation with elevations of serum IgG levels suggest that these levels are also nonspecific.[65]

Upper respiratory infection, trauma, and emotional stress are often cited as factors that may trigger the disease or a recurrence.[26,68] These situations occur with such frequency in children that their exact roles are difficult to assess. On the other hand, emotional conflicts may result from severe restrictions imposed by the disease. Consequently, psychologic evaluations should be routine in patients, so impending problems can be promptly identified and corrected.[57]

Genetic Factors

Twin studies give little support of any genetic influence because of the low concordance rates reported.[9] Recently, however, a genetic basis for JRA has been disclosed.[46] When patients with JRA were compared to healthy children, certain HLA antigens were found to occur with greater frequency among the major subgroups. Systemic onset was associated with the DR5 antigen, polyarticular onset with the DR4 antigen, and pauciarticular onset with the B27, DR5, and DR8 antigens.

Immunologic Parameters

Unlike in adults with RA, IgM rheumatoid factors are observed infrequently in the sera of children with JRA.[26,86] Moreover, in contrast to previous findings,[12] IgG rheumatoid factor levels are also normal in JRA, regardless of the type of onset.[86] On the other hand, antinuclear antibodies may be found in as many as 50% of patients with JRA.[2] Their presence may be linked to the evolution of chronic iridocyclitis.[74]

Serum immunoglobulin levels may be elevated in JRA.[13,41] When elevated levels are sustained, patients appear to have a poorer functional status and an increased incidence of hip involvement.[13] Selective IgA deficiency occurs in up to 4% of JRA patients, as compared to only 0.2% of controls.[41] IgA deficiency may thus be related to pathogenesis as a reflection of some unidentified immunologic disturbance.[41,63]

TYPES OF ONSET

Early diagnosis rests on the recognition of three distinct modes of onset, *systemic, polyarticular,* and *pauciarticular,* and is based on the character, frequency, and severity of systemic and articular manifestations observed during the first six months of disease (Table 51–2).[20,23,75] Each onset type has its own differential diagnosis and each its own major hazards (Table 51–2).

Systemic onset is accompanied by prominent systemic manifestations, particularly high fever, rash, generalized lymphadenopathy, splenomegaly, and cardiopulmonary involvement. Joint manifestations are variable; occasionally, only arthralgia is present. In polyarticular onset, defined as synovitis of more than four joints, the arthritis predominates; systemic manifestations are less frequent than in systemic onset, and fever is invariably of low grade. Pauciarticular onset, with arthritis confined to a single joint, usually a knee, or of two to four joints is the mildest form of the disease. Systemic signs are minimal or absent, with the notable exception of chronic iridocyclitis.

The major systemic manifestations of JRA are listed in Table 51–3. When viewed according to modes of onset, fever is high in patients with systemic onset and of low grade in those with polyarticular and pauciarticular onsets. Rash, generalized lymphadenopathy, splenomegaly, hepatomegaly, as well as cardiac and pleuropulmonary involvement are far more frequent in patients with

Table 51–2. American Rheumatism Association Onset Types: Differentiating Features

Onset Type	Systemic Features	Articular Findings	Major Hazard
Systemic (20%)	Frequent, including high fever	Variable, from arthralgia to florid polyarthritis	Cardiac failure from myocarditis
Polyarticular (30–40%)	Fewer, with low-grade fever	Arthritis of more than four joints	Deforming polyarthritis
Pauciarticular (40–50%)	Uncommon, except for iridocyclitis	Arthritis of one to four joints	Blindness from iridocyclitis

Table 51–3. Systemic Manifestations of 100 Patients with Juvenile Rheumatoid Arthritis According to Modes of Onset

Manifestation (No. Patients)	Frequency		
	Systemic (20)	Polyarticular (48)	Pauciarticular (32)
Fever:			
High	20	0	0
Low-grade	0	38	16
Rheumatoid rash	18	19	3
Lymphadenopathy	17	20	6
Splenomegaly	15	11	7
Hepatomegaly	4	2	4
Pericarditis	7	3	0
Myocarditis	2	0	0
Pneumonitis or pleuritis	6	2	0
Chronic iridocyclitis	1	1	7
Subcutaneous nodules	0	8	0

systemic onset. On the other hand, subcutaneous nodules occur only in patients with a polyarticular onset, whereas chronic iridocyclitis appears primarily in those with pauciarticular disease.

Systemic Onset

A predilection for boys is found only in this mode of onset, which occurs in about 20% of all patients with JRA.[26,75] Recognition of systemic onset is easy when the young patient has obvious arthritis in addition to characteristic systemic features (Fig. 51–1). Initially, however, when only arthralgia, fever, and an evanescent rash are present, diagnosis may be difficult. These children, frequently labeled as having fever of unknown origin, are often subjected to exhaustive diagnostic studies, trials of various antibiotics, and even exploratory laparotomy.[33]

When only arthralgia is present, the patient's appearance may provide the first diagnostic clue. Younger children usually appear toxic, listless, and irritable, with anorexia and weight loss. Even with high fever, shaking chills are rare, but seizures are unusual. Paradoxically, older children usually appear healthy, even at the time of fever spikes.

Cerebral signs, such as marked irritability, listlessness, seizures, and meningismus, may be so striking as to suggest primary central nervous system disease.[26,52] The cerebrospinal fluid is normal

in these patients, but their electroencephalographic tracings, unrelated to abnormalities from aspirin therapy,[15] disclose transient, nonspecific focal and diffuse abnormalities.[52]

Joint Involvement

Such involvement varies from arthralgia alone to a florid polyarthritis (Fig. 51–1). Synovitis should always be suspected when a child appears unusually inactive or refuses to walk for the examining physician. Moreover, children attempt to protect tender joints without complaining of pain. When in bed, for instance, they sit or lie in a position of generalized flexion to ease joint discomfort (Fig. 51–1). In patients with minimal or no objective arthritis, diagnosis then depends on detection of characteristic systemic signs.

Systemic Signs

Of the many systemic manifestations, fever and rash are of the greatest diagnostic value. Both may be associated with generalized lymphadenopathy, splenomegaly, hepatomegaly, pericarditis, myocarditis, pneumonitis, and a striking neutrophilic leukocytosis.

High Fever. Most often, the fever pattern is quotidian (intermittent) or double quotidian.[31] One or 2 temperature peaks above 102° F (39° C) occur daily, whereas hyperpyrexia (fever to 105° F or

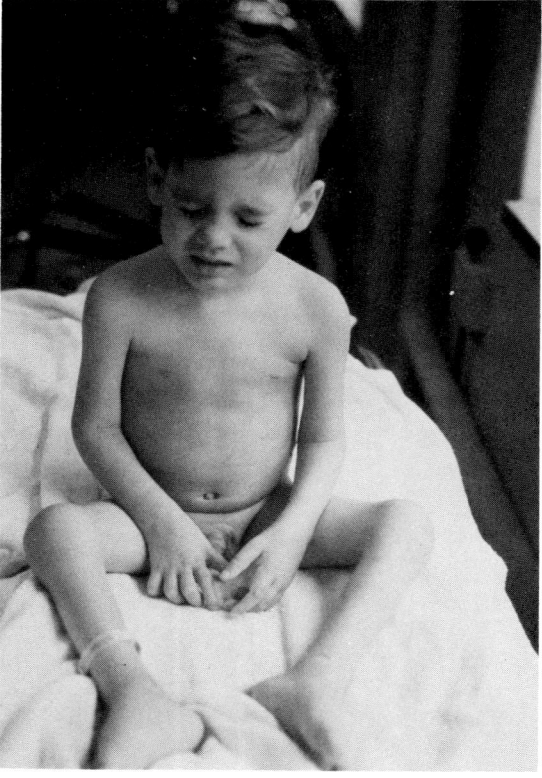

Fig. 51–1. A four-year-old boy with systemic onset who has obvious polyarthritis facilitating early diagnosis. The patient assumes a position of generalized flexion to ease the discomfort of tender, swollen joints.

40.5° C) is observed only occasionally (Fig. 51–2). Diurnal temperatures may range as widely as 9° F (5° C), so both hyperpyrexia and subnormal temperatures occur within the same day. Consequently, in patients without detectable joint swelling, careful plotting of the fever pattern may suggest the diagnosis, especially because high fever may antedate appreciable arthritis by weeks or months, even, rarely, by years.[31] High fever usually responds to aspirin, but the daily requirement varies from 60 to 130 mg/kg body weight. When the critical dose for an individual patient is reduced, fever may promptly recur.[31]

When fever is prolonged or recurs, the pattern may be relapsing (polycyclic) or even periodic. Rarely is the febrile pattern remittent.[31] In fact, the presence of remittent fever should suggest infection, drug reaction, or other causes.

Rash. A characteristic rash[29] occurs in as many as 90% of patients with systemic onset (Fig. 51–3).[26,75] It consists of discrete or confluent macules or maculopapules found on the trunk, face, or extremities, including the soles and palms.

The eruption is usually nonpruritic,[29] but it does itch, sometimes intensely,[76] in about 5% of patients.[36]

Occasionally constant, the rash is more often evanescent, usually appearing in conjunction with fever spikes. Individual macules migrate from day to day. The degree of erythema also varies; faint lesions may be intensified by massaging or by applying heat. The rash is most florid where the skin is rubbed or is subjected to microtrauma, such as the light pressure of underclothing. This characteristic is known as the Koebner phenomenon and may be diagnostically useful when parents report a rash that is not present when the child is examined. The typical rash may then be induced by rubbing or lightly scratching the skin at a susceptible site, an extremity or the lower abdomen.[29] Within several minutes, macules appear and often persist for a day or so.

The histologic features of the rash vary;[29] however, the preponderance of perivascular mononuclear cells, rather than neutrophils, differentiates the rheumatoid rash from that of rheumatic fever.

Carditis. Although fever may be misinterpreted and the rash overlooked, cardiac involvement of an untreated child may have serious, if not fatal, consequences.[21] Myocarditis is the most serious because it may rapidly induce cardiac enlargement and subsequent heart failure.[26,61] It should always be suspected in the presence of tachypnea, tachycardia disproportionate to the degree of fever, pericarditis, or pneumonitis.[22] Endocarditis does not seem to occur; cardiac murmurs suggesting its presence are believed to be functional.

Pericarditis, which is more frequent than myocarditis, is usually a benign manifestation that rarely produces acute cardiac tamponade,[58] but it may recur. The early detection of pericarditis is important because it may herald impending myocarditis.[26] Because precordial pain and dyspnea are rare, most attacks of pericarditis remain asymptomatic and undetected, unless the child is monitored regularly for evanescent friction rub, cardiomegaly, and electro- or echocardiographic abnormalities.[11]

Pleuropulmonary Signs. Pneumonitis or pleuritis frequently accompanies carditis, but also occurs independently.[88] Pleuritis is often asymptomatic and is detected as an incidental finding on chest roentgenogram. Chronic pulmonary fibrosis is rare.[54,88]

Lymphadenopathy. Generalized lymphadenopathy is frequent and may be prominent enough, particularly in epitrochlear and axillary lymph nodes, to suggest leukemia or lymphoma. Enlarged mesenteric lymph nodes may cause abdominal pain

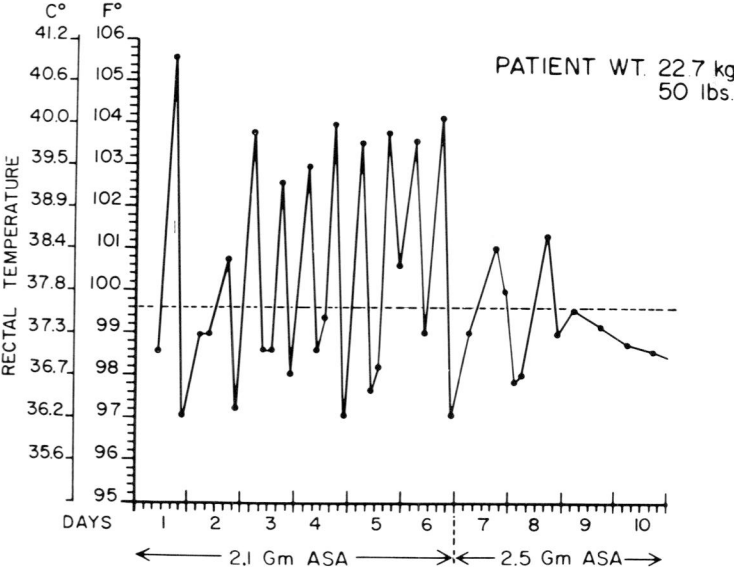

Fig. 51–2. Typical fever pattern of systemic onset has one (quotidian) or two daily peaks (double quotidian) and wide diurnal variations. Fever is suppressed with critical daily aspirin (ASA) dosage of 110 mg/kg.

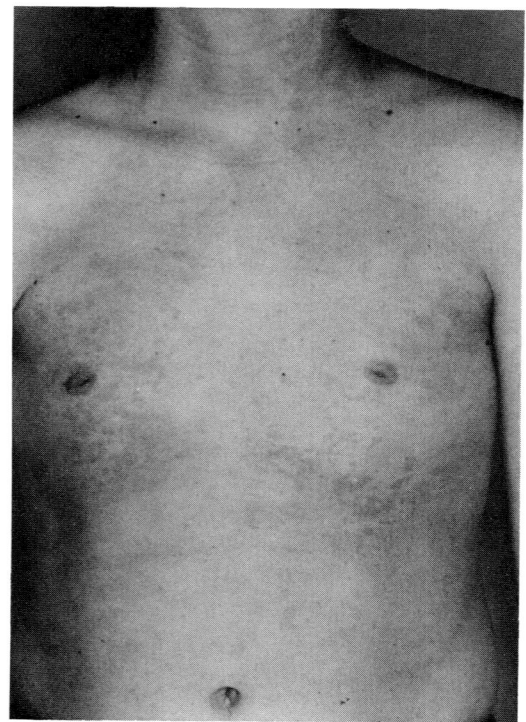

Fig. 51–3. The rheumatoid rash, present in 90% of systemic-onset patients, consists of faint macules or maculopapules occurring primarily on the trunk and extremities.

or distention, which may suggest an acute abdominal disorder requiring surgical intervention.

Hepatosplenomegaly. Splenomegaly occurs frequently, hepatomegaly less often.[26,75] Hepatomegaly may be accompanied by abdominal pain and distention as well as abnormalities of liver function and nonspecific histologic changes.[77] In addition to direct hepatic involvement,[66,77] abnormalities of liver function may result from therapy with aspirin.[7,67] Progressive hepatomegaly should arouse one's suspicion of secondary amyloidosis, but this complication is rare during the initial year of disease.

Other Systemic Signs. Encephalitis and vasculitis are rare in JRA. Their presence should suggest other diagnostic possibilities, particularly polyarteritis or other forms of systemic vasculitis. Serous peritonitis is rare, but constitutes another cause of abdominal pain and distention.

Differential Diagnosis

When arthritis is absent, the differential diagnosis may be difficult. Infection must always be ruled out first. Then, other causes of high fever, rash, and joint pain must be considered. Prominent among these are SLE, Kawasaki disease or another of the systemic vasculitides, leukemia, and inflammatory bowel disease.

Children with SLE, in contrast to adults, are more likely to have generalized lymphadenopathy, hepatosplenomegaly, and high fever,[60] features also typical of JRA. Oral mucosal lesions, renal involvement, and presence of antinative DNA antibodies support a diagnosis of SLE. Further clues include thrombocytopenia and leukopenia because these abnormalities are rare in JRA. On the other hand, the absence of antinuclear antibodies virtually excludes the diagnosis of SLE. Antinuclear antibodies may be detected in both JRA and SLE, but the titers are generally higher in SLE.[55]

Systemic vasculitis should be suspected in the presence of purpura, hypertension, or nephritis,[44] whereas profound anemia, purpura, or erosive changes on joint roentgenogram are clues to the possibility of malignant disease, particularly leukemia.[25,28,73] High spiking fever can be a prominent feature of inflammatory bowel disease, particularly regional enteritis,[72] as well as Kawasaki disease.[19] The presence of erythema nodosum and mucosal ulcers should suggest underlying inflammatory bowel disease; early features of Kawasaki disease include a strawberry tongue, red lips, conjunctivitis, erythema of the palms and soles, and an indurative edema of the hands and feet.

Polyarticular Onset

This presentation occurs in 30 to 40% of all affected children, mostly girls, and is characterized by arthritis of more than 4 joints that may begin either abruptly or insidiously. When abrupt, painful swelling of several joints occurs. When insidious, joint discomfort may be minimal; even early morning stiffness may be absent. Nevertheless, most patients appear ill. They are often listless, febrile, anorectic, and losing weight.

Articular Findings

Large joints such as knees, wrists, ankles, and elbows are the most frequent sites of initial involvement. Affected joints are usually swollen, tender, and restricted in motion, and warmth and redness may or may not be present. The pattern of arthritis varies. It may be generalized, as in adult RA, with symmetric involvement of multiple joints, including the hands and feet (Fig. 51–4). Polyarthritis may be confined to large joints and, when asymmetric or migratory, may be confused with other rheumatic disorders. Tenosynovitis may also occur, but it is rarely the sole presenting sign.

Hips are involved frequently, and when disease is progressive, ankylosis may ensue rapidly.[51] Affliction of the cervical spine, also frequent, causes tenderness and restriction of motion, particularly lateral flexion. Early radiographic changes include demineralization of vertebral bodies and apophyseal narrowing, primarily at C2 and C3 (Fig. 51–5).[59] Asymptomatic sacroiliitis is an early radiographic finding that appears to correlate with hip involvement, rheumatoid factors, and the onset of disease at ten years of age or older.[39] Axial

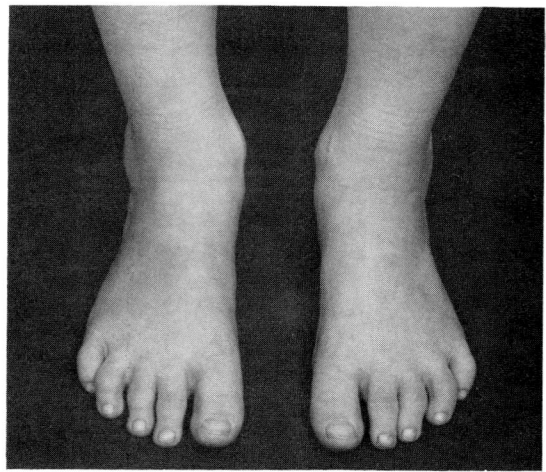

Fig. 51–4. Polyarticular onset in an 8-year-old girl with symmetric swelling of ankle, metatarsophalangeal, and proximal interphalangeal joints.

articulations other than cervical and sacroiliac are rarely involved. Transient temporomandibular complaints are frequent, and ankylosis is a rare but difficult problem.[69]

Systemic Signs

Fever is frequent; it is low grade, with one or two daily peaks under 102° F (39° C).[31] Tachycardia may be out of proportion to the degree of fever. Systemic signs are less frequent than in JRA of systemic onset, except for subcutaneous nodules, which occur only in patients with polyarticular onset (Table 51–3).

Subcutaneous Nodules. These nodules develop in areas of excessive pressure or friction and are most frequent at the olecranon process of the elbow, the proximal ulnar aspect of the forearm, or in back of the heel (Fig. 51–6). On histologic study, the nodules of JRA resemble those of rheumatic fever more closely than they do the nodules of adults with RA.[26] Nodules impart a poor prognosis, and their presence is often associated with progressive polyarthritis and deformity.

Subcutaneous nodules also occur in SLE, rarely in other connective tissue disorders. Nodules histologically indistinguishable from those observed in adult RA may also occur in otherwise healthy children and occasionally in conjunction with granuloma annulare.[81] Known as *pseudorheumatoid* or *benign rheumatoid nodules*, they are characterized by their predilection for the pretibial areas and the scalp, by their spontaneous regression, and by their frequent recurrence, particularly following surgical removal. Consequently, surgical excision and other forms of therapy are unnecessary in this self-limited and benign syndrome.

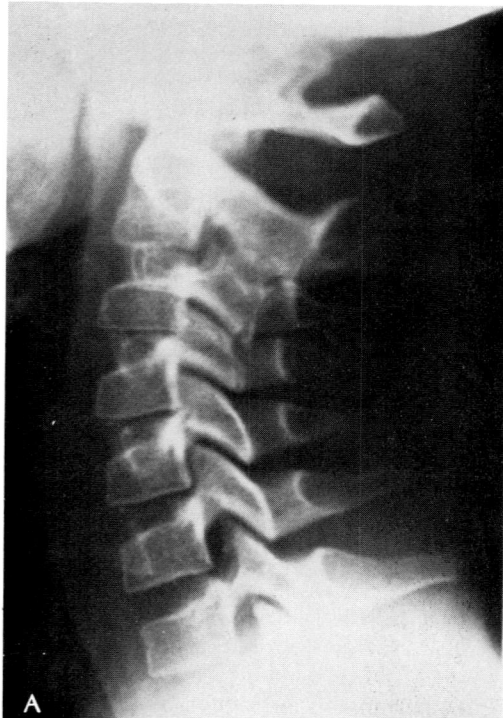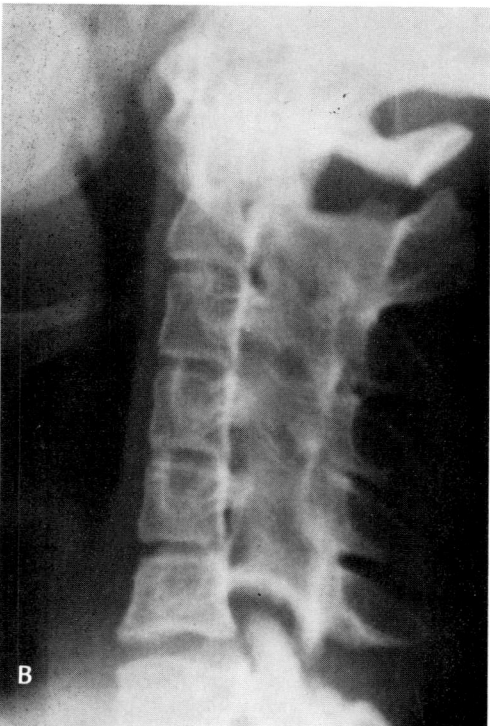

Fig. 51–5. Serial radiograms showing progressive cervical involvement. *A,* At age 12, early changes include diffuse demineralization of vertebral bodies and apophyseal fusion at C2 and C3. *B,* At age 16, one sees diffuse apophyseal fusion from C2 to C6 and underdeveloped vertebrae C2 to C6 from early closure of epiphyses.

Polyarticular Subtypes

Two subsets of polyarticular onset must be distinguished. The first includes primarily teenage-onset patients, usually girls, who frequently have rheumatoid nodules or rheumatoid factors.[21] As in adults with these findings, the course of arthritis is often progressive and deforming unless therapy with remission-inducing drugs, such as intramuscular gold, is instituted early.

The second subset consists of seronegative children, primarily girls, who have an atypical form of spondylitis characterized by rheumatoid-like joint swelling of the hands and limitation of neck motion from cervical apophyseal fusion that persists into adulthood.[6] In addition to the HLA-B27 antigen, cervical apophyseal fusion is associated with micrognathia, acute anterior uveitis, sacroiliitis, and spondylitis. Early recognition may be difficult because spondylitic features may be overshadowed by the prominence of peripheral joint involvement, including rheumatoid-like hand deformities.

Differential Diagnosis

Certain similarities make it difficult to distinguish polyarticular JRA from acute rheumatic fever.[35] Both disorders may manifest asymmetric and migratory arthritis of large joints, low-grade fever, pericarditis, abdominal pain, and elevation of ASO titers.[30] Remittent fever, in which the daily temperature does not fall to normal levels, should suggest rheumatic fever, whereas intermittent fever characterizes JRA.[31] Several other features that help to rule out rheumatic fever are onset under age four, cervical involvement, generalized lymphadenopathy, a poor mucin clot on synovial fluid analysis, and persistence of polyarthritis to or beyond the second month.

SLE must be considered in the differential diagnosis of polyarthritis. The salient features of this connective tissue disorder have already been cited. Serum sickness and drug reactions may also be confused with JRA because polyarthritis and fever are usually present. Presence of urticaria, remittent fever, and diminished serum complement levels favors these disorders, rather than JRA.

Viral arthritides have not been widely appreciated in the differential diagnosis of acute polyarthritis.[50,87] These disorders are usually self-limited. In viral hepatitis, for example, arthritis and urticaria disappear with the onset of clinical jaundice.

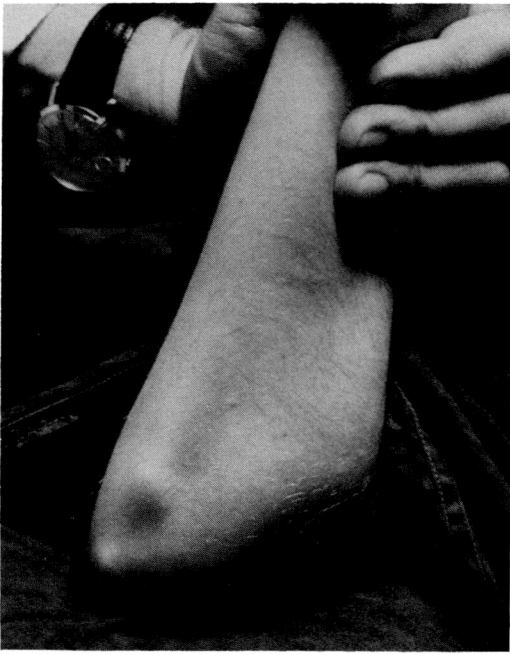

Fig. 51–6. Subcutaneous nodules occur most frequently at the olecranon process of the elbow and proximal ulnar aspect of the forearm.

The total serum hemolytic complement levels may be depressed in the presence of joint symptoms; hepatitis-associated antigen; and abnormalities of liver function may be found.[1] The arthritis that follows rubella[50] or rubella vaccination[85] may resemble JRA. Rising or falling hemagglutination-inhibition antibody titers in sera obtained during the acute phase and in convalescence, as well as the paucity of neutrophils in synovial fluid, differentiate these disorders from JRA.

Pauciarticular Onset

This mode of onset occurs in 40 to 50% of all cases and is manifest by arthritis of 1 to 4 joints. Girls are more frequently affected than boys. Children 5 years of age or under are often listless and irritable, have a low-grade fever, and fail to grow at a normal rate. On the other hand, constitutional symptoms are notably absent in older children.

Articular Findings

The onset of arthritis is usually insidious, with swelling and stiffness. The initial joint most often involved is the knee.[26,38,75] Joint pain is usually mild, but may be completely absent even in the presence of marked swelling and effusion.

Systemic Signs

Comparatively few systemic signs occur in this form of JRA (Table 51–3). Low-grade quotidian fever may be present, but cardiopulmonary involvement is notably absent. The most potentially serious manifestation is chronic iridocyclitis, which occurs in 20 to 40% of patients.[42,75,79]

Chronic Iridocyclitis. What makes this ocular manifestation so particularly treacherous is that it is so often asymptomatic, progressing quietly for weeks or months until failing vision alone compels medical attention.[27,79] This disorder may even occur months to years before the arthritis.

The course of iridocyclitis is usually chronic, with long periods of active ocular inflammation, remission, and subsequent recurrence. Initially, ocular pain and redness may be absent, and the process goes undetected until sight is impaired, first from synechiae or glaucoma, and later by cataract or band keratopathy (Fig. 51–7).

Pauciarticular Subtype

A subset of children with pauciarticular onset must be reclassified. It includes mostly teenage-onset boys with arthritis who are positive for the HLA-B27 antigen, but negative for both rheumatoid factors and antinuclear antibodies.[16,34,78] These patients usually have an asymmetric pauciarthritis of lower limb joints and are initially believed to have pauciarticular JRA. On long-term observation, however, some children eventually develop back complaints and other typical clinical and radiographic features of ankylosing spondylitis, whereas others develop Reiter's syndrome or still another of the seronegative spondyloarthropathies.[34,71]

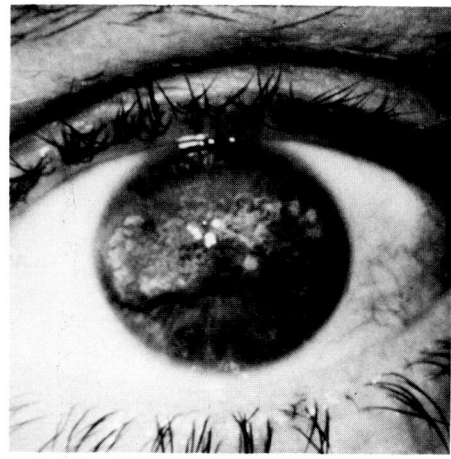

Fig. 51–7. Undetected iridocyclitis may lead to band keratopathy (as shown in the upper portion of the photograph) with calcific deposits in Bowman's membrane extending horizontally as a band across the cornea.

Differential Diagnosis

When a single joint is affected, arthrocentesis and synovial fluid analysis are essential to rule out septic arthritis. This approach also aids differentiation from traumatic and tuberculous arthritis. If tuberculosis is suspected, synovial biopsy to detect the presence of caseating granulomas may be needed. In JRA, histologic examination discloses nonspecific synovitis with hypertrophy, increased vascularity, and lymphocyte infiltration.

Pauciarticular arthritis may also be the initial manifestation of such diverse disorders as sarcoidosis, hemophilia, sickle cell anemia, inflammatory bowel disease, psoriasis, Reiter's syndrome, and Lyme disease.[26,82]

LABORATORY AND RADIOLOGIC FINDINGS

Laboratory Abnormalities

Although JRA has no consistent laboratory abnormality, each major presentation of the disease is associated with certain abnormalities that may provide additional clues for early diagnosis (Table 51–4). Elevation of the erythrocyte sedimentation rate (ESR), the presence of other acute-phase reactants, low-grade anemia, and thrombocytosis are frequently present, except in pauciarticular onset. A striking neutrophilic leukocytosis, with leukocyte values usually between 20,000 and 30,000/mm^3 and occasionally higher, is usual in systemic onset.[26] Leukocytosis is modest in polyarticular onset, whereas the white blood count is often normal in pauciarticular onset. Routine urinalysis reveals little, except febrile proteinuria.

A positive latex-fixation test is seen in 10 to 20% of children. Positive tests can be correlated with late onset (ages 12 to 16), polyarticular onset, subcutaneous nodules, and a poor functional outcome.[26,49,56] Elevated antinuclear antibody titers,

found in as many as 50% of patients, correlate with early onset (under age 6), pauciarticular onset, and chronic iridocyclitis.[2,74] Emergence of these antibodies may thus prove useful in identifying patients at risk for iridocyclitis.[74]

Serum protein electrophoresis may reveal low albumin levels and elevated levels of beta and gamma globulins. This test also excludes patients with the arthritis associated with agammaglobulinemia from those with JRA. The significance of serum immunoglobulin values, as well as elevated ASO titers, has already been cited. The presence of B27 on HLA typing, especially in teenage boys, may be a clue to ankylosing spondylitis.

Analysis of synovial fluid is variable and does not always correlate with the intensity of arthritis. The white blood cell count is usually between 10,000 and 20,000/mm^3, but it may range from 150 to 50,000/mm^3. Synovial fluid complement levels are often depressed.

Roentgenographic Features

Early roentgenographic abnormalities are nonspecific and include juxta-articular demineralization, radiodensities from soft tissue swelling or effusion, and, occasionally, periosteal proliferation (Fig. 51–8). Erosions are only late findings that occur primarily in patients with progressive polyarthritis. (See also Figs. 5–35 to 5–39.)

DISEASE COURSE AND PROGNOSIS

Course of Disease

Largely determined by the mode of onset, three patterns of disease course have been observed: polycyclic systemic, polyarthritic, and pauciarthritic.[23,26]

Children with systemic onset may pursue a polycyclic systemic course, with recurrent attacks, primarily consisting of high fever and rash, but with minimal or no arthritis. Most systemic-onset pa-

Table 51–4. Laboratory Findings in Each Major Presentation

	Systemic	*Polyarticular*	*Pauciarticular*
Erythrocyte sedimentation rate	Elevated, often to striking levels	Modest elevation	Usually normal or minimally elevated
Low-grade anemia	Frequent	Frequent	Rare
Thrombocytosis	Frequent	Frequent*	Frequent†
Leukocytosis	Common, often to marked levels	Modest	Rare
Rheumatoid factor‡	Rare	10–20%	Rare
Antinuclear antibodies	Rare	10–20%	30–50%§

*The highest values of one or more million/mm^3 occur with progressive polyarthritis or when secondary amyloidosis develops.

†Thrombocytosis (platelet count of 400,000/mm^3 or greater) may be the only laboratory abnormality in this presentation.

‡By the latex-fixation test, titer of 1:160 or greater.

§High correlation with chronic iridocyclitis.

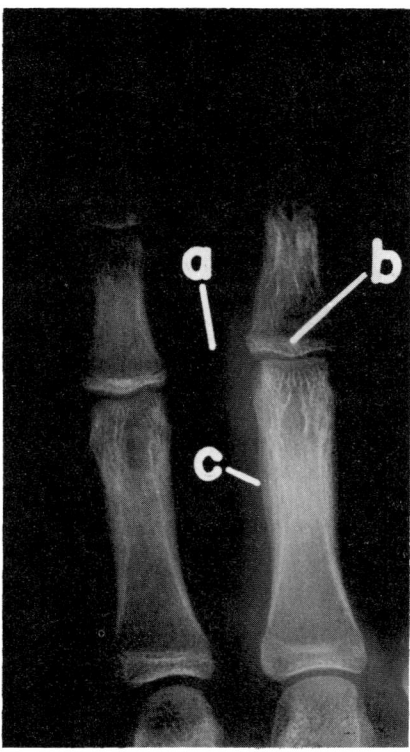

Fig. 51–8. Early roentgen features include soft tissue swelling (a), early closure of epiphysis (b), and periosteal new bone along shaft of third proximal phalanx (c).

tients develop polyarthritis or chronic arthritis of more than four joints; a few, however, continue to have superimposed attacks of high fever and other systemic manifestations. Patients with polyarticular onset remain polyarthritic; their course is usually characterized by flares and remissions, but occasionally by an unremitting and progressively downhill course. Of patients with pauciarticular onset, most pursue a course of pauciarthritis or chronic arthritis of one to four joints, but some develop polyarthritis. Regardless of the course, some patients may have to be reclassified when ankylosing spondylitis, psoriasis, or features of another rheumatic disorder eventually appear.

Growth Disturbances

General growth and development may be impaired in patients with JRA.[4,24,35,40] This impairment is related to progressively active disease as well as to the prolonged administration of corticosteroids. Once the disease becomes inactive, growth is resumed, and the child usually achieves normal proportions. If disease activity is prolonged and unremitting, however, permanent stunting of growth may occur from premature closure of epiph-

yses. The development of secondary sex characteristics may also be retarded.

Local abnormalities of growth include premature appearance and closure of epiphyses resulting in small hands or feet, as well as in isolated shortened metacarpals, metatarsals, or phalanges. Premature epiphyseal closure may be especially striking in the mandible, in which it produces micrognathia (Fig. 51–9). Occasionally, particularly in pauciarticular JRA, overgrowth of epiphyses and metaphyses may cause one limb to be longer than the other. Such a discrepancy usually reverts to normal once disease activity is suppressed or remits.

Prognosis

Of patients followed for up to 15 years, complete remission occurs in at least 50% whereas 70% regain normal function.[26,37,40,48] Remission can occur at any time and does not necessarily coincide with the onset of puberty. Occasionally, however, a child in prolonged remission may have an exacerbation of the disease as an adult that results in joint destruction and severe disability for the first time.[53]

The mortality rate of JRA is 2 to 4%.[10] Most deaths occur in children with prolonged active polyarthritis and are due primarily to infection and secondary amyloidosis.[26,84]

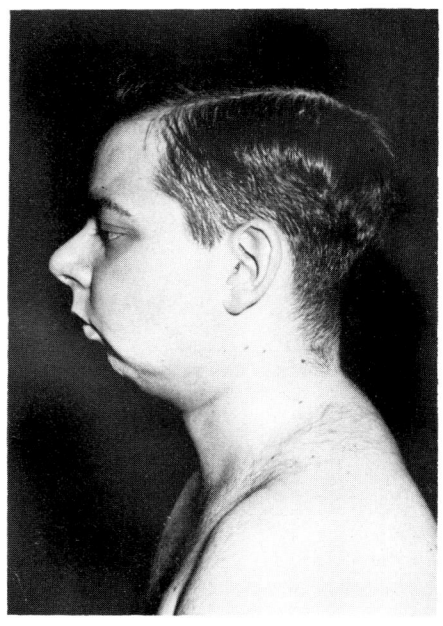

Fig. 51–9. Pronounced micrognathia in a young man with prolonged polyarthritis and progressive cervical involvement.

REFERENCES

1. Alpert, E., Isselbacher, K.J., and Schur, P.H.: The pathogenesis of arthritis associated with viral hepatitis. Complement-component studies. N. Engl. J. Med., 285:185–189, 1971.

2. Alspaugh, M.A., and Miller, J.J., III: A study of specificities of antinuclear antibodies in juvenile rheumatoid arthritis. J. Pediatr., 90:391–395, 1977.

3. Ansell, B.M.: Juvenile chronic polyarthritis. Series 3. Arthritis Rheum., 20(Suppl.):176–178, 1977.

4. Ansell, B.M., and Bywaters, E.G.L.: Growth in Still's disease. Ann. Rheum. Dis., 15:295–319, 1956.

5. Aptekar, R.G., et al.: Adult onset juvenile rheumatoid arthritis. Arthritis Rheum., 16:715–718, 1973.

6. Arnett, F.C., Bias, W.B., and Stevens, M.B.: Juvenile-onset chronic arthritis. Clinical and roentgenographic features of a unique HLA-B27 subset. Am. J. Med., 69:369–376, 1980.

7. Athreya, B.H., Gorski, A.L., and Myers, A.R.: Aspirin-induced abnormalities of liver function. Am. J. Dis. Child., 126:638–641, 1973.

8. Baum, J., Epidemiology of juvenile rheumatoid arthritis. Arthritis Rheum., 20 (Suppl.):158–160, 1977.

9. Baum, J., and Fink, C.: Juvenile rheumatoid arthritis in monozygotic twins: A case report and review of the literature. Arthritis Rheum., 11:33–36, 1968.

10. Baum, J., and Goutowska, G.: Death in juvenile rheumatoid arthritis. Arthritis Rheum., 20 (Suppl.):253–255, 1977.

11. Bernstein, G., Takahashi, M., and Hanson, V.: Cardiac involvement in juvenile rheumatoid arthritis. J. Pediatr., 85:313–317, 1974.

12. Bianco, N.E., et al.: Immunologic studies of juvenile rheumatoid arthritis. Arthritis Rheum., 14:685–696, 1971.

13. Bluestone, R., et al.: Juvenile rheumatoid arthritis: a serologic survey of 200 consecutive patients. J. Pediatr., 77:98–102, 1970.

14. Brewer, E.J., Jr., et al.: Current proposed revision of JRA criteria. Arthritis Rheum., 20 (Suppl.):195–199, 1977.

15. Brown, G.L., and Wilson, W.P.: Salicylate intoxication and the CNS with special reference to EEG findings. Dis. Nerv. Syst., 32:135–140, 1971.

16. Bywaters, E.G.L.: Ankylosing spondylitis in childhood. Clin. Rheum. Dis., 87:387–396, 1976.

17. Bywaters, E.G.L.: Still's disease in the adult. Ann. Rheum. Dis., 30:121–133, 1971.

18. Bywaters, E.G.L.: Diagnostic criteria for Still's disease (juvenile RA). In Population Studies of the Rheumatic Diseases. Edited by P.H. Bennett and P.H.N. Wood. Amsterdam, Excerpta Medica, 1968, pp. 235–240.

19. Calabro, J.J.: Kawasaki disease. Clin. Rheumatol. Pract., 1:29–35, 1983.

20. Calabro, J.J.: Juvenile rheumatoid arthritis. Mode of onset as key to early diagnosis and management. Postgrad. Med., 70:120–133, 1981.

21. Calabro, J.J.: Management of juvenile rheumatoid arthritis. Compr. Ther., 7:30–36, 1981.

22. Calabro, J.J.: Myocarditis in juvenile rheumatoid arthritis. Am. J. Dis. Child., 131:1306, 1977.

23. Calabro, J.J.: Clinical features of Still's disease: A general review and report of 100 patients observed for 15 years. In Still's Disease: Juvenile Chronic Polyarthritis. Edited by M.I.V. Jayson. London, Academic Press, 1971, pp. 1–45.

24. Calabro, J.J.: Rheumatoid arthritis: A potentially crippling disease that may attack at any age. CIBA Clin. Symp., 23:1–32, 1971.

25. Calabro, J.J.: Cancer and arthritis. Arthritis Rheum., 10:553–567, 1967.

26. Calabro, J.J., et al.: Juvenile rheumatoid arthritis. A general review and report of 100 patients observed for 15 years. Semin. Arthritis Rheum., 5:257–298, 1976.

27. Calabro, J.J., et al.: Chronic iridocyclitis in juvenile rheumatoid arthritis. Arthritis Rheum., 13:406–413, 1970.

28. Calabro, J.J., and Castleman, B.: Case records of the Massachusetts General Hospital. Multiple osteolytic lesions in a 16-year-old boy with joint pains. N. Engl. J. Med., 286:205–212, 1972.

29. Calabro, J.J., and Marchesano, J.M.: Rash associated with juvenile rheumatoid arthritis. J. Pediatr., 72:611–619, 1968.

30. Calabro, J.J., and Marchesano, J.M.: The early natural history of juvenile rheumatoid arthritis. A 10-year follow-up of 100 cases. Med. Clin. North Am., 52:567–591, 1968.

31. Calabro, J.J., and Marchesano, J.M.: Fever associated with juvenile rheumatoid arthritis. N. Engl. J. Med., 276:11–18, 1967.

32. Calabro, J.J., and Marchesano, J.M.: Medical intelligence. Current concepts. Juvenile rheumatoid arthritis. N. Engl. J. Med., 277:696–699, 746–749, 1967.

33. Calabro, J.J., Burnstein, S.L., and Staley, H.L.: Juvenile rheumatoid arthritis posing as fever of unknown origin. Arthritis Rheum., 20 (Suppl.):178–180, 1977.

34. Calabro, J.J., Gordon, R.D., and Miller, K.A.: Bechterew's syndrome in children: Diagnostic criteria. Scand. J. Rheumatol., 32 (Suppl.):45–46, 1980.

35. Calabro, J.J., Katz, R.M., and Maltz, B.A.: A critical reappraisal of juvenile rheumatoid arthritis. Clin. Orthop., 74:101–119, 1971.

36. Calabro, J.J., Katz, R.M., and Marchesano, J.M.: Pruritus in juvenile rheumatoid arthritis. Pediatrics, 46:322–323, 1970.

37. Calabro, J.J., Marchesano, J.M., and Miller, K.A.: Juvenile rheumatoid arthritis. In Prognosis: Contemporary Outcomes of Disease. Edited by J.F. Fries and E.G. Ehrlich. Bowie, MD, Prentice-Hall, 1981, pp. 347–349.

38. Calabro, J.J., Parrino, G.R., and Marchesano, J.M.: Monarticular-onset juvenile rheumatoid arthritis. Bull. Rheum. Dis., 21:613–616, 1970.

39. Carter, M.E.: Sacro-iliitis in Still's disease. Ann. Rheum. Dis., 21:105–120, 1962.

40. Cassidy, J.T.: Textbook of Pediatric Rheumatology. New York, John Wiley & Sons, 1982.

41. Cassidy, J.T., Petty, R.E., and Sullivan, D.B.: Abnormalities in the distribution of serum immunoglobulin concentrations in juvenile rheumatoid arthritis. J. Clin. Invest., 52:1931–1936, 1973.

42. Chylack, L.T., Jr., et al.: Ocular manifestations of juvenile rheumatoid arthritis. Am. J. Ophthalmol., 79:1026–1033, 1975.

43. Cornil, V.: Memoire sur les coincidences pathologiques du rhumatisme articulaire chronique. C. R. Soc. Biol. (Paris), ser. 4,3:2–25, 1864.

44. Cupps, T.R., and Fauci, A.S.: The vasculitides. In Major Problems in Internal Medicine. Edited by L.H. Smith, Jr. Philadelphia, W. B. Saunders, 1981./

45. Diamentberger, S.: Du rhumatisme noueux (polyarthrite déformante) chez les enfants. Paris, Lecrosnier & Babe, 1890.

46. Forre, O., et al.: HLA antigens in juvenile arthritis. Genetic basis for the different subtypes. Arthritis Rheum., 26:35–38, 1983.

47. Grossman, B.J., and Mukhopadhyay, D.: Juvenile rheumatoid arthritis. In Current Problems in Pediatrics. Vol. 5. Edited by L. Gluck, et al. Chicago, Year Book Medical Publishers, 1975, pp. 3–65.

48. Hanson, V., et al.: Prognosis of juvenile rheumatoid arthritis. Arthritis Rheum., 20 (Suppl.):279–284, 1977.

49. Hanson, V., Drexler, E., and Kornreich, H.: The relationship of rheumatoid factor to age of onset in juvenile rheumatoid arthritis. Arthritis Rheum., 12:82–86, 1969.

50. Hyer, F.H., and Gottlieb, N.L.: Rheumatic disorders associated with viral infection. Semin. Arthritis Rheum., 8:17–31, 1978.

51. Jacqueline, F., Boujot, A., and Canet, L.: Involvement of the hips in juvenile rheumatoid arthritis. Arthritis Rheum., 4:500–513, 1961.

52. Jan, J.E., Hill, R.H., and Low, M.D.: Cerebral complications in juvenile rheumatoid arthritis. Can. Med. Assoc. J., 107:623–625, 1972.

53. Jeremy, R., et al.: Juvenile rheumatoid arthritis persisting into adulthood. Am. J. Med., 45:419–434, 1968.

54. Jordan, J.D., and Snyder, G.H.: Rheumatoid disease of

the lung and cor pulmonale. Am. J. Dis. Child., *108*:174–180, 1964.

55. Kornreich, H.K., Drexler, E., and Hanson, V.: Antinuclear factors in childhood rheumatic diseases. J. Pediatr., *69*:1039–1045, 1966.

56. Laaksonen, A.-L.: A prognostic study of juvenile rheumatoid arthritis. Acta Paediatr. Scand., *166 (Suppl.)*:1–163, 1966.

57. McAnarney, E.R., et al.: Psychological problems of children with chronic juvenile arthritis. Pediatrics, *53*:523–528, 1974.

58. Majeed, H.A., and Kvasnicka, J.: Juvenile rheumatoid arthritis with cardiac tamponade. Ann. Rheum. Dis., *37*:273–276, 1978.

59. Martel, W., Holt, J.F., and Cassidy, J.T.: Roentgenologic manifestations of juvenile arthritis. Am. J. Roentgenol., *88*:400–423, 1962.

60. Meislin, A.G., and Rothfield, N.: Systemic lupus erythematosus in childhood. Analysis of 42 cases, with comparative data on 200 adult cases followed concurrently. Pediatrics, *42*:37–49, 1968.

61. Miller, J.J., III, and French, J.W.: Myocarditis in juvenile rheumatoid arthritis. Am. J. Dis. Child., *131*:205–209, 1977.

62. Ogra, P.L., and Herd, J.K.: Serologic association of rubella virus infection and juvenile rheumatoid arthritis. Arthritis Rheum., *15*:121, 1972.

63. Panush, R.S., et al.: Juvenile rheumatoid arthritis. Cellular hypersensitivity and selective IgA deficiency. Clin. Exp. Immunol., *10*:103–115, 1972.

64. Pazirandeh, M., Mackenzie, A.H., and Scherbel, A.L.: The natural course of juvenile rheumatoid arthritis. Cleve. Clin. Q., *36*:109–122, 1969.

65. Phillips, P., et al.: Virus antibody and IgG levels in juvenile rheumatoid arthritis. Arthritis Rheum., *16*:126, 1973.

66. Rachelefsky, G.S., et al.: Serum enzyme abnormalities in juvenile rheumatoid arthritis. Pediatrics, *58*:730–736, 1976.

67. Rich, R.R., and Johnson, J.S.: Salicylate hepatotoxicity in patients with juvenile rheumatoid arthritis. Arthritis Rheum., *16*:1–9, 1977.

68. Rimon, R., Belmaker, R.H., and Ebstein, R.: Psychosomatic aspects of juvenile rheumatoid arthritis. Scand. J. Rheumatol., *6*:1–10, 1977.

69. Ronning, O., Valiaho, M.-L., and Laaksonen, A.-L.: The involvement of the temporomandibular joint in juvenile rheumatoid arthritis. Scand. J. Rheumatol., *3*:89–96, 1974.

70. Ropes, M.W., et al.: 1958 Revision of diagnostic criteria for rheumatoid arthritis. Bull. Rheum. Dis., *9*:175–176, 1958.

71. Rosenberg, A.M., and Petty, R.E.: A syndrome of seronegative enthesopathy and arthropathy in children. Arthritis Rheum., *25*:1041–1047, 1982.

72. Schaller, J.G.: The arthritis of inflammatory bowel disease in children. Clin. Rheum. Dis., *2*:353–367, 1976.

73. Schaller, J.G.: Arthritis as a presenting manifestation of malignancy in children. J. Pediatr., *81*:793–797, 1972.

74. Schaller, J.G., et al.: The association of antinuclear antibodies with the chronic iridocyclitis of juvenile rheumatoid arthritis (Still's disease). Arthritis Rheum., *17*:409–416, 1974.

75. Schaller, J.G., and Wedgwood, R.J.: Is juvenile rheumatoid arthritis a single disease? A review. Pediatrics, *50*:940–953, 1972.

76. Schaller, J.G., and Wedgwood, R.J.: Pruritus associated with the rash of juvenile rheumatoid arthritis. Pediatrics, *45*:296–298, 1970.

77. Schaller, J.G., Beckwith, B., and Wedgwood, R.J.: Hepatic involvement in juvenile rheumatoid arthritis. J. Pediatr., *77*:203–210, 1970.

78. Schaller, J.G., Bitnum, S., and Wedgwood, R.J.: Ankylosing spondylitis with childhood onset. J. Pediatr., *74*:505–516, 1969.

79. Schaller, J.G., Kupfer, C., and Wedgwood, R.J.: Iridocyclitis in juvenile rheumatoid arthritis. Pediatrics, *44*:92–100, 1969.

80. Sievers, J., et al.: Serological patterns in juvenile rheumatoid arthritis. Rheumatism, *19*:88–93, 1963.

81. Simons, F.E.R., and Schaller, J.G.: Benign rheumatoid nodules. Pediatrics, *56*:29–33, 1975.

82. Steere, A.C., et al.: The early clinical manifestations of Lyme disease. Ann. Intern. Med., *99*:76–82, 1983.

83. Still, G.F.: On a form of chronic joint disease in children. Med. Chir. Trans., *80*:47–59, 1897. (Reprinted in Am. J. Dis. Child., *132*:195–200, 1978.)

84. Stoeber, E.: Prognosis in juvenile chronic arthritis. Follow-up of 433 chronic rheumatic children. Eur. J. Pediatr., *135*:225–228, 1981.

85. Thompson, G.R., Ferreyra, A., and Brachett, R.: Acute arthritis complicating rubella vaccination. Arthritis Rheum., *14*:19–26, 1971.

86. Wernick, R., et al.: Serum IgG and IgM rheumatoid factors by solid phase radioimmunoassay. A comparison between adult and juvenile rheumatoid arthritis. Arthritis Rheum., *24*:1501–1511, 1981.

87. West, R.J.: Acute polyarthritis: Diagnosis and management. Clin. Rheum. Dis., *2*:305–337, 1976.

88. Yousefzadeh, D.K., and Fishman, P.A.: The triad of pneumonitis, pleuritis, and pericarditis in juvenile rheumatoid arthritis. Pediatr. Radiol., *8*:147–150, 1979.

Chapter **52**

Treatment of Juvenile Rheumatoid Arthritis

Jane Green Schaller

Considerations in designing therapy for a child with juvenile rheumatoid arthritis (JRA) include the following: (1) recognition of the several disease subgroups of JRA; (2) identification of specific disease manifestations requiring therapy in the individual patient; (3) understanding of the long-term natural history of the disease and of its various manifestations; (4) cognizance of the overall favorable prognosis for most affected children; and (5) acknowledgment of the special burdens of chronic illness on children, adolescents, and their families.

Several subgroups can be distinguished within the "disease" now called JRA in the United States and Still's disease or juvenile chronic polyarthritis in other parts of the world.[1,6,15,17,19,42,48,49,53,54,59] Five possible subgroups and their characteristics are given in Table 52–1.[53,54,59] Whether these subgroups represent truly different diseases or only different host responses to one or more etiologic factors is not known. In any event, recognition of disease subgroups is helpful in diagnosis and in the selection of appropriate therapy in patients with JRA (see also Chap. 51).

Several distinct manifestations of JRA may require therapy. These should be identified accurately in the individual patient before planning any therapeutic program. These different disease manifestations are listed in Table 52–2 and are discussed separately in subsequent sections of this chapter.

The overall prognosis for children with JRA is better than had been previously assumed; at least 75% of affected children eventually have long remissions without significant residual damage and presumably lead normal adult lives.[1,3,6,15,17,19,42,49,53,59] Several long-term sequelae can follow JRA (Table 52–3). The risks of these sequelae vary according to disease subgroup. Children with rheumatoid-factor-positive or systemic-onset JRA are at greatest risk for chronic and destructive joint disease. Children with pauciarticular disease beginning in early childhood are at greatest risk for chronic iridocyclitis,[18,21,55,57,62] and those with pauciarticular disease beginning in later childhood are at some risk for subsequent ankylosing spondylitis

or another spondyloarthropathy.[31,34,46,49,51,53,57,61] Growth retardation occurs most frequently in children with chronic systemic-onset or polyarticular disease.[4,11,71]

Available therapy permits control of synovitis in many children with JRA, although chronic synovitis with joint destruction, a cause of ultimate morbidity in JRA, is not always preventable. Fortunately, fewer than 20% of children with JRA have relentlessly active synovitis with resultant severe joint destruction. Synovitis can be adequately controlled in many children, especially in those with seronegative polyarthritis or with pauciarticular disease. Much of the present therapy of JRA is focused on preventing lasting deformity, and this goal can often be reached. Such residual deformities can cripple the musculoskeletal system, the eye, and the child's psychosocial structure. Iatrogenic damage from the injudicious use of drugs and from overvigorous physical and surgical therapy must be prevented at all costs.

THERAPY OF ARTHRITIS AND MAINTENANCE OF MUSCULOSKELETAL FUNCTION

In planning therapy for the musculoskeletal manifestations of JRA, the physician must first assess the extent of joint involvement in the individual patient, the activity of the synovitis, the presence or absence of joint destruction, the status of muscle strength or weakness, and the amount of joint deformity and must determine whether observed joint deformities are due to active disease or are residua of inactive disease. In making these assessments, a careful history and physical examination, selected radiographs, and certain laboratory tests, such as the hematocrit and erythrocyte sedimentation rate, are of value.

Drug Therapy

To control active synovitis and the musculoskeletal manifestations of active JRA, drugs of the anti-inflammatory and antirheumatic classes are prescribed. None of these agents are curative, but synovitis can be satisfactorily suppressed with cur-

Table 52–1. Subgroups of Juvenile Rheumatoid Arthritis

Type of Disease	Ratio of Girls to Boys	Age at Onset	Joints Affected	Serology	Extra-articular Manifestations	Prognosis
Systemic onset	8/10	Any age	Any joints	ANA negative; RF negative; HLA-?	High fever, rash, organomegaly, polyserositis, leukocytosis	20% severe arthritis
Polyarticular: rheumatoid factor negative	8/1	Any age	Any joints	ANA 25%; RF negative; HLA-?	Low-grade fever, mild anemia, malaise	10% severe arthritis
Polyarticular: rheumatoid factor positive	6/1	Late childhood	Any joints	ANA 75%; RF 100%; HLA-DR4	Mild fever, anemia, malaise, rheumatoid nodules	>50% severe arthritis
Pauciarticular: early childhood onset, associated with chronic iridocyclitis	7/1	Early childhood	Scattered joints, predominantly large joints; hips and sacroiliac joints spared	ANA 60%; RF negative; HLA-DRW8, -DR5, -DRW6	Few constitutional complaints; chronic iridocyclitis in 50%	Severe arthritis uncommon; 10–20% ocular damage from iridocyclitis
Pauciarticular: late childhood onset, associated with sacroiliitis	1/10	Late childhood	Scattered large joints; hip girdle and sacroiliac involvement common	ANA negative; RF negative, HLA-B27	Few constitutional complaints; acute iridocyclitis in 5–10%	Some with ankylosing spondylitis at follow-up

ANA = Antinuclear antibodies; RF = rheumatoid factor.

Table 52–2. Manifestations of Juvenile Arthritis Requiring Therapy

Musculoskeletal effects
Active synovitis
Joint deformity
Muscle weakness or dysfunction
Systemic effects
Fever and other manifestations of systemic-onset disease
Constitutional manifestations of other subgroups
Iridocyclitis
Amyloidosis
Psychosocial Aspects

Table 52–3. Long-Term Sequelae of Juvenile Rheumatoid Arthritis

Persistent synovitis
Severe, with progressive joint destruction
Mild, with little progressive disability
Residual deformities from past disease
Musculoskeletal dysfunction
Ocular damage
Growth retardation
Amyloidosis
Psychosocial problems
Iatrogenic damage

rently available drug therapy in about 80% of affected children.

Salicylates

Salicylates provide the mainstay of therapy (see also Chap. 28).[1,7,16,24,50,58,59,69] They are effective as antipyretics, analgesics, and anti-inflammatory agents. Acetylsalicylic acid (aspirin) is most commonly prescribed. Other preparations occasionally used include sodium salicylate and choline salicylate; whether these are as effective as aspirin in suppressing inflammation has not been studied adequately. Appropriate doses of aspirin are 100 mg/kg body weight per day, in 4 to 6 divided doses, for children weighing 25 kg or less. For children weighing 25 kg or more, total daily doses of 2.4 to 3.6 g/day are usually sufficient. Serious salicylate intoxication can result if doses are calculated on the basis of 100 mg/kg body weight for children weighing more than 25 kg. Serum salicylate levels between 20 and 30 mg/dl are considered adequate for therapeutic effect; such blood levels are usually achieved with the aforementioned doses. Little benefit and great potential hazard exist in giving salicylates to the point of serious toxicity. Salicylates are effective in controlling synovitis in about 75% of patients. A full therapeutic response may not occur for several months.

The major hazard of salicylate therapy is salicylism resulting from overdosage. With careful adherence to dosages and measuring blood levels if necessary, serious toxicity should not result from therapeutic use of these agents. Most children do not note or complain of tinnitus, which usually occurs with serum levels of 20 to 30 mg/dl. The first signs of salicylism are central nervous system depression or excitation or hyperventilation, which occur with serum salicylate levels over 30 mg/dl. Such signs suggest overdosage. Parents, patients, and physicians should be alert to such signs of toxicity and should react to them immediately by decreasing the dose and by checking blood levels of the drug if possible.

Other problems with salicylates include gastrointestinal irritation with gastric distress or nausea. A few patients with JRA undergoing a prolonged course of salicylate therapy have developed peptic ulcers,[56] but the relationship of these ulcers to the drug is not clear. Gastrointestinal irritation can be minimized by giving salicylates with food, by using buffered preparations, by prescribing concomitant antacids, or by administering a preparation such as choline salicylate. Attention has been drawn to the "hepatotoxicity" of salicylates. Some children receiving salicylates in therapeutic dosages develop elevated serum transaminase levels, but not jaundice or other signs or symptoms of liver disease.[10,24,38,45,47,50] The hepatic involvement of systemic-onset JRA must be differentiated from that of other disorders.[33,60] Even with continuing use of drug, enzyme levels usually do not rise higher, and no later evidence of chronic liver disease appears. Few children develop severe acute liver disease after salicylate ingestion that precludes further salicylate usage. Although even low doses of aspirin affect platelet function and higher doses may lengthen the patient's prothrombin time,[43,70] serious bleeding problems are uncommon in aspirin-treated patients with JRA. It is wise to discontinue aspirin therapy several weeks before any surgical procedures and to substitute choline salicylate or sodium salicylate, neither of which affects hemostasis. Hypersensitivity reactions to aspirin such as hives are rare, and aspirin-related asthma and nasal polyps appear unusual in JRA patients.

Small numbers of red blood cells or tubular epithelial cells may be found in the urine.[41] Although chronic renal disease has not been associated with salicylate ingestion in children, a few instances of renal papillary necrosis have been reported in children with JRA who were receiving salicylates.[72] Recent epidemiologic surveys have suggested that an association may exist between salicylate ingestion and Reye's syndrome occurring with influenza or chicken pox.[68]

Other Nonsteroidal Anti-Inflammatory Agents

A number of other nonsteroidal anti-inflammatory agents are available for the treatment of arthritis in adults. These drugs seem to be similar to salicylates in efficacy, although some patients may respond better to one drug than to another (see also Chap. 28).

Although some of these drugs, particularly indomethacin, are widely used to treat JRA in various parts of the world, only tolmetin and naproxen are labeled for use in children in the United States.[12,35,39,40] In patients with pauciarticular JRA beginning in late childhood who may have ankylosing spondylitis, some of these drugs might be of therapeutic benefit. Some might provide useful alternatives to salicylates in selected cases, such as in patients who do not respond satisfactorily to salicylates.

Gold Compounds

In children with progressive loss of joint function due to active synovitis after 6 months of adequate salicylate and physical therapy, gold therapy may be indicated.[13,14,16,58,59] Such patients often have positive rheumatoid factors or chronic arthritis after a systemic onset. The gold preparations are the same as those used in adults. The dosage is 1 mg/kg body weight/week up to a body weight of 25 kg. For children weighing 25 to 50 kg, a dose of 25 mg/week is appropriate; for teenagers weighing more than 60 kg, doses of 25 to 50 mg/week are used. As in adults, small "test" doses of 10 or 20% of the full dose are given for 2 or 3 weeks.

Toxicity in children is similar to that in adults and is of no greater severity or frequency. Follow-up in children receiving gold therapy consists of weekly physical examination for evidence of rash or mucosal ulcers, a weekly white blood cell count, a hematocrit and smear for platelets, and a urinalysis for both red blood cells and protein levels. Any evidence of toxicity is cause for discontinuing the treatment with gold temporarily. When toxicity disappears, gold treatment may be resumed cautiously, perhaps at a lower dose initially. As in adults, after a six months' course of weekly doses, the patient's response to the drug is assessed. Children who respond are in full or partial remission and often have normal erythrocyte sedimentation rates. In such patients, the frequency of gold injections is reduced to once every two weeks, then once every three weeks, and then indefinitely on a once-monthly basis. It is imperative to continue surveillance for toxicity, including blood and urine tests, prior to each gold injection. Gold therapy probably should be abandoned in patients who do not appear to respond in six months. Patients with partial responses may be treated weekly for some months longer, or with doses administered at longer intervals, depending on the physician's evaluation of current status.

Oral gold has been used successfully in the treatment of JRA.[26]

Antimalarial Agents

As in adults, antimalarial drugs are a useful alternative to gold therapy in some patients. Hydroxychloroquine (Plaquenil) is the drug of choice. Doses should not exceed 200 mg/m^2 body surface area per day, and ophthalmologic examinations should be made every 3 months. The side effects of antimalarial agents in children are similar to those in adults, with ocular toxicity the chief hazard of prolonged administration. Antimalarial drugs are poisons with no antidote for overdosage,[20] so their inaccessibility to small children must be ensured.

Penicillamine

D-penicillamine is currently being tested in both adults and children with RA,[5] and may be of potential usefulness to patients with severe arthritis who do not respond to salicylates or other nonsteroidal agents and as an alternative to gold. Its toxicity is similar in children and adults, and it appears to be sometimes effective in both seronegative and seropositive childhood arthritis. This drug is not available for routine use in the treatment of arthritis. Toxic effects include rash, bone marrow suppression, nephritis, and Goodpasture's syndrome.

Corticosteroids

Although there was once great enthusiasm for these drugs,[32,63] corticosteroids are no more curative of JRA than they are of adult RA.[1,7,52] These agents may suppress symptoms for a time, but they do not prevent progression of joint damage in patients with severe JRA, and they may actually contribute to articular damage in some patients. Cushingoid side effects occur early after low doses of corticosteroids. Troublesome side effects other than cushingoid appearance are also common and include adrenal suppression, which may be fatal, growth suppression, osteoporosis, vertebral compression fractures, peptic ulcer disease, and corticosteroid cataracts. Few children with JRA gain much permanent benefit from corticosteroid therapy given for arthritis alone. Although the immediate relief of symptoms may be dramatic, the ultimate effect is not curative, and the long-term side effects are often horrendous. It is of little help to a patient to add chronic Cushing's syndrome and adrenal suppression to a severe destructive arthritis.

In the experience of clinics managing many children with JRA, corticosteroid therapy is rarely warranted for joint disease alone and, if given, is used in the lowest possible doses, preferably on alternate days[2] and for as short a time as possible. The use of large intravenous "pulse" doses of corticosteroids in patients with JRA remains experimental.[37]

Adrenocorticotropic hormone (ACTH) has been used to advantage in some clinics,[73] because it may have fewer long-term side effects than corticosteroids. Local corticosteroid injections into troublesome joints may suppress local synovitis, but no more than several injections should be made into any single joint, to avoid cartilage damage.

Immunosuppressive Drugs

Although drugs such as cyclophosphamide, azathioprine, and methotrexate have been tested and used in the therapy of adult RA,[36] no similar studies have been made in childhood arthritis.[30] The side effects of such drugs include increased susceptibility to potentially fatal and often untreatable infections with viruses, fungi, and other agents, possible future increased risk of malignant disease, and interference with future reproductive capacity.[30,44,65] Such side effects make the use of such drugs seem rarely warranted in JRA, a disease in which most patients have a favorable prognosis. Great care must be taken in interpreting anecdotal reports of successes with these agents in JRA. Some favorable experience in England and Europe has been reported with the use of chlorambucil[64] and azathioprine in patients with JRA and amyloidosis; concomitant improvement in arthritis has been noted in such patients during therapy. No evidence suggests that any of these drugs are efficacious in the treatment of chronic iridocyclitis.

Little experience exists with experimental measures such as plasmapheresis, lymphophoresis, or total lymph node irradiation in the therapy of children with JRA.

Physical and Occupational Therapy

In general, children with JRA should be encouraged to be active and to participate in normal activities of childhood (see also Chaps. 43 and 44). Activities such as tricycle riding and swimming may be valuable additions to physical therapy. Total bed rest is almost always contraindicated. Children should be trained and encouraged to function as normally as possible in a usual childhood environment.

Physical and occupational therapy are of great benefit in maintaining function and in preventing invalidism in patients with JRA.[13,16,23,58] Exercises to preserve joint range of motion and functional joint position, to maintain muscle strength, and to maintain normal function of the limbs and of the total child are vital. No evidence suggests that, with reasonable care, exercise damages inflamed joints. Physical and occupational therapy are invaluable, even in children with active arthritis.

All children with JRA should be instructed in range-of-motion and muscle-strengthening exercises, to be done once or twice daily at home. All joints should be put through a functional range of motion at least once daily, with particular attention to affected joints. Night splints may be useful in preserving functional joint positions, particularly in the knees and wrists. Joints should not be rigidly immobilized for long periods because loss of joint motion may be irreversible. Exercise programs should be taught to both the patient and the parents; children older than 6 years should be largely responsible for their own exercises with minimal parental supervision. Muscle-strengthening exercises should be done when necessary for the quadriceps, hip, or shoulder girdle muscles, the gastrocnemius-soleus muscles, and the peroneal muscles. Occupational therapy can improve hand function, and it may improve overall function. Heat, in the form of a hot morning bath at home, is often valuable in alleviating morning stiffness.

Inpatient medical, physical, and occupational therapy is usually justified for children with severe musculoskeletal dysfunction who are not self-sufficient or who cannot attend school regularly. Pool therapy may be a valuable adjunct. Heat from paraffin baths may help to restore motion of small hand joints. Splinting and traction may be useful in overcoming flexion contractures.

Orthopedic Therapy

Synovectomy plays a limited role in the early therapy of JRA.[25,28] Patients with pauciarticular disease, the most logical candidates for synovectomy, have a good prognosis for joint function without operative intervention. Synovectomy is useful occasionally in children with polyarthritis and one or few troublesome joints. Many children experience a recurrence of synovitis in operated joints, however.

Orthopedic surgery holds great promise in the late rehabilitation of children with serious disability from JRA.[8] Soft tissue release can alleviate contractures unresponsive to nonoperative therapy.[27] Osteotomies may be useful. Total joint replacement, particularly of the hips and knees, may be of great benefit to children with serious joint damage, but should be done only after adolescence and when full growth has been achieved.[8,9,22,66,67] Help is needed for younger children with serious disability, particularly from severe hip disease, because no routine surgical procedures that permit early rehabilitation are available at present.

THERAPY OF SYSTEMIC MANIFESTATIONS

Systemic-Onset Juvenile Rheumatoid Arthritis

The high fevers, malaise, polyserositis, organomegaly, and anemia of systemic-onset JRA can present major therapeutic problems. In the natural course of systemic-onset JRA, these manifestations usually subside spontaneously in about 6 months, regardless of treatment. Although the high fevers and malaise are debilitating, they are not generally life-threatening. Only rarely are severe pericarditis, myocarditis, or anemia potentially fatal. In treating systemic-onset JRA, it is thus imperative that the therapy be no worse than the disease. Salicylates, the drugs of choice, are effective in controlling systemic manifestations in more than half these patients. The doses used are similar to those described for treatment of arthritis: serum salicylate levels should not be higher than 40 mg/dl. Children who are seriously ill with systemic-onset JRA should be hospitalized and closely watched. If fever and other systemic symptoms remain severely incapacitating after 2 or 3 weeks of vigorous salicylate therapy, systemic corticosteroids are probably indicated. It is reasonable to begin with a high dose of corticosteroids, such as 30 to 60 mg prednisone a day, to control symptoms rapidly. A single, morning, corticosteroid dose regimen is often effective. The drug dosage can then be slowly tapered and discontinued within 6 months. Most children with severe systemic-onset disease respond rapidly to such a regimen, and corticosteroids can be withdrawn without incident. Arthritis appearing while the corticosteroid dose is being reduced should be treated with salicylates or with gold and not with more corticosteroids.

Alternate-day dosage schedules have been suggested.[2] These programs control symptoms less rapidly, but they may be effective in some patients. About half the children with systemic-onset disease experience later attacks of systemic complaints, and these should always be treated first with salicylates. Gold, antimalarial agents, and anticancer drugs are of little use in controlling systemic manifestations because all require several months for effect. The usefulness of nonsteroidal anti-inflammatory agents in controlling systemic manifestations has not been adequately explored. Because some of these drugs are effective antipyretics, some may prove effective.

Extra-Articular Manifestations of Other Subgroups

Patients with nonsystemic-onset JRA also may have low-grade fever, malaise, mild hepatosplenomegaly, and mild anemia. These extra-articular manifestations of disease usually respond to the therapy given for the arthritis and are rarely, if ever, indications for institution of vigorous therapy with systemic corticosteroids. Anemic children with JRA should be investigated for iron deficiency and should be treated appropriately with iron if necessary.

Growth Retardation

Growth retardation is concomitant with sustained disease during the growth period.[4,11,71] No therapy is effective except control of the underlying disease. Growth retardation also follows therapy with corticosteroids in daily doses of more than 3 to 5 mg prednisone daily or equivalent.[52,71]

THERAPY OF IRIDOCYCLITIS

Early detection of iridocyclitis is crucial to successful therapy. At highest risk are those young-onset patients with pauciarticular disease,[18,21,57,62] particularly those with positive tests for antinuclear antibodies.[55] Patients in this high-risk group should have screening slit-lamp examinations at least every three months by an ophthalmologist. Iridocyclitis should be treated initially with topical corticosteroids, dilating agents, and careful follow-up examinations. Should topical therapy fail, further treatment with injections of corticosteroids under the vagina bulbi or with systemic corticosteroids should be tried. Doses of systemic corticosteroids should be high enough to control ocular inflammation, as monitored by slit-lamp examinations; alternate-day dosage schedules may be effective. No evidence suggests that any of the other anti-inflammatory or antirheumatic agents, or any of the anticancer drugs, are effective in controlling chronic iridocyclitis. Surgical treatment sometimes helps to rehabilitate eyes severely damaged by chronic iridocyclitis. Band keratopathy can be chelated with topical edetate (EDTA) and may be removed surgically. Mature cataracts secondary to iridocyclitis may be extracted, but only by surgeons experienced in this procedure.

Children with older-onset pauciarticular disease with spondyloarthropathy sometimes have attacks of acute iridocyclitis.[55,57] This type of iridocyclitis is similar to that of ankylosing spondylitis in adults, as well as that of inflammatory bowel disease and Reiter's syndrome. Acute iridocyclitis is apparent early because of severe associated symptoms. Treatment with topical corticosteroids and dilating agents usually satisfactorily quiets the inflammation. Attacks are generally self-limited, and the prognosis for normal vision is excellent.

THERAPY OF AMYLOIDOSIS

Amyloidosis, a serious complication of childhood arthritis, is recognized in about 5% of patients with JRA in England, Europe, and most other parts of the world, but it is rare in the United States.[64] Reasons for this difference are not apparent. Amyloidosis is considered invariably fatal, generally from progressive renal disease. Therapy of amyloidosis with chlorambucil[64] and with azathioprine has been thought to be successful during short-term studies in several centers.

MANAGEMENT OF THE WHOLE CHILD

Appropriate management of the whole child is an important aspect of therapy.[30,42] The child and the family need to be educated about JRA and reassured that, although the disease may be chronic and unpredictable, the overall prognosis for the majority of patients is good. Children should be managed with optimism and encouragement. They should be helped to lead lives that are as full as possible, to attend regular schools, and to avoid thinking of themselves as chronic invalids. Bed rest and isolation from peers should be avoided. Children who are too ill or too disabled to be self-sufficient and to attend school should probably be hospitalized for rehabilitation. Children need constant support for the many problems of childhood and adolescence. Teenagers need appropriate counseling to help them to formulate and achieve realistic career goals.

Most children with JRA are cared for by primary physicians. For optimal care, however, the child with JRA should be seen at least periodically by a physician who understands the natural history of the disease and has had experience with needed drugs and physical therapy. Severely affected patients are best managed by such a physician directly. A team approach is optimal for care of affected children. A pediatrician or rheumatologist, a physiatrist, an orthopedist, an ophthalmologist, a physical therapist, and an occupational therapist are all needed at times. Consistent long-term follow-up of patients with JRA is crucial.

REFERENCES

1. Ansell, B.M.: Rheumatic disorders in childhood. *In* Postgraduate Paediatrics Series: Juvenile Chronic Arthritis. Edited by J. Apley. London, Butterworth, 1980, pp. 87–151.
2. Ansell, B.M., and Bywaters, E.G.L.: Alternate-day corticosteroid therapy in juvenile chronic polyarthritis. J. Rheumatol., *1*:176–186, 1974.
3. Ansell, B.M., and Bywaters, E.G.L.: Prognosis in Still's disease. Bull. Rheum. Dis., *9*:189–192, 1959.
4. Ansell, B.M., and Bywaters, E.G.L.: Growth in Still's disease. Ann. Rheum. Dis., *15*:295–319, 1956.
5. Ansell, B.M., and Hall, M.A.: Penicillamine in juvenile chronic polyarthritis. Arthritis Rheum., *20*:536, 1977.
6. Ansell, B.M., and Wood, P.H.N.: Prognosis in juvenile chronic polyarthritis. Clin. Rheum. Dis., *2*:397–412, 1976.
7. Ansell, B.M., Bywaters, E.G.L., and Isdale, I.C.: Comparison of cortisone and aspirin in treatment of juvenile rheumatoid arthritis. Br. Med. J., *1*:1075–1077, 1956.
8. Arden, G.P., and Ansell, B.M.: Surgical Management of Juvenile Chronic Polyarthritis. London, Academic Press, 1978, pp. 1–281.
9. Arden, G.P., Taylor, A.R., and Ansell, B.M.: Total hip replacement using the McKee-Farrar prosthesis in rheumatoid arthritis, Still's disease, and ankylosing spondylitis. Ann. Rheum. Dis., *29*:1–5, 1970.
10. Athreya, B.H., Gorski, A.L., and Meyers, A.R.: Aspirin-induced abnormalities of liver function. Am. J. Dis. Child., *126*:638–641, 1973.
11. Bernstein, B.H., et al.: Growth retardation in juvenile rheumatoid arthritis (JRA). Arthritis Rheum., *20*:212–216, 1977.
12. Brewer, E.J.: Nonsteroidal anti-inflammatory agents. Arthritis Rheum., *20*:513–525, 1977.
13. Brewer, E.J., Blattner, R.J., and Wing, H.: Treatment of rheumatoid arthritis in children. Pediatr. Clin. North Am., *10*:207–224, 1963.
14. Brewer, E.J., Giannini, E.H., and Barkley, E.: Gold therapy in the management of juvenile rheumatoid arthritis. Arthritis Rheum., *23*:404–411, 1980.
15. Bywaters, E.G.L.: Categorization in medicine: a survey of Still's disease. Ann. Rheum. Dis., *26*:185–193, 1967.
16. Calabro, J.J.: Management of juvenile rheumatoid arthritis. J. Pediatr., *77*:355–365, 1970.
17. Calabro, J.J., et al.: Juvenile rheumatoid arthritis: a general review and report of 100 patients observed for 15 years. Semin. Arthritis Rheum., *5*:257–298, 1976.
18. Calabro, J.J., et al.: Chronic iridocyclitis in juvenile rheumatoid arthritis. Arthritis Rheum., *13*:406–413, 1970.
19. Calabro, J.J., Katz, R.M., and Maltz, B.A.: A critical reappraisal of juvenile rheumatoid arthritis. Clin. Orthop., *74*:101–119, 1971.
20. Cann, H.M., and Verhulst, H.L.: Fatal acute chloroquine poisoning in children. Pediatrics, *27*:95–102, 1961.
21. Chylack, L.T.: The ocular manifestations of juvenile rheumatoid arthritis. Arthritis Rheum., *20*:217–223, 1977.
22. Colville, J., and Raunio, P.: Total hip replacement in juvenile rheumatoid arthritis. Analysis of fifty-nine hips. Acta Orthop. Scand., *50*:197–203, 1979.
23. Donovan, W.H.: Physical measures in the treatment of juvenile rheumatoid arthritis. Arthritis Rheum., *20*:553–557, 1977.
24. Doughty, R.A., Giesecke, L., and Athreya, B.: Salicylate therapy in juvenile rheumatoid arthritis: dose, serum level, and toxicity. Am. J. Dis. Child., *134*:461–463, 1980.
25. Eyring, E.J., Longert, A., and Bass, J.C.: Synovectomy in juvenile rheumatoid arthritis. J. Bone Joint Surg., *53A*:638–651, 1971.
26. Giannini, E.H., Brewer, E.J., and Person, D.A.: Auranofin in the treatment of juvenile rheumatoid arthritis. J. Pediatr., *102*:138–141, 1983.
27. Granberry, G.M.: Soft tissue release in children with juvenile rheumatoid arthritis. Arthritis Rheum., *20*:565–566, 1977.
28. Granberry, G.M.: Synovectomy in juvenile rheumatoid arthritis. Arthritis Rheum., *20*:561–564, 1977.
29. Hicks, R.M., Hanson, V., and Kornreich, H.K.: The use of gold in the treatment of juvenile rheumatoid arthritis (JRA). Arthritis Rheum., *13*:323, 1970.
30. Hollister, J.R.: Immunosuppressant therapy of juvenile rheumatoid arthritis. Arthritis Rheum., *20*:544–547, 1977.
31. Jacobs, J.C., Berdon, W.E., and Johnson, A.D.: HLA-B27 associated spondyloarthritis and enthesopathy in childhood: clinical, pathologic and radiographic observations in 58 patients. J. Pediatr., *100*:521–528, 1982.
32. Kelly, V.C.: Rheumatoid disease in childhood. Pediatr. Clin. North Am., *7*:435–456, 1960.
33. Kornreich, K.H., Malouf, N.N., and Hanson, V.: Acute

hepatic dysfunction in juvenile rheumatoid arthritis. J. Pediatr., 79:1, 27–33, 1971.

34. Ladd, J.R., Cassidy, J.T., and Martel, W.: Juvenile ankylosing spondylitis. Arthritis Rheum., 14:579, 1971.

35. Levinson, J.E., et al.: Comparison of tolmetin sodium and aspirin in the treatment of juvenile rheumatoid arthritis. J. Pediatr., 91:799–804, 1977.

36. Mainland, D., et al.: A controlled trial of cyclophosphamide in rheumatoid arthritis. Cooperating Clinics Committee of the American Rheumatism Association. N. Engl. J. Med., 283:883–889, 1970.

37. Miller, J.J.: Prolonged use of large intravenous steroid pulses in rheumatic diseases of children. Pediatrics, 65:989–994, 1980.

38. Miller, J.J., and Weissman, D.B.: Correlation between transaminase concentrations and serum salicylate concentrations in juvenile rheumatoid arthritis. Arthritis Rheum., 19:115–118, 1976.

39. Moran, H., et al.: Naproxen in juvenile chronic polyarthritis. Ann. Rheum. Dis., 38:152–154, 1979.

40. Pediatric Rheumatology Study Group: Methodology and studies of children with juvenile rheumatoid arthritis. J. Rheumatol., 9:107–155, 1982.

41. Prescott, L.F., and Cantab, M.B.: Effects of acetylsalicylic acid, phenacetin, paracetamol and caffeine on renal tubular epithelium. Lancet, 2:91–95, 1965.

42. Proceedings of the First American Rheumatism Association Conference on the Rheumatic Diseases of Childhood. Arthritis Rheum., 20:145–636, 1977.

43. Quick, A.J.: Salicylates and bleeding: the aspirin tolerance test. Am. J. Med. Sci., 252:265–269, 1966.

44. Reimer, R.R., et al.: Acute leukemia after alkylating-agent therapy of ovarian cancer. N. Engl. J. Med., 297:177–181, 1977.

45. Rich, R.R., and Johnson, J.S.: Salicylate hepatotoxicity in patients with juvenile rheumatoid arthritis. Arthritis Rheum., 16:1–9, 1973.

46. Rosenberg, A.M., and Petty, R.E.: A syndrome of seronegative enthesopathy and arthropathy in children. Arthritis Rheum., 25:1041–1047, 1982.

47. Russell, A.S., Sturge, R.A., and Smith, M.A.: Serum transaminases during salicylate therapy. Br. Med. J., 2:428–429, 1971.

48. Schaller, J.G.: Juvenile rheumatoid arthritis. Pediatrics, 2:163–174, 1980.

49. Schaller, J.G.: The seronegative spondyloarthropathies of childhood. Clin. Orthop., 143:76–83, 1979.

50. Schaller, J.G.: Chronic salicylate administration in juvenile rheumatoid arthritis: aspirin "hepatitis" and its clinical significance. Pediatrics, 62:916–925, 1978.

51. Schaller, J.G.: Ankylosing spondylitis of childhood onset. Arthritis Rheum., 20:398–401, 1977.

52. Schaller, J.G.: Corticosteroid therapy in childhood. Arthritis Rheum., 20:537–543, 1977.

53. Schaller, J.G.: The diversity of JRA: a 1976 look at the subgroups of chronic childhood arthritis. Arthritis Rheum., 20:1519–1527, 1977.

54. Schaller, J.G., et al.: Histocompatibility antigens in childhood-onset arthritis. J. Pediatr., 88:926–930, 1976.

55. Schaller, J.G., et al.: The association of antinuclear antibodies with the chronic iridocyclitis of juvenile arthritis (Still's disease). Arthritis Rheum., 17:409–416, 1974.

56. Schaller, J.G., and Christie, D.: Peptic ulcer disease in juvenile rheumatoid arthritis. In preparation.

57. Schaller, J.G., and Wedgwood, R.J.: Pauciarticular childhood arthritis: identification of two distinct subgroups. Arthritis Rheum., 19:820–821, 1976.

58. Schaller, J.G., and Wedgwood, R.J.: Rheumatic diseases. (Inflammatory diseases of connective tissue, collagen diseases.) In Nelson Textbook of Pediatrics. 10th Ed. Edited by V.C. Vaughan, R.J. McKay, and W.E. Nelson. Philadelphia, W.B. Saunders, 1975, pp. 522–524.

59. Schaller, J., and Wedgwood, R.J.: Is juvenile rheumatoid arthritis a single disease? A review. Pediatrics, 50:940–953, 1972.

60. Schaller, J.G., Beckwith, B., and Wedgwood, R.J.: Hepatic involvement in juvenile rheumatoid arthritis. J. Pediatr., 77:203–210, 1970.

61. Schaller, J.G., Bitnum, S., and Wedgwood, R.J.: Ankylosing spondylitis with childhood onset. J. Pediatr., 74:505–516, 1969.

62. Schaller, J.G., Kupfer, C., and Wedgwood, R.J.: Iridocyclitis in juvenile rheumatoid arthritis. Pediatrics, 44:92–100, 1969.

63. Schlesinger, B.E., et al.: Observations on the clinical course and treatment of one hundred cases of Still's disease. Arch. Dis. Child., 36:65–76, 1961.

64. Schnitzer, T.J., and Ansell, B.M.: Amyloidosis in juvenile chronic polyarthritis. Arthritis Rheum., 20:245–252, 1977.

65. Sieber, S.M., and Adamson, R.H.: Toxicity of antineoplastic agents in man: chromosomal aberrations, antifertility effects, congenital malformations, and carcinogenic potential. Adv. Cancer Res., 22:57–155, 1975.

66. Singsen, B.H., et al.: Total hip replacement in children with arthritis. Arthritis Rheum., 21:401–406, 1978.

67. Sledge, C.B.: Joint replacement surgery in juvenile rheumatoid arthritis. Arthritis Rheum., 20:567–572, 1977.

68. Starko, K.M., et al.: Reye's syndrome and salicylate use. Pediatrics, 66:859–864, 1980.

69. Stillman, J.S.: Salicylates—a review. Arthritis Rheum., 20:510–512, 1977.

70. Sutor, A.H., Bowie, E.J.W., and Owen, C.A.: Effect of aspirin, sodium salicylates and acetaminophen on bleeding. Mayo Clin. Proc., 46:178–181, 1971.

71. Ward, D.J., Hartog, M., and Ansell, B.M.: Corticosteroid-induced dwarfism in Still's disease treated with human growth hormone. Clinical and metabolic effects including hydroxyproline excretion in two cases. Ann. Rheum. Dis., 25:416–421, 1966.

72. Wortmann, D.W., et al.: Renal papillary necrosis in juvenile rheumatoid arthritis. J. Pediatr., 97:37–40, 1980.

73. Zutshi, D.W., Friedman, M., and Ansell, B.M.: Corticotrophin therapy in juvenile chronic polyarthritis (Still's disease) and effect on growth. Arch. Dis. Child., 46:584–593, 1971.

Chapter 53

Ankylosing Spondylitis

Rodney Bluestone

Ankylosing spondylitis (AS) is a disease characterized by inflammatory stiffening of the spine (from the Greek *spondylos,* meaning vertebrae). This inflammatory arthropathy, with its peculiar predilection for the cartilaginous joints of the axial skeleton, can be traced back to 3,000 B.C. Pathologic changes commensurate with the disease have been described in prehistoric crocodiles, monkeys, and horses, as well as in human skeletons dating back to the third Egyptian dynasty (2980–2900 B.C.). In these specimens, the tell-tale signs of ossification in ligaments and bony fusion of the spine indicate the probable pre-existence of AS. A classic pathologic study conducted in 1695 by Bernard Connor suggested the concept of an immovable and rigid patient. More detailed pathoclinical descriptions of the disorder became available in the late nineteenth century, including the first radiographic account by Velenti in 1899. The modern descriptions of the disease as a clinical syndrome with its radiographic and pathologic sequelae are accredited to Krebs, Buckley, Scott, and Forestier, all of whom presented well-defined clinical data during the 1930s.

All now agree that AS is *not* a form of rheumatoid arthritis (RA). Although these diseases may have features in common, the pathogenetic, clinical, pathologic, and radiographic features of AS are distinct and different from those of rheumatoid disease.[15] During recent years, a strong association between AS and the histocompatibility antigen HLA-B27 has been described and confirmed throughout the world. The recognition and further exploration of this association has broadened our understanding of this disease. Thus, it is now more apparent that AS exists as a spectrum of clinical presentations, ranging from the typical and fully expressed profile of spinal inflammation and stiffening to various "forme fruste" syndromes in which axial involvement may be inconspicuous. Moreover, AS shares many of its clinical, pathologic, and radiographic features with other related seronegative* spondyloarthropathies, such as Rei-

ter's syndrome and psoriatic arthritis. Many patients at some time possess features of any or all of these seronegative rheumatic syndromes.

The recent surge of interest in the pathogenesis of AS has refocused our attention on the pathologic process responsible for the common end-stage lesion in this disorder. Despite the dearth of pathologic material from patients with early disease, some revealing studies of the inflammatory process have been made. A collation of this data, combined with a keener appreciation of the pathoradiographic features, has increased our understanding of the natural history and evolution of AS. Moreover, the availability of a genetic marker for susceptibility to AS has already thrown into doubt the older prevalence and incidence figures for this disease among normal populations. Current evidence suggests that this rheumatic disorder is far more common than was previously supposed and frequently exists in a subclinical form. In addition, the strong familial incidence of AS can now be better explained on a genetic basis, coincident with the inheritance of the gene coding for HLA-B27 or other closely associated genetic material on the same chromosome.

PATHOLOGY

The *organ distribution* of the pathologic changes in AS follows a characteristic pattern. The major targets of this inflammatory disease appear to be the joints of the axial skeleton, including: (1) the nonsynovial (cartilaginous) synchondroses of the intervertebral spaces; (2) the diarthrodial synovial joints represented by the apophyseal, costovertebral, and neurocentral articulations; and (3) the sacroiliac joints, which are mixed joints possessing features of both nonsynovial and diarthrodial articulations.[7] The large anterior central joints of the body are also frequently involved, including the cartilaginous manubriosternal and symphysis pubis articulations, as well as the synovial but partly cartilaginous sternoclavicular joints. Inflammation of peripheral synovial joints, though less frequent, may also occur. In particular, the proximal synovial joints, notably the hips, shoulder, and knees, are often involved. More distal joints may become inflamed at any time during the natural history of AS, but severe involvement of small joints is un-

---

*For rheumatoid factor.

usual. Outside the skeleton, inflammatory foci may involve the anterior uveal tract or the aortic wall. Circumstantial evidence suggests that the spinal leptomeninges and the pulmonary upper lobe parenchyma also become targets of spondylitic disease in a few patients.

Within these organ systems, the *tissue distribution* of the inflammatory process is characteristic. The major target tissue within articular structures appears to be primarily cartilage, in particular fibrocartilage.[7] This process is often associated with a frank osteitis of the directly adjacent subchondral bone. The fibrous tissue of the joint capsule or anulus fibrosus, together with the periarticular ligamentous-bony junctions (enthesis) and periosteum, are also principal target tissues of the disease.[2] A true synovitis may occur, particularly in the large peripheral joints, but it is rarely as florid or clinically significant as the chondritis, osteitis, capsulitis, enthesopathy, and periostitis in and around the axial skeleton and centrally located joints.

Few detailed studies have been done on the early lesions of AS, before areas of involvement become encrusted and embedded in ossified scar tissue. In all the target organs and tissues mentioned, however, the initial cellular change appears to be an infiltration of lymphocytes and macrophages, perhaps suggesting an immune-mediated inflammatory lesion.[2,7,17,25] A brisk proliferative fibroplastic response soon emerges as a sequela of this inflammatory process, with the appearance of numerous plump and active fibroblasts, which progressively replace the inflammatory cell infiltrate. The fibroblastic tissue undergoes organization and develops into dense fibrous scars, which display a remarkable tendency to calcify and ossify. This fibrosis, calcification and ossification present the pathologists and clinician with a bland, apparently noninflammatory, fibrous and bony fusion of articular tissues. Proliferative synovitis is rarely as extensive as in RA, but it may erode joints, and it certainly can contribute to the progressive loss of normal skeletal architecture. Nevertheless, the inflammatory process of AS can result in the bony fusion of axial, central, or peripheral joints in the absence of a significant chronic synovitis.

MORPHORADIOGRAPHIC CHANGES

Sacroiliac Involvement

The sacroiliac joints are usually the most conspicuous areas of involvement in AS (see also Figs. 5–47, 5–48, 5–49, 5–50, 5–54). Although the lower anterior third of the sacroiliac joint is enclosed in a capsule lined by synovium, significant synovitis does not appear to be a feature of the disease at this site. Rather, inflammatory chondritis and subchondral osteitis involving the sacral and iliac cartilages in the inferior two-thirds of the joint, and a similar pathologic process arising within the ligamentous superior part of the joint, all have a characteristic morphoradiographic appearance.

The pathologic process results in a progressive destruction of the sacroiliac cartilage. Because the cartilage on the iliac side of the joint is thinner than that on the sacral side,[7] erosive destruction of the subchondral bone is typically most apparent on the iliac side of the joint. The erosions are seen radiographically as punched-out areas extending deep into the subchondral trabeculae and pathologically as areas filled with inflammatory granulation tissue. This destructive process leads to a radiographic "pseudowidening" of the joint space. The bone adjacent to the inflammatory foci undergoes a brisk osteoblastosis, producing the characteristic periarticular sclerotic appearance on the radiograph (Fig. 53–1,*A*). This juxta-articular sclerosis may become the most obvious radiographic sign of AS when bony erosion and joint space widening are no longer evident (Fig. 53–1,*B*). Because no cartilage is present in the superior third of the sacroiliac joint, where the bones are united by dense intra-articular ligaments, the early inflammatory changes are not radiographically distinct. The natural progression of the chondritis and ligamentous inflammation throughout the joint is one of intra-articular fibrotic scar formation, which then undergoes calcification and ossification, however. This process causes a variable degree of bony bridging of the joint (Fig. 53–2), which eventually has the radiographic appearance of mature and trabeculized osteoid tissue totally replacing the original joint space (Fig. 53–3). At any stage in this process, the periarticular bone may appear variably osteoblastic or osteopenic, but once the sacroiliac joint is completely fused by new bone formation, profound radiographic osteopenia is usual.

Because the pathologic changes within the sacroiliac joints take months or years to evolve, an inevitable lag between the morphologic and the radiographic expression of the disease ensues. Thus, the diagnostic changes of radiographic sacroiliitis do not become apparent until several years after the onset of disease. The recent application of computerized axial tomographic (CT) scanning to the sacroiliac region facilitates the display of the early and subtle, yet diagnostic, details of subchondral bone erosion and cyst formation.[20] The use of CT scanning is fully discussed in Chapter 6.

Pelvic Involvement

An equally brisk inflammatory process, with or without periostitis, is seen at the various liga-

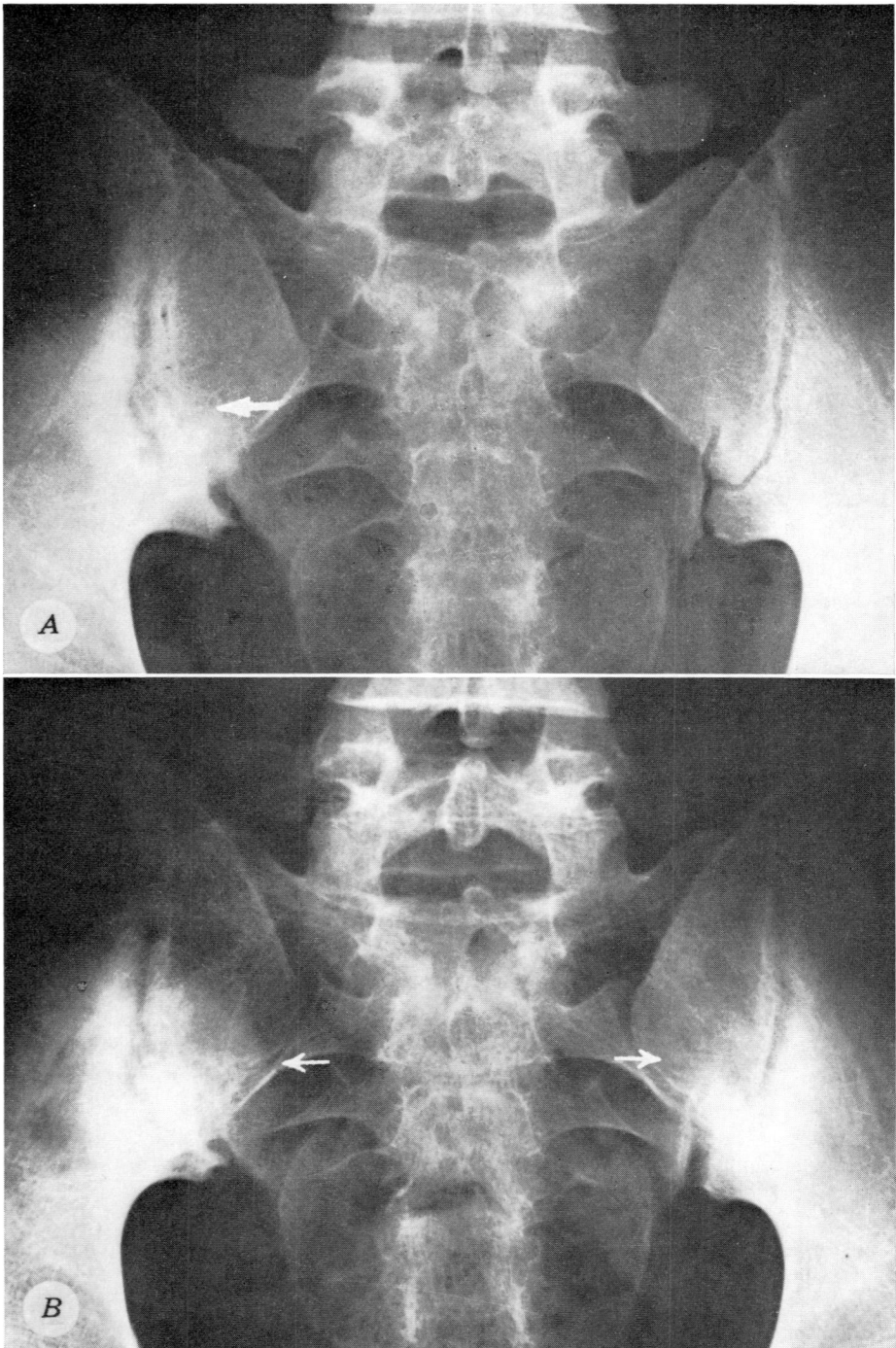

Fig. 53–1. Ankylosing spondylitis. *A,* Well-established sacroiliitis on the right, with erosions most marked on the iliac side of the joint and leading to a "pseudowidening" of the joint space (arrow). The left sacroiliac joint is virtually normal. *B,* A radiograph of the same patient, several years later, demonstrates a pronounced bilateral periarticular sclerosis with irregular loss of joint space (arrows).

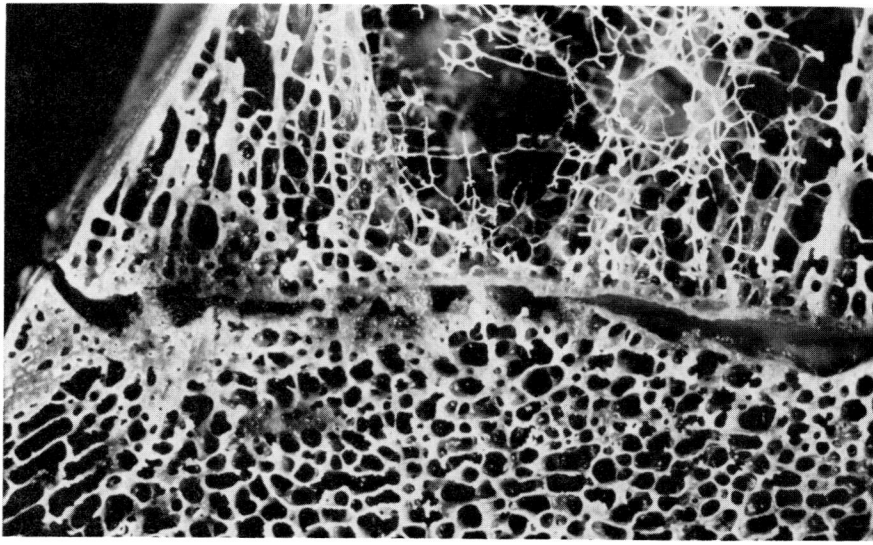

Fig. 53–2. Macerated sacroiliac joint obtained post mortem from a patient with ankylosing spondylitis. Irregular bony bridging of the joint space with mature osteoid tissue is visible. Note the patchy erosions of subchondral bone, most marked from the iliac (reader's right) side of the joint. (From Resnick, D., Niwayama, G., and Georgen, T.G.[74])

mentous-bony junctions of the pelvis. This involvement is most conspicuous around the insertions of the sacrotuberous and sacrospinous ligaments, as well as along the inferior rami of the ischium and pubis, along the superior iliac crests, and around the greater trochanters of the femora (Fig. 53–4). The healed lesions are detected radiographically as extension and roughening of bony margins and as frankly ossified soft tissue attachments. By the time these changes are seen, however, the sacroiliac joints are nearly always abnormal.

Vertebral and Intervertebral Disc Involvement

The chondritis of the intervertebral discs can occur anywhere in the disc substance, but it usually arises at their perimeter, underlying the attachment of the more vascular anulus fibrosus. The inflammatory process, which can destroy any amount of disc substance, generally undergoes early maturation, so complete loss of radiographic disc space is unusual. An adjacent subchondral vertebral osteitis is frequently seen (Fig. 53–5) and is characterized radiographically as a semilucent area within the vertebral body surrounded by a denser blastic zone (the Romanus lesion).[7] Because the chondritis heals by fibrosis, the secondary calcification and new bone formation attach to or replace the anulus fibrosus, thereby bridging the adjacent margins of one vertebral body to another. The subsequent healing of the adjacent osteitis is also as-

sociated with proliferative marginal spurs of new bone, which replace the outer layers of the anulus fibrosus and are seen radiographically as typical syndesmophytes (Fig. 53–6). The osteitis and destruction of the inferior and superior peripheral portions of the vertebral bodies, followed by syndesmophyte formation, are frequently associated with a low-grade periostitis of the anterior part of the vertebral body. This combined process blunts the vertebral corners and fills in the normally concave anterior vertebral margin. The result is radiographic "squaring" of the vertebral bodies (see Fig. 53–5). Thoracic vertebral squaring is often one of the earliest radiographic signs of AS and may be detectable before any other obvious ligamentous or bony abnormality is visible in the spine. Although less prominent, similar squaring of the cervical and lumbar vertebrae does occur.

The uniform development of widespread anulus fibrosus ossification and of syndesmophyte formation is largely responsible for the classic radiographic "bamboo spine" of end-stage AS (Fig. 53–7). A similar inflammatory process within the perispinal ligaments contributes to this bambooing. In particular, the closely applied posterior longitudinal ligament and the more remote interspinous ligament may become converted to continuous bony bars, augmenting the spinal rigidity. The initial changes within the disc and the vertebral bodies appear to be the key elements of the disease, however. Once the intervertebral discs are immobilized

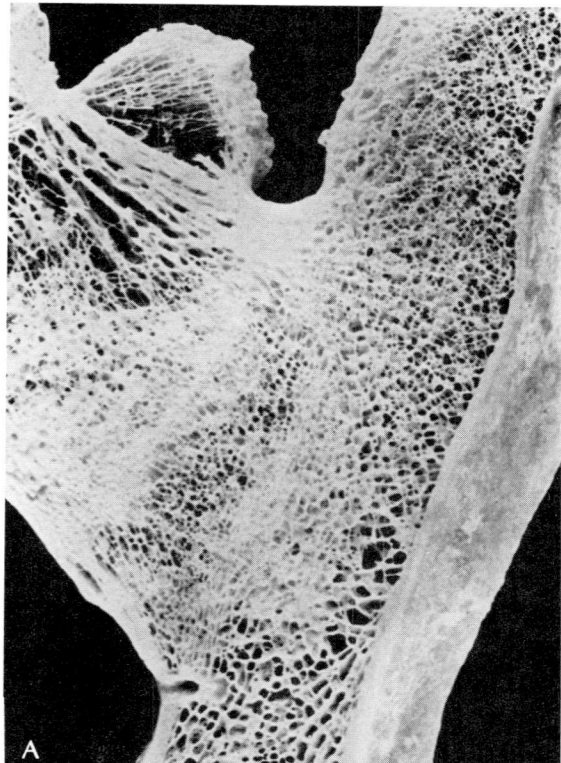

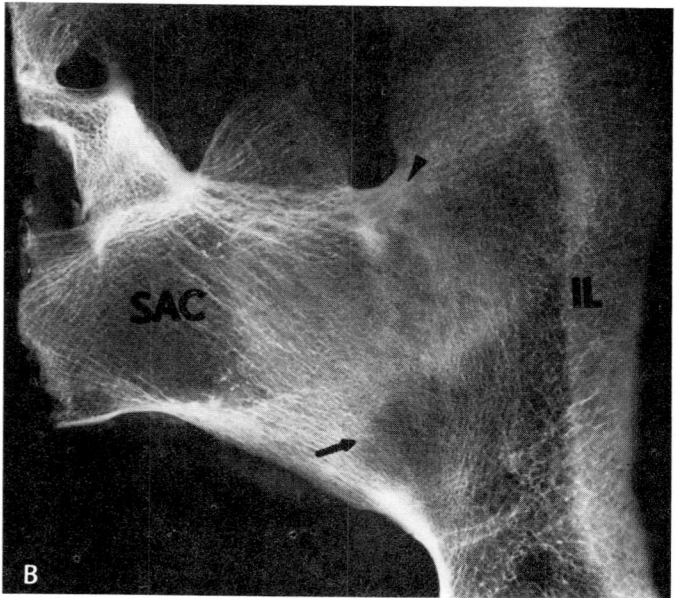

Fig. 53–3. *A*, Macerated specimen, and *B*, radiograph, of a sacroiliac joint removed at postmortem examination from a patient with end-stage ankylosing spondylitis. The joint is completely fused by mature trabeculized bone. *B* demonstrates complete loss of the lower joint space (arrow) and bony fusion of the upper, ligamentous portion of the joint (arrow head). (*A*, from Resnick, D., and Niwayama G.[71] *B*, from Resnick, D., Niwayama, G. and Georgen, T.G.[73])

by bony fusion, largely at their periphery, enchondral ossification of disc substance may ensue over the following decades, during which a greater amount of noninflamed disc cartilage becomes ossified.

Although the chondritis and adjacent osteitis are predominantly seen at the periphery of the discs and vertebral bodies close to the attachment of the anulus fibrosus, such is not always the case. The inflammatory foci can arise anywhere in the disc substance and may erode through the vertebral basal end plate with a destructive vigor reminiscent of septic discitis. The aggressive destruction of the disc and adjacent vertebral bodies may be associ-

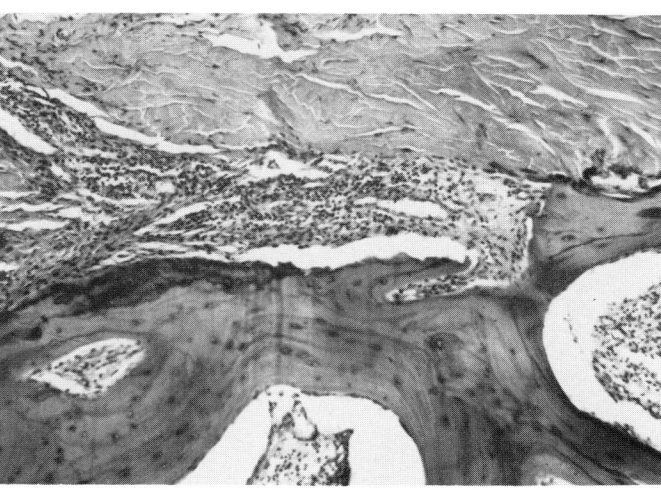

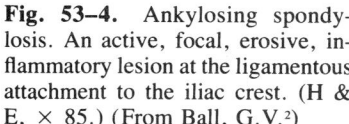

Fig. 53–4. Ankylosing spondylosis. An active, focal, erosive, inflammatory lesion at the ligamentous attachment to the iliac crest. (H & E, × 85.) (From Ball, G.V.[2])

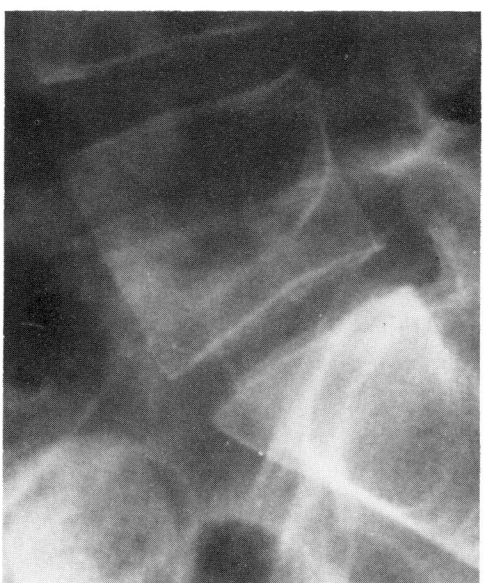

Fig. 53–5. Ankylosing spondylitis. Lateral radiograph of the lumbosacral spine showing an erosive osteitis at the posterior superior margin of the sacrum with surrounding sclerosis (Romanus lesion). Note that the anterior border of L5 is squared.

ated with an inapparent fracture of the neural arch or a solitary, unfused apophyseal joint at that level. The posterior instability might well permit inappropriate movement and shear stress on the central vertebral region in an otherwise completely fused and "protected" spine. This mechanism probably accounts for the occasional radiographic appearance of extensive disc and vertebral body destruction, which resembles osteomyelitis but is actually

due to the fundamental pathologic process of AS (Fig. 53–8).

The intervertebral and costovertebral synovial synchondroses may be extensively involved in the pathologic process. A modest amount of synovitis may prevail in these joints, and this disorder can contribute to joint destruction and fusion. The inflammatory process within the joint capsules appears to be an important cause of apophyseal joint fusion, however. Once the apophyseal and costovertebral joint capsules have become inflamed, fibrotic, and ossified, a secondary enchondral ossification of articular cartilage may follow, in the absence of true pannus. Radiographically, this situation is best seen in the cervical apophyseal joints, in which bony fusion of periarticular tissues leads to apparent loss of radiographic joint space, even though the encased articular cartilage may be preserved intact for many years (Fig. 53–9). Inflammatory disease in the superior cervical spine can lead to atlantoaxial subluxation comparable to that seen in RA. A patient may then display the paradoxic combination of an unstable atlantoaxial subluxation in an otherwise completely rigid cervical spine fused at both central and apophyseal junctions. The neurocentral joints of the cervical spine may also be involved in AS, but they have not been adequately studied either pathologically or radiographically.

Central Cartilaginous Joint Involvement

The central cartilaginous joints are commonly involved in AS. Both the manubriosternal and symphysis pubis articulations are notably prone to a subacute subchondral osteitis, with the inflammatory granulation tissue liable to replace the normal joint structures.[7] Later, fibrosis and ossification result in a complete synostosis. This process has a

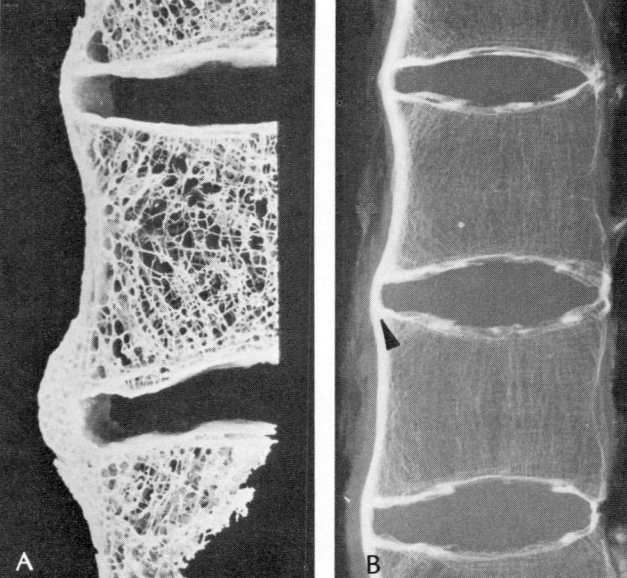

Fig. 53–6. Ankylosing spondylitis. Macerated portion, *A,* and radiograph, *B,* of lumbar spine showing typical syndesmophytes (arrow). (From Resnick, D.[70])

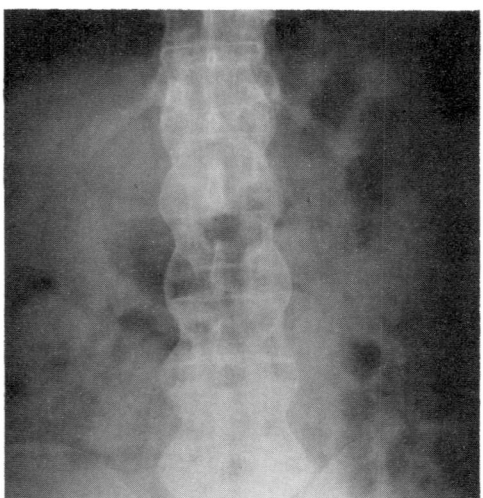

Fig. 53–7. Radiograph of the lumbosacral spine from a patient with long-standing ankylosing spondylitis. Note the uniform "bambooing" of the vertebral column.

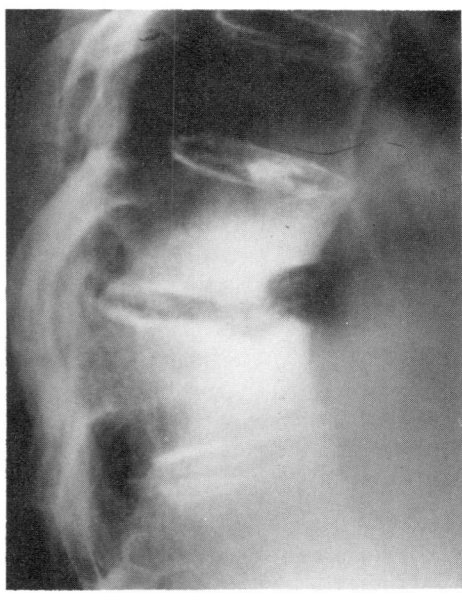

Fig. 53–8. Lateral radiograph of the lumbar spine from a patient with ankylosing spondylitis showing destructive osteitis with gross vertebral body erosion mimicking septic discitis. Note the posterior arch disruption leading to localized instability.

radiographic appearance of subchondral erosion with initial widening of the joint space and occasionally associated periostitis. Once healed, the articulations may still appear widened, with sclerotic new bone formation adjacent to the original joint. A similar process occurs less frequently in the sternoclavicular and costochondral junctions on the anterior chest wall. In all these sites, primary chondritis or subchondral osteitis is capable of destroying the normal joint architecture, with resolution by fibrosis or bony fusion.

Peripheral Joint Involvement

Involvement of the peripheral (diarthrodial) joints is seen in a variable proportion of patients with AS. In particular, the hips, shoulders, and knees may be affected by a chronic synovitis that grossly resembles the pannus seen in RA, but may

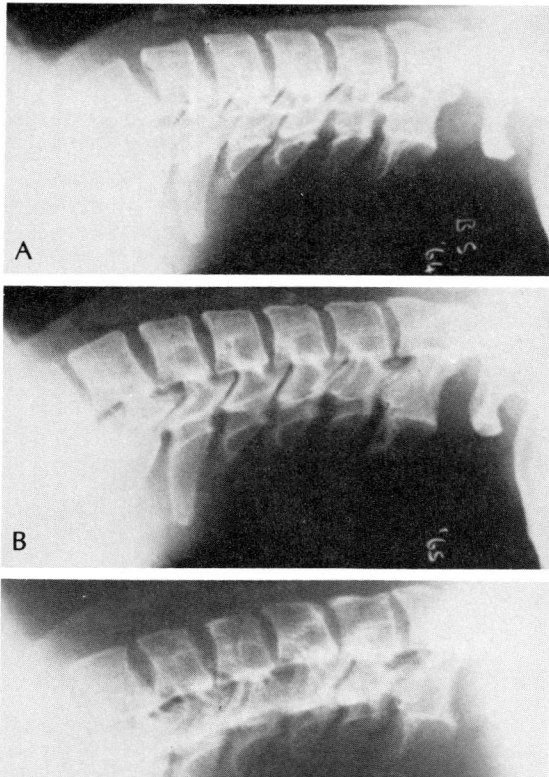

Fig. 53–9. Ankylosing spondylitis of the cervical spine. The progressive changes during a four-year period are shown from *A* to *C*. Irregular sclerosis and fusion of the apophyseal joints are seen posteriorly, with squaring of the vertebral bodies anteriorly.

differ from it in several respects.[7] Generally, one sees less surface necrosis of synovial tissue than in RA, but an equal amount of chronic inflammation with marked congestion, edema, and infiltration with small round cells. Much of this cellular infiltration appears to be perivascular in the subsynovial space, but only rarely are definite follicles with germinal centers seen. Not surprisingly, the synovial fluid is typically inflammatory in nature, with an elevated protein and white blood cell content, but normal hemolytic complement concentration. At a later stage, fibrosis of the inflammatory synovial tissue occurs, with focal metaplasia to cartilage and bone, and the perivascular fibrosis is often associated with endarteritis obliterans. The synovial pannus is capable of spreading over the articular cartilage, with gradual cartilage destruction and penetration to underlying bone. The process is not exclusively one of synovial inflammation, however. Independent foci of chronic inflamma-

tion, similar to those previously described, are found in the articular cartilage remote from areas of pannus, as well as in the subchondral bone. As fibrous and then bony fusion of the joint occurs, little normal tissue remains, its place taken by cancellous bone, which may even contain bone marrow. Inflammatory processes in and around the insertions of tendons and ligaments adjacent to the hips and shoulders promote the ankylosis of these large joints. Radiographically, the proximal joints can resemble those in rheumatoid disease, but with a greater tendency to central articular erosion (Fig. 53–10), and with the more obvious presence of proliferative new bone formation within periarticular structures. In addition, a greater tendency exists for fibrous and bony ankylosis to occur at an early stage of the disease. Occasionally, a destructive synovitis of smaller peripheral or temporomandibular joints is evident; however, such radiographic features as asymmetry, a lack of demineralization, small, "whiskery" erosions, an associated marginal periostitis, and a propensity for bony ankylosis all distinguish the changes from those of rheumatoid disease (Fig. 53–11).

Arteritis associated with AS is exceedingly rare.[3]

Scintigraphic Manifestations

Active skeletal inflammation anywhere, with its attendant increased vascularity, may be detected by scintigraphy (radionuclide bone survey) before radiographic changes are apparent (Fig. 53–12). This principle has been widely applied to the detection of early sacroiliitis mainly using

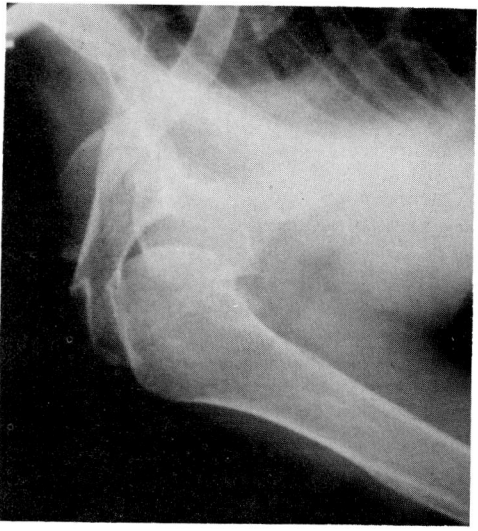

Fig. 53–10. Ankylosing spondylitis. Chronic synovitis of the shoulder joint has resulted in a large erosion destroying the superolateral humeral head.

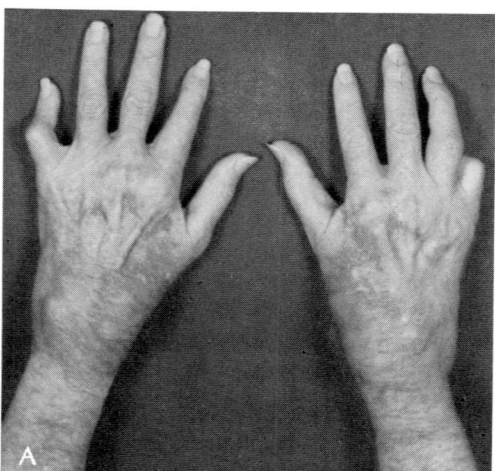

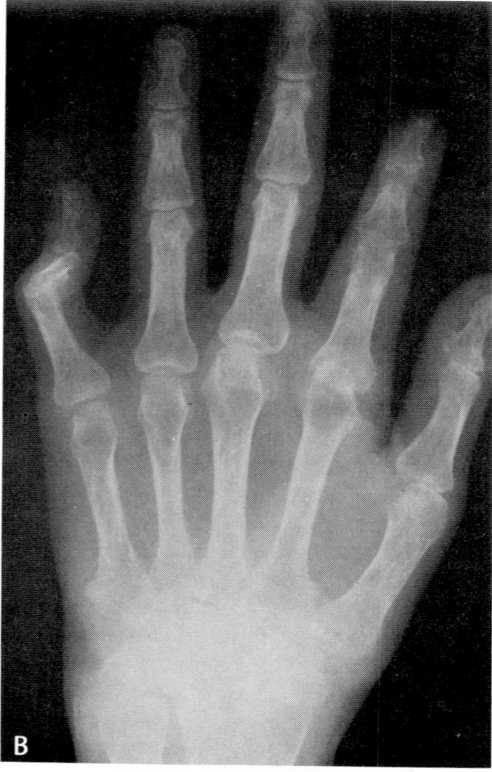

Fig. 53–11. Gross appearance, *A*, and radiograph, *B*, of the hands in a patient with ankylosing spondylitis and chronic peripheral joint involvement. The swollen wrists and finger deformities are obvious in *A*. The radiograph reveals postinflammatory bony fusion across the carpus and fifth proximal interphalangeal joint, with "whiskery" erosions affecting the first and second metacarpal joints.

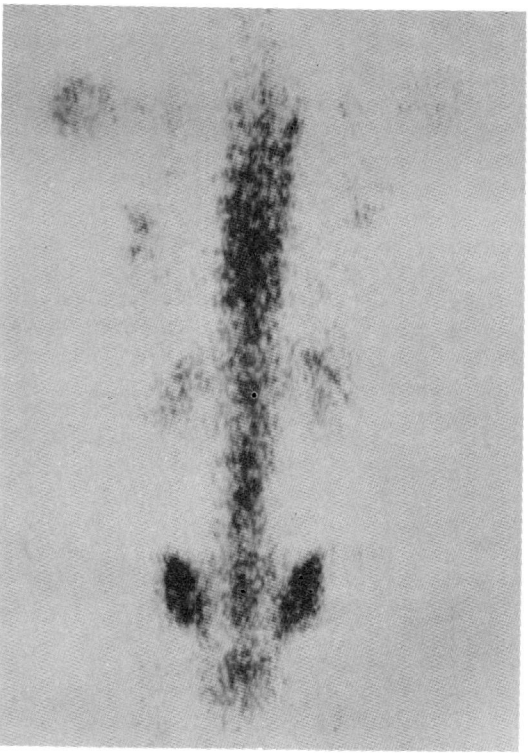

Fig. 53–12. Radionuclide bone scan (posterior image) in a patient with severe ankylosing spondylitis. Uptake in both sacroiliac joints, the entire thoracic spine, and costovertebral joints, discrete areas of the lumbar spin, and the right shoulder is moderately increased. The breadth and degree of thoracic spine uptake correlate with the clinical picture of severe costovertebral joint involvement. (Courtesy of Dr. Thomas Medsger.)

^{99m}technetium-tin-polyphosphate* (Tc-Sn-PP) for the performance of bone scans. Positive scans in patients with AS risk interpretation as evidence of metastatic disease. Scattered areas of active osteitis or postinflammatory osteoblastosis may be detected as "hot spots," even in patients presumed to have end-stage or inactive AS (Fig. 53–13).

The great sensitivity of modern radionuclide scanning techniques results in an inevitable loss of specificity when these methods are applied to the detection of preradiographic foci of articular inflammation. Hence the diagnostic role of scintigraphy in patients with suspected AS is limited. The detection of unsuspected axial microfractures or posterior pseudarthroses may be possible, how-

---

*Polyphosphate, pyrophosphate, or diphosphonate has been used. See Chapter 5 for details.

ever, using carefully matched radiographic and scintigraphic imaging.[29,69,75]

Several necropsy studies have revealed the presence of chronic aortitis in some patients with AS.[17,36] This inflammatory process appears to start as a perivascular lymphocytic infiltration of the adventitial vasa vasorum, followed by necrosis of medial tissue, with replacement of the normal muscle and elastic cells by dense scar formation. This process is associated with an overlying thickening and atrophy of the tunica intima. The process can occur throughout the entire aorta, but the long-term sequelae are most apparent in the proximal part of the vessel. Destruction of the tunica media near the aortic valve may dilate and stretch the aortic ring and may lead to a structurally intact but incompetent valve.[13] The final morphologic features are readily distinguishable from those of syphilis because the rheumatic disease extends to the aortic root inferior to the valve and results in a subvalvular mound of postinflammatory fibrous tissue, which

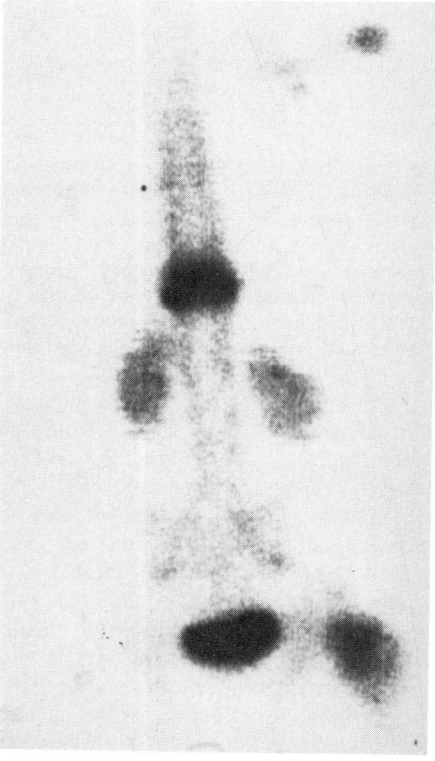

Fig. 53–13. Radionuclide bone scan (anterior image) in a patient presumed to have "burnt-out" ankylosing spondylitis. Foci of increased uptake are present in his left acromioclavicular and sacroiliac joints, as well as in a sharply localized region of his lower thoracic spine. The initial diagnosis of metastatic malignant disease was not substantiated on further evaluation.

may even be extensive enough to involve the anterior leaflet of the mitral valve. Because the valve leaflets are completely normal, one should have no difficulty in distinguishing this lesion from bacterial endocarditis, and the fibrous thickening of the aortic wall is entirely different from that observed in the thinned aorta of Marfan's syndrome. Radiographically, the usual sequelae of chronic aortic regurgitation may be evident on the chest film. This finding may be confirmed by angiography, which may also demonstrate the subaortic mound of scar tissue thought to be characteristic of AS. If the subaortic scarring becomes extensive enough, it may involve the cardiac conduction system and may thereby account for the incidence of all degrees of heart block complicating this rheumatic disease.

Iritis

The pathology of the acute iritis in AS has not been studied in great detail. This nongranulomatous inflammatory response appears to have few specific features, and only rarely does one see complete destruction of the anterior uveal tract. Recurrences are common, however, and some degree of scarring with secondary glaucoma can occur.

Any or all of the inflammatory lesions described can arise with a variable degree of severity at any time during the life span of a patient with AS. The symptoms, signs, radiographic changes, and necropsy findings at any stage of the disease depend on the extent to which the target tissues and organs are involved by the chronic inflammation, characteristic in its form and distribution. Acute anterior uveitis is per se also associated with HLA B-27.[9]

ETIOLOGY

The origin of AS is unknown, but recent studies may provide valuable pathogenetic clues. This disease is associated with the histocompatibility antigen B27 (HLA-B27) throughout the world.[15,79] Thus, approximately 90% of Caucasian patients with AS are HLA-B27-positive. The incidence of HLA-B27 in black Afro-Americans with AS appears to be lower (approximately 50%), but it is still higher than the prevalence of the antigen in control groups of 4 to 8%. The strength of the association is emphasized by Japanese surveys in which the normal prevalence of HLA-B27 is less than 1%, whereas the antigen is found in about 85% of patients with the disease. Moreover, this association holds for patients with AS complicating chronic inflammatory bowel disease, as well as those with the juvenile form of AS, which may mimic pauciarticular juvenile RA (JRA) in its clinical presentation. The possible role of HLA-B27 in arthropathy is further discussed in Chapter 24 and 25. Perhaps even more pertinent is the striking association between HLA-B27 and Reiter's syndrome.[7,11]

CRITERIA AND PREVALENCE

The diagnostic criteria for AS are customarily accepted as those first outlined by workers in Rome, and later modified in New York (Table 53–1). These criteria reflect the characteristic symptoms and signs of the disease, but are weighted toward the detection of radiographic sacroiliitis.[61] Unfortunately, mild or even moderate sacroiliitis may not be readily detectable on radiographic examination. Moreover, other diseases may affect the sacroiliac joints, and in particular, the minor degenerative joint changes found in an increasing proportion of elderly men render radiographic interpretation more difficult. In practice, a single posteroanterior radiograph centered on the pelvis is suitable for detecting sacroiliitis.[58] Only if a doubtful abnormality is detected, or if a surprisingly normal sacroiliac joint is apparent, are more detailed studies needed. A CT examination of the sacroiliac region then either confirms the normality of the joint or reveals the characteristic morphoradiographic changes of early sacroiliitis. The availability of CT scanning eliminates the need for oblique sacroiliac roentgenograms. It may be erroneous to interpret all radiographic sacroiliitis as evidence of AS, and such interpretations probably account for some of the confusion surrounding the true prevalence and incidence of the disease.

Most of the original prevalence data for AS were based on the detection of radiographic sacroiliitis, with or without historical or physical examination. These data supported a prevalence figure of 1.5 to 2 persons per thousand in several Caucasian populations studied, with a definite male:female preponderance of about 7:3. Family studies suggested the role of genetic factors in the development of AS because a strong familial aggregation of the disease was noted, either fully expressed or detected as radiographic sacroiliitis.[7] Although the mode of transmission was indeterminate, it seemed that expression of frank disease was more evident in men. Epidemiologic studies have confirmed the widespread geographic incidence of spondylitis, together with great racial variability. (See Chap. 2.)

All these epidemiologic data deserve re-evaluation in light of the association of AS with HLA-B27. Recent studies using HLA-B27 as a potential marker for susceptibility to AS suggest that the disease is far more prevalent in our society than was hitherto suspected. Thus, 2 independent studies detected historical and radiographic evidence of AS in 20 to 25% of all HLA-B27-positive "normal" individuals[18,24] Moreover, this incidence of subclinical spondylitis was equally distributed between the sexes. If these data are confirmed in larger studies, it would indicate a North American prevalence rate of AS approaching 2%, approximately equal to that for RA and with a more equal sex distribution than was realized previously.[41,52]

Armed with the detection of HLA-B27 as a marker for disease susceptibility, the epidemiology of AS clearly must be restudied. Even with the foregoing preliminary data, the racial prevalence and familial aggregation of the disease make more sense. Perhaps the previously accepted diagnostic criteria for AS may have to be modified to allow for a large population of subjects with lanthanic disease, but who nevertheless carry the means for transmitting susceptibility to future generations.

CLINICAL PROFILES

Typical Patient

The classic clinical presentation of AS usually occurs in a late adolescent or young adult male with persistent low back pain.[65] Although discomfort and stiffness may be felt in other parts of the spine, most symptoms are localized to the lumbosacral region, with the pain and stiffness often worse after prolonged resting and alleviated following physical exertion. Signs may include point tenderness localized directly over the posterior aspects of the sacroiliac joints and a variable degree of paraspinal muscle spasm with tenderness at any vertebral level.[82] A series of nonspecific clinical maneuvers are used to detect and to follow the loss of motion that is the outstanding feature of even early AS (Table 53–2). This initial loss of motion is more often associated with reflex muscle spasm secondary to the underlying inflammation rather than to true soft tissue or bony fusion. Thus, dramatic improvement in range of motion is common after treatment with anti-inflammatory drugs and physical therapy. Usually, symptoms precede obvious radiographic or even scintigraphic signs of the disease, although any degree of association between the clinical state and the radiographic

Table 53–1. Diagnostic Criteria* of Ankylosing Spondylitis

1. Low back pain of over three months' duration, unrelieved by rest
2. Pain and stiffness in the thoracic cage
3. Limited chest expansion
4. Limited motion in the lumbar spine
5. Past or present evidence of iritis
6. Bilateral radiographic sacroiliitis
7. Radiographic syndesmophytosis

*Diagnosis requires four of the five clinical criteria or No. 6 and one other criterion.

Table 53–2.   Clinical Examination for Ankylosing Spondylitis

Test	Method	Results
Occiput to wall (Flèche)	Patient places heels and back against the wall and tries to touch the wall with the back of the head, without raising the chin above carrying level	Inability to touch head to wall suggests cervical involvement; distance from occiput to wall is measured
Fingers to floor (forward flexion)	Patient bends forward with knees straight, and the distance from the fingertips to the floor is measured (lumbar curve observed)	Inability to touch toes is evidence of early lumbar disease
Schober test	Make a mark on the spine at the level of L5; then make another mark 10 cm directly above the patient, who is stranding erect; patient then bends forward maximally, and the distance between the two marks is measured	An increase of less than 5 cm indicate early lumbar involvement
Chest expansion	Measure maximum chest expansion at the nipple line	Chest expansion of less than 5 cm is a clue to early costovertebral involvement
Sacroiliac compression	Exert direct compression over sacroiliac joints	Tenderness or pain suggests sacroiliac involvement
Gaenslen's sign	Execute maneuver to stress sacroiliac joints	Maneuver evokes sacroiliac pain

From Neustadt, D.H.[65]

changes may be observed. Laboratory tests may reveal a low-grade normocytic anemia of the type associated with any chronic inflammatory disease; an elevated sedimentation rate more apparent in the early stage of the disease, but less reliable as an indicator of disease activity once established; and a moderate elevation of the serum alkaline phosphatase concentration thought to arise from release of the enzyme following osteitis immobilization, and bone resorption. Most patients are HLA-B27-positive.[46] If the disease persists and is left untreated, a typical sequence of events may develop over many years. These events reflect the progressive degree of fusion in axial, central, and proximal joints, with loss of motion and fixed flexion contractures of the involved areas. This process results in an early loss of the normal lumbar lordosis (Fig. 53–14), an increase in the thoracic and cervical kyphosis, restriction of chest wall expansion, and a position of increasing stoop with attendant flexion contractures of the hips. The classic end-stage picture is that of a cachectic man, imprisoned in a fetal position of flexion, walking with a shuffling gait, his eyes transfixed to the floor (Fig. 53–15).

Many patients with AS appear to have an eventual spontaneous remission, with subsidence of active focal inflammation and regression of systemic symptoms. Of course, the pre-existing contractures, bony fusion, and deformities perpetuate the physical signs and dysfunctional aspects of the disease. An active inflammatory process may persist indefinitely, however, or the disease can flare up after years of "end-stage" quiescence. Recrudescence of active skeletal inflammation in an elderly man with only modest old deformities may cause much diagnostic difficulty.

Asymptomatic Sacroiliitis

Demonstration of asymptomatic radiographic sacroiliitis in family members of probands with AS has hitherto been taken as presumptive evidence of subclinical disease. More recent surveys of HLA-B27-positive individuals for this radiographic sign have been offered as additional proof of a previously unsuspected increased frequency of AS. Nevertheless, it is possible that not all asymptomatic radiographic sacroiliitis is in fact due to AS. Other conditions may cause chronic changes in the sacroiliac joints that are radiographically indistinguishable from those due to the inflammatory disease described in this chapter.

Juvenile Ankylosing Spondylitis

In childhood, the usual clinical picture is that of a boy with an oligoarticular arthritis mimicking one form of JRA.[49] The pattern of joint involvement usually involves the large joints of the lower limb, with backache sometimes hardly evident. Nevertheless, like their adult counterparts, most children with AS are HLA-B27-positive.[80] Moreover, the patient eventually notices back pain and may develop recurrent acute iritis. As the child grows to a young adolescent, the typical clinical features of adult AS become more evident.

Colitic Spondylitis

The type of AS complicating chronic inflammatory bowel disease appears to be clinically, path-

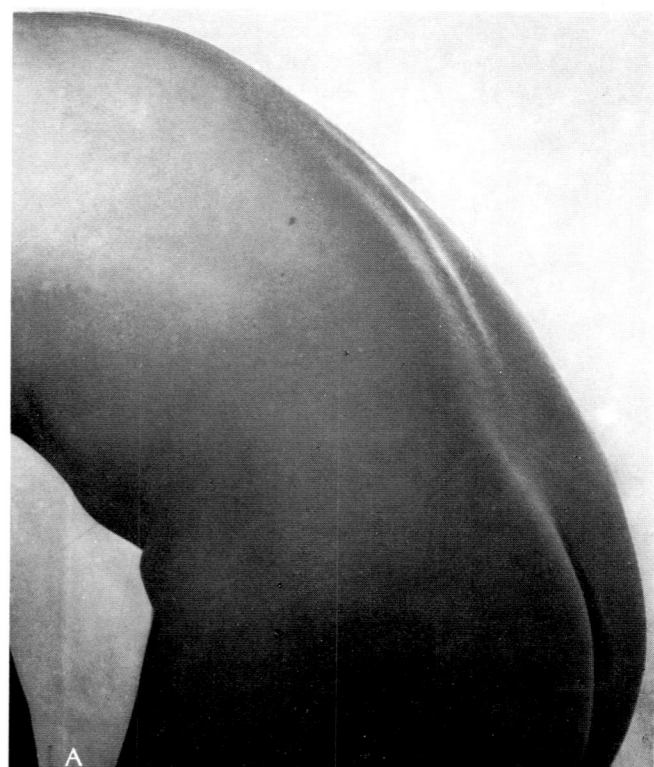

Fig. 53–14. Ankylosing spondylitis affecting the thoracolumbosacral spine. The normal contour in partial forward flexion, A, becomes ''ironed out'' in vertebral spondylitis, B.

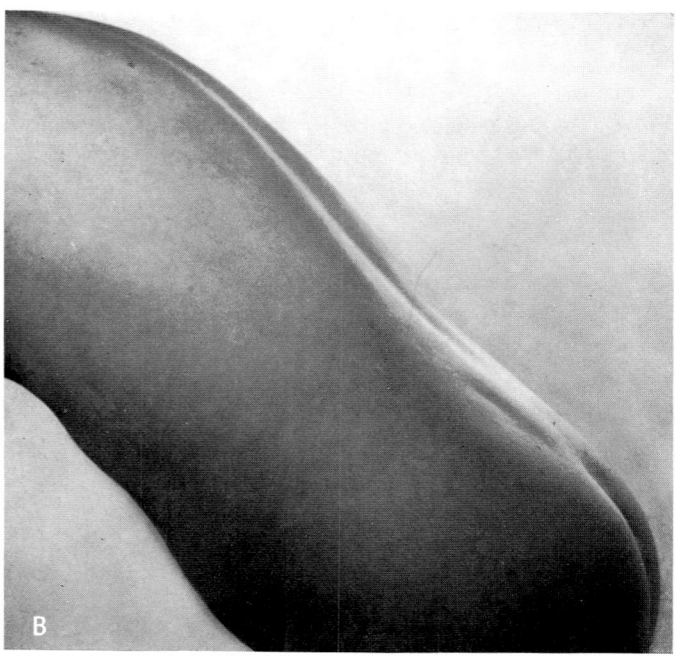

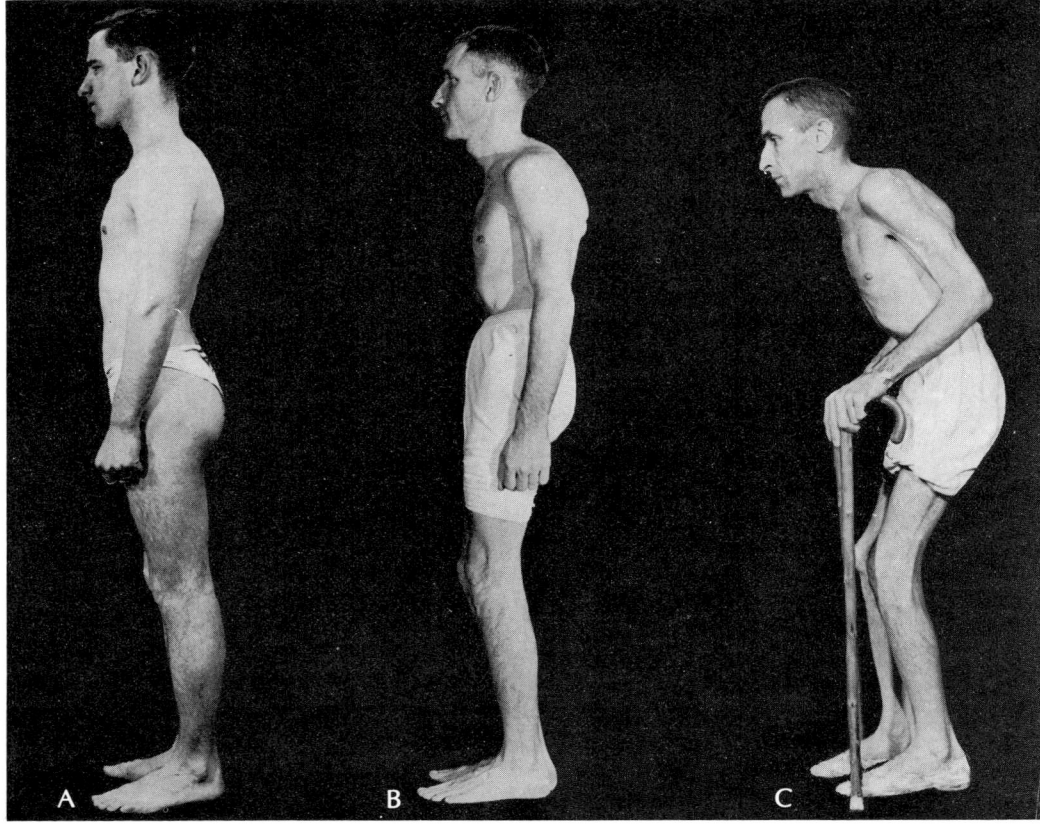

Fig. 53–15. Ankylosing spondylitis showing progression over 20 years. *A*, Normal posture at age 22 years; *B*, forward protrusion of neck and high dorsal kyphosis at age 32 years. *C*, Accentuation of deformity due to flexion contracture of hips and compensatory flexion of knees at age 42 years. (From Ogryzlo and Rosen. Courtesy of *Postgraduate Medicine*.)

ologically, and radiographically identical to idiopathic AS.[63] The rheumatic disease usually follows, but may precede, the intestinal manifestations.

Other Seronegative Spondyloarthropathies

Any of the seronegative spondyloarthropathies may show axial skeletal inflammation indistinguishable from that seen in classic AS.[7] Generally, the radiographic changes in the spine and sacroiliac joints in patients with chronic Reiter's disease or psoriatic arthropathy are less symmetric than those seen in AS. Moreover, the extra-articular features of those syndromes usually distinguish them from those of AS, although a continuous spectrum may be seen in any individual patient or in the patient's family members.[7,60] This pattern is understandable on the likely basis of common pathogenetic factors operative in these disorders.[11]

Lumbosacral Disc Syndrome

The symptoms and signs of an acute prolapsed, intervertebral disc are usually distinctive.[65] The low back pain of patients with AS may radiate along a radicular distribution, however, and may resemble a low-grade sciatica. Under such circumstances, no clinical or electrodiagnostic evidence of nerve root irritation should be present. Unfortunately, it is common to see young adults with obvious AS who have been subjected previously to myelography and spinal operations based on an erroneous diagnosis of a prolapsed intervertebral disc.

Peripheral Joint Disease

Occasionally, peripheral joint arthritis can dominate the clinical profile of adult AS. Although hip and shoulder joint involvement is common in the disease,[28] and severe central joint arthritis can be the first presenting feature of AS, it is unusual to see persistent and erosive synovitis of the smaller peripheral joints. Nevertheless, this type of presentation does occur, and then the radiographic features of involved peripheral joints resemble those of RA.[70] The axial changes retain their spondylitic character, however. Furthermore, the incidence of seronegative, HLA-B27-positive large-joint polyarthritis among middle-aged men has increased.[44] Careful radiographic and scintigraphic examinations of these individuals sometimes reveal subtle degrees of sacroiliitis, suggesting that AS-like disease can occur and may persist as a large-joint polyarthritis.

An increased incidence of HLA-B27 reported in patients with ''idiopathic'' frozen shoulder suggests that AS-like disease may cause an apparently nonspecific, chronic, proximal joint arthropathy in the absence of detectable sacroiliitis.[12]

Acute Iritis

About 25% of all patients with AS develop at least one episode of acute iritis at some time during the natural history of their disease. Many patients suffer from recurrent episodes of acute iritis, which may result in scarring and depigmentation of the iris with irregularity of the pupil. Rarely, advanced scarring and secondary glaucoma cause loss of vision. Studies in patients with ''idiopathic'' acute nongranulomatous iritis suggest that this, too, may be a solitary manifestation of the spondylitic diathesis, even in the absence of overt musculoskeletal disease.[10,78] Thus, almost half of such patients, mainly men, demonstrate subtle clinical, radiographic, or scintigraphic evidence of AS or of some other seronegative spondyloarthropathy;[76] and half of the remainder, both men and women, are HLA-B27-positive, but have no detectable arthropathy.

Aortic Regurgitation

The aortitis of AS can result in hemodynamically significant aortic valve regurgitation.[87,90] The clinical picture is then similar to that seen in other patients with aortic valve disease, with the additional possibility of widespread aortic dilatation and, rarely, an active arteritis affecting large, systemic vessels.[6,45] Additionally, fibrosis within the cardiac conduction tissue may result in any degree of heart block.[5,66] The cardiovascular manifestations of AS are invariably associated with obvious evidence of underlying chronic rheumatic disease.

Pulmonary Disease

Costovertebral and costochondral joint involvement can produce chest-wall pains simulating those of cardiopulmonary disease.[34] The eventual fusion of the costovertebral joints leads to a painless restriction of the thoracic cage, however.[39,62] Although the restricted ventilation and subsequent reduction of lung volume are readily detected on pulmonary function testing, rarely is gas exchange impaired.[23] Consequently, major surgical procedures in patients with AS do not usually give rise to undue anesthetic problems, unless the cricoarytenoid or temporomandibular joints are fused.[4] Another pulmonary manifestation of AS is a distinctive type of bilateral apical lobe fibrosis, probably secondary to a low-grade interstitial pneumonitis that has resolved by fibrosis and cavitation.[7,27,94] These pulmonary changes usually begin several years after the onset of skeletal symptoms. No evidence suggests that this upper zone process is due to tuberculous infection or to previous radiotherapy, although the cavities may eventually become colonized by opportunistic bacteria or fungi.

Spinal Cord and Root Damage

One feature of AS is the development of a fused, osteoporotic, and weakened spine. This rigid, bony bar is unduly vulnerable to fracture at any site, and traumatic paraplegias are well recognized as one disastrous consequence of even minor trauma in patients with the disease (Fig. 53–16).[43,64,88] In addition, a fused and immobile lower cervical spine may be associated with instability of C1 to C3.[38,86] This condition may result in atlantoaxial subluxation with subsequent spinal cord or brain stem compression, or it may irritate the posterior spinal roots and manifest as intense episodic pain referred over the occipital bone, partially relieved by local anesthetic infiltration of the affected dermatomes. Rarely, patients with established AS have lower-limb sensory and motor impairment, including loss of sphincter control, owing to the development of

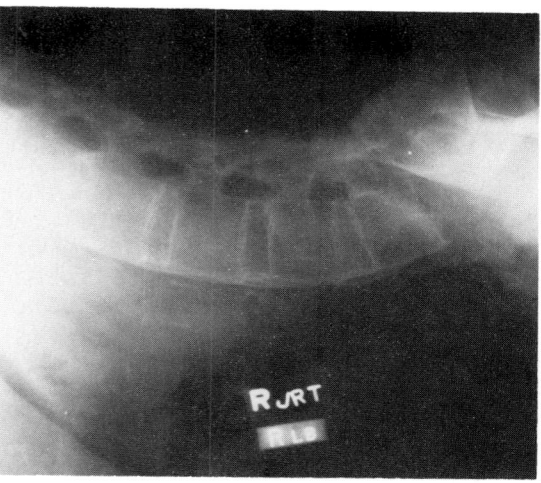

Fig. 53–16. Ankylosing spondylitis resulting in a totally fused and rigid spine. The complete fracture-dislocation at the lumbosacral region occurred following minor trauma.

spinal canal posterior lumbosacral arachnoidal diverticulae and leading to a cauda equina syndrome.[77,85,93,95] The mechanism of dural cyst development is unknown, but it might be the result of chronic arachnoiditis. Indeed, the moderate elevations of cerebrospinal fluid protein concentration detected in patients with AS suggest the presence of low-grade dural sac inflammation.[7] Alternatively, the theca might simply become passively adherent to the adjacent bony overgrowth and fibrosis that characterize the skeletal lesion.

Metabolic Bone Disease

Osteoporosis is an early and common feature of AS. This osteoporosis is usually most evident in the vertebral bodies and is detectable radiographically as marked osteopenia, often out of proportion to the other clinical and radiographic signs. This feature might account for the increased concentrations of serum alkaline phosphatase found in patients with the disorder,[48] as well as the inevitable hypercalciuria that develops when such patients are unduly immobilized. On this basis, the incidence of urinary tract calcium stones appears to be increased. Fully 9% of 132 patients with AS had stones in one controlled study.[93a] Suggestions of a true association between hyperparathyroidism and AS have not been confirmed, however, although the coexistence of both disorders is recognized.[14] On the other hand, subchondral resorption about the sacroiliac joint can occur in both primary and secondary hyperparathyroidism and can cause radiographic widening of the sacroiliac joint space.[72] The widened, eroded joint rarely looks sclerotic or abnormal in its noncartilaginous ligamentous portion, and healing is observed following cure of the endocrinopathy.

Chest Pain

Anterior chest-wall pain is an important mode of clinical presentation. The mechanism may be costovertebral joint inflammation with referred girdle pain or direct involvement of costochondral junctions with pain and tenderness elicited adjacent to the sternum. Recumbency aggravates either mechanism and often leads to disturbed sleep. Because this manifestation of AS occurs in middle-aged men with hitherto inconspicuous axial disease, a major diagnostic dilemma may ensue.[6]

Disease in Women

Because the wider recognition of the disease is in women, a more subtle and indistinct female clinical profile has emerged. The morphoradiographic changes of typical AS may not develop. Indeed, the accepted criteria for the disease do not ever become manifest in many women with AS. Strik-

ing symptoms, a strong family history, modest elevations in the Westergren erythrocyte sedimentation rate, the presence of HLA-B27, and subchondral erosions visible on sacroiliac CT scans all permit a valid diagnosis, however. Early data suggest that pregnancy has no deleterious effects on mothers with AS or on their infants.[8,35,68]

Amyloidosis

As with any other chronic inflammatory disease, patients with AS may develop secondary amyloidosis, particularly in the juvenile form of the disease. When systemic amyloidosis occurs, the clinical manifestations follow their usual pattern[51] (see Chap. 72).

DISEASES MIMICKING ANKYLOSING SPONDYLITIS

Low back pain, a common symptom among all segments of the population, may be due to many pathologic and psychologic factors. The diagnosis of lumbosacral disc disease, fibromyalgia (lumbago), lumbar strain, chronic pelvic disease with referred pain, or psychosomatic backache should only be considered once an inflammatory disease of the lumbosacral spine has been adequately excluded. This exclusion may be difficult, but a reliable method by which to distinguish between spondylitis and lumbar disc disorders is the measurement of lateral spinal flexion. This motion usually fails to provoke pain in patients with lumbar disc syndrome, but is usually limited and painful in patients with spondylitis. Nevertheless, the diagnosis of early AS often requires long-term observation because the clinical, radiographic, or scintigraphic changes may take many months to develop. Furthermore, recent epidemiologic data suggest that many women with chronic low backache previously ascribed to other causes may actually suffer from a "forme fruste" of AS.

Degenerative joint disease affecting the apophyseal and intervertebral joints of the lumbosacral spine is common. The clinical setting of an older individual with characteristic radiographic changes usually distinguishes this condition from inflammatory disease; however, the sacroiliac joint is not immune from osteoarthritis[74] especially in its inferior part, in which subchondral bony sclerosis, loss of joint space, and bridging anterior osteophytes may result in a radiographic appearance superficially resembling that of AS (Fig. 53–17). Nevertheless, the localization of these changes mainly to the inferior part of the joint with a largely spared superior ligamentous region is distinctive.[73]

The proliferative degenerative condition of the spine referred to as benign senile hyperostotic spondylosis, or Forestier's disease, may give rise

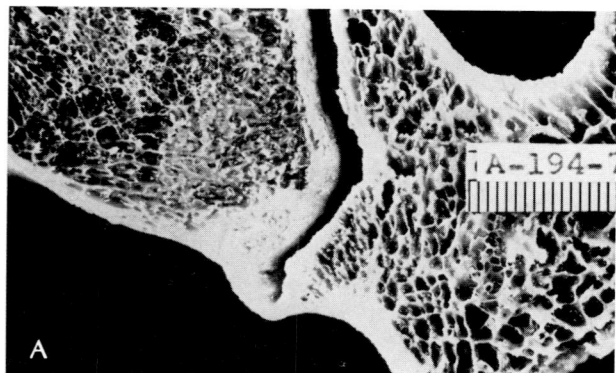

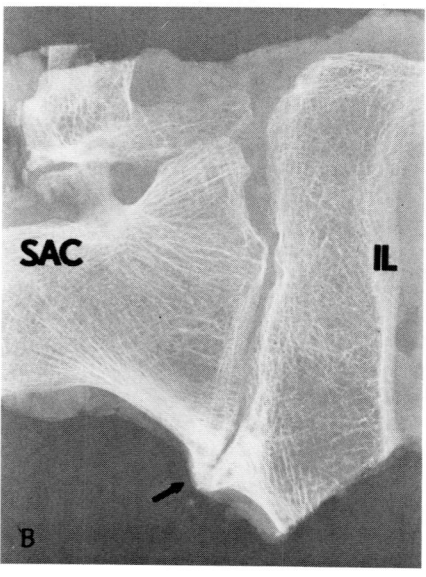

Fig. 53–17. Osteoarthrosis of the sacroiliac joint. The macerated specimen, *A,* and its radiograph, *B,* show irregular loss of the joint space interiorly with associated subchondral osteoblastosis and an osteophyte bridging the joint margin (arrow). The upper (cartilaginous) portion of the joint is normal. SAC = Sacrum; IL = ilium. (*A,* From Resnick, D., Niwayama, G., and Georgen, T.G.[74] *B,* from Resnick, D., and Niwayama, G.[71])

to diagnostic difficulties, especially if the perispinal hypertrophic new bone formation is extensive and uniform.[32] Patients with this disorder nearly always demonstrate intact vertebral bodies beneath the struts of new bone and have normal sacroiliac joints.[91] In addition, hypertrophic new bone formation at traction sites around the pelvis, knees, and elbows frequently accompanies the spinal changes of Forestier's disease.[71]

Postinflammatory fusion of the cervical spine resembling the radiographic appearance of AS can be seen in two forms of RA. First, the apophyseal joints of children with polyarticular JRA may fuse following persistent synovitis at this site.[21] These same children may develop radiographic changes around their sacroiliac joints, which probably reflect the abnormal stresses of altered weight bearing, as well as a low-grade erosive synovitis within the small amount of synovium lining the anterior capsule of the joint.[16] Postinflammatory fusion of the cervical spine has also been described in elderly patients with chronic RA who are institutionalized

by their disease.[37] The radiographs of the neck alone might suggest AS, but when viewed in the full clinical context, the correct diagnosis is obvious. AS and RA can undoubtedly occur together in the same patient, however.[30,54] Well-documented examples exist of patients with all the characteristic clinical, radiographic, and histologic features of both disorders, including the presence of rheumatoid nodules.[53] The coexistence of these two diseases probably occurs no more than would be expected by chance, and the presence of high titer rheumatoid factor, rheumatoid nodules, and widespread erosive peripheral joint arthropathy in a patient with obvious AS should suggest the diagnosis of two unrelated rheumatic diseases.

Several other forms of vertebral or paravertebral ossification may suggest inflammatory disease, but they are unrelated to AS. They include idiopathic calcification of the posterior longitudinal ligament of the spine, reported in elderly Japanese subjects,[42] and a florid paravertebral ossification or sacroiliac joint fusion, evident in patients with spinal cord injuries with variable degrees of paraplegia.[7] These changes in injured patients appear to be secondary to prolonged immobilization, with no evidence of preceding inflammation.[7]

A nonspecific, and probably noninflammatory, sclerosis of iliac subchondral bone is seen in parous women and is referred to as *osteitis condensans ilii*. It appears to be an innocent condition totally unrelated to AS, but may occasionally result in radiographic changes superficially resembling those of the inflammatory disease. Additionally, a painful erosive and sclerosing inflammatory disorder of the symphysis pubis is recognized in women who have undergone pelvic or urologic operations, and is referred to as *osteitis pubis*. The radiographic appearance of this condition may resemble that of AS, but osteitis pubis is not associated with skeletal disease elsewhere. Rarely, the arthropathies of both familial Mediterranean fever and Behçet's disease progress to erode large joints, including the sacroiliac regions. The systemic nature of these underlying inflammatory diseases, however, is usually evident. Intrabody disc herniations (Schmorl's nodes), reactive vertebral body sclerosis, and fractures of the vertebral endplate may all resemble various radiographic aspects of the spondylitic spine.[56] In addition, septic discitis with associated osteomyelitis of the adjacent vertebral bodies is usually a clear-cut infectious disease with its characteristic clinical and radiographic course;[57] however, the noninfective discitis and osteitis of AS may be destructive enough to mimic spinal osteomyelitis. In that situation, the obvious presence of the rheumatic disease should alert the physician to the probable course of events. Unfortunately, a needle exploration of the destroyed disc may still be necessary to exclude the possibility of sepsis, especially in young adults with a history of drug abuse.

Paget's disease can involve the bone on either side of the sacroiliac joint. The radiographic appearance may then mimic AS, especially because the intervening cartilage can undergo degenerative changes secondary to the subchondral process.[33] The consequent obliteration of the joint space, with a sclerotic subchondral boundary, may account for the reputed association of Paget's disease with AS. Finally, on examining any adult with pain and tenderness in the spine, one should consider the possibility of metastatic disease, particularly in elderly subjects, in whom the vertebral bodies are a favorite site for carcinomatous or myelomatous lesions. Usually, however, other features of malignant disease are evident on clinical, hematologic, or radiographic examination.

Several types of sports injuries may lead to radiographic changes suggestive of the postinflamma-tory sequelae of AS. The traumatic events include adduction insertion periostitis on the inferior pelvic rami, multiple vertebral basal plate fractures or herniations in adolescent weightlifters, and sacroiliac sclerosis or osteitis pubis in long-distance runners. The inciting physical activity, together with the absence of other diagnostic evidence, should lead to proper diagnosis.[40]

MANAGEMENT

At present, no specific therapy exists for AS. The central themes of management for patients with this disease are to maintain a maximal degree of skeletal mobility, to prevent the natural progression of increasing immobility and contracture, and to facilitate a completely normal life style within the patient's natural environment. These broad objectives are readily achieved in the majority of patients, but may require lifelong self-discipline in the pursuit of a structured exercise program, aided by the judicious recourse to surgical intervention for the relief of intractable deformities.[19,22,50,59,84]

Physical Therapy

The prevention of deformity and maintenance of an optimal range of pain-free motion, both in the spine and in the peripheral joints, inevitably requires a continuous program of physical therapy.[31,67] This program should permit general rest during active phases of the disease, when life style and work habits may have to be modified; however, complete immobilization or bed rest should be discouraged because of the high risks of accelerated bony fusion, increased osteopenia, and renal stone formation. The importance of maintaining good posture cannot be overemphasized, and the patient should be mentally trained always to hold himself erect when sitting or standing and to sleep stretched out on a firm mattress or stiff board with only one small pillow, to prevent undue flexion of any part of the spine. Active exercises designed to maintain chest expansion, full extension of all parts of the spine, and a complete range of motion of the proximal joints should be performed several times daily (Fig. 53–18). Before exercise, hot showers or hot and cold compresses can be used to alleviate local areas of discomfort or stiffness, but they are not a substitute for the exercises to follow. Natural sports activities that facilitate spinal extension and proximal joint movement, such as walking and swimming, should be encouraged. Some sports, such as road cycling, however, may maintain the patient in a position of flexion and are probably best avoided.

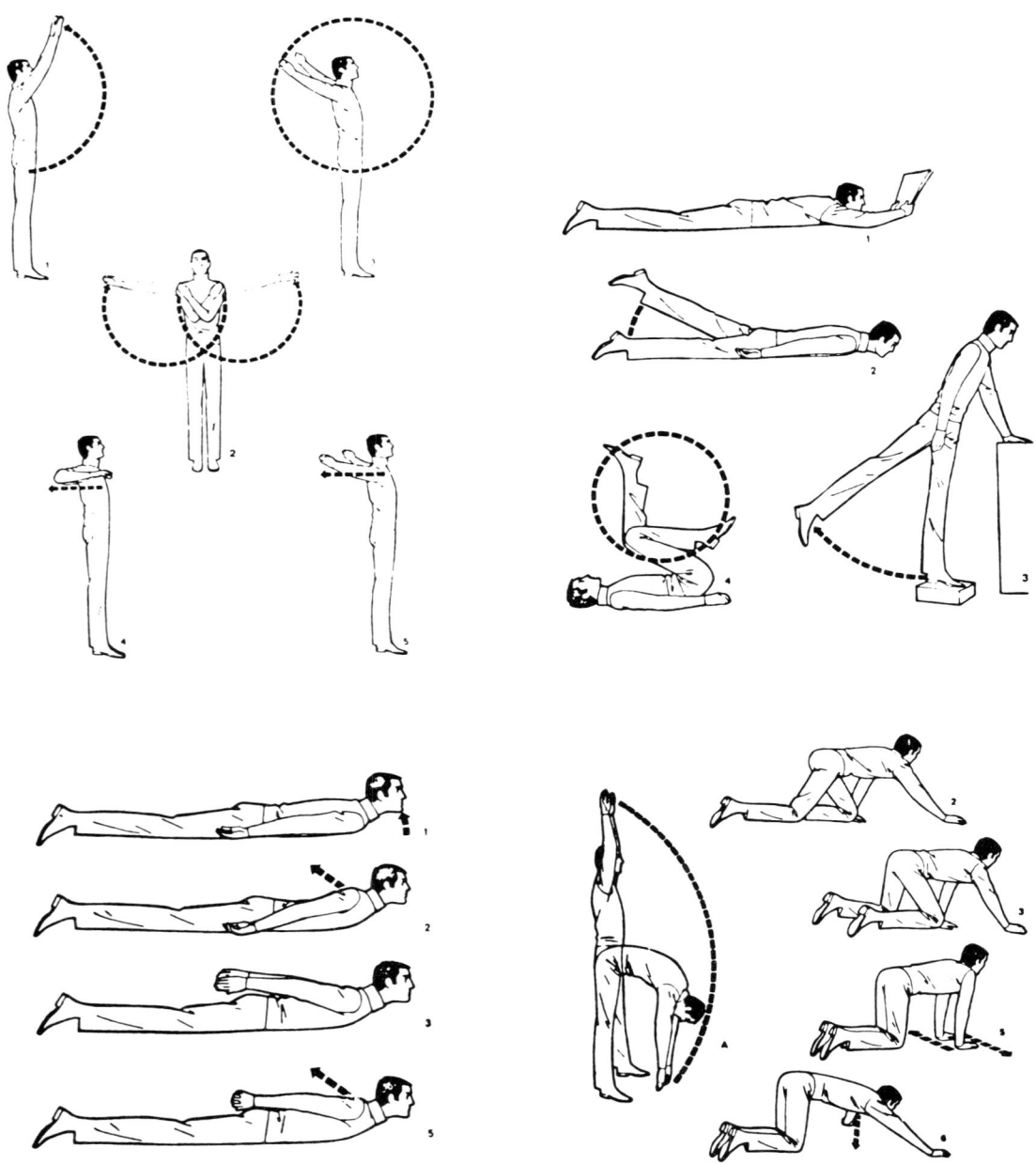

Fig. 53-18. Typical series of active exercises recommended for patients with ankylosing spondylitis.

Drug Therapy

The principal role of anti-inflammatory and analgesic agents in this disease is to suppress some of the pain and stiffness, to facilitate the exercise program. No clear evidence suggests that any of the drugs used in the treatment of AS influence the natural history of the disease, but symptomatic relief can be achieved.[92] The most popular and potent anti-inflammatory drug in most nations is phenylbutazone. When used at a maximum daily dose of 400 mg, with full awareness of its potential complications, this agent is invaluable in the management of patients with active disease. Bone marrow dyscrasia is only observed once in every 125,000 "patient-dose-months," with a fatality reported in every 250,000 dose-months, in contrast to the reported bone marrow toxicity of 1:25,000 patient-dose-months for chloramphenicol. Furthermore, most serious blood dyscrasias associated with phenylbutazone have been reported in patients with disorders other than AS.[7] Indeed, most of the fatal toxicity has been noted in patients with RA who may also be receiving numerous other agents, including gold, and may have a tendency to bone marrow suppression. Fortunately, most patients with AS are otherwise healthy young adults in whom the short- and long-term administration of phenylbutazone appears to be an effective and safe therapeutic measure. Even so, the onset of fever, rash, or a sore throat soon after initial treatment with phenylbutazone should immediately alert the patient and physician to the risk of agranulocytosis and should indicate immediate cessation of the drug. The symptoms are far more sensitive than a blood count for this early complication of the drug that is mainly seen in younger patients. The occult development of aplastic anemia, which is more usual in elderly patients and is likely to prove fatal, may be asymptomatic. Therefore, in patients undergoing long-term treatment with phenylbutazone, a full blood count every 4 to 6 weeks is advised, to detect incipient bone marrow failure at an early stage.

Indomethacin may be useful in some patients and is usually prescribed as a 25-mg capsule 4 times daily, often supplemented by a 50-mg suppository (not available in the United States) at night to help alleviate morning stiffness. Currently, it may be the drug of choice in the United States, where legal considerations can dominate prescription habits. For reasons that are unclear, a good therapeutic response to salicylate therapy is unusual in AS. Nevertheless, certain patients with the disease do benefit from this drug, and it should be considered as a therapeutic option. Data on the use of the newer nonsteroidal anti-inflammatory drugs in the treatment of AS are not sufficient now to formulate firm recommendations. In selected patients, ibuprofen, tolmetin, naproxen, or fenoprofen may be useful additives or substitutes for the older agents. No evidence indicates that corticosteroids or gold can control the symptoms or can mollify the outcome of AS. On the other hand, topical corticosteroids are an essential part of the management during an attack of acute iritis, and their prompt use can quickly suppress the ocular inflammation. Occasionally just as in other chronic inflammatory arthropathies, persistent synovitis of a peripheral joint requires the intrasynovial injection of corticosteroids.

Unfortunately, a few patients suffer from severe disease that is recalcitrant to orthodox anti-inflammatory therapy. Faced with intense pain and profound disability, the patient and physician may consider unproved, though rational, therapeutic techniques. Anecdotal (reported) measures include "pulse" corticosteroid infusions, long-term azathioprine administration, and weekly doses of parenteral methotrexate.

Radiotherapy

Radiotherapy directed at the spine and sacroiliac joints produces prompt symptomatic relief in many patients. Unfortunately, such courses were originally given on a repetitive basis resulting in a cumulative dose far in excess of safety. This overdosing almost certainly accounts for the increased incidence of acute leukemia noted among previously irradiated spondylitic individuals followed-up for many years.[47,83,89] The judicious use of a total dose of 600 to 700 rads applied during 1 or 2 exposures to the entire axial skeleton may still be recommended in controlling the pain and stiffness of severe AS. In particular, if the patient is unable to tolerate any oral agent, such as a patient with painful AS, severe inflammatory bowel disease, or short-bowel syndrome, this form of therapy can be useful. Unfortunately, adequate clinical trials comparing appropriately dosed radiation therapy to anti-inflammatory drugs in the treatment of AS have not been conducted.

Surgical Treatment

Some surgical procedures are of great potential benefit to certain patients with end-stage and intolerable deformity. In particular, total hip joint replacement has revolutionized the outlook for patients with fused hip joints, although a discouraging tendency to postoperative new bone formation with reankylosis is evident.[81] Totally ankylosed temporomandibular joints are best treated by condylar resection; adequate movement is sometimes achieved by operation on one side only.[26] Both cervical and lumbar osteotomies are well-described surgical procedures rarely indicated for the partial correction of devastatingly severe spinal kyphosis.[7,55] These procedures are difficult to perform, are potentially hazardous, and are usually reserved for carefully selected patients. If the aforementioned general principles of physical therapy and drug use are followed, few patients will progress to a stage requiring such heroic surgical measures. Reduction and stabilization of atlantoaxial subluxation are occasionally necessary and may be technically difficult to effect. Aortic valve replacement is sometimes required for the aortic regurgitation of AS. Under those circumstances, the operative procedure and perioperative risks appear to be no greater than in patients with other types of aortic valve disease.

Counseling

Family counseling may one day be an integral part in the management of an individual patient with AS. Data may soon become available that would permit a reasonable assessment of risk factors for the disease in HLA-B27-positive and HLA-B27-negative family members. It may then become desirable to counsel family members at a high risk of developing AS. Because this disease generally carries an excellent prognosis, however, prenatal counseling will probably not become important.

Although not curable, AS is one of the most rehabilitatable of all the chronic rheumatic diseases. Given appropriate efforts at education of the patient, self-disciplined exercise programs, and the selective use of anti-inflammatory drugs, it should be possible to enable most patients with this disease to live a completely normal life, with only minimal work adjustments. Occasionally, however, vocational alterations have to be recommended, depending on individual circumstances.

REFERENCES

1. Ansell, B.M., and Bywaters, E.G.L.: Juvenile chronic polyarthritis or Still's disease. Textbook of Rheumatic Diseases. 4th Ed. Edited by W.S.C. Copeman. Edinburgh, Livingstone, 1969.
2. Ball, G.V.: Enthesopathy of rheumatoid and ankylosing spondylitis. Ann. Rheum. Dis., 30:213–223, 1971.
3. Ball, G.V., and Hathaway, B.: Ankylosing spondylitis with widespread arteritis. Arthritis Rheum., 9:737–745, 1966.
4. Berendes, J., and Miehlke, A.: A rare ankylosis of the cricoarytenoid joints. Arch. Otolaryngol., 98:63–65, 1973.
5. Bergfeldt, L., et al.: Ankylosing spondylitis: an important cause of severe disturbances of the cardiac conduction system. Prevalence among 223 pacemaker-treated men. Am. J. Med., 73:187–191, 1982.
6. Bluestone, R.: Two cases of severe musculo-skeletal pain. Hosp. Pract., 17:114A–114G, 1982.
7. Bluestone, R.: Ankylosing spondylitis. In Arthritis and Allied Conditions, 9th Ed. Edited by D.J. McCarty. Philadelphia, Lea & Febiger, 1979.
8. Braunstein, E.M., Martel, W., and Martel, R.: Ankylosing spondylitis in men and women: a clinical radiographic comparison. Radiology, 114:91–94, 1982.
9. Brewerton, D.A., et al.: Acute anterior uveitis and HL-A27. Lancet, 2:994–996, 1973.
10. Brewerton, D.A., et al.: Ankylosing spondylitis and HL-A27. Lancet, 1:904–907, 1973.
11. Brewerton, D.A., and James, D.C.O.: The histocompatibility antigen HL-A27 and disease. Semin. Arthritis Rheum., 4:191–207, 1975.
12. Bulgen, D.Y., Hazelman, B.L., and Voak, D.: HLA-B27 and frozen shoulder. Lancet, 1:1042–1044, 1976.
13. Bulkley, B.H., and Roberts, W.C.: Ankylosing spondylitis and aortic regurgitation. Circulation, 48:1014–1027, 1973.
14. Bunch, T.W., and Hunder, G.G.: Ankylosing spondylitis and primary hyperparathyroidism. JAMA, 225:1108–1109, 1973.
15. Bywaters, E.G.L.: Clinico-pathological aspects of ankylosing spondylitis and comparison with the changes in sero-negative juvenile polyarthritis and sero-positive rheumatoid arthritis. Scand. J. Rheumatol., 9:61–66, 1980.
16. Bywaters, E.G.L.: Pathologic aspects of juvenile chronic polyarthritis. Arthritis Rheum., 20:271–276, 1977.
17. Bywaters, E.G.L.: A case of early ankylosing spondylitis with fatal secondary amyloidosis. Br. Med. J., 2:412–416, 1968.
18. Calin, A., and Fries, J.F.: Striking prevalence of anky-losing spondylitis in healthy W27 positive males and females. N. Engl. J. Med., 293:835–839, 1975.
19. Caretta, S., et al.: The natural disease course of ankylosing spondylitis. Arthritis Rheum., 26:186–190, 1983.
20. Carrera, G.F., et al.: Computerized tomography of sacroiliitis. AJR, 136:41–46, 1981.
21. Cassidy, J.T., and Martel, W.: Juvenile rheumatoid arthritis clinicoradiologic correlations. Arthritis Rheum., 20:207–211, 1977.
22. Chamberlain, M.A.: Socioeconomic effects of ankylosing spondylitis. Int. Rehabil. Med., 3:94–99, 1981.
23. Cirtin, D.L., Boyd, G., and Bradley, G.W.: Ventilatory function and transfer factor in ankylosing spondylitis. Scott. Med. J., 18:109–113, 1973.
24. Cohen, I.M., et al.: Increased risk for spondylitis stigmata in apparently healthy HL-AW27 men. Ann. Intern. Med., 84:1–7, 1976.
25. Cruickshank, B.: Pathology of ankylosing spondylitis. Bull. Rheum. Dis., 10:211–214, 1960.
26. Davidson, C., et al.: Temporomandibular joint disease in ankylosing spondylitis. Ann. Rheum. Dis., 34:87–91, 1975.
27. Davies, D.: Ankylosing spondylitis and lung fibrosis. Q. J. Med., 51:395–417, 1972.
28. Dwosh, I.L., Resnick, D., and Becker, M.A.: Hip involvement in ankylosing spondylitis. Arthritis Rheum., 19:683–692, 1976.
29. Esdaile, J., Hawkins, D., and Rosenthall, L.: Radionuclide joint imaging in the seronegative spondyloarthropathies. Clin. Orthop., 143:46–52, 1979.
30. Fallet, G.H., et al.: Rheumatoid arthritis and ankylosing spondylitis occurring together. Br. Med. J., 1:804–807, 1976.
31. Felts, W.R.: Ankylosing spondylitis: the challenge of early diagnosis. Postgrad. Med., 72:184–200, 1982.
32. Forestier, J., and Lagier, R.: Ankylosing hyperostosis of the spine. Clin. Orthop., 74:65–83, 1971.
33. Franck, W.A., Bress, N.M., and Singer, F.R.: Rheumatic manifestations of Paget's disease of the bone. Am. J. Med., 56:592–603, 1974.
34. Good, A.E.: The chest pain of ankylosing spondylitis. Ann. Intern. Med., 58:926–937, 1963.
35. Goodman, C.E., et al.: Ankylosing spondylitis in women. Arch. Phys. Med. Rehabil., 61:167–170, 1980.
36. Graham, D.C., and Smythe, H.A.: The carditis and aortitis of ankylosing spondylitis. Bull. Rheum. Dis., 9:171–174, 1958.
37. Grahame, R., et al.: Ankylosing rheumatoid arthritis. Rheumatol. Rehabil., 14:25–30, 1975.
38. Halla, J.T., Fallahi, S., and Havidin, J.G.: Non-reducible rotational head tilt and atlantoaxial lateral mass collapse. Clinical and roentgenographic features in patients with juvenile rheumatoid arthritis and ankylosing spondylitis. Arch. Intern. Med., 143:471–478, 1983.
39. Hart, F.D., Bogdanowitch, A., and Nichol, W.D.: The thorax in ankylosing spondylitis. Ann. Rheum. Dis., 9:116–131, 1950.
40. Helms, C.A.: Radiology of joggers injuries. Orthopedics, 5:1492–1504, 1982.
41. Hill, H.F.H., Hill, A.G.S., and Bodmer, J.G.: Clinical diagnosis of ankylosing spondylitis in women and relation to presence of HLA-B27. Ann. Rheum. Dis., 35:267–270, 1976.
42. Hiramatsu, Y., and Nobechi, T.: Calcification of the posterior longitudinal ligament of the spine among Japanese. Radiology, 100:307–312, 1971.
43. Hunter, T., and Dubo, H.I.C.: Spinal fractures complicating ankylosing spondylitis. Arthritis Rheum., 26:751–759, 1983.
44. Joliat, G., et al.: HLA-B27 antigen in diagnosis of atypical seronegative inflammatory arthropathy. Ann. Rheum. Dis., 35:531–533, 1976.
45. Kanasuji, M., et al.: Aortic valve replacement and ascending aorta replacement in ankylosing spondylitis: report of three surgical cases and review of the literature. Thorac. Cardiovasc. Surg., 30:310–314, 1982.
46. Khan, M.A., and Khan, M.K.: Diagnostic value of HLA-

B27 testing in ankylosing spondylitis and Reiter's syndrome. Ann. Intern. Med., 96:70–76, 1982.

47. Kaprove, R.E., et al.: Ankylosing spondylitis: survival in men with and without radiotherapy. Arthritis Rheum., 23:57–61, 1980.

48. Kendall, M.J., Lawrence, D.S., and Shuttleworth, G.R.: Haematology and biochemistry of ankylosing spondylitis. Br. Med. J., 2:235–237, 1973.

49. Ladd, J.R., Cassidy, J.T., and Martel, W.: Juvenile ankylosing spondylitis. Arthritis Rheum., 14:570–590, 1971.

50. Lehtinen, K.: Working ability of 76 patients with ankylosing spondylitis. Scand. J. Rheumatol., 10:263–265, 1981.

51. Lehtinen, K.: Cause of death in 79 patients with ankylosing spondylitis. Scand. J. Rheumatol., 9:145–147, 1980.

52. Levintin, P.M., Gough, W.W., and Davis, J.S.L.: HLA-B27 antigen in women with ankylosing spondylitis. JAMA, 235:2621–2623, 1976.

53. London, M.C., and Bland, J.H.: Ankylosing spondylitis with subcutaneous nodules. N. Engl. J. Med., 268:991–994, 1963.

54. Luthra, H.S., Ferguson, R.H., and Conn, D.L.: Coexistence of ankylosing spondylitis and rheumatoid arthritis. Arthritis Rheum., 19:111–114, 1976.

55. McMaster, M.J., and Coventry, M.B.: Spinal osteotomy in ankylosing spondylitis. Technique, complications and long-term results. Mayo Clin. Proc., 48:476–486, 1973.

56. Martel, W., et al.: Traumatic lesions of the discovertebral junction in the lumbar spine. AJR, 127:457–464, 1976.

57. Messer, H.D., and Litvinoff, J.: Pyogenic cervical osteomyelitis. Arch. Neurol., 33:571–576, 1976.

58. Mink, J.H., Gold, R.H., and Bluestone, R.: Radiographic arthritis survey. Arthritis Rheum., 20:1564, 1977.

59. Moll, J.M.H.: Ankylosing Spondylitis. New York, Churchill-Livingstone, 1980.

60. Moll, J.M.H., et al.: Associations between ankylosing spondylitis, psoriatic arthritis, Reiter's disease, the intestinal arthropathies and Behcet's syndrome. Medicine, 53:343–364, 1974.

61. Moll, J.M.H., and Wright, V.: New York clinical criteria for ankylosing spondylitis. Ann. Rheum. Dis., 32:354–363, 1973.

62. Moll, J.M.H., and Wright, V.: The pattern of chest and spinal mobility in ankylosing spondylitis. Rheumatol. Rehabil., 12:115–134, 1973.

63. Morris, R.I., et al.: HLA-W27. A useful discriminator in the arthropathies of inflammatory bowel disease. N. Engl. J. Med., 290:1117–1119, 1974.

64. Murray, G.C., and Persellin, R.H.: Cervical fracture complicating ankylosing spondylitis: a report of eight cases and review of the literature. Am. J. Med., 70:1033–1041, 1981.

65. Neustadt, D.H.: Ankylosing spondylitis. Postgrad. Med., 61:124–135, 1977.

66. Nitter-Hauge, S., and Otterstad, J.E.: Characteristics of atrioventricular conduction disturbances in ankylosing spondylitis. Acta Med. Scand., 210:197–200, 1981.

67. O'Driscoll, S.L., Jayson, M.I.V., and Baddeley, H.: Neck movements in ankylosing spondylitis and their response to physiotherapy. Ann. Rheum. Dis., 37:64–66, 1978.

68. Ostensten, M., Romberg, O., and Husby, G.: Ankylosing spondylitis and motherhood. Arthritis Rheum., 25:140–143, 1982.

69. Park, W.M., et al.: The detection of spinal pseudoarthroses in ankylosing spondylitis. Br. J. Radiol., 54:467–472, 1981.

70. Resnick, D.: Patterns of peripheral joint disease in ankylosing spondylitis. Radiology, 110:523–532, 1974.

71. Resnick, D., and Niwayama, G.: Radiographic and pathologic features of spinal involvement in diffuse idiopathic skeletal hyperostosis (DISH). Radiology, 119:559–568, 1976.

72. Resnick, D., Dwosh, J.L., and Niwayama, G.: Sacroiliac joint in renal osteodystrophy, roentgenographic-pathologic correlation. J. Rheumatol., 2:287–295, 1975.

73. Resnick, D., Niwayama, G., and Goergen, T.G.: Comparison of radiographic abnormalities of the sacroiliac joint in degenerative disease and ankylosing spondylitis. AJR, 128:189–196, 1977.

74. Resnick, D., Niwayama, G., and Goergen, T.G.: Degenerative disease of the sacroiliac joint. Invest. Radiol., 10:608–621, 1975.

75. Resnick, D., Williamson, S., and Alaziaki, N.: Focal spine abnormalities on bone scans in ankylosing spondylitis: a clue to the presence of fracture or pseudoarthroses. Clin. Nucl. Med., 6:213–217, 1981.

76. Russell, A.S., et al.: Scintigraphy of sacroiliac joints in acute anterior uveitis. Ann. Intern. Med., 85:606–608, 1976.

77. Russell, M.L., Gordon, D.A., and Ogryzlo, M.A.: The cauda equina syndrome of ankylosing spondylitis. Ann. Intern. Med., 78:551–554, 1973.

78. Scharf, J., et al.: HL-A27 antigen associated with uveitis and ankylosing spondylitis in a family. Am. J. Ophthalmol., 82:139–140, 1976.

79. Schlosstein, L., et al.: High association of HL-A antigen, W27 with ankylosing spondylitis. N. Engl. J. Med., 101:704–706, 1973.

80. Schaller, J.G., Ochs, H.D., and Thomas, E.D.: Histocompatibility antigens in childhood-onset arthritis. J. Pediatr., 88:926–930, 1976.

81. Shanahan, W.R., et al.: Assessment of long-term benefit of total hip replacment in patients with ankylosing spondylitis. J. Rheumatol., 9:101–104, 1982.

82. Sigler, J.W., et al.: The surgical correction of flexion deformity of the cervical spine in ankylosing spondylitis. Clin. Orthop., 86:132–143, 1972.

83. Smith, P.G., and Doll, R.: Mortality among patients with ankylosing spondylitis after a single treatment course with x-rays. Br. Med. J., 284:449–460, 1982.

84. Smythe, H.: Therapy of the spondyloarthropathies. Clin. Orthop., 143:84–89, 1979.

85. Soeur, M., Monseu, G., and Baleriaux-Waha, D.: Cauda equina syndrome in ankylosing spondylitis. Anatomical, diagnostic and therapeutic considerations. Acta Neurochir. (Wein), 55:303–315, 1981.

86. Sorin, S., Askari, A., and Moskowitz, R.W.: Atlantoaxial subluxation as a complication of early ankylosing spondylitis. Two case reports and a review of the literature. Arthritis Rheum., 22:273–276, 1979.

87. Thomas, L., et al.: Early detection of aortic dilatation in ankylosing spondylitis using echocardiography. Aust. N.Z. J. Med., 12:10–13, 1982.

88. Thorngren, K.G., Liedberg, E., and Aspelin, P.: Fractures of the thoracic and lumbar spine in ankylosing spondylitis. Arch. Orthop. Trauma Surg., 98:101–107, 1981.

89. Toolis, F., et al.: Radiation-induced leukemias in ankylosing spondylitis. Cancer, 48:1582–1585, 1981.

90. Tucker, C.R., et al.: Aortitis in ankylosing spondylitis: early detection of aortic root abnormalities with two-dimensional echocardiography. Am. J. Cardiol., 49:680–686, 1982.

91. Vernon-Roberts, B., Pirie, C.J., and Tenurth, V.: Pathology of the dorsal spine in ankylosing hyperostosis. Ann. Rheum. Dis., 33:281–288, 1974.

92. Washer, C., Briton, M.C., and Kraines, R.G.: Non-steroidal anti-inflammatory agents in rheumatoid arthritis and ankylosing spondylitis. JAMA, 246:2168–2172, 1981.

93. Weinstein, P.R., et al.: Spinal cord injury, spinal fracture and spinal stenosis in ankylosing spondylitis. J. Neurosurg., 57:609–616, 1982.

93a. Whalen, T.S., et al.: Increased incidence of nephrolithiasis in ankylosing spondylitis (abstract). Arthritis Rheum., 27:531, 1984.

94. Wolson, A.H., and Rohwedder, J.J.: Upper lobe fibrosis in ankylosing spondylitis. AJR, 124:466–471, 1975.

95. Young, A., et al.: Cauda eqina syndrome complicating ankylosing spondylitis: use of electromyography and computerized tomography in diagnosis. Ann. Rheum. Dis., 40:317–322, 1981.

Chapter 54

Reiter's Syndrome (Reactive Arthritis)

John T. Sharp

The development of arthritis in men with recently acquired urethral infections was observed at least as early as the sixteenth century. Pierre Van Forest described a patient who developed arthritis of the knee in association with urethritis in 1507,[7] and Martiniere referred to arthritis as a complication of urethritis in 1664.[9] John Hunter, in 1786, described a patient who had articular symptoms with several recurrences of urethral discharge.[7] In 1818, Brodie reported the association of urethritis, arthritis, and conjunctivitis in five patients.[6] Almost a century later, Hans Reiter described a patient who developed nongonococcal urethritis, conjunctivitis, and arthritis following an episode of bloody diarrhea.[23] In the same year, 1916, Fiessinger and LeRoy described four cases of mild diarrhea associated with a conjunctivourethrosynovial syndrome.[10] In 1942, Bauer and Engelman described the first case in the American literature and noted the previous report by Reiter.[4] Since that time, the combination of nongonococcal urethritis, arthritis, and conjunctivitis generally has been referred to as Reiter's syndrome.

During World War II in Finland, a large epidemic of dysentery due to *Shigella flexneri* was followed in several hundred patients by sterile arthritis, conjunctivitis, iritis, urethritis, and keratoderma.[21] A majority of affected individuals had combinations of these nonbacterial complications. In the 1960s and 1970s, nonbacterial arthritis was associated with *Yersinia* infections,[1,37] and complete Reiter's syndrome was observed in some of these patients.[29]

This experience has led to the concept that patients with *reactive arthritis* associated with dysentery or with nonbacterial urethritis have the same disease, whether or not the complete triad of Reiter's syndrome is present. A subcommittee of the American Rheumatism Association Diagnostic and Therapeutic Criteria Committee recognized this trend and proposed that Reiter's syndrome be defined as an episode of peripheral arthritis of more than one month's duration, occurring in association with urethritis or cervicitis.[36] This group defined Reiter's syndrome as reactive arthritis associated with genitourinary tract infection, but did not accept postdysenteric arthritis as synonymous with Reiter's syndrome. Studies are needed to clarify the relationship of reactive arthritis associated with dysentery with that occurring after urinary tract infection. Some distinctions between the two disorders are made in specific sections of this chapter, but generally, they are considered together because no evidence suggests otherwise.

EPIDEMIOLOGY

Reactive arthritis, with or without the complete Reiter's triad, may follow nonbacterial urethritis or dysentery due to a number of organisms. Reactive arthritis associated with either event occurs much more frequently in individuals who are HLA-B27 positive, but it is not limited to individuals who carry this gene marker[5,19] (see Chap. 25). Although nonbacterial urethritis may be due to trichomonads, chlamydiae, and probably ureaplasmas, a specific association of Reiter's syndrome with any of these agents has not been firmly established. Chlamydiae were grown from the synovial tissue or fluid of 6 patients with Reiter's syndrome among 84 studied.[25] Chlamydiae were isolated from synovial fluid of 1 patient with Reiter's syndrome and from the urethra of 5 additional patients, among 24 studied.[33] Other investigators have been unable to isolate chlamydiae from tissue or body fluids, and serologic studies have not shown elevated antichlamydial antibodies in patients with Reiter's syndrome.[14,27]

Among patients in whom diarrhea appears to be the precipitating event, reactive arthritis has been described in association with *Shigella flexneri*,[21,28] *Salmonella, Yersinia*,[29,37] and *Campylobacter* infections.[15,31,32] *Shigella sonnei* has not been associated with reactive arthritis, but that it is a common cause of dysentery suggests the importance of some specific property of the infecting organism.[28]

The incidence and prevalence of reactive arthritis associated with urethritis or diarrhea are not precisely established. The picture is confused by the use of multiple terms and varying diagnostic criteria. Nevertheless, some estimates are available.

Approximately 4 cases per 100,000 men per year were seen in United States Navy personnel over a 10-year period.[20] Interviews with 530 persons during a survey of chest roentgenograms disclosed that 13 individuals (1.3%), 6 men and 7 women, had a history of reactive arthritis associated with a genitourinary tract infection.[34]

Reactive arthritis occurred in 344 of an estimated 150,000 cases of dysentery on the Finnish front in World War II.[21] More recent studies indicate a higher frequency. A mailed questionnaire identified 6 individuals with reactive arthritis among 410 persons with *Shigella* infections in 2 epidemics, an incidence of 1.5%. Five persons had 2 or more features of Reiter's syndrome.[28]

A patient with Reiter's syndrome attributed to *Yersinia enterocolitica* was described in 1971.[29] This patient had diarrhea, arthritis, conjunctivitis, and dysuria with fever. Cultures were negative for *Yersinia*, but the patient had a high titer of agglutinins to this organism, and 4 members of the family had had diarrhea at the same time as the patient. Windblad studied sera from patients with acute arthritis that were submitted to the laboratory for antistreptolysin titers.[37] Seventy-four sera were found with *Yersinia enterocolitica* agglutinins of 1:320 or greater. Eighteen of these patients had positive stool cultures. Most of these patients developed diarrhea before arthritis, with an interval of 1 day to more than 12 days, and a median of about 7 days. Twelve patients had monoarticular arthritis, 25 had involvement of 2 joints, and the remaining 37 had arthritis in 3 or more joints. Tendinitis, conjunctivitis, urethritis, myocarditis, and myositis were all observed. *Yersinia* infections associated with reactive arthritis have not been as frequently reported in the United States as in Scandinavia. Whether this finding represents a greater frequency of *Yersinia* infections or a more careful search for these organisms in Scandinavia is unknown.

Campylobacter infections originally were reported to produce septic arthritis. Subsequently, reactive arthritis was described in association with enteritis caused by this organism. This form of Reiter's syndrome was first reported in a 41-year-old man with diarrhea, fever, arthralgia, mucosal lesions, keratoderma, and conjunctivitis.[31] In subsequent episodes, 3 years after the first, single blood cultures were positive for *Campylobacter* on 2 occasions during exacerbations of the Reiter's syndrome. Multiple other blood cultures were negative. Unfortunately, cultures of joint fluid were not obtained.

Van de Putte and his colleagues reported 6 patients with reactive arthritis associated with *Campylobacter* enteritis.[32] All had 1 or more positive stool cultures, although 1 of the 6 patients did not have diarrhea. One had a striking rise in agglutinin titer immediately after the episode of enteritis. The interval from enteritis to arthritis varied between 6 and 14 days, and the arthritis was polyarticular in 3 of these patients. Extra-articular manifestations occurred in 4 of the 6, and a complete Reiter's syndrome was observed in 1 patient.

Eight additional cases of reactive arthritis associated with *Campylobacter* enteritis were found during an 18-month observation.[15] Three of these patients had positive stool cultures, and 5 had decreasing titers of antibodies. Five of the 7 patients were HLA-B27 positive. In this study, the incidence of reactive arthritis following *Campylobacter* enteritis was 2.35%.

Because *Campylobacter fetus jejuni* is a particularly common cause of diarrhea, it may be one of the more frequent causes of reactive arthritis. One study of 514 patients with diarrhea showed that 5.1% had positive cultures for *Campylobacter* organisms.[3] In this study, *Campylobacter* species were more frequently isolated than *Salmonella* or *Shigella* species.*

Reiter's syndrome has generally been considered predominantly a disease of men, but several reports of reactive arthritis after dysentery note an equal sex distribution. The difficulty in making a clear-cut diagnosis of urethritis or cervicitis accounts for the less-frequent diagnosis of Reiter's syndrome in women.

PATHOGENESIS

The cause of reactive arthritis remains unknown. The occurrence of sterile synovitis after infection with an enteric organism or nongonococcal urethritis suggests that immune factors may play a prominent role in the pathogenesis, but no clues exist as to the specific mechanism. As noted previously, chlamydiae have been isolated from the synovial fluid in a few instances, but current data do not suggest that chlamydial infection accounts for more than a small fraction of all cases. A search for common antigens or other factors among the variety of organisms capable of precipitating postdysenteric reactive arthritis has not been successful, but studies have been far from comprehensive.

Early reports that HLA-B27 antigen is present in a high proportion of patients with reactive arthritis have been confirmed. An increased fre-

---

*Editor's note: A personal case of reactive arthritis in a 28-year-old nurse who was HLA-B27 positive followed an episode of culture-proved *Campylobacter* enteritis and was associated with painful aphthous stomatitis requiring local analgesics. Mildly painful aphthous stomatitis was found in 1 of 6 recorded cases.[32]

quency of HLA-B27 has been found in patients with reactive arthritis occurring after nongonococcal urethritis and *Shigella, Salmonella, Yersinia,* or *Campylobacter* infections. Individuals with Reiter's syndrome who were HLA-B27 negative were examined for the presence of antigens cross-reactive with HLA-B27; namely, HLA-B7, BW22, and BW42, and 7 of 10 of these persons tested positive.[2] This observation was interpreted as support for the hypothesis that the antigenic makeup of HLA-B27 was important in the pathogenesis of Reiter's syndrome, but in the absence of a 100% association with a specific antigen or hapten, the possibility that HLA-B27 is associated by linkage dysequilibrium with another gene determining susceptibility to arthritis following infection with the precipitating organism cannot be excluded. Such an association might reflect an immune response gene. The HLA-A2, B27 haplotype is present in increased frequency and seems to be associated with more severe disease, as well as with certain disease patterns, but the etiologic implications of this association are still not clear.[26]

CLINICAL MANIFESTATIONS

Patients with reactive arthritis may have a variety of clinical features[35] (Table 54–1). A history of sexual promiscuity and sexual deviation are elicited often. Common nonarticular manifestations include enthesopathies, ocular inflammation, and skin and mucous membrane lesions. Many patients are systemically ill, and most have fever. Weight loss is frequent and may be extensive in a few individuals. Lymphadenopathy and splenomegaly are occasionally seen, as is cardiovascular involvement. Neurologic and pulmonary involvement have been reported, but their specificity is uncertain.

Table 54–1.   Clinical Features Suggesting Reiter's Syndrome

History of diarrhea or extramarital sexual intercourse prior to attack
Fever
Arthritis, usually pauciarticular
Urethritis, possibly complicated by cystitis, prostatic abscess, or hydronephrosis
Conjunctivitis possibly complicated by keratitis, iritis, retinitis, or optic neuritis
Skin lesions, including keratoderma blennorrhagicum, circinate balanitis, and superficial ulcerations on tongue and buccal mucosa
Possible electrocardiographic changes; infrequently, pericarditis

Joints

Articular involvement is usually the second or third feature of the illness, with urethritis, diarrhea, or conjunctivitis, or a combination of these features, preceding synovitis. Arthritis is more frequent in the large joints, but toes and fingers are commonly involved. The weight-bearing joints are affected more frequently than those of the upper extremities. Arthritis is usually pauciarticular and asymmetric, but the number of joints involved varies. Arthritis may be mild or severe, with marked swelling, redness, heat, and pain. During the early phase of illness, synovitis may develop in new articulations every few days. In many patients, an initial period of polyarthritis is followed by more persistent inflammation in only a few joints for several weeks or longer. Back pain occurs in a few patients during the acute illness. Sacroiliac and vertebral tenderness may also occur. Vertebral joint involvement skips some segments ("skip pattern").

Enthesopathy

Inflammation at the site of tendinous insertion into bone has come to be known as enthesopathy. Such lesions are common and may be prominent among patients with Reiter's syndrome. Plantar fasciitis, manifested by heel tenderness and a fluffy calcification at the insertion of the plantar fascia into the calcaneus as seen radiographically, is common. Periostitis in a digit may give rise to a diffuse swelling that resembles a sausage. Other sites of enthesopathies include the lower tibia or shin bone, the insertion of the patellar tendon, and the insertion of the Achilles tendon. Although such lesions are not confined to the reactive arthritides, they are often prominent, particularly in spondyloarthropathy.

Genitourinary Tract

Urethral discharge is characteristic. In most men, the discharge is mucopurulent or mucoid. Dysuria may accompany the discharge, but urethritis is sometimes asymptomatic. In patients with a history of casual sexual relationships, the interval from sexual intercourse to the onset of urethritis varies from a few days to approximately a month.

Prostatis is frequently present in addition to urethritis. The prostatic gland is enlarged, soft, and tender, and prostatic secretions contain many pus cells. Prostatic abscesses occasionally develop.

In women, urethritis, cervicitis, or cystitis may be present. Symptoms are often minimal or are limited to dysuria or to a slight vaginal discharge.

Eye

Conjunctivitis is generally the first manifestation of eye involvement. Usually, inflammation is mild, accompanied by a slight burning sensation and some adhesiveness of the eyelids in the morning. Conjunctivitis may be unilateral, although in most cases, both eyes are involved. Iritis develops in 5 to 10% of patients during their first attack and eventually occurs or recurs in 20 to 50% of patients. Keratitis has been reported in several instances and may be a distinctive lesion.[18] Optic neuritis, retinitis, and macular edema have been reported, but are rare.

Skin and Mucous Membranes

Superficial ulcers on the penis, particularly around the urethral meatus, are common. Coalescence of lesions on the glans penis gives rise to a circular or scalloped border, called balanitis circinata (Fig. 54–1).

Small, painless, superficial ulcers with an erythematous base are frequently seen on the buccal mucosa and the tongue. The lesions vary from a few millimeters to more than a centimeter in diameter. Patients are often unaware of their presence. Ulcers occurring in the mouth of patients with enteritis following *Camplyobacter* infection can be painful.

Involvement of the skin is most common on the palms of the hands and the soles of the feet, but it may occur anywhere on the extremities, trunk or scalp. The initial skin lesion is a small papule that rapidly develops a pustular appearance, but when opened, this lesion contains only keratotic material. Individual lesions are a few millimeters in diameter, but when many are present, they may become confluent and may cover a large area with a thick, keratotic crust (Fig. 54–2). Eventually, the crust peels from the underlying skin and leaves no scar. Keratosis also occurs under the finger- and toenails

and may lead to separation of the nails from the nail beds (Fig. 54–3).

These skin lesions, referred to as keratoderma blennorrhagicum, usually develop several weeks after onset of other manifestations of Reiter's syndrome. The skin lesions are self-limiting, but generally last several weeks. Lesions on the skin are less common than mucous membrane lesions and frequently occur in patients who already have ulcers on the genitalia or in the oral cavity. Histologically, lesions of the skin and mucous membranes are the same, but the constant moisture on the mucous membranes prevents the keratosis, so the characteristic crusts do not form. These lesions are clinically and histologically identical to those of pustular psoriasis.

Gastrointestinal Tract

Diarrhea, which may be mild and brief or severe and prolonged, is typical. Occasionally, it is bloody. Diarrhea usually occurs one to three weeks before the onset of other manifestations of the illness, but it may follow other features of the syndrome.

Heart

Pericarditis occurs infrequently in the acute stage of Reiter's syndrome. Electrocardiographic abnormalities, including prolongation of the P-R interval and ST- and T-wave changes, may be seen, but cardiomegaly and congestive heart failure have not been observed in the initial attacks. Valvular heart disease has been reported as an infrequent sequela.[30]

Nerves

Peripheral neuritis has been reported in a few patients, but a clear association with Reiter's syndrome has not been established.

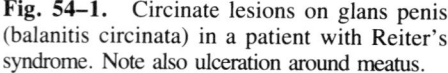
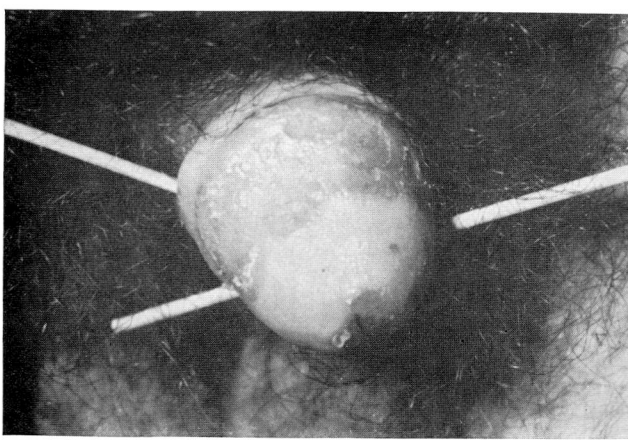

Fig. 54–1. Circinate lesions on glans penis (balanitis circinata) in a patient with Reiter's syndrome. Note also ulceration around meatus.

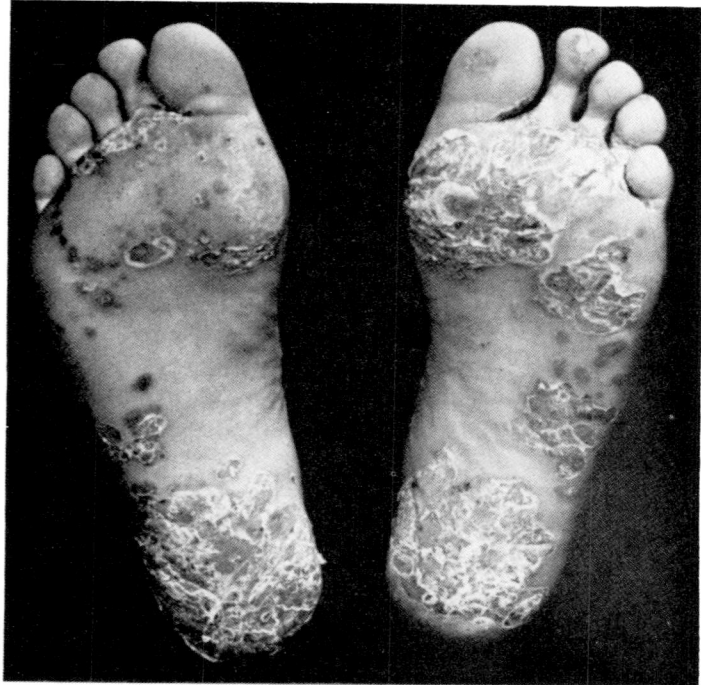

Fig. 54–2.   Keratodermia blennorrhagica of feet in a patient with Reiter's syndrome.

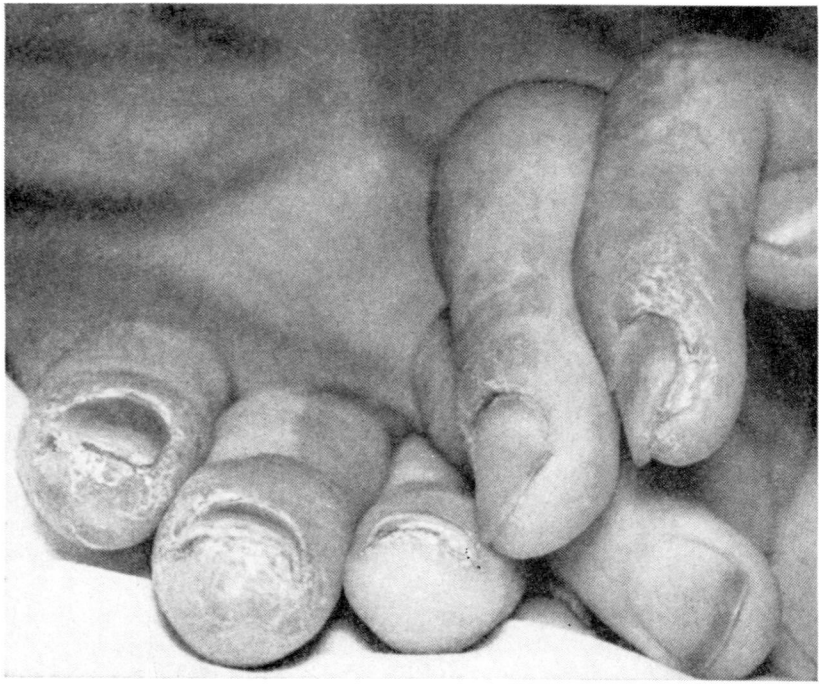

Fig. 54–3.   Keratotic lesions of fingernails in a patient with Reiter's syndrome.

Lung

Pleurisy and pneumonitis have been reported, but their rarity raises the question of coincidental infection.

PATHOLOGIC MANIFESTATIONS

In the early stages of this syndrome, the histologic changes in the synovium resemble a low-grade pyogenic infection.[16,35] The inflammatory reaction is localized to the superficial, vascular zone and is characterized by intense hyperemia and edema and by a cellular infiltrate dominated by neutrophilic leukocytes and lymphocytes. Plasma cells may be observed in lesions of more than two weeks' duration. Proliferation of connective tissue cells is variably present. Occasionally, necrosis of the synovial cell layer is seen. Focal areas of extravasation of red blood cells are found in many cases.

Chronic arthritis of several months' duration is characterized by villous synovial hypertrophy, pannus formation, and osseous erosions along the margins of the articular cartilage.[16,35] Microscopically, the inflammatory lesion is nonspecific, consisting of focal infiltrates of lymphocytes and plasma cells. Lymphoid nodules are observed in some cases. Foci of neutrophil infiltration (microabscesses) may also be present. Proliferation of connective tissue cells and of synovial cells is a regular feature of the syndrome. Histologically, the synovium in chronic disease often resembles rheumatoid arthritis (RA).

The skin lesions are characterized by thickening of the horny layer, parakeratosis, and acanthosis.[16,35] Vesicles are found in the epidermis as a result of lysis and vacuolization of the superficial prickle cells. The vesicles are filled with epithelial cells, polymorphonuclear leukocytes, and lymphocytes and often resemble microabscesses. The outer layer of the corium is infiltrated with lymphocytes and plasma cells. Histologically, the lesions on the mucous membranes resemble those on the skin, but without keratosis.

LABORATORY FINDINGS

The white blood cell count is usually elevated, in the range of 10,000 to 18,000 cells/mm³, but leukocytosis may exceed 20,000/mm³ and, in some instances, levels are not elevated. Anemia may develop in patients who have a prolonged course, but it is usually not present early in the illness. The sedimentation rate is regularly elevated and usually returns to normal as the patient recovers from the acute attack. The urethral discharge contains numerous white blood cells, most of which are polymorphonuclear cells. Pyuria is regularly present, and hematuria occurs in many patients.

The synovial fluid is turbid to a variable degree. In most instances, the joint fluid has a grossly purulent appearance. White blood cells in the synovial fluid usually number from 2000 to 50,000/mm³, but occasionally greater numbers are seen, even above 100,000/mm³. The majority of the white blood cells are polymorphonuclear leukocytes in the early, acute effusions, but their proportion falls as the inflammatory reaction subsides, and lymphocytes may become the predominant cells. The joint fluid sugar level is usually normal, but may be reduced, particularly when the leukocyte count is especially high.

The total hemolytic complement levels of the joint fluid are usually higher than in other types of effusions, but the synovial fluid protein level is also high and the synovial fluid protein complement-protein ratio is similar to that observed with degenerative joint disease and traumatic arthritis and contrasts with the reduction found in RA.

Cultures of the urethral and prostatic secretions are negative for gonococci, and the blood and synovial fluid are sterile. The conjunctival exudate is sterile or contains only nonpathogenic organisms. Some authors have claimed that they could distinguish cases of mixed infection, namely, gonococcal urethritis and nonspecific urethritis, coexisting in the same patient by the type of response to antibiotic therapy. Although many patients with gonorrhea respond rapidly and are completely free of the urethral discharge within several days of initial therapy, variability in response due to increasingly frequent penicillin-resistant strains makes it impossible to draw conclusions regarding cause from response to therapy.

Gonococcal and chlamydial antibodies are present in about the same frequency as in a clinic population of patients with venereal disease.

Stool cultures usually are negative in sporadic cases and frequently are negative even when associated with epidemic dysentery. In the latter instance, the results of stool cultures reflect the carrier rate for the interval between the onset of diarrhea and the time of culture.

RADIOLOGIC CHANGES

In the first few weeks of involvement, affected joints are radiographically normal, and milder cases may not exhibit radiologic abnormalities (see also Figs. 5–52, 5–53, 5–55, and 5–59). Osteoporosis of periarticular bone is common,[13] as early as three weeks after onset in severe cases.[35] Erosions in the small joints of the phalanges may be found when the articular inflammation persists for several weeks or longer.

Periosteal proliferation near involved joints is recognized as a frequent radiologic feature in Reiter's syndrome[13] (Fig. 54–4). Periostitis may be observed in the os calcis, ankles, metatarsals, phalanges of fingers and toes, knees, and elbows. Periostitis of the os calcis is usually seen as a diffuse, fluffy outline on the plantar surface, anterior to the calcaneal tuberosity. Such lesions have been reported in other forms of arthritis, but are much more frequent in Reiter's syndrome. Periostitis in fingers and toes may be indistinguishable from that seen in psoriatic arthritis.

COURSE OF ILLNESS

The clinical features of the syndrome may appear almost simultaneously or may evolve gradually over several weeks. Urethritis or diarrhea often precedes the second manifestations of the illness by several days to two or three weeks. New manifestations of the disease may develop at irregular intervals for weeks or months. Most patients recover from the initial episode within three or four months, but some have a chronic illness.

The majority of patients with Reiter's syndrome have recurrences.[8,11,17,24] In follow-up studies ex-

tending for 5 years or longer, as few as 20% of patients remain asymptomatic after recovery from the acute episode. Minor, minimally annoying symptoms occur in 20 or 30% of patients, and chronic or recurrent arthritis occurs in an additional 40 to 60%. Fifteen to 25% of patients become sufficiently disabled to alter their working conditions, to change jobs, or to stop working. Recurrent attacks may be characterized by single or multiple features of illness. Arthritis is most common, but recurrent ocular involvement and skin lesions also may be seen.

Chronic arthritis occasionally develops during the initial illness and persists for years. More often, chronicity becomes apparent during the second or third attack. Persistent inflammation in a peripheral joint may lead to deformities, flexion contractures, and extensive erosive changes. At times, marked destructive changes occur, particularly in the small joints of the hands and feet. Bony ankylosis is uncommon, but has been reported. Spinal involvement has been noted by many observers over the past 40 years. In one report, 8 of 26 patients, fol-

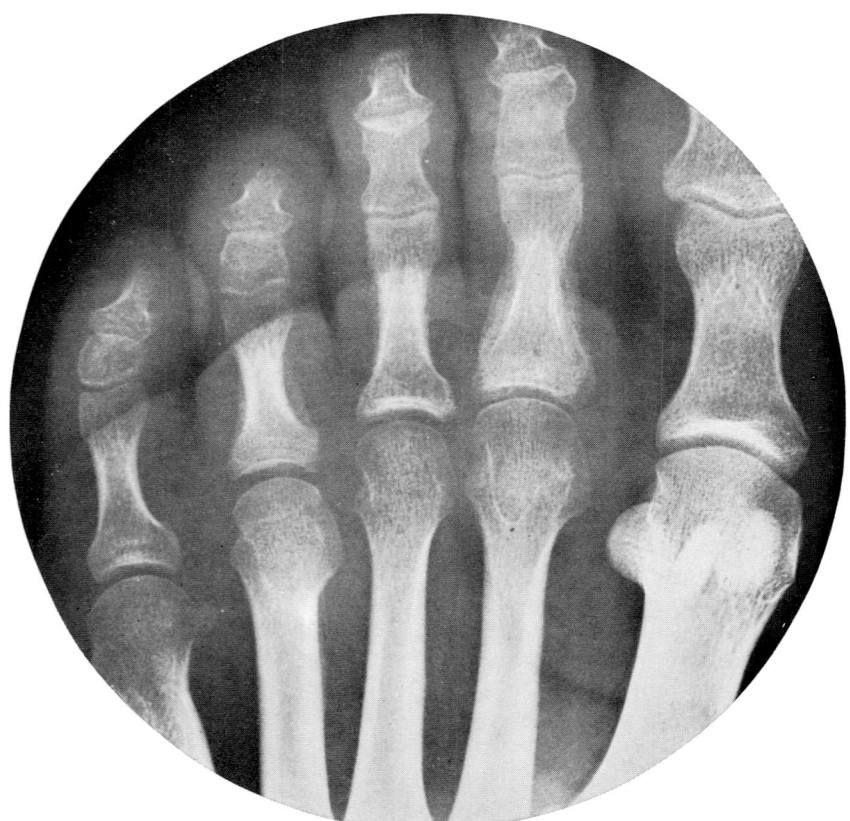

Fig. 54–4. Radiograph of the left foot of a patient with Reiter's syndrome who had complained of pain and swelling of the foot for the preceding 7 months. Periosteal new bone is visible in the shafts of the second, third, and fourth proximal phalanges and also on the medial aspect of the distal part of the shaft of the fourth metatarsal bone.

lowed for a mean of 14.5 years, had spondylitis.[12] Chronic back pain is common, and progressive limitation of spinal movement is observed in many patients. Radiographic abnormalities include syndesmophytes, extensive ankylosis of the apophyseal joints, paravertebral calcification, and dense bony bridging of vertebrae. In general, patients differ from those with classic ankylosing spondylitis by having shorter segments of involvement with asymmetry and "skip pattern."

Radiologic changes in the sacroiliac joints are observed frequently, even among patients lacking clinical evidence of spinal disease. The frequency of such changes in the sacroiliac joints is related to the duration of follow-up and the number of recurrent attacks, and it varies from 8 to 47%.

Aortic insufficiency was first described in a patient with Reiter's syndrome in 1959 and has subsequently been reported on a number of occasions.[30] The pathologic features are similar to those observed in the aortic insufficiency in ankylosing spondylitis, but prominent giant cells in the inflammatory lesion of a heart valve in one patient with Reiter's syndrome have been reported.[22]

DIFFERENTIAL DIAGNOSIS

The diagnosis is straightforward in patients with nonbacterial arthritis following nongonococcal urethritis or bacterial dysentery. The diagnosis is strengthened by an asymmetric, pauciarticular pattern and is further reinforced when the characteristic extra-articular manifestations are present as outlined previously. The differential diagnosis may include gonococcal arthritis, psoriatic arthritis, ankylosing spondylitis, enteropathic arthritis, and seronegative RA. In the early stages of acute arthritis associated with urethritis, appropriate cultures must be done from the genitourinary tract and the joints to exclude gonococcal infection. Because gonococcal arthritis may be limited to the synovial membrane without invasion of the joint cavity, joint fluid cultures may be negative, and many patients must be treated with an appropriate antibiotic on a presumptive diagnosis. Most patients with gonococcal arthritis still respond promptly to penicillin, but penicillin-resistant organisms are now spreading, and occasional patients with gonococcal arthritis require treatment with a penicillinase-resistant antibiotic. The presence of typical vesicular-pustular skin lesions helps one to make the diagnosis of gonococcal arthritis, and the occurrence of lesions characteristic of keratoderma blenorrhagicum confirms a diagnosis of Reiter's syndrome.

Enteropathic arthritis is almost always associated with a chronic form of diarrhea and, at times, with skin lesions of erythema nodosum.

Pustular psoriasis may be indistinguishable from keratoderma blenorrhagicum, both clinically and histologically. It is a moot point whether differential diagnosis is possible or whether it offers any advantage to the patient in such instances. In the majority of patients with psoriatic arthritis, the skin lesions are distinguishable, and the arthritis is chronic, often involving those digits with prominent nail involvement. Urethritis and dysentery are not features of psoriatic arthropathy, but frequent involvement of the conjunctiva in psoriasis may lead to confusion between the two entities.

One must differentiate between ankylosing spondylitis and Reiter's syndrome only in patients with chronic involvement of the spine. In such instances, a prior history of peripheral arthritis with urethritis may suggest the diagnosis of Reiter's syndrome. If keratoderma has been present, the diagnosis is reinforced. Because eye lesions are common to both disorders, the presence of such lesions is not helpful in the differential diagnosis. X-ray films of the spine usually show more limited involvement and asymmetry in patients with Reiter's syndrome, but they are not diagnostic.

TREATMENT

No specific treatment exists for Reiter's syndrome. Salicylates usually provide some relief from discomfort and fever, but the benefit is often limited. Indomethacin, in doses of 100 to 150 mg daily, may help, but only a few patients become asymptomatic. In most cases, a regimen of indomethacin combined with limited weight bearing or complete bed rest for a brief period provides relief during the early, acute stage of the illness, and the disease subsides in 2 to 16 weeks.

Some physicians have used antimetabolic or cytotoxic drugs in patients with more prolonged or chronic episodes. Because most patients with Reiter's syndrome are young men and because over 90% of patients recover completely from the initial episode in a few months, these potentially lethal and mitogenic drugs are not recommended. In patients with severe and prolonged episodes of Reiter's syndrome who develop permanent changes, antimetabolic and cytotoxic drugs might be considered, provided such patients are fully informed of the potentially serious side effects of such treatment. Azathioprine, cyclophosphamide, methotrexate, and 6-mercaptopurine all appear to be capable of suppressing the manifestations of Reiter's syndrome in doses that are tolerable, but the margin of safety in their use is limited. Serious reactions, including death, may occur with any of these drugs. A double-blind, placebo-controlled, cross-over trial of azathioprine (1 to 2 mg/kg) in refractory

Reiter's syndrome has shown the unequivocal beneficial effects of this drug.[7a]*

Antibiotics are not recommended in the treatment of Reiter's syndrome.

REFERENCES

1. Ahvonen, P., Sievers, K., and Aho, K.: Arthritis associated with *Yersinia enterocolitica* infection. Acta Rheumatol. Scand., *15*:232–253, 1969.
2. Arnett, F.C., Hochberg, M.D., and Bias, W.B.: Cross-reactive HLA antigens in B-27 negative Reiter's syndrome and sacroiliitis. Johns Hopkins Med. J., *141*:193–197, 1977.
3. Blaser, M.J., et al.: Campylobacter enteritis: clinical and epidemiologic features. Ann. Intern. Med., *91*:179–185, 1979.
4. Bauer, W., and Engleman, E.P.: Syndrome of unknown etiology characterized by urethritis, conjunctivitis and arthritis (so-called Reiter's disease). Trans. Assoc. Am. Physicians, *57*:307–313, 1942.
5. Brewerton, D.A., et al.: Reiter's Disease and HLA 27. Lancet, 2:996–998, 1973.
6. Brodie, B.D.: Pathologic and Surgical Observations on Diseases of Joints. London, Longman, 1818.
7. Burbacher, C.R., and Weiland, H.H.: Gonorrheal arthritis. An analysis of 200 cases. J. Fla. Med. Assoc., *24*:433–435, 1938.
7a. Burns, T., Marks, S., and Calin, A.: A double-blind, placebo-controlled cross over trial of azathioprine in refractory Reiter's syndrome. Arthritis Rheum., *26*:539, 1983.
8. Butler, M.J., et al.: A follow-up study of 48 patients with Reiter's syndrome. Am. J. Med., *67*:808–810, 1979.
9. Culp, O.S.: Treatment of gonorrheal arthritis. J. Urol., *43*:737–765, 1940.
10. Fiessinger, N., and LeRoy, E.: Contribution to the study of an epidemic of dysentery in the Somme. Bull. Mem. Soc. Med. Hop. (Paris), *40*:2051–2052, 1916.
11. Fox, R., et al.: The chronicity of symptoms and disability in Reiter's syndrome. Ann. Intern. Med., *91*:190–193, 1979.
12. Good, A.E.: Involvement of the back in Reiter's syndrome. Ann. Intern. Med., *57*:44–59, 1962.
13. Hollander, J.L., et al.: Arthritis resembling Reiter's syndrome. Observation of 25 cases. JAMA, *129*:593–595, 1945.
14. Kinsella, T.D., Norton, W.L., and Ziff, M.: Complement-fixing antibodies to bedsonia organisms in Reiter's syndrome and ankylosing spondylitis. Ann. Rheum. Dis., *27*:241–244, 1968.
15. Kosunen, T.U.: Reactive arthritis after *Campylobacter je-*

16. Kulka, J.P.: The lesions of Reiter's syndrome. Arthritis Rheum., *5*:195–201, 1962.
17. Leirisalo, M., et al.: Followup study on patients with Reiter's disease and reactive arthritis, with special reference to HLA-B27. Arthritis Rheum., *25*:249–259, 1982.
18. Mark, D.B., and McCulley, J.B.: Reiter's keratitis. Arch. Ophthalmol., *100*:781–784, 1982.
19. Morris, R., et al.: HL-A W27—a clue to the diagnosis and pathogenesis of Reiter's syndrome. N. Engl. J. Med., *290*:554–556, 1974.
20. Noer, H.R.: Am "experimental" epidemic of Reiter's syndrome. JAMA, *198*:693–698, 1966.
21. Paronen, I.: Reiter's disease: a study of 344 cases observed in Finland. Acta Med. Scand., *(Suppl. 212) 131*:1–112, 1948.
22. Podell, T.E., et al.: Severe giant cell valvulitis in a patient with Reiter's syndrome. Arthritis Rheum., *25*:232–234, 1982.
23. Reiter, H.: Uber eine bisher unerkannte Spirochaeteninfektion (Spirochaetosis arthritica). Dtsch. Med. Wochenschr., *42*:1535–1536, 1916.
24. Sairanen, E., Paronen, I., and Mahonen, H.: Reiter's syndrome: a follow-up study. Acta Med. Scand., *185*:57–63, 1969.
25. Schachter, J., et al.: Isolation of bedsoniae from the joints of patients with Reiter's syndrome. Proc. Soc. Exp. Biol. Med., *122*:283–285, 1966.
26. Schultz, J.S., et al.: HLA profile and Reiter's syndrome. Clin. Genet., *19*:159–167, 1981.
27. Sharp, J.T., Lidsky, M.D., and Riley, W.A.: Clinical studies on gonococcal arthritis and Reiter's syndrome and measurement of gonococcal and bedsonia antibodies. Arthritis Rheum., *11*:569–578, 1968.
28. Simon, D.G., et al.: Reiter's syndrome following epidemic shigellosis. J. Rheumatol., *8*:969–973, 1981.
29. Solem, J.H., and Lassen, J.: Reiter's disease following Yersinia enterocolitica infection. Scand. J. Infect. Dis., *3*:83–85, 1971.
30. Toone, E.C., Jr., Pierce, E.L., and Hennigar, G.R.: Aortitis and aortic regurgitation associated with rheumatoid spondylitis. Am. J. Med., *26*:255–263, 1959.
31. Urman, J.D., Zurrier, R.B., and Rothfield, N.F.: Reiter's syndrome associated with *Campylobacter fetus* infection. (Letter.) Ann. Intern. Med., *86*:444–445, 1977.
32. van de Putte, L.G.A., et al.: Reactive arthritis after *Campylobacter jejuni* enteritis. J. Rheumatol., *7*:531–535, 1980.
33. Vilppula, A.H., et al.: Chlamydial isolations and serology in Reiter's syndrome. Scand. J. Rheumatol., *10*:181–185, 1981.
34. Vilppula, A.H., Yli-Kerttula, U.I., and Terho, P.E.: Reiter' syndrome in the population: an interview study. Scand. J. Rheumatol., *11*:150–154, 1982.
35. Weinberger, H.W., et al.: Reiter's syndrome, clinical and pathologic observations. A long term study of 16 cases. Medicine, *41*:35–91, 1962.
36. Wilkens, R.F., et al.: Reiter's syndrome. Evaluation of preliminary criteria for definite disease. Bull. Rheum. Dis., *32*:31–34, 1982.
37. Winblad, S.: Arthritis associated with *Yersinia enterocolitica* infections. Scand. J. Infect. Dis., 7:191–195, 1975.

*Editor's note: I have used this regimen in patients with refractory cases for over a decade with excellent results. Complete remission can usually be obtained, although the required duration of treatment is often 12 to 15 months.

juni enteritis in patients with HLA B-27. Lancet, *1*:1312–1313, 1980.

Chapter 55

Psoriatic Arthritis

Robert M. Bennett

The association of psoriasis with inflammatory polyarthritis is generally credited to Baron Jean Louis Alibert (1768–1837). Reference to a connection with arthritis is mentioned in Alibert's *Maladies de la peau* in a brief passage, "affections arthritiques or rheumatismales," which appears under the title of "Lepre squammeuse."[2] In an early review of the subject in 1904, Menzen cites several mid-nineteenth-century case reports of a relationship between psoriasis and arthritis and describes five additional cases seen personally.[129]

The term "psoriasis arthritique" was introduced by the French dermatologist Pierre Bazin in his book entitled *Leçons théoriques et cliniques sur les affections cutanées de nature arthritique et arthreux.*[13] The first really detailed description of the disease appears in the doctoral thesis of Charles Bourdillon, entitled *Psoriasis et arthropothies,* published in 1888.[22]

During this same period, the realization that rheumatoid arthritis (RA) was a distinct clinical entity was largely a result of Garrod's differentiation of gout from "rheumatic gout" in terms of systemic hyperuricemia.[75] For about 30 years, the idea of psoriatic arthritis as a separate disease entity, as opposed to the coincidental occurrence of RA and psoriasis, was not generally accepted. From the 1920s on, various authors revived the concept of psoriatic arthritis, mainly in the form of individual case reports,[89,93,187,221] but other observers were not impressed with the association.[107,122,131,164] It was not until the demonstration of rheumatoid factor, by Waaler in 1940 and Rose et al. in 1948,[167] in the serum of most patients with typical RA, that much nosologic progress was made. This finding made possible a division of inflammatory arthritis into two major groups: the seropositive and the seronegative arthritides. The realization that the majority of patients with psoriasis and arthritis were "seronegative" and with the introduction of criteria for the diagnosis of RA[151,165,166] were important steps in interpreting data derived from several large epidemiologic surveys of patients with psoriasis. The familial aggregation of psoriatic arthritis, in common with some of the other seronegative arthritides, is a major factor in establishing the disease as a separate entity.

EPIDEMIOLOGY

Epidemiologic studies have been important in substantiating a statistically significant relationship between psoriasis and arthritis (see also Chap. 2). The most rigorously defined study to date is that of Baker,[9] who also provided an excellent critical review of the preceding contributions. The results of Baker's study are shown in Table 55–1, along with data on the prevalence of polyarthritis in psoriasis[112] and the prevalence of RA in the general population.[111]

It is apparent that the prevalence of psoriasis in seropositive arthritis (1.23%) is similar to that in the general population (1.22%), whereas the occurrence of psoriasis in seronegative arthritis (20.2%) is roughly 10 times that of control subjects. Furthermore, the prevalence of both seronegative and seropositive polyarthritis in patients with psoriasis (6.8%) is nearly double that of RA in the general population (3.8%). This strong association of psoriasis and seronegative arthritis has been confirmed by other workers,[109,118,136,183,184,207,208] and seronegativity is now regarded as an important criterion in defining psoriatic arthritis. Despite this persuasive epidemiologic evidence for the concept of psoriatic arthritis as a separate entity, some still disagree,[33,37,52,59] on the grounds that psoriatic arthritis is merely RA with certain features modified by the presence of psoriasis.

Family studies have demonstrated further differences between psoriatic arthritis and RA.[56] Shelley and Arthur have commented that "the fact of inheritance remains the single unchallenged fact

Table 55–1. Prevalence Data

	%	Reference
Psoriasis in general population	1.2	8
Psoriasis in seronegative polyarthritis	20.2	8
Psoriasis in seropositive polyarthritis	1.2	8
Polyarthritis in psoriasis	6.8	112
Rheumatoid arthritis in general population	3.8	111
Psoriatic arthritis in general population	0.1	205*

*Estimated prevalence in United Kingdom

about the psoriatic."[178] Variability in psoriatic pedigrees is remarkable, however, and a multifactorial pattern of inheritance is now generally considered to be the most likely mode of transmission.[60,139,199]

Histocompatibility typing has revealed increased frequencies of HLA-BW17 and HLA-B13 and a decrease in HLA-B12 in both uncomplicated psoriasis and psoriatic arthritis.[171,203] HLA-B17 is a useful genetic marker for detecting a subgroup of psoriatic patients characterized by a high rate of affected relatives and a slightly earlier age of onset. More recently, the frequency of HLA-BW16 has been found to be increased in uncomplicated psoriasis,[100] as well as in psoriatic arthritis.[46] In psoriatic patients with sacroiliitis or spondylitis, the incidence of HLA-B13 is decreased,[107] whereas the incidence of HLA-B27 is much increased.[24,25,127,130] Of particular interest is the association of certain HLA antigens with peripheral joint involvement. HLA-BW38 and HLA-CW6 are associated with peripheral joint involvement.[57,76] Within the spectrum of psoriatic arthritis, patients with HLA-DR4 and HLA-B40 have a higher incidence of a presentation similar to that of RA.[76] HLA-BW38 and HLA-B7, on the other hand, have been associated with a polyarticular, asymmetric form of the disease.[76] HLA-B7, HLA-A3, HLA-DR2, and HLA-DR7 have been linked with a milder disease course.[76] It is apparent from these studies that, apart from the well-known association of HLA-B27 with psoriatic spondylitis, the other HLA associations are of only limited use in defining subsets of psoriatic arthritis and in predicting the disease's severity. The differing incidence of at least four genetic markers in relation to the varying expression of psoriasis, the associated arthritis, and the presence of spondylitis are persuasive evidence for considering psoriatic arthritis as separate from RA.

The single most convincing study, to establish a definitive association between psoriasis and arthritis, was the report of Moll and Wright.[133] These workers studied 310 first- or second-degree relatives of 108 patients with peripheral psoriatic arthritis. Psoriasis alone was found in 21% of relatives, seronegative polyarthritis in 11%, sacroiliitis or spondylitis in 7.4%, and erosive polyarthritis in 1.8%. Compared to data from 83 spouses used as control subjects, these figures showed a statistically increased prevalence of disease, except for erosive polyarthritis, which had an incidence similar to that of RA in the general population. Using an index of familial aggregation, the value of the k factor*

for first-degree relatives was 48.8, as compared to 4.4 for spouses used as control subjects. These figures indicate an 80 to 90% chance of heritability in first-degree relatives of subjects with psoriatic arthritis.

PATHOLOGY

Psoriatic arthritis is characterized by an inflammatory synovitis macroscopically indistinguishable from RA.[206] Synovial biopsy and postmortem specimens show limited synovial cell proliferation and mononuclear cell infiltration similar to that seen in RA.[14,42,179] Fassbender found an excessive fibrous component in the articular soft tissues of patients with psoriasis,[63] and this finding has been noted by other workers.[42,179] In Gardner's experience, the only significant histologic difference between psoriatic arthritis and RA was the predilection to a more destructive arthropathy of the feet in psoriatic patients.[74] Immunofluorescent studies have demonstrated another similarity with RA, namely, the presence of rheumatoid factor in the synovium, albeit in smaller amounts than commonly encountered in a comparably inflamed rheumatoid synovium.[71] Psoriatic arthritis shows no characteristic histopathologic features; a similar picture is found in RA, enteropathic arthropathy, Reiter's disease, advanced joint lesions in systemic lupus erythematosus, and peripheral joint involvement in ankylosing spondylitis. Synovial biopsy may be of use in excluding diagnoses of arthritides of pyogenic, tuberculous, and traumatic origin, as well as pigmented villonodular synovitis.

ETIOLOGIC FACTORS

The importance of genetic factors in uncomplicated psoriasis, in peripheral psoriatic arthritis, and in psoriatic spondylitis has been discussed, but the "abnormal product" of this genetic background has not yet been characterized. Furthermore, the observed concordance of uncomplicated psoriasis in only 70% of monozygotic twin pairs[62] and the observed discordance of psoriatic arthropathy in monozygotic twins over 40 years[79] provide persuasive evidence that environmental factors also contribute to the disorder. Several interesting morphologic, biochemical, and, more recently, immunologic changes seen in uncomplicated psoriasis may have some bearing on the pathogenesis of the arthritis.

The concept of a generalized abnormality of capillaries in psoriatic skin, also expressed in the synovial membrane, may be relevant. Abnormal capillaries have been described in both affected and spared areas of skin in uncomplicated psoriasis.[169] These observations were extended to patients with psoriatic arthritis when meandering capillaries with

---

*The k factor indicates the prevalence of first-degree relatives divided by the expected prevalences in spouses used as control subjects.

tight terminal convolutions were noted in patients with psoriatic arthritis.[154] This feature was not noted in RA, scleroderma, morphea, systemic lupus erythematosus, or dermatomyositis. These changes appear to be a feature of psoriasis itself rather than of psoriatic arthritis, however.[219] Plethysmographic studies have shown that psoriatic patients have an enhanced response to reactive hyperemia in the small vessels of the phalanges that resembles the changes found in diabetes.[135] The relevance of this observation may be that acroosteolysis occurs in both diseases.[206]

Vascular changes consisting of prominent endothelial cells with a swollen appearance and a dilated rough endoplasmic reticulum have been recorded.[54] Inflammatory infiltrates, mainly lymphocytes and plasma cells, are generally perivascular. In contrast to RA, synovial hyperplasia is not a prominent feature (Figs. 55–1 and 55–2). These microvascular changes have stimulated a search for immunologic mechanisms that might mediate blood vessel damage. Circulating immune complexes have been noted in 29 to 58% of patients with either uncomplicated psoriasis or psoriatic arthritis,[26,96,110] but levels of these complexes are not elevated in patients with arthritis. Immunofluorescence studies have shown deposits of immunoglobulins and complement components in the blood vessels of both skin and synovium in patients with

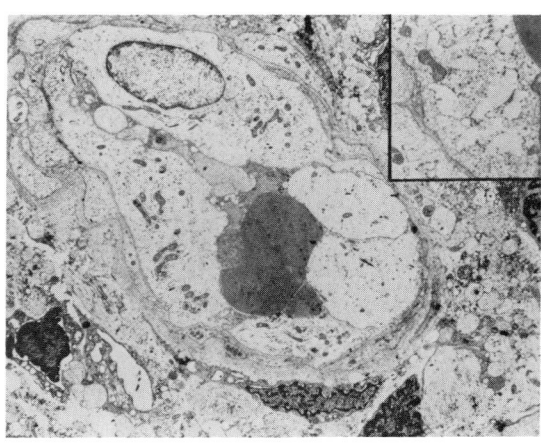

Fig. 55–2. Electron micrograph of synovial tissue taken from a patient with psoriatic arthritis (original magnification × 3,000). Dilation of the rough endoplasmic reticulum and marked swelling of the endothelial cells are visible. (From Espinoza, L.R., et al.[54])

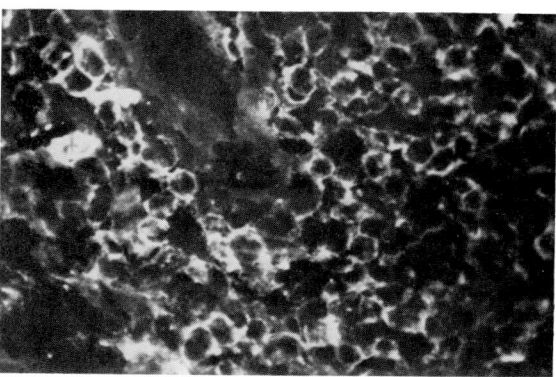

Fig. 55–3. Immunofluorescence staining with an anti-T-cell antiserum of synovial tissue from a patient with psoriatic arthritis. The majority of mononuclear cells are T-lymphocytes. (From Braathen, L.R., Fynard, O., and Mellbye, O.J.[23])

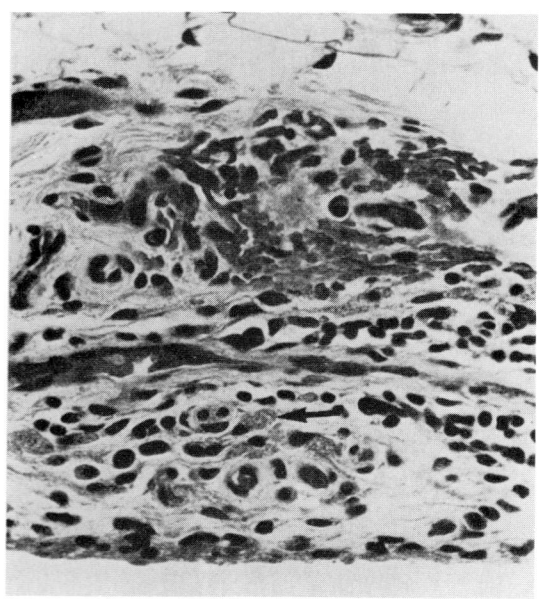

Fig. 55–1. Synovial biopsy from a patient with psoriatic arthritis (original magnification × 200). Limited synovial cell hyperplasia, increased vascularity, and mononuclear cell infiltration can be seen. (From Espinoza, L.R., et al.[54])

psoriasis and psoriatic arthritis,[72,192] and IgG-anti-IgG immune complexes have been eluted from the synovial membrane of patients with psoriatic arthritis.[138] Unlike in RA, however, in which such complexes fix complement and play an important role in joint inflammation, reduced levels of synovial fluid complement have not been observed in the effusions of psoriatic arthritis.[191] Recent work has failed to corroborate the presence of rheumatoid-factor-producing cells in the synovial tissue of patients with psoriatic arthritis.[65] The ratio of T to B cells in the synovial membrane of psoriatic arthritis has been examined, and T-cells predominate (Fig. 55–3), with a minority of cells staining for intra- and extracellular immunoglobulins.[23] Another apparent difference between psoriatic arthritis and RA is the demonstration of antibodies to native type II collagen in RA.[36]

No major abnormalities have been demonstrated in the peripheral blood lymphocytes of patients with psoriatic arthritis, although one study did show a statistically significant reduction in suppressor cell activity.[77] Another study showed a reduced response of peripheral blood lymphocytes to PHA, concanavalin A, and PWM, and clinical improvement was followed by an increased mitogen response.[55] The influence of therapy on these findings was not addressed.

Streptococcal infections are associated with flares of psoriasis, particularly guttate psoriasis in children.[40,60] Anti-DNase B antibodies, among several exotoxins produced by group A streptococci, were found in 51% of patients with psoriatic arthritis as compared to 10% of control subjects.[195] In a similar vein, increased reactivity to staphylococcal alpha-antitoxin was described in patients with psoriatic arthritis.[140] The speculation that bacterial cell wall peptidoglycans cause a reactive arthritis in some psoriatic patients has stimulated such studies.

Trauma localized to a joint can "trigger" osteolysis in psoriatic subjects. In one patient, generalized acro-osteolysis developed after needle puncture of one nail,[131] and similar associations have been reported by others.[19,206] Trauma may produce a "deep Koebner effect" on joint tissues.[206]

DIAGNOSIS

No single accepted definition of psoriatic arthritis exists, as emphasized by the wide variation of definitions[33] proposed over the years: (1) atrophic arthritis associated with psoriasis, having synchronous remissions and relapses of skin and joint changes;[93] (2) arthritis confined to the distal interphalangeal joints and associated with psoriasis;[14] (3) arthritis following long-standing, uncontrolled psoriasis;[89] (4) severely destructive arthritis associated with psoriasis;[38,64] (5) atypical arthritis accompanying atypical psoriasis;[47] and (6) psoriasis associated with erosive polyarthritis and usually a negative serologic test for rheumatoid factor.[213]

Most of these definitions describe certain distinguishing features of psoriatic arthritis, but a wider spectrum of disease is now appreciated, and such definitions are too restrictive and ignore the inflammatory aspect of the arthritis or the occurrence of sacroiliitis or spondylitis.

If other rheumatic diseases have been excluded, the presence of inflammatory arthritis in association with psoriasis is usually sufficient to diagnose psoriatic arthritis. Problems arise when the evidence of psoriasis is lacking or equivocal. The guidelines for the diagnosis of "borderline" psoriasis, as recommended by Baker,[9] are useful in such instances (Table 55–2). Errors may relate to seborrheic skin lesions and fungal infections of the nails. Nail pitting alone is nonspecific in differentiating between psoriasis and other diseases, such as exfoliative dermatitis and eczema. Isolated nail pitting is a normal occurrence. Twenty fingernail pits per person may suggest psoriasis, and more than 60 fingernail pits are rarely found in the absence of psoriasis.[52] Keratoderma blenorrhagicum of Reiter's syndrome is indistinguishable both clinically and histologically from pustular psoriasis; this skin lesion along with the nail changes encountered in Reiter's disease can lead to diagnostic confusion. Reiter's disease generally affects the joints of the lower limb, and the patient usually has an antecedent history of nonspecific urethritis or dysentery. A mild conjunctivitis can occur in psoriasis, but this finding is unreliable in differentiating Reiter's disease from psoriatic arthritis. Indeed attempts at differentiation may be pointless because some patients with well-defined Reiter's syndrome later develop psoriatic arthritis.[214]

Some cases of primary osteoarthritis of the hands, especially the erosive form, may be difficult to differentiate from psoriatic arthritis. The presence of bony thickening of the distal and proximal interphalangeal joints (Heberden's and Bouchard's nodes) and the involvement of the first carpometacarpal joint help to establish a diagnosis of osteoarthritis.

The onset of psoriatic arthritis may be acute, and when it involves a distal joint, gout is often suspected.[12,14,47] In such patients, joint aspiration for

Table 55–2. Criteria for Diagnosis of Borderline Psoriasis

1. Psoriasis of the scalp must be palpable.
2. Presumed scalp psoriasis, simulating dandruff, must exhibit normal skin between palques.
3. In the presence of eczema of seborrheic states, lesions other than classic psoriatic plaques cannot be accepted as psoriasis.
4. Toenail lesions alone cannot be accepted as evidence of psoriasis.
5. In the absence of psoriasis elsewhere, only the classic nail edge can be accepted as unequivocal psoriasis. In such patients, a diagnosis of infection should be excluded by microscopy and culture.
6. Flexural lesions can only be accepted if they have the classic appearance of a psoriatic plaque. In such cases, microscopy of scrapings should exclude diagnoses of tinea or *Candida* infection.
7. Pustular lesions of the palms and soles are not indicative of psoriasis unless accompanied by classic skin or nail lesions elsewhere.

detection of urate crystals is mandatory. Both gout and pseudogout may coincide with well-defined psoriatic arthritis.[113] A common anecdotal observation is a monoarticular form of psoriatic arthritis following trauma to a joint. If such a "traumatic" arthritis fails to resolve within the usual course of a few weeks, a diagnosis of psoriatic arthritis should be considered.

Distal joint involvement is not the usual finding in psoriatic arthritis; it occurs in only about 16% of patients.[160] By far the most common presentation is that of an inflammatory arthritis clinically similar to RA.[160] The persistent absence of rheumatoid factor and subcutaneous nodules and the presence of other features characteristic of psoriatic arthritis allow diagnosis (Table 55–3).

CLINICAL FEATURES

Age of Onset

In the United States, the mean age of onset of uncomplicated psoriasis was reported to be 28.7 years in men and 26.2 years in women.[61] In the Faroe Islands, with an apparently less favorable climate, the age of onset was 13 years for men and 12 years for women.[116] Psoriatic arthritis commonly occurs between 30 and 55 years of age,[11] a time of onset similar to that of RA.[181] In another study, the age of onset of psoriatic arthritis was 44 and 46 years for men and women, respectively.[113] In 3 recent studies, the age of onset in childhood was between 9 and 12 years.[102,180,184]

Sex Ratio

The ratio of males to females in psoriatic arthritis varies in different surveys. Moll and Wright pooled data from 10 different sources and computed a

Table 55–3. Clinical Characteristics Suggestive of Psoriatic Arthritis

1. Involvement of the distal interphalangeal joints in the absence of primary osteoarthritis.
2. Asymmetric arthritis.
3. The absence of rheumatoid factor and subcutaneous nodules.
4. The presence of a flexor tenosynovitis and "sausage" digits.
5. A family history of psoriatic arthritis.
6. The presence of significant nail pitting (>20 pits per person).
7. Axial radiographs showing one or more of the following: (1) sacroiliitis; (2) syndesmophytes (often "atypical"); and (3) paravertebral ossification.
8. Peripheral radiographs showing an erosive arthritis with a relative lack of osteopenia; in particular, erosions of the distal interphalangeal joints with expansion of the base of the terminal phalanx and terminal phalangeal osteolysis.

male-to-female ratio of 1:1.04,[134] contrasting sharply with the ratio of 1:3 found in RA (see also Chap. 2). The impression of male predominance in psoriatic arthritis[155] may reflect the increased frequency of distal phalangeal joint involvement in men.[205]

Patterns of Onset and Distribution

The classic view that the onset of arthritis coincides with the skin disease[93] has not been confirmed in subsequent studies.[11,197,207] A simultaneous onset is convincing evidence of a causal relationship, however. An isochronous onset is seen in about 10% of patients.[160] Wright has noted a close temporal relationship between distal interphalangeal joint involvement and psoriatic nail changes.[213] Although skin lesions usually precede arthritis, in 16% of patients, the arthritis appears first and can only be definitively diagnosed in retrospect. The view that psoriatic arthritis has a predilection for the distal interphalangeal joints should be revised.[14,148,179] Although predominant distal phalangeal joint involvement is important in differentiating psoriatic arthritis from RA, it only occurs in about 16% of cases,[160] and these joints are involved in about 25% of patients with RA.

It is now apparent from several broad clinical surveys that psoriatic arthritis has a wide spectrum of presentations, ranging from mild monoarticular involvement to rapidly destructive arthritis mutilans.[35,160,210,211] Five clinical patterns of psoriatic arthritis have been described, as follows:[206]

Group 1—"Classic" Psoriatic Arthritis

This uncommon form of the disease is characterized by predominant involvement of distal interphalangeal joints and nail lesions. Moll and Wright gave a figure of 5% in 1973.[134] This figure has been revised to 16.6% more recently.[160]

Group 2—Arthritis Mutilans

This form of psoriatic arthritis is due to osteolysis of the phalanges and the metacarpal joints (Fig. 55–4). Also called "doigt en lorgnette" or opera glass, this condition occurs in about 5% of patients and is often associated with sacroiliitis.

Group 3—Symmetric Polyarthritis

This form is similar to RA and is noted in about 15% of patients (Fig. 55–5). In long-standing cases, the predilection for bony ankylosis of the proximal and distal interphalangeal joints results in a poorly functional hand with a claw-like deformity (Fig. 55–6). In a recent long-term follow-up study of 131 such patients, 26% were seropositive at some time or other, 16% were consistently positive, and 10% fluctuated between positive and

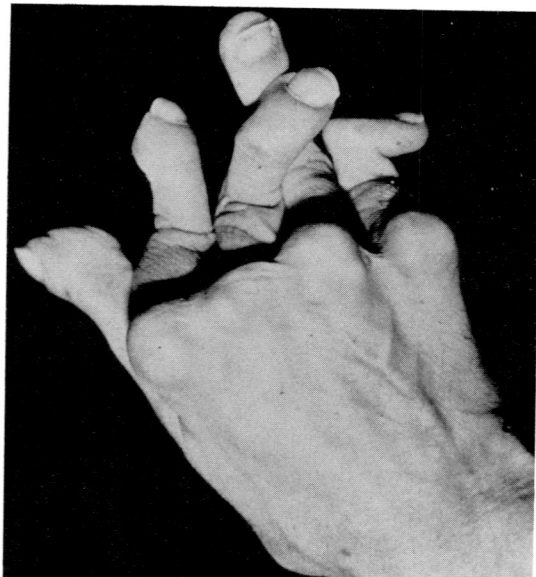

Fig. 55–4. Severe resorptive arthropathy resulting in arthritis mutilans. (From the ARA slide collection; with permission.)

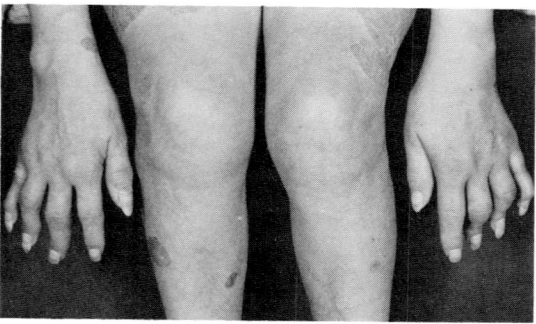

Fig. 55–5. Symmetric polyarthritis resembling rheumatoid arthritis in a patient with psoriasis.

negative.[160] It was concluded that the majority of these patients had true psoriatic arthritis.

Group 4—Oligoarticular Arthritis

This form is characteristically asymmetric in distribution, usually affecting scattered distal interphalangeal, proximal interphalangeal, and metatarsophalangeal joints. In some instances, involvement of a metacarpophalangeal or proximal interphalangeal joint is associated with a flexor tenosynovitis, giving the sausage-digit appearance (Fig. 55–7). This form of psoriatic arthritis is the most common and accounts for about 70% of all cases.

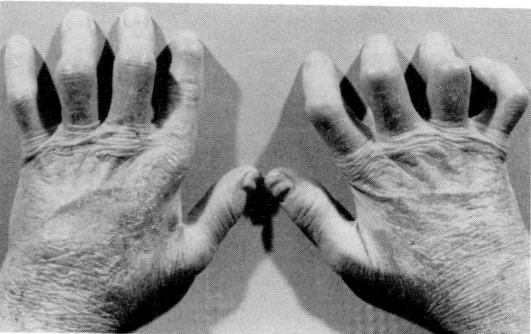

Fig. 55–6. Long-standing psoriatic arthritis of symmetric distribution. This patient has a "claw deformity" due to bony ankylosis of the proximal and distal interphalangeal joints.

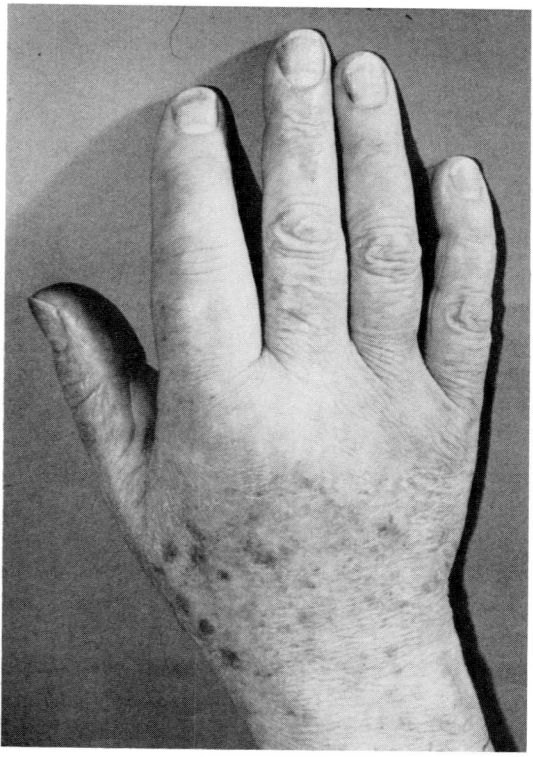

Fig. 55–7. Psoriatic arthritis involving the metacarpophalangeal and proximal interphalangeal joints of an index finger with an associated flexor tenosynovitis. This combination gives rise to the so-called "sausage digit."

Group 5—Ankylosing Spondylitis

Spinal joints may be involved with psoriatic arthritis.[47,156] The onset of psoriatic arthritis may be associated with a constitutional disturbance, malaise, and occasionally pyrexia.[160] It may be gout-like,[12,47,160,179] even involving the big toe initially.

In a few patients, a raised serum uric acid level and a favorable response to colchicine administration further complicate the diagnosis.[90] One study has indicated a higher association of gout and psoriatic arthritis than can be expected by chance alone,[222] and evidence suggests that the serum uric acid level is often elevated in psoriatic patients, especially in those with extensive skin disease.[16,78,113,190] One study has disputed the occurrence of hyperuricemia and has suggested that it may be due to the effect of concomitant drug therapy on urate excretion.[105]

Clinical Manifestations

Skin Findings

No evidence suggests that any particular pattern of dermal involvement is associated either with peripheral psoriatic arthritis or with spondylitis.[219] All patterns and gradations of severity of arthritis have been observed, ranging from patients with minimal psoriatic lesions to those with generalized exfoliative psoriasis. In patients with a seronegative arthritis compatible with psoriatic arthritis or with a positive family history, the clue to the diagnosis may lie in finding psoriatic lesions in one of the so-called "hidden" areas: scalp, perineum, natal cleft, or umbilicus. In attempting to make a diagnosis of minimal psoriasis, it is useful to bear in mind the criteria established by Baker[9] (see Table 55–2).

Nail Changes

A characteristic association between arthritis in the distal interphalangeal joints and psoriatic involvement of the adjacent nails is generally accepted[14,47,89,179] (Fig. 55–8). Wright reported an incidence of nail dystrophy of 80% among patients with psoriatic arthritis, as compared to an incidence of 20% among patients with uncomplicated psoriasis.[210] Baker found nail involvement in 83% of patients with psoriatic arthritis and noted that the changes were not necessarily related to the distribution of the joint involvement and patients with deforming arthritis had more extensive nail involvement.[10] Nail changes in psoriasis are summarized in Table 55–4. Lewin et al. more recently described the histopathologic features of these changes.[115] None of these nail changes are specific for psoriasis; other conditions to be considered are fungal and bacterial infections, dermatitis, alopecia areata, lichen planus, and trauma.

The most common differential diagnostic problem is fungal infection, which is usually caused by either *Trichophyton rubrum* or *T. mentagrophytes*. Although organisms can often be isolated from psoriatic nails, these are frequently found to be commensals,[218] possibly as a result of a glycoprotein

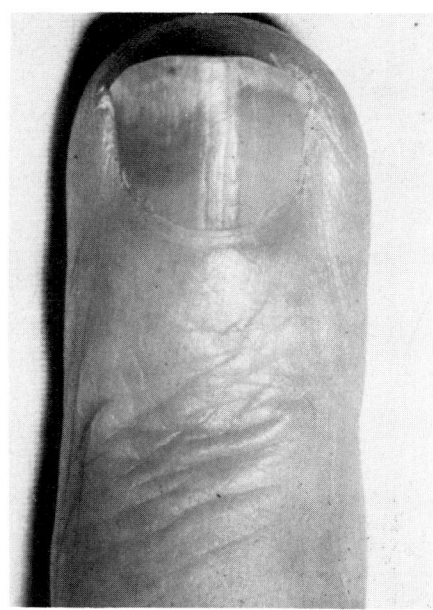

Fig. 55–8. Onycholysis in addition to psoriasis of the nail bed in a patient with an oligoarticular pattern of psoriatic arthritis.

dermatophyte inhibitor in psoriatic patients.[194] Up to 70% of normal subjects may show some nail pitting.[206] This phenomenon increases with age, and the pits, which are less densely distributed in normal subjects than in patients with psoriasis, are shallower and more irregular in outline.

Ankylosing Spondylitis

An association between psoriasis and ankylosing spondylitis was noted at a much later date than its association with peripheral arthritis.[47,58,201] In the 1950s, the concept of psoriatic spondylitis as a separate disease gained favor.[42,80,179,197,212] This concept has been strengthened by epidemiologic studies that show an increased incidence of ankylosing spondylitis and sacroiliitis in patients with psoriasis.[27,80,91,132,210] Further evidence of psoriatic spondylitis is found in some of its clinical and radiologic differences from classic ankylosing spondylitis. Jajic remarked on the distinct lack of back pain and stiffness, as well as a poor correlation between clinical and radiologic findings.[91] Distinctive radiologic features have been observed in some patients with psoriasis and spondylitis. The most impressive "atypical" radiologic appearance is paravertebral ossification;[29,31,189] other findings include vertebral fusion with disc calcification[108] and nonmarginal syndesmophytes.[58] The prevalence of these atypical features in a representative population of patients with psoriatic arthritis remains to

Table 55–4. Nail Changes in Psoriasis

Clinical Lesion	Original of Lesion
Nail	
Pitting	Psoriasis of proximal matrix
Transverse ridges	Psoriasis of proximal and medial matrix
Leukonychia	Psoriasis of proximal and medial matrix
Crumbling	Psoriasis of entire matrix
Nail Bed	
Splinter hemorrhages	Hemorrhages in nail bed
Large red patches	Psoriasis of nail bed
Horny mass	Long-standing psoriasis of nail bed
Hyponychium	
Subungual keratosis	Psoriasis of hyponychium
Discoloration of subungual debris	Colonization by yeasts or pseudomonas
Onycholysis	Air under separated nail plate

be determined. Paraspinal ossification, not unique to psoriasis, is also associated with senile ankylosing hyperostosis,[69] paraplegia,[1] fluorosis, hypoparathyroidism,[172] familial hypophosphatemia,[97] and heredofamilial articular and vascular calcification.[177] Nonmarginal syndesmophytes have also been observed in association with Reiter's disease.[120]

In a review of 130 patients with psoriatic arthritis,[104] spondylitis was noted in 40%. Only 21% had sacroiliitis, however, whereas 25% had radiologically evident syndesmophytes: 60% of this latter group had radiologically normal sacroiliac joints and were no more likely to have symptoms or signs of spinal disease than those with normal spinal radiographs. Patients with axial involvement are usually males (M:F ratio 6:1) who develop psoriasis later in life; the mean age of onset is 35 years, versus 27 years for all psoriatic patients.

Ocular Inflammation

Eye inflammation, a common accompaniment of the seronegative arthritides, is a feature of Reiter's disease,[44] ankylosing spondylitis,[21] Behçet's disease,[125] enteropathic arthropathy,[215] enteropathic arthropathy,[215] and Whipple's disease. Until the study of Lambert and Wright,[106] only passing references were made to eye involvement in psoriatic arthritis.[88,89] These investigators studied 112 patients with psoriatic arthritis and found an overall incidence of eye involvement in 31.2%. The diagnostic categories were conjunctivitis, 19.6%; iritis, 7.1%; episcleritis, 1.8% and keratoconjunctivitis sicca, 2.7%. Of the patients with iritis, 43% had sacroiliitis, and of those tested, 40% were positive for HLA-B27. Tests for antinuclear factor were negative in all patients with iritis. These findings are similar to those in juvenile rheumatoid arthritis, in which positive antinuclear factors are associated with chronic iritis, whereas negative tests are as-

sociated with acute iritis and a tendency to ankylosing spondylitis.[173]

Disease Interrelationships

The seronegative arthritides often have certain common features, the most frequently reported being sacroiliitis or spondylitis, ocular inflammation, and the presence of HLA-B27. Because HLA-B27 is associated with an inheritied susceptibility to both sacroiliitis[25,33] and iritis,[24] these common features seem to indicate a shared genetic background rather than specific "complications." Psoriatic arthritis has been described in association with all the seronegative arthritides, except Whipple's disease. The associated conditions are ulcerative colitis,[92,132,170] ankylosing spondylitis,[31,68,80,91,117,132,157,214] Crohn's disease,[4,70,87] Reiter's disease,[49,50,58,80,86,126,145,214] and Behçet syndrome.[124,125] Crystal-induced arthritis may be associated also.[196] Sometimes, the familial clustering of these diseases is striking, as shown in Figure 55–9. In this family, psoriasis, ulcerative colitis, and ankylosing spondylitis were grouped together in two generations.[18]

Other Features

A number of other interesting clinical associations have been reported in patients with psoriatic arthritis. Because these findings are, for the most part, isolated case reports, the associations cannot be regarded as true complications without further comprehensive studies. Such associated features include myopathy,[153] Sjögren' syndrome,[202] aortic incompetence,[37,137,156] gastrointestinal amyloidosis,[67,150,204] and fever.[164]

LABORATORY FINDINGS

No available blood tests diagnose psoriasis or psoriatic arthritis. The most important finding is an absence of rheumatoid factor, including "hidden"

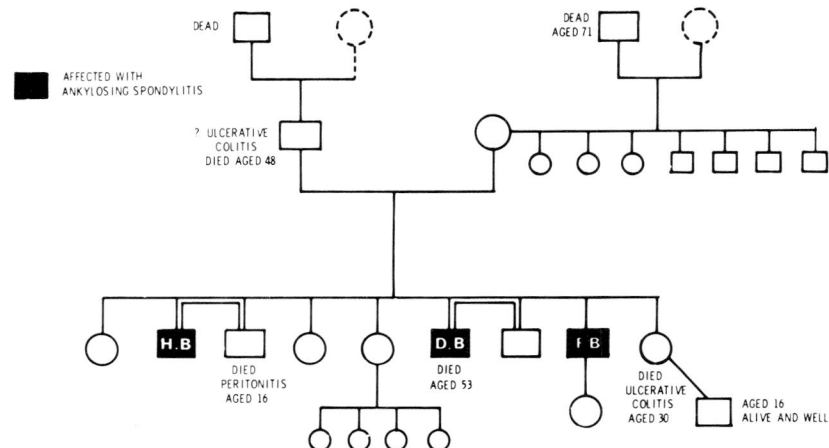

Fig. 55–9. Family study in which psoriasis, ulcerative colitis, and ankylosing spondylitis show a "clustering" phenomenon. Patients DB and FB had psoriasis in addition to ankylosing spondylitis.

rheumatoid factors.[43] A positive rheumatoid factor in a typical patient with psoriatic arthritis probably represents an association with the known occurrence of seropositivity in as many as 5% of the general population.[198] Positive tests in psoriatic patients with features of RA usually reflect the concurrent association of two common diseases, psoriasis and RA.

Nonspecific findings include an elevated acute-phase reactant level (fibrinogen, alpha-1-antitrypsin, the ninth component of complement, and C-reactive protein), a high sedimentation rate, anemia, and a transient leukocytosis.[11,110]

Hyperuricemia is found in 10 to 20% of patients,[11] and it appears to be related to the severity of the skin disease,[16,78,190] reflecting an increased purine metabolism due to a rapid turnover of epidermal cells.[53,193] Some workers, however, suggest that elevated uric acid levels may be due to concomitant drug therapy.[105] Other laboratory findings include elevated IgA levels in two-thirds of patients with psoriatic arthritis and in one-third with psoriasis;[45] decreased IgM levels in mild psoriatic arthritis and elevated levels in more severe disease;[146] elevated gamma and alpha-2-globulin levels;[161] normal erythrocyte phosphoglucose isomerase activity;[73] and an absence of antinuclear factors.[121,185] Circulating immune complexes have been described in up to 50% of patients with both psoriasis and psoriatic arthritis.[26,96,110] Other workers have not found any specific immunoglobulin disturbance in psoriatic arthritis[216] or any correlation between disease activity and the degree of plasma protein alteration.[11] An increased adherence of granulocytes to nylon fiber columns has been noted in both psoriasis and psoriatic arthritis,[174] but the relevance of this observation is unclear.

Synovial fluid is usually of an inflammatory type, but has been reported to have normal or elevated complement components.[99,191] This finding may be useful in distinguishing psoriatic arthritis from both seropositive and seronegative RA.

An association of psoriatic arthritis and psoriatic spondylitis with HLA antigens has already been mentioned. The work of Lambert et al. indicates a normal prevalence of HLA-B27 in patients with only peripheral arthritis.[107] All forms of axial involvement, including syndesmophytes without associated sacroiliitis, are associated with an increased incidence of HLA-B27. In HLA-B27-negative patients, females preponderate (M:F ratio is .06:1), the peripheral joint disease is more severe, and skin involvement is greater.

RADIOGRAPHIC FINDINGS

Radiographic findings in psoriatic arthritis have been important in delineating it as a separate disease[6,67,147,210] (see also Figs. 5–55 to 5–59). In the majority of patients, the findings are similar to those of RA, but with an asymmetric, oligoarticular distribution. Some less common findings in both the peripheral and the axial skeleton are more specific for psoriatic arthritis and spondylitis, however.

Findings in the peripheral joints include the following: (1) erosion of terminal phalangeal tufts (acro-osteolysis)[28] (Fig. 55–10); (2) "whittling" of phalanges and of metacarpal and metatarsal joints; (3) "cupping" of the proximal portion of the phalanges; when combined with "whittling," this condition is often referred to as the "pencil-in-cup" deformity (Fig. 55–11); (4) bony ankylosis (Fig. 55–12); (5) destruction of isolated small joints (Fig. 55–13); (6) predilection for distal and proximal interphalangeal joints, with relative sparing of metacarpophalangeal and metatarsophalangeal joints; (7) osteolysis of bones (arthritis mutilans), particularly the metatarsals (Fig. 55–14); in the hands, this osteolysis can give rise to the "opera glass" effect; and (8) a relative lack of osteoporosis, in comparison to the degree of joint involvement.

Findings in the axial skeleton include the following: (1) paravertebral ossification,[29,31,189] (2) atypical syndesmophytes, often present without sacroiliitis[58,104] (Fig. 55–15); (3) asymmetric sacroiliitis;[91,104] (4) solid fusion of thoracic vertebrae;[104] (5) rarity of the typical "bamboo" spine of ankylosing spondylitis;[104,220] (6) a tendency for cervical spinal disease to exhibit intervertebral disc-space narrowing, apophyseal sclerosis, and in-

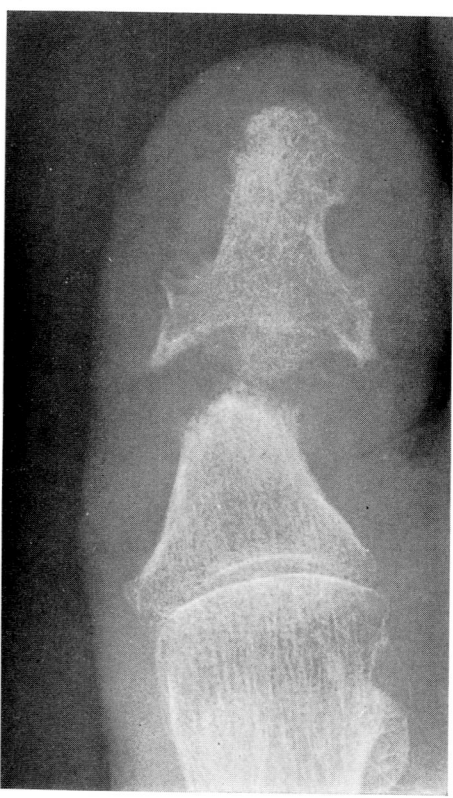

Fig. 55–11. "Whittling" of the middle phalanx and expansion of the base of the distal phalanx—the "pencil-in-cup" deformity.

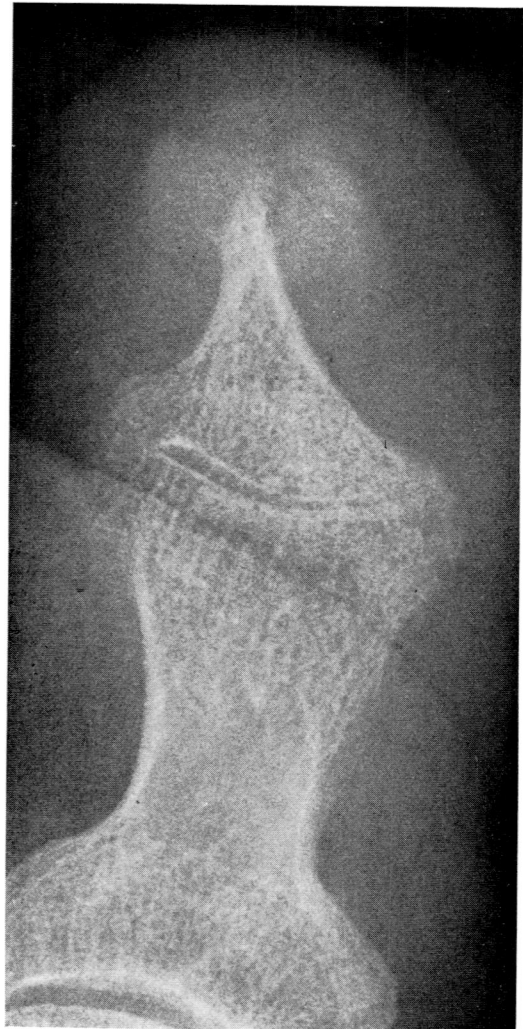

Fig. 55–10. Psoriatic arthritis with acro-osteolysis of the terminal phalanx of the great toe.

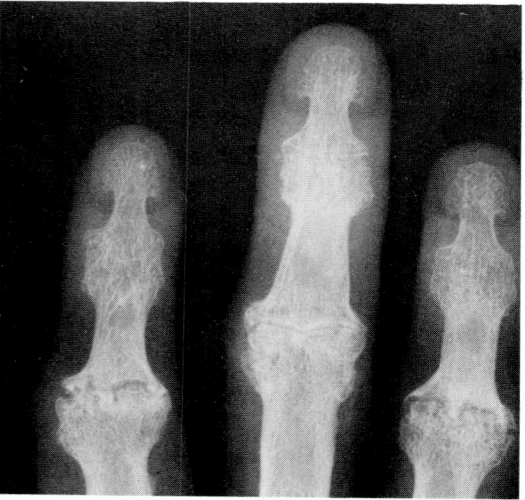

Fig. 55–12. Bony ankylosis of the distal interphalangeal joints in a patient with psoriatic arthritis.

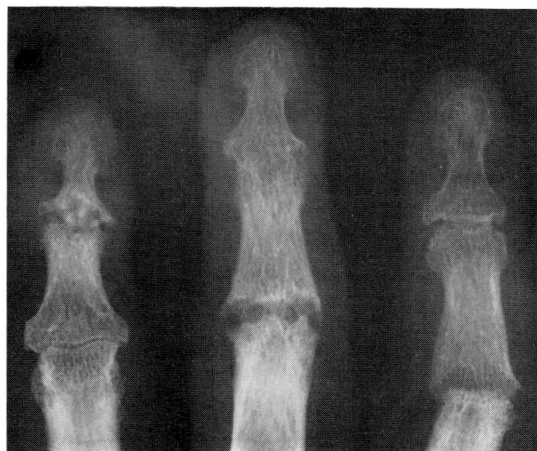

Fig. 55–13. Complete destruction of middle proximal interphalangeal joint; also note bony ankylosis of the corresponding distal interphalangeal joint.

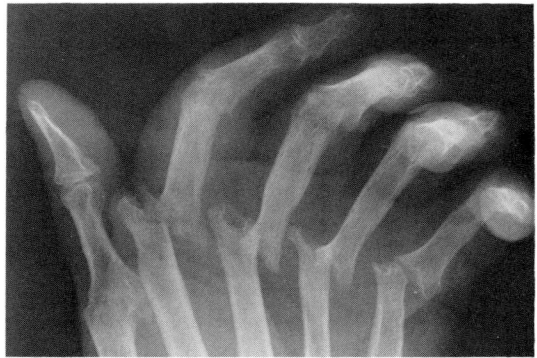

Fig. 55–14. Osteolysis of the bones of the metacarpophalangeal joints with resulting subluxations.

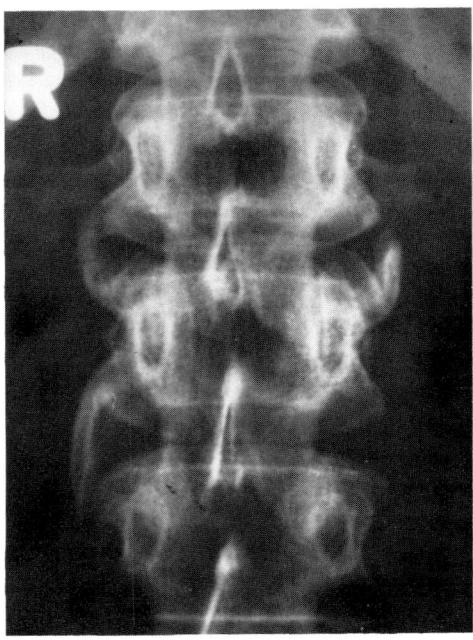

Fig. 55–15. Psoriatic arthritis with spinal involvement. The patient is HLA-B27 positive; syndesmophytes are present, but no evidence of sacroiliitis is seen.

terspinous or anterior ligamentous calcification[95,104] (Fig. 55–16).

JUVENILE PSORIATIC ARTHRITIS

Three recent studies have helped to delineate psoriatic arthritis as a further facet of the juvenile rheumatoid arthritis (JRA) syndrome.[102,180,184] Unlike in the adult form of the disease, a female predominance of about 3:2 is seen. The mean age of onset of both the psoriasis and the arthritis is 8 to 9 years, and in about 50% of patients, the arthritis antedates the skin changes. The mode of onset of the arthritis and its progression differ from the adult variety in that the onset is usually acute and is monoarticular in about one-third of cases. In contrast to the usual course of pauciarticular JCA, however, most patients develop arthritis in 5 or more additional joints, usually in an asymmetric pattern. Another feature at variance with adult psoriatic arthritis is hip involvement in 30 to 40% of cases; 6 patients in one series required bilateral hip arthroplasties.[180] A ''sausage'' digit, caused by flexor tenosynovitis with arthritis in contiguous joints, is the presenting feature in about 12% of patients and occurs in 23% of all patients at some stage of the disease. The pattern of skin and nail involvement is similar to that seen in adults.

As in the adult form of the disease, extra-articular manifestations are rare. The development of iridocyclitis (8% of Shore and Ansell's patients[180]). may cause confusion with pauciarticular JRA, especially because 17% of these patients, mostly girls, have positive test results for antinuclear antibodies. The presence of these antibodies was associated with an earlier onset of arthritis (mean of 4 years) and a poorer prognosis.[180] The course of the arthritis was benign in one series, and nonsteroidal anti-inflammatory agents provided adequate control.[184] None needed remittive agents. In contrast, a second series of patients had more severe disease; 35% required systemic corticosteroids at some point, and nearly 25% needed one or more slow-acting remittive drugs.

PROGNOSIS

The disease is usually mild, with an episodic course affecting only a few joints. If the arthritis

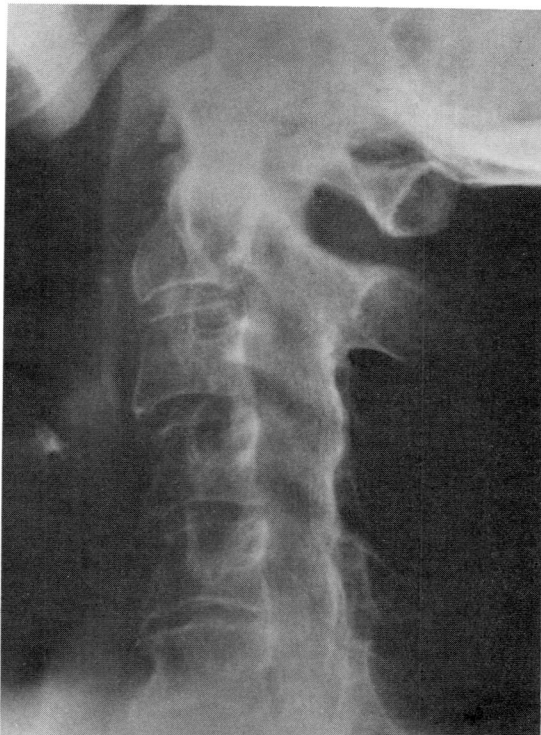

Fig. 55–16. Ankylosis of cervical apophyseal joints in patient with psoriatic spondylitis in association with bilateral sacroiliitis.

remains confined to small joints for a long period, the prognosis is favorable.[197] In a long-term study of 227 patients, only 5% developed a deforming arthritis, and 97% had lost less than a year of work throughout the entire period of their arthritis.[105] The arthritis or its treatment may have been a contributing factor in 3 of 18 fatal cases. One death from gastric hemorrhage could have been due to cytotoxic therapy, and 2 from bronchopneumonia were thought to be related to immobility. An earlier study reported 24 deaths; corticosteroids were implicated in 14, aminopterin in 1, and amyloidosis in another.[157] Death due to psoriasis itself is rare, but it has been reported as a complication of exfoliative dermatitis or amyloidosis. Rarely, patients with associated spondylitis may develop aortic incompetence or atrioventricular conduction defects.

In general, a correlation exists between the severity of the skin disease and the severity of the arthritis,[113] although in individual patients, such may not be true. Patients with psoriatic arthritis of juvenile onset appear to have a worse prognosis than adult-onset patients.[180] in particular, those with iridocyclitis or a positive test for antinuclear antibodies are predisposed to a potentially destructive form of arthritis.

MANAGEMENT

Psoriasis itself is a "socially difficult" affliction, and the prospect of disability from arthritis makes it even less tolerable. It is therefore important to explain the nature of the disease to the patient and to stress its benign course in the majority of cases and its lack of serious systemic complications, as compared to RA.

Mild Disease

The general principles of appropriate rest, splinting, range-of-motion exercises, joint protection, education, and use of adaptive devices, should be applied in these patients as in those with RA.[209] Many obtain satisfactory symptomatic control with high-dose aspirin therapy or another nonsteroidal anti-inflammatory agent (see Chap. 28). In patients with only a few involved joints, the local injection of corticosteroids into joints or tendon sheaths is an important therapeutic technique. In general, the relatively insoluble preparations such as triamcinolone hexacetonide (Aristospan), dexamethasone acetate (Decadron LA), and betamethasone acetate-phosphate (Celestone soluspan) are preferred because systemic absorption is minimal and the local effect is prolonged (see Chap. 34). A contraindication to local corticosteroid therapy may be the presence of psoriatic lesions around the joint. Pyogenic arthritis of an ankle following intra-articular injection through a psoriatic plaque has been reported.[206]

Severe or Potentially Severe Disease

A few patients, probably about 5%,[160] develop a severe, potentially crippling form of arthritis; physicians in referral centers, of course, see many of the more severe examples of psoriatic arthritis. For these patients, one must consider administering drugs that may alter the course of the disease.

Because of the relationship between the severity of the skin involvement and the severity of the arthritis, it seems logical to treat the skin lesions. Photochemotherapy using oral 8-methoxypsoralens, followed 2 hours later by long-wave ultraviolet-A light (PUVA) is successful in treating psoriasis.[128,143] Photochemotherapy may also benefit the patient's associated arthritis.[144] In this study, 27 patients with psoriatic arthritis received photochemotherapy for psoriasis and 86% achieved skin clearing. Eleven patients with peripheral joint involvement experienced a 50% improvement in articular index during the 6 months after skin clearing. In those patients with concomitant spondylitis, however, the peripheral arthritis was not generally improved. It seems reasonable to consider photo-chemotherapy in patients with serious disease.

Antimalarial agents have generally been contraindicated in the treatment of psoriatic arthritis because of possible exacerbation of the skin disease and even exfoliative dermatitis.[40,41,118,155,160] A recent, uncontrolled study, however, indicated that 72% of patients with psoriatic arthritis improved or their condition stabilized while taking hydroxychloroquine, 200 to 400 mg/day.[94] In this study, antimalarial therapy did not aggravate existing psoriasis or precipitate exfoliation.

Chrysotherapy, which had also been linked anecdotally with an exacerbation of skin lesions,[81,152] was thought to be more toxic in psoriatic arthritis than in RA.[163,183] Again, recent studies have shown that chrysotherapy is effective in psoriatic arthritis and is not accompanied by a worsening of the skin condition.[48,94,159,210] One report actually indicated a higher remission rate in psoriatic arthritis than in RA (remissions 71.4 and 59.5%, respectively), and less severe toxicity in patients with psoriasis.[48]

Caution in the use of systemic corticosteroids is urged because even when tapering low doses, the skin disease may be exacerbated, and ever-increasing doses are often required to exert a beneficial effect.

Penicillamine has been used occasionally in the treatment of psoriatic arthritis,[94,180] but not enough recorded experience exists with this drug to provide guidelines for indications or usefulness. Levamisole was used in 6 patients with psoriatic arthritis without improvement.[168]

Most now agree that cytotoxic drugs are of benefit and are indicated in recalcitrant cases of psoriatic arthritis. In a double-blind study of 21 patients, methotrexate was effective in suppressing both the skin and joint manifestations, but the incidence of side effects was 30%.[20] Other small trials have shown a beneficial response to methotrexate.[5,30,35,66,84,98] Liver damage, a potential problem with methotrexate,[3,39,149,176] occurs most often when the drug is given daily. An intermittent-dose regimen of 7.5 to 20 mg/week appears to be safer.[7] Methotrexate is ill advised in patients with pre-existing liver disease or alcoholism. No specific guidelines exist for monitoring the development of hepatotoxicity; liver function tests do not reliably predict adverse morphologic changes, as seen on biopsy.[200] It is the practice of most *dermatologists* to request a liver biopsy before initiating therapy, with biopsies repeated once or twice a year; this regimen has not been generally adopted by rheumatologists. Evidence suggests, however, that a liver biopsy is advisable in patients who have had a cumulative dose of methotrexate of 1.5 g and above.[162] Nonetheless, the progression of hepatic

fatty and cellular changes to frank cirrhosis is rare in patients treated with methotrexate.[217] Generalized adverse reactions to methotrexate include bone-marrow suppression, hemorrhagic enterocolitis, ulcerative stomatitis, alopecia, dermatitis, and hypersensitivity pneumonitis. Acute gouty arthritis has occurred within 24 hours of the administration of intravenous methotrexate.[123]

Intra-articular methotrexate (10 mg/knee) has a short-term beneficial effect in psoriatic arthritis, but not in RA.[85] It is unlikely, however, that such therapy has an advantage over the intra-articular injection of microcrystalline corticosteroid preparations. The intra-articular injection of radioactive colloids has generally been less effective than in RA,[188] as well as less effective than the injection of long-acting corticosteroids.[83]

Other cytotoxic agents used with varying success are as follows: aminopterin;[82,158] azathioprine;[51,66,114] and cyclophosphamide and triacetyl azauridine[32] (no longer available). Good results using 6-mercaptopurine in low doses 0.36 to 2.4 mg/kg/day have been reported in 13 patients;[15] the improvement is seen within 3 weeks, and the remission lasts as long as 10 months after cessation of treatment. Anecdotally, hydroxyurea, at a dose of 500 mg twice or 3 times a day, has ben used successfully by both Wright[205] and myself.

The indications for surgical intervention in psoriatic arthritis are similar to those in RA. Some surgeons are reluctant to operate on patients with psoriasis because of skin colonization with pathogenic bacteria[142] and the occasional anecdotal report of an infected prosthesis.[101] Although bacterial colonies are more numerous on psoriatic plaques, the standard preoperative skin preparations are as effective at sterilizing the psoriatic plaques as they are the uninvolved skin.[119] Another precautionary anecdotal note is the supposition that the tendency to ankylosis in psoriatic arthritis has an adverse effect on long-term surgical results.[42,179] These fears are ill founded; a recent report indicates that appropriate reconstructive surgical procedures should not be withheld from patients with psoriatic arthritis.[103] A review of hand surgery in psoriatic arthritis noted that the most useful procedures were arthroplasties of the metacarpophalangeal joints and fusion of fixed flexion contractures at the proximal and distal interphalangeal joints in positions of maximal function.[17]

REFERENCES

1. Abramson, D.J., and Kamberg, S.: Spondylitis, pathological ossification and calcification associated with spinal cord injury. J. Bone Joint Surg., *31A*:275–283, 1949.
2. Alibert, J.L.: Précis théorique et pratique sur les maladies de la peau. Paris, Caille et Ravier, 1818, p. 21.
3. Almeyda, J., et al.: Structural and functional abnormal-

ities of the liver in psoriasis before and during methotrexate therapy. Br. J. Dermatol., 87:623–631, 1972.
4. Ansell, B.M., and Wigley, R.A.D.: Arthritic manifestations in regional enteritis. Ann. Rheum. Dis., 23:64–72, 1964.
5. Auerbach, R., Orentreich, N., and Berger, R.: Diagnosis: psoriasis and psoriatic arthropathy treated with methotrexate administered intravenously. Arch. Dermatol., 90:115–116, 1964.
6. Avila, R., et al.: Psoriatic arthritis: a roentgenological study. Radiology, 75:691–702, 1960.
7. Baker, H.: Intermittent high dose oral methotrexate therapy in psoriasis. Br. J. Dermatol., 82:65–69, 1970.
8. Baker, H.: Epidemiological aspects of psoriasis and arthritis. Br. J. Dermatol., 78:249–261, 1966.
9. Baker, H.: The relationship between psoriasis, psoriatic arthritis and rheumatoid arthritis. An epidemiological, clinical and serological study. M.D. Thesis, University of Leeds, 1965.
10. Baker, H., Golding, N., and Thompson, M.: The nails in psoriatic arthritis. Br. J. Dermatol., 76:549–554, 1964.
11. Baker, H., Golding, N., and Thompson, M.: Psoriasis and arthritis. Ann. Intern. Med., 58:909–925, 1963.
12. Barber, H.W.: Psoriasis. Br. Med. J., 1:219–223, 1950.
13. Bazin, P.: Théoriques et cliniques sur les affections cutanées de nature arthritique et arthreux. (Monograph.) Paris, Delahaye, 1860, pp. 154–161.
14. Bauer, W., Bennett, G.A., and Zeller, J.W.: Pathology of joint lesions in patients with psoriasis and arthritis. Trans. Assoc. Am. Physicians, 56:349–352, 1941.
15. Baum, J., et al.: Treatment of psoriatic arthritis with 6-mercaptopurine. Arthritis Rheum., 16:139–147, 1973.
16. Baumann, R.R., and Jillson, D.F.: Hyperuricemia and psoriasis. J. Invest. Dermatol., 36:105–107, 1961.
17. Belsky, M.R., et al.: Hand involvement in psoriatic arthritis. J. Hand Surg., 7:203–207, 1982.
18. Bennett, R.M.: Familial spondylitis. Proc. R. Soc. Lond. (Biol.), 64:663–664, 1971.
19. Biernacki, R., Sadowska-Wroblewska, M., and Zabokrycki, J.: Acro-osteolysis in the course of ankylosing spondylitis. Rheumatologia, 6:163–168, 1968.
20. Black, R.L., et al.: Methotrexate therapy in psoriatic arthritis. JAMA, 189:743–747, 1964.
21. Blumberg, B., and Ragan, C.: The natural history of rheumatoid spondylitis. Medicine, 35:1–31, 1956.
22. Bourdillon, C.: Thèse de Paris, No. 298, 1888.
23. Braathen, L.R., Fynard, O., and Mellbye, O.J.: Predominance of cells with T-markers in the lymphocytic infiltrates of synovial tissue in psoriatic arthritis. Scand. J. Rheumatol., 8:75–80, 1979.
24. Brewerton, D.A., et al.: Ankylosing spondylitis and HL-A27. Lancet, 1:904–907, 1973.
25. Brewerton, D.A., Coffrey, M., and Nicholls, A.: HLA27 and the arthropathies associated with ulcerative colitis and psoriasis. Lancet, 1:956–958, 1974.
26. Braun-Falco, O., Manuel, C., and Sherer, P.: Demonstration of immune complexes of psoriatic patients using ^{125}I-C1q deviation test. Hautarzt, 28:658–660, 1977.
27. Bruhl, W., and Maldykowa, H.: Analiza klinicnza 50 przypadkow artropatii tuszczycowej. Pol. Tyg. Lek., 15:525–526, 1970.
28. Buckley, W.R., and Raleigh, R.L.: Psoriasis with acroosteolysis. N. Engl. J. Med., 261:539–543, 1959.
29. Bunim, J.J.: The syndrome of sarcoidosis, psoriasis and gout. Ann. Intern. Med., 57:1018–1022, 1962.
30. Burrows, D., and Kelly, A.: Methotrexate in psoriasis. Lancet, 1:1383, 1967.
31. Bywaters, E.G.L., and Dixon, A. St. J.: Paravertebral ossification in psoriatic arthritis. Ann. Rheum. Dis., 24:313–331, 1965.
32. Calabresi, P., and Turner, R.W.: Beneficial effects of triacetyl azauridine in psoriasis and mycosis fungoides. Ann. Intern. Med., 64:352–371, 1966.
33. Calin, A., and Fries, J.F.: Striking prevalence of ankylosing spondylitis in "healthy" W27 positive males and females. N. Engl. J. Med., 293:835–839, 1975.
34. Cats, A.: In Psoriasis (Proceedings of the International

Symposium, Stanford University). Stanford, Stanford University Press, 1971, p. 127.
35. Chaouat, Y., et al.: Le Rheumatisme psoriasique:traitement par le methotrexate. Rev. Rhum. Mal. Osteoartic., 38:453–460, 1971.
36. Clague, R.B., Shaw, M.J., and Holt, P.J.L.: Incidence and correlation between serum IgG and IgM antibodies to native type II collagen in patients with inflammatory arthritis. Ann. Rheum. Dis., 40:6–10, 1981.
37. Clark, W.S., Kulka, P.J., and Bauer, W.: Rheumatoid arthritis with aortic regurgitation. Am. J. Med., 22:580–592, 1957.
38. Clarke, O.: Arthritis mutilans associated with psoriasis. Lancet, 1:249, 1950.
39. Coe, R.O., and Bull, F.E.: Cirrhosis associated with methotrexate treatment of psoriasis. JAMA, 206:1515–1520, 1968.
40. Cohentervaest, W.C., and Esseveld, H.: A study of the incidence of hemolytic streptococci in the throat of patients with psoriasis vulgaris with reference to their role in pathogenesis of this disease. Dermatologica, 140:282–291, 1970.
41. Cornbleet, R.: Action of synthetic antimalarial drugs on psoriasis. J. Invest. Dermatol., 26:435–436, 1956.
42. Coste, F., and Solnica, J.: La polyarthrite psoriasique. Rev. Fr. Etudes Clin. Biol., 11:578, 1966.
43. Cracchiolo, A., Bluestone, R., and Goldberg, C.G.: Hidden antiglobulin in rheumatic disorders. Clin. Exp. Immunol., 7:651–656, 1970.
44. Csonka, F.W.: The course of Reiter's syndrome. Br. Med. J., 1:1088, 1958.
45. Danielsen, L.: Immuno-electrophoretic analysis of serum proteins in psoriasis and psoriatic arthritis. Acta Rheumatol. Scand., 11:112–118, 1965.
46. Dausset, J., and Hors, J.: Some contributions of the HLA complex to the genetics of human diseases. Transplant. Rev., 22:44–74, 1975.
47. Dawson, M.H., and Tyson, T.L.: Psoriasis arthropathia with observations on certain features common to psoriasis and rheumatoid arthritis. Trans. Assoc. Am. Physicians, 53:303, 1938.
48. Dorwart, B.B., et al.: Chryotherapy in psoriatic arthritis. Efficacy and toxicity compared to rheumatoid arthritis. Arthritis Rheum., 21:513–515, 1978.
49. Dryll, A., et al.: Les formes de passage l'oculo-uréthro-synovite de Fiessinger-Leroy-Reiter et le rhumatisme psoriasique. Sem. Hop. Paris, 8:499–515, 1969.
50. Dunlop, E.M., Harper, I.A., and Jones, B.R.: Sero-negative polyarthritis. The Bedsonia (Chlamydia) group of agents and Reiter's disease, a progress report. Ann. Rheum. Dis., 27:234–239, 1968.
51. duVivier, A., Munro, D.D., and Verbov, J.: Treatment of psoriasis with azathioprine. Br. Med. J., 1:49–51, 1974.
52. Eastmond, C.J., and Wright, V.: The nail dystrophy of psoriatic arthritis. Ann. Rheum. Dis., 38:226, 1979.
53. Eisen, A.Z., and Seegmiller, J.E.: Uric acid metabolism in psoriasis. J. Clin. Invest., 40:1486–1494, 1961.
54. Espinoza, L.R., et al.: Vascular changes in psoriatic synovium—a light and electron microscopic study. Arthritis Rheum., 25:677–684, 1982.
55. Espinoza, L.R., et al.: Cell mediated immunity in psoriatic arthritis. J. Rheumatol., 7:218–224, 1980.
56. Espinoza, L.R., et al.: Histocompatibility studies in psoriasis vulgaris: family studies. J. Rheumatol., 7:445–452, 1980.
57. Espinoza, L.R., et al.: Association between HLA-BW38 and peripheral psoriatic arthritis. Arthritis Rheum., 21:72–75, 1978.
58. Epstein, E.: Differential diagnosis of keratosis blenorrhagica and psoriatic arthropathy. Arch. Dermatol. Syphilol., 40:547–549, 1939.
59. Farber, E.M.: Proceedings of the Forty-fifth International Congress of Dermatology. Amsterdam, Excerpta Medica, 1972, p. 83.
60. Farber, E.M., and Noll, M.L.: In Psoriasis (Proceedings of the International Symposium, Stanford University). Stanford, Stanford University Press, 1971. pp. 7–13.

61. Farber, E.M., and Peterson, J.B.: Variations in the natural history of psoriasis. Calif. Med., 95:6–11, 1961.

62. Garber, E.M., Nall, M.L., and Watson, W.: Natural history of psoriasis in 61 twin pairs. Arch. Dermatol., 109:207–211, 1974.

63. Fassbender, H.G.: Pathology of Rheumatic Disease. Berlin, Springer-Verlag, 1975, p. 245.

64. Fawcitt, J.: Bone and joint changes associated with psoriasis. Br. J. Radiol., 23:440, 1950.

65. Fehr, K., et al.: Production of agglutinators and rheumatoid factors in plasma cells of rheumaotid and non-rheumatoid synovial tissues. Arthritis Rheum., 24:510–519, 1981.

66. Feldges, D.H., and Barnes, C.G.: Treatment of psoriatic arthropathy with either azathioprine or methotrexate. Rheumatol. Rehabil., 13:120–124, 1974.

67. Ferguson, A., and Downie, W.W.: Gastrointestinal amyloidosis in psoriatic arthritis. Ann. Rheum. Dis., 27:245–248, 1968.

68. Fletcher, E., and Rose, F.C.: Psoriasis spondylitica. Lancet, 1:695, 1955.

69. Forestier, J., and Rotes-Querol, J.: Senile ankylosing hyperostosis of the spine. Ann. Rheum. Dis., 9:321–330, 1950.

70. Fox, T.C., and McCleod, J.M.H.: On a case of parakeratosis variegata. Br. J. Dermatol., 13:319–346, 1901.

71. Frangione, B., Cooper, N.S., and McEwen, C.: Rheumatoid factor in rheumatoid "variants". Arthritis Rheum., 6:772, 1963.

72. Fyrand, O., Mellbye, O.J., and Natvig, J.B.: Immunofluorescence studies for immunoglobulin and complement C_3 in synovial joint membranes in psoriatic arthritis. Clin. Exp. Immunol., 29:422–427, 1977.

73. Gaedicke, H., and Kaiser Ward Mathies, H.: Die Bestimmung der Phosphoglucose-Isomerase-Aktivität in den Erythrocyten und ihre Bedeutung als diagnostisches Kriterium der Arthritis psoriatica. Klin. Wochenschr., 48:1456–1458, 1970.

74. Gardner, D.L.: Pathology of Connective Tissue Diseases. London, Arnold, 1965, p. 68.

75. Garrod, A.B.: The Nature and Treatment of Gout and Rheumatic Gout. London, Walton and Maberly, 1859.

76. Gerber, L.H., et al.: Human lymphocyte antigens characterizing psoriatic arthritis and its subtypes. J. Rheumatol., 9:703–707, 1982.

77. Gladman, D.D., et al.: Impaired antigen-specific suppressor cell activity in psoriasis and psoriatic arthritis. J. Invest. Dermatol., 77:406–409, 1981.

78. Goldthwait, J.C., Butler, C.F., and Stillman, S.: The diagnosis of gout. Significance of an elevated serum uric acid value. N. Engl. J. Med., 259:1095–1098, 1958.

79. Gottlieb, M., and Calin, A.: Discordance for psoriatic arthropathy in monozygotic twins. Arthritis Rheum., 22:805–806, 1979.

80. Graber-Duvernay, J.: A propos de la spondylarthrite psoriasique. Rev. Rhum., 24:288–294, 1957.

81. Graham, W.: Psoriasis and rheumatoid arthritis. In Comroe's Arthritis and Allied Conditions. 5th Ed. Edited by J.L. Hollander. Philadelphia, Lea & Febiger, 1953, pp. 164–170.

82. Gubner, R., August, S., and Ginsburg, V.: Therapeutic suppression of tissue reactivity effect of aminopterin in rheumatoid arthritis and psoriais. Am. J. Med. Sci., 221:176–182, 1951.

83. Gumpel, J.M.: Synoviorthesis with erbium 169: a double blind controlled comparison of erbium 169 with corticosteroids. Ann. Rheum. Dis., 38:341–343, 1979.

84. Haim, S., and Alroy, G.: Methotrexate in psoriasis. Lancet, 1:1165, 1967.

85. Hall, G.H., et al.: Intra-articular methotrexate. Clinical and laboratory study in rheumatoid arthritis and psoriatic arthritis. Ann. Rheum. Dis., 37:351–356, 1978.

86. Hall, W.H., and Finegold, S.: Study of 23 cases of Reiter's syndrome. Ann. Intern. Med., 38:533–550, 1953.

87. Hammer, B.P., Ashurst, P., and Naish, J.: Diseases associated with ulcerative colitis and Crohn's disease. Gut, 9:17–21, 1968.

88. Harkness, A.H.: Non-Gonococcal Arthritis. Edinburgh, Livingstone, 1950, p. 99.

89. Hench, P.S.: Arthropathia psoriatica—presentation of a case. Proc. Mayo Clin., 2:80–92, 1927.

90. Huskisson, E.C., and Balme, H.W.: Pseudopodagra—differential diagnosis of gout. Lancet, 2:269–271, 1972.

91. Jajic, I.: Radiological changes in the sacro-iliac joints and spine of patients with psoriatic arthritis and psoriasis. Ann. Rheum. Dis., 27:1–6, 1968.

92. Jayson, M.I.V., and Boucher, I.H.D.: Ulcerative colitis with ankylosing spondylitis. Ann. Rheum. Dis., 27:219–224, 1968.

93. Jeghers, H., and Robinson, L.J.: Arthropathia psoriatica: report of case and discussion of pathogenesis, diagnosis and treatment. JAMA, 108:949–952, 1937.

94. Kammer, G.M., et al.: Psoriatic arthritis: a clinical, immunologic and HLA study of 100 patients. Semin. Arthritis Rheum., 9:75–97, 1979.

95. Kaplan, D., et al.: Cervical spine in psoriasis and in psoriatic arthritis. Ann. Rheum. Dis., 24:313–319, 1965.

96. Karsh, J., et al.: Immune complexes in psoriasis with and without arthritis. J. Rheumatol., 5:514–519, 1978.

97. Kellgren, J.H., Stanbury, W., and Hall, L.: Proceedings of the Sixth European Congress of Rheumatology. Lisbon, Geigy, 1967.

98. Kersley, G.D.: Amethopterin (methotrexate) in connective tissue disease—psoriasis and polyarthritis. Ann. Rheum. Dis., 27:64–66, 1968.

99. Kim, H.J., et al.: Clinical significance of synovial fluid total hemolytic complement activity. J. Rheumatol., 7:143–152, 1980.

100. Krulig, L., et al.: Histocompatibility (HL-A) antigens in psoriasis. Arch. Dermatol., 111:857–860, 1975.

101. Kummerle, K., Wessinghage, D., and Schweikert, C.H.: Risk of alloplastic replacements in degenerative and inflammatory diseases of joints. Acta Orthop. Belg., 37:541–548, 1971.

102. Lambert, J.R., et al.: Psoriatic arthritis in childhood. Clin. Rheum. Dis., 2:339–342, 1976.

103. Lambert, J.R., and Wright, V.: Surgery in patients with psoriasis and arthritis. Rheumatol. Rehabil., 18:35–37, 1979.

104. Lambert, J.R., and Wright, V.: Psoriatic spondylitis: a clinical and radiological description of the spine in psoriatic arthritis. Q. J. Med., 46:411–425, 1977.

105. Lambert, J.R., and Wright, V.: Serum uric acid levels in psoriatic arthritis. Ann. Rheum. Dis., 36:264–267, 1977.

106. Lambert, J.R., and Wright, V.: Eye inflammation in psoriatic arthritis. Ann. Rheum. Dis., 35:354–356, 1976.

107. Lambert, J.R., Wright, V., and Rajah, S.M.: Histocompatibility antigens in psoriatic arthritis. Ann. Rheum. Dis., 35:526–530, 1976.

108. Langeland, N., and Roass, A.: Spondylitis psoriatica. Acta Orthop. Scand., 42:391, 1971.

109. Lassus, A., et al.: The lack of rheumatoid factor in psoriatic arthritis. Acta Rheumatol. Scand., 10:62–68, 1964.

110. Laurent, M.R., Panayi, G.S., and Shepperd, P.: Circulating immune complexes, serum immunoglobulins, and acute phase proteins in psoriasis and psoriatic arthritis. Ann. Rheum. Dis., 40:66–69, 1981.

111. Lawrence, J.S.: Prevalence of rheumatoid arthritis. Ann. Rheum. Dis., 20:11–17, 1961.

112. Leczinsky, C.G.: The incidence of arthropathy in a tenyear series of psoriasis cases. Acta Derm. Venereol. (Stockh.), 28:483–485, 1948.

113. Leonard, D.G., O'Duffy, J.D., and Rogers, R.S.: Prospective analysis of psoriatic arthritis in patients hospitalized for psoriasis. Mayo Clin. Proc., 53:511–518, 1978.

114. Levy, J., et al.: A double blind controlled evaluation of azathioprine treatment in rheumatoid arthritis and psoriatic arthritis. Arthritis Rheum., 15:116–117, 1972.

115. Lewin, K., DeWit, S., and Ferrington, R.A.: Pathology of the fingernail in psoriasis: a clinico-pathological study. Br. J. Dermatol., 86:555–563, 1972.

116. Lomholt, G.: Psoriasis, prevalence, spontaneous course, and genetics; a census study on the prevalence of skin

disease in the Faroe Islands. G.E.C. Gad, Copenhagen, 1963.

117. Lucherini, T., and Buratti, L.: Borsite reumatoide sottodeltoidea a granuli orizoidei. Rheumatismo, *17*:35–44, 1965.

118. Luzar, M.J.: Hydroxychloroquine in psoriatic arthropathy: exacerbations of psoriatic skin lesions. J. Rheumatol., *9*:462–464, 1981.

119. Lynfield, Y.L., Ostroff, G., and Abraham, J.: Bacteria, skin sterilization and wound healing in psoriasis. N.Y. J. Med., *72*:1247–1250, 1972.

120. McEwen, C., et al.: Ankylosing spondylitis accompanying ulcerative colitis, regional enteritis, psoriasis and Reiter's disease. Arthritis Rheum., *14*:291–298, 1971.

121. MacSween, R.N., et al.: A clinico-immunological study of serum and synovial fluid antinuclear factors in rheumatoid arthritis and other arthritides. Clin. Exp. Immunol., *3*:17–24, 1968.

122. Margolis, H.M.: Arthritis and Allied Disorders. New York, Hoeber, 1941, p. 125.

123. Martin, J.H., Gordon, M., and Wallace, R.: Methotrexate in psoriasis. Precipitation of gout. Arch. Dermatol., *96*:431–433, 1967.

124. Masheter, H.C.: Behçet's syndrome complicated by intracranial thrombophlebitis. Proc. R. Soc. Med., *52*:1039–1040, 1959.

125. Mason, R.M., and Barnes, G.C.: Behçet's syndrome with arthritis. Ann. Rheum. Dis., *28*:95–103, 1969.

126. Maxwell, J.D., et al.: Reiter's syndrome and psoriasis. Scott. Med. J., *11*:14–18, 1966.

127. Medsger, T.A., et al.: HL-A antigen B27 and psoriatic spondylitis. Arthritis Rheum., *17*:322–323, 1974.

128. Melski, J.W., et al.: Oral methoxsalen photochemotherapy for the treatment of psoriasis: a cooperative clinical trial. J. Invest. Dermatol., *68*:328–335, 1977.

129. Menzen, J.: Uber Gelenkerkrankungen bei Psoriasis. Arch. Dermatol. Syphilol., *70*:239–240, 1904.

130. Metzger, A.L., et al.: HL-AW 27 in psoriatic arthropathy. Arthritis Rheum., *18*:111–115, 1975.

131. Miller, J.L., Soltani, K., and Tourtellotte, C.D.: Psoriatic acro-osteolysis without arthritis. J. Bone Joint Surg., *53A*:371–374, 1971.

132. Moll, J.M.H.: D.M. Thesis, University of Oxford, 1971.

133. Moll, J.M.H., and Wright, V.: Familial occurrence of psoriatic arthritis. Ann. Rheum. Dis., *12*:181–201, 1973.

134. Moll, J.M.H., and Wright, V.: Psoriatic arthritis. Semin. Arthritis Rheum., *3*:55–78, 1973.

135. Monacelli, M.: *In* Psoriasis (Proceedings of the International Symposium, Stanford University). Stanford, Stanford University Press, 1971. p. 100.

136. Mongan, E.S., and Atwater, E.C.: A comparison of patients with seropositive and seronegative rheumatoid arthritis. Med. Clin. North Am., *52*:533–538, 1968.

137. Muna, W.F., et al.: Psoriatic arthritis and aortic regurgitation. JAMA, *244*:363–365, 1980.

138. Munthe, E.: Relationship between IgG complexes and anti IgG antibodies in rheumatoid arthritis. Acta Rheumatol. Scand., *16*:240–256, 1970.

139. Murray, C.: Histocompatibility alloantigens in psoriasis and psoriatic arthritis: evidence for the influence of multiple genes in the major histocompatibility complex. J. Clin. Invest., *60*:670–675, 1980.

140. Mustakallio, K.K., and Lassus, A.: Staphylococcal alpha-antitoxin in psoriatic arthropathy. Br. J. Dermatol., *76*:544–551, 1964.

141. Ohkawara, A., and Halprin, K.M.: *In* Psoriasis (Proceedings of the International Symposium, Stanford University). Stanford, Stanford University Press, 1971, p. 239.

142. Noble, W.C., and Sarin, J.A.: Carriage of staphylococcus aureus in psoriasis. Br. Med. J., *1*:417–418, 1968.

143. Parrish, J.A., et al.: Photochemotherapy of psoriasis with oral methoxsalen and long wave ultraviolet light. N. Engl. J. Med., *291*:1207–1211, 1974.

144. Perlman, S.G., et al.: Photochemotherapy and psoriatic arthritis. Ann. Intern. Med., *91*:717–722, 1979.

145. Perry, H.O., and Mayne, J.G.: Psoriasis and Reiter's syndrome. Arch. Dermatol., *92*:129–136, 1965.

146. Petres, J., and Majert, P.: Immunelektrophorese bei psoriatischer Arthropathie. Arch. Klin. Exp. Dermatol., *232*:398–401, 1965.

147. Petres, J., Klumper, A., and Majert, P.: Differentialdiagnose der psoriatischen Arthropathie auf Grund rontgenmorphologischer Befunde. Hautarzt, *21*:26, 1970.

148. Plenk, H.D.: Psoriatic arthritis—report of a case. Am. J. Roentgenol., *64*:635–639, 1950.

149. Podurgiel, B.J., et al.: Liver injury associated with methotrexate therapy for psoriasis. Mayo Clin. Proc., *48*:787–792, 1973.

150. Qureshi, M.S.A., et al.: Amyloidosis complicating psoriatic arthritis. Br. Med. J., *2*:302, 1977.

151. Ragan, C.: The clinical picture of rheumatoid arthritis. *In* Arthritis and Allied Conditions. 8th Ed. Edited by J.C. Hollander and D.J. McCarty. Philadelphia, Lea & Febiger, 1972, p. 333.

152. Ragan, C., and Tyson, T.L.: Chrysotherapy in rheumatoid arthritis. Am. J. Med., *1*:252–256, 1946.

153. Recordier, A.M., et al.: Les atteintes musculaires au cours du psoriasis arthropathique. Rev. Rhum., *36*:91–98, 1969.

154. Redisch, W., et al.: Capillaroscopic observations in rheumatic diseases. Ann. Rheum. Dis., *29*:244–253, 1970.

155. Reed, W.B.: Psoriatic arthritis. A complete clinical study of 86 patients. Acta Derm. Venereol. (Stockh.), *41*:396–403, 1961.

156. Reed, W.B., et al.: Psoriasis and arthritis—clinico pathological study. Arch. Dermatol., *83*:541–548, 1961.

157. Reed, W.B., and Wright, V.: *In* Modern Trends in Rheumatology. London, Butterworth, 1966.

158. Rees, R.B., et al.: Aminopterin for psoriasis. Arch. Dermatol., *90*:544–552, 1964.

159. Richter, M.B., Kinsella, P., and Corbet, M.: Gold in psoriatic arthropathy. Ann. Rheum. Dis., *39*:279–280, 1980.

160. Roberts, M.E.T., et al.: Psoriatic arthritis: a follow up study. Ann. Rheum. Dis., *35*:206–208, 1976.

161. Robillard, J.: Thesis, University of Lyon, 1968.

162. Robinson, J.K., et al.: Methotrexate hepatotoxicity in psoriasis. Arch. Dermatol., *116*:413–415, 1980.

163. Rodnan, G.P., McEwen, C., and Wallace, S.L.: Primer on the rheumatic diseases. JAMA, *224 (Suppl.)*:70–71, 1973.

164. Romanus, T.: Psoriasis from a prognostic and hereditary point of view. Acta Derm. Venereol. (Stockh.), *26 (Suppl. 12)*:6, 1945.

165. Ropes, M.W., et al.: Diagnostic criteria for rheumatoid arthritis. Bull. Rheum. Dis., *9*:175–176, 1959.

166. Ropes, M.W., et al.: Proposed diagnostic criteria for rheumatoid arthritis. Bull. Rheum. Dis., *7*:121–124, 1956.

167. Rose, H.M., et al.: Differential agglutination of normal and sensitized sheep erythrocytes by sera of patients with rheumatoid arthritis. Proc. Soc. Exp. Biol. Med., *68*:1–6, 1948.

168. Rosenthal, M.: A critical review of the effect of levamisole in rheumatic diseases other than rheumatoid arthritis. J. Rheumatol., *(Suppl. 4)*:97–100, 1978.

169. Ross, J.B.: The psoriatic capillary: its nature and value in the identification of the unaffected psoriatic patient. Br. J. Dermatol., *76*:511–517, 1964.

170. Rotstein, J., Entel, I., and Zeviner, B.: Arthritis associated with ulcerative colitis. Ann. Rheum. Dis., *22*:194–197, 1963.

171. Russell, T.J., Schultes, L.M., and Kuban, D.J.: Histocompatibility (HL-A) antigens associated with psoriasis. N. Engl. J. Med., *287*:738–740, 1972.

172. Salvesen, H.A., and Boe, J.: Idiopathic hypoparathyroidism. Acta Endocrinol., *14*:214–226, 1953.

173. Schaller, J.G., et al.: The association of antinuclear antibodies with the chronic iridocyclitis of juvenile rheumatoid arthritis. (Still's disease). Arthritis Rheum., *17*:409–416, 1974.

174. Sedgwick, J.B., Bergstresser, P.R., and Hurd, E.R.: Increased granulocyte adherence in psoriasis and psoriatic arthritis. J. Invest. Dermatol., *74*:81–84, 1980.

175. Serri, F., Cerimele, D., and Torsellini, A.: *In* Psoriasis (Proceedings of the International Symposium, Stanford

University). Stanford, Stanford University Press, 1971, p. 253.

176. Shapiro, H.A., et al.: Liver disease in psoriatics—an effect of methotrexate therapy? Arch. Dermatol., *110*:547–551, 1974.

177. Sharp, J.: Heredo-familial vascular and articular calcification. Ann Rheum. Dis., *13*:15–27, 1954.

178. Shelley, W.B., and Arthur, R.P.: Biochemical and physiological clues to the nature of psoriasis. Arch. Dermatol., *78*:14–29, 1958.

179. Sherman, M.: Psoriatic arthritis: observations on the clinical, roentgenographic and radiological changes. J. Bone Joint Surg., *34A*:831–852, 1952.

180. Shore, A., and Ansell, B.M.: Juvenile psoriatic arthritis—an analysis of 60 cases. J. Pediatr., *100*:529–535, 1982.

181. Short, C.L., Bauer, W., and Reynolds, W.E.: *In* Rheumatoid Arthritis. Cambridge, Harvard University Press, 1957, p. 38.

182. Shrank, A.B., and Blendis, L.M.: Folic acid antagonists in treatment of psoriasis. Br. Med. J., *2*:156, 1965.

183. Sigler, J.W.: Psoriatic arthritis. *In* Arthritis & Allied Conditions. 8th Ed. Edited by J.L. Hollander and D.J. McCarty, Jr. Philadlephia, Lea & Febiger, 1972, p. 732.

184. Sills, E.M.: Psoriatic arthritis in childhood. Johns Hopkins Med. J., *146*:49–53, 1980.

185. Sonnichsen, N.: Vergleichende immunologische Untersuchungen bei Lupus erythematodes, primar chronischer Polyarthritis und Psoriasis arthropathica. Allerg. Asthma, *15*:1–8, 1969.

186. Stossel, T.P., et al.: Regulations of glycogen metabolism in polymorphonuclear leukocytes. J. Biol. Chem., *245*:6228–6234, 1970.

187. Strom, S.: A case of arthropatia psoriatica. Acta Radiol., *1*:21–34, 1921.

188. Szanto, E.: Long term follow up of ⁹⁰Yttrium-treated knee joint arthritis. Scand. J. Rheumatol., *6*:209–212, 1977.

189. Theiss, B. von, et al.: Psoriasis-spondylarthritis. Z. Rheumaforsch., *28*:93–107, 1969.

190. Tickner, A., and Mier, P.D.: Serum cholesterol, uric acid and proteins in psoriasis. Br. J. Dermatol., *72*:132–144, 1960.

191. Townes, A.S., and Sowa, J.M.: Complement in synovial fluid. Johns Hopkins Med. J., *127*:23–37, 1970.

192. Ullman, S., et al.: Deposits of complement and immunoglobulins in dermal and synovial vessels in psoriasis. Acta Derm. Venereol., *58*:272–273, 1978.

193. Van Scott, E.J., and Ekel, T.M.: Kinetics of hyperplasia in psoriasis. Arch. Dermatol., *88*:373–381, 1963.

194. Vanbreuseghem, R.: The early diagnosis of mycetoma. Derm. Int., *6*:123–133, 1967.

195. Vasey, B.F., et al.: Possible involvement of group A streptococci in the pathogenesis of psoriatic arthritis. J. Rheumatol., *9*:719–722, 1982.

196. Venkatasubramaniam, K.V., Bluhm, G.B., and Riddle, J.M.: Psoriatic arthritis and crystal induced synovitis. J. Rheumatol., *7*:213–217, 1980.

197. Vilanova, X., and Pinol, J.: Psoriasis arthropathica. Rheumatism, *7*:197–200, 1951.

198. Waller, M., and Toone, E.C.: Normal individuals with positive tests for rheumatoid factor. Arthritis Rheum., *15*:348–359, 1968.

199. Watson, W.H., et al.: *In* Psoriasis (Proceedings of the

International Symposium, Stanford University). Stanford, Stanford University Press, 1971, p. 15.

200. Weinstein, G.D., Roenigk, H.H., and Maiback, H.: Psoriasis-liver methotrexate interactions: results of an international cooperative study. Arch. Dermatol., *108*:36, 1973.

201. Weissenbach, R.J.: Le psoriasis arthropathique. Arch. Dermatol. Syphilol. (Paris), *10*:13–17, 1938.

202. Whaley, K., et al.: Sjögren's syndrome in psoriatic arthritis, ankylosing spondylitis and Reiter's syndrome. Acta Rheumatol. Scand., *17*:105–114, 1971.

203. White, S.H., et al.: Disturbance of HL-A antigen frequency in psoriasis. N. Engl. J. Med., *287*:740–743, 1972.

204. Willoughby, C.P., et al.:Gastrointestinal amyloidosis complicating psoriatic arthritis. Postgrad. Med. J., *57*:663–667, 1981.

205. Wright, V.: Psoriatic arthritis. *In* Textbook of Rheumatology. Edited by W.N. Kelley, et al. Philadelphia, W.B. Saunders, 1980, p. 1060.

206. Wright, V., and Moll, J.M.H.: *In* Seronegative Polyarthritis. Amsterdam, North Holland, 1976.

207. Wright, V.: *In* Progress in Clinical Rheumatology. London, Churchill, 1965, p. 220.

208. Wright, V.: Proceedings of the 12th International Congress of Dermatology (Int. Congr. Series. No. 55). Amsterdam, Excerpta Medica, 1962, p. 176.

209. Wright, V.: Psoriasis and arthritis. Arch. Dermatol., *80*:27–32, 1959.

210. Wright, V.: Psoriatic arthritis: a comparative radiographic study of rheumatoid arthritis associated with psoriasis. Ann. Rheum. Dis.,*20*:123–132, 1959.

211. Wright, V.: Rheumatism and psoriasis—a re-evaluation. Am. J. Med., *27*:454–460, 1959.

212. Wright, V.: Psoriasis and arthritis—a study on the radiographic appearances. Br. J. Radiol., *30*:113–118, 1957.

213. Wright, V.: Psoriasis and arthritis. Ann. Rheum. Dis., *15*:348–353, 1956.

214. Wright, V., and Reed, W.B.: The link between Reiter's syndrome and psoriatic arthritis. Ann. Rheum. Dis., *23*:12–20, 1964.

215. Wright, V., and Watkinson, G.: The arthritis of ulcerative colitis. Br. Med. J., *2*:670–675, 1965.

216. Zachariae, H., and Zachariae, E.: Antinuclear factors, the antihuman globulin consumption test, and Wasserman reaction in psoriatic arthritis. Acta Rheumatol. Scand., *15*:62–66, 1969.

217. Zachariae, H., Kragballe, K., and Sogaard, H.: Methotrexate induced liver cirrhosis. Br. J. Dermatol., *102*:407–412, 1980.

218. Zaias, N.: Psoriasis of the nail—a clinico-pathological study. Arch. Dermatol., *99*:567–572, 1969.

219. Zaric, D., et al.: Capillary microscopy of the nail fold in patients with psoriasis and psoriatic arthritis. Dermatologica, *164*:10–14, 1982.

220. Zbojanova, M.F., et al.: The spine in psoriatic arthritis. *In* International Congress Series No. 299. Amsterdam, Excerpta Medica, 1973, p. 108.

221. Zellner, E.: Zur Kenntnis der Arthropathia psoriatica. Munchen Med. Wochenschr., *75*:903–911, 1928.

222. Zimmer, J.G., and Dennis, D.J.: Association between gout, psoriasis and sarcoidosis. Ann. Intern. Med., *64*:756–761, 1966.

Chapter 56

Enteropathic Arthritis

Richard H. Ferguson

Joint involvement complicating certain diseases of the bowel and some pancreatic diseases is discussed in this chapter. Arthritis is also associated with viral hepatitis, chronic active hepatitis, and acute enteric infections (see Chaps. 57 and 103). Conversely, bowel involvement is common in Behçet's and Reiter's syndromes (see Chaps. 54 and 58).

ARTICULAR MANIFESTATIONS OF CHRONIC ULCERATIVE COLITIS AND REGIONAL ENTERITIS

Arthritis was emphasized by Bargen in 1929 as the major extracolonic complication of chronic ulcerative colitis.[3] In 1935, Hench provided a clear description of the peripheral joint involvement in ulcerative colitis, which he regarded as distinct from rheumatoid arthritis (RA) on the basis of its clinical course.[25] The advent of tests for rheumatoid factor brought on a renaissance of interest in this subject and virtually unanimous agreement that it merited classification as a separate entity. Various terms have been suggested, including: "arthritis-ulcerative colitis,"[42] "colonic arthritis,"[55] and "acute toxic arthritis."[19]

An inordinately high prevalence of ankylosing spondylitis in ulcerative colitis was recognized by Steinberg and Storey in 1957,[45] and it has subsequently been confirmed by others.[1,23]

Regional enteritis, such as Crohn's disease, granulomatous colitis, and transmural colitis, exhibits many clinical, radiologic, and pathologic features that distinguish it from ulcerative colitis; however, it shares with ulcerative colitis an identical form of peripheral arthritis and an increased prevalence of ankylosing spondylitis. For the sake of brevity, the articular manifestations associated with these intestinal diseases are considered together.

Peripheral Arthritis

Prevalence

Peripheral arthritis occurs in about 12% of patients with chronic ulcerative colitis and in about 20% of patients with regional enteritis, excluding patients with spondylitis or other rheumatic diseases.[2,21,23] The higher prevalence rate in regional enteritis may reflect the involvement of the entire bowel, not just the colon. Proctocolectomy can eliminate ulcerative colitis and its associated peripheral arthritis, but it does not prevent recurrent bowel disease with recurrent bouts of arthritis in regional enteritis. The sex incidence of arthritis is approximately equal in both inflammatory bowel diseases. The usual age of onset is 25 to 45 years, but it ranges from childhood to old age.

Course

An episodic bout of arthritis with inflammatory bowel disease usually begins abruptly and reaches its zenith within 1 to 2 days in 84% of patients.[32] Oligoarticular involvement is characteristic; 8 or fewer joints are affected in most episodes. In one series, 85% of bouts were limited to 3 joints or fewer,[32] and 20 of 31 patients in another report had a monarticular onset in the initial attack.[55] The pattern of involvement is often migratory. Inflammatory signs are frequently striking, but the attack may be limited to localized or migratory arthralgia, with meager or no objective findings.

The small distal joints in both arms and legs are much less frequently affected than in RA, and the knees and ankles are the most commonly involved joints.[55] Joints in the lower extremities are more frequently involved than those in the upper extremities. An earlier suggestion that interphalangeal joint synovitis of the toe was a valuable diagnostic clue to ulcerative colitis[5] did not receive support in later studies.[32,55]

The duration of an individual attack was less than 1 month in 50% and less than 2 months in 75% of the episodes in a reported series.[32] Only 10% of the bouts lasted longer than 1 year, and even these often continued to exhibit partial remissions and flares paralleling the bowel disease.[32]

Although some individuals experience 1 or 2 attacks per year, recurrences are usually infrequent. An average of 1.4 attacks was reported in the first year after the onset of arthritis accompanying ulcerative colitis; the average was 2 attacks in patients observed for 5 years, 2.3 attacks in those observed for 10 years, and 2.5 attacks in those observed for 15 years.[32]

Relation to Bowel Disease

An arthritic flare shortly after an exacerbation of colitis has been recognized as a characteristic but inconstant phenomenon since Hench's description in 1935.[25] Recent authors have recognized a correlation of the bowel and joint inflammation in 60 to 74% of patients.[32,55] Even those patients whose arthritis antedates symptomatic colitis frequently have synchronous exacerbations and remissions later. Only 7 to 11% of patients studied experienced arthritis prior to bowel symptoms.[5,32] In one series, 25% of patients developed arthritis within 6 months of the onset of colitis, but another 25% did not experience joint symptoms until colitis had been present for over 10 years.[55]

Associated Features

Arthritis occurs four times as frequently in patients with chronic colitis as in those with acute fulminating disease or with proctitis alone.[55] Patients with ulcerative colitis who have perianal disease, pseudopolyps, uveitis, or aphthous stomatitis have a two- to fourfold increase in the incidence of arthritis.[32] These complications often occur concurrently in the wake of a flare in the bowel disease.

Erythema nodosum occurs in 5% of all patients with ulcerative colitis,[30] but it is found in about 25% of those with peripheral arthritis.[5,19,32,55] In regional enteritis, involvement of the colon is much more likely to be associated with arthritis than is small bowel involvement, but such complications as fistula formation or malabsorption do not predispose a patient to arthritis.[23]

Laboratory Studies

The histologic appearance of the synovial membrane may mimic that of RA. Synovial fluid cell counts range from 4,000 to 42,400, with 75 to 98% consisting of polymorphonuclear cells. The protein content of the synovial fluid may be low, but the relative viscosity may be higher than expected.[5] Blood leukocyte counts and erythrocyte sedimentation rates are usually high, and hemoglobin values are often reduced, probably because of the bowel disease rather than the articular reaction. Total complement in synovial fluid is normal.[24,26] Test results for rheumatoid factor and HLA-B27 antigen are positive only in the frequency expected for a normal population.[5,33] Antinuclear antibodies are rare. High levels of Raji cell-detectable circulating immune complexes have been reported in 20% of patients with ulcerative colitis or regional enteritis, but have not been found in patients with pseudomembranous colitis or bacterial colitis or in healthy control subjects.[29] Eight of 12 patients with active arthritis associated with Crohn's disease had elevated levels of circulating immune complexes in another study, but in only 3 did these levels remain elevated a year later, after regression of the arthritis.[16]

Radiologic Manifestations

Radiographic changes are usually nonspecific and minor. Soft tissue swelling and juxtoarticular osteoporosis may appear. Small bony erosions are seen at times, but these usually heal. Mild periostitis may be seen in patients with more persistent inflammation; this generally resolves or melds in with the bone.[5]

Differential Diagnosis

Diagnostic problems may arise, particularly when bowel disease is inapparent or mild. Migratory polyarthritis may result in confusion with rheumatic fever. Monarticular involvement of a knee or an ankle can suggest gout, pseudogout, or sepsis. Reiter's syndrome or reactive arthropathy with a diarrheal onset must be included in the differential considerations. Ankylosing spondylitis with peripheral joint manifestations must be kept in mind in patients with ulcerative colitis or regional enteritis because sacroiliac or spinal manifestations may not be evident for several years after the initial peripheral joint flares. A diagnosis of Whipple's disease may need to be excluded by appropriate studies.

The diagnosis of RA is occasionally impossible to exclude in those few patients in whom chronicity and some deformity ensue, and particularly when the courses of the joint disorder and the bowel disease do not correlate. Positive test results for rheumatoid factor may settle the issue in many instances, but even the passage of time may not eliminate uncertainty as to the most appropriate classification of patients who remain seronegative. In 3 extensive series of patients with colitis, the prevalence of the peripheral arthritis of ulcerative colitis was thought to be 8 to 25 times that of coexisting RA.[5,32,55] In a retrospective study of 550 patients, however, it was concluded that 18 patients had RA and 49 patients had arthritis of ulcerative colitis.[19] Most observers currently believe that the prevalence of RA in ulcerative colitis and regional enteritis is similar to that in the general population.

Prognosis

The prognosis in most patients is good with regard to articular function, even after repeated attacks. Perhaps one-fourth of those affected sustain residual limitation of contractures that are usually minor.[32]

Therapy

Treatment should be directed primarily at the underlying bowel disease. Joint symptoms can usually be managed adequately with a conservative regimen of rest, physical therapy, and nonsteroidal anti-inflammatory drugs. The intra-articular administration of corticosteroids may be useful, but *systemic corticosteroid therapy is rarely, if ever, indicated for the joint disease alone.* If corticosteroid therapy is required to control colitis, the arthritis, as a rule, is rapidly suppressed.

Arthritis accompanying ulcerative colitis or regional enteritis is *rarely the primary indication for surgical treatment,* although resection of diseased bowel is likely to prevent recurrent joint attacks, especially in patients with ulcerative colitis.[55]

Spondylitis

Prevalence

Ulcerative colitis and regional enteritis have a surprisingly frequent association with ankylosing spondylitis. Either of these inflammatory bowel diseases coexists with typical spondylitis in 4 to 7% of cases.[11,23,40,57] Epidemiologic studies indicate the prevalence of ankylosing spondylitis in Caucasian populations to be 0.13[8] to 1%.[6] HLA-B27 antigen in spondylitis associated with inflammatory bowel disease is present in 53 to 75% of patients,[10,37] a percentage distinctly less than the 90% association in uncomplicated ankylosing spondylitis. A study of 8 families of HLA-B27-negative individuals with both spondylitis and inflammatory bowel disease revealed 4 HLA-B27-negative first- or second-degree relatives with spondylitis or sacroiliitis, 1 with inflammatory bowel disease and sacroiliitis, and 1 with inflammatory bowel disease alone.[15] One reported family had HLA haplotypes completely dissociated from spondylitis and inflammatory bowel disease. The high association of spondylitis with inflammatory bowel disease, the lower frequency of HLA-B27 in these patients, and the family studies have suggested a non-HLA-linked genetic susceptibility to both inflammatory bowel disease and spondylitis.[15]

Course

The clinical picture of spondylitis occurring with colitis or regional enteritis is indistinguishable from that of spondylitis occurring without accompanying bowel disease with regard to age of onset, radiologic features, course, and response to therapy. The frequency of associated hip, shoulder, and knee involvement is increased in patients with spondylitis and colitis; other peripheral joints are affected to approximately the same degree and frequency as in idiopathic ankylosing spondylitis.[32]

Relation to Bowel Disease

Spondylitis often antedates the appearance of ulcerative colitis or regional enteritis. This sequence has been observed in 27% of patients reported in 5 series.[19,32,40,56,57] Furthermore, little correlation exists between the manifestations of the bowel disease and the spinal symptoms. About one-fourth of patients in one study had parallel flares and remissions of both spinal and bowel disease,[32] but most authors have concluded that no such relationship exists.[19,40,56] Colectomy and other surgical measures do not favorably influence the course of spondylitis, as a rule, even when the bowel disease is controlled.[19]

Sex Ratio

The usual ratio of men to women with idiopathic ankylosing spondylitis is in the neighborhood of 9:1.[38,50] Male predominance is much less striking in spondylitis associated with ulcerative colitis, however. Sixty-two men and 26 women have been reported to have both processes in 6 series, a sex ratio of only 2.4:1.[19,24,32,40,56,57]

Some prospective studies have reported radiographic sacroiliitis in about 18% of both men and women with ulcerative colitis or regional enteritis.[2,54,56] Only one-third of these patients had enough clinical evidence at the time of study to warrant a diagnosis of spondylitis, however; these patients were predominantly male.[2,56]

Therapy

The treatment and prognosis of spondylitis accompanying ulcerative colitis and regional enteritis are identical to those of ankylosing spondylitis. As mentioned earlier, the spinal and bowel processes run independent courses, in spite of their remarkable tendency to coexist.

Etiologic Considerations

Although some confusion existed in the past regarding colonic involvement in these two diseases, certain criteria to distinguish between the two entities have been accepted. In ulcerative colitis, rectal involvement is almost constant, with variable degrees of proximal spread in continuity with the remainder of the colon and, on occasion, the terminal ileum. Lesions are characteristically limited to the mucosa, which is universally inflamed and friable and frequently contains crypt abscesses. Toxic megacolon, massive hemorrhage, or spontaneous bowel perforation may complicate fulminating exacerbations, whereas shortening of the involved colon with loss of haustral markings, pseudopolyposis, and carcinoma are encountered later.[17] Regional enteritis may involve either the small or the large bowel, or both, in what is usually a segmental, discontinuous pattern. Transmural inflammation, featuring granulomas, fissuring, discrete ulceration, serositis, and mesenteric lymphadenitis, is common. Strictures, fistulas, and inflammatory masses are frequent complications, but carcinoma is not.[17,53]

Although the two diseases seem to be distinct entities on the basis of pathologic features and course, they share certain immunologic abnormalities in addition to some apparently identical extracolonic clinical manifestations. Circulating anticolon antibodies are found in both in similar incidence and titer; however, the presence of such antibodies is not constant in either condition, and they are also found in lesser frequency in lupus erythematosus and other autoimmune diseases.[12] In addition, lymphocytes from patients with chronic ulcerative colitis or regional enteritis have cytotoxic effects in vitro on colonic epithelial cells. This property can be induced in normal lymphocytes by incubation for four days in serum from patients with ulcerative colitis or by incubation with an extract of *Escherichia coli* 0119:B14.[44] Although this phenomenon has thus far been clearly identified only in chronic ulcerative colitis and regional enteritis, it may not prove to be specific and, for the present, cannot be assumed to represent delayed hypersensitivity.

The cause of these two enteric diseases remains unknown, but it is tempting to postulate a common basis for the associated arthritic syndromes. Pathogenetic hypotheses have included the following: (1) absorption from a damaged bowel of an endogenous or exogenous antigen, which stimulates an immune reaction producing peripheral inflammation; (2) a generalized autoimmune process with a common antigen in all the involved tissues; (3) an infectious disease with the same organism causing bowel and peripheral involvement; (4) an abnormal bowel mucosa allowing an enteric pathogen to reach the synovial membrane and other sites; and (5) the production of nonimmunologic toxin in the diseased bowel wall causing synovitis.[32,52]

WHIPPLE'S DISEASE

In 1907, Whipple reported a male patient "characterized by gradual loss of weight and strength, stools consisting chiefly of neutral fat and fatty acids, indefinite abnominal signs, and a peculiar multiple arthritis."[51] Since then, more than 125 patients have been recorded, with a male predominance of 9:1.[34] In addition to the findings in Whipple's patient, such features as fever, hypotension, hyperpigmentation of the exposed areas, peripheral lymphadenopathy, and pleural reactions have been noted frequently. The presence of granules in macrophages staining with periodic acid-Schiff (PAS) in the intestinal mucosa and lymph nodes was observed in 1949,[4] and this finding has facilitated the subsequent recognition of the disease. In recent

years, electron microscopy has demonstrated the constant presence of rod-shaped organisms infiltrating the lamina propria of the intestinal mucosa. This organism was originally described by Whipple using light microscopy in his remarkable case study. The PAS-staining granules are believed to represent incompletely digested components of the bacteria. Although it is not yet possible to transmit disease to experimental animals or to culture these rod-shaped structures, their disappearance with antibiotic therapy coincident with clinical recovery constitutes impressive evidence for a causal relationship.

Peripheral joint manifestations similar to those described in patients with ulcerative colitis and regional enteritis are a prominent feature in 65 to 90% of reported cases.[28,34] About half these patients have joint complaints antedating the development of diarrhea, and in one-third, articular signs or symptoms appear 5 years or more before bowel manifestations.[28,34] In one instance, arthritis persisted for 35 years before the other features of Whipple's disease appeared.[9] The onset of the illness commonly occurs between the ages of 30 and 50, with a range from 11 to 64 years.[28] Parallel exacerbations of arthritis and diarrhea have not impressed most observers in this disease; indeed, arthritis often regresses as bowel symptoms develop.

Arthritis, usually episodic and of abrupt onset, has a migratory pattern. Arthritic involvement lasts from hours to days in a given joint and is frequently interspersed with long remissions. Only 3% of patients with Whipple's disease and arthritis develop chronic or residual clinical signs, whereas 10% have some nonspecific roentgenologic changes.[28] Involvement is usually bilateral, but occasionally unilateral or monarticular disease occurs. The knees, ankles, fingers, hips, wrists, and elbows are involved, in descending order of frequency.[28]

In a review of reports of 95 patients with Whipple's disease, 2 had bilateral sacroiliac fusion, and 1 had unilateral fusion.[28] Five examples of associated ankylosing spondylitis associated have been reported.[7]

Tests for rheumatoid factor are uniformly negative. Histopathologic changes on synovial biopsies vary from mild, nonspecific inflammation to a dense, neutrophilic infiltrate resembling that of septic arthritis.[9,41] Macrophages containing PAS-staining granules have been noted in synovial tissue on occasion,[41] but not in synovial fluid smears. Cell counts range from 450 to 28,500 mm³ at different times in synovial fluid from the same knee and parallel the intensity of inflammation. Patients with low cell counts may have a preponderance of mononuclear cells, whereas those with high counts usually have predominantly polymorphonuclear cells.[41]

The diagnosis of this condition depends on the demonstration of PAS-positive inclusion bodies in macrophages in small intestinal mucosa, in mesenteric lymph nodes, or less constantly, in more peripheral tissues. Peroral jejunal biopsy is the most appropriate diagnostic approach because the disease is thought to be consistently present and most severe in the mucosa of the upper small intestine.

Prolonged treatment with antibiotics, most commonly 1 g tetracycline daily for 1 year, has resulted in an almost uniformly favorable response. Arthralgias usually clear in 5 to 30 days, along with other manifestations of the disease.[34] It is not yet known what effect such treatment may have on patients with spinal symptoms or findings.

The prolonged duration of articular symptoms prior to bowel manifestations is difficult to reconcile with current knowledge of the disease. One possibility might be that prolonged occult intestinal disease in some way produces arthritis. Alternatively, this disorder may prove to be a systemic infection that may affect the joints alone for many years.

ARTHRITIS FOLLOWING INTESTINAL BYPASS

Jejunocolic shunt for management of morbid obesity was introduced in 1956. This procedure has largely been superseded since 1963 by jejunoilial bypass, which is better tolerated. Intestinal bypass procedures, however, are complicated by arthritis in about 15% of patients and by dermatitis in 20%;[14,47] these manifestations commonly coexist and begin 2 weeks to 61 months postoperatively.[47]

Arthritis or arthralgia is usually polyarticular and is often symmetric. The onset is generally abrupt, with intense synovitis evolving over a period of several hours, often associated with fever and malaise. Tenosynovitis of the wrists and fingers is frequent. The duration varies and may range from 14 days to over 30 months. Multiple bouts may occur, but residual joint damage or limitation does not ensue.[13,14,20,27,31,35,43] One report has cited 9 patients who developed RA after 6 to 13 years of bypass disease, however.[48]

The initial manifestations of the characteristic skin lesion are as a group of erythematous macules that evolve into papules and then pustules. These lesions are clinically indistinguishable from those of gonococcal sepsis. The pustules may last a week and recur periodically in crops.[14,47] Occasionally, lesions resembling those of erythema nodosum have been reported on the lower extremities.[14,47]

Routine laboratory studies on blood, stool, and synovial fluid yield no distinctive findings.[20,47] Bowel biopsies are uniformly negative, and synovial biopsies show nonspecific chronic inflammation.[43] Roentgenograms are usually negative, but cortical erosions and demineralization have been reported rarely.[43]

Circulating immune complexes, detected in most patients during exacerbations, usually clear with remissions.[14,20,47,49] These complexes contain IgA, IgG, and IgM, in addition to elements of C3, C4, and C5. IgG antibodies specific for *Escherichia coli* and *Bacteroides fragilis* have been identified in complexes in a concentration much higher than in serum. Granular deposits of immunoglobulin and complement, as well as *E. coli* antigen, have been noted at the dermal-epidermal junction in some patients with arthritis and dermatitis.[14,47] Some have suggested that bacterial overgrowth in the blind loop may result in the antigenic invasion of the systemic circulation by an immune-complex-mediated arthropathy. Peptidoglycan, a bacterial cell wall antigen shared by multiple species of gram-negative bacteria as well as by group A streptococci, is suspected to play a causal role because it produces similar lesions in animal models. Furthermore, skin tests with multiple bacterial strains have reproduced local skin lesions and occasional joint exacerbations in patients with the bowel bypass syndrome.[14]

Nonsteroidal anti-inflammatory agents and antibiotics have met with variable success in management; corticosteroid therapy has been efficacious when used.[47] Transient improvement has been reported during pregnancy.[43] Lasting remissions consistently follow reanastomosis of the bowel.[31,35,43]

ARTHRITIS ASSOCIATED WITH PANCREATIC DISEASE

Nodular subcutaneous fat necrosis, which may clinically mimic erythema nodosum, is a rare manifestation of pancreatic carcinoma or pancreatitis. Analysis of isolated case reports reveals that 10 of 20 patients with fat necrosis complicating pancreatitis also had associated arthritis; arthritis was present in 7 of 9 patients studied with pancreatic carcinoma and subcutaneous fat necrosis. Other, less frequent features include pleuritis with effusion, eosinophilia, ascites, and pericarditis.[39]

Early biopsy of a subcutaneous lesion may yield a picture resembling that of erythema nodosum, but the characteristic necrosis with ''ghost'' fat cells later appears.

Synovial fluid analyses variably show inflammatory or noninflammatory changes, with or without free fat globules.[22,39,46] Biopsy demonstrates proliferation of lining cells and focal fat necrosis in joint capsule.[22] On serial observation, the synovial fluid lipase has been intermittently elevated without correlation with the clinical course.[22] Elevated synovial fluid amylase levels are also found inconstantly.[46] Finally, reduced synovial fluid C3 and C4, together with elevated synovial fluid prostaglandin E values, are noted on occasion.[22] Similar alterations have been reported in pleural, pericardial, and ascitic fluid, with elevated amylase and lipase values and depressed complement components in the presence of immune complexes. In the past, it was presumed that the fat necrosis, serositis, and polyarthritis were focal manifestations of pancreatic enzyme activity. The possibility that an immune complex pathogenesis might be involved in the pancreatitis as well as in some peripheral complications, however, has been suggested by the recognition of the immunologic phenomena.[18]

The ankles and knees are frequently affected, but any joint distal to the hips or shoulders may be involved. Monarticular or oligoarticular disease is common. The appearance of arthritis or serositis in the presence of a subcutaneous fat necrosis syndrome is ominous, with a 76% mortality rate in those with pancreatitis.[39] If the patient recovers, chronic joint sequelae are rare.[22]

REFERENCES

1. Acheson, E.D.: An association between ulcerative colitis, regional enteritis, and ankylosing spondylitis. Q. J. Med., 29:489–499, 1960.
2. Ansell, B.M., and Wigley, R.A.D.: Arthritic manifestations in regional enteritis. Ann. Rheum. Dis., 23:64–72, 1964.
3. Bargen, J.A.: Complications and sequelae of chronic ulcerative colitis. Ann. Intern. Med., 3:335–352, 1929.
4. Black-Schaffer, B.: The tinctorial demonstration of a glycoprotein in Whipple's disease. Proc. Soc. Exp. Biol. Med., 72:225–227, 1949.
5. Bywaters, E.G.L., and Ansell, B.M.: Arthritis associated with ulcerative colitis. Ann. Rheum. Dis., 17:169–183, 1958.
6. Calin, A., and Fries, J.F.: Striking prevalence of ankylosing spondylitis in "healthy" W27 positive males and females. N. Engl. J. Med., 293:835–839, 1975.
7. Canoso, J.J., Saini, M., and Hermos, J.A.: Whipple's disease and ankylosing spondylitis simultaneous occurrence in HLA-B27 positive male. J. Rheumatol., 5:79–84, 1978.
8. Carter, E.T., et al.: Epidemiology of ankylosing spondylitis in Rochester, Minnesota, 1935–1973. Arthritis Rheum., 22:365–370, 1979.
9. Caughey, D.E., and Bywaters, E.G.L.: The arthritis of Whipple's syndrome. Ann. Rheum. Dis., 22:327–335, 1963.
10. Dekker-Saeys, B.J., et al.: Clinical characteristics and results of histocompatibility typing (HLA B27) in 50 patients with both ankylosing spondylitis and inflammatory bowel disease. Ann. Rheum. Dis., 37:36–41, 1978.
11. Dekker-Saeys, B.J., et al.: Prevalence of peripheral arthritis, sacroiliitis, and ankylosing spondylitis in patients suffering from inflammatory bowel disease. Ann. Rheum. Dis., 37:33–35, 1978.
12. Deodhar, S.D., Michener, W.M., and Farmer, R.G.: A study of the immunologic aspects of chronic ulcerative colitis and transmural colitis. Am. J. Clin. Pathol., 51:591–597, 1969.
13. De Wind, L.T., and Payne, J.H.: Intestinal bypass surgery for morbid obesity: long term results. JAMA, 236:2298–2404, 1976.
14. Ely, P.H.: The bowel bypass syndrome: a response to bacterial peptidoglycans. J. Am. Acad. Dermatol., 2:473–487, 1980.
15. Enlow, R.W., Bias, W.B., and Arnett, F.C.: The spondylitis of inflammatory bowel disease: evidence for a non-HLA linked axial arthropathy. Arthritis Rheum., 23:1359–1365, 1980.
16. Espinoza, L.R., et al.: Circulating immune complexes in the seronegative spondyloarthropathies. Clin. Immunol. Immunopathol., 22:384–393, 1982.
17. Farmer, R.G., Hawk, W.A., and Turnbull, R.B., Jr.: Regional enteritis of the colon: a clinical and pathologic comparison with ulcerative colitis. Am. J. Dig. Dis., 13:501–514, 1968.
18. Foy, A., et al.: Immune complexes in acute pancreatitis. Aust. N.Z. J. Med., 11:605–609, 1981.
19. Fernandez-Herlihy, L.: The articular manifestations of chronic ulcerative colitis. N. Engl. J. Med., 261:259–263, 1959.
20. Ginsberg, J., et al.: Musculoskeletal symptoms after jejunoileal shunt surgery for intractable obesity. Am. J. Med., 67:443–448, 1979.
21. Hammer, B., Ashurst, P., and Naish, J.: Diseases associated with ulcerative colitis and Crohn's disease. Gut, 9:17–21, 1968.
22. Hammond, J., and Tesar, J.: Pancreatitis-associated arthritis: sequential study of synovial fluid abnormalities. JAMA, 244:694–696, 1980.
23. Haslock, I., and Wright, V.: The musculoskeletal complications of Crohn's disease. Medicine, 52:217–225, 1973.
24. Hedburg, H.: Studies on synovial fluid in arthritis. Acta Med. Scand., 479 (Suppl.):10–137, 1967.
25. Hench, P.S.: Nelson's Loose-Leaf Surgery. New York, Thomas Nelson and Sons, 1935, p. 104.
26. Hunder, G.G.: Personal communication.
27. Jewell, W.R., Hermreck, A.S., and Hardin, C.A.: Complications of jejunoileal bypass for morbid obesity. Arch. Surg., 110:1039–1042, 1975.
28. Kelly, J.J., and Weisiger, B.B.: The arthritis of Whipple's disease. Arthritis Rheum., 6:615–632, 1963.
29. Kemler, B.J., and Alpert, E.: Inflammatory bowel disease associated circulating immune complexes. Gut, 21:195–201, 1980.
30. Kirsner, J.B., Sklar, M., and Palmer, W.L.: The use of ACTH, cortisone, hydrocortisone and related compounds in the management of ulcerative colitis. Am. J. Med., 22:264–274, 1957.
31. Leff, R.D., Aldo-Benson, M.A., and Madura, J.A.: The effect of revision of the intestinal bypass on post-intestinal bypass arthritis. Arthritis Rheum., 26:678–681, 1983.
32. McEwen, C.: Arthritis accompanying ulcerative colitis. Clin. Orthop., 57:9–17, 1968.
33. McEwen, C., et al.: Arthritis accompanying ulcerative colitis. Am. J. Med., 33:923–941, 1962.
34. Maizel, H., Ruffin, J.M., and Dobbins, W.O.: Whipple's disease: a review of 19 patients from one hospital and a review of the literature since 1950. Medicine, 49:175–205, 1970.
35. Mir-Madjlessi, S.H., Mackenzie, A.H., and Winkelman, E.I.: Articular complications in obese patients after jejunocolic bypass. Cleve. Clin. Q., 41:119–125, 1974.
36. Mitchell, D.N., et al.: Further observations on the Kveim test in Crohn's disease. Lancet, 2:496–499, 1970.
37. Morris, R.I., et al.: HLA-W27—a useful discriminator in the arthropathies of inflammatory bowel disease. N. Engl. J. Med., 290:1117–1119, 1974.
38. Polley, H.F.: The diagnosis and treatment of rheumatoid spondylitis. Med. Clin. North Am., 39:509–528, 1955.
39. Potts, D.E., Mass, M.F., and Iseman, M.D.: Syndrome of pancreatic disease, subcutaneous fat necrosis and polyserositis. Am. J. Med., 58:417–423, 1975.
40. Rotstein, J., Entel, I., and Zeviner, B.: Arthritis associated with ulcerative colitis. Ann. Rheum. Dis., 22:194–197, 1963.
41. Rubinow, A., et al.: Arthritis in Whipple's disease. Isr. J. Med. Sci., 17:445–450, 1981.

42. Ruhl, M.J., and Sokoloff, L.: Thesaurus of rheumatology. Arthritis Rheum., 8:97–182, 1965.
43. Shagrin, J.W., Frame, B., and Duncan, H.: Polyarthritis in obese patients with intestinal bypass. Ann. Intern. Med., 75:377–380, 1971.
44. Shorter, R.G., et al.: Effects of preliminary incubation of lymphocytes with serum on their cytotoxicity for colonic epithelial cells. Gastroenterology, 58:843–850, 1970.
45. Steinberg, V.L., and Storey, G.: Ankylosing spondylitis and chronic inflammatory lesions of the intestines. Br. Med. J., 2:1157–1159, 1957.
46. Tan, A., et al.: Pancreatic arthritis syndrome. South. Med. J., 72:739–741, 1979.
47. Utsinger, P.D.: Systemic immune complex disease following intestinal bypass surgery: bypass disease. J. Am. Acad. Dermatol., 2:488–495, 1980.
48. Utsinger, P.D., et al.: Rheumatoid arthritis following the reactive arthritis of bypass disease. Arthritis Rheum., 25 (Suppl.):S24, 1982.
49. Wands, J.R., et al.: Arthritis associated with intestinal bypass procedure for morbid obesity. N. Engl. J. Med., 294:121–123, 1976.
50. West, H.F.: The aetiology of ankylosing spondylitis. Ann. Rheum. Dis., 8:143–148, 1949.
51. Whipple, G.H.: A hitherto undescribed disease characterized anatomically by deposits of fat and fatty acids in the intestinal and mesenteric lymphatic tissues. Bull. Johns Hopkins Hosp., 18:382–391, 1907.
52. Wilske, K.R., and Decker, J.L.: The articular manifestations of intestinal disease. Bull. Rheum. Dis., 15:362–365, 1965.
53. Wright, R.: Ulcerative colitis. Gastroenterology, 58:875–897, 1970.
54. Wright, R., et al.: Abnormalities of the sacro-iliac joints and uveitis in ulcerative colitis. Q. J. Med., 34:229–236, 1965.
55. Wright, V., and Watkinson, G.: The arthritis of ulcerative colitis. Br. Med. J., 2:670–675, 1965.
56. Wright, V., and Watkinson, G.: Sacro-iliitis and ulcerative colitis. Br. Med. J., 2:675–680, 1965.
57. Zvaifler, N.J., and Martel, W.: Spondylitis in chronic ulcerative colitis. Arthritis Rheum., 3:76–87, 1960.

Chapter 57

Arthritis and Liver Disease

Joseph Duffy and Doyt L. Conn

Until the discovery of the hepatitis B surface antigen as a serologic marker for viral hepatitis,[8] an association between arthritic disorders and liver diseases received little attention. An excellent review by Mills and Sturrock in 1982 described the numerous clinical associations between diseases of the liver and joints.[44]

The first recognition of coexistent arthritis and liver disease dates to the mid-nineteenth century. Graves, in 1843, reported polyarthritis and rash in patients with hepatitis.[27] In 1897, Still recorded a somewhat different observation, that of improvement in patients with juvenile polyarthritis who were also afflicted with catarrhal jaundice.[60] In the 1930s Hench confirmed and extended Still's observation in adults with rheumatoid arthritis and primary fibrositis. Partial or complete relief of joint symptoms appeared prior to or concurrent with spontaneous jaundice of diverse causes. Remissions lasted up to 45 months, but relapse usually occurred in a matter of weeks after resolution of jaundice.[27] Attempts to reproduce this phenomenon by Hench and others were unsuccessful[30] until Thompson and Wyatt administered an empiric combination of bilirubin and bile salts by infusion, which produced the desired beneficial effects.[63] New methods of producing jaundice were constantly being sought, and in 1945 it was shown that the deliberate transmittal of viral hepatitis to rheumatoid patients was also efficacious but the benefit was short-lived.[23]

Jaundice was neither easy to induce nor reproducible by any method, however. These findings led to the search for other remittive agents. During the same era, the analogy of the spontaneous, temporary ameliorating effects of pregnancy on rheumatoid arthritis garnered attention. It was postulated that perhaps jaundice and pregnancy shared similar pathways for their beneficial effects.[31] This theory eventually led to the investigation of possible derangements in hormone metabolism and culminated in the landmark decision to administer an adrenocortical steroid preparation, compound E, to a patient with rheumatoid arthritis in 1948.[32] Additional studies showed the hypothesis of hormonal disturbances to be incorrect, and the liver

has yet to reveal its secrets regarding its salutary effect on arthritis (see also Chap. 98).

In recent years arthritis has been described with several types of primary liver disease. This association has been observed with autoimmune and metabolic disorders as well as with viral hepatitis. We are, therefore, aware of remarkably disparate conditions wherein liver diseases may be associated with arthritis in some circumstances and may produce temporary remissions in others.

This chapter discusses primary liver disorders accompanied by arthritis or other connective tissue syndromes, primary articular diseases in which the liver may be affected, and liver dysfunction associated with the administration of anti-inflammatory drugs.

LIVER DISEASES

Primary Biliary Cirrhosis

Clinical Features. Primary biliary cirrhosis (PBC) is a rare, chronic progressive liver disease characterized by inflammatory destruction of septal and interlobular bile ducts resulting in intrahepatic cholestasis. The disease primarily affects middle-aged women, and there appears to be an increased familial incidence. Recognition of PBC has increased worldwide because of greater physician awareness, detection of elevated serum alkaline phosphatase values through chemistry screening profiles, greater expertise in liver histopathology, and the exclusion of extrahepatic biliary obstruction through newer endoscopic techniques.

The disease may be asymptomatic or may manifest itself with pruritus, fatigue, and slowly progressive jaundice. Although the cause remains obscure, numerous documented abnormalities in humoral and cellular immune functions suggest an autoimmune pathogenesis.[9] Increased concentrations of tissue copper, especially in the liver, are of indeterminate significance and probably reflect the degree and duration of cholestasis, since hepatobiliary clearance is crucial to the homeostasis of this trace metal.

In many patients PBC is clearly a multisystem disease. In the Mayo Clinic series of 113 patients, 84% had at least one associated autoimmune disorder, and 41% had two or more such conditions in addition to PBC (Tables 57–1, 57–2). The autoimmune diseases were more common in women with PBC.[14]

A unique arthropathy may be associated. Ansell

Table 57–1. Autoimmune Associations in 113 Patients With Primary Biliary Cirrhosis

	Patients	(%)
Keratoconjunctivitis sicca		66
Definite	46	
Incipient	20	
Polyarthritis		19
Rheumatoid arthritis	10	
Arthritis of PBC	9	
Scleroderma and variants		18
Scleroderma	3	
CREST syndrome*	7	
Raynaud's phenomenon	8	
Thyroid disorders		19
Hashimoto's thyroiditis	7	
Hypothyroidism and/or goiter	12	
Cutaneous disorders		11
Lichen planus	7	
Discoid lupus erythematosus	2	
Pemphigus	2	
Pernicious anemia		2
Inflammatory bowel disease		1

*CREST syndrome = calcinosis, Raynaud's phenomenon, esophageal dysfunction, sclerodactyly, and telangiectasia.
(From Culp, K.S., et al.[14])

Table 57–2. Patients With Primary Biliary Cirrhosis and Two or More Autoimmune Diseases

Type of Autoimmune Disease*	No. of Patients	% of Total
KCS, thyroid disease	8	17
KCS, arthritis of PBC	6	13
KCS, CREST	5	11
KCS, RA	5	11
KCS, Raynaud's	5	11
KCS, scleroderma	3	7
KCS, Hashimoto's	2	4
KCS, CREST, Hashimoto's	2	4
RA, KCS, Hashimoto's	2	4
LP, KCS, Hashimoto's	1	2
Raynaud's, KCS, RA, Hashimoto's	1	2
LP, Hashimoto's	1	2
Raynaud's, arthritis of PBC	1	2
PA, thyroid disease	1	2
RA, KCS, thyroid disease	1	2
RA, KCS, Raynaud's	1	2
KCS, Raynaud's, arthritis of PBC	1	2
Total	46	100

*KCS = keratoconjunctivitis sicca; CREST = calcinosis, Raynaud's phenomenon, esophageal dysfunction, sclerodactyly, and telangiectasia; RA = rheumatoid arthritis; LP = lichen planus; PA = pernicious anemia; Raynaud's = Raynaud's phenomenon; Hashimoto's = Hashimoto's thyroiditis.
(From Culp, K.S., et al.[14])

and Bywaters first reported erosive bone lesions affecting large and small joints with remarkably few symptoms in three patients with PBC. Hypercholesterolemia was present, and tissue from one osseous lesion showed xanthoma cells.[3] Mills et al. described a case of PBC with fleeting episodes of inflammatory arthritis involving hands, wrists, and shoulders in the presence of hypercholesterolemia.[43] They attributed the joint inflammation to the elevated cholesterol levels, although the report showed no clear-cut demonstration of cause and effect.

In the Mayo Clinic series, 9% of patients exhibited an atypical polyarthritis termed the arthritis of PBC. These patients did not meet the criteria for the diagnosis of definite or classic rheumatoid arthritis. Objective synovitis, usually symmetrical, affected interphalangeal joints of the hands, wrists, ankles, and knees in various combinations. Attacks generally lasted weeks to months, resolved without deformity, and did not recur. Morning stiffness varied in duration, but was significant in fewer than half the patients. In more than 80% the diagnosis of the liver disorder antedated the onset of arthritis. Most patients had or developed additional autoimmune disease features. There was no apparent relationship between the arthropathy and the histologic stage or progression of PBC.[14]

Distinctive radiographic features have been reported in some patients with PBC. In 1979 Marx and O'Connell described small, asymmetric, intracapsular, and nonarticular cortical bone erosions, mainly involving the distal small joints of the hands, accompanied by joint space narrowing in 6 of 12 PBC patients[39] (Figs. 57–1, 57–2). Subsequently, an extensive prospective radiologic survey of 42 patients with PBC confirmed the presence of

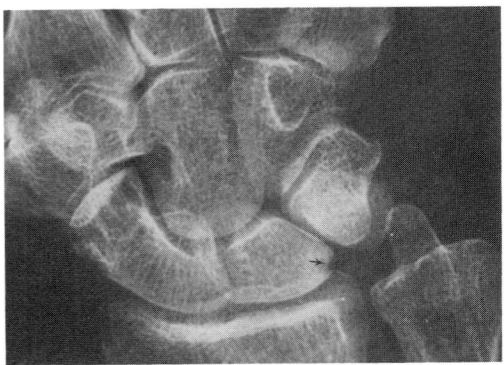

Fig. 57–1. Arthritis associated with primary biliary cirrhosis. Small cortical erosion in lunate. (From Marx, W.J., and O'Connell, D.J.: Arch. Intern. Med., *139*:213–216. Copyright 1979, American Medical Association.[39])

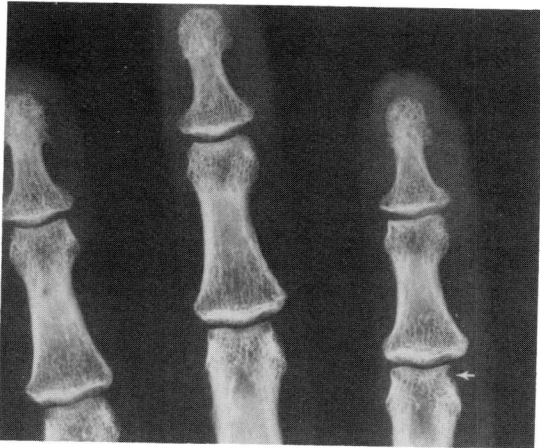

Fig. 57–2. Arthritic cortical erosion in proximal interphalangeal joint. (From Marx, W.J., and O'Connell, D.J.: Arch. Intern. Med., *139*:213–216. Copyright 1979, American Medical Association.[39])

articular erosions, usually in small joints, in 31% of cases. Additional significant radiographic findings in this study included hypertrophic osteoarthropathy in 38% of the cases, osteopenia, and lytic medullary bone defects typical of cholesterol deposition.[42] One report described a surprising number of patients with avascular necrosis of femoral or humeral heads.[10] Chondrocalcinosis has also been reported in a few patients.[39]

Rheumatoid arthritis (RA) coexists with PBC more often than expected by chance alone, with the prevalence ranging from 5 to 10% in several large series.[14,43,58] In the Mayo Clinic series, rheumatoid disease preceded the diagnosis of PBC in 45% of patients. All patients affected by RA had additional autoimmune disease features, usually keratoconjunctivitis sicca.[14]

The sicca complex of dry eyes and dry mouth is the most common extrahepatic autoimmune disorder in patients with PBC. The prevalence varies from 66 to 100% of cases depending upon the extent of testing to make the diagnosis. Sicca symptoms are usually mild and elicited only upon direct questioning. It is wise to include rose bengal staining in the ophthalmologic examinations of PBC patients because many cases of keratoconjunctivitis sicca may be discovered in a presymptomatic stage. The sicca syndrome is often associated with concurrent rheumatoid arthritis, scleroderma, and thyroid disease. It is usually preceded by the diagnosis of PBC (89%) and does not correlate with the duration or severity of liver disease.[1,14] The description of circulating Ro/anti-Ro (SSA) immune complexes and parotid deposition of anti-Ro in complexed form suggests a pathogenic potential for

circulating immune complexes in the development of the sicca syndrome in patients with PBC.[46]

Since the description of scleroderma in association with PBC in 1964,[4] there have been several confirmatory reports.[10,14,41,50] The full spectrum of scleroderma has been encountered, with the prevalence varying from 3 to 17% if patients with Raynaud's phenomenon alone are excluded.[10,14,58] Most cases are mild, nonprogressive, and constitute incomplete or complete expressions of the CREST variant. Although either liver disease or scleroderma may appear first, 50% of patients in one series exhibited one or more features of scleroderma prior to the diagnosis of PBC.[14]

A number of other autoimmune disorders have been described in patients with PBC. Renal tubular and pulmonary diffusion defects, perhaps due to an autoimmune process, occur in 52% and 40%, respectively, of patients with PBC when appropriate tests are performed.[26] Clinical features and overt or latent thyroid function abnormalities reveal a prevalence of thyroid disease in 19 to 26% of patients. Hashimoto's thyroiditis and antithyroid antibodies are most common.[13,14] Cases of discoid and systemic lupus erythematosus or lupus-like syndromes,[14,34,65] lichen planus, pemphigus, pernicious anemia, inflammatory bowel disease,[14] and polymyalgia rheumatica[51] have been reported. In addition, we reported an extraordinary case of Churg-Strauss vasculitis with temporal arteritis, polychondritis, and PBC in a single patient.[11]

Laboratory Features. The liver disease itself may account for nonspecific hematologic changes, including anemia, variable leukocyte and platelet counts, and an elevated sedimentation rate. Serum protein abnormalities show hypoalbuminemia and hyperglobulinemia. Liver function studies are usually dominated by a marked increase in serum alkaline phosphatase levels in contrast to lesser elevations of serum transaminase values. Elevation of serum cholesterol levels has been neither significant nor consistent in patients with articular complaints or peripheral joint erosive lesions.[14,39] Numerous autoantibodies have been detected (Table 57–3), the hallmark being antimitochondrial antibody in 96% of patients. Prevalence of other autoantibodies has varied from 22 to 70%.[14] Rheumatoid factor, antinuclear antibody, and antibody to extractable nuclear antigens have shown no clear-cut relationship with the arthropathy of PBC.[28,39] Serum concentrations of major immunoglobulins are elevated in almost all cases of PBC. IgM levels are increased in 95% of cases and occasionally are of monoclonal origin. Elevated IgG values are observed in about 40% of cases. In contrast, the percentage of patients with elevated IgA

Table 57–3. Autoantibodies in 113 Patients With Primary Biliary Cirrhosis

	Number Tested	Positive No.	%
Antimitochondrial antibodies	113	108	96
Rheumatoid factor	20	14	70
Smooth muscle antibody	29	19	66
Thyroid-specific antibodies	17	7	41
Extractable nuclear antigen	10	3	30
Antinuclear antibody	56	13	23
Antibody to native DNA	9	2	22

(From Culp, K.S., et al.[14])

levels increases with histologic evidence of disease progression.[14]

Circulating immune complexes, including cryoproteins, have been described in several large series of patients with or without extrahepatic features of PBC.[18,28,68] A longitudinal study, examining levels of immune complexes over three years, showed a subset of PBC patients with autoimmune disease and both a greater prevalence and higher mean levels of circulating immune complexes compared with those patients without autoimmune features.[28] This observation supports an earlier hypothesis that defective Kupffer cell-mediated clearance of complexes may result in higher circulating levels with potential for damage to organs besides the liver.[62] No particular target organ specificity seems associated with elevated levels of immune complexes, however. Antigens in these complexes include mitochondrial[45] and hepatic canalicular and ductular[2] components. These components indicate that more than one antigen-antibody system exists which, in turn, could have some bearing on the types of clinical manifestations. Use of the C1q binding assay in patients with PBC showed complexes in 31 of 50 (62%) patients, 17 of whom had arthritis. Most cases were rheumatoid factor-positive, but precise classification of the arthritic disorders was lacking.[12]

Evidence is abundant for activation of the complement cascade via the classic and alternative pathways.[36] Complement activation appears to be of little clinical significance, however, except for a report of reduced serum C4 levels in PBC patients with autoimmune features. C3 values in the same group of patients were normal.[28]

Chronic Active Hepatitis

Chronic active hepatitis is a continuous inflammatory disease of the liver lasting beyond the expected period of resolution. This condition may be idiopathic or induced by several diverse agents, and may progress to cirrhosis or liver failure.[15] The idiopathic disease, occurring primarily in young

women with multisystem involvement, forms the basis of this discussion. Lupoid hepatitis was a popular early term because many patients had lupus erythematosus (LE) cells and clinical features of a multisystem disorder resembling systemic lupus erythematosus.[38] No impressive clinical differences in LE cell-positive or LE cell-negative patients were found, however, that would characterize "lupoid" hepatitis as a distinct entity.[59] Smooth muscle antibody is reported to be a reliable serologic marker since it is detectable in most patients with chronic active hepatitis but is rarely found in systemic lupus erythematosus or in noninflammatory liver disease.[47] However, the demonstration of smooth muscle, antimitochondrial, and antinuclear antibodies may not enhance diagnostic accuracy of chronic active hepatitis since they may be undetectable in 15% of patients with severe disease.[15]

Multisystem involvement occurs in approximately 63% of patients.[26] Polyarthralgias and, less commonly, polyarthritis are observed in one-fourth to one-half of patients.[15,26] Large and small joints are affected. Periarticular swelling may be striking, but joint effusion is seldom encountered. Although occasional patients exhibit erosive rheumatoid-like disease, the arthropathy is usually transient and appears to coincide with episodes of relapse of the liver disease. Synovial histology is nonspecific, with findings of hypertrophy, plasma cell infiltration, fibrosis, and vascular proliferation.[26] Fibrinoid material on the synovial surface and IgG, IgM, and C3 deposits in the surface fibrinoid have been reported.[6]

Most organ systems have been affected to a variable degree and in various combinations in chronic active hepatitis, but renal disease and neurologic disorders are seldom serious.[47]

Cryptogenic Cirrhosis

In general, multisystem disease occurs less frequently in association with cryptogenic cirrhosis (38%) than in primary biliary cirrhosis or chronic active hepatitis. Essentially the same major organ systems are affected, however, as with the other chronic liver diseases. Although patient numbers are small in this group, the prevalence of pulmonary diffusion defects and peripheral neuropathy is surprisingly high. Arthralgia or arthritis is encountered only rarely (3%).[26]

Viral Hepatitis

Hepatitis B infection is an example of a disorder in which a single infectious agent, in combination with the host immune response, causes several immune complex syndromes. These syndromes are considered in detail in the chapter on viral arthritis (see Chap. 101).

The most common syndrome is an acute, often severe, symmetrical polyarthritis involving multiple joints simultaneously or less often in a migratory or additive pattern. Involvement of large and small joints is generally the rule. Synovial fluid is often inflammatory but nondiagnostic. The arthritis is short-lived, responding rapidly to aspirin. It usually disappears coincident with the appearance of jaundice.

Urticarial, petechial, and/or maculopapular rashes commonly appear with the arthritis and last days to weeks. Articular pain and rash usually precede the appearance of jaundice. Many patients, however, are never jaundiced, and the illness may be indistinguishable from other connective tissue syndromes unless serial liver function tests are performed.[19]

A less common but more serious illness is necrotizing vasculitis. Patients are usually profoundly ill and exhibit involvement of more than one major organ system. Fever, joint pain, mononeuritis multiplex, renal disease, and cardiac disease are the most prominent findings initially.[19,35,57] In one study, joint pain occurred in 100% of vasculitis patients with hepatitis B infection in contrast to only 55% of vasculitis patients who were hepatitis B negative.[57] These patients have a prolonged illness that is fatal in some cases in spite of treatment with corticosteroids alone or in combination with immunosuppressive drugs.[19,35,57]

Hemochromatosis

An arthropathy may be associated with hemochromatosis in 50% of the cases[40] (see also Chap. 96). The arthropathy may be the presenting complaint. In most cases the arthropathy accompanies hemochromatosis with clinical and histologic evidence of liver involvement and elevated serum iron and transferrin levels. Characteristically, it is a chronic degenerative polyarthritis. The joints that are commonly involved are the second and third metacarpophalangeal joints and the proximal interphalangeal joints of the hands, wrists, knees, and hips. This degenerative arthropathy accompanying hemochromatosis affects younger individuals with the average age 50, as compared to idiopathic primary osteoarthritis. The pattern of joint involvement is clearly different from that of "nodal" osteoarthritis. Roentgenographic changes of the involved joints include subchondral sclerosis, cyst formation, and joint space narrowing. Chondrocalcinosis may be seen in 70% of these patients along with increases in extent and number of joints involved with time. Chondrocalcinosis affects older patients predominantly. Attacks of acute pseudogout may occur and calcium pyrophosphate dihydrate crystals may be demonstrated in the synovial fluid of an involved joint. (see Chaps. 4 and 94).

Patients have presented with a chronic arthropathy and elevated serum iron and transferrin levels before any significant liver damage can be demonstrated.[37] In addition, a patient has been reported with the characteristic arthropathy, normal serum iron levels, but a liver biopsy consistent with hemochromatosis.[53] The chondrocalcinosis has not been shown to regress or to demonstrate control as a result of phlebotomy treatment of the hemochromatosis, which depletes the iron stores. However, this treatment has not been examined in those patients with arthropathy and mild or subclinical liver disease.[29]

Arthropathy has been most commonly reported in association with idiopathic hemochromatosis, but may also occur in secondary hemochromatosis (not necessarily the hemochromatosis secondary to alcoholic cirrhosis). There is a significant association of HLA A3 with idiopathic hemochromatosis.[48] Whether there is a closer association with certain of the clinical features of hemochromatosis, such as the arthropathy, is unknown.

Wilson's Disease

Osteoarthritis commonly accompanies Wilson's disease (see also Chap. 96) and involves the large joints and the spine.[25] Spinal osteophyte formation and squaring of the vertebral bodies may occur, simulating ankylosing spondylitis. A roentgenographic picture of osteochondritis dissecans may be present in the knee. Chondrocalcinosis has been seen, but is less common than in hemochromatosis. The loss of bone density, which is the most common roentgenographic abnormality noted in Wilson's disease, is commonly demonstrated in the hands, feet, and spine. Schmorl's nodes are present, involving the midthoracic and lumbar spine. The incidence of fractures in these patients is high. The bone loss results from loss of calcium and phosphorus in the urine due to a renal tubular defect. Rickets and osteomalacia may occur.

LIVER INVOLVEMENT SECONDARY TO CONNECTIVE TISSUE DISEASES

Rheumatoid Arthritis

Liver involvement, in the past, has not been thought to be a significant feature of rheumatoid arthritis. Hepatomegaly has been observed in about 10% of patients with rheumatoid arthritis. However, with the routine use of serum chemistry profiles in the evaluation of patients with rheumatoid arthritis, liver function abnormalities are noted frequently. From 25 to 50% of patients with rheumatoid arthritis have abnormal biochemical tests of liver function.[22] The abnormal tests are usually the liver alkaline phosphatase and the gamma glutamyl transpeptidase. These elevated serum enzymes have been correlated with the presence of associated Sjögren's syndrome and the activity of the arthritis.[69] The elevated liver alkaline phosphatase correlates with other laboratory indicators of disease activity, such as an elevated erythrocyte sedimentation rate, diminished serum albumin, elevated serum gamma globulins, and a diminished serum iron. Patients with rheumatoid arthritis have a 1.5% incidence of antimitochondrial antibodies. Those patients with antimitochondrial and smooth muscle antibodies have a higher prevalence of hepatomegaly, splenomegaly, and abnormal liver function tests. There have been case reports of liver rupture associated with rheumatoid vasculitis.[33] These patients have other clinical features indicating an underlying vasculitis. Study of the liver tissue in patients with rheumatoid arthritis and serum enzyme abnormalities has revealed nonspecific changes of Kupffer cell hyperplasia and infiltration of the periportal regions with mononuclear cells.

Patients with rheumatoid arthritis are treated with a variety of drugs that may be potentially hepatotoxic, particularly the nonsteroidal anti-inflammatory drugs. No association has been found between liver dysfunction and the use of a particular drug in rheumatoid arthritis. On the contrary, patients successfully treated with anti-inflammatory agents, specifically corticosteroids, usually demonstrate an improvement in liver function. Seronegative arthritis patients treated with similar nonsteroidal anti-inflammatory drugs are less likely to demonstrate liver function abnormalities than patients who are seropositive.[51]

Felty's Syndrome

Felty's syndrome is associated with a particular liver abnormality, *nodular regenerative hyperplasia,* which may lead to certain clinical manifestations, particularly gastrointestinal hemorrhage due to portal hypertension and esophageal varices.

Histologic evidence of liver damage may be present in 60% of patients with Felty's syndrome.[64] An equal number of patients show liver function abnormalities, and some patients with abnormal liver histology may have normal liver function tests. The histologic abnormalities include nodular regenerative hyperplasia, portal fibrosis, lymphocytic infiltration of the sinusoids, and Kupffer cell hyperplasia. Nodular regenerative hyperplasia has been found in about 25% of patients with Felty's syndrome, and is diagnosed histologically if there are two populations of hepatocytes, large cells, and small cells, and if the nodular regions contain the large cells. Fibrous septa are not present. The diagnosis of nodular regenerative hyperplasia may

not always be made by liver biopsy, because occasionally the nodule may not be sampled and the surrounding tissue will appear normal.

Portal hypertension, esophageal varices, and gastrointestinal bleeding occur most commonly in those patients with Felty's syndrome and associated nodular regenerative hyperplasia of the liver. The clinical, serologic, or extra-articular features of disease in patients with Felty's syndrome are no different in those with or without histologic abnormalities in the liver. Patients with Felty's syndrome and significant liver changes usually do not develop the serious clinical complications of ascites and deterioration of liver function that may occur in cirrhosis. Because of the gastrointestinal bleeding, however, some patients require splenectomy and a portal shunt to control the bleeding complications.[7]

Still's Disease

Juvenile arthritis and, particularly, the acute systemic form of the disease, Still's disease, have been associated with hepatomegaly and elevation of the serum transaminases.[55] This association has not led to chronic liver disease. Likewise, similar features may occur in adult Still's disease. Patients with adult Still's disease may have hepatomegaly, splenomegaly, and elevated serum transaminase.[20] The histologic abnormalities in the liver in juvenile and adult Still's disease are similar to those seen in rheumatoid arthritis with mononuclear cell infiltration of the sinusoids and portal tracts and Kupffer cell hyperplasia.

Systemic Lupus Erythematosus

Clinically, significant liver disease is uncommon in systemic lupus erythematosus, but subclinical liver involvement is being recognized more commonly. Approximately 50% of patients with systemic lupus erythematosus have elevated serum transaminase values.[24] Liver enlargement may be detected in over 30% of patients. In some of these patients, the serum biochemical abnormality is due to the effect of drugs, particularly the nonsteroidal anti-inflammatory drugs. Patients with active lupus erythematosus may be more susceptible to the hepatotoxic effect of nonsteroidal anti-inflammatory drugs, including aspirin. It has been estimated that in 20% of the cases, the elevated serum enzymes are caused by lupus-induced liver disease.

The most common histologic finding in the liver of patients with systemic lupus erythematosus is steatosis. In part, this condition may be related to the use of corticosteroids. A variety of nonspecific histologic abnormalities may be found in the liver of patients with systemic lupus erythematosus, including inflammatory cell infiltration of the portal tract, granulomatous hepatitis, chronic active hepatitis, and even cirrhosis.[54] Granulomatous hepatitis, chronic active hepatitis, and cirrhosis have been found in only a small number of patients in whom no other etiology could be determined. It is not known whether these patients have coincidental liver disease and systemic lupus erythematosus, liver disease as a manifestation of systemic lupus erythematosus, or autoimmune manifestations of chronic active hepatitis resembling those of systemic lupus erythematosus.

Some patients with chronic active hepatitis fulfill the American Rheumatism Association criteria for systemic lupus erythematosus. This group has been referred to as ''lupoid hepatitis.'' The presence of smooth muscle antibodies is more common in chronic active hepatitis than in systemic lupus erythematosus and may help in differentiation (vide supra). There does not appear to be an increased prevalence of hepatitis B surface antigen in systemic lupus erythematosus. As in rheumatoid arthritis, there are rare case reports of an arteritis causing liver infarction and rupture.

Polymyalgia Rheumatica and Giant Cell Arteritis

Liver function abnormalities, especially elevated serum liver alkaline phosphatase, occur in patients with giant cell arteritis[17] (see also Chaps. 59 and 63). These abnormalities occur in patients with more severe disease as indicated by constitutional features, including fever, weight loss, anorexia, and anemia. Liver function abnormalities occur less commonly in polymyalgia rheumatica without giant cell arteritis. The liver histologic abnormalities in patients with giant cell arteritis and liver function abnormalities include fatty changes, mild patchy liver necrosis, mononuclear cell infiltration, and granulomas.[67] The liver function abnormalities return to normal after corticosteroid therapy.

EFFECTS OF ANTIRHEUMATIC DRUGS ON THE LIVER

Salicylates

Serum transaminases may be elevated as a result of treatment with aspirin in patients with rheumatoid arthritis, systemic lupus erythematosus, and juvenile polyarthritis.[49] This elevation occurs most commonly in lupus erythematosus and juvenile polyarthritis. The serum transaminases are elevated more frequently when the salicylate level is greater than 25 mg/dl, but the transaminase elevation may occur at lower salicylate blood levels. The abnormalities are reversible on discontinuing the salicylates. Progression to significant liver disease has not been reported.

Because salicylates have been implicated as a causal factor in Reye's syndrome, they are not rec-

ommended for children with varicella or for those suspected of having influenza.[61] However, the studies that led to this conclusion were based on small numbers of cases, varying definitions of disease, and imprecise methods for determining the salicylate usage.[16]

Nonsteroidal Anti-Inflammatory Drugs

Liver function abnormalities, especially elevated serum transaminase levels, have been reported in patients taking sulindac, ibuprofen, naproxen, and fenoprofen. In some patients, such abnormalities occur as part of a toxic reaction manifest by fever and rash. Other patients show only an elevation of the serum transaminase levels without any associated clinical features. The laboratory abnormalities disappear with the discontinuation of the drug.

Phenylbutazone causes hypersensitivity-type liver damage and also has an intrinsic hepatotoxic potential. In most patients, the hepatic injury appears during the first six weeks of drug use and is accompanied by other features of hypersensitivity, including fever and a skin eruption.[66] The liver injury caused by phenylbutazone may result in intrahepatic cholestasis.[5] Hepatic granulomas have been detected in patients with phenylbutazone-induced hypersensitivity liver disease. Phenylbutazone is known to cause toxic hepatitis, sometimes with fatal outcome.

Gold and Penicillamine

Rare cases have been reported of hepatotoxicity in rheumatoid arthritis patients taking either gold or penicillamine.[21,52] It is usually manifest by cholestatic jaundice. The mechanism of the liver toxicity in most cases is hypersensitivity because the patients commonly have fever, skin eruption, and eosinophilia. The liver abnormalities resolve when the drug is withdrawn. It is important to recognize this rare complication of gold and penicillamine treatment and differentiate it from the surgical condition of extrahepatic biliary tract obstruction. The clinical appearance of the drug-induced cholestatic jaundice may simulate extrahepatic biliary tract obstruction.[56]

Azathioprine and Methotrexate

Liver function abnormalities may occur in patients treated with these drugs. Liver function abnormalities, especially elevated serum transaminase, occurs in rheumatoid patients taking azathioprine. This occurrence is infrequent, however, and does not result in significant liver disease.[70] This liver function abnormality returns to normal upon discontinuation of the drug.

Serum transaminase elevations may occur also in rheumatoid patients treated with methotrexate.

An elevated SGOT has been reported in 15% of the patients treated using doses of methotrexate of 7.5 to 15 mg per week.[72] Liver biopsy in these patients has not revealed significant pathologic changes. It is not known how many of these patients will eventually develop histologically significant liver disease, but caution must be observed because of the significant liver disease that has occurred in patients with psoriasis treated with methotrexate. *In these cases, liver function tests did not predict significant histologic liver damage.* Progression to cirrhosis in the methotrexate-treated psoriatic patients was related to risk factors such as alcohol consumption and total cumulative dose. Consequently, it has been suggested that a cumulative dose of methotrexate beyond 1.5 g needs tissue surveillance.[71]

REFERENCES

1. Alarcon-Segovia, D., Diaz-Jauonen, E., and Fishbein, E.: Features of Sjögren's syndrome in primary biliary cirrhosis. Ann. Intern. Med., 79:31–35, 1973.
2. Amoroso, P., et al.: Identification of biliary antigens in circulating immune complexes in primary biliary cirrhosis. Clin. Exp. Immunol., 42:95–98, 1980.
3. Ansell, B.M., and Bywaters, E.G.L.: Histiocytic bone and joint disease. Ann. Rheum. Dis., 16:503–510, 1957.
4. Bartholomew, L.G., et al.: Chronic diseases of the liver with systemic scleroderma. Am. J. Dig. Dis., 9:43–55, 1964.
5. Benjamin, S.B., et al.: Phenylbutazone liver injury: A clinical-pathologic survey of 23 cases and review of the literature. Hepatology, 1:255–263, 1981.
6. Bernardo, D.E., Vernon-Roberts, B., and Currey, H.L.F.: A case of active chronic hepatitis with painless erosive arthritis. Gut, 14:800–804, 1973.
7. Blendis, L.M., et al.: Oesophageal variceal bleeding in Felty's syndrome associated with nodular regenerative hyperplasia. Ann. Rheum. Dis., 37:183–186, 1978.
8. Blumberg, B.S., Alter, H.J., and Visrich, S.: A "new" antigen in leukemic sera. J.A.M.A., 191:541–546, 1965.
9. Bodenheimer, H.C., and Schaffner, F.: Primary biliary cirrhosis and the immune system. J. Gastroenterol., 72:285–296, 1979.
10. Clarke, A.K., et al.: Rheumatic disorders in primary biliary cirrhosis. Ann. Rheum. Dis., 37:42–47, 1978.
11. Conn, D.L., Dickson, E.R., and Carpenter, H.A.: The association of Churg-Strauss vasculitis with temporal artery involvement, primary biliary cirrhosis, and polychondritis in a single patient. J. Rheumatol., 9:744–748, 1982.
12. Crowe, J.P., et al.: Increased C1q binding and arthritis in primary biliary cirrhosis. Gut, 21:418–422, 1980.
13. Crowe, J.P., et al.: Primary biliary cirrhosis: The prevalence of hypothyroidism and its relationship to thyroid autoantibodies and sicca syndrome. Gastroenterology, 78:1438–1441, 1980.
14. Culp, K.S., et al.: Autoimmune associations in primary biliary cirrhosis. Mayo Clin. Proc., 57:365–370, 1982.
15. Czaja, A.J.: Current problems in the diagnosis and management of chronic active hepatitis. Mayo Clin. Proc., 56:311–323, 1981.
16. Daniels, S.R., Greenberg, R.S., and Ibrahim, M.A.: Scientific uncertainties in the studies of salicylate use and Reye's syndrome. J.A.M.A., 249:1311–1316, 1983.
17. Dickson, E.R., et al.: Systemic giant cell arteritis with polymyalgia rheumatica. J.A.M.A., 244:1496–1498, 1973.
18. Dienstag, J.L., et al.: Circulating immune complexes in primary biliary cirrhosis: Interactions with lymphoid cells. Clin. Exp. Immunol., 50:7–16, 1982.
19. Duffy, J., et al.: Polyarthritis, polyarteritis, and hepatitis B. Medicine, 55:19–37, 1976.
20. Esdaile, J.M., et al.: Hepatic abnormalities in adult onset Still's disease. J. Rheumatol., 6:673–679, 1979.
21. Favreau, M., Tannenbaum, H., and Lough, J.: Hepatic toxicity associated with gold therapy. Ann. Intern. Med., 87:717–719, 1977.
22. Fernandes, L., et al.: Studies on the frequency and pathogenesis of liver involvement in rheumatoid arthritis. Ann. Rheum. Dis., 38:501–506, 1979.
23. Gardner, F., Stewart, A., and MacCallum, F.O.: Therapeutic effect of induced jaundice in rheumatoid arthritis. Br. Med. J., 2:677–680, 1945.
24. Gibson, T., and Myers, A.R.: Subclinical liver disease in systemic lupus erythematosus. J. Rheumatol., 8:752–759, 1981.
25. Golding, D.N., and Walshe, J.M.: Arthropathy of Wilson's disease. Ann. Rheum. Dis., 36:99–111, 1977.
26. Golding, P.L., Smith, M., and Williams, R.: Multisystem involvement in chronic liver disease. Am. J. Med., 55:772–782, 1973.
27. Graves, R.J.: Clinical Lectures on the Practice of Medicine. Dublin, Fannin and Co., 1843, p. 937.
28. Gupta, R.C., et al.: Immune complexes in primary biliary cirrhosis. Am. J. Med., 73:192–198, 1982.
29. Hamilton, E.B.D., et al.: The natural history of arthritis in idiopathic haemochromatosis: Progression of the clinical and radiological features over ten years. Q. J. Med., 50:321–329, 1981.
30. Hench, P.S.: Effect of jaundice on chronic infectious (atrophic) arthritis and primary fibrositis. Arch. Intern. Med., 61:451–480, 1938.
31. Hench, P.S.: The ameliorating effect of pregnancy on chronic atrophic (infectious rheumatoid) arthritis, fibrositis, and intermittent hydrarthrosis. Mayo Clin. Proc., 13:161–167, 1938.
32. Hench, P.S., et al.: The effect of a hormone of the adrenal cortex (17-hydroxy-11-dehydrocorticosterone: Compound E) and of pituitary adrenocorticotropic hormone on rheumatoid arthritis. Mayo Clin. Proc., 24:181–197, 1949.
33. Hocking, W.G., et al.: Spontaneous hepatic rupture in rheumatoid arthritis. Arch. Intern. Med., 141:792–794, 1981.
34. Iliffe, G.D., Naidoo, S., and Hunter, T.: Primary biliary cirrhosis associated with features of systemic lupus erythematosus. Dig. Dis. Sci., 27:274–278, 1982.
35. Inman, R.D.: Rheumatic manifestations of hepatitis B infections. Semin. Arthritis Rheum., 11:406–420, 1982.
36. Jones, E.A., et al.: Primary biliary cirrhosis and the complement system. Ann. Intern. Med., 90:72–84, 1979.
37. M'Seffar, A., Fornasier, V.L., and Fox, I.H.: Arthropathy as the major clinical indicator of occult iron storage disease. J.A.M.A., 238:1825–1828, 1977.
38. Mackay, I.R., Taft, L.I., and Cowling, D.C.: Lupoid hepatitis. Lancet, 2:1323–1326, 1956.
39. Marx, W.J., and O'Connell, D.J.: Arthritis of primary biliary cirrhosis. Arch. Intern. Med., 139:213–216, 1979.
40. Milder, M.S., et al.: Idiopathic hemochromatosis, an interim report. Medicine, 59:34–49, 1980.
41. Miller, F., et al.: Primary biliary cirrhosis and scleroderma. Arch. Pathol. Lab. Med., 103:505–509, 1979.
42. Mills, P.R., et al.: A prospective survey of radiological bone and joint changes in primary biliary cirrhosis. Clin. Radiol., 32:297–302, 1981.
43. Mills, P.R., et al.: Hypercholesterolemic arthropathy in primary biliary cirrhosis. Ann. Rheum. Dis., 37:179–180, 1978.
44. Mills, P.R., and Sturrock, R.D.: Clinical associations between arthritis and liver disease. Ann. Rheum. Dis., 41:295–307, 1982.
45. Penner, E., et al.: Immune complexes in primary biliary cirhosis contain mitochondrial antigens. Clin. Immunol. Immunopathol., 22:394–399, 1982.
46. Penner, E., and Reichlin, M.: Primary biliary cirrhosis associated with Sjögren's syndrome: Evidence for circulating and tissue-desposited Ro/anti-Ro immune complexes. Arthritis Rheum., 25:1250–1253, 1982.
47. Plotz, P.H.: Autoimmunity in hepatitis. Med. Clin. North Am., 59:869–876, 1975.

48. Powell, L.W., Bassett, M.L., and Halliday, J.W.: Hemochromatosis: 1980 update. Gastroenterology, 78:374–381, 1980.
49. Prescott, L.F.: Hepatotoxicity of mild analgesics. Br. J. Clin. Pharmacol., 10:373S-379S, 1980.
50. Reynolds, T.B., et al.: Primary biliary cirrhosis with scleroderma, Raynaud's phenomenon, and telangiectasia. Am. J. Med., 50:302–312, 1971.
51. Robertson, J.C., Batstone, G.F., and Loebl, W.Y.: Polymyalgia rheumatica and primary biliary cirrhosis. Br. Med. J., 2:1128, 1978.
52. Rosenbaum, J., Katz, W.A., and Schumacher, H.R.: Hepatotoxicity associated with use of D-penicillamine in rheumatoid arthritis. Ann. Rheum. Dis., 39:152–154, 1980.
53. Rosner, I.A., et al.: Arthropathy, hypouricemia and normal serum iron studies in hereditary hemochromatosis. Am. J. Med., 70:870–874, 1981.
54. Rynyon, B.A., LaBrecque, D.R., and Anuras, S.: The spectrum of liver disease in systemic lupus erythematosus. Am. J. Med., 69:187–194, 1980.
55. Schaller, J.G., Beckwith, B., and Wedgwood, R.J.: Hepatic involvement in juvenile rheumatoid arthritis. J. Pediatr., 77:203–210, 1970.
56. Seibold, J.R., Lynch. C.J., and Medsger, T.A.: Cholestasis associated with D-penicillamine therapy: Case report and review of the literature. Arthritis Rheum., 24:554–556, 1981.
57. Sergent, J.S., et al.: Vasculitis with hepatitis B antigenemia. Medicine, 55:1–18, 1976.
58. Sherlock, S., and Scheuer, P.J.: The presentation and diagnosis of 100 patients with primary biliary cirrhosis. N. Engl. J. Med., 289:674–678, 1973.
59. Soloway, R.D., et al.: "Lupoid" hepatitis, a nonentity in the spectrum of chronic active disease. Gastroenterology, 63:458–465, 1972.
60. Still, G.F.: On a form of chronic joint disease in children. Med. Chir. Trans., 80:47–60, 1897.
61. Surgeon General's advisory on the use of salicylates and Reye's syndrome. Morbid. Mortal. Weekly Rep., 31:289–90, 1982.
62. Thomas, H.C., Potter, B.J., and Sherlock, G.: Is primary biliary cirrhosis an immune complex disease? Lancet, 2:1261–1263, 1977.
63. Thompson, H.E., and Wyatt, B.L.: Experimentally induced jaundice (hyperbilirubinemia). Arch. Intern. Med., 61:481–500, 1938.
64. Thorne, C., et al.: Liver disease in Felty's syndrome. Am. J. Med., 73:35–40, 1982.
65. Unpublished observations.
66. van de Merwe, J.P., van Blankenstein, M., and Wilson, J.H.P.: Intrahepatic cholestasis induced by phenylbutazone. Digestion, 22:317–320, 1981.
67. Von Knorring, J., and Wasatjerna, C.: Liver involvement in polymyalgia rheumatica. Scand. J. Rheumatol., 5:197–204, 1976.
68. Wands, J.R., et al.: Circulating immune complexes and complement activation in primary biliary cirrhosis. N. Engl. J. Med., 298:233–237, 1978.
69. Webb, J., et al.: Liver disease in rheumatoid arthritis and Sjögren's syndrome. Ann. Rheum. Dis., 34:70–81, 1975.
70. Whisnant, J.K., and Pelkey, J.: Rheumatoid arthritis: Treatment with azathioprine (Imuran®). Clinical side-effects and laboratory abnormalities. Ann. Rheum. Dis., 41 (Suppl. 1):44–47, 1982.
71. Willkens, R.F., and Watson, M.A.: Methotrexate: A perspective of its use in the treatment of rheumatic diseases. J. Lab. Clin. Med., 100:314–321, 1982.
72. Willkens, R.F., Watson, M.A., and Paxson, C.S.: Low dose pulse methotrexate therapy in rheumatoid arthritis. J. Rheumatol., 7:501–505, 1980.

Chapter 58

Intermittent and Periodic Arthritic Syndromes

George E. Ehrlich

Almost all the diseases considered in this book are characterized by intermittent manifestations of some of their symptoms. It is the symptom, however, superimposed on a progressive anatomic lesion, that is intermittent, and not the underlying disease. An example is the stiffness experienced by RA patients in the mornings and after rest. Although the stiffness may fluctuate, one cannot pretend that this manifestation represents a fluctuation of rheumatoid arthritis. The rhythmicity of symptoms thus reflects the patterns of nature, not the natural history of the disease itself. Nor are remissions and exacerbations exceptions to the rule in most disorders, not even in gout, where hyperuricemia and tophi often persist between attacks, unless altered by successful treatment.

A few disorders, however, produce intermittent symptoms, often with disease-free intercritical periods. Although some have been lumped together as *periodic disease,* others clearly present different pictures. The only link among these disorders seems to be their intermittency; they are relatively uncommon, their causes remain unknown, and their existence is controverted by some. With the possible exception of familial Mediterranean fever, which appears to be a heritable disease, these intermittent entities should be regarded as syndromes rather than diseases. Their definitions emphasize intermittently occurring symptom complexes, and for their diagnosis, a certain number of symptoms must occur concurrently. The more that is known about a disease, the fewer symptoms required for its diagnosis. If the etiology is known, no symptoms need be present for accurate diagnosis as long as the causative agents are recoverable. Syndromes aspiring to separate existence must establish their credentials and are not granted the luxury of *form fruste* existence. If *some* basic symptoms become unnecessary for the diagnosis of the syndrome, what is to prevent the diagnosis if only a single symptom is present? Is urethritis alone Reiter's syndrome? Is aphthous stomatitis alone Behçet's syndrome? Although some of the disorders discussed in this chapter may eventually be classified as diseases, the vexing problem of diagnosis can be eased if they are regarded as syndromes, a convenient way of grouping apparently related symptoms. Intermittent hydrarthrosis is characterized by periodic monarticular swelling with little pain. Palindromic rheumatism adds signs of local inflammation to swelling, with redness, tenderness, and heat over the joint. Familial Mediterranean fever may include joint symptoms only, but they are accompanied by fever; however, there are generally other systemic features as well. In Behçet's syndrome and the Stevens-Johnson syndrome, joint manifestations are overshadowed by more severe involvement of other areas of the body. Other syndromes often characterized by intermittency, such as Reiter's syndrome, the arthritis of ulcerative colitis, and the arthritis of sarcoidosis, are discussed elsewhere in this volume.

Feedback mechanisms seem to account for some periodic syndromes, such as cyclic neutropenia,[2] but as yet, these mechanisms have not been related to the syndromes discussed in this chapter.

INTERMITTENT HYDRARTHROSIS (PERIODIC ARTHROSIS)

This term refers to a recurrent pattern of joint effusions, usually of the knees, of long-term, even life-long, duration. These recurrent attacks usually maintain a predictable periodicity. For the diagnosis to be tenable, evidence of neither local inflammation nor systemic signs must develop. However, a similar pattern may characterize the early stages of rheumatoid arthritis or of other periodic syndromes.

Ragan attributed the first report to Perrin (in 1845).[3] A scant 200 cases have been reported since then,[4] probably because there have been few new developments. Most rheumatologists can recall a few such cases, often with the diagnosis made retrospectively. Perhaps because the condition is uncommon and benign, it has attracted little research interest.

Etiology. Nothing is known about the cause of intermittent hydrarthrosis. Even feedback mechanisms fail to explain the patterned rhythmicity.[2] Although in most cases, the syndrome begins early in life, it may begin at any time. Women are more susceptible than men,* and in many, the joint manifestations parallel the menses. Although familial occurrence has been claimed, other disorders may have been confused with intermittent hydrarthrosis. Because some patients have a strong allergic history, or develop giant urticaria, urticarial lesions of the joint have been suggested.[5] Unfortunately, antihistamines and other antiallergic medications have proved unsuccessful in controlling the disorder.

Symptoms. Regular periodic recurrence of effusion of joints is the rule. Usually a single knee is involved. Rarely, the disease may be bilateral, and some cases involving the elbow, hip, or ankle have been reported. Although the average interval between attacks is 1 to 2 weeks, intervals of as much as a month are not unusual, particularly when joint swelling accompanies the menses. The effusion is relatively painless, without local warmth, tenderness, or other signs of inflammation. Neither adjacent muscular spasm nor muscular atrophy occurs. However, because of the marked effusion, local mechanical difficulty in moving does occur. In some cases, the effusions cease about 20 years after onset, but in others, intermittent hydrarthrosis is a life-long condition. Generally, patients fail to consult physicians after the first few attacks because they have learned that little can or need be done about the swelling. The fluid rapidly accumulates over 12 to 24 hours, but it absorbs more slowly, a period of 2 to 4 days being required for restitution to the premorbid state.

Laboratory Data. Hemogram, erythrocyte sedimentation rate, and acute phase reactants all remain normal, even during the attack. Latex fixation and other rheumatoid factor tests remain negative, and antinuclear antibodies are absent. Serum uric acid is generally within normal limits, although elevations resulting from small doses of aspirin may lead to the erroneous presumptive diagnosis of gout. Development of abnormalities of acute phase reactants or serologic tests should cast some doubt on the validity of the diagnosis.

Joint fluid does not contain crystals. Cell counts vary from none to the low thousands (frequently polymorphonuclear leukocytes). The cells contain no characteristic inclusions. Serum and joint fluid complement levels are normal, although some authors claim a decrease in Cl esterase inhibitor.[4] Synovial fluid is of normal viscosity and forms a solid clump in acetic acid. Tests for rheumatoid

factor in joint fluid are likely to be positive unless the fluid is first digested with hyaluronidase.[6]

Typical Cases. It has become customary to illustrate this condition with case histories. One patient, aged 30, had her menarche at age 13. A year later, concurrent with the onset of a menstrual period, she experienced a swollen left knee, unaccompanied by pain or other signs of inflammation. After four days, the swelling disappeared, only to recur in 27 days, when the next menstrual period began. The pattern was thus set, with recurrent swelling of the left knee, unaccompanied by any signs of systemic disease or local inflammation. The numerous studies that her perplexed physicians ordered were always unrewarding; therapy with salicylates, gold, and corticosteroids proved unavailing. With the benefit of hindsight, the probable correct diagnosis of intermittent hydrarthrosis was finally made during the patient's thirtieth year. Watchful expectancy and optimism replaced drug therapy. At all times, synovial fluid removed from the joint was normal, and corticosteroids instilled into the joint failed to prevent the usual recurrence.

Not so fortunate was a 46-year-old man who had undergone 6 years of regularly recurring effusions of the left knee at 14-day intervals. The effusion, unaccompanied by other signs of inflammation or by pain, but interfering mechanically with the extremes of range of motion, contained normal fluid. Chrysotherapy, anti-inflammatory compounds, corticosteroids, and colchicine proved unavailing. Corticosteroids were instilled after the frequent aspirations and, ultimately, the effusion failed to subside even during the expected intercritical periods. Synovectomy ultimately was performed, the synovium displaying the features to be described in the following section. Even synovectomy, however, failed to halt the recurrent effusions.

Pathology. Only few cases have come to operation, providing a dearth of material for study. Villous proliferation of the synovium has been a constant feature, but the degree of round-cell infiltration has varied. Some portions of removed synovial membranes have resembled changes of early rheumatoid arthritis, with lymphocytic aggregates and large numbers of plasma cells; in a previous edition, Ragan called these findings consistent with the first stage of rheumatoid arthritis.[3] Nevertheless, pannus has never been described, and these nonspecific synovial changes, in the presence of normal joint fluid and normal acute phase reactants and serologic tests, make a diagnosis of rheumatoid arthritis untenable.

Roentgenography. The diagnosis of intermittent hydrarthrosis demands that no abnormalities more dramatic than soft tissue swelling be identified at the involved joint.

---

*Whereas many American authors would subscribe to this statement, Bywaters considers both sexes to be equally at risk,[1] and some series actually cite a preponderance of men.

Prognosis. In some patients, the disorder runs a finite course whose total length is unpredictable. In others, joint swelling recurs throughout the patient's lifetime. The similarity of intermittent hydrarthrosis to an early stage of rheumatoid arthritis or related rheumatic disease makes prognostic judgment difficult even if the disorder has recurred for some time. However, the longer recurrences continue without apparent conversion to a more serious disorder, the more likely that joint damage will be avoided.

Treatment. No satisfactory treatment is available. Most of the standard treatments have been recommended at some time, including those thought to be successful in aborting acute attacks or chronic progression of other rheumatic diseases. The constant possibility of spontaneous remission and the small number of total cases invalidate most claims for successful therapy. Unfortunately, as Ragan has pointed out, sustained effusions, sometimes with evidence of inflammation, may follow enthusiastic intra-articular corticosteroid instillation.[3] Observation and optimism ultimately serve these patients best.

PALINDROMIC RHEUMATISM

The safest way to make the diagnosis of palindromic rheumatism is by retrospection. The term *palindromic* comes from the Greek, meaning to run back or to recur. The term was chosen by Hench and Rosenberg to describe a type of rheumatism that recurs intermittently;[6,7] however, palindromes are more familiar to us as word games in which the word or sentence reads the same forward or backward.

Hench and Rosenberg published a detailed account of 34 cases in 1944,[7] and every investigator since then has essentially paraphrased their work. However, the definition has been made more precise, more has become known of the fate of some of the patients who have the disorder, and increased use of the diagnostic laboratory has led to speculations of etiology.

Clinical Picture. Palindromic rheumatism is characterized by intermittently recurring attacks of painful swelling of the joints. It differs from intermittent hydrarthrosis in that there are obvious signs of inflammation at the affected joint, but resembles the latter in that systemic manifestations are absent. Men are more likely to be affected, usually in mid or late life.[1]

Joint pain begins suddenly and resembles a gouty attack. Pain is variable, ranging from a dull ache in some patients to an intense bursting experience in others. The crescendo of pain reaches its maximum within a few hours to a few days, rarely more than three. The attack commonly begins late in the afternoon. Swelling consistently accompanies pain, at least in joints where it is clinically detectable, and warmth and redness may be found overlying the joint. The redness is fairly characteristic, varying from a bright pink to crimson.

The diagnosis of palindromic rheumatism should not be made merely because of the recurrence of arthralgias. The cardinal signs of inflammation are required: pain and tenderness, redness, heat and, particularly, swelling and dysfunction. Most authors have rejected the diagnosis when swelling has not been present. However, functional disability is usually mild and, in many patients, does not compromise their ability to work. Morning stiffness and gelling after rest rarely develop; when they do, they are confined to the involved joint at the time of acute involvement.[7] The occurrence of generalized stiffness should direct the clinician to another diagnosis.

The pattern of joint attacks tends to be characteristic in a given patient. One or a limited number of joints is involved at a time, although symptoms may wax in new joints while waning in those affected during the previous attack. Intervals between attacks, thus, may vary from none at all to months. On the whole, the established pattern continues relatively unchanged for the duration of the illness, thus satisfying both Greek definitions of palindromic: ''recurrence'' and ''reading the same, backward and forward.'' Although the original description claimed a distinct predilection for finger joints,[7] the knee is probably the most frequently involved joint, followed by wrist, dorsum of the hand, metacarpophalangeal and proximal phalangeal joints of the fingers, ankle, shoulder, elbow, temporomandibular or sternoclavicular joint, hip, small joints of the foot, and cervical vertebral articulations.[8]

Para-articular attacks also occur in about one-third of the patients. These attacks consist of painful swellings of variable size at the heels, finger pads, distal phalanges, and flexor and dorsal surfaces of the forearms, thumb pads, and Achilles tendons. Although they resemble angioneurotic edema, they are tender, do not pit on pressure, and do not cause itching or burning paresthesia. When present, these lesions are characteristic of palindromic rheumatism.[2,6]

Transient subcutaneous nodules are also a feature of this disorder. These nodules usually overlie the tendons in the hands and fingers, although some have been described at the proximal extensor surfaces of the forearm, the most common site for rheumatoid nodules. The main differentiating feature from rheumatoid nodules at these locations is the relatively short duration the nodules are present, in almost all cases less than a week. Isolated swelling of an olecranon bursa may also occur between attacks. Palindromic attacks occur frequently in a variant of rheumatoid arthritis called "rheumatoid nodulosis."[4] Mattingly reported a strong family history of palindromic rheumatism and a high incidence of joint disease in mothers of his patients.[8]

Laboratory Data. If palindromic rheumatism is to be considered as a separate entity, one should probably exclude patients with signs of systemic disease not otherwise explainable. Thus, most patients who bear this diagnosis evince no abnormalities of hemogram and, at most, *transient* abnormalities of acute phase reactants. Erythrocyte sedimentation rates, which are normal between attacks, may be modestly elevated during attacks (rarely above 35 mm/hr, Westergren method.)[8] Tests for LE cells and serum complement should be normal. No circulating immune complexes are found.[11] Uric acid likewise is normal, unless it is elevated as a result of small doses of salicylates taken for pain.

The findings in joint fluid are relatively unremarkable, with normal viscosity, mucin clot, cellular constituents, proteins,[8] and low collagenase.[5] Only few biopsy specimens have been examined, usually obtained by needle. During the acute attack, polymorphonuclear leukocyte invasion of synovial tissues characterizes the intense inflammation. The cell population changes to round cells during subsidence, and synovial tissues are normal between attacks.[2] The subcutaneous nodules and tendon nodules are nonspecific, although some investigators claim a similarity to rheumatoid nodules.[8] One synovial specimen obtained through open biopsy contained tuboreticular structures and much fibrin deposition.[9] In instances preceding rheumatoid arthritis, electron-dense deposits in vessel walls suggest circulating immune complexes, which are otherwise not demonstrable.[10]

Roentgenographic Findings. Except for soft tissue swelling at the time of the attack, no specific abnormalities result from palindromic rheumatism. Those patients who develop changes consistent with rheumatoid arthritis probably suffer from rheumatoid arthritis of episodic onset.

Prognosis. For the true syndrome of palindromic rheumatism, the prognosis in a given patient may be poor for recovery but good as far as potential crippling is concerned. In many patients, the attacks cease as abruptly as they began, with causes for their cessation as mysterious as those for their initiation. A follow-up of 140 patients with palindromic rheumatism for at least 5 years revealed that more than half (73) suffered continued attacks.[13] Eleven, or less than 10%, experienced complete remissions during the interval of obser-

vation, while more than a third (50) developed rheumatoid arthritis. Gout, systemic lupus erythematosus, and other diagnoses accounted for the remainder. The distribution of patients reflects the hazards of this diagnosis, as an appreciable number of patients who seem to have palindromic rheumatism actually have an episodic onset of rheumatoid arthritis, for which the prognosis is obviously not as favorable. A review of 39 patients diagnosed as having this syndrome disclosed that 17 cases evolved into typical rheumatoid arthritis while 22 remained palindromic.[12] Palindromic symptoms had lasted for as long as 20 years in one patient before rheumatoid arthritis supervened, and for two or more years in 8 of the 17 patients. No signal differences were noted between the two populations, although those whose palindromic pattern changed into fixed rheumatoid arthritis often were noted to have a raised erythrocyte sedimentation rate, a positive test for rheumatoid factor, or minor clinical or radiologic changes. The uncertainty of the diagnosis of palindromic rheumatism is thereby highlighted. Some patients develop a related rheumatic syndrome or even malignant diseases, such as multiple myeloma,[14] although it is doubtful that an episodic arthritis of such long duration can be regarded as heralding malignant tumors.

In occasional patients, palindromic rheumatism seems to be a response to an irritant or an allergen.[3] Whether such cases are perhaps examples of urticarial joint lesions remains unsettled. Ultimately, therefore, discussions of prognosis hinge upon the validity of the concept of palindromic rheumatism as a separate entity. The safest course appears to be to make the diagnosis only by exclusion and after a reasonable period of observation.

Treatment. Acute attacks may end before prophylactic treatment can become effective. Anti-inflammatory drugs, antiallergic medications, and colchicine have all been attempted and generally have been found wanting, although colchicine treatment has had a recent vogue based on analogies with disorders to be discussed later. Claims for various drugs have been made in individual cases, but the variability of this disorder makes such claims suspect. Vacations and administration of gold compounds[8] seem to promote the most benefit. Penicillamine, in uncontrolled trials, appears to suppress the attacks of arthritis. Various nonsteroidal anti-inflammatory drugs often seem effective prophylactically when taken daily, but again, no controlled experience is available. The attacks in a minority of patients are difficult to suppress with any anti-inflammatory drug except adrenal corticosteroids. As in most cases of acute arthritis, corticosteroids instilled into the joint may promote a more rapid return to normal, but their use is seldom justified in a disorder in which return to normal after a few days is the rule. Because of the expected recurrences, administration of narcotics is fraught with danger and should be avoided.

ARTHRITIS OF FAMILIAL MEDITERRANEAN FEVER

Familial Mediterranean fever (FMF) is a genetic disorder, apparently inherited as an autosomal recessive disorder with complete penetrance.[43] Although it occurs primarily in individuals originating in the greater Mediterranean area, chiefly Sephardic and Iraqi Jews,[19] Levantine Arabs,[35] Turks,[30] and Armenians,[36] it has been described in other groups and as isolated cases.[11,34,40,41] Many instances were undoubtedly included in series reported as periodic diseases, benign or familial paroxysmal peritonitis, or recurrent polyserositis.[31,32,36,41] The characteristic symptoms include intermittent fever and pain in the abdomen, chest, or joints. Amyloidosis (which is genetically determined) occurs in at least 40% of Sephardic Jews who have the disorder; in some, it may be the sole phenotypic expression of the disease (phenotype 2).[4] Amyloidosis develops only rarely when the disease occurs in patients other than Sephardic Jews or Turks,[20,30] and may occur early in life in predisposed groups.[24]

Clinical Picture. The disease first appears in childhood or adolescence, and recurs intermittently throughout life. No true sex predilection has as yet been determined, although more men than women seem to be affected.[43] The family history may reveal siblings or other close relatives who have the disease.[26,43] Often there is a history of consanguineous marriage among the forebears.[43]

Fever probably accompanies every attack, but does not give rise to shaking chills or other constitutional symptoms, and usually lasts only a few hours. Temperature elevations vary from persistent and low grade to spikes up to 103.1° F (39.5° C)[43] (Fig. 58–1).

The abdominal crises resemble acute peritonitis, last from 12 to 24 hours—in rare instances for 3 to 4 days.[43] Serous fluid in the abdominal cavity is the only abnormal finding on laparotomy. Occasionally, abdominal pain simulates pelvic inflammatory disease. Acute chest pain commonly involves only one hemithorax with referral to the corresponding shoulder. It is also of short duration, and is usually accompanied by minimal evanescent pleural effusion[43] or pericarditis.[7,33] Many patients experience recurrent attacks of intense tenderness and redness around the ankle. This erysipelas-like erythema is probably not related to underlying joint disease.[43] Intestinal obstruction of serious propor-

tion,[10,40] varying types of renal disease, and cyclic emotional states are sometimes considered part of the disease. Amyloidosis characteristically produces nephrotic syndrome progressing to early death in renal failure.[18,24] Periodic meningitis has been reported.[44] In some instances, Henoch-Schönlein purpura develops.[12]

The musculoskeletal attacks in FMF may occur together with, or independently of, other manifestations in approximately 70% of patients. When they occur alone, the later course or the family history confirms the diagnosis. The distribution of attacks is asymmetric, with large joints more commonly involved. The affected joints, in order of decreasing frequency, are knees, ankles, hips, shoulders, feet and toes, elbows, wrists and hands, and the remaining synovial joints.[17] Isolated disease of the temporomandibular joints[6] or the sacroiliac joints[17] has been described. Arthritis is commonly monarticular. Subsequent attacks tend to adhere to the established pattern. Attacks are intermittent, not periodic, and of varying duration. They generally last longer than other manifestations of this disease. All afflicted patients experience attacks that terminate in less than a week. Not infrequently, attacks may persist for 2 or 3 weeks, or rarely, for months.[11,17]

Localized pain is the predominant and, at times, the sole symptom. The joint and periarticular area are usually exquisitely tender, so that the slightest touch cannot be tolerated. At the knees, ankles, elbows, and shoulders, swelling is usually present, accompanied at times by massive effusion. However, it is usually not as pronounced as the dramatic pain would imply. Limitation of motion and severe functional impairment result. During an attack, the muscles around the joint are in spasm. However, morning stiffness in the involved or other joints does not occur. The patients do not develop gelling of joints and muscles after rest. Although the involved joints may be somewhat warm initially, the warmth does not persist as long as the pain or functional impairment. Except for the occasional erysipelas-like erythema, redness is notable by its absence. Thus, *an intermittent asymmetric monarthritis characterized primarily by pain, tenderness, and impaired joint function disproportionate to the amount of swelling and unaccompanied by warmth or redness should alert the physician to the possibility of arthritis of familial Mediterranean fever.*

Joint function recovers completely between attacks.[17] Disuse atrophy, which develops in prolonged attacks and may be marked, is also reversible. Demonstrable residua of attacks are extreme rarities, although occasionally destructive changes do develop.[21b] However, when the hip becomes

THE PATTERN OF FAMILIAL MEDITERRANEAN FEVER

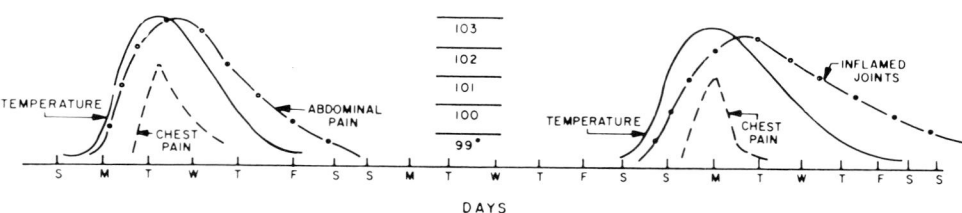

Fig. 58–1.   Typical clinical pattern of attacks of familial Mediterranean fever.

involved in a prolonged attack, functional recovery may not be as likely. In one study, 16 of 18 patients with affected hips developed moderate to marked anatomic and functional changes, with narrowing and sclerosis of the joint space and progressive limitation of motion. Destructive changes occasionally supervene, requiring surgical intervention.[26] Tendon contractures do not occur.[17]

During acute attacks, superficial vessels often dilate over the involved joints, especially at the knee, where they can be readily detected with infrared illumination.

Acute tenderness and swelling of the lower thigh or upper calf may mimic arthritis at the knee. Inflammation of bursal areas may be responsible, as has infrequently been the case at the hip.[17] Various types of trauma may precipitate attacks. In different patients, overexertion, bruising, heat, cold, and even paracentesis of joints have been implicated. The type of trauma is specific to the patient, but many attacks are not preceded by a recognizable precipitating event.[17]

Arthrodesis occasionally has been performed when FMF was so severe as to be mistaken for tuberculous arthritis. Surgical fusion thus prevented functional recovery, which might otherwise have been inevitable.[17]

Amyloidosis is probably the basis for the frequently encountered splenomegaly. Although many patients come from the area where infectious diseases result in enlarged spleens, patients who have familial Mediterranean fever rarely seem to develop intercurrent illnesses.[43]

Among the negative features that permit differential diagnosis are the absence of nodules, urethritis, stomatitis, balanitis, conjunctivitis, uveitis, choroiditis, and dermatitis.

Laboratory Data.   Most of the laboratory findings in FMF are nonspecific (Table 58–1). Erythrocyte sedimentation rate and fibrinogen level are elevated or at upper reaches of normal between attacks and soar precipitously with the onset of the attacks. Within days they return to previous levels.[13] Anemia may be a manifestation of chronic illness. Leukocytosis or leukopenia, the latter in the presence of splenomegaly, is an inconsistent feature. Urinary abnormalities appear only if there is amyloidosis and consist primarily of massive proteinuria. Serum albumin is often decreased. Gamma globulins may be normal or increased, but elevations of the alpha 2, alpha 2m, and beta 2m globulins, haptoglobin, and lipoproteins are common. The electrophoretic pattern is similar to that seen in amyloidosis even when this latter feature is not demonstrable.[43] Latex fixation tests for rheumatoid factor are negative, or only transiently positive in low dilutions (1:160 or less).[11,17] Other serologic tests are negative. Uric acid or etiocholanolone levels[5] are not elevated (but hypoaldosteronism has been unmasked after renal allotransplantation).[42] Whole serum complement and Cl esterase inhibitor may be deficient.[37] Levels of circulating immune complexes may be increased, as measured by Clq binding[23] (in one of four patients, but half the Sephardic patients). Cryofibrinogen was present in the plasma samples in one series.[29] Evidence has been presented for C5a inhibitor deficiency in peritoneal and synovial fluids.[24a] Lipoxygenase products have been identified in both serum and synovial fluid.[1]

Early in the attacks, the joint fluid contains many polymorphonuclear leukocytes, but these are later replaced by lymphocytes. Although viscosity is poor, the mucin clot is fairly adequate. Protein and sugar are unaltered, and cultures are negative.[11,17] Foamy cells have also been described.[43]

Roentgenography.   The bone age is generally younger than the chronologic age, leading to the paradoxic finding of degenerative changes with patent epiphyses. When the FMF is prolonged, coarse trabecular metaphyseal osteoporosis forms pseudocysts. Protracted involvement of the knee leads

Table 58–1. Laboratory Features in Arthritis of Familial Mediterranean Fever

Test	Results
Blood count	Variable
Urinalysis	Variable
Latex fixation	Negative
LE preparation	Negative
Uric acid	Normal
Fibrinogen	Elevated, spiking during attack
ESR	Elevated, spiking during attack
Circulating immune complexes	Increased in about one-fourth
Cryofibrinogen	Often present
Etiocholanolone	Not elevated
Roentgenograms	Degenerative changes, retarded bone age, osteoporosis, "eggshell line," sacroiliac changes
Biopsy	Nonspecific inflammatory changes, perireticulin amyloidosis

to enlargement of the femoral condyles (Fig. 58–2). All these findings are nonspecific features of long-term immobilization during bone growth, such as occurs in poliomyelitis or hemophilia arthritis.

During the acute phases, soft tissue enlargement can be seen. With chronicity, the joint space narrows and proliferative marginal bony changes develop. This development, which is particularly prevalent at hips and knees, is partly reversible. The changes may represent periosteal reaction to marginal destruction. True cysts are encountered only rarely. A triangular condensation of the ilium above the acetabulum characterizes chronic hip involvement[17,39] (Fig. 58–3).

In osteoporosis of the femur, the femoral condyles appear as thin eggshell lines separated from

Fig. 58–2. Roentgenogram of knee. The femoral condyles are large. Soft tissue swelling and osteoporosis are readily apparent. A double-contoured "eggshell" line outlines the femoral condyles. (Courtesy of Ezra Sohar, M.D., and Joseph Gafni, M.D.)

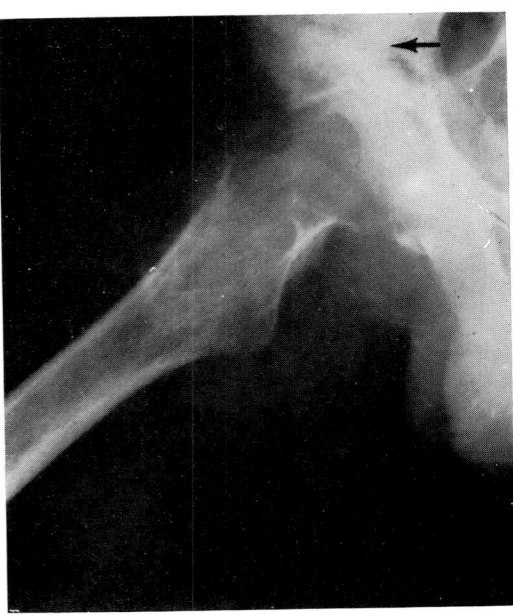

Fig. 58–3. Roentgenogram of hip (frog lateral). Marked degenerative changes include pseudocysts, periosteal proliferation and osteoporosis of the femur, and narrowing of the joint space, marginal spurs, and a triangular iliac density at the acetabulum. (Courtesy of Ezra Sohar, M.D., and Joseph Gafni, M.D.)

the trabecular pattern by a narrow radiolucent zone. With the arthritis of FMF, this eggshell line may be found on both sides of the radiolucent zone.[17] Although it has been described in only a few patients, it may be a specific finding. The line tends to remain even when other roentgenographic changes disappear (Fig. 58–4).

Although there is no clinical evidence of ankylosing spondylitis, some sacroiliac joints are widened and others are sclerosed.[26] Rarely, patchy calcified bridges can be seen in the lower spine. Osteitis condensans ilii is frequently present. In fact, because various sacroiliac abnormalities tend to be found in a disproportionate number of patients, FMF should always be included in the differential diagnosis of radiologic abnormalities of the sacroiliac joints.[16] However, the changes may reflect more the character of the population at risk than results of the disease. The occurrence of sacroiliac changes in populations in whom tropical diseases are prevalent[28] makes the significance of this finding questionable.

Pathologic Anatomy. The changes seen in

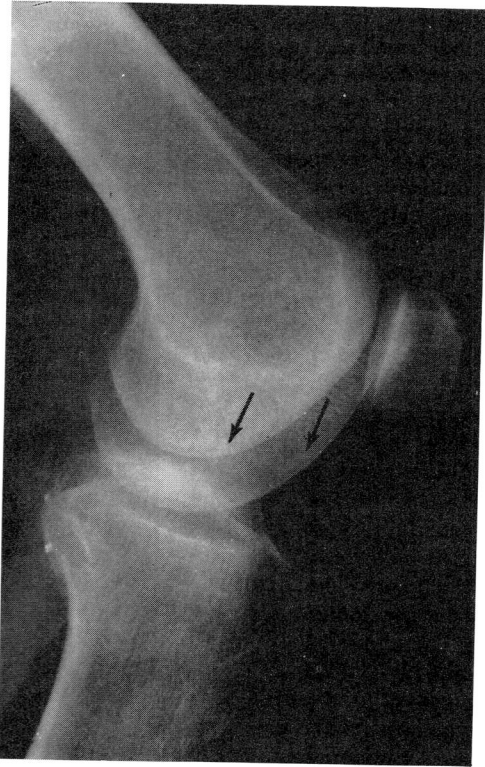

Fig. 58–4. Roentgenogram of knee. In this adult who no longer has symptoms of joint disease, the double-contoured "eggshell" line is present despite the recovery from osteoporosis. (Courtesy of Ezra Sohar, M.D., and Joseph Gafni, M.D.)

biopsies from inflamed joints are nonspecific. Irregular aggregates of round cells surround small blood vessels, but true perivascular cuffing does not occur. There is increased vascularity, and stromal fibroblasts and polymorphonuclear leukocytes are increased.[17] Lytic lesions of bone are filled with fibrous tissue. Postmortem examinations of joints that had been involved but had recovered reveal no abnormalities.[17]

The amyloidosis encountered in familial Mediterranean fever, though primary, is distributed as if it were of the secondary variety.[14] The amyloid is deposited in the perireticular areas of blood vessels, and is especially concentrated in spleen and kidney. It has occasionally been demonstrated around blood vessels in or near inflamed joints.[17]

Amyloidosis developed in a transplanted cadaver kidney after four years in an Armenian woman who had intermittently high levels of the serum precursor SAA, but renal function remained normal for at least an additional three years; defective degradation of amyloid precursor(s) may be important in fibril deposition as well.[3]

Treatment. Although no therapy has yet proved curative for FMF, consistent palliation has been achieved with colchicine,[8,15] perhaps because of effects on chemotaxis.[2] Long-term treatment with 0.6 mg of colchicine, two to three times daily, succeeded in reducing the number of attacks in controlled trials.[45] To avoid toxicity, intermittent colchicine therapy was attempted, but was successful only in some patients.[46] It was hoped that this regimen would be more acceptable in children, but long-term treatment has now been recommended even here.[22] Steatorrhea and other more minor problems can develop.[9]

Temporary relief of joint pain has sometimes followed use of analgesic preparations. Physical therapy is recommended to avoid disuse atrophy. Corticosteroids have proved singularly ineffective, and unresponsiveness to corticosteroids has been suggested as a differential diagnostic criterion.[17] Earlier intermittent courses of colchicine and immunosuppressive drugs have not stood the test of time.[10] Fat-free diets, once recommended, have been found wanting.[25] In view of the recurrent nature of this disorder, narcotics must be assiduously avoided. Because there is usually complete functional recovery from arthritis, operative intervention is rarely indicated. However, appendectomy should perhaps be performed early because appendicitis cannot readily be distinguished from the abdominal manifestations of this disease. When renal failure complicates amyloidosis of FMF, hemodialysis has extended life for a few years,[1a,21] as has renal transplantation.[21a] Amyloidosis seems to be prevented by timely administration of colchicine.[11a]

Prognosis. Functional recovery from individual attacks and asymptomatic remissions are the rule, except when the hip joint is involved during a protracted attack. Those with the greatest experience with this disease believe that the majority of patients in whom the occurrence is familial will succumb to amyloidosis at a relatively young age.[18] In ethnic groups other than those commonly affected, prognosis seems more favorable.

BEHÇET'S SYNDROME

Behçet's syndrome is a multisystem disorder, generally classified as an interface between vasculitis and systemic lupus erythematosus.[18] It was originally described as a triple symptom complex consisting of recurrent oral and genital ulcerations and relapsing iritis.[4] Other systemic manifestations were soon added.[45] The original cases were described in countries bordering the Mediterranean, especially Turkey, but large series have since been collected in the rest of Europe, the Middle East, Japan and, lately, the United States. Some superficial resemblances to Reiter's syndrome can be inferred from an uncritical description of the lesions, but obvious differences exist when all the manifestations are carefully defined. Arthralgias and arthritis have lately been recognized as frequent and prominent manifestations.[36]

Behçet's syndrome received its eponym in 1937, after a description of three patients by the Turkish dermatologist, Professor Hulusi Behçet.[4] A previous case described in Bulgaria by Adamantiades has caused his name to be added to the syndrome in some medical writings.[1] Individual cases were also described by Shigeta in Japan in 1924,[51] and Whitwell in England in 1934.[55] It is probable that a description of the disorder appeared in the writings of Hippocrates, who considered it an acute endemic disease and provided a fairly accurate clinical picture.[20]

The true prevalence of the disorder is difficult to estimate. Many cases go unrecognized, and others may be labeled Reiter's syndrome, Stevens-Johnson syndrome, or even periodic disease. However, Behçet's syndrome has been the subject of more medical articles than the number of cases diagnosed outside the two areas of greatest prevalence (Japan and the Middle East) would warrant.

Newer discoveries have provided some rationale for the two terms, Behçet's disease and Behçet's syndrome. Behçet's disease should be reserved for those cases that clearly meet all the criteria without the presence of some concomitant disorder that might account for certain manifestations; Behçet's syndrome, probably more common in the United States, describes cases in which the classic features are present, but in which an associated disease that could be responsible is also present (e.g., ulcerative colitis or granulomatous enteritis).[17]

Etiology is unknown. Proponents of allergic or "autoimmune" causation group the disorder among the connective tissue diseases,[32] whereas some investigators see evidence for a viral etiology,[12,13] a contention that has been challenged.[30] The possibility of viral precipitation of the disease in a receptive host may reconcile the various viewpoints. Earlier, there had been some interest in blaming various environmental chemicals for Behçet's syndrome; organophosphates and organochloride pesticides and polychlorinated biphenyls can produce a similar syndrome in swine.[52] Although chemicals and metals also have been implicated by some, substantive evidence remains elusive.[42]

Earlier reports linking HLA-B5 antigen with Behçet's syndrome were amplified, in that a split of this antigen, B-51, was found in 62% of patients compared with 21% of controls in Japanese studies.[43,44,50] Similar association has been proved in Turkish and British patients.[56] HLA-DR5 and MT2 are disproportionately represented among Japanese patients who have Behçet's syndrome.[44] DR7 is disproportionately represented in a British series.[30] These various antigenic markers are more common in patients who have ocular and neurologic manifestations; HLA-B12 and DR2 are frequently found in patients in whom mucocutaneous and arthritic manifestations predominate.[30] A defect in immunoregulation has been hypothesized, thought to be under HLA control, giving rise to changes in cell-mediated immunity and immune complexes that are ultimately responsible for the damage in the disease. Other studies have implicated HLA-AW31 and DRW6.[49] Because MT2 is present in half the Japanese population, its increased prevalence among Behçet's patients is not necessarily of diagnostic importance. HLA-B27 has at times been implicated in arthritic manifestations of Behçet's syndrome,[9] but the possibility remains that these patients might have had a seronegative spondyloarthropathy simulating the findings of Behçet's syndrome.

Clinical Picture. The combination of oral and genital ulcers and iritis is crucial to the diagnosis,[53] although some investigators have been satisfied with two of the three symptoms, with at least three other accompanying systemic involvements. The major and minor criteria are set forth in Table 58–2. These criteria do not refer to severity of the manifestations but rather to their almost certain appearance (major) and their relatively infrequent (50% or less minor) appearance. Because Behçet's syndrome is the leading cause of acquired blindness in Japan, a research committee has been formed.

Table 58–2.   **Diagnosis of Behçet's Syndrome**

MAJOR CRITERIA
1. Mouth (aphthous) ulcers
2. Iritis (with hypopyon)
3. Genital ulcers
4. Skin lesions
      pyoderma
      nodose lesions

MINOR CRITERIA
5. Arthritis
      of major joints
      arthralgias
6. Vascular disease
      migratory superficial phlebitis
      major vessel thrombosis
      aneurysms
      peripheral gangrene
      retinal and vitreous hemorrhage, papilledema
7. Central nervous system disease
      brain stem syndrome
      meningomyelitis
      confusional states
8. Gastrointestinal disease
      malabsorption
      colonic ulcers
      dilated intestinal loops
9. Epididymitis
10. Hemorrhagic pneumonitis
11. Glomerulonephritis

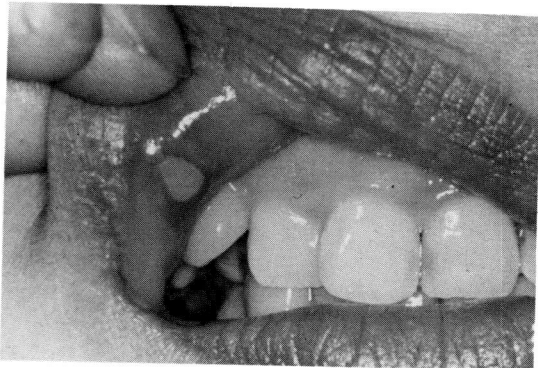

Fig. 58–5. Aphthous ulcer of the mucous membrane of the lip; note the distinct edges and the surrounding erythema. (Courtesy of Professor T. Shimizu.)

The following are the major criteria developed by this committee. (1) Recurrent aphthous ulcerations of the oral mucous membranes consist of painful round or oval ulcers with sharply defined borders, located on labial, buccal, gingival, and lingual mucous membranes (Fig. 58–5). These ulcers tend to occur in crops lasting 1 to 2 weeks and recur at frequent intervals. (2) Skin lesions include erythema nodosum, superficial thrombophlebitis, folliculitis, acne-like lesions, and cutaneous hyper-

sensitivity. This last named, a pathergy, is responsible for a sterile pustule with an erythematous margin that develops approximately one day after pricking of skin with a sterile needle. It is used as a diagnostic test, especially in Japan and Turkey (where it is positive in 90% of the patients) (Fig. 58–6). (3) Ocular symptoms include iridocyclitis, transient hypopyon iritis (Fig. 58–7), posterior uveitis, retinal detachment, chorioretinitis, and their sequels. (4) There are genital ulcers or painful punched out lesions of the scrotum (Fig. 58–8), vulva, bladder, cervix, or glans penis (associated with balanitis).

The minor criteria include: (1) arthritis resembling rheumatoid arthritis (Fig. 58–9) or asym-

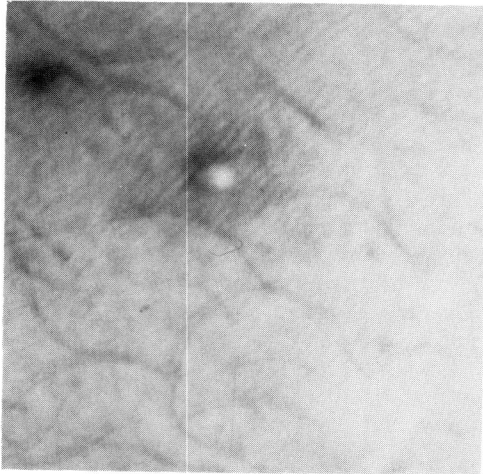

Fig. 58–6. Pin prick sign. When the sterile skin is pricked by a sterile needle, a pustule with surrounding erythema develops 24 hours later in many instances of Behçet's syndrome. (Courtesy of Professor T. Shimizu.)

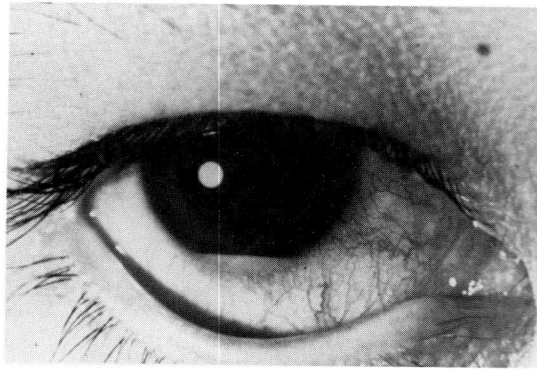

Fig. 58–7. Hypopyon iritis. Pus in the anterior chamber is a transient but important feature of Behçet's syndrome. (Courtesy of Professor T. Shimizu.)

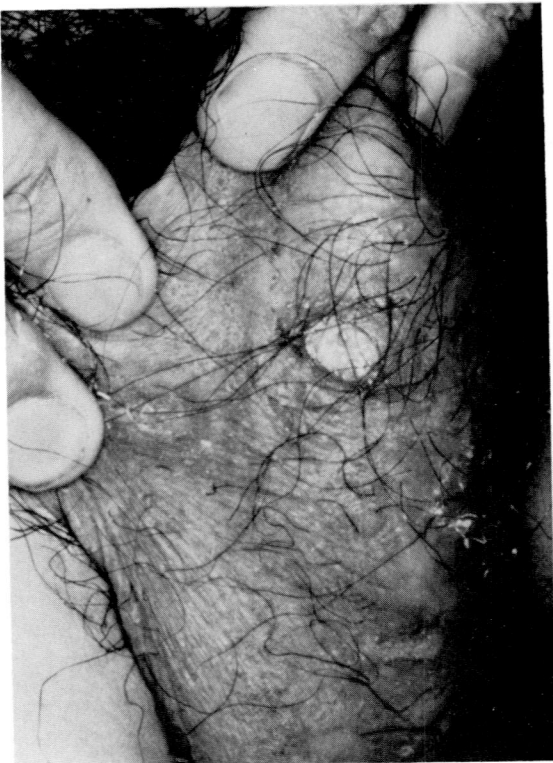

Fig. 58–8. Scrotal ulcer. Note resemblance to oral lesions. (Courtesy of Professor T. Shimizu.)

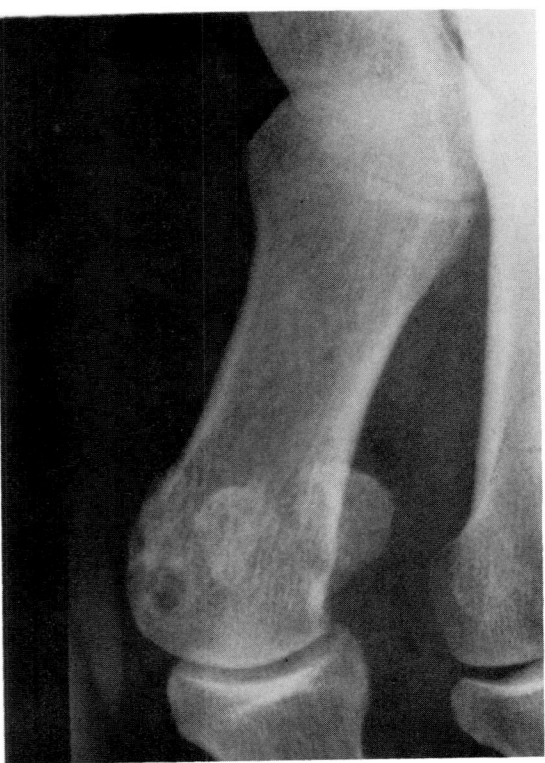

Fig. 58–9. Punched-out lesion of first metatarsal head in Behçet's syndrome. Roentgenographic changes of the joints are rare. (Courtesy of Professor T. Shimizu.)

metrical arthritis, such as Reiter's syndrome; (2) intestinal ulcerations, especially in the right colon; (3) epididymitis; (4) obliterating thrombophlebitis or arterial occlusions and aneurysms, especially of great vessels; and (5) neuropsychiatric symptoms, including demyelinating disease. According to this committee, the complete syndrome requires that the four main symptoms appear sometime during the clinical course, whereas in the incomplete type, three of the main symptoms and four minor symptoms suffice. Interestingly, HLA-B51 is found in most patients who have the complete syndrome, and only in a bare plurality of patients who have the incomplete syndrome.[42] From a diagnostic standpoint, the minor criteria assume increasing importance, as some of them are so characteristic as to point to the correct diagnosis, when the more frequent major criteria might not.

In the original series, men outnumbered women among those who developed the syndrome, but more recently, more women than men have been described.[27] The prevalence of the disorder in Japan ranges from 1 in 7,500 in Hokkaido to none among Japanese in Hawaii and only 6 cases in Okinawa.

The distribution favors appearance in cold regions. Attacks also tend to occur during cold spells.[35]

In addition to the ulcerative lesions of the mouth, clinical descriptions include scanty fungiform papillae of the tongue, plaque-like lesions of the pharynx and larynx,[31] and considerable oral fetor.[8] In the eye, in addition to the main features noted, papilledema,[46] exudates and hemorrhages,[38] and optic atrophy[10] are also encountered. Although the ulcerative lesions of the penis and scrotum tend to be painful, those of the vulva and vagina often are not, and may be missed.[52] The skin lesion can elaborate to pyoderma. Infection of surgical tracts to their full extent has been described, and is thought to be related to the pathergy tests.[57] Gangrene of fingertips and toes, thrombosis of superficial veins, thrombosis of the venae cavae (Fig. 58–10), aneurysms and thromboses of major arteries, small vessel vasculitis, and the consequences, including avascular necrosis of bone ends (Fig. 58–11), are dramatic manifestations of the syndrome.[17,52] In the digestive tract, nonspecific symptoms of vomiting, abdominal pain, flatulence, diarrhea, and constipation are usually noted.[28] Mal-

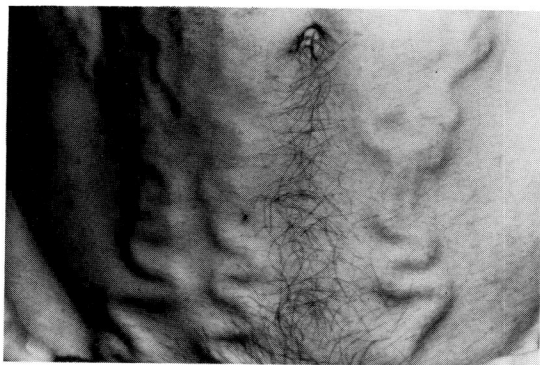

Fig. 58–10. Caput medusae secondary to inferior vena cava occlusion in Behçet's syndrome. (Courtesy of Professor T. Shimizu.)

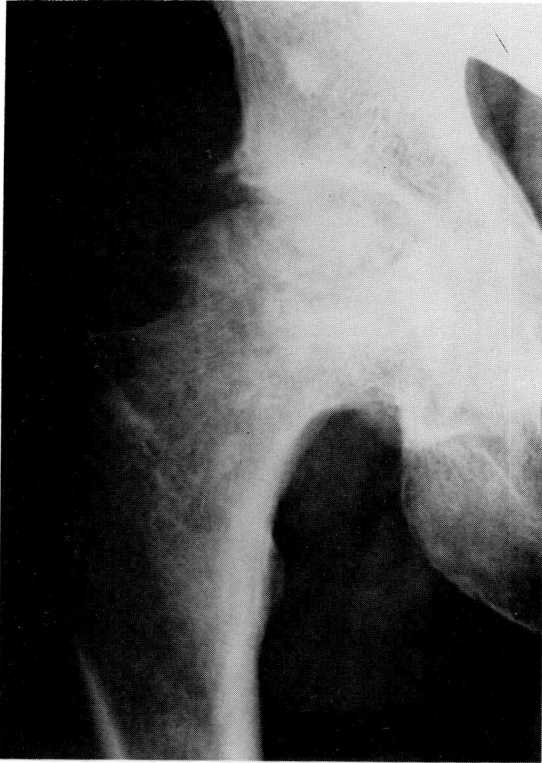

Fig. 58–11. Triangular aseptic necrosis of the femoral head secondary to occlusion of small arteries in Behçet's syndrome. (Courtesy of Professor T. Shimizu.)

absorption and abnormal digestion are commonly seen. Erosions and ulcers are found in the large bowel, predominantly in the cecum, right colon, and occasionally in the terminal ileum. Perforation, melena, and tumor may result. Thrombosis of pulmonary arteries has been described,[24] but is un-

common, as are pulmonary aneurysms[16] and hemorrhagic pneumonitis.[47] Renal involvement has been noted, especially focal glomerulonephritis,[26] but more serious forms of glomerulonephritis have also been encountered.[22,29] Almost any nervous system disorders, ranging from psychoneurosis through demyelinating disease, have accompanied the syndrome, but are particularly likely in Japanese patients.[52] Peripheral neuropathy and myositis can also occur.[2,3]

The prognosis is influenced by the sites of involvement, the severity, and the distribution of the lesions. Recurrent morbidity is likely. In some instances, where the disease settles in, destructive consequences to specific organs will result: enucleation of an eye may be necessary, gangrene may amputate a peripheral part, or perforation of a viscus may require surgical removal. Deaths due to Behçet's syndrome generally result from the central nervous system involvement, although glomerulonephritis or pulmonary involvement can also be blamed. In rare instances, amyloidosis may complicate the picture and also lead to fatality.[14]

Familial clustering has been reported frequently.[9,14,27] Although patients may belong to any racial grouping, the most likely examples come from inhabitants of the old silk route, extending from central Asia to Turkey and in the opposite direction to Japan via Korea. However, white and black subjects with no remote connection with these Altaic-speaking peoples develop more sporadic cases.[18]

As is true of most other intermittent and periodic syndromes, joint involvement in Behçet's syndrome tends to be monarticular or oligoarticular, although a symmetrical or asymmetrical polyarthropathy may also occur. Arthralgias are always more frequent than true arthritis, but arthritis itself develops in more than half the patients.[36] This arthritis often resembles palindromic rheumatism in the context of Behçet's syndrome.[52] The knee is most commonly involved, followed by the ankle, elbow, and wrist; small joints are less commonly involved. Destruction and atrophy of bone and cartilage have been described, but are exceedingly rare. Behçet's syndrome must be included in the differential diagnosis of sacroiliac joint disease, although sclerosis of the degree seen in ankylosing spondylitis rarely occurs. In some patients, little pain is registered, whereas in others, pain of the severity of gout is present.[23] Thus, intermittent hydrarthrosis, palindromic rheumatism, rheumatoid arthritis, gout and pseudogout, Reiter's syndrome, systemic lupus erythematosus, and enteroarthropathies figure prominently in the differential diagnosis. Onset tends to be insidious and duration variable, with arthritis remaining from a few weeks to several years. The intervals between arthritic attacks tend to be longer than those between attacks of extra-articular manifestations. The joints are warm, tender, and slightly reddened, and morning stiffness is present. Permanent changes and disability of the joints are rare.[52]

Fever and other constitutional signs are frequently encountered. Myalgias are common. Inner ear involvement with vertigo and hearing disturbances has been added to the list of symptoms.[7]

Laboratory Findings. Acute phase reactants tend to be abnormal during an attack, including rapid sedimentation rate, strongly positive C-reactive protein, and elevation of alpha-2 globulins.[52] Anemia is common. Chemotactic activity of neutrophils is markedly enhanced.[15,21,54] A polyclonal gammopathy is characteristically found in this disorder. Cryoglobulins can be found in most cases,[34,50] with significant increases of C3 in the arthritic and ocular types, and of IgM and IgG in the mucocutaneous type. In sequential studies, disease remissions or exacerbations correlated with a decrease or increase in serum IgM and IgG cryoglobulins.[34] The converse was found with IgA.[25] Serum complement level is usually high. B-lymphocytes are suppressed and T-lymphocytes are proportionately increased.[25,52] The in vitro response of T cells to mitogens is depressed.[25] Plasmin, plasminogen activator, and fibrin degradation products are present with greater frequency in the blood of patients who have Behçet's syndrome than in any controls. Enhanced fibrinolytic activity may therefore be present.[40] Antibodies against specific organs involved, including demyelinating antibodies and antimyelin serum factors, have also been reported. Inclusion bodies may be found in various cells from patients who have Behçet's syndrome, but are of uncertain significance.[13]

Neither rheumatoid factor nor antinuclear antibodies are generally present. Rosettes of platelets surrounding neutrophils are seen in Behçet's syndrome. They appear during attacks and are absent between attacks. EDTA-anticoagulated blood, incubated at room temperature for 2 or more hours, may show this phenomenon on an ordinary differential smear.[19] In supravital preparations, the addition of heparin does not alter the phenomenon, but a later addition of calcium abolishes it.[19] This test is relatively specific but insensitive, occurring in the minority of patients. Its sensitivity can be increased by adding sera from patients to donor granulocytes and platelets, and reproducing the rosette phenomenon.[52]

Roentgenography. Significant roentgenographic changes in the joints are rare, occurring in fewer than 1% of patients. These changes resemble the lesions of reactive spondyloarthropathies.

Chest radiographs often show infiltrates and rounded opacities, which may progress to excavation. The ulcers in the colon are large, discrete, and multiple, they may take ring shapes, and they often penetrate through the bowel wall. Venograms may reveal blockage of large and small vessels by thrombi, including thrombosis of renal veins and inferior and superior vena cava. Arteriograms show occlusion of major vessels, including the aorta and its branches, and aneurysms. The typical findings of aseptic necrosis of femoral heads may be seen.[52]

Differential Diagnosis. The various other oculocutaneous syndromes and the rheumatic diseases with somewhat similar manifestations have already been mentioned. There is no clear-cut way of differentiating Behçet's syndrome from other disorders it may resemble; the aphthous ulcers of the mouth, for example, are like ordinary aphthous ulcers, and only in context acquire additional significance. There may be regional differences in diagnosing Behçet's syndrome, with inclusion, in some areas, of cases that may be labeled differently in other parts of the world (especially Reiter's syndrome or systemic lupus erythematosus).

Pathology. Basic to all the ulcerative lesions of Behçet's syndrome is vasculitis. The vasculitis is so reminiscent of other autoimmune disorders that it has fueled claims for the inclusion of the disorder among the autoimmune connective tissue syndromes. Mucocutaneous lesions in rats resembling those of Behçet's syndrome in humans have been produced experimentally by injections of mycobacteria and Freund's adjuvant, which more commonly produce arthritis but can also result in dermal, genital, and ocular lesions. Organophosphate insecticides can produce similar lesions in swine. Lesions similar to those of Behçet's syndrome have been produced in man by sensitivities to English walnuts and to ginkgo-tree fruit. Skin hypersensitivity in general is found. Deep to the skin pustules, and to some of the other lesions, including nonspecific synovial involvement and arterial thromboses, are granulocyte-platelet thrombi.[17] The intestinal ulcers, even when perforating, contain minimal, if any, collections of neutrophilic leukocytes. There is superficial necrosis with signs of inflammation and prominent lymph follicles, but relatively uninvolved mucosa between lesions.[28,52] Vasculitis and platelet-granulocyte thrombi have been described in the intestines as well.[17,52]

Treatment. No uniformly effective treatment has been described. Because colchicine had proved effective in other intermittent syndromes, it was at first introduced empirically into the treatment of Behçet's syndrome, and showed much promise, although it was not capable of altering ocular or central nervous system manifestations.[39] Later, a rationale for the action of colchicine was found in its ability to reduce the enhanced granulocyte motility that is a feature of the syndrome.[40] Immunosuppressive compounds have been used; chlorambucil has fared best,[41] and is currently recommended for use, especially when the eye is involved.[6,42] Levamisole proves helpful in some cases, perhaps through its granulocyte suppressing actions.[48] Azathioprine, cyclophosphamide, and other immunosuppressive compounds seem not to be as effective. Corticosteroids provide indifferent results and, in the case of eye involvement, can actually worsen the disease.[37] Blood transfusions were at one time claimed to induce remissions, later shown to be of no value, but not before the probable active principle, transfer factor, was adduced as likely to prove helpful. In a limited series of cases, transfer factor has brought patients through large vessel thrombosis and other crises.[5] Fibrinolytic compounds have found some favor.[11,40] Overall, however, symptomatic therapy of the various expressions of the disease is required and is moderately successful. Major surgery may be necessitated by intractable involvement of vital organs.

Prognosis. Although Behçet's syndrome does not necessarily compromise life expectancy, the advent of nervous system symptoms and signs or of ocular involvement is an ominous event. This syndrome ought, therefore, to be considered as a benign disease subject to serious or fatal complications. Behçet's disease is more likely to be progressive and destructive than Behçet's syndrome occurring in the context of other diseases.

STEVENS-JOHNSON SYNDROME

In a sense, the Stevens-Johnson syndrome does not belong to the realm of rheumatology. Joint and muscle involvement consists of transient pains only, which may be mere reflections of the severity of the disease. Because there are so many similarities or potential points of confusion between the Stevens-Johnson syndrome and Behçet's syndrome or Reiter's syndrome, however, it will be discussed.

Stevens-Johnson syndrome is included among the oculocutaneous syndromes. Most clinicians regard it as a variant of erythema multiforme exudativum with systemic manifestations and a potentially grave prognosis. Although there seem to be earlier reports, the description by Hebra is considered to be the classic depiction of the cutaneous syndrome. In 1922, Stevens and Johnson elaborated the constitutional symptoms of the syndrome that now bears their name.[15]

The onset of Stevens-Johnson syndrome is heralded by high fever and extensive stomatitis. Although this onset may superficially resemble mon-

ilial stomatitis, it rapidly develops into a series of ulcerated lesions on the oral mucous membranes, the conjunctiva, the nasal mucosa, and the genitalia and anus. Within a few days, a bullous and erythematous skin eruption develops anywhere on the body (Fig. 58–12), and erythematous plaques form on the extremities.[3] Pneumonitis is frequently present, either as a precursor or as a concomitant finding. To make the diagnosis, the eruption of erythema multiforme accompanied by bullae or vesicles and stomatitis is required. Documented fever, balanitis, vaginitis or urethritis, and conjunctivitis also occur, although they need not all be present simultaneously in the same patients.

Widespread arthralgias and myalgias of relatively transient nature may be present. These symptoms are rarely accompanied by actual signs of arthritis.[7]

The syndrome is particularly prevalent in the pediatric age group, although it may occur at any age; the risk of developing the syndrome is greatly reduced after the age of 20. All reports emphasize a male preponderance.

The syndrome begins in one of three ways. It may suddenly appear in an individual of good health, without apparent exogenous factors. Second, there may be symptoms suggestive of an upper respiratory tract[8] or urinary tract infection, for which drug therapy is initiated.[3] Whereas only about one-fifth of the patients have the first pattern, half develop the syndrome after prodromata for which some treatment is afforded. In these cases, the prior illness occurs in bodily areas later to be affected by Stevens-Johnson syndrome. The third mode of presentation also follows drug treatment, but for disorders seemingly remote from the Stevens-Johnson syndrome. For example, epilepsy seems unrelated to Stevens-Johnson syndrome, but the administration of anticonvulsants may directly precede the onset of the syndrome.

Laboratory and Roentgenographic Features. No specific abnormalities of laboratory tests or roentgenographic examinations occur to support the diagnosis of Stevens-Johnson syndrome. However, in many cases, mycoplasma pneumoniae are recoverable from the pharynx,[8] sputum,[5] and exudates of the bullous lesions;[3] moreover, rises of specific hemagglutination inhibition and complement fixation antibodies are recorded during the disease, with fall of these antibodies during the recovery phase.[14] Leukocyte-bound immunoglobulin is also demonstrable.

Etiology. The causes of this syndrome are still the subject of controversy. Mycoplasma pneumoniae has a clear edge on other microorganisms as a provocative agent.[2,10] Other viruses, fungi, and bacteria have also been implicated. Most cases fol-

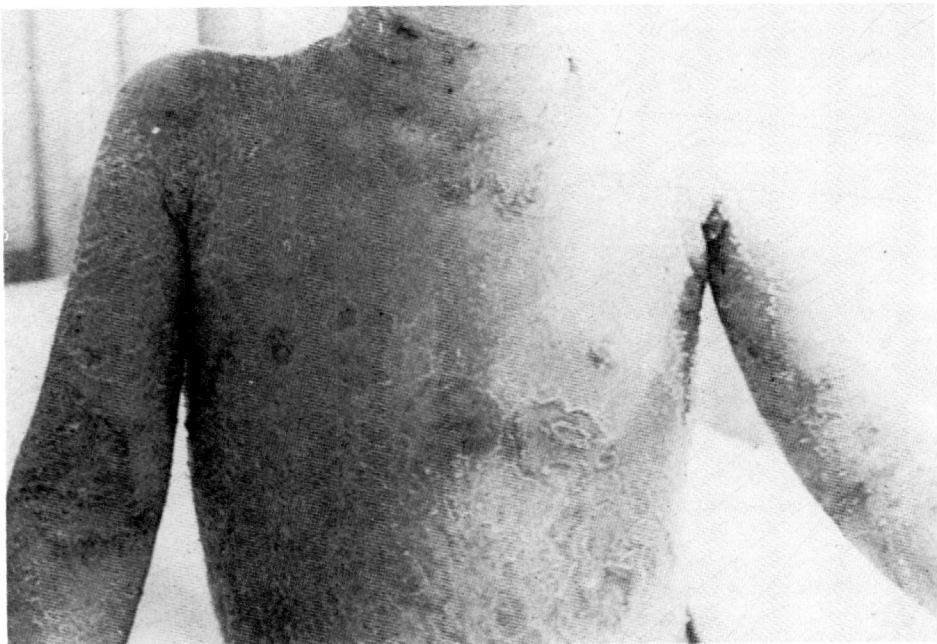

Fig. 58–12. Bullous and crusting cutaneous eruption in patient with Stevens-Johnson syndrome (erythema multiforme exudativum).

low drug therapy, with sulfonamides clearly the major cause.[1] Warning labels have been affixed to certain long-acting sulfa drugs, naming them as potential precursors of Stevens-Johnson syndrome,[6] but careful reviews of the evidence have found it wanting. A few recorded cases have followed administration of drugs in common use for treatment of rheumatic diseases, including aspirin and phenylbutazone.[1] Laxatives and sedatives, many nonprescription, are also culpable. Measles vaccination has preceded the onset. Antibiotics, including clindamycin,[9] have been implicated. Hypoglycemic drugs, most recently chlorpropamide, have also been incriminated.[11] In many cases, no causal relationship to a preceding event can be demonstrated. Antibodies at various sites of specific provocations may be responsible, and may account also for the neutropenia often seen at the same time.[13] Immune complexes then deposit in the superficial microvasculature of the skin and mucous membranes.[12]

Treatment. When a specific microorganism seems responsible for the syndrome, appropriate antibiotic therapy, usually with tetracycline, may prove beneficial.[10] In some cases, corticosteroids have been used with mixed success (it may be a matter of selection as some patients worsen while others improve). Nonspecific supportive measures should be taken.

Prognosis. Although fatalities have been re-

corded,[11] the outlook is not unfavorable, particularly in older patients. Infants and small children bear the greatest risk.

The *periodicity* of the syndrome results from renewed provocation by the offending factor. Multiple episodes are likely when the syndrome is precipitated by a nonprescription medication, because this is often beyond the physician's control. Other cases recur because the patient fails to give a complete history and the offending drug is prescribed again.

Because the Stevens-Johnson syndrome occurs in conjunction with ulcerative colitis[4] and disorders of the reticuloendothelial system, including leukemias (usually in response to some therapeutic agent used for these various disorders),[3] underlying diseases should always be sought.

Provocative tests with suspected drugs should never be attempted.

OTHER INTERMITTENT SYNDROMES

Many diseases exhibiting rheumatic symptoms and signs may recur after they have seemingly run their course. *Acute tropical polyarthritis,* an oligoarticular disorder affecting chiefly the large joints of adults, accompanied by fever and abnormalities of the acute phase reactants, is one such disease and is described by Greenwood.[1] Although the attack is usually single, and can be aborted with aspirin, recurrent attacks may develop after an indeterminate interval. Descriptions of this disease have thus far been limited to Africa, but they resemble the *epidemic polyarthritis of northern Australia,* which is associated with Group A arbovirus infection.

The overlapping manifestations of the syndromes discussed suggest that certain basic underlying mechanisms may be common to all. Because attention paid to esoterica often results in deeper understanding of more common problems, the periodic and intermittent syndromes may lead the way to better understanding of the mechanisms of joint inflammation and the rhythms of nature.

REFERENCES

General

1. Greenwood, B.M.: Acute tropical polyarthritis. Q. J. Med., *38*:295–306, 1969.
2. Morley, A., and Stohlman, F.: Cyclophosphamide-induced cyclical neutropenia: An animal model of a human periodic disease. N. Engl. J. Med., *282*:643–646, 1970.

Intermittent Hydrarthrosis

1. Bywaters, E.G.L., and Ansell, B.: Intermittent hydrarthrosis. *In* Textbook of the Rheumatic Diseases, 4th Ed. Edited by W.S.C. Copeman. London, E & S Livingstone, Ltd., 1968, p. 525.
2. Cronkite, E.P.: Granulopoietic models—effect on chemotherapy. N. Engl. J. Med., *282*:683–684, 1970.
3. Ragan, C.: Intermittent hydrarthrosis. *In* Arthritis and Allied Conditions, 7th Ed. Edited by J.L. Hollander, Philadelphia, Lea & Febiger, 1966, p. 755.
4. Reimann, H.A.: Periodic diseases in the aged. Geriatrics, *24*:146–149, 1969.
5. Schlesinger, H.: Die intermittirenden Gelenkschwellungen. Vienna, A. Holder, Nothnagel's Specielle Pathologie und Therapie, 7:3, 1903.
6. Weiner, A.D., and Ghormley, R.K.: Periodic benign synovitis: Idiopathic intermittent hydrarthrosis. J. Bone Joint Surg., *38A*:1039–1055, 1956.

Palindromic Rheumatism

1. Ansell, B.M., and Bywaters, E.G.L.: Palindromic rheumatism. Ann. Rheum. Dis., *18*:331–332, 1959.
2. Bywaters, E.G.L., and Ansell, B.M.: Palindromic rheumatism. *In* Textbook of the Rheumatic Diseases, 4th Ed. Edited by N.S.C. Copeman. London, E & S Livingstone, Ltd., 1958, p. 524.
3. Epstein, S.: Hypersensitivity to sodium nitrate: A major causative factor in case of palindromic rheumatism. Ann. Allergy, *27*:343–349, 1969.
4. Ginsberg, M.H., et al.: Rheumatoid nodulosis. Arthritis Rheum., *18*:49–58, 1975.
5. Harris, E.D., Jr., Cohen, G.L., and Krane, S.M.: Synovial collagenase: Its presence in culture from joint disease of diverse etiology. Arthritis Rheum., *12*:92–102, 1969.
6. Hench, P.S., and Rosenberg, E.F.: Palindromic rheumatism. Arch. Intern. Med., *73*:293–321, 1944.
7. Hench, P.S., and Rosenberg, E.F.: Palindromic rheumatism: New oft-recurring disease of joints (arthritis, periarthritis, para-arthritis) apparently producing no articular residues: report of 34 cases. Proc. Mayo Clinic, *16*:808–815, 1941.
8. Mattingly, S.: Palindromic rheumatism. Ann. Rheum. Dis., *25*:307–317, 1966.
9. Molnar, Z., Metzger, A.L., and McCarty, D.J.: Tubular structures in endothelium in palindromic rheumatism. Arthritis Rheum., *15*:553–556, 1972.
10. Schumacher, H.R.: Palindromic onset of rheumatoid arthritis. Arthritis Rheum., *25*:361–369, 1982.
11. Thompson, B., et al.: Palindromic rheumatism. II. Failure

to detect circulating immune complexes during acute episodes. Ann. Rheum. Dis., *38*:329–331, 1979.
12. Wajed, M.A., Brown, D.L., and Currey, H.L.F.: Palindromic rheumatism. Ann. Rheum. Dis., *36*:56–61, 1977.
13. Ward, L.E., and Okihiro, M.M.: Palindromic rheumatism: Follow-up report. Arch. Inter-Am. Rheum., *2*:208–222, 1959.
14. Zawadzki, Z.A., and Benedek, T.G.: Rheumatoid arthritis, dysproteinemic arthropathy, and paraproteinemia. Arthritis Rheum., *12*:555–568, 1969.

Familial Mediterranean Fever

1. Aisen, P., et al.: Lipoxygenase production in the serum and synovial fluid of patients with Familial Mediterranean fever (FMF) (abstract). Arthritis Rheum., *27*:546, 1984.
1a. Ari, J.B., et al.: Dialysis in renal failure caused by amyloidosis of familial Mediterranean fever. Arch. Intern. Med., *136*:449–451, 1976.
2. Bar Eli, M., et al.: Leukocyte chemotaxis in recurrent polyserositis (familial Mediterranean fever). Am. J. Med. Sci., *281*:15–18, 1981.
3. Benson, M.D., Skinner, M., and Cohen, A.S.: Amyloid deposition in a renal transplant in familial Mediterranean fever. Ann. Intern. Med., *87*:31–34, 1977.
4. Blum, A., et al.: Amyloidosis as the sole manifestation of familial Mediterranean fever (FMF): Further evidence of its genetic nature. Ann. Intern. Med., *57*:795–799, 1962.
5. Bondy, P.K., et al.: The possible relationship of etiocholanolone to periodic fever. Yale J. Biol. Med., *30*:395–405, 1958.
6. Cooksey, D.E., and Girard, K.: Temporomandibular joint synovitis with effusion in familial Mediterranean fever. Oral Surg., *47*:123–126, 1979.
7. Dabestani, A., et al.: Pericardial disease in familial Mediterranean fever: An echocardiographic study. Chest, *81*:592–595, 1982.
8. Dinarello, C.A., et al.: Colchicine therapy for familial Mediterranean fever. N. Engl. J. Med., *291*:934–937, 1974.
9. Ehrenfeld, M., et al.: Gastrointestinal effects of long-term colchicine therapy in patients with recurrent polyserositis (familial Mediterranean fever). Dig. Dis. Sci., *27*:723–727, 1982.
10. Ehrlich, G.E.: Periodic and intermittent rheumatic syndromes. Bull. Rheum. Dis., *24*:746–749, 1973.
11. Ehrlich, G.E.: Familial Mediterranean fever. Clin. Orthop., *57*:51–55, 1968.
11a. Eliakim, M., Levy, M., and Ehrenfeld, M.: Recurrent Polyserositis. Familial Mediterranean Fever, Periodic Disease. Amsterdam, Elsevier/North-Holland, 1981, pp. 119–121.
12. Flatau, E., et al.: Schonlein-Henoch syndrome in patients with familial Mediterranean fever. Arthritis Rheum., *25*:42–47, 1982.
13. Frensdorff, A., Sohar, E., and Heller, H.: Plasma fibrinogen in familial Mediterranean fever. Ann. Intern. Med., *55*:448–455, 1961.
14. Gafni, J., Sohar, E., and Heller, H.: The inherited amyloidoses: Their clinical and theoretical significance. Lancet, *1*:71–74, 1964.
15. Goldstein, R.C., and Schwabe, A.D.: Prophylactic colchicine therapy in familial Mediterranean fever: A controlled double blind study. Ann. Intern. Med., *81*:792–794, 1974.
16. Hart, F.D.: The stiff aching back: The differential diagnosis of ankylosing spondylitis. Lancet, *1*:740–742, 1968.
17. Heller, H., et al.: The arthritis of familial Mediterranean fever. Arthritis Rheum., *9*:1–17, 1966.
18. Heller, H., et al.: Amyloidosis in familial Mediterranean fever: An independent genetically determined character. Arch. Intern. Med., *107*:539–550, 1961.
19. Heller, H., Sohar, E., and Sherf, L.: Familial Mediterranean fever. Arch. Intern. Med., *102*:50–71, 1958.
20. Hurwich, B.J., Schwartz, J., and Goldfarb, S.: Record survival of siblings with familial Mediterranean fever: Phenotypes 1 & 2. Arch. Intern. Med., *125*:308–311, 1970.
21. Ilfeld, D., Weil, S., and Kuperman, O.: Correction of a

suppressor cell deficiency and amelioration of familial Mediterranean fever by hemodialysis. Arthritis Rheum., 25:38–41, 1982.

21a. Jacob, E.T., et al.: Renal transplantation in the amyloidosis of familial Mediterranean fever. Experience in ten cases. Arch. Intern. Med., 139:1135–1138, 1979.

21b. Kaushansky, K., Finerman, G.A., and Schwabe, A.D.: Chronic destructive arthritis in familial Mediterranean fever: The predominance of hip involvement and its management. Clin. Orthop., 155:156–161, 1981.

22. Lehman, T.J., et al.: Long term colchicine therapy of familial Mediterranean fever. J. Pediatr., 93:876–978, 1978.

23. Levy, M., et al.: Circulating immune complexes in recurrent polyserositis (familial Mediterranean fever, periodic disease). J. Rheumatol., 7:886–890, 1980.

24. Ludomirsky, A., Passwell, J., and Boichis, H.: Amyloidosis in children with familial Mediterranean fever. Arch. Dis. Child., 56:464–467, 1981.

24a. Matzner, Y., and Brzezinski, P.: C5a inhibitor deficiency in peritoneal fluids from patients with familial Mediterranean fever. N. Engl. J. Med., 311:287–290, 1984.

25. Mellinkoff, S.M., et al.: Familial Mediterranean fever: Plasma protein abnormalities, low fat diet, and possible implications in pathogenesis. Ann. Intern. Med., 56:171–181, 1962.

26. Meyerhoff, J.: Familial Mediterranean fever: Report of a large family, review of the literature, and discussion of the frequency of amyloidosis. Medicine (Baltimore), 59:66–77, 1980.

27. Michaeli, D., Pras, M., and Rozen, N.: Intestinal strangulation complicating familial Mediterranean fever. Br. Med. J., 2:30–31, 1966.

28. Mohr, W.: Spondylitis bei Tropenerkrankungen. Verh. Dtsch. Ges. Rheumatol., 1:70–80, 1969.

29. Mosesson, M.W., et al.: Evidence for circulating fibrin in familial Mediterranean fever. J. Lab. Clin. Med., 99:559–567, 1982.

30. Ozdemir, A.I., and Sokmen, C.: Familial Mediterranean fever among the Turkish people. Am. J. Gastroenterol., 51:311–316, 1969.

31. Priest, R.J., and Nixon, R.K.: Familial recurring polyserositis: A disease entity. Ann. Intern. Med., 51:1253–1274, 1959.

32. Rachmilewitz, M., Ehrenfeld, E.N., and Eliakim, M.: Recurrent polyserositis. J.A.M.A., 171:2355, 1959.

33. Raviv, U., Rubinstein, A., and Schonfeld, A.E.: Pericarditis in familial Mediterranean fever. Am. J. Dis. Child., 116:442–444, 1959.

34. Reich, C.B., and Franklin, E.C.: Familial Mediterranean fever in an Italian family. Arch. Intern. Med., 125:337–340, 1970.

35. Reimann, H.A.: Periodic disease. Medicine (Baltimore), 30:219–245, 1951.

36. Reimann, H.A.: Periodic disease. J.A.M.A., 136:239–244, 1948.

37. Reimann, H.A., Coppola, E.D., and Vellegos, G.R.: Serum complement defects in periodic diseases. Ann. Intern. Med., 73:737–740, 1970.

38. Schrager, G.J.: Intestinal obstruction complicating familial Mediterranean fever. Pediatrics, 74:968–996, 1969.

39. Shahin, N., Sohar, E., and Delith, F.: Roentgenological findings in familial Mediterranean fever (FMF). Am. J. Roentgenol., 84:269–283, 1960.

40. Siegal, S.: Familial paroxysmal polyserositis. Am. J. Med., 36:893–918, 1964.

41. Siegal, S.: Benign paroxysmal peritonitis. Ann. Intern. Med., 23:1–21, 1945.

42. Silver, J., et al.: Unmasking of isolated hypoaldosteronism after renal allotransplantation in familial Mediterranean fever. Isr. J. Med. Sci., 18:495–498, 1982.

43. Sohar, E., et al.: Familial Mediterranean fever: A survey of 470 cases and review of the literature. Am. J. Med., 43:227–253, 1967.

44. Vilaseca, J., et al.: Periodic meningitis and familial Mediterranean fever. Arch. Intern. Med., 142:378–379, 1982.

45. Wolff, S.M.: Familial Mediterranean fever: A status report. Hosp. Pract., 13:113–115, 1978.

46. Wright, D.E., et al.: Efficacy of intermittent colchicine therapy in familial Mediterranean fever. Ann. Intern Med., 86:162–165, 1977.

Behçet's Syndrome

1. Adamantiades, B.: Sur un cas d'iritis a hypopyon recidivante. Ann. Oculist, 168:271, 1931.

2. Afifi, A.K., et al.: The myopathology of Behçet's disease—a histochemical, light- and electron-microscopic study. J. Neurol. Sci., 48:333–342, 1980.

3. Arkin, C.R., et al.: Behçet syndrome with myositis: A case report with pathological findings. Arthritis Rheum., 23:600–604, 1980.

4. Behçet, H.: Über rezidivierende aphthöse, durch ein virus verursachte Geschwüre am Mund, am Auge und an den Genitalien. Dermatol. Wchnscr., 105:1152, 1937.

5. Bernhard, G.C., and Heim, L.R.: Transfer factor treatment of Behçet's syndrome (abstract). J. Rheumatol., 1:34, 1974.

6. Bonnet, M.: Immunosuppressive therapy of Behçet's syndrome: Long term follow-up evaluation. In Behçet's Disease. Edited by G. Inaba. Tokyo, University of Tokyo Press, 1982, pp. 487–498.

7. Brama, I., and Fainaru, M.: Inner ear involvement in Behçet's disease. Arch. Otolaryngol., 106:215–217, 1980.

8. Chajek, T., and Fainaru, M.: Behçet disease: Report of 41 cases and a review of the literature. Medicine (Baltimore), 54:179–196, 1975.

9. Chamberlain, M.A.: A family study of Behçet's syndrome. Ann. Rheum. Dis., 37:459–465, 1978.

10. Cotticelli, L., et al.: Behçet's disease: An unusual case with bilateral obliterating retinal panarteritis and ischemic optic atrophy. Ophthalmologica, 180:328–332, 1980.

11. Cunliffe, W.J., and Menon, J.S.: Treatment of Behçet's syndrome with phenformin and ethyl oestrenol. Lancet, 1:1239–1240, 1969.

12. Denman, A.M., et al.: Lymphocyte abnormalities in Behçet's syndrome. Clin. Exp. Immunol., 42:175–185, 1980.

13. Dilsen, N., et al.: Virus-like particles and tuboreticular structures in kidney and eye of patients with Behçet's syndrome. In Behçet's Disease. Edited by G. Inaba. Tokyo, University of Tokyo Press, 1982, pp. 3–14.

14. Dilsen, N., et al.: Preliminary family study on Behçet's disease in Turkey. In Behçet's Disease. Edited by G. Inaba. Tokyo, University of Tokyo Press, 1982, pp. 103–111.

15. Djawari, D., Hornstein, O.P., and Schotz, J.: Enhancement of granulocyte chemotaxis in Behçet's disease. Arch. Dermatol. Res., 270:81–88, 1981.

16. Durieux, P., et al.: Multiple pulmonary arterial aneurysms in Behçet's disease and Hughes-Stovin syndrome. Am. J. Med., 71:736–741, 1981.

17. Ehrlich, G.E.: Phagocytes and mediators of inflammation in Behçet's syndrome. In Behçet's Disease. Edited by G. Inaba. Tokyo, University of Tokyo Press, 1982, pp. 235–240.

18. Ehrlich, G.E.: Periodic and intermittent rheumatic syndromes. Bull. Rheum. Dis., 24:746–749, 1974.

19. Ehrlich, G.E., et al.: Further studies of platelet rosettes around granulocytes in Behçet's syndrome. Inflammation, 1:223–229, 1975.

20. Feigenbaum, A.: Description of Behçet's syndrome in the Hippocratic third book of endemic diseases. Br. J. Ophthalmol., 40:355–357, 1956.

21. Fordham, J.N., et al.: Polymorphonuclear function in Behçet's syndrome. Ann. Rheum. Dis., 41:421–425, 1982.

22. Gamble, C.N., et al.: The immune complex pathogenesis of glomerulonephritis and pulmonary vasculitis in Behçet's disease. Am. J. Med., 66:1031–1039, 1979.

23. Giacomello, A., Surgi, M.L., and Zoppini, A.: Pseudopodagra in Behçet's syndrome. Arthritis Rheum., 24:750–751, 1981.

24. Grenier, P., et al.: Pulmonary involvement in Behçet's disease. Am. J. Roentgenol., 137:565–569, 1981.

25. Haim, S., et al.: Leucocyte migration inhibition in Behçet's disease. Dermatologica, 159:302–306, 1979.

26. Herreman, G., et al.: Behçet's syndrome and renal involvement: A histological and immunofluorescent study of eleven renal biopsies. Am. J. Med. Sci., 284:10–17, 1982.

27. Jimi, S., et al.: Epidemiological studies on Behçet's dis-

ease. *In* Behçet's Disease. Edited by G. Inaba. Tokyo, University of Tokyo Press, 1982, pp. 51–56.

28. Kasahara, Y., et al.: Intestinal involvement in Behçet's disease: Review of 136 surgical cases in the Japanese literature. Dis. Colon Rectum, *24*:103–106, 1981.

29. Landwehr, D.M., Cooke, D.L., and Rodriguez, G.E.: Rapidly progressive glomerulonephritis in Behçet's syndrome. J.A.M.A., *244*:1709–1711, 1980.

30. Lehner, T.: Recent advances in cellular and humoral immunity in Behçet's syndrome. *In* Behçet's Disease. Edited by G. Inaba, Tokyo, University of Tokyo Press, 1982, pp. 357–369.

31. Lehner, T.: Progress report: Oral ulceration and Behçet's syndome. Gut, *18*:491–511, 1977.

32. Lehner, T.: Behçet's syndrome and autoimmunity. Br. Med. J., *1*:465–467, 1967.

33. Lehner, T., et al.: An immunogenetic basis for the tissue involvement in Behçet's syndrome. Immunology, *37*:895–900, 1979.

34. Lehner, T., Losito, A., and Williams, D.G.: Cryoglobulins in Behçet's syndrome and recurrent oral ulcerations: Assay by laser nephelometry. Clin. Exp. Immunol., *38*:436–444, 1979.

35. Maeda, K., Agata, T., and Nakae, K.: Recent trends of Behçet's disease in Japan and some of its epidemiological features. *In* Behçet's Disease. Edited by G. Inaba. Tokyo, University of Tokyo Press, 1982, pp. 15–24.

36. Mason, R.M., and Barnes, C.G.: Behçet's syndrome with arthritis. Ann. Rheum. Dis., *28*:95–103, 1969.

37. Mimura, Y.: Treatment of ocular lesions in Behçet's disease. *In* Behçet's Disease. Edited by G. Inaba. Tokyo, University of Tokyo Press, 1982, pp. 499–512.

38. Mishima, S., et al.: Behçet's disease in Japan: Ophthalmologic aspects. Trans. Am. Ophthalmol. Soc., *77*:225–279, 1979.

39. Miyachi, Y., et al.: Colchicine in the treatment of the cutaneous manifestations of Behçet's disease. Br. J. Dermatol., *104*:67–69, 1981.

40. Mizushima, Y., et al.: Colchicine and anti-thrombocytic drugs in the treatment of Behçet's disease. *In* Behçet's Disease. Edited by G. Inaba. Tokyo, University of Tokyo Press, 1982, pp. 513–518.

41. O'Duffy, J.D.: Treatment of Behçet's disease with chlorambucil. *In* Behçet's Disease. Edited by G. Inaba. Tokyo, University of Tokyo Press, 1982, pp. 479–486.

42. O'Duffy, J.D., Lehner, T., and Barnes, C.G.: Summary of the third international conference on Behçet's disease. J. Rheumatol., *10*:154–158, 1983.

43. Ohno, S., et al.: Close association of HLA-BW51 with Behçet's disease. Arch. Ophthalmol., *100*:1455–1458, 1982.

44. Ohno, S., et al.: Close association of HLA-BW51, MT2, and Behçet's disease. *In* Behçet's Disease. Edited by G. Inaba. Tokyo, University of Tokyo Press, 1982, pp. 73–74.

45. Oshima, Y., et al.: Clinical studies on Behçet's syndrome. Ann. Rheum. Dis., *22*:36–45, 1963.

46. Pamir, M.N., et al.: Papilledema in Behçet's syndrome. Arch. Neurol., *38*:643–645, 1981.

47. Reza, M.J., and Demanes, D.J.: Behçet's disease: A case with hemoptysis, pseudotumor cerebri, and arteritis. J. Rheumatol., *5*:320–326, 1978.

48. Sampson, D.: Studies on levamisole, a potentially useful drug in the treatment of Behçet's syndrome. J. Oral. Pathol., *7*:383–386, 1978.

49. Sazazuki, T., et al.: Genetic analysis of Behçet's disease. *In* Behçet's Disease. Edited by G. Inaba. Tokyo, University of Tokyo Press, 1982, pp. 33–40.

50. Scarlett, J.A., Kistner, M.L., and Yang, L.C.: Behçet's syndrome. Report of a case associated with pericardial effusion and cryoglobulinemia treated with indomethacin. Am. J. Med., *66*:146–148, 1979.

51. Shigeta, T.: Recurrent iritis with hypopyon and its pathological findings. Acta Soc. Ophthalmol. Japan, *28*:516, 1924.

52. Shimizu, T., et al.: Behçet's disease (Behçet's syndrome). Sem. Arthritis Rheum., *8*:223–260, 1979.

53. Shimizu, T., et al.: Behçet's disease: Guide to diagnosis of Behçet's disease. Jpn. J. Ophthalmol., *18*:291, 1974.

54. Takeuchi, A., et al.: The mechanism of hyperchemotaxis in Behçet's disease. J. Rheumatol., *8*:40–44, 1981.

55. Whitwell, G.P.B.: Recurrent buccal and vulvar ulcers with associated embolic phenomena in skin and eye. Br. J. Dermatol., *46*:414, 1934.

56. Yazici, H., et al.: HLA antigens in Behçet's disease: A reappraisal by a comparative study of Turkish and British patients. Ann. Rheum. Dis., *39*:344–348, 1980.

57. Yazici, H., et al.: The combined use of HLA-B5 and the pathergy test as diagnostic markers of Behçet's disease in Turkey. J. Rheumatol., *7*:206–210, 1980.

Stevens-Johnson Syndrome

1. Bianchine, J.R., et al.: Drugs as etiologic factors in the Stevens-Johnson syndrome. Am. J. Med., *44*:390–405, 1968.

2. Blattner, R.J.: Mycoplasma infection. J. Pediatr., *72*:554–555, 1968.

3. Bukantz, S.C.: Stevens-Johnson syndrome. DM, October 1968, pp. 1–36.

4. Cameron, A.J., Baron, J.H., and Priestley, B.L.: Erythema multiforme, drugs, and ulcerative colitis. Br. Med. J., *2*:1174–1178, 1966.

5. Cannell, H., Churcher, G.M., and Milton-Thompson, G.J.: Stevens-Johnson syndrome associated with mycoplasma pneumoniae infection. Br. J. Dermatol., *81*:196–199, 1969.

6. Carroll, O.M., Bryan, P.A., and Robinson, R.J.: Stevens-Johnson syndrome associated with long acting sulfonamides. J.A.M.A., *195*:691–693, 1966.

7. Coursin, D.B.: Stevens-Johnson syndrome. J.A.M.A., *198*:113–116, 1966.

8. Fleming, P.C., et al.: Febrile mucocutaneous syndrome with respiratory involvement associated with isolation of mycoplasma pneumoniae. Can. Med. Assoc. J., *97*:1458–1459, 1967.

9. Fulghum, D.D., and Catalano, P.M.: Stevens-Johnson syndrome from clindamycin. A case report. J.A.M.A., *223*:318–319, 1973.

10. Jones, M.C.: Arthritis and arthralgia in infection with mycoplasma pneumoniae. Thorax, *25*:748–750, 1970.

11. Kanefsky, T.M., and Medoff, S.J.: Stevens-Johnson syndrome and neutropenia with chlorpropamide therapy. Arch. Intern. Med., *140*:1543, 1980.

12. Kazmierowski, J.A., and Wuepper, K.D.: Erythema multiforme. Clin. Rheumat. Dis., *8*:415–426, 1982.

13. Safai, B., Good, R.A., and Day, N.K.: Erythema multiforme: Report of two cases and speculation on immune mechanisms involved in the pathogenesis. Clin. Immunol. Immunopathol., *7*:379–389, 1977.

14. Sieber, O.F., et al.: Mycoplasma pneumoniae infection associated with Stevens-Johnson syndrome. J.A.M.A., *200*:79–81, 1967.

15. Stevens, A.M., and Johnson, F.C.: A new eruptive fever associated with stomatitis and ophthalmia. Am. J. Dis. Child., *24*:526–533, 1922.

Chapter 59

Polymyalgia Rheumatica and Giant Cell Arteritis

Louis A. Healey

POLYMYALGIA RHEUMATICA

Polymyalgia rheumatica is a syndrome of older patients characterized by pain and stiffness in the neck, shoulders, and pelvic girdle, persisting for at least a month, without weakness or atrophy, accompanied by a rapid erythrocyte sedimentation rate (ESR), and dramatically relieved by adrenocorticosteroid treatment in low doses (Table 59–1).

History. In 1957, Barber introduced the name polymyalgia rheumatica for this illness. It had previously been reported as senile arthritis, myalgic syndrome of the aged, arthritic rheumatoid disease and, dating back to 1888, senile rheumatic gout. The rapid ESR suggested this disease might be a specific entity, and in 1951 Porsman pointed out the similarity to the prodrome of temporal arteritis. This relation was confirmed in 1963 by Alestig and Barr when they demonstrated giant cell arteritis on biopsy of asymptomatic temporal arteries in patients with polymyalgia rheumatica. This syndrome received little attention in the United States until 1966, but since then it has been widely recognized. The annual incidence has been estimated at 53 per 100,000 in persons over the age of 50.[2]

Clinical Picture. Polymyalgia rheumatica is rare in a patient less than 50 years old, and it has been reported twice as often in women as men. Racial predilection is striking; almost all reported patients have been Caucasian.

Patients complain of severe pain in the neck, back, shoulders, upper arms, and thighs. The onset is often abrupt. Patients may go to bed feeling well and awaken as uncomfortable as if they had chopped a cord of wood. Weakness is not prominent, but pain and gelling make rising from a chair

Table 59–1.   Definition of Polymyalgia Rheumatica

1. Patients at least 50 years old, usually Caucasian
2. Bilateral pain persisting for at least 1 month involving two of the following: neck, shoulder girdle, pelvic girdle Morning stiffness and gelling are marked
3. Erythrocyte sedimentation rate greater than 40 mm in 1 hour; often 100 mm or more

Exclusion: Any other diagnosis except giant cell arteritis

difficult. Morning stiffness is marked. In contrast to patients with rheumatoid arthritis, who describe difficulty with fine hand motions such as buttoning buttons, patients with polymyalgia rheumatica graphically describe how difficult it is to get out of bed. Some require help from a spouse, and others are forced to roll out of bed into a kneeling position and then push themselves erect. In some patients, symptoms are widespread; in others, one area, such as the pectoral or pelvic girdle, may predominate. Nonspecific symptoms may include fever, anorexia, weight loss (often marked), lassitude, apathy, and depression.

In view of the severity of the complaints, the paucity of physical findings is surprising. Patients show no rash, nodules, arteritis, muscle weakness, or atrophy. Shoulder joint tenderness may be detectable, and effusions are sometimes present in the knees. Radiographs are unrevealing. A clue to the diagnosis is found in the ESR, which is almost always elevated, often greatly so, and can exceed 100 mm/h (Westergren method). Other acute phase reactants, especially fibrinogen, are similarly increased. Anemia may be present as a result of a block in utilization of iron. Rheumatoid factor and antinuclear antibodies are not present. Muscle enzyme levels in serum and electromyograms are normal, reflecting normal muscle tissue found at biopsy.

Scintigrams using technetium pertechnetate have shown localization primarily in the shoulders and, to a lesser degree, in wrists and knees, suggesting the polymyalgia may be a form of synovitis.[5] Biopsies have also shown a mild nonspecific inflammation of synovial tissue. Such a synovitis is consistent with the marked morning stiffness and gelling so characteristic of the clinical picture. Synovitis at the wrist might explain why some of these patients also have carpal tunnel syndrome.

Differential Diagnosis. Since the constellation of findings in polymyalgia rheumatica is not specific, the diagnosis depends on differentiation from other diseases (Table 59–2). The pain and stiffness of polymyalgia persist for at least a month, in contrast to the myalgias seen with ''flu syndrome'' and

Table 59–2.   Conditions to be Distinguished from Polymyalgia Rheumatica

1. Viral myalgia	Duration is less than a month
2. Rheumatoid arthritis	Examination detects synovitis of small joints; rheumatoid factor is often present
3. Polymyositis	Muscle enzyme levels are elevated in serum; muscle biopsy and electromyogram are abnormal
4. Multiple myeloma	Gamma globulin spike on protein electrophoresis; plasma cells in bone marrow
5. Osteoarthritis	Erythrocyte sedimentation rate is usually normal
6. Fibrositis	Normal sedimentation rate
7. Depression and psychogenic symptoms	Normal sedimentation rate
8. Occult infection	Appropriate tests needed
9. Occult cancer	Appropriate tests needed

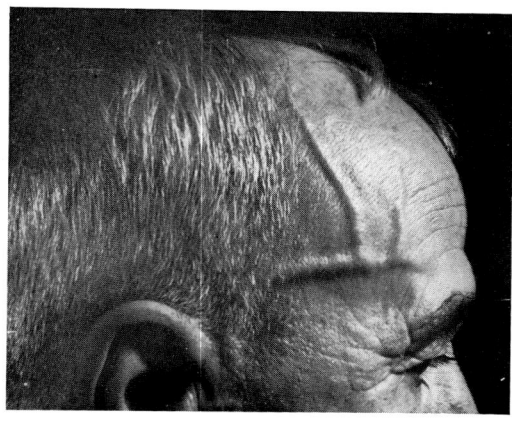

Fig. 59–1.   Temporal arteritis. The swollen temporal artery is tender and painful.

Table 59–3.   Manifestations of Giant Cell Arteritis

SYSTEMIC
Polymyalgia rheumatica
Fever
Anemia
Anorexia
Malaise
Weight loss
Abnormal liver function tests
LOCAL
Temporal headache
Blindness
Scalp necrosis
Tongue gangrene
Jaw claudication
Neuropathic manifestations—diplopia, paresthesia, brachial paralysis
Aortic arch syndrome—unequal pulses, claudication of arm or leg, aneurysm rupture, Raynaud's phenomenon

other viral illnesses, which last several days to a week. Apathy, depression, and lack of physical findings suggest depression of the aged, but the rapid ESR indicates that an additional factor is involved. The sedimentation rate also rules against a diagnosis of osteoarthritis. It may be difficult to differentiate muscle pain and stiffness from the weakness of polymyositis, but elevated muscle enzymes, abnormal electromyogram, and muscle biopsy are diagnostic of polymyositis.

Polymyalgia rheumatica may be difficult to distinguish from the onset of rheumatoid arthritis in the older patient when rheumatoid factor is not present. This similarity is not surprising, because both conditions are marked by synovitis. In rheumatoid arthritis, the small joints of hands and feet tend to be more involved, as opposed to the proximal distribution of polymyalgia. In some patients, only the subsequent course permits definite diagnosis.

Treatment.   The response of polymyalgia to corticosteroids is truly dramatic. Some patients are almost entirely well the next day. The improvement is so invariable that if response is not seen within a week, the diagnosis should be doubted. The usual initial dose is 10 to 30 mg of prednisone (or equivalent) a day. After several weeks, this dose is tapered to a daily maintenance dose of 5 to 7.5 mg while the clinical response is monitored. Aspirin and other anti-inflammatory drugs are less effective. The course is self-limited, lasting 1 to 2 years in approximately 50% of patients. Even those who require prednisone for longer periods eventually do well without joint destruction or disability.

Etiology.   The cause of polymyalgia rheumatica is not known. No infectious agent or toxin has been found. Hypocomplementemia, increased immu-

noglobulins, and other serologic tests often associated with "autoimmune diseases" are lacking. The striking preponderance of the disease in Caucasians suggests that a genetic predisposition is important. Studies have shown some association with the HLA antigens CW-3, DR-3, and DR-4. The predilection for older patients is unexplained. Long-term follow-up has not shown any association of polymyalgia with other disease, either rheumatic or neoplastic. Of great interest has been the relation to giant cell arteritis.

GIANT CELL ARTERITIS

In 1932, Horton described temporal arteritis in two elderly patients who had severe headache and high sedimentation rates. As he predicted, "this was a focal localization of an unknown systemic disease." It is now recognized that giant cell ar-

Table 59–4.   Symptoms Suggestive of Cranial Arteritis

Temporal headache
Scalp tenderness
Amaurosis fugax
Diplopia
Jaw claudication

teritis may involve medium-sized and large arteries throughout the body (see also Chap. 63). The temporal artery is only the most superficial and accessible (Fig. 59–1). The aorta and most of the larger arteries may be involved, but in contrast to polyarteritis, the small arterioles are spared. Thus, pulmonary and renal manifestations are not seen in giant cell arteritis. Stroke or myocardial infarction rarely occurs. The clinical manifestations can be divided into localized or systemic[4] (Table 59–3). The local manifestations (Table 59–4) depend on the artery involved and may include the typical temporal headache (temporal), sudden unilateral blindness (ophthalmic), transient diplopia due to paralysis of an extraocular muscle, pain in the jaw on chewing (facial), which is almost pathognomonic of cranial arteritis, and aortic arch syndrome, including claudication, aneurysm, and possibly rupture. In addition to polymyalgia, the systemic manifestations may include fever, anemia, weight loss, malaise, and abnormal liver function tests, particularly the *alkaline phosphatase*. At times, the systemic manifestations may predominate, posing a diagnostic problem such as fever of unknown origin, unexplained anemia, or simulation of an occult cancer.[3] In such patients, the rapid ESR may provide the clue that leads to biopsy of an asymptomatic temporal artery, and establishes the diagnosis.

Pathology. Inflammation is located on either side of the internal elastic lamina, which is fragmented. Infiltrate consists of histiocytes, lymphocytes, and the giant cells for which the lesion is named. The lumen is narrowed by the thickened edematous intima and at times may be occluded (Fig. 59–2). The histologic picture is indistinguishable from Takayasu's arteritis, but what relation might exist between the two is unknown. Electron microscopic examination reveals histiocytes and giant cells in close proximity to fragments of elastic lamina, whose ground substance is altered and appears dense and granular. Giant cell arteritis is distributed in skip fashion, interspersed with normal appearing artery, so that often biopsy of a sizable segment of artery is necessary for diagnosis.

Treatment. Giant cell arteritis responds to corticosteroids, but the dosage required is higher than that needed for treatment of polymyalgia rheumatica alone. Because of the risk of blindness, it

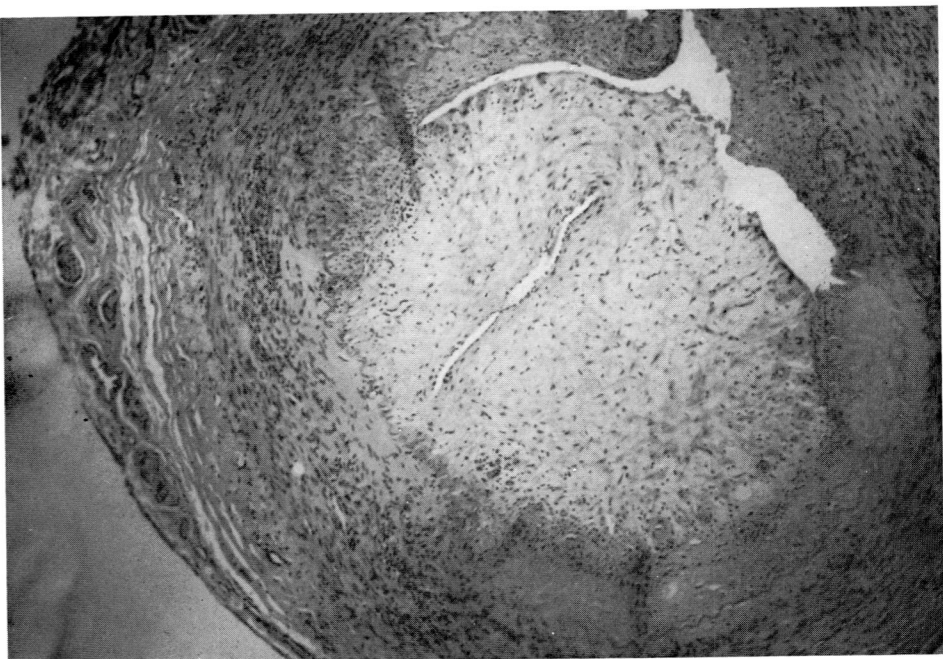

Fig. 59–2. Giant cell arteritis. Cross section of temporal artery showing inflammatory infiltrate, giant cells, fragmentation of elastic lamina, and intimal thickening; the lumen is almost occluded by thrombus. Separation at upper right is artifact.

is customary to treat with 60 mg (or equivalent) a day for 1 month. The dosage is then tapered following the symptoms, which are a better guide to tapering than the sedimentation rate. The primary side effect of steroid treatment in this older population is osteoporosis with vertebral collapse, which must be weighed against complications of the disease. Alternate-day steroids have not been effective in achieving control of the inflammation.

Etiology. The cause of giant cell arteritis is unknown. The histologic appearance suggests a cell-mediated immune response, but there has not been confirmatory evidence for this, whether in serologic tests, immunofluorescent staining of arterial tissue, or lymphocyte stimulation.

Relationship to Polymyalgia Rheumatica. It is evident that polymyalgia rheumatica is at times a manifestation of giant cell arteritis. Both have been noted in the same patient, either concurrently or at different times, and arteritis may be found in an asymptomatic temporal artery of a patient with polymyalgia rheumatica.[1] Whether polymyalgia is always a manifestation of occult arteritis is an important question because of the risk of blindness, but it has not yet been answered definitely. Many patients appear to have polymyalgia rheumatica alone. They respond well to low-dose steroid therapy and never develop headache, blindness, or any other sign of giant cell arteritis. At present, if a patient with polymyalgia rheumatica shows none of the clinical manifestations of cranial arteritis described, or if a temporal artery biopsy is negative, the chance of blindness is slight. Rather than risk corticosteroid toxicity, these patients might be treated with a lower dose. They should, however, be informed of the slight, but serious, risk of blindness, alerted to symptoms that are warning signals, and instructed to increase the steroid dose and to contact their physician if these symptoms appear.

REFERENCES

1. Bengtsson, B.-A., and Malmvall, B.-E.: Giant cell arteritis. Acta Med. Scand. [Suppl.], 658:1–102, 1982.
2. Chuang, T., Hunder, G.G., Ilstrup, D.M., and Kurland, L.T.: Polymyalgia rheumatica: A 10-year epidemiologic and clinical study. Ann. Intern. Med., 97:672–679, 1982.
3. Healey, L.A., and Wilske, K.R.: Occult giant cell arteritis. Arthritis Rheum., 23:641–643, 1980.
4. Healey, L.A., and Wilske, K.R.: The Systemic Manifestations of Temporal Arteritis. New York, Grune & Stratton, 1978.
5. O'Duffy, J.D., Hunder, G.G., and Wahner, H.W.: A follow-up study of polymyalgia rheumatica: evidence of chronic axial synovitis. J. Rheumatol., 7:685–693, 1980.

Systemic Rheumatic Diseases

Chapter 60

Introduction to Systemic Rheumatic Diseases: Nosology and Overlap Syndromes

Morris Reichlin

The diffuse connective tissue diseases are a group of syndromes of unknown etiology whose classification often presents formidable clinical problems. One cause of this classification problem is the large number of "overlap syndromes," which apparently exist among and between what are manifestly uncommon conditions. One experienced observer of the rheumatic diseases has stated that as many as 25% of all patients will have overlap features.[9] These findings include coexistent systemic lupus erythematosus (SLE) and scleroderma; an overlap of SLE, scleroderma, and polymyositis, which has been called mixed connective tissue disease (MCTD); scleroderma-polymyositis; coexistent SLE and rheumatoid arthritis; and the relationship that lymphocytic infiltration of the lacrimal and salivary glands bears to all the diffuse connective tissue diseases in what is recognized as Sjögren's syndrome.

Two current areas of investigation show promise for identifying specific biologic or biochemical markers that could be tightly linked with specific disease processes. These areas are (1) immunogenetics and (2) the identification of individual antigen-antibody reactions that exhibit disease specificity. The former subject is covered in Chapters 24 and 25, whereas the latter subject is discussed in many other chapters. Some specific aspects of this latter approach are explored here.

CLASSIFICATION OF POLYMYOSITIS

These problems are best illustrated by considering the classification of one group of these diseases, the polymyositis syndromes. A clinical diagnosis of polymyositis (PM) depends on the recognition of a pattern of proximal muscle weakness, on certain histopathologic findings in muscle biopsy specimens, on the demonstration of characteristic electromyographic findings, and on the presence in serum of elevated levels of muscle enzymes, notably creatine phosphokinase, transaminases, and aldolase (see Chap. 65). Further study of a given patient may also support the diagnosis

of another of the connective tissue diseases, such as rheumatoid arthritis, SLE, scleroderma, or Sjögren's (sicca) syndrome. If no connective tissue disease is present, one views the patient as having polymyositis or, if a characteristic dermatitis accompanies the muscle involvement, dermatomyositis (DM). It has long been believed that this group of patients carries an extraordinary risk for various carcinomas, although a critical analysis of this problem has raised questions about the extent of this relationship.[6]

The nosology is often complicated by the variable presence in the diffuse rheumatic diseases of shared clinical features. Polyarthritis and Raynaud's phenomenon may appear in PM patients without other clinical or serologic features suggesting the presence of other connective tissue diseases. In early evaluations, one may be erroneously led to the diagnosis of either SLE or scleroderma. Numerous opportunities for confusion can be cited at the time of the initial work-up of any of the connective tissue diseases.

Is PM one or many diseases with one or many pathogenetic mechanisms and one or many etiologies? PM occurring by itself is not distinguishable on clinical grounds from PM coincident with another connective tissue disease, and no solid clinical clues exist to differentiate the various forms of polymyositis. Although nothing is known of the etiologies of these diseases, something is known of their pathogenesis. A detailed exposition of the pathogenesis of muscle damage can be found in a review.[8] Evidence for humoral mechanisms, either immune complex-mediated or organ-specific, is sparse, whereas evidence supporting a cell-mediated immune attack on muscle is strong. Lymphocytes found in patients with PM are specifically cytotoxic for muscle cells and do not require serum factors for their activity. The presence and intensity of the activity of such cells correlate roughly with clinical activity. It is likely that such muscle-specific cytotoxic lymphocytes constitute the immunopathogenetic mechanism leading to muscle destruction and weakness in PM.

Data derivable from this work do not suggest possible heterogeneity of pathogenetic mechanisms in PM patients. In the future, the precise muscle antigens responsible for the activation of lymphocytes should be identified in patients with PM, and may shed light on the identity or nonidentity of immunopathogenetic pathways in these patients. If lymphocytes are activated by a single, unique muscle-specific antigen in all patients with PM, considerable importance will be given to the idea that a unitary immune mechanism exists in all polymyositis patients. If, however, each group of lymphocytes from patients with PM and DM or PM associated with a connective tissue disease reacts to a specific but different antigen, the alternative idea that PM is a collection of separate diseases in which the original sensitization process is characteristic for each "disease" would be more attractive. Finally, if such investigations reveal no pattern of antigenic specificity, then such studies will have failed to improve our ability to classify these diseases. The emergence of positive data for "marker" antibodies for the different connective tissue diseases lends encouragement to investigators engaged in such studies. A discussion of such data follows.

SPECIFIC ANTIGEN-ANTIBODY MARKERS

One of the major justifications underlying research on the immunology of the connective tissue diseases rests on the belief that specific antigen-antibody reactions exist which can serve as "markers" for specific diseases. Experience in the past decade has reinforced this belief. Serologic reactions shown to exhibit some disease specificity are listed in Table 60–1.

Until recently no antigen-antibody reaction had exhibited any specificity for the polymyositis syndromes. Although rheumatoid factors and antinuclear antibodies occur in moderate titers in about a third of such patients, these findings do not have an impact on diagnosis and are recognized as being nonspecific. At least three major antigen-antibody reactions are now recognized which show specificity for PM. The first of these involves a trypsin-sensitive nuclear antigen demonstrated by a modified complement fixation reaction with somewhat more specificity for DM than PM.[22] This antigen has been designated Mi, referring to the first two letters of the patient's name whose serum served as prototype for this reaction. In more recent studies utilizing an enzyme-linked immunoabsorbent assay (ELISA), the specificity for DM is even more apparent.[31a] The second antigen-antibody system described with specificity for patients with PM has been designated Jo_1.[16] Here again, Jo refers to the first two letters of the patient's name whose serum served as a prototype reagent for detection of this antibody by a precipitin reaction. This antibody occurs in 30% of uncomplicated PM and 10% or less of DM patients, and has thus far not been found in sera from patients with SLE, RA, progressive systemic sclerosis (PSS), Sjögren's syndrome, or normals. The antigen is a protein[16] that may be bound to histidyl tRNA.[26] Also of interest is the association of antibody to Jo_1 with the DRw3 antigen suggesting the involvement of specific immune response genes in its production.[5] Finally, a third reaction has been described. It involves a nucleolar antigen designated PM-Scl, since at least half the patients have PSS as well as PM.[20a] This latter system relates to a proportion of the patients (originally described by Wolfe, et al.[32]) whose sera contained antibody to an antigen designated PM_1. These authors reported that 60% of patients with PM had antibodies to PM_1, but did not comment on the marked heterogeneity that characterizes these reactions.[16] It is now apparent that while 60% of patients with PM have antibodies that precipitate

Table 60–1. Antigen-Antibody Reactions: "Markers" for Individual Connective Tissue Diseases

Antigen to which Specific Antibody Directed	Associated Disease*
Jo_1	PM
Mi	DM
PM-Scl	PM-PSS overlap
Native DNA	SLE
Sm	SLE
Nuclear ribonucleoprotein (nRNP)	SLE, MCTD
Ro/SSA	SLE, Sjögren's syndrome
La/SSB/Ha	SLE, Sjögren's syndrome
Scl_{70}	PSS
Centromere	PSS

*DM = dermatomyositis; PM = polymyositis; SLE = systemic lupus erythematosus; MCTD = mixed connective tissue disease; PSS = progressive systemic sclerosis (systemic scleroderma).

with crude extracts of thymus tissue, at least three major systems (Jo_1, PM-Scl, and nRNP) and a number of minor systems account for this reactivity.[18] Finally, more recent studies have shown that most patients without precipitins have antibodies, detectable by the indirect immunofluorescent method, that bind to Hep-2 cells (a human epithelial tissue culture line).[21]

Description of these antigen-antibody reactions not only signals the availability of tests that have diagnostic usefulness, but reemphasizes the finding that individual antigen-antibody reactions can serve as "markers" for specific connective tissue diseases. The presence of such reactions, which differentiate cases of polymyositis and dermatomyositis from cases of, for example, SLE and polymyositis, implies fundamental differences in the etiology or the pathogenesis of the myopathic process in these two situations. Continued study of these reactions should clarify our perception of polymyositis occurring in various clinical guises.

The best studied of such reactions concerns the disease specificity of antibodies to native DNA that occurs in SLE. Numerous reports attest to the high correlation of antibodies to native DNA with SLE,[23] but reports in the literature state that such antibodies do occur in the other connective tissue diseases. These reports must be interpreted with reservation because it has been well demonstrated that commercial "native" DNA (^{14}C-labeled KB DNA) has many single-stranded regions. Ablation of these single-stranded regions with a specific enzyme, S_1 nuclease, or removal of such partially denatured DNA fractions on modified DEAE columns leads to loss of apparent antinative DNA reactivity from non-SLE sera.[11] Thus, it is clear that the disease specificity of antibodies to native DNA rests on continued experience with impeccably native DNA. A technologic advance that should help greatly is the increasing use of a simple test for antibodies to native DNA: the crithidia lucilia assay.[1] The crithidia organism used as substrate in this immunofluorescent assay contains with its kinetoplast a giant molecule of circular double-stranded DNA.

The other antigen-antibody system exhibiting high specificity for SLE is that involving Sm, a soluble nuclear antigen, antibodies to which are detected by precipitation in agar gels.[17,31] Other antigen-antibody systems characteristically occur in SLE sera, but they are less specific, occurring to some extent in other diseases. Their disease specificity is under active investigation, and their ultimate usefulness as "markers" for SLE patients requires further study. These include antibodies to the soluble antigens Ro[7] and La[14] and nuclear ribonucleoprotein (nRNP).[14,23] Antibodies to Ro and La also occur in Sjögren's syndrome, and anti-nRNP occurs in mixed connective tissue disease (MCTD). Indeed, antibodies to nRNP constitute the only constant feature of patients with MCTD,[27-29] and the definition of this entity as distinct from its component diseases SLE, PM, and PSS remains a matter of discussion and study.[12,19,20] The classification problem can be illustrated by the following considerations: Many SLE patients lack overlap features (such as myositis and sclerodactyly), but show, as their sole precipitating serum antibody, anti-nRNP. Many such patients fulfill the preliminary criteria for the diagnosis of SLE. If they are classified as MCTD, the clinical criteria for the diagnosis are meaningless, since overlap features are absent. Yet these patients share with the MCTD patients a low frequency of serious renal disease and a similarly favorable prognosis.[24] Moreover, in our experience, such "SLE" patients with anti-nRNP outnumber those showing overlap features and serum anti-nRNP by 4 or 5 to 1.

A series of antigen-antibody reactions commonly associated with Sjögren's syndrome has been described by Alspaugh and Tan and designated SS-A and SS-B.[4] An antigen termed Ha has been characterized that reacts with antibodies in 13% of SLE sera as well as in 68% of sera with Sjögren's syndrome.[2,10] It is now known that Ro is antigenically identical to SSA, whereas La is antigenically identical to both SSB and Ha.[3] It is perhaps not surprising to find serologic links between the sicca syndrome and SLE that parallel the demonstrable genetic link between these diseases manifest by shared Ia antigens.[15,25]

Scleroderma is frequently recognized in overlap syndromes and is often difficult to recognize in the early phases of the disease. Biochemical, genetic, or serologic "markers" would be of great nosologic value in this disease.

Diverse antibodies have now been described in patients with PSS, and two of these promise to show high disease specificity.[30] One is demonstrated by precipitin reactions with a nuclear antigen of molecular weight of 70K daltons present in rabbit thymus extract. It has been designated Scl_{70} because of its disease specificity and molecular weight. It occurs in about 20% of patients with PSS. A second antibody that binds to the centromere of chromosomes of Hep-2 cells and is therefore designated anticentromere antibody occurs in 30% of PSS patients and seems to be more specific for the CREST variant of the disease (occurring in 57% of CREST patients) than for diffuse scleroderma (see Chap. 66). The apparent diagnostic specificity of these reactions for PSS patients awaits more extensive studies among large groups of patients.

Clearly, at least some of the reactions discussed here will take their place as standard tools in the nosology of the connective tissue diseases. Others, such as anti-nRNP, might prove less useful for diagnosis than for identifying a subset of patients with a lower frequency of serious nephritis and a more benign prognosis.

The ultimate resolution of the bewildering complexity and clinical overlapping that is so frequently encountered in the diffuse connective tissue diseases awaits better definition of pathogenetic and immunopathogenetic pathways as well as identification of etiologic agents.

REFERENCES

1. Aarden, L.A., de Groot, E.G.R., and Feltkamp, T.E.W.: Immunology of DNA. III. *Crithidia luciliae:* A simple substrate for the detection of antibodies to dsDNA with the immunofluorescence technique. Ann. N.Y. Acad. Sci., *254*:505–514, 1975.
2. Akizuki, M., Powers, R., Jr., and Holman, H.R.: A soluble acidic protein of the cell nucleus which reacts with serum from patients with systemic lupus erythematosus and Sjögren's syndrome. J. Clin. Invest., *59*:264–272, 1977.
3. Alspaugh, M.A., and Maddison, P.J.: Resolution of the identity of certain antigen-antibody systems in systemic lupus erythematosus and Sjögren's syndrome: An interlaboratory collaboration. Arthritis Rheum., *22*:796–798, 1979.
4. Alspaugh, M.A., and Tan, E.M.: Antibodies to cellular antigens in Sjögren's syndrome. J. Clin. Invest., *55*:1067–1073, 1975.
5. Arnett, F.C., et al.: The Jo$_1$ antibody system. Clinical and immunogenetic associations in myositis. J. Rheumatol., *8*:925–930, 1981.
6. Bohan, A., and Peter, J.R.: Polymyositis and dermatomyositis. N. Engl. J. Med., *292*:344–347, 1975.
7. Clark, G.C., Reichlin, M., and Tomasi, T.B.: Characterization of a soluble cytoplasmic antigen reactive with sera from patients with systemic lupus erythematosus. J. Immunol. *102*:117–122, 1969.
8. Dawkins, R.L.: Experimental autoallergic myositis, polymyositis, and myasthenia gravis. Clin. Exp. Immunol., *21*:185–201, 1975.
9. Dubois, E.L.: The relationship between systemic lupus erythematosus, progressive systemic sclerosis and mixed connective tissue disease. *In* Systemic Lupus Erythematosus. Edited by E.L. Dubois. Los Angeles, University Southern California Press, 1974, pp. 477–486.
10. Kassan, S.S., et al.: Antibody to a soluble nuclear acidic antigen in Sjögren's syndrome. Am. J. Med., *63*:328–335, 1977.
11. Locker, J.D., et al.: Characterization of DNA used to assay sera for anti-DNA antibodies. Determination of the specificities of anti-DNA antibodies in SLE and non-SLE rheumatic disease states. J. Immunol., *118*:694–701, 1977.
12. Maddison, P.J., Mogavero, H., and Reichlin, M.: Patterns of clinical diseases associated with antibodies to nuclear ribonucleoprotein. J. Rheumatol., *5*:407–411, 1978.
13. Mattioli, M., and Reichlin, M.: Heterogeneity of RNA-protein antigens reactive with sera of patients with systemic lupus erythematosus. Arthritis Rheum., *17*:421–429, 1974.
14. Mattioli, M., and Reichlin, M.: Characterization of a soluble nuclear ribonuclear protein antigen reactive with LE sera. J. Immunol., *107*:1281–1290, 1971.
15. Moutsopoulos, H.M., et al.: Genetic differences between primary and secondary sicca syndrome. N. Engl. J. Med., *301*:761–763, 1979.
16. Nishikai, M., and Reichlin, M.: Heterogeneity of precipitating antibodies in polymyositis and dermatomyositis. Characterization of the Jo$_1$ antibody system. Arthritis Rheum., *23*:881–888, 1980.
17. Notman, D.D., Kurata, N., and Tan, E.M.: Profiles of antinuclear antibodies in systemic rheumatic diseases. Ann. Intern. Med., *83*:464–469, 1975.
18. Reichlin, M.: Marker antibodies for polymyositis syndromes. *In* Antibodies to Nuclear Antigens. Amsterdam-Oxford-Princeton, Excerpta Medica, 1981, pp. 1–10.
19. Reichlin, M.: Mixed connective disease. *In* Modern Topics in Rheumatology. Edited by G.R.V. Hughes. London, Heinemann Ltd., 1976, pp. 157–162.
20. Reichlin, M.: Problems in differentiating SLE and mixed connective tissue disease. N. Engl. J. Med., *295*:1194, 1976.
20a. Reichlin, M., et al.: Antibodies to a nuclear/nucleolar antigen in patients with polymyositis overlap syndrome. J. Clin. Immunol., *4*:40–44, 1984.
21. Reichlin, M., and Arnett, F.C.: Antibodies to tissue antigens occur in most patients with polymyositis. Clin. Res., *31*:493A, 1983.
22. Reichlin, M., and Mattioli, M.: Description of serological reaction characteristic of polymyositis. Clin. Immunol. Immunopathol., *5*:12–20, 1976.
23. Reichlin, M., and Mattioli, M.: Antigens and antibodies characteristic of systemic lupus erythematosus. Bull. Rheum. Dis., *24*:756–761, 1974.
24. Reichlin, M., and Mattioli, M.: Correlation of a precipitin reaction to an RNA-protein antigen and a low prevalence of nephritis in patient with systemic lupus erythematosus. N. Engl. J. Med., *286*:908–911, 1972.
25. Reinertsen, J.L., et al.: B-lymphocyte alloantigens associated with systemic lupus erythematosus. N. Engl. J. Med., *299*:515–518, 1978.
26. Rosa, M.D., et al.: A mammalian tRNA histidyl-containing antigen is recognized by the polymyositis specific antibody anti-Jo-1. Nucleic Acids Res., *11*:853–870, 1983.
27. Sharp, G.C., et al.: Association of antibodies to ribonucleoprotein and Sm antigens with mixed connective tissue diseases, systemic lupus erythematosus, and other rheumatic diseases. N. Engl. J. Med., *295*:1149–1154, 1976.
28. Sharp, G.C., et al.: Mixed connective tissue disease. An apparently distinct rheumatic disease syndrome associated with a specific antibody to an extractable nuclear antigen. Am. J. Med., *52*:148–159, 1972.
29. Sharp, G.C., et al.: Association of autoantibodies to different nuclear antigens with clinical patterns of rheumatic disease and responsiveness to therapy. J. Clin. Invest., *50*:350–359, 1971.
30. Tan, E.M., et al.: Diversity of antinuclear antibodies in progressive systemic sclerosis: Anticentromere antibody and its relationship to CREST syndrome. Arthritis Rheum., *23*:617–625, 1980.
31. Tan, E.M., and Kunkel, H.G.: Characteristics of a soluble nuclear antigen precipitating with the sera of patients with systemic lupus erythematosus. J. Immunol., *96*:464–471, 1966.
31a. Targoff, I., and Reichlin, M.: Association of Mi-2 antibody with dermatomyositis (abstract). Arthritis Rheum., *27*:S26, 1984.
32. Wolfe, J.F., Adelstein, E., and Sharp, G.C.: Antinuclear antibody with distinct specificity for polymyositis. J. Clin. Invest., *59*:176–178, 1977.

Chapter 61

Systemic Lupus Erythematosus: Clinical Aspects and Treatment

Naomi F. Rothfield

Definition. Systemic lupus erythematosus (SLE) is a disease of unknown etiology that affects many organ systems; it is characterized by the presence of multiple autoantibodies that participate in immunologically mediated tissue injury.

Historical Aspects. During the nineteenth century, the term "lupus" described a skin disease that consisted of spreading ulcerations of the face. Acute and chronic types were distinguished in 1872 by Kaposi.[54] The concept of a systemic form of the disease was formulated by Osler in 1895 when he suggested that the basis of the disease was vasculitis.[71] He described a systemic disease with a variety of skin manifestations and recognized the involvement of joints, intestinal tract, serosal surfaces, and kidney. Osler also described the characteristic periods of exacerbation and remission. Later the pathologic abnormalities were described by Libman and Sacks,[62] Gross,[42] and Baehr, Klemperer, and Schrifrin,[5] who emphasized that changes in many organs occurred even in the absence of the typical skin lesions.

In 1948, Hargraves et al. described the LE cell.[45] This major advance soon led to an increased interest in the disease, to an increased frequency of diagnosis, and eventually to our understanding of the mechanism of the LE cell phenomenon and the concept that antibodies are directed against nuclear antigens. Soon after the discovery of the LE cell, corticosteroids and antimalarials were used for treatment. It became possible to prolong the life of patients and to follow the course of successfully treated patients. The discovery of antinuclear antibodies by means of the indirect fluorescence technique led to the recognition of a wide variety of antibodies and to an understanding of their clinical significance. The concept of SLE as an immune complex mediated disease evolved, and the role of complement in producing tissue damage was elucidated. More recently, various B cell, T cell, and macrophage functions have been noted to be abnormal in patients with active SLE.[100] Genetic factors have been elucidated and an abnormality of estrogen metabolism has been described.[100] However, no single abnormality can totally explain the disease. Additional environmental factors appear to be necessary for disease expression.

Incidence. SLE affects individuals of all races, but its incidence varies in different countries (see also Chap. 2). SLE appears to be less common in England than in the United States or the West Indies. In France, the disease appears to be more common among immigrants from Portugal, Spain, North Africa, and Italy than among natives. In Hawaii, the disease is more common in Orientals or Polynesians than in whites.[95] The average annual incidence in the United States has been estimated to be 27.5 per million population for white females and 75.4 per million for black females. The higher incidence of the disease in blacks in the U.S. is interesting because the disease is uncommon in Africa.[88] The prevalence of SLE in a prepaid health plan for 125,000 patients indicates that SLE affects approximately 1 in 1,000 women.[33] The incidence of new cases appears to be increasing, but this apparent increase is difficult to separate from a more widespread interest in the disease by physicians.

SLE occurs in children and in the elderly, but the peak age at onset of the first symptom is between 15 and 25 years. The mean age at diagnosis is 30 years (Fig. 61–1). In our own series of 433 patients, 90% are female. A higher percentage of males is affected among children and among the elderly SLE patients.

Genetic Factors. Several cases of SLE may occur within a family (see also Chap. 25).[2] Families with members who have chronic discoid lupus and others who have SLE have been reported. Family members of some SLE patients have isolated laboratory abnormalities, such as false positive tests for syphilis, antinuclear antibodies, hypergammaglobulinemia, and deposits of immunoglobulins in their skin.[2,65] Relatives of SLE patients have an increased frequency (5%) of the disease.[13] The frequency of DRw2 and DRw3 is high.[36,78] SLE is also associated with hereditary deficiencies of several complement proteins.[1] SLE and "lupus-like" syndromes have been found to be associated with genetic deficiencies of Clr, Cls, Cl, INH, C4, C2,

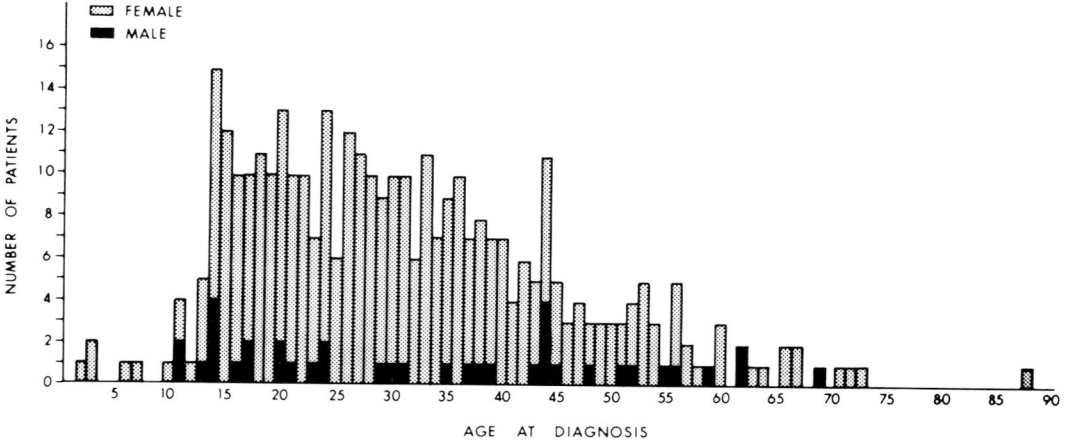

Fig. 61–1. Sex and age at diagnosis in 356 SLE patients. (From Tan, E., and Rothfield, N.: Lupus erythematosus. *In* Immunologic Disease. 3rd Ed. Edited by M. Samter. Boston, Little, Brown and Company, 1979.)

C5, and C8. The most commonly associated deficiency is C2. A total deficiency of C2 was found in 1 of 100 consecutive SLE patients studied by us and in 1 of 10,000 normal individuals studied by others.[1,40,113] Heterozygous (partial) deficiency of C2 is also common among patients with SLE, occurring in about 6% of patients as compared with 1% of normal individuals.[1] This genetic abnormality is associated with histocompatibility antigens HLA-A10 and HLA-B18.[1]

Sex Hormones. Studies have shown that both male and female SLE patients have an increased hydroxylation of estrogen to the urinary 16 alpha metabolite, which is a potent estrogenic hormone.[59] It is well known that the onset of SLE frequently occurs at menarche, during pregnancy, during the postpartum period, or with the use of oral contraceptives containing estrogen.[53]

Environmental Factors. A history of sun exposure before onset of the disease is obtained in about 36% of patients. The number of new cases of SLE usually increased during the late spring and summer months in southern New England and in New York. In other parts of the country with persistent year-round sun, the incidence of new cases may not vary in this fashion. The lack of sunlight in England has been postulated as an explanation for the rarity of the disease in that country. Sun exposure at the beach or swimming pools leads to rashes and the onset of multisystem disease.

SLE patients develop exacerbations of their disease during episodes of infection. Data show that bacterial products such as lipopolysaccharides can induce antibodies to single and double-stranded DNA in various strains of mice.[44] Lipopolysaccharide is a B cell activator. Thus, it is possible that during periods of infection, bacterial products

can produce similar changes in normal individuals with the appropriate genetic background and thereby lead to the development of SLE. A variety of drugs have been implicated as capable of producing the whole or partial clinical or serologic features of SLE.

CLINICAL FEATURES AND PATHOLOGY

General Features. Fatigue is present in nearly all SLE patients during periods of disease activity. It is frequently an early manifestation and may precede the appearance of objective findings such as rash or joint swelling. Corticosteroid treatment leads to a feeling of well-being and disappearance of fatigue. During subsequent periods of clinical exacerbation, fatigue usually reappears and may be the first symptom of an impending flare. The fatigue in SLE patients, not unlike that felt by patients with viral hepatitis, may be the patient's major symptom.

Fever is present in about 90% of patients at the time of diagnosis. In some, fever is low-grade, whereas in others it is spiking. It responds rapidly to corticosteroid therapy if the drug is given every 6 hours. A single daily dose of prednisone is usually not adequate to control fever, which will return 6 to 8 hours after the daily dose has been ingested. During the course of the disease, recurrence of fever is viewed with concern because it may be due to infection. *Fever in a treated SLE patient should be attributed to infection until proved otherwise.*

Weight loss has occurred in about 85% of patients at the time of diagnosis unless the nephrotic syndrome is present. Subsequent exacerbations may be preceded by a gradual loss of weight and accompanying fatigue.

Dermatologic Manifestations. Abnormalities of the skin, hair, or mucous membranes are the second most common manifestations of SLE, occurring in 85% of patients. The classic *butterfly "blush,"* nearly always located on both cheeks and across the bridge of the nose, was present at the time of diagnosis in 52% of our patients. It may be preceded by sun exposure at the beach and initially considered by the patient to be sunburn, but it may also occur without a history of sun exposure. The lesion heals well and leaves no scars. It may be confused with the erythematous rash of acne rosacea or seborrheic dermatitis. However, the erythema of seborrheic dermatitis is particularly marked in the nasolabial folds, an area characteristically spared by the SLE rash. Acne rosacea is characterized by the presence of papules and pustules. Pustules are not found in the facial rash of SLE.

The second most common skin finding is a *nonspecific maculopapular rash* resembling a drug eruption. It too may occur after sun exposure. The rash may be located anywhere on the body, but most often appears on the face and chest. Occasionally, scattered macules may also occur on the palms and fingers, less often on the soles. Such lesions heal without scarring or hyperpigmentation.

Occasionally, lesions persist, become crusted, and the skin may show hyperpigmentation and atrophy, although no scarring is noted. The occurrence of persistent lesions with central atrophy of the skin without true scarring has been called *subacute cutaneous lupus*. Subacute lesions differ from discoid lupus lesions in that they do not lead to scarring. They are erythematous at the edge and tend to be annular and widespread on the chest, back, arms, and occasionally, legs. These lesions are more common in patients with antibodies to Ro and La and in patients with HLA antigens B8 and Dr3.[38]

Lesions of *chronic discoid lupus* occurred in 19% of our patients. The lesions preceded the development of SLE by 2 to 35 years in about 40% of this group.[97] About half of those developing discoid lesions did so around the time of the initial diagnosis of SLE, and only about 10% developed discoid lesions after the diagnosis of SLE was established. Patients with discoid lesions showed a higher incidence of Raynaud's phenomenon and photosensitive rashes. Discoid lesions commonly involve the scalp and the external ear. They begin as erythematous plaques or papules and spread outward, leaving central areas of hyperkeratosis, follicular plugging, and atrophy. The edge of an active lesion is edematous and erythematous, whereas a healed lesion may show central depigmentation with scarring and hyperpigmentation at the margin.

Alopecia occurs in about 70% of patients. It is usually diffuse, but may be patchy (Fig. 61–2). In about 20% of patients, diffuse alopecia is so extreme that the patients buy wigs. The hair slowly regrows as the disease becomes inactive. As the new hair grows in, the scalp develops a "stubbled" look. It is important to reassure the patient that the hair loss is not permanent. Alopecia usually recurs at a time of disease exacerbation and, in some patients, may be an excellent first sign of an impending flare. In such patients, it is easy to pull out tufts of hair, and the severity of the alopecia can be followed quantitatively by repeated attempts to pull hairs. Patches of alopecia may occur temporarily if macular-papular lesions occur in the scalp. Lesions of discoid lupus in the scalp heal with scarring, permanent loss of hair follicles, and permanent alopecia.

Vasculitis is not uncommon in SLE patients. Ulcerative lesions may occur on the extensor surface of the forearm. *Palpable purpura* may occur, especially on the lower extremities. On biopsy, leukocytoclastic angiitis is seen. Less commonly, vasculitic lesions may be noted on the back of the hands, as blotchy, slightly purpuric lesions on the palms, near the small joints of the fingers, and as tender erythematous nodules on the finger pads. *Periungual erythema* or *palmar erythema* is each present in about 10% of patients. *Splinter hemorrhages* and *nailfold thrombi* are occasionally found. Atrophic "blanche" lesions similar to those seen in Degos' disease consist of erythematous papular or infiltrated lesions that gradually develop white centers and telangiectasis at the margins.[12] *Livedo reticularis* due to small vessel vasculitis is common in SLE patients, especially those with active disease. This condition is noted on the lower extremities and particularly around the knees, ankles, and elbows. When the legs are dependent, the toes take on a purplish hue. Livedo reticularis may precede gangrene in some patients.

Mucosal ulcers are common, occurring in about

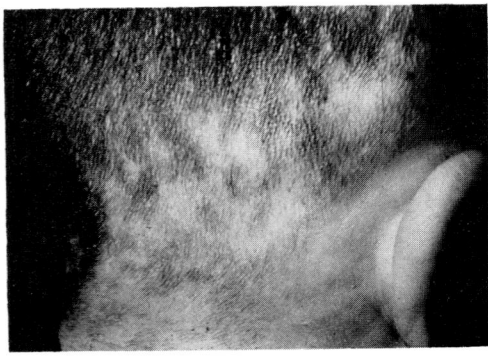

Fig. 61–2. Patchy alopecia in a man with systemic lupus erythematosus.

40% of patients.[110] These ulcers are most commonly found on the hard or soft palate and are asymptomatic (Fig. 61–3). Occasionally, a patient complains of pain on eating spicy foods or notes a tender area on the roof of the mouth. These palatal ulcers coincide with active disease and disappear after a few days of corticosteroid therapy. Nasal septal ulcerations are less common. These lesions are seen on the anterior aspect of the nasal septum and will be missed if the otoscope is inserted too far into the nares. Nasal septal perforations occur in some of these patients.[101] Such nasal ulcerations may produce epistaxis or nasal stuffiness due to secretions or crusts over the ulcerated areas.

Leg ulcers, most frequently located about the malleoli, are similar to those seen in patients with rheumatoid vasculitis. The "punched out" lesions are exquisitely tender. Such leg ulcers preceded the recognition of SLE by many years in a few of our patients.

Other less common dermatologic abnormalities occur in many patients. *Bullous* lesions may be present[87] and, in patients who are thrombocytopenic, the bullae may be hemorrhagic. *Periorbital edema, urticaria,* or *erythema multiforme* may be noted. *Ecchymoses* and *petechiae* may be observed in patients with severe thrombocytopenia. Many patients with SLE complain of easy bruisability prior to the diagnosis of SLE and treatment with corticosteroids. *Gangrene* of the fingers or toes, which is uncommon, may be preceded by severe Raynaud's phenomenon or by severe livedo reticularis. Occlusion of the medium-sized vessels of the legs has been noted in one such patient who eventually had a mid-calf amputation.

Lupus profundus or *panniculitis* is occasionally noted. *Soft tissue calcification* occurs rarely in SLE. The calcification appears in patients with and without myositis and is not associated with abnormalities of calcium or phosphorus metabolism.[76] *Rheumatoid nodules* are present in about 10% of patients, usually but not always associated with nonerosive deforming arthritis. The association of SLE with *porphyria cutanea tarda* has been reported.[26] *Dystrophic nail changes,* usually affecting only a few nails, occur in about 10% of patients, especially those with long-standing disease. In its most extreme form, the nails are lost. Nail bed erythema is found in most of these patients earlier in the course of the disease. *Hypermelanosis* of skin and/or mucous membranes is observed rarely in patients treated with antimalarial drugs.[109]

Histopathology of the skin lesions varies greatly.[82] Biopsies of the typical rash of acute SLE usually show (1) thinning of the epidermis, (2) liquefaction degeneration of the basal layer of the epidermis with disruption of the dermal-epidermal junction, and (3) edema of the dermis with a scattered infiltrate of lymphocytes concentrated around the upper dermal capillaries. Some biopsies reveal only a nonspecific vasculitis.

In some patients, the histologic picture lies between that of chronic discoid lupus and systemic lupus. Leukocytoclastic angiitis may be seen in biopsies of palpable purpuric lesions or urticaria.

Immunopathologic studies reveal deposits of immunoglobulins and complement components at the dermal-epidermal junction of lesional skin in 80 to 100% of patients (Fig. 61–4).[83,92,93,108] This finding is not specific for SLE. Similar deposits may be found in lepromatous leprosy,[18] in telangiectatic lesions from scleroderma patients, in lesions of

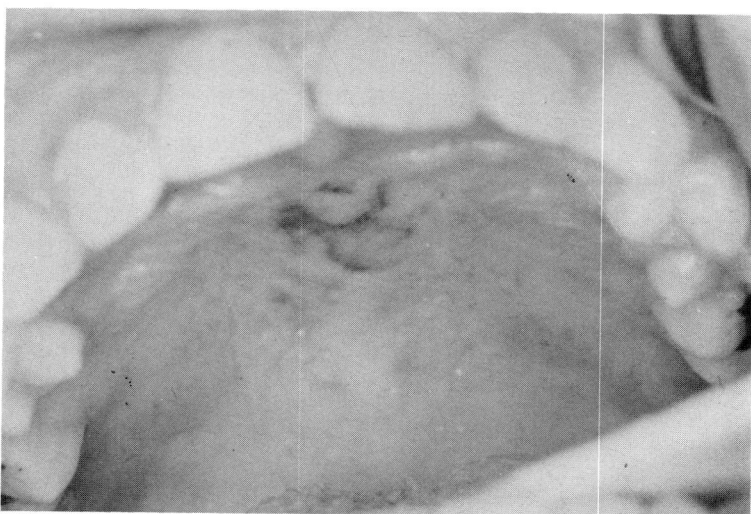

Fig. 61–3. Mucosal ulcer on hard palate.

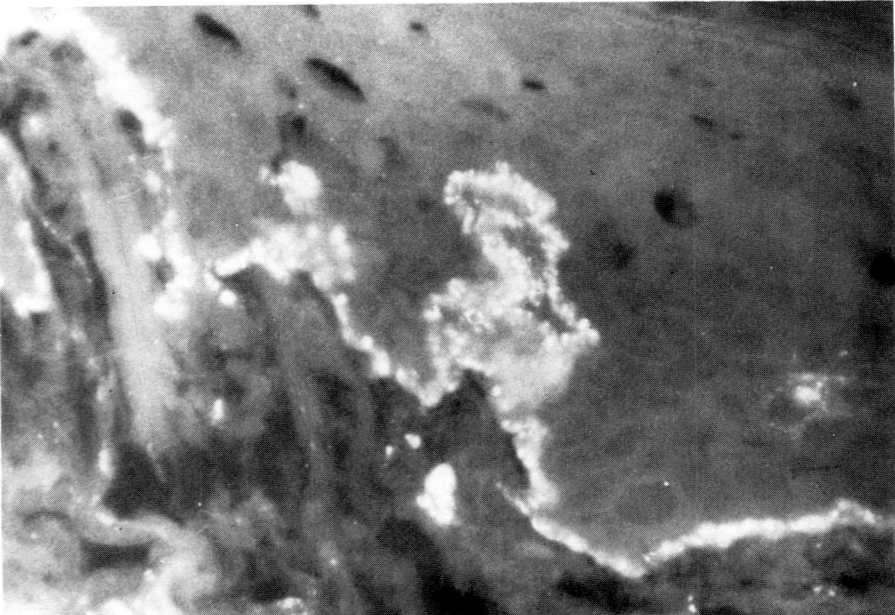

Fig. 61–4. Immunoglobulin deposits in the dermal-epidermal junction of the nonlesional skin from a patient with clinically active SLE. Anti-IgG fluorescein isothiocyanate (× 500).

rosacea,[49] and in lesions of active porphyria cutanea tarda.[4] Chronic discoid lupus from persons without clinical or serologic evidence of SLE also show deposits of immunoglobulins and complement proteins in the dermal-epidermal junction.[75,91] Thus, the diagnosis of SLE should not depend on the demonstration of immune protein deposits at the dermal-epidermal junction of skin lesions. Because rosacea is commonly confused with the butterfly blush of SLE, the finding of such deposits in 70% of lesions of rosacea is of particular importance.[49]

Immunopathologic studies of *nonlesional* skin from SLE patients also reveal the presence of immunoglobulins and complement proteins.[49,92,93,108] These deposits are more common in biopsies obtained during clinical and serologically active disease.[92] Repeated biopsies show that deposits present during active disease may disappear coincident with sustained remission.[86] Similar deposits in normal skin have been found in patients with rheumatoid arthritis, Sjögren's syndrome, scleroderma, Raynaud's syndrome, and poly-dermatomyositis,[99] and in patients with lepromatous leprosy.[18] We have found deposits intermittently in nonlesional skin of some patients with chronic discoid lupus who have no evidence of SLE. Similarly, deposits are found in nonlesional skin from one-third of patients with rosacea.[4]

Granular focal deposits have been noted in the normal skin of some relatives of SLE patients, including spouses,[65] and deposits have been found in skin of technicians handling SLE sera. The latter observation is similar to the finding of increased lymphocytotoxic antibodies, antinuclear antibodies, and positive LE cell preparations among workers in laboratories handling SLE sera.

Musculoskeletal Manifestations. Involvement of the joints is the most frequent manifestation of SLE.[58] At the time of diagnosis, 88% of the 209 SLE patients seen in New York had an undiagnosed rheumatic disease, and objective evidence of pain on motion, tenderness, effusion, or periarticular soft tissue swelling was present in 78%. During the course of the disease, additional objective evidence of joint disease developed so that 86% of all patients had arthritis at some time. Other patients have joint pain without objective arthritis; fully 95% of SLE patients have either arthralgia or arthritis.

A history of joint pain or objective evidence of arthritis may precede the onset of multisystem disease by many years. At the time of diagnosis, arthritis or arthralgia of the proximal interphalangeal joints was present in 82% of our patients. This finding was symmetric in all but two patients. The knees were the next most commonly involved joints (76%), followed by the wrists and metacarpophalangeal joints. Ankles, elbows, and shoulders were involved less frequently (55%, 54%, and 45%, respectively). The metatarsophalangeal joints and hips were affected in 20% of patients, and the distal interphalangeal joints of the hands in 14% of patients. Involvement was symmetric in nearly all patients. The temporomandibular joints were rarely involved, although severe malocclusion occurred in one patient owing to involvement of this joint.

In some patients, knee effusions are moderately severe. Joint aspiration usually reveals a clear (group 1) fluid, with leukocyte counts less than 3,000 per cubic millimeter. Most of the cells are small lymphocytes. Antinuclear antibodies and LE cells may be found in the synovial fluid. Serum complement proteins and total hemolytic complement are usually low, reflecting similar low levels in the serum. Occasionally, inflammatory fluids (group 2) may be found. These fluids should always be cultured, especially if the arthritis is monarticular. A single swollen joint should be viewed with suspicion to ensure that the arthritis is not due to SLE and should always be aspirated for appropriate cultures, including *N. gonorrhoeae*.

The histologic examination of the synovium reveals a fibrous villous synovitis. Typical pannus formation and erosions of bone and cartilage occur rarely in SLE patients.[34] Arthritis disappears completely within a few days when patients are treated with corticosteroids for their systemic disease.

Although joint deformities are an exclusion to the use of "arthritis" as one of the manifestations of SLE in the ARA Preliminary Criteria for the Classification of SLE (Table 61–1),[24] deformities do occur in some SLE patients. Typical swan neck deformities and ulnar deviation of the fingers developed in about 10% of our patients after three to four years of disease. In many of these patients, intermittent mild joint pain had been noted, but in others none had been present since the time of diagnosis. Radiograms of the hands revealed no bony erosions or loss of joint space, although osteoporosis and subluxation were seen. Surgical repair of the deformities has been performed on some of these patients and normal cartilage noted in the affected joints. The joint deformities are thought to be related to chronic involvement of the tendons of the hands and fingers and spasm of the intrinsic muscles. Because deformities do occur in SLE patients, but erosions of the bone do not, the "arthritis" manifestation has been changed in the 1982 Revised Criteria for the Classification of SLE (Table 61–2).[104] Deformities but not radiographic erosions permit the use of "arthritis" in the Revised Criteria.

Morning stiffness is present in 50% of patients. Typical subcutaneous nodules occur in 10% and tenosynovitis in 7%.

Involvement of muscles is not uncommon in SLE patients. Myalgia was present in 30% of our patients. Abnormalities of serum SGOT and SGPT were also present in 30% before any treatment. These enzyme abnormalities probably represent liver disease. The myalgia occurs with arthritis and, in some patients, the pain is "all over" and difficult to localize. These patients have pain in and between their joints. The muscle may be tender to palpation. Proximal muscle pain and tenderness are more common than distal pain. This muscle involvement rapidly disappears with corticosteroid doses needed to control the more significant systemic manifestations. Severe and prominent muscle involvement was noted in 8% of 228 patients studied by Tsokos et al.[106] Muscle biopsy usually reveals a nonspecific perivascular mononuclear infiltrate, but polymyositis with muscle necrosis can occur.[31] True polymyositis, with evidence of muscle weakness, electromyographic changes typical of polymyositis, vacuolar myopathy, and necrosis, has been reported in untreated SLE patients.[28] These abnormalities improved with corticosteroid therapy.

Cardiovascular Manifestations. *Pericarditis*, which occurs in about 25% of patients, varies from a transient friction rub to a massive pericardial effusion. LE cells are found frequently in pericardial fluid. A study using echocardiography revealed pericardial thickening in 29% of patients.[23] Pericardial tamponade is unusual. Transient electrocardiographic abnormalities due to myocardial ischemia may be seen and tachycardia may persist for many months after the subsidence of the acute episode. *Myocardial disease* usually accompanies pericarditis. Death due to *myocardial infarction* from arteritis has been reported early in the course of the disease in young patients. Studies of hearts of patients dying with SLE have revealed a high incidence of coronary atherosclerosis in the patients treated for more than one year with corticosteroids.[17] Myocardial infarction late in the course of the disease in corticosteroid-treated patients represents an important cause of late death.[112] One of our patients died suddenly of a myocardial infarction while in remission in the eighth year of disease. *Aortic and mitral insufficiency* due to scarring of leaflets and thickened or ruptured chordae tendineae has been reported.[9,72] Valve replacement has been used to treat these conditions.[60,77]

Verrucous endocarditis is present at autopsy in nearly all patients. The lesions are usually microscopic, but macroscopic vegetations are observed in nearly half the cases. Typical verrucous endocarditis is a pathologic diagnosis and does not correlate with the presence of cardiac murmurs. Both subacute and acute bacterial endocarditis have occurred on valves affected by lupus endocarditis.

Raynaud's phenomenon was present in 18% of our 365 patients. This condition may precede the

Table 61–1. Incidence of 14 Manifestations of the ARA Preliminary Criteria of the Classification of SLE[24]

Manifestation of the American Rheumatism Association Preliminary Criteria for the Classification of SLE[24]	Percentage Incidence			
	ARA Series[24]	Rothfield[82]	Davis et al.[26a]	Trimble et al.[104a]
1. Facial erythema (butterfly rash). Diffuse erythema, flat or raised, over the malar eminence(s) and/or bridge of the nose; may be unilateral.	64	55	64	40
2. Discoid lupus. Erythematous raised patches with adherent keratotic scaling and follicular plugging; atrophic scarring may occur in older lesions; may be present anywhere on the body.	17	19	31	32
3. Raynaud's phenomenon. Requires a two-phase color reaction, by patient's history or physician's observation.	20	20	19	44
4. Alopecia. Rapid loss of large amount of the scalp hair, by patient's history or physician's observation.	43	71	64	40
5. Photosensitivity. Unusual skin reaction from exposure to sunlight, by patient's history or physician's observation.	37	41	17	28
6. Oral or nasopharyngeal ulceration.	15	36	22	16
7. Arthritis without deformity. One or more peripheral joints involved with any of the following in the absence of deformity: (a) pain on motion, (b) tenderness, (c) effusion or periarticular soft tissue swelling. (Peripheral joints are defined for this purpose as feet, ankles, knees, hips, shoulders, elbows, wrists, and metacarpophalangeal, proximal interphalangeal, terminal interphalangeal, and temporomandibular joints.)	90	86	89	100
8. LE cells. Two or more classic LE cells seen on one occasion or one cell seen on two or more occasions, using an accepted published method.	92	86	75	48
9. Chronic false-positive STS. Known to be present for at least six months and confirmed by TPI or Reiter's tests.	12	26	8	12
10. Profuse proteinuria. Greater than 3.5 g per day.	20	25	25	16
11. Cellular casts. May be red cell, hemoglobin, granular, tubular, or mixed.	48	34	17	16
12. One or both of the following: (a) pleuritis, good history of pleuritic pain; or rub heard by a physician; or roentgenographic evidence of both pleural thickening and fluid, (b) pericarditis, documented by EKG or rub.	60 19	54	30 19	60
13. One or both of the following: (a) psychosis, (b) convulsions, by patient's history or physician's observation in the absence of uremia and offending drugs.	19	16	19	20
14. One or more of the following: (a) hemolytic anemia, (b) leukopenia, WBC less than 4,000 per cmm on two or more occasions, (c) thrombocytopenia, platelet count less than 100,000 per cmm.	16 40 11	54	14 47 14	52

A person shall be said to have systemic LE if any 4 or more of the above 14 manifestations are present, serially or simultaneously, during any period of observation.

Table 61–2.   The 1982 Revised Criteria for Classification of Systemic Lupus Erythematosus

Criterion*	Definition
1. Malar rash	Fixed erythema, flat or raised, over the malar eminences, tending to spare the nasolabial folds.
2. Discoid rash	Erythematous raised patches with adherent keratotic scaling and follicular plugging; atrophic scarring may occur in older lesions.
3. Photosensitivity	Skin rash as a result of unusual reaction to sunlight, by patient history or physician observation.
4. Oral ulcers	Oral or nasopharyngeal ulceration, usually painless, observed by a physician.
5. Arthritis	Nonerosive arthritis involving two or more peripheral joints, characterized by tenderness, swelling, or effusion.
6. Serositis	a) Pleuritis—convincing history of pleuritic pain or rub heard by a physician or evidence of pleural effusion. OR b) Pericarditis—documented by ECG or rub or evidence of pericardial effusion.
7. Renal disorder	a) Persistent proteinuria greater than 0.5 per day or greater than 3+ if quantitation not performed. OR b) Cellular casts—may be red cell, hemoglobulin, granular, tubular, or mixed.
8. Neurologic disorder	a) Seizures—in the absence of offending drugs or known metabolic derangements: e.g., uremia, ketoacidosis, or electrolyte imbalance. OR b) Psychosis—in the absence of offending drugs or known metabolic derangements, e.g., uremia, ketoacidosis, or electrolyte imbalance.
9. Hematologic disorder	a) Hemolytic anemia—with reticulocytosis. OR b) Leukopenia—less than 4,000/mm total on two or more occasions. OR c) Lymphopenia—less than 1,500/mm on two or more occasions. OR d) Thrombocytopenia—less than 100,000/mm in the absence of offending drugs.
10. Immunologic disorder	a) Positive LE cell preparation. OR b) Anti-DNA: antibody to native DNA in abnormal titer. OR c) Anti-SM: presence of antibody to Sm nuclear antigen: OR d) False positive serologic test for syphilis known to be positive for at least 6 months and confirmed by *Treponema pallidum* immobilization or fluorescent treponemal antibody absorption test.
11. Antinuclear antibody	An abnormal titer of antinuclear antibody by immunofluorescence or an equivalent assay at any time and in the absence of drugs known to be associated with "drug-induced lupus syndrome."

*The proposed classification is based on 11 criteria. For the purpose of identifying patients in clinical studies, a person shall be said to have systemic lupus erythematosus if any 4 or more of the 11 criteria are present, serially or simultaneously, during any interval of observation.

development of multisystem disease by many years. Cryoglobulinemia is common in patients who have the onset of Raynaud's phenomenon at the time of diagnosis, and such patients usually also have nephritis. Unlike systemic sclerosis, the Raynaud's phenomenon in SLE may gradually disappear after institution of corticosteroid therapy. Although *thrombosis* is unusual in SLE, it may involve large vessels. Thrombosis with occlusion of the femoral artery occurred in one patient necessitating mid-thigh amputation. These episodes of thrombosis occur during periods of clinical and serologic disease activity. *Thrombophlebitis* is also a manifestation of SLE and, in some patients, recurs with subsequent episodes of disease activity. A relationship between the lupus anticoagulant and deep vein thrombosis has been suggested.[102] Placental arterial thrombosis has been reported in association with a lupus anticoagulant.[20]

Thrombotic thrombocytopenic purpura (TTP) occurs rarely in patients with SLE.[28] We have observed this catastrophic event in 2 of 433 patients. In one patient, TTP occurred in the fourth month of pregnancy and resulted in massive brain infarcts. In the other, TTP was recognized earlier, and the patient responded to corticosteroid therapy and plasmapheresis.

Pulmonary Manifestations. Pleural involvement is more common than pericardial disease. Pleural effusions occur in 40% of patients. Most are small to moderate, but massive effusions occasionally occur. LE cells may be seen in those transudates that contain the same immunoglobulin and complement proteins as the peripheral blood. Occasionally, effusions persist for months after the institution of corticosteroid therapy, leading to concern regarding etiology. "Lupus pneumonitis," characterized by dyspnea, rales, and areas of plate-like atelectasis, associated with elevation and fixation of the diaphragm, occurs in about 10% of patients. Infiltrates may be bilateral and associated with pleural effusions.[67] It is important to remember that "lupus pneumonitis" is a diagnosis to be considered only after exclusion of an infectious etiology of lung abnormalities.[67] A study of the pathology of the lungs in SLE patients revealed that the most common cause of pulmonary infiltrates was infection.[46] Infectious pneumonias due to both bacterial and fungal agents are common in corticosteroid-treated SLE patients. The diagnosis of lupus pneumonitis should be made only after a rigorous search for an infectious agent.

Abnormalities of pulmonary function are common in SLE patients even when they do not have symptoms related to the respiratory system. Tests reveal a combination of pulmonary restriction, vascular obstruction, and airway obstruction.[37]

Nonspecific changes are found in the pleura. Deposits of immunoglobulins have been described in the alveolar walls.

Renal Disease. Clinical evidence of renal disease is present in about 50% of patients with SLE. On the other hand, pathologic abnormalities recognized by light microscopy are present in additional patients. Immunofluorescent studies of biopsy or autopsy material from nearly all patients reveal deposits of immunoglobulins or complement proteins. Therefore, the definition of lupus nephritis remains unclear. Additional studies of SLE patients without clinical evidence of renal involvement are needed to precisely define the incidence of pathologic and immunohistologic abnormalities. For practical purposes, however, persistent proteinuria occurs in about half of SLE patients. The pathologic and clinical forms of lupus nephritis in this discussion are based on a classification proposed by Andres, Pirani, and McCluskey.[73]

Mild (Focal) Lupus Nephritis. This condition is characterized by segmental proliferation of some glomerular tufts while others appear normal (Fig. 61–5). Mesangial proliferation may be present, but segmental proliferation is present in less than 50% of glomeruli. Immunofluorescence reveals immunoglobulins and C3 in the mesangium of all glomeruli. Fine scattered granules may be present along the capillary loops, especially in the areas of proliferation. The deposits are scattered and are not evenly distributed along all the capillary loops. Electron-dense deposits are noted by electron microscopy in the mesangium, and occasional deposits are also found in the subendothelial, subepithelial, and intra-basement membrane areas. Proteinuria occurs, but the nephrotic syndrome is uncommon.[6] Mild hematuria is usual, but renal insufficiency is either mild or absent. It is important to note that patients with mild (focal) lupus nephritis do not usually have mild systemic disease. They may be acutely ill with high fevers and severe extrarenal disease, including central nervous system disease. Anti-native DNA antibodies and low serum complement levels are present in patients with active systemic disease.

Treatment with corticosteroids in doses adequate to control the systemic manifestations of the disease usually leads to a clearing of the renal insufficiency if present and to clearing of the hematuria.[6] Proteinuria may persist for several months, but gradually the amount of protein is reduced and the urine is normal. Such patients do not usually develop severe renal disease or renal insufficiency if the serologic abnormalities return initially to the normal range and if the patient remains in serologic and clinical remission.[6,69] If an exacerbation of the disease does occur, it is usual to find the same focal

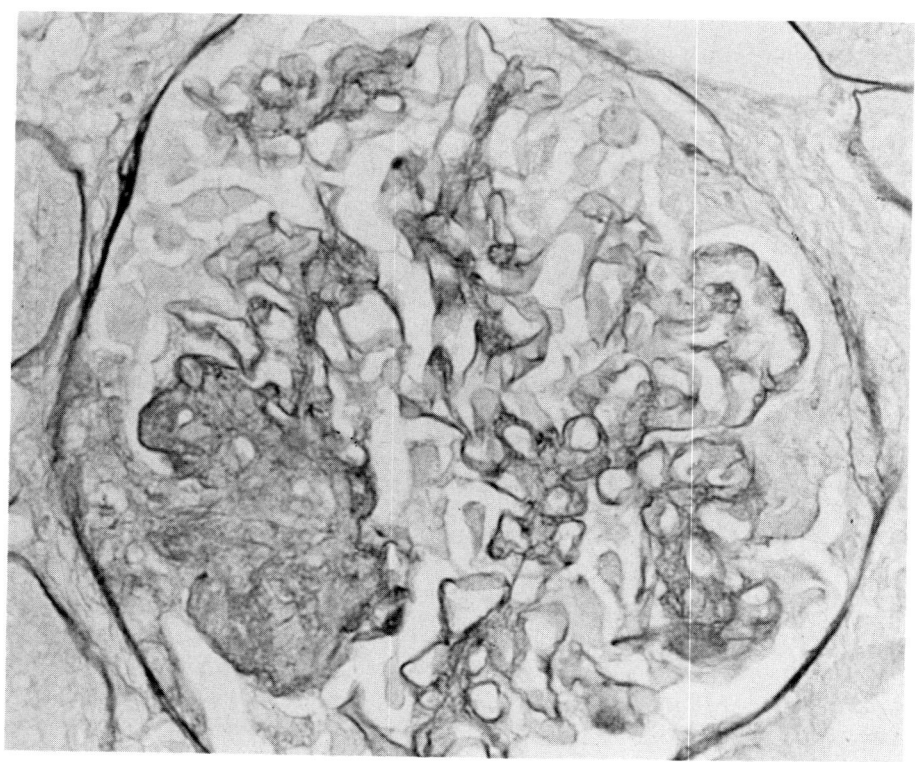

Fig. 61–5.   Focal proliferative lupus nephritis. (H&E × 500).

lesion. Prompt treatment again leads to remission. Death from renal disease or from other causes in the presence of renal insufficiency does not occur in these patients.

Progression from focal to diffuse lupus nephritis has been reported,[39,69,117] but has occurred in only two patients in our experience. In each, corticosteroid therapy had been abruptly discontinued and a full-blown exacerbation of the clinical and serologic disease occurred at the time that severe lupus nephritis was documented. The second renal biopsy, performed during the exacerbation, revealed diffuse proliferative lupus nephritis in both of these individuals. In a review of 22 patients with focal nephritis, there was an 82% five-year cumulative survival rate from the first sign of renal involvement. Deaths occurred in patients who had normal renal function.[69] This figure is similar to that previously found.[6] However, progression to diffuse lupus nephritis was more frequent in the series described by Ginzler et al.[39] and by Zimmerman et al.,[117] in which the progression occurred in 9 of 31 patients (29%) and 6 of 17 patients (38%) (Table 61–3). It is important to note that sclerosis may occur occasionally in patients with focal lupus nephritis, but the degree of sclerosis is minimal.[69] Minimal to mild sclerosis was noted in 8 of 16

patients with focal nephritis who had a stable course, and mild sclerosis was noted in the initial biopsy in half of the patients who later progressed to diffuse proliferative nephritis.[69]

Severe (Diffuse) Proliferative Lupus Nephritis. In this condition there are abnormalities of more than 50% of the total area of the glomerular tufts. Although the proliferation is irregular, all glomeruli are involved, and usually most of each glomerulus is abnormal (Fig. 61–6). Sclerosis may or may not be present in the initial biopsy. The activity of the proliferative lesion may be graded on a semiquantitative basis as originally suggested by Pirani et al.[74] The following are considered to be active glomerular lesions: fibrinoid necrosis, endocapillary proliferation, epithelial crescents, nuclear debris, hematoxylin bodies, wire-loops, and hyalin thrombi. Active interstitial lesions include: interstitial cell infiltration and acute tubular epithelial lesions.[69] Necrotizing angiitis is also considered to be an active lesion.

The pathologic index of activity is particularly useful if successive biopsies on the same patient are to be evaluated or if groups of patients with lupus nephritis are to be compared. Similarly, the amount of sclerosis in each biopsy can also be graded. Studies of repeated sequential biopsies in

Table 61–3.   Minimal Glomerular and Focal Lupus Nephritis: Clinical and Histologic Course

	Morel-Maroger et al.[69]	Ginzler et al.[39]	Zimmerman et al.[117]
No. patients	81	32	17
Stable course	77*	20†	11‡
Renal deterioration GN	4	11	5
Progression to diffuse	6(7.4%)	9(29%)	6(35%)

*GN remaining focal in 16/18 cases in which biopsy was repeated (mean time of 28 mos. between first and second biopsy), having progressed to a diffuse GN in the other cases.

†GN remaining focal in the two cases in which biopsy was repeated.

‡GN remaining focal in the five cases in which biopsy was repeated.

From Morel-Maroger, L., et al.: The course of lupus nephritis: Contribution of serial renal biopsies. *In* Advances in Nephrology. Vol. 6. Edited by J. Hamburger. Copyright © 1976 by Year Book Medical Publishers, Inc., Chicago. Used by permission.

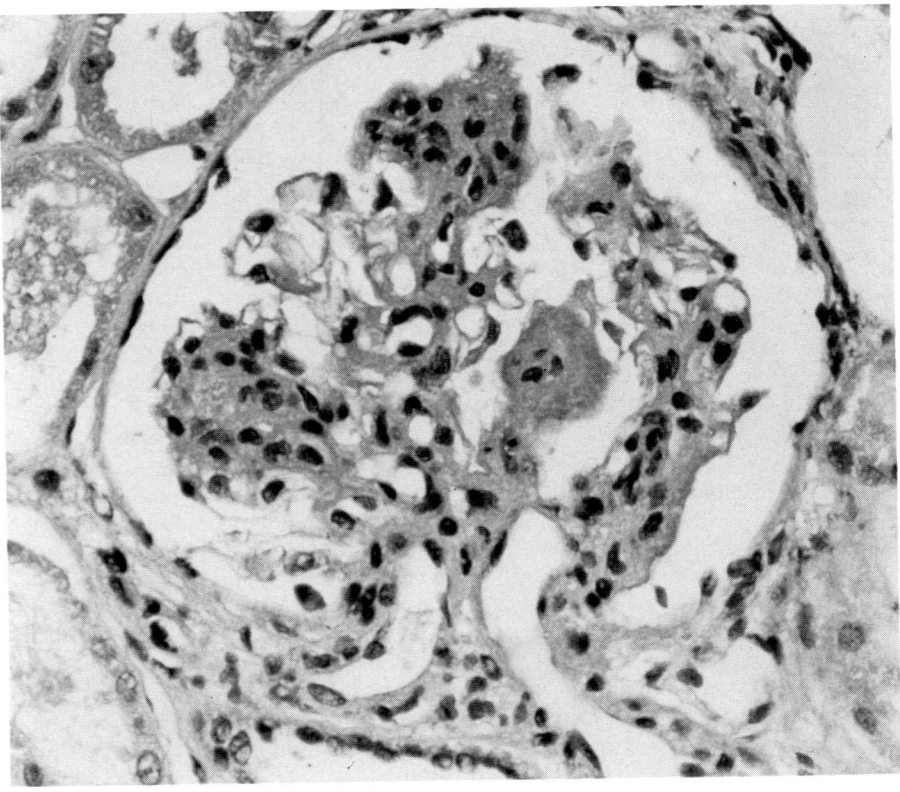

Fig. 61–6.   Diffuse proliferative lupus nephritis (H&E × 500).

40 patients with diffuse lupus nephritis were reported by Morel-Maroger et al.[69] These investigators found that the presence of extensive sclerotic lesions indicated a poor prognosis and that high doses of prednisone given to 14 patients after the first biopsy did not prevent progression of the sclerosis in 8 of the patients, even though active lesions diminished. These investigators also found that patients with active lesions had a good prognosis, responding to high doses of corticosteroids. In 19 of 25 patients in whom the active lesions were initially accompanied by only moderate sclerosis, the active lesions were considerably decreased in the repeated biopsies.

These conclusions are similar to those reported by Striker et al., who also noted an absence of correlation between the evolution of active lesions that respond to therapy and the evolution of the sclerotic lesions that progress unaffected by treatment.[103] The five-year survival of patients with diffuse proliferative nephritis appears to be improving. In our original report, the five-year survival was 41% of 24 patients prior to 1968.[6] The five-year survival in 22 patients with diffuse proliferative lupus nephritis followed since 1968 is 86%. It is clear that the renal biopsy should provide additional information besides the type of lupus nephritis. The prognosis in patients with diffuse proliferative lupus nephritis may depend greatly on the degree of activity and the degree of sclerosis noted in the biopsy.

The immunofluorescence findings in diffuse proliferative lupus nephritis are usually striking, with granules or clumps of immunoglobulins and complement proteins, as well as mesangial deposits noted along the peripheral capillary wall. Interstitial infiltrates and deposits of immunoglobulins and complement proteins may also be noted along the tubular basement membrane, within the walls of the peritubular capillaries, or in the interstitium.[15] Electron-dense deposits are noted in the mesangium, in the subendothelial and subepithelial areas, and within the basement membrane. The deposits are located all over the glomeruli but are not evenly distributed.

The clinical picture in these patients is one of moderate to heavy proteinuria with the nephrotic syndrome, hematuria, and mild to severe renal insufficiency. Red cell casts are not infrequent. Antibodies to native DNA and low serum C3 are usual unless the lesion is inactive with a predominance of sclerotic glomeruli. Many patients with severe sclerosis and inactive nonsclerotic glomeruli are in clinical remission and should be treated with small doses of corticosteroids or none at all. These individuals seem to have a prolonged serologic and clinical remission and do not require treatment for the SLE, although hemodialysis has been required in some.

Membranous Lupus Nephritis. The histologic appearance of this condition is similar to that of idiopathic membranous glomerulonephritis (Fig. 61–7). Although no proliferation is noted, slight irregular increases in mesangial cells and matrix may be present. Immunofluorescence is striking in that the immunoglobulins are located in a regular fashion along all the basement membranes (Fig. 61–8). It is possible to observe on immunofluorescence the spikes of the IgG that protrude on the epithelial side of the capillary loop. Electron microscopy confirms the presence of subepithelial deposits. Patients with this form of lupus nephritis have proteinuria and may or may not have hematuria. The nephrotic syndrome is usually present at onset or during the course of the disease.[6] Serologic evidence of disease activity may be absent if significant extrarenal disease activity is absent. Nor-

mal C3 levels and absence of antibodies to native DNA have been found in these patients at the time that the renal disease is first noted and the biopsy performed, but some patients do have hematuria, low serum C3 levels, and high titers of anti-DNA antibodies. The prognosis is variable, but is usually good. We have noted some patients with persistent nephrotic syndrome and slowly progressive renal insufficiency for as long as 10 years, and we have observed progression to severe renal insufficiency 14 years after the first biopsy.

Mesangial Lupus Nephritis. An additional form of lupus nephritis, called mesangial (minimal) lupus nephritis, has been recognized. The glomeruli appear normal or may merely show a slight irregular increase in mesangial cells and matrix (Fig. 61–9). The diagnosis depends on the demonstration of IgG and C3 in the mesangium and occasionally along the capillary walls. Electron-dense deposits may be noted in the mesangium. Patients either have normal urinary findings or have transient minimal proteinuria or minimal hematuria. A few instances of progression from the mesangial lesion to the diffuse proliferative form have been described.[41] In general, it is unlikely that patients with little or no clinical evidence of renal disease at the time of diagnosis will develop progression of the condition if the initial episode of active systemic disease is adequately treated and initial normalization of serologic abnormalities is sustained over the course of the disease. The presence of the IgG in the mesangium of these patients is similar to the findings of IgG in the nonlesional skin of patients with clinically active SLE. Deposits of immunoglobulins in the dermal-epidermal junction and in the mesangium of the kidney occur without inflammation in these areas.

Interstitial Nephritis. This condition has been described in approximately 50% of patients.[15] Focal or diffuse infiltrates of inflammatory cells, tubular damage, and interstitial fibrosis are observed. Immunoglobulins, complement, or both can be found in the peritubular capillaries, the interstitium, or the tubular basement membrane in a granular pattern. The interstitial abnormalities are more severe and frequent in patients with diffuse proliferative lupus nephritis, but severe interstitial nephritis with little or no glomerular abnormalities has been noted occasionally. Renal tubular acidosis occurs in some patients.

Nervous System Manifestations. *Peripheral Neuropathy.* This condition has occurred in 14% of our patients, an incidence similar to that reported by Feinglass.[32] The most common defect is sensory, but a mixed sensory-motor disturbance is seen in about 5% of patients with the typical asymmetric involvement of mononeuritis multiplex.

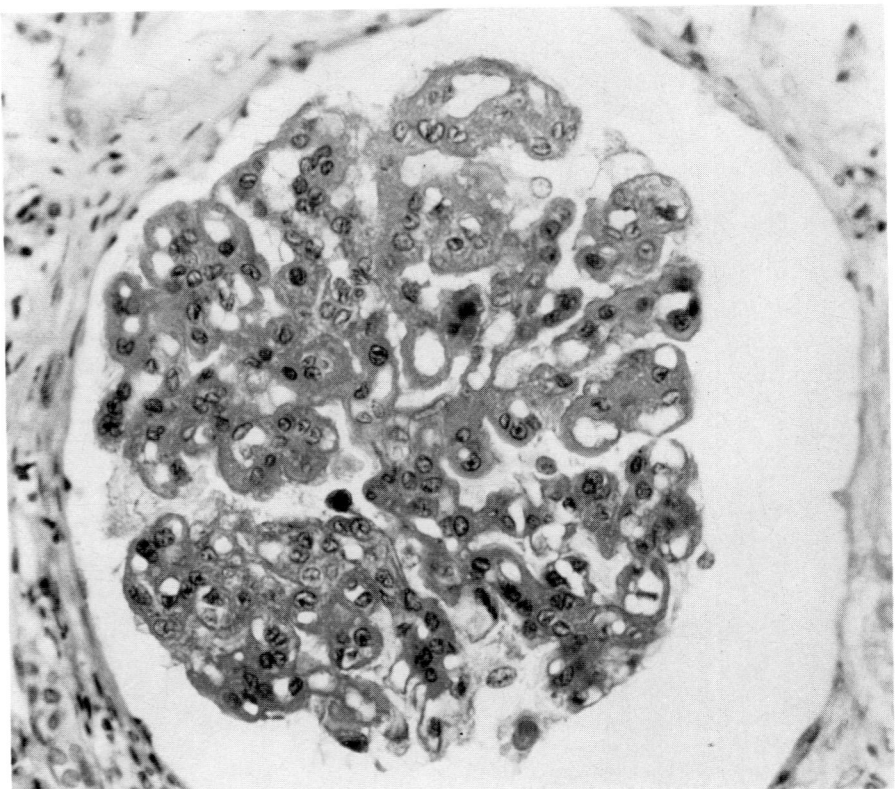

Fig. 61–7.   Membranous lupus nephritis. (H&E × 500).

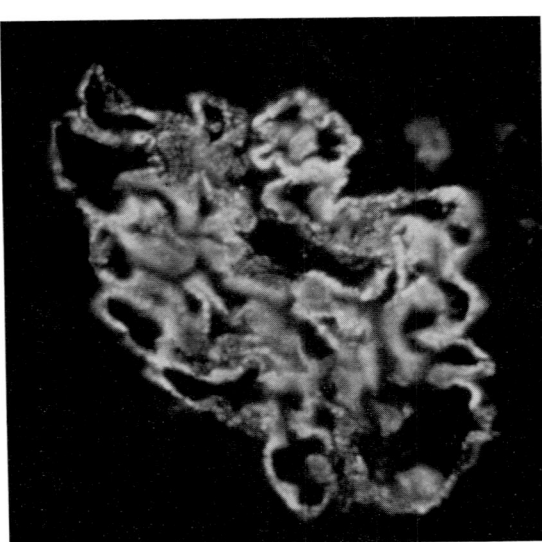

Fig. 61–8.   Membranous lupus nephritis with granular deposits on all capillary loops. Anti-IgG fluorescein isothiocyanate. (H&E × 500).

These episodes occur most often at the time of diagnosis along with evidence of active disease in other systems. In most patients, treatment of the systemic disease with corticosteroids leads to a gradual return of function to the affected extremities. Other less common abnormalities consist of a picture suggesting the Guillain-Barré syndrome and myelopathy. Some patients with peripheral neuropathy also have evidence of cranial neuropathy.

Cranial Nerve Signs.   These signs were noted in only 16 of the 140 SLE patients reported by Feinglass et al.[32] We have noted facial weakness, ptosis, diplopia, and other evidence of cranial nerve involvement. Optic neuritis may be the first manifestation of SLE.[98] These abnormalities most frequently occur concurrently with other neuropsychiatric features. One patient with optic neuritis, described by Feinglass, had transverse myelitis at the same time.[32] Peripheral neuropathy is common in patients with cranial neuropathy.

Long tract involvement occurred in 16 of 140 SLE patients described by Feinglass et al.[32] Five of his patients had cerebrovascular accidents. Long

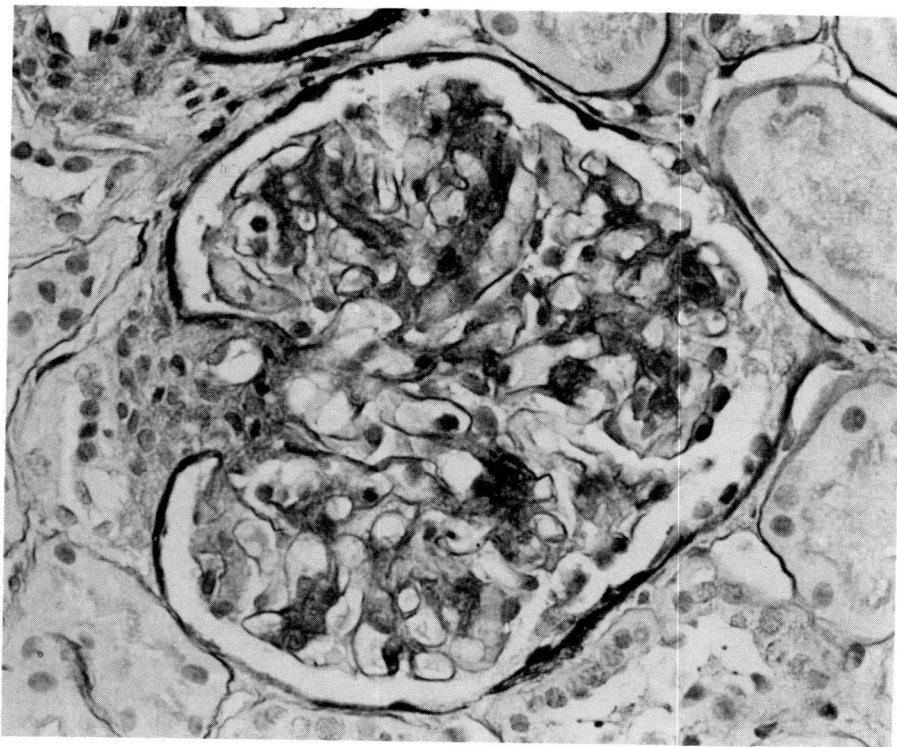

Fig. 61–9. Minimal (mesangial) lupus nephritis. (H&E × 500).

tract signs also usually occur along with other evidence of neuropsychiatric disease.

Involvement of Central Nervous System.[10,57]
More common and more serious than peripheral nervous system involvement, central nervous system disease occurs as two major forms: organic psychosis and seizures. Seizures in the absence of renal insufficiency, hypertension, or infection occur in about 15% of SLE patients[32] and are usually present at the time of the original diagnosis, accompanying active systemic disease. We have not noted the onset of seizures in our patients late in the course of the disease. Grand mal seizures are most common, but we have also seen patients with chorea, Jacksonian fits, petit mal, and temporal lobe seizures. Pseudotumor cerebri may also occur with acute disease. Nearly all of these manifestations occur at the time of disease onset and, in many cases, are accompanied by other neuropsychiatric abnormalities.[32] Chorea and petit mal seizures sometimes begin at the time of diagnosis of SLE along with other evidence of disease activity. These conditions persist for many years, even when no clinical evidence of disease activity elsewhere can be documented.

Central nervous system (CNS) involvement may also be manifested by organic brain disease. Organic syndromes are characterized by impairment of orientation, perception, and ability to calculate. Memory deficits are common, and the patient may have difficulty remembering the name of his physician. In our series of patients studied at the Bellevue Medical-Psychiatric wards, 21% of the total group of 209 patients had episodes of CNS disease during the year of diagnosis. These patients were acutely ill with multisystem disease and fever; 15% had CNS disease during the first year after diagnosis, but only 2% showed CNS findings during the fifth through the sixth years. No episodes of CNS disease occurred in 43 patients in their eighth year or in 24 patients during their ninth year. No episodes of psychosis occurred in 25 patients during their tenth through twelfth years, although two patients had cerebrovascular accidents, one 11 years, and one 12 years after diagnosis. Thus, CNS disease is a manifestation of severe active lupus, occurs early in the course of the disease, and coincides with evidence of disease activity in other systems.[32]

Complete recovery of the organic brain disease is usual, but some patients have residual impairment of mental processes, such as an inability to calculate as rapidly as they could before the disease episode. SLE patients with CNS disease are more likely to have evidence of vasculitis than those without CNS findings.[32] The five-year survival of our 82 patients with organic brain disease at the time of diagnosis was 71% as compared to a 77% survival of the 274 patients without organic brain disease.[99] The patients were treated with high doses of corticosteroids.[111]

Severe Headaches. At the time of diagnosis, 21 of our 209 SLE patients in New York complained of severe headache. In five of these patients, the headache was associated with organic brain disease and in eight others with seizures. Brandt and Lessel have described 11 patients with severe throbbing headaches or with wavy or zig-zag scotomata typical of the fortification specters of migraine.[14] These phenomena occurred either for the first time after the diagnosis of SLE or as an initial feature along with other manifestations of systemic disease. Migraine headaches or fortification specters have also occurred as an isolated symptom prior to the development of other clinical manifestations of SLE, but at a time when serologic abnormalities of SLE were found. Classic migraine headaches have an increased prevalence in SLE patients.[48] It is important to recognize these headaches as a manifestation of SLE because they disappear when prednisone is administered or when the dose of corticosteroid is increased, and they occur along with other manifestations of the disease during periods of exacerbation.

Psychologic Problems. It is important to recognize that most SLE patients have major psychologic problems in coping with their disease and the effects of the therapy they are receiving. Patients become depressed and anxious. The disfigurement caused by high doses of corticosteroids, which is especially difficult in young women and adolescents, may lead to a major depression. Because this type of mental abnormality is not part of the disease itself, it should not be called "CNS lupus." The corticosteroid dose should not be increased in such patients. These individuals need reassurance and may require psychotherapy.

Laboratory Findings. Abnormalities of the cerebrospinal fluid were present in 32% of episodes of neuropsychiatric illness in 37 patients studied by Feinglass.[32] Protein elevation was noted in about half the fluids, and in a few patients both protein and white cells were increased. Elevation of cerebrospinal fluid pressure may be associated with papilledema. Protein elevation may be absent, modest, or even significant. Rarely, the cerebrospinal fluid findings may suggest an infectious process. Feinglass et al. have noted that death was associated with cerebrospinal fluid abnormalities, but not with normal fluids.[32]

The electroencephalogram is frequently abnormal during an episode of neuropsychiatric disease. Abnormal electroencephalograms may also be noted in patients without any CNS abnormalities, but are more frequently abnormal in those with CNS disease. Diffuse slow wave activity is the most common abnormality, but focal changes may also be observed. Brain scans have been reported to correlate well with the presence of CNS disease.[8] It is probably wise to obtain a brain scan in a SLE patient with CNS disease. If findings are abnormal, the scan can be repeated later to determine whether the abnormalities disappear as the patient recovers. A new technique using oxygen-15 is capable of demonstrating temporary ischemia and may be of great help in the diagnosis and management of CNS lupus.[10] At present, computerized axial tomography is of more value than the brain scan. Major areas of infarction are visualized, especially in patients with localized findings. "Cerebral atrophy" is frequent and is a term describing enlargement of the ventricles and cortical sulci. This enlargement may be caused by loss of water or loss of nerve cells. "Cerebral atrophy" is not unique to CNS lupus but is noted in a variety of conditions, including non-SLE conditions in patients on corticosteroid therapy. Therefore, at present it is difficult to determine the significance of "cerebral atrophy" in an SLE patient with CNS manifestations.

Pathology. Pathologic abnormalities in patients with seizures usually consist of microinfarcts.[30,81] Vasculitis is found in 35% and intracerebral hemorrhages in 22%. Focal motor seizures are associated with findings of subarachnoid hemorrhage. Pathologic changes in 12 patients with hemiparesis were similar to the changes associated with seizures, except that intracerebral hemorrhage was present in 6,[30] and the hemorrhage was related to the presence of brain vasculitis. Vasculitis was also present in one-third of patients with subarachnoid hemorrhage and in 25% of those patients with microhemorrhages. In patients dying with lupus psychosis, researchers have found microinfarcts, vasculitis, and cerebral hemorrhages.[81]

Immunofluorescence studies have revealed deposits of immunoglobulins and C3 in the choroid plexus of SLE patients.[3]

C4 in the spinal fluid is lower than expected compared to other complement proteins, and repeated testing has revealed that C4 levels return to normal during remission.[43] Unfortunately, the assay must be performed immediately because the hemolytic activity of C4 decays rapidly. The presence of antineuronal antibodies in the spinal fluid is described elsewhere.

Gastrointestinal Manifestations. The most common gastrointestinal manifestation is abdominal pain. The pain may be accompanied by nausea and less often by diarrhea. In most patients, abdominal pain occurs in association with evidence of disease activity in other systems. The cause of abdominal pain usually is not clear. Mesenteric arteritis may be noted on arteriography. Patients with mesenteric arteritis have ileal and colonic ulcers, and colonic and ileal perforations may occur.[118] We have observed three deaths from intestinal perforation in our 365 patients. Zizic et al. described colonic perforations as the cause of 4 of 15 deaths occurring in 197 patients with SLE.[118] Thus, colonic perforations accounted for a significant percentage of deaths in SLE patients observed in recent years. The pain in patients with perforations is colicky and well localized to the lower abdomen or infra-umbilical area. Abdominal pain in SLE patients without perforations is less well localized or may be localized to the epigastrium or upper quadrants. It may be either sharp or colicky. Both rebound and direct tenderness were present in our patients with perforations and in four of the five patients reported by Zizic et al.[118] Neither rebound tenderness nor localized direct tenderness was present in SLE patients with abdominal pain without perforations. It is interesting to note that abdominal pain is more common in children with SLE than in adults, although perforations have not been observed. Abdominal pain in children is crampy and occurs during periods of disease activity, disappearing as other manifestations of the disease resolve.

It is important to recognize that patients with colonic perforation usually have evidence of severe active SLE in other systems. Both our patients and those described by Zizic et al. had highly active SLE. The only patient surviving received the earliest surgical intervention before radiologic evidence of perforation was apparent, even though she was a poor surgical risk because of lupus nephritis with uremia.[118] Thus, early surgical intervention is suggested if the diagnosis of perforation is suspected.

Some SLE patients have had regional enteritis[96] with erosions and ulceration of the intestinal mucosa at the time of operation for abdominal pain.[107]

In our series, abdominal pain of acute onset with evidence of peritonitis occurred in 16 patients. The pain was due to ruptured ovarian cyst, perforated gastric ulcer, appendicitis, diverticulitis, and abscess of the fallopian tubes. *It is wise to consider early surgical intervention in SLE patients.*

Pancreatitis occurred in 7 of our 365 SLE patients at a time that the disease was active in other systems. In one patient, pancreatitis was associated with organic brain disease as well as other clinical and serologic evidence of active SLE. In one anal-

ysis, elevated serum amylase was found in 26 SLE patients, and pancreatitis due to SLE was present in 4 patients. These four patients recovered with corticosteroid treatment.[105]

Liver and Spleen Abnormalities. Hepatomegaly occurs in about 30% of patients, more commonly among children than among adult-onset patients.[68] Clinical jaundice occurred in 9 of 365 patients, and hepatic insufficiency was the cause of death in one 8-year-old girl. Autopsy findings in this patient revealed acute fatty degeneration of the liver. In 4 of our 365 SLE patients, biopsy evidence of chronic active hepatitis was present. These patients all met the American Rheumatism Association Preliminary Criteria for the Classification of SLE.[24] Skin manifestations, central nervous system lupus, and mild lupus nephritis were present in these patients. Liver enzyme elevations are noted in about 30% of patients at the time of diagnosis when active disease is evident in many systems. In addition, aspirin may cause elevations of transaminase levels in patients with SLE. A review of the results of liver biopsies from SLE patients who had either clinical liver disease or had only liver enzyme abnormalities revealed findings of chronic active hepatitis, granulomatous hepatitis, cirrhosis, acute hepatitis, fatty change, or cholestasis.[90]

Slight to moderate splenomegaly is present in 20% of patients and is more common in children.[68] Splenomegaly is not usually associated with hemolytic anemia. Asplenism has been reported in SLE patients, including 2 of 65 patients whose functional asplenism was only detected by CAT scan.[27]

The "onion skin" appearance of the splenic arterioles is present in 15% of patients. This change is due to concentric periarterial fibrosis thought to be the end stage of an earlier focal arteritis.

Lymph Node Enlargement. Lymph node enlargement occurs in about half of all SLE patients at the time of disease activity. Lymphadenopathy is more common in children than in adults.[68] Enlargement is usually generalized but may be limited. Nodes are usually nontender. One of our patients has had two severe episodes of active disease, each associated with massive nontender enlargement of the occipital nodes.

Microscopic changes in lymph nodes are nonspecific. They consist of follicular hyperplasia, which may be associated with areas of necrosis, resembling a lymphoma (giant follicular lymphoma).

Ocular Manifestations. Conjunctivitis or episcleritis occurred in 15% of our patients. These conditions appear to be more common in patients with extensive cutaneous manifestations. Periorbital edema and subconjunctival hemorrhages have also been reported. Occlusion of the central retinal artery has been reported during periods of disease activity, but is a rare occurrence. Active retinal arteritis and arteriolar occlusion have been reported.[11,25] Blindness may be the first symptom of the disease.[116] Cytoid bodies, which occur in only 8% of patients, are retinal exudates appearing as hard white lesions adjacent to retinal vessels during periods of disease activity. These exudates disappear gradually as the disease becomes inactive. Cytoid bodies may be associated with organic brain disease and seizures.

Parotid Gland Enlargement. Enlarged parotid glands occurred in 8% of our patients. Xerostomia was not present in most of these patients. Typical keratoconjunctivitis sicca is uncommon. Unilateral enlargement of a parotid gland may be observed during periods of disease activity in a small number of patients. One prospective study reported a high incidence of Sjögren's syndrome, including a positive Schirmer's test in 21%, positive parotid scan in 58%, and positive lip biopsy in 50% of patients.[66]

Menstrual Abnormalities and Pregnancy. Cessation of menses during the initial 3 to 6 months of treatment of the disease occurs frequently. The menstrual periods return as the disease goes into remission and as the dose of corticosteroids is reduced. Menorrhagia occasionally occurs and may be due to thrombocytopenia or to an inhibitor of one of the clotting factors. Stillbirths and miscarriages are common in untreated patients with active disease. Normal deliveries are the rule in well-controlled patients taking low doses of corticosteroids for at least 6 months prior to conception.[53,119] This finding may be due to the suppression of maternal lupus anticoagulant.[65a] However, slight exacerbations of the disease are common in the immediate prepartum and postpartum periods.[53,70] Of four deliveries during 1977, mild thrombocytopenia occurred in two patients two weeks prior to delivery. Hemolytic anemia occurred in one patient a few days after delivery. In each instance, prompt remission occurred when the dose of corticosteroid was increased. We have not observed congenital abnormalities in the children of our patients, with the exception of complete heart block, which was present in two children of one of our patients.[22] This abnormality is associated with anti-Ro antibody passively transferred to the infant from the mother. The mothers of some affected infants had anti-Ro antibody, but were clinically asymptomatic. On the other hand, we have observed normal infants born to SLE mothers who had anti-Ro at the time of delivery.

Allergic Reactions. SLE patients do not have a higher than normal incidence of allergic dermatitis, rhinitis, asthma, or food or drug allergies. However, instances of severe exacerbations of the disease have been observed after treatment of urinary infections with sulfasoxazole. Hives are not uncommon and are probably a manifestation of the disease rather than of allergy.

LABORATORY FINDINGS

Hematologic Abnormalities. One or more hematologic abnormalities are present in nearly all SLE patients with active disease.[16] Most common is a mild-to-moderate normocytic, normochromic anemia due to retarded erythropoiesis. Hematocrit values of less than 30% occur in about half the patients during periods of clinical disease activity. On the other hand, Coombs-positive hemolytic anemia occurred in only 10% of our 365 patients, although positive Coombs' tests occur more frequently as an isolated abnormality owing to the presence of C3 or C4 on the erythrocyte surface without evidence of hemolysis or reticulocytosis.

Mild to moderate leukopenia is less common than anemia. Leukopenia of less than 4,000 cells/cmm was present in 17% of our patients. Lymphopenia is usually present during periods of disease activity.[80] Leukocytosis is occasionally noted during episodes of active disease and may be a confusing finding if spiking fever is also present. Leukocytosis due to corticosteroid therapy also occurs in SLE patients. White blood counts of 30,000, nearly all mature neutrophils, have occasionally been observed in corticosteroid-treated, noninfected patients.

Mild thrombocytopenia of between 100,000 and 150,000/cmm is present in about one-third of patients, but severe thrombocytopenia with purpura has occurred in only 5%. Thrombocytopenia may occur for the first time late in the course of the disease. It occurred as an isolated event in the last trimester of pregnancy in two well-controlled SLE patients taking low doses of prednisone. A factor is present on the surface of the platelets in most patients even without thrombocytopenia. This antiplatelet factor is present during periods of remission and during disease activity. Qualitative thrombocyte defects are also common and not clinically significant.[16,79]

The *lupus anticoagulant* can be identified by the presence of a slight prolongation of the thromboplastin time and more marked prolongation of the partial thromboplastin time.[79] The partial thromboplastin time prolongation is not corrected by the addition of equal volumes of normal plasma to the patient's plasma at dilutions of 1:50, 1:100, and 1:500. The lupus anticoagulant is not clinically significant; bleeding and clotting times are normal.

Renal biopsies have been performed on individuals with the lupus anticoagulant without any bleeding. The possible relationship between the lupus anticoagulant and thrombosis was discussed already. The anticoagulant disappeared in one of our newly diagnosed patients one week after corticosteroid therapy was instituted for systemic manifestations of the disease. *Anticoagulant activities, which specifically inactivate clotting factors, are more significant clinically.* These activities have been most frequently directed at factors VIII, IX, and XII. They must be identified because major bleeding episodes may result from renal biopsies or operative procedures. The action of these specific anticoagulants is also reversed by corticosteroid therapy. In general, bleeding problems in SLE patients usually occur in individuals with active disease, especially in those with evidence of vasculitis.

False positive serologic tests for syphilis were present in 25% of our patients. The test is frequently positive in patients with the lupus anticoagulant. It is probable that the anticoagulants arise as antibodies directed against the phospholipids necessary for blood coagulation. The test for syphilis is probably positive because the antigens used in these tests are phospholipids.

The erythrocyte sedimentation rate (ESR) is elevated in nearly all SLE patients and, in most patients, falls to normal when the disease becomes inactive. However, some SLE patients maintain a markedly elevated ESR for years in the absence of clinical or serologic evidence of active disease.

Cryoglobulins of the mixed IgG-IgM type may be found in about 11% of patients. They are usually associated with clinical and serologic disease activity, lower serum complement levels, and clinical nephritis.

A diffuse elevation of serum gamma globulin is observed in about 80% of patients with clinically active disease. Rheumatoid factor is present in 14% of SLE patients.

Serum Complement Levels. Serum complement levels are usually depressed in active disease.

DIFFERENTIAL DIAGNOSIS

The Preliminary Criteria for the Classification of SLE[24] have been used since 1971 and have been found to be a sensitive criteria for the diagnosis of the disease.[63] The Preliminary Criteria have also been of help in reminding physicians of the major laboratory and clinical manifestations of the disease. However, the Preliminary Criteria were established prior to the common use of tests, such as complement levels, antinuclear antibodies, anti-DNA, and anti-Sm antibodies. Therefore, the American Rheumatism Association appointed a subcommittee to review and revise the Preliminary

Criteria. For the purpose of establishing the new criteria, the subcommittee collected data from 20 centers on patients thought to have the diagnosis of SLE. The Revised Criteria were published in 1982 (see Table 61-2).[104] The Criteria were tested against the findings in series of scleroderma and rheumatoid arthritis patients for specificity and against the findings in a second group of SLE patients for sensitivity. To classify a patient as having SLE, 4 or more of 11 manifestations are required, whereas 4 of 14 manifestations were required in the Preliminary Criteria. As noted in Table 61-2, the Revised Criteria have the following major differences from the Preliminary Criteria: (1) The renal manifestations are grouped together, and the proteinuria item no longer requires 3.5 g per day of urinary protein; (2) alopecia has been deleted as a manifestation; (3) Raynaud's phenomenon has been deleted as a manifestation; (4) ANA has been added as a manifestation; (5) the LE preparation, which was a single manifestation, is included in the "Immunologic" manifestation; (6) the false positive test for syphilis, which was a single manifestation, is included in the "Immunologic" manifestation; and (7) anti-DNA antibodies and anti-Sm antibodies are included in the "Immunologic" manifestation. Thus, the Revised Criteria group all the relatively specific immunologic tests as one manifestation.

Although not included in the Revised Criteria, serum C3 levels are of major importance in the diagnosis of an individual patient with SLE. In one study, it was shown that the presence of a low serum C3, in addition to the presence of antibodies to native DNA, is highly specific for SLE.[115] The sensitivity of the anti-DNA antibody test was 72% and the specificity 96%. The sensitivity of a low serum C3 level was 38% and the specificity 90%. Thus, in addition to studies of serum antibodies to nuclear antigens, a serum C3 level should be performed in all individuals in whom a diagnosis of SLE is considered a possibility. The most common diagnosis made in patients before definitive diagnosis of SLE is rheumatoid arthritis or "nonspecific" arthritis. Approximately one-quarter of our SLE patients have had this diagnosis for at least one year prior to the diagnosis of SLE. Young women presenting with a history of arthritis or arthralgia should be studied carefully for the possibility of SLE. The onset of arthritis or arthralgia during pregnancy or the postpartum period should particularly alert the physician to the diagnosis of SLE. Diagnoses that may predate by 2 to 10 years a definitive diagnosis of SLE include rheumatic fever, chronic discoid lupus, idiopathic thrombocytopenic purpura, seizure disorder, Raynaud's phenomenon, psychosis, and hemolytic anemia.

It is important to remember that SLE can occur in elderly persons. These individuals are frequently not diagnosed early in the course of the disease because the possibility of SLE is overlooked. In addition, we found that some of these elderly patients were in nursing homes prior to admission to the hospital because they were confused and therefore considered to be senile. After SLE was finally diagnosed and the disease was treated with corticosteroids, the "senile" psychosis gradually cleared. The patients became alert and able to care for themselves.

Other diseases to consider in patients with multisystem disease include subacute bacterial endocarditis, gonococcal or meningococcal septicemia with arthritis and skin lesions, serum sickness, lymphoma and leukemia, thrombotic thrombocytopenic purpura, sarcoidosis, secondary syphilis, and bacterial septicemia.

MANAGEMENT

At the time the diagnosis of SLE is made, the physician should be able to evaluate the severity of the disease. This evaluation is accomplished by the history, physical examination, and laboratory workup. If the onset of the disease occurs rapidly, the patient should be considered to have a more severe condition. The presence of both anti-DNA antibodies and low serum complement (especially C3) levels suggests more severe disease.

Renal Biopsy. Urinary abnormalities, if present, should lead to complete workup for renal disease. This workup should include noninvasive studies, such as serum creatinine levels on two occasions, to determine whether renal insufficiency is present or impending. Patients with proteinuria and red cells in the urine should have a renal biopsy to determine the following: (1) the type of lupus nephritis, i.e., focal proliferative, diffuse proliferative, membranous, or mesangial; (2) the "activity" of the glomerular lesion; (3) the presence and extent of glomerular and/or tubular sclerosis; and (4) the presence and extent of tubular and interstitial disease. As described previously, the presence of sclerosis early in the course of the disease is a sign of poor prognosis. Extensive sclerosis does not respond to any kind of aggressive therapy. The management of the various forms of lupus nephritis is described in the section on renal disease.

The management of the patient with SLE is divided into four sections: (1) general measures that should be applied to most patients; (2) management of the patient with clinical evidence of active disease, particularly at the onset of the illness; (3) management of the period between control of the initial episode of active disease and clinical remis-

sion; and (4) management of the patient over an extended clinical remission.

General Measures. Both the patient and the physician should become familiar with the signs and symptoms during the time of onset of multisystem disease. The early clinical recurrence of disease activity may then be recognized by the patient, who should alert the physician. For example, some patients develop an erythematous rash as the first sign of an impending serious systemic exacerbation. If the patient merely waits until the next appointment to inform the physician of the rash, the delay may result in the appearance of more serious additional manifestations, such as hematuria or pericarditis.

The physician should be familiar with all the laboratory evidence of active disease in each patient and with the response of each laboratory test to corticosteroid therapy. Thus, if the erythrocyte sedimentation rate (ESR) is elevated initially and rapidly returns to normal after therapy, future marked increase in the ESR may be viewed with concern regarding exacerbation of the disease. Similarly, initial low C3 or C4 levels, which return to the normal range as the disease becomes inactive, usually fall again in the future, either just before or at the time of clinical disease activity.[94] It is also important, though, for the physician to know which laboratory tests were not abnormal during the initial episode of disease activity prior to treatment. Other patients have abnormal laboratory findings that do not resolve with treatment and clinical remission. For example, elevated antinative DNA antibodies have been noted over the course of five years in patients who are clinically well. Abnormal test results that do not respond initially to adequate treatment should probably be ignored in most patients. On the other hand, we have found that patients with persistently high anti-DNA antibody levels, who are well clinically and have otherwise normal laboratory tests, become acutely ill when their C3 levels fall.

All SLE patients need reassurance from the physician, adequate rest when the disease is active, and avoidance of sun exposure. Sunscreen creams and ointments, wide-brimmed hats, and long sleeves should be used by all SLE patients.

Birth Control. Pregnancy should be avoided during the first few years of disease. Oral contraceptives should be avoided. Pregnancy has been well tolerated in our patients who have no evidence of active renal disease or sclerotic glomeruli and who are in clinical remission while taking less than 15 mg prednisone daily for at least one year. Exacerbations of disease during pregnancy should be managed by vigorous treatment with corticosteroids rather than by therapeutic abortion.[120]

Infections. All SLE patients should be observed carefully for infections. Patients should be instructed to inform the physician immediately if any symptoms occur or if a fever is present. Urinalysis should be performed and cultures performed on specimens that show bacteria. Patients should be treated prophylactically with antibiotics if scaling of the gums, teeth extraction, or major dental surgery is performed.

Disease Severity. The treatment of SLE depends not only on the target organs involved but on the severity of the disease. Renal disease may be minimal or mild. Anemia may be slight or may be a severe hemolytic anemia. Mildly ill patients frequently are diagnosed at a time when arthritis and a butterfly rash are the only signs and symptoms of the disease. The laboratory evidence of severe disease is of great importance in such patients. A low serum C3 and high titers of anti-native DNA antibodies are considered by many, although not all investigators, to indicate that severe clinical and/or renal disease may ensue unless the patient is treated aggressively. Other laboratory parameters that may be present in patients whose signs and symptoms are mild include thrombocytopenia, hemolytic anemia, renal disease manifested by more than mild proteinuria, seizures, organic brain disease, and vasculitis of the skin or other organs. If present, these parameters indicate that the disease is severe and should be treated aggressively. In our experience, pericarditis and pleuritis are also considered "severe," but others do not agree.

Initial Treatment. Patients with severe disease should be treated with corticosteroids (see Chap. 32). Most patients respond to 60 mg of prednisone given in doses of 15 mg every 6 hours. Many severely ill patients without central nervous system or active renal disease require a similar high dose of prednisone initially. In most patients, evidence of disease activity disappears rapidly. Large pericardial or pleural effusions, hematuria, and occasionally central nervous system manifestations may respond more slowly and may require a higher daily dose of prednisone. In an analysis of 67 neuropsychiatric episodes, 84% had a favorable outcome, usually associated with initiation or increase in steroid dose.[32]

The use of pulse-therapy corticosteroids (intravenous infusion of large doses—usually 1 g methylprednisolone daily for 3 days) has been advocated in the management of severe SLE patients with rapidly advancing renal failure who have not responded to oral doses.[21,56] Although some investigators have described rapid fall of "nephrotic range" proteinuria, we have not found this to occur in a small number of patients so treated. Fessel described improvement in one of three patients with lupus cerebritis, in all three patients with lung disease, and in one patient with thrombocytopenia.[33a] In patients with pulmonary hemorrhage not due to infection, pulse therapy may be the treatment of choice because these patients need as rapid a therapeutic effect as possible. It is important to continue with high-dose oral corticosteroid therapy after the three-day pulse therapy in such an acutely ill patient. There are still no definite studies to determine whether pulse therapy provides a better long-term management of the disease. The question regarding long-term side effects, such as aseptic necrosis, is not clear at present. There have been acute side effects due to the IV pulse therapy. These side effects include bacteremia and sudden death, the latter presumably due to electrolyte effects on the myocardium. In addition, hyperglycemia, hypo- or hyperkalemia, sodium retention, hypotension, or hypertension have been described. In some centers, IV pulse therapy has been administered only in a setting where patients have cardiac monitors. Infusion over at least 30 minutes is recommended.[56] No controlled study of this form of therapy has been reported.

Plasmapheresis. Plasmapheresis is an experimental method of treatment and should be restricted to centers where controlled protocol studies are being conducted. Recorded data strongly suggest that plasmapheresis is followed by a serious rebound of both immunologic and clinical activity.[50,51] In addition, many of the reports in the literature describe a short-lived remission. Plasmapheresis together with corticosteroid therapy appears to be effective, but the response is also short-lived, as is the response to plasmapheresis and azathioprine. The most prolonged response followed plasmapheresis combined with both corticosteroids and cyclophosphamide. These patients responded, had no rebound, and the improvement lasted for at least 4 months. Thus, if plasmapheresis is to be used, it probably should be given with corticosteroids and cyclophosphamide.

Less severely ill patients respond to 20 to 40 mg of prednisone given in a regimen of 10 to 15 mg four times daily. The response is usually prompt, i.e., within 1 to 2 weeks with disappearance of symptoms and a change in abnormal laboratory tests toward a normal range.

Patients in whom SLE is diagnosed and who have mild disease without markedly abnormal laboratory tests may be treated with a combination of aspirin and hydroxychloroquine sulfate (Plaquenil). Aspirin is used in anti-inflammatory doses (see Chap. 28) and 200 mg of hydroxychloroquine is given twice daily (see Chap. 30). This regimen is adequate for most patients in whom arthritis and dermatologic abnormalities are the only clinical signs and symptoms and in whom laboratory tests are not "severe."

Management after Initial Response. Most SLE patients respond initially to high doses of oral corticosteroids. As the clinical disease responds, resolution of laboratory abnormalities is observed. The corticosteroid dose can then be lowered. Gradual tapering with frequent monitoring of laboratory values is usually successful until the daily dose of prednisone reaches 10 to 20 mg. At this dose, there may be evidence of serologic or clinical flare of the disease, and the prednisone dose should then be held constant temporarily or should be slightly increased.

Management on Low-Dose Prednisone. In patients controlled on small doses of prednisone, repeated attempts should be made to further reduce the dose. It may be necessary to lower the dose by small increments, e.g., 1 mg per week. In most patients, a daily dose of 10 mg or less is adequate to control the disease and to allow the patients to feel totally free of symptoms. Even in these individuals, the primary goal should be no medication or the lowest possible dose. Alternate-day therapy has been used successfully in some patients. In our own experience, daily small doses (2.5 to 10 mg) lead to better prolonged control.

Antimalarials. In patients with evidence of dermatologic manifestations, antimalarial therapy should be used. Hydroxychloroquine (Plaquenil) or chloroquine (Aralen) has been shown to significantly reduce the number of episodes of dermatologic abnormalities in SLE patients.[89] Retinal toxicity occurs in SLE patients who have taken the drugs for a significant length of time in high doses.[19,47] The incidence of retinopathy is related to the total ingested dose of the antimalarial drugs. Patients should be seen by an ophthalmologist before treatment and every 6 months while receiving therapy (see Chap. 30). Hydroxychloroquine, 400 mg daily, can be used initially with eventual decrease in daily dose to 200 mg when skin lesions are no longer present. An attempt should be made to further reduce the dose to alternate days, or three or two times per week, or to discontinue the drug. In some patients, however, relapses occur and the hydroxychloroquine must be restarted.

Aspirin and Nonsteroidal Anti-Inflammatory Drugs. Anti-inflammatory doses of aspirin are of value in control of the arthritis in patients who develop an exacerbation of this manifestation while receiving low doses of corticosteroids. Rapid control of pleural and/or pericardial effusions is sometimes achieved with indomethacin 25 mg TID.

Cyclophosphamide. The use of immunosuppressive agents in the treatment of SLE is still controversial. At present, their use should be confined to multicenter controlled studies or to those centers with extensive experience in their use. The toxicity and long-term side effects of these drugs and their use in the management of SLE have been reviewed in Chapter 33. In our experience, cyclophosphamide is of great value in SLE patients with medium or small vessel necrotizing vasculitis. Its efficacy is similar to that in patients with Wegener's vasculitis or periarteritis nodosa (see also Chaps. 33 and 63).

PROGNOSIS

Studies on the survival of SLE patients have shown improvement over time (Table 61–4).[28,29,31,55,61,111]

Corticosteroid-treated patients have shown five-year survivals of 93% and 94% in two reports.[32,111] It is therefore important to consider the period of observation when patients recently treated with immunosuppressive therapy are compared with patients treated 15 to 20 years ago with corticosteroids. The improved survival rate may be due to better use of serologic parameters and antibiotics, an increased awareness of the disease on the part of both patient and physician, or a change in the natural history of the disease.

RELATED OR ASSOCIATED CONDITIONS

Rheumatoid Arthritis and Other Connective Tissue Diseases. Only a small percentage of individuals who fulfill the American Rheumatism Association Preliminary or Revised Criteria have definite coincident rheumatoid arthritis with rheumatoid nodules, erosive arthritis, and rheumatoid factor.[34] Such individuals have at least 4 of the 14 manifestations of the Preliminary Criteria excluding the arthritis. Patients with classic or definite rheumatoid arthritis occasionally develop typical multisystem SLE including lupus nephritis. An occasional patient may have typical SLE along with one or more manifestations of another connective tissue disease. SLE patients with a typical violaceous rash of the V area of the chest and edematous violaceous upper eyelids have been observed. Necrotizing vasculitis typical of polyarteritis and plaques of scleroderma have also been observed in an occasional SLE patient.

Myasthenia Gravis. SLE has been reported in association with myasthenia gravis either before or after thymectomy.[35]

Porphyria Cutanea Tarda. This condition has been reported in association with SLE.[26]

Chronic Discoid Lupus. This benign skin disease is not rare and is thought to be more common than SLE itself. Discoid lupus has been reported

Table 61–4.   Reported Survival in Corticosteroid-Treated SLE Patients*

Series	No. of Cases	Years of Observation	Years After Diagnosis				
			1	3	5	7	10
Johns Hopkins	99	1949–1953	78	62	. .	. .	. .
Cleveland Clinic	299	1949–1959	89	75	69	59	54
University of Southern California	57	1950–1955	42	12	4	2	. .
Sweden	54	1955–1961	82	72	70	63	51
University of Southern California	100	1956–1962	63	32	16	12	4
Group 1	209	1957–1967	89	79	70	67	63
Columbia University	150	1963–1971	98	90	77	68	59
University of Southern California	92	1963–1973	98	91	79	65	41
Group 2	156	1968–1975	99	97	93	90	84
Johns Hopkins	140	1970–1975	. .	. .	94	. .	82

*For whom life-table analysis was employed.
From Urman, J.D., and Rothfield, N.F.[111]

in infants and in the elderly, but most patients are between the ages of 25 and 45 at the time of onset. Although women are affected more often than men, the sex ratio is only 2:1.[84] The disease occurs in all races. Family studies have revealed more than one case in the same family, and studies of relatives of SLE patients have revealed other family members with discoid lupus.[7] Studies of antinative DNA antibodies and complement proteins in discoid lupus patients show no increases compared to age-, sex-, and race-matched controls.[91] Complement proteins were normal in these studies except for increased levels of properdin found in nearly half the patients studied. It is of interest that a number of individuals with a hereditary deficiency of C2 have lesions of discoid lupus as their only clinical abnormality.[52]

It is clear that some patients with discoid lupus go on to develop SLE, but the percentage who do so is unknown. No serologic markers have been found that identify patients who eventually develop systemic disease.

Drug-Induced Lupus. This syndrome is caused by the chronic ingestion of several drugs and has been reviewed.[114] Prospective studies have revealed that procainamide-induced antinuclear antibodies develop in about 50% of individuals, about half of whom develop a lupus-like illness. Procainamide is therefore the most common drug inducing a lupus syndrome. Patients with this syndrome typically have joint pains and swelling, rashes, pleurisy, pericarditis, and pulmonary atelectasis. The disease clinically resembles the non-drug-induced disease in elderly individuals. In both the procainamide-induced syndrome and in elderly individuals with SLE, renal disease is uncommon and antibodies against native DNA are usually absent. Withdrawal of procainamide gradually leads to disappearance of the clinical syndrome and even-

tual disappearance of the serum antinuclear antibodies.

Although drug-induced clinical disease has been described rarely after isoniazid, the drug did induce antinuclear antibodies in 20% of individuals who received it.[85]

A prospective study on the immunologic effects of hydralazine was completed in a group of black patients. The results after two years revealed that antinuclear antibodies developed in 15 of the 25 patients. The antinuclear antibodies were detected in undiluted sera in 12, and a titer of 1:10 or greater occurred in 3 patients. Clinical symptoms of SLE developed in only 1 of the 25 patients.[64]

REFERENCES

1. Agnello, V.: Association of systemic lupus erythematosus and systemic lupus erythematosus-like syndromes with hereditary and acquired complement deficient states. Arthritis Rheum., 21:S146, 1978.
2. Arnett, F.C., and Shulman, L.E.: Studies in familial systemic lupus erythematosus. Medicine, 55:313–322, 1976.
3. Atkins, C.J., Kondan, J.J., and Quismorio, F.P.: The choroid plexus in systemic lupus erythematosus. Ann. Intern. Med., 76:65–72, 1972.
4. Baart de la Faille, H., and Baart de la Faille-Kuyper, E.H.: Immunofluorescence studies of the skin in rosacea. Dermatologica, 139:49–54, 1969.
5. Baehr, G., Klemperer, P., and Schrifrin, A.: A diffuse disease of the peripheral circulation usually associated with lupus erythematosus and endocarditis. Trans. Assoc. Am. Physicians, 50:139–155, 1935.
6. Baldwin, D.S., et al.: The clinical course of the proliferative membranous forms of lupus nephritis. Ann. Intern. Med., 73:929–942, 1970.
7. Belin, D.C., et al.: Familial discoid lupus erythematosus associated with heterozygous C2 deficiency. Arthritis Rheum., 23:898–903, 1980.
8. Bennahum, D.A., Messner, R.P., and Shoop, J.D.: Brain scan findings in central nervous system involvement by lupus erythematosus. Ann. Intern. Med., 81:763–765, 1974.
9. Bernhard, G.C., Lange, R.L., and Hensley, G.T.: Aortic disease with valvular insufficiency as the principal manifestation of systemic lupus erythematosus. Ann. Intern. Med., 71:81–87, 1969.
10. Bernstein, R.M., III: Cerebral lupus: A peep into Pandora's box. J. Rheumatol., 9:817–818, 1982.
11. Bishko, F.: Retinopathy in systemic lupus erythematosus.

A case report and review of the literature. Arthritis Rheum., *15*:57–63, 1972.

12. Black, M.M., and Hudson, P.M.: Atrophic and blanche lesions closely resembling malignant atrophic papulosis (Degos' disease) in systemic lupus erythematosus. Br. J. Dermatol., *95*:649–654, 1976.

13. Block, S.R., et al.: Immunologic observations on 9 sets of twins either concordant or discordant for systemic lupus erythematosus. Arthritis Rheum., *19*:545–554, 1976.

14. Brandt, K.D., and Lessel, S.: Migrainous phenomena in systemic lupus erythematosus. Arthritis Rheum., *21*:7–16, 1978.

15. Bretjens, J.R., et al.: Interstitial immune complex nephritis in patients with systemic lupus erythematosus. Kidney Int., *7*:342–358, 1975.

16. Budman, D.R., and Steinberg, A.D.: Hematologic aspects of systemic lupus erythematosus. Ann. Intern. Med., *86*:220–229, 1977.

17. Bulkley, B.H., and Roberts, W.C.: The heart in systemic lupus erythematosus and the changes induced in it by corticosteroid therapy. A study of 36 necropsy patients. Am. J. Med., *58*:243–256, 1975.

18. Bullock, W.E., Callerame, M.L., and Panner, B.J.: Immunohistologic alternational skin and ultrastructural changes in glomerular membrane in leprosy. Am. J. Trop. Med. Hyg., *23*:78–86, 1974.

19. Carr, R.E., et al.: Ocular toxicity of antimalarial drugs. Am. J. Ophthalmol., *66*:737–746, 1968.

20. Carreras, L.O., et al.: Arterial thrombosis, intrauterine death and "lupus anticoagulant": Detection of immunoglobulin interfering with prostacyclin formation. Lancet, *1*:244–246, 1981.

21. Cathcart, E.S., et al.: Beneficial effects of methylprednisolone "pulse" therapy in diffuse proliferative lupus nephritis. Lancet, *1*:163–166, 1976.

22. Chameides, L., et al.: Association of maternal systemic lupus erythematosus with congenital complete heart block. N. Engl. J. Med., *297*:1204–1207, 1977.

23. Chia, G.L., Mah, E.P.K., and Feng, P.H.: Cardiovascular abnormalities in systemic lupus erythematosus. J. Clin. Ultrasound, *9*:237–241, 1981.

24. Cohen, A.S., et al.: Preliminary criteria for the classification of systemic lupus erythematosus. Bull. Rheum. Dis., *21*:643–651, 1971.

25. Coppeto, J., and Lessell, S.: Retinopathy in systemic lupus erythematosus. Arch. Ophthalmol., *95*:794–797, 1977.

26. Cram, D.L., Epstein, J.H., and Tuffanelli, D.L.: Lupus erythematosus and porphyria. Arch. Dermatol., *108*:779–788, 1973.

26a. Davis, P., et al.: Br. Med. J., *3*:88, 1973.

27. Dillon, A.M., Stein, H.B., and English, R.A.: Splenic atrophy in SLE. Ann. Intern. Med., *96*:40–43, 1982.

28. Dubois, E.L.: Lupus Erythematosus, 2nd Ed. Univ. South Carolina Press, 1976.

29. Dubois, E.L., et al.: Duration and death in systemic lupus erythematosus. An analysis of 249 cases. J.A.M.A., *227*:1399–1402, 1974.

30. Ellis, S.G., and Verity, M.A.: Central nervous system involvement in systemic lupus erythematosus: A review of neuropathologic findings in 57 cases, 1955–1977. Semin. Arthritis Rheum., *8*:212–221, 1979.

31. Estes, D., and Christian, C.L.: The natural history of systemic lupus erythematosus by prospective analysis. Medicine, *50*:85–96, 1971.

32. Feinglass, E.J., et al.: Neuropsychiatric manifestations of systemic lupus erythematosus: Diagnosis, clinical spectrum and relationship to other features of the disease. Medicine, *55*:323–339, 1976.

33. Fessel, W.J.: Systemic lupus erythematosus in the community. Arch. Intern. Med., *134*:1027–1035, 1974.

33a. Fessel, W.J.: Megadose corticosteroid therapy in systemic lupus erythematosus. J. Rheumatol., *7*:486–500, 1980.

34. Fischman, A.S., et al.: The coexistence of rheumatoid arthritis and systemic lupus erythematosus. A case report and review of the literature. J. Rheumatol., *8*:405–415, 1981.

35. Gailbraith, R.F., Sümmerskill, W.H.J., and Murray, J.:

SLE, cirrhosis and ulcerative colitis after thymectomy for myasthenia gravis. N. Engl. J. Med., *270*:229–322, 1964.

36. Gibofsky, A., et al.: Contrasting patterns of newer histocompatibility determinants in patients with rheumatoid arthritis and systemic lupus erythematosus. Arthritis Rheum., *21*:134–138, 1978.

37. Gibson, G.E., Edmonds, J.P., and Hughes, G.R.V.: Diaphragm function and lung involvement in systemic lupus erythematosus. Am. J. Med. In press, 1984.

38. Gilliam, J.N., and Sontheimer, R.D.: Skin manifestations of SLE. Clin. Rheum. Dis., *8*:207–212, 1982.

39. Ginzler, E.M., et al.: Progression of mesangial and focal to diffuse lupus nephritis. N. Engl. J. Med., *291*:693–969, 1974.

40. Glass, D., et al.: Inherited deficiency of the second component of complement. J. Clin. Invest., *58*:853–861, 1976.

41. Grishman, E., et al.: Renal biopsies in lupus nephritis. Correlation of electron microscopic findings with clinical course. Nephron, *10*:25–31, 1973.

42. Gross, L.: The cardiac lesions in Libman-Sacks disease, with a consideration of its relationship to acute diffuse lupus erythematosus. Am. J. Pathol., *16*:375–408, 1940.

43. Hadler, N.M., et al.: The fourth component of complement in the cerebrospinal fluid in systemic lupus erythematosus. Arthritis Rheum., *16*:507–521, 1973.

44. Hang, L., et al.: Induction of murine autoimmune disease by chronic polyclonal B cell activation. J. Exp. Med., *157*:874–879, 1983.

45. Hargraves, M.M., Richmond, H., and Morton, R.: Presentation of two bone marrow elements: The "tart cell" and the "L.E." cell. Proc. Staff Meet. Mayo Clin., *23*:25–28, 1948.

46. Haupt, H.M., Moore, G.W., and Hutchins, G.M.: The lung in systemic lupus erythematosus. Analysis of the pathologic changes in 120 patients. Am. J. Med., *71*:791–803, 1981.

47. Henkind, P., and Rothfield, N.F.: Ocular abnormalities in patients treated with antimalarial drugs. N. Engl. J. Med., *269*:433–439, 1963.

48. Isenberg, D.A., et al.: A study of migraine in SLE. Ann. Rheum. Dis., *41*:30–32, 1982.

49. Jablonska, S., Chorzelski, T., and Maciejowska, E.: The scope and limitations of the immunofluorescence method in the diagnosis of lupus erythematosus. Br. J. Dermatol., *83*:242–247, 1970.

50. Jones, J.V.: Plasmapheresis in SLE. Clin. Rheum. Dis., *8*:243–260, 1982.

51. Jones, J.V., et al.: Plasmapheresis in the management of acute systemic lupus erythematosus. Lancet, *1*:709–711, 1976.

52. Jordon, R.E., and Provost, T.T.: The complement system and the skin. *In* Yearbook of Dermatology. Edited by F.D. Malkinson, and R.W. Pearson. Chicago, Yearbook Medical Publishers, 1976, pp. 7–37.

53. Jungers, P.J., et al.: Influence of oral contraceptive therapy on the activity of systemic lupus erythematosus. Arthritis Rheum., *25*:618–623, 1982.

54. Kaposi, M.K.: Neue Beitrage zur Kenntniss des Lupus erythematosus. Arch. Dermatol. Syph., *4*:36–78, 1872.

55. Kellum, R.E., and Haserick, J.R.: Systemic lupus erythematosus: A statistical evaluation of mortality based on a consecutive series of 299 patients. Arch. Intern. Med., *113*:200–211, 1964.

56. Kimberly, R.P.: Pulse methylprednisolone in SLE. Clin. Rheum. Dis., *8*:261–275, 1982.

57. Klippel, J.H., and Zvaifler, N.J.: Neuropsychiatric abnormalities in systemic lupus erythematosus. Clin. Rheum. Dis., *1*:621–638, 1975.

58. Labowitz, R., and Schumacher, H.R.: Articular manifestations of systemic lupus erythematosus. Ann. Intern. Med., *74*:911–921, 1971.

59. Lahita, R.G., et al.: Increased 16 alpha hydroxylation of estradiol in systemic lupus erythematosus. J. Clin. Endocrinol. Metab., *53*:174–178, 1981.

60. Laufer, J., Frand, M., and Milo, S.: Valve replacement for severe tricuspid regurgitation caused by Libman-Sachs endocarditis. Br. Heart J., *48*:294–297, 1982.

61. Leonhardt, T.: Long term prognosis of systemic lupus erythematosus. Acta Med. Scand., *445*:5440, 1966.

62. Libman, E., and Sacks, B.: A hitherto undescribed form of valvular and mural endocarditis. Arch. Intern. Med., 33:701–737, 1924.

63. Lie, T., and Rothfield, N.F.: An evaluation of the preliminary criteria for the diagnosis of systemic lupus erythematosus. Arthritis Rheum., 15:532–534, 1972.

64. Litwin, A., et al.: Prospective study of immunologic effects of hydralazine in hypertensive patients. Clin. Pharmacol. Ther., 29:447–456, 1981.

65. Lowenstein, M.B., and Rothfield, N.F.: Family study of systemic lupus erythematosus: Analysis of clinical history, skin immunofluorescence and serologic parameters. Arthritis Rheum., 20:1293–1303, 1977.

65a. Lubbe, W.F., et al.: Fetal survival after prednisone suppression of the lupus anticoagulant. Lancet, 1:1361–1363, 1983.

66. Matsopoulis, H.M., et al.: Correlative histologic and serologic findings of sicca syndrome in patients with systemic lupus erythematosus. Arthritis Rheum., 23:36–40, 1980.

67. Matthay, R.A., et al.: Pulmonary manifestations of systemic lupus erythematosus: Review of twelve cases of acute lupus pneumonitis. Medicine, 54:397–409, 1974.

68. Meislin, A.G., and Rothfield, N.F.: Systemic lupus erythematosus in childhood. Pediatrics, 42:37–49, 1968.

69. Morel-Maroger, L., et al.: The course of lupus nephritis: Contribution of serial renal biopsies. Adv. Nephrol., 6:79–86, 1976.

70. Mund, A., Simson, L., and Rothfield, N.F.: Effect of pregnancy on course of systemic lupus erythematosus. J.A.M.A., 183:917–920, 1963.

71. Osler, W.: On the visceral manifestations of the erythema group of skin diseases. Am. J. Med. Sci., 110:629–646, 1895.

72. Paget, S.A., et al.: Mitral valve disease of systemic lupus erythematosus. A cause of severe congestive heart failure reversed by valve replacement. Am. J. Med., 59:134–139, 1975.

73. Pirani, C.L., and Pollak, V.E.: Systemic lupus erythematosus glomerulonephritis. In Immunologically Mediated Renal Disease: Criteria for Diagnosis. Edited by G.A. Andres, and R.T. McCluskey. New York, Marcel Dekker, Inc. In press, 1984.

74. Pirani, C.L., Pollak, V.E., and Schwartz, F.D.: The reproducibility of semiquantitative analyses of renal histology. Nephron, 1:230–237, 1964.

75. Prystowsky, S.D., and Gilliam, J.N.: Discoid lupus erythematosus as part of a larger disease spectrum. Arch. Dermatol., 111:1448–1453, 1975.

76. Quismorio, F.P., Dubois, E.L., and Chandor, S.B.: Soft-tissue calcification in systemic lupus erythematosus. Arch. Dermatol., 111:352–356, 1975.

77. Rawsthorne, L., et al.: Lupus vasculitis necessitating double valve replacement. Arthritis Rheum., 24:561–564, 1981.

78. Reinertsen, J.H., et al.: B lymphocyte alloantigens associated with systemic lupus erythematosus. Arthritis Rheum., 21:586, 1978.

79. Rick, M.E., and Hoyer, L.W.: Hemostatic disorders in systemic lupus erythematosus. Clin. Rheum. Dis., 1:583–592, 1975.

80. Rivero, S.J., Diaz-Jouanen, E., and Alarcon-Segovia, D.: Lymphopenia in systemic lupus erythematosus. Clinical, diagnostic and prognostic significance. Arthritis Rheum., 21:205, 1978.

81. Ropes, M.: Systemic Lupus Erythematosus. Cambridge, Harvard University Press, 1976.

82. Rothfield, N.F.: Lupus erythematosus. In Dermatology in General Medicine, 2nd Ed. Edited by T.B. Fitzpatrick. New York, McGraw-Hill, 1979.

83. Rothfield, N.F., et al.: Glomerular and dermal deposition of properdin in systemic lupus erythematosus. N. Engl. J. Med., 287:681–685, 1972.

84. Rothfield, N.F., et al.: Chronic discoid lupus erythematosus: A study of 65 patients and 65 controls. N. Engl. J. Med., 269:1155–1161, 1963.

85. Rothfield, N.F., Bierer, W., and Garfield, J.: The introduction of antibodies by isoniazid: A prospective study. Ann. Intern. Med., 88:650–652, 1978.

86. Rothfield, N.F., and Marino, C.: Studies of repeat biopsies of non-lesional skin in patients with systemic lupus erythematosus. Arthritis Rheum., 25:624–628, 1982.

87. Rothfield, N.F., and Weissmann, G.: Bullae in systemic lupus erythematosus. Arch. Intern. Med., 107:174–180, 1961.

88. Rovers, M.J., and Coodvadia, H.M.: Systemic lupus erythematosus in children. A report of 3 cases. S. Afri. Med. J., 60:711–713, 1981.

89. Rudnicki, R.D., Gresham, G.E., and Rothfield, N.F.: The efficacy of antimalarials in systemic lupus erythematosus. J. Rheumatol., 2:323–330, 1975.

90. Runyon, B.A., LaBrecque, D.R., and Anuras, S.: The spectrum of liver disease in systemic lupus erythematosus. Am. J. Med., 69:187–194, 1980.

91. Schrager, M.A., and Rothfield, N.F.: Pathways of complement activation in chronic discoid lupus. Arthritis Rheum., 20:637–645, 1977.

92. Schrager, M.A., and Rothfield, N.F.: Clinical significance of serum properdin levels and properdin deposition in the dermal-epidermal junction in systemic lupus erythematosus. J. Clin. Invest., 57:212–221, 1976.

93. Schrager, M.A., and Rothfield, N.F.: The lupus band test in systemic lupus erythematosus. Clin. Rheum. Dis., 1:597, 1975.

94. Schur, P.H., and Sandson, J.: Immunologic factors and clinical activity in lupus erythematosus. N. Engl. J. Med., 278:533–540, 1968.

95. Serdula, M.K., and Rhoads, G.G.: Frequency of systemic lupus erythematosus in different ethnic groups in Hawaii. Arthritis Rheum., 22:328–333, 1979.

96. Shafer, R.B., and Gregory, D.H.: Systemic lupus erythematosus presenting as regional ileitis. Minn. Medicine, 53:789–792, 1970.

97. Shearn, M.A., and Pirofsky, B.: Disseminated lupus erythematosus. Analysis of 34 cases. Arch. Intern. Med., 90:790–807, 1952.

98. Smith, C.A., and Pinals, R.S.: Optic neuritis in SLE. J. Rheumatol., 9:963–966, 1982.

99. Smith, D., Marina, C., and Rothfield, N.F.: The clinical utility of the "lupus band test." Arthritis Rheum., 4:382–387, 1984.

100. Smith, H.R., and Steinberg, A.D.: Autoimmunity—a perspective. Annu. Rev. Immunol., 1:175, 1983.

101. Snyder, G.G., III, McCarthy, R.E., Toomey, J.M., et al.: Nasal septal perforation in systemic lupus erythematosus. Arch. Otolaryngol., 99:456–457, 1974.

102. St. Clair, W., et al.: Deep venous thrombosis and a circulating anticoagulant in systemic lupus erythematosus. Am. J. Dis. Child., 135:230–232, 1981.

103. Striker, G.E., et al.: The course of lupus nephritis. A clinical-pathological correlation of fifty patients. In Glomerulonephritis: Morphology, Natural History and Treatment. Vol. 2. Edited by P. Kincaid-Smith, T.H. Mathew, and L.E. Becker. New York, John Wiley & Sons, Inc., 1973, p. 1141.

104. Tan, E.M., et al.: Revised criteria for the classification of systemic lupus erythematosus. Arthritis Rheum., 25:1271–1277, 1982.

104a. Trimble, R.B., et al.: Preliminary criteria for the classification of systemic lupus erythematosus (SLE), evaluation in early diagnosed SLE and rheumatoid arthritis. Arthritis Rheum., 17:184, 1974.

105. Trynolds, J.C., et al.: Acute pancreatitis in systemic lupus erythematosus. Medicine (Baltimore), 61:25–32, 1982.

106. Tsokos, G.C., Moutsopoulos, H.M., and Steinberg, A.B.: Muscle involvement in SLE. J.A.M.A., 246:766–768, 1981.

107. Tsuchiya, M., et al.: Radiographic and endoscopic features of colonic ulcers in systemic lupus erythematosus. Am. J. Gastroenterol., 64:277–283, 1977.

108. Tuffanelli, D.L.: Cutaneous immunopathology; recent observations. J. Invest. Dermatol., 65:143–153, 1975.

109. Tuffanelli, D.L., Abraham, R.K., and Dubois, E.L.: Pigmentation associated with antimalarial therapy. Its possible relation to ocular lesions. Arch. Dermatol., 88:419–426, 1963.

110. Urman, J.D., et al.: Oral mucosal ulceration in systemic lupus erythematosus. Arthritis Rheum., 21:58–61, 1978.

111. Urman, J.D., and Rothfield, N.F.: Corticosteroid treatment in systemic lupus erythematosus: Survival studies. J.A.M.A., 238:2272–2276, 1977.

112. Urowitz, M.B., et al.: The bimodal mortality pattern of

systemic lupus erythematosus. Am. J. Med., *60*:221–225, 1976.

113. Walport, M.J., et al.: HLA linked complement allotypes and genetic susceptibility to systemic lupus erythematosus. Arthritis Rheum., *24*:S41, 1982.

114. Weinstein, A.: Drug-induced lupus erythematosus. *In* Progress in Clinical Immunology. Vol. 4. Edited by R. Schwartz. New York, Grune and Stratton, 1980, pp. 1–21.

115. Weinstein, A., et al.: Antibodies to native DNA and serum complement (C3) levels: Applications to the diagnosis and classification of systemic lupus erythematosus. Am. J. Med., *74*:206–216, 1983.

116. Wong, K., et al.: Visual loss as the initial symptom of systemic lupus erythematosus. Am. J. Ophthalmol., *92*:238–244, 1981.

117. Zimmerman, S.W., et al.: Progression from minimal or focal to diffuse proliferative lupus nephritis. Lab. Invest., *32*:665–672, 1975.

118. Zizic, T.M., Shulman, L.E., and Stevens, M.B.: Colonic perforations in systemic lupus erythematosus. Medicine, *54*:411–426, 1975.

119. Zulman, J.U., et al.: Problems associated with the management of pregnancies in patients with systemic lupus erythematosus. J. Rheumatol., *7*:37–49, 1980.

120. Zurier, R.B., et al.: Systemic lupus erythematosus—management during pregnancy. Obstet. Gynecol., *51*:178–189, 1978.

Chapter 62

Systemic Lupus Erythematosus: Immunologic Aspects

Eng M. Tan

Systemic lupus erythematosus (SLE) is a disease of multiple pathogenetic mechanisms affecting many organs of the body and characterized by abnormalities of the immune system. These abnormalities are manifested primarily by the presence of many autoantibodies in the serum. The autoantibodies of greatest clinical significance are those directed against nuclear antigens (ANA). In recent years, there has been an increasing awareness of the complexity of serum ANAs in SLE and a better understanding of how these play a role in pathogenetic mechanisms. The cumulative work of several investigators has shown that autoantibodies participate in immune complex-mediated tissue injury. Such injury may occur as immune complexes forming in the circulation or as immune complexes occurring at sites of tissue-fixed antigens (Fig. 62–1) (see Chap. 23).

ABNORMALITIES OF HUMORAL IMMUNITY

In a review by Kunkel, a pioneer in the study of immunologic aberrations in SLE, the types of autoantibodies encountered were discussed.[10] These autoantibodies are listed in Table 62–1. Autoantibodies in SLE can be divided into two classes. The first includes those antibodies that are not tissue-specific but react with antigens present in many tissues and organs. This class is exemplified in the autoantibodies to nuclear and cytoplasmic antigens. A second class of autoantibodies includes those that are tissue-specific, i.e., those directed against cellular elements of the hemopoietic system, such as red cells, white cells, and platelets and antibodies to tissue-specific antigens (thyroid, liver, muscle, stomach, and adrenal gland).

ANAs have received the most intensive scrutiny in SLE and can be classified in great detail, as shown in Table 62–2. ANAs can be divided into four main groups: (1) those directed against double-strand DNA; (2) those directed against single-strand DNA; (3) those directed against histones, a family of basic proteins present within the nucleus;

and (4) those directed against nonhistone nuclear proteins or nucleic acid-protein complexes.[21]

Antibodies to DNA were first reported in 1959.[3] Antibody to double-strand DNA reacts with an antigenic determinant present on both double-strand and single-strand DNA. This antibody is present in 60 to 70% of patients with SLE. It is generally agreed that antibody to double-strand DNA, when present in significant titer, is a diagnostic marker for SLE. It is rarely, if ever, present in high titers in other diseases. Antibody to single-strand DNA is antibody-reactive with antigenic determinants that are related to the exposed purines and pyrimidines in single-strand DNA. This antibody is present in 60 to 70% of patients with SLE, but may also be present in other rheumatic diseases as well as in nonrheumatic diseases. In the nonrheumatic diseases, antibody to single-strand DNA is most

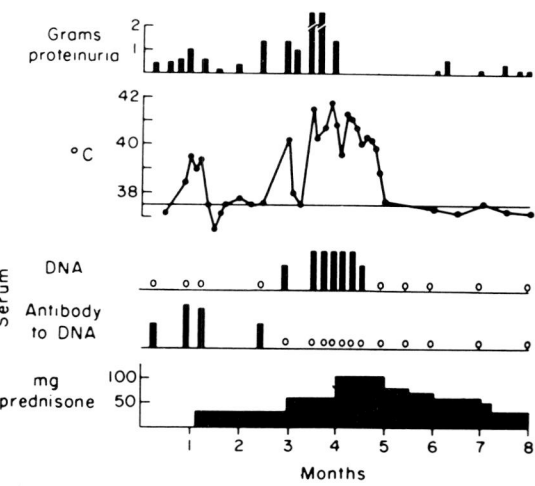

Fig. 62–1. Antibody to native DNA but no free DNA was detected in four consecutive serum samples of a patient with SLE. A relapse characterized by high fever and increased proteinuria coincided with disappearance of the antibody and the appearance of excess DNA antigen in the serum. The temporal sequence of DNA antibody followed by antigen strongly suggested immune complex formation during the period of relapse. (From Tan, E.M.[20a])

Table 62–1. Autoantibodies in SLE

Tissue Reactivity	Antibody Specificity
Nuclear antigens	DNA, nucleoprotein, histones, non-histone (acidic) proteins
Cytoplasmic antigens	RNA, ribosomes and other RNA-protein complexes, cytoplasmic protein and liquid antigens
Clotting factors	Lupus anticoagulants
Red cell antigens	
White cell antigens	T-lymphocyte cell surface antigens, B-lymphocyte cell surface antigens
Platelet antigens	
Other tissue-specific antigens (thyroid, liver, muscle, stomach, adrenal gland)	

Table 62–2. Autoantibodies to Nuclear Antigens in SLE

Antibody Specificity	Clinical Characteristics
1. *Double-strand (ds) DNA* Antigenic determinant present in both dsDNA and single-strand (ss) DNA.	60–70% of patients with SLE; when in high titer, practically a diagnostic marker
2. *ssDNA* Antigenic determinant related to exposed purines and pyrimidines.	60–70% of patients with SLE; however, present in other diseases, including nonrheumatic diseases.
3. *Histones* Antigenic determinants in all subclasses: H1, H2A, H2B, H3, H4 and H2A/H2B, H3/H4 complexes	70% of patients with SLE; >95% of patients with procainamide and hydralazine-induced LE.

4. *Nonhistone Antigens*
    1. *Sm antigen*
    Antigenic determinant is protein/s complexed to 6 species of small nuclear RNA(snRNA)
	30–40% of patients with SLE; diagnostic marker.

b. *Ul-RNP* Antigenic determinant is protein/s complexed to Ul-RNA	35–45% of patients with SLE; >95% of patients with mixed connective tissue disease.
c. *SS-A/Ro* Antigenic determinant unknown. Probably protein/s complexed to RNAs	30–40% of patients with SLE; 60–70% of patients with Sjögren's syndrome; related to neonatal lupus
d. *SS/B/La* Antigenic determinant is 43K protein complexed to RNAs	15% of patients with SLE; 45–60% of patients with Sjögren's syndrome
e. *Ma antigen* Antigenic determinant is trypsin sensitive, DNase and RNase resistant	20% of patients with SLE.
f. *PCNA* (proliferating cell nuclear antigen) Determinant is 33K protein	3% of patients with SLE.

often seen in patients with chronic infections. Because antibody to single-strand DNA is not restricted to SLE, it is not a useful serologic marker for diagnostic purposes. However, this should not be interpreted to mean that antibody to single-strand DNA is not pathogenetically important. Indeed, it has been shown that single-strand DNA antibody can be eluted from the glomeruli of patients with SLE and that it is present in the form of immune complexes in such tissues.[1,9]

Antibodies to histones are present in approximately 70% of patients with SLE. Currently, with the use of ELISA (enzyme-linked immunosorbent assay), it can be demonstrated that antibodies to histones are reactive with all the subclasses of histones, including H1, H2A, H2B, H3, and H4, as well as H2A/H2B and H3/H4 complexes.[16] Of great interest is the demonstration that patients with certain drug-induced lupus syndromes have antibodies to histones to the exclusion of other types of ANAs.[5]

Antibodies to nonhistone antigens have been reported with increasing frequency in SLE. Antibody to Sm antigen was the first such antibody reported.[23] Over the years, it has been confirmed repeatedly that this antibody is present almost exclusively in SLE and is a useful diagnostic marker, but it is present only in the 30 to 40% of patients with SLE. Antibody to nuclear ribonucleoprotein (RNP) was reported by Sharp et al.[19] as a characteristic feature of patients with mixed connective tissue disease (MCTD) (see Chap. 64). It was soon apparent that this antibody was similar to an antibody described by Mattioli and Reichlin in patients with SLE.[13] Studies have elucidated the chemical nature of this antigen and have shown that it is a complex of U1-RNA and proteins.[11] Hence, the current designation for nuclear RNP is U1-RNP. Antibody to U1-RNP is present in 35 to 45% of patients with SLE and in more than 95% of patients with MCTD.

Two classes of ANAs in patients with SLE are related to ANAs seen in patients with Sjögren's syndrome. These ANAs are antibodies to SS-A/Ro and SS-B/La. Anti-SS-A/Ro is present in 30 to 40% of patients with SLE, but in approximately 70% of patients with Sjögren's syndrome. Of great interest is the demonstration that anti-SS-A/Ro is related to neonatal lupus. Antibody to SS-B/La is present in only 15% of patients with SLE but in 45 to 60% of patients with Sjögren's syndrome. Finally, there are two other classes of ANAs: antibody to Ma antigen present in 20% of patients with SLE and antibody to PCNA (proliferating cell nuclear antigen) in 3% of patients with SLE.[14] The latter antibody, although present in low incidence, is unusual in that it reacts with a nuclear antigen

present in low concentrations in nondividing or interphase cells but in high concentrations in dividing cells or in cells undergoing blast transformation. Antibody to PCNA may be useful as a probe for the identification of blast-transformed or malignant cells.[20]

PROFILES OF ANAS IN SLE AND OTHER SYSTEMIC RHEUMATIC DISEASES

SLE is characterized by a multitude of ANAs. A striking feature of the profile of ANAs in SLE, which contrasts it with other systemic rheumatic diseases, is the simultaneous presence of three or four different types of ANAs in the same serum (Fig. 62–2).[15] In contrast, other systemic rheumatic diseases have two features that are different from SLE. One is the presence of antibodies of other specificities and the other is the presence of fewer types of ANAs in each individual serum. Table 62–3 describes the ANA profiles characteristic of MCTD, Sjögren's syndrome, scleroderma, and dermato/polymyositis. It is important to compare Table 62–3 with the profile of SLE in Table

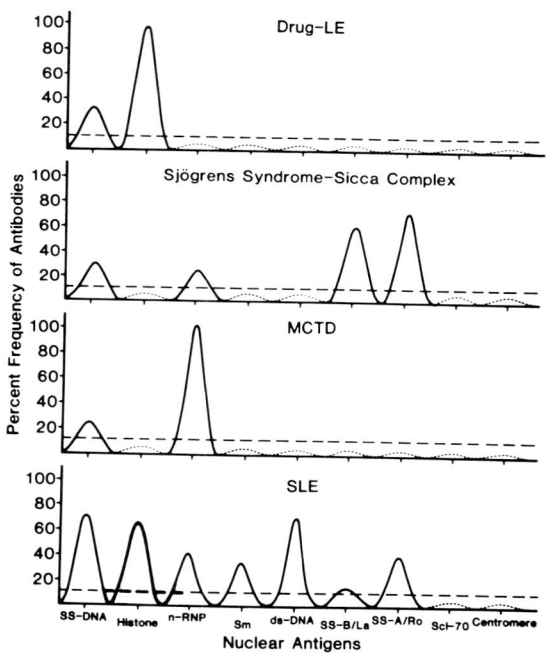

Fig. 62–2. Distinctive profiles of ANAs occur in various autoimmune diseases. SLE is characterized by a multiplicity of ANAs occurring in different frequencies. This is in contrast to other diseases, such as MCTD, Sjögren's syndrome, and drug-induced LE, in which the ANA profile is more restricted in heterogeneity. The broken lines indicate relative absence of antibodies. (From Tan, E.M.[20a])

Table 62–3. ANA Profiles in Certain Autoimmune Diseases

| | Percent Frequency in | | | | |
Antibodies to	SLE	MCTD	Sjögren's syndrome	Scleroderma	Dermato/ polymyositis
dsDNA	60–70	<5*	<5	<5	<5
ssDNA	60–70	10–20	10–20	10–20	10–20
Histones	70	<5	<5	<5	<5
Sm	30–40	<5	<5	<5	<5
U1-RNP	35–45	95–100	<5	20	<5
SS-A/Ro	30–40	<5	60–70	<5	<5
SS-B/La	15	<5	45–60	<5	<5
Scl-70	<5	<5	<5	20–30	<5
Centromere/kinetochore	<5	<5	<5	25–30	<5
Nucleolar antigen	<5	<5	5–10	50–60	5–10
PM-1	<5	<5	<5	<5	50†
Jo-1	<5	<5	<5	<5	30
Ku	<5	<5	<5	<5	55†

*<5% frequency is used to signify that the antibody is rarely observed.
†These reported frequencies are present in polymyositis-scleroderma overlap syndrome.

62–2. In certain syndromes, such as MCTD, antibody to U1-RNP is present in most patients, but this feature alone does not differentiate it from SLE, where it is present in 35–45% of patients. An equally important feature in MCTD is the absence of other ANAs, such as antibody to double-strand DNA, antibody to Sm antigen, and antibody to histones. Similarly, in Sjögren's syndrome, antibodies to SS-A/Ro and SS-B/La, characteristic of this disease, are also present in some patients with SLE. However, in Sjögren's syndrome as in MCTD, antibodies to double-strand DNA, Sm, and nuclear histones are absent.

The importance of ANAs in the clinical characterization and classification of SLE was recognized in the 1982 revised criteria for the classification of SLE.[22] In this scheme, ANA was recognized as an independent criterion, and anti-double-strand DNA and anti-Sm were included with the LE cell test and the biologically false-positive test for syphilis (anticardiolipin antibody—the "lupus anticoagulant") as four sub-items in a second immunologic criterion.

IDENTIFICATION AND CHARACTERIZATION OF NUCLEAR ANTIGENS

There has been a significant advance in the characterization of some of the nuclear antigens reactive with serum antinuclear antibodies. Both Sm antigen and U1-RNP antigen are proteins, as demonstrated by the use of transfer of electrophoretically separated antigens to nitrocellulose paper and the demonstration that specific polypeptide bands react with antibodies. There are several polypeptides reactive with anti-Sm and anti-U1-RNP, and these vary from 8,000 to 70,000 daltons in molecular weight.[2,11] The observation that anti-Sm antibody and anti-U1-RNP antibody immunoprecipitated highly specific sets of small nuclear RNAs was interesting.[11] Anti-U1-RNP immunoprecipitated only U1-RNA, whereas anti-Sm precipitated U1 as well as four other species of small nuclear RNAs: U2, U4, U5, and U6 (Fig. 62–3). These antibodies are not reactive with the small nuclear RNAs per se, but are reactive with polypeptides complexed to these small nuclear RNAs in highly specific associations. Such studies on the molecular biology of the nuclear antigens have clarified precisely the nature of nuclear antigens and have also shown that antinuclear antibodies can be used as useful probes to aid in identification of the structure and function of cellular constituents. Some studies have indicated that U1-RNA associated with its protein components (U1 ribonucleoprotein) is involved in processing heterogeneous nuclear RNA, the primary transcript of genomic DNA.[24]

Anti-SS-A/Ro and Neonatal Lupus

The relationship between anti-SS-A/Ro and neonatal lupus was studied in three infant-mother pairs.[4] All three infants and their mothers had serum anti-SS-A/Ro antibodies. Two years later, anti-SS-A/Ro antibody had disappeared from the sera of the children but was still present in the mothers, strongly suggesting transplacental passage of antibody from mother to infant. An interesting observation was the presence of a complete heart block in one of the infants. Following this initial study, several groups of investigators have confirmed these findings.[8,12,18] Clinical features include typical SLE skin lesions in the infants and a high association of congenital complete or partial heart block. It has been correctly pointed out that

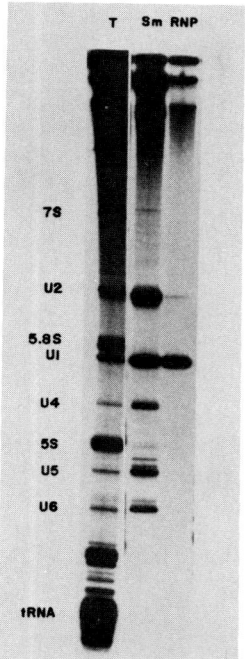

Fig. 62–3. Profiles of small nuclear RNAs immunoprecipitated by anti-Sm and anti-nuclear RNP sera. HeLa cells were labeled with ^{32}P and cell extract reacted with sera. The immunoprecipitates were solubilized and run on polyacrylamide gels to identify precipitated RNAs. Left lane represents total cellular RNA. Middle lane shows five major RNA bands precipitated by anti-Sm serum: U1, U2, U4, U5, and U6 RNAs. Right lane shows that only U1 RNA is precipitated by anti-RNP serum.

pregnant mothers with known SLE should be screened for the presence of anti-SS-A/Ro, so that there can be awareness of the possibility of cardiac problems in the infant. However, some of the mothers with anti-SS-A/Ro antibody may not have overt clinical disease at the time of gestation or delivery.

Drug-Induced Lupus and Anti-Histone Antibodies

There is a close association between anti-histone antibodies and drug-induced lupus, particularly those antibodies linked with ingestion of procainamide and hydralazine.[5] Owing to the increased use of sustained-release types of procainamide, the incidence of drug-induced lupus has increased.

Differentiation between drug-induced lupus and the idiopathic form of systemic lupus can be made serologically. In drug-induced lupus, ANAs are characterized by the presence of anti-histone antibodies, and the absence of anti-double-strand DNA, anti-Sm, or the other SLE-related ANAs listed in Table 62–2. Differentiation between drug-induced lupus and SLE has been notoriously difficult, and serologic analysis has helped to clarify the situation. Although both procainamide and hydralazine are characterized by anti-histone antibodies, there is a difference in the subclasses of histones that are reactive in the two conditions. Table 62–4 shows that procainamide-induced anti-histone antibodies are different from hydralazine-induced anti-histone antibodies. The former are more reactive with the H2A/H2B complex of histones. This involves both the IgG and IgM classes of antibodies. In contrast, hydralazine-induced anti-histone antibodies are characterized by IgM antibodies against histone H3 and H2A. In addition, hydralazine-induced anti-histone antibodies are primarily of the IgM class with few IgG antibodies. *Drug-induced ANAs are almost exclusively of the anti-histone type, and these are different anti-histone antibodies in procainamide- and hydralazine-induced ANAs.*

ANA-Negative Lupus

There has been some controversy concerning ANA-negative lupus. This controversy is probably associated with two features: (1) ANA as detected with the immunofluorescence technique varies in sensitivity from one laboratory to the next; and (2) many ANA-negative lupus patients have anti-SS-A/Ro.[17] Recent studies may have clarified some of these discrepancies. The SS-A/Ro antigen, unlike Sm and U1-RNP antigens, varies remarkably in concentration from one animal species to the next.[7] In man, monkey, and dog, SS-A/Ro antigen is present in higher concentrations than in the mouse, rat, and hamster. Therefore, when tissues from species such as rat or mouse are used as substrates in

Table 62–4. Types of Anti-Histone Antibodies Induced by Procainamide and Hydralazine

Antibody Class	Drug	Antibodies to			
		H2A	*H2B*	*H2A/H2B*	*H3*
IgM	Procainamide	0	0	+ +	0
	Hydralazine	+ +	+ / −	+ / −	+ +
IgG	Procainamide	+ +	+ / −	+ + +	+ / −
	Hydralazine	0	0	+ / −	+ / −

indirect immunofluorescence, a serum containing anti-SS-A/Ro may not show nuclear staining. When rabbit, human, or dog tissues are used as the substrate, however, this serum is positive. Some patients with anti-SS-A/Ro antibodies have been classified into a subset of lupus called *subacute cutaneous lupus*.[6] These individuals are highly photosensitive and have prominent skin lesions, but less involvement of other organ systems (see Chap. 61).

REFERENCES

1. Andres, G.A., et al.: Localization of fluorescein-labeled amino-nucleoside antibodies in glomeruli of patients with active systemic lupus erythematosus. J. Clin. Invest., 49:2106, 1971.
2. Conner, G.E., et al.: Protein antigens of the RNA-protein complexes detected by anti-Sm and anti-RNP antibodies found in serum of patients with systemic lupus erythematosus and related disorders. J. Exp. Med., 156:1475, 1982.
3. Deicher, H.R.G., Holman, H.R., and Kunkel, H.G.: The precipitin reaction between DNA and a serum factor in systemic lupus erythematosus. J. Exp. Med., 109:97, 1959.
4. Franco, H.L., et al.: Autoantibodies directed against sicca syndrome antigens in the neonatal lupus syndrome. J. Am. Acad. Dermatol., 4:67–72, 1981.
5. Fritzler, M.J., and Tan, E.M.: Antibodies to histones in drug-induced and idiopathic lupus erythematosus. J. Clin. Invest., 62:560, 1978.
6. Gilliam, J.N., and Sontheimer, R.D.: Distinctive cutaneous subsets in the spectrum of lupus erythematosus. J. Am. Acad. Dermatol., 4:471, 1981.
7. Harmon, C.E., et al.: The importance of tissue substrates in the SS-A/Ro antigen-antibody system. Arthritis Rheum., 27:166–173, 1984.
8. Kephart, D.C., Hood, A.F., and Provost, T.T.: Neonatal lupus erythematosus: New serologic findings. J. Invest. Dermatol., 77:331–333, 1981.
9. Koffler, D., et al.: The occurrence of single stranded DNA in the serum of patients with systemic lupus erythematosus and other diseases. J. Clin. Invest., 52:198, 1973.
10. Kunkel, H.G.: The immunologic approach to SLE. Arthritis Rheum., 20:S139, 1977.
11. Lerner, M.R., and Steitz, J.A.: Antibodies to small nuclear RNAs complexed with proteins are produced by patients with systemic lupus erythematosus. Proc. Natl. Acad. Sci. U.S.A., 765:5495, 1979.
12. Lockshin, D.D., et al.: Neonatal lupus erythematosus with heart block: Family study of a patient with anti-SS-A and anti-SS-B antibodies. Arthritis Rheum., 26:210–213, 1983.
13. Mattioli, M., and Reichlin, M.: Physical association of two nuclear antigens and mutual occurrence of their antibodies: The relationship of the Sm and RNA protein (Mo) systems in SLE sera. J. Immunol., 110:1318, 1973.
14. Miyachi, K., Fritzler, M.J., and Tan, E.M.: Autoantibody to a nuclear antigen in proliferating cells. J. Immunol., 121:2228, 1978.
15. Notman, D.D., Kurata, N., and Tan, E.M.: Profiles of antinuclear antibodies in systemic rheumatoid diseases. Ann. Intern. Med., 83:464, 1975.
16. Portanova, J.P., et al.: Reactivity of anti-histone antibodies induced by procainamide and hydralazine. Clin. Immunol. Immunopathol., 25:67, 1982.
17. Provost, T.T., et al.: Antibodies to cytoplasmic antigens in lupus erythematosus. Arthritis Rheum., 20:1457, 1977.
18. Scott, J.S., et al.: Connective tissue disease, antibodies to ribonucleoprotein, and congenital heart block. N. Engl. J. Med., 309:209–212, 1983.
19. Sharp, G.C., et al.: Mixed connective tissue disease—an apparently distinct rheumatoid disease associated with a specific antibody to an extractable nuclear antigen (ENA). Am. J. Med., 52:148, 1972.
20. Takasaki, Y., Robinson, W.A., and Tan, E.M.: Proliferating cell nuclear antigen (PCNA) in blast crisis cells of patients with chronic myeloid leukemia. J. Natl. Cancer Inst. In press, 1984.
20a. Tan, E.M.: The LE cell and antinuclear antibodies: A breakthrough in diagnosis. *In* Landmark Advances in Rheumatology. ARA Golden Anniversary Symposium. Edited by D.J. McCarty. Arthritis Foundation. In press, 1984.
21. Tan, E.M.: Autoantibodies to nuclear antigens. Their immunobiology and medicine. Adv. Immunol., 33:167, 1982.
22. Tan, E.M., et al.: The 1982 revised criteria for the classification of systemic lupus erythematosus. Arthritis Rheum., 25:1271, 1982.
23. Tan, E.M., and Kunkel, H.G.: Characteristics of a soluble nuclear antigen precipitating with sera of patients with systemic lupus erythematosus. J. Immunol., 96:464, 1966.
24. Yang, V.W., et al.: Proc. Natl. Acad. Sci. U.S.A., 78:1371, 1981.

Chapter 63

Vasculitis

Anthony S. Fauci

Vasculitis is a clinicopathologic process characterized by inflammation and damage to blood vessels. This process is usually associated with compromise of the vessel lumen and related ischemic changes in the tissues that are supplied by the involved vessels.[22,39] Vasculitis may be the primary manifestation of a disease and, in fact, may be its sole manifestation. Alternatively, vasculitis may be a secondary component of another primary disease. For example, Wegener's granulomatosis and classic polyarteritis nodosa are considered to be primary vasculitic syndromes, whereas the vasculitides associated with underlying connective tissue diseases such as rheumatoid arthritis (RA) or systemic lupus erythematosus (SLE) are classified as secondary vasculitic syndromes.[33]

PATHOGENESIS

Most of the vasculitic syndromes are mediated, at least in part, by immunopathogenic mechanisms.[22,39] Foremost among these mechanisms is the immune complex model whereby antigen-antibody complexes either circulate and deposit in the vessel walls or are formed in situ at the area of tissue damage.[17] Although circulating immune complexes can be demonstrated in most of the vasculitic syndromes,[22,39] and evidence suggests deposition of complexes in various tissues, the causal role of these mechanisms in the inflammatory response of involved vessels remains unclear. In few instances a causative antigen has been demonstrated in putative immune-complex-mediated disease. Hepatitis B antigen-associated systemic vasculitis is the prototype of immune-complex-mediated vasculitis in which an exogenous antigen is implicated.[97] In addition to the classic immune-complex-mediated vasculitis, other types of immunopathogenic mechanisms may damage vascular tissue. One of these is cell-mediated immune reactivity, a poorly documented form of damage to vascular tissue. Nonetheless, the histopathologic features of certain types of vasculitis suggest at least a component of cell-mediated immune injury. Granulomatous vasculitis may indeed represent a component of classic cell-mediated immune mechanisms in certain vasculitic syndromes,[22,39] and immune complexes themselves may trigger granu-

lomatous responses.[103] Therefore, the presence of granulomas in or proximal to vessels may indicate immune-complex mechanisms, cell-mediated immune responses, or both. Finally, although other mechanisms, such as tissue injury mediated directly by antibodies with specificity against the vessel itself or by cytotoxic effector cells in antibody-dependent cellular cytotoxicity, may play a role in vascular damage, little evidence supports their contribution to the pathogenesis of any of the recognized vasculitic syndromes.

CLASSIFICATION

The clinical spectrum of the vasculitides is characterized by heterogeneity as well as overlap among the various syndromes. Considerable confusion and difficulty have hindered the categorization of these diseases. Any categorization scheme is empiric but we have found an approach that is helpful in prognosis and in the design of therapeutic regimens.[22,30,39] This approach emphasizes the conceptual differences between disease that is predominantly systemic in nature and almost invariably causes irreversible organ system dysfunction and even death if untreated and those syndromes, with primarily cutaneous manifestations, that rarely result in irreversible dysfunction of vital organs. In addition, some syndromes may overlap these categories. A recently revised classification of the clinical spectrum of vasculitis is shown in Table 63–1.[30]

The first group in Table 63–1, systemic necrotizing vasculitis, has been the most difficult to categorize. The original *classic polyarteritis nodosa* is contained within this group.[68] Lung involvement, granulomas, eosinophilia, and a history of allergy are not characteristic of this syndrome. Another syndrome, however, called *allergic angiitis and granulomatosis or Churg-Strauss syndrome*,[16] resembles classic polyarteritis nodosa in many respects, except lung involvement is the rule and eosinophilia, granulomas, and allergy are common. The histopathologic features of these two syndromes also differ in that the vasculitic lesions of classic polyarteritis nodosa are confined to the small and medium-sized muscular arteries, whereas those of classic allergic angiitis and gran-

Table 63–1. Clinical Spectrum of Vasculitis

1. Systemic necrotizing vasculitis (polyarteritis nodosa group)
    - Classic polyarteritis nodosa
    - Allergic angiitis and granulomatosis
    - Polyangiitis overlap syndrome
2. Hypersensitivity vasculitis
    - Serum sickness and similar reactions
    - Other drug-related vasculitides
    - Vasculitis associated with infectious diseases
    - Henoch-Schönlein purpura
    - Vasculitis associated with connective tissue diseases
    - Vasculitis associated with neoplasms (mostly lymphoid)
    - Vasculitis associated with other underlying diseases
3. Wegener's granulomatosis
4. Lymphomatoid granulomatosis
5. Giant cell arteritides
    - Cranial or temporal arteritis
    - Takayasu's arteritis
6. Other vasculitic syndromes
    - Mucocutaneous lymph node syndrome (Kawasaki's disease)
    - Vasculitis isolated to the central nervous system
    - Behçet's disease
    - Thromboangiitis obliterans (Buerger's disease)
    - Miscellaneous vasculitides

(From Fauci, A.S.[30])

ulomatosis involve blood vessels of various types and sizes, including small and medium-sized muscular arteries as well as veins and venules.[22,39]

A form of systemic necrotizing vasculitis that is probably more common than classic polyarteritis nodosa or allergic angiitis and granulomatosis has been recognized recently. This syndrome may have features of both and also features of the predominantly cutaneous hypersensitivity small-vessel-vasculitis. My colleagues and I have termed this group the *polyangiitis overlap syndrome*[22,30,39] (Table 63–1). This group of systemic necrotizing vasculitides has a common denominator of involvement of multiple organ systems with the overriding tendency for irreversible organ-system dysfunction. In general, the prognosis for patients with this group of disorders is poor without appropriate and aggressive therapy.

This first group of syndromes is in contrast to the second broad category of predominantly cutaneous vasculitides, frequently referred to as the *hypersensitivity* vasculitides. Although these disorders may affect any organ system and so may be systemic in nature, they most frequently remain cutaneous and do not consistently pose a threat of irreversible dysfunction of vital organs.[2,95,113] If, indeed, the disease does remain confined to the skin and does not become systemic, aggressive therapy, such as with high doses of corticosteroids

or long-term administration of cytotoxic agents, is indicated only in unusual circumstances.

The broad category of "hypersensitivity vasculitis" has been applied to a heterogeneous group of disorders thought to represent a hypersensitivity reaction to an identifiable antigenic stimulus such as a drug or an infectious agent; hence the term "hypersensitivity."[22,30,34] The term is often a source of confusion because many, if not most, of the vasculitic syndromes represent hypersensitivity reactions of one form or another. As is discussed later, although the proved or suspected antigenic stimuli associated with this group are heterogeneous, these disorders generally share the characteristic involvement of small vessels and a predominant, often exclusive, involvement of the vessels of the skin. Confusion in the literature has resulted from the inclusion of this group with the more serious systemic varieties of vasculitis such as the true systemic necrotizing vasculitides and related disorders. This confusion probably arose from the variable degrees of organ system involvement other than cutaneous that can occur in the hypersensitivity vasculitides. Such involvement, however, is usually much less severe than in the systemic vasculitis of classic polyarteritis nodosa or Wegener's granulomatosis. The skin is exclusively involved, or if other organ systems are involved, the cutaneous disease dominates the clinical picture.[2,22,30,95,113] Finally, a vasculitic syndrome indistinguishable from hypersensitivity vasculitis can appear as a secondary component of another underlying disease, such as a connective tissue disease or neoplasm, and may thus lead to additional confusion concerning the hypersensitivity vasculitides.

Most of the remainder of the vasculitic syndromes have distinctive enough clinical and pathologic features that they can readily be grouped into separate categories (Table 63–1). Such is true of Wegener's granulomatosis, temporal arteritis, and Takayasu's arteritis. Several of these distinctive syndromes are also clearly systemic in nature, but they do not appear in the polyarteritis nodosa group because they warrant separate classification.

SYSTEMIC NECROTIZING VASCULITIS (POLYARTERITIS NODOSA GROUP)

This group includes the following: (1) classic polyarteritis nodosa; (2) allergic angiitis and granulomatosis; and (3) the polyangiitis overlap syndrome.

Classic Polyarteritis Nodosa

The first complete description of a vasculitic syndrome was made in 1866 by Kussmaul and Maier in an elegant clinicopathologic case report.[68] Classic periarteritis nodosa, as it was originally described[68] and further studied,[92,113] is a necrotizing vasculitis of small and medium-sized muscular arteries. The lesions are segmental, with a predilection for bifurcations of arteries with distal spread involving arterioles and, in some cases, circumferentially involving adjacent veins. This disorder is not primarily a venulitis. Histopathologically, in the acute stages, polymorphonuclear leukocytes infiltrate all layers of the vessel wall and perivascular areas (Fig. 63–1). Subsequently, mononuclear cell infiltration occurs as the lesions become subacute and chronic. Intimal proliferation, vessel wall degeneration with fibrinoid necrosis, thrombosis, ischemia, and infarction are seen in varying degrees. Generally, vascular lesions in various stages of development are found simultaneously. This finding may reflect the continuous deposition of immune complexes, such as one might expect in the vasculitis associated with persistent hepatitis B antigenemia.[97] Multiple organ systems are involved, and the clinicopathologic findings are consistent with the degree and location of vessel involvement and the resulting ischemic changes.[22,39]

Clinical Manifestations

The nature of the presenting problems may be nonspecific. Vague symptoms such as weakness, malaise, abdominal pain, extremity pain, headache, fever, and myalgias are frequent.[22,39] Less commonly, patients have signs and symptoms of neurologic and joint involvement. The nonspecific nature of the presentation and the uncommon oc-

currence of classic polyarteritis nodosa may contribute to the difficulty in establishing the diagnosis. The signs or symptoms and actual involvement may not correlate with those of documented vasculitis.

The clinical profile and manifestations in patients with classic polyarteritis nodosa are outlined in Table 63–2. These manifestations, together with the findings at autopsy summarized from several large series (Table 63–3), provide a striking witness to the scope and severity of the organ system involvement in this disease.

Variable degrees of renal involvement are seen in the majority of patients, and this complication is a major cause of death. The renal disease may be primarily vascular with secondary ischemic changes in the glomeruli, or it may be a primary glomerulitis, or a combination of both. Hypertension may compound the severity of the underlying renal disease or may itself be the predominant cause of renal dysfunction in the form of nephrosclerosis.[22,31] It was once thought that the hypertension of polyarteritis nodosa was almost exclusively associated with the healing stages of the renal polyarteritis nodosa or glomerulonephritis,[92] but it is now clear that hypertension may occur as an independent early finding before clinically apparent functional renal disease. In fact, the hypertension may itself dominate the clinical picture and may be directly responsible for certain of the associated cerebrovascular, cardiovascular, or renal manifestations.

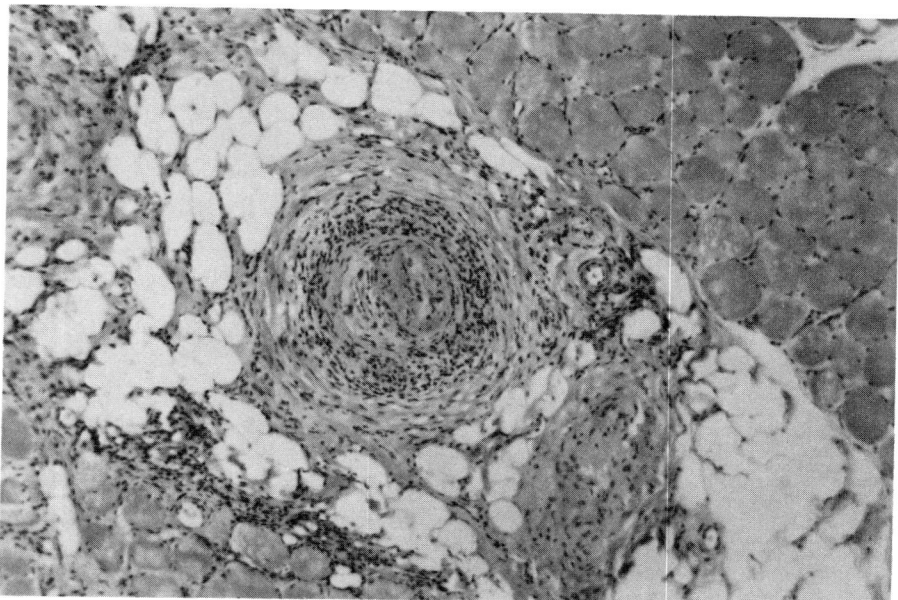

Fig. 63–1. Muscle biopsy in a 36-year-old patient with classic polyarteritis nodosa. A small muscular artery is involved, with fibrinoid necrosis and inflammatory cell infiltrate. (Hematoxylin and eosin stain; magnification × 130.)

Table 63–2. Clinical Profile and Manifestations in Patients with Classic Polyarteritis Nodosa

Clinical Parameter	Value
General considerations	
Age (mean)	45 years
Sex ratio (male to female)	2.5 to 1
	Percentage (%)
Fever	71
Weight loss	54
Organ involvement	
Kidney	70
Musculoskeletal system	64
Arthritis or arthralgia	53
Myalgias	31
Circulatory system (hypertension)	54
Peripheral nerves	51
Gastrointestinal tract	44
Abdominal pain	43
Nausea or vomiting	40
Cholecystitis	17
Bleeding	6
Bowel perforation	5
Bowel infarction	1.4
Skin	43
Rash or purpura	30
Livedo reticularis	4
Heart	36
Congestive failure	12
Myocardial infarction	6
Pericarditis	4
Central nervous system	23
Cerebral vascular accident	11
Altered mental status	10
Seizure	4

(From Cupps, T.R., and Fauci, A.S.[22])

Table 63–3. Organ Involvement at Autopsy in Classic Polyarteritis Nodosa

Organ System	Percentage (%)
Kidney	85
Heart	76
Liver	62
Gastrointestinal tract	51
Jejunum	37
Ileum	27
Mesentery	24
Colon	20
Rectosigmoid	10
Duodenum	10
Gallbladder	10
Appendix	7
Muscle	39
Pancreas	35
Testes	33
Peripheral nerves	32
Central nervous system	27
Skin	20

(From Cupps, T.R., and Fauci, A.S.[22])

In addition to hypertensive cardiovascular disease, primary involvement of the coronary arteries is a frequent finding, and cardiac involvement is a major cause of death.[31,52] Areas of myocardial infarction are frequently demonstrated at autopsy in the absence of a suggestive clear-cut clinical history.[99] Polyarteritis nodosa in children is associated with a high incidence of coronary artery involvement,[91] but most of the cases in the United States formerly reported as polyarteritis nodosa of children, with its characteristic and unusual selective involvement of the coronary arteries, were in fact the arteritis of unrecognized mucocutaneous lymph node syndrome (Kawasaki's disease).[69]

Gastrointestinal involvement is seen in over 50% of patients and usually relates to involvement of the visceral arteries.[22] Symptoms and signs include nausea, vomiting, diarrhea, ileus, abdominal pain, ulceration with bleeding, infarction, or perforation of intra-abdominal organs. Depending on the severity of involvement, manifestations range from abdominal angina or steatorrhea, associated with partial obstruction of the superior mesenteric artery or its branches, to massive bowel infarction, resulting from acute involvement of the superior mesenteric artery.[31] Bowel perforation with its attendant complications carries a high mortality rate. Significant abdominal involvement is often masked partially or completely in patients receiving daily corticosteroids, and an ischemic segment of bowel may go undetected until actual perforation has occurred.

Liver disease varies in classic polyarteritis nodosa. When hepatitis B antigenemia accounts for the vasculitis, hepatic involvement may relate to the underlying hepatitis and ranges from subclinical disease to chronic active hepatitis.[97] Liver disease related directly to the vasculitis may lead to massive hepatic infarction.[86]

Neurologic manifestations are common in classic polyarteritis nodosa. Mononeuritis multiplex resulting from vasculitis of the vasa nervorum is the most frequent finding. In a recent review of the neurologic manifestations of systemic necrotizing vasculitis (group 1, Table 63–1) including polyarteritis nodosa, 80% of patients had some form of nervous system disease.[85] The peripheral nervous system was involved in 60% of this subset. Four patterns of neuropathy were seen: mononeuritis multiplex, extensive mononeuritis, cutaneous neuropathy, and polyneuropathy. The central nervous system was involved in the remaining 40%, and these patients predominantly had diffuse and focal disturbances of cerebral, cerebellar, and brain stem function.

Cutaneous Involvement. The question of the precise type of cutaneous involvement in classic polyarteritis nodosa is controversial because many cases of small-vessel "hypersensitivity vasculitis" have been included in reports of groups of patients said to have polyarteritis nodosa. Furthermore, skin involvement in the polyangiitis overlap syndrome may have features of both classic polyarteritis nodosa and hypersensitivity venulitis.[22,30,34] Skin involvement in classic polyarteritis occurs in approximately 20 to 30% of patients and is usually confined to the small muscular arteries of the subcutaneous tissues.[43] The lesions are generally manifested as painful erythematous subcutaneous nodules, which may appear in crops and may range from a few millimeters to several centimeters in size.[9] Another characteristic of skin involvement is *livedo reticularis* (Fig. 63–2). *Cutaneous polyarteritis nodosa* is characterized by a necrotizing vasculitis of small arteries of subcutaneous tissue.[24] The disease is a localized process with sparing of visceral arteries and therefore is not a true systemic vasculitic syndrome. Cutaneous polyarteritis nodosa usually runs a chronic course and has a favorable long-term prognosis. Although the histologic lesion resembles that of classic polyarteritis nodosa, this disease is clinically similar to the hypersensitivity vasculitides.

Arthralgias are common in classic polyarteritis nodosa, but frank arthritis is rare. When small and medium-sized muscular arteries in skeletal muscle are involved, the muscles are almost invariably symptomatic (see Fig. 63–1). In addition, testicular or epididymal pain is characteristic, and testicular involvement is seen in approximately 30% of autopsies in classic polyarteritis nodosa (Table 63–3). Thus, when muscular or testicular pain is present, biopsy is likely to be helpful in making the diagnosis, whereas blind biopsies of asymptomatic organs have a low diagnositic yield.

Diagnosis

No diagnostic laboratory findings are indicative of classic polyarteritis nodosa, and the many abnormalities are outlined in Table 63–4. The finding of hepatitis B antigenemia has been reported in up to 30% of patients with systemic vasculitis of the polyarteritis nodosa type,[27,35,97] but this finding in itself does not establish the diagnosis, which depends on the appropriate characteristic clinical and pathologic manifestations.

The mainstay of the diagnosis of classic polyarteritis nodosa is the histopathologic demonstration of necrotizing vasculitis of small and medium-sized arteries in patients with compatible clinical manifestations.. It is preferable to perform a biopsy on accessible organs such as the skin, muscle, or testis, but these structures are not invariably involved, and "blind" biopsy has only limited value.

A characteristic feature of the polyarteritis no-

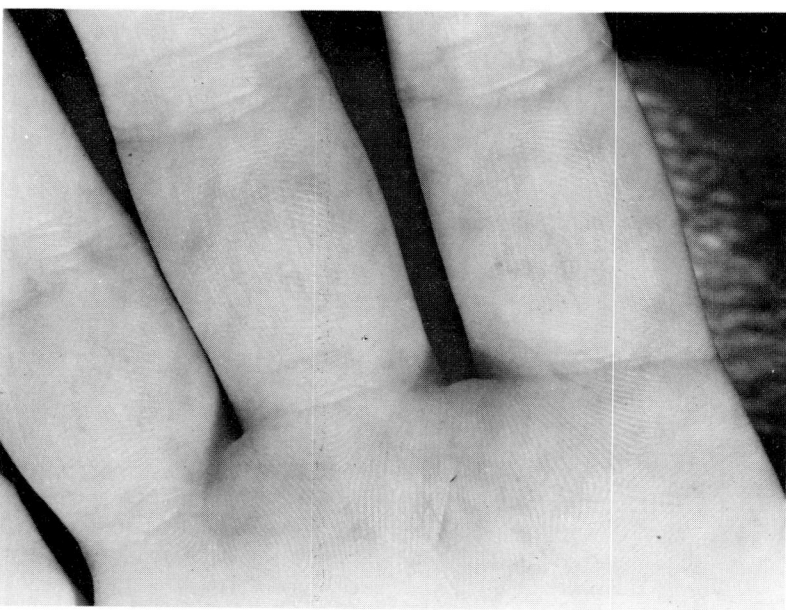

Fig. 63–2. Livedo reticularis of the volar aspect of the proximal phalanges and distal palm in a patient with systemic lupus erythematosus. The lesions are nonpalpable and may be seen in a variety of vasculitic syndromes.

Table 63–4. Laboratory Abnormalities in Patients with Classic Polyarteritis Nodosa

Laboratory Abnormality	Percentage (%)
Erythrocyte sedimentation rate >10 mm/hr	94
Leukocytosis (WBC >10,000/mm³)	74
Anemia (hematocrit <35%)	66
Thrombocytosis (>400,000/mm³)	53
Renal function abnormality	70
Proteinuria	64
Hematuria	45
Casts	34
Complement abnormality	
Depressed CH_{50}	21
Depressed C3	70
Depressed C4	30
Rheumatoid factor ≥1:160	40
Immune complexes present	62.5
Cryoglobulins present	25

(From Cupps, T.R., and Fauci, A.S.[22])

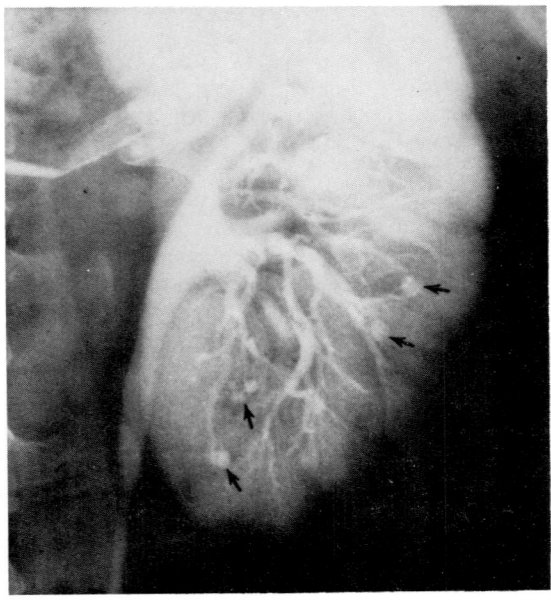

Fig. 63–3. Renal angiogram in a patient with classic polyarteritis nodosa. Note the multiple intraparenchymal aneurysms (arrows).

dosa type of necrotizing vasculitis is the finding of aneurysmal dilatations up to 1 cm in size in medium-sized arteries seen by angiogram in the renal, hepatic, and visceral vasculature (Fig. 63–3). It was formerly believed that this finding was virtually pathognomonic of classic polyarteritis nodosa;[10,26,40] however, multiple aneurysms of this type are seen in overlap syndromes in which vessels of various sizes are involved,[24,38] as well as in other disorders such as SLE[74] and fibromuscular dysplasia.[82] Nonetheless, demonstration of involved ves-

sels on a visceral angiogram is helpful in establishing the presence of systemic vascular disease and is valuable in clinical situations in which no involved organ is easily accessible for biopsy. If a patient has signs and symptoms suggestive of polyarteritis nodosa without readily accessible tissue for biopsy, the diagnosis can be made on the basis of a positive visceral angiogram.

Prognosis

The prognosis of untreated classic polyarteritis nodosa is poor. Although some cases have resolved spontaneously, the usual course of the disease is a relentless progression with intermittent acute flares.[22,39] The grave prognosis is reflected in the 5-year survival rate of 13% reported for untreated patients.[42] With the use of corticosteroids, survival rate has improved to 48%.[42] Survival rates are lower in patients with hypertension or renal disease initially. Death usually results from renal failure or cardiovascular or gastrointestinal involvement. Persistent and uncontrolled hypertension often contributes to the late morbidity and mortality of this disease by compounding the renal disease and by leading to late cardiovascular and cerebrovascular disorders. Treatment of classic polyarteritis nodosa is considered later in this chapter.

Allergic Angiitis and Granulomatosis (Churg-Strauss Syndrome)

The combination of allergic angiitis and granulomatosis is a disease characterized by granulomatous vasculitis of multiple organ systems.[16] Although the vascular lesions may be identical to those of classic polyarteritis nodosa, this disease is unique for the following reasons: (1) frequency of involvement of pulmonary vessels; (2) vasculitis of blood vessels of various types and sizes such as small and medium-sized muscular arteries, veins, arterioles, and venules; (3) intra- and extravascular granuloma formation; (4) eosinophilic tissue infiltrates; and (5) association with severe asthma and peripheral eosinophilia. In general, this disease can be thought of as a polyarteritis nodosa-like syndrome with strong allergic components and with pulmonary involvement as an essential element of the disease instead of a rarity.[39]

The clinical features of allergic angiitis and granulomatosis are listed in Table 63–5. Laboratory findings are similar to those in classic polyarteritis nodosa. An elevated erythrocyte sedimentation rate and leukocytosis are found in the majority of patients. An elevated total eosinophil count (greater than 1,000/mm³) is noted at some point in approximately 85% of patients. This peripheral eosinophilia is not seen in classic polyarteritis nodosa, but may be seen in the overlap syndromes described

Table 63–5.   Clinical Profile and Manifestations in Allergic Angiitis and Granulomatosis

Clinical Parameter	Value
General considerations	
Age (mean)	44 years
Sex ratio (male to female)	1.3 to 1
Duration (mean) of pulmonary symptoms prior to systemic symptoms	2 years
Fever	Majority of patients
Organ involvement	*Percentage (%)*
Lungs	96
Infiltrate on chest roentgenogram	93
Wheezing	82
Skin	67
Purpura	37
Nodules	35
Peripheral nerves	63
Circulatory system (hypertension)	54
Gastrointestinal tract	42
Heart	38
Kidney	38
Lower urinary tract	10
Musculoskeletal system	10
Arthritis or arthralgia	21

(From Cupps, T.R., and Fauci, A.S.[22])

below. Elevated serum IgE levels have also been described. Unlike with classic polyarteritis nodosa, no association exists between allergic angiitis and granulomatosis and hepatitis B antigenemia.

The degree of severity of allergic angiitis and granulomatosis varies from patient to patient, and so prognosis is also variable. The overall prognosis remains poor, however, and in untreated patients, it is similar to that of classic polyarteritis nodosa. Current treatment, which is similar to that of polyarteritis nodosa, is discussed below.

Polyangiitis Overlap Syndrome

Many systemic necrotizing vasculitides manifest clinicopathologic characteristics that overlap classic polyarteritis nodosa and allergic angiitis and granulomatosis, as well as the hypersensitivity small-vessel group of vasculitides. This subgroup has been referred to as the polyangiitis overlap syndrome.[22,30,39] This syndrome has caused the most difficulty in classification and has appeared under different designations and categories. A typical, perplexing case is that of a young person with a multisystem necrotizing vasculitis with renal involvement and mononeuritis multiplex. The patient may or may not have hypertension, and visceral and renal angiograms may or may not demonstrate multiple aneurysms. By most generally accepted criteria, this patient would be diagnosed as having classic polyarteritis nodosa.[68,113] This same patient, however, may also have significant lung involvement, a small-vessel cutaneous venulitis, or history of allergy with or without eosinophilia and gran-

uloma, all of which are not seen in classic polyarteritis nodosa, but rather are features of other vasculitis syndromes. The existence of this overlap syndrome avoids confusion as to appropriate diagnosis and therapy. This subgroup is indeed a "systemic" vasculitis with the same potential for irreversible organ system dysfunction. For this reason, we categorize all three of these subgroups under the major category of *systemic necrotizing vasculitis.*

Treatment

Corticosteroids are still the initial treatment of choice for the systemic necrotizing vasculitides, but the addition of a cytotoxic agent, such as cyclophosphamide, to the therapeutic regimen has resulted in striking remissions in a high percentage of patients within this category.[35,39] Early reports showed an increase in survival rates from 13% in untreated patients to 48% in corticosteroid-treated patients.[42] Unlike in Wegener's granulomatosis, in which corticosteroids alone are inadequate therapy and a cytotoxic drug such as cyclophosphamide is essential for the induction of remission,[33,35] treatment should be tailored to the degree, severity, and stage of the disease. Most patients require a combination of a cytotoxic agent and corticosteroids for maximal induction of remission, but some treated with corticosteroids alone have a complete remission. On the other hand, a few patients have such fulminant systemic vasculitis that they succumb to a devastating complication such as bowel perforation or infarction of other vital organs before any therapy has a chance to be effective. Patients with less severe forms of systemic vasculitis in whom irreversible organ system dysfunction does not appear to be imminent may be treated initially with corticosteroids alone. Initial therapy with prednisone is 1 mg/kg/day in divided doses, followed by consolidation in a few weeks to a single daily dose. Depending on the clinical response, the patient should be treated with daily prednisone for approximately one to two months, when one should attempt to convert to alternate-day therapy over one to two months. If the conversion is accomplished without relapse, the alternate-day regimen is maintained for several months to a year. The dose is then gradually tapered until the drug is discontinued or until a maintenance dose is reached.

If patients do not improve objectively after a month of corticosteroid therapy or if they initially have fulminant disease and deteriorating organ system function, a cytotoxic regimen should be started. My colleagues and I have had excellent results with oral cyclophosphamide at a dose of 2 mg/kg/day. A patient who cannot tolerate oral medication or a patient with bowel vasculitis in whom intestinal absorption is questionable should receive cyclophosphamide intravenously at the same dose. An aggressive surgical approach to the complications of ischemic bowel with early exploratory laparotomy, appropriate removal of necrotic bowel segments, and repeated operations for observation of the retained bowel may reduce the mortality rates associated with this most serious complication of systemic vasculitis. Prednisone should always be given together with cyclophosphamide during the induction phase of the therapeutic protocol because it usually takes two to three weeks to achieve an immunosuppressive effect from cyclophosphamide given at these doses. The combined regimen, which my associates and I use to treat the severe corticosteroid-resistant systemic vasculitides,[29] was originally developed for the treatment of Wegener's granulomatosis,[36] and it is outlined in Table 63–6. We have induced long-term clinical remissions in most patients with systemic necrotizing vasculitis using this therapeutic protocol.[35]

Although malignant diseases, chiefly leukemia and non-Hodgkin's lymphoma, have been noted in patients with polycythemia vera, Hodgkin's disease, or organ transplants treated with immunosuppressive drugs, only 1 instance of malignancy has occurred in over 200 patients treated by our group. This occurred in a patient with smoldering Wegener's granulomatosis treated for several years with cyclophosphamide. The patient developed an undifferentiated lymphoma and died of that disease.[3a]

Table 63–6. Combined Cyclophosphamide-Prednisone Therapy for Severe Systemic Vasculitis

> *Cyclophosphamide:* Initial dose of 2 mg/kg/day orally; adjust so that white blood cell count remains above 3,000 to 3,500/mm³ (neutrophil count 1,000 to 1,500/mm³); continue therapy with frequent downward adjustments of dosage, to prevent severe neutropenia; continue therapy for a year following induction of complete remission, and then taper dose by 25-mg decrements every 2 months until discontinued.
>
> *Prednisone:* Initial dose of 1 mg/kg/day in 3 to 4 divided doses for 7 to 10 days; consolidate to single morning dose by 2 to 3 weeks; continue single morning daily dose until patient has had 1 month's total corticosteroid treatment; convert to alternate-day regimen for the second month; maintain alternate-day regimen for the third month, followed by gradual tapering of alternate-day dose for the next 3 to 6 months.

(From Fauci, A.S.[29])

Other cytotoxic agents such as azathioprine, chlorambucil, and methotrexate have been used in vasculitic syndromes with variable success,[29] but cyclophosphamide is the most effective agent in the induction of long-term remission. Large, single bolus doses of corticosteroids or cyclophosphamide, or plasmapheresis,[62,73] have been administered to certain patients with vasculitic syndromes.[29] The efficacy of these regimens is not well established, however.

HYPERSENSITIVITY VASCULITIDES

This heterogeneous group of syndromes is characterized by inflammation of small vessels such as venules, capillaries, and arterioles.[2,43,95,109,113] The postcapillary venule is most commonly involved. Although hypersensitivity vasculitis may affect any organ system, cutaneous disease usually dominates the clinical picture. This type of vasculitic disease rarely progresses to life-threatening organ system dysfunction.

This type of vasculitis was first described in association with a recognized antigenic stimulus such as a microbe or a drug, accounting for the term "hypersensitivity."[2] The vasculitic component of serum sickness and similar reactions falls within the category of the hypersensitivity vasculitides.[22] The term is unfortunate because no inciting antigen can be identified or even suspected in most cases. Moreover, virtually all the recognized vasculitic syndromes have clinical and pathologic features that suggest underlying hypersensitivity or immunologic phenomena.

Other terms used synonymously with hypersensitivity vasculitis include *allergic vasculitis*[1] and *leukocytoclastic vasculitis*. The most common histopathologic pattern is the characteristic leukocytoclastic vasculitis involving the postcapillary venules (Fig. 63–4).[95,109] Mononuclear, predominantly lymphocytic, infiltrates have been described also, however.[102] The typical macroscopic appearance of the lesion is that of *palpable purpura* caused by a combination of endothelial swelling, infiltration by leukocytes, and extravasation of erythrocytes.[39] The lesions may range in size from pinpoint to several centimeters and may take the form of papules, nodules, vesicles, bullae, ulcers, or recurrent urticaria.

Although vasculitic skin lesions are the major features, the syndrome may be accompanied by systemic signs and symptoms such as fever, malaise, myalgia, and anorexia, similar to the systemic vasculitides. The disease may consist of a single acute episode lasting only a few weeks, or it may be recurrent or, less commonly, chronic, lasting for months or years. Weight loss and the anemia of chronic disease may be seen in chronic hypersensitivity vasculitis. The skin lesions may be pruritic or painful, with a stinging or burning sensation. Lesions are most common in dependent areas such as the lower extremities in ambulatory patients and over the sacrum in bedridden patients, most likely as a result of hydrostatic pressure. As

the lesions resolve or become chronic or recurrent, skin hyperpigmentation may result.

The hypersensitivity vasculitides comprise a number of subgroups (see Table 63–1), within which the extent of extracutaneous involvement varies. The approximate figures for extracutaneous involvement in the whole group include arthritis or arthralgias in 40%, renal involvement in 37%, gastrointestinal involvement in 15%, and peripheral neuropathy in 12% of patients.[22] Although pulmonary involvement is seen in up to 19% of patients with nonspecific patterns of infiltrates or effusions or both on chest roentgenograms, the significance of these findings is unclear because pulmonary vasculitis has not been demonstrated in several of these patients at autopsy.[109] In my opinion, those patients formerly diagnosed as having hypersensitivity vasculitis with significant extracutaneous involvement would now be categorized within the ''polyangiitis overlap'' group, in the broader category of systemic vasculitis.

Henoch-Schönlein Purpura

Henoch-Schönlein purpura, a distinctive subgroup of the hypersensitivity vasculitides, requires special mention not only because of its unique complex of manifestations, but also because it typifies vasculitis that is usually confined to the skin but may have significant extracutaneous manifestations. This disorder is characterized by the clinicopathologic complex of nonthrombocytopenic purpura, skin lesions, joint involvement, colicky abdominal pain sometimes associated with gastrointestinal hemorrhage, and renal disease.[2,4,5,20,72] The disease usually occurs in children; however, adults of any age may be affected. The male-to-female ratio is 1.5 to 1. This disease usually remits spontaneously within a week, but it may recur a number of times for some weeks to months before remission is complete. Rarely, patients have recurrent disease for years. The characteristic skin lesions are manifested as palpable purpura and represent leukocytoclastic venulitis (Fig. 63–5). Fever is seen in 75% of patients. Glomerulitis usually consists of microscopic hematuria without clinically significant functional renal impairment; rarely, renal failure occurs.[4] Hypertension is seen in 13% of patients. The organ system involvement and clinical manifestations in children with Henoch-Schönlein purpura are listed in Table 63–7.

Because of the excellent prognosis of this disease, immunosuppressive therapy rarely is indicated, and treatment usually consists of supportive and symptomatic therapy. In patients with recurrent disease, corticosteroids in daily doses of 1 mg/kg for limited periods are recommended; the dose is then tapered to an alternate-day regimen and is

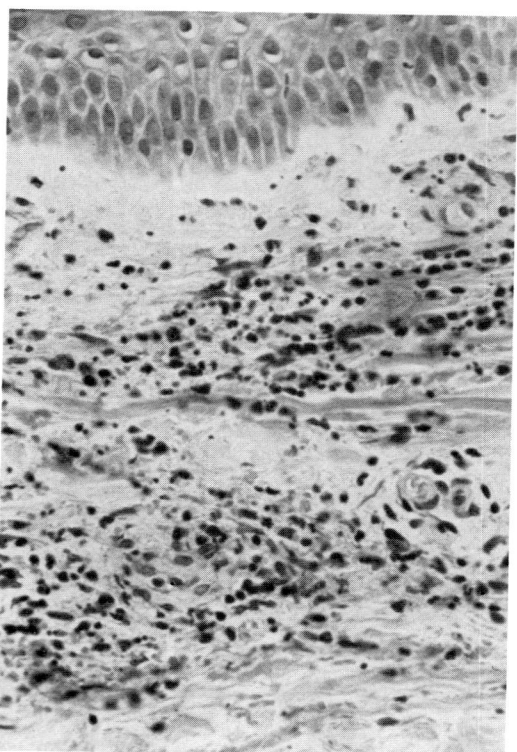

Fig. 63–4. Skin biopsy in a patient with hypersensitivity vasculitis. Note the involvement of postcapillary venules with leukocytoclasis, as manifested by nuclear debris.

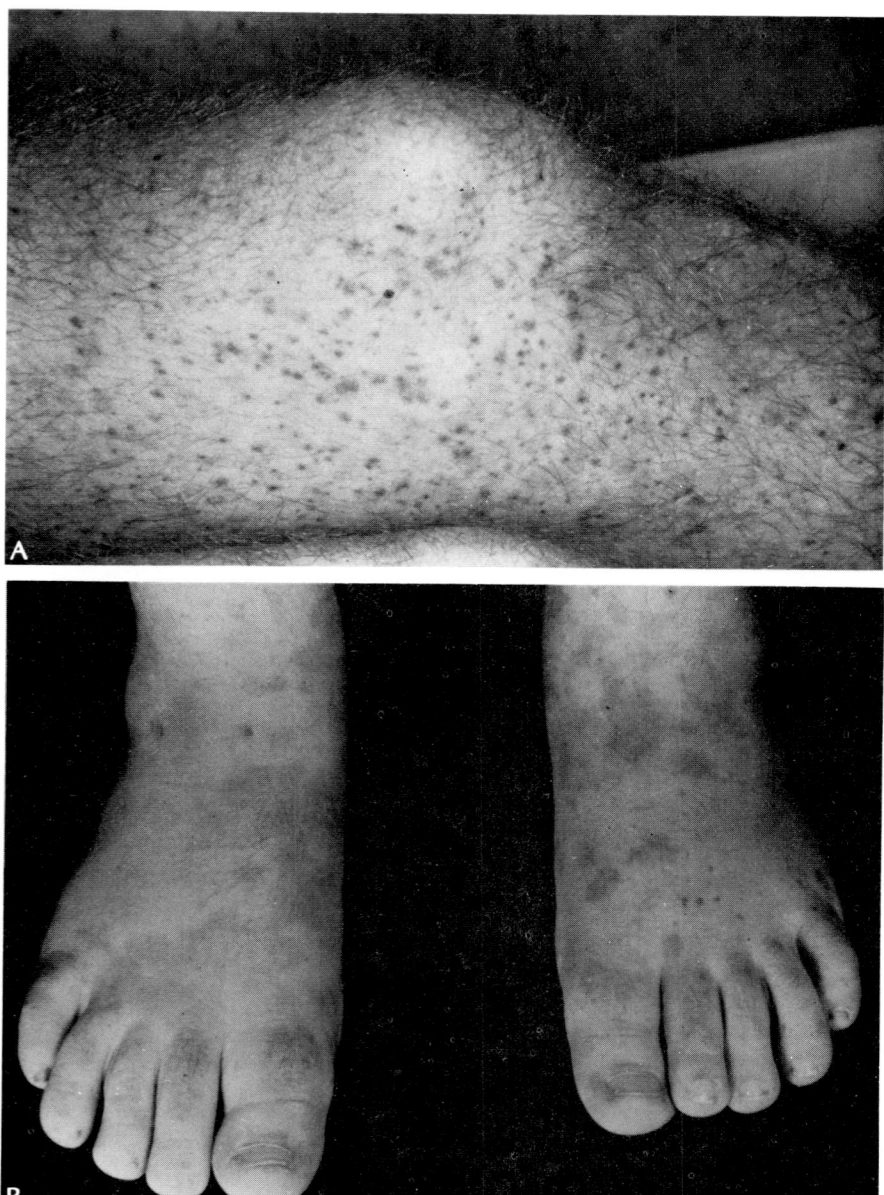

Fig. 63–5. *A*, Palpable purpura and flexion contracture of the knee in a patient with Henoch-Schönlein purpura. The flexion contracture is due to the periarthritis frequently seen with this disease. *B*, The larger, deeper, and more ecchymotic-appearing lesions seen in the dependent extremities in a patient with Henoch-Schönlein purpura. Also note the three more superficial palpable purpuric lesions over the dorsum of the distal left forefoot and the anterior aspect of the right ankle.

ultimately discontinued.[21,22] It has been difficult to evaluate the efficacy of corticosteroid therapy because of spontaneous remissions and recurrences. The few patients who develop significant renal disease may require cytotoxic therapy, according to the protocol for the systemic necrotizing vasculitides.

Vasculitis Associated with Connective Tissue Diseases

Vasculitis may be associated with the entire spectrum of connective tissue disorders,[2,14,43,113] as discussed in other chapters devoted to the individual connective tissue diseases. Vasculitis is most

Table 63–7. Organ Involvement and Clinical Manifestations in Pediatric Patients with Henoch-Schönlein Purpura

Involvement	Percentage (%)
Skin	100
Purpura	100
Ulceration	4
Joints	71
Gastrointestinal tract	68
Pain	57
Nausea or vomiting	50
Occult blood	42
Hematemesis or melena	35
Major bleeding	5
Intussusception	3
Kidney	
Hematuria	45
Microscopic	45
Macroscopic	26
Proteinuria	35
Functional impairment	9
Localized edema	32

(From Cupps, T.R., and Fauci, A.S.[22])

common in RA and in SLE.[14] Although we include the vasculitis associated with other systemic connective tissue diseases under the category of hypersensitivity vasculitis, implying small-vessel disease of the skin, vasculitis in these diseases may be indistinguishable from the fulminant multisystem disorder of the systemic necrotizing vasculitis group. Cutaneous small-vessel disease is the most common associated vasculitis.[102]

The vasculitis associated with RA usually consists of typical leukocytoclastic vasculitis of the postcapillary venules of the skin resulting in palpable purpura and cutaneous ulceration.[102] In addition, the synovium and early rheumatoid nodules can manifest vasculitis.[44] Less commonly, patients with RA, particularly those with severely erosive and nodular disease and high-titer seropositivity for rheumatoid factor,[84] develop a fulminant systemic vasculitis involving arterioles and medium-sized muscular arteries similar to that seen in the polyarteritis nodosa group of systemic necrotizing vasculitis.[11,101] Previously, it was believed that corticosteroid therapy either precipitated the development of or worsened the systemic vasculitis associated with RA;[65,96] it is now thought that systemic vasculitis merely reflects severe RA, a condition that may require corticosteroid therapy.[14]

Cutaneous vasculitis develops in approximately 20% of patients with SLE,[28] typically small-vessel vasculitis resulting in palpable purpura, although patients may develop cutaneous infarction and chronic ulceration. A serious, much less common, vasculitic complication of SLE is diffuse central

nervous system vasculitis and visceral involvement similar to that seen in the polyarteritis nodosa group of systemic vasculitis.[28,67,83]

The mechanism is most likely immune complex deposition. The evidence for immune complex-mediated tissue damage is ample.[18,43] Treatment of most vasculitides in the diffuse connective tissue diseases is that of the primary underlying disease. If the vasculitis threatens vital organs, the treatment is as described for systemic vasculitis.

Essential Mixed Cryoglobulinemia

Cryoglobulinemia may be present in a variety of disorders, with or without vasculitis. Indeed, cryoglobulinemia is present to a variable degree in many of the vasculitic syndromes under discussion. Several categories of cryoglobulinopathies exist, and vasculitis can be found in a number of them.[11,48] In the distinct syndrome called essential mixed cryoglobulinemia, identifiable underlying disease is not usually present.[75,81] In this syndrome, the vasculitis is generally confined to the skin, although some patients develop fulminant multisystem disease, particularly involving the kidney, with severe glomerulonephritis. Histopathologic examination of the purpuric skin lesions typically shows leukocytoclastic venulitis due to deposition of immune complexes, principally IgM rheumatoid factor directed against an IgG molecule; hence the term "mixed" cryoglobulinemia. Results of treatment are variable. When the disease remains confined to the skin, the prognosis is good. Patients with severe glomerulonephritis have a poor prognosis, however, because the disease has been reported to progress despite therapy with corticosteroids or even cytotoxic agents.[46,81] Plasmapheresis may be useful in this syndrome, but firm conclusions must await more extensive clinical trials.

Vasculitis Associated with Neoplasms and Other Primary Disorders

The association between small-vessel cutaneous vasculitis and certain malignant diseases is a well-recognized but rare phenomenon. Associated neoplasms usually are lymphoid or reticuloendothelial disorders such as Hodgkin's disease, other lymphomas, and multiple myeloma.[19,76,94] Although the vasculitis is usually a leukocytoclastic venulitis limited to the skin, systemic vasculitis in association with neoplasms also occurs rarely. Recent reports link hairy cell leukemia with systemic vasculitis of the polyarteritis nodosa type.[45,53] An interesting syndrome of granulomatous vasculitis of the central nervous system is associated with lymphoproliferative disorders, usually Hodgkin's disease, in which the vasculitis is found in areas not invaded by tumor.[90] Although the cause of vasculitis associated with neoplasms is not known, it may reflect a hypersensitivity reaction to tumor or tumor-related antigen with or without the formation and deposition of immune complexes. Treatment of the vasculitis should be directed at the underlying neoplasm.

An association exists between *atrial myxoma* and systemic vasculopathy.[70] Strictly speaking, this syndrome is not a true vasculitis because the arterial lesions result from embolization of myxomatous tissue and secondary inflammation of the arterial wall.[12,56,89]

Leukocytoclastic vasculitis may be a minor component of many other primary diseases.[43] Such diseases include subacute bacterial endocarditis, chronic active hepatitis, ulcerative colitis, retroperitoneal fibrosis, primary biliary cirrhosis, and Goodpasture's syndrome. As with other secondary vasculitides, therapy is directed at the underlying primary cause.

WEGENER'S GRANULOMATOSIS

Wegener's granulomatosis, a distinct clinicopathologic entity, is characterized by granulomatous vasculitis of the upper and lower respiratory tracts together with glomerulonephritis (Fig. 63–6). Variable degrees of disseminated vasculitis involving both small arteries and veins also may occur.[33,36] This disorder probably represents an aberrant hypersensitivity reaction to an unknown antigen, perhaps one that enters through the upper respiratory tract. No associations with allergic diatheses, geographic location, travel, or domestic or occupational exposure are known, however. The male-to-female ratio is 1.3 to 1, and the mean age of onset is 40.6 years.[33]

Clinical Manifestations

The presenting signs and symptoms of 85 cases of Wegener's granulomatosis in a series conducted by my colleagues and myself are listed in Table 63–8.[33] Clinical presentations varied widely, but the typical findings related to the upper respiratory tract and included rhinorrhea, severe sinusitis, nasal mucosal ulcerations, and otitis media, usually secondary to blockage of the eustachian tube resulting from upper airway disease. Some patients had primary middle ear disease. Hearing loss was the initial complaint of several patients. A few patients had pulmonary disease without any evidence of upper airway disease. Symptoms included cough, hemoptysis, and less frequently, chest discomfort. Chest roentgenograms usually demonstrated pulmonary infiltrates. Other organ systems affected by Wegener's granulomatosis were occasionally the focus of initial complaints, often associated with the foregoing respiratory tract findings. Rarely, patients had renal failure in the absence of significant and easily detectable disease in other organ systems. Arthralgias were often present initially, as were other generalized manifestations of systemic inflammatory disease such

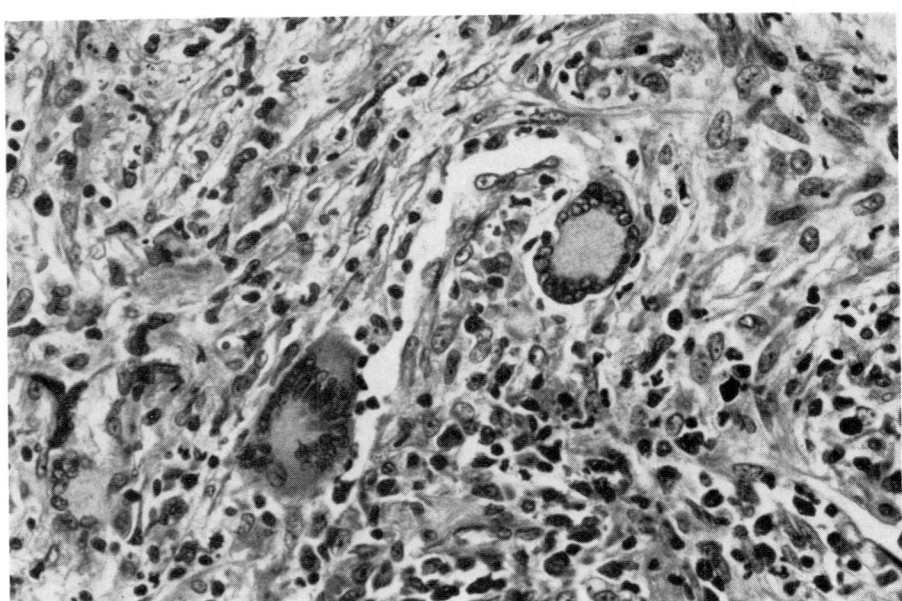

Fig. 63–6. Lung biopsy in a patient with Wegener's granulomatosis. Histopathologic study reveals granulomatous vasculitis with multinucleated giant cells infiltrating the vessel wall. (Hematoxylin and eosin stain; magnification × 200.)

Table 63–8. Presenting Signs and Symptoms in 85 Patients with Wegener's Granulomatosis

	Patients	
Sign or Symptom*	Number	Percentage (%)
Pulmonary infiltrates	60	71
Sinusitis	57	67
Arthralgia or arthritis	37	44
Fever	29	34
Otitis	21	25
Cough	29	34
Rhinitis or nasal symptoms	19	22
Hemoptysis	15	18
Ocular inflammation (conjunctivitis, uveitis, episcleritis, or scleritis)	14	16
Weight loss	14	16
Skin rash	11	13
Epistaxis	9	11
Renal failure	9	11
Chest discomfort	7	8
Anorexia or malaise	7	8
Proptosis	6	7
Shortness of breath or dyspnea	6	7
Oral ulcers	5	6
Hearing loss	5	6
Pleuritis or effusion	5	6
Headache	5	6

(From Fauci, A.S., et al.[33])

*Miscellaneous: hoarseness or stridor, saddle nose deformity, and mastoiditis, three patients each; cranial nerve dysfunction, and mastoiditis, three patients each; cranial nerve dysfunction, three patients; parotid mass or pain, two patients each; nasolacrimal duct obstruction, thyroiditis, liver function test abnormality, blindness, peripheral neuropathy, ear pinna mass, pedal edema, adenopathy, anosmia, pericarditis, asthma, diabetes insipidus, and Raynaud's phenomenon, one patient each.

Table 63–9. Organ or System Involvement in Wegener's Granulomatosis

	Patients	
Organ or System	Number	Percentage (%)
Lung	80	94
Paranasal sinuses	77	91
Kidney	72	85
Joints	57	67
Nose or nasopharynx	54	64
Ear	52	61
Eye	49	58
Skin	38	45
Nervous system	19	22
Heart	10	12

(From Fauci, A.S., et al.[33])

as fatigue, malaise, anorexia, and weight loss. Fever often occurred, perhaps from the underlying inflammatory disease, although it was more commonly associated with secondary bacterial infection of the involved paranasal sinuses.

Although Wegener's granulomatosis is a generalized systemic disease with certain cardinal and characteristic features reflected in multiple organ system involvement (Table 63–9), it is essentially a true pulmonary-renal syndrome, and these two organ systems are largely responsible for the clinical course of the disease.

The characteristic and typical lung findings consist of multiple, bilateral nodular infiltrates that usually cavitate. Pleural effusions occur in approximately 20% of patients, but hilar adenopathy is not seen, and pulmonary calcifications are rare.[36,79,111] Pulmonary function abnormalities are common and include obstruction to airflow as well as reduced lung volumes and diffusing capacity

abnormalities.[93] Small areas of atelectasis frequently occur adjacent to parenchymal infiltrates during active pulmonary disease. Patients with documented endobronchial disease may develop atelectasis related to scarred endobronchial tissue or smoldering endobronchial disease accompanying quiescent disease in other organs.

Renal lesions range from mild focal and segmental glomerulonephritis with minimal urinary findings and little, if any, renal functional impairment to fulminant diffuse necrotizing glomerulonephritis with proliferative and crescentic changes.[36,37,111] Granulomas and true arteritis are rarely found on renal biopsy. Once present, glomerulonephritis may rapidly progress from mild to severe and may lead to fulminant renal failure within weeks and even days of its inception. Because extrarenal manifestations precede functional renal disease, often by months, it is critical to establish the diagnosis early, to treat the patient appropriately, and to prevent irreversible renal failure.[33]

Most patients with Wegener's granulomatosis and serious sinus or nasal disease develop secondary infection of these tissues, almost surely because of mucosal damage and the subsequent impairment of host defenses.[33] *Staphylococcus aureus* is the predominant organism cultured from the nose or sinus of infected patients. Treated patients in complete remission often have an apparent relapse because of increased sinus symptoms together with an elevation of the erythrocyte sedimentation rate. Careful evaluation shows, however, that the symptoms and the erythrocyte sedimentation rate elevation are usually related to smoldering upper airway infection, and both respond promptly to antibiotics with or without drainage procedures. *This observation is important because increasing or reinstituting immunosuppressive therapy under these circumstances is obviously contraindicated.*

Treatment and Prognosis

Before the use of immunosuppressive therapy, the prognosis for patients with this disease was grave. Untreated, the disease usually ran a rapidly fatal course, particularly after the recognition of functional renal impairment. The mean survival rate of patients with untreated Wegener's granulomatosis was 5 months; 82% of patients died within a year, and more than 90% died within 2 years.[107] Wegener's granulomatosis was the first vasculitic syndrome in which the use of long-term, low-dose (2 mg/kg/day) cytotoxic agents, in this case cyclophosphamide, together with alternate-day corticosteroid administration, was effective in inducing remissions in most patients.[36] My colleagues and I recently recorded complete remissions in 79 of 85 patients (93%) using this protocol.[33] The mean duration of remission for survivors was over 4 years, and some patients maintained remission without therapy for more than 10 years. This striking response of a formerly fatal non-neoplastic disease to a combination of low-dose cyclophosphamide and alternate-day corticosteroids had led to its use in other severe systemic vasculitic syndromes, as previously discussed.

LYMPHOMATOID GRANULOMATOSIS

Lymphomatoid granulomatosis is characterized by infiltration of various organs with a polymorphic cellular infiltrate consisting of atypical lymphocytoid and plasmacytoid cells together with granulomatous inflammation in an angiocentric and angiodestructive pattern.[71] Strictly speaking, lymphomatoid granulomatosis is not a vasculitis because it is not a true inflammation of blood vessels, but it is rather an infiltration and invasion of blood vessel walls with atypical lymphoid cells in association with an intra- or extravascular granulomatous response. I include the disease here because it is often confused with certain vasculitic syndromes such as Wegener's granulomatosis.[32] The disease primarily involves the lungs, but skin, renal, and central nervous system disease has occurred in various patients. The characteristic inflammatory granulomas accompany lymphoproliferative disease; hence the term "lymphomatoid granulomatosis." The precise nature of this disorder remains unknown. It is unclear whether the disease represents a continuum from a more benign lymphocytic angiitis and granulomatosis to lymphomatoid granulomatosis and then to frank lymphoma, or whether these processes are indeed separate and should be so categorized.[32]

Patients generally have nonspecific signs and symptoms such as fever, malaise, weight loss, and fatigue. Chest roentgenograms reveal bilateral nodular infiltrates resembling metastatic cancer. The spectrum of organ system involvement in lymphomatoid granulomatosis is outlined in Table 63–10.

Untreated disease is almost uniformly fatal.[58,61,71] My colleagues and I recently described our experience in treating 15 patients with lymphomatoid granulomatosis with a regimen of cyclophosphamide and alternate-day prednisone administration.[34] Approximately half the patients had a complete remission, and therapy was ultimately discontinued. Patients who did not have a remission developed the lymphoproliferative phase of the disease and ultimately died. Thus, the prognosis remains poor.

GIANT-CELL ARTERITIDES

The giant-cell arteritides include temporal or cranial arteritis and Takayasu's arteritis. Both are pan-arteritides characterized by inflammation of medium and large arteries. The two are separable by the clear-cut differences in age range, by the distribution of involved vessels, by the associated syndromes, and by the response to therapy. The characteristics of these diseases are outlined in Table 63–11.

Temporal Arteritis

Temporal arteritis (see also Chap. 59) is well recognized by its classic clinical picture of fever, anemia, high erythrocyte sedimentation rate, and associated symptoms in a person more than 55 years old.[47,49] The diagnosis can often be made clinically and confirmed by biopsy of the temporal arteries. Because vessel involvement may be segmental and may be missed on routine biopsy, some authors have recommended local arteriography[55]

Table 63–10. Organ or System Involvement in 15 Patients with Lymphomatoid Granulomatosis

Organ or System	No. of Patients (%)
Lung	15 (100)
Skin	8 (53)
Kidney	6 (40)
Lymph nodes	6 (40)
Central nervous system	5 (33)
Bone marrow	5 (33)
Liver	4 (27)
Peripheral nervous system	3 (20)
Eyes	3 (20)
Muscle	2 (13)
Paranasal sinuses	1 (7)
Thyroid gland	1 (7)
Epididymis	1 (7)

(From Fauci, A.S., et al.[34])

Table 63–11. Characteristics of the Giant-Cell Arteritides

	Temporal Arteritis	*Takayasu's Arteritis*
Patients	Disease of the elderly; women more than men	More prevalent in young women; more common in the Orient, but neither racially nor geographically restricted
Blood vessels	Characteristically involves branches of carotid (temporal artery), but is a systemic arteritis and may involve any medium-sized or large artery	Large- and medium-sized arteries with predilection for aortic arch and its branches; may involve pulmonary artery
Histopathologic features	Panarteritis; inflammatory mononuclear cell infiltrates; frequent giant-cell formation within vessel wall; fragmentation of internal elastic lamina; proliferation of tunica intima	Panarteritis; inflammatory mononuclear cell infiltrates; intimal proliferation and fibrosis; scarring and vascularization of tunica media; disruption and degeneration of elastic lamina
Clinical manifestations	Classic complex of fever, anemia, high erythrocyte sedimentation rate, muscle aches in an elderly person; possible headache; strong association with polymyalgia rheumatica syndrome	Generalized systemic symptoms; local signs and symptoms related to involved vessels; occlusive phase
Complications	Ocular (sudden blindness)	Related to distribution of involved vessels; death usually occurs from congestive heart failure or cerebrovascular accidents
Diagnosis	Temporal artery biopsy; lesions may be segmental; multiple sections, arteriography, and bilateral biopsy may aid in diagnosis	Arteriography; biopsy of involved vessel
Treatment	Corticosteroids effective	Corticosteroids not of proved efficacy; cytotoxic agents currently being tested

(From Fauci, A.S., Haynes, B.F., and Katz, P.[39])

and examination of multiple sections of bilateral biopsies.[66]

Polymyalgia rheumatica syndrome, closely associated with temporal arteritis, is characterized by stiffness, aching, and pain in the muscles of the neck, shoulder, lower back, hips, and thighs.[15,49,50] This syndrome is detailed in Chapter 59.*

A well-recognized and serious complication of temporal arteritis, particularly in untreated patients, is ocular involvement, sometimes leading to sudden blindness.[106] Although the dramatic eye manifestations may appear suddenly, most patients have complaints relating to the head or eyes for months, and so one needs to pay careful attention to symptoms and rapid use of appropriate therapy. Temporal arteritis is generally exquisitely sensitive to corticosteroid therapy.[6,49,50] Treatment should begin with 40 to 60 mg prednisone daily, followed by gradual tapering to a daily maintenance dose of 7.5 to 10 mg, with upward readjustment of dosage if symptoms recur. Therapy should be continued for at least 1 to 2 years.[6,49,50,54] Although one should not attempt to induce initial remission of temporal arteritis with alternate-day therapy, many patients

can be given alternate-day therapy in preparation for discontinuing the drug after induction of remission.[54] The prognosis of this disorder is good with corticosteroid therapy, and remissions usually are maintained after withdrawal of therapy, although relapse can occur.

Takayasu's Arteritis

Usually seen in women in the second or third decade of life, this disease is characterized by inflammation and stenosis of large and intermediate-sized arteries with frequent involvement of the aortic arch and its branches.[41,57,78,87,105] Diagnosis is usually made angiographically. Takayasu's arteritis is often referred to as "pulseless disease" because of the frequent involvement of the subclavian artery (Fig. 63–7). Nonetheless, it has complex manifestations ranging from generalized, often vague, symptoms characteristic of a systemic inflammatory disease to local signs and symptoms relating to the involved vessels themselves, to the characteristic manifestations of compromised blood flow to the organs perfused by the involved vessels. Some patients experience no apparent inflammatory symptoms and signs, but have initial ischemic findings and changes related to the involved organ systems. The most common and obvious findings are absent pulses in the affected vessels. Bruits are

---

*Editor's note: We have reported three cases with onset before age 50.[23a]

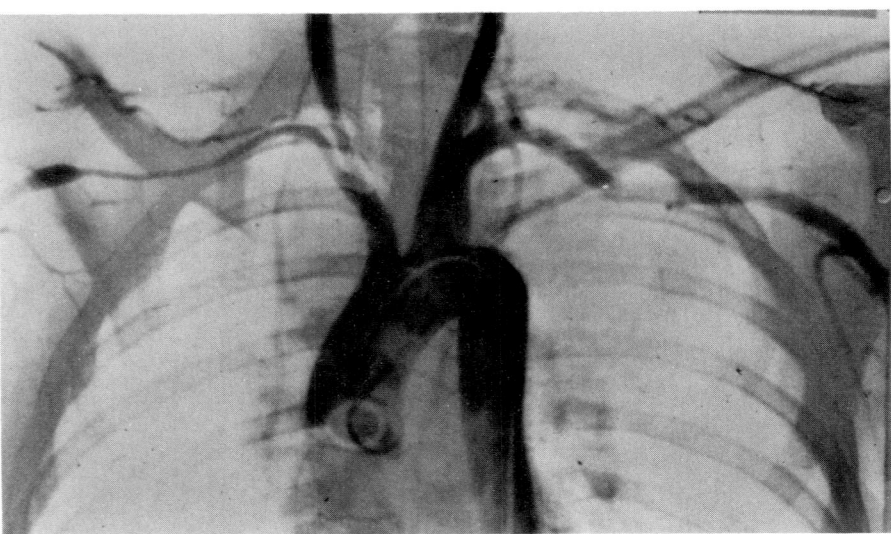

Fig. 63–7. Subtraction angiogram of the aortic arch in a 27-year-old woman with Takayasu's arteritis. Note the severe involvement along a large segment of the right subclavian artery, as well as involvement of the proximal portion of the right common carotid artery.

common. The clinical course of the disease varies. Gradual deterioration is the rule, but the process may spontaneously remit, stabilize temporarily, insidiously progress, or abruptly decompensate. This variability has made it difficult to evaluate therapy. Corticosteroids have been used with mixed results, and no convincing evidence suggests that they substantially improve the long-term prognosis. The role of cytotoxic agents remains unclear. Despite reports of spontaneous remissions, the course is generally progressive and fatal within a few years. Death usually occurs from congestive heart failure or cerebrovascular accidents.[87]

MUCOCUTANEOUS LYMPH NODE SYNDROME (KAWASAKI'S DISEASE)

The mucocutaneous lymph node syndrome is an acute febrile illness of infants and young children. The cause is completely unknown, and although an infectious agent has been suspected, no etiologic agent has been identified.[80] *Propionibacterium acnes* has been implicated as the most likely agent[58a] with house dust mites serving as its vector.[42a,48a,88a] The disease was originally described in Japan and is characterized by the following: nonsuppurative cervical adenitis; changes in the skin and mucous membranes such as edema; congested conjunctivae; erythema of the oral cavity, lips, and palms; and desquamation of the skin of the fingertips, all unresponsive to antibiotics.[63,64,104] The disease has recently been recognized with increasing frequency in the United States.[7] The clinical manifestations are listed in Table 63–12. Kawa-

Table 63–12. Clinical Manifestations of Mucocutaneous Lymph Node Syndrome (Kawasaki's Disease)

Manifestations	Percentage (%)
Fever	95
Changes of the extremity	
Desquamation from finger tips	94
Erythematous palms and soles	88
Indurated edema	76
Polymorphous exanthem of body and trunk	92
Changes in lips and oral cavity	
Dry, red lips	90
Erythematous oral mucosa	90
Prominent tongue papillae	77
Congested conjunctivae	88
Swelling of cervical lymph nodes	75

(From Cupps, T.R., and Fauci, A.S.[22])

saki's disease is usually self-limited, and most patients recover uneventfully. Approximately 1 to 2% of patients, however, develop severe and often fatal complications, resulting from vasculitic involvement of the coronary arteries. It is now generally agreed that most of the cases in the United States formerly reported as polyarteritis nodosa of children, with its characteristic and unusual selective involvement of the coronary arteries, were in fact the arteritis of unrecognized Kawasaki's disease.[63] Myocarditis, endopericarditis, myocardial infarctions, and cardiomegaly are also seen. Involvement of other vessels such as the aorta and the celiac, carotid, subclavian, and pulmonary arteries occurs much less frequently. Preliminary studies indicate that treatment with aspirin (30 mg/kg/day) lessens the incidence of cardiac complications. Furthermore, some evidence, as yet unconfirmed, suggests that corticosteroids are ineffective and may actually increase the incidence of cardiac complications.[59]

VASCULITIS ISOLATED TO THE CENTRAL NERVOUS SYSTEM

In addition to the granulomatous vasculitis of the central nervous system already discussed in association with certain lymphoproliferative malignant diseases, a syndrome of isolated vasculitis of the central nervous system also exists. This uncommon clinicopathologic entity is characterized by vasculitis restricted to the vessels of the central nervous system in the apparent absence of systemic vasculitis or other systemic disease.[23] Presenting manifestations include severe headaches, altered mental function, and focal neurologic defects. Systemic symptoms such as fever, myalgia, arthralgia, and arthritis, common in the systemic vasculitides, are usually not present in patients with isolated vasculitis of the central nervous system. Diagnosis is made by clinical presentation together with angiographic studies or biopsy of the brain parenchyma and leptomeninges, when feasible. Prognosis is generally poor, but corticosteroids together with cyclophosphamide used in the regimen described for systemic vasculitis may induce long-term remissions.[23]

BEHÇET'S DISEASE

This disease (see also Chap. 58) of unknown origin is characterized by recurrent episodes of oral ulcers, eye lesions, genital ulcers, and other cutaneous lesions.[88] The underlying pathologic lesion is a vasculitis predominantly involving venules, although vessels of any size in any organ system can be affected. No therapy for Behçet's disease is uniformly acceptable. A number of therapeutic regimens have been attempted with variable results, however. These treatments include topical and systemic corticosteroids, colchicine, indomethacin, transfer factor, blood transfusion, antifibrinolytic therapy, levamisole, chlorambucil, azathioprine, and sulfasalazine.[3]

THROMBOANGIITIS OBLITERANS (BUERGER'S DISEASE)

This rare inflammatory occlusive peripheral vascular disease involves the arteries and veins. The disease is seen predominantly in men, usually between the ages of 20 and 40 years.[78] It primarily involves medium-sized and small arteries as well as veins in a segmental fashion. The inflammatory process is associated with a thrombus and evolves through several stages. In the acute stage, the ves-

sel wall and thrombus are infiltrated by polymorphonuclear leukocytes. Microabscesses may be found within the thrombi.[80] A subacute stage follows, when mononuclear cells and giant cells may be seen, and ultimately a chronic stage develops, characterized by chronic inflammatory infiltrates, fibrosis, and recanalization of the vessel lumen. The entire process may be associated with migratory superficial thrombophlebitis.

Although the cause is unknown, the use of tobacco makes the disease much worse. Almost without exception, thromboangiitis obliterans occurs in heavy smokers.[78] No sufficient evidence suggests that immunologic phenomena play a role in pathogenesis.

The clinical presentation is variable and may be insidious or abrupt. Coldness of the distal extremities, color changes, dysesthesias, intense hyperemia, excruciating pain, ulceration, gangrene, and pulp atrophy are common.[51,77,78,108] Usually, acute attacks last one to four weeks, and the disease runs an indolent and recurrent course. Ultimately, the collateral circulation can no longer compensate for the progressive ischemia, and amputation of the involved distal extremities may be required. Various techniques such as anticoagulation, thromboendarterectomy, bypass operations, and sympathectomy have not improved the prognosis for the involved extremity.[51,100] The most effective approach to this disease seems to be meticulous local care of the involved area, together with complete abstinence from tobacco.

MISCELLANEOUS VASCULITIDES

In a number of other syndromes, vasculitis is either the primary disease process or a secondary component of an underlying disease entity. *Erythema nodosum* is a common syndrome well recognized as a hypersensitivity manifestation of underlying disorders.[8] Clinically, it is manifested as a painful, nodular, inflammatory process of the dermis and subcutaneous tissues. Vasculitis, predominantly of small venules, comprises a major component of its histopathologic picture.[110]

Other less common vasculitides that deserve mention are *erythema elevatum diutinum*,[60] *Cogan's syndrome*,[13] and *Eale's disease*.[98] Finally, some rare syndromes appear to be confined to single organs such as the vermiform appendix and the female breast.[104a]

GENERAL APPROACH TO THE PATIENT

The vasculitides comprise a broad spectrum of clinicopathologic syndromes. In certain disorders, vasculitis is the predominant and most obvious manifestation in the absence of an underlying disease process. Other disorders may be characterized

Table 63–13. General Approach to the Patient with Vasculitis

1. Categorize the syndrome correctly (specific syndrome; primary versus secondary; localized versus systemic).
2. Determine extent of disease activity.
3. Remove offending antigen if possible.
4. If associated with underlying disease, treat underlying disease when possible.
5. Use appropriate therapeutic agents immediately in diseases in which efficacy is clearly demonstrated, such as corticosteroids in temporal arteritis and cyclophosphamide and corticosteroids in Wegener's granulomatosis.
6. Avoid immunosuppressive therapy (corticosteroids or cytotoxic agents) in diseases that: (1) do not disseminate; (2) do not usually result in irreversible organ system damage; and (3) rarely respond dramatically to such agents.
7. Institute corticosteroids immediately in patients with systemic vasculitis; add a cytotoxic agent such as cyclophosphamide if response is not prompt or if disease is known to respond only to cytotoxic agents.
8. Continually attempt to taper corticosteroids to alternate-day regimens, and discontinue when possible.
9. Have a clear-cut understanding of goals and mechanisms of the long-term use of cytotoxic agents in the treatment of non-neoplastic diseases.
10. Use other agents when clinical situation dictates (nonsteroidal anti-inflammatory agents or plasmapheresis) based on results from therapeutic trials.

by a vasculitic syndrome secondary to a primary underlying disease. Most vasculitic syndromes can be associated directly or indirectly with immunopathologic mechanisms. Of particular importance is the role of immune complex-mediated damage, which plays a pathophysiologic role in some of these syndromes. Using various clinical, pathologic, and immunologic criteria, certain vasculitic syndromes can be clearly recognized and categorized as distinct entities, whereas others overlap different diseases within a broader category. It is important to categorize a vasculitic syndrome in a given patient, and particularly to identify disseminated systemic disease that will lead to irreversible organ system dysfunction if untreated or if inadequately treated. Such patients need prompt and aggressive treatment with corticosteroids and, in some cases, cytotoxic agents such as cyclophosphamide. In contrast, patients with predominantly cutaneous disease without a high risk of systemic involvement can be treated much less aggressively. Appreciation of the scope of the vasculitic syndromes is essential for an appropriate diagnostic and therapeutic approach to individual patients (Table 63–13).

REFERENCES

1. Ackroyd, J.F.: Allergic purpura, including purpura due to foods, drugs and infections. Am. J. Med., 14:605–632, 1953.
2. Alarcón-Segovia, D.: The necrotizing vasculitides. A new pathogenetic classification. Med. Clin. North Am., 61:241–260, 1977.
3. Allen, N., and Haynes, B.F.: Behçet's syndrome. In Current Therapy in Allergy and Immunology 1983–1984. Edited by L.M. Lichtenstein and A.S. Fauci. Philadelphia, B.C. Decker, 1983, pp. 147–151.
3a. Ambrus, J.L., and Fauci, A.S.: Diffuse histiocytic lymphoma in a patient treated with cyclophosphamide for Wegener's granulomatosis. Am. J. Med., 76:745–747, 1984.
4. Ansell, B.M.: Henoch-Schönlein purpura with particular reference to the prognosis of the renal lesion. Br. J. Dermatol., 82:211–215, 1970.
5. Ballard, H.S., Eisinger, R.P., and Gallo, G.: Renal manifestations of the Henoch-Schönlein syndrome in adults. Am. J. Med., 49:328–335, 1970.
6. Beevers, D.G., Harpur, J.E., and Turk, K.A.D.: Giant cell arteritis—the need for prolonged treatment. J. Chronic Dis., 26:561–570, 1973.
7. Bell, D.M., et al.: Kawasaki syndrome: description of two outbreaks in the United States. N. Engl. J. Med., 304:1568–1575, 1981.
8. Blomgren, S.E.: Erythema nodosum. Semin. Arthritis Rheum., 4:1–24, 1974.
9. Boyle, J.A., and Buchanan, W.W.: Polyarteritis nodosa. In Clinical Rheumatology. Philadelphia, F.A. Davis, 1971, pp. 519–541.
10. Bron, K.M., Stroot, C.A., and Shapiro, A.P.: The diagnostic value of angiographic observations in polyarteritis nodosa. Arch. Intern. Med., 116:450–453, 1965.
11. Brouet, J.C., et al.: The occurrence and nature of precipitating antibodies in anti-DNA sera. Clin. Immunol. Immunopathol., 2:310–324, 1974.
12. Burton, C., and Johnston, J.: Multiple cerebral aneurysms and cardiac myxoma. N. Engl. J. Med., 282:35–37, 1970.
13. Cheson, B.D., Bluming, A.Z., and Alroy, J.: Cogan's syndrome: a systemic vasculitis. Am. J. Med., 60:549–555, 1976.
14. Christian, C.L., and Sergent, J.S.: Vasculitis syndromes: clinical and experimental models. Am. J. Med., 61:385–392, 1976.
15. Chuang, T.-Y., et al.: Polymyalgia rheumatica. A 10-year epidemiologic and clinical study. Ann. Intern. Med., 97:672–680, 1982.
16. Churg, J., and Strauss, L.: Allergic granulomatosis, allergic angiitis and periarteritis nodosa. Am. J. Pathol., 27:277–301, 1951.
17. Cochrane, C.G., and Dixon, F.J.: Antigen-antibody complex induced disease. In Textbook of Immunopathology. 2nd Ed. Vol. 1. Edited by P.A. Meischer and H.F. Müller-Eberhard. New York, Grune & Stratton, 1976, p. 137.
18. Conn, D.L., McDuffie, F.C., and Dyck, P.J.: Immunopathologic study of sural nerves in rheumatoid arthritis. Arthritis Rheum., 15:135–143, 1972.
19. Copeman, P.W.M., and Ryan, T.J.: The problems of classification of cutaneous angiitis with reference to histopathology and pathogenesis. Br. J. Dermatol., 81:2–14, 1970.
20. Cream, J.J., Gumpel, J.M., and Peachy, R.D.G.: Schönlein-Henoch purpura in the adult. Q. J. Med., 39:461–484, 1970.
21. Cupps, T.R., and Fauci, A.S.: Cutaneous vasculitis. In Current Therapy in Allergy and Immunology 1983–1984. Edited by L.M. Lichtenstein and A.S. Fauci. Philadelphia, B.C. Becker, 1983, pp. 1–211.
22. Cupps, T.R., and Fauci, A.S.: The Vasculitides. Philadelphia, W.B. Saunders, 1981, pp. 1–211.
23. Cupps, T.R., Moore, P.M., and Fauci, A.S.: Isolated angiitis of the central nervous system. Prospective diagnostic and therapeutic considerations. Am. J. Med., 74:97–105, 1983.

23a. Dailey, M.D., and McCarty, D.J.: Polymyalgia rheumatica begins at 40. Arch. Intern. Med., *139*:743–744, 1979.

24. DeShazo, R.D., et al.: Systemic vasculitis with coexistent large and small vessel involvement. A classification dilemma. JAMA, *238*:1940–1942, 1977.

25. Diaz-Perez, J.L., and Winkelmann, R.K.: Cutaneous periarteritis nodosa. Arch. Dermatol., *110*:407–414, 1974.

26. Dornfeld, L., Lecky, L.W., and Peter, J.B.: Polyarteritis and intrarenal renal artery aneurysms. JAMA, *215*:1950–1952, 1971.

27. Duffy, J., et al.: Polyarthritis, polyarteritis and hepatitis B. Medicine, *55*:19–37, 1976.

28. Estes, D., and Christian, C.L.: The natural history of systemic lupus erythematosus by prospective analysis. Medicine, *50*:85–95, 1971.

29. Fauci, A.S.: Systemic vasculitis. *In* Current Therapy in Allergy and Immunology. Edited by L.M. Lichtenstein and A.S. Fauci. Philadelphia, B.C. Decker, 1983, pp. 129–136.

30. Fauci, A.S.: The vasculitic syndromes. *In* Cecil Textbook of Medicine, 16th Ed. Edited by J.B. Wyngaarden and L.H. Smith, Jr. Philadelphia, W.B. Saunders, 1982, pp. 1863–1866.

31. Fauci, A.S.: Vasculitis. *In* Clinical Immunology. Edited by E.W. Parker. Philadelphia, W.B. Saunders, 1980, pp. 473–519.

32. Fauci, A.S.: Granulomatous vasculitides: distinct but related. Ann. Intern. Med., *87*:782–783, 1977.

33. Fauci, A.S., et al.: Wegener's granulomatosis: prospective clinical and therapeutic experience with 85 patients for 21 years. Ann. Intern. Med., *98*:76–85, 1983.

34. Fauci, A.S., et al.: Lymphomatoid granulomatosis: prospective clinical and therapeutic experience over 10 years. N. Engl. J. Med., *306*:68–74, 1982.

35. Fauci, A.S., et al.: Cyclophosphamide therapy of severe systemic necrotizing vasculitis. N. Engl. J. Med., *301*:235–238, 1979.

36. Fauci, A.S., and Wolff, S.M.: Wegener's granulomatosis: studies in eighteen patients and a review of the literature. Medicine (Baltimore), *52*:535–561, 1973.

37. Fauci, A.S., Balow, J.E., and Wolff, S.M.: Effect of cytotoxic therapy on the renal lesions of Wegener's granulomatosis. *In* Proceedings of the Sixth International Congress of Nephrology. Edited by S. Giovannetti, V. Bonomini, and G. D'Amico. Basel, S. Karger, 1976, pp. 486–491.

38. Fauci, A.S., Doppman, J.L., and Wolff, S.M.: Cyclophosphamide-induced remissions in advanced polyarteritis nodosa. Am. J. Med., *64*:890–894, 1978.

39. Fauci, A.S., Haynes, B.F., and Katz, P.: The spectrum of vasculitis: clinical, pathologic, immunologic, and therapeutic considerations. Ann. Intern. Med., *89*:660–676, 1978.

40. Fleming, R.J., and Stern, L.Z.: Multiple intraparenchymal renal aneurysms in polyarteritis nodosa. Radiology, *84*:100–103, 1965.

41. Fraga, A., et al.: Takayasu's arteritis: frequency of systemic manifestations (study of 22 patients) and favorable response to maintenance steroid therapy and adrenocorticosteroids (12 patients). Arthritis Rheum., *15*:617–624, 1972.

42. Frohnert, P.P., and Sheps, S.G.: Long-term follow-up study of periarteritis nodosa. Am. J. Med., *43*:8–14, 1967.

42a. Fujimoto, T., et al.: Immune complex and mite antigen in Kawasaki disease. Lancet, *2*:980–981, 1982.

43. Gilliam, J.N., and Smiley, J.D.: Cutaneous necrotizing vasculitis and related disorders. Ann. Allergy, *37*:328–339, 1976.

44. Glass, D., Soter, N.A., and Schur, P.H.: Rheumatoid vasculitis. Arthritis Rheum., *19*:950–952, 1976.

45. Goedert, J.J., et al.: Polyarteritis nodosa, hairy cell leukemia and splenosis. JAMA, *71*:323–326, 1981.

46. Golde, D., and Epstein, W.: Mixed cryoglobulins and glomerulonephritis. Ann. Intern. Med., *69*:1221–1227, 1968.

47. Goodman, B.W.: Temporal arteritis. Am. J. Med., *67*:839–852, 1979.

48. Grey, H.M., and Kohler, P.F.: Cryoimmunoglobulins. Semin. Hematol., *10*:87–112, 1973.

48a. Hamashima, Y., et al.: Mite-associated particles in Kawasaki disease. Lancet, *2*:266, 1982.

49. Hamilton, C.R., Jr., Shelley, W.M., and Tumulty, P.A.: Giant cell arteritis: including temporal arteritis and polymyalgia rheumatica. Medicine (Baltimore), *50*:1–27, 1971.

50. Healey, L.A., Parker, F., and Wilske, K.R.: Polymyalgia rheumatica and giant cell arteritis. Arthritis Rheum., *14*:138–141, 1971.

51. Hill, G.L.: A rational basis for management of patients with the Buerger syndrome. Br. J. Surg., *61*:476–481, 1974.

52. Holsinger, D.R., Osmundson, P.J., and Edwards, J.E.: The heart in periarteritis nodosa. Circulation, *25*:610–618, 1962.

53. Hughes, G.R.V., et al.: Polyarteritis nodosa and hairy-cell leukemia. Lancet, *1*:678–681, 1978.

54. Hunder, G.G.: Temporal arteritis. *In* Current Therapy in Allergy and Immunology 1983–1984. Edited by L.M. Lichtenstein and A.S. Fauci. Philadelphia, B.C. Decker, 1983, pp. 140–143.

55. Hunder, G.G., et al.: Superficial temporal arteriography in patients suspected of having temporal arteritis. Arthritis Rheum., *15*:561–570, 1972.

56. Huston, K.A., et al.: Left atrial myxoma simulating peripheral vasculitis. Mayo Clin. Proc., *53*:752–756, 1978.

57. Ishikawa, K.: Natural history and classification of occlusive thromboaortopathy (Takayasu's disease). Circulation, *57*:617–624, 1978.

58. Israel, H.L., Patchefsky, A.S., and Saldana, M.J.: Wegener's granulomatosis, lymphomatoid granulomatosis, and benign lymphocytic angiitis and granulomatosis of lung: Recognition and treatment. Ann. Intern. Med., *87*:691–699, 1977.

58a. Kato, H., et al.: Variant strain of *Propionibacterium acnes*: A clue to the aetiology of Kawasaki disease. Lancet, *2*:1383–1388, 1983.

59. Kato, H., Koike, S., and Yokoyama, T.: Kawasaki disease: effect of treatment on coronary artery involvement. Pediatrics, *63*:175–179, 1979.

60. Katz, P., et al.: Erythema elevatum diutinum: skin and systemic manifestations, immunologic studies, and successful treatment with dapsone. Medicine (Baltimore), *56*:443–455, 1977.

61. Katzenstein, A.-L.A., Carrington, C.B., and Liebow, A.A.: Lymphomatoid granulomatosis: a clinico-pathologic study of 152 cases. Cancer, *43*:360–373, 1979.

62. Kauffmann, R.H., and Houwert, D.A.: Plasmapheresis in rapidly progressive Henoch-Schönlein glomerulonephritis and the effect on circulating IgA immune complexes. Clin. Nephrol., *16*:155–160, 1981.

63. Kawasaki, T., et al.: A new infantile acute febrile mucocutaneous lymph node syndrome (MLNS) prevailing in Japan. Pediatrics, *54*:271–276, 1974.

64. Kawasaki, T., et al.: Acute febrile mucocutaneous syndrome with lymphoid involvement with specific desquamation of the fingers and toes in children. Jpn. J. Allergy, *16*:178–222, 1967.

65. Kemper, J.W., Baggenstoss, A.H., and Slocumb, C.H.: The relationship of therapy with cortisone to the incidence of vascular lesions in rheumatoid arthritis. Ann. Intern. Med., *46*:831–851, 1957.

66. Klein, R.G., et al.: Skip lesions in temporal arteritis. Mayo Clin. Proc., *51*:504–510, 1976.

67. Klemperer, P., Pollack, A.D., and Baehr, G.: Pathology of disseminated lupus erythematosus. Arch. Pathol., *32*:569–631, 1941.

68. Kussmaul, A., and Maier, K.: Über eine bischer nicht beschriebene eigenthümliche Arterienerkrankung (Periarteritis nodosa), die mit Morbus Brightii und rapid fortschreitender allgemeiner Muskellähmung einhergeht. Dtsch. Arch. Klin., *1*:484–517, 1966.

69. Landing, B.H., and Larson, E.J.: Are infantile periarteritis nodosa with coronary artery involvement and fatal

mucocutaneous lymph node syndrome the same? Comparison of 20 patients from North America with patients from Hawaii and Japan. Pediatrics, 59:651–662, 1977.
70. Leonhardt, E.T.G., and Kullenberg, K.P.G.: Bilateral atrial myxomas with multiple arterial aneurysms—a syndrome mimicking polyarteritis nodosa. Am. J. Med., 62:792–794, 1977.
71. Liebow, A.A., Carrington, C.R.B., and Friedman, P.J.: Lymphomatoid granulomatosis. Hum. Pathol., 3:457–458, 1972.
72. Lindenauer, S.M., and Tank, E.S.: Surgical aspects of Henoch-Schönlein purpura. Surgery, 59:982–987, 1966.
73. Lockwood, C.M., et al.: Reversal of impaired splenic function in patients with nephritis or vasculitis (or both) by plasma exchange. N. Engl. J. Med., 300:524–530, 1979.
74. Longstreth, P.L., Lorobkin, M., and Palubinskas, A.J.: Renal microaneurysms in a patient with systemic lupus erythematosus. Radiology, 113:65–66, 1974.
75. LoSpalluto, J., et al.: Cryoglobulinemia based on interaction between a gamma macroglobulin and 75 gamma globulin. Am. J. Med., 32:142–147, 1962.
76. McCombs, R.P.: Systemic "allergic" vasculitis. Clinical and pathological relationships. JAMA, 194:157–164, 1965.
77. McKusick, V.A.: A form of vascular disease relatively frequent in the Orient. Bull. Johns Hopkins Hosp., 109:241–291, 1962.
78. McKusick, V.A., and Harris, W.S.: The Buerger syndrome in the Orient. Bull. Johns Hopkins Hosp., 109:241–291, 1961.
79. Maquire, R., et al.: Unusual radiographic findings of Wegener's granulomatosis. AJR, 130:133–138, 1978.
80. Melish, M.E.: Kawasaki syndrome: a new infectious disease? J. Infect. Dis., 143:317–324, 1981.
81. Meltzer, M., et al.: Cryoglobulinemia—a clinical and laboratory study. II. Cryoglobulins with rheumatoid factor activity. Am. J. Med., 40:837–856, 1966.
82. Meyers, D.S., Grim, C.E., and Kertzer, W.F.: Fibromuscular dysplasia of the renal artery with medial dissection. A case simulating polyarteritis nodosa. Am. J. Med., 56:412–416, 1974.
83. Mintz, G., and Fraga, A.: Arteritis in systemic lupus erythematous. Arch. Intern. Med., 116:55–66, 1965.
84. Mongan, E.S., et al.: A study of the relation of seronegative and seropositive rheumatoid arthritis to each other and to necrotizing vasculitis. Am. J. Med., 47:23–35, 1969.
85. Moore, P.M., and Fauci, A.S.: Neurologic manifestations of systemic vasculitis. A retrospective and prospective study of the clinicopathologic features and responses to therapy in 25 patients. Am. J. Med., 71:517–524, 1981.
86. Mowrey, F.H., and Lundberg, E.A.: The clinical manifestations of essential polyangiitis (periarteritis nodosa) with emphasis on the hepatic manifestations. Ann. Intern. Med., 40:1141–1155, 1967.
87. Nakao, K., et al.: Takayasu's arteritis. Clinical report of eighty-four cases and immunological studies of seven cases. Circulation, 35:1141–1155, 1967.
88. O'Duffy, J.D., Carney, J.A., and Deodhar, S.: Behçet's disease. Report of 10 cases, 3 with new manifestations. Ann. Intern. Med., 75:561–570, 1971.
88a.Patriarca, P.A., et al.: Kawasaki syndrome: Association with the application of rug shampoo. Lancet, 2:575–580, 1982.
89. Price, D.L., et al.: Cardiac myxoma. A clinicopathologic

and angiographic study. Arch. Neurol., 23:558–567, 1970.
90. Rewcastle, N.B., and Tom, M.I.: Non-infectious granulomatous angiitis of the nervous system associated with Hodgkin's disease. J. Neurol. Neurosurg. Psychiatry, 25:52–58, 1962.
91. Roberts, F.B., and Fetterman, G.H.: Polyarteritis nodosa in infancy. J. Pediatr., 63:519–529, 1963.
92. Rose, G.A., and Spencer, H.: Polyarteritis nodosa. Q. J. Med., 26:43–81, 1957.
93. Rosenberg, D.M., et al.: Functional correlates of lung involvement in Wegener's granulomatosis. Am. J. Med., 69:387–394, 1980.
94. Sams, W.M., Harville, D.D., and Winkelmann, R.K.: Necrotizing vasculitis associated with lethal reticuloendothelial diseases. Br. J. Dermatol., 80:555–567, 1968.
95. Sams, W.M., et al.: Leukocytoclastic vasculitis. Arch. Dermatol., 112:219–226, 1976.
96. Schmid, F.R., et al.: Arteritis in rheumatoid arteritis. Am. J. Med., 30:56–83, 1961.
97. Sergent, J.S., et al.: Vasculitis with hepatitis B antigenemia: long-term observations in nine patients. Medicine (Baltimore), 67:354–359, 1976.
98. Sheie, H.G., and Albert, D.M.: Textbook of Ophthalmology. 9th Ed. Philadelphia, W.B. Saunders, 1977, p. 32.
99. Sheps, S.G.: Vasculitis. In Peripheral Vascular Diseases. 4th Ed. Edited by J.F. Fairburn, J.L. Juergens, and J.A. Spittel. Philadelphia, W.B. Saunders, 1972, pp. 351–385.
100. Shionoya, S., et al.: Diagnosis, pathology, and treatment of Buerger's disease. Surgery, 75:195–199, 1974.
101. Sokoloff, L., and Bunim, J.J.: Vascular lesions in rheumatoid arthritis. J. Chronic Dis., 5:668–687, 1957.
102. Soter, N.A.: Clinical presentations and mechanisms of necrotizing angiitis of the skin. J. Invest. Dermatol., 67:354–359, 1976.
103. Spector, W.G., and Heesom, N.: The production of granulomata by antigen-antibody complexes. J. Pathol., 98:31–39, 1969.
104. Tanaka, N., Sekimoto, K., and Naoe, S.: Kawasaki disease. Relationship with infantile periarteritis nodosa. Arch. Pathol. Lab. Med., 100:81–86, 1976.
104a.Thaell, J.F., and Save, G.L.: Giant cell arteritis involving the breasts. J. Rheumatol., 10:329–331, 1983.
105. Vinijchaikul, L.: Primary arteritis of the aorta and its main branches (Takayasu's arteriopathy). Am. J. Med., 43:15–27, 1967.
106. Wagener, H.P., and Hollenhorst, R.W.: The ocular lesions of temporal arteritis. Am. J. Ophthalmol., 45:617–630, 1958.
107. Walton, E.W.: Giant-cell granuloma of the respiratory tract (Wegener's granulomatosis). Br. Med. J., 2:265–270, 1958.
108. Williams, G.: Recent views on Buerger's disease. J. Clin. Pathol., 22:573–578, 1969.
109. Winkelmann, R.K., and Ditto, W.B.: Cutaneous and visceral syndromes of necrotizing or "allergic" angiitis: A study of 38 cases. Medicine (Baltimore), 43:59–89, 1964.
110. Winkelman, R.K., and Förström, L.: New observations in the histopathology of erythema nodosum. J. Invest. Dermatol., 65:441–446, 1975.
111. Wolff, S.M., et al.: Wegener's granulomatosis. Ann. Intern. Med., 81:523–525, 1974.
112. Zeek, P.M.: Periarteritis nodosa and other forms of necrotizing angiitis. N. Engl. J. Med., 18:764–772, 1953.
113. Zeek, P.M.: Periarteritis nodosa: critical review. Am. J. Clin. Pathol., 22:777–790, 1952.

Chapter 64

Mixed Connective Tissue Disease

Gordon C. Sharp and Bernhard H. Singsen

For many years, clinicians have been aware that some patients have features of more than one rheumatic disease and thus do not fit into traditional classifications. Patients with a combination of clinical findings similar to those of systemic lupus erythematosus (SLE), progressive systemic sclerosis (PSS), polymyositis, and rheumatoid arthritis (RA), and with unusually high titers of a circulating antinuclear antibody with specificity for a nuclear ribonucleoprotein antigen, are considered to have *mixed connective tissue disease* (MCTD).[49]

Initial observations of MCTD suggested infrequent renal disease, a strong reponse to corticosteroids, and a favorable prognosis.[38,49] Further study has shown, however, that renal disease occurs in 10 to 20% of patients; some patients may require aggressive or prolonged pharmacologic intervention, and pulmonary involvement is common. Pulmonary hypertension, associated with proliferative vascular lesions, may be a serious complication, and the long-term outlook, therefore, is not always favorable.[22,31,54,56,59]

SEROLOGIC ALTERATIONS

When subjected to a sensitive passive hemagglutination test, all patients in the original study of MCTD had high titers of antibody to a nuclear antigen extractable in isotonic buffers (ENA).[49,51] Antibodies to ENA were detected in about half of a series of patients with SLE, although usually at reduced titers, and the reported incidence of ENA antibodies was also low in other rheumatic disorders.[49,51] Treatment of ENA-coated red blood cells with ribonuclease (RNase) reduced or eliminated the agglutination reaction in serum from patients with MCTD, but had little or no effect on serum from patients with SLE.[49]

Immunodiffusion studies subsequently revealed that ENA consisted of at least two distinct antigens, one sensitive to RNase and trypsin, which appeared to be a nuclear ribonucleoprotein, and the previously described Sm antigen,[33,38,42,50] which is resistant to RNase and trypsin. Sera that reacted with either the nuclear ribonucleoprotein antigen or the Sm antigen produced a speckled, fluorescent antinuclear antibody pattern.[33,48,49] Treatment of the tissue substrate with RNase eliminated the antinuclear antibody reaction when caused by the presence of ribonucleoprotein antibody, however.[33,48,49]

Most investigations have shown that sera containing ribonucleoprotein antibodies in high titer and no Sm antibodies are usually found in patients with MCTD, are uncommon in patients with SLE or PSS, and are rare in patients with polymyositis, RA, or other rheumatic diseases.[11,34,38,46,48,49,55,57,61] That some patients with high ribonucleoprotein antibody titers initially appear to have another rheumatic disorder and then in several years develop additional clinical features typical of MCTD suggests a predictive value of this serologic pattern for evolving MCTD.[26,48,49,55,56,61]

The typical serologic pattern in MCTD includes high titers of speckled antinuclear antibodies, often >1:1000, high levels of antibody to RNase-sensitive ENA by hemagglutination, frequently >1,000,000, and ribonucleoprotein antibody by immunodiffusion. Sm antibodies and high antinative DNA titers are infrequent in MCTD, and their appearance usually correlates with a severe flare of SLE-like features.[15,19,22,56] Rheumatoid agglutinins occur in over half the patients with MCTD, and titers are often high.[48,61] Diffuse hypergammaglobulinemia, ranging from 2 to >5 g/dl, may be present.[1,48,49] Serum complement levels are usually normal or only modestly reduced.[21,48,49,61]

Rarely, patients with clinical features of MCTD have no ribonucleoprotein antibody initially.[2,22,48,49] This test may subsequently become positive, sometimes following corticosteroid therapy.[2,48,49] Such a serologic evolution may relate to the presence of circulating immune complexes, often detected by Raji cell or C1q binding assays; these immune complexes may bind available ribonucleoprotein antibody, with subsequent dissociation. Once present, high titers of circulating ribonucleoprotein antibody usually persist during periods of active and inactive disease, but in some patients, these antibody levels fall or become undetectable in 5 to 11 years.[56] This phenomenon is more often seen after prolonged remission, and is less frequent in active disease.

CLINICAL FEATURES

These features include prevalence, course, and specific clinical manifestations.

Prevalence and Clinical Course

Patients with MCTD show an age range of 4 to 80 years, with a mean of 37 years; approximately 80% of patients are female.[47,48,55] MCTD may occur as frequently as scleroderma, more commonly than polymyositis, and less frequently than SLE. Typical clinical features of MCTD (Table 64–1) include polyarthritis, Raynaud's phenomenon, swollen hands or sclerodactyly, pulmonary disease, muscle disease, and esophageal hypomotility.[56] Lymphadenopathy, alopecia, malar rash, serositis, and cardiac and renal disease are less frequent findings. No particular racial or ethnic distribution has been noted.

In some patients, the typical overlapping pattern is fully expressed when they are first evaluated. As physicians more fully appreciate the association of ribonucleoprotein antibody with MCTD however, larger numbers of cases are identified at an early phase of disease. Initially, minimal symptoms such as Raynaud's phenomenon, arthralgias, myalgias, and swollen hands may be insufficient to make a definitive diagnosis. This constellation of clinical findings has been referred to as *undifferentiated connective tissue disease*.[30,56] Long-term follow-up study reveals that this pattern may persist for years in some patients; in others it may progress to PSS, whereas yet other patients develop additional manifestations resulting in MCTD.[21,22,26,55,56] In one

Table 64–1. Characteristics of 34 Patients with Mixed Connective Tissue Disease

Characteristic	Number	Percentage
Raynaud's phenomenon	31	91
Polyarthritis	29	85
Swollen hands or sclerodactyly	29	85
Pulmonary disease	29	85
Inflammatory myositis	27	79
Esophageal hypomotility	25	74
Lymphadenopathy	17	50
Alopecia	13	41
Pleuritis	12	35
Malar rash	10	29
Renal disease	9	26
Cardiac disease	9	26
Anemia	8	24
Leukopenia	7	21
Diffuse scleroderma	7	21
Sjögren's syndrome	4	12
Trigeminal neuropathy	2	6
Positive antinuclear antibody	34	100
Positive ribonucleoprotein antibody	34	100
Positive rheumatoid agglutinins	20	59
Hypergammaglobulinemia	18	53
Hypocomplementemia	11	32
Positive LE cell test	6	18

(From Sullivan, W.D., et al.[56])

prospective study, 60% of patients were initially thought to have RA, PSS, SLE, polymyositis, or undifferentiated connective tissue disease[56] (Table 64–2). At their most recent evaluation, 91% demonstrated typical overlapping features of MCTD, whereas 9% maintained their undifferentiated status.

Specific Manifestations

Skin

Swelling of the hands and fingers occurs in over two-thirds of patients with MCTD and results in a tapered or "sausage" appearance[16,21,38,48,49,55] (Fig. 64–1). The skin may be taut and thick, with histologic changes of marked edema and increased dermal collagen content.[49] Scleroderma-like changes are occasionally extensive, but diffusely involved or tightly bound skin with contractures is rare.[48,49] In 40% of patients, lupus-like rashes occur, including: (1) malar eruptions; (2) diffuse, nonscarring erythematous lesions; and (3) chronic, scarring discoid lesions.[21,48,49,55] Other findings include alopecia, areas of hyper- and hypopigmentation, periungual telangiectasia, "squared" telangiectasia over the hands and face, violaceous discoloration of the eyelids, and erythema over the knuckles, elbows, or knees.[21,48,49,55] Severe necrotic and ulcerative skin changes are seen only rarely.[48,49] Immunoglobulin deposits at the dermal-epidermal junction have been noted in some patients.[21,49]

Raynaud's Phenomenon

Paroxysmal vasospasm of the fingers and, less often, toes occurs in approximately 85% of patients with MCTD and may precede other manifestations of the disease by months to years.[11,16,21,48,49,55] Severe vasospasm and ischemic necrosis or ulceration of the fingertips, common in PSS, are rare in MCTD.[21,49] Angiographic and histologic studies of digital arteries have not been reported.

Joints

Polyarthralgias occur in most patients, and frank arthritis is seen in about three-quarters of those affected.[7,24,48,49,55] Although the arthritis is usually nondeforming, its features may be similar to those of RA.[7,24,49] The metacarpophalangeal, proximal interphalangeal, and carpal joints are frequently affected. Subcutaneous nodules and roentgenographic evidence of erosive changes are occasionally observed.[26,49]

Muscles

Proximal muscles are commonly tender and weak, and serum levels of creatine phosphokinase and aldolase may be elevated at some point in the

Table 64–2. Transitions in Mixed Connective Tissue Disease Over Longitudinal Study

Disease Classification	No. Classified at Initial Medical Evaluation	No. Classified at Latest Medical Evaluation
Polymyositis	1	0
Progressive systemic sclerosis	2	0
Adult or juvenile rheumatoid arthritis	4	0
Systemic lupus erythematosus	6	0
Undifferentiated connective tissue disease	7	3
Mixed connective tissue disease	14	31

(From Sullivan, W.D., et al.[56])

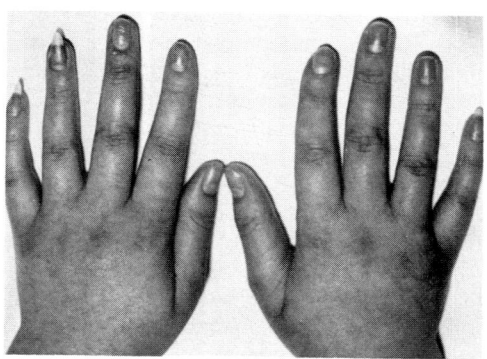

Fig. 64–1. Hands of a patient with mixed connective tissue disease demonstrating the tapered or sausage appearance of fingers and erythematous discoloration over the metacarpophalangeal, proximal interphalangeal, and distal interphalangeal joints.

course of MCTD.[37,38,48,49] Electromyographic findings are typical of inflammatory myositis, and biopsies reveal muscle fiber degeneration and perivascular and interstitial infiltration of plasma cells and lymphocytes.[37,48,49,54,55] Even in patients with only mild muscular weakness, histochemical and immunofluorescent analyses reveal perifascicular atrophy, type I fiber predominance, and immunoglobulin deposition within normal-appearing vessels, within normal fibers, around or on the sarcoplasmic membrane, or within the perimysial connective tissues.[37]

Esophagus

Esophageal abnormalities are frequent in MCTD.[16,48,49,60] Systematic studies of 35 patients by cine-esophagram or manometry revealed dysfunction in 80%, but 70% of these patients had no history of esophageal problems.[60] Decreased peristaltic amplitude in the distal two-thirds of the esophagus and reduced upper and lower esophageal sphincter pressures are characteristic changes. The severity of measured esophageal dysfunction appears to correlate with the duration of the disease, but not necessarily with the expression of symptoms.[55,60,61] Reflux esophagitis, sometimes leading to ulceration and stricture, may occur.

Lungs

Pulmonary dysfunction is usually clinically silent in the early phases of MCTD and may go undetected unless detailed evaluations are performed. A prospective study reported in 1976 showed that 80% of patients with MCTD had pulmonary disease, but 69% were asymptomatic.[25] Serial follow-up of those treated with corticosteroids revealed clinical and physiologic improvement in 12 of 14. It has since become apparent that pulmonary involvement in MCTD may lead to serious exertional dyspnea or to pulmonary hypertension, particularly in the later stages of the disease.[56]

Pulmonary hypertension associated with proliferative pulmonary vascular lesions was frequent and serious in a longitudinal evaluation of 34 individuals with MCTD.[56] The most common clinical finding was dyspnea, followed by pleuritic pain and bibasilar rales. Eight of 11 asymptomatic patients (73%) had abnormal pulmonary function tests or chest roentgenograms. Single-breath diffusing capacity (DLCO) was abnormal in 73%, and the vital capacity was reduced in 33%. Total lung capacity was low in 41%, and FEV_1 was abnormal in 17%; resting hypoxemia was present in 21% of patients. Thirty percent had *radiographic abnormalities* consisting of small, irregular opacities predominantly in the bases and middle regions.[56] These findings underscore that pulmonary involvement in MCTD is common and may be clinically inapparent until far advanced.

Right-heart catheterization was also performed on 15 of these patients. Ten had elevated pulmonary vascular resistance, and 10 had increased pulmonary artery pressure; wedge pressure was only abnormal in 1 patient. This study suggested that MCTD patients with features similar to those of PSS are more likely to develop pulmonary hypertension. Additionally, nailfold capillaroscopy in 3 of these patients showed severe capillary loop changes before pulmonary symptoms were present.

All 3 patients subsequently developed pulmonary vascular disease. Thus, *nailfold changes may predict pulmonary hypertension in MCTD*.

Heart

Cardiac involvement appears to be less common than pulmonary disease in adult MCTD, but it may be frequent in children.[48,49,55] Pericarditis is the most common cardiac abnormality reported.[5,35,55] In a prospective study of 37 adults with MCTD, pericarditis or pericardial effusion occurred in 10 patients, pulmonary hypertension was present in 10 of 15, and mitral valve prolapse occurred in 9 patients. Electrocardiographic abnormalities include arrhythmias, chamber enlargement, and conduction defects.[5] The prognostic significance of these cardiac findings is unclear.

Kidneys

Longer follow-up suggests that renal disease is more frequent in MCTD than initially thought. When isolated case reports are excluded, recent studies give a combined incidence of renal involvement of 28%, including children.[8,11,41,55] Glomerular deposition of immune complexes may be observed, although the patterns differ from those of SLE.[6,20] Patients with MCTD occasionally die of progressive renal failure.[8]

In a longitudinal study of MCTD, 6 patients had clinical evidence of renal disease manifested by proteinuria or hematuria; 1 developed the nephrotic syndrome.[56] Two renal biopsies showed focal glomerulonephritis. The kidney disease responded well to corticosteroid therapy, and renal failure did not occur. At autopsy, 3 patients who did not exhibit clinical manifestations of renal disease had proliferative vascular lesions similar to those noted in other organs; the glomeruli were normal in 2 of these patients, and mesangial thickening and hypercellularity were noted in the third. In a recent report,[54] 7 of 15 children with MCTD had clinical or histologic evidence of renal disease, and a patient in another study had died of "scleroderma kidney."[22] Comparable levels of circulating immune complexes in MCTD and SLE are observed,[19,23] but the clinical and histologic findings suggest that vascular lesions may represent a more serious problem than immune complex nephritis in MCTD.

Nervous System

Neurologic abnormalities, noted in only 10% of patients with MCTD, are not usually major management problems.[9,48,55] Trigeminal neuropathy is the most frequent finding.[48,61] Other observed problems include organic mental syndromes, "vascular" headaches, aseptic meningitis, seizures, encephalopathy, multiple peripheral neuropathies, and cerebral infarction or hemorrhage, probably related to hypertension and atherosclerosis.[9,10,13,48,55,61]

Blood

Anemia and leukopenia are found in a third of patients with MCTD.[16,48,49] Coombs-positive hemolytic anemia and significant thrombocytopenia are rare;[48,49] however, in a report of 14 children with MCTD, 6 had severe thrombocytopenia.[55] Two of these patients required splenectomy because persistent, severe thrombocytopenia, which had previously responded to corticosteroids, could only be controlled by 2 mg/kg/day prednisone. One child with thrombocytopenia died of an intracranial hemorrhage.

Other Findings

Sjögren's syndrome occurs frequently in MCTD,[18] and Hashimoto's thyroiditis and persistent hoarseness are observed occasionally in both children and adults.[54,61] Fever and lymphadenopathy occur in about one-third of patients.[21,47–49] Lymph nodes may be massively enlarged and may suggest a lymphoma, but biopsy reveals only lymphoid hyperplasia. Hepatomegaly and splenomegaly are possible, but serious liver function disturbances are uncommon. The intestinal tract may manifest hypomotility, pseudosacculation, dilatation, malabsorption, sclerosis, and perforation.[12,14,44] In one report, three patients with MCTD had extensive gastrointestinal changes similar to those found in PSS;[32] these changes have also been observed in children.[55]

CHILDHOOD DISEASE

Since 1973, 12 reports of pediatric MCTD have been published.[45,55] These studies encompass 39 children, with an additional 12 patients, <16 years of age, briefly mentioned in other reports but whose clinical features and treatment responses could not be isolated from the larger groups of adults. In a large pediatric rheumatic disease service, MCTD was 10% as frequent as SLE and occurred once for every 100 children with juvenile RA (JRA).[55] The median age of onset of MCTD in children is 10.8 years (range: 4 to 16 years); 29 girls and 10 boys have been reported.[27,39,53]

MCTD in children has several distinguishing features: (1) dermatomyositis and SLE-like rashes, which are more common than in adults;[6,55] (2) thrombocytopenia, which continues to be observed in about 25% of children with MCTD; (3) a higher frequency of cardiac disease, especially pericarditis, than in adult MCTD;[28,52,55] and (4) clinical and histologic evidence of renal disease, which is more common in pediatric MCTD.[28,36,55] In our experience, 5 of 16 children developed significant renal disease, including 2 who eventually required long-term hemodialysis.

Deforming but painless arthritis and the presence of rheumatoid factor are common in childhood MCTD.[6,36,55] The degree of synovitis is moderate, but complaints of discomfort are usually not marked in children; thus, responses to treatment may appear better than they actually are. Erosive disease is uncommon in children, but flexion contractures and deformity may occur.

Because Sjögren's syndrome is rare in children with rheumatic diseases, it is infrequently or incompletely sought in pediatric MCTD. At least half the children with MCTD have xerostomia, parotid gland enlargement, or keratoconjunctivitis sicca.[18,54] These findings suggest that salivary gland evaluation, Schirmer's test, and lip biopsy should be considered in all children with possible MCTD.

MCTD in children is frequently a sequential disease. The majority initially manifest Raynaud's phenomenon in association with polyarthritis. They then develop other features of MCTD, progressively, but not in any particular order. Serologic findings may also change over time, commensurate with the clinical situation. Thus, the absence of antinuclear antibodies and the presence of rheumatoid factor may be associated with early polyarthropathy, whereas anti-Sm antibodies may appear along with renal disease, hypocomplementemia, and other features of SLE.[54]

Many of the pediatric features of MCTD are initially clinically silent and may remain undetected unless carefully sought. The limited verbal skills, memory, and experiential understanding of children may magnify this observation. These asymptomatic features include the following: (1) minimal muscle disease with mild atrophy, moderate serum muscle enzyme elevations, and perhaps electromyographic changes, but with no significant proximal weakness; (2) esophageal dysfunction; (3) minimal alterations in bowel habits, related to early gastrointestinal tract involvement; and (4) pulmonary function test abnormalities found prior to complaints or roentgenographic changes. Children do not usually complain of dyspnea or shortness of breath. Thus, pulmonary function testing should be part of the routine evaluation of any child in whom a diagnosis of MCTD is considered. Pulmonary hypertension and idiopathic fibrosis must be recognized as potentially life-threatening in pediatric MCTD.[28,43,55]

HISTOLOGIC AND IMMUNOPATHOLOGIC FEATURES

Histologic Manifestations

The first comprehensive histologic investigation of MCTD reviewed material from 3 autopsies and from 5 additional renal biopsies.[54] The study group included 15 children with MCTD with a median age of disease onset of 10.7 years; the 3 who died had had the disease for 5.4 years before histologic evaluation. The age of these patients, the short duration of their disease, the absence of systemic or pulmonary hypertension, and the lack of corticosteroid treatment are relevant because, in adult patients, all would be variables that could cause, or reduce, the observed vasculopathy.

Widespread proliferative vascular lesions were the most prominent histopathologic features in the patients studied. All 3 children had diffuse vasculopathy; in combination, 9 organs (16%) revealed medial vessel wall thickening, and 31 of 58 organs (53%) had intimal proliferation (Fig. 64–2). These abnormalities occurred in large vessels such as the renal artery and aorta and within small arterioles. The frequency and severity of vascular compromise in organs without overt evidence of clinical involvement was striking and included coronary vessels, myocardium, aorta, lungs, intestinal tract, and kidney. Inflammatory infiltration of vessels was not a prominent feature.[54] Similar obstructive vascular lesions, particularly in the lungs, have now been described in MCTD in adults.[15,56,59] Thus, the presence of pulmonary hypertension in MCTD appears to be related to marked luminal vessel narrowing, rather than to interstitial fibrosis.

Other pathologic alterations in MCTD include prominent lymphocytic and plasmacytic infiltration of salivary glands, liver, and gastrointestinal tract, and a widespread inflammatory myopathy. Cardiac myopathy has been found in a few patients with MCTD,[5,54,58] but its prevalence is not yet known.

Our histopathologic understanding of MCTD is developing slowly. The absence of fibrinoid change, a predilection for large-vessel involvement, and minimal fibrosis all suggest fundamental differences from scleroderma. Evidence suggests a widespread but largely silent vasculopathy, cardiac and skeletal myopathy, membranoproliferative nephropathy, and pulmonary and gastrointestinal involvement in MCTD. Prospective histopathologic studies with serial treatment observations are necessary to determine whether current expectations of MCTD morbidity and mortality are overly optimistic.

Immunology

The immunologic aberrations identified in MCTD suggest that immune injury mechanisms are involved in the pathogenesis of the disease. The persistence of high titers of ribonucleoprotein antibody for many years and a marked polyclonal hypergammaglobulinemia indicate B-cell hyperactivity. In their studies of immune regulation in

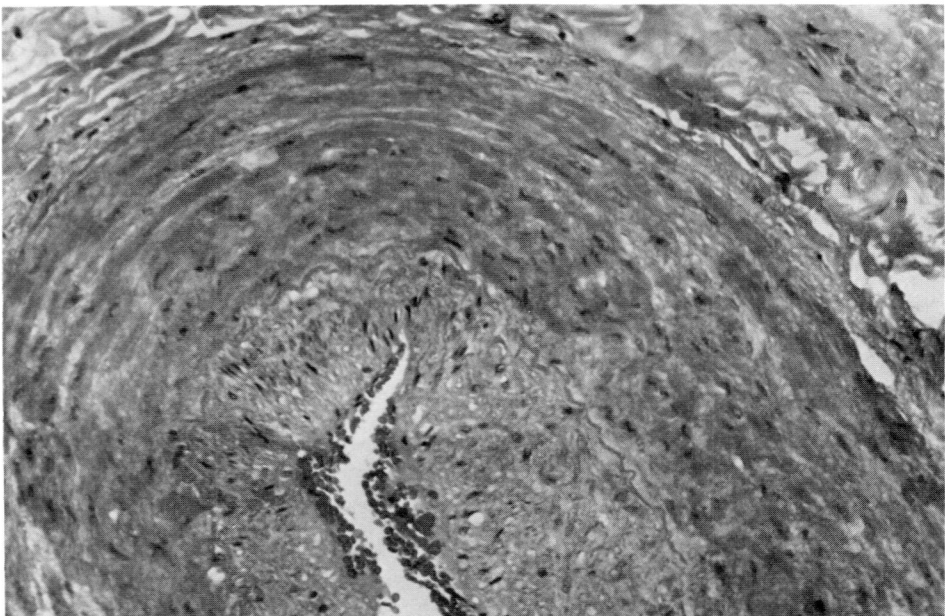

Fig. 64–2. Photomicrograph of a section of coronary artery from a 14-year-old boy with mixed connective tissue disease, showing intimal thickening, medial proliferation, and luminal narrowing. (Hematoxylin-eosin stain; magnification × 566.)

MCTD. Alarcon-Segovia and Palacios have demonstrated a defect at the level of helper T cells, either in their signaling to precursor cells for feedback inhibition or in the reception of suppressor signals from suppressor T cells.[3] Alarcon-Segovia and colleagues have also described a suppressor-T-cell defect possibly caused by a decreased stimulus from feedback inhibition or by the effect of anti-ribonucleoprotein antibodies, which can apparently penetrate living mononuclear cells through Fc receptors.[4] These abnormalities of immunoregulatory T-cell circuits in MCTD, different from those in SLE, Sjögren's syndrome, PSS, and RA, support the concept that MCTD is a distinct entity.[1] Other observations in patients with MCTD include reduced serum complement levels in about 25% of patients,[61] circulating immune complexes during active disease,[17,19,23] and deposition of IgG, IgM, and complement within muscle fibers, in the sarcolemmal-basement membrane region, in vascular walls, and along the glomerular basement membrane.[37,61]

Frank et al. recently studied 18 patients with MCTD. Most had active disease; only 4 had defective reticuloendothelial system Fc-specific immune clearance, although 17 had circulating immune complexes detected by Raji cell and C1q binding assays.[19] The 4 patients with defective clearance had an illness that, at that time, more closely resembled typical SLE, with antibodies to Sm or DNA, higher levels of immune complexes, glomerulonephritis, and severe skin lesions. Renal disease was absent in the 14 patients with normal clearance of the reticuloendothelial system. The maintenance of normal reticuloendothelial function in classic MCTD may enable these patients to clear immune complexes and thus to avoid serious renal damage.

TREATMENT AND PROGNOSIS

Treatment recommendations in MCTD have been based largely on anecdotal information because no controlled, long-term evaluations exist. Because MCTD is a progressive disease, different therapies may be appropriate for the same patient over a period of several years. For example, some children initially respond to intramuscular gold for JRA-like features, then improve with corticosteroids when proximal muscle weakness develops, and finally require cytotoxic agents for renal disease.[55]

Originally, MCTD was described as responsive to corticosteroids, although a few patients who did not respond to high doses of corticosteroids improved after the addition of cyclophosphamide. Further observations, however, do not support a uniformly optimistic outlook. In extended investigations, almost two-thirds of patients have responded favorably to treatment.[56] Patients with scleroderma-like features are the least likely to respond. A potentially good long-term prognosis for MCTD is demonstrated by the 13 of 34 (38%) patients studied who have inactive disease, including 10 who have not required therapy for 1 to 8 years (mean 5 years). Inflammatory changes are likely to respond to corticosteroids, whereas pulmonary, sclerodermatous, and esophageal lesions are less likely to respond.

Thirty-six percent of our patients have had less corticosteroid-responsive, more severe illness, including four patients who died. Pulmonary hypertension and widespread proliferative vasculopathy are major complications of MCTD that are emerging from several investigations. The pulmonary hypertension may or may not respond to corticosteroids or immunosuppressive agents, but without controlled studies, the most effective therapies remain uncertain.

Patterns of organ system involvement may be a useful way in which to consider treatment of MCTD. Arthritis may occur well before other overlapping manifestations suggest MCTD.[24] As the erosive and deforming potential of MCTD has been better recognized, so has the value of the early addition of remittive agents such as gold and penicillamine. The arthritis has responded to nonsteroidal anti-inflammatory drugs in some centers,[7] but others have not had similar success.[40] Rash, serositis, anemia, leukopenia, fever, and lymphadenopathy commonly improve within days to weeks of adding corticosteroids.[47] An inflammatory myopathy may require higher doses (1 to 2 mg/kg) or longer periods of treatment.*

The therapeutic response of other organ systems is more difficult to characterize. Pericarditis and pleuritis in MCTD apparently respond well to corticosteroids.[14] Pulmonary disease in general may improve with corticosteroids;[25] interstitial and restrictive lung disease may improve,[27] or it may not.[13] In addition, pulmonary hypertension does not uniformly respond to combinations of corticosteroids and cytotoxic agents.[28,43,56,59] Renal involvement due to MCTD may lead to the use of high doses of corticosteroids, possibly in association with cytotoxic agents. Most patients show at least some degree of response to corticosteroids, but the outcome is not uniformly predictable among the few patients treated with cytotoxic agents.

It is not clear whether gastrointestinal aspects of MCTD respond to therapy. One study showed improved esophageal motility in 8 of 14 cases as a result of corticosteroid therapy for other manifestations of the disease.[60] Several descriptions of the intestinal manifestations of MCTD exist, but indications of treatment response are lacking.[12,32,44]

Initial estimations of the prognosis of MCTD suggested a mild disease.[49] A more severe prognosis was first mentioned in the pediatric literature;[54,55] of particular concern were cardiac disease, life-threatening thrombocytopenia, and renal involvement. The proximate causes of death were infection in three, and cerebral hemorrhage in one patient. The infections, caused by encapsulated organisms (pneumococcal in two patients and meningococcal in one), were rapidly fatal and were not related to significant corticosteroid doses.

The current prognosis for MCTD can be projected from the data in 5 recent studies with long-term, sequential assessment.[22,31,48,54,56] Nimelstein et al. observed that 6 of 8 deaths were not directly related to a rheumatic disorder.[31] Pulmonary hypertension, other lung disease, and heart failure were major factors in another 4 reported deaths;[22] a fifth death was due to squamous cell carcinoma of the lung. In a recent investigation, 4 deaths were related to MCTD; contributing factors included pulmonary hypertension and cor pulmonale in 3 patients, pericardial tamponade in 1, perforated bowel in 2, and sepsis in 3. The combined mortality rate from these 5 reports (194 patients) was 13%, with the mean disease duration varying from 6 to 12 years.

As they have developed over time, the observations of MCTD morbidity and mortality suggest that early predictions must be modified. In both adults and children, the prognosis of MCTD is generally similar to that of SLE, but it is better than that of scleroderma. Our understanding of ideal therapy for MCTD, morbidity, and outcome all remain uncertain. Treatment protocols and longitudinal prospective assessments of this illness should all improve the care of patients with MCTD.

In conclusion, the debate over whether MCTD constitutes a distinct clinical entity has not been resolved, but some recent investigations support the unique nature of this disease. Features that appear to distinguish MCTD include the following: (1) abnormalities of immunoregulatory T-cell circuits in MCTD that differ from those found in other rheumatic diseases; (2) high titers of ribonucleoprotein antibody, usually in the absence of significant titers of other antibodies; (3) normal clearance of the reticuloendothelial system of immune complexes in most patients with MCTD, in contrast to SLE; (4) frequent pulmonary hypertension and a unique proliferative vasculopathy; and (5) other pathologic changes that may be restricted to MCTD such as widespread plasmacytic and lymphocytic

---

*Editor's Note: Intravenous methotrexate, 1 to 2 mg/kg/week, has effectively controlled myositis in our MCTD patients.

infiltration of tissues, an absence of fibrosis, and a distinctive hyalinization of the esophagus.

From our perspective, however, the current status of MCTD as a distinct entity is not the most critical issue. As clinical, serologic, and pathologic characteristics of these patients have become known and as reports of prognosis have begun to appear, certain repetitive patterns have emerged. First, the initially limited, undifferentiated connective tissue disease frequently becomes more widespread and typical of MCTD, and clinical and serologic transitions are observed during longitudinal study. Second, MCTD usually evolves gradually and, during the early phases, biopsies of tissues and functional tests often reveal abnormalities prior to the advent of clinical symptoms. Third, certain organs and tissues, such as the lung, the esophagus, and muscle, are at higher risk for pathologic involvement. Fourth, many manifestations of this disease initially respond to corticosteroids, but the scleroderma-like findings, which are the most resistant to treatment, may become the dominant clinical features later in the course of MCTD. Finally, although the prognosis remains favorable, a significant percentage of MCTD patients develop serious and sometimes fatal complications of pulmonary hypertension and proliferative vascular lesions.

The most significant outcome of the continuing controversy surrounding MCTD is the stimulus to further investigation. The numerous immunopathologic abnormalities of MCTD indicate that immune-injury mechanisms may play an important role in this disease. Environmental, genetic, hormonal, and immunologic factors probably determine whether patients will continue to have a prolonged, benign undifferentiated rheumatic disorder or will develop major organ-system involvement typical of MCTD, or whether the disease will become more typical of SLE or PSS. The MRL mouse model, which has some features in common with MCTD, may permit incisive investigation of some of these factors. The MRL mouse has already provided a means of producing monoclonal antibodies to ribonucleoprotein, Sm, and other nuclear antigens.

Finally, an unexpected but remarkable consequence of the investigations stimulated by MCTD has been the demonstration that Sm, ribonucleoprotein, and other nuclear acidic protein antigens may have central roles in cell biology, such as in the processing of messenger RNA.[29] Thus, just as the detection of the monoclonal proteins of multiple myeloma stimulated an elucidation of immunoglobulin structure and function, so the autoantibodies to ribonucleoprotein, Sm, and other nuclear acidic protein antigens occurring in MCTD and other rheumatic diseases have facilitated the purification, biochemical characterization, and study of these nuclear antigens and their biologic roles.

REFERENCES

1. Alarcon-Segovia, D.: Mixed connective tissue disease—a decade of growing pains. (Editorial). J. Rheumatol., 8:535–540, 1981.
2. Alarcon-Segovia, D.: Mixed connective tissue disease: appearance of antibodies to ribonucleoprotein following corticosteroid treatment. J. Rheumatol., 6:694–699, 1979.
3. Alarcon-Segovia, D., and Palacios, R.: Human postthymic precursor cells in health and disease. IV. Abnormalities in immunoregulatory T cell circuits in mixed connective tissue disease. Arthritis Rheum., 24:1486–1494, 1981.
4. Alarcon-Segovia, D., Ruiz-Arguelles, A., and Fishbein, E.: Antibody to nuclear ribonucleoprotein penetrates live human mononuclear cells through Fc receptors. Nature, 271:67–69, 1978.
5. Alpert, M.A., et al.: Cardiovascular manifestations of mixed connective tissue disease in adults. Circulation, 68:1182–1193, 1983.
6. Baldassare, A., et al.: Mixed connective tissue disease (MCTD) in children. Arthritis Rheum., 19:788, 1976.
7. Bennett, R.M., and O'Connell, D.J.: The arthritis of mixed connective tissue disease. Ann. Rheum. Dis., 37:397–403, 1978.
8. Bennett, R.M., and Spargo, B.H.: Immune complex nephropathy in mixed connective tissue disease. Am. J. Med., 63:534–541, 1977.
9. Bennett, R.M., Bong, D.M., and Spargo, B.H.: Neuropsychiatric problems in mixed connective tissue disease. Am. J. Med., 65:955–962, 1978.
10. Bernstein, R.F.: Ibuprofen-related meningitis in mixed connective tissue disease. Ann. Intern. Med., 92:206–207, 1980.
11. Bresnihan, B., et al.: Antiribonucleoprotein antibodies in connective tissue diseases: estimation by counter-immunoelectrophoresis. Br. Med. J., 1:610–611, 1977.
12. Cooke, C.L., and Lurie, H.I.: Case report: Fatal gastrointestinal hemorrhage in mixed connective tissue disease. Arthritis Rheum., 20:1421–1427, 1977.
13. Cryer, P.F., and Kissane, J.M. (Eds.): Clinicopathologic Conference. Mixed connective tissue disease. Am. J. Med., 65:833–842, 1978.
14. Davis, J.D., Parker, M.D., and Turner, R.A.: Exacerbation of mixed connective tissue disease during salmonella gastroenteritis–serial immunological findings. J. Rheumatol., 5:96–98, 1978.
15. Esther, J.H., et al.: Pulmonary hypertension in patients with mixed connective tissue disease and antibody to nuclear ribonucleoprotein. Arthritis Rheum., 24:S105, 1981.
16. Farber, S.J., and Bole, G.G.: Antibodies to components of extractable nuclear antigen. Arch. Intern. Med., 136:425–431, 1976.
17. Fishbein, E., Alarcon-Segovia, D., and Ramos-Niembro, F.: Free serum ribonucleoprotein (RNP) in mixed connective tissue disease (MCTD). In Proceedings of the Fourteenth International Congress on Rheumatology, San Francisco, 1977.
18. Fraga, A., et al.: Mixed connective tissue disease in childhood. Relationship with Sjögren's syndrome. Am. J. Dis. Child., 132:263–265, 1978.
19. Frank, M.M., et al.: Immunoglobulin G Fc receptor-mediated clearance in autoimmune disease. Ann. Intern. Med., 98:206–218, 1983.
20. Fuller, T.J., et al.: Immune-complex glomerulonephritis in a patient with mixed connective tissue disease. Am. J. Med., 62:761–764, 1977.
21. Gilliam, J.N., and Prystowsky, S.D.: Mixed connective tissue disease syndrome: the cutaneous manifestations of patients with epidermal nuclear staining and high titer antibody to RNAase sensitive extractable nuclear antigen (ENA). Arch. Dermatol., 113:583–587, 1977.
22. Grant, K.D., Adams, L.E., and Hess, E.V.: Mixed connective tissue disease—a subset with sequential clinical and laboratory features. J. Rheumatol., 8:587–598, 1981.

23. Halla, J.T., et al.: Circulating immune complexes in mixed connective tissue disease (MCTD). Arthritis Rheum., 21:562–563, 1978.
24. Halla, J.T., and Hardin, J.G.: Clinical features of the arthritis of mixed connective tissue disease. Arthritis Rheum., 21:497–503, 1978.
25. Harmon, C., et al.: Pulmonary involvement in mixed connective tissue disease (MCTD). Arthritis Rheum., 19:801, 1976.
26. Hench, P.K., Edgington, T.S., and Tan, E.M.: The evolving clinical spectrum of mixed connective tissue disease (MCTD). Arthritis Rheum., 18:404, 1975.
27. Hepburn, B.: Multiple antinuclear antibodies in mixed connective tissue disease: report of a patient with an unusual antibody profile. J. Rheumatol., 8:635–638, 1981.
28. Jones, M.B., et al.: Fatal pulmonary hypertension and resolving immune-complex glomerulonephritis in mixed connective tissue disease. A case report and review of the literature. Am. J. Med., 65:855–863, 1978.
29. Lerner, M.R., et al.: Are snRNP's involved in splicing? Nature, 283:220–224, 1980.
30. LeRoy, E.C., Maricq, H.R., and Kahaleh, M.B.: Undifferentiated connective tissue syndromes. Arthritis Rheum., 23:341–343, 1980.
31. Nimelstein, S.H., et al.: Mixed connective tissue disease: a subsequent evaluation of the original 25 patients. Medicine, 59:239–248, 1980.
32. Norman, D.A., and Fleischmann, R.M.: Gastrointestinal systemic sclerosis in serologic mixed connective tissue disease. Arthritis Rheum., 21:811–819, 1978.
33. Northway, J.S., and Tan, E.M.: Differentiations of antinuclear antibodies giving speckled staining patterns in immunofluorescence. Clin. Immunol. Immunopathol., 1:140–154, 1972.
34. Notman, D.D., Kurata, N., and Tan, E.M.: Profiles of antinuclear antibodies in systemic rheumatic diseases. Ann. Intern. Med., 83:464–469, 1975.
35. Oetgen, W.J., et al.: Cardiac abnormalities in mixed connective tissue disease. Chest, 2:185–188, 1983.
36. Oetgen, W.J., Boice, J.A., and Lawless, O.J.: Mixed connective tissue disease in children and adolescents. Pediatrics, 67:333–337, 1981.
37. Oxenhandler, R., et al.: Pathology of skeletal muscle in mixed connective tissue disease. Arthritis Rheum., 20:985–988, 1977.
38. Parker, M.D.: Ribonucleoprotein antibodies: frequencies and clinical significance in systemic lupus erythematosus, scleroderma and mixed connective tissue disease. J. Lab. Clin. Med., 82:769–775, 1973.
39. Peskett, S.A., et al.: Mixed connective tissue disease in children. Rheumatol. Rehabil., 17:245–248, 1978.
40. Ramos-Niembro, F., Alarcon-Segovia, D., and Hernandez-Ortiz, J.: Articular manifestations of mixed connective tissue disease. Arthritis Rheum., 22:43–51, 1979.
41. Rao, K.V., et al.: Immune complex nephritis in mixed connective tissue disease. Ann. Intern. Med., 84:174–176, 1976.
42. Reichlin, M., and Mattioli, M.: Correlation of a precipitin reaction to an RNA protein antigen and low prevalence of nephritis in patients with systemic lupus erythematosus. N. Engl. J. Med., 286:908–911, 1972.
43. Rosenberg, A.M., et al.: Pulmonary hypertension in a child with mixed connective tissue disease. J. Rheumatol., 6:700–704, 1979.
44. Samach, M., Brandt, L.J., and Bernstein, L.H.: Spontaneous pneumoperitoneum with pneumatosis cystoides intestinalis in a patient with mixed connective tissue disease. Am. J. Gastroenterol. 69:494–500, 1978.
45. Sanders, D.Y., Huntley, C.C., and Sharp, G.C.: Mixed connective tissue disease. J. Pediatr., 83:642–645, 1973.
46. Sharp, G.C.: Subsets of SLE and mixed connective tissue disease. Am. J. Kidney Dis., 2:201–205, 1982.
47. Sharp, G.C.: Mixed connective tissue disease. Bull. Rheum. Dis., 25:828–831, 1975.
48. Sharp, G.C., et al.: Association of antibodies to ribonucleoprotein and Sm antigens with mixed connective tissue disease, systemic lupus erythematosus and other rheumatic diseases. N. Engl. J. Med., 295:1149–1154, 1976.
49. Sharp, G.C., et al.: Mixed connective tissue disease. An apparently distinct rheumatic disease syndrome associated with a specific antibody to an extractable nuclear antigen (ENA). Am. J. Med., 52:148–159, 1972.
50. Sharp, G.C., et al.: Specificity of antibodies to extractable nuclear antigens (ENA) in mixed connective tissue disease (MCTD) and systemic lupus erythematosus (SLE). Arthritis Rheum., 15:125, 1972.
51. Sharp, G.C., et al.: Association of autoantibodies to different nuclear antigens with clinical patterns of rheumatic disease and responsiveness to therapy. J. Clin. Invest., 50:350–359, 1971.
52. Silver, T.M., et al.: Radiological features of mixed connective tissue disease and scleroderma-systemic lupus erythematosus overlap. Radiology, 120:269–275, 1976.
53. Singsen, B.H.: Mixed connective tissue disease, scleroderma and morphea in childhood. In Brenneman's Textbook of Pediatrics. Edited by R. Wedgwood. New York, Harper & Row Publishers, 1981.
54. Singsen, B.H., et al.: A histologic evaluation of mixed connective tissue disease in childhood. Am. J. Med., 68:710–717, 1980.
55. Singsen, B.H., et al.: Mixed connective tissue disease in childhood. A clinical and serologic survey. J. Pediatr., 90:893–900, 1977.
56. Sullivan, W.D., et al.: A prospective evaluation emphasizing pulmonary involvement in patients with mixed connective tissue disease. Medicine, 63:92–107, 1984.
57. Tan, E.M., et al.: Diversity of antinuclear antibodies in progressive systemic sclerosis. Arthritis Rheum., 23:617–625, 1980.
58. Whitlow, P.L., Gilliam, J.N., and Chubick, A.: Myocarditis in mixed connective tissue disease. Am. J. Med., 65:955–962, 1978.
59. Wiener-Kronish, J.P., et al.: Severe pulmonary involvement in mixed connective tissue disease. Am. Rev. Respir. Dis., 124:499–503, 1981.
60. Winn, D., et al.: Esophageal function in steroid treated patients with mixed connective tissue disease (MCTD). Clin. Res., 24:545A, 1976.
61. Wolfe, J.F., et al.: Disease pattern in patients with antibodies only to nuclear ribonucleoprotein (RNP). Clin. Res., 25:488A, 1977.

Chapter 65

Polymyositis/Dermatomyositis

Lawrence J. Kagen

Polymyositis and dermatomyositis are acquired, chronic, inflammatory muscle disorders of unknown cause. They occur in children and adults and are manifested by disability due to muscle weakness. A characteristic rash distinguishes dermatomyositis from polymyositis.

Although inflammation of muscle may develop in the course of other connective tissue disorders such as progressive systemic sclerosis, systemic lupus erythematosus, and Sjögren's syndrome, the terms polymyositis and dermatomyositis are reserved for the clinical situations in which chronic inflammatory myopathy is the dominant element in the absence of features diagnostic of other illness.

Symmetric proximal muscle weakness and histologic findings of inflammation and myofiber damage of muscle tissue, accompanied by evidence of increased amounts of certain sarcoplasmic constituents in the circulation and electrophysiologic signs of myopathy, are the chief clinical manifestations, along with characteristic changes of the skin in patients with dermatomyositis. In severe cases, impairment of deglutition and cardiorespiratory complications contribute to morbidity. Malignant neoplasms may be found in patients with myositis and may further complicate the outcome.

CLASSIFICATION

Several schemes for the classification of patients with inflammatory myopathy have been devised for the purpose of segregating patients into groups to study cause, prognosis and response to therapy more efficiently.[12,153] Patients with polymyositis are usually grouped separately from those with dermatomyositis, malignant diseases, and other connective tissue disorders. Because of factors discussed later in this chapter, dermatomyositis of childhood also has its own category. Attempts to classify a disease without knowledge of its cause and with incomplete knowledge of its pathogenesis may be flawed and are subject to revision, however. In this light, Table 65–1 presents a grouping of patients with polymyositis, for purposes of discussion and further study.

In general, a female preponderance exists in myositis, especially in patients with features of

Table 65–1. Classification of Inflammatory Muscle Disease

1. Polymyositis
2. Dermatomyositis
3. Dermatomyositis of childhood
4. Myositis with neoplasm
5. Myositis with other connective tissue disorders, such as progressive systemic sclerosis, systemic lupus erythematosus, Sjögren's syndrome, and rheumatoid arthritis

other connective tissue disorders. This preponderance is also present in the dermatomyositis and polymyositis groups, however (Table 65–2). No female preponderance is found in childhood dermatomyositis or in adults with myositis associated with neoplasia.

Although inflammatory muscle disease may occur at any age, most cases are noted in the fifth and sixth decades of life. In a survey of 380 reported cases, 17% were age 15 or younger, 14% were from age 15 to age 30, and 60% were between the ages 30 and 60. An additional 9% of patients were over age 60.[124]

Although rare, inflammatory myopathy has been reported in infants less than a year old.[148] In this situation, recognition of myositis and its distinction from congenital myopathies are important because corticosteroid therapy is valuable in the treatment of infants with myositis.

These disorders generally occur less frequently than certain other connective tissue syndromes. The incidence of dermatomyositis and polymyositis has been estimated at 0.5 cases per 100,000 population in a racially mixed area of Tennessee over a 22-year period. Ethnic or racial factors are important, and the highest frequency is noted in black women.[105] An English survey over a 20-year period indicated a prevalence of 8 cases per 100,000. The application of these figures to all populations is not precise; however, it is now estimated that 1 to 5 new cases per million population occur each year in the United States, with a frequency perhaps 4 times as great among black women.[37,105,122] As suggested in Table 65–2, the incidence in adults is greater than in children.

Table 65–2. Distribution of Patients by Group and Sex

Group	No. of Patients	Percentage of Total (%)	Percentage of Female Patients (%)
Polymyositis	52	34	69
Dermatomyositis	45	29	58
Dermatomyositis of childhood	11	7	36
Myositis with neoplasm	13	8.5	57
Myositis with overlap features of other connective tissue disorders	32	21	90

(Based on 153 patients reviewed by Bohan, A., et al.[11])

CLINICAL FEATURES

Muscle Weakness

Muscular weakness is the dominant feature of myositis syndromes, with symmetric involvement of proximal muscles of the extremities, trunk, and neck. Difficulty with the lower extremities is often first characterized by an inability to climb stairs, to arise from a low seat or a squat, and to cross the legs. Walking may be limited, and gait may become poorly coordinated and waddling. Weakness of the upper extremities limits lifting, hanging up clothes, and combing the hair. Weakness of the anterior neck flexor muscles interferes with lifting the head from the supine position, and arising from bed becomes difficult. Severely affected patients may have difficulty in swallowing and liquids may be regurgitated through the nose. Along with weakness and muscle pain, soreness with tenderness may be noted, particularly in patients whose disease progresses rapidly. Although weakness may be marked, little atrophy occurs initially. With time, affected muscles may lose volume, and involvement may become more generalized and may include distal muscles. The patient's speech may be altered and may assume a nasal quality. Whereas virtually all patients have proximal muscle weakness, few progress to distal involvement or have impaired swallowing or speech. Dysphagia occurs in approximately 10 to 15% of patients.[11] Facial involvement is rare.[121]

Because weakness is the central cause of morbidity in patients with myositis, ongoing assessment of muscle strength is of prime importance in clinical evaluation. One must therefore combine careful questioning, to record changes in functional capabilities, with muscle strength testing. The most common muscle testing schemes employ a semi-quantitative grading system (Table 65–3). The ability to assess muscle strength accurately is limited by several factors. First, one must be certain that the patient's effort is his best. Pain, fatigue, and malaise may interfere with full cooperation and may invalidate the results of the assessment. In

Table 65–3. Scheme for Testing Manual Muscle Strength

Grade	
0	No evident contraction
1	Trace of contraction
2	Poor—movement with gravity eliminated
3	Fair—movement against gravity
4	Good—movement against resistance
5	Normal

(Modified from Gardner-Medwin, D., and Walton, J.N.[60])

addition, variables related to the observer also can be a factor. The joint position in which the test is done should be recorded because it affects muscle length and mechanical advantage and the resultant tension. For example, knee extensor muscles tested at a 60° angle of knee flexion (full extension is 0°) have greater force than at a 30° position. The differences between grades 4 and 5 of muscle strength are significant, but they are difficult to quantify precisely. The position of the examiner's hand during the procedure should also be recorded, owing to considerations of mechanical advantage and lever arm length. Finally, tests of this nature are most useful for muscle groups of the extremities. For other muscles, such as of the torso, additional testing methods must be used.

To approach some of the observer-related variables, as well as to standardize and to increase reproducibility and sensitivity, several attempts have been made to introduce biomechanical methods and instruments into the clinical setting. The importance of such measurements has been stressed by Edwards and colleagues, who have reported that muscle strength correlates with metabolic studies of net losses and gains in total muscle mass and may be a better guide to progress than other laboratory measures.[45,159] Figure 65–1 demonstrates the use of biomechanical strength testing in a patient with polymyositis during initial therapy with prednisone. Torque production, an indicator of muscle strength, of the quadriceps mechanism rose after six to seven weeks of prednisone therapy and was associated with a fall in serum creatine kinase activity, as well as with gains in functional ability.

A rapid method for evaluation of lower extremity strength has been standardized for men and women of various ages.[23a] It permits "fine-tuning" of therapy for myositis.

Rash

The rash of dermatomyositis appears on the face, neck, chest, and extremities (Figs. 65–2 to 65–5). It is most common over the extensor surfaces of the extremities, particularly over the dorsum of the hands and the fingers. The rash is deep red and is slightly raised in small plaques over the wrists and knuckles. A whitish scale may be seen superficially. Similar patches occur over the elbows, the

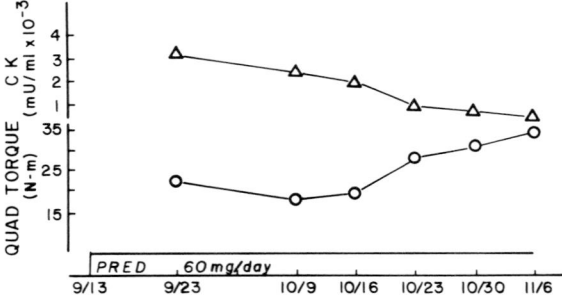

Fig. 65–1. The use of biomechanical measurement of muscle strength during the course of polymyositis. Strength is recorded as the torque (force × lever arm) produced by the knee extensors (quadriceps femoris). This patient demonstrates an increase in strength concomitant with a fall in serum creatine kinase (CK) level after treatment with prednisone (pred). (Data from Dr. J. Otis and Mr. M. Kroll.)

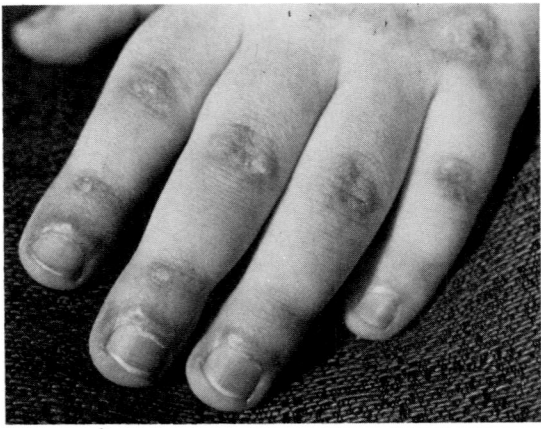

Fig. 65–2. The rash of dermatomyositis over the hand of a child. Patches of erythematous, scaly plaques over knuckles, as well as periungual changes, are evident.

knees, and the medial malleoli of the ankles. Involvement of the scalp, upper arms, and outer thighs also occurs. At the nail beds, one sees hyperemia, telangiectasia, and with more marked involvement, destruction of the architecture of the nail bed. Dilated capillary loops at the nail fold as well as over the knuckles and other areas of the fingers may be seen.[100] Cutaneous vasculitis, evidenced clinically by tender nodules, periungual infarctions, and digital ulcerations, has been noted in both adult and childhood dermatomyositis. In the adult, these lesions are less common and may be associated with an underlying malignant process. In a group of 76 adults studied, 7 had lesions of this nature, and 2 of these had an underlying malignant disease (28%). Of the total number of patients with malignant disease, 2 of 6 had these lesions.[50] A deep violet red rash may be present on the face, particularly in the periorbital areas, which may also be edematous. Involvement is most prominent over the upper eyelids, and scaling may also occur here. Lilac suffusion or *heliotrope rash* over the upper eyelids is characteristic of dermatomyositis. A similar deep red-to-violaceous rash may appear on the forehead, neck, shoulders, and chest.

Although the heliotrope rash is characteristic, it is not absolutely diagnostic. Similar changes may occur in patients with allergic manifestations and during the course of trichinosis. A characteristic rash of this type has also been described in a patient with sarcoidosis and myopathy.[76]

Rash may appear before other signs of myopathy become manifest. As extreme examples, six patients with classic heliotrope discoloration of the periorbital area with edema and a maculopapular violaceous rash over the interphalangeal joints with periungual telangiectasia did not develop clinical evidence of muscle involvement until months to years later.[92]

Histologic evaluation of skin biopsies in dermatomyositis reveals poikiloderma, that is, epidermal atrophy with liquefaction, degeneration of the basal cell layer, and vascular dilatation. Inflammatory infiltrates, composed of perivascular accumulations of lymphocytes and histiocytes in the upper dermis, are found along with few polymorphonuclear cells and occasional infiltrates around the pilosebaceous apparatus. Hyperkeratosis, dermal edema with increased deposits of mucin, and evidence of subcutaneous panniculitis may also be found.[79] Vascular endothelial changes characteristic of childhood dermatomyositis may be present in the skin (see the discussion on histology later in this chapter).

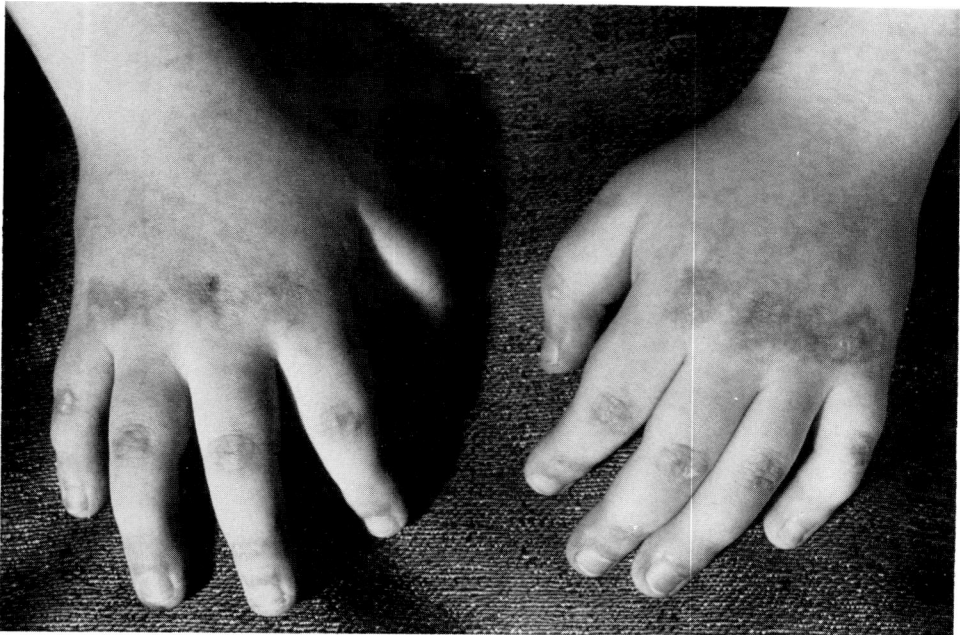

Fig. 65–3. Dermatomyositis, showing a raised, reddened rash over the dorsum of the hands.

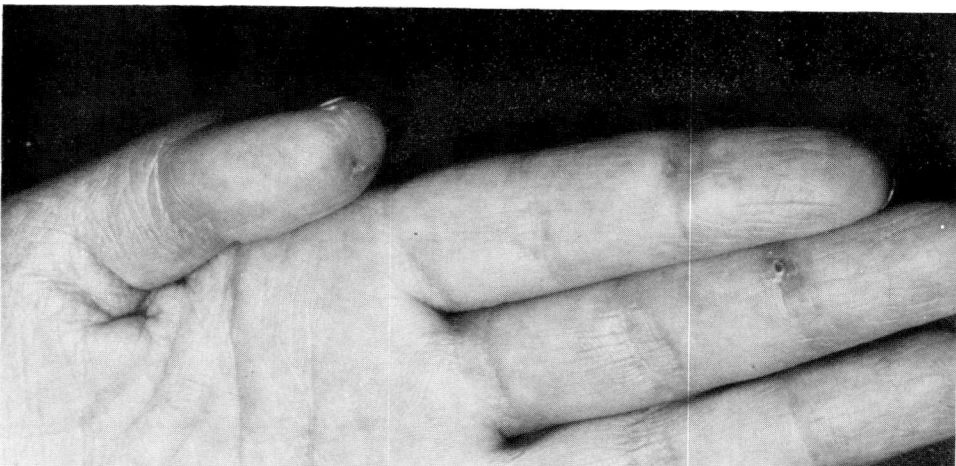

Fig. 65–4. Punched-out ulcerated skin lesions over the volar surface of the hands (at the tip of the thumb and at the terminal creases of the second and third fingers) in a patient with dermatomyositis and adenocarcinoma of the large intestine.

Dysphagia

Difficulty in swallowing may arise from several factors in patients with myositis. Decreased strength of pharyngeal contractions, disordered peristalsis, vallecular pooling, and weakness of the tongue may all interfere with normal swallowing. Patients with severe weakness of this type may also have difficulties in elevation of the palate and may have nasal speech. In addition, dysfunction of the cricopharyngeus muscle with spasm and improperly timed closure may occur in some patients and may accentuate symptoms. The importance of recognizing cricopharyngeal dysfunction due to constriction, fibrosis, or abnormal contraction lies in the possibility of surgical relief of obstruction. Appropriate investigation should be conducted in patients with dysphagia to determine to what extent cricopharyngeal dysfunction may be a complicating factor.[38]

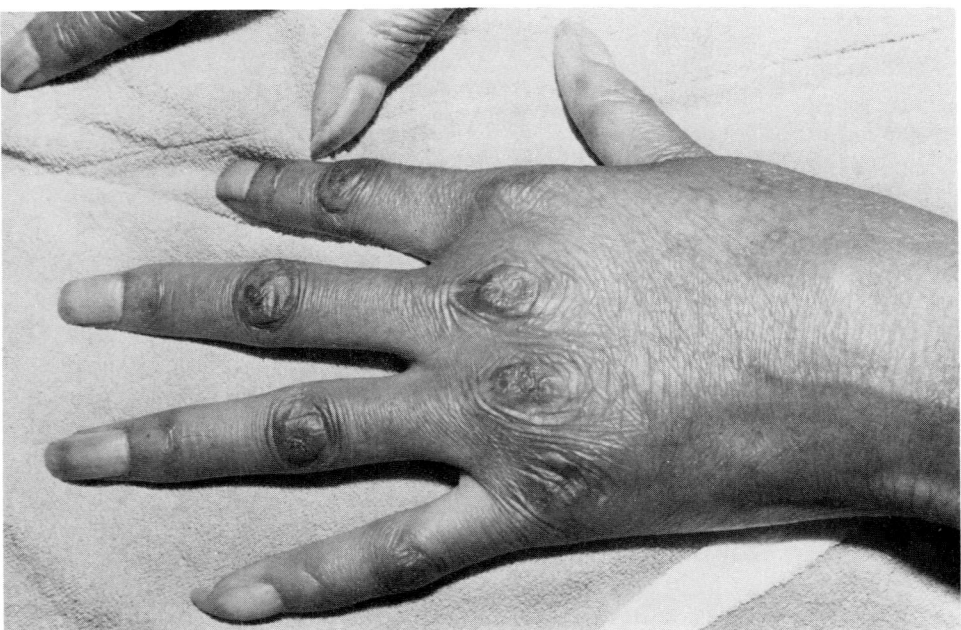

Fig. 65–5. Papular, raised rash of the knuckle above the metacarpophalangeal and proximal interphalangeal joints in a patient with chronic dermatomyositis.

Although found in only 10 to 15% of patients,[11] dysphagia is usually associated with severe disease and a poor prognosis.

Pulmonary Manifestations

Several factors, including hypoventilation secondary to muscular weakness, infectious agents, aspiration in association with abnormalities in swallowing, and rarely, drug hypersensitivity, such as related to methotrexate,[3] may play a role in the association of pulmonary disease and myositis. In addition to these factors, interstitial pulmonary fibrosis or fibrosing alveolitis may be a significant feature of myositis syndromes.

Pulmonary fibrosis has been noted in 5 to 10% of patients, generally by roentgenography. The frequency of this disorder seems unrelated to a previous history of cigarette smoking and does not have the female preponderance seen in adults with myositis. Pulmonary function tests indicate restriction of ventilation with reduction of total lung capacity and vital capacity. Hypoxemia may be characterized by a moderate reduction in diffusing capacity. Dyspnea and cough are the major symptoms, and physical examination may reveal the presence of fine, crepitant, basilar rales. In approximately half the affected patients, pulmonary abnormalities are noted prior to the appearance of myopathy.

Alveolar septal fibrosis, interstitial mononuclear cell infiltrates containing mainly lymphocytes with smaller numbers of large mononuclear cells and plasma cells, hyperplasia of the type I alveolar epithelial cells, and increased numbers of free alveolar macrophages are seen histologically. These findings may be irregularly distributed, intermixed with areas of apparently uninvolved lung. Interstitial edema and vascular change marked by intimal and medial thickening of arteries and arterioles may also be evident. Chest roentgenograms may show diffuse, linear, interstitial thickening, with an alveolar pattern of fibrosis. Patchy consolidation and "honeycomb" changes indicate more chronic and severe involvement. These changes may be associated with right-ventricular enlargement and with prominent hilar markings. Corticosteroid therapy may be followed by relief of dyspnea and by improvements in radiographic changes and abnormalities of pulmonary function, but some patients show no improvement. Therapeutic response may be better in patients with acute illness and lung biopsies showing inflammation of the alveolar wall, whereas fibrosis in the absence of inflammation is a sign of a poorer prognosis. Rapidly progressive, fatal pulmonary insufficiency may occur despite the early introduction of corticosteroid treatment. Carefully monitored therapy with these drugs is advisable, although generally applicable, statistically validated prognostic guides are still lacking. The progression of pulmonary dysfunction due to fibrosing alveolitis does stop in some patients.[42,52,56,135,141]

Cardiac Manifestations

Cardiac abnormalities in patients with polymyositis and dermatomyositis occur frequently, but are rarely clinically symptomatic. First-, second-, and third-degree heart block, left bundle branch block, left axis deviation, and atrial and ventricular dysrhythmias have been noted. Myocarditis and congestive heart failure occur less often. Approximately half, or more, of patients have electrocardiographic abnormalities, with an increased frequency of mitral valve prolapse noted in one report.[64] Uncommonly, conduction abnormalities are so severe that an artificial cardiac pacemaker is required.[69] It is not certain whether the tendency to cardiac abnormalities is greater in more severely or chronically ill patients.

Postmortem evaluations have demonstrated myocarditis, as well as myocardial fibrosis.[35,67] Myocarditis is associated with congestive heart failure. One patient with bundle branch block had inflammation and necrosis involving the conduction system. Overall, arrhythmia is estimated to occur in 6%, congestive heart failure in 3%, bundle branch block in 5%, and high-grade heart block in 2% of patients.[11] Cardiac involvement may occur in both polymyositis and dermatomyositis, but it may go unnoticed unless electrocardiographic examinations are performed.

Calcinosis

Soft tissue calcification can be a disabling complication of inflammatory muscle disease (Figs. 65–6 to 65–8). Most commonly, it occurs during the course of chronic childhood dermatomyositis. Calcification may invest the fascia surrounding muscle groups of the proximal extremities and may

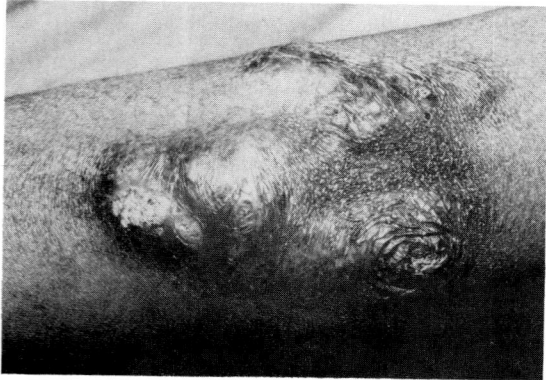

Fig. 65–6. Subcutaneous calcific masses nearing the skin surface at the elbow of a patient with dermatomyositis.

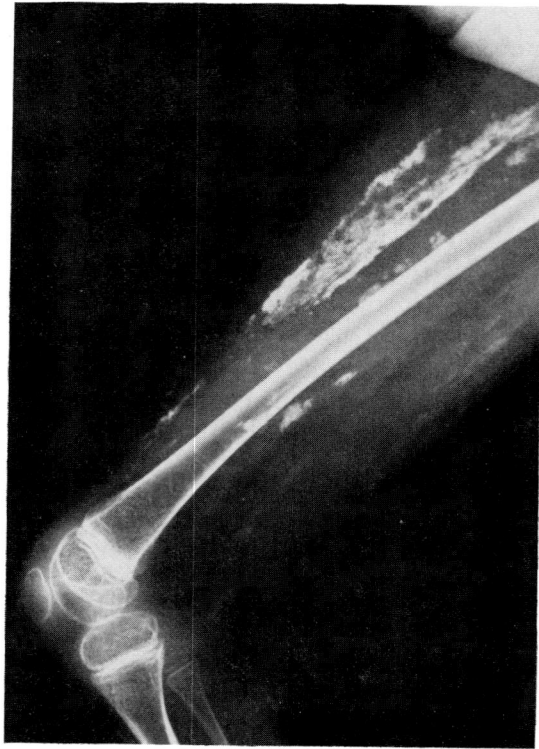

Fig. 65–7. Subcutaneous and perimuscular calcific masses in the thigh of a child with dermatomyositis in remission.

lead to diffuse "woody" induration that severely limits motion. Calcified masses may also appear under the skin and may open to the surface, to drain calcareous material. Diagnostic sensitivity in detecting this abnormality, prior to accumulation of masses large enough to be seen radiographically, may be increased by bone-scanning techniques with ^{99m}technetium diphosphonate.[136] Treatment methods for calcinosis are generally unsatisfactory. Localized masses may be removed surgically, but extensive or more generalized involvement is a distressing problem. A number of therapies, including corticosteroids, diphosphonates, ethylenediaminotetra-acetate, and aluminum hydroxide gel, have been unsuccessful. Probenecid has been reported to be useful.[36] Sometimes, the calcific deposits are resorbed spontaneously (see Chap. 95).

Renal Involvement

Renal disease is rare in patients with inflammatory myopathy. Renal insufficiency in patients with severe persistent myoglobinuria has been observed.[86] This complication may occur in both polymyositis and dermatomyositis. Although rare, glomerulonephritis of the focal-mesangial type or

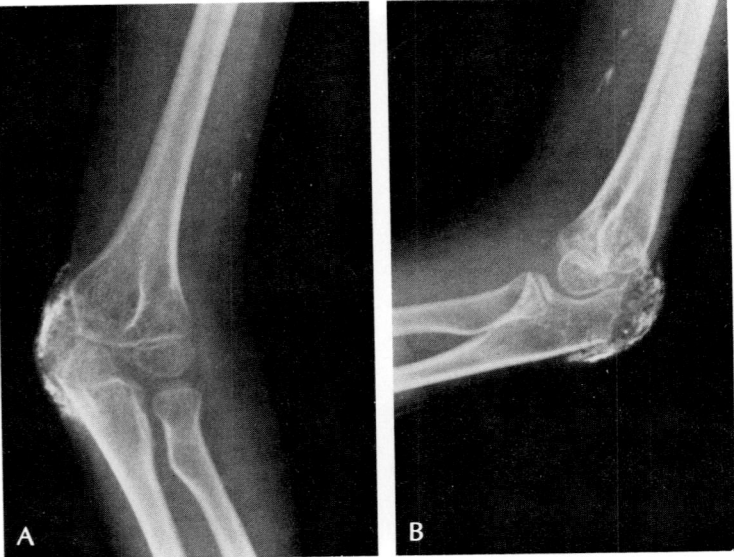

Fig. 65-8. *A* and *B,* Subcutaneous calcification at the elbow and other areas of calcification in the upper arm of a child with dermatomyositis in remission.

of the progressive-crescentic type has been recorded.[43,90]

Focal or Nodular Muscle Involvement

Polymyositis may begin with a single, localized, nodular swelling in muscle. This swelling may then progress over months to generalized inflammatory myopathy. This unusual variant has been described as focal or nodular myositis.[25,68] In some patients, focal myositis of the gastrocnemius muscle has simulated thrombophlebitis.[89]

Childhood Dermatomyositis

Although a female preponderance exists among adults with myositis, such is not the case in children.[120]

The signs of rash and myopathy are similar to those previously described. In addition, evidence of vascular involvement may be prominent. Abnormalities of nail fold capillaries, including dilatation, avascular areas, and tortuosity are present in over half the affected children, especially in those with severe disease.[144] Ulcerations of the gastrointestinal tract and hemorrhage related to vascular involvement of the digestive system are serious, life-threatening complications.[6] This manifestation was described prior to the use of corticosteroid agents and represents a result of dermatomyositis rather than a complication of therapy.[153] Although vascular involvement of the gastrointestinal tract is the most prominent visceral complication of dermatomyositis, other areas may also be involved, including, rarely, the retina, in

which exudates, macular edema, and visual impairment have been described.[157]

Histologic evaluation of dermatomyositis reveals distinctive abnormalities related to pathologic changes of the vessel walls, as discussed later in this chapter.

Arthralgia

Joint pains without overt synovitis commonly occur during periods of active disease. Overt synovitis is sufficiently rare that its presence suggests other connective tissue syndromes.

LABORATORY AND OTHER DIAGNOSTIC STUDIES

The laboratory studies most used during the course of inflammatory muscle disease involve measurement of sarcoplasmic constituents, enzymes, and myoglobin released into the circulation as a consequence of muscle damage.

Enzymes

Measurements of serum activities of creatine kinase, lactate dehydrogenase, aldolase, and aspartate aminotransferase (glutamic-oxaloacetic transaminase) are the most common enzyme tests. Elevations occur during periods of disease activity, and values return toward normal during remission or inactive disease.

An increase in serum creatine kinase activity is the most sensitive enzyme index of active muscle disease.[126] High creatine kinase activity is found in active disease, and the level falls during remission, sometimes weeks before clinically evident improvement. The level may then rise again if the therapeutic drug dosage is reduced too quickly or if a relapse is impending. Because aldolase, transaminase, and lactate dehydrogenase may be less consistently elevated in patients with myositis, estimation of creatine kinase levels is the most reliable enzyme test.[151]

In some situations, evaluations of serum enzyme activity are of limited use. From the technical point of view, the amount of enzyme is inferred from its activity and factors that inhibit or promote activity influence the interpretation of test results. Inhibitors of creatine kinase activity have been described in serum. Dilution of serum samples with elevated creatine kinase levels may produce artifactual increases in creatine kinase activity,[48] and certain pharmacologic agents, such as barbiturates, diazepam, and morphine may alter the removal rate of creatine kinase from the circulation and may increase its activity.[133] In addition, the question whether enzyme increases are due to tissue destruction, or whether cell membrane containment of enzyme is altered by disease or pharmacologic agents, is difficult to answer. For example, following exercise, elevations of creatine kinase levels may be observed in the absence of histologically demonstrable evidence of tissue necrosis. In neuromuscular disorders other than myositis, falls in creatine kinase activity may occur without clinical change,[115] so this index may not always correlate with disease activity.

Rarely, in 1 to 5% of patients with polymyositis and dermatomyositis, the serum creatine kinase level alone may be normal, and in other patients, all serum enzyme levels tested are normal throughout the course of illness.[11] One study measured serum creatine kinase levels prior to therapy and found these values to be normal in 5 of 15 patients. This finding may have been related to disease chronicity because high values were noted in all 7 patients with disease of under 3 years' duration, whereas in the 8 patients with a longer duration of illness, the creatine kinase level was normal in 5 and was only moderately elevated in 3 patients. No correlation was found between the magnitude of the enzyme elevation and the severity of the muscle weakness.[131] Taken together, therefore, the evidence suggests that serum enzyme evaluation is an important adjunct to the diagnosis and assessment of patients with myositis, but absolute correlations of strength and prognosis with the enzyme levels, particularly in patients with chronic illness, are often imprecise.

Creatine kinase exists as a dimer with three major isoenzymic forms: MM, MB, and BB. Creatine kinase-MM is the predominant form in skeletal muscle, where it represents approximately 95 to 98% of the total creatine kinase activity. The BB isoenzyme is the major component of brain and smooth muscle. The MB form is present in cardiac muscle to the extent of 20 to 30%, with the remainder as MM. The MB form may be present in skeletal muscle as well, in levels of 5% or less.[34,80,108] Creatine kinase-MB has been demonstrated in the circulation of patients with myositis in the absence of detectable, concomitant cardiac disease or dysfunction.[14,63,93,114] In these patients, creatine kinase-MB is probably synthesized in and released from skeletal muscle. Myofibers during embryologic development produce the B subunit and elaborate creatine kinase-MB, and skeletal muscle tissue in cell culture also produces this MB form.[47,97,150] These observations, combined with clinical information, suggest that regenerating myofibers within damaged skeletal muscle may be the source of the increased production of creatine kinase-MB.

Myoglobin

Myoglobin, the respiratory heme protein of the muscle cell, is found in both skeletal and cardiac muscle, but not in other tissues. During the course of muscle disease or disorder, myoglobin may enter the circulation and, following renal clearance, may appear in the urine.[84] Hypermyoglobinemia is seen in most patients with dermatomyositis and polymyositis. Myoglobinuria is less frequent.[85,86] From 70 to 80% of patients with active, untreated myositis have hypermyoglobinemia, with levels falling during periods of remission. Sequential determinations of serum myoglobin levels suggest rapid reductions with response to therapy, often before the activities of serum enzymes such as creatine kinase, lactic dehydrogenase, and glutamic-oxaloacetic transaminase return to normal. It is likely that the combined use of serum myoglobin determinations with the enzymes will offer advantages for the detection and assessment of myopathic states. In a study of patients with myositis,[118] 19% had hypermyoglobinemia in the absence of elevated creatine kinase levels. Myoglobinuria, although less frequent, also occurs in patients with inflammatory muscle disease, and persistent myoglobinuria has been associated with renal failure in these patients.[86] Because levels of myoglobin may undergo circadian variation, it is best to compare results from a standard time of day.[13]

Erythrocyte Sedimentation Rate

The erythrocyte sedimentation rate is often elevated in patients with active myositis in the range of 30 to 50 mm/hour as measured by the Westergren method. This value is normal, however, in many patients, and no correlation exists between the erythrocyte sedimentation rate and the grade of disability or degree of weakness.[37] During remission of the disease, this value generally returns toward normal.

Autoantibodies

Patients with dermatomyositis may have circulating antibodies to certain nuclear and cellular constituents. These are discussed later, in the section on serologic factors.

Electromyography

Patients with inflammatory muscle disease have evidence of myopathy on electromyographic examination; volitional contraction produces a pattern of activity characterized by short duration, low amplitude, and polyphasic potentials.[30] At rest, fibrillation potentials may be observed, presumably the result of involvement of terminal neural elements in the inflammatory process. Overall, 70 to 90% of patients studied have these findings; however, a few patients may have no demonstrable abnormalities. Generally, little or no correlation exists between the grade of disability at presentation and the electromyographic findings.[11,37]

Studies of patients with standard as well as single-fiber electromyography, a more specialized technique, indicate an increase in the number of muscle fibers in individual motor units, along with abnormal jitter and blocking. These findings also suggest changes in the pattern of terminal innervation of the muscle, perhaps related to involvement of intramuscular nerves by inflammation or anoxia or other factors coincident with inflammation, degeneration, and regeneration. In this connection, these changes may relate to the finding of fibrillation activity or to the occasional occurrence of fiber type grouping seen in affected tissues by histochemical techniques; these changes also suggest neural involvement.[71]

Muscle Biopsy

Muscle biopsy is indicated in nearly all patients with suspected myositis before proceeding with what may be a long course of potentially hazardous therapy. Demonstration of inflammation confirms the diagnosis.

The optimal procedure for obtaining and processing muscle tissue requires coordination among clinician, surgeon, pathologist, and technologists. The site selected should be one of active involvement, but not marked by advanced atrophic or end-stage disease. In addition, sites previously traumatized by electromyography needles, intramuscular injections, or surgical procedures should be avoided. In most cases, proximal muscle tissue of the extremity is usually selected. Cases of myositis with only spinal muscle involvement have been reported. Biopsy of the erector spinae muscles may be performed. Muscle is obtained at resting length for histologic processing.

In many cases, particularly when the clinician feels histologic evaluation is all that is desired, needle muscle biopsy may be employed. Its major advantages are ease of performance and low morbidity rate. A major drawback is the small size of the sample. If needed, however, multiple samples may be obtained. Expert handling of the small bits of tissue removed is critical to ensure their proper orientation for microtome sectioning. Contraction artifacts also may be encountered in needle biopsy samples. In a series of 30 patients, the overall diagnostic yield from needle biopsy was comparable to that expected with the open-surgical procedure. Inflammation, necrosis, and degeneration were noted in most specimens studied. Two had only myofiber atrophy, and one had no abnormality. In addition, sequential needle biopsies have been employed to demonstrate response to therapy. Definite correlation in this regard may be difficult, however, because of uneven involvement of muscle tissue and because of persistent abnormalities in otherwise stable patients. In one group of patients examined by needle biopsy, failure to respond to corticosteroid therapy was associated with an increased number of myofiber internal nuclei.[44,140]

Open-surgical biopsy, the present standard, is more time-consuming and is attended with more discomfort and morbidity than needle biopsy, but it obtains larger specimens with fewer chances for artifact, and it allows biochemical or electron-microscopic studies.

Histologic Examination

The major findings in muscle tissue of patients with inflammatory myopathy are necrosis, phagocytosis of necrotic muscle tissue, perivascular and interstitial inflammation, and myofiber regeneration (Figs. 65–9 to 65–12). Signs of regeneration include the presence of myoblasts, seen as crescentic cells with basophilic cytoplasm within the sarcolemmal sheath. Myoblasts of this type may contain one or two nuclei and either few coarse myofibrils or none. Syncytial masses of such presumed progenitor cells with basophilic cytoplasm and immature myofibrils, as well as myotubes, characterized by central nuclei, and large myofibers with peripheral basophilia may all be part of the regenerative process. Increased content of RNA and of certain enzymes such as lactate dehydrogenase and succinate dehydrogenase are noted in regenerating myofibers by histochemical techniques. The inflammatory infiltrate, the hallmark

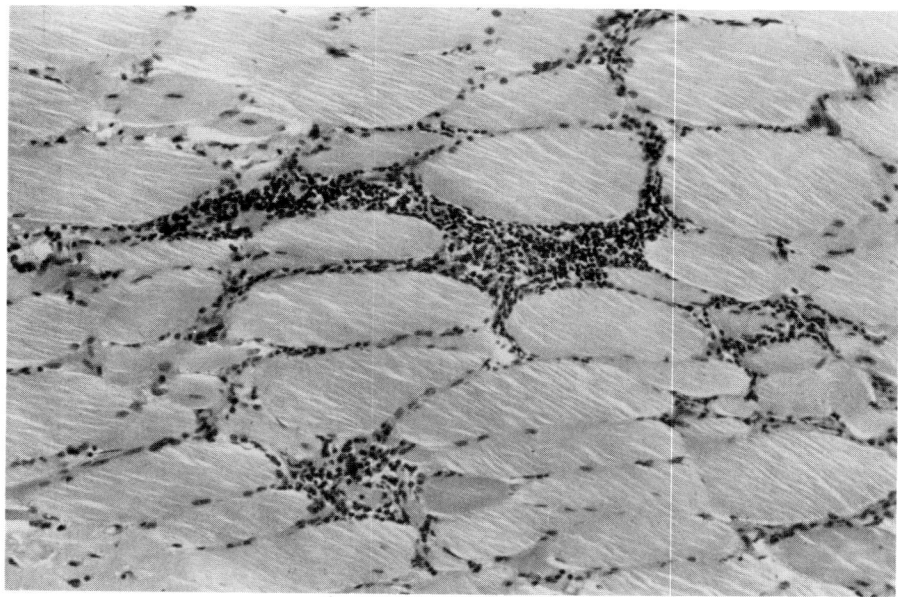

Fig. 65–9. Infiltration of inflammatory cells between fibers with necrosis and areas of loss of fibers seen on microscopic examination of a muscle biopsy specimen.

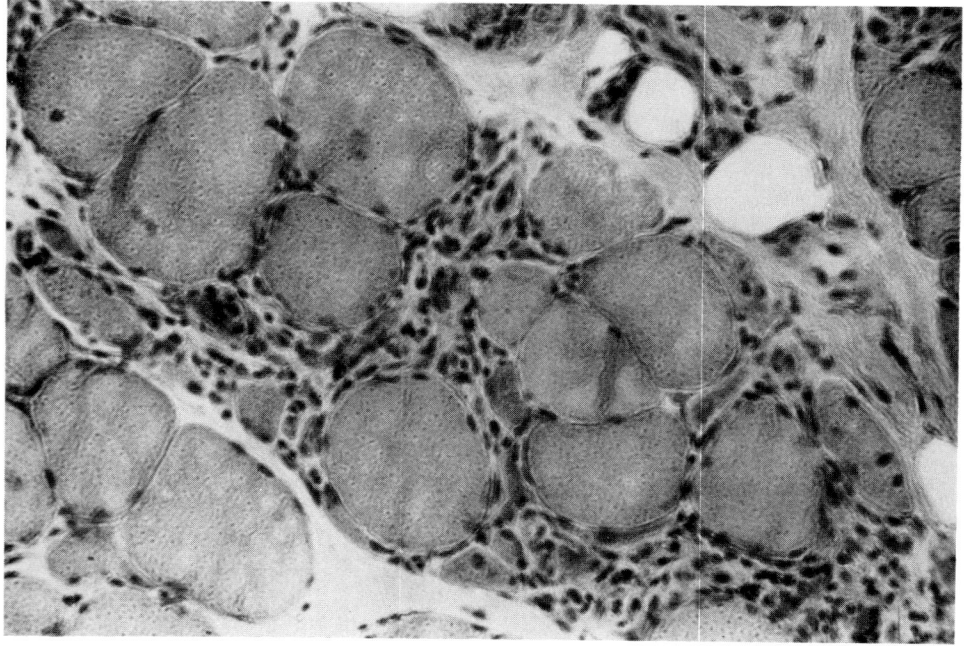

Fig. 65–10. Inflammatory cell infiltrate with areas of necrosis and an increase in connective tissue and lipid (upper right).

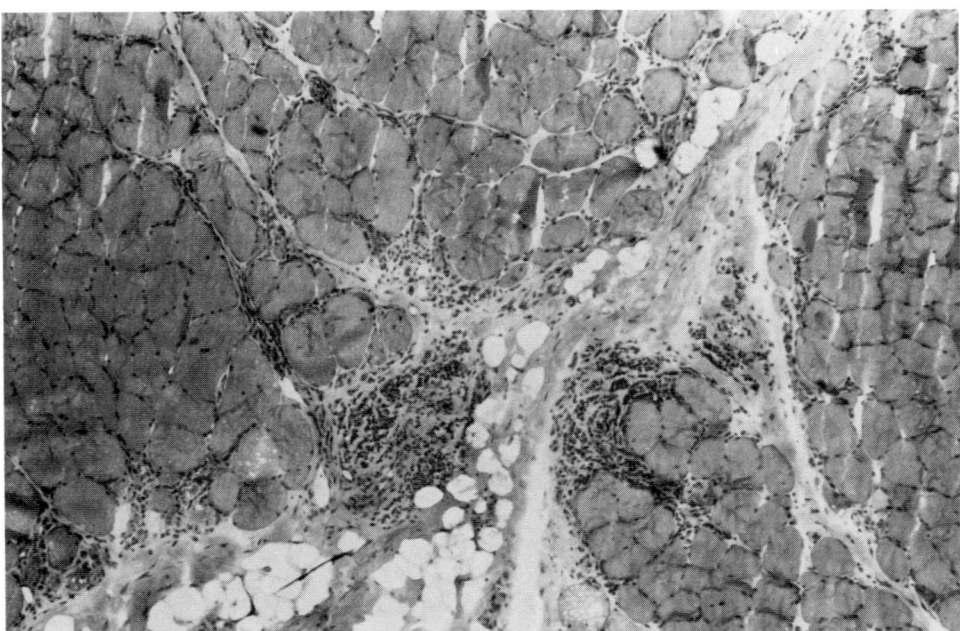

Fig. 65–11. Low-power microscopic view demonstrating zones of inflammation and an increase in connective tissue and lipid in a patient with chronic polymyositis.

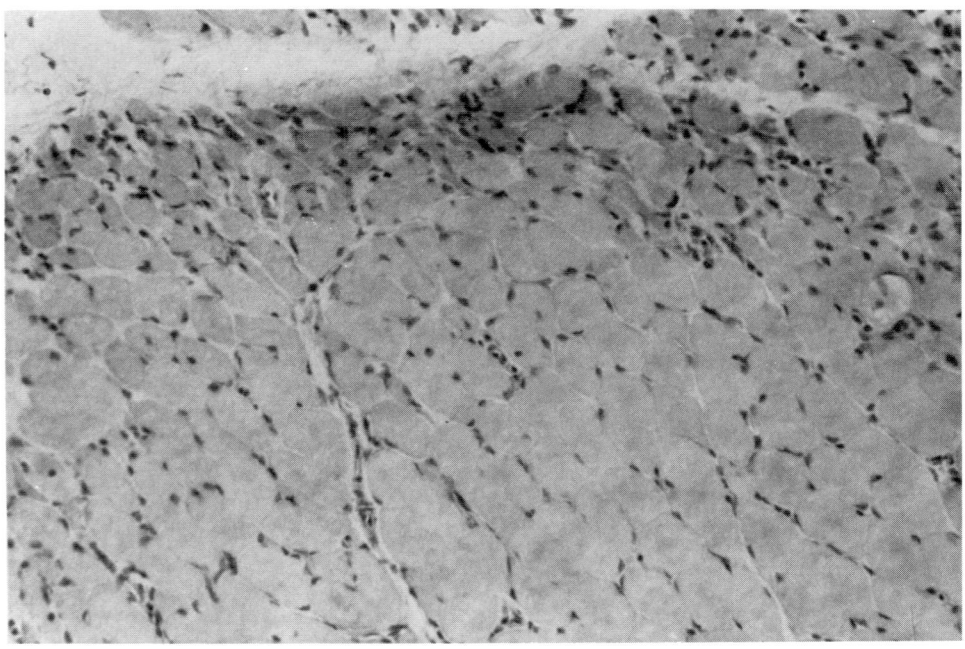

Fig. 65–12. Perifascicular atrophy in a biopsy from a child with dermatomyositis.

of myositis, consists of small and large lymphocytes, macrophages, and occasionally, plasma cells. Associated with the infiltrate of inflammatory cells, particularly in chronic cases, is an increase in collagen and connective tissue, which may separate bundles of myofibers as well as isolate and replace individual necrotic myofibers. Immunohistologic study has indicated that this connective tissue is rich in collagen types I to IV, and concentrations of the amino terminal propeptides of procollagen III, the precursor of type III collagen, are increased in blood serum of patients with polymyositis and dermatomyositis.[40,102,116,125]

Anastomoses between the terminal cisternae of the sarcoplasmic reticulum and the transverse tubules have been observed by electron-microscopic examination in myositis. These abnormal anastomoses may furnish pathways for the leakage of intracellular constituents such as enzymes to the extracellular space.[22]

In patients with chronic disease, inflammatory changes may be less marked, and the histologic picture may be characterized by myofiber atrophy, fibrosis, and increased deposits or accumulations of lipid.

Table 65–4 indicates the results of muscle biopsy of 103 patients, all of whom had clinical findings of polymyositis.[37] Sixty-five percent of the patients had findings of inflammation sufficient to be considered diagnostic of myositis (groups 1 and 2); however, 17% of patients had no demonstrable abnormalities. The experience therefore suggests that muscle biopsy is strong diagnostic evidence in most patients with active disease. A negative or nonspecific biopsy does not of itself exclude the diagnosis of polymyositis, however.

Childhood Dermatomyositis

The histologic findings of childhood dermatomyositis, characterized by zonal loss of capillaries,

Table 65–4. **Muscle Biopsy Findings in a Group of 103 Patients with Myositis**

Findings		Percentage of Total (%)
1. Fiber destruction, regeneration, perivascular and interstitial inflammation	46	65%
2. Perivascular and interstitial inflammatory infiltrate with minimal fiber destruction	19	
3. Myofiber destruction and regeneration without inflammatory cell infiltrates	8	
4. Fiber atrophy and other nonspecific changes	11	
5. Normal tissue	17	

(Data adapted from DeVere, R., and Bradley, W.G.[37])

muscle infarction, vasculopathy, and lymphocytic infiltration of blood vessels, set this entity apart from other types of inflammatory myopathy. Vasculopathy is the striking feature. In addition to an inflammatory component, swelling, necrosis, and obliteration of vessels also occur in the absence of nearby inflammatory cells. The endothelium of small vessels may appear prominent and hyperplastic.

Electron-microscopic evaluation of endothelial cells reveals necrosis, degeneration, and areas of regeneration. Affected endothelial cells appear pleomorphic and contain cytoplasmic inclusions made up of aggregates of tubular structures, both free and circumscribed by endoplasmic reticulum. The tubular structures are 250 to 280 Å in diameter, and the aggregate masses are 0.4 to 2.7 μ across. These inclusion aggregates appear to distort the endothelial cells. Gaps are present between endothelial cells. Changes in the endothelium and the loss of the normal covering of underlying collagen may be factors in the formation of thrombi in such affected vessels.

Thrombosis may be seen in capillaries, small arteries, and veins in muscle tissue obtained from children with dermatomyositis. Associated with these findings of small-vessel damage and occlusion are ischemic changes in muscle. Myofiber atrophy occurs as well as infarction, particularly at the periphery of the muscle fasciculus. In addition to the changes in the blood vessels and the muscle ischemia, changes in sarcolemmal nuclei and cytoplasmic inclusions of the muscle cells are present. Signs of muscle regeneration with enlarged satellite cells are present. Immunoglobulin, fibrin, and complement components have also been identified in or near blood-vessel walls, but these constituents have not been directly related to the presence of inflammation or to the degree of vascular damage. Vasculopathy may also occur in tissue other than skeletal muscle. Endarteropathy, marked by endothelial cell abnormalities with tubuloreticular inclusions, has been found in the superficial dermis, along with dermal infiltrates of mononuclear cells. Endarteropathy and vascular damage in the gastrointestinal tract are believed to be factors in perforation of the small intestine, a grave complication of childhood dermatomyositis.[5,23] Vascular lesions affecting the retina and skin were discussed already.

THEORIES OF PATHOGENESIS

The cause or causes of dermatomyositis and polymyositis are not known. Several areas, however, have served as foci for study and discussion in speculating on possible pathogenetic mechanisms. In this context, the following topics are discussed.: (1) the relation of the immune system to myositis; (2) the relation of infectious disease to myositis; and (3) the association of malignant disease with myositis.

Immune System

This discussion includes serologic factors, humoral and cell-mediated immunity, and genetics (see also Chap. 60).

Serologic Factors

Patients with myositis may have circulating antibodies to certain nuclear and cytoplasmic constituents of test cells. Several identified precipitins react with extracts of calf thymus. In one survey, 64% of patients with polymyositis and 80% of those with myositis associated with progressive systemic sclerosis had antibody to a thymic nuclear antigen, designated PM-1. Antibodies to other components may also be present. Sixty-five percent of blood sera from patients with polymyositis and 59% from patients with dermatomyositis had antibody of several specificities directed against whole thymus and thymic nuclear extracts. Jo-1, a protein of nuclear origin, is recognized by 31% of sera from patients with polymyositis and overlap syndromes. In another study, Jo-1 antibodies were present in 23% of adults with polymyositis or dermatomyositis. Another antigen, Mi, was recognized by the sera of some patients with dermatomyositis and polymyositis, as well as by others with inflammatory myopathy associated with systemic lupus erythematosus. The relation of these autoantibodies to the pathogenesis of disease remains a matter for study.[2,117,129,158]

Humoral Immunity

Most studies have not yet demonstrated humoral autoimmunity with specificity for muscle tissue or its components, although such autoantibodies have been found.[20,54,145] One interesting finding in this regard is the presence of immunoglobulin and complement components deposited in muscle during the course of myositis. The presence of immunoglobulin deposits is not always correlated with the presence of inflammation in the areas in which it is found, however, nor are these deposits found only in patients with myositis.[156] Further, not all investigators have found immunoglobulins or complement components in affected muscle.[54] This topic is controversial. One study concluded that immunoglobulin associated with blood vessels, connective tissue, and necrotic fibers may be nonspecifically deposited. Using the immunoperoxidase method, the mononuclear cells of the inflammatory infiltrate were found to contain IgG and IgM in most biopsies studied.[58]

In experimental myositis in animals, muscle-binding antibody may appear, but its presence is not correlated with the onset of illness, and no relationship exists between the titers of such antibody and the presence or severity of myositis. In this situation, muscle-binding antibody has not been demonstrated to be injurious to muscle,[33] although under other circumstances, antibody may be pathogenic.[91]

Little or no evidence exists for abnormalities in the humoral immune capabilities of most patients with inflammatory muscle disease, although the occurrence of myositis in certain patients with immunoglobulin or complement deficiency raises this issue. Hypogammaglobulinemic disorders of both the congenital and acquired types have been observed in association with dermatomyositis and polymyositis, and a patient with inflammatory myopathy associated with a deficiency of the second component of complement has been encountered.[61,78,95] Whether these associations suggest a relationship of myositis with a defective immune response against an unknown provoking agent is unknown at this time.

Cell-Mediated Immunity

A series of experimental studies in animals led to a proposed role for sensitized lymphocytes in the pathogenesis of inflammatory myopathy. Approximately three decades ago, it was observed that injections of emulsions of homologous or heterologous muscle preparations with Freund's adjuvant into guinea pigs led to the development of myositis manifested by infiltration of mononuclear cells, myofiber degeneration, and perivasculitis. In addition, affected animals demonstrated delayed skin sensitivity to the provocative muscle antigen preparations. Degeneration and atrophic changes persisted in these animals for at least six months. Focal myositis with arthritis has also been produced in rats after injection of skeletal muscle extracts emulsified in Freund's adjuvant. Our understanding of the relation of the immune system to disease production was strengthened with the observation that lymph node cells from affected animals were capable of destroying muscle cells in culture, as well as of transferring the disease to otherwise unimmunized, irradiated hosts. Lymphocytes from affected animals also underwent transformation to blast cell forms on exposure to autologous muscle proteins. Moreover, histologic evaluation suggested a close relationship between lymphocytes and the areas of muscle necrosis. Although the experimental illness was often patchy, focal, and mild, more severe disease associated with elevation of serum activities of creatine kinase, transaminase, and aldolase could be produced with greater quantities of sensitizing antigen. Antibody capable of binding muscle was present in these animals, but was not cytotoxic, although antibody to myosin, actin, and myofibrillar components has, under certain circumstances, induced myopathic changes.[31,88,91,103,112,123,143,146,154,155]

After these demonstrations of experimental myositis, several observations drew parallels to the human disease. Lymphocytes from patients with polymyositis underwent transformation accompanied by the release of lymphokines on exposure to muscle antigen preparations and caused the destruction of human and other animal muscle cells in culture. Cytotoxic lymphocytes of this type were not restricted to patients with polymyositis, however, but were observed also in certain other neuromuscular disorders. Cytotoxic lymphocytes are noted in some patients with active myositis, and the activity of these cells is reduced by successful treatment of the disease. The action of lymphocyte-mediated cytotoxicity in vitro is mediated by the release of lymphokines, or lymphotoxins, and it is possible to protect target muscle cells from these factors by the addition of methylprednisolone. Several different assays have demonstrated the presence of muscle-sensitized lymphocytes in the circulation of patients with polymyositis. Recently, by means of the technique of tritium-labeled carnitine release, cytotoxicity of peripheral blood lymphocytes against cultures of human fetal skeletal muscle cells was demonstrated with cells of patients with polymyositis, but not with cells of several patients with other muscle diseases or in normal individuals. These findings suggest that lymphocytes sensitized to antigens of skeletal muscle are in the circulation and tissues of patients with polymyositis and may participate in the inflammatory response and in muscle injury.[17,26,32,81,137]

Several matters remain unclear, however. It is still not known which factors initiate illness and give rise to lymphocytes of this sort. It is also unclear whether all patients with polymyositis have such sensitized lymphocytes. Although several studies have indicated a general relationship between disease and lymphocyte activity, such is not always the case. Active lymphocytes may be found in patients with stable disease and in those without clinical signs of active inflammation. In addition, patients with active inflammatory disease may not have demonstrably active lymphocytes. Active lymphocytes have been noted in patients with myasthenia gravis, with several forms of muscular dystrophy, and with polymyalgia rheumatica. In the last disorder, usually no evidence exists of muscle destruction or inflammation. These observations raise questions about the specificity of cytotoxic lymphocytes for myositis. Further, not all investigators who have studied this question have

been able to demonstrate cellular immunity to muscle in patients with polymyositis and dermatomyositis. Therefore, at present, the evidence is still incomplete. One important area that needs elaboration is the nature and stability of the muscle antigens. Further knowledge may help to explain the variation in experimental findings.[66,96]

Genetics

The possibility of a genetic influence in dermatomyositis and polymyositis has been suggested on the basis of studies of HLA associations, but this influence is not yet understood. HLA-B8 has been noted in increased frequency in many Caucasian children with dermatomyositis,[57,119] as well as in adults with polymyositis.[8,75] Associations of disease with HLA-B14 and B-40 have also been noted.[24] A recent study, of 33 patients, however, including children and adults, failed to confirm any HLA associations,[152] although the possible influence of genetic factors was supported by a high incidence of putative autoimmune diseases, such as rheumatoid arthritis (RA), thyroid disease, juvenile-onset diabetes, and pernicious anemia, in first-degree relatives of patients with polymyositis. None of the relatives had polymyositis.

Infectious Agents

Skeletal muscle may be the site of inflammation in a number of infectious disorders due to diverse agents including bacteria, protozoa, viruses, and parasites. None of these disorders have been linked to the development of chronic polymyositis; however, the possible role of infectious agents is considered in this section, particularly in relation to viruses and to toxoplasmosis.

Viruses

Several viruses may produce muscle damage and inflammation, usually of a transient nature. Among the best characterized of these are Coxsackie, echo- and influenza viruses. One such postviral syndrome of childhood is termed *benign acute myositis*. In this disorder, children develop severe lower extremity pain, usually in the calves, with soreness and cramps, 24 to 72 hours after an upper respiratory infection or apparent gastroenteritis. Boys are affected more frequently than girls. The average age is approximately nine years. The prodromal illness is marked by fever, occasionally headache, and gastrointestinal or respiratory symptoms. During the period of severe myalgia, muscles may swell. Biopsy is rarely performed; however, inflammation of muscle was observed in one girl, and in another child, no abnormalities were noted. Results of virologic studies in this syndrome are consistent with recent infection, usually with influenza virus of either type A or type B. On occasion, adenovirus and parainfluenza viruses are also implicated. Most children recover completely within a week. Creatine kinase activity of serum is elevated and returns to normal in two weeks.[1]

This disease has an epidemic form. In one such outbreak, 17 children developed acute myositis, chiefly involving the gastrocnemius and soleus muscles. Influenza B virus was isolated from 11 of the 17 patients. Complete recovery occurred in 4 to 5 days.[39]

Adults also have been affected with myositis following influenza virus infection. In some cases, myositis was transient; in others, severe and prolonged disease occurred with myonecrosis, myoglobinuria and renal failure. Although documentation of viral infection is most commonly serologic, virus has been isolated from respiratory secretions, and in a 65-year-old man with inflammatory myopathy following an influenza-like syndrome, influenza B virus was recovered from affected muscle and was seen in muscle by electron microscopy.[59]

Coxsackie virus has been seen by electron microscopy and has been isolated from muscle in children with inflammatory myopathy. Elevation of Coxsackie B neutralizing antibody titers was found in four patients with clinical syndromes of polymyositis and dermatomyositis.[149]

Hepatitis B virus also has been implicated in the pathogenesis of inflammatory muscle disease. Several instances of hepatitis B infection followed by myositis have been observed, with deposition of immunoglobulin, complement, and in one case, hepatitis surface antigen in muscle.[27]

Echovirus infection also has been associated with myositis including nine patients with X-linked hypogammaglobulinemia. Recovery of this virus has been reported from several sites. In one patient with weakness, elevated serum enzyme levels, a myopathic electromyographic pattern, and biopsy evidence of inflamed muscle and fascia, Echovirus 11 was recovered from muscle and cerebrospinal fluid. Treatment with immunoglobulin preparations containing specific antibody was followed by dramatic clinical recovery in this patient.[104]

Other viruses, including herpes and Epstein-Barr viruses, have been implicated in myopathy and myositis. Particles seen by electron microscopy, possibly related to picorna-type virus, have been noted in muscle in several patients with myositis, as well as in patients with Reye's syndrome. In such instances, viral identification has not been definite, and questions have been raised regarding other origins for these structures, such as degeneration of cellular components.

On the basis of available information, it is possible to conclude that viruses of several types may lodge in muscle and may lead to inflammation and myonecrosis. In some cases, as in patients with hypogammaglobulinemia, host factors may be important in viral infection and in disease severity.

Toxoplasma Gondii

This protozoan organism commonly infects individuals in the United States, and asymptomatic cysts may persist in muscle.[51,130] During the early invasion of muscle in man, it is not known whether an accompanying inflammatory response occurs; however, experimental murine infections are associated with mild focal myositis.[72] In certain cases, *Toxoplasma gondii* infection of muscle has been linked to severe myopathy. In some such patients, the diagnosis of toxoplasmosis was suggested by serologic tests, as well as by response to therapy. In others, in addition to serologic evidence, *Toxoplasma* organisms were seen in muscle biopsies. Of three patients with these organisms identified in muscle, polymyositis was the diagnosis in two, and dermatomyositis in one. Central nervous system disease and fever are common in such patients.[55,65,70]

Serologic evidence of toxoplasmosis has also been obtained in studies of patients with polymyositis. In an age-, sex-, and race-matched, controlled study, 60% of patients with polymyositis had positive Sabin-Feldman tests with titers higher than in control subjects. In addition, complement-fixing antibody, usually suggestive of recent infection, was present in greater frequency (35%) and at higher titers than in control subjects. Responses of this type were not found in the polymyositis patients tested for antibody against rubella, measles, parainfluenza, and Epstein-Barr viruses. Patients with serologic evidence of recent toxoplasmosis generally had polymyositis of less than 2 years' duration.[128] Declines in antibody titers over time and an improvement coincident with sulfa-pyrimethamine therapy have also been reported.[87] In addition, a high frequency of specific IgM anti-*Toxoplasma* antibody, suggestive of recent infection, is also found. In a recent study, 48% of patients with inflammatory muscle disease and positive Sabin-Feldman tests had IgM antibody.[98] Current evidence suggests high frequency of recent toxoplasmosis among certain patients with polymyositis of recent onset. It is not known, however, whether *Toxoplasma gondii* in such patients is the causative agent of polymyositis or whether dormant, persistent forms may be reactivated or reintroduced to the immune system concurrent with inflammation in muscle.

Malignant Disease

The association of malignant disease with inflammatory myopathy may offer an important clue to the pathogenesis of myositis. The basis for this association, initially noted over 100 years ago, is still poorly understood and remains controversial. The reported frequency of malignant disease in patients with dermatomyositis varies widely; however, several series reported a rate of approximately 15 to 20% of adults. Malignant disease in children with myositis is rare, although neoplasia and coincident dermatomyositis-like syndromes have been described. One review of this aspect listed 2 children with leukemia, 1 with agammaglobulinemia followed by lymphoma, and 1 with pituitary adenoma.

A retrospective survey of the literature to 1976 noted 258 cases of malignant disease concurrent with myositis. Most such cases were observed in the fifth and sixth decades of life, with a mean age of 52.6 years. The most frequent tumors were cancers of the breast and lung; malignant tumors of the ovary and stomach were also common. In this group, the temporal relation of the onset of the 2 disorders was reported in 167 patients. In 99 of these patients, myopathy was observed first, and the malignant process was discovered later, usually within a year. In 17 patients, both diseases were noted at the same time, and in 51, the tumor appeared first, and the myopathy was recognized later, usually within a year. The frequency of malignant disease in patients with myositis was 5 to 7 times that expected in the general population. Similar results have been noted in other retrospective surveys. One study over a 20-year period noted 7 of 27 patients with both dermatomyositis and malignant disease. This frequency, 26%, was not only greater than that expected in the general population, but also was greater than that reported in patients with RA or systemic lupus erythematosus. Of this group of 7 patients, 2 had breast cancer, 2 had cancer of the colon, and 3 had cancer of an unknown primary site. In most patients, the diagnosis of malignant disease was made at the same time as the diagnosis of dermatomyositis. Adding to the general impression of the significance of this relationship are case reports of patients with multiple neoplasms in whom recurrence of dermatomyositis-like signs were observed with the recurrence of the tumor or with the appearance of a new tumor.

In another group of 35 patients with dermatomyositis seen over a 20-year period, 12 had malignant disease. Of these, 6 of 9 showed improvement in the manifestations of dermatomyositis after treatment directed toward the neoplasm, and 3 had

exacerbations of dermatomyositis with progression of the neoplasm. The course of the 2 disorders is not always parallel, however. Although the course may not be predictable, the coexistence of these disorders generally bespeaks a grave prognosis. The types of associated malignant diseases vary, as previously indicated; most neoplasms are carcinomas originating in the lung, breast, gastrointestinal tract, nasopharynx, ovary, and uterus. Lymphomas, sarcomas, and other malignant diseases are also observed.

The reason for this concurrence is unknown. The retrospective method of enumerating published case reports may place undue emphasis on this association, and the lack of a prospective study leaves unanswered the question of the precise frequency of this association. Nonetheless, on the basis of available information, it is prudent to look for this coincidence, particularly in adults with dermatomyositis.

Because of the many kinds of malignant disorders noted, the varied times of the appearance of one disease relative to the other, and the lack of a predictable direct relationship in the short-term course of the illnesses, it seems unlikely that one illness is the direct cause of the other. It is possible that an alteration in host responsiveness, perhaps involving the immune apparatus, may underlie the mechanism of the expression of both illnesses.[4,7,16,105,142]

OTHER DISORDERS MARKED BY MYOSITIS

Drug-Related States

Drugs are not usually the cause of myositis, although toxic and myopathic effects of medications are known. Myositis-like states are reported rarely in patients receiving sulfonamides, penicillin, isoniazid, and azathioprine.[49,62] One agent that may produce inflammatory myopathy, however, is D-penicillamine. Most patients with this complication have received this agent for the treatment of RA. In one reported case, a patient had two muscle biopsies; myositis was not present prior to therapy and was seen after treatment with D-penicillamine.[53,113,127]

Other Connective Tissue Disorders

Myositis may be a prominent feature of other connective tissue disorders. Progressive systemic sclerosis, in particular, may begin in a manner indistinguishable from polymyositis and may later develop its own characteristic features. In undifferentiated or mixed connective tissue disorders, inflammatory myopathy is often a prominent element. Myositis also may complicate the course of systemic lupus erythematosus and of sarcoidosis.

Although patients with RA do not generally have clinical signs of inflammatory myopathy, histologic examination may reveal the presence of inflammation in skeletal muscle, particularly in severely affected patients.[66a] Myalgia and muscle weakness are noted in approximately one-third of patients with Sjögren's syndrome. Severe myositis with profound weakness and marked elevation of serum enzyme levels is less common.[101,132]

Inclusion Body Myositis

This recently recognized disorder is marked by chronic, progressive wasting and weakness with microscopic inclusions seen in both nuclei and cytoplasm of skeletal muscle cells. In contrast to dermatomyositis and polymyositis, this rare disorder has a male preponderance. The course is often prolonged and causes weakness of both proximal and distal musculature. No skin rash is present. Response to corticosteroids is generally poor. To date, 25 such patients have been recognized and reported. Eighteen have been men, mostly middle-aged. The proximal musculature has been involved in most, but in 7 patients, distal weakness predominated. Dysphagia occurred in four patients. Creatine kinase was elevated in most patients, and electromyographic testing has revealed myopathic signs with polyphasic potentials of brief duration as well as neuropathic features such as fibrillation and long-lasting, large amplitude potentials.

The distinguishing features of this disorder are seen on histologic examination of affected muscle tissues. Eosinophilic inclusions occur in both the sarcoplasm and the nucleus. Vascuoles may be present with mononuclear cell infiltration and myofiber degeneration and regeneration. Bluish or purplish granules may appear in the lined or rimmed vacuoles. These granules probably represent masses of cytomembranous structures. The number of capillaries is normal or increased. In some cases, group atrophy of myofibers is found.

By electron microscopy, the nuclear and cytoplasmic inclusions are seen to be masses of filamentous material. The diameters of the filaments range from 10 to 25 nm and are greater in the cytoplasm. The pathogenesis of the inclusions is not known. Similar inclusions may also be present in patients with other myopathic disorders.[19,21,28,83,160] Recently, adenovirus type 2 was isolated from muscle of a single patient after 14 years of illness.[110]

Tropical Pyomyositis

This disorder is marked by abscesses, apparently spontaneously occurring in skeletal muscle. Children and young adults chiefly in tropical areas of the world are affected. This disorder is rare in the United States; in some patients, it occurs after travel to or residence in the tropics. One or more skeletal muscles, such as biceps, pectoral, gluteal, or quadriceps become painful and tender. An accompanying fever is usually present. The involved area may resolve spontaneously or may swell and suppurate, yielding large numbers of micro-organisms, almost always *Staphylococcus aureus*. The presence of multiple abscesses suggests hematogenous spread. Occasionally, clinically involved areas may be bacteriologically sterile, and this observation has led to speculation that skeletal muscle may first be damaged by an unknown agent, and then colonized by *Staphylococcus*. Among candidates for such initiating agents have been tissue parasites, other bacteria and viruses, antecedent trauma, the presence of genetically variant hemoglobin, and nutritional deficiencies. The morbidity and mortality rates for tropical pyomyositis relate to the occurrence of staphylococcal septicemia and metastatic suppurative complications, such as osteomyelitis.[82,147]

Eosinophilic Myositis and Hypereosinophilic Syndromes

Myositis with eosinophilic infiltration may be part of hypereosinophilic syndromes, along with involvement of other organs and the central nervous system. In some patients, anemia, hypergammaglobulinemia, petechiae, Raynaud's phenomenon, and pulmonary and cardiac manifestations have been observed. Cardiac complications include endocardial and myocardial fibrosis, congestive heart failure, and arrhythmias. Peripheral neuropathy may be present. Circulating eosinophilia, which may not be constant in all cases, can be marked, with relative proportions of 20 to 60% of the circulating leukocytes. Leukocytosis is common. Response to corticosteroid therapy is inconsistent or poor. One patient responded after leukopheresis.[46,94] Myositis also may occur during the course of eosinophilic fasciitis.[10,139]

Granulomatous Myopathy

This entity may be associated with other disorders such as sarcoidosis or Crohn's disease of the bowel, or it may appear without the signs of other disease. Granulomatous myopathy occurring alone is generally observed in middle-aged women who have a chronically progressive, predominantly proximal pattern of muscle weakness, occasionally complicated by dysphagia. Histologic examination reveals groups of granulomas made up of loosely packed epithelioid cells and histiocytes, often in association with lymphocytes and a surrounding rim of collagenous fibers. Reticular fibers are present in the granuloma, as well as Langerhans-type giant cells.

Myositis may occur during the course of sarcoidosis, and granulomas have been observed in muscle tissue of patients with sarcoid myopathy, as well as in patients with sarcoidosis who have no muscular symptoms.[73,107,138]

TREATMENT

In considering the approach to therapy, two features should be accented: the first is accuracy of diagnosis, and the second, precision of assessment of disease activity.

It is important to secure as accurate a diagnosis as possible before initiating a treatment program that may be lengthy and possibly hazardous. In this connection, the presence of an associated malignant disease or of another connective tissue disorder may affect the patient's prognosis and response to treatment.

The assessment of disease activity and of response to therapy depends on evaluating elements of the patient's medical history, physical examination, and laboratory findings. Exacerbations of disease may have manifestations similar to those present at the disease's onset. Return of rash, arthralgia, and the spread of areas of telangiectasia may be early warnings of exacerbation and increased disease activity. Renewed weakness may be difficult to evaluate, and other factors, including therapy and the possibility of altered electrolyte balance, should be considered in the ongoing assessment of the patient's muscle strength and function. Laboratory findings, particularly increases in creatine kinase, lactate dehydrogenase, and serum myoglobin levels and, to a lesser extent, erythrocyte sedimentation rate, may accompany or may precede an exacerbation of inflammatory muscle disease. In the chronically ill patient, these laboratory findings may be less reliable than at the onset of disease. Active inflammation in muscle, as well as vasculitis, may be present and may continue in the absence of chemical evidence of active disease.[111] In addition, other factors such as trauma, injections, the performance of electromyographic studies, and exertion may lead to transient elevations of serum enzymes, unrelated to the progression of the disease. Patients returning to fuller schedules of activities after a period of bed rest, or those undertaking exercise programs too taxing for their clinical status, may experience muscle aching accompanied by serum enzyme elevations. All these considerations stress the need for careful analysis of changes in the patient's condition before adjusting the program of therapy.

The major approach to treatment involves the use of medications and physical measures, with a spirit of understanding and cooperation between physician and patient. The course of illness may be protracted, and periods of depression and frustration should be anticipated.

Physical Therapy

Rest during periods of active inflammation and physical therapy to rebuild muscle strength during periods of remission are indicated. Passive range-of-motion exercises are important to prevent the development of contractures. Despite daily therapy, however, contractures may occur and may progress in severely affected patients.

Pharmacologic Therapy

This form of treatment includes corticosteroids and immunosuppressive agents.

Corticosteroids

Corticosteroids are the mainstay of drug treatment for most patients (see Chap. 32). Although adequately controlled data are still insufficient to indicate the degree of effectiveness of agents of this class, corticosteroid therapy is generally considered beneficial and is recommended for both adults and children. One should be aware of spontaneous remissions of disease. Retrospective examinations of overall survival have not demonstrated the absolute value of corticosteroids; however, this information may be difficult to evaluate because of the lack of simultaneous comparison groups adequately matched for diagnostic classification, time of institution of therapy in relation to disease onset, variation of doses and types of treatment, and age and sex.

The usual practice is to begin oral corticosteroid therapy in the range of 40 to 80 mg/day prednisone for approximately 4 to 6 weeks or until the maximum benefit or remission of the disease is achieved. The dose may then be gradually reduced, with careful monitoring of symptoms, physical findings, and laboratory test results. For children, doses of 1 to 2 mg/kg body weight/day are used initially. Other approaches are possible; alternate-day therapy has been used. In general, corticosteroid dosage is reduced as clinical improvement is noted.[41, 134] Maintenance dosage and the need to increase therapy are decided by the patient's response and the ensuing course.

In both children and adults, one sees the usual potentially serious complications of corticosteroid therapy. Hypertension, cardiovascular decompensation, exacerbation of diabetes mellitus, gastrointestinal ulceration, sepsis, and osteoporosis, as well as changes in physical appearance and psychologic state, have been problems. Questions regarding corticosteroid-induced myopathy are sometimes difficult to analyze, although in many patients treated on a long-term basis, corticosteroid-induced weakness may cause protracted disability.

Most patients with myositis unassociated with malignant disease can be treated with corticosteroids alone; however, this treatment may not always be optimal. Two such situations are as follows: (1) life-threatening progressive illness without response to adequate corticosteroid therapy; and (2) partially responsive illness requiring doses of corticosteroids that have side effects difficult or impossible to tolerate. Under these circumstances, one should consider adding other forms of therapy, such as immunosuppressive agents.

Immunosuppressive Agents (see Chap. 33)

With regard to immunosuppressive agents, two general cautions should be observed. First, adequate and complete information about the effect of these drugs in myositis is lacking. The same problems mentioned in regard to corticosteroid therapy apply here, but because these agents have been less extensively used than corticosteroids, the amount of organized, controlled data on which to base judgments is even smaller. Second, although a number of different agents are classified together by virtue of immunosuppressive activity, current evidence is insufficient to relate this factor to therapeutic effectiveness. In addition, it is not known whether any two of these agents operate in a similar manner, through similar mechanisms.

A number of agents have been used, including 6-mercaptopurine and chlorambucil, but most experience has been gained with methotrexate, azathioprine, and cyclophosphamide.

Methotrexate was first employed in the treatment of dermatomyositis over 15 years ago;[99] since then, several reports have noted its usefulness, including its corticosteroid-sparing effects that allow reduction in corticosteroid dosage.[109] Methotrexate in conjunction with corticosteroid therapy is usually given intravenously, initially at doses of 10 to 15 mg at intervals of 5 to 7 days, then with gradually increasing doses up to 50 mg or higher. The frequency of administration is then reduced from weekly to biweekly and finally to monthly. Stomatitis is the most common side effect. Hepatotoxicity, bone-marrow suppression, usually evident as leukopenia, gastrointestinal hemorrhage, skin effects, nephropathy, and reduction of normal host defense against infection may be other complications of therapy. Drug-induced pneumonitis has been reported in patients receiving oral therapy.[3] Methotrexate, in biweekly injections of 2 to 3 mg/kg body weight or 7 mg/kg body weight with

citrovorum factor has been used in conjunction with corticosteroid therapy in children.[77]

Azathioprine has been added to corticosteroid treatment. A controlled study indicated that patients treated with azathioprine and corticosteroids showed improvements in functional ability and required less prednisone for maintenance than patients treated with prednisone alone.[15] The dose was 2 mg/kg/day until the concurrent prednisone dose could be reduced to less than 15 mg/day; then the azathioprine dose was reduced as tolerated. In general, doses for active disease in most studies are in the range of 100 to 150 mg/day orally, with a decrease to 50 to 75 mg/day for maintenance therapy after remission of the disease. Doses of 50 to 125 mg/day are prescribed for children.[77] Major areas of toxicity include bone-marrow suppression, chiefly leukopenia, gastrointestinal intolerance, and increased susceptibility to infections.

Cyclophosphamide has probably been used in fewer patients than either methotrexate or azathioprine. The dose has not been completely evaluated, but a range of 100 to 200 mg/day has been used. Toxicity includes bone-marrow suppression, increased susceptibility to infection, alopecia, and hemorrhage from the urinary bladder.

Other concerns relative to the use of these agents, except methotrexate, relate to possible genetic damage and the risk of malignant disease. These associations have not been completely evaluated in patients with myositis, but they should be considered, particularly in young patients. Overall, substantial corticosteroid-sparing effects have been noted in approximately 40 to 50% of patients treated with immunosuppressive agents.[124]

Plasmapheresis

Plasmapheresis is a newly developed mode of treatment in patients judged to have a poor response to corticosteroids and immunosuppressive agents. Patients undergoing plasmapheresis have continued to receive corticosteroids and immunosuppressive agents during the period of pheresis therapy, which has sometimes lasted several months or more. Most of a group of 35 patients treated in this manner were judged to be improved. Herpes zoster developed in 7 of 35 patients subjected to plasmapheresis.[9,29]

Other Therapeutic Considerations

Other areas of treatment include management of calcinosis, for which medical therapy has not been effective. Surgical removal of troublesome deposits may be helpful.

Several patients with evidence of recent *Toxoplasma gondii* infection have received therapy directed against this organism with sulfonamides, pyrimethamine, and folinic acid.

PROGNOSIS

Children

The prognosis of childhood dermatomyositis has been reviewed in several recent series. The outlook for complete remission is good in at least 50% of patients, and results are best in patients with early diagnosis and treatment. Although severe, unresponsive disease is less common, the course of such patients may be complicated by respiratory infection, cardiac failure, and gastrointestinal hemorrhage, all of which unfavorably influence prognosis. Fatalities have occurred. Approximately 30 to 40% of patients have chronic active disease and need protracted therapy. Calcinosis and joint contractures are sources of disability that, along with residual weakness, limit return to normal function when remission has occurred. Physical therapy, although not always effective, should be an early part of the therapeutic program to maximize chances for mobility and to decrease the likelihood of disabling contractures. The duration of disease activity in most children is generally 2 to 4 years.[74,111,134]

Adults

The outlook in adult patients does not appear to be as good as in children. In general, patients with malignant disease have a poor outcome. Patients under 20 years of age have better chances for survival than those over age 55. Intercurrent infections, particularly pneumonia, severe muscle weakness, chronically active disease, and dysphagia all unfavorably influence prognosis. The overall survival rate has varied in several studied groups. One retrospective survey, which did not include patients with malignant disease, indicated a mortality rate of 39% in the first year.[18] Another smaller study disclosed a similar mortality rate after 5 years.[131] A cumulative survival rate of 53% after 7 years was observed in a group of over 100 patients,[106] whereas a lower mortality rate, 28%, was noted in another group of similar size after 6 years.[37] Taken together, the experience indicates a substantial mortality rate in adults with inflammatory muscle disease, even in groups from which patients with cancer have been excluded. In addition, most surviving patients have long-term disability and need medication. Relapses are common, and many, perhaps 20 to 30% of patients, demonstrate disease activity with deterioration of strength or elevation of serum enzyme levels and erythrocyte sedimentation rate for over 10 years. Many patients have a static clinical state with elevated serum enzyme levels for long periods.

Histologic estimate of the severity of abnormalities demonstrated by muscle biopsy is not a generally reliable indicator of outcome.

The outlook in the future may not necessarily be as gloomy as these figures suggest. In a recent large series of patients, the mortality rate was 13.7% after a mean follow-up period of 4.3 years; 25% of the deaths were due to malignant disease, and 20% were due to sepsis. Recognition and prompt treatment of infections as well as careful monitoring and adjustment of medications may reduce the severity of complications and may improve the overall prognosis.[11]

REFERENCES

1. Antony, J.H., Procopis, P.C., and Ouvrier, R.A.: Benign acute childhood myositis. Neurology, 29:1068–1071, 1979.
2. Arnett, F.C., et al.: The Jo-1 antibody system in myositis: relationships to clinical features and HLA. J. Rheumatol., 8:925–930, 1981.
3. Arnett, F.C., et al.: Methotrexate therapy in polymyositis. Ann. Rheum. Dis., 32:536–546, 1973.
4. Arundell, F.D., Wilkinson, R.D., and Haserick, J.R.: Dermatomyositis and malignant neoplasms in adults. Arch. Dermatol., 82:772–775, 1960.
5. Banker, B.Q.: Dermatomyositis of childhood. J. Neuropathol. Exp. Neurol., 34:46–75, 1975.
6. Banker, B.Q., and Victor, M.: Dermatomyositis (systemic angiopathy) of childhood. Medicine, 45:261–289, 1966.
7. Barnes, B.E.: Dermatomyositis and malignancy. Ann. Intern. Med., 84:68–76, 1976.
8. Behan, W.M.H., Behan, P.O., and Dick, H.A.: HLA-B8 in polymyositis. N. Engl. J. Med., 298:1260–1261, 1978.
9. Bennington, J.A., and Dau, P.C.: Patients with polymyositis and dermatomyositis who undergo plasmapheresis therapy. Pathologic findings. Arch. Neurol., 38:553–560, 1981.
10. Bjelle, A., Henriksson, K.-G., and Hofer, P.-A.: Polymyositis in eosinophilic fasciitis. Eur. Neurol., 19:128–137, 1980.
11. Bohan, A., et al.: A computer-assisted analysis of 153 patients with polymyositis and dermatomyositis. Medicine, 56:255–286, 1977.
12. Bohan, A., and Peter, J.B.: Polymyositis and dermatomyositis. N. Engl. J. Med., 292:344–347, 403–407, 1975.
13. Bombardieri, S., et al.: Circadian variations of serum myoglobin levels in normal subjects and patients with polymyositis. Arthritis Rheum., 25:1419–1424, 1982.
14. Brownlow, K., and Elevitch, F.R.: Serum creatine phosphokinase iso-enzyme (CPK₂) in myositis. JAMA, 230:1141–1144, 1974.
15. Bunch, T.W.: Prednisone and azathioprine for polymyositis. Long-term followup. Arthritis Rheum., 24:45–48, 1981.
16. Callen, J.P., et al.: The relationship of dermatomyositis and polymyositis to internal malignancy. Arch. Dermatol., 116:295–298, 1980.
17. Cambridge, G., and Stern, C.M.M.: The uptake of tritium-labelled carnitine by monolayer cultures of human fetal muscle and its potential as a label in cytotoxicity studies. Clin. Exp. Immunol., 43:211–219, 1981.
18. Carpenter, J.R., et al.: Survival in polymyositis: corticosteroids and risk factors. J. Rheumatol., 4:207–214, 1977.
19. Carpenter, S., et al.: Inclusion body myositis: a distinct variety of idiopathic inflammatory myopathy. Neurology, 28:8–17, 1978.
20. Casparay, E.A., Gubbay, S.S., and Stern, G.M.: Cir-

culating antibodies in polymyositis and other muscle-wasting disorders. Lancet, 2:941, 1964.

21. Chou, S.-M.: Myxovirus-like structures and accompanying nuclear changes in chronic polymyositis. Arch. Pathol. Lab. Med., 86:649–658, 1968.

22. Chou, S.-M., Nonaka, I., and Voice, G.F.: Anastomoses of transverse tubules with terminal cisternae in polymyositis. Arch. Neurol., 37:257–266, 1980.

23. Crowe, W.E., et al.: Clinical and pathogenetic implications of histopathology in childhood polydermatomyositis. Arthritis Rheum., 25:126–139, 1982.

23a. Csuka, M.E., and McCarty, D.J.: A rapid method for measurement of lower extremity muscle strength. Am. J. Med. In press, 1984.

24. Cumming, W.J.K., et al.: HLA and serum complement in polymyositis. Lancet, 2:978–979, 1977.

25. Cumming, W.J.K., et al.: Localised nodular myositis: a clinical and pathological variant of polymyositis. Q. J. Med., 46:531–546, 1977.

26. Currie, S.: Destruction of muscle cultures by lymphocytes from cases of polymyositis. Acta Neuropathol., 15:11–19, 1970.

27. Damjanov, I., et al.: Immune complex myositis associated with viral hepatitis. Hum. Pathol., 11:478–481, 1980.

28. Danon, M.J., et al.: Inclusion body myositis. Arch. Neurol., 39:760–764, 1982.

29. Dau, P.C.: Plasmapheresis in idiopathic inflammatory myopathy. Arch. Neurol., 38:544–552, 1981.

30. Daube, J.R.: The description of motor unit potentials in electromyography. Neurology, 28:623–625, 1978.

31. Dawkins, R.L.: Experimental myositis associated with hypersensitivity to muscle. J. Pathol. Bacteriol., 90:619–625, 1965.

32. Dawkins, R.L., and Mastaglia, F.L.: Cell-mediated cytotoxicity to muscle in polymyositis. N. Engl. J. Med., 288:434–438, 1973.

33. Dawkins, R.L., Eghtedari, A., and Holborow, E.J.: Antibodies to skeletal muscle demonstrated by immunofluorescence in experimental autoallergic myositis. Clin. Exp. Immunol., 9:329–337, 1971.

34. Dawson, D.M., and Fine, I.H.: Creatine kinase in human tissues. Arch. Neurol., 16:175–180, 1967.

35. Denbow, C.E., et al.: Cardiac involvement in polymyositis. Arthritis Rheum., 22:1088–1092, 1979.

36. Dent, C.E., and Stamp, T.C.B.: Treatment of calcinosis circumscripta with probenicid. Br. Med. J., 1:216–218, 1972.

37. DeVere, R., and Bradley, W.G.: Polymyositis: its presentation, morbidity and mortality. Brain, 98:637–666, 1975.

38. Dietz, F., et al.: Cricopharyngeal muscle dysfunction in the differential diagnosis of dysphagia in polymyositis. Arthritis Rheum., 23:491–495, 1980.

39. Dietzman, D.E., et al.: Acute myositis associated with influenza B infection. Pediatrics, 57:255–258, 1976.

40. Duance, V.C., et al.: Polymyositis—an immunofluorescence study on the distribution of collagen types. Muscle Nerve, 3:487–490, 1980.

41. Dubowitz, V.: Treatment of dermatomyositis in childhood. Arch. Dis. Child., 51:494–500, 1971.

42. Duncan, P.E., et al.: Fibrosing alveolitis in polymyositis. Am. J. Med., 57:621–626, 1974.

43. Dyck, R.F., et al.: Glomerulonephritis associated with polymyositis. J. Rheumatol., 6:336–344, 1979.

44. Edwards, R.H.T., et al.: The investigation of inflammatory myopathy. J. R. Coll. Physicians Lond., 15:19–24, 1981.

45. Edwards, R.H.T., et al.: Muscle breakdown and repair in polymyositis. A case study. Muscle Nerve, 2:223–229, 1979.

46. Ellman, L., Miller, L., and Rappaport, J.: Leukopheresis therapy of a hypereosinophilic disorder. JAMA, 230:1004–1005, 1974.

47. Eppenberger, H.M., Richterich, R., and Aebi, H.: The ontogeny of creatine kinase isoenzymes. Dev. Biol., 10:1–16, 1964.

48. Farrington, C., and Chalmers, A.H.: The effect of dilution

49. in creatine kinase activity. Clin. Chim. Acta, 73:217–219, 1976.

49. Fayolle, J., et al.: Dermatomyosite déclenchée par l'isoniazide, avec syndrome biologique d'auto-immunisation de type lupique. Lyon Med., 233:135–138, 1975.

50. Feldman, D., et al.: Cutaneous vasculitis in adult polymyositis/dermatomyositis. J. Rheumatol., 10:85–89, 1983.

51. Feldman, H.A., and Miller, L.T.: Serological study of toxoplasmosis prevalence. Am. J. Hyg., 64:320–335, 1956.

52. Fergusson, R.J., et al.: Dermatomyositis and rapidly progressive fibrosing alveolitis. Thorax, 38:71–72, 1983.

53. Fernandes, L., Swinson, D.R., and Hamilton, E.B.D.: Dermatomyositis complicating penicillamine treatment. Ann. Rheum. Dis., 36:94–95, 1977.

54. Fessel, W.J., and Raas, M.C.: Autoimmunity in the pathogenesis of muscle disease. Neurology, 18:1137–1139, 1968.

55. Fonseca, R.C., et al.: Miositis toxoplasmica aguda en un adulto. Acta Med. Cost., 16:75–78, 1973.

56. Frazier, A.R., and Miller, R.D.: Interstitial pneumonitis in association with polymyositis and dermatomyositis. Chest, 65:403–407, 1974.

57. Friedman, J.M., et al.: Immunogenetic studies of juvenile dermatomyositis. Tissue Antigens, 21:45–49, 1983.

58. Fulthorpe, J.J., and Hudgson, P.: Immunocytochemical localization of immunoglobulins in the inflammatory lesions of polymyositis. J. Neuroimmunol., 2:145–154, 1982.

59. Gamboa, E.T., et al.: Isolation of influenza virus in myoglobinuric polymyositis. Neurology, 29:1323–1335, 1979.

60. Gardner-Medwin, D., and Walton, J.N.: The clinical examination of the voluntary muscles. In Disorders of Voluntary Muscle. Edited by J.N. Walton. Edinburgh, Churchill Livingstone, 1974, pp. 517–560.

61. Giuliano, V.J.: Polymyositis in a patient with acquired hypogammaglobulinemia. Am. J. Med. Sci., 268:53–56, 1974.

62. Goldenberg, D.L., and Stor, R.A.: Azathioprine hypersensitivity mimicking an acute exacerbation of dermatomyositis. J. Rheumatol., 2:346–349, 1975.

63. Goto, I.: Creatine phosphokinase isoenzymes in neuromuscular disorders. Arch. Neurol., 31:116–119, 1974.

64. Gottdiener, J.S., et al.: Cardiac manifestations in polymyositis. Am. J. Cardiol., 41:1141–1149, 1978.

65. Greenlee, J.E., et al.: Adult toxoplasmosis presenting as polymyositis and cerebellar ataxia. Ann. Intern. Med., 82:367–371, 1973.

66. Haas, D.C.: Absence of cell-mediated cytotoxicity to muscle cultures in polymyositis. J. Rheumatol., 7:671–676, 1980.

66a. Halla, J.T., et al.: Rheumatoid myositis: Clinical and histologic features and possible pathogenesis. Arthritis Rheum., 27:737–743, 1984.

67. Haupt, H.M., and Hutchins, G.M.: The heart and cardiac conducting system in polymyositis-dermatomyositis. Am. J. Cardiol., 50:998–1006, 1982.

68. Heffner, R.R., and Barron, S.A.: Polymyositis beginning as a focal process. Arch. Neurol., 38:439–442, 1981.

69. Henderson, A., et al.: Cardiac complications of polymyositis. J. Neurol. Sci., 47:425–429, 1980.

70. Hendrickx, G.F.M., et al.: Dermatomyositis and toxoplasmosis. Ann. Neurol., 5:393–395, 1979.

71. Henriksson, K.-G., and Stalberg, E.: The terminal innervation pattern in polymyositis: a histochemical and SFEMG study. Muscle Nerve, 1:3–13, 1978.

72. Henry, L., and Beverley, J.K.A.: Experimental myocarditis and myositis in mice. Br. J. Exp. Pathol., 50:230–238, 1969.

73. Hewlett, R.H., and Brownell, B.: Granulomatous myopathy: its relationship to sarcoidosis and polymyositis. J. Neurol. Neurosurg. Psychiatry, 38:1090–1099, 1975.

74. Hill, R.H., and Wood, W.S.: Juvenile dermatomyositis. Can. Med. Assoc. J., 103:1152–1156, 1970.

75. Hirsch, T.J., et al.: HLA-D related (DR) antigens in var-

ious kinds of myositis. Hum. Immunol., *3*:181–186, 1981.

76. Itoh, J., et al.: Sarcoid myopathy with typical rash of dermatomyositis. Neurology, *30*:1118–1121, 1980.

77. Jacobs, J.C.: Methotrexate and azathioprine treatment of childhood dermatomyositis. Pediatrics, *59*:212–218, 1977.

78. Janeway, C.A., et al.: "Collagen disease" in patients with congenital agammaglobulinemia. Trans. Assoc. Am. Physicians, *69*:93–97, 1956.

79. Janis, J.F., and Winkelmann, R.K.: Histopathology of the skin in dermatomyositis. Arch. Dermatol., *97*:640–650, 1968.

80. Jockers-Wretou, E., and Pfleiderer, G.: Quantitation of creatine kinase isoenzymes in human tissues by an immunological method. Clin. Chim. Acta, *58*:223–232, 1975.

81. Johnson, R.L., Fink, C.W., and Ziff, M.: Lymphotoxin formation by lymphocytes and muscle in polymyositis. J. Clin. Invest., *51*:2435–2449, 1972.

82. Joseph, S.C.: Pyomyositis. Am. J. Dis. Child., *130*:775–776, 1975.

83. Julien, J., et al.: Inclusion body myositis. J. Neurol. Sci., *55*:15–24, 1982.

84. Kagen, L.J.: Myoglobin: methods and diagnostic uses. CRC Crit. Rev. Clin. Lab. Sci., *9*:273–320, 1978.

85. Kagen, L.J.: Myoglobinemia in inflammatory myopathies. JAMA, *237*:1448–1452, 1977.

86. Kagen, L.J.: Myoglobinemia and myoglobinuria in patients with myositis. Arthritis Rheum., *14*:457–464, 1971.

87. Kagen, L.J., Kimball, A.C., and Christian, C.L.: Serologic evidence of toxoplasmosis among patients with polymyositis. Am. J. Med., *56*:186–191, 1974.

88. Kakulas, B.A.: Destruction of differentiated muscle cultures by sensitized lymphoid cells. J. Pathol. Bacteriol., *91*:495–503, 1966.

89. Kalyanaraman, K., and Kalyanaraman, U.P.: Localized myositis presenting as pseudothrombophlebitis. Arthritis Rheum., *25*:1374–1377, 1982.

90. Kamata, K., et al.: Childhood type polymyositis and rapidly progressive glomerulonephritis. Acta Pathol. Jpn., *32*:801–806, 1982.

91. Korenyi-Both, A., and Kelemen, G.: Damage of skeletal muscle in rats by immunoglobulins. Acta Neuropathol., *34*:199–206, 1976.

92. Krain, L.S.: Dermatomyositis in 6 patients without initial muscle involvement. Arch. Dermatol., *111*:241–245, 1975.

93. Larca, L.J., Coppola, J.T., and Honig, S.: Creatine kinase MB isoenzyme in dermatomyositis: a noncardiac source. Ann. Intern. Med., *94*:341–343, 1981.

94. Layzer, R.B., Shearn, M.A., and Satya-Murti, S.: Eosinophilic polymyositis. Ann. Neurol., *1*:65–71, 1977.

95. Leddy, J.P., et al.: Hereditary complement (C2) deficiency with dermatomyositis. Am. J. Med., *58*:83–91, 1975.

96. Lisak, R.P., and Zweiman, B.: Mitogen and muscle extract induced *in vitro* proliferative responses in myasthenia gravis, dermatomyositis and polymyositis. J. Neurol. Neurosurg. Psychiatry, *38*:521–524, 1975.

97. Lough, J., and Bischoff, R.: Differentiation of creatine phosphokinase during myogenesis. Quantitative fractionation of isoenzymes. Dev. Biol., *57*:330–334, 1977.

98. Magid, S.K., and Kagen, L.J.: Serological evidence for acute toxoplasmosis in polymyositis-dermatomyositis. Increased frequency of specific anti-toxoplasma IgM antibodies. Am. J. Med., *75*:312–320, 1983.

99. Malaviya, A.N., Many, A., and Schwartz, R.S.: Treatment of dermatomyositis with methotrexate. Lancet, *2*:485–488, 1968.

100. Maricq, H.R., and LeRoy, E.C.: Patterns of finger capillary abnormalities in connective tissue diseases by "wide-field" microscopy. Arthritis Rheum., *16*:619–628, 1973.

101. Martinez-Lavin, M., Vaughan, J.H., and Tan, E.M.: Autoantibodies and the spectrum of Sjögren's syndrome. Ann. Intern. Med., *91*:185–190, 1979.

102. Mastaglia, F.L., and Kakulas, B.A.: A histological and histochemical study of skeletal muscle regeneration in polymyositis. J. Neurol. Sci., *10*:471–487, 1970.

103. Mastaglia, F.L., Dawkins, R.L., and Papadimitriou, J.M.: Lymphocyte-muscle cell interactions *in vivo* and *in vitro*. J. Neurol. Sci., *22*:261–268, 1974.

104. Mease, P.J., Ochs, H.D., and Wedgewood, R.J.: Successful treatment of ECHO virus meningoencephalitis and myositis-fasciitis with intravenous immune globulin therapy in a patient with X-linked agammaglobulinemia. N. Engl. J. Med., *304*:1278–1281, 1981.

105. Medsger, T.A., Dawson, W.N., and Masi, A.T.: The epidemiology of polymyositis. Am. J. Med., *48*:715–723, 1970.

106. Medsger, T.A., Jr., Robinson, H., and Masi, A.T.: Factors affecting survivorship in polymyositis. Arthritis Rheum., *14*:249–258, 1971.

107. Menard, D.B., et al.: Granulomatous myositis and myopathy associated with Crohn's colitis. N. Engl. J. Med., *295*:818–819, 1976.

108. Mercer, D.W.: Separation of tissue and serum creatine kinase in human tissues. Arch. Neurol., *16*:175–180, 1967.

109. Metzger, A.L., et al.: Polymyositis and dermatomyositis: combined methotrexate and corticosteroid therapy. Ann. Intern. Med., *81*:182–189, 1974.

110. Mikol, J., et al.: Inclusion-body myositis: clinicopathological studies and isolation of an adenovirus type 2 from muscle biopsy specimen. Ann. Neurol., *11*:576–581, 1982.

111. Miller, J.J.: Late progression in dermatomyositis in childhood. J. Pediatr., *83*:543–548, 1973.

112. Morgan, G., Peter, J.B., and Newbould, B.B.: Experimental allergic myositis in rats. Arthritis Rheum., *14*:599–609, 1971.

113. Morgan, G.L., McGuire, J.L., and Ochoa, J.: Penicillamine-induced myositis in rheumatoid arthritis. Muscle Nerve, *4*:137–140, 1981.

114. Morton, B.D. III, and Statland, B.E.: Serum enzyme alterations in polymyositis. Am. J. Clin. Pathol., *73*:556–557, 1980.

115. Munsat, T.L., and Bradley, W.G.: Serum creatine phosphokinase levels and prednisone treated muscle weakness. Neurology, *27*:96–97, 1977.

116. Myllyla, R., et al.: Changes in collagen metabolism in diseased muscle. I. Biochemical studies. Arch. Neurol., *39*:752–755, 1982.

117. Nishikai, M., and Reichlin, M.: Heterogeneity of precipitating antibodies in polymyositis and dermatomyositis. Arthritis Rheum., *23*:881–888, 1980.

118. Nishikai, M., and Reichlin, M.: Radioimmunoassay of serum myoglobin in polymyositis and other conditions. Arthritis Rheum., *20*:1514–1518, 1977.

119. Pachman, L.M., et al.: HLA-B8 in juvenile dermatomyositis. Lancet, *2*:567–568, 1977.

120. Pachman, L.M., and Cooke, N.: Juvenile dermatomyositis: a clinical and immunological study. J. Pediatr., *96*:226–234, 1980.

121. Pearson, C.M.: Polymyositis and dermatomyositis. *In* Arthritis and Allied Conditions. 9th Ed. Edited by D.J. McCarty. Philadelphia, Lea & Febiger, 1979, pp. 742–761.

122. Pearson, C.M.: Polymyositis. Annu. Rev. Med., *17*:63–82, 1966.

123. Pearson, C.M.: Development of arthritis, periarthritis and periostitis in rats given adjuvants. Proc. Soc. Exp. Biol. Med., *91*:95–100, 1956.

124. Pearson, C.M., and Bohan, A.: The spectrum of polymyositis and dermatomyositis. Med. Clin. North Am., *61*:439–457, 1977.

125. Peltonen, L., et al.: Changes in collagen metabolism in diseased muscle. II. Immunohistochemical studies. Arch. Neurol., *39*:756–759, 1982.

126. Pennington, R.T.: Biochemical aspects of muscle disease. *In* Disorders of Voluntary Muscle. Edited by J.N. Walton. New York, Churchill Livingstone, 1981, pp. 415–447.

127. Petersen, J., et al.: Penicillamine-induced polymyositis-

dermatomyositis. Scand. J. Rheumatol., *7*:113–117, 1978.

128. Phillips, P.E., Kassan, S.S., and Kagen, L.J.: Increased toxoplasma antibodies in idiopathic inflammatory muscle disease. Arthritis Rheum., *22*:209–214, 1979.
129. Reichlin, M., and Mattioli, M.: Description of a serological reaction characteristic of polymyositis. Clin. Immunol. Immunopathol., *5*:12–20, 1976.
130. Remington, J.S., and Cavanaugh, E.N.: Isolation of the encysted form of *Toxoplasma gondii* from human skeletal muscle and brain. N. Engl. J. Med., *273*:1308–1310, 1965.
131. Riddoch, D., and Morgan-Hughes, J.A.: Prognosis in adult polymyositis. J. Neurol. Sci., *26*:71–80, 1975.
132. Ringel, S.P., et al.: Sjögren's syndrome and polymyositis or dermatomyositis. Arch. Neurol., *39*:157–163, 1982.
133. Roberts, R., and Sobel, B.E.: Effect of selected drugs and myocardial infarction on the disappearance of creatine kinase from the circulation in conscious dogs. Cardiovasc. Res., *11*:103–112, 1977.
134. Rose, A.L.: Childhood polymyositis. Am. J. Dis. Child., *127*:518–522, 1974.
135. Salmeron, G., Greenberg, D., and Lidsky, M.D.: Polymyositis and diffuse interstitial lung disease. Arch. Intern. Med., *141*:1005–1010, 1981.
136. Sarmiento, A.H., et al.: Evaluation of soft-tissue calcifications in dermatomyositis with ⁹⁹ᵐTc-phosphate compounds: case report. J. Nucl. Med., *16*:467–468, 1975.
137. Saunders, M., Knowles, M., and Currie, S.: Lymphocyte stimulation with muscle homogenate in polymyositis and other muscle-wasting disorders. J. Neurol. Neurosurg. Psychiatry, *32*:569–571, 1969.
138. Schimrigk, K., and Uldall, B.: The disease of Besnier-Boeck-Schaumann and granulomatous polymyositis. Eur. Neurol., *1*:137–157, 1968.
139. Schumacher, H.R.: A scleroderma-like syndrome with fasciitis, myositis and eosinophilia. Ann. Intern. Med., *84*:49–50, 1976.
140. Schwarz, H.A., et al.: Muscle biopsy in polymyositis and dermatomyositis. A clinicopathological study. Ann. Rheum. Dis., *39*:500–507, 1980.
141. Schwarz, M.I., et al.: Interstitial lung disease in polymyositis and dermatomyositis: analysis of six cases and review of the literature. Medicine, *55*:89–104, 1976.
142. Singsen, B.H., et al.: Lymphocytic leukemia, atypical dermatomyositis and hyperlipidemia in a 4-year-old boy. J. Pediatr., *88*:602–604, 1976.
143. Sobue, I., Watanabe, Y., and Matsui, T.: Experimental

studies on muscular allergy 1. Jpn. J. Med. Prog., *42*:22–30, 1955.
144. Spencer-Green, G., Crowe, W.E., and Levinson, J.E.: Nailfold capillary abnormalities and clinical outcome in childhood dermatomyositis. Arthritis Rheum., *25*:954–958, 1982.
145. Stern, G.M., Rose, A.L., and Jacobs, K.: Circulating antibodies in polymyositis. J. Neurol. Sci., *5*:181–183, 1967.
146. Takayanagi, T.: Immunohistological studies of experimental myositis in relation to human polymyositis. Folia Psychiatr. Neurol. Jpn., *21*:117–127, 1967.
147. Taylor, J.F., Fluck, D., and Fluck, D.: Tropical myositis: ultrastructural studies. J. Clin. Pathol., *29*:1081–1084, 1976.
148. Thompson, C.E.: Infantile myositis. Dev. Med. Child. Neurol., *24*:307–313, 1982.
149. Travers, R.L., et al.: Coxsackie B neutralisation titres in polymyositis/dermatomyositis. Lancet, *1*:1268, 1977.
150. Turner, D.C., Maier, V., and Eppenberger, H.M.: Creatine kinase and aldolase isoenzyme transitions in cultures of chick skeletal muscle cells. Dev. Biol., *37*:63–89, 1974.
151. Vignos, P.J., and Goldwin, J.: Evaluation of laboratory tests in diagnosis and management of polymyositis. Am. J. Med., *263*:291–308, 1972.
152. Walker, G.L., Mastaglia, F.L., and Roberts, D.F.: A search for genetic influence in idiopathic inflammatory myopathy. Acta Neurol. Scand., *66*:432–443, 1982.
153. Walton, J.N., and Adams, R.D.: Polymyositis. Edinburgh, E.S. Livingstone, 1958.
154. Watanabe, Y., Matsui, T., and Sobue, I.: Experimental studies on muscular allergy. 2. Jpn. J. Med. Prog., *42*:290–295, 1955.
155. Webb, J.N.: *In vitro* transformation of lymphocytes in experimental immune myositis. J. Reticuloendothel. Soc., *7*:445–452, 1970.
156. Whitaker, J.N., and Engel, W.K.: Vascular deposits of immunoglobulin and complement in idiopathic inflammatory myopathy. N. Engl. J. Med., *286*:333–338, 1972.
157. Winfield, J.: Juvenile dermatomyositis with complications. Proc. R. Soc. Med., *70*:548–551, 1977.
158. Wolfe, J.F., Adelstein, E., and Sharp, G.C.: Antinuclear antibody with distinct specificity for polymyositis. J. Clin. Invest., *59*:176–178, 1977.
159. Young, A., and Edwards, R.H.T.: Dynamometry and muscle disease. Arch. Phys. Med. Rehabil., *62*:295–296, 1981.
160. Yunis, E.J., and Samaha, F.J.: Inclusion body myositis. Lab. Invest., *25*:240–248, 1971.

Chapter 66

Systemic Sclerosis (Scleroderma), Eosinophilic Fasciitis, and Calcinosis

Thomas A. Medsger, Jr.

SYSTEMIC SCLEROSIS (SCLERODERMA)

Systemic sclerosis is a generalized disorder of connective tissue characterized by fibrosis and degenerative changes in the skin (scleroderma), synovium, muscles, and certain internal organs, notably the gastrointestinal tract, lung, heart, and kidney.[275] Raynaud's phenomenon and vascular lesions are prominent features. The recognition that its many manifestations represent a single systemic disease has been relatively recent.

Classification

The term scleroderma has traditionally been applied not only to the cutaneous changes of systemic sclerosis but to a heterogeneous group of conditions designated collectively as localized or focal scleroderma, in which there is more circumscribed dermal fibrosis. The hardening, tightening, and inelasticity of the integument may be indistinguishable from these same findings observed in systemic sclerosis, but certain pathologic as well as clinical differences separate these disorders. In our experience there has been no convincing evidence of internal involvement in the localized forms of scleroderma or of transition of these conditions to systemic sclerosis.

For these reasons, we have separated systemic sclerosis from the localized forms of scleroderma. We have divided the former into three major subtypes, dependent primarily on the degree and extent of cutaneous involvement and the presence of features commonly encountered in other connective tissue diseases (overlap syndromes) (Table 66–1). A similar spectrum of systemic sclerosis is recognized in the classification systems proposed by other authors.[16,108,149,357] Some of the many distinctive demographic, clinical, laboratory, and natural history differences between diffuse scleroderma, with distal and proximal extremity and truncal skin

Table 66–1. Classification of Scleroderma

I. SYSTEMIC SCLEROSIS (progressive systemic sclerosis; systemic scleroderma)

With diffuse scleroderma: symmetrical widespread (diffuse) skin involvement, affecting the trunk, face, and proximal as well as distal extremities; tendency to rapid progression and early appearance of visceral involvement.

With CREST syndrome: relatively limited (restricted) skin involvement, often confined to the fingers and face; prolonged delay in appearance of distinctive internal manifestations, e.g., pulmonary arterial hypertension and biliary cirrhosis; prominence of calcinosis and telangiectases.

With "overlap": having typical features of one or more members of the connective tissue disease family.

II. LOCALIZED SCLERODERMA

Morphea: single or multiple (generalized) plaques.

Linear scleroderma: with or without melorheostosis; includes scleroderma en coup de sabre (with or without facial hemiatrophy).

III. EOSINOPHILIC FASCIITIS

thickening, and the CREST* syndrome with cutaneous changes limited to the fingers and distalmost portions of the extremities and occasionally the face,[378] are shown in Table 66–2. Additional details concerning these two variants are provided in subsequent sections of this chapter.

Criteria for Classification of Systemic Sclerosis. A prospective multicenter study of the American Rheumatism Association compared 264 systemic sclerosis patients with 413 patients with polymyositis-dermatomyositis, systemic lupus erythematosus, or isolated Raynaud's phenomenon for the purpose of developing classification criteria.[214] Sclerodermatous skin changes in any location proximal to the digits were present in 91% of

---

*CREST: Calcinosis, Raynaud's phenomenon, Esophageal dysmotility, Sclerodactyly, and Telangiectasia.

994

Table 66–2. Comparison of Clinical and Laboratory Features at Time of First Evaluation for Systemic Sclerosis According to Extent and Location of Sclerodermatous Skin Changes (University of Pittsburgh, 1972–1983)

	Diffuse Scleroderma (N = 305)	CREST Syndrome (N = 265)
Demographic		
Age (<40 at onset)	36%	51%
Race (nonwhite)	11%	2%
Sex (female)	73%	83%
Duration of symptoms (yrs.)	4.0	11.5
Organ System Involvement		
Skin (total skin score)*	35.2	8.6
Telangiectases	32%	82%
Calcinosis	7%	43%
Raynaud's phenomenon	86%	95%
Arthralgias or arthritis	80%	58%
Tendon friction rubs	67%	6%
Contractures	84%	45%
Myopathy	19%	8%
Esophageal hypomotility	75%	77%
Pulmonary fibrosis	35%	37%
Pulmonary hypertension	<1%	11%
Congestive heart failure	10%	1%
Renal "crisis"	17%	1%
Laboratory Data		
ANA (1:16+)	54%	48%
Anticentromere antibody (1:40+)	3%	50%
Anti-Scl 70 (any titer)	38%	18%
Cumulative Survival (10 yrs from first diagnosis)	57%	75%

*As described in Steen, et al.[329]

systemic sclerosis patients and in fewer than 1% of the other group. With the addition of any two of three minor criteria, including sclerodactyly, digital pitting scars, and bibasilar pulmonary fibrosis on chest roentgenogram, sensitivity rose to 97% and specificity was maintained at 98%. However, fully 10% of our own systemic sclerosis patients, all with the CREST syndrome and other convincing evidence of the disease (e.g., esophageal or small bowel abnormalities, pulmonary hypertension, or cardiac involvement), did not satisfy these criteria. Modification of the preliminary criteria to more adequately accommodate individuals with the CREST syndrome presents a challenge for the future.

Clinical Features

Epidemiology

Systemic sclerosis has been described in all races and appears to be global in distribution. It occurs less frequently than systemic lupus erythematosus;

two community studies detected 4.5 and 12.0 new cases per million population at risk annually.[184,225] The disease is unusual in childhood, although it does occur. Women are affected approximately three times as often as men, and this sex difference is 15 to 1 in the childbearing years. No significant racial differences have been found.

Systemic sclerosis is more common among underground coal and gold miners and others occupationally exposed to silica dust.[82,278] Localized sclerodermatous cutaneous changes, a Raynaud's-like phenomenon, and osteolysis of the distal phalanges have been described in workers exposed to unfinished plastics in the manufacture of polyvinyl chloride; these individuals also develop an unusual form of hepatic and pulmonary fibrosis.[73,362] Nail fold microvascular abnormalities that mimic those seen in systemic sclerosis have been observed, but the relationship between these disorders is still uncertain.[206]

Occasionally, relatives of systemic sclerosis patients are affected by other connective tissue diseases, suggesting a heritable predisposition to those disorders. The number of reports of familial scleroderma has significantly increased[224,312] and includes instances of the disease in consanguineous kindreds.[112,238]

Initial Symptoms

The onset of systemic sclerosis is usually between 30 and 50 years of age, but onset in childhood and among the elderly is reported. In most cases of CREST syndrome, the initial complaint is Raynaud's phenomenon. In contrast, patients with diffuse scleroderma most often have skin thickening or arthritis as the first manifestation.[222] In the few remaining patients, the first clue is that of visceral involvement. Dysphagia or intestinal motility disturbances may long antedate the development of cutaneous changes (systemic sclerosis *sine* scleroderma).

Organ System Involvement

Skin. Edematous, indurative, and atrophic stages are recognized in the evolution of scleroderma. In the early or edematous phase, pitting edema of the fingers (''sausaging'') and hands occurs, which may also involve the forearms, legs, feet, and face. The edema may last indefinitely (e.g., fingers in CREST syndrome) or may be gradually replaced by thickening and tightening of the skin after several weeks or months. In the CREST syndrome, involvement of the skin is limited, generally restricted to the fingers and face. Diffuse scleroderma first affects the distalmost extremities and then spreads, in varying degree, to the upper arms, thighs, upper anterior chest, and abdomen (see Table 66–2). The affected skin becomes increasingly shiny, taut, and indurated. Facial changes may lead to the development of a characteristic pinched, immobile, expressionless appearance, with thin, tightly pursed lips and reduced oral aperture (Fig. 66–1). Microstomia may interfere with eating and with proper dental care.

Skin thickening is often accompanied, and in some instances preceded, by an impressive hyperpigmentation that spares the mucous membranes. Plasma levels of beta-melanocyte stimulating hormone are normal.[315] This pigmentation often coexists with tiny hypopigmented spots, leading to a "salt-and-pepper" appearance. Telangiectases consisting of dilated capillary loops and venules are frequent on the fingers, palms, face, and lips (Figs. 66–2, 66–3).

The skin overlying bony prominences, and especially that on the dorsum of the proximal interphalangeal joints, becomes tightly stretched as a result of contractures and is extremely vulnerable to trauma. Patients are often plagued by painful ulcerations at these sites and, less commonly, over the tip of the olecranon and malleoli of the ankles. Secondary infection may supervene. It should be noted that healing of skin is otherwise normal, including repair of surgical incisions.

Patients with systemic sclerosis, especially those with the CREST syndrome, are liable to develop subcutaneous calcification, which occurs chiefly in

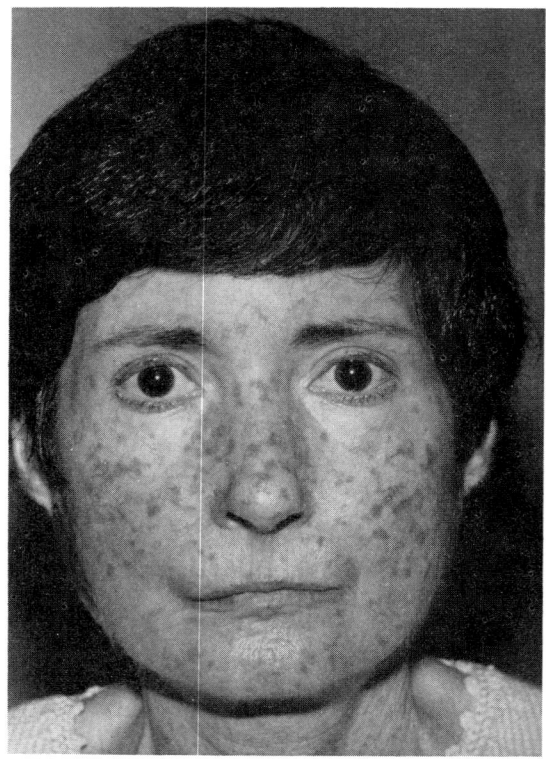

Fig. 66–2.   Face of a 45-year-old woman with systemic sclerosis and CREST syndrome showing multiple telangiectases.

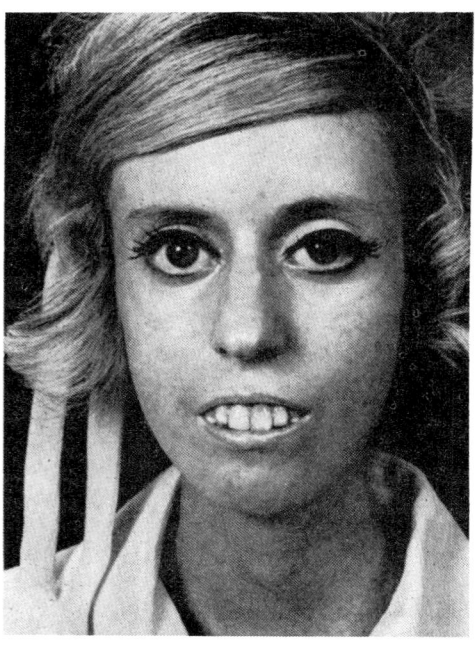

Fig. 66–1.   Face of a young woman with systemic sclerosis and diffuse scleroderma. Note loss of normal skin folds and retraction of lips.

the digital pads and periarticular tissues along the extensor surface of the forearms, in the olecranon bursae, and in the prepatellar area. These deposits vary in size from tiny punctate sites on the fingers (Fig. 66–4) to large conglomerate masses in the forearms. The latter may be complicated by ulceration of overlying skin and intermittent extrusion of calcium phosphate crystals (see Chap. 95).

Early in the disease, biopsy is less reliable for establishing a diagnosis than is careful physical examination of the skin. The weight and thickness of standard-diameter skin cores obtained by full-thickness punch biopsy during this stage of disease are significantly increased (Figs. 66–5, 66–6) and provide an accurate means of assessing the degree and progression of scleroderma.[279] Later, usually after several years, the dermis tends to soften and revert to normal thickness, or to atrophy. Specimens obtained during the active indurative phase of scleroderma disclose a striking increase of compact collagen fibers in the reticular dermis and other typical histopathologic changes, including thinning of the epidermis with loss of rete pegs, atrophy of dermal appendages, and hyalinization and fibrosis

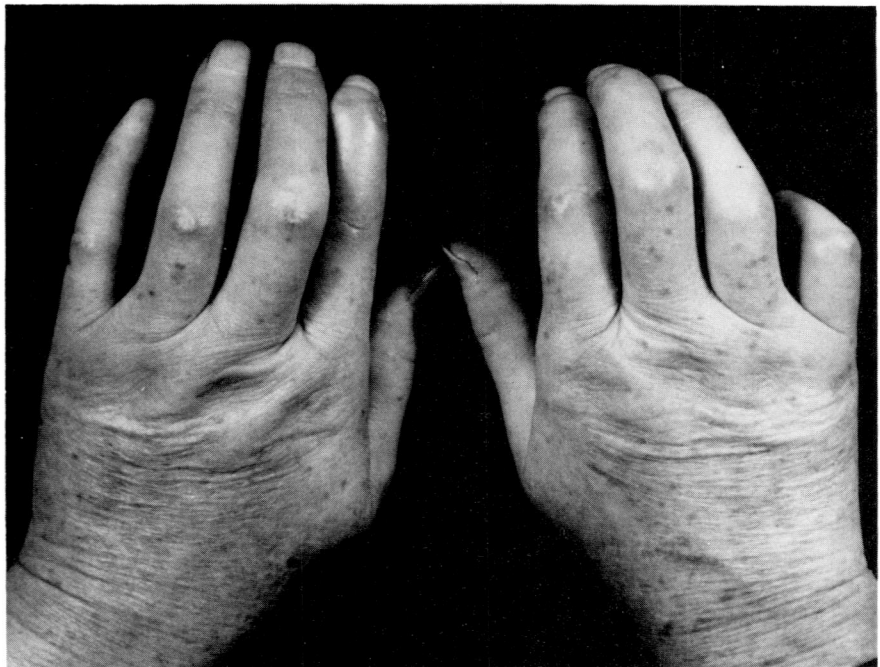

Fig. 66–3. Hands of a 76-year-old woman with systemic sclerosis and CREST syndrome. Note sclerodactyly, digital flexion contractures, and numerous telangiectases.

of arterioles (Fig. 66–7). Increased melanin is found in the basal layer of the epidermis. Variably large accumulations of mononuclear cells, chiefly T-lymphocytes, are encountered in the lower dermis and upper subcutis.[175,283] In typical cases of systemic sclerosis, direct skin immunofluorescence is absent, both at the dermal-epidermal junction and in blood vessels.[57]

Electron microscopic examination of sclerodermatous skin reveals numerous collagen fibers of narrow diameter and immature banding pattern. Also present are many double-stranded beaded filaments identical to those encountered in embryonic skin and believed to be precursors of extracellular collagen.[127,386] Fibronectin has been found in abundant quantity in the deep dermis of involved skin,[58,88] but plasma levels are normal.[322]

Raynaud's Phenomenon. Paroxysmal vasospasm of the fingers in response to cold exposure or emotional stress occurs in over 95% of patients with systemic sclerosis. Typically, the patient reports episodes of sudden pallor and/or cyanosis of the distal two-thirds of the fingers, which become cold, numb, and painful. During rewarming, reactive hyperemia is common. Small areas of ischemic necrosis or ulceration of the fingertip leaving pitted scars are frequent, and in some patients gangrene of the terminal portions of the phalanges ensues. The toes may also be affected and, rarely,

the tip of the nose, earlobes, or tongue. In most cases the Raynaud's phenomenon begins contemporaneously with skin changes and/or rheumatic complaints, or precedes these by a few months to a year. In patients with CREST syndrome, Raynaud's phenomenon may antedate other evidence of systemic sclerosis by many years.[222]

Patients with Raynaud's phenomenon with or without scleroderma have a persistently reduced digital pad temperature in the basal state and subnormal capillary blood flow in the fingers in both warm and cool environments.[54] Reduction in finger systolic blood pressure, unaltered by blockade of the sympathetic nervous system, has been observed.[132] These findings, together with delay in rewarming the fingers after cold exposure, suggest a persistent structural defect in the blood vessels. In systemic sclerosis, angiographic studies support this interpretation, disclosing narrowing and obstruction in the digital arteries (Fig. 66–8).

Concomitantly, the capillary circulation in patients with systemic sclerosis is altered by the appearance of "giant loops" and overall paucity of nail fold vessels on microscopy[209] (Fig. 66–9). Complete arrest of blood flow in these vessels has been observed following exposure to cold.[208] Capillary microscopic patterns are interpreted from photographs,[170] and a grading scale has been devised.[205] These observations may, therefore, be a

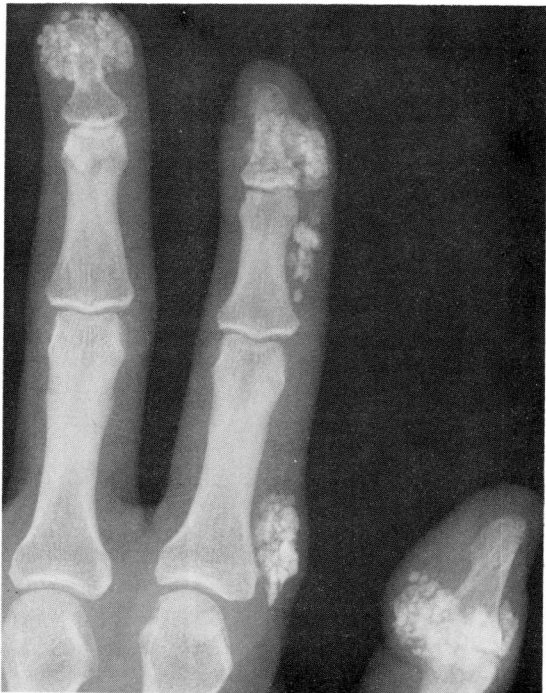

Fig. 66–4. Close-up hand roentgenogram in a 46-year-old woman with systemic sclerosis and CREST syndrome. Note extensive subcutaneous calcinosis.

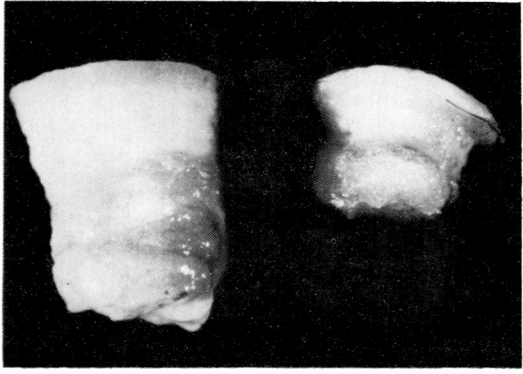

Fig. 66–5. Skin punch biopsies 7 mm in diameter obtained from the forearms of a 57-year-old woman with systemic sclerosis of one year's duration (right, 107.7 mg) and her 39-year-old unaffected sibling (left, 36.0 mg). The epidermal surface is at the top, and all subcutaneous tissue has been trimmed from the lower dermal surface (below). (From Rodnan, G.P., et al.[279])

useful permanent record of the state of the microvasculature. Such capillary changes may be an early predictor of evolution to scleroderma in individuals who clinically appear to have Raynaud's phenomenon alone.[122]

In systemic sclerosis with Raynaud's phenomenon, the viscosity of both blood and plasma has been reported to be increased.[220] In vivo platelet activation, presumably related to vascular injury and repair, was suggested by the finding of elevated levels of circulating platelet aggregates and beta-thromboglobulin.[162] Arteriolar smooth muscle displayed hypersensitivity to 5-hydroxytryptamine[376] and the reverse to catecholamine.[375] Resting venous plasma catecholamine concentrations and urine catecholamine excretion patterns were normal.[296]

Histologic examination of digital arteries at necropsy has revealed prominent intimal and adventitial fibrosis without evidence of inflammation. When severe, these changes led to considerable narrowing or occlusion of the lumen. Recent or old thrombosis was frequently found, and one-quarter of vessels examined had a distinctive lesion: telangiectases of the vasa vasorum[280] (Fig. 66–10).

Bone, Joints, and Tendons. Symmetrical polyarthralgias and joint stiffness affecting chiefly the fingers, wrists, knees, and ankles are frequent initial or early complaints in the course of systemic sclerosis. Such articular findings, with synovitis mimicking rheumatoid arthritis, are often the first manifestation of the disease, especially in individuals with diffuse scleroderma. Generalized swelling of the fingers also occurs. It may be difficult to ascertain the degree to which limitation of interphalangeal joint motion is caused by joint or tenosynovial disease, or to changes in the skin and periarticular connective tissues. Larger peripheral joints may show evidence of frank inflammation, including scanty synovial effusion. The synovial fluid in such cases is turbid and usually contains fewer than 2,000 cells/mm³ that are predominantly mononuclear. Pathologic examination of synovium reveals variable degrees of inflammation with hyperemia and infiltrates of lymphocytes and plasma cells, either in focal aggregates or scattered diffusely.[276]

Some patients are aware of creaking noises on movement. A peculiar type of coarse, leathery crepitus (tendon friction rub) may be palpated over such areas, particularly the elbows, wrists, fingers, knees, and ankles. These rubs, attributed to fibrinous deposits on the surfaces of the tendon sheaths and overlying fascia, are specific for systemic sclerosis with diffuse scleroderma. They occur only rarely in individuals with the CREST syndrome or with other inflammatory rheumatic conditions. Carpal tunnel syndrome may result from flexor

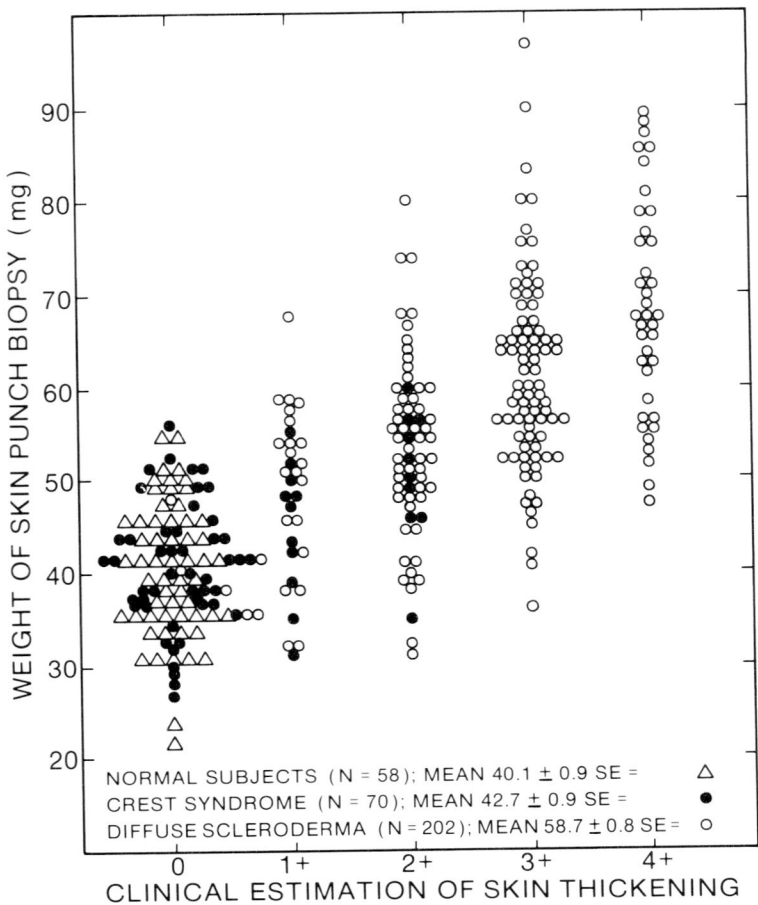

Fig. 66–6. Weight of 7-mm surface diameter skin punch biopsy cores, with subcutis trimmed off, from the midforearm (dorsal surface) of normal individuals and systemic sclerosis patients with CREST syndrome and diffuse scleroderma. The correlation with clinical estimation of skin thickening in the same area by physical examination is shown (Spearman's Rho = 0.69).

tenosynovitis at the wrist. The surface of the affected tenosynovium is covered by a thick coat of fibrin, which is later replaced by intense fibrosis of the lining tissue (Fig. 66–11).[299] Resulting flexion contractures (''bowed fingers'') are caused, at least in part, by tendinous and periarticular fibrosis and shortening.[255] These contractures, which occur commonly in the fingers, wrists, elbows, and ankles, usually become apparent within several months.

The most common radiographic abnormality is resorption of the tufts of the terminal phalanges of the fingers (and much less often, the toes), frequently accompanied by soft tissue atrophy and subcutaneous calcinosis. This resorption, generally limited to the tufts, may be severe, especially in individuals with the CREST syndrome, and may ultimately lead to complete dissolution of the terminal phalanx. Other examples of bone resorption

include ''notching'' of the ribs, which is limited to patients with diffuse scleroderma,[252] and dissolution of the condyle and ramus of the mandible.[251]

Most patients with systemic sclerosis have insignificant loss of articular cartilage and no destruction of subchondral bone. However, a considerably higher than expected frequency of severe erosive disease affecting the fingers, more typical of osteoarthritis than of rheumatoid arthritis, has been reported.[20,29] In our experience, but not that of others,[29] these erosions chiefly affect older women with the CREST syndrome. Patients with and without radiographic changes have similar degrees of joint deformity and skin changes as well as serologic findings. Some individuals with joint erosions are considered to have rheumatoid arthritis as the primary rheumatic disease, but they also have scleroderma.[8]

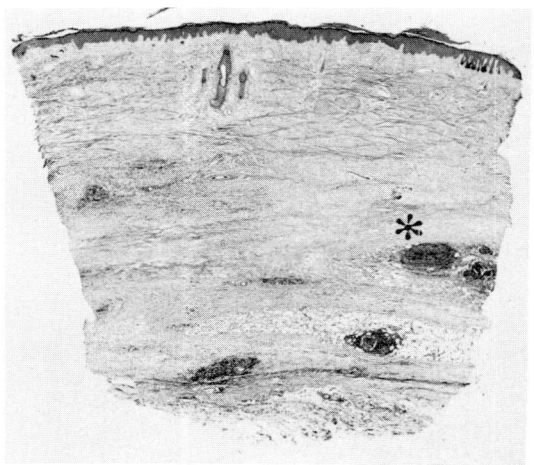

Fig. 66–7.   Photomicrograph of a skin punch biopsy obtained from the dorsum of the forearm of a 53-year-old woman with systemic sclerosis and severe diffuse scleroderma. Skin appendages are atrophic, the dermis is markedly thickened by the deposition of dense collagenous connective tissue, and there are prominent collections of small round cells (asterisk) that were identified as T-lymphocytes.

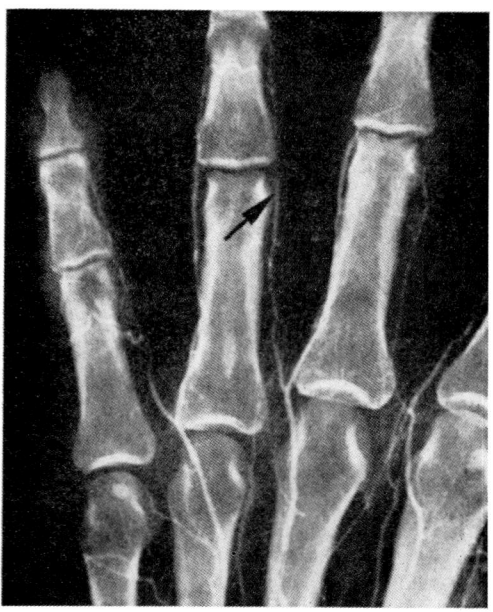

Fig. 66–8.   Brachial arteriogram of a man with systemic sclerosis and Raynaud's phenomenon. Note digital artery luminal narrowing, irregularity, and obstruction.

Patients with systemic sclerosis and calcinosis may develop widespread calcification of the synovium and tendon sheaths.[267] The synovial fluid in these cases has been described as being milky or chalky and containing large numbers of basic calcium phosphate crystals.[35] Thickening of the periodontal membrane, a collagenous structure, may lead to loss of the lamina dura and subsequent loosening of the teeth.

Skeletal Muscle. In many instances, weakness and atrophy of skeletal muscle found in systemic sclerosis are the result of disuse owing to joint contractures or chronic disease. Electromyographic and histologic abnormalities of skeletal muscle may be found in up to 75% of patients. These findings are more frequent among persons with diffuse scleroderma than in those with CREST syndrome.[124]

Approximately 20% of systemic sclerosis patients have a primary myopathy.[222] A few exhibit marked proximal muscle weakness and electrophysiologic, biochemical, and pathologic evidence of polymyositis.[50,223] These individuals may be classified as having "mixed connective disease" if serum anti-RNP antibodies are detected. In most cases, a more subtle myopathy occurs, with mild or no serum muscle enzyme elevation. A muscle biopsy shows replacement of myofibrils with collagenous connective tissue, and perimysial and epimysial fibrosis predominating over inflammatory changes (Fig. 66–12).

Electron microscopic examination of skeletal muscle has revealed a diminished number of capillaries, endothelial swelling of the remaining vessels, and reduplication and thickening of capillary basement membrane,[244,289] but some of these results have been disputed.[351]

Gastrointestinal Tract. *Esophagus.* Esophageal dysfunction eventually develops in nearly 90% of patients with systemic sclerosis, thus constituting the most common internal manifestation of disease. No predilection for diffuse scleroderma or CREST syndrome is obvious. In some cases, this abnormality occurs long before evidence of cutaneous disease, giving rise to a form of systemic sclerosis *sine* scleroderma.

At first, patients may complain only about mild retrosternal burning pain or postprandial fullness. Later, solid food tends to become "stuck" in the esophagus and requires fluids in order to pass. Patients often reduce food intake and may lose appreciable weight. Despite the frequency of peptic esophagitis, esophageal hemorrhage is surprisingly unusual.

Roentgenographic abnormalities are found in three-fourths of the patients, including many who are free from esophageal symptoms. Cinefluoroscopic examination, best performed in the recum-

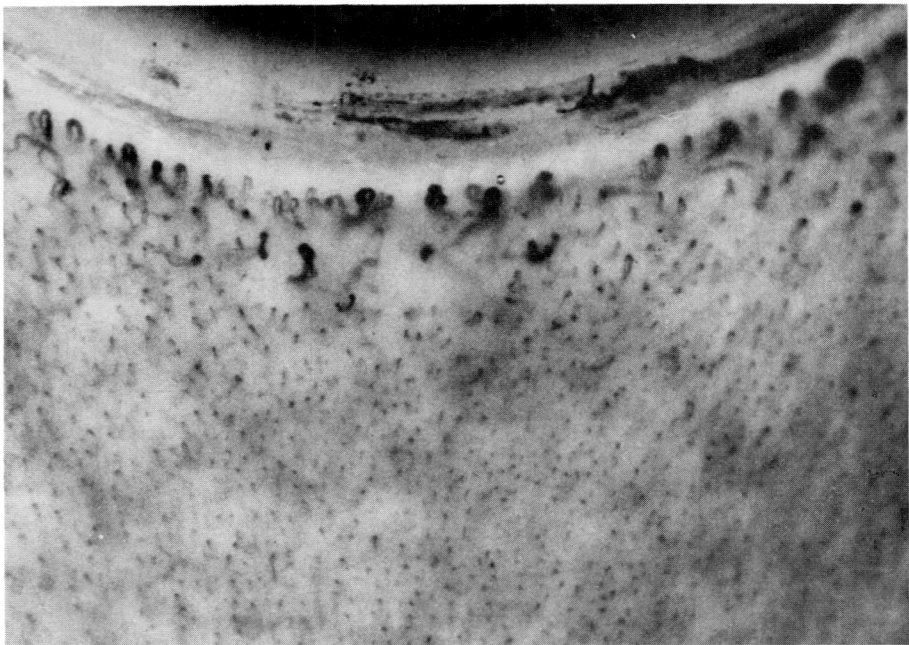

Fig. 66–9. Nailfold capillary pattern of a patient with systemic sclerosis (× 18). Note extensive avascular area along the edge of the nailfold and grossly enlarged capillary loops. (From Maricq, H.R.[204a])

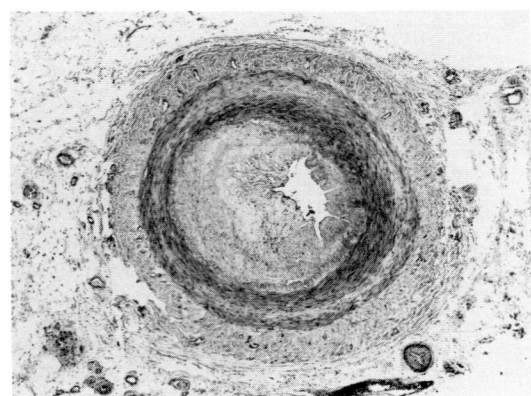

Fig. 66–10. Photomicrograph of a digital artery obtained at autopsy from a 45-year-old woman with systemic sclerosis and diffuse scleroderma who had Raynaud's phenomenon for over 20 years prior to her death. There is near occlusion of the lumen owing to subintimal proliferation and striking periadventitial fibrosis.

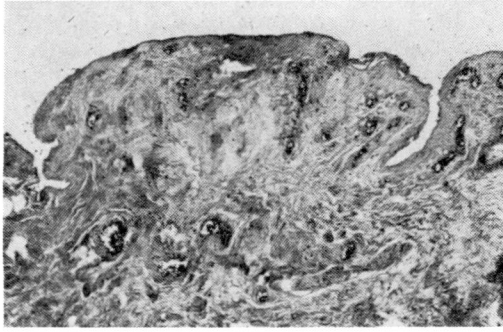

Fig. 66–11. Photomicrograph of the knee (suprapatellar bursa) synovium from a man with systemic sclerosis. Note dense fibrous replacement of the subsynovial tissue. (From Rodnan, G.P.[276])

bent position to eliminate the effect of gravity on emptying the organ, reveals a diminution or even total absence of peristaltic activity in the distal esophagus. Gastroesophageal reflux occurs because of incompetence of the lower esophageal sphincter, and in many cases, there is a small sliding hiatal hernia. With progression, the lower portion of the esophagus tends to become patulous and flaccid, but in some individuals, most often those with the CREST syndrome, peptic esophagitis is complicated by narrowing or stricture in this location (Fig. 66–13).

Manometric measurements reveal incoordination and loss of contractile power, affecting both primary and secondary waves, which may progress to complete, irreversible paralysis. These studies also confirm a reduction in the tone of the gastroesophageal sphincter.[102] This sphincter responds to direct muscle stimulation by metoclopramide,[262] a drug that blocks noradrenergic inhibitory nerves

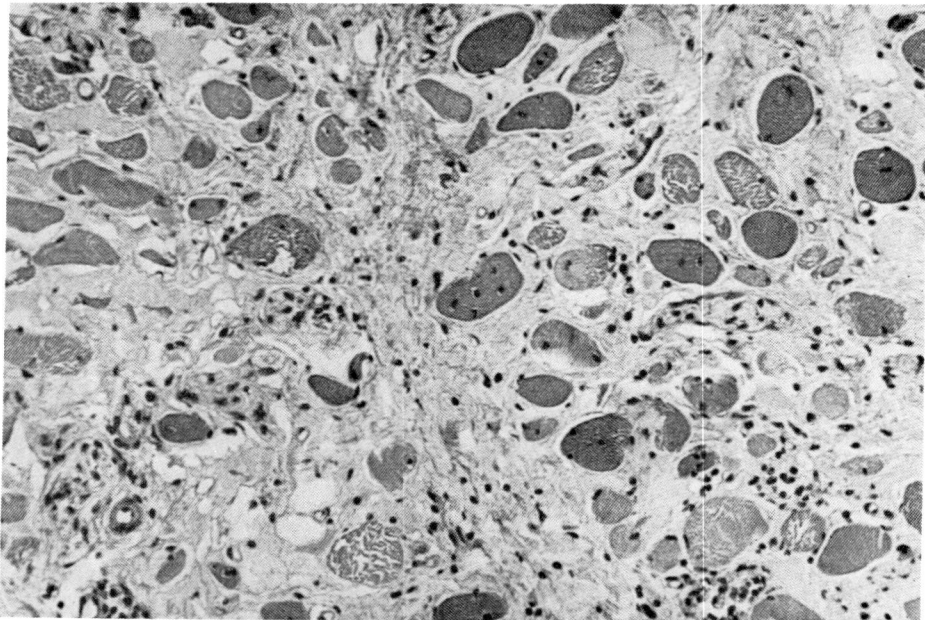

Fig. 66–12.   Photomicrograph of the deltoid muscle from a woman with systemic sclerosis. There is severe atrophy of myofibrils and extensive perimysial and epimysial replacement fibrosis. (From Medsger, T.A., et al.[223]).

with enhancement of the response to acetylcholine and also increases esophageal peristaltic activity. Unfortunately, use of this agent has not resulted in significant clinical improvement in patients with systemic sclerosis.

Upper (pharyngoesophageal) dysphagia with involvement of striated rather than smooth muscle is frequent in polymyositis, but has also been reported in systemic sclerosis.[261] Gastric atony and dilatation may occur, but involvement of the stomach is remarkably uncommon when compared to other portions of the alimentary tract. Gastric acid secretion is unimpaired in systemic sclerosis. Severe blood loss, believed to be secondary to telangiectases affecting the stomach or other upper gastrointestinal tract sites, has been reported.[281] In rare instances, telangiectases have been considered the source of serious bleeding in the gastrointestinal tract or bladder in individuals with CREST syndrome.[6,135]

Histologic changes are most marked in the lower two-thirds of the esophagus. Thinning of the mucosa, which is often ulcerated, may occur. Increased amounts of collagen are present in the lamina propria and submucosa. There is a variable degree of atrophy of the muscularis, which may be almost totally replaced by fibrous tissue. The walls of small arteries and arterioles are thickened and often surrounded by periadventitial deposits of collagen. Cellular infiltrates have been noted in the submucosa and also surround and infiltrate the myenteric plexuses of Auerbach, which may be conspicuously lacking in ganglion cells, but usually do not appear to be abnormal.

Small Intestine. In a small percentage of patients, most often those with the CREST syndrome, the illness is dominated by intestinal complaints, consisting of severe bloating, abdominal cramps, episodic diarrhea, and constipation. A few of these individuals develop malabsorption, which may result in extreme wasting. Striking hypomotility of the small intestine in these patients favors the overgrowth of intestinal microorganisms that consume large amounts of vitamin B_{12} and interfere with normal fat absorption as a result of their deconjugation of bile salts. Of 20 unselected systemic sclerosis patients in one study, 7 had jejunal bacterial cultures showing 10^6 organisms/ml or greater, and 4 had a positive bile acid breath test.[51] Dramatic symptomatic improvement has been observed following the administration of tetracycline or other broad-spectrum antibiotics, but the underlying motility disorder is not reversed by such therapy. Malabsorption most often recurs after variable periods of partial remission.

Myoelectric studies indicate that duodenal smooth muscle dysfunction is characterized by impaired activation by both mechanical and hormonal stimuli.[72] Duodenal and jejunal motor activity recorded manometrically is markedly reduced in symptomatic patients.[265] Radiographic studies may show a pronounced delay in intestinal transit, even in asymptomatic patients, with prolonged retention

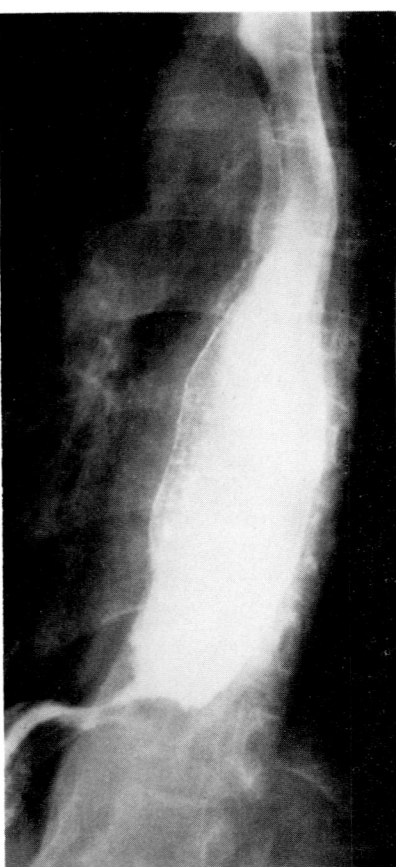

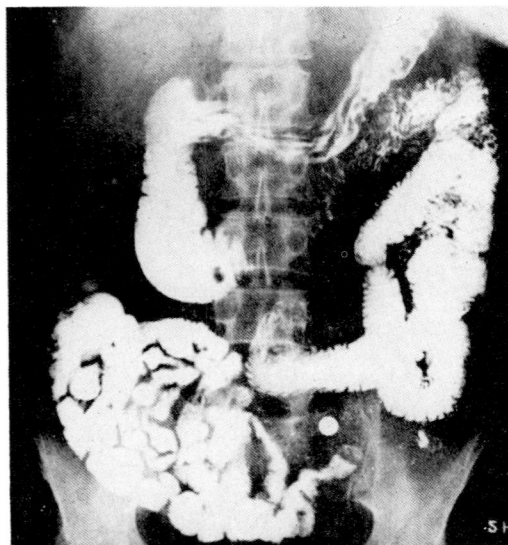

Fig. 66–14. Roentgenogram of the upper portion of the gastrointestinal tract of a 49-year-old man with systemic sclerosis and CREST syndrome. Film was obtained 2 hours after the ingestion of a barium meal. Contrast is retained in the stomach, and the duodenum is dilated (duodenal loop sign).

Fig. 66–13. Roentgenogram of the esophagus in a 49-year-old woman with systemic sclerosis and CREST syndrome who had increasing dysphagia for solid food for over 10 years. Midesophageal dilatation and a distal esophageal stricture are evident.

of barium in the second and third portions of the duodenum, which are often atonic and widely dilated ("loop sign") (Fig. 66–14). In the remainder of the small intestine one may find irregular flocculation of barium or localized areas of dilatation and hypersegmentation. The mucosal pattern of the distended jejunum contains prominent transverse folds (Fig. 66–15). The valvulae conniventes remain close to one another despite the marked dilatation of the lumen ("closed accordion sign"), presumably owing to excessive fibrosis of the submucosa. Similar changes are occasionally found in the ileum. Severe atony of the bowel produces a functional ileus (pseudo-obstruction) with symptoms simulating mechanical obstruction. Volvulus of the greatly dilated small intestine has been observed.[131]

There are several reports of pneumatosis intestinalis in systemic sclerosis. Gas entering from the lumen through small defects in the mucosa and muscularis mucosae appears as numerous radiolucent cysts or linear streaks within the bowel wall (Fig. 66–16). Rupture of subserosal cysts may lead to benign pneumoperitoneum. When rupture is accompanied by symptoms of partial small bowel obstruction, the clinical picture may mimic that of a perforated viscus. Instances of spontaneous small intestinal perforation with abscess formation have also been encountered.[24,266]

With the addition of serosal fibrosis, the chief pathologic changes in the intestine are similar to those described for the esophagus, i.e., normal mucosa or mild villous atrophy, extensive infiltration of the lamina propria by lymphocytes and plasma cells, fibrous thickening of the submucosa, and atrophy of the smooth muscle with collagenous replacement. The intrinsic ganglion cells and their processes have been found to be normal in number and appearance. Thickening of the walls of small arteries and arterioles has been observed, and on rare occasions larger mesenteric vessels have become occluded, with infarction of the pancreas[1] or portions of the ileum and colon.[78,139] Peroral biopsy specimens of the duodenum have revealed the presence of increased amounts of collagen surrounding and infiltrating Brunner's glands. Similar periglandular fibrosis is seen involving the esophageal,

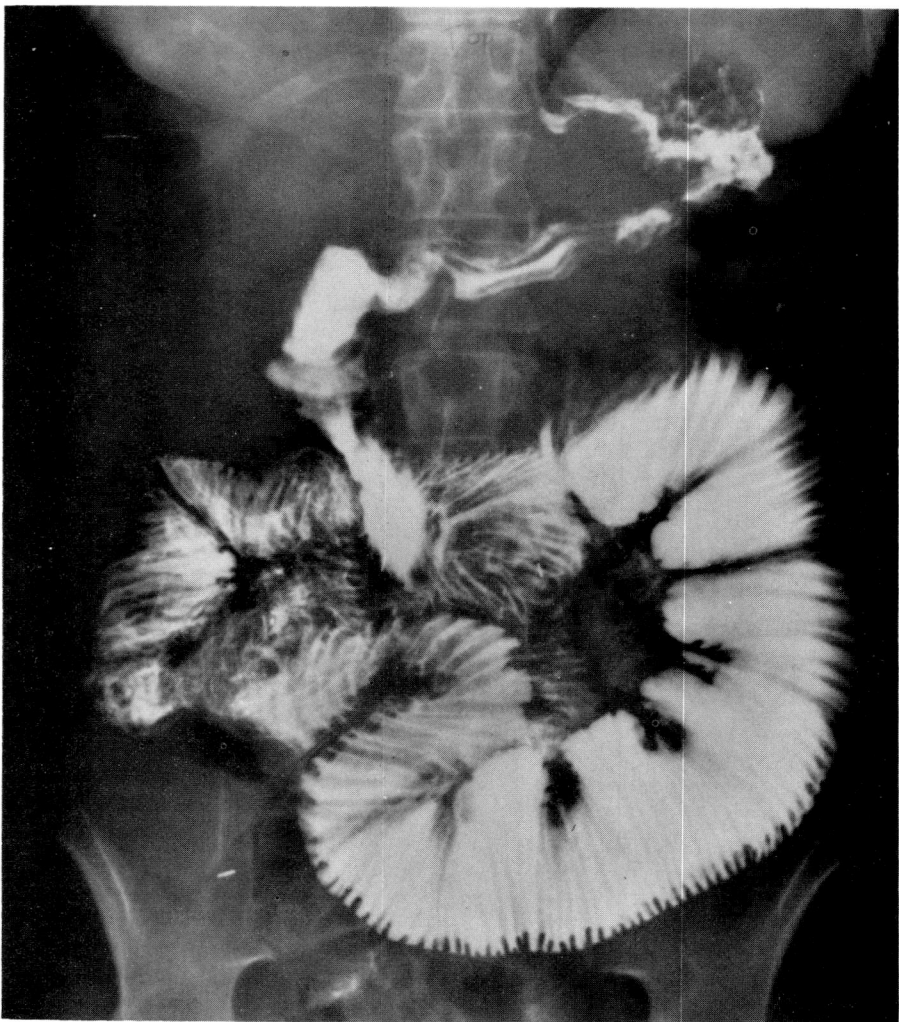

Fig. 66–15.   Upper gastrointestinal tract roentgenogram in a 46-year-old woman with systemic sclerosis and diffuse scleroderma. Although dilatation of the jejunum is striking, its valvulae conniventes remain closely approximated (closed accordion sign).

minor salivary, nasal mucosal, and thyroid glands.[48,109,345]

Colon. Constipation, either alone or alternating with diarrhea, may signal colonic involvement in systemic sclerosis. Reduced motility of this organ by manometry and decreased myoelectric activity have been reported.[23] Patchy atrophy of the muscularis leads to the development of wide-mouthed diverticula, which usually occur along the anti-mesenteric border of the transverse and descending colon (Figs. 66–17, 66–18). In time, these sacculations may disappear, to be replaced by generalized colonic dilatation.[309] Such sacculations may also be found in the jejunum and ileum. They are almost entirely unique to systemic sclerosis, having been described in only a single patient with

amyloidosis.[169] Ordinarily these outpouchings cause no difficulty, but rarely they may perforate or become impacted with fecal matter, producing obstruction.[273] Pneumatosis coli has been observed,[204] as well as volvulus[93] and stenosis[292] of the sigmoid colon and multiple telangiectases of the transverse colon.[212]

Lung. Lung involvement occurs in most patients with systemic sclerosis. The most prominent symptom is exertional dyspnea, which is present in nearly half the patients. Less often there is a chronic cough, which is nonproductive unless associated with superimposed infection, and rarely one or more episodes of pleuritic chest pain. Many patients remain entirely asymptomatic, however, despite evidence of pulmonary fibrosis, possibly

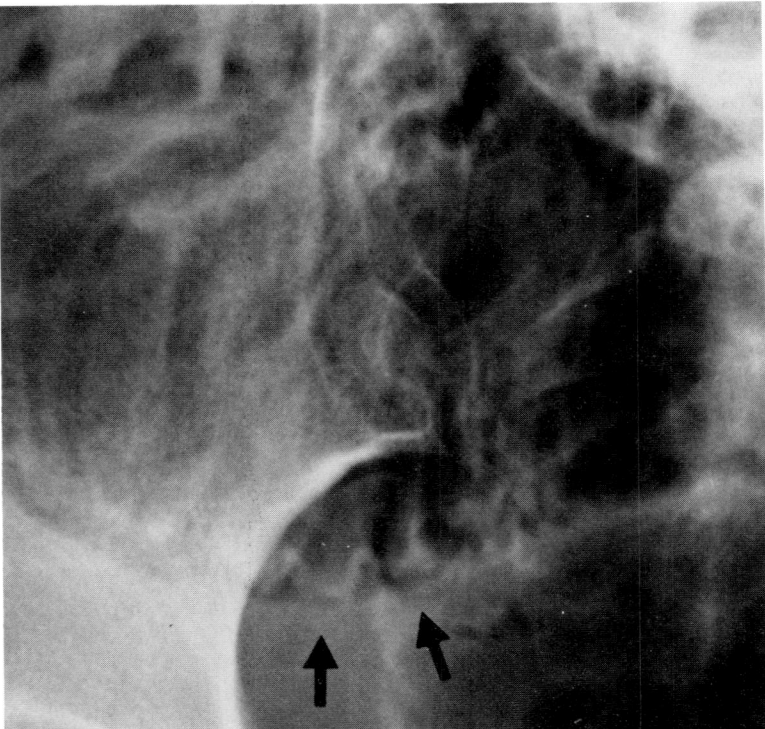

Fig. 66–16. Abdominal film of a patient with systemic sclerosis and CREST syndrome showing dilated loops of bowel and pneumatosis intestinalis (arrows).

because their physical activity is restricted. Physical examination may reveal tachypnea and dry basilar "fibrotic" rales. Intense pleural friction rubs have been noted in patients with pleurisy, but most often examination of the lungs proves unremarkable.

In over one-third of patients with both diffuse scleroderma and CREST syndrome subsets, the chest roentgenogram discloses a reticular pattern of linear, nodular, and lineonodular densities that are most pronounced in the lower lung fields. In some individuals the appearance is that of diffuse mottling or honeycombing, indicative of cystic lesions. Degeneration and rupture of septa lead to cyst-like cavities and small areas of bullous emphysema. Pleural thickening is frequent, whereas pleural effusion is unusual. In one study, calcified granulomata were noted more frequently in CREST syndrome than in diffuse scleroderma (67% vs. 10%), but rib notching was found exclusively in 6% of patients with diffuse scleroderma.[252]

Pulmonary function abnormalities occur in more than two-thirds of all patients with systemic sclerosis, irrespective of disease variant.[118,252] A restrictive ventilatory defect, indicated by a reduction in vital capacity and decreased lung compliance, is most common. Impairment in gas exchange, evidenced by a reduced diffusing capacity for carbon monoxide, is usually present in patients with restrictive lung disease. It is also common, however, as an isolated defect in the absence of both significant alteration in ventilation and roentgenographic evidence of fibrosis. Cold exposure produces an altered diffusing capacity response in systemic sclerosis patients with Raynaud's phenomenon compared to individuals with nonscleroderma-related Raynaud's phenomenon.[84,379] A few scleroderma patients have obstructive disease, but this finding is nearly always attributable to cigarette smoking.[28]

Serial studies of patients over a 10-year period have suggested that pulmonary disease in systemic sclerosis is progressive,[11] but compared with a normal population, no excessive deterioration occurred in these test results.[298]

The predominant histologic changes, present in nearly all cases at postmortem examination, consist of diffuse alveolar, interstitial, peribronchial, and pleural fibrosis (Fig. 66–19). The collagen type is not altered in these tissues.[308] In contrast, gallium scanning has been abnormal in many systemic sclerosis patients, suggesting that an inflammatory

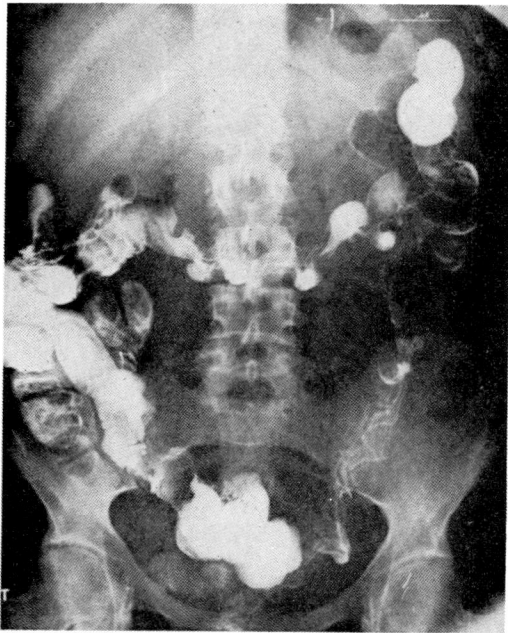

Fig. 66–17. Barium-filled colon of a woman with systemic sclerosis and CREST syndrome. Numerous large-mouthed diverticula are in the transverse and descending portions.

process may be present.[17,99] These results are consistent with the presence of circulating immune complexes in a high proportion of individuals with pulmonary involvement.[99,304] *Inflammatory fibrosing alveolitis* with increased proportions of neutrophils has now been documented by bronchoalveolar lavage.[175a]

Severe pulmonary arterial hypertension with cor pulmonale is encountered almost exclusively in some patients (fewer than 10%) with the CREST syndrome.[295,360] It is not uncommon for this complication to occur several decades after the onset of Raynaud's phenomenon. In this circumstance, there is a markedly accentuated pulmonic component of the second heart sound, and ultimately signs of right-sided cardiac failure. These changes occur in the presence of minimal or no pulmonary interstitial fibrosis.[295] The diffusing capacity is extremely low, consistent with impaired gas exchange across thickened small pulmonary blood vessels.[105,295,338,360] From first clinical detection until death, the mean time is two years, emphasizing the serious nature of this problem.[338] Pathologic signs include widespread narrowing and occlusion of small pulmonary arteries due to accumulation of subintimal mucopolysaccharide, and marked

medial smooth muscle hypertrophy[388] (Fig. 66–20). In contrast, a moderate degree of pulmonary hypertension, with a relatively slow progression, accompanies widespread pulmonary interstitial fibrosis, which gradually obliterates more and more of the pulmonary vascular bed. Pulmonary Raynaud's phenomenon may play a pathophysiologic role in the development of pulmonary arterial hypertension. Increased pulmonary artery pressure after cold challenge has been recorded.[285] Krypton perfusion lung scans showed a decrease in pulmonary perfusion[99] and the carbon monoxide diffusing capacity[379] after cold exposure.

Bronchiolar (alveolar cell) carcinoma has been reported in more than 20 systemic sclerosis patients, generally in the setting of long-standing and severe pulmonary fibrosis and intense bronchiolar epithelial proliferation and cellular atypia. Other types of pulmonary neoplasm may also be more frequent in non-smoking individuals with systemic sclerosis and pulmonary fibrosis.[284,346]

Heart. Cardiac involvement, one of the signs of a poor prognosis in systemic sclerosis, may be classified as primary or secondary.[32,41] Primary disease consists of either pericarditis with or without effusion, left ventricular or biventricular congestive failure, or serious supraventricular or ventricular arrhythmias.

Acute symptomatic pericarditis and pericardial effusion, leading on occasion to cardiac tamponade, have been appreciated with increasing frequency. Asymptomatic pericardial thickening and small effusions are readily detected using echocardiography.[317] The few reported aspirates of pericardial fluid have been exudates without evidence of immune complexes or complement activation.

Clinically apparent *congestive failure* due to myocardial fibrosis occurs in fewer than 10% of patients, nearly all of whom have systemic sclerosis with diffuse scleroderma. In one series, myocardial dysfunction was associated with typical polymyositis in three patients.[370] With the advent of new, noninvasive radionuclide studies, abnormalities of ventricular function have become more frequently recognized.[77,92,101] These changes are attributable to widespread replacement of functioning myocardium in the absence of angiographic evidence of coronary artery disease. Electrocardiographic evidence of *myocardial ischemia and/or necrosis* in the absence of the clinical syndrome of myocardial infarction has been noted.[352] The finding of contraction band necrosis of the myocardium has implied that heart damage in systemic sclerosis may be due to intermittent vascular spasm or "intramyocardial Raynaud's phenomenon."[41] A few such patients have exertional chest pain that mimics angina pectoris.

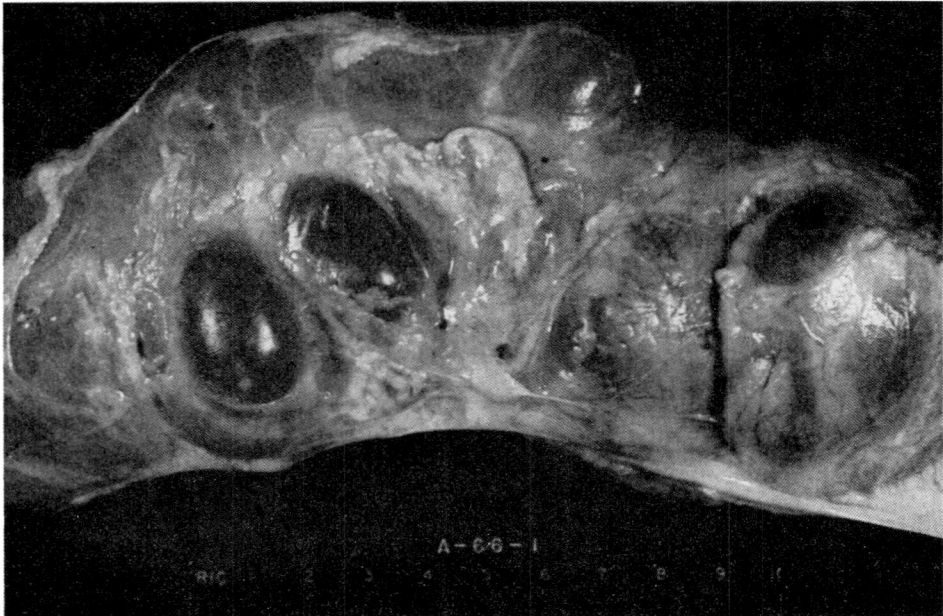

Fig. 66–18.   Gross appearance of the transverse colon from Figure 66–17. The diverticula (sacculations) are large and thin-walled owing to nearly complete absence of the muscularis layer.

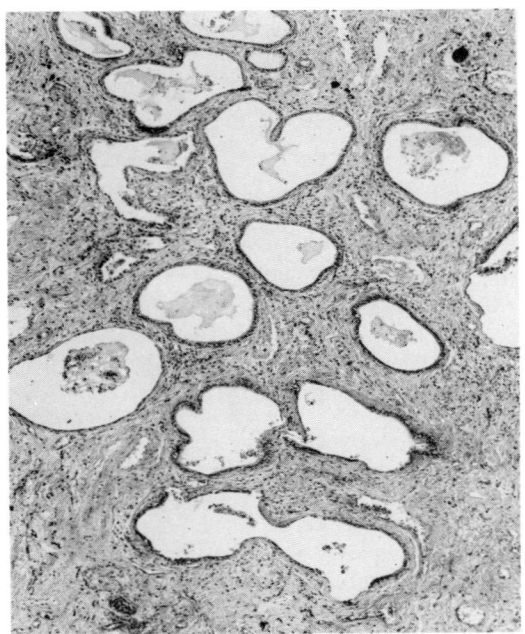

Fig. 66–19.   Photomicrograph of the lung of a 52-year-old woman with systemic sclerosis and diffuse scleroderma. She died as the result of respiratory insufficiency. Note the dramatic interstitial fibrosis and dilatation of air sacs (honeycomb lung).

Autopsy of individuals with diffuse scleroderma may show extensive degeneration of myocardial fibers with replacement by irregular patches of fibrosis that are prominent in, but not limited to, perivascular areas (Fig. 66–21). In addition, focal infiltrates of round cells and thickening of smaller coronary vessels may occur. Extensive disease of these arteries (1 mm diameter) has been reported,[153] but generally the large extramural coronary vessels are normal and myocardial infarction is unusual.

Cardiac arrhythmias, including complete heart block, and other electrocardiographic abnormalities are commonplace, as would be expected in the case of a myocardiopathy. Using the 24-hour continuous electrocardiogram (Holter monitor), 15 to 22% of patients had conduction defects in point prevalence studies.[49,271] Careful dissection of the conduction system of several patients with various rhythm disturbances, including complete heart block, has revealed fibrous replacement of the sinus node, atrioventricular node, particularly in its proximal segment,[270,272] and bundle branches.[156,269] In most cases, however, no specific morphologic changes have been identified in this tissue, and arrhythmias have been attributed to disturbance of the working myocardium.

Secondary causes of heart disease in patients with systemic sclerosis primarily involve the extracardiac stresses of pulmonary and systemic arterial hypertension. The former occurs almost exclusively in the CREST syndrome variant, as noted

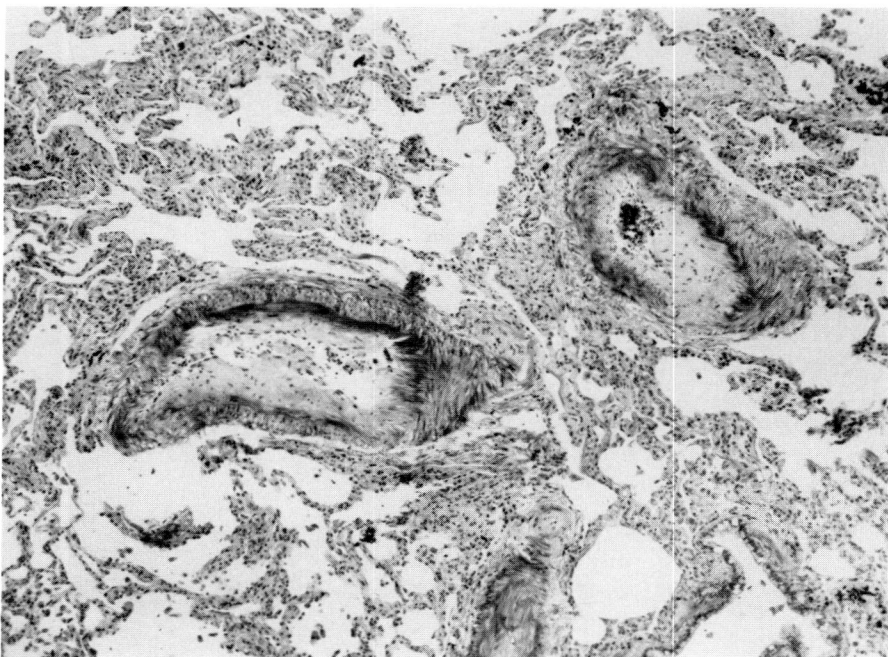

Fig. 66–20. Photomicrograph of the lung of a 61-year-old woman with systemic sclerosis and CREST syndrome who died as the result of pulmonary arterial hypertension with cor pulmonale. There is marked intimal proliferation and medial hypertrophy of small arteries, and no interstitial fibrosis.

previously. Another secondary cardiac disorder is the acute and/or chronic myocardial insufficiency attributable to severe arterial hypertension associated with renal involvement (to be discussed subsequently). The prevalence of valvular lesions is no greater than that found in age-matched controls,[66] and it is difficult to exclude coincidental rheumatic heart disease.

Kidney. Renal involvement is an important aspect of systemic sclerosis and, in the past, a major cause of death. The typical setting is one of severe and rapidly progressive diffuse scleroderma of less than 3 years duration.[328] Rarely is an individual with the CREST syndrome affected. This complication is characterized by the abrupt onset of highly malignant arterial hypertension associated with the early development of rapidly progressive renal insufficiency. The appearance of hypertension is often heralded by a variety of manifestations, including severe headache, visual difficulties resulting from striking hypertensive retinopathy and seizures or sudden left ventricular failure.

Within several days or weeks evidence of renal disease is indicated by microscopic hematuria and proteinuria, rapidly increasing azotemia, and terminally by oliguria or anuria. Proteinuria in the nephrotic syndrome range is unusual, but we and others[254] have noted this complication during the postpartum state, suggesting a contribution by preeclampsia. On occasion the blood pressure may remain within normal limits, but severe hypertension associated with extremely high plasma renin levels is the rule. Prior administration of ACTH or a corticosteroid preparation has been reported as an etiologic factor, but in most instances these drugs cannot be implicated. Their role in provoking or precipitating hypertensive crisis in patients with systemic sclerosis remains controversial.

Before the last decade, survival for more than 3 to 6 months after the onset of this most dreaded complication of systemic sclerosis was almost unknown, the patients succumbing to renal or cardiac failure, or to cerebral hemorrhage despite treatment with various antihypertensive agents. However, the recent aggressive use of potent drugs, including captopril and minoxidil, has dramatically improved the prognosis in so-called "scleroderma renal crisis."[355] Such therapy appears to be uniformly successful in controlling hypertension, but renal insufficiency may, nevertheless, progress.[373] However, in some instances, it has been possible to discontinue hemodialysis after several months.[188,232] Simultaneous remarkable reduction in skin thickness has been noted in patients who have survived renal crisis.[210,366]

Numerous small cortical infarcts are seen grossly

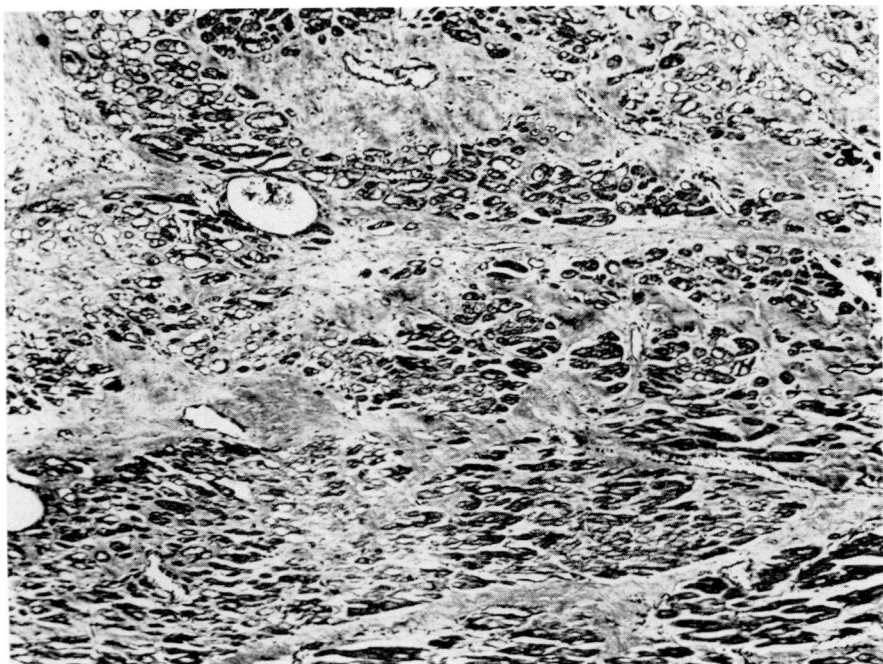

Fig. 66–21. Photomicrograph of myocardium of a 52-year-old woman with systemic sclerosis and diffuse scleroderma who died of congestive heart failure. Loss of normal myocardial fibers is extensive, and interstitial fibrosis is severe.

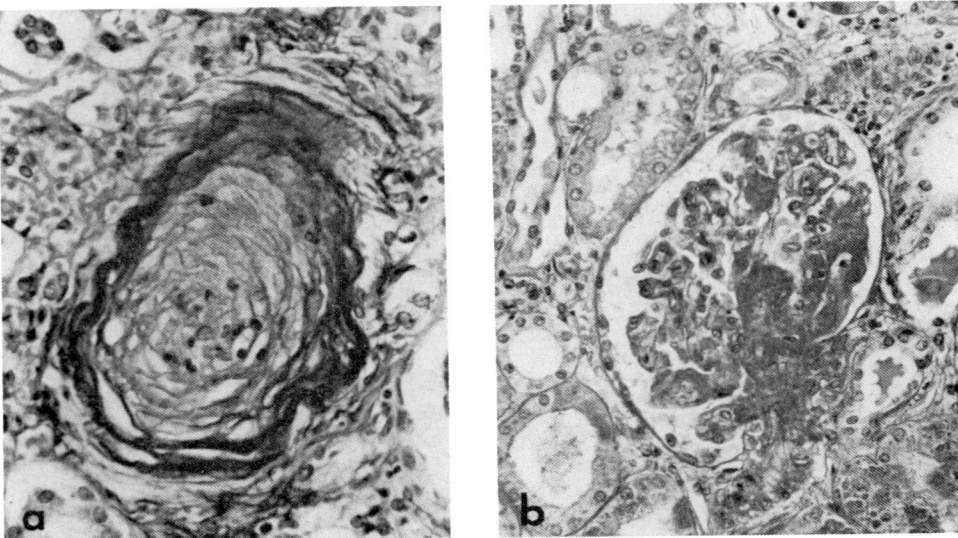

Fig. 66–22. Photomicrographs of kidneys of two women who died of malignant arterial hypertension and renal insufficiency complicating systemic sclerosis with diffuse scleroderma. *a*, Intimal hyperplasia with complete luminal occlusion of an interlobular artery. Note reduplication and fraying of the internal elastic lamina (orcein stain). *b*, Fibrinoid necrosis of blood vessels in the glomerulus.

in the affected kidneys. Focal microscopic alterations consist of (1) intimal hyperplasia with acid mucopolysaccharide deposition in inter- and intralobular and smaller arteries and (2) fibrinoid necrosis of the walls of these vessels, afferent arterioles, and glomerular tufts (Fig. 66–22). Only prominent fibrosis of the adventitia of the small vessels may distinguish this lesion from that of nonsclerodermatous malignant nephrosclerosis.[44] Identical histopathologic changes have been observed in the absence of hypertension.[66] These changes are reminiscent of those encountered in the digital vessels as discussed above.

Immunohistologic examination has revealed the regular presence of immunoglobulins (chiefly IgM), complement components (also reported in malignant hypertension not associated with systemic sclerosis), and antiglobulins, as well as fibrinogen in the walls of affected vessels.[190,219] The demonstration of antinuclear antibodies in the eluates of several kidneys has been construed as evidence for a role of immune complexes in the vessel injury.[217,219] However, electron microscopic examination has failed to reveal discrete electron-dense deposits or other features indicative of the presence of such complexes.[190]

Angiography during life and postmortem injection studies have demonstrated a striking constriction of the interlobular arteries and afferent arterioles and a sharp decrease in glomerular filling[44,146] (Fig. 66–23). In some cases, these changes in the small vessels give rise to a "spotted" nephrogram characterized by focal lucencies scattered throughout the kidneys without evidence of any changes in the major arteries.[377] This disturbance in the renal circulation may be likened to Raynaud's phenomenon in the digital circulation, but is nonspecific, also occurring in the kidneys of patients with malignant hypertension of other etiologies.

The pathogenesis of the renal circulatory abnormalities in systemic sclerosis remains unclear. Both efferent arteriolar constriction and arteriolar hyperreactivity to stimuli such as angiotensin have been proposed. Neither supine nor standing plasma renin elevations have been found to antedate the occurrence of renal involvement.[245,338] An exaggerated increase following cold pressor testing has been reported, especially in normotensive systemic sclerosis patients with prominent vascular changes on renal biopsy.[180] Diminished[65] and normal[116] sodium excretion have both been reported. Because no consistent physiologic changes have been observed, it is likely that mechanisms other than renin-angiotensin system dysfunction are responsible for hypertension in systemic sclerosis. Some, but not all, patients with frank renal involvement show evidence of increased intravascular coagulation and increased plasma fibrinogen turnover,[110] suggesting that intraluminal events play a role in the parenchymal damage.

The lower urinary tract may also be affected in systemic sclerosis. In addition to occasional fibrosis of the wall of the urinary bladder,[264] an instance of unilateral ureteral fibrosis and closure complicated by hydronephrosis has been reported.[179]

Liver and Pancreas. Primary biliary cirrhosis occurs in some women with the CREST syndrome.[268] These patients develop pruritus, jaundice, and hepatomegaly, with a marked elevation of serum alkaline phosphatase activity and antimitochondrial antibodies. Nodular regenerative hyperplasia of the liver has also been reported.[290] Although isolated instances of chronic pancreatitis[113] and arteritis involving this organ[1] have been described, there is no convincing clinical evidence of pancreatic exocrine or endocrine dysfunction in systemic sclerosis. The frequency of pancreatic fibrosis at autopsy has been similar in scleroderma patients,[52] and controls.[66]

Blood. In typical systemic sclerosis, hematologic studies are normal, and abnormalities suggest either a specific complication or an associated illness.[94] Anemia of chronic disease may be present with visceral involvement, e.g., renal failure with microangiopathic hemolysis, intestinal malabsorption, and peptic esophagitis with bleeding. The peripheral blood and bone marrow reflect these circumstances, and the latter is not fibrotic. Autoimmune hemolytic anemia[340] and neutropenia[368] have also been recorded. Leukopenia is often present when systemic sclerosis exists in overlap with SLE or with mixed connective tissue disease.[94] Eosinophilia is unusual; its presence should alert the physician to the possibility of eosinophilic fasciitis (discussed subsequently).

Nervous System. Primary disorders of the nervous system are rare in systemic sclerosis, and those problems that do occur either are purely coincidental or represent secondary manifestations of renal or cardiopulmonary involvement. Trigeminal sensory neuropathy, an occasional finding,[85,349] is associated most closely with myositis and anti-RNP antibodies.[85] Cerebral arteritis has been reported rarely.[83] Impotence without other obvious etiology has been described.[187]

Eye. Most ocular pathology in patients with systemic sclerosis is due to other conditions.[369] Hypertensive retinopathy found in individuals with scleroderma renal crisis has already been described. In addition, patchy areas of nonperfusion have been noted in the choroidal capillary bed in patients with both diffuse scleroderma and CREST syndrome.[106,114]

Sjögren's Syndrome. Xerostomia and kerato

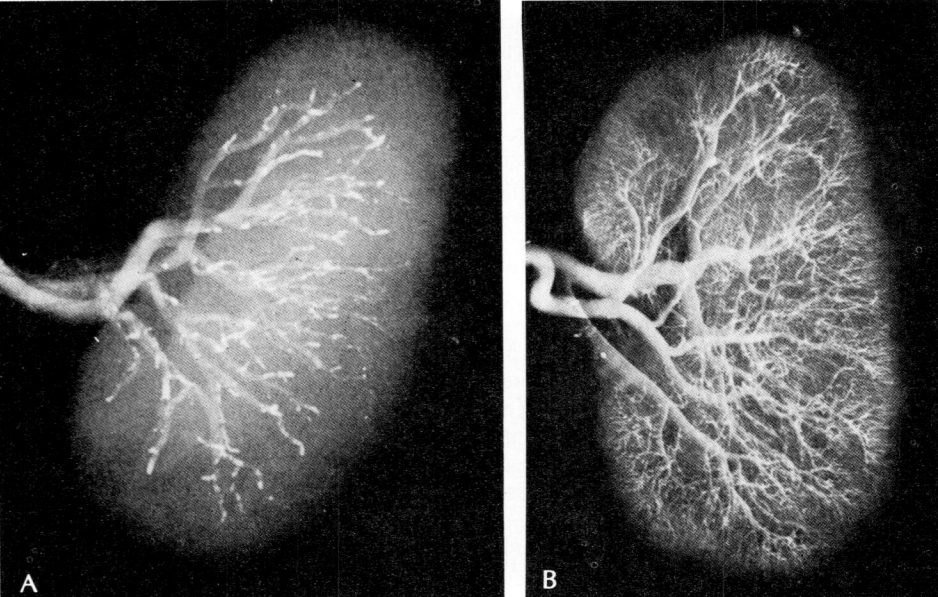

Fig. 66–23.   Roentgenograms of kidneys, injected post mortem, of two patients with systemic sclerosis and diffuse scleroderma. *a,* Kidney of man who died of cardiac disease without clinical evidence of renal involvement. Filling of the interlobular and smaller cortical vessels is normal. *b,* Kidney of man who developed "scleroderma renal crisis" with malignant hypertension and renal failure. There is irregular narrowing of the interlobular vessels, and little filling of smaller vessels supplying the renal cortex.

conjunctivitis sicca are frequent complaints in patients with systemic sclerosis. Based on the presence of lymphocytic infiltration of minor salivary glands on labial biopsy, Sjögren's syndrome is present in approximately 20 to 30% of patients.[98,250] Histologic evidence of periglandular and intraglandular fibrosis, changes believed to be characteristic of scleroderma,[48] are more frequent than inflammation. Nasal mucosal biopsies have shown similar fibrosis surrounding mucous-secreting glands, as well as blood vessel wall thickening, plasma cell infiltration, and electron-dense deposits.[345] Half the patients with systemic sclerosis and Sjögren's syndrome have serum anti-SSA and/or SSB antibodies, but these antibodies occur almost exclusively in patients with lymphocytic infiltration rather than fibrosis.[250] IgM is the dominant salivary and tissue immunoglobulin identified.[86]

Thyroid Gland. Hypothyroidism, often clinically unrecognized, occurs in one-fourth of patients with systemic sclerosis[165] and is frequently accompanied by serum antithyroid antibodies. As in the salivary glands, fibrosis is the dominant histologic finding.[109] Lymphocytic infiltration typical of Hashimoto's thyroiditis is unusual.

Disease Course

The course of systemic sclerosis is extremely variable. Early in the illness it is difficult to judge

prognosis with respect to both survival and disability. Many patients experience steadily increasing sclerosis of the hands and fingers, leading to deforming flexion contractures. In others, mobility is maintained despite the persistence of skin changes. Often, late in the disease, spontaneous improvement occurs, with the skin eventually returning to near normal thickness. In our experience, the most reliable early signs predicting subsequent severe diffuse skin and joint involvement are the appearance of cutaneous thickening prior to the onset of Raynaud's phenomenon, rapid and diffuse skin involvement with truncal changes, and palpable tendon friction rubs.

Most, if not all, patients eventually show evidence of visceral involvement, which can frequently be detected by appropriate testing (e.g., pulmonary function studies, esophageal manometry, and gastrointestinal radiographs) long before the appearance of symptoms. Internal organ dysfunction may occur in the face of minimal or apparently stable scleroderma, and its course may be independent of the latter. Although in many instances clear-cut progression of disease occurs over time, the prefix "progressive" is not uniformly applicable and should be abandoned.

Several large survival studies have been reported and summarized.[224] The 5-year cumulative survival rate after either first physician diagnosis or entry to study has ranged from 34 to 73%, and researchers agree that male sex, older age, and involvement of the kidneys, heart, and lungs adversely affect outcome (Fig. 66–24).

The CREST syndrome was initially considered to represent a benign variant of systemic sclerosis associated with a relatively favorable prognosis. Raynaud's phenomenon, alone or in combination with swollen, puffy fingers, is often present for a decade or more before the diagnosis of systemic sclerosis is entertained. The life span of patients with the CREST syndrome is significantly longer than that of individuals with systemic sclerosis and diffuse scleroderma, in part because the former rarely, if ever, develop myocardial or renal involvement. However, as noted, CREST patients are at higher risk to acquire severe pulmonary arterial hypertension and a peculiar form of biliary cirrhosis.

Pregnancy. Pregnancy appears to exert no consistent effect on the course of systemic sclerosis.[234] Conversely, the disease ordinarily does not interfere with pregnancy and parturition. However, instances of hypertension alone[12] and fatal third-trimester or postpartum renal involvement with severe hypertension (eclampsia?)[321] as well as a case of nephrotic syndrome,[254] have been observed.

Metabolism of Connective Tissue

Morphologic and biochemical evidence indicates that fibrosis of the skin and internal organs in systemic sclerosis is the result of overproduction of collagen. The weight and hydroxyproline content of uniform-diameter skin punch biopsy cores from systemic sclerosis patients are significantly greater in comparison with normal controls, confirming the marked increase in dermal thickness so obvious on clinical and histologic examination (see Figs. 66–5, 66–17).[279] Electron microscopic examination of the skin has revealed numerous collagen fibers of narrow diameter with an immature banding pattern and double-stranded periodic beaded filaments identical to those found in embryonic skin.[127,386] The ultrastructural appearance of dermal fibroblasts also suggests active fibrillogenesis.

Increased levels of protocollagen proline hydroxylase activity have been noted in both the affected[168,358] and unaffected[168] skin of patients with scleroderma. The values are twice as great, however, in the abnormal skin. Measurements of the activity of this enzyme in embryonic tissues and wound healing have correlated well with the rate of collagen synthesis. Additional evidence of the presence of newly synthesized collagen in scleroderma skin includes predominance of type III collagen,[74] an increased amount of readily soluble collagen,[359] and a high proportion of reducible aldimine-bond cross-links.[133]

Finally, dermal fibroblasts from patients with systemic sclerosis propagated in tissue culture synthesize glycosaminoglycans, chiefly hyaluronic

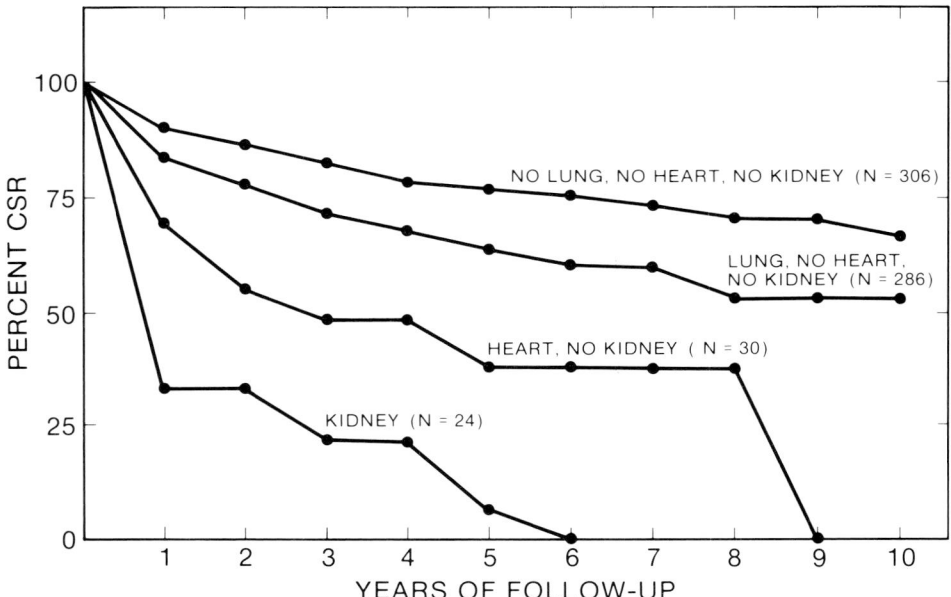

Fig. 66–24. Cumulative survival in patients with systemic sclerosis according to type of visceral involvement at first evaluation at the University of Pittsburgh from 1972 to 1983.

acid, even after many generations,[21,43] and accumulate abnormally large quantities of collagenase-sensitive protein (collagen).[38,195] Cells derived from the deeper portions of the dermis and subcutis are particularly active in this regard. Increased urinary excretion of acidic glycosaminoglycans, especially heparan sulfates, has been noted in patients with systemic sclerosis.[239]

The addition of serum from patients with systemic sclerosis enhances the synthesis of procollagen and hydroxyproline by cultured dermal fibroblasts, but this effect may be nonspecific.[22,347] Serum from patients with early scleroderma and more extensive skin involvement increases the rate of skin fibroblast proliferation.[258] Conflicting evidence has been presented regarding cytotoxic activity of sera from patients with systemic sclerosis for cultured human endothelial cells and fibroblasts.[56] Cloned human fibroblasts exposed to scleroderma sera show selective growth of high collagen-producing cells, suggesting that a selection of a subpopulation of cells underlies excessive collagen accumulation.[33] Other mechanisms, such as reduced collagen degradation, may also contribute to excessive accumulation of connective tissue components.[158]

Collagen in the skin of patients with systemic sclerosis appears to be qualitatively normal; studies have included the amino acid composition of the insoluble collagen fraction, collagen shrinkage temperature, and contractile qualities. Both type I and type III collagen, as well as procollagen, have been identified in the skin in the early stage of scleroderma. Later, when fibrosis dominates, the collagen is almost exclusively type I. Type V collagen, which is found frequently in vascular structures, has been identified in lower dermal tissues.[104]

Reports concerning serum glycosaminoglycan (mucopolysaccharide) and mucoprotein levels and urine glycosaminoglycan excretion in systemic sclerosis are conflicting, in part because of differences in methodology and case selection. Early stages show histologic evidence of an increase in acid mucopolysaccharides in the dermis. It appears likely that water binding by these substances accounts for the edema of the extremities, which is one of the first manifestations of the disease. Later in the course of scleroderma, however, there is a notable diminution or absence of such material in the skin.

Autografts of clinically normal abdominal skin transferred to the scleroderma-involved forearm have been reported to become progressively sclerodermatous, whereas forearm skin placed in the abdominal site remained thickened.[96] In contrast, the skin changes of localized scleroderma (morphea) proved reversible after transplantation into normal areas.[126] The importance of extracutaneous factors in determining the localization and severity of cutaneous involvement in systemic sclerosis is further suggested by the following case: A finger that had been reattached following accidental amputation many years prior to the development of scleroderma remained unaffected while Raynaud's phenomenon and the resorption of terminal phalangeal bone occurred in the remaining digits.[297]

Etiology and Pathogenesis

Systemic sclerosis has been linked with rheumatoid arthritis, systemic lupus erythematosus, polymyositis-dermatomyositis, and other connective tissue diseases because of certain epidemiologic similarities, overlapping clinical features, and involvement of blood vessels as a common target organ (see Chap. 2). The concept of immunologic and microvascular abnormalities as the common denominators in the pathogenesis of these diseases has been strengthened with respect to systemic sclerosis by evidence drawn from several different investigations.

Vascular Hypothesis

Widespread vascular disease affects the medium and small arteries and microvasculature of many organs, including the gastrointestinal tract, lungs, heart, and kidneys as well as the digital arteries. One popular concept is that systemic sclerosis is the end result of repeated insults to the vascular endothelium.[194]

Specific serum endothelial cell cytotoxic activity has been described[56,161] but not confirmed by all investigators.[229,310] The activity of products of these cells, factor VIII/von Willebrand factor antigen and von Willebrand factor, was increased under basal conditions (more so after cold exposure).[163] Decreased platelet serotonin content indicating platelet release[389] and raised levels of circulating platelet aggregates and plasma β-thromboglobulin, presumed to reflect vascular injury and repair, have been reported in patients with systemic sclerosis.[162]

At the level of the small artery, such platelet factors are capable of stimulating proliferation and connective tissue synthesis by smooth muscle (myointimal) cells in the vessel wall. Periadventitial fibrosis may be explained by increased vascular permeability and diffusion of platelet factors. In capillaries devoid of myointimal cells, devascularization occurs and existing vessels become dilated and telangiectatic, leading to the changes observed on capillary microscopy. Interstitial fibroblasts may be stimulated to produce collagen by escape of platelet factors from such compromised capillaries.

Vasoconstriction could also play an important

role because the aforementioned processes may be triggered by altered blood flow and resultant ischemia or intravascular coagulation. Cold exposure has been shown to cause capillary "standstill,"[207] decreased blood flow in the kidney,[44] and gastrointestinal,[333] pulmonary,[84] and myocardial[5] dysfunction.

Although a positive correlation appears to exist between the severity of skin capillary abnormalities and multisystem involvement,[209] the role of vascular disturbances in the pathogenesis of systemic sclerosis, including fibroblast activation, is unclear. For example, blood flow has been reported to be normal in the skin and subcutaneous tissue of the clinically involved forearm[53] and increased in areas of dense fibrosis from the dorsum of the hand.[182] Thus, mechanisms other than faulty nutritional blood flow must be invoked.

Immunologic Abnormalities

Association with Other Autoimmune Disorders. A variety of "overlap" conditions have been described in which patients with systemic sclerosis also have features of rheumatoid arthritis, polymyositis-dermatomyositis, and mixed connective tissue disease. In addition, the frequency of Sjögren's syndrome,[48] autoimmune thyroiditis,[109] and biliary cirrhosis[268] is unusually high in patients with systemic sclerosis.

Serologic Abnormalities. *Serum Proteins.* Moderate hypergammaglobulinemia (1.4 to 2.0 g/100 ml) occurs in over one-third of patients with systemic sclerosis, and is most often encountered in the setting of overlap conditions, such as mixed connective tissue disease. Typically, IgG is increased, but IgM elevation has also been observed.[15] Monoclonal gammopathy has been described in several cases of systemic sclerosis,[47,174,242] and a child with systemic sclerosis and myositis with IgA deficiency has been reported.[148] Mixed cryoglobulins[144] and circulating immune complexes have been either absent[246] or detected in only small amounts.[304]

Rheumatoid Factor and LE Cell Reactions. Between one-quarter and one-third of patients with systemic sclerosis have positive tests for rheumatoid factor, usually in low titer. Positive LE cell reactions and biologic false positive serologic reactions for syphilis have been reported most often in overlap syndromes.

Antinuclear Antibodies. With the use of multiple substrates, antinuclear antibodies have been found in the sera of over 90% of patients with systemic sclerosis.[25] The titers were typically low, as compared with those found in SLE, but titers of 1:1000 or greater were seen occasionally. In most instances, the pattern of nuclear fluorescence

was that of fine or large speckles or of threads, but occasionally diffuse (homogeneous) nuclear staining occurred. Both IgG and IgM antibodies occurred, but the predominant antinuclear (and antinucleolar) antibodies in patients with systemic sclerosis consisted of IgG, most often of the IgG3 subclass.[300] One recently identified antinuclear antibody, anti-Scl 70,[75] was found in 20% of systemic sclerosis sera, but rarely in control specimens.[46] It was associated more frequently with diffuse scleroderma and pulmonary involvement.[46]

Sera of individuals with systemic sclerosis contain either no antibody to native DNA, or only small quantities, and lack anti-Sm antibody; about 20% of patients have low titers of antibody to nuclear ribonucleoprotein (anti-nRNP). Antibody directed against a nuclear antigen (Ku), distinct from nRNP, has been found in a small proportion of Japanese patients, nearly all of whom had a scleroderma-polymyositis overlap syndrome.[231]

Little if any correlation appears to exist between the presence or titer of antinuclear antibody and the clinical severity or duration of disease, although there is some disagreement in this matter.

Anticentromere Antibodies. Antibodies morphologically appearing as fine, discrete speckles have been identified[42] as being directed against the centromeric portion of chromosomes observed in dividing cells (Fig. 66–25). Termed anticentromere antibodies, they have remarkable specificity (over 50%) for the CREST syndrome variant of systemic sclerosis[348] and occur in fewer than 5% of patients with diffuse scleroderma.[330] These antibodies are found in a few individuals with Raynaud's phenomenon alone, and those persons may be at increased risk to develop CREST syndrome eventually.[167] Anticentromere antibodies, primarily IgG, tend to persist in the serum for prolonged periods.[216,354] Immunoelectron microscopy has pinpointed the antigen as residing in the kinetocore region of chromosomes, but its precise identity is not yet known.[36]

Antinucleolar Antibodies. Nucleolar immunofluorescence or serologic evidence of antinucleolar antibodies has been reported in 10 to 54% of different series of cases. These antibodies, which are found more often in systemic sclerosis than in any other connective tissue disease, are particularly common in patients with associated Sjögren's syndrome. The responsible nucleolar antigens are still unknown.

Other Antibodies. Antibodies to centrioles have been detected in two patients with systemic sclerosis[233,249] and in one with Raynaud's phenomenon.[233] Cold-reactive anti-T-lymphocyte antibodies have been found by some[185,259] but not other[146a] investigators.

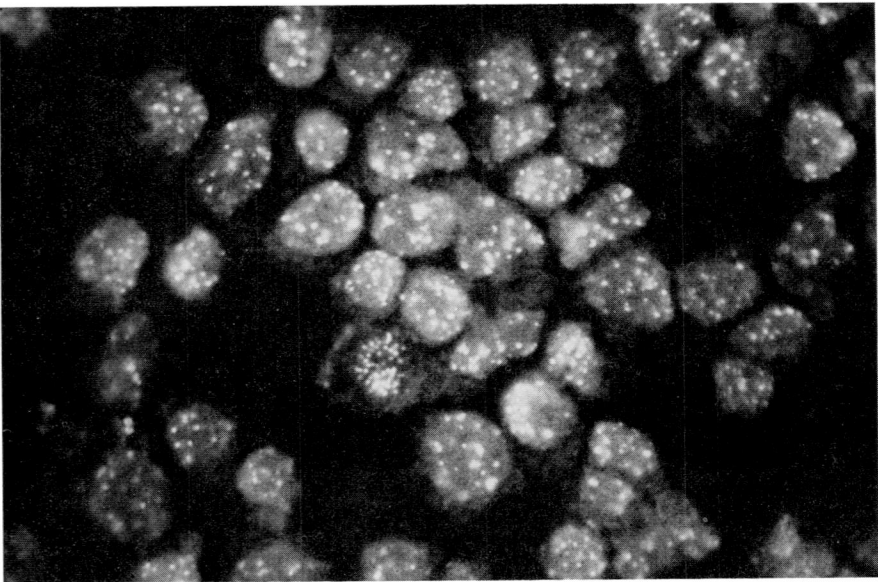

Fig. 66–25. Pattern of nuclear anticentromeric immunofluorescence on HEp-2 cells produced by serum from a patient with systemic sclerosis and CREST syndrome. (From the 1981 Revised Clinical Slide Collection on the Rheumatic Diseases. Reprinted with permission of the Arthritis Foundation, Atlanta.)

Antibodies to polyuridylic acid have been observed in patients with active diffuse scleroderma.[129] Antibodies to collagen types I and IV (basement membrane), found in most patients in one series, were correlated with a reduction in pulmonary diffusing capacity.[200]

Lymphocyte Abnormalities. Early in the course of disease, impressive collections of lymphocytes and plasma cells have been detected in the synovium, skin, gastrointestinal tract, lung, and other locations. The cells found in the dermis (see Fig. 66–7) have been identified, using monoclonal antibodies,[283] as consisting chiefly, if not wholly, of T-lymphocytes. In the peripheral blood, the number of T cells is most often reduced, with no consistent alteration in the number of B-lymphocytes. Further analysis of T cell subsets in the blood using monoclonal antibodies showed that the ratio of T-helper to T-suppressor cells is elevated in one-third of patients, owing to a decrease in circulating T-suppressor lymphocytes.[283,371] T-suppressor cells do not preferentially accumulate in the skin of patients with systemic sclerosis, whereas T-helper lymphocytes predominate regardless of the helper:suppressor ratio in the peripheral blood.[283] Both low[117] and high[3,172] T-helper to T-suppressor cell ratios and low[371] or normal[173] suppressor cell activity have also been found in peripheral blood.

With the exception of bacterial infections of the skin (especially fingertips and sites overlying bony prominences) and perhaps the lung, individuals with systemic sclerosis are not particularly prone to infections. In vitro leukocyte migration to casein is normal,[324] but phagocytosis has been found to be either normal[324] or reduced.[15] A normal response to antigenic stimulation with blood group substances has been reported.[335]

No clinical evidence of abnormal cell-mediated immunity is apparent in systemic sclerosis. Peripheral blood lymphocytes have reacted in a normal or near-normal manner to stimulation by phytohemagglutinin and other nonspecific mitogens. Exceptions include reports of impaired phytohemagglutinin-induced transformation response[137,142,198] and significantly decreased response to concanavalin A[294] and pokeweed mitogen.[19,294] Monocyte abnormalities may contribute to this hyporesponsiveness.[198] Serums from subjects with scleroderma have not inhibited blastogenesis of autologous lymphocytes.[138]

When challenged with a variety of antigens in vitro, peripheral leukocytes (lymphocytes) of patients with systemic sclerosis respond by blastogenesis. Lymphocytes of scleroderma patients with myositis have been stimulated strongly on incubation with a homogenate of muscle.[64] In other studies, these cells produced increased amounts of leukocyte migration inhibition factor[143] and a factor chemotactic for human monocytes.[337] Lymphocytes from systemic[337] and localized[98] scleroderma patients have undergone transformation in response to various human and animal skin collagen prep-

arations. The cells of patients with systemic sclerosis and diffuse scleroderma were stimulated to
produce macrophage migration inhibitory factor by
skin extracts of both normal and sclerodermatous
skin, whereas the lymphocytes of those with the
CREST syndrome were not.[175]

Peripheral blood mononuclear cells of patients
incubated with systemic sclerosis serum showed
selectively decreased spontaneous antibody-dependent and PHA-induced cell-mediated cytotoxicity against Chang liver cells,[59,382,384] but not
against chicken erythrocytes[59] or fibroblasts.[60,383]
These findings suggest a specific reduction or
blockade of certain effector cells in systemic sclerosis. Prostaglandin-producing but not concana-
valin-A-induced suppressor cell activity was found
to be increased,[181,301] whereas impaired primary in
vitro antibody response has been attributed to a
population of suppressor monocytes.[301]

These observations take on particular significance in view of other investigations that reveal
the influence of lymphokines on fibroblast activity.
Stimulated peripheral blood lymphocytes produce
a factor that is chemotactic for human dermal fibroblasts.[257] In addition, lymphokine-rich supernatants from activated normal human and scleroderma peripheral blood mononuclear cells enhance
collagen production by embryonic lung and foreskin fibroblasts.[45,160,323] Such fibroblast-stimulating
factors may be implicated in the fibrosis characteristic of chronic inflammation, which occurs in
many different disease states in addition to systemic sclerosis. These stimulatory effects of mononuclear cell supernatants may result in permanent
alteration of a certain subpopulation of fibroblasts;
i.e., these cells may acquire the ability to synthesize increased quantities of glycosaminoglycans
and may continue to do so for many generations,
even after mononuclear cell products are no longer
added to the cultures.[381] Alterations in the clonal
composition and phenotypic expression of these
fibroblasts have been hypothesized.[177]

Of interest in this regard is the development of
cutaneous fibrosis, joint contractures, and a Sjö-
gren-like syndrome in individuals with graft-vs.-
host disease following bone marrow transplantation.[100] However, infrequent Raynaud's phenomenon, atypical skin and esophageal changes, and
the presence of eosinophilia and hypergammaglobulinemia are features that suggest that this condition is different from systemic sclerosis.

**Family Studies and Histocompatibility Anti-
gens.** Although familial systemic sclerosis is unusual, reports have appeared with increasing frequency in recent years.[224] The disease has been
described in siblings, parent and child, and second-
degree relatives. Although such pairs have shown

a wide variety of clinical manifestations, strikingly
similar familial instances of fatal bowel
involvement[336] and the coexistence of CREST and
Sjögren's syndrome[95] have been encountered.
Serum antinuclear antibodies have been detected
in 7% of the first-degree relatives of patients with
systemic sclerosis and in over one-half of those
over age 60.[282]

Impaired responses to systemic sclerosis cells in
mixed lymphocyte culture experiments have been
found.[4,70,128] Although several small series of patients have been published with various A, B, and
DR locus histocompatibility antigen associations,
the number of patients studied has been embar-
rassingly small. Larger populations have shown no
such HLA correlations, but meaningful clinical
subsets may have been overlooked in these
analyses[27,372] (see Chap. 25).

Miscellaneous Abnormalities. The level of
serum complement is normal in all but a few patients with systemic sclerosis. An increase in random chromosomal breakage has been noted both
in patients and in their siblings and children.[80] It
has been suggested that this increase may constitute
evidence of a familial tendency toward autoimmune disease. Two cases on record demonstrate
an apparently fortuitous association between primary amyloidosis and systemic sclerosis.[199,293] Reported abnormalities in tryptophan metabolism are
discussed in the following section.

Experimental Models

In rats that develop homologous disease after the
injection of large numbers of lymphoid cells from
an unrelated strain of donor animals, a chronic
dermatitis develops, characterized by an increase
in dermal collagen, atrophy of the epidermis and
skin appendages, and minimal or no inflammatory
reaction. This circumstance is reminiscent of the
sclerodermatous skin change in patients with
chronic graft-vs.-host reaction after bone marrow
transplantation.

The TSK (tight skin) mutant mouse strain has
dermal thickening due to increased collagen, and
cardiac and pulmonary abnormalities atypical of
systemic sclerosis.[111,287] Scleroderma-like changes,
with abnormal skin physical and biochemical
characteristics[248] and metabolism,[157] have also been
noted. A disease with both clinical and serologic
abnormalities closely resembling systemic sclerosis has been described in white leghorn chickens;
manifestations include gangrenous changes in the
comb and digits and serum antinuclear antibodies.[107]

Whether such models will furnish important biochemical and immunologic insights into the pathogenesis of systemic sclerosis, or will provide a

mechanism for screening of potential therapeutic agents, is unclear.

Treatment

The first responsibility of the physician is to discuss the nature of the disease with the patient and his family, who are often unreasonably pessimistic. When possible, classification as diffuse scleroderma or CREST syndrome is helpful in understanding the future risk of developing visceral complications. Such classification helps to establish a good relationship between physician and patient which is particularly important in this chronic, demanding disease. Diagrams of the blood vessels, skin, esophagus, and other appropriate illustrations are useful in instruction.

A long list of vitamins, hormones, pharmaceuticals, and surgical procedures has been used to treat systemic sclerosis; nearly all of these have been abandoned after initial enthusiasm and later critical trial. Improvement can hardly be expected in those manifestations that are the result of far-advanced tissue fibrosis. Too often success has been claimed solely on the basis of a diminution in subjective complaints (e.g., a reduction in frequency of Raynaud's phenomenon, which occurs with virtually any new treatment) and poorly documented "softening" of the skin.

Evaluation of the effectiveness of treatment has proved difficult for several reasons.[221] Systemic sclerosis is variable in its severity and in its rate of progression; therefore, the classification of patients into subsets is important in understanding the results of therapy. Because spontaneous improvement often occurs after several years, controlled trials are necessary. There are limitations in the availability and application of objective criteria for ascertaining improvement (or deterioration) in the condition, particularly with respect to visceral changes. Finally, the influence of psychologic factors on many of the systems is important.

Drugs. Figure 66–26 summarizes current concepts of the pathogenesis of systemic sclerosis and indicates those points at which therapeutic intervention might be effective. *No drug or combination of drugs has been proved to be of value in adequately controlled prospective trials or is generally accepted as being useful.* Anti-inflammatory agents and corticosteroids have been disappointing. Because of potent side effects, we restrict the use of corticosteroids to patients with inflammatory myopathy or serositis characteristic of an overlap syndrome such as mixed connective tissue disease. The latter patients often respond favorably to relatively small doses of corticosteroids, i.e., prednisone 10 mg per day, with a reduction in the swelling or tightening of the skin, cessation of

fever, and improvement in arthritis. Myositis, however, may require higher doses.

In recent years, attention has been focused on D-penicillamine, a compound that interferes with the intermolecular cross-linking of collagen[241] and also possesses immunosuppressive activity (see Chap. 31). In several early studies, the results were generally disappointing, although in most of these cases D-penicillamine was given for less than a year.[30,374] Later reports from England,[156] Denmark,[9,10] and Russia[147] have been more optimistic. One study described 25 of 34 patients as improved after receiving an average total D-penicillamine dose of approximately 1,000 g during a mean of 2.3 years.[10] In a retrospective analysis of diffuse scleroderma patients with disease duration of less than 3 years, 73 patients treated with D-penicillamine for at least 6 months were compared with 45 not receiving this drug.[329] The treated group showed significantly reduced skin thickness and joint contractures after 18 to 30 months and also better survival, primarily owing to a considerably lower frequency of subsequent renal involvement. The use of D-penicillamine is accompanied by a disturbing plethora of side effects, including fever, loss of taste, nausea, anorexia, rash, leukopenia, thrombocytopenia, aplastic anemia, nephrotic syndrome, and myasthenia gravis.[353] Over one-fourth of patients may be forced to discontinue the drug.[329] A number of these undesirable side effects, particularly gastrointestinal intolerance, fever, and rash, occur with lower frequency when the drug is first taken in small amounts (250 mg per day) and slowly increased over many months to a full dose of 1.0 to 1.5 g per day. Careful monitoring of the white blood cell and platelet counts and urine protein are recommended. Despite the apparent clinical benefits, skin fibroblasts retain their potential for increased collagen synthesis.[311]

More recently, colchicine has been advocated.[2] This ancient remedy inhibits the accumulation of collagen by blocking the conversion of procollagen to collagen, probably through interference with microtubule-mediated transport,[71,79] or perhaps via stimulation of collagenase production.[123] In one long-term open trial (mean follow-up 39 months), improvement in skin thickening occurred in 17 of 19 patients.[2] However, another trial using similar dosage (10 mg/week), but only 1 year of treatment, resulted in no beneficial changes. In some patients, progression of skin, musculoskeletal, and pulmonary involvement was documented.[119] Several other negative studies have been published and reviewed.[221] In none of these trials was colchicine toxicity a serious limiting factor.

Considering the mounting evidence that immune processes, both humoral and cell-mediated, play

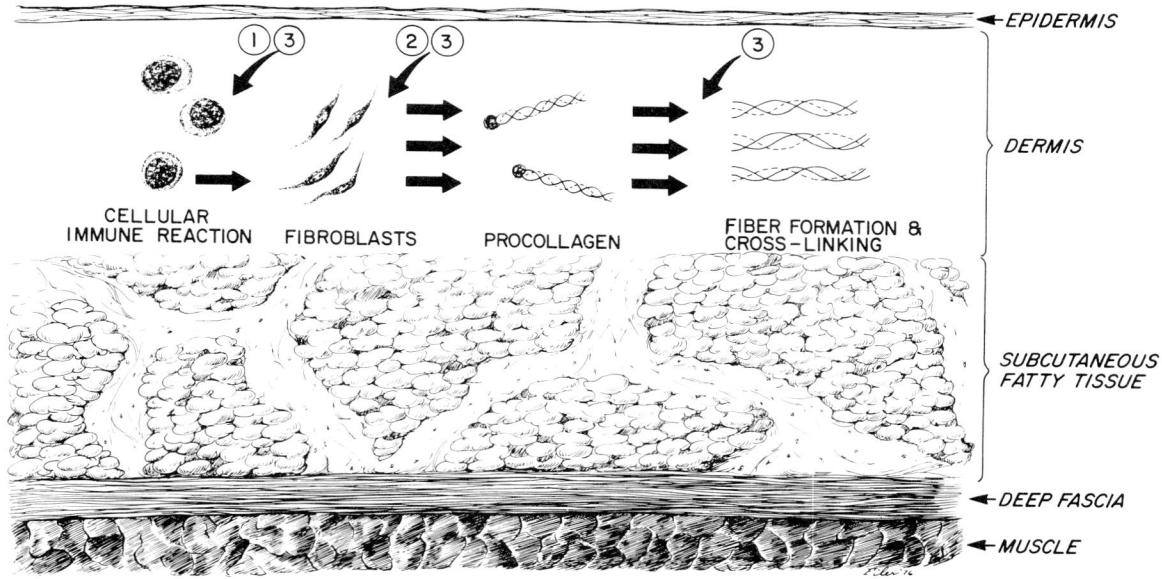

1   IMMUNOSUPPRESSIVE AGENTS
2   COLCHICINE
3   D-PENICILLAMINE

Fig. 66–26. Schematic representation of immune mechanisms in the pathogenesis of skin thickening in systemic sclerosis. The proposed location of action of certain drugs is indicated.

an important role in the pathogenesis of systemic sclerosis, various forms of immunosuppression have been proposed. Chlorambucil[202,331] and azathioprine[154] have been used in uncontrolled trials with mixed results. Plasmapheresis[67] has been attempted, but its effects are difficult to evaluate because of confounding immunosuppressive and corticosteroid therapy. To date, there is no general agreement on the effectiveness of immunosuppressive therapy, and adequately controlled therapeutic trials are urgently needed.[221] We believe the use of immunosuppressive measures is justified in patients with rapidly progressive, life-threatening, or disabling disease, provided there is informed consent and close surveillance for adverse effects.

Supporting Measures. A prominent role of the vasculature in systemic sclerosis is suggested by the nearly universal finding of Raynaud's phenomenon and morphologic changes in blood vessels.[280] Thoracic sympathectomy may be followed by partial (usually transient) improvement in Raynaud's phenomenon but not by significant or sustained influence on the course of cutaneous changes or visceral sclerosis.[31] Many patients with so-called "primary" Raynaud's disease have developed systemic sclerosis, usually the CREST syndrome, years after sympathectomy.

Accurate measurement of digital tissue blood

flow is technically difficult, results are not reproducible, and standardized cold challenge methods have not been developed. Such methodologic problems must be addressed before progress can be made in this area. Common-sense self-management includes avoiding undue cold exposure, dressing warmly, and abstaining from tobacco. Induced vasodilatation[159] and biofeedback[341] may also be helpful. Various vasodilating drugs have been employed in the past, including intra-arterial reserpine,[218,243] methyldopa,[361] adrenergic blocking agents, and alpha receptor blocking and beta receptor stimulating drugs.[31] In general, these agents have proved disappointing in systemic sclerosis. Low-molecular-weight dextran is said to increase digital capillary flow and relieve ischemic pain by reducing blood viscosity, but not all reports have been favorable.[189] Several promising new pharmacologic approaches include the use of the calcium channel blocking drug nifedipine,[164,274,316] an oral serotonin antagonist ketanserin,[305,334] and prostaglandin E_1.[18,213]

Reliable treatment of calcinosis in patients with scleroderma is not available. Low calcium diet and probenecid, chelating agents, and diphosphonates have a rational basis but disappointing results. Surgical excision of large calcareous masses may be helpful in selected instances.

Special lotions, soaps, and bath oils should be

used to relieve excessive skin dryness; taking unduly frequent baths and using household detergents may aggravate this condition. Digital tip ulcerations may be protected by a plaster finger cast. If these lesions become infected (almost always with staphylococci), half-strength hydrogen peroxide soaks and gentle local debridement are employed, and oral antibiotics are sometimes recommended. Deeper infections, especially septic arthritis or osteomyelitis, must be treated more radically, with excision of infected and devitalized tissue, joint fusion and, rarely, amputation. Articular symptoms may be helped by salicylates and other nonsteroidal anti-inflammatory drugs. Corticosteroids are seldom necessary for musculoskeletal involvement, although polymyositis with histologic evidence of chronic inflammatory cell infiltration should be so treated.

Patients who have difficulty in swallowing should learn to masticate carefully and to avoid foods likely to cause substernal dysphagia (e.g., meat, bread). Although metoclopramide improves esophageal motility,[262] its therapeutic usefulness is uncertain. Because nifedipine is capable of decreasing lower esophageal sphincter pressure and contraction amplitude in the body of the esophagus,[136] it thus, theoretically, could aggravate esophageal symptoms. Reflux esophagitis can be minimized by appropriate measures, such as antacids and histamine (H_2) receptor blockade,[256] but esophageal stricture may require periodic dilatation. Successful excision of strictures and correction of gastroesophageal reflux by gastroplasty, combined with fundoplication, have been reported.[34,130,247] Improvement in steatorrhea and other signs of intestinal malabsorption may follow the administration of tetracycline or other broad-spectrum antibiotics, but the underlying hypomotility is unaffected. Metoclopramide significantly increases small bowel motility, but the magnitude of this change is of dubious clinical impact.[265]

Patients with pulmonary fibrosis who have infectious bronchitis or pneumonitis require prompt and vigorous antibiotic treatment. No effective therapy is available for the pulmonary arterial hypertension associated with CREST syndrome. Because those who develop cardiac failure often respond poorly to digitalis and easily become intoxicated, greater reliance is placed on the use of diuretics. Symptomatic pericarditis should be treated with nonsteroidal drugs or corticosteroids.

The availability of new and more potent antihypertensive agents and of improved dialysis procedures and care has dramatically reduced mortality in renal involvement due to systemic sclerosis.[355] Early recognition of this complication and aggressive therapy with such agents as hydralazine, methyldopa, propranolol, minoxidil, and captopril may often, but not always,[37] reverse this process. A remarkable reduction in the degree of dermal thickening and induration has been observed in many of these patients during dialysis.[13,366] Whether edema confounds the skin examination, or the uremic state contributes to this finding, is unknown. Many instances of successful renal transplantation have now been reported, but typical ''scleroderma kidney'' histologic changes have been found in a transplanted organ[380] and in an allograft.[227]

LOCALIZED SCLERODERMA

Although the cause of localized scleroderma is obscure, in many cases the skin changes appear soon after trauma and originate at the site of injury. Familial occurrence has been observed.[343]

Morphea. This disorder begins at any age or site with discrete drop-like patches (guttate morphea) or plaques of erythematous or violaceous discoloration of the skin. The evolving lesions become sclerotic and waxy or ivory-colored and may increase to a diameter of many centimeters. The surface is smooth and hairless, and ceases to sweat. During this active phase, a surrounding violaceous border of inflammation occurs. After several months or years, spontaneous softening of the skin occurs with atrophy and hyper- or depigmentation; smaller patches may heal without trace. Morphea, which is confined entirely to the skin and subcutis, is ordinarily of little consequence unless the face is involved, or there is extensive dissemination of the lesions (generalized morphea). Rarely, localized patches of morphea may be present in individuals with otherwise typical systemic sclerosis.[145]

Early in the course the major histologic changes consist of new collagen deposition in the dermis and septa of the subcutaneous tissue, and variably heavy (often intense) infiltrations of lymphocytes, plasma cells, and histiocytes (Fig. 66–27). This inflammatory reaction is more marked than that usually encountered in systemic sclerosis. Inflammation and later fibrosis and atrophy of underlying striated muscle may be present, but in contrast to systemic sclerosis, muscle capillaries are normal. Treatment with D-penicillamine has been reported to be of value.[236]

Linear Scleroderma. In this form of localized scleroderma, which usually develops in childhood, a linear sclerotic band appears in the arm or leg (Fig. 66–28) and may extend the entire length of the extremity. Occasionally, multiple lesions may be present. Localized scleroderma in the frontoparietal area of the forehead and scalp (''en coup de sabre'') is associated frequently with ipsilateral facial hemiatrophy.[149] Some patients develop a non-

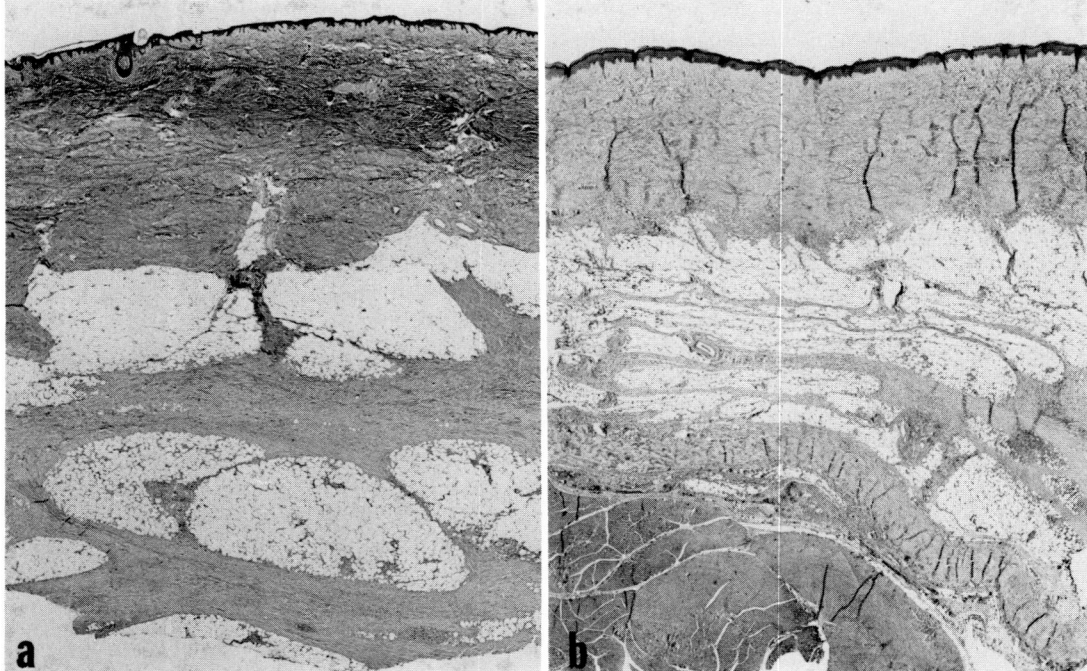

Fig. 66–27.   Photomicrographs of skin biopsies from patients with forms of localized scleroderma. *a,* Thigh of a 54-year-old man with morphea. *b,* Leg of a 3-year-old girl with linear scleroderma. Both have thickened dermis and thick fibrous septae coursing through the subcutis and involving the deep fascia. All layers are heavily infiltrated with lymphocytes.

erosive arthropathy, usually restricted to the small joints of the hands.

Severe fibrosis and inflammation, similar to the conditions found in morphea, occur in the dermis, subcutis, and deep fascia and extend into the underlying muscle (see Fig. 66–27), occasionally resulting in severely deforming fibrous contractures of the fingers, elbows, or knees. Physical therapy may prove useful in the prevention or reduction of these contractures, but they may require surgical correction. Linear scleroderma has been reported to coexist in the same extremity with melorheostosis, a peculiar linear fibrotic hyperostosis of bone.[319]

Laboratory Features of Localized Scleroderma. The clinical and histologic overlap between morphea and linear scleroderma is considerable, and patches of morphea are often found in individuals with linear scleroderma. The concurrence of linear scleroderma and other connective tissue diseases, especially systemic lupus erythematosus, has been reported.[76,201,356] Rheumatoid factor and antinuclear antibodies, including high titers of antibodies to single-stranded DNA, have been noted in the serum of patients with linear scleroderma[121,277,344] and morphea.[344] These serologic abnormalities, and modest degrees of periph-

eral eosinophilia, accompany active disease and disappear during remission. Lymphocytes from patients with linear scleroderma produce leukocyte migration inhibitory factors in response to RNA, human muscle, and human type I collagen, suggesting that immune mechanisms are involved in pathogenesis. The dermal fibroblasts of individuals with linear scleroderma produce excessive collagen in tissue culture.[39]

EOSINOPHILIC FASCIITIS

Eosinophilic fasciitis is a scleroderma-like disorder chiefly affecting adults, the onset of which is characterized by bilateral pain, swelling, and tenderness of the hands, forearms, feet, and legs. These symptoms are soon followed by the development of severe induration of the skin and subcutaneous tissues of these parts with marked limitation of motion of the hands and feet. Carpal tunnel syndrome is an early feature in many patients, and flexion contractures of the fingers may result. The induration often remains confined to the extremities, but spread to affect variably extensive areas of the trunk and the face may occur. Raynaud's phenomenon and internal manifestations of systemic sclerosis are conspicuously absent.

Striking peripheral eosinophilia, often 30% or

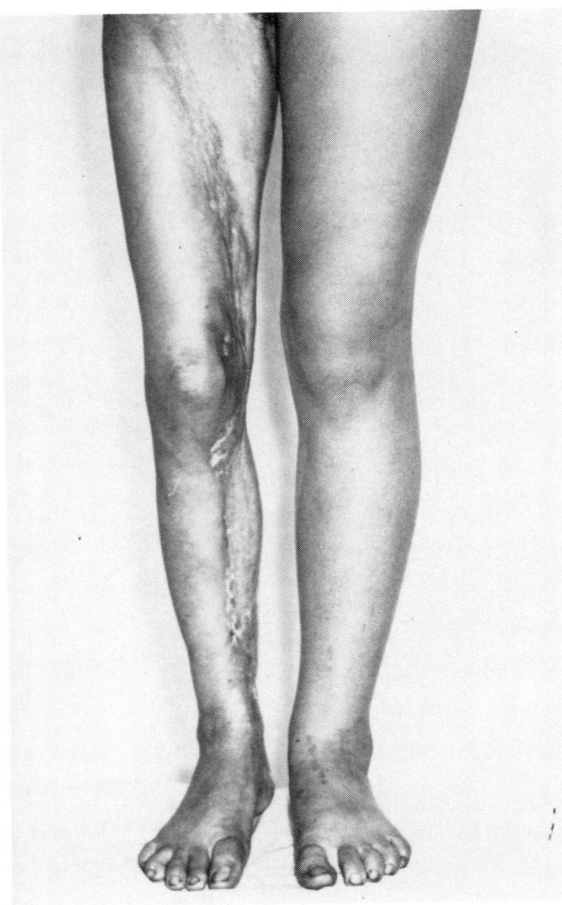

Fig. 66–28. Localized linear scleroderma in the thigh and leg of a 12-year-old girl. (Courtesy of Prof. Stephanie Jablonska.)

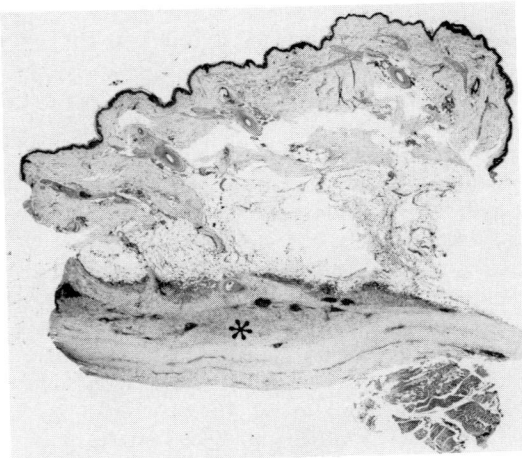

Fig. 66–29. Photomicrograph of the en-bloc biopsy from the leg of a 35-year-old woman with eosinophilic fasciitis. Note dermal thickening, thick subcutaneous fibrous septae, and markedly thickened deep fascia (asterisk). The latter is infiltrated by large collections of cells that were identified as lymphocytes, plasma cells, histiocytes, and eosinophils.

greater, is present during the early stages, but tends to decline later in the illness in parallel with serum eosinophil chemotactic activity.[367] Hypergamma-globulinemia (IgG) is common.[14,313] Circulating immune complexes have been detected in nearly half of patients.[303] These latter parallel disease activity more closely than other laboratory findings, including blood eosinophil concentration.

Histologic diagnosis is best confirmed using a deep wedge "en-bloc" biopsy that includes skin, subcutis, fascia, and muscle. Both inflammation and fibrosis are found in all layers, but they are most intense in the fascia, which may be thickened (Fig. 66–29). Large numbers of lymphocytes, plasma cells, and histiocytes are present in the affected areas, and eosinophil infiltration may be striking, particularly early in the disease.[14] Immunoglobulin and complement component C3 have been identified in the inflamed tissues.[14]

A variety of hematologic complications, including thrombocytopenia, aplastic anemia, and myelodysplastic syndromes have developed in patients with eosinophilic fasciitis.[11,49,134,230] These conditions, suspected to be of autoimmune cause, may occur at any time in the course of the fasciitis and do not correlate with its severity.

Eosinophilic fasciitis is self-limited in many patients, with spontaneous improvement and occasionally complete remission after two or more years. However, in our experience and that of others,[26] some patients have persistent or recurrent disease, and others are left with disabling fixed joint contractures. Corticosteroids, in small doses, often provide prompt and substantial symptomatic relief and readily obliterate the eosinophilia. Two reports suggest that cimetidine is another potentially effective form of therapy.[191,320]

The etiology of eosinophilic fasciitis is unknown. It has been preceded by unusually strenuous exertion, especially in younger men. The blood and tissue abnormalities described previously suggest an immune pathogenesis.[14,63,171] An association with autoimmune thyroiditis has been noted.[314] The diagnosis should be considered in an individual with scleroderma-like tightening and thickening of the skin, sparing the digits, who has peripheral eosinophilia and no Raynaud's phenomenon.

DIFFERENTIAL DIAGNOSIS

A number of other conditions exhibit scleroderma-like but often distinctive skin changes in the absence of typical visceral manifestations of systemic sclerosis[91] (Table 66–3).

Scleredema. Scleredema is characterized by firm, painless, symmetrical edematous induration of the skin of the face, scalp, neck, trunk, and proximal portions of the extremities. In contrast to systemic sclerosis, the distal parts are seldom affected. Recent streptococcal infection in childhood and diabetes mellitus[91] are the two most frequent associations of this condition, which may either resolve spontaneously after 6 to 12 months or persist for many years. Other manifestations include hydrarthrosis, pleural and pericardial effusions, widespread involvement of muscle, including the heart, and macroglossia. Histochemical studies have revealed swollen collagen bundles and the accumulation of mucopolysaccharide (probably hyaluronic acid) in the demis, subcutis, and skeletal muscle (Fig. 66–30).

Porphyria Cutanea Tarda. Hypopigmented plaque-like sclerodermatous induration of the skin and pigmentary changes occur in porphyria cutanea tarda usually, but not always, in sun-exposed areas.[176,263] Particularly on the face, long-standing lesions may ulcerate and contain dystrophic calcific deposits.[115] In contrast, bullae are rare in systemic sclerosis, and uroporphyrin excretion is normal.

Scleromyxedema. Scleromyxedema (lichen

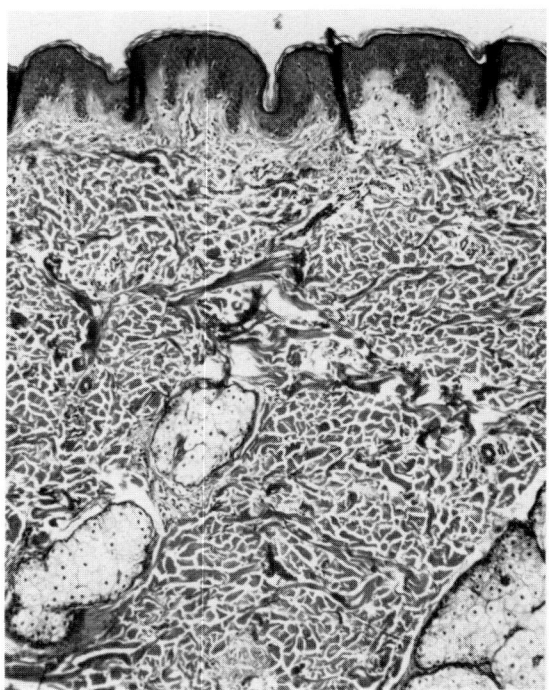

Fig. 66–30. Photomicrograph of upper back skin from an 18-year-old woman with scleredema of 10 years' duration. There is marked thickening of the dermis, and wide separation of its collagen bundles by clefts that contained mucopolysaccharide deposits.

Table 66–3. Disorders Associated with Skin Changes that may Resemble Scleroderma (Pseudoscleroderma)

Primary Cutaneous Diseases
Scleredema
Porphyria cutanea tarda; congenital porphyria
Scleromyxedema
Acrodermatitis chronica
Lichen sclerosus et atrophicus
Lipoatrophy
Primary Systemic Diseases in which Cutaneous Features are also Present
Amyloidosis
Juvenile onset diabetes mellitus
Acromegaly
Carcinoid syndrome
Phenylketonuria
Werner's syndrome
Progeria
Rothmund's syndrome
Graft-vs.-host disease
Chemical Agents Inducing Scleroderma-Like Conditions
Vinyl chloride
Organic solvents, epoxy resins
Trichloroethylene
L-hydroxytryptophan and carbidopa therapy
Bleomycin
Pentazocine
Silicone or paraffin implantation

myxedematosus, papular mucinosis) is a rare disorder in which widespread lichenoid eruption of soft pale red or yellowish papules is accompanied by diffuse thickening of the skin, including the face and hands. Dense deposits of acid mucopolysaccharide, without glycosaminoglycan subunits on electron microscopy,[203] are found in the upper portion of the dermis. Abnormal serum immunoglobulins (M components) have been detected in several patients, suggesting a relationship of this condition to myelomatosis.[192]

Acrodermatitis Chronica Atrophicans and Lichen Sclerosus et Atrophicus. Acrodermatitis chronica atrophicans and lichen sclerosus et atrophicus are uncommon diseases of unknown etiology, in which cutaneous inflammation is followed by atrophy. The latter shows a high frequency of organ-specific antibodies, e.g., to thyroid and gastric parietal cells.

Amyloidosis. Infiltration of the dermis may accompany amyloidosis of either the primary (multiple myeloma associated) or secondary type.[151,286] Firm, discrete, hemispherical brown or yellow papules are described, but when the deposition of amyloid is diffuse and involves the fingers, hands, and face, physical findings may mimic those of systemic sclerosis. Skin biopsies were positive for amyloid in involved skin in over one-half of cases and in clinically normal skin in over one-third.[286]

Juvenile Onset Diabetes Mellitus. Digital sclerosis and mild finger contractures occur in one-third of patients with insulin-dependent juvenile onset diabetes mellitus.[61,103,302] These findings are correlated better with disease duration than with microvascular (retinal and renal) complications.[61,302]

Acromegaly. Considerable thickening of the skin and subcutaneous tissues may appear in acromegaly as a result of connective tissue hyperplasia.[279]

Glycogen Storage Disease. Scleroderma-like skin induration has also been observed in individuals with glycogen storage disease of muscle.[150]

Carcinoid Syndrome. The occurrence of a peculiar localized scleroderma-like fibrosis in the skin of a few patients with the malignant carcinoid syndrome has suggested that 5-hydroxytryptamine (serotonin) metabolism might be deranged in systemic sclerosis.[97] There is, however, little evidence of any primary disturbance in serotonin metabolism in systemic sclerosis, and urinary excretion of 5-hydroxyindoleacetic acid is normal in these patients.[326] Patients with scleroderma (and also, in at least one case, unaffected relatives as well) have excreted excessive amounts of kynurenine and other intermediary metabolites of tryptophan. A partial deficiency in kynurenine hydroxylase may exist, but this finding appears to be nonspecific.[140] The intestinal absorption of tryptophan is normal in most patients with systemic sclerosis.[327] The finding that urinary levels of 5-hydroxyindoleacetic acid do not rise in response to increased dietary tryptophan in nearly half the cases indicates an impaired transformation of serotonin to 5-hydroxyindoleacetic acid. A disproportionately high ratio of total indoles to indoleacetic acid suggests the presence of excess tryptamine, presumably a result of impaired activity of monoamine oxidase.[326] Another abnormality in the conversion of tryptophan located at some point after the formation of hydroxyanthranilic acid also has been detected in some patients with systemic sclerosis.[120]

Phenylketonuria. Atypical scleroderma of the trunk and extremities without visceral stigmata has been reported in children with phenylketonuria,[152,178] a disorder in which the absence of the enzyme phenylalanine hydroxylase ultimately leads to excessive urinary excretion of indolic compounds, and decreased levels of plasma serotonin and urinary 5-hydroxyindoleacetic acid. Improvement follows conversion to a low phenylalanine diet. Studies of 9 children with scleroderma, from 3 to 14 years of age, however, revealed normal urinary levels of both phenylalanine and d-hydroxyphenylacetic acid.[178]

Werner's Syndrome, Progeria, and Rothmund's Syndrome. The classic findings of Werner's syndrome, a rare hereditofamilial disorder, include growth retardation, premature graying of the hair and baldness, juvenile cataracts, and a high frequency of diabetes mellitus. Additional manifestations also include atrophy and hyperkeratosis of the skin with chronic ulcerations over pressure points in the feet.[81,89] In progeria, a rare autosomal recessive syndrome, the corium and subcutis have been reported as being either thickened or atrophic,[90,363] and the thermal shrinkage and solubility of skin collagen resemble aged rather than normally growing connective tissue.[363] The nature of the primary defect in the development and metabolism of connective tissue in these conditions is unknown. Rothmund's syndrome is another heritable (recessive) disorder in which atrophy of the skin (poikiloderma), beginning in infancy, is associated with juvenile cataracts.

Vinyl Chloride Disease and Epoxy Resins. Workers who clean reactor-vessels containing the polymerizing agent vinyl chloride (CH_2CHCl) may acquire a systemic illness with some features of systemic sclerosis.[339] These individuals complain of soreness and tenderness of the fingertips and Raynaud's phenomenon. They develop nodular induration of the skin of the dorsum of the hands and forearms, clubbing, synovial thickening of the proximal interphalangeal joints, hepatic portal fibrosis, splenomegaly, and pulmonary fibrosis. Roentgenograms reveal varying degrees of acroosteolysis of the distal phalanges of the fingers, as well as erosive and sclerotic changes in the sacroiliac joints. Partial resorption of the mandible has been reported. Microvascular abnormalities similar to those encountered in systemic sclerosis are observed on capillary microscopy,[206] and luminal narrowing of the digital arteries has been seen on angiographic examination.[306] Circulating immune complexes have been reported in a high proportion of patients with polyvinyl chloride disease.[365] Cross-link analysis and measurement of hydroxyproline formation in skin grown in organ culture have indicated excessive new collagen production.[155] The vapor of epoxy resins is believed to lead to cutaneous sclerosis and muscle weakness.[387] A biogenic amine is the suspected causative agent. Similar compounds have been implicated in other pseudoscleroderma states, such as carcinoid syndrome[325] and L-5 hydroxytryptophan and carbidopa therapy.[332]

Bleomycin. Administration of the tumoricidal drug bleomycin often leads to the development of nodules and/or plaques of thickened skin, the result of an increase of dense collagen in the dermis.[55] Other manifestations may include more uniform induration of the skin, Raynaud's phenomenon,[350,364] and pulmonary fibrosis,[385] closely resembling the findings in systemic sclerosis. The dermal fibrosis tends to recede following discontinuation of bleomycin. Cultured fibroblasts from affected skin demonstrated increased collagen synthesis.[87]

Pentazocine. Nodular cutaneous sclerosis, often associated with ulceration, has been reported to follow intramuscular injection of the non-narcotic analgesic pentazocine.[253] "Woody" hard and occasionally calcified skin, subcutis, and muscle have resulted. Venous and/or arteriolar thrombosis and endarteritis are described in these patients, many of whom had a personal or family history of diabetes mellitus.

Foreign Substances. In Japan, systemic sclerosis has been reported to follow cosmetic surgery with injection of foreign substances (e.g., paraffin, silicone), chiefly for breast augmentation.[183]

CALCINOSIS

Calcinosis or pathologic calcification of the soft tissues occurs in a variety of local and systemic conditions (Table 66–4). Only a few of these disorders are discussed because most are considered in detail in Chapters 94 and 95. Classifications of ectopic calcification generally separate these conditions into those that are complications of long-continued hypercalcemia and/or hyperphosphatemia (metastatic calcification) and those that result from some local abnormality in the affected tissues (dystrophic calcification).

Metastatic Calcification

Calcareous deposits, which occur commonly in hypercalcemic states, are found in the kidney (nephrocalcinosis), stomach, lung, brain, eyes (band keratopathy), skin, subcutaneous and periarticular tissues, and arterial walls. Calcification of the articular cartilage (chondrocalcinosis), menisci, and joint capsules is a well-recognized feature of hyperparathyroidism. For many individuals, an attack of calcium pyrophosphate dihydrate crystal-induced synovitis (pseudogout) represents the first clinical manifestation of this disease. Accordingly, the possibility of parathyroid adenoma should be carefully considered in all patients with this arthropathy.

A similar pattern of soft tissue calcification without ocular involvement and seldom affecting skin[68] is also found in normocalcemic-hyperphosphatemic hyperparathyroidism secondary to renal insufficiency, although renal calculus formation is less frequent than in the hypercalcemic states. Acute episodes of articular and periarticular in-

Table 66–4. Diseases Associated with Calcification of the Soft Tissues in the Extremities

I. Metastatic Calcification
   Hypercalcemic conditions
      Primary hyperparathyroidism
      Hypervitaminosis D
      Milk-alkali syndrome
      Metastatic and other neoplasms of bone
      Sarcoidosis
   Hyperphosphatemic conditions
      Chronic renal failure with secondary hyperparathyroidism
      Hypoparathyroidism
      Pseudohypoparathyroidism
      Tumoral calcinosis (lipocalcinosis granulomatosis)
II. Dystrophic Calcification (Calcinosis)
   Connective tissue diseases
      Systemic sclerosis, with both diffuse scleroderma and CREST syndrome
      Dermatomyositis/polymyositis
      Ehlers-Danlos syndrome
      Pseudoxanthoma elasticum
   Metabolic disorders
      Chondrocalcinosis articularis (pseudogout)
      Gout
      Diabetes mellitus
      Alkaptonuria (ochronosis)
      Porphyria cutanea tarda
      Pseudopseudohypoparathyroidism
      Werner's syndrome
      Progeria
      Myositis (or fibrodysplasia) ossificans progressiva
   Vascular diseases
      Medial sclerosis of arteries (Mönckeberg's sclerosis)
      Venous calcifications
   Parasitic infestations
   Other diseases
      Neuropathic arthropathy
      Calcific tendinitis
      Para-articular limb joint ectopic calcification associated with paralysis and other neurologic disorders

flammation, which appear to be related to the local deposition of microcrystalline calcium phosphates (and, at times, monosodium urate), have been described in patients undergoing hemodialysis for chronic renal failure.[235] The finding of subperiosteal juxta-articular bone erosions following calcinosis in the same location suggests that the calcifications may induce erosions.[7] The removal of pyrophosphate, which appears to act as a physiologic inhibitor of calcification, may be responsible for this phenomenon.[288] Treatment with phosphate binding agents has resulted in a significant reduction of serum phosphorus levels, disappearance of cutaneous calcinosis, and relief from the articular attacks.[235] In hypoparathyroidism, pseudohypoparathyroidism, and pseudopseudohypoparathyroidism, calcification may occur in the brain, particularly in the basal ganglia, as well as in the subcutaneous tissues.

Tumoral Calcinosis. Although included in the category of metastatic calcification because of the frequent elevation in serum phosphorus levels and occasional elevation in serum calcium values, tumoral calcinosis is separable from other forms of metastatic calcification by the absence of visceral involvement (see also Chap. 95). This rare entity, which has also been called lipocalcinosis granulomatosis, is characterized by the rapid development of large, multilobulated calcific masses in the subcutaneous tissue and muscle overlying the hips, shoulders, and elbows in otherwise healthy young subjects. Smaller tumors occur adjacent to the spine, wrists, feet, lower ribs, sacrum, and ischium. These firm, nontender deposits may increase to a diameter of 20 cm or larger over a period of months to years. Little or no articular limitation occurs unless these masses become very large or are complicated by the development of fistulous tracts caused by either infection or attempts at surgical drainage. Curiously, a number of patients have angioid streaks of the retina. There is a notable lack of visceral calcification. Most patients with tumoral calcinosis have normal serum calcium and alkaline phosphatase, but hyperphosphatemia[186] and elevated levels of 1,25 dihydroxy vitamin D[390] have been noted in several cases. Rapid exchange of calcium between the serum and the masses is evident, along with an increased intestinal absorption of dietary calcium, with no defect in the turnover of skeletal calcium.[186] Approximately half the patients with tumoral calcinosis reported to date have had affected siblings. This observation, together with the occurrence of hyperphosphatemia, has led to the suggestion that this disorder may represent a heritable disturbance in the metabolism of phosphorus.[186]

On sectioning, the masses are found to be composed of multilocular cysts enclosing pockets of milky fluid or pasty microcrystalline calcareous matter. The tissue lining the walls of these cysts contains mononuclear cells that are rich in alkaline phosphatase and are believed to be responsible for the local accumulation of calcium phosphate, as well as foreign body giant cells. These mononuclear and multinuclear cells are structurally, and apparently functionally, similar to osteoblasts and osteoclasts, respectively.[186] The masses contain pure calcium carbonate, pure calcium phosphate, or a mixture of the two salts.

Treatment at present consists mainly of early surgical excision of the calcareous masses, which rarely recur at the same site. New deposits may appear in time around other joints. As a rule the prognosis is good, although in some instances sec-

ondary infection of the deposits has led to the development of multiple draining sinuses, cachexia, and amyloidosis. A low-calcium and low-phosphorus diet and large oral doses of antacids containing aluminum hydroxide have resulted in negative balances of both calcium and phosphorus with marked improvement.[237]

Dystrophic Calcification

Many restrict the use of the term calcinosis to those patients in whom the deposition of calcium salts in the soft tissues occurs in the absence of any generalized disturbance in calcium or phosphorus metabolism.

Calcinosis Associated with Connective Tissue Diseases. In systemic sclerosis, the calcareous deposits are generally confined to the extremities and are particularly frequent in the terminal phalanges, around joints, and near other bony eminences. Most of these cases and those with the most dramatic calcification are examples of the CREST syndrome (see Fig. 66–4). In contrast, widespread encasing calcification of the skin and subcutaneous and periarticular tissues, as well as involvement of the deeper structures, occurs later in the course of polymyositis-dermatomyositis (see Chap. 65). This process includes tendons, tendon sheaths, and muscles, forming irregularly shaped plaques and nodules, and is often associated with severe joint contractures and ankylosis. On microscopic examination, the precipitates of calcium in the skin appear as pleomorphic crystals, many in the shape of needles and large plates. They appear to develop in the elastic fibers of the connective tissue.[193,240]

As a rule, these individuals have normal concentrations of serum calcium, phosphorus, and alkaline phosphatase activity, with or without apparent calcinosis, but calcium balance studies have yielded conflicting data. In patients with cutaneous deposition (calcinosis cutis), increased absorption and retention of calcium have been evident, paradoxically with a more rapid disappearance rate of radio-labeled calcium injected intradermally.[5,211] When a woman with scleroderma and calcinosis was placed on a calcium-restricted diet, the bone resorption rate increased, and urinary excretion of calcium fell normally, but the net calcium accretion rate (which included extraosseous calcium deposition) remained constant.[166] Urinary excretion of a vitamin K-dependent calcium-binding protein (gamma-carboxyglutamic acid or Gla) is increased in patients with dermatomyositis and calcinosis, but it is premature to conclude that this substance plays a primary role in the etiology of calcinosis.[197]

The basis for the deposition of calcium salts in the dermis of patients with systemic sclerosis and dermatomyositis is unclear. A number of different

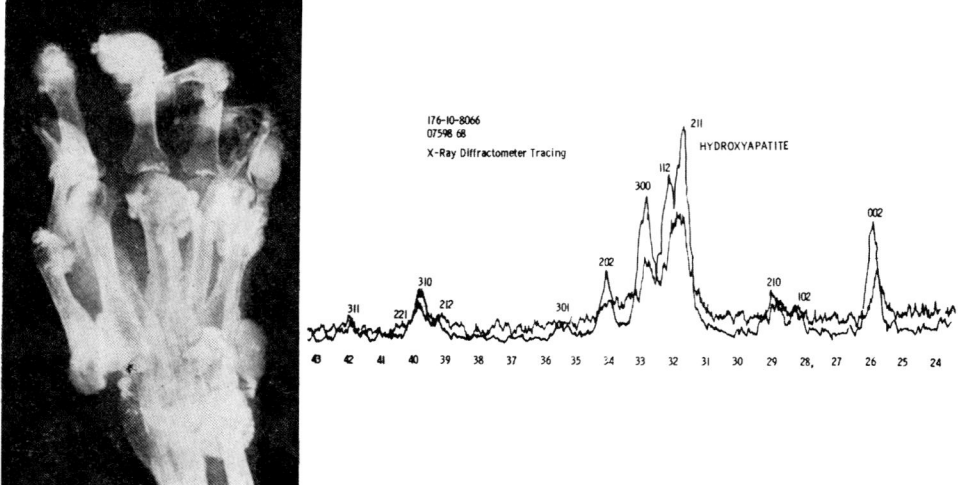

Fig. 66–31. Dystrophic calcinosis. *Left,* Roentgenogram of the hand of a woman with polymyositis, showing extensive calcinosis involving both subcutaneous tissues and tendon sheaths. *Right,* X-ray diffraction pattern of a sample of calcaneous matter from a nodule on this hand. The labeled spectra represent hydroxyapatite control, and the spectra with lower peak heights are those of the specimen. Correspondence of peak positions and their relative suggested the presence of hydroxyapatite (see Chap. 95 for additional information on identification of calcium phosphate crystals).

forms of cutaneous, subcuticular, periarticular, and visceral calcification have been produced experimentally in the rat by calciphylaxis and it has been suggested that this phenomenon may serve as a model of human calcinosis. During a critical period after "sensitization" by a systemic "calcifying factor" (e.g., vitamin D compounds, parathyroid hormone), topical treatment with a variety of "challengers," including metallic salts, leads to local calcification, followed by inflammation and fibrosis. In a related phenomenon termed "calcergy," no such pretreatment is necessary. Soft tissue calcification occurs wherever "direct calcifiers" or "calcergens," chiefly various metallic salts, come into contact with connective tissue.[307] The local injection of minute amounts of histamine or serotonin can elicit certain mast cell-dependent forms of this type of experimental calcinosis in which the "calcergen" is administered intravenously. In this respect, it is interesting that skin of patients with systemic sclerosis contains increased numbers of mast cells.[125]

The initial precipitation of calcium salts in the case of calciphylactic cutaneous calcinosis in the rat occurs in areas rich in mucopolysaccharides or, in some instances, collagen fibers, which appear to act as a matrix for this calcification. Because polysaccharides may "shield" reactive sites on collagen fibrils and block mineral nucleation, it is possible that the calcinosis that occurs in scleroderma may be related to the diminution of muco-

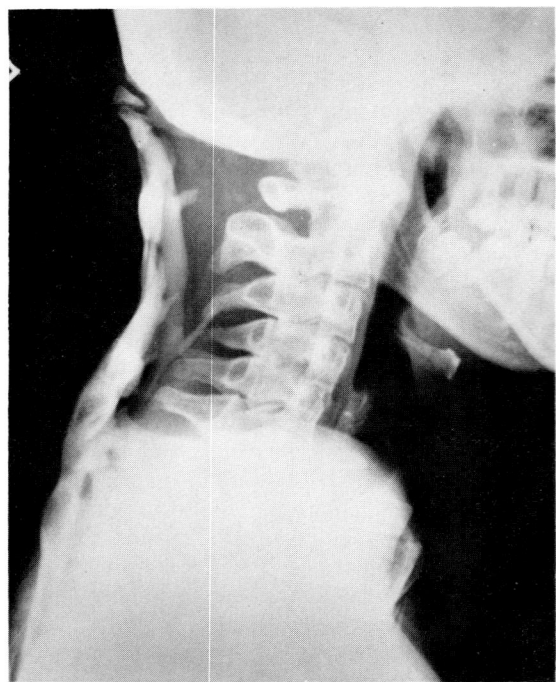

Fig. 66–32. Roentgenogram illustrating new bone formation in the cervical area of a 17-year-old woman with myositis ossificans progressiva. She first noted pain, swelling, and limitation of motion in this area after trauma 10 years previously.

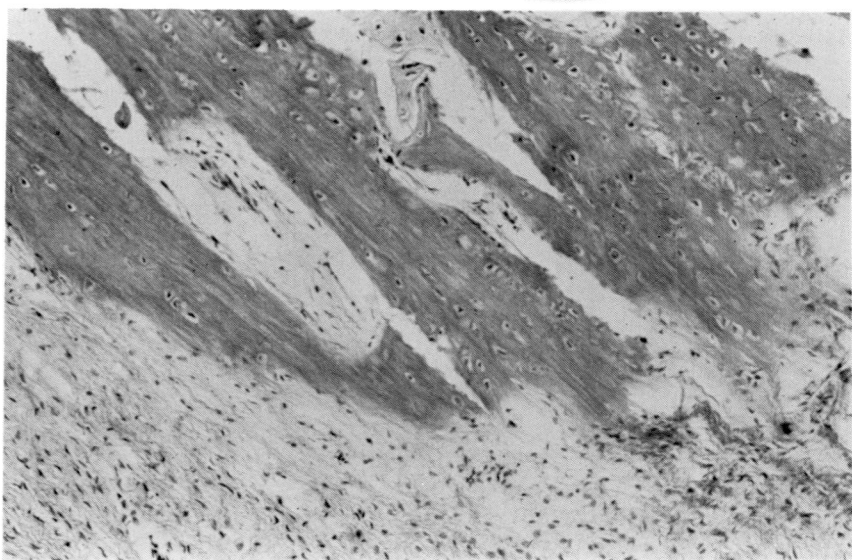

Fig. 66–33.   Photomicrograph of the masseter muscle of a 20-year-old woman with myositis ossificans progressiva. Note new bone formation within the substance of the muscle.

polysaccharides in the affected skin during later stages of the disease.

Numerous drugs, hormones, and a host of non-specific measures have been used unsuccessfully in the treatment of calcinosis. Intravenous sodium versenate (disodium ethylene-diamine-tetra-acetate) may be transiently effective, but its use is both difficult and impractical. The combination of probenecid (which induces hypophosphatemia) with a low calcium diet has seemed beneficial.[69] Diphosphonates, analogues of inorganic pyrophosphate, contain a P-C-P bond, inhibit the crystallization of calcium phosphates, and are capable of preventing various types of experimental pathologic calcification.[291] These compounds have proved disappointing, however, in the treatment of calcinosis in man.[62,228,260,291] Phosphate-binding antacids containing aluminum hydroxide are similarly ineffective.[141] Surgical excision of large calcareous masses may be helpful in selected instances.[226] See Chapter 95 for reports using coumadin therapy.

Myositis (or Fibrodysplasia) Ossificans Progressiva.   Patients with this uncommon disorder have widespread ectopic calcification and ossification in fascia, aponeuroses, and other fibrous structures related to muscle. The initial symptoms usually appear in early childhood, often preceded by local trauma (Fig. 66–32). The disease occurs in families and appears to be transmitted as an autosomal dominant trait with irregular penetrance. A number of associated congenital anomalies of the digits include microdactyly or total absence of

the thumbs and great toes. The initial manifestation usually consists of a localized area of swelling and redness and warmth in the neck or paravertebral area, often associated with extreme pain. After several days the signs of inflammation subside, leaving an area of residual doughy firmness that appears fibromatous, is rich in glycosaminoglycans,[215] and gradually ossifies over the following weeks (Fig. 66–33). Scanning with ^{99m}Tc pyrophosphate may be useful in the detection of areas of ossification prior to roentgenographic changes.[342] The replacement of the tendon and muscle by bone leads to characteristic contracture deformities. Once ossification occurs, further change is minimal. Recurring bouts of inflammation and ossification result in progressive damage to much of the striated musculature. Involvement of the muscles of the chest wall and back may lead to restrictive pulmonary disease.[40] Death usually results from respiratory failure and/or pulmonary infection due to involvement of the muscles of the thorax or from inanition as a result of damage to the muscles of mastication.

It has been suggested that myositis ossificans progressiva may result from an abnormal collagen or, alternatively, the deficiency of an inhibitor material (? proteoglycan), which normally prevents the crystallization and accretion of calcium salts on collagen fibers at sites other than bone. There is no evidence of any fundamental aberration in calcium metabolism per se in this disorder. The administration of diphosphonates may suppress, at least temporarily, the development of new areas of mineralization following surgical excision of ectopic bone, but the ultimate value of these agents is as yet uncertain.[291,318] Corticosteroids may relieve the acute symptoms of inflammation and may retard progression of the disease in some patients.[146]

REFERENCES

1. Abraham, A.A., and Joos, A.: Pancreatic necrosis in progressive systemic sclerosis. Ann. Rheum. Dis., 39:396–398, 1980.
2. Alarcon-Segovia, D.: Progressive systemic sclerosis: Management. Part IV. Colchicine. Clin. Rheum. Dis., 5:294–302, 1979.
3. Alarcon-Segovia, D., Palacios, R., and deKasep, G.I.: Human postthymic precursor cells in health and disease. VII. Immunoregulatory circuits of the peripheral blood mononuclear cells from patients with progressive systemic sclerosis. J. Clin. Lab. Immunol., 5:143–148, 1981.
4. Alcocer-Varela, J., et al.: Early proliferative response in the human autologous mixed lymphocyte reaction in scleroderma. J. Rheumatol., 11:48–52, 1984.
5. Alexander, E.L., et al.: Scleroderma heart disease: Evidence for cold-induced abnormalities of myocardial function and perfusion (abstract). Arthritis Rheum., 24 (Suppl. 4):S58, 1981.
6. Allende, H.D., Ona, F.V., and Noronna, A.I.: Bleeding gastric telangiectasia: Complication of Raynaud's phenomenon, esophageal motor dysfunction, sclerodactyly and telangiectasia (REST) syndrome. Am. J. Gastroenterol, 75:354–356, 1981.
7. Andresen, J., and Nielsen, H.E.: Juxta-articular erosions and calcifications in patients with chronic renal failure. Acta Radiol. [Diagn.], 22:709–713, 1981.
8. Armstrong, R.D., and Gibson, T.: Scleroderma and erosive polyarthritis: A disease entity? Ann. Rheum. Dis., 41:141–146, 1982.
9. Asboe-Hansen, G.: Treatment of generalized scleroderma: Updated results. Acta Derm.Venereol., 59:465–467, 1979.
10. Asboe-Hansen, G.: Treatment of generalized scleroderma with inhibitors of connective tissue formation. Acta Derm. Venereol., 55:461–465, 1975.
11. Bagg, L.R., and Hughes, D.T.D.: Serial pulmonary function tests in progressive systemic sclerosis. Thorax, 34:224–228, 1979.
12. Ballou, S.P., Morley, J.J., and Kushner, I.: Pregnancy and systemic sclerosis. Arthritis Rheum., 27:295–298, 1984.
13. Barker, D.J., and Farr, M.J.: Resolution of cutaneous manifestations of systemic sclerosis after haemodialysis. Br. Med. J., 1:501, 1976.
14. Barnes, L., et al.: Eosinophilic fasciitis. A pathologic study of twenty cases. Am. Assoc. Pathol., 96:493–507, 1979.
15. Barnett, A.J.: Some observations on the immunological status in scleroderma (progressive systemic sclerosis). Aust. N.Z. J. Med., 8:622–627, 1978.
16. Barnett, A.J., and Coventry, D.A.: Scleroderma: 1. Clinical features, course of illness and response to treatment in 61 cases. 2. Incidence of systemic disturbance and assessment of possible aetiological factors. Med. J. Australia, 1:992–1001, 1040–1047, 1969.
17. Baron, M., et al.: ^{67}Gallium lung scans in progressive systemic sclerosis. Arthritis Rheum., 26:969–974, 1983.
18. Baron, M., et al.: Prostaglandin E$_1$ therapy for digital ulcers in scleroderma. Can. Med. Assoc. J., 126:42–45, 1982.
19. Baron, M., et al.: Lymphocyte subpopulations and reactivity to mitogens in patients with scleroderma. Clin. Exp. Immunol., 46:70–76, 1981.
20. Baron, M., Lee, P., and Keystone, E.C.: The articular manifestations of progressive systemic sclerosis (scleroderma). Ann. Rheum. Dis., 41:147–152, 1982.
21. Bashey, R.I., et al.: Connective tissue synthesis by cultured scleroderma fibroblasts. II. Incorporation of ^{3}H-glu-

22. cosamine and synthesis of glycosaminoglycans. Arthritis Rheum., 20:879–885, 1977.
22. Bashey, R.I., and Jimenez, S.A.: Increased sensitivity of scleroderma fibroblasts in culture to stimulation of protein and collagen synthesis by serum. Biochem. Biophys. Res. Commun., 76:1214–1222, 1977.
23. Battle, W.M., et al.: Abnormal colonic motility in progressive systemic sclerosis. Ann. Intern. Med., 94:749–752, 1981.
24. Battle, W.M., et al.: Spontaneous perforation of the small intestine due to scleroderma. Dig. Dis. Sci., 24:80–84, 1979.
25. Bernstein, R.M., Steigerwald, J.C., and Tan, E.M.: Association of antinuclear and antinucleolar antibodies in progressive systemic sclerosis. Clin. Exp. Immunol., 48:43–51, 1982.
26. Bertken, R., and Shaller, D.: Chronic progressive eosinophilic fasciitis: Report of a 20-year failure to attain remission. Ann. Rheum. Dis., 42:103–105, 1983.
27. Birnbaum, N.S., et al.: Histocompatibility antigens in progressive systemic sclerosis (scleroderma). J. Rheumatol., 4:425–428, 1977.
28. Bjerke, R.D., et al.: Small airways in progressive systemic sclerosis (PSS). Am. J. Med., 66:201–209, 1979.
29. Blocka, K.L.N., et al.: The arthropathy of advanced progressive systemic sclerosis. A radiographic survey. Arthritis Rheum., 24:874–884, 1981.
30. Bluestone, R., et al.: Treatment of systemic sclerosis with D-penicillamine. A new method of observation of the effects of treatment. Ann. Rheum. Dis., 29:153–158, 1970.
31. Blunt, R.J., and Porter, J.M.: Raynaud's syndrome. Semin. Arthritis Rheum., 10:282–308, 1981.
32. Botstein, G.R., and LeRoy, E.C.: Primary heart disease in systemic sclerosis (scleroderma): Advances in clinical and pathologic features, pathogenesis and new therapeutic approaches. Am. Heart J., 102:913–919, 1981.
33. Botstein, G.R., Sherer, G.K., and LeRoy, E.C.: Fibroblast selection in scleroderma. An alternative model of fibrosis. Arthritis Rheum., 25:189–195, 1982.
34. Brain, R.H.F.: Surgical management of hiatal herniae and oesophageal strictures in systemic sclerosis. Thorax, 28:515–520, 1973.
35. Brandt, K.D., and Krey, P.R.: Chalky joint effusion: The result of massive synovial deposition of calcium apatite in progressive systemic sclerosis. Arthritis Rheum., 20:792–796, 1977.
36. Brenner, S., et al.: Kinetochore structure, duplication, and distribution in mammalian cells: Analysis by human autoantibodies from scleroderma patients. J. Cell Biol., 91:95–102, 1981.
37. Brown, E.A., MacGregor, G.A., and Maini, R.N.: Failure of captopril to reverse the renal crisis of scleroderma. Ann. Rheum. Dis., 42:52–53, 1983.
38. Buckingham, R.B., et al.: Increased collagen accumulation in dermal fibroblast cultures from patients with progressive systemic sclerosis (scleroderma). J. Lab. Clin. Med., 92:5–21, 1978.
39. Buckingham, R.B., et al.: Collagen accumulation by dermal fibroblast cultures of patients with linear localized scleroderma. Arthritis Rheum., 19:817, 1976.
40. Buhain, W.J., Rammohan, G., and Berger, H.W.: Pulmonary function in myositis ossificans progressiva. Am. Rev. Respir. Dis., 110:333–337, 1974.
41. Bulkley, B.H.: Progressive systemic sclerosis: Cardiac involvement. Clin. Rheum. Dis., 5:131–149, 1979.
42. Burnham, T.K., and Kleinsmith, D'A.M.: The "true speckled" antinuclear antibody (ANA) pattern: Its tumultuous history. Semin. Arthritis. Rheum., 13:155–159, 1983.
43. Cabral, A., and Castor, C.W.: Connective tissue activation. XXVII. The behavior of skin fibroblasts from patients with scleroderma. Arthritis Rheum., 26:1362–1369, 1983.
44. Cannon, P.J., et al.: The relationship of hypertension and renal failure in scleroderma (progressive systemic sclerosis) to structural and functional abnormalities of the renal cortical circulation. Medicine, 53:1–46, 1974.

45. Cathcart, M.K., and Krakauer, R.S.: Immunologic enhancement of collagen accumulation in progressive systemic sclerosis (PSS). Clin. Immunol. Immunopathol., 21:128–133, 1981.

46. Catoggio, L.J., et al.: Serological markers in progressive systemic sclerosis: Clinical correlations. Ann. Rheum. Dis., 42:23–27, 1983.

47. Cazalis, P., et al.: Rhumatismes inflammatories et gammopathies monoclonales benignes: Aspects cliniques at devinir. Rev. Rhum. Mal. Osteoartic., 41:698–702, 1974.

48. Cipoletti, J.F., et al.: Sjögren's syndrome in progressive systemic sclerosis (scleroderma). Ann. Intern. Med., 87:535–541, 1977.

49. Clements, P.J., et al.: The relationship of arrhythmias and conduction disturbances to other manifestations of cardiopulmonary disease in progressive systemic sclerosis (PSS). Am. J. Med., 71:38–46, 1971.

50. Clements, P.J., et al.: Muscle disease in progressive systemic sclerosis: Diagnostic and therapeutic considerations. Arthritis Rheum., 21:62–71, 1978.

51. Cobden, I., et al.: Small intestinal bacterial growth in systemic sclerosis. Clin. Exp. Dermatol., 5:37–42, 1980.

52. Cobden, I., Axon, A.T.R., and Rowell, N.R.: Pancreatic exocrine function in systemic sclerosis. Br. J. Dermatol., 105:189–193, 1981.

53. Coffman, J.D.: Skin blood flow in scleroderma. J. Lab. Clin. Med., 76:480–484, 1970.

54. Coffman, J.D., and Cohen, A.S.: Total and capillary fingertip blood flow in Raynaud's phenomenon. N. Engl. J. Med., 285:259–263, 1971.

55. Cohen, I.S., et al.: Cutaneous toxicity of bleomycin therapy. Arch. Dermatol., 107:553–555, 1973.

56. Cohen, S., Johnson, A.R., and Hurd, E.: Cytotoxicity of sera from patients with scleroderma. Effects on human endothelial cells and fibroblasts in culture. Arthritis Rheum., 26:170–178, 1983.

57. Connolly, S.M., and Winkelmann, R.K.: Direct immunofluorescent findings in scleroderma syndromes. Acta Derm. Venereol., 61:29–36, 1981.

58. Cooper, S.M., et al.: Increase in fibronectin in the deep dermis of involved skin in progressive systemic sclerosis. Arthritis Rheum., 22:983–987, 1979.

59. Cooper, S.M., et al.: Selective decrease in antibody-dependent cell-mediated cytotoxicity in systemic lupus erythematosus and progressive systemic sclerosis. Clin. Exp. Immunol., 34:235–240, 1978.

60. Cooper, S.M., and Friou, G.J.: Cytotoxicity in progressive systemic sclerosis: No evidence for increased cytotoxicity against fibroblasts of different origin. J. Rheumatol., 6:25–29, 1979.

61. Costello, P.B., Tambar, P.M., and Green, F.A.: The prevalence and possible prognostic importance of arthropathy in childhood diabetes. J. Rheumatol., 11:62–65, 1984.

62. Cram, R.L., et al.: Diphosphonate treatment of calcinosis universalis. N. Engl. J. Med., 285:1012–1013, 1971.

63. Cramer, S.F., et al.: Eosinophilic fasciitis: Immunopathology, ultrastructure, literature review and consideration of its pathogenesis and relation to scleroderma. Arch. Pathol. Lab. Med., 106:85–91, 1982.

64. Currie, S., Saunders, M., and Knowles, M.: Immunological aspects of systemic sclerosis: In vitro activity of lymphocytes from patients with the disorder. Br. J. Dermatol., 84:400–409, 1970.

65. D'Angelo, W.A., et al.: Functional renal involvement in normotensive patients with progressive systemic sclerosis. Impaired sodium excreton during isotonic saline infusion. Arthritis Rheum., 24:8–11, 1981.

66. D'Angelo, W.A., et al.: Pathologic observations in systemic sclerosis (scleroderma). A study of 58 autopsy cases and 58 matched controls. Am. J. Med., 46:428–440, 1969.

67. Dau, P.C., Kahalen, M.B., and Sagebiel, R.W.: Plasmapheresis and immunosuppressive drug therapy in scleroderma. Arthritis Rheum., 24:1128–1136, 1981.

68. deGraaf, P., et al.: Metastatic skin calcification: A rare

69. Dent, C.E., and Stamp, T.C.B.: Treatment of calcinosis circumscripta with probenecid. Br. Med. J., 1:216–218, 1972.

70. DiBartolomeo, A.G., Rabin, B.S., and Rodnan, G.P.: Common HLA-D antigen in patients with progressive systemic sclerosis. Arthritis Rheum., 19:794, 1976.

71. Diegelmann, R.F., and Peterkofsky, B.: Inhibition of collagen secretion from bone and cultured fibroblasts by microtubular-disruptive drugs. Proc. Natl. Acad. Sci. U.S.A., 69:892–896, 1972.

72. DiMarino, A.J., et al.: Duodenal myoelectric activity in scleroderma. Abnormal responses to mechanical and hormonal stimuli. N. Engl. J. Med., 289:1220–1223, 1973.

73. Dinman, B.L., et al.: Occupational acroosteolysis. I. An epidemiological study. Arch. Environ. Health, 22:61–73, 1971.

74. Dostal, G.O.: Heterogeneity in systemic scleroderma and other diseases. J. Clin. Chem. Clin. Biochem., 17:495–499, 1979.

75. Douvas, A.S., Achten, M., and Tan, E.M.: Identification of a nuclear protein (Scl-70) as a unique target of human antinuclear antibodies in scleroderma. J. Biol. Chem., 254:10514–10522, 1979.

76. Dubois, E.L., et al.: Progressive systemic sclerosis (PSS) and localized scleroderma (morphea) with positive LE cell test and unusual systemic manifestations compatible with systemic lupus erythematosus (SLE): Presentation of 14 cases including one set of identical twins, one with scleroderma and the other with SLE. Review of the literature. Medicine, 50:199–222, 1971.

77. Duska, F., et al.: Pyrophosphate heart scan in patients with progressive systemic sclerosis. Br. Heart J., 47:90–93, 1982.

78. Edwards, D.A.W., and Lennard-Jones, J.E.: Diffuse systemic sclerosis presenting as infarction of colon. Proc. R. Soc. Med., 53:877–879, 1960.

79. Ehrlich, H.P., and Bornstein, P.: Microtubules in transcellular movement of procollagen. Nature [New Biol.], 238:257–260, 1972.

80. Emerit, I.: Chromosomal abnormalities in progressive systemic sclerosis. Clin. Rheum. Dis., 5:201–214, 1979.

81. Epstein, C.J., et al.: Werner's syndrome. A review of its symptomatology, natural history, pathologic features, genetics and relationship to the natural aging process. Medicine, 45:177–221, 1966.

82. Erasmus, L.D.: Scleroderma in gold-miners on the Witwatersrand with particular reference to pulmonary manifestations. S. Afr. J. Lab. Clin. Med., 3:209–231, 1957.

83. Estey, E., et al.: Cerebral arteritis in scleroderma. Stroke, 10:595–597, 1979.

84. Fahey, P.J., et al.: Raynaud's phenomenon of the lung. Am. J. Med., 76:263–269, 1984.

85. Farrell, D.A., and Medsger, T.A., Jr.: Trigeminal neuropathy in progressive systemic sclerosis. Am. J. Med., 73:57–62, 1982.

86. Flessinger, J.N., et al.: Salivary immunoglobulins in progressive systemic sclerosis. Biomedicine, 28:298–303, 1978.

87. Finch, W.R., et al.: Bleomycin induced scleroderma. Unpublished observations, 1978.

88. Fleischmajer, R., et al.: Immunofluorescence analysis of collagen, fibronectin, and basement membrane protein in scleroderma skin. J. Invest. Dermatol., 75:270–274, 1980.

89. Fleischmajer, R., and Nedwich, A.: Werner's syndrome. Am. J. Med., 54:111–118, 1973.

90. Fleischmajer, R., and Nedwich, A.: Progeria (Hutchinson-Gilford). Arch. Dermatol., 107:253–258, 1973.

91. Fleischmajer, R., and Pollock, J.L.: Progressive systemic sclerosis: Pseudoscleroderma. Clin. Rheum. Dis., 5:243–261, 1979.

92. Follansbee, W.P., et al.: Physiologic abnormalities of cardiac function in progressive systemic sclerosis with diffuse scleroderma. N. Engl. J. Med., 310:142–148, 1984.

93. Fraback, R.C., et al.: Sigmoid volvulus in two patients

with progressive systemic sclerosis. J. Rheumatol., 5:195–198, 1978.

94. Frayha, R.A., Shulman, L.E., and Stevens, M.B.: Hematological abnormalities in scleroderma. A study of 180 cases. Acta Haematol., 64:25–30, 1980.

95. Frayha, R.A., Tabbara, K.F., and Gena, R.S.: Familial CREST syndrome with sicca complex. J. Rheumatol., 4:53–58, 1977.

96. Fries, J.F., Hoopes, J.E., and Shulman, L.E.: Reciprocal skin grafts in systemic sclerosis (scleroderma). Arthritis Rheum., 14:571–578, 1971.

97. Fries, J.F., Lindgren, J.A., and Bull, J.M.: Sclerodermalike lesions and the carcinoid syndrome. Arch. Intern. Med., 131:550–553, 1973.

98. Fritz, J., and Sandhofer, M.: Zellulare Immunophanomene bei der Sklerodermie. Dermatologica, 154:129–137, 1977.

99. Furst, D.E., et al.: Abnormalities of pulmonary vascular dynamics and inflammation in early progressive systemic sclerosis. Arthritis Rheum., 24:1403–1408, 1981.

100. Furst, D.E., et al.: A syndrome resembling progressive systemic sclerosis after bone marrow transplantation. A model for scleroderma? Arthritis Rheum., 22:904–910, 1979.

101. Gaffney, F.A., et al.: Cardiovascular function in patients with progressive systemic sclerosis (scleroderma). Clin. Cardiol., 5:569–576, 1982.

102. Garrett, J.M., et al.: Esophageal deterioration in scleroderma. Mayo Clin. Proc., 46:92–96, 1971.

103. Garza-Elizondo, M.A., et al.: Joint contractures and scleroderma-like skin changes in the hands of insulin-dependent juvenile diabetics. J. Rheumatol., 10:797–800, 1983.

104. Gay, R.E., et al.: Collagen types synthesized in dermal fibroblast culture from patients with early progressive systemic sclerosis. Arthritis Rheum., 23:190–196, 1980.

105. Germain, B.F.: Cardiopulmonary function in the CREST syndrome. Arthritis Rheum., 24 (Suppl. 1):S105, 1981.

106. Germain, B.F., et al.: Choroidal angiopathy in the CREST syndrome. Clin. Res., 29:164A. 1981.

107. Gershwin, M.E., et al.: Characterization of a spontaneous disease of white leghorn chickens resembling progressive systemic sclerosis (scleroderma). J. Exp. Med., 153:1640–1659, 1981.

108. Giordano, M.: La Sclerosi Sistemica Progressiva. Roma, Luigi Possi, 1977.

109. Gordon, M.B., et al.: Thyroid disease in progressive systemic sclerosis (PSS): Increased frequency of glandular fibrosis and hypothyroidism. Ann. Intern. Med., 95:431–435, 1981.

110. Gratwick, G.M., et al.: Fibrinogen turnover in progressive systemic sclerosis. Arthritis Rheum., 21:343–347, 1978.

111. Green, M.C., Sweet, H.O., and Bunker, L.E.: Tight-skin, a new mutation of the mouse causing excessive growth of connective tissue and skeleton. Am. J. Pathol., 82:493–507, 1976.

112. Greger, R.E.: Familial progressive systemic scleroderma. Arch. Dermatol., 111:81–85, 1975.

113. Greif, J.M., and Wolff, W.I.: Idiopathic calcific pancreatitis, CREST syndrome and progressive systemic sclerosis. Am. J. Gastroenterol., 71:177–182, 1979.

114. Grennan, D.M., and Forrester, J.A.: Involvement of the eye in SLE and scleroderma. Ann. Rheum. Dis., 36:152–156, 1977.

114a. Griffin, A.J.: Eosinophilic fasciitis with megakaryocyte aplasia. J. R. Soc. Med., 72:779–781, 1979.

115. Grossman, M.E., et al.: Porphyria cutanea tarda. Clinical features and laboratory findings in 40 patients. Am. J. Med., 67:277–286, 1979.

116. Guillevin, L., Godeau, P., and Leenhardt, A.: Renin-angiotensin system in normotensive and hypertensive patients with progressive systemic sclerosis: Hyporesponsiveness of renin during captopril test. Postgrad. Med. J., 59: (Suppl. 3):171–172, 1983.

117. Gupta, S., et al.: Subpopulations of human T lymphocytes. IX. Imbalance of T cell subpopulations in patients

with progressive systemic sclerosis. Clin. Exp. Immunol., 38:342–347, 1979.

118. Guttadauria, M., et al.: Pulmonary function in scleroderma. Arthritis Rheum., 20:1071–1079, 1977.

119. Guttadauria, M., Diamond, H., and Kaplan, D.: Colchicine in the treatment of scleroderma. J. Rheumatol., 4:272–275, 1977.

120. Hankes, L.V., et al.: Metabolism of ^{14}C-labelled L-tryptophan, L-kynurenine and hydroxy-L-kynurenine in miners with scleroderma. S. Afr. Med. J., 51:383–390, 1977.

121. Hanson, V., Drexler, E., and Kornreich, H.: Rheumatoid factor (anti-gammaglobulins) in children with focal scleroderma. Pediatrics, 53:945–947, 1974.

122. Harper, F.E., et al.: A prospective study of Raynaud phenomenon and early connective tissue disease. A five-year report. Am. J. Med., 72:883–888, 1982.

123. Harris, E.D., Evanson, J.M., and Krane, S.M.: Effects of colchicine on collagenase in cultures of rheumatoid synovium. Arthritis Rheum., 14:669–684, 1971.

124. Hausmanowa-Petrusewica, I., et al.: Electromyographic findings in various forms of progressive systemic sclerosis. Arthritis Rheum., 25:61–65, 1982.

125. Hawkins, R.A., et al.: Increased dermal mast cell populations in progressive systemic sclerosis (abstract). Arthritis Rheum., 27:S38, 1984.

126. Haxthausen, H.: Studies in pathogenesis of morphea, vitiligo and acrodermatitis atrophicans by means of transplantation experiments. Acta Derm. Venereol., 27:352–367, 1947.

127. Hayes, R.L., and Rodnan, G.P.: The ultrastructure of skin in progressive systemic sclerosis (scleroderma). I. Dermal collagen fibers. Am. J. Pathol., 63:433–442, 1971.

128. Hedberg, H., et al.: Impaired mixed leucocyte reaction in some different diseases, notably multiple sclerosis and various arthritides. Clin. Exp. Immunol., 9:201–207, 1971.

129. Heinzerling, R.H., et al.: Elevated levels of antibodies to polyuridylic acid detected and quantitated in systemic scleroderma patients by solid phase radioimmunoassay. J. Invest. Dermatol., 75:224–227, 1980.

130. Henderson, R.D., and Pearson, F.G.: Surgical management of esophageal scleroderma. J. Thorac. Cardiovasc. Surg., 66:686–692, 1973.

131. Hendy, M.S., Torrance, H.B., and Warnes, T.W.: Small-bowel volvulus in association with progressive systemic sclerosis. Br. Med. J., 1:1051–1052, 1979.

132. Henriksen, O., and Kristensen, J.K.: Reduced systolic blood pressure in fingers of patients with generalized scleroderma (acrosclerosis). Acta Derm. Venereol., 61:531–534, 1981.

133. Herbert, C.M., et al.: Biosynthesis and maturation of skin collagen in scleroderma and effect of D-penicillamine. Lancet, 1:187–192, 1974.

134. Hoffman, R., et al.: Diffuse fasciitis and aplastic anemia: A report of four cases revealing an unusual association between rheumatologic and hematologic disorders. Medicine, 61:373–382, 1982.

135. Holt, J.M., and Wright, R.: Anaemia due to blood loss from the telangiectases of scleroderma. Br. Med. J., 3:537–538, 1967.

136. Hongo, M., et al.: Effects of nifedipine on esophageal motor function in humans: Correlation with plasma nifedipine concentration. Gastroenterology, 86:8–12, 1984.

137. Horwitz, D.A., and Garrett, M.A.: Lymphocyte reactivity to mitogens in subjects with systemic lupus erythematosus, rheumatoid arthritis and scleroderma. Clin. Exp. Immunol., 27:92–99, 1977.

138. Horwitz, D.A., Garrett, M.A., and Craig, A.H.: Serum effects on mitogenic reactivity in subjects with systemic lupus erythematosus, rheumatoid arthritis and scleroderma. Technical considerations and lack of correlation with anti-lymphocyte antibodies. Clin. Exp. Immunol., 27:100–110, 1977.

139. Hoskins, L.C., et al.: Functional and morphologic alterations of the gastrointestinal tract in progressive systemic sclerosis (scleroderma). Am. J. Med., 33:459–470, 1962.

140. Houpt, J.B., Ogryzlo, M.A., and Hunt, M.: Tryptophan

metabolism in man (with special reference to rheumatoid arthritis and scleroderma). Semin. Arthritis Rheum., 2:333–353, 1973.

141. Hudson, P.M., Jones, P.E., and Dent, C.E.: Extensive calcinosis with minimal scleroderma: Treatment of ectopic calcification with aluminum hydroxide. Proc. R. Soc. Med., 67:1166–1168, 1974.

142. Hughes, P., et al.: The relationship of defective cell-mediated immunity to visceral disease in systemic sclerosis. Clin. Exp. Immunol., 28:233–240, 1977.

143. Hughes, P., Holt, S., and Rowell, N.R.: Leukocyte migration inhibition in progressive systemic sclerosis. Br. J. Dermatol., 91:1–6, 1974.

144. Husson, J.M., et al.: Systemic sclerosis and cryoglobulinemia. Clin. Immunol. Immunopathol., 6:77–82, 1976.

145. Ikai, K., et al.: Morphea-like cutaneous changes in a patient with systemic scleroderma. Dermatologica, 158:438–442, 1979.

146. Illingworth, R.S.: Myositis ossificans progressiva (Munchmeyer's disease). Brief review with report of two cases treated with corticosteroids and observed for 16 years. Arch. Dis. Child., 46:264–268, 1971.

146a. Inoshita, T., et al.: Abnormalities of T lymphocyte subsets in patients with progressive systemic sclerosis (PSS, scleroderma). J. Lab. Clin. Med., 97:264–277, 1981.

147. Ivanova, M.M., et al.: Treatment of systemic sclerosis with D-penicillin(sic). Ther. Arch., 7:91–99, 1977.

148. Ja, S., Helm, S., and Wary, B.B.: Progressive systemic scleroderma with IgA deficiency in a child. Am. J. Dis. Child., 135:965–966, 1981.

149. Jablonska, S.: Scleroderma and Pseudoscleroderma, 2nd Ed. Warsaw, Polish Medical Publishers, 1975.

150. Jablonska, S., and Stachow, A.: Pseudoscleroderma concomitant with a muscular glycogenosis of unknown enzymatic defect. Acta Derm. Venereol., 52:379–385, 1972.

151. Jablonska, S., and Stachow, A.: Scleroderma-like lesions in multiple myeloma. Dermatologica, 144:257–269, 1972.

152. Jablonska, S., Stachow, A., and Suffczynska, A.: Skin and muscle indurations in phenylketonuria. Arch. Dermatol., 95:443–450, 1967.

153. James, T.N.: De subitaneis mortibus: VIII. Coronary arteries and conduction system in scleroderma heart disease. Circulation, 50:844–956, 1974.

154. Jansen, G.T., et al.: Generalized scleroderma. Treatment with an immunosuppressive agent. Arch. Dermatol., 97:690–698, 1968.

155. Jayson, M.I.V., et al.: Collagen studies in acro-osteolysis. Proc. R. Soc. Med., 69:295–297, 1976.

156. Jayson, M.I.V., Lovell, C., and Black, C.M.: Penicillamine therapy in systemic sclerosis. Proc. R. Soc. Med., 70:82–88, 1977.

157. Jimenez, S.A., Millan, A., and Bashey, R.I.: Scleroderma-like alterations in collagen metabolism occurring in the TSK (tight skin) mouse. Arthritis Rheum., 27:180–185, 1984.

158. Jimenez, S.A., Yakowski, R.I., and Frontino, P.M.: Biosynthetic heterogeneity of sclerodermatous skin in organ cultures. J. Molec. Med., 2:423–430, 1977.

159. Jobe, J.B., et al.: Induced vasodilation as treatment for Raynaud's disease. Ann. Intern. Med., 97:706–709, 1982.

160. Johnson, R.L., and Ziff, M.: Lymphokine stimulation of collagen accumulation. J. Clin. Invest., 58:240–252, 1976.

161. Kahaleh, M.B., and Leroy, E.C.: Endothelial injury in scleroderma. A protease mechanism. J. Lab. Clin. Med., 101:553–560, 1983.

162. Kahaleh, M.B., Osborn, I., and LeRoy, E.C.: Elevated levels of circulating platelet aggregates and beta-thromboglobulin in scleroderma. Ann. Intern. Med., 96:610–613, 1982.

163. Kahaleh, M.B., Osborn, I., and LeRoy, E.C.: Increased factor VIII/von Willebrand factor antigen and von Willebrand factor activity in scleroderma and in Raynaud's phenomenon. Ann. Intern. Med., 94:482–484, 1981.

164. Kahan, A., et al.: Nifedipine and Raynaud's phenomenon (letter). Ann. Intern. Med., 94:546, 1981.

165. Kahl, L.E., et al.: Prospective evaluation of thyroid function in progressive systemic sclerosis (abstract). Arthritis Rheum., 26:S62, 1983.

166. Kales, A.N., and Phang, J.M.: Dietary calcium perturbation in patients with abnormal calcium deposition. J. Clin. Endocrinol. Metab., 31:204–212, 1970.

167. Kallenberg, C.G.M., et al.: Antinuclear antibodies in patients with Raynaud's phenomenon: Clinical significance of anticentromere antibodies. Ann. Rheum. Dis., 41:382–387, 1982.

168. Keiser, H.R., Stein, H.D., and Sjoerdsma, A.: Increased protocollagen proline hydroxylase activity in sclerodermatous skin. Arch. Dermatol., 104:57–60, 1971.

169. Kemp-Harper, R.A., and Jackson, D.C.: Progressive systemic sclerosis. Br. J. Radiol., 38:825–834, 1965.

170. Kenik, J.G., Maricq, H.R., and Bole, G.G.: Blind evaluation of the diagnostic specificity of nailfold capillary microscopy in the connective tissue diseases. Arthritis Rheum., 24:885–891, 1981.

171. Kent, L.T., Cramer, S.F., and Moskowitz, R.W.: Eosinophilic fasciitis. Clinical, laboratory and microscopic considerations. Arthritis Rheum., 24:677–683, 1981.

172. Keystone, E.C., et al.: Immunoregulatory T cell subpopulations in patients with scleroderma using monoclonal antibodies. Clin. Exp. Immunol., 48:443–488, 1982.

173. Keystone, E.C., et al.: Antigen-specific suppressor cell activity in patients with scleroderma. J. Rheumatol., 8:747–751, 1981.

174. Kogo, Y., et al.: A case of the progressive systemic sclerosis (PSS) with high serum concentration of M protein. Jpn. Soc. Intern. Med., 64:1167–1173, 1975.

175. Kondo, H., Rabin, B.S., and Rodnan, G.P.: Cutaneous antigen-stimulating lymphokine production by lymphocytes of patients with progressive systemic sclerosis (scleroderma). J. Clin. Invest., 58:1388–1394, 1976.

175a. König, G., et al.: Lung involvement in scleroderma. Chest 85:318–324, 1984.

176. Kordac, V., and Semradova, H.: Treatment of porphyria cutanea tarda with chloroquine. Br. J. Dermatol., 90:95–100, 1974.

177. Korn, J.H., Torres, D., and Downie, E.: Clonal heterogeneity in the fibroblast response to mononuclear cell derived mediators. Arthritis Rheum., 27:174–179, 1984.

178. Kornreich, H.K., et al.: Phenylketonuria and scleroderma. J. Pediatr., 73:571–575, 1968.

179. Korom, K., Sonkodl, S., and Ormos, J.: Scleroderma (progressive systemic sclerosis) inducing ureteral closure. Int. Urol. Nephrol., 5:261–269, 1973.

180. Kovalchik, M.T., et al.: The kidney in progressive systemic sclerosis. A prospective study. Ann. Intern. Med., 89:881–887, 1978.

181. Krawitt, E.L., et al.: Suppressor cell activity in progressive systemic sclerosis. J. Rheumat., 9:263–267, 1982.

182. Kristensen, J.K., and Wadskov, S.: Increased 133 xenon washout from cutaneous tissue in generalized scleroderma indicates increased blood flow. Acta Derm. Venereol., 58:313–317, 1978.

183. Kumagai, V., et al.: Clinical spectrum of connective tissue disease after cosmetic surgery. Observations on eighteen patients and a review of the Japanese literature. Arthritis Rheum., 27:1–12, 1984.

184. Kurland, L.T., et al.: Epidemiological features of diffuse connective tissue disorders in Rochester, Minnesota, 1951 through 1967, with special reference to systemic lupus erythematosus. Mayo Clin. Proc., 44:649–663, 1969.

185. Labro, M.T., Perianin, A., and Kahn, M.F.: Antilymphocyte antibodies in progressive systemic sclerosis. Clin. Exp. Rheumatol., 1:23–28, 1983.

186. Lafferty, F.W., Raynolds, E.S., and Pearson, O.H.: Tumoral calcinosis: A metabolic disease of obscure etiology. Am. J. Med., 38:105–118, 1965.

187. Lally, E.V., and Jiminez, S.A.: Impotence in progressive systemic sclerosis. Ann. Intern. Med., 95:150–153, 1981.

188. Lam, M., et al.: Reversal of severe renal failure in systemic sclerosis. Ann. Intern. Med., 89:642–643, 1978.

189. Lane, P.: Low molecular weight dextran infusions in systemic sclerosis with Raynaud's phenomenon: A report of nine cases. Br. Med. J., 4:657–659, 1970.

190. Lapenas, D., Rodnan, G.P., and Cavallo, T.: Immunopathology of the renal vascular lesion of progressive systemic sclerosis (scleroderma). Am. J. Pathol., 91:243–258, 1978.

191. Laso, F.J., Pastor, I., and deCastro, S.: Cimetidine and eosinophilic fasciitis. Ann. Intern. Med., 98:1026, 1983.

192. Lawrence, L.A., Tye, M.J., and Liss, M.: Immunochemical analysis of the basic immunoglobulin in papular mucinosis. Immunochemistry, 9:41–49, 1972.

193. Leroux, J-L., et al.: Ultrastructural and crystallographic study of calcifications from a patient with CREST syndrome. J. Rheumatol., 10:242–246, 1983.

194. LeRoy, E.C.: Pathogenesis of scleroderma (systemic sclerosis). J. Invest. Dermatol., 79 (Suppl. 1):87S–89S, 1982.

195. LeRoy, E.C.: Increased collagen synthesis by scleroderma skin fibroblasts in vitro. A possible defect in the regulation or activation of the scleroderma fibroblast. J. Clin. Invest., 54:880–889, 1974.

196. Lester, P.D., and Koehler, P.R.: The renal angiographic changes in scleroderma. Radiology, 99:517–521, 1971.

197. Lian, J.B., et al.: Gamma-carboxyglutamate excretion and calcinosis in juvenile dermatomyositis. Arthritis Rheum., 25:1094–1100, 1982.

198. Lockshin, M.D., et al.: Monocyte-induced inhibition of lymphocyte response to phytohemagglutinin in progressive systemic sclerosis. Ann. Rheum. Dis., 42:40–44, 1983.

199. Lowe, W.C.: Scleroderma and amyloidosis. Milit. Med., 134:1430–1433, 1969.

200. Mackel, A.M., et al.: Antibodies to collagen in scleroderma. Arthritis Rheum., 25:522–531, 1982.

201. Mackel, S.E., et al.: Concurrent linear scleroderma and systemic lupus erythematosus: A report of two cases. J. Invest. Dermatol., 73:368–372, 1979.

202. Mackenzie, A.H.: Prolonged alkylating drug therapy is beneficial in systemic sclerosis (abstract). Arthritis Rheum., 13:334, 1970.

203. Maeda, H., Ishikaw, H., and Onta, S.: Circumscribed myxedema of lichen myxedematosus as a sign of faulty formation of the proteoglycan macromolecule. Br. J. Dermatol., 105:239–245, 1981.

204. Mapp, E.: Colonic manifestations in the connective tissue disorders. Am. J. Gastroenterol., 75:386–393, 1981.

204a. Maricq, H.R.: The microcirculation in scleroderma and allied diseases. Adv. Microcirc., 10:17–52, 1982.

205. Maricq, H.R.: Widefield capillary microscopy: Technique and rating scale for abnormalities seen in scleroderma and related disorders. Arthritis Rheum., 24:1159–1165, 1981.

206. Maricq, H.R., et al.: Capillary abnormalities in polyvinyl chloride production workers. Examination by in vivo microscopy. J.A.M.A., 236:1368–1371, 1976.

207. Maricq, H.R., Downey, J.A., and LeRoy, E.C.: Standstill of nailfold capillary blood flow during cooling in scleroderma and Raynaud's syndrome. Blood Vessels, 13:338, 1976.

208. Maricq, H.R., and LeRoy, E.C.: Capillary blood flow in scleroderma. Bibl. Anat., 11:352–358, 1973.

209. Maricq, H.R., Spencer-Green, G., and LeRoy, E.C.: Skin capillary abnormalities as indicators of organ involvement in scleroderma (systemic sclerosis), Raynaud's syndrome and dermatomyositis. Am. J. Med., 61:862–870, 1976.

210. Markenson, J.A., and Sherman, M.L.: Renal involvement in progressive systemic sclerosis; prolonged survival with aggressive antihypertensive management. Arthritis Rheum., 22:1132–1134, 1979.

211. Marks, J.: Studies with ^{47}Ca in patients with calcinosis cutis. Br. J. Dermatol., 82:1–9, 1970.

212. Marshall, J.E., Moore, G.F., and Settles, R.H.: Colonic telangiectasias in scleroderma. Arch. Intern. Med., 140:1121, 1980.

213. Martin, M.F.R., and Tooke, J.E.: Effects of prostaglandin E$_1$ on microvascular haemodynamics in progressive systemic sclerosis. Br. Med. J., 285:1688–1690, 1982.

214. Masi, A.T., et al.: Clinical criteria for early diagnosed systemic sclerosis: Preliminary results of the ARA multicenter cooperative study. Arthritis Rheum., 21:576–577, 1978.

215. Maxwell, W.A., et al.: Histochemical and ultrastructural studies in fibrodysplasia ossificans progressiva (myositis ossificans progressiva). Am. J. Pathol., 87:483–492, 1977.

216. McCarty, G.A., et al.: Anticentromere antibody. Clinical correlations and association with favorable prognosis in patients with scleroderma variants. Arthitis Rheum., 26:1–7, 1983.

217. McCoy, R.C., et al.: The kidney in progressive systemic sclerosis. Immunohistochemical and antibody elution studies. Lab. Invest., 35:124–131, 1976.

218. McFayden, I.J., Housley, E., and MacPherson, A.I.S.: Intra-arterial reserpine administration in Raynaud's syndrome. Arch. Intern. Med., 132:526–528, 1973.

219. McGiven, A.R., deBoer, W.G.R.M., and Barnett, A.J.: Renal immune deposits in scleroderma. Pathology, 3:145–150, 1971.

220. McGrath, M.A., Peek, R., and Penny, R.: Blood hyperviscosity with reduced skin blood flow in scleroderma. Ann. Rheum. Dis., 36:569–574, 1977.

221. Medsger, T.A., Jr.: Progressive systemic sclerosis. Clin. Rheum. Dis., 9:655–670, 1983.

222. Medsger, T.A., Jr.: Progressive systemic sclerosis and associated disorders. In Principles of Rheumatic Diseases. Edited by R.S. Panush. New York, John Wiley & Sons, 1981, pp. 331–350.

223. Medsger, T.A., Jr.: Progressive systemic sclerosis: Skeletal muscle involvement. Clin. Rheum. Dis., 5:103–113, 1979.

224. Medsger, T.A., Jr., and Masi, A.T.: Epidemiology of progressive systemic sclerosis. Clin. Rheum. Dis., 5:15–25, 1979.

225. Medsger, T.A., Jr., and Masi, A.T.: Epidemiology of systemic sclerosis (scleroderma). Ann. Intern. Med., 74:714–721, 1971.

226. Mendelson, B.C., et al.: Surgical treatment of calcinosis cutis in the upper extremity. J. Hand Surg., 2:318–324, 1977.

227. Merino, G.E., et al.: Renal transplantation for progressive systemic sclerosis with renal failure. Am. J. Surg., 133:745–749, 1977.

228. Metzger, A.L., et al.: Failure of disodium etidronate in calcinosis due to dermatomyositis and scleroderma. N. Engl. J. Med., 291:1294–1296, 1974.

229. Meyer, D., et al.: Vascular endothelial cell injury in progressive systemic sclerosis and other connective tissue diseases. Clin. Exp. Rheumatol., 1:29–34, 1983.

230. Michet, C.J., Jr., Doyle, J.A., and Ginsburg, W.W.: Eosinophilic fasciitis. Report of 15 cases. Mayo Clin. Proc., 56:27–34, 1981.

231. Mimori, T., et al.: Characterization of a high molecular weight acidic nuclear protein recognized by autoantibodies in sera from patients with polymyositis-scleroderma overlap. J. Clin. Invest., 68:611–620, 1981.

232. Mitnick, P., and Feig, P.U.: Control of hypertension and reversal of renal failure in scleroderma. N. Engl. J. Med., 299:871–872, 1978.

233. Morol, Y., et al.: Human anticentriole autoantibody in patients with scleroderma and Raynaud's phenomenon. Clin. Immunol. Immunopathol., 29:381–390, 1983.

234. Mor-Yosef, S., et al.: Collagen diseases in pregnancy. Obstet. Gynecol. Surv., 39:67–84, 1984.

235. Moskowitz, R.W., et al.: Crystal-induced inflammation associated with chronic renal failure treated with periodic hemodialysis. Am. J. Med., 47:450–460, 1969.

236. Moynahan, E.J.: Morphoea (localized cutaneous scleroderma) treated with low-dosage penicillamine (4 cases, including coup de sabre). Proc. R. Soc. Med., 66:1083–1085, 1973.

237. Mozarfarian, G., Lafferty, F.W., and Pearson, O.H.: Treatment of tumoral calcinosis with phosphorus deprivation. Ann. Intern. Med., 77:741–745, 1972.

238. Muralidar, K., et al.: Familial scleroderma (case report). J. Assoc. Physicians India, 26:307–309, 1978.
239. Murata, K., and Takeda, M.: Compositional changes of urinary acidic glycosaminoglycans in progressive systemic sclerosis. Clin. Chim. Acta, 108:49–59, 1980.
240. Nielsen, A.O., et al.: Dermatomyositis with universal calcinosis. A histopathological and electron microscopic study. J. Cutan. Pathol., 6:486–491, 1979.
241. Nimni, M.: A defect in the intramolecular and intermolecular cross-linking of collagen caused by penicillamine: I. Metabolic and functional abnormalities in soft tissues. J. Biol. Chem., 243:1457–1466, 1968.
242. Nishikai, M., Funats, D., and Homma, M.: Monoclonal gammopathy, penicillamine-induced polymyositis and systemic sclerosis. Arch. Dermatol., 110:253–255, 1974.
243. Nobin, B.A., et al.: Reserpine treatment of Raynaud's disease. Ann. Surg., 187:12–16, 1978.
244. Norton, W.L., et al.: Evidence of microvascular injury in scleroderma and systemic lupus erythematosus: quantitative study of the microvascular bed. J. Lab. Clin. Med., 71:919–933, 1968.
245. Oliver, J.A., et al.: Renal vasoactive hormones in scleroderma (progressive systemic sclerosis). Nephron, 29:110–116, 1981.
246. O'Loughlin, S., Tappeiner, G., and Jordon, R.E.: Circulating immune complexes in systemic scleroderma and generalized morphea. Dermatologica, 160:25–30, 1980.
247. Orringer, M.B., et al.: Combined collis gastroplasty-fun-doplication operations for scleroderma reflux esophagitis. Surgery, 90:624–630, 1981.
248. Osborn, T.G., et al.: The tight-skin mouse: Physical and biochemical properties of the skin. J. Rheumatol., 10:793–796, 1983.
249. Osborn, T.G., et al.: Antinuclear antibody staining only centrioles in a patient with scleroderma. N. Engl. J. Med., 307:253–254, 1982.
250. Osial, T.A., Jr., et al.: Clinical and serologic study of Sjögren's syndrome in patients with progressive systemic sclerosis. Arthritis Rheum., 26:500–508, 1983.
251. Osial, T.A., Jr., et al.: Resorption of the mandibular condyles and coronoid processes in progressive systemic sclerosis (scleroderma). Arthritis Rheum., 24:729–733, 1981.
252. Owens, G.R., et al.: Pulmonary function in progressive systemic sclerosis: Comparison of CREST syndrome variant with diffuse scleroderma. Chest, 84:546–550, 1983.
253. Palestine, R.F., et al.: Skin manifestations of pentazocine abuse. J. Am. Acad. Dermatol., 2:47–55, 1980.
254. Palma, A., et al.: Progressive systemic sclerosis and nephrotic syndrome. Arch. Intern. Med., 141:520–521, 1981.
255. Palmer, D.G., et al.: Bowed fingers. A helpful sign in the early diagnosis of systemic sclerosis. J. Rheumatol., 8:266–272, 1981.
256. Petrokubi, R.J., and Jeffries, G.H.: Cimetidine versus antacid in scleroderma with reflux esophagitis. A randomized double-blind controlled study. Gastroenterology, 77:691–695, 1979.
257. Postlethwaite, A.E., Snyderman, R., and Kang, A.H.: The chemotactic attraction of human fibroblasts to a lymphocyte-derived factor. J. Exp. Med., 144:1188–1203, 1976.
258. Potter, S.R., et al.: Clinical associations of fibroblast growth promoting factor in scleroderma. J. Rheumatol., 11:43–47, 1984.
259. Pruzanski, W., et al.: Lymphocytotoxic and phagocytotoxic activity in progressive systemic sclerosis. J. Rheumatol., 10:55–60, 1983.
260. Rabens, S.F., and Bethune, J.E.: Disodium etidronate therapy for dystrophic cutaneous calcification. Arch. Dermatol., 111:357–361, 1975.
261. Rajapakse, C.N.A., et al.: Pharyngo-esophageal dysphagia in systemic sclerosis. Ann. Rheum. Dis., 40:612–614, 1981.
262. Ramirez-Mata, M., Ibanez, G., and Alarcon-Segovia, D.: Stimulatory effect of metoclopramide on the esophagus and lower esophageal sphincter of patients with PSS. Arthritis Rheum., 20:30–34, 1977.
263. Ramsay, C.A., et al.: The treatment of porphyria cutanea tarda by venesection. Q. J. Med., 43:1–24, 1974.
264. Raz, S., et al.: Scleroderma of lower urinary tract. Urology, 9:682–683, 1977.
265. Rees, W.D.W., et al.: Interdigestive motor activity in patients with systemic sclerosis. Gastroenteroloy, 83:575–580, 1982.
266. Regan, P.T., Welland, L.H., and Geall, M.G.: Scleroderma and intestinal perforation. Am. J. Gastroenterol., 68:566–571, 1977.
267. Resnick, D., et al.: Intra-articular calcification in scleroderma. Radiology, 124:685–688, 1977.
268. Reynolds, T.B., et al.: Primary biliary cirrhosis with scleroderma, Raynaud's phenomenon and telangiectasia. New syndrome. Am. J. Med., 50:302–312, 1971.
269. Ridolfi, R.L. Bulkley, B.H., and Hutchins, G.M.: The cardiac conduction system in progressive systemic sclerosis. Clinical and pathologic features of 35 patients. Am. J. Med., 61:361–366, 1976.
270. Roberts, N.K.: The morphology of the atrioventricular node in scleroderma—a three-dimensional reconstruction. Eur. Heart J., 1:361–367, 1980.
271. Roberts, N.K., et al.: The prevalence of conduction defects and cardiac arrhythmias in progressive systemic sclerosis. Ann. Intern. Med., 94:38–40, 1981.
272. Roberts, N.K., and Cabeen, W.R.: Atrioventricular nodal function in progressive systemic sclerosis: Electrophysiological and morphological findings. Br. Heart J., 44:529–533, 1980.
273. Robinson, J.C., and Teitelbaum, S.L.: Stercoral ulceration and perforation of the sclerodermatous colon: Report of two cases and review of the literature. Dis. Colon Rectum, 17:622–632, 1974.
274. Rodeheffer, R.J., et al.: Controlled double-blind trial of nifedipine in the treatment of Raynaud's phenomenon. N. Engl. J. Med., 308:880–883, 1983.
275. Rodnan, G.P.: Progressive systemic sclerosis. In Arthritis and Allied Conditions, 9th Ed. Edited by D.J. McCarty. Philadelphia, Lea & Febiger, 1979, pp. 762–809.
276. Rodnan, G.P.: The nature of joint involvement in progressive systemic sclerosis (diffuse scleroderma). Clinical study and pathological examination of synovium in twenty-nine patients. Ann. Intern. Med., 56:422–439, 1962.
277. Rodnan, G.P., et al.: Eosinophilia and serologic abnormalities in linear localized scleroderma. Arthritis Rheum., 20:133, 1977.
278. Rodnan, G.P., et al.: The association of progressive systemic sclerosis (scleroderma) with coal miners' pneumoconiosis and other forms of silicosis. Ann. Intern. Med., 66:323–334, 1967.
279. Rodnan, G.P., Lipinski, E., and Luksick, J.: Skin thickness and collagen content in progressive systemic sclerosis (scleroderma) and localized scleroderma. Arthritis Rheum., 22:130–140, 1979.
280. Rodnan, G.P., Myerowitz, R.L., and Justh, G.O.: Morphologic changes in the digital arteries of patients with progressive systemic sclerosis (scleroderma) and Raynaud's phenomenon. Medicine, 59:393–408, 1980.
281. Rosekrans, P.C.M., et al.: Gastrointestinal telangiectasia as a cause of severe blood loss in systemic sclerosis. Endoscopy, 12:200–204, 1980.
282. Rothfield, N.F., and Rodnan, G.P.: Serum antinuclear antibodies in systemic sclerosis (scleroderma). Arthritis Rheum., 11:607–617, 1968.
283. Roumm, A.D., et al.: Lymphocytes in the skin of patients with progressive systemic sclerosis: Quantification, subtyping and clinical correlations. Arthritis Rheum., 27:645–653, 1984.
284. Roumm, A.D., and Medsger, T.A., Jr.: Cancer in systemic sclerosis: An epidemiologic study. (abstract). Arthritis Rheum., 27:S19, 1984.
285. Rozkovec, A., et al.: Vascular reactivity and pulmonary hypertension in systemic sclerosis. Arthritis Rheum., 26:1037–1040, 1983.
286. Rubinow, A., and Cohen, A.S.: Skin involvement in generalized amyloidosis. A study of clinically involved and

uninvolved skin in 50 patients with primary and secondary amyloidosis. Ann. Intern. Med., *88*:781–785, 1978.

287. Russell, M.L.: The tight-skin mouse: Is it a model for scleroderma? (Editorial.) J. Rheumatol., *10*:679–681, 1983.

288. Russell, R.G.G., Bisaz, S., and Fleisch, H.: Pyrophosphate and diphosphonates in calcium metabolism and their possible role in renal failure. Arch. Intern. Med., *124*:571–577, 1969.

289. Russell, M.L., and Hanna, W.M.: Ultrastructure of muscle microvasculature in progressive systemic sclerosis: Relation to clinical weakness. J. Rheumatol., *10*:741–747, 1983.

290. Russell, M.L., and Kahn, J.J.: Nodular regenerative hyperplasia of the liver associated with progressive systemic sclerosis: A case report with ultrastructural observation. J. Rheumatol., *10*:748–752, 1983.

291. Russell, R.G.G., and Smith, R.: Diphosphonates. Experimental and clinical aspects. J. Bone Joint Surg., *55B*:66–86, 1973.

292. Sacher, P., Buchmann, P., and Burger, H.: Stenosis of the large intestine complicating scleroderma and mimicking a sigmoid carcinoma. Dis. Colon Rectum, *26*:347–348, 1983.

293. Sackner, M.A.: Scleroderma. New York, Grune & Stratton, 1966.

294. Salen, N.B., and Morse, J.H.: Lymphocyte response to mitogens in progressive systemic sclerosis. Arthritis Rheum., *19*:875–882, 1976.

295. Salerni, R., et al.: Pulmonary hypertension in the CREST syndrome variant of progressive systemic sclerosis (scleroderma). Ann. Intern. Med., *86*:394–399, 1977.

296. Sapira, J.L., et al.: Studies of endogenous catecholamines in patients with Raynaud's phenomenon secondary to progressive systemic sclerosis (scleroderma). Am. J. Med., *52*:330–337, 1972.

297. Scharer, L., and Smith, D.W.: Resorption of the terminal phalanges in scleroderma. Arthritis Rheum., *12*:51–63, 1969.

298. Schneider, P.D., et al.: Serial pulmonary function in systemic sclerosis. Am. J. Med., *73*:385–394, 1982.

299. Schumacher, H.R., Jr.: Joint involvement in progressive systemic sclerosis (scleroderma). A light and electron microscopic study of synovial membrane and fluid. Am. J. Clin. Pathol., *60*:593–600, 1973.

300. Schur, P.H., Monroe, M., and Rothfield, N.: The γG subclass of antinuclear and antinucleic acid antibodies. Arthritis Rheum., *15*:174–182, 1972.

301. Segond, P., et al.: Impaired primary in-vitro antibody response in progressive systemic sclerosis patients: Role of suppressor monocytes. Clin. Exp. Immunol., *47*:147–154, 1982.

302. Seibold, J.R.: Digital sclerosis in children. Skin changes in insulin-dependent diabetes mellitus. Arthritis Rheum., *25*:1357–1361, 1982.

303. Seibold, J.R., et al.: Circulating immune complexes in eosinophilic fasciitis. Arthritis Rheum., *25*:1180–1185, 1982.

304. Seibold, J.R., et al.: Immune complexes in progressive systemic sclerosis. Arthritis Rheum., *25*:1167–1173, 1982.

305. Seibold, J.R., and Jageneau, A.H.M.: Treatment of Raynaud's phenomenon with Ketanserin, a selective antagonist of the serotonin2 (5-HT2) receptor. Arthritis Rheum., *27*:139–146, 1984.

306. Selikoff, I.J., and Hammond, E.C.: Editors and Conference Chairmen: Toxicity of vinyl chloride—polyvinyl chloride. Ann. N.Y. Acad. Sci., *246*:1–337, 1975.

307. Selye, H., and Tuchweber, B.: Mast cell products and tissue calcification. Q. J. Exp. Physiol., *50*:196–202, 1965.

308. Seyer, J.M., Kang, A.H., and Rodnan, G.: Investigation of type I and type III collagens of the lung in progressive systemic sclerosis. Arthritis Rheum., *24*:625–631, 1981.

309. Shamberger, R.C., Crawford, J.L., and Kirkham, S.E.: Progressive systemic sclerosis resulting in megacolon. J.A.M.A., *250*:1063–1065, 1983.

310. Shanahan, W.R., Jr., and Korn, J.H.: Cytotoxic activity of sera from scleroderma and other connective tissue diseases. Lack of cellular and disease specificity. Arthritis Rheum., *25*:1381–1395, 1982.

311. Shapiro, L.S., et al.: D-penicillamine treatment of progressive systemic sclerosis (scleroderma): A comparison of clinical and in vitro effects. J. Rheumatol., *10*:316–318, 1983.

312. Sheldon, W.B., et al.: Three siblings with scleroderma (systemic sclerosis) and two with Raynaud's phenomenon from a single kindred. Arthritis Rheum., *24*:668–676, 1981.

313. Shulman, L.E.: Diffuse fasciitis with eosinophilia: A new syndrome? Trans. Assoc. Am. Physicians, *88*:70–86, 1975.

314. Smiley, A.M., Husain, M., and Indebaum, S.: Eosinophilic fasciitis in association with thyroid disease: A report of three cases. J. Rheumatol., *7*:871–876, 1980.

315. Smith, A.G., Holti, G., and Shuster, S.: Immunoreactive beta-melanocyte-stimulating hormone and melanin pigmentation in systemic sclerosis. Br. Med. J., *2*:733–734, 1976.

316. Smith, C.D., and McKendry, R.J.R.: Controlled trial of nifedipine in the treatment of Raynaud's phenomenon. Lancet, *2*:1299–1301, 1982.

317. Smith, J.W., et al.: Echocardiographic features of progressive systemic sclerosis (PSS). Correlation with hemodynamic and postmortem studies. Am. J. Med., *66*:28–33, 1979.

318. Smith, R.: Myositis ossificans progressiva: A review of current problems. Semin. Arthritis Rheum., *4*:369–380, 1975.

319. Soffa, D.J., Sire, D.J., and Dodson, J.H.: Melorheostosis with linear sclerodermatous skin changes. Radiology, *114*:577–578, 1975.

320. Solomon, G., Barland, P., and Rifkin, H.: Eosinophilic fasciitis responsive to cimetidine. Ann. Intern. Med., *97*:547–549, 1982.

321. Sood, S.V., and Kohler, H.G.: Maternal death from systemic sclerosis. (Report of a case of renal scleroderma masquerading as pre-eclamptic toxaemia.) J. Obstet. Gynecol. Br. Commw., *77*:1109–1112, 1970.

322. Soria, J., et al.: Normal level of plasma fibronectin and fibrin-stabilizing factor in progressive systemic sclerosis. Arthritis Rheum., *23*:1354–1355, 1980.

323. Spielvogel, R.L., Goltz, R.W., and Kersey, J.H.: Scleroderma-like changes in chronic graft vs. host disease. Arch. Dermatol., *113*:1424–1428, 1977.

324. Spisani, S., Lovigo, L., and Colamussi, V.: Leukocyte migration and phagocytosis in progressive systemic sclerosis. Scand. J. Rheumatol., *10*:299–300, 1981.

325. Stachow, A., Jablonska, S., and Skiendzielewska, A.: Biogenic amines derived from tryptophan in systemic and cutaneous scleroderma. Acta Derm. Venereol., *59*:1–5, 1979.

326. Stachow, A., Jablonska, S., and Skiendzielewska, A.: 5-hydroxy-tryptamine and tryptamine pathways in scleroderma. Br. J. Dermatol., *97*:147–154, 1977.

327. Stachow, A., Jablonska, S., and Skiendzielewska, A.: Intestinal absorption of L-tryptophan in scleroderma. Acta Derm. Venereol., *56*:257–264, 1976.

328. Steen, V.D.: Factors predicting the development of renal involvement in progressive systemic sclerosis. Am. J. Med., *76*:779–786, 1984.

329. Steen, V.D., Medsger, T.A., Jr., and Rodnan, G.P.: D-penicillamine therapy in progressive systemic sclerosis (scleroderma). Ann. Intern. Med., *97*:652–658, 1982.

330. Steen, V.D., et al.: Clinical and laboratory associations of anticentromere antibody ACA in patients with progressive systemic sclerosis scleroderma. Arthritis Rheum., *27*:125–131, 1984.

331. Steigerwald, J.C.: Progressive systemic sclerosis: Management. Part III: Immunosuppressive agents. Clin. Rheum. Dis., *5*:289–294, 1979.

332. Sternberg, E.M., et al.: Development of a scleroderma-like illness during therapy with L-5-hydroxytryptophan and carbidopa. N. Engl. J. Med., *303*:782–787, 1980.

333. Stevens, M.B., et al.: Aperistalsis of the esophagus in

patients with connective tissue disorders and Raynaud's phenomenon. N. Engl. J. Med., *270*:1218–1222, 1964.

334. Stranden, E., Roald, D.K., and Krong, K.: Treatment of Raynaud's phenomenon with the 5-HT2-receptor antagonist ketanserin. Br. Med. J., *285*:1069–1071, 1982.

335. Stringa, S.G., et al.: Immunologic response to blood group substance in scleroderma. Arch. Dermatol., *103*:394–399, 1971.

336. Strosberg, J.M., Peck, B., and Harris, E.D., Jr.: Scleroderma with intestinal involvement; fatal in two of a kindred. J. Rheumatol., *4*:46–52, 1977.

337. Stuart, J.M., Postlethwaite, A.E., and Kang, A.H.: Evidence for cell-mediated immunity to collagen in progressive systemic sclerosis. J. Lab. Clin. Med., *88*:601–607, 1976.

338. Stupi, A., et al.: Pulmonary hypertension (PHT) in the CREST syndrome variant of progressive systemic sclerosis (PSS). Arthritis Rheum., *25* (Suppl.):S4, 1982.

339. Sucio, I., et al.: Clinical manifestations in vinyl chloride poisoning. Ann. N.Y. Acad. Sci., *246*:53–69, 1975.

340. Sumithran, E.: Progressive systemic sclerosis and autoimmune haemolytic anemia. Postgrad. Med. J., *52*:173–176, 1976.

341. Surwit, R.S.: Biofeedback: A possible treatment for Raynaud's disease. Semin. Psychiatry, *5*:483–490, 1973.

342. Suzuki, Y., Bisada, K., and Takeda, M.: Demonstration of myositis ossificans by ^{99m}Tc pyrophosphate bone scanning. Radiology, *111*:663–664, 1974.

343. Taj, M., and Ahmad, A.: Familial localized scleroderma (morphoea). Arch. Dermatol., *113*:1132–1133, 1977.

344. Takehara, K., et al.: Antinuclear antibodies in localized scleroderma. Arthritis Rheum., *26*:612–616, 1983.

345. Talaat, A.M., et al.: Human respiratory nasal mucosa in progressive systemic sclerosis (scleroderma). An electron microscopic study. J. Laryngol. Otol., *94*:617–627, 1980.

346. Talbott, J.H., and Borrocas, M.: Progressive systemic sclerosis (PSS) and malignancy, pulmonary and non-pulmonary. Medicine, *58*:182–207, 1979.

347. Tan, E.M., et al.: Human skin fibroblasts in culture: Procollagen synthesis in the presence of sera from patients with dermal fibroses. J. Invest. Dermatol., *16*:462–467, 1981.

348. Tan, E.M., et al.: Diversity of antinuclear antibodies in progressive systemic sclerosis. Arthritis Rheum., *23*:617–625, 1980.

349. Teasdall, R.D., Frayha, R.A., and Shulman, L.E.: Cranial nerve involvement in systemic sclerosis (scleroderma): A report of 10 cases. Medicine, *59*:149–159, 1980.

350. Teutsch, C., Lipton, A., and Harvey, H.A.: Raynaud's phenomenon as a side effect of chemotherapy with vinblastine and bleomycin for testicular carcinoma. Cancer Treat. Rep., *61*:925–926, 1977.

351. Thompson, J.M., et al.: Skeletal muscle involvement in systemic sclerosis. Ann. Rheum. Dis., *28*:281–288, 1969.

352. Todesco, S., et al.: Cardiac involvement in progressive systemic sclerosis. Acta Cardiol., *5*:311–322, 1979.

353. Torres, C.F., et al.: Penicillamine-induced myasthenia gravis in progressive systemic sclerosis. Arthritis Rheum., *23*:900–908, 1980.

354. Tramposch, H.D., et al.: A long-term longitudinal study of anticentromere antibodies. Arthritis Rheum., *27*:121–124, 1984.

355. Traub, Y.M., et al.: Hypertension and renal failure (scleroderma renal crisis) in progressive systemic sclerosis. Report of a 25-year experience with 68 cases. Medicine, *62*:335–352, 1984.

356. Tuffanelli, D.L., Marmelzat, W.L., and Dorsey, C.S.: Linear scleroderma with hemiatrophy. Report of three cases associated with collagen-vascular disease. Dermatologica, *132*:51–58, 1966.

357. Tuffanelli, D.L., and Winkelmann, R.K.: Systemic scleroderma: A clinical study of 727 cases. Arch. Dermatol., *84*:359–371, 1961.

358. Uitto, J., Hanuksela, M., and Rasmussen, O.G.: Protocollagen proline hydroxylase activity in scleroderma and

other connective tissue disorders. Ann. Clin. Res., *2*:235–239, 1970.

359. Uitto, J., Ohlenschlager, K., and Lorenzen, I.B.: Solubility of skin collagen in normal subjects and in patients with generalised scleroderma. Clin. Chim. Acta, *31*:13–18, 1971.

360. Ungerer, R.G., et al.: Prevalence and clinical correlates of pulmonary arterial hypertension in progressive systemic sclerosis. Am. J. Med., *75*:65–74, 1983.

361. Varadi, D.P., and Lawrence, A.M.: Suppression of Raynaud's phenomenon by methyldopa. Arch. Intern. Med., *124*:13–18, 1969.

362. Veltman, G., et al.: Clinical manifestations and course of vinyl chloride disease. Ann. N.Y. Acad. Sci., *246*:6–17, 1975.

363. Villee, D.B., Nichols, G., and Talbot, N.B.: Metabolic studies in two boys with classical progeria. Pediatrics, *43*:207–216, 1969.

364. Vogelzang, N.J., et al.: Raynaud's phenomenon: A common toxicity after combination chemotherapy for testicular cancer. Ann. Intern. Med., *95*:288–292, 1981.

365. Ward, A.M., et al.: Immunological mechanisms in the pathogenesis of vinyl chloride disease. Br. Med. J., *1*:936–938, 1976.

366. Wasner, C., Cooke, C.R., and Fries, J.F.: Successful medical treatment of scleroderma renal crisis. N. Engl. J. Med., *299*:873–875, 1978.

367. Wasserman, S.I., et al.: Serum eosinophilotactic activity in eosinophilic fasciitis. Arthritis Rheum., *25*:1352–1356, 1982.

368. Waugh, D., and Ibels, L.: Malignant scleroderma associated with autoimmune neutropenia. Br. Med. J., *280*:1577–1578, 1980.

369. West, R.H., and Barnett, A.J.: Ocular involvement in scleroderma. Br. J. Ophthalmol., *63*:845–847, 1979.

370. West, S.G., Killian, P.J., and Lawless, D.J.: Association of myositis and myocarditis in progressive systemic sclerosis. Arthritis Rheum., *24*:662–667, 1981.

371. Whiteside, T.L., et al.: Suppressor cell function and T lymphocyte subpopulations in peripheral blood of patients with progressive systemic sclerosis. Arthritis Rheum., *26*:841–847, 1983.

372. Whiteside, T.L., Medsger, T.A., Jr., and Rodnan, G.P.: HLA-DR antigens in progressive systemic sclerosis (scleroderma). J. Rheumatol., *10*:128–131, 1983.

373. Whitman, H.H., III, et al.: Variable response to oral angiotensin-converting-enzyme blockade in hypertensive scleroderma patients. Arthritis Rheum., *25*:241–248, 1982.

374. Winkelmann, R.K., et al.: Management of scleroderma. Mayo Clin. Proc., *46*:128–134, 1971.

375. Winkelmann, R.K., Goldyne, M.E., and Linscheid, R.L.: Influence of cold on catecholamine response of vascular smooth muscle strips from resistance vessels of scleroderma skin. Angiology, *28*:330–339, 1977.

376. Winkelmann, R.K., Goldyne, M.E., and Linscheid, R.L.: Hypersensitivity of scleroderma cutaneous vascular smooth muscle to 5-hydroxytryptamine. Br. J. Dermatol., *95*:51–56, 1976.

377. Winograd, J., Schimmel, D.H., and Palubinskas, A.J.: The spotted nephrogram of renal scleroderma. Am. J. Roentgenol., *126*:734–738, 1976.

378. Winterbauer, R.H.: Multiple telangiectasia, Raynaud's phenomenon, sclerodactyly, and subcutaneous calcinosis: A syndrome mimicking hereditary hemorrhagic telangiectasia. Bull. Johns Hopkins Hosp., *114*:361–383, 1964.

379. Wise, R.A., et al.: The effect of cold exposure on diffusing capacity in patients with Raynaud's phenomenon. Chest, *81*:695–698, 1982.

380. Woodhall, P.B., et al.: Apparent recurrence of progressive systemic sclerosis in a renal allograft. J.A.M.A., *236*:1032–1034, 1976.

381. Worrall, J.G., et al.: Persistence of scleroderma-like phenotype in normal dermal fibroblasts following prolonged exposure to inflammatory mediators (abstract). Arthritis Rheum., *27*:S37, 1984.

382. Wright, J.K., et al.: Antibody-dependent and phytohae-

magglutinin-induced lymphocyte cytotoxicity in systemic sclerosis. Clin. Exp. Immunol., *36*:175–182, 1979.

383. Wright, J.K., Hughes, P., and Rowell, N.R.: Lymphocyte cytotoxicity in systemic sclerosis: No increase on short-term culture with established human cell lines. Ann. Rheum. Dis., *41*:414–416, 1982.

384. Wright, J.K., Hughes, P., and Rowell, N.R.: Spontaneous lymphocyte-mediated (NK cell) cytotoxicity in systemic sclerosis: A comparison with antibody-dependent lymphocyte (K cell) cytotoxicity. Ann. Rheum. Dis., *41*:409–413, 1982.

385. Yagoda, A., et al.: Bleomycin, an antitumor antibiotic. Clinical experience in 274 patients. Ann. Intern. Med., *77*:861–870, 1972.

386. Yakovleva, G.I., et al.: The ultrastructure of the skin in systemic sclerodermia. Arkh. Patol., *4*:32–37, 1975.

387. Yamakage, A., et al.: Occupational scleroderma-like disorder occurring in men engaged in the polymerization of epoxy resins. Dermatologica. *161*:33–44, 1980.

388. Young, R.H., and Mark, G.J.: Pulmonary vascular changes in scleroderma. Am. J. Med., *64*:998–1004, 1978.

389. Zeiler, J., et al.: Serotonin content of platelets in inflammatory rheumatic diseases. Correlation with clinical activity. Arthritis Rheum., *26*:532–540, 1983.

390. Zerwekh, J.E., et al.: Tumoral calcinosis: Evidence for concurrent defects in renal tubular phosphorus transport and in 1a,25-dihydrocholecalciferol synthesis. Calcif. Tissue Int., *32*:1–6, 1980.

Chapter 67

Sjögren's Syndrome and Connective Tissue Disease with other Immunologic Disorders

Norman Talal

SJÖGREN'S SYNDROME

Sjögren's syndrome is a chronic inflammatory disease characterized by diminished lacrimal and salivary gland secretion, the sicca complex, resulting in keratoconjunctivitis sicca and xerostomia. The glandular insufficiency is secondary to lymphocytic and plasma cell infiltrations. The term *autoimmune exocrinopathy* has recently been introduced for Sjögren's syndrome.[45] Both primary and secondary forms of this disease are recognized. Approximately half the patients with an associated rheumatoid arthritis (RA), are considered to have secondary Sjögren's syndrome; a small percentage may have another connective tissue disease accompanying the sicca complex. Primary Sjögren's syndrome is diagnosed in the absence of another connective tissue disease.

Sjögren's syndrome is particularly important among the autoimmune diseases for two reasons. First, perhaps two to three million individuals are affected in the United States, the majority undiagnosed. Second, Sjögren's syndrome is a disorder in which a benign autoimmune process can terminate in a malignant lymphoid disorder. Thus, it is a "crossroads" disease that offers potential insight into the mechanisms whereby immunologic dysregulation may predispose a person to a malignant transformation of B cells already involved in an autoimmune process.

Historical Background

A number of patients with various combinations of dry mouth, dry eyes, and chronic arthritis were described by European clinicians between 1882 and 1925. In 1892, Mikulicz reported a man with bilateral parotid and lacrimal gland enlargement associated with massive round-cell infiltration.[29] In 1925, Gougerot described 3 patients with salivary and mucous gland atrophy and insufficiency progressing to dryness. Two years later, Houwer emphasized the association of filamentary keratitis, the major ocular manifestation of the syndrome, with chronic arthritis. In 1933, Henrik Sjögren reported detailed clinical and histologic findings in 19 women with xerostomia and keratoconjunctivitis sicca, of whom 13 had chronic arthritis.[41] In 1953, Morgan and Castleman concluded that Sjögren's syndrome and Mikulicz's disease were the same entity.[32]

Etiologic Factors

Autoimmune disorders have a multifactorial origin with elements of: (1) genetic control related to the activity of specific immune-response genes; (2) immunologic control exerted by regulatory T-dependent lymphocytes (suppressor and helper T cells); (3) possible viral influences, although such influences are not yet clearly established; and (4) sex-hormone modulation of immune regulation in which estrogens enhance and androgens suppress autoimmunity.[36,48]

Sjögren's syndrome is one of several autoimmune diseases associated with the histocompatibility antigens HLA-B8 and HLA-DW3.[17,34] This genetic predisposition is seen in organ-specific autoimmune diseases such as celiac disease, dermatitis herpetiformis, myasthenia gravis, Graves' disease, chronic active hepatitis, idiopathic Addison's disease, and insulin-dependent diabetes mellitus. Moreover, certain Ia determinants occur more frequently in Sjögren's syndrome than in the general population. An animal model for Sjögren's syndrome has been described.[22]

The presence of multiple serum autoantibodies is a characteristic feature of Sjögren's syndrome. Some of these reactions are organ-specific, such as the antibody directed against salivary duct epithelium.[24] Others, such as antinuclear and rheumatoid factor, are not specific for salivary gland antigens. Three serum antibodies reacting with partially characterized nuclear antigens, SS-A, SS-B, and RAP, are present in high frequency in different clinical subsets of Sjögren's syndrome.[2,6]

The exact mechanism responsible for the glandular destruction is unknown. Both T- and B-lymphocytes are present in the tissue lesions,[1,49] and large amounts of immunoglobulin are synthesized locally;[50] β_2-microglobulin, a component of lymphocyte membranes that may play an immunologic role, is increased in serum and saliva of patients with Sjögren's syndrome.[28]

An imbalance of helper and suppressor T cells and the polyclonal activation of B cells are often features of autoimmunity. These abnormalities are less marked in Sjögren's syndrome than they are, for example, in systemic lupus erythematosus (SLE). The autologous mixed lymphocyte response, which may be a common denominator for the autoimmune and lymphoproliferative diseases of immunoregulation,[42] is abnormal in Sjögren's syndrome.[31]

Pathologic Features

The classic lesion is a lymphocytic and plasma-cell infiltrate of salivary, lacrimal, and other exocrine glands in the respiratory tract, gastrointestinal tract, and vagina. Major (parotid, submaxillary) and minor (gingival, palatine) salivary glands are affected.[11,20,50] The term "benign lymphoepithelial lesion" has been used to describe the characteristic histologic appearance in the salivary glands.[18] These lesions may be present without xerostomia and other features of Sjögren's syndrome.[14] The earliest infiltrates may be scattered around small, intralobular ducts. The histologic picture is varied and includes acinar atrophy, generally in proportion to the extent of lymphoid infiltration, occasional germinal center formation, and proliferative or metaplastic changes in the duct lining cells. The proliferation may progress to the characteristic epimyoepithelial islets (Fig. 67–1), which are seen in about 40% of parotid biopsy specimens.[10] In some patients, adipose replacement may be more prominent than lymphoid infiltration. Typically, the lobular architecture is preserved; some lobules may be spared while others are virtually destroyed.

When mucosal glands in the trachea and bronchi are involved, benign-appearing lymphoid infiltrates are again a prominent feature. More extensive lymphoid infiltrates may involve the lung, kidney, or skeletal muscle and may cause functional abnormalities of these organs.

In some patients, the lymphoid infiltrates in salivary glands, lymph nodes, or parenchymal organs are more pleomorphic, more primitive, or more invasive than in others, and these infiltrates suggest the possibility of a malignant disorder. Lymph node architecture can be destroyed, and malignant lymphoma may be diagnosed if such abnormal cells predominate. If it is not possible to distinguish a benign from a malignant process, then the term "pseudolymphoma" may be employed.[8,51] These patients may have a lymphoproliferative disorder of B-lymphocytes termed "immunoblastic lymphadenopathy,"[23] which can occur in Sjögren's syndrome.[35]

The recent discovery of natural killer (NK) cells reactive with virus-infected targets and important in immune defense against malignant disease may be particularly relevant to the association of lymphoma with Sjögren's syndrome. The diminished activity of NK cells in Sjögren's syndrome may contribute to the emergence of B-cell lymphomas in some individuals.

Clinical Features

More than 90% of patients are women; the mean age is 50 years. The disease occurs in all races and in children.[12] The two most common presentations are: (1) the insidious and slowly progressive development of the sicca complex in a patient with chronic RA; and (2) the more rapid development of a severe oral and ocular dryness, often accompanied by episodic parotitis, in an otherwise well patient.[27,38,53]

About 50% of patients with keratoconjunctivitis sicca have additional features of Sjögren's syndrome.[44] The most common ocular complaint is a sensation, described as "gritty" or "sandy," of a foreign body in the eye. Other symptoms include burning, accumulation of thick, ropy strands at the inner canthus, particularly on awakening, decreased tearing, redness, photosensitivity, eye fatigue, itching, and a "filmy" sensation that interferes with vision. Patients complain of eye discomfort and difficulty in reading or in watching television. Inability to cry is not a common complaint. Lacrimal gland enlargement occurs infrequently. Ocular complications include corneal ul-

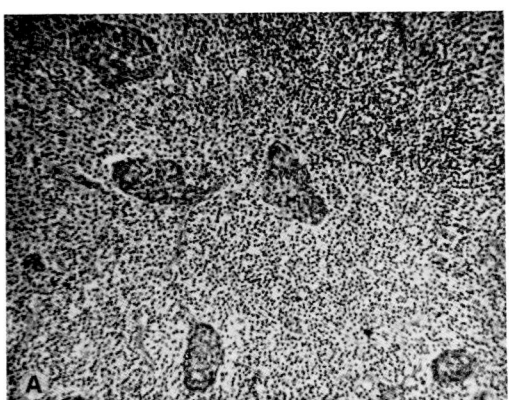

Fig. 67–1. Extensive lymphoid proliferation and formation of epimyoepithelial islets in the parotid gland of a patient with Sjögren's syndrome. (From Bloch, K.J.[10])

ceration, vascularization, or opacification, followed rarely by perforation.

The distressing manifestations of salivary insufficiency include the following: (1) difficulty with chewing, swallowing, and phonation; (2) adherence of food to buccal surfaces; (3) abnormalities of taste or smell; (4) fissures of the tongue, buccal membranes, and lips, particularly at the corners of the mouth; (5) frequent ingestion of liquids, especially at meal times; (6) and rampant dental caries. Patients are unable to swallow a dry cracker or toast without ingesting fluids and express displeasure at the suggestion. They may carry bottles of water or other lubricants with them, and they may awake at night for sips of water. The dentist may notice that fillings are loosening.

Dryness may also involve the nose, the posterior pharynx, the larynx, and the tracheobronchial tree and may lead to epistaxis, hoarseness, recurrent otitis media, bronchitis, or pneumonia.

Half these patients have parotid gland enlargement (Fig. 67–2), often recurrent and symmetric and sometimes accompanied by fever, tenderness, or erythema. Superimposed infection is rare. Rapid fluctuations in gland size are not unusual. A particularly hard or nodular gland may suggest a neoplasm.

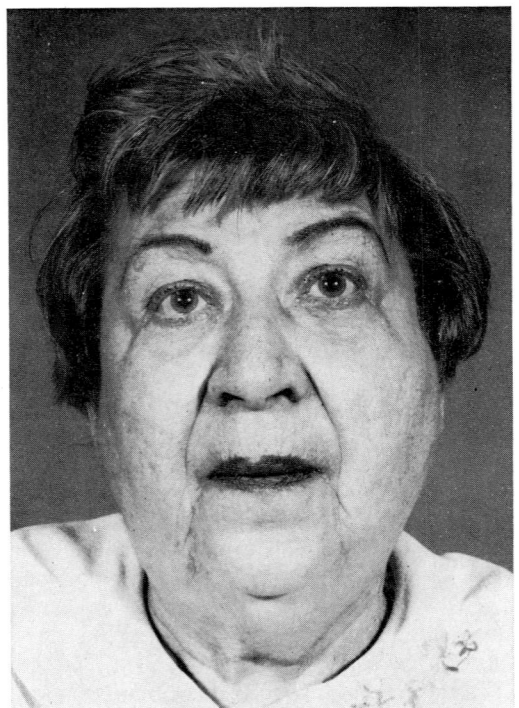

Fig. 67–2. Bilateral parotid gland enlargement in a patient with severe xerostomia and Sjögren's syndrome.

The arthritis of Sjögren's syndrome resembles classic RA in its clinical, pathologic, and roentgenographic features. Keratoconjunctivitis sicca develops in 10 to 15% of patients with RA. Arthralgias and morning stiffness without joint deformity may occur in patients with the sicca complex. Fluctuations in the course of the arthritis are not accompanied by parallel alterations in the symptoms of the sicca complex. Splenomegaly and leukopenia suggestive of Felty's syndrome, and vasculitis with leg ulcers and peripheral neuropathy, may appear even in the absence of RA. Raynaud's phenomenon occurs in 20% of patients.

Skin or vaginal dryness and allergic drug eruptions are frequent. Episodic lower-extremity purpura, sometimes preceded by itching or other prodromal signs, may be the presenting complaint. Glomerulonephritis develops rarely and should suggest either coexisting SLE or mixed (IgM-IgG) cryoglobulinemia. Overt or latent abnormalities of the renal tubules, such as in diabetes insipidus, renal tubular acidosis, and Fanconi's syndrome, occur with greater frequency.[33,40,52] A variety of pulmonary disorders may be present.[16,47]

Severe proximal muscle weakness and, rarely, tenderness may be early symptoms, leading to a diagnosis of polymyositis.[10] Weakness may also be associated with electrolyte imbalance, nephrocalcinosis, and the clinical findings of renal tubular acidosis. Peripheral or cranial neuropathy may cause symptoms of dysesthesia or paresthesia. Facial pain and numbness can accompany trigeminal neuropathy[21] and may contribute to the oral discomfort caused by the dryness. Focal or diffuse brain disease and spinal cord abnormalities have recently been reported.[5]

Although chronic thyroiditis of the Hashimoto type is present in 5% of patients, clinical hypothyroidism is rare. Sjögren's syndrome was found in 52% of patients with primary biliary cirrhosis and in 35% of patients with active chronic hepatitis.[19] Gastric achlorhydria, acute pancreatitis, and adult celiac disease have been reported in Sjögren's syndrome. Cervical or other lymph node enlargement may be the first indication of malignant lymphoma or pseudolymphoma (Fig. 67–3).

Physical Findings

The extreme picture of an elderly woman with joint deformities, reddened eyes, and parotid gland enlargement should immediately suggest the diagnosis. In many instances, however, findings are less obvious. The parotid glands may have any consistency, but are usually firm and nontender. Several bilateral parotid swellings may give rise to the so-called "chipmunk facies."

Gross inspection of the eyes may reveal nothing

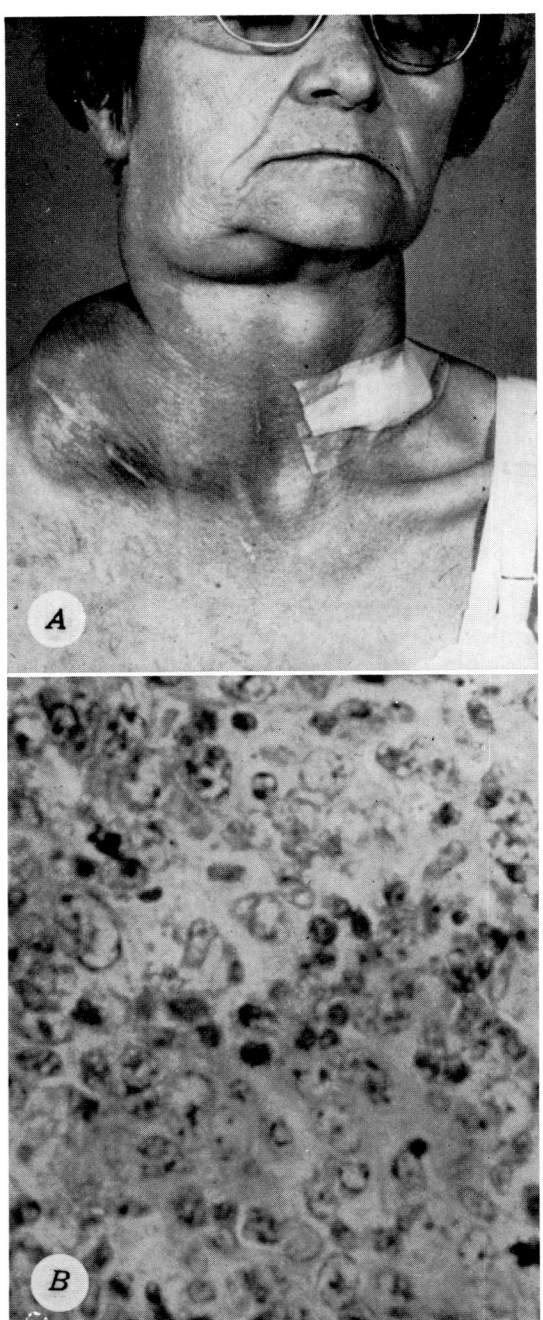

Fig. 67–3. *A,* Several hard, matted lymph nodes are present in the neck and submandibular region in this patient with Sjögren's syndrome of 20 years' duration. She has had intermittent, cervical lymphadenopathy for the last 6 years, with histologic diagnosis of pseudolymphoma made on 4 occasions. *B,* On biopsy, many abnormal reticulum cells with large nuclei and prominent nucleoli are found. The diagnosis is reticulum cell sarcoma. (Courtesy of Pediatric Clinics of North America.)

abnormal, a mucous thread, or conjunctival congestion. Lacrimal enlargement may not be apparent even when these glands are involved. The Schirmer test, in which a strip of Whatman No. 41 filter paper is folded and placed in the lower conjunctival sac, is a simple but crude measure of tear formation. Five minutes later, the moistened portion normally measures 15 mm or more. Most patients with Sjögren's syndrome moisten less than 5 mm of the test paper. More reliable diagnostic signs are obtained with rose bengal or fluorescein dye and biomicroscopic examination. Normally, no stain is visible a few minutes after dye instillation. Grossly visible or microscopic staining of the bulbar conjunctiva or cornea indicates the presence of small, superficial erosions. Biomicroscopic study may reveal increased amounts of corneal debris and attached filaments of corneal epithelium (filamentary keratitis).

The tongue and mucous membranes are characteristically dry, red, and "parchment-like." The lips may be dry and cracked. The tongue depressor adheres to oral surfaces, and the normal pool of saliva in the sublingual vestibule, visible when the tongue is elevated, is not present. A residual brownish pigmentation over the shins suggests past episodes of purpura (Fig. 67–4). Cervical or other lymph node enlargement may be the first indication of malignant lymphoma or pseudolymphoma. Splenomegaly occurs in 25% of patients.[51]

Laboratory Findings

Parotid salivary flow rates can be measured by means of Carlson-Crittenden cups placed over the orifices of the parotid ducts and secured by suction. Flow is stimulated by placing lemon juice on the tongue. Parotid secretion depends on age, sex, and other factors. Normal stimulated parotid flow rate should be about 0.5 to 1.0 ml/min/gland. Flow rates are reduced or unobtainable in Sjögren's syndrome.

Two techniques can be employed for visualization of the salivary glands. Secretory sialography is performed by introducing a radiopaque contrast medium through a small polyethylene catheter inserted into the orifice of the parotid duct.[10] Following injection of 0.5 to 1.0 ml contrast material, the catheter is plugged and radiographs are made (injection phase). The catheter is then removed, and emptying is encouraged by stimulation with lemon juice. Five minutes later, films are again taken (secretory phase). A normal sialogram shows fine arborization of parotid ductules with little retention of contrast medium. In patients with Sjögren's syndrome, one sees gross distortion of the normal pattern with marked retention. The sialectasis may appear punctate, globular, or cavitary (Fig. 67–5).

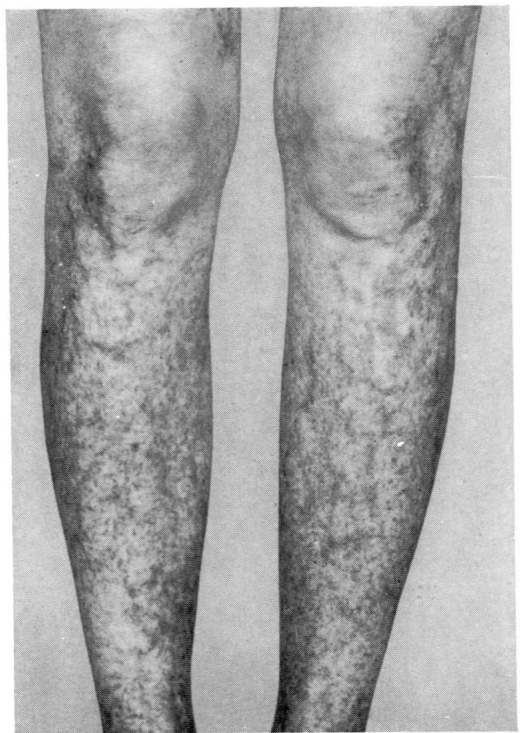

Fig. 67–4. Characteristic appearance of the legs of a patient with Sjögren's syndrome and intermittent, dependent, nonthrombocytopenic purpura.

This procedure is performed less frequently now than in the past.

The second method, developed more recently, depends on the uptake, concentration, and excretion of the radionuclide [99m]technetium (^{99m}Tc)-pertechnetate by the salivary gland. Patients are studied by sequential salivary scintigraphy in which the gland image is recorded visually on a gamma scintillation camera over a 60- to 80-minute period. Both uptake and release of radionuclide can be measured. The majority of patients have decreased glandular function.[37] The scintigraphic findings parallel the degree of xerostomia, the salivary flow rate determinations, and the results of secretory sialography (Fig. 67–6).

Involvement of minor salivary glands in the lower lip has made possible lower lip biopsies and histologic confirmation of the diagnosis in many patients. The procedure is performed, under local anesthesia, with the patient seated in a dental chair. The specimen is best obtained with a scalpel. An elliptic incision made in the labial mucosa parallels the vermilion border. Patients generally experience discomfort for 24 to 48 hours; approximately 1% complain of more persistent, localized numbness.

Lymphocytic infiltration can be measured by means of the focus-scoring method, in which the number of foci, defined as 50 or more round cells per 4 mm^2 of sectioned tissue, is determined on the biopsy specimen.[20] A focus score greater than 1 is a better criterion for the oral component of the syndrome than is the subjective evaluation of xerostomia.[15] The infiltrating cells synthesize large amounts of immunoglobulin and macroglobulin[50] and contain both T- and B-lymphocytes.[1,49] Although the diagnosis can often be made on the basis of clinical criteria alone, the complete evaluation of a patient should include a lip biopsy.

A mild normocytic, normochromic anemia occurs in about 25% of patients, leukopenia in 30%, eosinophilia (above 6% eosinophils) in 25%, and an elevated erythrocyte sedimentation rate (greater than 30 mm/hour by the Westergren method) in over 90%.

Half the patients have hypergammaglobulinemia, which is generally a diffuse elevation of all immunoglobulin classes. The most hyperglobulinemic patients may not have RA, but rather polymyopathy, purpura, or renal tubular acidosis. Monoclonal IgM may be seen. Cryoglobulinemia, often of the mixed IgM-IgG type, may be present, particularly in patients with glomerulonephritis or pseudolymphoma. Hyperviscosity associated with IgG rheumatoid factor[3] and intermediate complexes[9] have been reported. Some patients with lymphoma have hypogammaglobulinemia. A mild hypoalbuminemia is common.

Rheumatoid factor is detected in over 90% of sera when pooled human F II gamma globulin is used as antigen and in 75% when rabbit gamma globulin is employed. Thus, many patients who do not have RA have rheumatoid factor. Rheumatoid factor may disappear or may diminish in titer when lymphoma develops.[8]

The LE cell phenomenon occurs in 20% of patients who also have RA. This phenomenon is otherwise rare, unless SLE is also present.

Antinuclear factors, giving a homogeneous or speckled pattern of immunofluorescence, are seen in about 70% of patients.[10] Antibodies to native DNA are occasionally present in low titer. An antibody specific for salivary duct epithelium has been observed by indirect immunofluorescence in 50% of patients.[24] Thyroglobulin antibodies, detected by hemagglutination, are present in about 35% of patients.

The presence of multiple serum autoantibodies is a characteristic feature of Sjögren's syndrome. Rheumatoid factor and antinuclear factor, giving a homogeneous or speckled pattern of immunofluorescence, are seen in the majority of patients. An autoantibody to a nucleoprotein antigen called SS-

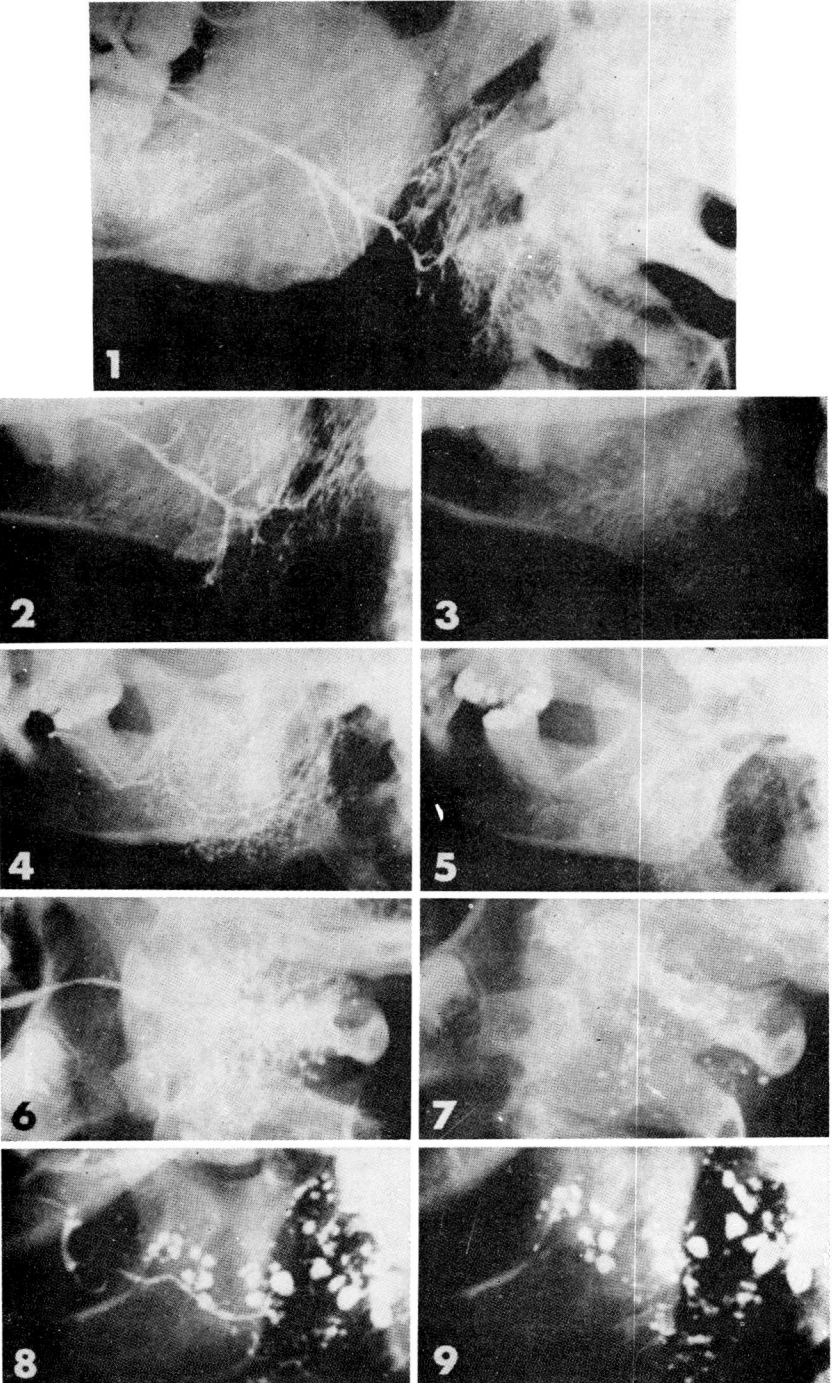

Fig. 67–5. Appearance of secretory sialography in normal individuals and in patients with Sjögren's syndrome. *1,* Injection phase, normal pattern. *2,* Injection phase, punctate sialectasis. *3,* Secretory phase, punctate sialectasis. *4,* Injection phase, punctate sialectasis with intermediate duct involvement. *5,* Secretory phase, punctate sialectasis with intermediate duct invovement. *6,* Injection phase, globular sialectasis. *7,* Secretory phase, globular sialectasis. *8,* Injection phase, cavitary and destructive sialectasis. *9,* Secretory phase, cavitary and destructive sialectasis. (From Bloch, K.J.[10])

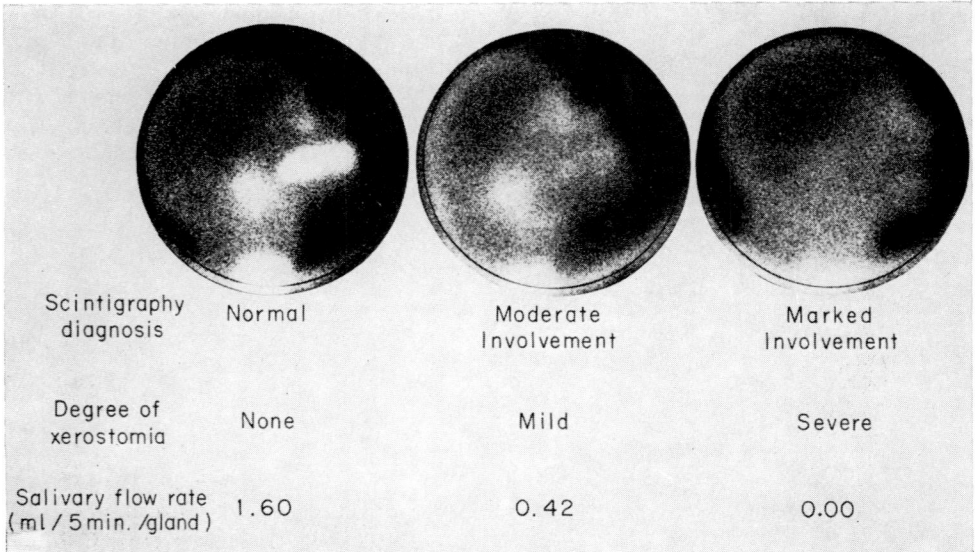

Scintigraphy diagnosis	Normal	Moderate Involvement	Marked Involvement
Degree of xerostomia	None	Mild	Severe
Salivary flow rate (ml / 5 min. /gland)	1.60	0.42	0.00

Fig. 67–6. Comparative studies of salivary function in Sjögren's syndrome illustrating the results achieved with scintigraphy employing [99m]technetium (pertechnetate).

B, also termed La, occurs in approximately 50 to 70% of patients with primary Sjögren's syndrome and to a lesser extent in Sjögren's syndrome accompanied by SLE.[6,26] Antibodies to a related nucleoprotein SS-A, also termed Ro, are less specific for Sjögren's syndrome; also they occur in patients with SLE and are associated with vasculitis.[4] An antibody, rheumatoid arthritis precipitin (RAP), to an Epstein-Barr virus-related nuclear antigen, rheumatoid arthritis nuclear antigen (RANA), occurs in secondary Sjögren's syndrome with RA. Levels of circulating immune complexes are increased, and reticuloendothelial clearance is defective in Sjögren's syndrome.[34]

Peripheral blood T-lymphocytes are decreased in about one-third of patients. The number of immunoglobulin-positive lymphocytes in peripheral blood may be increased. Abnormalities in T-cell function may be present, particularly in patients with lymphoproliferative or other systemic features. These patients often have alterations in T-cell subsets and decreased autologous mixed-lymphocyte responses.[31] NK cell activity is also diminished as a consequence of immunoregulatory abnormalities rather than intrinsic deficits.[30]

An increase in salivary β_2-microglobulin concentration correlates with the degree of lymphocytic infiltration found on labial biopsy. Serum β_2-microglobulin levels can be increased, particularly in patients with associated renal or lymphoproliferative complications.[28]

Lymphoma and Macroglobulinemia

As already indicated, lymphoid infiltration is a prominent feature of Sjögren's syndrome. In some

patients, lymphoproliferation is not benignly confined to glandular tissue, but becomes more generalized to involve regional lymph nodes or distant sites such as lung, kidney, spleen, bone marrow, muscle, or liver, as well as distant lymph nodes. When such "extraglandular" lymphoproliferation occurs, diagnosis is often difficult, and clinically and histologically the disease may simulate frankly malignant lymphoproliferative disorders such as Waldenström's macroglobulinemia or non-Hodgkin's lymphoma. Because the subsequent clinical course is frequently that of lymphoma, ending fatally, the early recognition of extraglandular lymphoproliferation in Sjögren's syndrome and the prompt institution of appropriate therapy are important.

In most patients, significant lymphoproliferation remains confined to salivary and lacrimal tissue and has a chronic, benign course of stable or progressive xerostomia and xerophthalmia. In some patients, however, after even 15 years or more of benign disease, evidence suggests the extension of lymphoproliferation to extraglandular sites. Persistent or massive parotid gland enlargement may also suggest lymphoma.

The extraglandular lymphoid infiltrates are of two general types. They may be highly pleomorphic and include small and large lymphocytes, plasma cells, and large reticulum cells. In a lymph node, the cells may distort the normal architecture and may extend beyond the capsule; the distinction between benign and malignant lesions is thereby made difficult. The term "pseudolymphoma" has been applied when the lesions show tumor-like aggregates of lymphoid cells, but do not meet histologic criteria for malignant disorders (Fig. 67–7). PAS-positive intranuclear inclusions and macroglobulins may be present, as in Waldenström's macroglobulinemia.[51]

In pseudolymphoma, the site of extraglandular lymphoproliferation determines the clinical presentation. Lymph nodes near salivary glands may be hyperplastic, and striking regional lymphadenopathy may be the predominant clinical feature. On the other hand, lymphoid infiltration may be

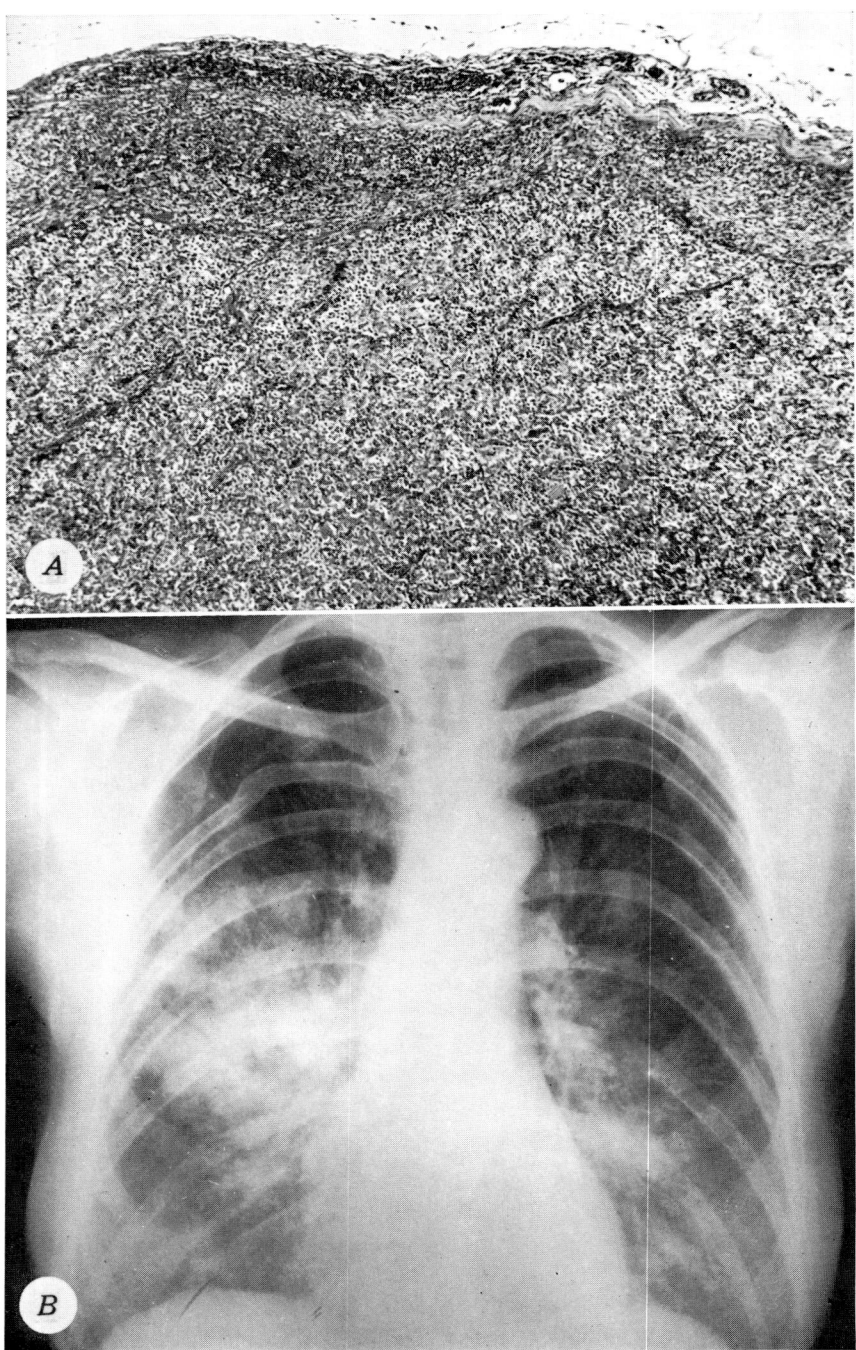

Fig. 67–7.   Pseudolymphoma can distort the normal lymph node architecture with penetration of cells through the capusle *(A)*, or it may appear as pulmonary infiltrates in chest radiogram *(B)*. (From Bloch, K.L.[10])

selectively excessive in a distant organ such as kidney or lung. These organs may become functionally impaired, giving rise to renal abnormalities or pulmonary insufficiency. Renal tubular acidosis may occur through such a mechanism.

Features that should alert the clinician to the possibility of extraglandular lymphoproliferation in a patient with Sjögren's syndrome are regional or generalized lymphadenopathy, hepatosplenomegaly, pulmonary infiltrates, renal insufficiency, purpura, leukopenia, hypergammaglobulinemia, and elevated serum β-2-microglobulin levels.[8,51] Vasculitis may be present, but arthritis is rare in such patients. The entity of pseudolymphoma cannot be clearly defined, but it occupies the middle portion of the spectrum of lymphoproliferation, merging with benign disease, such as hypergammaglobulinemic purpura, on the one end and frankly malignant disease, such as Waldenström's macroglobulinemia, on the other.

The other type of extraglandular lymphoid infiltrate is histologically malignant and enables one to make the specific diagnosis of lymphoproliferative neoplasm. These lesions may also appear after several years of apparently benign disease; they may or may not be preceded by pseudolymphoma, and they are often resistant to therapy. Although the histologic diagnosis may vary, the lymphoma belongs to the B-cell lineage and often contains intracellular IgMκ.[54]

A low IgM level may herald the presence or development of malignant lymphoproliferation and is a sign of a poor prognosis. A fall in the serum IgM level is often accompanied by a reduction in the rheumatoid factor titer and may precede the onset of generalized hypogammaglobulinemia.

Diagnosis

Clinically, a "sicca-like" syndrome may be caused by a number of other disease processes, including hyperlipoproteinemias IV and V, hemochromatosis, sarcoidosis, and amyloidosis.[45] The use of anticholinergic drugs as well as a number of other medications may cause xerostomia. Thus, it is essential to establish the presence of focal lymphoid infiltrates and autoimmunity in a patient suspected of having Sjögren's syndrome. The diagnosis, which should be suspected in any patient with RA, can be made when any two of the three major clinical features, that is, keratoconjunctivitis sicca, xerostomia, and RA, are present. Other connective tissue diseases such as scleroderma,[39] SLE,[43] and polymyositis, may substitute for RA in this definition. Generally, the arthritis precedes or is concurrent with the sicca complex.

Many patients have symptoms of oral or ocular dryness, but without an underlying connective tis-

sue disease. Such patients would appear to have primary Sjögren's syndrome. If arthritis does not develop within the first 12 months of the sicca complex, the chances are only 10% that it will appear later.

As with many diseases, obtaining the patient's medical history is the important first step in making the diagnosis of Sjögren's syndrome. Many patients, on casual questioning, reply that their mouths feel dry. More significant is the requirement for frequent fluids during the course of the day or the admission that they awake at night because of oral dryness. The dramatic negative response to the thought of ingesting a dry cracker is a helpful clue. Patients should be asked to describe their ocular complaints. They often use the expression "gritty" or "sandy" to characterize the discomfort of xerophthalmia.

Objective evidence of salivary or lacrimal gland insufficiency should be sought in any patient with a history suggestive of this syndrome. Such evidence includes a careful ophthalmologic examination with a biomicroscopic examination, measurement of salivary flow, and a labial salivary gland biopsy.

The varied clinical presentation and the multisystemic nature of Sjögren's syndrome may make the diagnosis obscure. As indicated in Table 67–1, the disease may become manifest in several different ways. Unilateral or asymmetric glandular enlargement may suggest a possible tumor. From 20 to 30% of patients with hyperglobulinemic purpura have other features of Sjögren's syndrome.[46] The initial symptoms may be related to a renal tubular disorder such as renal gravel or calculi, or they may suggest a severe degenerative or inflammatory muscle disease. Peripheral neuropathy may be a prominent feature, and trigeminal nerve involvement can cause facial discomfort. The disease may appear initially as chronic active hepatitis or biliary cirrhosis. Pulmonary disease may be related to dryness and infection or to lymphoid infiltration

Table 67–1. Clinical Presentation of Sjögren's Syndrome

1. Sicca complex—dry eyes and dry mouth
2. Rheumatoid arthritis—or other connective tissue disease
3. Salivary gland enlargement
4. Purpura—nonthrombocytopenic; hyperglobulinemic
5. Renal tubular acidosis—or other tubular disorder
6. Polymyopathy
7. Neuropathy—trigeminal
8. Chronic liver disease
9. Chronic pulmonary disease
10. Lymphoma—local or generalized
11. Immunoglobulin disorder—cryoglobulinemia; macroglobulinemia

of the lung. Malignant lymphoma or an immunoglobulin disorder is common.

Treatment

Most often, Sjögren's syndrome is a benign disease. Conservative management is therefore the best guide to therapy.

The sicca complex is treated with fluid replacement as often as necessary. Several readily available ophthalmic preparations, such as Tearisol, Liquifilm, and 0.5% methylcellulose, adequately replace the deficient tears. In severe situations, patients instill these drops as often as every half-hour to 1 hour. If corneal ulceration is present, patching of the eye and application of boric acid ointment may be necessary. Soft contact lenses are sometimes used to protect the cornea. Plastic-wrap occlusion or diving goggles may prevent tear evaporation at night. Topical corticosteroids are generally avoided unless specifically indicated because of the risk of corneal thinning and subsequent perforation. Diuretics, some antihypertensive drugs, and antidepressants may further diminish lacrimal and salivary gland function.

It is more difficult to compensate for the salivary insufficiency. Various saliva substitutes have not proved useful. Bromhexine, a mucolytic agent, has recently been used abroad.[25] The frequest ingestion of fluids, particularly with meals, is often the best treatment. Patients should see their dentists every four months and should pay scrupulous attention to proper oral hygiene. The careful use of a mouth-rinsing apparatus after eating may reduce the incidence of caries. Patients should avoid a high sucrose intake or the frequent ingestion of sugar-containing candies to decrease oral dryness. Vigorous dental plaque control and topical application of fluoride should be routine. Oral candidiasis may be treated with nystatin tablets for a prolonged course, with separate treatment of dentures.

Proper humidification of the home environment is helpful in reducing respiratory infections and other complications of the sicca complex. Patients should be encouraged to live with their disability. They require sympathetic understanding.

The management of RA or other associated disorders is not altered by the presence of Sjögren's syndrome. No controlled studies evaluating the efficacy of corticosteroids or immunosuppressive drugs in the treatment of the sicca complex have been reported. In view of the benign nature of this problem and the potential hazards of these agents, such therapy does not seem justified.

On the other hand, corticosteroids or immunosuppressive drugs seem indicated in the treatment of pseudolymphoma, particularly when the patient has renal or pulmonary involvement. Cyclophosphamide, at doses 75 to 100 mg daily, has diminished extraglandular lymphoid infiltrates and has restored salivary gland function in some patients.[7]

Malignant lymphoma should be treated with intensive chemotherapy, surgery, or radiotherapy as indicated by the location and extent of disease. These malignant and often fatal lesions require rapid and skilled intervention.

CONNECTIVE TISSUE DISEASE ASSOCIATED WITH OTHER IMMUNOLOGIC DISORDERS

Hypogammaglobulinemia

The functions of the immune system can be divided between those dependent on the secretion of antibody by plasma cells and those dependent on an intact thymus and specifically sensitized lymphocytes. One or both of these two functional systems, humoral and cellular immunity, respectively, may be defective in a variety of different immunodeficiency syndromes described in recent years.

A deficiency of humoral immunity results in a failure to produce specific antibody, a severe depression of serum gamma globulin concentration, and the absence of germinal center formation in lymph nodes and spleen. Five immunologically and structurally distinct classes of gamma globulin are known: IgG, IgM, IgA, IgD, and IgE. All immunoglobulin classes may be depressed simultaneously, or selective deficiencies may be present with normal or elevated levels of the remaining classes. The term "dysgammaglobulinemia" has been applied to describe the latter condition.

Hypogammaglobulinemia may be congenital or acquired. Congenital hypogammaglobulinemia is a sex-linked recessive disease usually heralded by recurrent pyogenic infections after the age of 6 months. Cellular immunity is generally intact, the level of IgG is usually less than 0.2 g/dl, and the other Ig classes are absent. These patients lack circulating B cells and tissue plasma cells.

Acquired hypogammaglobulinemia, also termed the common, variable-onset form, occurs in both sexes, often becomes symptomatic between the ages of 15 and 35 years, and is frequently associated with autoimmunity,[2] as well as with pyogenic infection. Cellular immunity can be defective, and thymomas may occur. Circulating B-lymphocytes are generally normal in number, but have a diminished ability to synthesize and to secrete immunoglobulin. Suppressor-T-cell function may be excessive.[39]

Selective IgA deficiency, the most common immunodeficiency disorder, appears to predispose persons to a variety of diseases. The incidence of IgA deficiency in the normal population varies between 1:800 and 1:600. The cause is unknown, but an arrest in B-cell maturation has been suggested. The other immunoglobulins are either normal or increased.

In addition to an enhanced susceptibility to bacterial and other infections, both congenital and acquired hypogammaglobulinemia may be accompanied by watery diarrhea and malabsorption producing a sprue-like syndrome, a chronic polyarthritis resembling RA, or other connective tissue or lymphoproliferative diseases. Frequently, the malabsorption is associated with infestation by *Giardia lamblia*.

Clinical and Diagnostic Features

The chronic polyarthritis associated with hypogammaglobulinemia often starts in the knees and then involves the ankles, wrists, and fingers.[19,27,41] Pain is infrequent, but joint effusion is common. Subcutaneous nodules are rare.[7] The incidence of arthritis in patients with hypogammaglubulinemia varies between 8 and 29%.[19,27]

Many characteristic features of RA, such as morning stiffness and symmetric joint swelling, are present in these patients. Radiograms show demineralization of the bones and narrowing of the joint spaces. Erosions are rare, and extensive joint destruction has not been reported. Rheumatoid factor is absent from the serum.

Synovial biopsies may show lymphocytic infiltration, but no B-lymphocytes or plasma cells are found.[1] An excessive suppressor-T-cell function has been reported in the synovium.[14] Other patients, however, may have chronic synovitis without these features.[21] The original suggestion that relatives of patients had a high incidence of RA[19] and hypergammaglobulinemia[7] has not been substantiated.[27]

In addition to polyarthritis, other disorders that may be associated with hypogammaglobulinemia include scleroderma,[37] SLE, dermatomyositis,[26] idiopathic thrombocytopenic purpura, Sjögren's syndrome,[22] hemolytic anemia, and pernicious anemia. Patients with the acquired form of this disorder may have marked lymphadenopathy and splenomegaly and, occasionally, autoantibodies associated with SLE or hemolytic anemia. Intestinal lymphoid nodular hyperplasia may accompany the malabsorption.[22] Lymphoreticular malignant tumors and thymomas have been reported. Two patients developed panhypogammaglobulinemia during the course of SLE.[4]

Some patients have a selective IgA deficiency associated with autoimmune disease or with serologic abnormalities suggestive of autoimmunity. Recurrent sinopulmonary infections are common in these patients. Allergies, ataxia-telangiectasia,

gastrointestinal tract disease, and malignant tumor may be present. Immunologic abnormalities include increased serum IgA and IgM concentrations, serum 7S IgM, abnormal κ-to-λ ratios, and antibodies reacting with IgG, IgA, milk, bovine proteins, and human tissue antigens.[3] The clinical presentations associated with selective IgA deficiency include RA,[13,24] SLE,[6,23] Sjögren's syndrome,[15,23] dermatomyositis, pernicious anemia, chronic active hepatitis, Coombs-positive hemolytic anemia, and thyroiditis. Cellular immunity is generally normal in this condition. Selective IgA deficiency occurs in approximately 4% of patients with SLE or juvenile RA (JRA).

Quantitative immunoglobulin determinations are essential for diagnosis. Immunoglobulin concentrations may be higher in the acquired form, but are still depressed. Isohemagglutinins either are absent or are present in low titers (1:10). A failure to make an antibody response to a specific antigenic challenge may help to establish the diagnosis if immunoglobulin levels are on the borderline. Live attenuated vaccines should not be used for immunization.

Abnormalities of cellular immunity may be seen, including absent delayed-hypersensitivity skin-test reactions, depressed responses to mitogenic stimulation, and decreased numbers of rosette-forming T-lymphocytes.[17]

Serum and secretory IgA may be selectively absent in IgA-deficient patients. Some subjects may have normal secretory IgA or increased amounts of serum and secretory 7S IgM.

Treatment

Commercial gamma globulin is given at regular intervals, starting at doses of 0.2 ml/kg and increasing progressively. The arthritis associated with hypogammaglobulinemia usually responds promptly to this treatment.[7,41] Anaphylactoid reactions to gamma globulin have been noted. Fresh frozen plasma may also be used. Patients with selective IgA deficiency should not be given gamma globulin because they may react to the foreign IgA and may develop anaphylactoid transfusion reactions.

Etiologic Factors

The immunologic events occurring locally in the synovium and joint space in these patients may be similar to those in typical RA, despite the hypogammaglobulinemia and impaired ability to produce specific antibody or rheumatoid factor.

The pathogenesis of the autoimmune and connective tissue diseases probably depends on genetic, immunologic, and viral factors. The immunologic deficiency present in these patients predisposes them to pyogenic respiratory tract infections and to unexplained diarrhea and malabsorption, as well as to autoimmunity. Perhaps their altered immune status renders them more susceptible to disorders induced by unusual pathogens such as latent viruses. The peculiar susceptibility of patients with selective IgA deficiency supports this concept. IgA, the major secretory immunoglobulin, may play an important host-defense role in the respiratory and gastrointestinal tract. Deficiency of IgA in these critical areas may permit the entry and establishment of foreign pathogens that induce antigenic alterations and contribute to the development of autoimmunity.

Knowledge of the role of suppressor cells in preventing normal B-cell maturation may help us to understand the cause of this disorder and may allow more specific immunotherapy.

Hyperglobulinemic Purpura

Clinical Features

This condition affects women predominantly and is characterized by hypergammaglobulinemia and episodes of purpura of the lower extremities. Described originally by Waldenström,[38] this disorder is not to be confused with another entity, Waldenström's macroglobulinemia. Patients often have no other associated illness, although myeloma,[33,34] arthritis, and Sjögren's syndrome may develop.[36] Prodromal symptoms such as burning or itching of the legs may precede the disorder by several hours and may announce the onset of another episode of purpura. A chronic brownish pigmentation of the skin often appears as the residue of these attacks.

Laboratory Findings

The erythrocyte sedimentation rate and gamma globulin concentration are elevated. Rheumatoid factor and antinuclear factor are frequently present in the serum.

Anti-gamma globulins of the IgG type are a feature of this disease and result in immune complexes with sedimentation properties intermediate between 7S and 19S immunoglobulins.[12] These "intermediate complexes" are formed by interactions of the IgG anti-IgG with itself and with other normal IgG molecules. The resulting pattern on serum paper electrophoresis is generally polydispersed, that is, polyclonal, but it may appear monoclonal. IgA complexes may also be involved, and the complexes may increase when the ambient temperature falls.[32]

Etiologic Factors

This disorder seems to occupy a middle ground between autoimmune and lymphoproliferative dis-

eases. It is distinguished immunologically from RA by the frequent presence of IgG rather than IgM rheumatoid factor, that is, anti-IgG antibody.

The exact relation of the hypergammaglobulinemia to the purpura is not understood. The circulating immune complexes become deposited in small blood vessels and give rise to vascular injury and extravasation of blood. The cooler skin temperature and orthostatic pressure changes may play a role in this process.

Cryoglobulinemia

Cryoglobulins are immunoglobulins with the physiochemical characteristic of precipitation in the cold followed by resolution on warming.

Three types of cryoglobulins have been defined,[8] as follows: (1) isolated monoclonal immunoglobulins produced by proliferating cells in Waldenström's macroglobulinemia or in multiple myeloma; (2) mixed cryoglobulins in which a monoclonal component, usually IgM, has antibody activity against polyclonal IgG; and (3) mixed polyclonal cryoglobulins, which are usually anti-immunoglobulin immune complexes, but may also contain other molecules such as $\beta1C$ or lipoprotein.

Cryoglobulins also occur in rheumatoid vasculitis,[42] cutaneous vasculitis,[16] and SLE.[43] They appear to represent circulating immune complexes and, in SLE, may contain antibodies to nucleoproteins and to lymphocyte antigens.

Clinical and Diagnostic Features

Cryoglobulins of either monoclonal or immune complex (mixed) nature may produce Raynaud's phenomenon, numbness, urticaria, vascular occlusions, tissue infarction, and digital ulcerations. Cutaneous and vasomotor symptoms are more severe in types 1 and 2 cryoglobulinemia. Types 2 and 3 are more often associated with renal and neurologic involvement, chronic vascular purpura, and Raynaud's phenomenon. Immunoproliferative disorders are associated with types 1 and 2, and autoimmunity with type 3.[8]

Mixed cryoglobulins may also be associated with a symptom complex, occurring predominantly in women, that includes arthralgias, purpura, especially involving the lower extremities, weakness, vasculitis, and diffuse glomerulonephritis.[29] Rheumatoid factor is present, and Sjögren's syndrome or thyroiditis may occur.

Forty patients with essential mixed cryoglobulins represented 32% of all cryoglobulinemic patients seen in an 18-year period.[20] Seventy percent had evidence of hepatic dysfunction, and 60% had serologic evidence of prior infection with hepatitis B virus. Many patients had severe renal disease with glomerular deposits of IgA, IgM, and complement. All cryoglobulins had rheumatoid factor activity. Renal involvement indicated a poor prognosis, and widespread vasculitis was frequently found during postmortem examination.

The laboratory finding that confirms the diagnosis is the cryoglobulin in the serum. It may require 24 to 48 hours in the cold to precipitate the cryoglobulin from serum. Anywhere from 20 to 60% of the mixed cryoprecipitate is IgM. It requires the presence of IgG to precipitate and behaves like an antibody to IgG. Cryoprecipitation occurs in the absence of complement, although complement may be associated with the complex, and serum complement levels are generally depressed. The IgM is a typical rheumatoid factor binding to the Fc portion of IgG. The IgM may be a monoclonal (Waldenström-type) paraprotein; mixed IgA-IgG cryoglobulinemia has also been reported.

One patient had mixed cryoglobulinemia, Sjögren's syndrome, and pulmonary lymphoid infiltrates, with an associated hypogammaglobulinemia and increased susceptibility to bacterial infection.[40] The IgM was monoclonal and reacted specifically with IgG subclasses 1, 2, and 4, but not with subclass 3. Serum concentrations of IgG 1, 2, and 4 were 10% of normal. These 3 subclasses also showed reduced synthesis and shortened survival times, whereas IgG 3 had a normal synthetic rate and survival time. The hypogammaglobulinemia was due in part to a rapid elimination of IgG through its interaction with the IgG-reactive monoclonal IgM.[40]

Hyperviscosity due to an IgM-IgG interaction has been reported in association with RA.[29]

Treatment

The treatment of mixed cryoglobulinemia has been reviewed.[28] Corticosteroids, immunosuppressive drugs, plasmaphoresis, penicillamine, and splenectomy have been employed with limited success.[31]

Etiologic Factors

The "mixed cryoglobulins" probably represent a special example of an immune-complex phenomenon with unusual physicochemical properties, both in vitro and in vivo. The cold precipitability in vitro makes it possible to identify, to isolate, and to characterize the individual components of the complex. The in vivo properties of the complex probably contribute to the findings of vascular insufficiency. The purpuric lesions may be caused by cryoprecipitation in the small skin capillaries, which reach a temperature (30° C) at which these aggregates are known to precipitate. The complexes may also induce glomerulonephritis and may be responsible for hypogammaglobulinemia with increased susceptibility to infection.

These cryoglobulins illustrate in an impressive way the dramatic pathologic consequences of immune-complex formation and deposition. They shed no light on the mechanism leading to their production, although their ready availability in serum may contribute to further investigation. If viral or tissue antigens are involved in the initial stages of production of these cryoglobulins, then the specificity of antibodies in the cryocomplex may conceivably be directed against such antigens.

Malignant Lymphoma

Enough published reports of this association of two rare conditions now exist that a mere coincidental relationship may not be the best explanation. A recent report notes an increased risk of lymphoma, leukemia, and multiple myeloma in patients with RA.[25] The association of Sjögren's syndrome with lymphoproliferation was discussed earlier in this chapter.

Patients with coexisting SLE and malignant lymphoma have been reported.[5,10,11,30,35] Four patients had Hodgkin's disease, two had lymphosarcoma, and one each had mixed-cell lymphoma, reticulum-cell sarcoma, and chronic lymphocytic leukemia. All but two died of the malignant disease. Two had hypogammaglobulinemia. One patient had hematoxylin bodies, onion-skin lesions in the spleen, and hypogammaglobulinemia with an increase in IgM. The IgM showed cryoprecipitability, was an anti-nuclear factor, and contained only λ light chains.[35]

The association of RA with monoclonal gammopathies is noteworthy. In a series of 16 patients with arthritis, 6 had multiple myeloma, 8 had asymptomatic monoclonal immunoglobulin "spike" on serum protein electrophoresis, and 1 each had Waldenström's macroglobulinemia or heavy-chain disease.[44] These patients had rheumatoid factor, and their arthritis antedated the development of the paraprotein by as much as 26 years. Such patients should be distinguished from those with multiple myeloma or Waldenström's macroglobulinemia in whom amyloid deposition or the bony lesions themselves can mimic RA.[9,18]

The connective tissue diseases may predispose patients to the subsequent development of lymphoid or plasma cell malignant disorders, possibly as a consequence of chronic viral infection or prolonged antigenic stimulation, perhaps coupled with impaired cellular immunity and immunologic surveillance.

REFERENCES

Sjögren's Syndrome

1. Adamson, T.C., III, et al.: Immunohistologic analysis of lymphoid infiltrates in primary Sjögren's syndrome using monoclonal antibodies. J. Immunol., 130:203–208, 1983.
2. Akizuki, M., Powers, R., and Holman, H.R.: A soluble acidic protein of the cell nucleus which reacts with serum from patients with systemic lupus erythematosus and Sjögren's syndrome. J. Clin. Invest., 59:264–272, 1977.
3. Alarcon-Segovia, D., et al.: Serum hyperviscosity in Sjögren's syndrome. Ann. Intern. Med., 80:35–43, 1974.
4. Alexander, E.L., et al.: Sjögren's syndrome: association of anti-Ro (SS-A) antibodies with vasculitis, hematologic abnormalities, and serologic hyperreactivity. Ann. Intern. Med., 98:155–159, 1983.
5. Alexander, E.L., et al.: Neurologic complications of primary Sjögren's syndrome. Medicine, 61:247–257, 1982.
6. Alspaugh, M.A., Talal, N., and Tan, E.M.: Differentiation and characterization of autoantibodies and their antigens in Sjögren's syndrome. Arthritis Rheum., 19:216–222, 1976.
7. Anderson, L.G., et al.: Salivary gland immunoglobulin and rheumatoid factor synthesis in Sjögren's syndrome. Am. J. Med., 53:456–463, 1972.
8. Anderson, L.G., and Talal, N.: The spectrum of benign to malignant lymphoproliferation in Sjögren's syndrome. Clin. Exp. Immunol., 10:199–221, 1972.
9. Blaylock, W.M., Waller, M., and Normansell, D.E.: Sjögren's syndrome: hyperviscosity and intermediate complexes. Ann. Intern. Med., 80:27–34, 1974.
10. Bloch, K.J., et al.: Sjögren's syndrome. A clinical, pathological, and serological study of sixty-two cases. Medicine, 44:187–231, 1965.
11. Chisholm, D.M., and Mason, D.K.: Labial salivary gland biopsy in Sjögren's syndrome. J. Clin. Pathol., 21:656–660, 1968.
12. Chudwin, D.S., et al.: Spectrum of Sjögren's syndrome in children. J. Pediatr., 98:213–217, 1981.
13. Chused, T.M., et al.: Sjögren's syndrome associated with HLA-Dw3. N. Engl. J. Med., 296:895–897, 1977.
14. Cruickshank, A.H.: Benign lymphoepithelial salivary lesion to be distinguished from adenolymphoma. J. Clin. Pathol., 18:391–400, 1965.
15. Daniels, T.E., et al.: The oral component of Sjögren's syndrome. Oral Surg., 39:875–885, 1975.
16. Fairfax, A.J., et al.: Pulmonary disorders associated with Sjögren's syndrome. J. Med., 199:279–295, 1981.
17. Fye, K.H., et al.: Association of Sjögren's syndrome with HLA-B8. Arthritis Rheum., 19:883–886, 1976.
18. Godwin, J.T.: Benign lymphoepithelial lesion of the parotid gland. Cancer, 5:1089–1103, 1952.
19. Golding, P.L., Smith, M., and Williams, R.: Multisystem involvement in chronic liver disease. Am. J. Med., 55:772–782, 1973.
20. Greenspan, J.S., et al.: The histopathology of Sjögren's syndrome in labial salivary gland biopsies. Oral Surg., 37:217–229, 1974.
21. Kaltreider, H.B., and Talal, N.: The neuropathy of Sjögren's syndrome. Ann. Intern. Med., 70:751–762, 1969.
22. Kessler, H.S.: A laboratory model for Sjögren's syndrome. Am. J. Pathol., 52:671–678, 1968.
23. Lukes, R.J., and Tindle, B.H.: Immunoblastic lymphadenopathy. N. Engl. J. Med., 292:1–8, 1975.
24. MacSween, R.N.M., et al.: Occurrence of antibody to salivary duct epithelium in Sjögren's syndrome, rheumatoid arthritis, and other arthritides. Ann. Rheum. Dis., 26:402–411, 1967.
25. Manthorpe, R., et al.: Sjögren's syndrome. A review with emphasis on immunological features. Allergy, 36:139–153, 1981.
26. Martinez-Lavin, M., Vaughan, J.H., and Tan, E.M.: Autoantibodies and the spectrum of Sjögren's syndrome. Ann. Intern. Med., 91:185–187, 1979.
27. Mason, A.M.S., Gumpel, J.M., and Golding, P.L.: Sjögren's syndrome—a clinical review. Semin. Arthritis Rheum., 2:301–331, 1973.
28. Michalski, J.P., et al.: Beta$_2$ microglobulin and lymphocytic infiltration in Sjögren's syndrome. N. Engl. J. Med., 293:1228–1237, 1975.
29. Mikulicz, J.: Concerning a peculiar symmetrical disease of the lacrymal and salivary glands. Medical Classics, 2:165–186, 1937.
30. Miyasaka, N., et al.: Natural killing activity in Sjögren's syndrome: An analysis of defective mechanisms. Arthritis Rheum., 26:954–960, 1983.
31. Miyasaka, N., et al.: Decreased autologous mixed lymphocyte reaction in Sjögren's syndrome. J. Clin. Invest., 66:928–933, 1980.
32. Morgan, W.S., and Castleman, B.: A clinicopathologic study of "Mikulicz's disease." Am. J. Pathol., 29:471–489, 1953.
33. Morris, R.C., and Fudenberg, H.H.: Impaired renal acidification in patients with hypergammaglobulinemia. Medicine, 46:57–69, 1967.
34. Moutsopoulos, H.M., et al.: Sjögren's syndrome (sicca syndrome): current issues. Ann. Intern. Med., 92:212–226, 1980.
35. Pierce, D.A.: Immunoblastic sarcoma with features of Sjögren's syndrome and systemic lupus erythematosus in a patient with immunoblastic lymphadenopathy. Arthritis Rheum., 22:911–916, 1979.
36. Roubinian, J.R., Papoian, R., and Talal, N.: Androgenic hormones modulate autoantibody responses and improve survival in murine lupus. J. Clin. Invest., 59:1066–1070, 1977.
37. Schall, G.L., et al.: Xerostomia in Sjögren's syndrome. JAMA, 216:2109–2116, 1971.
38. Shearn, M.A.: Major Problems in Internal Medicine. Vol. II. Edited by L.H. Smith. Philadelphia, W.B. Saunders, 1971.
39. Shearn, M.A.: Sjögren's syndrome in association with scleroderma. Ann. Intern. Med., 51:1352–1362, 1960.
40. Shearn, M.A., and Tu, W.H.: Latent renal tubular acidosis in Sjögren's syndrome. Ann. Rheum. Dis., 27:27–32, 1968.
41. Sjögren, H.: Histological examinations in keratoconjunctivitis sicca. Acta Ophthalmol., 11:1–2, 1933.
42. Smith, J.B., and Talal, N.: Significance of self-recognition and interleukin-2 for immunoregulation, autoimmunity and cancer. (Editorial.) Scand. J. Immunol., 16:269–278, 1982.
43. Steinberg, A.D., and Talal, N.: The coexistence of Sjögren's syndrome and systemic lupus erythematosus. Ann. Intern. Med., 74:55–61, 1971.
44. Stoltze, C.A., et al.: Keratoconjunctivitis sicca and Sjögren's syndrome. Arch. Intern. Med., 106:513–522, 1960.
45. Strand, V., and Talal, N.: Advances in the diagnosis and concept of Sjögren's syndrome (autoimmune exocrinopathy). Bull. Rheum. Dis., 30:1046–1052, 1980.
46. Strauss, W.G.: Purpura hyperglobulinemia of Waldenstrom. N. Engl. J. Med., 260:857–860, 1959.
47. Strimlan, V., et al.: Pulmonary manifestations of Sjögren's syndrome. Chest, 70:354–361, 1976.
48. Talal, N.: Sex hormones and modulation of immune response in SLE. Clin. Rheum. Dis., 8:23–28, 1982.
49. Talal, N., et al.: T and B lymphocytes in peripheral blood and tissue lesions in Sjögren's syndrome. J. Clin. Invest., 53:180–189, 1974.
50. Talal, N., Asofsky, R., and Lightbody, P.: Immunoglobulin synthesis by salivary gland lymphoid cells in Sjögren's syndrome. J. Clin. Invest., 49:49–62, 1970.
51. Talal, N., Sokoloff, L., and Barth, W.F.: Extrasalivary lymphoid abnormalities in Sjögren's syndrome (reticulum cell sarcoma, "pseudolymphoma," macroglobulinemia). Am. J. Med., 43:50–65, 1967.
52. Talal, N., Zisman, E., and Schur, P.H.: Renal tubular acidosis, glomerulonephritis and immunologic factors in Sjögren's syndrome. Arthritis Rheum., 11:774–786, 1968.
53. Whaley, K., et al.: Sjögren's syndrome. I. Sicca components. Q. J. Med., 42:279–304, 1973.
54. Zulman, J., Jaffe, R., and Talal, N.: Evidence that the malignant lymphoma of Sjögren's syndrome is a mono-

clonal B-cell neoplasm. N. Engl. J. Med., 229:1215–1220, 1978.

Connective Tissue Diseases Associated with Other Immunologic Disorders

1. Abrahamsen, T.G., et al.: Lymphocytes from synovial tissue of a boy with X-linked hypogammaglobulinemia and chronic polyarthritis. Arthritis Rheum., 22:71–78, 1979.
2. Ammann, A.J.: Immunodeficiency disorders and autoimmunity. In Autoimmunity: Genetic, Immunologic, Virologic, and Clinical Aspects. Edited by N. Talal. New York, Academic Press, 1977, pp. 479–508.
3. Ammann, A.J., and Hong, R.: Selective IgA deficiency: presentation of 30 cases and a review of the literature. Medicine, 50:223–238, 1971.
4. Ashman, R.F., et al.: Panhypogammaglobulinemia in systemic lupus erythematosus: in vitro demonstration of multiple cellular defects. J. Allergy Clin. Immunol., 70:465–473, 1982.
5. Agudelo, C.A., et al.: Non-Hodgkin's lymphoma in systemic lupus erythematosus. J. Rheumatol., 8:69–78, 1981.
6. Bachmann, R., Laurell, C.B., and Svenouius, E.: Studies on the serum $_{\gamma1A}$-globulin level. Scand. J. Clin. Lab. Invest., 17:46–50, 1965.
7. Barnett, E.V., Winkelstein, A., and Weinberger, H.J.: Agammaglobulinemia with polyarthritis and subcutaneous nodules. Am. J. Med., 48:40–47, 1970.
8. Brouet, J.C., et al.: Biologic and clinical significance of cryoglobulins. Am. J. Med., 57:775–788, 1974.
9. Calabro, J.J.: Cancer and arthritis. Arthritis Rheum., 10:553–567, 1967.
10. Cammarata, R.J., Rodman, G.P., and Jensen, W.N.: Systemic rheumatic disease and malignant lymphoma. Arch. Intern. Med., 111:330–337, 1963.
11. Canoso, J.J., and Cohen, A.S.: Malignancy in a series of 70 patients with systemic lupus erythematosus. Arthritis Rheum., 17:383–388, 1974.
12. Capra, J.D., Winchester, R.J., and Kunkel, H.G.: Hypergammaglobulinemic purpura. Medicine, 50:125–138, 1971.
13. Cassidy, J.T., Petty, R.E., and Sullivan, D.B.: J. Abnormalities in the distribution of serum immunoglobulin concentrations in juvenile rheumatoid arthritis. J. Clin. Invest., 52:1931–1936, 1973.
14. Chattopadhyay, J., Natvig, B., and Chattopadhyay, H.: Excessive suppressor T-cell activity of the rheumatoid synovial tissue in X-linked hypogammaglobulinaemia. Scand. J. Immunol., 11:455–459, 1980.
15. Claman, H.N., et al.: Isolated severe gamma A deficiency: immunoglobulin levels, clinical disorders, and chromosome studies. J. Lab. Clin. Med., 75:307–315, 1970.
16. Cream, J.J.: Clinical and immunological aspects of cutaneous vasculitis. Q. J. Med., 45:255–276, 1976.
17. Gajl-Peczalska, K.J., et al.: B and T lymphocytes in primary immunodeficiency disease in man. J. Clin. Invest., 52:919–928, 1973.
18. Goldberg, A., Brodksy, I., and McCarty, D.: Multiple myeloma with paramyloidosis presenting as rheumatoid disease. Am. J. Med., 37:653–658, 1964.
19. Good, R.A., and Rotstein, J.: Rheumatoid arthritis and agammaglobulinemia. Bull. Rheum. Dis., 10:203–206, 1960.
20. Gorevic, P.D., et al.: Mixed cryoglobulinemia: clinical aspects and long-term follow-up of 40 patients. Am. J. Med., 69:287–308, 1980.
21. Grayzel, A.I., et al.: Chronic polyarthritis associated with

hypogammaglobulinemia. Arthritis Rheum., 20:887–894, 1977.
22. Hermans, P.E., Diaz-Buzo, J.A., and Stobo, J.D.: Idiopathic late-onset immunoglobulin deficiency. Am. J. Med., 61:221–237, 1976.
23. Hobbs, J.R.: Immune imbalance in dysgammaglobulinemia type IV. Lancet, 1:110–114, 1968.
24. Huntley, C.C., et al.: Rheumatoid arthritis with IgA deficiency. Am. J. Dis. Child., 113:411–418, 1967.
25. Isomaki, H.A., Hakulinen, T., and Joutsenlahti, U.: Excess risk of lymphomas, leukemia and myeloma in patients with rheumatoid arthritis. J. Chronic Dis., 31:691–696, 1978.
26. Janeway, C.A., et al.: "Collagen disease" in patients with congenital agammaglobulinemia. Trans. Am. Assoc. Physicians, 69:93–97, 1956.
27. Lawrence, J.S., and Bremner, J.M.: Arthritis and hypogammaglobulinaemia. Scand. J. Rheumatol., 5:17–28, 1976.
28. Mathison, D.A., et al.: Purpura, arthralgia, and IgM-IgG cryoglobulinemia with rheumatoid factor activity. Ann. Intern. Med., 74:383–390, 1971.
29. Meltzer, M., et al.: Cryoglobulinemia—a clinical and laboratory study. Am. J. Med., 40:837–856, 1966.
30. Miller, D.G.: The association of immune disease and malignant lymphoma. Ann. Intern. Med., 66:507–521, 1967.
31. Ristow, S.C., et al.: Reversal of systemic manifestations of cryoglobulinemia. Arch. Intern. Med., 136:467–470, 1976.
32. Roberts-Thomson, P.J. and Kemp, A.S.: IgA and temperature dependent IgG complex formation in a patient with Waldenstrom's hypergammaglobulinaemic purpura. Clin. Exp. Immunol., 39:164–169, 1980.
33. Rogers, W.R., and Welch, J.D.: Purpura hyperglobulinemica terminating in multiple myeloma. Arch. Intern. Med., 100:478–483, 1957.
34. Savin, R.C.: Hyperglobulinemic purpura terminating in myeloma, hyperlipemia, and xanthomatosis. Arch. Dermatol., 92:679–686, 1965.
35. Smith, C.K., Cassidy, J.T., and Bole, G.G.: Type 1 dysgammaglobulinemia, systemic lupus erythematosus and lymphoma. Am. J. Med., 48:113–119, 1970.
36. Strauss, W.G.: Purpura hyperglobulinemia of Waldenstrom. N. Engl. J. Med., 260:857–860, 1959.
37. VanGelder, D.W.: Clinical significance of alterations in gamma globulin levels. South. Med. J., 50:43–50, 1957.
38. Waldenstrom, J.: Clinical methods for determination of hyperproteinemia and their practical value for diagnosis. Nord. Med., 20:2288–2295, 1943.
39. Waldmann, T.A., et al.: The role of suppressor cells in the pathogenesis of common variable hypogammaglobulinemia and the immunodeficiency associated with myeloma. Fed. Proc., 35:2067–2072, 1976.
40. Waldmann, T.A., Johnson, J.S., and Talal, N.: Hypogammaglobulinemia associated with accelerated catabolism of IgG secondary to its interaction with an IgG-reactive monoclonal IgM. J. Clin. Invest., 50:951–958, 1971.
41. Webster, A.D.B., et al.: Polyarthritis in adults with hypogammaglobulinaemia and its rapid response to immunoglobulin treatment. Br. Med. J., 1:1314–1316, 1976.
42. Weisman, M., and Zvaifler, N.: Cryoimmunoglobulinemia in rheumatoid arthritis. J. Clin. Invest., 56:725–739, 1975.
43. Winfield, J.B., Koffler, D., and Kunkel, H.G.: Specific concentration of polynucleotide immune complexes in the cryoprecipitates of patients with systemic lupus erythematosus. J. Clin. Invest., 56:563–570, 1975.
44. Zawadzki, Z.A., and Benedek, T.G.: Rheumatoid arthritis, dysproteinemic arthropathy, and paraproteinemia. Arthritis Rheum., 12:555–568, 1969.

Chapter **68**

Rheumatic Fever

Angelo Taranta

Once the most common cause of acute arthritis, rheumatic fever has become a rarity in industrialized countries in the West,[3,45,67] and physicians may complete their training without having seen a single case. Thus, when it does occur, rheumatic fever may be recognized late or not at all.[55] In other parts of the world, however, rheumatic fever continues to be a major health problem.[1,88,131] Several monographs are available on this subject,[79,117,131] as well as on streptococcal infections;[142,146] versions of this chapter in earlier editions of this book provide details omitted here.

CONCISE HISTORY AND GEOGRAPHY

The term "rheumatic fever" resulted from the fitting together of manifestations originally described independently of each other and thought to be unrelated: "acute articular rheumatism," valvular heart disease, and chorea (Fig. 68–1), in addition to subcutaneous nodules and erythema marginatum.[89a] In contrast to this process of synthesis, a number of entities have been recognized as mimics of rheumatic fever and have been separated from it[32] (Fig. 68–2).

While these conceptual changes took place, actual changes also occurred. Although records from the past are poor and details are lacking, the incidence of rheumatic fever seems to have increased with the industrialization and urbanization of a given society (Fig. 68–3) and decreased with subsequent affluence, a process completed in the industrialized West and still ongoing in the "developing" countries.[32,131]

Why these rises and falls? True believers claim the near disappearance of rheumatic fever in industrialized countries as another triumph of medicine; skeptics point out that although prevention is effective, the disease started to decline before the routine administration of preventive therapy. Economic determinists assign a leading role to "improved socioeconomic conditions," but skeptics again point out that conditions have worsened in the United States over the last dozen years, during which the incidence of rheumatic fever has declined dramatically.[45,67] A cumulative effect of many factors is probable[29] (Fig. 68–4).

In addition to becoming rarer, the disease has become milder in the industrialized Western world.

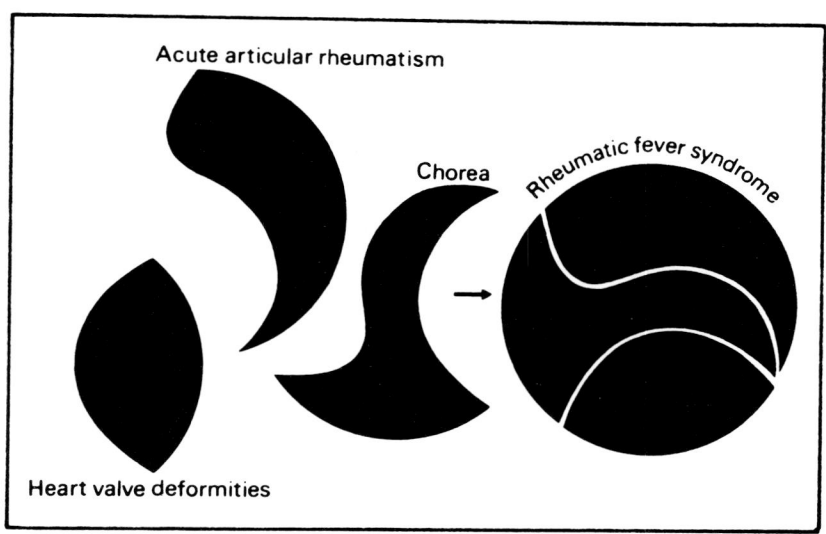

Fig. 68–1. Historical development of the concept of rheumatic fever syndrome from the fitting together of disease manifestations previously described independently of each other. (From Taranta, A., and Markowitz, M.[131])

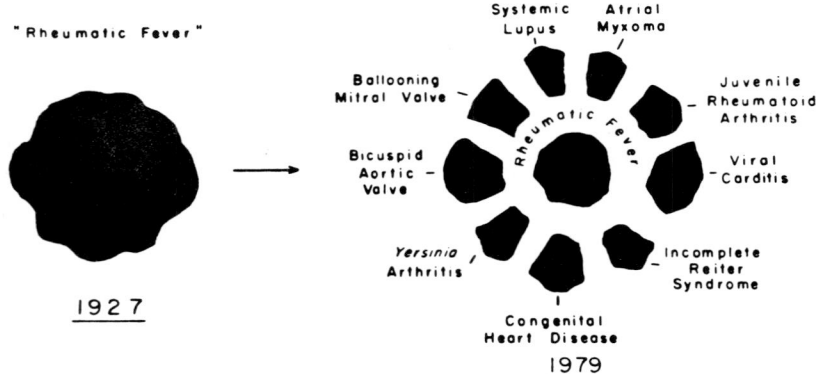

Fig. 68–2. The whittling away of rheumatic fever. Many diseases that had not been described or were difficult to diagnose in 1927 (the particular year is arbitrary) were "lumped" together as "rheumatic fever" (in the presence of fever) or as "rheumatic heart" disease (in its absence). They are now split off. What remains is a core, smaller but more homogeneous than the original lump. (From El-Sadr, W., and Taranta, A.[32])

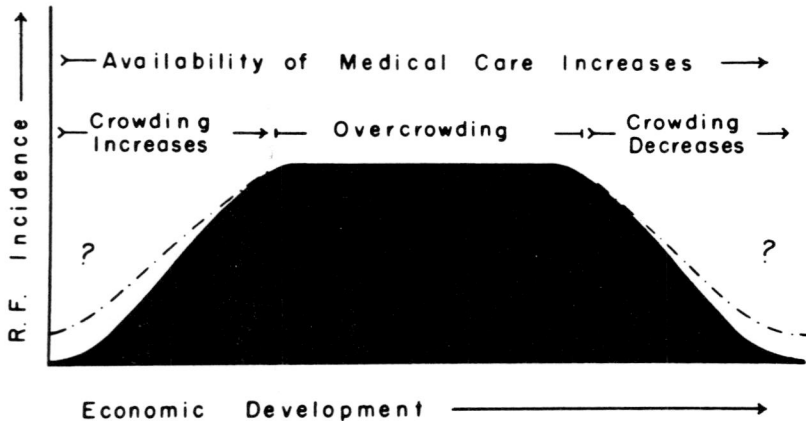

Fig. 68–3. Theoretical schema of the evolution of human societies indicated as "development" on the horizontal axis, in arbitrary units, and the prevalence of rheumatic fever, on the vertical axis, also in arbitrary units. In a first stage, primitive societies composed of small tribes isolated from each other may be unable to support a multitude of streptococcal types; hence, there is no rheumatic fever (perhaps). At the other, or postindustrialized, end of the spectrum, the individuals are isolated again by large houses and suburbia and (over-) treated with antibiotics; hence, rheumatic fever decreases and perhaps disappears. (From El-Sadr, W., and Taranta, A.[32])

This increasing mildness may be explained by a disproportionate decrease of recurrences, as compared to initial attacks of the disease, presumably because the prevention of recurrences is more effective than that of initial attacks and because the recurrent attacks are usually more severe than the initial one and more frequently affect the heart.

PATHOLOGIC AND IMMUNOPATHOLOGIC FEATURES

Rheumatic fever may "lick" other organs and tissues, but can be lethal only if it "bites" the heart. Therefore, the pathologist's view is biased, and statements true in the morgue, such as that rheumatic fever always affects the heart, may be false in the clinic.

In patients dying of acute rheumatic fever, pancarditis is usually present, affecting all the layers of the heart: endocardium, myocardium, and pericardium. Tiny translucent nodules or verrucae sit on the edges of the valves, one or more of which can no longer close properly: they are "regurgitant" or "incompetent." Above the base of the posterior leaflet of the mitral valve, the auricular endocardium may be thickened, furrowed, and gray (MacCallum's patch). The myocardium is pale, flabby, edematous, and mildly hypertrophic; the heart chambers are dilated. Fibrin and serosanguineous fluid may be present in the pericardial cavity.[111]

Microscopically, diffuse degeneration and swelling of muscle fibers may be apparent, with

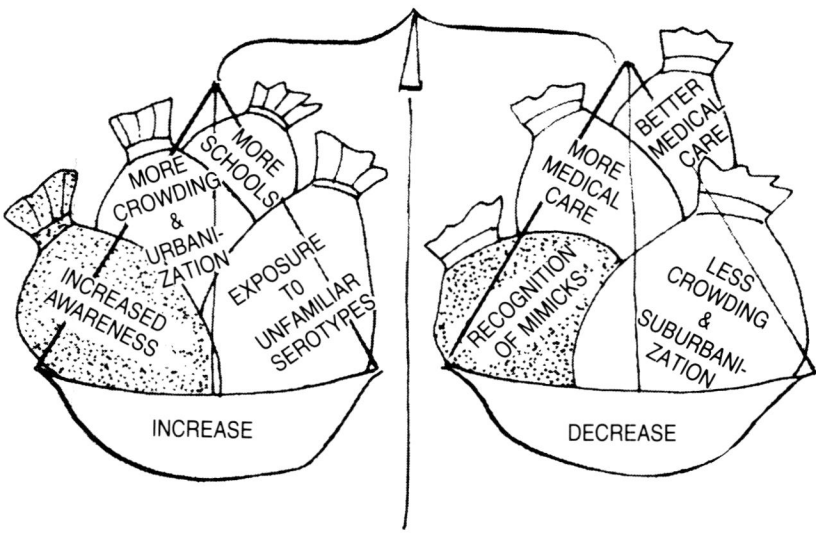

Fig. 68–4. Factors affecting the variations in incidence of rheumatic fever in the Western world and in "developing" countries. Stippling indicates the artifactual or biased nature of some of these factors. (From DiSciascio, G., and Taranta, A.[29])

fibrinoid degeneration of collagen. Perivascular foci of degeneration or necrosis may be surrounded by clusters of large mononuclear and giant multinuclear cells.[89,90] These clusters, known as Aschoff bodies or nodules, are considered specific for acute rheumatic fever, but they may persist long after any other evidence of active disease. Immunofluorescent study reveals deposits of immunoglobulins (IgG, IgA, and IgM) and of complement, specifically C3, in cardiac myofibers and in vessel walls; of IgG in heart valves;[59] and of IgG, IgM, and C3 in the pericardium.[96] Valvular lymphoid infiltrates contain a predominance of T cells;[98a] streptococcal antigens cannot be demonstrated.

In later stages of carditis, especially after recurrences of rheumatic fever, the valve leaflets are more grossly abnormal and are retracted, thickened, and deformed. Their commissures may be fused, and the chordae tendineae may be retracted and tangled. Scattered deposits of immunoglobulins in the myocardium may be found also in late stages, when the disease is clinically inactive, in patients who undergo cardiac surgery.[60] In the pericardium, fibrosis and adhesions may develop, but constrictive pericarditis does not.

Outside the heart, the pathologic features of the disease are sparse. A transient sterile exudate appears in the joints: complement components C3, C4, and C1q are decreased with respect to simultaneously determined serum levels,[121] but no synovial hypertrophy, bony erosions, or cartilage loss occurs. Chorea affects the basal ganglia, as one would expect, but also, diffusely, other parts of

the brain.[87] Subcutaneous nodules resemble the nodules of rheumatoid arthritis (RA) and consist of a central area of necrosis surrounded by parallel rows of elongated fibroblasts, as in a palisade ("palisading" fibroblasts), surrounded by loose connective tissue.[17] Erythema marginatum is not recognizable in biopsies or post-mortem.

CAUSE AND INCIDENCE

The evidence linking group A streptococcal infections of the throat to the subsequent development of rheumatic fever is based both on correlations and on experiments. Sore throats accompanied by scarlatiniform rash, that is, scarlet fever, have long been known to precede some attacks of rheumatic fever. In other patients, rheumatic fever may be preceded by a sore throat without rash or even by a pharyngitis without sore throat, both recognizable as streptococcal infections by antibody tests.[10,119]

The evidence is not based only on correlations, however. If streptococcal pharyngitis is treated, and streptococci are eradicated from the throat, rheumatic fever fails to appear;[141] if patients who have had previous attacks of rheumatic fever receive continual antibiotic prophylaxis, the disease does not recur.[22] In either case, the few failures to prevent rheumatic fever, whether initial or recurrent episodes, can be traced to failures to achieve the aims of prophylaxis, which are to eradicate the streptococci from the throat, in the case of initial occurrences,[18] and to prevent streptococcal infections, in the case of recurrences.[144]

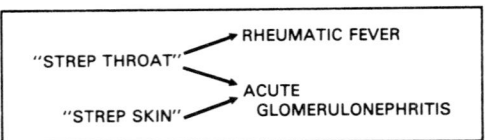

Fig. 68–5. Relation of streptococcal infections of the throat and of the skin to streptococcal sequels. Streptococcal infections of the throat ("strep throat") may lead either to glomerulonephritis or to acute rheumatic fever; streptococcal infections of the skin (impetigo; "strep skin") may lead only to glomerulonephritis. (From Taranta, A., and Markowitz, M.[131])

The other common site of streptococcal infection is the skin. Although skin infections can cause poststreptococcal glomerulonephritis, they do not cause rheumatic fever.[98] Streptococcal pharyngitis may lead to either disorder (Fig. 68–5). Group A streptococci that infect the skin usually differ in type from those that infect the throat,[140] but whether this variation accounts for the difference in rheumatogenicity is unclear. Immunologic, anatomic, or other factors may also be important. The antistreptolysin O antibody response that follows a skin infection is weaker than after a throat infection, possibly because of inhibition of streptolysin O by skin lipids;[58] this difference may play a role in pathogenesis.

Do all pharyngeal strains of group A streptococci carry the same risk of rheumatic fever? Yes, according to classic teaching, as long as the strain is capable of causing genuine pharyngitis;[99] no, according to some recent reports and an old, provocative observation. More than 40 years ago, Kuttner and Krumwiede reported that an epidemic of type 4 streptococcal pharyngitis among children convalescing from rheumatic fever failed, surprisingly, to reactivate the disease.[65] Recently, Bisno and co-workers have marshalled new evidence suggesting the existence of "rheumatogenic" and "nonrheumatogenic" streptococcal strains.[9]

The well-known correlation of rheumatic fever with poverty is of special interest because it appears to be mediated mainly by crowding. Figure 68–6 shows a linear relationship between the number of persons per room and the prevalence of rheumatic heart disease.[95] That this relationship is not purely coincidental, but rather is causal, is suggested by the observations in the military during World War II, when United States soldiers, who were well fed and well clothed, but overcrowded in their barracks, had an alarmingly high incidence of rheumatic fever.[141] In a civilian population, blacks have a higher incidence of rheumatic fever than whites, even within the same socioeconomic group. This finding at first suggested a genuine racial predilec-

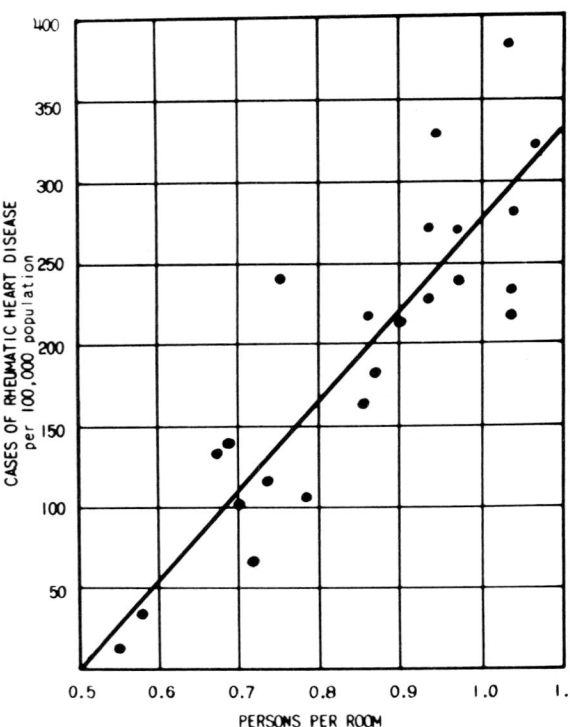

Fig. 68–6. The relationship between density of persons per room and incidence of rheumatic heart disease. (From Perry, B.C., and Roberts, M.A.F.[95])

tion, but on further analysis, the higher incidence was traced to greater crowding among blacks, even within the same socioeconomic group.[46] These "experiments of society" thus showed that, within the so-called constellation of poverty, crowding is necessary and sufficient for high rheumatic fever incidence rates. Crowding leads to multiple close contacts, which facilitate infection, not only because they increase the chances of contagion, but also because serial transfers of streptococci from patient to patient may lead to selection of mutants that produce more M protein and therefore are more able to resist phagocytosis, in a way similar to that accomplished in the laboratory by "passage" of a strain through a series of mice.

Although all attacks of rheumatic fever follow a streptococcal infection, only a few streptococcal infections are followed by rheumatic fever, and the reason is unknown. Adherence of streptococci to pharyngeal cells may be a factor.[103,111a] The severity of the infection bears some relation to the incidence of rheumatic fever. Although rheumatic fever follows 3% of infections accompanied by fever, exudate, swollen and tender cervical lymph nodes, persistence of positive streptococcal throat cultures and subsequent antistreptolysin O response,[99] only 0.3 to 0.1%, or even fewer, of the less severe infections develop into rheumatic fever.[120] This apparent relationship may be due simply to contamination of the "less severe" category with viral pharyngitides mistaken for streptococcal pharyngitis because of a coincidental streptococcal carrier state. Host factors may also be important because the concordance rate for rheumatic fever is 7 times higher in monozygotic twin pairs (18.7%) than in dizygotic twin pairs (2.5%).[129] The standard HLA antigens seem to have no reproducible relationship to susceptibility to rheumatic fever, but a recent preliminary report indicates that a novel B-cell alloantigen "883" carries an increase in the risk of developing rheumatic fever of 12.9%.[93,143a]

Recurrences

The attack rates of rheumatic fever after streptococcal pharyngitis are much higher in patients who have already had an attack than in those who have not. The recurrence rate per infection is highest in the first year after the rheumatic attack. This rate decreases sharply in the following two years, and then seems to level off[115] (Fig. 68–7). Little is known about the recurrence rate per infection many years after the latest rheumatic attack, but the few data available suggest that it remains elevated.[53] It thus appears that the decrease in the rate of recurrence of rheumatic fever per infection has two components, the first steep and the second much less steep or even flat (see Fig. 68–7). It is tempting to speculate that the first, fast-decaying component is a transient effect of the rheumatic fever attack and the second is either a permanent effect or the result of an inherent susceptibility of the host.

Rheumatic fever recurs only among patients who develop a streptococcal antibody response, and the recurrence rate per infection increases with the magnitude of the antibody rise. At each level of antibody response, streptococcal infections are more likely to lead to recurrences of rheumatic fever in patients with pre-existing rheumatic heart disease than in those with previous rheumatic fever but without heart disease (Table 68–1). In patients with heart disease, the rate of recurrence is higher in those with marked cardiomegaly than in those with little or no cardiomegaly.[127] The clinical severity of the pharyngitis is also a predictor of recurrence.[115]

PATHOGENESIS

Little is known about the chain of events that links streptococcal infections in the throat to the manifestations, distant in space and subsequent in time, that comprise rheumatic fever. The streptococci do not migrate from the throat to the heart or the joints, which are demonstrably sterile. Hence rheumatic fever is a nonsuppurative sequel to streptococcal infection, a poststreptococcal rather than a streptococcal disease.

Although streptococci remain localized at the site of infection, their products diffuse away. Some of these products are cardiotoxic in experimental animals and could be the mediators of tissue damage in rheumatic fever. The latent period between the streptococcal infections and the onset of rheumatic fever is a stumbling block in this hypothesis, but some toxins do act after such a latent period, as in tetanus or diphtheritic myocarditis.

As the streptococcal products diffuse from the throat, they encounter lymphoid cells and stimulate an antibody response. Several streptococcal antigens cross-react immunologically with human tissue antigens. As a result, the immune response to streptococci may be blunted because their antigens may be erroneously recognized as "self" by the lymphocytes, and whatever response is elicited may boomerang, in part, on the host because the host's antigens may now be mistaken as foreign. The latter "mistake," antoimmunity, may be the mechanism of tissue damage in rheumatic fever, especially in rheumatic carditis, as the well-studied cross-reactions of streptococcal antigens with heart antigens suggest.[102,146]

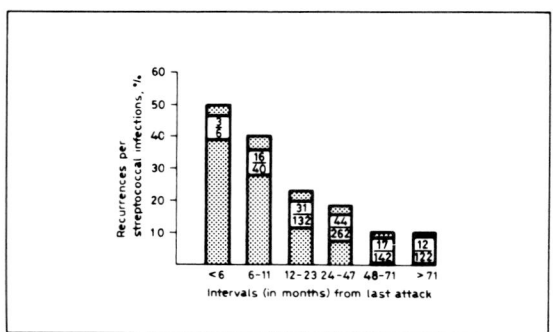

Fig. 68–7. Decrease of the rheumatic fever recurrence rate per infection with time lapsed since the latest rheumatic episode. (From Spagnuolo, M., et al.[115])

Table 68–1. Ratio of Rheumatic Fever Recurrences to Streptococcal Infections in Patients Stratified for Pre-Existing Rheumatic Heart Disease and for Rise in Antistreptolysin O (ASO)

ASO Rise in Number of Tube Dilutions	Pre-existing Heart Disease (%)	No Pre-existing Heart Disease (%)
0–1	3:24 (13)	1:79 (1)
2	10:38 (26)	3:50 (6)
3	6:16 (38)	5:34 (15)
4+	9:16 (56)	9:26 (35)

(Data from Taranta, A., et al.[127])

The nature of the group A streptococcal membrane antigen cross-reactive with human heart was reinvestigated recently by absorption of rheumatic fever sera with sarcolemmal sheets and subsequent elution. The purified antibody was used to follow the purification of the streptococcal membrane antigen, which turned out to consist of 4 distinct polypeptides with molecular weights ranging from 22,000 to 32,000 daltons.[138]

Attempts to demonstrate a state of delayed hypersensitivity against heart antigens in patients with rheumatic fever have yielded negative results.[76] In the guinea pig, however, sensitization to group A streptococcal antigens resulted in the acquisition by T-lymphocytes of the ability to kill guinea pig myocardial cells in vitro.[145]

A mechanism akin to that of serum sickness or the Arthus reaction has also been suggested. Streptococcal antigens might persist in the body of the patient who will develop rheumatic fever and might react with the corresponding antibodies, fix complement, and damage tissues. Countering this interpretation is that the latent period of rheumatic fever does not become shorter in recurrences,[100] whereas that of serum sickness characteristically does. In favor of this hypothesis is the recent finding of decreased complement components C1q, C3, and C4 in the synovial fluid of patients with rheumatic fever.[121]

Considering the variety of manifestations of the rheumatic fever syndrome, some fleeting, others chronic, some exudative, others proliferative, it would not be surprising if more than one mechanism is operative.

CLINICAL FINDINGS

The natural history of rheumatic fever may be said to start with the streptococcal pharyngitis that precedes it by an interval ("latent period") of 2 to 3 weeks (mean 18.6 days).[100] The latent period of rheumatic fever is a little longer than that of post-streptococcal glomerulonephritis,[101] and, as mentioned previously, it gets no shorter during recurrent episodes.[100]

The onset of the rheumatic attack is acute when the presenting manifestation is arthritis; it is usually gradual when the presenting manifestation is carditis alone, evidenced by heart failure. The onset of chorea may appear to be acute, but is often preceded by subtle behavioral changes interpreted as part of chorea only in retrospect. Subcutaneous nodules and erythema marginatum are rarely the presenting manifestations of rheumatic fever.

Joint Involvement

In the classic, untreated case, the arthritis of rheumatic fever affects several or many joints in quick succession, each for a short time (Fig. 68–8). This characteristic contributed much to the delineation of the clinical entity of rheumatic fever and to its separation from other "rheumatisms." The arthritis often affects the lower limbs first and later spreads to the arms. The terms "migrating" or "migratory" are often used to describe the polyarthritis of rheumatic fever, but these designations are not meant to signify that the inflammation necessarily disappears in one joint when it appears in another. Rather, the various localizations usually overlap in time, and the onset, as opposed to the full course of the arthritis, "migrates" from joint to joint. Because the arthritis is of short duration, the term "fleeting" is also used.

Joint involvement is more common, and also more severe, in teenagers and young adults than in children. This involvement occurs early in the rheumatic illness, and with the possible exception of abdominal pain, it is usually the earliest symptomatic manifestation of the disease, although asymptomatic carditis may precede it. Rheumatic polyarthritis may be excruciatingly painful, but is always transient. The pain is usually more prominent than the objective signs of inflammation; one often sees patients whose joints are painful, tender, and limited in their motions because of pain, yet have little swelling, redness, or heat. Conversely, one seldom sees a joint that is definitely swollen and only slightly tender.

When the disease is allowed to express itself fully, unchecked by anti-inflammatory treatment, the number of affected joints may be as high as

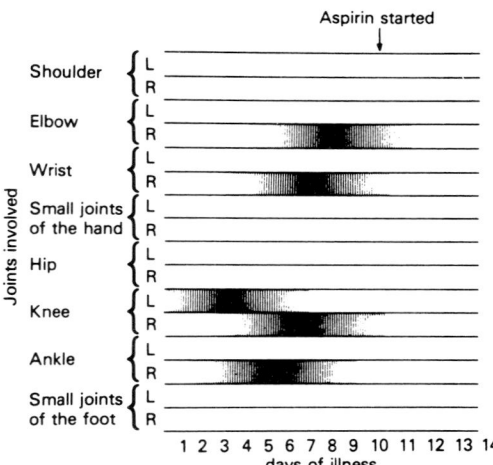

Fig. 68–8. Time course of the migratory polyarthritis of rheumatic fever. Notice that even in the absence of treatment, the involvement of each joint is short-lived, but the cumulative involvement of all joints is less so. Note also that arthritis rapidly responds to aspirin.

16, and about half these patients develop arthritis in more than 6 joints. Each joint is maximally inflamed for only a few days, or a week at the most, when the inflammation decreases. Milder and decreasing inflammation may linger for another week or so before disappearing completely. Considering all joints, the polyarthritis may be severe for a week in two-thirds of the patients, and for 2 or at the most 3 weeks in the others, and may then persist in a mild form for another week or two.[48] Radiologic examination shows only effusion.

Under the usual circumstances of medical practice, however, many patients with arthritis are treated empirically with aspirin or other drugs; arthritis subsides quickly in the joint(s) already affected and does not "migrate" to new joints: This therapy may deprive the diagnostician of a useful sign. In a large series of patients with rheumatic fever and associated arthritis, most of whom had been treated, involvement of only a single large joint was common (25%). One or both knees were affected in 76%, and 1 or both ankles in 50%. Elbows, wrists, hips, or small joints of the feet were involved in 12 to 15% of patients, and shoulders or small joints of the hand were affected in 7 to 8%. Joints rarely affected were the lumbosacral (2%), cervical (1%), sternoclavicular (0.5%), and temporomandibular (0.5%). Involvement of the small joints of the hands or feet alone occurred in only 1% of these patients.[37]

Some patients may have only the subjective manifestations of joint involvement, such as arthralgia or polyarthralgia. More often, objective evidence is present but is not detected, hence the quip: "arthralgia is arthritis minus a good physical examination."

Carditis

Rheumatic carditis is the most important manifestation of acute rheumatic fever, and when severe, death may result from acute heart failure. More commonly, rheumatic carditis has no symptoms and is later diagnosed in the course of the examination of a patient who comes to medical attention because of arthritis or chorea. Patients whose rheumatic illness consists only of asymptomatic carditis may develop rheumatic heart disease, despite the absence of a medical history of recognized rheumatic fever.

Clinically, patients with acute rheumatic fever may have endocarditis, myocarditis, pericarditis, or any combination of these findings. Important criteria for the clinical diagnosis of rheumatic carditis include organic heart murmur(s) not previously present, enlargement of the heart, congestive heart failure, and pericardial friction rubs or signs of effusion.

Organic murmurs are almost always audible in acute rheumatic carditis. The mitral valve is the most common site of involvement; a high-pitched, usually loud, long, blowing apical systolic murmur is a common finding and indicates acute mitral regurgitation.[71] Valvulitis may result from edema, cusp thickening, or verrucae. Depending on its extent, the murmur of mitral regurgitation may persist after treatment of the acute rheumatic episodes, or it may disappear, leaving little or no residua. A mid-diastolic or Carey-Coombs murmur, usually following a third heart sound, is common in patients with rheumatic fever and acute mitral regurgitation. This murmur does not indicate mitral stenosis and may disappear when the edema of the leaflets subsides during therapy with anti-inflammatory drugs.

The second most common valvular lesion during acute rheumatic fever is aortic regurgitation. This disorder produces a high-pitched decrescendo diastolic murmur that begins immediately after the second heart sound; it may be short and faint and therefore difficult to hear.[36] Once present, the murmur of aortic regurgitation usually persists.

Congestive heart failure is the most serious manifestation of rheumatic carditis. Usually, it develops in patients with combined, severe valvular involvement. It occurs in 5 to 10% of first episodes of rheumatic carditis and is more frequent during recurrences. The diagnosis is established by careful physical examination, history taking, and review of chest roentgenograms; hemodynamic monitoring may confirm it. Pericarditis can be detected clinically in up to 10% of patients with acute rheumatic fever. Pericardial effusion is occasionally striking, but cardiac tamponade is rare.

Electrocardiographic Findings

Prolongation of the P-R interval occurs in 28 to 40% of patients with rheumatic fever, much more frequently than in other febrile illnesses,[86] and therefore is useful in diagnosis. This prolongation does not correlate with residual heart disease,[39] however, and is not useful in prognosis. Second-degree atrioventricular block, atrioventricular dissociation, and even complete atrioventricular block may also occur.[27,70]

Chorea

Sydenham's chorea, chorea minor, or "St. Vitus' dance" is a neurologic disorder consisting of involuntary movements, muscular weakness, and emotional disturbances. The movements are abrupt and purposeless, not rhythmic or repetitive. They disappear during sleep, but may occur at rest and may interfere with voluntary activity. The movements can be suppressed by the will of the patient, for a while. They may affect all voluntary muscles, but the involvement of the hands and face is usually the most obvious. Grimaces and inappropriate smiles are common. Handwriting usually becomes clumsy and provides a convenient way of following the patient's course. Speech is often slurred. The movements are commonly more marked on one side and are occasionally completely unilateral (hemichorea).

The muscular weakness is best revealed by asking the patient to squeeze the examiner's hands. The examiner feels that the pressure of the patient's grip increases and decreases continuously and capriciously, a phenomenon known as relapsing grip, or milking sign.

The emotional changes manifest themselves in outbursts of inappropriate behavior, including crying and restlessness. Patients are frustrated by their inability to control their bodies and to perform the activities of daily living competently, and angry because they are made fun of by other children or scolded by adults. In exceptional cases, the psychologic manifestations may be severe and may result in transient psychosis.

The neurologic examination fails to reveal sensory losses or pyramidal tract involvement. Diffuse hypotonia may be present. The choreic movements can be elicited in doubtful cases by asking patients to stretch their hands in front of them, to stretch their fingers out, to close their eyes, and to stick their tongues out, one movement added to the other. By the time patients stick out their tongues, their fingers wiggle or their eyelids flutter. When the arms are projected straight forward, one sees flexion of the wrist, hyperextension of the metacarpophalangeal joints, straightening of the fingers, and abduction of the thumb ("spooning" or "dishing" of the hands; Fig. 68–9). When patients are asked to raise their arms above their heads, they also pronate one or both hands (pronator sign; Fig. 68–10).

Chorea may follow streptococcal infections after

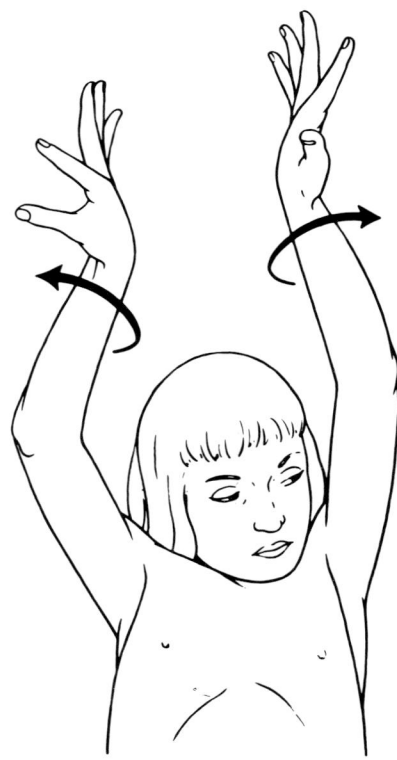

Fig. 68–10. "Pronator sign" in a patient with chorea. When the patient raises her hands above her head, she also pronates her hands.

a latent period, which is longer, on the average, than the latent period of other rheumatic manifestations.[125] Some patients with chorea have no other symptoms, but other patients develop chorea weeks or months after arthritis[132] (Fig. 68–11). In both cases, examination of the heart may reveal murmurs.

Subcutaneous Nodules

The subcutaneous nodules of rheumatic fever are firm and painless. The overlying skin is not inflamed and can usually be moved over the nodules. The diameter of these round lesions varies from a few millimeters to 1 or even 2 cm. They are located over bony surfaces or prominences, or near tendons (Fig. 68–12); their number varies from a single nodule to a few dozen and averages 3 or 4; when numerous, they are usually symmetric. These nodules are present for 1 or more weeks, rarely for more than a month. They thus are smaller and shorter-lived than the nodules of RA. Although in both diseases the elbows are most frequently involved, the rheumatic nodules are more common on the olecranon, and the rheumatoid nodules are usually found 3 or 4 cm. distal to it.[63] Rheumatic subcutaneous nodules generally appear only after

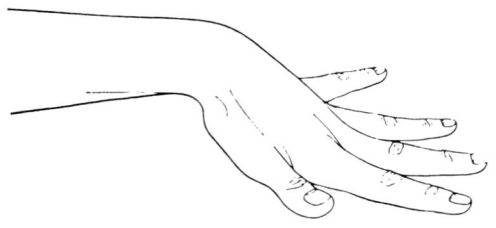

Fig. 68–9. "Spooning" or "dishing" of the hands in a patient with chorea. Notice the flexion of the wrists, the hyperextension of the metacarpophalangeal joints, the straightening of the fingers, and the abduction of the thumb.

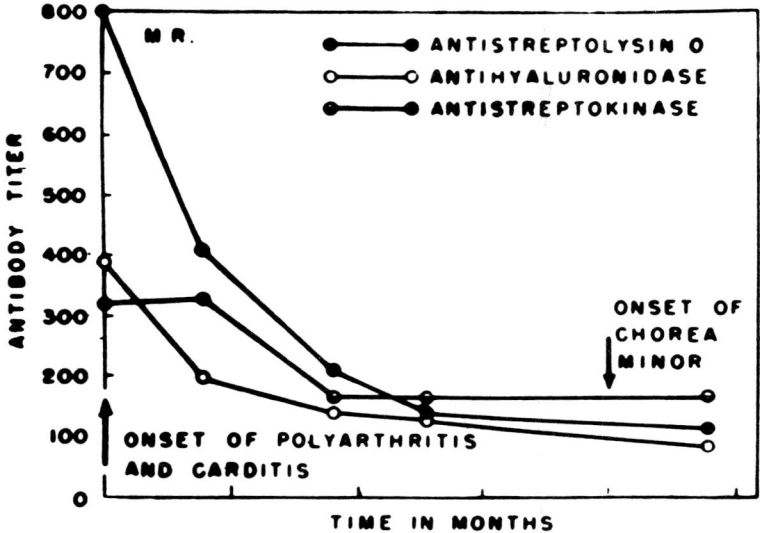

Fig. 68–11. Chorea appearing four months after the onset of polyarthritis and carditis. Intercurrent streptococcal infections were ruled out by the falling titers of three streptococcal antibodies. (From Taranta, A., and Stollerman, G.H.[132])

the first few weeks of illness, usually only in patients with carditis.[82]

Erythema Marginatum

Erythema marginatum is an evanescent, non-pruritic skin rash, pink or faintly red, affecting usually the trunk, sometimes the proximal parts of the limbs, but not the face. It is composed of a variable number of individual skin lesions, starting as a solid erythema that may be slightly raised. This lesion extends centrifugally while the skin in the center returns gradually to normal; hence the name "erythema marginatum." The outer edge of the lesion is sharp, whereas the inner edge is diffuse (Fig. 68–13). Because the margin of the lesion is usually continuous, making a ring, it is also known as "erythema annulare."[62,94]

The individual lesions may appear and disappear in a matter of hours, usually to return. They may change in shape and size almost as fast as smoke rings, which they resemble both in shape and in the centrifugal manner in which they expand and dissolve. The lesions may coalesce while expanding and may thus acquire a circinate, gyrate, or festooned pattern. A hot bath or shower may make them more evident or may even reveal them for the first time.

Erythema marginatum usually occurs in the early phase of the disease. It often persists or recurs, even when all other manifestations of disease have disappeared. On the other hand, the lesions occasionally appear for the first time, or perhaps are noticed for the first time, late in the course of the illness or even during convalescence. This disorder usually occurs only in patients with carditis.[37,82]

Other Manifestations

Fever is regularly present in rheumatic fever arthritis; it is often present in isolated carditis, but seldom in isolated chorea. It is a remittent type of fever without wide swings, usually does not exceed 104° F, and returns to normal or near normal in 2 or 3 weeks in most cases, even without treatment.[30,48,77]

Abdominal pain may occur in rheumatic fever as a manifestation of congestive heart failure, owing to distention of the liver. It may also occur in rare but important instances without heart failure and before any other manifestation has declared the rheumatic nature of the illness. In these patients, the pain may be periumbilical and severe, presumably because of mesenteric adenitis, and occasionally leads to an unnecessary appendectomy.[37]

Anorexia, nausea, and vomiting often occur, mostly as manifestations of congestive heart failure or salicylate intoxication. The incidence of epistaxis decreased from a maximum of 48% in the early 1930s,[21] to 4 to 9% in the late 1950s.[37] Fatigue is a vague and infrequent symptom, unless heart failure is present.

Other clinical manifestations, seldom seen now, include erythema nodosum, pleurisy, and "rheumatic pneumonia."[112] Congestive heart failure may simulate both pleurisy and pneumonia, with a pleural transudate and pulmonary congestion, respectively. Moreover, the old-time description of

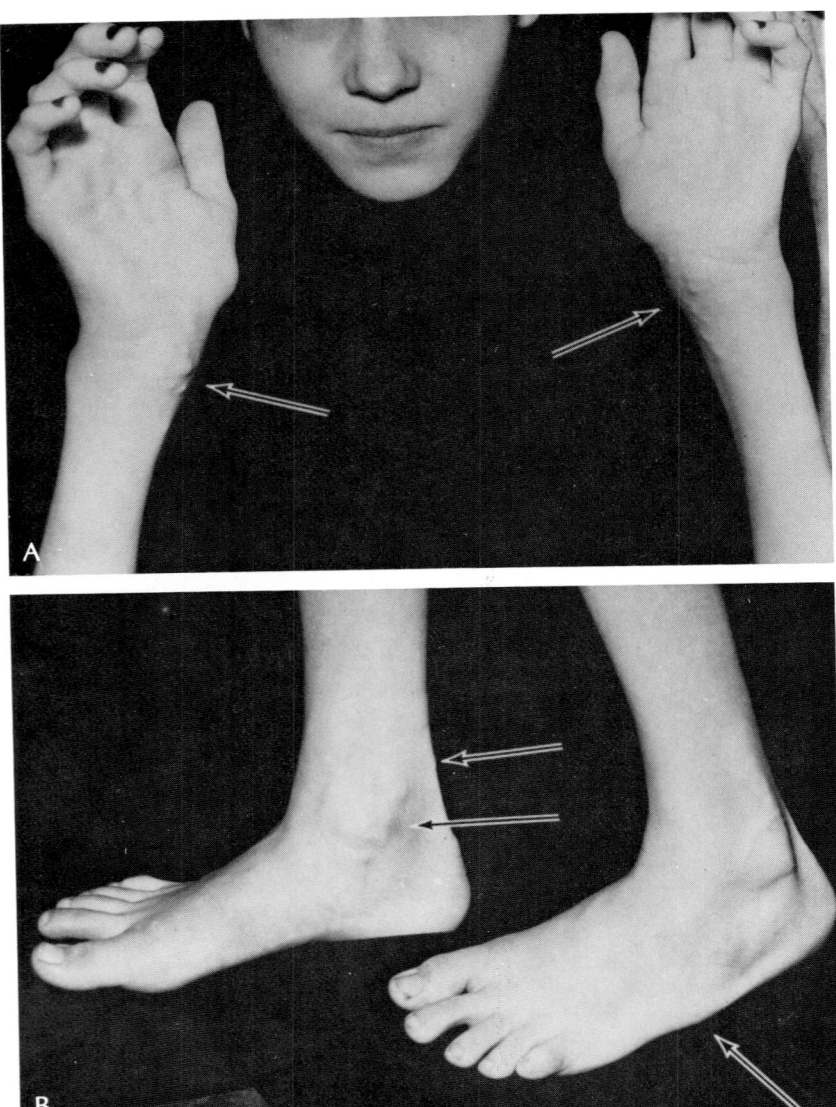

Fig. 68–12. *A* and *B*, Subcutaneous nodules (indicated by the arrows) in a child with rheumatic fever. Notice that some of them are difficult to see; they can often be more easily felt than seen. (Courtesy of Dr. Eugenie F. Doyle.)

rheumatic pneumonia, with patchy, shifting areas of infiltration,[104] is suspiciously similar to that of "viral" pneumonia.

Sequence of Appearance of Manifestations

Figure 68–14 summarizes schematically our current knowledge. Most episodes of rheumatic fever start with arthritis; in rare instances, abdominal pain precedes arthritis. When a physician is consulted, clinical evidence of carditis may or may not already be present. If not, it usually does not appear later; carditis usually appears in the first three weeks of the illness. Electrocardiographic altera-

tions may be detected during the latent period of rheumatic fever.

When seen initially, patients with chorea may have a significant heart murmur and no acute-phase reactant; these findings suggest a preceding carditis. Patients with polyarthritis may develop chorea later. Subcutaneous nodules usually appear after the first few weeks. Erythema marginatum is observed most frequently at the onset of a rheumatic attack, but it may also appear later.

Incidence of Clinical Manifestations

The incidence of arthritis, the most common major manifestation of rheumatic fever, increases

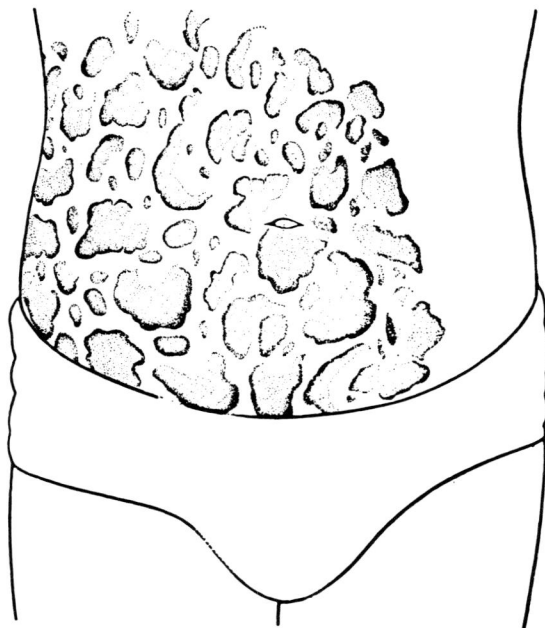

Fig. 68–13. Erythema marginatum in a child with rheumatic fever. Most individual lesions are outlined by closed rings. Some of the lesions have a circinate or festooned appearance.

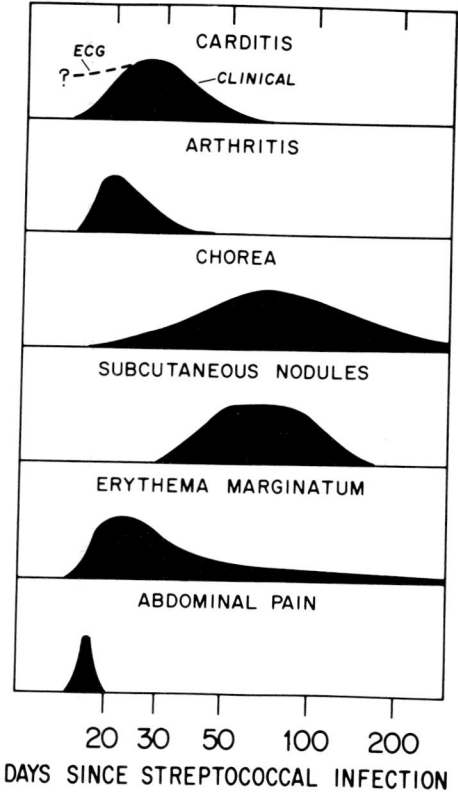

Fig. 68–14. Approximate schema of the sequence of appearance of the various rheumatic fever manifestations. The maximum height of each curve indicates the time at which most of the cases of a given manifestation "appear," that is, become known to a medical observer. Because of the concentration of events early in the attack, time is represented on a logarithmic scale.

with the age of the patient. Its incidence in first episodes of rheumatic fever increases from 66% in children aged 3 to 6 to 82% in teenagers;[37] it is nearly 100% in first attacks in adults.[5] In addition to being more frequent, arthritis is often more severe and lasts longer in adults[7,16,74] (Fig. 68–15). Arthritis was thought to be a less-frequent manifestation of rheumatic fever in the tropics, but more careful recent work has dispelled this notion.[98,110]

The incidence of carditis in rheumatic fever varies with age, but in a direction opposite to that of arthritis: it is present in 90 to 92% of children under the age of 3 years,[75,105] in 50% of children ages 3 to 6 years, in 32% of teenagers aged 14 to 17,[37] and in only 15% of adults with initial rheumatic fever.[5] In addition to being less frequent, carditis is less severe in adults with first attacks of rheumatic fever.[5]

The incidence of carditis, as well as its severity, may have decreased in recent years, but how much of this decrease is due to changed hospital admissions policies and to a disproportionate decline in recurrences of the disease is uncertain.

Chorea is the only major manifestation that has definitely decreased out of proportion to the others in recent decades, from 52%,[13] 43%,[81] and 41%,[84] of all the patients with rheumatic fever, to 22%,[97] 19%,[84] 15%,[81] and nil,[37,69] for reasons that are not understood. Chorea also occurs in the most limited

age range; it is not seen in children under 3 years of age,[4,75] is rare after puberty, and does not occur in adults,[4,92] with the exception of rare cases during pregnancy, termed chorea gravidarum.[72] Finally, it is the only manifestation with a marked sex preference. Chorea is twice as frequent in girls as in boys;[4] after puberty, this sex preference increases.[91]

Subcutaneous nodules are reported to be frequent in England (34%,[16] 21%[137]), common in Boston (10%),[82] but rare in New York (1%),[37] Baltimore (2%),[80] and New Delhi (2%).[110] Whether this incidence reflects a true geographic variation or whether it is due to differences in the thoroughness of physical examination is a matter for speculation. Subcutaneous nodules are certainly easy to miss and so is erythema marginatum, which has been reported in 13%,[137] 10%,[82] 4%,[37] and 2%[110] of patients with rheumatic fever. That this lesion may be difficult to see in dark-skinned patients may account for some of these reported variations.

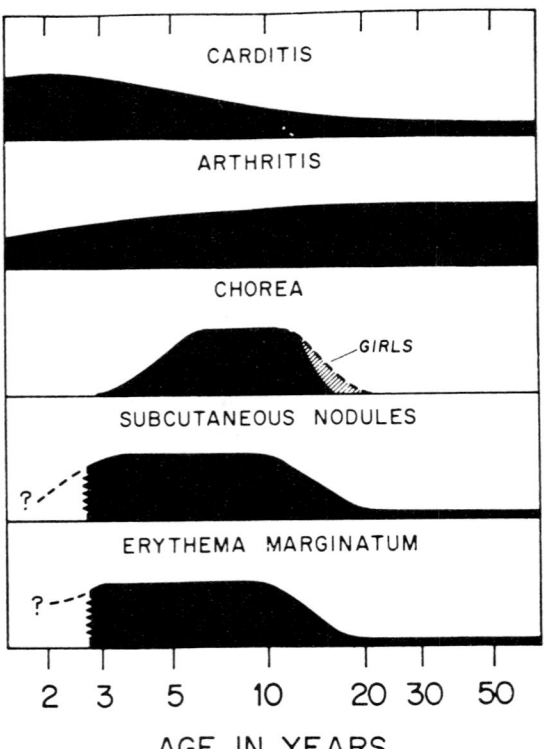

CARDITIS			
ARTHRITIS			
CHOREA			
		GIRLS	
SUBCUTANEOUS NODULES			
?			
ERYTHEMA MARGINATUM			
?			

2   3   5   10   20 30 50

AGE IN YEARS

Fig. 68–15. Schematic representation of the variations with age of the incidence of the major manifestations of rheumatic fever. The maximum height of each curve indicates the age at which a given manifestation attains its maximum incidence among patients with rheumatic fever.

Associations Among Clinical Manifestations

These may be positive or negative. Thus, subcutaneous nodules and erythema marginatum are much more frequent in the presence than in the absence of carditis,[63,68] and each is about twice as frequent in the presence of the other.[82] "Pure" chorea is, by definition, associated with no other clinical manifestations. Nevertheless, it may be associated with subclinical carditis, as suggested by the high incidence of delayed detection of heart disease among patients with chorea.[12] Carditis is more frequent when arthritis is absent or mild, but this difference arises in part by definition, because a patient without arthritis must have carditis or chorea to come to medical attention,[37] and in part to the opposite age variation of the incidence of arthritis and carditis.

Duration of the Attack and Sequelae

An episode of rheumatic fever is customarily considered to end when the patient's erythrocyte sedimentation rate returns to normal, usually sev-eral weeks after the subsidence of arthritis. By this criterion, the duration of the episode is 109 ± 57 days,[37] less than 12 weeks in 80% of cases and less than 15 weeks in 90%.[82] A few patients develop chronic rheumatic activity.[133]

Sequelae are limited to the heart and depend on the presence and severity of carditis. In addition, patients who have had rheumatic fever develop it again after streptococcal infections with an attack rate much higher than in the general population. This propensity can also be considered a sequela.

The structural and functional alterations of the heart caused by rheumatic fever and referred to collectively as "rheumatic heart disease" are described in detail in cardiology textbooks. They are dealt with here only in terms of their relation to the acute attack. Among large series of patients followed in recent years from the time of the acute illness, rheumatic heart disease has developed only in those who had clinical evidence of carditis, that is, in patients who at the time of the acute attack had "organic" or pathologic murmurs. Moreover, the severity of the residual rheumatic heart disease mirrors the severity of the previous acute carditis.[35,135–137] Patients whose first episode of rheumatic fever took the form of chorea without other clinical manifestations may also, however, develop rheumatic heart disease, usually mitral stenosis, gradually and insidiously over the years; up to 23% after 20 years.[12] Some of these patients may actually have had transient carditis shortly before the onset of chorea, as the outcome of the same streptococcal infection. The evidence of carditis may have disappeared by the time chorea appears, but a murmur may reappear later.

The mitral valve is the most frequently affected, followed by the aortic valve; involvement of the tricuspid valve is unusual, and that of the pulmonary valve is rare. Aortic and tricuspid valves are rarely affected unless the mitral valve is also affected. All affected valves are regurgitant at first; over the years and decades, some valves heal, the mitral more frequently than the aortic; others remain regurgitant, and still others become stenotic, either "purely" so or combined with regurgitation. In patients who receive continual and effective prophylaxis, mitral regurgitation disappears in as many as 70% over a 9-year period.[134]

Mitral stenosis may develop at a much earlier age among Indians, other Asians, and Africans than among Westerners ("juvenile mitral stenosis").[19,107] The same may be true of aortic stenosis.[139] Whether this phenomenon is due to the occurrence of streptococcal infections earlier in childhood, to nonstreptococcal cofactors, or even to a different cause of the disease remains uncertain.

Jaccoud's arthritis or arthropathy or syndrome, also called, more descriptively, chronic postrheumatic fever arthropathy, is a rare, indolent, slowly progressive process that deforms the fingers and sometimes the toes.[11,15,44,109,147] The deformity consists of ulnar deviation of the fingers, flexion of the metacarpophalangeal joints, and hyperextension of the proximal interphalangeal joints, just as in RA, but without the joint pains, heat, and swelling of the latter. The ulnar deviation occurs mostly in the fourth and fifth digits and is at first correctable, but later may become fixed. The toes may be affected similarly. Although no true erosions are present, notches or "hooks," thought to be due to the mechanical effect of ulnar deviation, are sometimes seen in roentgenograms on the ulnar side of each metacarpal head ("Bywater's hooks"). Rheumatoid factor is absent; the erythrocyte sedimentation rate is normal.

In classic cases, Jaccoud's arthropathy appears after multiple, prolonged, and severe attacks of rheumatic fever. It is thought to be the end result of the repeated inflammation caused by rheumatic fever in the small joints of the hand, perhaps depending on individual predisposition. Patients with systemic lupus erythematosus (SLE) may develop a similar arthropathy,[14,33] and some patients develop it without having either SLE or rheumatic fever.[54,90a] The prognosis of Jaccoud's arthropathy is good. Patients, alarmed by the deformity, may fear that it will extend to joints in other parts of the body, but this does not happen.

Recurrences

The same clinical manifestations present in the initial episode of rheumatic fever reappear in recurrences with a frequency greater than would be expected by chance[106] (Table 68–2). Conversely, manifestations absent in the first episode are usually absent in recurrent attacks. This characteristic is particularly important in the case of the most serious manifestation, carditis[38] (Table 68–3). Speculations on the reason(s) for this "mimetic" pattern are discussed elsewhere.[123]

In apparent contradiction to this pattern are the observations summarized in Table 68–4,[133] which indicate that the prevalence of heart disease increases with the number of previous episodes of rheumatic fever. Most likely, this finding is due to the increased tendency of patients with heart disease to develop recurrences,[127] rather than to the development of heart disease anew in patients originally free of it.

Mortality Rate

Of the many deaths ultimately caused by rheumatic fever, only a minority occur during an acute episode, and even fewer occur during the initial attack. Case-fatality rates of 0.36%,[37] 0.6%,[137] and 1.6%[82] have been reported in first episodes and rates of 2.3%[137] and 3%[37] have been noted in recurrences.

LABORATORY FINDINGS
Evidence of Recent Streptococcal Infection

Eighty percent of patients with acute rheumatic fever observed early in their course have elevated antistreptolysin O titers. The remaining 20% have elevation of one or more of the other streptococcal antibodies tested, such as antistreptokinase, antihyaluronidase, antideoxyribonuclease B, and antinicotinamide-adenine dinucleotidase.[119,128] All these antibody tests are based on the principle of inhibition of a specific toxic or enzymatic activity of streptococcal culture filtrate. Unfortunately, only the antistreptolysin O test is generally available, and all the tests are time-consuming.

In recent years, a simple, rapid test based on a different principle, the agglutination of sheep red blood cells coated with a mix of streptococcal antigens,[56] has become commercially available (Streptozyme). It is more sensitive than any other single streptococcal antibody test, simpler, and takes only a few minutes to perform. In small series, it was positive at a dilution of 1:200 in 100% of cases of rheumatic fever.[10]

The titer of streptococcal antibodies does not correlate with the severity of the illness, nor does their persistence correlate with its chronicity. An-

Table 68–2. Major Clinical Manifestations of Rheumatic Fever Recurrences According to Manifestations of the First Episode

Initial Manifestations (isolated or combined with others)	Manifestations of Recurrences (isolated or combined with others)		
	Polyarthritis No. (%)	Carditis No. (%)	Chorea No. (%)
Polyarthritis (N = 149)	110 (74)	51 (34)	18 (12)
Carditis (N = 89)	44 (49)	62 (70)	2 (2)
Chorea (N = 68)	11 (16)	10 (15)	54 (79)

(Data from Roth, I.R., Lingg, C., and Whittemore, A.[106])

Table 68–3. Appearance and Persistence of Rheumatic Heart Disease with Recurrent Rheumatic Fever in Patients Without Rheumatic Heart Disease During a Previous Episode of Rheumatic Fever

Studies	Patients with Rheumatic Fever Recurrences	Patients with Carditis During Recurrences	Patients with Persistent Rheumatic Heart Disease
Feinstein and Spagnuolo, 1960[38]	71	10 (14%)	10 (14%)
United Kingdom and United States Cooperative Study, 1965[135]	10	?	0
Feinstein et al., 1964[35]	11	2 (18%)	0

Table 68–4. Incidence of Rheumatic Heart Disease According to Number of Previous Attacks of Rheumatic Fever*

Previous Attacks	Number of Patients	Number of Patients with Heart Disease
0	797	264 (33%)
1	280	170 (60%)
2	57	43 (75%)
3	31	25 (81%)
4	4	4 (100%)

*Adapted from Taranta, A., et al.[127]

tibody titers are higher in groups of patients with rheumatic fever than in those with uncomplicated streptococcal infections, but considerable overlap of individual values occurs. By the time rheumatic fever develops, the patient's throat culture is often negative, especially if antibiotics have been given. A positive culture may provide presumptive evidence of streptococcal infection, but this should be confirmed by antibody determination to rule out a carrier state.

Laboratory Manifestations of a Systemic Inflammatory State

These manifestations include an elevated erythrocyte sedimentation rate, a positive test for C-reactive protein, and moderate leukocytosis. Anemia is also common.[83] Usually, changes in the C-reactive protein tests precede those in the erythrocyte sedimentation rate. With the exception of "pure" or isolated chorea, untreated rheumatic fever is consistently accompanied by an elevated erythrocyte sedimentation rate and a positive C-reactive protein test. These tests may be used in following the progress of healing when clinical signs of active illness are absent, but test results may become abnormal again for unrelated reasons and even after an injection of benzathine penicillin.[51]

Other Laboratory Abnormalities

Heart antibodies are demonstrable by a variety of techniques in the serum of patients with rheumatic fever. They are also found, however, in the serum of patients with uncomplicated streptococcal infections or with acute glomerulonephritis, although usually at a lower titer.[61] Because of this overlap and because of technical difficulties, these tests are not yet generally used.

Synovial fluid examination is useful to exclude other processes, especially septic, traumatic, and crystal-induced arthritis. The synovial fluid of patients with rheumatic fever is sterile and free from crystals, with glucose concentrations equivalent to those in simultaneously drawn plasma samples. The leukocytosis varies (from 600 to 80,000/mm³, with a mean of 16,000;[5] from 2,600 to 96,000/mm³, with a mean of 29,000[121]), polymorphonuclear leukocytes predominate (73 to 100%, with a mean of 90%;[5] 56 to 95%, with a mean of 83%[121]). The levels of C3, C4, and C1q are decreased with respect to simultaneously determined serum levels.[121]

Subclinical kidney involvement may be manifested by transient microscopic hematuria[5,23] and proteinuria.[5] Kidney biopsies may reveal glomerular changes[49] and even classic poststreptococcal glomerulonephritis,[43] but these findings are rare. Subclinical liver involvement, manifested by transient enzyme elevations, has long been known to occur in rheumatic fever patients treated with aspirin,[78] but it may also occur without therapy.[5]

DIAGNOSIS

No single manifestation is so characteristic as to be diagnostic; the greater the number of clearly recognized manifestations, the firmer the diagnosis. The most common presentation, but also the least specific, is arthritis without carditis. There is no diagnostic laboratory test.

Because the prognosis varies according to the manifestations of the acute attack, the diagnosis of rheumatic fever should be qualified by mention of the manifestations diagnosed, such as "rheumatic fever with polyarthritis only." An indication of the severity of carditis, in terms of congestive failure and cardiomegaly, is also useful for the same reason.[118]

Jones Criteria

T.D. Jones divided the manifestations of rheumatic fever into "major" and "minor" according to their diagnostic usefulness (Table 68–5). These criteria have been widely accepted and have proved useful, especially in preventing overdiagnosis. Jones proposed that the presence of two major or of one major and two minor manifestations indicates a high probability of rheumatic fever.

Patient's Medical History

Physicians who see patients early in the illness should be able to observe directly the various manifestations or to note their absence. In such patients, the role of history taking is limited to ascertaining whether they had scarlet fever two to four weeks previously. An affirmative answer to this question makes a diagnosis of rheumatic fever more likely. In the absence of scarlet fever, a history of recent pharyngitis is consistent with the diagnosis of rheumatic fever, but it is not specific enough to be taken as evidence of recent streptococcal infection. Many sore throats are viral; many streptococcal infections cause no sore throat, that is, are subclinical. Therefore, the diagnosis of recent streptococcal infection should be made serologically.

If the physician first sees the patient when the acute manifestations have subsided and therefore cannot be observed directly, the patient's medical history is of great and often critical importance.

Arthritis

Although the typical joint manifestation of rheumatic fever is migratory polyarthritis, arthritis is sometimes so short-lived, especially in treated patients, that it has no time to migrate. To facilitate diagnosis, anti-inflammatory treatment should be withheld or discontinued, so that the character of the arthritis may declare itself. Any arthritis that persists in the same joint for more than a week should make one think of another diagnosis, especially in children. In adults, arthritis may be more severe, and last longer. The arthritis of rheumatic fever responds readily to aspirin (mainly because its "migration" to new joints is stopped)[5] whereas many other arthritides do not respond.

Carditis

Rheumatic carditis is always associated with one or more of the three murmurs described earlier, organic apical systolic murmur, mid-diastolic apical murmur, or aortic diastolic murmur; hence the importance of careful auscultation.

Functional or innocent systolic murmurs may be mistaken for the organic systolic murmur of mitral regurgitation, especially when their loudness is increased by fever or anemia. Unlike the murmur of mitral regurgitation, however, most functional systolic murmurs, such as Still's murmur or innocent ejection-type murmurs, are heard best along the left sternal border, in the third to second interspace or at the lower left sternal border. The functional systolic murmurs are limited to the first two-thirds

Table 68–5. Jones Criteria (Revised) for Guidance in the Diagnosis of Rheumatic Fever

Major Manifestations	Minor Manifestations
Carditis	Clinical
Polyarthritis	Fever
Chorea	Arthralgia
Erythema marginatum	Previous rheumatic fever or rheumatic heart disease
Subcutaneous nodules	Laboratory
	Erythrocyte sedimentation rate, C-reactive protein, leukocytosis
	Prolonged P-R interval

PLUS

Supporting evidence of preceding streptococcal infection such as increased antistreptolysin O or other streptococcal antibodies; positive throat culture for group A streptococci; or recent scarlet fever.

The presence of two major criteria, or of one major and two minor criteria, indicates the probable presence of rheumatic fever if supported by evidence of a preceding streptococcal infection. The absence of the latter should make the diagnosis suspect, except when rheumatic fever is first discovered after a long latent period from the antecedent infection, as in Sydenham's chorea or low-grade carditis.

(Courtesy of the American Heart Association.)

of systole and usually have a midsystolic accentuation. Their pitch is generally low, and they lack the "blowing" or "steam-jet" quality of mitral regurgitation murmurs. Some functional murmurs have a "groaning" or "twanging-string" quality; they are often heard best along the lower left sternal margin or between it and the apex. At the apex, physiologic third heart sounds may be mistaken for mid-diastolic murmurs, Differentiation of the two rests mainly on the perceptible duration of the latter. The aortic diastolic murmur is notoriously easy to miss,[36] and good training in auscultation is essential to detect it. Overdiagnosis of aortic regurgitation, less commonly a problem, can be avoided if one remembers that this high-pitched, decrescendo murmur starts right at the end of the second heart sound and has a definite duration.

Role of Laboratory Findings in Diagnosis

The role of the laboratory is mainly to support the diagnosis by revealing evidence of a recent streptococcal infection and of a systemic inflammatory state. The lack of either throws doubt on the diagnosis, except in patients with isolated chorea and long-standing carditis. According to the revised Jones criteria, antistreptolysin O titers of at least 250 U in adults and 333 U in children over 5 years of age are considered indicative of a recent streptococcal infection.[118]

Differential Diagnosis

The differential diagnosis varies according to the presenting manifestations. It is always prudent to exclude bacteremia by blood cultures; polyarthralgia and polyarthritis, as well as heart murmurs, are frequent manifestations of infective endocarditis.[31,122] Gonococcal arthritis is a frequent cause of acute polyarthritis in adolescents and adults.[52,64] Polyarthralgia and polyarthritis occur in preicteric and anicteric viral hepatitis, which can be recognized by the accompanying urticarial rash, a high serum glutamic-oxaloacetic transaminase level, low complement levels, and positive tests for hepatitis B surface antigen.[41,113] RA of acute onset does not respond to aspirin as readily as rheumatic fever; in its juvenile form, RA is often accompanied by high antistreptolysin O titers, which may cause confusion;[108] rheumatoid factor tests are usually negative. Sometimes, only prolonged observation yields the diagnosis. Antinuclear antibody tests, regularly positive in patients with SLE, are negative in patients with rheumatic fever, and the clinical pictures usually differ. Particularly troublesome may be the differentiation from a serum-sickness type of reaction, with fever and polyarthritis, which may occur after administration of penicillin for a previous pharyngitis; urticaria or

angioneurotic edema, if present, may help in the diagnosis. Polyarthritis may follow a number of viral infections, especially rubella; rubella vaccination may also cause it.[26]

Isolated rheumatic carditis may be difficult to distinguish from viral carditis, with which it has many features in common, such as pericarditis, cardiomegaly, heart failure, and even heart murmurs.[143] In dubious cases, one should attempt viral isolation from stools and pharyngeal washings and look for an appropriate antibody response. Left atrial myxoma may also mimic isolated rheumatic carditis.[73]

Chorea must be differentiated from tics, which are repetitive, stereotyped, localized movements, and from benign familial chorea, a rare disorder transmitted as an autosomal dominant trait and beginning in childhood.[20]

Subcutaneous nodules must sometimes be differentiated from enlarged lymph nodes, especially in rubella. Rarely, these nodules clinically and histologically indistinguishable from rheumatic nodules occur in an isolated fashion and are benign.[124] Erythema marginatum must sometimes be differentiated from cutis marmorata, a fixed, reticular, bluish discoloration of the skin. Erythema marginatum has been reported in Lyme arthritis.

In Scandinavian countries, infections with *Yersinia enterocolitica* have been associated with acute polyarthritis, carditis, and abdominal pains, all of which may cause diagnostic confusion.[66,69] Febrile diarrhea, frequent in *Yersinia* infections, may help in the differentiation.[66] In doubtful cases, and maybe in all cases of acute polyarthritis in Scandinavia, the agglutination test for *Yersinia* should be performed.

Among blacks, another cause of diagnostic confusion is sickle cell anemia, which may mimic rheumatic fever because of heart murmurs and arthralgias, but may also coexist with it.[85]

TREATMENT

General Measures and Bed Rest

All patients with rheumatic fever should be examined daily for the first two or three weeks of the illness, primarily to watch for the development of carditis and to start treatment promptly should heart failure occur. Discussion at the patient's bedside concerning heart murmurs or cardiomegaly are better avoided; the patient often misunderstands and worries needlessly. Strict and prolonged bed rest, once the rule, appears useless.[50] Although no controlled studies exist, the recommendations in Table 68–6 seem reasonable.

Table 68–6.   Suggested Schedule of Bed Rest and Physical Activity in Rheumatic Fever

No Carditis	Carditis, but No Cardiomegaly and no Heart Failure	Carditis, With Cardiomegaly but no Failure	Carditis, With Cardiomegaly and Heart Failure
Bed rest for three weeks; then gradual ambulation, even if taking aspirin	Bed rest for a month once carditis is detected; then gradual ambulation, even if taking aspirin	Strict bed rest for first two weeks after detection of cardiomegaly; then modified bed rest for four weeks; then gradual ambulation, even if receiving treatment; modified bed rest again during the "rebound period" (first two weeks after cessation of treatment); then gradual ambulation	Strict bed rest as long as heart failure is present; if severe, patient should be washed and fed by aides; after subsidence or control of heart failure, modified bed rest until a month after cessation of treatment if no rebound ensues, or until two weeks after spontaneous subsidence of rebound; then gradual ambulation

Analgesics or Anti-Inflammatory Agents

Patients with arthralgia alone or with mild arthritis and no carditis, may be given analgesics only. This is particularly wise when the diagnosis is not definite. Patients with moderate or severe arthritis but no carditis, or with carditis but no cardiomegaly or fever, are treated with aspirin: 40 to 45 mg/lb/day for the first 2 weeks, and 20 mg/lb/day for the following 6 weeks. Larger doses may be necessary to control arthritis. In patients with carditis and cardiomegaly but without congestive heart failure, with or without polyarthritis, treatment should be started with aspirin. In patients with marked cardiomegaly, aspirin is often insufficient to control fever, discomfort, and tachycardia, or it does so only at toxic or near-toxic doses. These patients may then be treated with corticosteroids.

Patients with carditis and heart failure, with or without polyarthritis, should receive prednisone, starting with a dose of 40 to 60 mg/day, to be increased if heart failure is not controlled. In cases of extreme acuteness and severity, therapy should be started by intravenous administration of methylprednisone, 10 to 40 mg, followed by oral prednisone. In 2 or 3 weeks, prednisone may be slowly withdrawn; one should decrease the daily dose at the rate of 5 mg every 2 or 3 days. When the dose is tapered, aspirin at standard doses should be added and continued for 3 or 4 weeks after prednisone is discontinued. This "overlap" therapy reduces the incidence of post-therapeutic clinical rebounds.

The termination of anti-inflammatory treatment may be followed in all patients with rheumatic fever by the reappearance, within two or three weeks, of laboratory or clinical abnormalities.[40] All patients with "laboratory" rebounds and most with clinical rebounds are best left untreated or should be treated symptomatically with small doses of aspirin or other analgesics, lest the full treatment be followed by another rebound and the illness prolonged. Only patients with the most severe clinical rebounds require reinstitution of the full original treatment.[114]

Unfortunately, most well-controlled studies have failed to prove that treatment with corticosteroids decreases the incidence of residual rheumatic heart disease.[24,25,42,135–137] Nevertheless, such treatment is indicated in patients with severe carditis and heart failure because of the distinct impression that death may be averted during the acute attack.[28] One may "tide the patient over the acute attack."

Once rheumatic fever has subsided and more than two months have passed after discontinuing treatment with aspirin or corticosteroids, the disease will not reappear unless the patient contracts a new streptococcal infection.[119]

Patients with chorea may benefit from the administration of tranquilizers.

PREVENTION OF RECURRENCES ("SECONDARY PREVENTION")

For all its simplicity, secondary prevention is the finest achievement of medicine in this disease. Its importance is out of proportion to the reduction in the number of rheumatic fever attacks because recurrences are more dangerous than initial attacks.

Initial "Eradicating" Treatment

As soon as the diagnosis of rheumatic fever is made, but not sooner, lest other possible diagnoses be obscured, patients are customarily treated as if they had streptococcal pharyngitis, even though streptococci may not be cultured. One can then start continual prophylaxis with a "clean slate" and clearly identify new infections, should they occur.

Continual Parenteral Prophylaxis

Best results are obtained with the injection of 1.2 million U benzathine penicillin G every 4 weeks.[130,144] This treatment of choice is especially useful in high-risk patients, that is, those with rheumatic heart disease, a previous episode within the past 3 years, or multiple attacks, or in those unlikely to take daily medication. Additional risk factors are youth (childhood and adolescence), exposure to young people, and crowding in the home.

Continual Oral Prophylaxis

In patients intolerant of benzathine penicillin prophylaxis because of pain at the site of injection, continual oral medication may be prescribed. Its success depends on the compliance of the patient, which is often worse than one may think.[47] Sulfadiazine, at a dose of 0.5 g once daily in children weighing less than 60 pounds and 1 g in others, and oral penicillin, at a dose of 200,000 to 250,000 U twice a day, are about equally effective.[34]

Duration of Continual Prophylaxis

For maximum protection, continual prophylaxis may be maintained for the lifetime of the patient, particularly patients with rheumatic heart disease. The risk factors mentioned earlier may guide the physician in persuading each patient to comply with an individually tailored prophylactic drug regimen.[126]

Prevention of Infective Endocarditis

Rheumatic heart disease predisposes patients to infective endocarditis. It is advisable to administer appropriate antibiotics to patients with rheumatic heart disease whenever they are exposed to a procedure that causes bacteremia.[57,57a]

PREVENTION OF INITIAL EPISODE ("PRIMARY PREVENTION")

Although prevention of recurrences is both important and attainable, rheumatic fever can be eradicated only by preventing initial episodes. Moreover, the hearts of many patients are irreparably damaged by a first episode; for them, the triumphs of secondary prophylaxis are no consolation. This important field of medicine, however, pertains more to pediatricians, family physicians, emergency room physicians, and general internists than to rheumatologists. All are referred to the appropriate textbooks or to the American Heart Association Recommendations. Physicians with more than a casual interest may enjoy the proceedings of a recent conference.[45] A streptococcal vaccine, which is nearly ready, may provide a solution where needed.[6,116]

REFERENCES

1. Agarwal, B.L.: Rheumatic heart diseases unabated in developing countries. Lancet, 2:910, 1981.
2. Alexander, W.D., and Smith, G.: Disadvantageous circulatory effects of salicylate in rheumatic fever. Lancet, 1:768, 1962.
3. Annegero, J.F., et al.: Rheumatic fever in Rochester, Minnesota, 1935–1978. Mayo Clin. Proc., 57:753, 1982.
4. Aron, A.M., Freeman, J.M., and Carter, S.: The natural history of Sydenham's chorea. Review of the literature and long-term evaluation with emphasis on cardiac sequelae. Am. J. Med., 38:83, 1965.
5. Barnert, A.L., Jerry, E.E., and Persellin, R.H.: Acute rheumatic fever in adults. JAMA, 232:925, 1975.
6. Beachey, E.H., Stollerman, G.H., and Bisno, A.L.: A strep vaccine: how close? Hosp. Pract., 149:57, 1979.
7. Ben-Dov, I., and Berry, E.: Acute rheumatic fever in adults over the age of 45 years; an analysis of 23 patients together with a review of the literature. Semin. Arthritis Rheum., 10:100, 1980.
8. Bernstein, S.H., and Allerhand, J.: Abnormalities of serum proteins as criteria for the diagnosis of acute rheumatic fever. Am. J. Med. Sci., 247:431, 1964.
9. Bisno, A.L.: In Streptococcal Diseases and the Immune Response. Edited by S.E. Read and J.B. Zabriskie. New York, Academic Press, 1980.
10. Bisno, A.L., and Ofek, I.: Serologic diagnosis of streptococcal infection. Comparison of a rapid hemagglutination technique with conventional antibody tests. Am. J. Dis. Child., 127:676, 1974.
11. Bittl, J.A., and Perloff, J.K.: Chronic postrheumatic fever arthropathy of Jaccoud. Am. Heart J., 105:515, 1983.
12. Bland, E.F.: Chorea as a manifestation of rheumatic fever: a long term perspective. Trans. Am. Clin. Climatol. Assoc., 73:209, 1961.
13. Bland, E.F., and Duckett Jones, T.: Rheumatic fever and rheumatic heart disease—a twenty year report on 1000 patients followed since childhood. Circulation, 4:836, 1951.
14. Bywaters, E.G.L.: Jaccoud's syndrome: a sequel to the joint involvement of systemic lupus erythematosus. Clin. Rheum. Dis., 1:125, 1975.
15. Bywaters, E.G.L.: The relation between heart and joint disease including "rheumatoid heart disease" and chronic post-rheumatic arthritis (type Jaccoud). Br. Heart J., 12:101, 1950.
16. Bywaters, E.G.L., and Thomas, G.T.: Bed rest, salicylates, and steroid in rheumatic fever. Br. Med. J., 1:1628, 1962.
17. Bywaters, E.G.L., Glynn, L.E., and Zeldis, A.: Subcutaneous nodules of Still's disease. Ann. Rheum. Dis., 17:278, 1958.
18. Cantanzaro, F.J., Rammelkamp, C.H., Jr., and Chamovits, R.: Prevention of rheumatic fever by treatment of streptococcal infections. N. Engl. J. Med., 259:51, 1958.
19. Cherian, G., et al.: Mitral valvotomy in young patients. Br. Heart J., 26:157, 1964.
20. Chun, R.W.M., et al.: Benign familial chorea with onset in childhood. JAMA, 225:1603, 1973.
21. Coburn, A.F.: The Factor of Infection in the Rheumatic State. Baltimore, Williams & Wilkins, 1931.
22. Coburn, A.F., and Moore, L.V.: The prophylactic use of sulfanilamide in streptococcal respiratory infections, with especial reference to rheumatic fever. J. Clin. Invest., 18:147, 1939.
23. Cohen, S., et al.: The kidney in acute rheumatic fever. Clinicopathological correlations. Arch. Intern. Med., 127:245, 1971.
24. Combined Rheumatic Fever Study Group: A comparison of short-term, intensive prednisone and acetylsalicylic acid therapy in the treatment of acute rheumatic fever. N. Engl. J. Med., 272:63, 1965.
25. Combined Rheumatic Fever Study Group: A comparison of the effect of prednisone and acetylsalicylic acid on the incidence of residual rheumatic heart disease. N. Engl. J. Med., 262:895, 1960.

26. Cooper, L.A., et al.: Transient arthritis after rubella vaccination. Am. J. Dis. Child., 118:218, 1969.

27. Cristal, N., Stern, J., and Gueron, M.: Atrioventricular dissociation in acute rheumatic fever. Br. Heart J., 33:12, 1971.

28. Czoniczer, G., et al.: Therapy of severe rheumatic carditis. Comparison of adrenocortical steroids and aspirin. Circulation, 29:813, 1964.

29. DiSciascio, G., and Taranta, A.: Rheumatic fever in children. Am. Heart J., 99:635, 1980.

30. Dorfman, A., Gross, J.I., and Lorincz, A.E.: The treatment of acute rheumatic fever. Pediatrics, 27:692, 1961.

31. Doyle, E.F., et al.: The risk of bacterial endocarditis during antirheumatic prophylaxis. JAMA, 201:807, 1967.

32. El-Sadr, W., and Taranta, A.: The spectrum and the specter of rheumatic fever in the 1980's. Clin. Immunol. Update, 183–209, 1979.

33. Esdaile, J.M., et al.: Deforming arthritis in systemic lupus erythematosus. Ann. Rheum. Dis., 40:124, 1981.

34. Feinstein, A.R., et al.: Oral prophylaxis of recurrent rheumatic fever. Sulfadiazine vs. a double daily dose of penicillin. JAMA, 188:489, 1964.

35. Feinstein, A.R., et al.: Rheumatic fever in children and adolescents: a long-term epidemiologic study of subsequent prophylaxis, streptococcal infections, and clinical sequelae. VII. Cardiac changes and sequelae. Ann. Intern. Med., 60:87, 1964.

36. Feinstein, A.R., and Di Massa, R.: The unheard diastolic murmur in acute rheumatic fever. N. Engl. J. Med., 260:133, 1959.

37. Feinstein, A.R., and Spagnuolo, M.: The clinical patterns of acute rheumatic fever: a reappraisal. Medicine, 41:279, 1962.

38. Feinstein, A.R., and Spagnuolo, M.: Mimetic features of rheumatic-fever recurrences. N. Engl. J. Med., 262:533, 1960.

39. Feinstein, A.R., and Spagnuolo, M.: Prognostic significance of valvular involvement in acute rheumatic fever. N. Engl. J. Med., 260:1001, 1959.

40. Feinstein, A.R., Spagnuolo, M., and Gill, F.A.: The rebound phenomenon in acute rheumatic fever. 1. Incidence and significance. Yale J. Biol. Med., 33:259, 1961.

41. Fernandez, R., and McCarty, D.J.: The arthritis of viral hepatitis. Ann. Intern. Med., 74:207, 1971.

42. Friedman, S., Harris, T.N., and Caddell, J.L.: Long-term effects of ACTH and cortisone therapy in rheumatic fever. Pediatrics, 60:55, 1962.

43. Gibney, R., et al.: Renal lesions in acute rheumatic fever. Ann. Intern. Med., 94:322, 1981.

44. Girgis, F.L., Popple, A.W., Bruckner, F.E.: Jaccoud's arthropathy. A case report and necropsy study. Ann. Rheum. Dis., 37:561, 1978.

45. Gordis, L.: Changing risk of rheumatic fever in management of pharyngitis in an era of declining rheumatic fever. In Report on the Eighty-sixth Ross Conference on Pediatric Research. Columbus, Ohio, Ross Laboratories, 1984.

46. Gordis, L., Lilienfeld, A., and Rodriguez, R.: Studies in the epidemiology and preventability of rheumatic fever. II. Socio-economic factors and the incidence of acute attacks. J. Chronic Dis., 21:655, 1969.

47. Gordis, L., Markowitz, M., Lilienfeld, A.M.: The inaccuracy in using interviews to estimate patient reliability in taking medications at home. Med. Care, 7:49, 1969.

48. Graef, I., et al.: Studies in Rheumatic Fever. The natural course of acute manifestations of rheumatic fever uninfluenced by "specific" therapy. Am. J. Med. Sci., 185:197, 1933.

49. Grishman, E., et al.: Renal lesions in acute rheumatic fever. Am. J. Pathol., 51:1045, 1967.

50. Grossman, B.J.: Early ambulation in the treatment of acute rheumatic fever. A controlled study in children with acute rheumatic fever treated with prednisone. Am. J. Dis. Child., 115:557, 1968.

51. Haas, R.C., Taranta, A., and Wood, H.F.: Effect of intramuscular injections of benzathine penicillin G on some acute-phase reactants. N. Engl. J. Med., 256:152, 1957.

52. Handsfield, H.H., Wiesner, P.J., and Holmes, K.K.: Treatment of the gonococcal arthritis-dermatitis syndrome. Ann. Intern. Med., 84:661, 1976.

53. Houser, H. (Cited by Mortimer, E.A., and Rammelkamp, C.H.): Prophylaxis of rheumatic fever. Circulation, 14:1144, 1956.

54. Ignaczak, T., et al.: Jaccoud arthritis. Arch. Intern. Med., 135:577, 1975.

55. Jacobs, J.C.: Pediatric Rheumatology for the Practitioner. New York, Springer-Verlag, 1982.

56. Janeff, J., et al.: A screening test for streptococcal antibodies. Lab. Med., 2:38, 1971.

57. Kaplan, E., and Taranta, A. (Eds.): Infective Endocarditis—An American Heart Association Symposium. Dallas, American Heart Association, 1977.

57a. Kaplan, E.L., et al.: Prevention of bacterial endocarditis: AHA committee report. Circulation, 56:139A, 1977.

58. Kaplan, E.L., and Wannamaker, L.W.: Streptolysin O: suppression of its antigenicity by lipids extracted from skin. Proc. Soc. Exp. Biol. Med., 146:205, 1974.

59. Kaplan, M.H., et al.: Presence of bound immunoglobulins and complement in the myocardium in acute rheumatic fever. Association with cardiac failure. N. Engl. J. Med., 271:637, 1964.

60. Kaplan, M.H., and Dallenbach, F.D.: Immunologic studies of heart tissue. III. Occurrence of bound gamma globulin in auricular appendages from rheumatic hearts. Relationship to certain histopathologic features of rheumatic heart disease. J. Exp. Med., 113:1, 1961.

61. Kaplan, M.H., and Svec, K.H.: Immunologic relation of streptococcal and tissue antigens. III. Presence in human sera of streptococcal antibody cross-reactive with heart tissue: association with streptococcal infection, rheumatic fever, and glomerulonephritis. J. Exp. Med., 119:651, 1964.

62. Keil, H.: The rheumatic erythemas; a critical survey. Ann Intern. Med., 11:2223, 1938.

63. Keil, H.: The rheumatic subcutaneous nodules and simulating lesions, Medicine, 17:261, 1938.

64. Keiser, H., et al.: Clinical forms of gonococcal arthritis. N. Engl. J. Med., 279:234, 1968.

65. Kuttner, A.G., and Krumwiede, E.: Observations on the effect of streptococcal upper respiratory infections on rheumatic children: a three-year study. J. Clin. Invest., 20:275, 1941.

66. Laitinen, O., Leirisalo, M., and Allander, E.: Rheumatic fever and yersinia arthritis; criteria and diagnostic problems in a changing disease pattern. Scand. J. Rheumatol., 4:145, 1975.

67. Land, M.A., and Bisno, A.L.: Acute rheumatic fever: a vanishing disease in suburbia. JAMA, 249:895, 1983.

68. Lehndorff, H., and Leiner, C.: Erythema annulare. Ein typisches Exanthem bei Endokarditis. Kinderheilk., 32:46, 1922.

69. Leirisalo, M., and Laitinen, O.: Rheumatic fever in adult patients. Ann. Clin. Res., 7:244, 1975.

70. Lenox, C.C., et al.: Arrhythmias and Stokes-Adams attacks in acute rheumatic fever. Pediatrics, 61:599, 1978.

71. Levine, S., and Harvey, W.P.: Clinical Auscultation of the Heart. 2nd Ed. Philadelphia, W.B. Saunders, 1959.

72. Lewis-Johnson, J.: Chorea: J B nomenclature, etiology and epidemiology in a clinical material from Malmohus County. Acta Pediatr. Scand., 76:1, 1949.

73. Lortscher, R.H., et al.: Left atrial myxoma presenting as rheumatic fever. Chest, 66:302, 1974.

74. McDonald, E.C., and Weisman, M.H.: Articular manifestations of rheumatic fever in adults. Ann. Intern. Med., 89:917, 1978.

75. McIntosch, R., and Wood, C.L.: Rheumatic infections occurring in the first three years of life. Am. J. Dis. Child., 49:835, 1935.

76. McLaughlin, J.F., et al.: Rheumatic carditis: in vitro responses of peripheral blood leukocytes to heart and streptococcal antigens. Arthritis Rheum., 15:600, 1972.

77. McMinn, F.J., and Bywaters, E.G.L.: Differences between the fever of Still's disease and that of rheumatic fever. Ann. Rheum. Dis., 18:293, 1959.

78. Manso, C., Taranta, A., and Nydick, S.: Effect of aspirin administration on serum glutamic oxaloacetic and glu-

tamic pyruvic transaminase in children. Proc. Soc. Exp. Biol. Med., *93*:84, 1956.

79. Markowitz, M., and Gordis, L.: Rheumatic Fever. 2nd Ed. Philadelphia, W.B. Saunders, 1972.

80. Markowitz, M. and Kuttner, A.G.: Rheumatic fever: diagnosis, management and prevention. Philadelphia, W.B. Saunders, 1965.

81. Massell, B.G., Amezcua, F., and Pelargonio, S.: Evolving picture of rheumatic fever: data from 40 years at the House of the Good Samaritan. JAMA, *188*:287, 1964.

82. Massell, B.F., Fyler, D.C., and Rey, S.B.: The clinical picture of rheumatic fever. Diagnosis, immediate prognosis, course, and therapeutic implications. Am. J. Cardiol., *1*:436, 1958.

83. Mauer, A.M.: The early anemia of acute rheumatic fever. Pediatrics, *27*:707, 1961.

84. Mayer, F.E., et al.: Declining severity of first attack of rheumatic fever. Am. J. Dis. Child., *105*:146, 1963.

85. Mazzara, J.T., et al.: Coexistence of sickle-cell anemia and rheumatic heart disease. N.Y. State J. Med., *71*:2426, 1971.

85a. Meyers, O.L., and Chalmers, I.M.: Jaccoud's arthropathy. S. Afr. Med. J., *51*:753, 1977.

86. Mirowski, M., Rosenstein, B.J., and Markowitz, M.: A comparison of atrio-ventricular conduction in normal children and in patients with rheumatic fever, glomerulonephritis, and acute febrile illnesses. A quantitative study with determination of the P–R index. Pediatrics, *33*:334, 1964.

87. Mitkov, V.: Cerebral manifestations of rheumatic fever. World Neurol., *2*:920, 1961.

88. Mohs, E.: Infectious diseases and health in Costa Rica: the development of a new paradigm. Pediatr. Infect. Dis., *1*:2126, 1982.

89. Murphy, G.E.: The characteristic rheumatic lesions of striated and of non-striated or smooth muscle cells of the heart. Genesis of the lesions known as Aschoff bodies and those myogenic components known as Aschoff cells or as Anitschkow cells or myocytes. Medicine, *42*:73, 1963.

89a. Murphy, G.E.: Evolution of our knowledge of rheumatic fever: historical survey; with particular emphasis on rheumatic heart disease. Bull. Hist. Med., *14*:123, 1943.

90. Murphy, G.E., and Becker, C.G.: Occurrence of caterpillar nuclei within normal immature and normal appearing and altered mature heart muscle cells and the evolution of Anitschkow cells from the latter. Am. J. Pathol., *48*:931, 1966.

90a. Murphy, W.A., and Staple, T.W.: Jaccoud's arthropathy reviewed. AJR, *118*:300–307, 1973.

91. Osler, W.: On Chorea and Choreiform Affections. Philadelphia, P. Blakiston, Son, 1894.

92. Pader, E., and Elster, S.K.: Studies of acute rheumatic fever in the adult. I. Clinical and laboratory manifestations in thirty patients. Am. J. Med., *26*:424, 1959.

93. Patarroyo, M.E., et al.: Association of a B-cell alloantigen with susceptibility to rheumatic fever. Nature, *278*:173, 1979.

94. Perry, B.C.: Erythema marginatum (rheumaticum). Arch. Dis. Child., *12*:233, 1937.

95. Perry, B.C., and Roberts, M.A.F.: A study on the variability in the incidence of rheumatic heart disease within the city of Bristol. Br. Med. J., *154 (Suppl.)*:1937.

96. Persellin, S.T., Ramirez, G., and Moatamed, F.: Immunopathology of rheumatic pericarditis. Arthritis Rheum., *25*:1054, 1982.

97. Pilapil, V.R., and Watson, D.G.: Rheumatic fever in Mississippi: 104 cases seen over a decade. JAMA, *215*:1626, 1971.

98. Potter, E.V., et al.: Tropical acute rheumatic fever and associated streptococcal infections compared with concurrent acute glomerulonephritis. J. Pediatr., *92*:325, 1978.

98a. Raizada, V., et al.: Tissue distribution of lymphocytes in rheumatic heart valves as defined by monoclonal anti-T cell antibodies. Am. J. Med., *74*:90, 1983.

99. Rammelkamp, C.H., Jr.: Epidemiology of streptococcal infections. Harvey Lect., *15*:113, 1955–1956.

100. Rammelkamp, C.H., Jr., and Stolzer, B.L.: The latent period before the onset of acute rheumatic fever. Yale J. Biol. Med., *34*:386, 1961–1962.

101. Rammelkamp, C.H., Jr., and Weaver, R.S.: Acute glomerulonephritis. The significance of the variations in the incidence of the disease. J. Clin. Invest., *32*:345, 1953.

102. Reddy, K.S., Rao, P.S., and Bhatia, M.L.: Immunopathogenesis of rheumatic fever and rheumatic heart disease. Indian J. Pediatr., *49*:849, 1982.

103. Reed, W.P., et al.: Streptococcal adherence to pharyngeal cells of children with rheumatic fever. J. Infect. Dis., *142*:803, 1980.

104. Reimann, H.A.: Pneumonia. Springfield, IL, Charles C Thomas, 1954.

105. Rosenthal, A., Czoniczer, G., and Massell, B.F.: Rheumatic fever under 3 years of age. A report of 10 cases. Pediatrics, *41*:612, 1968.

106. Roth, I.R., Lingg, C., and Whittemore, A.: Heart disease in children. A. Rheumatic Group. I. Certain aspects of the age at onset and of recurrences in 488 cases of juvenile rheumatism ushered in by major clinical manifestations. Am. Heart J., *13*:36, 1937.

107. Roy, S.B., et al.: Juvenile mitral stenosis in India. Lancet, *2*:1193, 1963.

108. Roy, S.B., Sturges, G.P., and Massell, B.F.: Application of the antistreptolysin-O titer in the evaluation of joint pain and in the diagnosis of rheumatic fever. N. Engl. J. Med., *254*:95, 1956.

109. Ruderman, J.E., and Abruzzo, J.L.: Chronic postrheumatic-fever arthritis (Jaccoud's): report of a case with subcutaneous nodules. Arthritis Rheum., *9*:640, 1966.

110. Sanyal, S.K., et al.: The initial attack of acute rheumatic fever during childhood in North India: a prospective study of the clinical profile. Circulation, *49*:7, 1974.

111. Saphir, O., and Langendorf, R.: Nonspecific myocarditis in acute rheumatic fever. Am. Heart J., *46*:432, 1953.

111a. Selinger, D.S., et al.: Adherence of group A streptococci to pharyngeal cells: a role in the pathogenesis of rheumatic fever. Science: *201*:455, 1978.

112. Serlin, S.P., Rimsza, M.E., and Gay, J.H.: Rheumatic pneumonia: the need for a new approach. Pediatrics, *56*:1075, 1975.

113. Shumaker, J.B., et al.: Arthritis and rash: clues to anicteric viral hepatitis. Arch. Intern. Med., *133*:483, 1974.

114. Spagnuolo, M., and Feinstein, A.R.: The rebound phenomenon in acute rheumatic fever. II. Treatment and prevention. Yale J. Biol. Med., *33*:279, 1961.

115. Spagnuolo, M., Pasternak, B., and Taranta, A.: Risk of rheumatic fever recurrences after streptococcal infections. Prospective study of clinical and social factors. N. Engl. J. Med., *285*:641, 1971.

116. Stollerman, G.H.: Global changes in group A Streptococcal diseases and strategies for their prevention. Adv. Intern. Med., *27*:373, 1982.

117. Stollerman, G.H.: Rheumatic Fever and Streptococcal Infection. New York, Grune & Stratton, 1975.

118. Stollerman, G.H., et al.: Jones criteria (revised) for guidance in the diagnosis of rheumatic fever. Circulation, *32*:665, 1965.

119. Stollerman, G.H., et al.: Relationship of immune response to group A streptococci to the course of acute, chronic and recurrent rheumatic fever. Am. J. Med., *20*:163, 1956.

120. Stollerman, G.H., Siegel, A.C., and Johnson, E.E.: Variable epidemiology of streptococcal disease and the changing pattern of rheumatic fever. Mod. Concepts Cardiovasc. Dis., *34*:45, 1965.

121. Svartman, M., et al.: Immunglobulins and complement components in synovial fluid of patients with acute rheumatic fever. J. Clin. Invest., *56*:111, 1975.

122. Taranta, A.: Recent advances in the diagnosis and in the prevention of rheumatic fever. Bol. Assoc. Med. P.R., *69*:45, 1977.

123. Taranta, A.: Rheumatic fever made difficult: a critical review of pathogenetic theories. Pediatrician, *5*:74, 1976.

124. Taranta, A.: Occurrence of rheumatic-like subcutaneous nodules without evidence of joint or heart disease. N. Engl. J. Med., *266*:13, 1962.

125. Taranta, A.: Relation of isolated recurrences of Sydenham's chorea to preceding streptococcal infections. N. Engl. J. Med., *260*:1204, 1959.

126. Taranta, A., et al.: (Rheumatic fever and rheumatic heart disease study group) Resources for the management of patients with rheumatic heart disease. Circulation, *44*:273, 1971.

127. Taranta, A., et al.: Rheumatic fever in children and adolescents. A long-term epidemiologic study of subsequent prophylaxis, streptococcal infections, and clinical sequelae. V. Relation of the rheumatic fever recurrence rate per streptococcal infection to pre-existing clinical features of the patients. Ann. Intern. Med., *60*:58, 1964.

128. Taranta, A., et al.: Rheumatic fever in children and adolescents. A long-term epidemiologic study of subsequent prophylaxis, streptococcal infections, and clinical sequelae. IV. Relation of the rheumatic fever recurrence rate per streptococcal infection to the titers of streptococcal antibodies. Ann. Intern. Med., *60 (Suppl. 5)*:47, 1964.

129. Taranta, A., et al.: Rheumatic fever in monozygotic and dizygotic twins. *In* Proceedings of the Tenth International Congress of Rheumatology. Minerva Med., *96*, 1961.

130. Taranta, A., and Gordis, L.: The prevention of rheumatic fever: opportunities, frustrations, and challenges. Cardiovasc. Clin., *4*:1, 1972.

131. Taranta, A., and Markowitz, M.: Rheumatic Fever. Boston, MTP Press, 1981.

132. Taranta, A., and Stollerman, G.H.: The relationship of Sydenham's chorea to infection with group A streptococci. Am. J. Med., *20*:170, 1956.

133. Taranta, A., Spagnuolo, M., and Feinstein, A.R.: Chronic rheumatic fever. Ann. Intern. Med., *56*:367, 1962.

134. Tompkins, D.G., Boxerbaum, B., and Liebman, J.: Long-term prognosis of rheumatic fever patients receiving regular intramuscular benzathine penicillin. Circulation, *45*:543, 1972.

135. United Kingdom and United States Joint Report: The natural history of rheumatic fever and rheumatic heart disease: ten-year report of a cooperative clinical trial of ACTH, cortisone, and aspirin. Circulation, *32*:457, 1965.

136. United Kingdom and United States Joint Report: The evolution of rheumatic heart disease in children: five-year report of a cooperative clinical trial of ACTH, cortisone and aspirin. Circulation, *22*:503, 1960.

137. United Kingdom and United States Joint Report: The treatment of acute rheumatic fever in children: a cooperative clinical trial of ACTH, cortisone and aspirin. Circulation, *11*:343, 1955.

138. Van de Rijn, I., Zabriskie, J.B., and McCarty, M.: Group A streptococcal antigen cross-reactive with myocardium. Purification of heart-reactive antibody and isolation and characterization of the streptococcal antigen. J. Exp. Med., *146*:579, 1977.

139. Vijayaraghavan, G., et al.: Rheumatic aortic stenosis in young patients presenting with combined aortic and mitral stenosis. Br. Heart J., *39*:294, 1977.

140. Wannamaker, L.W.: T. Duckett Jones Memorial Lecture: The chain that links the heart to the throat. Circulation, *48*:9, 1973.

141. Wannamaker, L.W., et al.: Prophylaxis of acute rheumatic fever by treatment of the preceding streptococcal infection with various amounts of depot penicillin. Am. J. Med., *10*:673, 1951.

142. Wannamaker, L.W., and Matsen, J.M. (Eds.): Streptococci and Streptococcal Diseases. New York, Academic Press, 1972:

143. Ward, C.: Observations of the diagnosis of isolated rheumatic carditis. Am. Heart J., *91*:545, 1976.

143a. Williams, R.C.: Host factors in rheumatic fever and heart disease. Hosp. Pract., *17*:125, 1982.

144. Wood, H.F., et al.: Rheumatic fever in children and adolescents. A long-term epidemiologic study of subsequent prophylaxis, streptococcal infections, and clinical sequelae. III. Comparative effectiveness of three prophylaxis regimens in preventing streptococcal infections and rheumatic recurrences. Ann. Intern. Med., *60 (Suppl. 5)*:31, 1964.

145. Yang, L.C., et al.: Streptococcal-induced cell-mediated-immune destruction of cardiac myofibers in vitro. J. Exp. Med., *146*:344, 1977.

146. Zabriskie, J.B. (Ed.): Streptococcal Diseases and the Immune Response. New York, Academic Press, 1980.

147. Zvaifler, N.J.: Chronic postrheumatic-fever (Jaccoud's) arthritis. N. Engl. J. Med., *267*:10, 1962.

Chapter 69

Relapsing Polychondritis

David E. Trentham

Relapsing polychondritis is an uncommon entity whose manifestations are frequently widespread and dramatic. The essential features are inflammation with progressive loss of structural integrity of some cartilaginous tissues and involvement of organs of special sense such as the eye, the middle and inner ears, and the vestibular apparatus. Aortic insufficiency can also occur.

Prior to 1958, the medical literature contained only 10 single case reports, but since that time the condition has become widely recognized as a distinct clinical entity.[1,2,4,8,10] Many of the earlier authors did not realize that similar patients had been described before, and each invented his own descriptive terms for the disease. Thus, some of the terms used for relapsing polychondritis were "systemic chondromalacia," "panchondritis," and "chronic atrophic polychondritis." "Relapsing polychondritis" best describes the undulating clinical course that this syndrome follows, although admittedly it does not take into account the frequent involvement of some noncartilaginous structures.

CLINICAL FEATURES

The earliest identifiable report of relapsing polychondritis, published in 1923 by Jaksch-Wartenhorst,[9] still provides a clear picture of the disease. His patient, a 32-year-old brewer, first became ill with arthritic swellings and pain in several finger joints and then in the wrists, left hand, right knee, and toes of the right foot. There was also a febrile response. One-and-a-half months later, burning pain developed in both external ears, which slowly swelled and, within the next three months, receded and shrank, leaving a flabby deformity of both auricles. Two or three months later, without pain, the mid-segment of the nose slowly collapsed, leaving a saddle-nose deformity. At that time, there was nearly complete stenosis of both auditory canals and some diminution of hearing, even when the canals were held open. Associated dizziness and tinnitus also occurred. Somewhat later, crepitation developed in both knees and in the spine.

The disease occurs equally in both sexes. It is most common in the middle decades of life, but cases have been reported in children and the elderly. Although it is often fatal, the clinical course is highly variable and may be self-limited. One study reported a 7-year average life span in 11 patients from the time of appearance of symptoms to death, but the spectrum of survival ranged widely, from 10 months to over 20 years.[4] The causes of death were usually respiratory failure due to airway stenosis (or collapse) and complicating pulmonary infection and cardiovascular failure due to intractable aortic insufficiency.[1,4] Table 69–1 summarizes many of the clinical manifestations and their incidence.

Inflammation of isolated or multiple cartilages predominates, often with an initial febrile response and involvement of one or several structures of the eye. Onset is usually acute in the first and subsequent attacks unless the latter are modified by glucocorticoid therapy. Typically, the pinnas, or cartilaginous portions of the ears, swell and become purplish-red and exquisitely tender, so that it is impossible to rest them on a pillow. The soft earlobes are always spared. The external auditory canals, especially the meatus, also swell and may close almost completely; hearing is thereby reduced. Inflammation of the inner ear producing serous otitis media and obstruction of the eustachian tube from cartilage involvement in its nasopharyngeal portion can further impair hearing.[14] A labyrinthine type of vertigo may develop. Often, the episclerae are inflamed. Joint inflammation or simple arthralgias occasionally occur during these attacks. Sometimes, the cartilaginous portion of the bridge of the nose becomes inflamed during the first or later episodes.

An attack lasts from a few days to many weeks, and may, if left untreated, progress in a subacute or smoldering fashion to involve additional cartilaginous structures and special sense organs. As the inflammatory phase subsides, the external ear may shrink owing to the thinning of the cartilage or the loss of its structural integrity, so that the pinna droops forward from lack of support (Fig. 69–1). This condition may occur during the first episode or not until after several attacks. Similarly, the cartilaginous nasal septum may erode (Fig. 69–2), leaving a step-shaped or saddle nose, which is also characteristic for this conditon.

The two most serious complications of relapsing

Table 69–1.   Incidence of Various Clinical Features in Relapsing Polychondritis*

Manifestation	No. Affected/No. Reported	Frequency (%)
Ear cartilage involvement	45/51	88
Nasal cartilage involvement	40/49	82
Fever	21/26	81
Arthropathy	40/51	78
Laryngotracheal involvement	33/47	70
Episcleritis or conjunctivitis	29/48	60
Defective hearing	21/44	48
Costochondral cartilage involvement	21/45	47
Iritis	11/41	27
Labyrinthine vertigo†	—	25
Aortic valve lesion with insufficiency‡	10/74	14

*Modified from Dolan, D.L., et al.[4]
†Rough approximation of incidence. These organ systems were not always clearly described.
‡Data from Arkin, C.R., and Masi, A.T.[1] and others.

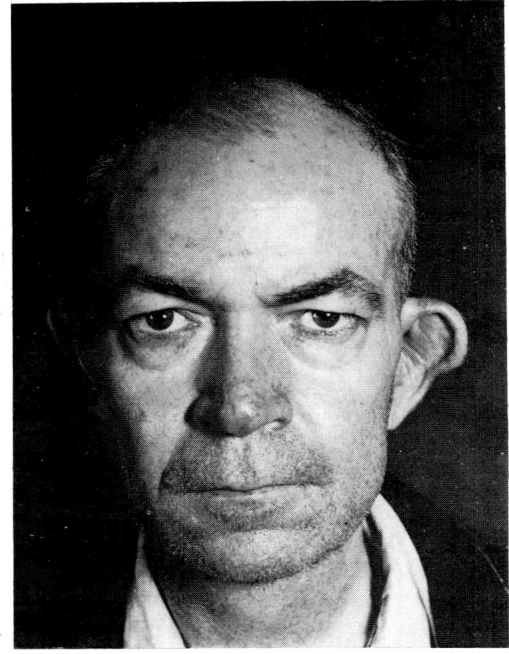

Fig. 69–1. Classic drooping of the left external ear in a man with recurrent episodes of polychondritis.

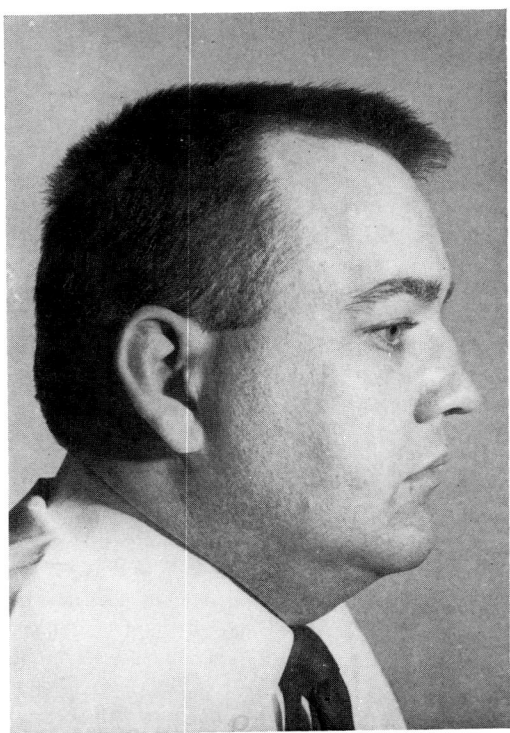

Fig. 69–2. The characteristic saddle-nose deformity had developed painlessly three months earlier.

polychondritis are: (1) an involvement of the cartilaginous structures of the respiratory tract, and (2) progressive aortic insufficiency. In the mildest forms of the disease, the respiratory tract involvement consists of hoarseness, slight cough, and minimal tenderness of the larynx and trachea. In more severe instances, there may be extensive inflammation and edema of the laryngeal and epiglottal cartilages, necessitating emergency tracheostomy. A similar process may also involve the tracheal and bronchial rings so that diffuse narrowing of the airways may ensue. This complication may be fatal, owing to asphyxia and/or superimposed respiratory infection. Moreover, in such circumstances, tracheostomy may be inadequate to maintain adequate pulmonary ventilation. If the patient survives one or more chondrolytic attacks on the air passages, the cartilages may be left with some loss of structural support in the involved regions. The trachea and bronchi may then become diffusely or focally narrowed because of varying degrees of stenosis, or the cartilages may lose all or nearly all of their architectural support. They then appear at autopsy as floppy collapsible tubes. In such patients, intubation is useless because of the collapse throughout even the smallest bronchi.[20] As if such serious involvement of the respiratory apparatus is not enough, further embarrassment to breathing may, on occasion, be caused by tenderness and swelling of one or several costosternal cartilages. In rare instances, partial or complete dissolution may result, leaving a flail anterior chest plate.

Aortic insufficiency, the other life-threatening complication, has been described in approximately 10 to 15% of cases.[1,2] The aortic regurgitation is due to progressive dilatation of the aortic ring and, often, the ascending aorta, rather than to inflammation of the valve leaflets. This pattern of involvement helps to differentiate the aortic insufficiency of relapsing polychondritis from the regurgitation that occurs in ankylosing spondylitis, Reiter's syndrome, and certain other rheumatic diseases (Table 69–2). Rarely, polychondritis can be associated with dilatation of the annulus of the mitral and tricuspid valves.[2] Prosthetic valves have been inserted successfully in some patients.[1]

Eye lesions are common and include episcleritis, conjunctivitis and, less frequently, iritis. Usually, the inflammation smolders at a low level or resolves as an attack subsides. Rarely have serious sequelae resulted, but proptosis, cataracts, severe keratitis, and even blindness have occurred in isolated instances.[2]

Articular involvement is variable, usually consisting of subacute swelling and pain in one or several large joints of the extremities. The articulations of the spine, either the true apophyseal cartilages or the intervertebral discs, are rarely involved. Serious peripheral joint damage has not been a common occurrence. However, it may resemble low-grade rheumatoid arthritis or, conversely, may culminate in osteophyte formation that even limits joint mobility. In a series of 23 patients, arthritis was the presenting symptom in 35% and was a significant clinical feature during the course of relapsing polychondritis in 85% of patients.[15]

Minor hematopoietic, hepatic, and renal involvement has been described,[4] but in some cases, this may have represented another associated disease process.

The most curious clinical feature is the selectivity of the chondritic process. Not only are some cartilages and cartilaginous structures spared while others are extensively involved, but there exists in some patients a remarkable unilaterality so that only one ear or one eye may be affected, even after multiple attacks. Other disorders to be considered in the differential diagnosis of relapsing polychondritis, such as a bacterial perichondritis, trauma or frostbite, Wegener's granulomatosis, lethal midline granuloma, or Cogan's syndrome,[2] do not produce multifocal chondritic lesions. However, polychondritis may develop in patients with a variety of connective tissue diseases, including systemic lupus erythematosus, vasculitis, adult or juvenile rheumatoid arthritis, and Sjögren's syndrome.[1,2]

LABORATORY OBSERVATIONS

As may be anticipated, aside from diagnostic biopsy findings, the laboratory features are nonspecific.[4] The most common findings are noted during the active disease process. They consist of an increased ESR, some degree of leukocytosis and anemia, occasional low titer positivity for rheumatoid factor or antinuclear antibody, and modest serum protein alterations, such as a decreased albumin and increased alpha and gamma globulins.

The roentgenographic finding that is of the greatest value, diagnostically, is tracheal stenosis. After

Table 69–2. Aortic Insufficiency

Condition	Disease Causing
Valvulitis	Rheumatic fever Rheumatoid arthritis Ankylosing spondylitis* Endocarditis Reiter's syndrome* Behçet's syndrome*
Congenital	Bicuspid aortic valve
Dilatation of valve ring	Marfan's syndrome Syphilis Relapsing polychondritis Secondary to dissecting aneurysm Idiopathic

*Also dilatation of valve ring

multiple inflammatory attacks, the external ears may show calcific deposits. This finding is not specific for relapsing polychondritis, however, because it may result from other inflammatory conditions such as frostbite. The joints may show moderate destructive changes, often spotty and asymmetric, but sometimes suggestive of rheumatoid arthritis. On a chest film, major airways may be narrowed. The closure may be focal or diffuse and is most clearly visualized by tracheal tomography (Fig. 69–3). In the presence of aortic insufficiency, cardiomegaly is commonly found.

PATHOLOGY

The histopathology of relapsing polychondritis is highly characteristic.[2,10,11,13,19,20] Acidophilic (pink) coloration of the cartilage matrix, in contrast to the usual basophilic (blue) hue, is seen by routine hematoxylin and eosin staining (Fig. 69–4). Focal or diffuse infiltration by predominantly mononuclear inflammatory cells, with occasional polymorphonuclear leukocytes and plasma cells in the perichondrial tissues, is associated with the dissolution of cartilage from its periphery inward (Fig. 69–5). Fibroblastic granulation tissue frequently coexists and leads to partial sequestration of the cartilage matrix (see Fig. 69–4). This vigorous re-

parative response may culminate in the production of new cartilage.[13] Evidence of necrotizing angiitis or thrombosis is lacking. Rarely, calcium salts are found in the cartilage. Examination of the ocular globe in one patient revealed mononuclear inflammatory cells and plasma cells scattered about the episcleral vessels.

In involved cardiac and aortic structures, the aortic valve leaflets are normal, whereas the ascending aorta, especially the aortic ring, is dilated, with a loss of basophilia and degeneration, necrosis, and fibrosis. The primary pathologic change in the aortic ring and ascending aorta is in the media, with a loss of elastic tissue, a decrease in basophilia, and fibrosis. Associated focal acute and chronic inflammation occurs in these areas as well as in the adventitial blood vessels and in the vasa vasorum.

Histochemical studies have confirmed these findings and have revealed a loss of metachromasia in the residual cartilage matrix, with some preservation of metachromasia in the cytoplasm and in the immediate perilacunar zones around chondrocytes.[20] In the aorta, there was a moderate loss in neutral or acidic polysaccharides by the toluidine blue, azure A (pH 2.0), or PAS-alcian blue methods. Hale's method for sulfated mucopolysaccharides showed marked depletion of these components in the abnormal aortas and aortic rings.

By electron microscopy, cartilage from patients with active relapsing polychondritis contains greatly increased numbers of "matrix granules."[7] These are small (below 10 nm in diameter) stellate granules of medium electron density and are compatible with particles of cartilage matrix composed primarily of proteoglycan. These granules are usually not membrane limited and are seen in normal cartilage in small numbers. "Matrix vesicles," also present in these specimens, are larger than the matrix granule, measure about 1,000 nm, and are located extracellularly. Ultrastructurally, the vesicles and dense granules found in the lesions are more compatible with lysosomes than typical matrix vesicles or granules, because they are usually larger and more irregular in shape, and because they often contain multiple myelin-like laminated structures. The matrix vesicles possess a significant amount of alkaline phosphatase and ATP-ase activities, but a low acid phosphatase activity, which is usually a marker for lysosomes. The origin of these cartilage matrix vesicles is uncertain. Because they are extracellular, it is likely that they are budding from cellular membranes containing cytoplasmic debris. Other investigators have recognized a few dense bodies, which they interpreted as lysosomes, in the chondrocytes of the lesion.[7] Furthermore, they observed a large number of extracellular dense

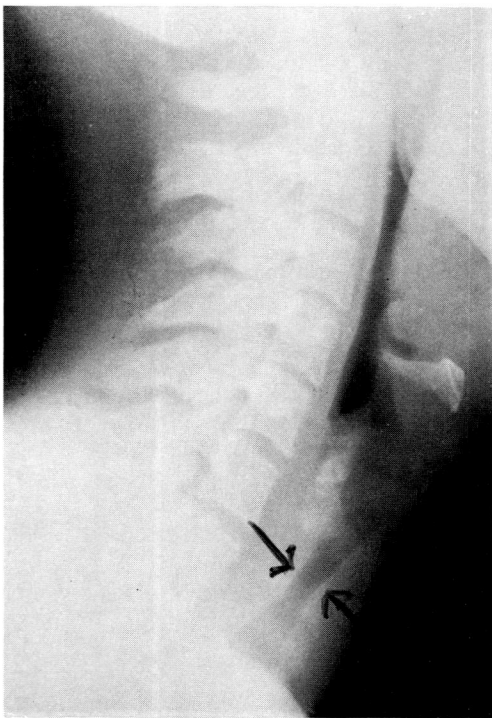

Fig. 69–3. Significant stenosis of the tracheal airway as demonstrated by air tomography in a 50-year-old woman with relapsing polychondritis.

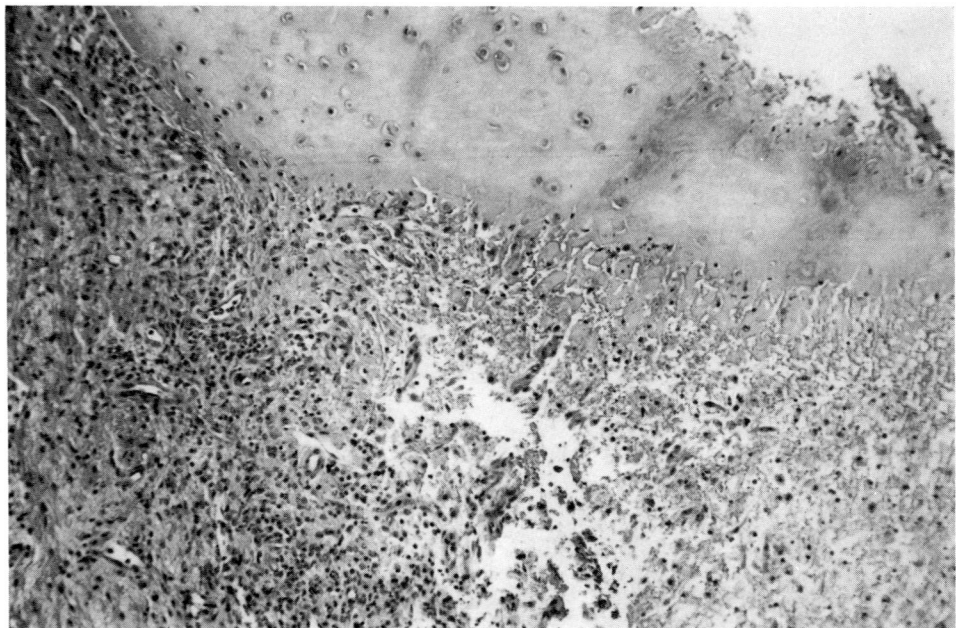

Fig. 69–4.   Chondrocyte necrosis, destruction of the matrix, and loss of basophilia in the elastic cartilage of the ear, sequestration of segments of cartilage by contiguous granulation tissue, and infiltration by inflammatory cells. These histopathologic features are characteristic of the cartilage lesion in relapsing polychondritis.

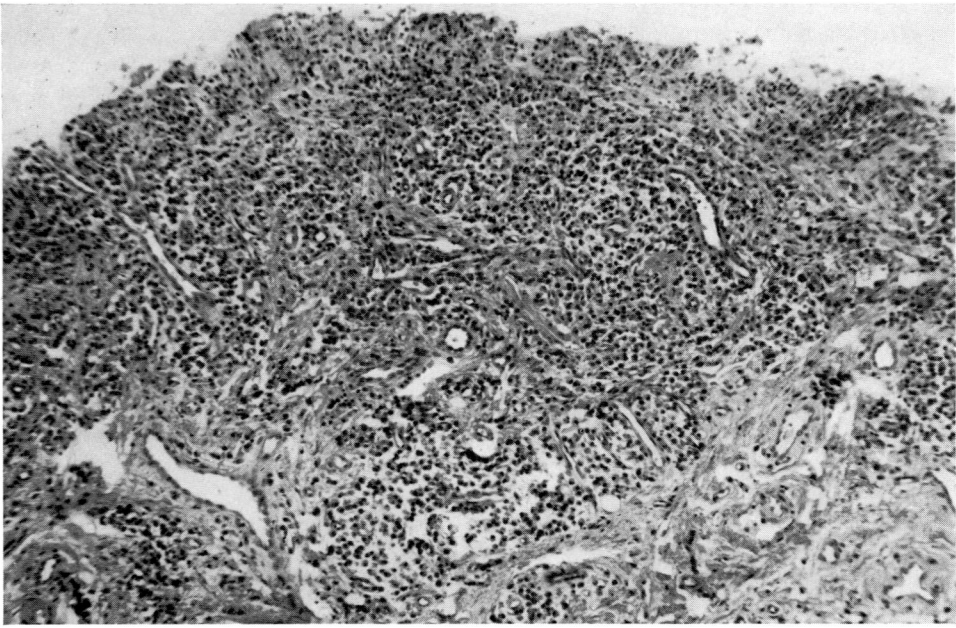

Fig. 69–5.   Marked cellular infiltration composed of mononuclear inflammatory cells, plasma cells, and histiocytes in the perichondrial tissues in relapsing polychondritis. Connective tissue and blood vessel elements have proliferated, but no vasculitis is present in this exuberant granulation tissue.

bodies containing multiple vesicles. Their significance is unknown.

Immunofluorescence studies of specimens from patients with relapsing polychondritis have identified granular deposits of IgG, IgA, IgM, and C3 at the lesional junction of fibrous and cartilaginous tissue, suggesting the presence of immune complexes.[2,13,16,19]

PATHOGENESIS

The etiology of relapsing polychondritis is unknown. The loss of acid mucopolysaccharides and many of the other cartilage changes that may be secondary events could be caused by release of lysosomal enzymes, especially proteases, either from chondrocytes or from other cellular elements. Thus, it is of potential interest that intravenously administered crude papain, a proteolytic enzyme, induced a noninflammatory dissolution of the ear cartilages of rabbits within 4 hours.[12] This reaction also involved a rapid loss of cartilage metachromasia. In addition, 3 to 6 weeks after a single intravenous injection of crude papain into rabbits, focal plaque lesions due to alterations of connective tissue of the media occurred in the ascending aorta and arch. Some of these lesions progressed by metaplasia into partially developed cartilage and bone.[18] It has been postulated that these lesions resulted from the release, by papain, of large amounts of sulfated mucopolysaccharides, which are then deposited in various organs and especially in the aortic wall. A similar mechanism may be operative in relapsing polychondritis, with an endogenous proteolytic enzyme, perhaps lysosomal, being responsible for the chondrolysis.

The identification of immunoglobulins in the lesions and the occasional coexistence of another systemic connective tissue disease are consistent with the possibility that autoimmune mechanisms cause the cartilage damage.[1–3,6,13,16,19] The ability of an autoimmune response to produce inflammation in both cartilage and ocular tissue could be explained by the reactivity being directed to a constituent shared by both structures. Type II collagen fulfills this requirement. Type II collagen is a brisk immunogen in rodents, and immunization with this protein can induce an inflammatory arthritis in rats or mice that resembles rheumatoid arthritis morphologically.[17] Recently, it has been observed that auricular chondritis, with immunoglobulin and complement deposits at the site of the lesion, occurred on occasion in rats with type II collagen-induced arthritis.[3,13] Because antibodies to type II collagen have been detected in the serum of patients during the acute stage of polychondritis, there is increasing, although indirect, evidence that immunologic responses to cartilage and ocular collagen participate in the pathogenesis of relapsing polychondritis.[5,6]

Based on these findings, a hypothetical scheme can be proposed to partially explain the pathogenesis of relapsing polychondritis. Clones of autoreactive T and/or B cells emerge, by as yet undefined mechanisms, that are sensitized to type II collagen. Autoantibodies and perhaps lymphokines induce inflammation in cartilage (and the eye), which leads to chondrocyte death and matrix dissolution. Fibroblasts and chondroblasts then attempt to repair the lesion. Occasionally, the cycle of injury and repair is repeated, accounting for the relapsing nature of the disease. Substances released into the blood during the destruction of cartilage are injurious to the structural integrity of major blood vessels and trigger the characteristic aortic lesion. Much remains to be learned about the pathogenesis of relapsing polychondritis.

THERAPY

Aside from prosthetic valve replacement for aortic insufficiency, therapy has consisted primarily of supportive measures and the use of glucocorticoids. An acute inflammatory attack on affected cartilages may be moderated or brought under complete control with prednisone, 20 to 60 mg a day.[1,2] As the attack subsides, the dosage may be reduced to a maintenance level of 10 to 15 mg daily. In some patients, the anti-inflammatory and abortive effects of prednisone diminish over months or years so that the maintenance dosage must be raised gradually in an effort to prevent further severe attacks. On occasion, it is necessary to eventually administer doses approximating 30 mg of prednisone daily in order to provide satisfactory suppression of inflammation of cartilages and episcleritis. Glucocorticoids have no obvious effect on inhibiting the development of the aortic lesions. In patients who are truly refractory to prednisone, other types of immunosuppressive drugs may be attempted.[1] Because the attacks are frequently self-limited and the response to prednisone is delayed, however, attempts to curtail the inflammation with glucocorticoids should not be abandoned prematurely.

REFERENCES

1. Arkin, C.R., and Masi, A.T.: Relapsing polychondritis: Review of current status and case report. Semin. Arthritis Rheum., 5:41–62, 1975.
2. Case Records of the Massachusetts General Hospital (Case 51-1982). N. Engl. J. Med., 307:1631–1639, 1982.
3. Cremer, M.A., et al.: Auricular chondritis in rats: An experimental model of relapsing polychondritis induced with type II collagen. J. Exp. Med., 154:535–540, 1981.
4. Dolan, D.L., Lemmon, G.B., and Teitelbaum, S.L.: Relapsing polychondritis: Analytical review and studies on pathogenesis. Am. J. Med., 41:285–299, 1966.
5. Ebringer, R., et al.: Autoantibodies to cartilage and type II collagen in relapsing polychondritis and other rheumatic diseases. Ann. Rheum. Dis., 40:473–479, 1981.

6. Foidart, J.-M., et al.: Antibodies to type II collagen in relapsing polychondritis. N. Engl. J. Med., 299:1203–1207, 1978.
7. Hashimoto, K., Arkin, C.R., and Kang, A.H.: Relapsing polychondritis: An ultrastructural study. Arthritis Rheum., 20:91–99, 1977.
8. Hughes, R.A.C., et al.: Relapsing polychondritis: Three cases with a clinico-pathological study and literature review. Q. J. Med., 41:363–380, 1972.
9. Jaksch-Wartenhorst, R.: Polychondropathia. Weiner Archive Innere Med., 6:93–100, 1923.
10. Kaye, R.L., and Sones, D.A.: Relapsing polychondritis: Clinical and pathologic features in fourteen cases. Ann. Intern. Med., 60:653–664, 1964.
11. Kindblom, L.-G., et al.: Relapsing polychondritis: A clinical, pathologic-anatomic and histochemical study of two cases. Acta Pathol. Microbiol. Scand. (A), 85:656–664, 1977.
12. McCluskey, R.T., and Thomas, L.: The removal of cartilage matrix, in vivo, by papain: The identification of crystalline papain protease as the cause of the phenomenon. J. Exp. Med., 108:371–384, 1958.
13. McCune, W.J., et al.: Type II collagen-induced auricular chondritis. Arthritis Rheum., 25:266–273, 1982.
14. Moloney, J.R.: Relapsing polychondritis—its otolaryngological manifestations. J. Laryngol. Otol., 92:9–15, 1978.
15. O'Hanlan, M., et al.: The arthropathy of relapsing polychondritis. Arthritis Rheum., 19:191–194, 1976.
16. Rogers, P.H., Boden, G., and Tourtellotte, C.D.: Relapsing polychondritis with insulin resistance and antibodies to cartilage. Am. J. Med., 55:243–248, 1973.
17. Trentham, D.E.: Collagen arthritis as a relevant model for rheumatoid arthritis: Evidence pro and con. Arthritis Rheum., 25:911–916, 1982.
18. Tsaltas, T.T.: Metaplasia of aortic connective tissue to cartilage and bone induced by the intravenous injection of papain. Nature, 196:1006–1007, 1962.
19. Valenzuela, R., et al.: Relapsing polychondritis: Immunomicroscopic findings in cartilage of ear biopsy specimens. Hum. Pathol., 11:19–22, 1980.
20. Verity, M.A., Larson, W.M., and Madden, S.C.: Relapsing polychondritis: Report of two necropsied cases with histochemical investigation of the cartilage lesion. Am. J. Pathol., 42:251–269, 1963.

Miscellaneous Rheumatic Diseases

Chapter 70

Nonarticular Rheumatism and Psychogenic Musculoskeletal Syndromes

Hugh A. Smythe

Many patients experience musculoskeletal pain that does not arise from the local joints. These symptoms may be caused by disease in other local structures, but often the origin of the complaints is not immediately obvious. Soreness and stiffness are described in tissues that seem normal to objective examination, except perhaps for local tenderness. The physician must make a working diagnosis, and must attribute the symptoms to subtle local pathology, to a referred pain syndrome, to "fibrositis," or to a psychogenic regional pain syndrome. In this situation, mature clinicians have differed so widely in their pronouncements that their patients, students, and colleagues are justifiably skeptical. Nevertheless, a scientific basis for the study of these patients is evolving. New data from a number of well-designed prospective studies[2,41,54,55] have validated and greatly extended our knowledge of local tenderness and its clinical associations. Problems of interpretation remain, but the most urgent challenge to rheumatologists is to ensure that this knowledge is spread to other physicians. Screening for nonarticular tenderness must become a necessary part of the routine assessment of the patient in pain, whatever other conditions are known to be present (Table 70–1).

When there is no visible evidence of inflammation, and no obvious and fresh distortion of local anatomy, the clinician is left with only three sources of information to help choose from these possibilities: the localization of individual site, the patterns of multiple sites, and the patient's reactions. Because many of the telltale sites are not known to the patient and not central to the areas of pain, the evidence is only available to a skilled examiner with a systematic approach. This account will begin with the "fibrositis" (polymyalgia) syndrome.

FIBROSITIS SYNDROME

This syndrome is the most common condition diagnosed in new patients seen by practicing rheumatologists.[14] It is essentially a disease of women in the childbearing years (20 to 50).[1,41] Only about 10% of patients are men.

Essential to the diagnosis of fibrositis is the discovery of localized sites of deep tenderness. Speculation as to the nature of these sites has a long history, and the early German literature has been splendidly reviewed by Simons.[45,46] Gowers in 1904 introduced the term "fibrositis" to describe hypothetical inflammatory changes in the fibrous structure of lumbar muscles.[11] Histologic studies have usually failed to reveal inflammatory lesions, or have shown similar minor changes in control materials. Many observers have described induration at the sites of tenderness. Hench said that these were "only accessible to the finger of faith";[17] They usually represent areas of muscle spasm, fatty lumps, or normal variations in muscle density found equally often in control subjects.

The fibrositis syndrome is a complex but highly characteristic blend of features summarized in Table 70–2. The syndrome is characterized by pain and stiffness felt in a widespread distribution through deep tissues. The symptoms are worse in the morning, are aggravated by fatigue, tension, excessive use, immobility, or chilling, and are

Table 70–1. Kinds of Nonarticular Tenderness

1. Normal variations in pain threshold
2. Local inflammation (e.g., bursitis, enthesopathy)
3. Referred and fibrositic tnderness
4. Diffuse regional tenderness, as in "steroid shins," or reflex dystrophy
5. Nerve tenderness (popliteal, femoral, carpal tunnel)
6. Tenderness in psychogenic regional pain

Table 70–2. Cardinal Features of Fibrositis

1. A rheumatic pain syndrome
2. Specific site tenderness
3. High sensitivity to internal and external stimuli
4. Nonrestorative sleep
5. The "fibrositic" personality

eased by heat, massage, gentle activity, or a holiday. The pain or aching is diffuse, generally in the broad regions of reference of the cervical and lumbar segments, including the shoulder and pelvic girdles, upper chest, elbow and knee regions, and hands. Subjective swelling may be firmly described, and a sense of numbness is common in the hands and feet. Morning stiffness lasting for 1 to 2 hours is a common feature.

The patients tend to be perfectionistic, demanding of themselves and of others, and effective in their chosen areas of activity. Unlike classic victims of civilized tension, they dislike the effects of tranquilizers, and use drugs and alcohol sparingly. Their vices are their virtues carried to excess. They hate to complain, they respectfully doubt, they forgivably fail to comply, they loyally reject. They are not abnormal, just characteristic. They are not depressed; commonly used personality inventories have demonstrated differences between "fibrositics" and controls,[1,2,41] Significant elevation in hysteria, hypochondriasis, psychopathic deviancy, paranoia, schizophrenia, and mania scales in hospitalized patients with fibrositis were found using the MMPI test.[41] This finding has been confirmed in ambulatory fibrositis patients, although 36% of patients fell within the normal range and 32% showed a pattern typical of pain patients.[1] Fibrositis patients also showed a significantly greater number of stressful life events. These workers previously showed an association with the irritable bowel syndrome.[55] I believe that the MMPI is an inadequate instrument for the evaluation of the psychologic status of rheumatic disease patients.[49a] Another study in fibrositis patients derived from a clinic population failed to show any psychologic factor vis-à-vis control, although there was a significant association with tension headaches and irritable bowel.[2] The syndrome tends to begin in middle life, but children[55] and the aged are not spared.

The patients relax poorly and are unhappy during examination. Their well-preserved musculature is in striking contrast to their account of chronic misery and disability. Active movements may be carried out slowly, with facial grimacing and spasmodic overactivity of antagonists as well as prime movers. Passive movements stimulate a variable plastic resistiveness, but a full range of joint motion is obtained with gentle persuasion. Grip testing reveals a weak and variable end point, approached slowly and irregularly.

Tender Points. These tender areas are often unknown to the patient, but are easily found by the examiner because of their precisely predictable location. Tenderness is not just reported, but often is dramatized by a characteristic sudden dramatic writhing leap, called the "jump sign."

Their predictability and association with the general pain-stiffness-fatigue syndrome have been confirmed in recent studies.[2,54,55] These sites are normally slightly tender, and their location can be verified and studied on normal subjects. Fourteen such sites have been described in detail (Fig. 70–1: Table 70–3).[49] These sites efficiently differentiate normal from fibrositic subjects.[2] With some loss of efficiency, the list could be extended to include medial epicondyles, tip of coracoid, occiput, infraspinatus origins, rhomboids, levator scapulae, greater trochanter, and lower soleus. As many as 53 sites were defined in one prospective study.[55]

Skinfold tenderness over the upper scapular region may be extreme and present in 85% of those with 12 or more tender points.[54] Testing for skinfold tenderness, or for costochondral or other deep tenderness, is often followed by a marked reactive hyperemia of the overlying skin, which speaks eloquently for the location and physiogenic nature of the pain. All these observations can and should be checked by similarly firm palpation of control areas, which have been shown to be normally tender in fibrositics[2] (Fig. 70–2). Blood studies are usually normal, including cell counts, erythrocyte sedimentation rates, serum proteins, and muscle enzyme studies—a defined requirement for the diagnosis of primary fibrositis.

Sleep Disturbance. Patients who met our criteria for the fibrositis syndrome[48] uniformly complained of sleep disturbance and intensification of

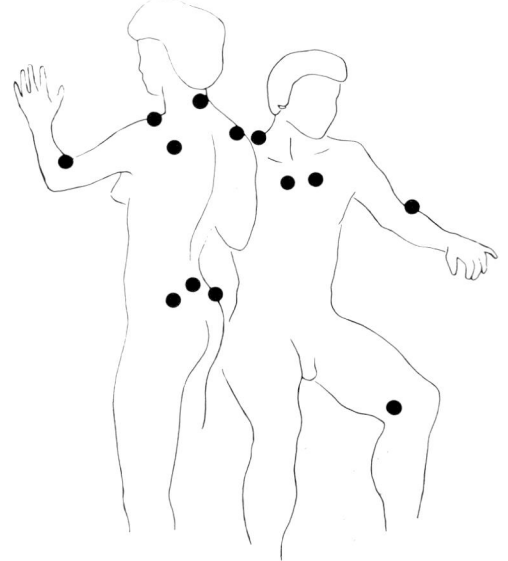

Fig. 70–1. Location of 13 typical sites of deep tenderness in "fibrositis." (From Smythe, H.A., and Moldofsky, H.[49])

Table 70–3.   Fourteen Sites of Tenderness in Fibrositis*

Site	Location of Tenderness
Trapezius (R and L)	The midpoint of the upper fold of trapezius in a somewhat firmer portion of muscle
Second costochondral junctions (R and L)	At or just lateral to the junction, often more marked on superior surface of rib, close to origin of pectoralis major. Overlying reactive hyperemia often develop (but costochondral junctions may also be tender).
Supraspinatus origins (R and L)	Above scapular spine, near the medial border of scapula.
Lateral epicondyles (R and L)	The "tennis elbow" sites, actually 1 to 2 cm distal to epicondyle, precisely located by extending and relaxing the third (long) finger. Medial epicondyle may also be tender.
Buttocks (R and L)	In the midpart of the upper outer quadrant of buttock, in anterior portion of gluteus medius.
Knees (R and L)	In the fat pad medial to the knee, proximal to the joint line, and overlying medial collateral ligament.
Neck	Actually several sites. Most marked tenderness is at anterior aspect of intertransverse ligaments at C4-C5 and C5-C6; interspinous tenderness less marked.
Low lumbar region	Again, several sites. Most marked usually at L4-L5 interspinous ligament, slightly less so at L5-S1.

*These sites are normally somewhat tender; thus, they should be palpated with about 80% of the force used in adjacent control areas. Overlying skin is not normally tender, but may be hyperesthetic if referred pain is present.

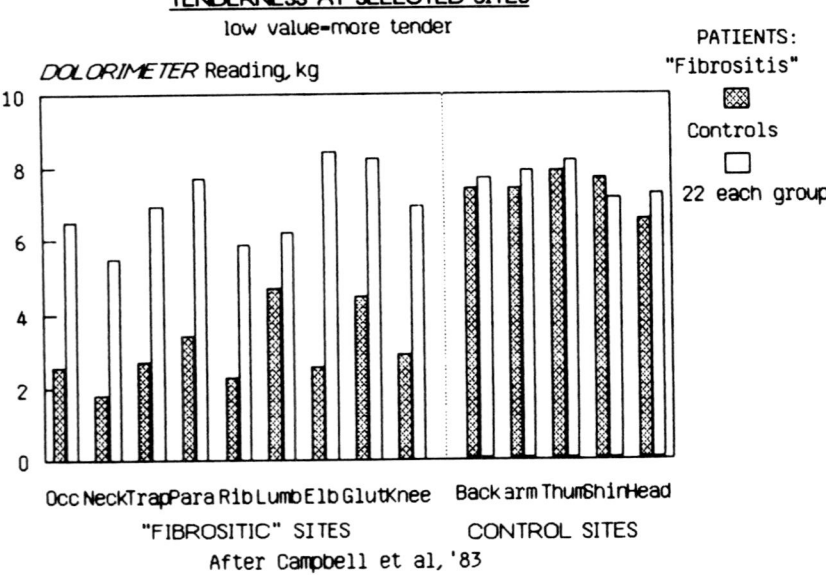

Fig. 70–2.   Tenderness at selected sites. (After Campbell, S.M., et al.[2])

pain, stiffness, and fatigue upon awakening. Key studies, still not confirmed, have provided evidence for a specific disturbance in sleep physiology. In the first study,[34] 10 fibrositic patients were observed, using standard EEG techniques. Before and after sleep, measurements of tenderness at the specific sites were made. All subjects showed an overnight increase in measures of tenderness, and all showed a disturbance in nonREM (non rapid eye movement) sleep (Fig. 70–3). No disturbance of REM (rapid eye movement) sleep was found. These observations have since been extended in a large number of additional patients.

In another study, experimental reproduction of the fibrositis symptoms was attempted in healthy university students.[36] After baseline studies, they

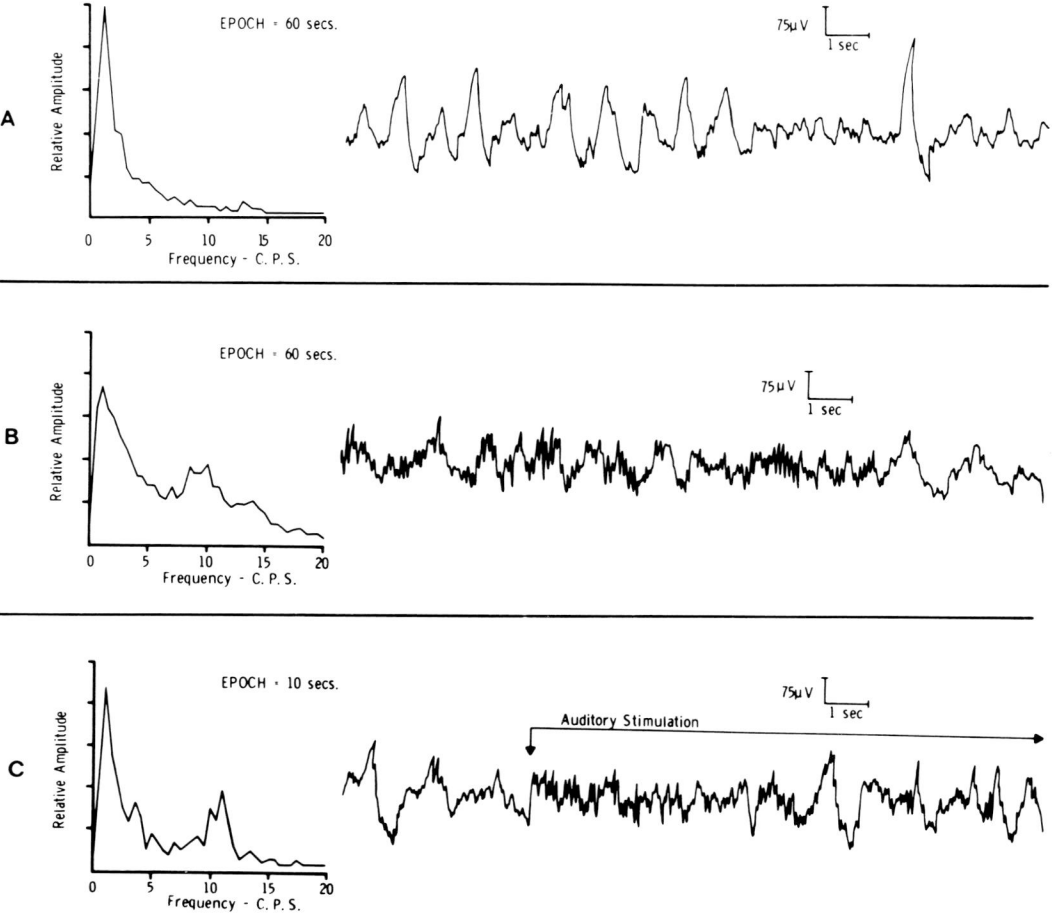

Fig. 70–3. Frequency spectra and raw EEG from *A*, NREM (stage 4) sleep in a healthy 25-year-old subject. The spectrum shows that most amplitude is concentrated at 1 cps (delta). *B*, NREM sleep in a 42-year-old "fibrositis" patient. The spectrum shows amplitude at both 1 cps (delta) and 8 to 10 cps (alpha). *C*, NREM sleep of a healthy 21-year-old subject during stage 4 sleep deprivation. In the EEG there is a clear association between external arousal (auditory stimulation) and alpha onset. Again the frequency spectrum (obtained by 10-sec analysis from stimulus onset) shows amplitude concentrated in the delta and alpha bands. (From Moldofsky, H., et al.[36])

were deprived during three nights of REM sleep (seven subjects) or stage 4 slow-wave nonREM sleep (six subjects), by means of a buzzer, supplemented when necessary by hand arousal. Only those who experienced slow-wave sleep deprivation showed a significant increase in tenderness, as measured by dolorimeter scores.[25] In addition, many of these patients suffered from anorexia, overwhelming physical tiredness, heaviness, or sluggishness to the point of experiencing difficulty with walking or standing. These symptoms disappeared during the recovery nights, and did not occur after REM sleep deprivation.

Physical fitness may be an important factor. In a pilot study, three subjects who were accustomed to running 2 to 7 miles per day did not develop pain symptoms or increases in dolorimeter scores while undergoing stage 4 deprivation.[36]

The auditory stimulus used to arouse the subjects from stage 4 to lighter stages of sleep caused an alpha rhythm to appear in the EEG, superimposed on the slow-wave (delta) rhythm, much like the pattern found in our fibrositis patients (see Fig. 70–3). The spontaneous alpha intrusion into the slow-wave nonREM rhythm of the fibrositis subjects was attributed to an arousal system, analogous to the external arousal stimulus used experimentally. In Moldofsky's studies, the frequency spectra were analyzed by computer, as illustrated in Figure 70–3. Alpha intrusion into delta sleep in high-energy bursts can be recognized by eye and was described as alpha-delta sleep.[13] The author described this pattern in one patient with aching, stiffness, and fatigue, relieved by amitriptyline.[12] In another study, this more florid pattern was recognized in only 8 of 26 chronic pain patients.[53]

Chlorpromazine has been claimed to facilitate slow-wave nonREM sleep. The effect of this agent on the manifestations of the fibrositis syndrome was explored in 8 subjects.[33] Chlorpromazine produced an increase in slow-wave sleep and a decrease in subjective pain and dolorimeter scores.[35] Symptoms rapidly returned when chlorpromazine was discontinued, and when subjects could not tolerate the untoward effects of this medication.

The fibrositis or fibromyalgia syndrome is now established as common and important, with a pattern of symptoms and signs validated by convergent, controlled, independent studies. Outside rheumatology, however, the concept still receives active rejection. Part of the problem is semantic; the names are archaic and unrelated to pathogenesis. In addition, the names have been applied to dissimilar patient groups. As our concepts evolve, it is difficult to restrict the application of the name to a single homogeneous entity.

The number of tender points was recorded in an unsorted group of patients presenting at an ambulatory rheumatic disease clinic (Fig. 70–4).[54]

Over 30% had at least one point, 19% at least four. Most of these patients did not have the exhaustion, morning stiffness, and "irritable everything" syndrome of the classic primary fibrositic patient. At least three groups were clearly perceived among the patients with tender points: referred pain syndromes, reactive fibrositis syndromes, and chronic fibrositis syndromes.

Referred pain syndromes exhibit a small number of points clustered regionally, the "localized fibrositis" of older literature. Systemic symptoms and a specific personality were not found. "Reactive fibrositis is situation-related, with exhaustion, stiffness, and pain, and a diffuse distribution of tender points. It may be part of a normal reaction to overwhelming pressure, grief, anger, fear or pain; possibly related to sleep disturbance. The prognosis is usually benign, and psychoactive drugs should be used gently. The *chronic fibrositic patient* has the intense, perfectionistic, neat but exhausting personality. They may have other diseases (secondary fibrositis) or not (primary). Inappropriate treatment is more likely and far more hazardous if they also have rheumatoid arthritis.[32]

The prevalence and clinical picture vary with the criteria employed. If one accepts the presence of 4 of 54 tender points as a key criterion,[55] nearly

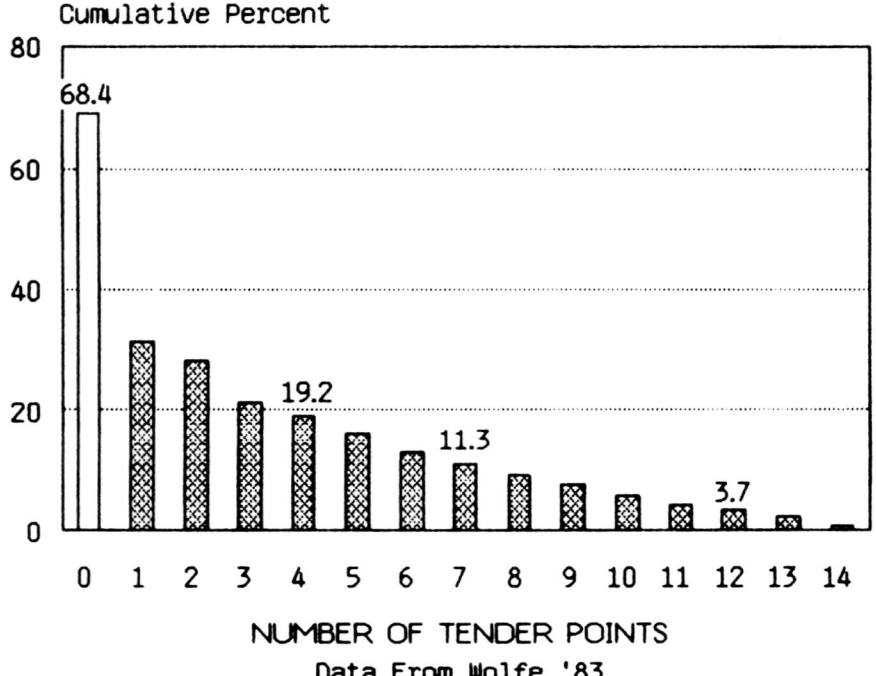

Fig. 70–4. Prevalence of "fibrositic" tender points. (Data from Wolfe, F.[54])

20% of clinic patients will be affected; if one demands 12 of 14,[48] 3.7% will be affected.[2,54] Information about its prevalence in the general population is not available. Strict criteria used in older studies helped define a classic picture of the chronic fibrositic;[48] these studies required (1) widespread aching of more than three months duration; (2) local tenderness at 12 of 14 specified sites; (3) skin roll tenderness over the upper scapular region; (4) disturbed sleep, with morning fatigue and stiffness; and (5) normal ESR, SGOT, rheumatoid factor test, ANA, muscle enzymes, and sacroiliac films.

These criteria also help to differentiate fibrositic pain from pain that is purely malingering pretense or neurotically symbolic. The specificity of location of the tender sites, many previously unknown to the patient, the reactive hyperemia accompanying skin fold tenderness, and the reproduction of the syndrome in normal volunteers by slow-wave sleep deprivation all indicate the importance of physiogenic mechanisms.

Prognosis. Objective evaluation continues to indicate excellent general health, and muscle bulk and range of passive joint movement remain normal. Temporary alleviation of discomfort can be obtained with a variety of programs, but loss of all symptoms is extremely unusual. Interruption of employment can be a disaster. Few of these patients ever return to full productive capacity if failing performance due to pain and exhaustion causes them to be fired or to resign. The meager effects of the most intensive multidisciplinary efforts at rehabilitation of these apparently fit patients is in striking contrast to the relative ease with which major functional improvement can be effected in most patients with rheumatoid arthritis. In general, the syndrome waxes and wanes for many years. Hench noted long ago that pregnancy or jaundice relieves the symptoms of fibrositis* completely and predictably.[15,16]

Pathogenesis. Four factors seem to interact to produce the syndrome: (1) local findings, (2) reflex phenomena associated with chronic pain of deep origin, (3) psychogenic factors, and (4) disturbed sleep.

It is hypothesized that local factors determine the sites of involvement, and that the extended duration and severity of the disability are due to the interactions of a chronic tension state, especially of a chronic nonrestorative sleep pattern, with the reflex phenomena that accompany deep pain.

Deep Pain. Exact knowledge of the position in space of such structures as the hand is essential to its function, and a mental image of the hand can be summoned at any time. Thus, a "body image" of the superficial parts of the body exists, and is based on specialized cerebral cortical representation.[20] However, no such image is formed of deeply lying structures. No part of the brain is assigned to keep an exclusive running account of events in these structures, and they do not lie within the "body image." Pain of deep origin must be referred, i.e., misinterpreted as arising in other areas within the body image. Lewis and Kellgren showed that pain localization after stimulation of deep ligaments, fascia, and muscles was grossly inaccurate, with spread of pain sensation distally to other tissues broadly sharing the same nerve supply, deep enough to share the quality of deep pain, but superficial enough to be included in the body image.[20–22,24]

Persistent pain of any origin gives rise to protective reflex changes. These changes include muscle spasm, inhibition of voluntary movement, increased blood flow, and cutaneous or deep hyperalgesia. Because neural localization may be wildly inaccurate when pain is of deep origin, these reflex effects may be found in areas far removed from the original site of pathologic change.

The patient with pain due to chronic cervical strain will have marked tenderness deep in the low anterior neck, but will also have referred tenderness of the unaffected intervertebral ligaments, often in the midtrapezius, spinal muscles, and epicondyles (Fig. 70–5). It is not a coincidence that these are the same sites found to be tender in the fibrositis syndrome. If reflex deep hyperalgesia is present, local anesthesia reults in abolition or marked diminution of pain. The pain associated with reflex hyperalgesia may be aggravated by many factors, of which cold is the best studied.[20]

Patients with referred pain commonly describe a heaviness, a swollen feeling, numbness, or even a prickling "pins-and-needles" sensation in some areas, particularly those distal in the limb. A pinprick is usually recognized as such, although less sharp than on the other side, and two-point discrimination is normal.

Sites of Origin of Referred Pain. Most deep pain is referred distally. Most fibrositic pain is in the areas of reference of the lower cervical and two lower lumbar levels. Acute cervical or lumbar syndromes are commonly associated with referred tenderness in the same local fibrositic points. Mechanical stresses in these two regions may therefore play a part in the production of symptoms in patients with fibrositis. These two sites are uniquely susceptible for excellent mechanical reasons. The

---

*Ed. Note: I have observed complete remission of classic fibrositis in five pregnancies in two patients. Symptoms invariably returned within six weeks after delivery.

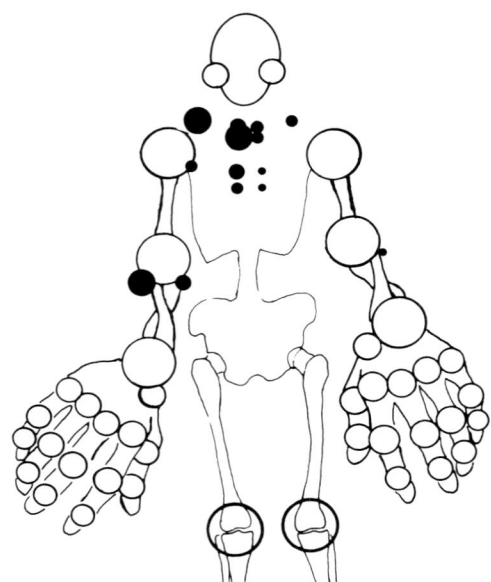

Fig. 70–5. Referred tenderness in the cervical syndrome. Clustered pattern in one patient with right sided neck and arm pain.

lower neck is vulnerable because of a number of factors, of which the most important and most neglected are the shearing and compressive forces arising in the unsupported arch of the neck during sleep. When upright, the lower lumbar spine is at the limit of hyperextension in virtually everyone with low back problems, and close to this limit in all of us. Locked at its extreme of range, the joints absorb shock into bone, ligament, and disc rather than into muscle.

Other Etiologic Considerations: Local Lesions. Some investigators believe that fibrositis exists as a pathologic entity, and a few detailed, carefully controlled studies of the pathology of this condition have been published. Miehlke and coworkers compared histologic and biochemical findings in muscle biopsy of several groups of patients with muscle pain and stiffness.[28,29] The "control" groups consisted of anxious, tense patients with diffuse and variable muscle aching, but no "trigger points" or palpable nodules. Biopsy was taken from the upper midportion of the trapezius muscle. The other groups consisted of patients with constantly located "trigger points" or tender indurations, and biopsies were taken from the most tender spot. Several differences were observed. The most common change was a mild "dusting" of fatty droplets through the muscle fibers, detected with fat stains. When a definite induration had been evident clinically, there was often an increase in interstitial connective tissue nuclei. Occasionally,

clumps of lymphocytes and plasma cells were seen, but never granulocytes. The muscle fibers did not show necrosis or loss of striation, although some variation in size and staining was apparent in the nodular lesions. The enzyme content of the muscles from the focal lesions was slightly reduced as compared with the controls. An agglutinating antibody against muscle antigen was described in some of these patients, but no controls were reported.

It seems possible that the observed histologic differences were due to variations in site of biopsy in patients vs. controls. The occasional presence of lymphoid cells is in accord with the control experience of others. A later report from this group was confused by the inclusion of patients with rheumatoid arthritis or other serious diseases.[29]

Trauma and Occupation. Trauma in the form of a single incident or repeated strain may be a cause of fibrositis, although adequate statistics regarding this point are not available. The discomfort after major trauma is usually of relatively short duration, but theoretically may be prolonged by a soft tissue lesion that results in mechanical instability of a pain-sensitive structure, by a tension state and associated sleep disturbance, or by consideration of secondary pain. The interrelations of these factors may be difficult to evaluate, but they have considerable significance.

Exposure. Exposure to cold, wet, drafts, and sudden changes in weather may precipitate or aggravate symptoms, by mechanisms not fully understood. Kellgren studied the effect of cooling on pain. He noted that when deep hyperalgesia is present, even slow cooling of the affected part causes severe and prolonged pain, and the analgesia that normally accompanies cooling develops imperfectly unless the tissues are cooled to low temperature (10° C).[20] This phenomenon may contribute to the weather effect noted by so many patients.

Secondary Fibrositis. Discomfort similar to that of primary fibrositis is common as an accompaniment to a wide variety of other disorders. These range from such well-known but pathologically ill-defined complaints as those following unaccustomed exercise or associated with influenza, to diseases such as rheumatoid arthritis in which lesions can be demonstrated histologically in muscles and connective tissues. The diagnosis in these instances is clarified by recognition of the primary disorder. The pain of polymyalgia rheumatica can easily be mistaken for fibrositis when the patient is first seen, but the inflammatory features, especially elevated erythrocyte sedimentation rate, permit rapid differentiation (see Chap. 59).

Many patients with secondary fibrositis lack the specific distribution of tender points characteristic of the fibrositis syndrome. Those who do share personality characteristics with primary fibrositic patients. The interaction of two sources of misery is possible and has important therapeutic implications.

Treatment of Fibrositis. The patient with the fibrositis syndrome comes to the physician feeling threatened by her illness and by her associated problems. She is on the defensive and will react negatively to any message she interprets as a further threat. The task of explanation may challenge all the physician's skill, training, and imagination. It is relatively easy to prescribe an analgesic regimen, but it can be extremely difficult to give the patient an adequate account of the origins of the symptoms, and in particular to deal with the relationship between pain and tension. Patients expect doctors to use euphemisms, and will examine words carefully for unfavorable underlying meanings. Thus, the suggestion that symptoms are of emotional origin, or the use of the word anxiety, may be translated by the patient into an accusation of inadequacy or willful malingering. The physician is further handicapped by the complexities of the explanation he must give, and he must assess the needs and the understanding of the patient with great care. The intelligent, curious patient may need a thorough, general discussion of referred pain and the origin of tension before her own problems are discussed. A simple extroverted patient may need only reassurance and a positive program (of almost any kind). The patient who is demoralized and no longer able to cope may need a brief hospitalization and a period of sympathetic protection before recovering sufficient strength of will to reconstruct her habits and attitudes.

A minimum initial discussion may cover: (1) referred pain and deep tenderness; (2) mechanical stresses in neck and low back; (3) the sleep disturbance; and (4) attitudes and expectations (Table 70–4).

No drug therapy has proved uniformly successful, although many rheumatologists believe that amitriptyline is helpful. I have prescribed aerobic exercises such as jogging or stationary bicycling for 30 minutes five to six times weekly with reasonable results in terms of symptomatic relief. Swimming in a heated pool is also useful. The patient must be encouraged to persevere because such exercise increases symptoms at first. The exercise program should begin at modest levels and be gradually increased. Whether the partial relief experienced is due to improved sleep, to release of substances such as beta endorphins,[10] or to other factors is unknown.

PSYCHOGENIC MUSCULOSKELETAL SYNDROMES

Four types of relationships, not mutually exclusive, between mental state and musculoskeletal symptoms may be seen: (1) psychosomatic production of symptoms or disease; (2) exaggeration (or denial): subconscious use of existing disease for secondary gain; (3) converion reactions: psychogenic regional pain and hysteria; and (4) malingering.

It is relatively easy to recognize organic disease in normally reacting individuals and relatively easy to recognize that a patient is odd, but it can be difficult to assess organic disease in a disturbed patient. Thus, major problems in diagnosis occur in all of the aforementioned four types.

Given accurate diagnosis, understanding the underlying processes in the last three categories is not difficult. Major controversy continues to exist about the existence and mechanisms involved in the psychosomatic production of structural changes in musculoskeletal syndromes.

Studies of Psychosomatic Factors in Rheumatoid Arthritis. An extensive literature exists,[3–6,23,27,32,37–41] including numerous original and disciplined studies of the psychology of rheumatoid patients, and excellent critical reviews. The various samples demonstrated a notably consistent finding of hidden anger, controlled by the patient because of insecurity in personal relations and expressed through "good" behavior, depression, and symptoms.[4,6,23,37] Physiologic differences have also been identified, including a lower blood pressure but faster pulse, increased sweating, and colder extremities, with exaggeration of these differences when the subjects were stressed by angry criticism.[23]

Few researchers claim that these differences are necessary for or specific for RA and intimately related to pathogenesis. The relevance of these phenomena to disease onset or exacerbations is controversial. Studies in identical twins discordant for RA suggested that stressful life events may be important,[27] but the one large controlled study of circumstances surrounding the onset of RA showed equal frequency of such events prior to disease onset of 532 patients and in matched controls.[7]

There is no doubt that disease course and personality interact. Moldofsky identified a subgroup of paradoxical responders among rheumatoid patients, whose moods worsen as their inflammation lessens.[32] Such patients arrived seemingly cheerful, brave, and compliant, but developed anxiety and new complaints as therapy progressed. They therefore selected themselves for alternative therapies, and were more likely to receive prolonged hospitalization, extensive investigation, and systemic steroid and surgical therapies with attendant increased morbidity and mortality.[32] The patient's need for care held family, friends, and therapists close to them, and they had much to fear from

Table 70–4. Management of Fibrositis

Technique	Explanation
Reassurance	Disease is not crippling or serious, but pain is "real" and follows usual pattern.

Explanation of origin of pain	In greater or lesser detail, depending on his needs, patient should be told:
	  pain of deep origin is necessarily referred.
	  referred tenderness is at constant, predictable sites.
	  exaggerated reflex hyperemia indicates tissue hyper-activity.
	  condition is aggravated by cold, sleep disturbance, tension, and depression.

Relief of mechanical stresses in neck and low back (probably the primary source of referred pain and tenderness)	Because neck is vulnerable to stresses during sleep, support is needed under arch of the neck. Because low back is vulnerable in hyperextension, strong abdominal muscles and flexed low back are needed. Abdominal support and unsagging mattress may help.
Medical therapies	Salicylates or other simple analgesics to break chronic pain cycles: need for compliance, persistence. Heat, massage, liniments, or other counterirritant and relaxation therapies. Amitriptyline, 10 to 75 mg h.s. or equivalent, for sleep disturbance.
Attitudes and expectations	Recognize perfectionist impatience. Challenges give life meaning; accept within limitations. Pursure fitness even if symptoms increase. Break tension with rest, diversion, exercise, or escape.

restored health. These patients were often perfectionists, depressed, sleepless, and exhausted, and felt tenderness at the fibrositic sites as well as in their joints. The paradoxical response pattern was seen in nearly half of one group of hospitalized rheumatoid patients. Recognition of this pattern is of great therapeutic importance. The push toward advanced therapies must be recognized and controlled. The patient tends to blame the therapies for many symptoms, and the unhappy therapist is tempted to cruelly lay bare all the personal dynamics at work, shifting blame back on the patient. These patients require more time, sympathetic support, explanations, and acceptance from their therapist before they can cope with their very real symptoms of exhaustion, depression, and stiffness—and rheumatoid arthritis.

Psychogenic Regional Pain Syndromes. The symbolic use of pain and disability may be symptomatic of depression, schizophrenia, various psychoneuroses, psychopathic personality, or even organic psychoses. The name "psychogenic regional pain" has been proposed for this large clinical group,[52] reserving the term "hysteria" for the small number of patients showing all the features of classic hysteria. The diagnosis of psychopathology by no means rules out the presence of organic disease, but greatly magnifies the difficulties in assessment and therapy.

The clinical presentation differs from the fibrositis syndrome. The distress tends to be concentrated in a single region that has emotional rather than segmental definition, such as the hand, back, anterior chest, or limbs. The distress is described dramatically: "The pain burns through my left breast and out my back." Spread to adjacent areas is common, subject to manipulation by the questioner, with sharp, nonsegmental, and varying boundaries at such sites as the root of a limb or the midline. The paradoxical association of tenderness and numbness is common. Hyperalgesia to traction on skin hairs may coexist with reported numbness to pinprick.

These bizarre features allow a positive diagnosis of psychopathology to be made, but unfortunately do not rule out the coexistence of organic disease. Resistance to movement may be quite stubborn, and reexamination after intravenous injection of thiopental (Pentothal), amobarbital (Amytal), or diazepam may be helpful. Such an examination usually requires informed consent, given in the presence of a qualified anesthesiologist and other witnesses and must be carefully described in the patient's records.

Anatomic Changes. Most patients with neurotic or psychotic complaints have no clinical or radiologic abnormalities. When diffuse swelling, osteopenia, restricted movement, or changes of sclerodactyly are attributed to "disuse" of functional origin, the burden of proof is heavy on the physician responsible for the diagnosis. In many cases, reflex dystrophic reactions or even major local disease is overlooked.

OTHER SOFT TISSUE PAIN SYNDROMES

Table 70–5 provides a partial list of the many syndromes that may be characterized by nonarticular pain. A full account of each of these syndromes is not possible here, but some discussion of the last group is in order.

Pain at bone-tendon junctions (enthesopathy) can occur in at least three apparently different clinical settings: in ankylosing spondylitis, Reiter's syndrome, or other HLA-B27 associated conditions. A painful heel may point strongly to the correct diagnosis. The pain most commonly occurs at the site of attachment of plantar fascia to medial calcaneal tubercle, and may precede radiologic change by a period of years. Similar lesions occur about the iliac crest, the greater trochanter, and many other sites.

Not all inferior heel pain is due to spondylitis. Athletes, especially runners, develop chronic pain at exactly the same site, with similar late ossification of the fascial insertion, presumably in response to chronic trauma. Again, similar lesions develop in many other sites, notably the patella, greater trochanter, and elbow. Most of these patients are B27-negative and have no other stigmata of spondylitis.

The third situation in which ossification of fibrous insertions occurs is in association with ankylosing hyperostosis, otherwise known as Forestier's syndrome[8,9] or diffuse idiopathic skeletal hyperostosis (DISH).[43,51] Extraspinal involvement in this syndrome was described by Forestier and involved sites including occiput, trochanters, is-

Table 70–5. Other Causes of Soft Tissue Pain

Bursitis
Tendonitis
Tenosynovitis
Phlebitis
Vasculitis
Panniculitis
Post-exercise myalgia
Hematoma in muscle
Myalgia in virus infections
Polymyalgia rheumatica
Referred pain syndromes
Reflex dystrophies
Nerve entrapment syndromes
Pain with CNS disease
Muscle-tendon junction syndromes
Bone-tendon junction syndromes
Tender shins with steroid therapy

chia, ilia, and calcanei. In these older patients, the relationship of late ossification to earlier symptoms may be difficult to ascertain and has not yet been studied systematically.

Pain at muscle-tendon junctions occurs under quite different circumstances. These lesions are not commonly associated with ankylosing spondylitis, and do not calcify or progress to ossification. The most typical example is the "tennis elbow" syndrome. Tenderness just distal to the lateral epicondyle may follow local trauma, may be associated with referred pain (usually of cervical origin), or may be associated with general hyperalgesia in the fibrositis syndrome or after experimental deep sleep deprivation. Similar lesions develop in the origins of the adductor muscles of the thigh in football and hockey players, or in the origin of the flexor hallucis brevis in ballet dancers. The bone-tendon and muscle-tendon lesions have in common a high tissue density, where a little swelling can cause much pain, as in a tooth socket or ear canal. If steroid injections are used in therapy, the patient should be warned that a flare of pain may occur for one to two days before relief follows.

TENDER SHINS OF STEROID THERAPY

Slocumb first described myalgias occurring after administration of large doses of cortisone.[47] Rotstein and Good described as "steroid pseudorheumatism" the occurrence of striking tenderness of the muscles of the extremities in 5 patients on high doses of oral steroids.[44] By dolorimetry, the tenderness is more marked in the lower than in the upper extremities. It is not confined to muscle, but is diffuse in the lower leg and over bone and tendon as well as muscle. It spares the feet. It is usually associated with a shiny atrophy of skin, but is usually not associated with edema, with evidence of neuropathy, or with tender fibrositic sites. The tenderness may lessen if the steroid can be decreased or withdrawn. Tender shins are commonly found in aged subjects of both sexes; the etiology is still obscure.

HYSTERIA

Overt conversion reactions are seen occasionally by rheumatologists, orthopedists, and others dealing with patients with musculoskeletal complaints. These reactions can be confusing and even alarming, especially to the younger physician. The most common of these are hysterical bent back (camptocormia), hysterical bent knee (Fig. 70–6), and an inability to use one or both hands (writer's cramp). The "restless legs" syndrome is considered by some to be a depressive expression. In my experience, it often has hysterical features. The typical patient complains of boring pains in the legs

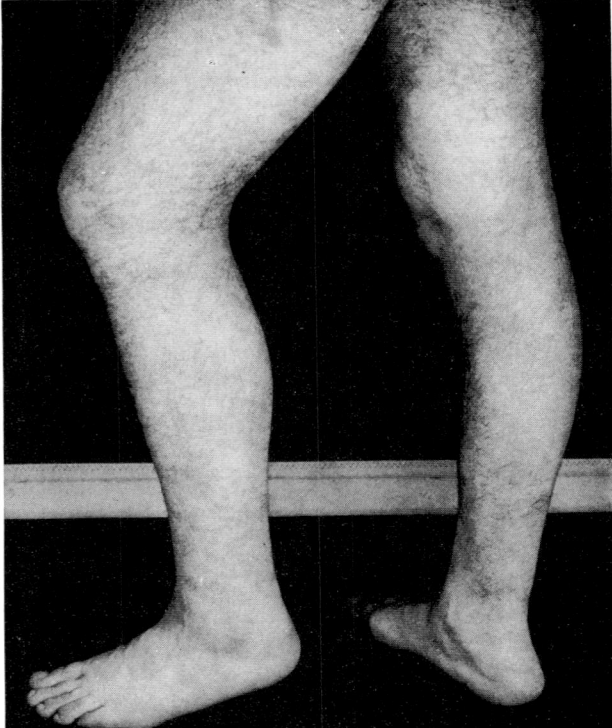

Fig. 70–6. Hysterical bent knee. The patient could straighten the knee fully while lying but not while standing. He had a bizarre gait, semi-squatting with each step. (From Boland, E.W.)

or thighs at night when recumbent, relieved by walking. Placebo therapy often relieves symptoms but nearly always produces side effects such as headache and nausea.

REFERENCES

1. Ahles, T.A., et al.: Psychological studies in primary fibromyalgia syndrome. (Abstract) Clin. Res., *31*:801, 1983.
2. Campbell, S.M., et al.: Clinical characteristics of fibrositis. Arthritis Rheum., *26*:817–824, 1983.
3. Cobb, S.: Contained hostility in rheumatoid arthritis. Arthritis Rheum., *2*:419–425, 1959.
4. Cobb, S., et al.: The interfamilial transmission of rheumatoid arthritis. An unusual study. J. Chronic Dis., *22*:193–194, 1969.
5. Cobb, S., et al.: Some psychological and social characteristics of patients hospitalized for rheumatoid arthritis, hypertension and duodenal ulcer. J. Chronic Dis., *18*:1259–1279, 1965.
6. Cobb, S., Miller, M., and Wieland, M.: On the relationship between divorce and rheumatoid arthritis. Arthritis Rheum., *2*:414–418, 1959.
7. Empire Rheumatism Council: Br. Med. J., *1*:799, 1950.
8. Forestier, J., and Lagier, R.: Vertebral ankylosing hyperostosis: Morphological basis, clinical manifestations, situation and diagnosis. *In* Modern Trends in Rheumatology. Vol. 2. Edited by A. Hill. London, Butterworths, 1971, pp. 323–337.
9. Forestier, J., and Rotes-Querol, J.: Senile ankylosing hyperostosis of the spine. Ann. Rheum. Dis., *9*:21, 1950.
10. Gambert, S.R., et al.: Effect of moderate exercise on plasma beta endorphin and ACTH in untrained human subjects. Proc. Soc. Exp. Biol. Med., *168*:1–4, 1981.
11. Gowers, W.R.: A lecture on lumbago: Its lessons and analogues. Br. Med. J., *1*:117–121, 1904.
12. Hauri, P.: The sleep disorders. Kalamazoo, The Upjohn Co., 1977, p. 51.
13. Hauri, P., and Hawkins, D.R.: Alpha-delta sleep. Electroencephalogr. Clin. Neurophysiol., *34*:233–237, 1973.
14. Healey, L.A., et al. (ARA Committee on Rheumatology Practice): A description of rheumatology practice. Arthritis Rheum., *20*:1278–1281, 1977.
15. Hench, P.S.: The ameliorating effect of pregnancy on chronic atrophic (infectious rheumatoid) arthritis, fibrositis, and intermittent hydroarthrosis. Proc. Staff Meet Mayo Clin., *13*:161–167, 1938.
16. Hench, P.S.: Effect of jaundice on chronic infectious (atrophic) arthritis and on primary fibrositis. Arch. Intern. Med., *61*:451–480, 1938.
17. Hench, P.S.: The problem of rheumatism and arthritis: review of American and English Literature from 1935. Ann. Intern. Med., *10*:880, 1936.
18. This reference has been deleted.
19. Hinoki, M., and Niki, H.: Role of the sympathetic nervous system in the formation of the traumatic vertigo of cervical origin. Acta Otolaryngol. (Suppl.), *330*:815, 1975.
20. Kellgren, J.H.: Deep pain sensibility. Lancet, *1*:943–949, 1949.
21. Kellgren, J.H.: On distribution of pain arising from deep somatic structures with charts of segmental pain areas. Clin. Sci., *4*:35–46, 1939.
22. Kellgren, J.H.: Observations on referred pain arising from muscles. Clin. Sci., *3*:174–190, 1938.
23. Kiviniemi, P.: Emotions and personality in rheumatoid arthritis. Scand. J. Rheumatol. (Suppl. 18), *6*:1–132, 1977.
24. Lewis, T., and Kellgren, J.H.: Observations relating to referred pain, visceromotor reflexes and other associated phenomena. Clin. Sci., *4*:47–71, 1939.
25. McCarty, D.J., Gatter, R.D., and Steele, A.D.: A twenty pound dolorimeter for quantification of articular tenderness. Arthritis Rheum., *11*:696–697, 1968.
26. This reference has been deleted.
27. Meyerowitz, S., Jacox, R.F., and Hess, D.W.: Monozygotic twins discordant for rheumatoid arthritis: A genetic, clinical and psychological study of 8 sets. Arthritis Rheum., *11*:1–21, 1968.

28. Miehlke, K., Schulze, G., and Eger, W.: Clinical and experimental studies on the fibrositis syndrome. Z. Rheumaforsch., *19*:310–330, 1960.

29. Miehlke, K.: Bull. Rheum. Dis., *12*:276, 1962.

30. Moldofsky, H.: Rheumatic pain modulation syndrome: The inter-relationships between sleep, central nervous system serotonin and pain. Adv. Neurol., *33*:51–57, 1982.

31. Moldofsky, H.: Occupational cramp. J. Psychosom. Res., *15*:439–444, 1971.

32. Moldofsky, H., and Chester, W.J.: Pain and mood patterns in patients with rheumatoid arthritis. Psychsom. Med., *32*:309–318, 1970.

33. Moldofsky, H., et al.: Comparison of chlorpromazine and L-tryptophan on sleep, musculoskeletal pain, and mood in fibrositis syndrome. Sleep Res., *5*:65–71, 1976.

34. Moldofsky, H., et al.: Musculoskeletal symptoms and non-REM sleep disturbance in patients with the "fibrositis" syndrome and healthy subjects. Psychosom. Med., *37*:341–351, 1975.

35. Moldofsky, H., and Lue, F.: Alpha and delta EEG frequencies. Pain and mood in "fibrositic" patients treated with chlorpromazine and L-tryptophan. Electroencephalogr. Clin. Neurophysiol., *50*:71–80, 1980.

36. Moldofsky, H., and Scarisbrick, P.: Induction of neurasthenic musculoskeletal pain syndrome by selective stage sleep deprivation. Psychosom. Med., *38*:35–44, 1976.

37. Moos, R.H.: Personality factor associated with rheumatoid arthritis: A review. J. Chronic Dis., *17*:41–55, 1964.

38. Moos, R.H., and Solomon, G.F.: Psychologic comparisons between women with rheumatoid arthritis and their non-arthritic sisters I. Personality test and interview data. Psychosom. Med., *27*:135–149, 1965.

39. Moos, R.H., and Solomon, G.F.: Personality correlates of the rapidity of progression of rheumatoid arthritis. Ann. Rheum. Dis., *23*:145–151, 1964.

40. Moos, R.H., and Solomon, G.F.: Personality correlates of rheumatoid arthritic patients' response to treatment. Arthritis Rheum., *7*:331, 1964.

41. Payne, T.C., et al.: Fibrositis and psychogenic disturbance. Arthritis Rheum., *25*:213–217, 1982.

42. Pomeranz, B.: Do endorphins mediate acupuncture analgesia? The endorphins. Adv. Biochem. Psychopharmacol., *18*:351–359, 1977.

43. Resnick, D., Shall, S.R., and Robbins, J.M.: Diffuse idiopathic skeletal hyperostosis (DISH): Forestier's disease with extraspinal manifestations. Radiology, *115*:513–524, 1975.

44. Rotstein, J., and Good, R.A.: Steroid pseudorheumatism. Arch. Intern. Med., *99*:545–555, 1957.

45. Simons, D.G.: Muscle pain syndromes—part 1. Am. J. Phys. Med., *54*:289–311, 1975.

46. Simons, D.G.: Muscle pain syndromes—part 2. Am. J. Phys. Med., *55*:15–42, 1976.

47. Slocumb, C.H.: Symposium on certain problems arising from the clinical use of cortisone. Mayo Clin. Proc., *28*:655–657, 1953.

48. Smythe, H.A.: Nonarticular rheumatism and the "fibrositis" syndrome. *In* Arthritis and Allied Conditions, 8th ed. Edited by J.L. Hollander, and D.J. McCarty. Philadelphia, Lea & Febiger, 1972, pp. 874–884.

49. Smythe, H.A.: Two contributions to understanding of the "fibrositis" syndrome. Bull. Rheum. Dis., *28*:928–931, 1977.

49a. Smythe, H.A.: Problems with the MMPI. J. Rheumatol., *11*:417–418, 1984.

50. Toglia, J.V.: Acute flexion-extension injury of the neck. Electronystagmographic study of 309 cases. Neurology, *26*:808–814, 1976.

51. Utsinger, P.D., Resnick, D., and Robins, J.M.: Diffuse skeletal abnormalities in Forestier's disease. Arch. Intern. Med., *136*:763–768, 1976.

52. Walters, J.A.: Psychogenic regional pain alias hysterical pain. Brain, *84*:1–18, 1961.

53. Wittig, R.M., et al.: Disturbed sleep in patients complaining of chronic pain. J. Nerv. Ment. Dis., *170*:429–431, 1982.

54. Wolfe, F.: The tender point count: Clinical significance in rheumatic disease. Personal communication, 1983.

55. Yunus, M., et al.: Primary fibromyalgia (fibrositis): Clinical study of 50 patients with matched normal controls. Semin. Arthritis Rheum., *11*:151–171, 1981.

Chapter 71

Neuropathic Joint Disease (Charcot Joints)

Gerald P. Rodnan

. . . Without any appreciable external cause we may see, between one day and the next, the development of a general and often enormous tumefaction of a member, most commonly without any pain whatever, or any febrile reaction. At the end of a few days the general tumefaction disappears, but a more or less considerable swelling of the joint remains, owing to the formation of a hydrarthus; and sometimes to the accumulation of liquid in the periarticular serous bursae also. On puncture being made, a transparent lemon-colored liquid has been frequently drawn from the joint.

One or two weeks after the invasion, sometimes much sooner, the existence of more or less marked cracking sounds may be noted, betraying the alteration of the articular surfaces which, at this period, is already profound. The hydrarthus becomes quickly resolved, leaving after it an extreme mobility in the joint. Hence consecutive luxations are frequently found, their production being largely aided by the wearing away of the heads of the bones which has taken place. I have several times observed a rapid wasting of the muscular masses of the members affected by the articular disorder. . . . Besides the wearing down of the articular surfaces . . . you may notice the presence of foreign bodies, of bony stalactites, and, in a word, of all the customary accompaniments of arthritis deformans. . . . I am led to believe that . . . they are produced in an accidental manner, and to all appearances chiefly by the more or less energetic movements to which the patient sometimes continues to subject the affected members. . .

—J.-M. Charcot, 1868[22]

Neuropathic joint disease (Charcot joints) is a form of chronic progressive degenerative arthropathy, affecting one or more peripheral or vertebral articulation, which develops as a result of a disturbance in normal sensory innervation of the joints. The arthropathy represents a complication of a variety of neurologic disorders, the most common of which are syphilitic tabes dorsalis, diabetic neuropathy, and syringomyelia.

Credit for the recognition of neuropathic arthropathy rests with J.-M. Charcot, who, in 1868, provided an incisive account of the indolent swelling and instability of the knees in patients with "l'ataxie locomotrice progressive," or tabes dorsalis.[22] The relationship between syringomyelia and neuropathic joint disease was established by Schultze and Kahler in 1888,[67] as well as by Sokoloff in 1892.[108] Clinical appreciation of diabetic neuropathy as a cause of this arthropathy dates from the report of Jordan in 1936.[59]

PATHOPHYSIOLOGIC FEATURES

It was apparent to Charcot that this condition was not a primary affection of the joints, but was rather a consequence of disease of the nervous system. He noted what he believed to be a similar disorder following other types of spinal cord injury and postulated that the articular disease was due to the damage or interruption of nerves that exerted a trophic influence on the tissues of the joint. This concept was soon challenged, and the hypothesis that the arthropathy resulted from trauma to a joint deprived of its sensory innervation was suggested.[31,126] This second view was supported by the studies in 1917 of Eloesser, who observed the occurrence of fractures and the development of an arthropathy corresponding to human neuropathic joint disease in cats that remained active, although ataxic after surgical section of posterior nerve roots.[35] Destructive change appeared rapidly in a number of animals in which rhizotomy was followed by cauterization of an area of femoral condyle. In another study, unilateral sensory denervation of the hind limb of rabbits resulted in progressive depletion of cells in all structures of the knee joint, even when protected in a plaster cast. That the initial change in the articular cartilage occurred in the middle layers suggests a nutritional deficiency.[40] Of interest with regard to pathogenesis is the frequent occurrence of fractures and of destructive arthropathy in children and young adults with congenital insensitivity to pain,[79,103,121] including that associated with familial dysautonomia.[16] The parts most often affected in this condition are the ankles and the tarsal joints. The knee may also be affected.[1,37,75,78,121,122] One report notes a pain-insensitive woman with severe degeneration of a knee and upper lumbar vertebrae at age 17 and, later, similar destructive changes in a hip and lower dorsal vertebrae.[87]

It appears that neuropathic arthropathy follows a loss of proprioceptive or pain sensation that leads to relaxation of supporting structures and chronic instability of the joint. Under these circumstances, the joint or, in the case of insensitivity to pain, the entire patient is deprived of normal protective reactions when exposed both to the stress of everyday motion and to the additional trauma caused by the underlying neurologic disease. Severe or cumulative injury damages articular cartilage and fractures subchondral bone; the results are degeneration and disorganization of the joint.

On occasion, affected joints undergo rapid disintegration, termed acute neuroarthropathy, with changes that suggest underlying linear "stress" or microfractures.[37,58,75,83,120] The swiftness of the bone destruction (resorption), combined with a lack of evidence of accompanying bone repair in these cases, has been considered evidence of a neurovascular mechanism in the pathogenesis of Charcot joint disease, whereby the changes result from a neurally initiated vascular reflex that leads to hyperemia and hyperactive resorption of bone by osteoclasts.[12,13] These changes occur most frequently in syringomyelia of the shoulder and in the vertebral neuroarthropathy associated with tabes dorsalis. The bone may shatter and fall apart within a few weeks to months. Microscopic examination reveals linear "hairline" or "stress" fractures that may be invisible on roentgenographic study. Such fractures may extend to the articular surface and are believed to play an important role in the development of neuropathic joint disease. The frequency of fractures in the various forms of neuropathic arthropathy and their importance in initiation and aggravation of joint destruction[58] are discussed later in this chapter.

The occurrence of severe degenerative joint disease in individuals deprived of protective proprioceptive sensibility suggests that repetitive, longitudinal, impulsive loading affects the pathogenesis of osteoarthritis.[90,91,93] Such loading, as occurs in all daily activities, places enormous stress on the articular structures in joints not protected by normal proprioceptive neuromuscular reflexes. This stress is especially great on the subchondral bone. This bone acts as the chief attenuator of the loading force or shock absorber in this system and thus protects the articular cartilage, which is sensitive to breakdown from tensile fatigue. Stiffening of the subchondral bone as a result of healing of trabecular fractures is probably the initial event in osteoarthritis and, from the foregoing evidence, can be implicated as a primary factor in the genesis of neuropathic joint disease. The loss of proprioceptive sensation increases stress on the articular cartilage on a long-term basis and can thereby initiate severe degenerative joint disease. Repetitive subluxation, which aggravates the stress of impulsive loading, would be expected to accelerate the breakdown of the Charcot joints.

Chondrocalcinosis, involving numerous joints and the presence of microcrystals of calcium pyrophosphate dihydrate in the knee joint fluid, has been described in four patients with late latent syphilis and polyarticular neuropathic joint disease.[7,55] Three of these individuals had evidence of tabes dorsalis: the fourth did not. In one of these patients, an episode of pseudogout in a knee was followed by the sudden collapse of the medial tibial plateau of that joint. The authors of these reports propose the existence of a pathogenetic synergism and suggest that neuropathic joint disease is more likely to develop in individuals with tabes dorsalis who have coincidental pre-existing chondrocalcinosis. They also postulate the release of calcium pyrophosphate crystals into the synovial cavity as a result of microfractures and progressive fragmentation of the articular cartilage and suggest that pseudogout may account for at least some of the intermittent joint effusions that are often early manifestations of Charcot joint disease. Others have noted roentgenographic changes resembling those found in neuropathic arthropathy in individuals with calcium pyrophosphate dihydrate deposition disease but without evidence of any underlying neurologic disturbance.[49,94]

PATHOLOGIC FINDINGS

In patients with advanced disease, the Charcot joint presents a combination of destructive and hypertrophic changes similar in many respects to those found in ordinary non-neuropathic degenerative joint disease. These changes include fibrillation and erosion of articular cartilage, destruction of menisci, formation of loose bodies, and the growth of marginal osteophytes.[57,64,88] Marginal osteophytes are more exuberant and grotesque in neuropathic arthropathy than in ordinary degenerative joint disease, perhaps because of the hypermobility of the joint.[26] New bone growth may extend up the shaft of the bone well beyond the confines of the joint and into ligaments and muscles.[88] Areas of dense bone formation also occur in the zone of provisional calcification beneath the articular surface, where one sees proliferation and calcification of cartilage. Subluxation is common, as are various intra- and juxta-articular fractures, which may involve articular facets, osteophytes, epicondyles, or condyles and may lead to the formation of additional callus.[58] Large or small fragments of bone lie free in the articular cavity. Metaplastic ossification takes place at the sites of attachment of ligaments and tendons.[57] The large masses of what appears to be metaplastic bone that are observed on roentgenographic examination are usually bits of osseous tissue that have broken off the condyles of the articulating bones and have become partly incorporated into the joint capsule and synovium.[53,57]

Neuropathic joint disease that affects large peripheral articulations is often accompanied by bulky, frequently sanguineous, effusions. The composition of the fluid is similar to that of other types of traumatic synovitis. When studied by means of the intra-articular injection of a tracer quantity of ^{131}iodine-labeled protein, the absorption of serum albumin from a Charcot knee joint was found to be the same as in a normal knee.[100] Villous transformation of the synovium occurs, and like the joint capsule, the synovium may be fibrotic. Numerous bits of cartilage and small bony fragments often adhere to the surface of the synovium and become incorporated into the substance of tissue. The synovium, which generally exhibits only a mild inflammatory reaction, may also contain bits of calcified cartilage and metaplastic bone, as well as deposits of hemosiderin[26,53,56,98] (Fig. 71–1). Although these abnormalities are not restricted to the Charcot joint, they suggest this diagnosis when found in synovium from patients with degenerative joint disease.

The pathologic changes in vertebral neuroarthropathy may be rapidly progressive and may involve degeneration of the intervertebral discs as well as the diarthrodial joints.[37] Subchondral sclerosis of the vertebral bodies has been attributed to reactive osteitis associated with the healing of multiple microfractures.[37,57,58] Gross fractures also occur. Severe fragmentation and extensive dissolution of bone may occur within a period of a few weeks to months.[37] Massive, bizarrely shaped marginal osteophytes are a characteristic finding. One sees narrowing of the intervertebral discs and malalignment of the spine in the form of lateral and anterior subluxations, gross dislocations, and deformity of vertebral bodies resulting from collapse of bone. Undue strain is thereby placed on the

diarthrodial articulations, which eventually undergo similar destructive changes.

CLINICAL FEATURES

Charcot joints occur more often in men than in women and usually develop after the age of 40 years; the distribution of affected joints is determined by the underlying neurologic lesion.[14,33,41,64,109,112,116,118,127] Changes characteristically commence in a single large joint or a group of neighboring small joints, such as the tarsus, and frequently follow trauma to the part. The onset of symptoms is usually insidious. The patient notes progressive enlargement of an effusion or increasing instability of the joint. Although the swelling is often painful, presumably because of stretching of the overlying soft tissue, the discomfort is disproportionately mild considering the degree of distention and destructive changes that may be present. Thus, the patient may continue to use the joint freely and may not seek medical attention. In some patients, an intra- or juxta-articular fracture causes symptoms with dramatic suddenness. About 50% of tabetic Charcot joints are painful.[63,115]

Spontaneous Fractures

Charcot first called attention to the frequency of spontaneous fractures in tabes dorsalis.[21] Such fractures, which are common,[5] were recorded 11 times in a report of 64 patients with tabes dorsalis and neuropathic joint disease.[115] Fractures may be the first evidence of tabes dorsalis,[46,57,115] and they usually occur early in the course of this disorder. The femur is broken most frequently,[5,115] followed by the tibia[5] and the bones of the forearm; fractures also occur in the small bones, especially in the tarsus.[5] Fractures of the tibia, fibula, tarsal bones, particularly the calcaneus, and the metatarsals (also frequent) have been recorded in patients with diabetic neuropathy and pseudotabes and often constitute the initial feature of neuropathic arthropathy.[28,34,59,66,77,104] Spontaneous dislocations in the foot and ankle may also occur in individuals with diabetic neuropathy. If unrecognized and untreated, this disturbance may provoke or may hasten the development of neuropathic arthropathy.[80] Spontaneous fractures may occur in the upper extremities in patients with syringomyelia.[46] The fractures of the long bones are most often transverse, especially fractures of the proximal portion of the femur, and heal quickly with proper management. On occasion, however, one may see striking fragmentation of bone (Fig. 71–2); if this occurs and if the fracture extends to the joint, recovery may be slow and considerable deformity may result. The basis for this tendency to pathologic fracture in these patients is unclear. The bone appears to be

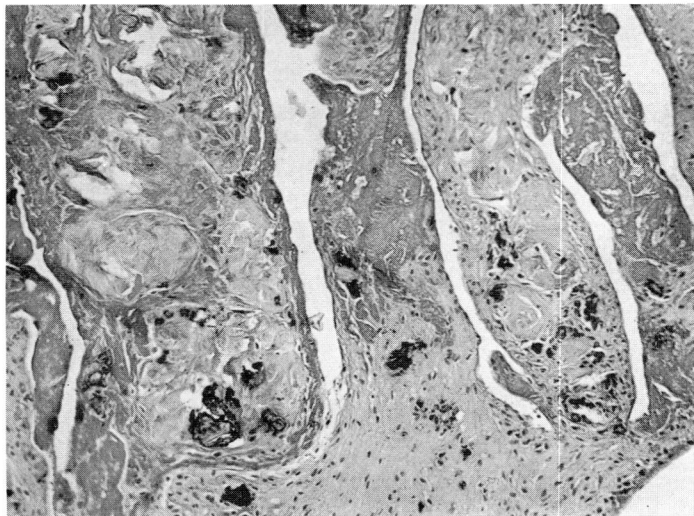

Fig. 71–1. Photomicrograph of synovium from the right hip of a 31-year-old man with neuropathic disease secondary to syphilitic tabes dorsalis resulting from congenital syphilis (See also Fig. 71–5). Note the surface hyalinization, dense fibrosis, and scattered areas of calcification. (Hematoxylin and eosin stain.)

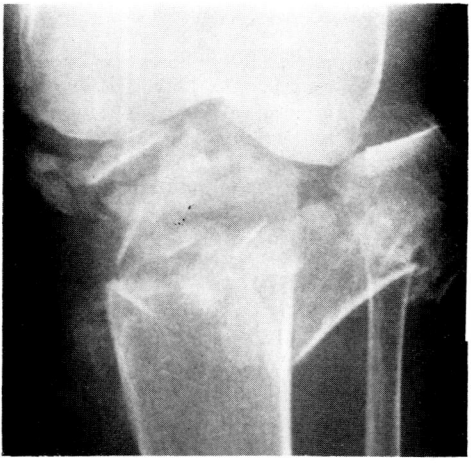

Fig. 71–2. Neuropathic arthropathy of the left knee of a 64-year-old woman with syphilitic tabes dorsalis who has a painless, comminuted fracture of the tibia.

normal on roentgenographic and microscopic examination.[57,115] Fractures also occurred in the cats studied by Eloesser following surgical section of the posterior nerve roots.[35]

Hypermobility and Effusion

Examination of the joint early in the course of the disease usually reveals hypermobility, always a possible sign of neuropathic arthropathy. In the presence of effusion, the joint is warmer than normal, and the patient often notes tenderness and pain

on motion, although these findings are much less intense than would be expected from the marked distention of the joint. Synovial effusions may persist for many weeks or months and may yield large amounts of fluid. Later, one sees increasing enlargement, deformity, and instability of the joint, as well as coarse crepitation resulting from the overgrowth of bone, the loss of articular cartilage, and the formation of loose bodies. Palpation of these loose bodies has been described as "feeling a bag of bones." When the feet, hips, or vertebrae are involved, abnormalities in articular form and function may be less apparent.

Vertebral Neuroarthropathy

Vertebral neuroarthropathy (Charcot spine), first reported by Kronig in 1884,[125] is most often associated with syphilitic tabes dorsalis, but it has also been described in patients with syringomyelia and diabetes mellitus.[17,29,37,51,119,125] It may be the initial manifestation of the underlying neurologic disease. Trauma has been implicated as a predisposing factor in many instances.[17] In tabes dorsalis, the most common site is the lumbar spine; less often, the lower thoracic region and, rarely, the cervical vertebrae are involved.[37] A single vertebra may be affected. In syringomyelia, changes occur most often in the cervical spine.[9] The initial symptom is usually low back pain, or pain in the lower extremities. This pain has been attributed to posterior nerve root compression resulting from malalignment of the vertebral bodies, disc protuberance, and hypertrophy of bone.[37] Anterior nerve root pressure may give rise to weakness of the leg or to footdrop.[3,37,119] The back may become deformed, with the development of lateral curvature and a kyphos.[125] In many instances, however, the patient with vertebral neuroarthropathy is asymptomatic or experiences only slight discomfort, and the diagnosis is suspected on circumstantial evidence, that is, the presence of tabes dorsalis, or it may be an incidental finding on radiographic examination.

The diagnosis of neuropathic arthropathy requires identificaiton of an underlying neurologic disorder. Suspicion should be aroused in cases of monarticular disease with marked joint effusion and hypermobility, especially if the patient has disproportionately little pain with respect to the degree of disorganization of the joint.

Tabes Dorsalis

Neuropathic joint disease was first associated with locomotor ataxia[22] and for many years recognition of this arthropathy was limited almost solely to its occurrence in patients with syphilitic tabes dorsalis. Typically, the onset of neuropathic arthropathy takes place between the ages of 40 and 60 years, but the disorder may be encountered much earlier in the uncommon individual with tabes dorsalis resulting from congenital syphilis. In view of the ease with which involvement of the vertebral column may be overlooked, previous estimates of an incidence rate of Charcot joints in 5% of tabetic patients may well be erroneously low.[63,115] With the decline in frequency of late syphilis, tabes dorsalis, once the most common cause of Charcot joint disease,[17,41,64,115,119,123] has become rare. The development of neuropathic joint disease may be one of the earliest manifestations of tabes dorsalis, and some patients may remain free of obvious ataxia or other complaints referable to neurologic dysfunction for long periods.[63,123]

Neither the classically complete form of Argyll Robertson pupils nor a positive serologic test result is essential to the diagnosis of syphilitic tabes dorsalis. The irregularity in pupillary size and reaction, described by D. Argyll Robertson in 1868, may be slight, and careful sensory examination is more important. The absence of deep pain sensation is the best single criterion of a neuroarthropathy. Conventional procedures measuring reagin often revert to negative, with treatment and time,[109,117,126] although reactions to more sensitive tests for specific antibody, using spirochetal antigen or treponemal immobilization, may remain positive indefinitely.

The neuropathic joint disease in tabes dorsalis is characteristically monarticular at the onset. Most frequently affected are the knee, the hip, the ankle,

and the joints between bodies of lumbar and lower dorsal vertebrae (Figs. 71–3, 71–4, 71–5, 71–6). Cervical vertebral arthropathy has been noted.[9] On occasion, polyarticular involvement may include joints of the upper as well as lower extremity.[6,109] In such cases, one must take care to exclude the possibility of other rheumatic disorders. The eventual involvement of more than a single joint is common, but seldom are more than three affected in one individual. Damage to the knee leads to an increase in lateral motion and to a varus, valgus, or genu recurvatum deformity. Partial or complete dislocation may occur. Pyemic staphylococcal infection of a Charcot knee has been reported.[71,99] Disease of the hip is often complicated by fracture,[111] and the absorption of bone may be striking. Vertebral osteoarthropathy leads to kyphosis or kyphoscoliosis; local tenderness may be lacking, and movement, although restricted, may be painless despite the deformity.

Diabetic Neuropathy

Diabetic neuropathy constitutes an increasingly frequent basis for Charcot joint disease and now outranks syphilitic tabes dorsalis in this respect.[18,25,36,37,68,72,104] The appearance of Charcot joint disease may be the first sign of the development of diabetic neuropathy. Patients who develop this arthropathy usually have diabetes mellitus of long standing and invariably show evidence of severe sensory impairment in the feet.[54,72,104]

The role of mechanical instability of the foot in the pathogenesis of this disorder has been stressed.[68] Although disruptive bacterial invasion is common in the diabetic Charcot foot, authorities believe that this infection probably plays little or no role in the pathogenesis of the joint disease.[68] The contributory or provocative role of pathologic fractures, which are especially frequent in the tarsal and metatarsal bones, has received considerable attention.[28,34,57,66,77,104]

Destructive changes, usually unilateral at first, occur chiefly in the metatarsal, tarsal, and phalangeal bones and in the metatarsophalangeal and tarsometatarsal joint.[25,36] Such changes occur much less often in the tibia, fibula, ankles, and knees. These patients, who seek medical attention because of soft tissue swelling or bony deformity, have instability and crepitus in the affected joints.[104] Individuals with tarsometatarsophalangeal joint involvement may have changes suggestive of inflammatory arthritis with local swelling, redness, and warmth, but they have little or no pain. Polyarticular disease is uncommon, but has been reported, including involvement of the fingers, wrists, and elbows.[6,38] Neuropathic osteoarthropathy in the upper extremities is uncommon;[18,104] however, in

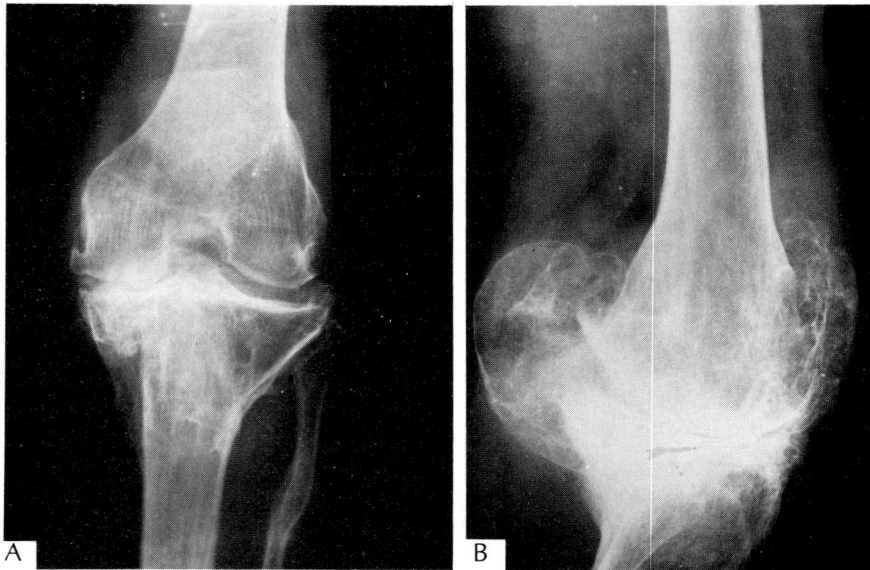

Fig. 71–3. *A,* Neuropathic arthropathy of the left knee of a 72-year-old man with tabes dorsalis. Note the fractures of the tibia and fibula, the loss of articular cartilage in medial compartment, and the large osteophytes. *B,* Neuropathic arthropathy of the right knee of a 76-year-old woman with tabes dorsalis. Note the exuberant new bone encasing the distal portion of the femur.

some cases, destructive changes in the shoulders have been associated with the presence of chondrocalcinosis. A few instances of vertebral neuroarthropathy associated with diabetic taboneuropathy have been recorded.[37] The development of tarsal or ankle disease is often preceded by trauma, with ligamentous injury or pathologic fracture of the calcaneus or other tarsal bones of the tibia.[36,104]

Faulty proprioception is associated with laxity of ligaments and instability of the intertarsal and tarsometatarsal joints and tendency toward talipes valgus. Microfractures of the bone occur,[36] and later, gross fragmentation is combined with dislocations. Bone destruction often progresses rapidly. As a result of progressive collapse of the tarsal and tarsometatarsal joints, the tarsal bones deviate and bulge medially, with marked convexity of the inner margin of the foot, which becomes shortened and thickened (cube foot).[104] Roentgenographic examination discloses erosion and sequestration of bone and osteolysis. Metatarsal fragments may fail to unite following fracture, especially if the patient has a superimposed infection of the part. Healing usually occurs, however, following prolonged immobilization.

The mutilation of the metatarsal and phalangeal bones is often striking in degree.[68,72] One may see complete absorption of the metatarsal heads and severe tapering of the shafts with pencil-point narrowing. The remaining bone becomes sclerotic.

The formation of synostoses of the tarsometatarsal and intertarsal joints accompanies the process of bone absorption. Loss of bone and remodeling of the bases of the proximal phalanges result in a variety of deformities of the metatarsophalangeal joints. In time, the proximal phalanges may be completely absorbed. The changes in the toes lead to foreshortening and are associated with the development of talipes cavus. Calcification of the blood vessels of the foot is common. Fracture of the tibia and fibula, as well as of tarsal and metatarsal bones, has been observed.[36,77,104] Increased uptake of both ^{99m}technetium-phosphate and ^{67}gallium-citrate was noted in the foot and ankle of a man with juvenile-onset diabetes mellitus who had advanced neuropathy. The positive scans were attributed to Charcot joint disease itself and not to infection.[44]

Typically, the patient has painless swelling of the foot, accompanied by little if any redness or warmth. Some cases are complicated by local infection, and in such circumstances, destructive changes may be partly the result of osteomyelitis.[50] Progressive disintegration of the joints leads to shortening and deformity of the foot, which becomes everted (Fig. 71–7).

Syringomyelia

Neuropathic joint disease develops in approximately one-fourth of patients with syringomyelia,

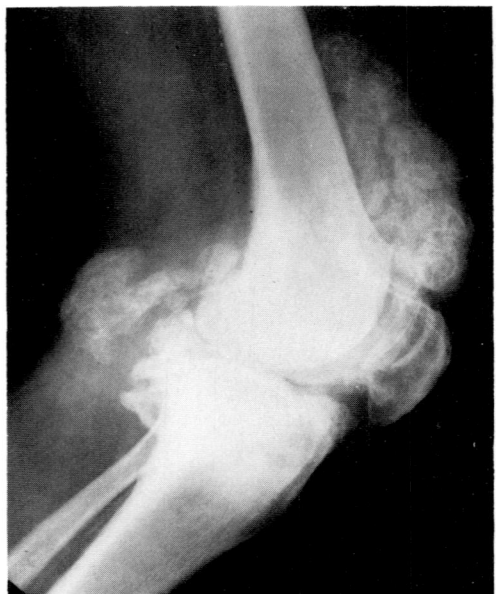

Fig. 71–4. Neuropathic arthropathy of the right knee of a man with tabes dorsalis. The suprapatellar and semi-membranosus bursae are filled and distended with numerous large, nodular, faceted ossifications. These lesions are partly or largely fused to each other, and those in the suprapatellar bursa have an internal structure simulating a cortex and medulla. The posterior surface of the patella and the surface of the tibia are grossly irregular, and several large osteophytes originate from the posterior portion of the tibia. Sclerosis of the subchondral bone is marked. An anteroposterior view of this knee revealed a fracture of the medial condyle of the tibia.

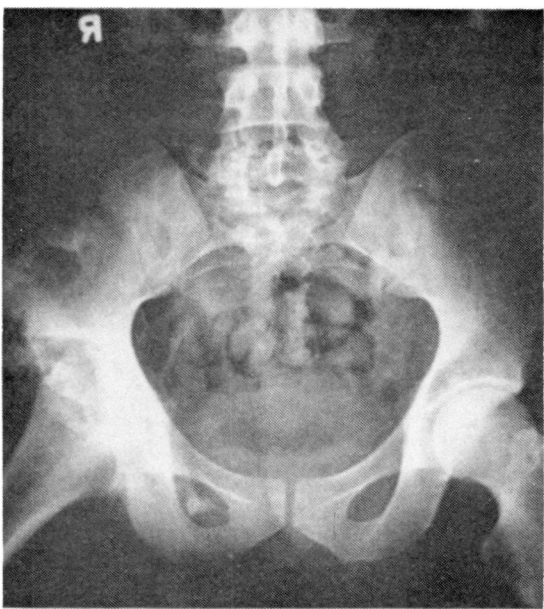

Fig. 71–5. Neuropathic disease of the right hip in a 31-year-old man with tabes dorsalis as a result of congenital syphilis. Note the loss of articular cartilage, the marked sclerosis of subchondral bone, and the deformity of the femur and the acetabulum.

usually involving a shoulder or elbow and less commonly the more distal joints of the upper extremity.[93,105,114] Brain and Wilkinson found roentgenographic evidence of cervical vertebral osteoarthropathy in nearly half their patients.[9] Other findings included osteoporosis and flattening of the vertebral bodies, narrowing of intervertebral discs, and a tendency to form florid osteophytes. All these findings represented the final stages of a process that had earlier appeared to be indistinguishable from ordinary cervical spondylosis. These workers concluded that these changes were due to the same causes as cervical spondylosis, but that the process of degeneration was intensified by the neurologic disease. When the shoulder and elbow are affected, the patient usually has large effusions and, later, severe disintegration of one joint, often with striking rapidity[74,82,105] (Fig. 71–8). In cases of neuropathic arthropathy associated with syringomyelia, affected joints are often painful.[124]

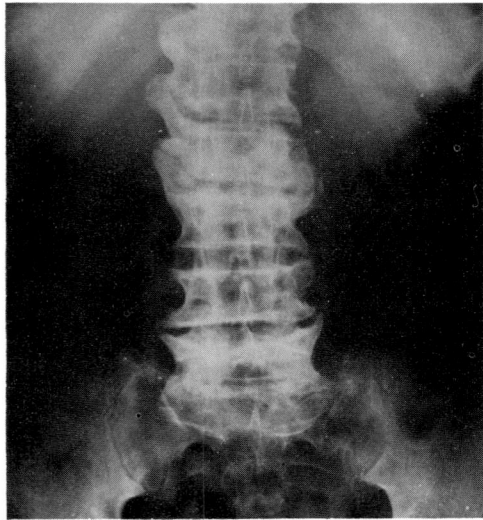

Fig. 71–6. Neuropathic osteoarthropathy of the lower portion of the vertebral column of a 78-year-old man with tabes dorsalis. Note the irregular narrowing of the disc spaces, the vertebral fracture, the subchondral sclerosis, and the bulky beaked osteophytes that resemble "les becs des perroquets."

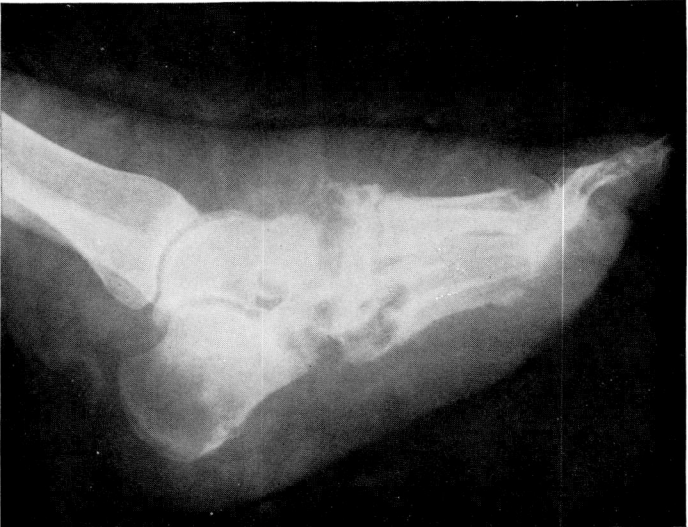

Fig. 71–7. Neuropathic joint disease of the foot in a 58-year-old woman with diabetic neuropathy. Note the almost complete destruction of the midtarsus and the proximal portions of the metatarsal bones.

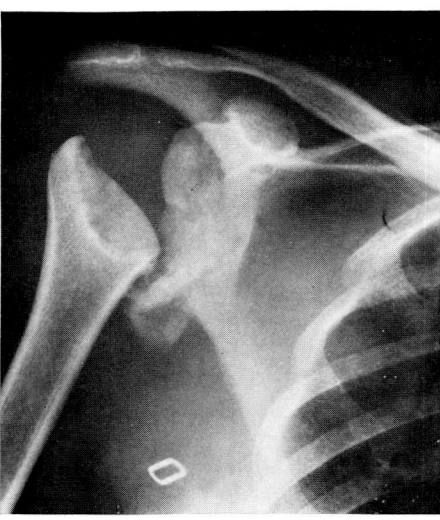

Fig. 71–8. Neuropathic disease of the shoulder in a 54-year-old woman with syringomyelia. Note the loss of bony substance of the humeral head and the cloud-like calcification in the periarticular soft tissues. The patient first noted painless swelling of the shoulder only 2 weeks prior to this roentgenogram.

Myelomeningocele

Sensory impairment resulting from myelomeningocele is the most frequent basis of neuropathic arthropathy in childhood, and the ankle and tarsal joints are affected.[19,41] Individuals who retain the power of locomotion are particularly liable to this complication, which has been observed in children a young as five years (Fig. 71–9).

Miscellaneous Features

Charcot joints have been described in patients with a variety of other spontaneous and traumatic disorders of the central and peripheral nervous system that cause sensory impairment in the limbs. These conditions include congenital insensitivity to pain and familial dysautonomia[1,16,75,78,87,103,120,121] (Fig. 71–10), myelopathy of pernicious anemia,[47] spinal cord injury and paraplegia,[62,110,116,125] tuberculous and other forms of adhesive arachnoiditis,[81] various forms of hereditary sensory neuropathy,[48,58,79,83] Charcot-Marie-Tooth disease, named for J.-M. Charcot, P. Marie, and H. H. Tooth who reported it in 1886,[15] familial interstitial hypertrophic polyneuropathy of Déjerine and Sottas, described by J.J. Déjerine and J. Sottas in 1890,[100] peripheral nerve injury,[41,62,116] amyloid neuropathy,[86,89,102] including familial amyloid polyneuropathy and amyloidosis associated with Waldenström's macroglobulinemia, the neuropathy of leprosy,[85] late yaws,[107] and acromegaly.[30]

Children with thalidomide disease have articular changes analogous to those encountered in adult neuropathic arthropathy,[69] and fetal sensory peripheral neuropathy may be responsible for these and other malformations seen in this disorder.

In rare instances, patients with joint disease that is otherwise typical of neuropathic arthropathy on clinical and radiographic examination fail to show evidence of any underlying neurologic disorder.[8,58]

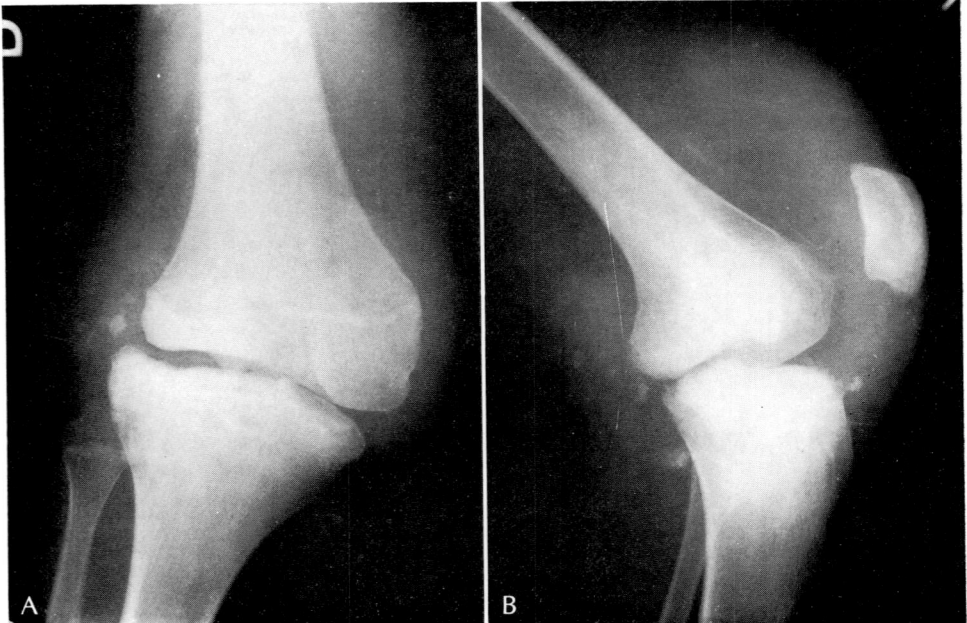

Fig. 71–9. *A* and *B,* Neuropathic disease of the right knee in an 18-year-old man with myelomeningocele. Note the erosion of the lateral condyle of the femur and the lateral portion of the tibial plateau, the numerous calcified bodies, and the evidence of a large effusion. Pathologic examination of the synovium revealed changes similar to those illustrated in Figure 71–1. Compression arthrodesis was performed and the joint has remained fused for more than 6 years.

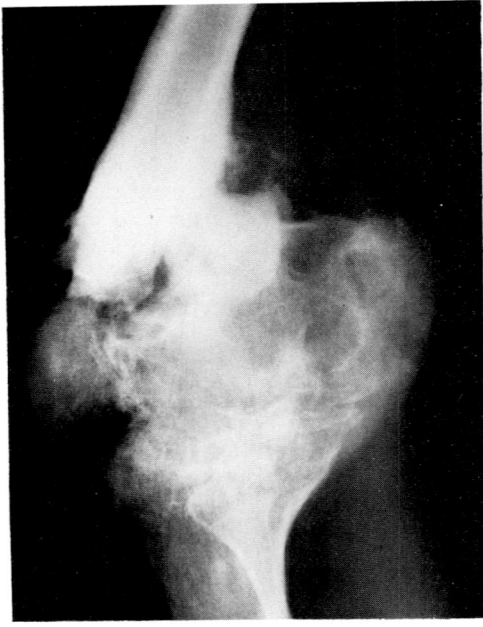

Fig. 71–10. Neuropathic arthropathy of the right knee of a 29-year-old man with congenital insensitivity to pain.

Progressive Arthropathy Following Intra-Articular Injection of Corticosteroids

A number of reports have noted the rapid deterioration of a hip or knee following the repeated intra-articular injection of hydrocortisone, with clinical and roentgenographic findings similar to those of neuropathic arthropathy.[2,20,113,118] One hypothesis is that the relief of pain provided by such treatment may permit excessive weight bearing and mobility and may interfere with normal protective processes, thereby accelerating the progress of the underlying joint disease, usually rheumatoid arthritis (RA) or osteoarthritis. Although this hypothesis may appear attractive, the question of a neuropathic basis for these joint changes remains controversial because corticosteroid-treated patients retain normal sensibility to pain. Moreover, evidence suggests that corticosteroids may directly inhibit the formation of protein polysaccharide (matrix) by articular cartilage.[70]

Hollander, Jessar, and Brown found that the extent of deterioration in injected knees of patients with RA or osteoarthritis was no greater over a 7-year period than that observed in untreated joints.[52] Instability of a weight-bearing joint developed in fewer than 1% of their patients and in only 4 joints, of approximately 4,000 patients, did they observe extensive absorption of bone. In at least one instance of so-called "cortisone arthropathy of the hip" in a patient receiving cortisone orally, the joint destruction appears to have been the result of staphylococcal infection.[76] Other instances of complicating infection, usually involving the staphylococci and termed septic arthritis, have been reported in individuals not receiving corticosteroids.[71,99]

ROENTGENOGRAPHIC FINDINGS

Roentgenographic examination is important in the evaluation of the degree of joint damage and is essential to the detection of involvement in such inaccessible articulations as those of the vertebral column. The roentgenographic findings in the early stages of the Charcot joint may be normal, however, except perhaps when changes are due to synovial effusion or when a patient has evidence of bony detritus in the para-articular soft tissue.[60,82]

In more advanced cases, roentgenograms show varying degrees and combinations of destructive and hypertrophic changes. One sees loss of articular cartilage, fragmentation and absorption of subchondral bone, and proliferation of new bone at the joint margins. The bony overgrowth, which is often bizarre in configuration, may be so great as to surround the joint like a spongy mass (see Fig. 71–3,B). The para-articular tissues are thickened and may contain numerous nodular or irregularly shaped calcifications and ossifications. These masses, which may fill the suprapatellar and other bursae, include fragments of fractured bone or appear to be the result of new, metaplastic bone formation (see Fig. 71–4).

Pathologic fractures are common and usually involve the articular surface. They vary from "chips" or minute fragments of the articular margins, which give rise to irregular free bodies within the joint, to transverse or comminuted fractures of the femur or tibia (see Figs. 71–2, 71–3). Destruction of epiphyseal substance, tapering, may be considerable, accompanied by fragmentation of bone, whereas the remaining subchondral bone is condensed (Fig. 71–4). Ultimately, the osseous structures may completely disintegrate. Findings such as these are present in Charcot joints, regardless of location or of the different primary neurologic disorders responsible for their development. Although the changes just described evolve slowly in some patients with neuropathic arthropathy of diverse origin, severe joint destruction has occurred within a few weeks to months.[7,82]

Similar changes encountered in the Charcot spine are narrowing of the disc spaces, destruction and collapse of the vertebral bodies, and formation of large, beaked osteopytes (les becs des perroquets), or massive paravertebral bone growths that may lead to ankylosis.[17,119,125] The most common deformity is kyphoscoliosis; spondylolisthesis may also occur (see Fig. 71–6).

The roentgenographic changes encountered in the pedal arthropathy complicating diabetic neuropathy, which have been described, are characterized by a combination of severe absorption and mutilation of the bones of the mid- and forefoot[34,36] (Fig. 71–7). Little or no new bone is formed in this type of neuropathic arthropathy.

In their general character, these abnormalities are similar to those encountered in non-neuropathic degenerative joint disease. The exaggerated degree of the changes lends distinctiveness to the radiographic appearance of the Charcot joint. In any event, suspicion aroused by roentgenographic findings must be carefully corroborated by clinical evidence before diagnosis can be established.

MANAGEMENT

The nature of most of the neurologic diseases responsible for neuropathic arthropathy is such that treatment of these conditions has little influence on the progression of the joint disease. Immobilization of the affected joint and restriction of weight bearing are basic principles in management. Mechanical devices should be fitted with great care and readjusted frequently because the patient may be unable to judge the efficiency of the appliance. Immobilization of the vertebral column is attempted by corset or brace. The patient with a Charcot joint of the lower extremity can be placed in a caliper walking splint. Crutches are helpful when the hips are involved. Conservative treatment with stress or prolonged non-weight bearing and prevention of pressure ulcers by proper weight distribution in the shoe and other measures has been beneficial in patients with diabetic neuroarthropathy involving the tarsal or tarsometatarsal joints, presumably by preventing further trauma.[4,54,66,68,104]

Operative procedures may include amputation or arthrodesis of weight-bearing joints. Amputation may become advisable in disease of the foot or knee, especially when this disorder is complicated by septic arthritis that fails to respond to appropriate treatment with antibiotics. Amputation in the case of genicular involvement should be considered only when disintegration of the joint is advanced and when the process has remained unilateral.

Arthrodesis of Charcot joints often proves difficult. Many surgeons failed in the past because of infection or nonunion, or both.[10,33,57,112,126] Reports exist of successful fusions of the hip, knee, ankle (extra-articular), and vertebrae, although the period of follow-up observation has often been brief.[11,24,53,101,112,123,125,126] The apparent improvement in efforts at arthrodesis of the knee, which is now successful more often than not,[42] has been attributed to the introduction of better methods of internal fixation and the use of a compression technique.[53,101] Other important factors include the following: (1) the careful removal of all cartilage and debris and sclerotic, poorly vascularized bone; (2) thorough debridement of the synovium and joint capsule;[32] and (3) the use of orthoses to protect the joint during the prolonged period of postoperative immobilization.[42,45]

Total knee arthroplasty and total hip replacement have been performed in a few patients,[27,43,69,96,106,111] but recurrent dislocation and other disastrous complications occur with such regularity that these procedures are generally contraindicated in individuals with Charcot joint disease,[14,23,39] who lack the proprioceptive and deep pain sensation that normally protect these unstable replacements against dislocation, subluxation, and subsequent loosening. Patients with hip pain subjected to other arthroplastic procedures, including cup arthroplasty, have been relieved of this pain, even though these joints have also subluxed, loosened, or dislocated.[43] Glenohumeral joint replacement has been performed in patients with syringomyelia.

Although gradual, progressive breakdown and lysis of bone are the general rule in the arthropathy of the foot secondary to diabetic neuropathy, an occasional patient shows improvement when placed in a walking cast or a short leg brace.[4] A patellar-tendon-bearing orthosis may help to protect the foot and ankle from trauma by partially relieving the lower extremity of weight; this device may assist in the healing of plantar and calcaneal ulcerations.[45] Bone destruction has beeen arrested in two cases following lumbar sympathectomy,[84] but such a result has not been reported by others.

REFERENCES

1. Abell, J.M., Jr., and Hayes, J.T.: Charcot knee due to congenital insensitivity to pain. J. Bone Joint Surg., 46A:1287–1291, 1964.
2. Alarcon-Segovia, D., and Ward, L.E.: Charcot-like arthropathy in rheumatoid arthritis. Consequence of overuse of a joint repeatedly injected with hydrocortisone. JAMA, 193:1052–1054, 1965.
3. Alergant, C.D.: Tabetic spinal arthropathy. Two cases with motor symptoms due to root compression. Br. J. Vener. Dis., 36:261–265, 1960.
4. Antes, E.H.: Charcot joint in diabetes mellitus. JAMA, 156:602–603, 1954.
5. Baum, E.W.: Knochenbruche bei Tabes und Deren atiologische Stellung. Dtsch. Z. Chir., 89:1–70, 1907.
6. Beetham, W.B., Jr., Kaye, R.L., and Polley, H.F.: Charcot's joints. A case of extensive polyarticular involvement and discussion of certain clinical and pathologic features. Ann. Intern. Med., 58:1002–1012, 1963.
7. Bennett, R.M., Mall, J.C., and McCarty, D.J.: Pseudogout in acute neuropathic arthropathy. A clue to pathogenesis? Ann. Rheum. Dis., 33:563–567, 1974.
8. Blanford, A.T., et al.: Idiopathic Charcot joint of the elbow. Arthritis Rheum., 21:723–726, 1978.
9. Brain, R., and Wilkinson, M.: Cervical arthropathy in syringomyelia, tabes dorsalis and diabetes. Brain, 81:275–289, 1958.
10. Brashear, H.R.:' The value of the intramedullary nail for knee fusion particularly for the Charcot joint. Am. J. Surg., 87:63–65, 1954.
11. Brigg, J.R., and Freehafer, A.A.: Fusion of the Charcot spine. Clin. Orthop., 53:83–93, 1967.
12. Brower, A.C., and Allman, R.M.: Pathogenesis of the neurotrophic joint: neurotraumatic vs. neurovascular. Radiology, 139:349–354, 1981.
13. Brower, A.C., and Allman, R.M.: The neuropathic joints: a neurovascular bone disorder. Radiol. Clin. North Am., 19:571–580, 1981.
14. Bruckner, F.E., and Howell, A.: Neuropathic joints. Semin. Arthritis Rheum., 2:47–70, 1972.
15. Bruckner, F.E., and Kendal, B.E.: Neuroarthropathy in Charcot-Marie-Tooth disease. Ann. Rheum. Dis., 28:577–583, 1969.
16. Brunt, P.W.: Unusual cause of Charcot joints in early adolescence (Riley-Day syndrome). Br. Med. J., 4:277–278, 1967.
17. Campbell, D.J., and Doyle, J.O.: Tabetic Charcot's spine. Br. Med. J., 1:1018–1020, 1954.
18. Campbell, W.L., and Feldman, F.: Bone and soft tissue abnormalities of the upper extremity in diabetes mellitus. AJR, 124:7–16, 1975.
19. Carr, T.L.: The orthopaedic aspects of one hundred cases of spinal bifida. Postgrad. Med. J., 32:201–210, 1956.
20. Chandler, G.N., et al.: Charcot's arthropathy following intra-articular hydrocortisone. Br. Med. J., 1:952–953, 1959.
21. Charcot, J.M.: Arthropathies, inxations et fractures spontanees chez une ataxique. Bull. Mem. Soc. Anat. Paris., 48:744–747, 1873.
22. Charcot, J.M.: Du Cerveau ou de la moelle épinière. Arch. Physiol. Norm. Pathol., 1:161–178, 379–399, 1868.
23. Charnley, J.: Present status of total hip replacement. Ann. Rheum. Dis., 30:560–564, 1971.
24. Cleveland, M., and Wilson, J.J., Jr.: Charcot disease of the spine. J. Bone Joint Surg., 41A:336–340, 1959.
25. Clouse, M.E., et al.: Diabetic osteoarthropathy. Clinical and roentgenographic observations in 90 cases. AJR, 121:22–34, 1974.
26. Collins, D.H.: The Pathology of Articular and Spinal Diseases. Baltimore, Williams & Wilkins, 1950.
27. Coventry, M., et al.: Geometric total knee arthroplasty. Clin. Orthop., 94:177–184, 1973.
28. Coventry, M.B., and Rothacker, G.W.: Bilateral calcaneal fracture in a diabetic patient. J. Bone Joint Surg., 61A:462–464, 1979.
29. Culling, J.: Charcot's disease of the spine. Proc. R. Soc. Med., 67:1026–1027, 1974.
30. Daughaday, W.H.: Extreme gigantism. Analysis of growth velocity and occurrence of severe peripheral neuropathy and neuropathic arthropathy (Charcot joints). N. Engl. J. Med., 297:1267–1269, 1977.
31. Delano, P.J.: The pathogenesis of Charcot's joints. AJR, 56:189–200, 1946.
32. Drennan, D.B., Fahey, J.J., and Maylahn, D.J.: Important factors in achieving arthrodesis of the Charcot knee. J. Bone Joint Surg., 53A:1180–1193, 1971.
33. Eichenholtz, S.N.: Charcot Joints. Springfield, IL, Charles C Thomas, 1966.
34. El-Khoury, G.Y., and Kathol, M.H.: Neuropathic fractures in patients with diabetes mellitus. Radiology, 134:313–316, 1980.
35. Eloesser, L.: On the nature of neuropathic affections of the joints. Ann. Surg., 66:201–207, 1917.
36. Esses, S., Langer, F., and Gross, A.: Charcot's joints: a case report in a young patient with diabetes. Clin. Orthop., 156:183–186, 1981.
37. Feldman, F., Johnson, A.M., and Walter, J.F.: Acute axial neuroarthropathy. Radiology, 111:1–16, 1974.
38. Feldman, M.J., et al.: Multiple neuropathic joints, in-

cluding the wrist, in a patient with diabetes mellitus. JAMA, *209*:1690–1692, 1975.

39. Fenlin, J.M., Jr.: Total glenohumeral joint replacement. Orthop. Clin. North Am., *6*:565–583, 1975.
40. Finsterbush, A., and Friedman, B.: The effect of sensory denervation on rabbits' knee joints. A light and electron microscopic study. J. Bone Joint Surg., *57A*:949–956, 1975.
41. Floyd, W., Lovell, W., and King, R.E.: The neuropathic joint. South Med. J., *52*:563–569, 1959.
42. Frymoyer, J.W., and Hoaglund, F.T.: The role of arthrodesis in reconstruction of the knee. Clin. Orthop., *101*:82–92, 1974.
43. Gerhart, T.N., and Scott, R.D.: Hip arthroplasty in patients with tabetic Charcot joints. Orthopedics, 6:179–183, 1983.
44. Glynn, T.P., Jr.: Marked gallium accumulation in neurogenic arthropathy. J. Nucl. Med., *22*:1016–1017, 1981.
45. Gristina, A.G., et al.: Neuropathic foot and ankle patellar-tendon-bearing orthosis. As an adjunct to patient management. Orthop. Rev., *6*:53–59, 1977.
46. Grunert: Uber pathologische Frakturen (Spontan-Frakturen). Dtsch. Z. Chir., *76*:254–289, 1905.
47. Halonen, P.I., and Jarvinen, K.A.J.: On the occurrence of neuropathic arthropathies in pernicious anaemia. Ann. Rheum. Dis., *7*:152–155, 1948.
48. Heller, I.H., and Robb, P.: Hereditary sensory neuropathy. Neurology, *5*:15–29, 1955.
49. Helms, C.A., Chapman, G.S., and Wild, J.H.: Charcot-like joints in calcium pyrophosphate dihydrate deposition disease. Skeletal Radiol., *7*:55–58, 1981.
50. Hodgson, J.R., Pugh, D.G., and Young, H.H.: Roentgenologic aspect of certain lesions of bone: neurotrophic or infections? Radiology, *50*:65–71, 1948.
51. Holland, H.W.: Tabetic spinal arthropathy. Proc. R. Soc. Med., *46*:747–752, 1953.
52. Hollander, J.L., Jessar, R.A., and Brown, E.M., Jr.: Intra-synovial corticosteroid therapy: a decrease of use. Bull. Rheum. Dis., *11*:239–240, 1961.
53. Horwitz, T.: Bone and cartilage debris in the synovial membrane. Its significance in the early diagnosis in neuroarthropathy. J. Bone Joint Surg., *30A*:579–588, 1948.
54. Jackson, W.P., and Louw, J.H.: The diabetic foot. S. Afr. Med. J., *56*:87–92, 1979.
55. Jacobelli, A., et al.: Calcium pyrophosphate dihydrate crystal deposition in neuropathic joints. Four cases of polyarticular involvement. Ann. Intern. Med., *79*:340–347, 1973.
56. Jaffe, H.L.: Metabolic, Degenerative, and Inflammatory Diseases of Bones and Joints. Philadelphia, Lea & Febiger, 1972.
57. Johnson, J.T.H.: Neuropathic fractures and joint injuries. Pathogenesis and rationale of prevention and treatment. J. Bone Joint Surg., *49A*:1–30, 1967.
58. Johnson, R.H., and Spalding, J.M.K.: Progressive sensory neuropathy in children. J. Neurol. Neurosurg. Psychiatry, *27*:125–130, 1964.
59. Jordan, W.R.: Neuritic manifestations in diabetes mellitus. Arch. Intern. Med., *57*:307–366, 1936.
60. Katz, I., Rabinowitz, J.G., and Dziadiw, R.: Early changes in Charcot's joints. AJR, *86*:965–974, 1965.
61. Kernwein, G., and Lyon, W.F.: Neuropathic arthropathy of the ankle joint resulting from complete severance of the sciatic nerve. Ann. Surg., *115*:267–279, 1942.
62. Kettunen, K.O.: Neuropathic arthropathy caused by spinal cord trauma. Ann. Chir. Gynaecol., *46*:95–100, 1957.
63. Key, J.A.: Clinical observations on Tabetic arthropathies (Charcot joints). Am. J. Syph., *16*:429–453, 1932.
64. King, E.J.S.: On some aspects of the pathology of hypertrophic Charcot's joints. Br. J. Surg., *18*:113–124, 1930.
65. Kraft, E., Spyropoulos, E., and Finby, N.: Neurogenic disorders of the foot in diabetes mellitus. AJR, *124*:17–24, 1975.
66. Kristiansen, B.: Ankle and foot fractures in diabetics provoking neuropathic joint changes. Acta Orthop. Scand., *51*:975–979, 1980.

67. Leede, C.S.: Arthropathen bei Syringomyelie. Munich, 1908.
68. Lipman, H.I., Perotto, A., and Farrar, R.: The neuropathic foot of the diabetic. Bull. N.Y. Acad. Med., *52*:1159–1178, 1976.
69. McCredie, J.: Thalidomide and congenital Charcot's joints. Lancet, *2*:1058–1061, 1973.
70. Mankin, H.J., and Conger, K.A.: The acute effects of intra-articular hydrocortisone on articular cartilage in rabbits. J. Bone Joint Surg., *48A*:1383–1388, 1966.
71. Martin, J.R., et al.: Staphylococcus suppurative arthritis occurring in neuropathic knee joints. A report of four cases with a discussion of the mechanisms involved. Arthritis Rheum., *8*:389–402, 1965.
72. Martin, M.M.: Diabetic neuropathy. A clinical study of 150 cases. Brain, *76*:594–624, 1953.
73. Mazas, F.B.: Guepar total knee prosthesis. Clin. Orthop., *94*:211–221, 1973.
74. Meyer, G.A., Stein, J., and Poppel, M.H.: Rapid osseous changes in syringomyelia. Radiology, *69*:415–418, 1957.
75. Mooney, V., and Mankin, H.J.: A case of congenital insensitivity to pain with neuropathic arthropathy. Arthritis Rheum., *9*:820–829, 1966.
76. Moynihan, F.J.: Cortisone arthropathy. Guy's Hosp. Rep., *111*:388–392, 1962.
77. Muggia, F.M.: Neuropathic fracture. Unusual complication in a patient with advanced diabetic neuropathy. JAMA, *191*:336–338, 1965.
78. Murray, R.O.: Congenital indifference to pain with special reference to skeletal changes. Br. J. Radiol., *30*:2–6, 1957.
79. Murray, T.J.: Congenital sensory neuropathy. Brain, *96*:387–394, 1973.
80. Newman, J.: Spontaneous dislocation in diabetes neuropathy. A report of six cases, J. Bone Joint Surg., *61*:484–488, 1979.
81. Nissenbaum, M.: Neurotrophic arthropathy of the shoulder secondary to tuberculous arachnoiditis. A case report. Clin. Orthop., *118*:169–172, 1976.
82. Norman, A., Robbins, H., and Milgra, J.E.: The acute neuropathic arthropathy—a rapid, severely disorganizing form of arthritis. Radiology, *90*:1159–1164, 1968.
83. Pallis, C., and Schneeweiss, J.: Hereditary sensory radicular neuropathy. Am. J. Med., *32*:110–118, 1962.
84. Parsons, H., and Norton, W.S.: The management of diabetic neuropathic joints. N. Engl. J. Med., *244*:935–938, 1951.
85. Paterson, D.E.: Radiological bone changes and angiographic findings in leprosy. With special reference to the pathogenesis of atrophic condition of the digits. J. Fac. Radiol. Lond., *7*:35–56, 1955.
86. Peitzman, S.J., et al.: Charcot arthropathy secondary to amyloid neuropathy. JAMA, *235*:1345–1347, 1976.
87. Petrie, J.G.: A case of progressive joint disorders caused by insensitivity to pain. J. Bone Joint Surg., *35B*:399–401, 1953.
88. Potts, W.J.: The pathology of Charcot joints. Ann. Surg., *86*:596–806, 1927.
89. Pruzanski, W., Baron, M., and Shopak, R.: Neuroarthropathy (Charcot joints) in familial amyloid polyneuropathy. J. Rheumatol., *8*:477–481, 1981.
90. Radin, E.L.: Mechanical aspects of osteoarthrosis. Bull. Rheum. Dis., *26*:862–865, 1976.
91. Radin, E.L.: The physiology and degeneration of joints. Semin. Arthritis Rheum., *2*:245–257, 1972–1973.
92. Radin, E.L., and Pa, I.L.: Response of joints to impact loading. Arthritis Rheum., *14*:356–362, 1971.
93. Rataj, R.: Artropatic w jamistorci rdzenia. Neurol. Neurochir. Pol., *14*:439–445, 1964.
94. Resnick, D., et al.: Clinical, radiographic, and pathologic abnormalities in calcium pyrophosphate dihydrate deposition disease (CPPD): pseudogout. Radiology, *122*:1–15, 1977.
95. Riley, L.H., Jr.: Geometric total knee replacement. Orthop. Clin. North Am., *4*:561–573, 1973.
96. Ritter, M.A., and DeRosa, G.P.: Total hip arthroplasty in a Charcot joint. A case report with a six-year follow-up. Orthop. Rev., *6*:51–53, 1977.

97. Rodnan, G.P., and Maclachlan, M.J.: The absorption of serum albumin and gamma globulin from the knee joint of man and rabbit. Arthritis Rheum., 3:152–157, 1960.
98. Rodnan, G.P., Yunis, E.J., and Totten, R.S.: Experiences with punch biopsy of synovium in the study of joint diseases. Ann. Intern. Med., 53:319–331, 1960.
99. Rubinow, A., Spark, E.C., and Canoso, J.J.: Septic arthritis in a Charcot joint. Clin. Orthop., 147:203–206, 1980.
100. Russell, W.R., and Garland, H.G.: Progressive hypertrophic polyneuritis with case reports. Brain, 53:376–384, 1930.
101. Samilson, R.L., et al.: Orthopedic management of neuropathic joints. Arch. Surg., 78:115–121, 1959.
102. Scott, R.B., et al.: Neuropathic joint disease (Charcot joints) in Waldenström's macroglobulinemia with amyloidosis. Am. J. Med., 54:535–538, 1973.
103. Silverman, F.N., and Gilden, J.J.: Congenital insensitivity to pain: a neurologic syndrome with bizarre skeletal lesions. Radiology, 72:176–189, 1959.
104. Sinha, S., Munichoodappa, C.S., and Kozak, G.P.: Neuro-arthropathy (Charcot joints) in diabetes mellitus. Medicine, 51:191–210, 1972.
105. Skall-Jensen, J.: Osteoarthropathy in syringomyelia. Analysis of seven cases. Acta Radiol., 38:382–388, 1952.
106. Skolnick, M.D., et al.: Polycentric total knee arthroplasty. J. Bone Joint Surg., 58A:743–748, 1976.
107. Smith, F.H.: Charcot-like joints in yaws. U.S. Naval Med. Bull., 46:1832–1843, 1946.
108. Sokoloff, N.A.: Die Erkrankungen der Gelenke bei Gliomatose des Ruckenmarks (Syringomyelia). Beut. Z. Chir., 34:505–549, 1892.
109. Soto-Hall, R., and Haldeman, K.O.: The diagnosis of neuropathic joint disease (Charcot joint). An analysis of forty cases. JAMA, 114:2076–2078, 1940.
110. Slabaugh, P.B., and Smith, T.K.: Neuropathic spine after spinal cord injury. J. Bone Joint Surg., 60A:1005–1006, 1978.
111. Sprenger, T.R., and Foley, C.J.: Hip replacement in a Charcot joint. A case report and historical review. Clin. Orthop., 165:191–194, 1982.
112. Stack, J.K.: Experiences with intramedullary fixation in knee fusion. Am. J. Surg., 83:291–299, 1952.
113. Steinberg, C.L., Duthie, R.B., and Piva, A.E.: Charcot-like arthropathy following intra-articular hydrocortisone. JAMA, 181:851–854, 1962.
114. Steinberg, V.L.: Syringomyelia with multiple neuropathic joints. Ann. Phys. Med., 3:103–104, 1956.
115. Steindler, A.: The tabetic arthropathies. JAMA, 96:250–256, 1931.
116. Stepanek, V., and Stepanek, P.: Changes in the bones and joints of paraplegics. Radiol. Clin., 29:28–36, 1960.
117. Storey, G.: Charcot joints. Br. J. Vener. Dis., 40:109–117, 1964.
118. Sweetnam, D.R., Mason, R.M., and Murray, R.O.: Steroid arthropathy of the hip. Br. Med. J., 1:1392–1394, 1960.
119. Thomas, D.F.: Vertebral osteoarthropathy or Charcot's disease of the spine. Review of the literature and report of two cases. J. Bone Joint Surg., 34B:248–255, 1952.
120. Thrush, D.C.: Congenital insensitivity to pain. A clinical, genetic and neurophysiological study of four children from the same family. Brain, 96:369–386, 1973.
121. Van der Houwen, H.: A case of neuropathic arthritis caused by indifference to pain. J. Bone Joint Surg., 43B:314–317, 1961.
122. Westphal, C.: Gelenkerkrankungen bei Tabes, Berl. Klin. Wochenschr., 18:413–417, 1881.
123. Wile, U.J., and Butler, M.G.: A critical survey of Charcot's arthropathy. Analysis of eighty-eight cases. JAMA, 94:1053–1055, 1930.
124. Williams, B.: Orthopaedic features in the presentation of syringomyelia. J. Bone Joint Surg., 61B:314–323, 1979.
125. Wirth, C.R., Jacobs, R.L., and Rolander, S.D.: Neuropathic spinal arthropathy. A review of Charcot spine. Spine, 5:558–567, 1980.
126. Wiseman, L.W.: Neurogenic arthritis and the problems of arthrodesis of the neurogenic knee. Clin. Orthop., 8:218–226, 1956.
127. Wolfgang, G.L.: Neurotrophic arthropathy of the shoulder. A complication of progressive adhesive arachnoiditis. Clin. Orthop., 87:217–221, 1972.
128. Zuckner, G., and Marder, M.J.: Charcot spine due to diabetic neuropathy. Am. J. Med., 12:118–124, 1952.

Chapter 72

Amyloidosis

Alan S. Cohen

In 1842, Rokitansky observed a unique disorder causing a waxy, enlarged liver and, occasionally, similar changes in the spleen.[95] Virchow noted the more widespread recurrence of this waxy material in other organs and subsequently observed that the "lardaceous" liver and spleen stained with iodine and sulfuric acid. Because he believed that it had a certain similarity to cellulose, Virchow named the material "amyloid."[33,35] This substance was studied for many years at the autopsy table or in experimental animals, usually with amyloid induced by infection, until direct biopsy procedures and the Congo red test and stain were introduced in the 1920s.[8,9,132] In the subsequent 30 years, many clinical and experimental studies were done on what was then considered to be a rare "degenerative" condition. It has become apparent, however, that amyloidosis is not as rare as was thought; it is often of great clinical significance, it is associated with many diseases, and as discovered in the past several decades, it is sometimes genetically determined.[30]

Amyloidosis may be defined as the extracellular deposition of the fibrous protein amyloid in one or more sites of the body. This protein has unique ultrastructural properties, x-ray diffraction, and biochemical characteristics. The substance may be local and isolated with no clinical consequences, it may grossly involve any organ system of the body and may thus lead to severe pathophysiologic changes, or the disorder may fall between these two extremes. The natural history is poorly understood, and the clinical diagnosis may not be made until the disease is far advanced.

CLASSIFICATION

Until recently, the diagnosis of amyloidosis was rarely made during the lifetime of the patient. It is therefore not surprising that most of the older systems of classification depended on the distribution of amyloid in the various organs and on the staining properties of the deposit. Patients with heart, gastrointestinal tract, skin, nerve, and tongue involvement were considered to have "primary" amyloidosis, and those with liver, spleen, kidney, and adrenal involvement, "secondary" amyloidosis. Amyloidosis of any type can involve any organ, however, with variable severity. Furthermore, routine stains do not enable one to distinguish "types" of amyloidosis. Pirani, who has extensively reviewed the complexities of the tissue distribution of amyloid, has pointed out that we still do not know the reason that this protein is deposited repetitively in certain organs in specific syndromes.[90]

The following clinical classification is accepted by most authors: (1) *primary amyloidosis*, in which one sees no evidence of pre-existing or coexisting disease; (2) *amyloidosis associated with multiple myeloma*; (3) *secondary*, or reactive or acquired, amyloidosis, with evidence of chronic infection, such as osteomyelitis, tuberculosis, or leprosy, or chronic inflammatory disease, such as rheumatoid arthritis (RA) or ankylosing spondylitis; (4) *heredofamilial amyloidosis*, which is the amyloidosis associated with familial Mediterranean fever and a variety of neuropathic, renal, cardiovascular, and other syndromes; (5) *local amyloidosis*, in which local deposits, often resembling tumors, are seen in isolated organs without evidence of systemic involvement; and (6) *amyloidosis associated with aging*.

With the recent progress in delineating the chemical composition of various amyloid proteins, a more exact clinicoimmunochemical classification is now possible. Each of several amyloid proteins has a serum protein precursor, as follows: (1) *the light chains of immunoglobulins* in AL (primary or myeloma associated) amyloidosis, (2) *the acute-phase reactant, serum amyloid A (SAA)* in AA (secondary or acquired) amyloidosis; and (3) *prealbumin* in AF (heredofamilial) amyloidosis (Table 72–1). Several forms of localized amyloidosis, especially those associated with endocrine organs and with the aged heart or brain, have also been identified.

Primary Amyloidosis and That Related to Multiple Myeloma (AL)

Although the term primary amyloidosis delineates disease in which no predisposing cause is found, it should not be misconstrued as a peculiar clinical type of amyloidosis easily distinguishable from the others. The classic distinctions between primary and secondary amyloidosis based solely

Table 72–1. Classification of Amyloidosis

Systemic Forms	Clinical Type	Chemical Composition
AA	Secondary or acquired or reactive	AA (amyloid protein A)
AF	Heredofamilial (dominant)	Prealbumin
AL	Primary; multiple myeloma associated	Immunoglobulin light chains or fragments
Localized Forms		
AE	Endocrine (thyroid)	Precalcitonin
	Endocrine (pancreas)	Unknown
AS	Senile (brain)	Prealbumin
	Senile (heart)	Prealbumin
AD	Skin	Keratin or precursor (?)

on organ distribution are not completely valid. Routine staining cannot distinguish the primary from the secondary type, and under the electron microscope, all types of amyloidosis have an identical fibrillar nature. Only in the early 1970s was the biochemical composition of the amyloid fibril in this form found to be unique and to consist of fragments of or whole immunoglobulin light chains (kappa or lambda) in both primary amyloidosis and that associated with multiple myeloma.[57,58]

Certain features that alert the clinician to the diagnosis of primary amyloidosis are unexplained proteinuria, peripheral neuropathy, progressive numbness and tingling of the feet, enlarged tongue, increased heart size, unexplained electrocardiographic abnormalities, malabsorption, hepatomegaly, and orthostatic hypotension. Laboratory abnormalities are nonspecific and may or may not include proteinuria, an elevated erythrocyte sedimentation rate, and Bence Jones protein or M component in the patient's serum or urine. The patient frequently has symptoms for several years before the correct diagnosis is made. A biopsy of an involved organ is necessary to confirm the diagnosis. All patients said to have primary amyloidosis should be thoroughly investigated for evidence of other disease, to rule out unsuspected inflammatory disorders and malignant tumors.

Multiple myeloma is a malignant condition with an increased prevalence of amyloid disease. From 6 to 15% of such patients have amyloidosis, the features of which are often indistinguishable from the primary type. Whereas organ involvement in the various types of amyloidosis usually overlaps, involvement of the synovial membrane is found almost exclusively in patients with multiple myeloma.[41] This joint disease may mimic the features of RA.

Secondary or Reactive (AA) Amyloidosis

The frequency of amyloidosis in the general population is not known. Most available data are based on postmortem studies, which are unreliable because they are performed on a selected group of patients and special staining for amyloidosis is not routine. The prevalence of amyloid at autopsy in many general hospitals around the world is about 0.5%. In Japan, it is low (0.1%), whereas in countries such as Portugal and Israel, where hereditary amyloid syndromes are known, the prevalence is much greater. Moreover, studies in patients with chronic infectious disease who have an increased risk of developing amyloidosis, such as patients with chronic tuberculosis or leprosy, have shown a high prevalence on postmortem examination, up to 50% in some series.

Patients with chronic inflammatory conditions treated by the rheumatologist may develop amyloidosis. These rheumatic conditions include RA, ankylosing spondylitis, juvenile RA (JRA), Reiter's syndrome, the arthritis associated with psoriasis, and other miscellaneous disorders. Currently, tuberculosis, leprosy, paraplegia, and RA have the greatest incidence.[90] The development of secondary amyloidosis in a patient with one of the aforementioned diseases is often heralded by proteinuria, hepatomegaly, or splenomegaly. The interval between the onset of the rheumatic disease and the appearance of amyloid is unpredictable. Secondary amyloid deposits are composed of a protein moiety termed protein AA, which has a unique amino acid sequence and is distinct from immunoglobulin light chains.

HEREDOFAMILIAL (AF) AMYLOIDOSIS

Hereditary amyloid syndromes have been described in a number of geographic locations; each family and each type described are associated with characteristic organ involvement and clinical manifestations. Generally, the mode of transmission is autosomal dominant, with the exception of familial Mediterranean fever, a condition common in the Near East and affecting Sephardic Jews, Armenians, Turks, and Arabs, for which autosomal recessive transmission has been described. The hereditary amyloidoses represent a new field in our knowledge of amyloid disease. Classification by organ involvement is perhaps the most useful at present. Multiple kinships with hereditary amyloidosis of the peripheral nervous system are especially prevalent. Reports of such hereditary syndromes have been appearing in the literature at a rate of about one new syndrome or kinship per year. The amyloid of familial Mediterranean fever is composed of AA protein, whereas the amyloid of all other familial syndromes studied to date is composed of prealbumin.

Localized Amyloidosis

In addition to systemic deposition, amyloid may be present in small, focal amounts, sometimes resembling tumors, in any area of the body. Common locations are the lung, skin, larynx, eye, and bladder. In these patients, one rarely sees evidence of systemic disease. Blood vessel involvement is common in primary and secondary amyloidosis. If such involvement is found in a local form, one should investigate further for more widespread disease.

Amyloidosis in Aged Persons

For reasons not completely understood, amyloidosis occurs more frequently with aging.[42,107] In one series, virtually all consecutive autopsies in individuals over 65 years of age demonstrated small deposits of amyloid.[140] Although usually clinically inapparent, small deposits are often found in the heart, brain, pancreas, and spleen of elderly patients. Occasionally, by virtue of its specific location, such as in the conducting system of the heart, symptoms are severe. Although the pathogenesis of amyloidosis in the process of aging is not clear, the staining properties and the ultrastructure of the amyloid found in the elderly are identical to those of the other types.

HISTOPATHOLOGIC FEATURES AND STRUCTURE

Gross Appearance

Amyloid is an amorphous, eosinophilic, glassy, hyaline extracellular substance ubiquitous in distribution. It may be identified by the classic iodine and dilute sulfuric acid stain first used by Virchow. When successful, this stain imparts a blue-purple color to the amyloid, but it is inconsistent and currently only of historical interest. Small amounts of amyloid do not produce gross organ abnormalities. With larger amounts, the involved organs take on a rubbery, firm consistency. They may have a waxy, pink or gray appearance. Organ enlargement, especially of the liver, kidney, spleen, and heart, may be prominent when the deposits are large. In patients with long-standing renal involvement, however, the kidneys may become small and

pale. The heart, in addition to being enlarged by the interstitial myocardial involvement, may have nodular elevations on its pericardial and endocardial surfaces, as well as lesions in the valves. Nerves are often normal, even when involved, but they may become thickened and nodular. Other gross findings are variable and depend on the presence or absence of local nodular deposits.

Tinctorial Properties

Microscopically, amyloid is pink when stained with hematoxylin and eosin, and shows crystal violet or methyl violet metachromasia, although it is orthochromatic when stained with toluidine blue. Collagen is stained red by the van Gieson stain, and most of the background appears yellow, but amyloid has a khaki appearance. The periodic-acid-Schiff (PAS) reagent gives amyloid a violaceous hue.

Congo red remains one of the most widely used stains. It is not completely specific because it stains elastic tissue and, unless carefully decolorized, stains dense bundles of collagen. When formalin-fixed, Congo-red-stained sections are viewed in the polarizing microscope, however, a unique green birefringence is present.[29] *This is the single most useful procedure for establishing the presence of amyloid.* Amyloid has also been stained with fluorochromes to produce a secondary fluorescence, and thioflavine dyes in particular are sensitive indicators of amyloid. The lack of specificity of these dyes, however, makes it mandatory to employ them primarily for screening and to follow with more specific stains. Cotton dyes, especially Sirius red, are also useful and specific. A comparative evaluation of these strains has borne out the high degree of sensitivity and specificity of the green birefringence after staining with Congo red or Sirius red.[48]

A histochemical method that is useful in differentiating AA from AL amyloid has been described by Wright,[141] who modified the Romhanyi amyloid stain. After incubation with potassium permanganate, AA amyloid, the amyloid of the secondary disorder, loses its affinity for Congo red, whereas AL amyloid, that of primary or myeloma-related amyloidosis, does not. In addition, immunocytochemical methods, using specific anti-AA, anti-AL, and antiprealbumin antisera, allow for even more precise delineation of the type of amyloid in a tissue section.[114]

Light-Microscopic Appearance

By light microscopy, amyloid is almost invariably extracellular in connective tissue. The deposits may be focal in almost any area of the body, but perivascular amyloid is most often present. The amyloid may involve bone marrow, spleen, capillaries, venules, veins, arterioles, or arteries. The heart may have focal or diffuse interstitial deposits in the myocardium, endocardium, or pericardium. In the kidney, the glomerulus is primarily affected, although interstitial, peritubular, and vascular amyloid may be prominent. In early lesions, small nodular or diffuse deposits appear near the basement membrane; as the disease progresses, the glomerulus may be massively laden, with apparent occlusion of the capillary bed. Atrophic glomeruli laden with amyloid may show marked thickening in the area of Bowman's capsule. Rarely, the glomerulus is replaced almost entirely by connective tissue. Tubular dilation, casts, and interstitial amyloid deposits may be found in the medulla.

In the gastrointestinal tract, one may see perivascular deposits alone, or irregular or diffuse deposits may be found in the submucosa, in the muscularis mucosa, or in the subserosa. The amyloid may appear at any level or portion of the gastrointestinal tract, including the gallbladder and pancreas. Hepatic deposits again may be perivascular only, but more commonly, diffuse amyloid is found between the Kupffer and parenchymal cells. In the nervous system, amyloid has been described along peripheral nerves, in autonomic ganglia, in senile plaques, and in vessels of the central nervous system. It may be found in any portion of the orbit including the vitreous humor and the cornea.

The bronchopulmonary tract may be involved focally or extensively. The unique aspect of pulmonary or pleural involvement is that although amyloid in virtually all areas of the body remains without evidence of resorption or foreign body reaction, pulmonary amyloid deposits may be accompanied by large numbers of macrophages about and within the lesions. These deposits may also contain islets of cartilage and of ossification. No area of the body is spared, and this ubiquitous distribution produces many clinical symptoms and signs.

Ultrastructure

In 1959, Cohen and Calkins found that, on direct examination of amyloid tissues under the electron microscope, the amyloid itself consisted of fine fibrils[40] (Fig. 72–1). This observation has been confirmed, and all types of human amyloid, whether primary, secondary, or heredofamilial no matter how classified, consist of these fine, nonbranching rigid fibrils that in tissue sections measure approximately 100 A in diameter.[40] When distant from the cell, these fibrils are usually arranged in random array, but close to cells, they may be parallel or perpendicular to the plasmalemma with which they occasionally appear to merge. Intra-

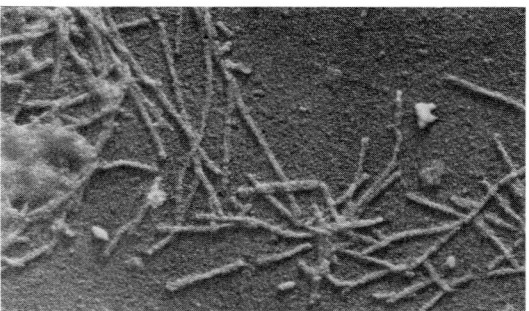

Fig. 72–1. Electron micrograph of isolated human secondary amyloid fibrils. Shadow-casted with platinum-palladium. (Magnification × 100,000.)

cellular fibrils of dimensions comparable to those outside the cell are sometimes observed. Their precise nature has not yet been established.

The amyloid fibrils are usually seen in earliest and closest relationship to the mesangial cell in the kidney,[111] although as deposits enlarge, they appear in comparable relationship to the endothelial and finally epithelial cell. In the liver, these fibrils first border the Kupffer cell, but they finally fill the space of Disse and are seen about the hepatic cell as well. In many other locations, amyloid fibrils have been found close to blood vessels, pericytes, and endothelial cells. Thus, although the cell processing amyloid fibrils may appear to be in the reticuloendothelial or macrophage family, this complex process involves, in AA amyloid, the macrophage, the hepatocyte, and probably the reticuloendothelial system or macrophage again.

The amyloid fibrils thus visualized can be extracted from amyloid-laden tissues for more definitive ultrastructural, chemical, and immunologic study. When isolated, these fibrils can be specially stained, either positively or negatively with phosphotungstic acid, and their delicate, thin, nonbranching fibrous character can thereby be illustrated. The individual fibril has a diameter of about 70 A, and the fibrils aggregate laterally. Each fibril is made up of filaments, and subunit protofibrils about 30 to 35 A in diameter have also been defined. The protofibril is beaded, may itself consist of two subunits, and exists in spirals of 5 protofibrils or multiples of 2 such subunits.[112] X-ray diffraction of isolated amyloid fibrils reveals a cross-beta pattern, the "pleated sheet" of Pauling and Corey, indicating that the polypeptide chain runs transversely to the fiber axis of the specimen.[19,50]

A second substance, P-component (plasma component or pentagonal unit) with different ultrastructure, x-ray diffraction pattern, and chemical characteristics, has also been isolated from amyloid and is identical to a circulating alpha globulin present in minute amounts. This substance is not responsible for the characteristic tinctorial properties or ultrastructure of amyloid.[17,31,122]

BIOCHEMISTRY OF AMYLOID FIBRILS

The bulk of amyloid deposits consists of fibrils. Once a purified amyloid fibril protein had been isolated, more precise identification of chemical and physical structure became possible. When solubility was studied as a function of pH, a point of maximum solubility at pH 4.5 was defined. The mucopolysaccharide and total carbohydrate content were 0.4 and 5%, respectively.[34] Amino acid analyses indicated the presence of all amino acids, except hydroxyproline and hydroxylysine, found in collagen, and desmosine and isodesmosine, found in elastin. Aspartic and glutamic acid constituted 20% of the total amino acid content.

Studies on this protein have been extensive, and purification methods have been improved. Amyloid was clearly insoluble in the usual media at various ionic strengths,[85] but was either soluble or formed a fine dispersion in distilled water.[93]

AL Amyloid

The first systemic form of amyloid to be defined biochemically was the immunoglobulin or primary type, identified in 1970,[58,59] by N-terminal sequence analysis as the variable (V_L) segment of a kappa I light chain in 2 amyloid fibril preparations. Over the subsequent 10 years, additional sequences on this type of amyloid were performed[36,78,84,124,125,129,135] (Table 72–2). These sequences have shown kappa I-, kappa II-, lambda IV-, and lambda VI-type light chains as amyloid fibril proteins. More than half of all isolated amyloid proteins have had a blocked N-terminus and have been suspected to be of a lambda type with a PCA amino terminus.[72] The purified amyloid proteins vary in size from 7,500 to 23,000 daltons, and although sequence data exist for only the N-terminal region, it is assumed that the primary amyloid fibril can consist of the variable part of the light chain, the variable part and a portion of the constant region, or the whole light chain (see Chap. 15). According to the accepted classification,[69] both kappa and lambda types of immunoglobulins have been identified as amyloid proteins. Three proteins in a lambda VI category are thought to be uniquely associated with amyloidosis, however.

In addition to the nine amyloid preparations that have undergone partial sequence analysis and the one that has undergone total sequence analysis, data are available on four Bence Jones proteins isolated from patients with amyloidosis.[18,55,94,126] Two of these have sequence data from both the Bence Jones and the protein amyloid fibril and are completely identified.[18,94] This finding supports the hypothesis that an underlying immunocyte dyscrasia, manifested by monoclonal proteins and increased bone marrow plasma cells, is of etiologic significance in this type of amyloidosis.

Because the primary proteins consist of the variable fragments of light chains, they also have idiotypic antigenic determinants. As a rule, no cross-reactivity has been noted between the amyloid proteins belonging to the different subgroups.[44,68] This lack of common antibody contributes to the diagnostic dilemma in identifying the type of amyloid in the patient with systemic disease. Tissue biopsy specimens are now analyzed for AA amyloid by radioimmunoassay or immunocytochemistry to rule out the secondary form of amyloid. If the test results are negative, the specimens can be examined for prealbumin by the same methods to exclude hereditary amyloidosis. If test results are still negative, one cannot precisely define primary amyloid short of postmortem isolation and sequence analysis of the fibrils.

AA Amyloid

Another protein unrelated to any known immunoglobulin has been described in secondary amyloid deposits.[5,13,52,67,77] Fibrils containing AA (amyloid A) protein can be isolated from patients with secondary amyloidosis, the disorder associated with familial Mediterranean fever, and the amyloid isolated from experimental animals following casein injections. It is a unique protein with the molecular weight of about 8,500 daltons made up of 76 amino acid residues arranged in a single chain, the amino acid sequence beginning arginine-serine-phenylalanine (ARG-SER-PHE). Heterogeneity among the different species has been described, showing that several additional residues may precede the first residue, possibly as the result of proteolysis of a larger precursor (Table 72–3).

Antisera to alkali-degraded amyloid fibrils of the AA protein have detected an antigenically related serum component, SAA.[1,13,81,96] Molecular weights of 80,000 to 100,000 daltons, and more recently of about 85,000, have been reported, although other techniques have suggested a molecular weight of 180,000. Several groups have isolated smaller subunits with molecular weights of 12,000 to 12,500, or 14,000 to 15,000. Amino acid analysis, peptide maps, and sequence studies suggest that AA protein is an amino terminal fragment of SAA and is derived from SAA by proteolysis. The precise relation of the fragment with a molecular weight of 12,000 or 12,500 to the species with a molecular weight of 85,000 or 180,000, however, has not been precisely determined. SAA behaves

Table 72–2. Primary Amyloid (AL) Sequence

AL	Type	1	2	3	4	5	6	7	8	9	10	Thru	M.W.	Ref.
10	AL$_{\kappa I}$	asp	ile	gln	met	thr	gln	ser	ala	ser	ser	(36)	7,500	57
8	AL$_{\kappa I}$	asp	ile	gln	met	thr	gln	ser	ala	ser	ser	(35)	18,300	57
MAG	AL$_{\kappa I}$	asp	ile	gln	met	thr	gln	ser	ala	ser	ser	(32)	11,000	38
LEP	AL$_{\kappa I}$	asp	ile	gln	met	thr	gln	ser	ala	ser	ser	(27)	23,000	78
TEW	AL$_{\kappa II}$	asp	ile	val	met	thr	glu	ser	pro	leu	ser	(27)	23,000	129
808	AL$_{IV}$	( )	tyr	asp	leu	thr	gln	(pro)	pro	ser	val	(21)		135
758	AL$_{IV}$	( )	tyr	asp	leu	thr	gln	pro	pro	ser	val	(27)		84
JAM	AL$_{IV}$	asp	phe	met	leu	thr	glu	pro	his	ser	val	(17)	16,000	124
AR	AL$_{IV}$	asp	phe	met	leu	thr	gln	pro	his	ser	val	(154)	16,000	125
RS	AL$_{IV}$	asp	phe	met	leu	thr	gln	pro	his	ser	val	(34)		84
LEP	BJP$_{\kappa I}$	asp	ile	gln	met	thr	gln	ser	ala	ser	ser	(29)	23,000	18
TEW	BJP$_{\kappa II}$	asp	ile	val	met	thr	gln	ser	pro	leu	ser	(214)	23,000	94
NIG-51	BJP$_I$	PCA	ser	val	leu	thr	gln	pro	pro	ser	ala	(214)	23,000	126
MCG	BJP$_V$	PCA	ser	ala	leu	thr	gln	pro	pro	ser	ala	(216)	23,000	55

(asp = aspartic acid; ile = isoleucine; tyr = tyrosine; phe = phenylalanine; ser = serine; gln = glutamine; val = valine; met = methionine; ala = alanine; leu = leucine; thr = thyroxine; glu = glutamic acid; pro = proline; his = histidine.)

Table 72–3. Amyloid A (AA) and Serum Amyloid A (SAA) Sequences

Species	1	2	3	4	5	6	7	8	9	10	Ref.
Human	arg	ser	phe	phe	ser	phe	lue	gly	glu	ala	35
Monkey	arg	ser	trp	phe	ser	phe	leu	gly	glu	ala	51
Mouse	(arg)	ser/ gly	phe	phe	ser	phe	ile	gly	glu	ala	108
Guinea pig	arg	ser	ile	phe	ser	phe	leu	lys	glu/ ala	ser/	69
	his	ala	lys	gly	glu						
					(Blocked N term-identity beginning res 17)						
Mink											54
Duck	arg	gly	gly	arg	phe	val	leu	asp	ala	ala	50
	asp	asn	pro	phe	thr						

(his = histidine; asp = aspartic acid; ala = alanine; asn = asparagine; lys = lysine; pro = proline; gly = glycine; phe = phenylalanine; glu = glutamic acid; thr = thyroxine; arg = arginine; ser = serine; trp = tryptophan; ile = isoleucine; val = valine; leu = leucine.)

as an acute-phase reactant and is elevated in infection and inflammation.[15,98] In patients with JRA, SAA is related more to the activity and seropositivity than to the presence of amyloid. Recent data suggest that SAA is not age related.[65] SAA levels have also been suggested as potential monitors of neoplastic disease.[97]

SAA has been studied in a variety of animal species including the mink, in which endotoxin was a potent stimulus for its generation prior to the appearance of detectable amyloid.[66] Casein given to CBA/J mice has induced SAA as well as amyloid composed of protein AA.[11,121] A study by McAdam and Sipe showed that murine SAA has a molecular weight of 160,000 and dissociated to a more stable 12,500 moiety on formic acid treatment.[82] These researchers found that SAA behaved as an acute-phase reactant and was elevated even in amyloid-resistant animals, either those pretreated with colchicine or a genetically resistant AJ strain, and suggested that amyloid resistance is related to the processing and catabolism of SAA. It has been suggested that SAA is a polymorphic serum protein and may not be a simple precursor of AA.[3] It has also been suggested that SAA suppresses antibody response and may regulate such response.[14] More extensive studies of murine SAA confirmed the human studies and showed that SAA is among the apoproteins of the high-density lipoprotein complex.[7]

Other Amyloid Moieties

In addition to the data on AA, and its serum counterpart SAA, and AL, the amyloid related to immunoglobulins, new and distinct types of amyloid fibril protein have recently been described. Most are in the stage of early identification, and definitive amino acid sequence studies are generally not available. In 1978, however, it was demonstrated that the major protein constituent in a Portuguese type of hereditary amyloid had antigenic determinants identical to those of prealbumin.[49] More recently, three separate reports of N-terminal sequence studies on the AF amyloid confirmed its prealbumin nature in familial amyloid polyneuropathy in persons of Swedish and Polish origin[10,70,91,123] (Table 72–4). In addition, the amyloid associated with medullary carcinoma of the thyroid may be related to thyrocalcitonin.[133] Senile cardiac amyloid is distinct immunologically from AA and AL,[137] and two types of this may exist.[136] Amyloid in the cerebral plaques, in the neurofibrillary tangles, and in the angiopathy of Alzheimer's disease appears to be prealbumin.[108] Clearly, studies on different amyloids will soon produce new and fascinating data.

P-Component of Amyloid

In addition to the characteristic fibrils described, a minor second component, the P-component, has been noted in most amyloid deposits.[17,31,122] P-component (AP) has been recognized by electron microscopy as a pentagonal unit measuring about 90 A in diameter on the outside and 40 A on the inside. It appears to consist of 5 globular subunits of 25 to 30 A, which may aggregate laterally to form short rods. On immunoelectrophoresis, this component migrates as an alpha globulin, and it possesses antigenic identity with a constituent of normal human plasma. The amino acid sequence is distinct from that of the amyloid fibrils. The N-terminal amino acid is histidine and contains large amounts of aspartic acid, glutamic acid, glycine, and leucine. Sequence to 23 residues has found the protein to be unique.[122] The molecular weight, probably that of a doublet, is about 180,000 to 220,000, and it has subunits of about 22,000 daltons. AP is associated with all types of amyloid, including that isolated from the pancreas of patients with long-standing diabetes.[138] The only exception is its absence from the amyloid plaques and neurofibillary tangles in the brain of patients with Alzheimer's disease. It has been found in the vascular amyloid in the brain, however.[134]

Human amyloid P-component has been isolated from plasma by affinity chromatography. Characterization and comparison of the isolated P-component proteins from tissue and plasma demonstrated immunologic and sequence identity[119] (Table 72–5). The AP N-terminal sequence compared from three amyloid fibril preparations, a primary kappa, a primary lambda, and a secondary lambda, has been found to be homologous. Electron-microscopic studies have revealed that the plasma P-component has a pentagonal ultrastructure identical to that of the tissue P-component.

Amyloid P-component also has substantial homology in amino acid sequence, molecular appearance, and subunit composition to C-reactive protein, but differences in molecular weight (C-reactive protein has about half the molecular weight of SAP) and in other parameters suggests that although these substances are analogous and may have evolutionary relationships to one another, they are indeed distinct.[86,118,119] SAP in humans does not usually behave as an acute-phase reactant, although it does become elevated in patients with malignant disease.[120] The unique relationship between SAP and amyloid fibrils, both AA and AL, is at least partly due to a calcium-dependent binding of SAP in vitro to isolated fibrils.[88,89]

Table 72–4. AF Amyloid Proteins

	1	2	3	4	5	6	7	8	9	10	11	12	Ref.
Prealbumin	gly	pro	thr	gly	thr	gly	glu	ser	lys	cys	pro	leu	57
Amyloid LIN	gly	pro	thr	gly	thr	gly	glu	ser	lys	cys	pro	leu	109
Amyloid GRO													
Amyloid SKO	gly	pro	(thr)	gly	( )	gly	glu	ser	lys	(cys)	pro	leu	83

	13	14	15	16	17	18	19	20	21	22	23	24
Prealbumin	met	val	lys	val	leu	asp	ala	val	arg	gly		pro
LIN	met	val	lys	val	leu	asp	ala	val	arg	gly	ser	
GRO	val	val	val	leu	asp	ala	val	arg	gly	thr	pro	
SKO	(met)	val	lys	val	leu	asp	asp					

(gly = glycine; met = methionine; val = valine; pro = proline; thr = thyroxine; lys = lysine; leu = leucine; asp = aspartic acid; ala = alanine; glu = glutamic acid; ser = serine; arg = arginine; cys = cystine.)

Table 72–5. Sequence Comparison of P-Component of Amyloid (AP). Serum P-Component (SAP), and C-Reactive Protein (CRP)

	1	2	3	4	5	6	7	8	9	10	Ref.
Human AP	his	thr	asp	leu	ser	gly	lys	val	phe	val	113
Human SAP	his	thr	asp	leu	ser	gly	lys	val	phe	val	113
Human CRP	PCA	thr	asp	met	ser	arg	lys	ala	phe	val	78
	11	12	13	14	15	16	17	18	20		
AP	phe	pro	arg	glu	ser	val	thr	asp	his	val	
SAP	phe	pro	arg	glu	ser	val	thr	asp	his	val	
CRP	phe	pro	lys	glu	ser	asp	thr	ser	tyr	val	

(his = histidine; phe = phenylalanine; thr = thyroxine; pro = proline; asp = aspartic acid; arg = arginine; lys = lysine; leu = leucine; met = methionine; glu = glutamic acid; ser = serine; gly = glycine; val = valine; ala = alanine; tyr = tyrosine.)

IMMUNOBIOLOGY OF AMYLOID

The origin and pathogenesis of amyloidosis are unknown. Advances in characterization of the chemical structure of amyloid may provide insight into these complex mechanisms. Ultrastructural studies of amyloid-laden tissues in an animal model have led to the concept that cytoplasmic invaginations, containing tufts of amyloid fibers, cell-amyloid interface, were the sites of amyloid formation.[46] Electron-microscopic autoradiographic studies have revealed high concentrations of fibrils adjacent to reticuloendothelial cells; this finding suggests that they may synthesize as well as degrade the fibrils. Unusual inclusions are found with the reticuloendothelial cells intimately associated with fresh amyloid deposits.[109] These inclusions are located in the areas rich in the primary lysosome type of dense bodies, and the cytoplasmic invaginations contain well-oriented fibrils. The inclusions may be transitional forms from the usual dense bodies and may constitute direct evidence of the involvement of lysosomes in amyloid fibril formation.

Excess antigenic stimulus has induced amyloid formation in animals. The basic conditions for the experimental induction have not been clearly defined, however. Marked depression of T cells with maintenance of normal B-cell function has been described, and administration of bovine thymus (thymosin) may suppress amyloid formation in mice.[104] These findings suggest that disturbances in immunoregulatory mechanisms may be important in the pathogenesis of amyloid disease.[106]

Additional studies of cellular and humoral immunity in amyloidosis have been performed.[27,63,105] The availability of animal models for acquired (secondary) systemic amyloidosis has advanced our understanding of this disease.[11] With these models, some important concepts regarding the pathogenesis of amyloid, such as the two-phase concept of amyloid induction,[128] transfer of amyloid,[63a,74] and involvement of the reticuloendothelial system in amyloid fibril formation,[46,109] were developed.

The mechanism of acute-phase SAA elevation has also been studied. The origin of SAA as an acute-phase reactant has become a prototype for the study of the regulation of acute-phase reactant synthesis. It is believed that acute-phase proteins are produced as part of the systemic host response to localized injury, and numerous studies suggest that circulating mediators are released at the site of injury. One of the functions of these mediators is to stimulate hepatic synthesis of acute-phase reactants. Endotoxin or lipopolysaccharide stimulates the acute-phase SAA response by interacting with macrophages to produce a substance, "SAA inducer," capable of eliciting an elevated SAA concentration in mice that do not mount an SAA response to the lipopolysaccharide itself. This mediator of SAA synthesis is similar, if not identical, to interleukin 1. Interleukin 1 is a soluble monokine elicited by inflammation and antigenic stimulation, with many target cells including T cells, hepatocytes, synovial cell fibroblasts, brain cells, and possibly B cells.[115,116] (see also Chap. 17).

An interesting but confusing concept, the "transfer of amyloid" studied by Hardt and Ranlov in the mid-1960s,[63a] as well as by many others later, has recently been refined.[2] A model of accelerated amyloidosis has made it possible to relate the formation of amyloid fibrils to the normal acute-phase response. A substance called amyloid-enhancing factor, extracted from spleens of preamyloidotic mice, can alter the acute-phase response such that amyloid fibrils are deposited in spleen. This factor is localized to the extracellular portion of spleen, where amyloid is deposited. It appears that amyloid-enhancing factor, produced by repeated episodes of inflammation, plays an essential role in the formaiton of AA fibrils from SAA. The role of this factor in the kinetics of amyloid deposition has been defined.[73,74] Amyloidogenesis has 2 phases, a predeposition phase that lasts from 7 to 21 days and a deposition phase that continues as long as inflammation persists. Amyloid-enhancing factor shortens the predeposition phase to under 2 days. The spleen, although the earliest and most heavily affected tissue, is not essential for production of this factor, and in any tissue to be affected, amyloid-enhancing factor is present 1 to 2 days prior to the appearance of fibrils. Furthermore, the deposition phase has been subdivided into rapid deposition and plateau stages. These stages are important in defining therapy. Colchicine and dimethyl sulfoxide are most effective during the rapid deposition period, but are ineffective in the plateau stage. These studies raise an important concept of staging and prophylaxis, as well as therapy, in secondary amyloidosis.

Among many treatments purported to influence the course of amyloidosis, colchicine has played an important role in studies of the acquired systemic variety that can occur in situations of chronic and recurrent acute inflammation. Since the observation that colchicine treatment of patients with familial Mediterranean fever lessens or prevents amyloid deposition, this drug has been used to treat all types of systemic amyloidosis. Colchicine has blocked or delayed the development of AA amyloidosis in the mouse model of the disease.[71,110] The therapeutic value of dimethyl sulfoxide in amyloidosis was first reported in a mouse model in 1976, and clinical trials have since been undertaken.[87]

Animals models for other than the AA type of amyloidosis are scarce.[44] Spontaneous amyloidosis has been reported in a few strains of mice and other species; however, in most cases, the models have been poorly defined with regard to reproducibility and the biochemical and immunologic characteristics of the amyloid. A mouse model for spontaneous amyloidosis seems valuable because of the high predictable incidence of amyloidosis, the absence of apparent predisposing conditions for acquired amyloidosis, and the preliminary biochemical and immunologic findings for the uniqueness of its amyloid protein.[127]

Thus, amyloidosis the disease and amyloid the substance have been more precisely defined in modern biochemical terms. Further categorization will doubtless be possible, with clinicopathologic implications concerning pathogenesis and diagnosis. A clearer delineation of the relation of animal models of acquired amyloidosis to the other systemic and localized forms of the disease in terms of mediators and amyloid-enhancing factor will also contribute to a better understanding of the origin and pathogenesis of this complex disorder.

CLINICAL ASPECTS

Diagnosis

Although the specific diagnosis of amyloidosis depends on tissue examination with appropriate stains,[40] the disease must first be suspected on clinical grounds. When a patient who has a disorder predisposing him to amyloid formation develops hepatomegaly, splenomegaly, malabsorption, cardiac disease, or, most important, proteinuria, amyloidosis should be suspected. Moreover, in heredofamilial syndromes,[27] especially those with an autosomal dominant mode of transmission and characterized by peripheral neuropathy, particularly that starting in the lower limb, nephropathy, or cardiopathy, the diagnosis of amyloidosis should be considered. Finally, primary systemic amyloidosis should be suspected in patients with a diffuse, noninflammatory, infiltrative disease involving either mesenchymal tissues such as blood vessels, heart, or gastrointestinal tract or parenchymal tissues such as kidney, liver, spleen, or adrenal gland.

For screening purposes, a subcutaneous abdominal fat-pad biopsy may be the simplest and most useful procedure[79,80] (Fig. 72–2). I have found complications to be almost nonexistent; no absolute contraindications exist, and with appropriate staining and interpretation, the overall sensitivity is in the range of 90%. Until this procedure is more generally used, however, it is good practice to perform a rectal biopsy for diagnosis (Fig. 73–3). If this procedure is contraindicated or if the patient refuses, gingival biopsy is recommended. Skin biopsy, of both involved and uninvolved skin, is also useful in all types of amyloidosis.[99] If results of the aforementioned procedures are negative in patients who have renal disease, hepatic disease, or other organ involvement, biopsy of the appropriate site is undertaken with the standard precautions against bleeding. All tissue obtained must be stained with Congo red and examined under a polarizing microscope for green birefringence. If a polarizing microscope is not available, a light microscope may be adapted.[29] If this is not possible, a crystal violet stain is useful. Electron-microscopic examination of tissue sections has been recommended when histochemical stains are negative. Such occasions, however, are rare, and the technique is not necessary for most routine studies.

If amyloidosis is still suspected even after negative biopsy results, a Congo red test may be performed. This test may be positive when the biopsy is negative, and vice versa.[23,139] The Evans blue test has been suggested as an alternative, but it does not add to results of the aforementioned test. My recommended procedures are outlined in Table 72–6, which lists the appropriate biopsy sites.

Amyloidosis as a Rheumatic Disease

Amyloid can directly involve articular structures and may be present in the synovial membrane (Figs. 72–4, 72–5), as well as in the synovial

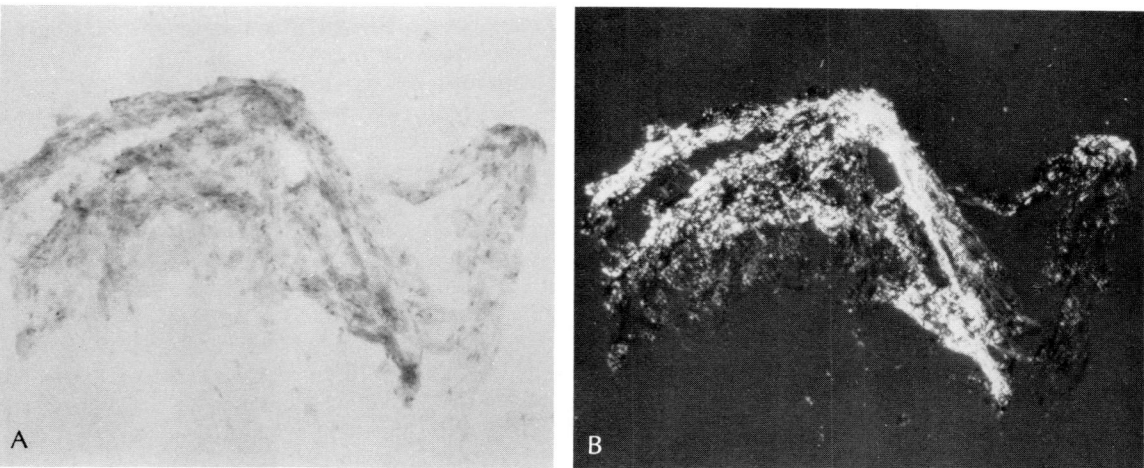

Fig. 72–2. Light micrographs of an abdominal fat biopsy stained with Congo red and hematoxylin nonpolarized (A) and polarized (B), the latter demonstrating green birefringence. (Magnification × 90.)

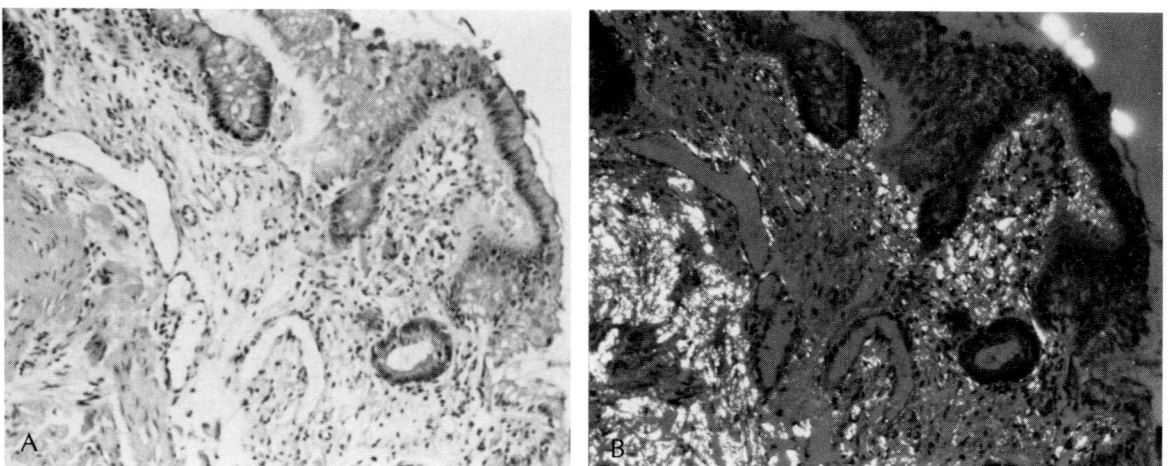

Fig. 72–3. Light micrographs of a rectal biopsy stained with Congo red and hematoxylin nonpolarized (A) and polarized (B), the latter demonstrating green birefringence. (Magnification × 90.)

Table 72–6.   Diagnosis of Amyloidosis

Biopsy		
Common Sites	*Occasional Sites*	*Rare Sites*
Subcutaneous abdominal fat	Small intestine	Kidney
Rectum	Muscle	Liver
Skin	Nerve	Bone marrow
Gingiva		Synovium
		Spleen
Appropriate Stain		
Congo red, viewed in polarizing microscope		
Others		
Cotton dyes (comparable to Congo red)		
Thioflavin (less specific)		
Crystal violet (less sensitive)		

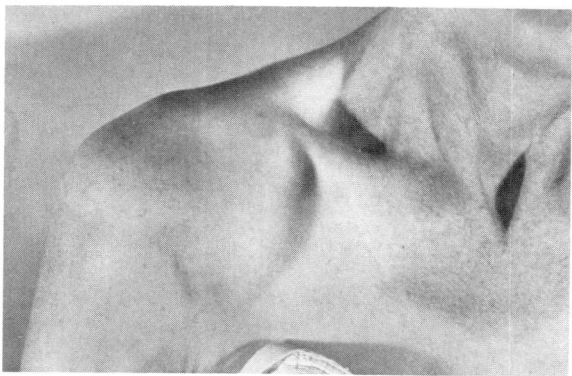

Fig. 72–4. "Shoulder pad" sign in a 52-year-old woman with primary amyloidosis and widespread amyloid arthropathy simulating rheumatoid arthritis.

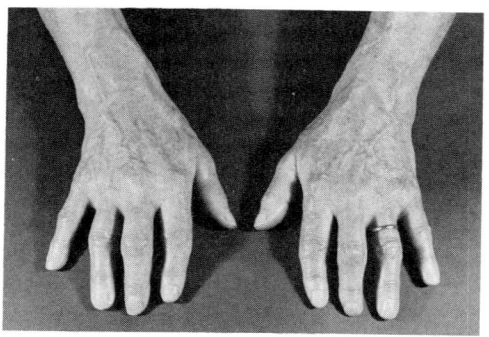

Fig. 72–5. The hands of the patient in Figure 72–4 showing flexion contractures of the fingers from synovial thickening of the metacarpophalangeal and proximal interphalangeal joints and flexor tendons.

fluid.[49] It may also occur in the articular cartilage.[22] Amyloid arthritis can mimic a number of rheumatic diseases because it can become manifest as a symmetric, small-joint arthritis associated with nodules, morning stiffness, and fatigue.[41] The diagnosis of RA can be made in error, and differentiation is imperative because of the great difference in prognosis. When diagnostic arthrocentesis is done and amorphous material is seen in the fluid, a Congo red stain should be used and the material viewed under a polarizing microscope. Individuals with nodules and no erosive disease, as well as patients whose nodules enlarge precipitously, should be looked at more critically. When excessive soft tissue boggy thickening is present, the patient may also have amyloid disease. Amyloidosis should be suspected in those patients with multiple myeloma with articular manifestations. Indeed, most patients with amyloid arthropathy do eventually seem to have multiple myeloma.[41,61]

One might expect that amyloidosis of the joints would not be limited to multiple myeloma and would be present in patients with systemic or generalized primary amyloidosis and with generalized secondary amyloidosis. Clinical arthropathy due to amyloid in generalized secondary amyloidosis is unusual, however. Few data are available from systemic analysis of joint disease for the presence of amyloid. In a report of 289 joint biopsies,[76] some suggestion of amyloid was found in 83 (28.7%). In most other autopsy series of patients with RA, either no mention is made of amyloid in joints or, in the few joints appropriately examined, none is found. Because of the widespread involvement of small blood vessels throughout the body in both primary and secondary disease, small amounts of perivascular amyloid may be found.

Amyloid has been found in association with degenerative joint disease,[26,60] as well as chondrocalcinosis.[103] Egan and associates found amyloid in 6 of 13 cartilage specimens, 4 of 18 articular capsules, and 2 of 16 synovial membranes from patients with osteoarthritis of the hip.[51] The clinical significance of such deposits is not known.

In summary, clinically significant amyloid arthritis can be characterized as follows.[69] The joints most frequently involved are shoulders, wrist, knees, and fingers.[41] The period of morning stiffness associated with the early lesions is shorter than in RA. The joints are often swollen and firm, and occasionally tender, but redness and severe tenderness have not been noted. Swelling of the shoulders may resemble shoulder pads (see Fig. 72–4). Subcutaneous nodules are present in almost 70% of cases, whereas rheumatoid factor is uncommon. Roentgenograms show soft tissue swelling. Erosions about the joints were noted only once among 20 patients studied. Generalized osteoporosis, with or without osteolytic lesions, however, is common and is seen in 80% of patients.

The synovial fluid is usually benign and appears to have the characteristics of a traumatic effusion or a low-grade inflammation. It is generally described as viscous, yellow, or xanthochromic; mucin clot is good to poor. The leukocyte count is usually low, with a median of about 1,000 cells/mm³ but counts as high as 10,000 cells/mm³ have been reported. Usually, one sees a predominance of mononuclear cells. Free-amyloid-containing bodies, presumably synovial villi, were found in the sediment of 3 fluids extensively studied, and possible free amyloid itself.[49] The synovial membrane may have lining-cell amyloid, subsynovial amyloid, or perivascular deposits. Multiple myeloma predominates. The carpal tunnel syndrome is common in association with amyloid arthritis.

General Manifestations

The clinical manifestations of amyloidosis vary and depend entirely on the affected structures.[20,33,75]

Renal Involvement

Renal involvement may consist of mild proteinuria or frank nephrosis, or in some cases, the urinary sediment may show only a few red blood cells.[28] The renal lesion is usually irreversible and in time leads to progressive azotemia and death. The prognosis does not appear to be related to the degree of the proteinuria. When azotemia finally develops, if it is due to the amyloid process and not to a reversible superimposed condition, the prognosis is grave. In a group of patients with secondary amyloidosis, those with some residual function remained comfortable for long periods, but once the patient's serum creatinine level was over 3 mg/dl, or the creatinine clearance was under 20 mg/ml, the prognosis was poor.[130] In another series, the mean survival after the time of biopsy was 29 months,[131] but in 5 cases, evidence showed regression of the disease. Hypertension is rare, except in long-standing amyloidosis. Serial films of the kidneys may or may not show a diminution in size. Renal tubular acidosis or renal vein thrombosis may occur. Localized accumulation of amyloid may be noted in the ureter, bladder, or other genitourinary tract tissue.

Hepatic Involvement

Although hepatomegaly is common, liver function abnormalities are minimal and occur late in the disease. The most useful tests of hepatic involvements with amyloid are the Bromsulphalein (BSP) extraction and the serum alkaline phosphatase level. Liver scans have variable, nonspecific results, but bone-seeking radionuclides, such as [99m]technetium diphosphonate, have recently shown increased liver uptake because of the high calcium content of amyloid.[143] Signs of intrahepatic cholestasis are uncommon.[101] In our series in which liver tissue from 54 patients was examined, whether the disorder was primary or secondary, all had some amyloid present, either in the parenchyma or in blood vessels.[45] The remarkable degree to which liver parenchyma can be replaced by amyloid was seen in a patient whose liver was palpable below the iliac crest and weighed 7,200 g; BSP extraction during life in this patient had been 17%, with only a modest elevation of the serum alkaline phosphatase level. Splenomegaly may be massive, although usually it does not cause symptoms unless traumatic rupture occurs. Amyloidosis of the spleen is not usually associated with leukopenia and anemia.

Cardiac Involvement

Cardiac manifestations consist primarily of enlargement and congestive heart failure, either with or without murmurs and arrhythmias.[21] Although these manifestations reflect predominantly diffuse myocardial amyloid deposition, the endocardium, valves, and pericardium may be involved. Pericarditis with effusion is rare, although one must frequently distinguish between constrictive pericarditis and restrictive myocardiopathy. The clinical features and the demonstration of a left ventricular end-diastolic pressure exceeding that of the right are useful in distinguishing restrictive myocardiopathy from constrictive pericarditis, but even left heart catheterization and quantitative left ventriculography are not always enough to make the differential diagnosis.[83] Echocardiographic study has demonstrated symmetric thickening of the left ventricular wall, hypokinesia, decreased systolic thickening of the interventricular septum and left ventricular posterior wall, and the small-to-normal size of the left ventricular cavities.[25]

Hearts heavily infiltrated with amyloid may or may not exhibit an enlarged silhouette. Fluoroscopic study shows decreased mobility of the ventricular wall; angiographic studies usually show a thickened ventricular wall, decreased ventricular mobility, and the absence of rapid ventricular filling in early diastole.

The first signs of cardiac amyloid are often those of intractable heart failure. Electrocardiographic abnormalities include a low-voltage QRS complex and abnormalities in atrioventricular and intraventricular conduction, often resulting in varying degrees of heart block. Electrocardiographic abnormalities are frequent, often without previous infarct.[52] Because of their propensity to conduction defects and arrhythmias, patients with cardiac amyloidosis appear to be especially sensitive to digitalis, and this drug should be used in small doses and with caution. Binding of digoxin by isolated amyloid fibrils may play a role in such sensitivity.[102]

Modern noninvasive techniques have added to our understanding of the extent of cardiac amyloid and the associated functional abnormalities. For example [99m]technetium pyrophosphate or diphosphonate scintigraphy is a sensitive and specific test for amyloid in patients with congestive heart failure of obscure origin. It is not useful, however, as an indicator of early cardiac amyloid in patients without electrocardiographic or other abnormalities.[53] Although M-mode echocardiography can, by the presence of thickened ventricular walls with a small or normal left ventricle, suggest amyloid, 2-dimensional echocardiography adds substantial new information. It demonstrates thickened ventricles with a normal left ventricular cavity and a unique diffuse hyperrefractile "granular" sparkling appearance.[117] Detailed 24-hour electrocardiographic monitoring of patients with amyloid heart disease has revealed a significant number of high-grade ventricular arrhythmias and a lesser incidence of clinically significant bradycardia.[54]

Skin Lesions

Involvement of the skin is one of the most characteristic manifestations of the so-called "primary" amyloidoses. The lesions may consist of raised, waxy, often translucent papules or plaques, usually clustered in the folds about the axillae, the anal or inguinal regions, the face and neck, or mucosal areas such as the ear or tongue. The patient may also have purpuric areas, nodules or tumefactions, alopecia, a yellowish waxy discoloration, glossitis, and xerostomia. The lesions are seldom pruritic. Involvement of the skin or mucosa may be inapparent, even on close inspection, yet may be disclosed at biopsy. Gentle rubbing of the skin with one's finger may induce bleeding (purpura). Skin involvement can also occur in secondary amyloidosis. Amyloid was demonstrated in biopsy of the skin, with or without clinical lesions, in 42% of a group of 12 patients with secondary disease and in 55% of a group of 38 patients with primary disease.[99] All of a group of 8 patients with hereditary amyloid neuropathy studied by our group had positive skin biopsies.

Gastrointestinal Involvement

Gastrointestinal findings in amyloidosis are common and may result from direct infiltration at any level or from infiltration of the autonomic nervous system. Symptoms and signs include those of obstruction, ulceration, malabsorption, hemorrhage, protein loss, and diarrhea. Infiltration of the tongue may lead to macroglossia, which may become incapacitating; alternatively, the tongue, although not enlarged, may become stiffened and firm to palpation. Infiltration of the tongue is especially characteristic of primary amyloidosis or amyloidosis accompanying multiple myeloma, but it may also occur in secondary amyloidosis.

Gastrointestinal bleeding may initiate from a number of sites, notably the esophagus, stomach, or large intestine, and may be severe or even fatal. Amyloid infiltration of the esophagus or small bowel may lead to clinical and radiologic changes of obstruction. A variable pattern has been observed in esophageal motility studies.[100] Malabsorption is sometimes seen. Amyloidosis may develop in association with other entities involving the gastrointestinal tract, especially tuberculosis, granulomatous enteritis, lymphoma, and Whip-

ple's disease. Differentiation of these conditions from diffuse amyloidosis of the small bowel may be difficult. Similarly, amyloidosis of the stomach may mimic gastric carcinoma, with obstruction, achlorhydria, and the radiologic appearance of tumor masses. Patients may also have alternating constipation and diarrhea.

Neurologic Involvement

Neurologic manifestations are common and include peripheral neuropathy, postural hypotension, inability to sweat, Adie's pupil, hoarseness, and sphincter involvement.[43] These manifestations are especially prominent in the heredofamilial amyloidoses.[30] Cranial nerves are generally spared, except for those involving the pupillary reflexes. The protein concentration of the cerebrospinal fluid may be increased. Infiltrates of the cornea or vitreous body may be present in hereditary amyloid syndromes. Amyloid may infiltrate the thyroid or other endocrine glands, but it rarely causes endocrine dysfunction. Local amyloid deposits almost invariably accompany medullary carcinoma of the thyroid. Amyloid infiltration of muscle may lead to pseudomyopathy.

Respiratory Tract Involvement

The nasal sinuses, larynx, and trachea may be involved by accumulations of amyloid that block the ducts, in the case of the sinuses, or the air passages. Amyloidosis of the lung may include diffuse involvement of the bronchi or alveolar septa. The lower respiratory tract is frequently involved in primary amyloidosis and in that associated with dysproteinemia.[24] Pulmonary symptoms attributable to amyloid are present in about 30% of patients, and in some individuals, these are the most serious disease manifestations. In secondary amyloidosis, pulmonary disease is a frequent histopathologic complication, but seldom gives rise to clinically significant symptoms. Amyloid may form a localized mass in the bronchi or alveolar tissue and may resemble a neoplasm. In such cases, local excision should be attempted; if successful, this procedure may be followed by a prolonged remission.

Hematologic Manifestations

Hematologic changes may include fibrinogenopenia, increased fibrinolysis, and selective deficiency of clotting factors, especially factor X.[56] Minor bleeding most often occurs in the absence of clotting abnormalities, however, and is due to local vessel amyloid infiltrates.[142]

Prognosis

The course of amyloidosis is difficult to document because it is rarely possible to date its time of onset. Amyloidosis seldom develops in patients with RA of less than 2 years' duration. The mean duration of arthritis in one series at the time of recognition of amyloidosis was 16 years.[32]

When amyloidosis develops in patients with multiple myeloma, manifestations leading to the initial hospitalization are more apt to be related to the amyloid than to the myeloma.[20] Life expectancy is less than a year in such cases.

In amyloidosis accompanying sepsis such as osteomyelitis, at least partial remission has been reported after treatment of the primary disease. Studies of experimental amyloidosis induced in rabbits by injections of sodium caseinate show that splenic amyloid accumulation, which peaks after about six months of injections, is resorbed over the next three to six months, despite continuance of the caseinate injections.

Established, generalized amyloidosis in man, although usually progressive and causing death in several years, may have a better prognosis than was once thought.[20] The chief cause of death is renal failure. The second most common cause is sudden death presumably from arrhythmias.[54] Occasionally, gastrointestinal hemorrhage, sepsis, respiratory failure, or intractable heart failure may cause death.

Treatment

No specific therapy exists for any variety of amyloidosis. Rational therapy should be directed at the following: (1) decrease of chronic antigenic stimuli producing amyloid; (2) inhibition of the synthesis of the amyloid fibril; (3) inhibition of its extracellular deposition; and (4) promotion of lysis or mobilization of existing deposits.

The progression of secondary amyloidosis is apparently retarded by eradication of the predisposing disease, although many such reports are not substantiated by biopsy proof of resorption. Conclusions have often been drawn on clinical grounds or on the basis of the Congo red test, although a few patients have had biopsy-proved improvement. Despite these occasional reports, amyloidosis is generally a progressive disease. Although the average survival in most large series is one to four years, I have been treating some patients with amyloidosis for five to more than ten years.

Among the most prominent of the many agents used to treat amyloidosis has been whole liver extract, but most clinicians have noted little effect on the course of the disease. Similarly, corticosteroids have little if any effect on amyloidosis. Ascorbic acid in large doses has been used, but proof of efficacy is lacking. The findings that immunoglobulin light chain fragments are incorporated into primary amyloid and its presumed synthesis from plasma cells have led to the use of alkylating agents. These agents cause bone marrow depression, however, and acute leukemia has developed in some patients receiving melphalan. Moreover, immunosuppressive agents used experimentally actually enhance amyloid deposition. Thus, conservative, supportive measures provide the mainstay of amyloidosis management. Rigid adherence to supportive and symptomatic therapy by these patients has led to a more optimistic outlook regarding their quality of life.

Two patients with severe renal amyloidosis and azotemia had bilateral nephrectomy and renal transplantation, followed by immunotherapy.[39] One patient died of infection five months later, and the donor kidney showed no evidence of amyloidosis. The second patient lived ten years after receiving a transplanted kidney. Biopsies of her kidney after two and four years showed no amyloid. Notwithstanding the hazards of operating on patients with systemic amyloidosis who may have cardiac involvement, carefully selected patients would probably benefit from kidney transplantation.

Colchicine is effective in preventing acute attacks in patients with familial Mediterranean fever. Amyloid deposition in the mouse model was inhibited by colchicine.[71,110] Colchicine may be effective in blocking amyloid deposition, but the mechanism of its action is not known. Although no prospective controlled human clinical study has been performed, comparision with retrospective controls suggests that colchicine treatment increases life expectancy in primary amyloidosis.[37]

HEREDOFAMILIAL AMYLOIDOSES

No generally accepted nosology exists for the heredofamilial amyloid syndromes. Some authors emphasize the site of predominant organ involvement, such as neuropathic versus nephropathic versus cardiopathic amyloid, whereas others stress genetic aspects. Most pedigree analyses, with one major exception, show autosomal dominant inheritance. The exception, amyloidosis of familial Mediterranean fever, is inherited as an autosomal recessive trait. Because no specific biochemical, hematologic, or immunologic tests exist to differentiate one type of amyloid from another, one must use specific, recognizable clinical patterns for classification. The classification used here is tentative and is based largely on the major site of organ involvement, in addition to genetic data and ethnic background when available[30,33,90] (Table 72–7).

A large group of these disorders primarily involves the nervous system. Among these, a lower limb neuropathy, first described in Portugal, has a poor prognosis and is characterized by progressively severe neuropathy including marked auto-

Table 72–7.   Heredofamilial Amyloidoses

Neuropathy
  Lower limb (Portuguese; Japanese; Swedish; Other)
  Upper limb (Swiss, Indiana; German, Maryland)
Nephropathy
  Familial Mediterranean fever
  Fever and abdominal pain (Swedish; Sicilian)
  Urticaria, deafness, and renal disease
  Renal disease and hypertension
Cardiopathy
  Progressive heart failure (Danish)
  Persistent atrial standstill
Miscellaneous
  Medullary carcinoma of the thyroid
  Lattice corneal dystrophy and cranial neuropathy
    (Finnish)
  Central hemorrhage (Icelandic)

nomic nervous system involvement. This variety has also been described in Japan, in a family of Greek origin in the United States, and in Sweden. A second type of neuropathy, seen in families of Swiss origin in Indiana and of German origin in Maryland, is a milder disease often associated with a carpal tunnel syndrome and vitreous opacities. A more severe generalized neuropathy with renal amyloid has been described in Iowa in a family of English-Irish-Scottish ancestry.[30]

Several types of severe familial renal disease associated with amyloid have been described. Possibly the most remarkable is familial Mediterranean fever, a disorder subdivided into phenotype I, with irregularly occurring fever and abdominal, chest, or joint pain, preceding or accompanying renal amyloid, and phenotype II, in which amyloidosis is the first or only manifestation of the disease. This disease is most commonly seen in Sephardic Jews, Armenians, Turks, and Arabs. Other hereditary renal amyloidoses have been sporadically, described, including the curious association of urticaria, deafness, and renal amyloid.

Severe familial amyloid heart disease has been described in a Danish family, and familial persistent atrial standstill has been reported in a family of Latin American origin. Miscellaneous hereditary amyloid syndromes include hereditary multiple endocrine neoplasia type 2, including medullary carcinoma of the thyroid with amyloid, and familial lattice corneal dystrophy associated with cranial neuropathy and renal disease in Finland. Finally, a syndrome of hereditary cerebral hemorrhage due to amyloid has been reported in Iceland.

REFERENCES

1. Anders, R.F., et al.: Amyloid-related serum protein SAA from three animal species: comparison with human SAA. J. Immunol., *118*:229–234, 1977.
2. Axelrad, M.A., and Kisilevsky, R.: Biological characterization of amyloid enhancing factor. *In* Amyloid and
Amyloidosis. Edited by G.G. Glenner, P.P. Costa, and A.F. Freitas. Amsterdam, Excerpta Medica, 1980, p. 527.
3. Bausserman, L.L., Herbert, P.N., and McAdam, K.P.W.S.: Heterogeneity of human serum amyloid protein. J. Exp. Med., *152*:641, 1980.
4. Benditt, E.P., et al.: SAA, an apoprotein of HDL: its structure and function. Ann. N.Y. Acad. Sci., *389*:183–189, 1982.
5. Benditt, E.P., et al.: Guideline for nomenclature. *In* Amyloid and Amyloidosis. Edited by G.G. Glenner, P.P. Costa, and A.F. Freitas. Amsterdam, Excerpta Medica, 1980, p. xi.
6. Benditt, E.P., et al.: The major proteins of human and monkey amyloid substance: common properties including unusual N-terminal amino acid sequences. F.E.B.S. Lett., *19*:169–173, 1971.
7. Benditt, E.P., Erikson, N., and Hanson, R.H.: Amyloid protein SAA is an apoprotein of mouse plasma high density lipoprotein. Proc. Natl. Acad. Sci. U.S.A., *76*:4092–4096, 1979.
8. Bennhold, H.: Eine spezifische Amyloidfarbung mit Kongorot. Munchen. Med. Wochenschr., *69*:1537–1538, 1922.
9. Bennhold, H.: Ueber die Ausscheidung intravenos einverleibter Farbstoffe bei Amyloidkranken. Verh. Dtsch. Ges. Inn. Med., *34*:313, 1922.
10. Benson, M.D: Partial amino acid sequence homology between a heredofamilial amyloid protein and human plasma prealbumin. J. Clin. Invest., *67*:1035–1041, 1981.
11. Benson, M.D., et al.: Kinetics of serum amyloid protein A in casein-induced murine amyloidosis. J. Clin. Invest., *59*:412–417, 1977.
12. Benson, M.D., et al.: P-component of amyloid. Isolation from human serum by affinity chromatography. Arthritis Rheum., *19*:749–754, 1976.
13. Benson, M.D., et al.: "A" protein of amyloidosis. Isolation of a cross-reacting component from serum by affinity chromatography. Arthritis Rheum., *18*:315–322, 1975.
14. Benson, M.D., et al.: Suppression of in vitro antibody response by a serum factor (SAA) in experimentally induced amyloidosis. J. Exp. Med., *142*:236–241, 1975.
15. Benson, M.D., et al.: Amyloid serum component: relationship to aging. Fed. Proc., *33*:618, 1974.
16. Benson, M.D., Skinner, M., and Cohen, A.S.: Antigenicity and cross-reactivity of denatured fibril proteins of primary, secondary, and myeloma associated amyloids. J. Lab. Clin. Med., *85*:650–659, 1975.
17. Bladden, H.A., Nylen, M.U., and Glenner, G.G.: The ultrastructure of human amyloid as revealed by the negative staining technique. J. Ultrastruct. Res., *14*:449, 459, 1966.
18. Block, P.J., et al.: The identity of peritoneal fluid immunoglobulin light chain and amyloid fibril in primary amyloidosis. Arthritis Rheum., *19*:755–759, 1976.
19. Bonar, L., Cohen, A.S., and Skinner, M.M.: Characterization of the amyloid fibril as a cross-B protein. Proc. Soc. Exp. Biol. Med., *131*:1373–1375, 1969.
20. Brandt, K., Cathcart, E.S., and Cohen, A.S.: A clinical analysis of the course and prognosis of 42 patients with amyloidosis. Am. J. Med., *44*:955–969, 1968.
21. Buja, L.M., Khoi, N.B., and Roberts, W.C.: Clinically significant cardiac amyloidosis. Am. J. Cardiol., *26*:394–405, 1970.
22. Bywaters, E.G.L., and Dorling, J.: Amyloid deposits in articular cartilage. Ann. Rheum. Dis., *29*:294–306, 1970.
23. Calkins, E., and Cohen, A.S.: The diagnosis of amyloidosis. Bull. Rheum. Dis., *10*:215–218, 1960.
24. Celli, B.R., et al.: Patterns of pulmonary involvement in systemic amyloidosis. Chest, *74*:543–547, 1978.
25. Child, J.S., et al.: Echocardiographic manifestations of infiltrative cardiomyopathy. A report of seven cases due to amyloid. Chest, *70*:726–731, 1979.
26. Christensen, H.E., and Sorenson, K.L.: Local amyloid formation of capsule fibrosa in arthritis coxae. Acta Pathol. Microbiol. Scand. [A], *233*:128–131, 1972.
27. Clerici, E., Pierpaoli, W., and Romussi, M.: Experimen-

tal amyloidosis in immunity. Pathol. Microbiol., 28:806–815, 1965.

28. Cohen, A.S.: Renal amyloidosis. *In* Textbook of Nephrology. Edited by S.G. Massry and R.J. Glassock. Baltimore, Williams & Wilkins, 1983, pp. 6.134–6.140.

29. Cohen, A.S.: Diagnosis of amyloidosis. *In* Laboratory Diagnostic Methods in the Rheumatic Diseases. 2nd Ed. Edited by A.S. Cohen. Boston, Little, Brown, 1975.

30. Cohen, A.S.: Inherited systemic amyloidosis. *In* The Metabolic Basis of Inherited Disease. Edited by J.B. Standbury, J.B. Wyngaarden, and D.S. Fredrickson. New York, McGraw-Hill, 1972, pp. 1,273–1,294.

31. Cohen, A.S.: Chemical and immunological characterization of two components of amyloid. *In* Chemistry and Molecular Biology of the Intercellular Matrix, Vol. 3. Edited by E.A. Balacz. New York, Academic Press, 1970, pp. 1,517–1,536.

32. Cohen, A.S.: Amyloidosis associated with rheumatoid arthritis. Med. Clin. North Am., 52:643–653, 1968.

33. Cohen, A.S.: Amyloidosis. N. Engl. J. Med., 277:522–530, 574–583, 628–638, 1967.

34. Cohen, A.S.: Preliminary chemical analyses of partially purified amyloid fibrils. Lab. Invest., 15:66–83, 1966.

35. Cohen, A.S.: The constitution and genesis of amyloid. *In* International Review of Experimental Pathology, Vol. IV. Edited by G.W. Richter and M.A. Epstein. New York, Academic Press, 1965, p. 159–243.

36. Cohen, A.S., et al.: Amyloid protein, precursors, mediator and enhancer. Lab. Invest., 48:1–4, 1983.

37. Cohen, A.S., et al.: Colchicine therapy in primary amyloidosis. A preliminary report. *In* Fifteenth International Congress of Rheumatology, June, 1981 (Abstract #1171). Rev. Rhum. Mal. Osteoartic.

38. Cohen, A.S., et al.: Ultrastructure and composition of amyloid—Variable or constant. *In* Protides of the Biological Fluids. 20th Colloquium. Edited by H. Peeters. New York, Pergamon Press, 1973, pp. 73–80.

39. Cohen, A.S., et al.: Renal transplantation in two cases of amyloidosis. Lancet, 2:513–516, 1971.

40. Cohen, A.S., and Calkins, E.: Electron microscopic observations on a fibrous component in amyloid of diverse origins. Nature [Lond.], 183:1,202–1,203, 1959.

41. Cohen, A.S., and Canoso, J.J.: Rheumatological aspects of amyloid disease. Clin. Rheum. Dis., 1:149–161, 1975.

42. Cohen, A.S., and Kneapler, D.: Senile amyloidosis. *In* Handbook of Diseases of Aging. Edited by H.T. Blumenthal. New York, VanNostrand Reinhold, 1983, pp. 466–501.

43. Cohen, A.S., and Rubinow, A.: Amyloid neuropathy. *In* Peripheral Neuropathy. 2nd Ed., Vol. 2. Edited by P.J. Kyck, P.K. Thomas, and E.H. Lambert. Philadelphia, W.B. Saunders, 1983.

44. Cohen, A.S., and Shirahama, T.: Amyloidosis, model no. 17, supplemental update. *In* Handbook: Animal Models of Human Disease. Edited by C.C. Capen, et al. Washington, D.C. Registry of Comparative Pathology, Armed Forces Institute of Pathology, 1980, fascicle 2.

45. Cohen, A.S., and Skinner, M.: Amyloidosis of the liver. *In* Diseases of the Liver. Edited by L. Schiff and E.R. Schiff. 5th Ed. Philadelphia, J.B. Lippincott, 1982, pp. 1,081–1,099.

46. Cohen, A.S., Gross, E., and Shirahama, T.: The light and electron microscopic authoradiographic demonstration of local amyloid formation in spleen explants. Am. J. Pathol., 47:1079–1111, 1965.

47. Cohen, A.S., Shirahama, T., and Skinner, M.: Electron-microscopy of amyloid. *In* Electron Microscopy of Proteins. Vol. 3. Edited by J.R. Harris. London, Academic Press, 1982, pp. 165–205.

48. Cooper, J.H.: An evaluation of current methods for the diagnostic histochemistry of amyloid. J. Clin. Pathol., 22:410–413, 1969.

49. Costa, P.P., Figueira, A.S., and Bravo, F.R.: Amyloid fibril protein related to prealbumin in familial amyloidotic polyneuropathy. Proc. Natl. Acad. Sci. U.S.A., 75:4499, 1978.

50. Eanes, E.D., and Glenner, G.G.: X-ray studies on amyloid filaments. J. Histochem. Chem., 16:673–677, 1968.

51. Egan, M.S., et al.: The association of amyloid deposits and osteoarthritis. Arthritis Rheum., 25:204–208, 1982.

52. Ein, C., Kimura, S., and Glenner, G.G.: An amyloid fibril protein of unknown origin: Partial amino-acid sequence analysis. Biochem. Biophy. Res. Commun., 46:498–500, 1972.

53. Falk, R.H., et al.: Sensitivity of technetium-99m-pyrophosphate scintigraphy for the diagnosis of cardiac amyloidosis. Am. J. Cardiol., 51:826–830, 1983.

54. Falk, R.H., et al.: Cardiac arrhythmias in patients with systemic amyloidosis. Arthritis Rheum., 255:558, 1982.

55. Fett, J.W., and Deutsch, H.F.: Primary structure of the MCG lambda chain. Biochemistry, 12:4102, 1974.

56. Furie, B., Greene, E., and Furie, B.C.: Syndrome of acquired factor X deficiency and systemic amyloidosis in vivo studies of the fate of factor X. N. Engl. J. Med., 297:81–85, 1977.

57. Glenner, G.G., et al.: Amyloid fibril proteins: proof of homology with immunoglobulin light chains by sequence analyses. Science, 172:1150–1151, 1971.

58. Glenner, G.G., et al.: Creation of "amyloid" fibrils from Bence Jones proteins in vitro. Science, 174:712–714, 1971.

59. Glenner, G.G., et al.: An amyloid protein: the amino terminal variable fragment of an immunoglobulin light chain. Biochem. Biophys. Res. Commun., 41:1287–1289, 1970.

60. Goffin, Y.A., Thoua, Y., and Potvliege, P.R.: Microdeposition of amyloid in the joints. Ann. Rheum. Dis., 40:27–33, 1981.

61. Gordon, D.A., et al.: Amyloid arthritis simulating rheumatoid disease in five patients with multiple myeloma. Am. J. Med., 55:142–154, 1973.

62. Gorevic, P.D., et al.: The amino acid sequence of such amyloid A (AA) protein. J. Immunol., 118:1113–1118, 1977.

63. Hardt, F., and Claesson, M.H.: Quantitative studies on the T cell populations in spleens from amyloidotic mice. Immunology, 22:677–683, 1972.

63a. Hardt, F., and Ranlov, P.: Transfer amyloidosis. Int. Rev. Exp. Pathol., 16:273, 1976.

64. Hermodson, M.A., et al.: Amino-acid sequence of monkey amyloid protein A. Biochemistry, 11:2934–2938, 1972.

65. Hijmans, W., and Sipe, J.D.: Levels of serum amyloid A protein (SAA) in normal persons of different age groups. Clin. Exp. Immunol., 35:96–100, 1979.

66. Husby, G., et al.: An experimental model in mink for studying the relation between amyloid fibril protein AA and the related serum protein SAA. Scand. J. Immunol., 4:811–816, 1975.

67. Husby, G., et al.: Amyloid fibril protein subunit, "Protein A": Distribution in tissue and serum in different clinical types of amyloidosis including that associated with myelomatosis and Waldenstrom's macroglobulinemia. Scand. J. Immunol., 2:395–404, 1973.

68. Isersky, C., et al.: Immunochemical cross reaction of human immunoglobulin light chains. J. Immunol., 8:486–493, 1972.

69. Kabat, E.A., Wu, T.T., and Bilofsky, H.: Sequences of Immunoglobulin Chains: Tabulation and Analysis of Amino Acid Sequences of Precursors, V-Regions, C-region, J-Chain B_2 Microglobulins. NIH Publication 80-2008. Bethesda, MD, National Institutes of Health, 1979.

70. Kanda, T., et al.: The amino acid sequence of human plasma prealbumin. J. Biol. Chem., 249:6796–6805, 1974.

71. Kedar, I., et al.: Colchicine inhibition of casein-induced amyloidosis in mice. Isr. J. Med. Sci., 10:787–789, 1974.

72. Kimura, S., et al.: Chemical evidence for lambda-type amyloid fibril proteins. J. Immunol., 109:891–892, 1972.

73. Kisilevsky, R., and Boudreau, L.: Kinetics of amyloid deposition. I. The effects of amyloid-enhancing factor and splenectomy. Lab. Invest., 48:53–59, 1983.

74. Kisilevsky, R., Boudreau, L., and Foster, D.: Kinetics of amyloid deposition. The effects of dimethylsulfoxide and colchicine therapy. Lab. Invest., 48:60–67, 1983.

75. Kyle, R., and Bayrd, E.: Amyloidosis: review of 236 cases. Medicine, 54:271–299, 1975.

76. Laine, V., Vaino, K., and Ritama, V.V.: Occurrence of amyloid in rheumatoid arthritis. Acta Rheumatol. Scand., 1:43–46, 1955.

77. Levin, M., Pras, M., and Franklin, E.C.: Immunologic studies of the major nonimmunoglobulin protein of amyloid. Identification and partial characterization of a related serum component. J. Exp. Med., 138:373–381, 1973.

78. Lian, J.B., et al.: Fractionation of primary amyloid fibrils: characterization and chemical interaction of the subunits. Biochim. Biophys. Acta, 491:167–176, 1977.

79. Libbey, C.A., et al.: Diagnosis of amyloidosis and differentiation of secondary amyloid by analysis of abdominal fat tissue aspirate. Arthritis Rheum., 24:5,125, 1981.

80. Libbey, C.A., Skinner, M., and Cohen, A.S.: The abdominal fat tissue aspirate for the diagnosis of systemic amyloidosis. Arch. Intern. Med., 143:1549–1552, 1983.

81. Linke, R.P., et al.: Isolation of low-molecular weight serum component antigenically related to an amyloid fibril protein of unknown origin. Proc. Natl. Acad. Sci. U.S.A., 72:1473, 1975.

82. McAdam, K.P.W.J., and Sipe, J.D.: Serum precursor of murine amyloid protein: an acute phase reactant in regard to polyclonal B cell mitogens. (Abstract.) Fed. Proc., 35:1500, 1976.

83. Meaney, E., et al.: Cardiac amyloidosis, constrictive pericarditis and restrictive cardiomyopathy. Am. J. Cardiol., 38:547–556, 1976.

84. Natvig, J.B., et al.: Further structural and antigenic studies of light-chain amyloid proteins. Scand. J. Immunol., 14:89–94, 1981.

85. Newcombe, D.S., and Cohen, A.S.: Solubility characteristics of isolated amyloid fibrils. Biochim. Biophys. Acta, 104:480–486, 1965.

86. Oliveira, E.B., Gotschlich, E.C., and Liu, L.: Primary structure of human C-reactive protein. J. Biochem. Chem., 254:489–502, 1979.

87. Osserman, E.F., Sherman, W.H., and Kyle, R.A.: Further studies of therapy of amyloidosis with dimethyl sulfoxide (DMSO). In Amyloid and Amyloidosis. Edited by G.G. Glenner, PP. Costa, and A.F. Freitas. Amsterdam, Excerpta Medica, 1980, p. 563.

88. Pepys, M.B., et al.: Binding of serum amyloid P-component (SAP) by amyloid fibrils. Clin. Exp. Immunol., 38:284–293, 1979.

89. Pepys, M.B., et al.: Isolation of amyloid P component (Protein AP) from normal serum as a calcium-dependent binding protein. Lancet, 1:1029–1032, 1977.

90. Pirani, C.L.: Tissue distribution of amyloid. In Amyloidosis. Proceedings of the Fifth Sigrid Juselius Foundation Symposium. Edited by O. Wegelius and A. Pasternack. New York, Academic Press, 1976, pp. 33–49.

91. Pras, M., et al.: A variant of prealbumin from amyloid fibrils in familial polyneuropathy of Jewish origin. J. Exp. Med., 154:989–993, 1981.

92. This reference has been deleted.

93. Pras, M., et al.: The characterization of soluble amyloid prepared in water. J. Clin. Invest., 47:924–933, 1968.

94. Putnam, F.W., et al.: Amino acid sequence of a kappa Bence-Jones protein from a case of primary amyloidosis. Biochemistry, 12:3763–3780, 1973.

95. Rokitansky, C.: Handbuch der Pathologischen Anatomie Vol. 3. Vienna, Braumuller and Seidel, 1842, p. 311.

96. Rosenthal, C.J., et al.: Isolation and partial characterization of SAA—an amyloid-related protein from human serum. J. Immunol., 116:1415–1418, 1976.

97. Rosenthal, C.J., and Sullivan, L.M.: Serum amyloid A to monitor cancer dissemination. Ann. Intern. Med., 91:383–390, 1979.

98. Rosenthal, C.J., and Franklin, E.C.: Variation with age and disease of an amyloid A protein-related serum component. J. Clin. Invest., 55:746–753, 1975.

99. Rubinow, A., and Cohen, A.S.: Skin involvement in generalized amyloidosis. A study of clinically involved and uninvolved skin in 50 patients with primary and secondary amyloidosis. Ann. Intern. Med., 88:781–785, 1978.

100. Rubinow, A., Burkoff, R.B., and Cohen, A.S.: Esophageal manometry in systemic amyloidosis. A study of 30 patients. Am. J. Med., 75:951–956, 1983.

101. Rubinow, A., Koff, R.S., and Cohen, A.S.: Severe intrahepatic cholestasis in primary amyloidosis. A report of 4 cases and a review of the literature. Am. J. Med., 64:937–946, 1978.

102. Rubinow, A., Skinner, M., and Cohen, A.S.: Digoxin sensitivity in amyloid cardiomyopathy. Circulation, 63:1285–1288, 1981.

103. Ryan, L.M., et al.: Amyloid arthropathy in the absence of dysproteinemia: a possible association with chondrocalcinosis. Arthritis Rheum., 21:587–588, 1978.

104. Scheinberg, M.A., and Cathcart, E.S.: Casein-induced experimental amyloidosis. VI. A pathogenic role for B cells in the murine model. Immunology, 31:443–453, 1976.

105. Scheinberg, M.A., and Cathcart, E.S.: Comprehensive study of humoral and cellular immune abnormalities in 26 patients with systemic amyloidosis. Arthritis Rheum., 19:173–182, 1976.

106. Scheinberg, M.A., Goldstein, A., and Cathcart, E.S.: Thymosin restores T cell function and reduces the incidence of amyloid disease in casein-treated mice. J. Immunol., 116:156–158, 1976.

107. Schwartz, P.: Senile cerebral, pancreatic insular and cardiac amyloidosis. Trans. N.Y. Acad. Sci., 27:393–413, 1965.

108. Shirahama, T., et al.: Senile cerebral amyloid: prealbumin as a common constituent in the neuritic plaque in the neurofibrillary tangle, and in the microangiopathic lesion. Am. J. Pathol., 107:41–50, 1982.

109. Shirahama, T., and Cohen, A.S.: Intralysosomal formation of amyloid fibrils. Am. J. Pathol., 81:101–116, 1975.

110. Shirahama, T., and Cohen, A.S.: Blockage of amyloid induction by colchicine in an animal model. J. Exp. Med., 140:1102–1107, 1974.

111. Shirahama, T., and Cohen, A.S.: Fine structure of the glomerulus in human and experimental renal amyloidosis. Am. J. Pathol., 51:869–911, 1967.

112. Shirahama, T., and Cohen, A.S.: High resolution electron microscopic analysis of the amyloid fibril. J. Cell Biol., 33:679–708, 1967.

113. This reference has been deleted.

114. Shirahama, T., Skinner, M., and Cohen, A.S.: Immunocytochemical identification of amyloid in formalin fixed paraffin sections. Histochemistry, 72:161–171, 1981.

115. Sipe, J.D., et al.: The role of interleukin I in acute phase serum amyloid A (AA) and serum amyloid P (SAP) biosynthesis. Ann. N.Y. Acad. Sci., 389:137–150, 1982.

116. Sipe, J.D.: Detection of a mediator derived from endotoxin-stimulated macrophages that induces the acute phase serum amyloid A response in mice. J. Exp. Med., 150:597–606, 1979.

117. Siqueira-Filho, A.G., et al.: M-mode and two-dimensional echocardiographic features in cardiac amyloidosis. Circulation, 63:188–196, 1981.

118. Skinner, M., et al.: Characterization of P-component (AP) isolated from amyloidotic tissue: half-life studies human and murine AP. Ann. N.Y. Acad. Sci., 389:190–198, 1982.

119. Skinner, M., et al.: Studies on amyloid protein AP. In Amyloid and Amyloidosis. Edited by G.G. Glenner, P.P. Costa, and A.F. Freitas. Amsterdam, Excerpta Medica, 1980, pp. 384–391.

120. Skinner, M., et al.: Serum amyloid P-component levels in amyloidosis. Connective tissue diseases, infection and malignancy as compared to normal serum. J. Lab. Clin. Med., 94:633–638, 1979.

121. Skinner, M., et al.: Murine amyloid protein AA in casein-induced experimental amyloidosis. Lab. Invest., 36:420–427, 1977.

122. Skinner, M., et al.: P-component (pentagonal unit) of amyloid: isolation, characterization and sequence analysis. J. Lab. Clin. Med., 84:604–614, 1974.

123. Skinner, M., and Cohen, A.S.: The prealbumin nature of the amyloid protein in familial amyloid polyneuropathy (FAP)—Swedish variety. Biochem. Biophys. Res. Commun., *99*:1326–1332, 1981.
124. Skinner, M., Benson, M.D., and Cohen, A.S.: Amyloid fibril protein related to immunoglobulin lambda-chains. J. Immunol., *114*:1433–1435, 1975.
125. Sletten, K., Husby, G., and Natvig, J.B.: N-terminal amino acid sequence of amyloid fibril protein AP. Prototype of a new lambda-variable subgroup, V lambda V. Scand. J. Immunol., *3*:833–836, 1974.
126. Takahashi, N., et al.: Amino acid sequence of a lambda Bence-Jones protein from a case of primary amyloidosis. Biomed. Res., *1*:321–333, 1980.
127. Takeda, T., et al.: A new murine model of accelerated senescence. Mech. Ageing Dev., *17*:183–194, 1981.
128. Teilum, G.: Pathogenesis of amyloidosis: The two phase cellular theory of local secretion. Acta Pathol. Microbiol. Scand., *61*:21–45, 1964.
129. Terry, W.D., et al.: Structural identity of Bence Jones and amyloid fibril proteins in a patient with plasma cell dyscrasia and amyloidosis. J. Clin. Invest., *52*:1276–1281, 1973.
130. Tribe, C.R.: Amyloidosis in chronic paraplegia. *In* Renal Failure in Paraplegia. London, Pitman Medical Publishing, 1969.
131. Triger, D.R., and Joekes, A.M.: Renal amyloidosis—a fourteen-year follow-up. Q. J. Med., *42*:15–40, 1973.
132. Waldenstrom, H.: On the formation and disappearance of amyloid in man. Acta Chir. Scand., *63*:479–507, 1928.
133. Westermark, P.: Amyloid of medullary carcinoma of the thyroid: partial characterization. Uppsala J. Med. Sci., *80*:88–92, 1975.
134. Westermark, P., et al.: Immunocytochemical evidence for the lack of protein AS in some intracerebral amyloids. Lab. Invest., *46*:457–460, 1982.
135. Westermark, P., et al.: Coexistence of protein AA and immunoglobulin light-chain fragments in amyloid fibrils. Scand. J. Immunol., *5*:31–36, 1976.
136. Westermark, P., Johansson, B., and Natvig, J.B.: Senile cardiac amyloidosis: evidence of 2 different amyloid substances in the aging heart. Scand. J. Immunol., *10*:303–308, 1979.
137. Westermark, P., Natvig, J.B., and Johansson, B.: Characterization of an amyloid fibril protein from senile cardiac amyloid. J. Exp. Med., *146*:631–636, 1977.
138. Westermark, P., Skinner, M., and Cohen, A.S.: The P-component of amyloid of human islets of Langerhans. Scand. J. Immunol., *4*:95–97, 1975.
139. Williams, R.C., Jr., et al.: Secondary amyloidosis in lepromatous leprosy. Possible relationships of diet and environment. Ann. Intern. Med., *62*:1000–1007, 1965.
140. Wright, J.R., et al.: Relationship of amyloid to aging. Medicine, *48*:39–60, 1969.
141. Wright, J.R., Calkins, E., and Humphrey, R.L.: Potassium permanganate reaction in amyloidosis: a histologic method to assist in differentiating forms of this disease. Lab. Invest., *36*:274–281, 1977.
142. Yood, R.A., et al.: Bleeding and impaired hemostasis in 100 patients with amyloidosis. JAMA, *49*:1322–1324, 1983.
143. Yood, R.A., et al.: Soft tissue uptake of bone seeking radionuclide in amyloidosis. J. Rheumatol., *8*:760–766, 1981.

Chapter 73

Sarcoidosis

H. Ralph Schumacher

Sarcoidosis is a systemic disease characterized by a noncaseating granulomatous reaction of unknown origin. Our present concept of this syndrome has evolved from the early descriptions by Hutchinson, Besnier, and Boeck,[2] as well as by Schaumann.[37] Symptoms and signs depend on the organs affected, most frequently the lymph nodes, lungs, liver, skin, and eyes. Muscle, spleen, bones, parotid glands, central nervous system, blood vessels, endocrine glands, and almost any other tissue including the joints may also be involved. Although generally a chronic disease, its onset can be acute, with hilar adenopathy, erythema nodosum, fever, and articular manifestations. This acute form is often termed Lofgren's syndrome.[25]

PATHOLOGIC FEATURES

The characteristic histopathologic features of epithelioid tubercles with minimal necrosis and no true caseation, in contrast to the lesions of tuberculosis, are the hallmark of sarcoidosis (Figs. 73–1, 73–2). Studies on skin (Kveim reactions) and pulmonary lesions have identified large numbers of T-lymphocytes around the epithelioid cells. At least in the lung lesions, these are enriched with T4 "helper" cells and activated cells.[11,19] Sarcoid granulomas often contain Langhans-type giant cells with three frequent types of cytoplasmic inclusions: (1) asteroid bodies, which appear to consist of criss-crossing bundles of collagen; (2) Schaumann bodies, which are round or oval, laminated calcifications containing hydroxyapatite (Fig. 73–3); and (3) irregular, poorly stained, anisotropic, glasslike fragments.[26] Such granulomas, even with the typical inclusions, are not pathognomonic for sarcoidosis. Similar granulomatous tissue reactions can be seen in histoplasmosis, coccidioidomycosis, tuberculosis, lymphoma, Hodgkin's disease, bronchogenic carcinoma, foreign body granuloma, drug reactions, beryllium poisoning, syphilis, and leprosy. Functional impairment in sarcoidosis appears to result from both the active granulomatous disease and the secondary fibrosis.

CAUSE AND PREVALENCE

Many have speculated on the possible causes of this unexplained disease. The incidence of tuberculosis in sarcoidosis is 4%, and an unusual reaction to *Mycobacterium tuberculosis* or to atypical mycobacteria is one suggested mechanism.[44] High

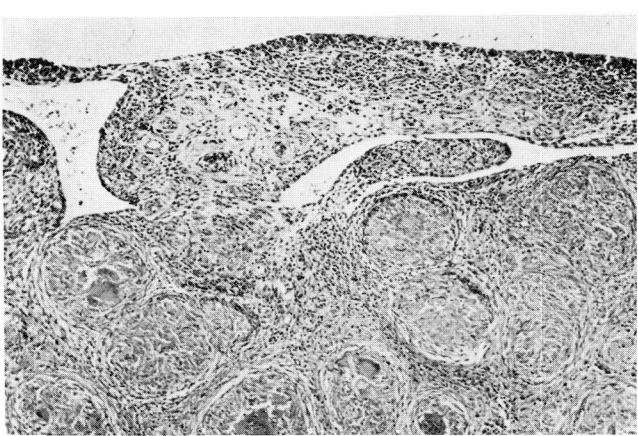

Fig. 73–1. Granulomatous synovitis of the elbow in chronic sarcoid arthritis. (Hematoxylin and eosin stain, × 60.) The synovial tissue is crowded with discrete, noncaseating miliary tubercles. At the surface, the villi are hypertrophied and infiltrated with leukocytes and fibroblasts. The articular cartilage of this joint is intact, and the subchondral bone (olecranon and lateral condyle of humerus) is free of tubercles. (From Sokoloff, L., and Bunim, J.J.[40])

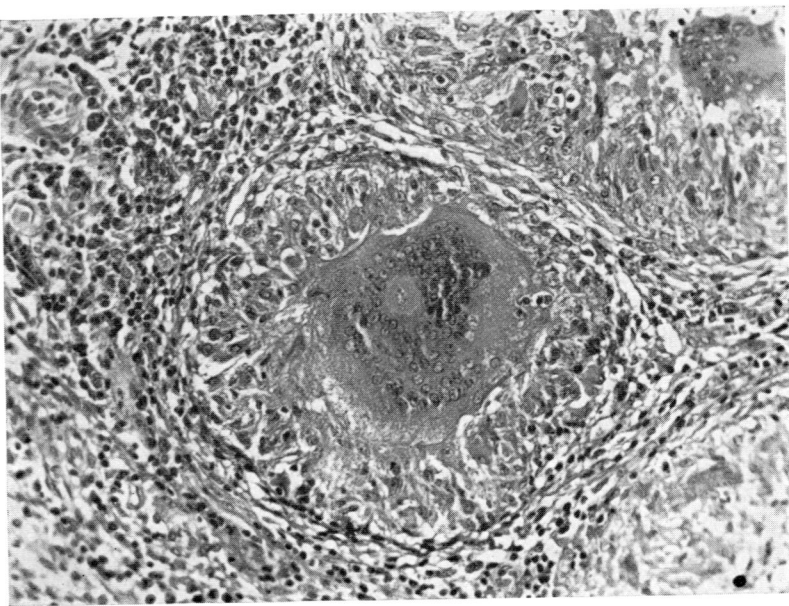

Fig. 73–2. Multinucleated giant cell in the center of a tubercle of epithelioid cells. Surrounding the tubercle is a layer of fibroblasts and a cuff of lymphocytes, plasma cells, and mononuclear cells. This figure is an area from Figure 73–1 under higher magnification. (× 175.) (From Sokoloff, L., and Bunim, J.J.[40])

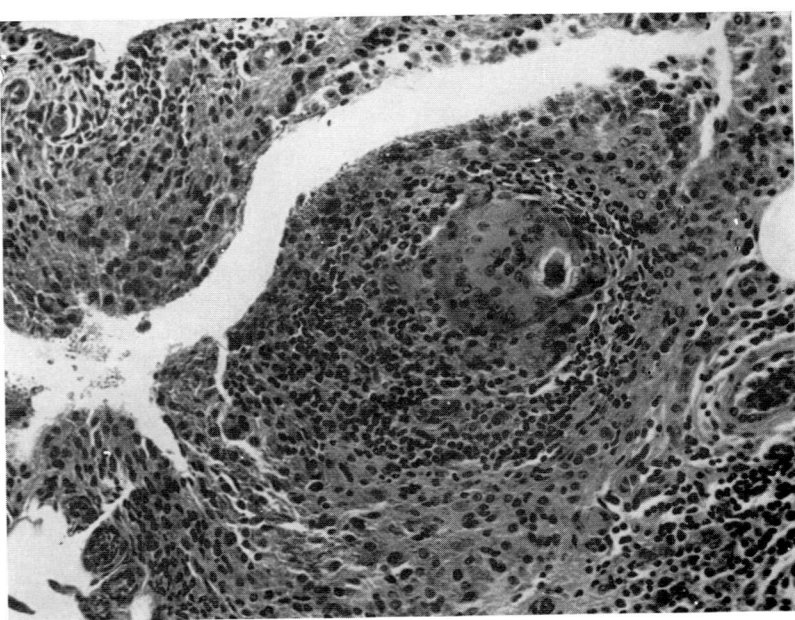

Fig. 73–3. Section of synovial tissue from the knee of a 33-year-old black woman with sarcoid polyarthritis of about 6 weeks' duration showing granulomatous synovitis and a Schaumann body. This Schaumann body appears in the cytoplasm of a giant cell as a circular clear space and consists of a colorless, crystalloid material that is doubly refractive. No bacteria or fungi are found with Brown-Brenn, Ziehl-Neelsen, or periodic-acid-Schiff stains. (From Sokoloff, L., and Bunim, J.J.[40])

titers of antibody to a number of viruses and other organisms have been reported in sarcoidosis.[14] Circulating immune complexes can be identified in up to 50% of cases, but their pathogenetic role is not clear.[14] Despite isolated reports of sarcoidosis in several members of a family and the familial coincidence of tuberculosis and sarcoidosis, no strong evidence supports a hereditary or contagious cause. Patients who have HLA antigens A1 and B8 may be more likely to express their sarcoidosis as erythema nodosum and acute arthritis.[8,14] Several series in this country show a higher incidence of sarcoidosis in black females than in the general population.[29] The disease may begin at any age, including infancy, but it is most commonly diagnosed in the third and fourth decades. Females predominate slightly over males. Sarcoidosis has a worldwide distribution, with the estimated incidence of the disease reaching as high as 64/100,000 in Sweden. American veterans after World War II had an incidence of 11/100,000.

GENERAL MANIFESTATIONS AND PROGNOSIS

The severity of manifestations can vary from an asymptomatic chest roentgenogram to death in approximately 4%. The most common symptoms and signs are fatigue (27%), malaise (15%), cough (30%), shortness of breath (28%), and chest pain (15%).[29] Ninety-two percent of patients have abnormal chest roentgenograms. Pulmonary parenchymal involvement is more ominous than the more frequent hilar adenopathy. Restrictive lung disease and cor pulmonale can develop. Granulomatous uveitis is the most frequent visual problem. Skin lesions occur in 30% of cases. They may be nondescript, but commonly are papular or nodular, erythematous or violaceous lesions, which show the typical granulomas on histologic examination. Erythema nodosum is common in sarcoidosis of acute onset. Liver involvement is almost always asymptomatic and is evidenced mainly by hepatomegaly. An elevated alkaline phosphatase level may suggest the presence of liver granulomas. The acute sarcoidosis, accompanied by erythema nodosum, hilar adenopathy, and arthralgia, generally has the best prognosis.

Despite the similar sarcoid tissue reaction, Truelove has urged physicians to distinguish this syndrome from sarcoidosis.[43] Certainly, most patients with this acute syndrome have a full remission within two years, but long-term follow-up has not been reported in such cases, and some caution is warranted.

DIAGNOSIS

The diagnosis of sarcoidosis is established by the demonstration of typical noncaseating granu-

lomas in the absence of other identifiable causes of such granulomas (Table 73–1). Impaired delayed hypersensitivity is characteristic, but not invariable. Impaired tuberculin sensitivity after bacille Calmette Guérin vaccination may persist even after apparent recovery from sarcoidosis. Antibody production is normal. The elevated immunoglobulins are of little help in the differential diagnosis. Leukopenia, anemia, eosinophilia, hypercalcemia, and elevated erythrocyte sedimentation rates may be seen. Hypercalciuria is found in most cases. The serum level of angiotensin-converting enzyme is typically elevated in active sarcoidosis.[24] Serum angiotensin-converting enzyme (ACE) activity is increased. ACE is produced by the granulomas, which also secrete 1,25 dihydrocholecalciferol, responsible for the absorptive hypercalciuria. Although increased ACE levels are seen in about 80% of patients, they are not unique to sarcoidosis and may also occur in inflammatory diseases of the liver,[28] Gaucher's disease, leprosy, silicosis, asbestosis, hyperthyroidism, and diabetes. Angiotensin-converting enzyme levels fall with successful therapy and may be useful in following treatment.[23] These levels can also be followed along with other findings in patients with mild disease who are not treated, to look for early clues to exacerbation.

Tissue diagnosis is most expeditiously established by biopsy of a skin lesion or an accessible superficial lymph node. With such superficial material, additional evidence of generalized disease is also needed because foreign body reactions can be difficult to distinguish from sarcoidosis. Liver samples also can show granulomas, especially if the liver is palpably enlarged, but a granulomatous liver reaction is common in other liver diseases,[7] and such granulomas are not as helpful in diagnosis as lymph node lesions. Mediastinoscopy in experienced hands is a safe and reliable method of obtaining lymph node tissue for diagnosis if hilar adenopathy is present. Transbronchial lung biopsy, using the fiberoptic bronchoscope, is an attractive initial biopsy procedure yielding diagnoses in about

Table 73–1. Diagnostic Features of Sarcoidosis

1. Noncaseating granulomas on biopsy; one must exclude other causes of granulomas.
2. Hilar and right paratracheal adenopathy in 90%.
3. Skin lesions, uveitis, or involvement of almost any tissue.
4. Onset most often in third and fourth decades, but cases reported at all ages.
5. Impaired delayed hypersensitivity in 85%.
6. Frequent hyperglobulinemia.
7. Increased angiotensin-converting enzyme levels in about 80%.
8. Hypercalciuria in most; hypercalcemia in some.

60% of cases in one series.[20] In typical Lofgren's syndrome with asymptomatic hilar and right paratracheal adenopathy, one can sometimes observe the patient without performing a biopsy.[46] Biopsies with serial sections often show granulomas in asymptomatic muscles.[42] Israel and Sones found muscle tissue positive in 89% of patients with erythema nodosum or arthralgia.[12]

An intradermal injection of 0.2 ml of a 10% saline suspension of sarcoid tissue (the Kveim test) has been used for diagnosis. A positive reaction consists of the development of a local sarcoid granuloma at the injection site. Positive test results can be obtained in 80% of patients with sarcoidosis, most often in those with prominent adenopathy, but standardization of preparations has been difficult, and reliable material is not generally available. Positive Kveim test results in patients with lymphadenopathy due to diseases other than sarcoidosis may be due to less-specific batches of antigen.[13]

[67]Gallium scintigrams can assist in evaluating activity of alveolitis,[23] and they may be abnormal even in patients with normal chest roentgenograms.[32] Bronchoalveolar lavage showing more than 35 to 45% T-lymphocytes also suggests active alveolitis.[5] Some patients without elevated numbers of lymphocytes in lavages have also responded to corticosteroid therapy, however.[23]

SPECIFIC MUSCULOSKELETAL MANIFESTATIONS

Muscle

Sarcoid granulomas in muscle are often asymptomatic, but they may be accompanied by local pain and tenderness or even palpable nodules. A symmetric proximal myopathy has also been described and has been reported to occur without evident sarcoidosis in other tissues.[10,39] Involved muscles show noncaseating granulomas as well as lymphocytic infiltration, muscle necrosis, and regeneration. Calcification of muscles and other soft tissues occasionally occurs in hypercalcemic patients.

Bone

Phalangeal cysts, often considered a helpful diagnostic clue in sarcoidosis (Fig. 73–4), were described in 14% of patients in one series.[29] Although some of these cysts are due to sarcoid granulomas, others may be unrelated to the sarcoidosis. A radiologic survey of the hands of 338 patients with sarcoidosis and 342 control subjects showed cystic changes in 5% of the patients with sarcoidosis, but also in 8% of the control subjects, a group that included normal persons and patients with a variety of diseases.[1] Other bones, including the skull and

vertebrae, may also develop cysts from sarcoid granulomas. Large lytic or sclerotic vertebral lesions can be seen.[36] Bone sarcoidosis is usually asymptomatic. The overlying cortex is almost always intact. The phalangeal lesions of sarcoidosis can also be associated with osteosclerosis.[27] Cystic bone lesions only occasionally extend into the joint, in which they may cause arthritis.[40] Rarely, destructive bony lesions are associated with overlying purplish red, nodular cutaneous masses, formerly termed *lupus pernio*.[26]

Joints

Arthritis was first described with sarcoidosis in 1936,[3] and since then, arthritis, periarthritis, or arthralgia has been reported in 2 to 38% of patients in various series.[9,29,38,41] Chronic sarcoidosis is associated less frequently with joint complaints. Table 73–2 outlines sarcoid arthropathy.

In acute sarcoidosis with hilar adenopathy, fever, and erythema nodosum, up to 89% of patients have articular symptoms, and 69 and 63% had articular or periarticular swelling in the series of Lofgren,[25] and James et al.,[15] respectively. Ankles and knee joints are most frequently involved in acute sarcoidosis. Most other joints are occasionally involved. Heel pad pain is common; monoarthritis is unusual.[9] The patient generally has a dramatic, tender, warm, erythematous swelling that often is clearly periarticular rather than synovial. Such changes are occasionally difficult to separate from adjacent cutaneous erythema nodosum, and the histologic appearance of the lesions is identical. Joint motion is often painless; pain is much less than one would expect, considering the inflammatory signs. The frequency of a severe, localized tenderness has been emphasized.[16]

Roentgenograms show only soft tissue swelling. Such articular findings may antedate erythema nodosum by as much as two weeks and suggest careful watch for the skin lesions. Both skin and joint lesions may antedate hilar adenopathy for up to several weeks. Ankle and knee involvement is often symmetric; joint involvement can be progressive. The acute inflammation often raises a suspicion of rheumatic fever, gonococcal or other infectious arthritis, and gout. Joint aspiration often yields no synovial fluid. When an effusion is aspirated, leukocyte counts can be as high as 42,500/mm[3], with 90% neutrophils.[34] Most effusions are only mildly inflammatory, however, with leukocyte counts of under 1,000/mm[3], predominantly lymphocytes and large mononuclear cells.[18]

Cultures are negative, and crystals cannot be identified by compensated, polarized light. Several patients with this syndrome, including an early case described by Hutchinson, had been thought to have

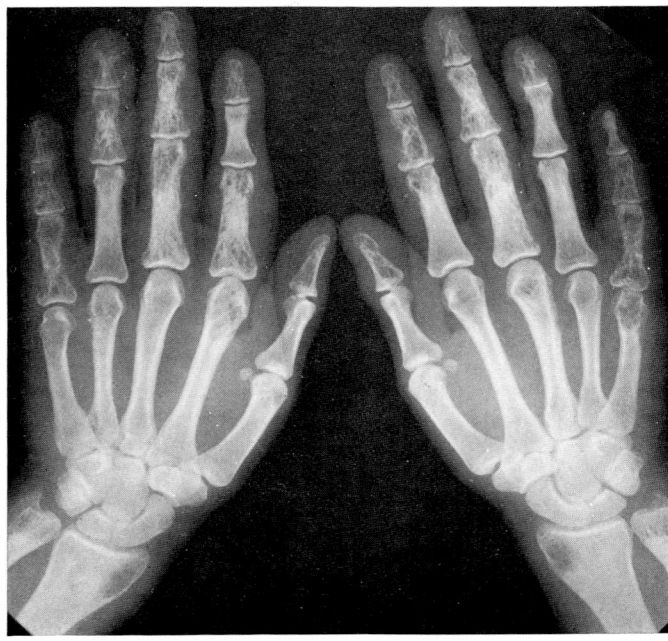

Fig. 73–4. Roentgenograms of the hands showing unusually severe bone lesions of sarcoidosis. The bone cysts have not broken through the articular cortex. The hands shown in Figure 73–5 have similar bone changes, but with extension into the distal interphalangeal joints.

Table 73–2. Sarcoid Arthropathy

Acute Sarcoidosis (Lofgren's Syndrome)
1. Often periarticular and tender, erythematous, warm swelling.
2. Ankles and knees almost invariably involved.
3. Joint involvement possibly the initial manifestation (chest film normal).
4. Joint motion possibly normal and pain absent or minimal.
5. Synovial effusions infrequent and generally only mildly inflammatory.
6. Usually nonspecific mild synovitis on synovial biopsy.
7. Self-limited in weeks to 4 months.

Chronic Sarcoidosis
1. Arthritis possibly acute and evanescent, recurrent, or chronic.
2. Noncaseating granulomas often demonstrable in synovium.
3. Usually nondestructive despite chronic or recurrent disease.

gout before synovial fluid crystal identification was available to confirm the presence of gouty arthritis.[17] That sarcoid arthritis may respond dramatically to colchicine further confuses the issue. Elevated uric acid levels have been noted in a small percentage of patients with sarcoidosis,[41] but recent studies suggest that hyperuricemia should not be anticipated unless due to drugs or renal failure.

Needle synovial biopsy specimens in acute sarcoidosis most often show only mild nonspecific synovitis and some lining-cell proliferation.[18] Although much of the inflammation in acute sarcoidosis may be periarticular, synovial granulomas are occasionally found during open surgical biopsy.[40] Caplan et al. have described an identical periarthritis in 19 patients with hilar adenopathy, none of whom had erythema nodosum.[4] These workers found sarcoid granulomas in the subcutaneous tissue over 3 of 7 inflamed ankles, but no granulomas in an open joint biopsy. Angiotensin-converting enzyme levels need not be elevated in patients with acute sarcoidosis without pulmonary parenchymal involvement.[8]

The joint manifestations of acute sarcoidosis subside in two weeks to four months, although rare patients may develop chronic sarcoid arthritis. Erythema nodosum and a similar arthropathy can also be seen in lepromatous leprosy, ulcerative colitis, regional enteritis, tuberculosis, coccidioidomycosis, histoplasmosis, oral contraceptive and possibly other drug use, pregnancy, and psittacosis and other infections. Other cases are idiopathic.

In sarcoidosis of more insidious onset, joint manifestations are less common. In such cases, even with widespread systemic granulomatous disease, the arthritis may still be mild and evanescent, as in acute sarcoidosis. Arthritis can also be recurring or protracted with polysynovitis, however. Even in patients with chronic synovitis, joint destruction is infrequent, and most roentgenograms show only soft tissue swelling. The destructive joint disease occasionally seen in sarcoidosis is illustrated in Figure 73–5. Such severe arthritis is most common in patients with multisystemic granulomatous disease. Arthritis may occur as an initial manifestation or after years of systemic disease. Thus, such a variety of patterns can be seen that a high index of suspicion is needed to lead to biopsy and other diagnostic studies to differentiate this disorder from rheumatoid or other types of arthritis.

Reports of synovial fluid analysis are infrequent. We recently found joint-fluid leukocyte counts of 250 to 6,250/mm³ with predominantly mononuclear cells in 6 patients with arthritis associated with chronic sarcoidosis.[35] Sokoloff and Bunim found noncaseating granulomas in 3 of 5 surgical synovial biopsy specimens from patients with chronic arthritis.[40] In addition, the synovium showed diffuse chronic inflammation including plasma cells. None of their patients, and only 3.3% of those studied by Owen et al.,[34] had any elevation of rheumatoid factor, but others have found rheumatoid factor in as many as 38% of patients with sarcoidosis.[33] The presence of rheumatoid factor does not correlate with the presence or severity of joint disease. Tenosynovitis at the wrists and elsewhere can also be seen.

Finger clubbing is an occasional complication of pulmonary sarcoidosis, but hypertrophic osteoarthropathy with joint effusions has not been re-ported.[45] Arthritis in early-childhood sarcoidosis has been described, with especially large, painless, boggy synovial and tendon sheath effusions.[31] The course of the disease is indolent, and constitutional symptoms are few. Despite prolonged synovitis, no erosive radiographic changes are seen. Synovial fluid findings are not described; synovial biopsy samples show either granulomas or nonspecific inflammation. Interestingly, the sarcoidosis reported in young children is associated with uveitis, but not with hilar adenopathy.

TREATMENT

Many patients with minimal symptoms require no treatment. No curative agent exists. Adrenal corticosteroids are commonly used to try to suppress potentially serious active inflammatory reactions, such as ocular disease, pulmonary parenchymal disease, and central nervous system involvement, and are often effective. Corticosteroids can also lower persistently elevated serum calcium levels. Initial doses of 20 to 60 mg prednisone are tapered to the lowest effective maintenance dose. Alternate-day dosage seems effective for maintenance therapy. Objective long-term benefits from corticosteroids have often been difficult to demonstrate,[47] but improved vital capacity even in severe disease has been shown in one series.[6] Spontaneous remission can occur. Active articular disease almost always shows at least temporary improvement with corticosteroid therapy. When these agents are used, isoniazid coverage may be needed. Because joint disease is often self-limited,

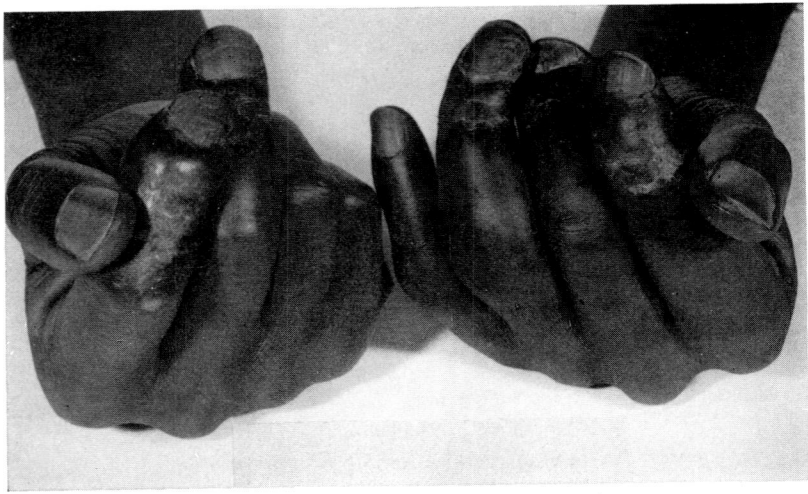

Fig. 73–5. The hands of a 33-year-old black male with sarcoidosis of 5 years' duration. Depigmented skin lesions are present on the dorsum of fingers, and the distal phalanx of the left fourth finger is displaced. Note the fusiform swelling of the proximal interphalangeal joint of the fourth and fifth fingers of left hand (asymmetric). This patient does not have psoriasis. (From Sokoloff, L., and Bunim, J.J.[40])

however, rest, salicylates, and other analgesics are often all that is required. Salicylates are not as dramatically effective as in rheumatic fever. Colchicine shortens attacks of acute arthritis in some patients,[16] but it is by no means invariably effective. Chloroquine has been reported to help cutaneous sarcoidosis.[30] Uncontrolled reports of methotrexate[22] and azathioprine[21] use in sarcoidosis have suggested benefit in these patients.

REFERENCES

1. Baltzer, G., et al.: Zur haufigkeit zystischer knochenveranderungen (Ostitis cystoides multiplex jungling) bei der Sarkoidose. Dtsch. Med. Wochenschr., 95:1926–1929, 1970.
2. Boeck, C.: Multiple benign sarkoid of the skin. J. Cutan. Genitourin. Dis., 17:543–550, 1899.
3. Burman, M.S., and Mayer, L.: Arthroscopic examination of knee joint: report of cases observed in course of arthroscopic examination, including instances of sarcoid and multiple polypoid fibromatosis. Arch. Surg., 32:846–874, 1936.
4. Caplan, H.I., Katz, W.A., and Rubenstein, M.: Periarticular inflammation, bilateral hilar adenopathy and a sarcoid reaction. Arthritis Rheum., 13:101–111, 1970.
5. Daniele, R.P., Dauber, J.H., and Rossman, M.D.: Immunologic abnormalities in sarcoidosis. Ann. Intern. Med., 92:406–416, 1980.
6. Emirgil, C., Sobol, B.J., and Williams, M.H.: Long-term study of pulmonary sarcoidosis. The effect of steroid therapy as evaluated by pulmonary function studies. J. Chronic Dis., 22:69–86, 1969.
7. Fagan, E.A., Moore-Gillon, J.C., and Turner-Warwick, M.: Multiorgan granulomas and mitochondrial antibodies. N. Engl. J. Med., 308:572–575, 1983.
8. Fitzgerald, A.A., and Davis, P.: Arthritis, hilar adenopathy, erythema nodosum complex. J. Rheumatol., 9:935–938, 1982.
9. Gumpel, J.M., Johns, C.J., and Shulman, L.E.: The joint disease of sarcoidosis. Ann. Rheum. Dis., 26:194–205, 1967.
10. Hinterbuchner, C.N., and Hinterbuchner, L.P.: Myopathic syndrome in muscular sarcoidosis. Brain, 87:355–366, 1964.
11. Hunninghake, G.W., and Crystal, R.G.: Pulmonary sarcoidosis: a disorder mediated by excess helper T-lymphocyte activity at sites of disease activity. N. Engl. J. Med., 305:429–434, 1981.
12. Israel, H.L., and Sones, M.: Selection of biopsy procedures for sarcoidosis diagnosis. Arch. Intern. Med., 113:255–260, 1964.
13. James, D.G.: Editorial: Kveim revisited, reassessed. N. Engl. J. Med., 292:859–860, 1975.
14. James, D.G., and Williams, W.J.: Immunology of sarcoidosis. Am. J. Med., 72:5–8, 1982.
15. James, D.G., Thomson, A.D., and Wilcox, A.: Erythema nodosum as a manifestation of sarcoidosis. Lancet, 2:218–221, 1956.
16. Kaplan, H.: Sarcoid arthritis with a response to colchicine. N. Engl. J. Med., 268:778–781, 1960.
17. Kaplan, H., and Klatskin, G.: Sarcoidosis, psoriasis, and gout: syndrome or coincidence? Yale J. Biol. Med., 32:335–352, 1960.
18. Kitridou, R.C., and Schumacher, H.R.: The arthritis of acute sarcoidosis. (Abstract.) Arthritis Rheum., 13:328–329, 1970.
19. Konttinen, Y.T., et al.: Inflammatory cells of sarcoid granulomas detected by monoclonal antibodies and an esterase technique. Clin. Immunol. Immunopathol., 26:380–389, 1983.
20. Koontz, C.H., Joyner, L.R., and Nelson, R.A.: Transbronchial lung biopsy via the fiberoptic bronchoscope in sarcoidosis. Ann. Intern. Med., 85:64–66, 1976.
21. Krebs, P., Abel, H., and Schonberger, W.: Behandling der boeckschan sarkoidose mit immunosuppressiven substanzen. Ertahrungen mit Azatioprin (Imurel). Munchen. Med. Wochenschr., 111:2307–2311, 1969.
22. Lacher, M.J.: Spontaneous remission or response to methotrexate in sarcoidosis. Ann. Intern. Med., 69:1247–1248, 1968.
23. Lawrence, E.C., et al.: Serial changes in markers of disease activity with corticosteroid treatment in sarcoidosis. Am. J. Med., 74:747–756, 1983.
24. Lieberman, J.: Elevation of serum angiotensin converting enzyme (ACE) level in sarcoidosis. Am. J. Med., 59:365–372, 1975.
25. Lofgren, S.: Primary pulmonary sarcoidosis. I. Early signs and symptoms. Acta Med. Scand., 145:424–431, 1953.
26. Longcope, W.T., and Freiman, D.G.: A study of sarcoidosis. Medicine, 31:1–32, 1952.
27. McBrine, C.S., and Fisher, M.S.: Acrosclerosis in sarcoidosis. Radiology, 115:279–281, 1975.
28. Matsuki, K., and Sakata, T.: Angiotensin-converting enzyme in disease of the liver. Am. J. Med., 73:549–551, 1982.
29. Mayock, R.L., et al.: Manifestations of sarcoidosis, analysis of 145 patients, with review of 9 series selected from literature. Am. J. Med., 35:67–89, 1963.
30. Morse, S.I., et al.: The treatment of sarcoidosis with chloroquine. Am. J. Med., 30:779–784, 1961.
31. North, A.F., et al.: Sarcoid arthritis in children. Am. J. Med., 48:449–455, 1970.
32. Nosal, A., et al.: Angiotensin-1-converting enzyme and gallium scan in non-invasive evaluation of sarcoidosis. Ann. Intern. Med., 90:328–331, 1979.
33. Oreskes, I., and Siltzbach, L.E.: Changes in rheumatoid factor activity during the course of sarcoidosis. Am. J. Med., 44:60–67, 1968.
34. Owen, D.S., et al.: Musculoskeletal sarcoidosis and rheumatoid factor. Med. Coll. VA Q., 8:217–220, 1972.
35. Palmer, D.G., and Schumacher, H.R.: Non-specific histologic changes in needle biopsy specimens of synovium in chronic sarcoidosis. Ann. Rheum. Dis. In press, 1984.
36. Perlman, S.G., et al.: Vertebral sarcoidosis with paravertebral ossification. Arthritis Rheum., 21:271–277, 1978.
37. Schaumann, J.N.: Etude sur le lupus pernio et ses rapports avec les sarcoides et la tuberculose. Ann. Dermatol. Syph., 6:357–373, 1916–1917.
38. Siltzbach, L.E., and Duberstein, J.L.: Arthritis in sarcoidosis. Clin. Orthop., 57:31–50, 1968.
39. Silverstein, A., and Siltzbach, L.E.: Muscle involvement in sarcoidosis. Asymptomatic myositis, and myopathy. Arch. Neurol., 21:235–241, 1969.
40. Sokoloff, L., and Bunim, J.J.: Clinical and pathological studies of joint involvement in sarcoidosis. N. Engl. J. Med., 260:842–847, 1959.
41. Spilberg, I., Siltzbach, L.E., and McEwen, C.: The arthritis of sarcoidosis. Arthritis Rheum., 12:126–137, 1969.
42. Stjernberg, N., et al.: Muscle involvement in sarcoidosis. Acta Med. Scand., 209:213–216, 1981.
43. Truelove, L.H.: Articular manifestations of erythema nodosum. Ann. Rheum. Dis., 19:174–180, 1960.
44. Vanek, J., and Schwartz, J.: Demonstration of acid-fast rods in sarcoidosis. Am. Rev. Respir. Dis., 101:395–400, 1970.
45. West, S.G., Gilbreath, R.E., and Lawless, O.J.: Painful clubbing and sarcoidosis. JAMA, 246:1338–1339, 1981.
46. Winterbauer, R.H., Belic, N., and Moores, K.D.: A clinical interpretation of bilateral hilar adenopathy. Ann. Intern. Med., 78:65–71, 1973.
47. Young, R.J., et al.: Pulmonary sarcoidosis: a prospective evaluation of glucocorticoid therapy. Ann. Intern. Med., 73:207–212, 1970.

Chapter 74

Arthritis Associated with Hematologic Disorders, Storage Diseases, Disorders of Lipid Metabolism, and Dysproteinemias

Robert B. Buckingham and Gerald P. Rodnan

In a number of hematologic diseases, diseases of lipid metabolism, storage diseases, and dysproteinemias, osteoarticular complaints play an important or even a dominant role.[83,85,152,267,277] These symptoms may be either the result of direct involvement of the bones and joints in the primary disease process or a consequence of secondary metabolic or immunologic disturbances. In either event, joint symptoms may be the first manifestation of the primary disease, and require proper identification to prevent serious delay in the recognition of the underlying disorder.

LEUKEMIA

The early manifestations of acute leukemia vary and often include symptoms indicative of rheumatic disease,[30,97,304,325] especially in children, who may be thought at first to have rheumatic fever, juvenile rheumatoid arthritis (JRA), or Still's disease.[11,30,141] Pain and tenderness of the bones may be present, and most patients have polyarticular disease with prominent involvement of the knees and ankles and, variably, large joint effusions. In some cases, the inflammation may be monoarticular or oligoarticular.[97,274,296,304,325] Synovial fluid leukocyte counts are also variable, ranging in one study from 50 cells/mm³ to 45,000 cells/mm³, with an average of 8,790 cells/mm³.[344] Although these findings occur most often in the larger peripheral joints, the small joints, including those in the fingers, may also be affected.

Severe bone pain out of proportion to the degree of arthritis has been stressed as a distinguishing feature of leukemia, in addition to the lymph node enlargement and hematologic abnormalities.[274] The occurrence of subcutaneous nodules resembling rheumatoid nodules and the presence of rheumatoid factor in some children with acute leukemia may further complicate diagnosis.[274] The joint symptoms are related in some instances to leukemic infiltrations in synovium, subperiosteum, and juxta-articular portions of the bones or to hemorrhage.[165,304,325] In such cases, bone scintigraphy may show increased juxta-articular uptake of radioactivity.[332] In other cases, one sees no infiltrate in synovium or bone and, therefore, no obvious cause of the articular inflammatory disease.[344] In these patients, disease may be mediated by an immune complex mechanism or by cell-mediated responses to a leukemic antigen within articular tissue.[207]

Articular involvement also occurs in the chronic forms of leukemia,[304] but it is seldom as dramatic and usually appears as a late manifestation of the disease. Biopsies have revealed leukemic infiltrations in the synovium in several instances.[304] Careful examination may reveal areas of bony tenderness, particularly in the sternum.[56] Patients with acute or chronic leukemia have an abnormally high frequency of positive tests for antinuclear antibodies,[282] as well as for rheumatoid factor, in titers up to 1:5,120.[196,274,288,304] Chronic lymphocytic leukemia of T-cell origin was associated with nodular polyarthritis in a woman with many T cells in the synovial fluid but no synovitis or synovial infiltrate.[333] Rare cases of acute polymyositis occurring in patients with leukemia have been recorded.[91] Septic arthritis may also complicate both acute and chronic leukemia, and osteomyelitis and disc space infections may occur. Arthritis in leukemia may be a result of hemorrhage in the joint or periarticular structures, or it may be a result of gout or pseudogout.

Roentgenograms reveal a variety of skeletal changes in acute leukemia.[226,244,325] In children, juxtaepiphyseal radiolucent bands are commonly seen in long bones, close to the site of rapid bone growth; this abnormality occurs in a number of other conditions associated with a disturbance in osteogenesis.[30,226] Other roentgenographic features of acute leukemia include osteoporosis, osteolytic lesions, cortical or periosteal defects, distortion of trabecular pattern, fractures, osteosclerosis, and subperiosteal new bone formation.[57,244,293,325]

Similar, although less frequent, roentgenographic abnormalities occur in patients with chronic leukemia.[57,178,226] The proximal portions of the femora and humeri, the bones of the pelvis, and the vertebrae are most often affected. Vertebral compression fractures are common, and osteolytic and sclerotic changes can be seen in the ribs, scapulae, long bones, and pelvis. Such bone lesions may represent an initial focus of blastic crisis.[332] Destruction of bone may be extensive, and osteonecrosis of the head of the femur may be seen.

Hairy cell leukemia has been reported in association with vasculitis, which may resemble classic polyarteritis nodosa. Although it is possible that the vasculitis is a result of the leukemia, it is also possible that the two diseases share a common pathogenetic or predisposing factor. Hepatitis B virus or cytomegalovirus infection may occur in individuals with leukemia and may lead to vasculitis.[87,118,249] Destructive bone involvement, also a complication of hairy cell leukemia, has been reported in at least 11 cases. Axial distribution of the lesions is most common, with involvement in the skull, vertebral bodies, and the femoral neck. One patient developed osteonecrosis of the femoral head. Radiation therapy is beneficial.[67]

The joint symptoms in patients with acute leukemia may be improved temporarily by salicylates and other anti-inflammatory agents. Such a therapeutic response has been cause for confusion in diagnosis.[325] The disappearance of bone and joint pain is often one of the first indications of improvement after antileukemic therapy.[325] Dramatic relief of bone pain and rapid resolution of knee joint inflammation have been described in a man with chronic myelomonocytic leukemia following the administration of cytosine arabinoside.[80]

MALIGNANT LYMPHOMAS

Skeletal involvement is common in the malignant lymphomas.[107,178,226,269] Bone defects, which can be seen roentgenographically in as many as 15% of patients with Hodgkin's disease, have been found at postmortem examination in up to 50% of such patients.[115,165,235] Sites of involvement include the spine, pelvis, ribs, femur, skull, and shoulder. Symptoms referable to these lesions include deep pain, which is unremitting and is worse at night, as well as pain due to pathologic fracture, particularly when the disease occurs within vertebrae. The five year survival is generally less than ten percent.

In one patient with reticulum cell sarcoma with articular involvement, the diagnosis was established by the demonstration of malignant cells in the synovial fluid at a time when these cells were absent from the peripheral blood and the initial bone marrow specimen.[88] We, too, have observed a man with a swollen, inflamed knee who had reticulum cell sarcoma that had invaded the synovium, but such direct involvement of the joints is unusual.[220] One patient with malignant lymphoma of a poorly differentiated, diffuse type initially had sternoclavicular joint arthritis. The joint was surrounded by grayish neoplastic tissue; marginal erosions and lysis of the adjacent clavicle and manubrium sterni were present.[4]

Reports exist of LE cells in patients with Hodgkin's disease[15] and of antinuclear antibodies with other lymphomas, as well as in other malignant neoplasms.[45,158] Many individuals with established systemic lupus erythematosus or RA have developed lymphoma or leukemia.[15,47,64,81,123,198,210,236,298] In some cases, the clinical and serologic evidence of lupus has disappeared during development of Hodgkin's disease.[15,236] Generally, however, antinuclear antibodies and rheumatoid factor are not found in patients with Hodgkin's disease or other types of lymphoma.[282] The increased susceptibility of patients with connective tissue disease to these malignant conditions remains hypothetic[240] (see also the following section of this chapter). Little question exists, however, concerning the increased frequency of malignant lymphomas in patients with Sjögren's syndrome.[316] Hodgkin's disease and other lymphomas are among the malignant neoplasms associated with the development of dermatomyositis in adults.[50,323]

Articular symptoms may also be associated with malignant lymphoma as the result of hypertrophic osteoarthropathy secondary to pleural or mediastinal involvement,[109] as well as because of secondary gout.[317] Children with neuroblastoma and widespread bone metastases often have severe bone and joint pain that may be mistaken for rheumatic fever or Still's disease.[36] Osteonecrosis of the femoral or humeral head has been reported uncommonly in patients receiving intermittent corticosteroid-containing multiple-drug chemotherapy (see Chap. 86). Most such patients have also received radiotherapy to the affected bones, however.[89,163,326] Malignant lymphomas of bone without involvement of regional lymph nodes or distant viscera are usually morphologically diverse, have been reported in the pelvis and the long bones of the upper and lower extremities, and are treated most often with radiotherapy with variable success.[77,78]

MULTIPLE MYELOMA

In most cases, pain in the back or extremities, perhaps the earliest symptom of multiple myeloma, is attributable to disease of the bone, and roentgenograms often reveal osteoporosis and osteolytic defects.[103,142,165,226] Individuals with multiple myeloma may develop *amyloid arthropathy* and may exhibit pain and swelling of the joints, most commonly the shoulders, wrists, knees, and fingers (see Chap. 72). One may note prominent enlargement of the shoulders (shoulder-pad sign) and a rubbery, hard consistency of the periarticular connective tissue from deposition of amyloid.[174,176,233] Amyloid deposits can be identified by histochemical and electron-microscopic techniques in articular cartilage, in perichondrocytic lacunae, in synovium (Fig. 74–1), and in synovial fluid debris including fragments of synovial villi.[131,150] The presence of morning stiffness, fatigue, polyarticular involvement, periosteal nodular deposits of amyloid, and occasional bony erosion and destruction may closely simulate the clinical features of RA.[53,120,130,142,150,233,321,347] The duration of morning stiffness is shorter and fatigue is more prominent than in RA, however, and the synovial fluid findings are completely incongruous with that disease. Synovial fluid in amyloid arthropathy is viscous and contains few leukocytes (200 to 4,500/mm³), which are predominantly mononuclear cells.[28,120,130,131,150,347] Synovial fluid pellets, stained with Congo red and viewed under polarized light, demonstrate intra- and extracellular amyloid (see also Chaps. 4 and 72).

Amyloidosis occurs in association with all forms of myeloma, including the IgD and pure Bence Jones varieties,[130,176,233] but it is found most frequently in patients with pure light-chain disease or with IgA myelomas.[53,130,310] Typical amyloid arthropathy is found most commonly in association with multiple myeloma, but it has also been reported with primary amyloidosis;[135] in contrast, it is rare, and indeed, may not occur, in those with generalized secondary amyloidosis.[53] The incidence of typical amyloid arthropathy in multiple myeloma is estimated to be about 5%.[150] Although small amounts of amyloid may be seen in synovial biopsy specimens of some patients with secondary amyloidosis,[191] prominent deposits resembling those of RA do not occur.

Amyloid may be deposited in the carpal tunnel and may compress the median nerve, to cause carpal tunnel syndrome.[22,120,134,142,347] A review of the literature from 1931 to 1975 revealed that 45% of patients reported with amyloid arthropathy also had carpal tunnel syndrome.[53] Thus, the concurrence of myeloma, symmetric polyarthropathy, and carpal tunnel syndrome suggests amyloidosis.

Amyloid fibrils in both primary generalized amyloidosis and myeloma-related amyloidosis consist of an immunoglobulin light chain or a fragment thereof.[115] In such cases, the amino acid sequence of the major component of the amyloid protein is homologous with that of the variable region of kappa or lambda light chains or, rarely, the intact Bence Jones protein[54,116,182] (see Chap. 72). Amyloid deposits of unknown origin occur in secondary amyloidosis, in association with familial Mediterranean fever, and in certain experimental animal models of amyloidosis. These proteins, designated AA proteins, are distinct from the AL proteins that appear to be derived from immunoglobulin light chain (L-chain amyloid).[161,162] The chemical identification of the components of amyloid and the variation in the composition of amyloid in the different clinical forms of amyloid disease are detailed in Chapter 72.

Skeletal involvement in multiple myeloma may be limited to diffuse osteoporosis, but one may also see circumscribed lytic areas, expansile lesions, or ill-defined diffuse areas of bone destruction ("moth-eaten" bone).[128] Scintigraphic examination of bone may be helpful in the diagnosis of

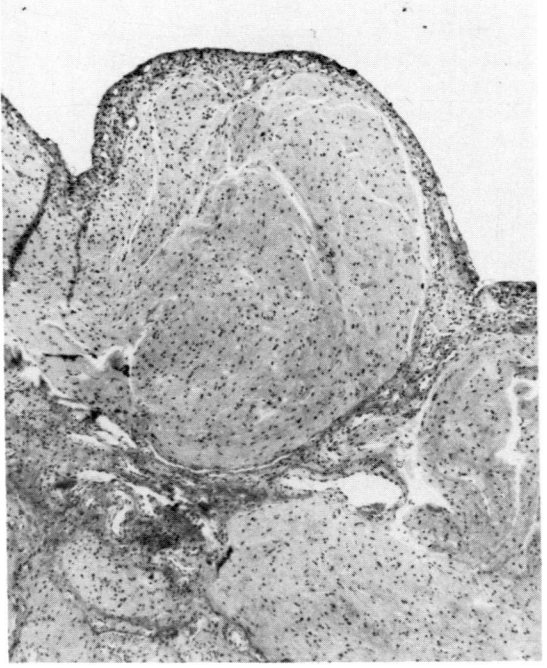

Fig. 74–1. Photomicrograph of synovium obtained from the right shoulder of a 56-year-old woman with multiple myeloma who had developed pain in this shoulder and inability to use her arm 10 days earlier, following a fall. The humerus was dislocated. At the time of open reduction of this dislocation, large deposits of amyloid were found in the glenoid fossa. Note the mass of amyloid covered by a thin rim of synovium. The material in this nodule stained metachromatically with crystal violet.

skeletal involvement by demonstrating osseous lesions not detected by conventional radiography.[234] In patients with amyloidosis, osteoporosis with or without lytic lesions is common.[53] When light-chain myeloma is accompanied by amyloidosis, the patient has fewer lytic lesions of bone and the prognosis is worse than when amyloid is absent.[310] Patients with Waldenström's macroglobulinemia may also exhibit bony changes including osteoporosis, isolated or multiple osteolytic defects resembling those seen in multiple myeloma, and multilocular cyst-like lesions found in the supra-acetabular portions of the iliac bones.[334] A single example of typical amyloid arthropathy has been described in a patient with Waldenström's macroglobulinemia,[121] and another case of Waldenström's disorder with neuropathic joint disease secondary to amyloid neuropathy has been reported.[280]

The course of myeloma, both IgG and IgA types, and Waldenström's macroglobulinemia may also be complicated by the *hyperviscosity syndrome*.[224,253] In patients with IgG myeloma, hyperviscosity develops when the serum concentrations of IgM components exceed 5 gm/dl, whereas in IgA myeloma and macroglobulinemia, hyperviscosity depends on the molecular size and shape of the abnormal proteins.[224,253]

Paraproteinemia, with or without myeloma or macroglobulinemia, may occur in patients with long-standing RA or systemic lupus erythematosus.[123,142,170,343,360] Neoplastic transformation may be a consequence of prolonged and intense immunologic activity associated with the primary connective tissue disease.[360] Multiple myeloma may also co-exist with Gaucher's disease. Again, chronic immunologic stimulation has been postulated to predispose patients to the malignant disorders.[113]

Several reports note an association between multiple myeloma and gout.[142,209,317] In many of these patients, gouty symptoms long preceded recognition of the myeloma.

SICKLE CELL DISEASE AND OTHER HEMOGLOBINOPATHIES

Sickle cell crisis is often associated with severe polyarthralgia and arthritis manifested by warmth, swelling, and tenderness in the joints and in periarticular areas.[277,278] Joint involvement is usually monoarticular or pauciarticular. The knees and elbows are most commonly involved. Synovial fluid is not usually inflammatory and is often clear, with a normal viscosity and a leukocyte count of fewer than 1,000 cells/mm³ with a low percentage of polymorphonuclear leukocytes.[278] Sickled erythrocytes can be seen in these effusions. A few reports note sterile inflammatory effusions with high

cell counts and no crystals.[74,90,122,146] Crystal-induced synovitis cannot be excluded by a single synovianalysis.

Synovial biopsies obtained at the time of acute joint disease show little cellular infiltrate, prominent congestion of small blood vessels, and, in a few cases, definite microvascular thrombosis.[278] Microvascular obstruction probably leads to infarction of synovium and adjacent bone and may account for joint effusions and inflammation. Bone scans using ^{99m}technetium sulfur colloid and other isotopes reveal diminished uptake in the bone marrow adjacent to painful joints; such a finding suggests infarction.[12,143] These defects occur in the absence of roentgenographic evidence of marrow or bone infarction and may precede such findings by many months. On occasion, however, joint inflammation is followed by rapid destruction of articular cartilage. The presence of prominent lymphocytic and plasma cell infiltrates in these patients suggests a possible immune mechanism. Cryoprecipitable immune complexes have been implicated in sickle cell nephropathy,[312] and an abnormality of the alternate pathway of complement activation has been demonstrated in the serum of patients wich sickle cell disease.[169] No direct evidence for the participation of immune mechanisms in sickle cell arthropathy has yet been found, however.

The skeletal lesions characteristic of this hemoglobinopathy may be separated into those related to hyperplasia of bone marrow and those resulting from local thrombosis and infarction.[48,74,126,149,226,258,259,260] Bone marrow proliferation is associated with widening of medullary cavities, thinning of cortices, coarsening and irregularity of trabecular markings, and cupping of vertebral bodies; on the other hand, lesions believed to result from sickle cell thrombosis and infarction include cortical bone infarcts with periostitis and periosteal elevation, bone marrow lysis, sclerosis and fibrosis, and most notably, avascular necrosis of the femoral and humeral heads (Figs. 74–2, 74–3, 74–4). Less commonly, one sees infarction in the distal portion of the femur, the radius, patella, and the vertebrae.[48,51,74,226,284,318]

Subchondral and intraosseous hemorrhages contribute to the destruction of articular cartilage in the hip.[287] Avascular necrosis of the femoral head has been reported in patients with S-S disease and sickle cell trait, as well as in those with S-C disease, sickle cell-thalassemia, and S-F disease.[51,124,160,164,232,272,299,300] Aseptic necrosis occurs in 20 to 68% of patients with S-C disease, but in only 4 to 12% of those with S-S disease.[51] In one study, the incidence of aseptic necrosis was not increased in patients with sickle cell trait, when compared with age-matched control subjects with

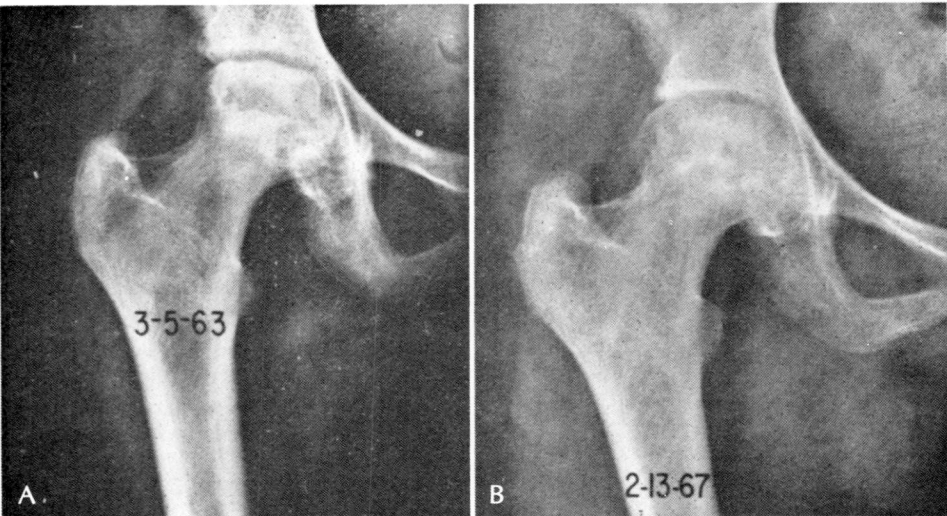

Fig. 74–2. *A,* Roentgenogram of the right hip of a 16-year-old girl with sickle cell anemia (S-S hemoglobin) who complained of pain and restricted movement in the joint. Note the changes indicative of avascular necrosis of the head of the right femur. *B,* The same hip 4 years later. Note the improvement, with evidence of regeneration of articular cartilage and subchondral bone. At this time, the patient was free of pain and had full motion of the joint.

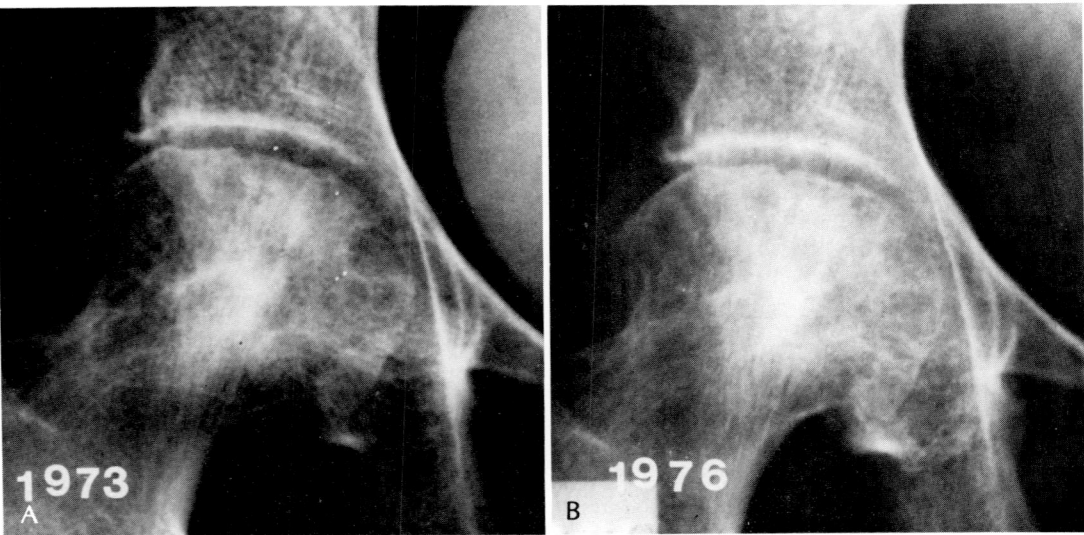

Fig. 74–3. *A* and *B,* Further follow-up of the patient whose hips are shown in Figure 74–2. Little change has taken place in the appearance of the head of the femur. In 1978, the patient experienced only occasional pain and stiffness in this hip, "with damp weather." The patient has full flexion and extension of the joint, but restriction in abduction (45°, as compared to 90° on her left side) as well as in both external rotation (60°, as compared to 90° on her left side) and internal rotation (45°, as compared to 60° on her left side). This young woman has also had osteomyelitis of the left fibula, presumably from salmonella infection, although cultures were sterile.

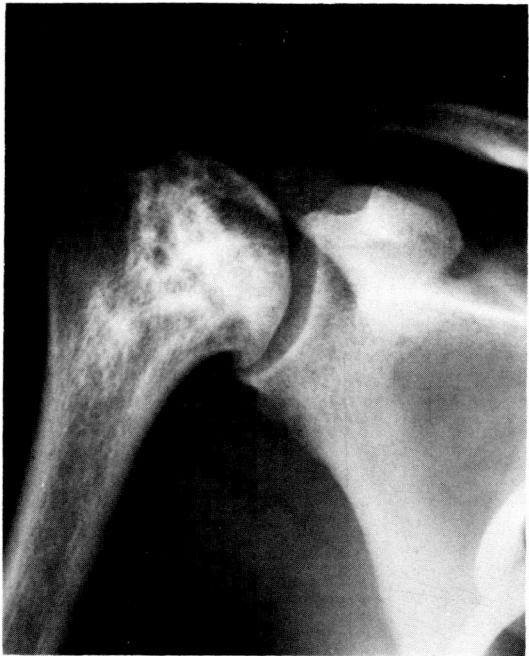

Fig. 74–4. Roentgenogram of the right shoulder of a 35-year-old woman with hemoglobin S-C disease illustrating avascular necrosis of the head of the humerus. This patient has had a 10-year history of pain and stiffness of this joint. She had bilateral avascular necrosis of the femoral heads as well.

A-A hemoglobin.[76] Total hip replacement has been successful in some patients with these hemoglobinopathies.[124,136]

Although it has generally been assumed that infarction of the femoral head is caused by sickle cell thrombosis of the fine epiphyseal vessels, it is tempting to speculate that occlusion may be the result of fat emboli. Systemic fat embolization, apparently originating in the necrotic bone marrow, has been reported in hemoglobin S-C disease, as well as in sickle cell (S-S) anemia[238,286] (see Chap. 86).

Young children with sickle cell disease may have transient swelling and tenderness of the hands and feet as a result of periostitis of the metacarpal, metatarsal, and proximal phalangeal bones, a condition known as sickle cell dactylitis.[48,74,90,226,341,353] Dactylitis may occur before the diagnosis of sickle cell disease is established. In addition to periosteal elevation and subperiosteal new bone formation, roentgenograms reveal radiolucent areas intermingled with areas of increased density, giving a moth-eaten appearance. These changes have been interpreted as representing infarction.[74] In most cases, the integrity of the affected bones is restored to

normal in several months without residual deformity or alteration in growth. The rarity of this "hand-and-foot" syndrome after the fourth year of life is explained by the recession of red marrow from the cool distal bones and its replacement by fibrous tissue.[74]

Another striking skeletal complication of sickle cell disease is *salmonella osteomyelitis*, which may be multifocal.[74,159,284] The first signs of this infection, which usually starts in the medullary cavity of the long and tubular bones, is periosteal proliferation. This process is followed by bone destruction extending throughout the shaft.[48] Septic arthritis, although less common than osteomyelitis, has been reported to be due to a number of organisms, including salmonellae,[74] staphylococci, *Escherichia coli, Fusobacterium varium,*[230] and *Serratia liquefaciens.*[147] Staphylococci and *Serratia* organisms have also been responsible for osteomyelitis in these patients.[74] After successful treatment with antibiotics, the bones usually heal with minimal deformity. Because the serum of many patients with sickle cell anemia is deficient in opsonins for salmonellae and pneumococci, the leukocytes of these patients are limited in their ability to phagocytose and to kill these pathogenic micro-organisms.[169] This impairment has been attributed to a defective alternative complement pathway.[145,350] Local vascular insufficiency associated with sickling may also affect the host response to infection and the efficacy of antibiotic treatment.[243]

Although 40% of patients with sickle cell disease have hyperuricemia,[262,337] only a few reports exist of suspected acute gouty arthritis, and even fewer case reports of crystal-proved gout are available.[19,200,273,317] Gout has been recorded in association with hemoglobin S-S, sickle cell trait, thalassemia, and hemoglobin C-C. Hyperuricemia results from impaired renal function (sickle cell kidney)[72,336] or overproduction of uric acid.[19,337] Evidence indicates increased tubular secretion of urate in young adults with sickle cell anemia and uric acid overproduction,[71] which permits these individuals to remain normouricemic and may account for the low frequency of secondary gout in this condition.

The development of a specific osteoarthropathy has been described in patients with beta-thalassemia major, as well as in those with thalassemia minor.[132,275] Twenty-five of 50 patients with beta-thalassemia major between the ages of 5 and 33 years had evidence of periarticular disease marked by pain and swelling of the ankles and pain on compression of the malleoli, calcaneus, and forefoot.[132] Synovial fluid obtained from the ankle joint in 2 of these patients was noninflammatory. Hyperplasia of the synovial lining and a heavy deposition of hemosiderin pigment were found. Radiographic changes included osteopenia, widened medullary spaces, thin cortices with coarse trabeculations, and evidence of microfractures. The presence of microfractures was confirmed histologically; and increased osteoblastic and resorptive (osteoclastic) surfaces, with iron deposits at the calcification front and cement lines, were found. The arthropathy in these individuals thus appears to be related to the underlying bone disease, although the role of iron overload in the pathogenesis remains to be fully evaluated. A similar form of pauciarticular, nonerosive, seronegative arthropathy was observed in individuals with thalassemia minor,[275] and bilateral avascular necrosis of the femoral heads has been reported in a patient with this condition.[2]

STORAGE DISEASES

The lysosomal storage diseases are uncommon inborn errors of metabolism resulting from the deficiency or absence of specific lysosomal hydrolytic enzymes. Most cases represent inherited autosomal recessive traits. Enzyme deficiency results in accumulation and storage of large amounts of substrate in lysosomes of cells in multiple organ systems and in connective tissues, including bones. Storage diseases include the mucopolysaccharidoses (see Chap. 75), the glycoproteinoses, the mucolipidoses, and the gangliosidoses. The skeletal features of many of these disorders resemble features of the Hurler syndrome and have been referred to collectively as *dysostosis multiplex*.[305] Characteristic radiographic abnormalities may be seen in the skull, chest, spine, pelvis, long bones, and hands. Skeletal features of the most common gangliosidoses and certain other storage diseases are discussed here.

Gangliosides are sphingolipids containing neuraminic acid. These substances were initially found in ganglion cells of the central nervous system. Much is now known regarding the enzyme deficiencies in these storage disorders. GM_1-gangliosidosis is a result of deficiency of β-galactosidase; in type 1 GM_2-gangliosidosis or *Tay-Sachs disease*, the patient lacks the isoenzyme A of total β-hexosaminidase; in type 2, Sandhoff's disease, the patient also lacks total β-hexosaminidase. Patients with *Fabry's disease* are deficient in galactosidase; *Gaucher's disease* results from a deficiency of β-glucocerebrosidase and β-glucosidase; *Farber's disease* occurs as a result of a deficiency of acid ceramidase; *Krabbe's disease* is associated with a deficiency of β-galactocerebrosidase; metachromatic leukodystrophy develops because of a deficiency of arylsulfatase A and sulfatidase; and *Neimann-Pick* disease, or sphingomyelin lipidosis,

results from a deficiency of the enzyme sphingomyelinase.[188,251] In the last decade, substantial progress has been made in detecting these enzyme deficiencies, initially by analysis of solid organ tissue and more recently by identification of enzyme deficiencies in leukocytes from the peripheral blood of affected individuals,[188,251] as well as in cultured dermal fibroblasts.[199] With fibroblast culture, it is now possible to diagnose storage diseases, to identify carriers, and to provide accurate prenatal diagnosis.

Gaucher's Disease

Gaucher's disease, described by P.C.E. Gaucher in 1882, is a heritable lysosomal sphingolipid storage disease characterized by the accumulation of the glycolipid glucocerebroside, or glucosylceramide, in reticuloendothelial cells in the bone marrow, spleen, liver, lymph nodes, and other internal organs.[37,245,322] Glucocerebroside, a complex glycolipid membrane constituent, accumulates because of a deficiency of the enzymes β-glucocerebrosidase and β-glucosidase, which catalyze the hydrolytic cleavage of glucocerebroside into ceramide and glucose.[37,245] Three clinical forms of Gaucher's disease are recognized.[37,245] Type 1, by far the most common, is the chronic, non-neuronopathic, "adult" form of the disease; type 2 is the infantile or acute neuronopathic form, with an average survival rate of less than a year; and type 3 is the juvenile or subacute neuronopathic form. All are transmitted as an autosomal recessive disorder. In the adult form, type 1, the patient is deficient in lysosomal glucocerebrosidase, whereas in type 2, both this enzyme and a soluble β-glucosidase are lacking.[245]

Osteoarticular complaints are an important feature in both type 1 and type 3 Gaucher's disease. These symptoms result from infiltration of the bone marrow by lipid-laden histiocytes (Gaucher's cells) and are often the earliest manifestation of Gaucher's disease.[14,37,267,295,322] The most common rheumatic complaint is acute, severe pain in the extremities, particularly in the hip, knee, and shoulder. Such painful bone crises are more common in children, but they occur in both juvenile and adult forms of the disease. When accompanied by signs of inflammation and fever, these episodes may mimic pyogenic osteomyelitis and have been called "*pseudo-osteomyelitis*."[14,276] In many ways, these crises resemble those of sickle cell anemia. The exact cause of these exacerbations is unknown, but vasospasm or vascular occlusion of end arteries within bone may result from deposition of Gaucher's cells and may increase the intramedullary pressure. This process may, in turn, lead to ischemia, necrosis, and local hemorrhage. Symptoms last from days to weeks, but they eventually resolve spontaneously.

The patient may also have pathologic fractures of long bones,[283] as well as compression deformity of vertebrae causing low back pain. In rare cases, the patient has migratory polyarthritis, the nature of which is poorly understood. Joint disease is usually mono- or pauciarticular and involves the large joints, in which it appears to be related to changes in adjacent bone.[226,295] Small joint involvement, including the proximal interphalangeal joints, is most uncommon.[354] A number of reports cite severe degenerative hip disease as a result of avascular necrosis and collapse of the head of the femur (Fig. 74–5).[133,226,295] Total hip arthroplasty has been successful in such patients, but it is associated with increased intraoperative blood loss; the likelihood of loosening of the prosthesis may also be greater, perhaps because infiltration of the medullary cavity by Gaucher's cells prevents adequate cement fixation.[189,192] Recurrent avascular necrosis of the capital femoral epiphysis has been observed.[14,74]

Changes in the femoral neck may lead to pathologic fracture or to coxa vara deformity. On occasion, invasion of the head of the humerus gives rise to degenerative arthropathy of the shoulder.[5,295]

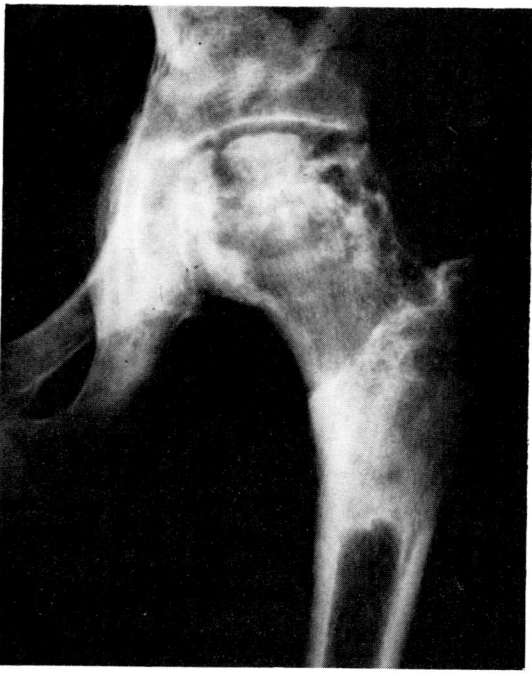

Fig. 74–5. Roentgenogram of the left hip joint of a 22-year-old man with Gaucher's disease illustrating avascular necrosis of the head of the femur. This roentgenogram was obtained 2 years after the onset of pain in the hip.

Splenectomy, performed on some individuals with hypersplenism or with mechanical problems resulting from the enlarged spleen, may be followed by accelerated skeletal manifestations.[268] Following splenectomy, cerebroside storage may occur at an increased rate in liver and bone and may lead more rapidly to osteoarthritis, aseptic necrosis, and pathologic fractures.[289] Many patients with longstanding disease have elevated serum immunoglobulin levels, often monoclonal.[252] Some patients with Gaucher's disease appear to progress from monoclonal dysproteinemia to overt multiple myeloma.[113,247]

One of the most consistent roentgenographic features of Gaucher's disease is widening of the distal portion of the femur. This process usually occurs just superior to the femoral condyles and creates the well-known "Erlenmeyer flask" appearance.[295] Similar flaring is less common in the tibia and humerus, together with changes in the other long bones, pelvis, skull, vertebrae, and mandible.[226,295,322] Characteristically, areas of rarefaction are mingled with patchy sclerosis and cortical thickening, resulting from new bone formation. With spondylar involvement, the intervertebral disc and the surfaces of adjacent vertebrae remain intact, and although there may be collapse with gibbus formation, the spinal cord escapes compression.[322]

The diagnosis of Gaucher's disease can be established by demonstrating large, kerasin-filled Gaucher cells in the bone marrow, as well as by analyzing peripheral blood leukocytes for residual β-glucocerebrosidase and β-glucosidase activities.[188,251] Angiotensin converting enzyme levels are elevated fivefold in patients with Gaucher's disease and may provide another means of substantiating the diagnosis.[294] Because enzyme levels are normal in cultured fibroblasts, the marked elevations in serum may be due to increased synthesis of angiotensin converting enzyme by stimulated Gaucher cells. Administration of purified glucocerebrase to patients with Gaucher's disease produces a significant reduction of glucocerebroside in the liver and a reduction to normal level of this substance in the erythrocytes.[25,37,38,245] Enzyme replacement therapy is under active study. In some patients, bone pain is relieved following x-irradiation or treatment with corticosteroids.[322]

Fabry's Disease

Fabry's disease, or glycolipid lipidosis, was first described by J. Fabry in 1898. This hereditary. X-linked disorder of glycosphingolipid metabolism is characterized by the progressive accumulation of birefringent deposits of a triglycosylceramide and, to a lesser extent, a diglycosylceramide and blood-group B substances in endothelial, perithelial, and smooth muscle cells of blood vessels, in ganglion and perineural cells of the autonomic nervous system, in epithelial cells of the cornea, and in kidney, bone marrow, and many other tissues.[70,315,351] This pathologic storage is due to a defect in the activity or absence of the lysosomal enzyme L-galactosidase A (ceramide trihexosidase), required for the normal catabolism of trihexosyl ceramide, which is derived from kidney and the membranes of senescent erythrocytes. Death usually occurs in the fifth or sixth decade, as a result of renal failure or from the cardiac and cerebral complications of arterial hypertension or vascular disease. Heterozygous women may exhibit the disease in an attenuated form.

The disorder is characterized by a typical rash, known as *angiokeratoma corporis diffusum universale*, consisting of widespread telangiectasia or angiokeratoma. These pinpoint lesions, which occupy the dermal papillae, are venules with multiple layers of basement membrane in the vascular walls and may represent the ectopic placement of small collecting veins. They are thought to arise by alteration of the existing microvasculature rather than as a result of newly proliferating microvessels (neovascularization).[41] Vasospasm similar to that seen in Raynaud's disease, induced by changes in temperature and associated with paresthesias and burning in the extremities, are seen in many patients and are caused by deposits in the cells of the autonomic nervous system.[281,351] A study of forearm hemodynamics in eight patients with Fabry's disease revealed increased vascular resistance, decreased venous capacitance, and decreased forearm blood flow.[281]

The patient may also have painful swelling of the fingers, elbows, and knees.[315] A characteristic deformity consisting of limitation in extension of the distal interphalangeal joints of the fingers has been described.[111,168,351] Avascular necrosis of the head of the femur[248] or talus[99] and multiple, small, infarct-like opacities in the femoral head may occur.[190] Involvement of the metacarpal and metatarsal bones and of the temporomandibular joint has been reported,[303] as well as osteoporosis of the dorsal vertebrae.[29] The diagnosis of Fabry's disease is established by demonstration of the characteristic birefringent lipid material in skin and also by enzymatic assay. Efforts have been made to determine whether an allograft, in the form of a kidney transplant, might provide a sufficient amount of L-galactosidase A to correct the metabolic defect. This question, as well as that of the value of other forms of enzyme replacement therapy, remains controversial.[10,39,52,246]

Farber's Disease

Farber's disease, or disseminated lipogranulomatosis, was first described in 1952 by S. Farber. This rare, progressive sphingolipidosis of early childhood is characterized by painful and swollen joints, periarticular and subcutaneous nodules, dysphonia, pulmonary infiltrations, and retardation of mental and motor development.[3,31,82,95,228,229] The patient has an accumulation of ceramide, a glycolipid, in the cytoplasm of neurons and certain other cells attributable to a heritable deficiency in the lysosomal enzyme acid ceramidase, which catalyzes the conversion of ceramide to sphingosine and fatty acids.[82,228] Ceramide may accumulate in lysosomes of cultured diploid fibroblasts from individuals with Farber's disease who are deficient in acid ceramidase.[49]

Articular disease, usually appearing between two weeks and four months of age, has been the dominant initial manifestation in the handful of patients recognized to date. Typically, the patient notes pain and swelling of the interphalangeal and metacarpophalangeal joints, the ankles, wrists, knees, and elbows. Nodular masses develop on tendon sheaths and in para-articular tissues, as well as at points of pressure such as the occiput and the lumbosacral region. Nodules have also been found in the conjunctiva, the external ear, and the external nares. These patients often develop flexion contractures of the fingers and other joints. Ankylosis may follow. Swelling and granuloma formation in the epiglottis and larynx are responsible for a disturbance in swallowing and episodes of lung infection. Few children survive past the age of two years, and the usual cause of death is pulmonary disease.

Fibroblasts, histiocytes, and macrophages with foamy cytoplasm-containing material with the staining properties of glycolipid are found in granulomatous deposits in the larynx, pleura, myocardium, pericardium, synovium, bones, liver, spleen, lymph nodes, cerebral cortex, and lung. Abnormal lipid is also present in the cytoplasm or neurons of the central nervous system. Roentgenographic changes consist of generalized bony demineralization, juxta-articular erosions of long bones, and irregular disruption of trabeculae in the metacarpal bones and phalanges.[31] Ceramide consists of a long-chain base, most commonly sphingosine, joined to a fatty acid by an amide linkage. Ceramide is a component of many important lipids, such as the gangliosides, sphingomyelin, cerebrosides, and other glycolipids.[228] Ceramidase, or acylsphingosine deacylase, is the enzyme that catalyzes ceramide degradation; it also catalyzes the reverse reaction and leads to the formation of ceramide from sphingosine and free fatty acid. A deficiency in acid ceramidase has been reported both in white blood cells and in cultured fibroblasts from several patients with Farber's disease.[228,229] In one patient, an accumulation of acid mucopolysaccharide, chiefly dermatan sulfate, was found in the tissue, and urinary excretion of this substance was increased.[31,228] The data on familial occurrence of Farber's disease are compatible with autosomal recessive inheritance.[228]

Lipochrome Histiocytosis

This rare, familial disorder is marked by pulmonary infiltrates, splenomegaly, hypergammaglobulinemia, increased susceptibility to infection, and lipochrome pigment granulation of the histiocytes. In the first report of this syndrome, one of three affected sisters had RA with typical nodules, and a second had transient episodes of joint inflammation; the serum of all three contained rheumatoid factor in high titer.[101] The peripheral blood leukocytes of these patients have impaired respiration and hexose monophosphate shunt activity after phagocytosis and are deficient in staphylocidal capacity.[263]

MULTICENTRIC RETICULOHISTIOCYTOSIS

Multicentric reticulohistiocytosis, or *lipoid dermatoarthritis,* is a rare disorder seen in adults and characterized by a profusion of histiocytic nodules in the skin and mucous membranes and by severe, often mutilating polyarthritis.[21,35,86,98,127,144,208,223,241,339] To date, approximately 80 cases have been reported.[26] The disease affects women 3 times as often as men and is usually insidious in onset. Although the disorder has been thought to represent a lipid storage disease,[187] definitive evidence for this classification has not been presented. It is possible that the histiocytes and giant cells contain a variety of nonspecifically accumulated lipid, but it is not clear whether this event is primary or secondary. There is no evidence that this disorder is heritable.[21] The disease appears to be inflammatory in nature, and the lesions in skin and synovium resemble experimentally produced granulomas, containing activated histiocytes that fuse to form cells of increasing size. These larger cells, or megalocytes, may eventually coalesce to form giant cells and may have granules that appear to contain a variety of lipids, including triglycerides, cholesterol esters, and phospholipids.[20,106,208,241,319] The severe bone and joint destruction is probably due to erosion of cartilage and bone by collagenase, elastase, and other degradative enzymes released by the proliferating, activated histiocytes.

Microscopic examination shows dense infiltrations of the dermis and synovium by a granulomatous proliferation of histiocytes and multinucleated giant cells containing large amounts of periodic acid-Schiff-positive material (Fig. 74–6). Similar cells have been observed in the bone marrow, lymph nodes, bone and periosteum, muscle, larynx, and endocardium.[339] Serum lipid abnormalities, including slight to moderate elevations in total lipid, cholesterol, phospholipid, and fatty acids, as well as lipoprotein abnormalities, have been found in a number of patients.

In approximately two-thirds of patients, the first sign of the disease is polyarthritis, followed months to years later, on the average three years later, by a nodular skin eruption. In the remaining patients, nodules appear first or are contemporaneous with joint symptoms. The polyarthritis is usually symmetric, often simulates RA, and may involve all the peripheral joints, including the distal interphalangeal joints of the fingers, as well as spinal and temporomandibular joints. Joint stiffness may be a prominent early complaint. The joints are swollen, tender, and may be inflamed. Large joint effusions may be present.[86]

The cell count in the few synovial fluid samples examined has varied from 1,800 to 93,000 cells/mm^3.[86,98,140,187] with predominance of either mononuclear[187] or polymorphonuclear cells.[98] Foamy giant cells have been noted in the synovial fluid as well as in the synovium.[106,187] The presence of these large cells, known as megalocytes, may be a helpful early diagnostic clue.[106] Pericardial or pleural effusions may occur.[140] Electron-microscopic study of these unusual macrophages reveals the presence of inclusions resembling the Golgi apparatus and seemingly developing from smooth endoplasmic reticulum.[187]

Both the course and severity of the arthritis vary. Although the patient may have a spontaneous remission, chronic active disease is usual. Many patients suffer severe destructive changes, particularly of the fingers (main en lorgnette) and less often of the hip and toe joints. The tendon sheaths on the flexor and extensor surfaces of the wrists may be involved,[86] and Dupuytren's contracture or carpal tunnel syndrome have been described in these patients.[98]

The skin lesions consist of firm, reddish brown or yellow papulonodules, most commonly on the face and hands, ears, forearms and elbows, scalp, neck, and chest.[21] Small tumefactions resembling *coral beads* are seen around the nail fold[21] (Fig. 74–7). These lesions may remain discrete, or they may coalesce into diffuse plaques. The lesions may also be pruritic.[140] The nodules usually wax and wane and may disappear without a trace. Xanthelasma is noted in a third of these patients. About

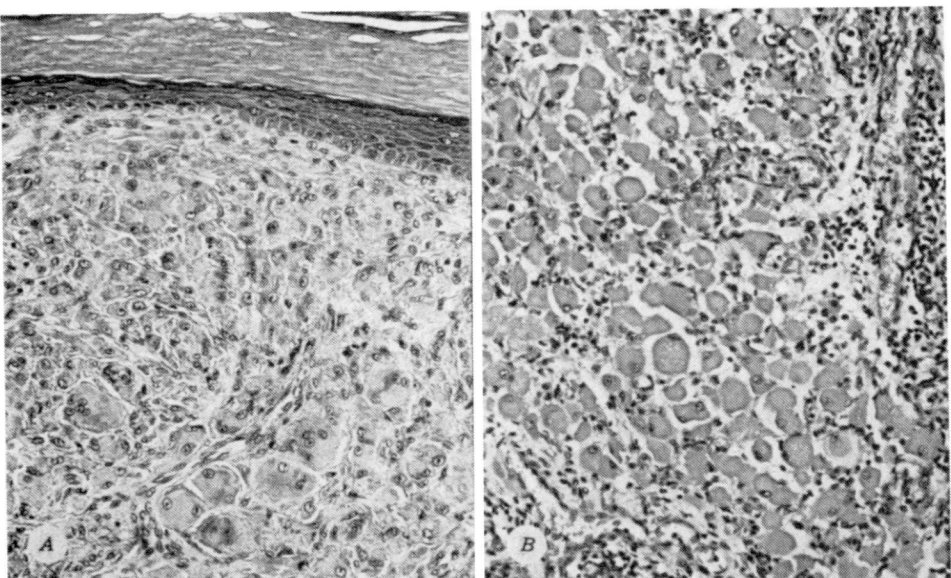

Fig. 74–6. Photomicrograph of *A*, a skin nodule, and *B*, synovium (knee) from a 54-year-old woman with multicentric reticulohistiocytosis. Numerous histiocytes and multinucleated giant cells contain large amounts of periodic-acid-Schiff-positive material. (× 185)

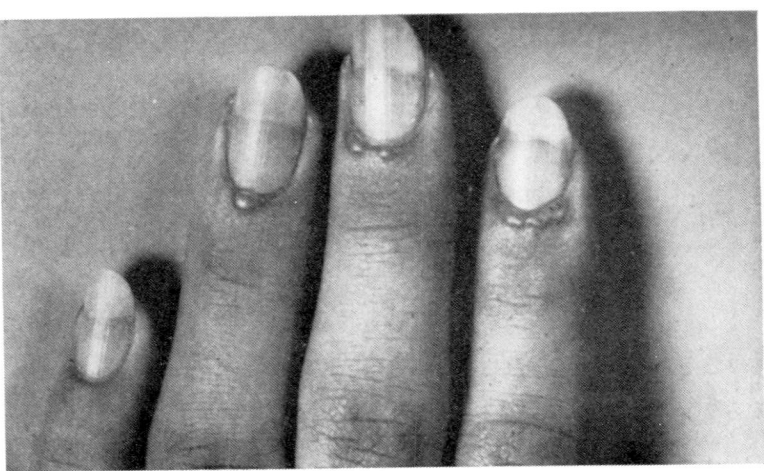

Fig. 74–7. The fingers of a 16-year-old girl who had polyarthritis for 8 months and these reddish brown "coral beads" for 5 months. Typical infiltrates of multicentric reticulohistiocytosis were found in biopsy specimens of both skin and synovium. (From Melton and Irby.[223])

half the patients develop mucosal papules on the lips, tongue, buccal membrane, nasal septum, and gingiva, as well as on the pharynx and larynx. Fever, weakness, and weight loss may occur during the course of this illness. Mild anemia, monoclonal gammopathy, or erythrocyte sedimentation rate elevation may occur.[140]

Roentgenograms reveal rapidly progressive, symmetric joint destruction with loss of cartilage and absorption of subchondral bone, disproportionately severe when compared to the mildness of the symptoms.[119] Characteristic features of the arthropathy of multicentric reticulohistiocytosis include the following: (1) Well circumscribed erosions spreading from the joint margins; (2) widened joint spaces; (3) predominance of interphalangeal, metacarpophalangeal, and metatarsophalangeal joint involvement; (4) early and severe atlantoaxial joint involvement with erosion of the odontoid process leading to subluxation;[219] (5) erosion of the distal ends of the clavicles; (6) absent or minimal periosteal reaction; (7) absent or disproportionately mild osteopenia when compared to the severity of erosive changes; and (8) prominent, uncalcified soft tissue nodules.[119]

Patients with multicentric reticulohistiocytosis have an increased incidence of co-existent malignant disease. Perhaps as many as 25% have a neoplasm.[106,140] The disease is not usually fatal, however, and may become spontaneously quiescent. Although the mucocutaneous nodules may shrink or may disappear completely, these patients are often left with serious joint disability and, at times, a disfigured, leonine facies.[21] Treatment with the anti-inflammatory corticosteroids may cause temporary regression of the cutaneous lesions, but these agents have little effect on the arthritis.[241] A few reports cite dramatic clinical response to cytotoxic drug therapy. Nodule formation and joint disease abated in one patient after treatment with cyclophosphamide,[144] and skin lesions were successfully treated with topical nitrogen mustard in another patient, who later responded to cyclophosphamide by an improvement in both joint and skin disease.[40] In other instances, treatment with nitrogen mustard and chlorambucil has been reported to be effective.[63] Two cases of co-existing multicentric reticulohistiocytosis and primary biliary cirrhosis, successfully treated with cyclophosphamide, have been reported.[75] In the first case, chlorambucil was substituted when the patient developed hematuria, and improvement continued. A patient with multicentric reticulohistiocytosis with salivary gland involvement and pericarditis with effusion responded to a regimen of prednisone, cyclophosphamide, and vincristine administered simultaneously.[108] In other cases, however, azathioprine controlled neither the arthritis nor the size and number of cutaneous nodules.[140,187]

In one report, four family members developed a reticulohistiocytosis-like disorder during childhood or adolescence.[361] The disease was characterized by a histiocytic papulonodular eruption on the face and hands, symmetric destructive polyarthritis, chiefly of the hands and wrists, and ocular involvement with cataract, uveitis, and glaucoma. The histologic changes in these patients differed from those of multicentric reticulohistiocytosis in a number of respects, however, including the absence of typical multinucleated giant cells and histiocytes with a ground-glass appearance of the cytoplasm.

SECONDARY GOUT

The term "secondary gout" has been applied to cases of gouty arthritis that occur as a complication of a variety of primary disorders involving a disturbance of purine or uric acid metabolism marked by prolonged hyperuricemia[112,137,138,355,357] (see also Chap. 91). The underlying disease is usually a myeloproliferative disorder with urate overproduction as a consequence of increased nucleic acid turnover.[19,186,209,317,355,356,357] Secondary gout is particularly frequent in patients with polycythemia, both primary and secondary, and in those with myeloid metaplasia.[46,68,138,209,302,317,340,357] This secondary form of gout has been noted less commonly in patients with acute leukemia, including children, in rare instances,[209,225,317,346] chronic granulocytic leukemia,[186,209,317] malignant lymphoma,[317] multiple myeloma,[142,209,317] sickle cell anemia,[19,302] thalassemia,[242,330] pernicious anemia after treatment,[302] and the megaloblastic anemia of tropical sprue.[302] The incidence of gout in patients with polycythemia vera varies in different series from 2 to 14%.[68,331] The initial episode may take place during the period of active polycythemia or during or after transition into its myeloproliferative phase.[356] The occurrence of hyperuricemia and of gout appears to be particularly frequent in patients with polycythemia vera in whom the renal clearance of uric acid is reduced to under 5 ml/min.[68] Secondary hyperuricemia and gout have also been reported in patients with disseminated carcinoma and sarcoma.[65,185,231,331]

Secondary gout is similar to primary gout in its clinical characteristics, although the average age of onset and the incidence in women are both greater.[209,317,356,357] A family history of the disorder is unusual in secondary gout, and the patient generally has higher serum urate levels and a greater rate of urinary uric acid excretion than patients with primary gout.[209,317,357] This excretion is often excessive in patients with adequate renal function. The frequency of uric acid nephrolithiasis is therefore higher in secondary than in primary gout,[357,358] and a number of patients develop urinary tract infection and uremia. Large tophaceous deposits may occur in patients whose primary disease permits prolonged survival.

Despite the clinical and pathologic similarities between primary (familial) and secondary gout, one basic difference exists in the origin of the hyperuricemia in the two conditions.[19,112,186,197,355] When patients with secondary gout due to polycythemia or myeloid metaplasia are given labeled purine precursors, the amount of isotope appearing in urinary uric acid is usually much greater than that observed in normal subjects. The rate at which this incorporation occurs is slower than the rapid enrichment of urinary uric acid often found in primary gout. This observation is consistent with the hypothesis that the hyperuricemia in these patients is the result of abnormally rapid catabolism of nucleoprotein incident to hyperactive erythropoiesis.

In the case of chronic granulocytic leukemia and myeloid metaplasia, the isotope enrichment of urinary uric acid after administration of sodium formate ^{14}C displays a diphasic pattern, with a first peak occurring 2 days after isotope administration and a second maximum in 12 days.[186] The initial peak has been attributed to renewed synthesis of uric acid, without prior incorporation of isotope into nucleic acids, and the second peak has been attributed to the release of purine from degenerating leukemic cells.

Striking increases in serum urate levels may occur in patients with leukemia and malignant lymphoma as a result of rapid breakdown of cellular nucleic acids following aggressive treatment with alkylating agents, x-irradiation, or adrenal corticosteroids.[185,209,261] The precipitation of uric acid in the renal tubules of such patients may lead to severe, sometimes fatal urinary obstruction. This hazard can be prevented or reversed by treatment with allopurinol (see Chap. 92). Allopurinol is effective in reducing hyperuricemia in patients with leukemia, lymphoma, and cancer.[65,140a,185,231,335,357,359] Dialysis may be a useful adjunct in the management of patients with acute obstructive uric acid nephropathy.[264]

HYPERLIPOPROTEINEMIA

Articular and tendinous manifestations are important features of certain heritable disorders of lipid transport or lipoprotein metabolism.[104,105,267] These articular signs and symptoms are often the first indication of the lipid disease and alert the physician to an underlying disorder that may respond to dietary modification or drug therapy.

Patients with *type II hyperlipoproteinemia* exhibit tendinous, tuberous, and periosteal xanthomas as well as xanthelasma, corneal ulcers, and early, rapidly progressive atherosclerosis. Tendinous xanthomas are located in Achilles and patellar tendons and in the extensor tendons of the hands and feet[94,104,285] (Fig. 74–8). Tendon xanthomas have also been found in the plantar aponeurosis, in the fascia, and in periosteum overlying the lower tibia and the peroneal tendons. Xanthomas are situated within the tendon fibers and not on the tendon sheath, and they cannot be separated from the tendon on movement. They contain large, lipid-lined histiocytes within the collagenous connective tissue (Fig. 74–9). Tendon xanthomas are composed of cholesterol and phospholipid.[94,148] Tuberous xanthomas are soft, subcutaneous masses occurring over extensor surfaces, especially of the elbows, knees, and hands, as well as on the buttocks. Individuals homozygous for type II hyperlipoproteinemia develop extensive xanthomas in childhood, whereas those who are heterozygous develop tendinous xanthomas after age 30 and lack tuberous xanthomas.

Tendinous and tuberous xanthomas also occur in type III and type IV hyperlipoproteinemia.[104,105] A distinctive clinical feature of the type III disorder is lipid deposition, or plane xanthomas, in the palms of the hands.[104,105] Types I, IV, and V hyperlipoproteinemia are characterized by eruptive xanthomas over the knees, buttocks, shoulders, and back.[105]

Several recent studies have described rheumatic syndromes associated with type II hyperlipoproteinemia.[117,181,266,338] Recurrent episodes of migratory polyarthritis have been reported in about 50% of patients homozygous for type II hyperlipoproteinemia.[181] Arthritis occurs chiefly in large peripheral joints, and inflammation varies from mild to severe. Severely inflamed joints are swollen, warm, and red, and joint involvement is symmetric. Episodes of arthritis are self-limited, lasting several days to two weeks. In many patients, the illness resembles rheumatic fever because of the evanescent arthritis, the presence of (atherosclerotic) aortic valvular disease, the elevated sedimentation rate, and the increased titer of antistreptolysin O. The valvular disease and the elevated erythrocyte sedimentation rate may occur in individuals without arthritis and are presumably a direct result of the hyperlipoproteinemia.

In patients heterozygous for type II hyperlipoproteinemia, recurrent Achilles tendinitis is a common problem (Fig. 74–10). This finding has been reported in adults, adolescents, and children.[117,266,285,338] In addition to Achilles tendinitis, monoarticular arthritis involving the knee or great toe is seen,[117] and in some heterozygous type II patients, migratory "polyarthritis" involving up to six joints has been reported.[266] Affected joints include the knee, the proximal interphalangeal joints, the ankle, the wrist, the elbow, the shoulder, and the hip. Some evidence suggests that the "polyarthritis" actually represents an inflammatory periarthritis or peritendinitis.[266] Synovial fluid from these joints contains no crystals, and the cell counts are low (less than 200 polymorphonuclear leukocytes/mm^3) (see also Chap. 4).

An arthropathy resembling that seen in type II hyperlipoproteinemia occurs in patients with type IV hyperlipoproteinemia.[44,125] These individuals have predominantly an asymmetric oligoarthritis involving both small and large joints, including the proximal interphalangeal and metacarpophalangeal joints in the hands, wrists, shoulders, knees, ankles, tarsus, and metatarsophalangeal joints. In some cases, the inflammatory disease is mild and persistent, and in others it is episodic and recurrent.

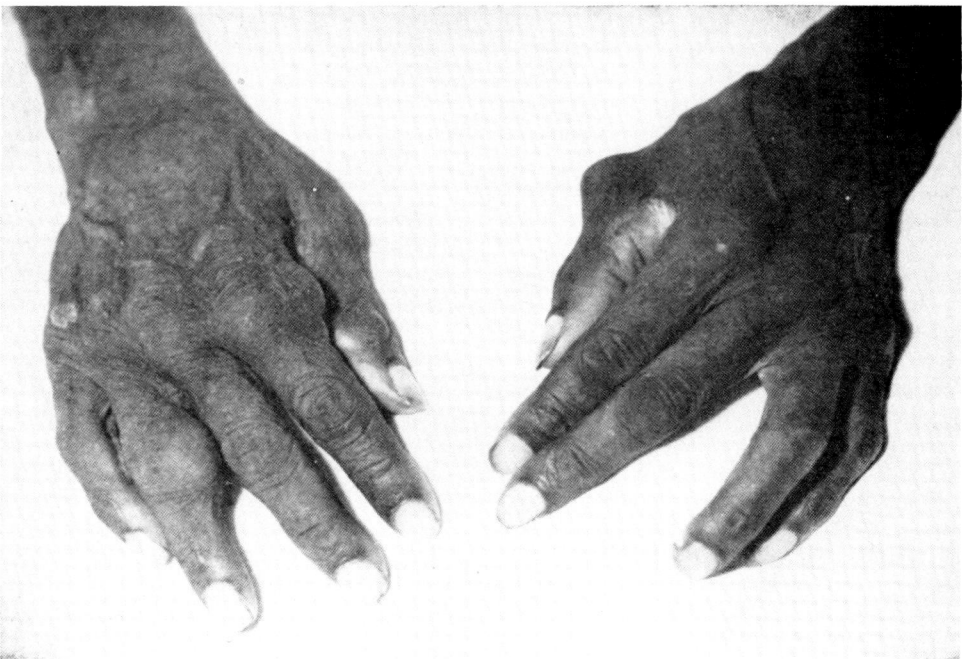

Fig. 74–8. Xanthoma tendinosum. The hands of a 75-year-old man with probable type II hyperlipoproteinemia, who has had nodular swellings involving extensor tendons of several fingers and both Achilles and infrapatellar tendons for more than 50 years. The patient's serum cholesterol concentration was 415 mg/dl.

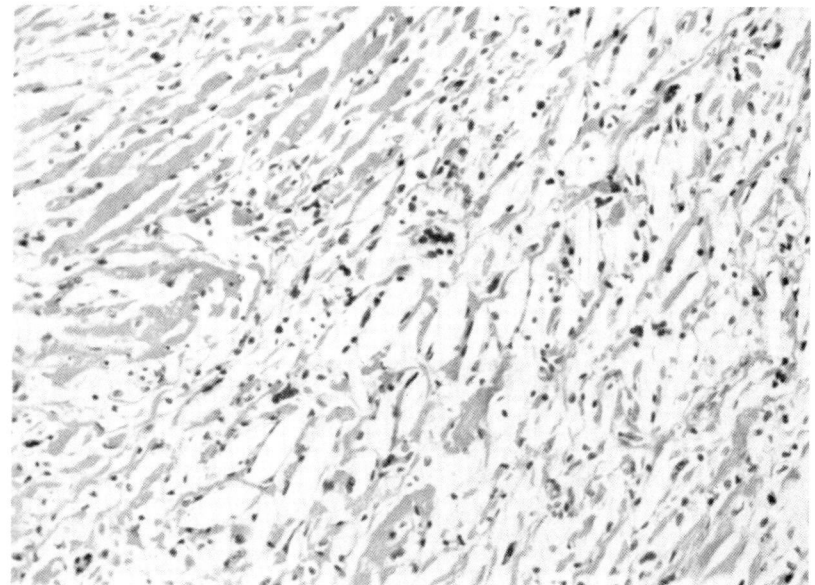

Fig. 74–9. Xanthoma tendinosum. Photomicrograph of a tendon nodule removed from the patient whose hands are shown in Figure 74–8. Numerous large lipid-filled histiocytes with pale, foamy cytoplasm are strewn about in a collagenous stroma. The clefts indicate the site of deposition of crystals of cholesterol. ($\times$ 175)

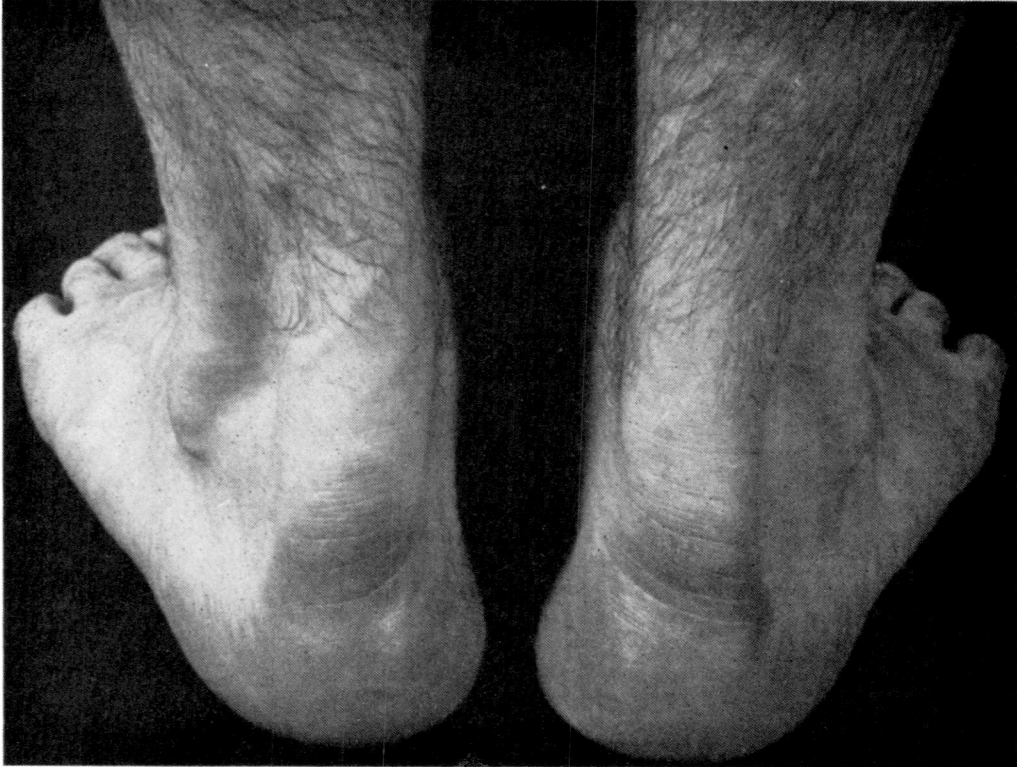

Fig. 74–10. Xanthoma tendinosum. The patient, a 34-year-old man with type II hyperlipoproteinemia, had repeated episodes of acute inflammation involving the Achilles tendons lasting from 1 to 3 days and leading to the mistaken diagnosis of gout. The tendons were enlarged, but no other xanthomas were present. This patient's serum cholesterol level varied from 330 to 485 mg/dl.

Morning stiffness and para-articular hyperesthesia have been described in these patients.[125] Synovial fluid is of the non-inflammatory (group I) type and is free of crystals. Radiographs in a number of these patients show prominent para-articular bone cysts (Fig. 74–11). One such cyst was grossly yellow and mucinous and on microscopic examination showed only fibrous tissue and fat cells (Fig. 74–12). There were no granulomata, no cholesterol deposits and no lipid-laden histiocytes. Synovial biopsy in one case revealed moderate hyperplasia of the synovial villi, prominent stomal vessels and a moderate mononuclear infiltrate. Four patients experienced decreased severity of articular symptoms after reduction or normalization of serum lipid levels.[44]

Some patients previously reported to have had arthropathy associated with types II and IV hyperlipoproteinemia might have had familial combined hyperlipidemia. Individuals within a single family who have this abnormality may exhibit any one of three apparent lipoprotein phenotypes, including type IIA, type IIB, and type IV hyperlipoprotein-emia. A given patient may convert from one abnormal lipoprotein pattern to another.

Other reports exist of skeletal lesions associated with hyperlipoproteinemia. An individual with probable type V hyperlipoproteinemia had cystic lesions in both proximal femurs. Curettage yielded yellowish fragments that on microscopic examination showed foamy histiocytes and a granulomatous reaction around cholesterol clefts.[292] Other investigators have noted joint changes secondary to infiltration of foam cells in subchondral bone in secondary hyperlipoproteinemia, such as that which develops in patients with biliary cirrhosis.[16] Secondary hyperlipoproteinemia can also be seen in association with the nephrotic syndrome, pancreatitis, alcoholism, hypothyroidism, and diabetes mellitus. Hyperlipoproteinemia may lead to musculoskeletal complaints in such cases.

Cerebrotendinous xanthomatosis is a rare, familial, apparently autosomal recessive disorder characterized by progressive cerebellar ataxia, dementia, and spinal cord paresis, subnormal intelligence, tendon xanthomas, and cataracts.[23,329] Cholestanol,

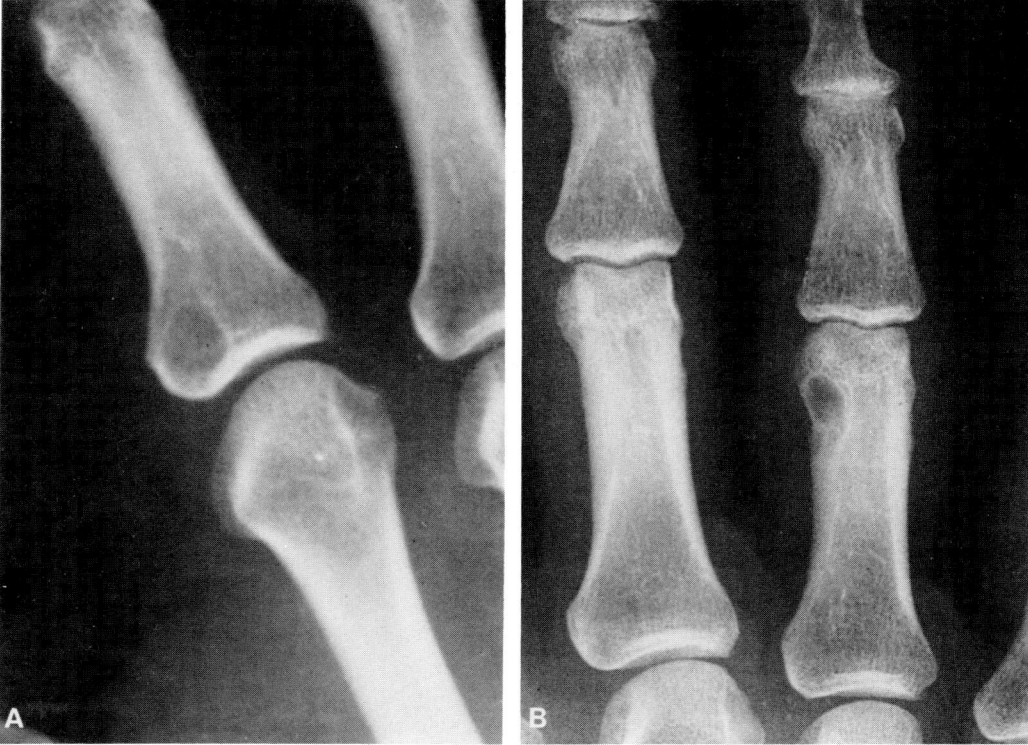

Fig. 74–11. *A,B,* Roentgenograms showing prominent para-articular bone cysts in the fingers of two patients with arthritis associated with type IV hyperlipoproteinemia. Both patients had polyarticular inflammatory disease.

or dihydrocholesterol, accumulates in the nervous tissue, tendons, and other tissues. The underlying defect has not been identified, and no specific treatment is available. Tendon xanthomas appear as early as the second decade, but they are usually first noted in the third or fourth decade. The Achilles tendons are the most common sites, but xanthomas may also occur in the triceps tendons, at the tibial tuberosities, and in the extensor tendons of the hands. Tuberous xanthomas and xanthelasma may occur also.

Tendon xanthomas also constitute a feature of β-sitosterolemia, another rare, newly recognized familial lipid storage disease marked by the accumulation of plant sterols in the blood and tissues.[23,24,291] These individuals have an increased intestinal absorption of dietary β-sitosterol, but the underlying metabolic defect has not yet been defined. The patient's serum cholesterol level may be normal or moderately elevated.[291] Inheritance is autosomal recessive. Tendon xanthomas indistinguishable histologically from those found in hyperlipoproteinemia appear during childhood, initially in the extensor tendons of the hands and later in the patellar, plantar, and Achilles tendons.

Tendinous, tuberous, and eruptive xanthomas have also been observed in patients with type II or type IV hyperlipoproteinemia associated with the development of multiple myeloma, as well as in some cases of myelomatosis without definite hyperlipoproteinemia.[105,234] Myeloma protein may interfere with lipid transport by at least two mechanisms, one involving heparin-paraprotein interaction and resulting in heparin resistance and impaired uptake of the remnant of glyceride-rich lipoproteins, and the other involving the formation of complexes among myeloma protein, lipoprotein, and cholesterol.[349]

HEMOPHILIC ARTHRITIS

Hemophilia is the collective designation for a group of hereditofamilial disorders in which the deficiency of a plasma coagulation protein results in faulty fibrin clot formation[32,33,34,205,257] (Table 74–1). Patients are subject to abnormal bleeding, the frequency and intensity of which varies with the severity of the clotting defect. In addition to easy bruising, present in nearly all patients, prolonged and excessive bleeding may follow minor injuries and the patient may have recurrent bleeding from the genitourinary and gastrointestinal tracts and hemorrhage into peripheral joints.[17,83,152] Hemarthrosis, the most frequent and most painful

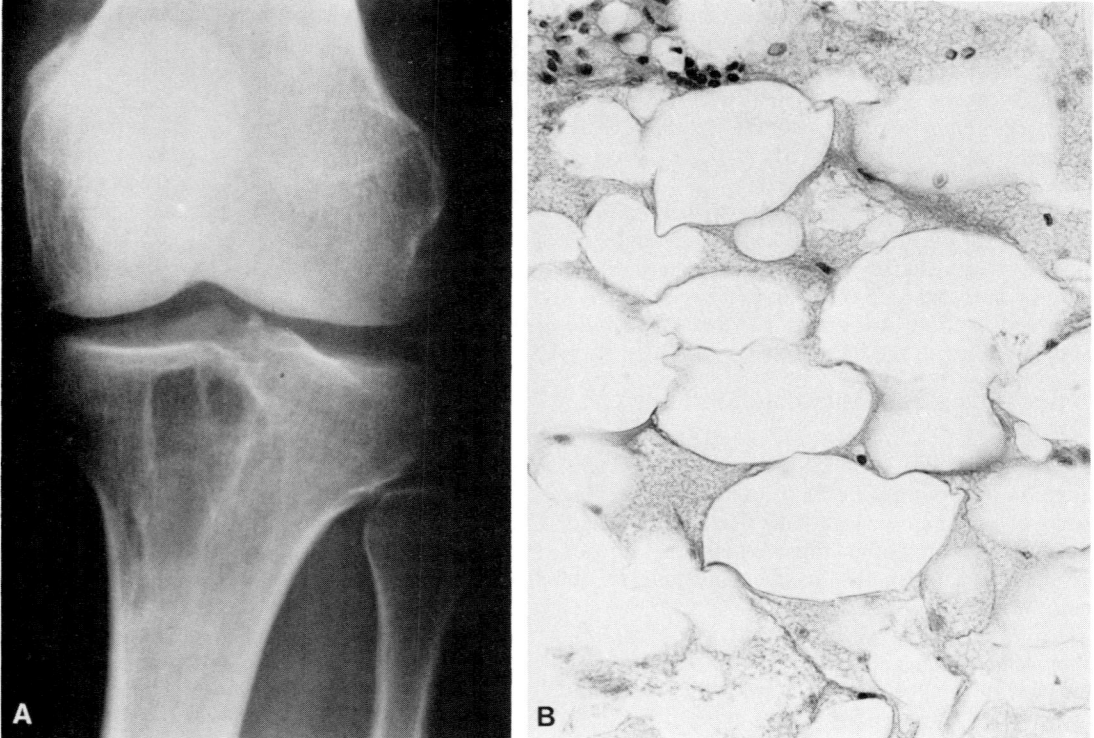

Fig. 74–12. A patient with arthritis associated with type IV hyperlipoproteinemia and prominent knee symptoms had a large cyst in the proximal tibia *(A)*. Tissue removed from the cyst at biopsy *(B)* was yellow and mucinous and on microscopic examination showed fibrous tissue and many fat cells (× 400).

Table 74–1. Heritable Disorders of Blood Coagulation (Hemophilias)*

Sex-linked recessive traits
Factor VIII (antihemophilic factor, AHF) deficiency (classic hemophilia)
Factor IX (plasma thromboplastin component, PTC) deficiency (Christmas disease)
Autosomal recessive traits
Factor I (fibrinogen) deficiency
Factor II (prothrombin) deficiency
Factor V (proaccelerin) deficiency (parahemophilia)
Factor VII (proconvertin) deficiency
Factor X (Stuart) deficiency
Factor XI (plasma thromboplastin antecedent, PTA) deficiency
Factor XII (Hageman) deficiency
Factor XIII deficiency
Autosomal dominant traits
Von Willebrand's disease (pseudohemophilia, vascular hemophilia)
Congenital dysfibrinogenemia

*Factor VIII deficiency (classic hemophilia) comprises approximately 70% of most large series of cases of hemophilia, whereas factor IX deficiency (Christmas disease), von Willebrand's disease, and factor XI (PTA) deficiency account for all but 1 to 2% of the remainder. The clinical manifestations in general, and the joint involvement in particular, of patients with factor IX deficiency are similar to those encountered in factor VIII deficiency.

manifestation of hemophilia, has been described in all the heritable coagulation disorders, except factor V deficiency, and may also occur as an unusual complication of anticoagulant drugs.[166,173,212,348] Repeated hemarthroses are often followed by permanent disability of one or more joints.[69,83,93,171,179,180,183,194,255,265,342]

The occurrence of joint disease in hemophilia, known also as bleeder's joints, has been recognized for well over a century and was considered originally to represent a form of atypical rheumatism. Volkman, in 1868, was one of the first to attribute the disturbance to the effects of hemorrhage.[180,342]

Pathogenesis and Anatomic Findings

Hemophilic hemarthrosis usually follows trauma. The injury is often trivial and is apparent neither to the young patient nor to his parents. The results of joint hemorrhage have been well studied in naturally hemophilic dogs, which develop an arthropathy comparable to that encountered in man.[314]

The initial lesion consists of synovial or subsynovial hemorrhage. Rupture of blood into the joint cavity provokes an inflammatory reaction characterized by effusion, villous hypertrophy, hyperplasia of the lining cells, and infiltration of lymphocytes and plasma cells. This reaction gradually subsides several days to weeks after the cessation of hemorrhage. Hemoglobin is released once lysis or erythrocytes in the joint cavity and synovial tissues has occurred. Hemosiderin remains in the synovium for an indefinitely long period, appearing as finely particulate matter within the phagocytic lining cells (Fig. 74–13). Additional coarser aggregates of this iron-containing pigment, lying free or within macrophages, are found in deeper portions of the synovium. The presence of large amounts of hemosiderin in this location distinguishes this variety of synovial siderosis from that found in hemochromatosis.

Repeated hemorrhage is marked by hyperplasia of the synovial lining cells and by gradually increasing synovial fibrosis and hemosiderosis, leading to rigidity of the subsynovial tissue and joint capsule. Although these changes may account for some degree of limitation in motion, the damage to cartilage and bone eventually is most harmful to the joint.[55,69,216] Marginal erosion of the cartilage due to encroachment of the hyperplastic synovium and more central, irregular, "map-like" degeneration attributable to subchondral hemorrhage occur.[180] The demonstration of plasmin, or fibrinolysin, in joint fluid during the course of acute hemarthrosis and the finding of numerous siderosomes suggest that the loss of cartilage may result from enzymatic degradation. Siderosomes are

membrane-bound bodies with aggregates of iron-containing particles, believed to be lysosomal organelles in which hemoglobin or its derivatives are digested.

One sees a marked increase in cathepsin-D and acid phosphatase activity in synovial tissue and a lesser increase in acid phosphatase activity in the joint fluid of patients with chronic hemophilic arthropathy.[17,152] These enzymes are inactive at neutral pH and probably contribute little to extracellular connective tissue degradation. Nevertheless, these findings indicate that the synovial tissue is "activated" and may release other degradative enzymes or may form pannus and directly invade and destroy contiguous cartilage and bone. Studies of synovium isolated from a young hemophilic boy with proliferative synovitis revealed secretion of latent collagenase in amounts equal to those secreted by rheumatoid synovium.[215] In addition, isolated hemophilic synovium and synovial cells secrete a proteinase, active at neutral pH, that can degrade the protein core of the glycosaminoglycan component of cartilage. Activated hemophilic synovium, therefore, appears to have the potential for considerable connective tissue destruction.

In experimental hemarthrosis in rabbits, the synthesis of both ribonucleic acid and protein by articular cartilage was initially unimpaired despite repeated daily intra-articular injection of autologous blood.[352] When such injections were continued for several weeks or months, however, definite alterations occurred in the cartilage matrix, consisting at first of altered metachromasia, followed by superficial and deep erosions,[216] accompanied by a reduction in proteoglycan concentration and a depression in the synthetic activity of the chondrocyte. The deposition of iron pigment in both synovium and cartilage plays a significant role in the pathogenesis of the degeneration of articular cartilage.[152,301] Degradation of ground substance surrounding chondrocytes containing iron suggests that local release of degradative enzymes may be prompted by the retained pigment.[156] Proteoglycan loss alters the resilience and compressibility of normal cartilage and may accelerate its destruction.

Articular cartilage damage due to repeated joint hemorrhage is accompanied by the development of cavities or "cysts" in the subchondral bone. These lesions can become large and have been thought to be the result of intraosseous bleeding (Fig. 74–14). In a study of hemophilic dogs, these "cysts" communicated with the synovial cavity at a point of cartilage and subchondral bone erosion, at the margin of the articular cartilage, or at the site of ligamentous attachments.[314] These and similar observations in human hemophilic joint disease suggest that the development of these "cysts" is

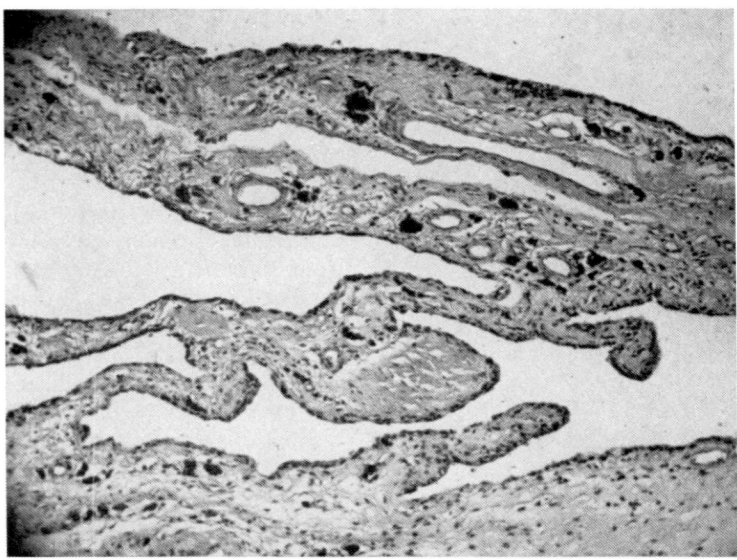

Fig. 74–13. Photomicrograph of synovium from the knee joint of a 76-year-old hemophilic man. Note the heavy deposits of iron-containing pigment (hemosiderin), present both in lining cells and in deeper portions of the synovium. Hematoxylin and eosin stain. (From Rodnan, et al.[264])

related more to degenerative changes in articular cartilage and subchondral bone than to intraosseous bleeding.[195,264] A striking finding in young patients is accelerated maturation and hypertrophy of the epiphyses adjacent to affected joints. Chronic hyperemia of the epiphyseal cartilage, induced by repeated hemarthrosis, may be responsible for this change.

In addition to hemarthrosis, bleeding into muscle and bone may occur. The terms "hemophilic pseudotumor" and "hemophilic cyst" have been applied to the destructive lesions that follow massive muscle, subperiosteal, or intraosseous hemorrhages. Such hematomas, if not optimally treated, subsequently organize, become vascular, and are locally destructive to soft tissue and bone. In the adult, these hematomas occur most often in the pelvis, thigh, or leg,[1,102,114,307,309,320,328] whereas in children, they occur distal to the elbow or knee and are less destructive.

Soft tissue bleeding may be dangerous because of neurovascular compression, severe destruction and contracture of muscle, including Volkmann's contracture,[93,307,324] cyst rupture, sinus formation, or chronic infection.[307] One of the most dramatic examples of hemophilic bleeding involves the iliopsoas muscle.[43,129] Hemorrhage into the closed fascial compartment that contains the iliopsoas muscle and the femoral nerve is marked by the development of sudden, severe pain in the groin and thigh, followed by the appearance of a tender mass, a hematoma, in the iliac fossa and the groin, flexion

contracture of the hip, and signs of femoral nerve palsy. Bleeding into the gastrocnemius or soleus muscle or both may lead to a talipes equinus deformity. Repeated bleeding in and about the joints and associated muscle atrophy lead to instability of the weight-bearing joints.

Clinical Features

Hemarthrosis occurs in approximately 80 to 90% of patients with hemophilia,[69,83,255,265,313,324] and it constitutes the most common major hemorrhagic event in the disease. Bleeding into the joints is particularly frequent when the patient's level of antihemophilic globulin is less than 1 to 2% of normal.[194,255,258,342] The majority of patients first experience articular symptoms between the ages of 1 and 5 years, and they usually have repeated hemarthroses during the remainder of the first decade of life; thereafter, these episodes ordinarily become less and less frequent.[93,313] Patients with levels of antihemophilic globulin greater than 5% of normal experience fewer episodes of hemarthrosis, and these occur only after severe trauma. Hemorrhage occurs most commonly in a knee, ankle, or elbow and less frequently in the shoulders, hips, wrists, fingers, and toes.[9,313] Generally, only a single joint is involved in each episode, but 2 joints may be affected simultaneously. The patient often has repeated hemorrhaging at the same site.[313] Involvement of a given joint may lead to chronic inflammatory synovitis and hypervascularity that

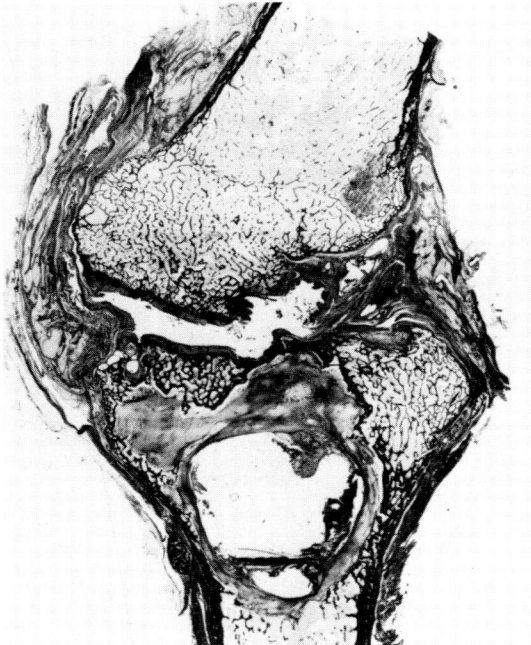

Fig. 74–14. Sagittal section of the knee joint of a 49-year-old man with advanced hemophilic arthropathy. The femoral condyle appears flattened, and the patella has virtually disappeared. The head of the tibia has undergone massive cystic resorption. The articular cartilage has disappeared from most of the joint surfaces, which have undergone partial fibrous ankylosis on the popliteal aspect on the right and have been replaced by fibrous tissue. The cyst in the tibia is lined by loose-textured fibrous tissue. The synovial and capsular tissues are thickened and infiltrated with many hemosiderin-laden mononuclear cells. (From Sokoloff.[301])

predispose the patient to recurrent hemorrhage in the same joint.

The affected joint is swollen, warm, and often exquisitely painful and tender. Associated muscle spasm leads to flexion of the extremity. When hemarthrosis is severe, the patient may have fever and peripheral leukocytosis. In instances of milder bleeding, the normal configuration and full motion of the joint may be restored within a matter of days, and the patient may experience little more than transient stiffness on reambulation. In the case of protracted bleeding, and particularly when repeated injury of the joint leads to renewed hemorrhage, symptoms may persist for many weeks to months. Thermograms and radionuclide scanning have been used to assess the effects of acute hemarthrosis,[100] and ultrasonographic studies have proved useful in demonstrating deeper bleeding, such as retroperitoneal hemorrhage.[213]

Following repeated severe hemarthrosis, the joint gradually fails to return to full, normal form

and function, and loss of muscle power and mass is progressive. Examination discloses thickening of the periarticular soft tissues, crepitation, atrophic muscle accentuating the bony enlargement of the joint, and various deformities, the most common of which are flexion contractures of the elbow and knee. Flexion contracture of the knee is frequently accompanied by posterior subluxation of the tibia. Occasionally, joints develop fibrous or (rarely) bony ankylosis.[69,93]

Bleeding into the hip joint during childhood may lead to dislocation,[93] as well as to flattening and destruction of the capital epiphysis and deformity of the femoral neck, with resultant shortening of the extremity. Synovial hyperemia may be accompanied by epiphyseal hyperemia and epiphyseal overgrowth. In growing children, this process causes axial deviations including cubitus valgus, coxa valga, genu valgum, and pes valgus, and any one of these structural abnormalities may be asymmetric.

Bleeding episodes necessitate long periods of bed rest, which, in turn, delay neuromotor maturation.[154] Approximately half of these patients have some permanent changes in the peripheral articulations, and only the rare individual with severe hemophilia, defined as less than 2% of the normal level of antihemophilic globulin, escapes some residual deformity.[342] In most cases, only a few joints are involved in this chronic arthropathy, usually knees and elbows, and many other joints remain normal despite repeated bleeding. In addition to muscle atrophy as a result of joint inflammation and disuse, hemophiliacs may demonstrate other features of a neuromyopathy. Electromyographic study shows reduced numbers of functioning motor units and "myopathic" motor unit potential; serum creatine phosphokinase levels are frequently increased, and muscle biopsies show type 2 fiber atrophy.[66]

Although the presence of hemophilia is suspected readily in the individual with a recognized bleeding tendency, the diagnosis may be much less obvious in the occasional child or adult in whom hemarthrosis is the initial symptom of the disease or in whom minor hemorrhagic episodes have been overlooked. It is especially important to recognize this condition before unsuspecting surgical intervention has disastrous consequences.[180]

For reasons not clear, septic arthritis is an extremely rare complication of hemophilia even though patients with the disorder have joints subjected to repeated damage by multiple episodes of hemarthrosis. One case of septic arthritis of the hip and three of the knee have been recorded.[157,227,271] This complication was not reported before 1977.

Roentgenographic Findings

In acute intra-articular hemorrhage, one sees distention of the joint capsule and increased density of the soft tissues. Evidence may indicate an accompanying subperiosteal hemorrhage, which is followed by thickening or, in some cases, by atrophy of the underlying cortex. Subchondral hemorrhage may lead to defects in epiphyseal ossification centers.

Chronic hemophilic joint disease is characterized by irregular narrowing or obliteration of the joint space and, later, by marginal spurring and sclerosis of bone, which often contains one or more areas of cystic translucency[69,171,226,309] (Figs. 74–15, 74–16, 74–17, 74–18, 74–19, 74–20, 74–21, 74–22). These cystic areas may be large. The periarticular soft tissues may be thickened and increased in density, and they occasionally contain fine opacities. These opacities were traditionally attributed to the deposition of hemosiderin in the synovium, a view that has been disputed. Certain roentgenographic features are characteristic but not pathognomonic of chronic hemophilic arthropathy. These findings include enlargement of the head of the radius in patients with elbow involvement,[69,342] flattening of the inferior portion of the patella, or squared-off patella, in advanced disease of the knee,[171,226] widening of the intercondylar notch of the femur, and flattening of the talus. Aseptic necrosis of the femoral head,[226] as well as of the talus,[69] may also be seen. In rare cases, chondrocalcinosis has been described in hemophiliacs,[167] and in one individual, an episode of acute pseudogout, masquerading as hemarthrosis, was proved by arthrocentesis and demonstration of calcium pyrophosphate dihydrate crystals.[201]

Management

The development of potent cryoprecipitates and other concentrated preparations of the plasma coagulation factors has revolutionized the treatment of joint and muscle bleeding.[17,152,153,221,274,290,308] Concentrates have been prepared from both human and animal plasma, particularly from cattle and pigs, whose blood contains factor VIII in much higher concentrations than human blood. Evidence suggests that maintenance of low levels, such as 3 to 5%, of factor VIII activity by the regular administration of small amounts of concentrate reduces the frequency of hemarthrosis and other serious hemorrhaging.[7,27,172] Moreover, chronic joint changes are uncommon in hemophilic patients with a coagulation factor content above 2 to 3% of normal.[7]

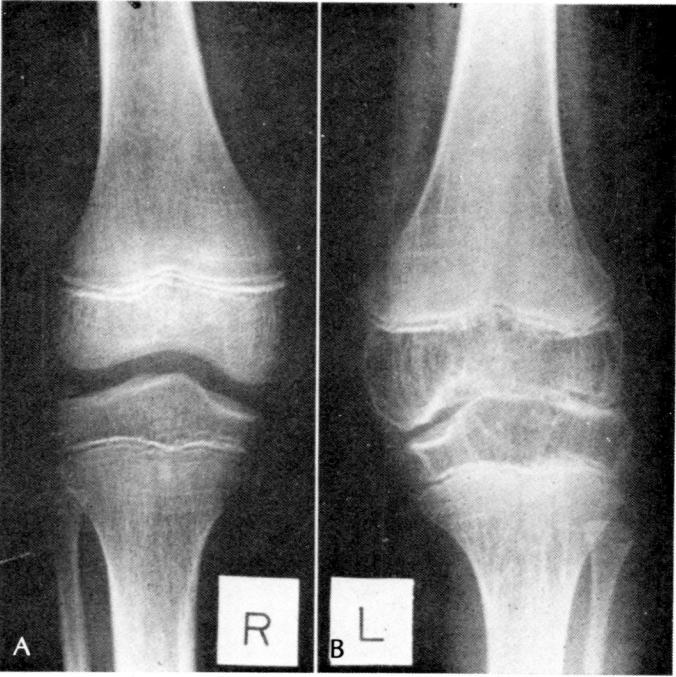

Fig. 74–15. *A* and *B*, Roentgenograms of the knee of a 9-year-old boy with hemophilia and repeated hemarthroses involving the left knee *(B)*. Note the loss of articular cartilage, the irregularity of bony surfaces, and the hypertrophy of the epiphyses of femur and tibia. The right knee *(A)* appears normal.

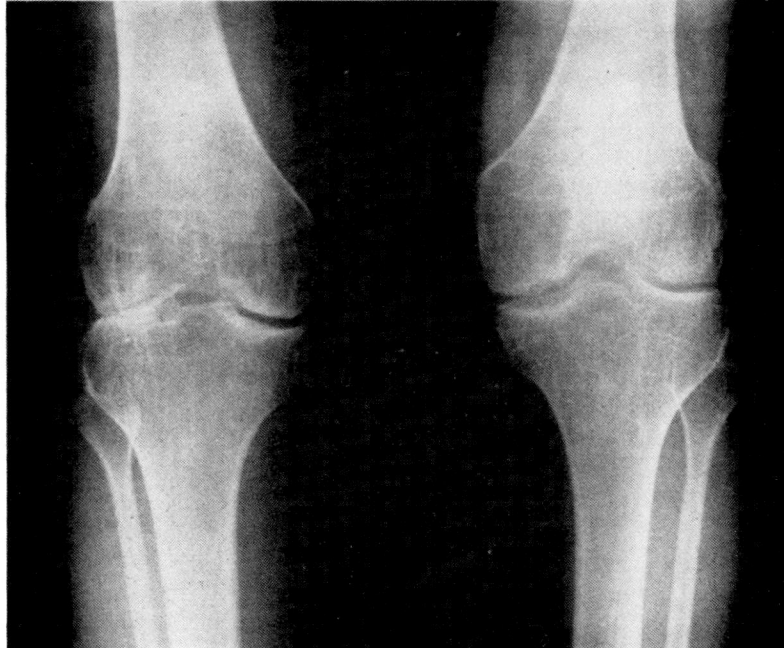

Fig. 74–16.   Roentgenograms of the knees of the patient in Figure 74–15 at the age of 17 years. During the 8 years since the roentgenograms in Figure 74–15 were obtained, the patient had many more episodes of joint hemorrhage involving both knees. Note the irregular narrowing of the joint space and early osteophyte formation.

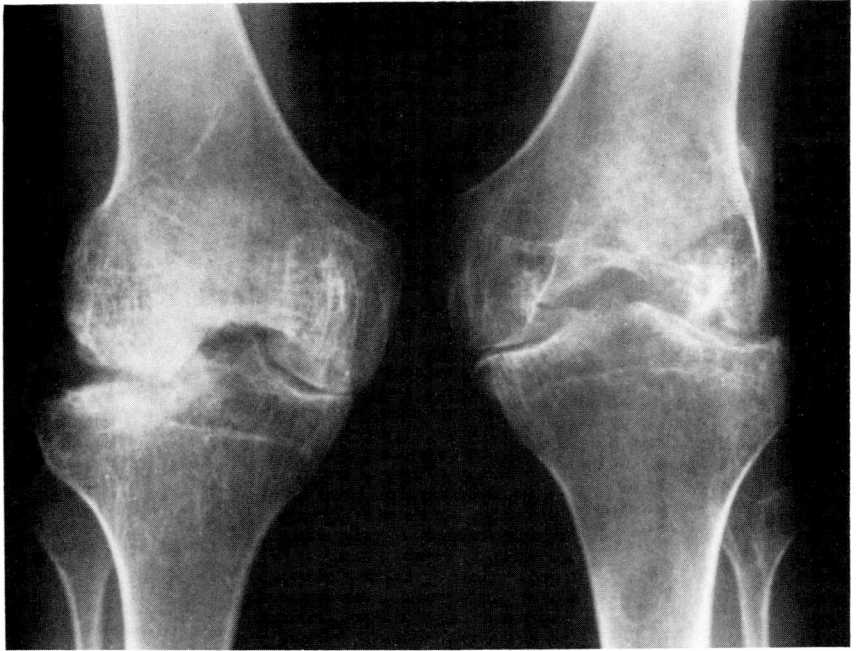

Fig. 74–17.   Roentgenogram of the knees of a 23-year-old man with hemophilia illustrating severe secondary degenerative joint disease.

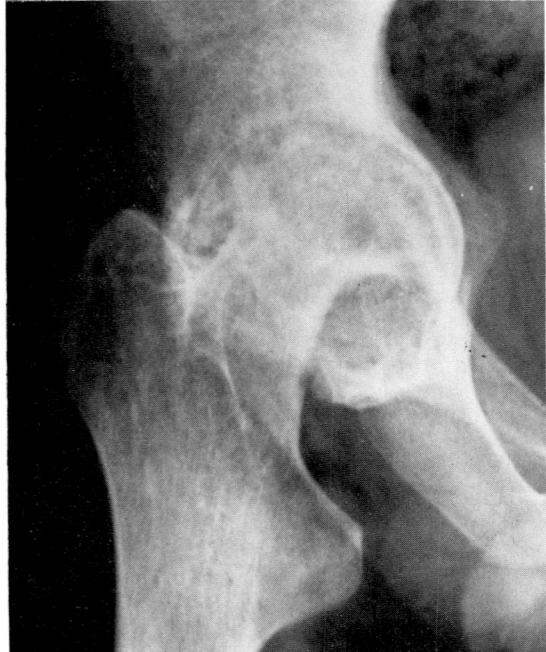

Fig. 74–18. Roentgenogram of the right hip of the patient in Figure 74–17 illustrating severe degenerative joint disease and protrusio acetabuli.

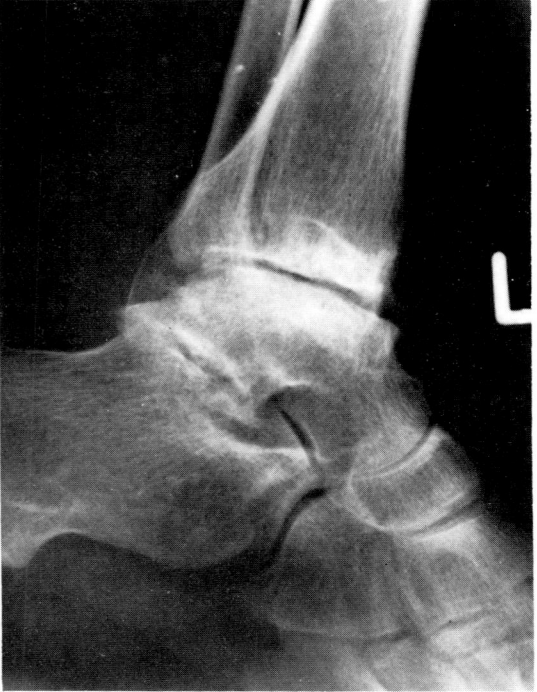

Fig. 74–19. Roentgenogram of the ankle of a 26-year-old man with hemophilia. Note the loss of cartilage and subchondral sclerosis in both ankle and subtalar joints.

Prophylaxis

Every reasonable attempt should be made to avoid joint trauma. Although it is wise to interdict football and other contact sports, one must keep in mind the psychologic needs of the child and the value of participation in group athletics. Patients with mild degrees of hemophilia, such as 5% or more of factor VIII and 10% or more of factor IX, are able to engage in strenuous activities with little or no difficulty. A program should be individualized for each child and each family, who must strive to maintain a balance between overprotection and unwarranted liberty.

Acute Hemarthrosis

It is essential that both patient and parents be instructed in the early recognition and immediate care of hemarthrosis, to minimize joint damage and loss of schooling. Home transfusion programs have been successful in relieving acute hemarthrosis promptly and in reducing the incidence of arthropathy.[17,152,202,203,254] Rapid treatment of hemarthrosis may prevent the chronic disability resulting from repeated joint bleeding.[193] When an episode of hemarthrosis begins, patients and their families can be prepared by having learned the principles of home therapy at one of the numerous hemophilia

treatment centers throughout North America. With proper education, early treatment, and good physical measures to maintain muscle tone and mass, progressive articular disease can largely be prevented. Most agree on the need for rest, which is best accomplished by bed rest and elevation of the affected extremity, maintained initially in a position of comfort. Ice packs lessen pain and inflammation. Aspirin should be avoided when prescribing analgesics because it may prolong the bleeding time by interfering with platelet aggregation by connective tissue[62,172,239,345] (see Chap. 28). Propoxyphene and acetaminophen can be used safely.[152,172]

Mild hemarthrosis is often treatable by immobilization alone. When the hemarthrosis is more severe, efforts should be made to correct the underlying defect in coagulation to prevent further bleeding.[13,34,42,59,69,183,256,308] The prompt infusion of active plasma preparations was found to reduce the duration of incapacity from hemarthroses by over half and the incidence of new deformities by 80%.[13] The patient with classic hemophilia should be given cryoprecipitate or another factor VIII concentrate; if these are not available, fresh frozen plasma or freshly drawn blood should be administered. Concentrates of factor IX, or plasma, are used to

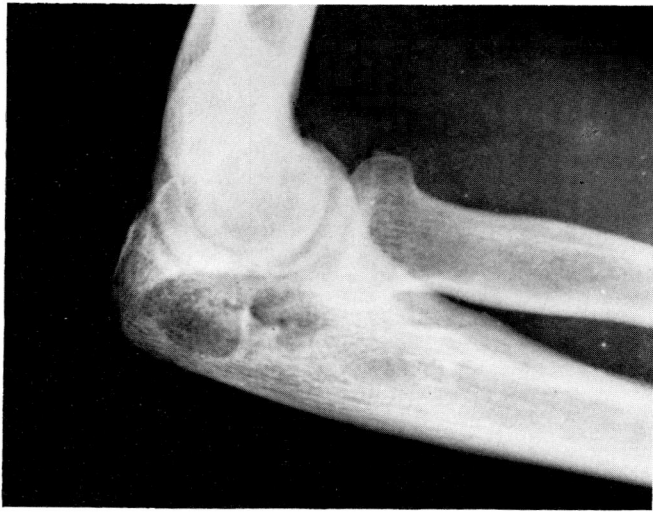

Fig. 74–20. Roentgenogram of the elbow of a 27-year-old man with hemophilla illustrating large subchondral erosion in the ulna.

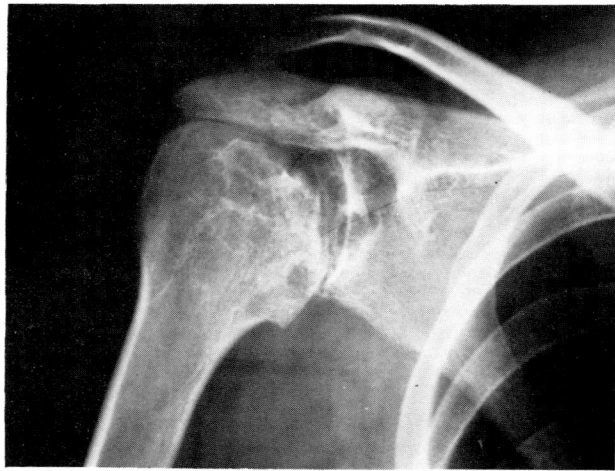

Fig. 74–21. Roentgenogram of the shoulder of a 24-year-old man with hemophilia illustrating the loss of articular cartilage and large defects in the subchondral bone of both the humerus and the glenoid fossa.

treat Christmas disease (factor IX deficiency).[7,13,34,42,69,256] Sufficient amounts of the appropriate clotting factor should be infused, to achieve levels of plasma activity equal initially to 10 to 20% of normal and to maintain a level of 5 to 10% of normal for at least 48 to 72 hours. Relief of pain, restoration of joint mobility, and cessation of further bleeding can be expected within a few hours. Prolonged treatment is often required in instances of severe hemorrhage.

When replacement therapy is restricted to whole blood or plasma, it is necessary to administer repeated infusions, every 6 to 12 hours in classic hemophilia and daily in Christmas disease, because of the short half-survival time of the coagulation factors, that is, 10 to 18 hours for factor VIII[290] and 18 to 35 hours for factor IX. The volume of fluid infused is limited to decrease the risk of hypervolemia. Levels of factor VIII greater than 20% of normal are only rarely attained with plasma alone.[155] This level is needed to maintain effective hemostasis for 48 hours.

Most,[69,73,83,93,221,307,328] but not all,[155] authorities favor aspiration in the case of large hemarthroses. Although some choose to intervene only after the initial infusion of plasma or concentrate has been completed,[69] it would seem preferable to aspirate immediately prior to or during replacement ther-

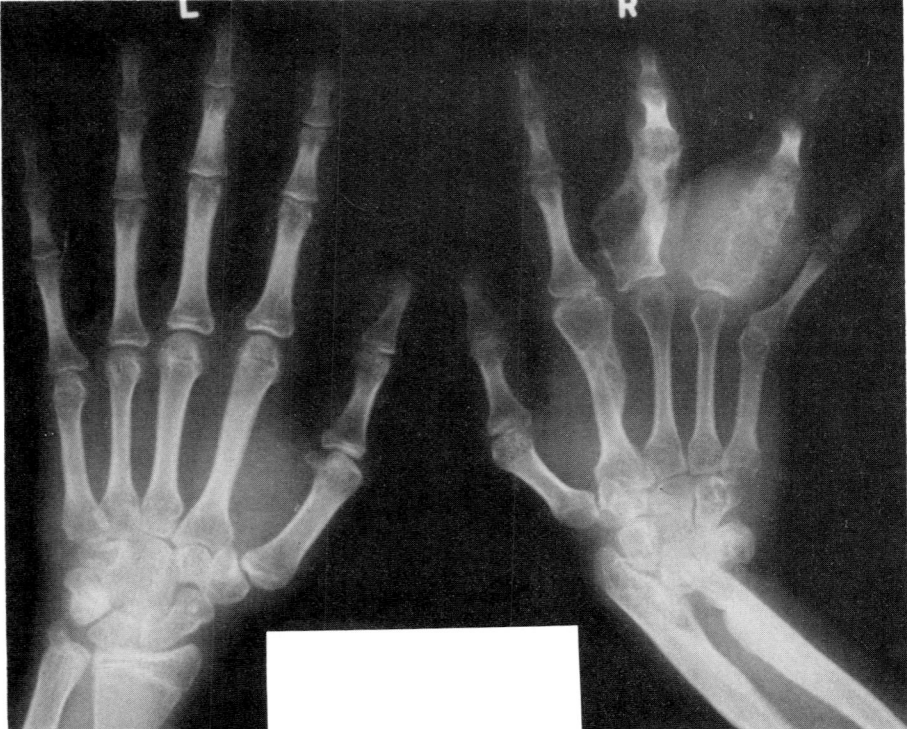

Fig. 74–22. Roentgenogram of the right hand of a 16-year-old boy with hemophilia illustrating the destruction of bone of the proximal phalanges of the fourth and fifth fingers resulting from hemophilic pseudotumor.

apy, to prevent clotting of blood within the joint cavity and to allow bleeding to cease soon after the optimal amount of the effusion has been withdrawn.[308,328] In any event, provided the coagulation defect is adequately corrected, aspiration can be performed without danger to the patient. Careful removal of the sanguineous fluid from the tense, distended joint relieves pain and stiffness, reduces the period of incapacity, and limits the damage to the synovium and cartilage.[69]

The intra-articular injection of corticosteroids or oral corticosteroid administration may facilitate the resolution of hemarthrosis. A 5-day course of prednisone, in doses of up to 80 mg/day, has reduced the amount of specific replacement factor necessary for the treatment of acute hemarthrosis and has increased the number of favorable responses to single infusions of factor VIII.[184]

As soon as pain and bleeding have been controlled, usually in three to five days, a normal, functional position should be restored, by serial cast changes if necessary, and muscle setting exercises should be prescribed. When the swelling and other signs of inflammation have subsided, active exercise is encouraged, to restore the normal range of motion because maintenance of this nor-

mal range is probably the single most important factor in the prevention of permanent contracture.[69,73] Excessively prolonged immobilization should be avoided because it leads to profound muscle atrophy. If a lower extremity is involved, the patient can ambulate on crutches, but weight bearing should be limited until the periarticular soft tissues return to near normal and muscle power is sufficient to stabilize the joint adequately.

Chronic Hemophilic Joint Disease

The knee is most often affected by the development of a chronic flexion contracture. This defect may be corrected, and stable weight bearing may be achieved by means of traction, wedging casts, quadriceps setting exercises, and later, active resistive exercises.[7,9,58,69,73,171] The use of a long leg-extension brace and crutches may be required for many months or years to prevent recurrence of the contracture.[17,69,320]

The use of surgical procedures for the correction of chronic joint deformities was limited because of the risk of uncontrollable postoperative hemorrhage until potent concentrates of antihemophilic factors became available. The prospect of orthopedic rehabilitation is now excellent.[320] Many procedures are now successful, including arthroplasty of the hip,[27] supracondylar wedge osteotomy for correction of valgus deformity of the knee,[7,9,17] wedge osteotomy of the tibia,[7] lengthening of the Achilles and other tendons of the feet for correction of equinus contracture,[7,17,93,222,313,328] compression athrodesis of the knee, hip, and ankle,[222,328] and total knee and total hip replacement.[17,60,83,211,218,297] Heroic operations, such as drainage or radical excision of hematoma and pseudotumor and the amputation of an extremity in cases of uncontrollable, life-threatening bleeding, or infection are now also possible.[139,204,250,270,306,307,320,328] An analysis of 76 individual operative procedures revealed 3 that were particularly successful: (1) supracondylar correction of knock knee; (2) intertrochanteric correction of coxa valga; and (3) evacuation of iliacus hematoma in patients with femoral nerve paralysis.[154]

Synovectomy of the knee has been performed to control repeated or intractable joint hemorrhage and has been considered useful in the prevention of recurrent bleeding.[17,84,152,206,217] Synoviorthesis with osmic acid is less effective than synovectomy in preventing recurrent hemarthrosis, but because of its simplicity, this operation has been recommended for use in younger patients.[110] Intra-articular radioactive gold (^{198}Au) also decreases the bleeding frequency and halts the progression of the disease if used early when the arthropathy is still reversible.[8] Hemophilic pseudotumor has been treated successfully surgically, as well as with x-irradiation;[6,17,151] a number of uncontrollable, destructive pseudotumors have now been excised successfully.[6,250,270] In the management of fractures in the hemophilic patient, rigid immobilization has been essential. In addition to the maintenance of hemostasis during healing, internal stabilization may be required.[96]

Before major surgical procedures are undertaken in the patient with classic hemophilia, the plasma should be examined for factor VIII inhibitor (antibody).[205,290] Preferably, both human and animal factor VIII should be used in such testing. If an inhibitor is found, elective operations should be avoided. If an operation is deemed necessary, the patient should be infused with massive doses of factor VIII as rapidly as possible, and the physician should choose a concentrate that is least affected by the inhibitor. An inhibitor has been found on rare occasions in Christmas disease. Sufficient factor VIII should be given to establish a level of approximately 30% of normal during the operation and 15 to 20% of normal in the postoperative period.[290] Because the potency of cryoprecipitates varies,[59,290] the patient's plasma must be assayed at regular intervals by means of the thromboplastin

generation test and partial thromboplastin time. Replacement therapy must be given without interruption until healing is well advanced, usually in 10 to 14 days. In extensive surgical procedures, however, infusions may have to be continued for 3 to 4 weeks or longer.[222]

The acquired immunodeficiency syndrome (AIDS) has now been reported in a number of patients with hemophilia, all of whom have been exposed to factor VIII or factor IX concentrates as well as other blood components. AIDS in hemophiliacs appears to be reaching epidemic proportions, and all evidence suggests that it is wise to attempt to limit further occurrence of the syndrome in this apparently high-risk group. The United States Public Health Service has asked potential carriers of AIDS to refrain from donating plasma or blood. Most of the patients with hemophilia who have acquired this syndrome have died of opportunistic infections within a short time. Hemophiliacs are more difficult to manage than the usual patients with AIDS because diagnostic and therapeutic procedures may be complicated by their bleeding diathesis.[92]

REFERENCES

1. Abell, J.M., Jr., and Bailey, R.W.: Hemophilic pseudotumor: two cases occurring in siblings. Arch. Surg., *81*:559–581, 1960.
2. Abou Rizk, N.A., Nasr, F.W., and Frayha, R.A.: Aseptic necrosis in thalassemia minor. Arthritis Rheum., *20*:1,147–1,148, 1977.
3. Abul-Haj, S.A., et al.: Farber's disease: report of a case with observations on its histogenesis and notes on the nature of the stored material. J. Pediatr., *61*:213–221, 1962.
4. Adamsky, A., Varetzky, A., and Klajman, A.: Malignant lymphoma presenting as sternoclavicular joint arthritis. Arthritis Rheum., *23*:1,330–1,331, 1981.
5. Adler, E., and Maybaum, S.: Rare features in a case of Gaucher's disease. Ann. Rheum. Dis., *13*:229–232, 1954.
6. Ahlberg, A.: On the natural history of hemophilic pseudotumor. J. Bone Joint Surg., *57A*:1,133–1,136, 1975.
7. Ahlberg, A.: Treatment and prophylaxis of arthropathy in severe hemophilia. Clin. Orthop., *53*:135–146, 1967.
8. Ahlberg, A., and Pettersson, H.: Synoviorthesis with radioactive gold in hemophiliacs. Acta Orthop. Scand., *50*:513–517, 1979.
9. Ahlberg, A., Nilsson, I.M., and Bauer, G.C.H.: Use of antihemophilic factor (plasma fraction I-O) during correction of knee-joint deformities in hemophilia A. J. Bone Joint Surg., *47A*:323–332, 1965.
10. Ahlmen, J., et al.: Clinical and diagnostic considerations in Fabry's disease. Acta Med. Scand., *211*:309–312, 1982.
11. Aisner, M., and Hoxie, T.B.: Bone and joint pain in leukemia, simulating acute rheumatic fever and subacute bacterial endocarditis. N. Engl. J. Med., *238*:733–737, 1948.
12. Alavi, A., et al.: Bone marrow scan evaluation of arthropathy in sickle cell disorders. Arch. Intern. Med., *136*:436–440, 1976.
13. Ali, A.M., et al.: Joint haemorrhage in haemophilia: is full advantage taken of plasma therapy? Br. Med. J., *3*:828–831, 1967.
14. Amstutz, H.C., and Carey, E.J.: Skeletal manifestations and treatment of Gaucher's disease: review of twenty cases. J. Bone Joint Surg., *48A*:670–701, 1966.

15. Andreev, V.C., and Ziatkov, N.B.: Systemic lupus erythematosus and neoplasia of the lymphoreticular system. Br. J. Dermatol, 68:503–508, 1968.
16. Ansell, B.M., and Bywaters, E.G.L.: Histiocytic bone and joint disease. Ann. Rheum. Dis., 16:503–510, 1957.
17. Arnold, W.D., and Hilgartner, H.W.: Hemophilic arthropathy: current concepts of pathogenesis and management. J. Bone Joint Surg., 59A:287–305, 1977.
18. Baldridge, C.W., and Awe, C.D.: Lymphoma: a study of one hundred and fifty cases. Arch. Intern. Med., 45:161–190, 1930.
19. Ball, G.V., and Sorensen, L.B.: The pathogenesis of hyperuricemia and gout in sickle cell anemia. Arthritis Rheum., 13:846–848, 1970.
20. Barrow, M.V., et al.: Identification of tissue lipids in lipoid dermatoarthritis (multicentric reticulohistiocytosis). Am. J. Clin. Pathol., 47:312–325, 1967.
21. Barrow, M.V., and Holubar, K.: Multicentric reticulohistiocytosis: a review of 33 patients. Medicine, 48:287–305, 1969.
22. Bastian, F.O.: Amyloidosis and the carpal tunnel syndrome. Am. J. Clin. Pathol., 61:711–717, 1974.
23. Battacharyya, A.K., and Conner, W.E.: Familial diseases with storage of sterols other than cholesterol (cerebrotendinous xanthomatosis and beta-sitosterolomemia and xanthomatosis). In The Metabolic Basis of Inherited Disease. 4th Ed. Edited by J.B. Stanbury, J.B. Wyngaarden, and D.S. Fredrickson. New York, McGraw-Hill, 1978, pp. 656–659.
24. Battacharyya, A.K., and Connor, W.E.: Beta-sitosterolemia and xanthomatosis: a newly described lipid storage disease in two sisters. J. Clin. Invest., 53:1,033–1,043, 1974.
25. Beichetz, P.E., et al.: Treatment of Gaucher's disease with liposome-entrapped glucocerebroside-beta-glucosidase. Lancet, 1:116–117, 1977.
26. Belaich, S.: Multicentric reticulohistiocytosis. J. Ital. Dermatol., 115:77, 1980.
27. Bellingham, A., et al.: Hip arthroplasty in a haemophiliac and subsequent prophylactic therapy with cryoprecipitate. Br. Med. J., 4:531–532, 1967.
28. Bernhard, G.C., and Hensley, G.T.: Amyloid arthropathy. Arthritis Rheum., 12:444–453, 1959.
29. Bethune, J.E., Landrigan, P.L., and Chipman, C.D.: Angiokeratoma corporis diffusum universale (Fabry's disease) in two brothers. N. Engl. J. Med., 264:1,280–1,285, 1961.
30. Bichel, J.: Arthralgic leukemia in children. Acta Haematol., 1:153–164, 1948.
31. Berman, S.M., et al.: Farber's disease: a disorder of mucopolysaccharide metabolism with articular, respiratory, and neurologic manifestations. Arthritis. Rheum., 9:620–630, 1966.
32. Biggs, R. (Ed.): The Treatment of Haemophilia A and B and von Willebrand's Disease. Oxford, Blackwell Scientific, 1978.
33. Biggs, R.: Human Blood Coagulation, Haemostasis and Thrombosis. 2nd Ed. Oxford, Blackwell Scientific, 1976.
34. Biggs, R., and Macfarlane, R.G.: Human Blood Coagulation and its Disorders. 3rd Ed. Philadelphia, F.A. Davis, 1962.
35. Bortz, A.L., and Vincent, M.: Lipoid dermato-arthritis and arthritis mutilans. Am. J. Med., 30:951–960, 1961.
36. Bond, J.V.: Clinical features of neuroblastoma. Br. J. Hosp. Med., 14:543–554, 1975.
37. Brady, R.O.: Glucosyl ceramide lipidosis: Gaucher's disease. In The Metabolic Basis of Inherited Disease. 4th Ed. Edited by J.B. Stanbury, J.B. Wyngaarden, and D.S. Fredrickson. New York, McGraw-Hill, 1978, pp. 731–746.
38. Brady, R.O., et al.: Replacement therapy for inherited enzyme deficiency: use of purified glucocerebrosidase in Gaucher's disease. N. Engl. J. Med., 291:989–993, 1974.
39. Brady, R.O., et al.: Replacement therapy for inherited enzyme deficiency: use of purified ceramidetrihexosidase in Fabry's disease. N. Engl. J. Med., 289:9–14, 1973.
40. Brandt, F., et al.: Topical nitrogen mustard therapy in multicentric reticulohistiocytosis. J. Am. Acad. Dermatol., 6:260–262, 1982.
41. Braverman, I.M., and Ken, Y.A.: Ultrastructure and three dimensional reconstruction of several macular and papular telangiectases. J. Invest. Dermatol., 81:489–497, 1983.
42. Breen, F.A., Jr., and Tullis, J.L.: Prothrombin concentrates in treatment of Christmas disease and allied disorders. JAMA, 208:1,848–1,852, 1969.
43. Brower, T.D., and Wilde, A.H.: Femoral neuropathy in hemophilia. J. Bone Joint Surg., 48A:487–492, 1966.
44. Buckingham, R.B., Bole, G.G., and Bassett, D.R.: Polyarthritis associated with type IV hyperlipoproteinemia. Arch. Intern. Med., 135:286–290, 1975.
45. Burnham, T.K.: Antinuclear antibodies in patients with malignancies. Lancet, 2:1,253–1,254, 1972.
46. Cameron, E.A.: Gout from cyanotic congenital heart disease. Br. Med. J., 1:34–35, 1961.
47. Cammarata, R.J., Rodnan, G.P., and Jensen, W.N.: Systemic rheumatic disease and malignant lymphoma. Arch. Intern. Med., 111:330–337, 1963.
48. Carroll, D.S.: Roentgen manifestations of sickle cell disease. South. Med. J., 50:1,486–1,490, 1957.
49. Chen, W.W., and Deeker, G.L.: Abnormalities of lysosomes in human diploid fibroblasts from patients with Farber's disease. Biochim. Biopys. Acta, 718:185–192, 1982.
50. Christianson, H.B., Brunsting, L.A., and Perry, H.O.: Dermatomyositis: unusual features, complications and treatment. Arch. Dermatol., 74:581–584, 1956.
51. Chung, S.M., and Ralston, E.L.: Necrosis of the femoral head associated with sickle-cell anemia and its genetic variants: a review of the literature and study of thirteen cases. J. Bone Joint Surg., 51A:33–58, 1969.
52. Clarke, J.T.R., et al.: Enzyme replacement therapy by renal allotransplantation in Fabry's disease. N. Engl. J. Med., 287:1,215–1,218, 1972.
53. Cohen, A.S., and Canoso, J.J.: Rheumatological aspects of amyloid disease. Clin. Rheum. Dis., 1:149–161, 1975.
54. Cohen, A.S., Cathcart, E.S., and Skinner, M.: Amyloidosis: current trends in its investigation. Arthritis Rheum., 21:153–160, 1978.
55. Convery, F.R., et al.: Experimental hemarthrosis in the knee of the mature canine. Arthritis Rheum., 19:59–67, 1976.
56. Craver, L.F.: Tenderness of the sternum in leukemia. Am. J. Med. Sci., 174:799–801, 1927.
57. Craver, L.F., and Copeland, M.M.: Changes of the bones in the leukemias. Arch. Surg., 30:639–646, 1935.
58. Crock, H.V., and Boni, V.: The management of orthopaedic problems in haemophiliacs: a review of 21 cases. Br. J. Surg., 48:8–15, 1960.
59. Dallman, P.R., and Pool, J.G.: Treatment of hemophilia with factor 8 concentrates. N. Engl. J. Med., 278:199–202, 1968.
60. D'Ambrosia, R.D., et al.: Total hip replacement for patients with hemophilia and hemorrhagic diathesis. Surg. Gynecol. Obstet., 139:381–384, 1974.
61. Damon, A., et al.: Polycythemia and renal carcinoma: report of ten new cases, two with long hematologic remission following nephrectomy. Am. J. Med., 25:182–197, 1958.
62. Davies, D.T., Hughes, A., and Tonks, R.S.: The influence of salicylate on platelets and whole blood adenine nucleotides. Br. J. Pharmacol., 36:437–447, 1969.
63. Davies, N.E.: Multicentric reticulohistiocytosis: report of a case with histochemical studies. Arch. Dermatol., 97:543–547, 1968.
64. Deaton, J.G., and Levin, W.C.: Systemic lupus erythematosus and acute myeloblastic leukemia: report of their coexistence and a survey of possible associating features. Arch. Intern. Med., 120:345–348, 1967.
65. DeConti, R.C., and Calabresi, P.: Use of allopurinol for prevention and control of hyperuricemia in patients with neoplastic disease. N. Engl. J. Med., 274:481–486, 1966.
66. Defaria, C.R., Demelo-Souza, S.E., and Pinheiro, E.D.: Haemophilic neuromyopathy. J. Neurol. Neurosurg. Psychiatry, 42:600–605, 1979.

67. Demames, D.J., Lane, N., and Beckstead, J.H.: Bone involvement in hairy-cell leukemia. Cancer, 49:1,697–1,701, 1982.

68. Denman, A.M., Szur, L., and Ansell, B.M.: Joint complaints in polycythaemia vera. Ann. Rheum. Dis., 23:139–144, 1964.

69. DePalma, A.F.: Hemophilic arthropathy. Clin. Orthop., 52:145–165, 1967.

70. Desnick, R.J., Kifonsky, B., and Sweeley, C.C.: Fabry's disease (a-galactosidase A deficiency). In The Metabolic Basis of Inherited Disease. 4th Ed. Edited by J.B. Stanbury, J.B. Wyngaarden, and D.S. Fredrickson. New York, McGraw-Hill, 1978, pp. 810–840.

71. Diamond, H.S., et al.: Hyperuricosuria and increased tubular secretion of urate in sickle cell anemia. Am. J. Med., 59:796–802, 1975.

72. Diamond, H.S., Meisel, A.D., and Holden, D.: The natural history of urate overproduction in sickle cell anemia. Ann. Intern. Med., 90:752–757, 1979.

73. Dietrich, S.L.: Rehabilitation and nonsurgical management of musculoskeletal problems in the hemophilic patient. Ann. N.Y. Acad. Sci., 240:328–337, 1975.

74. Diggs, L.W.: Bone and joint lesions in sickle-cell disease. Clin. Orthop., 52:119–143, 1967.

75. Doherty, M., Martin, M.F.R., and Dieppe, P.A.: Multicentric reticulohistiocytosis associated with primary biliary cirrhosis: successful treatment with cytotoxic agents. Arthritis Rheum., 27:344–348, 1984.

76. Dorwart, B.B., et al.: Absence of increased frequency of bone and joint disease with hemoglobin AS and AC. Ann. Intern Med., 86:66–67, 1977.

77. Dosovetz, D.E., et al.: Primary lymphoma of bone. Cancer, 51:44–46, 1983.

78. Dosovetz, D.E., et al.: Primary lymphoma of bone. Cancer, 50:1,009–1,014, 1982.

79. This reference has been deleted.

80. Douer, D., et al.: Successful treatment of severe bone pain and acute arthritis in chronic myelomonocytic leukaemia by cytosine arabinoside. Ann. Rheum. Dis., 36:192–193, 1977.

81. Druet, P., et al.: Rheumatoid polyarthritis and chronic lymphoid leukemia: studies of 7 cases of association of these 2 diseases. Sem. Hop. Paris, 45:489–498, 1969.

82. Dulaney, J.T., Moser, H.W., and Sidbury, J.: The biochemical defect in Farber's disease. In Current Trends in Sphingolipidoses and Allied Disorders. Edited by B.W. Volk and L. Schneck. New York, Plenum, 1976, pp. 403–411.

83. Duthie, R.B., and Rizza, C.R.: Rheumatological manifestations of the haemophilias. Clin. Rheum. Dis., 1:53–93, 1975.

84. Dyszy-Laube, B., et al.: Synovectomy in the treatment of hemophilic arthropathy. J. Pediatr. Surg., 9:123–125, 1974.

85. Easton, J.A.: Musculo-skeletal aspects of haematological disorders. Clin. Rheum. Dis., 2:459–491, 1976.

86. Ehrlich, G.E., et al.: Multicentric reticulohistiocytosis (lipoid dermatoarthritis): a multisystem disorder. Am. J. Med., 52:830–840, 1972.

87. Elkton, R.B., Hughes, G.R.V., and Catovsky, D.: Hairy cell leukemia with polyarteritis nodosa. Lancet, 2:280–282, 1979.

88. Emkey, R.D., et al.: A case of lymphoproliferative disease presenting as juvenile rheumatoid arthritis: diagnosis by synovial fluid examination. Am. J. Med., 54:825–828, 1977.

89. Engel, I.A., et al.: Osteonecrosis in patients with lymphoma: a review of twenty-five cases. Cancer, 48:1,245–1,250, 1981.

90. Espinoza, L.R., Spilberg, I., and Osterland, C.K.: Joint manifestations of sickle cell disease. Medicine, 53:295–305, 1974.

91. Evans, F.J., and Hilton, J.H.B.: Polymyositis associated with acute monocytic leukemia: case report and review of the literature. Can. Med. Assoc. J., 91:1,272–1,275, 1964.

92. Evatt, B.L., et al.: The acquired immunodeficiency syndrome in patients with hemophilia. Ann. Intern. Med., 100:499–504, 1984.

93. Eyring, E.J., Bjornson, D.R., and Close, J.R.: Management of hemophilia in children. Clin. Orthop., 40:95–112, 1965.

94. Fahey, J.J., et al.: Xanthoma of the Achilles tendon. J. Bone Joint Surg., 55A:1,197–1,211, 1973.

95. Farber, S., Cohen, J., and Uzman, L.: Lipogranulomatosis: a new lipo-glyco-protein "storage" disease. J. Mt. Sinai Hosp., 24:816–837, 1957.

96. Fell, E., Bentley, G., and Rizza, C.R.: Fracture management in patients with haemophilia. J. Bone Joint Surg., 56B:643–649, 1974.

97. Fink, C.W., Windmiller, J., and Sartain, P.: Arthritis as the presenting feature of childhood leukemia. Arthritis Rheum., 15:347–349, 1972.

98. Flam, M., et al.: Multicentric reticulohistiocytosis: report of a case with atypical features and electron microscopic study of skin lesions. Am. J. Med., 52:841–848, 1972.

99. Fone, D.J., and King, W.E.: Angiokeratoma corporis diffusum (Fabry's syndrome). Aust. Ann. Med., 13:339–348, 1964.

100. Forbes, C.D., et al.: A comparison of thermography, radioisotope scanning and clinical assessment of the knee joints in haemophilia. Clin. Radiol., 26:41–45, 1975.

101. Ford, D.K., et al.: Familial lipochrome pigmentation of histiocytes with hyperglobulinemia, pulmonary infiltration, splenomegaly, arthritis and susceptibility to infection. Am. J. Med., 33:478–489, 1962.

102. Fraenkel, G.J., Taylor, K.B., and Richards, W.C.D.: Haemophilic blood cysts. Br. J. Surg., 46:383–392, 1959.

103. Franklin, E.C., and Zucker-Franklin, D.: Current concepts of amyloid. Adv. Immunol., 15:249–304, 1972.

104. Fredrickson, D.S., Goldstein, J.L., and Brown, M.S.: The familial hyperlipoproteinemias. In The Metabolic Basis of Inherited Disease. 4th Ed. Edited by J.B. Stanbury, J.B. Wyngaarden, and D.S. Fredrickson. New York, McGraw-Hill, 1978, pp. 604–655.

105. Fredrickson, D.S., Levy, R.I., and Lees, R.S.: Fat transport in lipoproteins—an integrated approach to mechanisms and disorders. N. Engl. J. Med., 276:215–225, 1967.

106. Freemont, A.J., Jones, C.I.P., and Denton, J.: The synovium and synovial fluid in multicentric reticulohistiocytosis—a light microscopic, electron microscopic and cytochemical analysis of one case. J. Clin. Pathol., 36:860–866, 1983.

107. Fucilla, I.S. and Hamann, A.: Hodgkin's disease in bone. Radiology, 77:53–60, 1961.

108. Furey, N.D., et al.: Multicentric reticulohisticytosis with salivary gland involvement and pericardial effusion. J. Am. Acad. Dermatol., 8:679–685, 1983.

109. Galy, P.: Pierre Marie paraneoplastic syndrome and Hodgkin's disease (apropos of a case). Lyon Med., 217:715–722, 1967.

110. Gamba, G., Grignani, G., and Ascari, E.: Synoviorthesis versus synovectomy in the treatment of recurrent haemophilic haemarthrosis: long term evaluation. Thromb. Haemost., 45:127–129, 1981.

111. Garcin, R., et al.: Neurologic aspects of Fabry's angiokeratosis: apropos of 2 cases. Presse Med., 75:435–440, 1967.

112. Gardner, F.H., and Nathan, D.G.: Secondary gout. Med. Clin. North Am., 45:1,273–1,282, 1961.

113. Garfinkle, B., et al.: Coexistence of Gaucher's disease and multiple myeloma. Arch. Intern. Med., 142:2,229–2,230, 1982.

114. Ghormley, R.K., and Clegg, R.S.: Bone and joint changes in hemophilia: with report of cases of so-called hemophilic pseudotumor. J. Bone Joint Surg., 30A:589–600, 1948.

115. Glenner, G.G., Ein, D., and Terry, W.D.: The immunoglobulin origin of amyloid. Am. J. Med., 52:141–147, 1972.

116. Glenner, G.G., Terry, W.D., and Isersky, C.: Amyloidosis: its nature and pathogenesis. Semin. Hematol., 10:65–85, 1973.

117. Glueck, C.J., Levy, R.I., and Fredrickson, D.S.: Acute

tendinitis and arthritis: a presenting symptom of familial type II hyperlipoproteinemia. JAMA, 206:2,895–2,897, 1968.

118. Goedent, J., Neefe, R., and South, F.: Polyarteritis, hairy cell leukemia and splenosis. Am. J. Med., 71:323–326, 1981.

119. Gold, R.H., et al.: Multicentric reticulohistiocytosis (lipoid dermato-arthritis). An erosive polyarthritis with distinctive clinical, roentgenographic and pathologic features. AJR, 124:610–624, 1975.

120. Goldberg, A., Brodsky, I., and McCarty, D.: Multiple myeloma with paraamyloidosis presenting as rheumatoid disease. Am. J. Med., 37:653–658, 1964.

121. Goldberg, L.S., et al.: Amyloid arthritis associated with Waldenstrom's macroglobulinemia. N. Engl. J. Med., 281:256–257, 1969.

122. Goldberg, M.A.: Sickle cell arthropathy: analysis of synovial fluid in sickle cell anemia with joint effusion. South. Med. J., 66:956–958, 1973.

123. Goldenberg, G.J., Paraskevas, F., and Israels, L.G.: The association of rheumatoid arthritis with plasma cell and lymphocytic neoplasms. Arthritis Rheum., 12:569–579, 1969.

124. Golding, J.S.: Conditions of the hip associated with hemoglobinopathies. Clin. Orthop., 90:22–28, 1973.

125. Goldman, J.A., et al.: Musculoskeletal disorders associated with type-IV hyperlipoproteinaemia. Lancet, 2:449–452, 1972.

126. Goldring, J.S.R., MacIver, J.E., and Went, L.N.: The bone changes in sickle cell anaemia and its genetic variants. J. Bone Joint Surg., 41B:711–718, 1959.

127. Goltz, R.W., and Laymon, C.W.: Multicentric reticulohistiocytosis of the skin and synovia. Arch. Dermatol. Syphilol., 69:717–731, 1954.

128. Gompels, B.M., Votaw, M.L., and Martel, W.: Correlation of radiological manifestations of multiple myeloma with immunoglobulin abnormalities and prognosis. Radiology, 104:509–514, 1972.

129. Goodfellow, J., Fearn, C.B., and Matthews, J.M.: Iliacus haematoma: a common complication of haemophilia. J. Bone Joint Surg., 49B:748–756, 1967.

130. Gordon, D.A., et al.: Amyloid arthritis simulating rheumatoid disease in five patients with multiple myeloma. Am. J. Med., 55:142–154, 1973.

131. Gordon, D.A., Pruzanski, W., and Ogryzlo, M.A.: Synovial fluid examination for the diagnosis of amyloidosis. Ann. Rheum. Dis., 32:428–430, 1973.

132. Gratwick, G.M., et al.: Thalassemic osteoarthropathy. Ann. Intern. Med., 88:494–501, 1978.

133. Groen, J., and Garrer, A.H.: Adult Gaucher's disease with special reference to the variations in its clinical course and the value of sternal puncture as an aid to its diagnosis. Blood, 3:1,221–1,237, 1948.

134. Grossman, L.A., et al.: Carpal tunnel syndrome—initial manifestation of systemic disease. JAMA, 176:259–261, 1961.

135. Grossman, R.E., and Hensley, G.T.: Bone lesions in primary amyloidosis. AJR, 101:872–875, 1967.

136. Gunderson, C., D'Ambrosia, R.D., and Shoij, H.: Total hip replacement in patients with sickle-cell disease. J. Bone Joint Surg., 59A:760–762, 1977.

137. Gutman, A.B.: Primary and secondary gout. Ann. Intern. Med., 39:1,062–1,076, 1953.

138. Gutman, A.B., and Yu, T.F.: Secondary gout. Ann. Intern. Med., 56:675, 1962.

139. Hall, M.R.P., Handley, D.A., and Webster, C.U.: The surgical treatment of haemophilic blood cysts. J. Bone Joint Surg., 44B:781–789, 1962.

140. Hall, S., et al.: Multicentric reticulohistiocytosis. Arthritis Rheum., 27:S79, 1984.

140a. Hall, T.C.: Treatment of hyperuricemia of neoplastic disease. J. Clin. Pharmacol., 7:156–161, 1967.

141. Hallidie-Smith, K.A., and Bywaters, E.G.L.: The differential diagnosis of rheumatic fever. Arch. Dis. Child., 33:350–357, 1958.

142. Hamilton, E.B.D., and Bywaters, E.G.L.: Joint symptoms in myelomatosis and similar conditions. Ann. Rheum. Dis., 20:353–362, 1961.

143. Hammel, C.F., et al.: Bone marrow and bone mineral scintigraphic studies in sickle cell disease. Br. J. Haematol., 25:593–598, 1973.

144. Hanauer, L.B.: Reticulohistiocystosis: remission after cyclophosphamide therapy. Arthritis Rheum., 15:636–640, 1972.

145. Hand, W.L., and King, N.L.: Serum opsonization of Salmonella in sickle cell anemia. Am. J. Med., 64:388–395, 1978.

146. Hanissian, A.S., and Silverman, A.: Arthritis and sickle cell anemia. South. Med. J., 67:28–32, 1974.

147. Harden, W.B., et al.: Septic arthritis due to Serratia liquefaciens. Arthritis Rheum., 23:946–947, 1980.

148. Harlan, W.R., Jr., et al.: Familial hypercholesterolemia: a genetic and metabolic study. Medicine, 45:77–110, 1966.

149. Hewett, B.W., and Nice, C.M., Jr.: Radiographic manifestations of sickle cell anemia. Radiol. Clin. North Am., 2:249–259, 1964.

150. Hickling, P., Wilkens, M., and Newman, G.R.: A study of arthropathy in multiple myeloma. Q. J. Med., 200:417–433, 1981.

151. Hilgartner, M.W., and Arnold, W.D.: Hemophilic pseudotumor treated with replacement therapy and radiation: report of a case. J. Bone Joint Surg., 57A:1,145–1,146, 1975.

152. Hilgartner, M.W.: Hemophilic arthropathy. Adv. Pediatr., 21:139–165, 1974.

153. Hoag, M.S., et al.: Treatment of hemophilia B with a new clotting-factor concentrate. N. Engl. J. Med., 280:581–586, 1969.

154. Hofmann, P., Menge, M., and Brachman, H.H.: Reconstructive surgery in the lower limb in hemophiliacs. Isr. J. Med. Sci., 13:988–994, 1977.

155. Honig, G.R., et al.: Administration of single doses of AHF (factor VIII) concentrates in the treatment of hemophilic hemarthroses. Pediatrics, 43:26–33, 1969.

156. Hough, A.J., Banfield, W.G., and Sokoloff, L.: Cartilage in hemophilic arthropathy. Arch. Pathol. Lab. Med., 100:91–96, 1976.

157. Houghton, G.R.: Septic arthritis of the hip in a hemophiliac. Clin. Orthop., 129:223–224, 1977.

158. Howqua, J.A., and Mackay, I.R.: L.E. cells and lymphoma. Blood, 22:191–198, 1963.

159. Hughes, J.G., and Carroll, D.S.: Salmonella osteomyelitis complicating sickle cell disease. Pediatrics, 19:184–191, 1957.

160. Hurwitz, D., and Roht, H.: Sickle cell-thalassemia presenting as arthritis of the hip. Arthritis Rheum., 13:422–425, 1970.

161. Husby, G., Natvig, J.B., and Sletten, K.: New, third class of amyloid fibril protein. J. Exp. Med., 139:773–778, 1974.

162. Husby, G., Sletten, K.K., and Michaelsen, T.E.: Amyloid fibril protein subunit, protein AS: distribution in tissue and serum in different clinical types of amyloidosis including that associated with myelomatosis and Waldenstrom's macroglobulinemia. Scand. J. Immunol., 2:395–404, 1973.

163. Ihde, D.C., and DeVita, V.T.: Osteonecrosis of the femoral heads in patients with lymphoma treated with intermittent combination chemotherapy. Cancer, 36:1,585–1,588, 1975.

164. Jacob, G.F., and Raper, A.B., Hereditary persistence of foetal haemoglobin production, and its interaction with the sickle-cell trait. Br. J. Haematol., 4:138–149, 1958.

165. Jaffe, H.L.: Tumors and Tumorous Conditions of the Bones and Joints. Philadelphia, Lea & Febiger, 1958.

166. Jaffer, A.M., and Schmid, F.R.: Hemarthrosis associated with sodium warfarin. J. Rheumatol., 4:215–217, 1977.

167. Jensen, P.S., and Putnam, C.E.: Chondrocalcinosis and haemophilia. Clin. Radiol., 28:401–405, 1977.

168. Johnston, A.W., Weller, S.D., and Warland, B.J.: Angiokeratoma corporis diffusum: some clinical aspects. Arch. Dis. Child., 43:73–79, 1968.

169. Johnston, R.B., Jr., Newman, S.L., and Struth, A.G.: An abnormality of the alternate pathway of complement

activation in sickle cell disease. N. Engl. J. Med., *288*:803–808, 1973.

170. Jordan, E., et al.: Multiple myeloma complicating the course of seronegative systemic lupus erythematosus. Arthritis Rheum., *21*:260–265, 1978.

171. Jordan, H.H.: Hemophilic Arthropathies. Springfield, IL, Charles C Thomas, 1958.

172. Kasper, C.K., and Rapaport, S.I.: Bleeding times and platelet aggregation after analgesics in hemophilia. Ann. Intern. Med., *77*:189–193, 1972.

173. Katz, A.L., and Alepa, F.P.: Hemarthrosis secondary to heparin therapy. (Letter.) Arthritis Rheum., *19*:966, 1976.

174. Katz, G.A., et al.: The shoulder-pad sign—a diagnostic feature of amyloid arthropathy. N. Engl. J. Med., *288*:354–355, 1973.

175. Katz, J.F.: Recurrent avascular necrosis of the proximal femoral epiphysis in the same hip in Gaucher's disease. J. Bone Joint Surg., *49A*:514–518, 1967.

176. Kavanaugh, J.H.: Multiple myeloma, amyloid arthropathy, and pathological fracture of the femur: a case report. J Bone Joint Surg., *60A*:135–137, 1978.

177. Keeling, M.M., Lockwood, W.B., and Harris, E.A.: Avascular necrosis and erythrocytosis in sickle-cell trait. N. Engl. J. Med., *290*:442–444, 1974.

178. Kellerhouse, L.E., and Limarzi, L.R.: Bone manifestations of hematologic disorders. Med. Clin. North Am., *49*:203–228, 1965.

179. Kerr, C.B.: The fortunes of haemophiliacs in the nineteenth century. Med. Hist., *7*:359–370, 1963.

180. Key, J.A.: Hemophilic arthritis (bleeder's joints). Ann. Surg., *95*:198–225, 1932.

181. Khachadurian, A.K.: Migratory polyarthritis in familial hypercholesterolemia (type II hyperlipoproteinemia). Arthritis Rheum., *11*:385–393, 1968.

182. Kimura, S., et al.: Chemical evidence for beta-type amyloid fibril proteins. J. Immunol., *109*:891, 1972.

183. Kisker, C.T., Perlman, A.W., and Benton, C.: Arthritis in hemophilia. Semin. Arthritis Rheum., *1*:220–225, 1971.

184. Kisker, C.T., et al.: Double-blind studies on the use of steroids in the treatment of acute hemarthrosis in patients with hemophilia. N. Engl. J. Med., *282*:639–642, 1970.

185. Krakoff, I.H.: Use of allopurinol in preventing hyperuricemia in leukemia and lymphoma. Cancer, *19*:1,489–1,496, 1966.

186. Krakoff, I.H.: Studies of uric acid biosynthesis in the chronic leukemias. Arthritis Rheum., *8*:772–779, 1965.

187. Krey, P.R., Comerford, F.R., and Cohen, A.S.: Multicentric reticulohistiocytosis: fine structural analysis of the synovium and synovial fluid cells. Arthritis Rheum., *17*:615–633, 1974.

188. Kudoh, T., and Wenger, D.A.: Diagnosis of metachromatic leukodystrophy, Krabbe disease, and Farber's disease after uptake of fatty acid labeled cerebroside sulfate into cultured skin fibroblasts. J. Clin. Invest., *70*:89–97, 1982.

189. Lachiewicz, P.F., Lane, T.M., and Wilson, P.D.: Total hip replacement in Gaucher's disease. J. Bone Joint Surg., *53A*:602–608, 1981.

190. Lacroux, R.: Angiokeratome diffusum (angiokeratoma corporis diffusum) de Fabry. Bull. Soc. Fr. Dermatol. Syphilol., *67*:474–478, 1960.

191. Laine, V., Vaino, K., and Ritama, V.V.: Occurrence of amyloid in rheumatoid arthritis. Acta Rheumatol. Scand., *1*:43–46, 1955.

192. Lan, M.M., et al.: Hip arthroplasties in Gaucher's disease. J. Bone Joint Surg., *63A*:591–601, 1981.

193. Lancourt, J.E., Gilbert, M.S., and Posner, M.A.: Management of bleeding and associated complications of hemophilia in the hand and forearm. J. Bone Joint Surg., *59A*:451–460, 1977.

194. Landbeck, G., and Kurme, A.: Hemophilic arthropathy of the knee joint: treatment of hemorrhages of the knee-joint and their consequences. Monatsschr. Kinderheilkd., *118*:29–41, 1970.

195. Landells, J.W.: The bone cysts of osteoarthritis. J. Bone Joint Surg., *35B*:643–649, 1953.

196. Lane, J.J., Jr., and Decker, J.L.: Latex particle slide tests in rheumatoid arthritis. JAMA, *173*:982–985, 1960.

197. Laster, L., and Muller, A.F.: Uric acid production in a case of myeloid metaplasia associated with gouty arthritis, studied with ^{15}N-labeled glycine. Am. J. Med., *15*:857–861, 1953.

198. Lea, A.J.: An association between the rheumatic diseases and the reticuloses. Ann. Rheum. Dis., *23*:480–484, 1964.

199. Lee, R.E., Robinson, D.B., and Glew, R.H.: Gaucher's disease I. Modern enzymatic and anatomic methods of diagnosis. Arch. Pathol. Lab. Med., *105*:102–104, 1981.

200. Leff, R.D., Aldo-Bensen, M.A., and Fife, R.S.: Tophaecous gout in a patient with sickle cell-thalassemia: case report and a review of the literature. Arthritis Rheum., *26*:928–929, 1983.

201. Leonello, P.P., Cleland, L.G., and Norman, J.E.: Acute pseudogout and chondrocalcinosis in a man with mild hemophilia. J. Rheumatol., *8*:841–844, 1981.

202. LeQuesne, B., et al.: Home treatment for patients with haemophilia. Lancet, *2*:507–509, 1974.

203. Levine, P.H.: Efficacy of self therapy in hemophilia: a study of 72 patients with hemophilia A and B. N. Engl. J. Med., *291*:1,381–1,384, 1974.

204. Lewis, J.H., Cottington, M., and Brower, T.D.: The use of plasma fraction 1 to maintain hemostasis following amputation for hemorrhagic cysts of the thigh in a severe hemophiliac. J. Bone Joint Surg., *47A*:333–339, 1965.

205. Lewis, J.H., Spero, J.A., and Hasiba, U.: Coagulopathies. DM, *23*:1–64, 1977.

206. London, J.T., et al.: Synovectomy and total joint arthroplasty for recurrent hemarthroses in the arthropathic joint in hemophilia. Arthritis Rheum., *20*:543–545, 1977.

207. Luzar, M.J., and Sharma, H.M.: Leukemia and arthritis: including reports on light, immunofluorescent and electron microscopy of the synovium. J. Rheumatol., *10*:132–135, 1983.

208. Lyell, A., and Carr, A.J.: Lipoid dermatoarthritis (reticulohistiocytosis). Br. J. Dermatol., *71*:12–21, 1959.

209. Lynch, E.C.: Uric acid metabolism in proliferative diseases of the marrow. Arch. Intern. Med., *109*:639–655, 1962.

210. McCarty, G.A., et al.: Lymphocytic lymphoma and systemic lupus erythematosus. Arch. Pathol. Lab. Med., *106*:196–199, 1982.

211. McCollough, N.C., et al.: Synovectomy or total replacement of the knee in hemophilia. J. Bone Joint Surg., *61A*:69–75, 1979.

212. McLaughlin, G.E., McCarty, D.J., Jr., and Segal, B.L.: Hemarthrosis complicating anticoagulant therapy: report of three cases. JAMA, *196*:1020–1021, 1966.

213. McVerry, B.A., et al.: Ultrasonography in the management of hemophilia. Lancet, *1*:872–874, 1977.

214. Maner, J.F., Ratn, C.E., and Schreiner, G.E.: Hyperuricemia complicating leukemia: treatment with allopurinol and dialysis. Arch. Intern. Med., *123*:198–200, 1969.

215. Mainardi, C.L., et al.: Proliferative synovitis in hemophilia: biochemical and morphologic observations. Arthritis Rheum., *21*:137–144, 1978.

216. Mankin, H.J.: The reaction of articular cartilage to injury and osteoarthritis. N. Engl. J. Med., *291*:1,285–1,292, 1974.

217. Mannucci, P.M., et al.: Role of synovectomy in hemophilic arthropathy. Isr. J. Med. Sci., *13*:983–987, 1977.

218. Marmor, L.: Total knee replacement in hemophilia. Clin. Orthop., *125*:192–195, 1977.

219. Martel, W., Abell, M.R., and Duff, I.F.: Cervical spine involvement in lipoid dermato-arthritis. Radiology, *77*:613–617, 1961.

220. Martin, V.M., et al.: Lymphosarcomatous arthropathy. Ann. Rheum. Dis., *32*:162–166, 1973.

221. Mason, D.Y., and Ingram, G.I.: Management of the hereditary coagulation disorders. Semin. Hematol., *8*:158–188, 1971.

222. Mazza, J.J., et al.: Antihemophilic factor VIII in hemophilia: use of concentrates to permit major surgery. JAMA, *211*:1,818–1,823, 1970.

223. Melton, J.W., 3d and Irby, R.: Multicentric reticulohistiocytosis. Arthritis Rheum., *15*:221–226, 1972.

224. Mestecky, J., et al.: Properties of IgA myeloma proteins isolated from sera of patients with the hyperviscosity syndrome. J. Lab. Clin. Med., *89*:919–927, 1977.

225. Morley, C.J., Houston, I.B., and Morris-Jones, P.: Acute renal failure and gout as presenting features of acute lymphoblastic leukaemia. Arch. Dis. Child., *51*:723–725, 1976.

226. Moseley, J.E.: Bone Changes in Hematologic Disorders. New York, Grune and Stratton, 1963.

227. Moseley, P., et al.: Hemophilia, maintenance hemodialysis, and septic arthritis. Arch. Intern. Med., *141*:138–139, 1981.

228. Moser, H.W.: Ceramidase deficiency: Farber's lipogranulomatosis. *In* The Metabolic Basis of Inherited Disease. 4th Ed. Edited by J.B. Stanbury, J.B. Wyngaarden, and D.S. Fredrickson. New York, McGraw-Hill, 1978, pp. 707–717.

229. Moser, H.W., et al.: Farber's lipogranulomatosis: report of a case and demonstration of an excess of free ceramide and ganglioside. Am. J. Med., *47*:869–890, 1969.

230. Moxley, G.F., Owen, D.S., and Irby, R.: Septic arthritis due to Fusobacterium varium in patient with sickle-cell anemia. J. Rheumatol., *10*:161–162, 1983.

231. Muggia, F.M., Ball, T.J., Jr., and Ultmann, J.E.: Allopurinol in the treatment of neoplastic disease complicated by hyperuricemia. Arch. Intern. Med., *120*:12–18, 1967.

232. Nachamie, B.J., and Dorfman, H.D.: Ischemic necrosis of bone in sickle cell trait. Mt. Sinai. J. Med., *41*:527–536, 1974.

233. Nashel, D.J., Widerlite, L.W., and Pekin, T.J., Jr.: IgD myeloma with amyloid arthropathy. Am. J. Med., *55*:426–430, 1973.

234. Neufeld, A.H., Morton, H.S., and Halpenny, G.W.: Myelomatosis with xanthomatosis multiforme. Can. Med. Assoc. J., *91*:374–380, 1964.

235. Newcomer, L.N., et al.: Bone involvement in Hodgkin's disease. Cancer, *49*:338–342, 1982.

236. Nilsen, L.B., Missal, M.E., and Condemi, J.J.: Appearance of Hodgkin's disease in a patient with systemic lupus erythematosus. Cancer, *20*:1,930–1,933, 1967.

237. Nilsson-Ehle, H., et al.: Bone scintigraphy in the diagnosis of skeletal involvement and metastatic calcification in multiple myeloma. Acta Med. Scand., *21*:427–432, 1982.

238. Ober, W.B., et al.: Hemoglobin S-C disease with fat embolism. Am. J. Med., *27*:647–658, 1959.

239. O'Brien, J.R.: Effects of salicylates on human platelets. Lancet, *1*:779–783, 1968.

240. Oleinick, A.: Leukemia or lymphoma occurring subsequent to an autoimmune disease. Blood, *29*:144–153, 1967.

241. Orkin, M., et al.: A study of multicentric reticulohistiocytosis. Arch. Dermatol., *89*:640–654, 1964.

242. Paik, C.H., et al.: Thalassemia and gouty arthritis. JAMA, *213*:296–297, 1970.

243. Palmer, D.W.: Septic arthritis in sickle-cell thalassemia: pathophysiology of impaired response to infection. Arthritis Rheum., *18*:339–345, 1975.

244. Pear, B.L.: Skeletal manifestations of the lymphomas and leukemias. Semin. Roentgenol., *9*:229–240, 1974.

245. Peters, S.P., Lee, R.E., and Glew, R.H.: Gaucher's disease, a review. Medicine, *56*:425–442, 1977.

246. Philippart, M., Franklin, S.S., and Gordon, A.: Reversal of an inborn sphingolipidosis (Fabry's disease) by kidney transplantation. Ann. Intern. Med., *77*:195–200, 1972.

247. Pinkhas, J., Djaldetti, M., and Yaron, M.: Coincidence of multiple myeloma with Gaucher's disease. Isr. J. Med. Sci., *1*:537–540, 1965.

248. Pittelkow, R.B., Kierland, R.R., and Montgomery, H.: Angiokeratoma corporis diffusum. Arch. Dermatol., *72*:556–561, 1955.

249. Pope, A., et al.: Hairy cell leukemia and vasculitis. J. Rheumatol., *7*:895–899, 1980.

250. Post, M., and Telfer, M.C.: Surgery in hemophilic patients. J. Bone Joint Surg., *57A*:1,136–1,145, 1975.

251. Pouard, A.C., et al.: Enzymological diagnosis of a group of lysosomal storage diseases. Med. J. Aust., *2*:549–553, 1980.

252. Pratt, P.W., Estren, S., and Kochwa, S.: Immunoglobulin abnormalities in Gaucher's disease: report of 16 cases. Blood, *31*:633–640, 1968.

253. Pryzanski, W., and Watt, J.G.: Serum viscosity and hyperviscosity syndrome in IgG multiple myeloma: report on 10 patients and a review of the literature. Ann. Intern. Med., *77*:853–860, 1972.

254. Rabiner, S.F., and Telfer, M.C.: Home transfusion for patients with hemophilia A. N. Engl. J. Med., *283*:1,011–1,015, 1970.

255. Ramgren, O.: Haemophilia in Sweden. IV. Symptomatology, with special reference to differences between haemophilia A and B. Acta Med. Scand., *171*:237–242, 1962.

256. Ramgren, O. (ed.): Haemophilia in Sweden. Acta Med. Scand. (Suppl. 379), 1962.

257. Ratnoff, O.D., and Bennett, B.: The genetics of hereditary disorders of blood coagulation. Science, *179*:1,291–1,298, 1973.

258. Reynolds, J.: A re-evaluation of the "fish vertebra" sign in sickle cell hemoglobinopathy. AJR, *97*:693–707, 1966.

259. Reynolds, J.: The Roentgenological Features of Sickle Cell Disease, and Related Hemoglobinopathies. Springfield, IL, Charles C Thomas, 1965.

260. Reynolds, J.: An evaluation of some roentgenographic signs in sickle cell anemia and its variants. South. Med. J., *55*:1,123–1,128, 1962.

261. Rieselbach, R.E., et al.: Uric acid excretion and renal function in the acute hyperuricemia of leukemia: pathogenesis and therapy of uric acid nephropathy. Am. J. Med., *37*:872–884, 1964.

262. River, G.L., Robbins, A.B., and Schwartz, S.O.: S-C hemoglobin: a clinical study. Blood, *18*:385–416, 1961.

263. Rodey, G.E., et al.: Defective bactericidal activity of peripheral blood leukocytes in lipochrome histiocytosis. Am. J. Med., *49*:322–327, 1970.

264. Rodnan, G., et al.: Postmortem examination of an elderly severe hemophiliac, with observations on the pathologic findings in hemophilic joint disease. Arthritis Rheum., *2*:152–161, 1959.

265. Rodnan, G., et al.: Hemophilic arthritis. Bull. Rheum. Dis., *8*:137–138, 1957.

266. Rooney, P.J., et al.: Transient polyarthritis associated with familial hyperbetalipoproteinemia. Q. J. Med., *187*:249–259, 1978.

267. Rooney, P.J., Ballantyne, D., and Buchanan, W.W.: Disorders of the locomotor system associated with abnormalities of lipid metabolism and the lipoidoses. Clin. Rheum. Dis., *1*:163–193, 1975.

268. Rose, J.S., et al.: Accelerated skeletal deterioration after splenectomy in Gaucher type I disease. AJR, *139*:1,202–1,204, 1982.

269. Rosenberg, S.A., et al.: Lymphosarcoma: a review of 1269 cases. Medicine, *40*:31–84, 1961.

270. Rosenthal, R.L., Graham, J.J., and Selirio, E.: Excision of pseudotumor with repair by bone graft or pathological fracture of femur in hemophilia. J. Bone Joint Surg., *55A*:827–832, 1973.

271. Rosner, S.M., and Bhogal, R.S.: Infectious arthritis in a hemophiliac. J. Rheumatol., *8*:519–521, 1981.

272. Rothermel, J.E., and Raney, R.B.: The changing prognosis in hemophilic arthropathy. South. Med. J., *62*:1,340–1,342, 1969.

273. Rothschild, B.M., et al.: Sickle cell disease associated with uric acid deposition disease. Ann. Rheum. Dis., *39*:392–395, 1980.

274. Schaller, J.: Arthritis as a presenting manifestation of malignancy in children. J. Pediatr., *81*:793–797, 1972.

275. Schlumph, U., et al.: Arthritis in thalassemia minor. Schweiz. Med. Wochenschr., *107*:1,156–1,162, 1977.

276. Schubiner, H., Lefourdeau, M., and Murray, D.L.: Pyogenic osteomyelitis versus pseudo-osteomyelitis in Gaucher's disease. Clin. Pediatr., *20*:667–669, 1981.

277. Schumacher, H.R.: Rheumatological manifestations of

sickle cell disease and other hereditary haemoglobinopathies. Clin. Rheum. Dis., *1*:37–52, 1975.

278. Schumacher, H.R., Andrews, R., and McLaughlin, G.: Arthropathy in sickle-cell disease. Ann. Intern. Med., 78:203–211, 1973.

279. Schumacher, H.R., et al.: Chronic synovitis with early cartilage destruction in sickle cell disease. Ann. Rheum. Dis., *36*:413–419, 1977.

280. Scott, R.B., et al.: Neuropathic joint disease (Charcot joints) in Waldenstrom's macroglobulinemia with amyloidosis. Am. J. Med., *54*:535–538, 1973.

281. Seino, I., et al.: Peripheral hemodynamics in patients with Fabry's disease. Am. Heart J., *105*:783–787, 1983.

282. Seligmann, M., Cannat, A., and Hamad, M.: Studies on antinuclear antibodies. Ann. N.Y. Acad. Sci., *124*:816–832, 1965.

283. Seinsheimer, F., 3d, and Mankin, H.J.: Acute bilateral symmetrical pathologic fractures of the lateral tibial plateaus in a patient with Gaucher's disease. Arthritis Rheum., *20*:1,550–1,555, 1977.

284. Serjeant, G.R.: The clinical features in adults with sickle cell anaemia in Jamaica. West Indian Med. J., *19*:1–8, 1970.

285. Shapiro, J.R., et al.: Achilles tendinitis and tenosynovitis: a diagnostic manifestation of familial type II hyperlipoproteinemia in children. Am. J. Dis. Child., *128*:486–490, 1974.

286. Shelley, W.M., and Curtis, E.M.: Bone marrow and fat embolism in sickle cell anemia and sickle cell-hemoglobin C disease. Bull. Johns Hopkins Hosp., *103*:8–26, 1958.

287. Sherman, M.: Pathogenesis of disintegration of the hip in sickle cell anemia. South. Med. J., *52*:632–637, 1959.

288. Sherry, M.G.: The incidence of positive RA tests in Hodgkin's disease and leukemia. Am. J. Clin. Pathol., *50*:398–400, 1968.

289. Shiloni, E., et al.: The role of splenectomy in Gaucher's disease. Arch. Surg., *118*:929–932, 1983.

290. Shulman, N.R., et al.: The physiologic basis for therapy of classic hemophilia (factor VIII deficiency) and related disorders. Combined clinical staff conference at the National Institutes of Health. Ann. Intern. Med., 67:856–882, 1967.

291. Shulman, R.S., et al.: Beta-sitosterolemia and xanthomatosis. N. Engl. J. Med., *294*:482–483, 1976.

292. Siegelmann, S.S., et al.: Hyperlipoproteinemia with skeletal lesions. Clin. Orthop., *87*:228–232, 1972.

293. Silverman, F.N.: The skeletal lesions in leukemia: clinical and roentgenographic observations in 103 infants and children, with a review of the literature. AJR, *59*:819–844, 1948.

294. Silverstein, E., and Fiedland, J.: Angiotensin converting enzyme in cultured fibroblasts in Gaucher and Niemann-Pick disease. Proc. Soc. Exp. Biol. Med., *170*:251–253, 1982.

295. Silverstein, M.N., and Kelly, P.J.: Osteoarticular manifestations of Gaucher's disease. Am. J. Med. Sci., *253*:569–577, 1967.

296. Silverstein, M.N., and Kelly, P.J.: Leukemia with osteoarticular symptoms and signs. Ann. Intern. Med., 59:637–645, 1963.

297. Small, M., et al.: Total knee arthroplasty in hemophilic arthritis. J. Bone Joint Surg., 65:163–165, 1983.

298. Smith, C.K., Cassidy, J.T., and Bole, G.G.: Type I dysgammaglobulinemia, systemic lupus erythematosus and lymphoma. Am. J. Med., *48*:113–119, 1970.

299. Smith, E.W., and Conley, C.L.: Clinical features of the genetic variants of sickle cell disease. Bull. Johns Hopkins Hosp., *94*:289, 1954.

300. Smith, E.W., and Krevans, J.R.: Clinical manifestations of hemoglobin C disorders. Bull. Johns Hopkins Hosp., *104*:17–43, 1959.

301. Sokoloff, L.: Biochemical and physiological aspects of degenerative joint diseases with special reference to hemophilic arthropathy. Ann. N.Y. Acad. Sci., *240*:285–290, 1975.

302. Somerville, J.: Gout in cyanotic congenital heart disease. Br. Heart J., *23*:31–34, 1961.

303. Spaeth, G.L., and Frost, P.: Fabry's disease: its ocular manifestations. Arch Ophthalmol., *74*:760–769, 1965.

304. Spilberg, I., and Meyer, G.J.: The arthritis of leukemia. Arthritis Rheum., *15*:630–635, 1972.

305. Spranger, J.W., Langer, L.U., and Wiedemann, H.R.: Bone dysplasias—an atlas of constitutional disorders of skeletal development. Philadelphia, W.B. Saunders, 1974, p. 143.

306. Staas, W.E., Jr., et al.: Lower extremity amputation in hemophilia: case report and review of surgical principles. J. Bone Joint Surg., *54A*:1,514–1,522, 1972.

307. Steel, W.M., Duthie, R.B., and O'Connor, B.T.: Haemophilic cysts: report of five cases. J. Bone Joint Surg., *51B*:614–626, 1969.

308. Sterndale, H.: Haemarthrosis and haemophilia. Proc. R. Soc. Med., *60*:37–38, 1967.

309. Stoker, D.J., and Murray, R.U.: Skeletal changes in hemophilia and other bleeding disorders. Semin. Roentgenol., *9*:185–193, 1974.

310. Stone, M.J., and Frenkel, E.P.: The clinical spectrum of light chain myeloma: a study of 35 patients with special reference to the occurrence of amyloidosis. Am. J. Med., *58*:601–619, 1975.

311. Storti, E., et al.: Synovectomy in haemophilia arthropathy: a new approach to therapy and haemostasis. Schweiz. Med. Wochenschr., *100*:2,005–2,007, 1970.

312. Strauss, J., et al.: Cryoprecipitable immune complex nephropathy and sickle cell disease. Ann. Intern. Med., *81*:114–115, 1974.

313. Stuart, J., et al.: Haemorrhagic episodes in haemophilia: a 5-year prospective study. Br. Med. J., *2*:1,624–1,626, 1966.

314. Swanton, M.C.: Pathology of hemarthrosis in hemophilia. *In* Hemophilia and Hemophiloid Disease. Edited by K.M. Brinkous. Chapel Hill, University of North Carolina Press, 1957, pp. 219–224.

315. Sweeley, C.C., et al.: Fabry's disease; glycosphingolipid lipidosis. *In* The Metabolic Basis of Inherited Disease. 3rd Ed. Edited by J.B. Stanbury, J.B. Wyngaarden, and D.J. Fredrickson. New York, Blakiston-McGraw-Hill, 1972, pp. 663–687.

316. Talal, N., Sokoloff, L., and Barth, W.F.: Extrasalivary lymphoid abnormalities in Sjögren's syndrome (reticulum cell sarcoma, "pseudolymphoma", macroglobulinemia). Am. J. Med., *43*:50–65, 1967.

317. Talbott, J.H.: Gout and blood dyscrasias. 173–205. Medicine, *38*:173, 1959.

318. Tanaka, K.R., Clifford, G.U., and Axelrod, A.R.: Sickle cell anemia (homozygous S) with aseptic necrosis of femoral head. Blood, *11*:998–1,008, 1956.

319. Tani, M., et al.: Multicentric reticulohistiocytosis: electromicroscopic and ultracytochemical studies. Arch. Dermatol., *117*:495–499, 1981.

320. Tarnay, T.J.: Surgery in the Hemophiliac. Springfield, IL, Charles C Thomas, 1968.

321. Tarr, L., and Ferris, H.W.: Multiple myeloma: associated with nodular deposits of amyloid in the muscles and joints and with Bence Jones proteinura. Arch. Intern. Med., *64*:820–833, 1939.

322. Thannhauser, S.J.: Lipidoses: Disease of the Intracellular Lipid Metabolism. 3rd Ed. New York, Grune and Stratton, 1958.

323. Thiers, H., et al.: Acute dermatomyositis revealing Hodgkin's sarcoma. Lyon Med., *221*:954–957, 1969.

324. Thomas, H.B.: Some orthopaedic findings in ninety-eight cases of hemophilia. J. Bone Joint Surg., *18*:140–147, 1936.

325. Thomas, L.B., et al.: The skeletal lesions of acute leukemia. Cancer, *14*:608–621, 1961.

326. Thorne, J.C., et al.: Avascular necrosis of bone complicating treatment of malignant lymphoma. Am. J. Med., *71*:751–758, 1981.

327. Todd, R.M., and Keidan, S.E.: Changes in the head of the femur in children suffering from Gaucher's disease. J. Bone Joint Surg., *348*:447–453, 1952.

328. Trueta, J.: Orthopaedic management of patients with haemophilia and christmas disease. *In* Treatment of Haemophilia and Other Coagulation Disorders. Edited by R.

Biggs and R.G. Macfarlane. Oxford, Blackwell Scientific, 1966, pp. 279–323.

329. Truswell, A.S., and Pfister, P.J.: Cerebrotendinous xanthomatosis. Br. Med. J., *1*:353–354, 1972.

330. Tsachalos, P.: Gout secondary to thalassemia (minor form of Cooley's disease). Rev. Rheum., *27*:414–416, 1960.

331. Ultmann, J.E.: Hyperuricemia in disseminated neoplastic disease other than lymphomas and leukemias. Cancer, *15*:122–129, 1962.

332. Välimäki, M., Vuopio, P., and Liewendahl, K.: Bone lesions in chronic myelogenous leukemia. Acta Med. Scand., *210*:403–408, 1981.

333. Soebergen, E.M., et al.: T cell leukemia presenting as chronic polyarthritis. Arthritis Rheum., *25*:87–91, 1982.

334. Vermess, M., et al.: Osseous manifestations of Waldenstrom's macroglobulinemia. Radiology, *102*:497–504, 1972.

335. Vogler, W.R., et al.: Metabolic and therapeutic effects of allopurinol in patients with leukemia and gout. Am. J. Med., *40*:548–559, 1966.

336. Walker, B.R., et al.: Glomerular lesions in sickle cell nephropathy. JAMA, *215*:437–440, 1971.

337. Walker, B.R., and Alexander, F.: Uric acid excretion in sickle cell anemia. JAMA, *215*:255–258, 1971.

338. Walker, R.E.: Hyperlipoproteinemia and symptoms of the lower extremity. J. Am. Podiatry Assoc., *69*:370–375, 1979.

339. Warin, R.P., et al.: Reticulohistiocytosis (lipoid dermatoarthritis). Br. Med. J., *1*:1,387–1,391, 1957.

340. Wasserman, L.R., and Bassen, F.: Polycythemia. J. Mt. Sinai Hosp., *26*:1–49, 1959.

341. Watson, R.J., et al.: The hand-foot syndrome in sickle-cell disease in young children. Pediatrics, *31*:975–982, 1976.

342. Webb, J.B., and Dixon, A.St.J.: Haemophilia and haemophilic arthropathy: an historical review and a clinical study of 42 cases. Ann. Rheum. Dis., *19*:143–157, 1960.

343. Weglus, O., Skrifvars, B., and Anderson, L.: Rheumatoid arthritis terminating in plasmacytoma. Acta Med. Scand., *187*:133–138, 1970.

344. Weinberger, A., Schumacher, M.R., and Schimmer, B.M.: Arthritis in acute leukemia: clinical and histopathological observations. Arch. Intern. Med., *141*:1,183–1,187, 1981.

345. Weiss, H.J., Aledort, L.M., and Kochwa, S.: The effect of salicylates on the hemostatic properties of platelets in man. J. Clin. Invest., *47*:2,169–2,180, 1968.

346. Whitaker, J.A., et al.: Gout in childhood leukemia. J. Pediatr., *66*:961–963, 1963.

347. Wiernik, P.H.: Amyloid joint disease. Medicine, *51*:465–479, 1972.

348. Wild, J.H., and Zvaifler, N.J.: Hemarthrosis associated with sodium warfarin therapy. Arthritis Rheum., *19*:98–102, 1976.

349. Wilson, D.E., et al.: Multiple myeloma, cryoglobulinemia and xanthomatosis: distinct clinical and biochemical syndromes in two patients. Am. J. Med., *59*:721–729, 1975.

350. Wilson, W.A., Hughes, G.R., and Lachmann, P.J.: Deficiency of factor B of the complement system in sickle cell anaemia. Br. Med. J., *1*:367–369, 1976.

351. Wise, D., Wallace, H.J., and Jellinek, E.H.: Angiokeratoma corporis diffusum. Q. J. Med., *31*:177–206, 1961.

352. Wolf, C.R., and Mankin, H.J.: The effect of experimental hemarthrosis on articular cartilage of rabbit knee joints. J. Bone Joint Surg., *47A*:1,203–1,210, 1965.

353. Worrall, V.T., and Butera, V.: Sickle-cell dactylitis. J. Bone Joint Surg., *58A*:1,161–1,163, 1976.

354. Wrizman, Z., Tennenbaum, A., and Yatziv, S.: Interphalangeal joint involvement in Gaucher's disease, Type I, resembling juvenile rheumatoid arthritis. Arthritis Rheum., *25*:706–707, 1982.

355. Wyngaarden, J.B., and Kelley, W.N.: Gout. *In* The Metabolic Basis of Inherited Disease. 4th Ed. Edited by J.B. Stanbury, J.B. Wyngaarden, and D.S. Fredrickson. New York, McGraw-Hill, 1978, pp. 916–1,010.

356. Yu, T-F.: Secondary gout associated with myeloproliferative diseases. Arthritis Rheum., *8*:765–771, 1965.

357. Yu, T-F., et al.: Secondary gout associated with chronic myeloproliferative disorders. Semin. Arthritis Rheum., *5*:247–256, 1976.

358. Yu, T-F., and Gutman, A.B.: Uric acid nephrolithiasis in gout: predisposing factors. Ann. Intern. Med., *67*:1,133–1,148, 1967.

359. Yu, T-F., and Gutman, A.B.: Effect of allopurinol (4-hydroxypyrazolo-(3,4-d)pyrimidine) on serum and urinary uric acid in primary and secondary gout. Am. J. Med., *37*:885–898, 1964.

360. Zawadzki, Z.A., and Benedek, T.G.: Rheumatoid arthritis, dysproteinemic arthropathy, and paraproteinemia. Arthritis Rheum., *12*:555–568, 1969.

361. Zayid, I., and Farraj, S.: Familial histiocytic dermatoarthritis: a new syndrome. Am. J. Med., *54*:793–800, 1973.

Chapter 75

Heritable and Developmental Disorders of Connective Tissues and Bone

Victor A. McKusick and Reed E. Pyeritz

Theoretically, any disorder can be described or studied by two fundamental approaches: etiology and pathogenesis. Either can be useful, depending on the need. Understanding cause(s) leads to reliable classification, diagnosis, and prevention; understanding mechanisms leads to effective prognosis and treatment. Unfortunately, the two approaches are often thought to be similar or even interchangeable—misconceptions that confuse nosology, management, and clinical investigation. Knowledge of etiology, no matter how refined, may shed no light on how the clinical manifestations (the phenotype) develop. For example, the "cause" of sickle cell disease is known at the highest level of resolution possible, the specific nucleotide mutation, whereas the mechanisms by which the diverse clinical features appear remain largely obscure. Alternatively, the pathogenesis of acute gout is far better understood than is the etiology in most cases.

Consideration of the role of genetic factors in the disorders of a given system perforce focuses on etiology. The traditional approach has been to divide all disorders into mendelian, chromosomal, and multifactorial categories. This scheme retains some didactic utility, provided one recognizes that no disorder is purely genetic or environmental in cause, and that all involve some interaction of genes and environment to produce the phenotype that we recognize as abnormal.

In *mendelian disorders,* a single mutant gene is of overriding importance, although its effect may be modulated by other genetic and environmental factors. These conditions occur in families in simple inheritance patterns, i.e., autosomal dominant, autosomal recessive, or X-linked. Nearly all these disorders are individually rare (prevalences of $1/10^4$ to $1/10^6$ in the general population), but because so many are now known (3,368 in one tabulation[58]), in the aggregate they represent a substantial category of disease. The heritable disorders of connective tissue represent examples.

A *chromosomal disorder* is defined by the occurrence of an abnormal phenotype in association with a visible aberration of the karyotype. Heretofore, this category of disorders included complex malformations involving multiple organ systems, such as trisomy 21 (Down's syndrome) or the XO (Turner) syndrome. As improved cytogenetic techniques have greatly enhanced resolution, conditions once thought to be due to single gene mutations are being associated with miniscule defects in chromosome structure. Examples are retinoblastoma and the Prader-Willi syndrome, both caused by deletions of small parts of the long arms of chromosomes 13 and 15, respectively. The connective tissues are particularly affected in trisomy 8 (skeletal dysplasia, scoliosis, genu valgum); in most other disorders, connective tissue abnormalities are of relatively minor functional significance.

The term *multifactorial* has a specific and a general meaning. Disorders such as pyloric stenosis, clubfoot, and idiopathic scoliosis, which conform to empiric predictions of recurrence, concordance in monozygotic twins, and prevalence between sexes, are classified as multifactorial in the narrow sense.[37] On the other hand, any condition in which genes are a necessary, but insufficient, part of the cause and which are distributed in families in ways that do not fulfill any mendelian pattern can be described as multifactorial in the broad sense. Disorders in this latter category tend to be relatively common and include much of what is diagnosed as rheumatoid arthritis, osteoarthritis, and the "acquired" disorders of connective tissue (e.g., lupus and scleroderma).

Several excellent texts provide comprehensive coverage of genetic principles fundamental to an understanding of these concepts and those that will emerge from review of individual disorders.[22,59,66,78,92]

HERITABLE DISORDERS OF CONNECTIVE TISSUES AND BONE

The classification of these disorders reflects a varied appreciation of etiology and a reliance on purely descriptive aspects of the phenotypes. About 100 distinct, mendelian disorders of connective tissue are now known, and once the depths of genetic heterogeneity are plumbed, including allelic variations, the number will be many times greater. Nonetheless, only a handful warrant discussion because of their relevance to clinical rheumatology and their relative commonness (amyloidosis[56] and alkaptonuria are discussed in Chapters 72 and 96, respectively).

In Table 75–1 these disorders are grouped according to whether the known or suspected basic biochemical defect[44] involves primarily fibrous connective tissue elements (collagen or elastin), ground substance (mucopolysaccharide), cartilage and bone, or some other metabolic process that secondarily affects connective tissue.

Marfan Syndrome

Patients with the Marfan syndrome tend to have major abnormalities in the skeletal, ocular, cardiovascular, and pulmonary systems.[71,75] The diagnosis is based solely on the clinical features and the autosomal dominant inheritance pattern.[75] The basic defect is unknown, although individual patients with abnormalities of collagen and elastin have been studied. Unquestionably, the Marfan phenotype will prove to be due to a variety of single-gene mutations.[33,73,90]

Skeletal Features. Patients with the Marfan syndrome are excessively tall, or at least taller than unaffected relatives (Fig. 75–1). Body proportions are irregular (dolichostenomelia), with an abnormally low ratio of the upper segment to the lower segment (US/LS). In practice, two measurements are made with the patient standing: height and lower segment (top of the pubic symphysis to floor). In normal adult white persons, the mean ratio is about 0.92; in adult black persons, it is about 0.87. The excessive length of the lower extremities is primarily responsible for the abnormally low US/LS in the Marfan syndrome. The US/LS varies with age, race, sex, and degree of vertebral column deformity in all persons, so that an isolated determination in a suspected patient must be interpreted with caution. The arms also show excessive length, with the span of adult patients usually exceeding their height by more than 3%. The metacarpal index, based on the ratio of length to width of metacarpals, is said to be useful but requires a radiograph of the hands.

The ribs undergo the excessive longitudinal growth as well. Depression of the sternum (pectus excavatum), protrusion (pectus carinatum; see Fig. 75–1), or an asymmetric combination thereof often results.

The vertebral column is frequently deformed.

Most often, the normal thoracic kyphos is lost, resulting in a "straight back" or an outright thoracic lordosis. Scoliosis may involve multiple segments and may progress rapidly, particularly during the adolescent growth spurt.

Loose-jointedness is often striking in patients with the Marfan syndrome. Flat feet (pes planus), hyperextensibility at the knees (genu recurvatum), elbows, and fingers, and congenital dislocation of the hip are manifestations of the loose-jointedness. Because of both the joint laxity and the long limbs, the patient is often able to touch his umbilicus with his right hand passed around his back, and approaching his umbilicus from the left. A relatively narrow palm of the hand, long thumb, and longitudinal laxity of the hand are the bases for the Steinberg thumb sign (Fig. 75–2): the thumb apposed across the palm extends well beyond the ulnar margin of the hand. Another simple, but nonspecific, test is the wrist sign.[94] The first and fifth digits, when wrapped around the contralateral wrist, overlap appreciably in the Marfan syndrome (Fig. 75–3).

Joint laxity is a variable finding, even among relatives affected by the Marfan syndrome.[93] About 10% of patients have some *restriction* of extension at one or more joints, usually of congenital onset. Thus, while a separate congenital contractural arachnodactyly syndrome undoubtedly exists,[8] all patients with this signal feature should be evaluated as if they had the Marfan syndrome so that serious problems in other systems are not overlooked.[27]

Other Features. Most patients with the Marfan syndrome have myopia, and about half have subluxation of the lenses (ectopia lentis). The ascending aorta bears the main stress of ventricular ejection, leading to progressive dilatation beginning in the sinuses of Valsalva. Resultant dissection and/or aortic regurgitation are the main causes of death.[70] Before the development of reliable surgical procedures and their early application,[57,72] life expectancy was reduced, on average, one-third in patients with the Marfan syndrome. Mitral valve prolapse occurs in 80% of patients and leads to severe mitral regurgitation in about 10%.[70] Hernias are frequent, cystic changes in the lungs lead to pneumothorax, and striae distensae over the pectoral and deltoid areas and thighs are often seen in teen-age patients. Dural ectasia is usually an incidental finding on myelography or CT scanning of the vertebral column; occasional patients have problems with spinal fluid dynamics or spinal anesthesia as a consequence.

Management of the Skeletal Manifestations. Most Marfan patients can lead long and productive lives, especially now that the success of cardiovascular surgery in repairing the aorta has im-

Table 75–1. Common Heritable Disorders of Connective Tissue and Bone

Disorder	Major Skeletal Features	Other Features	Inheritance
Disorders of Fibrous Connective Tissue			
Marfan syndrome	arachnodactyly, tall stature, scoliosis, joint laxity, anterior chest deformity	ectopia lentis, aortic dilatation, mitral valve prolapse	AD
Ehlers-Danlos syndrome			
type I and II	joint hypermobility	skin hyperextensibility, poor wound healing	AD
type III	joint hypermobility		AD
type XI	joint instability		AD
Osteogenesis imperfecta			
type I	fractures, bone deformity, +/− short stature	blue sclerae, deafness, +/− opalescent teeth	AD
type II	multiple in utero fractures, ↓ calvarial calcification	blue sclerae, pulmonary hypertension, neonatal death	AR, AD
type III	severe bone deformity, short stature, kyphoscoliosis	variable	AR, AD sporadic
type IV	fractures, bone deformity, +/− short stature	normal sclerae, deafness, +/− opalescent teeth	AD
Disorders of Ground Substance			
Mucopolysaccharidoses	short stature, joint stiffness, dysostosis multiplex, odontoid hypoplasia	coarse facies, +/− mental retardation, cardiac disease	AR X-L (MPS II)
Mucolipidoses II and III	short stature, joint stiffness, dysostosis multiplex	coarse facies, mental retardation, cardiac involvement	AR
Osteochondrodysplasias			
Achondroplasia	rhizomelic dwarfism, genu varum, megalocranium, spinal stenosis, elbow contractures		AD
Multiple epiphyseal dysplasia	variable arthropathy (esp. hips) and short stature		AD
Spondyloepiphyseal dysplasia congenita tarada	severe dwarfism, odontoid hypoplasia, cleft palate, scoliosis	myopia, retinal detachment	AD
Diastrophic dysplasia	variable hip arthropathy symphalangism, club foot, scoliosis, dwarfism, "hitchhiker thumb"	calcified pinna	X-L AR
Larsen syndrome	marked joint hypermobility and instability, +/− short stature		AR, AD
Metabolic Defects with Secondary Effects on Connective Tissue			
Homocystinuria	dolichostenomelia, osteoporosis, joint stiffness, scoliosis	ectopia lentis, thromboembolism	AR
Alkaptonuria	spondylosis, ochronosis, degenerative arthropathy	aortic stenosis, pigmented sclerae	AR

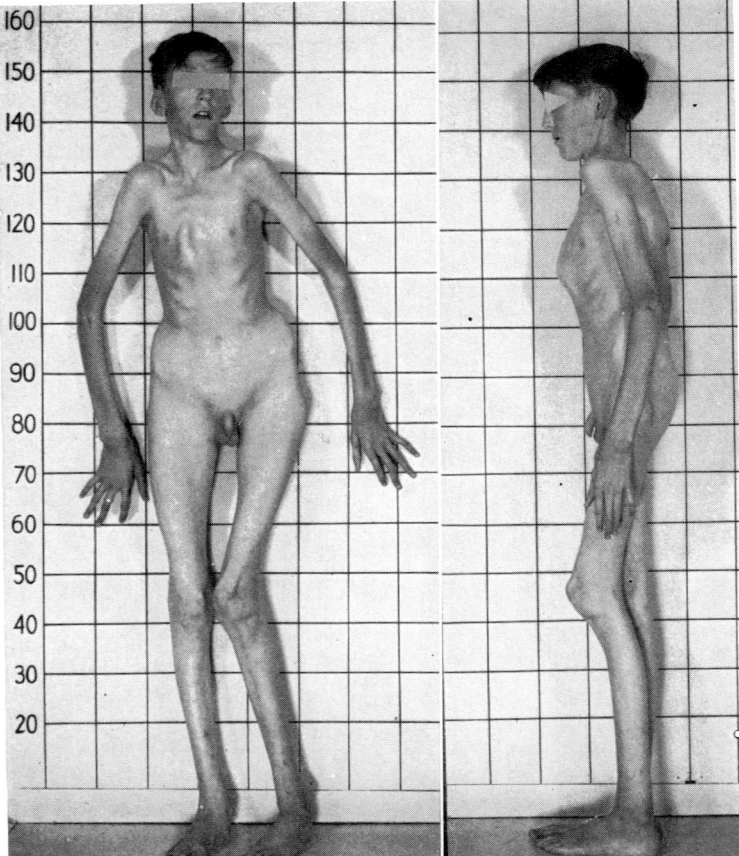

Fig. 75–1. Marfan syndrome in a 14-year-old boy. Note arachnodactyly, relatively long limbs (dolichostenomelia), pectus carinatum, sparse subcutaneous fat, unilateral genu valgum, and pes planus. Ectopia lentis and scoliosis were also present. This patient died of aortic rupture at 15 years of age.

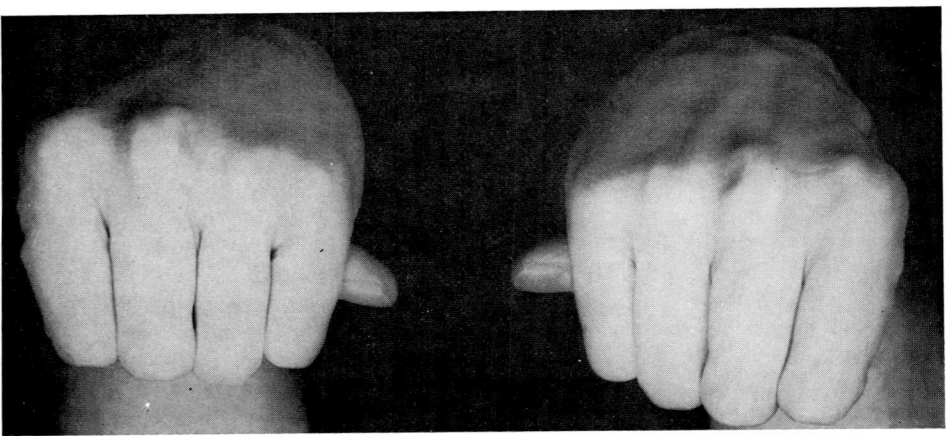

Fig. 75–2. The thumb sign in a patient with Marfan syndrome. A positive test, such as this, consists of the distal phalanx of the thumb protruding beyond the ulnar border of the clenched fist and reflects both longitudinal laxity of the hand and a long thumb.

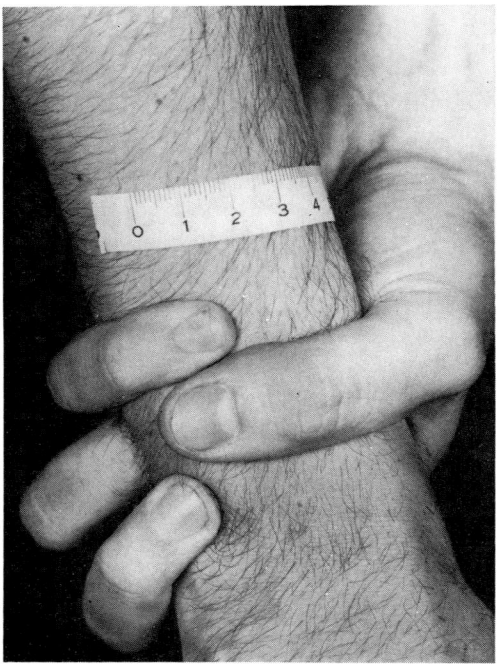

Fig. 75–3. The wrist sign in a patient with Marfan syndrome. In a positive test, the first phalanges of the thumb and fifth digit substantially overlap when wrapped around the opposite wrist.[94]

proved.[57,72] Thus, all patients deserve aggressive and appropriate management of all organ systems at risk. For the skeletal system, management must begin in childhood, because most problems are progressive during the years of growth.

Initial management of vertebral column deformity is by bracing. If abnormal curves can be stabilized, wearing the brace for 22 hours or more each day is necessary until the skeleton matures. The presence of thoracic lordosis, rather common in the Marfan syndrome, unfortunately limits the effectiveness of most braces. Whenever scoliotic curves exceed 40 to 45°, surgical stabilization and fusion are required.

Tall stature per se is usually not a problem in males. Girls, on the other hand, often suffer much psychosocial turmoil as a result of their height. Cross-sectional growth curves show that the average height for girls parallels the ninety-fifth percentile of the normal female growth curve; the average adult height is thus close to 6 feet.[71,75] Early induction of puberty by administration of ethinyl estradiol (0.05 mg/10 kg in a single oral dose daily) and medroxyprogesterone (2.5 mg/10 kg on days 25 to 28) results in accelerated skeletal maturation. If therapy is begun well before the age of physiologic menarche (we begin around 7 to 8 years of age), then adult height is clearly lessened.[71] Furthermore, by accelerating the "adolescent" growth spurt, there is less time for scoliosis to progress, and deformity is mitigated. Once the epiphyses are nearly fused or once the girl attains the age of physiologic menarche, hormonal therapy can be discontinued.

Deformity of the anterior chest also tends to worsen during adolescence as a result of rapid rib growth. Repair of either pectus excavatum or pectus carinatum for cosmetic indications should thus be delayed until mid-adolescence, when the defect is not likely to recur.

It is uncommon for disability to result from hyperextensibility at other joints. Dislocation of the patella and the first metacarpal-phalangeal joints, severe pes planus, and metatarsus valgus are the most frequent, often occurring in the same patient. Physical therapy, muscular strengthening, and well-fitted shoes are useful. Surgery for these problems should be avoided if possible.

Homocystinuria

Homocystinuria is an inborn error in the metabolism of methionine in which activity of the enzyme cystathionine synthase is deficient. Clinical features are superficially similar to those of the Marfan syndrome and include ectopia lentis, dolichostenomelia, arachnodactyly, and chest and spinal deformity (Fig. 75–4). Generalized osteoporosis, "tight" joints, arterial and venous thrombosis, malar flush, and mental retardation are features of homocystinuria usually not found in the Marfan syndrome.[59,63] Aortic aneurysm and mitral regurgitation are not features of homocystinuria. Back pain due to osteoporosis occurs in some patients. The hand in homocystinuria has none of the longitudinal laxity present in the Marfan syndrome, and the appendicular joints tend to have reduced mobility. Homocystinuria is an autosomal recessive disorder, like all other Garrodian inborn errors of metabolism and unlike the Marfan syndrome, which is a dominant trait.

The pathogenesis of the three cardinal groups of manifestations—mental retardation, connective tissue disorder (ectopia lentis, osteoporosis, reduced joint mobility), and thrombosis—is not understood. It is suspected that sulfhydryl groups of homocysteine or other substances that accumulate proximal to the block interfere with collagen cross-linking, thus accounting for the connective tissue manifestations. If true, this condition is a form of thiolism such as occurs from prolonged administration of penicillamine, a compound structurally similar to homocysteine (see Chap. 31).

Over half the patients with homocystinuria respond to large doses of vitamin B_6 (pyridoxine)

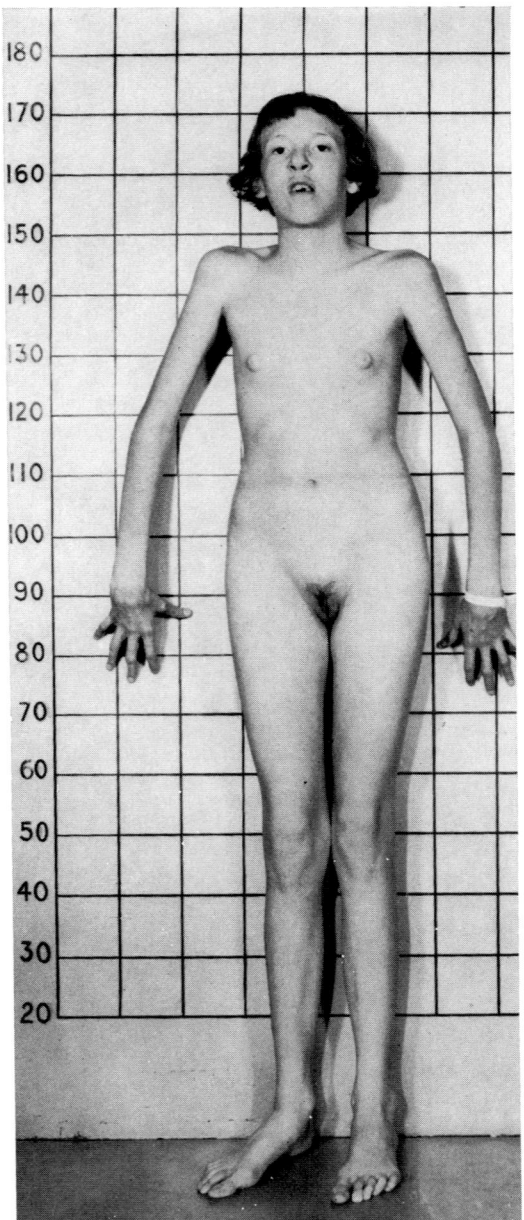

Fig. 75–4. Homocystinuria in a 12-year-old girl. Note the excessive height, long, narrow feet, and mild anterior chest deformity. The teeth were crowded, ectopia lentis was present, and the joints showed moderate restriction of motion. Despite several episodes of pulmonary embolism and thrombophlebitis, she was active at 35 years of age.

with clearing of homocystine from the urine, lowering of plasma methionine and raising of cystine to normal, and reducing the likelihood of developing clinical manifestations. Preexistent mental retardation and ectopia lentis are not improved by pyridoxine treatment in patients who show biochemical correction, emphasizing the need for early diagnosis and therapy. Because most states include testing for elevated blood methionine as part of the newborn screening program, early treatment is now feasible. With supplementary folic acid (1 mg daily), as little as 20 mg of vitamin B_6 daily may be effective, although usually a dosage of 100 or 300 mg or even more is required. In vitamin B_6 nonresponders, a low methionine diet is the mainstay of management,[91] although pyridoxine and folate should be included because of a tendency for unsupplemented patients to develop deficiency of these cofactors.[69] In addition, sulfinpyrazone, dipyridamole, or aspirin, singly or in combination, may be useful in preventing thrombotic episodes in all homocystinurics, even though platelet survival has proved to be normal in all patients.[29,32,63]

Weill-Marchesani Syndrome

The Weill-Marchesani syndrome is another systemic disorder with ectopia lentis as a conspicuous feature (Fig. 75–5). The skeletal features are the antithesis of those in the Marfan syndrome: The patients are short of stature, with particularly short hands and feet, and have stiff joints, especially in the hands. The hands sometimes show atrophy of the abductor pollicis brevis muscle consistent with carpal tunnel compression.[59] The Weill-Marchesani syndrome is autosomal recessive, but heterozygotes are shorter of stature than average.[45]

The Ehlers-Danlos Syndromes

The Ehlers-Danlos syndromes (EDS) are a group of disorders of wide phenotypic variability, largely due to extensive genetic heterogeneity. The cardinal features relate to the joints and skin: hyperextensibility of skin, easy bruisability, increased joint mobility, and abnormal tissue fragility. Internal manifestations, which include rupture of great vessels, hiatal hernia, diverticulum of the gastrointestinal and genitourinary tracts, spontaneous rupture of the bowel, and spontaneous pneumothorax, tend to occur only in specific types of EDS.

Eleven general EDS types are now accepted on the basis of phenotypic and inheritance characteristics (Table 75–2). Biochemical studies have, however, demonstrated considerable heterogeneity within individual types.[17,34,44,68] This extensive phenotypic and biochemical characterization nonetheless fails the clinician as often as it helps; nearly

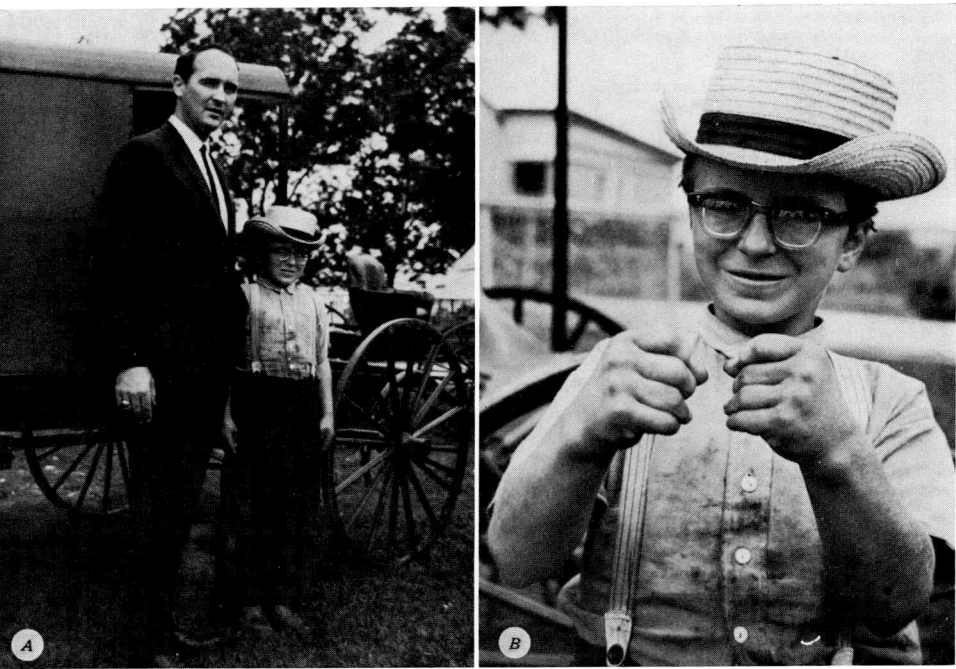

Fig. 75–5.   Weill-Marchesani syndrome in a 15-year-old Amish boy. *A,* Shown with normal adult male. Ectopia lentis was present, and attacks of acute glaucoma had occurred. *B,* The fingers were short with knobby joints and restricted flexion. Flattening of the thenar eminence was consistent with carpal tunnel compression.

half of all patients who have at least one "cardinal" manifestation defy categorization.[35]

EDS I (Gravis Form) and EDS II (Mitis Form).   Generalized hyperextensibility of joints (Fig. 75–6), together with stretchability of skin, leads to characterization of the affected persons as "India rubber men." Other features are bruising and fragility of the skin, with many gaping wounds from minor trauma and poor retention of sutures.[9,60] Congenital dislocation of the hips in the newborn, habitual dislocation of selected joints in later life, joint effusions, clubfoot deformity of the feet, and spondylolisthesis are all consequences of the loose-jointedness. Hemarthroses and "hemarthritic disability" have been described and are comparable to the bruising of the skin and bleeding at other sites, which occur in this syndrome. Scoliosis is sometimes severe. Severe leg cramps occurring at rest and of unclear cause are troublesome to some patients.

Both of these types are inherited as autosomal dominant traits, and tend to breed true within a family. They differ from one another only in severity; hence, the differentiation is somewhat more subjective than desired (Fig. 75–7). The biochemical defect(s) have not been characterized in either type, although abnormalities of collagen (probably type I collagen) undoubtedly will be found in most cases.

Management of both EDS I and II stresses prevention of trauma and great care in treating wounds. Some patients, particularly young boys, wear shin guards to protect their lower legs from the repeated minor injuries that lead to frequent hemorrhage, absence from school, and unsightly scars. Patients should be dissuaded from demonstrating their joint laxity as entertainment for their friends. Because the ligaments and joint capsules are lax, only the muscles can be developed to improve joint stability. Care must be employed, however, in weight lifting and other forms of exercise because of fragility of tendons.

EDS III (Benign Hypermobility Form).   This condition lacks the skin manifestations of the previous two types. The joint hyperextensibility ranges from the extreme to that which borders on the normal.[9] In fact, many patients with mild joint laxity without joint instability are often labeled as EDS III, particularly if relatives show a similar manifestation. In some cases, such labeling causes more harm than good, unless one makes it clear that little if any disability is likely to result.

EDS IV (Arterial Form).   This condition is by far the most serious type of EDS because of a propensity for spontaneous rupture of arteries and

Table 75–2. Ehlers-Danlos Syndromes

Type	Inheritance	Skeletal Features	Other Features	Basic Defect
I	AD	marked joint hypermobility	skin hyperextensibility and fragility	?
II	AD	less severe than type I		?
III	AD	marked joint hypermobility	none	?
IV	AR, AD	hypermobile digits	skin and bowel rupture	deficient type III collagen
V	X-L	similar to type II		?
VI	AR	marked joint hypermobility	rupture of globe	lysyl hydroxylase
VII	AR, AD	marked joint hypermobility and dislocations; short stature	minimal skin change	defect in procollagen cleavage
VIII	AD	variable joint hypermobility	periodontitis	?
IX	X-L	mild joint hypermobility	variable skin changes, bladder diverticula	defect in copper metabolism
X	AD	mild joint hypermobility	mild skin changes; MVP	defect in fibronectin
XI	AD	joint dislocations	mild or no skin change	?

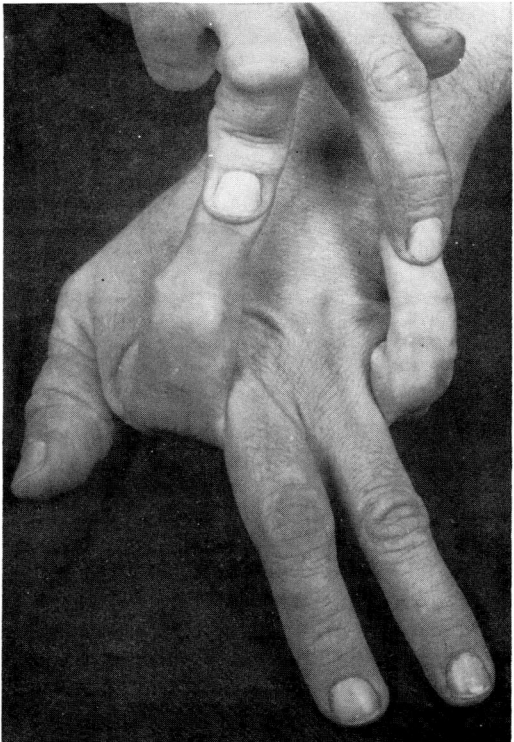

Fig. 75–6. Joint hypermobility in the Ehlers-Danlos syndrome, type I.

bowel. This type is particularly heterogeneous genetically, the unifying theme being abnormal production of type III collagen.[13] Skin involvement is variable, with thin, nearly translucent skin present in some, and mildly hyperextensible skin the only feature in others. Joint laxity is also variable, but is generally limited to the digitis. Inheritance can be either autosomal recessive or dominant.

EDS V. There is little question that an X-linked recessive form of EDS exists; it has been labeled type V.[10] The phenotype, not particularly distinctive, resembles EDS II most closely. Although a deficiency of lysyl oxidase was claimed in one pedigree,[19] this deficiency has not been confirmed or found in any other family.

EDS VI (Ocular-Scoliotic Form). Fragility of the ocular globe and a propensity to severe scoliosis, in addition to the skin and joint involvement seen in EDS I, are the hallmarks of this autosomal recessive form of EDS.[59] Collagen in this condition contains little hydroxylysine because of deficiency of the enzyme that hydroxylates selected lysyl residues in the nascent collagen chains.[46] Because hydroxylysine is normally involved, along with lysine, in cross-linking of collagen, the clinical feature of EDS VI is readily explained. Vitamin C

is a necessary cofactor of lysyl hydroxylase and, in high doses, may be beneficial in some cases of EDS VI[21] (comparable to the benefit of vitamin B_6 in some cases of homocystinuria).

EDS VII (Arthrochalasis Multiplex Congenita). Profound loose-jointedness with congenital dislocations dominates the clinical picture. The patients are moderately short of stature and the skin is variably, but usually mildly, involved.[30,59] An inability to convert type I procollagen to mature collagen has been found in the few patients who have been studied.[54] This defect, however, is genetically heterogeneous. Deficiency of procollagen N-peptidase, the enzyme that cleaves the propeptide from the amino-terminal end of type I procollagen, was said in one report to be deficient in fibroblasts from several patients.[54] One patient was subsequently found to have normal N-peptidase activity but an amino acid sequence alteration around the site of the procollagen molecule where cleavage occurs.[88] True deficiency of peptidase activity is likely an autosomal recessive trait, although direct proof is lacking. The amino acid sequence mutation occurred in only one of the alpha_1 (I) alleles. This finding suggested that the condition in that patient was an autosomal dominant trait resulting from a new mutation because the parents were unaffected.

EDS VIII (Periodontitis Form). This rare condition is characterized by severe periodontal disease, with early loss of both primary and permanent teeth. Presence of EDS I-like manifestations has varied in the few reported kindreds.[34,59] The basic defect is unknown, and inheritance is autosomal dominant.

EDS IX (Occipital Horn Form). The phenotype is defined by EDS II-like skin and joint involvement, bladder diverticula (often presenting as an obstructive uropathy), inferior cranial spurs (occipital horns), and a generalized skeletal dysplasia with osteoporosis. Only males have been found to be affected in kindreds, and X-linked recessive inheritance seems certain. Early reports of this condition affixed the name X-linked cutis laxa because of moderate skin laxity in some patients.[12] Deficient activity of lysyl oxidase was reported in several pedigrees.[12,34] Studies of a Finnish pedigree demonstrate a primary abnormality of copper metabolism (with low serum copper and ceruloplasmin as in Menkes syndrome) that results in secondarily diminished production of lysyl oxidase.[47]

EDS X (Fibronectin Deficiency). One pedigree was reported with a phenotype inherited as an autosomal recessive characterized by features of EDS II associated with abnormal platelet aggregation.[3] The platelet defect was corrected by exogenous plasma fibronectin; subsequent investi-

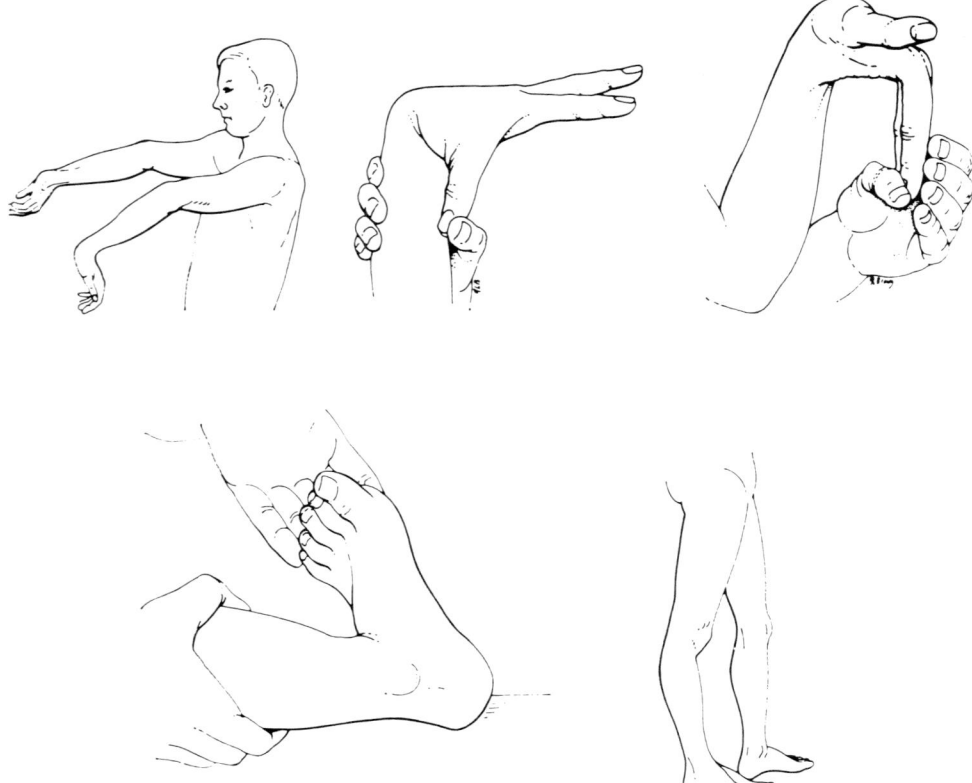

Fig. 75–7.   A method for evaluating joint mobility.[14,98] Excessive joint laxity is judged to exist when at least three of the following five conditions are present: (1) elbows and (2) knees extend beyond 180°; (3) thumb touches the forearm on flexing the wrist; (4) fingers are parallel to the forearm on extending the wrist and metacarpal joints; and (5) foot dorsiflexes to 45° or more.

gation of the patients' fibronectin has suggested a defect in glycosylation.

EDS XI (Familial Joint Instability).   The cardinal feature of this autosomal dominant condition is instability of multiple appendicular joints; recurrent dislocation is the usual clinical finding. Joint hyperextensibility is variable but usually mild, and skin involvement is uncommon.[39] EDS XI is one of the most common of the EDS variants. It is often associated with considerable disability. Clinical variability within a family is the rule, emphasizing the need for a comprehensive family history, including examination of close relatives if possible.

EDS XI is an extremely difficult condition to manage successfully. Most patients have had the diagnosis established only after multiple orthopedic surgical attempts (usually disappointing) to prevent recurrent dislocation of shoulders, knees, or elbows. As in EDS I and II, physical therapy of affected joints to increase periarticular muscle strength should be attempted first.

No basic biochemical defect has been elucidated in EDS XI, and its relationship to the Larsen syndrome has not been investigated.

The Larsen Syndrome

The Larsen syndrome is characterized by multiple congenital dislocations and characteristic facies: prominent forehead, depressed nasal bridge, and widely spaced eyes.[49] Dislocation occurs at the knees (characteristically anterior displacement of the tibia on the femur), hips, and elbows. The metacarpals are short, with cylindrical fingers lacking the usual tapering. Cleft palate, hydrocephalus, abnormalities of spinal segmentation, and moderate-to-severe short stature have occurred in some. Several instances of multiple affected sibs with normal parents are known, suggesting autosomal recessive inheritance, but parent-child involvement also occurs, consistent with dominant inheritance. Thus, two clinically indistinguishable forms of the Larsen syndrome may exist.[58]

Osteogenesis Imperfecta Syndromes

Several phenotypically distinct osteogenesis imperfecta (OI) syndromes, and even more classification schemes, exist.[23,24,59,84] The disorders share osseous, ocular, dental, aural, and cardiovascular involvement. The classification enjoying current application is based on clinical and inheritance pattern criteria[52,85] (Table 75–3). At the current rapid pace of defining basic biochemical defects in collagen, a nosology grounded in objective data is a reasonable expectation[6,7] (see Chap. 10).

Type I OI is the most common form and is associated with wide intrafamilial variability.[51,85] One patient might be markedly short of stature, with frequent fractures and much disability, whereas an affected relative leads an unencumbered, vigorous life. Type II encompasses the classic "OI congenita" variants, nearly all of which are lethal in infancy, if not in utero.[67] Molecular characterization of type II is progressing most rapidly, at both the collagen and the DNA level.[5] Some cases arise as the result of a new mutation (the phenotype thus being transmissible as a dominant, if the patient could live and reproduce) while others have affected sibs and normal but sometimes consanguineous parents, consistent with autosomal recessive inheritance.[59] Type III comprises miscellaneous phenotypes that cannot be classified better. Most cases include severe skeletal deformity and short stature as distinguishing features. Most occur sporadically. Type IV is similar to type I, only rarer and not associated with blue sclerae.

Skeletal Features. "Brittle bones" are a familiar and dramatic feature of all the OI variants. Sometimes fractures occur in utero, particularly in type II, and permit radiographic antenatal diagnosis. In such cases, the limbs are likely to be short and bent at birth. Multiple rib fractures give a characteristic "beaded" appearance on radiographs.

Other patients with types I or IV have few fractures or may escape them entirely, although blue sclerae or deafness indicates the presence of the mutant gene. Brittleness and deformability result from a defect in the collagenous matrix of bone. The skeletal aspect of OI is, therefore, a hereditary form of osteoporosis. "Codfish vertebrae" (scalloping of the superior and inferior vertebral bodies by pressure from the expansile intervertebral disc) or flat vertebrae are observed, particularly in older patients in whom senile or postmenopausal changes exaggerate the change, or young patients immobilized after fractures or orthopedic surgery. Usually the frequency of fractures decreases at puberty for patients with types I, III, and IV. Because of failure of union of fractures, pseudoarthrosis (e.g., of humerus or femur) occurs in some. Hypertrophic callus occurs frequently in patients with osteogenesis imperfecta and is often difficult to distinguish from osteosarcoma. Debate continues as to whether the risk of true osteosarcoma is increased in any form of OI; regardless, the risk is not great, but worthy of consideration whenever skeletal pain occurs in the absence of fracture, particularly in an older patient. Loose-jointedness is sometimes striking in type I OI; dislocation of joints can result from deformity secondary to repeated fracture, ligamentous laxity, or rupture of tendons (especially the Achilles and patellar).

Ocular Features. Blue sclerae are present in types I, II, and III and represent a valuable clue to the diagnosis. The cornea, like the sclera, is abnormally thin. The ocular features are usually not of great functional importance.

Aural Features. Hearing loss becomes detectable in many patients by the second or third decade of life. It was long assumed that deafness in OI was the result of precocious otosclerosis; alternatively, otosclerosis is such a common disorder that many OI patients are likely to develop it. A variety

Table 75–3. Osteogenesis Imperfecta Syndromes

Type	Inheritance	Skeletal Features	Other Features
IA	AD	variable bone fragility and short stature, wormian bones	blue sclerae, opalescent teeth, hearing loss
IB	AD	variable bone fragility and short stature, wormian bones	blue sclerae, normal teeth, hearing loss
II	AR, AD and sporadic	in utero fractures, little calvarial calcium	blue sclerae, pulmonary hypertension, neonatal death usual
III	most sporadic	variable fragility, marked deformity, scoliosis, joint laxity	variable sclerae, some with opalescent teeth
IVA	AD	variable bone fragility and short stature, wormian bones	normal sclerae, opalescent teeth, hearing loss
IVB	AD	variable bone fragility and short stature, wormian bones	normal sclerae and teeth, hearing loss

of aural abnormalities occur in OI, and symptomatic hearing loss is nearly always multifactorial.[11] The tympanic membrane may be thin, the pinna deformed, the ossicles disconnected, or the stapedial footplate thickened or degenerated. A surprisingly high percentage of patients have a sensorineural component, owing in part to cochlear deformity, cochlear hair loss, and tectorial membrane distortion.[11] Thus, each patient must be evaluated in considerable detail to determine whether hearing impairment is present and whether it is conductive, sensorineural, or mixed.

Dental Features. The characteristic dental manifestation of OI is opalescent teeth caused by a defect in dentin morphogenesis.[50] This finding is easily ascertained by direct observation of the blue or brown opalescent deciduous or permanent teeth or by the typical radiographic changes. This dental abnormality can be useful diagnostically because opalescent teeth, of all of the pleiotropic OI manifestations, breeds true in families.[52] It thus forms the basis for subdividing types I and IV into disorders with and without opalescent teeth. Affected teeth wear poorly; enamel loss is secondary to fracture of the underlying dentin.

Other Features. Unusual bruising occurs in some patients, probably owing to a defect in the connective tissue in the walls of small blood vessels or in the supporting connective tissues. No consistent defect of the coagulation mechanism has been demonstrated.

Mitral valve prolapse occurs in about 15% of patients with OI type I, several times more frequently than in the general population, and occasionally may progress to mitral regurgitation. Aortic dilatation and regurgitation also occur but are infrequent.[51]

The differential diagnosis of osteogenesis imperfecta includes idiopathic juvenile osteoporosis,[18] juvenile osteoporosis with ocular pseudoglioma and mental retardation,[65] Cheney syndrome (osteoporosis, multiple wormian bones, acroosteolysis),[2,96] pycnodysostosis (dwarfism, brittle bones, absent ramus of mandible, persistent cranial fontanelles, acro-osteolysis),[59] and hypophosphatasia.[77]

The Genetic Mucopolysaccharidoses

The conditions in this class are the result of inborn errors of mucopolysaccharide metabolism. Although phenotypically diverse, the individual disorders share mucopolysacchariduria and deposition of mucopolysaccharides in various tissues. Numerous distinct types of mucopolysaccharidoses (MPS) can be distinguished on the basis of combined phenotypic (i.e., clinical), genetic, and biochemical analysis, as well as allelic subtypes.[61,74]

Table 75–4 summarizes the distinctive features of each. Additional biochemical and clinical variants undoubtedly remain to be described. Furthermore, genetic disturbances of MPS metabolism without mucopolysacchariduria (e.g., mucolipidoses II and III) have been clearly identified. All these disorders are recessive, one being X-linked and the others autosomal.

Leading constituents of the ground substance, acid mucopolysaccharides (glycosaminoglycans),[42] are macromolecular substances, most of which consist of repeating units of hexosamine and a hexuronic acid bound to protein along a hyaluronic acid backbone (see Chap. 11). Excessive urinary secretion of three mucopolysaccharides—dermatan sulfate, heparan sulfate, and keratan sulfate—has been found in various types of genetic MPSs.

Mucopolysacchariduria can be identified by one of several standard screening tests, at least one of which is part of the standard battery performed when a "metabolic screen" is ordered. Fractionation and characterization of the urinary mucopolysaccharides are useful in separating the several types of MPSs. For example, MPS III (Sanfilippo syndrome—the heparan sulfate excretors) and MPS IV (Morquio syndrome—the keratan sulfate excretors) in young subjects may be distinguished from the other types, especially MPS IH (Hurler syndrome—dermatan sulfate excretors), mainly by chemical analysis.

Studies with radioactive sulfate indicate accumulation of label in cultured fibroblasts and delayed washout, compatible with the conclusion that these disorders are due to a degradative defect.[25] More specifically, they are lysosomal disorders. The specific lysosomal enzyme deficient in each is now known (see Table 75–4). Like other lysosomal disorders, the MPSs have six distinctive characteristics:

1. Intracellular storage of material occurs.
2. The storage material is heterogeneous because the degradative enzymes are not strictly specific. Ganglioside is deposited in brain and predominantly mucopolysaccharide in the liver, and two mucopolysaccharides are excreted in the urine.
3. Deposition is vacuolar, i.e., membrane-bound, when viewed with the electron microscope.
4. Many tissues are affected.
5. The disorder is clinically progressive.
6. Replacement therapy is at least theoretically possible, through replacing the missing enzyme by the process of endocytosis. The possibility of replacement therapy in the MPSs is more than theoretic. Normal cells or the medium in which they have grown, when mixed with MPS fibroblasts, correct the metabolic defect.[25,26] This finding in-

Table 75–4. The Genetic Mucopolysaccharidoses

Number	Eponym	Clinical Manifestations	Genetics	Urinary MPS	Enzyme-Deficient
MPS I H (25280)*	Hurler	Clouding of cornea, grave manifestations, death usually before age 10	Homozygous for MPS IH gene	Dermatan sulfate, heparan sulfate	α-L-iduronidase
MPS I S	Scheie	Stiff joints, cloudy cornea, aortic valve disease, normal intelligence and (?) lifespan	Homozygous for MPS I S gene	Dermatan sulfate, heparan sulfate	α-L-iduronidase
MPS I H/S	Hurler-Scheie	Intermediate phenotype	Genetic compound of MPS I H and MPS I S genes	Dermatan sulfate, heparan sulfate	α-L-iduronidase
MPS II-XR severe (30990)	Hunter, severe	No corneal clouding, milder course than in MPS IH, death before 15 years	Hemizygous for X-linked gene	Dermatan sulfate, heparan sulfate	Iduronate sulfatase
MPS II-XR, mild	Hunter, mild	Survival to 30s to 60s, fair intelligence	Hemizygous for X-linked allele	Dermatan sulfate, heparan sulfate	Iduronate sulfatase
MPS III A (25290)	Sanfilippo A	Indistinguishable phenotype: Mild somatic, severe central	Homozygous for Sanfilippo A gene	Heparan sulfate	Heparan N-sulfatase (sulfamidase)
MPS III B (25292)	Sanfilippo B		Homozygous for Sanfilippo B gene	Heparan sulfate	N-acetyl-α-D-glucosaminidase
MPS III C (25293)	Sanfilippo C	nervous system effects	Homozygous for Sanfilippo C gene	Heparan sulfate	Acetyl-CoA: α-glucosaminide N-acetyltransferase
MPS III D (25294)	Sanfilippo D		Homozygous for Sanfilippo D gene	Heparan sulfate	N-acetylglucosamine-6-sulfate sulfatase
MPS IV A (25300)	Morquio A	Severe, distinctive bone changes, cloudy cornea, aortic regurgitation, thin enamel	Homozygous for Morquio A genes	Keratan sulfate	Galactosamine-6-sulfate sulfatase
MPS IV B (25301)	Morquio B (O'Brien-Arbisser)	Mild bone changes, cloudy cornea, hypoplastic odontoid, normal enamel	Homozygous for Morquio B gene	Keratan sulfate	β-galactosidase
MPS V	No longer used	—		—	
MPS VI, severe (25320)	Maroteaux-Lamy, classic severe	Severe osseous and corneal change; valvular heart disease, striking WBC inclusions; normal intellect; survival to 20s	Homozygous for Maroteaux-Lamy (M-L) gene	Dermatan sulfate	Arylsulfatase B (N-acetylgalactosamine 4-sulfatase)
MPS VI, intermediate	Maroteaux-Lamy, intermediate	Moderately severe changes	Homozygous for allele at M-L locus or genetic compound	Dermatan sulfate	Arylsulfatase B (N-acetylgalactosamine 4-sulfatase)
MPS VI, mild	Maroteaux-Lamy, mild	Mild osseous and corneal change, normal intellect; aortic stenosis	Homozygous for allele at M-L locus	Dermatan sulfate	Arylsulfatase B (N-acetylgalactosamine 4-sulfatase)
MPS VII (25323)	Sly	Hepatosplenomegaly dysostosis multiplex, mental retardation WBC inclusions	Homozygous for mutant gene at β-glucuronidase locus	Dermatan sulfate, heparan sulfate	β-glucuronidase
MPS VIII (25323)	DiFerrante	Short stature, mild dysostosis multiplex, ring-shaped metachromasia of lymphocytes	Homozygous for MPS VIII gene	Keratan sulfate, heparan sulfate	Glucosamine-6-sulfate sulfatase

*Entry number in McKusick, V.A.[58]

(Adapted from Pyeritz, R.E., and McKusick, V.A.[74])

dicates the production of a diffusible correction factor by normal cells, which is found also in normal urine. The correction factor is the enzyme specially deficient in the given disorder. Several trials of enzyme replacement therapy, by plasma exchange and fibroblast transplantation, have been attended by limited success, however, particularly in reversing established neurologic defects.

The differential features of the MPSs are summarized in Table 75–4, and the clinical features of MPS IH, MPS IS, and MPS II are illustrated in Figures 75–8, 75–9, and 75–10, respectively. The nosologic validity of this classification is supported by the findings of cocultivation of fibroblasts. Mutual correction of their metabolic defects occurs when fibroblasts from MPS I and MPS II, MPS I and MPS III, and other combinations are mixed. Failure of cross-correction between cultured fibroblasts of two patients indicates that they have the same enzyme deficiency, and that the mutations underlying them at a minimum are allelic, if not identical.[26,61] Relatively easy methods for assay of the enzymes deficient in some of these conditions are also available.

MPS V does not exist in the present classification. It was previously the numeric designation for the Scheie syndrome, a disorder distinct clinically

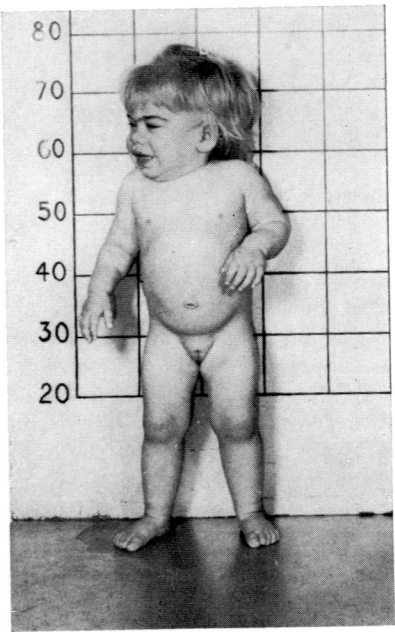

Fig. 75–8. Mucopolysaccharidosis I-H (Hurler syndrome) in a 2-year-old girl. Note the coarse facial features, prominent abdomen from hepatosplenomegaly, claw hands, and short stature. The joints generally had moderate restriction of motion. The patient died of congestive heart failure at 12 years of age.

from the other MPSs (Fig. 75–9). However, in vitro studies showed no cross-correction between Hurler and Scheie fibroblasts, and the same enzyme, α-L-iduronidase, was subsequently found deficient in the two disorders.[97] Our interpretation is that the Hurler and Scheie syndromes are due to homozygosity for two different mutations at the gene locus determining the structure of α-L-iduronidase. Thus, both are designated MPS I. The Hurler syndrome, MPS IH, is analogous to hemoglobin SS disease, a severe disorder, and the Scheie syndrome, MPS IS, to hemoglobin CC disease, a mild disorder. If the notion that MPS IH and MPS IS are due to allelic genes is correct, then a Hurler-Scheie genetic compound comparable to SC disease should exist. Indeed, patients with phenotypic features intermediate to MPS IH and MPS IS have been identified and are designated MPS IH/S. Some are likely true genetic compounds, whereas others are likely homozygotes (because of parental consanguinity) for other mutant alleles at the α-L-iduronidase locus. Allelic forms of MPS II and MPS VI presumably account for the severe and mild forms of those disorders.

Skeletal Features.   Relative short stature is the rule in all patients with the MPS disorders. This condition can be profound in MPS IH, MPS II, and MPS IV (the Morquio syndrome being the prototypic ''short trunk'' form of dwarfism), and severe in MPS VI. Radiographically, the skeletal dysplasia is similar in character in all but MPS IV, differing among the others largely in severity. The term dysostosis multiplex has been applied, but is not specific for the MPSs, similar changes occurring in a variety of storage disorders. The chief radiographic features are a thick calvaria, an enlarged J-shaped sella turcica, a short and wide mandible, biconvex vertebral bodies, hypoplasia of the odontoid, broad ribs, short and thick clavicles, coxa valga, metacarpals with widened diaphyses and pointed proximal ends, and short phalanges.[81,87]

For the disorders compatible with survival to adulthood without severe retardation (MPS IS, MPS II mild, MPS IV, MPS VI), progressive arthropathy and transverse myelopathy secondary to C1-C2 subluxation account for considerable disability. Cervical fusion should be considered whenever upper motor neuron signs appear. Joint replacement, particularly of the hips, has been beneficial in MPS IS.[74]

Stiff joints are a more or less striking feature of all forms except MPS IV. Like other somatic features, such as coarse facies, reduced joint mobility is less striking in MPS III. In the Scheie syndrome, stiff hands, together with clouding of the cornea, lead to the main disability. In that condition, as in

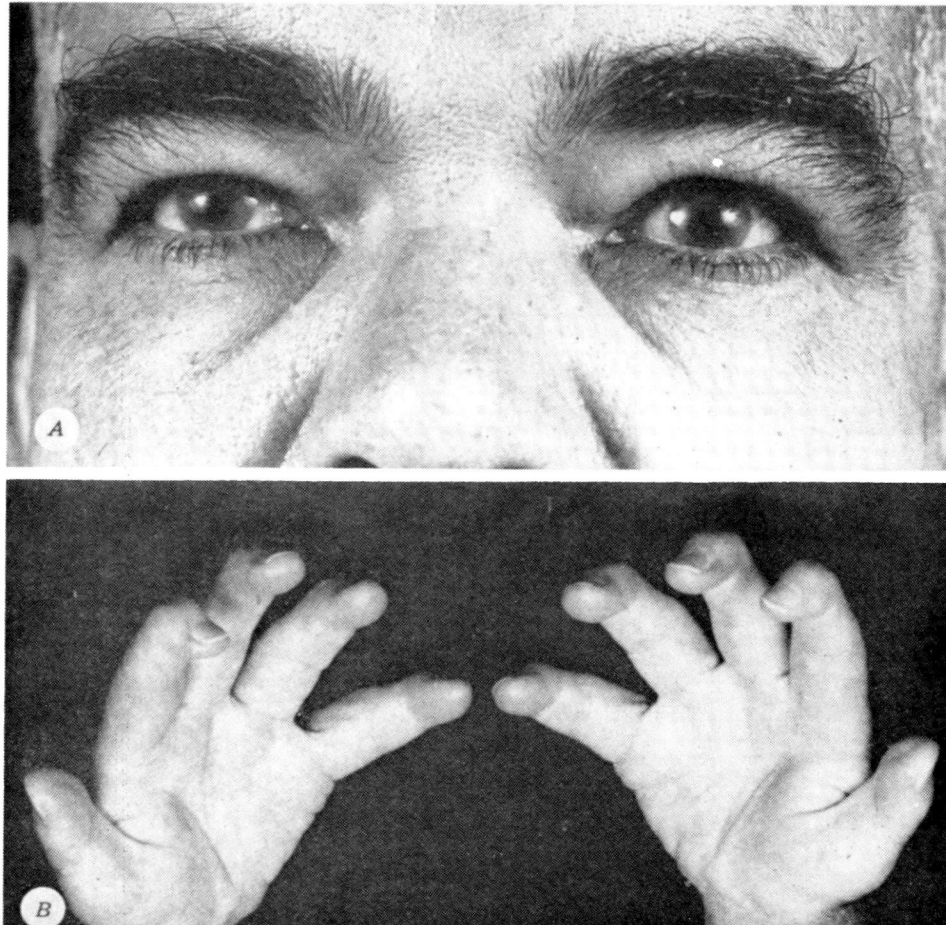

Fig. 75–9. Mucopolysaccharidosis I-S (Scheie syndrome) in a 54-year-old attorney. *A,* Clouding of the cornea was densest peripherally. *B,* The hands were clawed; atrophy of the lateral aspect of the thenar eminences indicated carpal tunnel compression.

the others, carpal tunnel syndrome contributes to the disability. Early decompression can be beneficial.

Mucolipidosis II and Mucolipidosis III

Mucolipidosis II (ML II) is also called I-cell disease (because of conspicuous inclusions in cultured cells). Mucolipidosis III (ML III) is also called pseudo-Hurler polydystrophy. Neither shows mucopolysacchariduria despite lysosomal storage of mucopolysaccharide and a demonstrable defect in degradation of mucopolysaccharides. Both are inherited as autosomal recessive conditions and are likely allelic. The basic biochemical defect rests with an enzyme, UDP-*N*-acetylglucosamine:lysosomal enzyme *N*-acetylglucosaminylphosphotransferase, responsible for posttranslational modification of lysosomal enzymes.[64]

This defect results in multiple enzyme deficiencies and accumulation in tissues of both mucopolysaccharides and mucolipids.

ML II is a severe Hurler-like disorder. ML III is a distinctive disorder with stiff joints, cloudy cornea, carpal tunnel syndrome, short stature, coarse facies, and sometimes mild mental retardation, compatible with survival to adulthood[43] (Fig. 75–11).

The Stickler Syndrome

The cardinal features of this relatively common, autosomal dominant condition are severe, progressive myopia, vitreal degeneration, retinal detachment, progressive sensorineural hearing loss, cleft palate, mandibular hypoplasia, hyper- and hypomobility of joints, variable epiphyseal dysplasia, and variable disability resulting from joint pain,

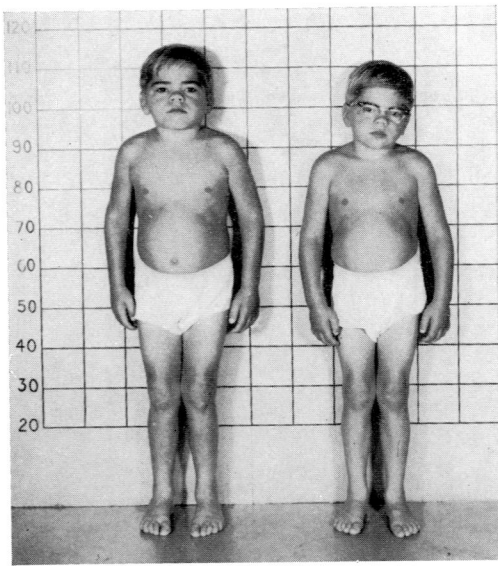

Fig. 75–10. Mucopolysaccharidosis II, mild (the Hunter syndrome, mild variant) in brothers, 7 and 6 years of age. Note the short stature, coarse facies, prominent abdomen, and clawed hands. Intellect was normal.

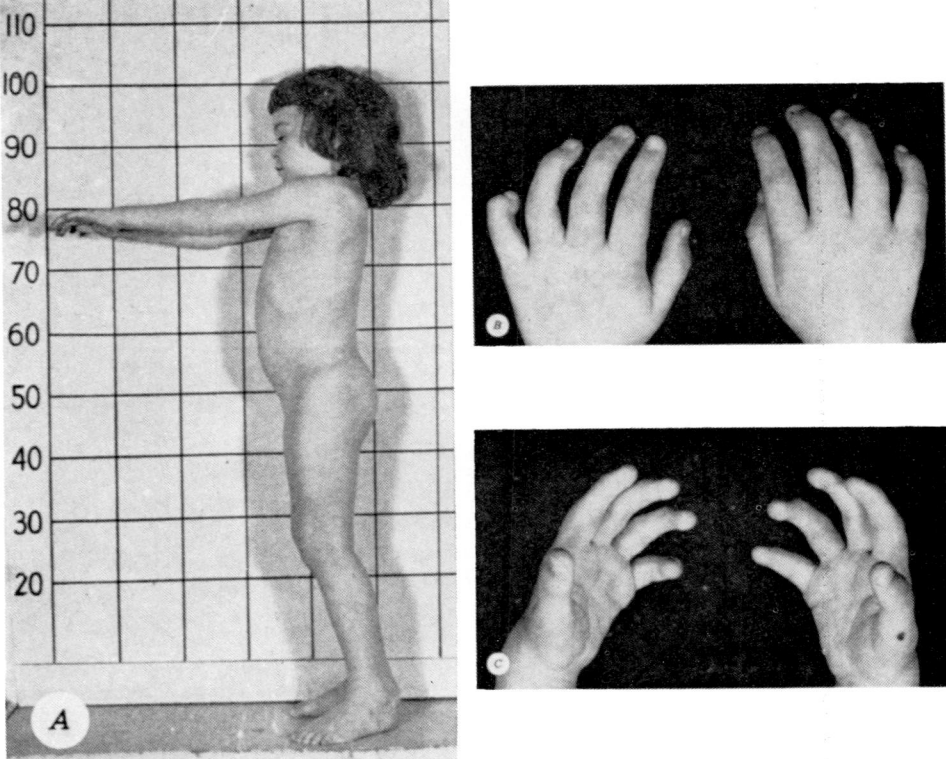

Fig. 75–11. Mucolipidosis III (pseudo-Hurler polydystrophy) in a 6-year-old girl. *A,* Note the short stature and coarse facies. The corneas were clouded, motion of all joints was restricted, a murmur of aortic regurgitation was present, and intellect was mildly deficient. *B, C,* The hands were clawed, and atrophy of the thenar eminences indicated carpal tunnel compression, for which operation was performed at 13 years of age, with some benefit.

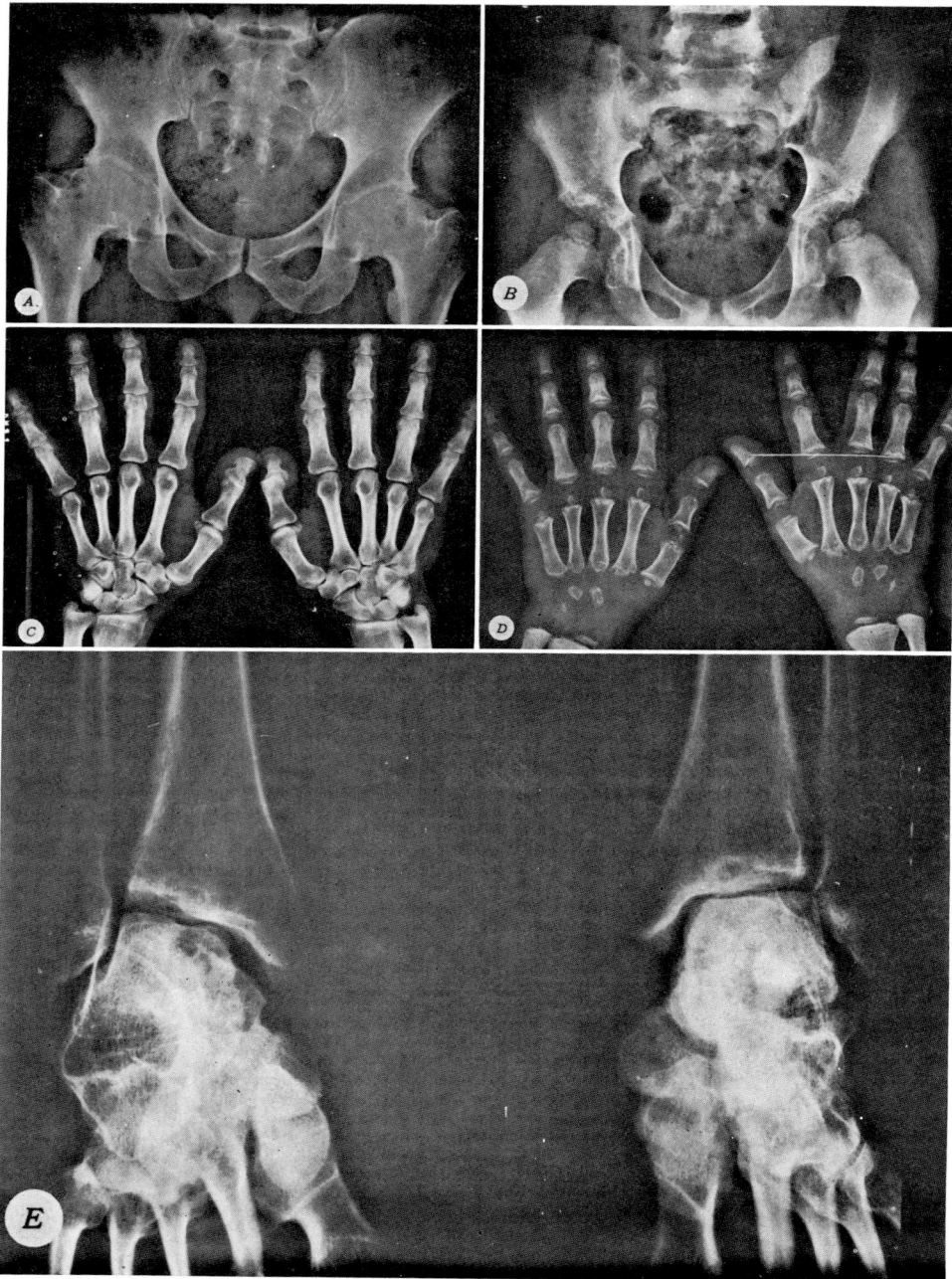

Fig. 75–12. Multiple epiphyseal dysplasia (MED) in father and son. Both were short of stature, the father being 61.5 inches tall. *A*, Hips in the father at 44 years of age showing advanced degenerative changes. *B*, Hips in the son at 10 years of age showing small femoral capital epiphyses and irregularities of the acetabula. *C*, Hands of the father showing brachydactyly, a short carpus, and degenerative joint disease. *D*, Hands of the son at 10 years of age showing dysplastic epiphyses and delayed development of the carpal bones. *E*, Sloping of the distal tibia is a clue to the diagnosis of MED in the adult.

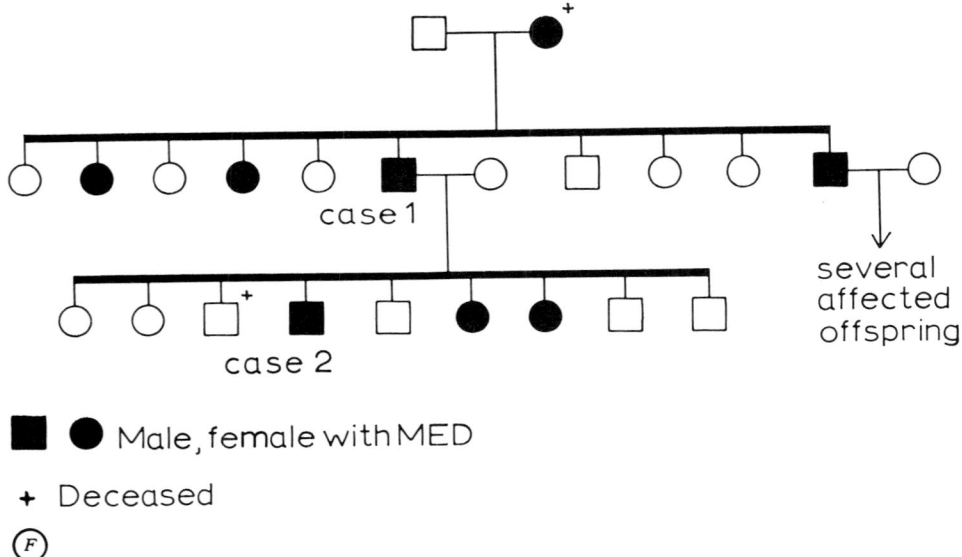

Fig. 75–12. (Cont'd)   *F*, Family pedigree, in which cases 1 and 2 are the father and son illustrated here, demonstrates typical autosomal dominant inheritance of MED.

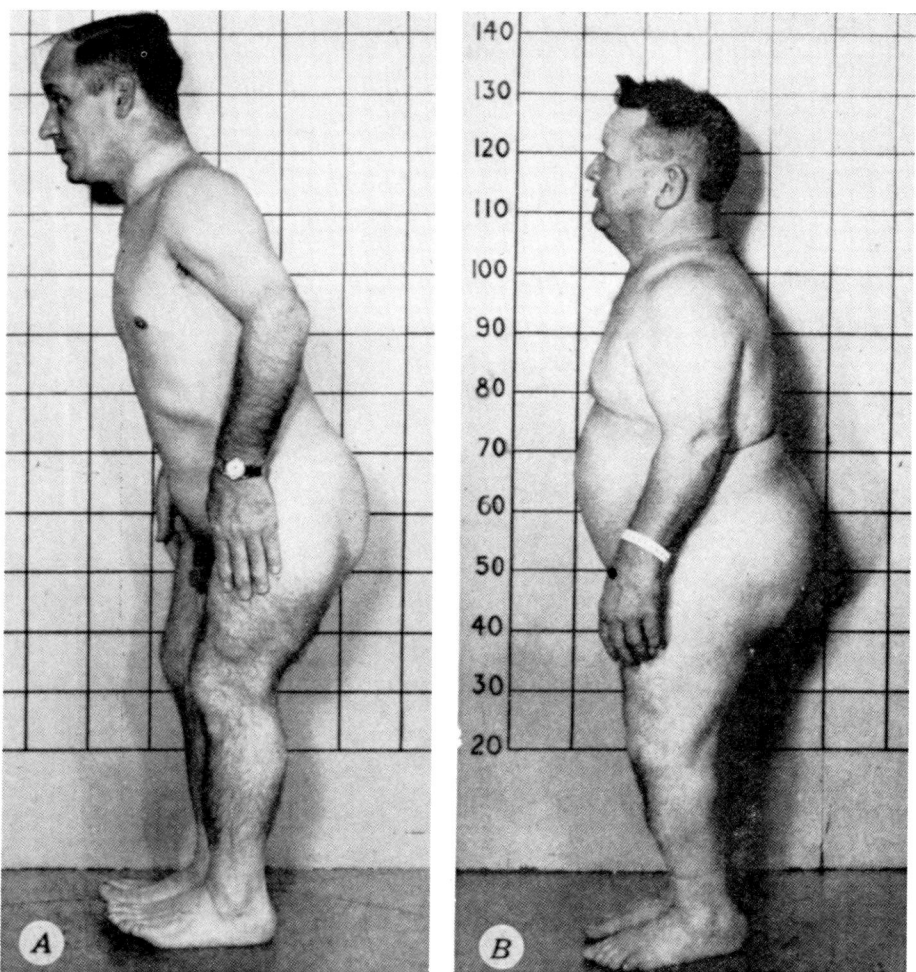

Fig. 75–13.   Ankylosing arthropathy in two men with vitamin D-resistant rickets. *A*, 41-year-old man. *B*, 61-year-old man. The younger man is the more severely affected, but both have almost complete ankylosis of the spine and similar changes in some peripheral joints. Note the short stature.

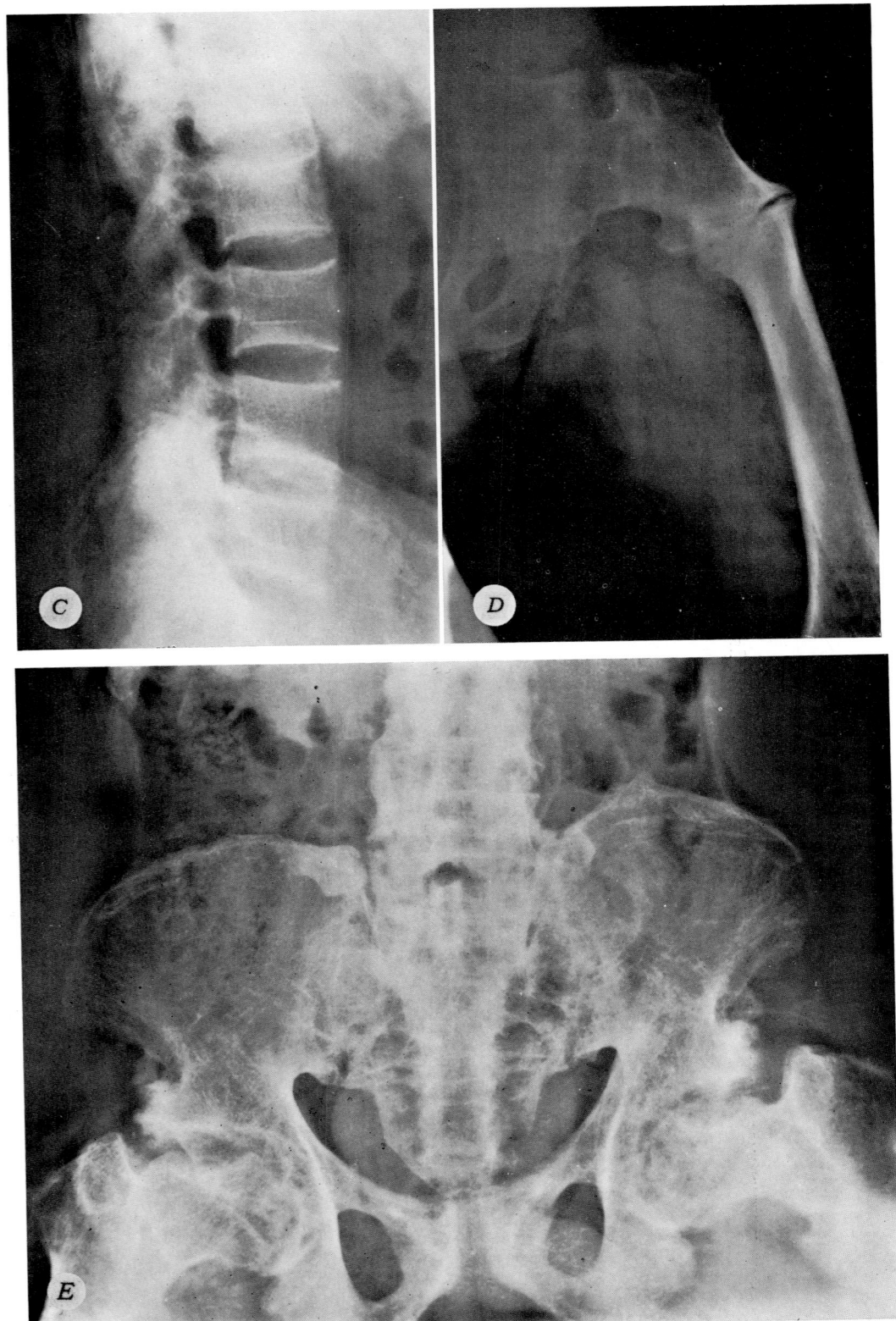

Fig. 75–13. (Cont'd) *C,* Lateral radiograph of the lower spine in the older patient. *D,* Left femur of the younger patient. Pseudofractures were situated symmetrically in the subtrochanteric area of both femurs. *E,* Pelvis of the 41-year-old patient.

dislocation, or degeneration.[31,53] The Stickler syndrome, also called progressive arthro-ophthalmopathy, is clearly underdiagnosed, in part because patients often do not have the full syndrome and in part because the physician fails to obtain a detailed family history that might suggest a hereditary condition. The diagnosis should be strongly considered in any infant with congenitally enlarged ("swollen") wrists, knees, or ankles, particularly when associated with the Robin anomalad (hypognathia, cleft palate, and glossoptosis).

SELECTED GENETIC DISORDERS SIMULATING ARTHRITIDES

Multiple Epiphyseal Dysplasia (MED)

The child comes to medical attention because of short stature or changes in the heads of the femurs, as in Legg-Perthes disease, leading to abnormality of gait. In the third and fourth decades, the patient develops osteoarthritis of the hips (Fig. 75–12) and, to a lesser extent, of other joints. The vertebral bodies may be involved, leading to mild platyspondyly, although not as severely as in the spondyloepiphyseal dysplasias. Suspicion that MED underlies precocious osteoarthritis of the hips may come from short stature and be corroborated by the finding of sloping at the distal end of the tibia. This condition is a mendelian dominant disorder of wide clinical variability. Some families with MED show especially striking changes in the hands, with short fingers and painless deformity at the proximal interphalangeal joints. This disorder may be the one that has been described as "familial osteoarthropathy of the fingers."[1]

Ankylosing Arthropathy in Vitamin D-Resistant Hypophosphatemic Rickets

Adults with this X-linked dominant disorder, especially untreated males, develop ankylosing spondylosis as well as ankylosis of some peripheral joints (Fig. 75–13). Some of these patients have been given x-ray therapy to the spine on the basis of a mistaken diagnosis. As in Reiter's disease, the patient with hypophosphatemia shows calcaneal spurs, roughening of the ischium, and capsular calcification at the hip.[59] The clinical picture also bears some similarity to that of Forrestier's disease (ankylosing hyperostosis or diffuse idiopathic skeletal hyperostosis—DISH).

Farber's Lipogranulomatosis

This autosomal recessive disorder appears in the first few weeks of life with irritability, hoarse cry, and nodular erythematous swelling of the wrists and other sites, particularly those subject to trauma.[62] Masses around the joints suggest rheumatoid nodules (Fig. 75–14). The basic defect is a deficiency of ceramidase, an enzyme involved in sphingolipid degradation.[15,62] The periarticular nodules and bone erosion, laryngeal obstruction, and mental retardation are due to abnormal storage of ceramide in granulomas and macrophages. A presumably allelic variant, associated with normal or mildly reduced intelligence, is compatible with survival to adulthood.[62]

Fibrodysplasia (formerly Myositis) Ossificans Progressiva (FOP)

Characterized by progressive ossification of ligaments, tendons, and aponeuroses, FOP begins an inexorable, progressive course in the first year or so of life, usually with a seemingly inflammatory process and nodule formation on the back of the thorax, neck, or scalp. Local heat, as well as leukocytosis and elevated sedimentation rate, is observed at this stage. Acute rheumatic fever is sometimes diagnosed. A valuable clue to the correct diagnosis is a short great toe with or without a short thumb; this is the leading cause of congenital hallux valgus.[82]

Most cases of this autosomal dominant disorder are the consequence of new mutation. Life expectancy is considerably reduced, with progressive restriction in lung capacity contributing to respiratory insufficiency and terminal pneumonia.[16]

Symphalangism

Harvey Cushing applied this term to a condition of hereditary ankylosis of the proximal interphalangeal joints.[89] Fusion of carpal and tarsal bones also occurs in this autosomal dominant disorder.

Camptodactyly

Limited extension of the digits is a feature of over 25 syndromes, including the Marfan syndrome, but occasionally is an isolated abnormality inherited as an autosomal dominant trait.[95] Permanent flexion contractures are present at the proximal interphalangeal joints without limitation of flexion, typically accompanied by hyperextension at the metacarpophalangeal joints, and sometimes at the distal interphalangeal joints. Camptodactyly may be limited to the fifth finger, or other fingers. Rarely the thumb may be involved as well, with severity decreasing in the radial direction. A contracture band can often be felt on the volar surface of the affected proximal interphalangeal joint, and the transverse skin crease is invariably absent there. Camptodactyly is present from birth or early childhood and shows little tendency to progression. Because of compensatory hyperextension at the metacarpophalangeal joints, the contracture causes little disability. As was pointed out by Archibald Garrod,

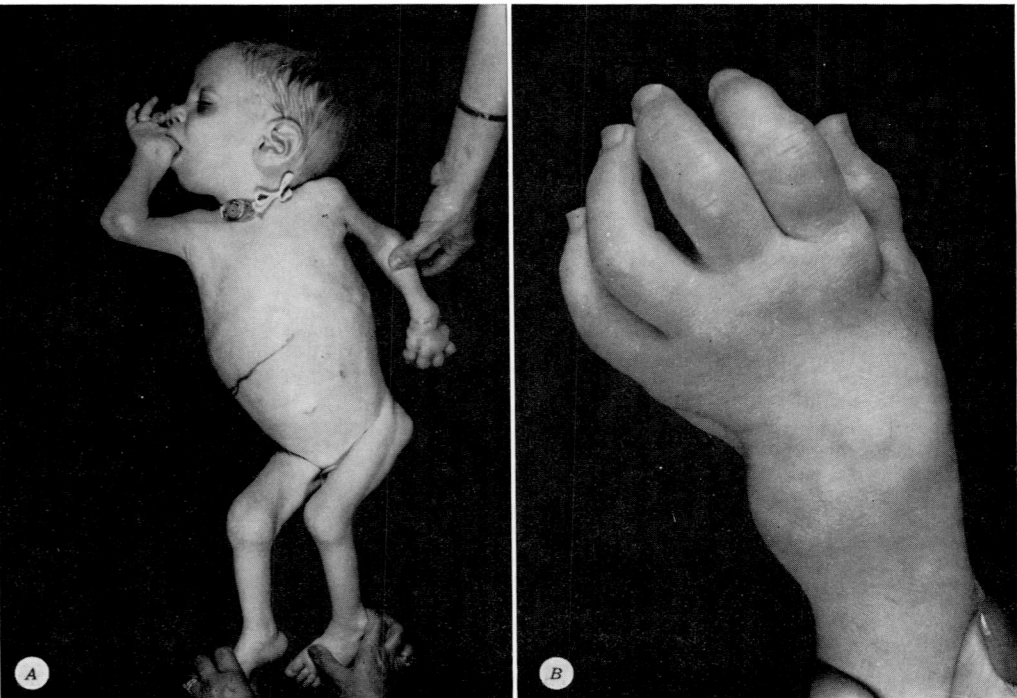

Fig. 75–14. Farber's lipogranulomatosis in an 18-month-old boy. Note the swelling and nodules on the wrists, hands, fingers, and elbows as well as the signs of grave illness. Tracheostomy was necessitated by laryngeal constriction. (From Abul-Haj, S.K., et al.: J. Pediatr., *61*:221, 1962.)

camptodactyly, when it involves multiple fingers, is often accompanied by "knuckle pads," thickened skin on the dorsal aspect of the proximal interphalangeal joints.[95] Camptodactyly is sometimes confused with Dupuytren's contracture, which is late in onset and has its primary site of contracture in the palm.

Genetic Disorders as Substrate for Precocious Osteoarthritis of the Hips

Lloyd-Roberts found that 26 of 124 cases of early osteoarthritis of the hips could be related to subluxation.[55] Of the 51 cases (of 124) in which an etiologic factor was evident, this condition was, then, a predominant one. Familial joint laxity, as in EDS III and XI discussed previously, is one factor in subluxation of the hip and acetabular dysplasia is another, apparently unrelated,[14] factor. Subluxation of the hip, which comes to light soon after birth, is usually related to familial joint laxity; that which is recognized later is related to acetabular dysplasia.

Genetic factors in primary osteoarthritis are discussed in Chapter 89.

Arthrogryposis Multiplex Congenita (AMC)

The syndrome of congenital rigidity of multiple joints is of complex etiology, pathogenesis, and phenotype.[20,28,41] In many instances, the disorder is a deformation of joints resulting from immobilization of the developing fetus, so that the proper stimulus for joint development is lacking.[20,41,86] The cause of the immobilization may be a prenatal disorder of the brain, spinal cord, peripheral nerves, vasculature, or muscle. The affected baby is born with the arms and legs fixed in postures dictated by the position of the embryo and fetus in development. In addition to joint rigidity, dislocation of the hips and micrognathia are frequent findings. The Drachman theory of fetal immobilization as the "cause" of AMC was developed from studies of the effects of neuromuscular blocking agents on chick embryos. His theory is supported by observation of AMC in an infant born of a mother who received tubocurarine in early pregnancy for treatment of tetanus.[20]

Disorders of the Bony Skeleton (Osteochondrodysplasias)

The osseous skeleton, the largest specialized connective tissue, participates in many of the gen-

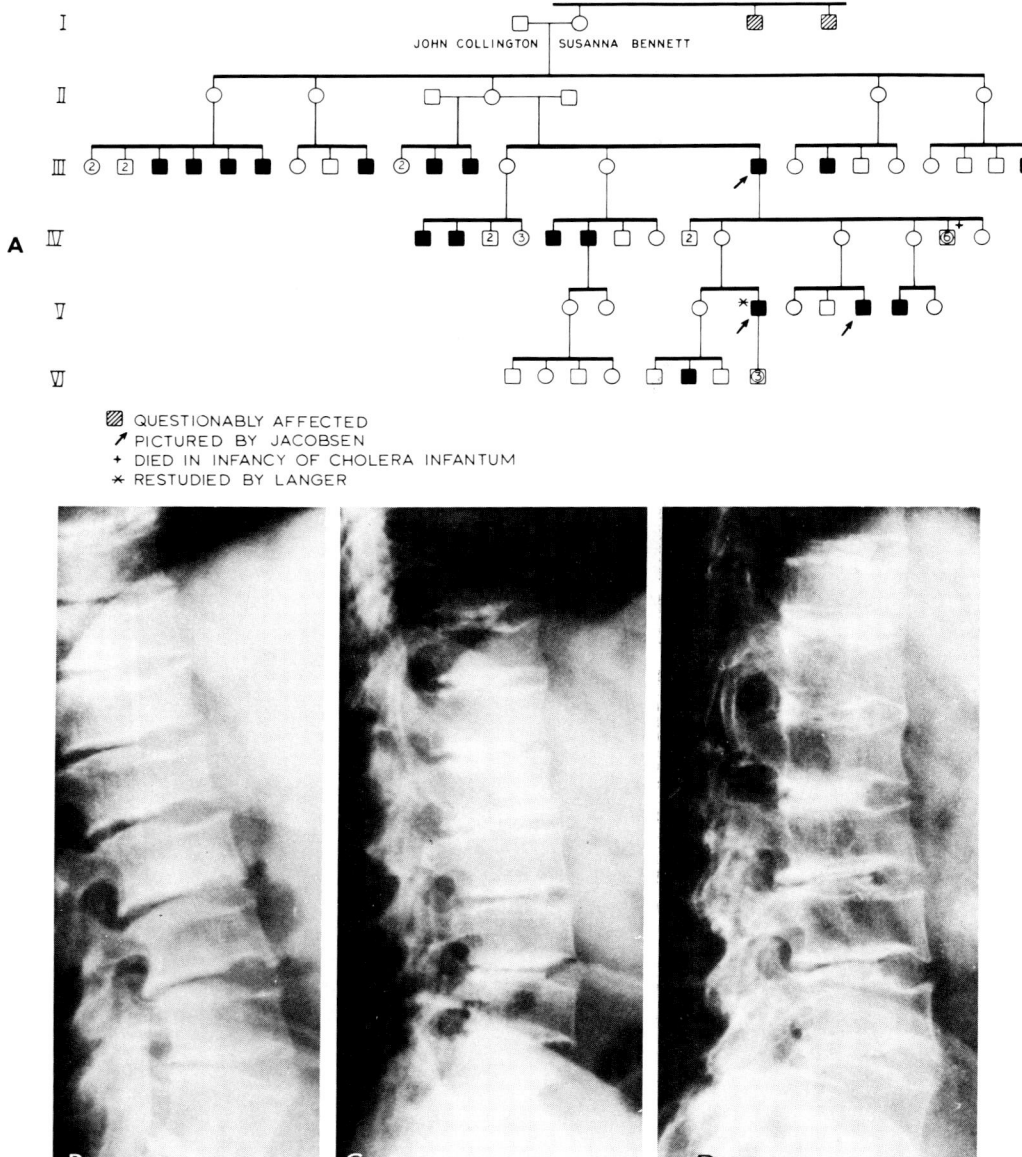

QUESTIONABLY AFFECTED
PICTURED BY JACOBSEN
DIED IN INFANCY OF CHOLERA INFANTUM
RESTUDIED BY LANGER

Fig. 75–15. X-linked spondyloepiphyseal dysplasia tarda. *A*, Partially updated pedigree of family reported by Jacobsen.[40] *B* to *D*, Radiographic changes in the spine are progressive; the heaping up of the posterior portion of the superior vertebral plate *(B)* is particularly distinctive. At first glance, the late changes *(D)* suggest those of alkaptonuria.

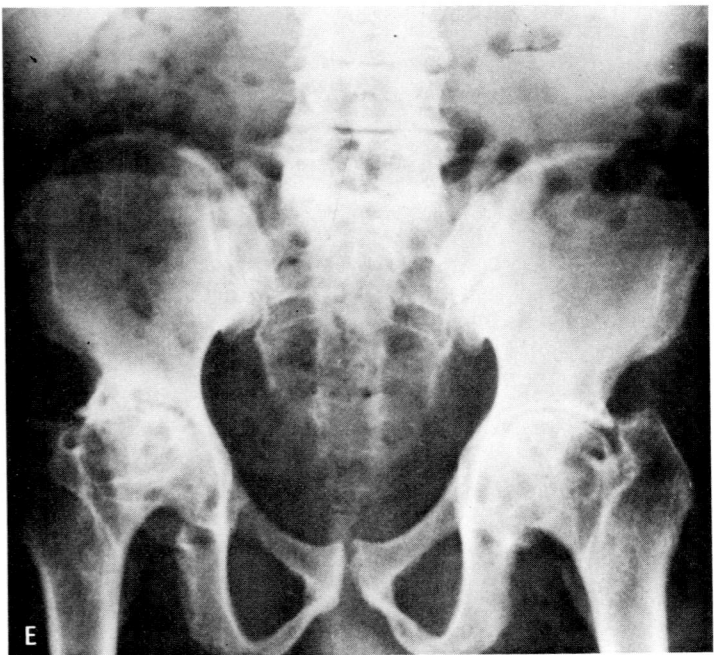

Fig. 75–15. (Cont'd) *E*, Late changes in the hips. Note the deep acetabula. (Radiographs courtesy of Dr. Leonard O. Langer, Jr., Minneapolis.)

eralized heritable disorders of connective tissue discussed earlier. In addition, it is subject to a large number of gene-determined derangements with primary effects apparently limited to bone and cartilage, exemplified by multiple epiphyseal dysplasia also discussed previously.

The osteochondrodysplasias represent a difficult category of hereditary disease because the types are legion; each is unusual, and most physicians, even specialists such as orthopedists, radiologists, and rheumatologists, encounter them rarely. Little is known of the etiopathogenesis[59] and, until recently, little was known even of their natural history[38] or histopathology.[22] No definite therapy is available for most, and nomenclature has been chaotic (see the nomenclature recommended by the Second Paris Conference convened in 1977).[22]

Most of the skeletal dysplasias fall into the category of disproportionate dwarfism (called "dwarfs" by the layman) contrasted with proportionate dwarfs (called "midgets" by the layman), who often have deficiency of growth hormone. Disproportionate dwarfs tend further to fall into short-limb or short-trunk groups, of which achondroplasia and the Morquio syndrome (MPS IV: see Table 75–2) are, respectively, prototypes. In individual patients, many different conditions have often been incorrectly labeled (and reported in the literature) as either achondroplasia or Morquio syndrome. In recent years, recognition of the heterogeneity in the osteochondrodysplasias,[22,59,87] delineation of many simulating but distinct disorders,[36,56,80] and better definition of the prototype disorders, achondroplasia[22,76,83] and Morquio syndrome,[62] have led to a better understanding of this category, although much remains to be learned.

For further information on osteochondrodysplasias, several useful monographs exist.[59,83,87] A grasp of this category of connective tissue disease will be provided by a familiarity with eight entities: achondroplasia (including its mild, probably allelic form, hypochondroplasia), Morquio syndrome, SED (spondyloepiphyseal dysplasia) congenita, X-linked SED tarda, pseudoachondroplastic dysplasia, diastrophic dysplasia, Ellis-van Creveld syndrome, and cartilage-hair hypoplasia.[61] Precocious hip arthritis occurs in several of these conditions, as illustrated by the examples of X-linked SED shown in Figure 75–15.[4,48]

REFERENCES

1. Allison, A.C., and Blumberg, B.S.: Familial osteoarthropathy of the fingers. J. Bone Joint Surg., *40B*:538, 1958.
2. Andren, L., et al.: Osteopetrosis acro-osteolytica. A syndrome of osteopetrosis, acro-osteolysis and open sutures of the skull. Acta Chir. Scand., *124*:496, 1962.
3. Arneson, M.A., et al.: A new form of Ehlers-Danlos syndrome: Fibronectin corrects defective platelet function. J.A.M.A., *244*:144, 1980.
4. Bannerman, R.M.: X-linked spondyloepiphyseal dysplasia tarda. Birth Defects, *5*:48, 1969.
5. Barsh, G.S., and Byers, P.H.: Reduced secretion of structurally abnormal type I procollagen in a form of osteogenesis imperfecta. Proc. Natl. Acad. Sci. U.S.A., *78*:5142, 1981.
6. Barsh, G.S., David, K.E., and Byers, P.H.: Type I osteogenesis imperfecta: A nonfunctional allele for proalpha₁ (I) chains of type I procollagen. Proc. Natl. Acad. Sci. U.S.A., *79*:3838, 1982.
7. Bauze, R.J., Smith, R., and Francis, M.J.O.: A new look at osteogenesis imperfecta. A clinical, radiological and biochemical study of 42 patients. J. Bone Joint Surg., *57B*:2, 1975.
8. Beals, R.K., and Hecht, F.: Congenital contractural arachnodactyly: A heritable disease of connective tissue. J. Bone Joint Surg., *53A*:987, 1971.
9. Beighton, P.: The Ehlers-Danlos Syndrome. London, William Heinemann Medical Books Ltd., 1970.
10. Beighton, P.: X-linked recessive inheritance in the Ehlers-Danlos syndrome. Br. Med. J., *3*:409, 1968.
11. Bergstrom, L.V.: Fragile bones and fragile ears. Clin. Orthop., *159*:58, 1981.
12. Byers, P.H., et al.: X-linked cutis laxa. N. Engl. J. Med., *303*:61, 1980.
13. Byers, P.H., et al.: Clinical and ultrastructural heterogeneity of type IV Ehlers-Danlos syndrome. Hum. Genet., *47*:141–150, 1979.
14. Carter, C.O., and Wilkinson, J.: Persistent joint laxity and congenital dislocation of the hip. J. Bone Joint Surg., *46B*:40, 1964.
15. Clausen, J., and Rampini, S.: Chemical studies of Farber's disease. Acta Neurol. Scand., *46*:313, 1970.
16. Conner, J.M., and Evans, D.A.P.: Fibrodysplasia ossificans progressiva: The clinical features and natural history of 34 patients. J. Bone Joint Surg., *64B*:76, 1982.
17. Cupo, L.N., et al.: Ehlers-Danlos syndrome with abnormal collagen fibrils, sinus of Valsalva aneurysms, myocardial infarction, panacinar emphysema, and cerebral heterotopias. Am. J. Med., *71*:1051, 1981.
18. Dent, C.E., and Friedman, M.: Idiopathic juvenile osteoporosis. Q. J. Med., *34*:177, 1965.
19. DiFerrante, N., et al.: Lysyl oxidase deficiency in Ehlers-Danlos syndrome type V. Connect. Tissue Res., *3*:49, 1975.
20. Drachman, D.B.: The syndrome of arthrogryposis multiplex congenita. Birth Defects, *7*:90, 1971.
21. Elas, L.J., II, Miller, R.L., and Pinnell, S.R.: Inherited human collagen lysyl hydroxylase deficiency: Ascorbic acid response. J. Pediatr., *92*:378–384, 1978.
22. Emery, A., and Rimoin, D.L.: Principles and Practice of Medical Genetics. London, Churchill Livingstone, 1983.
23. Francis, M.J.O., Bauze, R., and Smith, R.: Osteogenesis imperfecta: A new classification. Birth Defects, *11*:99, 1976.
24. Francis, M.J.O., and Smith, R.: Polymeric collagen of skin in osteogenesis imperfecta, homocystinuria and Ehlers-Danlos and Marfan syndromes. Birth Defects, *11*:15, 1976.
25. Fratantoni, J.C., Hall, C.W., and Neufeld, E.F.: The defect in Hurler's and Hunter's syndromes: Faulty degradation of mucopolysaccharide. Proc. Natl. Acad. Sci. U.S.A., *60*:699, 1968.
26. Fratantoni, J.C., Hall, C.W., and Neufeld, E.F.: Hurler and Hunter syndromes. Mutual correction of the defect in cultured fibroblasts. Science, *162*:570, 1968.
27. Gruber, M.A., et al.: Marfan syndrome with contractural arachnodactyly and severe mitral regurgitation in a premature infant. J. Pediatr., *93*:80–82, 1978.
28. Hall, J.G., Reed, S.D., and Greene, G.: The distal arthrogryposes: Delineation of new entities—review and nosologic discussion. Am. J. Med. Genet., *11*:185, 1982.
29. Harker, L.A., et al.: Homocystinemia: Vascular injury in arterial thrombosis. N. Engl. J. Med., *291*:537, 1967.
30. Hass, J., and Hass, R.: Arthrochalasis multiplex congenita: Congenital flaccidity of the joints. J. Bone Joint Surg., *40A*:663, 1958.

31. Herrmann, J., et al.: The Stickler syndrome (hereditary arthro-ophthalmopathy). Birth Defects, *11*:76, 1975.
32. Hill-Zobel, R.L., et al.: Kinetics and biodistribution of ¹¹¹In-labeled platelets in homocystinuria. N. Engl. J. Med., *307*:781, 1982.
33. Holbrook, K.A., and Byers, P.H.: Structural abnormalities in the dermal collagen and elastic matrix from the skin of patients with inherited tissue disorders. J. Invest. Dermatol., *79*:7s, 1982.
34. Hollister, D.W.: Clinical features of Ehlers-Danlos syndrome, types VIII and IX. *In* A.A.O.S. Symposium on Heritable Disorders of Connective Tissue. Edited by M.J. Glimcher, and P. Bornstein. St. Louis, C.V. Mosby Co., 1982.
35. Hollister, D.W.: Heritable disorders of connective tissue: Ehlers-Danlos syndrome. Pediatr. Clin. North Am., 25:575–591, 1978.
36. Hollister, D.W., et al.: The Winchester syndrome: A nonlysosomal connective tissue disease. J. Pediatr., *84*:701–709, 1974.
37. Holmes, L.B.: Inborn errors of morphogenesis: A review of localized hereditary malformations. N. Engl. J. Med., *291*:763, 1974.
38. Horton, W.A., et al.: Growth curves for height for diastrophic dysplasia, spondyloepiphyseal dysplasia congenita, and pseudoachondroplasia. Am. J. Dis. Child., *136*:316, 1982.
39. Horton, W.A., et al.: Familial joint instability syndrome. Am. J. Med. Genet., *6*:221–228, 1980.
40. Jacobsen, A.W.: Hereditary osteochondro-dystrophia deformans. J.A.M.A., *113*:121, 1939.
41. Jago, R.H.: Arthrogryposis following treatment of maternal tetanus with muscle relaxants. Arch. Dis. Child., *45*:277, 1970.
42. Jeanloz, R.W.: The nomenclature of mucopolysaccharides. Arthritis Rheum., *3*:233, 1960.
43. Kelly, T.E., et al.: Mucolipidosis III (pseudo-Hurler polydystrophy): Clinical and laboratory studies in a series of 12 patients. Johns Hopkins Med. J., *137*:156, 1975.
44. Kirsch, E., et al.: Molecular defects in inborn disorders of collagen metabolism. Enzyme, *27*:239, 1982.
45. Kloepfer, H.W., and Rosenthal, J.W.: Possible genetic carriers in the spherophakia-brachymorphia syndrome. Am. J. Hum. Genet., *7*:398, 1955.
46. Krane, S.M., Pinnell, S.R., and Erbe, R.W.: Lyso-protocollagen hydroxylase deficiency in fibroblasts from siblings with hydroxylysine deficient collagen. Proc. Natl. Acad. Sci. U.S.A., *69*:2899, 1972.
47. Kuivaniemi, H., et al.: Abnormal copper metabolism and deficient lysyl oxidase activity in a heritable connective tissue disorder. J. Clin. Invest., *69*:730, 1982.
48. Langer, L.O., Jr.: Spondyloepiphysial dysplasia tarda. Hereditary chondrodysplasia with characteristic vertebral configuration in the adult. Radiology, *82*:833, 1964.
49. Latta, R.J., et al.: Larsen's syndrome: A skeletal dysplasia with multiple joint dislocations and unusual facies. J. Pediatr., *78*:291, 1971.
50. Levin, L.S.: The dentition in the osteogenesis imperfecta syndromes. Clin. Orthop., *159*:64, 1981.
51. Levin, L.S., et al.: Dominant osteogenesis imperfecta: Heterogeneity and variation in expression (abstract). Am. J. Hum. Genet., *33*:66A, 1981.
52. Levin, L.S., Salinas, C.F., and Jorgenson, R.J.: Classification of osteogenesis imperfecta by dental characteristics. Lancet, *1*:332, 1978.
53. Liberfarb, R.M., Hirose, T., and Holmes, L.B.: The Wagner-Stickler syndrome: A study of 22 families. J. Pediatr., *99*:394, 1981.
54. Lichtenstein, J.R., et al.: Defect in conversion of procollagen to collagen in a form of Ehlers-Danlos syndrome. Science, *182*:298, 1973.
55. Lloyd-Roberts, G.C.: Osteoarthritis of the hip. J. Bone Joint Surg., *37B*:8, 1955.
56. Mahloudji, M., et al.: The genetic amyloidoses with particular reference to hereditary neuropathic amyloidosis type II (Indiana or Rukavina type). Medicine, *48*:1, 1969.
57. McDonald, G.R., et al.: Surgical management of patients with the Marfan syndrome and dilatation of the ascending aorta, J. Thorac. Cardiovasc. Surg., *81*:180, 1981.
58. McKusick, V.A.: Mendelian Inheritance in Man. Catalogs of Autosomal Dominant, Autosomal Recessive and X-linked Phenotypes, 6th Ed. Baltimore, Johns Hopkins Press, 1982.
59. McKusick, V.A.: Heritable Disorders of Connective Tissue, 5th Ed. St. Louis, C.V. Mosby Co., 1972.
60. McKusick, V.A., et al.: Dwarfism in the Amish. II. Cartilage-hair hypoplasia. Bull. Johns Hopkins Hosp., *116*:285, 1965.
61. McKusick, V.A., and Neufeld, E.F.: The mucopolysaccharide storage diseases. *In* The. Metabolic Basis of Inherited Disease. Edited by J.B. Stanbury, et al. New York, McGraw-Hill Book Co., 1983, pp. 751–777.
62. Moser, H.W., and Chen, W.W.: Ceramidase deficiency: Farber's lipogranulomatosis. *In* The Metabolic Basis of Inherited Disease. Edited by J.B. Stanbury, et al. New York, McGraw-Hill Book Co., 1983, pp. 820–830.
63. Mudd, S.H., and Levy, H.L.: Disorders of trans-sulfuration. *In* The Metabolic Basis of Inherited Disease. Edited by J.B. Stanbury, et al. New York, McGraw-Hill Book Co., 1983, pp. 522–559.
64. Neufeld, E.F., and McKusick, V.A.: Disorders of lysosomal enzyme synthesis and localization: I-cell disease and pseudo-Hurler polydystrophy. *In* The Metabolic Basis of Inherited Disease. Edited by J.B. Stanbury, et al. New York, McGraw-Hill Book Co., 1983, pp. 778–787.
65. Neuhauser, G., Kaveggia, E.G., and Opitz, J.M.: Autosomal recessive syndrome of pseudogliomatous blindness, osteoporosis, and mild mental retardation. Clin. Genet., *9*:324, 1976.
66. Nora, J.J., and Fraser,. F.C.: Medical Genetics Principles and Practice. Philadelphia, Lea & Febiger, 1974.
67. Penttinen, R.P., et al.: Abnormal collagen metabolism in cultured cells in osteogenesis imperfecta. Proc. Natl. Acad. Sci. U.S.A., *72*:586, 1975.
68. Pinnell, S.R.: Molecular defects in the Ehlers-Danlos syndrome. J. Invest. Dermatol., *798*:90s, 1982.
69. Pyeritz, R.E.: Unpublished data.
70. Pyeritz, R.E.: Cardiovascular manifestations of heritable disorders of connective tissue. Prog. Med. Genet., *5*:191, 1983.
71. Pyeritz, R.E.: The Marfan syndrome. *In* The Principles and Practice of Medical Genetics. Edited by A.E.H. Emery, and D.L. Rimoin. New York, Churchill-Livingstone, 1982.
72. Pyeritz, R.E., et al.: Surgical repair of the Marfan aorta: Techniques, indications and complications. Johns Hopkins Med. J., *150*:181, 1982.
73. Pyeritz, R.E., and McKusick, V.A.: Basic defects in the Marfan syndrome (editorial). N. Engl. J. Med., *305*:1011, 1981.
74. Pyeritz, R.E., and McKusick, V.A.: Genetic heterogeneity and allelic variation in the mucopolysaccharidoses. Johns Hopkins Med. J., *146*:71, 1980.
75. Pyeritz, R.E., and McKusick, V.A.: The Marfan syndrome: Diagnosis and management. N. Engl. J. Med., *300*:772, 1979.
76. Pyeritz, R.E., Sack, G.H., Jr., and Udvarhelyi, G.B.: Surgical intervention in achondroplasia: Cervical and lumbar laminectomy for spinal stenosis in achondroplasia. Johns Hopkins Med. J., *146*:203, 1980.
77. Rasmussen, H.: Hypophosphatasia. *In* The Metabolic Basis of Inherited Disease. Edited by J.B. Stanbury, et al. New York, McGraw-Hill Book Co., 1983, pp. 1497–1507.
78. Riccardi, V.M.: The Genetic Approach to Human Disease. New York, Oxford University Press, 1977.
79. Rimoin, D.L.: Pachydermoperiostosis (idiopathic clubbing and periostosis) genetic and physiologic considerations. N. Engl. J. Med., *272*:923, 1965.
80. Rovin, S., et al.: Mandibulofacial dysostosis, a familial study of five generations. J. Pediatr., *65*:215, 1964.
81. Rubin, P.: Dynamic Classification of Bone Dysplasias. Chicago, Year Book Medical Publishers, 1964.
82. Schroeber, H.W., Jr., and Zasloff, M.: The hand and foot malformations in fibrodysplasia ossificans progressiva. Johns Hopkins Med. J., *147*:73, 1980.

83. Scott, C.I., Jr.: The genetics of short stature. Prog. Med. Genet. (old series), 8:252, 1974.

84. Sillence, D.O.: Osteogenesis imperfecta: An expanding panorama of variants. Clin. Orthop., 159:11, 1981.

85. Sillence, D.O., Senn, A., and Danks, D.M.: Genetic heterogeneity in osteogenesis imperfecta. J. Med. Genet., 16:101, 1979.

86. Smith, D.W.: Recognizable Patterns of Human Deformation. Philadelphia, W.B. Saunders Co., 1981.

87. Spranger, J.W., Langer, L.O., Jr., and Wiedemann, H.R.: Bone Dysplasias. An Atlas of Constitutional Disorders of Skeletal Development. Stuttgart, Gustav Fischer Verlag, 1974.

88. Steinmann, B., et al.: Evidence for a structural mutation of procollagen type I in a patient with the Ehlers-Danlos syndrome type VII. J. Biol. Chem., 155:8887, 1980.

89. Strasburger, A.K., et al.: Symphalangism: Genetics and clinical aspects. Bull. Johns Hopkins Hosp., 117:108, 1965.

90. Uitto, J., et al.: Elastin in diseases. J. Invest. Dermatol., 79:160s-168s, 1982.

91. Valle, D., et al.: Homocystinuria due to cystathionine beta-synthase deficiency: Clinical manifestations and therapy. Johns Hopkins Med. J., 146:110, 1980.

92. Vogel, F., and Motulsky, A.G.: Human Genetics. New York, Springer-Verlag, 1979.

93. Walker, B.A., Beighton, P.H., and Murdoch, J.L.: The marfanoid hypermobility syndrome. Ann. Intern. Med., 71:349, 1969.

94. Walker, B.A., and Murdoch, J.L.: The wrist sign, A useful physical finding in the Marfan syndrome. Arch. Intern. Med., 126:276, 1970.

95. Welch, J.P., and Temtamy, S.A.: Hereditary contractures of the fingers (camptodactyly). J. Med. Genet., 3:104, 1966.

96. Weleber, R.G., and Beals, R.K.: The Hadju-Cheney syndrome. J. Pediatr., 88:243, 1976.

97. Wiesmann, U., and Neufeld, E.F.: Scheie and Hurler syndromes: Apparent identity of the biochemical defect. Science, 169:72, 1970.

98. Wynne-Davies, R.: Acetabular dysplasia and familial joint laxity. Two etiological factors in congenital dislocation of the hip. J. Bone Joint Surg., 52B:704, 1970.

Chapter 76

Hypertrophic Osteoarthropathy*

David S. Howell

Few clinical abnormalities manifest so ancient a vintage as clubbing, yet little more is known of its pathogenesis today than when it was recorded circa 400 B.C. by Hippocrates.[27,40] In addition to clubbing, bone and joint changes were noted by Bamberger and Marie (1889 and 1890, respectively).[6] The term *hypertrophic osteoarthropathy* refers to a syndrome that includes clubbing of fingers and toes, periostitis with new osseous formation at the ends of long bones, arthritis, and signs of autonomic disorders, such as flushing, blanching, and profuse sweating—most severe in hands and feet. The syndrome is classified as: (1) *secondary* to other diseases, (2) *hereditary,* or (3) *idiopathic* (pachydermoperiostosis).[11,69] The syndrome is to be distinguished from the isolated firm thickening of distal phalanges with clubbing of congenital origin; isolated clubbing deserves special consideration.[53] Clubbing associated with various extrathoracic diseases, discussed later in this chapter, wherein periosteal ossification and arthritis rarely develop,[28] may be, in some instances, a forme fruste of hypertrophic osteoarthropathy or may bear no direct relationship to it.

Pathology. Pathologic changes develop at the distal end of metacarpal, metatarsal, and long bones of the forearms and legs.[20] In severe disease, ribs, clavicles, scapulae, pelvis, and malar bones are sometimes afflicted. The earliest histologic alterations are round cell infiltration and edema of the periosteum, synovial membrane, articular capsule, and neighboring subcutaneous tissues. These changes are associated with lifting of the periosteum, deposition of osteoid matrix beneath it, and subsequent mineralization. After such foci enlarge, distal parts of the long bones eventually become ensheathed with a cuff of new bone (Fig. 76–1). Concurrent with thickening, there is accelerated resorption of endosteal and haversian bone. The resultant structure is thus weakened, and pathologic fractures may occur. With advancing disease, the pathologic alterations spread proximally along the shafts. Synovial membranes adjoining the involved bones are often edematous and infiltrated with lymphocytes, plasma cells, and a few polymorphonuclear leukocytes. Advancing proliferative fibrous tissue at joint margins is sometimes associated with cartilage degeneration.

Electron microscopic studies of the synovial membranes reveal alterations of the microcirculation, with dilatation of capillaries and venules, endothelial cell gaps, and multilamination of small vessel basement membranes.[57] Subendothelial electron-dense deposits have been described in the synovial membranes of five patients with secondary hypertrophic osteoarthopathy.[57] The significance of these deposits is not known. Negative immunofluorescent staining for gamma globulins and complement was reported in three studied hypertrophic osteoarthropathy synovia.[68]*

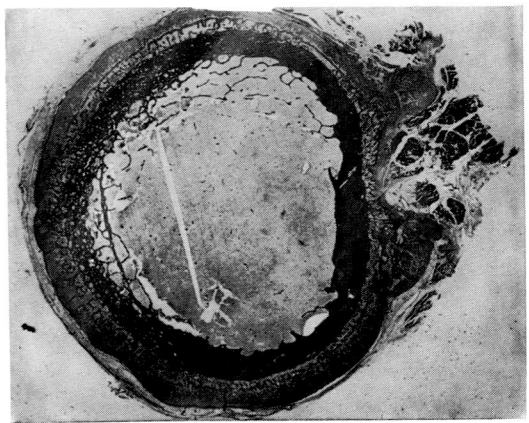

Fig. 76–1. Cross section through a metatarsal of a patient with hypertrophic osteoarthropathy. The periosteum shows thickening with an irregular cuff of new bone deposited over the cortex. (From Bartter, F.C., and Bauer, W.)

---

*Including familial idiopathic hypertrophic osteoarthropathy, Marie-Bamberger syndrome, osteoarthropathic hypertrophiante and pneumique, and secondary hypertrophic osteoarthropathy

*Recently, circulating tumor antigen-antibody complexes have been described in patients with a variety of tumors, including lung carcinomas. The electron microscopic findings seem equivocal but have made investigators question whether the synovitis seen in hypertrophic osteoarthropathy secondary to bronchogenic carcinoma might be immune complex-mediated.

In clubbed phalanges, there is edema of the soft parts, thickening of the blood vessel walls, cellular infiltration, fibroblastic proliferation, and growth of new collagenous tissue. These changes result in the uniform enlargement of terminal segments. Similar histopathologic changes have been found in the hereditary and secondary forms. Nail bed and finger pulp mast cell counts have been found to be lower in clubbed fingers as compared to controls.[41]

Etiology. This syndrome usually appears secondary to other systemic diseases, particularly neoplasms or suppurative conditions of the lungs, mediastinum, and pleura. In a small proportion of patients, the disorder is hereditary, whereas in others it is idiopathic. Hypertrophic osteoarthropathy has been observed in 5 to 10% of patients with intrathoracic neoplasms.[12,36,72] The most frequent associated tumor is bronchogenic carcinoma.[9,19] Tumors of the pleura[7] rank high, but metastatic lesions are an uncommon cause of osteoarthropathy.[73] The syndrome often accompanies lung abscess, bronchiectasis, and empyema, but with improved therapy of chronic infections, osteoarthropathy is now associated occasionally with chronic pneumonitis, pneumoconiosis, pulmonary tuberculosis, mediastinal Hodgkin's disease, and cystic fibrosis.[4,43]

For lack of convincing evidence of its separate nature, thyroid acropachy may be considered as a secondary form of hypertrophic osteoarthropathy.[15,35] The full syndrome of hypertrophic osteoarthropathy has been rarely documented in the presence of cyanotic heart disease[44] and various other extrathoracic diseases. Unless there is also periosteal and synovial involvement, the term "clubbing" rather than hypertrophic osteoarthropathy is preferable.[28]

Among diseases of the heart accompanied by clubbing, congenital malformations predominate, yet it seldom is seen in congenital heart disease without cyanosis, unless there is a complicating chronic pulmonary infection or bacterial endocarditis. Clubbing, a sign of the latter disease only with left-sided heart lesions, probably indicates embolization. Hypertrophic osteoarthropathy due to cyanotic congenital heart disease has been reported in up to 31% of patients and appears to be directly related to the degree of bypass of the lungs.[42] Hypertrophic osteoarthropathy sometimes appears with a rare disease, primary cholangiolitic cirrhosis.[8,34] Clubbing has been described in the presence of secondary hepatic amyloidosis, but a suppurative process may have been instrumental.[45] Among gastrointestinal diseases leading to osteoarthropathy, diarrheal states predominate. These conditions include ulcerative colitis, regional enteritis, intestinal tuberculosis, amebic or bacillary dysentery, idiopathic steatorrhea, sprue, neoplasms of the small intestine, multiple colonic polyposis, and carcinoma of the colon, esophagus,[50] and liver.[48] Clubbing has developed following thyroidectomy for Graves' disease, in hyperparathyroidism and, rarely, in a miscellaneous group of disorders in which the diagnosis of arthropathy is often questionable.[12,45,65] *Unilateral* clubbing results from aneurysms of the aorta, subclavian or innominate artery, as well as axillary tumors, subluxations of the shoulder, apical lung cancer, brachial arteriovenous aneurysm, and hemiplegia.[13,14] *Unidigital* clubbing has been reported after injury to the median nerve, in sarcoidosis, and in tophaceous gout. "Paddle fingers" occasionally develop in bass violin players. Osteoarthropathy confined to the lower extremity has been reported in association with an infected abdominal aneurysm.[64]

Pathogenesis. The nature of the genetic factors operative in the idiopathic form of hypertrophic osteoarthropathy is unknown, although angiographic studies have demonstrated hypervascularization of the finger pads.[32] In the secondary type, it has been postulated that the vascular proliferation and osteogenesis may be produced by: (1) obscure autonomic reflexes stimulated at the site of underlying disease, (2) a high local arteriolar pulse pressure, possibly also involving (1) or (3), (3) toxins liberated by primary malignant lesions, and (4) osteoblastic-stimulating agents released at the site of malignant pulmonary lesions or by the pluripotential cells of pleural membranes.*

Factors that might condition susceptibility of an individual with intrathoracic disease to develop the hypertrophic osteoarthropathy are unknown, but there is evidence for the participation of a local circulatory disorder.[45,47] A locally acting circulating vasodilator has been demonstrated in some patients.[61] Increased vascularity of clubbed fingers (secondary type) has been shown by measurement of skin temperature, infrared photography, nail bed capillarioscopy, and postmortem arteriography.[25,54] Mendlowitz clearly demonstrated elevated digital pulse pressure and blood flow in patients with the condition and a return to normal pressures following removal of pulmonary lesions.[45,46] Evidence for growth hormone production by bronchogenic carcinomas provides a possible explanation for joint marginal bony overgrowth observed in some af-

---

*Another theory implicates the development of pulmonary arteriovenous shunts. It is theorized that a hormone or toxin normally inactivated in the lungs is permitted escape into the systemic circulation, thereby causing the actual changes. One vasoactive substance thus implicated is reduced ferritin.

flicted patients.[10,17] Elevated urinary estrogens have been found in three patients with pulmonary lesions.[22] Audebert suggested that an amine precursor uptake and decarboxylation polypeptidic substance that differs from immunoreactive growth hormone but that is related to somatotropins may be responsible for hypertrophic pulmonary osteoarthropathy.[5] Ginsberg noted that abnormal vascular responses to intravenous infusion of epinephrine disappeared after excision of lung tumor.[21] Striking resolution of symptoms and signs in such cases follows simple denervation of the hilum or vagotomy on the same side as the lesion.[12,28,59] Thoracotomy alone is ineffective.

Clinical Description. Clubbing alone produces no symptoms except for occasional burning or warmth of fingertips. For this reason, the physician generally observes the deformity before the patient does. At the beginning of the disease, one observes increased convexity of the nail beds in sagittal and cross-sectional planes. Loss of the normal 15-degree angle between the proximal portion of the nail and dorsal surface of the phalanx also is an early sign. Another method of clinically evaluating clubbing is to measure the diameter of the finger at the base of the nail of the index finger and to divide it by the diameter at the distal interphalangeal joint. If the ratio is greater than one, it is abnormal and signifies clubbing. This ratio has been found to be independent of race, age, or sex.[63,71] A shadowgram technique has been proposed for measurement of the hyponychial angle.[62] Schamroth proposes placing the dorsal surfaces of the contralateral fingers together (the ring finger is preferred).[56] A gap appears in the normal nailbed; as the nailbed expands, this gap decreases and finally disappears. Excessive sweating or warmth of the fingertips, eponychia, paronychia, breaking or loosening of the nail, hangnails, and accelerated nail or cuticle growth are frequent. The nail base will rock on pressure owing to softening of the underlying proliferative tissue. In advanced stages, fingers may assume a drumstick appearance, and the distal interphalangeal joints show hyperextensibility (Fig. 76–2). Similar changes occur in the toes. A spade-like enlargement of the hands and feet may occur. In addition, coarsening of the facial features and thickened furrowed skin of the face (leonine facies) and scalp may develop.

In regard to bones and joints, symptoms range widely from mild arthralgias (often with asymptomatic periosteal reactions) to severe, deep-seated aching or burning pain and tenderness over the long bones, progressive clumsiness of hands, and awkwardness of gait. Concomitant with these symptoms is variable heat, erythema, restricted joint motion, ankylosis, and swelling with effusion of the wrists, elbows, metacarpophalangeal joints, knees, ankles, and other regions discussed under pathology. Alcohol may worsen joint pain and swelling.[49] Aggravation of bone pain on dependency of the limbs is a unique feature suggesting that local vascular stasis may play a role in production of pain. Excessive distal phalangeal resorption of fingers and toes may lead to acrolysis.[26] Gynecomastia, as well as elevation of urinary estrogen excretion, is noted sometimes in patients with hypertrophic osteoarthropathy, but the significance is obscure.[21,33] Cranial suture defects have also been noted.[53] Hypopigmentation of the skin and induration of the subcutaneous tissue around the active joint may be suggestive of scleroderma.[23] Insidious development of symptoms and signs over a period of months or years generally characterizes osteoarthropathy associated with suppurative disease of the lungs, and rheumatic complaints are mild. In contrast, a rapidly progressing syndrome with prominent joint pain and stiffness is common with malignant diseases and chronic infections.

Laboratory and Roentgenographic Findings. Synovial fluids in this condition have been generally ''noninflammatory,'' clear and of high viscosity. Leukocyte counts are usually below 2,000/mm³, with less than 50% polymorphonuclear leukocytes.[9,57,68]

Serum and synovial fluid C3 and C4 levels were normal in three reported cases of hypertrophic osteoarthropathy secondary to bronchogenic carcinoma.[68]

The fluorescent antinuclear antibody and latex fixation tests for rheumatoid factor have been negative in most patients, while the sedimentation rate is often elevated.

The roentgenogram is important in the diagnosis of hypertrophic osteoarthropathy. Subperiosteal new bone layering characteristically appears in the distal diaphyseal regions of long bone, especially of the legs and forearms, and less commonly of the phalanges. The involvement is usually symmetrical. Rarely, a few patients will have florid clinical disease in the absence of any radiologic changes.[31]

The diagnosis of hypertrophic pulmonary osteoarthropathy can also be suggested by the characteristic abnormal pattern seen on skeletal imaging using ^{99m}Tc pyrophosphate or diphosphonate.[16,55] A pericortical linear accumulation of tracer along the long bones and proximal phalanges is seen along with increased periarticular uptake disclosing the synovitis also present in this illness. Involvement of the skull, scapulae, clavicles, and patellae is frequently noted. Asymmetric and/or irregular distribution may be seen in fewer than 20% of patients. Differentiation of hypertrophic

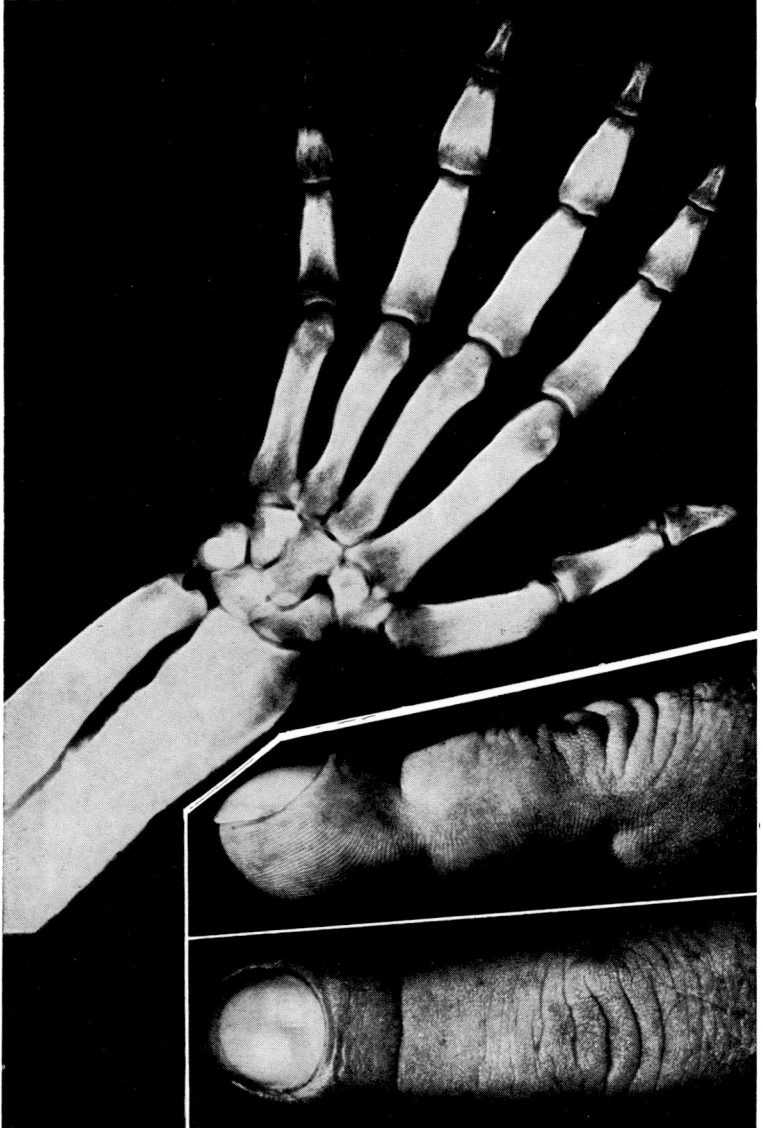

Fig. 76–2. Hippocratic finger and roentgenogram of hand showing the characteristic features of hypertrophic osteoarthropathy. (From Campbell et al.)

osteoarthropathy from metastatic disease by bone scanning is not difficult because the patterns of radionuclide distribution vary considerably. After tumor removal, a resolution of the abnormal tracer accumulations may be seen.[1]

Differential Diagnosis. The presence of clubbing, which almost always accompanies hypertrophic osteoarthropathy, simplifies diagnosis, and a primary disease is sought. Yet, if acute polyar-

thritis precedes clubbing by months or years, search for an asymptomatic pulmonary neoplasm may be neglected and the case may be mislabeled as rheumatoid arthritis.[30,51] In most instances, roentgenograms reveal elevation of the periosteum and evidence of new bone growth[24] (Fig. 76–3). To be differentiated are periosteal elevations resulting from tumors, lymphangitis, syphilis, and the hemorrhages of trauma or scurvy (Fig. 76–4).

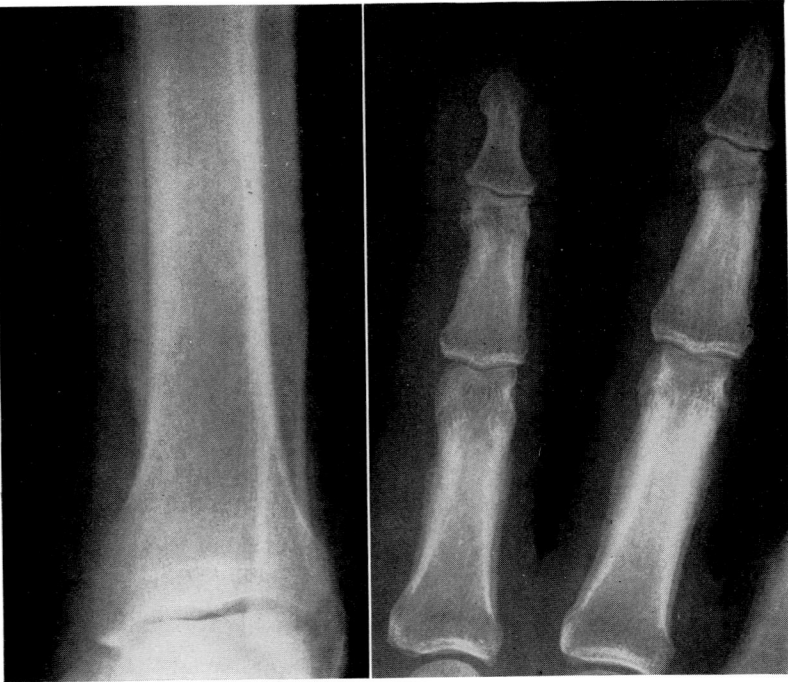

Fig. 76–3. Hypertrophic osteoarthropathy. Radiodense bands along a margin of the shaft indicate new osseous formation beneath the elevated periosteum. Appearance of these typical lesions is similar in phalanges *(right)* to that of long bones *(left)*. (Courtesy of the late Dr. J. J. Bunim.)

Swelling and tenderness of the lower legs may falsely suggest thrombophlebitis, and bony pains may be misinterpreted as peripheral neuritis. The spoon-shaped nails of hypochromic anemia should be readily distinguishable.

Care should be exerted to exclude primary disease before assigning patients to the ill-defined hereditary or idiopathic groups. This point is emphasized because of the danger of overlooking a resectable tumor or other treatable lesions. In hereditary or idiopathic osteoarthropathy, also known as the Touraine-Solente-Golé syndrome, there is often onset of the clinical manifestations after puberty, a self-limited course after one to two decades, and detection in other members of the family.[67] Males are affected more often than females. Findings in these cases range from clubbing alone, to widespread periosteal thickening of the long bones, metacarpals, metatarsals, and distal phalanges, with limitation of joint motion and ankle edema. Bone and joint pain is usually absent. Some of these patients have shown gynecomastia, thickening, furrowing, and excessive oiliness of the skin over the face and limbs *(cutis verticis gyrata)*,

feminine distribution of hair, striae, acne vulgaris, and hypertrophy or atrophy of the ungual tufts of the fingers, all of which become manifest at adolescence.[67,69,70] The hereditary form is transmitted as a mendelian dominant trait. Thyroid acropachy is manifested by (present or past) hyperthyroidism, pretibial myxedema, exophthalmos, clubbing, and periosteal elevation of phalanges, metacarpals, and metatarsals.[15,35] When measured, long-acting thyroid stimulator (LATS) has been present in these cases.[39]

Treatment. Clubbing is usually asymptomatic and usually requires no treatment. Disabling symptoms related to joints and bones respond with dramatic promptness to removal of the primary pulmonary lesion or to intrathoracic vagotomy.[12,28,37] Chemical vagotomy by atropine[13,38] or propantheline bromide may provide benefit in the treatment of symptoms.[58] Supportive analgesic measures or, in some instances, treatment with adrenocortical steroid derivatives may be useful.[28] Complete disappearance of hypertrophic osteoarthropathy is described after appropriate therapy for empyema, lung abscess, bronchiectasis, pneumonia, and bac-

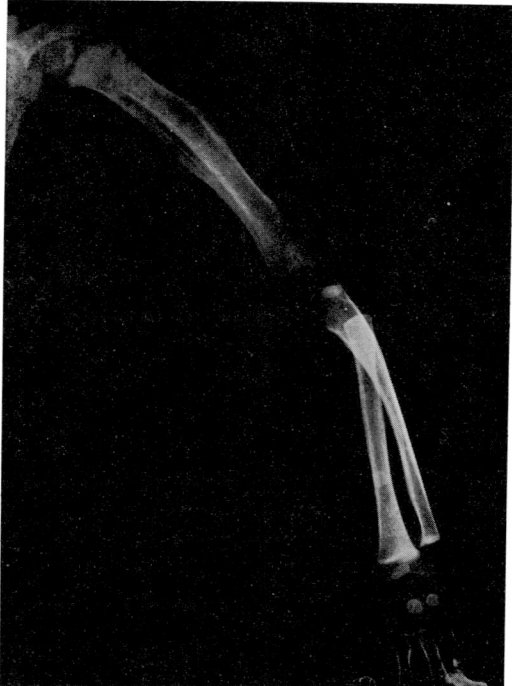

Fig. 76–4. Periosteal reaction in a patient with scurvy (following recent antiscorbutic treatment). Trauma, syphilis, or scurvy, although a cause of proliferative periostitis, should rarely be confused with hypertrophic osteoarthropathy. (From Stein, Stein, and Beller)

terial endocarditis.[60] Treatment of the idiopathic form is symptomatic. Radiotherapy to the primary tumor site[66] or to metastatic lesions,[52] as well as chemotherapy,[18] has been reported to relieve joint symptomatology.

REFERENCES

1. Ali, A., et al.: Distribution of hypertrophic pulmonary osteoarthropathy. Am. J. Roentgenol., *134*:771–780, 1980.
2. Allison, N.L., et al.: Pulmonary osteoarthropathy preceding evidence of metastases from hypernephroma (letter). Lancet, *1*:950, 1981.
3. Alvarez, A.S., et al.: Unilateral clubbing of the fingernails in patients with hemiplegia. Gerontologia Clinica, *17*:1–6, 1975.
4. Athreya, B.H., Gorske, A.L., and Myers, A.R.: Aspirin-induced abnormalities of liver function. Am. J. Dis. Child., *129*:638–641, 1973.
5. Audebert, A.A., et al.: Osteoarthropathie hypertrophiante pneumique associee a une quadruple secretion hormonale paraneoplastique. Sem. Hop. Paris, *458*:529–530, 1982.
6. von Bamberger, E.: Uber Knochen veranderungen bei chronischen Lungenund. Herzkran Kenheiten Klin. Med., *18*:193, 1890–1891.
7. Briselli, M., Mark, E.J., and Dickersin, G.R.: Solitary fibrous tumors of the pleura: Eight new cases and review of 360 cases in the literature. Cancer, *1;47*:2678–2689, 1981.
8. Buchan, D.J., and Mitchell, D.M.: Hypertrophic osteoarthropathy in portal cirrhosis. Ann. Intern. Med., *66*:130–135, 1967.
9. Calabro, J.J.: Cancer and arthritis. Arthritis Rheum., *10*:553–567, 1967.
10. Cameron, D.P., et al.: On the presence of immunoreactive growth hormone in a bronchogenic carcinoma. Aust. Ann. Med., *18*:143–146, 1969.
11. Camp, J.D., and Scanlan, R.L.: Chronic idiopathic hypertrophic osteoarthropathy. Radiology, *50*:581–593, 1948.
12. Christian, C.L.: Chairman Editorial Committee. 19th Rheumatism Review. Arthritis Rheum., *13*:615, 1970.
13. Day, W.H., and Hagelsten, J.O.: Blocking of the vagus nerve relieving osteoarthropathy in lung diseases. Dan. Med. Bull., *11*:131–133, 1964.
14. Denham, M.J., Hodkinson, H.M., and Wright, B.M.: Unilateral clubbing in hemiplegia. Gerontologia Clinica, *17*:7–12, 1975.
15. Diamond, M.T.: The syndrome of exophthalmos, hypertrophic osteoarthropathy and localized myxedema: A review of the literature and report of a case. Ann. Intern. Med., *50*:206–213, 1959.
16. Donnelly, B., and Johnson, P.M.: Detection of hypertrophic pulmonary osteoarthropathy of skeletal imaging with 99m Tc-labeled diphosphonate. Radiology, *114*:389–391, 1975.
17. Dupont, B.: Plasma growth hormone and hypertrophic osteoarthropathy in carcinoma of the bronchus. Acta Med. Scand., *188*:25–30, 1970.
18. Evans, W.K.: Reversal of hypertrophic osteoarthropathy after chemotherapy for bronchogenic carcinoma. J. Rheumatol., *7*:93–97, 1980.
19. Freeman, M.H., and Tonkin, A.K.: Manifestations of hypertrophic pulmonary osteoarthropathy in patients with carcinoma of the lung. Demonstration by ^{99m}Tc-pyrophosphate bone scans. Radiology, *120*:363–365, 1976.
20. Gall, E.A., Bennett, G.A., and Bauer, W.: Generalized hypertrophic osteoarthropathy. Am. J. Pathol., *27*:349–381, 1951.
21. Ginsburg, J.: Observations on the peripheral circulation in hypertrophic pulmonary osteoarthropathy. Q. J. Med., *27*:335–352, 1958.
22. Ginsburg, J., and Brown, J.B.: Increased oestrogen excretion in hypertrophic pulmonary osteoarthropathy. Lancet, *2*:1274–1276, 1961.
23. Gray, R.G., and Gottlieb, N.L.: Pseudoscleroderma in hypertrophic osteoarthropathy. J.A.M.A., *246*:2062–2063, 1981.
24. Greenfield, G.B., Schorsch, H.A., and Ahkoln, A.: The various roentgen appearances of pulmonary hypertrophic osteoarthropathy. Am. J. Roentgenol. Rad. Ther. Nucl. Med., *101*:927–931, 1967.
25. Harter, J.S.: Joint manifestations (discussion). J. Thorac. Surg. *9*:505, 1939–1940.
26. Hedayati, H., Barmada, R., and Skosey, J.L.: Acrolysis in pachydermoperiostosis. Arch. Intern. Med., *140*:1087–1088, 1980.
27. Hippocrates (c. 400 B.C.): The Genuine Works of Hippocrates. Vol. 1. Translated by F. Adams. Sydenham Society, 1849, p. 249.
28. Holling, H.E., and Brodey, R.S.: Pulmonary hypertrophic osteoarthropathy. J.A.M.A., *178*:977–982, 1961.
29. Holling, H.E., Brodey, R.S., and Boland, H.C.: Pulmonary hypertrophic osteoarthropathy. Lancet, *2*:1269–1274, 1961.
30. Holmes, H.H., Bauman, E., and Ragan, C.: Symptomatic arthritis due to hypertrophic pulmonary osteoarthropathy in pulmonary neoplastic disease. Report of seven cases. Ann. Rheum. Dis., *9*:169–173, 1950.
31. Horn, C.R.: Hypertrophic pulmonary osteoarthropathy with radiographic evidence of new bone formation. Thorax, *35*:479, 1980.
32. Jajic, I., et al.: Primary hypertrophic osteoarthropathy (PHO) and changes in the joints. Scand. J. Rheumatol., *9*:89–96, 1980.
33. Jao, J.Y., Barlow, J.J., and Krant, M.J.: Pulmonary hypertrophic osteoarthropathy, spider angiomata, and estrogen hyperexcretion. Ann. Intern. Med., *70*:581–584, 1969.
34. Kieff, E.D., and McCarty, D.J.: Hypertrophic osteoar-

thropathy with arthritis and synovial calcification in a patient with alcoholic cirrhosis. Arthritis Rheum., 12:261–268, 1969.

35. Kinsella, R.A., Jr., and Back, D.K.: Thyroid acropachy. Med. Clin. North Am., 52:393–398, 1968.

36. Lansbury, J.: Connective tissue manifestations of neoplastic disease. Geriatrics, 9:319–324, 1954.

37. LeRoux, B.T.: Bronchial carcinoma with hypertrophic pulmonary osteoarthropathy. S. Afr. Med. J., 42:1074–1075, 1968.

38. Lopez-Enriquez, E., Morales, A.R., and Robert, F.: Effect of atropine sulfate in pulmonary hypertrophic osteoarthropathy. Arthritis Rheum., 23:822–824, 1980.

39. Lynch, P.J., Maize, J.C., and Sisson, J.C.: Pretibial myxedema and nonthyrotoxic thyroid disease. Arch. Dermatol., 107:107–111, 1973.

40. Marie, P.: De l'osteoarthropathie hypertrophiante pneumique. Rev. Med., 10:1–36, 1890.

41. Marshal, R.: Observations of the pathology of clubbed fingers with special reference to mast cells. Am. Rev. Respir. Dis., 113:395–397, 1976.

42. Martinez-Lavin, M., et al.: Hypertrophic osteoarthropathy in cyanotic congenital heart disease. Arthritis Rheum., 25:1186–1192, 1982.

43. Matthay, M.A., et al.: Hypertrophic osteoarthropathy in adults with cystic fibrosis. Thorax, 31:572–575, 1976.

44. McLaughlin, G.E., McCarty, D.J., Jr., and Downing, D.F.: Hypertrophic osteoarthropathy associated with cyanotic congenital heart disease. Ann. Intern. Med., 67:579–587, 1967.

45. Mendlowitz, M.: Clubbing and hypertrophic osteoarthropathy. Medicine, 21:269–306, 1942.

46. Mendlowitz, M.: Measurement of blood flow and blood pressure in clubbed fingers. J. Clin. Invest., 20:113–117, 1941.

47. Mendlowitz, M., and Leslie, A.: Experimental simulation in dogs of cyanosis and hypertrophic osteoarthropathy which are associated with congenital heart disease. Am. Heart J., 24:141–152, 1942.

48. Morgan, A.G., et al.: A new syndrome associated with hepatocellular carcinoma. Gastroenterology, 63:340–345, 1972.

49. Mueller, M., and Trevarthen, D.: Pachydermoperiostosis: Arthropathy aggravated by episodic alcohol abuse. J. Rheumatol., 8:862–864, 1981.

50. Peirce, T.H., and Weir, D.G.: Hypertrophic osteoarthropathy associated with a non-metastasizing carcinoma of the oesophagus. J. Ir. Med. Assoc., 66:160–162, 1973.

51. Polley, H.F., et al.: Articular reactions with localized fibrous mesothelioma of the pleura. Ann. Rheum. Dis., 11:314, 1952.

52. Rao, G.M., et al.: Improvement in hypertrophic pulmonary osteoarthropathy after radiotherapy to metastases. Am. J. Radiol., 133:944–946, 1979.

53. Reginato, A., Jr., Schinpachasse, Y., and Guerrero, R.: Familial idiopathic hypertrophic osteoarthropathy and cranial suture defects in children. Skeletal Radiol., 8:105–109, 1982.

54. Rominger, E.: Ein fall von morbus caeroleus mit demonstration der hautkapillaren am lebenden nach weibund elek-

tro kardiographischen untersuchungen. Dtsch. Med. Wochenschr., 46:168, 1920.

55. Rosenthal, L., and Kirsh, J.: Observations on radionuclide imaging in hypertrophic pulmonary osteoarthropathy. Radiology, 120:359–362, 1976.

56. Schamroth, L.: Personal experience. S. Afr. Med. J., 50:297–300, 1976.

57. Schumacher, H.R.: Articular manifestations of HPO in bronchogenic carcinoma. A clinical and pathologic study. Arthritis Rheum., 19:629–636, 1976.

58. Schwartz, H.A.: Pro-Banthine for hypertrophic osteoarthropathy. Arthritis Rheum., 23:1588, 1981.

59. Semple, T., and McCluskie, R.A.: Generalized hypertrophic osteoarthropathy in association with bronchial carcinoma. Br. Med. J., 1:754–759, 1955.

60. Shapiro, C.M., and Mackinnon, J.: The resolution of hypertrophic pulmonary osteoarthropathy following treatment of subacute bacterial endocarditis. Postgrad. Med. J., 56:513–515, 1980.

61. Shneerson, J.M.: Digital clubbing and hypertrophic osteoarthropathy: The underlying mechanisms. Br. J. Dis. Chest, 75:113–131, 1981.

62. Sinniah, D., and Omar, A.: Quantitation of digital clubbing by shadowgram technique. Arch. Dis. Child., 54:145–146, 1979.

63. Sly, R.M., et al.: Objective assessment for digital clubbing in Caucasian, Negro, and Oriental subjects. Chest, 64:687–689, 1973.

64. Sorin, S.B., Askari, A., and Rhodes, R.S.: Hypertrophic osteoarthropathy of the lower extremities as a manifestation of arterial graft sepsis. Arthritis Rheum., 23:768–770, 1980.

65. Souders, C.R., and Manuell, J.L.: Skeletal deformities in hyperparathyroidism. N. Engl. J. Med., 250:594–597, 1954.

66. Steinfeld, A.D., and Munzenrider, J.E.: The response of hypertrophic pulmonary osteoarthropathy to radiotherapy. Radiology, 113:709–711, 1974.

67. Touraine, A., Solente, A., and Golé, L.: Un syndrome osteo-dermo pathique: La pachydermie plicaturee avec pachyperiostose des extremités. Presse Med., 43:1820–1824, 1935.

68. Vidal, A.F., et al.: Structural and immunologic changes of synovium of hypertrophic osteoarthropathy (HPO). Arthritis Rheum., 20:139, 1977.

69. Vogl, A., Blumenfeld, S., and Gutner, L.B.: Diagnostic significance of pulmonary hypertrophic osteoarthropathy. Am. J. Med., 18:51–65, 1955.

70. Vogl, A., and Goldfischer, S.: Pachydermoperiostosis. Primary or idiopathic hypertrophic osteoarthropathy. Am. J. Med., 33:166–187, 1962.

71. Waring, W.W., et al.: Quantitation of digital clubbing in children. Measurements of casts of the index finger. Am. Rev. Respir. Dis., 104:166–174, 1971.

72. Wierman, W.H., Clagett, O.T., and McDonald, J.R.: Articular manifestations in pulmonary diseases: An analysis of their occurrence in 1,024 cases in which pulmonary resection was performed. J.A.M.A., 155:1459–1463, 1954.

73. Yacoub, M.H., Simon, G., and Ohnsorge, J.: Hypertrophic pulmonary osteoarthropathy in association with pulmonary metastases from extrathoracic tumours. Thorax, 22:226–231, 1967.

Regional Disorders of Joints and Related Structures

Chapter 77

Traumatic Arthritis and Allied Conditions

Robert S. Pinals

In its broadest sense, the term "traumatic arthritis" circumscribes a diverse collection of pathologic and clinical states that develop after single or repetitive episodes of trauma (Table 77–1). Although these conditions may be encountered frequently by the rheumatologist, interest in the area has been casual, and studies of basic mechanisms of disease have been few as compared with those in the other rheumatic diseases. Because surgeons are more likely to deal with the sequelae of trauma, it is not surprising that the most significant contributions are to be found in the orthopedic literature. The credulous assignment of etiologic roles to trauma in early writings stands in sharp contrast to modern attitudes on the subject. Rheumatoid arthritis, tuberculous arthritis, gout, and other rheumatic diseases were formerly attributed to trauma, which might alter the structural integrity of joints, predisposing them to inflammation.[98] As other pathogenetic mechanisms have been revealed, it has become less necessary to invoke "unrecognized trauma," which was previously such a convenient explanation for poorly understood disorders. Even in osteoarthritis, once the bellwether of traumatic disorders, considered by some to be synonymous with traumatic arthritis, increasing emphasis is being placed on altered cartilage metabolism, leaving an even smaller role for "multiple microtraumata."

ACUTE TRAUMATIC SYNOVITIS

Following a direct blow or forced inappropriate motion to a joint, swelling and pain may develop. Because the knee is most commonly affected, the following discussion will be directed at that joint, but one might follow a similar approach for a traumatic synovitis in the elbow, shoulder, or ankle. On examination, an effusion is usually evident, which should be aspirated to determine whether hemarthrosis is present and to aid in further examination of the joint. Hemarthrosis is usually present if fluid appears within two hours after the injury.[106] In about half the cases, swelling occurs within 15 minutes.[22] On the other hand, nonbloody effusions generally appear 12 to 24 hours after injury.[22] With hemarthrosis there is usually more pain, and at times a low-grade fever. Fractures, internal derangements, or major ligamentous tears must be ruled out by examination and radiographs, which should include stress, skyline, and intercondylar views. In one series of patients with traumatic hemarthrosis, 66 had fractures or ligamentous rupture, and 20 did not.[106] Detachment or laceration of cartilage and capsular tears may not be discovered in this manner. It has been suggested, on the basis of calcification that developed later in the median parapatellar area, that lateral subluxation of the patella, tearing the medial retinaculum, may be the source of joint hemorrhage in some cases.[106] The presence of fat globules floating on the surface of bloody fluid usually indicates a fracture. At times, sufficient fat may be present to be detectable on a lateral knee radiograph as a radiolucent layer in the suprapatellar pouch[5] (Fig. 77–1). A similar appearance has been described in the anterior compartment of the elbow.[114] Hemorrhagic fluid usually does not clot; coagulation may indicate more profound tissue damage and a poorer prognosis.

In the absence of gross bleeding, examination of the fluid reveals a variable number of red blood cells and 50 to 2,000 white blood cells, of which only a few are neutrophils. The protein content, mostly albumin, is two or three times that of normal fluid. Viscosity is slightly reduced, but the mucin clot is good.[87] Synovial biopsy reveals some vasodilatation, edema, and an occasional small focus of synovial cell proliferation with mild lymphocytic infiltration. An electron-microscopic study has shown evidence of increased protein synthesis by synovial cells, perhaps accounting for a portion of the excessive protein content in post-traumatic effusions.[89]

Rarely, a high leukocyte count in traumatic synovial effusions is accompanied by intra- and extracellular lipid globules, suggesting that lipid droplet phagocytosis might have provoked an inflammatory reaction.[37] This hypothesis was supported by studies of dog knees subjected to blunt trauma, which resulted in clear effusions containing fat globules. Intra-articular injection of autolo-

Table 77-1. Classification of Traumatic Arthritis and Allied Conditions

I.   Articular trauma, single episode.
    A. Traumatic synovitis, without disturbance of articular cartilage or disruption of major supporting structures. This type includes acute synovitis, with or without hemarthrosis, and most sprains. Healing is expected within several weeks, without permanent tissue damage.
    B. Disruptive trauma, with infraction of the articular cartilage or complete rupture of major supporting structures. This type includes intra-articular fractures, meniscal tears, and severe sprains.
    C. Post-traumatic osteoarthritis. This type includes cases of disruptive trauma in which major residual damage is present. Patients may have deformity, limited motion, or instability of joints.
II. Repetitive articular trauma. This type includes a variety of conditions related to occupation or sports and results in localized chronic arthritis.
III. Induction or aggravation of another specific rheumatic disease by acute or repetitive trauma.
IV. Conditions in which trauma may be one of several etiologic factors, or in which a relationship has been suggested but not established: osteochondritis dissecans, osteitis pubis, Tietze's syndrome, and hypermobility syndrome.

V.   Disorders of extra-articular structures, such as tendons, bursae, and muscles, in which trauma commonly plays an etiologic role.
VI. Nonmechanical types of trauma, such as arthropathy following frostbite, radiation, and decompression.

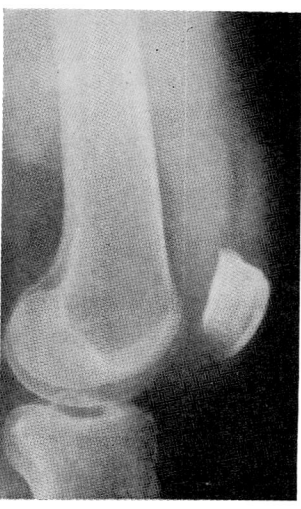

Fig. 77-1. Traumatic hemarthrosis. Liquid fat and a fat-blood level are visible in the joint. (From Berk, R.N.[5])

gous fat was shown to induce phagocytosis and mild inflammation[105] (see Chap. 4).

Treatment may include such measures as cold packs initially and heat later; compression dressings or posterior splints; graded quadriceps exercises; repeated aspiration if significant volumes of fluid reaccumulate; and a period of bed rest or partial weight-bearing, depending upon the severity of the injury. Prognosis is excellent in the absence of improper treatment, such as cylinder cast immobilization, which may result in muscle atrophy and loss of motion, or premature weight-bearing, which may lead to an extended duration of synovitis. A study of experimental hemarthrosis in rabbits has shown that there is no deleterious effect on articular cartilage, even from repeated hemarthroses, although the synovium may show a mild inflammatory process and iron accumulation.[110]

SPRAINS

A sprain may be defined as a stretching or tearing of a supporting ligament of a joint by forced movement beyond its normal range. In its simplest form, there is minimal disruption of fibers, swelling, pain, and dysfunction. Severe sprains may cause total rupture of ligaments, marked swelling and hemorrhage, and joint instability, which may be permanent if untreated. Sprains occur most frequently in the ankle, but are also common in the knee, low back, and neck.

Ankle Sprains. Most ankle sprains result from unintentional weight-bearing on the inverted, plantar-flexed foot. There is partial or total disruption of one or more of the three main lateral supporting structures, which unite the fibula above with the calcaneus and talus below (Fig. 77-2). Rupture of the anterior talofibular ligament is most common; this structure prevents anterior displacement of the talus out of the ankle joint mortise. With additional force, the calcaneofibular ligament, which prevents excessive inversion, may also rupture. The third ligament, the posterior talofibular ligament, is seldom torn with the usual type of injury. If it also tears, a completely unstable ankle results. Stretching of the medial supporting structures usually results in fracture and avulsion of the medial malleolus rather than a sprain.

The patient presents with severe pain and swelling on the outer aspect of the foot and ankle. Much of the early swelling is due to hemorrhage, resulting in ecchymosis several hours later. A history of something snapping, giving away, or slipping out of place may suggest a complete ligament rupture.

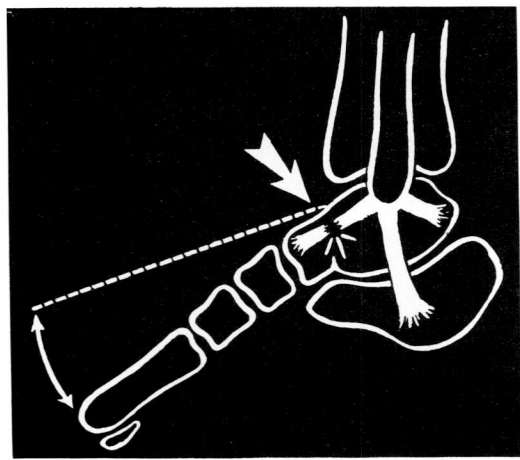

Fig. 77–2. A severe ankle sprain, occurring in equinus and inversion, may result in rupture of the anterior talofibular ligament. (From Pipkin, G.: Clin. Orthop., *3*:8, 1954.)

The nature of the treatment is largely dependent upon assessment of the integrity of these ligaments. This is most easily accomplished soon after the injury, before swelling and pain make forced motion difficult. Local anesthesia may be required for proper examination. Some orthopedists insist upon stress roentgenograms after all severe sprains.

Early treatment of simple sprains may include elevation, ice packs, and compression dressing to prevent swelling; injection of local anesthetics to permit early motion; and adhesive strapping. Full weight-bearing is permitted on the following day. A lift on the outer border of the heel will maintain eversion and prevent strain on the injured ligament. Strapping or, later, an elastic support is continued until healing is complete, usually for 3 to 6 weeks.[2]

Severe sprains may demand additional treatment, such as walking plaster for 4 to 6 weeks when the anterior talofibular ligament is ruptured, and early surgical repair when, in addition, the calcaneofibular ligament is torn.[2] A follow-up study of patients with long-standing lateral ligament instability demonstrated a high incidence of degenerative changes in the articular cartilage of the medial joint surface.[41]

Other Sprains. Knee sprains are considered in Chapter 78, and low back sprains in Chapter 82. Shoulder ''sprain'' is actually a subluxation of the acromioclavicular joint, commonly seen in body contact sports. Wrist ''sprain'' is usually a fractured navicular bone, often missed on initial roentgenograms. Traumatic torticollis may be called a neck sprain. Following a sudden twist or wrenching of the neck, pain and muscle spasm may result in involuntary assumption of a ''wry neck'' position. Spontaneous remission occurs after 1 to 2 weeks. Such measures as a cervical collar, traction, and heat may be helpful. The actual structures involved in neck sprain have not been well defined.

PELLEGRINI-STIEDA SYNDROME; PERIARTICULAR OSSIFICATION

A linear calcific density may develop in the area of the medial collateral ligament after acute knee trauma. A hematoma may be the initial event. Calcification is noted on roentgenograms obtained as early as 3 or 4 weeks after the injury.[71] Few biopsies have been obtained in the early stages; those performed later show bone rather than a calcific deposit. The initial injury may be minor or may produce a fracture, torn meniscus, or ligamentous rupture. Initial signs and symptoms, as well as subsequent disability, are related more to this associated trauma than to the Pellegrini-Stieda lesion itself.[35] However, persistent tenderness and some swelling are often found on the medial aspect of the knee. Local corticosteroid injections have been advocated for these patients.

ECTOPIC BONE FORMATION AFTER SPINAL CORD INJURY

Paraplegic and quadriplegic patients may develop ossification in soft tissues adjacent to joints that are located below the level of the neurologic lesion. The hips and knees are most commonly involved. This complication occurs in 16 to 53% of patients with spinal cord injury[103] and occasionally in other neurologic conditions.[31] Although some of the milder cases may not be detected by physical examination, many patients have swelling, warmth, and erythema in the affected area, suggesting alternative diagnoses, such as cellulitis and thrombophlebitis. These signs may appear as early as three weeks after the injury, when radiographic findings are minimal or absent.[72] At this stage, serum alkaline phosphatase may be elevated, and soft tissue uptake of radionuclide may be increased on a bone scan.[31] Over a period of weeks or months a firm mass of trabeculated bone may be detected on physical examination and demonstrated radiologically. This finding is often accompanied by loss of joint motion and occasionally by complete ankylosis. Serious functional impairment may result; for instance, the patient may be unable to sit because hip flexion is lost. The osseous deposit may be excised when it reaches maturity, but it recurs in most patients.

The pathogenesis of this condition is unknown, but it has been suggested that these immobile patients develop areas of ischemic tissue necrosis at pressure points near joints, leading to an inflammatory reaction and subsequent bony metaplasia.[93] The areas of ectopic bone formation correlated with decubitus ulcerations of the overlying skin in one report.[43] Vigorous passive exercise, advocated to prevent loss of joint motion, does not appear to increase the ossification process.[93] Patients with spinal cord injury may also develop hydrarthrosis or hemarthrosis of the knee,[72,102] presumed to be of traumatic origin.[102]

DISRUPTIVE ARTICULAR TRAUMA: POST-TRAUMATIC OSTEOARTHRITIS

Permanent joint damage may be the end result of various types of trauma, including fractures through the articular surface, dislocations, internal derangements, major ligamentous ruptures, and wounds, often with sepsis and foreign body implantation (Fig. 77–3). There may be permanent or progressive structural alterations, e.g., deterioration of articular cartilage, limitation of joint motion, instability, or angular deviation. Detailed consideration of these injuries and their treatment is beyond the scope of this book. Pathologically and radiographically the condition has most of the characteristics of osteoarthritis. However, a specific traumatic episode should not be definitely accepted as etiologically related to osteoarthritis unless there is evidence establishing the following points: (1) the joint was normal prior to injury; (2) records document either an effusion or structural damage shortly after the injury; and (3) similar disease has not occurred in nontraumatized joints. Other points favoring a traumatic origin are the occurrence of significant isolated osteoarthritis in a joint not usually involved by the idiopathic variety (such as ankle, wrist, elbow, or metacarpophalangeal joint) and radiologic demonstration of foreign bodies and healed fractures near the joint in question.

REPETITIVE ARTICULAR TRAUMA

Osteoarthritis may develop in joints that are repeatedly traumatized as a result of certain occupations and sports. Radiographic abnormalities, such as joint space narrowing, subcortical cysts, and marginal osteophytes, are common in some groups studied, but many of the affected individuals are asymptomatic. These changes occur in the hands and wrists of boxers and stone workers using pneumatic hammers, in the ankles of soccer players, in the first metatarsophalangeal joints of ballet dancers, and in the elbows of foundry workers.

ROLE OF TRAUMA IN OTHER TYPES OF ARTHRITIS

Trauma plays an important role in the development of neuropathic joint disease (see Chap. 71). Attacks of gouty arthritis often develop in recently injured joints. Rheumatoid arthritis occasionally begins in a joint that has been injured or subjected to a surgical procedure. In a follow-up study of patients who had sustained a serious fracture, the incidence of rheumatoid arthritis was found to be greater than in control subjects.[50] A history of recent or old trauma to the affected joint is sometimes obtained from patients with septic or tuberculous arthritis. However, the evidence in these situations is anecdotal and difficult to evaluate. Data have not been gathered in an organized fashion, and the mechanisms involved are not well understood. In many instances, the trauma has been minimal, perhaps representing an unrelated antecedent to the joint disease.[32]

Williams and Scott have reported three patients in whom trauma to a finger joint was followed by chronic polyarthritis with most prominent involvement of the injured joint.[107] On reviewing the literature, they concluded that trauma is a precipitating factor in about 5% of patients with rheumatoid arthritis. The mechanism may be sim-

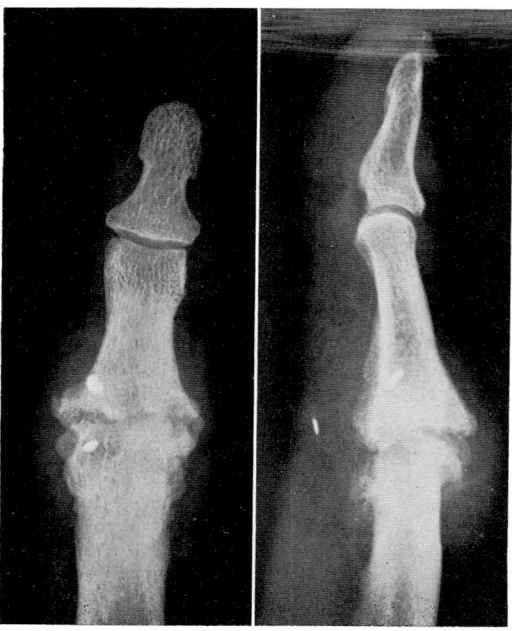

Fig. 77–3. Arthritis due to foreign body. A piece of steel lodged in this index finger of the patient four years earlier. Swelling of the finger began about two years later and has continued to date. Roentgenograph shows marked deformity of the proximal interphalangeal joint of the right index finger. This consists of marked hypertrophic changes with possible ankylosis of the joint. There are two small opaque foreign bodies in relation to the palmar and radial aspects of the joint.

ilar to that in experimental arthritis in rabbits, induced by intra-articular fibrin injections.[28]

Preexisting arthritis may certainly be aggravated by trauma, but the dimensions of this statement are an unknown quantity, and each case must be considered on its own merits.[30] Only minor force would be required to cause rupture of a frayed wrist extensor tendon or collateral ligament in a patient with rheumatoid arthritis. Other acute episodes, such as abrupt increase in joint swelling or rupture of the posterior knee joint capsule, are commonly associated with unusual resistive exercise. Sanguineous joint fluid is sometimes aspirated from a knee or shoulder in patients with rheumatoid arthritis who report sudden increase in pain and swelling following relatively minor trauma. It is presumed that pinching or compression of the hypertrophied synovium may result in bleeding. In such cases, the synovial fluid hematocrit is fairly low, usually less than 10%.

BENIGN HYPERMOBILITY SYNDROME

Generalized joint hypermobility due to ligamentous laxity occurs in about 5% of the population. The condition is regarded by some as a familial disorder that predisposes the affected individual to articular injuries, leading to chronic or recurrent arthralgia. The term "hypermobility syndrome" was introduced by Kirk et al. to describe healthy subjects with joint laxity in the absence of major features of the Marfan or Ehlers-Danlos syndromes, and arthralgia for which no other explanation could be found.[52] The syndrome has a marked female preponderance. Symptoms first appear in children or young adults. Hypermobile individuals are often able to hyperextend the knee and elbow beyond 10°, to achieve sufficient lumbar flexion to place both palms on the floor without bending the knees, and to passively oppose the thumb to the flexor aspect of the forearm. Lacking the stability afforded by normal ligaments, hypermobile subjects are said to be more vulnerable to the adverse effects of injury and overuse, including sprains, traumatic synovitis, recurrent dislocations, tendinitis, and premature degenerative arthritis.[4] An associated systemic connective tissue abnormality is possible. A group of patients with mitral valve prolapse in one study had a higher frequency of joint hypermobility than controls.[82] A marfanoid habitus,[38] thin skin, and uterine prolapse[1] may also be associated with hypermobility.

The relationship between benign hypermobility and joint symptoms or systemic features is not universally accepted. In one study of healthy blood donors, no differences were found between hypermobile individuals and controls in the frequency of arthralgias, dislocations, mitral valve prolapse, or thin skin.[49]

ACUTE BONE ATROPHY (SUDECK'S ATROPHY; REFLEX DYSTROPHY)

After trauma to an extremity, a few patients develop severe pain, edema, vasomotor abnormalities, and atrophy of bone, muscle, and skin. Many labels have been applied to this syndrome, depending upon the feature of particular interest to the describer: *Sudeck's atrophy, Leriche's post-traumatic osteoporosis, Weir Mitchell's causalgia, peripheral trophoneurosis, reflex dystrophy,* and *chronic traumatic edema.* The term "causalgia" should probably be reserved for cases in which there has been injury to a major nerve trunk, but the resulting intense burning pain is not confined to the distribution of the nerve and may not differ from that which occurs in reflex dystrophy without nerve injury.[27] Another variant, the "shoulder-hand syndrome," is usually not related to trauma and is described in detail in Chapter 85.

The antecedent injury may be a fracture, but it is often fairly trivial, such as a sprain or laceration, and it may occur with about equal frequency in an upper or lower extremity.[27] Pain, of a quality and degree inappropriate for the injury, may begin immediately or not until several weeks after the trauma.[90] Disinclination to move the extremity is also an early feature that is inextricably linked to the pain. The limb is painful on motion and may have striking cutaneous hyperalgesia and cold sensitivity. A hyperemic stage may be noted in some cases, but a cold, moist, cyanotic, edematous hand or foot is more typical after 2 or 3 months. Roentgenograms, usually normal during the first month, later show patchy osteopenia, often periarticular in distribution initially, but diffuse later. With continued immobility, muscle and skin atrophy occur and joint motion is lost.

Pathogenesis and management are discussed in Chapter 85. It should be emphasized that early identification of patients and restoration of active motion are the keys to successful treatment. Early treatment with simple, conservative measures, including graded active exercises, heat, and elevation,[83] may produce good results. Long-standing disease, with advanced atrophy of skin, muscle, and bone, may be largely irreversible. One study of patients with fractures suggested that active exercise to joints that do not require immobilization may prevent Sudeck's atrophy. Osteopenia developed in only 0.6% of the exercised group and in 17.4% of those who were not so instructed.[13]

Another syndrome characterized by pain and osteopenia has been described in several reports since 1959[19,29,47,59,95] under the following titles: *migratory osteolysis, regional migratory osteoporosis,* and *transient osteoporosis of the hip.* The condition was first described during pregnancy,[19] but subsequently has been noticed most often in middle-aged men, who develop a painful swelling in one region of a lower extremity, rarely with preceding trauma.[95] Either the hip, knee, or foot may be involved. Pain is often severe, especially on motion and weight-bearing. Although radiographs may be normal during the first 2 or 3 weeks of symptoms, severe osteoporosis in the painful region is readily apparent thereafter. This condition is unlikely to be related to disuse because uptake of a bone-seeking radioisotope is increased in the affected area during the first week, prior to immobilization of the extremity.[76] The disorder is self-limited, with resolution of signs and symptoms in several months and eventual return of bone density to normal. Subsequent attacks may occur in other areas but not in previously involved joints. Nothing is known of the pathogenesis of this syndrome, but its resemblance to Sudeck's atrophy has been noted.[59,95]

OSTEOCHONDRITIS DISSECANS

This local disorder of subchondral bone is most commonly found in the knees of adolescents and young adults. A devitalized fragment of bone, with its articular cartilage still present, demarcates from its original site, usually on the lateral portion of the medial femoral condyle. Partial or complete detachment may occur eventually, with resulting signs and symptoms of a "loose body" in the joint; less frequently, the fragment may lodge in the intercondylar notch and may remain clinically silent.

Antecedent trauma, though common, seems to be only one of several etiologic factors. Smillie,[91] who has reviewed this controversial topic in great detail, believes that anomalous ossification centers, locally deficient blood supply, and genetic factors[40] are particularly important in the younger age group, whereas trauma plays a greater role in adults. However, in histologic studies, no evidence of ischemic necrosis was found.[15,69] The trauma involved may be "endogenous," such as repeated contact between an unusually prominent tibial spine or aberrantly situated cruciate ligament and the femoral condyle.

The clinical picture in patients with knee involvement consists of mild discomfort rather than pain. This pain is aggravated by exercise, but there may also be some aching at rest. With separation of the fragment, the patient may complain of instability or "giving-way." Often an unusual stance, due to external rotation of the tibia, may be noted.[108] This stance diminishes contact between the tibial spine and the usual site of osteochondritis on the medial condyle, near the intercondylar

notch. A sign that correlates with this may be demonstrated by forcing the tibia into internal rotation while slowly extending the knee from 90° of flexion. At about 30°, the patient complains of pain, which is relieved immediately by external rotation of the tibia.

Roentgenograms may be normal for as long as 6 months after the injury; the typical picture is that of a bony sequestrum lodged in a sharply defined cavity (Fig. 77–4). The lesion has a similar appearance when it occurs in other locations such as the elbow (capitellum), ankle (talus), hip, and metatarsal head.[61,78] Occasionally, multiple sites are involved, particularly in individuals from predisposed families.[40]

Treatment is conservative if the fragment remains in place. Loose fragments may be treated surgically, with either removal or fixation.[78,91] The immediate prognosis is good, but some patients may develop osteoarthritis later in life.

Epiphyseal Osteochondritis. Necrosis of an entire epiphysis is a common localized disorder in childhood. Vascular insufficiency is thought to be the most significant etiologic factor; trauma is often mentioned but seldom established as a primary cause. Experimental evidence suggests that compression fractures may lead to disorderly epiphyseal ossification characteristic of osteochondritis.[26] In the hip *(Legg-Calvé-Perthes disease),* osteochondritis occurs in younger children (2 to 10 years of age), usually presenting with a limp rather than with pain. In the knee *(Osgood-Schlatter disease),* older children (9 to 15 years of age) develop pain and swelling in the tibial tubercle; this con-

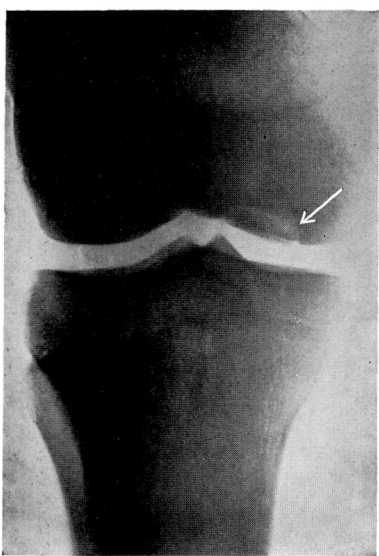

Fig. 77–4. Osteochondritis dissecans.

dition may result from a traction injury.[26] Osteochondritis of the vertebrae *(Scheuermann's disease)* presents with kyphosis and is described in Chapter 82.

Generalized osteochondritis involving small joints in the hands and wrists, as well as the joints already mentioned, is a rare but definite entity. This condition must be differentiated from the polyarthritides.[25]

TIETZE'S SYNDROME; COSTOCHONDRITIS

Tietze's syndrome is a benign condition in which painful enlargement develops in the upper costal cartilages.[99] The syndrome occurs with the same frequency in both sexes and on both sides of the chest. Involvement of only a single costal cartilage is found in 80% of patients, the second and third being most affected. Onset of pain is either acute or insidious, usually without prior injury, with the exception of trauma, which may have occurred during vigorous coughing in a minority of cases. Pain is sometimes severe, is aggravated by motion of the rib cage, and may radiate to the shoulder and arm. Palpation of a firm tender fusiform swelling of the costal cartilage confirms the diagnosis. Biopsy usually shows normal cartilage, occasionally some edema of the perichondrium, and rarely nonspecific chronic inflammation in the surrounding tissues. The duration is variable, from a week to several years. Some patients have multiple episodes, but spontaneous remission is the rule. The swelling has been attributed to cartilaginous hypertrophy by some and to abnormal angulation by others, but nothing is known of the pathogenesis. Treatment may include analgesics, heat, local infiltration with corticosteroids, intercostal nerve block, and reassurance that symptoms are not due to heart disease.

Other disorders may produce pain, tenderness, or evidences of inflammation in the costochondral joints, but not a hard swelling as in Tietze's syndrome. They include rheumatoid arthritis, fibrositis, gout, pyogenic infection, and the anterior chest wall syndrome that may follow myocardial infarction.

The most common cause of chest wall pain in individuals who do not have a generalized rheumatic disease is an ill-defined condition usually called *costochondritis*.[111] The pain may be severe, radiating widely, but is often worse on the left side. In some cases it is aggravated by coughing, deep respiration, and motion of the thorax. Anxiety and hyperventilation are common accompaniments. Some episodes are brief and self-limited but others are chronic, recurrent, and disabling. Tenderness over the costal cartilages, simulating or accentuat-

ing the spontaneous pain, is the main physical finding. The xiphoid may be tender in patients with generalized costochondritis, but there is also a syndrome of *isolated xiphoidalgia,* which may result in epigastric pain suggestive of various intra-abdominal disorders. Reproduction of the pain by pressing over the xiphoid is the essential diagnostic maneuver. Little is known of the etiology and pathology of these conditions. In most cases there is no evidence for a traumatic cause, but emotional factors are frequently involved. Care must be taken to rule out coronary artery disease, which may occasionally be associated with chest wall hyperalgesia.

Sudden episodes of sharp pain at the costal margin may be caused by the *rib-tip syndrome*.[66,112] This condition is due to hypermobility of the anterior end of a costal cartilage, usually that of the tenth rib, as a result of past trauma. The patients, usually middle-aged of either sex, complain of upper abdominal pain, precipitated by movement and by certain postures. A snapping sensation and point tenderness at the rib tip, relieved by a local anesthetic injection, will confirm the diagnosis.

OSTEITIS PUBIS

Surgical trauma in the retropubic area may occasionally provoke an inflammatory process in the pubic symphysis and adjacent bone.[16] Osteitis pubis may occur after prostate or bladder surgery and, more rarely, following herniorrhaphy or childbirth. Several weeks postoperatively, the patient develops pain over the symphysis radiating down the inner aspects of the thighs, often aggravated by coughing and straining. Physical findings include an antalgic gait, point tenderness over the symphysis, spasm in the abdominal and hip adductor muscle groups, and a low-grade fever. Radiographs may be normal initially but rarefaction and osteolysis develop around the symphysis within 2 to 4 weeks. A sterile chronic inflammatory process is usually noted on biopsy,[16] but a true osteomyelitis may be discovered in a minority of patients, generally those with more marked bone destruction and fever.[88] Tuberculosis and metastatic disease must also be considered in the differential diagnosis. Similar radiographic findings may be observed in ankylosing spondylitis and occasionally in chondrocalcinosis or in other types of polyarthritis, but pain is minimal or absent. Although spontaneous remission may be expected in osteitis pubis, disabling symptoms may persist for many months. The gamut of anti-inflammatory drugs has been used with varying success. Other measures, such as immobilization, wearing a tight pelvic belt, surgical debridement, and radiotherapy, have been advocated. The pathogenesis is uncertain, but there is general agreement that one or more factors, in addition to trauma, must contribute.

SYNOVIAL CYSTS OF THE POPLITEAL SPACE: "BAKER'S CYSTS"

Six primary bursae are associated with muscles and tendons on the posteromedial aspect of the knee. Communications between two bursae and between a bursa and the knee joint are common. Popliteal cysts may arise in three ways: (1) accumulation of fluid in a noncommunicating bursa; (2) distention of a bursa by fluid originating as a result of a lesion in the knee joint; and (3) posterior herniation of the joint capsule in response to increased intra-articular pressure. The communication between joint and cyst is generally narrow and the anatomy such that a flap-valve mechanism may be operative, allowing free passage of fluid from knee to cyst, but not in the opposite direction.[84]

Popliteal cysts may be seen at all ages. Those in children are usually unassociated with joint disease and are often bilateral. Most disappear spontaneously.[24] In about half of all cases, some abnormality is evident in the knee joint. In one study of 198 patients, 40 had osteoarthritis, 27 had rheumatoid arthritis, 11 had cartilage tears or osteochondromatosis, and 11 had a variety of other conditions.[9] Only 10 patients had a history of trauma. In most patients with knee joint disease, a connection between the cyst and joint could be demonstrated. The cyst itself usually causes only mild discomfort; other symptoms may be related to the associated joint lesions. A fluctuant swelling is present in the popliteal area, occasionally extending well into the calf and presenting superficially at the medial border of the gastrocnemius. The differential diagnosis includes aneurysms, benign neoplasms, varicosities, and thrombophlebitis. Arthrograms may be helpful if the cyst communicates with the knee joint.[42] The histopathologic characteristics of the cysts are varied, and do not particularly correspond to the presumed origin, bursal or hernial.[9] Most have a thin fibrous wall, lined by a single layer of flat cells. Others have structural characteristics of a synovial membrane, particularly those occurring in patients with rheumatoid arthritis. A few have a thickened, inflamed wall coated with fibrin, but no villus formation.

Definitive treatment is essentially surgical. In some cases, correction of knee joint pathology (such as synovectomy in a patient with rheumatoid arthritis) may result in spontaneous disappearance. Aspiration of the cyst and corticosteroid injections are often palliative.

Synovial cysts in rheumatoid arthritis are seen in many other joints.[77] Occasionally a communicating cyst of traumatic or nonspecific origin may be seen elsewhere. For instance, a cyst connecting with the hip joint may present anteriorly as a mass in the groin or posteriorly with sciatic pain.

GANGLION

A ganglion is a cystic swelling that may be found near and often attached to a tendon sheath or joint capsule, and is believed to be derived from these structures.[67] A slender connection may be demonstrated histologically[101] and radiographically.[3] The thick mucoid material within the ganglion contains hyaluronic acid, although no true synovial membrane lines the cavity.[33] The most common location is on the dorsum of the wrist (Fig. 77–5), but ganglia are also frequently noted on the fingers and dorsum of the foot. Ganglia of the flexor tendon sheaths, at the base of the fingers, are common in typists.[64] They have been reported near many other joints and also attached to the tibial periosteum.[10] In most instances, there has been no definite relationship to trauma. There are few symptoms other than unsightly swelling and slight discomfort on motion.

Ganglia may disappear spontaneously.[14] Treatment is not necessarily required, but is often demanded by the patient for cosmetic reasons. Successful treatment in about 80% of cases has been reported after multiple punctures of the cyst wall with a large bore needle, aspiration of the contents, and injection of a corticosteroid preparation.[23,57] If the ganglion recurs after this procedure, surgical excision may be performed.

TENOSYNOVITIS; STENOSING TENOVAGINITIS

Tenosynovitis is an inflammation of the cellular lining membrane of the fibrous tube (vagina) through which a tendon moves. It may be produced by various diseases (e.g., rheumatoid arthritis, gout, gonococcal arthritis), but even more commonly by trauma. Such trauma may occur from a direct blow, from abnormal pressure upon a tendon (such as from the stiff counter of a new shoe on the Achilles tendon) or, most often, from a short period of unusual activity involving a certain muscle-tendon unit. In one industrial study of 88 cases, the wrist and thumb extensors were involved in 71% and the dorsiflexors at the ankle in 18%. Most were related to a new type of repetitive work or to resumption of work after vacation.[109] The condition is identified by tenderness, swelling, and palpable crepitus over the tendon as it is moved (peritendinitis crepitans). Remission usually occurs if the affected part is rested for a few days.

Stenosing tenovaginitis is primarily a disorder of the fibrous wall of the tendon sheath, particularly

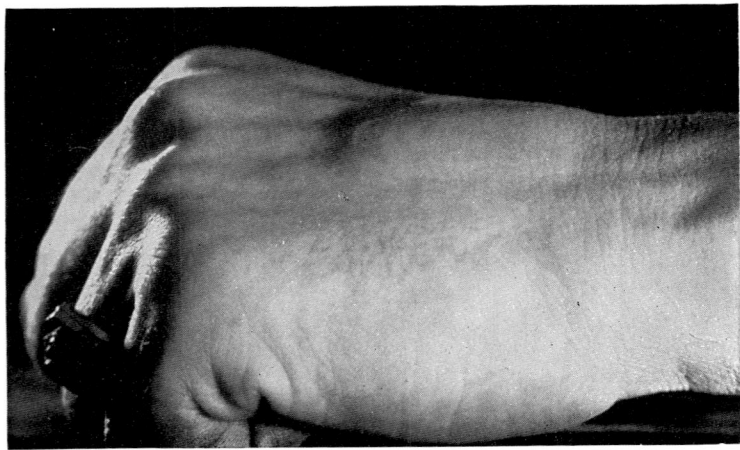

Fig. 77–5. Ganglion arising from extensor tendon sheaths. An oval and flattened cystic mass is on the dorsum of hand.

at locations where the tendon passes through a fibrous ring or pulley. Generally, an osseous groove comprises part of the ring, which is completed by a thickening of the tendon sheath. Such arrangements are found over bony prominences such as the radial styloid and the flexor surfaces of the metacarpal and metatarsal heads. With prolonged mechanical stress from either tendon motion under an excessive load or external pressure, such as from the handles of pruning shears, abnormal proliferation of fibrous tissue in the ring constricts the lumen of the tendon sheath. Secondary changes may then occur in the tendon, usually with enlargement distal to the constriction. There may be a snapping sensation with movement of the enlarged segment of tendon through the narrowed ring ("trigger finger" and "snapping thumb"). Further progression may produce locking in flexion; the tendon may be pulled through the constriction by its own flexor muscle but not by its weaker extensor antagonist. When extension is forced, the bulbous portion suddenly pops back through the constriction, and the digit "unlocks." Tenosynovitis due to mechanical stress may also contribute to pain and loss of motion.

Stenosing tenovaginitis of the abductor pollicis longus and extensor pollicis brevis at the radial styloid is known as *de Quervain's disease*.[70,113] It is a common disorder among women who perform repetitive manual tasks involving grasping with the thumb accompanied by movement of the hand in a radial direction (Fig. 77–6). Symptoms include pain in the area of the radial styloid and weakness of grip. Examination reveals tenderness and thickening over the involved tendons and limited ex-

cursion of the thumb; locking and snapping seldom occur. The classic test is the demonstration of *Finkelstein's sign*. The thumb is placed in the palm of the hand and grasped by the fingers; ulnar deviation of the wrist elicits a sharp pain if inflammation of the tendon sheath is present.

The most common locations for stenosing tenovaginitis are the thumb flexor and extensor tendons and the finger flexors, but occasionally other sites are involved. These sites include the flexor carpi radialis tendon, resulting in pain at the base of the thenar eminence,[104] the common peroneal sheath, causing pain on the lateral aspect of the ankle,[74] and the tibialis posterior tendon,[74] presenting with pain below and behind the medial malleolus after prolonged standing and walking.

Treatment of Stenosing Tenovaginitis. Conservative measures such as (1) cessation of the repetitive activity thought to have provoked the condition, (2) immobilization with splints, and (3) local corticosteroid injections often result in improvement, but recurrences are common. Tenosynovitis may subside, but the area of fibrous constriction is unlikely to be greatly altered by this approach. It is sometimes necessary to resort to surgical excision of this portion of the sheath. In all the locations, the operation is simple and results in permanent remission, even allowing resumption of full activity in most cases.

Carpal Tunnel Syndrome. Tenosynovitis in the flexor compartment of the wrist, where the tendons are enclosed in a bony canal, roofed by a rigid transverse carpal ligament, may result in compression and degeneration of the median nerve that shares this space.[86] Trauma is only one of many

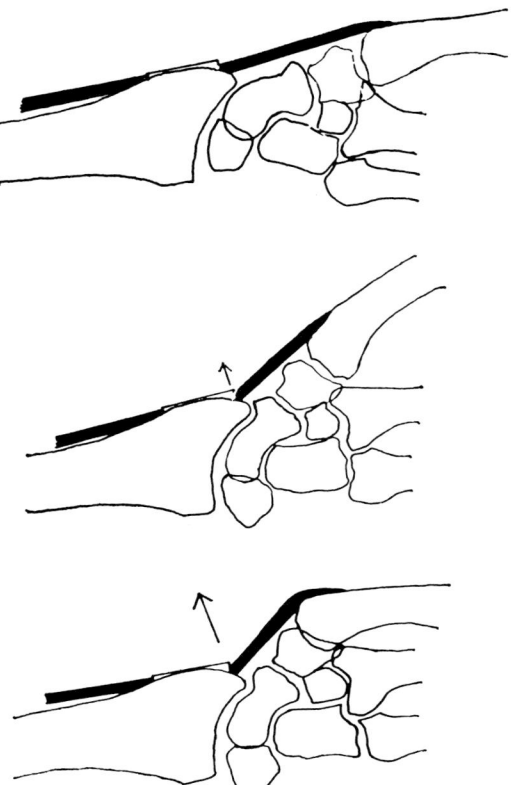

Fig. 77–6. *Top,* Wrist and thumb in neutral position, tendons relaxed. *Center,* Radial deviation of wrist and thumb relaxed, minor tearing stress applied to retinaculum. *Bottom,* Radial deviation of wrist while gripping, strong tearing stress applied to retinaculum. (From Muckart, R.D.[70])

causes of this syndrome; others include rheumatoid arthritis, amyloidosis, myxedema, benign tumors, pregnancy, acromegaly, polymyalgia rheumatica, and diabetes.[18,81,96] In one report, about half of the patients had been engaged in prolonged activity involving forceful flexion of the fingers with the wrist held in flexion or moving through an arc of flexor motion.[96] In another larger series, only 16% of patients had a history of possible related trauma, including fractures and sprains, as well as excessive use.[81]

The patient complains of paresthesias and pain, usually worse at night, in the first three fingers of the hand. At times the pain may radiate proximally as far as the shoulder. Physical findings may include sensory loss in the median nerve distribution, weakness in abduction and opposition of the thumb, atrophy of the thenar musculature, and a tender swelling on the volar aspect of the wrist. Symptoms may be reproduced by light finger percussion over the median nerve at the volar surface

of the wrist *(Tinel's sign)* and by forced flexion of the wrist by the examiner for at least one minute *(Phalen's sign)*. Nerve conduction time across the wrist is often prolonged. Motor latency is most often measured, but sensory latency may be a more sensitive indicator of median nerve compression. In one study, motor latency and EMG studies were normal in 25% of patients, but sensory conduction was delayed.[8] These electrodiagnostic methods are of value in confirming the diagnosis in atypical cases. The typical syndrome can be present only at night, in which case the physical findings may be equivocal and the electrical testing may be negative when performed during the day. Immobilization of the wrist with a rest splint in slight dorsiflexion and local corticosteroid injections often bring about a remission, but surgical division of the transverse carpal ligament is the definitive treatment.[17]

Tarsal Tunnel Syndrome. An entrapment neuropathy of the posterior tibial nerve behind and below the medial malleolus may be caused by tenosynovitis of the tendons that accompany the nerve through an osseofibrous tunnel.[55] The patient experiences burning pain and numbness of the toes and sole of the foot, reproduced by direct pressure behind the medial malleolus and by forced valgus deviation of the heel.

Other nerve entrapment syndromes are described in a monograph by Kopell and Thompson.[54]

OTHER FORMS OF TENDINITIS AND BURSITIS

Painful conditions attributed to strain or injury of tendons and their attachments to bone are often loosely described by the term tendinitis. The supraspinatus and bicipital tendons of the shoulder, which are commonly affected, are discussed in Chapter 85. Frequently, tendinitis is related to a particular occupation or sport. For instance, a baseball pitcher, at the end of his delivery, stretches the attachment of the long head of the triceps to the inferior glenoid rim. This movement results in pain in the posterior axillary fold. It is presumed that inflammatory changes occur in the tendon attachment; treatment includes rest, local corticosteroid injections, and ultrasound.[68] Baseball pitchers and golfers may also develop a similar condition at the *medial* epicondyle of the elbow. Jumper's knee refers to tendinitis of the patellar tendon, usually at its attachment to the lower pole of the patella.[62]

Injections of corticosteroid ester crystals into the tendon substance should be avoided, especially in athletes, because subsequent severe loading may result in a tear and severe disability.

TENNIS ELBOW (EPICONDYLITIS)

This is a common condition, most often found in middle-aged men, in which pain derives from the origin of the wrist and finger extensors at the lateral epicondyle. Although first described in tennis players, most cases are not related to that sport, but may be provoked by any exercise or occupation that involves repeated and forcible wrist extension or pronation-supination. The right elbow is involved more often than the left; the condition is seldom bilateral.[56] Pain is usually gradual in onset, but is sometimes related to a specific traumatic incident. It often radiates to the forearm and dorsum of the hand. Physical examination reveals point tenderness at or near the lateral epicondyle, with little or no swelling. Elbow joint motion is unrestricted and painless, but resisted wrist extension results in accentuation of pain. Many possibilities have been expressed for the pathogenesis,[36] including tendon rupture, radiohumeral synovitis, periostitis, neuritis, aseptic necrosis, and displacement of the orbicular ligament. A detailed pathologic study, including a control group of individuals with apparently normal elbows, revealed no evidence of a bursa in the area of the common extensor insertion, but rather a subtendinous space containing loose areolar connective tissue. In patients with tennis elbow, this space showed granulation tissue, increased vascularity, and edema. Periostitis and tendon tears were not noted.[36]

Many treatments have been proposed, including massage, ultrasound, anti-inflammatory drugs, braces, and several surgical procedures.[6] However, the most common approach, local corticosteroid injection, is usually successful.[56]

BURSITIS

Bursae are closed sacs, lined with a cellular membrane resembling synovium. They serve to facilitate motion of tendons and muscles over bony prominences. There are over 80 bursae on each side of the body.[11] Many are nameless, and additional ones may form at almost any point subjected to frequent irritation. Excessive frictional forces or, at times, direct trauma may result in an inflammatory process in the bursal wall, with excessive vascularity, exudation of increased amounts of viscous bursal fluid, and fibrin-coating of the lining membrane. Only small numbers of inflammatory cells are found in bursal fluid in traumatic bursitis, but there may be a greater leukocyte response in bursitis secondary to other rheumatic diseases, such as rheumatoid arthritis or gout. Septic bursitis is usually caused by organisms introduced through punctures, wounds, or cellulitis in the overlying skin. Traumatic bursitis may be complicated by infection or hemorrhage. "Beat knee" and "beat

shoulder" in miners are examples of this condition. Continuous abrasion of the skin with stone dust results in cellulitis, and repeated scraping of the bursa against rough stone surfaces leads to hemorrhage. With modification of occupations and habits, many of the classic forms of bursitis are encountered less frequently, e.g., "housemaid's knee," "weaver's bottom," and "policeman's heel."

Subdeltoid bursitis, which is described in detail in Chapter 85, is the most common bursitis. The following other types are also frequently seen.

Trochanteric Bursitis. Trochanteric bursitis is an inflammation of one or more of the bursae about the gluteal insertion on the femoral trochanter. This condition is usually insidious in onset, preceded by apparent trauma in only about a fourth of the cases. Aching pain on the lateral aspect of the hip and thigh is aggravated by lying on the affected side. The patient experiences tenderness posterior to the trochanter and pain with external rotation of the hip and with active abduction against resistance, but not with flexion and extension.

Olecranon Bursitis. An inflammation with effusion at the point of the elbow occurs frequently with rheumatoid arthritis and gout as well as after trauma. Pain is usually minimal, except when pressure is exerted on the swollen bursa. Elbow motion is unimpaired and usually painless. The swelling often subsides if additional trauma is prevented with a sponge ring. Fluid from the bursa is often serosanguineous with a low leukocyte concentration. Septic bursitis here is common.

Achilles Bursitis. In this condition, an inflammation of the bursa occurs just above the attachment of the Achilles tendon to the os calcis. Achilles bursitis is often related to trauma from tight shoes ("pump bumps") and perhaps to an unusual configuration of the posterior calcaneus (see Chap. 79).

Calcaneal Bursitis. An inflammation of a bursa occurs at the point of attachment of the plantar fascia to the os calcis (see Chap. 79).

Bunion. A painful bursitis occurs over the medial surface of the first metatarsophalangeal joint, usually with a hallux valgus (see Chap. 79).

Ischial Bursitis. An inflammation of the bursa separating the gluteus maximus from the underlying ischial tuberosity is usually produced by prolonged sitting on hard surfaces ("weaver's bottom").

Prepatellar Bursitis. This type of bursitis is a swelling between the skin and lower patella or patellar tendon, resulting from frequent kneeling (Fig. 77-7). Pain is usually slight unless there is direct pressure on the swollen area.

Anserine Bursitis. This inflammation of the

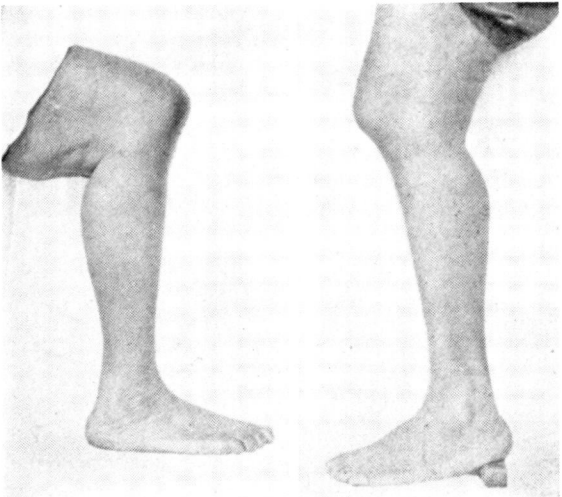

Fig. 77–7. Bilateral prepatellar bursitis (housemaid's knee) in a scrubwoman. (From Lewin: Orthopedic Surgery for Nurses. Philadelphia, W.B. Saunders Co.)

sartorius bursa on the medial aspect of the tibia is said to occur in women whose legs are disproportionately large. The characteristic complaint is pain with stair climbing. Inflammation in another, nameless bursa located at the anterior edge of the medial collateral ligament also gives pain on the inner aspect of the knee, but with point tenderness in a different area.

Iliopectineal Bursitis. With this inflammation of a bursa between the iliopsoas and inguinal ligament, the patient complains of groin pain radiating to the knee. He often adopts a shortened stride to prevent hyperextension of the hip while walking. Examination reveals tenderness just below the inguinal ligament, lateral to the femoral pulse, and pain on hyperextension of the hip.

Treatment. In general, therapy includes protection from irritation and trauma, either by modifying the patient's activities or by using appropriate padding. Anti-inflammatory drugs, heat, and ultrasound are also commonly employed. Local corticosteroid injections are usually successful. Surgical excision is reserved for refractory cases.

Calcific Tendinitis and Periarthritis

Some cases of tendinitis and bursitis are associated with calcific deposits, most commonly with subdeltoid bursitis and trochanteric bursitis, but occasionally with tendinitis, bursitis, or periarthritis around the wrist, knee, or elbow. In these instances, the attacks are less likely to be preceded by recognized trauma. The attacks tend to be abrupt in onset, with intense local inflammatory signs resembling an attack of gout. These episodes, which

may be examples of crystal-induced inflammation, are described further in Chapters 85 and 93.

INJURIES TO MUSCLES AND TENDONS

The following clinical features are suggestive of rupture of muscles and tendons:

1. The patient has a history of sudden sharp pain or a snapping sensation that occurs during vigorous muscular effort.

2. The patient is unable to perform certain definite movements following this pain or snapping sensation.

3. The diagnosis is more certain if a defect is apparent in the belly of the muscle or in the tendon, with subsequent ecchymosis.

4. Roentgenogram of soft tissues often reveals a defect in the shadow cast by the muscle; in some cases, a small chip of bone is seen attached to a tendon that has been torn from its insertion.

5. Electrical stimulation of the muscle causes it to contract and produce pain at the site of a tear in either the muscle or tendon.

6. Local anesthetic injection eliminates pain and permits testing of muscular function in those patients in whom the diagnosis is difficult.

The supraspinatus muscle or tendon is the most likely to be torn in the upper extremity. The calf muscles and the quadriceps are the most vulnerable in the lower extremity.

Because of their great tensile strength, rupture seldom occurs in the tendons, but rather at the muscle-tendon junction or at the bony insertion.[11] Attrition of the musculotendinous cuff, secondary to local trauma by pulley systems and bony prominences, may lead to necrobiotic changes that predispose to rupture.[7] Trauma is the immediate and direct cause of rupture; sudden application of a stretching force on a strongly contracting muscle results in tearing of muscle fibers, followed by hemorrhage, edema, and localized spasm ("charley horse"). In some cases, the primary mechanism is extreme passive stretching of a tendon attachment, such as the avulsion of the adductor insertion in the groin in a water skier falling with widely abducted hips. Muscle fatigue results in incomplete relaxation and predisposes to stretch injuries. Therefore, these injuries are more likely to occur in poorly conditioned athletes.[7]

Tendon rupture, common in rheumatoid arthritis, is caused by the lytic effect of tenosynovial inflammation and, in addition, mechanical abrasion of tendons due to disruption of the contiguous bone. Injection of corticosteroids for tendinitis has also been said to predispose to tendon rupture, especially in the Achilles tendon.[94]

Tears in the supraspinatus tendon occur in older

individuals. It is presumed that attrition and trauma both contribute to the rupture (see Chap. 85).

Rupture of the long head of the biceps may be the final result of chronic frictional attrition of the tendon within the bicipital groove (see Chap. 85). The rupture may be accompanied by transient pain over the anterior aspect of the shoulder. The belly of the muscle assumes a spherical shape and lies closer to the elbow than normal. Surgical repair is often possible, but not mandatory since disability is generally mild.

The greater or lesser rhomboid muscles may be strained by a sudden uncoordinated movement of the shoulder. This injury occurs frequently in industrial practice. These muscles arise from the ligamentum nuchae and the spinous process of the seventh cervical to the fifth dorsal vertebrae, and they insert into the vertebral border of the scapula. Contraction of these muscles draws this border of the scapula upward.

Following injury to the rhomboid muscles, there is a localized tenderness between the mid-dorsal spine and the scapula. Pain occurs at this point if the shoulder is passively flexed forward or if it is extended against resistance. Treatment consists of partial immobilization of the scapula by drawing it backward and upward with adhesive. Physical therapy (heat and light massage) should be started when the signs of injury have disappeared.

Other muscles arising from the spinous processes and inserting on the scapula or humerus include the levator scapulae, latissimus dorsi, and trapezius muscles. Strains of these muscles give a clinical picture somewhat similar to that for injury to the rhomboids.

Rupture of the pectoralis major muscle is usually caused by an abrupt traction injury, with sudden sharp pain in the shoulder and a snapping sensation.[79] A tender mass is felt in the muscle, and there is ecchymosis of the overlying skin. Evacuation of the hematoma and surgical repair are the treatments of choice.

Rupture of the rectus abdominis muscle may at times be mistaken for intraperitoneal disease (such as appendicitis). Rupture of this muscle may occur following a severe bout of coughing or sneezing, during pregnancy or labor, or following influenza or typhoid fever (with degeneration of the muscle fibers). A large hematoma may form as a result of tears of branches of the epigastric vessels. The hematoma may require evacuation surgically.

Rupture of the quadriceps muscle or tendon is relatively common. This injury occurs at the point of attachment of the tendon to the patella or at the musculotendinous junction; occasionally, a tear may occur through the purely tendinous or muscular portions. The usual cause of this condition is a violent contraction of the muscle, such as falling on a flexed knee. The injury occurs in both young and aged individuals. The patient is unable to actively extend the knee, and a hiatus is seen in the tendon or muscle. Partial tears of the muscle may leave only a depression in the muscle substance without permanent disability. These depressions usually heal readily following splinting of the leg in full extension for 3 or 4 weeks, followed by gradual mobilization. Complete tears of the quadriceps muscle or tendon should be repaired surgically.

When the patellar tendon is ruptured, the patella lies higher than usual, a gap is noted, active knee extension is lost, and joint effusion is usually present. A roentgenogram will confirm the diagnosis.

Partial rupture of one of the calf muscles, termed "tennis leg," usually involves a belly of the gastrocnemius muscle. Symptoms include a snap with sudden burning pain in the calf during a strong muscular contraction. The pain may extend to the popliteal space; it is aggravated by passive dorsiflexion of the ankle. Treatment includes adhesive strapping to immobilize the ankle in plantar flexion for several weeks, followed by heat, massage, and exercises.

Spontaneous rupture of the posterior tibial tendon results in pain, tenderness, and swelling behind and below the medial malleolus, with loss of stability of the foot. This injury is usually preceded by chronic symptoms suggestive of tenosynovitis and is often associated with planovalgus feet. Treatment is either surgical repair, in cases diagnosed early, or an arch support.[51]

Injury to the Achilles tendon may occur in runners or in middle-aged men, unaccustomed to exertion, who indulge in weekend athletics involving jumping (such as basketball and volleyball). There may be rupture at the musculotendinous junction or avulsion at the attachment to the calcaneus. Examination reveals a depression over the tendon and inability to flex the ankle against resistance. In partial rupture, the pain may be mild. Swelling and ecchymosis may conceal the depression usually noted with complete tears. Partial rupture may be treated conservatively with immobilization of the foot in plantar flexion; complete tears usually require surgical intervention.[34]

The anterior tibial compartment syndrome is an ischemic necrosis of muscle caused by swelling after unaccustomed exercise. The muscles in this compartment are confined by a tight fascial sheath, resulting in a compromised blood supply when swelling occurs. Examination shows a marked weakness of the involved muscle and local swelling and erythema. Sensation in the first two toes is often lost because of compression of the deep peroneal nerve. Immediate fasciotomy must be performed to prevent irreversible destruction of the muscle. Less frequently, similar problems may arise from high pressure in other muscle compartments of the lower leg.[63]

Fibrotic Induration and Contracture Owing to Repeated Intramuscular Injections

Certain drugs may cause local destruction of muscle tissue at injection sites, leading to fibrosis and contracture.[39] Self-administration of pentazocine (Talwin) by patients with chronic pain has resulted in the most striking examples of this condition.[75] Woody induration of the quadriceps, deltoids, and other muscles, needle marks and ulcerations in the overlying skin, and marked muscle shortening are the characteristic features.

RUNNING INJURIES

The extraordinary popularity of running has engendered special interest in associated injuries and increased awareness of biomechanical aspects, including running techniques, conditioning, and equipment. These activities are often centered in special runners' clinics, in which the therapeutic goals may differ from those of conventional medicine. Emphasis is placed on continued participation and enhanced performance, in addition to the traditional aims of symptomatic relief and prevention of permanent tissue damage. The spectrum of running injuries encompasses virtually all the categories of musculoskeletal trauma (Table 77–2). About one-third of running injuries involve the knee; heel pain is next in frequency. Certain preexisting conditions may predispose the runner to injury. For instance, a high-arched foot (pes cavus) does not pronate sufficiently to absorb shock during running, leading to Achilles tendinitis or plantar fasciitis. Running on a hyperpronated or flat foot may result in lateral ankle pain. Incongruity, faulty tracking, or laxity in the patellofemoral joint may predispose to patellar pain or chondromalacia. Recrudescent symptoms from virtually any previous

articular derangement may develop when the individual begins to run regularly. Ill-fitting or poorly constructed footwear, hard or irregular running surfaces, poor running posture or technique, and inadequate warm-up or tendon stretching also increase the likelihood of injury. Detailed discussion of these matters is available elsewhere.[21,48]

Stress fractures, also called fatigue fractures, are partial, cortical fractures related to prolonged, repetitive mechanical loading. A complete fracture may eventually result if the activity is continued. Currently, running is probably the most common cause. The presenting symptom is pain, which is generally aggravated by weight-bearing and relieved by rest. In some areas, such as the tibia and fibula, tenderness, warmth, and swelling may occur over the fracture. The diagnosis is usually made radiographically, but typical findings of a linear cortical radiolucency or a localized area of periosteal new bone formation may not be present during the first week or two of symptoms. Therefore, negative radiographs should be repeated if a stress fracture is strongly suspected. A radionuclide scan shows increased uptake at the stress fracture site at this early stage,[73] but this expensive procedure is seldom justified in typical cases. The treatment of stress fractures depends upon their location and severity. If the fibula is involved, continuation of running at a reduced level may be possible. At the other extreme, femoral fractures occasionally require surgical intervention.

Knee problems represent about a third of running injuries. They most frequently involve tracking abnormalities of the patella, often in relation to underlying anatomic and biomechanical factors (see Chap. 78). Internal derangements are seldom caused by running, but patients with preexisting, asymptomatic lesions are likely to develop pain and swelling under the stress of running. *"Overuse" synovitis* in the apparent absence of intra-articular pathology is noted occasionally with rapid increases in mileage. This condition should be managed with temporary cessation until the effusion

Table 77–2. Common Disorders in Runners

Disorder	Sites of Involvement
Stress fracture	tibia, fibula, metatarsus, femur
Compartmental syndromes	
Sprains	
Bursitis	retrocalcaneus, anserine, ischium, trochanter
Fasciitis	plantar area, iliotibial band
Tendinitis	Achilles, anterior and posterior tibial, peroneal, quadriceps, patella
Tendon and muscle rupture	Achilles, hamstrings
Intra-articular disorders	chondromalacia, meniscal tears, plica, "overuse" synovitis, osteoarthritis
Cervical and lumbar disc degeneration	

resolves, with gradual resumption of the running program later. Lateral knee pain may be due to the *iliotibial band friction syndrome*.[85] A thick strip of fascia lata, which inserts into the lateral tibial condyle, may impinge on the femoral condyle during repeated flexion and extension of the knee, particularly in individuals with tibia vara and hyperpronated feet.

Heel pain, the second most frequent complaint among runners, results from various conditions that can usually be distinguished by physical examination and radiographs. These conditions include plantar fasciitis, calcaneal bursitis, Achilles tendinitis and/or rupture, and calcaneal stress fractures. Treatment includes instruction in running technique to avoid excessive heel strike, heel pads and orthotic devices, stretching exercises, temporary cessation or reduction in running, and anti-inflammatory drugs.

Degenerative arthritis and disc disease may produce pain and limited activity among older runners, but the role of running in the initiation of articular cartilage or disc attrition is difficult to assess at the present time in the absence of prospective controlled studies. Substitution of an alternative exercise program with less impact loading, such as swimming or walking, may be recommended in such cases.

RADIATION ARTHROPATHY FOLLOWING NONMECHANICAL TRAUMA

Because articular cartilage is relatively radioresistant, the effects of radiation on joints are usually secondary to destruction of osteoblasts.[20,46] Vascular damage (endarteritis) may also contribute to osteonecrosis. Since the field of radiotherapy is more likely to include the axial skeleton than the extremities, radiation arthropathy is usually seen in the hips, shoulder, spine, and sacroiliac and temporomandibular joints. Radiation changes are dose-related; the threshold is 3,000 rads, with cell death occurring at 5,000 rads. Their occurrence depends not only on dosage, but on age, various technical factors, and superimposed trauma or infection. The time of onset of clinical manifestations is generally greater than one year, and is often several years after irradiation. Adults may present with aseptic necrosis, fracture, or protrusio acetabuli[44] (Fig. 77–8). Children may develop slipped capital femoral epiphysis,[60] and scoliosis or kyphosis[65] due to injury of the epiphyseal plates, leading subsequently to wedge deformities of the vertebral bodies.

Changes resembling degenerative arthritis are occasionally found only in joints that had been included in the field of radiation many years previously.[53] Radiographic findings include narrowing

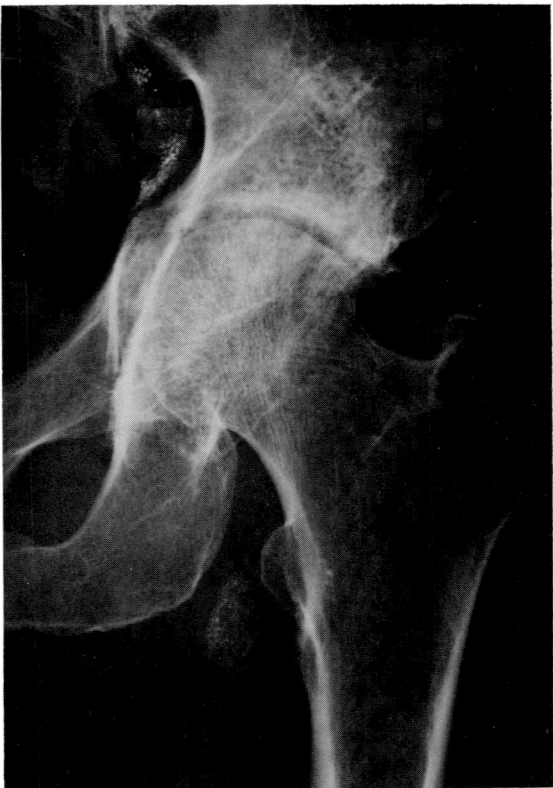

Fig. 77–8. Radiation necrosis of acetabulum with protrusio acetabuli due to pathologic fractures.

of the joint space, marginal new bone formation, and periarticular osteoporosis. Occasionally, chondrocalcinosis and ankylosis may occur. A few examples of "rheumatoid-like" arthritis with soft tissue swelling have been noted. The spine may be involved, showing narrowing and calcification of intervertebral discs.

Irradiation of the rib cage may result in osteochondritis, with pain and swelling in the costal cartilages. These symptoms may suggest cancer or Tietze's syndrome but, in contrast to these conditions, erythema exists in the tender area.[58] High-dose ultrasound[100] and diathermy have been reported to cause exacerbations of synovitis in rheumatoid arthritis (see Chap. 44).

FROSTBITE ARTHROPATHY

Frostbite injury to the distal extremities may occasionally involve the joints, in addition to overlying soft tissues. Skeletal changes are not apparent until several months after frostbite, and include demineralization, juxta-articular cysts, and joint space narrowing. The late development of osteophytes results in a clinical picture closely resembling that of osteoarthritis, with Heberden's and Bouchard's nodes.[35] In children, destruction of the phalangeal epiphyses may lead to premature closure and digital growth impairment.[12] These changes may be the result of direct chondrocyte injury during cold exposure.

REFERENCES

1. Al-Rawi, Z.S., and Al-Rawi, Z.T.: Joint hypermobility in women with genital prolapse. Lancet, *1*:1439–1441, 1982.
2. Anderson, K.J., LeCocq, J.F., and Clayton, M.L.: Athletic injury in the fibular collateral ligament of the ankle. Clin. Orthop., *23*:146–161, 1972.
3. Andren, L., and Eiken, O.: Arthrographic studies of wrist ganglions. J. Bone Joint Surg., *53A*:299–302, 1971.
4. Beighton, P.H., Grahame, R., and Bird, H.: Hypermobility of Joints. New York, Springer-Verlag, 1983.
5. Berk, R.N.: Liquid fat in the knee joint after trauma. N. Engl. J. Med., *277*:1411–1412, 1967.
6. Boyd, H.B., and McLeod, A.C., Jr.: Tennis elbow. J. Bone Joint Surg., *55A*:1183–1187, 1973.
7. Brewer, B.J.: Athletic injuries; musculotendinous unit. Clin. Orthop., *23*:30–38, 1972.
8. Buchthal, F., Rosengalck, A., and Trojaborg, W.: Electrophysiological findings in entrapment of the median nerve at the wrist and elbow. J. Neurol. Neurosurg. Psychiatry, *37*:340–360, 1974.
9. Burleson, R.J., Bickel, W.H., and Dahlin, D.C.: Popliteal cyst: A clinicopathological survey. J. Bone Joint Surg., *38A*:1265–1274, 1956.
10. Byers, P.D., and Wadsworth, T.G.: Periosteal ganglion. J. Bone Joint Surg., *52B*:290–295, 1970.
11. Bywaters, E.G.L.: Lesions of bursae, tendons and tendon sheaths. Clin. Rheum. Dis., *5*:883–925, 1979.
12. Carrera, G.F., Kozin, G., and McCarty, D.J.: Arthritis after frostbite injury in children. Arthritis Rheum., *22*:1082–1087, 1979.
13. Carstensen, E., and Giebel, M.G.: Does active exercise therapy diminish the incidence of Sudek's atrophy after fractures of the extremities. Dtsch. Med. Wochenschr., *86*:2114–2116, 1961.
14. Cherry, J.H., and Ghormley, R.K.: Bursa and ganglion. Am. J. Surg., *52*:319–330, 1941.
15. Chiroff, R.T., and Cooke, C.P.: Osteochondritis dissecans: A histologic and microradiographic analysis of surgically excised lesions. J. Trauma, *15*:689–696, 1975.
16. Coventry, M.B., and Mitchell, W.C.: Osteitis pubis: Observations based on a study of 45 patients. J.A.M.A., *178*:898–905, 1961.
17. Cracchiolo, A.: The carpal tunnel syndrome. Semin. Arthritis Rheum., *1*:87–95, 1971.
18. Cseuz, K.A., et al.: Long-term results of operation for carpal tunnel syndrome. Mayo Clin. Proc., *41*:232–241, 1966.
19. Curtiss, P.H., Jr., and Kincaid, W.E.: Transient demineralization of the hip in pregnancy: A report of three cases. J. Bone Joint Surg., *41A*:1327–1333, 1959.
20. Dalinka, M.K., and Bonavita, J.A.: Radiation changes. *In* Diagnosis of Bone and Joint Disorders. Edited by D. Resnick, and G. Niwayama. Philadelphia, W.B. Saunders Co., 1981, pp. 2341–2362.
21. D'Ambrosia, R., and Drez, D., Jr.: Prevention and Treatment of Running Injuries. Thorofare, New Jersey, Charles B. Slack, Inc., 1982.
22. Davie, B.: The significance and treatment of haemarthrosis of the knee following trauma. Med. J. Aust., *1*:1355–1359, 1969.
23. Derbyshire, R.C.: Observations on the treatment of ganglia with a report on hydrocortisone. Am. J. Surg., *112*:635–636, 1966.
24. Dinham, J.M.: Popliteal cysts in children, the case against surgery. J. Bone Joint Surg., *57B*:69–71, 1975.
25. Duthie, R.B., and Houghton, G.R.: Constitutional aspects of the osteochondroses. Clin Orthop., *15B*:19–27, 1981.
26. Douglas, G., and Rang, M.: The role of trauma in the pathogenesis of the osteochondroses. Clin. Orthop., *158*:28–32, 1981.
27. Drucker, W.R., et al.: Pathogenesis of post-traumatic sympathetic dystrophy. Am. J. Surg., *97*:454–465, 1959.
28. Dumonde, D.C., and Glynn, L.E.: The production of arthritis in rabbits by an immunological reaction to fibrin. Br. J. Exp. Pathol., *43*:373–383, 1962.
29. Duncan, H., et al.: Migratory osteolysis of the lower extremities. Ann. Intern. Med., *66*:1165–1173, 1967.
30. Durman, D.C.: Arthritis and injury. J. Mich. Med. Soc., *51*:301–303, 1955.
31. Furman, R., Nicholas, J.J., and Jivoff, L.: Elevation of the serum alkaline phosphatase coincident with ectopic bone formation in paraplegic patients. J. Bone Joint Surg., *52A*:1131–1137, 1970.
32. Gelfand, L., and Merliss, R.: Trauma and rheumatism. Ann. Intern. Med., *50*:999–1009, 1959.
33. Ghadially, F.N., and Mehta, P.N.: Multifunctional mesenchymal cells resembling smooth muscle cells in ganglia of the wrist. Ann. Rheum. Dis., *30*:31–42, 1971.
34. Gillies, H., and Chalmers, J.: The management of fresh ruptures of the tendo Achillis. J. Bone Joint Surg., *52A*:337, 1970.
35. Glick, R., and Parhami, N.: Frostbite arthritis. J. Rheumatol., *6*:456–460, 1979.
36. Goldie, I.: Epicondylitis lateralis humeri (epicondylalgia or tennis elbow). A pathogenetical study. Acta Chir. Scand. (Suppl.), *339*:1+, 1964.
37. Graham, J., and Goldman, J.A.: Fat droplets and synovial fluid leukocytosis in traumatic arthritis. Arthritis Rheum., *21*:76–80, 1978.
38. Grahame, R., et al.: A clinical and echocardiographic study of patients with the hypermobility syndrome. Ann. Rheum. Dis., *40*:541–546, 1981.
39. Groves, R.J., and Goldner, J.L.: Contracture of the deltoid muscle in the adult after intramuscular injections. J. Bone Joint Surg., *56A*:817–820, 1974.
40. Hanley, W.B., McKusick, V.A., and Barranco, F.T.: Osteochondritis dissecans with associated malformations in two brothers. J. Bone Joint Surg., *49A*:925–937, 1967.
41. Harrington, K.D.: Degenerative arthritis of the ankle secondary to longstanding lateral ligament instability. J. Bone Joint Surg., *61A*:354–361, 1979.
42. Harvey, J.P., Jr., and Corcos, J.: Large cysts in lower leg originating in the knee occurring in patients with rheumatoid arthritis. Arthritis Rheum., *3*:218–228, 1960.
43. Hassard, G.H.: Heterotopic bone formation about the hip and unilateral decubitus ulcers in spinal cord injury. Arch. Phys. Med. Rehabil., *56*:355–358, 1975.
44. Hasselbacher, P., and Schumacher, H.R.: Bilateral protrusio acetabuli following pelvic irradiation. J. Rheumatol., *4*:189–196, 1977.
45. Houston, A.N., et al.: Pellegrini-Stieda syndrome: Report of 44 cases followed from original injury. South. Med. J., *61*:113–117, 1968.
46. Howland, W.J., et al.: Postirradiation atrophic changes of bone and related complications. Radiology, *117*:677–685, 1975.
47. Hunder, G.G., and Kelly, P.J.: Roentgenologic transient osteoporosis of the hip. A clinical syndrome? Ann. Intern. Med., *68*:539–552, 1968.
48. James, S.L., Bates, B.T., and Ostering, L.R.: Injuries to runners. Am. J. Sports Med., *6*:40–50, 1978.
49. Jessee, E.F., Owen, D.S., and Sagar, K.B.: The benign hypermobility joint syndrome. Arthritis Rheum., *23*:1053–1056, 1980.
50. Julkunen, H., Rasanen, J.A., and Kataja, J.: Severe trauma as an etiologic factor in rheumatoid arthritis. Scand. J. Rheumatol., *3*:97–102, 1974.
51. Kettelkamp, D.B., and Alexander, H.H.: Spontaneous rupture of the posterior tibial tendon. J. Bone Joint Surg., *49A*:759–764, 1969.
52. Kirk, J.A., Ansell, B.M., and Bywaters, E.G.L.: The hypermobility syndrome. Ann. Rheum. Dis., *26*:419–425, 1967.
53. Kolar, J., Vrabec, R., and Chyba, J.: Arthropathies after irradiation. J. Bone Joint Surg., *49A*:1157–1166, 1967.

54. Kopell, H.P., and Thompson, W.A.L.: Peripheral Entrapment Neuropathies. Huntington, New York, R.E. Krieger Publishing Co., 1976.
55. Lam, S.J.S.: Tarsal tunnel syndrome. J. Bone Joint Surg., *49B*:87–92, 1967.
56. Lapidus, P.W., and Guidotti, F.P.: Lateral and medial epicondylitis of the humerus. Industr. Med., *39*:171–173, 1970.
57. Lapidus, P.W., and Guidotti, F.P.: Report on the treatment of 102 ganglions. Bull. Hosp. Joint Dis., *28*:50–57, 1967.
58. Lau, B.P.: Postirradiation costal osteochondritis simulating metastatic cancer. Radiology, *89*:1090–1092, 1967.
59. Lequesne, M.: Transient osteoporosis of the hip. A nontraumatic variety of Sudek's atrophy. Ann. Rheum. Dis., *27*:463–471, 1968.
60. Libshitz, H.I., and Edeiker, B.S.: Radiotherapy changes of the pediatric hip. Am. J. Roentgenol., *137*:585–588, 1981.
61. Lindholm, T.S., Osterman, K., and Vankka, E.: Osteochondritis dissecans of the elbow, ankle and hip. Clin. Orthop., *148*:245–253, 1980.
62. Martens, M., et al.: Patellar tendinitis: Pathology and results of treatment. Acta Orthop. Scand., *53*:445–450, 1982.
63. Matsen, F.A., Winquist, R.A., and Klugmire, R.B.: Diagnosis and management of compartmental syndromes. J. Bone Joint Surg., *62A*:286–291, 1980.
64. Matthews, P.: Ganglia of the flexor tendon sheaths in the hand. J. Bone Joint Surg., *55B*:612–617, 1973.
65. Mayfield, J.K.: Postradiation spinal deformity. Orthop. Clin. North Am., *10*:829–844, 1979.
66. McBeath, A.A., and Keene, J.S.: The rib-tip syndrome. J. Bone Joint Surg., *57A*:795–797, 1975.
67. McEvedy, B.V.: Simple ganglia. Br. J. Surg., *49*:585–594, 1962.
68. Middleman, I.C.: Shoulder and elbow lesions of baseball players. Am. J. Surg., *102*:627–632, 1961.
69. Milgram, J.W.: Radiological and pathological manifestations of osteochondritis dissecans of the distal femur. Radiology, *126*:305–311, 1978.
70. Muckart, R.D.: Stenosing tendovaginitis of abductor pollicis longus and extensor pollicis brevis at the radial styloid (de Quervain's disease). Clin. Orthop., *33*:201–207, 1964.
71. Nachlas, I.W.: The Pellegrini-Stieda para-articular calcification. Clin. Orthop., *3*:121–127, 1954.
72. Nicholas, J.J.: Ectopic bone formation in patients with spinal cord injury. Arch. Phys. Med. Rehabil., *54*:354–359, 1973.
73. Norfray, J.F., et al.: Early confirmation of stress fractures of joggers. J.A.M.A., *243*:1647–1649, 1980.
74. Norris, S.H., and Mankin, H.J.: Chronic tenosynovitis of the posterior tibial tendon with new bone formation. J. Bone Joint Surg., *60B*:523–526, 1978.
75. Oh, S.J., Rollins, J.I., and Lewis, I.: Pentazocine-induced fibrous myopathy. J.A.M.A., *231*:271–273, 1975.
76. O'Mara, R.E., and Pinals, R.S.: Bone scanning in regional migratory osteoporosis. Radiology, *97*:579–581, 1970.
77. Palmer, D.G.: Synovial cysts in rheumatoid disease. Ann. Intern. Med., *70*:61–68, 1969.
78. Pappas, A.M.: Osteochondrosis dissecans. Clin. Orthop., *158*:59–69, 1981.
79. Park, J.Y., and Espiniella, J.L.: Rupture of pectoralis major muscle. J. Bone Joint Surg., *52A*:577–581, 1970.
80. Parvin, R.W., and Ford, L.T.: Stenosing tenosynovitis of the common peroneal tendon sheath. J. Bone Joint Surg., *38A*:1352–1357, 1956.
81. Phalen, G.S.: The carpal tunnel syndrome. J. Bone Joint Surg., *48A*:211–228, 1966.
82. Pitcher, D., and Grahame, R.: Mitral valve prolapse and joint hypermobility: Evidence for a systemic connective tissue abnormality? Ann. Rheum. Dis., *41*:352–354, 1982.
83. Plewes, L.W.: Sudek's atrophy in the hand. J. Bone Joint Surg., *38B*:195–203, 1956.
84. Rauschning, W.: Anatomy and function of the communication between knee joint and popliteal bursae. Ann. Rheum. Dis., *39*:354–358, 1980.
85. Renne, J.W.: The iliotibial band friction syndrome. J. Bone Joint Surg., *57A*:1110–1111, 1975.
86. Robbins, H.: Anatomical study of the median nerve in the carpal tunnel and etiologies of the carpal tunnel syndrome. J. Bone Joint Surg., *45A*:953–966, 1963.
87. Ropes, M.W., and Bauer, W.: Synovial Fluid Changes in Joint Disease. Cambridge, Harvard University Press, 1953.
88. Rosenthal, R.E., et al.: Osteomyelitis of the symphysis pubis: A separate disease from osteitis pubis. J. Bone Joint Surg., *64A*:123–128, 1982.
89. Roy, S., Ghadially, F.N., and Crane, W.A.J.: Synovial membrane in traumatic effusion. Ultrastructure and autoradiography with tritiated leucine. Ann. Rheum. Dis., *25*:259–271, 1966.
90. Shumaker, H.B., and Abramson, D.I.: Post-traumatic vasomotor disorders. Surg. Gynecol. Obstet., *88*:417–434, 1949.
91. Smillie, I.S.: Osteochondritis Dissecans. Edinburgh, E. & S. Livingstone Ltd., 1960.
92. Stark, W.A.: Anterior compartment syndrome. Clin. Orthop., *62*:180–182, 1969.
93. Stover, S.L., Hataway, C.J., and Zeiger, H.E.: Heterotopic ossification in spinal cord injured patients. Arch. Phys. Med. Rehabil., *56*:199–204, 1975.
94. Sweetnam, R.: Corticosteroid arthropathy and tendon rupture. J. Bone Joint Surg., *51B*:397–398, 1969.
95. Swezey, R.L.: Transient osteoporosis of the hip, foot and knee. Arthritis Rheum., *13*:858–868, 1970.
96. Tanzer, R.C.: The carpal tunnel syndrome: A clinical and anatomical study. J. Bone Joint Surg., *41A*:626–634, 1959.
97. Taylor, A.R., and Rana, W.A.: An explanation of the formation of popliteal cysts. Ann. Rheum. Dis., *32*:419–421, 1973.
98. Thomas, H.O.: Diseases of the Hip, Knee and Ankle Joints, with their Deformities, Treated by a New and Efficient Method, 3rd Ed. London, H.K. Lewis, 1878.
99. Tietze, A.: Ueber eine eigenartige häufung von fällen mit dystrophie der rippenknorpel. Berlin, Klin. Wochenschr., *58*:829–831, 1921.
100. Tiliakos, N.A., and Wilson, C.H., Jr.: Ultrasound-induced arthritis (abstract). Arthritis Rheum., *26*:549, 1983.
101. Tophoj, K., and Henriques, U.: Ganglion of the wrist— a structure developed from the joint. Acta Orthop. Scand., *42*:244–250, 1971.
102. Varghese, G., and Chung, T.: Benign hydrarthrosis of the knee in patients with spinal cord injury. Arch. Phys. Med. Rehabil., *57*:468–469, 1976.
103. Venier, L.H., and DiTunno, J.F.: Heterotopic ossification in the paraplegic patient. Arch. Phys. Med. Rehabil., *52*:475–479, 1971.
104. Weeks, P.M.: A cause of wrist pain: Non-specific tenosynovitis involving the flexor carpi radialis. Plast. Reconstr. Surg., *62*:263–266, 1978.
105. Weinberger, A., and Schumacher, H.R.: Experimental joint trauma: Synovial response to blunt trauma and inflammatory reaction to intra-articular injection of fat. J. Rheumatol., *8*:380–389, 1981.
106. Wilkinson, A.: Traumatic haemarthrosis of the knee. Lancet, *2*:13–15, 1965.
107. Williams, K.A., and Scott, J.T.: Influence of trauma on the development of chronic inflammatory polyarthritis. Ann. Rheum. Dis., *26*:532–537, 1967.
108. Wilson, J.N.: A diagnostic sign in osteochondritis dissecans of the knee. J. Bone Joint Surg., *49A*:477–480, 1967.
109. Wilson, R.N., and Wilson, S.: Tenosynovitis in industry. Practitioner, *178*:612–615, 1957.
110. Wolf, C.R., and Mankin, H.J.: Effect of experimental hemarthrosis on articular cartilage of rabbit knee joints. J. Bone Joint Surg., *47A*:1203–1210, 1965.
111. Wolf, E., and Stern, S.: Costosternal syndrome: Its frequency and importance in differential diagnosis of coronary heart disease. Arch. Intern. Med., *136*:189–191, 1976.

112. Wright, J.T.: Slipping-rib syndrome. Lancet, 2:632–634, 1980.

113. Younghusband, O.Z., and Black, J.D.: DeQuervain's disease: Stenosing tenovaginitis at the radial styloid process. Can. Med. Assoc. J., 89:508–512, 1963.

114. Yousefzadeh, D.K., and Jackson, J.H., Jr.: Lipohemarthrosis of the elbow joint. Radiology, 128:643–645, 1978.

Chapter 78

Mechanical Disorders of the Knee

Roger Paul Johnson and Bruce J. Brewer

A mechanical disorder of the knee is defined as any condition that interferes with normal joint motion or mobility. Strictly speaking, an internal derangement of the knee is a mechanical disorder due to an intra-articular pathologic process. An external derangement, a term not commonly used but certainly appropriate, implies a disorder external to the joint proper that creates abnormalities in motion and function. Examples include cruciate and collateral ligamentous tears, quadriceps or hamstring insufficiency or contractures, masses outside the joint cavity such as popliteal cysts and tumors, and extensor tendon malalignment. Many of these external disorders can cause sudden or long-term loss of motion of the knee and they may mimic or may even cause internal derangements, such as ligamentous instability leading to meniscal tears.

DEFINITIONS OF INTERNAL DERANGEMENT OF THE KNEE

William Hey, of Leeds, England, coined the term "internal derangement of the knee" in the late 1700s.[83] He noted that "trifling accidents" could unexpectedly lock the knee and lead to an inability to "freely bend or extend the limb in walking." If the knee remained locked for months or even years, Hey indicated that it could become a "serious misfortune" leading to a "considerable degree of lameness," a condition he suffered with himself for almost 50 years. He reasoned that "some slight derangement of the semilunar cartilages may probably be sufficient to bring on the complaint," and if caught in the joint, would prevent the "os femoris from moving truly in the hollow formed by the semilunar cartilages and articular depression of the tibia."[83]

Hey also stated that a loose body or fragment of meniscus locked in the joint could cause "an unequal tension of the lateral (collateral) or cross (cruciate) ligaments of the knee." He advised manipulation "without surgical assistance." In a case presentation of a young lady who suffered from a locked knee, Hey noted that three days after manipulation, "she danced at a private ball without inconvenience."[83]

From this statement, we conclude that Hey clearly understood the essential features of internal derangement of the knee, as follows: (1) incarceration or entrapment of bony or soft tissue fragments between the condyles and the tibial plateau causing the knee to lock; (2) circumscription by the tibia of an abnormal arc about the femur causing painful stretching of the ligaments of the knee and capsule; (3) sudden loss of motion, usually of full extension; (4) sudden loss of function of the knee, often associated with a minor injury; (5) possible restoration of the knee to normal function by manipulation; and (6) significant long-term disability if the condition remains uncorrected. To these features we add: (7) recurrent locking; (8) the reflex "pseudoparalysis" of the hamstring and quadriceps muscles at the time of locking causing the knee to buckle during weight bearing; (9) subjective complaints of "something moving around in the knee," the "knee skipping over one track" and "jumping out of the groove;" and finally (10) the history of a remote, more severe injury, such as a "sprain" of the knee or patellar dislocation, that left the patient disabled for at least a few weeks, followed by a return to normal or near-normal activities.

A fragment of bone or soft tissue that suddenly becomes interposed between the articular surfaces is the classic cause of internal derangement. This misplaced fragment can be radiolucent or radiopaque. The most frequent cause of locking is entrapment of the radiolucent meniscus. Osteochondritis dissecans and patellar disorders are the most common conditions that generate radiopaque osteocartilagenous loose bodies. Other causes of fragment generation with incarceration and internal derangement are discussed briefly in this chapter. Current methods used to define accurately the precise cause of mechanical disorders of the knee are also discussed in this chapter.

MENISCAL TEARS AND INSTABILITY

The best-known internal derangement of the knee is the torn meniscus.[12,30,43,69,96] Partial rings of fibrocartilage fill the marginal triangular space between the convex condyles and the flat posterior sloping tibial plateaus. As load-dispersing structures and stabilizers of the knee, the menisci are subject to considerable compression.[104] The medial meniscus is typically narrower and less mobile and is torn three to six times more commonly than the lateral meniscus.

Subtle instability, often secondary to old anterior cruciate ligament insufficiency,[4,17,19,27,70,71,101] previously diagnosed as a "sprained knee," allows the condyle to deviate from its normal plane of motion and to encroach on the margin of the meniscus. Because its peripheral attachments are stretched, the meniscus migrates closer to the center of the knee and renders it more susceptible to trapping and peripheral tears, the so-called "hypermobile meniscus."

Such stretching tugs on the joint capsule and peripheral attachments with minute bleeding, irritation, and synovitis that causes joint-line tenderness, an important sign noted in patients with trapping, tearing, or shredding of a meniscus. Condylar or tibial plateau degeneration or other causes of knee irritation with synovitis may also produce joint-line tenderness, a sign that becomes less reliable when these chronic conditions antedate the meniscal tear.

The many types of tears are classified as longitudinal, vertical, transverse, "parrot-beak," horizontal or cleavage, or pedunculated[69] (Figs. 78–1, 78–2, 78–3, 78–4). Under direct vision through an arthroscope, rotation of the knee can produce wrinkles in a meniscus. If the condyle should impinge on a wrinkled meniscus, a transverse or parrot-beak tear can occur. External rotation of the tibia brings the medial tibial plateau anteriorly and the posterior horn of the medial meniscus under the condyle (Fig. 78–4). This characteristic explains the posterior medial horn tears of the medial meniscus commonly associated with anteromedial instability.

Longitudinal vertical tears can involve the knife-like edge of the meniscus or a major portion of its body (see Fig. 78–3). When torn and separated, the inner margin displaces into the intercondylar notch, a condition referred to as a "bucket-handle tear" (see Fig. 78–4). This tear locks the knee in flexion. The patient may notice that the knee is becoming progressively straighter. Such a finding indicates anterior extension of the tear.

Locking is classically defined as sudden loss of extension. A torn meniscus may also block flexion, but the end point may be more difficult to define because the knee is less restrained in flexion.

Loss of extension should be assessed by comparing the affected and normal knees. With the patient supine, the legs are lifted by the heels to equal levels. The patella is higher on the side with a loss of extension. Any passive attempt to straighten the knee is resisted. The mechanical block forces the tibia to circumscribe an abnormal arc, to stretch the ligaments and joint capsule, and to cause pain. Effusion and protective muscle spasm can also suddenly prevent full extension. Usually, one notes a soft, spongy feeling at extension, which we call "soft locking." When the extension stop is abrupt, definite, and repeatable, we call this "hard locking."

The relationship between a torn meniscus and knee instability becomes clear when we recognize that the primary purpose of the ligaments of any joint is to direct the motion of one articular surface in a prescribed plane or planes about another articular surface.[105] Instability is said to be present when joint motion occurs outside this normal domain. As Hey noted,[83] the condyles normally ride "in the hollow formed by the semilunar cartilages and articular depression of the tibia." When insta-

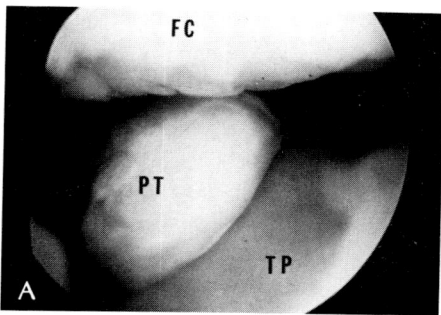
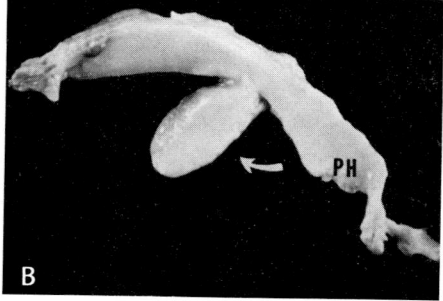

Fig. 78–1. *A,* This arthroscopic view demonstrates pedunculated tear (PT) of the medial meniscus incarcerated between the femoral condyle (FC) and the tibial plateau (TP). The patient is a 27-year-old athletically active man who had to give up all sports because of sudden locking and giving way of his knee. Note the damage to the cartilage covering the femoral condyle, as evidenced by the irregularity of the surface, which is normally perfectly smooth. *B,* This surgical specimen demonstrates the pedunculated tear shown in *A.* This pedunculated part (arrow) arose from a longitudinal tear of the posterior horn (PH), which became detached and protruded into the joint cavity, to become intermittently caught between the femoral condyle and the tibial plateau.

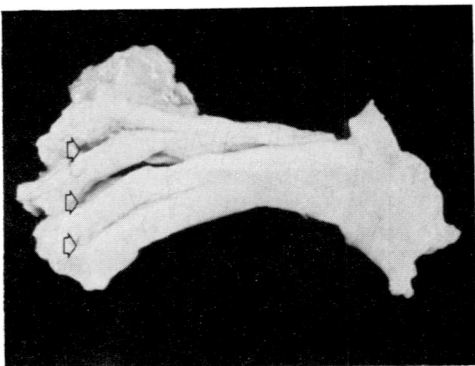

Fig. 78–2. This specimen is from a 27-year-old man who had three painful incidents of locking of his left knee in one year. Three longitudinal tears (arrows) of the lateral meniscus were found at operation.

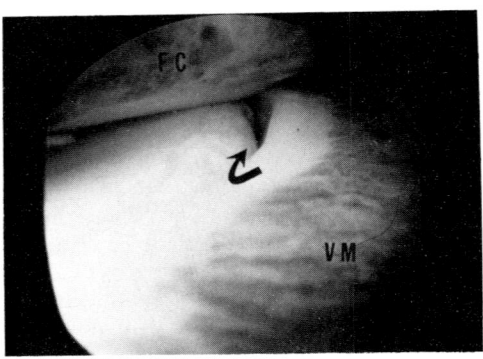

Fig. 78–3. This arthroscopic view of a longitudinal tear of a medial meniscus demonstrates the smoothness of the femoral condyle (FC), the vascular margin of the meniscus (VM), and the longitudinal tear of the meniscus (arrow).

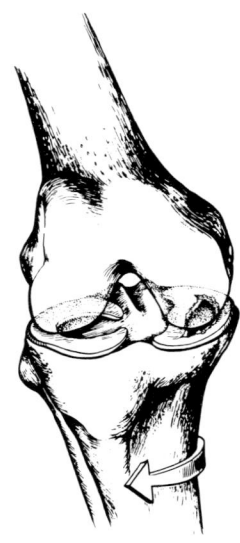

Fig. 78–4. Anteromedial instability is the most common form of instability of the knee. It has components of valgus and anterior motion of the medial tibial plateau, which is a manifestation of external rotation of the tibia on the femur (arrow). For this reason, tears of the medial meniscus typically start posteromedially and extend anteriorly into bucket-handle tears with forceful extension of the knee when the meniscus is trapped.

bility is present, and it is often subtle, the femoral condyle rides out of the meniscal hollow and over the meniscus. Should weight bearing occur and the meniscus not slide out from under the condyle, it will be torn. A torn fragment free on one end is called a pedunculated tear (see Fig. 78–1). Such fragments can be easily trapped in the joint without any abnormal motion of the condyle or the body of the meniscus. If the joint is then forced into extension, it will be pried apart, stretching the ligaments and further aggravating instability and damaging the articular surfaces.

The complex interplay between instability, torn menisci, athletic activities, muscle control, and repeated trauma ultimately leads to a degenerative knee. It is difficult to evaluate studies of meniscectomy and instability because it is often unclear whether the original injury, the repeated locking, the instability, the high athletic demands of the patient, the powerful muscular contractions, the repeated microtrauma, or the altered mechanics,[21] (most likely a combination of these factors) caused the disabled knee.

Terminology describing instability of the knee is as for dislocations, that is, according to the motion or abnormal position of the distal articulation or bone (Table 78–1).[34,35,58,59] *Anterior instability* indicates anterior displacement of the tibia on the femur and generally means at least anterior cruciate insufficiency. *Posterior instability* means posterior displacement of the tibia on the femoral condyles and usually indicates at least posterior cruciate ligament insufficiency. *Medial instability* means that the medial compartment opens with valgus stress, and *lateral instability,* opening laterally with varus stress. A comparison of mobility of affected and opposite knees is important because considerable ''normal'' variation occurs.

Basically, two types of rotational instability exist, internal and external. *Anteromedial*[76] and *posterolateral*[35] instability are forms of external rotational instability. When the tibia rotates externally,[68] the medial tibial plateau moves anteriorly, and the lateral moves posteriorly to an excessive degree. Excessive *posteromedial* and *anterolateral* mobility can be thought of as internal rotational instability. In the anterolateral disorder, a ''pivot shift''[23] or sudden anterior subluxation of the tibial

Table 78–1. Tests of Knee Instability

ANTERIOR INSTABILITY
Anterior drawer test[8,15,34,35,60]
Ritchey-Lachman test[86,101]

POSTERIOR INSTABILITY
Posterior drawer test[15,34,35]

MEDIAL INSTABILITY
Abduction stress test (20–30° flexion)[15,33,34,35]

LATERAL INSTABILITY
Adduction stress test (20–30° flexion)[15,33,34,35]

INTERNAL ROTARY INSTABILITY
Pivot shift[23]
Losee test[53]
ALRI test[93]
Jerk test[34,35]
Crossover test[4]
Flexion-rotation drawer test[72,79]
Posterior medial displacement of medial tibial plateau
    with valgus stress[48]

EXTERNAL ROTATORY INSTABILITY
Posterolateral drawer test[5,37]
External rotational recurvatum test[5,37]
Reversed pivot shift[39]
Anterior drawer with foot externally rotated[15,48]

plateau occurs as the knee is extended. Another sign of anterior cruciate ligament insufficiency is the anterior "drawer sign" with the knee at 90°.[58] *The Ritchey-Lachman* test,[86,101] which consists of anterior subluxation of the tibia with the knee at 0 to 20°, is a more sensitive sign of anterior cruciate ligament damage, especially if no anterior drawer sign is present at 90° of flexion.

Obviously, many combinations, degrees, and variations in anatomic involvement can accompany instability.[8,58] Although most students of the knee acknowledge that instability is "bad," it is difficult to say whether the injury, the "scrubbing" action of the articular surfaces, the indentation of the articular surface by the loose fragment, the loss of muscular control, or the ligamentous laxity is the ultimate cause of articular cartilage degeneration, the final common denominator of most arthritides.[21]

The relationship between instability and torn menisci is inherent in understanding the concept of the knee with a deficient anterior cruciate ligament.[17] An acute injury, usually of the internal or external rotational type, bowstrings the anterior cruciate ligament across the medial or lateral femoral condyles and attenuates or ruptures this ligament. The injury, often diagnosed as a "sprained knee," is the most common cause of hemarthrosis in the active adolescent or young adult.[13,72] In two or three weeks, the hemarthrosis subsides, and many patients return to normal activities within a

month or two. Often, no clinical instability or evidence of knee dysfunction is present at that time. Usually, a few years later, the burden of stabilization, formerly borne by the anterior cruciate ligament, is absorbed by the remaining ligamentous structures, which gradually stretch, especially if the patient participates in competitive athletics without adequate muscular control. Trivial injuries or simple twisting start to produce fleeting sensations of giving way, "skipping over one track," or sudden loss of control. These clinical manifestations suggest instability and trapping, but not necessarily cutting or tearing of the meniscus.

When the meniscus is ultimately torn, repair[30] or meniscectomy[96] is considered. Meniscectomy, which removes the "spacer effect" of the meniscus, can aggravate or potentiate the instability[36] and may hasten degeneration of the femoral condyle and, secondarily, the tibial plateau. With this series of events in mind, Allman has dubbed anterior cruciate ligament rupture as "the beginning of the end" of the knee.[101]

OSTEOCHONDRITIS DISSECANS

Osteochondritis dissecans is a prototype for conditions producing osteocartilaginous loose bodies. It was named by Konig in 1887,[67] but had been described by Sir James Paget in 1870 as "quiet necrosis" as compared with the more dramatic suppurative necrosis of bacterial infection. Although the term denotes inflammation of bone and cartilage, little inflammation is present. The term as used here means an island in the femoral condyle consisting of subchondral bone with its articular cartilage. This island, usually 1 to 2 cm in diameter, often "dissects" from the main condylar mass and can be thought of as a small fracture that develops chronic nonunion. Eighty-five percent of such lesions are found in the knee, but they have been reported in many sites,[3,85] including the femoral head, the dome of the talus, and the capitulum humeri.

Osteochondritis dissecans is a condition of unknown origin in which 85% of the lesions appear on the medial or central portion of the medial femoral condyle and 15% occur laterally.[3] These lesions are possibly shear fractures, but their occasional "mirror-image," bilateral occurrence suggests other anatomic or developmental disorders. Prominent tibial spines have been associated with the condition and have been implicated as sites of impingement with rotation of the tibia against the condyles.[24] Fairbank failed to find any evidence to dispute the hypothesis that the separation is caused by "trauma and trauma alone."[16]

This lesion is most common in adolescents and young adults, less common in patients in their thirties and forties, and rare in the elderly, in whom degeneration overshadows the primary cause. In the skeletally immature, the lesions heal without surgical intervention if the affected area is immobilized for a long enough time.[26] In children, we prefer multiple drilling of these lesions transversely through the femoral condyle distal to the epiphyseal plate with immobilization. This process seems to hasten the healing time if the articular surface is intact, as it usually is. In adults, excision gives favorable results,[51,52,74] although some prefer to pin the fragment in place.[40,94]

Osteochondritis dissecans is three times more common in males than in females. Shed or free fragments of bone loose in the knee joint are common in adults and rare in children. Smillie called it a "mysterious condition . . . never seen in the recent state."[94] True spontaneous healing was not observed in his five pediatric patients.

The small bony island is probably alive at the time of separation or fracture. The edges of the bony fragment become necrotic, but the overlying articular cartilage remains alive.[2] Studies on the blood supply of the condyles indicate a rich, anastomotic arterial network that makes localized infarction an unlikely cause.[16] The lesion has been reported in families as an autosomal dominant condition.[97,98,102] Osteochondritis dissecans of the patella, at least in some cases, appears to be due to a tangential or shear fracture secondary to subluxation. Osteochondritis dissecans of the femoral condyles, patellar fractures, and lateral femoral condylar fractures secondary to patellar dislocation are the three most common generators of "loose bodies," also called arthrophytes, "joint mice," corpora mobile, or arthroliths, in the knee (Fig. 78–5).

Long-term follow-up studies have revealed that many patients with osteochondritis dissecans develop degenerative arthritis. Thirty-eight of 48 patients seen at an average of 33 years after diagnosis had arthritis.[51] At least 20 years of observation are often required before arthritis is manifest. The process is accelerated in athletes.[3]

LATERAL FACET SYNDROME OF THE PATELLA

Malalignment of the extensor mechanism can be manifested by chronic lateral patellar pain or lateral patellar subluxation or dislocation. Acute dislocation causes acute patellar pain, but many patients have little or no pain in a few weeks. Those with the lateral facet syndrome have chronic lateral patellar pain and tenderness, but they rarely have a dislocation. Both conditions can cause crepitation of the patella clinically, which indicates chondro-

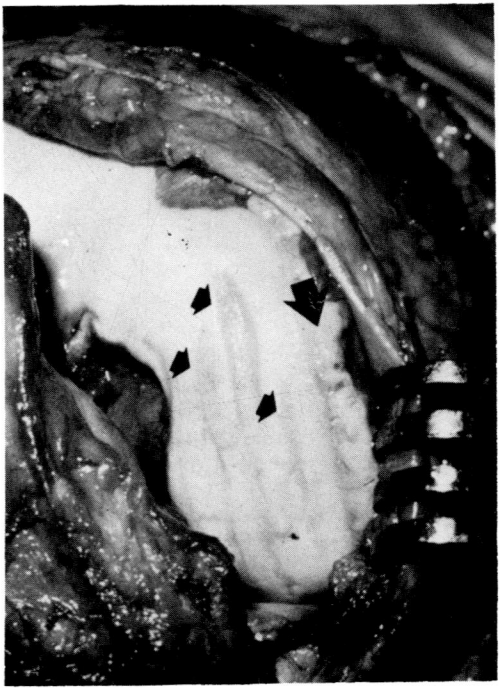

Fig. 78–5. The three small arrows point to longitudinal grooves or excoriations in the medial femoral condyle in this 21-year-old dock worker. These lesions were the result of repeated trapping with impingement of a single loose body. The large arrow points to early osteophyte formation along the medial border of the femoral condyle.

malacia patellae, and is due to the excessive forces across the patella by extensor malalignment.

The lateral facet syndrome is characterized by a gradual onset of lateral patellar pain while on stairs or during athletic activity, particularly running, jumping, squatting, or doing progressive resistive exercises. It is most common in a teenage female athlete and is erroneously diagnosed as "chondromalacia patellae."

An increase in lateral force in flexion of the combined lateral knee structures, that is, the vastus lateralis, the lateral retinaculum, and the patellofemoral and patellotibial ligaments, posterior migration of the iliotibial band, and lateral fat pad contractures, drives the lateral patellar facet into the lateral slope of the intercondylar groove. The exact mechanism of pain as a result of this increased pressure remains unclear.[20] The cause of pain may be increased intraosseous venous pressure[103] or marginal synovitis with capsular swelling. If the intercondylar groove is shallow, or if terminal lateral deviation of the patella occurs at full extension with quadriceps contraction, dislocation is more likely. This dislocation decompresses the patellofemoral joint and loosens the medial restraints, to cause patellar "tilting" and to decrease the likelihood of lateral facet syndrome and patellar pain. This process explains why many patients with recurrent patellar dislocations have little or no pain between dislocations.

The physical findings of the lateral facet syndrome include; (1) lateral patellar marginal tenderness; (2) resistance to medial displacement of the patella with the knee in 30° of flexion; and (3) vastus lateralis obliquus tenderness. Conservative measures include aspiration or nonsteroidal anti-inflammatory drugs, modification of the patient's activities, quadriceps muscle stretching, such as heel-to-buttock exercises, and occasional patellar bracing. Surgical treatment consists of complete resection of all the structures attaching to the lateral patellar surface, especially the vastus lateralis obliquus muscle.[41]

SYNOVIAL PLICA SYNDROME

A plica is a synovial fold, pleat, or band that is usually soft, mobile, thin, pliable, asymptomatic, and more prominent in flexion.[31,81,82] Occasionally, embryonic remnants of intrasynovial septa persist into adult life and become thickened, fibrotic, and often hemorrhagic cords causing snapping, clicking, or "catching" along the medial or lateral side of the patella.

The medial suprapatellar plica and the less-common lateral suprapatellar plica are the most prominent. These structures can also cause localized tenderness or a click as they snap over the anterior femoral condyles, usually at repeatable positions when the knee is extended or flexed.

Double-contrast arthrography can identify these folds[89,90] (Fig. 78–6), although arthroscopic visualization with documentation of synovitis, hemorrhage, and thickening and actual catching over the condyle is more conclusive evidence that the plica is the cause of the symptoms. Initially, nonoperative management consisting of rest, heat, and anti-inflammatory drugs may control the patient's symptoms. If this regimen fails, partial resection of the cord arthroscopically or through arthrotomy cures the condition.

RECURRENT LATERAL DISLOCATION OF THE PATELLA

Sudden "giving way" of the knee mimicking locking can occur with subluxation of the patella. True locking can result from an osteochondral fracture of the patella (Fig. 78–7) or of the lateral femoral condyle (Fig. 78–8) from a recent or remote dislocation of the patella.[49] We agree with Macnab that most patellar subluxations and dislocations begin at or near full extension.[55] When

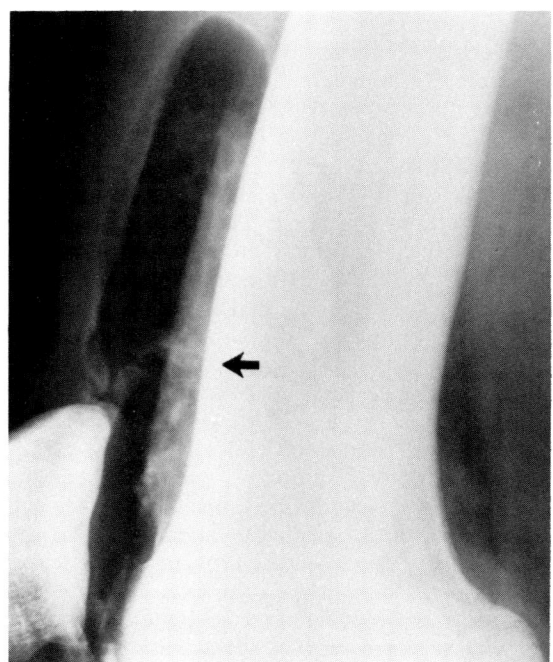

Fig. 78–6. Double-contrast arthrographic study documents a suprapatellar plica (arrow).

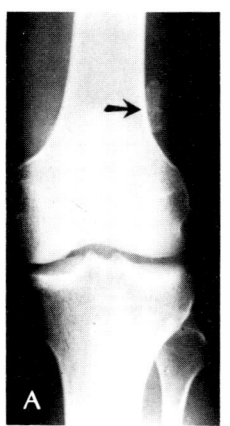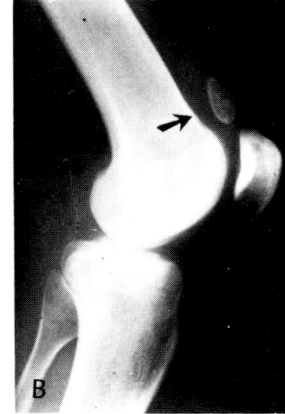

Fig. 78–7. The large radiopaque loose body (arrows) can be seen in both the anteroposterior *(A)* and lateral *(B)* projections in the suprapatellar pouch. Note the sclerotic margin on the undersurface of the patella in the lateral view, the site of origin of the loose body.

the patella is subluxed laterally at full extension and sudden uncontrolled flexion occurs, the patella is drawn along the lateral femoral condyle. With progressive flexion, the vastus medialis muscle and the medial retinaculum can become progressively taut, so as the patella is forcibly returned to the sulcus, fracture of the medial facet of the patella or lateral condylar margin can occur. If the patella

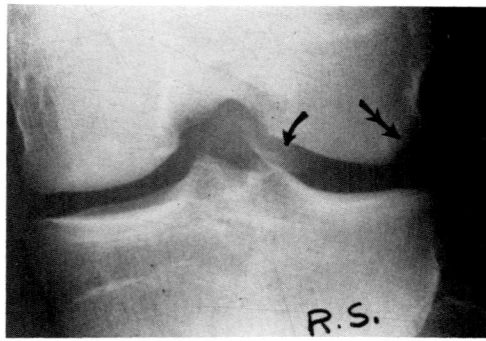

Fig. 78–8. The single arrow points to a loose body in the intercondylar notch from a "corner fracture" of the lateral femoral condyle (double arrows).

does not snap back but continues to ride the lateral margin of the condyle to full flexion, the medialis muscle and retinaculum will be torn or severely stretched. When this process occurs and the scar does not retract to repair it, medialis muscle insufficiency ensues. With the medial restraints gone and further contracture laterally, patellar tilt becomes evident.[50,62]

Many factors have been implicated in the cause of malalignment of the extensor mechanism of the knee.[38,41,45,49] We divide them into *intrinsic* factors, those directly located to the patellofemoral articulation, and *extrinsic* factors.

The intrinsic factors, usually more evident in severe forms of patellofemoral instability, include the following: (1) hypoplasia of the patella;[91] (2) high-riding patella, also called patella alta; (3) enlarged lateral patellar facet; (4) flat articular surface of the patella; (5) flat lateral femoral condyle; and (6) shallow intercondylar groove.

Extrinsic factors that may contribute to instability of the patella include the following: (1) insufficiency of the vastus medialis muscle, from disuse, prior rupture, or an anomalous high position of insertion on the patella; (2) over-pull or contracture of the vastus lateralis muscle;[41] (3) contracture of the iliotibial band; (4) contracture of the lateral retinaculum; (5) tethering through the patellofemoral and patellotibial ligaments; (6) lateral fat pad scarring from repeated arthroscopy; (7) an excessive "Q" angle (line of quadriceps force) creating a "bowstring" effect on the patella accentuated by external rotation of the tibia near full extension; (8) a laterally positioned tibial tubercle; (9) a valgus deformity of the knee; and (10) generalized hyperlaxity. Turner's syndrome, nail-patella or Fong's disease, and Down's syndrome[95] are three genetic conditions of which patellar dislocation is a clinical manifestation.

Surgical treatment progresses from lateral re-

lease to medial reefing or plication and, finally, to tibial tubercle transplantation medially if severe malalignment is present. Occasionally, patellar and intercondylar groove reshaping are necessary if the groove is shallow, flat, or convex and the patella is flat.

CHONDROMALACIA PATELLAE

Chondromalacia patellae is a morbid softening, fissuring, degenerative process of the articular surface of the knee cap owing to many causes[38] (Fig. 78–9). It can result from overuse during athletic activity,[28] from disuse following prolonged traction or cast immobilization, from direct injury such as a blow to the patella from a car dashboard, or from an old patellar fracture with imperfect reduction. The disorder is accompanied by quadriceps muscle contractures with loss of flexion, frequently with malalignment of the quadriceps muscles and a laterally riding or chronically dislocating patella.[38] This common form of internal derangement of the knee is present in the majority of patients over the age of 30 who have a history of one of the aforementioned conditions. Athletic adolescent girls seem especially prone to chondromalacia.

Symptoms consist of bone pain on ascending or descending stairs. Localized aching also occurs after periods of immobility with the knee in the flexed position, such as while watching television or working at a desk. The symptoms of crepitation and grinding usually correspond directly to the degree of surface cartilaginous disruption. We grade this into three degrees: I, fine fibrillation with yellowing (xanthochromia) and softening; II, surface degeneration with a "crabmeat" appearance; and III, exposure of the subchondral bone.

Crepitation, a sound resembling that of dry leaves underfoot, and grating, a palpatory sensation of roughness, are best demonstrated by active extension of the knee against resistance. These signs can be enhanced by direct manual compression of the patella against the femoral groove, with active resistive extension of the knee. Tenderness is often elicited along the inferior patella on the medial and lateral margins of the patellar ligament. We think that this sign is caused by a mild synovitis from the chips of chondromalacic fragments.

If chondromalacia is secondary to quadriceps muscle malalignment, the frightening "apprehension test" will be positive; this test produces a feeling of uneasiness with passive medial or lateral displacement of the patella. It is unusual to see an effusion of the knee due to chondromalacia patellae, unless the fibrillated surface has rapidly degenerated and has shed many fragments into the joint cavity over a short time, a phenomenon called "snowstorm knee." Therefore, an effusion in a

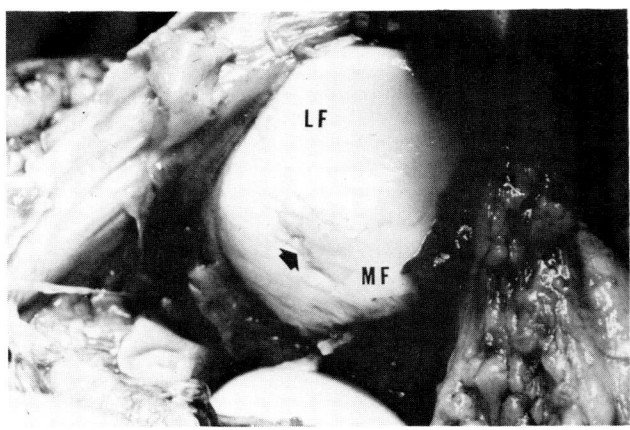

Fig. 78–9. This operative view of the undersurface of the patella shows typical chondromalacia with fissuring (arrow) of the medial facet (MF). The surface of the lateral facet (LF) appears unaffected.

patient with chondromalacia patellae is an ominous sign. These patients often obtain dramatic relief when the fragments and their products of digestion are arthroscopically irrigated from the joint.

The pathologic changes in chondromalacia may be precursors to osteoarthritis and may consist of a localized softening, discoloration, and loss of normal off-white sheen[56] (see also Chap. 87). Surface signs of progressive degeneration include fine fibrillation, fissuring, fragmentation, and finally, exposure of subchondral bone. The exact relationship between chondromalacia, primarily seen in the central and inferior part of the patella, and patellar osteoarthritis, which is primarily lateral facet degeneration, remains unclear. Few of our patients with severe chondromalacia have developed severe lateral facet arthritis without concomitant medial or lateral compartment degeneration. The roentgenographic findings of a degenerative patellofemoral joint include loss of mainly lateral facet cartilage space and roughening on the superficial surface, the so-called "hair-on-end" appearance of the patella seen best in the "sunrise view."[62] The lateral projection shows superior and inferior pole osteophytes adjacent to the articular surface. If the compartments of the knee have moderate-to-severe degeneration in comparable degrees, the medial compartment will be the most symptomatic, the lateral compartment will be less symptomatic, and the patellofemoral compartment will be symptomatic in 20 to 30% of patients.

The treatment of chondromalacia patellae is difficult because of the multiple causes and the general irreversibility of this degenerative process. The inherent constant loading of the patellar articular surface with three to six times body weight during athletic activity further frustrates recovery.

Repair of identifiable mechanical defects such as malalignment of the extensor mechanism, lateral capsular release, and tibial tubercle elevation

(Maquet technique) can be helpful.[18,57] Chondroplasty or debridement of the patellar articular surface is a nonphysiologic operation. Other than narrowing the articular surface by patellar decompression and preventing debris from falling into the joint cavity, this procedure offers little long-term relief. Patellectomy results in a 30 to 40% loss of quadriceps muscle power and is the last resort.

DIAGNOSTIC METHODS

An adequate medical history, physical examination,[79] and a roentgenographic evaluation of the knees consisting of at least anteroposterior and lateral views should be obtained. One may also consider patellar axial, sunrise or sunset, views for further evaluation of malalignment of the patella,[50,62] oblique views for occult lesions or fractures, and tunnel views to see the posterior portion of the femoral condyles more clearly, when looking for osteochondritis dissecans. Arthrography has been especially useful in demonstrating posterior horn tears of the medial meniscus and has been used to document anterior cruciate ligament tears.[22]

Ultrasound has been used to delineate Baker's cysts.[7] Computed-tomographic (CT) scanning is helpful in showing the size and anatomic configuration of masses about the knee,[78,80] as well as in evaluating the configuration and anatomic features of the patellofemoral joint.[14] Recently, triple-phase bone scintigraphy has been especially useful in determining the presence of active bony lesions of the condyles, tibial plateaus, and patella, as well as synovial hyperemia.[61] This technique has also been helpful in determining industrial and legal cases in which claims of serious dysfunction do not seem to correspond to the physical examination and the physician does not feel arthroscopy is indicated.

Aspiration of the knee to look for free fat in a

patient with acute hemarthrosis may aid in discovering an occult fracture not radiographically visible, but of all diagnostic procedures, arthroscopy has added more to our understanding of the knee than any other technique.[9,11,44,54,64,77] Its great diagnostic usefulness lies in the direct vision of the articular surfaces of the knee, the synovium, the anterior cruciate ligament, and the menisci. Various selections in angle of viewing with scopes of 0, 30, 70, and 110° are available. Many portals including suprapatellar, medial, lateral, and transpatellar tendon, and posterior have been described. The use of fiberoptics with more intense illumination has led to the ability to document intraarticular disorders in color. Miniature television cameras have expanded the capabilities of arthroscopy as an educational and operative tool.

Intra-articular arthroscopic surgery, without formal arthrotomy,[73,106] permits lateral plica release, patellar shaving, irrigational debridement, removal of loose bodies, debridement of the lesions of osteochondritis, synovectomy, plical resection,[31,66] meniscectomy,[73] and closed fixation of small intraarticular fractures.

The complications of arthroscopy are few. With sterile, continuous irrigation, small portals, minimal tissue retraction, and limited dissection, infections are rare. Leakage of irrigation fluid from the synovial cavity into the soft tissues about the knee and transient swelling and discomfort are occasionally encountered. Intra-articular seeding of extra-articular tumor arthroscopically has been reported.[44]

We can say without reservation that the arthroscope has taught us more about the knee than any other development in diagnosis. Nevertheless, it is not what is seen but what is understood that counts.

MECHANICAL DISORDERS AND OSTEOARTHRITIS

Many osteoarthritic knees began with a minor insult leading to degeneration of one of its three compartments, that is, the medial, patellofemoral, or lateral. The injured compartment sheds debris and spreads the "seeds" of arthritis ("wear particles") to the other compartments; the result is triple-compartment disease. Most commonly, the first affected knee compartment in women is the patellofemoral joint, and in men, it is the medial compartment.[47]

The lateral compartment can be injured by instability, meniscal tear, or lateral tibial plateau fracture, but degeneration beginning in this compartment is much less common than in the other two compartments. It is known as the "silent compartment" both because degeneration does not start

there and because it is often asymptomatic even in the presence of a significant pathologic process.

The following case history illustrates a typical course of a degenerative knee:

Case History

A 16-year-old boy sprained his right knee while playing football; he was clipped from the "blind side." The knee became massively swollen a few hours after injury, it was wrapped in an elastic bandage, and crutches were obtained from a friend. Three weeks later, the patient's knee felt much improved, and he resumed playing football without seeking medical attention.

Interpretation

The twisting injury resulted in a tear of the anterior cruciate ligament, the most common cause of hemarthrosis in young athletes.[13] Because the knee was swollen, no tear could have been present in the capsule. With acute anterior cruciate ligament rupture, signs of knee instability are often absent, and the patient thereby had the impression that nothing was seriously wrong.

Case History Continued

Four years later, while playing basketball in college, the same patient turned to throw the ball. His knee suddenly gave way and he fell to the floor. He tried to extend the knee, but could not. The trainer applied traction, and the knee suddenly became free, but the patient was unable to return to the game because of pain. Two weeks later, the same thing occurred again when the patient simply turned to talk to a friend. This time, he could straighten his knee to a greater degree. Once again, traction and slight twisting of the leg suddenly "released it." For the first time, the patient saw a physician, who made the diagnosis of a torn medial meniscus and surgically removed it. The patient returned to sports with no further problems.

Interpretation

The insufficiency of the torn anterior cruciate ligament led to increased loading and attenuation of the other ligamentous structures stabilizing the knee. The combined ligamentous insufficiency caused an instability manifested by a subtle anterior motion of the medial tibial plateau in relation to the femoral condyle, with the knee in flexion and the leg and foot in external rotation. This aberrant motion brought the posterior horn of the medial meniscus forward underneath the femoral condyle during most turning or "cutting" activities, eventually trapping the meniscus and finally causing a longitudinal tear (see Fig. 78-4). Repeated incidents of trapping and progressive tearing, allowing greater extension with each episode, gave the false impression that the knee was improving with each locking event.

Case History Continued

At age 46, the patient was still active in athletics, refereeing basketball and coaching soccer. He noticed that his right knee was beginning to bow, and the inner medial side of the knee ached after standing on it all day. The patient also noted intermittent swelling, heat, and deep bone pain with weather changes. He had tried some of the new "antiarthritic medications," which took the edge off the discomfort but did not seem to halt the progression of the disorder. His physician recommended "taking a wedge out of the tibia," to shift some of the weight to the lateral compartment and to correct the bowing.

Interpretation

Medial femoral condylar degeneration is common after meniscectomy.[99] Progressive degeneration with wearing of the medial condylar cartilage places more stress on the medial compartment of the knee and causes further varus. This process initiates the vicious cycle of medial compartment overload-further degeneration-greater compartment overload, and it ultimately leads to a "loss of medial joint space" on standing anteroposterior views of the knee. Proximal valgus tibial osteotomy shifts the weight from the medial to the lateral compartment and is often effective in controlling most of the symptoms of medial compartment degeneration.

Table 78–2. Conditions That Mimic or Produce Symptoms of Internal Derangement of the Knee

Avascular necrosis of the femoral condyles[1,88]
Chondromalacia patellae[38]
Cystic degeneration of the lateral meniscus[6]
Discoid lateral meniscus[29,84]
Heterotopic calcification[100]
Lipoma arborescens[32]
Localized pigmented villonodular synovitis[25]
Osteochondromatosis[63]
Pigmented villonodular synovitis[87]
Posterior cruciate ligament rupture[10]
Segond fracture[92]
Synovial cyst[46]
Synovial hemagioma[65]
Tibiofibular instability[75]
Tumors about the knee[42]

Case History Continued

The patient was relieved of pain by the osteotomy until age 65, when he retired as a school teacher. He continued to golf, but had to ride a cart because he was unable to walk 18 holes, owing to severe right knee discomfort. The patient had almost continual swelling, heat, grinding, and discomfort during minimal activity (Fig. 78–10). Soon thereafter, he underwent total knee replacement.

In summary, we have reviewed internal and external derangements of the knee, using the torn meniscus and its relationship to instability as the prototype for soft tissue entrapment and osteochondritis and patellar dislocation as prototypic conditions that generate osteochondral loose bodies. Other conditions can mimic internal derangements (Table 78–2). Finally, we have reviewed current diagnostic methods and have presented a typical case history of degenerative osteoarthritis of the knee.

REFERENCES

1. Ahlback, S., Bauer, G.C.H., and Bohne, W.H.: Spontaneous osteonecrosis of the knee. Arthritis Rheum., *11*:705–733, 1968.
2. Ahuja, S.C., and Bullough, P.G.: Osteonecrosis of the knee: a clinico-pathological study in twenty-eight patients. J. Bone Joint Surg., *60A*:191–197, 1978.
3. Aichroth, P.: Osteochondritis dissecans of the knee: a clinical survey. J. Bone Joint Surg., *53A*:440–447, 1971.
4. Arnold, J.A., et al.: Natural history of anterior cruciate tears. Am. J. Sports Med., 7:305–313, 1979.
5. Baker, C.L., Norwood, L.A., and Hughston, J.C.: Acute posterolateral rotatory instability of the knee. J. Bone Joint Surg., *65A*:614–618, 1983.
6. Barrie, H.J.: The pathogenesis and significance of meniscal cysts. J. Bone Joint Surg., *61B*:184–189, 1979.
7. Beals, R.K., et al.: Ultrasound as a diagnostic aid in the evaluation of popliteal swelling. Clin. Orthop., *149*:220–223, 1980.
8. Brantigan, O.C., and Voshell, A.F.: The mechanics of the ligaments and menisci of the knee joint. J. Bone Joint Surg., 23:44–66, 1941.
9. Casscells, S.W.: The place of arthroscopy in the diagnosis

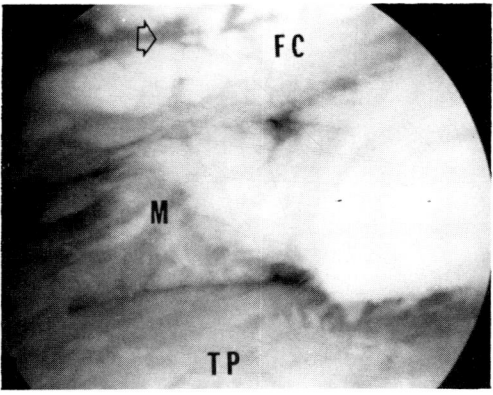

Fig. 78–10. This arthroscopic picture demonstrates end-stage degeneration of the femoral condyle (FC), the meniscus (M), and the tibial plateau (TP). The arrow points to an ulceration of the articular cartilage extending to subchondral bone.

and treatment of internal derangement of the knee: an analysis of 1000 cases. Clin. Orthop., *151*:135–142, 1980.

10. Clancy, W.G., et al.: Treatment of knee joint instability secondary to rupture of the posterior cruciate ligament. J. Bone Joint Surg., *65A*:310–322, 1983.

11. Curran, W.P., and Woodward, E.P.: Arthroscopy: its role in diagnosis and treatment of athletic knee injuries. Am. J. Sports Med., *8*:415–418, 1980.

12. Daniel, D., Daniels, E., and Aronson, D.: The diagnosis of meniscus pathology. Clin. Orthop., *163*:218–224, 1982.

13. DeHaven, K.E.: Diagnosis of acute knee injuries with hemarthrosis. Am. J. Sports Med., *8*:9–14, 1980.

14. Delgado-Martins, H.: A study of the position of the patella using computerized tomography. J. Bone Joint Surg., *61B*:443–444, 1979.

15. Ellison, A.E.: Skiing injuries. Ciba Symp., *29*:2–40, 1977.

16. Fairbank, H.A.T.: Osteochondritis dissecans. Br. J. Surg., *21*:67–82, 1933.

17. Feagin, J.A.: The syndrome of the torn anterior cruciate ligament. *In* Symposium on disorders of the knee joint. Orthop. Clin. North Am., *10*:81–90, 1979.

18. Ferguson, A.B., Jr., et al.: Relief of patellofemoral contact stress by anterior displacement of the tibial tubercle. J. Bone Joint Surg., *61A*:159–172, 1979.

19. Fetto, J.F., and Marshall, J.L.: The natural history and diagnosis of anterior cruciate ligament insufficiency. Clin. Orthop., *147*:29–38, 1980.

20. Ficat, R.P., and Hungerford, D.S. (Eds.): Disorders of the Patellofemoral Joint: The Excessive Lateral Pressure Syndrome. Baltimore, Williams & Wilkins, 1977, pp. 123–148.

21. Frankel, V.H., Burstein, A.H., and Brooks, D.B.: Biomechanics of internal derangement of the knee—pathomechanics as determined by analysis of the instant centers of motion. J. Bone Joint Surg., *53A*:945–962, 1971.

22. Freiberger, R.H., and Kaye, J.J.: Arthrography. New York, Appleton-Century-Crofts, 1979.

23. Galway, H.R., and MacIntosh, D.L.: The lateral pivot shift: a symptom and sign of anterior cruciate ligament insufficiency. Clin. Orthop., *147*:45–50, 1980.

24. Giorgi, B.: Morphologic variations of the intercondylar eminence of the knee. Clin. Orthop., *8*:209–217, 1956.

25. Granowitz, S.P., and Mankin, H.J.: Localized pigmented villonodular synovitis of the knee: report of five cases. J. Bone Joint Surg., *49A*:122–218, 1967.

26. Green, W.T., and Banks, H.H.: Osteochondritis dissecans in children. J. Bone Joint Surg., *35A*:26–47, 1953.

27. Grove, T.P., et al.: Non-operative treatment of the torn anterior cruciate ligament. J. Bone Joint Surg., *65A*:184–192, 1983.

28. Gruber, M.A.: The conservative treatment of chondromalacia patellae. *In* Symposium on disorders of the knee joint. Orthop. Clin. North Am., *10*:105–115, 1979.

29. Hall, F.M.: Arthrography of the discoid lateral meniscus. AJR, *128*:993–1002, 1977.

30. Hamberg, P., Gillquist, J., and Lysholm, J.: Suture of new and old peripheral meniscus tears. J. Bone Joint Surg., *65A*:193–197, 1983.

31. Hardaker, W.T., Whipple, T.L., and Bassett, F.H., III: Diagnosis and treatment of the plica syndrome of the knee. J. Bone Joint Surg., *62A*:221–225, 1980.

32. Hermann, G., and Hockberg, F.: Lipoma arborescens: arthrographic findings. Orthopedics, *3*:19–21, 1980.

33. Hoppenfeld, S.: Physical examination of the knee joint by complaint. Orthop. Clin. North Am., *10*:3–20, 1979.

34. Hughston, J.C., et al.: Classification of knee ligament instabilities. Part I. The medial compartment and cruciate ligaments. J. Bone Joint Surg., *58A*:159–172, 1976.

35. Hughston, J.C., et al.: Classification of knee ligament instabilities, Part II. The lateral compartment. J. Bone Joint Surg., *58A*:173–179, 1976.

36. Hughston, J.C., and Barrett, G.R.: Acute anteromedial rotatory instability. J. Bone Joint Surg., *65A*:145–153, 1983.

37. Hughston, J.C., and Norwood, L.A.: The posterolateral drawer test and external rotational recurvatum test for posterolateral rotatory instability of the knee. Clin. Orthop., *147*:82–87, 1980.

38. Insall, J.: Current concepts review: patellar pain. J. Bone Joint Surg., *64A*:147–152, 1982.

39. Jakob, R.P., Hassler, H., and Staeubli, H.U.: Observations on rotatory instability of the lateral compartment of the knee. Acta Orthop. Scand., Suppl 191, *52*:1–32, 1981.

40. Johnson, E.W., and McLeod, T.L.: Osteochondral fragments of the distal end of the femur fixed with bone pegs. J. Bone Joint Surg., *59A*:677–679, 1977.

41. Johnson, R.P.: Lateral resection for moderate patellofemoral instability. Orthop. Trans., *7*:196, 1983.

42. Johnston, A.D., and Parisien, M.V.: Soft tissue tumors about the knee. Symposium on disorders of the knee joint. Orthop. Clin. North Am., *10*:263–284, 1979.

43. Jones, R.E., Smith, E.C., and Resich, J.S.: Effects of medial meniscectomy in patients older than forty years. J. Bone Joint Surg., *60A*:783–786, 1978.

44. Joyce, M.J., and Mankin, H.J.: Caveat arthroscopos: extra-articular lesions of bone simulating intra-articular pathology of the knee. J. Bone Joint Surg., *65A*:289–292, 1983.

45. Kettelkamp, D.B.: Current concepts review: management of patellar malalignment. J. Bone Joint Surg., *63A*:1,344–1,348, 1981.

46. Kilcoyne, R.F., Imray, T.J., and Stewart, E.T.: Ruptured Baker's cyst simulating acute thrombophlebitis. JAMA, *240*:1,517–1,518, 1978.

47. Klunder, K.B., Rud, B., and Hansen, J.: Osteoarthritis of the hip and knee joint in retired football players. Acta Orthop. Scand., *51*:925–927, 1980.

48. Larson, R.L.: The Knee—the physiological joint. (Editorial.) J. Bone Joint Surg., *65A*:143–144, 1983.

49. Larson, R.L.: Subluxation-dislocation of the patella. *In* The Injured Adolescent Knee. Edited by J.C. Kennedy. Baltimore, Williams & Wilkins, 1979, pp. 161–204.

50. Laurin, C.A., et al.: The abnormal lateral patellofemoral angle: a diagnostic roentgenographic sign of recurrent patellar subluxation. J. Bone Joint Surg., *60A*:55–60, 1978.

51. Linden, B.: Osteochondritis dissecans of the femoral condyles. J. Bone Joint Surg., *59A*:769–776, 1977.

52. Linden, B., and Nilsson, B.E.: Strontium-85 uptake in knee joints with osteochondritis dissecans. Acta Orthop. Scand., *47*:668–671, 1976.

53. Losee, R.E., Johnson, T.R., and Southwick, W.O.: Anterior subluxation of the lateral tibial plateau. J. Bone Joint Surg., *60A*:1,015–1,030, 1978.

54. McGinty, J.B., and Freedman, P.A.: Arthroscopy of the knee. Clin. Orthop., *121*:173–180, 1976.

55. Macnab, I.: Recurrent dislocation of the patella. J. Bone Joint Surg., *34A*:957–967, 1952.

56. Mankin, H.J.: Biochemical changes in articular cartilage in osteoarthritis. *In* Symposium on Osteoarthritis. St. Louis, C.V. Mosby, 1976, pp. 1–22.

57. Maquet, P.G.J.: Biomechanics of the Knee: With Application to the Pathogenesis and the Surgical Treatment of Osteoarthritis. Berlin, Springer-Verlag, 1976, p. 137.

58. Marshall, J.L., and Baugher, W.H.: Stability examination of the knee: a simple anatomic approach. Clin. Orthop., *146*:78–83, 1980.

59. Marshall, J.L., Getto, J.F., and Botero, P.M.: General orthopaedics: knee ligament injuries: a standardized evaluation method. Clin. Orthop., *123*:115–129, 1977.

60. Marshall, J.R., Warren, R., Fleiss, D.F.: Ligamentous injuries of the knee in skiing. Clin. Orthop., *108*:196–199, 1975.

61. Mauer, A.H., et al.: Utility of three-phase skeletal scintigraphy in suspected osteomyelitis: concise communication. J. Nucl. Med., *22*:941–949, 1981.

62. Merchant, A.C., et al.: Roentgenographic analysis of patellofemoral congruence. J. Bone Joint Surg., *56A*:1,391–1,396, 1974.

63. Milgram, J.W.: Synovial osteochondromatosis: a histopathological study of thirty cases. J. Bone Joint Surg., *59A*:792–801, 1977.

64. Minkoff, J.: The philosophy and application of arthros-

copy in non-meniscal problems of the knee. *In* Symposium on disorders of the knee joint. Orthop. Clin. North Am., *10*:37–50, 1979.

65. Moon, N.F.: Synovial hemangioma of the knee joint. Clin. Orthop., *90*:183–190, 1973.

66. Munzinger, U., et al.: Internal derangement of the knee joint due to pathologic synovial folds: the mediopatellar plica syndrome. Clin. Orthop., *155*:59–64, 1981.

67. Nagura, S.: The so-called osteochondritis dissecans of Konig. Clin. Orthop., *18*:100–122, 1960.

68. Nicholas, J.A.: The five-one reconstruction for antero-medial instability of the knee: indications, technique, and the results in fifty-two patients. J. Bone Joint Surg., *55A*:899–922, 1973.

69. Noble, J., and Erat, K.: In defense of the meniscus. J. Bone Joint Surg., *62B*:7–11, 1980.

70. Noyes, F.R., et al.: The symptomatic anterior cruciate-deficient knee. Part II. The results of rehabilitation activity modification and counseling on functional disability. J. Bone Joint Surg., *65A*:163–174, 1983.

71. Noyes, F.R., et al.: The symptomatic anterior cruciate-deficient knee. Part I. The long term functional disability in athletically active individuals. J. Bone Joint Surg., *65A*:154–162, 1983.

72. Noyes, F.R., et al.: Arthroscopy in acute traumatic hemarthrosis of the knee. J. Bone Joint Surg., *62A*:687–695, 1980.

73. O'Connor, R.L.: Arthroscopy. Philadelphia, J.B. Lippincott, 1977.

74. O'Donoghue, D.H.: Chondral and osteochondral fractures. J. Trauma, *6*:469–481, 1966.

75. Ogden, J.A.: Subluxation and dislocation of the proximal tibiofibular joint. J. Bone Joint Surg., *56A*:145–154, 1974.

76. Parker, H.G.: Chronic anteromedial instability of the knee. Clin. Orthop., *142*:123–130, 1979.

77. Patel, D., Fahmy, N., and Sakayan, A.: Isokinetic and functional evaluation of the knee following arthroscopic surgery. Clin. Orthop., *167*:84–91, 1982.

78. Paul, D.F., Morrey, B.F., and Helms, C.A.: Computerized tomography in orthopedic surgery. (Section II. General orthopaedics.) Clin. Orthop., *139*:142–149, 1979.

79. Paulos, L., Noyes, F.R., and Malek, M.: A practical guide to the initial evaluation and treatment of knee ligament injuries. J. Trauma, *20*:498–506, 1980.

80. Pavlov, H., et al.: Computer-assisted tomography of the knee. Invest. Radiol., *13*:57–62, 1978.

81. Pitkin, G.: Knee injuries: the role of the suprapatellar plica and suprapatellar bursa in simulating internal derangement. Clin. Orthop., *74*:161–174, 1971.

82. Pitkin, G.: Lesions of the suprapatellar plica. J. Bone Joint Surg., *32A*:363–369, 1950.

83. Rang, M. (Ed.): Anthology of Orthopaedics. Internal Derangement of the Knee: William Hey. London and Edinburgh, E. and S. Livingstone Ltd., 1966, pp. 30–32.

84. Resnick, D., and Niwayama, G.: Discoid meniscus. *In* Diagnosis of Bone and Joint Disorders. Vol. I. Arthrography, Tenography, and Bursography. Philadelphia, W.B. Saunders, 1981, pp. 579–582.

85. Ribbing, S.: The hereditary multiple epiphyseal disturbance and its consequences for the aetiogenesis of local malacias—particularly the osteochondrosis dissecans. Acta Orthop. Scand., *24*:286–299, 1955.

86. Ritchey, S.J.: Ligamentous disruption of the knee. U.S. Armed Forces Med. J., *11*:167–176, 1960.

87. Rosenthal, D.I., Coleman, P.K., and Schiller, A.L.: Pigmented villonodular synovitis: correlation of angiographic and histologic findings. Am. Roentgen Ray Soc., *135*:581–585, 1980.

88. Rozing, P.M., Insall, J., and Bohne, W.H.: Spontaneous osteonecrosis of the knee. J. Bone Joint Surg., *62A*:2–7, 1980.

89. SanDretto, M.A., et al.: Suprapatellar plica synovialis: a common arthrographic finding. J. Can. Assoc. Radiol., *33*:163–166, 1982.

90. SanDretto, M.A., and Carrera, G.F.: The double fat fluid level: lipohemarthrosis of the knee associated with suprapatellar plica synovialis. Skeletal Radiol., *10*:30–33, 1983.

91. Scott, J.E., and Taor, W.S.: The "small patella" syndrome. J. Bone Joint Surg., *61B*:172–175, 1979.

92. Segond, P.: Pathologie externe. Recherches cliniques et experimentales sur les epanchements sanguins du genou par entorse test. *7*:319–321, 1879.

93. Slocum, D.B., et al.: Clinical test for anterolateral rotary instability of the knee. Clin. Orthop., *118*:63–69, 1976.

94. Smillie, I.S.: Treatment of osteochondritis dissecans. J. Bone Joint Surg., *39B*:248–260, 1957.

95. Smith, D.W.: Recognizable Patterns of Human Malformation. Vol. 7. Major Problems in Clinical Pediatrics. Philadelphia, W.B. Saunders, 1970, pp. 33–35, 57–59, 234–235.

96. Sonne-Holm, S., Fledelius, I., Ahn, N.: Results after meniscectomy in 147 athletes. Acta Orthop. Scand., *51*:303–309, 1980.

97. Stougaard, J.: Familial occurrence of osteochondritis dissecans. J. Bone Joint Surg., *46B*:542–543, 1964.

98. Stougaard, J.: The hereditary factor in osteochondritis dissecans. J. Bone Joint Surg., *43B*:256–258, 1961.

99. Tapper, E.M., and Hoover, N.W.: Late results after meniscectomy. J. Bone Joint Surg., *51A*:517–526, 1969.

100. Tibone, J., et al.: Heterotopic ossification around the hip in spinal cord-injured patients. J. Bone Joint Surg., *60A*:769–775, 1978.

101. Torg, J.S., Conrad, W., and Kalen, V.: Clinical diagnosis of anterior cruciate ligament instability in the athlete. Am. J. Sports Med., *4*:84–93, 1976.

102. Wagoner, G., and Cohn, B.N.E.: Osteochondritis dissecans: a resume of the theories of etiology and the consideration of heredity as an etiologic factor. Arch. Surg., *23*:1–25, 1931.

103. Waisbrod, H., and Treiman, N.: Intraosseous venography in patellofemoral disorders—a preliminary report. J. Bone Joint Surg., *62B*:454–456, 1980.

104. Walker, P.S., and Erkman, M.J.: The role of the menisci in force tranmission across the knee. Clin. Orthop., *109*:184–192, 1975.

105. Warren, R.F., and Levy, I.M.: Meniscal lesions associated with anterior cruciate ligament injury. Clin. Orthop., *172*:32–37, 1983.

106. Watanabe, M.: Arthroscopy: the present state. Orth. Clin. North Am., *10*:505–522, 1979.

Chapter 79

Painful Feet

N. Noel Testa and Theodore A. Potter

Over 90% of painful feet are caused by static disabilities. The other 10% may be due to trauma, infection, inflammatory conditions, congenital deformities, or disturbances of growth or circulation. Static disabilities are caused by weak muscles, relaxed ligaments, and deformity. These static disabilities usually begin as mild weakness and slowly progress, if untreated, to serious disability with deformities in the bones, muscles, and ligaments.

Traumatic disabilities are easily diagnosed and usually require immediate treatment. In most instances, recovery is prompt. Serious congenital disabilities usually come under the care of orthopedic surgeons early. Infections anywhere in the foot usually require avoidance of weight bearing, except in the mildest cases. Antibiotics are often indicated. Most developmental disabilities are self-limited, and treatment is necessary only if the patient has symptoms. Circulatory disturbances are most commonly found in the aged. Although most of these disorders can be treated, few of them can be cured, and treatment is at best palliative.[2] Neoplasms are rare in the feet.[9]

NORMAL PHYSIOLOGY OF THE FEET

The center of gravity of the body is normally balanced over the triangular weight-bearing area of the foot, with its apex posteriorly. This weight is divided equally among the heads of the metatarsal bones and the tuberosity of the os calcis. Physicians desiring detailed anatomic or physiologic data on this subject are referred to the works of DuVries,[5] Kelikian,[10] and Giannestras.[7]

The foot is like a spring, composed of a bony framework with arches maintained by the physiologic tone of muscles, ligaments, and fascia. The whole weight of the body in walking and in standing is borne by an elastic arch composed of small bones joined by ligaments and connected by muscles. Unfortunately, this complicated structure is not left free to perform its function, but is encased from childhood in a distorting leather covering that may compress and deform the forefoot and may weaken its muscles. Inasmuch as the shape of a shoe seldom correponds to the shape of the adult foot, shoes are one of the most important contributors to foot strain.[15]

The longitudinal arch runs anteroposteriorly along the inner border of the foot from the tuberosity of the os calcis to the heads of the metatarsal bones and centers about the inner three metatarsal bones, the cuneiform bones, and the navicular, astragalus, and calcaneus bones (Fig. 79–1). The medial portion of the longitudinal arch rests on the os calcis and on the head of the first metatarsal bone. The anterior transverse metatarsal arch passes through the necks of the second, third, and fourth metatarsal bones and through the heads of the first and fifth metatarsal bones. This arch becomes flattened on weight bearing, but returns to its arched position when the weight is removed.[3] All the heads of the metatarsal bones rest on the ground in weight bearing, so no transverse arch is present at that time.[16]

The longitudinal and transverse arches form a composite system. The longitudinal arch blends into the transverse arch proximal to the metatarsal heads, and the transverse arch passes imperceptibly into the longitudinal arch as one approaches the base of the metatarsal bones. When the feet are brought together and are viewed from inferiorly, the feet resemble a shallow, inverted bowl (Figs. 79–2, 79–3).

The ligaments that aid in maintaining the integrity of the longitudinal arch include the "spring" ligament, or inferior calcaneonavicular, which is the main ligamentous support on the inner side, and the long and short calcaneocuboid or plantar ligaments, which support the middle and outer parts.

The strength and importance of the plantar fascia are demonstrated in paralysis of the extensor muscles of the foot, in which extreme contracture of the plantar fascia results in a pes cavus deformity.

The muscles are important structures in the foot. The plantar flexor muscles are approximately five times as strong as the dorsal flexors, and the gastrocnemius and soleus muscles are three times as powerful as the remainder of the foot muscles combined. The chief movements of the foot are performed by the tibial and peroneal muscles. The tibialis anterior muscle elevates and the peroneus longus muscle depresses the first metatarsal bone. The tibialis posterior muscle produces inversion

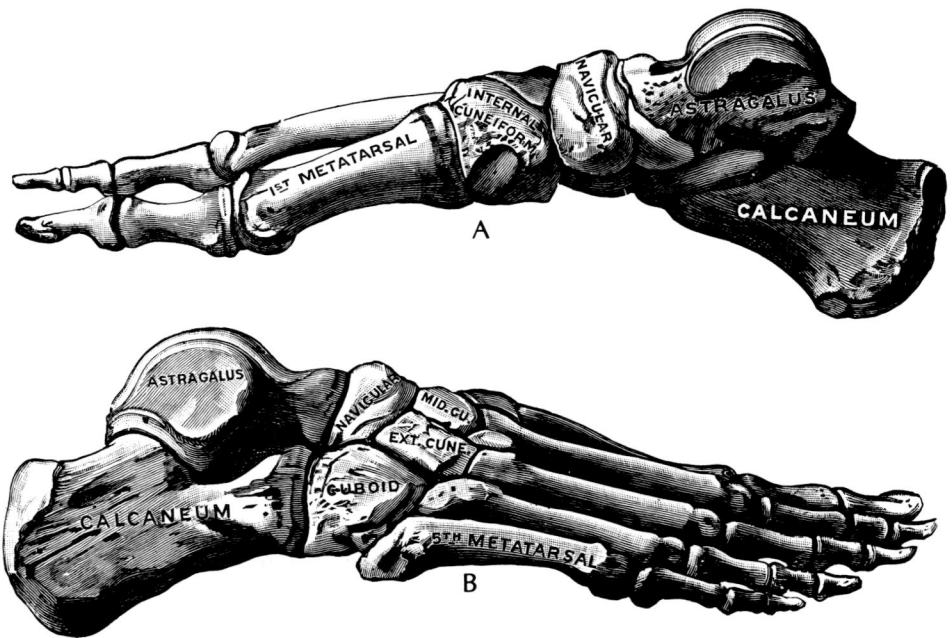

Fig. 79–1. *A*, The bones of the right foot, viewed from the inner side; *B*, the bones of the right foot, viewed from the outer side.

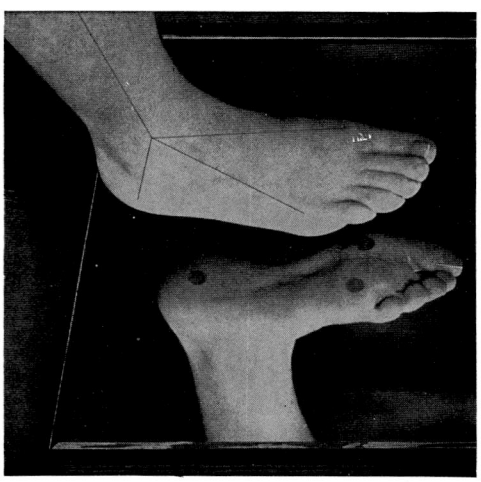

Fig. 79–2. Distribution of weight to the foot. (Courtesy of the George E. Keith Company.)

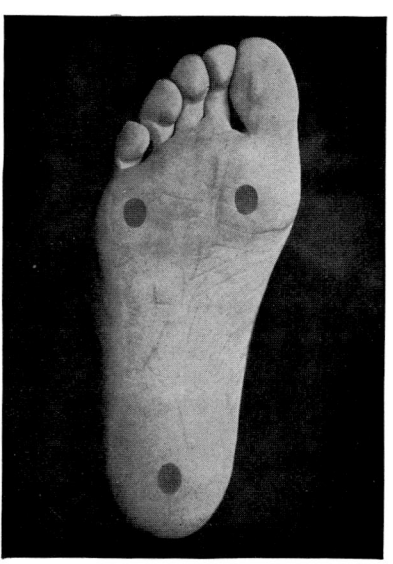

Fig. 79–3. Weight-bearing points of the foot. (Courtesy of the George E. Keith Company.)

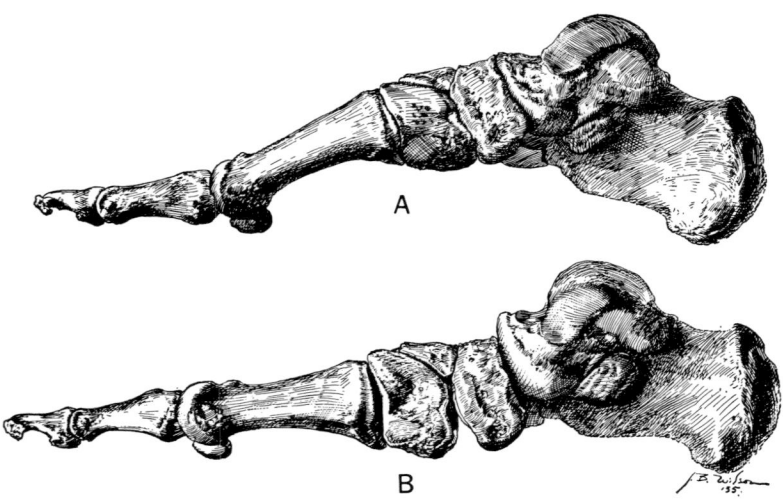

Fig. 79–4. Medial aspect of the foot. *A,* Normal longitudinal arch; *B,* arch in flat foot. (From Shands, A.: Orthopedic Surgery. St. Louis, C. V. Mosby Co.)

and adduction. The peroneal muscles aid eversion and abduction. The chief evertors of the foot are the peroneus longus and brevis muscles. The invertors are chiefly the tibialis anterior and posterior muscles. The normal ratio of strength of the invertors to the evertors should be six to five.

PAINFUL FLAT (WEAK) FEET

Flat feet may be congenital or acquired. The acquired disorder may be classified as flaccid or static, spastic, or rigid. In the flaccid type of flat foot, the main or longitudinal arch is depressed only during weight bearing and assumes a normal contour when weight is removed. If the flaccid foot is untreated, peroneal muscular spasm may occur. The result is a spastic flat foot with tenderness over the peroneal tendons and painful limitation of inversion.

The rigid flat foot is an end-stage disorder, with the foot firmly fixed in eversion by contractures and adhesions; simple measures do not restore the normal balance of the foot. Many of these patients have severe pain, which can only be alleviated by appropriate correction (Fig. 79–4).

The causes of painful, weak feet can be congenital, developmental, occupational, systemic, traumatic, neurologic, or circulatory. Patients seen in early childhood usually have a congenital relaxation or weakness of muscles and ligaments (Fig. 79–5). In the developmental group, in addition to faulty posture, abnormal development in tarsal or metatarsal bones is sometimes seen. Obesity leads to a slow tiring and overstretching of muscles and ligaments. Systemic diseases involving the bones

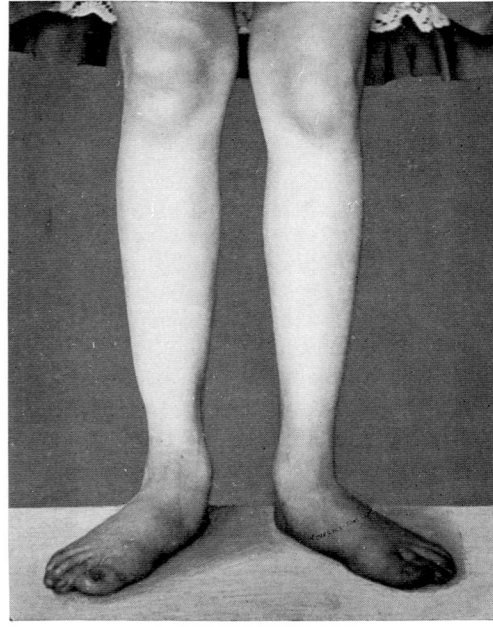

Fig. 79–5. The ordinary type of weak foot in a child. The degree of abduction is indicated by the relation of the patellae to the feet.

and joints of the feet lead to weakening, distortion, and limitation of motion in these structures.

Traumatic causes include fractures and their sequelae, such as favoring of the "good" foot. Vocational flat feet may develop from prolonged standing on a hard surface, as is required of dentists, policemen, and nurses. Failure of the tibialis anterior and posterior muscles, which maintain the longitudinal arch of the foot, strains and stretches the ligaments during weight bearing; this stress causes pain in early flat foot.

Painful flat feet are caused mainly by improper shoes, overweight, and muscle strain. Foot strain may be alleviated by proper shoes and well-fitted supports. Exercises and training in correct walking are required, however, to develop the foot muscle and to relieve symptoms entirely.

Ligamentous strain is preceded by muscular strain and weakness. Only after muscles and ligaments give way do flat feet occur. Strain of the transverse arch is due mainly to cramping of the forefoot; treatment includes raising the arch by pads, a metatarsal bar, and exercises.

Most patients with symptomatic flat feet develop a moderate degree of pronation.[4] Normal feet may be strained by excessive loads, such as by long hours of standing or walking, because of the assumption of a neutral position with the toes turned outward about 15°. This overuse produces ligamentous strain on the inside of the foot. In the strained foot, overstretching of the inferior calcaneonavicular ligament, of the plantar fascia, and of the plantar ligaments, and straining of the muscles controlling the inner side of the foot occur (Tables 79–1, 79–2, 79–3).

Treatment

Pain and impaired function are indications for treatment. If pain is present at rest or if the patient has associated arthritis, weight bearing should be proscribed until pain subsides. One should apply a light, removable plaster cast to maintain the foot in inversion and the forefoot in adduction and to support the longitudinal arch. This cast may be removed each day to permit exercise of the invertor muscles of the foot; exercises must not cause muscular fatigue or pain. Exercises and postural aids useful in treatment are summarized in Table 79–4. Other treatment considerations are listed in Table 79–5.

Many individuals with weak, pronated, painful feet may be benefited by a longitudinal rubber arch pad (average 3/16 inch beveled to 1/32 inch on the lateral side) or by a heel wedge at the rand of the shoe (Fig. 79–6). One should insist that the entire heel of the shoe be removed, and the wedge placed next to the sole (heel rand); the heel should then be replaced. Wedges average 1/4 inch anteromedially and taper to 1/32 inch posteriorly and laterally.

In cases of painful feet associated with knock knee, the weight should be thrown toward the outer side of the foot, by means of a medial heel wedge.

Patients with flexible weak feet often obtain greater comfort by the use of a pronatory inner

Table 79–1. Examination of the Foot

Medical History
  Determine extent of pain or pre-existing arthritis, relation of pain to standing and walking, pain while resting, stiffness on arising, and relation of pain to work.
  Include duration and course of the disability and the type and result of treatment.

Gait
  Observe gait.

Shoes
  See that the patient's shoe is not too short, long, narrow, or wide.
  Note the points of greatest wear on the shoe; in patients with a short Achilles tendon, the tips of the soles are scuffed and worn; in simple eversion, the inner side of the heel is worn; with depression of the metatarsal bones, a hole may be worn in the anterior part of the sole.
  If any part of the foot is displaced, a distortion will show in that part of the shoe.

Posture
  Examine the posture of the body, particularly excessive lordosis and flexion and rotation at the hip and flexion or genu valgum at the knee; are the patient's legs of equal length?

Foot
  Examine the foot at rest and during weight bearing; Look for prominences on the inner side of the foot, the spread of the forefoot, and the shape and position of the toes.
  See whether the heel or forefoot is held in a varus or valgus position.
  Look for corns and calluses, prominence of the metatarsal heads on the sole of the foot, bony prominences at the side or dorsum of the foot, swelling about the malleoli, thickening over any tendon, plantar warts, varicose veins, ulceration, and blueness or coldness of feet.
  Palpate the joints for swelling or tenderness.
  Examine for peroneal muscle spasm or clonus.
  Look for tenderness under the calcaneal fat pad, in the plantar fascia, and on the inner and outer sides of the ankle.
  See to what extent the longitudinal and transverse arches are depressed during weight bearing.
  Examine the range of motion at the ankle, tarsal, and toe joints; if the ankle joint dorsiflexes to a right angle when the knee is straight, the Achilles tendon will not have a contracture.
  Examine the skin for color, warmth, and excessive perspiration; look for epidermophytosis between the toes.
  Palpate the dorsalis pedis and posterior tibial arteries.
  Look for deformities of the nails and irritation at the sides of the nails.

Further Study
  Radiographic examination is indicated if any gross variation from normal is found.

Table 79–2. Positions of the Foot

Position	Definition
Adduction*	Forefoot displaced inward in relation to midline of limb.
Abduction*	Forefoot displaced outward in relation to midline of limb.
Inversion*	Sole of foot turned inward.
Eversion*	Sole of foot turned outward.
Valgus	Deformity of the foot in abduction and eversion.
Varus	Deformity of the foot in adduction and inversion.
Calcaneus	Deformity of the foot in dorsiflexion.
Equinus	Deformity of the foot in plantar flexion.
Supination	Same as inversion.
Pronation	Same as eversion.

*Adduction and inversion and abduction and eversion are often combined.

wedge under the heel and a supinatory outer wedge under the little toe (Fig. 79–7). The wedge raises the inner border of the heel and places the os calcis squarely on the ground. In addition, to equalize any tendency to excessive supination in the fore-foot, a short cleat is applied to the outer side of the forepart of the shoe.

In patients with short Achilles tendons, the whole heel must be raised temporarily to relieve strain.

An arch support, if necessary, is used temporarily when the patient becomes ambulatory. The altered heel or arch supports are used for several months after the patient can perform a day's work or exercise without fatigue or pain in the feet. In severely deformed feet and in elderly individuals, the supports must often be used permanently.

Arch Supports

Two types of arch support exist, tempered steel plates and leather inlays, with raises of felt, sponge rubber, or cork. About half of all steel arch supports are manufactured in a small number of standard sizes (Figs. 79–8, 79–9). These can be obtained readily from a surgical supply house, but they rarely fit accurately and do not give as much relief as those made from plaster impressions of the patient's foot.

Leather inlays fit in the shoe like insoles, and arches are supported by felt, sponge rubber, or cork molds. These types of arch support have the advantage of being adjustable, to fit the changing needs of support as the foot becomes less strained and fatigued. In this regard, they are superior to any rigid support.

The rationale of arch support is the relief of strained muscles and ligaments. When relief has occurred, one should pay attention to proper po-

Table 79–3. Signs of the Painful Flat (Weak) Foot

Primary Signs

Abduction, dorsiflexion, and supination of the forefoot. The weight-bearing line, dropped from the middle of the patella, comes between the first and second toes in the normal foot; in flat feet, this line often falls medial to the great toe.

Prominence of the internal malleoli with a prominent convex curve along the inner and inferior aspects of the arch.

Pain and tenderness beneath the navicular bone, the head of the astragalus, the sustentaculum tali, and the internal malleolus and along the plantar surface of the inner border of the foot and over the central portion of the plantar fascia.

Lengthening of the inner borders of the feet from separation of the os calcis and navicular bone, stretching of the spring ligament, and dropping of the head of the astragalus between these bones.

A downward and outward position of the Achilles tendon, instead of the normal directly downward position.

Swelling of the feet, especially anterior to the internal and external malleoli. List of the foot to the inner side; apparent medial displacement of the leg.

Marked wear of the soles of the shoes along the inner side. Weight is borne on the inner side of the foot.

Knock knee, as a possible early sign of flat foot.

In weak feet with peroneal spasm, limitation to adduction or turning in of the foot when the leg is extended. The flat foot is actually a valgus foot, that is abducted and everted.

Secondary Signs

Tenderness and callus formation under the first metatarsophalangeal joint and the inner side of the heel; callus formation beneath the prominent scaphoid bone, if marked relaxation of the longitudinal arch occurs; and an awkward gait.

Course and Sequelae

If not relieved, eversion and abduction leading to osseous, irreducible flat foot. When rigid flat foot has occurred, the gait has no spring, and patients use their lower extremities like pedestals.

Deformities secondary to flat feet including hallux valgus, hallux rigidus, and hammer toe.

Radiographic Findings

Roentgenographic examinations of the feet aiding in establishing an accurate diagnosis. Findings of importance in such films include:

Shortness of the first metatarsal bone; one should note the position of its head in comparison to the head of the second metatarsal bone.

Partial union of the astragalus bone and the os calcis, or other bony union.

Navicular-cuneiform sag.

Supernumerary bones, especially an accessory navicular bone.

Loss of cartilage and development of bony ridges and deformities in the intertarsal and metatarsophalangeal joints in most cases.

Table 79–4.   Exercises and Postural Aids for the Painful (Weak) Foot

Rationale and Principles

Exercise is important in the treatment of the weak foot. Exercises strengthen the lifting muscles on the medial border and transverse portion of the arch. Proper function of the foot muscles assists in maintaining the arch, so mechanical support is unnecessary. Exercises must not be instituted in the acute stages of foot strain because they may aggravate the condition.

Foot exercises aim to strengthen plantar flexors and adductor muscles and to stretch the dorsiflexors and pronator muscles. Plantar flexor muscles are strengthened by rising on the toes, whereas rolling onto the outer sides of the feet strengthens the supinator muscles.

Schedule

Foot exercises should be performed barefooted. Exercises are instituted gradually, are done slowly and regularly, and must not cause fatigue or pain. At the onset, 1 or 2 exercises may be performed 5 times once or twice a day. Exercises should be done first without weight bearing. As symptoms become less severe, sitting and standing exercises should be done. Later, the exercises are performed less frequently as normal strength returns.

Exercise Regimen
1. Spread and flex the toes sharply downward with the shoes off or on.
2. Stand on the toes with these turned inward, roll out on the sides, and return to a flat position.
3. Place about 12 small marbles on the floor. While sitting, pick up 1 marble at a time with the bare foot and place it in the opposite hand, that is, right foot to left hand and vice versa. Repeat several times a day using a dozen marbles each time with each foot. This exercise is particularly useful in children.
4. Walk on the outer borders of the bare feet along a straight line.
5. Stand with the toes pointing inward and attempt to externally rotate the knees without lifting the big toe from the floor.
6. While seated on the floor, bring one sole into contact with the other as much as possible.
7. Sit with feet pointing forward, curl all toes slowly, relax.
8. Sit squarely, roll feet outward until soles are almost parallel, relax.
9. Sitting cross-kneed, push foot downward, roll foot inward, and then pull foot upward to describe a circle with the foot.
10. For stretching a tight Achilles tendon, stand facing the wall, 2 feet away, and sway toward the wall with heels on the floor; do not bend the knees.

Table 79–5.   Treatment of the Early, Flaccid Flat (Weak) Foot

1. Prohibition of weight bearing if pain is present at rest.
2. Proper shoes, with heel and sole wedges, if indicated.
3. Temporary use of arch supports in some cases, especially in overweight patients and those required to stand or walk for long periods.
4. Correct posture in standing and walking.
5. Physical therapy and exercises for foot and leg muscles.
6. Foot baths, particularly contrast baths.
7. Reduction of weight if indicated.
8. Plaster boot worn at night, with ankle at right angle and foot in slight inversion if persistent muscular spasm exists.

sitioning of the foot in walking. The elevation of the arch support should extend from the anterior portion of the heel, the sustentaculum tali, to the head of the first metatarsal bone and laterally about three-quarters of the width of the foot. These elevations should extend only to the fifth metatarsal bone, and the height should conform, in both longitudinal and transverse arches, to the height of these regions when no weight is borne.

Proper Shoes

Well-fitting shoes of proper construction are necessary for walking under present-day conditions. To fit the shoes properly and to order modifications intelligently, one must know something about the various parts of a shoe (see Fig. 79–6).[19] The last of a shoe is a wooden model, similar to the shape of a foot, over which the shoe is built. Shoes with a combination last are made with several different combinations of widths, that is, at the heel, waist, tread measurements, and ball measurement. The heel is narrower than the ball of the foot. The toe box is the part covering the toes and may be either soft or firm. The vamp is the upper part of the shoe anterior to the laces. The quarter is the remainder of the upper behind the vamp. The waist is the portion of the upper immediately to the front of the heel. This part is often too tight in high-arched feet. The shank is a thin, supportive bar, usually made of steel, placed above the sole and running from the anterior third of the heel forward almost to the metatarsal heads.

A Thomas heel, often combined with a raise of the front runner corner of the heel, is a ½- to ¾-inch forward extension of the heel on the medial side (Fig. 79–10). This apparatus gives added support to the shank of the shoe and lessens fatigue in the region of the longitudinal arch.

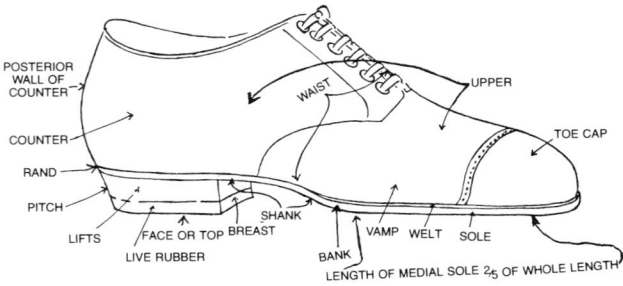

Fig. 79–6. External parts of a shoe. (From Ashley: Med. Rec.)

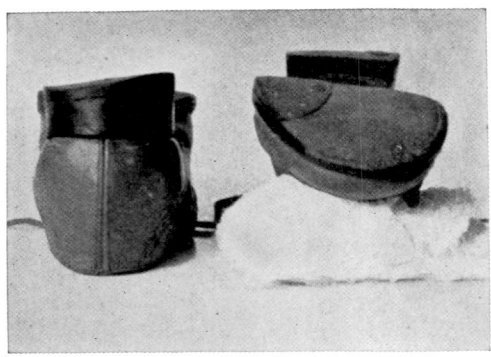

Fig. 79–7. Shoes corrected with cleats; inner wedge heel and outer patch over toes. (From Steindler, A.: J. Bone Joint Surg.)

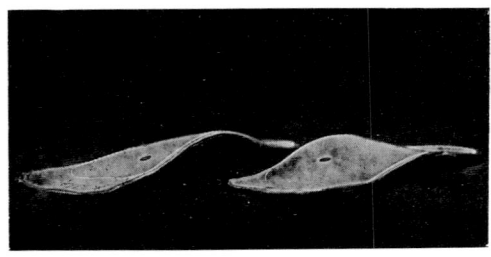

Fig. 79–8. Metal foot plates of the type sometimes used to support the arches. (From Kuhns, J.G.: Rheumatism.)

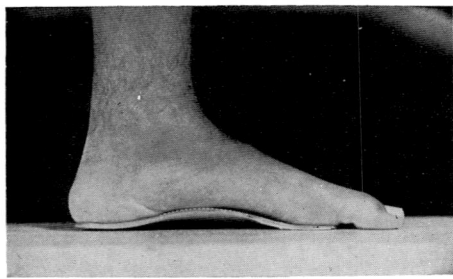

Fig. 79–9. Metal plate beneath the foot. (From Kuhns, J.G.: Rheumatism.)

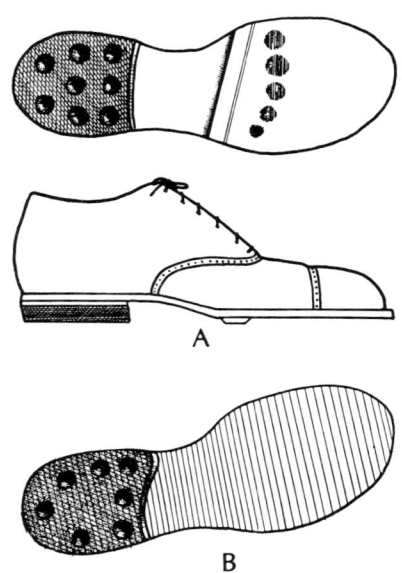

Fig. 79–10. *A,* Metatarsal bar. *B,* Thomas heel; note the forward extension of the heel along the inner margin. (From Shands, A.: Orthopedic Surgery. St. Louis, C.V. Mosby Co.)

A metatarsal bar is a strip of leather* fixed externally to the sole of the shoe transversely just behind the metatarsal heads (Fig. 79–10). It is usually ⅛ to ¼ inch thick and about ⅜ inch wide. To prevent tripping, the metatarsal bar may be placed between the outer and the inner sole. It is used chiefly in rigid depressions of the transverse arch associated with contracture of the extensor tendons and hammer toe deformity. It shifts the weight back to the bar from the metatarsal heads and usually affords comfort from severe anterior arch strain. The toe box can be made double the normal height, to provide relief from severe hammer toe deformities. A bunion pocket can be cre-

---

*Editor's note: These bars are now often man-made of the same material in a composition sole. They can be cemented to the sole or can be an integral part of the sole.

ated by stretching the upper medially to the appropriate degree.

Corrections should not be applied in pumps or high-heeled shoes. Corrections on shoes or firm corrective shoes are worn until symptoms subside and examination shows disappearance of the weakness or deformity.

Under certain conditions, molded shoes, which are made from a mold taken of the bottom of the foot during weight bearing, control symptoms in the painful flat foot. These shoes are expensive, but may be useful for severely deformed arthritic feet.

OTHER COMMON ABNORMALITIES

Deficiency of the First Metatarsal Segment

The main disturbance in disorders of the longitudinal arch and of the anterior portion of the foot is a functional deficiency of the first metatarsal segment, in which excessive load and strain are placed on the second metatarsal segment and its tarsal joints.

To treat this condition, one places a support of sufficient height under the head of the first metatarsal bone, to allow contact to be made by this metatarsal bone at the same time as by the others. Thus, the first metatarsal segment again carries its portion of the burden,[13] and it allows the second metatarsal segment to support only its normal share of body weight. For this purpose, a compensating insole can be fit into the shoe with a platform-like projection, just under the head of the first metatarsal bone. This insole may also be useful in cases of foot strain caused by a congenitally short first metatarsal bone. The height of the small platform thus placed can be determined only by trial; the "compensating insole" can be removed easily for adjustment of the height of this portion. In some patients, however, any support under the first metatarsal head causes midtarsal pain, throws weight to the outer aspect of the foot, and thereby irritates the fifth metatarsal bone.

Sprains of the Transverse Arch of the Foot

The transverse arch of the foot, the space proximal to the distal ends of the metatarsal bones, is frequently depressed and sprained. This condition often accompanies flat foot. The anterior arch acts as a shock absorber for the anterior part of the foot. Its integrity depends chiefly on the normal strength of the flexor muscles of the toes. This condition occurs most often in adults, especially in women who wear high-heeled, poorly fitted shoes. The usual symptoms are pain in the forefoot and toes, often with swelling about the metatarsophalangeal

joints. Tenderness and callus formation under the metatarsal heads are present. Hallux valgus and hammer toe deformity usually accompany sprain of the anterior arch of the foot.

Treatment includes the following: (1) removal of the painful callus under the metatarsal heads; (2) heat, particularly in the form of foot soaks, if the tissues are tender; (3) felt or sponge rubber metatarsal pads, $\frac{1}{4}$ to $\frac{1}{2}$ inch thick, as a temporary measure; (4) strapping of the anterior arch or an elastic or leather cuff around the foot behind the metatarsal heads; (5) a metatarsal bar; (6) properly fitted shoes; and (7) exercises to strengthen the flexor and extensor muscles of the toes and thus to aid the metatarsal arch.

Many individuals with tender second, third, and fourth metatarsal heads are relieved by a metatarsal bar, particularly in the presence of contracture of the extensor muscles of the toes.[8,18] A strip of leather approximately $\frac{3}{4}$ inch wide and $\frac{3}{16}$ inch thick, running across the outer sole from just proximal to the first metatarsal head to a point proximal to the fifth metatarsal head, is attached to the sole or inserted between the layers of the sole. Selective osteotomy of the depressed metatarsal head is sometimes necessary.

Hammer Toe

This condition, which may begin in childhood, is most common in the second toe. It consists of extension at the metatarsophalangeal joint with flexion at the proximal interphalangeal joint. This disorder is usually caused by pressure of a short, narrow shoe. Pain results from the development of a callus or corn on the top of the proximal joint. Therapy consists of the use of felt pads about or behind the affected joints in early, mild cases and surgical resection combined with fusion in more advanced cases. Occasionally, syndactyly of the adjoining toe is necessary.

Hallux Valgus

The great toe is abducted to lie on top of, or under, the other toes. Marked prominence of the first metatarsophalangeal joint occurs, with bony enlargement of the inner side of the first metatarsal head, over which a bursa may form. This bursa is commonly called a bunion (Fig. 79–11). Inflammation may occur in the bursa, occasionally with suppuration.[11]

Hallux valgus may be present without the formation of a bunion and without marked discomfort, even in the presence of marked deformity.[14] Short, narrow, pointed shoes are a common cause of this disorder. A congenital metatarsus varus may precede hallux valgus. It is often associated with a depressed metatarsal arch. In mild cases in which

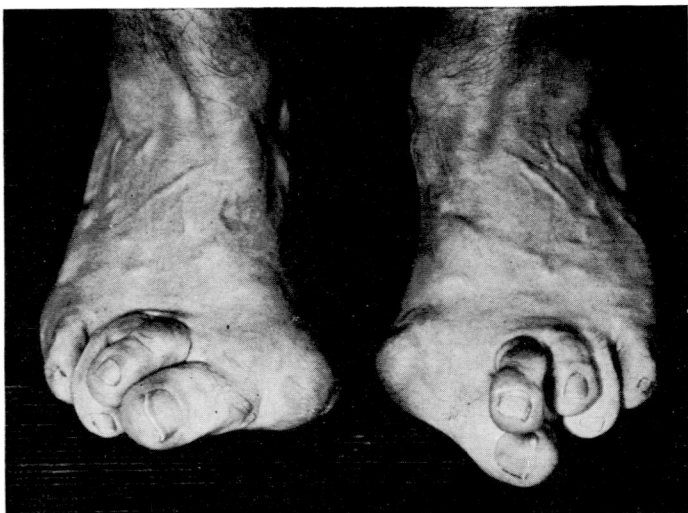

Fig. 79–11. Hallux valgus, with marked spread of the forefoot, exostosis, and bursa at first metatarsophalangeal joint.

discomfort is slight, relief may be obtained by the use of proper shoes and insertion of a pad between the first and second toes.

Severe deformity of hallux valgus and hallux rigidus can be corrected, usually by removal of the exostoses from the metatarsal head and by excision of a small portion of the proximal phalanx. Many surgical procedures exist for the correction of this deformity.

Hallux Rigidus

This disorder limits plantar flexion or dorsiflexion of the great toe and results from degenerative joint disease at the metatarsophalangeal joint (Fig. 79–12). Permanent subjective relief may be obtained in early cases by a properly made shoe with pads, supports, and a metatarsal bar. A stiff sole

or a long arch support may relieve symptoms. A shoe with a soft toe cap should be worn. Resection arthroplasty and insertion of Silastic implants may be beneficial and are the surgical treatments of choice (see Chap. 50).

Metatarsalgia and Morton's Neuroma

This condition may occur in the foot with a high longitudinal arch, the foot with a short Achilles tendon, the abducted foot, or the foot without evident pathologic change. It is often seen in persons with a depressed metatarsal arch. This disorder is characterized by the sudden onset of a severe crampy pain in the anterior portion of the foot forcing the patient to remove the shoe at once and to move and rub the toes until the pain is eased.

This disorder is often unilateral and affects

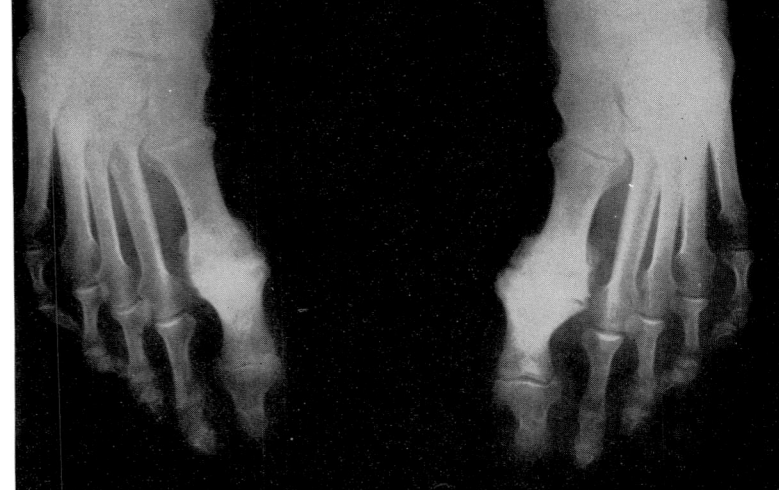

Fig. 79–12. Severe hallux rigidus, with osteoarthritis in the first metatarsophalangeal joint.

women more frequently than men.[1] It is due mainly to lateral compression of the forefoot that forces the head of the fifth metatarsal bone medially and posterior to the head of the fourth and thus causes pressure on the large superficial branch of the external plantar nerve, which lies between the heads of these two bones. This process results in a neuralgic pain. With prolonged irritation of the nerve, a neuroma may develop.[4]

Symptoms of this disorder include the following: (1) burning, numbness, tingling, or cramplike pain in the forepart of the foot, often under the fourth metatarsal head, when shoes are worn; (2) pain so intense as to require sudden removal of the shoes and rubbing of the foot to obtain relief; this pain is often relieved by squeezing the metatarsal bones together; soreness may persist at night and may keep the patient awake; in long-standing cases, a traumatic neuritis develops and causes pain whether or not the shoe is worn; (3) tenderness and numbness persisting for several days in the forepart of the foot or toes, especially about the head of the second, third, and fourth metatarsal bones; (4) pain radiating up the foot or leg or to the end of the toe; (5) in some cases, only an aching across the metatarsal arch; (6) painful callus under the metatarsal head;[12] and (7) sensory disturbance in the web between the fourth and fifth or third and fourth toes.

Treatment consists of the use of felt pads placed just proximal to the head of the fourth metatarsal bone and a metatarsal elastic strap to decrease splaying of the foot; if the pain persists, a metatarsal bar may be prescribed. In some patients, it may be necessary to inject 2 to 3 ml 1% procaine hydrochloride into the dorsum of the foot or to the painful area near the sole of the foot.

Morton's metatarsalgia is possibly caused by a tumor involving the most lateral branch of the medial plantar nerve; these tumors are neurofibromas or angioneurofibromas. The tumor should be excised if symptoms become severe.[17]

Achillodynia

This disorder is due to inflammation of the bursa between the os calcis and the point of attachment of the Achilles tendon. Symptoms include localized pain and swelling, especially during walking. Treatment consists mainly of rest, removal of pressure from shoes, and application of heat to the bursa. It may be necessary to inject the part with procaine for relief. A felt or sponge rubber pad under the heel affords some relief. Surgical removal of the bursa or rheumatoid nodules within it may be indicated.[6]

Painful Heel

This problem may be caused by traumatic rupture of the Achilles tendon, inflammation of the retrocalcaneal bursa, exostoses, degenerative joint disease, strain on the attachment of the plantar fascia, inflammation of a bursa between the Achilles tendon and the skin, or degeneration of the calcaneal fat pad.

Pain on the sole at the center of the heel on walking may be due to an exostosis, an inflamed bursa, or trauma to the tissues in this area. Relief may be obtained by injections of 1 to 3 ml 1% procaine into the painful region and insertion into the heel of the shoe of a soft rubber doughnut, that is, a piece of rubber approximately ¼ inch thick with an area about 1½ inches in diameter cut out in its center portion of the heel and padding around the edge of the heel. Use of a broad-jumper's heel cup, obtainable at a sporting goods store, is also an effective way to treat a painful heel.

Bony Spurs

Bony spurs occur on the anterior plantar surface of the os calcis or on the dorsal surface of the foot. Many of these result from chronic strain at points of ligamentous attachments. Relief of strain and procaine infiltration usually cause symptoms to disappear. Surgical treatment is rarely necessary.

Miscellaneous Causes of Painful Feet

In many patients, painful feet are not the result of static disturbances. The largest group comprises those with traumatic lesions, such as contusions,

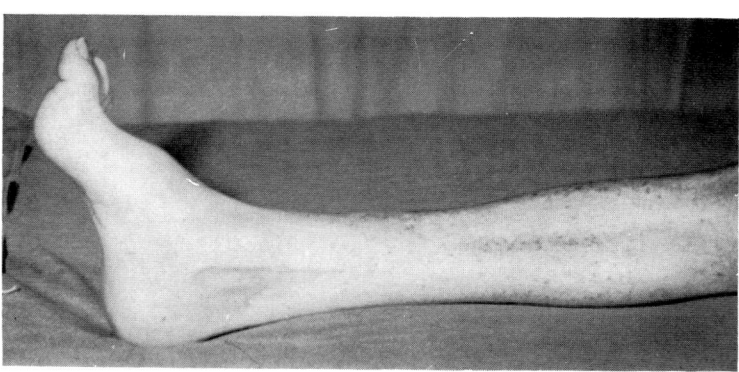

Fig. 79–13. Cavus of the foot with contracture of the plantar fascia. The dorsal portion of the midfoot is prominent. The toes are held in extension.

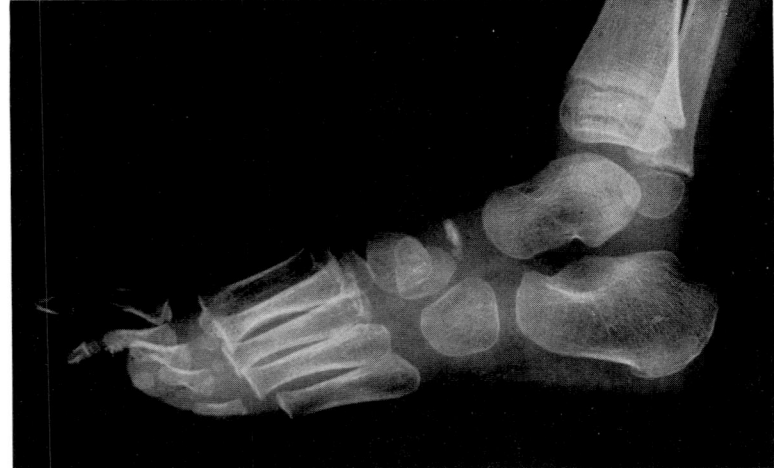

Fig. 79–14. Köhler's disease. Note the thin, dense tarsal navicular bone.

sprains, and fractures, in which a definite history of injury to the foot is usually present. Other articulations are not involved, and these lesions usually respond promptly to treatment. Inflammatory lesions include infections of the bones or soft tissue, various forms of articular inflammation, and inflammation of the skin. Congenital deformities, the most common of which are clubfoot, deformities of the toes, metatarsus primus varus, and cavus deformity (Fig. 79–13), can usually be diagnosed by their characteristic appearance and a history of their presence since infancy. All these conditions become progressively worse if untreated. The great majority of them are corrected in early childhood.

Disturbances in the venous return of blood are observed in many patients with arthritic deformities of the legs. Stasis dermatitis, eczema, and finally, ulceration of the skin occur usually over the lower leg and dorsum of the foot. An elastic stocking may be necessary. Correction of flexion deformities improves the circulation. If ulceration has occurred, elevation of the foot, an Unna paste boot, sterile wet dressings, or skin grafting may be required.

Brief mention should be made of disturbances of growth, particularly epiphyseal disturbances, which may be precursors of arthritic disabilities in the feet. Growth disturbances of the tarsal navicular bone, called Köhler's disease (Fig. 79–14), osteochondritis of the second metatarsal bone, called Freiberg's disease, and involvement of the epiphysis of the os calcis are common. Temporary protection of these areas is usually all that is necessary, but deformity sometimes occurs anyway.

REFERENCES

1. Brattstrom, H., and Brattstrom, M.: Resection of metatarsophalangeal joint in rheumatoid arthritis. Acta Orthop. Scand., *41*:213–223, 1970.
2. Calabro, J.J.: A critical evaluation of the digits of the feet in rheumatoid arthritis. Arthritis Rheum., *5*:19–29, 1962.
3. Carlsoo, S., and Wetzenstein, H.: Change of form of the foot and the foot skeleton upon momentary weight-bearing. Acta Orthop. Scand., *39*:413–423, 1968.
4. Duthie, J.J.: Arthritis of the hands and feet. Practitioner, *186*:729–736, 1961.
5. DuVries, H.: Surgery of the Foot. St. Louis, C.V. Mosby, 1973.
6. Gerster, J.C.: Plantar fasciitis and achilles tendinitis among 150 cases of seronegative spondarthritis. Rheumatol. Rehabil., *19*:218–222, 1980.
7. Giannestras, N.J.: Foot disorders: Medical and Surgical Management. Philadelphia, Lea & Febiger, 1967.
8. Harty, M.: Metatarsalgia. Surg. Gynecol. Obstet., *136*:105–106, 1973.
9. Jahss, M.H.: Unusual diagnostic problems of the foot. Clin. Orthop. Rel. Res., *85*:42–49, 1972.
10. Kelikian, H.: Hallux Valgus, Allied Disorders of the Forefoot and Metatarsalgia. Philadelphia, W.B. Saunders, 1965.
11. Kirkup, J.R.: The hallux and rheumatoid arthritis. Acta Orthop. Scand., *48*:527–544, 1977.
12. Mann, R.A., and DuVries, H.L.: Intractable plantar keratosis. Orthop. Clin. North Am., *4*:67–73, 1973.
13. Montgomery, R.M.: Painful feet—modern ways to manage old problems. N.Y. State J. Med., 1301–1305, 1969.
14. Rose, G.K.: Correction of the pronated foot. J. Bone Joint Surg., *44B*:647, 1962.
15. Stewart, S.F.: Footgear—its history, uses and abuses. Clin. Orthop. Rel. Res., *88*:119–130, 1972.
16. Stott, J.R.R., Hutton, W.C., and Stokes, I.A.F.: Forces under the foot. J. Bone Joint Surg., *55B*:335–344, 1973.
17. Thompson, T.C.: Surgical treatment of disorders of the forefoot. J. Bone Joint Surg., *46A*:1117–1128, 1964.
18. Viladot, A.: Metatarsalgia due to biomechanical alterations of the forefoot. Clin. Orthop. North Am., *4*:165–178, 1973.
19. Wickstrom, J.: Shoe corrections and orthopaedic foot supports. Clin. Orthop. Rel. Res., *70*:30–42, 1970.

Chapter 80

Syndrome of Cervical Nerve Root Compression

Ruth Jackson

The syndrome of cervical nerve root compression includes a group of symptoms and clinical findings resulting from compression or irritation of the nerve roots before the nerve trunks, formed by the coalition of sensory and motor fibers, divide into anterior and posterior primary rami, as well as compression of the accompanying vascular and sympathetic structures.

ANATOMIC CHARACTERISTICS

A knowledge of the anatomic features of the spine is imperative for adequate interpretation and treatment of the cervical spinal disorders that contribute to symptoms and signs of irritation or compression of the nerve roots and their accompanying structures.

Bones and Joints

The cervical spine, the most mobile part of the spinal column, is placed vulnerably between the less-mobile thoracic spine and the 8- to 12-lb head that must be balanced on it and held in place by the supporting ligamentous, capsular, muscular, and fibrocartilaginous structures. The cervical spine is composed of 7 vertebrae, 34 joints, and 94 muscles, all of which contribute to its great mobility. The slight flexibility of the intervertebral discs, the shape and inclination of the apophyseal joints and their incomplete apposition, the lateral interbody joints, the laxity of the capsules, and the inherent elasticity and tensile properties of the ligaments contribute to the functional capacity of this structure.

The special architectural design of the atlas and axis permits nodding, rotation, and lateral bending. The head and atlas move as one unit on the axis. The shape of the atlantooccipital articulations and the laxity of their capsules permit free nodding movements, backward more than forward, but minimal side-to-side motion and no rotary motion.

As the head and atlas rotate on the axis, the inferior facets of the atlas slip forward and backward over the superior facets on the lateral masses of the axis; however, in radiographs made with the head rotated, the lateral masses of the atlas main-

tain a contant relationship to the odontoid process of the axis, provided all the ligaments are intact and functioning.

Motion in the other cervical joints consists of flexion, hyperextension, lateral bending, and rotation. The plane of the articular surfaces prevents lateral bending without some degree of rotation and rotation without some degree of lateral bending. Any undue laxity of the joint structures allows subluxations of the joints or an abnormal range of motion between the articular surfaces (Fig. 80–1).

The apophyseal joints and the fibrocartilaginous disc joints are characteristic of all areas of the spine inferior to the atlantoaxial articulations. The cervical spine, in addition, has two lateral interbody joints. These small articulations are formed by the superior posterolateral projections on the superior surfaces of the vertebral bodies and the adjacent beveled surfaces on the inferior portion of the vertebral bodies from C2 to C7 (Fig. 80–2).

Luschka described these joints between the bodies of the cervical vertebrae in 1858, and they are often called the joints of Luschka.[12] Trolard called them *articulations uncovertébrales* in 1892.[21] These terms are used interchangeably. I prefer to call these small articulations the lateral interbody joints, a correct anatomic description that avoids confusion. Many controversies have arisen concerning these joints, but these have no foundation when one recalls that these joints develop from the primary centers of ossification of the neural arches, as do the transverse processes, and not from the ossification center of the centrum.[11] These joints are cartilaginous until they become ossified at the age of six or seven years, as revealed by radiographs.

The lateral interbody joints are significant because their presence prevents the exposure of the intervertebral discs at the posterolateral margins of the vertebral bodies. Moreover, these joints and the adjacent surfaces of the bodies of the vertebrae form the anterior walls of the intervertebral canals through which the cervical nerve roots and their accompanying structures pass. Some motion in all planes occurs in these joints. Their capsular liga-

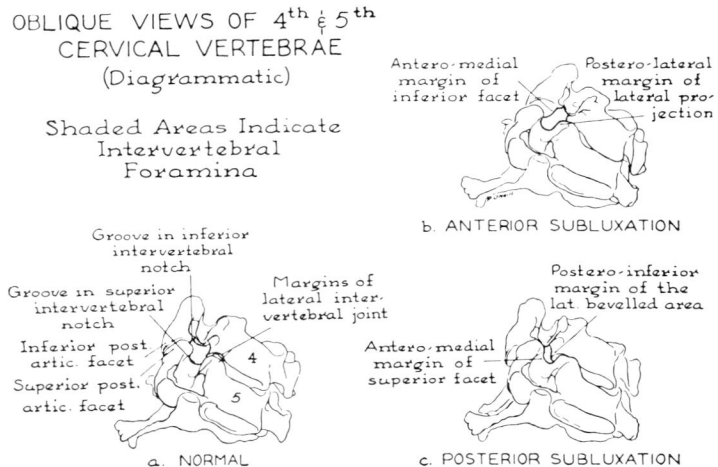

Fig. 80–1. A normal intervertebral canal and its boundaries *(a)*. Foraminal changes from subluxations of the cervical vertebrae *(b and c)*, resulting from ligamentous injury or instability. (From Jackson.[8])

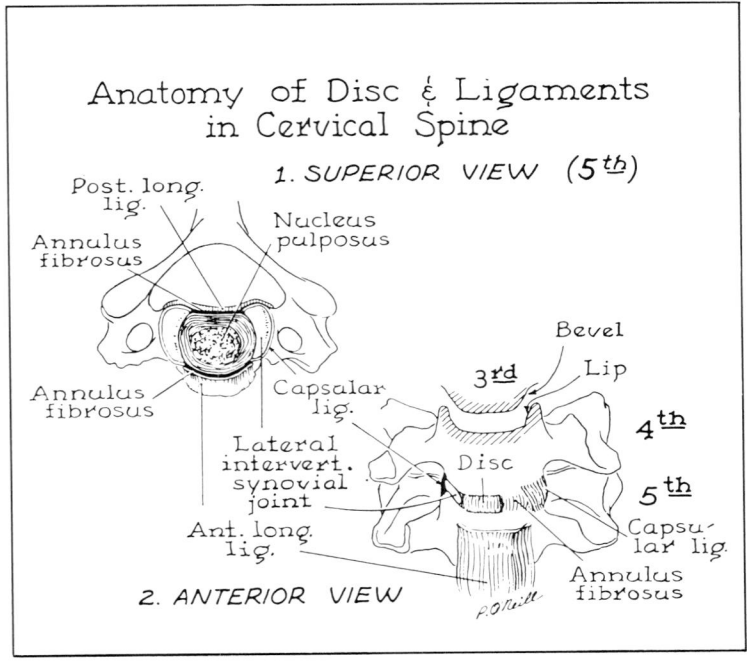

Fig. 80–2. The lateral interbody joints and their relation to the cervical discs. (From Jackson.[8]).

ments are short and taut, and they are therefore vulnerable to sprains. The greatest amount of arthrosis or osteoarthritic change occurs at the margins of these joints. The close proximity of the cervical nerve roots and their accompanying vascular and sympathetic structures makes them susceptible to irritation or compression from any derangement in or about these joints. The lateral interbody joints prevent the extrusion of disc material posterolaterally, the favorite site of extrusion in other areas of the spine. If the seventh and the sixth vertebrae do not have well developed superior

posterolateral projections, disc material may be extruded posterolaterally.[8]

The bodies of the cervical vertebrae are flat posteriorly, and their anterior surfaces are curved, with the inferior margins jutting inferiorly. Their posterior vertical diameters are greater than their anterior vertical diameters, but the vertical diameter of the posterior portion of the intervertebral discs is 5 to 10 mm less than the anterior diameter; this characteristic ensures the normal forward curve of the cervical spine.[8]

The intervertebral foramina from C2 to C3 to

C6 to C7 are bony canals that are ovoid in shape and have greater vertical than anteroposterior diameters. They decrease inferiorly in overall size. The grooves in the vertebral arches form the roofs and floors of the canals. The apophyseal joints form the posterior walls, and the lateral interbody joints form the anterior walls[8] (see Figs. 80–1, 80–2).

Nerves

The nerve roots, the spinal branches of the vertebral arteries, and the spinal meningeal nerves lie on the floor of the intervertebral canals and fill their anteroposterior diameter. The superior one-eighth to one-fourth of the canals is filled with areolar and fatty tissues and with small veins.

The ventral and dorsal nerve roots arise from the corresponding surfaces of the spinal cord on a level with the vertebral bodies. Small intervals, on a level with the intervertebral discs, exist between the origin of the nerve root fibers from the spinal cord, to prevent the nerve root fibers from crossing the intervertebral discs, as they do in other areas of the spine (see Fig. 80–6). As the nerve root fibers leave the spinal canal, they carry with them a dural covering from the dura spinalis, and they enter the intervertebral canals immediately, where they join to form the nerve trunks. These fibers are, therefore, well protected from posterior extrusion of disc material, but they are vulnerable to any derangement within the intervertebral canals.[8]

The nerve roots lack a perineural sheath, and the nerve fibers are more exposed than those of peripheral nerves. Because some fibers are better protected than others, all nerve root fibers do not suffer the same amount of compressive forces. The arteries of the nerve roots may be blocked by compression within the intervertebral canals, to cause ischemia.[18]

The autonomic nervous system, an integral part of the central nervous system, is linked to it by afferent and efferent fiber systems. It is divided topographically into the sympathetic and parasympathetic systems. The parasympathetic system is connected with the central nervous system in the cervical area through the oculomotor, facial, glossopharyngeal and vagus nerves and through the cranial nerve roots of the spinal accessory nerves.[11] The sympathetic system in the cervical area originates in the mediolateral gray matter at the base of the anterior horns of the spinal cord, as shown by Laurelle.[10]

The fibers of both nervous systems run side by side to the same structures, in which normally a harmonious, although antagonistic, interaction occurs. Their reactions depend on substances liberated at their ganglia or at their endings. The sympathetic fibers, which release a substance similar to epinephrine, are known as adrenergic fibers. The parasympathetic fibers release acetylcholine and are called cholinergic fibers.[11]

Laurelle has demonstrated the presence of sympathetic cell bodies in the cervical portion of the spinal cord in the mediolateral gray matter at the base of the anterior horns from C4 through C8. The preganglionic sympathetic fibers leave the spinal cord with the somatic motor nerve fibers in the ventral roots of C5 through T1.[10] One part of the preganglionic neurons forms a synaptic connection with the postganglionic neurons in the small ganglia of a deep sympathetic chain. This connection has been described by Delmas and his associates.[5] The other preganglionic neurons traverse the deep chain of small sympathetic ganglia situated in the transverse canals and join the vertebral nerve that is formed by the afferent branches. The deep chain consists of a tangled web of sympathetic fibers and of macroscopically visible ganglia. It ascends along the posterior aspect of the vertebral artery from C7 to C4 and is the continuation in the neck of the thoracolumbar ganglionated nerve trunk.[5]

The sympathetic nerve trunk in the cervical area is composed of the superior, middle, and inferior ganglia, connected by intervening cords. The efferent branches proceed to the viscera of the neck and chest, and the afferent branches, as stated, form the vertebral nerve. Communicating rami connect the superior ganglion with the ninth, tenth, and twelfth cranial nerves. Gray rami communicantes join the anterior rami of the superior four cervical nerves. The internal carotid nerve passes superiorly with the internal carotid artery and forms a plexus about the artery. Pharyngeal branches communicate with the superior laryngeal nerve and join the pharyngeal plexus. The external carotid nerve forms a plexus around the external carotid artery. On the left side, cardiac branches follow the carotid artery into the thorax, and on the right side, branches follow the trachea and end in the deep cardiac plexus.[11]

From the middle ganglion, postganglionic fibers are given to the inferior thyroid artery and the thyroid gland. A cardiac branch ends in the cardiac plexus, and another branch, the ansa subclavia, descends to the subclavian artery and then ascends to join the inferior ganglion.

The inferior ganglion sends fine filaments to the subclavian plexus and larger filaments to the vertebral artery, to form the vertebral plexus. A cardiac branch reaches the deep cardiac plexus.[11]

According to Tinel, the fifth cervical nerve root carries sympathetic fibers, which join the carotid plexus to give sympathetic innervation to the arteries of the head and neck.[19] The sixth nerve root carries sympathetic fibers to the subclavian artery and the brachial plexus. From the seventh nerve root, fibers reach the cardioaortic plexus and the subclavian and axillary arteries, as well as the phrenic nerve.

Other postganglionic fibers communicate with the recurrent spinal meningeal nerves. Fibers that invest the internal carotid arteries give branches to the back of the orbit, the dilator muscle of the pupil, and the smooth muscle of the upper eyelid. Some of the branches that surround the vertebral arteries supply the vestibular portion of the auditory complex.[11]

Pain-conducting, afferent spinal nerve fibers from the blood vessels of the head, neck, and upper extremities traverse the sympathetic trunk and communicating rami.[11]

With these characteristics in mind, it is easy to understand that stimulation of the sympathetic fibers gives rise to symptoms and clinical findings that may confuse the picture of cervical nerve root compression. Stimulation of the cervical sympathetic nerve fibers may result in vasoconstriction and aggravation of pain caused by irritation of the cervical nerve roots. Interruption or paralysis of the sympathetic fibers may relieve pain either by paralyzing the afferent pain-conducting spinal nerve fibers that traverse the sympathetic trunk and the communicating rami or by relieving vasoconstriction.

Other Structures

The dural covering of the spinal cord is firmly fixed to the margins of the foramen magnum, to the second and third cervical vertebrae, and to the periosteum of the coccyx. It is separated from the walls of the vertebral canal by the cavum epidurale, which is filled with soft fat and a plexus of thin-walled veins. The spinal dura is, therefore, free within the spinal canal, and its attachments do not interfere with the free movement of the vertebral column. As the spinal nerve roots pierce the dura, they carry with them a tubular covering of the dura spinalis (Fig. 80–3). Injuries or inflammatory reactions of the dural sleeves of the nerve roots may cause adhesions to form between the sleeves and the adjacent capsular ligaments. In dissecting anatomic specimens, I have found this to be true, and the spinal dura may be bound completely to the posterior longitudinal ligament at definite areas of localized pathologic changes.[8]

The relationship of the vertebral arteries and their branches to the spinal nerves and the bony structures is important. These arteries and their surrounding plexuses of sympathetic fibers may be injured by subluxation of the vertebrae or by changes in the anterior portions of the lateral in-

terbody joints and in the intertransverse muscles. Angiographic studies have shown obliteration of these arteries by changes in position of the head and neck.[17] Actual constrictions of these arteries may occur, especially at the level of the upper two cervical vertebrae.[8]

The posterior longitudinal ligament in the cervical area is composed of two distinct layers, in contradistinction to its structure inferior to this area. The superficial layer, which is absent inferior to the cervical area, is a strong ligamentous structure that extends vertically inferiorly from the skull, dorsal to the deep layer. It extends laterally to the intervertebral foramina (Fig. 80–4), and it adheres to the deep layer and to the capsules of the lateral interbody joints. The deep layer has the denticulated appearance of the posterior ligament distal to the cervical area. Some of the fibers of the capsular ligaments of the lateral interbody joints originate in the deep layer, as well as in the adjacent bone of the vertebral bodies. This strong ligament acts as a barrier to extrusion of disc material in the midline posteriorly, although disc extrusion can occur here, depending on the severity of an injury and the integrity of the ligament.[8]

The greatest amount of stress and strain in the cervical spine occurs at the level of the fourth and fifth cervical vertebrae when the neck is in hyperextension and at the level of the fifth and sixth cervical vertebrae when the neck is in hyperflexion. Limitation of motion from muscle spasm or arthrosis alters the points of greatest stress and strain, depending on the degree and level of arthrosis. Thus, the greatest amount of degenerative change in the intervertebral discs and in the lateral interbody joints occurs at these levels, but such changes may take place at any level.[8]

CAUSATIVE FACTORS

The cervical spine, because of its position, structure, and great mobility, is much more vulnerable to injury than any other portion of the spine and hence is more vulnerable to the changes initiated by trauma, as well as by unusual stresses and strains.

SPRAIN INJURIES

Approximately 90% of all cervical nerve root irritation is the result, either directly or indirectly, of sprain injuries of the ligamentous and capsular structures of the cervical spine. Sprain injuries of these structures permits vertebral subluxations. Anteroposterior narrowing of the intervertebral canals results in immediate or delayed irritation or compression of the cervical nerve roots. Sixty percent of these injuries give rise to some immediate

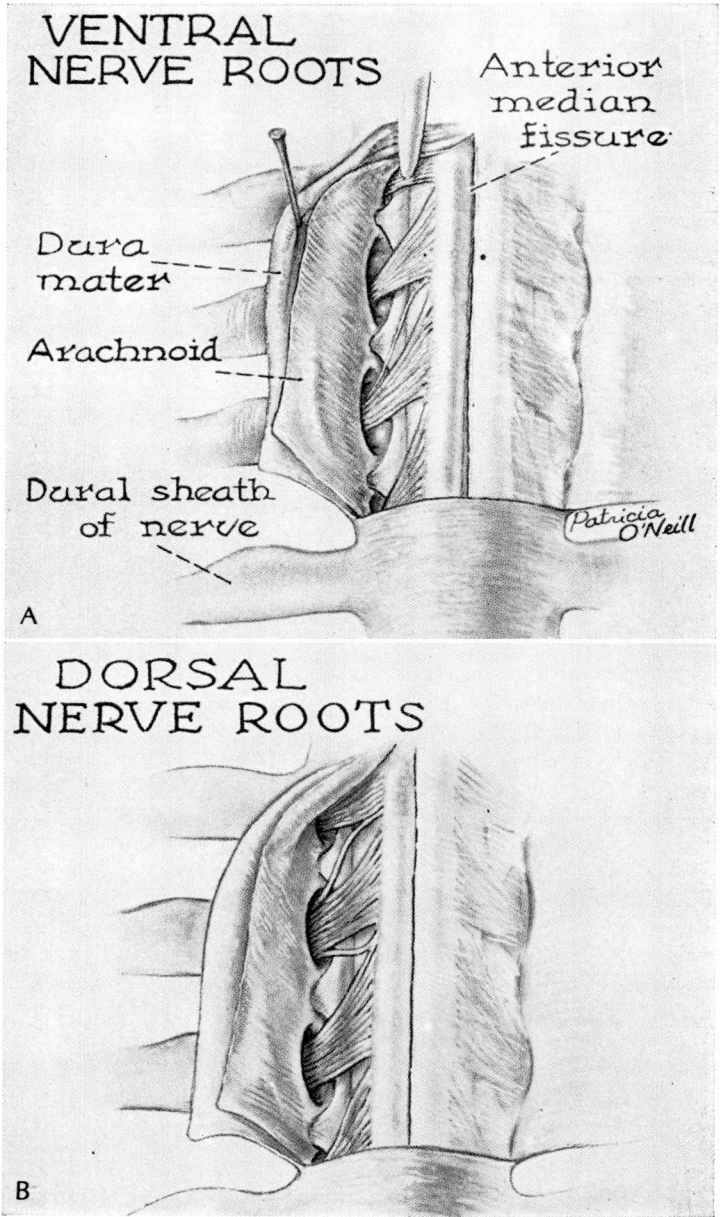

Fig. 80–3.   The origin of the ventral *(A)* and dorsal *(B)* nerve roots from the spinal cord and their exit through the dura spinalis. (From Jackson, R.[8])

symptoms, whereas the other 40% produce symptoms days, weeks, or months later.

Symptoms that occur immediately or within a few hours following injury may be due to actual compression of the nerve roots within their bony canals as the joints are subluxated, or they may be due to swelling and hemorrhage of the adjacent capsular ligaments or to injury of the vascular and sympathetic structures.

Delayed symptoms are the result of foraminal narrowing initiated by the original trauma and by repeated stress and strain of continued movement of the joints. The ligamentous and capsular structures become hypertrophied and lose their normal elasticity. Such foraminal encroachment may cause gradual compression of the nerve roots and fibrosis. Eventually, osteophytic formations, or spurs, develop at the margins of the lateral interbody and/or

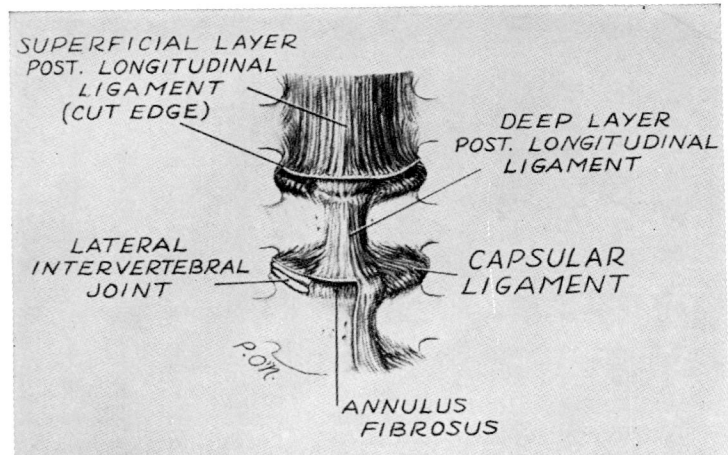

Fig. 80–4. The two-layered posterior longitudinal ligament and the capsular ligaments of the lateral interbody joints. (From Jackson, R.[8])

apophyseal joints. Inasmuch as these changes are gradual, the nerve roots may adjust to, or may tolerate, their narrowed canals, until some apparently trivial incident sets off a response manifested by pain and functional impairment.[8]

Vehicular crash accidents are responsible for the greatest percentage of neck injuries. The "whiplash" mechanism, which may be described as any sudden forceful movement of the neck in any direction with a recoil in the opposite direction, accounts for 80 to 90% of these sprain injuries (Fig. 80–5). The lashing effect is greatest when the muscles are caught off guard, as occurs frequently in rear-end, side, and head-on collisions. The element of torque that is often present adds to the injuries. Sprain injuries also occur from strenuous sports, from falls, from sudden forceful pulls on the arms, from sudden thrusting forces against the arms, and from blows to the head or chin.[8]

A diagnosis of "cervical disc" is made frequently following sprain injuries with nerve root involvement. This term implies pressure on a nerve root from posterolateral disc extrusion; however, the nerve roots are protected by the lateral interbody joints, and the nerve root fibers are protected by safety zones, the vertebral bodies (Fig. 80–6). Disc extrusion occurring posteriorly in the cervical spine causes pressure on the spinal cord itself. Some of the upper or lower fibers of the ventral portion of the nerve roots may suffer compression if the disc material is large or if it is forced superiorly or inferiorly in the spinal canal. The cervical discs do not extend to the posterolateral margins of the vertebral bodies because of the presence of the lateral interbody joints (see Fig. 80–2). Thickening of the capsular ligaments and osteo-

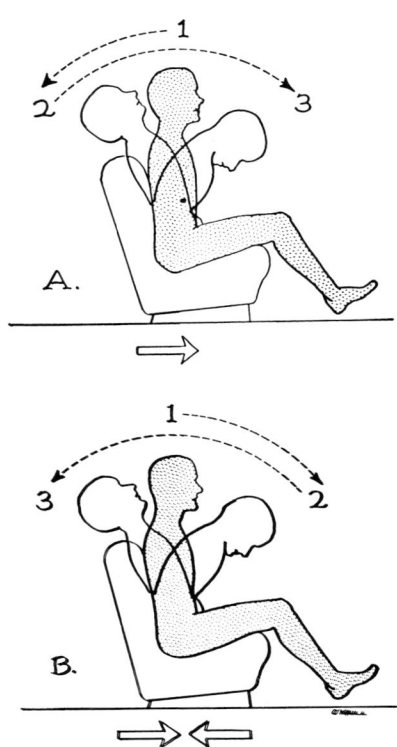

Fig. 80–5. The "whiplash" mechanism. Rear-end collision *(A)* and head-on collision *(B)*. (From Jackson, R.[8])

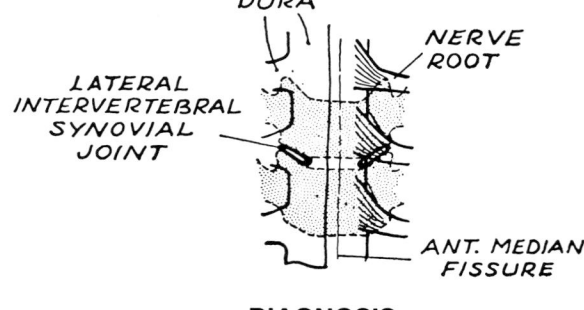

Fig. 80–6. The "safety zone" for the cervical nerve roots, which is the corresponding vertebral body. The nerve roots do not pass over the intervertebral discs. (From Jackson, R.[8])

phytic formations at the margins of a lateral interbody joint give the appearance of a bulging disc ventral to the nerve root. This condition is the so-called "hard disc," which is removed frequently by surgical measures. The projecting spurs are lined on their adjacent surfaces by cartilage, but this cartilage has neither the microscopic nor the macroscopic characteristics of disc cartilage.[8]

Sprain injuries damage the cervical discs and cause disc degeneration and narrowing, which impose greater stress on the lateral interbody joints. Osteoarthrosis and chondromalacia occur as motion is continued. Osteophytic formations may develop at the anterior margins of the vertebral bodies at the attachments of the anterior longitudinal ligament. These formations may bridge the vertebral bodies. This bridging, however, is unlike the ossification of the joints and ligaments seen in ankylosing spondylitis (Fig. 80–7). In ankylosing spondylitis, foraminal narrowing does not usually occur, except by swelling of the adjacent capsular and ligamentous structures from inflammation.

Other Causes

Arthritis, fractures of the articular processes, of the vertebral arches, and of the vertebral bodies, and developmental anomalies produce symptoms of cervical nerve root irritation in approximately 10% of cases. Other conditions that may aggravate symptoms and clinical findings associated with irritation of the cervical nerve roots include emotional tension, fatigue, poor posture, unusual activities, and weather changes.

In general, foraminal narrowing from mechanical derangements and from inflammatory changes may irritate the cervical nerve roots. The degree of mechanical derangement, as evidenced by radiographic studies, indicates neither the severity of the symptoms, nor the extent of the clinical findings. The problem is made more complex by virtue of the involvement of the sympathetic nerve supply, as well as by the associated injury or involvement of the vertebral arteries and their branches.[8]

DIAGNOSIS

Diagnosis is based on an adequate and detailed medical history, on a meticulous physical examination, and on adequate radiographic studies.

Medical History

What are the patient's symptoms, when did they first occur, are they constant or intermittent, has the patient had recent or past trauma, what aggravates and what relieves the symptoms, what treatment has the patient undergone, and what medications is the patient taking? Moreover, it is important to obtain a detailed past medical history, including injuries, surgical procedures, serious illnesses, and marital and family histories.

Physical Examination

Motion of the neck should be determined first. The normal range of active motion is shown in Figure 80–8. Head compression and shoulder depression tests should then be done. One must palpate the neck muscles, which are often in spasm. Then, the apophyseal joints, the spinous processes, and the shoulder, back, and arm muscles are palpated for tender areas and muscle spasm. Muscle spasm with localized deep tenderness means cervical nerve root irritation. Shoulder, elbow, and wrist motion are then determined. The radial pulses are felt with the patient's arms elevated. Spasm of the scalene muscles or a cervical rib may obliterate the pulse when the patient's arm is elevated above the head.

The shoulders and upper extremities should be examined for decreased sensory changes, and the reflexes should be tested, remembering that sensory distribution overlaps. Reflexes may be normal, absent, or decreased, and they may vary from time to time, depending on the extent of the irritation of the motor fibers of the nerve roots. The circumference of the patient's arms and forearms should be measured, and the grip in each hand should be checked with a dynamometer.

The pupils should be examined. Dilatation of one pupil indicates involvement of the sympathetic nerve supply through the branches of the internal carotid artery that supply the pupillary muscle.

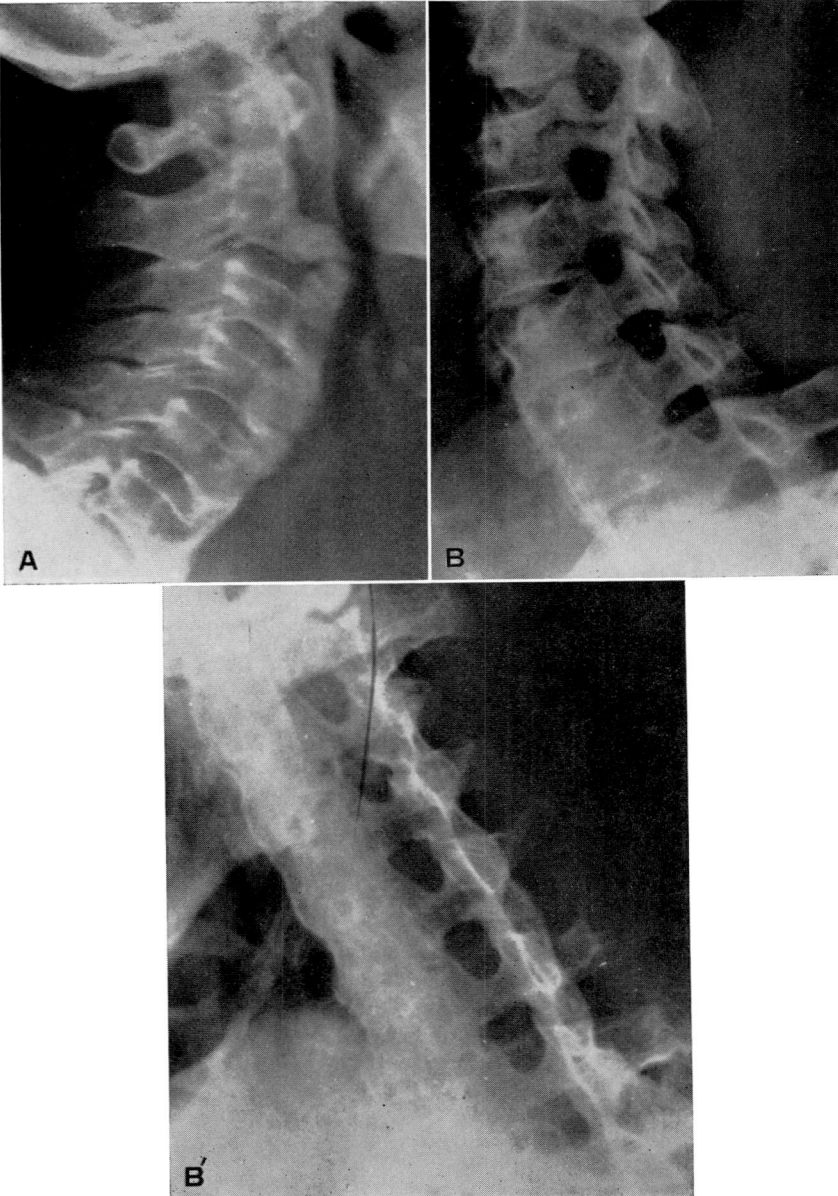

Fig. 80–7.   Ankylosing spondylitis involving the anterior portion of the vertebral bodies *(A)*, the anterior longitudinal ligament *(B)*, and the joints *(B')*. Note the lack of foraminal narrowing in *B* and *B'*. (From Jackson, R.[8])

If the patient complains of loss of balance, tinnitus, or light-headedness, electronystagmography may be necessary, provided conservative treatment does not give relief.[16] This test differentiates between peripheral and central nervous causes. Symptoms referable to the ear are usually the result of irritation of the autonomic supply of the vertebral artery that may cause vasospasm, vasodilation, and edema of the labyrinth of the inner ear.

The blood pressure in both arms should be de-termined. One may find a variance of 10 to 20 mm Hg. Involvement of the cervical sympathetic nerves or the presence of muscle spasm in one arm may account for such variation.[8] Auscultation for a bruit in the arteries of the neck should be done, especially if the patient complains of vertigo and blurred vision.

Radiographic Findings

Adequate studies should be made in all cases. Correct interpretation is impossible unless the clin-

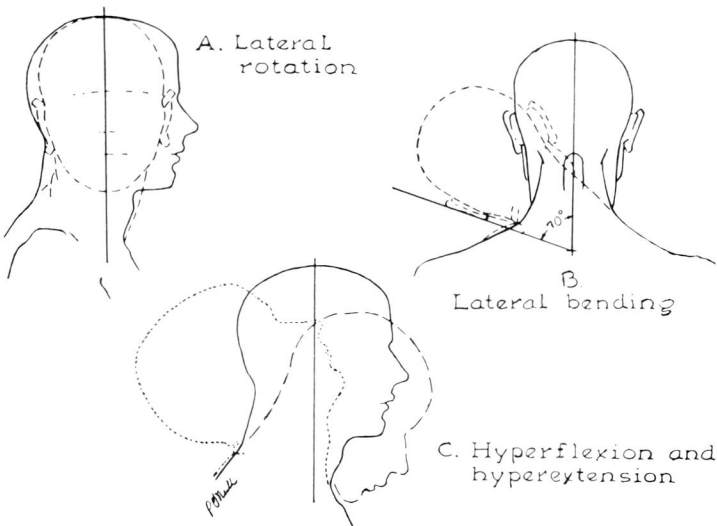

A. Lateral rotation

B. Lateral bending

C. Hyperflexion and hyperextension

Fig. 80–8. The range of normal neck motion. The head can be rotated so the chin is parallel with the shoulder *(A)*. It can be bent laterally 70 to 80° *(B)*. It can be flexed so the chin rests on the superior portion of the sternum, and it can be extended so the occiput touches the spinous process of the first thoracic vertebra *(C)*. (From Jackson, R.[8])

ical findings are correlated. Minimal changes may give rise to severe symptoms, and marked changes may be associated with minimal symptoms and clinical findings.

If the patient is seen in a hospital emergency room, a cross-table lateral film should be made first, and an anteroposterior view should be obtained to rule out any gross fracture or dislocation.

The following radiographic views should be obtained: (1) an anteroposterior view of the upper 2 cervical vertebrae; (2) an anteroposterior view of the lower 5 vertebrae, made with the x-ray tube angled cephalad 15 to 25°; (3) an anteroposterior caudad-angled view with the x-ray tube angled 30 to 35° toward the feet, as described by Abel;[1] (4) a lateral view with the patient sitting upright, looking straight ahead, and holding a sandbag in each hand to pull the shoulders inferiorly to bring the C7 to T1 vertebrae into view; (5) a similar lateral view made with the head flexed forward as far as possible; (6) a third lateral view with the neck in hyperextension; and (7) left and right oblique views made with the patient sitting upright and turned at a 45° angle away from the film and toward the x-ray tube. As suggested by Abel, it may be important to make 2 caudad-angled views with the neck in right and left lateral bending positions, to localize capsular disruption or instability. These positions are called "pillar" views.[1] The anteroposterior view of the upper 2 cervical vertebrae may reveal fractures, subluxations, rotational deformities, and congenital anomalies.

The anteroposterior view of the lower cervical vertebrae shows the superior posterolateral projections of the vertebral bodies and widening or narrowing of the lateral interbody joint spaces, osteophytic formations at their margins, and compression of or absence of the posterolateral projections of the bodies, usually at C6–7 and C5–6 (see Fig. 80–10). Even a narrowed intervertebral disc, or discs, can be seen, as well as rotation of one or more vertebral bodies.

The caudad-angled view showing the posterior elements is important, although seldom obtained. It shows narrowing of an interarticular isthmus and fractures of the laminae and of the apophyseal joints, if present.

The straight lateral view shows a loss of the normal forward curve in approximately 90% of the cases, with a reversal of the curve in 50% of these patients (Fig. 80–9). Spasm or contraction of the muscles that straighten the neck causes the loss of the forward curve. A sharp posterior angulation at a specific level may be noted, indicating a tear of the interspinous and/or posterior longitudinal ligament. Forward subluxation of the apophyseal joints with widening of the joint spaces and unusual separation of the contiguous spinous processes may account for this condition (Fig. 80–9). Retropharyngeal swelling or osteophytic formations of the anterior vertebral bodies may produce pharyngeal narrowing.

The forward flexion and the hyperextension views show the amount and location of motion and

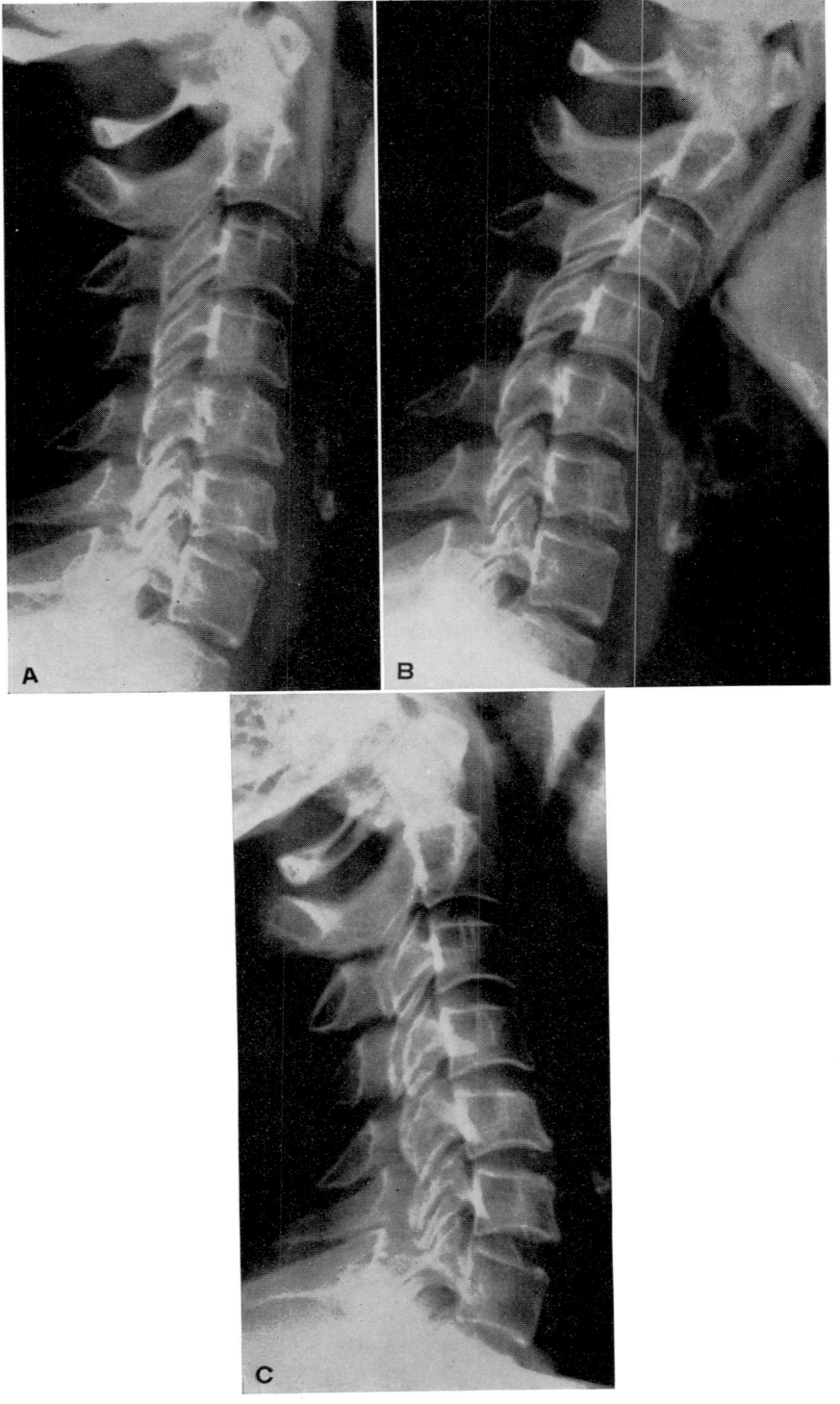

Fig. 80–9. *A* to *C*, The Davis series of lateral radiographs, which show posterior angulation at C4 to C5. (From Jackson, R.[8])

the presence of subluxations. These radiographs also confirm other abnormalities noted in the straight lateral view. One may see a separation of the anterior arch of the atlas from the odontoid process if the patient has relaxation from tearing or stretching of the transverse ligament or destructive lesions, as sometimes found in rheumatoid arthritis (RA). The usual separation is usually 3 to 4 mm; if greater, the transverse ligament is involved.

The oblique radiographic views may show foraminal narrowing if the patient has ligamentous instability or if osteophytic formations are present at the margins of the lateral interbody or apophyseal joints. The exact degree of foraminal narrowing cannot always be determined. Dissection of anatomic specimens has shown that the greatest amount of osteophytic formation occurs at the margins of the lateral interbody joints. In the lateral radiographic views, these osteophytes may appear to be projections on the posterior margins of the vertebral bodies, when in reality, they are on the margins of the lateral interbody joints (Fig. 80–10).

If spinal stenosis or a space-occupying lesion is suspected, myelographic studies may be indicated. This invasive procedure should be performed only if specific indications for differential diagnosis exist. Metrizamide has replaced Pantopaque. This newer agent is recommended because it enhances computerized tomography (CT), but its use is associated with complications (see Chap. 82). Nuclear magnetic resonance, a revolutionary diagnostic imaging procedure, augments CT scanning (see Chap. 5).[22]

Arteriograms may be indicated in the event of vascular insufficiency. Discography is of little value.[6] I do not recommend it. The routine radiographs described give adequate information for interpretation by the experienced examiner.

Radiographs of a recently injured cervical spine that show osteoarthrosis should be regarded with respect. Cervical spines showing such changes are more vulnerable to injuries than are normal cervical spines. Motion is limited, and any sudden movement or unusual activity, such as painting a ceiling, beyond the tolerance of these joints may exacerbate quiescent symptoms and clinical findings.

Other Diagnostic Techniques

Electromyographic examination may be indicated to differentiate between myogenic and neurogenic disorders.[3,4] I have found this procedure helpful in the differentiation of peripheral nerve involvement and constant localized nerve root compression not responding to conservative treatment. Electroencephalograms may be helpful in differentiating organic brain disorders from cervical involvement. After cervical spinal trauma, about 50% of patients have electroencephalographic changes similar to those seen in closed head injuries.[20] Electronystagmography is used to distinguish between central and peripheral involvement of the vestibular apparatus. If dizziness, loss of balance, tinnitus, and hearing deficits occur or persist after conservative treatment, then electronystagmography should be done.[16] Thermography may be useful in the diagnosis of nervous system dysfunction.[15]

TREATMENT

Treatment must be individualized, and the patient must be taught to live with the altered mechanics of his neck. Heat is gratifying to most patients; hot moist packs or diathermy give the best results. In those with an acute injury, cold packs block the conduction of pain impulses and may be helpful.

Traction

Traction is indicated in most instances of nerve root irritation. Skeletal traction is indicated for patients with certain fractures and fracture dislocations for a period of six to eight weeks. Brace or collar immobilization may then be used for three to six weeks and then discontinued gradually, supplemented by resistive exercises to strengthen the muscles.

Some patients with acute neck sprains may be treated best in a hospital with constant, 15–20 lb. head-halter traction for a few days. The patient should be in a jack-knife position, both for comfort and for effectiveness of traction (Fig. 80–11). After ambulation, brace or collar immobilization, to keep the neck straight and to avoid hyperextension, is indicated for a few weeks (Fig. 80–12). In the event of marked disruption of the posterior ligamentous structures or in certain fractures, hyperextension braces may be indicated.

In patients with acute sprain injuries, collar or brace immobilization should be used for a period of six to eight weeks. Patients with chronic sprain injuries may need such immobilization only for short intervals, usually 10 to 20 days, or when engaging in unusual activities.

Motorized intermittent traction, which can be given in the doctor's office or in a hospital physical therapy department, gives the best results because its amount and duration can be controlled, and it provides maximal pull with minimal discomfort to the patient's jaw and chin (see Fig. 80–11A,C). I have shown by cineradiography that 15 lb traction on normal spines lifts the weight of the head from the neck, but produces no visible distraction of the

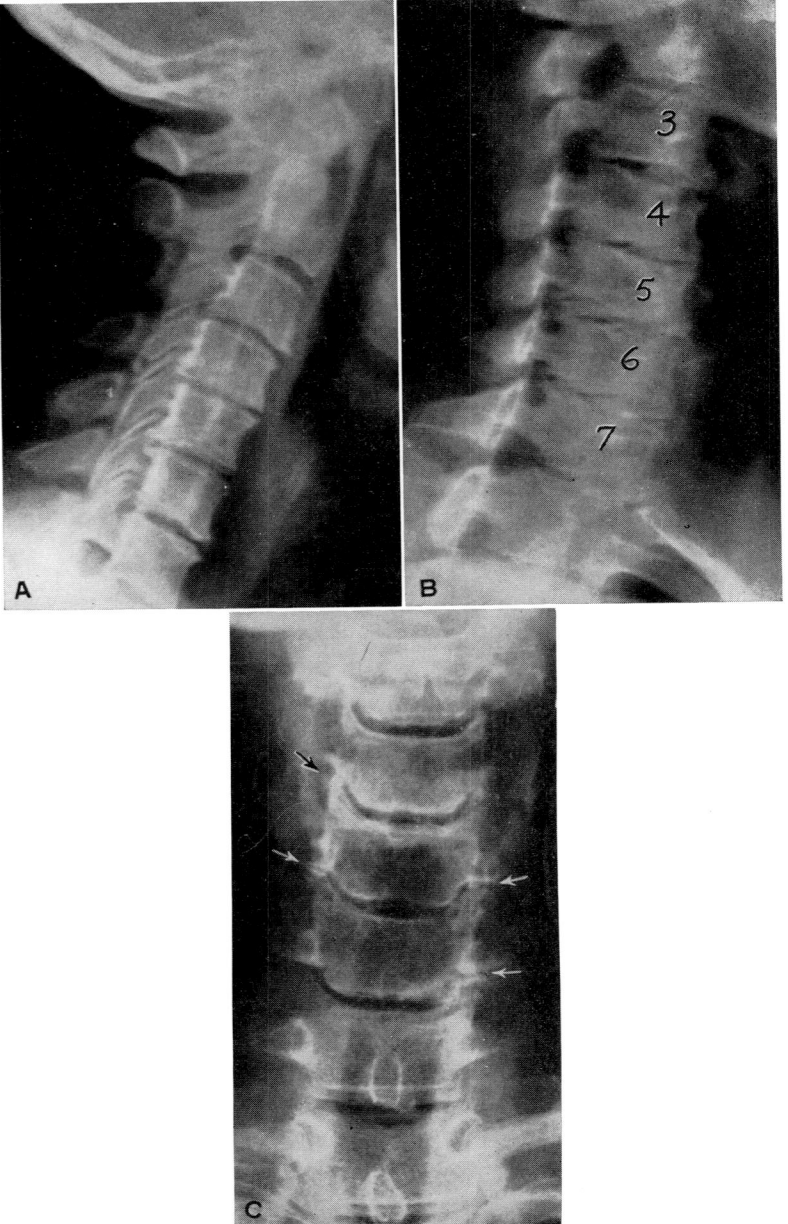

Fig. 80–10. Lateral *(A)*, oblique *(B)*, and anteroposterior *(C)* views of a cervical spine, showing hypertrophic changes with marked spur formation at the margins of the lateral interbody joints. (From Jackson, R.[8])

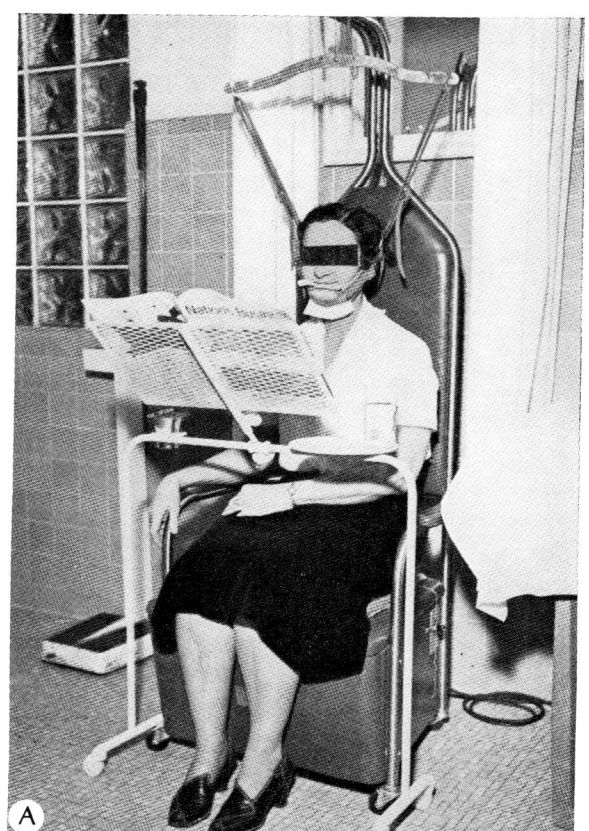

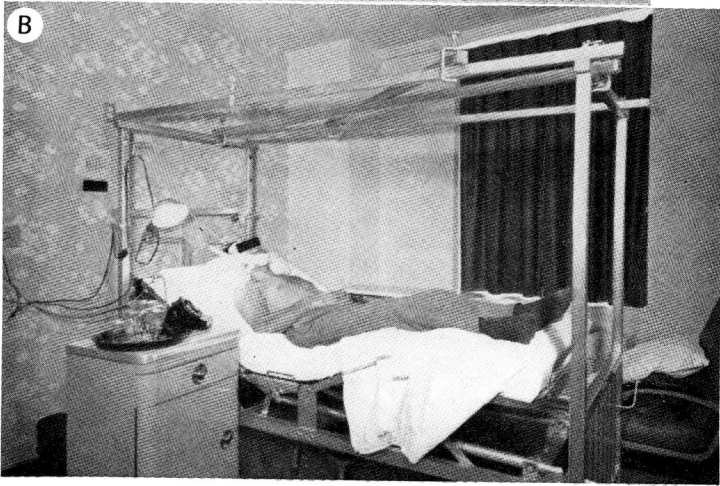

Fig. 80–11. Motorized intermittent traction *(A)* and constant bed traction *(B)*, *C*, Tru-eze motorized intermittent traction. *D*, Tru-eze on-the-door traction for home use (hot pack not shown). (*A* and *B* from Jackson.[8] *C* and *D* courtesy of Tru-eze Manufacturing Company, Temecula, CA.)

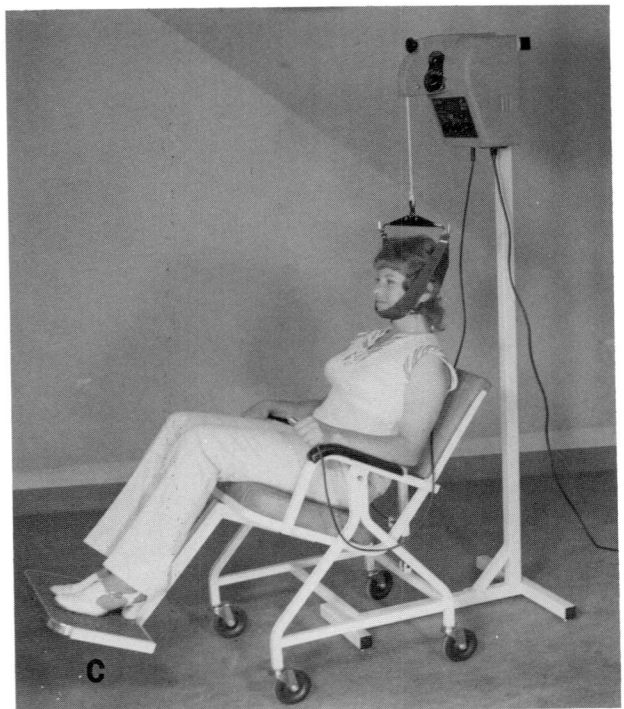

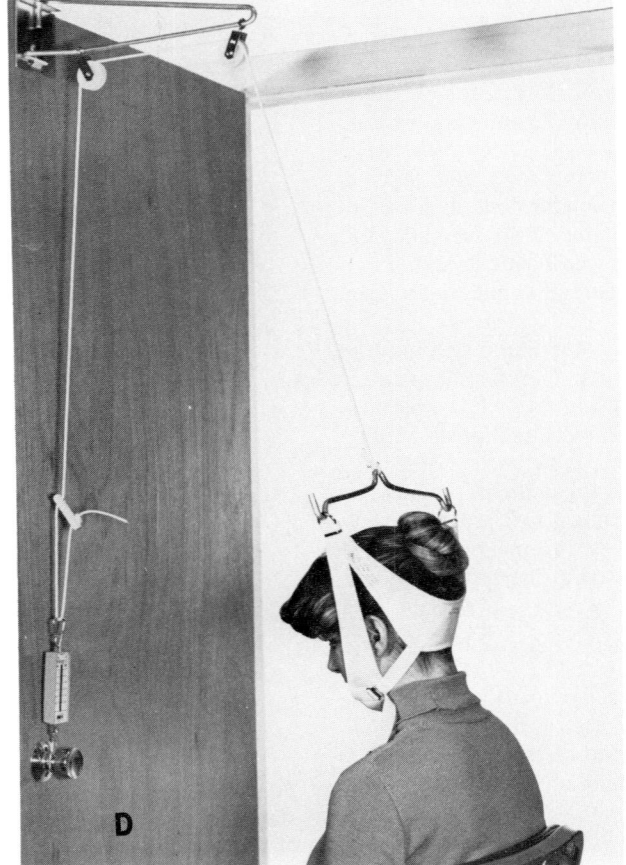

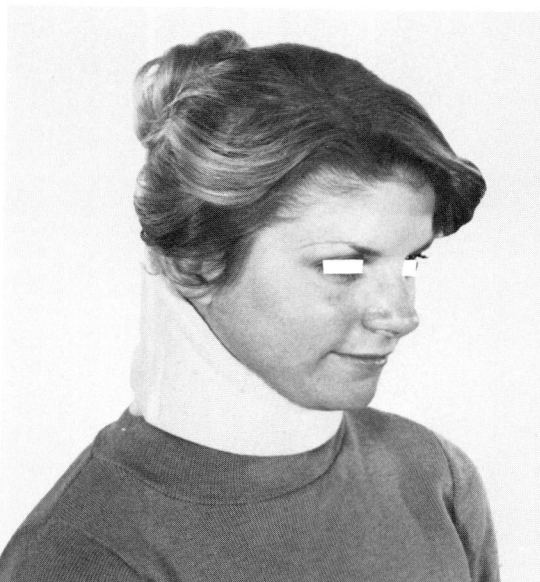

Fig. 80–12. Tru-FLEX collar provides adequate immobilization for most cervical disorders and prevents hyperextension of the head and neck, as shown. The neck is in neutral position, which maximizes the size of the intervertebral foramina. (Courtesy of the Tru-eze Manufacturing Company, Temecula, CA.)

vertebrae, whereas 25 to 35 lb traction produces definite vertebral distraction. This method of traction prevents the formation of adhesions between the dural sleeves of the nerve roots and adjacent structures; and it may free adhesions in some instances. It also relieves muscle spasm and pain. Many patients fall asleep during treatment. Traction should be continued at regular intervals as long as indicated.

"On-the-door" traction for home use may be indicated for some patients. I prefer the Tru-eze model with the scale (see Fig. 80–11,*D*), because the patient can see how much traction is applied and does not have to use cumbersome water bags or weights. Moreover, the patient can produce intermittent traction by leaning forward for a few seconds and then back to the original position. The patient should be instructed in the proper amount and duration of traction.

Drug Therapy

Medication for the relief of pain is usually indicated. I prefer buffered aspirin, 0.9 g q.i.d., because of its anti-inflammatory and analglesic actions. Narcotics should be used sparingly, if at all. If localized pain and muscle spasm persist, dramatic relief can often be obtained by the injection of 0.5% local anesthetic, such as procaine, into either the myalgic areas or the cervical joint capsules. Paralysis of the pain receptors and conductors breaks the pain reflex and may provide relief for days, weeks, or months.

Posture and Related Apparatus

Poor postural habits should be corrected. The patient should be taught to avoid hyperextension and hyperflexion of the neck in everyday activities because the intervertebral canals are of maximum caliber when the neck is straight. Shoulder braces may be indicated to correct drooping shoulders and to help straighten the cervical spine. Resistive exercises are important to strengthen the muscles.

The cervical contour pillow, Cervipillo, which I designed, is an important adjunct to the treatment of cervical spinal conditions (Fig. 80–13). It ensures correct positioning of the neck during sleep, whether the patient sleeps supine or on his side. Sleeping in the prone position is contraindicated because it keeps the neck turned to one side for prolonged periods and aggravates symptoms.

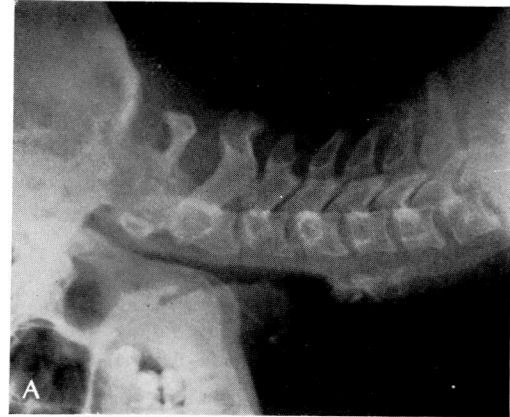

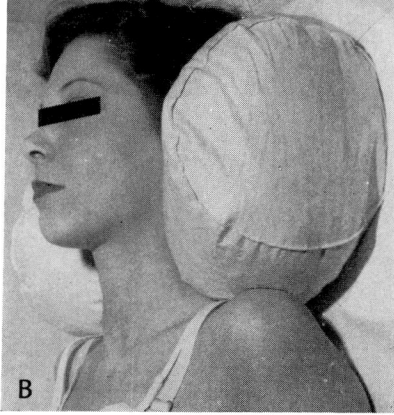

Fig. 80–13. *A*, The cervical contour pillow for correct sleeping posture. *B*, The radiograph shows the position of the vertebrae with the neck on the pillow. (From Jackson, R.[8])

Surgical Procedures

Surgical procedures are reserved for patients not responding to conservative measures or for those with definite spinal cord compression from epidural or subarachnoid space-occupying lesions. Overriding spinous processes may require removal in some instances.

Persistent and resistant nerve root irritation may be relieved by a simple facet fenestration, which removes the posterior wall of the intervertebral canal and decompresses the nerve root.[8]

Removal of degenerated disc material and spurs by the anterior (transvertebral) route, followed by an intervertebral body bone graft fusion, has gained popularity, but it should be performed only when specific indications exist. Most surgeons who fuse the cervical spine by the anterior route use discographic examination to localize the disc and to determine the site for fusion. A degenerated or narrowed disc may not be the true cause of the symptoms, however, and so second and third operations are often performed to relieve these persistent symptoms. Removal of foraminal osteophytes by facetectomy followed by fusion by the posterior route is much preferred by some surgeons, in spite of the putative advantages of the anterior approach.

Other Techniques

Transcutaneous nerve stimulators have become popular. In my experience, they may work well for short periods. Acupuncture and acupressure are used frequently by many physicians, with questionable results.

Injections of corticosteroids intradurally and intrathecally and/or ice solutions are being used with variable results.

In conclusion, a detailed medical history, clinical examination, and adequate radiographs of any patient with head, neck, chest, upper back, shoulder, or arm pain are imperative for proper diagnosis and treatment. Diagnoses of arthritis, bursitis, neuritis, muscular rheumatism, fibrositis, fasciitis, tendonitis, pseudoangina, and migraine should be avoided until cervical nerve root involvement has been eliminated.

Conservative measures give gratifying results in the majority of patients. Treatment should be individualized and definitive. Surgical measures are rarely necessary and should be reserved for those patients not responding to adequate conservative treatment and who have definite indications for operative procedures.

REFERENCES

1. Abel, M.: Occult Traumatic Lesions of the Cervical Spine. St. Louis, Green, 1970, pp. 17, 45–47.
2. Basmajian, J.V.: Muscles Alive: Their Function Revealed by Electromyography. Baltimore, Williams & Wilkins, 1962, pp. 97–124.
3. Campion, D.S.: Electromyography in Orthopaedic Surgery. Vol. 13, No. 12. South Pasadena, CA. Orthopaedic Audio Symposium Foundation, 1982.
4. Craun, G.G., and Riley, L.H.: Evaluation of neck and associated arm pain. Surg. Pract. News, 2:13-16, 26-27, 31, 1982.
5. Delmas, J., et al.: Comment atteinde les préganglionaires Luschka. Gaz. Med. Franc., 54:703, 1947.
6. Hall, M.C.: Luschka Joints. Springfield, IL, Charles C Thomas, 1965, pp. 133–141.
7. Holt, E.P., Jr.: Further reflections on cervical discography. JAMA, 231: 613–644, 1975.
8. Jackson, R.: The Cervical Syndrome. 4th Ed. Springfield, IL, Charles C Thomas, 1977.
9. Kaplan, L., and Kennedy, F.: Brain, 73:337–345, 1950.
10. Laurelle, L.L.: Les Bases Anatomi ques Du systèmes Autonomes, Cortical, et Bulbospinalis. Rev. Neurol., 72:349, 1940.
11. Lockhart, R.D., et al.: Anatomy of the Human Body. Philadelphia, J.B. Lippincott, 1959, pp. 66–71, 143, 322–327.
12. Luschka, Von H.: Die Halbergelenke des Menshiechen Korpes. 1958.
13. Neuwirth, E.: Current concepts of the cervical portion of the sympathetic nervous system. Jr. Lancet, 80:337–338, 1960.
14. Norris, F.H.: The EMG. New York, Grune & Stratton, 1963.
15. Pochaczesky, R.: Assessment of back pain by contact thermography of extremity dermatomes. Orthop. Rev., 12:45–58, 1983.
16. Rubin, W., and Norris, C.H.: Electronystagmography. Springfield, IL, Charles C Thomas, 1974, pp. 52–59.
17. Sheehan, et al.: Vertebral artery compression in cervical spondylosis: arteriographic demonstration during life of vertebral artery insufficiency due to rotation, flexion, and extension of the neck. Neurology, 10:1,968–1,986, 1960.
18. Sunderland, S.: Nerves and Nerve Injuries, 2nd Ed. Edinburgh, Churchill Livingstone, 1978.
19. Tinel, J.: Le système nerveux Végátatif. Paris, Masson, 1937.
20. Torres, F.H., and Shapiro, S.K.: Electroencephalograms in whiplash injuries: a comparison of EEG abnormalities with those in closed head injuries. Arch. Neurol., 5:28–35, 1961.
21. Trolard, A.: Quelques articulations de la colonne vertébrale. Int. Monatsschr. Anat. Physiol., 10:3, 1893.
22. Willcott, M.R., III: Nuclear magnetic resonance. Baylor Med., 8:3, 1982.

Chapter 81

Painful Temporomandibular Joint

Eugene J. Messer and Doran E. Ryan

The temporomandibular joint is specialized and is different from other joints of the body because it is paired and cannot function alone. This rotating, sliding joint must function in total harmony with its counterpart on the opposite side of the "horseshoe-shaped" mandible. The articulating surfaces of the bone are not covered by hyaline cartilage as are most other joints of the body, but rather by an avascular fibrous connective tissue that may contain cartilage cells, when it is designated fibrocartilage.[15] The fifth cranial nerve, which supplies the muscles that move the joint, also provides sensory protection and innervates the overlying skin.

ANATOMIC FEATURES

This joint is complex, with an articulating fibrocartilaginous disc interposed between the temporal and the mandibular bones, separating the articular space into superior and inferior compartments. The articulating surface of the mandible is the anterosuperior surface of the condylar head. This surface measures approximately 16 to 20 mm mediolaterally and 8 to 10 mm anteroposteriorly. The disc (meniscus) is essentially ovoid in shape with distinct anterior, central, and posterior zones and is firmly attached to the medial and lateral poles of the condylar head. Its average measurements are 27.5 mm mediolaterally and 9 mm anteroposteriorly. The posterior band is its thickest part (3 mm). The central zone is only 1 mm thick, and the anterior band is about 2 mm thick.

The fibrous capsule is frail, although its lateral surface is strengthened into a distinct temporomandibular ligament. The joint capsule is attached to the border of the temporal articulating surface and to the neck of the mandible. It is directly fused to the medial anterior and lateral circumference of the articulating disc. Posteriorly, however, the disc and the capsule become integrated into the posterior attachment or "bilaminar zone." This area is generously innervated and vascularized with large sinusoids that fill and empty during joint function. The zone is termed "bilaminar" because it splits, with one attachment on the posterior condyle neck and the other on the anterior wall of the auditory canal.

The only muscle directly attached to the temporomandibular joint is the lateral (external) pterygoid muscle. It has two points of origin, the superior portion from the infratemporal crest and the undersurface of the greater wing of the sphenoid bone. Its bundles converge to attach to the capsular ligament and directly into the articular disc. The inferior portion of the muscle is larger and arises from the lateral surface of the pterygoid process, from the pyramidal process of the palatine bone, and from the maxillary tuberosity. Its bundles converge to insert on the condylar head and neck. As the head rotates and then translates, the interior belly of the muscle contracts, helping to pull the condyle forward and inferiorly along the posterior slope of the eminentia articularis. The superior belly of the muscle remains flaccid on opening and the meniscus moves in concert with the head of the condyle by mechanical action. On closing, the superior belly of this muscle contracts to maintain the meniscus in proper relation to the head of the condyle.

PHYSICAL EXAMINATION

Examination of the patient with temporomandibular joint symptoms begins when the patient enters the room. Note should be made of the posture, stride, and general carriage.

When did symptoms first appear and under what circumstances? Was the onset acute or insidious? Was there a specific incident, or did the patient simply wake up one morning with symptoms? How do the symptoms relate to time of day and physical activity? What can be accomplished to increase or decrease the severity of symptoms? Where are the symptoms located? Has treatment of any kind been instituted? If so, has the treatment helped?

The examiner should put the patient at ease and should watch mandibular function as the conversation proceeds, noting particularly thrusting, limited function, or deviation of the mandible. Once normal or abnormal function of the mandible has been established, specific voluntary movements are requested. The interincisal distance is measured at the midline with the patient's mouth open. A range of approximately 38 to 42 mm is normal, although this distance varies with sex and general physical build. Lateral excursions are requested, and measurements are made as the jaw moves into right lateral, left lateral, and protrusive positions. Normal lateral excursions are 5 to 10 mm, and normal protrusion is 4 to 6 mm. Function of the mandible is then ascertained while the joints are palpated. A smooth rotation followed by translation of the condylar head without pops, clicks, or crepitus is normal. At the same time, the patient is questioned about pain and local tenderness determined by digital pressure over the joint.

A stethoscope is used to auscultate the joints during function; one should listen for the character of the noise, if noise is present. A pop or click signifies malposition of the disc, whereas grating or crepitus usually indicates bone-on-bone contact. The muscles of mastication are then palpated, beginning with the temporalis muscle and proceeding to the masseter, digastric, and medial and lateral pterygoid muscles. Accessory muscles of mastication such as the supra- and infrahyoid, digastric, and sternocleidomastoid muscles are also palpated. Muscle spasm in the sternocleidomastoid or the hyoid muscles or in the muscles of mastication may occur in patients with limited mandibular function. Spasm in some or all of the vertebral muscles may cause the patient to have difficulty in moving the head.

Examination of the dentition follows, with special attention to the skeletal relationship of the arches, as well as the tooth-bone relationship. This determination is important because individuals with a class II (retrognathia) skeletal and dental malocclusion frequently have temporomandibular joint symptoms. Internal joint derangements are rare in patients with class I (normal) and class III (prognathic) skeletal relationships. Finally, the patient is asked to point to the area of pain. The pointing finger frequently distinguishes between muscle disorders and internal joint derangements.

RADIOGRAPHIC EXAMINATION

Roentgenograms of the painful temporomandibular joint give a wealth of information and are particularly useful in patients with possible internal joint derangements. Screening films are important, but definitive diagnosis should not be attempted using these alone. The most common views are the panoramic and the transcranial or transpharyngeal views in both opened and closed positions. These views reveal the general shape and condition of the bony condylar head, but they do not show its position relative to the glenoid fossa. It is possible to obtain these data with corrected tomograms but, in our opinion, other studies give more information. If the clinical examination and screening radiographic examination suggest internal joint de-

rangement, further specific radiographic studies are indicated.

ARTHROGRAPHY

Arthrography is the standard diagnostic tool for internal temporomandibular joint derangement.[1,3,4] An iodized dye is injected into the inferior joint spaces or into both the inferior and superior spaces. If both joint spaces are injected, the meniscus will be outlined between the two concentrations of dye (Fig. 81–1). With a single inferior joint space injection, the meniscus is outlined by dye between the inferior compartment and the eminentia articularis (Fig. 81–2). As multiple sequential films are exposed with the patient opening and closing the mouth, the dye shifts from anterior to posterior as the condyle first rotates and then translates. In an individual with an anterior displacement of the meniscus, the dye concentrates anterior to the condylar head. As the disc is captured by forward movement of the condyle, the dye flows rapidly posterior to the condylar head. At maximal joint opening, little dye is evident in the anterior portion of the inferior joint space. In the anterior closed lock, the meniscus is not recaptured, and a pool of dye remains in the anterior compartment of the inferior joint space, with the meniscus bunched superior to the dye concentrations and inferior to the eminentia articularis (Fig. 81–3).

Arthrographic views of the temporomandibular joint are now recorded dynamically on videotape and are far easier to interpret because the action of the condylar head in relation to the meniscus and dye is viewed in its entirety. One can watch the immediate and rapid shift of dye from anterior to posterior as the meniscus is captured, or the concentrated anterior pools of dye with forced displacement of the meniscus anterior to the eminentia articularis. In a static arthrogram, in which the disc is recaptured at midfunction, the series of pictures may well show abnormal position of the meniscus on two or three views, followed by normal position of the meniscus on the remaining views.

Scintigraphy

Single-photon-emission computerized tomography is an excellent technique for determining the presence or absence of temporomandibular joint disorders.[2] When internal joint derangement is present, bone scintiscans using ^{99m}technetium MDP are positive before either conventional radiographs or x-ray tomograms demonstrate joint space narrowing, bony sclerosis, or meniscal degeneration. Therefore, when it is necessary to distinguish between temporomandibular joint disease and other causes of facial pain, bone scanning is the noninvasive test of choice for localizing the abnormality.[2]

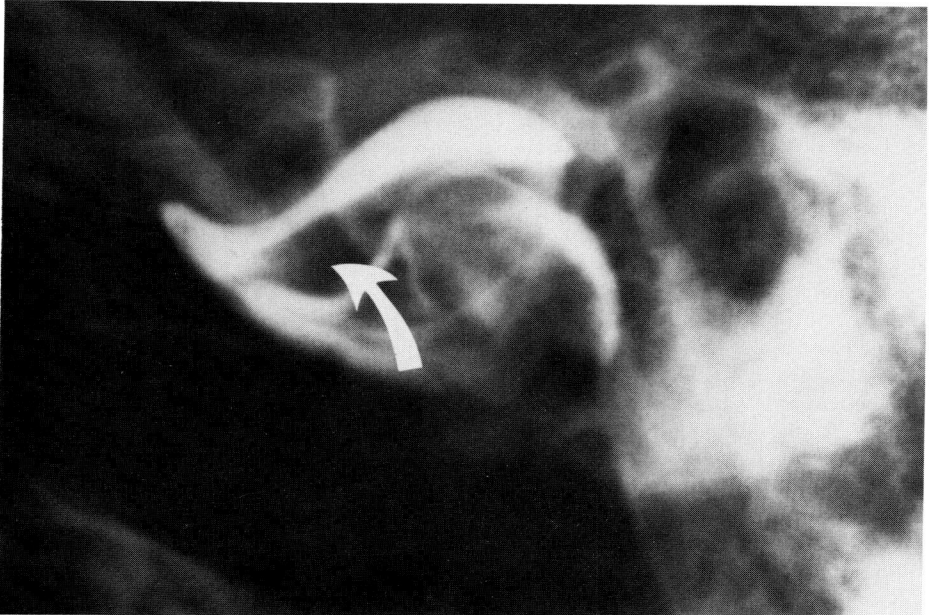

Fig. 81–1.   Meniscus (arrow) outlined by dye in both the superior and inferior joint compartments.

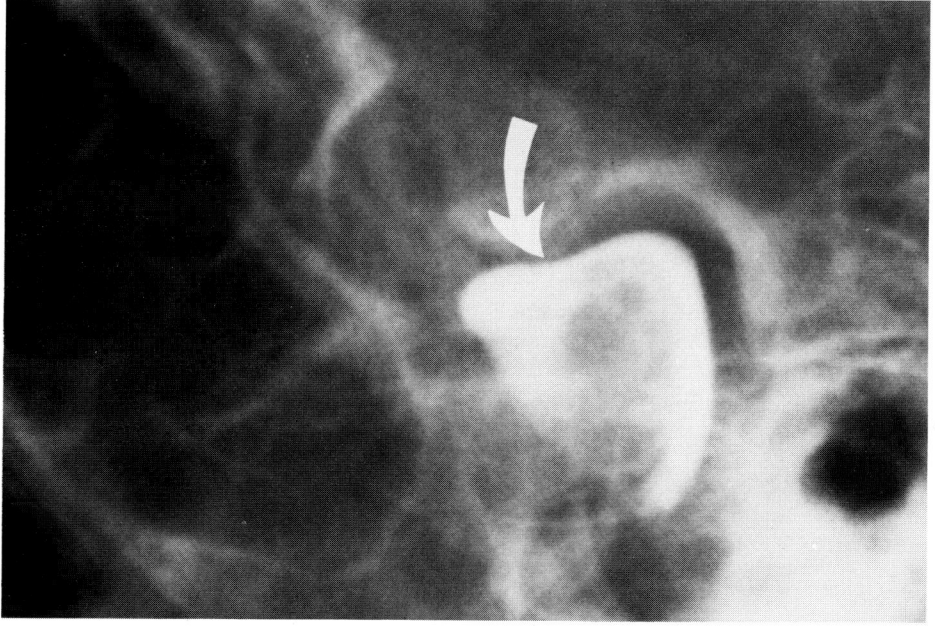

Fig. 81–2.   Meniscus (arrow) outlined by dye between the inferior joint compartment and the eminentia articularis.

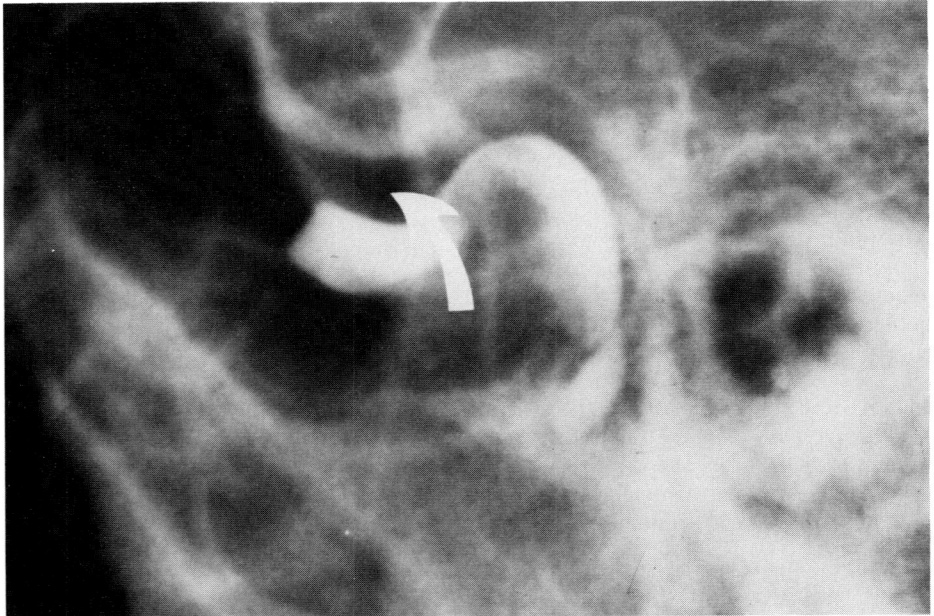

Fig. 81–3. Meniscus bunching ahead of the condyle as the condyle head attempts to move anteriorly (arrow).

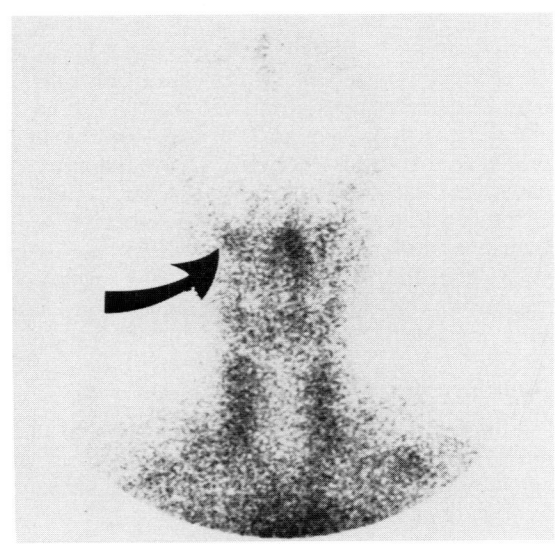

Fig. 81–4. Increased radionuclide activity (arrow) over the right temporomandibular joint.

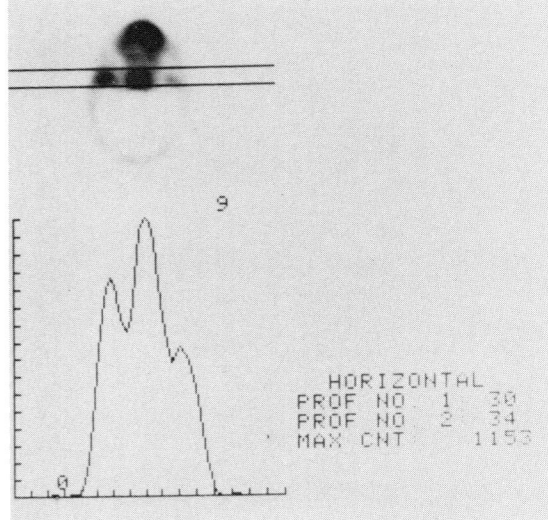

Fig. 81–5. Coronal slice through the head of the temporomandibular joint showing a marked increase in activity on the right side (arrow).

Radionuclide angiography is performed with 10 sequential 3-second anterior-view images of the head, followed by a 50,000-count image 3 hours later. Anterior, right-lateral, and left-lateral planar bone scintigrams (500,000 count) of the head are obtained using a large-field-of-view gamma camera equipped with a high-resolution collimator. A right lateral view demonstrates increased bone uptake over the right temporomandibular joint (Fig. 81–4). Tomographic studies in the coronal and transaxial planes can confirm the marked increase in radionuclide activity over the right temporomandibular joint (Figs. 81–5, 81–6). Quantitative analysis of the bone uptake over both joints and intervening bony structures also shows the sharp peak of increased activity over the right temporomandibular joint (Fig. 81–6), caused by subchondral bone changes from anterior displacement of the meniscus noted on clinical examination.

DIFFERENTIAL DIAGNOSIS AND TREATMENT

Determining the source of pain from the temporomandibular joint and its surrounding structures is complex because the maxillofacial region has the highest sensory innervation density in the body, and the cranial nerves do not follow the orderly segmentation typically found in other joints of the body. Because of this complicated innervation, the diagnosis of diseases of this joint can be difficult.

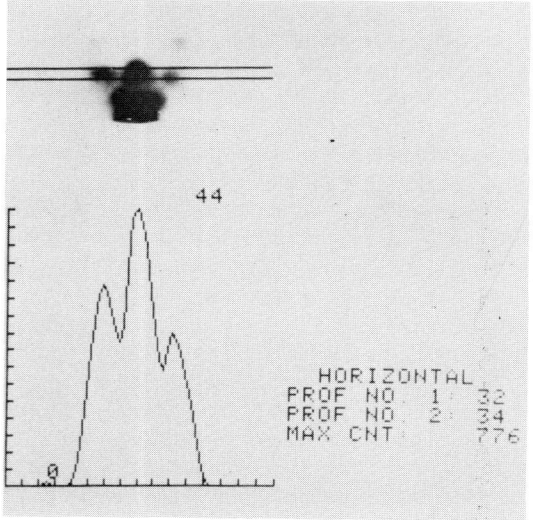

Fig. 81–6. Transaxial slice in a single-photon-emission computerized tomogram confirms increased radioactivity in the right temporomandibular joint (upper part of the figure). Quantitative analysis shows a sharp peak of activity in the right temporomandibular joint (lower part of the figure).

Referred Otalgia and Odontalgia

The symptom of "earache" is common with lesions of the temporomandibular joint. The auricle, external auditory canal, and tympanum are supplied by sensory fibers from the fifth, seventh, ninth, and tenth cranial nerves, in addition to the second and third cervical nerves. Earache due to pain referred from other sites is more common than that due to disorders of the ear itself. Because the sensory innervation varies widely and overlaps, it is often difficult for the patient to localize the pain to a particular area of the ear. For these reasons, diagnosis of lesions of both the external and the inner ear is made mainly by clinical evaluation. If the patient's pain is localized within the meatus of the auditory canal and if pain is produced by palpation or passive movement of the auricle, a lesion of the external ear or auditory canal should be suspected. Diseases of the middle ear usually produce symptoms of hearing impairment, low-pitched tinnitus, and pain that runs from mild discomfort or pressure sensation, as seen with an early, acute serous or purulent otitis media, to a deep, boring pain, as seen late in these diseases. If the earache is modified in any way by movement of the lower jaw, and if the auricle, external auditory canal, and tympanic membrane appear normal on examination, the diagnosis of temporomandibular joint disease should be considered.

Pain from dental origin is commonly referred to the temporomandibular joint through the fifth cranial nerve, primarily the auriculotemporal branch. It is often difficult for the patient to determine whether the offending tooth is in the mandible or the maxilla, and the pain may be felt diffusely throughout the teeth, jaw, face, and head. Because of the variability and the diffuse nature of the pain, it is wise to consider all diffuse pain in the head and neck, including the oral cavity, to be of dental origin until proved otherwise. In the majority of cases, clinical evaluation reveals a large carious lesion or a fractured tooth to be the source of pain. Palpation of the affected tooth with a tongue blade elicits pain and is thereby a dependable means of diagnosis. The surrounding soft tissues may also show signs of inflammation.

Radiographic Findings

In dental disease, radiographs are helpful and most often diagnostic. The panogram and the periapical radiograph taken in a dental office are most frequently used.

Laboratory Findings

Except in the case of acute infection, in which the patient's white blood cell count is elevated, the laboratory examination does not contribute to the diagnosis.

Myofascial Pain Dysfunction Syndrome

As many as 85% of all patients seen with "temporomandibular joint syndrome" really have myofascial pain dysfunction of the muscles of mastication. The joint is implicated because pain occurs when it is mobilized. The female-to-male sex ratio is 8 to 1, with an age range from puberty to 40 years, although it does occur at any age. The cardinal signs and symptoms of this syndrome include pain on movement of the jaw, limited ability to open the jaw, deviation of the open jaw toward the affected side, and "clicking" or "popping" in the temporomandibular joint during motion. Two negative findings are important: (1) *No tenderness on palpation of the joint; and (2) normal bony radiographic findings.*[8] Classically, the patient describes the pain by placing the whole hand over the affected side of the face. The description of pain varies from a sensation of pressure to severe and lancinating, occurring both spontaneously and in response to movement of the involved muscles. Pain occurs when chewing and when clenching the teeth. The pain is often more severe in the morning, on awakening, secondary to nocturnal bruxism. A period of emotional stress precedes the onset of symptoms.

Clinical Findings

No pain is present in the temporomandibular joints during movement or on palpation of the condylar head. The "clicking" sometimes felt during early movement of the joint is related to spasm of the superior belly of the lateral pterygoid muscle. If clicking is detected during extreme excursion, a diagnosis of internal joint derangement should be considered. At least one of the muscles of mastication is tender to palpation on the painful side, and when the patient bites, pain is experienced in the same muscles. If a tongue blade is placed between the incisors and the patient is asked to bite, the pain should decrease. If the tongue blade is placed on the posterior teeth, and the patient is asked to bite, the pain will probably increase.

TREATMENT

Initial treatment consists of analgesic or anti-inflammatory drugs, moist heat, and a soft diet. If the symptoms persist for more than 2 weeks, the patient should be referred to a dentist for construction of an acrylic splint to help to disocclude the teeth. Because bruxism or clenching of the teeth is a primary cause of this syndrome, the splint may interrupt the cycle of jaw clenching and muscle spasm. Psychologic counseling may be indicated

because emotional stress often initiates the problem. If these measures are not successful, physical therapy, biofeedback, hypnosis, and formal psychotherapy may be tried.

Internal Temporomandibular Joint Derangement

By definition, this disorder is an abnormal relationship of the meniscus with the condyle when the teeth are in maximal occlusion.[3] The abnormal position of the meniscus is usually anteromedial because of the direction of contraction of the superior belly of the lateral pterygoid muscles toward the pterygoid plates. Internal derangements are subdivided into the following categories: (1) *anteromedial displacement of the meniscus with reduction; (2) anteromedial displacement of the meniscus without reduction (close lock); and (3) perforation of the meniscus or the posterior attachment of the meniscus.* These derangements are also classified by the amount of movement of the mandible necessary to reposition or "capture" the meniscus, as evidenced by the clicking sound. Thus, *early, midphase,* or *late reductions* are classified by measurement of the interincisal opening. If the reduction takes place during the first 15 mm of interincisal opening, it is considered an early reduction; if it takes place during 15 to 30 mm of interincisal opening, it is a midphase reduction; and if it happens after 30 mm, it is classified as a late reduction. If the patient can open the mouth only to 27 to 30 mm with deviation toward the affected side and no clicking is heard or palpated, a close lock must be considered. With close lock, the meniscus is wedged in front of the condyle and prevents forward motion of the mandible. The pathophysiologic features of the abnormality are compared to its unpredictable clinical progression[3,5,14] (Table 81–1). The disorder may progress in a period of several months to years, or it may not follow the full sequence of clinical events.

Clinical Findings

The ratio of women to men affected with the disorder is 8 to 1, and the condition is most commonly seen in the second or third decade, but it can occur at any age. The cardinal signs and symptoms of internal joint derangement include pain on palpation of the condylar head, and popping, clicking, or crepitus in the temporomandibular joint. One also sees limited range of motion, as in close lock, deviation toward the affected side before the pop takes place, and finally, return to midline at maximal opening. Other, more variable symptoms include temporal or frontal headaches, retro-orbital pain, otalgia, tinnitus, dizziness, and varying de-

Table 81-1. Internal Temporomandibular Joint Derangement

Clinical Progression of Disease	Pathophysiology
Clicking	Stretching of lateral attachment Stretching and loss of elasticity of posterior attachment
Clicking with intermittent locking	Thickening of posterior ridge of disc
Close-lock	Metaplasia of disc tissue to cartilage or permanent deformation of disc
Crepitus	Perforation of posterior attachment

grees of myofascial pain dysfunction syndrome. A history of asymptomatic clicking is important, especially when the patient has limited and noiseless joint opening.

Radiographic Findings

Routine radiographic examination is not diagnostic. Arthrography is invaluable in the diagnosis of internal joint derangement and is the definitive test of choice.[1,3] More recently, scintigraphy has become a useful diagnostic tool.[2]

Treatment

Treatment depends on the severity of the condition. The patient with painless joint clicking is informed of the possible progression of the disease, but no treatment is indicated. If a patient has early clicking and pain, nonsurgical techniques are used, including splint therapy to recapture the meniscus followed by alteration of the occlusion to hold that position.[4,9,10] With late reduction or with nonreduction (close lock) of the meniscus or in patients unsuccessfully treated by nonsurgical means, a surgical procedure is indicated. If the meniscus is of normal shape and texture and is easily pulled posteriorly and laterally into a normal relationship with the condyle head, then a meniscoplasty is performed. The posterior and lateral attachments are shortened, and the meniscus is reattached to the condyle.[3,9] If the meniscus has undergone metaplasia or is scarred in an anteromedial position, a menisectomy is indicated, with implantation of a soft Silastic implant.[2] Patients tolerate these surgical procedures well; meniscoplasty is successful in 80 to 90%; the success rate of the menisectomy with implantation is about 85 to 95%.

Degenerative Joint Disease

Unlike other diarthrodial joints, the articular surface of the temporomandibular joint is covered with fibrocartilage rather than with hyaline cartilage. The progression of degenerative disease in this joint is also different from that in other joints. Initially, erosion is seen in the subchondral bone, followed by thinning and destruction of the fibro-

cartilage, with some attempts at repair. Degenerative joint disease is traditionally divided into primary and secondary types.[16] Primary disease is idiopathic, whereas secondary disease is related to trauma or, most important, to chronic internal joint derangement. In patients with primary disease, with an intact articular meniscus, the clinical course of pain and dysfunction is short and is usually followed by repair, with diminution or resolution of symptoms. In secondary disease, the meniscus is either destroyed or damaged beyond repair, symptoms become chronic, and natural repair is only partial.

Clinical Findings

The onset of this disorder is usually insidious. The initial symptom is stiffness of the involved joint. Pain on motion of the affected joint becomes worse by progressive activity during the day. Patients are least symptomatic on arising in the morning. Coarse crepitus is often felt in the affected joint late in the disease process, especially in secondary degenerative joint disease.[7]

Radiographic Findings

A screening radiograph is initially used to evaluate the patient. Tomograms can be used to delineate the extent of the bony changes if a surgical procedure is contemplated. Arthrograms are of great value in determining whether the meniscus is displaced or torn, a finding that determines therapy. Bone scanning with tomography is also of diagnostic value and can be used in follow-up to evaluate the effectiveness of treatment. Early radiographic changes include thinning or loss of the cortical bone in the area of articulation. As the disease progresses, one sees a roughened and irregular bony surface, which can lead to loss of normal condylar anatomic features. Flattening of the superior and anterior aspects with anterior lipping of the condyle are evidence of natural repair, and cortical margins develop when repair is complete.

Treatment

Primary degenerative joint disease is usually a self-limiting process, often treated symptomatically and nonsurgically. If the meniscus remains intact, normal healing by fibrocartilaginous proliferation will take place on the condylar surface, and the disease generally runs its course in approximately two years. In secondary disease, in which the meniscus is destroyed or torn and displaced, the condition progresses, and surgical treatment is indicated. This treatment consists of meniscectomy, smoothing of the articular surfaces, and placement of an implant between the condylar head and glenoid fossa. Corticosteroid injections have been used to create a chemical smoothing of the articular surfaces of the condyle with moderate success.[12]

Rheumatoid Arthritis (RA)

Involvement of the temporomandibular joint varies from 1 to 60%. Women outnumber men, almost 3 to 1, with the usual age of onset. The disease usually affects both temporomandibular joints. Only the condylar head is affected, and the glenoid fossa is seldom involved. Initial bony destruction occurs in the neck of the condyle inferior to the fibrocartilaginous cover of the head. It then involves the cartilaginous surface and the subchondral spaces of the bone.[11] The meniscus is usually destroyed in the process.

Clinical Findings

Signs and symptoms of RA in the temporomandibular joint are similar to those in any other affected joint. Pain and stiffness on arising in the morning are prominent features. These symptoms decrease with moderate activity, and stiffness recurs with inactivity. Pain becomes more severe during strenuous activity. On palpation, the patient notes tenderness over the joint, and limitation of motion becomes progressive as the disease develops. Later in the disease process, crepitus may be found.

Radiographic Findings

A screening radiograph is used for initial evaluation. Erosions of the neck and head, marginal proliferations of bone, flattening of the superior and anterior surfaces of the condylar head, and eventually, gross deformities are evident. Although not as diagnostic, limitation of joint excursions and narrowing of the joint space are also seen. More detailed evaluation can be accomplished by the use of tomography or corrected tomography. Tomographic bone scanning is specifically diagnostic for RA, and arthrograms can be valuable in determining the status of the meniscus.

Laboratory Findings

The rheumatoid factor test is positive in 70 to 80% of patients, and other findings are identical to those described in Chapter 40.

Treatment

The usual treatment is conservative, as described in Chapter 42. With successful management of the systemic disease, symptoms in the temporomandibular arthritic joint usually subside. Rest is prescribed for the joints during the acute phase of the illness, along with mild exercises to maintain function. Occasionally, acrylic splint therapy is useful to remove the mandible from tooth function, thereby decreasing trauma to the joint. Ankylosis of the temporomandibular joint is rare. If it does occur, the procedure of choice consists of creating a joint space, lining the joint space with a Silastic implant, and the institution of motion soon after the operation. Occasionally, a total joint replacement is necessary to maintain a functioning mandible.

Gouty Arthritis

Gout of the temporomandibular joint is rare but painful. As in other joints of the body, urate crystals precipitate in the synovial tissues and fluid. Left untreated, degenerative joint disease develops.[6,13]

Clinical and Laboratory Findings

Sudden onset of symptoms, frequently at night and for no apparent reason, is characteristic. A warm sensation over the joint is common, and the patient notes limitation of mandibular movement because of the acute pain and swelling. The patient may also experience headache, fever, and general malaise (see Chap. 91).

Radiographic Findings

In the acute phase of the disorder, no radiographic changes ae seen. If the disease becomes chronic, radiographic changes are similar to those seen in degenerative joint disease.

Treatment

Aspiration of the joint gives temporary symptomatic relief; medical management of the acute attack is uniformly successful (see Chap. 93).

Other Diseases

The temporomandibular joints can be affected by any disease that involves the joints. Short- or long-term symptoms in this joint may be due to the deposition of calcium pyrophosphate dihydrate crystals, as discussed in Chapter 94. Crystal masses may occur in areas of chondroid metaplasia in the synovium as an isolated finding, resembling osteochondromatosis. Acute temporomandibular gout or pseudogout was thought to be precipitated by bruxism in one patient.[5a]

Two other categories, only mentioned here, that cause extreme joint symptoms are trauma and both benign and malignant tumors. Trauma can cause pain and may limit movement in the temporomandibular joint, but diagnosis is straightforward, by medical history, clinical examination, and standard facial radiographs. Tumors that occur in other joints can also affect this joint, but such tumors are rare. Pain usually occurs late in the course of the disease. Limited function and grossly abnormal radiographic changes often precede pain. Biopsy is needed for diagnosis, and treatment is determined by the nature of the lesion.

In summary, pain in the temporomandibular joint is often misdiagnosed and is frequently attributed to a psychologic cause. With the recent introduction of arthrography, scintigraphy, and a better understanding of the anatomy and physiology of this joint, many patients can now be helped.

REFERENCES

1. Bronstein, S.L., Tomasetti, B.J., and Ryan, D.E.: Internal derangement of the temporomandibular joint: correlation of arthrographic and surgical findings. J. Oral Surg., 39:572–584, 1982.
2. Collier, D., et al.: Detection of internal derangement of the temporomandibular joint by single photon emission computed tomography. Radiology, 149:557–561, 1983.
3. Dolwick, M.F.: Surgical management in internal derangements of the temporomandibular joint. Edited by C.A. Helms, R.W. Katzberg, and M.F. Dolwick. San Francisco, Radiology Research and Education Foundation, 1983.
4. Dolwick, M.F., et al.: Arthrotomographic evaluation of the temporomandibular joint. J. Oral Surg., 37:793–799, 1979.
5. Farrar, W.B.: Diagnosis and treatment of anterior dislocation of the articular disc. N.Y. J. Dent., 41:348–351, 1971.
5a. Good, A.E., and Upton, L.G.: Acute temporomandibular arthritis in a patient with bruxism and calcium pyrophosphate deposition disease. Arthritis Rheum., 25:353–355, 1982.
6. Kleinman, H.Z., and Ewbank, R.L.: Gout of the temporomandibular joint: report of three cases. Oral Surg., 27:281–282, 1969.
7. Kreutziger, K.L., and Mahan, P.E.: Temporomandibular degenerative joint disease. I. Anatomy, pathophysiology and clinical description. Oral Surg., 40:165–182, 1975.
8. Laskin, D.M.: Etiology of pain dysfunction syndrome. J. Am. Dent. Assoc., 79:147–153, 1969.
9. McCarty, W.L., Jr., and Farrar, W.B.: Surgery for internal derangement of the temporomandibular joint. J. Prosthet. Dent., 42:191–196, 1979.
10. McNeill, C., et al.: Craniomandibular (TMJ) disorders—the state of the art. J. Prosth. Dent., 44:434, 1980.
11. Ogus, H.: Rheumatoid arthritis of the temporomandibular joint. Br. J. Oral Surg., 12:275–284, 1975.
12. Poswillo, D.: Experimental investigation of the effects of interarticular hydrocortisone and high condylectomy on the mandibular condyle. Oral Surg., 30:161, 1970.
13. Rodnan, G.P.: Gout and other crystalline forms of arthritis. Postgrad. Med., 58:6, 1978.
14. Scapino, R.P.: Histopathology associated with malposition of the human temporomandibular joint disc. Oral Surg., 55:382–397, 1983.
15. Sicher, H.: Oral Anatomy. 2nd Ed. St. Louis, C.V. Mosby, 1952, p. 157.
16. Toller, P.A.: Osteoarthrosis of the mandibular condyle. Br. Dent. J., 134:223–231, 1973.

Chapter 82

The Painful Back

David B. Levine

The syndrome of low back pain, with or without radiation, is one of the most common disorders affecting man. Although great strides have been made in understanding the complexities of the pathogenesis of this syndrome, medical knowledge is still not advanced sufficiently to clarify the origin of low back pain.

In considering the painful low back, anatomic focus is on the lower lumbar spine (L3 to L5), the lumbosacral junction, the sacrum, the sacroiliac joints, and finally, the sacral-coccygeal region. Although symptoms in these regions often stem from local disease, etiologic factors may be present elsewhere.

Physicians should plan an orderly approach to the patient with low back syndrome. They should first attempt to determine whether the cause is primarily musculoskeletal, neurologic, or visceral. A differential diagnosis should then be established by medical history, physical examination, routine radiograms, and laboratory analysis. Precise diagnosis may be reached by repeated examinations and special tests. Only then can logical management be formulated.

PREVALENCE

From studies the world over, the prevalence of low back pain is becoming known. It has been estimated that 80% of the population will experience low back pain at some time.

The painful low back is a major cause of loss of time from work. Work days lost are reported to be 1,400 per thousand workers in the United States and 2,600 per thousand workers in Great Britain.

Because of our changing society, the prevalence of low back pain is directly influenced by various social and psychologic factors. Consequently, psychologic evaluation has become a necessary part of the clinical examination.

DIFFERENTIAL DIAGNOSIS

The list of possible diagnoses of the low back syndrome seems endless. Yet the physician must make every effort to arrive at a specific presumptive diagnosis. Although such terms as "lumbago" and "sciatica" were common labels in the past, they should be avoided because of their ambiguity.

The diagnosis of "strain" alone is meaningless unless applied to a certain anatomic part.

The differential diagnosis may be reached by a logical and reasonable approach, based on appropriate anatomic and potential etiologic factors. The following outline provides a basis for differential diagnosis:

ANATOMIC FACTORS
    Vertebra (hard)
        Body
        Neural arch
        Spinous process
        Lamina
        Facet
        Pedicle
        Transverse process
    Vertebra (soft)
        Supraspinous ligament
        Infraspinous ligament
        Ligamentum flavum
        Posterior longitudinal ligament
        Anterior longitudinal ligament
        Intervertebral disc
        Minor ligaments
    Vertebra (articulation)
        Anterior (disc)
        Posterior (facets)
        Lateral (sacroiliac joints)
    Vertebra (orifices)
        Neural canal
        Intervertebral foramina
    Vertebra (alignment)
    Paravertebra (muscular)
        Anterior
        Posterior
        Lateral
ETIOLOGIC FACTORS
    Traumatic
        Acute
        Chronic
    Congenital
    Degenerative
    Inflammatory
        Infectious
        Noninfectious
    Neoplastic
    Developmental

Metabolic
Toxic
Psychoneurotic
Nerves
    Primary (local)
    Primary (general)
    Coverings
Vessels
    Arterial
    Venous
Visceral organs

ANATOMIC CONSIDERATIONS

Vertebral Column

Each vertebra is composed of an anterior portion, the body, and a posterior portion, the neural arch (Fig. 82–1). From the neural arch, several processes are important: the transverse processes, one on each side; the superior and inferior articular processes (facets), one above and one below on each side; and one spinous process. The portion of the neural arch connected to the body and anterior to the articular processes is called the root or pedicle; that posterior to it is called the lamina; that part between the superior and inferior articular facets has come to be known as the pars interarticularis or isthmus.

The vertebrae are articulated together by a system of joints, three for each level. The disc lies between two adjacent vertebral bodies and is composed of a tough fibrocartilaginous outer ring, the annulus fibrosus, with a central viscous core, the nucleus pulposus. It is bounded superiorly and inferiorly by hyaline cartilaginous plates that blend with the annulus fibrosus. The transitions from cartilaginous plate to annulus and from annulus to nucleus are gradual. The fibers of the annulus fibrosus are arranged concentrically and in multiple layers. In the lumbar discs, the layers are thicker anteriorly and laterally than posteriorly, and the nucleus pulposus is closer to the posterior aspect of the disc. Posteriorly, one for each side, are true diarthrodial joints, which lie between the inferior facets of one vertebra above and the superior facets of the next below.

The ligamentous support of the spine is provided by the massive anterior longitudinal and the narrow posterior longitudinal ligaments. In a study of 35 autopsy specimens at the level of the L5 vertebral body, the average width of the anterior longitudinal ligament was 2 cm and the average thickness 1.9 mm, whereas the average width of the posterior longitudinal ligament was 0.7 cm and the average thickness 1.3 mm. These ligaments are situated

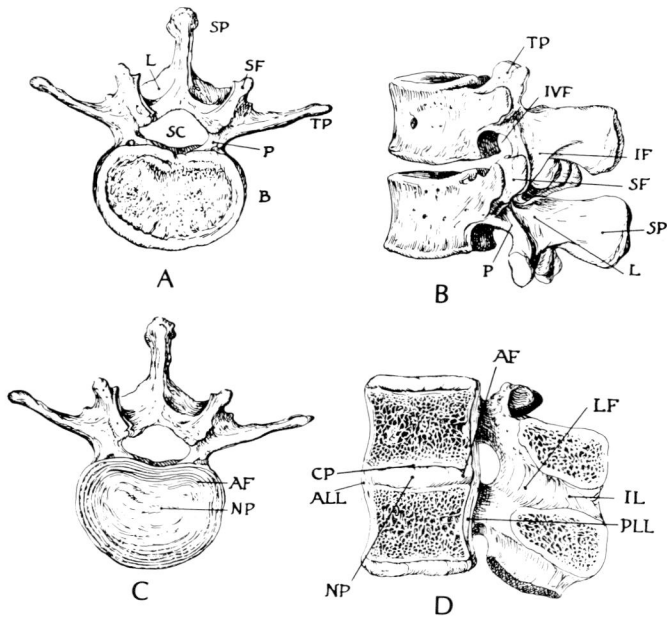

Fig. 82–1. Anatomy of the lumbar vertebrae and their articulations. *A,* Superior view of a stripped lumbar vertebra. *B,* Lateral view of two articulated lumbar vertebrae. *C,* Superior view of a horizontal section of a lumbar disc. *D,* Lateral view of a sagittal section of two articulated lumbar vertebrae. B = Body of the vertebra; SC = spinal column; IVF = intervertebral foramen; IF = inferior articular facet; SF = superior articular facet; P = pedicle; TP = transverse process; SP = spinous process; L = lamina; AF = anulus fibrosus; NP = nucleus pulposus; CP = cartilage plate; ALL = anterior longitudinal ligament; PLL = posterior longitudinal ligament; LF = ligamentum flavum; IL = interspinous ligament.

around the margins of the vertebral bodies and lend strong support to the discs, except posteriorly on either side of the midline, where their fibers are much attenuated or nonexistent. In contrast to the anterior ligaments, which can be easily separated from the underlying anulus fibrosus, the posterior longitudinal ligament is strongly attached to the annulus fibers. Additional support is provided by the ligamentum flavum, an elastic structure that bridges the interlaminar spaces and reinforces the facet joint capsules, and the interspinous, inter-transverse, and iliolumbar ligaments.

Embryology

The anlage of the spine forms in a right and left column on each side of the primitive notochord, just anterior to the neural tube. At a later stage of development, the two halves fuse anteriorly and posteriorly around the developing spinal cord. A failure of this process accounts for the frequent incidence of fusion defects, various degrees of spina bifida when posteriorly, and various degrees of platyspondylisis and butterfly vertebrae when anteriorly. Anterior fusion defects are much rarer than posterior defects.

At the same time, the vertebrae are formed, also from a fusion of two embryonic parts in another plane, that is, the inferior portion of one sclerotome with the subjacent superior part of another. Disturbances of this stage of development produce incomplete and asymmetric segmentation and hemivertebrae.

As the lateral halves of the vertebral body fuse in the midline, the notochord is forced superiorly and inferiorly, where its remnants concentrate to aid in the formation of the nucleus pulposus. This process, when imperfect, leads to defects in the cartilaginous plates. The annulus fibrosus, which encloses the nucleus pulposus, originates in the mesenchyme left as the cephalad and caudad portions of the sclerotome separate to form the vertebral bodies.

Sacrum and Pelvis

The anatomic details of the sacrum do not warrant special description. The articulation between it and the fifth lumbar vertebra follows the pattern previously described. The sacrum articulates with the pelvis by means of the two sacroiliac joints, which are partly fibrous and partly diarthrodial. The surfaces of the fibrous portion of these joints are irregular and fit closely together. The female pelvis has less bony apposition than the male, and the ligaments are stronger. The cartilaginous surface of the sacrum is thicker and hyaline, that of the ilium thinner and fibrous. In both sexes, some motion can and does take place, but with the ex-

ception of the late stages of pregnancy, the range is small and physiologically insignificant. The motion is in a rotary plane and is resisted in one direction by the wedge shape of the sacrum and in the other by the sacrotuberous and sacrospinous ligaments. Increased compensatory motion can occur at the sacroiliac joints in patients who have had surgical fusions of the lumbar spine. Because the joint is supported by some of the densest ligaments of the body, it is doubtful that sacroiliac strain or ''slipping'' can occur without extensive injury, pregnancy, or disease. That portion of the joint lined, although imperfectly, by synovium is subject to all the diseases of diarthrodial joints, however, and is a common site of involvement for arthritic disease, whether infectious, rheumatoid, or degenerative.

Coccyx

This part is composed of four segments, the first one of which is often free from the others. Motion can and does take place between the sacrum and the coccyx. This joint has little ligamentous support and it is vulnerable to injury, but its anatomic situation protects it.

Neural Structures

The neural arch of each vertebra encloses the spinal cord, together with its supporting structures. Originally, the distal end of the spinal cord extends to the caudal end of the dural sac at about the level of the third sacral segment, but it retracts superiorly as the spine grows in length to reach a final adult position at the level of the first lumbar vertebra. The nerve roots of the lumbosacral plexus are drawn up with the spinal cord and lie within the dura, to form the cauda equina. A slender filament, the filum terminale, loosely anchors the distal end of the spinal cord to the coccyx. Cephalad, the spinal cord is held by its origin from the brain. It is also fixed by the succession of spinal nerves, which pass out through the intervertebral foramina. It is supported everywhere by its dural and arachnoidal membranes. Over this immobile neural tube, the spinal segments must move smoothly to perform their physiologic functions.

Each nerve root leaves the spinal canal inferior to its corresponding vertebral arch, except in the cervical spine, where it leaves superiorly. That is, the first cervical nerve root passes out superior to the first cervical vertebral arch, whereas the fifth lumbar nerve root leaves the canal inferior to the fifth lumbar vertebral arch. The difference is made up by the presence of eight cervical nerves, as opposed to seven cervical vertebrae, the eighth cervical nerve passing out of the intervertebral foramen between C7 and T1.

A nerve root is in an intimate relationship with several parts of the vertebra and discs as it passes from the dural sac to outside the neural canal. In the lower lumbar spine, each nerve root, together with a sheath of dura, becomes separated from the remainder of the cauda equina at the level of the superior disc, courses laterally as it passes distally across its corresponding vertebral body, and reaches the intervertebral foramen at a point opposite its disc of the same numerical designation. For instance, the fifth lumbar nerve leaves the cauda equina just superior to the level of the fourth lumbar disc (the disc between L4 and L5) and passes diagonally laterally, posterior to the fifth lumbar body to reach the intervertebral foramen between L5 and the sacrum. In the foramen, it is held against the medial and inferior surfaces of the pedicle (in this case, of L5) lying in a groove called the sulcus nervi spinalis. Anteriorly lies the body (of L5), inferiorly the bulging fifth lumbar disc, and posteriorly, shielded by ligamentum flavum, the inferior facet (of L5). Although the nerve root moves freely in the intervertebral foramen, pathologic or traumatic disturbances of any of these structures (pedicle, body, or facet) can obstruct its passage and may cause pressure. More recently, transforaminal ligaments, reducing available space for passage of the nerve root through the lumbar intervertebral foramina, have been described. The extradural courses of the lower lumbar nerve roots are related to two discs: the one superior to and the one inferior to their corresponding vertebrae.

Vascular Supply

Arnoldi reported that interosseous hypertension may be a cause of lumbar spine pain.[2] The blood supply of the lumbar spine is derived from four lumbar arteries, arising in pairs from the abdominal aorta and traversing close to the anterior and lateral portions of the vertebral bodies.[8] The middle sacral artery, a small vessel, arises from the back of the aorta superior to the bifurcation and occasionally produces a fifth pair of segmental vessels. Each lumbar artery divides into three main branches: anterior, intermediate, and posterior.

The anterior branches supply the abdominal wall. The intermediate branches divide and supply mainly the neural structures, including the nerve roots and the cauda equina. The posterior branches come in contact with the laminae and enter the sacrospinalis muscles. The division of the segmental arteries occurs at the "distribution point" at the level of the intervertebral foramina. This anatomic landmark is important when anterior spinal surgical procedures are contemplated.

The veins draining the vertebral column form intricate plexuses, which may be divided into external and internal, according to their position inside or outside the vertebral canal. Lumbar veins accompany the lumbar arteries and drain into the venae cavae and the left common iliac vein. Through ascending lumbar veins, drainage continues into the lumbar azygous or hemiazygous system. Because the vertebral plexuses have few valves and communicate with veins in the body wall and pelvis, they are a potential pathway by which metastasis from other areas may involve the vertebral column. Variations in pressure on arteries, veins, and capillaries may interfere with nerve conduction.

BIOMECHANICAL CONSIDERATIONS

In utero, the spine is formed in one long curve, with its convexity directed posteriorly. After birth and with the gradual assumption of vertical posture, this curve is altered. Because of the immobility of the thoracic segment and because of its attached ribs, the kyphosis (curve with convexity posteriorly) persists in this area. As strength develops to allow the infant to raise his head and then to sit and finally to stand, however, lordoses (curves with their convexities directed anteriorly) develop first in the cervical segment and then in the lumbar segment. By this means, balance is achieved, and the weight of the trunk is carried directly over its base. As long as the curves anteriorly and posteriorly balance each other, the erect position can be maintained with surprisingly little muscular effort. The lordotic curves are entirely functional and can be reversed by bending forward, in contrast to the kyphotic thoracic curve, which is structural.

Two essential forces are responsible for the development of these curves. One is the anterior tilt of the pelvis produced by the downward pull of the iliopsoas muscles and the hip capsules, and the other is the extending force of the massive erector spinae muscle. Once the spine is balanced in the erect position, however, the muscular forces in various directions become purely stabilizing. Thus, if the normal erect posture is not disturbed, it is possible to stand with little or no muscular effort, and the ligaments act mainly as check-reins to prevent excessive motion.

Lordosis of the lumbar spine varies among different races, age groups, and sexes. Standardized values of lumbar lordosis in the normal population for these different groups are not available. An average value for the "lumbosacral angle" is about 135°[20] (Fig. 82–2). Of course, the angle depends on the load on the spine and the position at the time of measurement, whether recumbent, sitting, or standing.

Because of the relative fixation of the pelvis, the

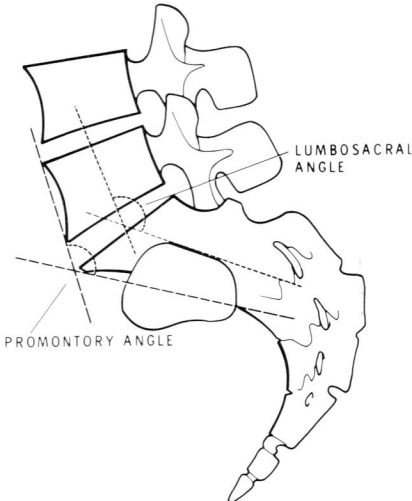

LUMBOSACRAL ANGLE

PROMONTORY ANGLE

Fig. 82–2. The angle between L5 and the sacrum is commonly known as the *lumbosacral angle*, obtained by measuring the intersection of two lines drawn through the midbodies of L5 and the sacrum and perpendicular to their end plates. The intersection of vertical lines parallel to the anterior border of L5 and the sacrum is known as the promontory angle.

lumbosacral junction is subject to a high level of stress. Axial compression can cause flexion, lateral bend, and rotation. Similarly, deformation such as lateral bend may cause rotation, flexion, and axial compression. Most important, depending on the lumbosacral angle, such forces promote shear. The amount of shear is related to the stiffness of the area. The load on the third lumbar disc is four times greater in an upright than in a recumbent patient. This load becomes six times greater when the patient is standing and is partially bent forward. More recently, lumbar disc pressure and myoelectric activity of spinal muscles have been recorded in subjects in different sitting positions.[1] In the lumbar spine, motion is largely flexion and extension. On bending forward, lumbar lordosis is reversed, and on extension, it is increased. Lateral inclination and rotation occur mainly at the thoracolumbar junction.

Generally speaking, muscles that lie anterior to the small posterior articulations, especially the abdominal muscles, act as flexors, and those posterior act as extensors. The actions of the muscle groups on one side result in lateral inclination. Rotation is produced by more complex muscle combinations. Because many of the spinal motions are performed in the erect position, however, the force of gravity cannot be discounted, and once the motion is started, the opposing muscles are called into play to prevent loss of balance. For instance, on bending to the right, the muscles on the left side of the spine

must act to prevent falling to the right. This description of function represents a great oversimplification of spinal kinesiology, but it serves as a basis for understanding the principles discussed elsewhere in this chapter.

PHYSIOLOGICAL CONSIDERATIONS

Another basic consideration is the source and character of the pain itself. Pain from deep skeletal structures and pain from direct nerve pressure must be differentiated. Almost everyone is familiar with direct nerve pressure as the "funny or crazy bone" sensation when the ulnar nerve is suddenly bumped. Faradic stimulation of a peripheral mixed nerve causes the same sensation. The onset of pain is rapid; it follows the distribution of the sensory portion of the ulnar nerve and is associated with numbness and tingling when severe. Stimulation of a single spinal nerve root produces a sensation that is the same in character, but is confined to the peripheral representation or dermatome of that nerve root. The pain is sharp, lancinating, and accompanied by paresthesia and numbness. It may also be accompanied by muscle cramps. This condition is *"neuralgia."*

If the pressure is severe and prolonged, the nerve will be deadened, and the property of conduction will be lost even though the fibers are still in continuity. The larger nerve fibers, which mediate touch and motor stimuli, lose their function first, followed by the progressively smaller nerve fibers. Pain fibers, although both large and small, are in general smaller than those for touch and motor conduction, and their function may be unimpaired if pressure is relieved soon enough.

The foregoing properties hold only for sudden forceful pressure on a nerve. In the case of gradual or intermittent pressure, the stimulus may not be sufficient at any time to excite the nerve tissue, and its presence may remain undetected until paresis develops. Such is frequently the case in gradually developing gibbus consequent to tuberculosis.

The pain produced by stimuli within deep skeletal structures, such as ligaments, fascia, muscle, and periosteum, is different. Here the pain is vaguely localized, aching in character, radiating over great distances, slow in onset, and long in duration. When severe, it is often accompanied by sweating, nausea, and vomiting. The patterns of radiation are consistent for one point of stimulation, but the extent of radiation depends on the intensity of stimulation. According to results of experiments, the pattern of radiation is consistent from one individual to another. Although these "sclerotomes" appear to have a segmental representation, they do not follow the patterns of corresponding dermatomes. The sclerotome and dermatome coincide more nearly in the midportion of the trunk than they do in the extremities.

The pain thresholds of different somatic structures are variable. The periosteum is most sensitive, followed by ligaments and fibrous joint capsules, tendons, fascia, and muscle. Ligaments and capsules are particularly sensitive at points close to their osseous attachments. Bone is usually insensitive, although its endosteal surface apparently contains some pain-perceptive nerves.

The difference between this "deep" pain and the "superficial" pain of skin is important. This difference can be readily demonstrated by pinching a small piece of skin (superficial pain) and by squeezing a web space between the fingers (deep pain). This simple experiment is not completely accurate because touching the skin helps to localize the deep pain elicited. Experimental evidence suggests that the more superficially situated deep structures allow accurate localization of a pain source. Thus, stimulation of periosteum overlying the subcutaneous surface of the tibia can be identified accurately by the subject. Pain from deeply situated periosteum, however, as in the spine, is poorly localized and is diffuse, with radiation to areas distant from the source.

Various kinds of pain may be mediated by changes in the intervertebral disc itself and may result from a decrease in pH or leakage of connective tissue breakdown products. Naylor et al. have reported that lysosomal enzymes present in the nucleus pulposus of the prolapsed intervertebral disc degrade protein polysaccharides,[17] and they postulated a possible autoimmune basis for these biochemical changes. Others have suggested a cellular immune response in patients who have sequestrated discs.[12] The relationship of pain originating from pathologic intervertebral discs with local biochemical changes needs further investigation.

MEDICAL HISTORY AND PHYSICAL EXAMINATION

A general appraisal should include sex, age, race, economic and social background, family and past medical history, and a general review. The patient's type of work and daily habits are important.

Analysis of the Patient's Pain

An analysis of the pain should proceed along two lines: one concerned with the chronologic aspect, such as onset, development, and reaction to previous treatment, the other with the character of this pain. Chronologically, one should ascertain when and where the pain began. Was its onset associated with injury or illness? If the patient was injured, was it on the job or involving liability? Has the pain remained the same, worsened, or lessened? Is it intermittent, or has the patient had periods of amelioration or exacerbation? Has the site of pain changed, or has it extended to involve hitherto painless areas? Have any aggravating incidents occurred since its onset? Has the patient had any kind of treatment, self-administered or otherwise, and with what effect?

The character of the pain may be analyzed in various ways, as follows:

1. *Severity,* an individually variable factor that should be interpreted with caution. Useful indices include inability to work, confinement to bed, and sleeplessness.

2. *Quality,* which is variable and depends much on previous experience. Therefore, its usefulness is questionable. One should differentiate somatic from nerve root pain insofar as possible.

3. *Localization,* a most important criterion, although it is often difficult for the patient to locate the pain accurately. A point of origin is usually recognized. Distal radiation is often present. The extent of radiation in many instances may be used as a rough index of the severity of the lesion. The type of radiation should be distinguished again, whether it is a nerve root type or the vaguely localized, deep, aching pain so characteristic of irritation of skeletal structures.

4. *Duration,* whether steady or intermittent. If steady, is it at all times the same, or does it have periods of exacerbation? If intermittent, at what times does pain seem to occur? Is it a night or early morning pain suggesting a joint source? Is it a pain associated with work or with activity, suggesting strain, or does it occur only during certain movements?

5. *Reduplication,* either by the patient or by some technique of examination.

6. *Aggravation.* Is the pain aggravated by coughing or sneezing or by bending or lifting, and if so, is it reproduced in full or only in part?

7. *Alleviation.* Is the pain relieved by rest or by any particular types of medication? Is it relieved by manipulation, by gentle activity, or by vigorous exercise?

General Physical Appraisal

In general, it is sufficient to note whether the individual is stocky and heavy-set with heavy musculature, strong ligaments, and tight joints, or whether he is sthenic, tall, and lithe, with a relaxed joint structure, ligaments, and muscles. Are the legs well aligned? Are the feet pronated? Are the knees bowed, straight, or in some valgus position? Are abnormal or suggestive skin pigmentations visible? A café-au-lait mark may signify an underlying neurofibromatosis.

If, in taking the patient's medical history, any points of suspicion have come up relative to systemic diseases, these should be investigated before proceeding with the specific examination of the back.

Stance and Posture

The posterior aspect of the back is first viewed. It should be noted whether the iliac crests are level, whether the spine is straight or curved, and whether the patient lists to one side or the other. Humans have a strong reflex to keep the head centered over the feet and the eyes level. Thus, in the normal individual, a deviation of the spinal column from the vertical is compensated by an opposite deviation elsewhere whenever possible (Fig. 82–3). From the point of view of the spine, full compensation signifies that the first thoracic vertebra is centered over the sacrum, no matter what the spine does in between. If the spine is uncompensated, that is, if the first thoracic vertebra is not centered over the sacrum, the patient is spoken of as having a *list*. A convenient measurement of list is to drop a perpendicular line from the first thoracic spine and to measure how far to right or left of the gluteal cleft it falls. If a list is present, a lateral curvature

of the spine (scoliosis) must also be present. Scoliosis may be classified as structural or nonstructural. In the former, intrinsic structural changes of the vertebral column and thoracic rib cage are present and may be detected by asking the patient to bend forward and by viewing the trunk from posteriorly. Asymmetry is then noted, with the high side on the convex side of the curve. In nonstructural scoliosis, no intrinsic anatomic changes occur, and no asymmetry is found on forward bending. Nonstructural scoliosis commonly occurs secondary to pain and may be termed "sciatic scoliosis."

Scoliosis is designated right or left, depending on the direction of its convexity; right scoliosis indicates a curve convex to the right. The curve pattern of the scoliosis is designated by the apex of the curve. A thoracic curve has its apex at the thoracic level; a thoracolumbar curve has its apex at the junction of the thoracic and lumbar spine; and a lumbar curve has its apex at the lumbar level. Usually, the pelvis is level in nonstructural and structural scoliosis. If not, some other causes for the pelvic obliquity should be sought, such as a gross decompensation of the curves or a short leg or a hip contracture.

The patient is then viewed from the side, and the posture is noted. It is normal to stand with a

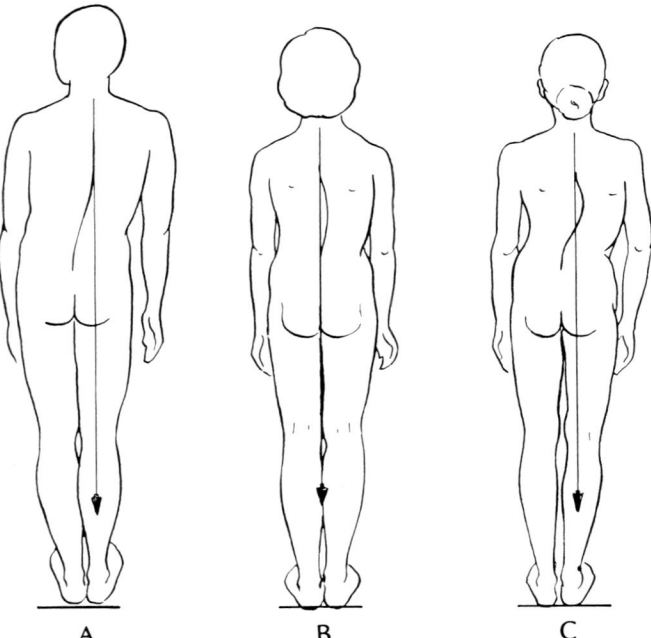

Fig. 82–3. Compensated and uncompensated deviations of posture. *A*, A plumb line dropped from the first thoracic spinal process indicates a right list. *B*, A compensated right thoracolumbar scoliosis. *C*, An uncompensated right thoracic, left lumbar scoliosis with right list. List or decompensation causes prominence of the hip opposite to the direction of the list.

slight degree of lumbar lordosis and thoracic kyphosis. Increase or decrease of these curves should be noted. Muscle spasm in acute low back pain often causes flattening of the lumbar lordosis. In the sagittal plane, as well as in the transverse plane, man usually maintains balance, that is, has the head centered over the feet. The curves in between generally balance one another. Thus, if the thoracic kyphosis is increased, the lumbar lordosis is usually increased. Sometimes, such a state of affairs does not exist, and to balance an increased thoracic kyphosis, the patient stands with a posterior *overcarriage*, that is, leaning backward. Overcarriage is to the sagittal plane what list is to the transverse.

The degree of forward inclination of the pelvis should be noted. Is the abdomen pendulous and is the chest well developed, or does the patient stand with a narrow anteroposterior thoracic diameter? Persons of the thin body type often have a narrow chest, and those of the heavy body type often have just the opposite.

An analysis of stance is completed by a brief survey from anteriorly. Again, list may be noted, and the anterior superior iliac spines should be palpated to check whether the pelvis is level. Slight degrees of curvature of the spine are difficult to detect, especially in heavy-set individuals. Certain signs may lead one to suspect the presence of a structural scoliosis, that is, a prominent hip, a flank crease on one side or the other, prominence of one side of the chest or of the opposite shoulder blade, or a high shoulder.

Spinal Motions

The spine is now analyzed in motion (Figs. 82–4, 82–5). One again views the patient from posteriorly. He is asked to bend forward. The lordotic curve of the lumbar spine should first flatten and should then reverse slightly as the degree of forward bending increases. If it does not do so, motion will be limited, even though the patient is able to touch the floor. The patient should be watched to see whether he bends straight forward or whether he lists to one side as he bends forward. Listing may suggest restriction of straight-leg raising on the opposite side. If scoliosis has been detected in the erect position, the flexed position should be checked to determine whether it is structural. The associated rotation of the vertebrae produces a prominence of the thorax and overlying scapula on the side of convexity. In lumbar scoliosis, the rotation is not so readily evident, but it can be detected by prominence of the paravertebral muscles on the side of the convexity and a depression of those on the opposite side. In patients with a slight degree of scoliosis, forward flexion is the best position for detection because it accentuates the deformity. When the patient is bent forward, it is also wise to view his back from the side. Usually, one sees a smooth curve with its convexity posteriorly extending from the base of the skull to the sacrum. If the curve is broken and becomes more sharply angular at any point, it should be recorded. Such is often the case in structural round back, that is, ''epiphysitis'' of the spine.

Fig. 82–4. Measurement of spinal motion. *A*, Zero starting position, the correct standing position. *B*, Flexion. Four clinical methods of estimating the range of spinal flexion are used: (1) by measuring the degrees of forward inclination of the trunk in relation to the longitudinal axis of the body; the examiner should ''fix'' the pelvis with his hands; the loss (or not) of lordosis should also be noted; (2) by indicating the level the fingertips reach along the patient's leg; for instance, fingertips to the patella or fingertips to the midtibia; (3) by measuring the distance in inches or centimeters between the fingertips and the floor; and (4) by the steel or plastic tape measure method. *C*, The steel tape measure method (4), perhaps the most accurate clinical method of measuring true motion of the spine in flexion. The flexible steel or plastic tape adjusts accurately to the thoracic and lumbar contours of the spine. *D*, As the patient bends forward, the reversal of the lumbar curve and the spread of the spinous processes can be indicated by lengthening the tape measure. The normal healthy adult has an average increase of 4 inches in forward flexion. If the patient bends forward with his back straight (as in ankylosing spondylitis), the tape measure will not record motion. One is able to record motion of the thoracic spine itself by taping from the spinous process of C7 to T12. Similarly, motion of the lumbar spine can be measured from the spinous process of T12 to S1. Usually, if the increase in the total spine in flexion is 4 inches, the examiner will find that 1 inch occurs in the dorsal spine and 3 inches occur in the lumbar spine. *E* and *F*, Lateral bending. The vertical steel tape, if held firmly and straight, may also aid in measuring the motion of lateral bending. This can be estimated by: (1) the degrees of lateral inclination of the trunk; (2) noting the position of spinous process of C7 with relation to the pelvis; (3) using the level of lumbar spine as a reflection of the base of lateral motion; this level may be lumbosacral or higher and may vary from right to left in the same patient; and (4) using the knee joint as a fixed point; one should record the distance of the fingertips from the knee joint on lateral bending. *G*, Extension standing. The range of extension is recorded by degrees. *H*, Extension lying prone. The range of motion in this position is measured by degrees, in relation to the position of the spinous process of C7.

THE DORSAL AND LUMBAR SPINE (FLEXION)

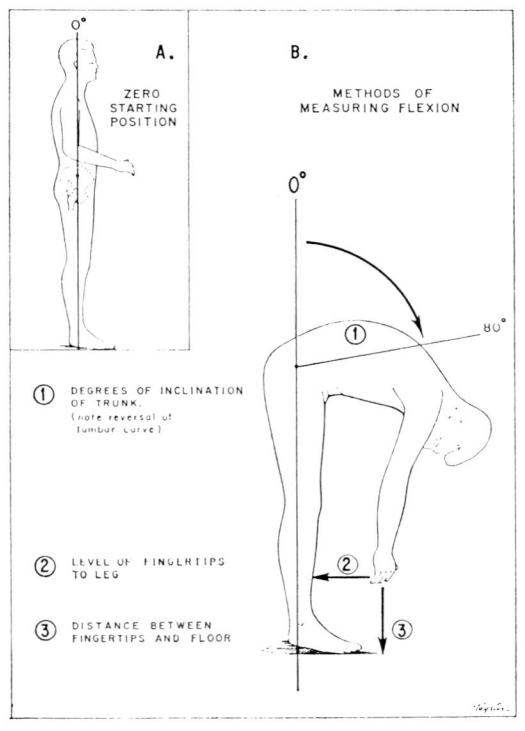

A. ZERO STARTING POSITION

B. METHODS OF MEASURING FLEXION

① DEGREES OF INCLINATION OF TRUNK.
(note reversal of lumbar curve)

② LEVEL OF FINGERTIPS TO LEG

③ DISTANCE BETWEEN FINGERTIPS AND FLOOR

(Contination)
METHODS OF MEASURING SPINAL FLEXION

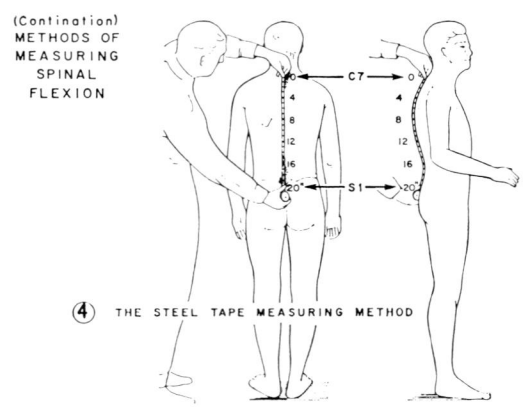

④ THE STEEL TAPE MEASURING METHOD

C. THE PATIENT STANDING ERECT

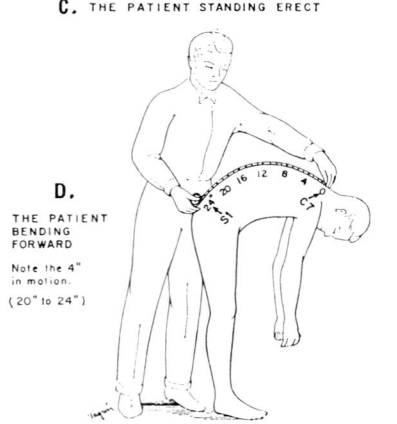

D. THE PATIENT BENDING FORWARD
Note the 4" in motion.
(20" to 24")

THE DORSAL AND LUMBAR SPINE
LATERAL BENDING

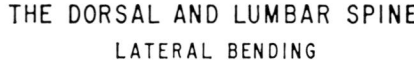

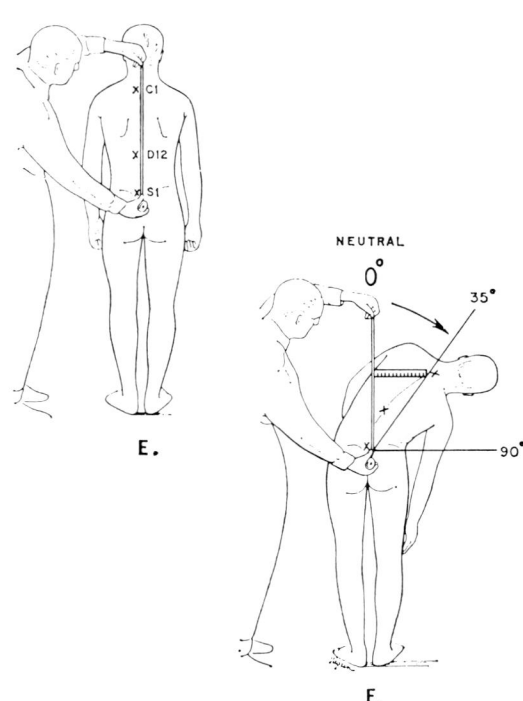

E.

NEUTRAL

F.

THE DORSAL AND LUMBAR SPINE (EXTENSION)

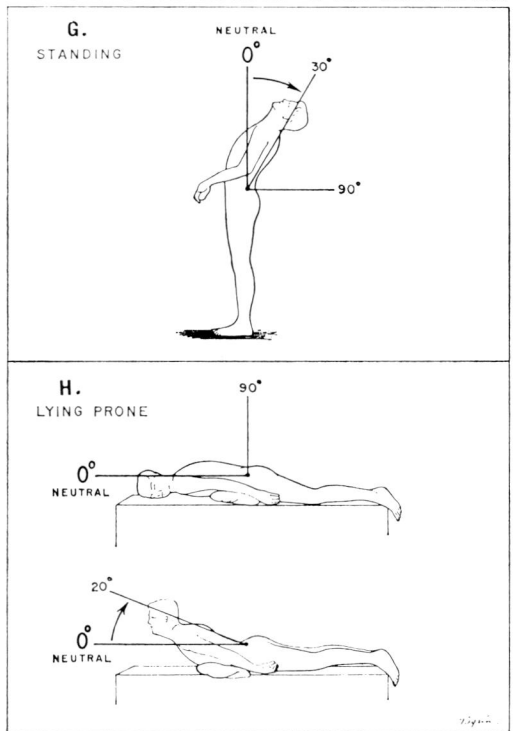

G. STANDING

NEUTRAL

H. LYING PRONE

I. THE SPINE — ROTATION

Fig. 82–4 (Cont.). *I,* Rotation. To estimate the degrees of rotation of the spine, the pelvis must be held firmly by the examiner's hands, and the patient is instructed to rotate to the right or left. This motion is recorded in degrees, or in percentages of motion, as compared to individuals of similar age and physical build.

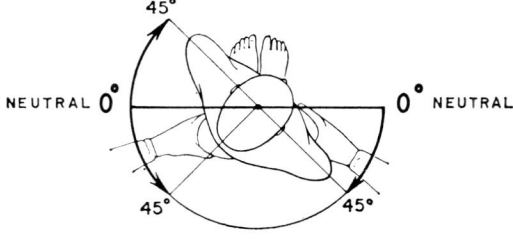

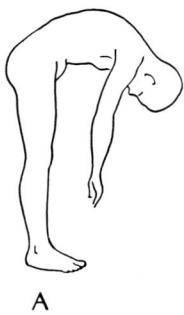 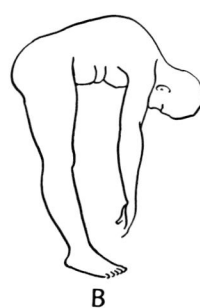 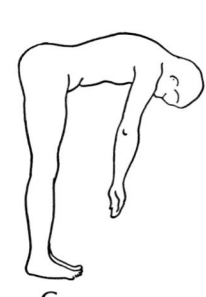 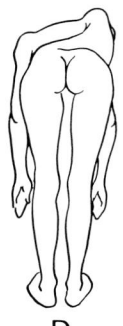

A   B   C   D

Fig. 82–5. Forward bending. *A,* Normally on forward bending, one sees an even contour of the spine when viewed laterally. *B,* An accentuation of the thoracic kyphosis indicates a thoracic round back, especially when the apex of the curve is sharp and angular. *C,* A persistence of the angular lordotic curve in the position of forward bending indicates that the lumbar spine has lost its flexibility. The flexion is all taking place at the hip joints. *D,* When viewed posteriorly, minor degrees of structural scoliosis can readily be detected in the position of forward bending. The convex rotation of the thoracic vertebrae is easily recognized because it is accentuated by the rib deformity or hump. Similar rotation of the lumbar segment is more difficult to detect.

The degree of backward bending is then determined. This bending is accompanied by an increase in the lordotic curve. If the degree of lordosis does not increase, the motion is limited. On returning to the upright position, the patient is asked to bend to one side and then to the other. The normal spine has an equivalent degree of bending to both sides with a smooth curve starting at the sacrum. Limitation of motion can be detected in one of two ways. The maximal degree of motion may not be as much to one side as to the other, or the curve on bending to one side may be broken and may begin at a higher level than it does to the other side.

In examination of the lower back, the motions of flexion, extension, and lateral bending are the most important. It is often wise, however, to check the whole spine, and the patient should be asked to demonstrate the degree of rotation by lacing his fingers behind his neck. This motion occurs chiefly in the thoracic region. The degree of cervical lordosis and cervical motions should also be noted. The findings are rechecked in the sitting position, where normally the lordosis flattens and scoliosis, if functional, disappears.

Measurements

The patient is next asked to lie supine on the examining table. A patient in acute pain can be made more comfortable if a pillow is placed under the knees. Measurements of the thigh and calf at equivalent points superior and inferior to the patellae should be made and recorded. Atrophy may be due to disuse or to neuromuscular disease. The patient is next carefully positioned so that the pelvis is level and the hips are placed in a neutral degree of abduction and adduction. The leg lengths are then recorded, using the bony landmarks of the anterior superior iliac spine and medial malleolus. In the presence of a fixed deformity of one hip, the measurement loses some significance. For measurements to be accurate, the lower extremities must have equivalent relationships with the pelvis.

Hip Motions

The hip movements are now analyzed (Fig. 82–6). Flexion contracture is noted by maximally flexing the opposite hip to flatten the lumbar lordosis and by measuring the degree of the angle between the horizontal surface of the table and the maximally extended extremity. The movements of

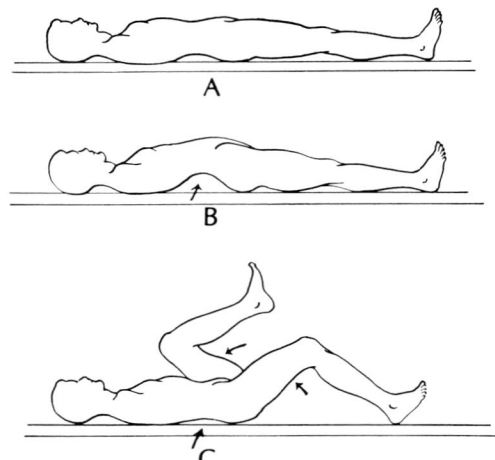

Fig. 82–6. Lumbar lordosis and hip flexion contracture. An inability to fully extend one or both hips may produce an increase in the lumbar lordosis in the standing or lying positions. The angle of the deformity can be determined by flattening the lordosis, by maximum flexion of the opposite hip. *A,* Normal. *B,* Flexion deformity of the hip masked by an increase in the lumbar lordosis. *C,* Flexion of the opposite hip flattening the lumbar spine to the table and indicating the true situation.

each hip in abduction, adduction, and internal and external rotation should be measured. The arcs of rotation are usually most easily obtained by rotating the foot and leg inward (external rotation) and outward (internal rotation) with the hips flexed to 90°.

Passive Spinal Movements

Movements of the lumbar spine are now performed passively by grasping the patient's legs with the knees bent and by flexing the spine maximally. With the patient's hips flexed to 90°, the pelvis is then inclined laterally and is rotated on the spine. Note is made if these motions produce pain.

Palpation and Tenderness

The patient is next asked to lie prone with a pillow under his abdomen (Fig. 82–7). The thickness of the pillow should be sufficient to flatten the lumbar lordosis. The lower spine and the structures of the back are carefully palpated. Tightness or spasm of paravertebral muscles is noted. At all times, the patient must be fully relaxed. Just as in examination of the abdomen, the anatomic structures under the examining finger must constantly be kept in mind. The spine of each lumbar vertebra is pressed, and the interspaces between are palpated. It is sometimes advantageous to examine the flexed patient lying on his side, to palpate more easily the bony spinous processes and the inter-

spinous ligaments. Adjacent spinous processes can be grasped from the side by the examiner and can be rotated in opposite directions to determine the source of pain. Useful landmarks are the iliac crests, a horizontal line from which usually runs across the fourth lumbar process, and the posterior superior iliac spines, which lie opposite the second sacral spine. The sacrosciatic notch is palpated when tenderness may indicate irritation of one or more roots of the sciatic nerve. The patient's thighs and calves must also be palpated when pain extends into the legs. The region of the trochanters should also be examined.

Percussion Tenderness

Pressure or percussion over the interlaminal spaces may, in patients with disc herniation, produce sharp, lancinating pain radiating to the lower extremities. Because lumbar lordosis is increased in the position of extension, the vertebral spinous processes are brought closer together, and it is difficult to distinguish the separate processes. For this reason, it is most important to have the patient's back flattened or the lumbar lordosis reversed. If this effect cannot be achieved in the prone position with a pillow under the abdomen, the patient may be asked to bend over the examining table (Fig. 82–8). He can usually do this despite the presence of pain, if the knees are flexed and the weight is borne on the abdomen.

Rectal Examination

A rectal examination is usually advisable, especially in patients with coccygeal pain. The coccyx may be grasped between the finger in the rectum and the thumb outside, and it can be moved about. One should note the angle of inclination of the coccyx, its freedom of movement, and the presence of pain on movement. The levator ani and coccygeus muscles and the sacrotuberous and sacrospinalis ligaments are palpated on either side of the sacrum, and tenderness is noted. In thin individuals, the region of the sacrosciatic notch can often be reached, and bimanual palpation of this region is possible. The rectal examination is completed with palpation of the pelvic viscera. Tenderness in the sacroiliac joint may be elicited by pressure exerted over it. This joint lies between the posterior inferior spine and superior border of the sciatic notch. Bimanual vaginal examination with cytologic smear should be performed when indicated.

Neurologic Examination

It is important to analyze the knee and ankle jerks. The best position for eliciting knee jerks is with the patient sitting with the legs hanging free;

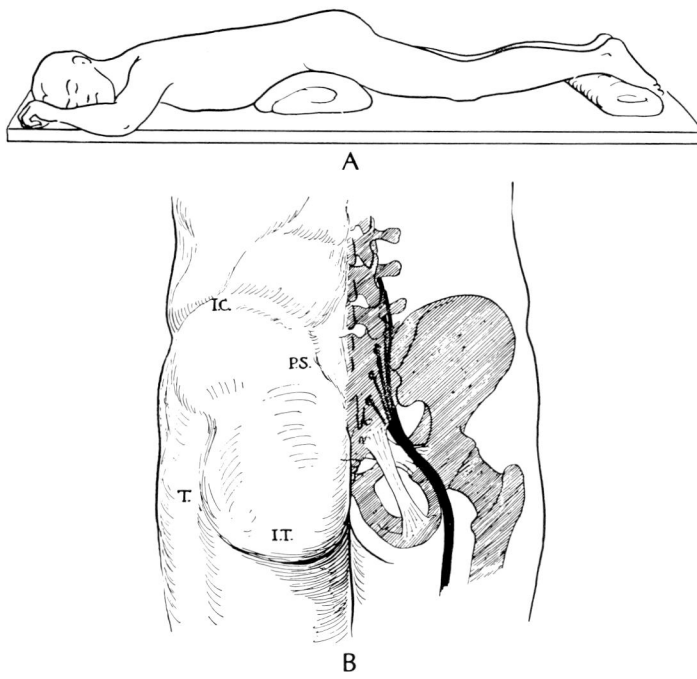

Fig. 82–7. Palpation of the back. *A*, Proper positioning is necessary for adequate examination. When the lumbar spine is flat, the bony elements are more easily distinguished from one another. The interspinous and interlaminal spaces are opened. *B*, Useful landmarks include the iliac crest (I.C.), the posterior superior iliac spine (P.S.), the greater trochanters (T.), and the ischial tuberosities (I.T.). The position of the sacrosciatic notch and the course of the sciatic nerve should be kept in mind. The lumbar roots are shielded from palpation in their extraspinal course.

that for ankle jerks is with the patient kneeling on a chair with a pillow under the legs and the feet projecting outward from the edge of the seat. If necessary, the reflexes can be reinforced if the patient contracts the muscles of the upper extremities with the fingers locked together. In reflexes tested carefully in this fashion, small discrepancies are of much greater significance than when testing is done casually. Gluteus maximus, medial hamstring, and posterior tibial reflex responses should also be determined, but they are more difficult to elicit and, therefore, are most significant when absent on one side and present on the other. Babinski's sign is also tested.

Sensory examination is performed with the point of a pin and light stroke of the finger or cotton. Significant zones of sensory disturbance may be found in this manner, and if so, the examination can be repeated in more detail, including heat and cold sensation.

Atrophy of the buttocks is determined by inspection and palpation. Although atrophy of thigh and calf muscles may be seen, circumferential measurements are helpful to document the degree of atrophy and to follow the response to therapeutic exercises. The ability to walk on tiptoe and on the heel, the ability to do a deep knee bend, and the

ability to stand on one leg alone should be tested. The manner of walking should be observed, and the cause of limp, if one is present, should be determined. More accurate analysis of motor function is done by testing the strength of muscle action in various planes, but such an evaluation may be omitted for practical purposes unless some previous point of the patient's medical history or physical examination leads one to suspect nerve root compression. The power of dorsiflexion of the great toe, of the lateral four toes, and of the entire foot should be analyzed and should be compared on the two sides. Similarly, the forces of inversion, eversion, and plantar flexion of the foot and of the toes can be tested. Powers of hip flexion when sitting and of knee extension when supine are easily determined. When the patient is in pain or when movement is accompanied by pain, weakness of function should be given less significance. Moreover, the inability of some patients, especially older ones, to coordinate may interfere with muscle examinations of this kind.

Special Tests

Straight Leg Raising Test of Lasegue

This test is one of the most useful maneuvers in analysis of low back disorders (Fig. 82–9). First,

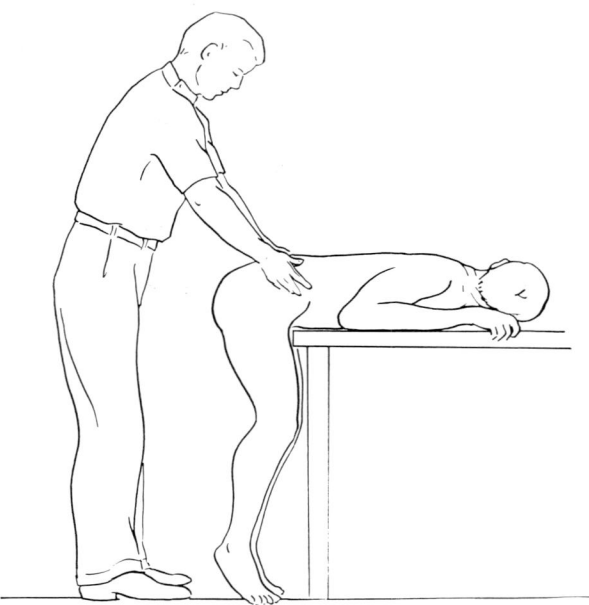

Fig. 82–8. Percussion test. With the patient positioned as shown, the interlaminal spaces are opened as much as possible. In the case of irritation of a nerve root, sharp percussion or deep pressure may reproduce the sciatic distribution of pain, especially in the presence of disc herniation because the nerve root is forced posteriorly in the spinal cord. This position is also useful for palpation of the back, particularly for examination of the sacroiliac joints.

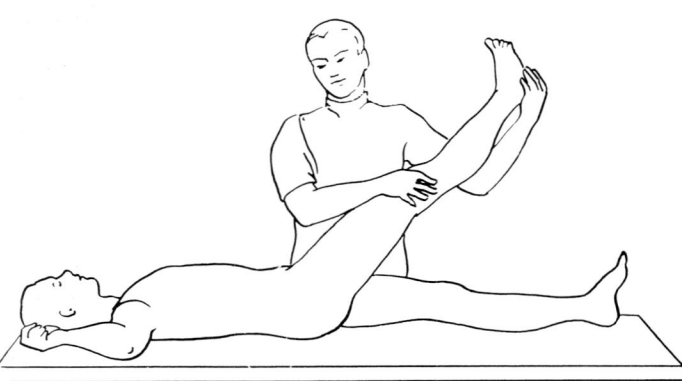

Fig. 82–9. Straight leg raising. The leg being tested should be relaxed and should rest in the examiner's hand. The knee is fully extended and is kept from flexing by gentle pressure against the patella.

it stretches the roots of the lumbosacral plexus by putting tension on the sciatic nerve, a tension that increases as the leg is raised higher. Second, it flattens the lumbar spine by putting tension on the extensor muscles of the hip and hamstrings as they pass from the pelvis to the femur and tibia. Thus, a nerve root lesion is not prerequisite for painful or restricted leg raising. On the other hand, restriction of straight leg raising is usually much more marked in lesions affecting the nerve roots than it is in purely skeletal disorders. The angle of straight leg raising, which is limited by tightness of the hamstring muscles, is normally less in sthenic than it is in asthenic individuals.

The test is performed by the examiner, and the patient must relax. The knee is held extended, and the leg is raised gradually from the table until the point of pain is reached. This point is recorded, and the patient is asked to describe the extent and radiation of the pain. In nerve root lesions, the typical pattern of radiation may be reproduced.

Sitting Knee Extension Test

While the patient is sitting, one knee is extended. The patient should be observed to see whether and at what angle of extension he leans backward. If the patient finds the test painful, he should be asked whether the pain is localized to his back or whether it radiates. The maneuver is repeated on the other side, and the two sides are then compared. Occasionally, extension of one knee aggravates "sciatica" in the opposite leg. This test is similar to straight leg raising, but with one major difference; that is, in the sitting position, the lumbar lordosis is usually largely obliterated.

Popliteal Compression Test

Radiating pain produced either by sitting knee extension or by straight leg raising can often be aggravated by pressure over the course of the tibial nerve through the popliteal space. This finding also suggests nerve root compression.

Jugular Compression Test (Naffziger Test)

This test should be performed whenever one suspects involvement of the spinal cord or nerve roots. A blood pressure cuff about the neck is inflated to 40 mm Hg and is held in place for a minute. The cerebrospinal fluid pressure is increased. The patient is asked to indicate when and if the pain is reproduced and if it is reproduced accurately. When the exact pattern of the patient's leg pain is reproduced, the test is practically pathognomonic of an intraspinal lesion. A negative test result, however, is not as significant.

Iliac Compression Test

Of all the tests described as pathognomonic of sacroiliac disease, the test of iliac compression is the most sensitive. It is performed most easily with the patient lying on his side. The examiner applies firm pressure against the uppermost iliac crest. When the test is positive, pain will be produced in the region of the involved, sacroiliac joint. Other signs of sacroiliac disease are pain in the region of that joint on passive abduction of one or both hips while flexed, tenderness along the superior bony margin of the sacroiliac notch, lower quadrant abdominal tenderness, and tenderness in the region of the joint on rectal examination. (See also Chap. 3 for the technique of determining tenderness in this joint.)

Passive Extension Test

This test is performed with the patient lying on his back at the foot of the examining table. The extremities are supported by the examiner with the hips and knees flexed. First, the uninvolved lower extremity is lowered. No pain is produced. The involved leg is then gradually lowered, to extend the spine, and pain develops. The unaffected extremity is then flexed maximally, thus flattening the lumbar spine, and the pain is relieved. If this test produces pain with radiation similar to that which the patient experiences spontaneously, it is suggestive of nerve root compression. Other lesions of the back, however, may be associated with pain on hyperextension.

The back examination is now finished. It requires considerable exertion by the patient and may not be possible to complete. After a day or two of rest and sedation, a more satisfactory analysis can often be made, however.

RADIOGRAPHIC EXAMINATION

A routine examination of the back is not complete unless roentgenograms have been made. To the trained observer, anteroposterior and lateral views of the entire lumbar spine and sacrum often suffice. First, anteroposterior and lateral views are made of the lumbar spine, with the x-ray tube centered at the upper lumbar region and inclined slightly distally (10°) (Fig. 82–10). A true or 45° anteroposterior view of the lumbosacral region is then obtained (Fig. 82–11). For this view, the direction of the x-ray tube is adjusted to the inclination of the sacrum. The actual angle of the tube is usually nearer 30° than 45°. The x-ray tube itself is centered opposite the third or fourth lumbar vertebra. Details of the vertebral bodies, the sacrum, and the sacroiliac and intervertebral joints should be adequate to detect significant abnormalities, including defects of the neural arch and facets.

Special roentgenographic views are used to obtain better detail of spinal parts or to detect the presence of specific pathologic processes. Oblique views show the intervertebral foramina and lesions of the neural arch and facets exceptionally well, but the technique is difficult (Fig. 82–12). A posteroanterior film made with the patient standing, bending first to the right and then to the left, is often helpful in diagnosing the level of a disc lesion. If the restriction of lateral movement is diffuse throughout the lumbar spine, such views are of no help, but if the restriction of lateral bending is confined to one disc space and to one side only, it suggests a pathologic condition at this level. Lateral roentgenograms of the lumbosacral spine in full flexion and extension are occasionally useful to demonstrate an anteroposterior instability in the early stages of disc degeneration, but they are mainly indicated for postoperative study of spinal lesions.

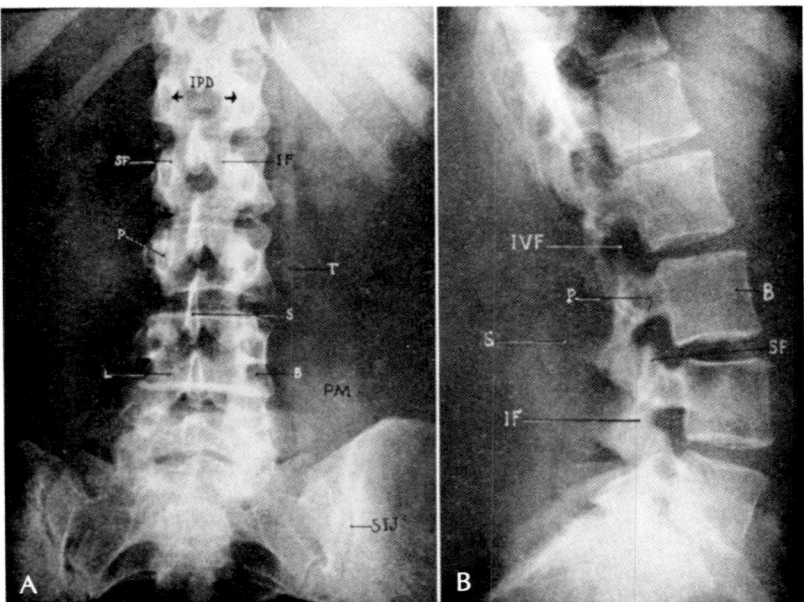

Fig. 82–10. Roentgenograms of the normal spine. *A*, Anteroposterior and *B*, lateral films of the lumbar spine. Note the detail of most of the lumbar spine, but the obscurity of the lumbosacral region. B = Body; D = disc space; I = isthmus or pars interarticularis; IF = inferior facet; IVF = intervertebral foramen; L = lamina; P = pedicle; PM = psoas margin; S = spinous process; SF = superior facet; SIJ = sacroiliac joint; T = transverse process; and IPD = interpedicular diameter.

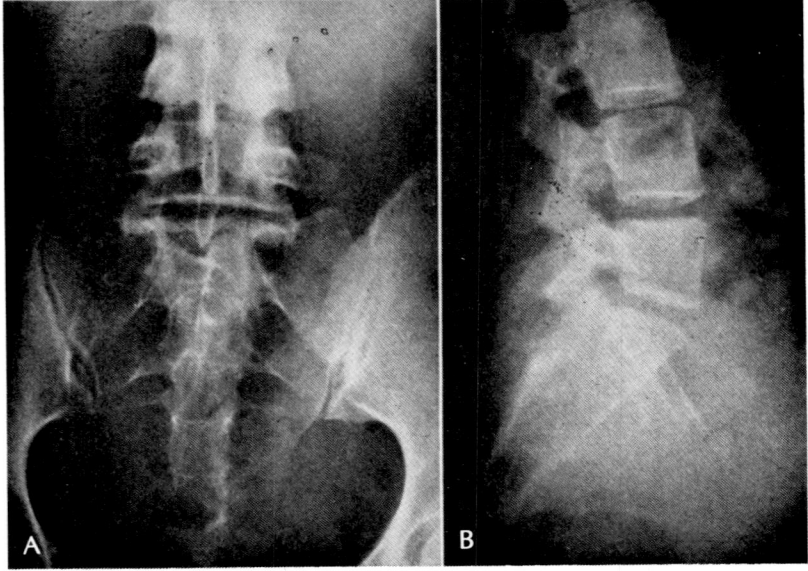

Fig. 82–11. Forty-five degree anteroposterior *(A)* and lateral *(B)* roentgenograms of the lumbosacral level and the sacrum. Note the detail of the fifth lumbar vertebra, sacrum, lumbosacral disc space, and sacroiliac joints.

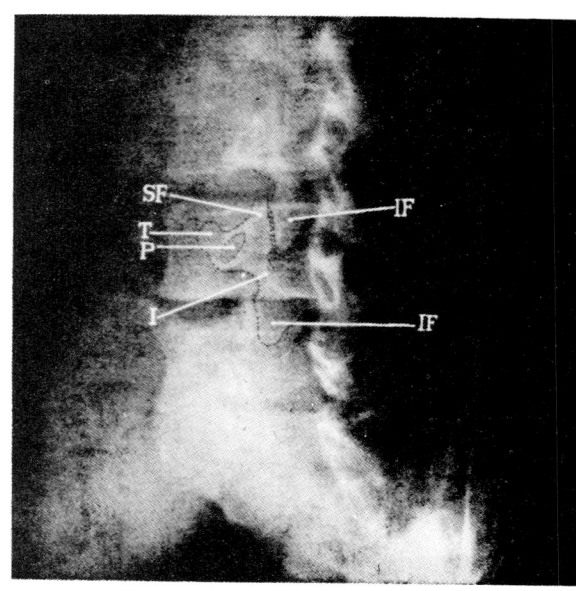

Fig. 82–12. Oblique roentgenogram of the lumbar spine. Note the detail of the facets and the pars interarticularis. SF = Superior facet; T = transverse process; P = pedicle; I = isthmus or pars interarticularis; and IF = inferior facet.

Myelography

Radiologic visualization of neural structures of the spinal canal is obtained by myelographic examination. Myelograms are used to determine compression of the spinal cord or nerve roots by tumor, intervertebral disc herniation, osteophyte formation, or other bony ridges. Complete blocks or narrowing of the neurocanal by spinal stenosis may also be seen. The accepted technique in the past was to introduce an oil-contrast medium into the subarachnoid space (Pantopaque myelography) (Fig. 82–13). The oil-contrast medium has a minimal immediate neurotoxic effect, but if allowed to remain in the spinal canal for extended periods, it may cause arachnoiditis. Consequently, at the end of the procedure the contrast material is generally removed. The dye is usually introduced by injection into the lower lumbar spine and may be used to visualize the neurocanal from the lumbar to the cervical spine. Few side effects occur other than transient headaches. The technique is safe when performed by experienced physicians. Usually, myelograms are indicated only when surgical treatment is considered.

Because oil has a high density, the nerve root sheaths may be incompletely filled. Water-soluble contrast agents have a lower viscosity and allow better filling of the nerve root sheaths. Such agents do not have to be removed because they are rapidly absorbed from the subarachnoid space. Recently a water-soluble medium, metrizamide, has been used (Fig. 82–14).

Metrizamide Myelography

Of the many water-soluble agents used as contrast media in myelography today, metrizamide

(Amipaque) is the most popular (Fig. 82–14). Metrizamide was developed by the Norwegian company Nyegaard on the theory that a nonionic compound would result in lower osmolarity and would produce fewer adverse effects. Nonetheless, the two major possible complications are grand mal seizures and arachnoiditis.[5]

We prepare patients for metrizamide myelography by hydration the night before and after the procedure. Phenothiazine derivatives, which interact with this contrast medium by lowering the convulsion threshold, should be withheld for at least 48 hours prior to the myelogram. Other drugs with similar effects are monoamine oxidase inhibitors, tricyclic antidepressants, analeptic agents, and central nervous system stimulants. Patients are positioned with their head elevated at least 30° following the procedure. If the patient has to be supine, the neck is maintained flexed to prevent the agent from traveling above the cervical spine. An aqueous technique may be used for lumbar myelograms as well as for thoracic and cervical myelograms. The agent provides less contrast ability in the superior spine, but it is satisfactory.

The use of computerized tomography (CT) with aqueous myelograms has been rewarding in establishing more definitive diagnoses of tumors, spinal stenosis, and congenital anomalies.

Discography

Visualization of the internal structures of a disc by the injection of radiopaque absorbable compounds may be helpful in the diagnosis of disc degeneration. Lumbar discography is still controversial, but is used by many physicians. The ex-

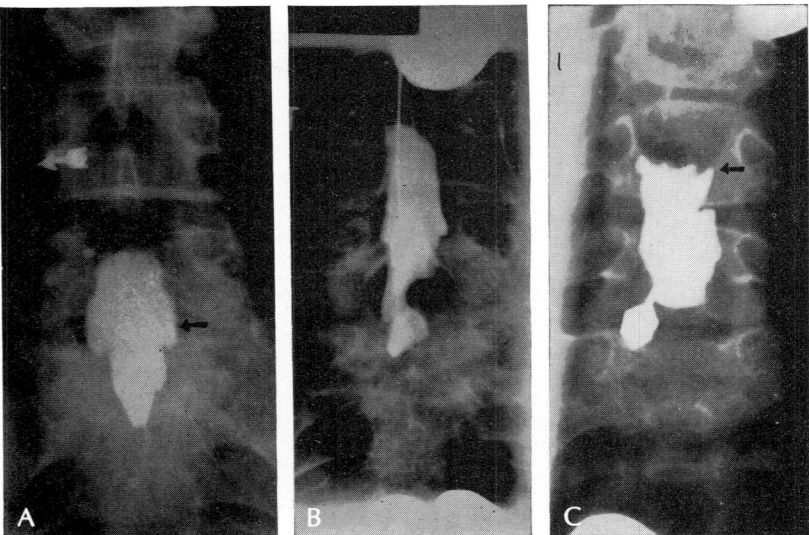

Fig. 82–13. Myelogram. *A,* Normal filling of the lower end of the dural sac. The axillary pouches (nerve root sheaths) are well visualized at the lumbosacral level (black arrow). To complete the examination, each intervertebral level must be similarly visualized until the inferior end of the spinal cord is reached. *B,* A filling defect on the left side at the level of the fifth lumbar disc. A disc herniation is likely, although a cyst or a tumor is possible. *C,* Complete block of the spinal canal (arrow) through which the contrast material cannot pass. Such a block indicates a tumor of the cauda equina. It is rarely seen in disc herniation.

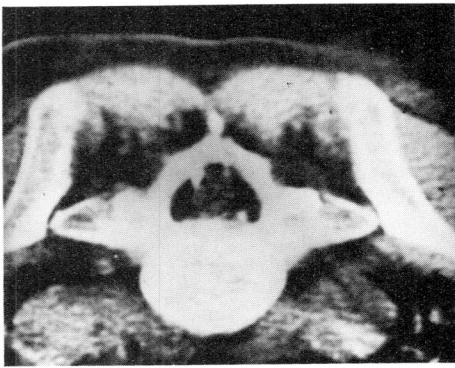

Fig. 82–15. A cross section of a thoracic level of the vertebral spine is depicted by computerized axial transverse tomography.

amination is performed under local anesthesia with premedication. The contrast medium is a mixture of 50% diatrizoate (Hypaque) and 1% procaine. The normal disc accepts as much as 2 ml fluid, depending on its size. If the disc is ruptured, the contrast material escapes. The technique and interpretation vary according to experience.

Computerized Axial Tomography

Computerized transverse axial tomography of the spine developed as an extension of CT scanning

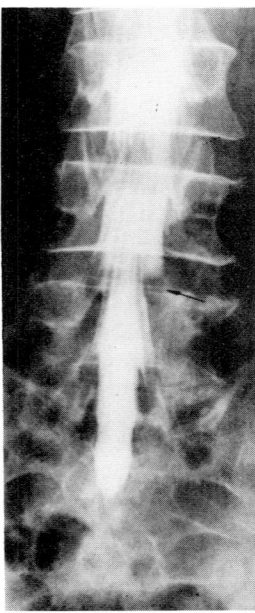

Fig. 82–14. Metrizamide myelogram. A filling defect is noted at the L4 to L5 interspace. The arrow points to blunting of the L5 nerve root sleeve from a protruding disc.

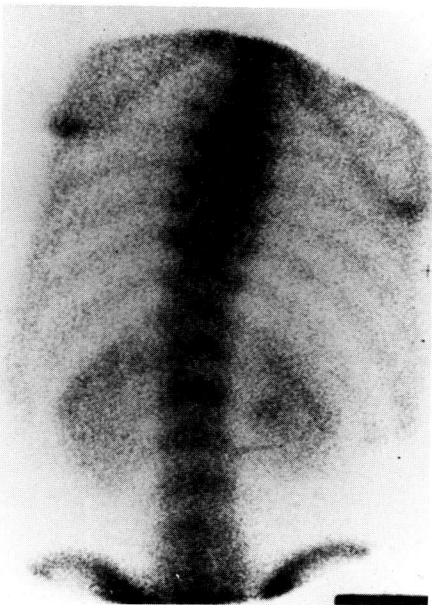

Fig. 82–16. ^{99m}Technetium diphosphonate scan of the vertebral column. The dark area in the upper spine illustrates an area of increased radioactive uptake confirming an osteoid osteoma of the thoracic spine. Note the spinal curvature (scoliosis) characteristically associated with this lesion.

of the skull. This newer technique shows a cross section of the spinal canal and is helpful in the diagnosis of bony encroachment of neural structures, such as spinal stenosis, spondylosis, and spondylolisthesis (Fig. 82–15) (see also Chap. 6).

CT scanning of the spine is now used extensively in the United States and has become a routine diagnostic procedure in evaluation of the patient with a spinal problem.[19] This type of study is changing as new generations of scanners are brought onto the market. New CT data provide diagnostic insights previously unavailable. Except for its radiation effects, the procedure is essentially noninvasive.

Radioactive Scanning

Radionuclides have been used extensively in the diagnosis of bone diseases associated with increased calcium turnover. Scanning agents such as ^{85}strontium (^{85}Sr) and ^{18}fluorine (^{18}F) have been used.[4] The diagnosis of osteoid osteoma has been facilitated by scintimetric examination.[6] At present, the scanning agent of choice is ^{99m}technetium-tin-polyphosphate (or diphosphonate) (Fig. 82–16) (see Chap. 5).

Electromyography

Electromyography is the study of spontaneous involuntary electric waves generated in a motor unit and recorded by a coaxial electrode attached to an oscilloscope. In a typical nerve root compression syndrome, muscles innervated by the involved roots show fibrillation potentials. The technique is a useful adjunct in the diagnosis of nerve root compression and in localizing its level. It may be particularly helpful in patients with questionable neurologic findings.

Somatosensory Evoked Potentials

The technique of stimulating peripheral nerves in the extremities and recording electrical potentials in the scalp was first described by Dawson.[9] In the past 10 years, this technique has been used by Nash and his colleagues for monitoring spinal cord function during spinal operations on patients with scoliosis.[14,15] Modifications of this technique using surface electrodes on the spine provide spinal evoked potentials that may be helpful as a noninvasive test for evaluating spinal cord and cauda equina lesions. We have used this technique in a small group of patients with congenital spinal deformities as a screening test in evaluating spinal cord or peripheral nerve lesions. Once greater familiarity with this technique is gained, it should help physicians to localize low back pain with nerve root involvement.

CONDITIONS PREDISPOSING PATIENTS TO SPRAIN SYNDROMES

Faulty Posture

Poor posture is prevalent and can be classified into two groups. The first type is *functional*, in which the position of faulty posture is correctable. It is common in children and is progressively less frequent in older age groups. The second is a *structural* group in which the deformity is fixed. The cervical lordosis is increased; the thoracic spine is rounded, and its motion is limited. An exaggerated lordotic lumbar curve may become fixed owing to shortening of the sacrospinalis muscles. If so, the interspinous ligaments become contracted so that the tips of the spinous processes and facets "kiss." Conversely, the abdominal muscles overstretch and relax, a process that may be accelerated by pregnancies and obesity. The pelvis tilts more anteriorly than normal, and the hip flexor muscles shorten. The lumbosacral angle increases. When the patient is asked to bend forward, he cannot obliterate his lumbar curve as he normally would. Often, one sees secondary degenerative changes on x-ray examination.

In the purely functional state, faulty posture is

rarely painful; at most, it may cause fatigue and backache. When the position becomes fixed, however, the symptoms are more likely to be bothersome.

Spondylolisthesis

Generically, this term means a slipped vertebra, but clinically it is associated only with anterior displacement of one vertebra on the next inferior vertebra (Figs. 82–17, 82–18). The classification of spondylolisthesis that is now generally accepted is dysplastic, degenerative, traumatic, and pathologic.

Dysplastic Type

A congenital dysplasia of the upper sacrum or neural arch of L5 allows the upper lumbar vertebra to slip forward.

Isthmic defects are present in the portions of the vertebral arch lying between the superior and inferior articular processes (pars defects). The defect may be unilateral or bilateral. Three types of defects have been recognized: (1) lytic, with fatigue fracture of the pars interarticularis; (2) with an elongated but intact pars; and (3) involving acute fracture of the pars interarticularis.

When bilateral defects are present, the anterior vertebral body may slip forward while the posterior arch remains behind; the result is a true spondy-

lolisthesis. If the pars defect occurs without forward slip, the condition is termed *spondylolysis*.

The cause of the basic neural arch defect is still the subject of some controversy. Willis found spondylolysis in 4% of adult skeletal specimens, but not in fetal skeletons.[25] We have encountered it in identical twins and in several members of the same family. These findings indicate a predisposing factor, such as vulnerability of the pars interarticularis, which is congenital and may be genetically determined, whereas the final condition is produced by wear and tear or trauma.

Spondylolisthesis is usually qualified by the amount of forward displacement, first degree for one-quarter anteroposterior-vertebral-diameter displacement and fourth degree for full-diameter displacement. Although it is uncommon to see the condition progress in adults, it is not unusual in children. The fibrous tissue bridging the defects, the structure of the disc, and the intervertebral ligaments must give and stretch, so the vertical body, pedicles, and superior facets can slip away from the detached portion of the neural arch, which includes the laminae, spinous process, and inferior facets. Pseudoarthroses may develop in the sites of defective ossification if the degree of slipping is minimal because movements of the spine cause false motion between the two vertebral segments.

Several syndromes are caused by spondylolis-

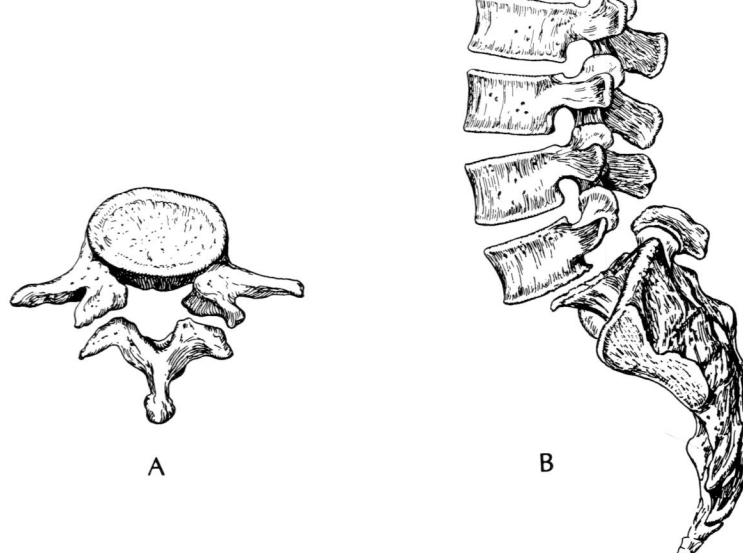

A   B

Fig. 82–17.   Spondylolisthesis. *A,* Vertebra showing failure of ossification of the interarticular portions of the neural arch. Without forward slip of the involved vertebra, this disorder is called spondylolysis. (From Willis.[25]) *B,* The deformity (spondylolisthesis), which may occur as the result of the foregoing disorder. The defect is in the arch of L5. The posterior portion of the arch including the inferior facets remains with the sacrum while the rest of the fifth lumbar vertebra slips forward, carrying with it the entire spine. All degrees of slipping are seen.

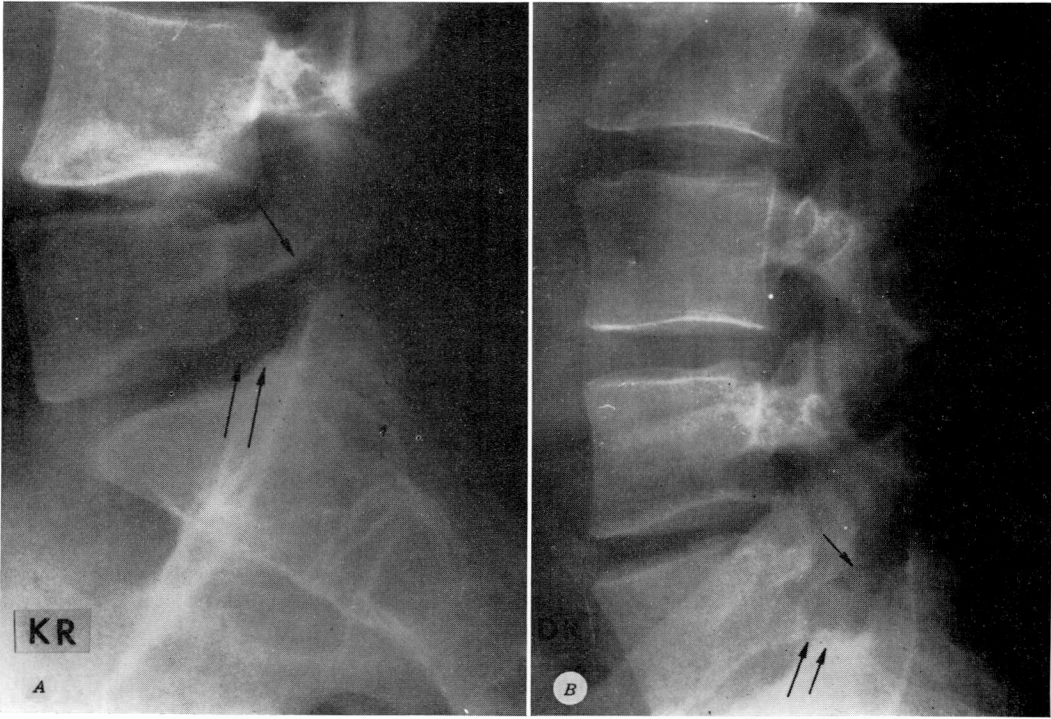

Fig. 82–18.   Identical twins with spondylolisthesis of L5 to S1. *A,* Lateral roentgenogram of the lumbosacral area of K.R., who had progressive back pain requiring spinal fusion. *B,* Lateral roentgenogram of twin, D.R., who had no back symptoms.

thesis. First, the condition may be silent or the symptoms associated with it may be inconsequential. Second, back pain may arise from the pseudoarthrosis or from the wear and tear of the disc joint, which has slipped. In this connection, herniation of such a disc has been described, but we have not encountered it. Third, unilateral or bilateral sciatica may be caused by root impingement due to hypertrophy of the fibrous tissue in one or both defects, or by traction on the roots secondary to forward displacement, especially when the defects are situated low in the superior articular processes. Fourth, the displacement may be so severe that a lesion of the whole cauda equina is produced, in part from traction and in part from compression. The most severe syndrome is usually seen in adolescents.

Although the astute clinician can often make the diagnosis from a visible or palpable prominence of the spine of the affected vertebra, noticed most readily when the patient is bent forward, final diagnosis depends on radiographic demonstration of the neural arch defects. When slipping is sufficient, these defects may be visible in a routine lateral film if the x-ray tube is well centered (Fig. 82–18). In the presence of minimal slipping, however, oblique views are necessary (see Fig. 82–12). Occasion-

ally, although a defect is present, slippage may not be evident on the routine lateral recumbent film of the lumbosacral junction, but if the films are taken with the patient standing, slippage becomes apparent.

Treatment varies with the syndrome. Postural measures sometimes suffice for patients with minimal symptoms, especially if no nerve involvement has occurred. Spinal fusion is indicated when the symptoms of sprain are severe, persistent, or begin before maturity, however. When the nerve roots or the cauda equina are involved, decompression is the most important part of the operation and is indicated at the time of, or before, spinal fusion. Occasionally, simple removal of the loose neural arch and hypertrophic tissue in the defects, that is, foraminotomy, affords relief, but the outcome in our experience is too uncertain to recommend this procedure routinely.

Degenerative Type

The most common acquired form is one in which osteoarthritic changes of the facets combined with disc degeneration result in forward displacement. This condition is diagnosed radiographically, especially by oblique views (Fig. 82–19). Treatment is much the same as for dysplastic spondylolis-

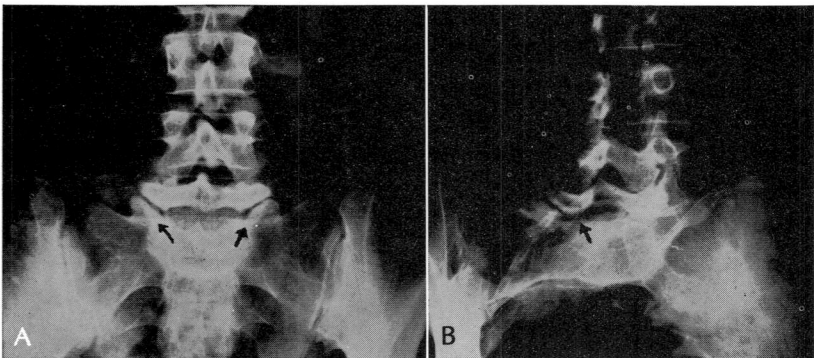

Fig. 82–19. Abnormal facets. Anteroposterior *(A)* and oblique *(B)* films in a patient with low back pain. Note the abnormal plane of the facets between the fifth lumbar vertebra and the sacrum. Less bony stability is present, and actual spondylolisthesis may occur. The instability may sometimes be detected roentgenographically only during flexion or extension of the spine.

thesis. Complicating compression of nerve roots or cauda equina should be looked for and should be given precedence in the therapeutic plan.

Traumatic Type

This type is secondary to an acute injury with a fracture of some portion of the posterior arch. Treated early with immobilization, these injuries often heal.

Pathologic Type

Because of local or generalized bone disease, the posterior arches may become incompetent and may allow spondylolisthesis.

Trauma

Each spinal injury weakens the spine and predisposes the patient to further injury, regardless of type and extent of damage. This phenomenon is especially true when protection of the injured part is not adequate. Ligaments and muscles heal only by scar formation, and the anulus fibrosus is almost powerless to heal tears of its substance. These circumstances, unfortunately, are beyond the control of the physician, but the patient should be warned to protect his back following injury.

Disc Degeneration

The pathologic aspects of this condition are also discussed later in this chapter. Besides predisposing a patient to herniation, disc degeneration also weakens the structure of the intervertebral joint and increases the risk of sprain syndromes. When the degeneration is localized, little stability is lost, and the normal width of the disc space may be pre-

served. A patient with such a condition may have few or no symptoms, and some patients therefore do well after simple removal of herniated disc material.

When the degeneration is more massive, however, narrowing of disc space follows. If this condition occurs slowly over the course of years, the patient may have little pain or few other symptoms. Stability and vertebral alignment are preserved by marginal spur formation and by adaptive changes in the facets and intervertebral ligaments. Occasionally, such patients have a history of several acute episodes of back pain many years prior to examination, but frequently they are unaware of any previous back trouble.

Massive disc degeneration occurring rapidly is likely to be continuously painful, whether or not herniation and root compression are associated. Instability of such joints leads to either backward shift of the superior vertebra on the inferior as the facets telescope on each other (Fig. 82–20) or forward displacement as the structure of the articular facets gives way, that is, degenerative spondylolisthesis.

During the course of collapse of the disc space, not only the disc itself but also the intervertebral joint is *unstable* and is therefore prone to give symptoms of sprain. When the intervertebral space becomes narrowed and arthritic, however, it again become stable, and back pain may subside, although later symptoms may develop from projection of marginal osteophytes against the nerve roots, either posteriorly in the neural canal or laterally in the narrowed intervertebral foramina.

Phylogenetic Shortening of the Spine

The structure of the lowest lumbar vertebra and of the first sacral segment is variable. Either may

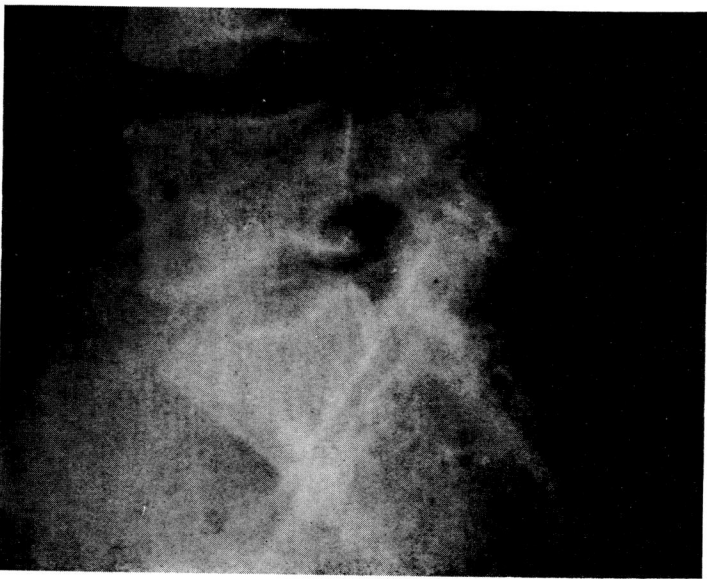

Fig. 82–20. Retrodisplacement. Lateral roentgenogram showing slight narrowing of the fifth lumbar disc and retrodisplacement of the fifth lumbar vertebra on the sacrum. This condition, often called reverse spondylolisthesis, is generally painful.

take on some or all of the characteristics of the other. When this happens the vertebrae are spoken of as *transitional*. Certainly, complete fusion or sacralization of the fifth lumbar vertebra does not predispose a patient to strain. It is also difficult to see how complete lumbarization of the first sacral segment could cause strain.

When the changeover is incomplete, however,

the situation is different. One finds a unilaterally enlarged transversed process articulating with the sacrum and asymmetric facets (Fig. 82–21); that is, the facets are in different planes on the two sides. These changes reduce intervertebral mobility and therefore may predispose a patient to sprain. They are not incompatible, on the other hand, with normal existence, and if trouble occurs, the su-

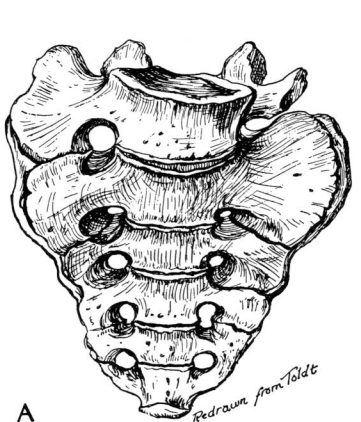
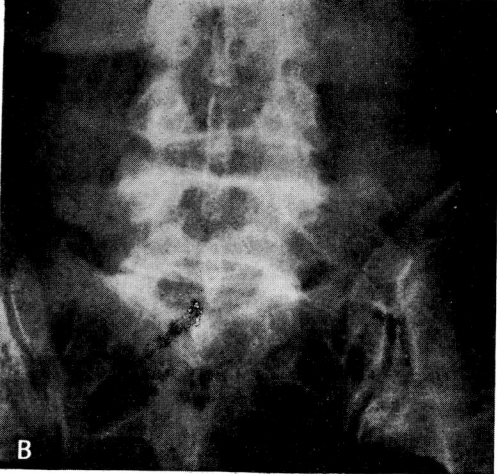

Fig. 82–21. Articulating transverse process. *A,* An incompletely sacralized fifth lumbar vertebra is shown with an articulating transverse process on the right. The intervertebral disc is usually congenitally narrow in these patients. *B,* An articulating transverse process on the left side of the fifth lumbar vertebra. The articulation is usually fibrous. This common congenital anomaly is not necessarily associated with pain.

periorly placed joint is often involved. Pain from a transitional vertebra itself probably arises from sclerosing osteitis of the pseudoarthrosis between the enlarged transverse process and the sacrum.

Spina Bifida Occulta

This condition is a failure of fusion between the right and left halves of the neural arch and may occur at any level of the vertebral column. The most common site for spinal bifida occulta is S1, where the incidence has recently been reported to be 9% in women and 13% in men. The condition is in no way a predisposing factor to low back pain. When spina bifida occulta occurs at L5, further evaluation should be made to rule out a spondylolisthesis or spondylolysis.

CLINICAL PICTURE OF SPRAIN SYNDROMES

Low back sprain may be acute, subacute, or chronic. The acute syndrome usually follows an injury or a trivial strain, is of short duration, and is self-limited enough to respond well to treatment of any type. The chronic form, on the other hand, is usually of long duration, often occurs without an initiating trauma, and is refractory to treatment. Recurrences of the acute form are common.

Acute Sprain

The pain is usually severe and diffuse over the lower back and is associated with paravertebral muscle spasm. The patient adopts a protective attitude of moderate flexion and perhaps some list. Any motion is painful and aggravates the spasm.

Examination obviously cannot be complete, but is carried as far as possible. Roentgenograms should be made if the patient can cooperate well enough. If not, they can be safely deferred until later.

The patient should be put to bed, preferably a bed with a thin sponge-rubber or hair mattress reinforced by an underlying board (Fig. 82–22). If such a board is not available, shifting the mattress to the floor often substitutes. A pillow behind the knees may assist in relaxation. "Muscle relaxants" and salicylates are usually helpful, but narcotics are sometimes necessary. No particular drug combination is effective in all patients. Heat in the form of hot moist packs applied to the back relieves muscle spasm. Light massage is often helpful, but deep massage should be avoided. Sometimes, procaine infiltration of the tight muscles is effective, but injection of a locally acting corticosteroid into the disc has questionable value. Traction has been used for acute low back symptoms for many years, to keep a restless patient still. If applied directly to the pelvis, such forces no doubt may be trans-

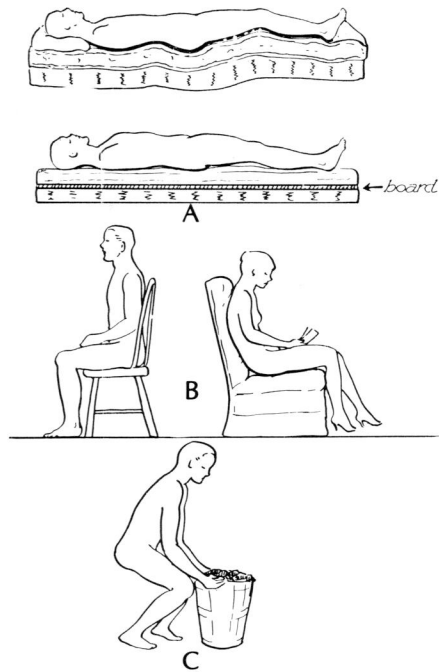

Fig. 82–22. Postural principles. Patients should be instructed in some simple principles to avoid unnecessary back strain. *A*, The bed should be hard, to avoid sagging of the buttocks with increase in the lumbar lordosis. *B*, A hard, straight-back chair is desirable. Arm rests are not contraindicated. *C*, Lifting should be avoided whenever possible. When it is unavoidable, the legs should do most of the work; the elbows can be buttressed by the thighs.

mitted to the spine and may have a stretching effect. Countertraction may be provided by positioning the patient with the foot of the bed elevated or by applying countertraction on the head. In the routine management of scoliosis, the effects of head and pelvic traction have been documented by x-ray films of the spine showing the stretching effect. Constant pelvic traction may be used with weights up to 35 to 40 lb, whereas intermittent pelvic traction of 65 to 70 lb has been of value in treating patients with acute back symptoms. If traction is necessary, I believe that it should be instituted while the patient is hospitalized. It is difficult to instruct a patient initially in the correct use of traction unless he is in the hospital.

As the pain subsides, a complete examination can be done. As soon as straight leg raising is free through an arc of 45° or more, the patient may be allowed up. His back must be protected until symptoms have subsided completely. If the sprain has been severe, a brace or lumbosacral corset may be advisable. Before normal activities are resumed, the patient should be checked to see whether he has regained full motion. Exercises should be instituted not only to restore motion and strength, but also to stretch contracted muscles and ligaments. Exercises must be started gradually and gauged to pain tolerance.

Many acute episodes are not so severe as the one described. In less-severe cases, ambulatory treatment may be sufficient. Immobilization with a brace or adhesive strapping, procaine injection, and heat and massage are all useful measures. Again, one should watch for developing contractures, which should be corrected with exercises.

Chronic Sprain

This syndrome, probably the most common of low back conditions, has variable clinical manifestations. In its milder form, it is characterized by a mild low backache aggravated by bending and lifting and improved by rest. On the other hand, the pain may be more severe and may cause true discomfort. Rarely is it severe for more than short periods, and it subsides to a nagging, diffuse low backache with radiation into one or both thighs. It is aggravated by activity and is improved by rest.

The physical signs of this syndrome are also variable. In patients with mild cases, motion may not be limited, but the extremes of motion are usually painful. The patient notes tenderness at some point over the lower spine. As the severity of the syndrome increases, one notes additional signs such as partial restriction of straight leg raising, loss of motion, abnormal postural attitudes, and muscle spasm, particularly in response to movement.

In patients with severe cases, a period of bedrest may be indicated; therapeutic measures are as described for acute low back pain. In milder cases, the patient should be instructed in proper postural principles. Proper sleeping and sitting positions should be demonstrated, and he should be taught to avoid bending and lifting or to bend and lift in such a way as to minimize the pressure on his back. He is instructed in postural exercises, which have as their principles the reduction of lumbar lordosis and the strengthening of the trunk. Stretching of shortened hamstring and sacrospinal muscles may be advisable, but should be done cautiously.

Frequently, external support is helpful, and many different types of braces have been designed to achieve the desired goals of abdominal compression and restricted spinal movement (Fig. 82–23). In principle, these braces should reach from the pubic level to the lower costal margins and should support the abdomen, particularly the lower abdomen. The central back uprights, if present, should be contoured to fit comfortably when the patient is seated erect. Pressure into the lumbosacral hollow is not necessary and in fact should be avoided.

When conservative therapy fails, lumbosacral fusion should be considered. In this operation, two or more vertebrae are induced to grow together, to put the intervening joint at rest. Many techniques have been devised. Although newer methods have shortened the period of morbidity, the incidence of pseudoarthroses is still bothersome; and rarely, following a successful fusion, the intervertebral joint superior to the operation site may become painful as a result of the additional wear and tear placed on it. Because the operation is elective, the decision should be left up to the patient, once the advantages and disadvantages have been explained.

NERVE ROOT COMPRESSION SYNDROMES

Degenerative Disc Disease and Herniated Disc

Since Mixter and Barr first clearly described the syndrome of nerve root compression due to herniated disc in 1934, it has become clear that lesions of the disc are responsible for much of idiopathic low back pain (Fig. 82–24).

Pathogenesis

Although a single trauma, if severe enough, can rupture a hitherto normal anulus fibrosus and can allow prolapse of disc substance with disastrous effect on the cauda equina, this occurence is rare. More commonly, the trauma or strain acts only as a triggering mechanism. Underlying asymptomatic biomechanical and biochemical changes usually first weaken the disc structure. The course of these changes has been traced anatomically, and alteration and weakening of the discs are part of the aging process. Because the discs have no innervation and no blood supply, such degeneration can take place silently and with little appreciable repair. When the annulus has weakened enough, the interior disc substance, that is, the nucleus pulposus and the degenerating annular fibers, prolapse in the direction of greatest weakness. Because of these forces and certain anatomic factors already described, the directions of greatest weakness for the lumbar discs are to right and left of the posterior midline. Lumbar disc herniations, therefore, follow these two directions. They are favored by radially oriented annular tears or fissures, which develop either as a result of normal wear and tear or as the result of one or more excessive strains.

Herniations that approach the surface distend the superficial fibers and longitudinal ligaments, where pain-perceptive nerve endings are situated. This

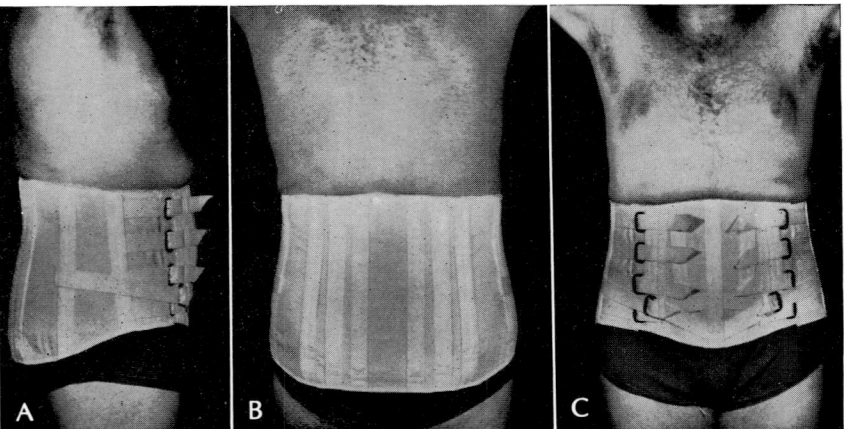

Fig. 82–23. *A, B, C,* Lumbosacral corset. Steel stays are incorporated into the back of the support, which must extend from the iliac crests to just over the costal margins.

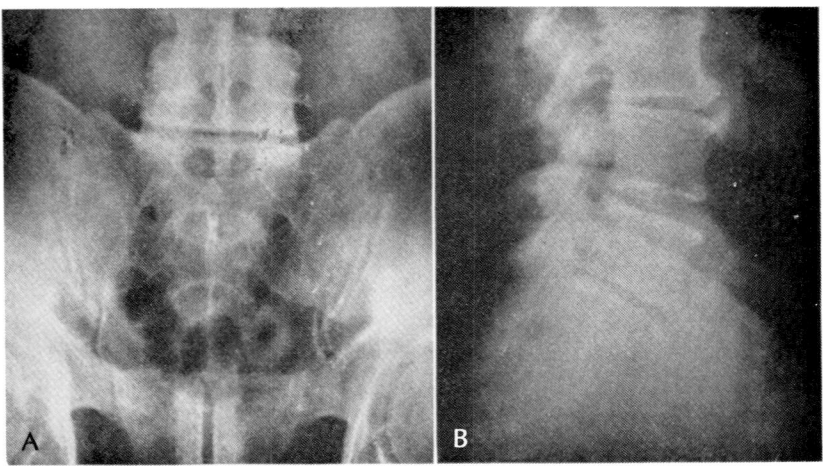

Fig. 82–24. *A* and *B,* Roentgenograms showing an advanced stage of degenerative disc disease.

deep pain is poorly localized and can radiate into the buttocks and perhaps even into the lower extremities. The source of the pain is further obscured by the frequent development of spasm of the lumbar and hamstring muscles, and this spasm in itself is painful. If herniation proceeds, the lumbar nerve roots or the cauda equina may next become involved; the smaller the diameter of the neural canal and the larger the herniation, the more likely this disorder is to occur and to affect nerve root functions. If the herniation does not rupture through the longitudinal ligament, it is called *protrusion,* and if it does, *extrusion.* In either case, the nerve root or roots are displaced and compressed. Disc fragments may herniate from the disc space and may lie superior or inferior to it and still not extrude.

Because of all these variables, the manifestations of disc herniation differ from one patient to the next. Most commonly, nerve root compression is localized, and the neurologic deficit is minor. In rare instances, however, the prolapse may be massive and may involve several nerve roots or the entire cauda equina. As the site of herniation comes closer to the midline, the more likely is multiple nerve root involvement; as the site shifts laterally, the more likely is involvement confined to one nerve root.

Clinical Picture

Although any of the lumbar discs can herniate, one or both of the most inferior (L4 to L5 and L5 to S1) are usually responsible for symptoms. The level L3 to L4 is involved occasionally; other lumbar levels, rarely.

Minimal nerve root compression may have no localizing physical or roentgenographic manifestations, and conclusive diagnosis depends on CT or myelographic findings. In many instances, however, symptoms and signs may subside with bedrest, and these studies can be deferred. I recommend myelograms only when the syndrome is atypical or operative intervention is contemplated. In any event, CT study is preferred, as it is safe and noninvasive.

Classic cases of root compression due to herniated disc are difficult to overlook. Patients are otherwise healthy and are often vigorous men or women in middle age. Patients often have a previous history of backache or of one or more acute lumbosacral sprains from which recovery has been complete. Usually, the onset of the present pain follows a back injury, but not necessarily a severe injury; in fact, it is sometimes so minor that it is difficult for the patient to recall it. Frequently, a snap is felt before the back pain begins. Once started, the pain increases in intensity and, after an interval, radiates distally into one or the other lower extremity. As radiation begins, the back pain may subside, but the radiating pain typically increases and is associated with numbness and paresthesia. The patient cannot stand straight, and the involved leg is too sensitive to bear weight. Examination shows a patient in great pain, with paravertebral muscle spasm, who stands with a flattened lumbar lordosis and a list to the side opposite the pain and who walks only with difficulty. All spinal movements are limited, particularly bending to the side of the pain. Straight leg raising is restricted on the involved side, and often this leg cannot be straightened. The patient prefers the sitting or flexed position to any other. In addition, the patient has marked paravertebral tenderness with reproduction of sciatica on percussion or deep palpation.

Neurologic signs are variable for the reasons already described, but certain combinations suggest specific nerve root involvements. Loss or suppression of ankle jerk, sensory deficit in the lateral border and sole of the foot and toes, and weakness and atrophy of the calf suggest S1 nerve root compression. Unchanged reflexes, sensory deficit in the lateral leg and mediodorsal aspect of the foot, and weakness of the toe extensors suggest L5 nerve root compression. Loss or suppression of the knee jerk, sensory deficit along the shin, and weakness of knee extension suggest L4 nerve root compression. Most commonly, S1 nerve root compression is the result of herniation of the L5 to S1 disc, L5 root compression of the L4 to L5 disc, and L4 root compression of the L3 to L4 disc. When neurologic findings are profound, however, it is wise to suspect multiple nerve root involve-

ment. CT and (perhaps) myelography are obtained to confirm the level of involvement when an operation is contemplated.

Treatment

Thanks to improvement of diagnostic technique, diagnosis can be definitely established in most patients. Operative intervention is elective unless the patient has an important nerve deficit or is in intractable pain. Even in the presence of definite signs of nerve root compression, the majority of patients respond to conservative treatment. A trial of two to three weeks of bedrest in the hospital is indicated for most patients with acute symptoms before operation is recommended. When the syndrome is subacute, bedrest may be less valuable, but a sustained course of outpatient treatment is indicated before operation is considered.

When pain is relieved by conservative treatment, the relief is probably due to subsidence of root edema and to limited repair of the superficial layers of the annulus fibrosus and the posterior longitudinal ligament. It is doubtful that the herniated disc material is ever fully absorbed, but it may shrink or become pocketed in the neural canal, no longer compressing nerve tissue. This phenomenon is more likely when the lumbar neural canal is proportionately larger than the cauda equina. Along with subsidence of pain, the neurologic picture often improves, but some neurologic changes of little functional significance may persist.

Chymopapain and Chemonucleolysis. Intradiscal injection of chymopapain or chemonucleolysis is a technique reported by Lyman Smith in 1964 to treat herniated lumbar intervertebral discs.[22] Chymopapain, derived from papaya latex, is a proteolytic enzyme that catalyzes rapid hydrolysis of the noncollagen ground substance of the nucleus pulposus.[23] Based on this pharmacologic effect, chemonucleolytic treatment of low back pain with nerve root irritation was used in clinical trials in this country and in Canada until 1975, when the efficacy and safety of the method came into question. The technique was discontinued in this country, but it was still used by Canadian orthopedic and neurologic surgeons. In 1980, a double-blind, randomized trial was conducted to compare the efficacy of chymopapain injection with placebo injection in patients with a herniated lumbar disc.[13] Based on these clinical trials, the United States Food and Drug Administration (FDA) approved the use of this enzyme for intradiscal injections in this country in January 1983. The American Academy of Orthopaedic Surgeons and the American Association of Neurological Surgeons then began a cooperative educational program to instruct their members in the clinical use of chymopapain injections.

Patients considered suitable for intradiscal injection are as follows: (1) those with clear-cut lumbar radiculopathy who have had an appropriate trial of conservative treatment for two to four weeks and who have not responded well; and (2) those with an abnormal myelogram confirming disc protrusion; patients with a large, extruded fragment are not likely to benefit.

Certain contraindications are as follows: (1) major weakness in a muscle group; (2) sphincter disturbance; (3) extensive spondylosis or spinal stenosis; (4) pregnancy; and (5) allergy to papaya or to any meat tenderizer.

Less clear-cut contraindications include patients who: (1) have had previous operations at the current symptomatic level; and (2) have workmen's compensation claims, are in litigation related to their back disorder, or have a psychiatric disturbance.

The major adverse effect of this treatment is anaphylaxis. In a worldwide series of 40,000 cases, the incidence of this complication was 1%, with 2 deaths reported.[18] The incidence of anaphylaxis in women was approximately 2.5%, whereas in men it was approximately 0.18%. Women had a greater risk of reaction if their erythrocyte sedimentation rate was above 20 or if treatment occurred during the menstrual period.

Intradiscal injection of chymopapain may open new avenues to patients with low back pain and radiculopathy.

Operative Treatment. When operative treatment is advised, the question is whether to be content with nerve root decompression only or whether to proceed with spinal fusion. Should the degenerative disc process be controlled by fusing the involved joint at the same time that loosened disc tissue is removed? On this point opinion still differs, and arguments on both sides are convincing. In cases of rupture of the intervertebral discs in adolescence, in acute ruptures for the first time, and in intervertebral disc ruptures with a previous history of symptoms but with little radiologic change, when operation becomes necessary I prefer to decompress the involved disc space without fusion. If a repeat operation is necessary or if the patient has advanced changes of degenerative arthritis, however, spinal fusion may be considered. In questionable cases, I prefer not to perform spinal fusion because the decompression operation is less extensive, convalescence is usually easier, and if a fusion fails to heal properly and a pseudoarthrosis develops, the situation may be worse than if no fusion had been done. I review these various aspects of the problem with the patient and, if he is still uncertain, I request his permission to make the final decision at the time of operation (see also Chap. 47).

Complications

If the indications for operative intervention are conservative, and if the type of operation is precisely fitted to the circumstances, the results will be satisfying. Complications are rare, but one deserves particular mention. Spondylitis or discitis sometimes develops in the operated disc space. It is manifested by recurrence of back pain, which begins three or four weeks after operation, and elevation of the patient's erythrocyte sedimentation rate. Other manifestations of inflammation such as fever and leukocytosis are absent, and infection, the primary concern, cannot be demonstrated. In time, roentgenograms show sclerosis of the adjacent vertebral margins and localized areas of bone absorption. The cause of this complication has not been definitely established, but the condition is usually self-limited and subsides with bedrest.

Recurrences of nerve root compression from fresh herniation of degenerated disc tissue can occur, but are infrequent. Because the mobility of the nerve root and the dura is reduced by postoperative scarring, such herniations do not have to be large to irritate the nerve tissue. In such cases, treatment by bedrest is well worth a trial. If it fails, however, reoperation for decompression is indicated, and a spinal fusion should be carefully reconsidered. It is probably wise to advise a fusion operation, especially if the degenerative disease is still localized to one disc level.

Spinal Stenosis

The frequency of diagnosis of a condition known as lumbar spinal stenosis has increased dramatically. This condition includes any narrowing of the spinal canal or of the intervertebral foramina. The following is a current classification of lumbar spinal stenosis.

Classification

1. Congenital Developmental Stenosis
   a. Idiopathic
   b. Achondroplastic
2. Acquired Stenosis
   a. Degenerative
      1. Central portion of spinal canal
      2. Peripheral portion of canal, lateral recesses, and nerve root canal
      3. Degenerative spondylolisthesis
   b. Combined
      Any possible combinations of congenital or developmental stenosis, degenerative stenosis, and herniations of the nucleus pulposus

   c. Spondylolisthetic or spondylolytic
   d. Iatrogenic
     1. Following laminectomy
     2. Following fusion (anterior and posterior)
     3. Following chemonucleolysis
   e. Post-traumatic, including late changes
   f. Miscellaneous
     1. Paget's disease
     2. Fluorosis

The clinical picture depends on the site of the stenosis. If the encroachment involves only one nerve root, the symptoms may mimic those of a herniated intervertebral disc. Multiple levels may be involved, making clinical evaluation more complicated. If the central neural canal is affected, the patient may complain of varied symptoms. Pain in both thighs, worse during walking and improved at rest, such as seen in patients with *intermittent claudication,* may occur. The patient often complains of generalized weakness or peculiar feelings in the upper legs. Night pain while in bed may be relieved by a change of position, such as walking. This disorder can be confused with the syndrome of restless legs.

Clinical findings are variable, with or without patchy neurologic changes. Extension of the back may exaggerate the pain. Provisional diagnosis depends on a strong suspicion; myelography or transaxial tomography is used to confirm the diagnosis.

The treatment of spinal stenosis is often conservative at the beginning. Eventually, decompression laminectomy or surgical enlargement of the area of the bony stenosis is indicated.

OTHER CONDITIONS PRODUCING LOW BACK PAIN

Infections

Backache may occur as part of the toxemia of a generalized infection. In these cases, diagnosis usually is not a problem. Except for muscle soreness, few if any localizing signs exist. More important is the back pain that accompanies meningeal irritation. Usually, one may detect a generalized spasm of the erector spinae muscle by Kernig's maneuver or by limitation of straight leg raising. When severe, as in infectious meningitis, this spasm produces opisthotonos.

Infections may cause backache by direct involvement of spinal structures. Nontubercular infections are now more prevalent and are seen most commonly in the aged. The infection usually begins in the disc space and spreads to involve the bone secondarily. Roentgenographic changes may be slow to develop. At first, the shadow of an abscess may appear, followed by gradual destruction of the contiguous vertebral margins, with final obliteration of the disc space.

The infecting organism may be obtained from culture of blood or from aspiration biopsy of the disc space itself. Sometimes, the spine may be involved by an infection elsewhere, such as the urinary tract; culture from the suspected source may reveal the organism. Treatment by bedrest, spinal bracing, and suitable chemotherapy is best. Operation is rarely necessary because the involved vertebrae often undergo spontaneous fusion.

Perhaps of greater interest in the differential diagnosis are the granulomatous infections. By far the most important of these is tuberculosis, although brucellosis and fungal, particularly coccidioidomycosis, infections also occur (see Chap. 102).

Pott's Disease (Tuberculosis)

Symptoms vary because of the marked individual patterns of resistance. Back pain may be present for several months before other characteristic changes of the disease occur. Systemic signs, particularly otherwise *unexplained weight loss,* should make one suspicious. Night pain, night cries, fever, and previous pulmonary tuberculosis all help one to make the diagnosis. Paraplegia is a common complication. *Elevation of the erythrocyte sedimentation rate* is the most helpful laboratory clue. A tuberculin test should always be done. Even though a positive test result is not conclusive evidence, a negative result excludes this diagnosis.

Roentgenographic changes are usually present, although early in the disease they may be difficult to find (Fig. 82–25). Tomograms may be helpful as are bone scans. Narrowing of the disc space with destruction of neighboring vertebrae and *soft tissue abscess* are the most typical changes. Diagnosis can be made from culture of aspirated pus.

This disease often involves the sacroiliac joints. Here again, roentgenographic evidence of bone destruction is the most important diagnostic finding.

Herpes Zoster

Infection of the dorsal lumbar root ganglions by the herpes zoster virus may cause severe sciatica. Early diagnosis is difficult, but the absence of trauma and the presence of fever should make one suspicious. As soon as the vesicular eruption appears, the diagnosis becomes evident.

Fractures and Dislocations

Characteristic wedge fractures of the vertebral bodies caused by injuries of flexion are not difficult to recognize or to treat. Fractures of the posterior elements, such as the pedicles, laminae, and articular processes, may be complicated by severe

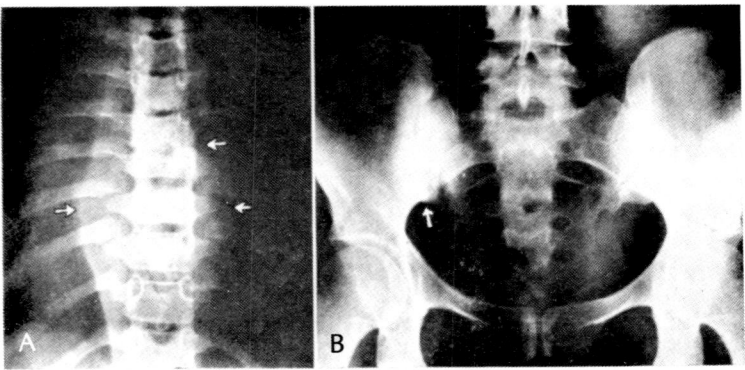

Fig. 82–25. Tuberculosis. *A,* Tuberculous spondylitis; note the abscess (arrow). Destruction of the sixth dorsal intervertebral disc space has occurred. This case is too high to cause pain in the lower back. When involvement is in the lumbar spine, the abscesses frequently follow the plane of the psoas muscle, and roentgenograms show distention of the muscle border. *B,* Sacroiliac tuberculosis; note the sclerosis and irregularity (arrow) of the right sacroiliac joint.

spinal cord or nerve root damage, however, especially when such fractures are accompanied by subluxation or dislocation. Immediate exploration and fixation of the region of injury are indicated, and these patients require around-the-clock care to avoid pressure sores, urinary tract infection, and increased neurologic damage, all of which can take place quickly with improper management. Later, rehabilitation is also necessary.

Fractures of the spinous processes are rare in the lumbar spine. Separations of the posterior elements, with or without fractures of the vertebral body or neural arch, have occurred in persons involved in automobile accidents when wearing the lap-type seat belt. Fractures of one or more transverse processes are common, however. These injuries are usually caused by simultaneous local contusion and strain and generally respond well to supportive treatment such as rest, sedation, and strapping. Sometimes, injection of the injured area with procaine provides remarkable relief.

Fractures of the sacrum usually result from direct trauma. Localized tenderness and superficial hematomata help one to make the diagnosis. These fractures are difficult to demonstrate roentgenographically. Fractures of the pelvic ring are sometimes associated with dislocation of the sacroiliac joints; proper roentgenographic evaluation is not difficult.

Pathologic Fractures

Because of the great forces brought to bear on the spine, it is not surprising that destruction or weakening of the vertebral trabecular structure is followed by vertebral fracture. It is surprising, however, that much bone substance may be lost without roentgenographic evidence. The pain of the fracture is frequently the first indication of the pathologic process. Lack of adequate trauma should cause one to suspect this diagnosis. The following lesions are most likely to lead to collapse of a vertebra: (1) *metastatic malignant disease,* such as breast, kidney, thyroid, or lung cancer in the adult, or neuroblastoma in children; occasionally the primary source cannot be found; (2) *primary neoplasms,* such as multiple myeloma; (3) *metabolic dyscrasias,* particularly senile, postmenopausal, or "steroid-induced" osteoporosis; rarely, osteomalacia or hyperparathyroidism; (4) *tuberculosis;* and (5) *other conditions,* such as Gaucher's disease and eosinophilic granuloma.

Differential diagnosis of these conditions depends on a complete medical history and physical examination and full use of laboratory and radiographic techniques. As previously discussed, radioactive bone scanning is effective in distinguishing various lesions of the spine. Differentiation can now be made between recent and old compression fractures, one can now detect occult metastasis to the spine, and activity of an infectious spondylitis may be evaluated.[10] Biopsy of the lesion itself should be performed whenever possible. If the lesion is accessible without hazard to adjacent viscera, blood vessels, or nerves, needle biopsy is a practical method of obtaining material for section. If not, open biopsy is necessary unless clinical, laboratory, and radiographic findings are conclusive.

Rheumatic Diseases

Ankylosing Spondylitis

This common cause of low back pain in young men involves the sacroiliac joints early in the disease. It can be diagnosed by diminished chest expansion and reduced spinal mobility. A useful sign is the contraction of the ipsilateral spinal musculature when bending to the side (Forestier's bowstring sign). Normally, the contralateral musculature tightens (see also Chap. 53).

Osteitis Condensans Ilii

This term is applied to the roentgenographic demonstration of sclerotic changes on the iliac sides of the sacroiliac joints. It is particularly common post partum and may be related to the strain that delivery places on these joints. When such changes occur, however, a more exact diagnosis should be sought because these lesions are also seen in osteoarthritis, in early ankylosing spondylitis, and in the presence of a nearby osteoid osteoma. Osteitis condensans ilii is not associated with the HLA-B27 antigen.[21] The clinical picture is not characteristic, and the condition is said to respond to conservative therapy identical to that for low back sprain.

Occasionally, late in pregnancy, women develop low back pain as the result of relaxation of the sacroiliac joints. The pubic symphysis is also involved and is tender. The syndrome can be troublesome, and the pain may be severe enough to force the patient to bed. Although it may be aggravated during delivery, such pain usually subsides afterward, and the joints resume their former stability. Rarely this pain and instability may persist, requiring sacroiliac fusion for relief.

Metabolic Bone Disease

Metabolic disorders of bone are discussed in Chapter 97.

Neoplastic Disease

Certain tumors show a predilection for the spine.

Intraspinal Lesions

Those experienced in spinal surgery have, at one time or another, encountered an intraspinal tumor causing backache and sciatica. A report from the Mayo Clinic has shown the incidence of various lesions. Neurofibroma and ependymoma each occurred 3 times in over 1,000 cases. Carcinoma metastatic to the spinal cord and its supporting structures occurs, as do primary tumors. These conditions develop frequently in the *absence* of neurologic signs. Myelographic or CT examination is needed for diagnosis.

Lesions of Vertebral Column

Of the malignant tumors, by far the most common are *multiple myeloma* and *metastatic carcinoma*. Both often have a similar roentgenographic

appearance and can cause extensive bone destruction. Myeloma spares the neural arch, which does not contain red bone marrow. Both diseases are often widespread. Differentiation depends on the demonstration of a primary source such as prostate, breast, kidney, thyroid, and lung, most frequently, in the case of metastatic disease and of abnormal gamma globulins in the case of multiple myeloma. Plasma electrophoresis is valuable in the early diagnosis of multiple myeloma. One often sees an associated anemia. Rarely, both metastatic carcinoma and multiple myeloma cause spinal cord and nerve root compression (Fig. 82–26). Chordoma, a rare malignant tumor largely confined to the sacrococcygeal and cranial portions of the axial skeleton, arises from remnants of the primitive notochord and is locally invasive. It is resistant to both surgical treatment and radiotherapy.

Benign tumors of the spine are less common. Giant cell tumor, bone cysts, osteochondromas, and chondromas may occur, but hemangiomas, aneurysmal bone cysts, and osteoid osteomas are seen more frequently. It is probably wrong to classify all hemangiomas as benign because some lead to extensive bone destruction. Many of these tumors respond favorably to irradiation, however. The typical roentgenogram is easily recognized and has vertical striations in the vertical body, which is often partially crushed and broadened in all dimensions but the vertical. Aneurysmal bone cysts involve the posterior vertebral elements and form large paraspinal masses with scattered calcific deposits. Although biopsy is required for definitive diagnosis, these cysts are radiosensitive and are therefore best treated by irradiation.

Osteoid osteoma is a painful tumor in which a small focus of osteogenetic activity develops and leads to extensive surrounding sclerosis of bone.[11] This tumor usually arises in the posterior vertebral elements and is therefore difficult to demonstrate roentgenographically. Tomograms are helpful to demonstrate the typical lesion, a zone of dense bone surrounding a small, radiolucent nidus. The pain, which may be severe and often occurs at night, is so dramatically relieved by aspirin or other NSAIDs that this response is a helpful diagnostic test.

Epiphysitis

Also known as Scheuermann's disease, epiphysitis is a painful back condition of adolescence, the cause of which is obscure. It is more common in boys than in girls and involves the thoracic spine much more frequently than the lumbar. Although structural round back, increased anteroposterior diameter of the chest, and tight hamstrings form part of the syndrome, this triad frequently occurs with-

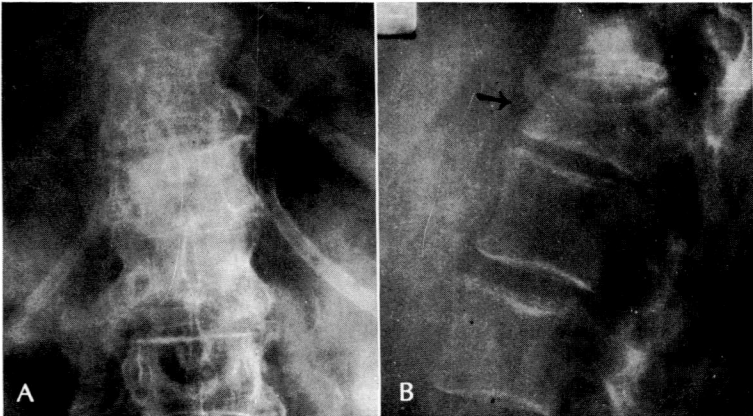

Fig. 82–26. *A* and *B,* An osteolytic metastasis with a pathologic compression fracture of D12 (arrow). These lesions may be difficult to recognize before collapse occurs. The source of the metastasis was carcinoma of the breast, surgically treated 20 years previously.

out pain. I have seen it most often without pain, and the usual presenting complaint is poor posture. The so-called typical roentgenographic findings of several mildly wedged vertebrae, narrowed disc spaces, and irregular vertebral margins are also not exclusively limited to patients in pain. These radiographic lesions are caused by faults in the cartilaginous end plates and permit herniation of the disc material into the spongiosa.

Treatment for patients whose primary problem is deformity differs from therapy for those who are in pain. A firm mattress, a bed board, and postural exercises are recommended when the deformity is mild. When thoracic kyphosis is significant and the patient has not completed growth, the use of a Milwaukee brace is gratifying. Frequently, after wearing this brace full time for only six months and part time for six months more, one sees a noticeable improvement of the round back. In patients in pain but with little deformity, more simplified bracing or the use of a plaster jacket for a few months may be all that is necessary.

The intent of postural treatment is not to correct deformity, but to prevent its progression. Whether this end can actually be achieved is open to question because the condition is often self-limiting. The problem of such treatment is actually to reduce the thoracic or thoracolumbar kyphosis and not merely to increase the lumbosacral lordosis. When an exercise program is considered, therefore, the usual lumbar flattening exercises are recommended, but in addition, a special one is added to extend the thoracic spine. The patient is asked to flatten his lumbar spine by flexing his hips over the end of a hard table and to hold this position while he raises his head and shoulders.

If a plaster jacket or brace is used, the same principles again apply: the lumbar lordosis must first be flattened and then the thoracic kyphosis extended. Immobilization of this kind is more likely to be helpful to patients with subacute pain. For those whose pain is severe, however, spinal fusion should not be delayed because it is not only the best way of relieving the pain, but also the most effective means of controlling progression of deformity. Operative reduction of kyphosis is difficult, but it may take place with further spinal growth, once a strong fusion is obtained.

Scoliosis

I have found that 40% of patients with adolescent idiopathic scoliosis are in pain.[16] The problem of pain in the older patient with scoliosis can sometimes be most challenging. Pain may exist at the level of the apex of the curve secondary to osteoarthritis, which occurs in the growing child. In lumbar curves, low back pain with leg radiation simulates disc symptoms. The usual operative management of excision of the disc fails. Such patients should be treated by external support with lumbosacral corsets. If no relief is obtained, a course of traction, supplemented by a more rigid brace, is often helpful. In patients not responding to conservative treatment, reduction of the curve and spinal fusion relieve the pain.

Although idiopathic scoliosis does not usually progress after full maturation of the spine. I have seen several patients in whom lumbar curves worsened during middle age. Such symptomatic curves may best be treated initially by correction and fusion because they continue to progress throughout life. Patients with untreated, progressive, painful scoliosis over the age of 65 are the most difficult to manage.

Coccygodynia

Pain in the coccygeal area is often difficult to diagnose and to treat. It may be of three separate types.

Primary Coccygeal Abnormality

As the result of direct trauma or childbirth, the coccyx may be fractured or the sacrococcygeal joint may be severely strained.

Primary Low Back Disorder

Coccygodynia commonly develops as a secondary phenomenon in a patient with low back pain. The mechanism is not understood, but the pain is most likely to be referred.

Visceral Lesion

It is common for patients with rectal or genitourinary disease to develop coccygeal pain. This pain is of a referred type and is sometimes associated with "spasm" of the muscles of the pelvic floor.

It is only by careful evaluation that these three entities may be separated. The back must always be examined because trauma to the coccyx cannot usually occur without simultaneously involving the low back. Rectal examination should include palpation of pelvic structures as well as of the coccyx and its adjacent structures, that is, the coccygeus and levator ani muscles and the sacrospinous and sacrotuberous ligaments.

Proctologic, gynecologic, and urologic evaluations may be indicated. When examination points to primary disease in the sacrococcygeal articulation, coccygectomy may be effective if conservative therapy fails. Every effort should be made to avoid irritation of the painful area. Soft chairs are usually worse than hard, and the patient should sit with good posture. A rubber ring may be necessary. Sometimes, a strapping or "sacroiliac belt" helps by pulling fatty tissues over the nonpadded coccygeal region.

Camptocormia

Hysterical back pain characterized by extreme flexion of the spine and by pain in the lumbar area has been termed "camptocormia." The diagnosis is made by normal findings on orthopedic and neurologic examinations and a deformity that disappears in recumbency or by suggestion.

Although this condition is not common, psychologic overlay in the patient with back pain is almost always present. Such anxiety frequently confuses the clinical picture and is often transferred to the treating physician; this phenomenon makes diagnosis and successful treatment difficult (see Chap. 70).

When evaluating the patient with low back pain, the physician must be aware of the possibility of secondary gain, as with liability cases, compensation cases, avoidance of military draft, and malingering.

Stenosis of the Aortic Bifurcation and Iliac Arteries

When pain is centered in the buttocks, groin, and thighs and is brought on by walking, but relieved quickly by rest, one should consider the possibility of intermittent claudication due to stenosis of the iliac arteries. Palpation of the femoral arteries should provide a quick diagnosis. The condition is common enough so that palpation of the arterial trunks should be included as part of the routine back examination.

Hip Joint Disease

Occasionally, it is difficult to distinguish the pain of hip disease from that of the spine because both may radiate along the same pathways. Intra-articular disease often causes pain radiating down the inner aspects of the thighs to the knees, whereas the pain of trochanteric bursitis may follow the more usual "sciatic" distribution. For this reason, it is important to analyze hip joint movements in all patients with sciatica and especially those in whom the findings in the lower back are equivocal.

Referred Pain from Visceral Structures

A lesion in one of the pelvic organs or the retroperitoneal structures can cause pain referred to the back. In women, the most usual condition is a retroverted uterus, but disease of the ovaries and fallopian tubes may also be the cause. The pain is usually worse during menses. In men, referred low back pain is usually the result of a prostatic lesion. Stones within the urinary tract are easily diagnosed in the presence of typical ureteral colic, but at other times, they may be a more obscure cause of back pain. In the presence of associated anorexia and weight loss, a retroperitoneal neoplasm must be considered. In most such patients, the back findings are insufficient to explain the symptoms, but in elderly patients, associated lower back lesions may complicate the picture and may test the diagnostic acumen of the attending physician.

Herniated Fat Syndrome

As pointed out by Copeman many years ago, fibrofatty nodules may develop by herniation through the dense fascia of the lower back. These nodules may become tender, especially in patients lying in bed for prolonged periods. Symptomatic relief may be obtained by infiltration with corticosteroid ester crystal suspensions diluted 1:10 in 1% procaine.

REFERENCES

1. Andersson, B.J., et al.: The sitting posture: an electromyographic and discometric study. Orthop. Clin. North Am., *6*:105–120, 1975.
2. Arnoldi, C.C.: Intraosseous hypertension: a possible cause of low back pain? Clin. Orthop., *115*:30–34, 1976.
3. Arnoldi, C.C., et al.: Lumbar spinal stenosis and nerve root entrapment syndromes: definition and classification. Clin. Orthop., *115*:4–5, 1976.
4. Asnis, S., Blau, L., and Bohne, W.: A comparison of ^{18}F and ^{85}Sr scintimetric patterns by computerized data analysis and display. Radiology, *106*:607–614, 1973.
5. Baker, R.A., et al.: Sequelae of metrizamide myelography in 200 examinations. A.J.R., *130*:499–502, 1978.
6. Bohne, W.H., Levine, D.B., and Lyden, J.P.: ^{18}F scintimetric diagnosis of osteoid osteoma of the carpal scaphoid bone. Clin. Orthop., *107*:156–158, 1975.
7. Cowell, M.J., and Cowell, H.R.: The incidence of spina bifida occulta in idiopathic scoliosis. Clin. Orthop., *118*:16–18, 1976.
8. Crock, H.V., and Hoshizawa, H.: The blood supply of the lumbar vertebral column. Clin. Orthop., *115*:6–21, 1976.
9. Dawson, G.D.: Cerebral responses to electrical stimulation of peripheral nerve in man. J. Neurol. Neurosurg. Psychiatr., *10*:137–140, 1947.
10. DeFiore, J.C., Lindberg, L., and Ranawat, N.S.: ^{85}Strontium scintimetry of the spine. J. Bone Joint Surg., *52A*:21–38, 1970.
11. Freiberger, R.H.: Osteoid osteoma of the spine. Radiology, *75*:232–236, 1960.
12. Gertzbein, S., et al.: Autoimmunity in degenerative disc disease of the lumbar spine. Orthop. Clin. North Am., *6*:67–73, 1975.
13. Javid, M.J., et al.: Safety and efficacy of chymopapain (chymodiatin) in herniated nuclear pulposus with sciatica. J.A.M.A., *249*:2,489–2,498, 1983.
14. Nash, C.L., Brodsky, J.S., and Croft, T.J.: A model for electrical monitoring of spinal cord function in scoliosis patients undergoing correction. *In* Proceedings of the Scoliosis Research Society. J. Bone Joint Surg., *54A*:197–198, 1982.
15. Nash, C.L., Schatzinger, L., and Lorig, R.: Intraoperative monitoring of spinal cord function during scoliosis spine surgery. J. Bone Joint Surg., *56A*:1,765, 1974.
16. Nastasi, A.J., Levine, D.B., and Veliskakis, K.P.: Pain patterns associated with adolescent idiopathic scoliosis. (Abstract of paper presented at the sixth Annual Meeting of the Scoliosis Research Society, Hartford, CT, 1971.) J. Bone Joint Surg., *54A*:199, 1972.
17. Naylor, A., et al.: Enzymic and immunological activity in the intervertebral disk. Orthop. Clin. North Am., *6*:51–58, 1975.
18. Nordby, E.J., Long, D.M., and Dawson, E.G.: Postgraduate Syllabus on Intradiscal Therapy. Chicago, American Academy of Orthopaedic Surgeons and American Association of Neurological Surgeons, 1983.
19. Pettersson, H., and Harwood-Nash, D.C.F.: CT and Myelography of the Spine and Cord. New York, Springer-Verlag, 1982.
20. Schmorl, G., and Junghanns, H.: The Human Spine in Health and Disease. New York, Grune & Stratton, 1971.
21. Singal, D.P., et al.: HLA antigens in osteitis condensans ilii and ankylosing spondylitis. J. Rheumatol., *4*:105–108, 1977.
22. Smith, L.: Enzyme dissolution of the nucleus pulposus in humans. J.A.M.A., *187*:137–140, 1964.
23. Stern, I.J.: Biochemistry of chymopapain. Clin. Orthop., *67*:42–46, 1969.
24. Weis, E.B.: Stresses at the lumbosacral junction. Orthop. Clin. North Am., *6*:83–91, 1975.
25. Willis, T.A.: The separate neural arch. J. Bone Joint Surg., *13*:709–721, 1931.
26. Wilson, P.D., and Levine, D.B.: Compensatory pelvic osteotomy for ankylosing spondylitis: a case report. J. Bone Joint Surg., *51A*:142–148, 1969.
27. Wiltse, L.L.: American Academy of Orthopaedic Surgeons Symposium on Spine. St. Louis, C.V. Mosby, 1969.
28. Wiltse, L.L., Newman, P.H., and MacNab, I.: Classification of spondylolisis and spondylolisthesis. Clin. Orthop., *117*:23–29, 1976.

Chapter 83

Dupuytren's Contracture

John W. Sigler and Alexander P. Kelly, Jr.

Contraction of the palmar fascia involving the digits was first described by Plater in 1614.[27] Sir Astley Cooper described its correction by subcutaneous fasciotomy in 1823.[3] Dupuytren's classic description of fascial contracture, flexion deformities of the fingers, and loss of function appeared in the *Lancet* in 1834.[4] In the century and a half since these initial publications, the tremendous body of literature created has been out of all proportion to the disability caused by this entity.

ETIOLOGIC FACTORS

The origin of this condition remains unknown. Numerous factors have been implicated, among which the most important are heredity, race, sex, trauma, focal hypertrophy of connective tissues originating in the vessel walls, fibroblastic proliferation disturbances, changes in sympathetic tone, central and peripheral nervous system lesions, ruptures of the fibers of the palmar aponeurosis with subsequent iron pigment deposition, and various chronic disease states. Histologic similarity to other fibrodysplasias such as desmoids, plantar fibromatosis, and induratio penis plastica (Peyronie's disease) have been noted frequently.

Trauma is no longer considered to cause Dupuytren's contracture, but it may represent an aggravating factor in individuals with a predisposition to the disease. Surgeons who see many of these patients note an occasional case in which an acute traumatic event seems causally related to the onset of Dupuytren's contracture. The importance of trauma was probably exaggerated in the past, both because of Dupuytren's original observations and because patients associated the onset of their disease with an explicit injury or with occupational wear and tear.

Dupuytren's contracture has been observed in several generations of the same family, usually in men, and a high familial incidence has been noted in several large series.[5,20,30] The role of heredity in Dupuytren's contracture is increasingly acknowledged. Evidence of heredity varies proportionally with the effort of the examiner to pursue the disorder through the various members of the patient's family. On examining 832 relatives of 50 patients, Ling found a familial incidence in 68% and strong

hearsay evidence of an even higher percentage.[20] In Skoog's group of 50 patients with Dupuytren's contracture, 44% of other members of the patients' families were affected.[30] In this series, men were affected 9 times as frequently as women. More recent work indicates the male-to-female ratio to be approximately 6:1.[13] One might assume hard manual labor to be related, in view of this sex disproportion, but most authors discount occupational trauma. Moreover, the sex disproportion diminishes in the older age groups.[20] The normal aging process may relate to Dupuytren's contracture because the incidence gradually increases with age. Dupuytren's contracture is found with increasing frequency in each decade over age 40. After 60 years of age, 25% of all persons examined have palmar thickening suggesting Dupuytren's contracture.[11,12,13]

Chronic invalids have a higher incidence of Dupuytren's contracture regardless of their general health. Diseases associated with Dupuytren's contracture include epilepsy, pulmonary tuberculosis, chronic alcoholism, and diabetes. The increased incidence of Dupuytren's contracture in these groups is thought to be related to constant observation of an aging patient population. The high incidence of diabetic glucose tolerance curves in association with palmar contractures is worthy of further investigation.[31] Barbiturate usage has been suspected as a common factor in many of these chronic diseases.[30] Other studies have noted an association of Dupuytren's contracture with abnormal liver function (excretory enzymes) in patients with alcoholism or epilepsy.[28]

A curious and perhaps significant association between Dupuytren's contracture and epilepsy has been described by Lund,[22] who reported contractures of the hand in 50% of 190 epileptic men and in 25% of 171 women. Skoog studied 207 epileptic men and found palmar contractures in 42%. Concurrent hereditary predisposition to both conditions may be a common denominator. Barbiturates were again mentioned as a possible contributing factor in these studies.[30] Use of newer anticonvulsive agents may better define the role of barbiturates in these patients.

Numerous studies have attempted to associate

Dupuytren's contracture with various diseases of the central and peripheral nervous systems, especially the reflex dystrophies involving the shoulder and the hand.[22]

SYMPTOMS AND SIGNS

One or both hands may be affected, but bilateral involvement is more common in the experience of most observers. The right hand is affected more often than the left in unilateral disease. The ring finger is most frequently involved; the little, middle, and index fingers follow, in that order. When several fingers are affected, the involvement may not occur at the same time and may not progress at the same rate. Occasionally, the nodules are dorsal in the proximal interphalangeal area, and rarely, they have a puckering of the skin characteristic of this condition (Table 83–1).

DIAGNOSIS

The diagnosis is made by inspection and palpation of the hand (Fig. 83–1). Congenital or spastic contractures or those following injury or infection can be differentiated by having the patient flex his wrist; this maneuver shortens the flexor tendons and permits full extension of the fingers. In Dupuytren's contracture, extension of the digits is unchanged by flexion of the wrist, and if the metacarpophalangeal joints are also flexed, one can rule out flexion deficiencies due to intrinsic muscle contracture.

Hypertrophic scarring of the palms secondary to burns or other injury may occasionally be confused with Dupuytren's contracture. Deformities due to such trauma can be determined by the patient's medical history. Small solid tumors in the palm can be distinguished by their lack of fixation to the overlying skin. Knuckle pads, plantar fibromatosis (Fig. 83–2), and Peyronie's disease are associated

Table 83–1.   Signs of Dupuytren's Contracture

1. Small nodules or plaque-like thickening of the palmar connective tissues overlying the tendons of the digits, usually the fourth and fifth digits.
2. Puckering of the palmar skin.
3. Appearance of fibrous bands extending longitudinally from the palmar nodule.
4. Extension of fascial bands from the concavity of the palm to the metacarpophalangeal and proximal interphalangeal joints.
5. Progressive involvement of the palmar skin and fingers.
6. Possible progressive involvement of the greater portion of the palmar fascia and all the fingers, leading to marked flexion contracture of the fingers.
7. Course of illness often remaining stationary for months or years, without affecting the palmar fascia beyond the distal palmar crease.

processes that should be sought in patients with Dupuytren's contracture.

PATHOLOGIC FEATURES

Normally, the palmar fascia or aponeurosis is a triangular membrane consisting of four layers, with its apex at the transverse carpal ligament.[16] The dense superficial layer separates into four bundles, one for each finger fusing into the flexor tendon sheath. It is attached to the deeper layers of the skin proximal to the webs and extends into the bases of the fingers. Some fibers run vertically and obliquely, bind the skin to the aponeurosis, and give rise to creases at the level of the metacarpal heads. Transverse fasciculi communicate with the deeper fascial layers, the metacarpal bones, the phalanges, and the interphalangeal joints. All the components of the fascia can be affected by the disease except the deep transverse portion. Some of the fine fascial structures are rarely identified until they become involved in this fibroplasia. The palmar aponeurosis protects the important compartments of the hand and stabilizes the skin, so it does not slide loosely when the hand is used for grasping.

Early changes consist of a small palmar nodule or a plaque-like thickening arising in the palmar connective tissues overlying the tendons of the fourth and fifth fingers. The process may extend to the third, first, and second digits sequentially. Nodule formation is the first or cellular phase.[21] The overlying skin becomes puckered and adheres to the fascia. In many instances, the fibrosis may remain stationary for months or years and may not affect the palmar fascia beyond the distal palmar crease. McCallum and Hueston have adopted the view expressed by Goyrand that the nodule arises primarily in the fibrofatty tissues overlying the palmar fascia rather than in the fascia proper.[8,23] The arguments for this thesis are strong, but the palmar fascia becomes involved so rapidly in the process that, from a clinical point of view, the origin of the nodule appears to be unimportant. Electron microscopic study has identified myofibroblasts in the nodular areas.[6] The cells appear to be contractile, based on the presence of actin. Their origin is unclear; they may arise from the blood vessel walls. Similar cells have been identified in the granulation tissue of healing wounds. The myofibroblast is not found in the band.[6,14,19,29] These findings may explain the progress of the disease as it is observed clinically. Histochemical studies indicate that the levels of enzymes of glucose metabolism of palmar fascia in Dupuytren's contracture are much higher than in normal palmar fascia.[10] Our understanding of this disease will depend on advances in cellular

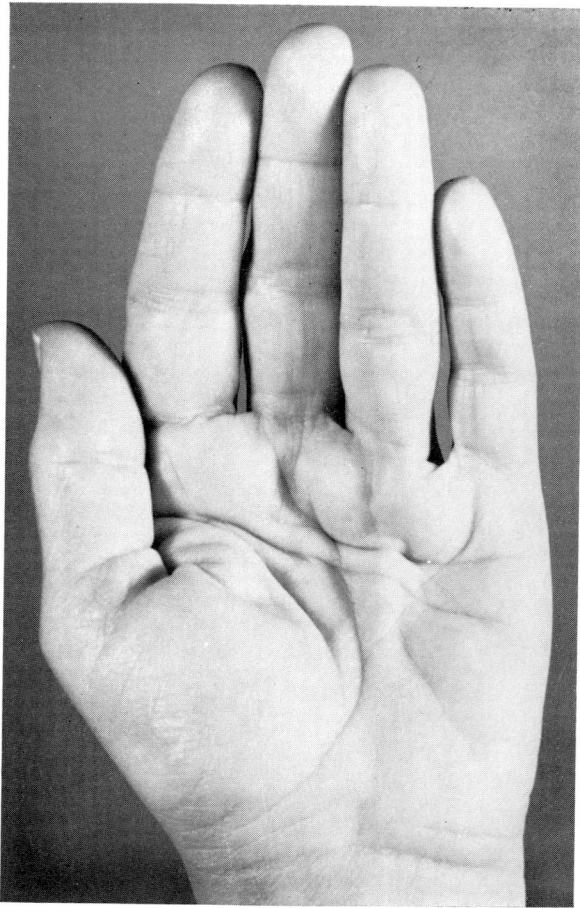

Fig. 83–1. Dupuytren's contracture. Puckering of the palmar skin and contraction of the palmar fascial bands extending to the base of the fourth metacarpophalangeal joint cause an early flexion contracture of the fourth finger.

biology because other approaches have been found wanting.[26]

In the second or involutional phase of the disease, the cellularity of the nodule decreases, and the fibrous bands extend centrifugally from the nodule. Once the fascial bands extend to the base of the fingers, contractures of the metacarpophalangeal and proximal interphalangeal joints occur (see Fig. 83–1).

In the third or residual phase, the nodule involutes and leaves dense fibrous bands connecting the skin and palmar fascia along the lines of maximal tension. Whether the fibrous cord is an actively formed structure or whether it represents a scar contracture developing secondary to finger motion is not certain. Both nodule formation and the various stages of involution may be present simultaneously in several areas of the affected hand.

TREATMENT

Therapy should first be directed toward reassuring the patient of the benign nature of the disease. The patient with a primary complaint of a painful nodule in the palm most often finds the discomfort negligible after an adequate explanation. In the occasional patient with persistent pain, a single ten-day course of ultrasonic therapy may prove effective. Local corticosteroid injections into the painful nodule may give symptomatic relief. Heat therapy together with stretching exercises may also relieve symptoms. Corticosteroids, either systemic or local, other drugs, and radiation therapy do not alter the course of Dupuytren's contracture.

Surgical management of Dupuytren's contracture is indicated when and if contracture begins. The patient is instructed to return when limitation of extension of the fingers is first noted. Patients are advised that metacarpophalangeal joint contracture needs to be corrected only when it becomes physically annoying, but proximal interphalangeal joint contracture is an indication for early surgical intervention. Less-reliable patients should be examined at regular intervals to determine the extent

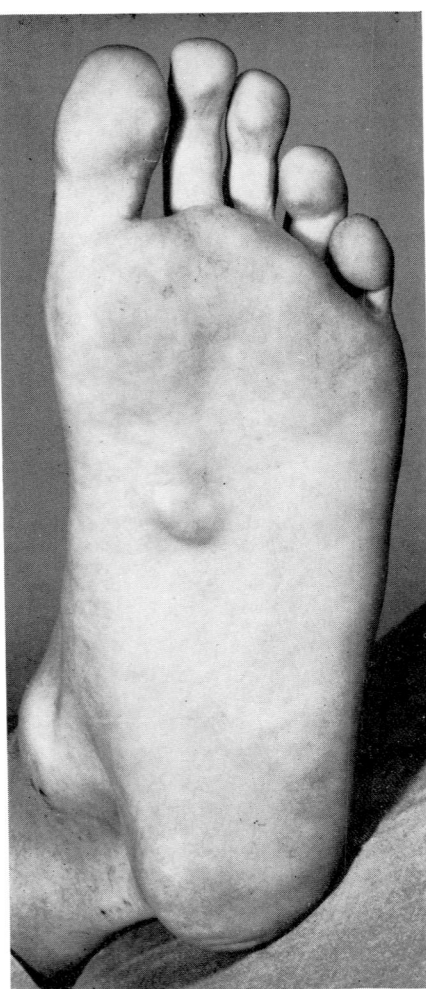

Fig. 83–2. Plantar fibromatosis associated with Dupuytren's contracture histologically may be mistaken for fibrosarcoma, prompting unnecessary radical surgical procedures and even amputation in isolated instances.

of the contracture. The presence of nodules, puckering, and skin involvement may remain static for a number of years and do not represent an indication for surgery.

Surgical Procedures

Surgical treatment includes the following: (1) subcutaneous fasciotomy; (2) limited fasciectomy; (3) radical fasciectomy; (4) open palm fasciectomy; (5) division of contracture and skin graft; and (6) digital amputation. The type and extent of involvement and the overall health and needs of the patient determine which procedure is most suitable. The simplest procedure offering the most function with the lowest risk of complication and reasonable freedom from recurrence is chosen. The marked de-

crease in extension and recurrence of the disease after the sixth decade should influence the choice of procedure.

Subcutaneous fasciotomy, reported by Sir Astley Cooper in 1823, is most suitable for the single-band contracture, particularly when active disease has subsided.[3] Nodule excision from the palm or proximal finger, combined with fasciotomy, represents adequate and definitive treatment for many patients.[21] The rate of recurrence is not much higher than after more radical forms of treatment. Fasciotomy has a distinct place in the treatment of patients with contractures less suitable to this operation but in whom the severity of concomitant disease makes a minimal procedure desirable.[17]

Limited fasciectomy is suitable for most patients seeking surgical relief of Dupuytren's contracture. The procedure, probably introduced by Kocher in the last century, was revived by Iselin and Dieckmann with their multiple Z-plasty operations.[15,18] The current use of this approach began with Hamlin and his studies, who demonstrated the prolonged morbidity of the more radical procedures.[9] Visualization of important structures, especially the digital nerves, is excellent, and undermining of skin, with the threat of hematoma or skin slough, is minimal. Postoperative morbidity is only a few days longer than after fasciotomy, and light work is permitted in four to five days.

The goal of radical fasciectomy, the procedure of choice of surgeons for several decades, is the complete removal of the palmar fascia. Ideally, this operation reverses the contracture and eliminates the prospect of recurrence. Unfortunately, recurrences and extension into unoperated areas were common in the past. The morbidity was prolonged, and many hands never recovered mobility. The result was more disabling than the original complaint, and many referring physicians therefore became disenchanted with surgical interventions. Reports from discontented surgeons followed.[1,2] Clarkson detailed the case against radical fasciectomy.[2] The radical procedure, however, still has a definite place in the treatment of Dupuytren's contracture. We now remove all diseased fascia in the palm and fingers in a single operative session. Closure may be a problem because of the sacrifice of damaged skin or inelasticity when it is retained. Skin grafts or rotated dorsal flaps are sometimes necessary for closure. Most surgeons reserve the procedure for younger patients with a rapid course and widespread involvement. Postoperative edema may be severe and slow to resolve, but if patients are properly selected, this problem is less formidable. Seldom is the patient able to return to any but the most sedentary occupation in less than two months and to manual labor in about four months.

Gonzalez has proposed dividing the contracting band at the point of maximum stress and closing the defect with a full-thickness skin graft. The procedure offers minimal morbidity and loss of joint motion and probably the lowest recurrence rate of any of these surgical procedures.[7]

McCash has reported a series wherein the palm was left open to heal secondarily, and primary attention was directed to maintaining finger motion.[24] The open-palm technique is similar to the Baron Dupuytren's original operative approach. Several recent series attest to the low morbidity and the efficacy of this technique.

Finger amputation is indicated in the patient with severe digital deformity. In some cases, the proximal interphalangeal joint is destroyed by severe flexion deformities. An extensive procedure restoring excellent metacarpophalangeal joint mobility fails to clear the finger from its obstructing position. In such patients, simple amputation of one digit can make the hand more useful than can the more radical operations. Filleting a finger to create a pedicle flap to cover a palmar defect may allow excellent release of the remaining digits. The little finger is important to hand function, and efforts to preserve it by cross-finger flaps, arthroplasty, arthrodesis, and intramedullary pegs have been proposed.[25]

In summary, treatment of Dupuytren's contracture producing hand dysfunction is surgical. The proper selection of patient and procedure affords excellent relief of disability. Surgical treatment is not curative any more than insulin cures diabetes mellitus. Physicians who think of the surgical treatment of this disorder in this context can better prepare their patients for the repeated, limited procedures that have gained favor over a single, radical operation.

Postoperative Care

The majority of our postoperative patients are ambulatory. They are placed in a compression dressing for 48 to 72 hours and then in a light dressing, to allow freedom of movement. Patients are encouraged to move their fingers actively and passively as much as comfort permits. Occupational therapists treat some patients in the first weeks if the correction obtained surgically is lost.

REFERENCES

1. Bruner, J.M.: The selective treatment of Dupuytren's contracture with special reference to complications and indications for treatment. *In* Transactions of the International Society of Plastic Surgeons Second Congress. Edited by A.B. Wallace. London, E. & S. Livingstone, 1959.

2. Clarkson, P.: The radical fasciectomy operation for Dupuytren's disease: a condemnation. Br. J. Plast. Surg., 16:273–279, 1963.
3. Cooper, A.: Treatise on Dislocations and on Fractures at the Joints. 2nd Ed. London, Longmans, 1823.
4. Dupuytren, G.: Permanent retraction of the fingers, produced by an affection of the palmar fascia. Lancet, 2:222–225, 1834.
5. Early, P.F.: Population studies in Dupuytren's contracture. J. Bone Joint Surg., 41B:602–612, 1962.
6. Gabbiani, G., and Majno, G.: Dupuytren's contracture: fibroblast contraction? Am. J. Pathol., 66:131–146, 1972.
7. Gonzalez, R.I.: Dupuytren's contracture of the fingers: a simplified approach to the surgical treatment. Calif. Med., 115:25–31, 1970.
8. Goyrand, G.: Nouvelles recherche sur la rétraction permanente des doigts. Mem. Acad. R. Med., 3:489, 1833.
9. Hamlin, E.: Limited excision of Dupuytren's contracture. Ann. Surg., 135:94–97, 1952.
10. Hoopes, J.E., et al.: Enzymes of glucose metabolism in palmar fascia and Dupuytren's contracture. J. Hand Surg., 2:62–65, 1977.
11. Hueston, J.T.: Dupuytren's Contracture. Baltimore, Williams & Wilkins, 1963.
12. Hueston, J.T.: Further studies on the incidence of Dupuytren's contracture. Med. J. Aust., 49:586–588, 1962.
13. Hueston, J.T.: The incidence of Dupuytren's contracture. Med. J. Aust., 2:999–1,002, 1960.
14. Hueston, J.T., Hurley, J.V., and Whittinghan, S.: The contracting fibroblast as a clue to Dupuytren's contracture. Hand, 8:10–12, 1976.
15. Iselin, M., and Dieckmann, D.G.: Traitement de la maladie de dupuytren par plastie en z totale. Presse Med., 59:1394–1395, 1951.
16. Kaplan, E.B.: Functional and Surgical Anatomy of the Hand. Philadelphia, J.B. Lippincott, 1953.
17. Kelly, A.P.: Subcutaneous fasciotomy in the treatment of Dupuytren's contracture. Plast. Reconstr. Surg., 24:505–510, 1959.
18. Kocher, T.: Behandlung der retraction der palmar-apponeurose. Zentralbl. Chir., 14:481–487, 1887.
19. Legge, J.W.H., Finlay, J.B., and McFarlane, R.M.: A study of Dupuytren's tissue with the scanning electron microscope. J. Hand Surg., 6:482–492, 1981.
20. Ling, R.S.M.: The genetic factor in Dupuytren's disease. J. Bone Joint Surg., 45B:709–718, 1963.
21. Luck, J.V.: Dupuytren's contracture: a new concept of the pathogenesis correlated with surgical management. J. Bone Joint Surg., 41A:635–664, 1959.
22. Lund, M.: Dupuytren's contracture and epilepsy. Acta Psychiatr. Neurol. Scand., 16:465–492, 1941.
23. McCallum, P., and Hueston, J.T.: The pathology of Dupuytren's contracture. Ann. Surg., 135:94–97, 1952.
24. McCash, C.R.: The open palm technique in Dupuytren's contracture. Br. J. Plast. Surg., 17:271–280, 1964.
25. Moberg, E.: Three useful ways to avoid amputation in advanced Dupuytren's contracture. Orthop. Clin. North Am., 4:1,001–1,005, 1973.
26. Peacock, E.E.: Dupuytren's disease: controversial aspects of management. Clin. Plast. Surg., 3:29–37, 1976.
27. Plater, F.: Observationem in Hominis Affectibus. Basel, Konig, 1614.
28. Pojer, J., Radivojevic, M., and Williams, T.F.: Dupuytren's disease: its association with abnormal liver function in alcoholism and epilepsy. Arch. Intern. Med., 129:561–566, 1972.
29. Salamon, A., and Hamori, J.: The role of myofibroblasts in the pathogenesis of Dupuytren's contracture. Handchirurgie, 12:113–117, 1980.
30. Skoog, T.: Dupuytren's contraction. Acta Chir. Scand., 96 (Suppl. 139):1–190, 1948.
31. Spring, M., Fleck, H., and Cohen, B.D.: Dupuytren's contracture: warning of diabetes. N.Y. State J. Med., 70:1,037–1,041, 1970.

Chapter 84

Tumors of Joints and Related Structures

Alan S. Cohen and Juan J. Canoso

Neoplasms and other tumorous conditions of the articular structures are uncommon in rheumatologic practice. Nevertheless, it is important to give these disorders prominent consideration in patients with monarticular disease, lest proper diagnosis and treatment be delayed. The diagnosis of these lesions has been facilitated by techniques such as arthroscopy,[49,50,55] arteriography,[138] and computerized tomography (CT).[39,62,85,121]

BENIGN TUMORAL CONDITIONS

This category comprises a heterogeneous group of disorders of joints, bursae, and tendon sheaths. It includes pigmented villonodular synovitis, which is a chronic inflammatory lesion of unknown origin, synovial chondromatosis and other cartilaginous metaplasias of the subsynovial tissue, vascular malformations, fat growths, and fibromas.

Pigmented Villonodular Synovitis

The term "pigmented villonodular synovitis" denotes a group of interrelated, benign, tumorous disorders that involve the lining of joints, bursae, and tendon sheaths.[20,42,51,52,83,105] These lesions consist of villous or nodular growths, which are covered by a thin layer of synovial lining cells. The connective tissue stroma contains a heterogeneous and variably dense collection of cells, collagen bundles, and blood vessels. The cellular infiltrate consists of polyhedral, histiocytic-like cells, lipid-laden cells appearing as foam cells on routine histologic preparations, hemosiderin-laden macrophages, and multinucleated giant cells (Fig. 84–1). Early lesions are highly vascular, whereas old lesions are less vascular, exhibit more fibrosis and hyalinization, and may contain cholesterol crystals.[52,99] The color of the lesion, ranging from yellow to tan to dark brown, depends on the proportion of lipid and hemosiderin. Bone invasion results from direct penetration through vascular foramina,[108] as well as from pressure erosion.

Electron-microscopic studies in both villous[1,33,36,107] and nodular[1,91] forms usually revealed a predominance of cells resembling fibroblasts, and a lesser number both of cells resembling macrophages and of intermediate cells, consistent with a derivation from normal synovium. So far, pigmented villonodular synovitis has only been detected in humans. Reported cases in horses bear little resemblance to the human disease.[2,82]

Clinical Findings

Involvement of the affected joint, tendon sheath, or bursa may be either diffuse or localized. The condition is typically monotopic and lacks systemic symptoms or findings. The patient's erythrocyte sedimentation rate is usually normal.[21,54,81] Rarely are two or more joints affected.[4,7,34,61,66,131] Several cases have been observed in association with rheumatoid arthritis (RA).[81,91,125] It is unclear whether this connection represents a true association or whether it is the result of a detection bias.

It is useful to classify pigmented villonodular synovitis according to its location, articular, tenosynovial, or bursal, and to the lesional type, either diffuse or nodular.

Articular, Diffuse. This condition occurs chiefly in young adults and is equally frequent in both sexes.[54,81] The joint usually affected is the knee; much less commonly involved are the hip, ankle, elbow, carpus, hand, and tarsus.[16,30,83,105] Rare locations include the temporomandibular joint[60] and the vertebral facet joint.[11] The principal symptoms are pain and swelling, which may be mild and intermittent for a long period, and gradual swelling of the joint due to effusion and synovial proliferation. Focal masses are usually palpable in or about the joint. A popliteal cyst often develops.[107] The joint fluid is usually sanguineous or dark brown, not viscous, and does not usually clot.[81,95,107] One report noted an average white blood cell count of 3,110/mm^3, with an average of 26% polymorphonuclear cells. The red blood cell count varied from 43,000 to 1,780,000/mm^3. Results of the mucin test varied from fair to good.[95] The glucose content was normal.[81,95]

Roentgenographic examination, in addition to demonstrating increased amounts of joint fluid, may reveal lobulation and thickening of the synovial tissues. Narrowing of the joint space and peri-

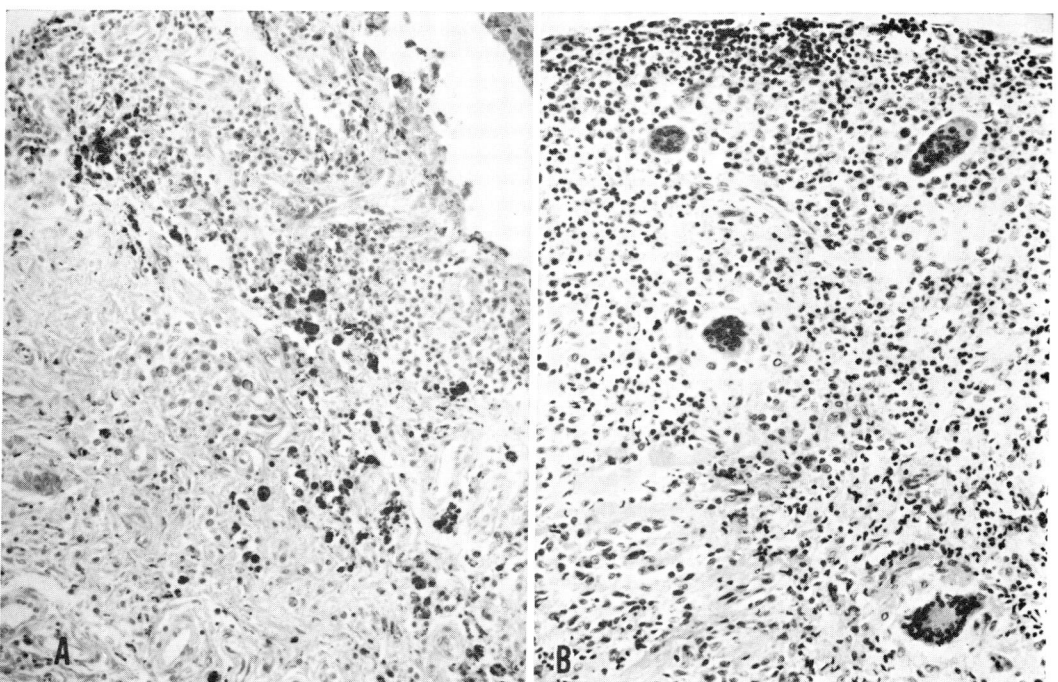

Fig. 84–1. Circumscribed nodular synovitis; photomicrographs of a nodular lesion. *A,* Large deposits of hemosiderin pigment in richly cellular connective tissue stroma. *B,* Multinucleated giant cells amid dense infiltrate of small round cells and large cells with pale, spindle-shaped nuclei (× 175).

articular demineralization occur late in the disorder.[134] In the hip, elbow, and shoulder, and on occasion the wrist, finger, and temporomandibular joint, one may see considerable narrowing of the joint space, bony erosions, and uni- and multiloculated cysts in the subchondral bone.[16,54,60,134] Erosions and cysts usually involve both sides of the joint, and their peripheral location around and just proximal to the articulating surfaces parallels the distribution of the perforating blood vessels.[53,64,108] Arthrograms, preferably with double contrast, demonstrate enlargement and distortion of the suprapatellar pouch with numerous recesses and filling defects.[134] Similar features have been shown by sonography.[57] The high iron content of the lesion can be determined by CT scanning, although the specificity of this finding is still unknown.[98] The diagnostic procedure of choice is arthroscopy.[49,50,55] The synovium is stained brown and appears shaggy and proliferative. Representative biopsies can be obtained for pathologic and bacteriologic studies, including mycobacterial and fungal cultures.

Articular, Circumscribed (Nodular). Localized involvement of the synovium occurs less frequently than the diffuse form of the disease, with a ratio of 1 to 4.[54,81] Here again, the knee is most commonly affected, and the patient is usually an adult with symptoms for many months or years

before the diagnosis is established. The symptoms are often episodic and consist of pain, swelling, locking, and "giving way" of the joint.[81] Small to moderate effusions and occasional limited range of motion are found. The synovial fluid is less likely to be sanguineous. Radiograms of the joint usually show no abnormalities.[41,54,81] Arthrographic examination may demonstrate an intra-articular bulge.[37,68] The true nature of the process is not suspected until one or more sessile or stalked, yellow-brown nodular growths are found at arthroscopy or at operation.

Tenosynovial, Circumscribed (Nodular). This type constitutes by far the most common form of the disorder,[81,105] and it is ten times more common than circumscribed nodular synovitis.[81] It is the second most common soft tissue tumor of the hand, outnumbered only by ganglia.[5] The majority of patients are young or middle-aged adults. Women are affected more often than men, and the incidence is higher in the dominant hand. Most frequently involved is a finger, more often the index or middle, on the volar (60%) or dorsal or lateral aspect of which a firm, slow-growing, painless nodular mass develops. Less often, this lesion is found near a metacarpophalangeal joint, wrist, ankle, or toe. Larger lesions may cause extensive pressure erosion of adjacent bone.[134] The origin of lesions arising in sites devoid of tendon sheaths, such as the lateral or dorsal aspect of fingers, is controversial. Some authors believe that they represent outgrowths of silent joint lesions.[14]

Tenosynovial, Diffuse. Occasionally, one sees diffuse involvement of the tendon sheaths of the hand and foot, in which the lesions may grow to a large size and may erode neighboring bone.[51]

Bursal. This uncommon lesion, usually diffuse, may be found in a deep bursa such as the gastrocnemius-semimembranosus and the iliopsoas.[51,105] No instances have been described involving the subcutaneous bursae.

Pathogenesis

Whether this condition represents a true neoplasm of synovial tissue or some form of obscure chronic inflammation is still not clear. The frequent erosion of adjacent bone by these lesions, their recurrence after synovectomy, and the presence of clefts and spaces surrounded by synovial lining cells have been thought to support the theory of neoplasm. In fact, many lesions have been considered neoplastic at operation, leading to amputation.[53,83] Strict histologic criteria of malignant lesions are lacking, however, and no case has been known to metastasize.

Fragments of the lesion grown in culture have shown a metabolic rate far in excess of rheumatoid synovium and a significant rise in the activity of glycolytic and lysosomal enzymes.[46] Such tissue, similar to hemophilic synovitis,[72] may produce large amounts of collagenase or other proteolytic enzymes, and such a finding would further explain the destructive nature of many of these lesions.

Similarities between pigmented villonodular synovitis and the findings in hemophilia and intra-articular hemangioma have led many to consider that the lesion might result from recurrent hemarthrosis.[22,45] In support of this view, changes resembling those of the human disease have been produced experimentally in dogs and in rhesus monkeys by repeated intra-articular injection of blood and colloidal iron.[101,119] Moreover, multiple lesions in children have been associated with cutaneous or synovial hemangiomas; this finding suggests a pathogenetic role of recurrent hemarthrosis.[4,61,66] No evidence of vascular malformation exists in most instances of pigmented villonodular synovitis, however, and foam cells do not occur in hemosideric synovitis induced experimentally[119] or in hemophilic joints.[22] It has been suggested that recurrent lipohemarthrosis would explain the deposition of both hemosiderin and lipids.[36] This view is supported by the finding that, in over 50% of patients, acute or repetitive local trauma seemingly precedes the appearance of the lesion.[81]

A microbial cause of the lesion has been sought, but not found. Cultures are routinely negative. Tubular structures resembling myxovirus nucleoprotein were found in only one of many cases studied by electron microscopy.[77] A primary proliferation of synovial cells has also been proposed.[107] Although the exact nature of pigmented villonodular synovitis is unknown at present, the condition appears to be an inflammatory granuloma, rather than a true neoplasm. The possibility still remains that the lesion, defined on clinical, radiologic, and histopathologic grounds, may result from more than one causative mechanism.[107]

Treatment

Although pigmented villonodular synovitis appears to be a benign lesion usually confined to a single joint or soft tissue structure, the results of surgical treatment are often disappointing. Resection of nodular synovitis of tendon sheath has a recurrence rate of approximately 20%, presumably owing to incomplete removal of the lesion.[42] In localized nodular synovitis of the knee, results have been better.[21,41,42,54] Major difficulties are encountered in the treatment of the diffuse form of pigmented villonodular synovitis in the knee. Extensive synovectomy has been followed by a 30 to 40% recurrence rate.[42,54] In the event of recurrence, radiotherapy has been instituted, but the response to this therapeutic technique is also uncertain.[29,42] Arthroscopic surgical procedures[50,55] and intra-articular administration of radiocolloids[93,136] hold promise in the treatment of recurrent disease. In the hip, the destructive lesions of pigmented villonodular synovitis can be eradicated by total hip arthroplasty,[54,124] but the youth of the patients raises questions about the long-term results of the prosthesis. Follow-up studies have shown that chronic pain and limitation of motion are frequent sequelae of the disease.[21,54]

Synovial Chondromatosis

Synovial chondromatosis arises from focal metaplasia of subsynovial tissue producing nodules of normal-appearing cartilage, or rarely in bursa, tendon sheath, joint capsule, or para-articular connective tissue.[51,79,105,115] These nodules become pedunculated and often detach from the synovium and grow as viable loose bodies within the joint cavity.[75] These cartilage nodules may calcify or even ossify, leading to the term osteochondromatosis. The origin of the disorder is unknown. The lesion is benign and rarely undergoes malignant change.[105]

Synovial chondromatosis occurs most often as a monarticular disturbance in young or middle-aged adults and is more common in men than in women.[79,105] The joint most frequently involved is the knee, followed by the hip, the elbow, and the shoulder.[18,79,86,105] Osteochondromatosis of the temporomandibular joint has been reported.[97] In the uncommon cases of multiple joint involvement, both knees are usually affected.

Clinical Findings

Patients may have pain, swelling, and limitation of joint motion, or they may be asymptomatic, with the lesion discovered by accident. Examination of the joint often reveals the presence of loose bodies and increased amounts of synovial fluid, which is viscous and normal in all other characteristics.[95]

The diagnosis, usually established by roentgenographic examination, discloses multiple stippled calcifications within the confines of the joint capsule in approximately 90% of patients.[105,134] The joint otherwise appears normal, although patients with advanced disease may exhibit evidence of osteoarthritis. The differential diagnosis of synovial chondromatosis includes several other conditions associated with loose joint bodies, such as severe osteoarthritis with intra-articular osteophytic fragments, osteochondritis dissecans, neuropathic arthropathy, and the "Milwaukee" shoulder.[69,134] Synovial calcification mimicking osteochondromatosis can also occur in calcium pyrophosphate dihydrate deposition disease.[24]

Pathogenesis

Gross examination of the affected joint reveals variably large and compact clusters of flat or pedunculated cartilaginous nodules protruding from the thickened synovial membrane, as well as loose bodies within the joint cavity. Microscopic study indicates that the cartilage found in synovial chondromatosis develops as a result of metaplastic transformation of the subsynovial connective tissue (Fig. 84–2). An imperceptible transition between subsynovial fibrocytes and fully developed chondrocytes has been shown by electron microscopy.[70] Predictably, the collagen of the nodules is type II.[104]

Detailed analysis of operative and histologic findings in loose bodies and synovial membrane has permitted a reconstruction of the natural history of the disease.[75] At first, cartilage metaplasia occurs in the subsynovial tissue in a multifocal fashion. In a later stage, some of the growing nodules become pedunculated and are finally released as loose joint bodies, whereas others remain buried in the membrane. Finally, the synovial membrane resumes its normal morphologic features, probably by resorption of residual foci of cartilaginous metaplasia, while the loose bodies undergo further remodeling. Calcification and ossification of the nod-

ules can occur prior to or following their release into the joint cavity.[75,76] Although this view is based on pathologic findings rather than a longitudinal study of individual cases, it has gained wide acceptance. Spontaneous regression of calcified bodies has been reported in one patient.[87]

Treatment

When the condition is suspected, arthroscopy or arthrotomy should be undertaken to remove the loose bodies, to determine the condition of the synovial membrane, and to assess the integrity of the articular cartilage. Synovectomy is indicated in extensive synovial disease.[79] Minor synovial metaplasia can be treated arthroscopically,[55] provided the articular cartilage is still normal.

Intracapsular, Extrasynovial Chondroma

This unusual lesion occurs most frequently in the knee. The patient has discomfort and a firm mass distal to the patella and deep to the patellar tendon.[120] Lateral radiographs reveal a calcified lesion within the infrapatellar fat pad.[134] Treatment is surgical excision.

Hemangioma

The tissue usually affected is the synovial membrane of the knee.[44,51,63,96,105] When the joint capsule is diseased, the adjacent soft tissues and bone may become involved. Hemangiomas occur most often in adolescents or in young adults, many of whom have had symptoms since childhood; this feature suggests that the lesion may represent a congenital vascular malformation.[45] The affected joint is periodically painful and swollen and often contains bloody fluid. In fact, intra-articular hemangioma should be suspected when a patient is subject to recurrent episodes of hemarthrosis of the knee in the absence of a clear explanation.[45] Hemangiomas may be seen in the skin overlying the affected joint.

An arteriovenous shunt in a patient with a hemangioma may be associated with increased leg length. In some cases, a tender, doughy joint mass decreases in size on elevation of the limb. The roentgenographic examination may show a tumor that contains phlebolithic densities of differential diagnostic value. Patients with a hemangioma of long standing can exhibit enlarged epiphyses, joint-space narrowing, and enlargement of the intercondylar notch resembling hemophilic arthropathy.[92] When hemangioma is suspected, arteriography or phlebography may help to localize the lesion and to rule out arteriovenous shunt.[28,92,138]

A hemangioma within the joint can be localized in the form of a dark, grape-like mass, or it can be diffuse. Circumscribed lesions commonly originate from the infrapatellar fat pad. It may be dif-

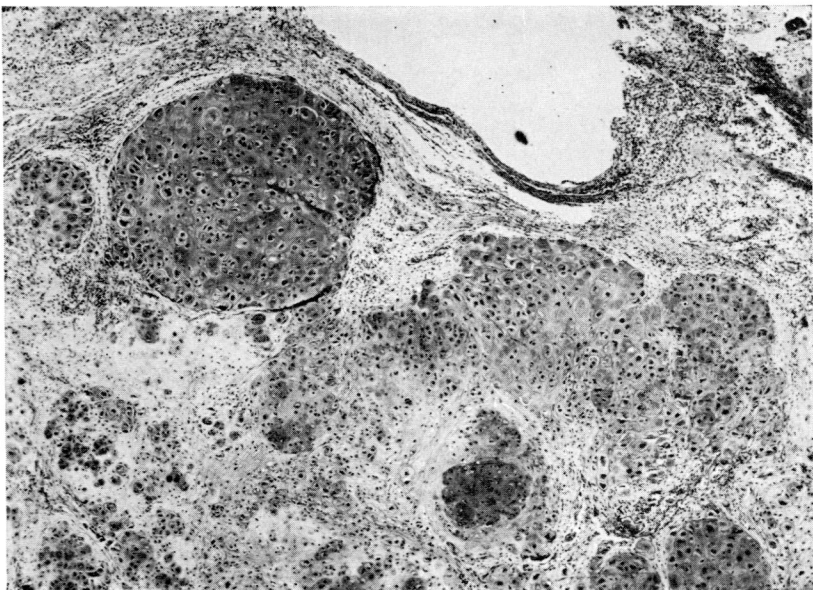

Fig. 84–2. Synovial chondromatosis; photomicrograph of synovium showing several small islands of cellular cartilage lying just beneath the surface of the membrane (× 25).

ficult to differentiate diffuse hemangiomatous involvement of the synovium from hemorrhagic villonodular synovitis.[4,61,66] In circumscribed lesions, the histologic pattern is usually that of a capillary or cavernous hemangioma, whereas in the diffuse variety, the vascular channels appear to be venous. Surgical excision, which is usually simple and effective in patients with a circumscribed hemangioma, is often unsatisfactory in patients with diffuse involvement of the synovial membrane and regional soft tissues, and the likelihood of recurrence is high.

Hemangiomas may also occur in tendon sheaths and may grow to involve both the tendon itself and the surrounding structures.[105] One usually notes a soft, compressive swelling, which changes when the limb is elevated or when a tourniquet is placed proximal to the mass. The roentgenographic examination frequently reveals many calcified phleboliths. The hand, forearm, and ankle are the sites favored by this lesion, which is treated by surgical excision.

Fat Tumor

Intra-articular lipomas are rare. Almost all examples have been found in the knee joint in relation to the subsynovial fat on either side of the patellar ligament or the anterior surface of the femur.[51,89,105] Lipomas are also found in the tendon sheaths of the hand, wrist, feet, and ankles.[94] Extensor tendons appear to be affected more often than flexor tendons, and involvement may be bilateral.

The term "lipoma arborescens" represents a villous or polypoid synovial proliferation in response to chronic mechanical irritation of the synovium. This disorder can also occur in seemingly normal joints.[51,133] Arthrographic examination reveals sharply marginated filling defects.[9]

The term "Hoffa's disease" designates the traumatic inflammation of the infrapatellar fat pad.[47] Patients are in pain and the usual finding is swelling in the infrapatellar region, deep to the patellar tendon. The differential diagnosis includes pretendinous bursitis, deep infrapatellar bursitis, and intracapsular chondroma. Hoffa's disease is now classified in the broader category of plica syndromes, as defined arthroscopically (see Chap. 78).[50]

Fibroma

Jaffe has suggested that most reported cases of fibromas of joint and tendon sheaths in the older literature were probably examples of the late fibrous stage of pigmented villonodular synovitis.[51] True fibromatous lesions appear to be rare.

MALIGNANT NEOPLASMS OF JOINTS

These neoplasms may be either primary or secondary. Primary tumors are uncommon and are represented almost solely by synovial sarcoma. Other malignant tumors with an origin in the fascial tissues of the extremities, and probably related to synovial sarcoma, are the clear cell sarcoma of tendons and aponeuroses and the epithelioid sarcoma. Secondary involvement of joints occurs as a complication of the contiguous spread of malignant bone tumors, metastases of carcinoma, or leukemia. Rheumatologic manifestations of hematologic malignant diseases are discussed in Chapter 74.

Synovial Sarcoma

Clinical Findings

This malignant and histologically complex neoplasm of connective tissue is generally found near a large joint. The tumor seldom originates within the joint itself. This lesion has been described by many different names, including malignant synovioma, synovial fibrosarcoma, sarcoendothelioma, and mesothelioma, and has been observed in certain domestic animals, such as the dog and cow.

Synovial sarcoma occurs most often in adolescents or in young adults, but it has been observed at all ages from birth to 80 years. A preponderance is seen in men. The lower limb (thigh, leg, foot, and knee) is more commonly the site of primary involvement than the upper limb (arm, forearm, and hand).[8,10,15,43] Other primary sites include the buttock, trunk (back), chest or abdominal wall, retroperitoneum,[112] neck,[100] mouth and face,[113] and orbit.[137] The characteristic history is that of a slowly growing mass that, in the case of a deeply situated lesion, may reach a considerable size before detection. When located on the hand or foot, the tumor may resemble a ganglion or a distended tendon sheath. Pain is not marked, except in unusual lesions or when the tumor interferes with the normal movement of the joint.

The typical roentgenographic appearance of malignant synovioma is that of a para-articular soft tissue mass of homogeneous water density,[134] possibly lobulated, with a sharp, discrete border. Less often, the mass is irregular in outline and is not clearly separable from the surrounding tissues. In 30% of patients, the tumor contains clusters of small foci of calcification. Secondary invasion of contiguous bone produces osteolytic defects in 10 to 20% of patients. A nearby periosteal reaction may occur. Increased uptake of bone-seeking radionuclides has been shown in a partially calcified lesion,[48] but this finding is probably nonspecific. Arteriographic examination has shown increased vascularity, particularly in rapidly growing tumors.[138] Angiography and CT scanning are both useful in the initial evaluation of patients with synovial as well as other types of soft tissue sarcoma, prior to biopsy.[65] Angiography gives better information when tumors are placed distally, where little fat is present.[62] CT scanning provides more precise information in the assessment of size, location, axial extent, and relationships of more centrally placed primary or locally recurrent lesions,[85] as well as in the detection of metastases.[39]

Although the rate of growth and the rapidity of metastatic spread vary, the disease characteristically follows a malignant course.[102] As is true of other connective tissue sarcomas, the synovial sarcoma spreads by direct extension along tissue planes, by invasion of regional lymph nodes (possibly a later phenomenon), and by way of the vascular system. The rate of local recurrence, particularly after simple excision, is high.[111] The most common site of visceral metastasis is the lung,[43,103] in which the lesions take the form of multiple large densities or a diffuse infiltrate. The pleura, diaphragm, pericardium, and skin are also frequently involved. Osteolytic lesions are more common than sclerotic changes in skeletal metastases.

Histopathologic Findings

Synovial sarcomas most commonly originate in peri- and para-articular tissues including the joint capsule, tendon sheaths, intermuscular septa, and fascia separating muscles and ligaments.[10,43,127]

Rarely does this neoplasm lie within a joint cavity, and joint involvement is usually secondary.[10,105,134] Unequivocal origin in a synovial structure is rare.[17] In most cases, the tumor probably arises from neoplastic mesenchymal cells with a characteristic pattern of differentiation that resembles synovium.[43] The gross appearance of a synovial sarcoma depends on its place of origin, the duration and rapidity of its growth, and its cellular composition. The color of the tumor, which may be 1 to 20 cm or more in diameter, varies from a pale gray-yellow to a deep red, usually the result of hemorrhage. The tumor may feel uniformly firm when spindle cell elements predominate, or it may be soft and contain cystic spaces filled with mucoid secretions when epithelial-like cells predominate. Compression of the surrounding tissue may give rise to the mistaken belief that the tumor is encapsulated.

Synovial sarcomas are pleomorphic tumors. Some are characterized by a biphasic cellular pattern that includes epithelial-like cells arranged in nests, tubules and acini, and a stroma of spindle cells and abundant reticulin fibers with the appearance of a fibrosarcoma (Fig. 84–3). Other tumors are monophasic, most commonly of the spindle-cell type and less commonly of the epithelial-like type, in which the cells are arranged in sheaths and cords in a tenuous reticular stroma.[43,127,137]

The most distinctive histologic feature of synovial sarcoma is the presence of clefts and cystic spaces, which are lined by cuboidal or columnar

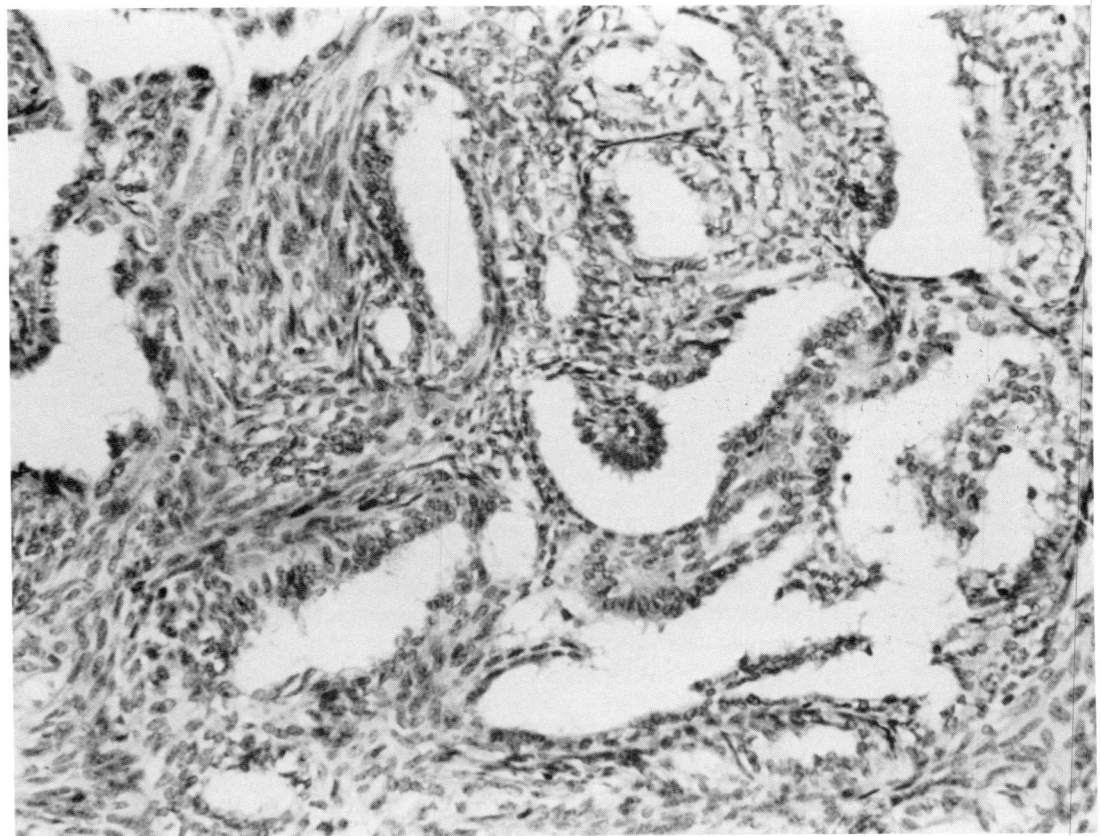

Fig. 84–3. Biphasic synovial sarcoma. Note the irregular spaces lined with columnar cells, in addition to the spindle-cell stroma (× 100).

cells and contain a mucin-rich secretion that stains intensely with periodic acid-Schiff, mucicarmine, colloidal iron, and alcian blue and is resistant to hyaluronidase.[127] The ultrastructural characteristics of these tumors are intriguing.[19,32,73,127] For instance, the epithelial-like cells, which under light microscopy resemble the synovial lining cells, are connected by desmosomes and maculae adherentes, which are not present in normal synovial tissue. In addition, most observations reveal the presence of a basal lamina at the epithelial-stromal junction, a structure also absent from normal synovial tissue. To complicate the issue, anti-intermediate filament antibodies demonstrate keratin in the epithelial-like cells, and vimentin, specific for fibroblasts, in the spindle-cell stroma. This feature has led Miettinen and co-workers to conclude that "keratin positivity of tumor cells can be used as evidence against sarcoma, except in cases of biphasic synovial sarcoma."[74]

The random location of synovial sarcoma in relation to joints, the lack of effect of hyaluronidase on the tinctorial characteristics of the mucinous material, and the presence of structures that do not occur in normal synovial tissue raise questions regarding the histogenesis of these tumors, although some nonmalignant inflammatory lesions of synovial tissue also share some of these characteristics, probably from cellular crowding.[35]

Diagnosis and Treatment

The principles of therapy in synovial sarcoma are based on current concepts of growth and spread of soft tissue sarcomas. These tumors are poorly circumscribed, and even if invested by a pseudo-capsule, their enucleation inevitably leaves behind microscopic tumor. In addition, their rapid extension along soft tissue planes explains the local recurrence rates of 18% after "en bloc" soft part resection and of 4% after amputation.[111] The possibility of synovial sarcoma should be suspected in patients with any tumor in the soft parts of the hand or foot or in the vicinity of the knee, elbow, and shoulder joints, especially. Once considered, the diagnosis should be confirmed by histologic examination. Plain roentgenograms of the region should be followed by angiographic examination or CT scanning; only then should biopsy be performed.[102] Although surgical and needle biopsies both have advocates, a surgical biopsy has the advantage of a larger sample, which can be used for prognostic studies, such as the mitotic index.

If the results of biopsy are positive, a wide resection is undertaken, depending on the extent and location of the tumor. In superficial lesions of the hands and feet and in lesions emerging from extra-articular connective tissues and tendons, a wide local excision with a margin of at least 6 cm normal tissue has been recommended. The entire muscle group in which the tumor grows should be resected. Deeper tumors of hands and feet and tumors developing in the vicinity of joints usually require amputation. Radical dissection of regional lymph nodes is optional, except when nodal metastases are obvious or in proximal lesions, as part of the "en bloc" resection.[111] Interest in preserving a functional limb has stimulated the use of adjuvant perfusion chemotherapy as well as radical radiotherapy in association with local excision in various types of soft tissue sarcoma,[12,23] and short-term results are encouraging. Postoperative chemotherapy may also hold promise.

Prognosis

Features of the tumor or the host that may affect prognosis have been investigated. The most important determinant of prognosis appears to be the size of the tumor at the time of initial therapy. For patients with tumors under 5 cm in diameter, the 5-year survival rate is much better than for patients with larger tumors. Other favorable features include: (1) the extremes of age; (2) occurrence in an "exposed" area such as the foot, ankle, forearm, wrist, and neck; (3) female sex; (4) biphasic histologic pattern;[43,137] and (5) calcification within the tumor.[130] Recent experience has indicated overall 5- and 10-year actuarial survival rates of 58% and 48%, respectively, in patients treated with "en bloc," wide, soft part resection and amputation.[111] The possible beneficial effects of newer techniques for the control of the primary tumor, such as isolation-perfusion chemotherapy and radical radiotherapy in association with surgical excision, as well as prevention of recurrence and metastasis by postoperative chemotherapy, remain to be determined.

Clear Cell Sarcoma of Tendons and Aponeuroses

A neoplasm arising from tendons or aponeuroses is termed clear cell sarcoma.[26] This painless mass is usually present for long periods. Many such tumors arise from the lower limb in the region of the

foot (Achilles tendon, ankle, and plantar fascia) and the knee (patellar tendon and aponeuroses about the knee). The tumor is peculiarly composed of compact nests and fascicles of round or fusiform, pale-staining cells with vesicular nuclei and prominent nucleoli. Electron-microscopic studies have raised questions about the histogenesis of this neoplasm. Some lesions contain melanosomes and have tentatively been reclassified as melanomas of soft parts, whereas others have features consistent with a synovial derivation.[126] Keratin filaments are absent from these tumors.[74] Surgical excision is only temporarily beneficial, and the prognosis is generally poor.[43,126]

Epithelioid Sarcoma

This distinctive sarcoma occurs predominantly in young adults. Common sites include the hand, wrist, forearm, and lower leg, where the lesion arises from tendon and fascial structures. Necrosis of the tumor nodule with skin ulceration often leads to the erroneous diagnosis of a chronic inflammatory process, granuloma, or squamous cell carcinoma. Microscopically, the tumor includes large, acidophilic polygonal cells and spindle cells arranged in irregular nodules, where central necrosis frequently occurs.[25] Electron-microscopic findings resemble those of synovial sarcoma.[31,84]

Involvement of Joints by Primary Bone Tumors

Metaphyseal bone tumors, chiefly osteosarcoma, fibrosarcoma, and chondrosarcoma, often invade joints.[117] Articular (hyaline) cartilage is thought to act as a barrier to local tumor extension by means of tissue factors that inhibit tumor angiogenesis.[6] Tumor penetration eventually occurs, however, whether peripherally beneath the joint capsule, at the bone attachment of intracapsular ligaments such as the cruciate ligaments of the knee, or across cartilage itself.[117] Bland synovial effusions may indicate early invasion of the joint.[59]

Carcinomatous Synovitis

That metastases to synovium are clinically rare is surprising given the high frequency of disseminated carcinomas and the rich vascular supply of synovial tissue.[64] Knees are most commonly affected.[27,80] Other evidence of disseminated tumor is usually present, but, rarely, joint metastases are the first indication of malignant disease or of tumor dissemination.[27,132] Radiographic studies of such joints demonstrate lytic lesions of the patella, femur, or tibia, but patients with early cases may lack abnormal findings.[38,132]

Bone scanning may reveal increased local radionuclide uptake.[58,122] Multiple focal lesions of increased activity throughout the skeleton provide further evidence of metastatic disease. Synovial fluid is hemorrhagic, with 100 to 8,000 white blood cells/mm³, predominantly mononuclear cells. The fluid of one patient reported exhibited eosinophilia.[38] Tumor cells are found in synovial fluid in 80% of patients;[27,58,122,132] arthrotomy or closed synovial biopsy reveals carcinomatous involvement of the synovium. Arthroscopy is valuable in the diagnosis of synovial metastases when the results of other tests are inconclusive.

Metastases to Bones of the Hands and Feet

This unusual form of "arthritis" occurs in patients with disseminated carcinoma. Metastases occur in small bones, particularly the distal phalanges and the tarsal bones. The clinical syndromes resemble paronychia or gout. Lytic lesions, sometimes with pathologic fractures, are usually present.[13,129,139]

NONMETASTATIC SYNDROMES

This category comprises a variety of conditions.

Hypertrophic Osteoarthropathy

This well-known association of intrathoracic tumors and hypertrophic osteoarthropathy is discussed separately (see Chap. 76). It can be considered the prototype of tumor-associated arthritis; its onset often leads to the discovery of an unsuspected intrathoracic malignant process.[106,109, 114]

Pancreatic Cancer with Arthropathy and Fat Necrosis

Panniculitis resembling erythema nodosum accompanied by synovitis and serositis is a well-known accompaniment of pancreatic carcinoma, particularly of the acinar-cell type, as well as of pancreatitis. The pathogenesis of this disorder includes fat necrosis in subcutaneous tissue, bone marrow, and subsynovial fat, as a result of high levels of pancreatic lipase.[40,78,116,135]

Cancer Arthritis

Several observers have described a syndrome resembling RA with typical or atypical features,[71,110,123] having its onset a few months before the discovery of a tumor. The atypical form is characterized by explosive onset, asymmetry of joint involvement, sparing of wrists and small joints of the hand, absence of subcutaneous nodules, and seronegativity. All patients in one series were in their fifth decade or older. Removal or successful treatment of the tumor was associated with remission of the arthritis in approximately half these patients. Remission was more frequent in the atyp-

ical than in the typical RA-like arthritis. The validity of these associations has not been definitely established by epidemiologic methods.

Supporting evidence of a causal association between carcinoma and rheumatic disease has been provided by individual observations, in which removal of carcinoma has been followed by complete clinical and serologic remission of the syndrome. The cases included: (1) an epidermoid carcinoma of lung associated with nodular RA with eosinophilia and a high titer of rheumatoid factor;[67] (2) an ovarian dysgerminoma associated with arthritis, pleuropericarditis, and a positive antinuclear antibody test;[56] (3) an ovarian adenocarcinoma associated with arthritis, fever, mental confusion, anemia, leukocytosis, positive test for rheumatoid factor, and the presence of antinuclear antibodies;[3] and (4) a colonic carcinoma associated with RA-like arthritis and a positive rheumatoid factor.[118]

Hyperuricemia and Gout

The degree of hyperuricemia in patients with carcinoma correlates with extensiveness of the disease, involvement of the liver, and presence of hypercalcemia. Gout was not common and occurred in 5 of 70 patients studied. In 2 of these patients, the gout preceded the tumor.[128] The frequency of hyperuricemia and gout in a cancer patient population remains to be elucidated. Interestingly, hypouricemia has also been described in association with disseminated carcinoma.[90]

Carcinoid Arthropathy

This peculiar form of arthropathy characterized by arthralgias, juxta-articular demineralization, erosions, and subchondral cysts was observed in four of five consecutive patients with the carcinoid syndrome.[88]

Lymphomatoid Granulomatosis

Arthralgia may be associated with this peculiar lymphoproliferative disorder, which is characterized by angiodestructive lymphoreticular proliferative granulomata. A case presenting with polyarthritis has been recorded.[2a]

Palmar Fasciitis and Polyarthritis Associated with Ovarian Carcinoma

Medsger et al. have described a unique syndrome including palmar fasciitis and polyarthritis in six patients with ovarian carcinoma predominantly of the endometrioid type.[72a] The palmar changes ranged from diffuse, globular swelling with warmth and erythema to typical Dupuytren's contracture. The shoulders and the metacarpophalangeal and proximal interphalangeal joints were most frequently involved and exhibited painful limitations of motion and flexor contractures. Morning stiffness was prominent. Although two of these patients had the carpal tunnel syndrome, none had Raynaud's phenomenon, dermal or pulmonary fibrosis, or evidences of myositis. In five patients, the articular symptoms preceded the diagnosis of malignant disease by several months to two years. In the remaining patient, the articular symptoms preceded tumor recurrence. In all patients, the ovarian tumor was extensive and gave evidence of intra- and extraperitoneal spread. The median survival time after diagnosis of the tumor was six months. The pathogenesis of this syndrome, which resembled reflex sympathetic dystrophy, remains unexplained.

Other Rheumatologic Syndromes

Polymyositis (dermatomyositis) and other muscle syndromes associated with tumors are discussed in Chapter 65. Other nonmetastatic rheumatologic or neuromuscular syndromes associated with malignant disease are listed in Table 84–1.

Complications of Cancer Treatment

Tumor involvement of joints is occasionally suggested when a patient is receiving corticosteroid or immunosuppressive therapy, which alone can be associated with secondary joint manifestations. These manifestations include *aseptic necrosis of bone* (see Chaps. 32 and 86), *septic arthritis* (see Chaps. 101 and 102) and *steroid myopathy* (see Chap. 32). In addition, chemotherapy with bleomycin can give rise to a *fibrotic syndrome* resembling systemic sclerosis (see Chap. 66).

Table 84–1.   Rheumatologic Syndromes Associated with Nonhematologic Malignant Diseases

> *By Direct Extension or Metastatic*
>   Primary bone tumors
>   Carcinomatous (metastatic) synovitis
>   Metases to small bones
>
> *Nonmetastatic (Paraneoplastic)*
>   Articular
>   Hypertrophic osteoarthropathy
>   Subcutaneous nodules, arthritis, and serositis (fat necrosis) in pancreatic cancer (as in pancreatitis)
>   Cancer arthritis
>   Hyperuricemia and gout; hypouricemia
>   Carcinoid arthropathy
>   Palmar fasciitis and polyarthritis associated with ovarian carcinoma
>   Coincidental arthritis of any type
>   Muscular
>   Polymyositis (dermatomyositis)
>   Eaton-Lambert syndrome
>   Carcinoid myopathy
>   Type II muscle fiber atrophy
>   Coincidental myopathy of any type
>   Cutaneous
>   Carcinoid ''scleroderma''
>
> *As Complications of Therapy*
>   Aseptic necrosis of bone
>   Septic arthritis
>   Corticosteroid myopathy
>   Chemotherapy-induced fibrotic syndromes

REFERENCES

1. Alguacil-García, A., Unni, K.K., and Goellner, J.R.: Giant cell tumor of tendon sheath and pigmented villonodular synovitis: an ultrastructural study. Am. J. Clin. Pathol., 69:6–17, 1978.
2. Barclay, W.P., White, K.K., and Williams, A.: Equine villonodular synovitis: a case survey. Cornell Vet., 70:72–76, 1980.
2a. Bergin, C., et al.: Lymphomatoid granulomatosis presenting as polyarthritis. J. Rheumatol., 11:537–539, 1984.
3. Bennett, R.M., Ginsberg, M.H., and Thomsen, S.: Carcinomatous polyarthritis: the presenting symptom of an ovarian tumor and association with a platelet activating factor. Arthritis Rheum., 19:953–958, 1976.
4. Bobechko, W.P., and Kostuik, J.P.: Childhood villonodular synovitis. Can. J. Surg., 11:480–486, 1968.
5. Bogumill, G.P., Sullivan, D.J., and Baker, G.I.: Tumors of the hand. Clin. Orthop., 108:214–222, 1975.
6. Brem, H., and Folkman, J.: Inhibition of tumor angiogenesis mediated by cartilage. J. Exp. Med., 141:427–439, 1975.
7. Brown-Crosby, E., Inglis, A., and Bullough, P.G.: Multiple joint involvement in pigmented villonodular synovitis. Radiology, 122:671–672, 1977.
8. Buck, P., Mickelson, M.R., and Bonfiglio, M.: Synovial sarcoma: a review of 33 cases. Clin. Orthop., 156:211–215, 1981.
9. Burgan, D.W.: Lipoma arborescens of the knee: another cause of filling defects on a knee arthrogram. Radiology, 101:583–584, 1971.
10. Cadman, N.L., Soule, E.H., and Kelly, D.J.: Synovial sarcoma: an analysis of 134 tumors. Cancer, 18:613–627, 1965.
11. Campbell, A.J., and Wells, I.P.: Pigmented villonodular synovitis of a lumbar vertebral facet joint. J. Bone Joint Surg., 64A:145–146, 1982.
12. Carson, J.H., et al.: The place of radiotherapy in the treatment of synovial sarcoma. Int. J. Radiat. Oncol. Biol. Phys., 7:49–53, 1981.
13. Colson, G.M., and Willcox, A.: Phalangeal metastases in bronchogenic carcinoma. Lancet, 1:100–102, 1948.
14. Crawford, G.P., and Offerman, R.J.: Pigmented villonodular synovitis in the hand. Hand, 12:282–287, 1980.
15. Crocker, D.W., and Stout, A.P.: Synovial sarcoma in children. Cancer, 12:1123–1133, 1959.
16. Danzig, L.A., Gershuni, D.H., and Resnick, D.: Diagnosis and treatment of diffuse pigmented villonodular synovitis of the hip. Clin. Orthop., 168:42–47, 1982.
17. Dardick, I., et al.: Synovial sarcoma arising in an anatomical bursa. Virchows. Arch. (Pathol. Anat.), 397:93–101, 1982.
18. De Benedetti, M.J., and Schwinn, C.P.: Tenosynovial chondromatosis in the hand. J. Bone Joint Surg., 61A:898–903, 1979.
19. Dische, F.E., Darby, A.J., and Howard, E.R.: Malignant synovioma: electron microscopical findings in three patients and review of the literature. J. Pathol., 124:149–166, 1978.
20. Docken, W.P.: Pigmented villonodular synovitis: a review with illustrative case reports. Semin. Arthritis Rheum., 9:1–22, 1979.
21. Donde, R., and Funding, J.: Pigmented villonodular synovitis: a follow-up study. Scand. J. Rheumatol., 9:172–174, 1980.

22. Duthie, R.B., and Rizza, C.R.: Rheumatological manifestations of the haemophilias. Clin. Rheum. Dis., *1*:53–93, 1975.
23. Eilber, F.R., et al.: Is amputation necessary for sarcomas? A seven-year experience with limb salvage. Ann. Surg., *192*:431–438, 1980.
24. Ellman, M.H., Krieger, M.I., and Brown, N.: Pseudogout mimicking synovial chondromatosis. J. Bone Joint Surg., *57A*:863–865, 1975.
25. Enzinger, F.M.: Epithelioid sarcoma: a sarcoma simulating a granuloma or a carcinoma. Cancer, *26*:1029–1041, 1970.
26. Enzinger, F.M.: Clear-cell sarcoma of tendons and aponeuroses: an analysis of 21 cases. Cancer, *18*:1163–1174, 1965.
27. Fam, A.G., Kolin, A., and Lewis, A.J.: Metastatic carcinomatous arthritis and carcinoma of the lung: a report of two cases diagnosed by synovial fluid cytology. J. Rheumatol., *7*:98–104, 1980.
28. Forrest, J., and Staple, T.W.: Synovial hemangioma of the knee. Demonstration by arthrography and arteriography. AJR, *112*:512–516, 1971.
29. Friedman, M., and Schwartz, E.E.: Irradiation therapy of pigmented villonodular synovitis. Bull. Hosp. Joint Dis., *18*:19–32, 1957.
30. Fyfe, I.S., and MacFarlane, A.: Pigmented villonodular synovitis of the hand. Hand, *12*:179–188, 1980.
31. Gabbiani, G., et al.: Epithelioid sarcoma: a light and electron microscopic study suggesting a synovial origin. Cancer, *30*:486–499, 1972.
32. Gabbiani, G., et al.: Synovial sarcoma: electron microscopic study of a typical case. Cancer, *28*:1031–1039, 1971.
33. Gaucher, A., et al.: Pigmented villonodular synovitis of the hip: ultrastructure and scanning electron microscopy. Rev. Rheum. Mal. Osteoartic., *43*:357–362, 1976.
34. Gehweiler, J.A., and Wilson, J.W.: Diffuse biarticular pigmented villonodular synovitis. Radiology, *93*:845–851, 1969.
35. Ghadially, F.N.: Diagnostic Electron Microscopy of Tumours. London, Butterworths, 1980, pp. 51–67.
36. Ghadially, F.N., Lalonde, J.M., and Dick, C.E.: Ultrastructure of pigmented villonodular synovitis. J. Pathol., *127*:19–26, 1979.
37. Goergen, T.G., Resnick, D., and Niwayama, G.: Localized nodular synovitis of the knee: a report of two cases with abnormal arthrograms. AJR, *126*:647–650, 1976.
38. Goldenberg, D.L., Kelley, W., and Gibbons, R.B.: Metastatic adenocarcinoma of synovium presenting as acute arthritis: diagnosis by closed synovial biopsy. Arthritis Rheum., *18*:107–110, 1975.
39. Golding, S.J., and Husband, J.E.: The role of computed tomography in the management of soft tissue sarcomas. Br. J. Radiol., *55*:740–747, 1982.
40. Good, A.E., et al.: Acinar pancreatic tumor with metastatic fat necrosis. Dig. Dis. Sci., *21*:978–987, 1976.
41. Granowitz, S.P., and Mankin, H.J.: Localized pigmented villonodular synovitis of the knee. J. Bone Joint Surg., *49A*:122–128, 1967.
42. Granowitz, S.P., D'Antonio, J., and Mankin, H.J.: The pathogenesis and long-term end results of pigmented villonodular synovitis. Clin. Orthop., *114*:335–351, 1976.
43. Hajdu, S.I., Shiu, M.H., and Fortner, J.G.: Tendosynovial sarcoma: a clinicopathological study of 136 cases. Cancer, *39*:1201–1217, 1977.
44. Halborg, A., Hansen, H., and Sneppen, H.O.: Haemangioma of the knee joint. Acta Orthop. Scand., *39*:209–216, 1968.
45. Hawley, W.L., and Ansell, B.M.: Synovial haemangioma presenting as monarticular arthritis of the knee. Arch. Dis. Child., *56*:558–560, 1981.
46. Henderson, B., et al.: Metabolic alterations in human synovial lining cells in pigmented villonodular synovitis. Ann. Rheum. Dis., *38*:463–466, 1979.
47. Hoffa, A.: The influence of the adipose tissue with regard to the pathology of the knee joint. JAMA, *43*:795–796, 1904.
48. Horne, T., et al.: Increased uptake of ^{99m}Tc-MDP in cal-cified synovial sarcoma. Eur. J. Nucl. Med., *8*:75–76, 1983.
49. Jackson, R.W.: Current concepts review: arthroscopic surgery. J. Bone Joint Surg., *65A*:416–420, 1983.
50. Jackson, R.W., and Dandy, D.J.: Arthroscopy of the Knee. New York, Grune and Stratton, 1976.
51. Jaffe, H.L.: Tumors and Tumorous Conditions of the Bones and Joints. Philadelphia, Lea & Febiger, 1958.
52. Jaffe, H.L., Lichtenstein, L., and Sutro, C.J.: Pigmented villonodular synovitis, bursitis and tenosynovitis. Arch. Pathol., *31*:731–765, 1941.
53. Jergesen, H.E., Mankin, H.J., and Schiller, A.L.: Diffuse pigmented villonodular synovitis of the knee mimicking primary bone neoplasm. J. Bone Joint Surg., *60A*:825–829, 1978.
54. Johansson, J.E., et al.: Pigmented villonodular synovitis of joints. Clin. Orthop., *163*:159–166, 1982.
55. Johnson, L.L.: Diagnostic and Surgical Arthroscopy. 2nd Ed. St. Louis, C.V. Mosby, 1981.
56. Kahn, M.F., et al.: Systemic lupus erythematosus and ovarian dysgerminoma: remission of the systemic lupus erythematosus after extirpation of the tumor. Clin. Exp. Immunol., *1*:355–359, 1966.
57. Kaufman, R.A., et al.: Arthrosonography in the diagnosis of pigmented villonodular synovitis. AJR, *139*:396–398, 1982.
58. Khan, F.A., Garterhouse, W., and Khan, A.: Metastatic bronchogenic carcinoma: an unusual cause of localized arthritis. Chest, *67*:738–739, 1975.
59. Lagier, R.: Synovial reaction caused by adjacent malignant tumors: anatomopathological study of three cases. J. Rheumatol., *4*:65–72, 1977.
60. Lapayowker, M.S., et al.: Pigmented villonodular synovitis of the temporomandibular joint. Radiology, *108*:313–316, 1973.
61. Leszczynski, J., et al.: Pigmented villonodular synovitis in multiple joints: occurrence in a child with cavernous hemangioma of hip and pulmonary stenosis. Ann. Rheum. Dis., *34*:269–272, 1975.
62. Levine, E., et al.: Comparison of computed tomography and other imaging modalities in the evaluation of musculoskeletal tumors. Radiology, *131*:431–437, 1979.
63. Lewis, R.C., Coventry, M.B., and Soule, E.H.: Hemangioma of the synovial membrane. J. Bone Joint Surg., *41A*:264–270, 1959.
64. Liew, M., and Carson-Dick, W.: The anatomy and physiology of blood flow in a diarthrodial joint. Clin. Rheum. Dis., *7*:131–148, 1981.
65. Lindell, M.M., Jr., et al.: Diagnostic technique for the evaluation of the soft tissue sarcoma. Semin. Oncol., *8*:160–171, 1981.
66. Lindenbaum, B.L., and Hunt, T.: An unusual presentation of pigmented villonodular synovitis. Clin. Orthop., *122*:263–267, 1977.
67. Litwin, S.D., Allen, J.C., and Kunkel, H.G.: Disappearance of the clinical and serological manifestations of rheumatoid arthritis following a thoracotomy for a lung tumor. Arthritis Rheum., *9*:865, 1966.
68. Lowenstein, M.B., Smith, J.R.V., and Cole, S.: Infrapatellar pigmented villonodular synovitis: arthrographic detection. AJR, *135*:279–282, 1980.
69. McCarty, D.J., et al.: "Milwaukee shoulder"—Association of microspheroids containing hydroxyapatite crystals, active collagenase, and neutral protease with rotator cuff defects. 1. Clinical aspects. Arthritis Rheum., *24*:464–473, 1981.
70. McCarty, E.F., and Dorfman, H.D.: Primary synovial chondromatosis. An ultrastructural study. Clin. Orthop., *168*:178–186, 1982.
71. MacKenzie, A.H., and Scherbel, A.L.: Connective tissue syndromes associated with carcinoma. Geriatrics, *18*:745–753, 1963.
72. Mainardi, C.L., et al.: Proliferative synovitis in hemophilia: biochemical and morphological observations. Arthritis Rheum., *21*:137–144, 1978.
72a. Medsger, T.A., Jr., Dixon, J.A., and Garwood, V.F.: Palmar fasciitis and polyarthritis associated with ovarian carcinoma. Ann. Intern. Med., *96*:424–431, 1982.

73. Mickelson, M.R., et al.: Synovial sarcoma: an electron microscopic study of monophasic and biphasic forms. Cancer, *45*:2109–2118, 1980.
74. Miettinen, M., et al.: Expression of intermediate filaments in soft-tissue sarcomas. Int. J. Cancer, *30*:541–546, 1982.
75. Milgram, J.W.: Synovial osteochondromatosis. J. Bone Joint Surg., *59A*:792–801, 1977.
76. Milgram, J.W.: The development of loose bodies in human joints. Clin. Orthop., *124*:292–303, 1977.
77. Molnar, Z., Stern, W.H., and Stoltzner, G.H.: Cytoplasmic tubular structures in pigmented villonodular synovitis. Arthritis Rheum., *14*:784–787, 1971.
78. Mullin, G.T., et al.: Arthritis and skin lesions resembling erythema nodosum in pancreatic disease. Ann. Intern. Med., *68*:75–87, 1968.
79. Murphy, F.P., Dahlin, D.C., and Sullivan, C.R.: Articular synovial chondromatosis. J. Bone Joint Surg., *44A*:77–86, 1962.
80. Murray, G.C., and Persellin, R.H.: Metastatic carcinoma presenting as monoarticular arthritis: a case report and review of the literature. Arthritis Rheum., *23*:95–100, 1980.
81. Myers, B.W., Masi, A.T., and Feigenbaum, S.L.: Pigmented villonodular synovitis and tenosynovitis: a clinical epidemiologic study of 166 cases and literature review. Medicine, *59*:223–238, 1980.
82. Nickels, F.A., Grant, B.D., and Lincoln, S.D.: Villonodular synovitis of the equine metacarpophalangeal joint. J. Am. Vet. Med. Assoc., *168*:1043–1046, 1976.
83. Nilsonne, U., and Moberger, G.: Pigmented villonodular synovitis of joints: histological and clinical problems in diagnosis. Acta Orthop. Scand., *40*:448–460, 1969.
84. Patchefsky, A.S., Soriano, R., and Kostianovsky, M.: Epithelioid sarcoma: ultrastructural similarity to nodular synovitis. Cancer, *39*:143–152, 1977.
85. Paul, D.F., Morrey, B.F., and Helms, C.A.: Computerized tomography in orthopedic surgery. Clin Orthop., *139*:142–149, 1979.
86. Paul, G.R., and Leach, R.E.: Synovial chondromatosis of the shoulder. Clin. Orthop., *68*:130–135, 1970.
87. Pelker, R.R., Drennan, J.C., and Ozonoff, M.D.: Juvenile synovial chondromatosis of the hip: a case report. J. Bone Joint Surg., *65A*:552–554, 1983.
88. Plonk, J.W., and Feldman, J.M.: Carcinoid arthropathy. Arch. Intern. Med., *134*:651–654, 1974.
89. Pudlowski, R.M., Gilula, L.A., and Kyriakos, M.: Intraarticular lipoma with osseous metaplasia: radiographic-pathologic correlation. AJR, *132*:471–473, 1979.
90. Ramsdell, C.M., and Kelley, W.N.: The clinical significance of hypouricemia. Ann. Intern. Med., *78*:239–242, 1973.
91. Reginato, A., et al.: Giant cell tumor associated with rheumatoid arthritis. Ann. Rheum. Dis., *33*:333–341, 1974.
92. Resnick, D., and Oliphant, M.: Hemophilia-like arthropathy of the knee associated with cutaneous and synovial hemangiomas. Radiology, *114*:323–326, 1975.
93. Robert D'Eshoughes, J., Delcambre, B., and Delbart, P.: Pigmented villonodular synovitis and radioisotopic synoviorthesis. Lille Med., *20*:438–446, 1975.
94. Rodriguez, J.M.: Lipomas in the hand and wrist. Cleve. Clin. Q., *37*:201–205, 1970.
95. Ropes, M.W., and Bauer, W.: Synovial Fluid Changes in Joint Disease. Cambridge, Harvard University Press, 1953.
96. Rosales Wynne-Roberts, C., et al.: Synovial hemangioma of the knee: light and electron microscopic findings. J. Pathol., *123*:247–254, 1977.
97. Rosen, P.S., et al.: Synovial chondromatosis affecting the temporomandibular joint. Arthritis Rheum., *20*:736–740, 1977.
98. Rosenthal, D.I., Aronow, S., and Murray, W.T.: Iron content of pigmented villonodular synovitis detected by computed tomography. Radiology, *133*:409–411, 1979.
99. Rosenthal, D.I., Coleman, P.K., and Schiller, A.L.: Pigmented villonodular synovitis: correlation of angiographic and histologic findings. AJR, *135*:581–585, 1980.
100. Roth, J.A., Enzinger, F.M., and Tannenbaum, M.: Syn-ovial sarcoma of the neck: a followup study of 24 cases. Cancer, *35*:1243–1253, 1975.
101. Roy, S., and Ghadially, F.N.: Synovial membrane in experimentally produced chronic hemarthrosis. Ann. Rheum. Dis., *28*:402–414, 1969.
102. Russell, W.O., et al.: Staging system for soft tissue sarcoma. Semin. Oncol., *8*:156–159, 1981.
103. Ryan, J.R., Baker, L.H., and Benjamin, R.S.: The natural history of metastatic synovial sarcoma. Clin. Orthop., *164*:257–260, 1982.
104. Ryan, L.M., et al.: Predominance of type II collagen in synovial chondromatosis. Clin. Orthop., *168*:173–177, 1982.
105. Schajowicz, F.: Tumors and Tumorlike Lesions of Bone and Joints. New York, Springer-Verlag, 1981.
106. Schumacher, H.R., Jr.: Articular manifestations of hypertropic pulmonary osteoarthropathy in bronchogenic carcinoma. Arthritis Rheum., *19*:629–636, 1976.
107. Schumacher, H.R., Lotke, P., and Rothfuss, S.: Pigmented villonodular synovitis: light and electron microscopy studies. Semin. Arthritis Rheum., *12*:32–43, 1982.
108. Scott, P.M.: Bone lesions in pigmented villonodular synovitis. J. Bone Joint Surg., *50B*:306–311, 1968.
109. Segal, A.M., and MacKenzie, A.H.: Hypertrophic osteoarthropathy: a 10-year retrospective analysis. Semin. Arthritis Rheum., *12*:220–232, 1982.
110. Sheon, R.P., et al.: Malignancy in rheumatic disease: interrelationships. J. Am. Geriatr. Soc., *25*:20–27, 1977.
111. Shiu, M.H., et al.: Surgical treatment of tendosynovial sarcoma. Cancer, *43*:889–897, 1979.
112. Shmookler, B.M.: Retroperitoneal synovial sarcoma. Am. J. Clin. Pathol., *77*:686–691, 1982.
113. Shmookler, B.M., Enzinger, F.M., and Brannon, R.B.: Orofacial synovial sarcoma: a clinicopathologic study of 11 new cases and review of the literature. Cancer, *50*:269–276, 1982.
114. Shneerson, J.M.: Digital clubbing and hypertrophic osteoarthropathy: the underlying mechanisms. Br. J. Dis. Chest, *75*:113–131, 1981.
115. Sim, F.H., Dahlin, D.C., and Ivins, J.C.: Extra-articular synovial chondromatosis. J. Bone Joint Surg., *59A*:492–495, 1977.
116. Simkin, P.A., et al.: Free fatty acids in the pancreatic arthritic syndrome. Arthritis Rheum., *26*:127–132, 1983.
117. Simon, M.A., and Hecht, J.D.: Invasion of joints by primary bone sarcomas in adults. Cancer, *50*:1649–1655, 1982.
118. Simon, R.D., and Ford, L.E.: Rheumatoid-like arthritis associated with colonic carcinoma. Arch. Intern. Med., *140*:698–700, 1980.
119. Singh, R., Grewal, D.S., and Chakravarti, R.N.: Experimental production of pigmented villonodular synovitis in the knee and ankle joints of rhesus monkeys. J. Pathol., *98*:137–142, 1969.
120. Smillie, I.S.: Diseases of the Knee Joint. 2nd Ed. Edinburgh, Churchill Livingstone, 1980.
121. Soye, I., et al.: Computed tomography in the preoperative evaluation of masses arising in or near the joints of the extremities. Radiology, *143*:727–732, 1982.
122. Speerstra, F., et al.: Arthritis caused by metastatic melanoma. Arthritis Rheum., *25*:223–226, 1982.
123. Strandberg, B.: Rheumatoid arthritis and cancer arthritis. Scand. J. Rheumatol., *5 (Suppl.)*:1–14, 1974.
124. Tartaglia, L., and Chiroff, R.T.: Diffuse pigmented villonodular synovitis: an indication for total hip replacement in the young patient. Clin. Orthop., *115*:172–176, 1976.
125. Torisu, T., and Watanabe, H.: Pigmented villonodular synovitis occurred in a rheumatoid patient. Clin. Orthop., *91*:134–140, 1973.
126. Tsuneyoshi, M., Enjoji, M., and Kubo, T.: Clear cell sarcoma of tendons and aponeuroses: a comparative study of 13 cases with a provisional subgrouping in the melanotic and synovial types. Cancer, *42*:243–252, 1978.
127. Tsuneyoshi, M., Yokoyama, K., and Enjoji, M.: Synovial sarcoma: clinicopathologic and ultrastructural study of 42 cases. Acta Pathol. Jpn., *33*:23–36, 1983.
128. Ultman, J.E.: Hyperuricemia in disseminated neoplastic

disease other than lymphomas and leukemias. Cancer, 15:122–129, 1962.

129. Vaezy, A., and Budson, D.C.: Phalangeal metastases from bronchogenic carcinoma. JAMA, *239*:226–227, 1978.
130. Varela-Duran, J., and Enzinger, F.M.: Calcifying synovial sarcoma. Cancer, *50*:345–352, 1982.
131. Wagner, M.L., et al.: Polyarticular pigmented villonodular synovitis. AJR, *136*:821–823, 1981.
132. Weinblatt, M.E., and Karp, G.I.: Monarticular arthritis: early manifestations of a rhabdomyosarcoma. J. Rheumatol., *8*:685–688, 1981.
133. Weitzman, G.: Lipoma arborescens of the knee: report of a case. J. Bone Joint Surg., *47A*:1030–1033, 1965.

134. Wilner, D.: Radiology of Bone Tumors and Allied Disorders. Philadelphia, W.B. Saunders, 1982.
135. Wilson, H.A., et al.: Pancreatitis with arthropathy and subcutaneous fat necrosis. Arthritis Rheum., *26*:121–126, 1983.
136. Wiss, D.A.: Recurrent villonodular synovitis of the knee: successful treatment with Yttrium-90. Clin. Orthop., *169*:139–144, 1982.
137. Wright, P.H., et al.: Synovial sarcoma. J. Bone Joint Surg., *64A*:112–122, 1982.
138. Yaghmai, I.: Angiography of Bone and Soft Tissue Lesions. Berlin, Springer-Verlag, 1979.
139. Zindrick, M.R., et al.: Metastatic tumors of the foot. Clin. Orthop., *170*:219–225, 1982.

Painful Shoulder and the Reflex Sympathetic Dystrophy Syndrome

Franklin Kozin

Evolutionary development of the prehensile upper extremity and upright posture in man was accompanied by structural changes in the shoulder girdle and its musculature. Unlike the weight-bearing lower extremity, which remained firmly fixed to the axial skeleton, the upper extremity became loosely joined to the trunk at the small sternoclavicular joint. The result was a tremendous increase in mobility providing a wide range of efficient hand function. This freedom of motion was achieved only by sacrificing stability.

EVOLUTIONARY CHANGES

The origins of the upper limb and shoulder girdle can be traced to the lateral fin folds of early fish.[66,100,116] The first true pectoral girdle is found in later fish, however, in which it is attached to the skull and buttresses the bilateral pectoral fins and their cartilaginous radials (limb forerunners). As these structures were adapted for weight bearing and terrestrial locomotion in amphibians and reptiles, the shoulder girdle separated from the skull and migrated to a more caudal position to provide increased support. Failure of scapular separation and descent in human ontogeny is reflected in congenital anomalies such as Sprengel's deformity.

Acquisition of prehensile function in mammals and upright posture in primates evoked new changes in the shoulder. The greatest change occurred in the structure and position of the scapula. The scapular spine appeared, creating the infra- and supraspinous segments, and gradually the infraspinous segment elongated. The distal end of the scapular spine, the acromion, enlarged in size and mass to accommodate a growing deltoid muscle. With these changes, the scapula migrated from its lateral position on the chest wall to a posterior position and, at the same time, rotated, maintaining the anterior and lateral planes of arm movement. A new bone, the clavicle, developed and assumed its present position in the shoulder girdle, where it functions primarily as a buttress to prevent medial and forward displacement of the scapula and arm. The humerus elongated and twisted along its shaft,

to bring the hand into a more functional position relative to the arm and trunk.

Parallel modifications evolved in the shoulder musculature. The scapulohumeral muscles, that is, the supraspinatus, infraspinatus, teres major and minor, subscapularis, and deltoid, which subserve arm rotation and elevation, underwent the most pronounced changes. The deltoid muscle doubled in relative mass while its insertion on the humerus migrated distally. These factors increased its leverage and established the deltoid muscle as a prime abductor and extendor of the arm. The lower fibers of the deltoid gave rise to a new muscle not found in lower animals, the teres minor. It and the other short rotator muscles formed the musculotendinous cuff of the shoulder, so important in stabilizing the joint. Less-pronounced changes occurred in the axioscapular (trapezius, rhomboids, levator scapulae) and axiohumeral (pectoralis major and minor, latissimus dorsi) muscles, which help to suspend the arm and to fix the scapula during movement.

FUNCTIONAL ANATOMY

Normal shoulder motion is the result of complex, integrated movement in four separate joints: the glenohumeral, acromioclavicular, sternoclavicular, and scapulothoracic joints. This last structure, although not a true joint anatomically, is concerned with scapular motion around the thoracic wall. The three diarthrodial joints allow movement of the shoulder girdle as a whole and a wide range of glenohumeral motion. Although these joints are considered individually, all four joints normally move simultaneously and synchronously to produce smooth, uninterrupted shoulder motion or "scapulothoracic rhythm," after Codman.

The sternoclavicular joint unites the shoulder girdle to the trunk and is formed by the first rib, the clavicle, and the manubrium sterni. A fibrocartilaginous disc is interposed between the bones to provide stability and to ensure a smooth articulation. A thick, fibrous capsule and several surrounding ligaments strengthen this important joint. The acromioclavicular joint also has an intra-articular fibrocartilaginous disc, but unlike that of the sternoclavicular joint, it is inconstant and often rudimentary and may predispose the joint to degenerative arthritis.[66] Adjacent to this joint is the coracoacromial arch (Fig. 85–1), which consists of the acromium and coracoacromial ligaments and protects the humeral head and rotator cuff superiorly. The sternoclavicular and acromioclavicular joints allow the clavicle to rotate along its long axis and permit elevation or depression, as in shrugging the shoulders, and extension or flexion, as in forward or backward thrusting of the shoulders, of the entire shoulder girdle[54,66,100,116] (Fig. 85–2). These movements are essential to full elevation of the arm in abduction or extension.

The glenohumeral joint is formed by the articulation of the humerus and scapula at the shallow glenoid fossa, which is deepened by an encircling rim of fibrocartilage, the labrum glenoidale or glenoid lip. The articular capsule is loose and redundant inferiorly (Fig. 85–3); its surface area is twice that of the humeral head.[66,238] Anteriorly, it is usually thickened into two or three glenohumeral ligaments that support the humerus at its least stable point.[244] The coracohumeral ligament and the long bicipital tendon, which passes through the capsule and functions as an accessory ligament,[100] further support the joint. Despite this organization, most of the dynamic stability of the joint is derived from the surrounding short rotator muscles of the humerus, the supraspinatus superiorly, the infraspinatus and teres minor posteriorly, and the subsca-

pularis anteriorly. The relative position of these muscles may change with glenohumeral motion,[283] although no stabilizing structures are present inferiorly. The short rotator muscle tendons insert radially on the proximal humerus (Fig. 85–4); they are joined by loose connective tissue to form a layer, the rotator cuff, that is closely applied to the underlying capsule. Overlying the rotator cuff, and separated from it by the subacromial bursa, is a second layer of muscle composed of the deltoid and teres major (see Fig. 85–3). Thus, the joint capsule is supported and protected by two musculotendinous layers: the inner rotator cuff and the outer deltoid and teres minor.

Normal movement in the glenohumeral joint is accompanied by scapulothoracic motion. During the initial 30 to 60° of humeral elevation, that is, abduction or extension, scapular motion is variable and apparently unique to each individual.[116] Thereafter, depending on the precise plane in which it is studied, the ratio of glenohumeral to scapulothoracic movement is constant and ranges from 1.25 to 2.00; in other words, for every degree of glenohumeral motion is 0.5 to 0.8° scapulothoracic motion.[116,219] It is possible to fix or to immobilize the scapula and still elevate the arm 90° actively or 120° passively, when further movement is blocked by the acromion. This movement results in a significant loss of power, however, and is not physiologically important.[116,159]

The chief muscles producing glenohumeral joint motion are the deltoid, pectoralis major and minor,

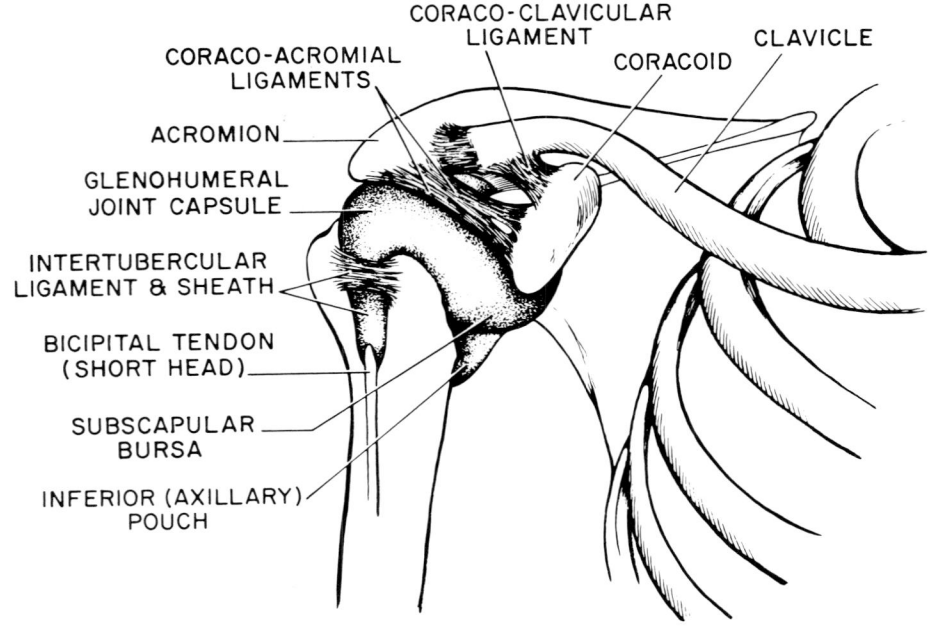

Fig. 85–1. The glenohumeral joint capsule and surrounding structures.

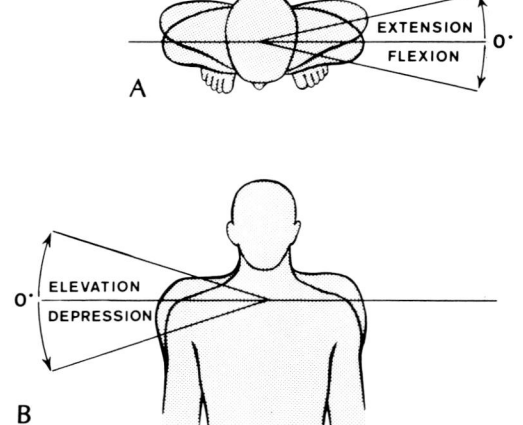

Fig. 85–2. *A* and *B,* Movements of the sternoclavicular and acromioclavicular joints.

teres major, latissimus dorsi, and those in the rotator cuff.[14] Abduction is accomplished by the rotator cuff muscles acting in concert with the deltoid and, occasionally, the long head of the biceps. The down-and-in action of the rotator muscles and the up-and-down action of the deltoid muscle produce a "force couple," in which the off-setting vertical forces stabilize the humeral head within the glenoid while the lateral forces cause abduction.[116,159,244] During abduction, maximum forces on the glenohumeral joint are attained at 90° of elevation.[218] The chief adductors are the pectoralis major and latissimus dorsi, with assistance from the deltoid

muscle. Internal and external rotation are produced by the short rotator (cuff) muscles and the latissimus dorsi and deltoid muscles, respectively. Flexion is due primarily to the action of the pectoralis major and deltoid muscles, although both heads of the biceps muscle also are active, and extension is produced by the deltoid, pectoralis major, and latissimus dorsi muscles.

PHYSICAL EXAMINATION OF THE PATIENT

A detailed medical history and physical examination are essential in all patients with shoulder complaints, to determine whether these symptoms arise from local injury, from systemic disease, or from pain referred from another location.[18,30,66,189,258] Particular attention should be given to a patient's occupation or avocation, the presence of chronic illness, and general mental attitude.

The shoulder is examined with the patient standing or sitting and undressed to the waist, to permit a thorough inspection and comparison of both sides. Joint swelling, abnormality of bony structure, such as inequality or malposition, or muscle fasciculation or atrophy may be apparent. Atrophy of the infraspinatus or supraspinatus muscles, detected as diminished fullness of the respective scapular fossae, usually indicates chronically painful shoulders or acute, severe rupture of the rotator cuff. Arthritis involving the synovial joints of the shoulder may produce soft tissue or bony swelling or effusions; in the glenohumeral joint, an effusion may be detected by swelling along the bicipital

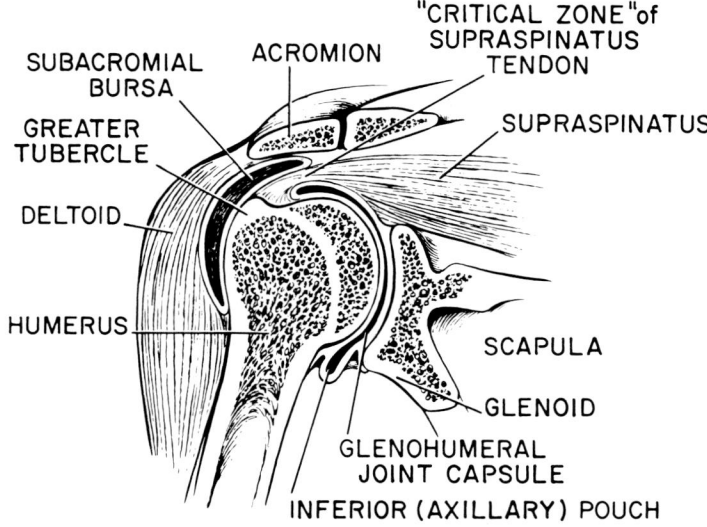

Fig. 85–3. Coronal section of the shoulder, illustrating the relationships of the glenohumeral joint, the joint capsule, the subacromial bursa, and the rotator cuff (supraspinatus tendon).

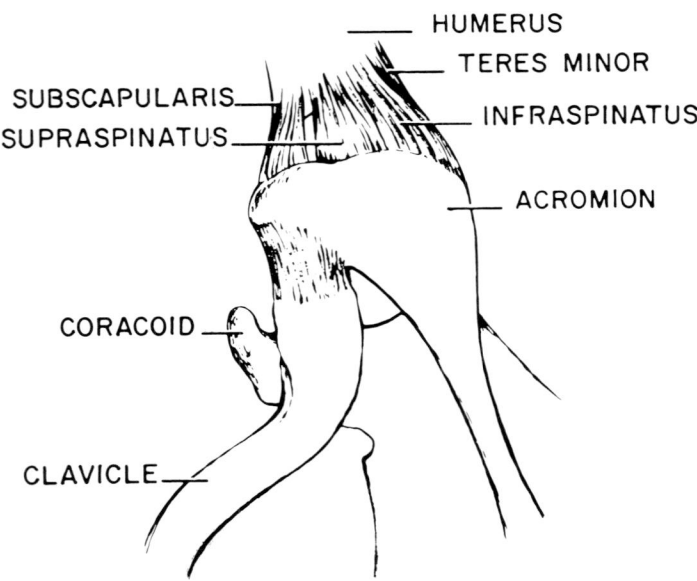

Fig. 85–4. The rotator (musculotendinous) cuff viewed from above.

tendon as it traverses the bicipital groove. Fullness or fluctuance beneath the deltoid muscle suggests subacromial (subdeltoid) bursitis. The patient's posture should be noted.

Shoulder motion is next evaluated. The normal shoulder is capable of a wide range of movement including abduction and adduction (raising or lowering the arm in the coronal plane), flexion and extension (backward or forward movement of the arm in the sagittal plane), internal and external rotation, circumduction, and other remarkable combinations of these motions (Fig. 85–5). Movements of the shoulder girdle as a unit include elevation and depression, as in shrugging, or extension and flexion, as in protrusion (see Fig. 85–2). Active range of motion may be determined quickly and accurately by asking the patient to perform the following movements, keeping in mind that minor variations of the "normal range" exist, depending on the age and sex of the patient[4]: (1) raise both arms to the side until the hands touch overhead, return them to the side, and cross them in front (abduction and adduction); (2) extend both arms forward until the hands touch overhead and extend them behind the back (flexion and extension); (3) place both hands behind the neck (external rotation) and behind the back, as high as possible (internal rotation) (Fig. 85–6); and (4) shrug and protrude the shoulders (sternoclavicular and acromioclavicular joints). Careful observation during these movements is essential because patients with shoulder pain often learn to achieve full abduction or

extension by hunching the shoulder to reverse the normal scapulohumeral rhythm.

Assessment of passive shoulder motion may provide additional diagnostic clues when active movements are limited. As with active motion, particular attention is given to abduction and rotation because these movements are frequently the best indicators of early glenohumeral disease. Passive abduction is measured by fixing the scapula with one hand while the other supports the arm at the partially flexed elbow and abducts it; normally, 90 to 120° of abduction is possible. To measure passive rotation, the arm is abducted with the elbow flexed to 90° and is slowly rotated (see Fig. 85–5,*B*); a 180° arc can usually be achieved.

Patients who complain of pain during arm elevation, usually from 60 to 120° of abduction or extension, a "painful arc," should be assessed with several specific maneuvers. The *impingement sign* is elicited by immobilizing the scapula while forcibly elevating the arm. Subjects with the impingement syndrome experience pain when the greater tuberosity impinges against the coracoacromial arch;[192] on occasion, concomitant popping or "clunking" can be palpated or heard. Injection of 10 ml 1% procaine beneath the acromium may produce relief during this maneuver, thereby conferring some specificity to this test.[192] The *supraspinatus test* is performed by placing the arm in 90° of abduction and internal rotation and by angling the arm 30° forward to isolate the supraspinatus muscle. Muscle strength is tested against resistance to indicate weakness or pain in the

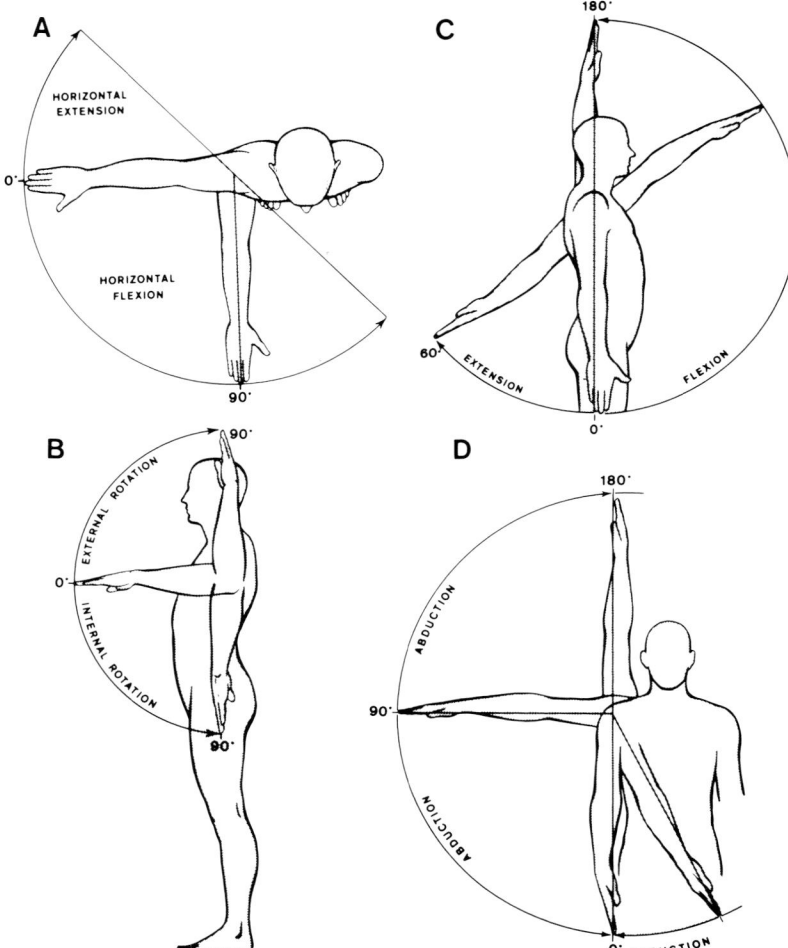

Fig. 85–5. Movements of the shoulder. *A,* "Horizontal" flexion and extension. *B,* Internal and external rotation. *C,* "Vertical" flexion and extension. *D,* Abduction and adduction.

supraspinatus. A *subluxability test* also may be useful, especially in elderly individuals with poorly localized pain. Patients are asked to lie supine with the shoulder over the edge of the examination table; the shoulder is then tested for ease of subluxation.[119] During this test, the glenoid lip should be palpated to disclose tenderness, which may be the only physical finding in tears of this structure.

Cyriax and Bland and others have advocated testing resisted movements in the arm extensively as a method of isolating the painful structure(s).[29,60] Thus, pain on resisted abduction suggests supraspinatus tendinitis; pain on resisted external rotation, infraspinatus tendinitis; pain on resisted internal rotation, subscapularis tendinitis. This approach may be helpful in diagnosis of difficult shoulder problems, especially when pain is not reproduced by simple active range of motion.

Finally, the shoulder must be palpated to deter-

mine the exact site of tenderness and to identify areas of increased heat, swelling, fluctuation, muscle spasm or atrophy, or, on occasion, frank tears within the rotator cuff. Although shoulder pain may be deep and widely radiating, the patient often suggests the diagnosis by identifying a specifically painful point.

RADIOLOGIC EXAMINATION

A general discussion of radiologic examination in rheumatic diseases is provided in Chapter 5. Certain studies that should be considered in many patients with shoulder pain are discussed in this chapter.

Plain Radiography

Proper positioning is essential in visualizing specific structures such as the glenohumeral, sternoclavicular, and acromioclavicular joints, the sca-

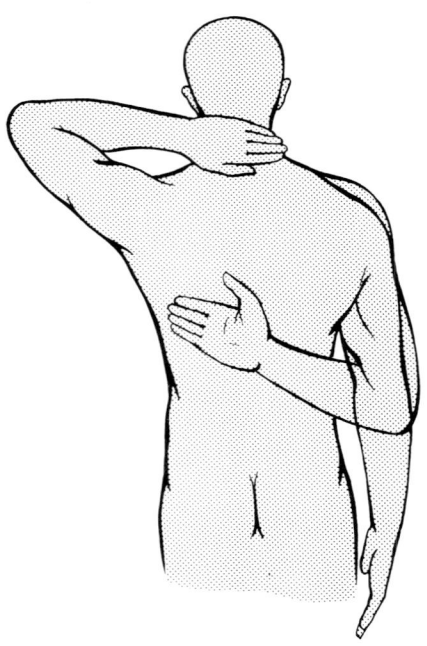

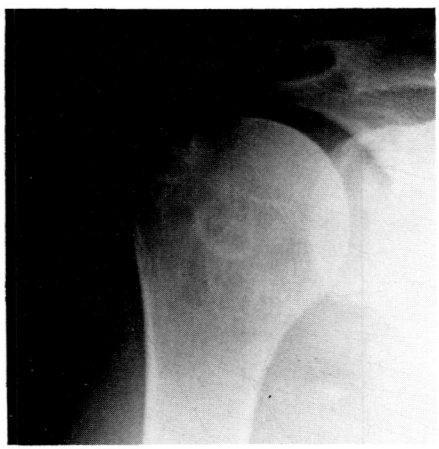

Fig. 85–7. Plain radiograph of the shoulder, illustrating humeral cysts and sclerosis, particularly about the greater tuberosity.

Fig. 85–6. Internal and external rotation of the shoulder (active).

pula and clavicle, the humeral head or greater tuberosity, and the bicipital groove.[118] Arthritic changes, fractures and dislocation, and soft tissue calcification may be identified and localized more readily when the appropriate projection is used. Although of little direct benefit in the diagnosis of soft tissue lesions such as tendinitis, bursitis, or rotator cuff tears, plain radiography may show degenerative changes in the tuberosities or the humeral head and avulsion fractures at tendon insertions, which frequently accompany these conditions (Fig. 85–7). Soft tissue xeroradiography may be of considerable value in the recognition of soft tissue lesions and localized areas of tendon calcification.[92,228]

Arthrography

Contrast studies of the glenohumeral joint are helpful in diagnosing adhesive capsulitis, bicipital tenosynovitis or tendon rupture, rotator cuff tears, and shoulder dislocations.[82,97,195,227] The normal arthrogram demonstrates the bicipital sheath, the redundant inferior joint capsule, and the subscapular bursa (Fig. 85–8, A). The cartilage of the glenoid lip appears as a negative shadow. Because no communication normally exists between the joint cavity and the subacromial bursa, the bursa is not visible.

Complete rotator cuff tears (full-thickness tears) are seen readily as extravasation of contrast material into the subacromial bursa or, occasionally, soft tissues (Fig. 85–8, B). Incomplete tears (par-

tial-thickness tears) are more difficult to recognize, although they may be suggested by irregularities or small clefts in the rotator cuff. Bicipital tendon tenosynovitis or rupture may produce irregularity in the bicipital sheath or leakage of the contrast material into the soft tissues of the upper arm. Shoulder dislocations and subluxations that tear the capsule away from the glenoid lip may be demonstrated by excessive capsule laxity (ballooning) or by leakage of dye.

The arthrogram in adhesive capsulitis is characteristic. Joint volume is reduced, and the normal anterior and inferior pouches are obliterated. As a result, *the volume of contrast material that can be injected is reduced from the usual 15 to 35 ml to only 5 to 10 ml.*

Double-contrast arthrography, in which a small amount of radiopaque contrast material and a larger amount of air are instilled into the glenohumeral joint, improves the resolution of the rotator cuff structures and the articular cartilage,[97] and it may cause less joint irritation than other methods.[105] This technique is more difficult to perform and to interpret than the conventional method, however.[229] When this technique is combined with tomography (arthrotomography), it is possible to visualize abnormalities of the glenoid lip effectively and to diagnose avulsion or tears of the cartilaginous rim.[33,166]

Subacromial bursography is used with increasing frequency, particularly for diagnosis of adhesive subacromial bursitis, in which the bursal volume is reduced, from 4 to 6 ml to 1 to 2 ml,[151] and in the shoulder impingement syndrome discussed later in this chapter.[151,227]

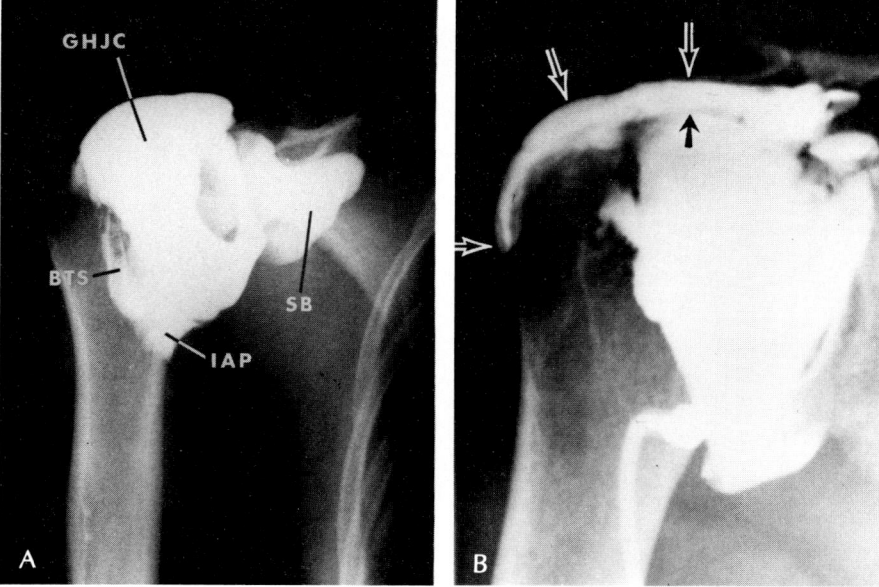

Fig. 85–8. *A,* Arthrogram of the normal shoulder, showing the glenohumeral joint capsule (GHJC), the subscapular bursa (SB), the inferior axillary pouch (IAP), and the bicipital tendon sheath (BTS). *B,* Arthrogram of the shoulder in a patient with a complete rotator cuff rupture, demonstrating contrast in the subacromial bursa (arrows).

Scintigraphy

Inflamed joints can be readily detected by this method,[177] and it may be useful in mild or even noninflammatory articular disease.[19,202] Studies in adhesive capsulitis[300] and polymyalgia rheumatica[202] show abnormal shoulder uptake, but such findings must be interpreted cautiously because increased local radioactivity is common in patients without symptoms or radiographic abnormalities relating to the shoulder,[91,247] or in patients with injury of the rotator cuff.[264]

Other radiologic techniques, including ultrasound[7,249] and computed tomography (CT),[61] may prove useful in assessing patients with shoulder pain, but these methods have not been adequately evaluated.

PAINFUL SHOULDER

Shoulder pain is among the most common complaints in medical practice. Such pain may be caused by local problems within the shoulder region or by remote disorders, especially heart, lung, and cervical spinal disease, or systemic conditions. A variety of classifications have been devised to aid in differential diagnosis; it seems most useful to divide shoulder pain into two broad etiologic categories[30,42,258]: intrinsic (local) and extrinsic (remote and systemic) disorders (Table 85–1). Intrinsic conditions, which account for most shoulder complaints,[258] are emphasized here.

Impingement Syndrome

The coracoacromial arch (see Fig. 85–1) protects the humeral head and the rotator cuff from direct trauma. The arch is rigid and may limit full arm elevation. The "impingement syndrome" occurs when the supraspinatus tendon is caught between the humerus and the coracoacromial arch.[192,193] Repeated impingement may result in attrition of rotator cuff tendons or frank rotator cuff tears. A number of sports appear to increase the incidence of impingement.[211]

Subjects with the impingement syndrome often complain of a "painful arc" in the range of 60 to 120° of arm elevation. The impingement sign, described previously in this chapter, is a specific test for diagnosis.[192] Radiographs frequently show bony spurs on the undersurface of the acromion,[193] and subacromial bursography demonstrates reduced volume and abnormal configuration of the bursa.[266]

Conservative therapy is sufficient to control symptoms and to limit progression in early cases.[192] Later, bursectomy or acromioplasty may be necessary for symptomatic relief.[103,193] It is not clear how often or when recurrent impingement may cause degenerative or calcific tendinitis.

Degenerative Tendinitis ("Supraspinatus Syndrome")

Origin and Pathogenesis

Degenerative changes in the rotator cuff tendons appear to represent the "normal" aging proc-

Table 85–1. Differential Diagnosis of the Painful Shoulder

Intrinsic Disorders
  Impingement Syndrome
  Specific Lesions of the Rotator Cuff
    Degenerative tendinitis
    Calcific tendinitis
    Subacromial bursitis
    Rotator cuff rupture
  Lesions of the Bicipital Tendon
  Adhesive Capsulitis ("Frozen Shoulder")
  Fibrositis and Fibromyalgia
  Arthritis
    Degenerative
    "Milwaukee shoulder"
    Neurotrophic
  Traumatic and Athletic Injuries
    Subluxation or dislocation
  Neurologic
    Peripheral neuropathy
    Brachial plexus injury
  Postural Effects
  Infection
  Neoplasia, Benign and Malignant

Extrinsic Disorders
  Inflammatory Conditions
    Rheumatoid arthritis
    Spondyloarthritides
    Myopathies
    Polymyalgia rheumatica
  Avascular Necrosis
  Metabolic and Endocrine
    Gout and pseudogout
    Diabetes mellitus
    Hyperparathyroidism
    Other
  Neurologic
    Cervical nerve root compression (C4, C5, C6)
    Lesions of the spinal cord
    "Viscerosomatic" and referred pain
    Peripheral neuropathy
  Neurovascular
    Thoracic outlet syndrome
    Axillary arterial and venous thrombosis
  Reflex Sympathetic Dystrophy Syndrome(s)

ess.[42,189] Twenty-five percent of unselected subjects have attritional changes in the rotator cuff by their fifth decade, and the incidence increases progressively thereafter.[189] The supraspinatus tendon is affected most frequently, especially in the so-called critical zone of Codman, a site approximately 1 to 2 cm medial to its insertion at the greater tuberosity. Several factors may combine to explain the increased susceptibility of this region[173,190,225,239]: (1) it is a relatively avascular zone where the osseous and tendinous blood supplies anastomose; (2) the few blood vessels in this area are compressed when the arm is hanging down normally;[225] and (3) re-peated impingement of this area may occur between the acromion and the humeral head during abduction. In contrast, the vascular supply of the other flat tendons of the rotator cuff is greater, nonanastomotic, and unimpeded by arm motion.[225] These observations also may explain the high frequency of degenerative tendinitis in subjects with repeated occupational stresses to the shoulder, such as carpenters, painters,[189] and welders,[111] or with a compromised neurologic or vascular supply, such as alcoholics and diabetics.[43,189,217,281] Experimentally, it is difficult to tear a normal tendon, but it is easy to tear an ischemic tendon.

Clinical Features

The patient with degenerative tendinitis is most likely to be a man in his fifth decade or older, to work as a laborer, and to localize his complaints to the dominant side. The condition is generally asymptomatic until provoked by minor trauma or exertion; however, careful questioning often elicits a history of recurrent shoulder problems.

The patient complains of a dull ache in the shoulder that is not easily localized. It may be more severe at night and may interfere with sleep. On examination, active shoulder movements are restricted, especially abduction. A painful arc from 70 to 100° of abduction is characteristic, probably reflecting supraspinatus involvement because at this range supraspinatus activity is maximal and greatest force is applied across the glenohumeral joint.[14,116,218] Many patients learn to avoid this painful arc by reversing the scapulohumeral rhythm, that is, by hunching their shoulder to position the scapula before initiating glenohumeral motion. Often, passive movements are normal because force across the joint is minimal when the arm is supported. Weakness is uncommon unless the pain is chronic, of more than 3 weeks' duration, or an associated rotator cuff tear is present. In patients with severe pain, it may be necessary to inject an anesthetic agent into the rotator cuff before attempting to assess strength.[126a] Palpation is helpful in identifying the source of pain. Tenderness over the bicipital groove suggests bicipital tendinitis. Subscapularis tendinitis may be detected by tenderness at its insertion on the lesser tuberosity. Similarly, tenderness localized to the superior or inferolateral aspects of the greater tuberosity suggests supraspinatus tendinitis or injuries of the infraspinatus or teres minor tendons, respectively. Location of the area of maximal tenderness is important in guiding therapy.[128]

Radiologic Examination

A radiograph of a shoulder with an early tendon lesion generally is normal. In patients with chronic disease, degenerative changes such as bony fragments, pseudocysts, sclerosis, and osteophytes may develop in the greater tuberosity and the humeral head (see Fig. 85–7).[66,189] Unless the disorder has progressed to a frank rotator cuff tear, the arthrogram is usually normal, although small irregularities on the undersurface of the tendon may be noted.

The treatment of this disorder is discussed later in this chapter, under "Bursitis."

Calcific Tendinitis

Origin and Pathogenesis

Many have assumed that tendon calcification occurs as a consequence of degenerative tendinitis.[66,171,189,210] Yet considerable evidence from studies in experimental animals,[165,250] as well as from observations of patients with uremia,[207] hypervitaminosis D,[47,50] and multiple sites of "calcific periarthritis,"[44,163,214] suggests that calcium deposits in tendon may occur in the apparent absence of local degeneration.

Most studies of the pathogenesis of this condition have focused on local factors that predispose tendons to calcification. Although the precise mechanism still remains uncertain, a number of hypotheses have evolved.[63,148,157,158,187,277,287,288] Altered tendon physiologic features, possibly produced by changes in blood flow, minor trauma, or mild inflammation, promote a direct interaction between tendon matrix and calcium ion.[157,158] Phospholipids and various proteins have been implicated in the process of calcification in bone,[24,194,276,303] and they may subserve this function in tendon as well. The resultant calcium complex then may react with phosphorus, to produce a series of intermediate salts until hydroxyapatite is formed.[63,277,289] This crystalline substance has been identified in shoulder tendons,[66,221] just as in other forms of calcific periarthritis.[163]* Four histologic phases have been described in "primary" calcific tendinitis which occurs typically in the aforementioned critical zone.[154,168,287] These phases are: (1) "precalcific," in which metaplastic fibrocartilage is observed within the tendon; (2) "calcific," in which deposits of calcium are found within a fibrocartilaginous nodule in a close relationship with matrix vesicles, without reactive changes; (3) "resorptive," in which reactive changes consist of phagocytic cells and increased vascularity; and (4) "repair," which is characterized by the appearance of abundant mesenchymal

cells within the tendon. The natural history of primary calcific deposits is spontaneous resorption. The majority of patients in a recent study had no reactive or reparative changes associated with tendon calcification.[168] "Secondary" calcification occurs at the torn edges of the rotator cuff or in a degenerated tendon insertion into the greater trochanter, that is, an enthesopathy distal to the critical zone. Such calcific deposits do not resorb spontaneously and elicit little repair reaction.[287]

Once deposited, the calcified material exists in two states, or possibly phases, that seem to correlate with the clinical stage of the condition. In the chronic stage, the deposits are usually hard and dry (inspissated), with a gritty consistency; in the acute stage, the material is creamy white and pastelike (hydrated).[168,189]

Clinical Features

The prevalence of calcific tendinitis is high, occurring in 2.7 to 8.0% of the general population.[31,222] The highest incidence appears to be in the fifth decade, and the association with various chronic diseases, particularly diabetes mellitus, is strong.[43,189,217] Unlike degenerative tendinitis, this condition is seen in both sexes equally and often affects subjects in sedentary occupations.[31,66,189] Like degenerative tendinitis, the supraspinatus tendon is most commonly involved (approximately 50% of cases), followed by the infraspinatus, teres minor, and subscapularis tendon and the subacromial bursa. Multiple sites of calcification and bilateral involvement are also common.[31,66,215]

Three clinical states are recognized and resemble those of the other crystal-induced arthritides (see Chaps. 91, 94, 95).[66,171,189,254] The first, asymptomatic stage is found incidentally on radiographs usually obtained for other reasons.[31] Little or no inflammatory reaction is present, possibly because the calcium deposit is small and located in the avascular critical zone.[66,171] Radiologically, the borders of the deposit are smooth. The calcium may be resorbed spontaneously, often correlating with symptoms of pain and inflammation.[28] The borders of the calcific deposit appear scalloped. Other symptoms develop later. These stages might be likened to acute or "tophaceous" gout, both clinically and pathologically, because a granulomatous reaction with chronic inflammation and giant cells is present as part of the resorptive process.[153,189] Chronic symptoms and physical signs are indistinguishable from those of degenerative tendinitis, previously described, and the course of the disorder is characterized by exacerbations and remissions. The acute stage resembles the acute gouty or pseudogouty attack: pain is sudden and severe, often following minimal trauma or effort.

Editors' Note: Such calcifications contain hydroxyapatite, partly substituted by carbonate, and octacalcium phosphate (see Chap. 95).

This diffuse pain may radiate into the subdeltoid (bursa) area; a few patients develop features of a reflex sympathetic dystrophy in the ipsilateral hand.[66,189] Because the rotator cuff muscles are in spasm, the arm is held rigidly in a neutral or an adducted position. Even the slightest movement evokes a painful outcry. Complete examination of the patient is virtually impossible, although gentle palpation may reveal a point of maximal tenderness. As in acute gout and pseudogout, colchicine therapy often has dramatic results. The relation of calcific tendinitis to a more advanced form of crystal-induced shoulder disease, "Milwaukee shoulder" (see Chap. 95), is uncertain.

Standard radiographs show the typical ovoid calcific deposit (Fig. 85–9,*A*), although special views may be needed to identify the exact site of calcification.[215,291] Rupture into the subacromial bursa is noted in about 5% of cases (Fig. 85–9,*B*).[31] When rupture occurs, the calcium salt is usually rapidly resorbed. Such rupture may leave a hole in the rotator cuff, which is now officially "torn."[126]

The treatment of this disorder is discussed in the following section, "Bursitis."

Bursitis

Origin and Pathogenesis

A number of bursae or thin-walled, usually closed, sacs lined with synovial tissue strategically placed to minimize friction between moving parts are found in the shoulder region. The largest and most constant is the subacromial bursa, located between the rotator cuff inferiorly and the deltoid and teres major muscles superiorly (see Fig. 85–3). Its lateral extension beneath the deltoid muscle is termed the subdeltoid bursa. Other bursae include the subscapular, supracoracoid, and those found in relation to the insertion of various muscles, such as the trapezius, pectoralis major, teres major, and latissimus dorsi muscles. Except for the systemic arthritides, which may affect the bursae primarily, bursitis of the shoulder area usually is secondary to traumatic, degenerative, or calcific disease in the rotator cuff. The subacromial bursa is most commonly involved because of its large size and its anatomic position.

Clinical Features

Symptoms of subacromial bursitis or "deal-runner's shoulder" are similar to those of the primary disease. Pain and tenderness may extend distally to the superior third of the arm because of the subdeltoid extension of the bursa. Active and passive abduction are usually reduced, but active motion is disproportionately limited, probably because of the added force of the contracting abductor muscles on the bursa.[60]

Depending on the primary disease, plain radiographs may demonstrate bony changes,[137,298] calcific deposits,[22,31,215] or actual enlargement of the bursa.[295] An arthrogram may show a communication with the glenohumeral joint capsule when bursitis is caused by complete rupture of the rotator cuff.[126a,131,195] Bursography may be useful in demonstrating the impingement syndrome, adhesive bursitis, or rotator cuff tears.[151]

Treatment

Treatment of degenerative or calcific tendinitis and subacromial bursitis is directed at pain relief, maintenance of maximal shoulder function, prevention of complications such as adhesive capsulitis or the reflex sympathetic dystrophy syndrome, early rehabilitation, and education of the patient in methods of avoiding recurrent attacks.[16,66,189,258,278] The vast numbers of therapeutic programs that have been advocated attest to their lack of specificity and to the unavailability of a uniformly successful program.

A standard conservative program should first be instituted (Table 85–2). Rest of the acutely painful

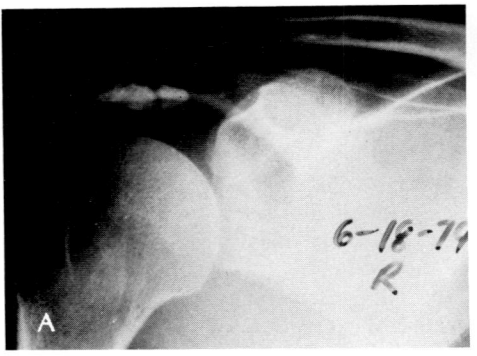
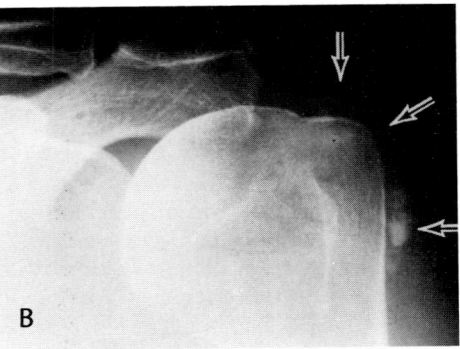

Fig. 85–9. Plain radiographs of the shoulder in a patient with calcification in the supraspinatus tendon, *A*, and in the subacromial bursa, *B*. Note the calcium extending into the subdeltoid area in *B* (arrows).

Table 85–2. Conservative Treatment Program for Painful Shoulder*

---

1. Limited use of extremity during acute painful period
    Complete rest for hyperacute symptoms
    Arm in adduction sling; hand and forearm elevated
2. Anti-inflammatory and analgesic agents (and muscle relaxants)
    Salicylates and other nonsteroidal anti-inflammatory drugs
    Acetaminophen and propoxyphene derivatives
    Narcotic analgesics for severe pain only
    Muscle relaxants not recommended
3. Physical Therapy
    Heat or cold (cold for acute conditions; heat for subacute or chronic symptoms)
        Home: heating pad, hot packs, ice packs
        Physician's office or hospital: ultrasound, diathermy, hydrocollator packs
    Exercises
        Initially, as acute pain subsides: passive range of motion
        Later, when pain is mild to moderate: pendulum swinging (Codman), when possible; active exercises with resistance or assistance
4. Treatment of associated or underlying condition
5. Psychologic support in the form of reassurance and encouragement
6. Education for self-help and avoidance of provocative activities

---

*Objectives: Relief of pain and muscle spasm, maintenance and restoration of motion, and prevention of secondary changes.

shoulder is essential. Immobilization of the arm in partial adduction with a sling may help. Salicylates or other nonsteroidal anti-inflammatory drugs in adequate doses (see Chap. 28) are useful for their analgesic and anti-inflammatory properties,[256] although concomitant administration of simple analgesics, such as acetaminophen or propoxyphene, or narcotic analgesics may be required. Muscle relaxants are of doubtful value. Any of a variety of local physical techniques that provide heat or cold to the affected area may assist in reducing pain. These techniques include moist hot packs, such as hydrocollator packs, ultrasound,[20,26,99,223] short-wave diathermy,[114] other such methods,[278] or simple ice packs.[20] These techniques may raise the local pain threshold,[20] promote local blood flow,[71,114] enhance tissue repair,[108,232] reduce muscle spasm, or simply exert a placebo effect.[187] Controlled studies suggest that some of these approaches have no effect.[72] Treatment with local radiotherapy, dimethyl sulfoxide (DMSO),[273] or acupuncture,[187] although recommended by some, does not appear to be any more effective than treatment with the other measures discussed and is not recommended.

Early mobilization of the painful extremity is important in minimizing disability and the risk of adhesive capsulitis or reflex dystrophy. Passive movements immediately after local heat or cold applications or one to two hours after analgesic drug administration may be instituted. These movements may be extended gradually, and active exercises may be started as symptoms subside. Often, the simple pendulum exercise of Codman, which uses the effect of gravity, is a good starting point. The trunk is flexed at the hips and lumbar spine,

and the arm allowed to hang in approximately 90° of flexion; by swinging the body, the arm moves back and forth like a pendulum. This exercise is done first in the sagittal plane (flexion-extension) and later in the coronal plane (abduction-adduction). Eventually, full, active range-of-motion exercises can be encouraged, with or without assistance or resistance.[172]

Failure of these basic measures to control symptoms and to restore movement requires a more aggressive approach. The usual first step is the local instillation of corticosteroids. One should mix 25 to 100 mg hydrocortisone acetate or equivalent amounts of the newer preparations (see Chap. 34) with 5 to 10 ml 1% procaine and inject into the point(s) of maximal tenderness. Local corticosteroids are not without potentially serious side effects, however.[81,96,232,240,261] In addition to the possible complication of systemic adsorption and the risk of infection,[133] intra- or peritendinous corticosteroids may interfere with healing,[10,23] may reduce the tensile strength of unaffected tendon, and ultimately may cause tendon rupture.[117,179,271,304] A transient, 24- to 48-hour increase in symptoms may follow local injection.[164] Little critical evidence suggests that corticosteroid injections are more or even equally effective than the basic conservative measures.[62] Empirically, however, when conservative treatment fails to produce satisfactory results, corticosteroid injections may be useful. Systemic administration of corticosteroids or adrenocorticotrophic hormone (ACTH) has also been advocated, but it should be reserved for the most difficult therapeutic problems, in view of serious potential side effects. Operative intervention for degenerative tendinitis is rarely necessary.

In most cases, considerable improvement occurs within two to six weeks of therapy. Persistence of pain beyond this time should suggest a serious rotator cuff tear, and a thorough re-evaluation, including arthrographic study, is indicated. After improvement, every effort should be made to identify the source(s) of shoulder trauma, such as employment or avocational abuse, and to suggest appropriate modifications in these activities, to prevent recurrence.

Calcific tendinitis or bursitis presents a special problem. Acute symptoms probably represent a form of crystal-induced synovitis, so local corticosteroids early in the disease appear justified,[221] especially if conservative therapy, including nonsteroidal anti-inflammatory agents, proves ineffective within the initial 24 to 72 hours of symptoms. Spontaneous resolution occurs in at least 30 to 40% of such patients, however. In those with chronic symptoms or recurrent attacks, removal of the calcific deposit may be indicated, by needling the affected area, with or without concomitant instillation of corticosteroids and local anesthetics.[53,66] On occasion, surgical removal of the deposit is useful in providing relief,[168,188] but this procedure should be delayed as long as possible because recovery with resorption of the deposits is the rule in most patients.[31,66]

Rupture of the Rotator Cuff

Origin and Pathogenesis

Because of its critical role in stabilizing the glenohumeral joint, the musculotendinous (rotator) cuff may be torn by a variety of forces applied to the joint.[66,189,199] In younger individuals, considerable force is necessary, so tears usually follow direct trauma, unexpected falls on an outstretched arm, or the extreme stress of modern athletics. Much less force is required in older individuals, possibly as a result of pre-existent degenerative tendinitis and decreased vascularity that weakens the tendon structure. In such patients, tears are usually idiopathic or follow minor falls or the lifting of a weight with the arm fully extended or abducted.

Lesions of the rotator cuff are divided into complete or partial tears. Complete tears involve the full thickness of the cuff and the overlying subacromial bursa. As in degenerative tendinitis, the supraspinatus tendon is affected most commonly. Partial tears produce incomplete rents in the cuff, usually on the undersurface of the tendon near its insertion, and communication with the subacromial bursa does not occur.

Both conditions are more common than generally believed; partial tears are found in as many as 30% of cadavers.[66,189] The condition frequently goes unrecognized because the clinical and radiographic features of other forms of rotator cuff disease are so similar.

Clinical Features

The classic history of a fall or direct shoulder trauma in a patient complaining of shoulder pain and limitation of motion generally suggests the diagnosis of rotator cuff tear. Often, however, a specific event is not apparent, even after careful questioning. Persistence of symptoms in the shoulder of a patient who was previously diagnosed as having tendinitis, bursitis, or "strain" for more than six to eight weeks should suggest a rotator cuff tear, especially in an older patient.

Acute full-thickness rupture produces immediate pain and muscle spasm. Weakness of the arm may be marked within hours to days of the injury, and both pain and weakness may persist for many months. On examination, motion is limited by pain and muscle spasm; in mild cases, pain may be present during active abduction in an arc between 70 and 100°. Local infiltration of an anesthetic agent abolishes pain, but not weakness. Although this finding is not entirely specific, it is suggestive of a rotator cuff tear. Frequently, the *drop arm sign* is positive: the arm is passively abducted to 90°, but it falls to the side when no longer supported by the examiner.[189,196] The patient cannot usually hold the arm in abduction at 90°, or the arm collapses to the side with just a little push downward by the physician. Occasionally, the actual tear can be palpated directly by an experienced examiner.

Diagnosis of the small complete tear or partial tear is more difficult. Persons engaged in overhead work, such as paperhangers and painters, or in lifting with extended arms, such as nurses and waitresses, appear to be predisposed to those lesions, just as they are to degenerative tendinitis. Although shoulder pain or discomfort is often present, it may be minimal. Frequently, the only complaint or physical finding is weakness in elevation of the arm, an important clue to diagnosis.

The symptoms and signs of rotator cuff rupture are similar to those of other "degenerative diseases" of the rotator cuff, but persistent pain and, especially, weakness in arm elevation, often with early (two to four weeks) muscle atrophy, suggest this diagnosis. Full-thickness tears can be present for years without any symptoms, especially in the elderly person who demands little from his body.

Radiologic Examination

The plain radiograph in rotator cuff ruptures in younger individuals is usually normal. That it is abnormal in as many as 60% of older individuals may reflect pre-existent degenerative tendinitis.[137,298] Changes consist of erosion sclerosis, pseudocysts, and osteophytes about the greater tuberosity at the site of insertion of the supraspinatus tendon. These changes are indistinguishable from those of degenerative tendinitis (see Fig. 85–7). Narrowing of the space between the humeral head and the acromion is a useful radiologic sign of superior subluxation of the humerus. This condition may be so extreme as to produce a "pseudoarticulation."

Complete ruptures of the rotator cuff may be confirmed by arthrography.[82,126a,131,195] Leakage of contrast material into surrounding soft tissues or into the subacromial bursa is diagnostic of this condition (see Fig. 85–8,*B*). In partial ruptures, however, the arthrogram is normal, although, rarely, small irregularities or clefts are seen.[199] Partial rotator cuff tears or degenerative changes in the cuff are best visualized by double-contrast arthrography[97] or bursography.[151]

Treatment

Early surgical repair of the acute, complete rupture, before granulation tissue forms and the edges of the torn capsule retract or calcify, appears to provide the best long-term result.[13,41,66,189,196,245,298] Treatment of patients with chronically torn rotator cuffs remains an unresolved problem.[104,245] Conservative therapy, as outlined in Table 85–2, may be effective, especially when supplemented with local corticosteroid injection.[294] Sixty percent of patients so treated show significant improvement,[245] although this figure may depend on which factors are assessed.[62] Newer surgical approaches have produced more satisfactory results,[104,220] but complete alleviation of pain and restoration of full function are still uncommon.[127,220]

Bicipital Syndromes
Origin and Pathogenesis

The long head (tendon) of the biceps brachii extends from its origin on the supraglenoid tubercle and posterior rim of the glenoid lip, through the articular capsule and intertubercular (bicipital), groove, and inserts on the posterior portion of the radial tuberosity. Within the joint capsule, the tendon functions as an accessory ligament and prevents upward and outward displacement of the humeral head. The tendon remains ensheathed in synovial tissue as it leaves the articular capsule until it traverses the bicipital groove (see Fig. 85–1). The biceps supinates the forearm and assists in abduction and flexion of the arm.

The following four conditions are included in the category of bicipital syndromes: (1) tendinitis and tenosynovitis; (2) elongation of the tendon; (3)

rupture; and (4) dislocation and subluxation.[189] Bicipital tendinitis or tenosynovitis is usually produced by constant friction within the intertubercular groove that causes attrition and inflammation of the tendon and its sheath. When these attritional changes are severe, the tensile strength of the tendon is lost, and elongation occurs. This condition may progress to frank rupture following even minimal effort. Dislocation or subluxation of the bicipital tendon is usually related to a congenitally shallow intertubercular groove or to traumatic disruption of the intertubercular ligaments that hold the tendon in the groove (see Fig. 85–1).

Clinical Features

Bicipital tendinitis produces pain in the anterior shoulder that may radiate along the biceps into the forearm. Limitation of abduction or internal rotation may be present. Occasionally, a history of repetitive arm movements can be elicited, but it is not generally possible to identify a specific cause. On examination, a number of signs are useful in differential diagnosis. Manual side-to-side displacement of the bicipital tendon ("twanging") or simple palpation of the tendon in the bicipital groove during arm rotation may be associated with marked tenderness, indicating bicipital tendinitis. Pain along the course of the tendon produced by resisted supination of the forearm (Yergason's supination sign) or by resisted flexion at the elbow also suggests bicipital tendinitis. When elongation has occurred, pain may be minimal, but bicipital weakness is prominent. Absence of a palpable tendon and loss of normal bicipital contraction during resisted supination confirm this diagnosis. This syndrome can be differentiated from frank rupture, which causes persistent swelling of the biceps in the upper arm; in acute rupture, extravasation of blood is noted in the upper arm. Dislocation and subluxation are recognized by palpation of the tendon as it snaps or slides in and out of the bicipital groove.

Radiologic Examination

Radiographic studies of the shoulder in this condition are usually normal. Special views of the bicipital groove may show irregularity or osteophytes of the tuberosities in tendinitis or a shallow groove in a case of subluxation of the tendon. Arthrograms are rarely abnormal, but they may demonstrate irregularity or blockage of contrast medium within the tendon sheath.

Treatment

The initial program consists of the measures outlined in Table 85–2. In resistant cases, local instillation of corticosteroids into the tendon sheath is indicated and often produces a good result. Operative intervention is rarely necessary, but in persistent cases it may prove beneficial.[198] When a lax, elongated tendon does not respond to conservative therapy, resection of the intra-articular portion of the tendon with fixation of the distal end may restore useful function.

Pain from a dislocating or subluxing tendon may also respond to a conservative program and exercises. Surgical treatment may be necessary, however, to fix the tendon within the groove or to the proximal humerus. In acute bicipital rupture in younger patients, early surgical repair is indicated. If several weeks have passed or if the patient is elderly, a conservative approach may be better.

Adhesive Capsulitis

This disorder is also known as frozen shoulder, scapulohumeral periarthritis, periarthritis of Duplay, periarthritis of the shoulder, and check-rein shoulder.

Origin and Pathogenesis

Adhesive capsulitis is a clinical entity apparently unique to the shoulder. It is characterized by pain and stiffness in the absence of any recognized intrinsic abnormality, although it may complicate any of the conditions previously discussed. In addition to following local soft tissue injuries, adhesive capsulitis may result from such problems as other trauma, coronary artery disease, chronic lung disease, pulmonary tuberculosis, diabetes mellitus, and cervical spinal syndromes.[34,302] The common denominator appears to be prolonged immobility of the arm.[66,145] A third factor, the "periarthritic personality," has been suggested as a necessary component for the development of the full syndrome, but psychologic testing of a large group of patients has failed to confirm this hypothesis.[302] Recently, a possible immunologic basis for adhesive capsulitis has been suggested,[39,40,173] but the putative association of this syndrome with HLA-B27 has not been confirmed.[39,40,201,248]

The pathologic findings have been described by several investigators.[57,66,120,197] The joint capsule is thickened and is loosely adherent to the underlying humeral head; the normal capsular folds are obliterated. Microscopic changes include proliferation of synovial lining cells, fibrosis, and a mild, chronic inflammatory cell infiltrate. Such findings are inconstant, and at least 20% of cases have a normal histologic appearance.[197] As in other immobilized joints,[3] biochemical studies of the joint capsule have shown diminished glycosaminoglycan and water content.[3,160]

Clinical Features

Adhesive capsulitis is more common in women than in men, occurs in the fifth decade or later, and bears no relation to occupation.[66,189,258,302] The associated clinical conditions have already been enumerated. Both shoulders may be affected simultaneously or successively in some patients.[66,226]

The patient characteristically complains of the insidious onset of a diffusely painful and stiff shoulder. A specific precipitating event is rarely identified. The patient is unable to sleep because of pain and, perhaps as a result, is often anxious and irritable; hence the "periarthritic personality." Objective findings include diffuse tenderness about the glenohumeral joint and restricted active and passive motion in all planes. Injection of anesthetic agent locally may reduce pain but it fails to improve mobility.

Three phases of the disease have been described.[66,226] The first, characterized primarily by pain and by gradually increasing stiffness, usually lasts 2 to 9 months. In the second phase, pain is less severe, and the patient often describes a vague discomfort in the shoulder, but stiffness is marked ("frozen shoulder"). This phase persists from 4 to 12 months. The final phase, lasting an additional 5 to 26 months, is one of gradual recovery of function ("thawing") and resolution of pain. *The natural history of a frozen shoulder is a thaw.* The majority of patients are often fully improved within 12 to 18 months of the onset of this disorder,[109,146,156,226] although symptoms may persist for many more months.[189,226]

Radiologic Examination

Except for localized osteopenia in the shoulder after one to two months of disuse,[161] the plain radiograph in adhesive capsulitis is generally normal.[109,197,258,301] An arthrogram may be useful in differentiating this from other painful conditions, however.[82,195] The joint capsule typically appears contracted, with absence of the normal inferior reflection (axillary pouch), bicipital tendon sheath, and subscapular bursa.[131,189,195,227] The injectable volume of contrast material may be reduced by 60 to 90%.[195] One report demonstrated some volume loss in 67% of cases, but marked volume loss ($\geq$ 50%) was found in only 43%.[102] Intra-articular adhesions were not observed. It was recently suggested that scintigraphy of the shoulder may be helpful in the diagnosis of adhesive capsulitis and related conditions and in predicting response to local corticosteroid injection.[202,300] Confirmatory studies and further characterization of scintigrams in normal shoulders,[199,247] as well as in injured shoulders,[264] are needed before this approach can be recommended, however.

Treatment

The best treatment of adhesive capsulitis is prevention. Early mobilization of the shoulder(s) in any painful condition or chronic illness is essential, although this approach may not be effective in patients with hemiparesis.[35,151] Once the disorder is established, little critical evidence suggests that any therapeutic approach shortens the natural course of the disease.[59,107] A conservative program should be instituted as early as possible (see Table 85–2); however, if symptoms persist or worsen, a variety of therapeutic techniques have been advocated. These include local corticosteroid injections,[59,146,240,251,259,296] stellate ganglion blockade,[296] systemic corticosteroids or ACTH,[222] antidepressant medications,[284] and exercises combined with transcutaneous nerve stimulation.[234]

In the patient with a resistant case or in those who have had symptoms for several months, I have achieved good to excellent responses with injection into the joint of a mixture containing 2.5 to 3.0 ml 1% procaine, 20 to 40 mg of prednisolone tertiary butyl acetate microcrystalline suspension, and 20 ml sterile saline solution, using maximum pressure on the injecting syringe, followed immediately by exercises.[138] A similar procedure, termed "infiltration brisement," has been used successfully by others,[254] and simple pressure distention during arthrography appears to yield similar gratifying results.[7,93,204] Unfortunately, none of these regimens have been studied under controlled conditions. Manipulation of the shoulder under general anesthesia has been used in refractory cases with varied success,[279] but this form of therapy remains controversial because of the risk of considerable soft tissue damage, shoulder dislocation, or even humeral fracture.[254]

Fibrositis (Fibromyopathy)

Fibrositis, a poorly defined entity of unknown cause, appears to be most common in women between the ages of 35 and 50 years who are anxious and often fatigued. An aching pain, usually aggravated by stress or cold, damp weather, is reported in soft tissues between the shoulder and neck. Frequently, painful trigger points or actual small nodules can be found on careful palpation. Treatment by injection of local anesthetic agents with or without corticosteroids may be helpful, especially when accompanied by considerable reassurance and support. This condition is more fully discussed in Chapter 70.

Arthritis

Although arthritis is an uncommon cause of isolated shoulder pain,[232] each of the shoulder girdle joints and bursae can be affected by the various arthritides described in this book. By far the most frequent is degenerative arthritis, which is found in the shoulders of approximately 30% of elderly subjects.[189,299] This disorder is almost always asymptomatic and is an incidental radiographic abnormality,[174,305] but unless considered in the differential diagnosis of shoulder pain, especially in patients of advanced age, error in diagnosis and treatment may occur.

Acromioclavicular Joint

The acromioclavicular joint is particularly prone to degenerative arthritis because of its rudimentary intra-articular disc,[66] which apparently has a protective function, and because of the repeated stresses to which this joint is exposed during overhead arm movements. The patient usually complains of shoulder pain, but often cannot localize it specifically; sleeping on the affected side may increase the pain. That elevation of the arm above shoulder level produces pain is an important clue to diagnosis because rotator cuff lesions cause pain at or below this level.

Inspection of the shoulder may reveal a distorted contour with prominence of the affected joint. Direct palpation over this area elicits tenderness. Active shrugging of the shoulder, passive adduction and flexion of the arm across the chest, and forcing of the humerus by passively raising the arm against a fixed clavicle are maneuvers that isolate the movement of this joint and aid in diagnosis when pain or crepitus is found. Confirmation of the diagnosis by plain radiography is helpful, but degenerative changes, although frequently present, are often asymptomatic.

Treatment consists of the standard conservative approach (see Table 85–2) and restriction of the patient's movements to a painless, and usually functional, arc. Occasionally, intra-articular corticosteroid injections are of benefit. In difficult cases, arthroplasty may be necessary; this procedure generally provides a satisfactory result.[16,66]

Sternoclavicular Joint

Arthritis in this small but important joint is rare. Post-traumatic, degenerative, and rheumatoid arthritis (RA) are the most common forms, although this joint is also affected in ankylosing spondylitis and related diseases. Two unusual forms of arthritis, pustulotic arthro-osteitis,[257] reported in Japanese patients, and sternoclavicular hyperostosis,[230] appear to involve the sternoclavicular joint particularly frequently.

Patients complain of pain, tenderness, and swelling and often localize these findings to the joint, so diagnosis is readily established. On examination, maximal pain is present during the midrange of arm elevation or on protrusion of the shoulders. The plain radiograph may be difficult to interpret because of overlying shadows; tomography is often necessary, and scintigraphy may be helpful.

Conservative therapy or intra-articular corticosteroid injection is generally sufficient for symptomatic relief, although surgical intervention is occasionally indicated, particularly in patients with post-traumatic lesions.[212]

Glenohumeral Joint

Degenerative arthritis of the glenohumeral joint, which is uncommon, generally involves the glenoid rather than the humeral side of the joint.[66,178] This feature may be due to its non-weight-bearing nature, although considerable force is exerted across the joint.[66] On occasion, ischemic (avascular) necrosis or neurotropic arthropathy, usually secondary to syringomyelia, causes identical symptoms. Pain is rarely severe, and the patient is more likely to be concerned by the cosmetic appearance of the joint, such as after fracture and malunion, or by the restricted motion. Functional limitation can usually be overcome by increased movement in accessory joints and by avoidance of painful motion. Examination discloses a crepitant joint with diminished mobility, but minimal pain. Radiography may reveal an old fracture site or characteristic changes of osteoarthritis. Severe degenerative arthropathy is often associated with calcium pyrophosphate or basic calcium phosphate crystal deposits in synovial tissues or in shoulder joint cartilage; the shoulder is not involved in primary generalized osteoarthritis.

Again, treatment is conservative and symptomatic for the most part. Arthrodesis or arthroplasty may be indicated in certain instances, but the results, except pain relief, are less than ideal.

"Milwaukee shoulder" is a recently described form of advanced degenerative arthritis involving the glenohumeral joint,[162] as well as other large joints. Patients usually are elderly women who complain of weakness and loss of motion in the dominant shoulder, but who are in little pain. Massive rotator cuff tears are present. Microcrystalline basic calcium phosphates are found in synovial fluids and have been implicated in the pathogenesis of this syndrome (see Chap. 95). This arthropathy resembles *dislocation arthropathy* in some respects,[246] and both conditions seem related to shoulder joint instability.

Other "Intrinsic" Causes of Shoulder Pain

Athletic and Other Traumatic Injuries

A detailed discussion of traumatic injuries to the shoulder, whether produced by blunt or by penetrating forces, is beyond the scope of this chapter.

Although such injuries are diagnosed with relative ease from the patient's medical history, cautious examination is essential to avoid overlooking associated soft tissue, bony, or neurovascular complications.

In addition to many of the conditions discussed previously, trauma may result in capsular ruptures with or without associated hemarthrosis, subluxation or dislocation, fractures, tendon avulsion, especially in adolescents, nerve injuries, and a variety of sprains and contusions. Obviously, knowledge of the type and mechanism of injury provides important clues to diagnosis; several of the more common injuries are considered briefly.

Falls. During unexpected falls, the arm is usually extended to cushion the impact, thereby transmitting the force upward to the shoulder and either anteriorly, as in backward falls, or posteriorly, as in forward falls.[16,66] As a result, the rotator cuff or the joint capsule itself can be torn, or if sufficient force is applied, subluxation (dislocation), neurovascular injury, or actual fracture may be present.

Dislocation of the glenohumeral joint is common, especially in athletic young men. Anterior dislocation occurs in 95% of these cases because the humeral head is usually thrust forward against the weak anteroinferior portion of the joint capsule. Posterior dislocations, although rare, are more likely to be overlooked.[16]

Acute dislocation is readily diagnosed. The patient provides a history of recent injury followed by sudden, severe pain in the shoulder. He supports the injured arm at the forearm with the elbow angled outward. The deltoid muscle is often tense on palpation. A depression is observed on palpation just inferior to the acromion. Neurovascular injuries may accompany shoulder dislocation in up to 25% of cases;[208] careful examination of the neurologic and vascular systems is essential whenever dislocation is suspected. Characteristic radiographic changes are present, although special views may be required.

Treatment consists of closed reduction within the first hours after dislocation. Thereafter, increasing restriction in shoulder motion may necessitate surgical repair.

Recurrent or habitual dislocations may follow the acute dislocation, especially in subjects under 20 years of age. Each subsequent dislocation may require less and less force, so even routine tasks, such as combing the hair, may cause it. A number of reasons for recurrent dislocation have been proposed, including an incompetent glenoid labrum, poor capsular ligament development, an enlarged humeral head, or a shallow glenoid fossa. A number of surgical approaches have been advocated for this problem.[16,66]

Direct Impact. The shoulder girdle is a prime target for falling objects, in part because of the protective flexion reflex of the neck and head.[16,66] Depending on the point of impact, fractures, severe contusions, or nerve root or neurovascular injuries may occur.

Throwing. The overhead throw in baseball or football is a complex, coordinated series of movements.[16,66] The shoulder girdle acts first as a base and then as a fulcrum to support and propel the object. The throw has four phases: (1) the preparation, in which the arm is extended, abducted, and externally rotated; (2) the phase of forward flexion and release; (3) the follow through; and (4) the braking phase. Shoulder pain may result from repeated impingement,[119] as well as from injury during the last or braking phase, because the joint capsule and rotator cuff are maximally stretched to prevent humeral dislocation. Tears may result, and when they occur repeatedly or are not allowed to heal, a periosteal reaction and, later, osteophytes develop.

The underhand throw, as in softball, bowling, or curling, is not as forceful, and injuries to the shoulder are far less common. Because this motion brings the anterior capsular mechanism and the bicipital apparatus into play, injuries to these structures may result. They are rarely serious, and rest is sufficient for complete healing in most cases.

Golfing. Usually considered a "safe" sport, golfing may result in injuries to the shoulder girdle. The most common injuries, because of recurrent stress at or superior to the horizontal plane, are those of the acromioclavicular joint. Symptoms and findings relating to this joint have previously been discussed; rest and other conservative measures are usually adequate.

Contact Sports. The causes of injury in the various contact sports, such as football, hockey, basketball, and soccer, are apparent.[16,66] In addition to those already discussed, fracture and dislocation, subluxation, and soft tissue tears are common.

Congenital and Developmental Anomalies

Many bony, muscular, and articular anomalies of the shoulder region have been recognized.[16,52,66,274] Although they rarely cause serious pain, they may produce functional or cosmetic problems requiring medical intervention.

The most common congenital anomaly of the shoulder, *Sprengel's deformity* or congenital elevation of the scapula, is often associated with other skeletal and soft-tissue abnormalities. It is caused by a failure of the scapula to descend normally during ontogeny. Surgical treatment is arduous and is often less than satisfactory, and it is warranted only if the deformity produces serious functional disability or psychologic problems.[52]

Another congenital anomaly that occasionally produces shoulder pain is the Klippel-Feil syndrome or congenital brevicollis, in which failure of segmentation or fusion of two or more cervical vertebrae may be associated with a cervical rib, other bony abnormalities, or an anomalous nerve and blood supply to the head, neck, and upper extremities.[12]

Posture

Poor posture, a frequent cause of shoulder and neck pain, often goes unrecognized.[16] It may result from working in a slumped position, from spinal malformation such as kyphosis or spondyloarthritis, from psychologic difficulties, from chronic illness with reduced muscle tone, or from a combination of these and other factors. Whatever the cause, abnormal posture places undue stress on the suspensory or mooring muscles of the upper extremity, especially the trapezius, rhomboid, and latissimus dorsi muscles. It may be difficult to identify this cause of shoulder pain because symptoms often develop hours after the patient has left work, and only a careful medical history reveals the source. Chronic aberrant posture is readily apparent. The patient complains of pain in the shoulder girdle, although this pain may radiate widely.

Correction of work or living habits, postural instruction, and physiotherapy usually produce improvement, but braces or supports are occasionally required.

Neurologic Causes of Shoulder Pain
Brachial Plexus Injuries

Trauma is the most common cause of isolated brachial plexus lesions.[66,147,175,282] These injuries may result from penetrating wounds such as stab or gunshot wounds, blunt trauma, as from falling objects, external pressure, such as from backpacks, or stretch injuries, either obstetric or from machines. The clinical picture varies, depending on the specific site and branch affected; however, loss of motor function, rather than pain, is usually the predominant complaint. Involvement of cervical roots 5 and 6 is common and produces weakness in the deltoid, biceps, and rotator cuff muscles, so abduction and rotation of the arm are altered. When pain does occur in brachial plexus injuries, it often has a burning or causalgic quality, which represents an adverse prognostic sign.[147]

Peripheral Neuropathy

Localized peripheral nerve lesions are usually traumatic in origin, but other factors may contribute to or may produce them directly, such as vasculitis, metabolic derangements, heavy-metal toxicity, and vitamin deficiencies.[66,175] As with brachial plexus injury, peripheral neuropathies generally result in loss or decrease in motor function, but rarely in pain. The *suprascapular nerve* may be *entrapped* during scapular fractures or by compression of the nerve as it traverses the notch of the scapula.[84,85] Lesions of the axillary nerve are most often produced by blunt or penetrating trauma,[27] as well as by traumatic shoulder dislocation. Injuries of the suprascapular nerve, which supplies the infra- and supraspinatus muscles, or of the axillary nerve, which supplies the deltoid muscle, weaken abduction, but do not eliminate it.

Neuralgic Amyotrophy (Brachial Plexitis, Parsonage-Turner Syndrome)

This rare disorder has received scant attention in the literature in the United States.[30,86,175] It appears to be an actual peripheral neuropathy with "causalgic" features in patients recovering from a variety of serious illnesses. Characteristically, the patient has sudden pain in and about the shoulder, followed in several days to weeks by muscle weakness or paralysis, again usually in the shoulder region. Spontaneous recovery generally occurs, and no specific treatment exists.

Extrinsic Causes of Shoulder Pain

Few causes of shoulder pain are truly "extrinsic," except "referred" pain. A variety of systemic inflammatory or metabolic diseases are considered under this category because shoulder pain or disability is a single manifestation of the broader disease process. Such diseases in fact produce "intrinsic" shoulder lesions.

Arthritis

Virtually all forms of generalized arthritis can, and often do, affect the shoulder girdle joints and the bursae. RA and osteoarthritis are most common. These and the other arthritides are discussed elsewhere and need not be considered here. Up to 30 to 40% of unselected patients with RA have erosive disease in the glenohumeral, acromioclavicular, and sternoclavicular joints.[125,174] Similarly, radiographic evidence of osteoarthritis in these joints is common, especially in patients with osteoarthritis in other joints.[174]

Avascular Necrosis

Avascular (ischemic, aseptic) necrosis of the humeral head is rarely an isolated finding in the shoulder. It usually occurs in patients with other diseases, as discussed in Chapter 86.

Polymyalgia Rheumatica

Polymyalgia rheumatica, a chronic systemic disease of unknown origin, primarily affects individuals in their sixth decade or older[115] and is discussed in Chapter 59. Pain and stiffness occur in both the shoulder and the pelvic girdles, but symptoms may be present in only one girdle.

Muscular Diseases

Polymyositis, the muscular dystrophies, and various other myopathies frequently affect the upper limb girdle muscles. Pain is rarely a major symptom, but weakness and disability may cause the patient to seek medical attention.

Metabolic Diseases

Diabetes Mellitus. The incidence of certain disorders of the shoulder, such as degenerative and calcific tendinobursitis,[43,124,279,281] degenerative arthritis,[43] and adhesive capsulitis,[34,302] is increased in patients with diabetes mellitus. It remains unclear whether these changes are a consequence of the vascular, neurologic, or other metabolic features of this disease.

Gout and Pseudogout. Crystal-induced synovitis may occur in any of the shoulder girdle joints. Gouty arthritis is rare,[101] whereas pseudogout is seen in 25 to 50% of affected subjects, at least by the radiographic findings of calcium pyrophosphate deposition (see Chap. 94).[203]

Hyperparathyroidism. Patients with hyperparathyroidism may develop a number of musculoskeletal complaints. In addition to a distinct hyperparathyroid arthropathy, these patients may have pseudogout, resorption of the distal clavicle, or formation of cystic brown tumors in the clavicle, humerus, or other long bones. With the greater use of biochemical screening studies and the earlier recognition of this disease, articular complications are far less common than formerly.[90]

Other Disorders. Shoulder arthropathy may be found in patients with other metabolic diseases including hemachromatosis, alkaptonuria, ochronosis, Wilson's disease, and amyloidosis.

Neurologic Diseases

Perception of pain at a site remote from the area of irritation is considered "referred pain." Attention was focused on this cause of pain by the classic experiments of Kellgren and Lewis, who injected hypertonic saline solution into interspinous ligaments or specific muscle groups and mapped out the location and extent of resulting pain. These researchers found that pain frequently radiated distally, but always within the same sensory root segment. The various causes of neurologic pain to be discussed under the category of "extrinsic" are all examples of referred pain.[36]

Cervical Nerve Root Compression. Compression of a cervical nerve root is commonly a result of degenerative arthritis or spondylopathy.[16,32,37,175] Other causes include spinal infection, especially tuberculosis, primary or secondary neoplasms, spondyloarthritis, fractures, subluxations, or congenital anomalies.

Because the fifth and sixth cervical vertebrae are usually affected, complaints of shoulder and neck stiffness and aching are common. Pain may be increased by moving the neck and by coughing and sneezing, which stretch the affected nerve root. Objective evidence of motor or sensory nerve involvement, of changes in tendon reflexes, and of muscle wasting provides clues to diagnosis.

Radiographic evidence of degenerative arthritis is common in subjects beyond the age of 50 years and must be interpreted cautiously unless definite neuroforaminal encroachment is present. In patients with a herniated disc, the plain radiograph may be entirely normal, and diagnosis depends on myelographic or CT study.

These and other features of the cervical syndrome, which represents the most common "extrinsic" cause of shoulder pain, are discussed fully in Chapter 80.

Spinal Cord Lesions. Other lesions of the cervical spine and of the spinal cord itself may cause pain to be referred to the shoulder.[16] These lesions include traumatic injuries, infections such as tuberculosis, herpes zoster, and poliomyelitis, syringomyelia, tumors, and various vascular anomalies. Patients with herpes zoster also may lack shoulder abduction when the C5 to C6 nerve roots are affected.

Viscerogenic (Viscerosomatic) Pain. Pain is referred to the shoulder from deeper somatic or visceral structures by intrasegmental transmission.[175,258] Most common are lesions along the course of the phrenic nerve, originating from C4 primarily, with fibers from C3 and C5, or from the diaphragm, which it supplies. The diaphragm can be irritated by many conditions involving the mediastinum, the pericardium, the inferior pulmonary segments, the liver, and, especially the biliary tract. Other visceral diseases that refer pain to the shoulder are myocardial ischemia, pulmonary infarction or neoplasm, perforated intra-abdominal or pelvic viscera, peptic esophagitis or esophageal spasm, and dissecting aortic aneurysm (Fig. 85–10). Referred pain to the shoulder may be the sole symptom of serious distant disease.

Thoracic Outlet Syndrome(s)

The region through which the neurovascular supply of the upper extremity exits the neck and thorax to enter the axilla constitutes the thoracic outlet.[175,235,285] It actually represents a series of narrow, fixed passages, each of which affords opportunity for compression of the neurovascular bundle. Symptoms and signs vary, depending on the nature and position of the obstruction. These manifestations include a cervical rib, anomalies of the first rib, interscalene muscle compression, and other rarer entities collectively termed the "thoracic outlet syndrome."

Anatomy and Pathophysiology

The anatomic relationships of the thoracic outlet are complex, but are considered briefly.[66,235] The clavicle conveniently divides the region into three segments, supraclavicular, retroclavicular, and infraclavicular. Each is associated with certain structural or functional abnormalities that may compress the neurovascular bundles.

In the supraclavicular segment, in the posterior triangle of the neck, the subclavian artery and the brachial plexus lie between the anterior and posterior scalenic muscle masses. The subclavian vein is situated in front of the anterior scalene muscle here and therefore is separated from the artery and the plexus; it joins them at the level of the clavicle. Two major sources of neurovascular compression are seen in this segment. Interscalenic compression, also known as scalenus anterior syndrome or Naffziger's syndrome, is caused by minor variations in the size, contour, or sites of insertion of the scalene muscles, with resultant narrowing of the already small interscalenic triangle. The presence of a cervical rib, found in approximately 0.6% of the population,[235] may also compromise the neurovascular supply in this segment by angulating the bundle or by narrowing the interscalene triangle (Fig. 85–11).

In the retroclavicular space, the neurovascular bundle, now joined by the subclavian vein, passes between the clavicle anteriorly and the first or thoracic rib posteriorly (Fig. 85–11). Compression in this segment is produced by a variety of conditions that narrow this space, such as clavicular fracture or its complications of malunion or exuberant callus formation, congenital anomalies of the clavicle or first rib, external pressure from heavy weights or packs, and poor posture. These conditions are termed the *"costoclavicular disorders."*

The infraclavicular segment of the neurovascular bundle is situated behind (beneath) the pectoralis minor tendon and the clavipectoral fascia and in front of the subscapularis, from which it is separated by abundant areolar tissue. The considerable variation in the structural relationships of this region that occurs with normal arm motion may result in neurovascular compression, the so-called "cla-

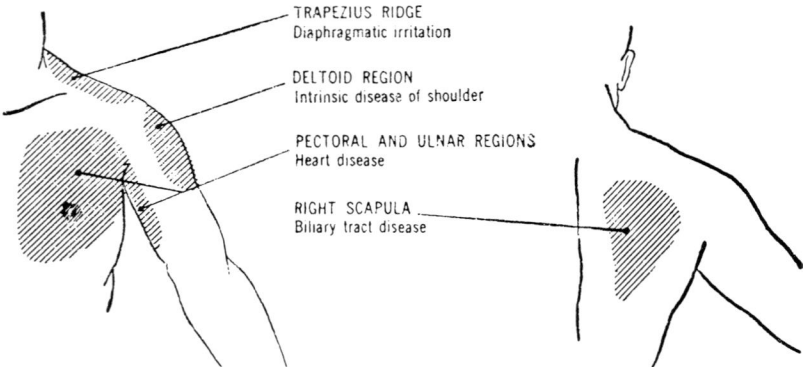

Fig. 85–10. Sites of reference about the shoulder in viscerogenic pain. (From Morgan. Courtesy of Modern Medicine.)

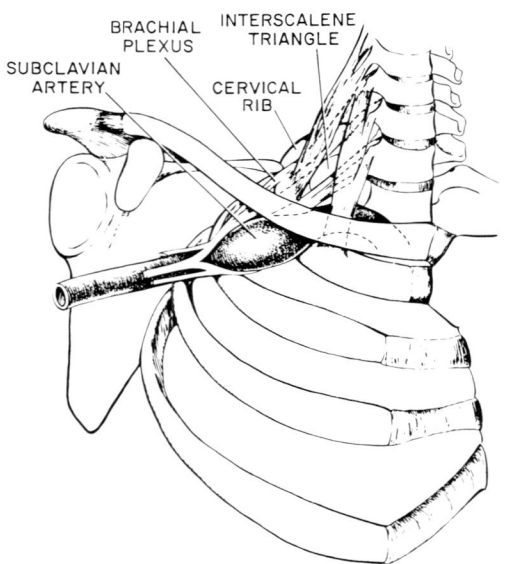

Fig. 85–11. Thoracic outlet syndrome produced by a cervical rib; poststenotic dilatation of the subclavian artery is present.

vipectoral disorders.'' The most common is the hyperabduction syndrome, in which the neurovascular bundle is pulled around the pectoralis minor tendon during abduction, to create a pulley-like effect (Fig. 85–12). This hyperabducted position was well known to soldiers in the past as a method of controlling upper extremity bleeding. It is usually seen in patients who sleep with arms hyperabducted, that is, folded under the head, or who are engaged in occupations requiring this position for prolonged periods, such as automobile mechanics and painters.

Clinical Features

Symptoms of the thoracic outlet syndrome may be variable and intermittent, depending on the role of fixed anatomic abnormalities, shoulder movement, or combinations of these factors.[74,235,285,290] Pain in the shoulder or arm is characteristic of the syndrome, although it is present in only 70% of patients.[74] When neural in origin, the pain is segmental in distribution, usually in the ulnar segment because its roots, C8 and T1, are lowermost and more readily compressed, and is often described as a dull aching or burning sensation. This pain is almost always associated with paresthesias and numbness. Objective findings include diminished sensation, muscle weakness, or atrophy. When the pain is vascular in origin, it is vague and poorly localized and is described as a fullness or numbness. One may see associated objective findings of edema, color, and temperature change, Raynaud's phenomenon, and dilatation of the superficial veins of the arm, shoulder, and neck.

A careful medical history may reveal typical patterns of aggravation and relief of symptoms. For example, symptoms present on awakening may be produced by placing the hands beneath the head or pillow during sleep. Occupation may be a factor when symptoms develop during the day or early evening in those who work overhead, such as automobile mechanics and painters. Symptoms that occur on weekends or vacations may be traced to sporting habits, as with backpackers who compress their costoclavicular space with heavy shoulder weights. Certain large-breasted women also may experience compressive symptoms as a consequence of brassiere-strap pressure.

The presenting complaint may represent a complication of neurovascular compression. A cool, cyanotic, or pallid extremity, with or without Ray-

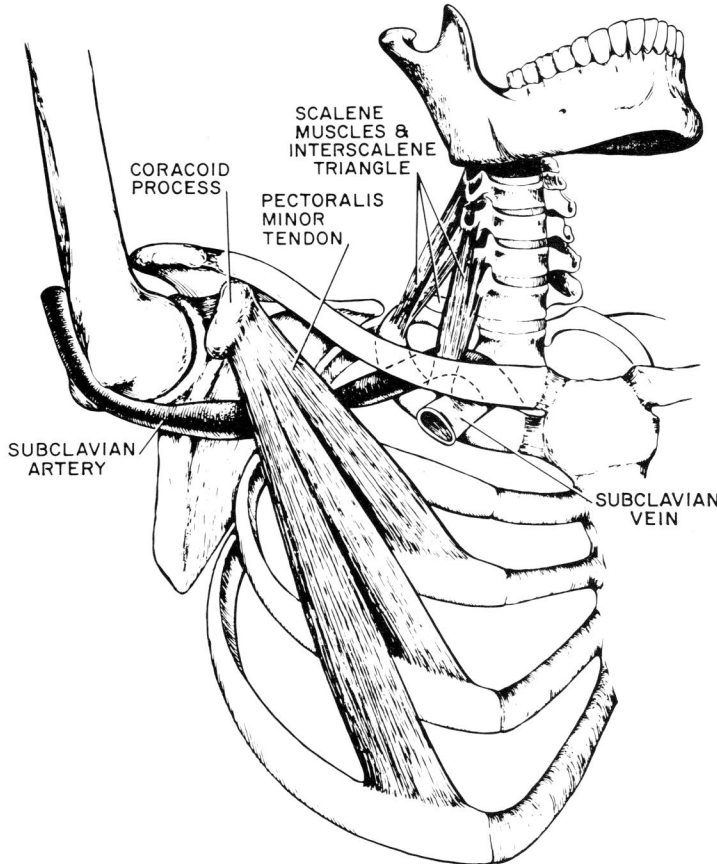

Fig. 85–12. Thoracic outlet syndrome produced by hyperabduction maneuver; note compression beneath the pectoralis minor tendon.

naud's phenomenon, ulceration, or frank gangrene, may occur consequent to arterial obstruction or thrombosis. Postobstructive arterial dilatation may be recognized as a supraclavicular mass. Venous obstruction produces edema, an increased girth in the affected arm, dilation and tortuosity of superficial veins, or venous thrombosis (Paget-Schroetter syndrome).

Diagnosis and Differential Diagnosis

Diagnosis depends on a thorough medical history and physical examination to reveal the typical clinical features of neurovascular compression.[205,235,285,290] Several special tests may be helpful in confirming the diagnosis and in localizing the site of obstruction. The *Adson maneuver,* which narrows the interscalene triangle, is performed with the patient holding his breath in full inspiration and then fully extending his neck and rotating it toward the side examined. The *costoclavicular maneuver* diminishes the costoclavicular space and is effected by bracing the shoulders posteriorly and inferiorly,

the exaggerated military posture. The *hyperabduction maneuver* for hyperabduction syndrome is performed by abducting the arms 180° in external rotation. A "positive" test result produced by these maneuvers reproduces the patient's symptoms and obliterates or dampens the radial artery pulse. Because the radial pulse is often reduced in normal subjects during these maneuvers,[74,285,297] this sign alone is insufficient for diagnosis.

Other studies may be useful in diagnosis and differential diagnosis. The plain radiograph of the chest, cervical spine, and entire shoulder area may disclose specific bony abnormalities, such as cervical rib or clavicular fracture, that explain the patient's symptoms. Doppler studies, venography, arteriography, and plethysmography may be useful as well, especially when performed during the foregoing postural maneuvers.[74,144,237,297] Determination of nerve conduction velocities across the thoracic outlet, elbow, and wrist may also help in diagnosis and differential diagnosis.

Depending on whether neurologic or vascular

signs predominate, a number of conditions may enter into the differential diagnosis. Some of these are listed in Table 85–3. When the thoracic outlet syndrome is suspected, it is essential that the diagnosis be established promptly, so appropriate therapy can be initiated.

Treatment

Unless the disorder is complicated by serious obstructive vascular disease or neurologic findings, initial therapy of the thoracic outlet should be conservative. Reassurance, education, and postural retraining to reduce thoracic outlet compression are of prime importance and are sufficient in most patients.[74,285,290,297] Usually, these measures are combined with physiotherapy to reduce muscle spasm and to strengthen the suspensory muscles, such as the rhomboid, levator scapulae, and trapezius muscles. In patients with severe or refractory disease, operative intervention is indicated. Careful preoperative assessment is imperative, however, because more than one site of obstruction may be present.

REFLEX SYMPATHETIC DYSTROPHY SYNDROME

The unusual complex of symptoms comprising this syndrome was first isolated by S. Weir Mitchell and his colleagues Moorehouse and Keen during the American Civil War,[185] although several cases with similar features had been reported earlier.[231] Later, Mitchell introduced the term "causalgia,"

derived from the Greek words for "heat" and "pain," to describe the peculiar burning pain so characteristic of this disorder.[184,231] Unfortunately, the confusing array of terms and designations for the syndrome that appeared in the years following Mitchell's classic studies created considerable uncertainty as to its very nature and existence (Table 85–4).

The exact prevalence of the reflex sympathetic dystrophy syndrome is unknown. Data from several studies suggest that it is frequent in patients with coronary artery disease (5 to 20%),[120,138,242] in patients with hemiplegia (12 to 21%),[64,78] in patients with Colles' fracture (0.2 to 11%),[11,55,75] and in patients with peripheral nerve (3%) or other forms of traumatic injury (0.05%).[216] Although emphasis on early mobilization following fractures, myocardial infarction, and stroke has reduced the frequency of this complication, it has not been eliminated.[55,64,206]

Origin

A number of diseases, precipitating events, or drugs have been associated with this syndrome (Table 85–5). They are thought to provoke the syndrome through reflex neurologic mechanisms, although their exact role in its pathogenesis remains obscure. It is difficult, if not impossible, to determine the relative frequency of these factors in initiating the syndrome because of selection factors in reported series. In surgical practice, trauma is clearly the most common precipitant, especially fractures or peripheral nerve injuries. In medical practice, although trauma, often minor, still ranks as the leading provocative event, myocardial ischemia, cervical spinal or spinal cord disorders, and a variety of cerebral lesions are also common. These findings are shown in Table 85–6, in which

Table 85–3.   Differential Diagnosis of Thoracic Outlet Syndrome

Primarily Neurologic Symptoms
Cervical Spine Syndromes
Spinal Cord Tumors
Syringomyelia
Entrapment Neuropathy
Ulnar nerve (elbow)
Medial nerve (carpal tunnel)
Peripheral Neuropathy
Brachial Plexus Neuropathy
Herpes Zoster and Postherpetic Neuralgia
Primarily Vascular Symptoms
Arterial
Granulomatous arteritis, Takayasu's disease
Atherosclerosis
Embolic disease
Arterial aneurysms
Raynaud's phenomenon or disease
Venous
Thrombophlebitis
Obstruction, benign or malignant
Neurovascular Symptoms
Reflex Sympathetic Dystrophy Syndrome

Table 85–4.   Synonyms for the Reflex Sympathetic Dystrophy Syndrome

Causalgia, major or minor
Acute atrophy of bone
Sudeck's atrophy
Sudeck's osteodystrophy
Peripheral acute thrombophoneurosis
Traumatic angiospasm
Traumatic vasospasm
Post-traumatic osteoporosis
Postinfarctional sclerodactyly
Shoulder-hand syndrome
Shoulder-hand-finger syndrome
Reflex dystrophy
Reflex neurovascular dystrophy
Reflex sympathetic dystrophy
Algodystrophy
Algoneurodystrophy

Table 85–5. Conditions Associated with the Reflex Sympathetic Dystrophy Syndrome

Trauma, major or minor
Fractures, especially Colles' fracture
Primary central nervous system disorders
Cerebrovascular disease with hemiplegia
Hemiplegia of other causes
Convulsive disorders (?)
Spinal cord lesions
Cervical spine disease, such as arthritis or discogenic disorders
Peripheral neuropathy
Herpes zoster with postherpetic neuralgia
Ischemic heart disease
Painful lesions of the rotator cuff
Pulmonary tuberculosis
Antituberculous drug administration
Barbiturate and other anticonvulsive drug administration
Hysterical personality (?)

several studies are compared. Two points are worthy of note. First, in over 25% of patients, a definitive precipitating event could not be identified. Second, cervical discogenic disease is so common in this age group that its significance remains uncertain; before considering this as an "associated disease," definite evidence of nerve root impingement should be present.

Clinical Features

Both sexes are affected equally in this syndrome, except when the provocative cause is sex-related, such as myocardial ischemia in men. No predilection exists for the dominant side. In medical practice, the syndrome is far more common in patients over the age of 50 years (Table 85–6), probably because of the foregoing disease associations. Children and younger individuals are not spared,[17,25,46,80,143,216] although only recently has the syndrome been described in large series of children.[25,241]

The fully developed syndrome is usually characterized by pain and swelling in the distal extremity, trophic skin changes, and signs and symptoms of vasomotor instability (Table 85–7). The pain is often severe and burning, or causalgic, and it generally involves the entire hand or foot. Other sites are less commonly affected; the syndrome may be segmental in distribution, involving one or two rays of the hand or foot (radial form),[110,150] knee,[56,132] or hip,[87,145] or a portion of bone (zonal form), such as part of the femoral head.[150] Patients may wrap an extremity in wet dressings to protect it and to reduce the pain. Objective examination may disclose an exquisitely tender hand or foot, which the patient withdraws at the slightest touch. Tenderness is generalized, but is most severe in the periarticular tissues.[142] Pitting or nonpitting edema is usu-

ally present and is localized to the painful and tender region; again, this feature appears to be more pronounced in the periarticular areas.[142,183,185] When the reflex sympathetic dystrophy syndrome occurs in the upper extremity, the patient may have associated pain and limitation of motion in the ipsilateral shoulder (*shoulder-hand syndrome*) (Fig. 85–13).

Vasomotor disturbances vary from patient to patient or within the same patient at different times. Occasionally, frank Raynaud's phenomenon occurs, but vasodilation or vasoconstriction is more common. Locally, increased sweating, hyperhidrosis, may be noted or reported by the patient and is an important diagnostic sign. Dystrophic changes in the skin gradually develop (Table 85–7). Ultimately, atrophy of the skin and of the subcutaneous tissue produces a shiny, thinned appearance. Contractures of the fingers and palmar fascia, Dupuytren's contracture, may eventually occur, leaving a claw-like, deformed hand.

The clinical course of this syndrome has been divided into three overlapping stages.[183,260] The first, "acute" stage lasts three to six months and is characterized primarily by pain, tenderness, swelling, and vasomotor disturbances. In the second, "dystrophic" stage, these features resolve completely or partially, and trophic changes develop in the skin. This phase persists an additional three to six months. A third, "atrophic" stage then gradually evolves, in which skin and subcutaneous tissue atrophy and contractures predominate. Once this stage occurs, substantial reversal is uncommon, and the patient is left with a shiny, cool, contracted, and usually painless extremity.

Although staging of this syndrome is useful, it is often difficult to distinguish specific stages in an individual patient. More often, fluctuation between the first two stages occur for weeks or months, until the atrophic and contractural changes gradually supervene. Therapy during the "active" period (stages 1 and 2) is essential, whereas therapy during the last stage is rarely of benefit.

Incomplete (partial, limited, abortive, circumscribed) forms of this syndrome exist.[263] These types may include such diverse conditions as transient painful osteoporosis or osteolysis,[56,87,145,275] juvenile osteoporosis,[65,123] major or minor causalgia, segmental causalgia as in postherpetic syndromes, adhesive capsulitis or frozen shoulder, and idiopathic carpal tunnel syndrome or Dupuytren's contracture, especially when associated with a painful shoulder. Until the pathogenic mechanisms are understood and until more specific diagnostic tests are developed, the relation of these conditions to the reflex sympathetic dystrophy syndrome must remain uncertain. The incomplete category also in-

Table 85-6. Estimated Frequency of Associated Conditions in the Reflex Sympathetic Dystrophy Syndrome

Study	No. of Patients	Age	Bilateral Involvement (%)	Fracture	Peripheral Nerve Injury	Other Trauma	Myocardial Ischemia	Central Nervous System Disease	Spinal Injury or Discogenic Disease	Idiopathic or Miscellaneous Conditions
Acquaviva et al.[2]*	585	51	10	216	23	179	3	16	0	148
Evans[79]	57	—	—	12	1	26	0	1	2	15
Johnson and Pannozzo[121]	76	59†	18	6	0	15	10	18	13	14
Kozin et al.[142]	11	56	18	0	0	1	1	2	3	4
Kozin et al.[140]	32‡	—	—	4	3§	10§	0	6	2	7
Pak et al.[206]	140	54	—	28	0	40	12	3	3	43
Patman et al.[209]	113	44†	—	41	0	57	0	0	0	15
Rosen and Graham[236]	73	63	30	1	0	5	27	9	14	17
Steinbrocker and Argyros[260]	146	>50	25	0	0	15	30	11	29	61
Subbarao and Stillwell[267]	125	54||	10	31	24	25	4	6	0	35
Thompson[280]	17	>50	47	0	0	1	2	7	1	6
Totals										
Number:	1,375	—	—	339	51	374	89	79	67	376
Percentage:	—	—	23	25	4	27	6	6	5	27

*Patients diagnosed as "algodystrophy"; number with "definite" diagnosis uncertain
†Estimated average age
‡Definite and probable diagnosis
§Two patients had peripheral nerve injury associated with fractures
||Median age

Table 85-7. Classification and Clinical Criteria for the Reflex Sympathetic Dystrophy Syndrome

Definite
1. Pain and tenderness in an extremity
2. Symptoms or signs of vasomotor instability
   Raynaud's phenomenon
   Cool, pallid skin (vasoconstriction)
   Warm, erythematous skin (vasodilatation)
   Hyperhidrosis
3. Swelling of the extremity
   Pitting or nonpitting edema
4. Dystrophic skin changes
   Atrophy
   Scaling
   Hypertrichosis or hair loss
   Nail changes
   Thickened palmar fascia

Probable
1. Pain and tenderness
2. Signs or symptoms of vasomotor instability
3. Swelling of the extremity

Possible
1. Symptoms or signs of vasomotor instability
2. Swelling of the extremity

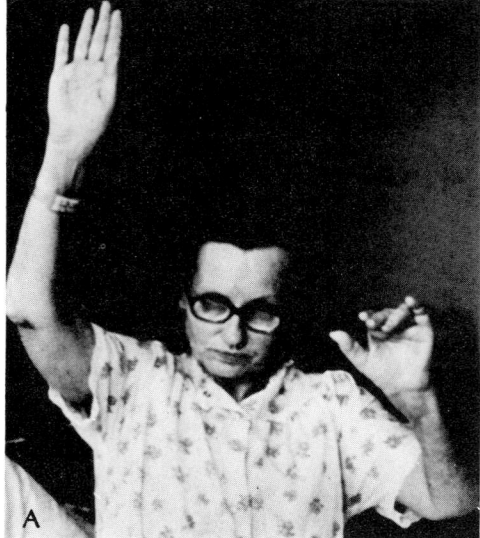

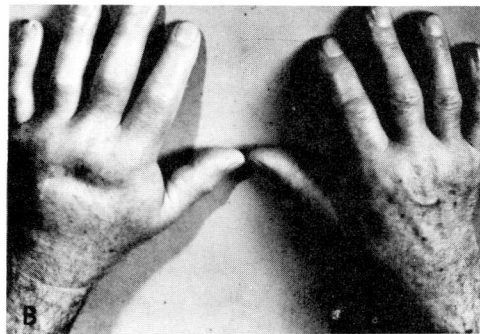

Fig. 85-13. *A,* A patient with shoulder-hand syndrome who has limited shoulder motion and diffuse swelling of the hand. *B,* Note the flexion contractures of the hands and the presence of pitting edema.

cludes patients who do not manifest all four clinical features evident in the classic syndrome (see Table 85–6).[140] My colleagues and I have proposed criteria that allow such patients to be distinguished clinically and to be compared with others having overlapping symptoms or signs (see Table 85–7).[140]

Bilateral involvement is generally thought to be present in 18 to 50% of patients (see Table 85–6). Careful analysis of a small group of patients with the fully developed syndrome, however, has disclosed bilateral changes in all instances by clinical and radiologic methods.[141,142] This finding supports the concept that the syndrome is, in fact, "reflex" and is mediated by central neurologic mechanisms.

Laboratory studies, such as blood counts and erythrocyte sedimentation rate, and other special studies are usually normal or show changes consistent with other associated conditions. The prevalance of hyperlipoproteinemia may be increased.[6,213] Reports of frequent abnormal electromyography have not been confirmed[1,142,286] For the most part, unless the patient has had a specific nerve injury, electromyography and nerve condition velocity studies are normal. Thermography,[76,113,272,286] as well as skin potential measurements,[58] have been advocated as diagnostic tests for this disorder.

Radiologic Features

These features include those evident on plain roentgenograms, as well as those requiring newer radiographic techniques.[5,9,88,112,122,139,140,141,150]

Plain Radiography

The characteristic radiographic appearance of the reflex sympathetic dystrophy syndrome is a patchy or mottled osteopenia (Fig. 85–14), a finding recognized since the early descriptions of Sudeck[268,269] and Kienbock.[130] This appearance is not found in all cases,[9,135,139,140,236] however, nor is it pathognomonic of the syndrome because it may be present in simple disuse osteopenia, such as from hemiparesis or immobilization, or in other conditions.[5,9] Its patchy character is caused by irregular resorption of cancellous or trabecular bone.[5,88] In addition, fine-detail radiographic techniques have disclosed resorption of subperiosteal, intracortical, endosteal, and subchondral and marginal bone.[88] Subchondral bone resorption produces a form of "erosive" articular disease manifested either as cortical breaks, surface erosions, as may be seen in early RA, or a peculiar frag-

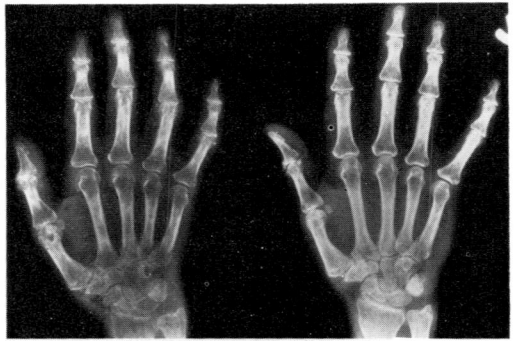

Fig. 85–14. Fine-detail radiographs of a patient with the reflex sympathetic dystrophy syndrome illustrating progressive osteopenia at three months (right) and eight months (left) after the onset of symptoms.

mentation of marginal bone, "crumbling" erosion (Fig. 85–14).[88,141] Late in the course of the illness, diffuse osteopenia occurs and gives the radiograph a ground-glass appearance.

Once these changes are established in adults, they appear to be irreversible, although this feature may depend on the duration of the disease.[9,122] In children, the potential for healing appears to be greater.[143]

Quantitative Bone Mineral Analysis

In this syndrome, one sees an average loss of one-third of the entire bone mineral content or cortical thickness in the affected extremity.[88] Treatment halts progression of the osteopenia, but it does not reverse it.

Scintigraphic Studies

The use of ^{99m}technetium (^{99m}Tc) as the pertechnetate, which depends on the local "blood pool,"[15,48,169] demonstrates increased periarticular uptake in the affected extremity.[88,134,140,141] Frequently, uptake in the contralateral extremity is also increased, suggesting subclinical bilateral involvement.[141] ^{99m}Tc labelled diphosphonate or polyphosphate uptake, which depends on local blood flow immediately after injection and on adsorption to bone later on, is also increased in the metaphysial regions of the bones on the affected, and to a lesser extent, on the contralateral side. Other bone-seeking radionuclides, such as strontium, have demonstrated enhanced uptake on the affected side, but without apparent localization.[28] In several reported cases, diminished radionuclide uptake was found in the affected extremity.[69,140] Scintigraphy may also be valuable in detecting incipient or subclinical reflex dystrophy.[45,88]

Rapid-sequence imaging immediately after radionuclide injection often demonstrates enhanced uptake in the affected extremity in patients with this syndrome,[139,140] and these findings indicate increased local blood flow.[68,89]

A number of studies have confirmed the value of scintigraphy in the diagnosis,[134,139,140,253] and possibly in the therapy,[140] of this syndrome. Studies are abnormal in 68 to 87% of subjects,[139,140,253] as well as in virtually all patients with transient osteoporosis syndromes, which often are clinically indistinguishable from the reflex sympathetic dystrophy syndrome.[87] Nuclide uptake was reported to be normal in certain patients responsive to corticosteroid therapy.[139]

Pathology and Pathophysiology

The skin and subcutaneous tissues are usually normal or exhibit minor, nonspecific changes. Dupuytren's contracture is frequently present.[258] Affected bone is hyperemic, and prominent osteoclastic activity is seen in the areas of patchy osteoporosis.[8,149,183,268,269] Fibrosis of the surface of affected cartilage may be observed.[8] Synovial tissue is abnormal and generally resembles that of the shoulder in adhesive capsulitis.[142] The histologic changes consist of proliferation of synovial lining cells and small blood vessels, synovial edema, and subsynovial fibrosis (Fig. 85–15). Little or no inflammatory cell infiltrate is present.

Any explanation of the pathophysiologic features of the reflex sympathetic dystrophy syndrome must account for its peculiar clinical features, such as nonsegmental pain, trophic skin changes, and vasomotor instability, its radiographic findings of patchy osteopenia, and its evidence of increased local blood flow.[49,183,265,272] Although a number of theories have been proposed, most suggest a disturbance of autonomic nervous system regulation to explain these diverse findings. Little true evidence of autonomic nerve dysfunction exists, however.

Moberg attributes the reflex sympathetic dystrophy syndrome primarily to a mechanical disturbance of venous and lymphatic flow.[186] He suggests that shoulder and hand movements are essential for fluid removal from the extremity, and any interference in this mechanism produces edema, further limitation of motion, disuse osteopenia, and, eventually, contracture formation. A second factor, sympathetic nervous system stimulation, occasionally contributes to the pain and limitation of motion when the syndrome is initiated by a traumatic, usually painful, injury. Although intriguing, especially with regard to the shoulder-hand syndrome, this hypothesis fails to account for the syndrome after painless, nonimmobilizing events, such as drug ingestion,[98,136] after myocardial ischemia with pain

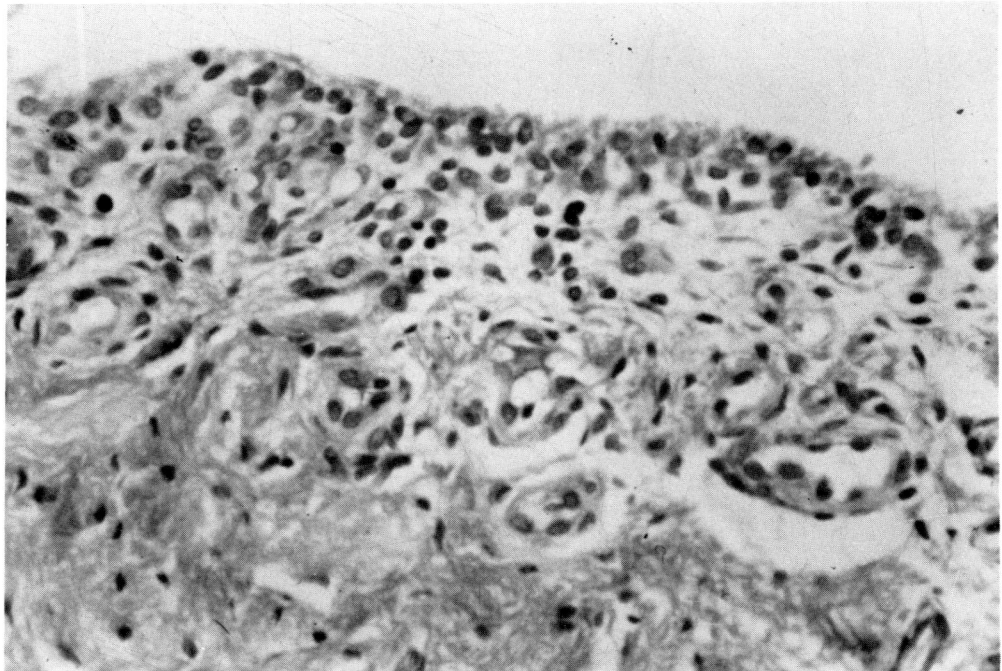

Fig. 85–15. Photomicrograph of synovium of a metacarpophalangeal joint from a patient with the reflex sympathetic dystrophy syndrome, illustrating synoviocyte and vascular proliferation.

in the opposite arm,[236] or in isolated regions, for example, the hand or the patella.[56]

Theories that suggest that the sympathetic nervous system is affected primarily are more popular. DeTakats and Miller,[67,183] and later Steinbrocker and co-workers,[258,260,263] have championed the theory of Livingston,[155] who originally proposed that a painful peripheral stimulus produced excessive, repetitive excitation of the internuncial neuron pool in the spinal cord. Spread of these impulses to adjacent areas in the spinal cord then activates efferent autonomic and motor nerves and results in increased blood flow, vasomotor changes, and other "dystrophic" changes in bone and soft tissues. These factors, in turn, produce further sensory input and establish a "vicious cycle" between central and peripheral mechanisms of pain and response. Livingston's theory may explain the reflex sympathetic dystrophy syndrome in any location and may be extended to precipitants other than pain because changes in the central regulatory mechanism may be caused by drugs, stroke, or other provocative stimuli.

Noordenhos and others have offered an intriguing variant of this mechanism.[200] Two types of nerve fibers are suggested to exist: small fibers that carry the painful impulse and large fibers that inhibit its transmission. Normally, a delicate balance exists under central control, but a shift in this bal-

ance may result in excessive pain, either real or imagined, and may establish the vicious cycle already described. The beneficial effects of selective large-fiber stimulation in certain patients with causalgia support this proposal.[182,233]

More recently, the gate-control theory of pain, which combines many features of the aforementioned mechanisms, has achieved prominence.[180,181] In this model, a dynamic balance that exists between large, inhibitory and small, effector neurons is influenced by cognitive and perceptual processes in the central nervous system. Because the sympathetic nervous system impulses also feed into the same receptor center(s), stimulation of efferent sympathetic fibers may produce the reflex sympathetic dystrophy syndrome, by ascending "painful" sources such as trauma, by descending cognitive or perceptual mechanisms such as stroke, drugs, or trauma, or by direct irritation of the receptor center(s) such as by stroke, drugs, or cervical spine or spinal cord lesions.

Treatment

Because the natural history of this syndrome is so variable and unpredictable, results of the usual therapeutic approaches are difficult to interpret. Therapy appears to have little relation to the initiating or provocative event, the severity of trauma, or the stage of disease. It is generally thought that the earlier the institution of therapy, the better the result.[206,236,258] Rosen and Graham examined this problem carefully and found that only 20% of patients symptomatic for 6 months or longer had a good or excellent response to treatment, as compared with 43% of those with symptoms of shorter duration.[236] The overall response rate was poor, however; over 50% of their patients had significant pain or disability 2 to 6 years later. Other authors suggest that most patients recover in 6 to 24 months.[70,135]

Clearly, avoidance of the syndrome is the best treatment. Early mobilization following trauma,[83] or myocardial infarction,[242] may be helpful in this regard, although even this concept is controversial.[35,152] Once the disease process is established, a number of therapeutic approaches have been advocated, including exercises, various physical therapeutic techniques, sympathetic blockade, local or systemic corticosteroids, vasodilator drugs, alpha- or beta-adrenergic drugs, and continuous elevation of the involved extremity. None are specific; all are most effective when used early. Unfortunately, even today, prolonged delays in recognition of the syndrome and in institution of therapy are common.[209]

The basic treatment program should consist of analgesic medications, local heat or cold packs, and exercises of the affected and contralateral extremities to improve motion. A favorable result may be expected in a majority of patients with these conservative measures if treatment is started early in the course of the disease,[77,121,206] especially in children.[25,241] More aggressive therapy is indicated if a satisfactory result is not obtained within one to four weeks. The most effective therapeutic measures are sympathetic blockade and administration of systemic corticosteroids.

Sympathetic blockade represents a rational attempt to block the vicious cycle of pain at an accessible site in the efferent pain pathway. Results of this approach are variable, although the patient may have partial or transient relief of pain.[79,129,209,252,262] Satisfactory control of symptoms, defined as a 50% relief of pain or a significant reduction in disability, can be expected in only 14 to 25% of patients,[73,79,84,209,234,242] although several authors report response rates as high as 75 to 100%.[75,224,262] My own experience with stellate ganglion blockade has been discouraging,[140] and Patman et al. found that all 41 causalgic patients treated with sympathetic blockade later required surgical sympathectomy.[209] Frequently, a series of daily or alternate-day sympathetic blocks are required;[252,258,262] this approach should be abandoned if 3 to 5 successive blocks fail to provide lasting symptomatic relief. Patients who benefit from sympathetic blockade appear to be excellent candidates for surgical sympathectomy. Results of this procedure appear to be rewarding, both in reduction of pain and in restoration of motion.[38,79,209]

Other methods for interrupting sympathetic tone appear to be effective as well, including regional intravenous reserpine,[21,51] or guanethidine, which is not approved by the United States Food and Drug Administration.[29a,106,107,167] Beta-adrenergic blocking agents have been beneficial in some,[255,292] but not all[21] patients.

Systemic corticosteroids are effective in controlling the reflex sympathetic dystrophy syndrome,[64,95,140,142,191,236,243] although the use of these agents is not without controversy.[94] Studies of high-dose corticosteroid treatment, using sensitive, quantifiable methods of assessment, showed improvement in a majority of patients with a reflex dystrophy.[140,142,191] These findings have been confirmed.[49] Although not all patients had a complete recovery, most experienced marked, lasting pain relief and restoration of function. Furthermore, progression of osteopenia appeared to be reduced in adults,[141] as well as reversed in a child.[143] Patients with positive scintigraphic evidence of the disease appeared to respond best to corticosteroids.[139]

Initial therapy should consist of 60 to 80 mg prednisone or an equivalent preparation daily *in 4 divided doses*. In 1 to 2 weeks, one can rapidly reduce the dose, with the aim of discontinuing corticosteroids entirely after 3 to 4 weeks of treatment. One often sees a mild, "poststeroid" exacerbation, which usually resolves within 10 days.[140,142] Occasionally, patients require retreatment, in which case a longer period of high-dose therapy, lasting 2 to 4 weeks, and a more gradual tapering program, lasting 4 to 8 weeks, are indicated. Rarely, a maintenance dose of prednisone, 5 to 10 mg on alternate days or 5 mg daily, is required to control symptoms permanently. Lower doses have been used successfully.[49] Intravenous injection of corticosteroids into the affected extremity may be an effective approach.[217a]

Unlike the interruption of sympathetic pathways, no currently known theoretic mechanisms explain the efficacy of corticosteroids in the reflex sympathetic dystrophy syndrome. It is possible that these agents interfere with the action of peripheral mediators, which perhaps are prostaglandin-like substances, or they may modulate the transmission of neural impulses in the gate-control system or the internuncial pool.

Other agents, including griseofulvin and calcitonin, have been used effectively in patients with algodystrophy;[70] it is not clear whether all patients with this diagnosis fulfill the rigorous criteria of the reflex sympathetic dystrophy syndrome.

Recent studies employing transcutaneous nerve stimulation in patients with causalgia following nerve injuries have been encouraging,[233,293] although this technique has failed on occasion.[21] Again, the best responses were obtained in patients symptomatic for brief periods prior to treatment.

REFERENCES

1. Abe, S.: Electromyographic and immunoserological studies on the shoulder-hand syndrome coming after myocardial infarction. (English summary). Jpn. Circ. J., 35:994, 1971.
2. Acquaviva, P., et al.: Reflex dystrophies: background and etiological factors. Rev. Rhum. Mal. Osteoartic., 49:761, 1982.
3. Akeson, W.H., et al.: The connective tissue response to immobility: biochemical changes in periarticular connective tissue of the immobilized rabbit knee. Clin. Orthop., 93:356, 1973.
4. Allander, E., et al.: Normal range of joint movements in shoulder, hip, wrist and thumb with special reference to side: a comparison between two populations. Int. J. Epidemiol., 3:253, 1974.
5. Allman, R.M., and Brower, A.C.: Circulatory patterns of deossification. Radiol. Clin. North Am., 19:553, 1981.
6. Amor, B., et al.: Algodystrophies et hyperlipemies. Rev. Rhum. Mal. Osteoartic., 47:353, 1980.
7. Andren, L., and Lundberg, B.J.: Treatment of rigid shoulders by joint distension during arthrography. Acta Orthop. Scand., 36:45, 1965.
8. Arlet, J., et al.: Histopathology of bone and cartilage lesions in reflex sympathetic dystrophy of the knee: report of 16 cases. (French.) Rev. Rhum. Mal. Osteoartic., 48:315, 1981.
9. Arnstein, A.R.: Regional osteoporosis. Orthop. Clin. North Am., 3:585, 1972.
10. Asboe-Hansen, G.: Influence of corticosteroids on connective tissue. Dermatologica, 152:127, 1976.
11. Bacorn, R.W., and Kurtzke, J.F.: Colles' fracture: a study of two thousand cases from the New York State Workman's Compensation fund. J. Bone Joint Surg., 35A:643, 1953.
12. Bailey, R.W.: The Cervical Spine. Philadelphia, Lea & Febiger, 1974.
13. Bakalim, G., and Pasila, M.: Rotator cuff tears. Acta Orthop. Scand., 46:751, 1975.
14. Basmajian, J.V.: Muscles Alive: Their Functions Revealed by Electromyography. Baltimore, Williams & Wilkins, 1962.
15. Bassett, L.W., Gold, R.H., and Webber, M.M.: Radionuclide bone imaging. Radiol. Clin. North Am., 19:675, 1981.
16. Bateman, J.: The Shoulder and Neck. 2nd Ed. Philadelphia, W.B. Saunders, 1978.
17. Bayles, T.B., Judson, W.E., and Potter, T.A.: Reflex sympathetic dystrophy of the upper extremity (hand-shoulder syndrome). JAMA, 144:537, 1950.
18. Beetham, W.P., et al.: Physical Examination of the Joints. Philadelphia, W.B. Saunders, 1965.
19. Bekerman, C., et al.: Radionuclide imaging of the bones and joints of the hand: a comparison of normal and a comparison of sensitivity using ^{99M}Tc-pertechnetate and ^{99M}Tc-diphosphonate. Radiology, 118:653, 1976.
20. Benson, T.B., and Copp, E.P.: The effects of therapeutic forms of heat and ice on the pain threshold of the normal shoulder. Rheumatol. Rehabil., 13:101, 1974.
21. Benzon, H.T., Chomka, C.M., and Brunner, E.A.: Treatment of reflex sympathetic dystrophy with regional intravenous reserpine. Anesth. Analg., 59:500, 1980.
22. Berger, L.S., and Ziter, F.M.H.: Calcifications within enlarged subdeltoid bursae in rheumatoid arthritis. Br. J. Radiol., 45:530, 1972.
23. Berliner, D., et al.: Decreased scar formation with topical corticosteroid treatment. Surgery, 61:619, 1967.
24. de Bernard, B.: Glycoproteins in the local mechanism of calcification. Clin. Orthop., 162:233, 1982.
25. Bernstein, B.H., et al.: Reflex neurovascular dystrophy in childhood. J. Pediatr., 93:211, 1978.
26. Berry, H., et al.: Clinical study comparing acupuncture, physiotherapy, injection and oral-anti-inflammatory therapy in shoulder-cuff lesions. Curr. Med. Res. Opin., 7:121, 1980.
27. Berry, H., and Bril, V.: Axillary nerve palsy following blunt trauma to the shoulder region: a cervical and electrophysiological review. J. Neurol. Neurosurg. Psychiatry, 45:1027, 1982.
28. Besseler-Winterthus, W.: Bedantung Szintigraphiscer untersuchengen fur die Beurteilung von Folgen zustanden nach Frakturen und Knochenoperationen. Langenbecks Arch. Chir., 327:146, 1970.
29. Bland, J.H., Merrit, J.A., and Boushey, D.R.: The painful shoulder. Semin. Arthritis Rheum., 7:21, 1977.
29a. Bonelli, S., Conocente, F., et al.: Regional intravenous guanethidine vs. stellate ganglion block in reflex sympathetic dystrophies: a randomized trial. Pain, 16:297, 1983.
30. Booth, R.E., and Marvel, J.P.: Differential diagnosis of shoulder pain. Orthop. Clin. North Am., 6:353, 1975.
31. Bosworth, B.M.: Calcium deposits in the shoulder and subacromial bursitis: a survey of 12,122 shoulders. JAMA, 116:2477, 1941.
32. Brain, L., and Wilkinson, M. (Eds.): Cervical Spondylosis. Philadelphia, W.B. Saunders, 1967.
33. Braunstein, E.M., and O'Connor, G.: Double-contrast arthrotomography of the shoulder. J. Bone Joint Surg., 64A:192, 1982.
34. Bridgeman, J.F.: Periarthritis of the shoulder and diabetes mellitus. Ann. Rheum. Dis., 31:69, 1972.
35. Brockelhurst, J.C., et al.: How much physical therapy for patients with stroke? Br. Med. J., 1:1307, 1978.
36. Brown, C.: Compressive, invasive referred pain to the shoulder. Clin. Orthop., 173:55, 1983.
37. Bucy, P.C., and Oberhill, H.R.: Pain in the shoulder and arm from neurological involvement. JAMA, 169:798, 1950.
38. Buker, R.H., et al.: Causalgia and transthoracic sympathectomy. Am. J. Surg., 124:724, 1972.
39. Bulgen, D.Y., et al.: Immunological studies in frozen shoulder. Ann. Rheum. Dis., 37:135, 1978.
40. Bulgen, D.Y., Hazelman, B.L., and Voak, D.: HLA-B27 and frozen shoulder. Lancet, 1:1042, 1976.
41. Bush, L.F.: The torn shoulder capsule. J. Bone Joint Surg., 57A:256, 1975.
42. Calliet, R.: Shoulder Pain. Philadelphia, F.A. Davis, 1966.
43. Campbell, H.L., and Feldman, F.: Bone and soft tissue abnormalities of the upper extremity in diabetes mellitus. AJR, 124:7, 1975.
44. Caner, J.R.Z., and Decker, J.L.: Recurrent acute (gouty) arthritis in chronic renal failure treated with periodic hemodialysis. Am. J. Med., 36:571, 1964.
45. Carlson, D.H., Simon, H., and Wegner, W.: Bone scanning and diagnosis of reflex sympathetic dystrophy secondary to herniated lumbar discs. Neurology, 27:791, 1977.
46. Carron, H., and McCue, F.: Reflex sympathetic dystrophy in a ten year old. South. Med. J., 65:631, 1972.
47. Chaplin, H., Clarke, L.D., and Ropes, M.W.: Vitamin D intoxication. Am. J. Med. Sci., 221:369, 1951.
48. Charkes, N.D.: Skeletal blood flow: implications for bone-scan interpretation. J. Nucl. Med., 21:91–98, 1980.
49. Christensen, K., Jensen, E.M., and Noer, I.: The reflex dystrophy syndrome: response to treatment with systemic corticosteroids. Acta Chir. Scand. 148:653, 1982.
50. Christensen, W.R., Liebman, C., and Sosman, M.C.: Skeletal and periarticular manifestations of hypervitaminosis D. AJR, 65:27, 1951.
51. Chuinard, R.G., et al.: Intravenous reserpine for treatment

of reflex sympathetic dystrophy. South. Med. J., 74:1481, 1981.

52. Chung, S.M.K., and Nissenbaum, M.M.: Congenital and developmental defects of the shoulder. Orthop. Clin. North Am., 6:381, 1975.

52a.Codman, E.A.: The Shoulder. Boston, Thomas Todd Co., 1934.

53. Comfort, T.H., and Arafiles, R.P.: Barbotage of the shoulder with image-intensified fluoroscopic control of needle placement for calcific tendinitis. Clin. Orthop., 135:171, 1978.

54. Conway, A.M.: Movements in the sternoclavicular and acromioclavicular joints. Phys. Ther. Rev., 41:421, 1975.

55. Cooney, W.P., Dobyns, J.H., and Linscheid, R.L.: Complications of Colles' fracture. J. Bone Joint Surg., 62A:613, 1980.

56. Corbett, M., Colston, J.R., and Tucker, A.K.: Pain in the knees associated with osteoporosis of the patella. Am. Rheum. Dis., 36:188, 1977.

57. Crenshaw, A.H., and Kilgore, W.E.: Surgical treatment of bicipital tenosynovitis. J. Bone Joint Surg., 48A:1946, 1966.

58. Cronin, K.D., and Kirsner, R.L.G.: Diagnosis of reflex sympathetic dysfunction: use of skin potential response. Anaesthesia, 37:847, 1982.

59. Crosson, E.W., and Heltz, J.E.: Non-tuberculous shoulder disabilities in sanatorium patients. Can. Med. Assoc. J., 92:1110, 1965.

60. Cyriax, J.: Textbook of Orthopaedic Medicine. Vol. I. 6th Ed. Baltimore, Williams & Wilkins, 1975.

61. Danzig, L., Resnick, D., and Greenway, G.: Evaluation of unstable shoulders by computed tomography. Am. J. Sports Med., 10:138, 1982.

62. Darlington, L.G., and Coombs, E.N.: The effects of local steroid injection for supraspinatus tears. Rheumatol. Rehabil., 16:172, 1977.

63. Davis, N.R., and Walker, T.E.: The role of carboxyl groups in collagen calcification. Biochem. Biophys. Res. Comm., 48:1656, 1972.

64. Davis, S.W., et al.: Shoulder-hand syndrome in a hemiplegic population: 5-year retrospective study. Arch. Phys. Med. Rehabil., 58:3553, 1977.

65. Dent, C.E., and Friedman, M.: Idiopathic juvenile osteoporosis. Q. J. Med., 34:177, 1965.

66. DePalma, A.F.: Surgery of the Shoulder. 2nd Ed. Philadelphia, J.B. Lippincott, 1973.

67. DeTakats, G.: Reflex sympathetic dystrophy of the extremities. Arch. Surg., 34:939, 1937.

68. Deutsch, S.D., Gandsman, E.J., and Spraragen, S.C.: Quantitative regional blood-flow analysis and its clinical application during routine bone-scanning. J. Bone Joint Surg., 63A:295, 1981.

69. Doury, P., et al.: Algodystrophy with hypofixation of technetium 99m pyrophosphate on bone scintigraphy. (French.) Sem. Hop. Paris, 57:1325, 1981.

70. Doury, P., Dirheimer, Y., and Pattin, S.: Algodystrophy. New York, Springer-Verlag, 1981.

71. Downey, J.A., Frewin, D.B., and Whelan, R.F.: Vascular responses in the forearm to heating by shortwave diathermy. Arch. Phys. Med. Rehabil., 51:354, 1970.

72. Downing, D., and Weinstein, A.: Ultrasound therapy of subacromial bursitis: a double blind trial. (Abstract.) Arthritis Rheum., 26:S87, 1983.

73. Drucker, W.R., et al.: Pathogenesis of post-traumatic sympathetic dystrophy. Am. J. Surg., 97:454, 1979.

74. Dunant, J.H.: The diagnosis of thoracic outlet syndrome. In Pain in the Shoulder and Arm. Edited by J.M. Greep, et al. The Hague, Martinus Nijhoff, 1979.

75. Dunningham, T.H.: The treatment of Sudeck's atrophy in the upper limb by sympathetic blockade. Injury, 12:139, 1981.

76. Ecker, A.: Personal communication.

77. Edeiken, J.: Shoulder-hand syndrome following myocardial infarction with special reference to prognosis. Circulation, 16:14, 1957.

78. Eto, F., et al.: Shoulder-hand syndrome as a complication of hemiplegia. Jpn. J. Geriatr., 12:245, 1977.

79. Evans, J.A.: Reflex sympathetic dystrophy: report on 57 cases. Ann. Intern. Med., 26:417, 1947.

80. Fermaglich, D.R.: Reflex sympathetic dystrophy in children. Pediatrics, 60:881, 1977.

81. Fitzgerald, R.H.: Intrasynovial injection of steroids: uses and abuses. Mayo Clin. Proc., 51:655, 1976.

82. Freiberger, R.H., and Kaye, J.J.: Arthrography. New York, Appleton-Century-Crofts, 1979.

83. Frykman, G.: Fracture of the distal radius including sequelae—shoulder-hand-finger syndrome, disturbance in the distal radioulnar joint, and impairment of nerve function. Acta Orthop. Scand., 108 (Suppl.):1, 1967.

84. Ganzhorn, R.W., et al.: Suprascapular nerve entrapment. J. Bone Joint Surg., 63A:492, 1981.

85. Garcia, G., and McQueen, D.: Bilateral suprascapularnerve entrapment syndrome. J. Bone Joint Surg., 63A:491, 1981.

86. Gathier, J.C., and Bruyn, G.W.: Neuralgic amyotrophy. In Handbook of Clinical Neurology. Vol. 8. Diseases of Nerves. Part II. Edited by P.J. Vinkin and G.W. Bruyn. New York, American Elsevier, 1970.

87. Gaucher, A., et al.: The diagnostic value of ^{99m}Tc-diphosphonate bone imaging in transient osteoporosis of the hip. J. Rheumatol., 6:774, 1979.

88. Genant, H.K., et al.: The reflex sympathetic dystrophy syndrome: a comprehensive analysis using fine-detail radiography, photon absorptiometry and bone and joint scintigraphy. Radiology, 117:21, 1975.

89. Genant, H.K., et al.: Bone-seeking radionuclides: an in vivo study of factors affecting skeletal uptake. Radiology, 113:373, 1974.

90. Genant, H.K., et al.: Primary hyperparathyroidism: a comprehensive study of clinical, biochemical and radiographic manifestations. Radiology, 109:513, 1973.

91. Genoe, G.A., and Moeller, J.A.: Normal shoulder variations in the technetium 99m polyphosphate bone scan. South. Med. J., 67:659, 1974.

92. Gerster, J.C., et al.: Tendon calcification in chondrocalcinosis. Arthritis Rheum., 20:717, 1977.

93. Gilula, L.A., Schoenecker, P.C., and Murphy, W.A.: Shoulder arthrography as a treatment modality. AJR, 131:1047, 1978.

94. Glick, E.N.: Reflex dystrophy (algoneurodystrophy): results of treatment by corticosteroids. Rheumatol. Rehabil., 12:84, 1973.

95. Glick, E.N., and Helal, B.: Post-traumatic neurodystrophy: treatment by corticosteroids. Hand, 8:45, 1976.

96. Goldie, I.: Local steroid therapy in painful orthopaedic conditions. Scott. Med. J., 17:176, 1972.

97. Goldman, A.B., and Ghelman, B.: The double-contrast shoulder arthrogram. Radiology, 127:655, 1978.

98. Good, A.E., Green, R.A., and Zorafonetis, C.J.D.: Rheumatic symptoms during tuberculosis therapy: a manifestation of isoniazid toxicity. Ann. Intern. Med. 63:800, 1965.

99. Goodman, C.R.: Ultrasonic therapy for chronic acromioclavicular separation with calcific deposits. N.Y. State J. Med., 72:2884–2886, 1972.

100. Boileau Grant, J.C., and Basmajian, J.V.: Grant's Method of Anatomy. 7th Ed. Baltimore, Williams & Wilkins, 1965.

101. Hadler, N.M., et al.: Acute polyarticular gout. Am. J. Med., 56:715, 1974.

102. Ha'eri, G.B., and Maitland, A.: Arthroscopic findings in the frozen shoulder. J. Rheumatol., 8:149, 1981.

103. Ha'eri, G.B., and Wiley, A.M.: Shoulder impingement syndrome. Clin. Orthop., 168:128, 1982.

104. Ha'eri, G.B., and Wiley, A.M.: Advancement of the supraspinatus muscle in the repair of ruptures of the rotator cuff. J. Bone Joint Surg., 61A:232, 1981.

105. Hall, F.M., et al.: Morbidity from shoulder arthrography: etiology, incidence, and prevention. AJR, 136:59, 1981.

106. Hannington-Kiff, J.G.: Relief of causalgia in limbs by regional intravenous guanethidine. Br. Med. J., 2:367, 1979.

107. Hannington-Kiff, J.G.: Relief of Sudeck's atrophy by regional intravenous guanethidine. Lancet, 1:1132, 1977.

108. Harvey, W., et al.: The stimulation of protein synthesis in human fibroblasts by therapeutic ultrasound. Rheumatol. Rehabil., 14:237, 1975.

109. Hazelman, B.L.: The painful stiff shoulder. Rheum. Phys. Med., *11*:413, 1972.

110. Helms, C.A., O'Brien, E.T., and Katzberg, R.W.: Segmental reflex sympathetic dystrophy syndrome. Radiology, *35*:67, 1980.

111. Herberts, P., et al.: Shoulder pain in industry: an epidemiological study on welders. Acta Orthop. Scand., *52*:299, 1981.

112. Herrmann, L.G., Reincke, H.G., and Caldwell, J.A.: Post-traumatic painful osteoporosis: a clinical and roentgenological entity. AJR, *47*:353, 1942.

113. Hindler, N., Uematesu, S., and Long, D.: Thermographic validation of physical complaints in "psychogenic pain" patients. Psychosomatics, *23*:283, 1982.

114. Hovind, H., and Nielsen, S.L.: Local blood flow after short-wave diathermy: preliminary report. Arch. Phys. Med. Rehabil., *55*:217, 1974.

115. Hunder, G.G., Disney, T.F., and Ward, L.E.: Polymyalgia rheumatica. Mayo Clin. Proc., *44*:849, 1969.

116. Inman, V.T., Saunders, J.B., and Abbott, L.C.: Observations on the function of the shoulder joint. J. Bone Joint Surg., *26*:1, 1944.

117. Ismail, A.M., Balakrishnan, R., and Rajahumar, M.K.: Rupture of patellar ligament after steroid infiltration. J. Bone Joint Surg., *51B*:503, 1969.

118. Jean, J.P.: Radiologic aspects of shoulder lesions. *In* Shoulder Lesions. 3rd Ed. Edited by H.F. Moseley. Edinburgh, Churchill Livingstone, 1972.

119. Jobe, F.W., and Jobe, C.M.: Painful athletic injuries of the shoulder. Clin. Orthop., *173*:117, 1983.

120. Johnson, A.C.: Disabling changes in the hands resembling sclerodactylia following myocardial infarction. Ann. Intern. Med., *19*:443, 1943.

121. Johnson, E.W., and Pannozzo, A.N.: Management of shoulder-hand syndrome. JAMA, *195*:1552, 1966.

122. Jones, G.: Radiological appearances of disuse osteoporosis. Clin. Radiol., *20*:345, 1969.

123. Jowsey, J., and Johnson, K.A.: Juvenile osteoporosis: bone findings in seven patients. J. Pediatr., *81*:511, 1972.

124. Kaklamanis, P., et al.: Calcification of the shoulders and diabetes mellitus. N. Engl. J. Med., *293*:1266, 1975.

125. Kalliomaki, J.L., Viitanen, S.-M., and Virtama, P.: Radiological findings of sternoclavicular joints in rheumatoid arthritis. Acta Rheumatol. Scand., *14*:233, 1968.

126. Kerwein, G.A.: Roentgenographic diagnosis of shoulder dysfunction. JAMA, *194*:1081–1085, 1965.

126a.Kerwein, G.A., Roseberg, B., and Sneed, W.R.: Aids in differential diagnosis of the painful shoulder syndrome. Clin. Orthop., *20*:11–20, 1961.

127. Kessel, L.: Injuries around the shoulder. Proc. R. Soc. Med., *65*:1030, 1972.

128. Kessel, L., and Wastson, M.: The painful arc syndrome: clinical classification as a guide to management. J. Bone Joint Surg., *59B*:166, 1977.

129. Kiaer, A.: Remarks on the prognosis of the post-traumatic dystrophy of the extremities. Acta Orthop. Scand., *17*:253, 1948.

130. Kienbach, R.: Uber akute knochenatrophie bie Enuyndung-processen an den Extrematatun (Falschlich sagenannage inactivitats atrophie die Knochen) und ihre Diagnose nach dem Roentgen-Bild. Wien Med. Wochenschr., *5*:1345, 1901.

131. Killoran, J.R., Marcone, R.C., and Freiberger, R.H.: Shoulder arthrography. AJR, 103:658, 1968.

132. Kim, H.J., et al.: Reflex sympathetic dystrophy of the knee following meniscectomy: report of three cases. Arthritis Rheum., *22*:177, 1979.

133. Koehler, B.E., Urowitz, M.B., and Killinger, D.W.: The systemic effects of intra-articular corticosteroid. J. Rheumatol., *1*:117, 1974.

134. Koppers, V.B.: Three-phase scintigraphy in the Sudeck syndrome: comparison of the radiological and clinical examination. (German.) Fortschr. Röntgenstr., *137*:564, 1982.

135. van der Korst., J.B.: Shoulder-pain as a rheumatologic problem. *In* Pain in the Shoulder and Arm. Edited by J.M. Greep, et al. The Hague, Martinus Nijhoff, 1979.

136. van der Korst, J.K., Colenbrauder, H., and Cats, A.:

137. Kotzen, L.M.: Roentgen diagnosis of rotator cuff tear: report of 48 surgically proven cases. AJR, *112*:507, 1971.

138. Kozin, F.: Painful shoulder and the reflex sympathetic dystrophy syndrome. *In* Arthritis and Allied Conditions. Edited by D.J. McCarty. 9th Ed. Philadelphia, Lea & Febiger, 1979.

139. Kozin, F., et al.: Bone scintigraphy in the reflex sympathetic dystrophy syndrome. Radiology, *138*:437, 1981.

140. Kozin, F., et al.: The reflex sympathetic dystrophy syndrome (RSDS) III. Scintigraphic studies, further evidence for the therapeutic efficacy of systemic corticosteroids, and proposed diagnostic criteria. Am. J. Med., *70*:23, 1981.

141. Kozin, F., et al.: The reflex sympathetic dystrophy syndrome. II. Roentgenographic and scintigraphic evidence of bilaterality and periarticular accentuation. Am. J. Med., *60*:332, 1976.

142. Kozin, F., et al.: The reflex sympathetic dystrophy syndrome. I. Clinical and histologic studies: evidence for bilaterality, response to corticosteroids, and articular involvement. Am. J. Med., *60*:321, 1976.

143. Kozin, F., Houghton, V., and Ryan, L.N.: The reflex sympathetic dystrophy in a child. Pediatrics, *90*:417, 1977.

144. Lang, E.K.: Roentgenographic diagnosis of the neurovascular compression syndromes. Radiology, *79*:78, 1962.

145. Langloh, N.D., et al.: Transient painful osteoporosis of the lower extremities. J. Bone Joint Surg., *55A*:1188, 1973.

146. Lee, P.N., et al.: Periarthritis of the shoulder, trial of treatments investigated by multivariate analysis. Ann. Rheum. Dis., *33*:116, 1974.

147. Leffert, R.D.: Brachial plexus injuries. N. Engl. J. Med., *291*:1059, 1974.

148. LeGeros, L.Z., Contiguglia, S.R., and Alfrey, A.C.: Pathological calcifications associated with uremia: two types of calcium phosphate deposits. Calcif. Tissue Res., *13*:173, 1973.

149. Lenggenhager, K.: Sudeck's osteodystrophy: its pathogenesis, prophylaxis and therapy. Minn. Med., *54*:967, 1971.

150. Lequesne, M., et al.: Partial transient osteoporosis. Skeletal Radiol., *2*:1, 1977.

151. Lie, S. and Mast, W.A.: Subacromial bursography. Radiology, *144*:626, 1982.

152. Lind, K.: A synthesis of studies on stroke rehabilitation. J. Chronic Dis., *35*:133, 1982.

153. Lippmann, R.K.: Observations concerning the calcific cuff deposit. Clin. Orthop., *20*:49, 1961.

154. Litchman, H.M., et al.: The surgical management of calcific tendinitis of the shoulder. Int. Surg., *50*:474, 1968.

155. Livingston, W.K.: Pain Mechanisms. New York, MacMillan, 1943.

156. Lloyd-Roberts, G.C., and French, P.R.: Periarthritis of the shoulder: a study of the disease and its treatment. Br. Med. J., *1*:1569, 1959.

157. Luben, R.A., and Wadkins, C.L.: Studies of the relationship of proton production and calcification of tendon matrix in vitro. Biochemistry, *10*:2183, 1971.

158. Luben, R.A., Sherman, J.K., and Wadkins, C.L.: Studies of the mechanism of biological calcification. IV. Ultrastructural analysis of calcifying tendon matrix. Calcif. Tissue Res., *11*:39, 1973.

159. Lucas, D.B.: Biomechanics of the shoulder joint. Arch. Surg., *107*:425, 1973.

160. Lundberg, B.J.: Glycosaminoglycans of the normal and frozen shoulder-joint capsule. Clin. Orthop., *69*:279, 1970.

161. Lundberg, B.J., and Nilsson, B.E.: Osteopenia in the frozen shoulder. Clin. Orthop., *60*:187, 1968.

162. McCarty, D.J., et al.: "Milwaukee shoulder"—association of microspheroids containing hydroxyapatite crystals, active collagenase, and neutral protease with rotator cuff

defects. I. Clinical aspects. Arthritis Rheum., *24*:464, 1981.

163. McCarty, D.J., and Gatter, R.A.: Recurrent acute inflammation associated with focal apatite crystal deposition. Arthritis Rheum., *9*:804, 1964.

164. McCarty, D.J., and Hogan, J.: Inflammatory reaction after intrasynovial injection of microcrystalline adrenocorticosteroid esters. Arthritis Rheum., *7*:359, 1964.

165. McClure, J., and Gardner, D.L.: The production of calcification in connective tissue and skeletal muscle using various chemical compounds. Calcif. Tissue Res., *22*:129, 1976.

166. McClynn, F.J., El-Khoury, G., and Albright, J.P.: Arthrotomography of the glenoid labrum in shoulder instability. J. Bone Joint Surg., *64A*:506, 1982.

167. McKay, N.N.S., Woodhous, N.J.Y., and Clarke, A.K.: Post-traumatic sympathetic dystrophy syndrome (Sudeck's atrophy): effects of regional guanethidine infusion and salmon calcitonin. Br. Med. J., *1*:1575, 1977.

168. McKendry, R.J.R., et al.: Calcifying tendinitis of the shoulder: prognostic value of clinical, histologic, and radiologic features in 57 surgically treated cases. J. Rheumatol., *9*:75, 1982.

169. McKinstry, P., et al.: Relationship of 99m Tc-MDP uptake to regional osseous circulation in skeletally immature and mature dogs. Skeletal Radiol., *8*:115, 1982.

170. McLaughlin, H.L.: The "frozen shoulder." Clin. Orthop., *20*:126, 1961.

171. McLaughlin, H.L.: Lesions of the musculotendinous cuff of the shoulder. III. Observations on the pathology, course, and treatment of calcific deposits. Ann. Surg., *124*:354, 1946.

172. McMillan, J.A.: Therapeutic exercise for shoulder disabilities. J. Am. Phys. Ther. Assoc., *46*:1052, 1966.

173. MacNab, I.: Rotator cuff tendinitis. Ann. R. Coll. Surg. Engl., *53*:271, 1973.

174. McNair, M.M., et al.: A clinical and radiological study of rheumatoid arthritis with a note on the findings in osteoarthrosis. I. The shoulder joint. Clin. Radiol., *20*:269, 1969.

175. McNaughton, F.L.: Neurological aspects of shoulder lesions. *In* Shoulder Lesions. 3rd Ed. Edited by H.F. Moseley. Edinburgh, Churchill Livingstone, 1972.

176. Matles, A.I.: Reflex sympathetic dystrophy in a child: a case report. Bull. Hosp. Joint. Dis., *32*:193, 1971.

177. Maxfield, W.S., Weiss, T.E., and Shirler, S.E.: Synovial membrane scanning in arthritic disease. Semin. Nucl. Med., *2*:50, 1972.

178. Meachim, G.: Effect of age on the thickness of adult articular cartilage at the shoulder joint. Ann. Rheum. Dis., *30*:43, 1971.

179. Melmed, E.P.: Spontaneous bilateral rupture of the calcaneal tendon during steroid therapy. J. Bone Joint Surg., *47B*:105, 1965.

180. Melzack, R.: The Puzzle of Pain. New York, Basic Books, 1973.

181. Melzack, R., and Wall, P.D.: Pain mechanisms: a new theory. Science, *150*:971, 1965.

182. Meyer, G.A., and Fields, H.L.: Causalgia treated by selective large fibre stimulation of peripheral nerve. Brain, *95*:163, 1972.

183. Miller, D.S., and de Takats, G.: Post-traumatic dystrophy of the extremities. Surg. Gynecol. Obstet., *125*:558, 1941.

184. Mitchell, S.W.: Injuries of Nerves and Their Consequences. Philadelphia, J.B. Lippincott, 1872.

185. Mitchell, S.W., Moorehouse, G.R., and Keen, W.W.: Gunshot Wounds and Other Injuries of Nerves. Philadelphia, J.B. Lippincott, 1864.

186. Moberg, E.: The shoulder-hand-finger syndrome. Surg. Clin. North Am., *40*:367, 1960.

187. Moore, M.E., and Berk, S.N.: Acupuncture for chronic shoulder pain: an experimental study with attention to the role of placebo and hypnotic susceptibility. Ann. Intern. Med., *84*:381, 1976.

188. Moseley, H.F.: The natural history and clinical syndromes produced by calcified deposits in the rotator cuff. Surg. Clin. North Am., *43*:1505, 1963.

189. Moseley, H.F.: Shoulder Lesions. 3rd Ed. Edinburgh, Churchill Livingstone, 1960.

190. Moseley, H.F., and Goldie, I.: The arterial pattern of the rotator cuff of the shoulder. J. Bone Joint Surg., *45B*:780, 1963.

191. Mowat, A.G.: Treatment of the shoulder-hand syndrome with corticosteroids. Ann. Rheum. Dis., *33*:120, 1974.

192. Neer, C.S.: Impingement lesions. Clin. Orthop., *173*:70, 1983.

193. Neer, C.S.: Anterior acromoplasty for the chronic impingement syndrome in the shoulder. J. Bone Joint Surg., *54A*:41, 1972.

194. Neuman, W.F., et al.: Blood:bone disequilibrium. VI. Studies of the solubility characteristics of brushite:apatite mixtures and their stabilization by noncollagenous proteins of bone. Calcif. Tissue Int., *34*:149, 1982.

195. Neviaser, J.S.: Arthrography of the Shoulder. Springfield, IL, Charles C Thomas, 1975.

196. Neviaser, J.S.: Ruptures of the rotator cuff of the shoulder. Arch. Surg., *102*:483, 1971.

197. Neviaser, J.S.: Adhesive capsulitis of the shoulder: a study of the pathological findings in periarthritis of the shoulder. J. Bone Joint Surg., *27*:211, 1945.

198. Neviaser, T.J., et al.: The four-in-one arthroplasty for the painful arc syndrome. Clin. Orthop., *163*:107, 1983.

199. Nixon, J.E., and DiStefano, V.: Ruptures of the rotator cuff. Orthop. Clin. North Am., *6*:423, 1975.

200. Noordenhos, W.: Pain. Amsterdam, Elsevier, 1959.

201. Noy, S., et al.: HLA-B27 and frozen shoulder. Tissue Antigens, *17*:251, 1981.

202. O'Duffy, J.D., Wahner, H.W., and Hunder, G.G.: Joint imaging in polymyalgia rheumatica. Mayo Clin. Proc., *51*:519, 1976.

203. Okazaki, T., et al.: Pseudogout: clinical observations and chemical analysis of deposits. Arthritis Rheum., *19*:293, 1976.

204. Older, M.W.J., McIntyre, J.L., and Lloyd, G.J.: Distension arthrography of the shoulder joint. Can. J. Surg., *19*:203, 1976.

205. Overton, L.M.: The causes of pain in the upper extremities: a differential diagnosis study. Clin. Orthop., *51*:27, 1967.

206. Pak, T.J., et al.: Reflex sympathetic dystrophy—a review of 140 cases. Minn. Med., *53*:507, 1970.

207. Parfitt, A.M., et al.: Disordered calcium and phosphorus metabolism during maintenance hemodialysis. Am. J. Med., *51*:319, 1971.

208. Pasila, M., et al.: Recovery from primary shoulder dislocation and its complications. Acta Orthop. Scand., *51*:257, 1980.

209. Patman, R.D., Thompson, J.E., and Perrson, A.V.: Management of post-traumatic pain syndromes: report of 113 cases. Ann. Surg., *177*:780, 1973.

210. Pedersen, H.E., and Key, J.A.: Pathology of calcareous tendinitis and subdeltoid bursitis. Arch. Surg., *62*:50, 1951.

211. Penny, J.N., and Welch, R.P.: Shoulder impingement syndromes in athletes and their surgical management. Am. J. Sports Med., *9*:11, 1981.

212. Pierce, R.: Internal derangement of the sternoclavicular joint. Clin. Orthop., *141*:247, 1979.

213. Pinals, R.S., and Jabbs, J.M.: Type IV hyperlipoproteinemia and transient osteoporosis. Lancet, *2*:929, 1972.

214. Pinals, R.S., and Short, C.L.: Calcific periarthritis involving multiple sites. Arthritis Rheum., *9*:566, 1966.

215. Plenk, H.P.: Calcifying tendinitis of the shoulder: a critical study of the value of X-ray therapy. Radiology, *59*:384, 1952.

216. Plewes, L.W.: Sudeck's atrophy in the hands. J. Bone Joint Surg., *38B*:195, 1956.

217. Podolsky, S.: *In* Diabetes Mellitus. Edited by A. Karkle, et al. Philadelphia, Lea & Febiger, 1971.

217a. Poplawski, E.J., Wiley, A.M., and Murray, J.F.: Post-traumatic dystrophy of the extremities. J. Bone Joint Surg., *65A*:642, 1983.

218. Poppen, N.K., and Walker, P.S.: Forces at the glenohumeral joint in abduction. Clin. Orthop., *135*:165, 1978.

219. Poppen, N.K., and Walker, P.S.: Normal and abnormal motion of the shoulder. J. Bone Joint Surg., *58A*:195, 1976.

220. Post, M., Silver, R., and Singh, M.: Rotator cuff tear: diagnosis and treatment. Clin. Orthop., *173*:78, 1983.

221. Quigley, T.B.: The nonoperative treatment of symptomatic calcareous deposits in the shoulder. Surg. Clin. North Am., *6*:1495, 1963.

222. Quigley, T.B., and Renold, A.E.: Acute calcific tendinitis and "frozen shoulder": their treatment with ACTH. N. Engl. J. Med., *246*:1012, 1952.

223. Quin, C.E.: Humeroscapular periarthritis: observations on the effects of X-ray therapy and ultrasonic therapy in cases of "frozen shoulder." Ann. Phys. Med., *10*:64, 1969.

224. Rasmussen, T., and Freedman, H.: Treatment of causalgia: an analysis of 100 cases. J. Neurosurg., *8*:165, 1945.

225. Rathburn, J.B., and Macnab, I.: The microvascular pattern of the rotator cuff. J. Bone Joint Surg., *52B*:540, 1970.

226. Reeves, B.: The natural history of the frozen shoulder syndrome. Scand. J. Rheumatol., *4*:193, 1975.

227. Reeves, B.: Arthrographic changes in frozen and posttraumatic stiff shoulders. Proc. R. Soc. Med., *59*:827, 1966.

228. Reichmann, S., et al.: Soft tissue xeroradiography of the shoulder joint. Acta Radiol. (Diagn.), *21*:572, 1975.

229. Resnick, D.: Shoulder arthrography. Radiol. Clin. North Am., *19*:243, 1981.

230. Resnick, D., Vint, V., and Poteshman, N.L.: Sternoclavicular hyperostoses. J. Bone Joint Surg., *63A*:1329, 1981.

231. Richards, R.L.: The term 'causalgia.' Med. Hist., *11*:97, 1967.

232. Richardson, A.T.: The painful shoulder. Proc. R. Soc. Med., *68*:731, 1975.

233. Richlin, D.M., et al.: Reflex sympathetic dystrophy: successful treatment by transcutaneous nerve stimulation. J. Pediatr., *93*:84, 1978.

234. Rizk, T.E., et al.: Adhesive capsulitis (frozen shoulder): a new approach to its management. Arch. Phys. Med. Rehabil., *64*:29, 1983.

235. Rosati, L.M., and Lord, J.W.: Neurovascular Compression Syndromes of the Shoulder Girdle. New York, Grune and Stratton, 1961.

236. Rosen, P.S., and Graham, W.: The shoulder-hand syndrome: historical review with observations on seventy-three patients. Can. Med. Assoc. J., *77*:86, 1957.

237. Rosenberg, J.C.: Arteriographic demonstration of compression syndromes of the thoracic outlet. South. Med. J., *59*:400, 1966.

238. Rothman, R.H., Marvel, J.P., and Heppenstall, R.B.: Anatomic considerations in the glenohumeral joint. Orthop. Clin. North Am., *6*:341, 1975.

239. Rothman, R.H., and Parke, W.W.: The vascular anatomy of the rotator cuff. Clin. Orthop., *41*:176, 1965.

240. Roy, S., and Oldham, R.: Management of painful shoulder. Lancet, 1:1322, 1976.

241. Rugeri, S.B., et al.: Reflex sympathetic dystrophy in children. Clin. Orthop., *103*:225, 1982.

242. Russek, H.I.: Shoulder-hand syndrome following myocardial infarction. Med. Clin. North Am., *42*:1555, 1958.

243. Russek, H.I., et al.: Cortisone treatment of shoulder-hand syndrome following acute myocardial infarction. Arch. Intern. Med., *91*:487, 1953.

244. Saha, A.K.: Dynamic stability of the glenohumeral joint. Acta Orthop. Scand., *42*:491, 1971.

245. Samilson, R.L., and Bruder, W.F.: Symptomatic full thickness tears of the rotator cuff: an analysis of 292 shoulders in 276 patients. Orthop. Clin. North Am., *6*:449, 1975.

246. Samilson, R.L., and Preito, V.: Dislocation arthropathy of the shoulder. J. Bone Joint Surg., *65A*:456, 1983.

247. Sebes, J.I., Vasinrapee, P., and Friedman, B.I.: The relationship between radiographic findings and asymmetrical radioactivity in the shoulder. Radiology, *120*:139, 1976.

248. Seignalet, J., et al.: Lack of association between HLA-B27 and frozen shoulder. Tissue Antigens, *18*:364, 1981.

249. Seltzer, S.E., et al.: Arthrosonography: gray-scale ultrasound evaluation of the shoulder. Radiology, *132*:467, 1979.

250. Selye, H., Goldie, I., and Strebel, R.: Calciphylaxis in relation to calcification in periarticular tissues. Clin. Orthop., *28*:151, 1963.

251. Sheldon, P.J.H.: A retrospective survey of 102 cases of shoulder pain. Rheum. Phys. Med., *11*:422, 1972.

252. Schumacker, H.B., Spiegel, I.J., and Upjohn, R.H.: Causalgia. I. The role of sympathetic interruption in treatment. Surg. Gynecol. Obstet., *86*:76, 1948.

253. Simon, H., and Carlson, D.H.: The use of bone scanning in the diagnosis of reflex sympathetic dystrophy. Clin. Nucl. Med., *5*:116, 1980.

254. Simon, W.H.: Soft tissue disorders of the shoulder. Orthop. Clin. North Am., *6*:521, 1975.

255. Simson, G.: Propanolol for causalgia and Sudeck's atrophy. JAMA, *227*:327, 1974.

256. Soave, G., et al.: Indoprofen versus indomethacin in acute painful shoulder and other soft-tissue rheumatic complaints. J. Int. Med. Res., *10*:99, 1982.

257. Sonozaki, H., et al.: Clinical features of 53 cases with pustulotic arthro-osteitis. Ann. Rheum. Dis., *40*:541, 1981.

258. Steinbrocker, O.: The painful shoulder. *In* Arthritis and Allied Conditions. 7th Ed. Edited by J.L. Hollander and D.J. McCarty. Philadelphia, Lea & Febiger, 1972.

259. Steinbrocker, O., and Argyros, T.G.: Frozen shoulder: treatment by local injections of depot corticosteroids. Arch. Phys. Med. Rehabil., *55*:209, 1974.

260. Steinbrocker, O., and Argyros, T.G.: The shoulder-hand syndrome: present status as a diagnostic and therapeutic entity. Med. Clin. North Am., *42*:1533, 1958.

261. Steinbrocker, O., and Neustadt, D.H.: Aspiration and Injection Therapy in Arthritis and Musculo-Skeletal Disorders. Hagerstown, MD, Harper & Row, 1972.

262. Steinbrocker, O., Neustadt, D., and Lapin, L.: Sympathetic block compared with corticotropin and cortisone therapy. JAMA, *153*:788, 1953.

263. Steinbrocker, O., Spitzer, N., and Friedman, H.H.: The shoulder-hand syndrome in reflex dystrophy of the upper extremity. Ann. Intern. Med., *29*:22, 1947.

264. Stodell, M.A., et al.: Radio-isotope scanning in the painful shoulder. Rheumatol. Rehabil., *19*:163, 1980.

265. Stolte, B.H., Stolte, J.B., and Leyten, J.F.: De pathofysiologie van het shoulder-handsyndroom. Ned. Tijdschr. Geneeskd., *114*:1208, 1980.

266. Strizak, A.M., et al.: Subacromial bursography. J. Bone Joint Surg., *64A*:196, 1982.

267. Subbarao, J., and Stillwell, G.K.: Reflex sympathetic dystrophy syndrome of the upper extremity: analysis of total outcome of management of 125 cases. Arch. Phys. Med. Rehabil., *62*:549, 1981.

268. Sudeck, P.: Uber die akute (reflektorishe) Knockenatrophie nach Entzundungen und Verletzungen an den Extrematation und ihre Klinischen Ersheinungen. Fortschr. Gebd. Roentgen., *5*:277, 1901–1902.

269. Sudeck, P.: Uber die akute entzundlicke Knockenatrophie. Arch. Klin. Chir., *62*:147, 1900.

270. Sullivan, J.D.: Painful shoulder syndrome. (Letter.) Can. Med. Assoc. J., *111*:505, 1974.

271. Sweetham, R.: Corticosteroid arthropathy and tendon rupture. J. Bone Joint Surg., *51B*:397, 1969.

272. Sylvest, J., et al.: Reflex dystrophy: resting blood flow and muscle temperature as diagnostic criteria. Scand. J. Rehabil. Med., *9*:25, 1977.

273. Symposium: DMSO in musculoskeletal conditions. Ann. N.Y. Acad. Sci., *141*:493, 1967.

274. Tachdjian, M.O.: Pediatric Orthopedics. Philadelphia, W.B. Saunders, 1972.

275. Targ, J.S., and Steel, H.H.: Sequential roentgenographic changes occurring in massive osteolysis. J. Bone Joint Surg., *51A*:1649, 1969.

276. Termine, J.D., Eanes, E.D., and Conn, K.M.: Phosphoprotein modulation of apatite crystallization. Calcif. Tissue Int., *31*:247, 1980.

277. Termine, J.D., Peckauskas, R.A., and Posner, A.S.: Calcium phosphate formation in vitro. II. Effects of environment on amorphous-crystalline transformation. Arch. Biochem. Biophys., *140*:318, 1970.

278. Thistle, H.G.: Neck and shoulder pain: evaluation and conservative management. Med. Clin. North Am., *53*:511, 1969.

279. Thomas, D., Williams, R.A., and Smith, D.S.: The frozen shoulder: a review of manipulative treatment. Rheumatol. Rehabil., *19*:173, 1980.

280. Thompson, M.: Shoulder-hand syndrome. Proc. R. Soc. Med., *54*:679, 1961.

281. Trapp, R.G., Soler, N.G., and Spencer-Green, G.: Musculoskeletal abnormalities of the upper extremities and neck in insulin dependent diabetics: symptomatology and physical findings. (Abstract.) Arthritis. Rheum., *26*:547, 1983.

282. Tsairis, P.: Brachial plexus neuropathies. *In* Peripheral Neuropathy. Vol. I. Edited by P.J. Dyck, P.K. Thomas, and E.H. Lambert. Philadelphia, W.B. Saunders, 1975.

283. Turkel, S.J., et al.: Stabilizing mechanisms preventing anterior dislocation of the gleno-humeral joint. J. Bone Joint Surg., *63A*:1208, 1981.

284. Tyler, M.A.: Treatment of the painful shoulder syndrome with amitriptyline and lithium carbonate. Can. Med. Assoc. J., *111*:137, 1974.

285. Tyson, R.R., and Kaplan, G.F.: Modern concepts of diagnosis and treatment of the thoracic outlet syndrome. Orthop. Clin. North Am., *6*:507, 1975.

286. Uematsu, S., et al.: Thermography and electromyography in the differential diagnosis of chronic pain syndromes and reflex sympathetic dystrophy. Electromyogr. Clin. Neurophysiol., *21*:165, 1981.

287. Uhthoff, H.K., Sarkar, K., and Maynard, J.A.: Calcifying tendinitis. A new concept of its pathogenesis. Clin. Orthop., *118*:164, 1976.

288. Urist, M.R., Moss, M.J., and Adams, J.M.: Calcification of tendon: a triphasic local mechanism. Arch. Pathol., *77*:594, 1964.

289. Urry, D.W.: Natural sites for calcium ion binding to elastin and collagen: a charge neutralization theory for calcification and its relationship to atherosclerosis. Proc. Natl. Acad. Sci., *68*:810, 1971.

290. Urschel, H.D., Paulson, D.L., and McNamara, J.J.: Thoracic outlet syndrome. Ann. Thorac. Surg., *6*:1, 1968.

291. ViGario, G.D., and Keats, T.E.: Localization of calcific deposits in the shoulder. AJR, *108*:806, 1970.

292. Visitsunthorn, U., and Prete, P.: Reflex sympathetic dystrophy of the lower extremity. West. J. Med., *135*:62, 1981.

293. Wall, P.D., and Sweet, W.H.: Temporary abolition of pain in man. Science, *155*:108, 1967.

294. Weiss, J.J.: Intra-articular steroids in the treatment of rotator cuff tear: reappraisal by arthrography. Arch. Phys. Med. Rehabil., *62*:555, 1981.

295. Weston, W.J.: The enlarged subdeltoid bursa in rheumatoid arthritis. Aust. Radiol., *17*:214, 1973.

296. Williams, N.E., et al.: Treatment of capsulitis of the shoulder. Rheumatol. Rehabil., *14*:236, 1975.

297. Windsor, T., and Brow, R.: Costoclavicular syndrome: its diagnosis and treatment. JAMA, *196*:109, 1966.

298. Wolfgang, G.L.: Surgical repair of tears of the rotator cuff or the shoulder. J. Bone Joint Surg., *56A*:14, 1974.

299. Worcester, J.N., and Green, D.P.: Osteoarthritis of the acromioclavicular joint. Clin. Orthop., *58*:69, 1968.

300. Wright, M.G., Richards, A.J., and Clarke, M.B.: ⁹⁹mTc-pertechnetate scanning in capsulitis. Lancet, *2*:1264, 1975.

301. Wright, V., and Haq, A.M.M.M.: Periarthritis of the shoulder. II. Radiological features. Ann. Rheum. Dis., *35*:220, 1976.

302. Wright, V., and Haq, A.M.M.M.: Periarthritis of the shoulder. I. Aetiological considerations with particular reference to personality factors. Ann. Rheum. Dis., *35*:213, 1976.

303. Yaari, A.M., Shapiro, I.M., and Brown, C.E.: Evidence that phosphatidylserine and inorganic phosphate may mediate calcium transport during calcification. Biochem. Biophys. Res. Comm., *105*:778, 1982.

304. Zachariae, L.: Tendinitis calcarea supraspinati: 41 operated cases. Acta Orthop. Scand., *36*:126, 1965.

305. Zanca, P.: Shoulder pain: involvement of the acromioclavicular joint. AJR: *112*:493, 1971.

Chapter 86

Osteonecrosis

John Paul Jones, Jr.

The term "osteonecrosis," or avascular necrosis or osseous ischemia, indicates death of the cellular constituents of bone and bone marrow. Axhausen, who first used the term "aseptic necrosis" in 1907, postulated that the presence of dead bone was due to an anemic infarct caused by bland emboli.[8]

PATHOPHYSIOLOGIC FEATURES

These features include traumatic and atraumatic damage.

Traumatic (Macrovascular) Damage

Traumatic osteonecrosis usually involves bones covered extensively by cartilage, with few vascular foramina and limited collateral circulation. For example, 8% of posterior hip dislocations without fractures develop femoral necrosis.[162] The incidence increases to 13 to 18% with associated fractures of the acetabulum or the femoral head.[134] Dislocations usually rupture the ligamentum teres.[84]

Rarely does necrosis of the femoral head complicate *extracapsular*, intertrochanteric hip fractures, noted in only 11 of 3,839 (0.29%) reported cases.[104] *Intracapsular* femoral neck fractures, however, interrupt most blood flow through the subsynovial retinacular vessels, including the important lateral epiphyseal arteries to the femoral head. Because blood to the superolateral two-thirds of the femoral head comes almost entirely from these lateral epiphyseal arteries, this area is particularly susceptible to osteonecrosis. The only other blood available to the femoral head flows through the ligamentum teres (medial epiphyseal artery),[145] which anastomosed with the lateral epiphyseal vessels in only 5 of 17 (29.4%) reported cases.[147] Reestablishment of blood flow through the ligamentum teres to a portion of the femoral head may occur in 50 to 60% of patients, but rarely does this process supply the entire femoral head. Osteonecrosis (28 to 32% total; 46% partial) occurs in about 78% of displaced femoral neck fractures.[9,22]

Nontraumatic (Microvascular) Damage

In nontraumatically induced osteonecrosis, the precise mechanism(s) and location(s) of vascular interruption have been partially elucidated, particularly in patients with hypercortisonism. One epidemiologic study, for example, cited 89% of 269 patients with disorders known to be complicated by disturbed fat metabolism or fat embolism.[68]

Embolism

Fat Embolism. Death from fat embolism has been documented in corticosteroid-treated patients with fatty livers.[58,76] Systemic fat embolism was found in 6 of 11 patients treated with corticosteroids; fat globules were seen in glomeruli on renal biopsy, and 2 patients had intravascular fat globules in their necrotic femoral heads.[72]

Cushing's syndrome may result in fatty liver.[153] Hepatocytes may rupture, releasing fat globules and causing fat embolism.[54,119] In another series, probable fat emboli were identified in subchondral arterioles in 12 of 25 necrotic femoral head specimens.[42] In another report, 4 of 8 femoral heads with corticosteroid-induced osteonecrosis showed intravascular fat in the subchondral vessels in regions of necrotic bone.[31] Intraosseous fat emboli were found at autopsy of an alcoholic patient (Fig. 86–1).[72]

Vascular obstruction by aggregates of sickle cells has not been demonstrated in resected femoral heads,[150] but reports exist of fat embolism in sickle cell crises. In one series, 5 of 8 patients with hemoglobinopathies had co-existent disorders, such as alcoholism, liver disease, or hyperlipemia.[68] Necrosis of bone marrow may lead to mobilization of fat,[114] and particles of cellular marrow trabeculae may lodge in pulmonary arteries.[139] Fat embolism is more frequent in patients with sickle cell trait (AS) or SC disease than in those with sickle cell anemia (SS). Although the bone marrow in the former variants contains more fat, sickle cell anemia produces extensive erythroid hyperplasia but little fat.[49] Sickled cell occlusion of the intramedullary capillary-sinusoidal circulation probably results in bone marrow infarctions and in fat necrosis, but the juxta-articular lesions are probably due to subchondral fat embolism.

Experimental Embolism. Experiments in corticosteroid-treated rabbits from 5 laboratories showed hyperlipemia, fatty liver, and fat embolism in lung, kidney, and femoral heads.[31,41,46,70,167]

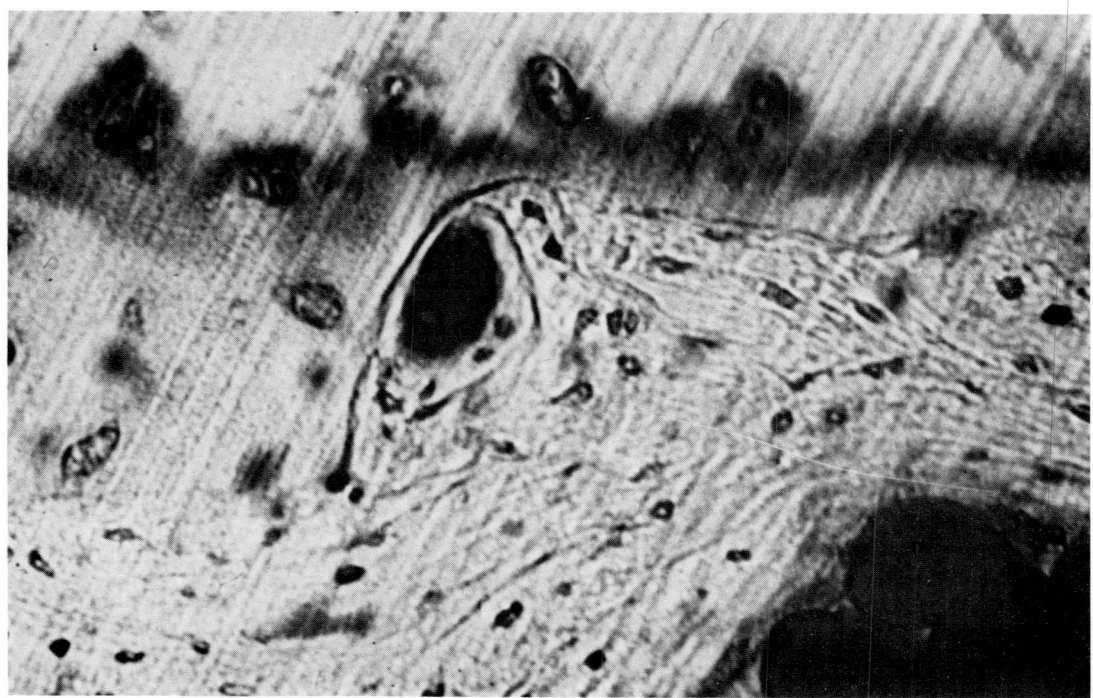

Fig. 86–1. Photomicrograph of the right femoral head of an autopsy specimen from an alcoholic patient with a large (4,600 mg) fatty liver and a pulmonary and, apparently, a systemic (intraosseous) fat embolism of an isolated subchondral vessel, without necrosis of normal-appearing marrow lipocytes (lower right). (Oil red O stain × 450.)

Focal osteocyte death in the femoral heads was also recorded. Hyperlipemia, especially increased levels of very-low-density pre-beta-lipoproteins (VLDL), occurred in 4 to 7 days. Fatty liver[102] and systemic fat embolism in the subchondral arterioles and capillaries of femoral heads developed in 2 to 3 weeks. Increased intrafemoral head pressures appeared in 6 to 8 weeks. Focal osteocytic death began in 2 weeks, with frank osteonecrosis appearing in 1 femoral head at 18 weeks.[46]

Rieger suggested in 1920 that traumatic fat embolism was the cause of osteochondritis dissecans.[132] Vascular obstruction by fat emboli as a possible cause of nontraumatic osteonecrosis was proposed in 1939.[80] A direct relationship of fat embolism with osteonecrosis was first demonstrated clinically in 1965,[73] and it was shown experimentally in 1966.[75,77] Focal regions of necrosis in the metaphysis and epiphysis of rabbit femoral heads were induced by a single infusion of fat into their distal aortas. Fat emboli persisted for as long as five weeks, especially in the subchondral vessels of the femoral heads. It was theorized that intraosseous fat embolism was followed by focal intravascular coagulation, fibrin thrombus propagation, focal bone marrow necrosis, osteon anoxia, intramedullary inflammation with edema and second-

arily increased intraosseous pressure and venous obstruction, and osteocytic death. Peripheral osteoclastic bone resorption causes trabecular thinning and results in gross trabecular fragmentation, especially after weight bearing, and eventual segmental subchondral bony collapse.

Emboli may produce osteonecrosis experimentally in conditions other than hypercortisonism and alcoholism. Aseptic bacterial emboli (agglutinated killed staphylococci) produced aseptic subarticular infarctions in the rabbit femur.[90] Anemic infarcts of the femoral head were produced by charcoal embolism.[91] Osteonecrosis did not follow gas embolism alone,[80] but it did occur in 12 femoral heads and in 14 femoral shafts of 46 rabbits after injection of leaded glass microspheres, 65 μ or smaller, into the iliac artery.[27] Microspheres localized in the upper metaphyseal region and in the lower half of the shaft of the rabbit femur.[51] In another study, glass microspheres, 50 to 70 μ, were introduced into the external iliac artery. By 12 weeks, 10 of 14 rabbits had abnormal scintigrams and histologic evidence of necrosis of bone and marrow.[50]

Gas and Fat Embolism. Possible mechanisms causing dysbaric osteonecrosis include: (1) intraosseous vessel compression by extravascular bubbles; (2) vessel obliteration by bubbles, fibrin thrombi, platelet aggregates, clumped erythrocytes, or coalesced lipids; (3) narrowing of arterial lumina by bubble-induced myointimal thickening; and (4) fat embolism resulting from blood-bubble interface reactions or marrow fat intravasation.[24,105] Experimentally increasing intraosseous pressure to 50 to 100 mm H_2O produced liquid fat intravasation into torn vessels and pulmonary fat embolism.[170] The sequence of intravascular bubble formation, endothelial damage, and platelet thrombosis with fibrin deposition has also been described using a hyperbaric swine model.[152]

Examination of bones from fatalities involving divers or compressed-air workers frequently reveals intramedullary gas surrounded by compressed bone marrow. Despite this compression and the probably increased intraosseous pressure, no cellular reaction occurs, and adjacent bone and marrow are not usually necrotic,[23] although the femoral head of one patient who died five days after diving did show extensive hemorrhage, edema, and bone marrow necrosis.[82]

Fat embolism is a common postmortem finding in human deaths from decompression sickness. Autopsy studies of two patients with histologic evidence of extensive fat embolism showed a patent foramen ovale in each patient.[56] One Japanese fisherman who died ten hours after diving had pulmonary fat embolism, air bubbles within the femoral head, red blood cell aggregation, and sludging.[82] Lipid macromolecules which coalesce after significant overcompression and decompression are also a source of fat emboli.[26,126] Furthermore, plasma lipids subjected to progressively lengthened periods of exposure to a blood-gas interface show increasing aggregation and coalescence. The contribution of marrow fat to systemic embolism may be less than that of lipids extruded from the liver as a result of tissue damage by bubbles.[122] Furthermore, the paradoxic lipid-clearing effect following severe decompression sickness may be due to lipid coalescence and entrapment in terminal (intraosseous) vessels.[81]

Although metadiaphyseal intramedullary lesions have been reported after a single sickle cell crisis or dysbaric exposure, juxta-articular (epiphyseal) lesions probably require repetitive or continuous ischemic events. The possibility of ''silent involvement'' of an opposite hip or shoulder can be as high as 40 to 50%, and it often takes over 2 years to develop. Such a delay is difficult to explain if only a single ischemic event were necessary. Double infarction studies in dogs suggest that Legg-Calvé-Perthes disease, which is osteonecrosis of the capital femoral epiphysis in children, may also arise from multiple infarctions. That more than a single infarction probably occurs in nontraumatic

osteonecrosis in adults is evidenced by dead granulation tissue, dead appositional bone on dead trabecular bone,[67,71] and other pathologic changes characteristic of recurrent necrosis, as reported in 83% of 40 femoral heads.[67,109,159] Complete revascularization of the femoral head in dogs failed after 2 or more episodes of infarction.[141]

Emboli can enter the systemic circulation through various bypasses. Pulmonary arteriovenous communications in dogs allow passage of glass spheres that are 20 to 40 times the average capillary size.[112] Moreover, 29% of the human population has a probe-patent foramen ovale.[160]

Intravascular Coagulation

A common, subclinical form of fat embolism is associated with disseminated intravascular coagulation. Fifty-eight of 110 patients with fractures developed evidence of this disorder.[133] Platelets and fibrin thrombi are closely associated with fat emboli.[17] This coagulation disorder may be precipitated by endothelial damage and fat embolism.[93] Fibrin microthrombi, similar to those encountered in disseminated intravascular coagulation, may also propagate after decompression sickness.[125] Elevated plasma lipids may accelerate blood clotting and may favor thrombogenesis, increased platelet adhesiveness, and red blood cell and platelet aggregation.[126,151]

Intraosseous Hypertension

Intraosseous hypertension and impaired venous drainage have been demonstrated in nontraumatic osteonecrosis, although a widespread process would be necessary if this were the primary cause. Increasing bone marrow pressure directly affects vascular resistance and, therefore, bone blood flow. Because bone marrow circulation is sinusoidal, and fat is rigidly encased in bone, increased marrow fat cell volume or marrow inflammation with edema may compress the capillary-sinusoidal circulation and may increase the intraosseous pressure until it further infarcts the bone marrow and any contained bone.[71] Experimentally, Wang et al. demonstrated an increase in intraosseous fat cell volume of up to 25% in mature rabbits treated chronically with corticosteroids. This change may further decrease blood supply to the femoral head, which has already been impaired three to four weeks earlier by fat embolism.[167]

The precise relationship among blood flow, fat cell hypertrophy, inflammatory edema, and intramedullary pressure is not yet well defined.[61,167] Osteonecrosis does not occur in the *intraosseous engorgement pain syndrome*, despite interruption of venous drainage and intraosseous hypertension.[7,97] Elevation of intraosseous pressure is at least an early secondary, if not a primary, factor in the pathogenesis of ischemic necrosis.

Other Factors

Free Fatty Acids. Such acids, liberated as a result of lipase activity, have been suggested as the cause of an inflammatory response in the fat embolism syndrome. Free fatty acids may also act as toxins in bone and may give rise to other mediators of inflammation, such as prostaglandins, some of which are potent stimulators of bone resorption. Dead bone stimulates a massive invasion by osteoclasts and subsequent bone resorption. This may predispose to microscopic fractures and, later, segmental collapse.

Vascular Occlusive Disease. Arteriographic studies showed stenosing lesions in 4 of 17 patients with osteonecrosis.[40] Thrombotic arterial obliteration has been reported, and a patient with Leriche's syndrome developed bilateral necrosis of the femoral head.[60] Localized medullary infarcts are also occasionally associated with peripheral gangrene.[19] Venous insufficiency or thrombophlebitis occurred in 11 of 15 reported patients with osteonecrosis.[40] Some believe that venous stasis can be the primary precipitating event.[69]

Radiation Necrosis. This disorder is linked to cellular cytotoxicity and to endarteritis because preferential bone absorption increases with secondary irradiation during orthovoltage therapy. Osteonecrosis may occur in patients with leukemia or lymphoma after irradiation or after radiotherapy for carcinoma of the prostate.

POPULATION AT RISK

Dysbarism-Related Osteonecrosis

Those exposed to changes in atmospheric pressure in the course of their occupations, principally compressed-air workers, divers, and, to a lesser extent, aviators, are at risk.

Compressed-Air Workers (Tunnel or Caisson)

"Caisson disease" was first described in 1911.[14] Virtually all caisson and tunnel workers in the United States were once decompressed according to modifications of the New York code of 1922, which required workers to split shifts. Unfortunately, inadequate surface time permitted considerable nitrogen gas to remain dissolved in the workers' tissues at the start of their second shift, with a resultant high incidence of decompression sickness and osteonecrosis.

The Washington State Decompression Tables were used first in 1964 during the Seattle tunnel construction and later in the San Francisco Bay

Area Rapid Transit (BART) project. These tables became the United States Occupational Safety and Health Administration (OSHA) standard in 1971 and have minimized the development of osteonecrosis at pressures up to 34 psig (pounds per square inch gauge pressure), but the incidence of the disorder at pressures over 36 psig is still unacceptable. Roentgenograms and bone scans of 23 men working at pressures up to 43 psig using the OSHA schedules revealed 9 (39%) with osteonecrosis.[89] The risk of decompression sickness is minimal if working pressures are maintained below 11 psig, but pressures greater than 17 psig increase the incidence of this illness and the risk of osteonecrosis.[74]

Femoral lesions are distributed differently in compressed-air workers than in commercial divers. Only 38% of 977 lesions in 383 compressed-air workers appeared in the lower femoral shaft, as compared to 54% of 114 lesions in 60 commercial divers; the compressed-air workers developed 12% of their lesions in the femoral head, as compared to only 0.9% in the divers. Of the lesions in both compressed-air workers and commercial divers, 24% involved the humeral head, however.[34] Therefore, the skeletal distribution of lesions in dysbaric, in contrast to other causes of, osteonecrosis involves the humeral head(s) much more frequently than the femoral head(s). The shoulder regions are most often involved, with petechial hemorrhages caused by systemic fat emboli blocking dermal capillaries,[146] whereas the knee is not involved, and the elbow rarely. Paradoxically, both the knee and the elbow are the commonest sites of symptoms in decompression sickness (type I bends), but even the presence of intramedullary shaft lesions does not increase one's susceptibility to juxta-articular lesions.

Dysbaric osteonecrosis may be prevented by a combination of proper engineering and recommended medical practices. Pre-employment examinations, including a body-composition analysis with hydrostatic weighing, special radiographic procedures, bone scans, and laboratory studies, are essential to disqualify applicants with significant obesity, prior juxta-articular osteonecrosis, or other conditions known to predispose persons to osteonecrosis (Table 86–1).[74]

Divers

In 1941, Grutzmacher first described osteonecrosis in a diver.[52] Today, advances in diving research and operations permit safe and effective underwater work in depths to 1,600 feet. Four groups of divers are considered: (1) skin divers, in whom osteonecrosis is nonexistent, and sport scuba divers, in whom it is virtually nonexistent; (2) United

Table 86–1. Conditions Associated with Osteonecrosis (risk increases with number of conditions)

Alcoholism†	Gaucher's disease†	Pancreatitis*
Arthropathy	Gout	Peripheral vascular disease
Neuropathic	Hemoglobinopathy†	Pregnancy
Carbon tetrachloride poisoning	Hepatitis	Systemic lupus erythematosus*
Chemotherapy	Histiocytosis	Thermal injuries†
Congenital malformation	Hypercortisonism†	Burns
Clotting defects	Hyperlipemia*	Electrical injuries
Convulsive disorders	Hyperuricemia*	Frostbite
Cushing's syndrome†	Irradiation†	Thrombophlebitis
Diabetes*	Leriche's syndrome	Trauma†
Dysbaric phenomena†	Microfractures	Fractures
Endocarditis	Myxedema	Dislocations
Fat embolism*	Obesity	

*Commonly reported associated factor
†Generally accepted contributory factor
(Modified from Park, W.M.: *In* Aseptic Necrosis of Bone. Edited by J.K. Davidson. Amsterdam, Excerpta Medica, 1976.)

States, British, French, Japanese, and Canadian navy divers, who have a 1 to 3% incidence of osteonecrosis using standard tables;[55,64,116] (3) commercial divers, who have a 4.2% overall and a 1.2% juxta-articular incidence; and (4) Hawaiian and Japanese diving fishermen, who have a 50 to 65% incidence of osteonecrosis. Dysbaric osteonecrosis is not a risk at depths of less than 30 m. Divers with the most experience and "saturation" divers, rather than "bounce" divers, are more prone to develop bone lesions. Thirteen of 30 saturation divers, exposed to depths between 100 and 540 m sea water, exhibited scintigraphic changes after diving, and 3 of these divers subsequently developed radiographic changes characteristic of osteonecrosis in sites corresponding to the previously noted scintigraphic changes.

The British Decompression Sickness Panel studied 4,980 commercial divers. At least 1 definite bone lesion was found in each of 207 divers (4.2%), but only 62 divers (1.2%) had juxta-articular lesions.[34] In contrast, 13 of 20 Hawaiian diving fishermen neither following conventional diving procedures nor using standard oxygen decompression schedules had 43 osteonecrotic lesions, 44% of these in juxta-articular regions.[163] Osteonecrosis was found in 268 of 450 (59.5%) Japanese diving fishermen.[82,117]

Osteonecrosis Associated With Other Conditions

Hemoglobinopathies

Femoral-head abnormalities in patients with sickle cell disease were first recognized in 1937.[36] Bone necrosis due to combined sickle cell-thalassemia disease was reported in 1953,[130] and it was reported later in patients with sickle cell anemia.[47] Osteonecrosis was also associated with sickle cell

trait. The incidence of femoral-head involvement in sickle cell anemia (SS) varied from 0% in 120 cases studied in West Africa to 12% in 51 cases studied in the United States,[161] whereas hip involvement in hemoglobin SC disease varied from 20 to 68%.[10] The prevalence of SS hemoglobin in the American black population is approximately 3 times greater than that of other sickle cell variants, but the incidence of osteonecrosis is higher in hemoglobin SC disease, in which, paradoxically, hemolytic crises are fewer and milder.[10,25]

At arterial oxygen tensions below 60 mm Hg in sickle cell anemia, or below 15 mm Hg in sickle cell trait, hemoglobin undergoes a conformational change with erythrocyte deformation, increased blood viscosity, stasis, thrombosis in small vessels, and finally, infarction. These events are initially reversible with adequate oxygen, but eventually, the red blood cells become damaged, and the process becomes irreversible.[131] Small intraosseous vessels are conceivably occluded many times, although revascularization from collateral blood supply often circumvents overt necrosis.

Bony infarction, probably in the painful crises of sickle cell disorders, occurs one to three days after the onset of pain. Indeed, necrotic bone marrow and liquid fat can be aspirated from the area of the infarct.[3] Within one month, however, the bone marrow is usually repopulated by normal hematopoietic tissue.[110]

Hyperlipemia

This disorder was first linked with osteonecrosis in 1960,[98,148] with hypertriglyceridemia in 18 of 22 patients. Type IV, or rarely type II or type V, is present. Type IV hyperlipemia is characterized by increased pre-beta-lipoprotein, elevated triglyceride, and normal or slightly elevated cholesterol levels. Patients with osteonecrosis often had increased pre-beta-lipoproteins[12,111] and other type II and type IV abnormalities.[137] Eight members of a family had type IV hyperlipidemia and osteonecrosis of the femoral heads. Seven were affected bilaterally.[120]

Hyperlipidemia is accompanied frequently by hypothyroidism, diabetes, obesity, or hyperuricemia. Hyperuricemia is a frequent finding in both osteonecrosis and hyperlipidemia. Obesity, which increases the risk of osteonecrosis and contributes to hyperlipidemia, was reported in 20% of 150 patients with osteonecrosis. Of 23 patients with osteonecrosis and hyperlipidemia not associated with alcohol ingestion or corticoids, 6 were obese and 3 were diabetic.[68] Fat embolism in diabetes has been observed since 1880.[155]

Autopsies of patients with definite type II and IV hyperlipidemia have shown no bone marrow involvement, but cholesterol accumulation is well documented in necrotic and ischemic areas.[159] Eighteen necrotic femoral heads showed elevated total lipid levels in the affected superolateral region.[15]

The most dramatic elevations of serum triglycerides occur in types I and V; osteonecrosis is most common in type IV. Management of the type IV disorder includes diet, treatment of diabetes or hypothyroidism, restriction of alcohol, avoidance of corticoids and oral contraceptives, and a therapeutic trial of clofibrate.[115] Used experimentally, clofibrate tempered the rise of serum cholesterol and the degree of fatty liver, but barely reduced fatty emboli in subchondral arteries.[166,168]

Hypercortisonism

Corticosteroid treatment[127,144] and Cushing's disease[43] have been complicated by osteonecrosis. One patient developed osteonecrosis after only 700 mg prednisolone in 7 days.[4] Osteonecrosis of both femoral heads occurred in another patient 9 months after a 16-day course of corticotropin, during which he received a total dose of 1,070 U.[48] Still another patient received only 16 mg prednisolone daily for 30 days.[42]

A series of 75 patients with corticosteroid-associated osteonecrosis reported that 30.6% were females and 42.6% had bilateral hip disease.[68] In another series, 91 of 95 patients had involvement of the femoral head; 49 of these patients developed a subchondral osteolytic defect that healed, whereas in 38 others with similar lesions, the underlying bone collapsed.[29]

Osteonecrosis was found in 26 of 520 (5%) patients with systemic lupus erythematosus;[37,38] an even higher incidence (40%) occurs in childhood. No relationship exists between osteonecrosis and the severity of systemic lupus erythematosus. A more recent series of 365 lupus patients showed osteonecrosis in 17 (4.7%). More prednisone was consumed during the initial 6 months of therapy by patients who developed osteonecrosis (6.4 g) than by those who did not (3.0 g).[1] Vasculitis was not found in 13 resected femoral heads from patients with systemic lupus erythematosus and is no longer considered an etiologic mechanism.[99] The capitellum, carpal scaphoid and capitate, metacarpal and metatarsal heads, distal femoral condyles, patella, talus, and tibial plateau, as well as the femoral and humeral heads, have been involved in systemic lupus erythematosus. Osteonecrosis complicating renal transplantation was reported in 1964.[156] Osteonecrosis occurred in 299 of 2,285 (13%) patients from 18 renal-transplant centers.[65] Kidney transplant recipients frequently have osteoporosis, osteomalacia, and secondary hyperparathyroidism, but heart-transplant recipients with osteonecrosis do not have these co-existent diseases; these findings further implicate corticosteroids.[21,32]

As with treatment for systemic lupus erythematosus, a correlation exists between the total steroid dose during the first few weeks after transplantation and the incidence of osteonecrosis. Osteonecrosis developed in 16 of 50 (32%) patients receiving higher doses (2,960 mg prednisone in 3 weeks), as compared with only 2 of 101 (2%) patients receiving lower doses (1,180 mg prednisone in 3 weeks).[53]

Pregnancy

In two instances, osteonecrosis of the femoral head developed in an otherwise uncomplicated pregnancy,[83] and this disorder has been found by biopsy in six instances.[40] Acute fatty liver, first noted in 1934, occurs regularly in the third trimester of pregnancy.[124,154] A number of recorded deaths associated with fatty livers are now known to be associated with increased plasma cortisol and aggravated by high-dose tetracycline administration.[79] Fat embolism during childbirth was originally thought to result from injury of the pelvic fat by the fetal head,[118] but it is now recognized that plasma lipid levels increase after the third month of gestation. Femoral head osteonecrosis has been linked to the use of *oral contraceptives*.[68] A possible sequence of events may be hyperlipidemia, fatty liver, fat embolism, and, finally, osteonecrosis.

Pancreatitis

Bone marrow involvement was found in a fatal case of acute pancreatitis in 1872.[128] Pancreatitis may be associated with subcutaneous fat necrosis, polyarthritis, and bone lesions.[44,96] Macroscopic evidence of fat necrosis in bone was found in

10.4% of 67 necropsied cases of acute pancreatitis.[16,142]

Alcoholism

The first report of osteonecrosis in an alcoholic patient appeared in 1928. Two series of patients with bone necrosis showed a signifcant incidence of alcoholism, 19% and 17%, respectively.[121,143] Thirty-eight hips in 26 alcoholic patients with osteonecrosis of the femoral head, even in the earliest stages, showed elevated intraosseous pressures.[63] Twenty-four of 38 (63%) alcoholics with osteonecrosis had type II or type IV hyperlipidemia and biopsy-proved fatty livers.

Although no well-established pathogenetic link exists between osteonecrosis and hyperuricemia or gout, a relationship between all of these factors and alcoholism is known. Hip radiographs of 370 patients with gout revealed no evidence of osteonecrosis.[136] One patient with exposure to carbon tetrachloride developed osteonecrosis.[68]

MANAGEMENT

Early diagnosis has been a serious obstacle to treating potentially reversible lesions. This discussion focuses on management of lesions affecting the juxta-articular or epiphyseal regions because metadiaphyseal lesions, including calcified intramedullary fat necrosis or bone infarction,[20] are neither symptomatic nor disabling. Four stages of osteonecrosis are considered.

Stage I Lesion

The patient is asymptomatic, with no physical findings. Routine roentgenograms are normal, but scintigraphy, and occasionally tomography, often suggest focal avascularity.

Pathologic Features

Because they are three-dimensional dead-space lesions, infarcts can be subdivided into four zones, consisting of a central zone of cell death and, surrounding it, three successively milder zones of ischemic injury, active hyperemia, and, finally, normal tissue. Once ischemic necrosis begins, the breakdown products of dying cells provoke an inflammatory response, characterized by vasodilatation, transudation of edema fluid, fibrin precipitation, and local infiltration of inflammatory cells in the hyperemic zone.[23]

All the osseous tissues do not die simultaneously. Hematopoietic marrow cells die first because they are the most sensitive to acute anoxia. Death of hematopoietic cellular elements, especially capillary endothelial cells and, later, bone marrow lipocytes, is the most reliable evidence of osteonecrosis.[85] Over 200 core biopsy specimens of early

lesions indicated interstitial edema and necrosis of fatty and hematopoietic marrow and rupture of lipocytes that produced large fatty cysts and liquefaction necrosis, amorphous debris, sinusoidal distention, and arteriolar thrombosis.[40] Bone marrow changes occur before alterations in the trabecular architecture. Osteocytes are the last cells to show histologic and cytologic changes.

Bone ischemia lasting longer than 6 to 12 hours produces cellular death,[135,171] although osteocytes may retain radioactive amino acids and glucose for 48 hours after their blood supply is obliterated.[86] Thus, the presence or absence of osteocytes (empty lacunae) is variable because of differences in their rates of autolytic reduction following functional death.

Noninvasive Diagnostic Procedures

Laboratory Tests. Certain laboratory tests are recommended for persons suspected of having an associated condition (Table 86–1). These tests include a complete blood count, urinalysis, erythrocyte sedimentation rate, rheumatoid factor, antinuclear antibody, serum uric acid, hemoglobin and lipoprotein electrophoreses, liver and thyroid function, serum amylase and lipase, serum cholesterol, triglycerides, free fatty acids, four-hour glucose tolerance, platelet count, prothrombin time, partial thromboplastin time, fibrinogen, fibrin split products, and serum cortisol determinations.

Radiography. Because osteonecrotic damage is selective, radiographs should concentrate on the shoulder, hip, and knee joints, with two rotational views of each shoulder and an anteroposterior and lateral projection of each hip and knee. Conventional radiography is not satisfactory for early diagnosis of osteonecrosis, however, because the death of bone and marrow, without repair, produces no radiologic abnormality.

Scintigraphy. If routine radiographs and tomograms have not resolved the diagnosis, [99m]technetium (^{99m}Tc)-diphosphonate radionuclide bone scans are useful (Fig. 86–2). Because interpretation of the scintigram is generally based on asymmetric radioisotope uptake, diagnosis becomes difficult in patients with bilateral involvement; the less affected side is often overlooked.[113] Abnormal scintigrams usually precede the earliest radiographic changes by 3 to 4 months. Experimental osteonecrosis has been detected consistently within 12 weeks by these scans.[51]

Bone marrow scans, using ^{99m}Tc-sulfur colloid, are effective in the early detection of intramedullary bone infarctions in sickle hemoglobinopathies and dysbaric phenomena.[3] Fifty patients with osteonecrosis affecting 70 hips were effectively studied.[108] Thirty-two patients underwent [99m]Tc-

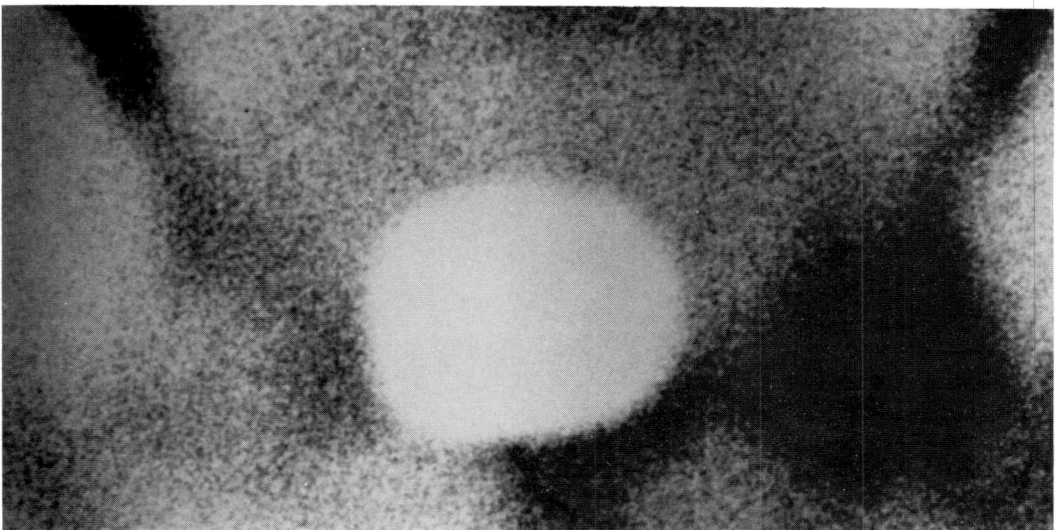

Fig. 86–2. A [99m]technetium-diphosphonate bone scintigram of the pelvis showing asymmetrically increased uptake in a necrotic left femoral head.

sulfur colloid medullary scans, as an index of perfusion, and ^{99m}Tc-diphosphonate cortical scans, as an index of osteoblastic activity, to detect early osteonecrosis following organ transplantation. If both cortical and medullary studies demonstrate a compromised blood supply, as evidenced by decreased uptake of the radioisotope, then the patient's circulation has been obliterated.[35] Studies performed a few days after sickle cell crises indicate "cold" defects without activity, but if the scan is repeated 10 to 14 days later, increased uptake will surround the developing infarct.[101]

Invasive Diagnostic Procedures

Intramedullary Pressure Determinations. These are usually elevated in the intertrochanteric region on the side of the lesion.[6] In one series, no cases of osteonecrosis went undetected when bone marrow pressures were 30 mm Hg or greater, when this procedure was combined with intraosseous venography.[172]

Intraosseous Venography. Because veins and arteries follow a nearly parallel course, venography provides indirect information about the arterial blood supply of the femoral head. If a typical venous pattern is present, it is likely that the corresponding arterial tree is also present. Generally, about 10 ml contrast fluid is injected in 15 seconds into the femoral head, although some have injected the material into the trochanteric region.[6] Radiographs are taken during and after injection. Poor filling of extraosseous veins, diaphyseal reflux, and delayed clearance of dye with intramedullary stasis 5 minutes after injection suggest osteonecrosis. In high-risk patients with obvious involvement in a single femoral head, the apparently unaffected side should be evaluated for an early lesion.[95]

Biopsy Drilling Procedure. Biopsy drilling should be performed to confirm a diagnosis of osteonecrosis if hemodynamic and/or venographic test results are abnormal.[6] A trephine is introduced into the subchondral bone of the femoral or humeral head under radiologic control, and the tissue is examined both microscopically and microroentgenographically.

Stage II Lesion

The patient is aymptomatic and still has no physical findings.

Pathologic Features

The repair process begins. Because the osteonecrotic segment is avascular, repair can only begin along its outer perimeter, at the junction between the ischemic zone surrounding the dead area and the viable area with intact circulation, the hyperemic zone. Primitive, undifferentiated, mesenchymal cells and capillary buds containing live endothelial cells proliferate and differentiate to fibroblasts, which begin synthesizing collagen. Subsequently, these mesenchymal cells differentiate to osteoblasts. This process is reduced in corticoid-treated transplant patients. Next, the central core of dead trabeculae is partially or completely resorbed by osteoclasts and is replaced or covered with new appositional bone, resulting in thickened, reinforced trabeculae.

Reossification usually occurs distal to the revascularization and resorption front. The revascularization front, including osteoclasts, fibroblasts, and capillaries, has been estimated to progress about 30 μ a day.[71] Narrowed, attenuated, and serrated trabeculae appear resorbed. The osteoclast, derived from a fusion of progenitor cells of the mononuclear phagocytic system, is the major agent of bone resorption.

Radiographic Features

In some cases, suspicious early lesions spontaneously heal. About 20% of divers' suspicious lesions (17 of 86) become definite, whereas 28% of compressed-air workers' suspicious lesions (25 of 91) become definite. The presence of one or more small, sclerotic areas, with indistinct margins, adjacent to the articular surface of the head of the humerus or femur, varying in diameter from 3 to 15 mm, may indicate necrosis. The increased density results from thickened trabeculae following reossification of the necrotic segment.[33]

Radiographic changes produced by infarcted bone and marrow vary according to location.[57] Areas of focal demineralization beneath an intact articular surface first appear, on radiographic examination, as less dense areas, the result of subchondral bone resorption (radiolucency) and surrounding appositional new bone formation (radiosclerosis). Metaphyseal lesions often appear as irregular lucencies or linear or mottled densities. Shaft or diaphyseal lesions often show serpentine calcification. Focal necrotic lesions may coalesce into a single, larger lesion, but without rupture or focal incongruity of the osteochondral joint surface. No evidence suggests secondary subchondral fracture; the radiolucent crescent-line sign is negative. These lesions are potentially reversible if their maximal diameter is less than 15 mm and no chondro-osseous rupture is found on tomographic examination (Fig. 86–3).

Noninvasive Treatment

Therapeutic measures are instituted in stages I and II to prevent articular collapse, by prolonged nonweight bearing, and to increase juxta-articular strength, by decreasing osteoclastic bone resorption and increasing osteoblastic new bone formation.

Electricity. A relationship exists among mechanical forces, bioelectricity, and enhanced osteogenesis. Direct-current electrical stimulation of bone as a supplement to core decompression and grafting is currently being compared to surgical treatment alone in the management of disorders of the femoral head. A single cathode is coiled around the graft and is connected to a subcutaneous power pack. Of 18 hips so treated, 5 showed healing of

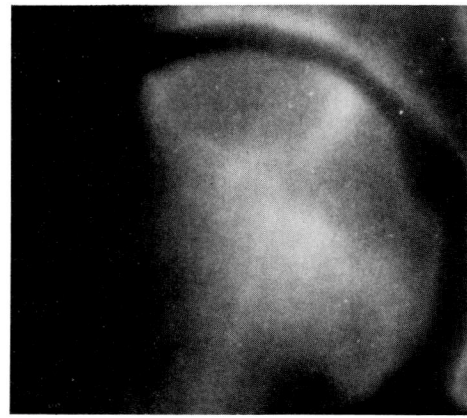

Fig. 86–3. Anteroposterior tomograms of a necrotic right femoral head showing a sclerotic-marginated, and a V-shaped superior, subchondral-based lesion without structural collapse (stage II lesion).

cystic areas, and only 1 became worse.[157] A decrease in oxygen tension near the cathode may stimulate osteogenesis.

Pulsing electromagnetic fields diminish abnormal levels of resorption in disuse osteoporosis and increase the rate of bone formation.[30] Patients with osteonecrosis have been treated with repeated, single, quasirectangular pulse bursts of these electromagnetic fields, which have 3 major effects[11]: (1) increasing blood flow and ingrowth of small vessels under 0.03 mm in diameter; (2) decreasing osteolysis by decreasing lysosomal activity, that is, decreasing collagenase, beta-gluconidase, and acid-phosphatase activity; and (3) probably most important, inhibiting, by 90%, parathyroid hormone and osteoclast-activating factor on bone-cell responsiveness in vitro. The earliest enzyme involved in the action of parathyroid hormone, membrane adenylate cyclase, is inhibited by these fields. Because the effects of short-term treatment with parathyroid hormone are osteolytic, blocking of the effects of this hormone in vivo should lead to a net increase in the rate of bone formation.[100]

Currently, a multicenter study of osteogenesis stimulation to heal early necrotic lesions of the femoral head is underway using pulsing electromagnetic fields, applied through electromagnetic, Helmholtz coils. This noninvasive treatment promotes calcification of fibrocartilage, vascular penetration, and bone formation. These pulsing electromagnetic fields were applied anteriorly and posteriorly to 28 necrotic hips for 10 hours a day at home for a minimum of 6 months. All patients in this study had radiographs demonstrating stage II (11 hips) and Stage III (17 hips) lesions. Only

2 of the 11 hips collapsed, advancing from stage II to III while under treatment. The majority of patients improved or showed no evidence of deterioration.[39]

Invasive Treatment

Core decompression was performed in 11 of 12 patients with early disease. All remained asymptomatic and without radiologic progression after 45 months. Eight additional patients remained free of symptoms and without radiologic progression 24 months after core decompression.[62] Because of its deleterious effects on the distribution of stress to the femoral head, core biopsy decompression without cortical grafting is discouraged.[123] Revascularization of segmental necrotic lesions of the femoral head from the cancellous region is possible, within certain limits, if the patient has no evidence of secondary subchondral fracture. To augment intrinsic revascularization, the necrotic area in the femoral head is excavated without dislocating the hip joint. Although some surgeons fill the excavated cavity with iliac bone grafts,[164] others advocate introducing square, autogenous bone pegs from the tibial cortex through round holes created in the femoral neck and head (Phemister-type graft);[13] 70% of stage II hip lesions so treated responded satisfactorily in 2 separate studies.[169]

The Judet musculo-osseous pedicle transfer operation,[78] for osteosynthesis of femoral-neck fractures, has been modified in an attempt to revascularize the femoral head.[72] Ten patients with osteonecrosis of the femoral head were treated with this technique, and 7 showed progressive healing of the hip lesion.[94] Muscle-pedicle grafts were performed in another 23 patients; results were good in the 8 patients with stage I and stage II lesions.[107]

Stage III Lesions

The patient is asymptomatic until the articular surface undergoes late segmental collapse, when a

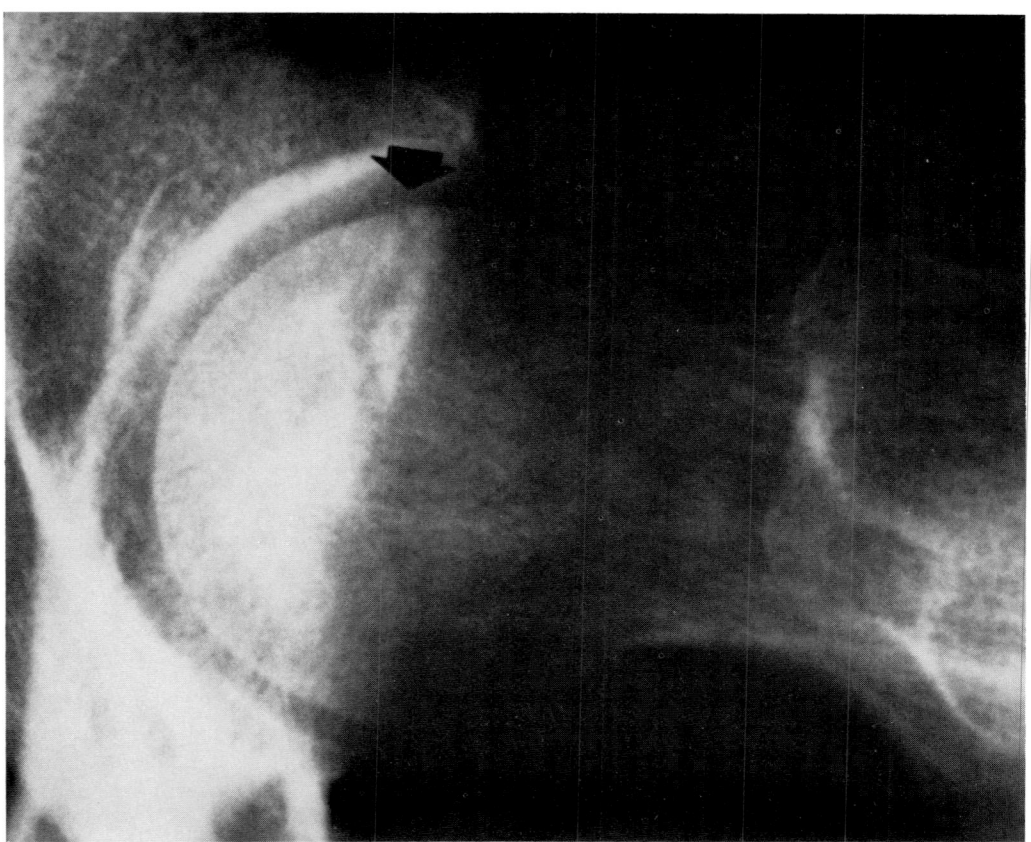

Fig. 86–4. Lateral roentgenogram of the left hip with an early stage III lesion in an alcoholic patient. Secondary fractures through necrotic subchondral bone begin from a focal area (stress riser) of resorption (radiolucency) at the anterolateral chondro-osseous junction (arrow).

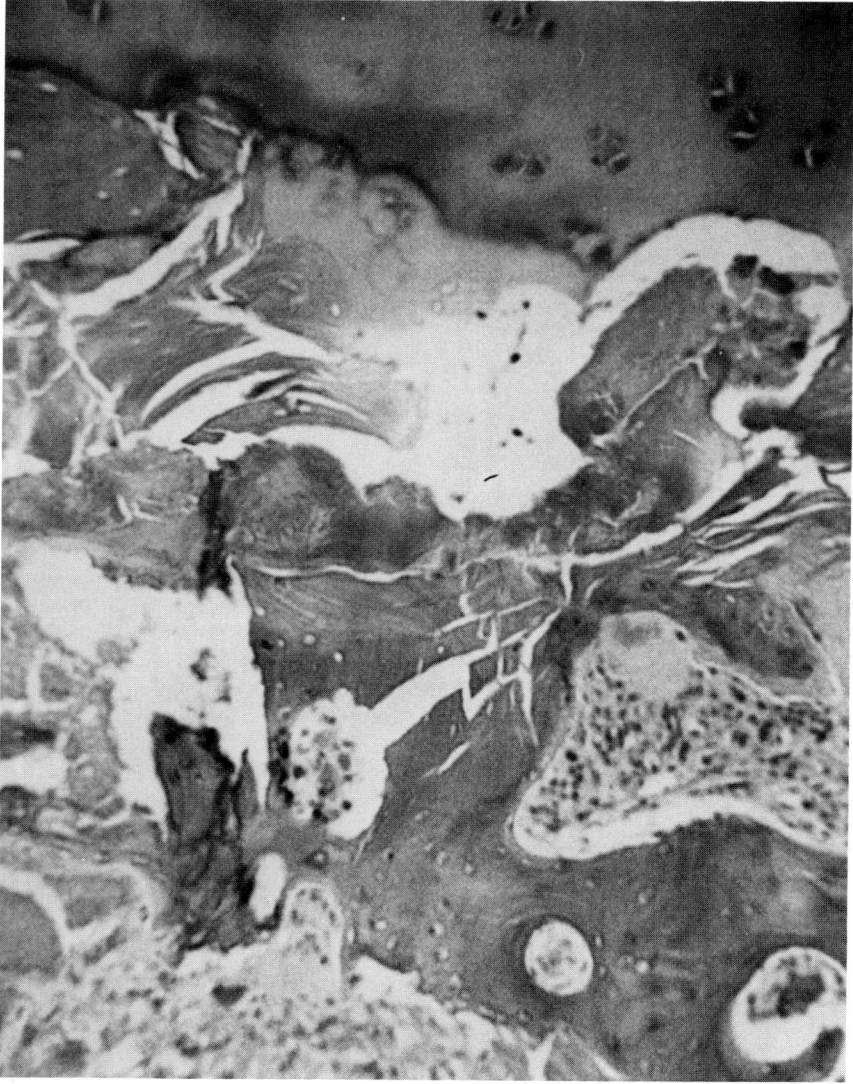

Fig. 86–5. Photomicrograph of the left femoral head of an alcoholic patient showing the initiation of trabecular delamination and microfracture propagation, through resorbed subchondral bone anterolaterally and focal cartilaginous resorption extending through the tide mark (boxed area, Fig. 86–6).

stage II lesion becomes a stage III lesion. At this point, the patient first reports symptoms of acute joint pain, and occasionally spasm, usually aggravated by weight bearing and relieved by rest. Joint tenderness and slight limitation of motion are often present.

Pathologic Features

Late segmental collapse is a result of the repair process. If repair were prevented altogether, one would see a necrotic femoral or humeral head, cov-

ered with viable cartilage, which theoretically would not collapse because dead (unrepaired) bone is essentially as strong as living bone. In Stage III lesions, however, the radiolucent revascularization front progressively resorbs subchondral bone and uncalcified articular cartilage. The subchondral-based femoral head lesion usually assumes a V-shaped configuration (Fig. 86–3), the limbs of which appear banded by lucent (proximal) and sclerotic (distal) margins. The medial limb of the V begins just superior to the fovea capitis and is

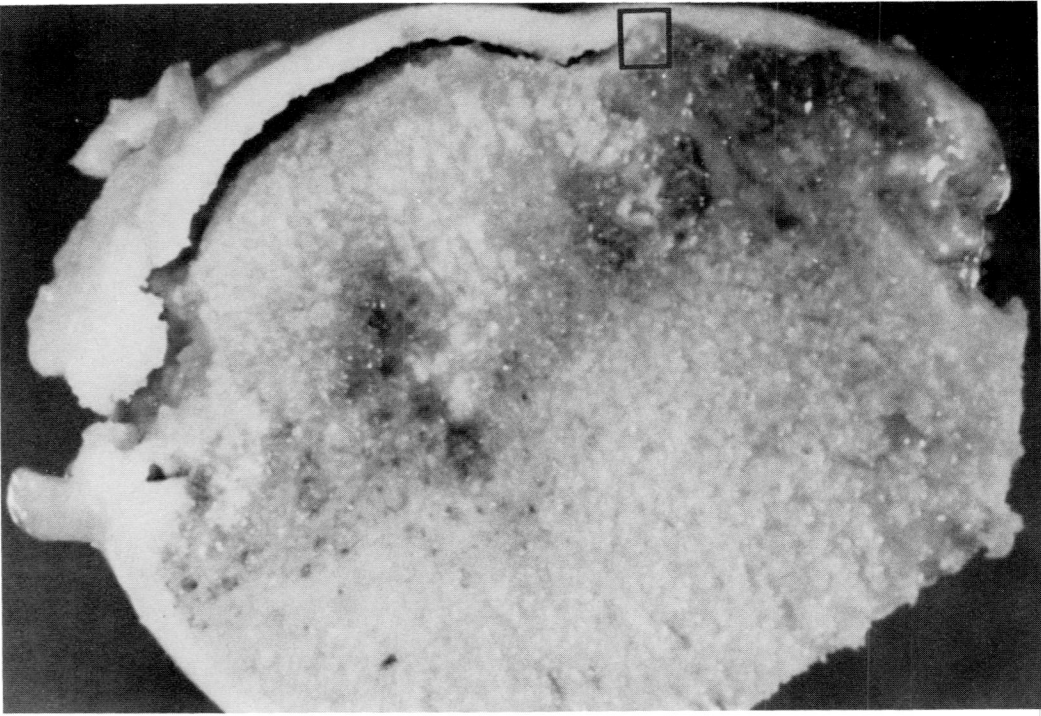

Fig. 86–6. Gross sagittal section of the left femoral head showing a stage III lesion with chalky, necrotic subchondral bone separated from normal tissue by the dark, hyperemic zone. Fracture through the necrotic subchondral bone with articular incongruity is evident. (The boxed area is magnified in Figure 86–5.)

caused by resorption and subsequent reossification from vessels within the ligamentum teres; the lateral limb is derived from lateral epiphyseal vessels. Intracapital fractures invariably begin from a focal area of osteoclastic resorption at the chondro-osseous junction of the lateral limb. Stress risers are created by this focal resorption of the subchondral plate (Fig. 86–4, arrow).

Impulse loading of the hip, especially if the load is applied while the hip is in abduction,[18] leads to shear-induced microfractures (Fig. 86–5) of the pre-existing necrotic trabeculae, beginning at the stress risers, which propagate into the femoral head as a subchondral saucer (Fig. 86–6). In post-traumatic osteonecrosis, these intracapital fractures usually propagate deeper into the femoral head than in the nontraumatic disease.[87] Finally, one sees buckling and collapsing of the anterosuperior portion of the femoral head or the central portion of the humeral head.[45]

Fibrocartilaginous metaplasia often occurs beneath the subchondral fracture and blocks further revascularization. This metaplasia probably develops as a result of micromotion or terminal hypoxia at the revascularization front. Articular hyaline cartilage overlying severely osteonecrotic femoral heads, even with gross deformity of the underlying bone structure, shows surprisingly few histologic, biochemical, or metabolic changes because joint cartilage in mature adults derives most of its nutrition from synovial fluid.[103]

When the patient is standing on both legs, the force across the femoral head is directed vertically, resulting in strong shearing forces. When weight is borne on one leg, as in walking, the trunk is stabilized on the femur by the abductor muscles. Because the hip is a pivoting, gimbal-type joint, its limited, primary, anterosuperior, contact area is subjected to more stress than the rest of the femoral head. In one-legged stance, or in walking downstairs, the hip compression force is 2.5 times body weight; when walking upstairs, it is about 3 times body weight, and when running, the force is about 4.5 to 5 times body weight.[138] The glenohumeral joint is frequently considered to be nonweight bearing, but Inman et al. calculated a maximal compressive and shear force 10 times the weight of the extremity at 90° of abduction.[66] Re-

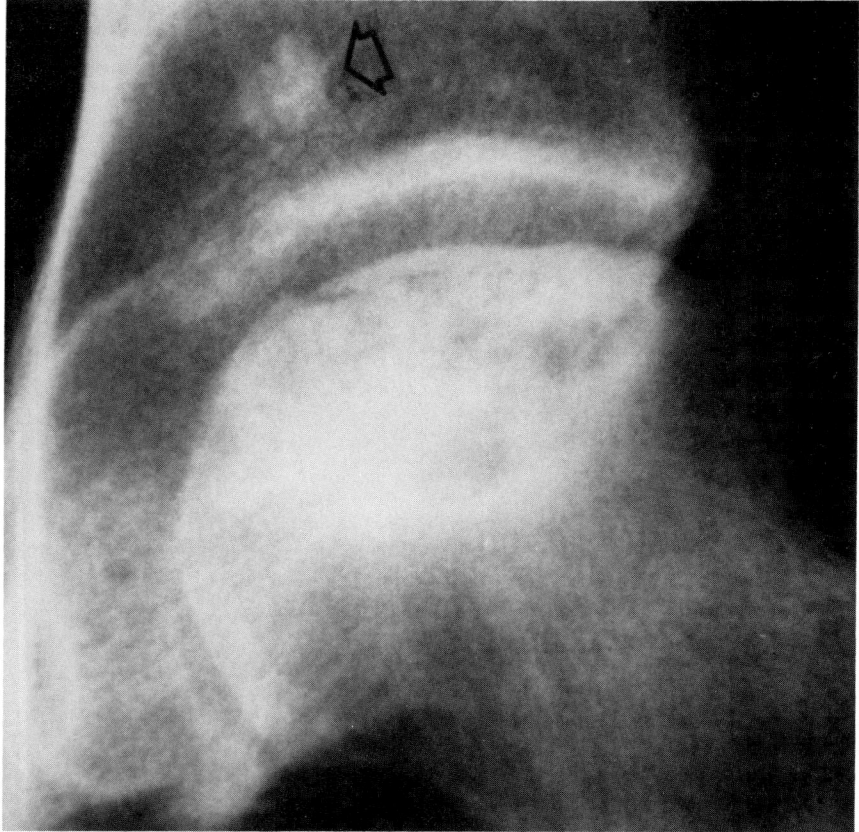

Fig. 86–7. Anteroposterior roentgenogram of the left hip of an alcoholic patient showing a positive, crescent-line sign (translucent subcortical band, or meniscus, sign) of late segmental collapse with preservation of joint-space width; a focal sclerotic infarct is also present in the supra-acetabular region (arrow).

sultant forces also reach a maximum of 0.89 times body weight at 90° of abduction.[129]

The conditions required to produce late segmental collapse are persistent osteonecrosis and mechanical loading, by weight bearing. Perhaps this combination is also the mechanism of spontaneous osteonecrosis of the knee, especially the medial femoral condyle, which appears to be a discrete clinical entity:[2] 80% of these patients are women, only 10% of patients are under age 60, and bilateral involvement is rare.[59]

Radiographic Features

Radiographic examination, particularly external rotation views of the shoulder in the Grashey projection and lateral views of the hip, indicate architectural failure and structural collapse. Often, a unipolar or bipolar subchondral fracture is apparent. A traction force applied to each leg prior to and during x-ray exposure may accentuate this cur-

vilinear radiolucent shadow; a positive radiolucent crescent-line (meniscus) sign (Fig. 86–7) indicates a stage III lesion.[165] Once a break has occurred in the smooth, spherical articular cartilage and in subchondral bone, the necrotic lesion is *irreversible*, inevitably progressing to further collapse, with articular incongruity and secondary degenerative changes.

This subchondral infarction and subarticular collapse must not be confused with the faint, subchondral, osteolytic lucent area that may be detected in stage II lesions. In one report, a radiolucent subcortical band was visible in the femoral head in 84% of renal-transplant patients after 14 months. The earliest subcortical radiolucency appeared a month after transplantation.[5]

Treatment

The humeral or femoral head is not salvageable at this point. The humeral head can be replaced by

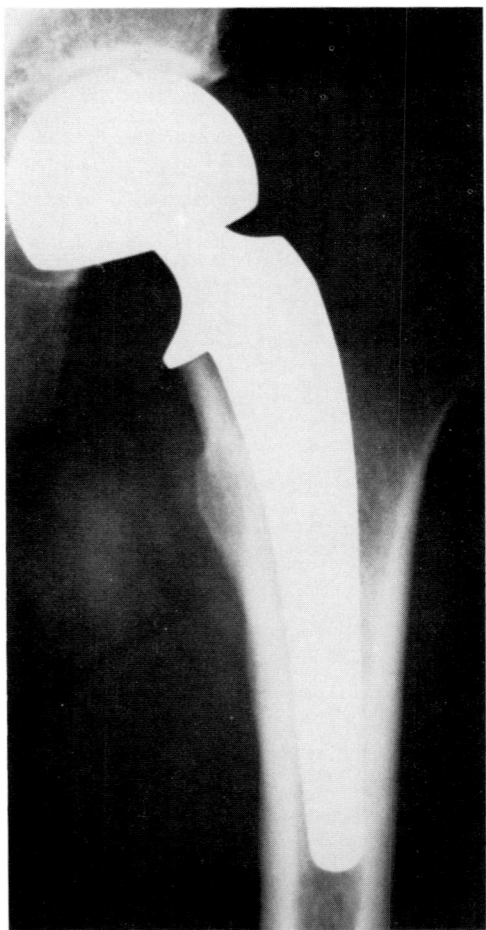

Fig. 86–8. Anteroposterior roentgenogram of the left hip showing an articulated, inner-bearing endoprosthesis (Bateman type) installed as a hemiarthroplasty, to replace a stage III lesion.

a metal prosthesis held in the humeral shaft by a stem (hemiarthroplasty), if the glenoid is normal.[28]

Five patients with stage III lesions have been treated successfully by replacement of the collapsed segment with fresh osteochondral allografts.[106] A 4-year follow-up study of bone-cartilage homografts of the femoral head in 29 adults has shown encouraging results.

Computed tomography, in conjunction with linear tomography, is useful to determine spacially the degree of involvement of the femoral head. If the lesion involves less than 25% of the femoral head and is confined entirely to the anterosuperior quadrant, a transtrochanteric osteotomy may be successful. Although excellent results were obtained in 98 of 128 (77%) hips in one study, progressive collapse in the newly created weight-bearing area occurred in 25 hips in which the lesions

had been more extensive.[92,158] Using a varus intertrochanteric osteotomy, the necrotic area is moved inferiorly and medially, so maximal stress may fall on the uninvolved, posterolateral surface of the femoral head. About 60% of 92 patients in one report were free of pain 5 years postoperatively.[88]

Hemiarthroplasty is indicated for patients with severe, extensive involvement of the femoral head when the acetabulum is normal. Evaluation of 195 patients with noncemented femoral-head replacements for an average of 9.6 years showed best results in patients with intact acetabular cartilage.[140] If the lesion involves more than 25% of the femoral head, however, an articulated endoprosthesis (Bateman) is recommended (Fig. 86–8). The potential advantages of articulated endoprostheses include decreased shear stress on acetabular cartilage, reduced acetabular wear by impact load absorption, decreased stem loosening, and improved inner-bearing action (70% of motion at the inner-bearing).

Stage IV Lesions

These patients have continuous joint pain, limp, stiffness, and weakness. Physical findings include tenderness, deformity, crepitation, contracture, and limited motion.

Pathologic Features

As subchondral collapse continues, joint destruction occurs with advanced changes typical of degenerative arthritis, including a narrowed, incongruous joint space, diffuse hypertrophy with extensive marginal osteophytic proliferation, and degenerative cyst formation on either side of the joint. Malignant fibrous histiocytoma and osteogenic sarcomas are also, although rarely, associated with bone infarcts.

Treatment

Resection (Girdlestone) arthroplasty or arthrodesis are not recommended, nor is hip resurfacing in young, active patients with osteonecrosis.[149] Total joint replacement is the recommended treatment for stage IV lesions.

REFERENCES

1. Abeles, M., Urman, J.D., and Rothfield, N.F.: Aseptic necrosis of bone in systemic lupus erythematosus: relationship to corticosteroid therapy. Arch. Intern. Med., *138*:750–754, 1978.
2. Ahlback, S., Bauer, G.C.H., and Bohne, W.H.: Spontaneous osteonecrosis of the knee. Arthritis Rheum., *11*:705–733, 1968.
3. Alavi, A., McCloskey, J.R., and Steinberg, M.E.: Early detection of avascular necrosis of the femoral head by 99m technetium diphosphonate bone scan: a preliminary report. Clin. Orthop., *127*:137–141, 1977.
4. Anderton, J.M., and Helm, R.: Multiple joint osteonecrosis following short-term steroid therapy: case report. J. Bone Joint Surg., *64A*:139–141, 1982.

5. Andresen, J., and Nielsen, H.E.: Osteonecrosis in renal transplant recipients: early radiological detection and course. Acta Orthop. Scand., *52*:475–479, 1981.

6. Arlet, J., and Ficat, P.: Biopsy drilling as a means of early diagnosis. *In* Idiopathic Ischemic Necrosis of the Femoral Head in Adults. Edited by W.M. Zinn. Stuttgart, Thieme, 1971, pp. 152–157.

7. Arnoldi, C.C., Lemperg, R., and Linderholm, H.: Intraosseous hypertension and pain in the knees. J. Bone Joint Surg., *57B*:360–364, 1975.

8. Axhausen, G.: Histologische Untersuchungen uber Knochentransplantation am Menschen. Dtsch Z. Chir., *91*:388, 1907.

9. Barnes, R., et al.: Subcapital fractures of the femur: a prospective review. J. Bone Joint Surg., *58B*:2–24, 1976.

10. Barton, C.J., and Cockshott, W.P.: Bone changes in hemoglobin SC disease. AJR, *88*:523–532, 1962.

11. Bassett, C.A.L.: Biomedical implications of pulsing electromagnetic fields. Surg. Rounds, *6*:22–31, 1983.

12. Blotman, F., et al.: Epreuve d'hyperlipémie, provoquée en crus, et ostéonécrose. Rev. Rhum. Mal. Osteoartic., *43*:419–424, 1976.

13. Bonfiglio, M., and Bardenstein, M.B.: Treatment by bone-grafting of aseptic necrosis of the femoral head and non-union of the femoral neck (Phemister technique). J. Bone Joint Surg., *40A*:1329–1346, 1958.

14. Bornstein, A., and Plate, E.: Chronic joint changes due to compressed air sickness. Fortschr. Gabiete Roentgenstr., *18*:197–206, 1911.

15. Boskey, A.L., et al.: Changes in the bone tissue lipids in persons with steroid- and alcohol-induced osteonecrosis. Clin. Orthop., *172*:289–295, 1983.

16. Boswell, S.H., and Baylin, G.J.: Metastatic fat necrosis in lytic bone lesions in a patient with painless acute pancreatitis. Radiology, *106*:85–86, 1973.

17. Bradford, D.S., Foster, R.R., and Nossel, H.L.: Coagulation alterations, hypoxemia, and fat embolism in fracture patients. J. Trauma, *10*:307–321, 1970.

18. Brown, T.D., and Ferguson, A.B., Jr.: The development of a computational stress analysis of the femoral head: mapping tensile, compressive, and shear stress for the varus and valgus positions. J. Bone Joint Surg., *60A*:619–629, 1978.

19. Bullough, P.G., et al.: Bone infarctions not associated with caisson disease. J. Bone Joint Surg., *47A*:477–491, 1965.

20. Burton, C.C., and Phemister, D.B.: Aseptic necrosis of bone. II. Infarction of bones of undetermined etiology resulting in encapsulated calcified areas in diaphyses and in arthritis deformans. Surg. Gynecol. Obstet., *68*:631–641, 1939.

21. Burton, D.S., Mochizuki, R.M., and Halpern, A.A.: Total hip arthroplasty in the cardiac transplant patient. Clin. Orthop., *130*:186–190, 1978.

22. Calandruccio, R.A.: Comparison of specimens from nonunion of neck of femur with fresh fractures and avascular necrosis specimens. J. Bone Joint Surg., *49A*:1,471–1,472, 1967.

23. Catto, M.: Pathology of aseptic bone necrosis. *In* Aseptic Necrosis of Bone. Edited by J.K. Davidson. Amsterdam, Excerpta Medica, 1976, pp. 3–100.

24. Chryssanthou, C.P.: Dysbaric Osteonecrosis: etiological and pathogenetic concepts. Clin Orthop., *130*:94–106, 1978.

25. Chung, S.M.K., and Ralston, E.L.: Necrosis of the femoral head associated with sickle cell anemia and its genetic variants: a review of literature and study of 13 cases. J. Bone Joint Surg., *51A*:33–58, 1969.

26. Cockett, A.T.K., et al.: Pathophysiology of bends and decompression sickness: an overview with emphasis on treatment. Arch. Surg., *114*:296–301, 1979.

27. Cox, P.T.: *In* Aseptic Bone Necrosis. Proceedings of a Symposium of the European Undersea Biomedical Society, Newcastle-Upon-Tyne, England. Edited by A. Evans and D. N. Walder. Newcastle-Upon-Tyne University, 1977, pp. 65–72.

28. Cruess, R.L.: Experience with steroid-induced avascular necrosis of the shoulder and etiologic considerations regarding osteonecrosis of the hip. Clin. Orthop., *130*:86–93, 1978.

29. Cruess, R.L.: Cortisone-induced avascular necrosis of the femoral head. J. Bone Joint Surg., *59B*:308–317, 1977.

30. Cruess, R.L., Kan, K., and Bassett, C.A.L.: The effect of pulsing electromagnetic fields on bone metabolism in experimental disuse osteoporosis. Clin. Orthop., *173*:245–250, March 1983.

31. Cruess, R.L., Ross, D., and Crawshaw, E.: The etiology of steroid-induced avascular necrosis of bone: a laboratory and clinical study. Clin. Orthop., *113*:178–183, 1975.

32. Danzig, L.A., Coutts, R.D., and Resnick, D.: Avascular necrosis of the femoral head following cardiac transplantation. Clin. Orthop., *117*:217–220, 1976.

33. Davidson, J.K.: The earliest radiographic evidence of dysbaric osteonecrosis. *In* Underwater Physiology V. Proceedings of the Fifth Symposium on Underwater Physiology. Edited by C.J. Lambertson. Bethesda, MD, Federation of American Societies for Experimental Biology, 1976, pp. 133–139.

34. Decompression Sickness Panel, Medical Research Council: Aseptic bone necrosis in commercial divers. Lancet, *8243*:384–388, 1981.

35. Deutsch, S.D., Gandsman, E.J., and Spraragen, S.C.: Quantitative regional blood-flow analysis and its clinical application during routine bone-scanning. J. Bone Joint Surg., *63A*:295–305, 1981.

36. Diggs, L.W., Pulliam, H.N., and King, J.C.: Bone changes in sickle cell anemia. South. Med. J., *30*:249–259, 1937.

37. Dubois, E.L.: Lupus Erythematosus. 2nd Ed. Los Angeles, University of Southern California Press, 1974, pp. 332–342.

38. Dubois, E.L., and Cozen, L.: Avascular (aseptic) bone necrosis associated with systemic lupus erythematosus. JAMA, *174*:966–971, 1960.

39. Eftekhar, N.S., et al.: Osteonecrosis of the femoral head treated by pulsed electromagnetic fields: a preliminary report. *In* Orthopaedic Transactions. Anaheim, CA, American Academy of Orthopaedic Surgeons, 1983.

40. Ficat, R.P., and Arlet, J.: Ischemia and Bone Necrosis. Baltimore, Williams & Wilkins, 1980.

41. Fisher, D.E., et al.: Corticosteroid-induced aseptic necrosis. II. Experimental study. Clin. Orthop., *84*:200–206, 1972.

42. Fisher, D.E., and Bickel, W.H.: Corticosteroid-induced avascular necrosis: a clinical study of seventy-seven patients. J. Bone Joint Surg., *53A*:859–873, 1971.

43. Frost, H.M., and Villanueva, A.R.: Human osteoblastic activity. III. Effect of cortisone on lamellar osteoblastic activity. Henry Ford Hosp. Med. Bull., *9*:97–99, 1961.

44. Gerle, R.D., et al.: Osseous changes in chronic pancreatitis. Radiology, *85*:330–337, 1965.

45. Glimcher, M.J., and Kenzora, J.E.: The biology of osteonecrosis of the human femoral head and its clinical implications. I. Tissue biology. Clin. Orthop., *138*:284–309, 1979.

46. Gold, E.W., et al.: Corticosteroid-induced avascular necrosis: an experimental study in rabbits. Clin. Orthop., *135*:272–280, 1978.

47. Golding, J.S.R., MacIver, J.E., and Went, L.N.: The bone changes in sickle cell anemia and its genetic variants. J. Bone Joint Surg., *41B*:711–718, 1959.

48. Good, A.E.: Bilateral aseptic necrosis of femur following a 16-day course of corticotropin. JAMA, *228*:497, 1974.

49. Graber, S.: Fat embolization associated with sickle-cell crisis. South. Med. J., *54*:1,395–1,398, 1961.

50. Gregg, P.J., and Walder, D.N.: Regional distribution of circulating microspheres in the femur of the rabbit. J. Bone Joint Surg., *62B*:222–226, 1980.

51. Gregg, P.J., and Walder, D.N.: Scintigraphy versus radiography in the early diagnosis of experimental bone necrosis, with special reference to caisson disease of bone. J. Bone Joint Surg., *62B*:214–221, 1980.

52. Grutzmacher, K.T.: Changes of the shoulder as a result of compressed air sickness. Roentgenpraxis, *13*:216–218, 1941.

53. Harrington, K.D., et al.: Avascular necrosis of bone after

renal transplantation. J. Bone Joint Surg., *53A*:203–215, 1971.

54. Hartroft, W.S., and Ridout, J.H.: Pathogenesis of the cirrhosis produced by choline deficiency: escape of lipid from fatty hepatic cysts and into the biliary and vascular systems. Am. J. Pathol., *27*:951–989, 1951.

55. Hauteville, D., et al.: Les lésions ossseuses latentes des plongeurs: resultats, comparés d'une enquête portant sur 105 plongeurs et 105 sujets temoins. Rev. Rhum. Mal. Osteoartic., *43*:635–643, 1976.

56. Haymaker, W., Johnston, A.D., and Downey, V.M.: Fatal decompression sickness during jet aircraft flight. J. Aviat. Med., *27*:2–17, 1956.

57. Heard, J.L., and Schneider, C.S.: Radiographic findings in commercial divers. Clin. Orthop., *130*:129–138, 1978.

58. Hill, R.B.: Fatal fat embolism from steroid-induced fatty liver. N. Engl. J. Med., *265*:318–321, 1961.

59. Houpt, J.B., et al.: Spontaneous osteonecrosis of the medial tibial plateau. J. Rheumatol., *9*:81–90, 1982.

60. Hughes, E.C., Shumacher, H.R., and Sbarbaro, J.L.: Bilateral avascular necrosis of the hip following Leriche syndrome. J. Bone Joint Surg., *53A*:380–382, 1974.

61. Hungerford, D.S.: Pathogenetic considerations in ischemic necrosis of bone. Can. J. Surg., *24*:583–590, 1981.

62. Hungerford, D.S., and Zizic, T.M.: The treatment of ischemic necrosis of bone in systemic lupus erythematosus. Medicine, *59*:143–148, 1980.

63. Hungerford, D.S., and Zizic, T.M.: Alcoholism associated ischemic necrosis of the femoral head: early diagnosis and treatment. Clin. Orthop., *130*:144–153, 1978.

64. Hunter, W.L., Jr., et al.: Aseptic bone necrosis among U.S. Navy divers: survey of 934 nonrandomly selected personnel. Undersea Biomed. Res., *5*:25–36, 1978.

65. Ibels, L.S., Alfrey, A.C., and Huffer, W.E.: Aseptic necrosis of bone following renal transplantation: experience in one hundred and ninety-four transplant recipients and review of the literature. Medicine, *57*:25–45, 1978.

66. Inman, V.T., Saunders, J.B., and Abbott, L.C.: Observations of the function of the shoulder joint. J. Bone Joint Surg., *26*:1–30, 1944.

67. Inoue, A., and Ono, K.: A histological study of idiopathic avascular necrosis of the head of the femur. J. Bone Joint Surg., *61B*:138–143, 1979.

68. Jacobs, B.: Epidemiology of traumatic and nontraumatic osteonecrosis. Clin. Orthop., *130*:51–67, 1978.

69. Jacqueline, F., and Rutishauser, E.: Idiopathic necrosis of the femoral head. (Anatomo-pathological study). *In* Idiopathic Ischemic Necrosis of the Femoral Head in Adults. Edited by W. M. Zinn. Stuttgart, Georg Thieme, 1971, pp. 34–48.

70. Jaffe, W.L., et al.: The effect of cortisone on femoral and humeral heads in rabbits: an experimental study. Clin. Orthop., *82*:221–228, 1972.

71. Johnson, L.C.: Histogenesis of avascular necrosis. *In* Proceedings of the Conference on Aseptic Necrosis of the Femoral Head. St. Louis, United States Public Health Service, 1964, pp. 55–79.

72. Jones, J.P., Jr.: Alcoholism, hypercortisonism, fat embolism and osseous avascular necrosis. *In* Idiopathic Ischemic Necrosis of the Femoral Head in Adults. Edited by W. M. Zinn. Stuttgart, Georg Thieme, 1971, pp. 112–132.

73. Jones, J.P., Jr., et al.: Fat embolization as a possible mechanism producing avascular necrosis. Arthritis Rheum., *8*:449, 1965.

74. Jones, J.P., Jr., and Behnke, A.R., Jr.: Prevention of dysbaric osteonecrosis in compressed-air workers. Clin. Orthop., *130*:118–128, 1978.

75. Jones, J.P., Jr., and Sakovich, L.: Fat embolism of bone: a roentgenographic and histological investigation, with use of intra-arterial Lipiodol, in rabbits. J. Bone Joint Surg., *48A*:149–164, 1966.

76. Jones, J.P., Jr., Engleman, E.P., and Najarian, J.S.: Systemic fat embolism after renal homotransplantation and treatment with corticosteroids. N. Engl. J. Med., *273*:1,453–1,458, 1965.

77. Jones, J.P., Jr., Sakovich, L., and Anderson, C.E.: Experimentally produced osteonecrosis as a result of fat embolism. *In* Dysbarism-Related Osteonecrosis. Edited by E.L. Beckman, D.H. Elliott, and E.M. Smith. Washington, D.C. United States Department of Health, Education and Welfare, 1974, pp. 117–131.

78. Judet, R.: Traitement des fractures du col du fémur par greffe pediculée. Acta Orthop. Scand., *32*:421–427, 1962.

79. Kahil, M.E., et al.: Acute fatty liver of pregnancy: report of two cases. Arch. Intern. Med., *113*:63–69, 1964.

80. Kahlstrom, S.C., Burton, C.C., and Phemister, D.B.: Aseptic necrosis of bone. II. Infarction of bones of undetermined etiology resulting in encapsulated and calcified areas of diaphyses and in arthritis deformans. Surg. Gynecol. Obstet., *68*:631–641, 1939.

81. Kalberer, J.T., Jr.: Dysbarism: role of fat embolization to the lung. Aerospace Med., *40*:1,068–1,075, 1969.

82. Kawashima, M., et al.: Pathological review of osteonecrosis in divers. Clin. Orthop., *130*:107–117, 1978.

83. Kay, N.R.M., Park, W.M., and Bark, M.B.: The relationship between pregnancy and femoral head necrosis. Br. J. Radiol., *45*:828–831, 1972.

84. Kelly, R.P., and Yarbrough, S.H., III: Posterior fracture-dislocation of the femoral head with retained medial head fragment. J. Trauma, *11*:97–108, 1971.

85. Kenzora, J.E., et al.: Experimental osteonecrosis of the femoral head in adult rabbits. Clin. Orthop., *130*:8–46, 1978.

86. Kenzora, J.E., et al.: Tissue biology following experimental infarction of the femoral heads. Part I. Bone studies. J. Bone Joint Surg., *51A*:1,021, 1969.

87. Kenzora, J.E., and Glimcher, M.J.: Osteonecrosis. *In* Textbook of Rheumatology. Edited by Kelley, et al. Philadelphia, W.B. Saunders Co., 1981, pp. 1,755–1,779.

88. Kerboul, et al.: The conservative surgical treatment of idiopathic aseptic necrosis of the femoral head. J. Bone Joint Surg., *56B*:291–296, 1974.

89. Kindwall, E.P., Nellen, J.R., and Spiegelhoff, D.R.: Aseptic necrosis in compressed air tunnel workers using current OSHA decompression schedules. J. Occup. Med., *24*:741–745, 1982.

90. Kistler, G.H.: Sequences of experimental bacterial infarction of the femur in rabbits. Surg. Gynecol. Obstet., *60*:913–925, 1935.

91. Kistler, G.H.: Sequences of experimental infarction of the femur in rabbits. Arch. Surg., *29*:589–611, 1934.

92. Kotz, R.: Avascular necrosis of the femoral head: a review of the indications and results of Sugioka transtrochanteric rotational osteotomy. Int. Orthop., *5*:53–58, 1981.

93. Lasch, H.G.: Therapeutic aspect of disseminated intravascular coagulation. Thromb. Diath. Haemorrh., *36 (Suppl.)*:281–293, 1969.

94. Lee, C.K., and Rehmatullah, N.: Muscle-pedicle bone graft and cancellous bone graft with "silent hip" of idiopathic ischemic necrosis of the femoral head in adults. Clin. Orthop., *158*:185–194, 1981.

95. Lee, C.K., Hansen, H.T., and Weiss, A.B.: The "silent hip" of idiopathic ischemic necrosis of the femoral head in adults. J. Bone Joint Surg., *62A*:795–800, 1980.

96. Lee, P.C., and Howard, J.M.: Fat necrosis. Surg. Gynecol. Obstet., *148*:785–789, 1979.

97. Lempberg, R.K., and Arnoldi, C.C.: The significance of intraosseous pressure in normal and diseased states with special reference to the intraosseous engorgement-pain syndrome. Clin. Orthop., *136*:143–156, 1978.

98. Lequesne, M., Cloarec, M., and DeSeze, S.: Le terrain bioloqique de la nécrose primitive de la tête fémorale: hyperuricémie, hyperlipidémie. Dixième Congrés de la ligue internationale contre la rhumatism, Rome, 1961. Turin, Minerva Medica, 1961.

99. Leventhal, G.H., and Dorfman, H.D.: Aseptic necrosis of bone in systemic lupus erythematosus. Semin. Arthritis Rheum., *4*:73–93, 1974.

100. Luben, R.A., et al.: Effects of electromagnetic stimuli on bone and bone cells *in vitro*: inhibition of responses to parathyroid hormone by low-energy low-frequency fields. Proc. Natl. Acad. Sci. U.S.A., *79*:4,180–4,184, 1982.

101. MacLeod, M.A., et al.: Functional imaging in the early diagnosis of dysbaric osteonecrosis. Br. J. Radiol., 55:497–500, 1982.

102. Mahley, R.W., et al.: Lipid transport in liver. II. Electron microscopic and biochemical studies of alterations in lipoprotein transport induced by cortisone in the rabbit. Lab Invest., 19:358–369, 1968.

103. Mankin, H.J., Thrasher, A.Z., and Hall, D.: Biochemical and metabolic characteristics of articular cartilage from osteonecrotic human femoral heads. J. Bone Joint Surg., 59A:724–728, 1977.

104. Mann, R.J.: Avascular necrosis of the femoral head following intertrochanteric fractures. Clin. Orthop., 92:108–115, 1973.

105. Meek, R.N., Woodruff, M.B., and Allardyce, D.B.: Source of fat macroglobules in fractures of the lower extremity. J. Trauma, 12:432–434, 1972.

106. Meyers, M.H.: Allografts with the muscle pedicle technique. Clin. Orthop., 130:202–209, 1978.

107. Meyers, M.H., Harvey, J.P., Jr., and Moore, T.M.: The muscle pedicle bone graft in the treatment of displaced fracture of the femoral neck: indications, operative technique and results. Orthop. Clin. North Am., 5:779–792, 1974.

108. Meyers, M.H., Telfer, N., and Moore, T.M.: Determination of the vascularity of the femoral head with technetium 99ᵐ-sulphur colloid: diagnostic and prognostic significance. J. Bone Joint Surg., 59A:658–664, 1977.

109. Mickelson, M.R., et al.: Legg-Calve-Perthes disease in dogs: a comparison to human Legg-Calve-Perthes disease. Clin. Orthop., 157:287–300, 1981.

110. Middlemiss, H.: Aseptic necrosis and other changes occurring in bone in the haemoglobinopathies. In Aseptic Necrosis of Bone. Edited by J.K. Davidson. New York, American Elsevier, 1976.

111. Mielants, H., et al.: Avascular necrosis and its relation to lipid and purine metabolism. J. Rheumatol., 2:430–436, 1975.

112. Niden, A.H., and Aviado, D.M.: Effects of pulmonary embolism on the pulmonary circulation with special reference to arteriovenous shunts in the lungs. Circ. Res., 4:67–72, 1956.

113. Nishioka, J.: The diagnostic value of bone scintiscanning in aseptic osteonecrosis of femur—comparative study between bone scintigram and histological finding. J. Jpn. Orthop. Assoc., 53:429–440, 1979.

114. Ober, W.B., et al.: Hemoglobin S-C disease with fat embolism: report of a patient dying in crisis; autopsy findings. Am. J. Med., 27:647–658, 1959.

115. O'Driscoll, M., and Powell, F.J.: Injury, serum lipids, fat embolism and clofibrate. Br. Med. J., 4:149–151, 1967.

116. Ohiwa, H., and Itoh, A.: Aseptic bone necrosis in Japanese navy divers. In Underwater Physiology VI. Proceedings of the Sixth Symposium on Underwater Physiology. Edited by C.W. Schilling and M.W. Beckett. Bethesda, MD, Federation of American Societies for Experimental Biology, 1978, pp. 299–305.

117. Ohta, Y., and Matsunaga, H.: Bone lesions in divers. J. Bone Joint Surg., 56B:3–16, 1974.

118. Olbrycht, J.: Experimentelle Beitrage zur Lehre von der Fettembolie der Lungen mit besonderer Berucksichtigung ihrer gerichtsarztlichen Bedeutung. Dtsch. Z. Gessamte Gerichtl. Med., 1:642, 1922.

119. Owens, G., and Northington, B.A.: Liver lipid as a source of post-traumatic embolic fat. J. Surg. Res., 2:283–290, 1962.

120. Palmer, A.K., et al.: Osteonecrosis of the femoral head in a family with hyperlipoproteinemia. Clin. Orthop., 155:166–171, 1981.

121. Patterson, R.J., Bickel, W.H., and Dahlin, D.C.: Idiopathic avascular necrosis of the head of the femur: a study of 52 cases. J. Bone Joint Surg., 46A:267–282, 1964.

122. Pauley, S.M., and Cockett, A.T.K.: Role of lipids in decompression sickness. Aerospace Med., 41:56–60, 1970.

123. Penix, A.R., et al.: Femoral head stress following cortical bone grafting for aseptic necrosis: a finite element study. Clin. Orthop., 173:159–165, 1983.

124. Peters, R.L., Edmondson, H.A., and Kunelis, C.T.: Acute fatty metamorphosis of the liver in pregnancy. JAMA, 180:767, 1962.

125. Philp, D., Schachan, P., and Gowdey, C.W.: Involvement of platelets and microthrombi in experimental decompression sickness: similarities with disseminated intravascular coagulation. Aerospace Med., 42:494–502, 1971.

126. Philp, R.B.: A review of blood changes associated with compression-decompression: relationship to decompression sickness. Undersea Biomed. Res., 1:117–150, 1974.

127. Pietrograndi, V., and Mastromario, R.: Osteopathia de proluregato trattamento cortisonico. Ital. J. Orthop. Traumatol., 25:791–810, 1957.

128. Ponfick, E.: Ueber die sympathischen Erkrankungen des Knochenmarkes bei inneren Krankheiten. Virchows Arch. (Pathol. Anat.), 56:534, 1872.

129. Poppen, N.K., and Walker, P.S.: Forces at the glenohumeral joint in abduction. Clin. Orthop., 135:165–170, 1978.

130. Reich, R.S., and Rosenberg, N.J.: Avascular necrosis of bone in Caucasians with chronic hemolytic anaemia due to combined sickling and thalassemia traits. J. Bone Joint Surg., 35A:894–904, 1953.

131. Rickles, F.R., and O'Leary, D.S.: Role of coagulation system in pathophysiology of sickle cell disease. Arch. Intern. Med., 133:635–640, 1974.

132. Rieger, H.: Zur Pathogenese von Gelenkmaueuen. Munch. Med. Wochenschr., 67:719–720, 1920.

133. Riseborough, E.J., and Herndon, J.H.: Alterations in pulmonary function, coagulation and fat metabolism in patients with fractures of the lower limbs. Clin. Orthop., 115:248–267, 1976.

134. Roeder, L.F., Jr., and DeLee, J.C.: Femoral head fractures associated with posterior hip dislocations. Clin. Orthop., 147:121–130, 1980.

135. Roesingh, G.E., and James, J.: Early phases of avascular necrosis of the femoral head in rabbits. J. Bone Joint Surg., 51B:165–176, 1969.

136. RotesQuerol, A.J., and Munoz-Gomez, G.J.: Gota en la cadera. Rev. Esp. Reum. Enferm. Osteoartic., 11:89–98, 1965.

137. Roux, H., et al.: Exploration lipidique d'un groupe d'ostéonécroses. Rev. Rhum., 41:393–398, 1974.

138. Rydell, N.: Biomechanics of the hip-joint. Clin. Orthop., 92:6–15, 1973.

139. Rywlin, A.M., Block, A.L., and Werner, C.S.: Hemoglobin C and S disease in pregnancy: a report of a case with bone marrow and fat emboli. Am. J. Obstet. Gynecol., 86:1,055–1,059, 1963.

140. Salvati, E.A., and Wilson, P.D., Jr.: Long-term results of femoral-head replacements. J. Bone Joint Surg., 54A:1,355–1,356, 1972.

141. Sanchis, M., Zahir, A., and Freeman, M.A.R.: Experimental simulation of Perthes's disease by consecutive interruptions of the blood supply to the capital femoral epiphysis in the puppy. J. Bone Joint Surg., 55A:335–342, 1973.

142. Scarpelli, D.G.: Fat necrosis of bone marrow in acute pancreatitis. Am. J. Pathol., 32:1,077–1,087, 1956.

143. Serre, H., and Simon, L.: L'ostéonécrose de la tête fémorale chez l'adulte. Rev. Rhum., 29:527, 1962.

144. Serre, H., and Simon, L.: Le rôle de la corticothérapie dans l'ostéo-nécrose primitive de la tête fémorale chez l'adulte. Presse Med., 69:1,995–1,998, 1961.

145. Sevitt, S.: Avascular necrosis and revascularization of the femoral head after intracapsular fracture: a combined arteriographic and histological study. J. Bone Joint Surg., 46B:270–296, 1964.

146. Sevitt, S.: In Fat Embolism. London, Butterworths, 1962, pp. 168–169.

147. Sevitt, S., and Thompson, R.G.: The distribution and anastomoses of arteries supplying the head and neck of the femur. J. Bone Joint Surg., 47B:560–573, 1965.

148. DeSeze, S., Welfling, J., and Lequesne, M.: L'ostéo-

nécrose primitive de la tête fémorale chez l'adulte: étude de 30 cas. Rev. Rhum., 27:117–127, 1960.

149. Shea, W.D.: Indications and contraindications in surface replacement arthroplasty of the hip. Orthop. Clin., 13:729–737, 1982.

150. Sherman, M.: Pathogenesis of disintegration of hip in sickle-cell anemia, South. Med. J., 52:632, 1959.

151. Sikorski, J.M.: Venous thrombosis produced by the local injection of fat. J. Bone Joint Surg., 65B:340–345, 1983.

152. Slichter, S.J., et al.: Dysbaric osteonecrosis: a consequence of intravascular bubble formation, endothelial damage and platelet thrombosis. J. Lab. Clin. Med., 98:568–590, 1981.

153. Soffer, L.J., Iannoccone, A., and Gabrilove, J.L.: Cushing's syndrome: a study of fifty patients. Am. J. Med., 30:129–146, 1961.

154. Stander, H.J., and Cadden, J.F.: Acute yellow atrophy of the liver in pregnancy. Am. J. Obstet. Gynecol., 28:61, 1934.

155. Starr, L.: Lipemia and fat embolism in diabetes mellitus. Med. Rec., 17:477–481, 1880.

156. Starzl, T.E., et al.: Renal homotransplantation. Late function and complications. Ann. Intern. Med., 61:470–497, 1964.

157. Steinberg, N.E., et al.: Treatment of avascular necrosis of the femoral head with electrical stimulation—a preliminary report. Orthop. Rev., 12:76, 1983.

158. Sugioka, Y., Katsuki, I., and Hotokebuchi, T.: Transtrochanteric rotational osteotomy of the femoral head for the treatment of osteonecrosis: follow-up statistics. Clin. Orthop., 169:115–126, 1982.

159. Sweet, D.E., and Madewell, J.E.: Pathogenesis of osteonecrosis. In Diagnosis of Bone and Joint Disorders. Vol. 3. Edited by D. Resnick and G. Niwayama. Philadelphia, W.B. Saunders, 1981, p. 2,781.

160. Taber, R.E., Maraan, B.M., and Tomatis, L.: Prevention of air embolism during open-heart surgery: a study of the role of trapped air in the left ventricle. Surgery, 68:685–691, 1970.

161. Tanaka, K.R., Clifford, G.O., and Axelrod, A.R.: Sickle cell anemia with aseptic necrosis of the femoral head. Blood, 11:998, 1956.

162. Upadhyay, S.S., Moultoj, A., and Srikrishnamurthy, K.: An analysis of the late effects of traumatic posterior dislocation of the hip without fractures. J. Bone Joint Surg., 65B:150–152, 1983.

163. Wade, C.E., et al.: Incidence of dysbaric osteonecrosis in Hawaii's diving fishermen. Undersea Biomed. Res., 5:137–147, 1978.

164. Wagner, H.: Treatment of idiopathic necrosis of the femoral head. In Idiopathic Ischemic Necrosis of the Femoral Head in Adults. Edited by W.M. Zinn. Stuttgart, Georg Thieme, 1971, pp. 202–204.

165. Waldenstrom, H.: The first stages of coxa plana. J. Bone Joint Surg., 20:559–566, 1938.

166. Wang, G.-J., et al.: Steroid-induced femoral head pressure changes and their response to lipid-clearing agents. Clin. Orthop., 174:298–302, 1983.

167. Wang, G.-J., et al.: Cortisone-induced intrafemoral head pressure change and its response to a drilling decompression method. Clin. Orthop., 159:274–278, 1981.

168. Wang, G.-J., et al.: Cortisone induced bone changes and its response to lipid clearing agents. Clin. Orthop., 130:81–85, 1978.

169. Wang, G.-J., and Thompson, R.C.: Treatment of aseptic necrosis of the femoral head with Phemister-type bone grafts. South. Med. J., 69:305–308, 1976.

170. Whitenack, S.H., and Hausberger, F.X.: Intravasation of fat from the bone marrow cavity. Am. J. Pathol., 65:335–345, 1971.

171. Woodhouse, C.F.: Anoxia of the femoral head. Surgery, 52:55–63, 1962.

172. Zizic, T.M., Hungerford, D.S., and Stevens, M.B.: Ischemic bone necrosis in systemic lupus erythematosus. I. The early diagnosis of ischemic necrosis of bone. Medicine, 59:134–148, 1980.

Section IX

Osteoarthritis

Chapter 87

Pathology of Osteoarthritis

Leon Sokoloff and Aubrey J. Hough, Jr.

Despite the almost ubiquitous occurrence of osteoarthritis in the adult population, many elements of its pathogenesis are not understood. Although the term *osteoarthritis* is a misnomer because it implies an inherently inflammatory process, it has been in common use in the English speaking world for many years and will probably continue to be because it has greater appeal than the more accurate term, *degenerative joint disease*. The term *arthrosis* or *osteoarthrosis,* frequently employed in Europe, offers certain advantages. Osteoarthritis is an inherently noninflammatory disorder of movable joints characterized by deterioration and abrasion of articular cartilage, as well as by formation of new bone at the joint surfaces. Two different views of the relationship between the bone changes and the joint changes have been argued over the years.

OSTEOARTHRITIS AS A REMODELING PROCESS

Remodeling is the alteration of the internal and external architecture of the skeleton, as dictated by Wolff's law, in response to variation in mechanical loading. It involves removal of bony tissue at certain points and simultaneous formation of new bone elsewhere. The concept has been expanded to include changes in shape of joints with age and osteoarthritis.[14] These mechanisms in bone have been the subject of much thought. Only recently has the question even been formulated in the case of the remodeling of cartilage. Changes in the shape of joints from loading have been shown by Thompson and Bassett,[130a] who produced abnormal pressures on the articular surfaces of the knees in rabbits by excising one of the femoral condyles. In the joint compartment with the reduced pressure, the calcified layer of the tibial cartilage was resorbed by invading blood vessels. On the side subjected to increased pressure, the articular cartilage proper showed loss of metachromasia and necrobiosis of its chondrocytes.

The usual accounts of the pathologic features of degenerative joint disease state that the lesions begin with fibrillation of articular cartilage. Fibrillation is the earliest gross change seen on the surface of the opened joint (Fig. 87–1). It is not necessarily the first change, however, if the adja-

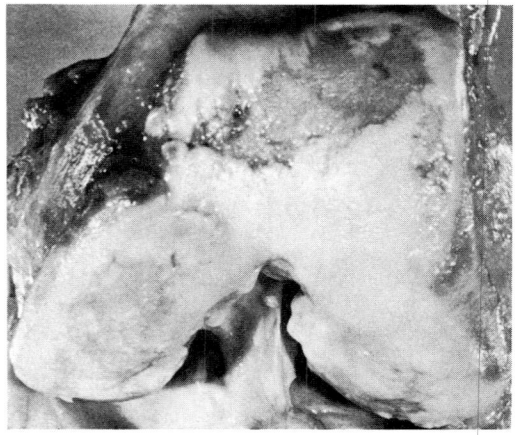

Fig. 87–1. Degenerative joint disease of the knee. Large areas of erosion of articular cartilage are present on the patellar facet and on the condyles of the femur. These erosions occupy principally the central portions of the joint surfaces and spare the marginal regions. The cartilage at the eroded edges is fibrillated. The irregular elevations at the periphery of the surfaces are osteophytic.

cent bony structure is also examined. The sequences in the remodeling of osteoarthritis can be reconstructed only hypothetically. The recognition of the complexity of the pathologic sequences is important because several pharmacologic strategies for treatment of osteoarthritis are based on the assumption that loss of cartilage is at its heart.[69]

Three general hypotheses of the relationships between cartilaginous and bony changes have been proposed at various times, but all seem overly simple. First, osteoarthritis is a *degeneration of articular cartilage that progressively leads to denudation of the joint surface*. If this statement were valid, little or no remodeling of bone would occur. Only rarely is extensive eburnation seen in surgically resected femoral heads that retain their sphericity.[118] Concentric osteoarthritis has been attributed to inflammatory lysis, as distinct from mechanical overloading of the cartilage.[38,122] The degree of deformity in surgically resected femoral heads is generally greater in degenerative arthritis than in rheumatoid arthritis (RA).[69] Lagier has made analogous observations on the sparing of the contour of the hip joint in ochronotic arthropathy, in which the destruction of the cartilage is related to inherent metabolic deterioration of the cartilage rather than to mechanical remodeling.[77]

The second hypothesis states that osteoarthritis begins as *fibrillation of articular cartilage that leads to secondary remodeling of the bony components of the joint*. This view is most commonly held (see Fig. 87–3,*A*). A principal difficulty with the concept is that it is difficult to isolate any individual finding as a unique morphologic event that precedes others in the complicated changes seen in histologic section. It does not take into account, for example, the remodeling of the osteochondral junction as an early age-related change in the cartilage.[15,78] The changes ordinarily coexist.

The third hypothesis is that osteoarthritis is the *consequence of changes in the stiffness of subchondral bone*. Radin et al. proposed that microfractures of subchondral bone precede cartilage damage.[101] This idea is predicated on the observations that bone, rather than cartilage, absorbs most of the energy of impact stress on the extremities. Repair of the fractures leads to a net local increase in stiffness of the bone that, in turn, causes the overlying cartilage to absorb excess energy. This process, it is argued, leads to the degeneration of the cartilage. This hypothesis has a distinct mechanical logic as well as some experimental support, but it suffers from the same limitations as the preceding hypothesis.

The degenerative and remodeling changes are so intimately associated that it seems unrealistic to attempt to identify a unique initial event in the osteoarthritic process. The structural disintegration of the osteoarticular junction and abrasion lead to the loss of substance of the articular surface. These processes are also responsible for the proliferative phenomena, including the formation of new cartilage at the surface of the osteoarthritic joint (Fig. 87–2). The generation of new cartilage in defects in the joint surface that penetrate into the subjacent bone marrow has been documented experimentally.[21,44]

In advanced osteoarthritis, overt microfractures and osteoclastic resorption of the subchondral plate are seen together with osteoblastic foci and sclerotic new bone. Irregularity of the accretion lines indicates that the sclerotic process occurs in bursts, at least some of which arise through repair of microfractures. Islands of cartilaginous proliferation interdigitate with new bone formation in the subchondral marrow.[89] These changes represent abortive attempts at repair of infractions of the joint surfaces.

It would be an error to conclude that osteophytes represent late changes in the evolution of the lesions. In osteoarthritis produced experimentally in canine knee joints by incising the anterior cruciate ligament, remodeling of the bone occurs by the end of the first week, no later than changes in the composition of the cartilage.[50] Osteoarthritis in this sense is not so much an inherent biologic inability of the joint surface to repair itself as it is a failure of the repair to be successful.

ARTICULAR CARTILAGE

Early Changes

The earliest changes observed microscopically in the cartilage have been described differently by various investigators.

Focal Chondromucoid Softening

In their historic study of the knee joint, Bennett and co-workers concluded that the initial abnormality is a focal swelling of cartilage matrix associated with increased affinity for hematoxylin.[11] This mucoid transformation takes place close to the surface of the cartilage. Cellular changes are also present in relation to this alteration: chondrocytes adjacent and superficial to the softened matrix are more numerous than normal.

Focal Loss of Metachromasia

Loss of metachromatic material, presumably chondroitin sulfate, from all but the deepest portion of the radial zone of the articular cartilage, has been proposed as the morphologic counterpart of chondromalacia followed by osteoarthritis. The diminution of metachromasia corresponds to a loss, rather than an increase, of affinity for hematoxylin, as proposed in the preceding view.

Proliferation of Chondrocytes

Small clusters of chondrocytes are common at the margin of minute fissures in the surface of the cartilage. These chondrocytes have proliferated in response to the dehiscence of the tissue (Fig. 87–3).

Diminution of Chondrocytes

The unit number of chondrocytes is lower in adult than in young joint cartilage, but the cell count alters little in aging articular cartilage once adulthood is reached, unless osteoarthritis is present.[135] Electron-microscopic evidence of chondrocyte loss has been found in all layers of aging human and other mammalian articular cartilage. This evidence takes the form of microscars in which relics of disintegrated cells are associated with fragmentation, disarrangement, and great variation in the girth of adjacent collagen fibrils.[139] Lipid droplets are often present in these foci.

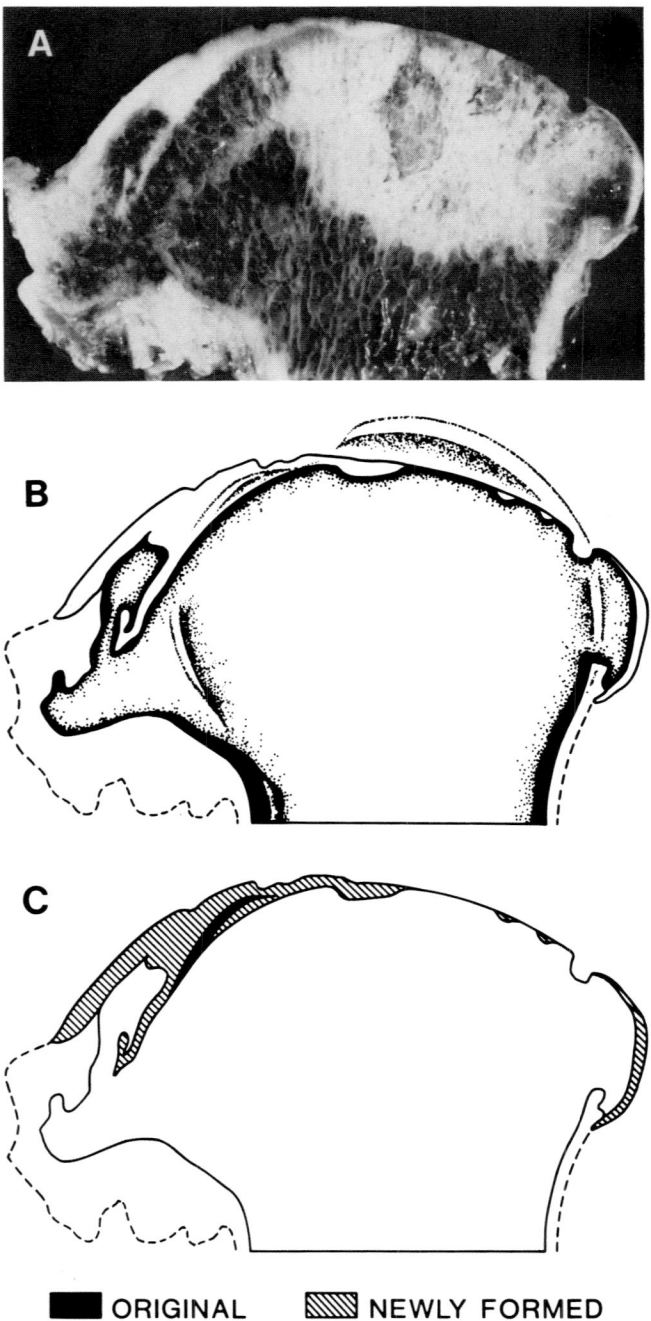

ORIGINAL   NEWLY FORMED

Fig. 87–2.   Advanced osteoarthritis of the head of the femur. *A,* The contour has been deformed both by abrasion of the bearing surface and by formation of marginal osteophytes. The large inferomedial spur at the left has grown not only to the side, but also into the original joint cartilage. Subchondral pseudocysts approach the eroded surface through slender crevices. The pallor of the eburnated zone reflects the condensation of bony trabeculae and compact fibrous tissue, in contrast to the darker, vascular hematopoietic marrow. *B,* Schematic representation of the remodeling. The outline of the gross specimen is superimposed on a best-fit contour of a normal femoral head of corresponding size. Bone appears black; cartilage, white outlined by a solid line. The broken line demarcates retinacular synovium. The loss of substance affects both articular cartilage and the immediately subjacent bone. *C,* Newly formed cartilage as deduced from the difference in the corresponding outlines in *B.* Only a minute residue of the original cartilage (black) persists at the base of the inferomedial osteophyte. The bulk of the cartilage must have therefore formed in the retinaculum or the subchondral bone marrow.

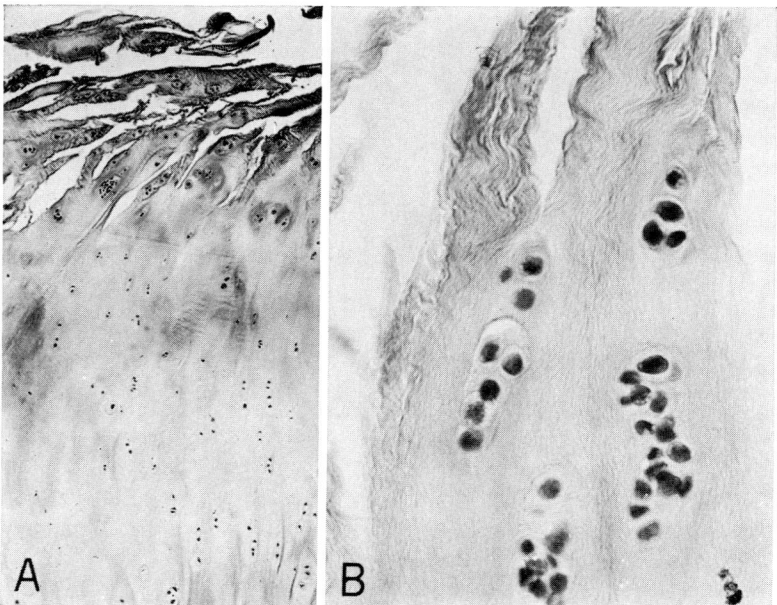

Fig. 87–3. Fibrillation of articular cartilage, *A,* The most superficial dehiscences are oriented parallel to the surface and then arch downward in a more vertical direction. This pattern corresponds to the fibrous planes of the cartilage. (Hematoxylin and eosin stain, × 40) *B,* Higher magnification (× 240) of the fibrillated edge. The collagen fibrils at the surface have been "unmasked" from the hyaline matrix and appear frayed. Clusters of chondrocytes have proliferated to form so-called "brood capsules."

Fatty Degeneration

Fine fat deposits in the interterritorial matrix have been described as an early degenerative change in cartilage; these deposits may become larger and may form coarse droplets at the "capsule" of the chondrocytes. The content of triglyceride and complex lipids increases with age in the cells and the matrix of cartilage even prior to fibrillation. The increase of arachidonic acid, the precursor of prostaglandins, is confined to the tangential layer.

Alteration of Collagen Fibrils

In aging articular cartilage, the general architecture and appearance of the collagen fibrils are preserved, although looser packing and occasional fragmentation are sometimes seen in the superficial layers. The aforementioned microscars increase in number as osteoarthritis evolves. Some of the fragmented fibrils in these areas have a large diameter. A progressive radial reorientation of the collagen has been noted, both by electron-microscopic study and by x-ray diffraction methods. Although *amianthoid* (asbestos-like) degeneration of the matrix has been described as a late feature of the disorder,[48] this process is typical of costal and other extra-articular cartilage rather than of joint cartilage.[66]

Surface Irregularities

Age-dependent irregularities in the surface of articular cartilage have been proposed to evolve into fibrillation.[81] Although several types of evidence support this concept, data are inconclusive because the various analytic procedures themselves may involve technical artifacts.[47]

Weichselbaum's Lacunar Resorption

Focal dissolution of matrix by chondroclastic cells in the cartilage lacunae was once regarded as a feature of osteoarthritis (Fig. 87–4). This change is more characteristic of RA, however.

Gross Changes

Localized areas of softening of the cartilage are associated with a fine, velvety disruption of the surface. In these areas, one sees a dehiscence of the cartilage along the axis of the matrix collagen. When the disruption is confined to the tangential layer of the surface, the process is referred to as *flaking;* when the process extends to the deeper radial layer, it is described as *fibrillation* (see Fig. 87–3). Because these minute discontinuities in the surface are readily stained grossly by India ink,[86] they lend themselves to quantitative study. Abrasion of the fibrillated cartilage takes place with progressive denudation of the underlying bony cor-

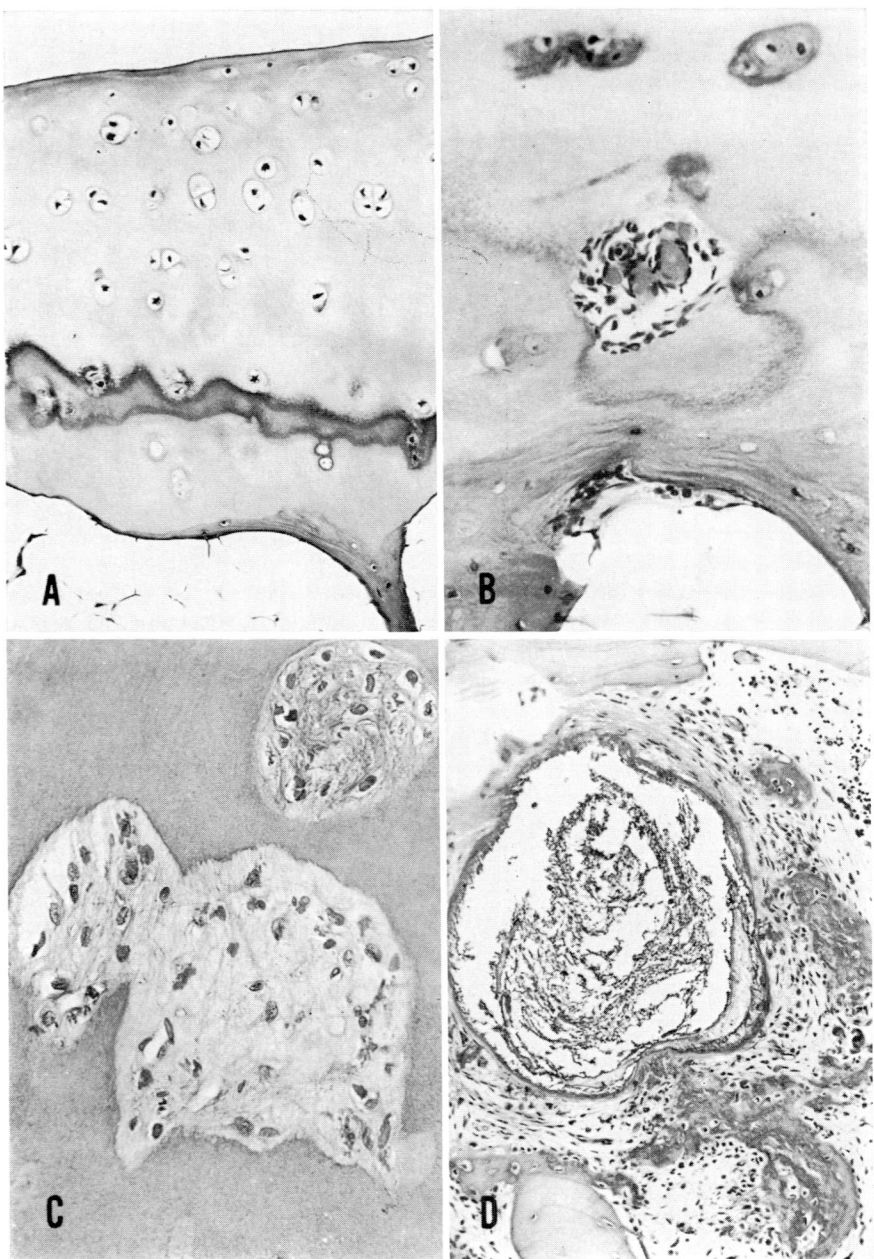

Fig. 87–4. Miscellaneous remodeling and degenerative changes; all sections are stained with hematoxylin and eosin. *A*, Reduplication of calcification "tidemark." (×95) *B*, Vascularization of base of articular cartilage; the dark-stained material in the capsules of the chondrocytes is calcific. (×183) *C*, Weichselbaum's lacunar resorption; small, geographic areas of hyaline cartilage are replaced by loose-textured, cellular fibrous tissue. (×210) *D*, Early subchondral "cystic" degeneration; a small true cyst, filled with mucoid material, has a fibrous border. New bone formation is seen in the adjacent marrow. (×90)

tex (see Fig. 87–1). The sites of predilection for destruction of the joint surface are those subject to greatest load bearing or shearing stress. Earliest fibrillation, however, is often present in regions with presumably low compressive stress, such as the infrafoveal portion of the femoral head. In the patella, the central facets are the sites most prone to erosion.[85] Although not a weight-bearing joint, the patella is subjected to enormous loads by leverage when the knee is flexed, such as while climbing stairs or in the squatting position.

Late Histologic Changes

In fibrillated regions, continuity of the surface of the articular cartilage is disrupted. The height of the fronds is in the range of 20 to 150 μm.[92] Ground-substance metachromasia is reduced, and the matrix has a fibrillary, disheveled appearance. Birefringence of the collagen is increased. Clusters of chondrocytes, long known as ''brood capsules,'' are located close to the margins of the clefts (see Fig. 87–3,*B*). The proliferative and proteoglycan-producing activities of these cells have been amply documented by autoradiography. Little or no collagen is seen within the clones, and it must be presumed that chondrolytic enzymes, including collagenases, have been generated to make room for the new cells (see Chap. 88). Some investigators regard these cellular clusters as doomed to fail and die.[32] Only small segments of necrobiosis are seen, however, and these segments are not necessarily confined to the cell clusters. Focal proliferation of chondrocytes is also seen in deeper areas of disrupted cartilage in severe lesions. The matrix in such lesions has a pale, myxoid appearance.

Mitrovic and others have described *activation* of articular chondrocytes in osteoarthritis; that is, a generalized increase of biosynthetic activity in the same joint even at a distance from overt damage to the tissue.[93] This judgment is based on advanced lesions in which the bulk of the cartilage studied is of a new, immature type. The morphologic character of early lesions indicates that activation is a focal rather than a generalized phenomenon. Reparative cartilage has a mixed hyaline and fibrocartilaginous character. Fibrillary collagen typically is more conspicuous than normal. In osteophytes, much of the covering is fibrocartilaginous, and overt fibrous tissue covers segments of the latter. Variable degrees of secondary degenerative change and fibrillation are superimposed in reparative cartilage. The histochemical features of the matrix, accordingly, are heterogeneous.[24,46]

Reduplication of the tidemark is exaggerated in the vicinity of the fibrillated cartilage and, more remotely, at the margin of the joint. Calcium-containing crystals are deposited in the territorial ma-

trix of the adjacent chondrocytes as forward remodeling occurs. These crystals appear as basophilic granules in demineralized sections (see Fig. 87–4,*B*) and within or around matrix vesicles in electron micrographs.[4,15]

BONE

New bone formation takes place in two separate locations in relation to the joint surface: in exophytic growths at the margins of the articular cartilage and in the immediately subjacent bone marrow (see Fig. 87–2). Marginal osteophytes have two patterns of growth. One is a protuberance into the joint space; the other develops within capsular and ligamentous attachments to the joint margins. In each circumstance, the direction of the osteophyte is governed by the lines of mechanical force exerted on the area of growth and generally corresponds to the contour of the joint surface from which the osteophyte protrudes. The osteophyte consists in large part of bone that merges imperceptibly with the other cortical and cancellous tissue of the subchondral bone. The osteophyte is capped by a layer of hyaline and fibrocartilage, continuous with the adjacent synovial lining. In advanced lesions, the landmarks are obliterated because the osteophyte itself is caught up in the degenerative process. Not only does the proliferative tissue occupy the fovea of the ligamentum teres, but also it extends along the femoral neck to form buttress osteophytes.[70] In most resected specimens, little or no demonstrably native articular cartilage is present.

The proliferation of bone in the subchondral tissue is most marked in areas denuded of their cartilaginous covering.[22,60,103,104] In these regions, the articulating surface consists of bone that has been rubbed smooth. The glistening appearance of this polished sclerotic surface suggests ivory, hence the name *eburnation*. Nubbins of newly proliferated cartilage usually protrude through minute gaps in the eburnated bone.[89] Most of the osteocytes in the eburnated surface undergo necrobiosis, as indicated by empty lacunae. Perhaps this process results from frictional heat. In addition to this alteration, two other variants of new bone formation are also seen in relation to the articular cartilage.

''Cystic'' areas of rarefaction of bone are commonly seen immediately beneath the eburnated surfaces in the hip joint (see Fig. 87–2), but they are much less frequent in other joints. Both femoral and acetabular components are affected. Most often, the lesions are present on the superolateral weight-bearing surface, but in severe instances, they involve other regions of the hip as well.[107] In a few cases, these lesions appear roentgenographically before narrowing of the joint space, which is evidence of cartilage destruction. The lesions only infrequently contain pockets of mucoid fluid and thus are not truly cystic (see Fig. 87–4,D). The trabeculae in the affected areas disappear, and the bone marrow undergoes fibromyxoid degeneration. Fragments of dead bone, cartilage, and amorphous debris are often interspersed within them. In time, the entire area is encircled by a rim of reactive new bone and compact fibrous tissue (see Fig. 87–2). Minute gaps in the overlying articular cortex, resulting from microfractures, are commonly seen at the apex of the pseudocysts (Fig. 87–5). These findings are consistent with an intrusion of pressure, if not of synovial fluid, from the joint cavity through a defect in the articular cortex into the subchondral bone marrow. Intra-articular pressures exceeding 1,000 mm Hg have been calculated to occur in hip joints with effusions. The increased pressure is dissipated radially into the adjacent bone marrow, compresses the medullary

blood vessels, and thereby leads to the retrogressive changes. This mechanism is not contradicted by observations that the intraosseous pressure is not elevated in osteoarthritic femoral heads at the time of arthroplasty.[130] In these specimens, bulk pressures, rather than localized gradients, are measured. Furthermore, internal remodeling compensates for the presumptive pressure gradients. The "punched-out" lesions observed roentgenographically in gout and the bone "cysts" in hemophilic arthropathy correspond pathologically to the pseudocysts in osteoarthritis, except the specific exudates of the former arthropathies also lie within the degenerated bone marrow space.

The other type of new bone formation in this location is a focal ossific metaplasia of the base of the articular cartilage. This metaplasia is part of the remodeling of the joint contour through which bone is added to a portion of the articular cortex, whereas other areas in the joint surface undergo focal resorption. The junction between the articular cartilage and the subchondral plate of bone is occupied by a zone of calcified cartilage. During the years of skeletal growth, the epiphysis and the articular cartilage participate in the enlargement of the bone. During this period, the epiphysis is expanded by endochondral ossification of the calcified cartilage. The interface between calcified and noncalcified hyaline articular cartilage is demarcated in usual histologic preparations by the *tidemark,* which is a thin, wavy hematoxyphil line (see Fig. 87–4,A). In joints of older persons, it is common to find a number of such discontinuous parallel lines in this region. Their presence is clear evidence of progression of calcification of the basal portion of the articular cartilage.[15,57] The possibility that basilar calcification may lead to a thinning of articular cartilage (senile atrophy) has received no support in a recent study.[78]

Much of the deformity in symptomatic osteoarthritis results from collapse of the joint surface. Localized areas of necrosis are seen frequently in this location, and occlusion of minute intramedullary arteries has been demonstrated by angiography. Small secondary infarcts of eburnated bone are seen in approximately 6% of surgically resected femoral heads.[68,87,89] Nevertheless, Streda's suggestion that all osteoarthritis of the hip is secondary to osteonecrosis goes beyond the evidence.[127] The new bone formation of the remodeling process is accompanied by increased vascularity and is the basis for scintigraphic studies using bone-seeking radionuclides in this disorder.[23]

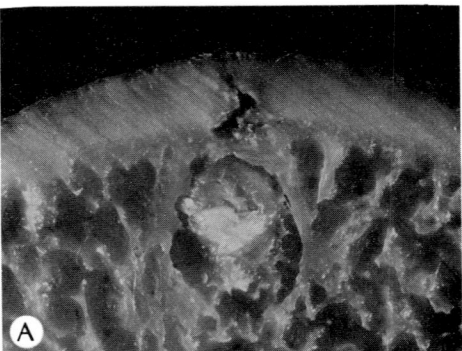

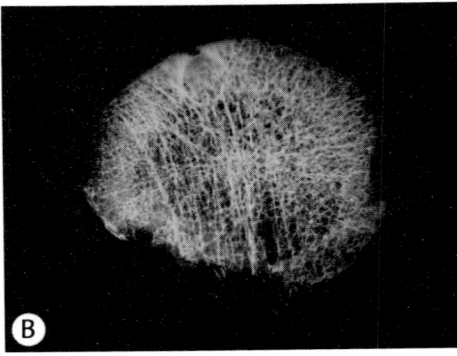

Fig. 87–5. Relationship between a pseudocyst and a microfracture of the subchondral plate. This fortuitous slab section is from a recently fractured femoral head of a 77-year-old woman. Although moderate fibrillation is present elsewhere in the cartilage surface, the sole pseudocyst is located immediately beneath the minute discontinuity in the otherwise intact cartilage and osteochondral junction. A, Gross appearance (approximately ×4); B, Roentgenogram, showing the gap in the subchondral plate and the sclerotic wall of the "cyst."

CHANGES IN SOFT TISSUE

During recent years, the inflammatory aspects of osteoarthritis have aroused discussion.[8,31,54,123]

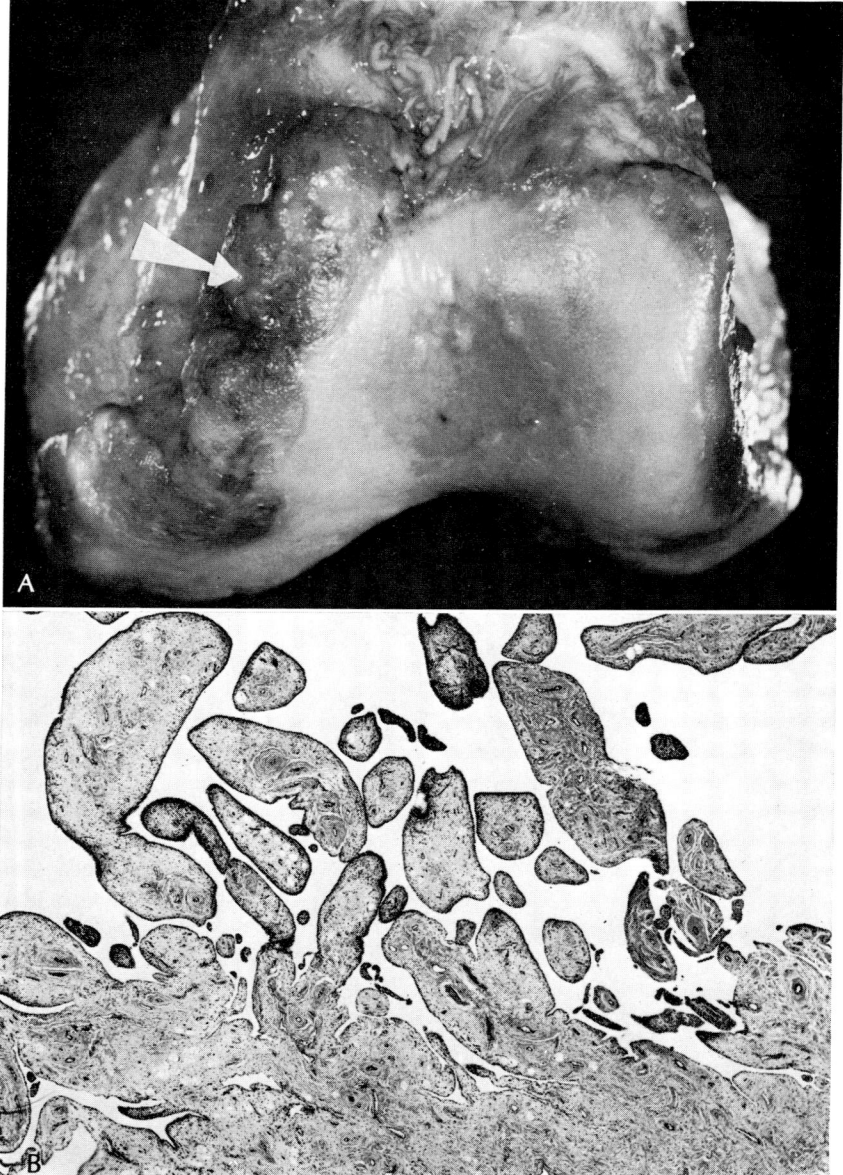

Fig. 87–6. Synovial hypertrophy in severe osteoarthritis. The patient is a 63-year-old man whose left knee had been enlarged for 23 years following an automobile accident. *A,* A massive osteophyte (arrow) is seen at the medial border of the articular surface. The adjacent synovial tissue has undergone prominent papillary thickening. *B,* Histologically, the villous processes are made up of compact fibrous tissue not infiltrated by inflammatory cells. (Hematoxylin and eosin stain, ×16)

Although degenerative joint disease is inherently not inflammatory by definition, villous hypertrophy and fibrosis are the rule in clinically symptomatic cases (Fig. 87–6). Moderate, focal, chronic synovitis is seen in about one-fifth of surgically resected specimens.[87] This synovitis is characterized by hyperplasia and enlargement of lining cells and by mild infiltration of lymphocytes and mononuclear cells. Polyclonal B cells comprise part of the infiltrate, and extracellular deposits of C3 have also been described.[43,49,100] Fibronectin is deposited in exudative foci.[113] Hemosiderin,[96] foreign-body reaction to joint detritus, and even xanthoma-cell aggregation about foci of fat necrosis may be seen.

Occasionally, the inflammation is severe enough to raise the question of RA. Some observers suggest that, in one or more subsets of osteoarthritis, anti-inflammatory medication may be helpful. The inflammatory reaction probably is a secondary phenomenon. It is seen equally in other deforming joint diseases in which no primary phlogistic origin is likely, such as acromegalic arthropathy.[72] Auto-sensitization to joint detritus is an attractive possibility and receives some experimental support from studies in rabbits.[20] Lymphokines are occasionally found in the synovial fluid and constitute supportive evidence for such a mechanism.

Cooke has emphasized the presence of immune complex components in the surface of the cartilage in primary, but not in secondary, osteoarthritis.[27] Doyle relates the inflammation to calcific crystals.[31] Minute quantities of hydroxyapatite and calcium pyrophosphate dihydrate occur both in the synovium and in the synovial fluid (see Chap. 95). Such crystals may arise as part of the basilar remodeling of the cartilage that accompanies the osteoarthritis. Synovitis must be responsible for the effusion as well as some of the accompanying pain. Minute tears in capsular tissue appear as slender, fibrovascular seams disrupting the principal axis of the collagen bundles. Secondary osteochondromatosis occurs only infrequently. The ligamentum teres commonly disintegrates. In the knee joint, cruciate ligaments and menisci also become frayed. Although substantial clinical evidence suggests that meniscectomy leads to osteoarthritis, no correlation has been found in autopsy material between tears or other lesions of the semilunar cartilages and degenerative joint disease.[39] Fibrillation and fibrosis of the synovial surface and even mild cartilaginous metaplasia of patellar tendon occur at times in such cases. Analysis of hand and bilateral knee radiographs of 150 subjects who had undergone unilateral meniscectomy 19 or more years earlier showed a striking correlation between degeneration in the finger joints and in both operated and opposite knees.[30a] Degeneration was more severe on the operated side and was independent of age and sex. This study suggests that the predisposition to primary osteoarthritis influences the development of secondary degeneration and makes a clear distinction between these 2 subsets of the disease more difficult.

Amyloid deposits have been reported in the joint capsule in osteoarthritis, but they also occur in nonosteoarthritic joint capsules, in articular cartilage, and in intra-articular discs of older individuals.[35,51,75,76,131] It may not be entirely gratuitous to question whether green birefringence following alkaline Congo red staining, the usual histochemical method for demonstrating amyloid, is a reliable measure for this material in cartilage.

A progressive increase in the amount of fibrous tissue separating the synovial capillaries from the joint space has been described as an age-related finding, but it is unlikely that this condition interferes with the nourishment of the cartilage. Hyaline sclerosis of minute vessels is a common, although focal, finding in joints even of young individuals that is not directly related to osteoarthritis. Periarticular muscle undergoes atrophy; type 2 myofibers are affected primarily.[116]

COMPARATIVE PATHOLOGIC FEATURES

Osteoarthritis occurs widely in the vertebrate kingdom, regardless of the position of the species in the taxonomic scale.[121] Osteophytic lesions, sometimes leading to ankylosis, were common in certain giant dinosaurs a hundred million years ago. The disorder has been observed in large and small mammals, in animals that swim (cetaceans) rather than bear their weight on their extremities, and also, to a mild degree, in birds. It is of considerable economic importance in livestock commerce, the horse-racing industry, and veterinary practice.

In small laboratory animals, it has been possible to study a number of pathogenetic concepts of degenerative joint disease. The importance of genetic factors has been established in mice.[121,140] The inheritance appears to be polygenic and the overall behavior, recessive. No evidence suggests major sex linkage. Male mice consistently develop more severe osteoarthritis than do females. Obesity is not an important factor.[137] In laboratory rodents, the knee and elbow joints are most commonly severely affected, and the hips rarely. That heritable biochemical defects are major factors in the development of osteoarthritis is indicated by the frequency of osteoarthritic lesions in blotchy (BLO) mice, in which a mutant gene leads to inadequate cross-linking of collagen.[114] In another strain of mouse, STR/ORT, widely studied for its predisposition to degenerative joint disease, Walton attributes osteoarthritis of the knee to spontaneous subluxation of the patella.[138] By containing the subluxation surgically, this investigator prevented the development of the osteoarthritis, and implies that the susceptibility to degenerative joint disease in these animals is due to abnormal mechanical loading rather than to some metabolic peculiarity of the cartilage. These data are impressive, but difficult to reconcile with our observations that lesions in STR/1N mice are not confined to the knee, but are more generalized. The broader principle is that *genetic factors that influence the development of os-*

teoarthritis may operate at many levels, local and generalized, mechanical and metabolic.

The genetic aspect of the disorder is also manifested by the variable susceptibility of different species to its development. Rats, for example, are generally resistant, whereas another rodent, *Mastomys natalensis,* develops severe generalized, degenerative joint disease by the time it is two years old. Genetic contributions also are found in certain breeds of cattle and swine. The fundamental pathogenetic problem is whether these genetic factors are local and articular, related to the configuration and mechanical forces exerted on the joint, as in the dysplastic hips of German shepherd dogs, or whether they are more generalized metabolic properties of the articular tissues.

DEGENERATIVE DISEASE OF THE SPINAL COLUMN

Degenerative changes in the spine affect two discrete intervertebral articular systems: the diarthrodial or apophyseal joints and the synchondroses or intervertebral discs. The term *spinal osteoarthritis* describes the changes in the apophyseal joints, whereas the term *spinal osteophytosis* or *spondylosis deformans* applies to degenerative disc disease. This distinction should not lead to a fundamental dichotomy between the pathologic processes in these two sets of joints. It is common, in the cervical region, to find both lesions, albeit on neighboring rather than the same vertebrae. The pathologic findings in the two sets of joints are similar. The nucleus pulposus becomes fissured and deformed. Fibrillary disintegration of the hyaline cartilage plates, through which the disc is attached to the vertebral bodies, cannot be distinguished histologically from the changes in diarthrodial osteoarthritis. Eburnation of the subchondral bony plate develops in like manner. Marginal osteophytes arise under the mechanical stimulus of horizontal pulsion of the anulus fibrosus and its periosteal attachments attending collapse and spreading out of the nucleus pulposus. Traction forces of spinal muscles on the tendinous insertions in this region also have been implicated in this disorder. These mechanisms are not qualitatively different from those in the more movable joints.

Although the marginal osteophytes develop most often on the anterolateral aspects of the vertebral bodies, posterior osteophytic protrusions also occur and may affect the spinal cord and its roots. In the cervical region, antecedent spondylosis constitutes a principal neurosurgical hazard of injuries among older patients.[141] Osteophytes in the Luschka (uncovertebral, neurocentral) joints have been shown by anatomic and angiographic means to compromise the neighboring vertebral arteries (see Chap.

80). The narrowing of the vascular lumen is most marked during rotation of the head and provides the basis for the posterior cervical sympathetic or *Barre-Lieou* syndrome.

Degenerative joint disease does not characteristically lead to ankylosis; however, in at least three forms of segmental disease of the senescent spine, bony bridges unite the vertebral bodies. The proclivity for ankylosis may be related to the inherent limited mobility of the intervertebral disc.

Hyperostotic Spondylosis

The best-known entity goes by several names: *hyperostotic spondylosis, senile ankylosing hyperostosis of Forestier and Rotés-Querol, spondylorheostosis.* Hyperostotic spondylosis nominally is distinguished from ordinary spondylosis by the absence of disc degeneration.[133] The distal thoracic spine is the site of predilection. The ankylotic bridges are located on the anterolateral portions of the vertebral bodies and extend into the anterior longitudinal ligaments. The appearance has often led to confusion with ankylosing spondylitis, also known as Marie-Strümpell disease. In some instances, at least, the vertebral lesion is accompanied by excessive osteophyte formation in peripheral joints. From this feature comes still another term for this condition, *diffuse idiopathic skeletal hyperostosis* (DISH).[106,132] Currently, no consensus exists on the bounds of the DISH syndrome.

Ankylosis

Ankylosis may accompany severe spondylosis in man and other species (Fig. 87–7). The disc space is narrowed. Destructive changes are present in the cortex of the anterior portion of the vertebral bodies. Dense new bone formation is seen in the anterior longitudinal ligament. The appearance suggests that the ligament is first avulsed from the osteophyte and then is repaired.

Other Segmental Disease

Several patterns of dorsal protrusion and bridging of cervical vertebrae (posterior spondylotic osteophytes) may cause life-threatening cervical myelopathy. The relation of *physiologic vertebral ligamentous ossification* to the preceding disorder and to hyperostotic spondylosis is uncertain. It occurs in 7% of Japanese[97] and 0.3% of U.S. adults.[41] These lesions are asymptomatic in individuals with large spinal canals, but they require surgical decompression when spinal canals are small.

Baastrup's syndrome, an osteoarthritis-like change in the distal portions of "kissing" dorsal spinous processes,[18] is usually associated with se-

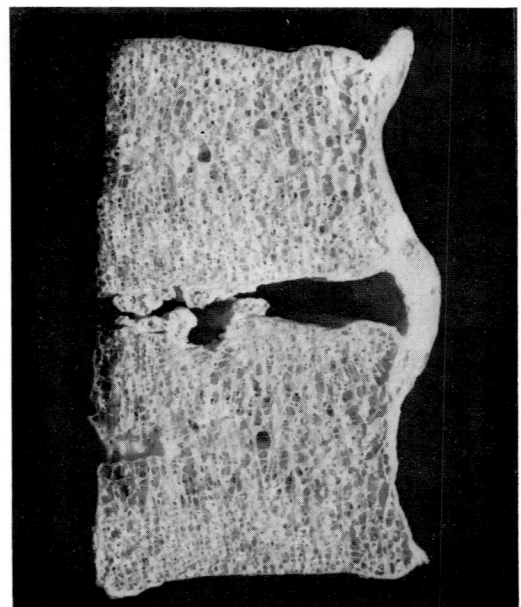

Fig. 87–7. Hyperostotic ankylosing spondylosis in thoracic vertebrae of a 72-year-old man. Unlike the Marie-Strümpell lesion, marked degenerative changes occur in the intervertebral disc: the space between the vertebral bodies is narrowed, and the articular lamella is irregular as a result of both focal resorption and protrusion of new bone into the disc. The cortex on the anterolateral surface of the vertebra (right) has blended with the bony bridge.

vere spondylosis and is primarily of roentgenographic interest.

Degeneration of intervertebral discs takes place normally with aging and apparently is exaggerated in instances of herniation. It is characterized microscopically by a depletion of metachromatic ground substance from the matrix and partial fibrous transformation of the nucleus pulposus. In electron micrographs of herniated nucleus pulposus, the collagen fibers are disorderly and attenuated; the cross-striations are often indistinct, and the periods are shortened. Although swelling of the nucleus pulposus has sometimes been considered to cause acute herniation, evidence suggests that the water content and the swelling pressure of the disc are reduced, rather than increased, in the disorder.[7] The herniation ultimately depends on the development of tears in the anulus fibrosus. The direction of displacement of the nucleus pulposus in quadrupeds differs from that in man. In dogs, for example, displacement often occurs dorsally and, particularly in chondrodysplastic breeds, leads to spinal cord paralysis. In man, the upright posture leads more characteristically to displacement to-

ward the vertebral bodies. The common development of nodules of cartilaginous and fibrous tissue beneath the subchondral plate of the veterbral bodies, the *Schmorl nodes,* is usually attributed to the displacement of nucleus pulposus into the vertebral body.[62] These islands are often surrounded by a shell of bone and, except for their greater content of cartilage, are reminiscent of the subchondral "cysts" in osteoarthritic peripheral joints. Schmorl's nodes are not a particular feature of vertebral osteoporosis.

SPECIAL FORMS OF OSTEOARTHRITIS

Heberden's Nodes

Despite the great frequency of these nodes, little systemic information is available on the morbid anatomic features of these common marginal osteophytes at the base of the distal finger phalanges. In advanced cases, the lesions cannot be distinguished from osteoarthritis in other locations (Fig. 87–8). Some specimens have, however, a different appearance and are of considerable theoretic interest. In these, the articular cartilage, rather than displaying degenerative fibrillation and erosion, is actually hypertrophic. Ossific transformation of the insertion of the tendons into joint capsule and periosteum accounts for the exophytosis. Whether these two forms correspond, as has been suggested,[125] to two clinically different types of Heberden node, the traumatic acquired and the genetically governed, cannot be determined without further clinicopathologic information. In other instances, mucoid transformation of the periarticular fibroadipose tissue is associated with proliferation of myxoid fibroblasts and cyst formation. Hyaluronic acid has been found in the cyst fluid. This finding is not a unique anatomic feature of Heberden nodes. Indistinguishable changes may be present in other osteoarthritic joints in other species. The process has certain morphologic similarities to ganglion formation or to cystic degeneration of the semilunar cartilages and the subchondral pseudocysts of osteoarthritis. Unilateral sparing from Heberden node formation following hemiplegia has been reported on numerous occasions,[53] and this observation suggests the possibility of neurovascular contributions to the development of the lesion without excluding a biomechanical explanation.

The association of the para-articular mucoid cysts ("synovial cysts") of the distal interphalangeal joints with osteophytes has been emphasized because the cysts are likely to recur following excision unless the osteophytes are also removed.[34]

The term "erosive osteoarthritis" has been applied to a disorder resembling osteoarthritis in its predilection for the DIP and PIP joints, but in which

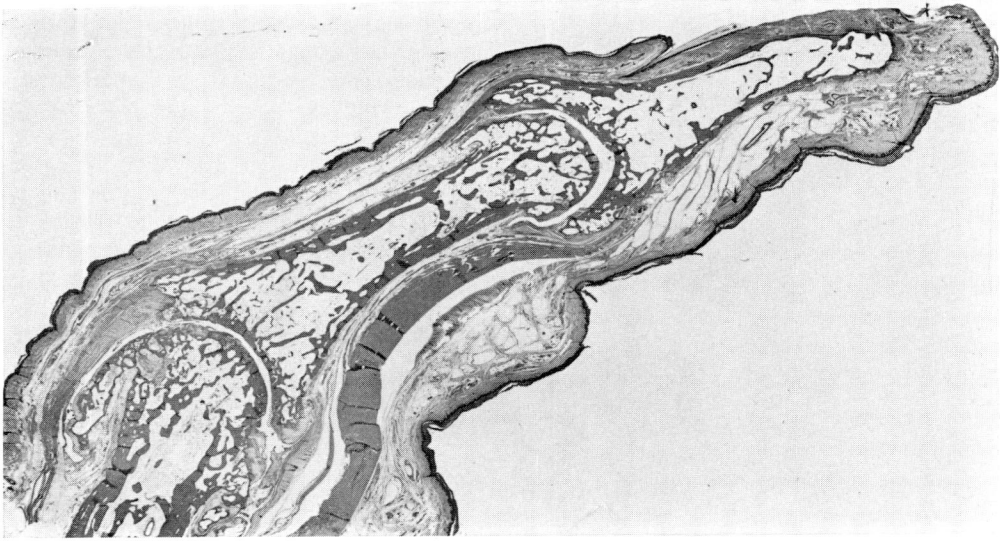

Fig. 87–8. Heberden's node. The articular cartilage has completely disappeared from the surfaces of the distal interphalangeal joint. Bony osteophytes, directed toward the base of the finger, are present on the dorsal and palmar aspects of both articulating surfaces. Advanced osteoarthritic changes also are present in the proximal interphalangeal joint and form a so-called Bouchard node. (Hematoxylin and eosin stain, × 20)

a distinct inflammatory component exists.[134] A nonspecific, chronic, lymphocytic and mononuclear cell infiltrate is present in the synovium. The nosologic status of the disorder is uncertain. One possibility is that this entity represents osteoarthritis with a prominent, detritic synovitis. In a few cases, the lesion is disseminated to other joints and may evolve into RA.[36]* We may therefore be dealing with two separate conditions. Bony ankylosis occurs in rare instances in association with Heberden's nodes.[117]

Primary Generalized Osteoarthritis

The concept of a pattern of primary osteoarthritis affecting multiple joints was first formulated by Kellgren and colleagues.[73] These workers found that Heberden node formation was a conspicuous feature of this disorder, as was involvement of the first carpometacarpal and knee joints; the hip was less often affected. Inflammatory manifestations were common, and the onset often occurred at menopause. Radiologic examination of the joints suggested that the primary events were not erosion of the articular cartilage, but proliferation of adjacent bone. Only limited anatomic material was available to document the nature of the pathologic process.

The status of primary osteoarthritis remains controversial. The pattern is encountered far more often in rheumatologic than in orthopedic practice. The association of Heberden's nodes with osteoarthritis of the hips has been affirmed by some,[30,84,87,126] but denied by others.[143] Discrimination of subsets of osteoarthritis may resolve some of these contradictions. Heberden's nodes, particularly those associated with inflammatory manifestations, more often co-exist with concentric or nondeforming than with deforming osteoarthritis of the hip. This form of hip disease has been referred to by some as postinflammatory,[38,122] whereas others consider it to be part of primary generalized osteoarthritis.[26,84]

Malum Coxae Senilis

A variety of structural abnormalities of the hip joint in childhood, such as congenital dysplasia, Legg-Perthes disease, slipped capital epiphysis, and congenital coxa vara, lead to premature osteoarthritic degeneration. In other patients, however, no precursors are clinically overt. Roentgenographic analysis of the contour of the hip joint has suggested to some investigators that low-grade dysplasia is actually the basis for most of these cases.[128] The validity of this retrospective view may be questionable because subluxation has been documented roentgenographically as a late manifestation of the joint deformity.

---

*Editor's Note: Such patients are generally seronegative and radiologically different from seropositive RA in that osteophyte formation is prominent.

Osteoarthritis Associated with Heritable Articular Diseases

Precocious osteoarthritis develops with great frequency in *multiple epiphyseal dysplasias*. In these rare diseases, epiphyseal growth and maturation of variable portions of the axial and appendicular skeleton are defective.[124] Allison and Blumberg have reported the development of osteoarthritis in patients with a rare form of heritable osteochondrosis of the digits.[5] The *nail-patella syndrome (hereditary osteo-onychodysplasia, Turner-Kieser syndrome, iliac horn syndrome)* is also frequently complicated by osteoarthritis. The hereditary component of *congenital dysplasia of the hip* has been argued several ways. In dogs, evidence seems to support a significant genetic contribution to the disorder because certain breeds, such as German shepherds, commonly develop it, whereas others, such as American greyhounds, do not. Shepherd dogs are also prone to dysplasia and secondary osteoarthritis of the elbows.

Chondromalacia Patellae

This term is used loosely to describe a clinically distinctive, post-traumatic softening of the articular cartilage of the patella in young persons (see Chap. 78). It is usually difficult to distinguish the anatomic lesions from those of early osteoarthritis. Subtle differences have been described by some authors. The changes are not confined to the cartilage, but also involve subchondral bone.[1,56] Softening, swelling, and an increased water content of the cartilage have been reported in early chondromalacia. These changes presumably result from localized dehiscence of the collagen in the cartilage.

Charcot Joints

The morphology of neuropathic arthropathies varies with the duration and underlying sensory defect.[13] Extensive dentritic synovitis is characteristic and may be accompanied by secondary osteochondromatosis. Advanced lesions resemble severe osteoarthritis in which the destructive and hypertrophic elements are exaggerated by trauma. The often postulated primary role of neurovascular reflexes on the para-articular circulation has received some support from experimental studies.[40] In the diabetic foot, currently the most frequent form of Charcot joint, landmarks of tarsal bones are often obliterated.[102] The pattern thus differs from the characteristically nonankylosed lesions in other joints and may reflect inflammatory complications in the diabetic foot (see Chap. 71).

Associated Osteonecrosis

A considerable literature describes osteoarthritis as a late sequela of bone infarction (see also Chap.

86). The epiphyseal ends of the bones are involved primarily in osteonecrosis. Articular cartilage, deriving nutrition from synovial fluid, does not become infarcted, whereas the subchondral bone does. Nevertheless, weakening of the bony support of the joint over the course of a year or so leads to mechanical fracture and collapse of the joint surface. Proliferative remodeling results in variable osteophyte formation. In late stages of this disorder, the articular cartilage is sloughed off, and the apposed articulating member remodels. In some patients, overt osteoarthritis ensues, but eburnation is ordinarily inconspicuous. Evidence suggests that when osteonecrosis is associated with osteoarthritis of the hip, the arthritis is the primary and the necrosis is the secondary event.[68,87,89] Thus, ischemic necrosis of bone must be an infrequent cause of osteoarthritis.

"Gonarthrosis," supervening on a special form of osteonecrosis of the medial femoral condyle, is a frequent finding in elderly persons.[10] Clinical onset is sudden, and the initial event may be segmental fracture with depression of the articular cortex. Norman and Baker have associated this disorder with a torn medial meniscus.[95] Osteoarthritis has been described as a late consequence, but the available data are not persuasive. When segmental infarction occurs in osteoarthritic knee specimens,[3] it probably is a secondary phenomenon, as in the hip.

Osteonecrosis is a common occupational disease in sandhogs, pearl divers, and submariners. Dysbaric release of dissolved gases from the adipose tissue in the bone marrow is responsible for the death of bone tissue. Despite this association, a history of "bends" (caisson disease) often cannot be elicited. Several cases of authentic osteoarthritis have been reported, but in most published accounts, eburnation has not been documented.

Gout

The articular lesions of gout are related to the deposition of monosodium urate monohydrate crystals in or about the joint tissues (see Chaps. 91 and 93). The form that these lesions take varies with the amount, location, and duration of the deposits. Aside from massive disorganization of the articular structures by tophaceous deposits, the most common lesion is osteoarthritis. Urate crystals are deposited not only on and in the surface of the articular cartilage, but also in the subchondral cysts, where they constitute the so-called "punched-out" lesions. In the areas of crystal deposition in the cartilage, chondrocytes are characteristically necrotic, and the matrix is exceptionally oxyphilic.

Ochronotic Arthropathy

The articular and spinal lesions associated with alkaptonuria are similar to those of degenerative joint disease (see Chap. 96). External remodeling is less prominent than in ordinary osteoarthritis.[77] The hyaline articular cartilage and the nucleus pulposus become discolored by the ochronotic pigment, and their material properties are grossly altered. These structures become remarkably brittle despite a normal water content. Necrosis of chondrocytes is more conspicuous than in degenerative joint disease. Splitting off of fragments of the brittle cartilage is much more evident in ochronotic than in nonochronotic osteoarthritis, and these fragments may be found in joint fluid (see Chap. 4). With these exceptions, the processes are similar. Although "calcification" of the nucleus pulposus is frequently described in ochronosis, probably ossific replacement of degenerated, pigmented tissue, is seen, rather than calcium deposition in the disc. Furthermore, the radiologically recognized, so-called "loose bodies" in the peripheral joints actually represent a reactive polypoid, secondary osteochondromatous response of the synovial tissue to the articular detritus. Both calcium pyrophosphate and basic calcium phosphate (apatite) crystals have been identified in ochronotic cartilage (see Chaps. 94, 95, and 96).

Endemic Osteoarthritis

Special types of noninflammatory deforming joint disease occur frequently in several parts of the world. These disorders share several features with generalized osteoarthritis, but they are distinguished from the latter by, among other things, stunted growth. Despite extensive research, their cause is obscure. These diseases are discussed in the following paragraphs.

Kashin-Beck Disease

This disease, also known as endemic osteoarthrosis deformans, is common in parts of eastern Siberia, Manchuria, and northern China. The changes are not present at birth and develop with variable severity in different individuals. To some observers, the clinical features indicate that the basic problem resides in the growth plate, and articular cartilage is subsequently damaged nonspecifically.[9] Available histologic data show, however, that articular cartilage shares with the growth plate a focal, apparently episodic, necrosis of chondrocytes.[25] For many years, the predominant Soviet view has been that Kashin-Beck disease results from poisoning by a fungal toxin. Contemporary Chinese investigators more often attribute the condition to a dietary deficiency of selenium.

Mseleni Disease

This arthropathy is endemic in northern Zululand.[33] It resembles multiple epiphyseal dysplasia, but genetic investigations fail to support its heritability. The hip is particularly susceptible to the disease, and total joint replacements have been successful. The lesions in the resected femoral heads differ from those of ordinary osteoarthritis in that the joint surface is covered by a heterogeneous regenerated and degenerated cartilage. Eburnation is conspicuously absent in the material we have examined. du Toit also cites a little-known endemic osteoarthritis in southern India, Handigodu disease, which bears some resemblance to the preceding disease.[33]

Hemophilic Arthropathy

The joint disease that complicates the hemophilias may also be regarded as a variation of osteoarthritis. Erosion of articular cartilage occurs early and is accompanied by eburnation and marginal osteophyte formation. The subchondral pseudocysts are filled with hemorrhagic material, but otherwise are analogous to those of degenerative joint disease. Although hemosiderin deposition in synovial tissue reaches great proportions, only minute quantities are found in articular chondrocytes.[65,108] How the iron enters the chondrocytes is unknown because excessive iron is not detectable in the matrix. The pathogenesis of the cartilage destruction is not understood, although it obviously is related to the articular hemorrhages (see also Chap. 74).

Two general hypotheses are entertained currently: (1) elaboration of chondrolytic enzymes by hemosiderin-laden synovial cells;[83] and (2) damage to the cartilage by toxic products of hemoglobin degradation. For example, free radicals, generated from ionic hemoglobin-derived iron, may damage the cartilage. The iron may also chelate with proteoglycans and may thereby alter the elastic properties of the matrix.[65,108] In advanced lesions, destruction of the joint passes beyond osteoarthritic limits; disintegration and fibrous ankylosis are then seen.

CHEMICAL CHANGES

The biochemistry of osteoarthritis has made rapid strides in recent years and is reviewed in Chapter 88. Several comments from the perspective of the pathologist are necessary to avoid making erroneous conclusions from the chemical findings. These comments principally concern problems of sampling and a discrimination between changes associated with osteoarthritis and those simply related to chronologic age in the cartilage.

Living tissue is required for studies involving incorporation of metabolic tracers or in vitro culture. Surgically resected femoral heads are most often used. Major discrepancies in published data have arisen from the sampling of reparative rather than degenerated native cartilage. How else does one account for the disparity in the biochemical data of Santer et al.,[111] based on cartilage obtained at routine necropsy, with data from numerous reports (reviewed in the following chapter) based on cartilage taken from surgically resected specimens? A warning concerning the use of fractured femoral heads as a source of control cartilage is also in order because this tissue undergoes secondary changes following the injury.[63]

Changes should be studied in articular rather than in other types of cartilage because important biologic differences exist among various types of cartilage. For example, the vascularity, amianthoid degeneration,[66] and pigmentation that occur in adult costal cartilage are not characteristic of old articular cartilage.[118] Although the costal cartilage of human adults has approximately 20% less water by weight than that of children, the difference in patellar cartilage is only about 2% less. Corresponding differences are found in the histochemical, elastic, and chemical properties of the two tissues.

Even within a single joint, areas that are fibrillated or are otherwise disintegrated differ from those that are not. It is therefore necessary to denote as aging changes only those found in the intact portions of such cartilage.

REPAR OF ARTICULAR CARTILAGE AND POTENTIAL REVERSIBILITY

The persistent erosion of articular cartilage in osteoarthritis has long aroused interest in the limited ability of this tissue to grow. By all aspects studied, the metabolic activity of hyaline cartilage is low. In general, experimentally induced gaps in articular cartilage show little tendency to be filled in with new cartilage, as long as they do not penetrate into the subchondral vascular bone marrow. These observations provide the basis for the common view that the inability of cartilage to repair itself is responsible for the irreversible development of osteoarthritis.

A number of reasons for re-examining the validity of this concept exist. The cornerstone of the wear-and-tear theory of degenerative joint disease is a putative inability of articular chondrocytes to undergo mitotic division. Nevertheless, these cells, isolated from mature individuals, divide, grow, and synthesize phenotypic glycosaminoglycans and collagen under proper conditions of culture in vitro.[119] The clue to this process is the release of the chondrocytes from their imprisoning matrix by enzymatic means. The matrix thus serves ordinarily

to switch off the cell-replicative mechanism. The clones of chondrocytes illustrated in Figure 87–3 are analogous to the in vitro cell division previously described. Autoradiographic studies demonstrate that the proliferating cells in osteoarthritis not only incorporate thymidine as a precursor of DNA synthesis,[59,64] but also show an increased rather than a diminished uptake of sulfate.[88] The rate of repair of articular cartilage by this mechanism is low, but it may not be negligible over time.

A more obtrusive mechanism of repair exists, that is, formation of new cartilage from pluripotential granulation tissue in subchondral bone marrow. The experimental data,[21,44] as well as the morphologic features of osteoarthritis already described, illustrate this mechanism. Surgical experience offers two sorts of limited evidence relevant to this potential for restoring the joint surface. First, following arthroplasties in which devitalized tissue is removed, a new articular surface forms beneath the prosthesis. The metallic device presumably protects the reparative granulation tissue from mechanical abrasion. Most such reparative tissue is bony and fibrous,[91] but foci of hyaline and fibrocartilaginous metaplasia also are seen.[118] Second, wedge osteotomies and other procedures designed to relieve mechanical stresses on osteoarthritic hips have frequently widened the radiologic joint space. Although much of the radiologic change may be an artifact caused by the repositioning of the weight-bearing surface, in a few, well-documented anatomic instances, fibrocartilaginous recovering of the joint surface has been noted.

EXPERIMENTAL INDUCTION

Numerous efforts have been made to establish possible mechanisms in the pathogenesis of degenerative joint disease through induction of osteoarthritis by diverse local manipulations,[2] as discussed in the following paragraphs.

Surgical Discontinuity in the Articular Surface

Although the literature on the subject is not wholly consistent, minute defects in the articular cartilage generally do not result in osteoarthritis. On the other hand, larger defects, which deform the joint contour, may.

Physical or Chemical Injury to Articular Cartilage

Heat, freezing,[115] and traumatic insults to the cartilage may also cause osteoarthritis. Necrosis of chondrocytes and associated degenerative changes have also been induced by the topical application of caustic agents. Synovitis, induced by intra-articular instillation of acids or other irritants or infectious materials, may also be accompanied by certain osteoarthritic changes, but these same agents may act on the cartilage as well as on the synovium.

Subluxations and Luxations

Protracted displacements of the patella and of the hip have resulted in early remodeling and in later degenerative changes in the articular tissues.

Instability

Surgical disruption of the cruciate ligaments or partial excision of the menisci result in the rapid development of lesions that are frequently used as experimental models of osteoarthritis.

Prolonged Compression

When the articular cartilages remain compressed for even a few days, death of chondrocytes may be followed by the development of osteoarthritis. Under these circumstances, the compression is presumed to hinder the normal percolation of interstitial fluid on which the nutrition of the chondrocytes depends.

Restriction of Joint Motion

Altered mobility is often associated with changes in the loading of joints. Failure to distinguish between the two phenomena accounts for some of the contradictions in the literature. Older studies indicated that experimental restriction of motion leads to degenerative changes with varying similarities to osteoarthritis, but Palmoski et al. found that motion in the absence of weight-bearing does not maintain normal articular cartilage.[98] Immobilization itself leads to reversible depletion of aggregatable proteoglycan. In humans immobilized for prolonged periods by paralysis or by other means, contracture and fibrous ankylosis occur, rather than osteoarthritis.[37]

Impulsive Loading

Minor degenerative changes have been produced in rabbit joints by repetitive-impact forces. These findings support the contention that the destruction of cartilage in osteoarthritis results from compressive insults to subchondral bone, rather than from shearing of the surface cartilage.

Foreign Body Abrasion

Degenerative changes in the superficial layer of articular cartilage have resulted from the intra-articular instillation of carborundum. These particles, like cartilage detritus, also evoke a foreign-body reaction in the synovium and joint capsule. Ex-

ostoses develop in the vicinity of the attachments of the joint capsule to the articular surface.

Injection of Chondrolytic Enzymes

Intra-articular injection of papain into rabbits causes degenerative changes in articular cartilage associated with low-grade synovitis, and then eburnation of the surface.

It thus appears that a variety of procedures that impair the viability of articular chondrocytes and the integrity of the collagenous framework can lead to osteoarthritic changes. The procedures placing abnormal mechanical stresses on the cartilage also evoke structural remodeling of the joint contours.

PATHOGENESIS

With this background, we can attempt to formulate some concepts on the nature of osteoarthritis.

Primary versus Secondary Osteoarthritis

Osteoarthritis often supervenes on a pre-existing structural abnormality of joints. Such instances are classified as secondary, in contradistinction to primary osteoarthritis, in which no traumatic origin or predisposition can be assigned. In primary osteoarthritis, intrinsic aging or other alteration of the articular tissue is presumed to underlie development of the disease. The previously noted paucity of external remodeling in ochronotic or postinflammatory arthropathies is consistent with the idea that cartilage damage is responsible for concentric osteoarthritis, whereas biomechanical overloading is responsible for the common varieties in which one sees much joint deformity. The localization of the areas of greatest joint-space narrowing in the hip, such as the superolateral or medial area, and the configuration of osteophytes have been proposed as guides to a particular etiologic abnormality in roentgenograms,[52] as well as in excised specimens.[105] In surgically resected femoral heads, however, the changes are usually so far advanced and so diverse that it is difficult to sustain these interpretations.[87] Stulberg et al. are confident that they can identify a structural basis for at least 85% of cases of osteoarthritis of the hip.[128] They speculate that the bulk of osteoarthritis in other joints is also of a secondary type. Other workers report a much lower percentage and recognize primary osteoarthritis as a valid and frequent entity.[27,84,87,122] The recent study of Doherty et al., previously cited, complicates the traditional classification of osteoarthritis as either "primary" or "secondary."[30a]

Does Osteoarthritis Begin Primarily in the Bone or in Cartilage?

If the view that the earliest events in osteoarthritis take place in articular cartilage is correct, then the bony remodeling results from the loss of energy-absorbing function of the cartilage. Transmission of mechanical forces to more labile para-articular tissues transduces the abortive attempts at repair. A different view emphasizes primary alteration in the bone. One formulation is that growth does not completely cease at the articular ends of bones in the adult; furthermore, remodeling takes place, under the aegis of functional demand, independently of degeneration of the cartilage.[15] Accordingly, only when the rate of remodeling exceeds that of orderly cartilage repair would osteoarthritis develop. Evidence supporting the view that bony changes underlie the deterioration of the cartilage includes the following: (1) articular cartilage is so much thinner than the length of bone that it has little measurable impact-absorbing function; (2) in experimental and clinical lesions, microfractures and sclerosis of subchondral trabeculae precede measurable changes in the cartilage; and (3) the cartilage is mechanically more susceptible to disintegration by impact-loading than by shearing stresses.[101]

Ordinarily, the degree of osteophyte formation corresponds to that of cartilage damage, but such is not always the case. Osteophytes themselves are not reliable indicators of the prognosis of osteoarthritis in the hip or knee.[61] Nevertheless, even in early osteoarthritis of the hip with joint-space narrowing, marginal osteophytosis is present.[142] This finding corresponds with the experimental data of Gilbertson described earlier.[50]

In the absence of more-definitive methods for resolving these divergent concepts, it seems useful to attempt to reconcile them: both are likely true and are intimately related to each other. This formulation denies neither the possible role of metabolic factors in deterioration of the cartilage nor the significance of mechanical factors in inducing or treating osteoarthritis. The relative importance of the cartilage degeneration to bone remodeling may, of course, vary in different joints and in the different types of osteoarthritis.

Systemic Contributions

These factors include age, metabolic and genetic influences, and obesity, among others.

Age

An outstanding feature of degenerative joint disease is its relation to age. As an etiologic factor, senescence can have two different meanings. It may simply represent a series of cumulative insults to the articular tissue or, more biologically, it may suggest time-dependent molecular alterations that take place independent of acquired lesions. In the case of the articular cartilage, for example, a long-protracted, low-grade thermal degradation of the collagen or interaction of the collagen with cross-linking metabolites might represent such a biologic aging of cartilage. Dehydration does not occur as a progressive phenomenon of aging in articular cartilage. Chemical alterations presumably would change the biomechanical properties of the cartilage on which its functional integrity depends.

One way in which to assess the contribution of aging is to compare the severity of the clinically obtrusive lesions with the changes found in a general, aging population.[19] A quantitative time curve of the severity of degenerative joint disease in routine necropsies is not readily obtained. The available data are limited, but they indicate that the deterioration of the joint surfaces progresses linearly with age.[118] The slope is greater in the patellofemoral than in the hip joint. The changes in surgically resected specimens fall far outside the scatter in the natural history of the aging hip. This finding suggests that some local or systemic factors aside from aging itself are of major etiologic importance, at least in the hip.[17]

Metabolic Factors

Other differences in the occurrence of osteoarthritis have aroused speculation about systemic modifying factors. Ochronotic arthropathy is a striking prototype of a metabolic factor. We can easily conceive of metabolic patterns of degenerative joint disease that remain unknown because the metabolites are colorless. Endocrine factors have been invoked. The arthropathy complicating acromegaly is an extreme example of damage to articular cartilage by somatotropin, through somatomedin-induced stimulation.[72] In one report, fasting levels of growth hormone were higher in patients with primary osteoarthritis than in control subjects.[30] Little convincing evidence suggests that thyroidal dysfunction plays a role in human degenerative joint disease. In addition to favoring neurogenic arthropathy, diabetes mellitus has been found to predispose patients to the development of degenerative joint disease.[136] Although gonadal hormones contribute to osteoarthritis in mice, menopausal changes probably do not affect the development of osteoarthritic lesions. Osteoarthritis of the hip, however, is twice as frequent in women as in men.

Genetic Factors

Genetic factors that contribute to osteoarthritis in other species may have systemic, metabolic, or, as in the case of the dysplasias, simply local effects on the joint disease. In man, one investigation has yielded evidence of a genetic influence on the development of Heberden's nodes. The data were interpreted as indicating involvement of a single gene; its behavior in females appeared to be dominant, whereas it was recessive in males.[125] This type of inheritance is different from that described previously in mice. In another study in man, degenerative joint disease of other peripheral and spinal joints also gave evidence of genetic influence, but of a recessive, polygenic type.[73] Several remarkable familial occurrences of chondromalacia patellae have also suggested heritable factors.

Obesity

Obesity has generally been accepted as a definite contributory factor because it seems self-evident that excessive weight imposes a mechanical burden on the joints undergoing abrasion. Several studies indicate that the situation is not so simple. In mice, obesity itself does not have an important, harmful effect on osteoarthritis.[120,137] Obesity does not contribute to the formation of Heberden's nodes,[125] nor apparently to osteoarthritis of the hip.[71,112] Some reports affirm a degree of correlation between overweight and degenerative disease of the knee,[80] whereas others deny this association.[55,94] In certain epidemiologic studies, osteoarthritis and spondylosis were more common in obese persons than in those of normal weight.[79] In these studies, the affected joints were not necessarily those that bear weight, and the contribution of overloading was unclear. Perhaps the impact of obesity was greater on the symptomatic than the anatomic expressions of osteoarthritis.[71]

Ligamentous Laxity

In addition to congenital dysplasia of the hip, a variety of postural abnormalities of joints associated with laxness of the ligamentous structures also predispose patients to osteoarthritis. These abnormalities include recurrent luxations of the patella and shoulder, genu recurvatum or back-knee, and genu valgum or knock-knee. Laxness has been described as a feature of several systemic disorders, including Ehlers-Danlos and Marfan's syndromes. Howorth observed that general relaxation of the ligaments is common in children growing up in New York City, but not in youngsters in many less-privileged parts of the world.[67] Whether this finding reflects different genetic substrates or is an untoward acquired consequence of urban life remains to be determined.

"Unmasking" of Collagen

One feature common to osteoarthritic alteration of joint cartilage, degeneration of intervertebral discs, and senescent change in costal cartilage is a diminution of chondroitin sulfate content relative to the collagen in the matrix. This chemical change has its histologic counterpart in the depletion of metachromatic ground substance and in a more conspicuous fibrillary appearance under polarized light. One would anticipate that this change would alter the material properties of the cartilage with respect to wear and tear: the matrix sol ordinarily dissipates applied stresses hydrostatically. In the absence of such protection, flexural and torsional forces might lead the unmasked collagen fibrils to rupture. Several processes probably are involved. Enzymatic mechanisms for selective removal of proteoglycan are reviewed in Chapter 88. Escape of interfibrillar components must be facilitated by disruption of the collagen. It has also been suggested that excessive percolation of fluid associated with vascularization of the base of the cartilage may enhance the leaching process. Another contributor may be synthesis of collagen types not usually found in cartilage. Minute amounts of abnormal (type I) collagen have been found by immunohistochemical means in the immediate vicinity of some chondrocytes in osteoarthritic cartilage.[45]

Mechanical Factors

Medicolegal agencies deal constantly with occupational injuries as mechanical factors in osteoarthritis. In many publications on this subject opinions differ widely. The type of loading, for example, sustained rather than impulsive, does not itself account for the disparities of the findings. Osteoarthritis of the elbow has been observed in foundry workers who use long tongs to lift hot metals and so exert great leverage on this joint. Some investigators affirm,[12] and others deny,[16] that vibratory pressure causes osteoarthritis in the hands and arms of pneumatic drill workers. The occurrence of osteoarthritis of the hip is less among long-distance runners than in the general population; on the other hand, retired soccer players had more radiologically visible osteoarthritis of the hips than an age- and weight-matched control group.[74] Single injuries probably do not cause osteoarthritis unless they are severe enough to disorganize the joint surface or its major stabilizing components (see Fig. 87–6).

It is not known whether articular cartilage turns over normally through desquamation of its surface layer. Electron-microscopic studies have not disclosed a progressive death of cells proceeding toward the tangential layer. Evidence for mechanical abrasion of the cartilage in osteoarthritis is provided by the anatomic findings in the joint surface and by the demonstration of shards of cartilage in the synovial fluid. Information on the mechanics of such changes is sparse.

The articular cartilage of animal joints that is

oscillated in vitro in the absence of synovial fluid undergoes rapid frictional destruction. Instillation of testicular hyaluronidase also leads to in vitro scoring of the joint surface. Although the results of this second group of experiments suggested that depolymerization of synovial mucin accounted for the friction, it is possible that the hyaluronidase may also have acted on the cartilage. Recently developed concepts of lubrication make untenable the widely accepted views of the importance of the viscosity of synovial fluid in maintaining the low friction.[28,82]

The volume, hyaluronate content, and relative viscosity of synovial fluid are usually normal in osteoarthritis and may even be greater than normal. Several studies have shown diminished polymerization of synovial mucin in osteoarthritis, as measured by the intrinsic and dynamic viscosities, as well as a reduction of the hyaluronate content.[120] The contradictory data arise in part because truly normal synovial fluids are not readily obtained for comparison. Synovial fluid obtained at necropsy differs from that aspirated clinically because the clinical specimen is often complicated by synovitis.

The principal contribution of synovial fluid to joint lubrication, other than the simple supply of water and salts to the cartilage, is the provision of a specific lubricating glycoprotein,[129] which adheres to the cartilage surface and makes it slippery. Using a synthetic bearing test system, no deficiency in the boundary-lubricating ability of synovial fluid has been found in degenerative joint disease.[29]

The stresses on diarthrodial joints have never been measured directly. Rough estimates have been made in artificial models,[110] as well as through analyses of the forces between the feet and the ground, in concert with the rate and magnitude of excursion of the center of gravity of the body during walking.[99] The computation of moments from roentgenograms provides a clinical approximation of the distribution and magnitude of compressive loading of the hip and knee and underlies the design for osteotomy in the surgical treatment of osteoarthritis. Direct measurement of the stress in intervertebral discs has been made in vivo and in vitro.[7] The nucleus pulposus, through its hydrostatic properties, distributes the loads uniformly on the surrounding tissues. This purpose is effectively preserved even in the presence of moderate degenerative changes in the disc; only in severe disease is the hydrostatic function of the disc decreased.

The elastic properties and the strength of the articular cartilage are important factors governing its resistance to wear. The elasticity is determined largely by the water-binding capacity of the matrix. Neither the water content nor the elasticity, meas-

ured either as stiffness or recovery from a standard deformation, is altered in aging, as long as fibrillation is absent.[120]

The stiffness of the underlying bone has also been considered in relation to the development of degenerative joint disease. Although osteoporosis and osteoarthritis affect the same age groups, no association exists between these two common senescent processes. Indeed, osteoporosis seems to militate against development of the joint disease.[30,42] Considerable veterinary evidence suggests that metabolic states in which mineralized bone is insufficient may adversely affect the articular cartilage.[121] The arthropathy that complicates hyperparathyroidism may, in part, reflect a lack of mechanical support from the subchondral, articular lamella.[120] This interpretation is complicated by the additional joint lesions: infractions of the surface and calcification of the cartilage. The obverse bone disease, osteopetrosis, also favors premature osteoarthritic degeneration.[90] The excessive stiffness of the bone may interfere with the normal nutritive movement of fluid in the cartilage during joint function.

In Paget's disease, the pathologic process sometimes extends into the base of the articular cartilage and wrinkles its surface. Mixed patterns of Paget's disease and osteoarthritis are frequently present in the hip.[6,109] Protrusio acetabuli develops in approximately 25% of such patients.

PATHOLOGIC BASIS OF CLINICAL COMPLAINTS

A general correlation exists between the clinical features and the anatomic manifestations of peripheral degenerative joint disease.[58,71] Patients' complaints fall into two groups: pain and loss of motion. The sources of pain include synovitis, localized circulatory disturbances associated with subchondral microfractures, capsular tears, and impingement of the deformed bony structures on adjacent soft tissues. Loss of mobility must be attributed to the abnormal configuration of the joints, to muscle atrophy, and to capsular fibrosis. Anterolateral osteophytes in lumbosacral spondylosis are quite asymptomatic. Spurs located close to the neural foramina do, however, account for radicular pain.

CONCLUDING REMARKS

In conclusion, we have progressed in recent years in our understanding of the pathogenesis of osteoarthritis, as in other fields of rheumatic disease. This progress has largely taken the form of inquiry into an area of disease formerly regarded as incomprehensible to the pathologist and hopeless for the patient. Apparently divergent biomechanical and biochemical concepts of the nature of the lesions seem to reaffirm an interdependence between the wear-and-tear process and the metabolic state of the articular tissues.[120] The pathologic findings should not be interpreted as proof that degenerative joint disease is an inevitable concomitant of aging or that the lesions have no biologic potential for reversibility. By the same token, clinical trials of medications for osteoarthritis, based on the biologic features of articular cartilage, are premature and are conceivably hazardous.[69]

REFERENCES

1. Abernethy, P.J., et al.: Is chondromalacia patellae a separate clinical entity? J. Bone Joint Surg., 60B:205–210, 1978.
2. Adams, M.E., and Billingham, M.E.: Animal models of degenerative joint disease. Curr. Top. Pathol., 71:265–297, 1982.
3. Ahuja, S.A., and Bullough, P.G.: Osteonecrosis of the knee: a clinicopathological study in twenty-eight patients. J. Bone Joint Surg., 60A:191–197, 1978.
4. Ali, S.Y.: Matrix vesicles and apatite nodules in arthritic cartilage. In Perspectives in Inflammation. Edited by D.A. Willoughby, J.P. Giroud, and G.P. Velo. Baltimore, University Park Press, 1978, pp. 211–223.
5. Allison, A.C., and Blumberg, B.S.: Familial osteoarthropathy of the fingers. J. Bone Joint Surg., 40B:538–545, 1958.
6. Altman, R.D., and Collins, B.: Musculoskeletal manifestations of Paget's disease of bone. Arthritis Rheum., 23:1121–1127, 1980.
7. Andersson, G.B.J.: Measurements of loads on the lumbar spine. In American Academy of Orthopaedic Surgeons Symposium on Low Back Pain. Edited by A.A. White, III, and S.L. Gordon. St. Louis, C.V. Mosby, 1982, pp. 220–251.
8. Arnoldi, C.C., Reimann, I., and Bretlau, P.: The synovial membrane in human coxarthrosis. Light and electron microscope studies. Clin. Orthop., 148:213–220, 1979.
9. Basilevksaja, Z.V.: Pathogenese orthopädischer Deformitäten bei der Kaschin-Beckschen Krankheit (Osteoarthrosis endemica deformans). Beitr. Orthop. Traumatol., 26:427–433, 1979.
10. Bauer, G.C.H.: Osteonecrosis of the knee. Clin. Orthop., 130:210–217, 1978.
11. Bennett, G.A., Waine, H., and Bauer, W.: Changes in the Knee Joint at Various Ages. New York, Commonwealth Fund, 1942.
12. Bovenzi, M., Petronio, L., and Di Marino, F.: Epidemiological survey of shipyard workers exposed to hand-arm vibration. Int. Arch. Occup. Environ. Health, 46:251–266, 1980.
13. Brower, A.C., and Allman, R.M.: The neuropathic joint: a neurovascular bone disorder. Radiol. Clin. North Am., 19:571–580, 1981.
14. Bullough, P.G.: The geometry of diarthrodial joints, its physiological maintenance and the possible significance of age-related changes in geometry to load distribution and the development of osteoarthritis. Clin. Orthop., 156:61–66, 1981.
15. Bullough, P.G., and Jagannath, A.: The morphology of the calcification front in articular cartilage. J. Bone Joint Surg., 65B:72–78, 1983.
16. Burke, M.D., Fear, E.C., and Wright, V.: Bone and joint changes in pneumatic drillers. Ann. Rheum. Dis., 36:276–279, 1977.
17. Byers, P.D., Contempomi, C.A., and Farkas, T.A.: Postmortem study of the hip joint. III. Correlations between observations. Ann. Rheum. Dis., 35:122–126, 1976.
18. Bywaters, E.G.L.: The pathology of the spine. In The Joints and Synovial Fluid. Vol. 2. Edited by L. Sokoloff. New York, Academic Press, 1980, pp. 428–547.

19. Casscels, S.W.: Gross pathological changes in the knee joint of the aged individual: a study of 300 cases. Clin. Orthop., 132:225–232, 1978.
20. Champion, B.R., Sell, S., and Poole, A.R.: Immunity to homologous collagens and cartilage proteoglycans in rabbits. Immunology., 48:605–616, 1983.
21. Cheung, H.S., et al.: In vitro synthesis of tissue specific type II collagen by healing cartilage. 1. Short term repair of cartilage in mature rabbits. Arthritis Rheum., 23:211–219, 1980.
22. Christensen, P., et al.: The subchondral bone of the proximal tibial epiphysis in osteoarthritis of the knee. Acta Orthop. Scand., 53:889–896, 1982.
23. Christensen, S.B., and Arnoldi, C.C.: Distribution of 99mTc-phosphate compounds in osteoarthritic femoral heads. J. Bone Joint Surg., 62A:90–96, 1980.
24. Christensen, S.B., and Reimann, I.: Differential histochemical staining of glycosaminoglycans in the matrix of osteoarthritic cartilage. Acta Pathol. Microbiol. Scand., 88:61–68, 1980.
25. Chu, C.J., and Tsui, T.Y.: Pathological study of metacarpophalangeal joints in Kaschin-Beck disease. Chin. Med. J., 4:309–318, 1978.
26. Cooke, T.D.V.: The polyarticular features of osteoarthritis requiring hip and knee surgery. J. Rheumatol., 10:288–290, 1983.
27. Cooke, T.D.V.: The interactions and local disease manifestations of immune complexes in articular collagenous tissues. Stud. Joint Dis., 1:158–200, 1980.
28. Davis, W.H., Jr., Lee, S.L., and Sokoloff, L.: A proposed model boundary lubrication by synovial fluid: structuring of boundary water. J. Biomech. Eng., 101:185–192, 1979.
29. Davis, W.H., Jr., Lee, S.L., and Sokoloff, L.: Boundary lubricating ability of synovial fluid in degenerative joint disease. Arthritis Rheum., 21:754–760, 1978.
30. Dequeker, J., et al.: Aging of bone: its relation to osteoporosis and osteoarthrosis in post-menopausal women. Front. Horm. Res., 3:117–130, 1975.
30a. Doherty, M., Watt, I., and Dieppe, P.A.: Influence of primary generalized osteoarthritis on development of secondary osteoarthritis. Lancet, 2:8–11, 1983.
31. Doyle, D.V.: Tissue calcification and inflammation in osteoarthritis. J. Pathol., 136:199–216, 1982.
32. Dustmann, H.O., Puhl, W., and Krempien, B.: Phänomen der Cluster im Arthroseknorpel. Arch. Orthop. Unfallchir., 79:321–333, 1974.
33. duToit, G.T.: Hip disease of Mseleni. Clin. Orthop., 141:223–228, 1979.
34. Eaton, R.C., Dobranski, A.I., and Littler, J.W.: Marginal osteophyte excision in treatment of mucous cysts. J. Bone Joint Surg., 55A:570–574, 1973.
35. Egan, M.S., et al.: The association of amyloid deposits and osteoarthritis. Arthritis Rheum., 25:204–208, 1983.
36. Ehrlich, G.E.: Pathogenesis and treatment of osteoarthritis. Compr. Ther., 5:36–40, 1978.
37. Enneking, W.F., and Horowitz, M.: The intra-articular effects of immobilization on the human knee. J. Bone Joint Surg., 54A:973–985, 1972.
38. Fabry, G., and Mulier, J.C.: Biochemical analyses in osteoarthritis of the hip: a correlative study between glycosaminoglycan loss, enzyme activity and radiologic signs. Clin. Orthop., 153:253–264, 1980.
39. Fahmy, N.R., Williams, E.A., and Noble, J.: Meniscal pathology and osteoarthritis of the knee. J. Bone Joint Surg., 65B:24–28, 1983.
40. Finsterbush, A., and Friedman, B.: The effect of sensory denervation on rabbits' knee joints: a light and electron microscopic study. J. Bone Joint Surg., 57A:949–956, 1975.
41. Firooznia, H., et al.: Calcification and ossification of posterior longitudinal ligament of spine. N.Y. State J. Med., 82:1193–1198, 1982.
42. Foss, M.V.L., and Byers, P.D.: Bone density, osteoarthrosis of the hip, and fracture of the upper end of the femur. Ann. Rheum. Dis., 31:259–264, 1972.
43. Fritz, P., et al.: Beitrage zum enzymhistochemischen Nachweis von Immunoglobulinen in Gelenkkapsel bei

chronischer Polyarthritis und entzündlich aktivierter Arthrose. Z. Rheumatol., *39*:331–342, 1980.

44. Furukawa, T., et al.: Biochemical studies on repair cartilage resurfacing experimental defects in the rabbit knee. J. Bone Joint Surg., *62A*:79–89, 1980.

45. Gay, S., et al.: Immunohistologic study on collagen in cartilage-bone metamorphosis and degenerative osteoarthrosis. Klin. Wochenschr., *54*:969–976, 1976.

46. Getzy, L., et al.: Factors influencing metachromatic staining in paraffin-embedded sections of rabbit and human articular cartilage: a comparison of the safranin O and toluidine blue O techniques. J. Histotechnol., *5*:111–116, 1982.

47. Ghadially, F.N.: Fine structure of joints. *In* The Joints and Synovial Fluid. Vol. 1. Edited by L. Sokoloff. New York, Academic Press, 1978, pp. 105–176.

48. Ghadially, F.N., Lalonde, J.M., and Yong, N.K.: Ultrastructure of amianthoid fibers in osteoarthrotic cartilage. Virchows Arch. (Cell Pathol.), *31*:81–86, 1979.

49. Ghose, T., et al.: Immunopathological changes in rheumatoid arthritis and other joint diseases. J. Clin. Pathol., *28*:109–117, 1975.

50. Gilbertson, E.M.M.: Development of periarticular osteophytes in experimentally induced osteoarthritis in the dog. Ann. Rheum. Dis., *34*:12–25, 1975.

51. Goffin, Y.A., Thoua, Y., and Potvliege, P.R.: Microdeposition of amyloid in the joints. Ann. Rheum. Dis., *40*:27–33, 1981.

52. Gofton, J.P.: Studies in osteoarthritis of the hip. Part I. Classification. Can. Med. Assoc. J., *104*:679–683, 1971.

53. Goldberg, R.P., Zulman, J.I., and Genant, H.K.: Unilateral primary osteoarthritis of the hand in monoplegia. Radiology, *135*:65–66, 1980.

54. Goldenberg, D.L., Egan, M.S., and Cohen, A.S.: Inflammatory synovitis in degenerative joint disease. J. Rheumatol., *9*:204–209, 1982.

55. Goldin, R.H., et al.: Clinical and radiological survey of the incidence of osteoarthrosis among obese patients. Ann. Rheum. Dis., *35*:349–353, 1976.

56. Goodfellow, J., Hungerford, D.S., and Wood, C.: Patello-femoral joint mechanics and pathology. 2. Chondromalacia patellae. J. Bone Joint Surg., *58B*:291–299, 1976.

57. Green, W.T., Jr., et al.: Microradiographic study of the calcified layer of articular cartilage. Arch. Pathol., *90*:151–158, 1970.

58. Gresham, G.E., and Rathery, U.K.: Osteoarthritis in knees of aged persons. Relationship between roentgenographic and clinical manifestations. JAMA, *233*:168–170, 1975.

59. Havdrup, T., and Telhag, H.: Mitosis of chondrocytes in normal adult cartilage. Clin. Orthop., *153*:248–252, 1980.

60. Havdrup, T., Hulth, A., and Telhag, H.: The subchondral bone in osteoarthritis and rheumatoid arthritis of the knee: a histological and microradiographical study. Acta Orthop. Scand., *47*:345–350, 1976.

61. Hernborg, J.S., and Nilsson, B.E.: The relationship between osteophytes in the knee joint, osteoarthritis and aging. Acta Orthop. Scand., *44*:69–74, 1973.

62. Hilton, R.C., Ball, J., and Benn, R.T.: Vertebral endplate lesions (Schmorl's nodes) in the dorsolumbar spine. Ann. Rheum. Dis., *35*:127–132, 1976.

63. Hirotani, H., and Ito, T.: The fate of the articular cartilage in intracapsular fractures of the femoral neck. Arch. Orthop. Unfallchir., *86*:195–199, 1976.

64. Hirotani, H., and Ito, T.: Chondrocyte mitosis in the articular cartilage of femoral heads with various diseases. Acta Orthop. Scand., *46*:979–986, 1975.

65. Hough, A.J., Banfield, W.G., and Sokoloff, L.: Cartilage in hemophilic arthropathy: ultrastructural and microanalytical studies. Arch. Pathol. Lab. Med., *100*:91–96, 1976.

66. Hough, A.J., Mottram, F.C., and Sokoloff, L.: The collagenous nature of amianthoid degeneration of human costal cartilage. Am. J. Pathol., *73*:201–216, 1973.

67. Howorth, M.B.: General relaxation of the ligaments with special reference to the knee and shoulder. Clin. Orthop., *30*:133–143, 1963.

68. Ilardi, C.F., and Sokoloff, L.: Secondary osteonecrosis in osteoarthritis of the femoral head: a pathological study. Hum. Pathol., *15*:79–83, 1984.

69. Ilardi, C.F., and Sokoloff, L.: The pathology of osteoarthritis: ten strategic questions for pharmacologic management. Semin. Arthritis Rheum., *11 (Suppl. 1)*:3–7, 1981.

70. Jeffery, A.K.: Osteophytes and the osteoarthritis femoral head. J. Bone Joint Surg., *57B*:314–324, 1975.

71. Jerring, K.: Osteoarthritis of the hip: epidemiology and clinical role. Acta Orthop. Scand., *51*:523–530, 1980.

72. Johanson, N.A., et al.: Acromegalic arthropathy of the hip. Clin. Orthop., *173*:130–139, 1982.

73. Kellgren, J.H., Lawrence, J.S., and Bier, F.: Genetic factors in generalized osteoarthritis. Ann. Rheum. Dis., *22*:237–255, 1963.

74. Klünder, K.B., Rud, B., and Hansen, J.: Osteoarthritis of the hip and knee in retired football players. Acta Orthop. Scand., *51*:925–927, 1980.

75. Ladefoged, C.: Amyloid in osteoarthritis hip joints: a pathoanatomical and histological investigation of femoral head cartilage. Acta Orthop. Scand., *53*:581–586, 1982.

76. Ladefoged, C., Christensen, H.E., and Sorensen, K.H.: Amyloid in osteoarthritis hip joints: deposition in cartilage and capsule. Acta Orthop. Scand., *53*:587–590, 1982.

77. Lagier, R.: The concept of osteoarthrotic remodeling as illustrated by ochronotic arthropathy of the hip: an antomico-radiological approach. Virchows Arch. (Pathol. Anat.), *385*:293–298, 1980.

78. Lane, L.B., and Bullough, P.G.: Age-related changes in the thickness of the calcified zone and the number of tidemarks in adult human articular cartilage. J. Bone Joint Surg., *62B*:372–375, 1980.

79. Lawrence, J.S.: Rheumatism in Populations. London, William Heinemann, 1977, p. 572.

80. Leach, R.E., Baumgard, S., and Broom, J.: Obesity: its relationship to osteoarthritis of the knee. Clin. Orthop., *93*:271–273, 1973.

81. Longmore, R.B., and Gardner, D.L.: The surface structure of aging human articular cartilage: a study by reflected light interference microscopy (RLIM). J. Anat., *126*:353–365, 1978.

82. McCutchen, C.W.: Lubrication of joints. *In* The Joints and Synovial Fluid. Vol. 1. Edited by L. Sokoloff. New York, Academic Press, 1978, pp. 437–483.

83. Mainardi, C.L., et al.: Proliferative synovitis in hemophilia: biochemical and morphological observations. Arthritis Rheum., *21*:137–144, 1978.

84. Marks, J.S., Stewart, I.M., and Hardinge, K.: Primary osteoarthrosis of the hip and Heberden's nodes. Ann. Rheum. Dis., *38*:107–111, 1979.

85. Meachim, G.: Age-related degeneration of patellar articular cartilage. J. Anat., *134*:365–371, 1982.

86. Meachim, G.: Light microscopy of Indian ink preparations of fibrillated cartilage. Ann. Rheum. Dis., *31*:457–464, 1972.

87. Meachim, G., et al.: An investigation of radiological, clinical and pathological correlations in osteoarthrosis of the hip. Clin. Radiol., *31*:565–574, 1980.

88. Meachim, G., and Collins, D.H.: Cell counts of normal and osteoarthritic articular cartilage in relation to the uptake of sulphate ($^{35}SO_4$) *in vitro*. Ann. Rheum. Dis., *21*:45–50, 1962.

89. Milgram, J.W.: Morphologic alterations in the subchondral bone in advanced degenerative arthritis. Clin. Orthop., *173*:293–312, 1983.

90. Milgram, J.W., and Jasty, M.: Osteopetrosis: a morphological study of twenty-one cases. J. Bone Joint Surg., *64A*:912–929, 1982.

91. Milgram, J.W., and Rana, N.A.: The pathology of the failed cup arthroplasty. Clin. Orthop., *158*:159–179, 1981.

92. Minns, R.J., Steven, F.S., and Hardinge, K.: Osteoarthrotic articular cartilage lesions of the femoral head observed in the scanning electron microscopy. J. Pathol., *122*:63–70, 1977.

93. Mitrovic, D., et al.: Metabolism of human femoral head cartilage in osteoarthrosis and subcapital fracture. Ann. Rheum. Dis., 40:18–26, 1981.

94. Mohing, M.: Die Arthrose Deformans des Kniegelenkes. New York, Springer Verlag, 1966.

95. Norman, A., and Baker, N.D.: Spontaneous osteonecrosis of the knee and medial meniscal tears. Radiology, 129:653–656, 1978.

96. Ogilvie-Harris, D.J., and Fornasier, V.L.: Synovial iron deposition in osteoarthritis and rheumatoid arthritis. J. Rheumatol., 7:30–49, 1980.

97. Ono, K., et al.: Ossified posterior longitudinal ligament: a clinicopathological study. Spine, 2:128–138, 1977.

98. Palmoski, M.J., Colyer, R.A., and Brandt, K.D.: Joint motion in the absence of normal loading does not maintain normal articular cartilage. Arthritis Rheum., 23:325–334, 1980.

99. Paul, J.P.: Joint kinetics. In The Joints and Synovial Fluid. Vol. 2. Edited by L. Sokoloff. New York, Academic Press, 1980, pp. 139–176.

100. Pringle, J.A., Byers, P.D., and Brown, M.E.A.: Immunofluorescence in osteoarthritis and rheumatoid arthritis. Nature, 274:84, 1978.

101. Radin, E.L., et al.: Response of joints to impact loading. III. Relationship between trabecular microfractures and cartilage degeneration. J. Biomech., 6:51–57, 1973.

102. Raju, U.B., Fine, G., and Partemian, J.O.: Diabetic neuroarthropathy (Charcot's joint). Arch. Pathol. Lab. Med., 106:349–351, 1982.

103. Reimann, I., and Christensen, S.B.: A histochemical study of alkaline and acid phosphatase activity in subchondral bone from osteoarthrotic human hips. Clin. Orthop., 140:85–91, 1979.

104. Reimann, I., Mankin, H.J., and Trahan, C.: Quantitative histological analysis of articular cartilage and subchondral bone from osteoarthritic and normal human hips. Acta Orthop. Scand., 48:64–73, 1977.

105. Resnick, D.: Patterns of migration of the femoral head in osteoarthritis of the hip: roentgenographc-pathologic correlation and comparison with rheumatoid arthritis. AJR, 124:62–74, 1975.

106. Resnick, D., et al.: Diffuse idiopathic hyperostosis (DISH) (ankylosing hyperostosis of Forestier and Rotes-Querol). Semin. Arthritis Rheum., 7:153–187, 1978.

107. Resnick, D., Niwayama, G., and Coutts, R.D.: Subchondral cysts (geodes) in arthritic disorders: pathologic and radiographic appearance of the hip joint. AJR, 128:799–806, 1977.

108. Rippey, J.J., et al.: Articular cartilage degradation and the pathology of hemophilic arthropathy. S. Afr. Med. J., 53:345–351, 1978.

109. Roper, B.A.: Paget's disease involving the hip joints. Clin. Orthop., 80:33–38, 1971.

110. Rushfeldt, R.D., Mann, R.W., and Harris, W.H.: Improved techniques for measuring in vitro the geometry and pressure distribution in the human acetabulum. II. Instrumental endoprosthesis measurement of articular surface pressure distribution. J. Biomech., 14:315–323, 1981.

111. Santer, V., White, R.J., and Roughley, P.J.: Proteoglycans from normal and degenerate cartilage of adult human tibial plateau. Arthritis Rheum., 24:691–700, 1981.

112. Saville, P.D.: Age and weight in osteoarthritis of the hip. Arthritis Rheum., 11:635–644, 1968.

113. Scott, D.L., et al.: Significance of fibronectin in rheumatoid arthritis and osteoarthrosis. Ann. Rheum. Dis., 40:142–153, 1981.

114. Silberberg, R.: Epiphyseal growth and osteoarthrosis in blotchy mice. Exp. Cell Biol., 45:1–8, 1977.

115. Simon, W.H., Lane, J.M., and Beller, P.: Pathogenesis of degenerative joint disease produced by in vivo freezing of rabbit articular cartilage. Clin. Orthop., 155:259–268, 1981.

116. Sirca, A., and Sucec-Michieli, M.: Selective type II fibre muscular atrophy in patients with osteoarthritis of the hip. J. Neurol. Sci., 44:149–159, 1980.

117. Smukler, N.M., Edeiken, J., and Giuliano, V.J.: Ankylosis in osteoarthritis of the finger joints. Radiology, 100:525–530, 1971.

118. Sokoloff, L.: Aging and degenerative diseases affecting cartilage. In Cartilage. Vol. 3. Edited by B.K. Hall. New York, Academic Press, pp. 109–142.

119. Sokoloff, L.: In vitro culture of joints and articular tissues. In The Joints and Synovial Fluid: Vol. 2. Edited by L. Sokoloff. New York, Academic Press, 1980, pp. 1–26.

120. Sokoloff, L.: The Biology of Degenerative Joint Disease. Chicago, University of Chicago Press, 1969.

121. Sokoloff, L.: Comparative pathology of arthritis. Adv. Vet. Sci., 6:193–250, 1960.

122. Solomon, L.: Patterns of osteoarthritis of the hip. J. Bone Joint Surg., 58B:176–183, 1976.

123. Soren, A.: Osteoarthritis—an arthritis? Z. Rheumatol., 41:1–6, 1982.

124. Spranger, J.: The epiphyseal dysplasias. Clin. Orthop., 114:46–60, 1976.

125. Stecher, R.M.: Heberden's nodes: a clinical description or osteoarthritis of the finger joints. Ann. Rheum. Dis., 14:1–10, 1955.

126. Stewart, I.M., Marks, J.S., and Hardinge, K.: Generalized osteoarthrosis and hip disease. In Epidemiology of Osteoarthritis. Edited by J. Peyron. Paris, Geigy, 1981, pp. 193–197.

127. Streda, A.: Participation of osteonecrosis in the development of severe coxarthrosis. Acta Univ. Carol. (Med. Monogr.), 46:103–153, 1971.

128. Stulberg, S.D., et al.: Unrecognized childhood hip disease: a major cause of osteoarthritis of the hip. In The Hip. St. Louis, C.V., Mosby, 1975, pp. 212–218.

129. Swann, D.A.: Macromolecules of synovial fluid. In The Joints and Synovial Fluid. Vol. 1. Edited by L. Sokoloff. New York, Academic Press, 1978, pp. 407–435.

130. Termansen, N.B., et al.: Primary osteoarthritis of the hip: interrelationship between intraosseous pressure, x-ray changes, clinical severity and bone density. Acta Orthop. Scand., 52:215–222, 1981.

130a. Thompson, R.C., Jr., and Bassett, C.A.L.: Histological observations on experimentally induced degeneration of articular cartilage. J. Bone Joint Surg., 52A:435–443, 1970.

131. Uchino, F., et al.: Amyloid-like substance in cartilage of the sternoclavicular joints. In Amyloid and Amyloidosis. Edited by G. Glenner, P. Pinho e Costa, and A. Falcao de Freitas. Amsterdam, Excerpta Medica, 1980, pp. 55–59.

132. Utsinger, P.D., et al.: Roentgenologic, immunologic, and therapeutic study of erosive (inflammatory) osteoarthritis. Arch. Intern. Med., 138:693–697, 1978.

133. Utsinger, P.D., Resnick, D., and Shapiro, R.: Diffuse skeletal abnormalities in Forestier disease. Arch. Intern. Med., 136:763–768, 1976.

134. Vernon-Roberts, B., Pirie, C.J., and Trenwith, V.: Pathology of the dorsal spine in ankylosing hyperostosis. Ann. Rheum. Dis., 33:281–288, 1974.

135. Vignon, E., Arlot, M., and Vignon, G.: Etude de la densité cellulaire du cartilage de la tête femoral en fonction de l'age. Rev. Rhum. Mal. Osteoartic., 43:403–405, 1976.

136. Waine, H., et al.: Association of osteoarthritis and diabetes mellitus. Tufts Fol. Med., 7:13–19, 1961.

137. Walton, M.: Obesity as an aetiological factor in the development of osteoarthrosis. Gerontology, 25:165–172, 1979.

138. Walton, M.: Patella displacement and osteoarthrosis of the knee joint in mice. J. Pathol., 127:165–172, 1979.

139. Weiss, C.: Ultrastructural characteristics of osteoarthritis. Fed. Proc., 32:1459–1466, 1973.

140. Wigley, R.D., et al.: Degenerative arthritis in mice: study of age and sex frequency in various strains with a genetic study of NZB/B1, NZY/B1, and hybrid mice. Ann. Rheum. Dis., *36*:249–253, 1977.

141. Wilkinson, M.: Pathology. *In* Cervical Spondylosis. Its Early Diagnosis and Treatment. Edited by M. Wilkinson. Philadelphia, W.B. Saunders, 1971.

142. Wroblewski, B.M., and Charnley, J.: Radiographic morphology of the osteoarthritic hip. J. Bone Joint Surg., *64B*:568–569, 1982.

143. Yazici, H., et al.: Primary osteoarthrosis of the knee or hip. JAMA, *231*:1256–1260, 1975.

Chapter 88

Etiopathogenesis of Osteoarthritis

David S. Howell

Our understanding of the etiopathogenic pathways in primary and, to a lesser extent, secondary osteoarthritis has been advanced over the last two decades. In this chapter, some recent concepts that depend on expanding information on the cell biology, metabolism, and biochemical structure of cartilage are emphasized, and some biomechanical aspects are considered. I presuppose the reader's familiarity with the terminology and concepts presented in the section of this volume on the scientific basis for the study of arthritis.

Problems multiply when one obtains scientific data on a given osteoarthritic lesion from living tissues. Careful morphologic data are needed on the site and stage of the lesion, its depth in the cartilage, and the presence or absence of inflammation. Many of the hypotheses on which studies of the origin or the pathogenesis of osteoarthritis have been based stem from combined morphologic, biomechanical, and epidemiologic observations, as reviewed in Chapters 87, 8, and 2, respectively. Biochemical etiologic errors have been considered in relation to disorders of cartilage matrix expressed as a failure of its biomaterial properties or a failure in the biomechanical aspects of joint development. Such errors may occur during pre- or postnatal growth, maturation, or aging. We need to know more about the biology of the chondrocyte (see Chap. 14). Metabolic control by local and systemic hormones, feedback control from matrix products regulating molecular synthesis, and types and numbers of membrane receptors are biochemical subjects currently in their infancy.

EARLY BIOCHEMICAL EVENTS AND THE "FINAL COMMON PATHWAY"

At the present early stage of biochemical research in osteoarthritis, we have more information on pathogenesis than on etiologic factors. Both morphologic and biochemical data so far seem to indicate a similar pattern by which the cartilage expresses a degenerative response, in both natural disease and in animal models. Working hypotheses linking these observations have been described by Bollet,[4] as well as by George and Chrisman.[24] Multiple etiologic factors are thought to result in cartilage cell injury leading to a disturbance in syn-

thetic and degradative processes (Fig. 88–1). The net result of these changes is accelerated matrix breakdown by chondrocytic and perhaps synovial enzymes, followed by altered repair. Products of this tissue response stimulate new chondrocytic proliferation and further matrix synthesis at the local site. Breakdown products from cartilage are absorbed and are phagocytized by the surrounding tissues, synovia, and joint marginal cartilage. This process induces a remodeling phenomenon involving new cartilage and bone production. Various theories have been advanced concerning the so-called "final common pathway" as follows: (1) injurious stimuli might lead to faulty cartilage matrix metabolism and inadequate repair as the major defective mechanism; (2) trauma or other factors, such as hormonal influences, may directly initiate the hypertrophic remodeling at marginal synovial membrane and ligament attachment sites, with accelerated cartilage breakdown as a secondary event; and (3) direct traumatic injury of the collagen network could lead to unraveling of proteoglycans and secondary tissue breakdown.

In *secondary osteoarthritis* from a variety of causes, cartilage breakdown may be the result of abnormal biochemical products accumulating in the cartilage matrix, such as ochronosis or blood products in hemophilia, discussed in Chapters 96 and 74, respectively.

Chondromalacia or the development of soft spots in unloaded or non-weight-bearing margins of articular cartilage probably results from lack of normal physical stimulus to the regionally affected chondrocytes, as well as reduced local nutrition. The biochemical changes and histologic appearance are similar to those of early, aggressive lesions. *Chondromalacia patellae* develops most often on the medial patellar facet, an unloaded surface. Such lesions usually appear in young adults and may: (1) spontaneously heal; (2) remain as localized spots; or (3) progress to patellofemoral osteoarthritis, depending on the applicable biomechanical factors, such as the degree of lateral pull of the quadriceps tendon, the shallowness of the intertrochlear fossa, or inadvertent injury during unusual load carriage by the medial facet. Factors that permit advancement or restriction of such

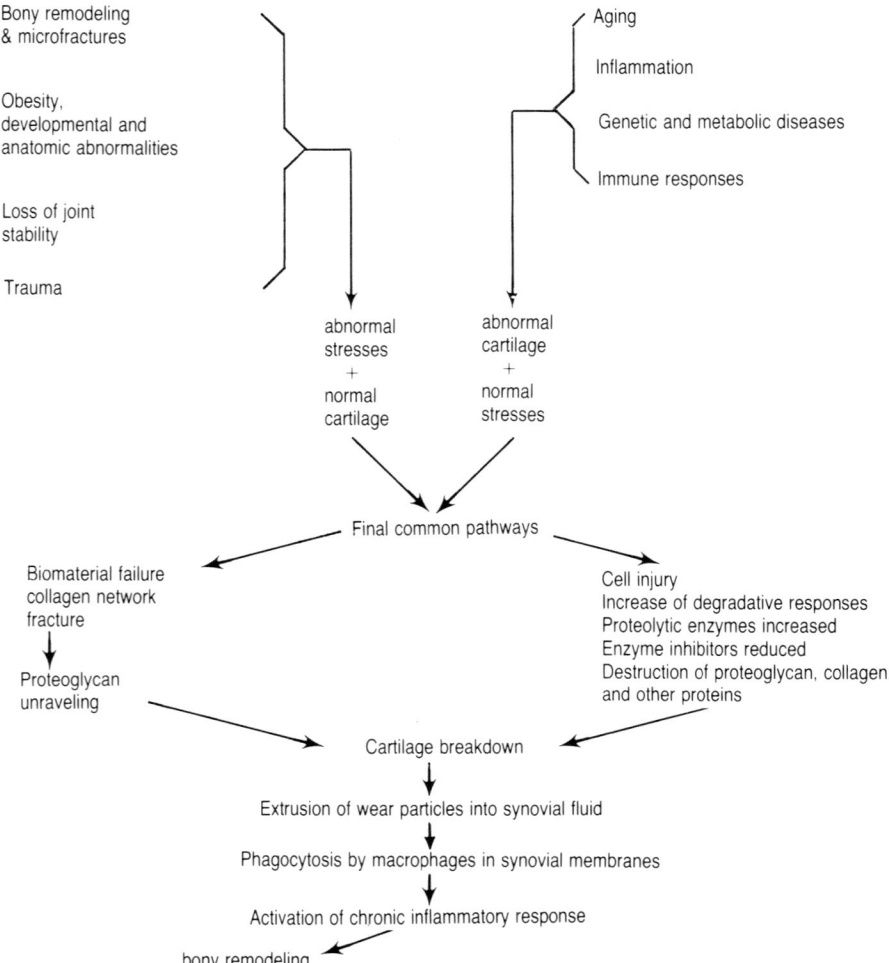

Fig. 88–1. Etiopathogenic factors in osteoarthritis.

lesions probably involve a balance of injury and repair responses and are both biomechanical and biochemical.

BIOCHEMICAL STRUCTURE OF ARTICULAR CARTILAGE AND OSTEOARTHRITIC CHANGES

Throughout a lifetime, cartilage maintains an unusual isolation from exposure to endogenous and exogenous agents normally carried to extracellular tissues by the circulation. This isolation stems largely from an absence of capillaries and from an abundance of proteoglycans, which are huge molecules with strong negative charges. The diffusion of other macromolecules into the cartilage is thereby limited. On a dry-weight basis, cartilage contains about 35% proteoglycan and electrolytes, 60% collagen, and 5% noncollagenous, nonproteoglycan protein.[48] Its water content varies from 65 to 80% of the wet weight of the tissue. More

detailed reviews of the subject of proteoglycan and collagen metabolism in cartilage appear in the literature.[27,43,52]

Striking verification of the structure of the proteoglycan molecules predicted by biochemical analysis was observed by electron microscopy. These molecules looked like a cluster of Christmas trees.[65] The "trunk" of each "tree" comprised a hyaluronate molecule, with branches of core protein of the proteoglycan subunits; linear glycosaminoglycans make up the secondary branches and are attached to the protein cores. Along with the glycosaminoglycans are O-linked and mannose-containing oligosaccharides attached at intervals along the protein core. The proteoglycan subunits are attached to the hyaluronate molecule, stabilized by a "link" glycoprotein (see Chap. 11). The subunit proteoglycan units contain a core protein of about 250,000 daltons, to which the linear glycosaminoglycan molecules weighing 11,000 to 36,000 daltons are attached. In adult articular cartilages, about 90% of these glycosaminoglycan molecules are a mixture of chondroitin-6 sulfate and keratan sulfate and a small remainder of chondroitin-4 sulfate. The existence of such aggregates in vivo has been established by their associative extraction from cartilage and by their presence in samples of extracellular fluid obtained from cartilage by micropuncture. In such samples, ultramicrobiochemical analysis has demonstrated the existence of these aggregates.[58]

The importance of the aggregates to the function of normal articular cartilage has been shown in studies in which compressive and tensile moduli of the aggregates were much higher than those of monomers.[39] In fact, the biomechanical properties of cartilage depend partly on the presence of these aggregates. Without proteoglycans, such as following protease degradation, the shape of cartilage is still maintained by the collagen network, but all elastic properties are lost.[26] The elastic properties conferred by proteoglycans are due to their large size and to their high level of sulfation. The resultant high density of negative charges repels the molecules and keeps the branches of glycosaminoglycans extended, thereby encompassing water and contained solutes. Such properties make the proteoglycans excellent "stuffing material" for the interstices in the collagen fiber network of cartilage. Although large, linear macromolecules such as the monomers themselves can slowly diffuse through cartilage, plasma proteins, except for traces of albumin, are excluded under normal conditions.[47]

Normal nutrition of cartilage requires delivery of nutrients almost completely through the synovial fluid,[38] with passage of low-molecular-weight compounds such as glucose and amino acids directly to the cartilage cells[47] (see Chaps. 8 and 9). Cyclic loading of joints probably increases the flow of nutrients to the cartilages; conversely, the supply of nutrients is reduced during immobilization.

Changes have been observed in the composition of cartilage in osteoarthritis;[43] the total proteoglycan content was reduced in rough proportion to the severity of the lesion sampled. The ratio of keratan sulfate and chondroitin-6 sulfate to chondroitin-4 sulfate was decreased. Other important changes included a shortened length of the proteoglycan subunit core protein, either in the chondroitin sulfate or the HA binding region, a shortened glycosaminoglycan chain length, decreased hyaluronic acid polymer size, incapacity to form aggregates by some isolated subunits, and increased concentrations of nonproteoglycan, noncollagen proteins. Whether the size of the macromolecules and their component subunits was reduced by enzymatic

degradation or by errors of synthesis is unclear. Reviews of these studies appear in the literature.[30,43,52]

Whether osteoarthritic cartilage is characterized by low, normal, or increased metabolism of key matrix constituents remains controversial. The rates of glycosaminoglycan and DNA synthesis, measured by the uptake of small precursor molecules, was positively correlated with the severity of the osteoarthritic processes in one study.[42] This correlation abruptly failed when severe osteoarthritic changes were noted histologically. These findings were corroborated in a subsequent study from the same laboratory,[46] and partial confirmation was obtained from other laboratories.[79] Other investigators have found no increase of metabolism or of lowered metabolic turnover rates of macromolecules in osteoarthritic cartilage, however.[6,37]

Reports suggesting that collagen might be increasingly cross-linked with aging were not supported by a study of reducible cross-links.[22] The hydroxypyridinium cross-link has been examined as a promising candidate for possible pathologic alteration in osteoarthritis, however.[18] Moreover, a change in the type of collagen synthesized to type I was postulated as a biochemical response in osteoarthritic lesions, but other researchers, using different biochemical techniques,[21] or using immunochemical techniques,[23] have found type II collagen still predominant in osteoarthritic cartilage, although tiny amounts of type I and type V collagen were seen around cartilage cells. In addition, small amounts of newly discovered minor collagen types have been detected in cartilage.[22,53] Fibronectin and type III collagen have also been discovered in human osteoarthritic cartilages (G. Lust and M. Adams, personal communications).

Important reviews of cartilage collagen types have appeared.[22,53] Repair of osteoarthritic ulcerations seems to be almost impossible for nature to accomplish. For example, the arcade of collagen fibers visualized by polarizing light microscopy, or to some extent by scanning electron microscopy, is not duplicated in the healing lesions. This failure to recreate the correct "basketweave" of tissue collagen may account for the inadequate biomechanical properties of repair cartilage. After experimentally damaging knee cartilage in rabbits, it was noted that repair cartilage lacked the mechanical strength of the original tissue, despite elaborate measures to promote healing.[68] Clinical and laboratory experience with the fibrocartilage layers formed after tenotomy and osteotomy, however, indicates that a functional weight-bearing surface may develop under defined conditions, despite the aforementioned limitations.[63] Thus, hope remains that even the weaker tissue arising from a limited repair response may suffice as a resurfaced weight-bearing joint, and many such experiments have been performed. Proper pharmaceutical or physical stimulation might encourage such regenerated cartilage to function satisfactorily.

A prototype of this approach to treatment is seen in patients with acromegaly, in whom a thickened layer of apparently normal articular cartilage results from overproduction of growth hormone.[10] Although this disease is often attended by arthritis resulting from mechanical stresses due to over-thickened joint cartilage, control of cartilage thickness seems a necessary prerequisite to adequate cartilage replacement. Growth hormone is inactive in direct stimulation of articular cartilage cell proliferation or increased matrix synthesis.[41] Growth hormone treatment seems feckless, but somatomedins stimulated in part by growth hormone are potential candidates for such experimentation because they are partly responsible for the effects of growth hormone on cartilage. Certainly, other cartilage-growth-stimulating factors have been demonstrated.[31,33,61]

Our understanding of the role of growth factors is changing as a result of new information gained largely from studying the effect of these factors on chondrocytes in cell culture. The response of these cells seems to depend on the matrix adhesion of the cells believed to be partly dependent on such factors as anchorin and fibronectin. Repair responses are conditioned first by matrix hindrance of diffusion of growth factors to reach chondrocytes. Theoretically, hindrance to permeability of growth factors, such as CTAP's (connective-tissue activating peptides), platelet-derived growth factor, pituitary-fibroblast growth factor, and somatomedin C, is reduced as the matrix becomes degraded in osteoarthritis. Depending on local conditions, these factors then may amplify repair responses (see Chap. 12).

Insulin appears to be essential for adequate synthetic responses. Somatomedin C appears to amplify such responses and reacts with its own receptors, as well as with insulin receptors on chondrocytes. Pituitary-fibroblast growth factor appears to stimulate chondrocyte proliferation, but not matrix production. Certain lymphokines appear to enhance and others to inhibit, repair responses.[28,31,32,61,75]

Chondroitin sulfate injected into canine knee joints has stimulated the production of peripheral cartilage and of bony spurs.[24] Obviously, therapeutic use of such factors must result in healing of osteoarthritic erosions without promoting marginal bony and cartilaginous overgrowth.

CARTILAGE DEGRADATIVE MECHANISMS

No consistent findings have been recorded with regard to breakdown products of collagen in osteoarthritic tissues, but in cultures of osteoarthritic human cartilages, a small but significant elevation of collagenase activity has been found.[14,15] Incubates of human osteoarthritic cartilage elaborated hydroxyproline-containing products into the culture medium, and these products could be used to assess the activity of endogenous collagenolytic enzymes.[54] In these experiments, collagenase enzyme activity was positively correlated with the severity of human osteoarthritic lesions based on histologic criteria. Activity was higher in the erosion sites than in the margins or in sites distant from the erosions. In the Pond-Nuki dog model of osteoarthritis, the same methods showed elevated collagenolytic enzyme activity in the erosive lesions.[55] The collagenase itself was postulated to be the cause of these changes on the basis of the response to a number of inhibitors.[55] Whether the collagenolytic enzymes produce the eosions themselves, or whether they enlarge the lacunae to accommodate proliferating chondrocytes, remains unknown.

Proteoglycans are major constituents believed to be degraded early in the genesis of osteoarthritis. Although lysosomes of cultured chondrocytes contain exo-B-n-D-hexosaminidase and exo-B-d-glucuronidases capable of degrading oligosaccharides, no enzyme capable of cleaving the chains of chondroitin sulfate and of releasing sulfated oligosaccharides has been found in adult cartilage. Hyaluronidase has been isolated from adult articular cartilage but it was not active at physiologic pH.[76] This enzyme failed to break down chondroitins, which seem to be largely cleaved to monomers in the liver.[82]

Protein degradation proceeds principally in relation to chondrocytes. The major enzymes available for such a function are cathepsins B and D. These enzymes are localized in chondrocytic lysosomes and have been implicated in the breakdown of cartilage in man and in various animals. Other acid hydrolases have also been detected, one of which is cathepsin F.[81] The proteolytic activity of cathepsin D was found to be two or three times greater in osteoarthritic than in normal cartilage.[72] Human cathepsin D has been carefully distinguished from that of animals; it is localized in lysosomes from osteoarthritic cartilage.[1] Antibodies to purified cathepsin D showed that the enzyme was localized within the cell and about the cell-limiting membranes,[60] this finding supports the concept that cathepsin D has a role at least in the later steps of cartilage degradation. Nevertheless, because cathespin D and such hydrolases act at a low pH, they probably can degrade only those substrates taken into the cartilage cells or perhaps those located in the immediate environment of the cell membranes. In organ cultures, it has not been possible to block cartilage degradation with inhibitors of cathepsin D.[81]

The mechanism by which proteoglycan degradation occurs at a distance from the nearest chondrocytes is an important issue. The pH of the extracellular fluid in cartilage matrix is almost neutral, not the appropriate condition for the foregoing acid hydrolases.[19,74] A metal-binding neutral protease in multiple forms from human articular cartilage was purified 2,000-fold and was found to be a potent proteoglycanase.[71,73] This enzyme appears similar to that partially characterized by Ehrlich et al. from articular and growth plate cartilage.[16] Little controversy has arisen over the source of this enzyme because no pannus invades osteoarthritic cartilage, and no lymphocytic or other cellular infiltrates occur within the osteoarthritic cartilages from which these proteases have been extracted. A chondrocytic origin was confirmed by the finding of these neutral metal-binding proteases in chondrocyte cultures.[40,70]

Although these enzymes are considered to play some role in early cartilage destruction, the picture becomes more complicated once an osteoarthritic erosion develops and thereby permits an influx of synovial fluid. Despite its content of potent enzyme inhibitors, such as alpha-2-macroglobulin, synovial fluid could deliver enzymes deleterious to the matrix originating from leukocytes or from synovial lining cells. Synovial lining cells can elaborate a metal-binding neutral protease, cathepsin D, and collagenase, as recently reviewed.[81]

Protease tissue degradation must be a closely regulated process. Evidence indicates that collagenase is secreted as a proenzyme and is activated by another factor of about the same molecular weight.[80] Treatment with a mercurial organic compound, APMA, or trypsin can reduce the molecular weight of the enzyme from studies on synovial culture, but the activation requires the presence of this new factor. Thus, the reduction of molecular weight by about 11,000 daltons still occurs with APMA, but procollagenase activator is required. The activated enzyme can then bind irreversibly to the inhibitors of neutral metalloprotease that have recently been purified from bovine and human cartilage. Inhibitors of other proteases, particularly serine protease and collagenase, as well as an antitumor invasion factor, have been discovered in cartilage.[35,49,67] Once cartilage is degraded by protease, its permeability to large molecules, hitherto effectively excluded, is lost, and exogenous enzymes can readily penetrate and continue the cartilage degradation.

The cationic protein lysozyme is abundantly present in cartilage. Regardless of whether its origin is endogenous or exogenous, growing evidence suggests that lysozyme can regulate the size of proteoglycan aggregates.[34,57,59] The presence of aggregates appears to reduce the vulnerability of proteoglycans to enzymatic attack. Once a minute amount of neutral protease attacks a proteoglycan monomer, it may remove selectively the HA-binding region.[17] Such fragments can readily diffuse from an incubated piece of cartilage and can selectively leave behind the normal proteoglycans capable of aggregation.[69] This important finding may explain why so few breakdown products of proteoglycans have been found in osteoarthritic cartilage; as fast as this degradation occurs, the products are further degraded by the chondrocytes, or they diffuse into the synovial fluid. The wear products are then carried to the synovial membrane.

Water Content and the Collagen Network

The actual role of proteases in cartilage breakdown in osteoarthritis remains controversial because remodeling phenomena cannot be separated from genuine primary tissue breakdown. It is still possible that most cartilage destruction proceeds mechanically.[2] Increased water content, one of the earliest changes in osteoarthritis, is apparently caused by disruption of collagen network and exposure of water-binding proteoglycans.[2] The collagen network in articular cartilage is a "sealed type," that is, one in which the proteoglycan aggregates are confined in a concentrated, semidehydrated state.[6] After rupture of this network, by enzymes or by physical forces or by both, the proteoglycans expand and imbibe water.[6] The collagen fibers may take up some water as well.[45] As a result, not only do proteoglycans become more exposed to enzyme attack, but also their cushioning effect is lost, and the cell and matrix are injured further.

Role of Inflammatory Products

As osteoarthritis progresses, wear particles gain access to synovial fluid and are phagocytized by synovial membrane macrophage-like cells. These cells have been grown in tissue culture, and their responses to these particles have been studied. Such studies may relate to clinical work showing a frequent component of inflammatory change in osteoarthritis. Nearly 75% of a series of osteoarthritic joints showed some component of inflammatory response.[11] This finding might explain the remarkable improvement of most patients with osteoarthritis treated with nonsteroidal anti-inflammatory agents. Chondroitin sulfate may activate Hageman factor in vivo, with activation of the kinin pathway.[51] Vascular and synovial cell hyperplasia and spotty, low-grade infiltration with mononuclear cells have been commonly observed in osteoarthritic synovium. Studies on leukocytes from human patients with osteoarthritis have provided clear evidence that lymphokines stimulate or suppress chondrocyte synthesis of proteoglycans.[28]

A delayed immune response to proteoglycan protein fractions in osteoarthritis has been suggested, based on studies of cartilage in patients with idiopathic chondrolysis.[29] Additional studies indicate that a systemic autoantibody response may be involved in some subsets of osteoarthritis. Cooke et al. found C3, IgG, and IgA deposits within the surfaces of osteoarthritic cartilage,[8] and heterologous serum antibodies to proteoglycan antigens have been detected.[25] Clinical characterization of such patients, in comparison to those lacking these deposits, has not led to any well-defined syndrome, but most of these studies were conducted on patients with osteoarthritis involving the hips or knees. Wear particles stimulate synovial cells to produce collagenase.[17] Mononuclear cell factor, interleukin-1, and catabolin are factors that stimulate chondrocytes to produce degradative enzymes in organ culture. These factors may have overlapping identity,[9,12,13,56,64] and their role in osteoarthritis has not yet been demonstrated. Nevertheless, such factors may trigger the elaboration of collagenase, prostaglandins, and neutral proteoglycanases.

Crystals may play an important role in causing secondary inflammation in secondary osteoarthritis involving calcium pyrophosphate crystal deposition disease or basic calcium phosphate arthropathy. For a discussion of the role of crystals in synovial inflammation, see Chapters 93, 94, and 95. Certainly, crystals destabilize plasma membranes of leukocytes, engender synthesis or release of prostaglandin E_2, elaborate and activate collagenase, and may effect such processes without a classic inflammatory response. An example is the Milwaukee shoulder syndrome reviewed in Chapter 95. This syndrome is a unique form of osteoarthritis that lacks involvement of polymorphonuclear leukocytes or other inflammatory cells, but is associated with synovial cell proliferation.[36] One usually sees severe bilateral osteoarthritis of the shoulder joints, microaggregates of basic calcium phosphate crystals in the synovial membranes, and synovial fluid and lysis of rotator cuff and other tendons, probably by active collagenase. High levels of collagenolytic and neutral protease activity in the synovial fluid have been associated with this secondary form of osteoarthritis.

Endocrine Factors

Animal models of osteoarthritis have been studied extensively for effects of hormones, but direct application of findings to the human disease is difficult. Adrenocorticosteroids in dosages comparable to those injected into human joints had no effect on osteoarthritic erosions in the Moskowitz rabbit model, but these agents seemed to prevent spur formation.[50] When delivered in larger doses, corticosteroids cause severe cartilage damage by interfering with matrix repair.[3,44] An estrogen antagonist, tamoxifen, has blocked osteoarthritic erosions in this animal model, but whether through reduced degradation or through improved synthetic repair is unclear.[66] Most nonsteroidal anti-inflammatory agents, including the currently marketed proprionic acid derivatives, fenamates, salicylates, and some acetic acid derivatives, appear to reduce synthetic rates of proteoglycans in incubates of articular cartilage from normal dogs and from Pond-Nuki dogs with osteoarthritis.[5] The possibility of unfavorable effects on cartilage repair of these agents remains to be demonstrated by in vivo studies, but these results certainly deserve further consideration (see Chap. 90).

Recent studies indicate that hyaluronic acid, previously considered the main lubricant in joints, is a poor lubricant of cartilage-to-cartilage bearings and, hydrolysis of synovial hyaluronic acid with hyaluronidase does not lessen synovial fluid lubrication.[62] A hyaluronate-free glycoprotein called *lubricin* probably contributes the most to lubrication of joints by its adsorption on cartilage surfaces.[78] In contrast, in periarticular soft tissues in which resistance to joint motion predominates, hyaluronic acid still seems to be an effective lubricant[77] (see Chaps. 8 and 87). Whether abnormalities exist in joint lubrication in osteoarthritis is unknown.

REFERENCES

1. Ali, S.Y., and Evans, L.: Enzymic degradation of cartilage in osteoarthritis. Fed. Proc., 32:1494–1498, 1973.
2. Baylis, M.T., and Venn, M.: Chemistry of human articular cartilage. *In* Studies in Joint Disease 1. Edited by A. Maroudas and E.J. Holborow. Tunbridge Wells, Pitman Medical, 1980, pp. 2–58.
3. Behrens, F., Shepard, N., and Mitchel, N.: Alterations of rabbit articular cartilage by intra-articular injections of glucocorticoids. J. Bone Joint Surg., 57A:70–76, 1977.
4. Bollet, A.J.: Connective tissue polysaccharide metabolism and the pathogenesis of osteoarthritis. Adv. Intern. Med., 13:33–60, 1967.
5. Brandt, K.D., and Palmoski, M.: Effects of nonsteroidal anti-inflammatory drugs on proteoglycan metabolism in articular cartilage. Semin. Arthritis Rheum., 11 (Suppl. 1):133–134, 1981.
6. Byers, P.D., et al.: Histological and biochemical studies on cartilage from osteoarthritic femoral heads with special reference to surface characteristics. Connect. Tissue Res., 5:41–49, 1977.
7. Castor, C.W., et al.: Regulation of articular cell metabolism by CTAP mediators. Semin. Arthritis Rheum., 11 (Suppl. 1):95–96, 1981.
8. Cooke, T.D., et al.: Relationships of immune deposits in osteoarthritis (OA) cartilage to disease site pattern and syn-

ovial reaction. *In* Epidemiology of Osteoarthritis. Edited by J.G. Peyron. Paris, Ciba-Geigy, 1981, pp. 113–123.

9. Dayer, J.-M., Robinson, D.R., and Krane, S.M.: Prostaglandin production by rheumatoid synovial cells: stimulation by factor from human mononuclear cells. J. Exp. Med., *145*:1,399–1,404, 1977.

10. Detenbeck, L.C., et al.: Peripheral joint manifestations of acromegaly. Clin. Orthop., *91*:119–127, 1973.

11. Dieppe, P.A.: Inflammation in osteoarthritis and the role of microcrystals. Semin. Arthritis Rheum., *11 (Suppl. 1)*:121–122, 1981.

12. Dingle, J.T.: The role of catabolin in arthritic damage. Semin. Arthritis Rheum., *11*:82–83, 1981.

13. Dingle, J.T., et al.: A cartilage catabolic factor from synovium. Biochem. J., *184*:177–180, 1979.

14. Ehrlich, M.G., et al.: Correlation between articular cartilage collagenase activity and osteoarthritis. Arthritis Rheum., *21*:761–766, 1981.

15. Ehrlich, M.G., et al.: Collagenase inhibitors in osteoarthritic and normal human cartilage. J. Clin. Invest., *59*:226–233, 1977.

16. Ehrlich, M.G., Mankin, H.J., and Davis, M.N.: Human epiphyseal plate proteoglycanases and degradation patterns. Trans. Orthop. Res. Soc., *4*:139, 1979.

17. Evans, C.H.: Cellular mechanisms of hydrolytic enzyme release in osteoarthritis. Semin. Arthritis Rheum., *11 (Suppl. 1)*:93–95, 1981.

18. Eyre, D.R.: Collagen: molecular diversity in the body's protein scaffold. Science, *207*:1,315–1,322, 1980.

19. Fessel, J.M., and Chrisman, O.D.: Enzymatic degradation of chondromucoprotein by cell-free extracts of human cartilage. Arthritis Rheum., *7*:398–405, 1964.

20. Freeman, M.A.R.: Adult Articular Cartilage. 2nd Ed. Tunbridge Wells, Pitman Medical, 1979.

21. Fukae, M., et al.: Chromatographically different type II collagens from human normal osteoarthritic cartilage. Biochem. Biophys. Res. Commun., *67*:1,575–1,580, 1975.

22. Gay, S., Gay, R., and Miller, E.J.: The collagen of the joint. Arthritis Rheum., *23*:937–941, 1980.

23. Gay, S., et al.: Immunohistological study on collagen in cartilage—bone metamorphoses and degenerative arthritis. Klin. Wochenschr., *54*:969–976, 1976.

24. George, R.C., and Chrisman, O.D.: The role of cartilage polysaccharides in osteoarthritis. Clin. Orthop., *57*:259–265, 1968.

25. Glant, T., Csongor, J., and Szucs, T.: Immunopathologic role of proteoglycan antigens in rheumatoid joint disease. Scand. J. Immunol., *11*:247–252, 1980.

26. Harris, E.D., Jr., et al.: Effects of proteolytic enzymes on structural and mechanical properties of cartilage. Arthritis Rheum., *15*:497–503, 1972.

27. Hascall, V.C.: *In* Biology of Carbohydrates. Vol. I. Edited by V. Ginsburg. John Wiley & Sons, 1981, pp. 1–49.

28. Herman, J.H., et al.: Potential role in the immunopathogenesis of osteoarthritis. Semin. Arthritis Rheum., *11 (Suppl. 1)*:104–107, 1981.

29. Herman, J.H., et al.: Idiopathic chondrolysis—an immunopathologic study. J. Rheumatol., *7*:694–705, 1980.

30. Howell, D.S., and Talbott, J.H. (Eds.): Osteoarthritis Symposium. Vol. 2, Suppl. 1. New York, Grune and Stratton, Inc., 1981.

31. Kato, Y., et al.: Cartilage-derived factor (CDF). 1. Stimulation of proteoglycan synthesis in rat and rabbit costal chondrocytes in culture. Exp. Cell Res., *130*:73–82, 1980.

32. Kempson, G.E., et al.: Correlations between stiffness and the chemical constituents of cartilage of the human femoral head. Biochim. Biophys. Acta, *215*:70–77, 1970.

33. Klagsburn, M., et al.: Stimulation of DNA synthesis and cell division in chondrocytes and 3T3 cells by a growth factor isolated from cartilage. Exp. Cell Res., *105*:99–108, 1977.

34. Kuettner, K.E., et al.: Lysozyme in preosseous cartilage. VII. Evidence for physiological role of lysozyme in normal endochondral calcification. Biochim. Biophys. Acta, *372*:335–344, 1974.

35. Kuettner, K.E., Harper, E., and Eisenstein, R.: Protease

36. McCarty, D.J., et al.: Milwaukee shoulder: association of microspheroids containing hydroxyapatite crystals, active collagenase and neutral protease with rotator cuff defects. Arthritis Rheum., *24*:464–491, 1981.

37. McKenzie, L.S., et al.: Sulphated glycosaminoglycan synthesis in normal and osteoarthritic hip cartilage. Ann. Rheum. Dis., *36*:369–373, 1977.

38. McKibbin, B.: The nutrition of articular cartilage and its relationship to development. *In* Normal and Osteoarthrotic Articular Cartilage. Edited by S.Y. Ali, N.W. Elves, and D.H. Leaback. London, Institute of Orthopaedics, 1974, pp. 3–8.

39. Mak, A.F., et al.: Assessment of proteoglycan-proteoglycan interactions from solution biorheological behaviors. Trans. Orthop. Res. Soc., *7*:169, 1982.

40. Malemud, C.J., et al.: Neutral proteinases from articular chondrocytes in culture. 1. A latent collagenase that degrades human cartilage type II collagen. Biochim. Biophys. Acta, *657*:517–529, 1981.

41. Mankin, H.J., et al.: Dissociation between the effect of bovine growth hormone in articular cartilage and in bone of the adult dog. J. Bone Joint Surg., *60A*:1,071–1,075, 1978.

42. Mankin, H.J., et al.: Biochemical and metabolic abnormalities in articular cartilage from osteoarthritic human hips. II. Correlation of morphology with biochemical and metabolic data. J. Bone Joint Surg., *53*:523–537, 1971.

43. Mankin, H.J., and Brandt, K.: *In* Textbook of Osteoarthritis. Edited by R. Moskowitz, et al.: Philadelphia, W.B. Saunders, 1983.

44. Mankin, H.J., and Conger, K.A.: The acute effects of intraarticular hydrocortisone on articular cartilage in rabbits. J. Bone Joint Surg., *48A*:1,383–1,388, 1966.

45. Mankin, H.J., and Thrasher, A.Z.: Water content and binding in normal and osteoarthritic human cartilage. J. Bone Joint Surg., *57A*:76–80, 1975.

46. Mankin, H.J., Johnson, M.E., and Lippiello, L.: Biochemical and metabolic abnormalities in articular cartilage from osteoarthritic human hips. II. Distribution and metabolism of amino sugar containing macromolecules. J. Bone Joint Surg., *63A*:131–134, 1981.

47. Maroudas, A.: Transport through articular cartilage and some physiologic implications. *In* Normal and Osteoarthrotic Articular Cartilage. Edited by S.Y. Ali, M.W. Elves, and D.H. Leaback. London, Institute of Orthopaedics, 1974, pp. 33–45.

48. Maroudas, A., and Holborow, E.J. (Eds.): Studies in Joint Disease. Vols. 1 and 2. Tunbridge Wells, Pitman Medical, 1980.

49. Morales, T.I., et al.: Regulation of cartilage metalloproteinases. (Abstract 89.) Arthritis Rheum., *25 (Suppl.)*, 1982.

50. Moskowitz, R.W., et al.: Specific drug therapy of experimental osteoarthritis. Semin. Arthritis Rheum., *11 (Suppl. 1)*:127–129, 1981.

51. Moskowitz, R.W., et al.: Generation of kinin-like agents by chondroitin sulfate, heparin, chitin sulfate, and human articular cartilage: possible pathophysiologic implications. J. Lab. Clin. Med., *76*:790–798, 1970.

52. Muir, H.: Heberden oration: molecular approach to the understanding of osteoarthrosis. Ann. Rheum. Dis., *36*:199–208, 1977.

53. Nimni, M.E.: Collagen: structure, function, and metabolism in normal and fibrotic tissues. Semin. Arthritis Rheum., *13*:1–86, 1983.

54. Pelletier, J.-P., et al.: Collagenase and collagenolytic activity in human osteoarthritic cartilage. Arthritis Rheum., *26*:63–68, 1983.

55. Pelletier, J.-P., et al.: Collagenolytic activity and collagen matrix breakdown of the articular cartilage in the Pond-Nuki dog model of osteoarthritis. Arthritis Rheum., *26*:1,193–1,202, 1983.

56. Phadke, K.D., and Lawrence, M.N.: Synthesis of collagenase and neutral protease by articular chondrocytes: stimulation by a macrophage-derived factor. Biochem. Biophys. Res. Commun., *85*:490, 1978.

57. Pita, J.C., et al.: Proteoglycans from normal and experimentally induced osteoarthritic (OA) articular cartilage from rabbits. (Abstract 90.) Arthritis Rheum., *25 (Suppl.)*: 1982.

58. Pita, J.C., et al.: Ultracentrifugation characterization of proteoglycans from rat growth cartilage. J. Biol. Chem., *254*:10,313–10,320, 1979.

59. Pita, J.C., Howell, D.S., and Kuettner, K.: Regulation of epiphyseal cartilage maturation. *In* Extracellular Matrix Influences on Gene Expression. Edited by H.C. Slavkin and R.C. Greulich. New York, Academic Press, 1975.

60. Poole, A.R., Hembry, R.M., and Dingle, J.T.: Cathepsin D in cartilage: the immunohistochemical demonstration of extracellular enzyme in normal and pathological conditions. J. Cell Sci., *14*:139–161, 1974.

61. Prins, A.P.A., Lipman, J., and Sokoloff, L.: Effect of purified growth factors on rabbit articular chondrocytes in monolayer culture. I. DNA synthesis. Submitted for publication.

62. Radin, E.L.: The physiology and degeneration of joints. Semin. Arthritis Rheum., *2*:245–257, 1972.

63. Radin, E.L., Maquet, P., and Parker, H.: Rationale and indications for the ''hanging hip'' procedure: a clinical and experimental study. Clin. Orthop., *112*:221–230, 1975.

64. Ridge, S., Oransky, A.L., and Kerwar, S.S.: Induction of the synthesis of latent collagenase and latent neutral protease in chondrocytes by a factor synthesized by activated macrophages. Arthritis Rheum., *23*:448–454, 1980.

65. Rosenberg, L., Hellman, W., and Kleinschmidt, A.K.: Electron microscope studies of proteoglycan aggregates from bovine articular cartilage. J. Biol. Chem., *250*:1,877, 1975.

66. Rosner, I.A., et al.: Pathologic and metabolic responses of experimental osteoarthritis to estradiol and an estradiol antagonist. Clin. Orthop., *171*:280–286, 1982.

67. Roughley, P.J., Murphy, G., and Barrett, A.J.: Proteinase inhibitors of bovine nasal cartilage. Biochem. J., *169*:721, 1978.

68. Salter, R.B., et al.: The effects of continuous passive motion on the healing of articular cartilage defects—an experimental investigation in rabbits. J. Bone Joint Surg., *57*:570, 1975.

69. Sandy, J.D., Brown, H.L.G., and Lowther, D.A.: Degradation of proteoglycan in articular cartilage. Biochim. Biophys. Acta, *543*:536–544, 1978.

70. Sapolsky, A.I., et al.: Neutral proteinases from articular chondrocytes in culture. 2. Metal-dependent latent neutral proteoglycanase, and inhibitory activity. Biochim. Biophys. Acta, *658*:138–147, 1981.

71. Sapolsky, A.I., et al.: Metalloproteases of human articular cartilage that digest cartilage proteoglycan at neutral and acid pH. J. Clin. Invest., *58*:1,030–1,041, 1976.

72. Sapolsky, A.I., et al.: The action of cathepsin D in human articular cartilage on proteoglycans. J. Clin. Invest., *52*:624–633, 1973.

73. Sapolsky, A.I., and Howell, D.S.: Further characterization of a neutral metalloprotease isolated from human articular cartilage. Arthritis Rheum., *25*:988, 1983.

74. Sapolsky, A.I., Howell, D.S., and Woessner, J.F., Jr.: Neutral proteases and cathepsin D in human articular cartilage. J. Clin. Invest., *53*:1,044–1,053, 1974.

75. Sokoloff, L. (Ed.): The Joints and Synovial Fluid. Vols. 1 and 2. New York, Academic Press, 1980.

76. Stack, M.T., and Brandt, K.D.: Identification and characterization of articular cartilage hyaluronidase (HAase). (Abstract 70.) Arthritis Rheum., *25 (Suppl.)*: 1982.

77. Swann, D.A.: Micromolecules of synovial fluid. *In* The Joints and Synovial Fluid. Vol. 1. Edited by L. Sokoloff. New York, Academic Press, 1978, pp. 407–432.

78. Swann, D.A.: The lubricating activity of synovial fluid glycoproteins. Arthritis Rheum., *24*:22–30, 1981.

79. Thompson, R.C., Jr., and Oegema, T.R., Jr.: Metabolic activity of articular cartilage in osteoarthritis: an in vitro study. J. Bone Joint Surg., *61A*:407–416, 1979.

80. Vater, C.A., Nagase, H., and Harris, E.D., Jr.: Procollagenase activator: a regulatory protein essential for rabbit synovial collagenase activation. (Abstract 135.) Arthritis Rheum., *26*:S31, 1983.

81. Woessner, J.F., Jr., and Howell, D.S.: Hydrolytic enzymes in cartilage. *In* Studies in Joint Disease 2. Edited by A. Maroudas and E.J. Holborow. Tunbridge Wells, Pitman Medical, 1983, pp. 106–152.

82. Wood, K.M., Wusterman, F.S., and Curtis, C.G.: The degradation of intravenously injected chondroitin-4 sulfate in the rat. Biochem. J., *134*:1,009–1,013, 1973.

Chapter 89

Clinical and Laboratory Findings in Osteoarthritis

Roland W. Moskowitz

Osteoarthritis is a slowly evolving articular disease characterized by the gradual development of joint pain, stiffness, and limitation of motion. The terms *degenerative joint disease* or *osteoarthrosis* may be more precise because degeneration of cartilage is the most prominent pathologic change. Both experimental[89] and clinical[100] studies have shown mild to moderate synovitis, however. Some favor a particular form of nomenclature, but at present, the terms osteoarthritis, osteoarthrosis, and degenerative joint disease are used interchangeably. Although this disease is often benign, severe degenerative changes may cause serious disability. Newer concepts of pathogenesis suggest that osteoarthritis is not an inevitable consequence of aging itself, and raise the possibility of rational preventive and therapeutic methods in the future.

CLASSIFICATION

Classification of osteoarthritis is difficult because of its varying forms of presentation. Increasing support exists for the concept that osteoarthritis may represent a number of disease subsets leading to similar clinical and pathologic alterations, rather than one specific disorder. The disease is classified as *primary* or idiopathic when it occurs in the absence of any known underlying predisposing factor. In contrast, *secondary* osteoarthritis is that form of the disease following an identifiable underlying local or systemic pathogenetic factor. The distinctions on which this simple classification are based may be artificial, however. Studies on osteoarthritis of the hip, for example, show that many cases of ''primary'' osteoarthritis are actually secondary to anatomic abnormalities that result in articular incongruity and premature cartilage degeneration, such as congenital hip dysplasia and slipped capital femoral epiphysis of childhood.[90] Various forms of the disease, such as primary generalized osteoarthritis, erosive inflammatory osteoarthritis, diffuse idiopathic skeletal hyperostosis, and chondromalacia patellae, have different clinical, pathologic, and radiologic findings and are generally considered distinct syndromes. Alternatively, because of fundamental ignorance in pathogenesis,

these syndromes may merely reflect various clinical extremes of the disease. A working classification of osteoarthritis based on known anatomic and etiologic mechanisms is presented in Table 89–1.

PRIMARY OSTEOARTHRITIS

Interpretation of data regarding the natural history of primary osteoarthritis is complicated by the

Table 89–1. Classification of Osteoarthritis

Primary (Idiopathic)
  Peripheral joints
  Spine
    Apophyseal joints
    Intervertebral joints
  Subsets
    Generalized osteoarthritis
    Erosive inflammatory osteoarthritis
    Diffuse idiopathic skeletal hyperostosis
    Chondromalacia patellae
Secondary
  Trauma
    Acute
    Chronic (occupational, sports)
  Underlying joint disorders
    Local (fracture, infection)
    Diffuse (rheumatoid arthritis)
  Systemic metabolic or endocrine disorders
    Ochronosis (alkaptonuria)
    Wilson's disease
    Hemochromatosis
    Kashin-Beck disease
    Acromegaly
    Hyperparathyroidism
  Crystal deposition disease
    Calcium pyrophosphate dihydrate (pseudogout)
    Basic calcium phosphate (hydroxyapatite-octacalcium phosphate-tricalcium phosphate)
    Monosodium urate monohydrate (gout)
  Neuropathic disorders (Charcot joints)
    Tabes dorsalis
    Diabetes mellitus
  Intra-artcular corticosteroid overuse
  Miscellaneous
    Bone dysplasia (multiple epiphyseal dysplasia; achondroplasia)
    Frostbite

different case-finding techniques, whether clinical, radiologic, or pathologic, used in many of the reported studies. Moreover, studies focused on different joints cannot be compared, even when similar case-finding methods are used. Variations due to interobserver error may be significant, despite the use of essentially identical protocols. Nevertheless, sufficient data permit a reasonable approximation of the natural course of the disease.

Epidemiologic Features

A comparison of epidemiologic surveys undertaken to characterize the prevalence and clinical characteristics of osteoarthritis requires close attention to variations in analytic techniques and populations studied[101] (see also Chap. 2). Such variations may have a major impact on the data obtained. Studies derived from autopsy analyses, for example, define earlier disease than clinical studies based on symptoms that develop later. In clinical surveys, disease definitions must be clear, and the use of prospective or retrospective techniques must be taken into account. Data obtained from roentgenographic studies depend on the number and location of joints studied.[12,66] Surveys of hospitalized patients, in contrast to those in the general population, are narrow in scope, but they may be useful in identifying certain disease subsets.

Prevalence

Autopsy studies show that degenerative joint changes begin in the second decade.[78] By age 40, 90% of all persons have such changes in their weight-bearing joints, even though clinical symptoms are generally absent. Roentgenographic manifestations of the disease are common in the third decade, and involvement increases progressively with age. In a survey of roentgenograms of the hands and feet, 40.5 million (37 of each 100) adult United States citizens living outside institutions had some evidence of osteoarthritis.[111] The prevalence rate increased from 4 per 100 among persons 18 to 24 years of age to 85 per 100 at age 75 to 79 years. In addition, 23% of those with osteoarthritis had moderate or severe disease. Under age 45, nearly all cases were mild. A roentgenographic survey of a larger number of joints showed osteoarthritis in approximately 52% of an adult English population.[75] When minimal disease was excluded, the prevalence of osteoarthritis was about 20%. In persons aged 55 to 64 years, 85% of those studied had some degree of osteoarthritis in one or more joints.

In all studies, the relation of osteoarthritis to aging is striking. When individuals with severe grades of osteoarthritis only are considered, the increase in osteoarthritis with age is exponential.[75] Several possible explanations have been advanced. Release of cartilage matrix molecules from their normally isolated locale relative to the vascular system may lead to a progressively enhanced autoimmune response. Alternatively, mild, early degeneration may be augmented by superimposed mechanical instability.

Sex, Race, and Heredity

Men and women were equally affected by osteoarthritis in one study when all ages were considered.[111] Under age 45, prevalence was greater among men, whereas prevalence was greater in women than in men after age 55. Moderate and severe grades of osteoarthritis were seen to a greater extent in women than in men. In radiographic studies in Great Britain on population samples from the age of 15 years,[69] the number of joints involved and severity were similar in men and women to age 54; thereafter, the disease was more severe and more generalized in women. The pattern of joint involvement was also similar in men and women under age 55, but in older persons, distal interphalangeal, proximal interphalangeal, and first carpometacarpal joints were more frequently affected in women, and hips were more commonly affected in men. The sex difference in patterns of joint involvement suggests that, although the same basic etiologic mechanisms may be involved in osteoarthritis in both sexes, the pattern in men may be affected by trauma, occupational stress, and mechanical factors. Clinical symptoms appear to be more common in women.

Differences in the prevalence of osteoarthritis in black and white races have been noted, particularly when patterns of joint involvement are analyzed.[15,127] Heberden's nodes are rare in the black populations of South Africa, Nigeria, Liberia, and the United States.[71,126] The differences can often be attributed to variations in occupation and life style. Differences in certain predisposing genetic factors, such as congenital subluxation of the hip, may also play a role.

Studies in China and India have documented a lower incidence of hip osteoarthritis in these populations than in Caucasians.[17,61] In the Chinese, the hip joint may be protected by the extreme range of motion required for frequent squatting. A decreased frequency of predisposing factors such as rheumatoid arthritis (RA), congenital dysplasia of the hip, and slipped capital femoral epiphysis, all believed to be uncommon in the Chinese, may also explain some of the differences.[61] Degenerative joint disease was more prevalent in American Indians than in the general population.[111]

The prevalence of osteoarthritis of the hips is

greater in white populations than in black and American Indian populations.[74] A study of osteoarthritis of the knees, in contrast, revealed less difference among ethnic groups. A lower prevalence of knee osteoarthritis in women from the west coast of Greenland, who are from a mixed Eskimo-European stock, than in women from the east coast, who are pure Eskimo, may be related to occupational factors.[5]

Genetic factors in generalized osteoarthritis have been evaluated in a detailed series of studies by Kellgren and Lawrence and their co-workers in England.[67,69,72,73] Patients with generalized osteoarthritis comprise two clinical groups, differentiated by the presence or absence of osteoarthritis of the distal interphalangeal joints of the hands (Heberden's nodes). Patients with generalized disease and involvement of these hand joints are said to have "nodal" osteoarthritis. Involvement of proximal interphalangeal, first carpometacarpal, spinal apophyseal, hip, knee, first tarsometatarsal, and first metatarsophalangeal joints is frequent. Nodal generalized osteoarthritis is more common in women than in men and has an inheritance pattern similar to that described by Stecher and colleagues for Heberden's nodes alone.[134] The inheritance pattern is consistent with a single autosomal gene, dominant in females and recessive in males. Generalized osteoarthritis in the absence of Heberden's nodes, "non-nodal osteoarthritis," appears to show polygenic inheritance. Statistically significant associations with seronegative inflammatory polyarthritis,[69] hyperuricemia,[73] and hypertension[72] have been observed.

Climate

On the basis of geographic studies in Northern Europe and America, it has been suggested that osteoarthritis is less frequent farther north.[15] To support these observations are the findings that the prevalence of osteoarthritis may be lower in Alaskan Eskimos,[14] as well as less prevalent in Finland than in the Netherlands.[76] Studies comparing populations in Jamaica and Great Britain, however, revealed an equal frequency in the two climates.[15] Factors such as race, culture, and environment complicate comparisons of climatic effects on disease prevalence. Clinical symptoms may be less severe in a warmer climate, related perhaps to higher temperatures, greater amounts of sunshine, and lighter-weight clothes.

Obesity, Body Somatotype, and Bone Density

The role of obesity as an etiologic factor in osteoarthritis remains controversial. Some experimental[124] and clinical[48,113,119] studies have

suggested that obesity itself is not a factor in the induction or aggravation of degenerative joint disease; other studies have demonstrated an increased frequency of osteoarthritis in the obese, particularly in weight-bearing joints.[64,65,77] Obese persons have an increased incidence of osteoarthritis in non-weight-bearing joints, such as the sternoclavicular and distal interphalangeal joints.[65] It has also been suggested that obesity in osteoarthritic patients may be a secondary phenomenon caused by the relative inactivity brought on by joint pain and limitation of motion.[48]

In addition to the possible biomechanical effects of obesity in the origin of osteoarthritis, a metabolic role for fat in disease pathogenesis has been suggested.[121] Studies in certain strains of mice that develop osteoarthritis showed that diets enriched with lard, a saturated fat, increased the frequency and severity of the osteoarthritic lesions. When unsaturated fat was fed to achieve the same body weight, however, no adverse effect was noted. Perhaps obesity in humans is related to osteoarthritis not only through its biomechanical effects, but also as a result of still obscure metabolic changes in cartilage.

Osteoarthritis has been associated with specific somatotypes; its prevalence is greater in stout individuals than in thin ones.[2] When patients with osteoarthritis of the hip or femoral neck fractures were compared, 94% of the osteoarthritic patients were endomorphic mesomorphs, whereas the majority of patients with fractures were ectomorphic.[128]

Data from several studies now support the concept that bone density is associated with osteoarthritis. In studies of the femoral head, a diminished bone mass was associated with femoral neck fracture; increased bone mass, on the other hand, showed a positive correlation with osteoarthritis of the hip.[45,112,125,128,143] Quantitative bone density by photon-absorption study of the proximal phalanx of both hands was greater than normal in a group of 25 patients with degenerative arthritis of the hip or knee associated with calcium pyrophosphate dihydrate crystal deposition and in a group of 22 patients with similar degenerative changes not associated with crystal deposition.[79a] It has been suggested that reduction in bone mass increases the shock-absorbing capacity of subchondral bone and thus protects articular cartilage against stress. Conversely, the stiffer, denser subchondral bone increases the mechanical forces acting through cartilage, with a resultant predisposition to degenerative change.

Increased ligamentous laxity correlates positively with joint degeneration. A study of patients with joint hypermobility revealed an increased prevalence of generalized osteoarthritis over age- and sex-matched control subjects.[11] Conversely, when patients with osteoarthritis were evaluated, the prevalence of generalized joint hypermobility was higher than in matched control subjects.[145] Synovial effusions and chondrocalcinosis were common.

Occupation and Sports

Stress related to occupation or sports activities has been implicated in the induction of osteoarthritis. In one study, osteoarthritis of the hips, knees, and shoulders was more common in miners than in porters or clerks.[114] Dock workers showed a higher prevalence of osteoarthritis of the fingers, elbows, and knees than age-matched civil servants.[97] The joints in the right hand are more commonly involved than those in the left hand. Repetitive handwork peformed by women in a weaving factory confirmed that the right hand was more severely involved; this study also noted that the pattern of hand and finger lesions could be directly related to the type of work done by each group, and the joints used most repetitively were also the most involved by disease.[53] Prolonged or repeated, heavy overuse of joints has been related to an increased frequency of osteoarthritis in bus drivers[73] and foundry workers.[87]

Other studies, however, have failed to demonstrate a consistent relationship between osteoarthritis and trauma. Studies of pneumatic hammer drillers showed no increased risk of osteoarthritis of the elbow, and studies of Finnish running champions revealed no increase in degenerative joint disease of the hip over age- and sex-matched control subjects.[105] An evaluation of knee joints of veteran marathon runners confirmed the relative absence of osteoarthritis.[82] Osteoarthritis was not seen as a complication of free-fall or military parachute jumping.[146]

A number of studies have suggested that osteoarthritis is common in soccer players.[16,99,129] Many of these studies, however, used osteophytes alone as an indication of osteoarthritis. Little evidence suggests that exercise itself is deleterious to normal joints when the criterion is the loss of roentgenographic joint space.[3,105]

Symptoms and Signs

The symptoms of osteoarthritis are localized to the affected joints (Table 89–2). Involvement of a number of joints may suggest a systemic form of arthritis. Frequently, little or no correlation exists between the joint symptoms and the extent or degree of pathologic or radiologic change. This disparity was noted in the previously mentioned autopsy study wherein, by age 40, 90% of all persons

had degenerative changes in weight-bearing joints, even if clinical symptoms were absent.[78] Cobb, Merchant, and Rubin reported that only about 30% of persons with roentgenographic evidence of degenerative joint disease complained of pain at the relevant sites.[20] Studies by Lawrence, Bremner, and Bier showed that, except for lumbar apophyseal joints, persons with radiographic osteoarthritis were predisposed to develop related symptoms.[75] Similarly, a positive correlation between clinical symptoms and roentgenographic evidence of osteoarthritis of the knee was noted by Gresham and Rathey.[52] Some of the apparent disparity between symptoms and radiologic abnormalities may relate to the roentgenologic definitions of osteoarthritis. For example, the use of osteophytes alone as a diagnostic feature of osteoarthritis has been questioned. Long-term radiographic studies of the hip and knee suggest that the presence of osteophytes does not imply later development of other structural changes of osteoarthritis, such as joint space narrowing, subchondral bone cysts, and eburnation.[25,26,60] Correlation of symptoms with these more definitive structural abnormalities might well provide evidence of a positive interrelationship.

The cardinal symptom of osteoarthritis is pain, which at first occurs after joint use and is relieved by rest. The pain is usually aching in character and is poorly localized. As the disease progresses, pain may occur with minimal motion or even at rest. In advanced cases, pain may awaken the patient during sleep because of the loss of protective muscular joint splinting, which limits painful motion during the waking hours. Because cartilage has no nerve supply and is insensitive to pain, the pain in osteoarthritis must arise from noncartilaginous intra- and periarticular structures. The pain is usually multifactorial and may result from elevation of the periosteum accompanying marginal bony proliferation, pressure on exposed subchondral bone, trabecular microfractures, involvement of intra-articular ligaments, capsular distention, and pinching or abrasion of synovial villi. Additional contributory factors may be synovitis and capsulitis. Although prostaglandins released from synovial tissues and chondrocytes theoretically may contribute to pain response, a parallel between the inflammatory response and joint fluid prostaglandin concentrations has not been described.[137] Periarticular tissues such as tendons and fascia are supplied with sensory nerves and are an important source of pain. Spasm of muscles around the joint or pressure on contiguous nerves may be more painful than the pain of articular origin. Frequently, as with other types of joint disease, the pain is intensified just before changes in weather.

Osteoarthritis is sometimes associated with acute

Table 89–2.   **Clinical Profiles of Osteoarthritis**

Factor	Characteristics and Occurrence
Age	Usually advanced; symptoms uncommon before age 40, unless due to secondary cause
Joint involvement	Commonly, distal interphalangeal, proximal interphalangeal, first carpometacarpal, hip, knee, first metatarsophalangeal joints and lower lumbar and cervical vertebrae
	Rarely, metacarpophalangeal, wrist, elbow, or shoulder joints, except after trauma
Joint effusion	Little or none
Onset	Usually insidious
Systemic manifestations	Rarely
True bony ankylosis	Uncommon
Symptoms	Pain on motion (early); pain at rest (later); pain aggravated by prolonged activity, relieved by rest; localized stiffness of short duration relieved by exercise; possibly painful muscle spasm; limitation of motion; "flares" associated with crystal-induced synovitis
Signs	Localized tenderness; crepitus and crackling on motion; mild joint enlargement with firm consistency from proliferation of bone and cartilage; synovitis (less common), gross deformity (later)

or subacute inflammation. This response is most common in erosive (inflammatory) osteoarthritis of the hands, but it may occur in other peripheral joints. When seen in peripheral joints other than the hands, such inflammatory "acute flares" have been attributed to various degrees of trauma or to crystal-induced synovitis in response to calcium pyrophosphate or other crystals.[30,116,117]

Stiffness on awakening in the morning and after periods of inactivity during the day is a common complaint. Such stiffness is of short duration, rarely lasting for more than 15 minutes. Limitation of motion develops as the disease progresses, owing to joint-surface incongruity, muscle spasm and contracture, capsular contracture, and mechanical block from osteophytes or loose bodies. In weight-bearing joints, abrupt *giving way* may occur. Objectively, joints may show *localized tenderness*, especially if synovitis is present. *Pain on passive motion* may be a prominent finding even without local tenderness. *Crepitus*, a crackling or grating sound as the joint is moved, may result from cartilage loss and joint-surface irregularity. Enlargement of the joint may be caused by secondary synovitis, an increase in synovial fluid, or marginal proliferative changes in cartilage or bone (osteophytes). Osteophytes can be readily palpated along the margins of the affected joint. Late stages of the disease are associated with gross deformity and subluxation due to cartilage loss, collapse of subchondral bone, formation of bone cysts, and gross bony overgrowth. Although these symptoms and signs are common to osteoarthritis in general, the clinical picture and course depend on the particular joint involvement.

Specific Joint Involvement

Heberden's Nodes

One of the most common manifestations of primary degenerative joint disease is the *Heberden's*

node[58] (Figs. 89–1, 89–2). This cartilaginous and bony enlargement of the dorsolateral and dorsomedial aspects of the distal interphalangeal joints of the fingers is often associated with flexion and lateral deviation of the distal phalanx. Similar nodes may be seen in the proximal interphalangeal joints, where they are called *Bouchard's nodes* (Fig. 89–3). Heberden's nodes may be single, but they usually are multiple. They begin most often after age 45. Women are affected much more frequently than men, at a ratio of approximately 10 to 1.[133] Stecher and co-workers found that heredity plays a large part in the origin of these lesions, particularly in the female side of the family, in mothers, daughters, and sisters.[132] Heberden's nodes were twice as common in mothers and 3 times as common in sisters of affected women than in the general population.[134] Stecher postulated a single autosomal gene, sex-influenced, dominant in females and recessive in males, with complete penetrance by age 70, because all who have this gene develop the disease. Although idiopathic Heberden's nodes undoubtedly have a genetic origin, the exact mode of transmission remains open to question because several genetic patterns fit the available data.

Clinically, Heberden's nodes may develop gradually with little or no pain and may progress essentially unnoticed for months or years. In other cases, they appear rapidly with redness, swelling, tenderness, and aching, particularly after use. Afflicted individuals may complain of paresthesias and loss of dexterity. A number of joints may be involved almost simultaneously, or one or two joints may be involved for a long time before others develop similar changes. The swollen joints may feel either soft and fluctuant or hard. Small, gelatinous cysts may appear, generally on the dorsal

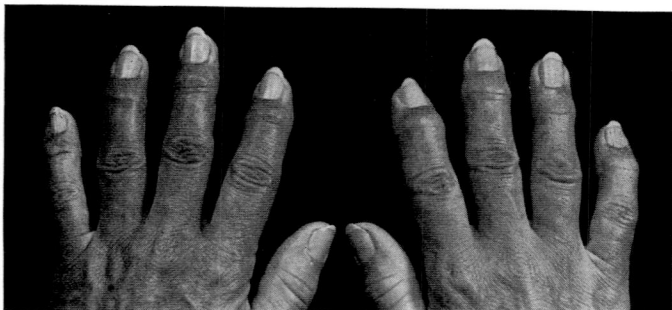

Fig. 89–1. Typical Heberden's nodes, the cardinal sign of primary osteoarthritis. Note their characteristic position at the distal interphalangeal joints. The proximal interphalangeal joints may be involved later.

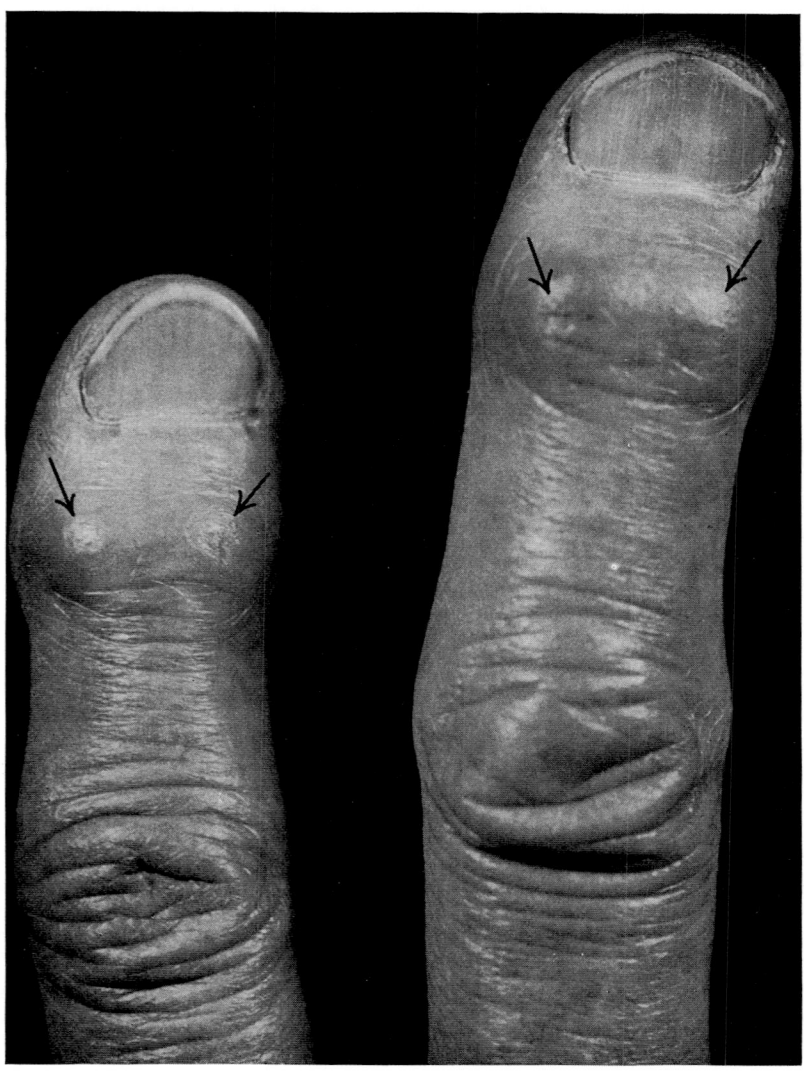

Fig. 89–2. Close-up view of Heberden's nodes (arrows) affecting the index and middle fingers.

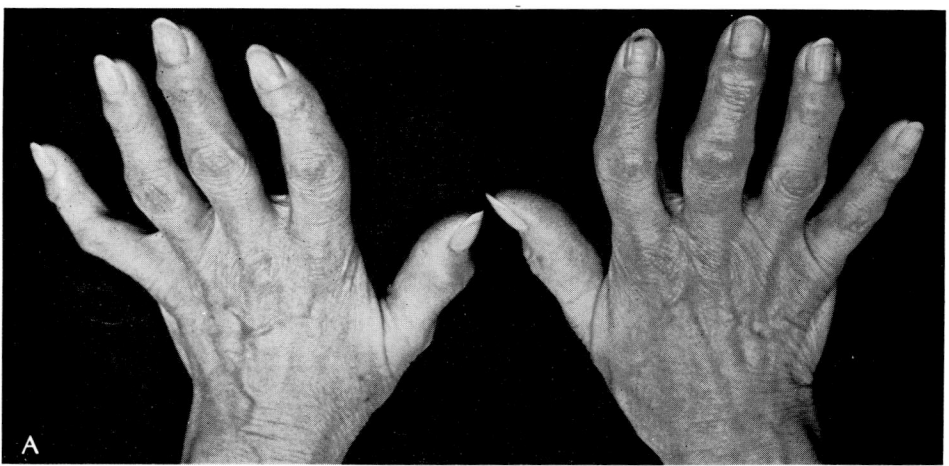

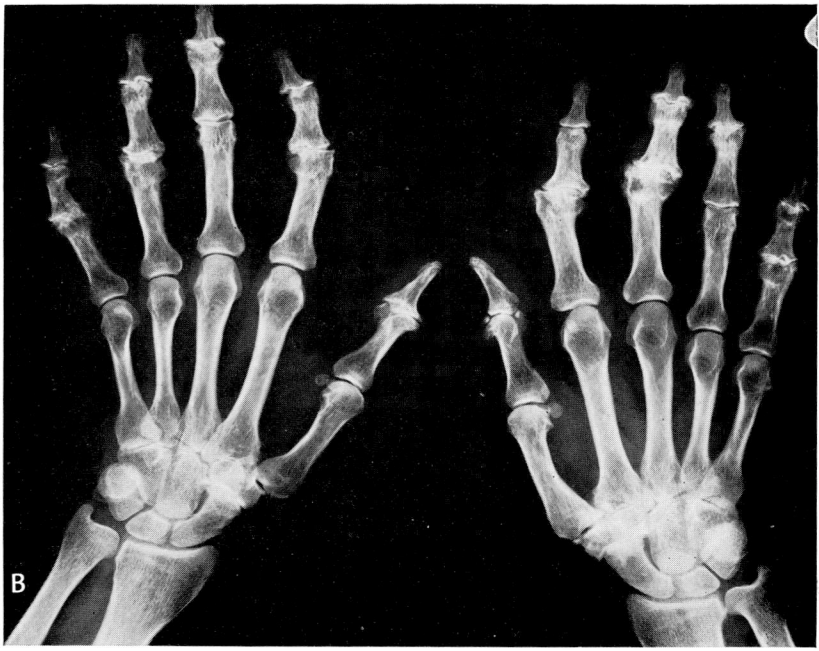

Fig. 89–3. *A,* Primary osteorarthritis of the hands with marked proximal interphalangeal joint involvement (Bouchard's nodes), as well as distal interphalangeal joint involvement (Heberden's nodes). *B,* Roentgenographic appearance of the same hands.

aspects of the joint or just proximal to it. These cysts, which are often attached to tendon sheaths and resemble ganglia, may recede spontaneously or may persist indefinitely. At times, they precede the appearance of the Heberden's node itself. Their cause is uncertain. Studies have demonstrated communication of the cyst with the distal interphalangeal joint space.[33] Later, this communication may be pinched off, but at some stage in development the cyst is in direct communication with the joint space. As stated, the *proximal interpha-*

langeal joints of the fingers may also be involved, usually after several distal joints are affected. Horizontal deviation of the distal and proximal interphalangeal joints may lead to a snake-like configuration of the hands. Metacarpophalangeal joint involvement is rare.

Carpometacarpal Joint. Degenerative changes involving the first carpometacarpal joint are often present. Pain and localized tenderness may suggest a stenosing tenosynovitis. The patient often has a tender prominence at the base of the first metacarpal bone, and the joint in this area may have a squared appearance (shelf sign) (Fig. 89–4). Motion is often limited and painful. Radiographic examination may reveal subluxation of the base of the first metacarpal bone in addition to joint space narrowing and osteophyte formation. The occurrence of osteoarthritic changes in the *trapezioscaphoid joint* of the wrist is common.[98] Changes may occur in association with osteoarthritis of the first carpometacarpal and distal interphalangeal joints, or they may be an isolated finding. Symptoms and signs include pain in the wrist and thumb base, radial and volar swelling, and tenderness over the scaphoid bone.

Metatarsophalangeal Joints. One of the most common sites of primary osteoarthritis is the first metatarsophlangeal joint of the foot. The onset is usually insidious, with gradual progression of swelling and pain. Symptoms may be aggravated by wearing tight shoes. A sudden increase in swelling and pain may accompany inflammation of the bursa at the medial aspect of the joint (bunion). The irregular contour of the involved joint can be felt. Foot symptoms may also result from osteoarthritis of the subtalar and other tarsal joints. Pain of subtalar origin is aggravated by inversion and eversion of the foot, and symptoms may make walking difficult.

Acromioclavicular Joint. Degenerative arthritis of the acromioclavicular joint is frequently overlooked as a cause of shoulder pain and disability. Symptoms are usually poorly localized to the joint, and shoulder motion is nearly normal, although painful. Roentgenographic changes of degeneration are often minimal. Osteoarthritis of the manubriosternal joint is rare, but it may result in chest pain and tenderness.

Temporomandibular Joint. Osteoarthritis occurs in the temporomandibular joint and produces symptoms of crepitus, stiffness, and pain (see also Chap. 81). Similar symptoms may be caused by disturbances in temporomandibular joint dynamics (temporomandibular dysfunction syndrome), rather than by structural degenerative change. The patient may complain of joint noise and pain, masticatory muscle tenderness, limited motion, and deviation of the jaw to the affected side. The distinction between osteoarthritis and temporomandibular dysfunction is primarily established by objective roentgenographic findings of degenerative change. Panoramic jaw films with the mouth first closed and then opened should be obtained, to assess condylar motion. Polytomographic studies, with or without arthrograms, are helpful for further, detailed evaluation.

Knee. The knee joints are frequently affected by primary degenerative joint disease (Fig. 89–5). One should try to localize the clinical findings to the medial femorotibial, lateral femorotibial, and patellofemoral compartments, its three anatomic components. Symptoms consist of pain on motion, relieved by rest; stiffness, particularly after sitting or rising in the morning; and crepitus on motion. Little objective change might be found on examination. At times, the patient has localized tenderness over various aspects of the joint and pain on passive motion. Irregular, hard enlargement due to osteophytes may be seen and felt. Mild synovitis and joint effusion may be present. Crepitus can often be detected when the examiner's hand is held over the patella as the knee is flexed. Pain may be elicited by the examiner, by holding the patella tight against the femur with the quadriceps relaxed and then requesting that the patient contract this muscle. Limitation of joint motion, usually extension, on both active or passive motion may be noted. Muscle atrophy about the knee may occur rapidly, especially with disuse. Disproportionate degenerative changes localized to the medial or lateral compartment of the knee may lead to secondary genu varus or, much less commonly, to genu valgus with joint instability and subluxation. Instability is further aggravated by laxity of the collateral ligaments. Isolated patellofemoral compartment or tricompartmental involvement should alert the clinician to underlying calcium pyrophosphate dihydrate crystal deposition. Calcium pyrophosphate dihydrate and basic calcium phosphate crystal deposition are commonly associated with disease of the lateral tibiofemoral compartment and genu valgus.[54a]

Hip. Osteoarthritis of the hip, also known as malum coxae senilis or morbus coxae senilis, may be disabling (Fig. 89–6). Symptoms usually first appear in older individuals. This condition occurs more frequently in men than in women and may be unilateral or bilateral. In a study of the natural history of hip osteoarthritis, Evarts noted that over

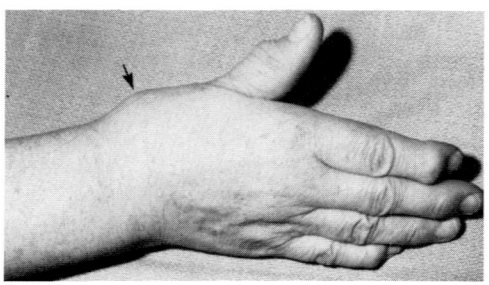

Fig. 89–4. Severe osteoarthritis of the first carpometacarpal joint leads to a prominent squaring (shelf sign) at the base of the thumb (arrow). Heberden's nodes are also seen.

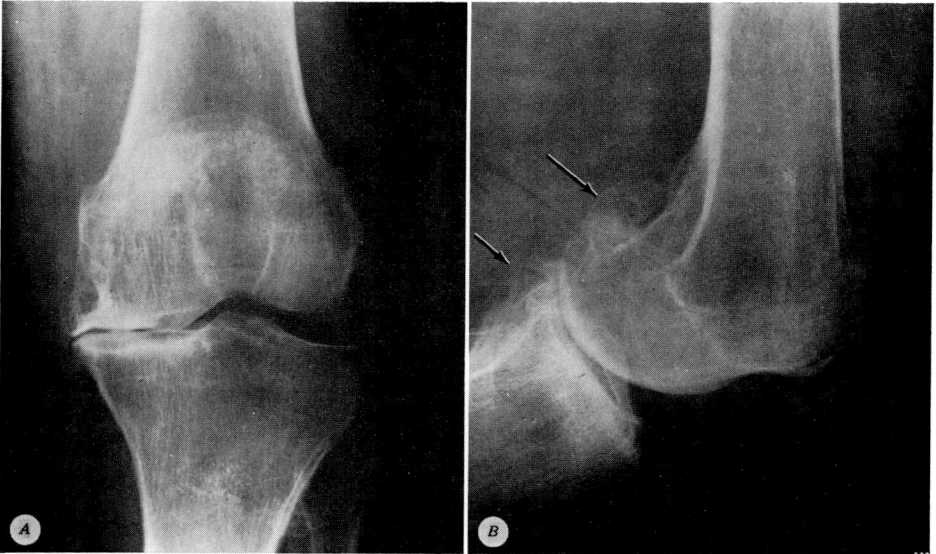

Fig. 89–5. *A,* Osteoarthritis of the knee; medial joint space narrowing is prominent and is associated with subchondral bony sclerosis (eburnation) and osteophyte formation. *B,* Lateral view of the same knee; large osteophytes can be seen at the posterior aspects of the femur and tibia (arrows).

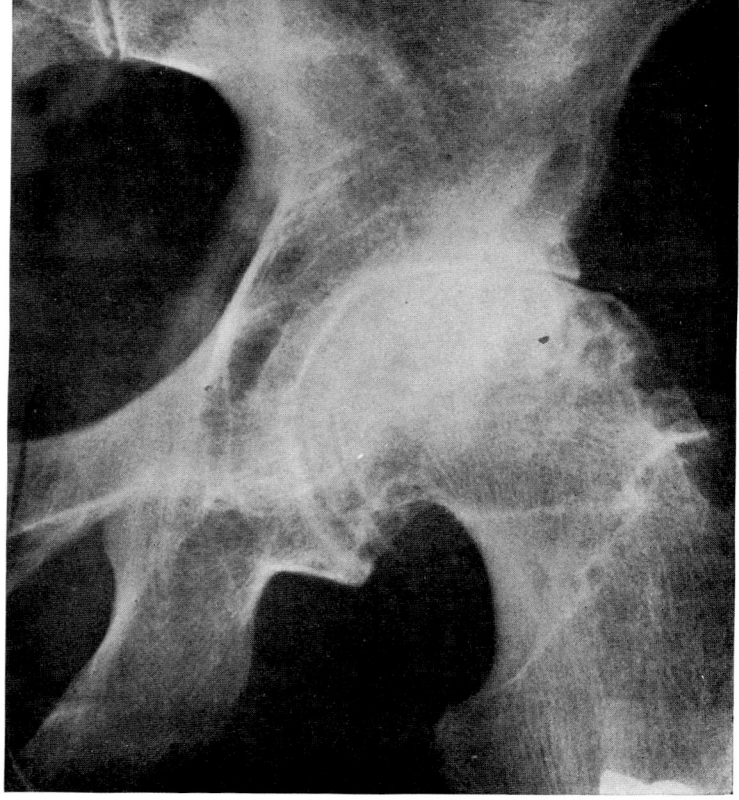

Fig. 89–6. Osteoarthritis of the hip. Note the almost complete loss of articular cartilage, flattening of the femoral head, and small cystic areas in the head and neck of the femur. Subchondral bone is sclerotic.

a period of 8 years, 10% of patients with unilateral hip degeneration developed bilateral disease.[37]

Data on the frequency of right and left hip involvement in unilateral disease are conflicting. In a study of 54 patients with idiopathic osteoarthritis of the hip, Meachim and colleagues noted that the right and left hip were affected with equal frequency when hip disease was unilateral.[84] In a study of 175 patients, Macys et al. noted that 13% of males and 29% of females had unilateral disease.[82] The female patients had a significant predilection for a particular side. Twenty right and 10 left hips were involved, a 2:1 ratio. In those with the onset of symptoms after age 60, the ratio of right to left hip involvement was even more marked, 7:1.

The main symptom of degenerative joint disease of the hip is insidious pain followed by a characteristic limp *(antalgic gait).* Pain in the hip may not originate there, and pain actually arising in the hip joint may be referred to other areas. Hip pain may arise in the lower back and may be referred to the iliac crest or buttock. True hip pain is usually felt on its outer aspect, in the groin, or along the inner aspect of the thigh. It may be referred to the buttocks or sciatic region and is often referred along branches of the obturator nerve down to the knee. Occasionally, most of the pain is in the knee, and its true origin is overlooked. The degree of pain varies widely and does not always correlate with the extent of cartilaginous and osseous changes. Trochanteric bursitis, caused by inflammation of the bursa between the gluteus maximus muscle and the greater trochanter, produces pain and tenderness at the lateral aspect of the hip; symptoms and physical findings may simulate these seen in patients with osteoarthritis of the hip. Pain is exaggerated by weight bearing, and a mild limp is common. Hip motion is normal, in contrast to the limitation of motion seen in osteoarthritis of the hip joint itself. Localized tenderness over the area of bursitis is characteristic. Rapid relief of symptoms following bursal injection with local corticosteroids and procaine is diagnostically helpful.

Stiffness is common and increases after inactivity. Examination reveals varying degrees of limitation of motion. The leg is often held in external rotation with the hip flexed and adducted. Severe backache may result from the compensatory lordosis accompanying flexion contracture. Functional shortening of the extremity may occur. The gait is frequently awkward and shuffling or waddling. Sitting is difficult, as is rising from this position, owing to limitation of motion.

Spine. Degenerative joint disease of the spine is common (Fig. 89–7). It may result from degenerative changes in the intervertebral fibrocartilag-

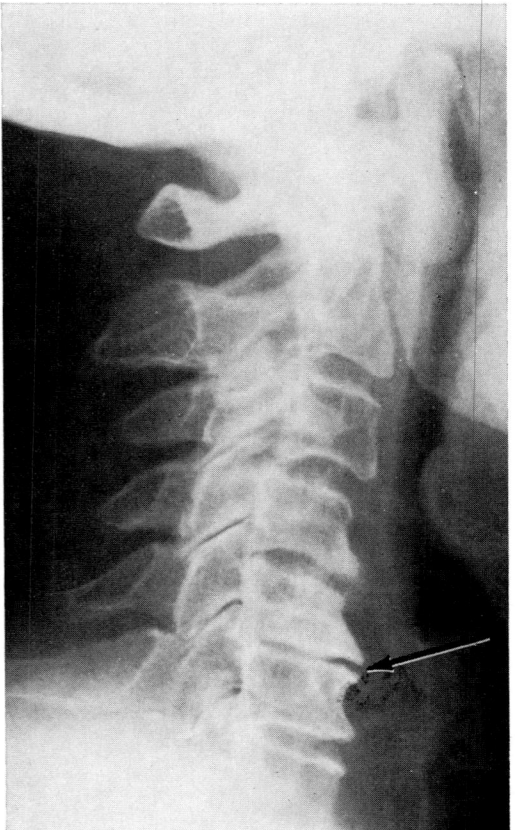

Fig. 89–7. Osteoarthritic changes in the lower cervical spine. Spur formation is prominent. Note the marked narrowing of the intervertebral disc between C5 and C6 vertebrae (arrow).

inous discs, from vertebral bodies, or from posterior apophyseal articulations. Disc narrowing may cause subluxation of the posterior apophyseal joints (see also Chap. 80). Lipping or spur formation (osteophytosis) on the vertebral bodies is a prominent finding (Fig. 89–8). Anterior spurs are most prevalent. Although usually asymptomatic, large anterior osteophytes in the cervical spine may give rise to symptoms of dysphagia.[85,104] Respiratory symptoms such as hoarseness, coughing, and aspiration may be noted. Degenerative changes consisting of joint-space narrowing, bony sclerosis, and spur formation are seen in apophyseal joints. Some authors make a distinction between degenerative changes involving the discs and vertebral bodies, for which they use the term *spondylosis,* and degenerative changes of the apophyseal joints, which are classified as true osteoarthritis, because radiologic abnormalities more closely resemble those seen in other diarthrodial joints.

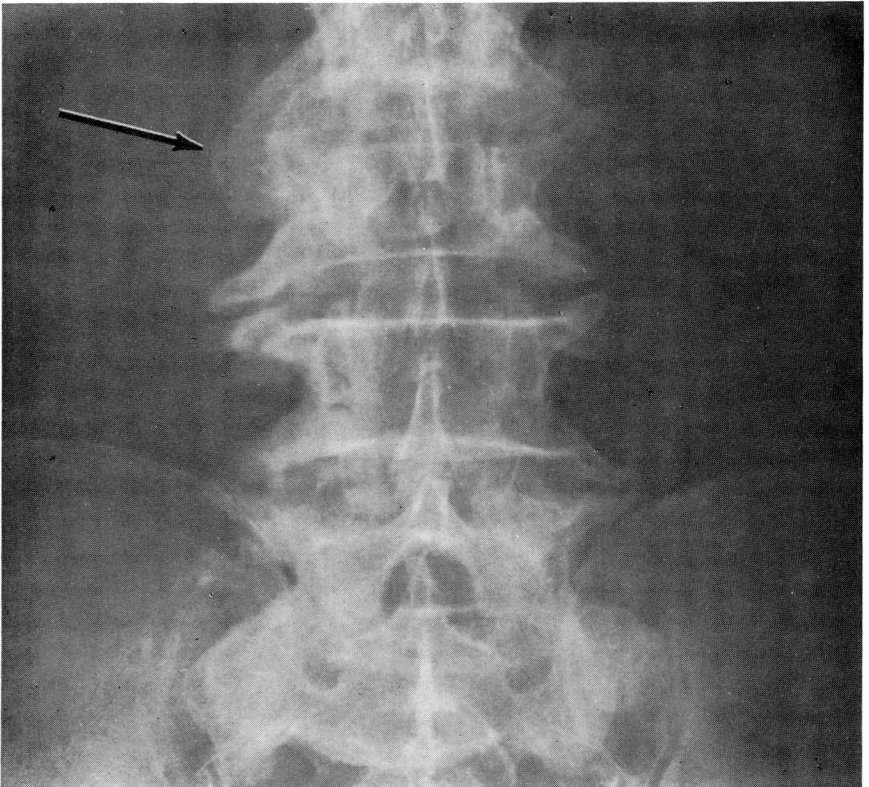

Fig. 89–8. Osteoarthritis of the lumbar spine. Note the marked osteophyte formation with bridging of spurs between L2 and L3 on the right (arrow).

Degenerative changes of all types are most frequent in the areas of the lordotic and kyphotic apices, C5, T8, and L3 to L4, and correlate in general with the areas of maximal spine motion. In some older individuals, however, osteophytes may extend along the entire length of the spine, with prominent involvement of the thoracic region (Fig. 89–9). These osteophytes may be striking, and coalescence with fusion may occur (Fig. 8–10). Forestier et al. have suggested the name *ankylosing vertebral hyperostosis* for these severe cases, which may be associated with moderate-to-severe spinal limitation.[43] The frequent extraspinal manifestations of Forestier's disease have led to the term *diffuse idiopathic skeletal hyperostosis*,[108,141] discussed later in this chapter.

Symptoms of spinal osteoarthritis include localized pain and stiffness and radicular pain. Localized pain has been assumed to originate in paraspinal ligaments, joint capsules, and periosteum. Such changes may explain spontaneous fluctuations of symptoms in the presence of persistent or progressive cartilage degeneration and spur formation. Spasm of paraspinal muscles is common

and may be a major cause of pain. Radicular pain may be due to compression of nerve roots, or it may represent pain referred along dermatomes related to the primary local lesion.

Nerve root compression causing neuropathy is common. This disorder may result from impingement on the nerve root by spurs that compromise the foraminal space (Fig. 89–11), by lateral prolapse of a degenerated disc, or by foraminal narrowing from apophyseal joint subluxation. Pressure on nerve roots may cause radicular pain, paresthesias, and reflex and motor changes in the distribution of the involved root. Neurologic complications of this type occur most frequently in the neck because of its small spinal canal and intervertebral foramina, but they can occur in other areas of the spine. Nerve root compression in the dorsal spine may result in radicular pain radiating around the chest wall in a girdle distribution, and it must be differentiated from symptoms caused by other disorders. Involvement of nerve roots in the lumbosacral area is associated with low back pain and neurologic signs and symptoms, which frequently allow localization of specific nerve root

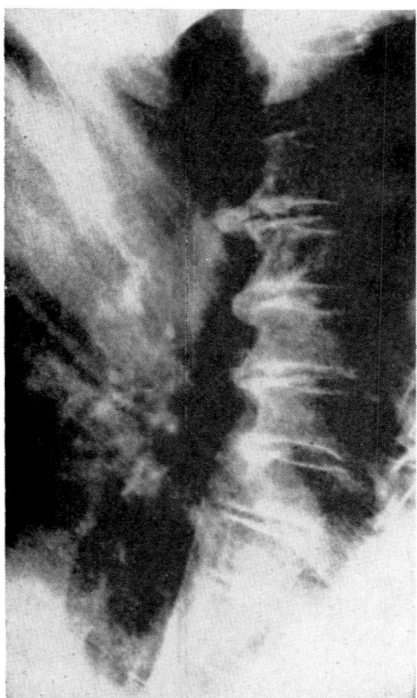

Fig. 89–9. Osteoarthritis of the thoracic spine. Note the pronounced exostoses at the anterior vertebral margins and the narrowed intervertebral disc spaces.

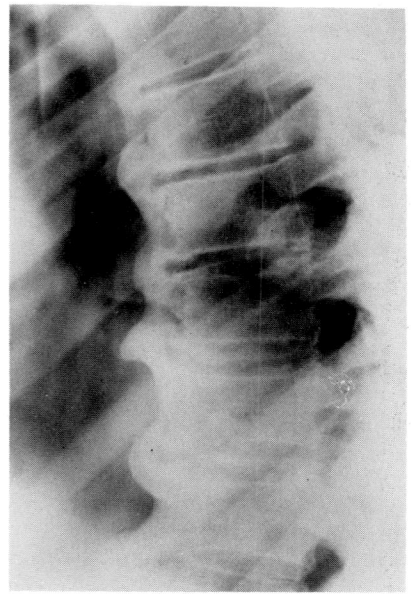

Fig. 89–10. Florid hyperostosis of the spine in a patient with Forestier's disease (diffuse idiopathic skeletal hyperostosis). A flowing mantle of ossification from ligamentous calcification and coalescence of osteophytes is seen at the anterior aspect of the spine. (Courtesy of Dr. Donald Resnick.)

involvement. Involvement of the L3 or L4 nerve roots is associated with a diminished or absent patellar reflex; an absent ankle jerk indicates involvement of the S1 nerve root. Sensory loss over the anteromedial aspect of the leg is consistent with L4 nerve root compression. A lesion at L5 causes sensory changes at the anterolateral aspect of the leg and the medial aspect of the foot and weakness of dorsiflexion of the foot and great toe. S1 nerve root compression results in sensory changes at the posterolateral aspect of the calf and the lateral foot. Gastrocnemius muscle weakness may be evident.

Further neurologic symptoms may be associated with cervical osteoarthritis if large posterior spurs or protruded discs compress the spinal cord. In these cases, upper-motor-neuron and other long-tract signs may be observed. Compression of the anterior spinal artery may produce a central cord syndrome. The blood supply to the brain may be compromised if large spurs compress the vertebral arteries. The spectrum of clinical signs and symptoms is similar to that in basilar artery insufficiency. Dizziness, vertigo, and headaches are frequent complaints. Visual symptoms include blurring of vision, diplopia, field defects, and scotomata. Nystagmus and ataxia may be observed. A characteristic feature of this clinical entity is its intermittent

nature, frequently described by the patient as "attacks." Abrupt loss of leg strength may be noted. Exacerbations are often associated with postural neck changes from compression of vertebral arteries by osteophytes. Angiographic studies of carotid and vertebral arteries are diagnostically helpful.

Osteoarthritis of the atlantoaxial joint has been described in 31 patients.[56] Radiologic signs in these patients consisted of narrowing of the joint space, marginal cortical thickening, and osteophyte formation. Roentgenograms revealed involvement of the lateral atlantoaxial joint or the articulation of the atlas with the odontoid, or they showed mixed involvement. Patients complained of occipital pain, stiffness of the shoulder, and paresthesias of the fingers. Conservative treatment provided satisfactory relief of symptoms, except in one patient who required a transoral atlantoaxial fusion.

Spinal cord lesions as a result of osteoarthritis of the dorsal spine are rare. Spinal cord compression is not seen in patients with lumbosacral lesions because the spinal cord ends at the level of L1. *Cauda equina syndrome* with sphincter dysfunction may, however, be produced. In addition, symptoms suggestive of intermittent vascular claudication have been described, owing to mechanical and vascular factors that compromise the cauda equina.

Spinal stenosis of the lumbar spine may produce

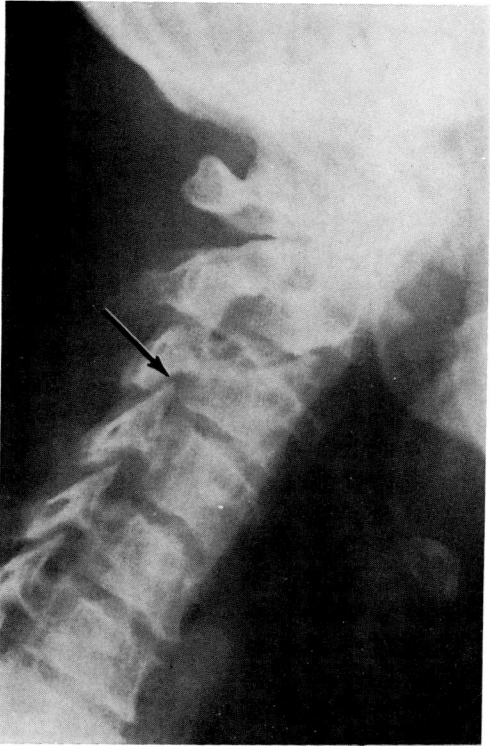

Fig. 89–11. Osteoarthritis of cervical spine, oblique radiologic view. The foraminal space between C3 and C4 (arrow) is compromised by marked posterior spur formation.

symptoms in the lower back and the lower extremities. Pain may be constant or intermittent. It is often worsened by exercise, thereby simulating intermittent claudication. Hyperextension of the spine often exacerbates symptoms; relief is noted with flexion. The patient may stand with knees, hips, and lumbar spine flexed (simian stance). Sensory changes may be present, and motor power in the legs may be diminished. Stenosis is usually caused by combined anatomic abnormalities because congenital narrowing alone is generally asymptomatic.[7] Commonly associated causes include degenerative spurs, disc herniation, ligamentous hypertrophy, and spondylolisthesis. Trauma, postoperative fibrosis, Paget's disease, and fluorosis are associated less commonly.

Radiologic evidence of degenerative disease in the spine may be extensive but may still bear little relation to the patient's symptoms. On the other hand, severe symptoms may develop with minor spur formation if the spur is located in a critical area. Roentgenographic changes of marginal lipping, sclerosis of the articular margins, and narrowing have been found in sacroiliac joints with

increasing age, but it is unlikely that these changes themselves lead to symptoms.

Laboratory Findings

No specific diagnostic laboratory abnormalities exist in primary osteoarthritis (Table 89–3). The erythrocyte sedimentation rate is normal in most patients. Results of routine blood counts, urinalyses, and blood chemical determinations are normal in patients with primary disease. Blood chemistries and serologic studies, urine findings, and synovial fluid analyses are important in excluding other forms of arthritis considered in the differential diagnosis, and they identify systemic metabolic disorders associated with secondary osteoarthritis. For example, patients with associated calcium pyrophosphate dihydrate crystal deposition disease may have evidence of underlying primary hyperparathyroidism with elevation of serum calcium and an increase in serum parathyroid hormone level. Patients with Paget's disease of bone exhibit elevated serum alkaline phosphatase levels and increased urinary hydroxyproline excretion. In patients with joint disease associated with ochronosis, the presence of homogentisic acid metabolites in the urine darkens the urine on standing or causes a false-positive Benedict's test result for glycosuria.

Synovial fluid in primary osteoarthritis is "noninflammatory." When synovial effusions are present, study of synovial fluid reveals few abnormalities with a slight increase in cells. Viscosity is good, and the mucin clot formed after addition of glacial acetic acid is normal in appearance. Synovial fluid fibrils morphologically indistinguishable from sloughed collagen fibers are often seen.[70] The collagen fibers seen in synovial fluid in osteoarthritis appear to be type II, derived from articular hyaline cartilage.[19] Calcium pyrophosphate dihydrate or basic calcium phosphate crystals may be present. Cholesterol crystals have been identified by light microscopy in synovial fluids of patients with recurrent osteoarthritic knee effusions.[38] Although evidence of altered cellular and humoral immune mechanisms has been described,[81,131,144] its significance remains to be determined. Immune complexes have been detected in hyaline articular cartilage of osteoarthritic joints, but they have not yet been reported in synovial fluid.[23]

Synovial histologic examination in primary osteoarthritis reveals nonspecific changes of chronic mild inflammation, particularly in more advanced disease.

Radioisotopic bone and joint scintigraphy is associated with variable increases in uptake of isotope tracer, related to mild inflammatory synovitis or stimulated bone reaction.[136] Intraosseous phle-

Table 89–3. Laboratory and Radiologic Findings in Primary Osteoarthritis

Laboratory Tests	Results
Erythrocyte sedimentation rate	Usually normal
Routine blood counts	Normal
Rheumatoid factor	Negative
Antinuclear antibody	Negative
Serum calcium, phosphorus, alkaline phosphatase, serum protein electrophoresis	Normal
Synovial fluid analysis	Good viscosity with normal mucin clot; possible increase in number of cells
	Presence of fibrils and debris (wear particles)

Radiologic Findings	Causes
Narrowing of joint space	Destruction and loss of articular cartilage
Subchondral bony sclerosis (eburnation)	New bone formation
Marginal osteophyte formation	Proliferation of cartilage and bone
Bone cysts and subchondral microfractures	
Gross deformity with subluxation and loose bodies	

bography reveals impaired drainage from the juxta-articular bone marrow.[6,8] Venous stasis and engorgement are generally associated with intramedullary hypertension. Thermography, a method of constructing photographic images of surface temperatures, may be normal or, in the presence of mild synovitis, may show a pattern of heat emission. Arthrography and arteriography may be useful in the differential diagnosis. The role of these techniques in the routine diagnosis of osteoarthritis remains limited and poorly defined. They usually add little to observations evident on routine physical examination.

Roentgenographic Appearance

The roentgenographic appearance may be normal if the pathologic changes leading to clinical symptoms are sufficiently mild (see also Chap. 5). Many gradations of abnormality may be noted as the disease progresses (Table 89–3). *Joint space narrowing* occurs as a result of degeneration and disappearance of articular cartilage. *Subchondral bony sclerosis* (eburnation) is noted as increased bone density. *Marginal osteophyte formation* takes place as a result of proliferation of cartilage and bone. *Cysts,* varying in size from several millimeters to several centimeters, are seen as translucent areas in periarticular bone. Gross *deformity* and *subluxation* and *loose bodies* may occur in advanced cases.

Although osteophytes are usually regarded as a manifestation of osteoarthritis, the use of this feature alone in diagnosis has been questioned, as noted earlier in this chapter. Osteophytes correlate with aging and are not necessarily an early sign of osteoarthritis.[59,60] Some suggest that the diagnosis of osteoarthritis of the peripheral joints should be based on radiologic findings of structural abnormalities in cartilage (decreased joint space) or in subchondral bone (cysts and eburnation) or both.

The origin of the subchondral "detritus" cysts has been explained as follows: (1) a failure in the bone remodeling process, in which local osteoclastic activity outstrips that of osteoblasts; or (2) the result of pressure transmitted from the joint surface to subarticular bone through cracks in the subchondral plate (trabecular microfractures). The cysts may contain fluid, nonspecific detritus, or a primitive mesenchymal tissue that undergoes fibrosis. These cysts may be prominent even in joints with adequately preserved joint space when seen radiographically.

Ankylosis in osteoarthritis is uncommon. A form of ankylosis may be seen in the spine when marginal osteophyte formation is extensive and leads to coalescence of spurs (ankylosing hyperostosis). Ankylosis is also seen occasionally in osteoarthritis of the hands,[80] especially in the erosive inflammatory form of the disease.

Osteophytes are usually located on the anterior and anterolateral borders of the vertebral bodies and are best visualized on lateral roentgenograms. The amount of bony overgrowth varies. Spurs arising from the posterior margins of the vertebral bodies or from the margins of the articular facets are less common but are of greater clinical importance, owing to their proximity to neural structures. Narrowing of intervertebral joint spaces results from disc degeneration; this is most frequent and usually most marked in the lower cervical and lower lumbar regions. Sclerosis of adjacent bone is common, and one sometimes sees wedging of the anterior borders of the vertebral bodies. Apophyseal joints may show joint space narrowing, sclerosis, and associated spur formation. Osteoporosis is not a component of degenerative change.

Many of the previously mentioned radiologic abnormalities may be visualized on routine posteroanterior and lateral views. Oblique views of the cervical and lumbar spine should be routinely performed, if degenerative changes involving intervertebral foramina and apophyseal joints are to be accurately delineated. Myelography may be of help when symptoms are severe and a surgical procedure is contemplated. Computed axial tomography (CT scanning) is particularly useful diagnostically in patients with osteoarthritis of the spine, especially when spinal stenosis or lumbar facet disease is suspected (see Chap. 6). Diagnostic evaluation of disc herniation is enhanced, especially when the procedure is combined with myelography.

Roentgenographic study of Heberden's and Bouchard's nodes reveals joint space narrowing, bony sclerosis, and cyst formation. Spur formation, best seen radiologically on routine posteroanterior views, is prominent and appears to develop at the attachments of the flexor and extensor tendons to the distal phalanx. In some patients, however, spurs may be directed anteroposteriorly rather than mediolaterally, and lateral views with the fingers spread may be necessary to demonstrate changes. Although the nodes may feel hard, only minimal spur formation may be visible radiographically, and the enlargement may consist of soft tissue and cartilage. Degenerative joint disease of metacarpophalangeal joints is uncommon, but *hook-like osteophytes* were noted on the radial side of the head of the metacarpal bones in 7 of 100 patients with osteoarthritis of the hands.[135] These changes, seen primarily in patients over 65 years of age, may result from tension on capsular ligaments caused by contraction of interosseous muscles at the radial side of the metacarpal head.

Anteroposterior views of the pelvis should be obtained routinely when osteoarthritis of the hip is suspected. This view is especially informative in that the hips, sacroiliac joints, symphysis pubis, and pelvic bones are visualized. Special views of the hips, including lateral views and tomograms, may be of value when pathologic changes are suspected but are not seen by routine techniques. Advanced degenerative disease may demonstrate striking abnormalities such as *protrusio acetabuli* (arthrokatadysis), a condition in which the floor of the acetabulum is displaced medially by the head of the femur, so it bulges into the pelvis ("Otto's pelvis").

Although degenerative changes of the knee are usually readily seen on routine anteroposterior and lateral views, special views are often diagnostically helpful. Tunnel views taken with the knee in flex-

ion expose the intercondylar notch and enable one to identify loose bodies, intra-articular spurs, and changes in the tibial spines. In addition, recent studies suggest that the tunnel view most dramatically reveals loss of the joint space.[107] The effectiveness of this view in delineating cartilage loss may be related to the ability of this projection to profile a more posterior portion of the femoral condyles, where cartilage loss may be significant. Skyline or Hughston views taken from superiorly allow more detailed study of the patellofemoral compartment. Films obtained when the patient is bearing weight allow optimal demonstration of genu varus or valgus and medial or lateral compartment narrowing. Roentgenograms of the contralateral joint are helpful in evaluating observed degenerative changes.

Variant Forms

The clinical, radiologic, and pathologic findings in certain patients with primary degenerative joint disease are sufficiently different from those usually seen to warrant consideration of these cases as distinct symptom complexes.[24,35,36,41,42,57,67,100,108,141] One such group, characterized by diffuse polyarticular involvement, has been termed "primary generalized osteoarthritis."[67] A second group demonstrating similar features of degenerative joint disease has been given the name ankylosing hyperostosis or diffuse idiopathic skeletal hyperostosis.[41,42,57,108,141] A third group, characterized by inflammatory synovitis of interphalangeal joints of the hands in association with juxta-articular bone erosions, has been termed "erosive" inflammatory osteoarthritis.[24,35,36,100] Finally, a fourth group of patients may exhibit evidence of chondromalacia patellae with variable degrees of progression to full forms of osteoarthritic change.[27,40,50]

Primary Generalized Osteoarthritis

This pattern of "nodal" osteoarthritis has been seen predominantly in middle-aged women.[67] Distal and proximal interphalangeal joints and first carpometacarpal joints are sites of predilection and are often affected in succession. Other peripheral joints including knees, hips, and metatarsophalangeal joints are frequently involved, as are joints of the spine. An acute inflammatory phase commonly precedes chronic articular symptoms. The erythrocyte sedimentation rate is normal or slightly elevated; serum rheumatoid factor is absent. Although the overall pattern of radiologic changes is similar to that usually seen in localized osteoarthritis, certain differences are notable. Articular facets, neural arches, and spinous processes of the vertebral column are often enlarged and lead to the radiologic designation of "kissing spines." Knee films show marked joint space narrowing with "molten wax" osteophytes instead of the ordinary, sharply pointed osteophytes. Patients with advanced cases show radiologic changes in excess of the clinical findings. Joint function is often only mildly affected despite severe anatomic changes.

The concept of primary generalized osteoarthritis as a distinct subset is still controversial. This form of osteoarthritis may simply reflect more severe disease differentiated only by polyarticular involvement.[21]

In some patients with generalized osteoarthritis, chondrocalcinosis has been noted.[29,32,115,116] Studies have demonstrated the presence of diffuse deposits of calcium pyrophosphate dihydrate,[4,28,142] with associated findings of generalized osteoarthritis and evidence of crystals in material obtained from synovial fluid of involved joints. A familial form of chondrocalcinosis associated with apatite crystal deposition has been described in patients exhibiting symptoms indistinguishable from those seen in generalized osteoarthritis alone.[83]

Erosive Inflammatory Osteoarthritis

Erosive inflammatory osteoarthritis,[24,35,100,139] another variant of "nodal" osteoarthritis, involves primarily the distal and proximal interphalangeal joints. The metacarpophalangeal joints may also be involved. The disease is usually hereditary. Painful inflammatory episodes eventually lead to joint deformity and sometimes to ankylosis. Postmenopausal women are most frequently affected. Acute flares may occur for years, but eventually, the affected joints often become asymptomatic. Gelatinous cysts, variably painful and tender, are seen at the site of the involved joints. Inflammation and swelling may be sufficiently severe to support a diagnosis of RA. Roentgenographic examination reveals loss of joint cartilage, spur formation, and subchondral bony sclerosis. Bony erosions are prominent. Bony ankylosis, commonly seen, may be the result of synovial inflammation and pannus formation, healing of denuded cartilage surfaces, or coalescence of adjacent osteophytes. Studies of synovium may reveal an intense proliferative synovitis, often indistinguishable from that of RA. The erythrocyte sedimentation rate is usually normal or only slightly elevated. In one study of this disorder,[35] later changes more characteristic of RA were noted in 15% of cases.

Rheumatoid factor and antinuclear antibodies are absent. The presence of abnormal immune mechanisms has been suggested, however, by the demonstration of immune complexes in involved synovium.[22,23,95] Synovial fluid and synovial specimens from patients with erosive osteoarthritis have increased numbers of Ia+ T-lymphocytes, similar to those seen in specimens from patients with RA.[140] These findings, which are present in patients with erosive osteoarthritis but not in those with osteoarthritis of other types, suggest that erosive osteoarthritis represents a subset of patients with osteoarthritic disease. Evidence of sicca syndrome in 17 of 22 patients with erosive osteoarthritis has been described,[122] and it further suggests the presence of some immunologic abnormality.

Diffuse Idiopathic Skeletal Hyperostosis; Ankylosing Hyperostosis

In 1950, Forestier and Rotes-Querol described an unusual type of florid hyperostosis of the spine, characterized by large spurs or marginal bony proliferations in the form of anterior osseous ridges.[42] Fusion of these ridges often has a flowing appearance (see Fig. 89–10). Ossification occurs in the connective tissue surrounding the spine, involving the anterior longitudinal ligament and peripheral disc margins. A predilection exists for involvement of the dorsal spine, although all levels of the spine may be affected. Lesions are most marked at the anterior and right lateral aspects of the vertebral column. The observation of left-sided vertebral bridging in patients with situs inversus suggests that the descending thoracic aorta plays a role in the location of vertebral calcification.[10] Although most common in older patients, the disease has been noted in younger persons. Despite extensive anatomic abnormalities, pain is often minimal or absent, and spinal motion is only moderately limited. Physiologic vertebral ligamentous calcification is probably a variant of this same process.[123]

Subsequent studies have further defined the clinical and pathologic features of this syndrome[57,108,141] and, in addition, they have demonstrated extraspinal manifestations.[108] Resnick and co-workers defined specific criteria for vertebral involvement, to allow differentiation of this disorder from degenerative disc disease and ankylosing spondylitis.[106] The criteria include "flowing ossification along the anterolateral aspect of at least four contiguous vertebral bodies, preservation of disc height, absence of vacuum phenomena or vertebral body marginal sclerosis, and absence of apophyseal joint ankylosis or sacroiliac joint erosions, sclerosis, or fusion. Frequently, radiolucency is apparent between the abnormal calcification and the underlying vertebral body. Extraspinal manifestations include irregular new bone formation or "whiskering," large bony spurs, seen particularly on the olecranon process and the calcaneus (Fig. 89–12), and severe ligamentous calcification, seen mainly in the sacrotuberous, iliolumbar (Fig. 89–13), and patellar ligaments. Periarticular osteophytes were conspicuous.

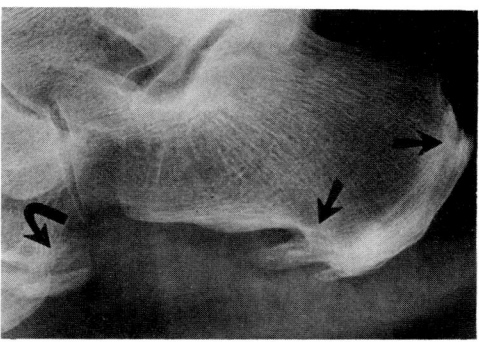

Fig. 89–12. Diffuse idiopathic skeletal hyperostosis. The calcaneus demonstrates large, irregular spurs at its posterior and plantar aspects (straight arrows). Associated irregularity at the area of the cuboid and fifth metatarsal bones is seen (curved arrow). (Courtesy of Dr. Donald Resnick.)

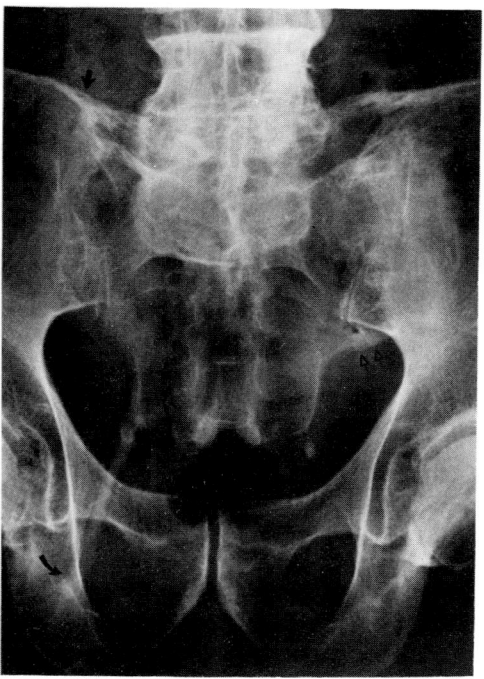

Fig. 89–13. Radiogram of the pelvis in a patient with diffuse idiopathic skeletal hyperostosis reveals iliolumbar (straight arrow) and sacrotuberous (curved arrow) ligament ossification and para-articular sacroiliac osteophyte formation (open arrows). (From Resnick, D., et al.[108])

Clinical findings related to the spine as described in the diffuse idiopathic skeletal hyperostosis syndrome are similar to those initially described by Rotes-Querol and Forestier. Spinal stiffness is a prominent complaint despite surprising maintenance of spinal motion with minimal pain. Dysphagia related to severe cervical osteophytosis has been reported. Peripheral joint symptoms include pain in involved elbows, ilium, shoulders, hips, knees, and ankles. Heel pain related to calcaneal spur formation is common. The diffuse radiographic findings involving both spinal and extraspinal structures have led some to suggest that this disorder represents a diffuse "ossifying diathesis," rather than merely a localized disorder of the spine.

Hyperglycemia is the commonest laboratory abnormality noted in patients with this syndrome, with an incidence of abnormal glucose tolerance tests about twice that seen in an age-, sex-, and weight-matched populations. In a recent study, diabetes mellitus was present in 40% of these patients.[110] Serum levels including those of calcium, phosphorous, and alkaline phosphatase are characteristically normal, as are studies of serum growth hormone and parathyroid hormone.

The etiopathogenesis of the diffuse idiopathic skeletal hyperostosis is unknown. In one report, 16 of 47 patients with this syndrome were HLA-B27 positive.[120] In other studies, however, a statistically significant increase in HLA-B27 has not been confirmed. Studies of Pima Indians have shown this syndrome to be present in 50% of all individuals, with a 20% frequency of HLA-B27.[130] No significant association was seen, however, with B-locus antigens when Pima Indians with the syndrome were compared to age-matched control subjects. Recent studies indicate that patients with diffuse idiopathic skeletal hyperostosis have increased levels of serum vitamin A.[1] Of special interest in this regard is the recent observation that patients receiving high doses of synthetic vitamin A derivative, 13-cis-retinoic acid, developed an ossification disorder resembling diffuse idiopathic skeletal hyperostosis.[102] In a limited report, 5 patients with this hyperostosis syndrome were noted to have elevated plasma and urine fluoride levels.[86] Abnormal levels of fluoride were, however, not noted in other studies.[138,141]

A syndrome characterized by *ossification of the posterior longitudinal ligament* has been described, occurring mainly in the Japanese population.[96] It has been estimated that over 4,000 patients in Japan are afflicted with this disorder. Roentgenographic study of the spine reveals lumpy or linear bony masses across one or more disc spaces, sometimes extending from the superior cervical spine to the thoracic region. Ankylosing hyperostosis of the type seen in the diffuse idiopathic skeletal hyperostosis syndrome may be associated. Clinical manifestations may be severe because of serious spinal cord compression.

Chondromalacia Patellae (see also Chaps. 78 and 87)

This disorder is characterized by degenerative changes of the cartilage of the patella and is included in those conditions associated with osteoarthritic changes in the knee. Although in the past it was identified as a specific entity, chondromalacia patellae is now thought to result from many conditions affecting the knee that lead to cartilage degeneration.[27,40,50] The malacic changes in the patellar articular cartilage are considered to be simply the final common pathway through which articular cartilage of the patella degenerates. The specific conditions effecting these changes, such as primary meniscal disease, knee laxity, or abnormal patellar positions such as patella alta, may lead to a similar end-stage complex of symptoms. The syndrome is often associated with repeated trauma, as occurs in recurrent lateral subluxation of the patella. Radiologic changes may be minimal or absent. Pain is present about the patella and is aggravated by activity. Paradoxically, vague knee pain may occur after periods of inactivity in the flexed position, such as watching a movie. The disease is typically seen in young adults, especially women, and may be a precursor to the development of patellofemoral osteoarthritis.

Although the findings described in the foregoing discussion support the existence of various forms of osteoarthritis, the validity of classifying these forms as distinct symptom complexes or entities remains open to question. Osteoarthritis may affect one or a number of joints in any given patient, so generalized involvement may merely reflect one end of the clinical spectrum of severity of this disease. Acute inflammation may occur in early osteoarthritis,[80,100] whether localized or generalized, and its use as a differentiating characteristic is not definitive. In some patients, it is difficult to rule out the co-existence of seronegative RA and osteoarthritis.[35] Ankylosing hyperostosis has many characteristics that appear to distinguish it from the more common forms of osteoarthritis. The pathologic changes may be indistinguishable, however, especially in the early course of the disease.

Prognosis

The outlook for patients with primary osteoarthritis is variable. Involvement of the distal interphalangeal joints, for example, may be associated with a moderate amount of pain, but it usually causes little limitation of essential function unless fine finger motion is required occupationally. Involvement of weight-bearing joints, on the other hand, may lead to marked disability as the disease progresses. Similarly, osteoarthritis of the cervical spine may not only give rise to distressing symptoms, but may also lead to severe objective neurologic deficits and disability.

Studies of progression of the disease in specific joints suggest that not all cases of osteoarthritis inevitably deteriorate.[93,119] In a study of 6,321 patients who had undergone roentgenographic examination of the colon, 4.7% had osteoarthritis of the hip.[62] Only half of these patients with roentgenographic evidence of hip osteoarthritis actually needed treatment, however; 20% were entirely free of symptoms. Occasional patients may develop a rapidly progressive, destructive osteoarthritis of the hip.[34,63,103] Severe changes are seen both in the acetabulum and in the femoral head. Degenerative pseudocysts and lack of osteophyte formation are characteristic findings. Synovitis noted at operation is of a low grade.

Some studies of the natural course of osteoarthritis of the knee suggest a worse prognosis than in disease of the hip.[59] Most patients worsened during the 10- to 18-year period of follow-up, with increased pain, deformity, and instability and decreased function. Most patients were unable to use public transportation because of pain on walking. Marked radiologic deterioration was noted, usually limited to the compartment first affected. Varus deformity and early development of pain were unfavorable prognostic factors. Other data suggest that osteoarthritis of the knee affects only a limited portion of the population and is not inevitably progressive.[44]

Treatment may retard the progression of the disease and is of further value in protecting the contralateral joints exposed to increased stress. Patients should be reassured that the general outlook is favorable and disability is uncommon, in contrast to the threat of crippling seen in patients with RA. When necessary, however, these patients should be told that involvement of certain joints may be associated with localized pain, stiffness, and limitation of motion. Osteoarthritis is not always benign.

Differential Diagnosis

The differentiation of primary osteoarthritis from other disorders of the musculoskeletal system depends on a correlation of clinical, laboratory, and roentgenographic findings. Osteoarthritis may be confused with other forms of arthritic disease because pain, stiffness, and limitation of motion are common features in all these disorders. The differential diagnosis is further complicated by the high radiologic prevalence of osteoarthritis in the general population that often bears no relation to the musculoskeletal complaints of a given patient.

In most patients, the diagnosis of osteoarthritis is simple. In other patients, however, atypical disease presentation and behavior may require extensive differential diagnostic considerations. Examples of such presentations include osteoarthritis occurring in an atypical site such as the shoulder, association with a significant inflammatory element, co-existence with other entities such as calcium pyrophosphate dihydrate crystal deposition disease, precocious occurrence in young individuals, and osteoarthritis of the spine with neurologic findings that simulate other underlying neurologic disorders.

RA can usually be differentiated on the basis of its more inflammatory nature and the characteristic pattern of joint involvement. When RA occurs as monarticular disease of the knee or hip, however, differentiation from osteoarthritis may be difficult without prolonged follow-up study. An increase in the erythrocyte sedimentation rate and a positive test result for rheumatoid factor are of value because they are not characteristic of degenerative joint disease. Synovial fluid analysis is also important (see Chap. 4). RA may be particularly difficult to differentiate from the so-called erosive form of osteoarthritis. The pattern of joint involvement is of diagnostic value because erosive osteoarthritis is limited mainly to the distal and proximal interphalangeal joints of the hands; RA usually affects the metacarpophalangeal and the proximal interphalangeal joints as well as the peripheral joints elsewhere. *Joints afflicted with active seropositive RA rarely develop osteophytes.* Some patients with Heberden's nodes or erosive osteoarthritis may later develop RA, in which case osteophytes precede rheumatoid involvement, and a careful clinical history is necessary to identify the presence of a "mixed" arthritis. Mixed disease may also be present when RA leads to secondary degenerative change, but bony overgrowth only occurs in "burned out" disease and even then, the osteophytes are abortive.

Rheumatic syndromes characterized by involvement of the distal interphalangeal joints of the hands, such as psoriatic arthritis, Reiter's syndrome, and the arthritis of chronic ulcerative colitis, may be confused with osteoarthritis of the Heberden's type. The associated clinical findings of the underlying disease in these patients usually suffice to clarify the diagnosis. Pseudogout syndrome, or chondrocalcinosis articularis, may simulate osteoarthritis when low-grade arthralgias result from the presence of calcium pyrophosphate dihydrate crystals in synovial fluid. The pattern of arthritis is clearly different in these patients; the metacarpophalangeal joints, wrists, elbows, shoulders, knees, hips, and ankles are often affected. Symptoms related to early manifestations of localized joint disorders such as aseptic osteonecrosis, pigmented villonodular synovitis, and chronic infectious arthritis may be mistakenly attributed to degenerative changes seen as coincidental radiographic findings. Neurologic symptoms secondary to spinal osteoarthritis must be differentiated from those that result from other neurologic disorders. The symptoms of osteoarthritis of the cervical spine may simulate those of multiple sclerosis, syringomyelia, amyotrophic lateral sclerosis, progressive spinal atrophy, and spinal cord tumors.

SECONDARY OSTEOARTHRITIS

The term "secondary osteoarthritis" describes those cases of osteoarthritis that appear to occur in response to some recognizable underlying local or systemic factor. Some of these factors are noted in Table 89–1. A diagnosis of secondary osteoarthritis should be particularly considered when the disease develops at an early age.

Secondary to Acute Trauma

Joint degeneration may follow acute injury. The usual medical history includes trauma followed by redness, soft tissue swelling, and pain over the involved joint. In several months, the acute inflammatory changes subside and are replaced by a hard, painless enlargement. The deformity is localized to the injured joint. The anatomic changes are similar to those seen in primary osteoarthritis. Injury of this nature involving the distal interphalangeal joints of the hands may lead to traumatic Heberden's nodes.[133] Acute trauma to any of the interphalangeal joints of the hands may lead to the common "baseball finger" (Fig. 89–14).

Secondary to Chronic Trauma

An increased prevalence of osteoarthritis is associated with chronic trauma related to certain occupations. Although exposure of a joint to subtle chronic trauma, or microtrauma, has been suggested as an etiologic factor in the development of primary osteoarthritis, the relationship between trauma and joint changes, as described previously, seems more clear cut and supports the classification of such lesions as secondary forms of osteoarthritis.

Secondary to Other Joint Disorders

Such disorders may be either local or diffuse. Secondary localized osteoarthritis may follow local joint disorders of other cause, such as old fractures, aseptic necrosis, or acute or chronic infection.

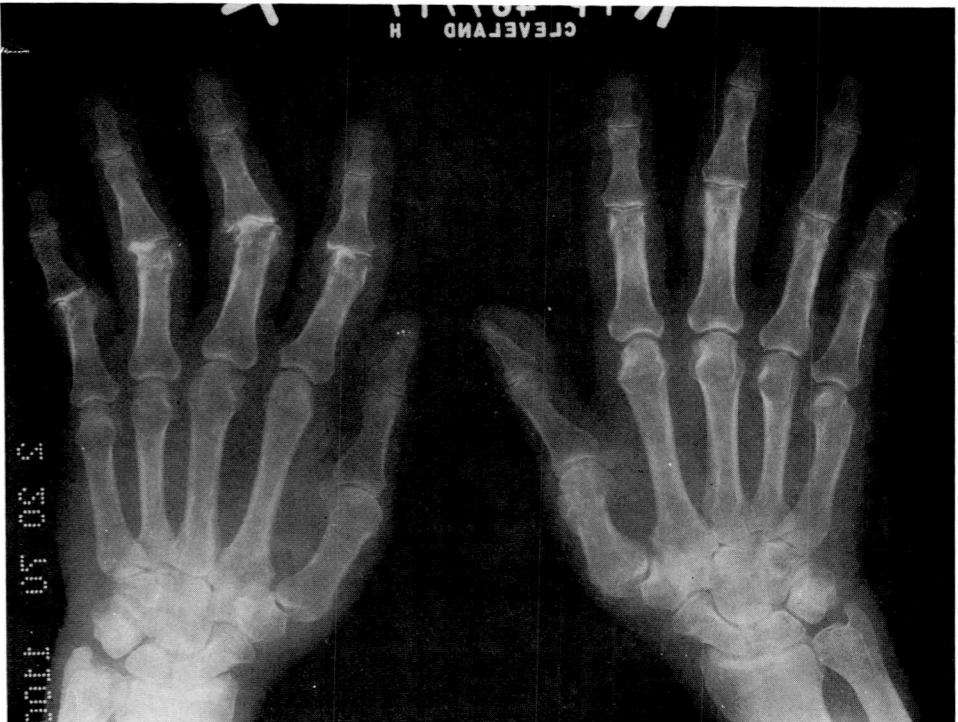

Fig. 89–14. Secondary osteoarthritis of the second, third, fourth, and fifth proximal interphalangeal joints of the left hand ("baseball fingers") in a patient with recurrent episodes of acute trauma while a semiprofessional baseball player.

Early onset of osteoarthritis in the knee may be the result of torn menisci, patellar dislocation, strain resulting from obesity, or poor mechanics due to genu varus, genu valgus, or tibial torsion. Localized osteoarthritis of the hip may follow childhood disorders such as congenital dysplasia of the hip, slipped capital epiphysis, and Legg-Perthes' disease. Osteoarthritis of the mid- or hindfoot may result in patients with congenital calcaneonavicular and talocalcaneal coalition.

Diffuse secondary degenerative changes may supervene in patients with RA, in patients with bleeding dyscrasias in whom repeated hemarthroses may occur, or in dwarfs with achondroplasia.

Secondary to Systemic Metabolic or Endocrine Disorders

Osteoarthritis is associated with several metabolic or endocrine disorders (see also Chaps. 96, 98).

Alkaptonuria (Ochronosis)

This inherited metabolic disease, associated with an absence of homogentisic acid oxidase and characterized by excretion of homogentisic acid in the urine and by a binding of its metabolic products to connective tissue components, is associated with generalized osteoarthritis.[94] Tissue deposition of brown-black pigment, or ochronosis, is seen primarily in cartilage, skin, and sclera. Degenerative joint disease of the spine occurs frequently; calcification of numerous intervertebral discs is a characteristic finding. Arthritis of peripheral joints such as hips, knees, and shoulders is less common and develops later.

Wilson's Disease

Hepatolenticular degeneration, or Wilson's disease, is an inherited disorder characterized by excessive retention of copper, with degenerative changes in the brain and hepatic cirrhosis. Premature osteoarthritis has been described as one component of associated articular manifestations of this disorder.[39,49] Chondromalacia patellae was a prominent finding in one reported series.[39] Chondrocalcinosis has also been described in these patients.

Hemochromatosis

This chronic disease is associated with excessive deposition of iron and fibrosis in a variety of tissues. Although it can result from long-term over-ingestion of iron and from multiple transfusions, the disease is most often idiopathic. Osteoarthritic changes occur in 20 to 50% of patients.[55] Hands, knees, and hips are most commonly involved, although virtually any joint, including those in the feet, can be affected. Involvement of the second and third metacarpophalangeal joints of the hands is particularly characteristic. Synovial tissue shows a striking deposition of iron, most prominently in the synovial lining cells. Roentgenograms reveal joint-space narrowing and irregularity, subchondral sclerosis, cystic erosions, bony proliferation, and at times, subluxation. Chondrocalcinosis with deposits of calcium pyrophosphate dihydrate is seen in up to 60% of patients.

Kashin-Beck Disease

This disorder, characterized by disturbances in growth and maturation in children, is endemic in eastern Siberia, northern China, and northern Korea.[91] Abnormalities in enchondral bone growth lead to dystrophic changes in epiphyseal and metaphyseal areas. Severe secondary osteoarthritis involves the peripheral joints and the spine. Various causes have been suggested, including a relation to a fungus ingested with cereal grains.

Acromegaly

Hypersecretion of growth hormone by the anterior pituitary gland in adults leads to a slowly progressive overgrowth of soft tissue, bone, and cartilage. Peripheral and spinal osteoarthritis is common. Peripheral joint symptoms occur in about 60% of patients.[13,68] Most commonly involved are the knees, hips, shoulders, and elbows. Carpal tunnel syndrome is frequently seen. Backache is common, but back motion is often normal or increased because of the thickened intervertebral discs and the laxity of acromegalic ligaments. Early, increased cartilage thickness gives wide joint spaces on roentgenograms. Later, joint-space narrowing, osteophyte formation, and subchondral sclerosis occur.

Hyperparathyroidism

Increased levels of parathyroid hormone, whether primary or secondary, can produce many rheumatic problems, one of which is degenerative joint disease. It has been postulated that degenerative changes result from damage to cartilage related either to calcium pyrophosphate dihydrate crystal deposition or to subchondral bony erosion from the resorptive effects of parathyroid hormone. Roentgenograms classically show subperiosteal bone resorption, cystic or sclerotic changes in bones, and chondrocalcinosis.

Secondary to Crystal Deposition Disease

Generalized osteoarthritis has been reported in patients with idiopathic articular chondrocalcinosis.[9] Large joints of the lower limbs and intervertebral joints of the lumbar spine are especially involved. Although a destructive arthropathy has been described in patients with articular chondrocalcinosis,[109] these destructive changes appear to be much more common when generalized osteoarthritis and chondrocalcinosis co-exist.[46] Weight-bearing joints are frequently affected, but involvement of non-weight-bearing joints such as the elbow, shoulders, wrist, and metacarpophalangeal joints is also common. Osteoarthritis and chondrocalcinosis appear to be related to generalized joint hypermobility.[11]

Several mechanisms have been postulated to relate the increased association of calcium pyrophosphate dihydrate crystal deposition to osteoarthritis. In certain patients, obvious crystal deposition antedates significant osteoarthritis; alterations in calcium matrix in these patients may predispose them to degenerative changes. In other patients, osteoarthritis is present for a prolonged period and crystal deposition disease occurs later in the disorder. Changes in cartilage matrix due to osteoarthritis may favor the precipitation and deposition of these crystals.

An association between hydroxyapatite crystal deposition and osteoarthritis has been described.[30,117,118] Osteoarthritis in patients with identifiable apatite crystals in synovial fluid is similar to other forms of osteoarthritis, except the presence of crystals correlates with more severe roentgenographic change. Whether apatite crystals are a result of or a cause of osteoarthritis is unknown. Severe degenerative changes of the shoulder in association with apatite deposition have recently been described by Halverson and McCarty and colleagues and have been termed "Milwaukee shoulder."[54,79] Similar changes have been seen in other joints, such as the knee.[31,54a]

Secondary to Neuropathic Disorders

Severe degenerative joint disease occurs in association with neuropathic disorders, as first described by Charcot.[18] The loss of proprioceptive or pain sensation, or both, relaxes the normal protective mechanisms of the joint and leads to articular instability and an exaggerated response to normal daily stresses. Although first described in patients with tabes dorsalis, similar lesions may be seen in other diseases associated with neuropathy including diabetes mellitus, syringomyelia, meningomyelocele, and peripheral nerve section (see Chap. 71).

Secondary to Overuse of Intra-articular Corticosteroid Therapy

The development of localized osteoarthritis has been ascribed to the repeated use of intra-articular injections of adrenal corticosteroids.[51] In these patients, pain relief may allow overuse of already damaged joints and may thereby promote degenerative change. Studies that have demonstrated a direct, deleterious effect of corticosteroids on cartilage suggest a second mechanism for the development of those degenerative changes.[88]

Miscellaneous Associations

Osteoarthritis, often polyarticular, is associated with a number of bone dysplasias. These disorders are uncommon and include multiple epiphyseal dysplasia, spondyloepiphyseal dysplasia, and osteo-onychodystrophy or nail-patella syndrome. Mechanisms for osteoarthritis are related to the severe distortion of articulating bone. The primary defects leading to bone dysplasia and the possible contributions of the primary metabolic defect to osteoarthritis are as yet unknown.

Severe cold injury with frostbite may lead to premature osteoarthritis when cold exposure occurs prior to epiphyseal closure.[47] Joint pain may begin months to years later.

Symptoms and signs, laboratory findings, and roentgenographic abnormalities of secondary osteoarthritis are generally similar to those seen in the primary form of the disease. Additional findings related to associated underlying disease states are also present. The management of patients with secondary osteoarthritis is similar to that outlined for patients with primary osteoarthritis.

REFERENCES

1. Abiteboul, M., et al.: Hyperostose vertébral ankylosante et métabolisme de la vitamine A. Rev. Rhum., 9:8–9, 1981.
2. Acheson, R.M., and Collart, A.B.: New Haven survey of joint diseases. XIII. Relationship between some systemic characteristic and osteoarthrosis in a general population. Ann. Rheum. Dis., 34:379–387, 1975.
3. Adams, I.D.: Osteoarthrosis of the Knee Joint in Sportsmen. M.D. thesis, University of Leeds, 1973.
4. Alexander, G.M., et al.: Pyrophosphate arthropathy: a study of metabolic associations and laboratory data. Ann. Rheum. Dis., 41:377–381, 1982.
5. Anderson, S.: The epidemiology of primary osteoarthrosis of the knee in Greenland. Scand. J. Rheumatol., 7:109–112, 1978.
6. Arnoldi, C.C., et al.: Intraosseous phlebography, intraosseous pressure measurements and ^{99m}TC-polyphosphate scintigraphy in patients with various painful conditions in the hip and knee. Acta Orthop. Scand., 51:19–28, 1980.
7. Arnoldi, C.C., Brodsky, A.E., and Cauchoix, J.: Lumbar spinal stenosis and nerve root entrapment syndromes—definition and classification. Clin. Orthop., 115:4–5, 1976.
8. Arnoldi, C.C., Linderholm, H., and Müssbichler, H.: Venous engorgement and intraosseous hypertension in osteoarthritis of the hip. J. Bone Joint Surg., 54B:409–421, 1972.
9. Atkins, C.J., et al.: Chondrocalcinosis and arthropathy: studies in haemochromatosis and in idiopathic chondrocalcinosis. Q. J. Med., 39:71–82, 1970.
10. Bahrt, K.M., Nashal, D.J., and Haber, G.: Diffuse idiopathic skeletal hyperostosis in a patient with situs inversus. Arthritis Rheum., 26:811–812, 1983.
11. Bird, H.A., Tribe, C.R., and Bacon, P.A.: Joint hypermobility leading to osteoarthrosis and chondrocalcinosis. Ann. Rheum. Dis., 73:203–211, 1978.
12. Bland, J.H., et al.: A study of inter- and intra-observer error in reading plain roentgenograms of the hands: 'to err is human'. AJR, 105:853–859, 1969.
13. Bluestone, R., et al.: Acromegalic arthropathy. Ann. Rheum. Dis., 30:243–258, 1971.
14. Blumberg, B.S., et al.: A study of the prevalence of arthritis in Alaskan Eskimos. Arthritis Rheum., 4:325–341, 1961.
15. Bremner, J.M., Lawrence, J.S., and Miall, W.E.: Degenerative joint disease in a Jamaican rural population. Ann. Rheum. Dis., 27:326–332, 1968.
16. Brodelius, A.: Osteoarthrosis of the talar joints in footballers and ballet dancers. Acta Orthop. Scand., 30:309–314, 1961.
17. Byers, P.D., et al.: Articular cartilage changes in Caucasian and Asian hip joints. Ann. Rheum. Dis., 33:157–161, 1974.
18. Charcot, J.M.: Sur quelques arthropathies qui paraissent dépendre d'une lésion du cerveau ou de la moelle épinière: arthrites dans l'hémiplégie de cause cérébrale. Arch. Physiol. Norm. Pathol., 2:379–400, 1868.
19. Cheung, H.S., et al.: Identification of collagen subtypes in synovial fluid sediments from arthritic patients. Am. J. Med., 68:73–79, 1980.
20. Cobb, S., Merchant, W.R., and Rubin, T.: The relation of symptoms to osteoarthritis. J. Chronic Dis., 5:197–204, 1957.
21. Cooke, T.D.V.: The polyarticular features of osteoarthritis requiring hip and knee surgery. J. Rheumatol., 10:288–290, 1983.
22. Cooke, T.D.V., et al.: Identification of immunoglobulins and complement in rheumatoid articular collagenous tissues. Arthritis Rheum., 18:541–551, 1975.
23. Cooke, T.D.V., Bennett, E.L., and Ohno, O.: Identification of immunoglobulin and complement components in articular collagenous tissues of patients with idiopathic osteoarthritis. In The Aetiopathogenesis of Osteoarthritis. Edited by G. Nuki. Kent, Pitman Medical, 1980, pp. 144–154.
24. Crain, D.C.: Interphalangeal osteoarthritis. JAMA, 175:1049–1053, 1961.
25. Danielsson, L.G., and Hernborg, J.: Clinical and roentgenologic study of knee joints with osteophytes. Clin. Orthop., 69:302–312, 1970.
26. Danielsson, L.G., and Hernborg, J.: Morbidity and mortality of osteoarthritis of the knee (gonarthrosis) in Malmö, Sweden. Clin. Orthop., 69:224–226, 1970.
27. DeHaven, K.E., Dolan, W.A., and Mayer, P.J.: Chondromalacia patellae in athletes. Am. J. Sports Med., 7:1–5, 1979.
28. Dieppe, P.A., et al.: Pyrophosphate arthropathy: a clinical and radiological study of 105 cases. Ann. Rheum. Dis., 41:371–376, 1982.
29. Dieppe, P.A., et al.: Mixed crystal deposition disease in osteoarthritis. Br. Med. J., 1:150–152, 1978.
30. Dieppe, P.A., et al.: Apatite deposition disease: a new arthropathy. Lancet, 1:266–269, 1976.
31. Dieppe, P.A., Doherty, M., and Watt, I.: Apatite associated large joint lysis. (Abstract.) Arthritis Rheum., 26:S18, 1983.
32. Doyle, E.V., Huskisson, E.C., and Willoughby, D.A.: A histological study of inflammation in osteoarthritis: the role of calcium phosphate crystal deposition. Ann. Rheum. Dis., 28:192, 1979.
33. Eaton, R.G., Dobranski, A.I., and Littler, J.W.: Marginal osteophyte excision in treatment of mucous cysts. J. Bone Joint Surg., 55A:570–754, 1973.
34. Edelman, J., and Owen, E.T.: Acute progressive osteoar-

thropathy of large joints: report of three cases. J. Rheumatol., 8:482–485, 1981.

35. Ehrlich, G.E.: Inflammatory osteoarthritis. II. The superimposition of RA. J. Chronic Dis., 25:635–643, 1972.

36. Ehrlich, G.E.: Inflammatory osteoarthritis. I. The clinical syndrome. J. Chronic Dis., 25:317–328, 1972.

37. Evarts, C.M.: Challenge of the aging hip. Geriatrics, 24:112–119, 1969.

38. Fam, A.G., et al.: Cholesterol crystals in osteoarthritic joint effusions. J. Rheumatol., 8:273–280, 1981.

39. Feller, E.R., and Schumacher, H.R.: Osteoarticular changes in Wilson's disease. Arthritis Rheum., 15:259–266, 1972.

40. Ficat, P., and Hungerford, D.S.: Disorders of the Patello-Femoral Joint. Baltimore, Williams & Wilkins, 1977.

41. Forestier, J., and Lagier, R.: Ankylosing hyperostosis of the spine. Clin. Orthop., 74:65–83, 1971.

42. Forestier, J., and Rotes-Querol, J.: Senile ankylosing hyperostosis of spine. Ann. Rheum. Dis., 9:321–330, 1950.

43. Forestier, J., Jacqueline, F., and Rotes-Querol, J.: Ankylosing Spondylitis: Clinical Considerations, Roentgenology, Pathologic Anatomy, Treatment. Springfield, IL, Charles C Thomas, 1956.

44. Forman, M., Malamet, R., and Kaplan, D.: A survey of osteoarthritis of the knee in the elderly. J. Rheumatol., 10:283–287, 1983.

45. Foss, M.V.L., and Byers, P.D.: Bone density, osteoarthrosis of the hip and fracture of the upper end of the femur. Ann. Rheum. Dis., 31:259–264, 1972.

46. Gerster, J.C., Vischer, T.L., and Fallet, G.H.: Destructive arthropathy in generalized osteoarthritis with articular chondrocalcinosis. J. Rheumatol., 2:265–269, 1975.

47. Glick, R., and Parhami, N.: Frostbite arthritis. J. Rheumatol., 6:456–460, 1979.

48. Goldin, R.H., et al.: Clinical and radiological survey of the incidence of osteoarthrosis among obese patients. Ann. Rheum. Dis., 35:349–353, 1976.

49. Golding, D.N., and Walshe, J.M.: Arthropathy of Wilson's disease: study of clinical and radiological features in 32 patients. Ann. Rheum. Dis., 36:99–111, 1977.

50. Goodfellow, J.W., Hungerford, D.S., and Woods, C.: Patello-femoral mechanics and pathology. II. Chondromalacia patellae. J. Bone Joint Surg., 58B:291–299, 1976.

51. Gottlieb, N.L., and Risken, W.G.: Complications of local corticosteroid injections. JAMA, 243:1547–1548, 1980.

52. Gresham, G.E., and Rathey, U.K.: Osteoarthritis in knees of aged persons: relationship between roentgenographic and clinical manifestations. JAMA, 233:168–170, 1975.

53. Hadler, N.M., et al.: Hand structure and function in an industrial setting: influence of three patterns of stereotyped repetitive usage. Arthritis Rheum., 21:210–220, 1978.

54. Halverson, P.G., et al.: "Milwaukee shoulder"—association of microspheroids containing hydroxyapatite crystals, active collagenase, and neutral protease with rotator cuff defects. II. Synovial fluid studies. Arthritis Rheum., 24:474–483, 1981.

54a. Halverson, P.B., et al.: Milwaukee shoulder syndrome: eleven additional cases with involvement of the knee in seven (basic calcium phosphate crystal deposition disease). Sem. Arthritis. Rheum., 14:36–44, 1984.

55. Hamilton, E., et al.: Idiopathic hemochromatosis. Q. J. Med., 145:171–182, 1968.

56. Harata, S., Tohno, S., and Kawagishi, T.: Osteoarthritis of the atlanto-axial joint. Int. Orthop., 5:277–282, 1981.

57. Harris, J., et al.: Ankylosing hyperostosis. I. Clinical and radiological features. Ann. Rheum. Dis., 33:210–215, 1974.

58. Heberden, W.: Commentaries on the History and Cure of Diseases. 2nd Ed. London, T. Payne, 1803, p. 148.

59. Hernborg, J.S., and Nilsson, B.E.: The natural course of untreated osteoarthritis of the knee. Clin. Orthop., 123:130–137, 1977.

60. Hernborg, J.S., and Nilsson, B.E.: The relationship between osteophytes in the knee joint, osteoarthritis and aging. Acta Orthop. Scand., 44:69–74, 1973.

61. Hoaglund, F.T., Yau, A.C.M.C., and Wong, W.L.: Osteoarthritis of the hip and other joints in Southern Chinese in Hong Kong. J. Bone Joint Surg., 55A:645–657, 1973.

62. Jorring, K.: Osteoarthritis of the hip: epidemiology and clinical role. Acta Orthop. Scand., 51:523–530, 1980.

63. Keats, T.E., Johnstone, W.H., and O'Brien, W.M.: Large joint destruction in erosive osteoarthritis. Skeletal Radiol., 6:267–269, 1981.

64. Kellgren, J.H.: Osteoarthrosis in patients and populations. Br. Med. J., 2:1–6, 1961.

65. Kellgren, J.H., and Lawrence, J.S.: Osteo-arthrosis and disk degeneration in an urban population. Ann. Rheum. Dis., 17:388–397, 1958.

66. Kellgren, J.H., and Lawrence, J.S.: Radiological assessment of osteo-arthrosis. Ann. Rheum. Dis., 16:494–502, 1957.

67. Kellgren, J.H., and Moore, R.: Generalized osteoarthritis and Heberden's nodes. Br. Med. J., 1:181–187, 1952.

68. Kellgren, J.H., Ball, J., and Tutton, G.K.: The articular and other limb changes of acromegaly. Q. J. Med., 21:405–424, 1952.

69. Kellgren, J.H., Lawrence, J.S., and Bier, F.: Genetic factors in generalized osteo-arthrosis. Ann. Rheum. Dis., 22:237–255, 1963.

70. Kitridou, R., et al.: Identification of collagen in synovial fluid. Arthritis Rheum., 12:580–588, 1969.

71. Lawrence, J.S.: Rheumatism in Populations. London, Heinemann, 1977.

72. Lawrence, J.S.: Hypertension in relation to musculoskeletal disorders. Ann. Rheum. Dis., 34:451–456, 1976.

73. Lawrence, J.S.: Generalized osteoarthrosis in a population sample. Am. J. Epidemiol., 90:381–389, 1969.

74. Lawrence, J.S., and Sebo, M.: The geography of osteoarthrosis. In The Aetiopathogenesis of Osteoarthrosis. Edited by G. Nuki. London, Pitman, 1981, pp. 155–183.

75. Lawrence, J.S., Bremner, J.M., and Bier, F.: Osteoarthrosis: prevalence in the population and relationship between symptoms and x-ray changes. Ann. Rheum. Dis., 25:1–24, 1966.

76. Lawrence, J.S., DeGraff, R., and Laine, V.A.I.: Degenerative joint disease in random samples and occupational groups. In The Epidemiology of Chronic Rheumatism. Vol I. Edited by J.H. Kellgren, M.R. Jeffrey, and J. Ball. Oxford, Blackwell, 1963, pp. 98–119.

77. Leach, R.E., Baumgard, S., and Broom, J.: Obesity: its relationship to osteoarthritis of the knee. Clin. Orthop., 93:271–273, 1973.

78. Lowman, E.W.: Osteoarthritis. JAMA., 157:487–488, 1955.

79. McCarty, D.J., et al.: "Milwaukee shoulder"—association of microspheroids containing hydroxyapatite crystals, active collagenase, and neutral protease with rotator cuff defects. I. Clinical aspects. Arthritis Rheum., 24:464–473, 1981.

79a. McCarty, D.J., et al.: Diseases associated with calcium pyrophosphate dihydrate crystal deposition—a controlled study. Amer. J. Med., 56:704–714, 1974.

80. McEwen, C.: Osteoarthritis of the fingers with ankylosis. Arthritis Rheum., 11:734–744, 1968.

81. MacSween, R.N.M., et al.: Antinuclear factors in synovial fluids. Lancet, 1:312–314, 1967.

82. Macys, J.R., Bullough, P.G., and Wilson, P.D., Jr.: Coxarthrosis: a study of the natural history based on a correlation of clinical, radiographic, and pathologic findings. Semin. Arthritis Rheum., 10:66–80, 1980.

83. Marcos, J.C., et al.: Idiopathic familiar chondrocalcinosis due to apatite crystal deposition. Am. J. Med., 71:557–564, 1981.

84. Meachim, G., et al.: An investigation of radiological, clinical and pathological correlations in osteoarthrosis of the hip. Clin. Radiol., 31:565–574, 1980.

85. Meeks, L.W., and Renshaw, T.S.: Vertebral osteophytosis and dysphagia: two case reports of the syndrome recently termed ankylosing spondylitis. J. Bone Joint Surg., 55A:197–201, 1973.

86. Mills, D.M., et al.: Association of diffuse idiopathic skeletal hyperostosis and fluorosis. (Abstract.) Arthritis Rheum., 26 (Suppl.):S11, 1983.

87. Mintz, G., and Fraga, A.: Severe osteoarthritis of the

elbow in foundry workers. Arch. Environ. Health, 27:78–80, 1973.

88. Moskowitz, R.W., et al.: Experimentally induced corticosteroid arthropathy. Arthritis Rheum., 13:236–243, 1970.

89. Moskowitz, R.W., Goldberg, V.M., and Berman, L.: Synovitis as a manifestation of degenerative joint disease: an experimental study. Arthritis Rheum., 19:813, 1976.

90. Murray, R.O.: The aetiology of primary osteoarthritis of the hip. Br. J. Radiol., 38:810–824, 1965.

91. Nesterov, A.I.: The clinical course of Kashin-Beck disease. Arthritis Rheum., 7:29–40, 1964.

92. Nettles, J.L., Whelan, E., and Filson, E.: Does long term long distance running cause osteoarthritis. (Abstract.) In Fifteenth International Congress on Rheumatism. Rev. Rhum. Mal. Osteoartic., 794, 1981.

93. Nilsson, B.E., Danielsson, L.G., and Hernborg, S.A.J.: Clinical features and natural course of coxarthrosis and gonarthrosis. Scand. J. Rheumatol., 43 (Suppl.):13–21, 1982.

94. O'Brien, W.M., La Du, B.N., and Bunim, J.J.: Biochemical, pathologic and clinical aspects of alcaptonuria, ochronosis and ochronotic arthropathy: review of world literature (1584–1962). Am. J. Med., 34:813–838, 1963.

95. Ohno, O., and Cooke, T.D.: Electron microscopic morphology of immunoglobulin aggregates and their interaction in rheumatoid articular collagenous tissues. Arthritis Rheum., 21:516–517, 1978.

96. Ono, K., et al.: Ossified posterior longitudinal ligament, a clinicopathologic study. Spine, 2:126–138, 1977.

97. Partridge, R.E.H., and Duthie, J.J.R.: Rheumatism in dockers and civil servants: a comparison of heavy manual and sedentary workers. Ann. Rheum. Dis., 27:559–568, 1968.

98. Patterson, A.C.: Osteoarthritis of the trapezioscaphoid joint. Arthritis Rheum., 18:375–379, 1975.

99. Pelligrini, P., Nibbio, N., and Piffanelli, A.: Artropatie croniche da attivate sportiva: il piede e il ginocchio del calciatore professionista. Archispedale S. Anna di Ferrara, 17:879, 1964.

100. Peter, J.B., Pearson, C.M., and Marmor, L.: Erosive osteoarthritis of the hands. Arthritis Rheum., 9:365–388, 1966.

101. Peyron, J.G.: Epidemiologic and etiologic approach of osteoarthritis. Semin. Arthritis Rheum., 8:288–306, 1979.

102. Pittsley, R.A., and Yoder, F.W.: Retinoid hyperostosis. N. Engl. J. Med., 308:1,012–1,025, 1983.

103. Postel, M., and Kerboull, M.: Total prosthetic replacement in rapidly destructive arthrosis of the hip joint. Clin. Orthop., 72:138–144, 1970.

104. Prince, D.S., et al.: Osteophyte-induced dysphagia: occurrence in ankylosing hyperostosis. JAMA, 234:77–78, 1975.

105. Puranen, J., et al.: Running and primary osteoarthrosis of the hip. Br. Med. J., 2:424–425, 1975.

106. Resnick, D., et al.: Diffuse idiopathic skeletal hyperostosis (DISH) [ankylosing hyperostosis of Forestier and Rotes-Querol]. Semin. Arthritis Rheum., 7:153–187, 1978.

107. Resnick, D., and Vint, V.: The ''tunnel'' view in assessment of cartilage loss in osteoarthritis of the knee. Radiology, 137:547–548, 1980.

108. Resnick, D., Shaul, S.R., and Robins, J.M.: Diffuse idiopathic skeletal hyperostosis (DISH): Forestier's disease with extraspinal manifestations. Radiology, 115:513–524, 1975.

109. Richards, A.J., and Hamilton, E.B.D.: Destructive arthropathy in chondrocalcinosis articularis. Ann. Rheum. Dis., 33:196–203, 1974.

110. Robbes-Ruy, E., et al.: Diffuse idiopathic skeletal hyperostosis: clinical and radiologic manifestations in 50 patients. Arthritis Rheum., 25:101, 1982.

111. Roberts, J., and Burch, T.A.: Prevalence of osteoarthritis in adults by age, sex, race, and geographic area, United States—1960–1962. [National Center for Health Statistics: vital and health statistics: data from the national health survey.] United States Public Health Service Publication No. 1000, Series 11, No. 15, 1966. Washington, D.C.: United States Government Printing Office.

112. Roh, Y.S., Dequeker, J., and Mulier, J.C.: Bone mass in osteoarthrosis, measured in vivo by photon absorption. J. Bone Joint Surg., 56:587–591, 1974.

113. Saville, P.D., and Dickson, J.: Age and weight in osteoarthritis of the hip. Arthritis Rheum., 11:635–644, 1968.

114. Schlomka, G., Schroter, G., and Ocherwal, A.: Uber der Bedeutung der beruflischer Belastung fur die Entsehung der degenerativen Gelenkleiden. Z. Gesamte Inn. Med., 1:447; 10:993, 1955.

115. Schmidt, K.L., Leber, H.W., and Schutterle, G.: Arthropathie bei primärer oxalose—Kristallsynovitis oder Osteopathie. Dtsch. Med. Wochenschr., 106:19–22, 1981.

116. Schumacher, H.R., et al.: Osteoarthritis, crystal deposition, and inflammation. Semin. Arthritis Rheum., 11 (Suppl.):116–119, 1981.

117. Schumacher, H.R., et al.: Arthritis associated with apatite crystals. Ann. Intern. Med., 87:411–416, 1977.

118. Schumacher, H.R., et al.: Hydroxyapatite-like crystals in the synovial fluid cell vacuoles: a suspected new cause for crystal-induced arthritis. (Abstract.) Arthritis Rheum., 19:821, 1976.

119. Seifert, M.H., Whiteside, C.G., and Savage, O.: A 5-year follow-up of fifty cases of idiopathic osteoarthritis of the hip. Ann. Rheum. Dis., 28:325–326, 1969.

120. Shapiro, R., Utsinger, P.D., and Wiesner, K.B.: The association of HLA-B27 with Forestier's disease (vertebral ankylosing hyperostosis). J. Rheumatol., 3:4–8, 1976.

121. Silberberg, M., and Silberberg, R.: Osteoarthritis in mice fed diets enriched with animal or vegetable fat. Arch. Pathol., 70:385–390, 1960.

122. Singleton, P.T., Cervantes, A.G., and McKoy, J.: Sicca complex and erosive osteoarthritis: immunologic implications of a new osteoarthritis subset. Arthritis Rheum., 25:S33, 1982.

123. Smith, C.F., Pugh, D.G., Polley, H.F.: Physiologic vertebral ligamentous calcification: aging process. AJR, 74:1,049–1,058, 1955.

124. Sokoloff, L., et al.: Experimental obesity and osteoarthritis. Am. J. Physiol., 198:765–770, 1960.

125. Solomon, L.: Osteoarthritis of the hip and femoral neck fracture: a mutual exclusive diad. In Studies in Joint Diseases. Edited by Arthritis and Rheumatism Council. London, 1978.

126. Solomon, L., Beighton, P., and Lawrence, J.S.: Osteoarthrosis in a rural South African Negro population. Ann. Rheum. Dis., 35:274–278, 1976.

127. Solomon, L., Beighton, P., Lawrence, J.S.: Rheumatic disorders in the South African Negro. Part II. Osteoarthrosis. S. Afr. Med. J., 49:1,737–1,740, 1975.

128. Solomon, L., Schnitzler, C.M., and Browett, J.P.: Osteoarthritis of the hip: the patient behind the disease. Ann. Rheum. Dis., 41:118–125, 1982.

129. Solonen, K.A.: The joints of the lower extremities of football players. Ann. Chir. Gynaecol. Fenn., 55:176, 1966.

130. Spagnole, A., Bennett, P., and Terasaki, P.: Vertebral ankylosing hyperostosis (Forestier's disease) and HLA antigens in Pima Indians. Arthritis Rheum., 21:467–472, 1978.

131. Stastny, P., et al.: Lymphokines in the rheumatoid joint. Arthritis Rheum., 18:237–243, 1975.

132. Stecher, R.M.: Heberden's nodes: heredity in hypertrophic arthritis of finger joints. Am. J. Med. Sci., 201:801–809, 1941.

133. Stecher, R.M., and Hauser, H.: Heberden's nodes: roentgenological and clinical appearance of degenerative joint disease of fingers. AJR, 59:326–327, 1948.

134. Stecher, R.M., Hersh, A.H., and Hauser, H.: Heberden's nodes: family history and radiographic appearance of large family. Am. J. Hum. Genet., 5:46–60, 1953.

135. Swezey, R.L., Peter, J.B., and Evans, P.L.: Osteoarthritis of the metacarpophalangeal joint: hook-like osteophytes. Arthritis Rheum., 12:405–410, 1969.

136. Tanaka, S., et al.: Clearance of technetium pertechnetate from the hip joint with arthrosis deformans. AJR, *118*:870–875, 1973.

137. Tokunaga, M., et al.: Change of prostaglandin E level in joint fluids after treatment with flurbioprofen in patients with rheumatoid arthritis and osteoarthritis. Ann. Rheum. Dis., *40*:462–465, 1981.

138. Utsinger, P.D.: A clinical and laboratory analysis of 200 patients with DISH. Clin. Exp. Rheumatol. In press.

139. Utsinger, P.D., et al.: Roentgenologic, immunologic, and therapeutic study of erosive (inflammatory) osteoarthritis. Arch. Intern. Med., *138*:693–697, 1978.

140. Utsinger, P.D., and Fite, F.L.: Immunologic evidence for inflammation (I) in osteoarthritis (OA): high percentage of Ia$^+$ T lymphocytes (L) in the synovial fluid (SL) and synovium (S) of patients with erosive osteoarthritis (EOA). Arthritis Rheum., *25*:S44, 1982.

141. Utsinger, P.D., Resnick, D., and Shapiro, R.: Diffuse skeletal abnormalities in Forestier disease. Arch. Intern. Med., *136*:763–768, 1976.

142. Utsinger, P.D., Resnick, D., and Zvaifler, N.J.: Wrist arthropathy in calcium pyrophosphate dihydrate deposition disease. Arthritis Rheum., *18*:485–491, 1975.

143. Weintroub, S., et al.: Osteoarthritis of the hip and fractures of the proximal end of the femur. Acta Orthop. Scand., *53*:261–264, 1982.

144. Wordsworth, P., et al.: Thyroid antibodies in synovial effusions. Lancet, *1*:660, 1980.

145. Wright, V.: Biomechanical factors in the development of osteoarthrosis, epidemiological studies. *In* Epidemiology of Osteoarthritis. Edited by J. G. Peyron. Paris, Geigy, 1981, pp. 140–146.

146. Wright, V.: Osteoarthrosis-epidemiology. Presented at a Conference of the International Symposium on Epidemiology of Osteoarthrosis. Paris, June 30, 1980.

Chapter 90

Treatment of Osteoarthritis

Kenneth D. Brandt

Management of a patient with osteoarthritis begins appropriately with an assessment of the goal of treatment. Is it to relieve pain, to increase mobility, to prevent progression of disease in the involved joint, or to reduce disability? Each of these aims is not equally relevant to all patients with osteoarthritis. Obviously, success in attaining any of these objectives requires accurate analysis of the pathogenetic factors underlying the patient's problems. All patients with osteoarthritis were not poured from a single mold, and optimal management cannot be based on a "cookbook" approach to treatment. Is the patient's pain due to synovitis, to periarticular muscle spasm, to mechanical instability of the joint, or to end-stage disease, with bone rubbing against bone? Or, perhaps, is the pain due to bursitis, rather than to intra-articular disease? The type of treatment is influenced by the answers to these questions.

Is loss of joint motion due to soft tissue contracture or to a restrictive osteophyte? Does sufficient cartilage remain on the osteoarthritic joint so that measures to prevent further damage are reasonable? Or is the joint so badly destroyed that such measures can accomplish nothing? The approach to treatment cannot be the same in both cases.

Because disability is defined in terms of the handicapped person's ability to relate to his environment,[55] can treatment reduce the patient's handicap and thus enable him to deal more effectively with obstacles presented by the workplace or home? Or can the environment be altered to lessen the consequences of the handicap? Both patient and physician must understand what can and what cannot be accomplished. The physician needs to know what the patient expects from treatment, and the patient needs to know whether these expectations are realistic. The chances of successful management,[50,51] and of the patient's satisfaction,[26] are greatest when both patient and physician agree about the importance of various facets of a treatment program.

For the individual with advanced disease, especially in the hip or knee, with chronic pain and disability, an aggressive, multidisciplinary, comprehensive program of management is warranted.[18,44] For many patients with mild osteoarthritis, however, reassurance that the disease is not likely to become generalized or crippling, instruction in principles of joint protection, and prescription of a mild analgesic are all that is required. Such reassurance is important; patients with mild osteoarthritis involving only one or two joints are often unnecessarily concerned that their disease will become increasingly painful and limiting. These patients contemplate a life of pain, confinement, and dependence. Indeed, a recent survey of elderly persons in Indianapolis showed that some believed that osteoarthritis may be fatal.[46]

Conservative management of the patient with mild disease can be fully justified in view of the following considerations: (1) the drugs prescribed today for treatment of osteoarthritis are analgesic or anti-inflammatory, and although they may provide effective symptomatic relief, they do not arrest or reverse the pathologic changes of the disease in articular cartilage or bone; indeed, some agents may contribute to these changes; and (2) joint pain in individuals with osteoarthritis is often episodic and not necessarily crippling;[23] the natural history of osteoarthritis is not one of inevitable progression of pain or disability. Thus, although radiographic evidence of osteoarthritis of the knee was present in about 10% of a group surveyed at age 50 and rose steadily to about 50% at age 80, only about half those persons with radiologic changes reported episodic knee pain at any age. Few in any age group reported crippling knee pain, and the proportion of those with crippling pain showed no tendency to increase between the ages of 60 and 80.[23]

Similarly, a recent study of nearly 700 elderly people surveyed for signs and symptoms of osteoarthritis of the knee indicated that neither the prevalence of these features nor their severity increased with age, but remained constant between the seventh and ninth decades.[14] A lack of progressive degeneration of the knee was also noted in an autopsy study.[8] Moreover, a longitudinal radiologic analysis emphasized the slow rate of progression of osteoarthritis of the hand, especially in the proximal interphalangeal joints.[45]

DRUG THERAPY

Various types of drugs are prescribed for patients with osteoarthritis.

Analgesics

Although articular cartilage lacks pain receptors, pain in osteoarthritis may arise from the fibrous capsule, from the subchondral bone, owing to microfractures or to venous congestion caused by remodeling of subchondral trabeculae,[28] or from periarticular muscle or ligaments. Ligamentous sprains are common, especially in the unstable joint, and local pain receptors may become hypersensitive.[22]

In patients with osteoarthritis and mild or intermittent pain without clinical evidence of inflammation, such as joint warmth or synovial effusion, an analgesic, taken as needed, and instruction of the patient in general measures of joint protection may be sufficient to relieve symptoms.

Acetylsalicylic acid, or aspirin, in a dose of 650 mg every 4 to 6 hours, as needed, is an effective analgesic for many patients with osteoarthritis. At this dose, the drug usually has little or no anti-inflammatory effect. Aspirin should always be taken with food. Even when taken with meals, however, or as a buffered preparation or with antacids, aspirin may produce dyspepsia. Enteric-coated aspirin, such as Zorprin, which is aspirin encapsulated in a special matrix to control its rate of release, and the nonacetylated salicylate preparations, such as Disalcid, Trilisate, or Arthropan, cause less gastric distress than standard aspirin. Although enteric-coated aspirin has been criticized for years for lack of efficacy, the newer preparations no longer have shellac coatings, and they now dissolve reliably and provide excellent bioavailability of acetylsalicylic acid[34] (see Chap. 28).

Nonetheless, some individuals with osteoarthritis are unable to tolerate salicylate in any form because of dyspepsia or ototoxicity. For these patients, acetaminophen (Tylenol), 650 mg every 4 to 6 hours as needed, or propoxyphene hydrochloride (Darvon), 32 to 65 mg every 4 to 6 hours as needed, provides comparable analgesia. Taken in excess, however, acetaminophen may cause toxic hepatitis. It is thus contraindicated in patients with prior liver disease.[2,4,20] Propoxyphene may cause drowsiness, lightheadedness, or gastrointestinal upset. Drug dependence may develop from long-term propoxyphene therapy. Codeine or other narcotics are rarely required in osteoarthritis and, if used, they should be prescribed for only a brief period.

Two recently marketed analgesic preparations have been reported to be useful in osteoarthritis, zomepirac (Zomax) and naproxen sodium (Anaprox). These agents may provide more effective analgesia than aspirin, with a longer duration of action. Each is, in fact, a weak nonsteroidal anti-inflammatory drug that inhibits the cyclo-oxygenase pathway of arachidonate metabolism. In patients who are also taking salicylate or another cyclo-oxygenase inhibitor, the analgesic effect of these new drugs seems less obvious than when they are given alone. Furthermore, because undesirable side effects, such as gastric irritation or renal insufficiency, may be additive, zomepirac or naproxen sodium should not be given concurrently with aspirin or other cyclo-oxygenase inhibitors.

Anti-Inflammatory Drugs

Synovial inflammation, although usually much less intense than that seen in RA, for example, occurs in osteoarthritis and may contribute to the patient's pain. Perhaps for this reason patients with osteoarthritis prefer anti-inflammatory drugs to comparably analgesic agents that lack anti-inflammatory properties.[10] Thus, if the patient's pain is not alleviated by an analgesic, or if signs of joint inflammation are present, one should prescribe an anti-inflammatory drug, that is, a higher dose of salicylate, such as 975 mg aspirin 4 times daily, or another cyclo-oxygenase inhibitor.

Since ototoxicity may develop in the elderly with a low salicylate dose, maintenance therapy with anti-inflammatory levels of *any* salicylate preparation is sometimes precluded in the older individual. Furthermore, older patients may develop gastrointestinal upset from salicylate more readily than younger persons.

Several nonsteroidal anti-inflammatory drugs currently available in the United States, such as fenoprofen, ibuprofen, indomethacin, meclofenamic acid, naproxen, piroxicam, tolmetin sodium, and sulindac, are effective in osteoarthritis. The average daily dose for treatment of osteoarthritis is often only half, or less, of the required dose for the treatment of RA. Because these agents are generally well tolerated and produce dyspepsia less frequently than aspirin, it is argued by some that they should be the drugs of first choice for the patient with osteoarthritis. They are considerably more expensive than aspirin, however.

Because gastrointestinal and neurologic side effects are more frequent with indomethacin than with the other foregoing agents, this drug should be considered separately. Indomethacin may produce dyspepsia and peptic ulcer, headache, depression, and a variety of other symptoms of central nervous dysfunction, including muzziness, that is, altered sensory perception.

Despite these limitations of higher doses of indomethacin, a low dose, such as 25 to 50 mg, is usually well tolerated and, if taken at bedtime, may be particularly helpful for patients with nocturnal pain. The sustained-release formulation of indomethacin that has recently become available appears to produce fewer side effects than the standard preparation.

Salicylate and all other cyclo-oxygenase inhibitors are contraindicated in patients with peptic ulcer disease. All these agents also affect platelet aggregation to some extent, although the inhibition of platelet function by the other nonsteroidal anti-inflammatory drugs is reversible and may be clinically less profound than the irreversible inhibition of platelet cyclo-oxgenase caused by aspirin. In patients at particular risk of bleeding, nonacetylated salicylate preparations, which appear to have no effect on platelets, may be preferable to the foregoing agents.

Certain risk factors, such as cardiac decompensation, cirrhosis and ascites, administration of diuretics, and clinically apparent renal disease,[6] are clearly associated with the development of reversible renal insufficiency in patients taking nonsteroidal anti-inflammatory drugs. Even in the osteoarthritic patient who exhibits none of these risk factors, however, age alone, presumably because of the presence of subclinical glomerulosclerosis,[21] may cause renal blood flow to depend on local prostaglandin production and hence to be vulnerable to the effects of cyclo-oxygenase inhibitors.[6] In such patients, serum creatinine and urea nitrogen concentrations may rise rapidly after initiation of treatment. The serum potassium concentration may also rise, occasionally to alarming levels, reflecting inhibition of the renin-angiotensin-aldosterone mechanism.[16,53] Body weight may increase because of fluid retention, which may precipitate congestive heart failure.

Phenylbutazone and its derivative oxyphenylbutazone, which are not cyclo-oxygenase inhibitors, are potent anti-inflammatory agents and may relieve symptoms in patients with osteoarthritis, especially during acute flares. One may prescribe 100 mg of either compound to be taken 3 or 4 times daily with meals for a few days; then the dose is tapered, to terminate treatment with the drug in 7 to 10 days. When these drugs are given for only brief periods, their ulcerogenic potential is usually not a concern. These drugs are aldosterone agonists and may cause fluid retention. They may also potentiate the action of warfarin derivatives, and may enhance the activity of oral hypoglycemic agents. Thus, they may cause problems, particularly in elderly patients with osteoarthritis, who are often predisposed to the above side effects and drug interactions. Furthermore, some cases of agranulocytosis or aplastic anemia associated with phenylbutazone and oxyphenylbutazone, although uncommon, may be idiosyncratic and thus may be unrelated to the dose or duration of treatment. The

risk of serious side effects with these agents and the availability of the previously mentioned alternatives, which, although less potent are less toxic, limit the role of phenylbutazone and oxyphenylbutazone in the treatment of osteoarthritis.

All the foregoing cyclo-oxygenase inhibitors were designed principally for use as anti-inflammatory compounds for patients with RA, without consideration of the pathophysiologic features of osteoarthritis. Recently, attempts have been made to develop compounds to treat osteoarthritis that take into account our current understanding of the mechanisms of cartilage damage in this disease.[13] Thus, compounds that stimulate chondrocyte metabolism or inhibit enzymes capable of degrading articular cartilage matrix have been produced. Some have achieved a certain popularity, particularly in Europe. Unfortunately, none of these agents have yet been shown in a controlled study to alter the natural history of osteoarthritis in man. This area of research can be expected to receive much more attention over the next few years.

Can anti-inflammatory drugs aggravate osteoarthritis? A retrospective radiographic analysis of osteoarthritis of the hip has suggested that indomethacin administration may be associated with greater joint destruction than that seen in control subjects.[47] It is conceivable that the relief of symptoms produced by indomethacin, and perhaps by other analgesic or anti-inflammatory drugs as well, may lead the patient to overuse the osteoarthritic joint, inciting further damage. On the other hand, indomethacin and other agents that inhibit prostaglandin synthetase may interfere with the repair of microfractures in subchondral bone.[52] This interference could account for the increases in subchondral cyst formation and joint destruction observed radiologically in patients treated with indomethacin.[47]

In vitro studies employing organ cultures of normal canine articular cartilage have shown that salicylates,[36] as well as several other nonsteroidal anti-inflammatory drugs that inhibit prostaglandin synthetase,[37] may suppress proteoglycan biosynthesis. Not all prostaglandin synthetase inhibitors have exhibited this effect, however, because indomethacin and sulindac sulfide did not reduce proteoglycan metabolism under identical experimental conditions. Furthermore, benoxaprofen, a long-acting propionic acid derivative, stimulated net proteoglycan and protein synthesis in normal canine knee cartilage in vitro.[40] Stimulation was also observed with nordihydroguaiaretic acid,[40] and this finding suggests that the effect of benoxaprofen may have been related to inhibition of the lipoxygenase pathway in cartilage.

Notably, the suppressive effect of salicylate in

the foregoing in vitro studies was much greater in osteoarthritic cartilage, in which basal levels of proteoglycan synthesis are increased three- to five-fold, than in normal cartilage.[43] Furthermore, it did not reflect a general toxic effect on the chondrocyte because net protein synthesis was unaffected by salicylate concentrations that suppressed proteoglycan synthesis. Presumably, this effect of salicylate is due to inhibition of enzymes involved in the early stages of chondroitin sulfate synthesis, such as uridine diphosphoglucose dehydrogenase, which is required for conversion of uridine diphosphoglucose to uridine diphosphoglucuronic acid.[38]

Recent evidence indicates that salicylate may inhibit proteoglycan metabolism in articular cartilage in vivo as well as in vitro. Thus, the feeding of aspirin in reasonable doses to dogs developing osteoarthritis,[41] or to dogs in which atrophy of articular cartilage was induced by immobilization of the ipsilateral limb,[39] aggravated the degeneration of articular cartilage. Salicylate had no apparent in vivo effect, however, on normal articular cartilage.

Additional studies indicate that the proteoglycan content of the matrix may be related to the vulnerability of articular cartilage to the effects of nonsteroidal anti-inflammatory drugs.[42] Furthermore, the effects of these agents on proteoglycan metabolism may be unrelated to their actions on prostaglandin biosynthesis.[35] Notably, the data suggest that differences among various nonsteroidal anti-inflammatory agents with respect to their effects on joint cartilage may be related to variations in the synovial fluid concentration of these agents. This difference, in turn, is related to the dose administered, which is based on the clinical potency of the drug.

Although these experimental data are interesting, they have been derived only from studies in animals. Although they suggest that long-term administration of salicylates and perhaps of other nonsteroidal anti-inflammatory drugs may be injurious to articular cartilage in arthritic joints, the effects of these drugs on the pathophysiologic features of the human osteoarthritic joint cannot confidently be deduced from these animal data.

Adrenal Corticosteroids

No place exists for systemic corticosteroids or adrenal corticotrophic hormones in the management of osteoarthritis. The side effects associated with prolonged use of these agents outweigh any potential benefits.

Intra-articular injection of adrenal corticosteroids may be helpful, however. In a review of nearly 1,000 patients with osteoarthritis of the knee who were treated with repeated intra-articular corticosteroid injections, as needed, over a 9-year period, Hollander found that almost 60% became sufficiently free of pain to require no further injections, and about 20% achieved sufficient temporary benefit to continue to receive intra-articular injections; the remainder either did not benefit from the treatment or were lost to follow-up.[19] These data must be judged against the results of other studies, which have shown similar benefits following a single injection of procaine,[54] saline solution,[54] or the suspending vehicle.[56] Furthermore, pain relief following intra-articular corticosteroid injection is usually temporary; 4 weeks later, the response of patients who received an intra-articular corticosteroid injection may be indistinguishable from that of control subjects.[15]

Although some evidence suggests that intra-articular corticosteroid injections may lessen the severity of the pathologic changes of osteoarthritis in experimental animals,[7,32] no such evidence exists in man. On the other hand, amelioration of pain may lead to overuse of the damaged joint and may aggravate the breakdown of cartilage. Furthermore, corticosteroids may cause direct cartilage injury. Repeated injections of corticosteroid into the joints of normal rabbits depressed the biosynthesis of collagen and proteoglycans[5] and caused cartilage degeneration.[33] Although histologic change in the non-weight-bearing joints was minimal, fibrillation and cystic degeneration were prominent in weight-bearing cartilage. For these reasons, intra-articular corticosteroids should generally be administered at intervals of at least four to six months for a given joint. In addition, on the basis of the foregoing evidence, *one should caution the patient to minimize joint loading for a time following an intra-articular corticosteroid injection.* Notably, injection of corticosteroids into ligaments and painful pericapsular sites may produce excellent relief of symptoms in patients with osteoarthritis, and this type of injection is not associated with the potential hazards of the intra-articular route.

REDUCTION OF JOINT LOADING

Analysis of the vocational and avocational demands on the arthritic joint is an integral part of the patient's evaluation, and joint usage must be taken into account in designing the treatment program. Indeed, the pattern of usage may have influenced the development of osteoarthritis. Activities that lead to excessive loading of the involved joint should be avoided when possible. Rest periods, for 30 to 60 minutes in the morning and afternoon, may help to reduce pain in the lower extremity joints or in the lumbar spine. Activities requiring loading of the diseased joint should be fractionated, rather than performed in a sustained fashion. Several short periods of standing or walking are preferable to a single prolonged one for the patient with osteoarthritis of the lower extremity.

Recommendations for modification of activities in the work place may be considered impractical by the patient. One of the goals of treatment should be to assist the patient to maximize his potential for employment. As an initial step, this goal requires an assessment of the functional capacity of the patient. Occupational and physical therapists may provide valuable input regarding a feasible type of employment.

In many instances, the solution to employment problems may be simple, such as having the patient use principles of joint protection or modifying the pace of work. It may be helpful for the physician or other health-care professional to contact the patient's employer to discuss modifications of the work place that may be desirable. Some patients may benefit by referral to a state department of vocational rehabilitation for job counseling, retraining, aid in establishing an independent business, or assistance in seeking further formal education. The physician should inform the vocational rehabilitation counselor of the patient's limitations and disease diagnosis.

Poor body mechanics may, in some cases, be etiologic in the development of osteoarthritis; in other patients, they are an aggravating factor. Poor posture should be corrected. For the excessively lordotic lumbar spine, or for the pendulous abdomen or breast, supports are useful. Pronated feet and varus and valgus deformities of the knee, all of which create excessive loading on the tibiofemoral joint, may be corrected with orthotics or by osteotomy. A cane, held in the contralateral hand, is helpful if hip or knee involvement is unilateral. If involvement is bilateral, crutches or a walker are preferable.

Obesity contributes to the excessive loading of articular cartilage. It may aggravate symptoms and may accelerate cartilage breakdown in the lumbar spine and in the joints of the lower extremity. The obese osteoarthritic patient should be instructed in a weight-reduction diet, although such patients often find it difficult to lose weight because of the degree of inactivity imposed by their disease. Participation in a mutual support group, such as Weight Watchers or TOPS, may be helpful.

For the patient with osteoarthritis who feels guilty because of a belief that obesity is the cause of the joint disease, it may be helpful to point out that no evidence suggests that obesity itself produces osteoarthritis in lower extremity joints except, perhaps, when the obesity is so marked that the patient is unable to appose the thighs. Under those circumstances, genu varus develops to maintain the feet under the center of gravity and osteoarthritis of the medial compartment of the knee may result.[27] The United States Health and Nutrition Examination Survey (HANES) found an association between obesity and osteoarthritis of the hands and knees, but not of the hips or ankles.[1]

PHYSICAL THERAPY
(see also Chap. 44)

The recommendation to reduce the use of an osteoarthritic joint, to minimize wear and tear, may not be accepted readily by the patients, because of concern that the joint will become stiffer unless it is used. Some of this concern arises because patients with osteoarthritis, especially of lower extremity joints, often experience "gelling" in the involved joint after inactivity, such as after an automobile trip or an airplane ride. One should advise the patient to put the involved joint through its range of motion intermittently during such periods of inactivity to minimize gelling. Moreover, emphasizing the importance of prescribed exercises as an integral component of the treatment program reassures some individuals who balk at a recommendation to curtail activities that stress the diseased joint.

Physical therapy is an indispensable component of the treatment plan for most patients with osteoarthritis. It involves, principally, the use of heat or cold and an exercise program tailored to the individual. Usually, it is helpful to precede each exercise session with applications of moderate heat for 15 to 20 minutes to relieve joint pain and to diminish stiffness. Liniment should be removed from the skin prior to application of heat, and the patient should be instructed not to lie on the heat source because this may impede blood flow to the skin and may lead to a burn. A variety of forms of heat are available, such as electric pads, paraffin baths, hydrocolator packs, ultrasound, diathermy, and infrared bakers. Practicality and cost should be considered. Often, with respect to selection of the heat modality, the simpler the better. Many patients find moist heat more effective than dry heat; a warm bath or shower may be the most convenient form of providing heat to the involved joint. For deep-seated joints, such as the hips or spine, ultrasound or diathermy may be especially helpful, although they often provide no greater benefit than cheaper, simpler techniques. Occasionally, pain is aggravated by the use of heat, and ice packs provide more effective analgesia.

The exercise program is designed to preserve or to improve range of motion and to strengthen periarticular muscles. Periarticular muscle atrophy is common in osteoarthritis, probably because of decreased activity.[48] Isometric exercises, which minimize joint stress, are preferable to isotonic exercises.

For the patient with lower extremity involvement who requires an ambulatory aid, such as a cane, crutches, or a walker, consultation with a physical therapist is desirable. The therapist can educate the patient concerning the mechanical advantages of the assistive device and can oversee its initial use, to demonstrate pain relief and to ensure that the patient uses the device correctly. The physical therapist may also assist the physician in educating the patient about the principles of joint protection.

ORTHOPEDIC SURGERY

For patients with advanced disease who have intractable pain or impaired function, surgical treatment may be helpful (see also Chaps. 45 through 50). For example, tibial or femoral osteotomy in the patient with genu varus or valgus and osteoarthritis of the knee may be of value, especially when the disease is only moderately advanced. These procedures often relieve pain by altering the stresses of loading and by creating a more normal alignment of the opposing cartilage surfaces. Debridement of the joint, with removal of free cartilage fragments, known as joint mice, may prevent locking, may eliminate pain, and may reduce the wear of joint surfaces. Resection of large osteophytes may also improve the range of motion. In advanced disease, arthroplasty or arthrodesis may be required. Both procedures generally relieve pain; often, arthroplasty also improves the joint's range of motion. Arthrodesis is generally not indicated in weight-bearing joints, such as the hip or knee. In patients whose future activities will necessitate heavy usage of the diseased joint, however, arthroplasty is associated with a high failure rate, so that arthrodesis may be preferable even though it eliminates joint motion permanently.

TREATMENT OF SPECIFIC JOINT INVOLVEMENT

Hand

The patient with osteoarthritis in the first carpometacarpal joint may obtain considerable relief of symptoms by an occasional intra-articular injection of corticosteroids. A simple hand splint to immobilize the first carpometacarpal and metacarpophalangeal joints of the thumb often reduces pain during functional activities.[30] In more severe cases, when the pain is not diminished by these measures, arthroplasty or arthrodesis may be indicated. Arthroplasty permits retention of motion, but results in subnormal grip strength. On the other hand, arthrodesis provides excellent grip strength, but eliminates motion.

In many patients, Heberden's nodes develop insidiously and asymptomatically and are of no consequence. In others, however, they develop rapidly and are associated with localized swelling, erythema, acute pain, and marked tenderness. Such patients often require reassurance that they do not have a crippling form of arthritis or a disease that is likely to become more generalized. Most patients are grateful for the reassurance that the nodes will eventually become painless and will cause minimal disability. For relief of pain from Heberden's nodes, heat is usually helpful, in the form of hot soaks, paraffin baths, contrast baths, and electric pads. Analgesic or nonsteroidal anti-inflammatory drugs may be useful. Occasionally, local injection of a corticosteroid preparation into or around the joint may be of benefit, especially when the node is acutely inflamed. Trauma to the hands, which may exacerbate the pain and may aggravate deformity, should be avoided or reduced.

One should instruct the patient in measures to reduce stress on the involved joints. An occupational therapist can often provide a useful analysis of the patient's activities of daily living and may recommend measures to minimize joint trauma during such activities. Nylon-spandex stretch gloves, worn at night, may relieve pain and stiffness in patients with osteoarthritis of the interphalangeal joints.[12] If lateral deviation of the distal interphalangeal joints limits function, arthrodesis in the functional position of mild flexion, 10 to 15°, is indicated.

Foot

Osteoarthritis of the metatarsophalangeal joint of the great toe is a common problem. It produces pain, limits mobility, and causes bony enlargement from proliferation of osteophytes at the joint margins. In patients with only mild or moderate discomfort, metatarsal pads or metatarsal bars may be helpful. The use of metal to stiffen the sole of the shoe and thereby to minimize dorsiflexion of the joint during walking may also be useful. Inflammation of the bursa medial to the first metatarsophalangeal joint may be treated effectively by a local corticosteroid injection. If the foregoing measures are ineffective, surgical intervention may be required. Silastic prosthetic replacement often leads to a pain-free, functional forefoot.

Osteoarthritis of the subtalar joint is often resistant to the general measures described. When pain is aggravated by weight bearing, a cane or crutches may be helpful. Triple arthrodesis may be indicated in patients with severe disease of the subtalar joint.

Knee

A program of analgesic or anti-inflammatory medication, heat and prescribed exercises, periods of rest, and adherence to principles of joint protection often provides effective relief of pain and stiffness. If the patient is obese, weight reduction is indicated. Other measures to decrease joint loading should also be recommended. For example, jogging and participation in racket sports should be discouraged. Swimming is an excellent alternative. The patient should be advised to avoid climbing stairs whenever possible and, in general, to sit rather than to stand. The use of a high stool is helpful if the patient is required to work at a counter. Chairs with high seats should be used rather than low sofas. The patient should avoid kneeling or squatting. Pillows should not be placed behind or under the knees at night, because this practice may lead to flexion contractures. Isometric quadriceps exercises should be prescribed. Knee cages, which are hinged braces that lace up the front, or elastic supports may increase stability.

Often, the patient with knee osteoarthritis complains of "knee" pain actually due to anserine bursitis. Injection of corticosteroid into the bursa often eliminates the discomfort. In acute flares of the joint disease, with increased pain, warmth and tenderness, or effusion, one should eliminate weight-bearing by bedrest or by the temporary use of an assistive device such as a cane. Aspiration of the effusion and an intra-articular injection of corticosteroid may also be beneficial.

In advanced cases, surgical treatment may be warranted. Total knee arthroplasty is not generally as successful as total hip arthroplasty. Nonetheless, in selected patients, it may afford excellent pain relief, as well as increasing mobility and function.

Hip

Measures to reduce loading of the involved joint should be considered an integral component of the treatment program. A cane, crutches, or a walker should be recommended if the patient finds walking painful. Canes are particularly effective in unloading the hip joint because of their great mechanical advantage. The obese patient should be encouraged to lose weight. Principles of joint protection should be outlined. Those described for osteoarthritis of the knee apply equally to the patient with arthritis of the hip. Rest, heat, analgesic and anti-inflammatory drugs, and isometric exercises to strengthen the supporting muscles in the lower extremity, as well as exercises to maintain normal range of motion, are indicated. Flexion contractures may be prevented, and mild ones may be corrected, by the patient lying prone for 30 minutes 2 or 3 times daily. Elevated toilet seats help the patient who has difficulty with a low commode because of limited motion. If muscle spasm is severe, traction may be required. Because capsular fibrosis is a significant cause of loss of motion in patients with hip osteoarthritis, exercises to strength abduction, extension, and external rotation are indicated. Intra-articular injections of corticosteroids may be helpful during flares.

For the patient with severe disease who is otherwise a candidate for surgical treatment, total hip arthroplasty is generally the procedure of choice. It usually relieves pain and restores hip motion. Intertrochanteric osteotomy may also be effective.[25,31] That later conversion to total hip replacement may not be technically feasible limits the role of this procedure, however. Pain at night and an inability to cut one's toenails are useful, simple clues leading to a consideration of surgical intervention.

Spine

Pain from osteoarthritis of the cervical spine may also respond to local heat and to analgesic or anti-inflammatory drugs. If acute muscle spasm or evidence of nerve root irritation is present, a cervical collar may be helpful. Occasionally, severe muscle spasm or nerve root compression requires traction. To decrease stress on the cervical spine, the patient should avoid postures in which the neck is maintained in a fixed position for prolonged periods, as during shampooing, sitting near the screen in a movie theater, or watching television while lying on a sofa. Patients whose neurologic complications fail to respond to the foregoing measures may require surgical treatment.

Pain from osteoarthritis of the lumbar spine also generally responds to heat, rest, and analgesic or anti-inflammatory drug therapy. Adherence to joint protection principles is particularly important. In general, patients should avoid prolonged leaning over a desk or work surface. When driving a car they may find it helpful to move the seat forward sufficiently to flex the knees and to diminish lumbar lordosis. A lumbosacral corset with abdominal support, and weight reduction if the patient is obese, are advisible. A firm mattress or a board placed beneath the mattress is often helpful. Local heat, massage, or muscle relaxants may be administered to relieve spasm. An exercise program to strengthen the anterior abdominal muscles and to correct faulty posture should be instituted after acute symptoms subside. Surgical procedures. such as laminectomy, discectomy, or fusion, may be indicated when symptoms are severe of if neurologic deficits occur (see also Chaps. 47, 82).

MANAGEMENT OF PSYCHOSOCIAL PROBLEMS

Emotional Issues

Osteoarthritis often causes major changes in life style and imposes losses of mobility, function, and independence. To the extent that the patient's identity depends on his body image, major impairment in physical function may also result in a loss of self-esteem. Notably, patients with osteoarthritis are less satisfied with their present life than patients undergoing renal dialysis.[24] The emotional reactions to these losses experienced by people with osteoarthritis are similar to those of people with other chronic illnesses,[17] and include denial, depression, and anger.

Denial serves as a buffer against threatening information, such as the initial diagnosis of arthritis. It is marked by minimization of the severity of the symptoms, the chronicity of the disease, or the importance of following medical recommendations. It may lead the patient to "shop around" for an alternate diagnosis, or to search for a miracle cure through quackery.

The denying patient should be approached supportively. Questions should be answered truthfully, but with only minimal detail. Because the denying patient may have a limited ability to absorb information about his treatment, the physician should be prepared to repeat instructions during subsequent appointments.

Depression may occur as the patient with osteoarthritis recognizes the full impact of his situation and the extent of his limitations. Mild, temporary depression is normal. Low self-esteem is a factor in depression, and the patient may believe that he has nothing of value to contribute to others. In addition, isolation and withdrawal are characteristic at this stage. Regression is evidenced by dependent behavior.

Because the depressed patient may be unable to relate to the hope of future improvement, immediate positive feedback is more appropriate than discussion of the long-term goals of treatment. To counteract low self-esteem, the physician might encourage the patient to emphasize valuable traits not affected by the disease, such as: "You may not be able to climb the steps in the football stadium any longer, but your terrific tenor voice can still enhance the church choir." Isolation from others should be discouraged. If depression is severe or if it interferes with function, one should consider antidepressant drugs or psychiatric referral.

The realization that a quick cure does not exist may lead to anger, which may be projected outward toward physically healthy people. Other patients may blame God or fate, saying: "Why me?" If anger is not expressed openly, it may be manifested indirectly through passive-aggressive, manipulative behavior.

Before a meaningful discussion of treatment can begin, it may be necessary to allow the patient to ventilate feelings of anger. Focusing on the patient's feelings is often preferable to reacting to the content of a hostile comment. When confronted with a patient who is angry about his slow improvement, for example, a response such as, "What you are really telling me is that you are concerned about your future," may be more helpful than a lecture concerning the nature of the patient's medications. Passive-aggressive patients who manifest their anger by refusing to comply with treatment plans and by failing to keep appointments should be confronted, and the feelings behind their behavior should be discussed.

Sexuality

Sexuality is a normal lifetime phenomenon for many, perhaps most, people. Disease and disability do not preclude sexual needs.[11] Because patients are often reluctant to express sexual concerns, the physician should initiate a discussion of sexual functioning. This discussion is an appropriate component of the physical examination, as the physician ascertains the impact of the disease on other aspects of function. For example, during the hip examination, the physician may include such questions as: Can you raise and lower yourself from a toilet seat? Can you engage comfortably in sexual intercourse? Can you climb a flight of stairs?

Because of pain and mechanical problems, sexuality may be particularly problematic for patients with osteoarthritis of the hips, knees, or spine. Results of a survey of 121 patients with osteoarthritis of the hip indicated that 67% expressed sexual difficulties, the most frequent of which were joint pain (40%) and stiffness (75%).[9] For the patient with reduced mobility or joint pain, a side-by-side position for sexual intercourse may be the most comfortable. The Arthritis Foundation's pamphlet, "Living and Loving with Arthritis," describes a variety of sexual problems and provides patients with suggestions for their solution.[3]

FINANCIAL ASPECTS

Financial concerns may lead patients with osteoarthritis to refuse certain treatment recommendations. If the patient is unable to work and is ineligible for retirement benefits, disability benefits may be obtained through the Social Security Administration. Patients with osteoarthritis may be eligible for Social Security disability or Supplemental Security Income (SSI) disability benefits if their disabling condition is expected to last for at least 12 months and if they are unable to engage in any substantial gainful employment. Laboratory and radiographic findings, functional ability, age, and educational and vocational background all may be considered in determining the patient's eligibility. The Social Security Administration provides a booklet for physicians that describes in detail the medical criteria used to assess the extent of disability.[49] To reduce the likelihood that patients who are legitimately disabled by osteoarthritis will be denied disability benefits, the physician must provide the Social Security Administration with specific information about the claimant's ability to perform work-related tasks and must document the objective clinical findings.[29]

Patients who have received Social Security disability benefits for 2 years, or who are age 65 or over, may receive Medicare benefits. With the exception of a deductible and certain copayments, Medicare hospital insurance, Part A, pays the "allowable" charges, which are based on the average cost of a service in the locale, for inpatient hospital care, including physical and occupational therapy, laboratory tests and radiograms, and skilled home health care following hospitalization. Medicare medical insurance, Part B, pays the allowable charges for physicians' services and outpatient treatment, including diagnostic tests and procedures, roentgenograms, drugs that cannot be self-administered, durable medical equipment, physical and occupational therapy, and skilled home health care. Medicare does not pay for drugs that can be self-administered, for education, or for orthopedic shoes, unless they are a component of a leg brace.

Patients who are "medically indigent," that is, those whose income beyond a certain subsistence allowance is less than their medical expenses, may qualify for Medicaid (MedCal in California). This program is administered by county departments of human services or departments of welfare or public assistance. Although the services paid for by Medicaid vary from state to state, this program generally pays for a large proportion of many medical expenses, such as hospital and outpatient care, prescribed medication, home care, nursing home care, and transportation to medical care providers.

REFERENCES

1. Acheson, R.M.: Epidemiology and the arthritides. Ann. Rheum. Dis., *41*:325, 1982.
2. Ameer, B., and Greenblatt, D.J.: Acetaminophen. Ann. Intern. Med., *87*:202, 1977.
3. Arthritis Foundation: Living and Loving with Arthritis: Information About Sex. Atlanta, Arthritis Foundation, 1982.
4. Barker, J.D., deCarle, D.J., and Anuras, S.: Chronic excessive acetaminophen use and liver damage. Ann. Intern. Med., *87*:299, 1977.
5. Behrens, F., Shepard, H., and Mitchell, N.: Alteration of rabbit articular cartilage by intra-articular injections of glucocorticoids. J. Bone Joint Surg., *58A*:1157, 1976.
6. Blackshear, J.L., Davidman, M., and Stillman, T.: Identification of risk for renal insufficiency from nonsteroidal anti-inflammatory drugs. Arch. Intern. Med., *143*:1130, 1983.
7. Butler, M., et al.: A new model of osteoarthrosis in rabbits. III. Evaluation of antiarthrosic effects of selected drugs administered intraarticularly. Arthritis Rheum., *26*:1380, 1983.
8. Casscells, S.W.: Gross pathological changes in the knee joint of the aged individual. Clin. Orthop., *132*:225, 1978.
9. Currey, H.L.F.: Osteoarthrosis of the hip joint and sexual activity. Ann. Rheum. Dis., *29*:488, 1970.
10. Doyle, D.V., et al.: An articular index for the assessment of osteoarthritis. Ann. Rheum. Dis., *40*:75, 1981.
11. Ehrlich, G.E.: Sexual problems of the arthritic patient. *In* Total Management of the Arthritic Patient. Edited by G.E. Ehrlich. Philadelphia, J.B. Lippincott, 1973, pp. 193–208.
12. Ehrlich, G.E., and DiPierro, A.M.: Stretch gloves: nocturnal use to ameliorate morning stiffness in arthritic hands. Arch. Phys. Med. Rehabil., *52*:479, 1971.
13. Fife, R., and Brandt, K.: Experimental modes of therapy in osteoarthritis. *In* Osteoarthritis: Diagnosis and Management. Edited by R.W. Moskowitz, et al., Philadelphia, W. B. Saunders Co., 1984, pp. 549–559.
14. Forman, M.D., Malamet, R., and Kaplan, D.: A survey of osteoarthritis of the knee in the elderly. J. Rheumatol., *10*:282, 1983.
15. Friedman, D.M., and Moore, M.A.: The efficacy of intraarticular corticosteroid for osteoarthritis of the knee. Arthritis Rheum., *21*:556, 1978.
16. Galler, M., Folkert, V.W., asnd Schlondorff, D.: Reversible acute renal insufficiency and hyperkalemia following indomethacin therapy. JAMA, *246*:154, 1981.
17. Gross, M.: Psychosocial aspects of osteoarthritis: helping patients cope. Health Soc. Work, 6:40, 1981.
18. Gross, M., et al.: Team care for patients with chronic rheumatic disease. J. Allied Health, *11*:239, 1982.
19. Hollander, J.L.: Treatment of osteoarthritis of the knees. Arthritis Rheum., *3*:564, 1960.
20. Johnson, G.K., and Tolman, K.G.: Chronic liver disease and acetaminophen. Ann. Intern. Med., *87*:302, 1977.
21. Kaplan, C., et al.: Age-related incidence of sclerotic glomeruli in human kidneys. Am. J. Pathol., *80*:227, 1975.
22. Kellgren, J.H.: Some painful joint conditions and their relation to osteoarthritis. Clin. Sci., *4*:193, 1939.
23. Kellgren, J.H., and Lawrence, J.S.: Osteoarthrosis and disc degeneration in an urban population. Ann. Rheum. Dis., *17*:388, 1958.
24. Laborde, J.M., and Powers, M.J.: Satisfaction with life for patients undergoing hemodialysis and patients suffering from osteoarthritis. Res. Nurs. Health, *3*:19, 1980.
25. Langlais, F., Roure, J.L., and Maquet, P.: Valgus osteotomy in severe osteoarthritis of the hip. J. Bone Joint Surg., *61B*:424, 1979.
26. Larsen, D.E.: Physician role performance and patient satisfaction. Soc. Sci. Med., *10*:29, 1976.
27. Leach, R.E., Baumgard, S., and Broom, J.: Obesity: its relationship to osteoarthritis of the knee. Clin. Orthop., *93*:271, 1973.
28. Lemberg, R.K., and Arnoldi, C.C.: The significance of intraosseous pressure in normal and diseased states with special reference to intraosseous engorgement pain syndrome. Clin. Orthop., *136*:143, 1978.
29. Meenan, R.F., Liang, M.H., and Hadler, N.M.: Social Security disability and the arthritis patient. Bull. Rheum. Dis., *33*:1, 1983.
30. Melvin, J.L.: Splinting for arthritis of the hand. *In* Rheumatic Disease, Occupational Therapy and Rehabilitation. 2nd Ed. Philadelphia, F.A. Davis, 1982, pp. 315–350.
31. Mogensen, B.A., Zoega, H., and Marinko, P.: Late results of intertrochanteric osteotomy for advanced osteoarthritis of the hip. Acta Orthop. Scand., *51*:85, 1980.
32. Moskowitz, R.W., et al.: Effects of intraarticular corticosteroids and exercise in experimental models of inflammatory and degenerative arthritis. Arthritis Rheum., *18*:417, 1975.

33. Moskowitz, R.W., et al.: Experimentally induced corticosteroid arthropathy. Arthritis Rheum., *134*:236, 1970.

34. Orozlo-Alcala, J.J., and Baum, J.: Regular and enteric coated aspirin: a reevaluation. Arthritis Rheum., *22*:1034, 1979.

35. Palmoski, M., and Brandt, K.: Effects of salicylate and indomethacin on glycosaminoglycan and prostaglandin E_2 synthesis in intact canine knee cartilage *ex vivo*. Arthritis Rheum., *27*:398, 1984.

36. Palmoski, M., and Brandt, K.: Benoxaprofen stimulates proteoglycan synthesis in normal canine knee cartilage in vitro. Arthritis Rheum., *26*:771, 1983.

37. Palmoski, M., and Brandt, K.: *In vivo* effect of aspirin on canine osteoarthritic cartilage. Arthritis Rheum., *26*:994, 1983.

38. Palmoski, M., and Brandt, K.: Proteoglycan content determines the susceptibility of articular cartilage to salicylate-induced suppression of proteoglycan synthesis. J. Rheumatol., *10 (Suppl. 9)*:78, 1983.

39. Palmoski, M., and Brandt, K.: Aspirin aggravates the degeneration of canine joint cartilage caused by immobilization. Arthritis Rheum., *25*:1333, 1982.

40. Palmoski, M., and Brandt, K.: Partial reversal by beta-D-xyloside of salicylate-induced inhibition of glycosaminoglycan synthesis in articular cartilage. Arthritis Rheum., *25*:1084, 1982.

41. Palmoski, M., and Brandt, K.: Effects of some nonsteroidal anti-inflammatory drugs on articular cartilage proteoglycan metabolism and organization. Arthritis Rheum., *23*:1010, 1980.

42. Palmoski, M., and Brandt, K.: Effects of salicylate on proteoglycan metabolism in normal canine articular cartilage *in vitro*. Arthritis Rheum., *22*:746, 1979.

43. Palmoski, M., Colyer, R.A., and Brandt, K.: Marked suppression by salicylate of the augmented proteoglycan synthesis (? matrix repair) in osteoarthritic cartilage. Arthritis Rheum., *23*:83, 1980.

44. Pigg, J.S.: Beyond the Platitude: The Team Approach to Arthritis Care and How to Prepare for its Delivery. Presentation at the Forum on Arthritis Research and Education in Nursing and Allied Health, National Arthritis Advisory Board, Washington, D.C., April, 1980.

45. Plato, C.C., and Norris, A.H.: Osteoarthritis of the hand: longitudinal studies. Am. J. Epidemiol., *110*,740, 1979.

46. Potts, M., et al.: Educational needs of ambulatory arthritics attending senior citizens centers. Clin. Rheumatol. Pract. In press.

47. Ronninger, H., and Langeland, N.: Indomethacin treatment in osteoarthritis of the hip joint. Does the treatment interfere with the natural course of the disease? Acta Orthop. Scand., *50*:169, 1979.

48. Sirca, A., and Susec-Michieli, M.: Selective type II fibre muscular atrophy in patients with osteoarthritis of the hip. J. Neurol. Sci., *44*:149, 1980.

49. Social Security Administration: Disability Evaluation under Social Security: A Handbook for Physicians. United States Department of Health and Human Services, Social Security Administration, Publication No. (SSA) 79-10089, 1979.

50. Starfield, B., et al.: The influence of patient-practitioner agreement on outcome of care. Am. J. Public Health, *71*:127, 1981.

51. Starfield, B., et al.: Patient-doctor agreement about problems: influence on outcome for care. JAMA, *242*:344, 1979.

52. Sudmann, E., et al.: Inhibition of fracture healing by indomethacin in rats. Eur. J. Clin. Invest., *9*:333, 1979.

53. Tan, S.A.Y., et al.: Indomethacin-induced prostaglandin inhibition with hyperkalemia. Ann. Intern. Med., *90*:783, 1979.

54. Traut, E.F.: Procaine and procaine amide hydrochloride in skeletal pain. JAMA, *150*:785, 1952.

55. World Health Organization: Technical Report No. 419. Geneva, World Health Organization, 1969.

56. Wright, V., et al.: Intra-articular therapy in osteoarthritis: comparison of hydrocortisone acetate and hydrocortisone tertiary butylacetate. Ann. Rheum. Dis., *19*:257, 1960.

Metabolic Bone and Joint Diseases

Chapter 91

Clinical Gout and the Pathogenesis of Hyperuricemia

Edward W. Holmes

Gout is a metabolic disease manifested by the following: (1) an increase in the serum urate concentration; (2) recurrent attacks of a characteristic type of acute arthritis in which crystals of monosodium urate monohydrate are demonstrable in synovial fluid leukocytes; (3) aggregated deposits of monosodium urate monohydrate (tophi), which occur chiefly in and around the joints of the extremities and sometimes lead to joint destruction and severe crippling; (4) renal disease involving glomerular, tubular, and interstitial tissues and blood vessels, and in which hypertension is common; and (5) urolithiasis. These manifestations can occur in different combinations.

Many gouty patients do not develop visible urate deposits, but few patients with gout escape without some renal damage. This damage is generally slowly progressive, and without a noticeable effect on life expectancy. Severely affected patients may manifest all the foregoing features, and in some patients renal disease or cardiovascular accidents may lead to premature death.

HISTORICAL BACKGROUND

Ancient Greek and Roman physicians possessed an intimate knowledge of gout. As early as the fifth century B.C., Hippocrates described gout as podagra, cheiagra, or gonagra, depending on whether the foot, wrist, or knee was involved. Tophi were first described by Galen (A.D. 131 to 200). The term gout, introduced in the thirteenth century, is derived from the Latin *gutta*, a drop, and reflects an early belief that a *noxa*, a poison, falling drop by drop into the joint was responsible for the disease.

Colchicine, the classic agent used to treat gout, was known to Byzantine physicians in the fifth century under the name "hermadactyl" (finger of Hermes). A drug probably identical to colchicine was described in Ebers Papyrus (1500 B.C.). *Colchicum autumnale*, or meadow saffron, was introduced into Europe in 1763 by Baron Anton von Storch, physician to Empress Maria Theresa.[247] The term "colchicum" probably originates from the ancient district of Colchis in Asia Minor.

The modern clinical history of gout began with Thomas Sydenham, whose unsurpassed description of the disease, authoritatively drawn from 34 years of personal affliction, clearly differentiated gout from other articular disorders.[232,233] The chemical history of gout began a century after Sydenham, when Scheele discovered uric acid as a constituent of a kidney stone in 1776.[197] Shortly thereafter, Wollaston in 1797,[257] and Pearson in 1798,[170] demonstrated urate in the tophi of patients with gout. Leeuwenhoek, the inventor of the microscope, had first described these crystals in 1679 when examining material obtained from a tophus, but the chemical composition of the crystal was not recognized at this time.[149] In 1848, A.B. Garrod performed the historic experiments in which he demonstrated, first by the murexide test,[81] and later by his famous "thread" test (1854),[80] an increased amount of uric acid in the blood of gouty subjects. The first specific enzymatic defect responsible for one rare subtype of hereditary gout, hypoxanthine-guanine phosphoribosyltransferase deficiency, was discovered by Seegmiller, Rosenbloom, and Kelley in 1967.[207] The introduction of the first effective and well-tolerated uricosuric agent, probenecid, in 1950 and the xanthine-oxidase inhibitor, allopurinol, in 1963 opened the way to successful clinical management of gout. Through the centuries, gout has enjoyed a royal patronage, and victims of gout have been favored subjects of caricature, novels, and biography. Among the illuminating articles on the history of gout are those by Rodnan,[190a] Hartung,[109] Bywaters,[44] and Copeman.[53]

DEFINITION OF HYPERURICEMIA

The limit of solubility of sodium urate in solutions with the sodium content of extracellular fluid is about 6.4 mg/dl.[171] Although the percentage of urate bound to plasma proteins in vivo is unknown, an additional 0.3 to 0.4 mg/dl may be bound to plasma proteins at 37° C, so saturation of plasma may be reached at approximately 6.8 mg/dl. Table 91–1 gives the known causes of hyperuricemia.

The traditional definition of hyperuricemia is based on the statistical range of values, mean ± 2

Table 91–1. Causes of Hyperuricemia in Man

Increased purine biosynthesis or urate production
  Inherited enzymatic defects
    Hypoxanthine-guanine phosphoribosyltransferase
      deficiency
    Phosphoribosylpyrophosphate synthetase overactivity
    Glucose-6-phosphatase deficiency
  Clinical disorders leading to purine overproduction
    Myeloproliferative disorders
    Lymphoproliferative disorders
    Polycythemia vera
    Malignant diseases
    Hemolytic disorders
    Psoriasis
    Obesity
    Myocardial infarction
  Drugs or dietary habits
    Ethanol
    Diet rich in purines
    Pancreatic extract
    Fructose
    Nicotinic acid
    Ethylamino-1,3,4-thiadiazole
    4-Amino-5-imidazole carboxamide riboside
    Vitamin B_{12} (patients with pernicious anemia)
    Cytotoxic drugs
Decreased renal clearance of urate
  Clinical disorders
    Chronic renal failure
    Lead nephropathy
    Polycystic kidney disease
    Hypertension
    Dehydration
    Salt restriction
    Starvation
    Diabetic ketoacidosis
    Lactic acidosis
    Obesity
    Hyperparathyroidism
    Hypothyroidism
    Diabetes insipidus
    Sarcoidosis
    Toxemia of pregnancy
    Bartter's syndrome
    Chronic beryllium disease
    Down's syndrome
  Drugs or dietary habits
    Ethanol
    Diuretics
    Low doses of salicylates
    Ethambutal
    Pyrazinamide
    Laxative abuse (alkalosis)
    Levodopa
    Methoxyflurane

S.D., with a given analytic method in a normal population. With modern colorimetric,[70,225] as well as enzymatic spectrophotometric,[110,160] methods, the upper limits of normal, thus defined, are 6.9 to 7.5 mg/dl in adult males and 5.7 to 6.6 mg/dl in adult premenopausal females. Automated analyzer (colorimetric) methods give values about 0.4 to 1.0 mg/dl higher than enzymatic methods.[55] The values in males averaged 19% higher than in females in 11 studies.[260] The sex difference is in part attributable to a greater renal clearance of uric acid in the premenopausal female.

The physicochemical definition of hyperuricemia is preferable to the statistical definition for a number of reasons, some theoretic, others pragmatic, as follows: (1) The distribution of plasma urate values are not symmetric about the mean, but are skewed to the right, so the majority of values outside the 2 S.D. range are high; (2) some frequency histograms show bimodality; (3) serum urate values are positively correlated with body weight, surface area, ponderal index, social class, academic achievement, leadership qualities, aptitude test scores, and hemoglobin and plasma protein values—the ''associates of plenty;'' and (4) in some populations, mean values are higher or lower than in the United States. Thus, a true serum urate level above 7.0 mg/dl is abnormal. In physicochemical terms, it represents supersaturation; in epidemiologic terms, it carries an increased risk of gout or renal stone.

Asymptomatic Hyperuricemia

A distinction should be drawn between a chemical abnormality, which is usually innocent, and a disease, which by definition produces symptoms. Thus, asymptomatic hyperuricemia alone is not a disease. Hyperuricemia with nephrolithiasis is a disease, but in my opinion it should not be called gout. The term gout is reserved for the disease marked by urate crystal deposition and an associated inflammatory tissue response, that is, articular manifestations or tophus formation.

Serum urate levels average 3.5 mg/dl in both males and females prior to puberty. Serum urate levels rise in normal males at puberty and in normal females after menopause. Alterations in urate clearance account for a portion of these changes in serum urate levels at puberty and at menopause.[255] The onset of hyperuricemia in males often occurs at puberty, and in females it occurs at menopause. Asymptomatic hyperuricemia may last a lifetime without recognizable consequences. The incidence of gout increases, however, as the serum urate concentration increases. In most instances, gout is not noted until the patient has had hyperuricemia for 20 to 30 years. Nephrolithiasis may precede articular symptoms in as many as 10 to 40% of gouty subjects.[272]

Few epidemiologic studies have assessed the risks of asymptomatic hyperuricemia. The data reported by Fessel suggest that asymptomatic hyperuricemia of <13 mg/dl in males and <10 mg/dl in females sustained for 40 years is not associated with an accelerated rate of renal deterioration, but the risk of urolithiasis is increased with asymptomatic hyperuricemia.[75] The data do not indicate that a reduction in the serum urate concentration, even in gouty subjects, necessarily prevents deterioration of renal function.[26,75] Because the major reason for treating it is to prevent renal damage, the limited data available do not justify therapy for most patients with asymptomatic hyperuricemia, although elimination of underlying causes of hyperuricemia, such as obesity and alcoholism, is appropriate. The apparently benign nature of asymptomatic hyperuricemia should not lead the physician to overlook the obvious, that is, that hyperuricemia predisposes persons to both articular gout and nephrolithiasis. Once the hyperuricemic patient experiences one of these complications, the asymptomatic phase is ended, and medical management of the hyperuricemia may be indicated.

CLINICAL DESCRIPTION OF GOUT

In the full development of its natural history, gout passes through three stages: (1) acute gouty arthritis; (2) intercritical gout; and (3) chronic tophaceous gout.

Acute Gouty Arthritis

The basic pattern of clinical gout is one of acute attacks of exquisitely painful arthritis, usually monoarticular at first and associated with few constitutional symptoms, and later often polyarticular and febrile, lasting a variable but limited time and separated by completely asymptomatic intervals. Attacks then recur at progressively shorter intervals and eventually resolve incompletely, leaving in their train chronic arthritis, which slowly progresses to a crippling disease with acute exacerbations superimposed with decreasing frequency and severity. The peak age of onset of acute gouty arthritis was in the fourth,[58] fifth,[36,89] or sixth[108] decade in various studies. Onset before the age of 30 years should raise the question of an unusual form of gout, perhaps related to a specific enzymatic defect causing overproduction of purines, or rarely to an unusual form of parenchymal renal disease.

In about 85 to 90% of first attacks, a single joint is involved. In at least half the initial acute attacks, the first metatarsophalangeal joint is the site of the paroxysm (podagra). In Scudamore's series of 516 cases collected in the early nineteenth century, 60% of initial attacks involved the great toe of one foot only.[202] Both great toes were involved simultaneously in 5% of subjects in the first attack. The percentage of patients in whom the initial attack is polyarticular varies. In the study of Delbarre et al., only 3% of initial attacks were polyarticular in 143 males, whereas 26% were polyarticular in 40 females.[58] Salzman et al. reported that 14.5% of first attacks in 76 patients, only 71% of whom were male, involved multiple joints.[195]

Ninety percent of patients with gout experience acute attacks in the great toe at some time during the course of their disease. Next in order of frequency as site of initial involvement are the insteps, ankles, heels, knees, wrists, fingers, and elbows. Acute gout is predominantly a disease of the lower extremity, but any joint may be involved. Acute episodes may affect the shoulders, hips, spine, and the sacroiliac, sternoclaviclar, and temporomandibular joints, but such sites are rare.* *The more distal the site of the involvement, the more typical is the character of the attack.*

Some patients report numerous short, trivial episodes of "ankle sprains," or sore heels, or twinges of pain in the great toe, prior to the first dramatic gouty attack, sometimes going back over several years. The patient may "walk these off" in a few hours. In most patients, however, the initial manifestation of gout occurs with explosive suddenness during apparent excellent health. Commonly, the first attack begins at night. Some patients first detect symptoms when they place their feet on the floor after awakening. In others, the pain awakens the victim. Within a few hours, the skin over the affected joint becomes hot and dusky red, and the joint becomes tender. Initially, the joint is only slightly swollen, but signs of inflammation may progress to resemble those of bacterial cellulitis, and on occasion, a joint is incised by an unwary physician intent on draining pus. Lymphangitis may be evident. Systemic signs of inflammation may include leukocytosis, fever, and elevation of the erythrocyte sedimentation rate. When the big toe is involved, the site of maximum sensitivity is on the medial aspect of the first metatarsophalangeal joint, where even the slightest pressure may produce exquisite pain. The tenderness is so severe that the patient takes voluntarily to bed, and not even the weight of a sheet can be borne on the affected part. It is difficult to improve on Sydenham's classic description of the acute attack:

Editor's note: I have never seen acute gout in the temporomandibular joints. The few reported cases cited in Chapter 81 seem incompletely documented.

The victim goes to bed and sleeps in good health. About two o'clock in the morning he is awakened by a severe pain in the great toe; more rarely in the heel, ankle, or instep. This pain is like that of a dislocation, and yet the parts feel as if cold water were poured over them. Then follow chills and shivers, and a little fever. The pain, which was at first moderate, becomes more intense. With its intensity the chills and shivers increase. After a time this comes to its height, accommodating itself to the bones and ligaments of the tarsus and metatarsus. Now it is a violent stretching and tearing of the ligaments—now it is a gnawing pain and now a pressure and tightening. So exquisite and lively meanwhile is the feeling of the part affected, that it cannot bear the weight of bedclothes nor the jar of a person walking in the room. The night is passed in torture, sleeplessness, turning of the part affected, and perpetual change of posture; the tossing about of the body being as incessant as the pain of the tortured joint, and being worse as the fit comes on. Hence the vain effort by change of posture, both in the body and the limb affected, to obtain an abatement of the pain.[232]

The course of untreated acute gout is variable. Mild attacks may subside in several hours or may persist for only a day or two, and they may not reach the intensity described by Sydenham. Severe attacks may last many days to several weeks. "With age and impaired habits gout may last two months."[232] The skin over the joint may desquamate as the episode subsides. On recovery, the patient re-enters an asymptomatic phase termed the intercritical period. Even though the attack may have been incapacitating, with excruciating pain and marked swelling, resolution is usually complete, and the patient is once again well. The freedom from symptoms during this stage, an important diagnostic feature, was noted by Areteus 17 centuries ago; he records that an athlete had won the Marathon in the Olympic Games between gouty attacks.

The mechanism by which crystals of sodium urate monohydrate cause the acute attack of gout and the management of this illness are discussed in Chapter 93.

Provocative or Possible Etiologic Factors

The acute gouty attack may be triggered by a specific event recognizable by the patient or the physician. The most commonly cited are trauma, alcohol ingestion, administration of certain drugs, and surgical procedures. These factors play some part in determining individual attacks of gouty arthritis and its site, but their relation to the disease is not usually clear.

Trauma. Acute gouty arthritis commonly results from trauma. The first metatarsophalangeal joint is subject to chronic strain; in walking, it is exposed to the greatest pressure, as defined as force per unit area, of any joint in the body. Gouty episodes may follow such minor trauma as that from long walks, from golf, or from hunting trips. Occupational trauma may predispose a person to certain localizations of acute attacks. In automobile mechanics, attacks of specific joints of fingers may occur at sites of injury; in truck drivers, gout may favor the right knee; in treadle workers, such episodes may affect the ankle. The signs of gouty arthritis are out of proportion to the severity of injury, an important point in differentiation from traumatic arthritis or fracture.

Alcohol Ingestion. Alcohol ingestion is both a predisposing and a provocative factor in gout. In his classic review on gout, Garrod wrote: "There is no truth in medicine better established than the fact that the use of fermented liquors is the most powerful of all the predisposing causes of gout; nay, so powerful, that it may be a question whether gout would ever have been known to mankind had such beverages not been indulged in."[79] The mechanisms by which ethanol contributes to hyperuricemia are discussed later in this chapter.

Drugs. Various drugs may be associated with acute gouty episodes. In some instances, the response is an idiosyncrasy, such as with attacks precipitated by thiamine chloride, insulin, penicillin,[234] mercurial diuretics,[177] or adrenocorticotropic hormone withdrawal.[112,256] Other episodes may be related to transient hyperuricemia, such as when they follow administration of liver or vitamin B_{12} to patients with untreated pernicious anemia,[203] or of thiazides in the treatment of hypertension.[3] In still others, an apparent relation exists to suddenly induced hypouricemia, such as in patients given probenecid or allopurinol.[3] It has been suggested that a rapid lowering of the serum urate concentration following a temporary elevation, as seen during overindulgence of food and alcohol, for example, is responsible for the release of microcrystals of sodium urate from intra-articular tophi leading to the development of acute gouty arthritis.[190] Thus, a sudden change in serum urate concentration in either direction is capable of leading to an acute attack of gout in a predisposed individual.

Medical and Surgical Illnesses. The patient with hyperuricemia is at risk of developing an attack of gout in association with the stress of an acute medical illness or during the postoperative period. In patients with known gout, the risk of a postoperative episode is high in the absence of preventive therapy. Linton and Talbott reported an incidence of 86% of acute gout in 22 gouty patients subjected to surgical procedures without prophylactic colchicine therapy.[146] Acute arthritis often occurs between the third and fifth postoperative days and, less commonly, is seen as late as the tenth day.* Attacks of gout in predisposed hyper-uricemic persons are also common during acute medical illnesses.[248] Factors leading to episodes of gout in these medical and surgical patients are not identified and may be complex.

Other Factors. Gout has been precipitated by dietary excess, diuresis, hemorrhage, venisection, foreign protein therapy, infection, and x-ray therapy.

Prevalence and Incidence

The prevalence of gout varies in different parts of the world. A figure of 0.3% in Europe was recorded,[141] and in the United States, the prevalence has been estimated to be 275 per 100,000 (0.27%).[262] In the Heart Disease Epidemiology Study conducted in Framingham, Massachusetts, a prevalence of gouty arthritis of 0.2% was found in a population of 5,127 subjects, 2,283 men and 2,844 women, aged 30 to 59 years (mean age 44). Fourteen years later, the prevalence had increased to 1.5% of this population (mean age 58), 2.8% in men and 0.4% in women.[106] The prevalence appears to be even higher among Filipino males in northwestern North America, and it is much higher among the Chamorros and the Carolinians in the Mariana Islands and the Maori of New Zealand. In the Maori, the mean serum urate value is 7.1 mg/dl in males, and the prevalence of gout is 10%.[142,153] The relation of prevalence to the serum urate level is shown in Table 91–2, which summarizes the situation in the Framingham population.

During World Wars I and II, acute gouty arthritis was uncommon in Europe. When protein again became plentiful, the prevalence of gout returned to prewar levels.[275] In Japan, where protein intake per capita has doubled since World War II, gout is becoming increasingly prevalent. These and other observations underscore the importance of dietary and environmental influences in determining the expression of genetic factor(s) in persons at risk.

Primary* gout is pre-eminently a disease of the adult male. Physicians have known that gout is uncommon in women since the time of Hippocrates. In large series, only 3 to 7% of cases of primary gout are found in women, and these women are chiefly postmenopausal.[11,100,118] In limited series, higher percentages of women are occasionally noted. These series may include patients with secondary* gout complicating hypertension, renal disease, especially lead nephropathy, or diuretic therapy.

Primary gout is uncommon before the third decade, and its peak incidence in various series is in the thirties, forties, or fifties.[108,242] In general, the higher the serum urate level, the earlier the onset of gouty arthritis.[106] In the Framingham study, the cumulative incidence of gouty arthritis in men appeared to approach a plateau at mean age 58 years, although only one-third of the men with urate levels of 8 mg/dl or more had experienced an attack of gout.[106] Age may explain the low fraction of 21 patients with gout among 5,400 cases of arthritis (0.4%) in a United States Army Arthritis Center during World War II,[119] as compared with the usual frequency of 4 or 5% of gout among all arthritic patients in civilian clinic populations in this country.[163,215]

Editor's note: Acute pseudogout is also often precipitated by surgical procedures or an acute medical illness; postsurgical bouts are most common on the second postoperative day.

Primary indicates gout or hyperuricemia occurring in the absence of a predisposing disorder; *secondary* refers to gout or hyperuricemia occurring as a complication of such disorder.

Table 91–2. Prevalence of Gouty Arthritis in Relation to Serum Uric Acid Level (admitted at a mean age of 44 and followed for 14 years)

Serum Uric Acid Level (mg/dl)	Men			Women		
	Total No. Examined	Gouty Arthritis Developed I		Total No. Examined	Gouty Arthritis Developed I	
		No.	Percentage (%)		No.	Percentage (%)
6	1,281	8	0.6	2,665	2	0.08
6–6.9	790	15	1.9	151	5	3.3
7–7.9	162	27	16.7	23	4	17.4
8–8.9	40	10	25.0	4	0	0
9+	10	9	90.0	1	0	0
Total	2,283	65	2.8	2,844	11	0.4

(From Hall, A.P., et al.[106])

Intercritical Gout and Recurrent Episodes

The intervals between gouty attacks are called intercritical periods. Some patients do not have a recurrence. In others, a second attack occurs 5 to 10 years later, but most patients experience a second episode within 6 months to 2 years. In Gutman's series, 62% had recurrences within the first year, 16% in 1 to 2 years, 11% in 2 to 5 years, 4% in 5 to 10 years, and 7% not for 10 or more years.[97] The frequency of attacks usually increases with time in any untreated patient. Later episodes are often polyarticular, more severe, longer lasting, and are accompanied by fever. Roentgenographic changes may develop, and the attacks may abate more gradually than before, but the affected joints often recover complete, asymptomatic function.

One-third of patients with late polyarticular attacks report that their initial episode was also polyarticular.[105] In polyarticular gout, 83% of all joints involved are of the lower extremity. In one-third of patients with this pattern, the foot is spared. Various joints may be affected in sequence in a migratory attack, which may involve the subdeltoid or olecranon bursae, the Achilles tendon, or other para-articular sites. Eventually, the patient may enter a phase of chronic polyarticular gout without pain-free intercritical periods. At this stage, gout may be easily confused with degenerative or rheumatoid arthritis (RA).

The previously described course of illness is usual. If the patient is seen late in the disease, the physician can usually obtain a clear and detailed description of the initial attacks and of the completely asymptomatic intervals between attacks of sudden onset and rapid offset, and this history is valuable in making the correct diagnosis. Not all patients follow this course, however. Rarely, the disease runs a fulminant, febrile course, and it may then be misdiagnosed as rheumatic fever, especially in a young patient. In addition, some patients progress directly from the initial acute attack to a subchronic and then a chronic illness, with no remissions and early development of tophi and incapacity. On occasion, the clinical course of gout mimics that of RA, and the joint deformities and tophi may be mistaken for nodular rheumatoid disease.* The subcutaneous nodules in patients with rheumatoid nodulosis are also easily confused with tophi.[82a]

One helpful clue in distinguishing nodular rheumatoid disease from tophaceous gout is a positive test result for rheumatoid factor in the patient with rheumatoid nodules. Nonetheless, 10% of gouty patients had positive tests for rheumatoid factor,[248] and fully one-third of patients with tophaceous gout had positive results, although the titers were generally lower than in RA.[138a] Another study also found a similar prevalence of low-titer rheumatoid factor in gouty patients and demonstrated a correlation between the presence of liver disease and seropositivity in these individuals.[183]

Chronic Tophaceous Gout

The time from the initial attack to the occurrence of chronic symptoms or visible tophaceous involvement ranges, in the experience of Hench, from 3 to 42 years, with an average of 11.6 years.[113] A retrospective analysis by Gutman of 1,165 patients with primary gout before appropriate drug therapy showed that 1 to 5 years after the first attack of arthritis, 70% were free of demonstrable tophi, and few of the remainder had more than minimal deposits.[96] Ten years after the first acute attack, about half the patients were still free of tophi, and most of the remainder had only minimal deposits. Thereafter, the proportion of nontophaceous cases slowly declined to 28% in 20 years. The percentage of patients with severe crippling disease was appreciable, 24%, only 20 years after the initial attack. Gutman pointed out that even these figures for tophaceous and chronic gout may be higher than should be expected in the gouty population at large because his series contained a disproportionate percentage of severe cases. A recent study has documented the following profile for the typical patient with tophaceous gout: early age of onset, long duration of disease, long period of active but untreated gout, frequent attacks, high serum urate values, and increased tendency to upper extremity and polyarticular episodes.[162a] Occasional startling exceptions to these general rules are encountered, however.

The rate of urate deposition in and about the joints correlates with the patient's serum urate level. In Gutman's series, the mean serum urate concentration was 9.1 mg/dl (uricase method) in 722 nontophaceous patients, 10 to 11 mg/dl in 456 patients with minimal to moderate tophaceous deposits, and greater than 11.0 mg/dl in 111 patients with extensive tophaceous involvement.[96] The rate of formation of tophaceous deposits in primary gout is thus a direct function of the degree and duration of hyperuricemia. The rate of formation of tophi also correlates with the severity of renal disease, which, in turn, is related to the duration of hyperuricemia and is a factor in determining its degree.[102]

Tophaceous gout is a consequence of a progres-

---

*Editor's note: This situation is especially common in patients treated with systemic corticosteroids. In gout, however, involved joints are inflamed out of phase with each other, a differential point from RA, in which the inflammation in multiple joints is synchronous.

sive inability to dispose of urate as rapidly as it is produced. The urate pool expands, and crystalline deposits of urate appear in cartilage, synovial membranes, tendons, soft tissues, and elsewhere. Occasionally, tophi are present at the time of the initial acute attack. This situation is unusual in primary gout, but it has been recorded by Yu in nearly 0.5% of patients with gout secondary to myeloproliferative disease,[270] and it may also occur in juvenile gout, such as that complicating glycogen storage disease[217] or the Lesch-Nyhan syndrome.[259] Tophi rarely develop in gout secondary to primary renal disease.

A classic location of tophi is the helix, or less commonly, the anthelix of the ear (Fig. 91–1). Tophaceous deposits may produce irregular, asymmetric, discrete tumescences of fingers, hands (Fig. 91–2), knees, or feet that require the patient

to wear larger gloves or shoes. The classic gouty shoe is one with a "window" cut to accommodate an irregularly prominent joint, usually the first metatarsophalangeal joint. Tophi commonly form lumps along the ulnar surface of the forearm (Fig. 91–3), or saccular distentions of olecranon bursae, or fusiform, or lumpy enlargements of the Achilles tendon. Occasionally, they develop subcutaneously along the tibial surface. The predilection for developing tophi in the distal part of the extremities and the helix of the ear may be related to the relative coolness of these regions of the body and the decreasing solubility of urate at lower temperatures.[146a] The frequent involvement of the ulnar surface of the forearm has been related to repeated trauma and pressure in this area.

As tophi and renal disease advance, acute attacks recur less frequently and are milder; later in the

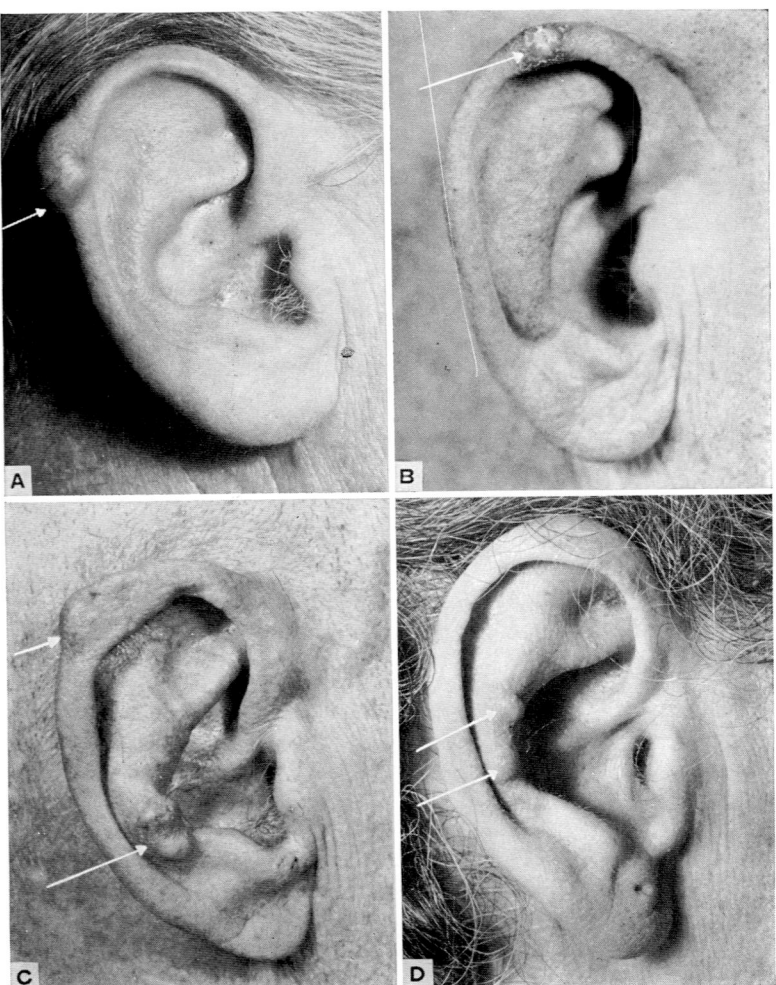

Fig. 91–1. Tophi in ears. *A*, Large cystic tophus on the helix. *B*, Ulcerated tophus. *C*, Two tophi in ear, on the helix and the antihelix. *D*, Subcutaneous nodules of rheumatoid arthritis, *not* gouty tophi, in a female patient.

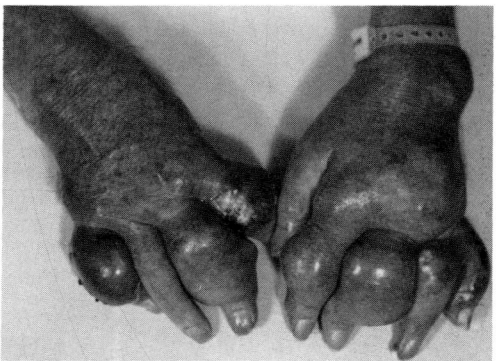

Fig. 91–2.   Chronic tophaceous gout of severe degree, with bulbous enlargement of several fingers. Note sparing of the fourth finger of the right hand. (From Wyngaarden, J.B., and Kelley, W.N.[267])

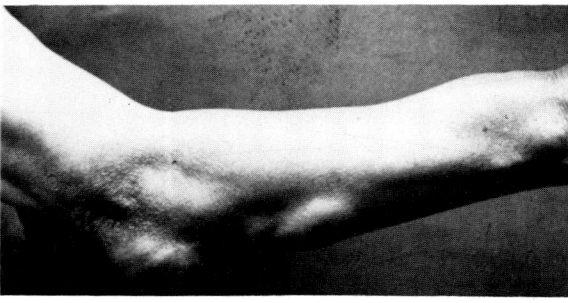

Fig. 91–3.   Lumpy tophi of the olecranon bursa, the ulnar surface, and the wrist. (From Wyngaarden, J.B., and Kelley, W.N.[267])

illness, they may disappear altogether. Acute episodes may be superimposed on the indolent soreness of the involved joint, or they may affect previously uninvolved sites.

The process of tophaceous deposition advances insidiously, and although the tophi themselves are painless, the patient often notes progressive stiffness and persistent aching of affected joints. Eventually, extensive destruction of joints and large subcutaneous tophi may lead to grotesque deformities, particularly of the hands and feet, and to progressive crippling. The tense, shiny, thin skin overlying the tophus may ulcerate and may extrude white, chalky or pasty material composed of myriad fine, needle-like crystals. Rarely, tophi suppurate. Ulcerated tophi may become secondarily infected, but such a diagnosis is difficult to establish because open lesions are usually contaminated with skin flora, and cultures are positive but difficult to interpret. Tophi may limit joint movement by the direct involvement of the joint structure or of tendons serving the joint. Any joint may be involved,

although those of the lower extremity are chiefly affected. Spinal joints do not escape urate deposition, but acute gouty spondylitis is unusual. Tophaceous involvement of the sacroiliac joint and aseptic necrosis of the hip have been reported as manifestations of gout.[151] Monosodium urate crystals were identified in one case in avascular bone.[128a] No cases of avascular necrosis of the femoral head were found in a series of 138 gouty patients, however.[229a]

Prior to the advent of uricosuric agents, 50 to 70% of patients with gout developed visible tophi, permanent joint changes, or chronic symptoms.[13,16] With the introduction of prophylactic colchicine therapy and uricosuric drugs, the incidence of tophi dropped to less than 35%.[236,269] A further drop since 1968 reflects the introduction of allopurinol into general use. At the Mayo Clinic, the incidence of tophi decreased from 11 to 3% between 1959 and 1972 without an appreciable change in the prevalence of acute gout in their patients.[167] With the ever increasing awareness of gout, future incidence figures should be lower still.

DIAGNOSIS OF GOUTY ARTHRITIS

The preceding discussion provides the basis for a rational approach to diagnosis. The diagnosis of gout should be established on firm criteria, to ensure that expensive and potentially toxic medications are not prescribed. Available data do not support therapy for most patients with asymptomatic hyperuricemia (see Chap. 92). I diagnose gout only in patients who fulfill one of the following three criteria: (1) demonstration of intracellular sodium urate monohydrate crystals in synovial fluid leukocytes; (2) demonstration of sodium urate monohydrate crystals in an aspirate or biopsy of a tophus; or (3) in te absence of specific crystal identification, a history of monoarticular arthritis followed by an asymptomatic intercritical period, rapid resolution of synovitis following colchicine administration, and the presence of hyperuricemia.

In a study conducted by the American Rheumatism Association Subcommittee on Diagnostic and Therapeutic Criteria, approximately 85% of patients with gouty arthritis had demonstrable intracellular crystals of sodium urate monohydrate in acutely inflamed joints,[248] and this finding had absolute specificity for gout. Such specificity should not lead the physician to overlook the rare patient in whom gout co-exists with another type of arthritis, however, such as infectious arthritis or RA. Extracellular urate crystals have been described in the synovial fluid of approximately 70% of patients with gout when these individuals are asymptomatic.[193] Only 1 of 19 asymptomatic hyperuricemic control subjects had synovial fluid urate crystals, whereas 2 of 9 patients with renal failure and no history of synovitis had extracellular urate crystals. Thus, extracellular urate crystals in synovial fluid are common in patients with intercritical gout, but this finding does not carry the specificity of intracellular urate crystals for establishing the diagnosis of gout.

The finding of urate crystals in tophi is almost as specific as the demonstration of intracellular urate crystals in synovial fluid in establishing that the patient has gouty arthritis.[248] In the absence of specific crystal identification, I have found the following combination of findings useful in making the diagnosis: (1) a classic history of monoarticular arthritis following an intercritical period free of symptoms; (2) rapid resolution of synovitis following administration of colchicine, as opposed to the patient's response to nonsteroidal anti-inflammatory agents, which does not have this specificity; and (3) demonstration of hyperuricemia. Arthralgia or synovitis alone in a hyperuricemic patient is not sufficient to establish the diagnosis of gouty arthritis. Episodes of pseudogout, the most difficult disease to differentiate,[248] may also respond to colchicine therapy, especially if given intravenously (see Chaps. 93 and 94).

ROENTGENOGRAPHIC FINDINGS IN GOUT

The diagnosis of gout does not depend on roentgenographic findings. Perhaps the major value of radiographic examination in gouty patients is to exclude other diagnoses from serious consideration and to detect bony tophi in those with an established diagnosis.

Erosions

Well-defined "punched-out" areas of bone lysis suggest gout. These lesions are usually 5 mm or more in diameter and are most often observed in subchondral bone in the bases or heads of the phalanges. Erosions, which are more common in the feet than in the hands, may be present in regions that have not been inflamed clinically. These erosions begin as punched-out lytic lesions, most typically located on the medial aspect of the head of the first metatarsophalangeal joint. They may progress to lysis of the entire phalanx (Fig. 91–4).

A characteristic lesion is the sharply marginated lucent pocket (Fig. 91–5). Martel noted that 40% of 78 gouty patients with erosions exhibited a "thin shell-like configuration continuous with adjacent bone contour" (Fig. 91–4,A), referred to as the "overhanging margin."[157] Although bony erosions occur in other diseases, such as RA, degenerative joint disease, tuberculosis, sarcoidosis, syphilis, leprosy, and yaws, outward displacement of the overhanging margin from the bone contour by new bone formation (Fig. 91–6) is characteristic of gout and is its most specific radiographic feature. The radiologic findings must be interpreted in the setting of the clinical history and findings. Marginal bone reaction or subchondral decalcification with increased prominence of the trabecular pattern suggests other diagnoses, although a "lobulated" bone response is a characteristic finding in gout (see Fig. 5–78). Even though erosions are "early" roentgenographic changes, they usually occur late in the disease. Many patients with repeated attacks of acute gouty arthritis have no radiographic evidence of bony or soft tissue lesions.

The bony defects, which are the result of deposits of sodium urate in bone (tophi), are directly related to the severity and the duration of the disease. Radiographic changes characteristic of bony urate deposition, namely, erosive changes with sclerotic or overhanging margins, usually occur before subcutaneous tophi are identifiable on physical examination.[162a] In patients with advanced, chronic tophaceous gout, one may see extensive lytic lesions of bone, asymmetrically dispersed among the phalanges, the metatarsal and metacarpal bones, and the bones of the ankles and wrists (Fig. 91–7), at times disseminated throughout the long bones, axial skeleton, sacroiliac joints, hips, shoulders, and clavicle. Joint destruction may be extensive, the cartilage may be destroyed, the articular margins may be eroded, the joint spaces may be narrowed, and the joint margins may be enlarged with osteophytes. Rarely, one sees bony ankylosis. Pathologic fractures may occur, requiring wiring. In some cases, the cortex is raised and displaced, and in extreme instances, the lesions may suggest an expanding lytic bone tumor (see Fig. 91–6). Such advanced roentgenographic changes are so characteristic of gout that they can scarcely be mistaken for any other condition.

Radiologic assessment of the extent of damage is important in establishing a basis for therapy, and substantial repair of lytic lesions occurs with sustained control of serum urate levels.

Soft Tissue Swelling

Acute gout is frequently accompanied by an effusion of fluid into the joint space and surrounding tissues. Radiographic examination of the involved joint usually reveals only soft tissue swelling, but the roentgenogram may help to exclude other causes of pain and swelling such as fracture, osteomyelitis, or chondrocalcinosis with pseudogout.

In the patient with long-standing gout and tophi, soft tissue swelling is readily apparent (Fig. 91–7), because tophi have the same density as soft tissue and thus exhibit no distinctive radiographic prop-

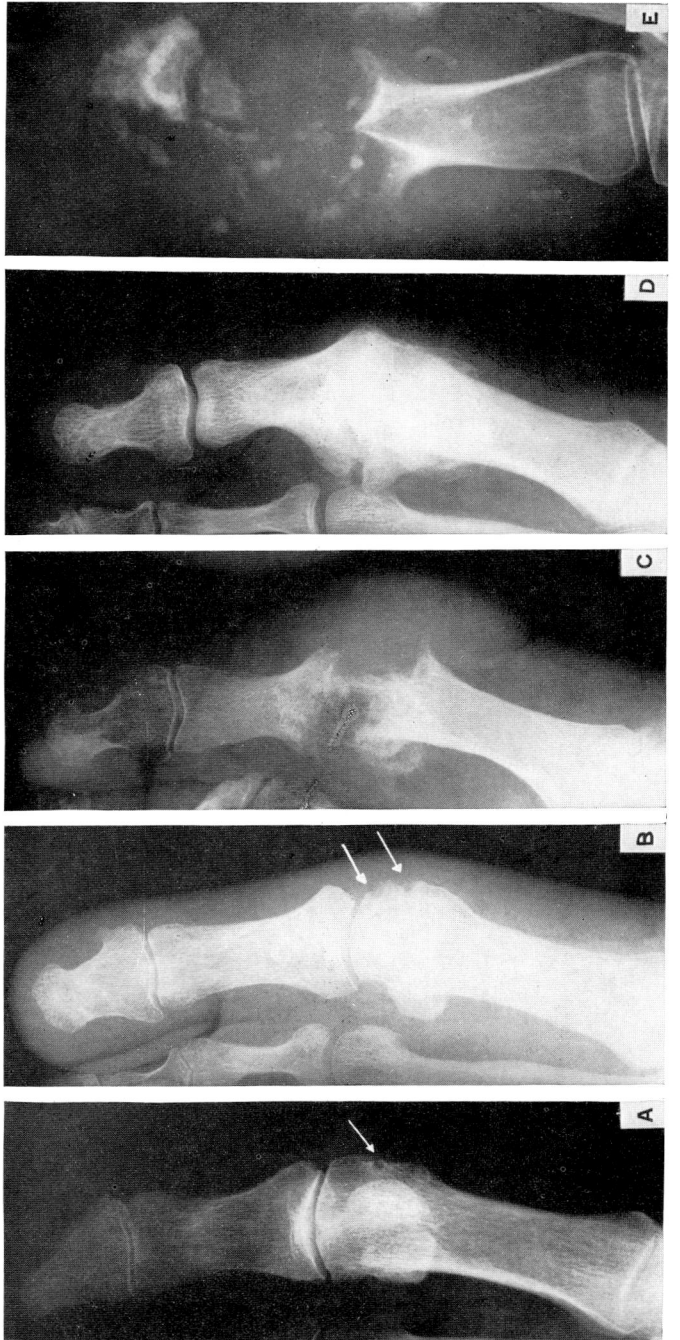

Fig. 91–4. Roentgenograms of the first metatarsophalangeal joint of five gouty patients; progressive erosions and joint destruction are illustrated from left to right. *A.* Punched-out area. *B.* More marked erosive changes. *C.* More marked destructive changes. *D.* Secondary hypertrophic changes. *E.* Far advanced destruction.

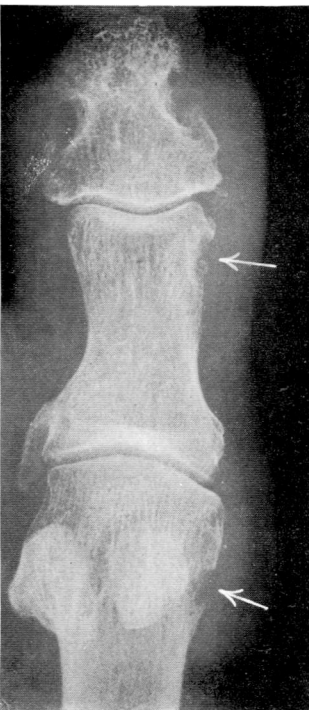

Fig. 91–5. Sharply marginated lucent pockets with cortical erosions of the bones of the great toe of a 62-year-old brewmaster with gout. This toe had suffered repeated episodes of podagra.

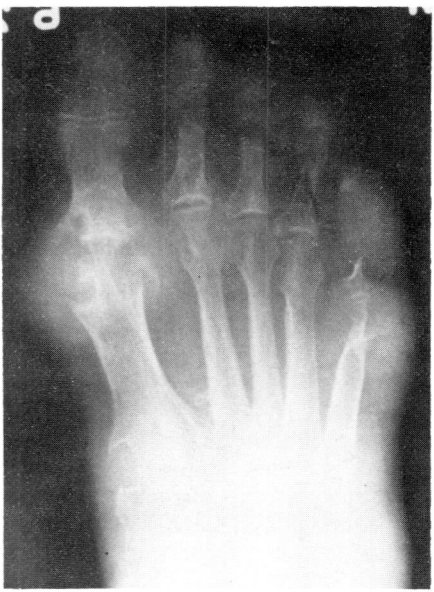

Fig. 91–6. Gouty arthritis of many years' duration. Roentgenogram demonstrates a large cystic area in first metatarsophalangeal joint with an overhanging margin. The outward displacement is characteristic of gout. A tumor-like tophus is also present at the first metatarsophalangeal joint.

erties. That the lesions are usually asymmetric and the swelling is often accompanied by the typical erosions in adjacent bone helps one to distinguish tophi from the swelling associated with RA and other types of arthritis.

Xerography may provide enough soft tissue detail to allow visualization of the tophaceous material.

Calcification

Dodds and Steinbach reported that 10 of 31 patients with gout had meniscal calcification usually associated with pseudogout.[62] Demonstration of this high incidence of calcification required the use of special radiographic techniques. Using routine clinical films analyzed blindly, Good and Rapp found lamellar or punctate calcification of 1 or more menisci in only 2 of 43 patients with gout,[88] roughly the incidence of chondrocalcinosis observed in elderly populations (5%), but higher than that observed in the general adult population (0.3%). Because of the high incidence of gout in patients with pseudogout (5%) and vice versa, the presence of such calcification in the patient with gout should suggest the possible co-existence of calcium pyrophosphate dihydrate crystal deposi-

tion and pseudogout. The finding of calcification of menisci has no specificity with respect to the diagnosis of gout.

Tophi may also calcify as an extension of the overhanging margin (see Fig. 91–6), and calcification may occur in tophaceous masses (see Fig. 5–79).

Osteopenia

Periarticular osteopenia may occur (Fig. 91–7), although this disorder is less common early in the course of the disease than in RA. Although the mechanism responsible has not been extensively evaluated, osteopenia has been attributed to disuse in some cases. The demonstration that monosodium urate crystal interaction with synovial cells leads to the production of prostaglandin E_2,[109a] which can stimulate calcium mobilization from bone,[187] suggests that subchondral osteopenia in gout may be related to active synovitis in some patients.

Narrowing of Joint Space

Destruction of articular cartilage as a result of repeated attacks of gouty arthritis or deposition of tophaceous material may lead to progressive narrowing of the joint space (see Fig. 91–4,*B*). Collagenase, as well as prostaglandin E_2, is secreted

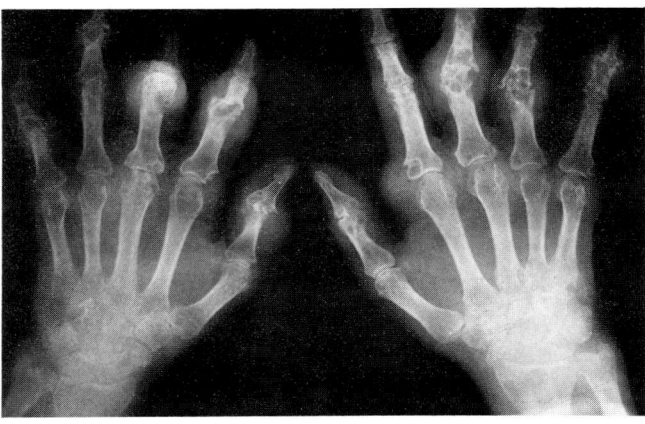

Fig. 91–7. Advanced chronic gouty arthritis of the hands. Note the extensive destructive changes, especially of the proximal interphalangeal joints, and the large soft tissue tophi. Also present is marked subchondral bone resorption of several metacarpal heads and bases of the proximal phalanges. Cystic lesions are seen in several metacarpal bases and heads, as well as in the wrist bones. (From Wyngaarden, J.B., and Kelley, W.N.[267])

by synovial fibroblasts exposed to monosodium urate, and this process many lead to bone erosion and joint destruction in chronic gouty arthritis.[109a] Fibrosis and ankylosis are unusual.[128]

Aseptic Necrosis

Aseptic necrosis of the femoral head has been reported in a few patients with gout. In a series of 48 patients with idiopathic aseptic necrosis, half were hyperuricemic.[152] The finding of urate crystals in synovium obtained from the hip at the time of operation led the researchers to postulate that hyperuricemia may have played a causative role. Whatever the relationship, no specific radiographic finding in aseptic necrosis suggests the presence of gout or hyperuricemia. Bone infarcts also occur in gouty patients (see Fig. 5–80).

Sacroiliac Joint Involvement

Subchondral lesions may be found near the sacroiliac joints in patients with generalized tophaceous disease. Bauer and Klemperer published one of the first examples.[16] Sclerotic-rimmed, punched-out cystic lesions were found in the sacroiliac joints in 7 of 95 patients with gout.[154] In at least 6 of the 7 patients, advanced tophaceous deposits were present in the extremities, and in 2 patients, the presence of monosodium urate crystals in the cystic spaces was documented post mortem. In a prospective study, radiographic sacroiliac changes were found in 24 of 143 patients (17%).[2] The findings included sclerosis of joint margins (16%), irregularity of margins (16%), focal osteoporosis (10%), and cysts with sclerotic rims (10%). All 24 subjects had peripheral tophi. Sclerosis alone, an earlier and less-specific finding, occurred in the absence of peripheral tophi.

Uric Acid Stones

These stones are especially common in patients with gout, and renal calculi are one of the roent-genographic manifestations of the disease. The radiolucent nature of the pure uric acid stone requires use of radiopaque contrast media. Uric acid stones appear as a filling defect, which may be confused with a blood clot, a tumor, or some other radiolucent space-filling mass. Although xanthine and 2,8-dihydroxyadenine stones are also radiolucent, most radiolucent stones are composed of uric acid.*

Radiopaque stones may also occur in gouty subjects. Such stones may be composed largely of calcium, but they often contain a small amount of uric acid or urate, which presumably serves as a nidus for the deposition of calcium. These stones may be identified on a "flat plate" of the abdomen without contrast dye.

HEREDITY IN GOUT

The familial nature of gout has been recognized since antiquity. Galen ascribed gout to "debauchery, intemperance, and an hereditary trait." English observers have reported a familial incidence of gout in 38 to 80% in their cases.[52] In series reported from the United States, the familial incidence has generally been from 6 to 22%,[64] but the true familial incidence may be higher, as reflected in an incidence figure of 75%,[237] obtained after persistent and diligent questioning. Among hyperuricemic relatives of gouty patients, the incidence of gout averaged 20% in 5 series reviewed by Smyth.[214]

Serum Urate Concentrations

Impressive evidence for heredity in the determination of hyperuricemia has come from studies of serum urate values in families of gouty patients

---

*Editor's note: Uric acid stones or gravel may be white or pink ("brick-dust" urine) because of absorption of an unidentified pigment. Some patients with this sign may believe that they have hematuria.

and in certain populations, particularly those of some isolated ethnic groups.

In 1940, Talbott reported that 5% of 136 asymptomatic blood relatives of 27 gouty perons had hyperuricemia.[238] Similar incidences of 24 and 27% were found in groups of 87 and 261 relatives.[110,216] In other studies, incidences from 11%[225] to 72% have been recorded.[252]

Patterns of Transmission of Hyperuricemia

Older studies suggested that hyperuricemia in families of gouty subjects was determined by a single autosomal dominant gene, which had a much lower penetrance in women than in men.[216,225] A major factor in this interpretation was the apparent bimodality of the frequency histogram, a feature much less evident when the families in a series were restudied 18 years later.[165,216] Hauge and Harvald confirmed the influence of heredity in the determination of hyperuricemia, but concluded that their data were not compatible with a single gene difference, and that several, perhaps many, genes were involved.[110]

Subsequent studies have supported both genetic patterns. A study of 2,000 Blackfeet and Pima Indians showed strong hereditary determinants of serum urate levels, which appeared to be polygenic. Transmission patterns suggested that some of the genes were autosomal dominant, others possibly X-linked.[166] The studies of Mikkelsen et al. in 6,000 residents of Tecumseh, Michigan,[160] and of Hall et al. in 5,000 residents of Framingham, Massachusetts,[106] also favored multifactorial inheritance. The frequency histograms showed a prevalence of high values without evidence of bimodality.

In contrast, the population studies of Lawrence in England,[141] of Cobb in Pittsburgh executives and medical students,[50] of Decker et al. in Filipino males living in northwest North America,[56] and of Burch et al. in the Chamorros and Carolinians of the Mariana Islands,[42] all showed bimodal distributions of serum urate values. These studies support the single-dominant-gene hypothesis.

An alternate view of these data is that the serum concentration is controlled by multiple genes, but in any selected group one genetic factor predominates. The probability of selecting a single genetic factor increases when the basis of selection is racial, when the group is an isolate, or when the study concerns several generations of families in which gout occurs, as in the older studies of Smyth[216] and Stecher.[225] Evidence for polygenic control is more prominent when the population is heterogeneous or when only siblings of gouty patients are studied, as in the investigations of Hauge and Harvald.[110]

These genetic concepts imply that although multiple metabolic aberrations may be responsible for hyperuricemia, a single defect may characterize a given hyperuricemic family. Strong evidence is now available within the types of hyperuricemia associated with specific enzyme abnormalities. Hypoxanthine-guanine phosphoribosyltransferase deficiency is an X-linked condition.[133] Phosphoribosylpyrophosphate synthetase overactivity is also inherited as an X-linked condition,[20,223] which may be expressed as a dominant trait for some mutations. Glucose-6-phosphatase deficiency is an autosomal recessive trait.[126] No doubt, additional specific subtypes of gout remain to be recognized within and separated from the large category of idiopathic primary gout.

PATHOLOGIC FEATURES OF GOUT

In gout, urate salts deposit in cartilage, epiphyseal bone, periarticular structures, and kidneys. Release of urate crystals into synovial fluid is the initiating event in the acute attack of synovitis characteristic of gouty arthritis (see Chap. 93 for a description of the mechanism of the acute attack). Urate deposits in these tissues produce local necrosis and, unless the tissue is avascular, an ensuing foreign body reaction with proliferation of fibrous tissue. The characteristic tophaceous nodule consists of a multicentric deposit of urate crystals and intercrystalline matrix together with the inflammatory reaction and foreign body granuloma it has evoked (Fig. 91–8). The crystals, which have been shown by x-ray crystallography to be monosodium urate monohydrate,[32,127] are acicular and are arranged radially in small clusters. Granular and amorphous deposits have also been described. Calcific material deposited in the matrix may render the tophus radiopaque; this process rarely reaches the proportions of heterotopic ossification.[143] Protein, lipid, and polysaccharide components have been found in the tophi.[218]

Tophi commonly occur in the helix or antihelix of the ear, the olecranon and patellar bursae, and the tendons. Less commonly, they occur in skin of fingertips, palms, or soles, the tarsal plates of the eyelids, the nasal cartilages, or the cornea or sclerotic coats of the eye. Rarely, they occur in the corpus cavernosum and prepuce of the penis, the aorta, the myocardium, the aortic or mitral valves, the tongue, the epiglottis, the vocal cords, and the arytenoid cartilages. Tophi may cause nerve compressions, carpal and tarsal tunnel syndromes, and paraplegia.

Affected joints may undergo cartilaginous degeneration, synovial proliferation, destruction of

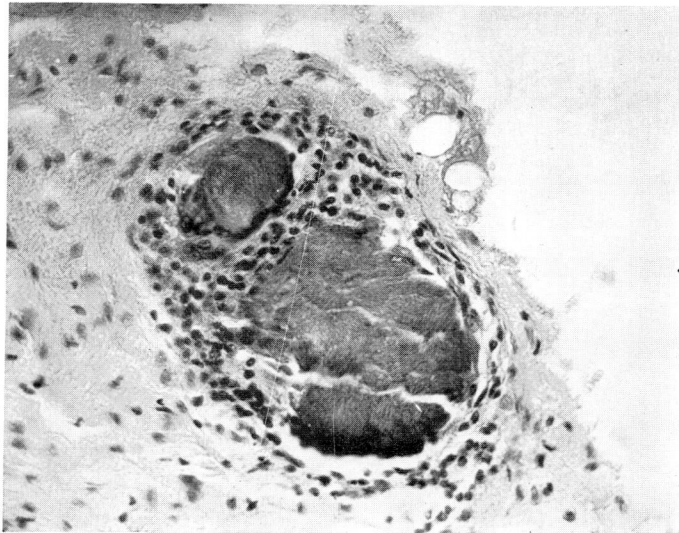

Fig. 91–8. Gouty tophaceous deposit in synovial membrane obtained by closed needle-punch biopsy.

subchondral bone, proliferation of marginal bone, often synovial pannus, and sometimes fibrous or bony ankylosis.[147] No joint is exempt, although those of the lower extremity are most commonly involved. Spinal joints do not escape urate deposition, but acute gouty spondylitis is rare. Tophaceous involvement of the sacroiliac joint,[154] as well as aseptic necrosis of the hip,[150] are well-documented but uncommon complications of gout. In vertebral bodies, urate deposits are found in bone marrow spaces adjacent to intervertebral discs, as well as in disc tissue itself. The punched-out lesions of bones commonly seen in roentgenograms of gouty patients represent bone marrow tophus deposits, which generally communicate with the urate crust on the articular surface through erosions and defects in articular cartilage (Fig. 91–9).

The tissues in which urates deposit are avascular.[109] Sokoloff has pointed out that several sites of urate deposition in gout, such as articular and other cartilages, synovial tissues, interstitial tissue of the renal pyramid, and sclerae and heart valves, are rich in ground substance containing acid mucopolysaccharide.[218] Cartilage has an affinity for absorbing urates in vitro,[39] and the tarsal bones of swine cause the precipitation of needles such as are seen in gout when suspended in saturated solutions of urate.[186] Katz and Schubert have identified substances from bone nasal cartilage that are protein polysaccharides composed of protein and chondroitin sulfate and that augment urate solubility.[132] Unbound chondroitin sulfate or trypsin-digested material fails to exhibit this property. These investigators suggested that when, as a result of normal or accelerated connective tissue turn-over, protein polysaccharides are destroyed, urate crystals may precipitate from saturated tissue fluids. Perricone and Brandt have presented data that question the physiologic role of proteoglycans in enhancing urate solubility, however.[170a] These investigators did not find that aggregated proteoglycan sustained supersaturated solutions of the sodium salt of urate and questioned whether the exchange of potassium for sodium ions in prior experiments could have accounted for some of the effects noted by Katz and Schubert.

Kidney in Gout

Renal disease is the most frequent complication of gout apart from arthritis.[10,241,263] Hyperuricemia may affect the kidney through (1) the deposition of monosodium urate monohydrate crystals in the renal interstitium, an entity referred to as *urate nephropathy;* (2) the deposition of uric acid crystals in the collecting tubules, an entity referred to as *uric acid nephropathy;* or (3) *uric acid stone* formation. The distinction between these first two entities is often unclear, and the term ''gouty kidney'' has been used for both. Uric acid nephropathy is uncommon in the absence of malignant disease or enzymatic defects leading to the overproduction and overexcretion of uric acid; urate nephropathy is more common in patients with gout unassociated with the overproduction of uric acid. In addition to these direct effects of hyperuricemia, other causes of renal dysfunction such as hypertension and lead nephropathy, are also prevalent in the gouty population.

Ordinarily, urate nephropathy is only slowly progressive and does not materially reduce life ex-

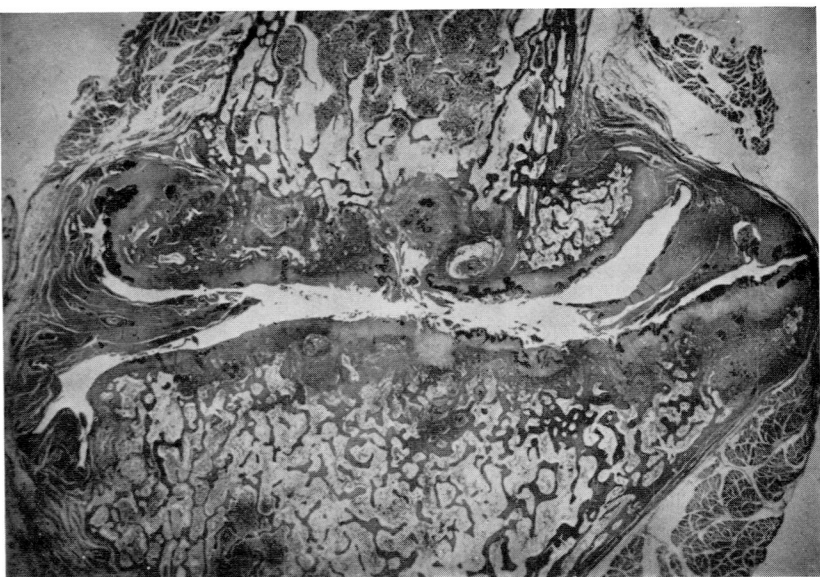

Fig. 91–9. Urate crystals in the synovial membrane, articular cartilages, and subchondral bone appear black. Erosion of cartilage, advanced osteoarthritic changes, and marginal osteophyte formation are seen. (From Sokoloff, L., and Gleason, I.O.[219])

pectancy.[240,244] The incidence of proteinuria varies from 20 to 40%. It may be intermittent or persistent; only rarely is the quantity great. Hypertension is approximately as common as albuminuria.[241] It is not clear whether hypertension is the result of hyperuricemia and urate nephropathy, or whether it is the cause of renal dysfunction observed in gouty patients.[158] The experience of the Mount Sinai group suggests that uncontrolled hypertension is responsible for a significant amount of the renal dysfunction observed in gouty patients,[26] and other studies also support this concept.[75,158]

The only distinctive histologic feature of urate nephropathy is the presence of urate crystals and the surrounding giant-cell reaction (Fig. 91–10). These crystals may be associated with interstitial or vascular changes or both.[218] That some of the vascular changes may be related to concomitant hypertension emphasizes the difficulty of attributing pathologic changes to a single origin. In a review of 191 gouty patients of whom clinical information and postmortem renal tissue permitted adequate evaluation, only 3 showed neither urate crystals nor pyelonephritic or vascular changes.[241] These features were present in variable proportions and severity. A strong correlation existed between the clinical severity of gout and the severity of the renal lesions, both in patients with predominantly pyelonephritic changes and in those whose kidneys had predominantly vascular changes. Such vascular lesions included arterial and arteriolar scle-

rosis, and in 11 instances, the findings were of malignant hypertension. Kidneys from 30 patients revealed both well-developed vascular changes and pyelonephritis with extensive structural alterations from urate deposits.

A few notable exceptions from the correlated severity of clinical symptoms and renal disease were found. Some patients with severe tophaceous gout showed only minimal clinical evidence of renal insufficiency; conversely, some patients with severe renal disease had only minimal articular distress. In this second type of patient, renal disease may have been the cause of premature death. The extreme degree of this phenomenon may be represented by the few reports of "gouty nephrosis" occurring without clinical evidence of gout. In four patients purported to have this syndrome,[38,65,234] however, no serum uric acid levels had been obtained during life.

A number of mechanisms have been proposed to explain the various pathologic findings reported in urate nephropathy. The renal lesions may stem from deposition of uric acid in collecting tubules with resultant obstruction, atrophy of the more proximal tubules, and secondary necrosis and fibrosis.[38,161] The associated interstitial inflammatory process has been attributed to complicating pyelonephritis.[38,78] Other studies have shown that an early structural abnormality is tubular damage associated with interstitial reaction; this finding suggests a relationship between the interstitial and the

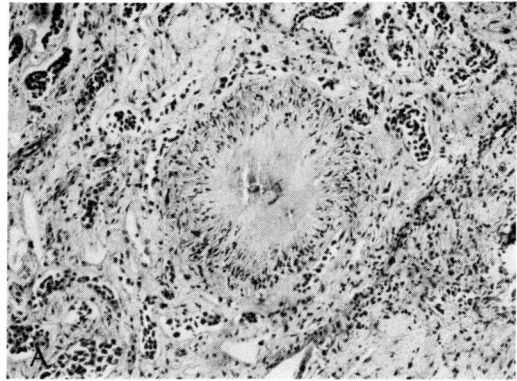

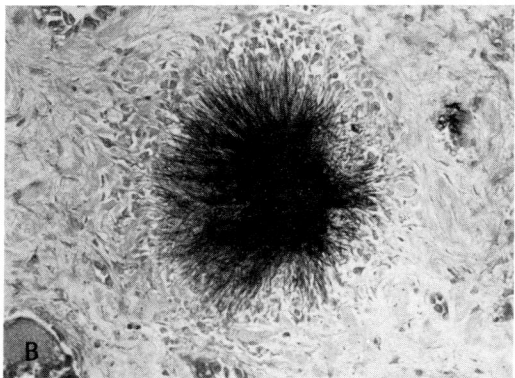

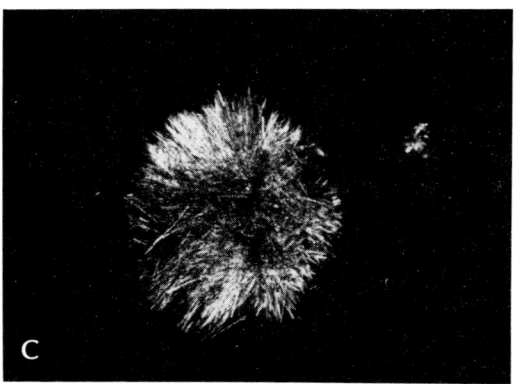

Fig. 91–10. *A,* Urate deposit in the medulla of kidney, as seen in alcohol-fixed section stained with hematoxylin and eosin. (× 150) *B,* Adjacent section of deposit shown in *A,* stained with methanamine silver. (× 150) *C,* Adjacent section of deposit shown in *A,* as seen under polarized light. (From Wyngaarden, J.B., and Kelley, W.N.[267])

tubular changes.[87,90] The epithelial cells of Henle's loop show early atrophy and dilatation, occasionally associated with brown-pigment degeneration of the epithelium.[87] The interstitial reaction is maximal in the region near the changes in the loops of Henle, and the changes in the epithelial cells precede the interstitial reaction. In kidneys without

tophi, this reaction usually spares the medulla and the juxtamedullary cortex. Thus, the changes labeled as chronic pyelonephritis may not be of infectious origin, but may rather be a manifestation of urate nephropathy itself.[87] According to Gonick et al., a distinctive glomerulosclerosis in urate nephropathy also exists, with uniform fibrillar thickening of glomerular capillary basement membranes, different from that of nephrosclerosis or diabetic glomerulosclerosis,[87] but Heptinstall does not agree that this lesion is distinctive.[116]

In addition to urate nephropathy, hypertension, renal vascular disease, and nephropathy from other causes may contribute to renal dysfunction in gouty patients. A long-term study of a large population of patients with gout found that the onset of hypertension correlated with a reduction in glomerular filtration rate, and nephrosclerosis associated with hypertension was postulated as a common cause of renal damage.[26] The excessive lead stores associated with decreased creatinine clearance found in a group of gouty patients at the East Orange, New Jersey Veterans Administration Hospital suggest that lead nephropathy may be an unrecognized cause of renal dysfunction in gout.[15] These studies underscore the need for keeping an open mind in evaluating renal dysfunction in patients with gout and suggest that multiple etiologic factors may produce the renal lesions observed in biopsy and postmortem specimens.

Renal failure is the eventual cause of death in 18 to 25% of patients with gout,[157a,241] and this statistic emphasizes the need to follow renal function and to treat commonly associated and preventable causes of renal dysfunction, such as hypertension, aggressively in the gouty population.

Pathogenesis of Hyperuricemia in Primary Gout

For convenience in discussing pathogenetic mechanisms, hyperuricemia is considered either as a primary process, that is, an innate defect in purine metabolism, or as a secondary process, that is, the consequence of an associated disorder that may have several clinical manifestations, one of which is a derangement in purine metabolism. Gout as a consequence of primary hyperuricemia is referred to as primary gout, whereas that associated with secondary hyperuricemia is referred to as secondary gout.

Potential Mechanisms

In theory, hyperuricemia could result from increased absorption of precursor purines, or decreased excretion, decreased destruction, or increased production of uric acid, or from a combination of these factors. A purine-free diet resulted in an average reduction of serum urate level of 1 to 1.2 mg/dl in gouty subjects,[103,205] but it did not correct hyperuricemia. Hyperuricemia cannot be attributed to abnormal absorption of precursor purines.

Uricolysis in man is accounted for by the action of intestinal flora on uric acid entering the gastrointestinal tract in gastric, biliary, pancreatic, and intestinal secretions, which may amount to 200 or 300 mg/day.[222,268] Thus, under normal conditions, one-fourth to one-third of the uric acid produced each day may be eliminated by this route. No evidence indicates that the extrarenal disposal of uric acid is diminished in gout. On the contrary, it is increased in nearly all hyperuricemic subjects,[174,222] and it may constitute the chief route of disposal of urate in gouty patients with reduced renal urate excretion.[221] Impairment of uricolysis is not a cause of hyperuricemia. Considerable evidence suggests, however, that both increased production and reduced renal clearance of uric acid play important roles in the pathogenesis of hyperuricemia.

Production of Uric Acid

Chemical Balance. The rate of purine synthesis is theoretically assessed by measuring the difference between purine excretion and intake in the dynamic steady state. Because urinary excretion of uric acid represents a variable fraction of total purine excretion, only gross estimates of purine production are possible by urinary measurements. Purine intake may be reduced as much as 3 mg purine-N/day by dietary restriction, and urinary uric acid then becomes a minimal estimate of purine production. Values in normal men ranged from 278 to 558 mg/day (mean 418 $\pm$ 70 mg),[102] or from 264 to 588/day (mean 426 $\pm$ 81 mg).[206]

The distribution of urinary uric acid values in men with gout extends from 150 mg/day or less to 1,500 mg/day or more. Low values are found in patients with overt renal damage. In some referral centers, 21 to 28% of patients with gout consistently excreted quantities of urate exceeding the mean ± 2 S.D.;[102,206] in the general population of gouty patients, this percentage is lower, and a generous estimate would be no more than 10 to 15%. Such patients have arbitrarily been classified as overexcretors of uric acid. The possibility that augmented urinary excretion is secondary to a decreased extrarenal disposal of urate has been excluded by normal urinary recoveries of injected labeled uric acid in many such overexcreting patients.[206] Therefore, sustained overexcretion of uric acid is evidence for excessive de novo synthesis of purines. A normal urinary excretion of uric acid does not exclude overproduction of uric acid in gouty subjects, however, because in the hyperuri-

cemic subject with reduced renal urate clearance, the extrarenal, or gastrointestinal, disposal of urate may be increased and may account for over 80% of the urate turnover.[206]

Turnover of Uric Acid. The isotope-dilution technique for measuring the miscible pool of uric acid and the rate of its turnover was introduced by Benedict et al. in 1949.[25] Isotopic uric acid is injected intravenously, and isotope concentration of uric acid isolated from urine is determined during succeeding days. From these data, the size of the "miscible pool" of uric acid and the rate of its turnover may be calculated.

In 25 normal men, the rapidly miscible pool of uric acid averaged 1,200 mg (range 866 to 1,587 mg), and its turnover averaged 695 mg/day (range 513 to 1,108 mg/day).[200,206,260] In patients with gout, the miscible pool was generally enlarged to 2,000 to 4,000 mg in those without tophi,[25,30,222] and 18,000 to 31,000 mg in patients with severe tophaceous gout.[24] Even so, the miscible pool may represent only a small fraction of the total urate in the body, because only the peripheral layers of tophi are readily exchangeable with urate in solution in body fluids.[24] In one patient, the amount of urate in the tophaceous compartment participating in a slow exchange with soluble urate was estimated to be 300 times the size of the rapidly miscible pool.

Because of the possibility of exchange of labeled urate of the miscible pool with unlabeled urate of the solid phase, the rate of change of isotope concentration of the soluble phase may not be a dependable measure of the synthesis of new urate in subjects with tophaceous gout. The derived values for urate turnover often agree well with values from another calculation of synthesis rate, however, as follows:

$$\frac{\text{Basal urinary uric acid, mg/day}}{\begin{array}{c}\text{Urinary recovery of injected isotopic uric acid,}\\ \text{fraction of administered dose}\end{array}}$$

In gouty patients whose miscible pool is within or just above the normal range, it is sometimes possible to calculate that all the urate measured in the miscible pool is in solution. In two patients meeting these criteria, Sorensen found an excessive turnover of uric acid.[222] In five patients also meeting these criteria, however, Seegmiller et al. found a normal turnover of uric acid, and these five patients also demonstrated a normal incorporation of isotopic glycine into uric acid.[206]

Incorporation of Labeled Precursors into Uric Acid. The rate of generation of uric acid has also been studied by measuring the rate of incorporation of isotopically labeled precursors into urinary uric acid. The purine ring is synthesized in the body from various low-molecular-weight precursors, which are identified in Figure 91–11. When glycine-[^{15}N] or [^{14}C] was fed to normal men, the isotopic enrichment of urinary uric acid reached a maximum on the second or third day and thereafter declined.[23,264] In gouty patients, the pattern of incorporation was abnormal.[22,23,206,264] Particularly in overexcretors, the peak enrichment values were higher, occurred earlier, and were followed by a more rapid decline; these findings signify an accelerated rate of urate synthesis.

The results of published studies conducted under standardized conditions are presented in Figure 91–12, in which the data are expressed in terms of cumulative incorporation into urinary uric acid in seven days. The results show an overincorporation of precursor glycine into urinary uric acid in all overexcreting patients, as well as in more than half the normal-excreting patients with primary gout.

Several patients with apparently normal incorporation values had extensive tophaceous deposits and impaired renal function. Theoretically, these factors could completely mask overincorporation by lowering the isotope values in urinary uric acid. Seegmiller and co-workers have corrected their statistics for that fraction of intravenously injected uric acid, labeled with a different isotope, not recovered in the urine.[206] Two of five gouty subjects whose uncorrected glycine-[^{14}C] incorporation values were normal then showed excessive incorporation, but in the others, the values were still normal. These glycine incorporation studies in subjects with primary gout showed a spectrum of urate production rates ranging from normal to four- or fivefold the normal rate.

Control of de novo Purine Biosynthesis

Studies performed in vivo as well as in vitro with isolated enzymes and cells grown in tissue culture have documented an important role for phosphoribosylpyrophosphate and purine ribonucleotides in the control of de novo purine biosynthesis.[120,226] Figure 91–13 illustrates some of the important steps in the purine biosynthetic pathway and indicates a common site at which phosphoribosylpyrophosphate and purine ribonucleotides may help to regulate purine biosynthesis. This point is the first step unique to the pathway, and this reaction is catalyzed by the enzyme amidophosphoribosyltransferase. Phosphoribosylpyrophosphate is a substrate for this enzyme, and purine ribonucleotides inhibit catalytic activity through an allosteric feedback mechanism. Amidophosphoribosyltransferase activity and the rate of purine biosynthesis are regulated either by the availability of its substrate or by the concentration of its ribonucleotide inhibitors.

The mechanisms controlling the activity of amidophosphoribosyltransferase have been studied extensively.[121,124,129,258] The apparent Km of human amidophosphoribosyltransferase for phosphoribosylpyrophosphate is approximately 0.5 mM,[121,258] a value 10 to 100 times greater than the intracellular concentration of phosphoribosylpyrophosphate,[17] and it is unlikely that amidophosphoribosyltransferase is saturated with this substrate in vivo. Consequently, any change in phosphoribosylpyrophosphate concentration could lead to a corresponding change in the rate of purine biosynthesis.

Purine ribonucleotides inhibit the catalytic activity of human amidophosphoribosyltransferase (Fig. 91–13), and the molecular features of this inhibitory process have been clarified.[121,124,129,258]

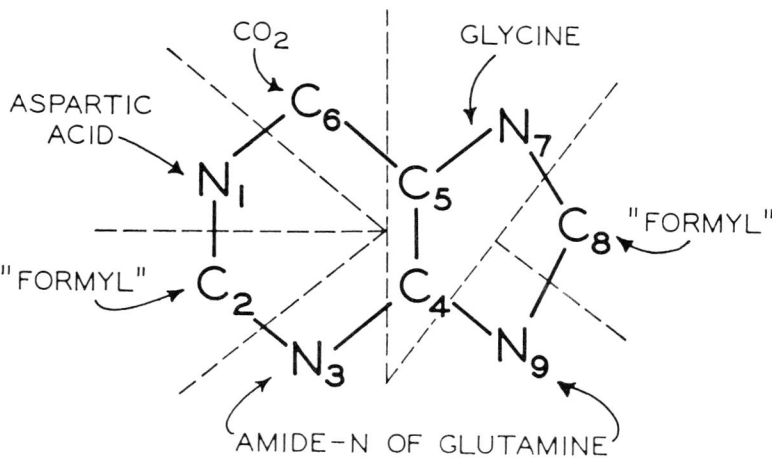

Fig. 91–11.   Origins of the atoms of the purine ring.

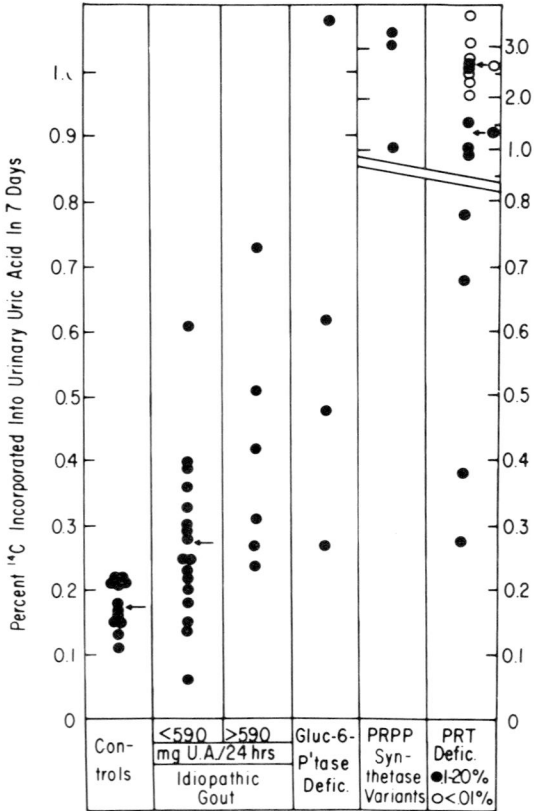

Fig. 91–12. Summary of values of cumulative incorporation of ¹⁴carbon (¹⁴C) into urinary uric acid (U.A.) in control and gouty subjects reported from 1957 through 1973. PRPP = phosphoribosylpyrophosphate; PRT = phosphoribosyltransferase. (From Wyngaarden and Kelley.[267])

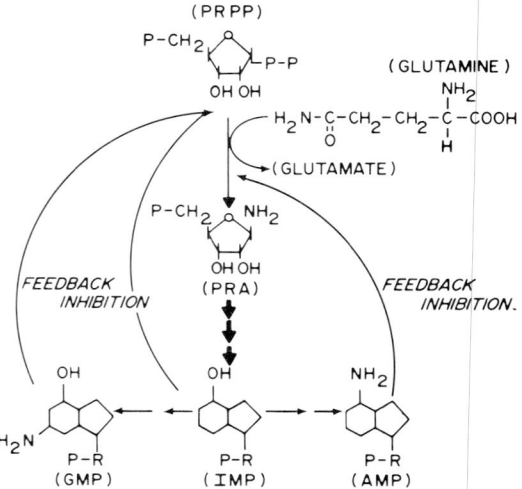

Fig. 91–13. Abbreviated pathway of purine biosynthesis. PRPP = phosphoribosylpyrophosphate; GMP = guanosine monophosphate; IMP = inosine 5′-monophosphate; AMP = adenosine monophosphate.

The enzyme displays molecular heterogeneity, as shown by the demonstration of a small form of 133,000 daltons and a large form of 270,000 daltons (Fig. 91–14). The small form is converted to the large form by incubation of the enzyme with purine ribonucleotides, and the large form is converted to the small form by incubation with phosphoribosylpyrophosphate. Enzyme catalytic activity is directly proportional to the amount of amidophosphoribosyltransferase present in the small form.[124] Experiments in an animal model confirmed that interconversion between the small and large forms of amidophosphoribosyltransferase occurs in vivo when the intracellular concentrations of phosphoribosylpyrophosphate and purine ribonucleotides are altered.[129] Thus, the model illustrated by Figure 91–14 provides an explanation at the molecular level for the regulation of human amidophosphoribosyltransferase by the relative concentrations of phosphoribosylpyrophosphate and purine ribonucleotides.

Enzymatic Abnormalities Leading to Purine Overproduction in Man

Some patients with primary gout exhibit an increased rate of de novo purine biosynthesis. In clinical practice, one can detect the florid overproducer of uric acid by quantifying the 24-hour urinary excretion. Individuals who excrete more than 600 mg uric acid on a low purine diet,[102,206] or more than 800 to 1000 mg on the average unrestricted North American diet, synthesize purines at an excessive rate and consequently overproduce uric acid. More sensitive tests, such as the isotopic-incorporation techniques previously outlined, however, are required to detect this abnormality in individuals with less-pronounced overproduction of uric acid.

A specific enzymatic abnormality has been identified in only a small proportion of patients who overproduce uric acid. The demonstrated or proposed enzymatic abnormalities can be categorized into two groups on the basis of the regulatory mechanisms already reviewed: (1) those that lead to an increase in the concentration or availability of phosphoribosylpyrophosphate; and (2) those that lead to a decrease in the intracellular pool of purine ribonucleotides.

Increase in Phosphoribosylpyrophosphate. The enzymatic alterations that have been documented or postulated to result in an increased availability of this substance are illustrated in Figure 91–15. For each example listed here, it has been proposed that the concentration or availability of phosphoribosylpyrophosphate is increased, but

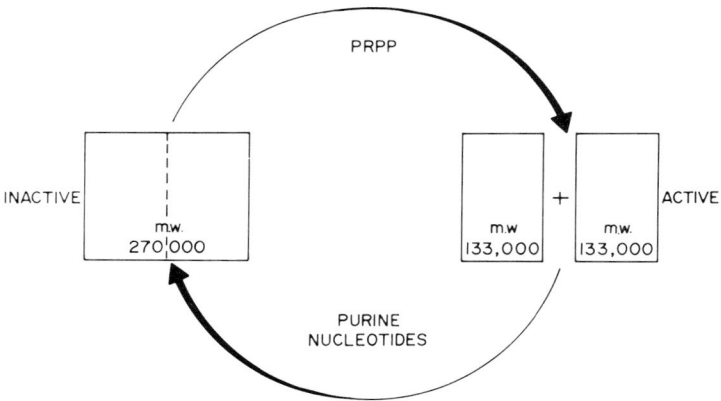

Fig. 91–14. Model illustrating the control of human amidophosphoribosyltransferase by phosphoribosylpyrophosphate (PRPP) and purine ribonucleotide.

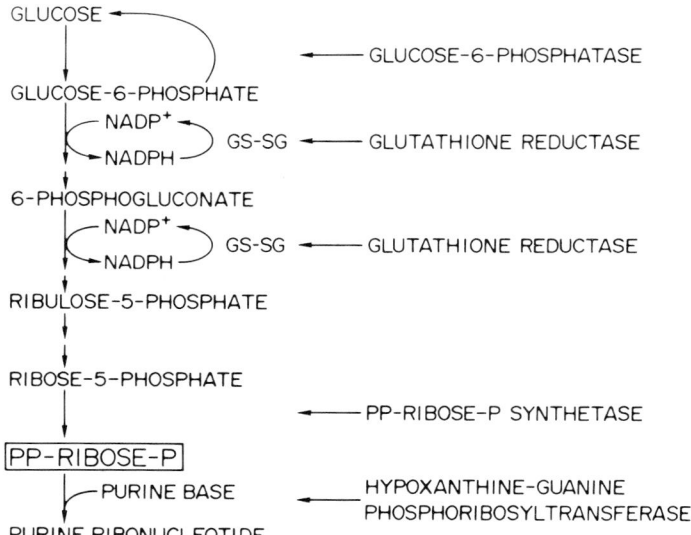

Fig. 91–15. Enzymatic abnormalities that could lead to an increase in phosphoribosylpyrophosphate (PP-ribose-P). NADP = nicotinamide-adenine dinucleotide phosphate.

such has been established only in the hypoxanthine-guanine phosphoribosyltransferase and phosphoribosylpyrophosphate synthetase mutants. All the enzymatic abnormalities indicated in Figure 91–15 are associated with an increase in the rate of purine biosynthesis, except the glutathione reductase variant. The significance of the observed increase in glutathione reductase activity has been questioned because dietary manipulation, such as change in content of riboflavin, alters glutathione reductase actvity in man,[28,29] and a study of 52 gouty patients did not detect an abnormality in glutathione reductase activity or electrophoretic mobility.[249]

This group of enzymatic defects can be divided into those leading to an increase in the rate of

synthesis or a decrease in the rate of use of phosphoribosylpyrophosphate in the salvage pathway. Glucose-6-phosphatase deficiency, increased activity of glutathione reductase, and increased activity of phosphoribosylpyrophosphate synthetase fall into the first category. *Glucose-6-phosphatase* hydrolyzes glucose-6-phosphate to glucose, and a *deficiency* of this enzyme causes the intracellular accumulation of glucose-6-phosphate,[91] which could lead to an increase in phosphoribosylpyrophosphate production by augmenting the substrate availability for the pentose phosphate pathway (Fig. 91–15). Glucose-6-phosphatase deficiency could increase phosphoribosylpyrophosphate production by an additional mechanism. Fasting depletes the purine nucleotide pools in the liver of these patients,[91] and depletion of certain purine nucleotides, such as adenosine diphosphate, in the liver of experimental animals may decrease the inhibition of phosphoribosylpyrophosphate synthetase.[129] *Glutathione reductase* catalyzes the reaction in which the hydrogenated form of nicotinamide-adenine dinucleotide phosphate (NADPH) reduces oxidized glutathione (Fig. 91–15). An *increase* in the activity of this enzyme could augment phosphoribosylpyrophosphate production as a consequence of an increase in the NADP-NADPH ratio.

In a report of two gouty patients, concentrations of ribose-5-phosphate and phosphoribosylpyrophosphate were increased in fibroblasts grown in vitro.[18] The mechanism responsible for the increase in ribose-5-phosphate in these patients is unknown, but both had greater rates of de novo purine biosynthesis than normal and hyperuricemia. These data suggest that metabolic abnormalities leading to an increase in the availability of ribose-5-phosphate speed the rate of purine biosynthesis. In addition, an increase in the activity of phosphoribosylpyrophosphate synthetase leads to an increase in the rate of synthesis of this substance. The reaction catalyzed by phosphoribosylpyrophosphate synthetase is depicted in Figure 91–17.

Hypoxanthine-guanine phosphoribosyltransferase deficiency is classified in the group of abnormalities that lead to an accumulation of phosphoribosylpyrophosphate as a consequence of

decreased use in the salvage pathway. The reaction catalyzed by hypoxanthine-guanine phosphoribosyltransferase is depicted in Figure 91–16; the substrates for this enzyme are phosphoribosylpyrophosphate and hypoxanthine (or guanine), and the products are inosine 5'-monophosphate and inorganic pyrophosphate. A high-grade deficiency of this enzyme results in decreased use of both substrates, phosphoribosylpyrophosphate and hypoxanthine. The accumulation of phosphoribosylpyrophosphate leads to an increase in the rate of purine biosynthesis for the reasons already cited, and the unused hypoxanthine is oxidized by xanthine oxidase to uric acid. Purine nucleoside phosphorylase deficiency (Fig. 91–16) also leads to purine overproduction, probably as a result of decreased use of phosphoribosylpyrophosphate in the salvage pathway.[51] This disorder leads to hypouricemia rather than to hyperuricemia, however, because no hypoxanthine is formed and consequently the substrate for oxidation to urate is decreased (Fig. 91–16).

The deficiencies of hypoxanthine-guanine phosphoribosyltransferase and glucose-6-phosphatase and the increased activity of phosphoribosylpyrophosphate synthetase deserve special mention because they are the best-characterized enzymatic abnormalities leading to purine overproduction and gout. The deficiency of hypoxanthine-guanine phosphoribosyltransferase catalytic activity, an X-linked disorder, has been ascribed to several en-

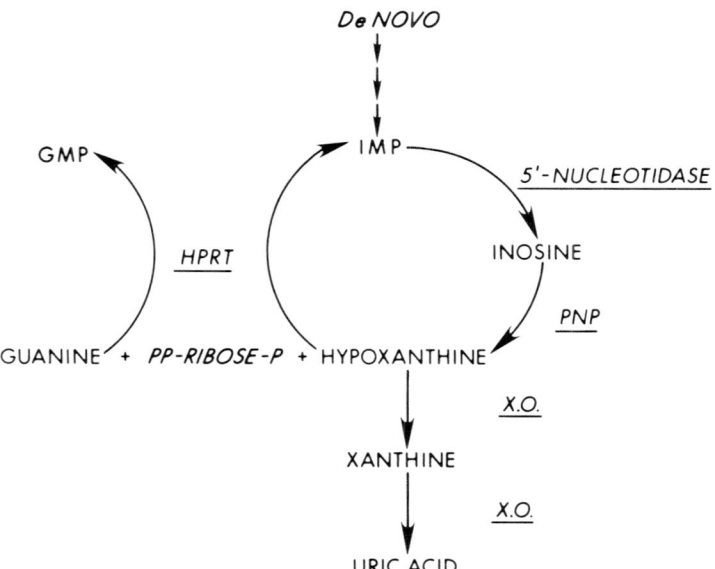

Fig. 91–16.   Pathways illustrating purine ribonucleotide catabolism, purine base reuse, or oxidation to uric acid. HPRT = Hypoxanthine-guanine phosphoribosyltransferase; PNP = purine nucleoside phosphorylase; X.O. = xanthine oxidase; GMP = guanosine monophosphate; IMP = inosine 5'-monophosphate; PP-RIBOSE-P-phosphoribosylpyrophosphate.

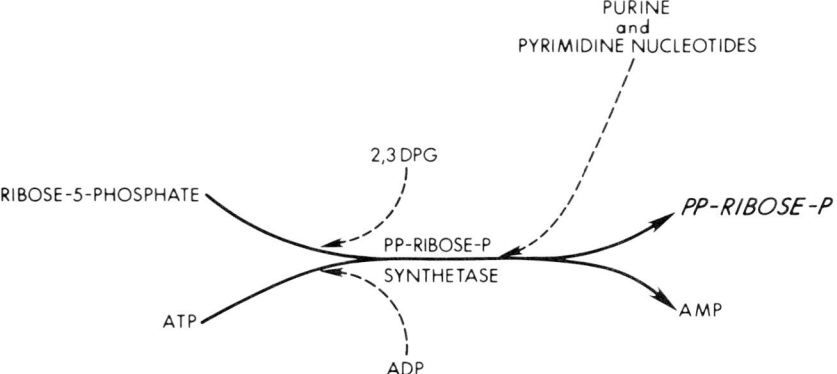

Fig. 91–17. Control of phosphoribosylpyrophosphate (PP-ribose-P) synthetase activity by substrates and feedback inhibition. ATP = adenosine triphosphate; ADP = adenosine diphosphate; AMP = adenosine monophosphate; DPG = diphosphoglycerate.

zymatic abnormalities. Extracts from cells of most patients have no demonstrable hypoxanthine-guanine phosphoribosyltransferase cross-reactive material.[135] In others, a decreased affinity for substrates or increased sensitivity to inhibition by reaction products accounts for the reduced catalytic activity. Specific amino acid substitutions have been found in some of these mutations,[253] and the presumed defect in the hypoxanthine-guanine phosphoribosyltransferase gene is confirmed by direct study of DNA isolated from these patients.[254] This disorder is seen as one of two clinical phenotypes.[133,135] The *Lesch-Nyhan syndrome* occurs in males with a complete deficiency of enzyme catalytic activity. In addition to hyperuricemia, hyperuricaciduria, and a tendency to form uric acid calculi, these individuals develop a devastating neurologic disorder characterized by compulsive self-mutilation, choreoathetosis, spasticity, and mental retardation. In patients with only a *partial deficiency of hypoxanthine-guanine phosphoribosyltransferase* activity, the neurologic manifestations may be minimal or nonexistent. In such patients, the major clinical manifestations are hyperuricemia, with serum urate concentrations often greater than 10 mg/dl, excessive uric acid excretion, often more than 1,000 mg/day, gouty arthritis beginning in the second or third decade, and renal calculi in 75% of patients.

Patients with glucose-6-phosphatase deficiency or glycogen storage disease type I have hyperuricemia from infancy, ranging from 10 to 16 mg/dl.[126] Gouty arthritis may develop by the end of the first decade, and chronic tophaceous gout and gouty nephropathy may be responsible for the major morbidity in these patients as they become adults.

In patients with *increased phosphoribosylpyrophosphate synthetase* activity, considerable genetic heterogeneity occurs.[17,21a] As shown in Figure 91–17, phosphoribosylpyrophosphate synthetase is a complex enzyme subject to several different types of regulation. The availability of its substrate, ribose-5-phosphate, may be important in determining the rate of synthesis of phosphoribosylpyrophosphate, and it is subject to inhibition by a number of different compounds. In one family, increased phosphoribosylpyrophosphate synthetase activity was the result of a decrease in sensitivity of the enzyme to inhibition by the purine ribonucleotides, adenosine diphosphate and guanosine diphosphate. In another family, the increased phosphoribosylpyrophosphate synthetase activity was attributed to an increase in catalytic activity per enzyme molecule with no demonstrable abnormalities in kinetic properties of the mutant protein. In yet another family, a preliminary report has attributed the change in activity to an increased affinity of phosphoribosylpyrophosphate synthetase for its substrate, ribose-5-phosphate. Like hypoxanthine-guanine phosphoribosyltransferase, phosphoriboslpyrophosphate synthetase is encoded on the X chromosome.[20,223] This group of gouty patients has no distinguishing clinical characteristics, but all individuals have marked overproduction of purines, hyperuricemia, and hyperuricaciduria. Gouty arthritis and renal calculi have often occurred at an early age, but at least one patient, a young girl, has remained asymptomatic at seven years of age.

Decrease in Purine Ribonucleotides. It has been postulated that a deficiency of hypoxanthine-guanine phosphoribosyltransferase could lead to a decrease in the rate of synthesis of inosine 5′-monophosphate or guanosine monophosphate from the respective purine bases (Fig. 91–16), but quantification of purine ribonucleotide concentrations in extracts from cells that are deficient in hypoxanthine-guanine phosphoribosyltransferase has not documented a reduction in nucleotide content.[19] In contrast, the hepatic content of purine ribonucleotides falls in association with fasting or glucagon administration in patients with glucose-6-phosphatase deficiency.[91] Studies in human volunteers and in animal models using fructose administration, which mimics the hepatic purine nucleotide depletion seen in patients with glucose-6-phosphatase deficiency, have provided insight into the pathogenesis of hyperuricemia and increased purine biosynthesis in these conditions. The reduction in hepatic content of purine nucleotides following fructose administration, and presumably in glucose-6-phosphatase deficiency, leads to hyperuricemia due initially to an increase in catabolism of endogenous purine ribonucleotides and subsequently to an increase in the rate of de novo purine biosynthesis.[182] The decreased hepatic content of purine nucleotides and the increased purine biosynthesis following fructose administration are associated with a shift of amidophosphoribosyltransferase, the rate-limiting enzyme in the purine biosynthetic pathway, from the large, inactive to the small, active form of this enzyme (see Fig. 91–14).[129] In addition, a lowered hepatic content of purine nucleotides is associated with an increase in the phosphoribosylpyrophosphate content of the liver,[129] and this process may contribute to the shift in amidophosphoribosyltransferase to the active conformation and increase in purine biosynthesis (see Fig. 91–14). Thus, conditions such as glucose-6-phosphatase deficiency, which lead to intracellular nucleotide depletion, may secondarily increase purine biosynthesis through complex allosteric effects on amidophosphoribosyltransferase activity.

Additional studies are needed to determine whether other enzymatic defects increase purine biosynthesis through a similar mechanism. A regulatory defect in adenosine monophosphate deaminase may be responsible for an accelerated rate of purine nucleotide catabolism in some patients with gout and purine overproduction.[245] Fibroblasts from another reported patient with gout catabolized adenine nucleotides at an excessive rate,[114] but a specific enzymatic defect was not defined.

Excretion of Uric Acid

Approximately two-thirds to three-fourths of the uric acid produced each day is excreted by the kidney, and one-fourth to one-third is eliminated through the gastrointestinal tract.[43,222,268] In patients with gout, it is clear that decreased renal clearance commonly leads to hyperuricemia, but gastrointestinal excretion is increased,[174,212,222] and consequently it is not responsible for hyperuricemia.

Control of Renal Uric Acid Excretion. According to present concepts, uric acid excretion is regulated by a three-component system, comprising glomerular filtration, tubular reabsorption, and tubular secretion of uric acid.[101]

Glomerular ultrafiltration of uric acid has been conclusively demonstrated in animals by the analysis of fluid obtained from Bowman's space,[31] and presumably a similar process occurs at the human glomerulus. It is often assumed that urate is freely filterable at the glomerulus, but the reported studies are conflicting with regard to urate binding to human serum proteins in vivo. One in vitro study suggested that as much as 30% of urate may be bound to serum protein,[46] whereas other in vitro studies have been unable to document significant binding of urate to human serum proteins at 37° C.[74,138,209] Few studies have been performed in vivo, and the limited available data do not indicate that a significant amount of urate is bound to albumin,[122] or to other plasma proteins.[136]

Even assuming the highest figures reported for the percentage of urate bound to plasma protein in vitro, urate is clearly reabsorbed by the human nephron because, on the average, only $7.6 \pm 2.4\%$ of the filtered load of uric acid is excreted in the urine.[102] The site of uric acid reabsorption has not been defined in man, but micropuncture studies in rats,[1,93,94,139,188] and in primates,[189] have documented a proximal tubular reabsorptive site. In the primate, in which uric acid handling by the kidney closely approximates that seen in man,[73] reabsorption of uric acid is limited to the proximal nephron.[189] Some studies in rats have revealed a distal reabsorptive site,[93,94] however, and one report has suggested a reabsorptive site in the ascending limb of Henle's loop[92] (Fig. 91–18). Clearance studies in man have been interpreted to indicate yet another reabsorptive site for uric acid in the collecting duct[60] (Fig. 91–18). The processes that control urate reabsorption are not known, but this process is thought to be mediated by active transport.[139,189] Indirect data suggest that the urate ion, rather than uric acid, is the transported species because proximal tubular fluid pH is greater than 6.7,[155] and the pKa of uric acid is 5.75. Although many questions remain concerning the control of urate reabsorption in the human nephron, available studies suggest that the major site of urate reabsorption is the proximal tubule.

Tubular secretion of uric acid was first clearly demonstrated in a patient whose serum urate concentration was less than 0.6 mg/dl and in whom the clearance of uric acid was 1.46 times greater than the clearance of inulin.[176] Uric acid secretion was subsequently confirmed in normal subjects after urate loading, mannitol diuresis, and large

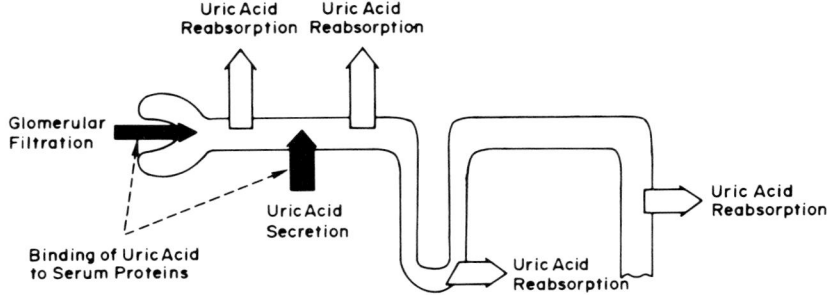

Fig. 91–18. Model illustrating three components of urate handling by the kidney, glomerular filtration, reabsorption, and secretion.

doses of probenecid.[104] In the only direct study in man, the proximal, but not the distal, nephron transported urate from the plasma to the tubular fluid.[173] The design of this study did not distinguish between active and passive transport of uric acid. Micropuncture studies in rats have documented net urate secretion in the proximal nephron,[1,94] whereas the single micropuncture study performed in primates did not find any evidence for net urate secretion under experimental conditions.[189] Uric acid secretion is thought to be mediated by one of the pathways common to several organic acids because pyrazinoic acid, lactate, beta-hydroxybutyrate, acetoacetate, salicylate, and other organic acids decrease uric acid excretion in man,[250] and micropuncture studies have demonstrated directly that organic acids inhibit uric acid secretion.[93] Experiments with metabolic inhibitors such as 2,4-dinitrophenol documented that uric acid secretion was an energy-dependent process.[250]

Considering this information, each of the three components proposed by Gutman and Yu[101] is operative in the renal excretion of uric acid in man, although the relative contribution of each to the final urinary excretion of uric acid has been difficult to evaluate. In the case of glomerular filtration, a controversy exists regarding urate binding to plasma proteins. Even more perplexing is the relative contribution of secreted and nonreabsorbed urate to urinary uric acid excretion. On the basis of the pyrazinamide suppression test, it was originally proposed that 98% of the filtered load of uric acid was reabsorbed in the proximal nephron and uric acid excreted in the urine was largely due to secretion at a more distal site.[229] For reasons reviewed elsewhere,[123] the pyrazinamide suppression test is no longer considered to be a valid tool for distinguishing between the relative contributions of nonreabsorbed and secreted urate to urinary uric acid excretion. Moreover, studies performed with pyrazinamide in combination with other drugs cannot be explained by the previous model.[61,227] To

accommodate these observations, a model proposing two sites for uric acid reabsorption in the proximal nephron, separated by a uric acid secretory site, has been developed (Fig. 91–18). This "postsecretory reabsorptive" model represents the best attempt so far to accommodate all the observations on the renal handling of uric acid in man. The relative flux of uric acid through the proposed transport processes is unknown, and documentation of their existence requires more direct techniques, such as micropuncture and isolated nephron studies.

Decreased Uric Acid Clearance in Gout. A reduction of uric acid clearance may contribute to hyperuricemia in 75 to 85% of patients with gout. The importance of this pathogenic mechanism was deduced by Wyngaarden through a comparison of uric acid excretion rates and plasma urate concentrations in gouty patients and in control subjects.[261] Uric acid excretion increased as the plasma urate concentration increased in both groups, but a plasma urate concentration 2 to 3 mg/dl higher was required for the patients with gout to achieve equivalent rates of uric acid excretion. Simkin has also shown that, on the average, the gouty individual excretes 41% less urate than normal for any given plasma concentration of urate (Fig. 91–19).[210] In both these studies, the renal clearance of uric acid was lower in the gouty patients than in the control subjects. Patients with primary hyperuricemia but without gout also had a greater increment in plasma urate in response to the oral ingestion of purines than did normouricemic control subjects[276] (Fig. 91–20). Because uric acid excretion was comparable in both groups, the disproportionate increase in plasma urate in the hyperuricemic subjects following the oral ingestion of a purine load was attributed to decreased urate clearance.

One of three mechanisms operating alone or in conjunction might explain the decrease in uric acid clearance observed in gouty patients: (1) decreased

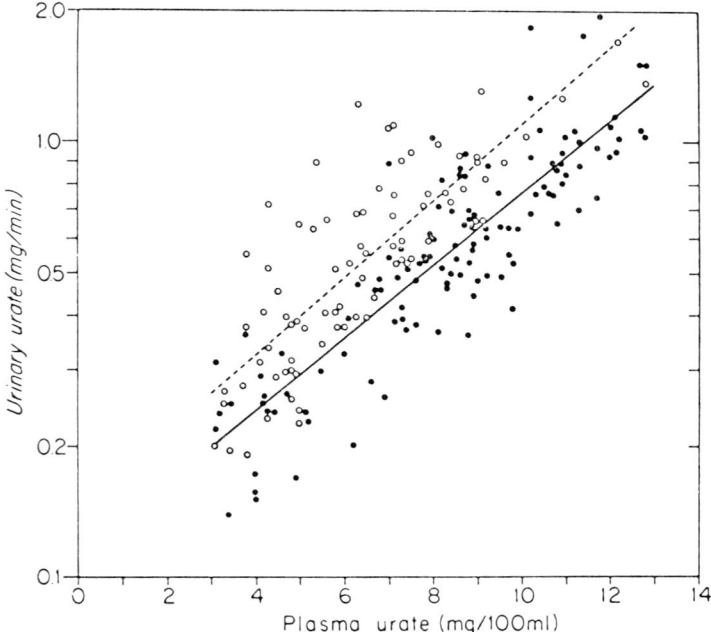

Fig. 91–19. Urate excretion at varying plasma urate concentrations in normal (○) and gouty (●) men. (From Simkin, P.A.[210])

filtered load of urate; (2) increased urate reabsorption; or (3) decreased urate secretion.

The filtered load of urate is influenced by the glomerular filtration rate and by the extent to which urate is ultrafilterable. Consequently, the filtered load of urate could be reduced even in patients with normal glomerular filtration rates if urate binding to plasma proteins were increased. Such an increased binding of urate to plasma proteins was found in a group of hyperuricemic patients from New Zealand,[45] but the clearance of uric acid in these subjects was not reported. Until the question of urate binding to plasma proteins is resolved in these and other individuals with primary gout, the decreased ultrafiltration of urate remains a speculative mechanism.

Increased reabsorption and decreased secretion of uric acid have both been proposed to account for the lowered uric acid clearance observed in patients with gout. In one study of six gouty individuals, a decrease in uric acid clearance, documented by isotopic incorporation techniques, was the only cause of hyperuricemia.[185] The pyrazinamide suppression test was used to distinguish between increased reabsorption and decreased secretion. Using the older interpretation of this test, it was concluded that the decreased clearance of uric acid was due to a lower secretion, but this report appeared before some of the problems associated with the pyrazinamide suppression test were ap-

preciated. Using the postsecretory reabsorptive site model, interpretation of these data leads to the conclusion that either increased reabsorption or decreased secretion of urate was responsible for the observed decrease in uric acid clearance.

Metabolic Defects in Idiopathic Gout

Increased production and decreased renal clearance of uric acid have been considered separate pathogenetic mechanisms, but many patients with gout exhibit both. For example, patients with glucose-6-phosphatase deficiency have both a higher de novo purine biosynthesis and a lower uric acid clearance, owing to increased availability of phosphoribosylpyrophosphate or decreased intracellular concentrations of purine ribonucleotides,[91] and from hyperlactacidemia and decreased urate secretion, respectively.[126] The concurrence of both pathogenetic mechanisms leading to hyperuricemia is also found in patients with idiopathic gout. Patients with primary gout are usually overweight, and Emmerson has found evidence for hyperuricemia, hyperuricaciduria, increased urate turnover, and decreased renal clearance of uric acid in obese subjects.[67,68] In addition, hyperuricemia and alcohol intake are positively correlated, and alcohol consumption is exaggerated in those with gout.[71,153,194] Alcohol ingestion reduces urate clearance,[144] as well as accelerates purine nucleotide catabolism,[72] with a resultant increase in de novo

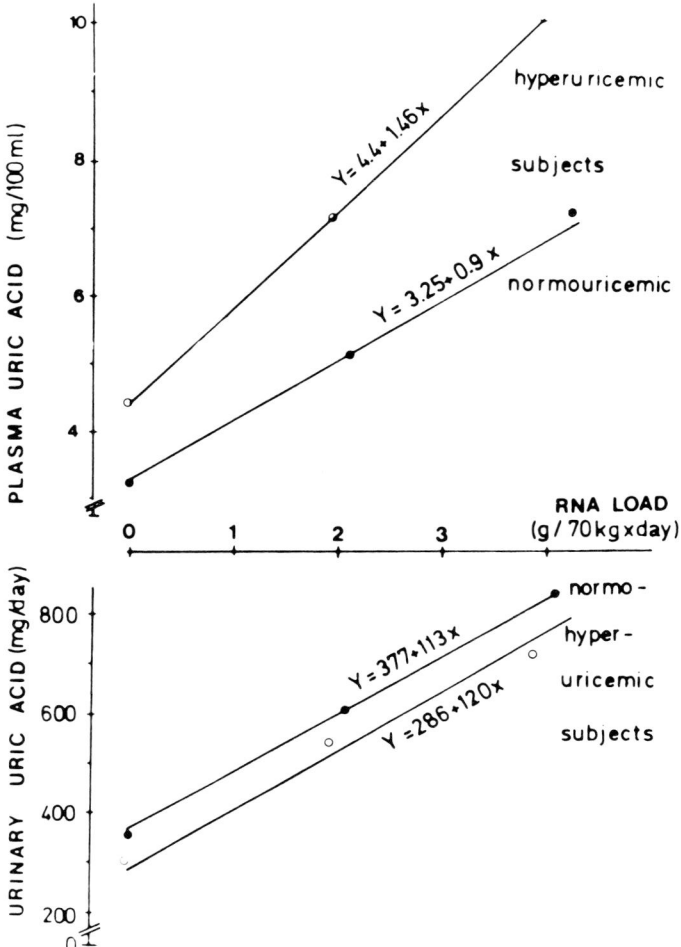

Fig. 91–20. Change in plasma uric acid concentration and in urinary uric acid excretion in response to increments in dietary purine. *Top,* Change in plasma uric acid concentration (mg/100 ml); *Bottom,* change in urinary uric acid excretion (mg/day). (From Zollner., and Griebsch, A.[276]).

purine biosynthesis.[57,153] Such studies emphasize the complex nature of the possible metabolic defects in patients with idiopathic gout. Clinical observations and studies of various populations have long implicated both nongenetic, namely, dietary, and genetic factors in the development of hyperuricemia and gout. As our understanding of the control of purine biosynthesis and of the renal excretion of uric acid continues to grow, the defective metabolic controls responsible for the development of hyperuricemia in many patients with gout may become more evident.

HYPERURICEMIA AND GOUT ASSOCIATED WITH OTHER DISORDERS
Hematologic Disorders

Hyperuricemia and secondary gout occur in lymphoproliferative and myeloproliferative disor-

ders,[98,117,236,270] multiple myeloma,[37] secondary polycythemia,[220,274] certain hemoglobinopathies, thalassemia, and pernicious anemia. All these conditions are associated with a long-term increase in bone marrow activity.[235]

In a large series of patients with leukemia, myeloid metaplasia, polycythemia vera, and multiple myeloma, hyperuricemia was noted in 66% of 113 men and 69% of 73 women. Only 10 patients had a history of gouty arthritis,[148] and 6 of them were found among the 22 patients with myeloid metaplasia. In other series, gouty arthritis has occurred in 2 to 14% (mean 6%) of patients with polycythemia vera. Curiously, 84% of these gouty patients were men, although the disease is almost as common in women.

An underlying mean urinary uric acid excretion value of 634 mg/24 hours was found in 27 patients with secondary gout complicating hematologic disorders, as compared to a mean value of 497 mg/ 24 hours in a control group.[100] Urate excretion was either normal or increased in these individuals, and the incorporation of labeled precursors into urinary purine bases and uric acid has revealed a striking labeling of the bases during the first day, followed by secondary maxima in bases and uric acid between 7 and 12 days. Cumulative incorporation of isotope into uric acid is near normal during the first few days, but it exceeds normal in 1 to 2 weeks; this finding indicates an exaggerated turnover of nucleic acid purines as the cause of hyperuricemia in these subjects.[265]

Gouty arthritis may also complicate sickle cell disease,[7,84] hemoglobin SC disease, beta-thalassemia, and other chronic hemolytic anemias.[156,168]

Drug Ingestion

The list of drugs that induce hyperuricemia include the potent diuretics, alcohol, pyrazinamide, and salicylates in low doses.

Diuretics

In a study of hyperuricemia in men admitted to a Veterans Administration hospital, diuretics were considered to be the cause in 20%.[169] Of new cases of gout in Framingham, Massachusetts, 50% developed in persons taking thiazides or ethacrynic acid. Hyperuricemia has been noted in as many as 75% of patients treated with diuretics.[59]

Potent diuretic agents may produce hyperuricemia by several mechanisms. The work of Steele and Oppenheimer,[226,228] and of Suki et al.,[231] suggests that a prerequisite is sufficient salt and water loss to produce volume contraction. The administration of diuretics increases the tubular reabsorption of filtered urate. In addition, the inhibition of the tubular secretion of urate seems likely. Neither effect appears to represent a direct action of the diuretic agent on tubular transport of urate because urate excretion values remain near control values when volume depletion is prevented by replacement of urinary salt and water losses with intravenous saline solution. Thus, secondary extrarenal influences on the kidney may be responsible for the hyperuricemia. Volume contraction leads to a generalized increase in solute reabsorption, perhaps mediated by changes in factors such as oncotic pressure or intrarenal blood flow.[226] In addition, furosemide induces sufficient hyperlactacidemia to suppress the tubular secretion of urate.

Ethanol

Epidemiologic studies have reported a strong correlation between serum urate levels and habitual alcohol intake.[71,194] Hyperuricemia is common in inebriated patients,[145] and infusion of ethanol results in hyperuricemia.[144] Patients with gout consume more alcohol than the nongouty population.[71,153,194] At Duke University Medical Center, 55% of patients followed in the gout clinics gave a history of consuming more than a pint of alcohol per week.[183]

Both pathophysiologic mechanisms discussed earlier play a role in the production of hyperuricemia in patients who consume alcohol. As ethanol is metabolized by alcohol dehydrogenase, the level of nicotinamide-adenine dinucleotide (NAD) is reduced, and this change may account in part for the excessive conversion of pyruvate to lactate. The levels of hyperlactacidemia in some patients consuming ethanol are adequate to suppress the renal excretion of uric acid and to induce hyperuricemia.[144] In addition, the daily ingestion of alcohol in significant but tolerated amounts, such as 100 ml/24 hours, may be associated with hyperuricemia and increased urinary uric acid excretion, both of which may return to normal during days of abstinence and normal diet.[57] These cycles are not explained by the reduced urinary clearance of uric acid. Increased catabolism of purine nucleotides occurs after oral or intravenous ethanol administration,[72] a significant amount of which occurs in the liver.[95] Because other agents, such as fructose,[129,182] also induce hepatic purine nucleotide catabolism, it is reasonable to assume that purine biosynthesis is increased in liver and possibly other tissues by ethanol. Thus, patients consuming significant amounts of ethanol probably go through periods of accelerated nucleotide catabolism and increased purine biosynthesis, and this process may account for the observed increase in uric acid production.

Other Drugs

In addition to diuretics and ethanol, a number of other drugs produce hyperuricemia. Although ingestion of these agents has not been correlated with the development of gout, the hyperuricemia resulting from their administration may lead to confusion in the evaluation of patients with acute arthritis. Low doses of salicylates at a plasma concentration of less than 5 mg/dl,[273] antituberculosis agents such as pyrazinamide[251] and ethambutol,[175] nicotinic acid,[21,82] fructose,[182] methoxyflurane,[107] and levodopa[125] lead to hyperuricemia. Low doses of salicylates, pyrazinamide, and ethambutol decrease the renal clearance of uric acid. Nicotinic acid decreases the renal clearance of uric acid and also stimulates de novo purine biosynthesis. Ethylamino-1,3,4-thiadiazole, an agent that arrests tumor growth in mice, causes a striking increase in de novo purine bioynthesis and hyperuricemia in man.[204]

Body Weight

Epidemiologic studies document a strong positive correlation between body weight and serum urate concentration.[33,76,77,83,199,230] The relationship between body weight and serum urate concentration is complex and probably multifactorial. Fessel and co-workers have alluded to many factors, including hyperuricemia, obesity, hypertension, and diabetes.[77] In a study by Reynolds, myself and our colleagues, 52% of our patients with gout were more than 20% over ideal body weight, 85% were hypertensive, and 48% had abnormal glucose tolerance tests and hypertriglyceridemia.[183] Obesity has a number of effects on urate metabolism, such as decreasing urate clearance and increasing urate production.[67,68] Other factors such as muscle mass also play a role in producing hyperuricemia,[33,76] and Fessel and Barr have reported that nonadipose body weight exhibits the most important correlation with serum uric acid concentration in multiple regression analyses.[76] Weight reduction is associated with a modest lowering of the serum urate concentration.[199]

Hyperlipidemia

The relationship between hypertriglyceridemia and hyperuricemia is well established. As many as 80% of patients with hypertriglyceridemia have hyperuricemia, and 50 to 75% of patients with gout have hypertriglyceridemia.[9,27,199] No correlation exists between hyperuricemia and isolated hypercholesterolemia, but hypercholesterolemia in association with hypertriglyceridemia is common in patients with gout.[191,199] The relationship between hyperuricemia and hypertriglyceridemia is not clear, but it is not simply the result of obesity because data from the foregoing studies on different populations of patients with gout are conflicting on the contributory role of obesity in producing hypertriglyceridemia.

Hypertension

In untreated hypertensive patients without discernible renal disease, the incidence of hyperuricemia ranges from 22 to 27%.[34,48] When therapy and renal disease are not excluded, the incidence increases to 47 to 67%.[63,130,137] Hyperuricemia is equally common in essential and renovascular hypertension.[48] The overall incidence of gout in hypertensive patients is 2 to 12%.[34,48] From another perspective, the incidence of hypertension in the gouty population varies from 30 to 52%.[181]

In most hypertensive patients, hyperuricemia appears to be related to reduced renal clearance of uric acid, attributed to a lower ratio of uric acid clearance to glomerular filtration rate than in non-hyperuricemic hypertensive persons.[211] Some have suggested that tubular dysfunction may be a consequence of vascular disease, tissue hypoxia, and local lactic acid excess, but attempts to relate hyperuricemia to hyperlacticacidemia have been controversial.[48,130] Although the mechanism underlying the common association between gout and hypertension has not been defined, the importance of this association should not be overlooked in the management of gout because uncontrolled hypertension may be a major contributor to renal dysfunction in these patients.[26]

Chronic Renal Insufficiency

Hyperuricemia is common in renal insufficiency, but in spite of high serum urate concentrations in some patients, gouty arthritis is rare. In a study of 496 patients with chronic renal insufficiency, Sarre found only 6 with gout, in 4 of whom the disease appeared to be primary.[196] The incidence of gout in lead nephropathy and in polycystic and medullary cystic disease of the kidney is higher than in other, more common forms of chronic renal disease. The low incidence of gouty arthritis in patients with renal insufficiency has been attributed to: (1) shortened life span of these patients; and (2) their decreased ability to respond to an inflammatory stimulus.[40]

Recurrent episodes of acute arthritis or periarthritis may occur in patients with chronic renal failure treated with periodic hemodialysis. The clinical features of the acute inflammatory episodes, their response to colchicine, and the tendency for their frequency to vary directly with the plasma urate level have led to the diagnosis of acute gouty arthritis.[47] An examination of the involved tissues may reveal the presence of calcium phosphate (apatite) crystals in addition to monosodium urate crystals, however.[150] Crystals in muscle of patients with renal failure have been identified as calcium phosphate (apatite and possibly dicalcium phosphate), not urate[162] (see Chaps. 4, 95).

Lead Intoxication

The association of gout with chronic lead poisoning led many years ago to the concept of "saturnine gout," in which gout was regarded as a complication of the nephritis of plumbism. Reduced renal clearance of uric acid is the primary mechanism of hyperuricemia in patients with saturnine gout.[8] This type of gout has been well documented in Queensland, Australia,[69a] in France,[184] and in the southeastern United States.[6,8] In Australia, the patients studied had been exposed to leaded paint in childhood. In this type of saturnine gout, the incidence of affected females is greater than in the population of patients with primary gout, the mean age of onset is younger, incidence of renal calculi is lower, hyperlipoproteinemia is absent, and a family history of gout is unlikely. In the southeastern United States, the primary source of lead exposure in the patients studied was illicit or "moonshine" alcohol, which became contaminated with lead during distillation or storage. This form of saturnine gout is more common in males of lower socioeconomic status because this is the primary population at risk.

Unrecognized lead intoxication may be a more common cause of renal dysfunction in the general population of patients with gout in the United States than the foregoing examples might suggest.[15] One should be cautious in ascribing renal dysfunction to lead nephropathy in any population, including gouty patients, simply on the basis of eliciting a history of lead exposure and demonstrating excessive lead stores. Studies have shown that individuals with gout may excrete more than 1,000 μg lead following calcium edetate (EDTA) administration in the absence of any measurable reduction in creatinine or urate clearance.[183]

Starvation

Total caloric restriction results in extreme degrees of hyperuricemia,[54,64] attributable in part to a reduced renal clearance of uric acid and in part to the overproduction of uric acid. The retention of uric acid is correlated best with ketosis and with the serum concentration of beta-hydroxybutyrate.[85,111,208] Refeeding of carbohydrate corrects the ketosis, causes a temporary, excessive excretion of uric acid, and reduces serum urate levels.

Episodes of gouty arthritis may occur during periods of starvation, but they are unusual except in patients with a prior history of gout.[153]

Hyperparathyroidism

The incidence of hyperuricemia in hyperparathyroidism is high.[201] Scott et al. noted hyperuricemia in 11 of 12 patients, and 5 of these had a medical history consistent with gout.[201] Synovial fluid examination is required to differentiate urate gout in these patients from the calcium pyrophosphate dihydrate crystal deposition of pseudogout.

Psoriasis and Sarcoidosis

The relationship between hyperuricemia and psoriasis is not clear. Some series report that 21 to 50% of psoriatic patients have hyperuricemia, whereas in others, the incidence of hyperuricemia is no greater in patients with psoriasis.[66,140] Urinary uric acid in selected hyperuricemic patients with psoriasis given 1-[14C]-glycine showed peak enrichment values intermediate in time between those of primary gout and those of secondary gout due to myeloproliferative disease; this finding is interpreted as evidence of increased nucleotide and nucleic acid turnover in the psoriatic lesions as probable pathogenetic factors.[66]

A high percentage of patients with sarcoidosis have been reported to have hyperuricemia.[41,274] The association of sarcoidosis, psoriasis, and gout has been reported and is regarded as a syndrome by some, as a chance concurrence by others, or possibly as sarcoid arthritis in a hyperuricemic subject with psoriasis but without true gout.

Bartter's Syndrome

In a study of 9 patients with Bartter's syndrome, 50% were found to be hyperuricemic, and 20% had episodes of acute gouty arthritis.[159] These patients all had a subnormal clearance of uric acid, and it is postulated that the reduction in urate clearance and hyperuricemia in these patients is the consequence of systemic alkalosis.

UROLITHIASIS IN GOUT

The incidence of renal calculi in various American or European series of gout is 5 to 33%;[5,236] it is 75% in Israel.[5] The incidence was 22% in a series of 1,258 patients with primary gout and 42% in 59 patients with secondary gout, or at least 1,000 times that of the general population.[272] In 40% of patients with primary gout, lithiasis antedated acute arthritis, occasionally by more than 20 years. Uric acid nephrolithiasis may be associated with hyperuricemia without acute arthritis. About one-third of such patients have a family history of gout. Over 80% of calculi in gouty patients are composed of uric acid.[272] Occasionally they are mixed, they may have only a central nidus of uric acid,[178] or they may contain only calcium oxalate or phosphate.[272] Studies from several laboratories have demonstrated the predisposition of hyperuricosuric persons to the development of calcium oxalate stones.[50a] Sodium urate or uric acid may act as a heterogeneous nucleus for calcium oxalate, or the urate or uric acid crystal may adsorb macromolecular growth inhibitors for calcium oxalate crystals. Whatever the mechanism, a reduction in urinary urate excretion by dietary manipulation or allopurinol administration decreases calcium oxalate stone formation in hyperuricosuric patients.

Factors that predispose patients to uric acid nephrolithiasis in gout include undue acidity of the urine, increased urinary excretion of uric acid, increased urinary concentration, and perhaps qualitative or quantitative abnormalities of urinary constituents that affect the solubility of uric acid.[5]

Patients with gout often have unusually acid

urine, both in fasting morning specimens and throughout the day,[272] as well as a substandard rise of urinary pH in response to oral alkali. No correlation exists between urine pH and urinary uric acid excretion. This situation, in turn, is a reflection of a low ratio of NH_4 to titratable acidity, attributed by some to a subnormal ammonium excretion at a given acid load,[99,115,172] and by others to high values of titratable acidity.[14] In the 75% of patients with gout whose urinary uric acid values fall within the normal range, the high incidence of renal stones is probably related to low urinary pH. The pK_{a1} and pK_{a2} values of uric acid are 5.75 and 10.3, respectively. At urinary pH values of 4.5 to 5, the predominant form should be uric acid, not sodium urate, as established by x-ray crystallographic studies.[127,178] The solubility or uric acid is only one-seventeenth that of sodium urate in water at 37° C. The prevalence of renal stones rises with increasing plasma urate levels in the general population and approximates 50% when serum urate levels exceed 12 mg/dl in patients with gout.[272] The major influence of hyperuricemia is probably the effect it has on urinary uric acid excretion. The prevalence of urolithiasis increases from 11% in patients with excretion values under 300 mg/day to 50% in patients with values over 1,100 mg/day.[272]

Uric Acid Nephrolithiasis in Nonhyperuricemic Subjects

Only about 20% of patients without clinical gout who form uric acid stones are hyperuricemic.[236] In idiopathic uric acid nephrolithiasis, by definition occurring in patients with normal plasma and urinary uric acid values, a consistent finding, as in gouty and in otherwise asymptomatic hyperuricemic subjects, is a tendency to a low urine pH. The risk of uric acid stones is also increased in patients with ileostomies, who have an increased renal conservation of sodium, a decreased urinary sodium-to-potassium ratio, increased urinary acid excretion, and low urinary pH values.[49]

Uric acid stones are sometimes dissolved with protracted fluid and alkali therapy,[4] but allopurinol is the treatment of choice.

HYPOURICEMIA

It is difficult to give a precise number below which the serum concentration of urate is abnormal. This problem relates in part to the different methods used to determine urate and in part to the non-Gaussian distribution of serum urate concentrations in the population. To obviate these problems, investigators have adopted a conservative definition of hypouricemia: a serum urate concentration of 2.0 mg/dl or less.[160,180,246] The prevalence of hypouricemia in normal subjects[160]

Table 91–3. Potential Causes of Hypouricemia

Decreased production
  Congenital xanthine oxidase deficiency
  Liver disease
  Allopurinol administration
  Low phosphoribosylpyrophosphate synthetase activity
  Purine nucleoside phosphorylase deficiency
Increased excretion
  "Isolated" defect in renal transport of uric acid
  Idiopathic
  Neoplastic diseases
  Liver disease
  Generalized defect in renal tubular transport (Fanconi's syndrome)
  Idiopathic
  Wilson's disease
  Cystinosis
  Multiple myeloma
  Heavy metals
  Galactosemia
  Hereditary fructose intolerance
  Outdated tetracyclines
  Bronchogenic carcinoma and other neoplasms
  Liver disease and alcoholism
  Drugs
    Acetohexamide
    Azauridine
    Benzbromarone
    Benziodarone
    Calcium ipodate
    Chlorprothixene
    Cinchophen
    Citrate
    Dicumarol
    Diflumidone
    Estrogens
    Ethyl biscoumacetate
    Ethyl p-chlorophenoxyisobutyric acid
    Glyceryl guaiacolate
    Glycine
    Glycopyrrolate
    Halofenate
    Iodopyracet
    Iopanoic acid
    Meglumine iodipamide
    p-Nitrophenylbutazone
    Orotic acid
    Outdated tetracyclines
    Phenindione
    Phenolsulfonphthalein
    Phenylbutazone
    Probenecid
    Salicylates
    Sodium diatrizoate
    Sulfaethidole
    Sulfinpyrazone
    W 2354
    Zoxazolamine
Mechanism unknown
  Pernicious anemia
  Acute intermittent porphyria

and hospitalized patients[160,180,246] varies from 0.7 to 1.0%. Table 91–3 lists the potential causes of hypouricemia. Hypouricemia may be due either to a low rate of uric acid production or to a high renal clearance of urate. Congenital deficiency of xanthine oxidase activity, producing and termed xanthinuria, is an autosomal recessive trait. Xanthine nephrolithiasis has been noted in approximately half the patients with this disorder, and a few have been reported to have myopathy. Decreased activity of phosphoribosylpyrophosphate synthetase has been described in one patient, a male infant who was mentally retarded. Purine nucleoside phosphorylase deficiency is associated with T-cell dysfunction and an immunodeficiency state. Increased renal clearance of uric acid may also be an inherited abnormality, or it may be secondary to one of the acquired conditions listed in Table 91–3. The clinical significance of hypouricemia is determined by the underlying condition that produces this abnormal biochemical finding because no pathologic consequence of hypouricemia is recognized. No therapy is required for the hypouricemia, and management is directed to the underlying illness. The detection of a low serum urate concentration during routine laboratory screening may be the initial clue that ultimately leads to the diagnosis of one of these conditions.

REFERENCES

1. Abramson, R.G., and Levitt, M.F.: Micropuncture study of uric acid transport in rat kidney. Am. J. Physiol., *228*:1597–1605, 1975.
2. Alarcon-Segovia, D.A., Cetina, J.A., and Diaz-Jouanen, E.: Sacroiliac joints in primary gout: clinical and roentgenographic study of 143 patients. AJR, *118*:438–443, 1973.
3. Aronoff, A.: Acute gouty arthritis precipitated by chlorothiazide. N. Engl. J. Med., *262*:767–769, 1960.
4. Atsmon, A., et al.: Dissolution of renal uric acid stones by oral alkalinization and large fluid intake in a patient suffering from gout. Am. J. Med., *27*:167–171, 1959.
5. Atsmon, A., De Vries, A., and Frank, M.: Uric Acid Lithiasis. Amsterdam, Elsevier, 1963.
6. Ball, G.V., and Moran, J.M.: Chronic lead ingestion and gout. South. Med. J., *61*:21–24, 1968.
7. Ball, G.V., and Sorensen, L.B.: The pathogenesis of hyperuricemia and gout in sickle cell anemia. Arthritis Rheum., *13*:846–848, 1970.
8. Ball, G.V., and Sorensen, L.B.: Pathogenesis of hyperuricemia in saturnine gout. N. Engl. J. Med., *280*:1199–1202, 1969.
9. Barlow, K.A.: Hyperlipidemia in primary gout. Metabolism, *17*:289–299, 1968.
10. Barlow, K.A., and Beilin, L.J.: Renal disease in primary gout. Q. J. Med., *37*:79–96, 1968.
11. Bartels, E.C.: Gout as a complication of surgery. Surg. Clin. North Am., *38*:845–848, 1957.
12. Bartels, E.C.: Gout. Postgrad. Med., *15*:255–264, 1954.
13. Bartels, E.C., and Matossian, G.S.: Gout: six-year follow-up on probenecid (Benemid) therapy. Arthritis Rheum., *2*:193–202, 1959.
14. Barzel, U.S., et al.: Renal ammonium excretion and urinary pH in idiopathic uric acid lithiasis. J. Urol., *92*:1–5, 1964.
15. Batuman, V., et al.: The role of lead in gout nephropathy. N. Engl. J. Med., *304*:520–523, 1981.
16. Bauer, W., and Klemperer, F.: Gout. *In* Diseases of Metabolism. 2nd Ed. Edited by G. Duncan. Philadelphia, W.B. Saunders, 1947, p. 611.
17. Becker, M.A.: Abnormalities of PRPP metabolism leading to an overproduction of uric acid. *In* Uric Acid: Handbook of Experimental Pharmacology. Vol. 51. Edited by W.N. Kelley and I.M. Weiner. New York, Springer-Verlag, 1978, pp. 155–183.
18. Becker, M.A.: Patterns of phosphoribosylpyrophosphate and ribose-5-phosphate concentration and generation in fibroblasts from patients with gout and purine overproduction. J. Clin. Invest., *57*:308–313, 1976.
19. Becker, M.A.: Regulation of purine nucleotide synthesis: effects of inosine on normal and hypoxanthine-guanine phosphoribosyltransferase-deficient fibroblasts. Biochim. Biophys. Acta, *435*:132–144, 1976.
20. Becker, M.A.: Regional localization of the gene for human phosphoribosylpyrophosphate synthetase on the X chromosome. Science, *203*:1,016–1,019, 1979.
21. Becker, M.A., et al.: The effects of nicotinic acid on human purine metabolism. (Abstract.) Clin. Res., *21*:616, 1973.
21a. Becker, M.A., and Seegmiller, J.E.: Genetic aspects of gout. Annu. Rev. Med., *25*:15–28, 1974.
22. Benedict, J.D., et al.: A further study of the utilization of dietary glycine nitrogen for uric acid synthesis in gout. J. Clin. Invest., *32*:775–777, 1953.
23. Benedict, J.D., et al.: Incorporation of glycine nitrogen into uric acid in normal and gouty man. Metabolism, *1*:3–12, 1952.
24. Benedict, J.D., et al.: The effect of salicylates and adrenocorticotropic hormone upon the miscible pool of uric acid in gout. J. Clin. Invest., *29*:1,104–1,111, 1950.
25. Benedict, J.D., Forsham, P.H., and Stetten, DeW., Jr.: The metabolism of uric acid in the normal and gouty human studied with the aid of isotopic uric acid. J. Biol. Chem., *181*:183–193, 1949.
26. Berger, L., and Yu, T.-F.: Renal function in gout. IV. An analysis of 524 gouty subjects including long-term follow-up studies. Am. J. Med., *59*:605–613, 1975.
27. Berkowitz, D.: Blood lipid and uric acid interrelationships. JAMA, *190*:856–858, 1964.
28. Beutler, E.: Effect of flavin compounds on glutathione reductase activity: in vivo and in vitro studies. J. Clin. Invest., *48*:1,957–1,966, 1969.
29. Beutler, E.: Glutathione reductase: Stimulation in normal subjects by riboflavin supplementation. Science, *165*:613–615, 1969.
30. Bishop, C., Garner, W., and Talbott, J.H.: Pool size, turnover rate, and rapidity of equilibration of injected isotopic uric acid in normal and pathological subjects. J. Clin. Invest., *30*:879–888, 1951.
31. Bordley, J., III, and Richards, A.N.: Quantitative studies of the composition of glomerular urine. VIII. The concentration of uric acid in glomerular urine of snakes and frogs, determined by an ultramicroadaptation of Folin's method. J. Biol. Chem., *101*:193–221, 1933.
32. Brandenberger, E., De Quervain, F., and Schinz, H.R.: Roentgenographische und Mikroskopish-Kristalloptische Untersuchungen an Harnsteinen. Helv. Med. Acta, *14*:195–211, 1947.
33. Brauer, G.W., and Prior, I.A.M.: A prospective study of gout in New Zealand maoris. Ann. Rheum. Dis., *37*:466–472, 1978.
34. Breckenridge, A.: Hypertension and hyperuricaemia. Lancet, *1*:15–18, 1966.
35. Brochner-Mortensen, K.: Review of diagnostic criteria and known etiological factors in gout. *In* Epidemiology of Chronic Rheumatism. Vol. 1. Edited by J.H. Kellgren, M.R. Jeffrey, and J. Ball. Philadelphia, F.A. Davis, 1963, pp. 140–155.
36. Brochner-Mortensen, K.: 100 Gouty patients. Acta Med. Scand., *106*:81–107, 1941.
37. Bronsky, D., and Bernstein, A.: Acute gout secondary to multiple myeloma: a case report. Ann. Intern. Med., *41*:820–823, 1954.
38. Brown, J., and Mallory, G.K.: Renal changes in gout. N. Engl. J. Med., *243*:325–329, 1950.

39. Brugsch, T., and Citron, J.: Ueber die Absorption der Harnsaure durch Knorpel. Z. Exp. Pathol. Ther., 5:401–405, 1908.
40. Buchanan, W.W., Klinenberg, J.R., and Seegmiller, J.E.: The inflammatory reponse to injected microcrystalline monosodium urate in normal, hyperuricemic, gouty and uremic subjects. Arthritis Rheum., 8:361–367, 1965.
41. Bunin, J.J., et al.: The syndrome of sarcoidosis, psoriasis, and gout. Ann. Intern. Med., 57:1,018–1,040, 1962.
42. Burch, T.A., et al.: Hyperuricaemia and gout in the Mariana Islands. Ann. Rheum. Dis., 25:144–119, 1966.
43. Buzard, J., Bishop, C., and Talbott, J.H.: The fate of uric acid in the normal and gouty human being. J. Chronic Dis., 2:42–49, 1955.
44. Bywaters, E.G.L.: Gout in the time and person of George IV: a case history. Ann. Rheum. Dis., 21:325–338, 1962.
45. Campion, D.W., et al.: Does increased free serum urate concentration cause gout? (Abstract.) Clin. Res., 23:261A, 1975.
46. Campion, D.W., Bluestone, R., and Klinenberg, J.R.: Uric acid: characterization of its interaction with human serum albumin. J. Clin. Invest., 52:2,383–2,387, 1973.
47. Caner, J.E.Z., and Decker, J.L.: Recurrent acute (?gouty) arthritis in chronic renal failure treated with periodic hemodialysis. Am. J. Med., 36:571–582, 1964.
48. Cannon, P.J., et al.: Hyperuricemia in primary and renal hypertension. N. Engl. J. Med., 275:457–464, 1966.
49. Clarke, A.M., and McKenzie, R.G.: Ileostomy and the risk of urinary uric acid stones. Lancet, 2:395–397, 1969.
50. Cobb, S.: Hyperuricemia in executives. In The Epidemiology of Chronic Rheumatism. Vol. 1. Edited by J.H. Kellgren, M.R. Jeffrey, and J. Ball. Philadelphia, F.A. Davis, 1963, pp. 182–186.
50a. Coe, F.L.: Hyperuricosuric calcium oxalate nephrolithiasis. In Nephrolithiasis: Contemporary Issues in Nephrology. Vol. 5. 1980, pp. 116–135.
51. Cohen, A., et al.: Abnormal purine metabolism and purine overproduction in a patient deficient in purine nucleoside phosphorylase. N. Engl. J. Med., 295:1,449–1,454, 1976.
52. Cohen, H.: Gout and other metabolic disorders producing joint disease. In Textbook of the Rheumatic Diseases. Edited by W.S.C. Copeman. Edinburgh, Livingstone, 1955, p. 361.
53. Copeman, W.S.C.: A Short History of the Gout and the Rheumatic Diseases. Berkeley, University of California Press, 1964.
54. Cristofori, F.C., and Duncan, G.G.: Uric acid excretion in obese subjects during periods of total fasting. Metabolism, 13:303–311, 1964.
55. Crowley, L.V., and Alton, F.I.: Automated analysis of uric acid. Am. J. Clin. Pathol., 49:285–288, 1968.
56. Decker, J.L., Lane, J.J., Jr., and Reynolds, W.E.: Hyperuricemia in a male Filipino population. Arthritis Rheum., 5:144–155, 1962.
57. Delbarre, F., et al.: Action de l'éthanol dans la goutte et sur le métabolisme de l'acide urique. Sem. Hôp. Paris, 43:659–664, 1967.
58. Delbarre, F., Braun, S., and St. George-Chaumet, F.: La goutte: problémes cliniques, biologiques et thérapeutiques. Sem. Hôp. Paris, 43:623–633, 1967.
59. Demartini, F.E., et al.: Effect of chlorothiazide on the renal excretion of uric acid. Am. J. Med., 32:572–577, 1962.
60. Diamond, H.S., and Meisel, A.D.: Collecting duct urate reabsorption in man. (Abstract.) Clin. Res., 23:360A, 1975.
61. Diamond, H.S., and Paolino, J.S.: Evidence for a post-secretory reabsorptive site for uric acid in man. J. Clin. Invest., 52:1,491–1,499, 1973.
62. Dodds, W.J., and Steinbach, H.L.: Gout associated with calcification of cartilage. N. Engl. J. Med., 275:745–749, 1966.
63. Dollery, C.T., Duncan, H., and Schumer, B.: Hyperuricaemia related to treatment of hypertension. Br. Med. J., 2:832–835, 1960.
64. Drenick, E.J., et al.: Prolonged starvation as treatment for severe obesity. JAMA, 187:100–105, 1964.
65. Ebstein, W.: Die Natur und Behandlung der Gicht. Wiesbaden, Bergmann, 1906.
66. Eisen, A.Z., and Seegmiller, J.E.: Uric acid metabolism in psoriasis. J. Clin. Invest., 40:1,486–1,494, 1961.
67. Emmerson, B.T.: Alteration of urate metabolism by weight reduction. Aust. N.Z. J. Med., 3:410–412, 1973.
68. Emmerson, B.T.: The clinical differentiation of lead gout from primary gout. Arthritis Rheum., 11:623–634, 1968.
69. Emmerson, B.T.: Symposium on allopurinol: biochemistry and metabolism. Ann. Rheum. Dis., 25:622, 1966.
69a. Emmerson, B.T.: Chronic lead neuropathy: the diagnostic use of calcium EDTA and the association with gout. Aust. Ann. Med., 12:310–324, 1963.
70. Emmerson, B.T., and Sandilands, P.: The normal range of plasma urate levels. Aust. Ann. Med., 12:46–52, 1963.
71. Evans, J.G., Prior, I.A.M., and Harvey, H.P.B.: Relation of serum uric acid to body bulk, haemoglobin, and alcohol intake in two South Pacific Polynesian populations. Ann. Rheum. Dis., 27:319–324, 1968.
72. Faller, J., and Fox, I.H.: Ethanol-induced hyperuricemia: evidence for increased urate production by activation of adenine nucleotide turnover. N. Engl. J. Med., 307:1,598–1,602, 1982.
73. Fanelli, G.M., Jr., et al.: Renal urate transport in the chimpanzee. Am. J. Physiol., 220:613–620, 1971.
74. Farrell, P.C., Popovich, R.P., and Babb, A.L.: Binding levels of urate ions in human serum albumin and plasma. Biochim. Biophys. Acta, 243:49–52, 1971.
75. Fessel, W.J.: Renal outcomes of gout and hyperuricemia. Am. J. Med. 67:74–82, 1979.
76. Fessel, W.J., and Barr, G.D.: Uric acid, lean body weight, and creatinine interactions: results from regression analysis of 78 variables. Semin. Arthritis Rheum., 7:115–121, 1977.
77. Fessel, W.J., Siegelaub, A.B., and Johnson, E.S.: Correlates and consequences of asymptomatic hyperuricemia. Arch. Intern. Med., 132:44–54, 1973.
78. Fineberg, S.K., and Altschul, A.: The nephropathy of gout. Ann. Intern. Med., 44:1,182–1,194, 1956.
79. Garrod, A.B.: The Nature and Treatment of Gout and Rheumatic Gout. London, Walton and Maberly, 1859, p. 251.
80. Garrod, A.B.: On the blood and effused fluids of gout, rheumatism, and Bright's disease. Med. Chir. Soc. Trans., 37:49–60, 1854.
81. Garrod, A.B.: Observations on certain pathological conditions of the blood and urine, rheumatism, and Bright's disease. Med. Chir. Soc. Trans., 31:83–98, 1848.
82. Gershon, S.L., and Fox, I.H.: Pharmacologic effects of nicotinic acid on human purine metabolism. J. Lab. Clin. Med., 84:179–186, 1974.
82a. Ginsberg, J.H., et al.: Rheumatoid nodulosis: an unusual variant of rheumatoid disease. Arthritis Rheum., 26:49–58, 1975.
83. Glynn, R.J., Campion, E.W., and Silbert, J.E.: Trends in serum uric acid levels 1961–1980. Arthritis Rheum., 26:87–93, 1983.
84. Gold, M.S., et al.: Sickle cell anemia and hyperuricemia. JAMA, 206:1,572–1,573, 1968.
85. Goldfinger, S., Klinenberg, J.R., and Seegmiller, J.E.: Renal retention of uric acid induced by infusion of beta-hydroxybutyrate and acetoacetate. N. Engl. J. Med., 272:351–355, 1965.
86. Goldthwait, J.C., Butler, C.F., and Stillman, J.S.: The diagnosis of gout: significance of an elevated serum uric acid value. N. Engl. J. Med., 259:1,095–1,099, 1958.
87. Gonick, H.C., et al.: The renal lesion in gout. Ann. Intern. Med., 62:667–674, 1965.
88. Good, A.E., and Rapp, R.: Chondrocalcinosis of the knee with gout and rheumatoid arthritis. N. Engl. J. Med., 277:286–290, 1967.
89. Grahame, R., and Scott, J.T.: Clinical survey of 354 patients with gout. Ann. Rheum. Dis., 29:461–468, 1970.
90. Greenbaum, D., Ross, J.H., and Steinberg, V.L.: Renal biopsy in gout. Br. Med. J., 1:1,502–1,504, 1961.
91. Greene, H.L., et al.: ATP depletion, a possible role in

the pathogenesis of hyperuricemia in glycogen storage disease type I. J. Clin. Invest., *62*:321–328, 1978.

92. Greger, R., Lang, F., and Deetjen, P.: Urate handling by the rat kidney. IV. Reabsorption in the loops of Henle. Pfluegers Arch., *352*:115–120, 1974.

93. Greger, R., Lang, F., and Deetjen, P.: Handling of uric acid by the rat kidney. II. Microperfusion studies on bidirectional transport of uric acid in the proximal tubule. Pfluegers Arch., *335*:257–265, 1972.

94. Greger, R., Lang, F., and Deetjen, P.: Handling of uric acid by the rat kidney: I. Microanalysis of uric acid in proximal tubular fluid. Pfluegers Arch., *324*:279–287, 1971.

95. Grunst, J., Dietze, G., and Wicklmayr, M.: Effect of ethanol on uric acid production of human liver. Nutr. Metab., *21 (Suppl. 1)*:138–141, 1977.

96. Gutman, A.B.: The past four decades of progress in the knowledge of gout, with an assessment of the present status. Arthritis Rheum., *16*:431–445, 1973.

97. Gutman, A.B.: Gout and gouty arthritis. In Textbook of Medicine. Edited by P.B. Beeson and W. McDermott. Philadelphia, W.B. Saunders, 1958, p. 595.

98. Gutman, A.B.: Primary and secondary gout. Ann. Intern. Med., *39*:1,062–1,076, 1953.

99. Gutman, A.B., and Yu, T.-F.: Urinary ammonium excretion in primary gout. J. Clin. Invest., *44*:1,474–1,481, 1965.

100. Gutman, A.B., and Yu, T.-F.: Secondary gout. (Abstract.) Ann. Intern. Med., *56*:675, 1962.

101. Gutman, A.B., and Yu, T.-F.: A three-component system for regulation of renal excretion of uric acid in man. Trans. Assoc. Am. Physicians, *74*:353–365, 1961.

102. Gutman, A.B., and Yu, T.-F.: Renal function in gout: with a commentary on the renal regulation of urate excretion, and the role of the kidney in the pathogenesis of gout. Am. J. Med., *23*:600–622, 1957.

103. Gutman, A.B., and Yu, T.-F.: Gout, a derangement of purine metabolism. Adv. Intern. Med., *5*:227–302, 1952.

104. Gutman, A.B., Yu, T.-F., and Berger, L.: Tubular secretion of urate in man. J. Clin. Invest., *38*:1,778–1,781, 1959.

105. Hadler, N.M., et al.: Acute polyarticular gout. Am. J. Med., *56*:715–719, 1974.

106. Hall, A.P., et al.: Epidemiology of gout and hyperuricemia: a long-term population study. Am. J. Med., *42*:27–37, 1967.

107. Hamilton, W.F.D., and Robertson, G.S.: Changes in serum uric acid related to the dose of methoxyflurane. Br. J. Anaesth., *46*:54–58, 1974.

108. Harth, M., and Robinson, C.E.G.: Gouty arthritis in a D.V.A. hospital: a retrospective study. Med. Serv. J. Can., *18*:671–674, 1962.

109. Hartung, E.F.: Symposium on gout: Historical considerations. Metabolism, *6*:196–208, 1957.

109a. Hasselbacher, P., et al.: Monosodium urate monohydrate crystals stimulate secretion of collagenase and PGE_2 by synovial fibroblasts: a model of joint destruction in chronic gouty arthritis. Arthritis Rheum., *24*:577, 1981.

110. Hauge, M., and Harvald, B.: Heredity in gout and hyperuricemia. Acta Med. Scand., *152*:247–257, 1955.

111. Healey, L.A.: The effect of fasting and ketosis on uric acid excretion. (Abstract.) Arthritis Rheum., *7*:313, 1964.

112. Hellman, L.: Production of acute gouty arthritis by adrenocorticotropin. Science, *109*:280–281, 1949.

113. Hench, P.S.: Diagnosis of gout and gouty arthritis. J. Lab. Clin. Med., *22*:48–55, 1936.

114. Henderson, J.F., et al.: Variations in purine metabolism of cultured skin fibroblasts from patients with gout. J. Clin. Invest., *47*:1,511–1,516, 1968.

115. Henneman, P.H., Wallach, S., and Dempsey, E.F.: The metabolic defect responsible for uric acid stone formation. J. Clin. Invest., *41*:537–542, 1962.

116. Heptinstall, R.H.: Gout. In Pathology of the Kidney. 2nd Ed. Boston, Little, Brown, 1966, p. 495.

117. Hickling, R.A.: Gout, leukaemia, and polycythaemia. Lancet, *1*:57–59, 1953.

118. Hoffman, W.S.: Some unsolved problems of gout. Med. Clin. North Am., *43*:595–606, 1959.

119. Hollander, J.L.: Introduction to arthritis and the rheumatic diseases. In Arthritis and Allied Conditions. 8th Ed. Edited by J.L. Hollander and D.J. McCarty, Jr. Philadelphia, Lea & Febiger, 1972, pp. 13–14.

120. Holmes, E.W.: Regulation of purine biosynthesis de novo. In Uric Acid: Handbook of Experimental Pharmacology. Vol. 51. Edited by W.N. Kelley and I.M. Weiner. New York, Springer-Verlag, 1978, pp. 21–41.

121. Holmes, E.W.: Human glutamine phosphoribosylpyrophosphate amidotransferase: kinetic and regulatory properties. J. Biol. Chem., *248*:144–150, 1973.

122. Holmes, E.W., and Blondet, P.: Update binding to serum albumin: lack of influence on renal clearance of uric acid. Arthritis Rheum., *22*:737–739, 1979.

123. Holmes, E.W., and Kelley, W.N.: Renal pathophysiology of gout. In Renal Pathophysiology. Springfield, IL, Charles C Thomas, 1976.

124. Holmes, E.W., Wyngaarden, J.B., and Kelley, W.N.: Human glutamine phosphoribosylpyrophosphate amidotransferase: two molecular forms interconvertible by purine ribonucleotides and phosphoribosylpyrophosphate. J. Biol. Chem., *248*:6,035–6,040, 1973.

125. Honda, H., and Gindin, R.A.: Gout while receiving levodopa for Parkinsonism. JAMA, *219*:55–57, 1972.

126. Howell, R.R., and Williams, J.C.: The glycogen storage diseases. In The Metabolic Basis of Inherited Diseases. 5th Ed. Edited by J.B. Stanbury, et al. New York, McGraw-Hill, 1983, pp. 141–166.

127. Howell, R.R., Eanes, E.D., and Seegmiller, J.E.: X-ray diffraction studies of the tophaceous deposits in gout. Arthritis Rheum., *6*:97–103, 1963.

128. Hughes, G.R., Barnes, C.G., and Mason, R.M.: Bony ankylosis in gout. Ann. Rheum. Dis., *27*:67–70, 1968.

128a. Hunder, G.G., Worthington, J.W., and Bickel, W.H.: Avascular necrosis of the femoral head in a patient with gout. JAMA, *203*:47–49, 1968.

129. Itakura, M., et al.: Basis for the control of purine biosynthesis by purine ribonucleotides. J. Clin. Invest., *67*:994–1,002, 1981.

130. Itskovitz, H.D., and Sellers, A.M.: Gout and hyperuricemia after adrenalectomy for hypertension. N. Engl. J. Med., *268*:1,105–1,108, 1963.

131. Jacobson, B.M.: The uric acid in the serum of gouty and of non-gouty individuals: its determination by Folin's recent method and its significance in the diagnosis of gout. Ann. Intern. Med., *11*:1,277–1,295, 1937.

132. Katz, W.A., and Schubert, M.: The interaction of monosodium urate with connective tissue components. J. Clin. Invest., *49*:1,783–1,789, 1970.

133. Kelley, W.N., et al.: Hypoxanthine-guanine phosphoribosyltransferase deficiency in gout. Ann. Intern. Med., *70*:155–206, 1969.

134. Kelley, W.N., et al.: Excessive production of uric acid in type I glycogen storage disease. J. Pediatr., *72*:488–496, 1968.

135. Kelley, W.N., and Wyngaarden, J.B.: Clinical syndromes associated with hypoxanthine-guanine phosphoribosyltransferase deficiency. In The Metabolic Basis of Inherited Diseases. 5th Ed. Edited by J.B. Stanbury, et al. New York, McGraw-Hill, 1983, pp. 1,115–1,143.

136. Kelton, J.G., et al.: A method for monitoring dialysis patients and a tool for assessing binding to serum proteins in vivo. Ann. Intern. Med., *89*:67–70, 1978.

137. Kinsey, D.: Gout and hyperuricemia in hypertensive patients 15–25 years following lumbodorsal splanchnicectomy. (Abstract.) Arthritis Rheum., *6*:778–779, 1963.

138. Kovarsky, J., Holmes, E.W., and Kelley, W.N.: Absence of significant urate binding to human serum proteins. J. Lab. Clin. Med., *93*:85–91, 1979.

138s. Kozin, F., and McCarty, D.J.: Rheumatoid factors in the serum of gouty patients. Arthritis Rheum., *20*:1,559, 1977.

139. Kramp, R.A., Lassiter, W.E., and Gottschalk, C.W.: Urate-2-^{14}C transport in the rat nephron. J. Clin. Invest., *50*:35–48, 1971.

140. Lambert, J.R., and Wright, V.: Serum uric acid levels in psoriatic arthritis. Ann. Rheum. Dis., *36*:264–267, 1977.

141. Lawrence, J.S.: Heritable disorders of connective tissue. Proc. R. Soc. Med., 53:522–526, 1960.

142. Lennane, G.A.Q., Rose, B.S., and Isdale, I.C.: Gout in the Maori, Ann. Rheum. Dis., 19:120–125, 1960.

143. Lichtenstein, L., Scott, H.W., and Levin, M.H.: Pathologic changes in gout: survey of 11 necropsied cases. Am. J. Pathol., 32:871–895, 1956.

144. Lieber, C.S., et al.: Interrelation of uric acid and ethanol metabolism in man. J. Clin. Invest., 41:1,863–1,870, 1962.

145. Lieber, C.S., and Davidson, C.S.: Some metabolic effects of ethyl alcohol. Am. J. Med., 33:319–327, 1962.

146. Linton, R.R., and Talbott, J.H.: The surgical treatment of tophaceous gout. Ann. Surg., 117:161–182, 1943.

146a. Loeb, J.N.: The influence of temperature on the solubility of uric acid and monosodium urate. Arthritis Rheum., 15:189, 1972.

147. Ludwig, A.P., Bennett, G.A., and Bauer, W.: A rare manifestation of gout: widespread ankylosis simulating rheumatoid arthritis. Ann. Intern. Med., 11:1,248–1,276, 1938.

148. Lynch, E.C.: Uric acid metabolism in proliferative diseases of the marrow. Arch. Intern. Med., 109:639–653, 1962.

149. McCarty, D.J., Jr.: A historical note: Leeuwenhoek's description of crystals from a gouty tophus. Arthritis Rheum., 13:414–418, 1970.

150. McCarty, D.J., Jr.: The inflammatory reaction to microcrystalline sodium urate. Arthritis Rheum., 8:726–735, 1965.

151. McCollum, D.E., Mathews, R.S., and O'Neil, M.T.: Aseptic necrosis of the femoral head: associated diseases and evaluation of treatment. South. Med. J., 63:241–253, 1970.

152. McCollum, D.E., et al.: Aseptic necrosis of the femoral head: associated diseases and evaluation of treatment. J. Bone Joint Surg., 49A:1,019–1,020, 1967.

153. MacLachlan, M.J., and Rodnan, G.P.: Effects of food, fast and alcohol on serum uric acid and acute attacks of gout. Am. J. Med., 42:38–57, 1967.

154. Malawista, S.E., et al.: Sacroiliac gout. JAMA, 194:954–956, 1965.

155. Malnic, G., Aires, M.M., and Giebisch, G.: Micropuncture study of renal tubular hydrogen ion transport in the rat. Am. J. Physiol., 222:147–158, 1972.

156. March, H.W., Schlyen, S.M., and Schwartz, S.E.: Mediterranean hemopathic syndromes (Cooley's anemia) in adults: study of a family with unusual complications. Am. J. Med., 13:46–57, 1952.

157. Martel, W.: The overhanging margin of bone: a roentgenologic manifestation of gout. Radiology, 91:755–756, 1968.

157a. Mayne, J.G.: Patholoical study of the renal lesions found in 27 patients with gout. Ann. Rheum. Dis., 15:61–62, 1956.

158. Messerli, F.H., et al.: Serum uric acid in essential hypertension: an indicator of renal vascular involvement. Ann. Intern. Med., 93:817–821, 1980.

159. Meyer, W.J., III, Gill, J.R., Jr., and Bartter, F.C.: Gout as a complication of Bartter's syndrome: a possible role for alkalosis in the decreased clearance of uric acid. Ann. Intern Med., 83:56–59, 1975.

160. Mikkelsen, W.M., Dodge, H.J., and Valkenburg, H.: The distribution of serum uric acid values in a population unselected as to gout or hyperuricemia: Tecumseh, Michigan 1959–1060. Am. J. Med., 39:242–251, 1965.

161. Modern, F.W.S., and Meister, L.: The kidney of gout, a clinical entity. Med. Clin. North Am., 36:941–951, 1952.

162. Moskowitz, R.W., et al.: Crystal-induced inflammation associated with chronic renal failure treated with periodic hemodialysis. Am. J. Med., 47:450–460, 1969.

162a. Nakayama, D.A., et al.: Tophaceous gout: a clinical and radiographic assessment. Arthritis Rheum., 27:468–471, 1984.

163. Nathan, L.A., Kubota, C.K., and Turnbull, G.C.: Relative incidence of gout in Negro and white males at Cook County Hospital (1944–1950). (Abstract.) J. Lab. Clin. Med., 42:927, 1953.

164. Neel, J.V.: The clinical detection of the genetic carriers of inherited disease. Medicine, 26:115–153, 1947.

165. Neel, J.V., et al.: Studies on hyperuricemia. II. A reconsideration of the distribution of serum uric acid values in the families of Smyth, Cotterman, and Freyberg. Am. J. Hum. Genet., 17:14–22, 1965.

166. O'Brien, W.M., Burch, T.A., and Bunim, J.J.: Genetics of hyperuricaemia in Blackfeet and Pima indians. Ann. Rheum. Dis., 25:117–119, 1966.

167. O'Duffy, J.D., Hunder, G.G., and Kelly, P.J.: Decreasing prevalence of tophaceous gout. Mayo Clin. Proc., 50:227–228, 1975.

168. Paik, C.H., et al.: Thalassemia and gouty arthritis. JAMA, 213:296, 1970.

169. Paulus, H.E., et al.: Clinical significance of hyperuricemia in routinely screened hospitalized men. JAMA, 211:277–281, 1970.

170. Pearson, G.: Philos. Trans. Lond., 88:15, 1798.

170a. Perricone, E., and Brandt, K.D.: Enhancement of urate solubility by connective tissue. Arthritis Rheum., 21:453–460, 1978.

171. Peters, J.P., and Van Slyke, D.D.: Quantitative Clinical Chemistry. Vol. 1. 2nd Ed. Baltimore, Williams & Wilkins, 1946, p. 937.

172. Plante, G.E., Durivage, J., and Lemieux, G.: Renal excretion of hydrogen in primary gout. Metabolism, 17:377–385, 1968.

173. Podevin, R., et al.: Etude chez l'homme de la cinétique d'apparition dans l'urine de l'acide urique 2¹⁴C. Nephron, 5:134–140, 1968.

174. Pollycove, M., et al.: Uric acid metabolism: the oxidation of uric acid in normal subjects and patients with gout, polycythemia and leukemia. (Abstract.) Clin. Res., 5:38, 1957.

175. Postlethwaite, A.E., Bartel, A.G., and Kelley, W.N.: Hyperuricemia due to ethambutol. N. Engl. J. Med., 286:761–763, 1972.

176. Praetorius, E., and Kirk, J.E.: Hypouricemia: with evidence for tubular elimination of uric acid. J. Lab. Clin. Med., 35:865–868, 1950.

177. Price, N.L.: Gout following salyrgan diuresis. Lancet, 1:22–23, 1939.

178. Prien, E.L., and Prien, E.L., Jr.: Composition and structure of urinary stone. Am. J. Med., 45:654–672, 1968.

179. Prior, I.A.M., and Rose, B.S.: Uric acid, gout and public health in the South Pacific. N.Z. Med. J., 65:295–300, 1966.

180. Ramsdell, C.M., and Kelley, W.N.: The clinical significance of hypouricemia. Ann. Intern. Med., 78:239–242, 1973.

181. Rapado, A.: Relationship between gout and arterial hypertension. Adv. Exp. Med. Biol., 41B:451–459, 1974.

182. Ravio, K.O., et al.: Stimulation of human purine synthesis de novo by fructose infusion. Metabolism, 24:861–869, 1975.

183. Reynolds, P.P., et al.: Moonshine and lead: relationship to the pathogenesis of hyperuricemia in gout. Arthritis Rheum., 26:59–67, 1983.

184. Richet, G., et al.: Le rein du saturnisme chronique. Rev. Fr. Etudes Clin. Biol., 9:188–196, 1964.

185. Rieselbach, R.E., et al.: Diminished renal urate secretion per nephron as a basis for primary gout. Ann. Intern. Med., 73:359–366, 1970.

186. Roberts, W.: The Croonian Lectures on the chemistry and therapeutics of uric acid gravel and gout. Br. Med. J., 2:61–65, 1892.

187. Robinson, D.R., Tashjian, A.H., Jr., and Levine, L.: Prostaglandin induced bone resorption by rheumatoid synovia. (Abstract.) Clin. Res., 23:443A, 1975.

188. Roch-Ramel, F., and Boudry, J.F.: Tubular fate of 2-¹⁴C urate: microperfusion experiments. (Abstract.) Fed. Proc., 30:338, 1971.

189. Roch-Ramel, F., and Weiner, I.M.: Excretion of urate by the kidneys of Cebus monkeys: a micropuncture study. Am. J. Physiol., 224:1,369–1,374, 1973.

190. Rodnan, G.P.: The pathogenesis of aldermanic gout: procatarctic role of fluctuations in serum urate concentrations

in gouty arthritis provoked by feast and alcohol. (Abstract.) Clin. Res., 28:359A, 1980.

190a. Rodnan, G.P.: A gallery of gout: being a miscellany of prints and caricatures from the 16th century to the present day. Arthritis Rheum., 4:27–46, 1961.

191. Rondier, J., et al.: Gout and hyperlipidaemia effect of overweight on the levels of circulating lipids. Ann. Clin. Res., 9:239, 1977.

192. Rosenbloom, F.M., et al.: Biochemical bases of accelerated purine biosynthesis de novo in human fibroblasts lacking hypoxanthine-guanine phosphoribosyltransferase. J. Biol. Chem., 243:1,166–1,173, 1968.

193. Rouault, T., Caldwell, D.S., and Holmes, E.W.: Aspiration of the asymptomatic metatarsophalangeal joint in gout patients and hyperuricemic controls. Arthritis Rheum., 25:209–212, 1982.

194. Saker, B.M., et al.: Alcohol consumption and gout. Med. J. Aust., 1:1,213–1,216, 1967.

195. Salzman, R.T., Howell, D.S., and Ricca, L.R.: Aberrancy in clinical hallmarks of gouty arthritis: brief clinical report. Arthritis Rheum., 8:998–1,001, 1965.

196. Sarre, H. (Ed.): Congrès International de la Goutte et de la Lithiase Urique. Evian, France, 1964.

197. Scheele, K.W.: Examen chemicum calculi urinarii. Opuscula, 2:73, 1776.

198. Schirmeister, J., Man, N.K., and Hallauer, W.: Study on renal and extrarenal factors involved in the hyperuricemia induced by furosemide. In Progress in Nephrology. Edited by G. Peters and F. Roch-Ramel. Berlin, Springer-Verlag, 1969, pp. 59–63.

199. Scott, J.T.: Obesity and hyperuricaemia. Clin. Rheum. Dis., 3:25–355, 1977.

200. Scott, J.T., et al.: Studies of uric acid pool size and turnover rate. Ann. Rheum. Dis., 28:366–373, 1969.

201. Scott, J.T., Dixon, A. St. J., and Bywaters, E.G.L.: Association of hyperuricaemia and gout with hyperparathyroidism. Br. Med. J., 1:1,070–1,073, 1964.

202. Scudamore, C.: A Treatise on the Nature and Cure of Gout and Rheumatism, Including General Considerations on Morbid States of the Digestive Organs: Some Remarks on Regimen; and Practical Observations on Gravel. 2nd Ed. London, Lomgman, 1817, p. 592.

203. Sears, W.G.: The occurrence of gout during the treatment of pernicious anaemia. Lancet, 1:24, 1933.

204. Seegmiller, J.E., et al.: The effect of 2-ethylamino-I,3,4,-thiadiazole on the incorporation of glycine into urinary purines and uric acid in man. Metabolism, 12:507–515, 1963.

205. Seegmiller, J.E., et al.: The renal excretion of uric acid in gout. Clin. Invest., 41:1,094–1,098, 1962.

206. Seegmiller, J.E., et al.: Uric acid production in gout. J. Clin. Invest., 40:1,304–1,314, 1961.

207. Seegmiller, J.E., Rosenbloom, F.M., and Kelley, W.N.: Enzyme defect associated with a sex-linked human neurological disorder and excessive purine synthesis. Science, 155:1,682–1,684, 1967.

208. Shapiro, J.R., et al.: Hyperuricemia associated with obesity and intensified by caloric restriction. (Abstract.) Arthritis Rheum., 7:343, 1963.

209. Sheikh, M.I., and Moller, J.F.: Binding of urate to proteins of human and rabbit plasma. Biochim. Biophys. Acta, 158:456–458, 1968.

210. Simkin, P.A.: Urate excretion in normal and gouty men. Adv. Exp. Med. Biol., 76B:41–45, 1977.

211. Simon, N.M., et al.: Differential uric acid excretion in essential and renal hypertension. Circulation, 39:121–125, 1969.

212. Skupp, S., and Ayvazian, J.H.: Oxidation of 7-methylguanine by human xanthine oxidase. J. Lab. Clin. Med., 73:909–916, 1969.

213. Smyth, C.J.: Diagnosis and treatment of gout. In Arthritis and Allied Conditions. 8th Ed. Edited by J.L. Hollander and D.J. McCarty, Jr. Philadelphia, Lea & Febiger, 1972, pp. 1,112–1,139.

214. Smyth, C.J.: Hereditary factors in gout: a review of recent literature. Metabolism, 6:218–229, 1957.

215. Smyth, C.J., and Huffman, E.R.: Gouty arthritis: diagnosis and treatment. Rocky Mt. Med. J., 52:513–518, 1955.

216. Smyth, C.J., Cotterman, C.W., and Freyberg, R.H.: The genetics of gout and hyperuricemia—an analysis of nineteen families. J. Clin. Invest., 27:749–759, 1948.

217. Smythe, C.M., and Cutchin, J.H.: Primary juvenile gout. Am. J. Med., 32:799–804, 1962.

218. Sokoloff, L.: The pathology of gout. Metabolism, 6:230–243, 1957.

219. Sokoloff, L., and Gleason, I.O.: The sternoclavicular articulation in rheumatic diseases. Am. J. Clin. Pathol., 24:406–414, 1954.

220. Somerville, J.: Gout in cyanotic congenital heart disease. Br. Heart Med., 23:31–34, 1961.

221. Sorensen, L.B.: The pathogenesis of gout. Arch. Intern. Med., 109:379–390, 1962.

222. Sorensen, L.B.: Degradation of uric acid in man. Metabolism, 8:687–703, 1959.

223. Sperling, O., et al.: Superactivity of phosphoribosylpyrophosphate synthetase, due to feedback resistance, causing purine overproduction and gout. Ciba Found. Symp., 48:143–164, 1977.

224. Sperling, O., and Wyngaarden, J.B.: In preparation.

225. Stecher, R.M., Hersh, A.H., and Solomon, W.M.: The heredity of gout and its relationship to familial hyperuricemia. Ann. Intern. Med., 31:595–614, 1949.

226. Steele, T.H.: Evidence for altered renal urate reabsorption during changes in volume of the extracellular fluid. J. Lab. Clin. Med., 74:228–299, 1969.

227. Steele, T.H., and Boner, G.: Origins of the uricosuric response. J. Clin. Invest., 52:1,368–1,375, 1973.

228. Steele, T.H., and Oppenheimer, S.: Factors affecting urate excretion following diuretic administration in man. Am. J. Med., 47:564–574, 1969.

229. Steele, T.H., and Rieselbach, R.E.: The renal mechanism for urate homeostasis in normal man. Am. J. Med., 43:868–875, 1967.

229a. Stockman, A., Darlington, L.G., and Scott, J.T.: Frequency of chondrocalcinosis in the knees and avascular necrosis of the femoral head in gout: a controlled study. Ann. Rheum. Dis., 39:7–11, 1980.

230. Sturge, R.A., et al.: Serum uric acid in England and Scotland. Ann. Rheum. Dis., 36:420–427, 1977.

231. Suki, W.N., et al.: Mechanism of the effect of thiazide diuretics on calcium and uric acid. (Abstract.) J. Clin. Invest., 46:1,121, 1967.

232. Sydenham, T.: The Works of Thomas Sydenham. Vol. II. Translated from the Latin edition of Greenhill. London, Sydenham Society, 1850, p. 214.

233. Sydenham, T.: Tractatus de Podagra et Hydrope. London, G. Kettilby, 1683.

234. Talbott, J.H.: Gout. 2nd Ed. New York, Grune and Stratton, 1964.

235. Talbott, J.H.: Gout and blood dyscrasias. Medicine, 38:173–205, 1959.

236. Talbott, J.H.: Gout. New York, Grune and Stratton, 1957.

237. Talbott, J.H.: Gout. J. Chronic Dis., 1:338–345, 1955.

238. Talbott, J.H.: Serum urate in relatives of gouty patients. J. Clin. Invest., 19:645–648, 1940.

239. Talbott, J.H., and Coombs, F.S.: Metabolic studies on patients with gout. JAMA, 110:1,977–1,982, 1938.

240. Talbott, J.H., and Lilienfeld, A.: Longevity in gout. Geriatrics, 14:409–420, 1959.

241. Talbott, J.H., and Terplan, K.L.: The kidney in gout. Medicine, 39:405–468, 1960.

242. Turner, R.E., et al.: Some aspects of the epidemiology of gout: sex and race incidence. Arch. Intern. Med., 106:400–406, 1960.

243. Umber, F.: Ernahrung und Stoffwechselkrankheiten. 2nd Ed. Vienna, Urban und Schwarzenberg, 1914.

244. Ungerleider, H.E.: The internist and life insurance. Ann. Intern. Med., 41:124–130, 1954.

245. Van Den Berghe, G., and Hers, H.G.: Abnormal AMP deaminase in primary gout. Lancet, 2:1,090, 1980.

246. Van Peenen, H.J.: Causes of hypouricemia. Ann. Intern. Med., 78:977–978, 1973.

247. Von Storch, A.: An Essay on the Use and Effects of the Root of the Colchicum autumnale, or Meadow Saffron.

Translated from the Latin by T. Becker and P.A. de Honet, 1764.

248. Wallace, S.L., et al.: Preliminary criteria for the classification of the acute arthritis of primary gout. Arthritis Rheum., *20*:895–900, 1977.

249. Wasserzug, O., Szeinberg, A., and Sperling, O.: Altered physical properties of glutathione reductase in G-6PD deficiency. (Abstract.) Hum. Hered., *27*:220, 1977.

250. Weiner, I.M., and Mudge, G.H.: Renal tubular mechanisms for excretion of organic acids and bases. Am. J. Med., *36*:743–762, 1964.

251. Weiner, I.M., and Tinker, J.P.: Pharmacology of pyrazinamide: metabolic and renal function studies related to the mechanism of drug-induced urate retention. J. Pharmacol. Exp. Ther., *180*:411–434, 1972.

252. Wilson, D., Collins, D.H., and Mason, R.M.: Gout. Proc. R. Soc. Med., *44*:285–292, 1951.

253. Wilson, J.M., and Kelley, W.N.: Molecular basis of hypoxanthine-guanine phosphoribosyltransferase deficiency in a patient with the Lesch-Nyhan syndrome. J. Clin. Invest., *71*:1,331–1,335, 1983.

254. Wilson, J.M., and Kelley, W.N.: Molecular characterization of hypoxanthine-guanine phosphoribosyltransferase deficiency in man. (Abstract.) Clin. Res., *31*:479A, 1983.

255. Wolfson, S.Q., et al.: The transport and excretion of uric acid in man. V. A sex difference in urate metabolism. J. Clin. Endocrinol. Metab., *9*:749–767, 1949.

256. Wolfson, S.Q., Cohn, C., and Levine, R.: Rapid treatment of acute gouty arthritis by concurrent administration of pituitary adrenocorticotrophic hormone. (Abstract.) J. Lab. Clin. Med., *34*:1766, 1949.

257. Wollaston, W.H.: On gouty and urinary concretions. Philos. Trans. Lond., *87*:386–400, 1797.

258. Wood, A.W., and Seegmiller, J.E.: Properties of 5-phosphoribosyl-1-pyrophosphate amidotransferase from human lymphoblasts. J. Biol. Chem., *248*:138–143, 1973.

259. Wood, M.H., et al.: The Lesch-Nyhan syndrome: report of three cases. Aust. N.Z. J. Med., *1*:57–64, 1972.

260. Wyngaarden, J.B.: Gout. *In* The Metabolic Basis of Inherited Disease. 2nd Ed. Edited by J.S. Stanbury, J.B. Wyngaarden, and D.S. Fredrickson. New York, McGraw-Hill, 1966, pp. 667–728.

261. Wyngaarden, J.B.: Gout. Adv. Metab. Disord., *2*:1–78, 1965.

262. Wyngaarden, J.B.: Gout. *In* The Metabolic Basis of Inherited Disease. Edited by J.B. Stanbury, D.S. Fredrickson, and J.B. Wyngaarden, New York, McGraw-Hill, 1960, pp. 679–760.

263. Wyngaarden, J.B.: The role of the kidney in the pathogenesis and treatment of gout. Arthritis Rheum., *1*:191–203, 1958.

264. Wyngaarden, J.B.: Overproduction of uric acid as the cause of hyperuricemia in primary gout. J. Clin. Invest., *36*:1,508–1,515, 1957.

265. Wyngaarden, J.B., et al.: Utilization of hypoxanthine, adenine, and 4-amino-5-imidazolecarboxamide for uric acid synthesis in man. Metabolism, *8*:455–464, 1959.

266. Wyngaarden, J.B., and Kelley, W.N.: Gout. *In* The Metabolic Basis of Inherited Disease. 4th Ed. Edited by J.B. Stanbury, J.B. Wyngaarden, and D.S. Fredrickson. New York, McGraw-Hill, 1978, pp. 916–1,010.

267. Wyngaarden, J.B., and Kelley, W.N.: Gout and Hyperuricemia. New York, Grune and Stratton, 1976.

268. Wyngaarden, J.B., and Stetten, D., Jr.: Uricolysis in normal man. J. Biol. Chem., *203*:9–21, 1953.

269. Yu, T.-F.: Milestones in the treatment of gout. Am. J. Med., *56*:676–685, 1974.

270. Yu, T.-F.: Secondary gout associated with myeloproliferative diseases. Arthritis Rheum., *8*:765–771, 1965.

271. Yu, T.-F., et al.: A simultaneous study of glycine-N[15] incorporation into uric acid and heme, and of Fe[59] utilization, in a case of gout associated with polycythemia secondary to congenital heart disease. Am. J. Med., *15*:845–856, 1953.

272. Yu, T.-F., and Gutman, A.B.: Uric acid nephrolithiasis in gout: predisposing factors. Ann. Intern. Med., *67*:1,133–1,148, 1967.

273. Yu, T.-F., and Gutman, A.B.: Study of the paradoxical effects of salicylate in low, intermediate and high dosage on the renal mechanisms for excretion of urate in man. J. Clin. Invest., *38*:1,298–1,315, 1959.

274. Zimmer, J.G., and Demis, D.J.: Associations between gout, psoriasis, and sarcoidosis: with consideration of their pathologic significance. Ann. Intern. Med., *64*:786–796, 1966.

275. Zollner, N.: Modern gout problem: etiology, pathogenesis, clinical manifestations. Ergeb. Inn. Med. Kinderheilkd., *14*:321–389, 1960.

276. Zollner, N., and Griebsch, A.: Diet and gout. Adv. Exp. Med. Biol., *41B*:435–442, 1974.

Chapter 92

Management of Hyperuricemia

Robert L. Wortmann

Hyperuricemia is a common clinical state with many possible causes. Progress in the understanding of purine metabolism, knowledge of the potential consequences of this condition, and the availability of excellent therapeutic measures have rendered hyperuricemia one of the most rationally manageable conditions in medicine. Because of these factors, the treatment of hyperuricemia should be safe, effective, and satisfying for both patient and physician.

GENERAL PRINCIPLES

Hyperuricemia refers to an elevated serum urate concentration. This laboratory finding is present in 2% of adult males in the United States,[53] and 17% in France.[132] The incidence of hyperuricemia was 13.2% in a large series of hospitalized adult male patients.[90] Hyperuricemia does not represent a specific disease, nor is it an indication for therapy. Rather, the finding of hyperuricemia is an indication to determine its origin, and a decision to treat this condition is based on the cause and the consequences in each hyperuricemic patient. Rational management requires that the physician answer the following questions: (1) Is the individual truly hyperuricemic? (2) What is the cause of the hyperuricemia? (3) Should the serum urate concentration be lowered?

Definition of Hyperuricemia (see also Chap. 91)

Hyperuricemia is defined as a serum urate concentration greater than 7.0 mg/dl measured by the specific uricase method. The physicochemical saturation of urate in plasma occurs at this concentration, and in epidemiologic studies of healthy adults not selected for gout or hyperuricemia, 95% of the individuals had serum urate concentrations below this value.[84] The method used for urate determination is important because obsolete nonspecific colorimetric methods are still used and may detect reducing substances other than urate and may provide artificially high values, when compared to those obtained by the specific uricase method.* It is therefore important to know the method employed, to interpret laboratory results properly.

Because the decision to treat hyperuricemia is usually a commitment to therapy for life, it is essential to document that the hyperuricemia is real and sustained. Certainly, the decision should not be based solely on the result of one test. Serum urate concentrations vary with age and sex, fluctuate throughout the day in some individuals, and may be subject to seasonal variation. Other factors such as recent weight loss, heavy physical exertion, or renal functional impairment may alter the serum urate concentration. The ingestion of many substances, such as alcohol, diuretics, or salicylates in doses under 2 g/day, may cause hyperuricemia.

Workup of Hyperuricemia

Although the finding of hyperuricemia is not necessarily an indication for treatment, one must determine the cause. Hyperuricemia may be easily explained and judged clinically insignificant, or it may reflect a serious medical problem. Knowledge of the cause helps one to decide whether and how the condition should be treated. Fortunately, the cause can be easily determined in 70% of patients by means of medical history and physical examination alone.[90]

Traditionally, hyperuricemia has been classified as either primary or secondary. Primary hyperuricemia refers to an elevated serum urate concentration the cause of which is not understood, or if it is known, hyperuricemia is its first manifestation, as for example, hypoxanthine-guanine phophoribosyltransferase deficiency. Secondary hyperuricemias are those ascribed to some other disorder or therapy in which the basic defect is understood. A more practical classification of hyperuricemia is based on the underlying pathophysiologic features. As reviewed in Chapter 91, hyperuricemia results from urate overproduction, from decreased uric acid excretion, or from a combination of these two mechanisms.

---

*Automated specific enzymatic methods are now used in most modern hospital clinical chemistry laboratories.

A 24-hour urinary uric acid measurement should be obtained to determine whether hyperuricemia in a given patient is the consequence of overproduction or of decreased excretion.[117] On a purine-free diet, normal men excrete 164 to 588 mg uric acid/day.[99] Hyperuricemic individuals who excrete more than 600 mg uric acid/day while on a purine-free diet are hyperuricemic because of purine overproduction, and those excreting less than 600 mg are most often hyperuricemic because of inadequate excretion. If the assessment is performed while the patient is on a regular diet, then a value of 800 mg/24 hours can be used.

Interpretation of 24-hour urine uric acid excretion requires attention to three factors. First, the foregoing values were determined in subjects with normal renal function. Because impaired renal function decreases the amount of urate filtered in the glomeruli, less uric acid appears in the urine. Consequently, a 24-hour urinary uric acid value of under 600 mg, or under 800 mg with regular diet, does not necessarily rule out urate overproduction in a patient with renal failure. On the other hand, elevated values in the presence of renal failure are strong evidence of purine overproduction. Second, it is essential to know the method employed by the laboratory to measure the uric acid in urine. The normal values given previously are for the specific uricase method. Colorimetric methods are even less specific in urine than they are in serum because drugs and chromogens normally found in urine often cause spuriously high values. These normal chromogens are increased in patients with renal failure. Third, one must ascertain that the patient is not taking a uricosuric agent at the time of urine collection. Corticosteroids, ascorbic acid, phenylbutazone, salicylates in doses greater than 2 g/24 hours, and other agents (Table 92–1) promote urate excretion and interfere with the interpretation of results.

It is useful to know whether the hyperuricemia is due to overproduction or to decreased excretion because it narrows the list of conditions that may have caused the hyperuricemia (Table 92–2). If such a factor or disease is identified, then the hyperuricemia should be considered secondary, and initial attempts at management should be directed to treating or eliminating the primary cause. In addition, knowing whether hyperuricemia is due to overproduction or to decreased excretion helps in the choice of drug, if one is indicated.

Exactly when hyperuricemia should be treated is a complex, much debated question. In patients, with frequent attacks of acute gouty arthritis or tophi, therapy is clearly indicated. Similarly, if the serum urate concentration can be lowered by treatment of an underlying disease or by removing an etiologic factor, then such steps should be taken. The use of specific urate-lowering drugs to treat asymptomatic hyperuricemia, whether primary or secondary in origin, or in patients who have had only a single acute episode, is controversial.

Treatment with urate-lowering medications is inconvenient, costly, and potentially toxic. Moreover, because these drugs are prescribed for the rest of the patient's life, they should not be used without definite indication. The decision to treat should be based on the needs of each patient.*

The potential benefit-to-risk ratio should be weighed for each patient individually. Hyperuricemia can lead to gouty arthritis and renal disorders, and it is considered by some authors to be a risk factor for cardiovascular disease. Obviously, if evidence indicated that keeping serum urate concentrations within normal limits prevented renal failure or heart disease, no debate concerning treatment would exist, but such evidence is not available.

COMPLICATIONS OF ASYMPTOMATIC HYPERURICEMIA

Few data exist concerning the benefits of treatment of asymptomatic hyperuricemia. Thus, in deciding on a therapeutic regimen, one must evaluate

---

*Editor's note: A mistake made in the treatment of a chronic disease is a chronic mistake.

Table 92–1.   Drugs with Uricosuric Activity

Acetohexamide	Estrogens
Adrenocorticotropic hormone (ACTH) and glucocorticoids	Glyceryl guaiacolate
Allopurinol	Glycopyrrolate
Ascorbic acid	Halofenate
Azauridine	Meclofenamate
Benzbromarone	Phenylbutazone
Calcitonin	Probenecid
Chlorprothixene	Salicylates
Citrate	Sulfinpyrazone
Dicumarol	X-ray contrast agents
Diflunisol	Zoxazolamine

Table 92–2.   Classification of Hyperuricemia (see also Table 91–1)

	Primary causes	*Secondary causes*

Overexcretion
(24-hour urinary uric acid concentration greater than 600 mg on purine-restricted diet; 800 mg on unrestricted diet)
	Idiopathic
	Hypoxanthine-guanine phosphoribosyltransferase deficiency
	Increased phosphoribosylpyrophosphate synthetase activity
		Hemolytic process
		Myeloproliferative disease
		Lymphoproliferative disorder
		Psoriasis
		Paget's disease
		Exercise
		Glucose-6-phosphatase deficiency
		Artifactual
		    nonspecific method to measure
		      uric acid
		    patient taking uricosuric agent

Underexcretion
(24-hour urinary uric acid concentration less than 600 mg on purine-restricted diet; 800 mg on unrestricted diet)
	Idiopathic	Renal insufficiency
		Hypertension
		Acidosis
		Drug ingestion
		    salicylates (<2 g/24 hr)
		    diuretics
		    alcohol
		    levodopa
		    phenylbutazone (<200 mg/24 hr)
		    ethambutol
		    pyrazinamide
		    nicotinic acid
		Sarcoidosis
		Lead intoxication
		Berylliosis

the chance of the following complications if therapy is withheld.

Gout

The risk of gouty arthritis rises both with the degree of hyperuricemia and with age.[53,87] In most cases, gout develops only after 20 or more years of sustained hyperuricemia. Although certain individuals may be at high risk for developing gouty arthritis, it is unwise to treat asymptomatic hyperuricemia simply to prevent the first episode of acute gouty arthritis. No evidence indicates that structural kidney damage occurs before the first attack of gouty arthritis,[30,68] nor are tophi identifiable prior to that occurrence. Moreover, first attacks of gout are easily treated. It is best to withhold hypouricemic therapy until arthritis becomes manifest and the diagnosis is confirmed; this form of therapy is long term, and the drugs used are potentially toxic. The cost of the medication and the generally poor compliance in the treatment of asymptomatic problems both reinforce this position.

Renal Disease

Chronic renal disease is an important potential consequence of hyperuricemia. Progressive renal failure, a major cause of death in patients with gout,

accounts for 6.6 to 25% of the overall mortality.[110,131] An important question is whether asymptomatic hyperuricemia adversely affects renal function over time.

Hyperuricemia can affect the kidneys in three ways (see Chap. 91): (1) urate nephropathy, with deposition of sodium urate crystals in the medullary interstitium and pyramids and a giant-cell inflammatory response; (2) nephrolithiasis; and (3) uric acid nephropathy, a reversible form of acute renal failure caused by the precipitation of uric acid crystals in the tubules, collecting ducts, pelvis, and ureters and obstructing the flow of urine.

Urate nephropathy leading to renal failure is difficult to document and rarely encountered today. Concern about this manifestation does not warrant treatment of asymptomatic hyperuricemia. Urate nephropathy is a late event in the natural history of gout and has not been reported in the absence of previous gouty arthritis.[12,81,102] No evidence suggests that renal function is compromised at the time of the first gouty attack.[30,68]

The risk of renal failure from hyperuricemia alone is low. One study of 113 patients with asymptomatic hyperuricemia and of 193 normouricemic control subjects followed for 8 years found that azotemia, defined as a serum creatinine greater than

1.6 mg/100 ml in males and 1.3 mg/100 ml in females, occurred in 1.8 and 2.1%, respectively.[38] Thus azotemia attributable to hyperuricemia alone is infrequent, mild, and probably of little clinical significance.

No evidence indicates that treatment of asymptomatic hyperuricemia alters the progression of renal disease. A study of 116 patients, followed for 2.5 or more years, compared the effects of allopurinol versus placebo therapy in nongouty patients matched for serum urate concentration, mean creatinine clearance, blood pressure, and size. No statistically significant differences were found among the groups, and it was concluded that normalization of the plasma urate did not alter renal function.[95]

Even in patients with gout, strong evidence indicates that hyperuricemia alone is rarely damaging to renal function.[13] Long-term follow-up of renal clearance in 149 gouty patients suggested that various, independently co-existing diseases with associated nephropathy have the most significant impact on renal function, with aging itself a second important factor.[127] Studies of renal hemodynamics in 624 gouty patients confirmed that hyperuricemia alone did not adversely affect renal function. Associated cardiovascular disease, especially hypertension, independently occurring intrinsic renal disease, and aging did correlate with decreased renal function, however. Reduced inulin clearance was attributed to hyperuricemia only in patients with extensive tophaceous deposits, and even in this group, renal dysfunction was greater in patients with associated hypertensive vascular disease.[128]

The relationship between hyperuricemia and nephrolithiasis is complex.[124] Renal stones are 1,000 times more prevalent in patients with primary gout than in the general population, but uric acid nephrolithiasis occurs in patients without manifestations of gout, only 20% of whom are hyperuricemic.[4,109] Moreover, some nongouty patients with calcium oxalate stones also have hyperuricosuria.[15,89]

In gouty patients, the risk of nephrolithiasis is related to the magnitude of the urinary uric acid excretion and, to a lesser degree, to the extent of serum urate elevation.[129] Such data are not available for individuals with asymptomatic hyperuricemia, but the risk of nephrolithiasis in such patients was assessed in one study. The rate of stone formation was 2.8 times higher in asymptomatic hyperuricemic individuals than in normouricemic control subjects; 1 stone per 295 asymptomatic hyperuricemic patients per year, as opposed to 1 stone per 825 control subjects per year.[38] This risk is sufficiently low to justify withholding therapy until the occurrence of the first stone.

Acute uric acid nephropathy is rare and occurs almost exclusively in patients receiving chemotherapy for hematologic malignancies. It is of little or no concern in the context of asymptomatic hyperuricemia, and its treatment is discussed later in this chapter.

Cardiovascular Disease

Whether hyperuricemia is an independent risk factor for atherosclerotic cardiovascular disease is unknown. Hyperuricemic individuals, with or without gout, have a high incidence of hypertension and coronary artery disease. In the Framingham study, patients with gout had twice the risk of coronary artery disease compared to normal subjects,[52] but the risk was not increased for hyperuricemic individuals without gouty arthritis. No correlation was observed between hyperuricemia and coronary artery disease in the Tecumseh Community Health study.[85] A Finnish health examination survey showed that hyperuricemia was associated with more advanced heart disease, but was not an independent cause of cardiovascular disease.[92] Attempts to relate hyperuricemia and heart disease have been complicated by the frequent co-existence of obesity and hypertension. One study demonstrated that the hypertension and atherosclerosis observed in gouty and hyperuricemic individuals were not simply the consequence of obesity.[37]

Therefore, hyperuricemia itself cannot be labeled a direct risk factor for cardiovascular disease, and it is best considered an indicator. In patients with essential hypertension, hyperuricemia most likely reflects early renal vascular involvement, that is, nephrosclerosis,[83] and persistence of hyperuricemia following myocardial infarction is a sign of a poor prognosis.[116] No evidence indicates that lowering the serum urate concentration in either an asymptomatic hyperuricemic person or a patient with gout prevents cardiac disease.

In conclusion, probably no indication exists to screen asymptomatic individuals for hyperuricemia, but if hyperuricemia is found, its cause should be determined. The available data suggest that: (1) renal function is not adversely affected by elevated serum urate concentrations; (2) renal disease accompanying hyperuricemia is often related to poorly controlled hypertension; (3) correction of hyperuricemia has no apparent effect on renal function; and (4) hyperuricemia is not a true risk factor for coronary artery disease. For these reasons and because of the inconvenience, cost, and potential toxicity of antihyperuricemic drugs, it is reasonable not to treat, but merely to observe patients with asymptomatic hyperuricemia, regardless of the serum urate level. Correction of causal factors, if the condition is secondary, and control of associated problems such as obesity, hypercholesterolemia, diabetes, and particularly hypertension, are definitely indicated.

SYMPTOMATIC HYPERURICEMIA

Gout

The most common indication for lowering the serum urate concentration is articular gout. Because treatment is costly, lifelong, and potentially toxic, and because the differential diagnosis of acute monoarticular arthritis is extensive, accurate diagnosis must precede therapy. The finding of negatively birefringent crystals in polymorphonuclear leukocytes in synovial fluid or in subcutaneous tophi by compensated polarized light microscopy is definitive. The triad of acute monoarticular arthritis, hyperuricemia, and a dramatic response to colchicine* is presumptive evidence of gouty arthritis in the absence of crystal identification. Nevertheless, one should perform joint aspiration to search for crystals whenever possible until the diagnosis is proved.

Much debate exists concerning the appropriate moment to begin hypouricemic therapy in the course of gout. All authors agree that hyperuricemia should be treated in patients with recurrent attacks of gout, tophi, classic radiographic changes (bone tophi), or gout combined with nephrolithiasis. Some maintain that the first attack of acute gouty arthritis is sufficient indication to initiate therapy. Others argue that first attacks are easily, inexpensively, and effectively treated, and these physicians postpone urate-lowering therapy. Some individuals experience only a single gouty episode and may not have another for up to 42 years (mean 11.4 years).[56] In the Framingham study, 25% of the patients with acute gouty arthritis had only a single attack in 12 years of observation.[53]

A gouty patient should be educated about the disease and the logic and risks of therapy. Weight control is recommended for obese patients, and meticulous attention should be given to blood pressure control. A 24-hour urinary uric acid measurement helps determine the cause of the hyperuricemia and aids in selecting the most appropriate hypouricemic agent.[8,117,119] This measurement also influences the decision whether to start hypouricemic therapy after a first gouty attack because the prevalence of renal stones in gouty subjects correlates with the amount of urinary uric acid. One

study reported that 35% of patients excreting 700 to 900 mg uric acid/24 hours had nephrolithiasis; 50% of patients excreting more than 1,100 mg/24 hours had renal stones.[129]

If hypouricemic therapy is withheld from the patient with gout, a definite risk of destruction to bone and cartilage exists from the sustained hyperuricemia. All patients with gout have deposits of monosodium urate in their tissues. If hyperuricemia is not controlled, these deposits enlarge and are radiographically evident before subcutaneous tophi are found. In a study of patients with intercritical gout, 42% without subcutaneous tophi had radiographic changes characteristic of bony tophi.[86] One could not predict from the frequency of acute attacks, the history of therapy, or the serum urate levels at the time of evaluation which patient would show bony changes. Thus, if urate-lowering therapy is withheld from patients with gout. radiographic assessment is useful in defining the severity of the disease and provides useful information concerning the advisability of treatment.[7]

Before giving specific hypouricemic agents, the following criteria apply: (1) all signs of acute inflammation should be absent; (2) the patient should be counseled regarding factors capable of precipitating an acute attack and its prevention; (3) treatment with prophylactic colchicine should be started; (4) the patient should be advised that additional episodes of gouty arthritis are possible; and (5) he should be provided with anti-inflammatory medication with instructions concerning dosage should such an episode occur.

The goal of hypouricemic therapy is the reduction of the total body urate pool. The serum urate concentration, which reflects this pool, is lowered either with a uricosuric agent or with a xanthine oxidase inhibitor. Because any sudden increase or decrease in the serum urate concentration can prolong or trigger an acute attack, such therapy should be withheld until all signs of inflammation have resolved completely. Low doses of colchicine, 0.6 mg 1 to 3 times/day, are successful in preventing acute gouty attacks.[17,123] Prophylactic colchicine is most effective if started at least a week before the first dose of the hypouricemic agent is given and if continued until the serum urate concentration has been under control and the patient has been free of acute gouty attacks for a year.

Hypouricemic therapy, regardless of the agent employed, should be entirely successful, but it can succeed only if the dosage is adequate. Dosage is adequate when it is sufficient to maintain the serum urate concentration below 5.0 mg/dl. Extracellular fluid is saturated with urate at a concentration of approximately 6.4 mg/dl, and if the serum urate

---

*Rigid criteria for improvement as a result of colchicine therapy have been established: (1) major subsidence of objective joint inflammatory changes within 48 hours of colchicine therapy; and (2) no recrudescence of inflammatory joint manifestations within 7 days.[113]

concentration remains above this level, urate may still be deposited in tissues.

Nephrolithiasis

Medical prophylaxis of either uric acid or calcium stones in hyperuricemic patients is effective. Both types of stones occur in association with hyperuricosuria. The chemical composition of the stone should be identified whenever possible. Regardless of the nature of the calculi, patients should dilute their urine by ingesting fluid sufficient to produce a daily urine volume greater than 2 L. Alkalinization of the urine with sodium bicarbonate or acetazolamide may be justified for patients with uric acid stones because this process increases the solubility of uric acid. At pH 5.0, urine is saturated at a uric acid concentration of 15 mg/dl; at pH 7.0, saturation occurs with 200 mg/dl.[68]

Specific treatment of uric acid calculi is achieved by reducing urinary uric acid concentration with allopurinol, an inhibitor of xanthine oxidase. Allopurinol is also useful in reducing the recurrence of calcium oxalate stones in gouty subjects and in nongouty individuals with hyperuricemia or hyperuricosuria because uric acid may nucleate calcium stones.[16,88]

Uric Acid Nephropathy

This reversible form of acute renal failure is due to the precipitation of uric acid in renal tubules and collecting ducts resulting in obstruction. Uric acid nephropathy may follow sudden urate overproduction with marked hyperuricosuria, dehydration, and acidosis. Autopsy studies have demonstrated intraluminal uric acid precipitates accompanied by dilated proximal tubules and normal glomeruli.[100] Work in animals suggests that the primary early pathogenetic events include obstruction of the collecting ducts by un-ionized uric acid and obstruction of the distal renal vasculature.[18,104] This form of acute renal failure develops most often in patients undergoing an aggressive or "blastic" phase of leukemia or lymphoma prior to or during cytotoxic therapy,[42,94] but it has also been observed in patients with disseminated adenocarcinoma,[19] after vigorous exercise with heat stress,[69] and following epileptic seizures.[114]

Uric acid nephropathy is important because it is often preventable and because immediate, appropriate therapy reduces the mortality rates associated with this condition from 47% to practically nil.[94] In addition to hyperuricemia, ranging from 12 to 80 mg/dl,[23,66] and oliguria, the distinctive clinical finding is probably the urinary uric acid concentration. In most forms of acute renal failure with decreased urine output, uric acid excretion is normal or reduced,[106] and the ratio of uric acid to

creatinine is less than 1.0. A ratio of uric acid to creatinine greater than 1 in a random urine sample or in a 24-hour specimen may be diagnostic of uric acid nephropathy.[65]

Factors that favor uric acid precipitation should be reversed, and uric acid production should be blocked. Vigorous hydration by the intravenous route and furosemide administration are used to promote urine flow to 100 ml/hour or more. Acetazolamide, 240 to 500 mg every 6 to 8 hours, and sodium bicarbonate, 89 mEq/L, given intravenously, maximize the likelihood of achieving an alkaline urine.[63] It is important to monitor the patient's urine frequently to ensure that the pH remains above 7.0 and to watch for signs of circulatory overload.

Allopurinol, 8 mg/kg, is given as a single dose to inhibit uric acid production and thereby to decrease the concentration of urinary uric acid. If renal insufficiency persists, the daily dose should be reduced to 100 to 200 mg because allopurinol and its active metabolites are excreted primarily in the urine. Despite these measures, dialysis may be required. Hemodialysis should be employed because it is 10 to 20 times more effective than peritoneal dialysis in removing uric acid.[66]

THERAPEUTIC TECHNIQUES

Diet

Dietary considerations now play a minor role in the treatment of hyperuricemia, despite a fascinating history and abundant literature on the subject.[108] Strict restriction of purine intake reduces the mean serum urate concentration by only 1.0 mg/dl and urinary uric acid excretion by 200 to 400 mg/day.[50] Fortunately, modern therapeutic agents render attention to dietary purines rarely necessary.

Dietary counseling is important, however, and it should address the use of alcohol and associated medical problems such as obesity, hyperlipidemia, diabetes, or hypertension. Heavy alcohol consumption should be discouraged. An episode of excessive alcohol ingestion may cause temporary hyperlacticacidemia, may elevate the serum urate concentration, and may provoke an attack of gouty arthritis.[73] Long-term alcohol use increases uric acid production, hyperuricemia, and hyperuricosuria.[32,78]

Uricosuric Agents

Candidates for uricosuric agents are gouty patients who meet all the following criteria: (1) hyperuricemia attributable to decreased uric acid excretion (less than 800 mg uric acid/24-hour urine specimen while the patient is on a regular diet; or less than 600 mg on a purine-restricted diet); (2) age under 60 years; (3) satisfactory renal function (a creatinine clearance greater than 80 ml/min is ideal, but it should be at least 50 ml/min); and (4) no history of nephrolithiasis.

Uricosuric agents reduce the serum urate concentration by enhancing the renal excretion of uric acid. This process occurs by the partial inhibition of proximal tubular reabsorption of filtered and secreted urate from the luminal side of the tubule at a site distal to the point of uric acid secretion.[34,72,82,105] If employed at a dosage sufficient to maintain the serum urate concentration at around 5.0 mg/100 ml, which is well below the level at which urate is saturated in extracellular fluid, these agents not only prevent urate deposition, but also allow dissolution of existing tophi.[49]

During the initial treatment period, the patient has a negative urate balance, and urinary uric acid excretion is elevated above pretreatment levels. Once the excess urate has been mobilized and excreted, urinary uric acid values return to original levels. At this point, the patient excretes uric acid at the pretreatment rate, but at a lower serum urate concentration.[51] Early in the course of treatment, before a steady state is re-established, however, the risk of developing renal calculi is as high as 9%.[49]

Uricosuric agents may be effective in 70 to 80% of patients. In addition to drug intolerance, failure to control a serum urate concentration can be attributed to poor compliance, concomitant salicylate ingestion, or impaired renal function. Salicylates block the uricosuric effects of these agents, possibly by inhibiting urate secretion.[55] These agents lose effectiveness as the creatinine clearance falls, and they are completely ineffective when glomerular filtration reaches 30 ml/min.[118,125]

Figure 92–1 illustrates the chemical structures of the three uricosuric agents discussed in the following paragraphs.

Probenecid

The "era of hypouricemic therapy" began in 1949 with the introduction of probenecid and the observations that sustained use of this agent controlled hyperuricemia, could mobilize tophi, and was well tolerated.[47,49,111] Probenecid is readily absorbed in the gastrointestinal tract. Its half-life ranges from 6 to 12 hours, is dose-dependent,[21] and is prolonged by allopurinol.[112] This drug is extensively bound to plasma proteins, is largely confined to extracellular fluid, and is rapidly metabolized, with less than 5% of the administered dose recoverable in the urine in 24 hours.[20,49,112] Probenecid increases the half-life of penicillin, ampicillin, dapsone, acetazolamide, indomethacin, and sulfinpyrazone by decreasing renal excretion,

and rifampin by impairing hepatic uptake; and of heparin by retarding its metabolism.[120]

Therapy is begun at 250 mg twice a day and is increased as necessary up to 3.0 g/day. A dose of 1 g/day is appropriate for about 50% of patients.[49,125] Because the half-life is 6 to 12 hours, probenecid should be taken in 2 to 3 evenly spaced doses.

The potential complications of probenecid most likely to occur early in the course of therapy include precipitation of acute gouty arthritis and nephrolithiasis. Gouty arthritis is prevented by the use of prophylactic colchicine. Nephrolithiasis is prevented by starting therapy at low doses and by increasing the dose at a rate of 0.5 g every 1 to 2 weeks, by liberally ingesting fluids, and possibly by alkalinizing the urine. Hypersensitivity, skin rash, and gastrointestinal complaints are the major side effects. Serious toxicity is rare, but hepatic necrosis[93] and the nephrotic syndrome have been reported.[36,57]

Sulfinpyrazone

This analogue of a uricosuric metabolite of phenylbutazone possesses no anti-inflammatory activity and is a potent uricosuric agent. It is well absorbed through the gastrointestinal tract, with peak serum levels observed within an hour. The half-life of this agent is 1 to 3 hours.[14,22] Sulfinpyrazone is 98% bound to plasma proteins and is largely distributed in extracellular fluids. Although 20 to 45% of this drug is excreted unchanged in the urine, the majority is excreted as the parahydroxyl metabolite, which is also uricosuric.[14,48] In addition to the uricosuric properties, sulfinpyrazone has antiplatelet activity, mediated by thromboxane synthesis inhibition, rather than by its hypouricemic effect.[2]

Sulfinpyrazone therapy is initiated at a dose of 50 mg twice a day. The usual maintenance level is 300 to 400 mg/day in 3 or 4 divided doses, but 800 mg/day may be required for satisfactory results.

Sulfinpyrazone has side effects similar to those of probenecid, and the drug is generally well tolerated. Bone marrow suppression can occur, but is rare.[31,91] Because of the rapid absorption and extreme potency of this drug, renal calculi are potentially more common early in the course of its use than with probenecid.

Benzbromarone

Benzbromarone is a new halogenated uricosuric agent currently available outside the United States. This agent is debrominated in the liver and is excreted free or in the conjugated form primarily in the bile. Although a weak inhibitor of xanthine oxidase activity in vitro, the drug acts in vivo by

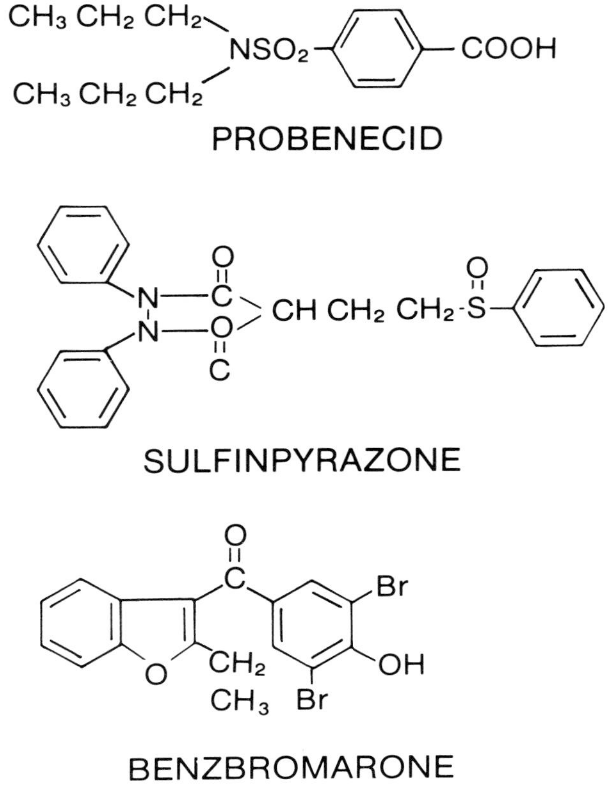

Fig. 92–1. Structures of uricosuric agents effective in the treatment of hyperuricemia.

inhibiting the tubular reabsorption of uric acid.[24,59,101]

Benzbromarone is effective and is well tolerated at daily doses of 25 to 120 mg.[24,79] This agent has been effective in patients with serum creatinine concentrations greater than 2.0 mg/dl and therefore may be useful for patients with renal insufficiency.[133]

Inhibitors of Uric Acid Synthesis

Another approach for controlling the patient's serum urate concentration is the use of agents that decrease uric acid formation. Such agents are effective in the treatment of all types of hyperuricemia but are specifically indicated for the following: (1) patients with gout and: (a) evidence of urate overproduction (24-hour urinary uric acid greater than 800 mg on a general diet; 600 mg on a purine-restricted diet); (b) nephrolithiasis; (c) renal insufficiency (creatinine clearance less than 80 ml/min); (d) tophaceous deposits; (e) age over 60 years; or (f) inability to take uricosuric agents because of ineffectiveness or intolerance; (2) patients with nephrolithiasis of any type and urinary uric acid excretion greater than 600 mg/24 hours; (3) patients

with renal calculi composed of 2,8-dihydroxy-adenine; and (4) patients with, or at risk for, acute uric acid nephropathy.

The most widely used compound in this group is allopurinol, which inhibits xanthine oxidase. Oxipurinol, the major metabolite of allopurinol, is available outside the United States. Although useful in some patients who are sensitive to allopurinol,[74,96] the clinical utility of this drug is limited by its poor absorption from the gastrointestinal tract.[25] Thiopurinol, which probably inhibits de novo purine synthesis,[5] has had limited clinical use.

Allopurinol

This analogue of hypoxanthine originally synthesized to be an antitumor agent is a potent competitive inhibitor of xanthine oxidase. It is also a substrate for that enzyme.[35] Oxipurinol is an analogue of xanthine and also effectively inhibits xanthine oxidase[80,97] (Fig. 92–2).

Allopurinol is completely absorbed from the gastrointestinal tract and has a half-life of 3 hours or less. Most oxipurinol formed is excreted unchanged in the urine and has a half-life of 14 to 28 hours.[28,54] Oxipurinol excretion is enhanced by

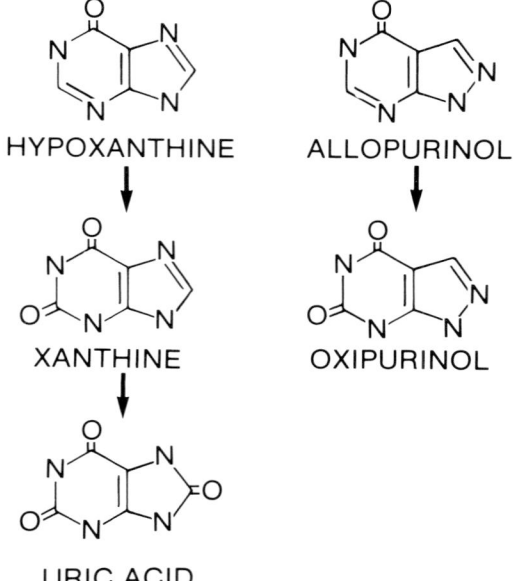

HYPOXANTHINE ALLOPURINOL

XANTHINE OXIPURINOL

URIC ACID

Fig. 92–2. Xanthine oxidase catalyzes the conversion of hypoxanthine to xanthine, of xanthine to uric acid, and of allopurinol to oxipurinol. Note the structural similarity of hypoxanthine to allopurinol and of xanthine to oxipurinol.

uricosuric agents and is reduced by renal insufficiency.[27]

By inhibiting xanthine oxidase, these compounds block the conversion of hypoxanthine to xanthine and of xanthine to uric acid. The administration of allopurinol leads to decreases in serum urate concentration and in the urinary excretion of uric acid in the first 24 hours, and a maximum reduction occurs within 4 days to 2 weeks.[98,121] This change is accompanied by increased quantities of the oxypurines,* hypoxanthine and xanthine, which are the more readily excreted uric acid precursors, in serum and urine.[67] Total purine excretion declines by 10 to 60% of pretreatment levels when allopurinol is taken.[25,67,98] This decline is due to increased salvage of hypoxanthine to inosine 5'-monophosphate and to the concomitant reduction in the rate of de novo purine biosynthesis, the metabolic consequences of allopurinol conversion to allopurinol ribonucleotides[26,40,62] (Fig. 92–3). Allopurinol is also a potent inhibitor of de novo pyrimidine biosynthesis,[64] but the significance of this observation is uncertain.

Between 100 and 800 mg/day allopurinol is required to control the serum urate concentration ad-

equately, and the dose for a specific patient depends on the severity of the tophaceous disease and on renal function. The average effective dose for most individuals is 300 mg/day.[126] The failure of an 800-mg dose to produce an adequate hypouricemic effect is rare and should cause one to question the patient's compliance. Allopurinol is effective in patients with renal insufficiency, but the dose should be reduced because of the prolonged half-life of oxipurinol. Therapy may be initiated at a low dose and may gradually be increased, to minimize precipitation of acute gouty attacks or to find the lowest effective dose, but this regimen is not necessary for most patients. Because of the long half-life of oxipurinol, allopurinol need be taken only once a day.[11]

Allopurinol is clinically effective. Resolution of tophi is generally obvious, the frequency of gouty attacks is reduced, and the patient's functional status improves when the serum urate concentration has been controlled for 6 to 12 months. Although the incidence of recurrent gouty arthritis is low in patients who discontinue allopurinol therapy after 2 years despite the return of their serum urate concentrations to pretreatment levels,[75] patients should continue to take the hypouricemic agent indefinitely once treatment is initiated.

Side effects, serious complications, and toxicity of allopurinol are unusual. Prophylactic colchicine is 85% effective in preventing episodes of acute arthritis that might be triggered by a sudden fall in serum urate concentration induced by allopurinol.[123] Because of the increased concentrations of oxypurines in the urine, xanthine renal calculi are possible. This complication is rare and has been demonstrated only 4 times, in patients with Lesch-Nyhan syndrome,[46,103] lymphosarcoma,[6] and Burkitt's lymphoma.[1] Microcrystalline deposits of oxipurinol, as well as of hypoxanthine and xanthine, have been demonstrated in muscle biopsy specimens from gouty patients taking allopurinol.[115] No clinical sequelae are known to result from that deposition, however.

The overall incidence of side effects from allopurinol is 5 to 20%, but only half the affected patients consider these effects sufficient to warrant discontinuing the medication.[77,112] The most frequent side effects include skin rash, gastrointestinal distress, diarrhea, and headache.[98,130] The most common rash is a maculopapular erythema, but exfoliative dermatitis and toxic epidermal necrolysis have been reported.[70,107] A mild rash is not a contraindication for further use of allopurinol. The drug should be stopped, but it may be reinstituted once the rash has cleared. Desensitization with low doses may be required in some individuals.[33]

More serious adverse effects include alopecia,

---

*Uric acid itself is the most "oxy" purine, but the term is usually meant to include only its "oxy" precursors.

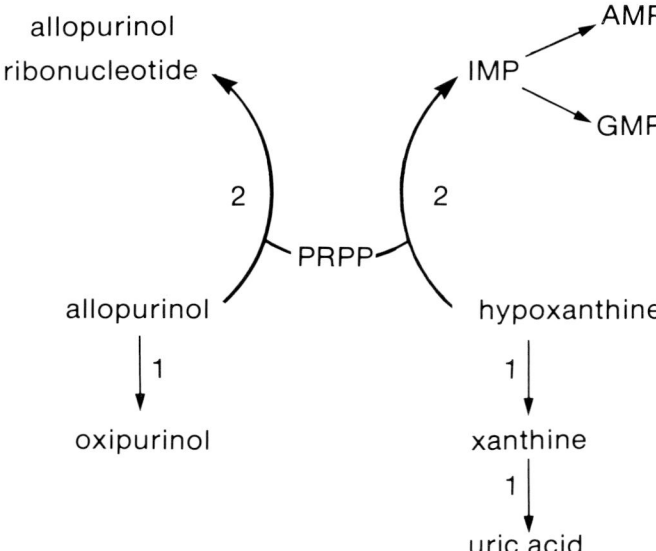

Fig. 92–3. Abbreviated scheme of allopurinol and hypoxanthine metabolism. The inhibition of xanthine oxidase (enzyme 1) by allopurinol and oxipurinol lowers uric acid formation by blocking the conversion of hypoxanthine to xanthine and xanthine to uric acid. Xanthine oxidase inhibition also results in the accumulation of hypoxanthine and allopurinol, which are converted to their respective ribonucleotide monophosphates by the action of hypoxanthine-guanine phosphoribosyltransferase (HGPRTase, enzyme 2). The formation of these ribonucleotides further decreases uric acid production by diminishing de novo purine biosynthesis (see Chap. 91) by three mechanisms: (1) inhibition of amidophosphoribosyltransferase activity by allopurinol ribonucleotide; (2) inhibition of both amidophosphoribosyltransferase and phosphopyrophosphate (PRPP) synthetase activity by inosine 5'-monophosphate (IMP), adenosine 5'-monophosphate (AMP), and guanosine 5'-monophosphate (GMP); and (3) depletion of phosphoribosylpyrophosphate. PRPP is not only a substrate for HGPRTase, but also is an essential and rate-limiting substrate for de novo purine synthesis.

fever, lymphadenopathy, bone marrow suppression,[45] hepatic toxicity,[3] interstitial nephritis,[44] renal failure, hypersensitivity vasculitis, and death.[76,122] Some data also suggest that allopurinol may cause or may worsen existing cataracts.[41,71] Serious toxicity is fortunately rare, but it is most often seen in patients with renal insufficiency or in those taking thiazide diuretics. Unfortunately, the majority of serious reactions have occurred in patients whose medical problems did not require allopurinol in the first place.

Potentially important drug interactions must be considered when allopurinol is prescribed. Because 6-mercaptopurine and azathioprine are inactivated by xanthine oxidase, allopurinol prolongs the half-life of these agents and thus potentiates their therapeutic and toxic effects.[29] Cyclophosphamide toxicity may be enhanced,[9] and a threefold increase in the incidence of ampicillin- and amoxicillin-related skin rashes has been reported in patients taking allopurinol.[10,60] On the other hand, allopurinol can reduce the toxicity of 5-fluorouracil.[58]

Allopurinol and a uricosuric agent may be used simultaneously in the rare patient whose hyperuricemia cannot be controlled by a single medi-

cation.[61] Although uricosuric agents increase the urinary excretion of oxipurinol,[27] this effect is balanced because allopurinol increases the half-life of probenecid by inhibiting microsomal drug-metabolizing enzymes.[112] Clinically, the drugs can be used in combination without modifying the dosage schedule of either agent. The addition of a uricosuric drug to a therapeutic program including allopurinol usually increases the patient's urinary uric acid excretion and further lowers the serum urate concentration.[98]

The use of allopurinol in acute uric acid nephropathy and in the hyperuricemic individual with nephrolithiasis has been discussed in previous sections. One additional indication for the use of this agent is in the treatment of 2,8-dihydroxyadenine kidney stones. Individuals with this condition have a homozygous deficiency of adenine phosphoribosyltransferase,[43] an enzyme that catalyzes the conversion of adenine to adenosine 5'-monophosphate. In the absence of this activity, adenine is converted by xanthine oxidase to the insoluble 2,8-dihydroxyadenine, which is excreted in the urine. Reports of 2,8-dihydroxyadenine stones are rare, most likely because of the chemical similarity between this compound and uric acid. X-ray powder diffraction analysis is necessary for correct identification. Stones of this type, however, may be more common than previously thought because the prevalence of heterozygous state for this enzyme deficiency in the general population may be as high as 1%.[39]

REFERENCES

1. Albin, A., et al.: Nephropathy, xanthinuria, and orotic aciduria complicating Burkitt's lymphoma treated with chemotherapy and allopurinol. Metabolism, *21*:771–778, 1972.
2. Ali, M., and McDonald, W.D.: Effects of sulfinpyrazone on platelet prostaglandin synthesis and platelet release of serotonin. J. Lab. Clin. Med., *89*:868–875, 1977.
3. Al-Kawas, F.H., et al.: Allopurinol hepatotoxicity: report of two cases and review of the literature. Ann. Intern. Med., *95*:588–590, 1981.
4. Armstrong, W.A., and Greene, L.F.: Uric acid calculi with particular reference to determinations of uric acid content of blood. J. Urol., *70*:545–547, 1953.
5. Auscher, C., et al.: Allopurinol and thiopurinol: effect in vivo on urinary oxypurine excretion and rate of synthesis of their ribonucleotides in different enzymatic deficiencies. Adv. Exp. Med. Biol., *41B*:657–662, 1974.
6. Band, P.R., Silverberg, D.S., and Henderson, J.F.: Xanthine nephropathy in a patient with lymphosarcoma treated with allopurinol. N. Engl. J. Med., *283*:354–357, 1970.
7. Barthelemy, C.R., et al.: Gouty arthritis: a prospective radiographic evaluation of sixty patients. Skeletal Radiol., *11*:1–8, 1984.
8. Boss, G.R., and Seegmiller, J.E.: Hyperuricemia and gout: classification, complications and management. N. Engl. J. Med., *300*:1,459–1,468, 1979.
9. Boston Collaborative Drug Surveillance Program: Allopurinol and cytotoxic drugs: interactions in relation to bone marrow depression. JAMA, *227*:1,036–1,040, 1974.
10. Boston Collaborative Drug Surveillance Program: Excess of ampicillin rashes associated with allopurinol or hyperuricemia. N. Engl. J. Med., *286*:505–507, 1972.
11. Brewis, I., Ellis, R.M., and Scott, J.T.: Single daily dose of allopurinol. Ann. Rheum. Dis., *34*:256–259, 1975.
12. Brown, J., and Mallory, G.K.: Renal changes in gout. N. Engl. J. Med., *243*:325–329, 1950.
13. Burger, L., and Yu, T.-F.: Renal function in gout. IV. An analysis of 524 gouty subjects including long-term follow-up studies. Am. J. Med., *59*:605–613, 1975.
14. Burns, J.J., et al.: A potent new uricosuric agent, the sulfoxide metabolite of the phenylbutazone analogue, G-25671. J. Pharmacol. Exp. Ther., *119*:418–426, 1957.
15. Coe, F.L.: Hyperuricosuric calcium oxalate nephrolithiasis. Kidney Int., *13*:418–426, 1978.
16. Coe, F.L.: Treated and untreated recurrent calcium nephrolithiasis in patients with idiopathic hypercalciuria, hyperuricosuria, or no metabolic disorder. Ann. Intern. Med., *87*:404–410, 1977.
17. Cohen, A.: Gout. Am. J. Med. Sci., *192*:448–493, 1936.
18. Conger, J.D., et al.: A micropuncture study of the early phase of acute urate nephropathy. J. Clin. Invest., *58*:681–689, 1976.
19. Crittenden, D.R., and Ackerman, G.I.: Hyperuricemic acute renal failure in disseminated carcinoma. Arch. Intern. Med., *137*:97–99, 1977.
20. Dayton, P.G., et al.: Studies of the fate of metabolites and analogs of probenecid: the significance of metabolic sites, especially lack of ring hydroxylation. Drug Metab. Dispos., *1*:742–751, 1973.
21. Dayton, P.G., et al.: The physiological disposition of probenecid, including renal clearance in man, studied by an improved method for its estimation in biological material. J. Pharmacol. Exp. Ther., *140*:278–286, 1963.
22. Dayton, P.G., et al.: Metabolism of sulfinpyrazone (An-
turane) and other thio analogues of phenylbutazone in man. J. Pharmacol. Exp. Ther., *132*:287–290, 1961.
23. Deger, G.E., and Wagoner, R.D.: Peritoneal dialysis in acute uric acid nephropathy. Mayo Clin. Proc., *47*:189–192, 1972.
24. deGery, A., et al.: Treatment of gout and hyperuricemia by benzbromarone, ethyl-2 (dibromo-3,5-hydrox-4-benzoyl)-3 benzofuran. Adv. Exp. Med. Biol., *41B*:683–689, 1974.
25. Delbarre, F., et al.: Treatment of gout with allopurinol: a study of 106 cases. Ann. Rheum. Dis., *25*:627–633, 1966.
26. Edwards, N.L., et al.: Enhanced purine salvage during allopurinol therapy: an important pharmacologic property in humans. J. Lab. Clin. Med., *98*:673–683, 1981.
27. Elion, G.B., et al.: Renal clearance of oxypurinol, the chief metabolite of allopurinol. Am. J. Med., *45*:69–77, 1968.
28. Elion, G.B., et al.: Metabolic studies of allopurinol, an inhibitor of xanthine oxidase. Biochem. Pharmacol., *15*:863–880, 1966.
29. Elion, G.B., et al.: Potentiation by inhibition of drug degradation: 6-substituted purines and xanthine oxidase. Biochem. Pharmacol., *12*:85–93, 1963.
30. Emmerson, B.T.: The clinical differentiation of lead gout from primary gout. Arthritis Rheum., *11*:623–634, 1968.
31. Emmerson, B.T.: A comparison of uricosuric agents in gout, with special reference to sulfinpyrazone. Med. J. Aust., *1*:839–844, 1963.
32. Faller, J., and Fox, I.H.: Ethanol-induced hyperuricemia: evidence for increased urate production and activation of adenine nucleotide turnover. N. Engl. J. Med., *307*:1,598–1,602, 1982.
33. Fam, A.G., Paton, T.W., and Chaiton, A.: Reinstitution of allopurinol therapy for gouty arthritis after cutaneous reactions. Can. Med. Assoc. J., *123*:128–129, 1980.
34. Fanelli, G.M., Jr.: Uricosuric agents. Arthritis Rheum., *18 (Suppl.)*:853–858, 1975.
35. Feigelson, P., Davidson, J.K., and Robins, P.K.: Pyrazolopyrimidines as inhibitors and substrates of xanthine oxidase. J. Biol. Chem., *226*:993–1,000, 1957.
36. Ferris, T.F., Morgan, W.S., and Levitin, H.: Nephrotic syndrome caused by probenecid. N. Engl. J. Med., *256*:592–596, 1957.
37. Fessel, W.J.: High uric acid as an indicator of cardiovascular disease: independence from obesity. Am. J. Med., *68*:401–404, 1980.
38. Fessel, W.J.: Renal outcomes of gout and hyperuricemia. Am. J. Med., *67*:74–82, 1979.
39. Fox, I.H.: Partial deficiency of adenine phosphoribosyltransferase in man. Medicine, *56*:515–526, 1977.
40. Fox, I.H., Wyngaarden, J.B., and Kelley, W.N.: Depletion of erythrocyte phosphoribosylpyrophosphate in man: a newly observed effect of allopurinol. N. Engl. J. Med., *283*:1,177–1,182, 1970.
41. Fraunfelder, F.T., et al.: Cataracts associated with allopurinol therapy. Am. J. Ophthalmol., *94*:137–140, 1982.
42. Frei, E., et al.: Renal complications of neoplastic disease. J. Chronic Dis., *16*:757–776, 1963.
43. Gault, M.H., et al.: Urolithiasis due to 2,8-dihydroxyadenine in an adult. N. Engl. J. Med., *305*:1,570–1,572, 1981.
44. Gelbart, D.R., Weinstein, A.B., and Fajardo, L.F.: Allopurinol-induced interstitial nephritis. Ann. Intern. Med., *86*:196–198, 1977.
45. Greenberg, M.S., and Zambrano, S.S.: Aplastic agranulocytosis after allopurinol therapy. Arthritis Rheum., *15*:413–416, 1972.
46. Greene, M.L., Fujimoto, W.Y., and Seegmiller, J.E.: Urinary xanthine stones—a rare complication of allopurinol therapy. N. Engl. J. Med., *280*:426–427, 1969.
47. Gutman, A.B.: Uric acid metabolism and gout: combined staff clinic. Am. J. Med., *9*:799–817, 1950.
48. Gutman, A.B., et al.: A study of the inverse relationship between pK_a and rate of renal excretion of phenylbutazone analogs in man and dog. Am. J. Med., *29*:1,017–1,033, 1960.

49. Gutman, A.B., and Yu, T.-F.: Protracted uricosuric therapy in tophaceous gout. Lancet, 2:1,258–1,260, 1957.

50. Gutman, A.B., and Yu, T.-F.: Gout, a derangement of purine metabolism. Adv. Intern. Med., 5:227–302, 1952.

51. Gutman, A.B., and Yu, T.-F.: Benemid (p-[di-n-propylsulfamyl] benzoic acid) as uricosuric agent in chronic gouty arthrits. Trans. Assoc. Am. Physicians, 64:279–287, 1951.

52. Hall, A.P.: Correlations among hyperuricemia, hypercholesterolemia, coronary disease and hypertension. Arthritis Rheum., 8:846–851, 1965.

53. Hall, A.P., et al.: Epidemiology of gout and hyperuricemia: a long term population study. Am. J. Med., 42:27–37, 1967.

54. Hande, K., Reed, E., and Chabner, B.: Allopurinol kinetics. Clin. Pharmacol. Ther., 23:598–605, 1978.

55. Hansten, P.D.: Drug Interactions. 4th Ed. Philadelphia, Lea & Febiger, 1979, p. 255.

56. Hench, P.S.: The diagnosis of gout and gouty arthritis. J. Lab. Clin. Med., 22:48–55, 1936.

57. Hertz, P., Yager, H., and Richardson, J.A.: Probenecid induced nephrotic syndrome. Arch. Pathol., 94:241–243, 1972.

58. Howell, S.B., et al.: Modulation of 5-fluorouracil toxicity by allopurinol in man. Cancer, 48:1,281–1,289, 1981.

59. Jain, A.K., et al.: Effect of single oral doses of benzbromarone on serum and urinary uric acid. Arthritis Rheum., 17:149–157, 1974.

60. Jick, H., and Porter, J.B.: Potentiation of ampicillin skin reactions by allopurinol or hyperuricemia. J. Clin. Pharmacol., 21:456–458, 1981.

61. Kelley, W.N.: Pharmacologic approach to the maintenance of urate homeostasis. Nephron, 14:99–115, 1975.

62. Kelley, W.N., et al.: An enzymatic basis for variation in response to allopurinol: hypoxanthine-guanine phosphoribosyltransferase deficiency. N. Engl. J. Med., 278:287–293, 1968.

63. Kelley, W.N., et al.: Acetazolamide in phenobarbital intoxication. Arch. Intern. Med., 117:64–69, 1966.

64. Kelley, W.N., and Beardmore, T.D.: Allopurinol: alteration in pyrimidine metabolism in man. Science, 169:388–390, 1970.

65. Kelton, J., Kelley, W.N., and Holmes, E.W.: A rapid method for the diagnosis of acute uric acid nephropathy. Arch. Intern. Med., 138:612–615, 1978.

66. Kjellstrand, C.M., et al.: Hyperuricemic acute renal failure. Arch. Intern. Med., 133:349–359, 1974.

67. Klinenberg, J.R., Goldfinger, S.E., and Seegmiller, J.E.: The effectiveness of the xanthine oxidase inhibitor allopurinol in the treatment of gout. Ann. Intern. Med., 62:639–647, 1965.

68. Klinenberg, J.R., Gonick, H.C., and Dornfield, L.: Renal function abnormalities in patients with asymptomatic hyperuricemia. Arthritis Rheum., 18 (Suppl.):725–730, 1975.

69. Knochel, J.P., Dotin, L.N., and Hamburger, R.J.: Heat, stress, exercise, and muscle injury: effects on urate metabolism and renal function. Ann. Intern. Med., 81:321–328, 1974.

70. Lang, P.G.: Severe hypersensitivity reactions to allopurinol. South. Med. J., 72:1,361–1,368, 1979.

71. Lerman, S., Megaw, J.M., and Gardner, K.: Allopurinol therapy and cataractogenesis in humans. Am. J. Ophthalmol., 94:141–146, 1982.

72. Levinson, D.J., and Sorensen, L.B.: Renal handling of uric acid in normal and gouty subjects: evidence for a 4-component system. Ann. Rheum. Dis., 39:173–179, 1979.

73. Lieber, C.S., et al.: Interrelations of uric acid and ethanol metabolism in man. J. Clin. Invest., 41:1,863–1,870, 1962.

74. Lockard, O., Jr., et al.: Allergic reaction to allopurinol with cross-reactivity to oxypurinol. Ann. Intern. Med., 85:333–335, 1976.

75. Loebl, W.Y., and Scott, J.T.: Withdrawal of allopurinol in patients with gout. Ann. Rheum. Dis., 33:304–307, 1974.

76. Lupton, G.P., and Odon, R.B.: The allopurinol hyper-

77. McInnes, G.T., Lawson, D.H., and Jick, H.: Acute adverse reactions attributed to allopurinol in hospitalized patients. Ann. Rheum. Dis., 40:245–249, 1981.

78. MacLachlan, M.J., and Rodnan, G.P.: Effect of food, fast, and alcohol on serum uric acid and acute attacks of gout. Am. J. Med., 42:38–57, 1967.

79. Masbernard, A. and Giudicelli, C.P.: Ten year's experience with benzbromarone in the management of gout and hyperuricemia. S. Afr. Med. J., 59:701–706, 1981.

80. Massey, V., Komai, H., and Palmer, G.: On the mechanism of inactivation of xanthine oxidase by allopurinol and other pyrazolo(3,4-d)pyrimidines. J. Biol. Chem., 245:2,837–2,844, 1970.

81. Mayne, J.G.: Pathological study of renal lesions found in 27 patients with gout. Ann. Rheum. Dis., 15:61–62, 1965.

82. Meisel, A.D., and Diamond, H.S.: Inhibition of probenecid uricosuria by pyrazinamide and para-aminohippurate. Am. J. Physiol., 232:F222–F226, 1977.

83. Messerli, F.H., et al.: Serum uric acid in essential hypertension: an indicator of renal vascular involvement. Ann. Intern. Med., 93:817–821, 1980.

84. Mikkelsen, W.M., Dodge, H.J., and Valkenburg, H.: The distribution of serum uric acid values in a population unselected as to gout or hyperuricemia: Tecumseh, Michigan, 1959–1960. Am. J. Med., 39:242–251, 1965.

85. Meyers, A.R., et al.: The relationship of serum uric acid to risk factors in coronary heart disease. Am. J. Med., 45:520–528, 1968.

86. Nakayama, D.A., et al.: Tophaceous gout: a clinical and radiographic assessment. Arthritis Rheum., 27:468–471, 1984.

87. O'Sullivan, J.B.: The incidence of gout and related uric acid levels in Sudbury, Massachusetts. In Population Studies of the Rheumatic Diseases. Edited by P. Bennett and P. Wood. New York, Excerpta Medica, 1968, pp. 371–376.

88. Pak, C.Y.C., et al.: Is selective therapy of recurrent nephrolithiasis possible? Am. J. Med., 71:615–622, 1981.

89. Pak, C.Y.C., et al.: Mechanism for calcium urolithiasis among patients with hyperuricosuria. Supersaturation of urine with respect to monosodium urate. J. Clin. Invest., 59:426–431, 1977.

90. Paulus, H.E., et al.: Clinical significance of hyperuricemia in routinely screened hospitalized men. JAMA, 211:277–281, 1970.

91. Persellin, R.H., and Schmid, F.R.: The use of sulfinpyrazone in the treatment of gout reduces serum uric acid levels and diminishes severity of arthritis attacks, with freedom from significant toxicity. JAMA, 175:971–975, 1961.

92. Reunanen, A., et al.: Hyperuricemia as a risk factor for cardiovascular mortality. Acta Med. Scand., 668 (Suppl.):49–59, 1982.

93. Reynolds, E.S., et al.: Fatal massive necrosis of the liver as a manifestation of hypersensitivity to probenecid. N. Engl. J. Med., 256:592–596, 1957.

94. Rieselbach, R.E., et al.: Uric acid excretion and renal function in the acute hyperuricemia of leukemia. Am. J. Med., 47:872–884, 1964.

95. Rosenfeld, J.B.: Effect of long-term allopurinol administration on GFR in normotensive and hypertensive subjects. Adv. Exp. Biol. Med., 41B:581–596, 1974.

96. Rundles, R.W.: Metabolic effects of allopurinol and alloxanthine. Ann. Rheum. Dis., 25:615–620, 1966.

97. Rundles, R.W., et al.: Drugs and uric acid in man. Annu. Rev. Pharmacol., 9:345–362, 1969.

98. Rundles, R.W., Metz, E.N., and Silberman, H.R.: Allopurinol in the treatment of gout. Ann. Intern. Med., 64:229–258, 1966.

99. Seegmiller, J.E., et al.: Uric acid production in gout. J. Clin. Invest., 40:1,304–1,314, 1961.

100. Seegmiller, J.E., and Frazier, P.D.: Biochemical considerations of the renal damage of gout. Ann. Rheum. Dis., 25:668–672, 1966.

101. Sinclair, D.S., and Fox, I.H.: The pharmacology of hy-

pouricemic effect of benzbromarone. J. Rheumatol., 2:437–445, 1975.

102. Sokoloff, L.: The pathology of gout. Metabolism, 6:230–243, 1957.

103. Sorenson, L., and Seegmiller, J.E.: Seminars on the Lesch-Nyhan syndrome: management and treatment, discussion. Fed. Proc., 27:1,097–1,104, 1968.

104. Stavric, B., Johnson, W.J., and Grice, H.C.: Uric acid nephropathy: an experimental model. Proc. Soc. Exp. Biol. Med., 130:512–519, 1969.

105. Steele, T.H., and Boner, G.: Origins of the uricosuric response. J. Clin. Invest., 52:1,368–1,375, 1973.

106. Steele, T.H., and Rieselbach, R.E.: The contribution of residual nephrons within the chronically diseased kidney to urate homeostasis in man. Am. J. Med., 43:876–886, 1967.

107. Stratigos, J.D., Bartsokas, S.K., and Capetanakis, J.: Further experience of toxic epidermal necrolysis incriminating allopurinol, pyrazoline, and derivatives. Br. J. Dermatol., 86:564–567, 1972.

108. Talbott, J.H.: Solid and liquid nourishment in gout: selected historical excerpts, largely empiric or fashionable and current scientific(?) concepts in the management of gout and gouty arthritis. Semin. Arthritis Rheum., 11:288–306, 1981.

109. Talbott, J.H.: Gout. New York, Grune and Stratton, 1957, p. 205.

110. Talbott, J.H., and Terplan, K.L.: The kidney in gout. Medicine, 39:405–467, 1960.

111. Talbott, J.H., Bishop, C., and Norcross, M.: The clinical and metabolic effects of Benemid in patients with gout. Trans. Assoc. Am. Physicians, 64:372–377, 1951.

112. Tjandramaga, T.B., et al.: Observations on the disposition of probenecid on patients receiving allopurinol. Pharmacology, 8:259–272, 1972.

113. Wallace, S.L., Berstein, D., and Diamond, H.: Diagnostic value of colchicine therapeutic trial. JAMA, 199:525–528, 1967.

114. Warren, D.J., Leitch, A.G., and Leggett, R.J.E.: Hyperuricemic acute renal failure after epileptic seizures. Lancet, 2:385–387, 1975.

115. Watts, R.W.E., et al.: Microscopic studies on skeletal muscle in gout patients treated with allopurinol. Q. J. Med., 40:1–14, 1971.

116. Woolliscroft, J.O., Colfer, H., and Fox, I.H.: Hyperuricemia in acute illness: a poor prognostic sign. Am. J. Med., 72:58–62, 1982.

117. Wortmann, R.L. and Fox, I.H.: Limited value of uric acid to creatinine ratios in estimating uric acid excretion. Ann. Intern. Med., 93:822–825, 1980.

118. Wyngaarden, J.B.: Metabolic and clinical aspects of gout. Am. J. Med., 22:819–824, 1957.

119. Wyngaarden, J.B., and Kelley, W.N.: Gout and Hyperuricemia. New York, Grune and Stratton, 1976, pp. 284–289.

120. Wyngaarden, J.B., and Kelley, W.N.: Gout and Hyperuricemia. New York, Grune and Stratton, 1976, pp. 430–438.

121. Wyngaarden, J.B., Rundles, R.W., and Metz, E.N.: Allopurinol in the treatment of gout. Ann. Intern. Med., 62:842–847, 1965.

122. Young, J.L., Jr., Boswell, R.B., and Nies, A.S.: Severe allopurinol hypersensitivity: association with thiazides and prior renal compromise. Arch. Intern. Med., 134:553–558, 1974.

123. Yu, T.-F.: The efficacy of colchicine prophylaxis in articular gout—a reappraisal after 20 years. Semin. Arthritis Rheum., 12:256–264, 1982.

124. Yu, T.-F.: Urolithiasis in hyperuricemia and gout. J. Urol., 126:424–430, 1981.

125. Yu, T.-F.: Milestones in the treatment of gout. Am. J. Med., 56:676–685, 1974.

126. Yu, T.-F.: The effect of allopurinol in primary and secondary gout. Arthritis Rheum., 8:905–906, 1965.

127. Yu, T.-F., et al.: Renal function in gout. V. Factors influencing the renal hemodynamics. Am. J. Med., 67:766–771, 1979.

128. Yu, T.-F., and Berger, L.: Impaired renal function in gout: its association with hypertensive vascular disease and intrinsic renal disease. Am. J. Med., 72:95–100, 1982.

129. Yu, T.-F., and Gutman, A.B.: Uric acid nephrolithiasis in gout. Predisposing factors. Ann. Intern. Med., 67:1,133–1,148, 1967.

130. Yu, T.-F., and Gutman, A.B.: Effect of allopurinol (4-hydroxypyrazolo-(3,4-d) pyrimidine) on serum and urinary uric acid in primary and secondary gout. Am. J. Med., 37:885–898, 1964.

131. Yu, T.-F., and Talbott, J.H.: Changing trends of mortality in gout. Semin. Arthritis Rheum., 10:1–9, 1980.

132. Zalokar, J., et al.: Serum uric acid in 23,923 men and gout in a subsample of 4,257 men in France. J. Chronic Dis., 25:305–312, 1972.

133. Zollner, N., Griebsch, A., and Fink, J.K.: Uber die Wirkung von Benzbromarone auf den Serumharnsauerespiegel und die Harnsaureausscheidung des Gichtkranken. Dtsch. Med. Wochenschr., 95:2,405–2,411, 1970.

Chapter 93

Pathogenesis and Treatment of Crystal-Induced Inflammation

Daniel J. McCarty

Information pertaining to the cellular and molecular mechanisms of the inflammatory host response to several microcrystals characteristic of human rheumatic diseases is considered here. Although many questions remain unanswered, inflammation due to monosodium urate monohydrate (MSU) crystals is now one of the best understood types of inflammation in medicine. Other crystals related to arthritis include calcium pyrophosphate dihydrate (CPPD) and adrenocorticosteroid esters. That inflammation can be induced by basic calcium phosphate crystal aggregates in joints, skin, tendons, and bursae also seems clear. Basic calcium phosphate (BCP) crystals, comprising mixtures of carbonate-substituted hydroxyapatite, octacalcium phosphate, or tricalcium phosphate,[129] are associated with clinical syndromes discussed in Chapter 95. A summary of crystals identified in human joints appears in Table 4–7.

HISTORICAL ASPECTS

The constant presence of microcrystalline MSU in gouty joint fluid was reported in 1961.[126] Needle-shaped MSU crystals can often be seen under ordinary light microscopy, but compensated polarized light microscopy is much more sensitive and specific. The inventor of the microscope, van Leeuwenhoek, born in 1633, was the first to describe these crystals, having obtained them from a draining tophus[116] (Figs. 93–1, 93–2). Van Leeuwenhoek was unaware of their chemical composition because uric (lithic) acid was not discovered until 1776 by Scheele.[181] A.B. Garrod used polarized light microscopic inspection of fresh tissue sections, cut by hand with a razor blade, to identify urate crystals; he wrote in 1876 that ". . . in the constancy of such deposition lies the clue that has long been wanting; the occurrence of the deposit is at once pathognomonic and separates gout from every other disease which at first sight may appear allied to it."[60]

Phagocytosis of MSU crystals by both polymorphonuclear and mononuclear cells was described in recently erupted human skin tophi by the Viennese dermatologist Gustav Riehl in 1897,[174] a phenomenon rediscovered later in gouty joint fluid[120] (Fig. 93–3).

At the turn of the century, Swiss investigators Wilhelm His, Jr. and Max Freudweiler, working in Germany, reported an inflammatory response to injected synthetic MSU and other crystals in man and in several other species (Fig. 93–4).[19,20] Subcutaneous injections of crystals produced inflammation initially, and later developed into tophi that were histologically indistinguishable from those seen in natural gout.

An acute, inflammatory response associated with crystal phagocytosis after injection of synthetic urate crystals and control crystals composed of other substances into normal human and canine joints was described in 1962,[55] and a similar response to crystals injected into the joints of gouty patients was found the same year.[192] The terms "crystal deposition diseases" and "crystal-induced inflammation" were coined; the latter was characterized as dose-related, completely reversible, and nonspecific with reference both to host species and to chemical composition of the crystals.[123] Diamond and cholesterol crystals were not phlogistic in canine joints. Inflammation in human and canine joints after injection of microcrystalline adrenocorticosteroid esters was postulated as responsible for the "poststeroid injection flare" sometimes observed after the therapeutic use of such preparations.[125]

Recent Discoveries

Dicalcium phosphate dihydrate crystals, $CaHPO_4 \cdot 2H_2O$, have been found in patients with arthritis.[61,232] These relatively soluble orthophosphate crystals (brushite) were originally found in cadaver cartilage.[122] Dicalcium phosphate dihydrate appeared as punctate deposits in multiple cartilages of 2.3% and CPPD deposits were found in 3.2% of the 215 cadavers studied. With a single exception, these substances were mutually exclusive.

Gaucher and colleagues identified dicalcium phosphate dihydrate in cartilage removed surgically from a patient with radiologic chondrocal-

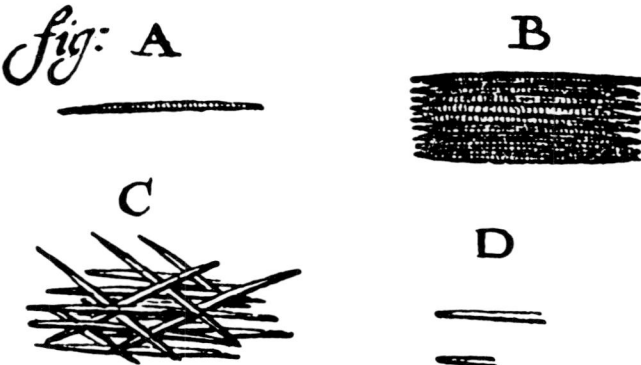

Fig. 93–1. *A* to *D*, Urate crystals from a draining tophus as seen in the seventeenth century by Antoni van Leeuwenhoek, inventor of the microscope. (Courtesy of *Arthritis and Rheumatism.*)

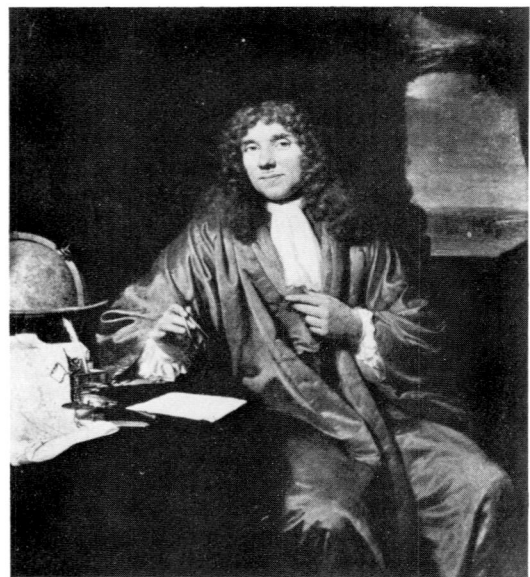

Fig. 93–2. Antoni van Leeuwenhoek, a draper from Delft, born 1633. (Courtesy of *Arthritis and Rheumatism.*)

cinosis and destructive arthropathy.[61] By scanning electron microscopy, these crystals appeared pyramidal (Fig. 93–5). Utsinger identified this substance by x-ray diffraction of crystals obtained from one patient with acute and two patients with chronic arthritis.[232] All three were men, and two of them had radiographic chondrocalcinosis. Dicalcium phosphate dihydrate only was identified in two instances, and they co-existed with CPPD crystals in one synovial fluid and CPPD was found once. Whether dicalcium phosphate dihydrate crystal deposition disease and crystal-induced inflammation are true entities is still unclear.

The term "apatite deposition disease" was suggested by Dieppe and colleagues in 1976,[42] but as indicated previously, the more precise term *basic calcium phosphate (BCP) crystal deposition* disease seems appropriate to describe their associated clinical syndromes.

A single case of cystinosis with intermittent pain involving both large and small joints was reported as "cystinosis with crystal-induced synovitis and arthropathy."[220] Crystals were found in bone marrow macrophages and histiocytes. Such crystals have been found in polymorphonuclear leukocytes of peripheral blood in this disease.[99] Whether *cystine* crystals induce clinically significant inflammation remains questionable. The reported case had radiologic evidence of epiphysitis in two joints. No crystals were found in joint tissues, much less inside joint fluid leukocytes.

Tyrosine crystals have been found within cells in the destructive corneal lesions in children with tyrosinosis and crystals, presumably tyrosine, formed within corneal epithelial cells in tyrosine-fed rats.[62] Moreover, some species of tyrosine crystals are membranolytic.[72,73] *Charcot-Leyden* crystals, some intracellular, have been found in inflammatory joint fluid associated with eosinophilia[46] (see Chap. 4). *Cholesterol* crystals may be found in fluid from either degenerative or inflammatory types of arthritis, especially in effusions of long standing.[15,42,52,56,57,254] Although cholesterol crystals obtained commercially have activated complement through the alternate pathway,[43,79] and injection into animal tissues has caused inflammation associated with phagocytosis,[168,231] cholesterol crystals have not been found within polymorphonuclear leukocytes in human joint effusions. Endotoxin contamination or the presence of cholesterol oxidation products not found in vivo in commercial preparations may invalidate any extrapolation of

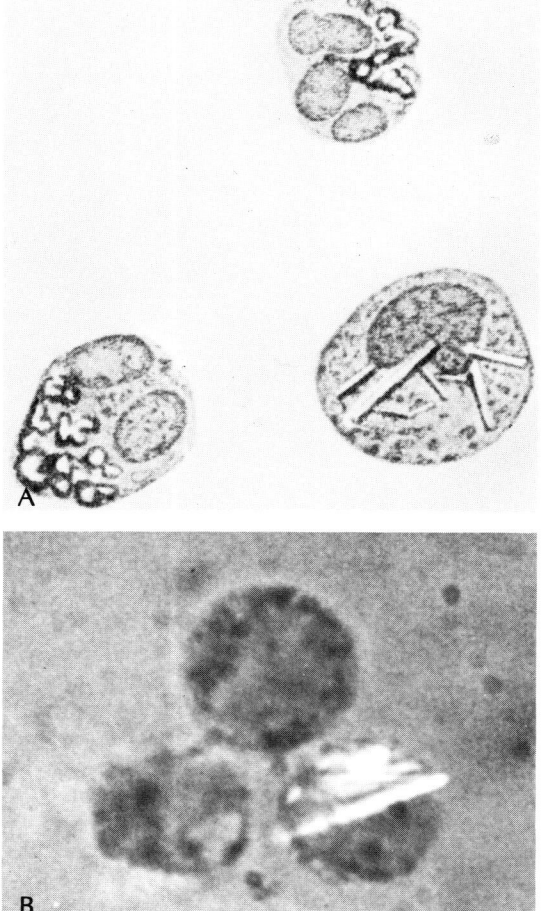

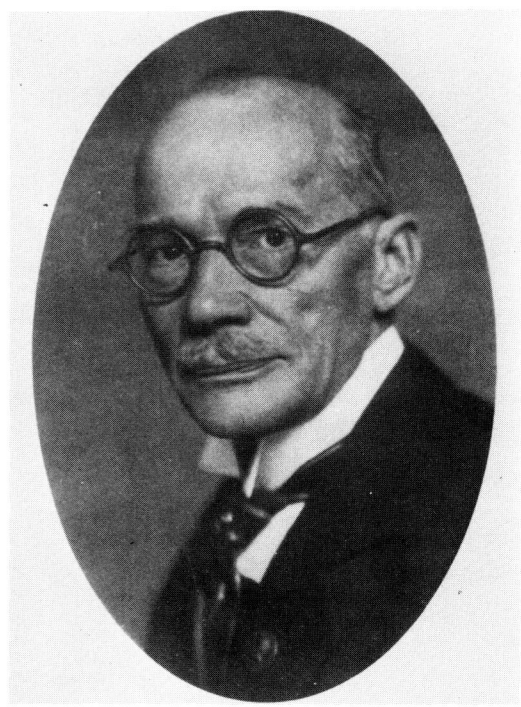

Fig. 93–4.   Wilhelm His, Jr.

Fig. 93–3. *A,* Synthetic monosodium urate crystals phagocytosed by a monocyte and two polymorphonuclear leukocytes. (From Freudweiler, 1901.) *B,* Natural monosodium urate crystals in a polymorphonuclear leukocyte (polarized light × 1,250). The lysosomes have been stained supravitally with neutral red.

these experimental data to human arthritis. The question of a possible relation of cholesterol crystals to joint symptoms in familial type II hyperlipoproteinemia remains enigmatic.[96,176,222] Treatment by lowering serum cholesterol levels decreased the frequency and severity of episodes of arthritis in one reported case.[27] Additional clinical studies and experimental work with better-characterized crystals are needed.

Similarly, the possible pathogenetic role of *calcium oxalate* or *aluminum phosphate* crystals, both described in long-term dialysis patients, requires further clinical and experimental studies (see Chap. 4).

IDENTIFICATION OF CRYSTALS

Techniques useful in routine clinical practice and in experimental work are discussed in Chapters 4 and 95.

SOURCES OF CRYSTALS

The following discussion focuses on the problems associated with the nucleation and growth of crystals in joint tissues.

Monosodium Urate Monohydrate (MSU)

In most instances, urate crystallizes as its sodium salt from oversaturated joint fluids. MSU crystals found in joint fluid at the time of the acute attack may derive from rupture of preformed synovial deposits, or they may have precipitated de novo (Fig. 93–6). The recognition of urate spherulites and of ultramicroscopic MSU crystals is discussed in Chapter 4. Acute attacks of gout have been correlated with the rate of change of serum uric acid, either up or down, rather than with a sustained high or sustained low level.[132] Rodnan found that acute gout precipitated by an oral purine load, especially when ethanol was ingested, occurred 18 to 80 hours afterward, when serum urate levels were falling rapidly to prefast levels.[175] This observation may account for the clinical finding of the occasional acute gouty patient with a normal serum urate level.

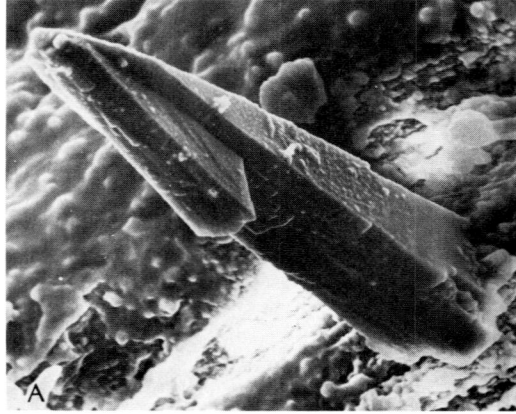

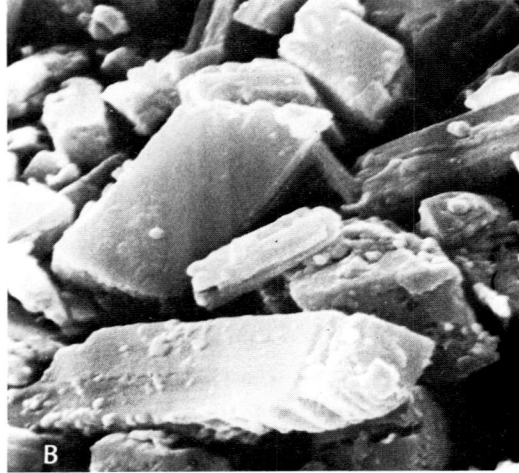

Fig. 93–5. *A*, Dicalcium phosphate dihydrate crystal from cartilage (scanning electron microscope × 1,900); *B*, Calcium pyrophosphate dihydrate from cartilage (scanning electron microscope × 10,000). (Courtesy of Dr. Gilbert Faure.)

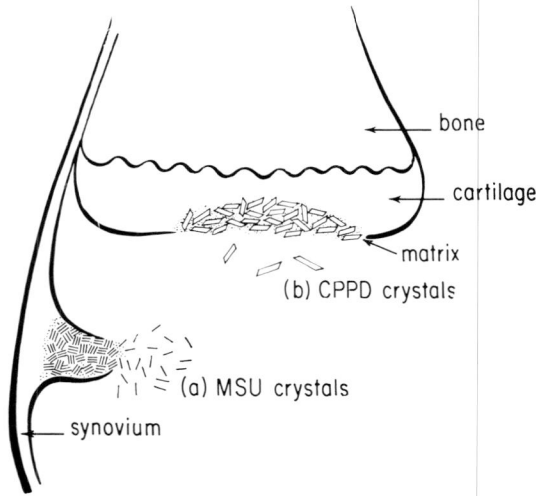

Fig. 93–6. "Autoinjection" of monosodium urate (MSU) crystals (a) from preformed tophus in synovium into adjacent joint space; and "autoinjection" of calcium pyrophosphate dihydrate (CPPD) crystals (b) from preformed cartilaginous deposit into adjacent joint space, due to "crystal shedding." Both concepts are still hypothetic and have only indirect supportive evidence. See text for details.

Treatment with allopurinol commonly produces this situation, an abrupt decline in urate levels and an acute attack of gout.

The consensus of arthroscopists convening at the Thirteenth International Congress of Rheumatology in Kyoto, Japan in 1973 was that the earliest urate crystal deposits were in the synovium, rather than in cartilage, were they appeared as white furuncles with an erythematous base. Several investigators have found tophi in synovial membrane at the time of the first gouty attack.[21,182] Urate crystals were found in 6 of 9 asymptomatic metatarsophalangeal joints that had not been involved in an acute attack of gout, despite MSU crystal-proved attacks in other joints.[246] This observation was confirmed in another study in which aspirates from 11 of 15 metatarsophalangeal joints of gouty patients

had extracellular crystals.[171] In addition, 1 of 8 asymptomatic hyperuricemic patients had MSU crystals in a metatarsophalangeal joint. These findings are not surprising because they merely confirm that gout, like CPPD crystal deposition, can exist in a lanthanic (asymptomatic) state.

Simkin has shown convincingly that the rate of diffusion of urate molecules from synovial space to plasma is only half that of water.[196] He envisions that the urate level in a small effusion in a dependent joint, such as the great toe, would equilibrate with plasma urate during the day. As the effusion resorbs during recumbency, a localized increase in urate level should occur. This phenomenon could account for those few patients who develop MSU crystals and acute gout in the absence of hyperuricemia, as well as for the usual nocturnal onset of symptoms in a dependent joint,[195] but it cannot explain why only some hyperuricemic individuals develop clinical gout.[112]

The decreased solubility of sodium urate at the lower temperatures of peripheral structures such as the toes and ears has been suggested as a reason why MSU crystals deposit in these areas.[97,109,250]

The recent finding by Katz of threefold elevations of serum uronic acid levels in patients with articular gout, but not in those with hyperuricemia or other inflammatory diseases, provides the first clue to the specificity of MSU crystal deposition.[90] The normalization of these elevated levels by the usual therapeutic doses of colchicine lent further credence to this finding and suggests that the prophylactic mechanism of colchicine may be different from that operative in the treatment of established acute gouty arthritis.[89] Katz was prompted to measure serum uronic acid levels, an index of serum glycosaminoglycans, because he and Schubert had found earlier that cartilage proteoglycans enhanced urate solubility.[91] These workers speculated that enzymes degrading proteoglycans might lead to local sodium urate crystallization. The elevated serum uronic acid levels in gout were thought to represent accelerated connective tissue turnover. The time- and dose-related suppression to normal levels of serum uronic acid by colchicine, but not by probenecid or allopurinol, suggests a presumed, as yet undefined, metabolic abnormality specific for gouty expression and unrelated to hyperuricemia.[89]

The increased urate solubility in proteoglycans is due to their aggregation by hyaluronic acid.[154] The original results of Katz and Schubert were probably caused by the potassium used to precipitate the proteoglycan, rather than by the proteoglycan itself, because potassium urate is more soluble than sodium urate.

The fundamental mechanism of MSU crystal formation in joint and other tissues remains unclear. The lack of tophi in gout secondary to the hyperuricemia of renal disease is well documented but unexplained.[50,201] The suggestion that lactate production by leukocytes in gouty joint fluid lowers the pH and causes further urate crystal formation[192] has received support by in vitro studies showing that lowering of pH enhances nucleation by the formation of protonated solid phases.[107,108] But the solubility of sodium urate, as opposed to that of uric acid, actually increases as pH decreases from 7.4 to 5.8.[98] Actual measurements of both pH and buffering capacity in gouty joints, however, failed to demonstrate significant acidosis;[217] pH changes therefore are unlikely to significantly influence MSU crystal formation, certainly not influences of the magnitude of the temperature effects already referenced.

Another series of studies examined the onset of MSU crystal nucleation by lengthy incubation of soluble sodium urate solutions.[223,224,225,250] The appearance of crystals was observed microscopically; the critical-threshold MSU concentration increased as the ratio of sodium to uric acid increased. Unfortunately, the physical instability of uric acid over time was ignored.[23] Although these data may indicate critical supersaturation levels, they give no information about the kinetics of crystal formation. The possible participation of a calcium urate phase was suggested by the finding that calcium only affected MSU nucleation when the solutions were also supersaturated with calcium urate.[223] Lead, at 1,000 μg/L, effectively nucleated MSU from normal saline solution containing 10 mg/dl urate.[225] Such high levels are found only in acute lead poisoning, so it remains unlikely that lead acts as a nucleating agent even in saturnine gout. The possible existence of joint fluid supernatant nucleating substances in MSU crystal formation was explored; fluids from gouty joints enhanced nucleation, those from osteoarthritic joints had less activity, and rheumatoid joint fluids had almost none.[224] The possible participation of ultramicrocrystals in the gouty fluids as "seeds" was not definitely excluded.

Calcium Pyrophosphate Dihydrate (CPPD)

The initial site of CPPD crystal formation is probably articular cartilage. Precipitation de novo in synovial fluid or synovium has not been ruled out, and CPPD crystals are found frequently in these sites. In hyaline cartilage, such crystals often lie in a granular matrix,[14,61,172] which stains more densely than surrounding cartilage with periodic acid-Schiff, alcian blue, colloidal iron,[100] and ruthenium red.[183] These features suggest the presence of abnormal proteoglycan (Fig. 93–6).

The generation of inorganic pyrophosphate (PPi) from cartilage and the nucleation and growth of CPPD crystals from solution and from gels are discussed in Chapter 94.

Assuming that the CPPD crystals lying in their cartilaginous mold of peculiar proteoglycan are in thermodynamic equilibrium with (Ca^{++} and $P_2O_7^{-4}$), the ions from which they were formed, conditions that either lower ionized calcium or reduce ($P_2O_7^{-4}$) should increase the solubility of these crystals and should free them from their mold. This still hypothetic phenomenon has been called "crystal shedding."[10] The marked effect of even small changes in ionized calcium level on crystal solubility in vitro,[11] the onset of acute pseudogout after lavage of joints with solubilizers of CPPD crystals such as edetate (EDTA) or Mg^{++}-containing buffers,[10] and the clinical correlation of acute arthritis with falling serum calcium concentrations recorded by O'Duffy,[151] as well as by Bilezikian and coworkers,[13] all support this hypothesis, however (Fig. 93–6). Joint fluid PPi levels are often higher than plasma levels.[6,113,121,179,194] Fluid PPi levels are lower during the acute attack,[194] owing to a more rapid clearance into the blood.[25] Thus, once an acute attack begins, the fall in ambient PPi may further increase crystal solubility and shedding.

Other postulated mechanisms for the "autoinjection" of CPPD crystals, which is presumed to precede acute pseudogout, are summarized in

Table 93–1. Mechanical disruption of cartilage accompanying subchondral microfracture was implicated in an acute attack developing for the first time in a knee joint with acute neuropathic changes,[12] and trauma is a common antecedent of acute pseudogout.[128] "Enzymatic strip mining" of crystals from preformed cartilaginous deposits was proposed to explain the occurrence of CPPD and MSU crystals in an osteoarthritic joint with superimposed acute pyogenic arthritis.[199] Numerous reports of this phenomenon have appeared and are reviewed in Chapter 4. Presumably, any significant intrasynovial discharge of inflammatory proteases might digest the components of the "mold" and might thereby release crystals into the joint space. CPPD crystals were readily released from cartilage by synovial cell collagenase, for example.[77] Thus, the mere presence of these or MSU crystals in joint fluid must be interpreted cautiously because they might be a result, as well as a cause of, joint inflammation.

Finally, the reported association of silent CPPD crystal deposition and hypothyroidism with the onset of acute pseudogout after thyroid hormone therapy suggests that metabolically induced changes in cartilage matrix may also release crystals.[45]

Basic Calcium Phosphates (BCP)

These ultramicrocrystals generally occur as aggregates, appearing as microspheroidal "snowballs" by scanning electron microscopy. Hydroxyapatite, partially substituted with carbonate, and octacalcium phosphate or tricalcium phosphate have been identified in these aggregates in synovial fluid and in a subcutaneous calcification from a patient with dermatomyositis.[129] The aggregates may appear purple with Wright's stain.[186] These crystals are discussed in detail in Chapters 4 and 95.

BCP crystals, like MSU[200] and CPPD[14,183] crystals, lie within a connective tissue matrix, the com-position of which is poorly understood.[124,169] They seem intimately associated with particulate collagen.[129] These crystals may gain access to joints or tendon spaces by rupture of preformed deposits,[18,37,124] or they may provoke extra-articular inflammation.[124,228] The clinical syndromes associated with BCP crystals are discussed in Chapter 95.

Corticosteroid Ester

Synovitis occurs after some but not all injections,[114,125] probably because of the anti-inflammatory effect of that portion of the dose that is in solution. The appearance of these crystals varies with the type of ester, with the batch, and with the storage conditions.[87]

MECHANISM OF CRYSTAL-INDUCED INFLAMMATION

The interaction of MSU crystals with various cells and molecules is summarized diagrammatically in Figure 93–7. The other crystals found in arthritis have not been as well studied, but they probably share some of these reactivities.

Protein Adsorption

Clearly, many of the biologic phenomena associated with crystals found in joint fluids are attributable to molecules adsorbed to their surfaces. Immunoglobulin G (IgG) was strongly adsorbed from serum to MSU, CPPD, and silicon dioxide microcrystals,[104] and it is found in gouty tophi.[83] Small amounts of albumin and other unidentified proteins were also adsorbed. Kinetic study of adsorption under physiologic conditions suggested that a monomolecular layer exists at the IgG levels found in joint fluid. Moreover, the adsorbed IgG was oriented with the Fc ends functionally available.[103] Crystal phagocytosis by human polymorphonuclear leukocytes was expedited when they were coated with IgG;[66] these cells have Fc receptors in their membranes.[147] In addition, IgG-

Table 93–1. Proposed Mechanisms of "Autoinjection" of Calcium Pyrophosphate Dihydrate (CPPD) Crystals from Cartilage to Vascular Joint Tissue Space

Trigger	Hypothetic Mechanism	Clinical Circumstances of Acute Attack
Fall in synovial fluid (Ca^{++}) or inorganic pyrophosphate level	Partial dissolution "crystal shedding"	Postoperatively or during acute medical illness
Mechanical disruption of cartilage architecture	Microfractures of subchondral bone	Trauma
Increased activity of enzymes degrading cartilage matrix	"Crystal shedding" due to removal of matrix by "enzymatic strip mining"	Pseudogout superimposed on another type of arthritis; i.e., pyogenic infection, acute gout, or osteoarthritis
Hypothyroidism with treatment	Altered cartilaginous "mold" with crystal shedding	Joint symptoms after thyroid hormone replacement

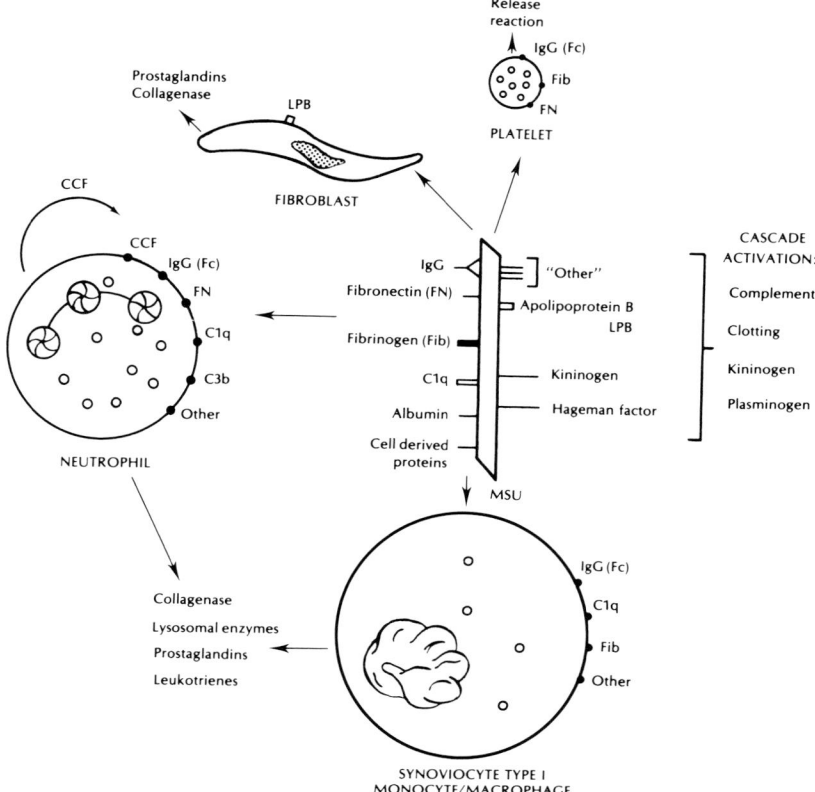

Fig. 93–7.   Schematic representation of interaction of monosodium urate (MSU) crystals with various cells and molecules. See text for details of how these interactions may lead to acute gout and to chronic destructive (tophaceous) gout.

coated MSU or CPPD crystals activated the release reaction from human platelets, but not from rabbit platelets, which lack Fc membrane receptors.[65,67,68,102] The reactivity of naked MSU crystals with human platelet membranes was shown to be due to four glycoproteins.[86] Enzymatic digestion of the proteins or use of specific F(ab')$_2$ antibodies against them abrogated the release reaction stimulated by crystals, but not by collagen or thrombin. The adsorption of IgG was thought to be ionic, based on elution studies.[104] Electrophoretic studies confirmed that adsorption of IgG to MSU and other crystals which, like most suspensoids, are negatively charged, was proportional to their cationic behavior.[79] Similar monomolecular adsorption of IgG from serum by latex beads was related to opsonization and phagocytosis by polymorphonuclear leukocytes through complement activation.[38] Immunoelectron-microscopic study showed large amounts of IgG and lesser amounts of IgM, IgA, C3, and fibrinogen adsorbed to natural MSU crystal surfaces in gouty joint fluids. Intralysosomal and extracellular crystals showed similar

amounts of adsorbed proteins.[33] Two-dimensional gel electrophoresis of eluates from MSU crystals exposed to plasma showed that more than 30 species of polypeptides had been adsorbed; both anionic and cationic molecules were found. Proteins increased relative to the starting whole plasma included C1q, C1r̄, C1s̄, fibronectin, fibrinogen, and kininogen.[227] Direct evidence for crystal activation of both complement and coagulation cascades was provided by the finding of activation fragments of C1 and kininogen. That C1 was activated even in immunoglobulin-deficient plasma confirmed previous evidence of direct C1q adsorption and activation on the surface of MSU crystals.[63] MSU crystal activation of the coagulation cascade by the contact system has been well characterized,[92,93,94,95] and it is associated with prekallekrein and high-molecular-weight kininogen.[64] An abundance of the cleaved form of kininogen was also eluted from MSU crystals.[227] Kininogen activation should result in the formation of bradykinin, which has been generated by MSU crystals in vitro,[92,245] and has been found in gouty synovial fluid.[148]

Immunoautoradiographic and SDS gel studies on eluates from synthetic MSU crystals exposed to gouty synovial fluid showed C1q, C3, IgM, and fibronectin; traces of albumin and variable amounts of IgG and C3 activation products were also found.[8] Products of polymorphonuclear leukocytes, such as acid phosphatase[182] and beta-glucuronidase,[66] were also adsorbed.

Finally, molecules are adsorbed to crystal surfaces that have antiphlogistic properties. Hyaluronate interferes with crystal phagocytosis.[17] More recently, Terkeltaub et al. have discovered that apolipoprotein B molecules adsorb to MSU crystal surfaces and have a profound and specific inhibiting effect on polymorphonuclear leukocyte function.[226] Apolipoprotein B accounted for nearly all the inhibitory activity of whole plasma. This large molecule exists only in trace amounts in normal synovial fluid, but its concentrations may approach 50% of the plasma level in inflammatory fluids. Thus, inflammation due to an "autoinjection" of MSU crystals may gradually subside as the concentration of crystal-associated lipoprotein rises. Tophaceous gout occurring in the absence of acute attacks and the presence of milky, crystal-laden joint fluid in the absence of leukocytes may be explicable in light of this new discovery. Because synovial fluid crystals are exposed to fibroblasts, platelets, monocytes, lymphocytes, and the various types of synovial cells in vivo, many of which have receptors for the adsorbed proteins, the complexity of the host reaction to MSU and other crystals is readily apparent (Fig. 93–7).

Inflammatory Mediators

Like nearly all colloids and suspensoids, MSU crystals are electronegative.[94] Like glass surfaces, these crystals bind, denature, and cleave Hageman factor (clotting factor XII). This process, in turn, activates the clotting, kininogen, and plasminogen cascades.[94] Hageman factor has been found in synovial fluid, and factors increasing vascular permeability were induced by adding activated Hageman factor to normal joint fluid.[92,93] Because acute inflammation followed the intrasynovial injection of MSU crystals into chickens, which lack Hageman factor, this molecule may not be a critical feature of the host response, however.[202]

Synovial fluid kinin levels were elevated by bioassay both in natural gout and in arthritis induced in a human volunteer by the intra-articular injection of MSU crystals,[148] but no diminution of inflammation was noted in a canine model of MSU crystal-induced inflammation when carboxypeptidase B, which hydrolyzes bradykinin to an impotent octapeptide, was injected into the joint along with the crystals.[166] Nor was an increase in ornithokinin

found in chicken synovial fluid,[202] although an anti-inflammatory effect of trypsin-kallikrein inhibitor on crystal-induced inflammation in rabbits was noted.[210] Thus, kinins do not appear to be a prereguisite for crystal synovitis, at least not in experimental models.

Pretreatment of dogs[161] and rabbits[203] with cobra venom factor lowered total serum hemolytic complement ($C'H_{50}$) levels, but it did not suppress inflammation induced by urate or CPPD crystals detectably. Complement depletion partially inhibited edema of rat paws injected with MSU crystals, however.[245]

Earlier work showing that MSU crystals deplete hemolytic complement when added to serum,[24,81,149,161] by activation of the classic pathway has been extended by the demonstration of adsorption and activation of C1q.[63,223] Complement activation was enhanced by prior IgG adsorption to the crystals and was much less evident in IgG-deficient serum.[178] Complement activation was restored by adding either IgG or C-reactive protein to the deficient serum. MSU crystals also activate complement through the alternative pathway.[43,80,81]

Joints are exquisitely sensitive to pyrogen, and amounts of pyrogen not detected by the usual intravenous test in the rabbit have produced marked synovitis.[85] My colleagues and I had always heated MSU and CPPD crystals to 180 to 200° C for 2 hours to destroy pyrogens that may have been trapped in the crystal from the mother liquor during its growth. This treatment totally destroys bacterial pyrogen deliberately added to the solution from which crystals are prepared. Such pyrogen is taken up by the crystals, which are then extraordinarily potent when tested in the dog model.[115,160] It is now clear that heating dehydrates MSU crystals to the anhydrous form,[23,32,41,139] and it affects the crystalline surface with respect to its zeta potential (net surface charge),[23,41] membranolytic potential,[21] and complement activation potency.[24,81,149,161] MSU crystals stimulated human blood monocytes to release endogenous pyrogen (interleukin 1), and this factor may account for fever accompanying acute gouty arthritis.[48] Calcium pyrophosphate and hydroxyapatite crystals failed to release pyrogen, however.[47] A synergistic effect of intravenously administered bacterial pyrogen and MSU crystals given intra-articularly has been demonstrated.[233]

The striking, complete suppression of tenderness, out of proportion to effects on swelling, local heat, and volume of local effusion, in synovitis induced by MSU crystals in normal human volunteers pretreated with aspirin suggests that prostaglandins may play a role as mediators of pain.[218,219] Rats on a diet deficient in prostaglandin precursors showed a diminished response to injected MSU crystals that was restored by the addition of prostaglandin E_1 (PGE$_1$).[39]

MSU crystals generated PGE$_2$ when added to either human or rabbit synovial fibroblasts in tissue culture.[78,82,133,249] This reaction was also produced by calcium oxalate,[78] calcium pyrophosphate, and hydroxyapatite crystals.[34] Chondrocytes[34] and macrophages[123] behaved similarly. The stable metabolite of prostacyclin (6 keto PGF$_1\alpha$) and 5 HETE, a product of the lipoxygenase pathway, were also released by MSU crystals.[249] Leukotrienes and hydroxy acids were released from human neutrophils or platelets exposed to these crystals.[193] The release of the potent chemotactic factor leukotriene B$_4$ was blocked by colchicine, as described later in this chapter.

Uric acid itself may have the ability to potentiate inflammation. Random motility of neutrophilic leukocytes,[230] and protein adsorption by the membranes of neutrophils,[135] may be increased and decreased, respectively, as ambient urate levels are elevated.

Crystal Interaction with Neutrophils

The neutrophil seems inextricably linked to the pathogenesis of acute inflammation mediated by MSU, CPPD, or basic calcium phosphate crystals. Intracellular crystals are a regular feature of gout, pseudogout, and acute calcific tendinitis.[115,120,124,128,192]

Phagocytosis

Synovial fluids from either acute gout or pseudogout show average leukocyte counts of 19,500 cells/mm^3, and 90% or more of these cells are neutrophils. A range of 1,000 to 70,000 cells/mm^3 was found in a large series of acute gout,[177] and others have reported up to 100,000 cells/mm^3 in pseudogout.[59] Crystals are often found within joint fluid phagocytes in residual effusions for months after apparent clinical termination of the acute attack or in chronically symptomatic joints that have not been the site of an acute episode, but the leukocyte counts in such patients are generally lower, and the total leukocyte response (concentration × effusion volume) is much less. The increased turnover of synovial fluid inorganic phosphate and pyrophosphate pools in the presence of even a few CPPD crystals is probably due to increased synovial blood flow and to low-grade inflammation.[25]

Most series report a few fluids from putative cases of acute gout or pseudogout in which no crystals are found despite an increased leukocyte concentration.[126,198,255] A collection of nine such fluids has been recorded.[187] Conjectural explanations include the following: (1) the presence of the primary inflammation in a contiguous bursa, with

needling of a "sympathetic" synovial effusion;[119] (2) dissolution or clearing of the crystals by fixed synovial phagocytes;[130] (3) the inability to detect crystals because they are below the resolving power of light microscopy (<0.5 μm); (4) the settling of crystals in a joint immobilized by pain; or (5) another cause for arthritis.

The converse phenomenon, the findings of crystals but few leukocytes in an inflamed joint, has also been recorded.[145,152] The release of eicosenoids from synovial cells by MSU crystals has been offered as a possible explanation,[249] but in view of the absence of inflammation after intrasynovial crystal injection in neutropenic experimental animals,[29,164,203] this hypothesis seems unlikely. MSU, CPPD, and basic calcium phosphate crystals are often found in the virtual absence of leukocytes in fluids from chronically symptomatic joints, sometimes in quantities sufficient to render a milky appearance. My long-held suspicion that molecules adsorb to the crystal surface and thereby reduce their phlogistic potency has been reinforced by the foregoing apolipoprotein B discovery. Whether such molecules are also responsible for apparently effete CPPD or basic calcium phosphate crystals remains to be explored.

Certainly, the number of CPPD or MSU crystals per unit volume of aspirated joint fluid does not correlate with the clinical severity of arthritis. In experimental canine crystal synovitis, which is clearly dose-related,[55] the host response has correlated with the number of crystals injected and not with their subsequent concentration in aspirated joint fluid. Crystal dissolution, clearance by synovial cell endocytosis, clumping of crystals, settling within the joint cavity, or sequestration in synovial recesses may all contribute to this poor correlation.

Although polymorphonuclear leukocytes predominate in acute attacks of crystal-induced synovitis, phagocytosis of both CPPD and MSU by monocytes occurs,[120,128,182] as does phagocytosis by synovial cells.[183,184,185] Phase-contrast and polarized light microscopic study of supravitally stained joint fluid leukocytes from inflamed gouty joints, and of buffy-coat leukocytes that had engulfed MSU crystals in vitro, failed to show the expected phagosome (sac) about the ingested particles.[120] CPPD crystals in joint leukocytes from patients with pseudogout were often inside phagosomes, and such sacs were seen in nearly all buffy-coat leukocytes that had ingested CPPD.[128] Polymorphonuclear leukocytes rapidly disintegrated after ingestion of MSU and released crystals into the ambient medium, often with shreds of adherent cytoplasm.[120,190,197] CPPD crystal phagocytosis also resulted in death and disintegration of the phagocyte, sometimes releasing intact phagosomes with crystals still inside.[128]

Electron-microscopic studies confirmed that the MSU crystals in polymorphonuclear leukocytes in gouty exudate had no surrounding membranous sac, leading to speculation that they had formed intracellularly.[173] Sequential electron microscopy of phagocytes exposed to synthetic MSU crystals for varying times showed that a phagosome was formed initially by inversion of the plasma membrane, but breaks soon occurred[190] (Fig. 93–8). These crystals were often liberated into the cytoplasm. The plasma membrane of the polymorph also fragmented eventually, and the crystal was again extracellular. Similar study of synthetic CPPD crystal phagocytosis with incubation periods as long as two hours showed phagolysosome formation, but few breaks in their integrity, although cell death was greater (23%) than in cells incubated without crystals (8%).[188] Electron-microscopic examination of leukocytes from acutely inflamed pseudogout joints confirmed that most crystals were inside membranous sacs, and similar inspection of the synovium from patients with pseudogout revealed CPPD crystals mostly within synoviocyte phagosomes.[185]

Protein-coated MSU crystals, unlike naked crystals, were not membranolytic.[106] When IgG-coated crystals had been phagocytosed by neutrophils, the IgG was rapidly degraded,[101] presumably exposing the naked crystal to the phagolysosomal membrane. Lysozyme, neutral protease, and collagenase release from neutrophils occurred after MSU crystal phagocytosis.[36] This phagocytosis by neutrophils stimulated the formation of superoxide anion (O_2^-) and other reactive oxygen species,[1,195] but as the death rate of cells from patients with

chronic granulomatous disease, who are deficient in NADH oxidase, was no different from that of normal cells, O_2^- is probably not responsible for cell death due to MSU crystals.[195]

Characterization of MSU and CPPD crystals from patients with gout and pseudogout, synthesis of crystals with identical properties, and production of inflammation in the normal joints of man and several species of experimental animls fulfill Koch's postulates. Polymorphonuclear leukocytes appear to be an absolute requirement of the host response to crystals for the following reasons: (1) they are constantly associated with crystals during the acute attack;[120,128,192] (2) their depletion in experimental animals with drugs or antisera completely inhibited the inflammatory response to crystals;[29,164,203] (3) restoration of leukocytes by perfusion of the crystal-containing limb of a leukopenic dog with fresh dog blood, restored the inflammatory response.[164]

Membranolysis

Studies by several groups of investigators showed that silica crystals hemolyzed erythrocytes,[31] and after phagocytosis, they induced the rupture of macrophage phagolysosomes.[5] Such lysis was blocked by potent hydrogen acceptors such as the synthetic polymer polyvinylpyridine N-oxide (PVPNO), which was thought to be due to the formation of pre-emptive hydrogen bonds with the surface of silica crystals. PVPNO was adsorbed by both MSU and silica crystals, but not by erythrocytes or CPPD crystals. MSU crystals behaved much like silica and produced brisk hemolysis of washed erythrocytes.[242] CPPD crystals induced much slower destruction of red blood cells and exceeded control values only after 2 hours, but

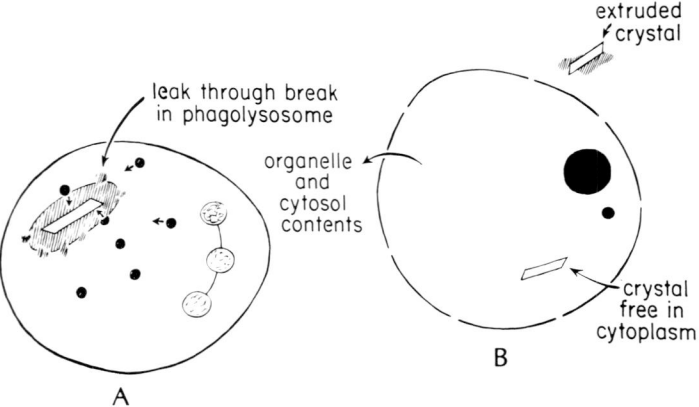

Fig. 93–8. *A,* Breaks occur in the phagosome and allow lysosomal materials to escape into the cytoplasm, producing autolysis and cell death. *B,* Monosodium urate crystal lies in the cytoplasm, and the cell membrane leaks potassium, lactic dehydrogenase, and other cytosol contents into the ambient medium. The crystal, now extracellular and with adherent parts of the dead cell, may again be phagocytosed by a fresh leukocyte.

reached 50% of MSU-induced hemolysis after (or by) 21 hours. The hemolytic effects of silica and MSU were blocked completely by PVPNO and were inhibited by normal plasma. These observations and the aforementioned electron-microscopic findings led to the following hypothesis: "Protein-coated crystals are phagocytosed, and subsequent fusion of lysosomes with the phagosome produces a phagolysosome that contains enzymes. These digest the protein coat on the crystal, allowing hydrogen bond-mediated membranolysis to occur. Phagolysosome lysis is accompanied by the release of hydrolytic enzymes into the cytoplasm, resulting in cellular autolysis, increased permeability of the outer membrane, and release of enzymes into the extracellular medium."[242] This scheme is depicted diagrammatically in Figure 93–8.

The adsorbed proteins may be removed by elution at the more acid pH within the phagolysosome,[103] or they may be digested by lysosomal proteases, as has been demonstrated in vitro.[58,110] This second mechanism has been found by Kozin.[101]

MSU and silica crystals present an ordered array of positively charged hydrogen atoms at their surface, available for bonding with a complementary array of negatively charged groups, as occur in proteins and phospholipids of cell membranes and in anionic polymers, such as PVPNO. The combined energy of thousands of such bonds could produce a strong union between complementary surfaces. How this union leads to breaks in membrane continuity is not known. The mechanism of the much slower membranolytic effect of CPPD is also unknown. A direct relationship between the solubility of urate crystals prepared with different mono- and divalent cations and their membranolytic potential suggested an osmotic effect on membranes by rapid crystal dissolution.[111]

The single crystal (lattice) structures of both MSU and triclinic CPPD, the predominant crystal in pseudogout, are known.[141,143] Both these crystals, as well as silicon dioxide crystals, have irregular surfaces at the atomic level, as opposed to nonmembranolytic crystals, such as diamond, and several rarer types of silica crystals that have a flat lattice structure. Mandel believes that an ionic mechanism of binding is at least as likely on theoretic grounds as is hydrogen bonding, and the irregular lattice structure of membranolytic crystals results in forces that deform the bound membrane phospholipids.[140]

The pattern of release of polymorphonuclear lysosomal enzymes and of the cytoplasmic marker enzyme lactate dehydrogenase after ingestion of MSU or CPPD crystals has been studied by several groups.[144,243,248] Both crystals induced the release of lysosomal enzymes into the extracellular medium, but only MSU crystals caused the release of lactate dehydrogenase; this finding indicates the loss of integrity of the cell membrane (Fig. 93–8). Lactic dehydrogenase release peaked five hours after MSU crystals had been incubated with the leukocytes.[243] Release of lactoferrin, an iron-binding cytosol protein, from polymorphonuclear leukocytes was much greater after MSU than after CPPD crystal phagocytosis, and lactoferrin levels in gouty synovial fluid were high.[9]

Synthetic MSU and CPPD have been tested against the following: (1) isolated heavy granule fraction of rabbit liver cells, containing both mitochondria and lysosomes; (2) isolated human neutrophil lysosomes; and (3) artificial lipid membranes (liposomes), which had a precisely defined composition and contained marker anions.[247] MSU crystals produced a dose-related release of lysosomal, but not mitochondrial, marker enzymes; 20 mg/ml MSU doubled the rate of enzyme release compared to control after a 60-minute incubation. CPPD crystals failed to release enzymes from either lysosomes or mitochondria. Isolated human leukocyte lysosomes released acid phosphatase into the supernatant on contact with MSU crystals; 40 mg/ml caused a 40% increase in liberated enzyme over the control after a 15-minute incubation. The lack of release of marker enzyme from cholesterol-poor mitochondrial membranes suggested a requirement for this molecule for membrane vulnerability. Marker anion release from liposomes by MSU crystals was doubled when cholesterol was incorporated into the membrane, and essentially no anion release over the control was found when cholesterol was omitted. Liposomes were made "female" with 1% 17-estradiol or "male" with 1% testosterone; 20 mg/ml MSU crystals, incubated for 4 hours with liposomes of each "sex," released only 20% more marker than the control from the "female" liposomes, but the increase over the control from the "male" liposomes was 100%. "Packing" of membrane phospholipids controlled by corticosteroid "spacer" was suggested by these authors, who speculated that the observed "sex" difference may account for the increased incidence of gouty arthritis in men.[247]

The evidence of a cholesterol requirement for membrane vulnerability to MSU appears stronger than that for estrogen protection, because at least one natural cholesterol-poor (mitochondrial) membrane was spared, in addition to the demonstrated lack of effect on cholesterol-free liposomes. There is no evidence that natural membranes are protected by estrogen from MSU crystals. The estrogen effect even in liposomes is not specific for crystals, but stabilizes them against other types of perturbation as well.

The sensitivity of the erythrocyte system is greater than that of systems using lysosome or liposome suspensions. MSU crystal hemolysis was consistently 6 times greater than control lysis in the erythrocyte system, as compared to a maximum of twice greater for the smaller control particles, even though higher crystal concentrations were used in the latter experiments.[247] The much longer incubation periods in the red cell incubations showed unequivocal hemolysis with synthetic CPPD crystals, although the rate of lysis was 8 times slower than that of MSU and 42 times slower than that of silica. Both monoclinic and triclinic CPPD, as well as hydroxyapatite, were membranolytic in the erythrocyte system.[142] Grinding the CPPD crystals completely abolished membranolysis. Moreover, the finding of some of these crystals free, as well as membrane-bound, in the cytoplasm of synovial cells and synovial fluid neutrophils by electron microscopy suggests that membranolysis caused by CPPD crystals may actually occur in vivo. Hydrogen bonding can hardly be the mechanism because PVPNO offered no greater protection than afforded control erythrocytes incubated without crystals.[242]

Further studies have demonstrated direct visual disruption of phagosomes after MSU crystal ingestion by dogfish leukocytes, and peroxidase staining material was shown escaping into the adjacent cytoplasm of human neutrophils through breaks in the phagosome by electron microscopy; this direct evidence supports the "suicide sac" hypothesis outlined already.[84,197]

Chemotactic Factors

In addition to the complement-derived factors discussed in the section on inflammatory mediators, a unique glycopeptide was discovered by Phelps and colleagues in 1969 (see also Chap. 19).[156,157,165,229,230] This substance was the first cell-derived chemotactic factor ever described and was released from human, dog, or rabbit neutrophils after MSU or other crystal phagocytosis. It was released into the ambient medium within 7 minutes of crystal exposure to the cells.[157] This crystal-induced chemotactic factor, termed CCF by Spilberg et al.,[207,209] is released by a number of particulates, including latex beads and aggregated gamma globulin.[175,253] The release of CCF by neutrophils exposed to CPPD crystals[229] has been confirmed.[214]

The generation of CCF was inhibited by actinomycin D,[211,213] and newly synthesized CCF was found in the lysosomal fraction of the cell, in addition to its extracellular release. CCF was not released from neutrophils exposed to MSU or CPPD crystals in the presence of cytochalasin B, which blocks phagocytosis, although lysosomal discharge occurred.[206,211,212] The molecular weight of CCF has been estimated at 8,500 daltons[165] by one group and at 11,500 daltons by another.[208]

Scatchard analysis suggested the presence of about 600,000 receptor sites for CCF per neutrophil.[209] Injection of purified CCF into rabbit joints provoked a marked accumulation of neutrophilic leukocytes with severe inflammation, but without change in capillary permeability.[215] These data challenge traditional concepts of inflammation, which invariably envision the development of soluble inflammatory mediators before cellular exudation occurs. But (or nevertheless) they conform to previous work showing a complete lack of inflammatory response to MSU crystals in severely neutropenic dogs, with restoration of such response after neutrophil repletion.[164]

Diamond crystals were phagocytosed, but did not release CCF or cause inflammation in dogs;[164] they released CCF from rabbit neutrophils and caused inflammation in rabbit joints, however.[216]

Colchicine, $10^{-6}M$, a level approximating that obtained with the usual therapeutic doses given to patients with gout,[53,54] predictably blocked the release of CCF by at least 50% after MSU crystal phagocytosis, but its effects on the release of CCF after CPPD crystal phagocytosis were much less predictable.[229] These in vitro studies parallel the effects of colchicine used to treat patients with acute attacks of gout and pseudogout. Oral colchicine is nearly always effective in gout, but in pseudogout, the effects range from dramatic to none.[115,117] Injection of 1 mg colchicine intravenously, which provides higher plasma levels, predictably suppresses acute attacks of pseudogout,[204] however, including polyarticular episodes.[146]

The inflammatory response to MSU crystals injected into rabbit joints was abrogated by colchicine in doses that did not affect the response to injected CCF.[205] Unfortunately, these data were obtained using heated MSU crystals, which are ineffective activators of complement, as already discussed. CCF, like synthetic and complement-derived chemotactic factors, caused lysosomal discharge from neutrophils.[215] The membrane changes and lysosomal degranulation, noted in neutrophils within synovial capillaries in gout,[2,189] may be caused by the diffusion of such factors from the site of crystal phagocytosis in the joint space. This phenomenon may explain the warmth, redness, and swelling of the skin and periarticular tissues so typical of acute gouty arthritis.

Natural MSU crystals activate complement,[101] and complement-derived chemotactic factors have been found in gouty joint fluid.[244] Data relative to complement activation by synthetic crystals have already been discussed. The lack of a suppressive effect of C3 depletion by cobra venom factor in experimental crystal-induced synovitis in dogs and rabbits,[161,203] suffers from the same criticism as the CCF data just discussed, that is, the crystals used were heated first. Whether complement-derived chemotactic factors are critical to the genesis of crystal-induced inflammation is an unsettled issue.

Leukotriene B_4 has been found by radioimmunoassay,[170] as well as by high-performance liquid chromatography,[193] in ambient medium about neutrophils exposed to MSU crystals. This extraordinarily potent chemotactic factor and other products of the lipoxygenase pathway such as 5-HETE were released. The generation of leukotriene B_4, but not of 5-HETE, was blocked by $10^{-5}M$ colchicine.[193]

Because leukotriene B_4 is a highly charged molecule, it may be bound to proteins. Generation of both leukotriene B_4 and CCF are blocked by colchicine, so it is conceivable that CCF is actually leukotriene B_4 bound to a cell-derived glycopeptide. On the other hand, Phelps found that CCF release from neutrophils exposed to MSU crystals was blocked to a significant extent by colchicine in concentrations of $10^{-9}M$,[157] 4 orders of magnitude lower than those that effectively blocked leukotriene B_4 generation.[193]

Thus, colchicine appears to interfere with the formation of two cell-derived chemotactic factors, one more potent (leukotriene B_4) and one weaker (CCF) than those derived from complement. The inter-relationship of these two factors and the precise mechanism of the colchicine effect remain to be determined.

EXPERIMENTAL MODELS

Crystal-induced inflammation has been used as an experimental model both in animals and in man.

Animal

After the initial demonstration of urate crystal-induced synovitis in man, a similar reaction was found in unanesthetized dogs, using the time of onset of a 3-legged gait as a sharply defined end point.[55] The model developed in the dog permitted serial measurement of a number of physiologically meaningful parameters simultaneously. Mongrel dogs of medium to large size were lightly anesthetized with barbiturates. A stifle (knee) joint was catheterized with a polyethelyene catheter, which was attached by a 3-way stopcock to a pressure transducer.[131] The joint was fixed with tape in 90° of flexion because intra-articular pressure varies with the position of the joint. Normal intra-articular pressure is slightly subatmospheric. Change in this

pressure, once the position of the joint is constant, reflects volume change in the joint and is an index of the fluid phase of the exudative inflammatory response. The rise in intra-articular pressure is driven by the hydrodynamic pressure within the arterial circulation, and in severe inflammation, it may equilibrate with the diastolic blood pressure.

The gradual fall in synovial fluid pH is entirely due to leukocyte exudation and represents an index of the cellular phase of the exudative inflammatory response.[131] The leukocyte concentration can be determined serially in small samples obtained through the indwelling catheter. The estimated total synovial exudative response could be calculated by aspiration of the joint to zero pressure with direct measurement of volume. Although it is unlikely that true synovial membrane blood flow can be measured because of the many assumptions required,[167] [133]xenon clearance from the joint does provide an index of such flow and increases after urate crystal injection. Other advantages of this model are the ability to perform histologic studies concurrently,[191] and because the inflammation is completely reversible, control experiments can be performed on the same joint four or more weeks later.

Intravenous indomethacin effectively lowered the leukocyte and pressure responses to MSU crystals in this model, which has been used also to determine the effects of exercise, heat, cold, and other drugs on the inflammatory response.[3,7,29,30,44,153,162,163] The failure of non-leukopenia-producing doses of colchicine to suppress the inflammatory response to MSU crystals in dogs suggests that the experimental model differs from natural gout and from the synovitis induced in man by these crystals.[30,219]

Animal models of crystal-induced inflammation have also used rabbit joints,[204,205,210,215,216] rat paws,[39,40,234] rat pleural spaces,[69] and birds.[22,202]

Man

Crystal-induced inflammation was first used as an experimental model testing for drug effectiveness in humans in 1965.[138] The response to subcutaneous injection of crystals was evaluated by measuring the diameter of induration and erythema. The response to intra-articular crystals was gauged by an inflammatory index, which was the sum of clinical rating of local heat, swelling, tenderness, and erythema on a 0 to 4+ scale. The effectiveness of pretreatment with colchicine, phenylbutazone, or corticosteroids was shown.

Urate crystal-induced synovitis in humans proved to be a safe measure of drug efficacy.[219] An indwelling polyethylene catheter was inserted into normal knee joints through a small skin wound and was sewn in place with a single suture. Intra-articular volume, tenderness of selected areas of the overlying skin, skin temperature over the joint, and joint circumference were useful empiric measurements of the inflammatory response. The effect of anti-inflammatory drugs given in usual doses was invariably detectable.[218,219]

Although the model systems of crystal-induced inflammation have been useful in the dissection of some critical features of the host response to crystals, the precise mode of action of drugs effective in the treatment of acute crystal synovitis in everyday clinical practice is not known. The model systems in man and in animals have been used for this purpose only in a preliminary way. Even if further experimental work is done with regard to the mechanism of action of anti-inflammatory drugs, one must remember that the experimental models using synthetic crystals are at best analogues of their natural counterparts.

TREATMENT OF CRYSTAL-INDUCED INFLAMMATION

The aims of therapy in gout are: (1) to alleviate pain, which is often excruciating; and (2) to restore the inflamed joint to useful function. After protection of the joint by splinting and after administration of analgesics, a choice of effective drugs is at hand. Thorough aspiration of the joint, often possible at the time of diagnostic arthrocentesis to obtain fluid for crystal identification, may be followed by local injection of microcrystalline adrenocorticosteroid esters. Such therapy is ideal in a single large joint; inflammation subsides predictably within 12 hours of treatment, regardless of the prior duration of the acute attack.

Colchicine

Colchicine remains a useful drug in the average patient, especially when small joints are involved, or in polyarticular inflammation. It may be given orally, 0.5 mg every hour until relief or side effects occur. About 10 tablets are generally required. Diarrhea is almost always produced. Signs and symptoms of inflammation subside in 12 to 24 hours, and pain is gone in over 90% of patients in 24 to 48 hours.[235,240] Electrolyte imbalances in the elderly may be severe. The bone marrow may be fatally depressed, especially in persons with hematologic malignant disease who are receiving chemotherapy. The drug often cannot be given orally in persons with postoperative acute gout. The intravenous route must be used in these instances; 2 mg are given as a single dose, with care to avoid extravasation because of the irritating properties of the drug. Gastrointestinal effects are prevented completely, and the anti-inflammatory effects are more rapid, noticeable in 6 to 8 hours and affording complete relief in 24 hours.[235] The effectiveness of intravenous colchicine in acute pseudogout has already been discussed.[146,204]

Prophylactic Use

Acute gouty attacks are effectively prevented by small daily doses of colchicine. Doses of 0.5 to 2 mg daily are given; the average patient takes about 1 mg. Such doses either completely prevented attacks or greatly reduced their frequency in 93% of a large series of gouty patients during many years of follow-up.[252] Only 4% had gastrointestinal toxicity, and many of these patients had underlying intestinal disease. The mechanism of prophylaxis may be different from the effects of the drug in treatment, as discussed previously in connection with the elevated serum uronic acid levels in gouty arthritis.

Diagnostic Use

The natural history of the diagnostic use of therapeutic trials is one of abandonment as better tests are developed. The time-honored colchicine therapeutic trial is no exception. Wallace and colleagues treated 58 patients with acute gout and 62 patients with other types of arthritis using rigidly defined criteria for clinical response;[240] 44 of 58 gouty patients (75%) and 3 of 62 (5%) control subjects showed major improvement. Colchicine was a weak general anti-inflammatory drug in suppressing inflammation in rodent skin induced by staphylococcal toxin,[137] and so it is not surprising that "false-positive" trials occur. Patients with sarcoid arthritis,[88] calcific tendinitis (apatite),[228] and pseudogout[59,204,238] sometimes show dramatic response to colchicine treatment.

Metabolism

Recent use of a radioimmunoassay for colchicine with a sensitivity of 0.05 ng showed measurable plasma levels in 5 of 7 patients given a single 2-mg dose intravenously 24 hours earlier.[54] Mean plasma half-life was 58 ± 20 minutes; zero time plasma concentration was 2.9 ± 1.5 μg/dl. Although maximal urinary excretion occurred 2 hours after drug administration, colchicine was found in the urine up to 10 days later. No breakdown products were noted[239] despite published in vitro evidence of microsomal degradation.

Colchicine has been measured in human serum, urine, and peripheral blood neutrophils after the intravenous administration of usual therapeutic doses.[53,241] The highest plasma concentration (zero time extrapolation of decay curve) was 7×10^{-7} M. Drug concentration in peripheral blood leukocytes was much greater, ranging from 1 to $2 \times$

10^{-5} M; at 72 hours, leukocyte colchicine levels approximated 5×10^{-6} M, and detectable drug levels were still found in cells isolated from the blood 10 days later. The increased concentration in leukocytes is probably related to their content of labile microtubules (tubulin), each dimer subunit of which specifically binds one molecule of colchicine.[16] Absorption after a single oral dose of 1 mg was variable; peak concentrations an order of magnitude lower than when the drug was given intravenously $(0.3 \pm 0.17 \ \mu g/dl)$ were reached in 0.5 to 2 hours. Interestingly, vinblastine also binds to tubulin dimers, produces metaphase arrest, and is effective in the treatment of gouty arthritis.

Mechanism of Action

Parameters of neutrophilic function suppressed by colchicine include random motility, adherence, chemotaxis, chemotactic factor (CCF and leukotriene B_4) release, lysosomal discharge, and perhaps, lysosomal fusion with phagosomes.[115,117,155]

Two schools of thought on the mode of action of this venerable drug exist. Malawista favors the concept that the anti-inflammatory and antimitotic effects of colchicine share a common mechanism.[136] The stabilization of labile microtubules normally needed for leukocyte motility may decrease chemotaxis, may inhibit phagocytosis, may lessen adhesiveness, and may suppress leukocyte chemotactic factor release. Inhibition of the mitotic spindle, which is largely tubulin, arrests mitosis in metaphase. Wallace has pointed out certain paradoxes not explicable by this unitary theory, however.[235] Trimethylcolchicinic acid (TMCA), an experimental analogue of colchicine not now available, is as effective in treating acute gout as is colchicine itself, although it has no effect on microtubules and is not metabolized to colchicine in humans. Comparison of the ability of various colchicine analogues to suppress polymorphonuclear leukocytic motility in vitro showed the same order of effectiveness as their clinical potency in treating gout.[161,237] On the other hand, lumicolchicine, which does not block mitosis, is ineffective in the treatment of gout.[138a] Colchicine binds to other proteins in living cells besides microtubules, especially membrane proteins,[221] which might be tubulin-like protein providing attachment points for microtubules. Moreover, colchicine is effective in preventing attacks of familial Mediterranean fever,[7] but not in their treatment.[49]

On the cellular level, colchicine probably acts by inhibiting leukocyte-derived chemotactic factors because potent effects were seen in vitro with concentrations as low as $10^{-9}M$. Detectable effects on phagocytosis in the same experiments required much larger levels of the drug.[157]

Phenylbutazone and Oxyphenbutazone

These drugs, which are as effective orally as colchicine is intravenously, are still popular drugs for acute gout (see Chap. 28). About 600 mg are given in the first 24 hours, followed by 100 mg 4 times daily for about a week. Nearly all attacks of acute gout can be controlled with these drugs. Fluid retention and gastritis are common side effects. Phenylbutazone blocked the phagocytosis of CPPD crystals by polymorphonuclear leukocytes and indirectly lessened the release of CCF.[206]

Other Drugs

Indomethacin, at initial doses of 400 mg in the first 24 hours and 100 mg daily in divided doses over the next 4 to 5 days, is as effective as phenylbutazone. It, too, has been shown to interfere with CPPD crystal phagocytosis,[206] and with the phagocytosis of starch granules.[28] Release of CCF is again inhibited indirectly.

Naproxen, at 0.3 to 1.5 g/24 hours, followed by smaller maintenance doses, suppressed acute gout in 75% of 40 patients.[251] Fourteen of 19 patients with acute gout responded satisfactorily to fenoprofen.[236] Either drug provides alternate therapy for acute gout.

Adrenocorticotropic hormone and corticosteroids are reportedly effective agents in acute gout, although corticosteroids may control pain while inflammation continues at a subdued level. Corticosteroids are often given on a long-term basis for polyarticular gout misdiagnosed as rheumatoid arthritis. Additional joints become inflamed, and the patient looks more and more as though he has the disease for which he is being treated. I doubt whether the systemic use of corticosteroids or of adenocorticotropic hormone is ever indicated for the treatment of gouty or other types of crystal-induced inflammation.

Pseudogout

Supportive measures are useful, as outlined previously. Thorough aspiration of a large joint often effectively reverses acute inflammation even without local corticosteroid injection.[128,198] This effect is presumably due to removal of sufficient crystals to control what is an experimentally demonstrable dose-related response. Concomitant use of local steroid esters is virtually 100% effective in control of acute pseudogout in a single large joint.

Phenylbutazone, oxyphenbutazone, and indomethacin are effective in doses previously outlined for the treatment of acute gout. Colchicine effectiveness is less predictable when the drug is given orally, perhaps because of its variable suppressive effects on the release of the cell-derived chemotactic factor. Intravenous colchicine (1 mg) predictably controls acute pseudogout,[204] probably because it produces much higher blood levels, as outlined previously.

REFERENCES

1. Abramson, S., Hoffstein, S.T., and Weissmann, G.: Superoxide anion generation by human neutrophils exposed to monosodium urate: effect of protein adsorption and complement activation. Arthritis Rheum., 25:174–180, 1982.
2. Agudelo, C.A., and Schumacher, H.R.: The synovitis of acute gouty arthritis. Hum. Pathol., 4:265–279, 1973.
3. Agudelo, C.A., Schumacher, R.F., and Phelps, P.: Effect of exercise on urate crystal-induced inflammation in canine joints. Arthritis Rheum., 15:609–616, 1972.
4. Ali, S.Y., and Wisby, A.: Ultrastructural aspects of normal and osteoarthritic cartilage. Ann. Rheum. Dis., 34 (Suppl.):21–23, 1975.
5. Allison, A.C., Harrington, J.S., and Berbeck, M.: An examination of the cytotoxic effects of silica on macrophages. J. Exp. Med., 124:141–153, 1966.
6. Altman, R.D., et al.: Articular chondrocalcinosis. Arthritis Rheum., 16:171–178, 1973.
7. Andrews, R., and Phelps, P.: Release of lysosomal enzymes from polymorphonuclear leukocytes (PMN) after phagocytosis of monosodium urate (MSU) and calcium pyrophosphate dihydrate (CPPD) crystals: effects of colchicine and indomethacin. Arthritis Rheum., 14:368, 1971.
8. Antomattei, O., et al.: Protein adsorption to monosodium urate crystals (MSUC): analysis by SDS polyacrylamide gel electrophoresis (Page) and immunoautoradiography. (Abstract.) Arthritis Rheum., 26:S12, 1983.
9. Bennett, R.M., and Skosey, J.L.: Lactoferrin and lysozyme levels in synovial fluid. Arthritis Rheum., 20:84–90, 1977.
10. Bennett, R.M., Lehr, J.R., and McCarty, D.J.: Crystal shedding and acute pseudogout: an hypothesis based on a therapeutic failure. Arthritis Rheum., 19:93–97, 1976.
11. Bennett, R.M., Lehr, J.R., and McCarty, D.J.: Factors affecting the solubility of calcium pyrophosphate dihydrate crystals. J. Clin. Invest., 56:1,571–1,579, 1975.
12. Bennett, R.M., Mall, J.C., and McCarty, D.J.: Pseudogout in acute neuropathic arthropathy. A clue to pathogenesis? Ann. Rheum. Dis., 33:563–567, 1974.
13. Bilezikian, J.P.: Pseudogout after parathyroidectomy. Lancet, 1:445–446, 1973.
14. Bjelle, A.: Morphological study of articular cartilage of pyrophosphate arthropathy. Ann. Rheum. Dis., 31:449–456, 1972.
15. Bland, J.H., Gierthy, J.F., and Suhre, E.D.: Cholesterol in connective tissue joints. Scand. J. Rheumatol., 3:199–203, 1974.
16. Borisy, G.G., and Taylor, E.W.: The mechanism of action of colchicine. J. Cell Biol., 34:525–548, 1967.
17. Brandt, K.D.: The effects of synovial hyaluronate on the ingestion of monosodium urate crystals by leukocytes. Clin. Chim. Acta, 55:307–315, 1974.
18. Brandt, K.D., and Krey, P.R.: Chalky joint effusion. Arthritis Rheum., 20:792–796, 1977.
19. Brill, J.M., and McCarty, D.J.: Translation of "Experimental Investigations into Origin of Gouty Tophi" by Max Freudweiler, Deutsch Arch. fur Klin. Med., 69:155, 1901. Arthritis Rheum., 8:267–288, 1965.
20. Brill, J.M., and McCarty, D.J.: An abridged translation with comments on "Studies on the Nature of Gouty Tophi" by Max Freudweiler and Wilhelm His, Jr., 1899. Ann. Intern. Med., 60:486–505, 1964.
21. Brochner-Mortensen, K.: Heberden Oration—1957. "Gout." Ann. Rheum. Dis., 17:1–8, 1958.
22. Brune, K., and Glatt, M.: The avian microcrystal arthritis. IV. The impact of sodium salicylate, acetaminophen and colchicine on leukocyte invasion and enzyme liberation in vivo. Agents Action, 4:101–106, 1974.
23. Burt, H., Kalkman, P.H., and Mauldin, D.: Membranolytic effects of crystalline monosodium urate monohydrate. J. Rheumatol., 10:440–448, 1983.
24. Byers, P.H., et al.: Complement as a mediator of inflammation in acute gouty arthritis. II. Biological activities generated from complement and sodium urate crystals. J. Lab. Clin. Med., 81:761–769, 1973.
25. Camerlain, M., et al.: Inorganic pyrophosphate pool size and turnover rate in arthritis joints. J. Clin. Invest., 55:1,373–1,381, 1975.
26. Cannon, R.B., and Schmid, F.R.: Calcific periarthritis involving multiple sites in identical twins. Arthritis Rheum., 16:393–396, 1973.
27. Carroll, G.J., and Bayliss, C.E.: Treatment of the arthropathy of familial hypercholesterolemia. Ann. Rheum. Dis., 42:206–209, 1983.
28. Chang, Y.H.: Studies on phagocytosis. II. The effect of non-steroidal anti-inflammatory drugs on phagocytosis and on urate crystal induced canine joint inflammation. J. Pharmacol. Exp. Ther., 183:235–244, 1972.
29. Chang, Y.H., and Gralla, E.J.: Suppression of urate crystal induced canine joint inflammation by heterologous anti-polymorphonuclear leukocyte serum. Arthritis Rheum., 11:145–150, 1968.
30. Chang, Y.H., and Malawista, S.E.: Mechanism of action of colchicine. IV. The failure of non-leukopenic doses of colchicine to suppress urate crystal-induced canine joint inflammation. Inflammation, 1:143–156, 1976.
31. Charache, P., MacLeod, C.M., and White, P.: Effects of silicate polymers on erythrocytes in presence of and absence of complement. J. Gen. Physiol., 45:1,117–1,143, 1962.
32. Cheng, P.T., and Pritzker, K.P.H.: Effect of heat on crystals. Arthritis Rheum., 24:637–638, 1981.
33. Cherian, P.B., et al.: Immunoelectron microscopic identification of protein coatings on intracellular monosodium urate (MSU) crystals. (Abstract.) Arthritis Rheum., 26:S60, 1983.
34. Cheung, H.S., Halverson, P.B., and McCarty, D.: Phagocytosis of hydroxyapatite or calcium pyrophosphate dihydrate crystals by rabbit articular chondrocytes stimulates release of collagenase, neutral protease and prostaglandins E_2 and $F_2\alpha$. Proc. Soc. Exp. Biol. Med., 173:181–189, 1983.
35. Cheung, H.S., Halverson, P.B., and McCarty, D.J.: Release of collagenase, neutral protease and prostaglandins from cultured mammalian synovial cells by hydroxyapatite and calcium pyrophosphate dihydrate crystals. Arthritis Rheum., 24:1,338–1,344, 1981.
36. Cheung, H.S., Bohan, S., and Kozin, F.: Kinetics of collagenase and neutral protease release by neutrophils exposed to microcrystalline sodium urate. Connect. Tissue Res., 11:78–85, 1983.
37. Codman, E.A.: The Shoulder. Boston, Thomas Todd, 1934.
38. Davies, W., et al.: Phagocytosis and the gamma globulin monolayer: analysis by particle electrophoresis. J. Reticuloendothel. Soc., 18:136–148, 1975.
39. Denko, C.W.: Phlogistic action of prostaglandins in urate crystal inflammation. (Abstract.) J. Rheumatol., 1:24, 1974.
40. Denko, C.W., and Whitehouse, M.W.: Experimental inflammation induced by naturally occurring microcrystalline calcium salts. J. Rheumatol., 3:54–61, 1976.
41. Dieppe, P.A., et al.: Changes in monosodium urate monohydrate crystals on heating or grinding. Arthritis Rheum., 24:975–976, 1981.
42. Dieppe, P.A., et al.: Apatite deposition disease. Lancet, 1:266–270, 1976.
43. Doherty, M., Whicker, J.T., and Dieppe, P.A.: Activation of the alternative pathway of complement by monosodium urate monohydrate crystals and other inflammatory particles. Ann. Rheum. Dis., 42:285–291, 1983.
44. Dorwart, B.B., Hansell, J.R., and Schumacher, H.R.: Effects of cold and heat on urate crystal-induced synovitis in the dog. Arthritis Rheum., 17:563–571, 1974.
45. Dorwart, B.B., and Schumacher, H.R.: Joint effusion chondrocalcinosis and other rheumatic manifestations in hypothyroidism. Am. J. Med., 59:780–789, 1975.
46. Dougados, M., et al.: Charcot-Leyden crystals in synovial fluid. Arthritis Rheum., 26:1416, 1983.

47. Duff, G.W., et al.: Crystal induced endogenous pyrogen production. Clin. Res. Arthritis Rheum., 27:S50, 1984 (abstract).

48. Duff, G.W., Atkins, E., and Malawista, S.E.: The fever of gout. Clin. Res., 31:361A, 1983.

49. Ehrlich, G.E.: Colchicine for familial Mediterranean fever. N. Engl. J. Med., 288:798, 1973.

50. Emmerson, B.T., Stride, P.J., and Williams, G.: The clinical differentiation of primary gout from primary renal disease in patients with both gout and renal disease. Adv. Exp. Med. Biol., 122A:9–13, 1980.

51. This reference has been deleted.

52. Ettlinger, R.E., and Hunder, G.C.: Synovial effusions containing cholesterol crystals. Mayo Clin. Proc., 54:366–374, 1979.

53. Ertel, N.H., and Wallace, S.L.: Measurement of colchicine in urine and peripheral leukocytes. Clin. Res., 19:348–357, 1971.

54. Ertel, N.H., Mittler, J.C., and Akgun, S.: Radioimmunoassay for colchicine in plasma and urine. Science, 193:233–239, 1976.

55. Faires, J.S., and McCarty, D.J.: Acute arthritis in man and dog after intrasynovial injection of sodium urate crystals. Lancet, 2:682–685, 1962.

56. Fam, A.G., et al.: Cholesterol crystals in osteoarthritic joint effusions. J. Rheumatol., 8:273–280, 1981.

57. Fam, A.G., et al.: Cholesterol associated synovitis: a clinico-pathologic study of 8 cases. Ann. R. Coll. Phys. Surg. Can., 12:94–103, 1979.

58. Fehr, K., LoSapalluto, A., and Ziff, M.: Degradation of immunoglobulin G by lysosomal acid proteases. J. Immunol., 105:973–983, 1970.

59. Frischknecht, J., and Steigerwald, J.C.: High synovial fluid white blood cell counts in pseudogout. Arch. Intern. Med., 135:298–307, 1975.

60. Garrod, A.B.: A Treatise on Gout and Rheumatic Gout and Rheumatic Gout (Rheumatoid Arthritis) 3rd Ed. London, Longmans, Green, 1876.

61. Gaucher, A., et al.: Identification des cristaux observés dans les arthropathies destructrices de la chondrocalcinose. Rev. Rhum. Mal. Osteoartic., 44:407–414, 1977.

62. Gibson, I.K., Burns, R.P., and Wolfe-Lande, J.D.: Crystals in corneal epithelial lesions of tyrosine fed rats. Invest. Ophthalmol., 14:937–941, 1975.

63. Giclas, P.C., Ginsberg, M.H., and Cooper, N.R.: Immunoglobulin G independent activation of the classical complement pathway by monosodium urate crystals. J. Clin. Invest., 63:759–764, 1979.

64. Ginsberg, M.H., et al.: Urate crystal-dependent cleavage of Hageman factor in human plasma and synovial fluid. J. Lab. Clin. Med., 95:497–506, 1980.

65. Ginsberg, M.H., et al.: Mechanisms of platelet response to monosodium urate crystals. Am. J. Pathol., 94:549–568, 1979.

66. Ginsberg, M.H., et al.: Adsorption of polymorphonuclear leukocyte lysosomal enzymes to monosodium urate crystals. Arthritis Rheum., 20:1,538–1,542, 1977.

67. Ginsberg, M.H., et al.: Release of platelet constituents by monosodium urate crystals. J. Clin. Invest., 60:999–1,007, 1977.

68. Ginsberg, M.H., and Kozin, F.: Mechanisms of cellular interaction with monosodium urate crystals: IgG dependent and IgG independent platelet stimulation by urate crystals. Arthritis Rheum., 21:896–903, 1978.

69. Glatt, M., Dieppe, P., and Willoughby, D.: Crystal-induced inflammation, enzyme release and the effects of drugs in the rat pleural space. J. Rheumatol., 6:251–257, 1979.

70. Glueck, C.J., Levy, R.I., and Fredrickson, D.S.: Acute tendinitis and arthritis. A presenting symptom of familial type II hyperlipoproteinemia. JAMA, 206:2,895–2,897, 1968.

71. Goldfinger, S.E.: Colchicine for Mediterranean fever. N. Engl. J. Med., 228:1,301, 1973.

72. Goldsmith, L.A.: Haemolysis induced by tyrosine crystals. Biochem. J., 158:17–22, 1976.

73. Goldsmith, L.A.: Hemolysis and lysosomal activation by solid state tyrosine. Biochem. Biophys. Res. Commun., 64:558–565, 1975.

74. Gondos, B.: Observations on periarthritis calcarea. Am. J. Roentgenol., 77:93–108, 1957.

75. Graham, R., Sutor, D.J., and Mitchener, M.B.: Crystal deposition in hyperparathyroidism. Ann. Rheum. Dis., 30:597–604, 1971.

76. Halverson, P.B., and McCarty, D.J.: Identification of hydroxyapatite crystals in synovial fluid. Arthritis Rheum., 21:723–726, 1978.

77. Halverson, P.B., Cheung, H.S., and McCarty, D.J.: Enzymatic release of microspheroids containing hydroxyapatite crystals from synovium and of calcium pyrophosphate dihydrate crystals from cartilage. Ann. Rheum. Dis., 41:527–531, 1982.

78. Hasselbacher, P.: Stimulation of synovial fibroblasts by calcium oxalate and monosodium urate monohydrate: a mechanism of connective tissue degradation in oxalosis and gout. J. Lab. Clin. Med., 100:977–985, 1982.

79. Hasselbacher, P.: Activation of the alternative pathway of complement by microcrystalline cholesterol. Atherosclerosis, 37:239–245, 1980.

80. Hasselbacher, P.: Binding of IgG and complement protein by monosodium urate monohydrate and other crystals. J. Lab. Clin. Med., 94:532–541, 1979.

81. Hasselbacher, P.: C3 activation by monosodium urate monohydrate and other crystalline material. Arthritis Rheum., 22:571–578, 1979.

82. Hasselbacher, P., et al.: Stimulation of the secretion of collagenase and prostaglandin E_2 by synovial fibroblasts in response to crystals of monosodium urate monohydrate: a model for joint destruction in gout. Trans. Assoc. Am. Physicians, 94:243–252, 1981.

83. Hasselbacher, P., and Schumacher, H.R.: Immunoglobulin in tophi and on the surface of monosodium urate crystals. Arthritis Rheum., 21:353–361, 1978.

84. Hoffstein, S., and Weissmann, G.: Mechanisms of lysosomal enzyme release from leukocytes. Arthritis Rheum., 18:153–165, 1975.

85. Hollingsworth, J.W., and Atkins, E.: Synovial inflammatory response to bacterial endotoxin. Yale J. Biol. Med., 38:241–256, 1965.

86. Jaques, B.C., and Ginsberg, M.H.: The role of cell surface proteins in platelet stimulation by monosodium urate crystals. Arthritis Rheum., 25:508–521, 1982.

87. Kahn, C.B., Hollander, J.L., and Schumacher, H.R.: Corticosteroid crystals in synovial fluid. JAMA, 211:807–809, 1970.

88. Kaplan, H.: Sarcoid arthritis with a response to colchicine. N. Engl. J. Med., 263:778–781, 1960.

89. Katz, W.A.: Abstract 137. In Proceedings of the Fourteenth International Rheumatology Congress. Edited by International League Against Rheumatism. San Francisco, 1977.

90. Katz, W.A.: Deposition of urate crystals in gout. Arthritis Rheum., 18:751–756, 1975.

91. Katz, W.A., and Schubert, M.: The interaction of monosodium urate with connective tissue components. J. Clin. Invest., 49:1,783–1,789, 1970.

92. Kellermeyer, R.W.: Inflammatory process in acute gouty arthritis. III. Vascular permeability-enhancing activity in normal human synovial fluid; induction by Hageman factor activators; and inhibition by Hageman factor antiserum. J. Lab. Clin. Med., 70:372–383, 1967.

93. Kellermeyer, R.W., and Breckenridge, R.T.: The inflammatory process in acute arthritis. II. The presence of Hageman factor and plasma thromboplastin antecedent in synovial fluid. J. Lab. Clin. Med., 67:455–460, 1966.

94. Kellermeyer, R.W., and Breckenridge, R.T.: The inflammatory process in acute gouty arthritis. I. Activation of Hageman factor by sodium urate crystals. J. Lab. Clin. Med., 65:307–315, 1965.

95. Kellermeyer, R.W., and Naff, G.F.: Chemical mediators of inflammation in acute gouty arthritis. Arthritis Rheum., 18:765–770, 1975.

96. Khachadurian, A.K.: Migratory polyarthritis in familial hypercholesterolemia (type II hyperlipoproteinemia). Arthritis Rheum., 11:385–393, 1968.

97. Kippen, I., et al.: Factors affecting urate solubility in vitro. Ann. Rheum. Dis., *33*:313–317, 1974.
98. Klinenberg, J.R., et al.: Urate deposition disease. Ann. Intern. Med., *78*:99–111, 1973.
99. Korn, D.: Demonstration of cystine crystals in peripheral white blood cells in a patient with cystinosis. N. Engl. J. Med., *262*:545–548, 1960.
100. Kowai, K., and McCarty, D.J.: Unpublished data.
101. Kozin, F.: Unpublished data.
102. Kozin, F., et al.: Protein binding to monosodium urate crystals and its effect on platelet degranulation. Adv. Exp. Med. Biol., *76B*:201–207, 1976.
103. Kozin, F., and McCarty, D.J.: Molecular orientation of immunoglobulin G adsorbed to microcrystalline monosodium urate monohydrate. J. Lab. Clin. Med., *95*:49–58, 1980.
104. Kozin, F., and McCarty, D.J.: Protein binding to monosodium urate monohydrate calcium pyrophosphate and silicon dioxide crystals. I. Physical characteristics. J. Lab. Clin. Med., *89*:1,314–1,325, 1977.
105. Kozin, F., and McCarty, D.J.: Rheumatoid factors in serum of gouty patients. Arthritis Rheum., *20*:559–560, 1977.
106. Kozin, F., Ginsberg, M.H., and Skosey, J.: Polymorphonuclear leukocyte responses to monosodium urate crystals: modification by adsorbed serum protein. J. Rheumatol., *6*:519–528, 1979.
107. Lam-Erwin, C.Y., and Nancollas, G.H.: The crystallization and dissolution of sodium urate. J. Crystal Growth, *53*:215–223, 1981.
108. Lam-Erwin, G.Y., Nancollas, G.H., and Ko, S.J.: The kinetics of formation and dissolution of uric acid crystals. Invest. Urol., *15*:473–481, 1978.
109. Loeb, J.N.: The influence of temperature on the solubility of monosodium urate. Arthritis Rheum., *15*:189–192, 1972.
110. LoSpaulluto, J.J., Fehr, K., and Ziff, M.: Degradation of immunoglobulin by intercellular proteases in the range of neutral pH. J. Immunol., *105*:886–897, 1970.
111. Lussier, A., and deMedicis, R.: Mechanism of phagolysosome membranolysis by urate crystals. (Abstract.) J. Rheumatol., *1 (Suppl.)*:23, 1974.
112. McCarty, D.J.: The gouty toe—a multifactorial condition. Ann. Intern. Med., *86*:234–238, 1977.
113. McCarty, D.J.: Calcium pyrophosphate dihydrate crystal deposition disease—1975. Arthritis Rheum., *19 (Suppl.)*:275–285, 1976.
114. McCarty, D.J.: Treatment of rheumatoid joint inflammation with triamcinolone hexacetonide. Arthritis Rheum., *15*:157–173, 1972.
115. McCarty, D.J.: Urate crystal phagocytosis by PMN leukocytes and the effects of colchicine. *In* Phagocytic Mechanisms in Health and Disease. Edited by R.C. Williams and H.H. Fudenberg. New York, Intercontinental Medical Book, 1972, pp. 107–121.
116. McCarty, D.J.: A historical note: Leeuwenhoek's description of crystals from a gouty tophus. Arthritis Rheum., *13*:414–418, 1970.
117. McCarty, D.J.: Pathogenesis and treatment of the acute attack of gout. Clin. Orthop., *71*:28–39, 1970.
118. McCarty, D.J.: The inflammatory reaction to microcrystalline sodium urate. Arthritis Rheum., *8*:726–735, 1965.
119. McCarty, D.J.: Diagnosis of gouty arthritis—18 months experience with a pathognomonic test. Postgrad. Med., *33*:142–148, 1963.
120. McCarty, D.J.: Phagocytosis of urate crystals in gouty synovial fluid. Am. J. Med. Sci., *243*:288–295, 1962.
121. McCarty, D.J., et al.: Inorganic pyrophosphate concentrations in the synovial fluid of arthritis patients. J. Lab. Clin. Med., *78*:216–229, 1971.
122. McCarty, D.J., et al.: Studies on pathological calcifications in human cartilage. I. Prevalence and types of crystal deposits in the menisci of two hundred and fifteen cadavera. J. Bone Joint Surg., *48*:309–325, 1966.
123. McCarty, D.J., et al.: Crystal deposition diseases: sodium urate (gout) and calcium pyrophosphate (chondrocalcinosis, pseudogout). JAMA, *193*:129–132, 1965.
124. McCarty, D.J., and Gatter, R.A.: Recurrent acute inflam-

mation associated with focal apatite crystal deposition. Arthritis Rheum., *9*:804–819, 1966.
125. McCarty, D.J., and Hogan, J.M.: Inflammatory reaction after intrasynovial injection of microcrystalline adrenocorticosteroid esters. Arthritis Rheum., *7*:359–367, 1964.
126. McCarty, D.J., and Hollander, J.: Identification of urate crystals in gouty synovial fluid. Ann. Intern. Med., *54*:452–460, 1961.
127. Reference has been omitted.
128. McCarty, D.J., Kohn, N.N., and Faires, J.S.: The significance of calcium phosphate crystals in the synovial fluid of arthritis patients: the "pseudogout syndrome." I. Clinical aspects. Ann. Intern. Med., *56*:711–737, 1962.
129. McCarty, D.J., Lehr, J.R., and Halverson, P.B.: Crystal populations in human synovial fluid: identification of apatite, octacalcium phosphate and beta tricalcium phosphate. Arthritis Rheum., *26*:1,220–1,224, 1983.
130. McCarty, D.J., Palmer, D.W., and James, C.: Clearance of calcium pyrophosphate dihydrate (CPPD) crystals in vivo II. Studies using triclinic crystals doubly labelled with ^{45}Ca and ^{85}Sr. Arthritis Rheum., *22*:1,122–1,131, 1979.
131. McCarty, D.J., Phelps, P., and Pyenson, P.: Crystal induced inflammation in canine joints. I. An experimental model with quantification of the host response. J. Exp. Med., *124*:99–114, 1966.
132. Maclachlan, M.J., and Rodnan, G.P.: Effects of food, fast and alcohol on serum uric acid and acute attacks of gout. Am. J. Med., *42*:38–57, 1967.
133. McMillan, R.M., et al.: Induction of collagenase and prostaglandin synthesis in synovial fibroblasts treated with monosodium urate crystals. J. Pharm. Pharmacol., *33*:382–383, 1981.
134. McMillan, R.M., et al.: Interactions of murine macrophages with monosodium urate crystals: stimulation of lysosomal enzyme release and prostaglandin synthesis. J. Rheumatol., *8*:555–562, 1981.
135. Malawista, S.E.: Gouty inflammation. Arthritis Rheum., *21*:S241–248, 1977.
136. Malawista, S.E.: The action of colchicine in acute gouty arthritis. Arthritis Rheum., *18*:835–846, 1975.
137. Malawista, S.E., and Andriole, V.T.: Colchicine: antiinflammatory action of low doses in a sensitive bacterial system. J. Lab. Clin. Med., *72*:933–942, 1968.
138. Malawista, S.E., and Seegmiller, J.E.: The effect of pretreatment with colchicine of the inflammatory response to microcrystalline urate. Ann. Intern. Med., *62*:648–657, 1965.
138a. Malawista, S.E., Chang, Y.H., and Wilson, L.: Lumicolchicine—lack of anti-inflammatory effect. Arthritis Rheum., *15*:641–643, 1972.
139. Mandel, N.S.: Structural changes in sodium urate crystals on heating. Arthritis Rheum., *23*:772–776, 1980.
140. Mandel, N.S.: The structural basis of crystal-induced membranolysis. Arthritis Rheum., *19*:439–445, 1976.
141. Mandel, N.S.: The crystal structure of calcium pyrophosphate dihydrate. Acta Crystallogr., *B31*:1,730–1,734, 1975.
142. Mandel, N.S., et al.: Crystal mediated membranolysis in pseudogout. (Abstract.) Arthritis Rheum., *22*:637, 1979.
143. Mandel, N.S., and Mandel, G.S.: Monosodium urate monohydrate: the gout culprit. J. Am. Chem. Soc., *98*:2,319–2,323, 1976.
144. Mandell, B.F., Spilberg, I., and Lichtman, J.: Inhibition of polymorphonuclear leukocyte capping by a chemotactic factor. J. Immunol., *118*:1,375–1,379, 1977.
145. Mattham, M., et al.: Acute pseudogout in the absence of synovial fluid leukocytes. J. Rheumatol., *4*:303–306, 1977.
146. Meed, S.D., and Spilberg, I.: Successful use of colchicine in acute polyarticular pseudogout. J. Rheumatol., *8*:689–691, 1981.
147. Messner, R.P., and Jelenek, J.: Receptors for human γ globulin on human neutrophils. J. Clin. Invest., *49*:2,165–2,171, 1970.
148. Melmon, K.L., et al.: The presence of a kinin in inflammatory synovial effusion from arthritides of varying etiologies. Arthritis Rheum., *10*:13–20, 1967.

149. Naff, G.F., and Byers, P.H.: Complement as a mediator of inflammation in acute gouty arthritis. I. Studies on the reaction between human serum complement and sodium urate crystals. J. Lab. Clin. Med., 81:747–760, 1973.

150. Nash, T., Allison, A.C., and Harrington, J.S.: Physiochemical properties of silica in relation to its toxicity. Nature, 210:259–265, 1966.

151. O'Duffy, J.D.: Clinical studies of acute pseudogout attacks: comments on prevalence, predisposition and treatment. Arthritis Rheum., 19:349–352, 1976.

152. Ortel, R.W., and Newcombe, D.S.: Acute gouty arthritis and response to colchicine in the virtual absence of synovial fluid leukocytes. N. Engl. J. Med., 290:1,363–1,364, 1974.

153. Paul, H., Clayburne, G., and Schumacher, H.R.: Lidocaine inhibits leukocyte migration and phagocytosis in monosodium urate crystal induced synovitis in dogs. J. Rheumatol., 10:434–439, 1983.

154. Perricone, E., and Brandt, K.: Enhancement of urate solubility by connective tissue. Arthritis Rheum., 21:453–460, 1978.

155. Pesante, E.L., and Axline, S.G.: Colchicine effects on lysosomal enzyme induction and intracellular degradation in the cultivated macrophage. J. Exp. Med., 141:1,030–1,046, 1976.

156. Phelps, P.: Appearance of chemotactic activity following intraarticular injection of monosodium urate crystals: effect of colchicine. J. Lab. Clin. Med., 76:622–631, 1970.

157. Phelps, P.: Polymorphonuclear leukocyte motility in vitro. IV. Colchicine inhibition of chemotactic activity formation after phagocytosis of urate crystals. Arthritis Rheum., 131:1–9, 1970.

158. Phelps, P.: Polymorphonuclear leukocyte motility in vitro. III. Possible release of a chemotactic substance following phagocytosis of urate crystals. Arthritis Rheum., 12:197–204, 1969.

159. Phelps, P.: Polymorphonuclear leukocyte motility in vitro. II. Stimulatory effect of monosodium urate crystals and urate in solution: partial inhibition by colchicine and indomethacin. Arthritis Rheum., 12:189–196, 1969.

160. Phelps, P., and McCarty, D.J.: Unpublished data.

161. Phelps, P., and McCarty, D.J.: Animal techniques for evaluating anti-inflammatory agents. In Animal and Clinical Pharmacology Techniques in Drug Evaluation. Vol. 2. Edited by P. Siegler and J.H. Moyer. Chicago, Yearbook, 1969.

162. Phelps, P., and McCarty, D.J.: Crystal induced arthritis. Postgrad. Med., 45:87–94, 1969.

163. Phelps, P., and McCarty, D.J.: Suppressive effects of indomethacin on crystal induced inflammation in canine joints and on neutrophilic motility in vitro. J. Pharmacol. Exp. Ther., 158:546–553, 1967.

164. Phelps, P., and McCarty, D.J.: Crystal induced inflammation in canine joints. II. Importance of polymorphonuclear leukocytes. J. Exp. Med., 124:115–126, 1966.

165. Phelps, P., Andrews, R., and Rosenbloom, J.: Demonstration of chemotactic factor in human gout: further characterization of occurrence and structure. J. Rheumatol., 8:889–894, 1981.

166. Phelps, P, Prockop, D.J., and McCarty, D.J.: Crystal induced inflammation in canine joints. III. Evidence against bradykinin as a mediator of inflammation. J. Lab. Clin. Med., 68:433–444, 1966.

167. Phelps, P., Steele, A.D., and McCarty, D.J.: Significance of Xenon-133 clearance rate from canine and human joints. Arthritis Rheum., 15:360–370, 1972.

168. Pritzker, K.P.H., et al.: Experimental crystal arthropathy. J. Rheumatol., 8:281–290, 1981.

169. Pritzker, K.P.H., and Luk, S.C.: Proceedings of Workshop on Techniques for Particulate Matter Studies in Scanning Electron Microscopy. Chicago., IIT Research Institute, 1976, p. 493.

170. Rae, S.E., Davidson, E.M., and Smith, M.J.H.: Leukotriene B$_4$, an inflammatory mediator in gout. Lancet, 2:1,122–1,138, 1982.

171. Rauault, T., Caldwell, D., and Holmes, E.W.: Re-evaluation of aspiration of asymptomatic metatarsophalangeal

joints in the diagnosis of gout. Arthritis Rheum., 23:740, 1980.

172. Reginato, A.S., Schumacher, H.R., and Martinez, V.A.: The articular cartilage in familial chondrocalcinosis: light and electron microscopic study. Arthritis Rheum., 17:977–992, 1974.

173. Riddle, J.M., Bluhm, G.B., and Barnhart, M.I.: Ultrastructural study of leukocytes and urates in gouty arthritis. Ann. Rheum. Dis., 26:389–400, 1967.

174. Riehl, G.: Wien. Klin. Wochenschr., 10:761, 1897.

175. Rodnan, G.P.: The pathogenesis of aldermanic gout: procatartic role of fluctuation in serum urate concentrations in gouty arthritis provoked by feast and alcohol. Arthritis Rheum., 23:737, 1980.

176. Rooney, P.J., et al.: Transient polyarthritis associated with familial hyperbetalipoproteinaemia. Q. J. Med., 187:249–259, 1978.

177. Ropes, M.W., and Bauer, W.: Synovial Fluid Changes in Joint Diseases. Cambridge, Harvard University Press, 1953.

178. Russell, I.J., et al.: Effect of IgG and C-reactive protein on complement depletion by monosodium urate crystals. J. Rheumatol., 10:425–433, 1983.

179. Russell, R.G.G., Bisaz, S., and Fleisch, H.: Inorganic pyrophosphate in plasma, urine and synovial fluid of patients with pyrophosphate arthropathy (chondrocalcinosis or pseudogout). Lancet, 2:899–902, 1970.

180. Sandstrom, C.: Peritendinitis calcarea. Am. J. Roentgenol., 40:1, 1938.

181. Scheele, C.W.: The Chemical Essays. Translated from Transactions of Academy of Sciences of Stockholm. London, J. Murray, 1787, p. 199.

182. Schumacher, H.R.: Pathogenesis of crystal-induced synovitis. Clin. Rheum. Dis., 3:105–131, 1977.

183. Schumacher, H.R.: Ultrastructural findings in chondrocalcinosis and pseudogout. Arthritis Rheum., 19:413–425, 1976.

184. Schumacher, H.R.: Pathology of the synovial membrane in gout. Arthritis Rheum., 18:771–782, 1975.

185. Schumacher, H.R.: The synovitis of pseudogout: electron microscopic observations. Arthritis Rheum., 11:426–435, 1968.

186. Schumacher, H.R., et al.: Arthritis associated with apatite crystals. Ann. Intern. Med., 87:411–416, 1977.

187. Schumacher, H.R., et al.: Acute gouty arthritis without urate crystals identified on initial examination of synovial fluid. Arthritis Rheum., 18:603–612, 1975.

188. Schumacher, H.R., et al.: Comparison of sodium urate and calcium pyrophosphate crystal phagocytosis by polymorphonuclear leukocytes. Arthritis Rheum., 18:783–792, 1975.

189. Schumacher, H.R., and Agudelo, C.A.: Intravascular degranulation of neutrophils, an important factor in inflammation? Science, 175:1,139–1,140, 1972.

190. Schumacher, H.R., and Phelps, P.: Sequential changes in human polymorphonuclear leukocytes after urate crystal phagocytosis. Arthritis Rheum., 14:513–526, 1971.

191. Schumacher, H.R., Phelps, P., and Agudelo, C.A.: Urate crystal induced inflammation in dog joints: sequence of synovial changes. J. Rheumatol., 1:102–110, 1974.

192. Seegmiller, J.E., Howell, R.R., and Malawista, S.E.: The inflammatory reaction to sodium urate. JAMA, 180:469–476, 1962.

193. Serhan, C.N., et al.: Formation of leukotrienes and hydroxy acids by human neutrophils and platelets exposed to monosodium urate. Clin. Res., 31:521A, 1983.

194. Silcox, D.C., and McCarty, D.J.: Elevated inorganic pyrophosphate concentrations in synovial fluid in osteoarthritis and pseudogout. J. Lab. Clin. Med., 83:518–531, 1974.

195. Simchowitz, L., Atkinson, J.P., and Spilberg, I.: Stimulation of the respiratory burst in human neutrophils by crystal phagocytosis. Arthritis Rheum., 25:181–188, 1982.

196. Simkin, P.A.: The pathogenesis of podagra. Ann. Intern. Med., 86:230–233, 1977.

197. Sirahama, T., and Cohen, A.: Ultrastructural evidence for leakage of lysosomal contents after phagocytosis of

monosodium urate crystals. Am. J. Pathol., 76:500–511, 1974.

198. Skinner, M., and Cohen, A.S.: Calcium pyrophosphate dihydrate crystal deposition disease. Arch. Intern. Med., 123:636–644, 1969.

199. Smith, R.J., and Phelps, P.: Septic arthritis, gout, pseudogout and osteoarthritis in the knee of a patient with multiple myeloma. Arthritis Rheum., 15:89–96, 1972.

200. Sokoloff, L.: The pathology of gout. Metabolism, 6:230–243, 1957.

201. Sorensen, L.B.: Gout secondary to chronic renal disease: studies on urate metabolism. Ann. Rheum. Dis., 39:424–430, 1980.

202. Spilberg, I.: Urate crystal arthritis in animals lacking Hageman factor. Arthritis Rheum., 17:143–148, 1974.

203. Spilberg, I.: Studies on the mechanism of inflammation induced by calcium pyrophosphate crystals. J. Lab. Clin. Med., 82:86–91, 1973.

204. Spilberg, I., et al.: Colchicine and pseudogout. Arthritis Rheum., 23:1,062–1,063, 1980.

205. Spilberg, I., et al.: Mechanism of action of colchicine in acute urate-crystal induced arthritis. J. Clin. Invest., 64:775–780, 1979.

206. Spilberg, I., et al.: A mechanism of action for non-steroid anti-inflammatory agents in calcium pyrophosphate dihydrate (CPPD) crystal induced arthritis. Agents Actions, 7:153–160, 1977.

207. Spilberg, I., et al.: Urate crystal-induced chemotactic factor: isolation and partial characterization. J. Clin. Invest., 58:815–819, 1976.

208. Spilberg, I., and Mandell, B.: Crystal induced chemotactic factor. Adv. Inflamm. Res., 5:57–65, 1983.

209. Spilberg, I, and Mehta, J.: Demonstration of a specific neutrophil receptor for a cell-derived chemotactic factor. J. Clin. Invest., 63:85–88, 1979.

210. Spilberg, I., and Osterland, C.K.: Anti-inflammatory effect of the trypsin kallikrein inhibitor in acute arthritis induced by urate crystals in rabbits. J. Lab. Clin. Med., 76:472–479, 1970.

211. Spilberg, I, Gallacher, A., and Mandell, B.: Calcium pyrophosphate dihydrate (CPPD) crystal-induced chemotactic factor: subcellular localization, role of protein synthesis and phagocytosis. J. Lab. Clin. Med., 9:817–822, 1977.

212. Spilberg, I., Gallacher, A., and Mandell, B.: Studies on crystal-induced chemotactic factor. II. Role of phagocytosis. J. Lab. Clin. Med., 85:631–636, 1975.

213. Spilberg, I., Mandell, B., and Wochner, R.D.: Studies on crystal-induced chemotactic factor. I. Requirement for protein synthesis and neutral protease activity. J. Lab. Clin. Med., 83:56–63, 1974.

214. Spilberg, I, Mehta, J., and Simchowitz, L.: Induction of a chemotactic factor from human neutrophils by diverse crystals. J. Lab. Clin. Med., 100:399–404, 1982.

215. Spilberg, I, Rosenberg, D., and Mandell, B.: Induction of arthritis by purified cell-derived chemotactic factor. J. Clin. Invest., 59:582–585, 1977.

216. Spilberg, I., Rosenberg, D., and Mehta, J.: Induction of cell-derived chemotactic factor (CF) and of arthritis by amorphous diamond crystals. (Abstract.) Arthritis Rheum., 20:136, 1976.

217. Spilberg, I., Tanphaichitr, K., and Kantor, P.: Synovial fluid pH in acute gouty arthritis. Arthritis Rheum., 20:142, 1977.

218. Steele, A.D., and McCarty, D.J.: Suppressive effects of indoxal in crystal-induced synovitis in man. Ann. Rheum. Dis., 26:39–42, 1967.

219. Steele, A.D., and McCarty, D.J.: An experimental model of acute inflammation in man. Arthritis Rheum., 9:430–442, 1966.

220. Stepan, J., Petrova, S., and Pozderka, V.: Cystinosis with crystal-induced synovitis and arthropathy. Z. Rheumatol., 35:347–355, 1976.

221. Stodler, J., and Franke, W.: Colchicine binding of proteins in chromatin and membranes. Nature, 237:237–238, 1972.

222. Struthers, G.R., et al.: Musculoskeletal disorders in pa-

tients with hyperlipidemia. Ann. Rheum. Dis., 42:519–523, 1983.

223. Tak, H.K., and Wilcox, W.R.: Crystallization of monosodium urate and calcium urate at 37° C. J. Coll. Int. Sci., 77:195–201, 1980.

224. Tak, H.K., Cooper, S.M., and Wilcox, W.R.: Studies on the nucleation of monosodium urate at 37° C. Arthritis Rheum., 23:574–580, 1980.

225. Tak, H.K., Wilcox, W.R., and Cooper, S.M.: The effect of lead upon urate nucleation. Arthritis Rheum., 24:1,291–1,295, 1981.

226. Terkeltaub, R., et al.: Lipoproteins containing apoprotein B are a major regulator of neutrophil responses to monosodium urate crystals. J. Clin. Invest., 73:1719–1730, 1984.

227. Terkeltaub, R., et al.: Plasma protein binding by monosodium urate crystals: analysis by two-dimensional gel electrophoresis. Arthritis Rheum., 26:775–783, 1983.

228. Thompson, G.R., et al.: Calcific tendinitis and soft tissue calcification resembling gout. JAMA, 203:464–472, 1968.

229. Tse, R.L., and Phelps, P.: Polymorphonuclear leukocyte motility in vitro. V. Release of chemotactic activity following phagocytosis of calcium pyrophosphate crystals, diamond dust and urate crystals. J. Lab. Clin. Med., 76:403–411, 1970.

230. Tse, R.L., Phelps, P., and Urban, D.: Polymorphonuclear leukocyte motility in vitro. VII. Effect of purine and pyrimidine analogues: possible role of cyclic AMP. J. Lab. Clin. Med., 80:264–281, 1972.

231. Ulrich, F., abnd Zilversmit, D.B.: Release from alveolar macrophages of in inhibitor of phagocytosis. Am. J. Physiol., 217:1,118–1,126, 1970.

232. Utsinger, P.D.: Abstract 448. In Proceedings of the Fourteenth International Congress of Rheumatology. San Francisco, 1977.

233. Van Arman, C.G., et al.: Experimental gouty synovitis caused by bacterial endotoxin adsorbed onto urate crystals. Arthritis Rheum., 17:439–450, 1974.

234. Van Arman, C.G., Carlson, R.P., and Risley, E.H.: Inhibitory effects of indomethacine, aspirin and certain other drugs of inflammations induced in rat and dog by carrageenan sodium urate-ellagic acid. J. Pharmacol. Exp. Ther., 175:459–468, 1970.

235. Wallace, S.L.: The treatment of the acute attack of gout. Clin. Rheum. Dis., 3:133–143, 1977.

236. Wallace, S.L.: Colchicine and anti-inflammatory drugs for treatment of acute gout. Arthritis Rheum., 18:847–851, 1975.

237. Wallace, S.L.: Colchicine analogs in the treatment of acute gout. Arthritis Rheum., 2:389–395, 1959.

238. Wallace, S.L., et al.: Preliminary criteria for the classification of the acute arthritis of primary gout. Arthritis Rheum., 20:895–900, 1977.

239. Wallace, S.L., and Ertel, N.H.: Plasma levels of colchicine after oral administration of a single dose. Metabolism, 22:749–753, 1973.

240. Wallace, S.L., Bernstein, D., and Diamond, H.: Diagnostic value of the colchicine therapeutic trial. JAMA, 199:525–528, 1967.

241. Wallace, S.L., Omokoku, B., Ertel, N.H.: Colchicine plasma levels—implications as to pharmacology and mechanisms of action. Am. J. Med., 48:443–448, 1970.

242. Wallingford, W.R., and McCarty, D.J.: Differential membranolytic effects of microcrystalline sodium urate and calcium pyrophosphate dihydrate. J. Exp. Med., 133:100–112, 1971.

243. Wallingford, W.R., and Trend, B.: Phagolysosome rupture after monosodium urate (MSU) but not calcium pyrophosphate dihydrate (CPPD) phagocytosis in vitro. Arthritis Rheum., 14:420–421, 1971.

244. Ward, P.A., and Zvaifler, N.J.: Complement derived leukotactic factors in inflammatory synovial fluids of humans. J. Clin. Invest., 50:606–616, 1971.

245. Webster, M.E., Maling, H.M., and Williams, M.A.: Urate crystals induced inflammation in the rat: Evidence of the combined actions of kinins, histamine and components of complement. Immunology, 1:185–198, 1972.

246. Weinberger, A., Schumacher, H.R., and Agudelo, C.A.: Urate crystals in asymptomatic metatarsophalangeal joints. Ann. Intern. Med., *56*:56–57, 1979.

247. Weissmann, G., and Rita, G.: Molecular basis of gouty inflammation. Interaction of monosodium urate crystals with lysosomes and liposomes Nature (New Biol.), *240*:167–172, 1972.

248. Weissmann, G., Zurier, R.B., and Spieler, P.G.: Mechanisms of lysosomal enzyme release from leukocytes exposed to immune complexes and other particles. J. Exp. Med., *134 (Suppl.)*:149S–165S, 1971.

249. Wigley, F.M., Fine, I.T., and Newcombe, D.S.: The role of human synovial fibroblast in monosodium urate crystal induced synovitis. J. Rheumatol., *10*:602–611, 1983.

250. Wilcox, W.R., and Khalaf, A.A.: Nucleation of mono-sodium urate crystals. Ann. Rheum. Dis., *34*:332–339, 1975.

251. Willkens, R.F., Case, J.B., and Huix, F.J.: Treatment of gout with naproxen. J. Clin. Pharmacol., *15*:363–372, 1975.

252. Yu, T.F., and Gutman, A.B.: Efficiency of colchicine prophylaxis in gout. Ann. Intern. Med., *55*:179–192, 1961.

253. Zigmond, S.H., and Hirsch, J.G.: Leukocyte locomotion and chemotaxis. J. Exp. Med., *137*:387–410, 1973.

254. Zuckner, J., et al.: Cholesterol crystals in synovial fluid. Ann. Intern. Med., *60*:436–446, 1964.

255. Zvaifler, N.J., and Perkin, T.J.: Significance of urate crystals in synovial fluids. Arch. Intern. Med., *111*:99–102, 1963.

Chapter **94**

Calcium Pyrophosphate Crystal Deposition Disease; Pseudogout; Articular Chondrocalcinosis

Lawrence M. Ryan and Daniel J. McCarty

Microscopic examination of wet preparations of synovial fluid under compensated polarized light has provided a rapid, specific, and sensitive method for identification of crystals in gout, which might be called monosodium urate (MSU) crystal deposition disease.[134] Both monoclinic (unit cell with one obtuse and two right angles) and triclinic (unit cell with three obtuse angles) MSU crystals are seen, and "twinning" or pairing of crystals is observed frequently. Digestion with purified uricase has established the specific chemical composition of these crystals. See Chapters 4 and 95 for a discussion of various techniques of crystal identification.

Application of these methods to examination of synovial fluids led to the discovery of nonurate crystals in patients with a gout-like syndrome termed "pseudogout."[136] These biaxial crystals were identified as calcium pyrophosphate dihydrate ($Ca_2P_2O_7 \cdot 2H_2O$ or CPPD)[112] (Fig. 94–1,*A*). These crystals also exhibited monoclinic and triclinic dimorphism, and they frequently showed twinning. Polariscopically, they had a weakly positive birefringence and inclined extinction. Some of these crystals were isotropic under polarized light (nonrefractile). Urate crystals, on the other hand, were negatively birefringent under compensated polarized light and showed axial extinction. Fluid removed from acutely inflamed joints of patients with pseudogout invariably showed phagocytosed CPPD crystals (Fig. 94–1,*B*).

Both MSU and CPPD crystals with morphologic features identical to natural crystals were synthesized.[16,29,132] Injection of such crystals into normal human and canine joints was followed by an acute inflammatory response. The phrase "crystal-induced synovitis" was coined to describe the tissue reaction provoked by either type of crystal,[128] and the responsible mechanisms are discussed in Chapter 93.

NOMENCLATURE

We initially termed the syndrome associated with CPPD deposition "pseudogout" because of the obvious parallel with true (urate) gout.[136] Subsequent study has revealed that many patients with symptomatic arthritis do not have acute attacks, so this term should be reserved for the acute episodes associated with CPPD crystals. "Chondrocalcinosis" was coined by Zitnan and Sitaj, based on the characteristic radiologic features.[239] Because subsequent analysis of cartilage calcifications showed at least three distinct mineral phases, this term is too broad and nonspecific, although it may suffice to indicate radiologic cartilage calcifications when crystal identification is lacking. "Pyrophosphate arthropathy" was coined in 1969 by H.L.F. Currey and is widely used in the United Kingdom.[125] No reason appears to justify blaming pyrophosphate for the arthropathy. Indeed, recent studies indicate that the calcium component of the crystal is responsible for profound biologic effects (see Chap. 95). It appears most prudent to use the specific term "CPPD crystal deposition disease" unless some good reason can be found to abandon it.

EARLY REPORTS

Initially, seven arthritic patients were studied over a two-year period, and the presence of microcrystalline CPPD was used as a common denominator (Figs. 94–1,*A*, 94–2). Table 94–1 compares the interplanar spacings and the relative intensities of x-ray diffraction powder patterns prepared from clinical material with those of pure monoclinic and triclinic CPPD prepared by Brown et al.[29] The radiographic appearance of calcification of fibroarticular and hyaline articular cartilage was noted (see Fig. 94–1,*C*). Analysis of such deposits showed CPPD crystals identical to those seen in joint fluid. Figure 94–3 shows the basic features of the x-ray diffraction powder technique.

In addition to pseudogout attacks and a chronic degenerative arthropathy, other findings in this initial group of patients were confirmed by subsequent separate reports. For example, a destructive arthropathy resembling Charcot joints, radiologic le-

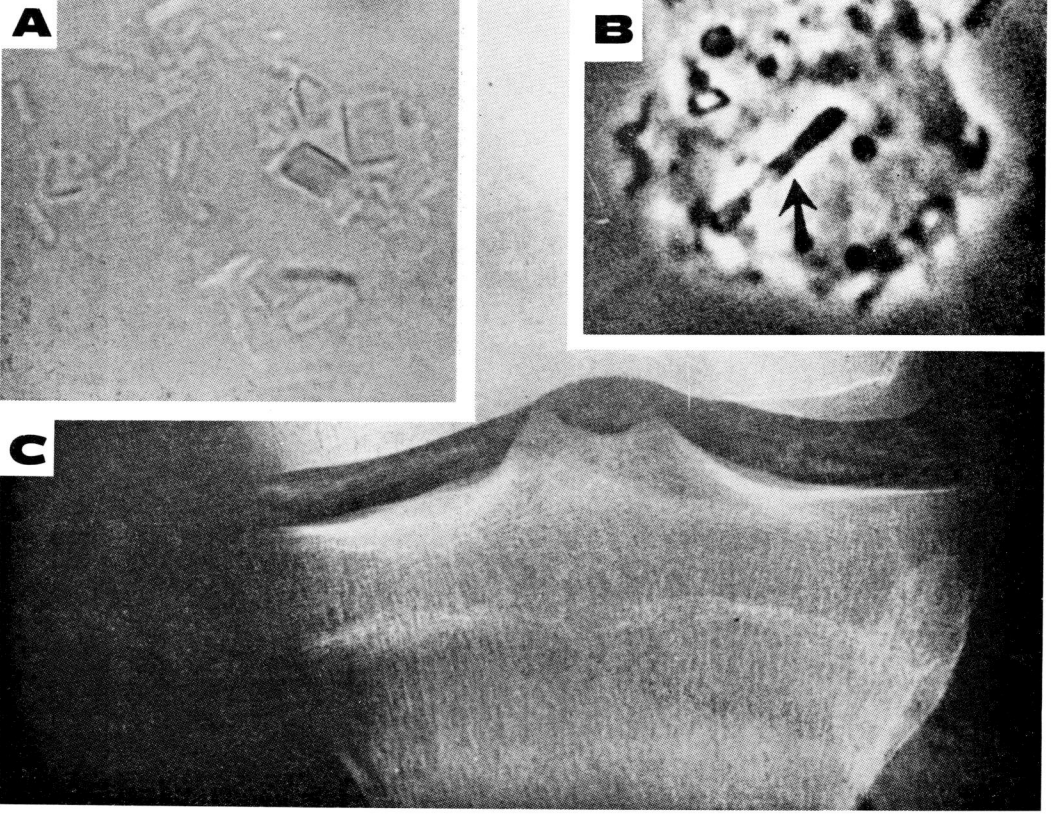

Fig. 94–1. *A,* Weakly birefringent monoclinic and triclinic calcium pyrophosphate dihydrate (CPPD) microcrystals in synovial fluid removed from a chronically symptomatic knee (polarized light × 1,250). *B,* Phagocytosed crystal (arrow) in a polymorphonuclear leukocyte (phase contrast × 1,250). *C,* Anteroposterior roentgenogram of the knee showing typical punctate and linear deposits of CPPD in the menisci and articular cartilage.

sions resembling osteochondromas, hemorrhagic joint fluids, prominent subchondral cysts, and urate crystals associated with gouty arthritis were all documented at least once in our initial series. When the clinical and roentgenographic findings in this group were analyzed, a review of the literature revealed a similarity to chondrocalcinosis polyarticularis (familiaris), as described in 1958 by the Czechoslovakian authors, Zitnan and Sitaj.[239] These workers used the characteristic roentgenographic appearance as the unifying diagnostic feature. They pointed out that the menisci of the knee were most commonly involved (see Fig. 94–1,*C*). These authors later reported 27 cases, 21 from 5 Hungarian families living in a single village in Slovakia.[238] Many patients in our present series have crystallographically proved familial disease.

Perhaps the first report of CPPD deposition was made in 1903 by Bennett.[13] He described autopsy findings in an elderly man of mineral deposits in cartilages of the hips, shoulders, sternoclavicular

joints, and temporomandibular joints. Chemical analysis indicated a substantial calcium and carbonate content, but no urates by the murexide test. The individual crystals were described as smaller than urate crystals and rhomboidal in shape under an ordinary light microscope.

Two types of meniscal calcification were differentiated on gross and microscopic pathologic grounds in 1927 by the Viennese surgeon Mandl,[140] who is best remembered for having performed the first parathyroidectomy for hyperparathyroidism. A "primary" type predominated in the elderly and involved all four menisci with diffuse focal deposits of calcium salts; meniscal surfaces were smooth; the disorder occurred without antecedent trauma and was frequently asymptomatic. Microscopically, punctate deposits of granular calcific material and a striking hypocellularity of the involved cartilage were noted. A "secondary" type, found in a younger age group, involved a localized deposit in a single meniscus and usually followed

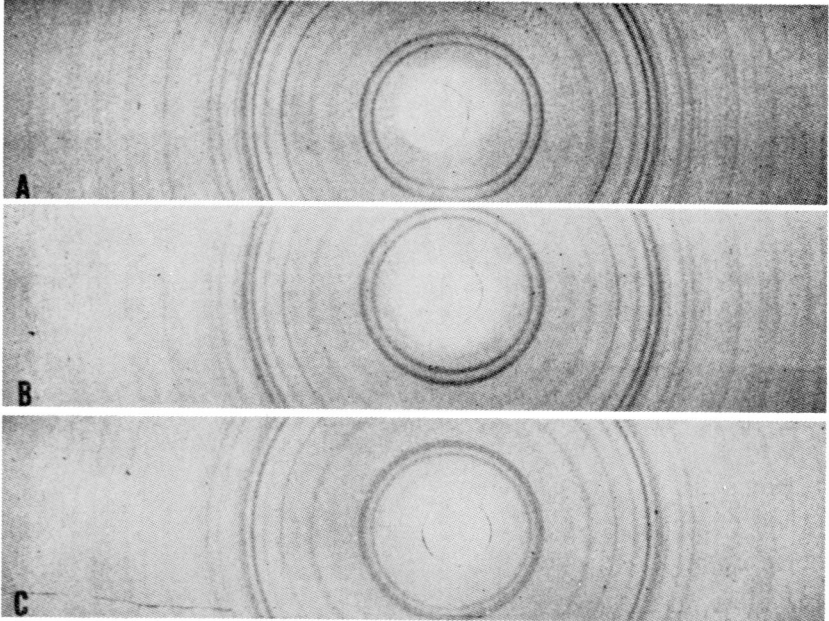

Fig. 94–2. X-ray diffraction powder patterns of crystals harvested from fluid aspirated from the knees of three patients; the interplanar spacings of the crystal populations are identical. The powder pattern is known as the "fingerprint" of the crystal and is ideal for the specific identification of small crystals such as these.

trauma to the joint. The cartilage surface over the deposit was roughened, and the condition was symptomatic, frequently requiring meniscectomy.

A well-studied case reported by Werwath in 1926 contained the first roentgenogram showing the characteristic pattern of "primary" calcification; the author correlated this pattern with the pathologic findings.[229] Calcifications were found in the menisci, hyaline articular cartilage, ligaments, and joint capsule; Werwath thought that the condition was due to a metabolic disorder and that it led to arthritis deformans (osteoarthritis). In 1929, Tobler systematically examined 400 menisci from 100 necropsies of cadavers ranging in age from several days to 86 years.[221] He found degenerative changes in 75% and calcification in 25% of menisci.

In their classic monograph on the effect of aging in the knee, Bennett, Waine, and Bauer described small deposits of "granular material" in semilunar cartilages showing interstitial matrix altered by degenerative changes.[14] Marked calcifications of the "primary" type were found in the lateral meniscus of a 90-year-old man; the medial meniscus, similarly involved, had been almost completely destroyed. Thus, 3 of 63 cadavers studied showed "primary" calcification (4.1%). None in their series had had symptomatic arthritis during life.

PREVALENCE

A summary of reported anatomic and radiologic studies of the prevalence of knee joint calcification is given in Table 94–2. The study of elderly Jewish subjects by Ellman and Levin, using high-resolution film, is of particular interest.[66] Fully 27.6% of their ambulatory volunteers showed calcific deposits. Assuming that all were CPPD deposits, this finding implicated age itself as a factor in the expression of the condition. These findings have been confirmed by a recent French report using standard radiograms of the knee in 108 women over 80 years of age.[145] Meniscal calcification was found in 16% of the 55 women aged 80 to 89, and in 30% of 53 women aged 89 to 99; 22 of 25 with knee chondrocalcinosis had deposits in other joints as well. Similarly, a radiographic survey of unselected patients admitted to a geriatric unit in the United Kingdom disclosed a 44% prevalence of chondrocalcinosis in patients over 84 years of age, when films of the hands and wrist, pelvis, and knees were examined.[232] The prevalence was 15% in patients between 65 and 74 years of age and 36% in those between 75 and 84 years.

X-ray diffraction powder patterns were obtained from at least 1 tissue deposit or from crystals harvested from synovial fluid in 51 of our first 80 cases; all were CPPD crystals. A study of over 800 menisci from 215 anatomic cadavers was undertaken, using the CPPD crystal as a "marker"[131] (Fig. 94–4). At least 1 tiny deposit was seen in the type-M roentgenogram of 22% of excised menisci; most were too small to permit dissection,

Table 94–1. Summary of Major Interplanar Spacings and Relative Intensities of Natural Calcium Pyrophosphate Dihydrate (CPPD) (Mean of 78 Patterns*) Compared With Those of Synthetic CPPD

Natural		Synthetic			
		Monoclinic		Triclinic	
d†	i‡	d	i	d	i
8.04	100			7.94	90
7.37	30	7.37	90		
7.01	90			6.95	90
		6.12	35		
5.50	20			5.50	20
		5.40	30		
5.25	20			5.27	20
4.61	40	4.62	100		
4.50	25			4.49	50
4.02	30			4.03	50
3.74	10	3.72	75	3.74	10
3.45	50	3.45	50	3.48	70
3.24	100	3.25	100	3.24	100
3.12	90			3.11	100
3.06	40	3.05	100	3.06	25
2.98	50			2.98	60
2.78	50	2.79	40	2.78	60
2.67	50	2.65	90	2.67	60
2.59	20	2.57	100	2.59	30
2.52	25			2.53	40
2.44	15	2.42	40		
2.40	10			2.40	35
2.34	15			2.34	25
2.30	5	2.31	40		
2.26	25			2.26	50
2.18	10	2.21	35	2.20	25
2.11	15	2.11	35	2.11	30
2.06	10			2.07	25
2.01	20	2.01	40	2.01	40
		1.91	40		
1.90	15			1.90	20
1.84	15	1.85	25	1.84	30
1.81	10			1.81	30
		1.77	30		
1.75	10	1.74	25	1.75	25
1.72	10	1.71	25	1.72	40
1.66	10			1.66	30
1.63	10			1.63	20
1.57	15	1.57	20	1.57	25

*All patterns obtained with a 114.59-mm diameter Debye-Scherrer powder camera using nickel-filtered copper K alpha radiation ($\lambda = 1.54050$ Å).

†d = Interplanar spacings in Angstroms.

‡i = Relative intensities estimated visually by assigning the value of 100 to the strongest line and comparing the other lines to this standard.

(From Brown, et al.[30])

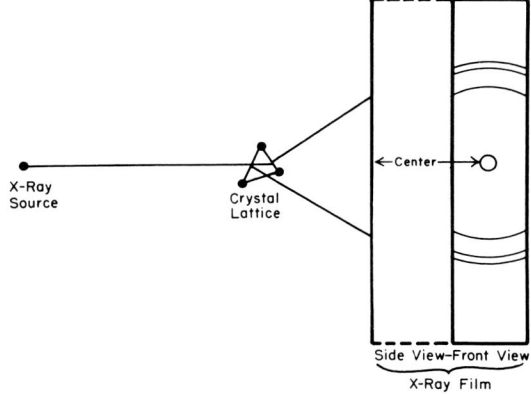

Fig. 94–3. Diagram showing the essential features of the powder pattern technique. Low-energy x rays are diffracted by sheets of atoms the arrangement of which is specific for a given crystal. The diffracted beams are recorded on a strip of x-ray film, located at a fixed distance from the crystals. When the film is developed. a series of arcs is obtained. The interplanar spacings between the atomic sheets may then be calculated simply from measurements made on the arcs.

much less identification. Seven sets of menisci (3.2% of cadavers) showed linear and punctate deposits of CPPD; 5 sets (2.3% of cadavers) showed multiple punctate deposits of dicalcium phosphate dihydrate ($CaHPO_4 \cdot 2H_2O$ or DCPD) (Fig. 94–5); 3 single menisci (1.4% of cadavers) showed solitary deposits of "hydroxyapatite." Studies now suggest the term "basic calcium phosphate" (BCP) instead of hydroxyapatite (see Chapter 95). Thus, 2 types of "primary" pathologic cartilaginous calcifications were mutually exclusive in a given cadaver, with a single exception. Most cadavers with "primary" meniscal deposits had them in avascular articular structures in other joints as well. Four cadavers in this series had sodium urate deposits in the menisci.

Two reports have identified DCPD crystals in cartilage (Fig. 94–5) and in synovial fluid.[77,222] The crystals in synovial fluid were both free and intraleukocytic, so they too might be inflammatory. Still other reports of apatite-like crystals in joint fluids,[50] and in joint fluid leukocytes,[204] have appeared (see Chap. 95). At times, synovial fluids contain both apatite-like and CPPD crystals, leading to the term, "mixed crystal deposition disease."[49,58] CPPD crystals were also seen in joint fluids in 6 of 15 patients with Milwaukee shoulder/knee syndrome (see Chap. 95),[94] which is characterized by the presence of synovial BCP crystals.

A survey of a large number of pathologic nonarticular calcifications from necropsy and surgical specimens using crystallographic techniques

Table 94–2. Prevalence of Calcific Deposits in Knee Joints

Anatomic Studies (Authors)	Cadavers (No.)	Positive for Calcium Pyrophosphate Dihydrate (%)	
Bennett et al.[14]	63	4.1*	
McCarty et al.[131]	215	3.2	
Lagier and Baud[116]	320	6.8	
Mitrovic et al.[151]	108	18.5	

Radiologic Studies (Authors)	Subjects (No.)	Average Age (Yr.)	Positive for Calcific Deposits (%)
Bocher et al.[26]	455	80	7.0
Cabanel et al.[35]	200	—	6.5
Zinn et al.[236]	131	65	4.6
Schmied et al.[201]	52	66 (diabetic)	5.8
	45	61 (control)	2.2
Ellman and Levin[66]	58	83	27.6
Mezard et al.[147]	299	65	12.5
Glimet et al.[87]	50	73	14
DeLauche et al.[42a]	62	85	32
Memin et al.[145]	108	88	23
Wilkins et al.[232]	100	79	34

*Crystals not identified specifically.

showed no CPPD crystals and thus established their relative specificity for articular tissue.[75] Identification of crystals in aortic plaques, costal cartilages, pancreas, and pineal glands obtained from pseudogout patients at necropsy showed only apatite. Periarticular deposits of crystallographically proved CPPD, however, have been reported in tendons,[82] dura mater,[93] ligamenta flava,[34,65,109,111] and the olecranon bursa,[97] as well as in isolated "tophi."[119,122]

Joint Fluid Findings

Nearly all fluids aspirated from inflamed joints showed phagocytosed CPPD microcrystals (Fig. 94–1*B*). Unlike urate crystals, they were often within phagolysosomes.[136] CPPD crystals are much more difficult to see by polarized light microscopy than are MSU crystals, and we routinely use phase-contrast in addition to polarized light at thousand-fold magnification for crystal identification. Even using these sensitive techniques, ultramicrocrystals cannot be detected.[23] The number of crystals bears some relation to the acuteness of inflammation because pellets from joint fluid taken during acute attacks contained much more pyrophosphate on chemical analysis, after acid treatment to dissolve the crystals, than did pellets from noninflamed joints.[126] Exceptions occur, however. Some fluids from inflamed joints have few CPPD crystals, and some fluids from noninflamed joints are milky on gross inspection because of the large number of crystals present. This same phenomenon has been noted in true gout. The mean leukocyte concentra-

tion in acute attacks is exactly the same as in urate gout, about 20,000/mm³, with over 90% polymorphonuclear cells. The addition of acetic acid is more likely to yield a "good" mucin clot in pseudogout than in gout.[40] As already noted, the fluid in pseudogout may be tinged with blood, especially early in the acute episode.[136,161,217] In at least one case, such fluid was associated with subchondral bony fractures.[17]

DIAGNOSTIC CRITERIA

A diagnostic classification, based on the premise that CPPD crystals are the specific feature of the disease,[128] has been modified to include radiographic clues suggested by Resnick[177] and Martel[142] (Table 94–3). A case is considered "definite" if CPPD crystals are demonstrated in tissues or synovial fluid by definitive means, such as by x-ray diffraction, or if crystals compatible with CPPD are demonstrated by compensated polarized light microscopy and typical calcifications are seen on roentgenograms. If only one of these criteria is found, a "probable" diagnosis is made. The clinical findings or the radiologic clues given in Table 94–3 should alert the clinician to the possible presence of underlying CPPD crystal deposition disease. Most of our cases are now suspected on clinical grounds, with subsequent confirmation by joint fluid and roentgenographic study.

CLINICAL FEATURES

The features of two crystal deposition diseases, gout and pseudogout, are compared in Table 94–4.

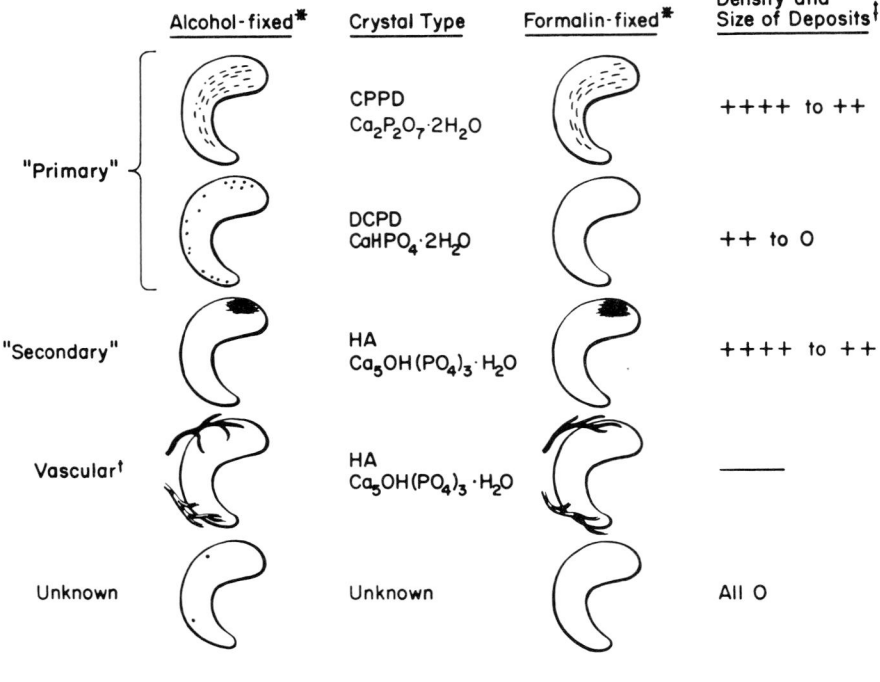

Alcohol-fixed*	Crystal Type	Formalin-fixed*	Density and Size of Deposits†

"Primary" — CPPD $Ca_2P_2O_7 \cdot 2H_2O$ — $++++$ to $++$

DCPD $CaHPO_4 \cdot 2H_2O$ — $++$ to 0

"Secondary" — HA $Ca_5OH(PO_4)_3 \cdot H_2O$ — $++++$ to $++$

Vascular† — HA $Ca_5OH(PO_4)_3 \cdot H_2O$ — ——

Unknown — Unknown — All 0

* Roentgenographic appearance
† No systematic attempt was made to study vascular deposits
‡ Estimated from gross inspection of alcohol-fixed menisci

Fig. 94–4. Summary of pathologic calcifications found in over 800 menisci removed from 215 anatomic cadavers. The 2 types of "primary" calcification found were, with a single exception, mutually exclusive in a given cadaver. Calcium pyrophosphate dihydrate (CPPD) crystal deposits were found in 3.3% of cadavers, dicalcium phosphate dihydrate (DCPD) in 2.3%. Both involved other cartilaginous structures in the same cadavers. Calcification of the vessels supplying the outer third of the menisci occurred frequently and usually affected all 4 menisci. Tiny radiopaque deposits, occurring in at least 1 meniscus in 30% of cadavers, were too small to permit identification. (Calcium oxalate crystals, now known to occur in the cartilage of uremic patients, should be added.) HA = Hydroxyapatite.

In our present series of over 450 "definite" and "probable" cases, men predominate in a ratio of 1.5 to 1. A similar sex ratio was recorded at the Mayo Clinic.[156] Female predominance has been reported in 2 surveys of patients with symptomatic CPPD deposition.[48,69] Our patients' ages averaged 72 years at the time of diagnosis. The average age at the time of diagnosis was lower in the Czechoslovakian and Chilean series because these studies included familial and asymptomatic cases detected radiographically. The absence of the putative associated diseases, such as hyperparathyroidism, hemochromatosis, and urate gout, in the familial cases is noteworthy.

The various patterns of arthritis encountered clinically are summarized graphically in Figure 94–6. We now regard CPPD deposition as a great mimic because it often superficially resembles not only gout, but also rheumatoid arthritis (RA), osteoarthritis, and other types of joint disease. An expanded version of this clinical classification, to include hemarthrosis, monoarthropathy, solitary tophaceous deposits, and other clinical presentations, has been published.[125]

Type A—Pseudogout

This pattern is marked by acute or subacute arthritic attacks lasting approximately one day to four weeks (Fig. 94–7A). These episodes are self-limited and generally involve only one or a few appendicular joints. Such attacks can be as severe as those of true gout, but they usually take longer to reach peak intensity and are less painful and disabling than gouty episodes. Inflammation may begin in a single "mother" joint with spread to involve other nearby "daughter" joints, the so-called "cluster" attack of the crystal deposition diseases. Mild "petite" attacks also occur, as in urate gout, and these may often outnumber full-blown attacks.

Provocation of acute episodes by a surgical procedure or by medical illness is common in both

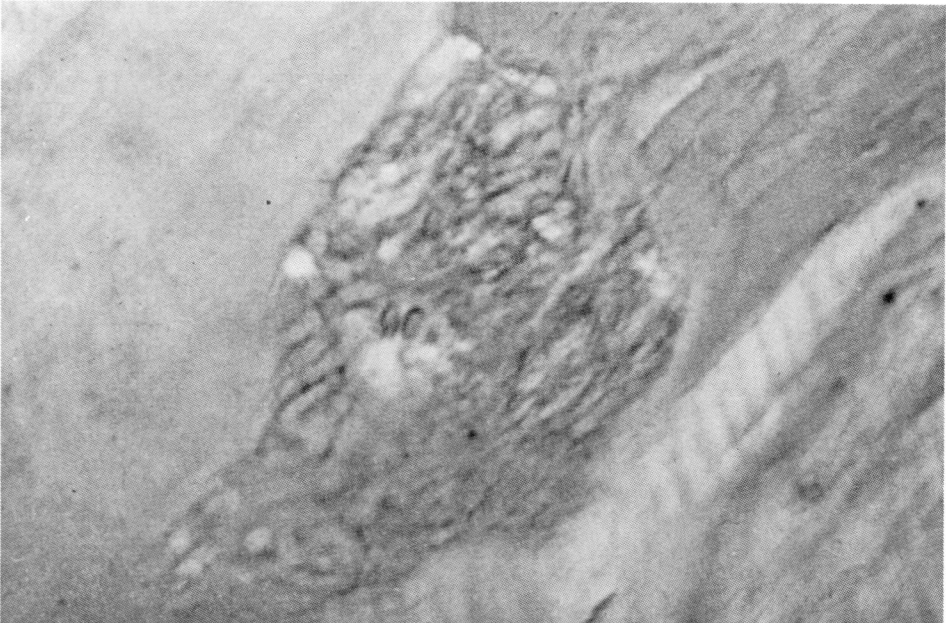

Fig. 94–5. A focal deposit of dicalcium phosphate dihydrate (Brushite) microcrystals in fibrocartilage. These birefringent crystals are relatively soluble in water and were not found in specimens fixed in aqueous formalin (unstained section by polarized light × 1,250; linear magnification × 3.5 when printed).

gout and pseudogout. One study reported that the percentage of patients with either disease who had at least a single episode after operation was virtually identical: 8.3% of 168 gouty patients and 9.4% of 106 patients with pseudogout.[127,225] Parathyroidectomy is particularly likely to precipitate acute arthritis.[19,156] Similarly, severe medical illness, particularly vascular occlusion such as stroke or myocardial infarction, provoked attacks in 20.3% of 167 gouty subjects, as opposed to 24% of 104 patients with pseudogout. Trauma may provoke acute arthritis in patients with either gout or pseudogout. Because both types of crystals are often found in the same subject, and because either may cause self-limited attacks under identical clinical circumstances and may respond similarly to treatment, joint aspiration and specific crystal identification are essential for precise differential diagnosis.

The knee joint is to pseudogout as the bunion joint is to gout, and it is the site of over half of all acute attacks. At least nine crystal-proved instances of first metatarsophalangeal joint involvement, "pseudopodagra," are known to us.

Although not nearly as predictably effective as in urate gout, oral colchicine may provide dramatic relief in pseudogout. The release of a chemotactic factor by polymorphonuclear leukocytes after phagocytosis of either MSU or CPPD crystals[162] (see Chap. 93) is inhibited by colchicine in concentrations easily reached in serum by the usual therapeutic doses. That the inhibition of urate crystal-induced release was more predictable than that induced by CPPD crystals provides an in vitro parallel to the clinical experience in patients. Spilberg and associates found that colchicine, 1 to 2 mg, given intravenously predictably controls acute attacks of pseudogout[215] (see Chap. 93).

Approximately 20% of patients with CPPD deposits have hyperuricemia, and about 5% have MSU crystal deposits as well. About 25% of our series of patients show this gout-like, type A pattern. Men predominate. As in gout, the patients are usually completely asymptomatic between attacks. Radiographic evidence of CPPD deposits is found in most patients with this pattern of disease.

Type B—Pseudorheumatoid Arthritis

Approximately 5% of patients have multiple joint involvement with subacute attacks lasting 4 weeks to several months. Nonspecific symptoms of inflammation, such as morning stiffness and fatigue, are common; signs such as synovial thickening, localized pitting edema, limitation of joint motion due to inflammation or to flexion contractures, and elevated erythrocyte sedimentation rates are found. Such patients are often thought to have RA.[45,152] In addition, because about 10% of patients

Table 94–3.   Revised Diagnostic Criteria for Calcium Pyrophosphate Dihydrate (CPPD) Crystal Deposition Disease (Pseudogout)

Criteria
  I. Demonstration of CPPD crystals, obtained by biopsy, necropsy, or aspirated synovial fluid, by definitive means; e.g., characteristic "fingerprint" by x-ray diffraction powder pattern or by chemical analysis.
 II. A. Identification of monoclinic or triclinic crystals showing a weakly positive, or a lack of birefringence by compensated polarized light microscopy.
      B. Presence of typical calcifications on roentgenograms.*
III. A. Acute arthritis, especially of knees or other large joints, with or without concomitant hyperuricemia.
      B. Chronic arthritis, especially of knees, hips, wrists, carpus, elbow, shoulder, and metacarpophalangeal joints, particularly if accompanied by acute exacerbations; the chronic arthritis shows the following features helpful in differentiating it from osteoarthritis:[177]
          1. Uncommon site for primary osteoarthritis; e.g., wrist, metacarpophalangeal joints, elbow, or shoulder.
          2. Radiographic appearance; e.g., radiocarpal or patellofemoral joint space narrowing, especially if isolated (patella "wrapped around" the femur†); femoral cortical erosion superior to the patella on the lateral view of the knee.[115]
          3. Subchondral cyst formation.
          4. Severe progressive degeneration, with subchondral bony collapse (microfractures), and fragmentation, with formation of intra-articular radiodense bodies.
          5. Variable and inconstant osteophyte formation.
          6. Tendon calcifications, especially of Achilles, triceps, and obturator tendons.
          7. Involvement of the axial skeleton with subchondral cysts of apophyseal and sacroiliac joints, multiple levels of disc calcification and vacuum phenomenon, and sacroiliac vacuum phenomenon.[142]

Categories
     A. Definite—criteria I or II(A) and (B) must be fulfilled.
     B. Probable—criteria IIA or IIB must be fulfilled.
     C. Possible—criteria IIIA or B should alert the clinician to the possibility of underlying CPPD deposition.

*Heavy punctate and linear calcifications in fibrocartilages, articular (hyaline) cartilages, and joint capsules, especially if bilaterally symmetric; faint or atypical calcifications may be due to DCPD ($CaHPO_4 \cdot 2H_2O$) deposits or to vascular calcifications; both are also often bilaterally symmetric.
†Also described as a feature of the arthritis of hyperparathyroidism.

with CPPD-related arthritis have positive tests for rheumatoid factor,[127,225] albeit usually in low titer, the opportunities for confusion abound. The presence of high titers of rheumatoid factor and typical radiographic erosions favor a diagnosis of "true" RA.[176] Interestingly, urate gout may also present with polyarticular involvement, rheumatoid factors in 10% of cases, and symptoms mimicking those of RA.[225]

CPPD deposits have been described both histologically[31] and radiographically[90] in patients with presumably bona fide RA. By chance alone, at least 1% of patients with CPPD joint deposits would be expected to have RA. This figure agrees with the finding of 4 cases of true RA in our series. A lower incidence (3%) of joint cartilage calcification in RA subjects was found in one study as compared to normal controls (14%) but the high incidence in the latter group, whose average age was 64.8 years, is hard to believe.[54a] Conversely, we studied over 600 cases of crystal-proved urate gout and only 1 showed a coincidence with RA.[159] This patient had rheumatoid nodules and factor, hyperuricemia, and an ear tophus; the articular disease was unequivocally RA. The apparent negative

association of urate gout and RA probably does not hold for CPPD deposits and RA.

The type-B pattern is intended to apply only to patients: (1) whose joints are inflamed "out of phase" with one another, as in gout, rather than "in phase," as in RA; (2) who form osteophytes; (3) who do have CPPD crystals in joint fluid leukocytes; and (4) who do not have typical radiographic erosive disease. When RA and CPPD crystal deposition do coexist, the typical radiographic appearance of the former is said to be atypical for RA.[54a] Asymmetric disease, retained bone density, prominent osteophytes, well-corticated cysts and paucity of erosions were found in 7 of 10 patients thought to have both diseases. It seems possible that those 7 patients actually had the "pseudorheumatoid" pattern of CPPD crystal deposition.

A variant of "pseudorheumatoid" arthritis (type B) is worth mention because it can cause confusion clinically. The patient, usually elderly, when first seen has multiple acutely inflamed joints, marked leukocytosis, fever of 102 to 104° F, and mental confusion or disorientation.[27a] Systemic sepsis is suspected by the attending physicians, and antibiotics have usually been prescribed despite neg-

Table 94–4. Clinical Features of Two Crystal Deposition Diseases

Features	Monosodium Urate (MSU)	Calcium Pyrophosphate Dihydrate (CPPD)
Synonyms	Gout	Pseudogout, chondrocalcinosis
Sex ratio (male:female)	20:1	1.5:1
Hereditary tendency	Sometimes middle decades; rare but severe in young; incidence with age	Sometimes; middle or late decades; rare but severe in young; incidence rises with age
Prevalence	4 of 215 cadavers	7 of 215 cadavers
Asymptomatic deposition of crystals in joints	Probable*	Frequent
Acute attacks	Almost always	Common
Time from onset to peak intensity	Abrupt (2 to 12 hours)	Abrupt or gradual (2 to 72 hours)
Site	Small peripheral joints especially in feet; all other joints occasionally, except temporomandibular joint	Large joints, especially knees; all other joints occasionally
Precipitating factors	Surgical procedures, medical stress, trauma, alcohol ingestion, exercise, dietary excesses	Surgical procedures, trauma, medical stress
Duration	12 hours to 3 weeks	12 hours to 4 weeks or longer
Colchicine therapy	Usually dramatically effective	Sometimes effective
Serum urate levels	Almost always elevated	Elevated in 20% of cases
"Petite" (abortive) attacks	Common; may outnumber classic attacks	Much more common than severe attacks
Synovianalysis		
(Acute symptoms)		
Gross	Inflammatory (group II)†	Inflammatory (group II)†
Microscopic	Mostly intracellular crystals	Mostly intracellular crystals
(Chronic or no symptoms)		
Gross	Noninflammatory (group I)†	Noninflammatory (group I)†
Microscopic	Extracellular crystals (not always)	Extracellular crystals (not always)
Associated diseases‡	Hypertension, diabetes mellitus, hyperparathyroidism, CPPD deposition disease, hypothyroidism	Hyperparathyroidism, sodium urate deposition disease, osteoarthritis, hemochromatosis, hypothyroidism, hypomagnesemia, hypophosphatasia
Chronic arthritis	Common (chronic tophaceous gouty arthritis)	Common, especially in hip, knee, metacarpophalangeal joints, wrist
Gross cartilaginous deposits	Almost invariable	Invariable, especially in fibrocartilaginous menisci
Microscopic appearance	In superficial hyaline (articular) cartilage and often in fibrocartilaginous structures, tendons, ligaments, joint capsules, and synovium	In midzone, and with erosion, in superficial hyaline cartilage, ligaments, tendons, joint capsules, synovium; most marked in fibrocartilage
Roentgenograms of affected joints	Sometimes, nonspecific punched-out lesion in subchondral bone	Often, characteristic appearance Punctate and linear radiodensities in cartilage

*Garrod found sodium urate deposits in 2 of 40 first metatarsophalangeal joints from cadavers not known to have had gout during life.[173]

†Group designations of Ropes and Bauer.[184]

‡No causal relationships established or implied.

ative cultures. The entire clinical picture reverses with anti-inflammatory drug therapy.

Types C and D—Pseudo-osteoarthritis

Approximately half of our patients have progressive degeneration of multiple joints (see Figs. 94–12 through 94–15). Women predominate. The knees are most commonly affected, followed by the wrists, metacarpophalangeal joints, hips, spine, shoulders, elbows, and ankles. Involvement is generally bilaterally symmetric, although the degenerative process may be much further advanced on one side, especially in joints that have been subjected to fracture or trauma. Flexion contractures of the involved joints are common. CPPD crystal deposition should be suspected in patients with bilateral varus deformities, unilateral valgus deformity, or flexion contractures of the knees, especially

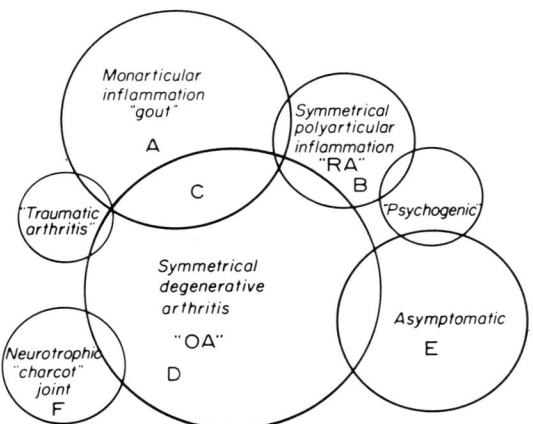

Fig. 94–6. Diagrammatic representation of clinical pattern seen in patients with calcium pyrophosphate dihydrate deposition disease. RA = Rheumatoid arthritis; OA = osteoarthritis. See text for details. (From McCarty, D.J.[127])

if accompanied by osteophytes and flexion contractures of other joints not usually affected by primary osteoarthritis, such as the wrists, elbows, shoulders, and metacarpophalangeal joints.

About 28% of the total series, or about half of those with types C and D disease, have a history of episodic, superimposed acute attacks and have been classified as "type C." Those without an apparent inflammatory component have been classified as "type D."

Characteristic CPPD deposits may or may not be visible on radiographs of involved joints. CPPD crystals are often found in radiographically negative joints, especially those with extensive degenerative change.[133,223] The elegant serial radiographic studies by Zitnan and Sitaj contain examples of joints with obvious CPPD deposits at an early phase of the disease that may be difficult to discern when severe degeneration has supervened.[237] "Fine-detail" roentgenograms are helpful in the detection of small or faint deposits.[66,80,160]

Martel and co-workers,[141] as well as Hamilton and his colleagues,[97] have described squaring of bone ends, subchondral cystic changes, and hook-like osteophytes, especially in the metacarpophalangeal joints. Atkins et al. compared the radiographic features of metacarpophalangeal degeneration in sporadic CPPD crystal deposition disease with that associated with hemochromatosis; they found more severe changes in a greater proportion of patients with hemochromatosis.[10]

Resnick and his colleagues have studied patients with CPPD deposition in a Veterans Hospital population, using age- and sex-matched control subjects. Certain differences in the radiographic appearance and the pattern of joint degeneration provided useful diagnostic clues and have been incorporated into the criteria outlined in Table 94–3. Axial skeleton involvement is frequent and is characterized by anular calcification, multiple levels of disc degeneration with vacuum phenomenon and subchondral erosions, and vacuum phenomenon of the sacroiliac joints.[142]

In any event, the pattern of joint degeneration in types C and D, that is, wrists, metacarpophalangeal joints, elbow, and shoulder, is clearly different from that of primary osteoarthritis, that is, proximal and distal interphalangeal and first carpometacarpal joints. The knee is commonly affected in both conditions. Concomitant Heberden's and Bouchard's nodes,[28a] as well as other stigmata of primary osteoarthritis, often co-exist with the pattern of joint involvement peculiar to CPPD crystal deposition, probably a chance association of two common conditions in elderly persons.

Type E—Lanthanic (Asymptomatic) Calcium Pyrophosphate Dihydrate Crystal Deposition

This type may be the most common of all. Most joints with CPPD deposits plainly visible on roentgenograms are not symptomatic, even in patients with acute or chronic symptoms in other joints. As previously mentioned, a recent study in a Jewish home for the aged showed CPPD deposits in 27.6% of volunteer subjects. Wrist complaints and genu varus deformities, but not acute joint inflammation, were more common in the group with CPPD deposits than in control subjects from the same population.[66]

Type F—Pseudoneuropathic Joints

One of the patients in our original report had a Charcot-like arthropathy of a knee in the absence of neurologic abnormality.[136] Subsequently, four cases of "neuropathic" arthritis of the knees associated with polyarticular CPPD deposition were reported; three of the patients had mild tabes dorsalis and tertiary syphilis; the fourth also had late syphilis, but no neurologic abnormality.[106] One of these patients later developed an acute Charcot joint with hemorrhagic joint fluid and acute pseudogout (see Figs. 5–75, 94–15).[17] Other reports of destructive arthropathy similar to neurotrophic arthropathy in patients with CPPD deposits and normal neurologic examinations underscore this association.[84,98,146,174] Severe degeneration of the neuropathic type has even been reported in the temporomandibular joints.[166]

In all reported series of patients with tabes dorsalis, Charcot knee joints developed in only 5 to 10%.[182] Because our 3 cases were seen consecu-

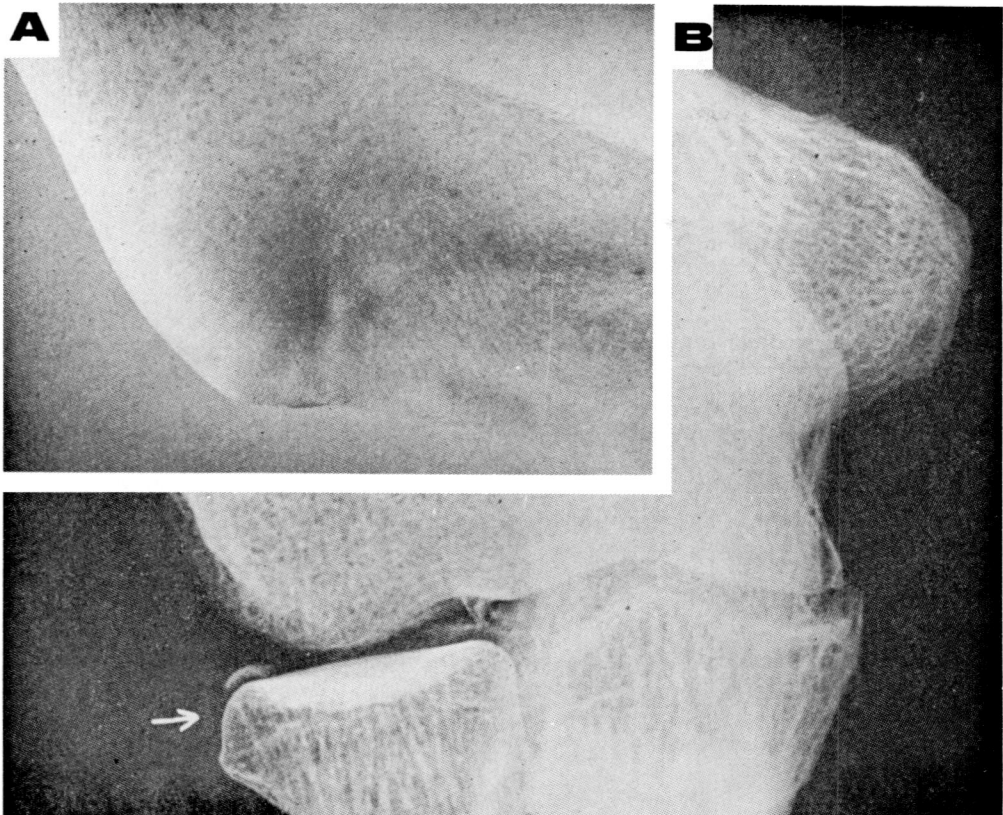

Fig. 94–7. *A,* Acute arthritis of the right elbow. Severe pain, tenderness, swelling, warmth, and erythema of the overlying skin were noted; 25 ml inflammatory-type fluid with a leukocytic content of 65,000/mm³ were aspirated, and many phagocytosed calcium pyrophosphate dihydrate crystals were found. *B,* Roentgenogram of elbow showing calcific deposits in articular cartilage of the humerus and the radial head; deposits, less well visualized, are also present in the articular capsule (arrow).

tively and because CPPD deposition affects about 5% of the adult population (see Table 94–2), the 2 conditions might be expected to co-exist by chance alone in only 1 of 20 tabetics with Charcot joints. For the 2 conditions to co-exist in 3 of 3 consecutive cases, however, the odds are only one in 8,000. Thus, it was postulated that neurotrophic joints actually develop in that 5% of the tabetic population that has underlying CPPD crystal deposition.[106] That CPPD crystals alone can be associated with a destructive arthropathy, without the help of a neurologic deficit, reinforces this hypothesis (see Figs. 5–75, 94–15).

Other Patterns of Crystal Deposition

Multiple other patterns of disease have been described.[125] Stiffening of the spine that mimics ankylosing spondylitis or diffuse idiopathic skeletal hyperostosis has been observed, particularly in two kindreds with familial CPPD deposition.[174,238] True bony ankylosis was observed in the Chilean series of familial cases, and none of the affected individuals were HLA-B27 positive.[173] Predominant symptoms of meningeal irritation[118] or radiculopathy[65,109,111] have been reported and may be related to involvement of spinal joints or to CPPD deposits in the ligamentum flavum. Mono-articular inflammation or degeneration may occur in CPPD secondary to trauma or attendant operations. This presentation is particularly common in the knee, years after meniscectomy,[55] after operations to remove osteochondral fragments in osteochondritis dissecans,[121] or in disc fibrocartilage after lumbar surgical procedures.[8,64]

The frequent finding (8%) of polymyalgia rheumatica in a series from the United Kingdom suggests that: (1) CPPD deposition may mimic the proximal stiffness, pain, and elevated erythrocyte sedimentation rate of polymyalgia rheumatica; (2) the two diseases are associated; or (3) corticosteroid treatment may predispose persons to CPPD deposition.[48] Rarely, a localized, progressively destructive, solitary, "tophaceous" mass of CPPD crystals occurs in synovial tissue with chondroid metaplasia. Five cases have been reported, 4 in humans,[47,117,122] and 1 in the paw of a 12-year-old golden retriever.[85]

It is clear from the long-term observations of the natural history of CPPD joint deposition in familial cases by Zitnan and Sitaj that a given patient may show one pattern of arthritis early in the course of the disease and a different pattern later on; many type-A patients may eventually have pattern C, D, or F, for example.[237]

Systemic findings during an acute attack are frequent but not invariable.[136] These include a fever of 99 to 103° F, leukocytosis of 12 to 15,000/mm^3 with a "left shift," and an elevated erythrocyte sedimentation rate and serum acute phase reactants.

Calcium Pyrophosphate Dihydrate Deposits in Animals

In addition to the previously mentioned dog, CPPD crystals have been identified in the cartilages of a barbary ape[180] and in elderly monkeys.[179] Calcifications in old rabbits have also been found, but were composed of apatite rather than of CPPD.[235]

ETIOLOGIC CLASSIFICATION

A tentative classification is given in Table 94–5. The genetic aberrations responsible for each of the nine largest reported series of *hereditary* cases probably differ.[76,79,155,172,181,183,200,224] Table 94–6

Table 94–5. Etiologic Classification of Calcium Pyrophosphate Dihydrate Crystal Deposition Disease

I. Hereditary (see Table 94–6)
II. Sporadic (idiopathic)
III. Associated with metabolic disease (see Table 94–7)
IV. Associated with trauma or surgical procedures

lists the evidence for this statement. Most of the families show disease transmission as an autosomal dominant trait. The Hungarian group has an HLA association, no male-to-male transmission, and symptomatic heterozygotes. Five of the other series showed male-to-male transmission of disease, indicating autosomal inheritance. Because nearly half the offspring of a heterozygote in all series developed radiographic evidence of CPPD crystal deposition, penetrance is nearly complete. Associated metabolic conditions such as hyperparathyroidism were rare in any of these kindreds. Phenotypic manifestations of the disease were severe in some kindreds and were mild in others. The Hungarian homozygotes had severe disease, and the heterozygotes developed milder disease.[155]

The so-called "*sporadic*" or "*idiopathic*" cases deserve comment. Generally, no systematic search for the condition has been conducted among blood relatives, and none of the putative metabolic disease associations have been found. We examined 1 or more relatives clinically and radiologically in 12 of the first 18 cases and found 3 examples of familial disease. Such a study is difficult in the United States in view of the extreme mobility of our citizens and the widespread psychologic resistence to submit to study because of possible discovery of abnormality. In Spain, a study of 46 apparently "sporadic" cases revealed a familial incidence in 5 (11%).[183] This finding could represent a coincidence of sporadic cases in aged subjects. It is likely that a thorough study of "sporadic cases" would result in reclassification of many as either hereditary or as associated with metabolic disease.

ASSOCIATED DISEASES

A number of metabolic diseases and physiologic stresses, such as aging and joint trauma, have been associated with CPPD deposition. None of these except aging and surgery have yet been statistically proved to occur with increased frequency in pa-

Table 94–6. Characteristics of Hereditary Calcium Pyrophosphate Dihydrate Crystal Deposition Disease

Series	Type	Male-to-Male Transmission	Associations		
			Arthritis	Onset	HLA Antigens
Slovakian[155] (Hungarian gene)		No	Severe	Early	Yes
Chilean[172] (Spanish gene)	Autosomal dominant	Yes	Severe	Early	No
French[76]	Autosomal dominant	Yes	Severe	Early	No
Japanese[200]	Autosomal dominant	Yes	Severe	Early	NA*
Swedish[24]	Autosomal dominant	Yes	Severe	Early	No
Dutch[224]	Autosomal dominant	Yes	Mild	Early	No
Mexican-American[181]	Autosomal dominant	Yes	Mild	Early	No
French-Canadian[79]	Autosomal dominant	?	Mild	Early	No
Spanish[183]			Mild	Late	NA*

*NA = Not available.

tients with CPPD deposition by controlled, prospective studies. Nonetheless, strong circumstantial evidence suggests that many of these associations are "true," and the converse has often been proved; that is, that chondrocalcinosis occurs more frequently in patients with several of these conditions, notably gout,[102] hemochromatosis,[96] and hyperparathyroidism,[198] than in age- and sex-matched control populations. Even when associations seem significant, however, a cause-and-effect relationship should not be inferred. If it is assumed that the putative associations are real, an immediate generalization is that all the metabolic diseases listed in Table 94–7 affect connective tissue metabolism in some way.

Analysis of the first seven cases and a review of the literature suggest that a number of metabolic and degenerative diseases are more prevalent than might be expected by chance.[136] Reported associations between CPPD deposition and other diseases

must be interpreted with caution. Because CPPD deposits occur in about 5% of the adult population, they are associated with nearly all diseases on the basis of chance alone. The conditions listed in Table 94–7 are grouped according to an estimated likelihood of a real association. Thus, CPPD crystal deposits associated with rare conditions such as hypophosphatasia and hypomagnesemia are more likely to be "real" than associations with diabetes mellitus or hypertension. Pragmatically, the clinician is well advised to keep the diseases listed in Table 94–7 in mind when confronted with a case of CPPD crystal deposition disease. Unsuspected hyperparathyroidism, hypothyroidism, and other metabolic abnormalities have been found repeatedly when appropriate laboratory studies were performed in such patients. Conversely, when arthritis supervenes in a patient with one of these metabolic conditions, the possibility of CPPD deposition disease should be considered in the differential diagnosis.

Hyperparathyroidism

Numerous reports of CPPD crystal deposition in patients with hyperparathyroidism have appeared,[3,32,240] and most series of patients with CPPD deposition show an incidence of 2 to 15%.[42,45,146,212] Conversely, 20 to 30% of patients with hyperparathyroidism have radiologic chondrocalcinosis.[51,198] Hyperparathyroid patients with CPPD deposits are older than those without such deposits.[51,198] In most surgically treated cases, parathyroid adenoma rather than hyperplasia is found. Following parathyroidectomy, acute attacks of pseudogout are common.[19,156] During long-term postoperative follow-up study, the calcific deposits persist despite normalization of the serum calcium level.[86,99,164] An important effect of persistent hypercalcemia on the development of CPPD crystal deposits is reinforced by the reported associations of joint symptoms and radiologic chondrocalcinosis suggestive of CPPD crystal deposits in persons with a benign lifelong condition called hypocalciuric hypercalcemia.[143,144] A better rheumatologic analysis of such patients would be helpful.

Elevated parathyroid hormone levels were found in 10 of 26 patients with CPPD deposition, only 4 of whom were hypercalcemic.[163] This finding had been confirmed, but its significance was obscured by the discovery of elevated parathyroid hormone levels in control patients with osteoarthritis of weight-bearing joints.[129] Nearly 75% of both groups had elevated levels of parathyroid hormone. One case of hypercalcemia was found in each group, but 2 additional patients with CPPD deposits had already undergone parathyroidectomy. Serum calcium levels showed a positive correlation

Table 94–7. Conditions Reported as Associated with Calcium Pyrophosphate Dihydrate Crystal Deposition Disease*

Group A	*True association probable*
	Hyperparathyroidism
	Familial hypocalciuric hypercalcemia
	Hemochromatosis
	Hemosiderosis
	Hypophosphatasia
	Hypomagnesemia
	Hypothyroidism
	Gout
	Neuropathic joints
	Aging
	Amyloidosis
	Trauma, including surgical trauma
Group B	*True association possible*
	Hyperthyroidism
	Renal stone
	Ankylosing hyperostosis
	Ochronosis
	Wilson's disease
	Hemophiliac arthritis
Group C	*True association unlikely*
	Ankylosing spondylitis
	Diabetes mellitus
	Hypertension
	Mild azotemia
	Hyperuricemia
	Gynecomastia
	Rheumatoid arthritis
	Paget's disease of bone
	Acromegaly
	Corticosteroid treatment

*Degenerative arthritis, included in our initial list, was deleted because it is probably an integral part of the basic disease process.

with parathyroid hormone levels in both groups, rather than the expected inverse correlation, suggesting glandular autonomy. This relationship was not confirmed in a subsequent study using a different antibody in the parathyroid hormone assay.[67] Knee joint degeneration, as graded radiologically, correlated with the level of parathyroid hormone, and a positive correlation was seen between calcium levels and bone density, as quantified by radiodensitometry in both groups.[129] Normocalcemic hyperparathyroidism has been reported,[233] but most patients had renal stones containing calcium.

Although the situation is far from clear, it now appears that hyperparathyroidism may correlate with degenerative arthritis, rather than with the more obvious CPPD deposition. A well-known action of low doses of parathyroid hormone is to increase bone density; some patients with primary hyperparathyroidism may even have osteosclerosis.[3,41] It is possible that increased bone density, secondary to chronic, sustained, low-grade hyperparathyroidism, predisposes patients to osteoarthritis by the mechanism of subchondral microfractures of dense, less-compliant bone, as proposed by Pugh and colleagues.[167] Patients with osteoarthritis of the hip have increased bone density.[73]

Hemochromatosis

The original report of arthritis in patients with hemochromatosis noted one example of articular cartilage calcification.[203] Many subsequent reports have documented this association.[9,10,12,34,43,44,56,59,60,91,97,107,228] Nearly half the patients with hemochromatosis have arthritis, and half of these have radiologic chondrocalcinosis.[56,60] Again, these are the older patients in the series.[60,95] CPPD deposition and related joint complaints are often present in patients with asymptomatic hemochromatosis. Involvement of metacarpophalangeal joints is more common in patients with hemochromatosis than in those with idiopathic chondrocalcinosis,[10] but the appearance of "squared off" bone ends, joint-space narrowing, and subchondral cysts in these joints was identical to that described by Martel and colleagues in patients with idiopathic chondrocalcinosis.[141] Appropriate treatment of the iron overload did not prevent the development of new calcifications over a 10-year period.[96] Radiologic evidence of CPPD crystal deposition increased from 7 to 13 of the 18 male patients followed over that 10-year interval.

That the iron itself may be directly related to the calcific deposits is suggested by reports of CPPD deposition in patients with transfusion hemosiderosis.[1,18,60,222] Moreover, patients with hemophilia arthritis and chondrocalcinosis have been recorded.[108,120]

Just how tissue iron predisposes to CPPD crystal deposits is unclear. Ferrous, but not ferric, ions inhibited some inorganic pyrophosphatases;[135] ferric ions promoted CPPD crystal growth in vitro at lower inorganic pyrophosphate concentrations.[101] Synovial hemosiderosis slowed the metabolic clearance of radiolabeled CPPD crystals from rabbit joints by about 50%.[137] But whether any of these mechanisms relate to the association of local tissue iron overload with CPPD crystals is still conjectural.

Other Disorders

O'Duffy reported a patient with *hypophosphatasia* and CPPD deposits,[157] and subsequently several others have been described.[62,230] Inorganic pyrophosphate is a natural substrate of alkaline phosphatase,[188] and as urinary and plasma inorganic pyrophosphate levels are elevated in hypophosphatasia,[187,189] it is not surprising that hypophosphatasa may be associated with CPPD crystal deposition. Attempts at replacing alkaline phosphatase by infusing plasma from patients with Paget's disease of bone into a patient with infantile hypophosphatasia had no appreciable effect on the urinary excretion of inorganic pyrophosphate, but may have improved the bony abnormalities.[231]

Hypomagnesemia associated with CPPD crystal deposition was first reported in 1974;[129] at least five cases have been reported since.[67,149,171,186] This association makes sense teleologically because magnesium increases the solubility of CPPD crystals,[16] and is also an important co-factor for alkaline phosphatase,[130] as well as for many inorganic pyrophosphatases.[135] In most reported instances, the defect appeared to be a failure of renal conservation of magnesium. In one case, magnesium replacement therapy decreased radiologic calcification.[186] A controlled study of oral magnesium therapy in patients with CPPD crystal deposits showed statistically significant beneficial effects.[53] CPPD deposition has also been reported in *Bartter's syndrome*,[11,92] perhaps secondary to the associated hypomagnesemia.

Hypothyroidism is associated with asymptomatic CPPD deposits, with frequent onset of joint inflammation after treatment with thyroid hormone.[57] One survey reported that 11% of 105 consecutive patients with CPPD deposition were hypothyroid.[4]

Periarticular and intra-articular *amyloid* deposits have been noted in association with CPPD deposition since the first report in 1976.[110] Four of five elderly patients with amyloid arthropathy, most of whom had carpal tunnel syndrome and pitting edema of the hands, had chondrocalcinosis.[192,196]

Subsequent histologic studies have shown frequent amyloid deposits in cartilage and synovium, often in close proximity to the CPPD crystals.[39,63,213,219] Because most such patients are elderly, this association may represent the chance concurrence of two age-related processes. Amyloid is known to bind pyrophosphate analogues,[234] as well as calcium, however, and local sequestration could favor CPPD crystal formation. Amyloid has also been recently described in osteoarthritic cartilage,[63,114] and has been reported in joints of senescent mice.[207]

Hyperuricemia, often accompanying mild azotemia, hypertension, or diuretic use, is common in the elderly population. The co-existence of pseudogout and *urate gout* varies from 2 to 8% in most reported series;[42,45,153,212,228] 5% of our series had both CPPD and MSU crystals. If the prevalence of MSU crystal deposition were 2% of the adult male population, as it might be,[131] then this association could be one of chance. Although 32% of a series of 31 gouty patients had radiologically evident chondrocalcinosis,[52] only 5% of another series of 43 gouty patients showed such deposits, a percentage no greater than in control subjects.[90] In carefully controlled prospective studies, the prevalence of chondrocalcinosis in patients with gout was 8 of 138; in age-matched normal control patients and in asymptomatic hyperuricemic patients, the prevalence was 0 of 142 and 1 of 84, respectively.[102,218] These results imply an association of CPPD with gout but not with hyperuricemia.

Diabetes mellitus, as defined by glucose intolerance, is common in the elderly. Controlled studies have not supported an association of CPPD deposition with diabetes.[182,201] A 26.5% incidence of diabetes in 49 patients with chondrocalcinosis was lower than that found (32.6%) in 46 control patients. If insulin requirement is used as a definition of diabetes, then the problem of small numbers in both patients and control groups supervenes.[129]

Ankylosing hyperostosis has been noted in serial studies of hereditary cases of CPPD deposition in Slovakia.[237] It appeared in one-third of 18 Japanese patients,[158] and it was found in a number of hereditary cases studied in the Netherlands.[224] Conversely, CPPD deposits were found in 6% of 34 patients with ankylosing hyperostosis.

The association of chondrocalcinosis with acromegaly is probably fortuitous,[25,117] despite the high plasma inorganic pyrophosphate levels in this disease.[210] The incidence of Paget's disease of bone is not increased in patients with CPPD deposits.[170] Definite crystal identification is still lacking in patients reported with Wilson's disease.[28,72] The calcification in some patients with ochronosis appears to be CPPD.[33,175,199,216]

None of the other conditions listed in Table 94–7 are likely to have more than a chance association with CPPD deposition.

The routine examination of a newly diagnosed patient with CPPD deposition should probably include determinations of the following: serum calcium, magnesium, phosphorus, alkaline phosphatase, ferritin, iron and total iron-binding capacity, glucose, thyroid-stimulating hormone, T_4, and uric acid, with further metabolic study if abnormalities are found.

Trauma/Surgery

Mounting evidence links CPPD deposition with antecedent joint trauma or surgical procedures. A traumatic cause of cartilage calcification was first postulated by Mandl in 1927,[140] when he reported a "secondary" type of cartilage calcification in menisci of previously traumatized knees, without involvement of the contralateral knee. Other observers have confirmed monoarticular calcific deposition following trauma, as summarized by Weaver.[227] Arthroscopic findings in such joints have been described.[6] Since then, radiographic chondrocalcinosis has been recognized in hypermobile joints,[20] in unstable joints,[206] and in neuropathic joints.[106] The most compelling evidence was presented by Linden and Nilsson[121] and by Doherty et al.[55] In the Linden and Nilsson study, 25 of 42 knees previously treated operatively for osteochondritis dissecans of the femoral condyle developed chondrocalcinosis in the operated knee, but not in the contralateral knee. A control group of meniscectomy patients developed chondrocalcinosis in 14 of 41 operated knees. In the Doherty study of postmeniscectomy patients, knee radiographs were obtained a mean of 25 years after operation; at that time, 20% of operated, but only 4% of contralateral, knees showed chondrocalcinosis.

ROENTGENOGRAPHIC FEATURES

Heavy CPPD crystal deposits in fibrocartilaginous structures, hyaline (articular) cartilage, ligaments, and joint capsules have a characteristic appearance that is diagnostically helpful[133,239] (see also Figs. 5–81 and 5–85). Punctate and linear radiodensities are most frequently seen in the fibrocartilaginous menisci of the knee and usually involve both menisci of both knees (Figs. 94–1,*C*, 94–8,*B*). Other fibrocartilaginous structures often calcified in this miliary fashion are the articular discs of the distal radioulnar joint (Fig. 94–9), the symphysis pubis (Fig. 94–10), the glenoid and acetabular labra, and the anulus fibrosus of the intervertebral discs. The articular discs of the ster-

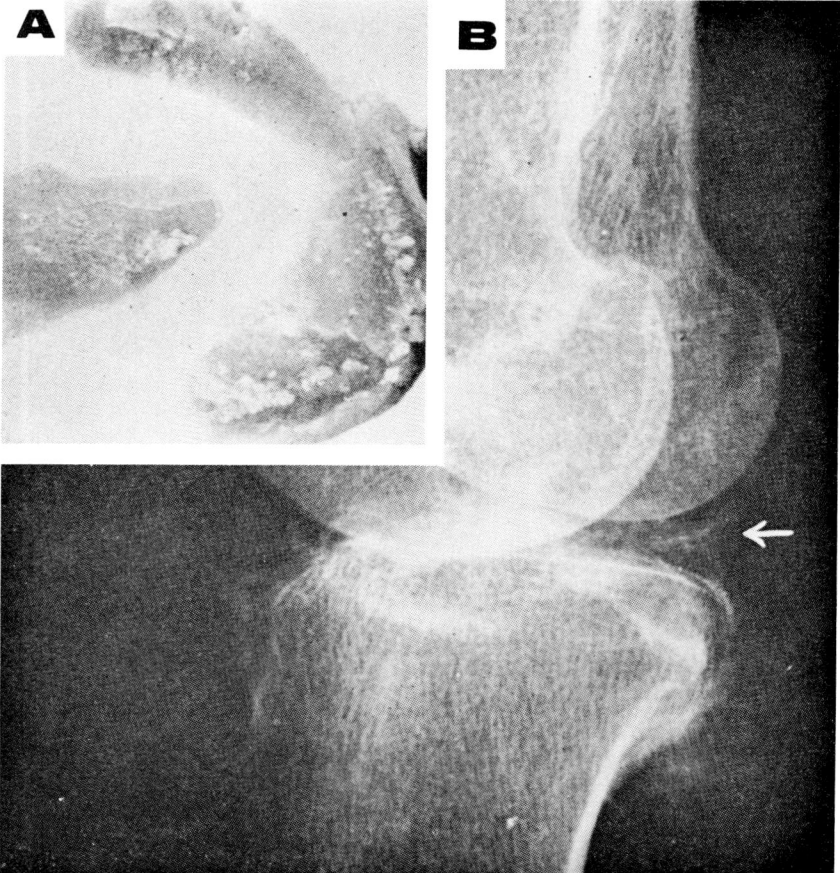

Fig. 94–8. *A,* Meniscus excised at necropsy showing punctate and linear aggregates of calcium pyrophosphate dihydrate microscrystals; a wedge of articular cartilage from the tibial plateau shows similar deposits. *B,* Lateral roentgenogram of the knee showing the typical Y-shaped appearance of meniscal calcification (arrow).

noclavicular joints are often involved, but those of the temporomandibular joint are usually spared.

Calcification of the hyaline articular cartilage is common; the deposits in the midzonal layer appear as a radiopaque line paralleling the density of the underlying bone (see Figs. 94–7,*B*, 94–9). The larger joints show these deposits most frequently, although they are observed in nearly every diarthrodial joint. Calcifications of articular capsules or synovium, especially of the elbow, shoulder, hip, and knee, are frequent; the deposits appear as a broader, more diffuse, faintly opaque line (Figs. 94–7,*B*, 94–11, 5–82, 5–84).

Calcification of bursae, tendons, and ligaments also occurs in CPPD deposition disease. This calcification may represent BCP crystal deposition in some patients, but crystal-proved CPPD deposits have been reported in all the aforementioned sites. Synovial deposits may be so large as to mimic synovial chondromatosis,[68] and ligamentous or ten-

dinous deposits may produce local compressive symptoms, such as carpal tunnel syndrome[81] or myelopathy, as already outlined.

Subchondral bone cysts are common and can attain a large size. Histologic examination of the walls of the lesion shown in Figure 94–12 confirmed that it was only a bone cyst. How such lesions are related to CPPD deposition disease is unknown, but they occur frequently enough to be a diagnostic clue.[177]

A number of distinct regional radiographic abnormalities may suggest CPPD deposition. A peculiar erosion of the femoral cortex superior to the patella has been reported.[2,115] This lesion appears to correlate with osteoarthritis of the patellofemoral compartment (Fig. 94–14). Carpal instability reported in association with CPPD deposits resembles that of RA.[178] A particular propensity for radiocarpal involvement has been observed. Navicular-lunate dissociation is thought to result from

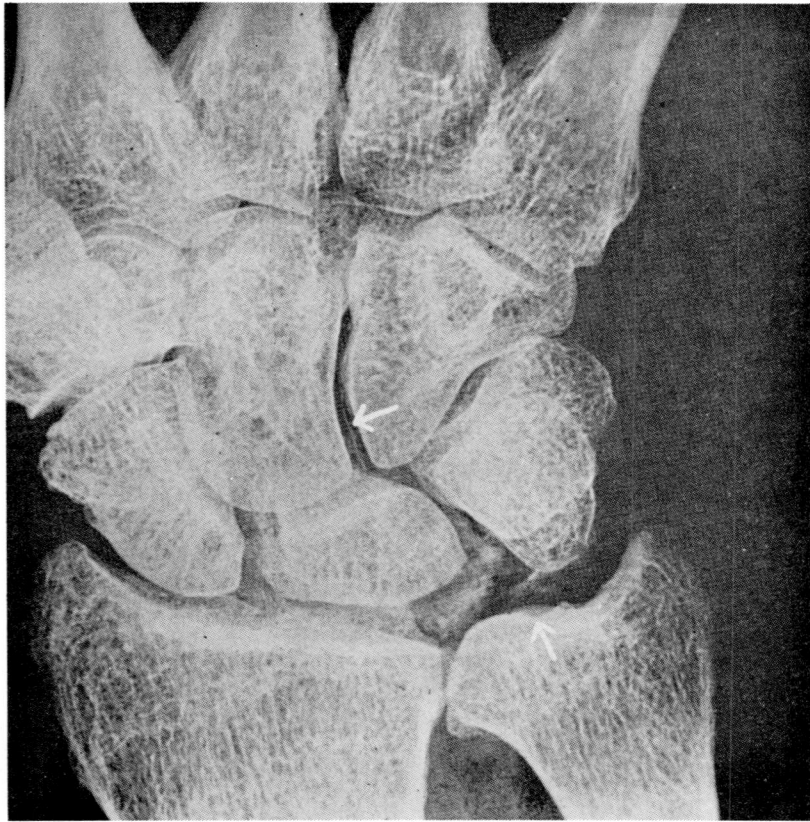

Fig. 94–9. Anteroposterior roentgenogram of the wrist showing calcification of the fibrocartilaginous articular disc and a fine line of calcification parallel to the radiodensity of the underlying bone indicative of articular cartilage calcification (arrow).

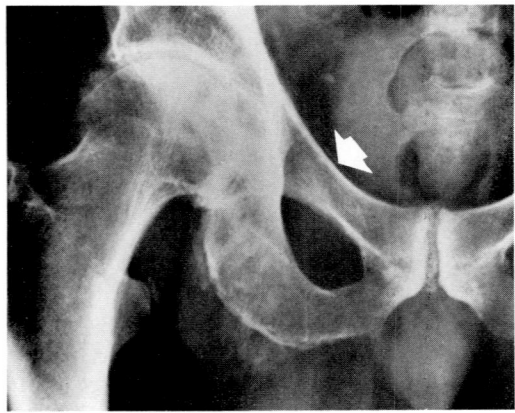

Fig. 94–10. Calcific deposits in the symphysis pubis, the hyaline cartilage, and the acetabular labrum of the hip, the origin of the adductor tendons on the ischium and lesser trochanter, and Cooper's ligament (arrow). (Courtesy of Harry K. Genant, M.D.)

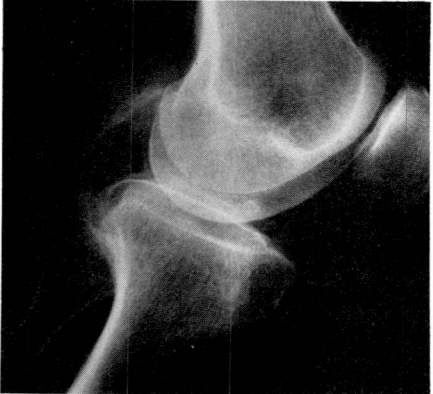

Fig. 94–11. Capsular calcification is prominent; deposits are also visible in the hyaline articular cartilage of the knee and in the proximal tibiofibular joint.

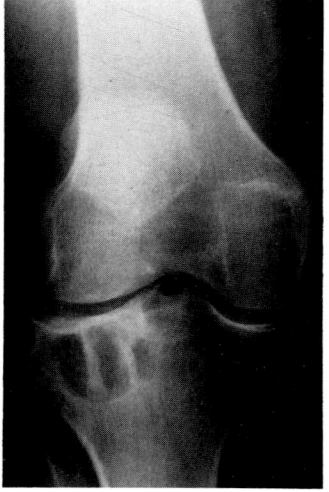

Fig. 94–12. Subchondral bone cyst under the lateral tibial plateau in a patient with generalized calcium pyrophosphate dihydrate deposition.

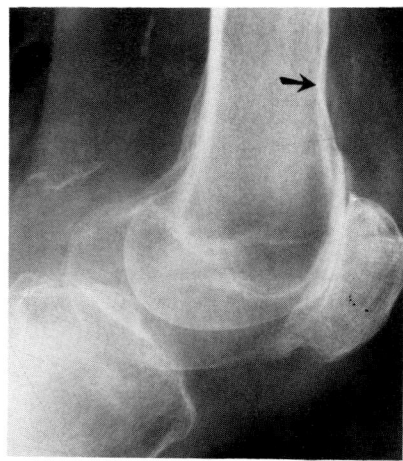

Fig. 94–14. Lateral roentgenograms of the knee showing peculiar erosion of the femoral cortex superior to the patella (arrow), as described by Ahlgren[2] and Lagier.[115] Note the patella "wrapped around" the femur. (Courtesy of Harry K. Genant, M.D.)

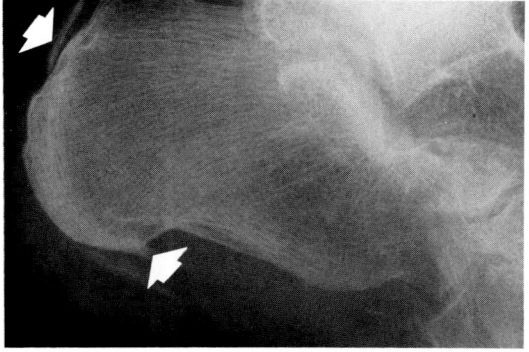

Fig. 94–13. Calcifications in the insertion of the Achilles tendon and of the plantar fascia are seen in this lateral roentgenogram of the heel. Such deposits are particularly prominent in patients with hyperparathyroidism. (Courtesy of Harry K. Genant, M.D.)

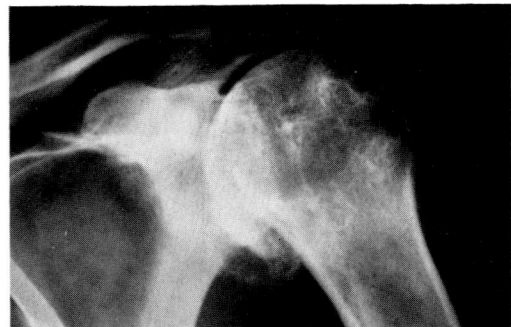

Fig. 94–15. Anteroposterior roentgenogram of the shoulder showing neurotrophic joint appearance with extensive cystic bone lesions and powdered bony fragments in the synovial recesses inferiorly.

degeneration of the ligamentous structures. Features of axial skeleton involvement have recently been described.[142] In the lumbar spine, multiple levels of anulus fibrosus calcification, vacuum disc phenomena, and disc narrowing are emphasized. Sacroiliac joint abnormalities include subchondral erosions, reactive sclerosis, and bilateral vacuum phenomena. Axial skeletal involvement is particularly prominent in uremic patients with secondary hyperparathyroidism.[73a]

Features that may accompany CPPD deposition include degenerative joint disease, tibial stress fractures, and avascular necrosis of the medial or lateral femoral condyle. Some of these features are pe-

culiar to and may suggest CPPD deposition disease even in the absence of radiographically detectable chondrocalcinosis. Degenerative changes appear in joints not commonly involved in primary osteoarthritis, such as the metacarpophalangeal, radiocarpal, elbow, and shoulder joints. Subchondral cysts, bone and cartilage fragmentation, and variable osteophyte formation are characteristic (Fig. 94–15). The best serial studies are those of Hungarian familial cases.[237] CPPD deposits first appeared in radiographically normal cartilage, and degeneration inevitably followed. Tibial stress fractures were reported in 5 elderly patients with CPPD deposition and severe degenerative knee disease.[185] Because their knees were usually painful prior to the fractures, the source of increased pain was not readily apparent. Interestingly, 4 of 14 patients with osteonecrosis of the medial femoral condyle had CPPD knee deposits,[103] an association subsequently confirmed.[226]

Practically, an arthritic patient may be screened for CPPD deposition with four suitably exposed roentgenograms: (1 and 2) an anteroposterior view of each knee; (3) an anteroposterior view of the pelvis; and (4) a posteroanterior view of the wrists. If nothing diagnostic is seen on these films, a more extensive survey is unlikly to be helpful.

The deposits visualized roentgenographically were extensively studied by crystallographic techniques in three necropsies; all were CPPD. The chemical composition of the crystal deposits may be inferred with confidence from typical roentgenograms. Caution must be exercised when the calcifications are faint or atypical, however, because of the possibility of DCPD, basic calcium phosphate, or calcium oxalate crystal deposits or vascular calcifications, all of which are symmetric.[131]

PATHOLOGIC FEATURES

The joints of 3 cases at necropsy and 7 anatomic cadavers were extensively examined.[131] The distribution of calcification generally paralleled that seen on radiogram. Joint capsules, especially in the hip and shoulder, and the hyaline articular cartilages, were often affected, but the heaviest deposits were in fibrocartilaginous structures. The menisci of the knee were involved in all cases (see Fig. 94–8,A). Heavy deposits were often noted in tendons and in intra-articular ligaments, such as the cruciate ligaments in the knee. Microscopically, the deposits were composed of various-sized microcrystalline aggregates of CPPD (Fig. 94–16). Their diameters varied from 15 μ to 0.6 cm; the larger ones appeared grossly as white chalky deposits. It was difficult on gross inspection to distinguish these deposits (see Fig. 94–8,A) from the white chalky lesions of true gout. These lesions were distributed diffusely in fibrocartilage, mainly in the midzonal or superficial areas of hyaline cartilage (Fig. 94–17).

The smallest, and presumably the earliest, crystals appeared at the lacunar margin of chondrocytes. When adjacent chondrocytes were damaged, pericellular matrix vesicles were often seen. Increased glycogen islands and rough endoplasmic reticulum were observed in the chondrocytes.[5] The surrounding matrix may appear normal or granular. Collagen fibril fragmentation in uncalcified areas of CPPD cartilage has been described in familial cases.[21] Larger superfical deposits occur in degenerative cartilages, usually at sites of surface ulcerations and fissuring and often associated with chondrocyte ''cloning.''

Still unpublished studies by Ishikawa have shown convincing evidence of abnormal proteoglycan deposition within chondrocytes in the immediate vicinity of small, presumably early, CPPD crystal deposits. These deposits, stained with safranin-0, were not seen if the tissue was first exposed to either papain or chondroitinase ABC, which confirms their proteoglycan nature (Fig. 94–18,A,B). These abnormal ''red cells'' were a constant feature of evolving, but not of ''mature,'' CPPD crystal deposits in fibrocartilage, in hyaline cartilage, and in synovium showing chondroid metaplasia. They were seen in tissue from both sporadic and familial cases. In these samples, Ishikawa also found the following: (1) absence of normal safranin-0 staining in the matrix in areas of early crystal deposition; (2) ''packing'' of the proteoglycan-denuded collagen fibers in these same areas; (3) hypertrophy and mitotic activity of the ''red cells'' (Fig. 94–18,B); and (4) the appearance of CPPD crystals in empty chondrocyte lacunae, (5) ''mature'' deposits were ringed with dense, proteoglycan-free collagen, as shown in Figure 94–18,C, but the crystals were coated with a thin film of proteoglycan. No collagen or cells could be identified within these crystal masses by light or electron microscopy. The surrounding matrix now contained normal-appearing cells and stained normally.

Ishikawa speculates that the cell-associated proteoglycan may indicate faulty release from the chondrocytes after synthesis, or that it may enter these cells by endocytosis. His findings deserve further exploration and must be taken into account in any scheme of the pathogenesis of CPPD crystal deposition.

In three patients, superficial amyloid deposits were adjacent to CPPD crystals.[63] Two isolated descriptions of CPPD crystals within chondrocytes have been reported,[27,150] indicating that chondrocytes may phagocytose crystals with attendant biologic consequences (see Chap. 95).

In no case has a cause-and-effect relationship been established between crystal deposits and morphologic changes.

Synovial biopsy material obtained with the Polley-Bickel needle showed inflammatory and reparative changes consistent with the clinical state of the joint at the time of biopsy. Early in an acute attack, the edematous synovium was infiltrated with polymorphonuclear leukocytes; later, mononuclear infiltration and fibroblastic proliferation were seen. Synovial proliferation and infiltration with chronic inflammatory cells in chronically symptomatic joints can resemble rheumatoid pannus (Fig. 94–19). Crystals have been identified in

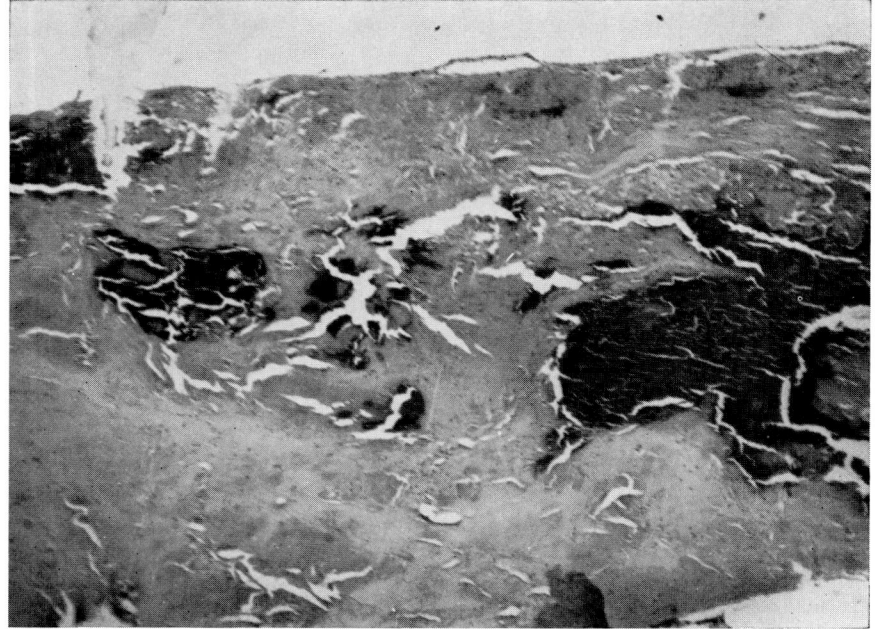

Fig. 94–16.   Photomicrograph of a section through the meniscus shown in Figure 94–8,*A*; various-sized aggregates of calcified material are distributed throughout (hematoxylin and eosin stain, × 26).

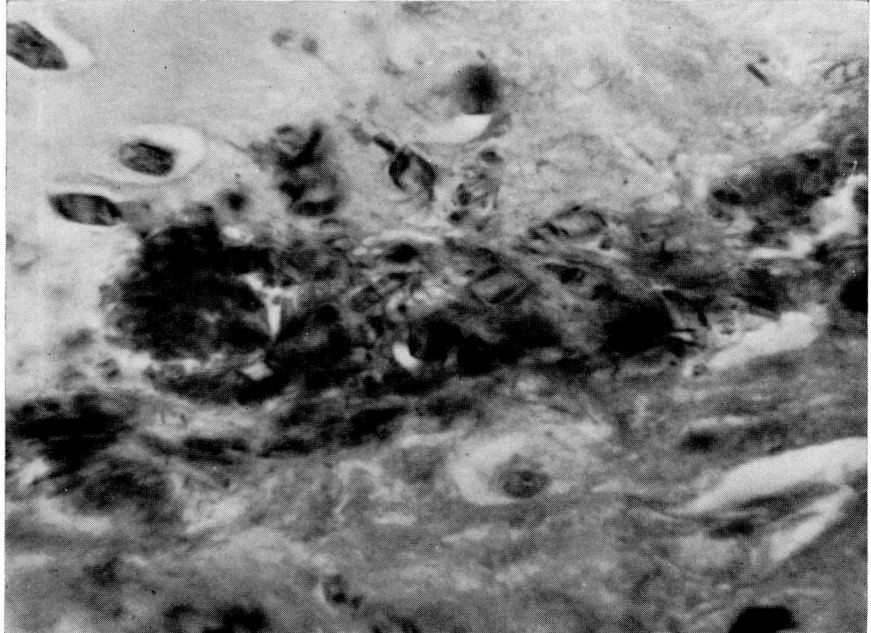

Fig. 94–17.   Photomicrograph of the smallest deposits found shows them surrounding the lacunae of the chondrocytes. This process begins in the midzonal layer of articular cartilage, more diffusely in fibrocartilage. Individual crystals of calcium pyrophosphate dihydrate are visible in this section (alizarin red, × 800; linear magnification × 3).

Fig. 94–18. *A,* Transitional zone articular cartilage from a 63-year-old man with sporadic calcium pyrophosphate dihydrate (CPPD) crystal deposition showing a small crystal deposit. The chondrocytes about the deposit have a characteristic loss of dark nuclear staining. Instead, they appear red because of their proteoglycan content. The matrix about the crystal deposit has lost its proteoglycan. (safranin-O-fast green-iron hematoxylin × 370). *B,* Fibrocartilaginous meniscus from a 73-year-old woman with sporadic CPPD crystal deposition showing normal-appearing cartilage on the right. The area on the left, showing fibrillation and no matrix proteoglycan, contains the crystals. Again, the chondrocytes stain red and are hypertrophic, with some mitotic activity (same stains as *A,* × 370). *C,* Mature deposits in the same tissue showing crystal masses encapsulated by dense proteoglycan-free collagen. The crystals are coated with proteoglycan, but neither cells nor collagen exists among them. The surrounding matrix and chondrocytes now stain normally (same stains as *A,* × 370). (Courtesy of Koichiro Ishikawa, M.D.)

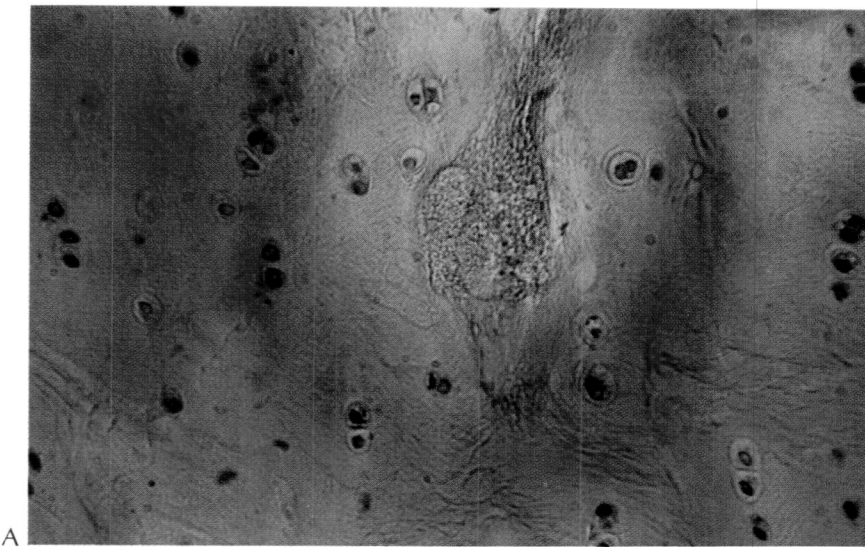

A

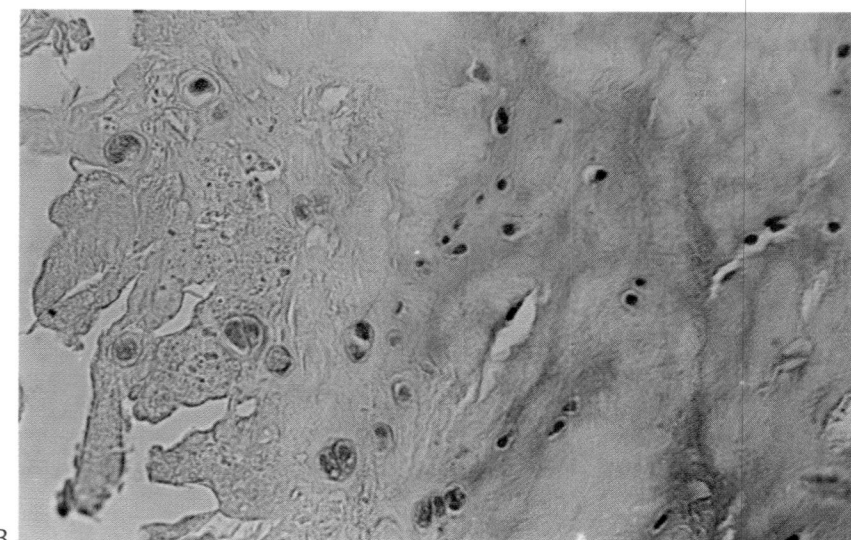

B

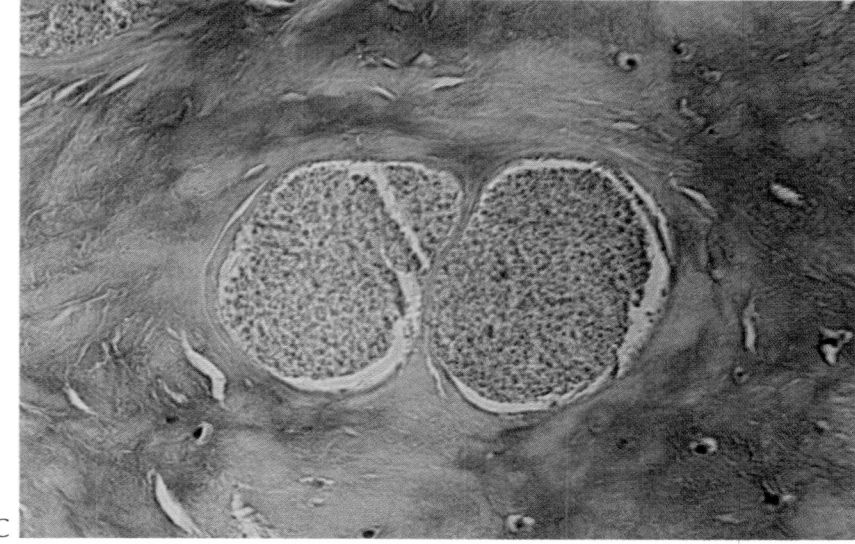

C

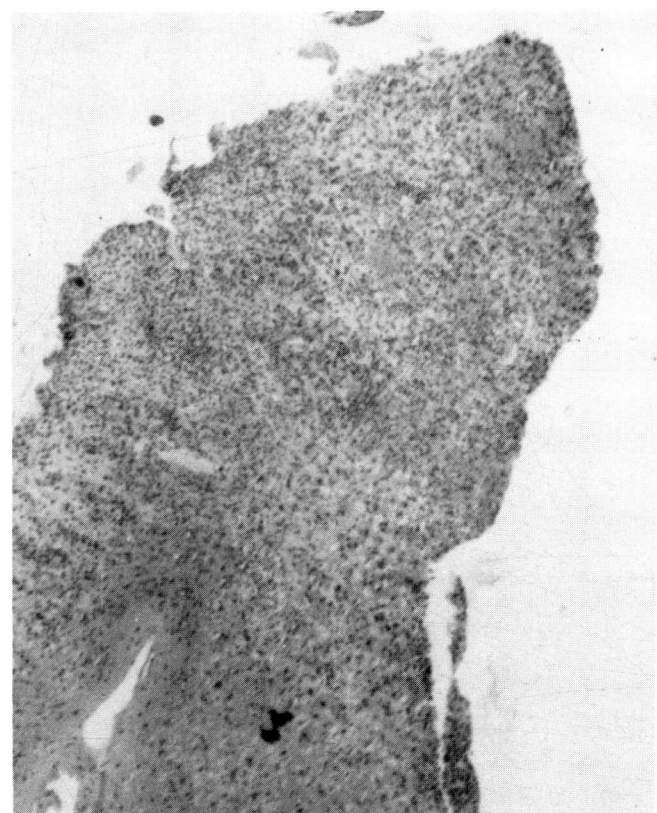

Fig. 94–19. Biopsy of knee joint synovium in a patient with chronic arthritic symptoms showing marked infiltration of chronic inflammatory cells (hematoxylin and eosin stain, ×40).

the superficial synovium under polarized light and by electron microscopy.[27,88,202]

PATHOGENESIS

The cause of CPPD crystal deposition is unknown. Conceptually, formation of CPPD crystals in cartilage may result from elevated levels of either calcium or inorganic pyrophosphate (PPi), from changes in the matrix that promote crystal formation, or from combinations of these factors (Fig. 94–20). Because CPPD crystal deposition is a clinically heterogeneous disorder, different factors probably predominate in individual cases, much as hyperuricemia and MSU crystal deposition may have different causes.

Bjelle favors the hypothesis that matrix changes antedate and predispose persons to CPPD crystal formation.[22] In studies of Swedish patients with familial CPPD deposition, he found weakly staining midzonal matrix with decreased collagen content, some fragmentation of collagen fibers, and abnormal hexosamine profile.[21] The proportions of keratan sulphate and chondroitin-6-sulfate were increased, and those of chondroitin-4-sulfate were decreased. A decrease in mucin-like oligosaccharides was found. Because these changes were in-

dependent of the amount of crystal deposits and because morphologically abnormal crystal-free areas in midzonal cartilage were seen by electron microscopy, Bjelle postulated a primary role of a matrix abnormality in promoting CPPD mineral phase.

The ionic composition of matrix may also affect CPPD crystal formation. Ferrous ions inhibit some pyrophosphatases;[135] ferric ions lower the formation product for CPPD crystals in vitro[101] and slowed the intracellular degradation of CPPD crystals injected into rabbit joints.[137] Hypomagnesemia, both primary and secondary to Bartter's syndrome, has also been associated with chondrocalcinosis. Magnesium is a co-factor for many pyrophosphatases and increases the solubility of CPPD crystals.[16] Therefore, its deficiency may decrease hydrolysis of PPi, and may slow crystal dissolution. Profound hypomagnesemia induced by dietary magnesium deprivation did not change the rate of CPPD crystal clearance from rabbit joints, however.[138] Elevations of inorganic phosphate have promoted CPPD crystal nucleation and growth in vitro and may act similarly in vivo.[100] That such an aberration may exist is suggested by the finding

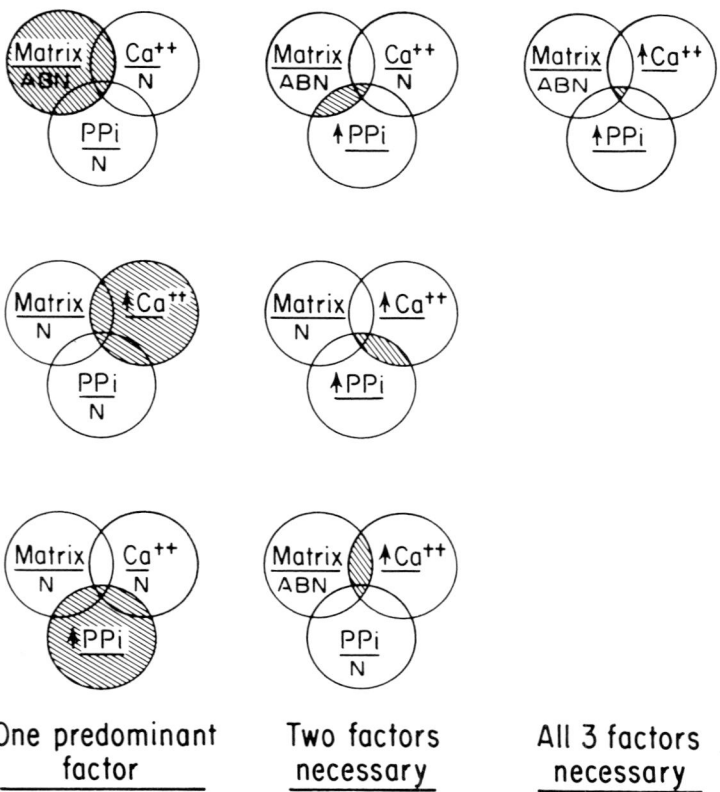

One predominant factor

Two factors necessary

All 3 factors necessary

Fig. 94–20. CPPD crystal deposition theoretically may result from abnormalities of matrix, calcium metabolism, or PPi metabolism. Possibilities are shown in the shaded areas of these Venn diagrams. ABN = Abnormal; N = normal; ↑ = elevated.

of elevated levels of inorganic phosphate in synovial fluid in pseudogout.[209]

Studies of crystal formation in gels provide indirect evidence that matrix components may play a role as nucleating agents in CPPD crystal formation. In aqueous solutions, standard CPPD crystal synthesis occurs at acid pH and at high ionic concentrations.[29,138] In model collagen gels, however, crystals are formed at neutral pH,[165] and at PPi concentrations between 2 and 20 μM.[139] Formation of amorphous calcium pyrophosphate and orthorhombic calcium pyrophosphate tetrahydrate preceded formation of monoclinic and triclinic CPPD crystals identical to those observed in vivo.[139] These studies seem particulary relevant because cartilage is a gel.

No systematic study has been made of abnormalities of cartilage interstitial fluid calcium in patients with CPPD deposition. Clearly, some of these patients have hyperparathyroidism, usually due to parathyroid adenoma, with associated hypercalcemia. CPPD deposition has also been noted in patients with familial hypocalciuric hypercal-

cemia,[143,144] a finding that further supports the role of calcium in promoting CPPD deposition.

PPi is produced by most biosynthetic reactions in macromolecular synthesis.[186] It has been thought that the ubiquitous pyrophosphatases, hydrolyzing PPi to inorganic orthophosphate, drive these reactions in the direction of synthesis, but the intracellular enzymatic hydrolysis of PPi does not go to completion, for unknown reasons, and detectable amounts are measurable in cells,[187] including fibroblasts and chondrocytes.[124]

The amount of PPi produced in the body is immense. It has been calculated that 30 g are made daily in the human liver as a by-product of the synthesis of serum albumin alone.[187] Only a small amount of that synthesized appears in the urine (approximately 10 to 100 μmol daily), where it acts as a powerful inhibitor of crystal nucleation and growth. That the turnover rate of plasma PPi in dogs is only about two minutes further complicates the interpretation of static plasma values of this substance. Neither the source nor the fate of plasma PPi is known.

Much PPi is absorbed to bone mineral,[113] where it is thought to act as a regulator of mineralization. In addition to its effect on crystal precipitation, it retards the conversion of amorphous calcium phosphate into crystalline hydroxyapatite, inhibits crystal aggregation, and slows the dissolution rate of hydroxyapatite crystals. The diphosphonates, which have P-C-P bonds, instead of P-O-P bonds, are nonhydrolyzable analogues of PPi. These compounds have similar biologic effects and are used experimentally as therapeutic agents in various diseases of mineral metabolism and, coupled with tin and [99m]technetium, as bone-scanning agents.[187]

Studies of PPi metabolism were stimulated by recognition of this substance as a constituent of the crystal deposits. Because urinary levels are much higher and are easier to quantify than those in plasma, these were measured earliest and were found to be normal.[190] Blood levels of PPi were later measured, and serum contained two to three times the concentration of plasma.[21] This increase resulted from the release of PPi by platelets during clotting. Plasma levels were higher in venous blood than in arterial blood, were increased with systemic exercise, and were spuriously elevated by application of a venous tourniquet prior to phlebotomy.[194,195] Plasma concentrations in sporadic cases of CPPD deposition were similar to those in osteoarthritic or normal control subjects.[7,190,195] In patients with hypophosphatasia, a disease associated with CPPD deposition, however, both urinary and plasma levels of PPi were elevated,[189,214] presumably as a result of decreased hydrolysis of this substance.

Abnormal local metabolism of PPi was suggested by reports of elevated levels in synovial fluids from patients with CPPD crystal deposition, although elevations were also observed in synovial fluids from patients with gout, osteoarthritis, and even RA.[7,130,148,190,209] The highest joint fluid levels were found in the most severely degenerated joints, as judged radiographically[209] (Fig. 94–21). PPi levels were lower during acute attacks and rose as the episode subsided[209] (Fig. 94–22), probably because of increased synovial blood flow during acute attacks with more rapid equilibration with plasma PPi. The elevated synovial fluid levels could not be explained by dissolution of crystals in the fluid. The gradient between synovial fluid and plasma implied a local origin of PPi.[7,209] The site of the synovial fluid production of this substance was expected to be the chondrocyte, based on the histologic observation that the smallest and presumably the earliest crystals are seen adjacent to chondrocytes. Subsequent studies by Howell et al.[104] and Ryan et al.[193] indicated that articular hyaline and fibrocartilages in organ culture liberated PPi into

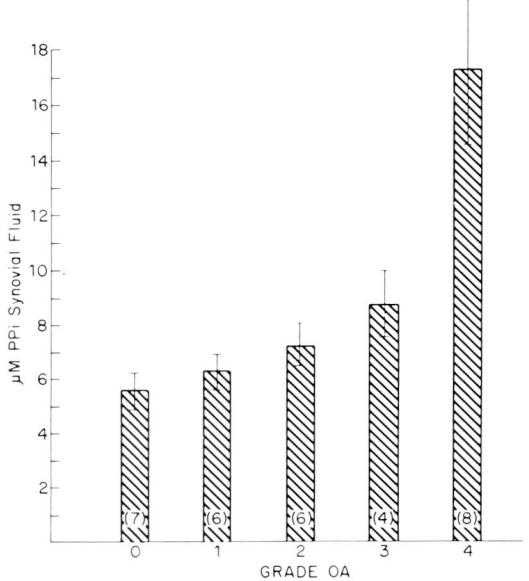

Fig. 94–21.   The concentration of PPi in synovial fluid is plotted for each radiologic grade of osteoarthritis. The number of fluids in each group is given in parentheses. (From Silcox, D.C., and McCarty, D.J.[209])

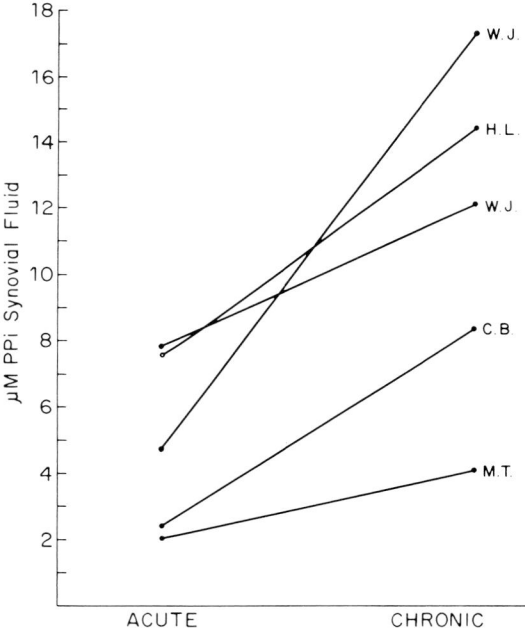

Fig. 94–22.   The inorganic pyrophosphate (PPi) concentration in the synovial fluids of five patients with acute attacks of pseudogout is compared with the concentration in fluids from the same joints once the acute signs and symptoms had subsided. (From Silcox, D.C., and McCarty, D.J.[209])

the ambient media, whereas synovium, subchondral bone, and nonarticular (elastic) cartilages did not. Liberation of PPi correlated directly with uronic acid secretion.[193] Extrapolation of the amount produced by incubated slices to the amount of cartilage in a whole knee joint yielded figures for local production of the same order of magnitude as estimated from in vivo kinetic experiments.[36,104] Thus, cartilage is the most likely source of locally elevated concentrations of PPi in CPPD deposition.

Recently, Tenenbaum and associates described augmented PPi generation in the presence of adenosine triphosphate by extracts of cartilages from patients with CPPD deposition, as compared with generation in extracts of osteoarthritic or normal cartilages.[220] These workers postulated that adenosine triphosphate was enzymatically hydrolyzed to adenosine monophosphate and PPi by adenosine triphosphate pyrophosphohydrolase. A similar activity had been described in calcifying sheep cartilage.[37] Subsequent reports have verified the presence of this enzyme in matrix vesicle fractions of epiphyseal cartilage.[105,208] We have characterized this activity as a chondrocyte nucleoside triphosphate pyrophosphohydrolase with broad substrate reactivity and as an ectoenzyme.[191]

Because CPPD crystals appear to form extracellularly adjacent to chondrocytes, and because PPi does not passively cross cell membranes,[71] the extracellular position of this enzyme might allow the generation of PPi at the site of crystal formation in the presence of suitable substrate. Levels of nucleoside triphosphate pyrophosphohydrolase activity were also higher in the synovial fluid of patients with CPPD deposition and osteoarthritis than in fluids from patients with RA or gout.[168] Enzyme activity correlated directly with the concentration of PPi in synovial fluid. In addition to elevated nucleoside triphosphate pyrophosphohydrolase activity in detergent extracts of cartilages with CPPD deposition, Tenenbaum et al. also described higher levels of 5'nucleotidase activity and lower levels of alkaline phosphatase and inorganic pyrophosphatase activity than in osteoarthritic cartilages.[220] All these aberrations would favor the accumulation of PPi in the ectoenzyme system shown in Figure 94–23. A naturally occurring substrate for nucleoside triphosphate pyrophosphohydrolase in cartilage has not yet been demonstrated, but cellular secretion of adenosine triphosphate has been described in other tissues.[38]

Lust et al. found intracelluar PPi levels twice those of control subjects in cultured skin fibroblasts and in lymphoblasts obtained from affected members of a French kindred with familial CPPD deposition.[123,124] A generalized metabolic abnormality phenotypically expressed only in chondrocytes was postulated. The PPi total and releasable content of platelets in 5 patients with sporadic or familial CPPD deposition was similar to that of 17 control subjects,[197] but a significant positive correlation was found between platelet PPi content and the age of the donor.

We have confirmed and extended the data of Lust et al.[123] PPi levels in cultured skin fibroblasts from patients with both sporadic and familial CPPD crystal deposition were significantly elevated compared to those from normal persons or subjects with osteoarthritis. Activity of ectonucleoside triphosphate pyrophosphohydrolase was elevated in fibroblasts from sporadic, but not familial, CPPD crystal deposition.[197a] Lastly, intracellular PPi levels and ectonucleoside triphosphate pyrophosphohydrolase activity were positively correlated in fibroblasts from each of the groups studied.

Although these biochemical changes cannot yet be directly related to the pathogenesis of CPPD crystal deposition, it is clear that they represent the earliest biochemical correlates of this metabolic arthropathy.

THERAPY

Acute attacks of pseudogout are readily treated by a number of methods, including: (1) thorough aspiration of the joint to remove crystals; (2) administration of nonsteroidal anti-inflammatory agents, particularly indomethacin and phenylbutazone; (3) joint immobilization; and (4) local injection of microcrystalline corticosteroid esters. Intravenous colchicine works as well in pseudogout as it does in gout.[84] Currently, the prophylactic efficacy of oral colchicine in the prevention of acute attacks is under study.

No known way exists to halt the progressive deposition of crystals or to remove those already deposited. Correction of associated metabolic disorders such as hyperparathyroidism, myxedema, and hemochromatosis has not resulted in the disappearance of radiographic cartilage calcification. In fact, new calcifications have developed in some such patients.[96] Attempts at lavage of affected joints with magnesium chloride were unsuccessful in removing significant amounts of crystal, and acute attacks were precipitated.[15] Several examples of spontaneous disappearance of calcific deposits have been reported. Wrist calcification disappeared in one case after immobilization and subsequent development of reflex sympathetic dystrophy.[70] The increased blood flow may have increased the clearance of pyrophosphate from the wrist. Another case associated with familial hypomagnesemia showed radiologic evidence of decreased meniscal calcification two years after institution of magnesium treatment.[186] In a double-blind, placebo-con-

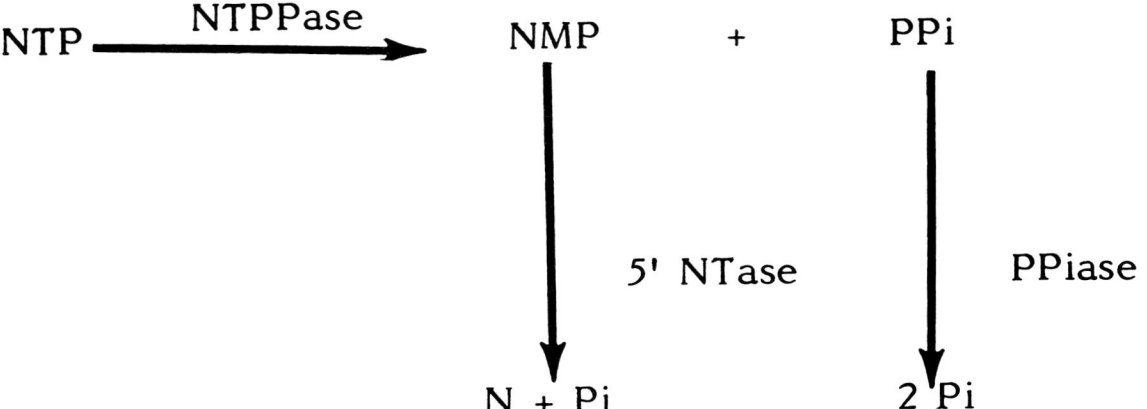

Fig. 94–23. Postulated enzymatic cascade of inorganic pyrophosphate (PPi) production from nucleotide triphosphate (NTP). Elevated NTP pyrophosphohydrolase and 5′nucleotidase activities and decreased inorganic pyrophosphate activity in chondrocalcinosic cartilages all favor PPi accumulation. 5′NTase = 5′nucleotidase; PPiase = inorganic pyrophosphatase; Pi = inorganic phosphate; N = nucleotide; NMP = nucleotide monophosphate.

trolled trial of magnesium carbonate treatment for sporadic CPPD crystal deposition, radiographic calcification did not change over six months, although symptoms improved significantly.[53]

Treatment of the frequently associated degenerative disease is the same as for osteoarthritis. Intra-articular injection with [90]yttrium was reported to ameliorate pain and stiffness and to decrease the size of effusion in knee joints over a six-month period.[54] Joint deformity and radiographic changes were not better than in the contralateral, uninjected knee, however.

Even if effective treatment were available, two problems would remain. First, no biochemical marker identifies those patients who will develop CPPD crystal deposition. We must await radio-

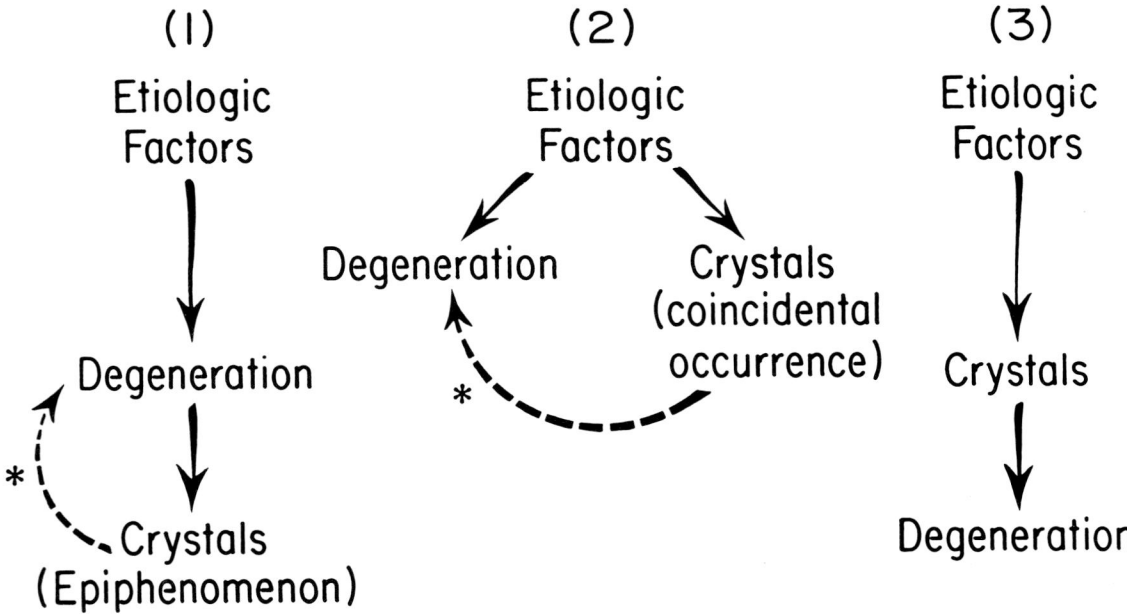

Fig. 94–24. Prevention of crystal formation or dissolution of CPPD crystals would have little effect on cartilage degeneration except in schema number 3 or if an amplification loop exists.
*amplification loop.[55]

graphic evidence of cartilage calcification or identification of crystals in joint fluids, both of which probably signal long-standing disease. Therapeutic interventions at this stage may be much less effective. Second, although treatment of the crystal deposition would probably ameliorate or would prevent acute pseudogout attacks, it might have no effect on the much more significant degenerative joint disease. Figure 94–24 illustrates three potential pathogenetic sequences relating degenerative disease to crystal deposition. Only in sequence 3, which is analogous to the pathogenesis of tophaceous gout, would removal or prevention of crystal formation affect cartilage degeneration. Dieppe has postulated that the biologic phenomena induced by crystals may act as an amplification loop, as shown by the hatched lines in sequences 1 and 2, which envision crystal formation as an epiphenomenon or a coincidental phenomenon, respectively. If an amplification loop exists, then prevention of crystal formation or crystal removal would also have a salutary effect. Perhaps each of the paradigms shown here actually occurs in patients with CPPD crystal deposition, with varying sequences in different patients. Because the clinical importance of CPPD crystals will rise as the population ages, these therapeutic considerations will be of more than theoretic interest.

REFERENCES

1. Abbott, D.J., and Gresham, G.A.: Arthropathy in transfusional siderosis. Br. Med. J., *1*:418–419, 1972.
2. Ahlgren, P.: Chondrocalcinois og knogleusurer. Nord. Med., *73*:309–313, 1965.
3. Aitken, R.E., Kerr, J.L., and Lloyd, H.M.: Primary hyperparathyroidism with osteosclerosis and calcification in articular cartilage. Am. J. Med., *37*:813–820, 1964.
4. Alexander, G.M., et al.: Pyrophosphate arthropathy: a study of metabolic associations and laboratory data. Ann. Rheum. Dis., *41*:377–381, 1982.
5. Ali, S.Y., et al.: Ultrastructural studies of pyrophosphate crystal deposition in articular cartilage. Ann. Rheum. Dis., *42 (Suppl.)*:97–98, 1983.
6. Altman, R.D.: Arthroscopic findings of the knee in patients with pseudogout. Arthritis Rheum., *19*:286–292, 1976.
7. Altman, R.D., et al.: Articular chondrocalcinosis: microanalysis of pyrophosphate (PPi) in synovial fluid and plasma. Arthritis Rheum., *16*:171–178, 1973.
8. Andres, T.L., and Trainer, T.D.: Intervertebral chondrocalcinosis: a coincidental finding possibly related to previous surgery. Arch. Pathol. Lab. Med., *104*:269–271, 1980.
9. Angevine, C.D., and Jacox, R.F.: Unusual connective tissue manifestations of hemochromatosis. Arthritis Rheum., *17*:477–485, 1974.
10. Atkins, C.J., et al.: Chondrocalcinosis and arthropathy: studies in haemochromatosis and in idiopathic chondrocalcinosis. Q. J. Med., *39*:71–79, 1970.
11. Bauer, F.M., et al.: Syndrome de Bartter, chondrocalcinose et hypomagnésemie. Schweiz. Med. Wochenschr., *109*:1,251–1,256, 1979.
12. Bauer, G.C., and Jeffries, G.H.: Articular chondrocalcinosis in a case of hemochromatosis. Acta Med. Scand., *179*:434–439, 1966.
13. Bennett, E.H.: Abnormal deposits in joints. Dublin J. Med. Sci., *65*:161–163, 1903.
14. Bennett, G.A., Waine, H., and Bauer, W.: Changes in the Knee Joint At Various Ages. New York, Commonwealth Fund, 1942, pp. 20–39.
15. Bennett, R.M., Lehr, J.R., and McCarty, D.J.: Crystal shedding and acute pseudogout: a hypothesis based on a therapeutic failure. Arthritis Rheum., *19*:93–97, 1976.
16. Bennett, R.M., Lehr, J.R., and McCarty, D.J.: Factors affecting the solubility of calcium pyrophosphate dihydrate crystals. J. Clin. Invest., *56*:1,571–1,579, 1975.
17. Bennett, R.M., Mall, J.C., and McCarty, D.J.: Pseudogout in acute neuropathic arthropathy: a clue to pathogenesis? Ann. Rheum. Dis., *33*:563–567, 1974.
18. Berry, E.M., and Miller, J.P.: Hereditary spherocytosis, haemochromatosis, diabetes mellitus and chondrocalcinosis. Proc. R. Soc. Med., *66*:9–10, 1973.
19. Bilezikian, J.P., et al.: Pseudogout after parathyroidectomy. Lancet, *1*:445–449, 1973.
20. Bird, H.A., Tribe, C.R., and Bacon, P.A.: Joint hypermobility leading to osteoarthrosis and chondrocalcinosis. Ann. Rheum. Dis., *37*:203–211, 1978.
21. Bjelle, A.: Cartilage matrix in hereditary pyrophosphate arthropathy. J. Rheumatol., *8*:959–964, 1981.
22. Bjelle, A.: Morphological study of articular cartilage in pyrophosphate arthropathy. Ann. Rheum. Dis., *31*:449–456, 1972.
23. Bjelle, A., Crocker, P., and Willoughby, D.: Ultra-microcrystals in pyrophosphate arthropathy. Acta Med. Scand., *207*:89–92, 1980.
24. Bjelle, A., Edvinsson, U., and Hagstam, A.: Pyrophosphate arthropathy in two Swedish families. Arthritis Rheum., *25*:66–74, 1982.
25. Bluestone, R., Bywaters, E.G.L., and Hartog, M.: Acromegalic arthropathy. Ann. Rheum. Dis., *30*:243–258, 1971.
26. Bocher, J., et al.: Prevalence of calcified meniscal cartilage in elderly persons. N. Engl. J. Med., *272*:1,093–1,097, 1965.
27. Boivin, G., and Lagier, R.: An ultrastructural study of articular chondrocalcinosis in cases of knee osteoarthritis. Virchows Arch. (Pathol. Anat.), *400*:13–29, 1983.
27a. Bong, D., and Bennett, R.: Pseudogout mimicking systemic disease. JAMA, *246*:1,438–1,440, 1981.
28. Boudin, G., Pepin, B., and Hubault, A.: Les arthropathies de la maladie de Wilson. Soc. Med. Hôp. Paris, *114*:617–622, 1963.
28a. Bourqui, M., et al.: Pyrophosphate arthropathy in the carpal and metacarpophalangeal joints. Ann. Rheum. Dis., *42*:626–630, 1983.
29. Brown, E.H., et al.: Preparation and characterization of some calcium pyrophosphates. J. Agric. Food Chem., *11*:214–222, 1963.
30. Brown, W.E., et al.: Crystallography of octacalcium phosphate. J. Am. Chem. Soc., *79*:5,318, 1957.
31. Bywaters, E.G.L.: Calcium pyrophosphate deposits in synovial membrane. Ann. Rheum. Dis., *31*:219–220, 1972.
32. Bywaters, E.G.L., Dixon, A. St. J., and Scott, J.T.: Joint lesions of hyperparathyroidism. Ann. Rheum. Dis., *22*:171–187, 1963.
33. Bywaters, E.G.L., Dorling, J., and Sutor, J.: Ochronotic densification. Ann. Rheum. Dis., *29*:563, 1970.
34. Bywaters, E.G.L., Hamilton, E.B.D., and Williams, R.: The spine in idiopathic haemochromatosis. Ann. Rheum. Dis., *30*:453–465, 1971.
35. Cabanel, G., et al.: Communication No. 667/776 Piestany, October 13, 1969.
36. Camerlain, M., et al.: Inorganic pyrophosphate pool size and turnover rate in arthritic joints. J. Clin. Invest., *55*:1,373–1,381, 1975.
37. Cartier, P., and Picard, J.: La mineralisation du cartilage ossifiable. III. Le mécanisme de la réaction atpasique du cartilage. Bull. Soc. Chim. Biol., *37*:1,159–1,168, 1955.
38. Chaudry, I.: Does ATP cross the cell membrane? Yale J. Biol. Med., *55*:1–10, 1982.
39. Christensen, E.G., and Sorensen, K.H.: Local amyloid formation of capsula fibrosa in arthrosis coxae. Acta Pathol. Microbiol. Scand., *80 (Suppl. 223)*:128–131, 1972.
40. Cohen, A.S., Brandt, K.D., and Krey, P.R.: *In* Labo-

ratory Diagnostic Procedures in the Rheumatic Diseases, 2nd Ed. Edited by A.S. Cohen. Boston, Little, Brown, 1975.

41. Connor, T.B., et al.: Generalized osteosclerosis in primary hyperparathyroidism. Trans. Am. Clin. Climatol. Assoc., *85*:185–196, 1976.

42. Currey, H.L.F., et al.: Significance of radiological calcification of joint cartilage. Ann. Rheum. Dis., *25*:295–306, 1966.

42a.DeLauche, M.C., et al.: Fréquence de la chondrocalcinose radiologique aprés 80 ans. Rev. Rhum. Mal. Osteoartic., *44*:555–557, 1977.

43. Delbarre, F.: Les manifestations ostéo-articulares de hémochromatose. Presse Méd., *72*:2,973–2,978, 1964.

44. DeSeze, S., et al.: Joint and bone disorders and hypoparathyroidism in hemochromatosis. Semin. Arthritis Rheum., *2*:71–83, 1972.

45. DeSeze, S., et al.: Les chondrocalcinoses articulaires. Sem. Hop. Paris, *42*:2,461–2,470, 1966.

46. DeSeze, S., et al.: Les arthropathies de hémochromatoses: hémochromatose and "chondrocalcinose" articulaire. Rev. Rhum. Mal. Osteoartic., *31*:479–485, 1964.

47. deVos, R.A., et al.: Calcium pyrophosphate dihydrate of the temporomandibular joint. Oral Surg., *51*:497–502, 1980.

48. Dieppe, P.A., et al.: Pyrophosphate arthropathy: a clinical and radiological study of 105 cases. Ann. Rheum. Dis., *41*:371–376, 1982.

49. Dieppe, P.A., et al.: Mixed crystal deposition disease and osteoarthritis. Br. Med. J., *1*:150–151, 1978.

50. Dieppe, P.A., et al.: Apatite deposition disease. Lancet, *1*:266–270, 1976.

51. Dodds, W.J., and Steinbach, L.: Primary hyperparathyroidism and articular cartilage calcification. AJR, *104*:884–892, 1968.

52. Dodds, W.J., and Steinbach, H.L.: Gout associated with calcification of cartilage. N. Engl. J. Med., *275*:745–749, 1966.

53. Doherty, M., and Dieppe, P.A.: Double blind, placebo controlled trial of magnesium carbonate in chronic pyrophosphate arthropathy. (Abstract.) Ann. Rheum. Dis., *42 (Suppl.)*:106–107, 1983.

54. Doherty, M., and Dieppe, P.A.: Effect of intra-articular yttrium-90 on chronic pyrophosphate arthropathy of the knee. Lancet, *1*:1,243–1,246, 1981.

54a.Doherty, M., Dieppe, P., Watt, I.: Low incidence of calcium pyrophosphate dihydrate crystal deposition in rheumatoid arthritis, with modification of radiographic features in coexistent disease. Arthritis Rheum., *27*:1002–1009, 1984.

55. Doherty, M., Watt, I., and Dieppe, P.A.: Localised chondrocalcinosis in post-meniscectomy knees. Lancet, *1*:1,207–1,210, 1982.

56. Dorfmann, H., et al.: Les arthropathies des hémochromatoses: résultats d'une enquète prospective portant sur 54 malades. Sem. Hôp. Paris, *45*:516–523, 1969.

57. Dorwart, B.B., and Schumacher, H.R.: Joint effusions, chondrocalcinosis and other rheumatic manifestations in hypothyroidism. Am. J. Med., *59*:780–789, 1975.

58. Doyle, D.V., et al.: Mixed crystal deposition in an osteoarthritic joint. J. Pathol., *123*:1–4, 1977.

59. duLac, Y., Deloux, G., and Deuil, R.: Arthropathies et chondrocalcinose au cours des hémochromatoses. Rev. Rhum. Mal. Osteoartic., *34*:758–769, 1967.

60. Dymock, I.W., et al.: Arthropathy of hemochromatosis. Ann. Rheum. Dis., *29*:469–476, 1970.

61. Eade, A.W.T., Swannell, A.J., and Williamson, N.R.: Abstract 424. In Proceedings of the Fourteenth International Rheumatology Congress, San Francisco, June, 1977.

62. Earde, A.W., Swannell, A.J., and Williamson, N.R.: Pyrophosphate arthropathy in hypophosphatasia. Ann. Rheum. Dis., *40*:164–170, 1981.

63. Egan, M.S., et al.: The association of amyloid deposits and osteoarthritis. Arthritis Rheum., *25*:204–208, 1982.

64. Ellman, M.H., et al.: Calcium pyrophosphate dihydrate deposition in lumbar disc fibrocartilage. J. Rheumatol., *8*:955–958, 1981.

65. Ellman, M.H., et al.: Calcium pyrophosphate deposition in ligamentum flavum. Arthritis Rheum., *21*:611–613, 1978.

66. Ellman, M.H., and Levin, B.: Chondrocalcinosis in elderly persons. Arthritis Rheum., *18*:43–47, 1975.

67. Ellman, M.H., Brown, N.L., and Porat, A.P.: Laboratory investigations in pseudogout patients and controls. J. Rheumatol., *7*:77–81, 1980.

68. Ellman, M., Krieger, M.I., and Brown, N.: Pseudogout mimicking synovial chondromatosis. J. Bone Joint Surg., *57A*:863–865, 1975.

69. Fam, A.G., et al.: Clinical and roentgenographic aspects of pseudogout: a study of 50 cases and review. Can. Med. Assoc. J., *124*:545–550, 1981.

70. Fam, A.G., and Stein, G.: Disappearance of chondrocalcinosis following reflex sympathetic dystrophy. Arthritis Rheum., *24*:747–749, 1981.

71. Felix, R., and Fleisch, H.: The effect of pyrophosphate and diphosphonates on calcium transport in red cells. Experientia, *33*:1,003–1,005, 1977.

72. Feller, E.R., and Schumacher, H.R.: Osteoarticular changes in Wilson's disease. Arthritis Rheum., *15*:259–266, 1972.

73. Foss, M.V.L., and Byers, P.D.: Bone density, osteoarthritis of the hip and fracture of the upper end of the femur. Ann. Rheum. Dis., *31*:259–264, 1972.

73a.Frederick, N., et al.: Chondrocalcinosis in primary and in renal hyperparathyroidism. Kidney Int. In press.

74. Garrod, A.B.: A Treatise on Gout and Rheumatic Gout. London. Longmans, Green, 1876.

75. Gatter, R.A., and McCarty, D.J.: Pathological tissue calcification in man. Arch. Pathol., *84*:346–353, 1967.

76. Gaucher, A.: Hereditary diffuse articular chondrocalcinosis. Scand. J. Rheumatol., *6*:216–221, 1977.

77. Gaucher, A., et al.: Identification des cristaux observés dans les arthropathies destructives de la chondrocalcinose. Rev. Rhum. Mal. Osteoartic., *44*:407–414, 1977.

78. Gaucher, A., et al.: Les chondrocalcinose articulaires diffusés héréditaires. Rev. Rhum. Mal. Osteoartic., *44*:589–598, 1977.

79. Gaudreau, A., et al.: Familial articular chondrocalcinosis in Quebec. Arthritis Rheum., *24*:611–615, 1981.

80. Genant, H.K.: Roentgenographic aspects of calcium pyrophosphate dihydrate crystal deposition disease (pseudogout). Arthritis Rheum., *19*:307–328, 1976.

81. Gerster, J.C., et al.: Carpal tunnel syndrome in chondrocalcinosis of the wrist. Arthritis Rheum., *23*:926–931, 1980.

82. Gerster, J.C., et al.: Tendon calcifications in chondrocalcinosis. Arthritis Rheum., *20*:717–722, 1977.

83. Gerster, J.C., Lagier, R., and Boivin, G.: Olecranon bursitis related to calcium pyrophosphate dihydrate crystal deposition disease. Arthritis Rheum., *25*:989–996, 1982.

84. Gerster, J.C., Vischer, T.L., and Fallet, G.H.: Destructive arthropathy in generalized osteoarthritis with articular chondrocalcinosis. J. Rheumatol., *2*:265–269, 1975.

85. Gibson, J.P., and Roenijk, W.J.: Pseudogout in a dog. J. Am. Vet. Med. Assoc., *161*:912–915, 1972.

86. Glass, J.S., and Grahame, R.: Chondrocalcinosis after parathyroidectomy. Ann. Rheum. Dis., *35*:521–525, 1976.

87. Glimet, T., Masse, J.P., and Ryckewaert, A.: Etude radiologique: genoux indolores de 50 femmes plus de 65 ans. Rev. Rhum. Mal. Osteoartic., *46*:589–592, 1979.

88. Goldenberg, D.L., and Cohen, A.S.: Synovial membrane histopathology in the differential diagnosis of rheumatoid arthritis, gout, pseudogout, systemic lupus erythematosus, infectious arthritis and degenerative joint disease. Medicine, *57*:239–252, 1978.

89. Goldenberg, D.L., Egan, M.S., and Cohen, A.S.: Inflammatory synovitis in degenerative joint disease. J. Rheumatol., *9*:204–209, 1982.

90. Good, A.E., and Rapp, R.: Chondrocalcinosis of the knee with gout and rheumatoid arthritis. N. Engl. J. Med., *277*:286–290, 1967.

91. Gordon, D.A., Clarke, P.V., and Orgyzlo, M.A.: The chondrocalcific arthropathy of iron overload. Arch. Intern. Med., *134*:21–28, 1974.

92. Goulon, M., Raphael, J.C., and deRohan, P.: Syndrome de Bartter et chondrocalcinose. Nouv. Presse Méd., 9:1,291–1,295, 1980.
93. Grahame, R., Sutor, D.J., and Mitchener, M.B.: Crystal deposition in hyperparathyroidism. Ann. Rheum. Dis., 30:597–604, 1971.
94. Halverson, P.B., et al.: Milwaukee shoulder syndrome: report of eleven additional cases with concomitant involvement of the knee in seven instances. Semin. Arthritis Rheum., 14:36–44, 1984.
95. Hamilton, E.B.D.: Diseases associated with CPPD deposition disease. Arthritis Rheum., 19 (Suppl.):353–357, 1976.
96. Hamilton, E.B.D., et al.: The natural history of arthritis in idiopathic haemochromatosis: Progression of the clinical and radiological features over ten years. Q. J. Med., 50:321–329, 1981.
97. Hamilton, E.B.D., et al.: The arthropathy of idiopathic haemochromatosis. Q. J. Med., 37:171–182, 1968.
98. Hamilton, E.B.D., and Richards, A.J.: Destructive arthropathy in chondrocalcinois articularis. Ann. Rheum. Dis., 33:196–203, 1974.
99. Harris, J., et al.: Ankylosing hyperostosis. Ann. Rheum. Dis., 33:210–215, 1974.
100. Hearn, P.R., Guilland-Cumming, D.F., and Russell, R.G.G.: Effect of orthophosphate and other factors on the crystal growth of calcium pyrophosphate in vitro. Ann. Rheum. Dis., 42 (Suppl.):101, 1983.
101. Hearn, P.R., Russell, R.G.G., and Elliott, J.C.: Formation product of calcium pyrophosphate crystals in vitro and the effect of iron salts. Clin. Sci. Mol. Med., 54:29–33, 1978.
102. Hollingworth, P., Williams, P.L., and Scott, J.T.: Frequency of chondrocalcinosis of the knees in asymptomatic hyperuricemia and rheumatoid arthritis: a controlled study. Ann. Rheum. Dis.,41:344–346, 1982.
103. Houpt, J.B., and Sinclair, D.S.: Spontaneous osteonecrosis of the medial femoral condyle. (Abstract.) J. Rheumatol., 1 (Suppl.):117, 1974.
104. Howell, D.S., et al.: Extrusion of pyrophosphate into extracellular media by osteoarthritic cartilage incubates. J. Clin. Invest., 56:1,473–1,480, 1975.
105. Hsu, H.: Purification and partial characterization of ATP pyrophosphohydrolase from fetal bovine epiphyseal cartilage. J. Biol. Chem., 258:3,463–3,468, 1983.
106. Jacobelli, S.G., et al.: Calcium pyrophosphate dihydrate crystal deposition in neuropathic joints: four cases of polyarticular involvement. Ann. Intern. Med., 79:340–347, 1973.
107. Jaffres, R., and Kerbat, G.: Calcinose articulaire diffusé chez deux frères atteints d'hémochromatose. Rev. Rhum. Mal. Osteoartic., 32:431–438, 1965.
108. Jensen, P.S., and Putnam, C.E.: Chondrocalcinosis and haemophilia. Clin. Radiol., 28:401–405, 1977.
109. Kamakura, K., Manko, S., and Furakawa, T.: Cervical radiculomyelopathy due to calcified ligamenta flava. Ann. Neurol., 5:193–195, 1978.
110. Kaplinski, N., Biran, D., and Frankl, O.: Pseudogout and amyloidosis. Harefuah, 91:59, 1976.
111. Kawano, N., et al.: Cervical radiculomyelopathy caused by deposition of calcium pyrophosphate dihydrate crystals in the ligamenta flava. J. Neurosurg., 52:279–283, 1980.
112. Kohn, N.N., et al.: The significance of calcium phosphate crystals in the synovial fluid of arthritis patients: the "pseudogout syndrome." II. Identification of crystals. Ann. Intern. Med., 56:738–745, 1962.
113. Krane, S.M., and Glimcher, M.J.: Transphosphorylation from nucleoside di- and tri-phosphates by apatite crystals. J. Biol. Chem., 237:2,991–2,998, 1962.
114. Ladefoged, C.: Amyloid in osteoarthritic hip joints: a pathoanatomical and histological investigation of femoral head cartilage. Acta Orthop. Scand., 53:581–586, 1982.
115. Lagier, R.: Case report: rare femoral erosions and osteoarthritis of the knee associated with chondrocalcinosis. A histological study of this cortical remodeling. Virchows Arch. (Pathol. Anat.), 364:215–223, 1974.
116. Lagier, R., and Baud, C.A.: In Rapports et communications au quatrième symposium européen des tissus cal-

117. cifiés, Bordeaux, 1967. Edited by J. Melhaud, M. Owen, and H.J.J. Blackwood. Paris, Sedes, 1968, p. 109.
117. Lamotte, M., Segresta, J.M., and Krassinine, G.: Arthrite microcristalline calcifique (pseudo-goutte) chez un acromégale. Sem. Hôp. Paris, 42:2,420–2,424, 1966.
118. LeGoff, P., Penunec, Y., and Youinou, P.: Signes cervicaux aigus pseudoméninge, relateurs de la chondrocalcinose articulaire. Sem. Hop. Paris, 56:1,515–1,518, 1980.
119. Leisen, J.C., et al.: The tophus in calcium pyrophosphate deposition disease. JAMA, 244:1,711–1,712, 1980.
120. Leonello, P.P., Cleland, L.G., and Norman, J.E.: Acute pseudogout and chondrocalcinosis in a man with mild hemophilia. J. Rheumatol., 8:841–844, 1981.
121. Linden, B., and Nilsson, B.E.: Chondrocalcinosis following osteochondritis dissecans in the femur condyle. Clin. Orthop., 130:223–227, 1978.
122. Ling, D., Murphy, W.A. and Kyriakos, M.: Tophaceous pseudogout. Radiology, 138:162–165, 1982.
123. Lust, G., et al.: Evidence of a generalized metabolic defect in patients with hereditary chondrocalcinosis. Arthritis Rheum., 24:1,517–1,521, 1981.
124. Lust, G., et al.: Increased pyrophosphate in fibroblasts and lymphoblasts from patients with hereditary diffuse articular chondrocalcinosis. Science, 214:809–810, 1981.
125. McCarty, D.J.: The Heberden Oration, 1982. Crystals, joints and consternation. Ann. Rheum. Dis., 42:243–253, 1983.
126. McCarty, D.J.: Calcium pyrophosphate dihydrate crystal deposition disease (pseudogout syndrome): clinical aspects. Clin. Rheum. Dis., 3:61–89, 1977.
127. McCarty, D.J.: Diagnostic mimicry in arthritis: patterns of joint involvement associated with calcium pyrophosphate dihydrate crystal deposits. Bull. Rheum. Dis., 25:804–809, 1975.
128. McCarty, D.J.: Crystal-induced inflammation: syndromes of gout and pseudogout. Geriatrics, 18:467–478, 1963.
129. McCarty, D.J., et al.: Diseases associated with calcium pyrophosphate dihydrate crystal deposition: a controlled study. Am. J. Med., 56:704–714, 1974.
130. McCarty, D.J., et al.: Inorganic pyrophosphate concentrations in the synovial fluid of arthritis patients. J. Lab. Clin. Med., 78:216–229, 1971.
131. McCarty, D.J., et al.: Studies on pathological calcifications in human cartilage. I. Prevalence and types of crystal deposits in the menisci of two hundred fifteen cadavera. J. Bone Joint Surg., 48A:308–325, 1966.
132. McCarty, D.J., and Faires, J.S.: A comparison of the duration of local anti-inflammatory effect of several adrenocorticosteroid esters: a bioassay technique. Curr. Ther. Res., 5:284–290, 1963.
133. McCarty, D.J., and Haskin, M.: The roentgenographic aspects of pseudogout (articular chondrocalcinosis): an analysis of 20 cases. Am. J. Roentgenol. Radium Ther. Nucl. Med., 90:1,248–1,257, 1963.
134. McCarty, D.J., and Hollander, J.L.: Identification of urate crystals in gouty synovial fluid. Ann. Intern. Med., 54:452–460, 1961.
135. McCarty, D.J., and Pepe, P.F.: Erythrocyte neutral inorganic pyrophosphate in pseudogout. J. Lab. Clin. Med., 79:277–284, 1972.
136. McCarty, D.J., Kohn, N.N., and Faires, J.S.: The significance of calcium phosphate crystals in the synovial fluid of arthritis patients": the "pseudogout syndrome." I. Clinical aspects. Ann. Intern. Med., 56:711–737, 1962.
137. McCarty, D.J., Palmer, D.W., and Garancis, J.C.: Clearance of calcium pyrophosphate dihydrate crystals in vivo. III. Effects of synovial hemosiderosis. Arthritis Rheum., 24:706–710, 1981.
138. McCarty, D.J., Palmer, D.W., and James, C.: Clearance of calcium pyrophosphate dihydrate crystals in vivo. II. Studies using triclinic crystals doubly labeled with ^{45}Ca and ^{85}Sr. Arthritis Rheum., 22:1,122–1,131, 1979.
139. Mandel, N.S., and Mandel, G.S.: Nucleation and growth of CPPD crystals and related species in vitro. In Calcium in Biological Systems. Edited by R.P Rubin, G. Weiss, and J.W. Putney. New York, Plenum. In press.

140. Mandl, F.: Zur pathologie und therapie der Zwischen-knorpilerkrankungen des Kniegelenks. Arch. Klin. Chir., *146*:149–214, 1927.

141. Martel, W., et al.: A roentgenologically distinctive arthropathy in some patients with pseudogout syndrome. AJR, *109*:587–605, 1970.

142. Martel, W., et al.: Further observations on the arthropathy of calcium pyrophosphate crystal deposition disease. Radiology, *141*:1–15, 1981.

143. Marx, S.J., et al.: The hypocalciuric or benign variant of familial hypercalcemia: clinical and biochemical features in fifteen kindreds. Medicine, *60*:397–412, 1981.

144. Marx, S.J., et al.: An association between neonatal severe primary hyperparathyroidism and familial hypocalciuric hypercalcemia in three kindreds. N. Engl. J. Med., *306*:257–263, 1982.

145. Memin, Y., Monville, C., and Ryckewaert, A.: La chondrocalcinose articulaire aprés 80 ans. Rev. Rheum. Mal. Osteoartic., *45*:77–82, 1978.

146. Menkes, C.J., Simon, F., and Chourki, M.: Les arthropathies destructrices de la chondrocalcinose. Rev. Rhum. Mal. Osteoartic., *40*:115–123, 1973.

147. Mezard, M., et al.: Etude de la chondrocalcinose articulaire dans une population de 200 vieillards. Lyon Med., *245*:365–370, 1981.

148. Micheli, A., Po, J., and Fallet, G.H.: Measurement of soluble pyrophosphate in plasma and synovial fluid of patients with various rheumatic diseases. Scand. J. Rheumatol., *10*:237–240, 1981.

149. Milazzo, S.C., et al.: Calcium pyrophosphate dihydrate deposition disease and familial hypomagnesemia. J. Rheumatol. *8*:767–771, 1981.

150. Mitrovic, D.: Pathology of articular deposition of calcium salts and their relationship to osteoarthritis. Ann. Rheum. Dis., *42 (Suppl.)*:19–26, 1983.

151. Mitrovic, D., et al.: Fréquence anatomique de la menisco-chondrocalcinose du genou. Rev. Rhum. Mal. Osteoartic., *49*:495–499, 1982.

152. Moskowitz, R.W., et al.: Chronic synovitis as a manifestation of calcium crystal deposition disease. Arthritis Rheum., *14*:109–116, 1971.

153. Moskowitz, R.W., and Garcia, F.: Chondrocalcinosis articularis (pseudogout syndrome). Arch. Intern. Med., *132*:87–91, 1973.

154. M'Seffar, A., Fornasier, V.L., and Fox, I.H.: Arthropathy as a major clinical indicator of occult iron storage disease. JAMA, *238*:1,825–1,828, 1977.

155. Nyulassy, S., et al.: HL-A system in articular chondrocalcinosis. Arthritis Rheum., *19 (Suppl.)*:391–393, 1976.

156. O'Duffy, J.D.: Clinical studies of acute pseudogout attacks. Arthritis Rheum., *19 (Suppl.)*:349–353, 1976.

157. O'Duffy, J.D.: Hypophosphatasia associated with calcium pyrophosphate dihydrate deposits in cartilage. Arthritis Rheum., *13*:381–388, 1970.

158. Okazaki, T., et al.: Pseudogout: clinical observations and chemical analyses of deposits. Arthritis Rheum., *19*:293–305, 1976.

159. Owen, D.S., Toone, E., and Irby, R.: Coexistent rheumatoid arthritis and chronic tophaceous gout. JAMA, *197*:953–956, 1966.

160. Parlee, D.E., Freundlich, I.M., and McCarty, D.J.: A comparative study of roentgenographic techniques for detection of calcium pyrophosphate dihydrate deposits (pseudogout) in human cartilage. Am. J. Roentgenol. Radium Ther. Nucl. Med., *99*:688–694, 1967.

161. Phelip, X., Verrier, J.M., and Gras, F.P.: Les hémarthroses de la chondrocalcinose articulaire. Rev. Rhum., Mal. Osteoartic., *43*:259–268, 1976.

162. Phelps, P.: Polymorphonuclear leukocyte motility in vitro. IV. Colchicine inhibition of chemotactic activity formation after phagocytosis of urate crystals. Arthritis Rheum., *13*:1–9, 1970.

163. Phelps, P., and Hawker, C.D.: Serum parathyroid hormone levels in patients with calcium pyrophosphate crystals deposition disease (chondrocalcinosis, pseudogout). Arthritis Rheum., *16*:590–596, 1973.

164. Pritchard, M.H., and Jessop, J.D.: Chondrocalcinosis in primary hyperparathyroidism. Ann. Rheum. Dis., *36*:146–151, 1977.

165. Pritzker, K.P.H., et al.: Calcium pyrophosphate dihydrate crystal formation in model hydrogels. J. Rheumatol., *5*:469–473, 1978.

166. Pritzker, K.P.H., et al.: Pseudotumor of temporomandibular joint: destructive calcium pyrophosphate hydrate arthropathy. J. Rheumatol., *3*:70–81, 1976.

167. Pugh, J., Rose, R., and Radin, E.: Elastic and viscoelastic properties of trabecular bone: dependence on structure. J. Biomech., *6*:475–485, 1973.

168. Rachow, J.W., and Ryan, L.M.: Adenosine triphosphate pyrophosphohydrolase and pyrophosphatase activities in human synovial fluids. Clin. Res., *31*:806A, 1983.

169. Radi, J., et al.: Chondrocalcinose articulaire primaire: ses rapports avec le sexe des malades, l'age des patients au debut de l'affection, le diabète. Rev. Rhum. Mal. Osteoartic., *37*:263–279, 1970.

170. Radi, J., Epiney, J., and Reiner, M.: Chondrocalcinose et maladie osseuse de Paget. Rev. Rhum. Mal. Osteoartic., *37*:385–388, 1970.

171. Rapado, A., et al.: Condrocalcinosis de hypomagnesemia: un nuevo síndrome. Rev. Esp. Reum. Enferm. Osteoartic., *3*:283–291, 1976.

172. Reginato, A.J.: Articular chondrocalcinosis in the Chiloe islanders. Arthritis Rheum., *19 (Suppl.)*:395–404, 1976.

173. Reginato, A.J., et al.: HLA antigens in chondrocalcinosis and ankylosing chondrocalcinosis. Arthritis Rheum., *22*:928–932, 1979.

174. Reginato, A.J., et al.: Polyarticular and familial chondrocalcinosis. Arthritis Rheum., *13*:197–213, 1970.

175. Reginato, A.J., Schumacher, H.R., and Martinez, V.A.: Ochronotic arthropathy with calcium pyrophosphate crystal deposition. Arthritis Rheum., *16*:705–714, 1973.

176. Resnick, D., et al.: Rheumatoid arthritis and pseudo-rheumatoid arthritis in calcium pyrophosphate dihydrate crystal deposition disease. Radiology, *140*:615–621, 1981.

177. Resnick, D., et al.: Clinical, radiographic and pathologic abnormalities in calcium pyrophosphate dihydrate deposition disease (CPPD) pseudogout. Diagn. Radiol., *122*:1–15, 1977.

178. Resnick, D., and Niwyama, G.: Carpal instability in rheumatoid arthritis and calcium pyrophosphate deposition disease. Ann. Rheum. Dis., *36*:311–318, 1977.

179. Renlund, R.C., et al.: Calcium pyrophosphate dihydrate crystal deposition disease in aged non-human primates. Am. J. Pathol. In press.

180. Renlund, R.C., et al.: Calcium pyrophosphate dihydrate crystal deposition disease with concurrent diffuse idiopathic skeletal hyperostosis in Barbary ape. Arthritis Rheum., *26*:682–683, 1983.

181. Richardson, B., et al.: Hereditary chondrocalcinosis (CPPD) in a Mexican-American family. Arthritis Rheum., *26*:1,387–1,396, 1983.

182. Rodnan, G.P.: Arthritis with hematologic disorders, storage diseases and dysproteinemias. *In* Arthritis and Allied Conditions. 8th Ed. Edited by J.L. Hollander and D.J. McCarty. Philadelphia, Lea & Febiger, 1972, pp. 1,303–1,328.

183. Rodriquez-Valverde, V., et al.: Familial chondrocalcinosis: prevalence in northern Spain and clinical features in five pedigrees. Arthritis Rheum., *23*:471–478, 1980.

184. Ropes, M.W., and Bauer, W.: Synovial Fluid Changes in Joint Disease. Cambridge, Harvard University Press, 1953.

185. Ross, D.J., et al.: Tibial stress fracture in pyrophosphate arthropathy. J. Bone Joint Surg., *65B*:474–477, 1983.

186. Runeberg, L., et al.: Hypomagnesemia due to renal disease of unknown etiology. Am. J. Med., *59*:873–881, 1975.

187. Russell, R.G.G.: Metabolism of inorganic pyrophosphate (PPi). Arthritis Rheum., *19 (Suppl.)*:463–478, 1976.

188. Russell, R.G.G.: Pyrophosphate metabolism and pseudogout. Lancet, *2*:461–476, 1976.

189. Russell, R.G.G., et al.: Inorganic pyrophosphate in plasma in normal persons and in patients with hypophos-

phatasia, osteogenesis imperfecta and other disorders of bone. J. Clin. Invest., *50*:961–969, 1971.

190. Russell, R.G.G., Bisaz, S., and Fleisch, H.: Inorganic pyrophosphate in plasma, urine and synovial fluid of patients with pyrophosphate arthropathy (chondrocalcinosis or pseudogout). Lancet, *2*:899–902, 1970.

191. Ryan, L.M., et al.: Cartilage nucleoside triphosphate (NTP) pyrophosphohydrolase. I. Identification as an ectoenzyme. Arthritis Rheum., *27*:913–918, 1984.

192. Ryan, L.M., et al.: Amyloid arthropathy in the absence of dysproteinemia: possible association with chondrocalcinosis. (Abstract.) Arthritis Rheum., *21*:587, 1978.

193. Ryan, L.M., Cheung, H.S., and McCarty, D.J.: Release of pyrophosphate by normal mammalian articular hyaline and fibrocartilage in organ culture. Arthritis Rheum., *24*:1,522–1,527, 1981.

194. Ryan, L.M., Kozin, F., and McCarty, D.J.: Quantification of human plasma inorganic pyrophosphatase. II. Biologic variables. Arthritis Rheum., *22*:892–895, 1979.

195. Ryan, L.M., Kozin, F., and McCarty, D.J.: Quantification of human plasma inorganic pyrophosphatase. I. Normal values in osteoarthritis and calcium pyrophosphate dihydrate crystal deposition disease. Arthritis Rheum., *22*:886–891, 1979.

196. Ryan, L.M., Liang, G., and Kozin, F.: Amyloid arthropathy: possible association with chondrocalcinosis. J. Rheumatol., *9*:273–278, 1982.

197. Ryan, L.M., Lynch, M.P., and McCarty, D.J.: Inorganic pyrophosphate levels in blood platelets from normal donors and patients with calcium pyrophosphate dihydrate crystal deposition disease. Arthritis Rheum.,*26*:564–566, 1983.

197a.Ryan, L.M., et al.: Elevated intracellular pyrophosphate (PPi) and ecto-nucleoside triphosphate pyrophosphohydrolase activity (NTPPH) in fibroblasts of patients with calcium pyrophosphate dihydrate (CPPD) crystal deposition disease. Clin. Res., *32*:792A, 1984 (abstract).

198. Rynes, R.I., and Merzig, E.G.: Calcium pyrophosphate crystal deposition disease and hyperparathyroidism: a controlled prospective study. J. Rheumatol., *5*:460–468, 1978.

199. Rynes, R.I., Sosman, J.L., and Holdsworth, D.E.L.: Pseudogout in ochronosis. Arthritis Rheum., *18*:21–25, 1975.

200. Sakaguchi, M., et al.: Familial pseudogout with destructive arthropathy in Japan. Ryumachi, *22*:4–13, 1982.

201. Schmied, P., et al.: Etude radiologique sur la fréquence de l'association entre la chondrocalcinose articulaire et le diabéte. Schweiz. Med. Wochenschr., *101*:272–274, 1971.

202. Schumacher, H.R.: The synovitis of pseudogout: electron microscopic observations. Arthritis Rheum., *11*:426–435, 1968.

203. Schumacher, H.R.: Hemochromatosis and arthritis. Arthritis Rheum., *7*:41–50, 1964.

204. Schumacher, H.R., et al.: Arthritis associated with apatite crystals. Ann. Intern. Med., *87*:411–416, 1977.

205. Sella, E.J., and Goodman, A.H.: Arthopathy secondary to transfusion hemochromatosis. J. Bone Joint Surg., *55A*:1,077–1,083, 1973.

206. Settas, L., Doherty, M., and Dieppe, P.: Localized chondrocalcinosis in unstable joints. Br. Med. J., *285*:175–176, 1982.

207. Shimizu, K., et al.: Amyloid deposition in the articular structures of AKR senescent mice. Arthritis Rheum., *24*:1,540–1,543, 1981.

208. Siegel, S.A., Hummel, C.F., and McCarty, R.P.: The role of nucleoside triphosphate pyrophosphohydrolase in *in vitro* nucleoside triphosphate-dependent matrix vesicle calcification. J. Biol. Chem., *258*:8,601–8,607, 1983.

209. Silcox, D.C., and McCarty, D.J.: Elevated inorganic pyrophosphate concentrations in synovial fluid in osteoarthritis and pseudogout. J. Lab. Clin. Med., *83*:518–531, 1974.

210. Silcox, D.C., and McCarty, D.J.: Measurement of inorganic pyrophosphate in biological fluids, elevated levels in some patients with osteoarthritis, pseudogout, acro-

megaly and uremia. J. Clin. Invest., *52*:1,863–1,870, 1973.

211. Silcox, D.C., Jacobelli, S.G., and McCarty, D.J.: The identification of inorganic pyrophosphate in human platelets and its release on stimulation with thrombin. J. Clin. Invest., *52*:1,595–1,600, 1973.

212. Skinner, M., and Cohen, A.S.: Calcium pyrophosphate dihydrate crystal deposition disease. Arch. Intern. Med., *123*:636–644, 1969.

213. Sorensen, K.H., et al.: Pyrophosphate arthritis with local amyloid deposition. Acta Orthop. Scand., *52*:129–133, 1981.

214. Sorensen, S.A., Flodgaard, H., and Sorensen, E.: Serum alkaline phosphatase, serum pyrophosphatase, phosphorylethanolamine, and inorganic pyrophosphate in plasma and urine: a genetic and clinical study of hypophosphatasia. Monogr. Hum. Genet., *10*:66–69, 1978.

215. Spilberg, I., et al.: Colchicine and pseudogout. Arthritis Rheum., *23*:1,062–1,063, 1980.

216. Steiger, U., and Lagier, R.: Combined anatomical and radiological study of the hip joint in alcaptonuric arthropathy. Ann. Rheum. Dis., *31*:369–373, 1972.

217. Stevens, L.W., and Spiera, H.: Hemarthrosis in chondrocalcinosis (pseudogout). Arthritis Rheum., *15*:651–652, 1972.

218. Stockman, A., Darlington, L.G., and Scott, J.T.: Frequency of chondrocalcinosis of the knees and avascular necrosis of the femoral heads in gout: a controlled study. Ann. Rheum. Dis., *39*:7–11, 1980.

219. Teglbjaerg, P.S., et al.: Local articular amyloid deposition in pyrophosphate arthritis. Acta Pathol. Microbiol. Scand., *87*:307–311, 1979.

220. Tenenbaum, J., et al.: Comparison of phosphohydrolase activities from articular cartilage in calcium pyrophosphate deposition disease and primary osteoarthritis. Arthritis Rheum., *24*:492–500, 1981.

221. Tobler, T.H.: The normal and pathological histology of the meniscus of the knee joint. Schweiz Med. Wochenschr., *59*:10–21, 1929.

222. Utsinger, P.D.: Abstract 448. *In* Proceedings of the Fourteenth International Congress of Rheumatology, San Francisco, June, 1977.

223. Utsinger, P.D., Resnick, D., and Zvaifler, N.J.: Wrist arthropathy in calcium pyrophosphate dihydrate deposition disease. Arthritis Rheum., *18*:485–491, 1975.

224. Vander Korst, J.K., Geerards, J., and Driessens, F.C.M.: A hereditary type of idiopathic articular chondrocalcinosis. Am. J. Med., *56*:307–314, 1974.

225. Wallace, S.L., et al.: Preliminary criteria for the classification of the acute arthritis of primary gout. Arthritis Rheum., *20*:895–900, 1977.

226. Watt, I., and Dieppe, P.: Medial femoral condyle necrosis and chondrocalcinosis: A causal relationship? Br. J. Radiol., *56*:7–11, 1983.

227. Weaver, J.B.: Calcification and ossification of the menisci. J. Bone Joint Surg., *24*:873–882, 1942.

228. Webb, J., Corrigan, A.B., and Robinson, R.G.: Haemochromatosis and pseudogout. Med. J. Aust., *2*:24–29, 1972.

229. Werwath, K.: Abnormal depositions of calcium within the knee joints, an addition to the question of primary "meniscopathy." Acta Radiol., *37*:169–171, 1926.

230. Whyte, M.P., et al.: Infantile hypophosphatasia: enzyme replacement therapy by intravenous infusion of alkaline phosphatase-rich plasma from patients with Paget's bone disease. J. Pediatr., *101*:379–386, 1982.

231. Whyte, M.P., Murphy, W.A., and Fallon, M.D.: Adult hypophosphatasia with chondrocalcinosis and arthropathy: variable penetrance of hypophosphatemia in a large Oklahoma kindred. Am. J. Med., *72*:631–641, 1982.

232. Wilkins, E., et al.: Osteoarthritis and articular chondrocalcinosis in the elderly. Ann. Rheum. Dis., *42*:280–284, 1983.

233. Wills, M.R., Pak, C.Y., and Hammond, W.G.: Normocalcemic primary hyperparathyroidism. Am. J. Med., *47*:384–391, 1969.

234. Yood, R.A., et al.: Soft tissue uptake of bone seeking

radionuclide in amyloidosis. J. Rheumatol., *8*:760–766, 1981.

235. Yosipovitch, Z., and Glimscher, M.J.: Chondrocalcinosis in adult rabbits. Metab. Bone Dis. Relat. Res., 7:503–504, 1971.

236. Zinn, W.M., Currey, H.L.F., and Lawrence, J.S.: Communication No. 779, Piestany, October 13, 1969.

237. Zitnan, D., and Sitaj, S.: Natural course of articular chondrocalcinosis. Arthritis Rheum., *19 (Suppl.)*:363–390, 1976.

238. Zitnan, D., and Sitaj, S.: Chondrocalcinosis articularis. Section I. Clinical and radiological study. Ann. Rheum. Dis., *22*:142–169, 1963.

239. Zitnan, D., and Sitaj, S.: Mnohopocentna familiarna kalcifikacin articularnych chrupiek. Bratisl. Lek. Listy, *38*:217–228, 1958.

240. Zvaifler, N.J., Reefe, W.E., and Black, R.L.: Articular manifestations in primary hyperparathyroidism. Arthritis Rheum., *5*:237–249, 1962.

Chapter **95**

Basic Calcium Phosphate (Apatite, Octacalcium Phosphate, Tricalcium Phosphate) Crystal Deposition Diseases

Daniel J. McCarty
Paul Halverson

There are hundreds of reports of pathologic calcium phosphate mineral phase deposition in various human tissues. These reports are largely descriptive, and most present no clear pattern of disease. Basic calcium phosphate (BCP) crystals, formerly termed hydroxyapatite (HA), have long been associated with periarticular diseases such as calcific periarthritis and tendonitis.[27,56,75,91,92] Recently, BCP crystals have been found in synovial fluid by scanning electron microscopy (SEM) or transmission electron microscopy (TEM).[27,87]

CRYSTAL IDENTIFICATION

The study of BCP crystal-associated arthritis has been relatively difficult because of the lack of a simple, reliable diagnostic test (see also Chap. 4). Heterogeneity of crystal species in periarticular shoulder joint calcifications was first established by Faure et al., who directly measured the interplanar spacings of individual apatite crystals using high-resolution-transmission electron microscopy.[35] These crystals were largely carbonate-substituted, and other nonapatite calcium phosphates were found. Intensive study of a subcutaneous calcification from a patient with scleroderma showed amorphous and poorly crystallized calcium phosphate in nodular aggregates with internodular apatite crystals.[23] Fourier transform infrared (FTIR) analysis of shoulder joint fluid crystals, of rabbit synovium calcified by calciphylaxis, and of subcutaneous calcifications from a girl with dermatomyositis showed that each contained partially carbonate-substituted HA, octacalcium phosphate (OCP), and particulate collagens[59] (Table 95–1). Samples from one patient had tricalcium phosphate (TCP) (Whitlockite) instead of OCP. BCP is therefore used here to designate these crystal mixtures. Perhaps "BCP crystal deposition disease" is the most appropriate term for the associated clinical syndromes.

Radiography. Radiography of BCP crystal deposits has shown rounded or fluffy calcifications that vary in size from a few millimeters to several centimeters. They may occur either as solitary nodules or as multiple deposits. Although radiography is a useful diagnostic tool, it is both relatively insensitive and nonspecific in the diagnosis of BCP crystal arthropathies.[41] Asymptomatic periarticular calcific deposits are frequently observed as incidental findings.

Synovial Fluid. Phase contrast-polarized light microscopy, invaluable for the detection of the larger monosodium urate monohydrate and calcium pyrophosphate dihydrate crystals, provides little help with BCP crystals, because their size is below the limits of resolution of optical microscopy. Although these crystals have a marked tendency to aggregate, their orientation within an aggregate is random. Birefringence is rarely noted.[58] Individual needle- or plate-shaped crystals are usually less than 0.1 μm long (Fig. 95–1). BCP crystal aggregates may be visible by light microscopy as shiny laminated "coins" (Fig. 4–5,B).[8,20,58] Alizarin red S staining of synovial fluid pellets has been suggested as a screening technique for BCP crystals.[74] The method is sensitive to 0.005 μg of HA standard/ml, but it is not specific for calcium phosphates, and in our hands, led to many false positive results.

A technique for semiquantitation of BCP in synovial fluids utilizing the binding of (^{14}C) ethane-1-hydroxy-1, 1-diphosphonate (EHDP) to BCP crystals has proved useful as a screening test.[45] The protocol for this method, sensitive to about 2 μg HA standard/ml, is shown in Table 95–2. Positive and negative controls are included routinely, and a detergent is added if many cells are present to release intracellular crystals. Diphosphonate binding in synovial fluids strongly correlated with the

Table 95–1.   Chemical Formulas and Molar Ratios of Calcium (Ca) to Phosphorus (P) of Calcium-Containing Crystals Found in Human Synovial Fluid, Cartilage or Synovium

Crystal	Formula	Ca/P
BCP		
Hydroxyapatite (HA)	$Ca_5(PO_4)_3OH2H_2O$	1.67
Octacalcium phosphate (OCP)	$Ca_8H_2(PO_4)_65H_2O$	1.33
Tricalcium phosphate (TCP) (Whitlockite)	$Ca_3(PO_4)_2$	1.5
OTHER		
Dicalcium phosphate dihydrate (Brushite)	$CaHPO_42H_2O$	1.0
Calcium pyrophosphate dihydrate	$Ca_2P_2O_72H_2O$	1.0
Calcium oxalate	$CaC_2O_4\text{-}H_2O$	∞

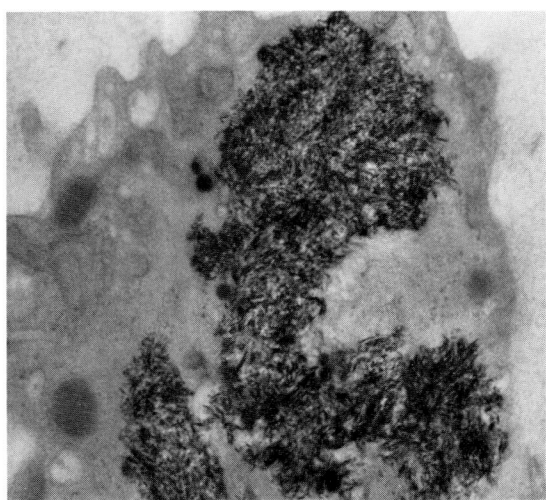

Fig. 95–1.   Aggregate of needle-shaped crystals within a synovial fibrocyte. No limiting membrane can be identified ($\times$ 43,800). (From Garancis, J.C., et al.[36])

Table 95–2.   Protocol for (^{14}C) Diphosphonate (EHDP) Binding

1. Collect 1–10 ml joint fluid in plastic tube containing 250 μl heparin and 1 mg hyaluronidase (300–800 units/mg). Incubate 30 min at room temperature. Transfer to plastic centrifuge tube with pipette. Record volume transferred.
2. Centrifuge 27,000 $\times$ g/20 min. Discard supernatant; resuspend in same volume of 0.1M tris Cl buffer pH 8.0.
3. Store at $-20°$ or proceed with assay.
4. Thaw and centrifuge 27,000 $\times$ g/20 min, resuspend in 0.5 ml tris Cl containing trypsin (180–220 units/ml), incubate 37° $\times$ 30 min. This step permits scanning EM and x-ray energy dispersive analysis to be performed on the pellet.
5. Centrifuge at 37,000 $\times$ g/20 min, discard supernatant, and resuspend in 1 ml of 20-mM phosphate buffer in normal saline containing 2 $\times$ 10^{-3}μCi (^{14}C) EHDP.
6. Rotate tube in roller drum $\times$ 2 h, remove two 100-μl aliquots before and after centrifugation at 37,000 $\times$ g/20 min.
7. Count (^{14}C) in liquid scintillation spectrophotometer.
8. Calculate % binding of radionuclide. This can be related to a standard curve relating binding to various concentrations of a hydroxyapatite standard to express results in μg/ml.

$$\frac{\text{Initial CPM} - \text{post centrifuge CPM}}{\text{Initial CPM}} \times 100 = \% \text{ bound}$$

radiographic grade of osteoarthritis present[45,74] (Fig. 95–2). Synovial fluid pellets that bound EHDP were examined routinely by SEM. Microspheroidal aggregates approximately 1 to 19 μm in diameter were generally found (Fig. 95–3,*A*). These aggregates were then further characterized by x-ray energy dispersive analysis.[42] The spectrum is analyzed for calcium and phosphorus, and the relative molar amounts of each element are calculated using an on-line computer (Fig. 95–3,*B*). Schumacher has suggested routine use of TEM[12] which, while not quantitative, has the advantage of better definition of crystal morphology and location (e.g., in cells).

X-ray diffraction of BCP mineral by the powder method is relatively insensitive. Such small, poorly crystallized material yields broad diffraction minima that cannot differentiate between closely related calcium phosphate compounds. Electron diffraction, high-resolution TEM, and FTIR spectrophotometry are useful research tools, but are

not practical for everyday clinical use. A thick section technique for BCP crystal deposition in tissues that prevents dislodgement of crystals by the microtome has been described.[22]

Direct chemical analysis for calcium and phosphorus of several pellets from joint fluids that bound (^{14}C) EHDP showed levels of 12 to 45 μg BCP mineral per ml.[42]

DISEASES

Several articular and periarticular conditions associated with BCP crystals have been described (Table 95–3). Calcific tendonitis and calcific bursitis are discussed in Chapters 77 and 85, and calcinosis in Chapter 66. Calcific periarthritis has long

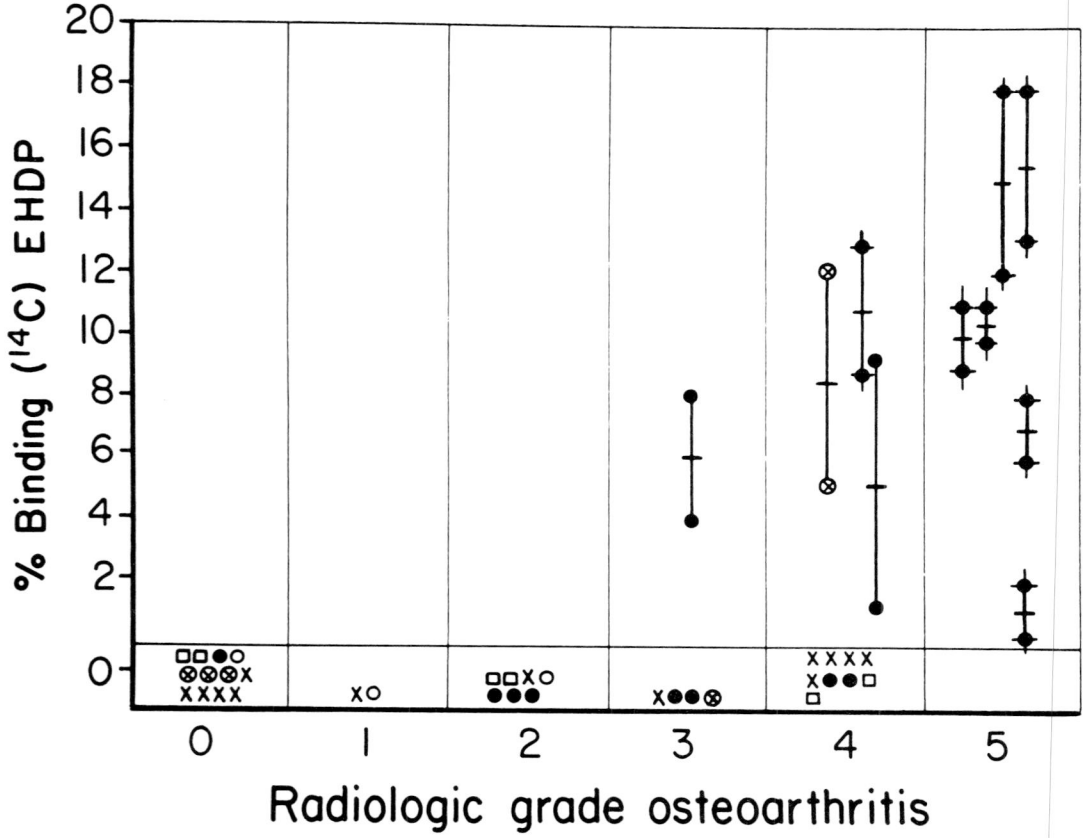

Fig. 95–2. Fluids that bound (^{14}C) EHDP generally were obtained from joints with advanced degenerative changes (radiologic grades 4 and 5). □ = internal derangement of knee; ● = osteoarthritis; ● = osteoarthritis with few CPPD crystals in fluid; × = inflammatory arthritis with WBC concentration >3,000 cmm; ⊗ = inflammatory arthritis with WBC concentration <3,000 cmm; ○ = miscellaneous arthritis. Positive results are shown in duplicate. (From Halverson, P.B., and McCarty, D.J.[45])

been recognized, but acute and chronic synovitis associated with intra-articular BCP crystal deposition are recent discoveries. The so-called secondary BCP arthropathies are known to predispose to articular and/or periarticular BCP crystal deposition.

Rotator Cuff Calcifications

In the shoulder, the location of rotator cuff calcifications has been related to etiopathogenesis, natural history, and prognosis.[93] Sarkar and Uhthoff found that calcifications at the tidemark of the rotator cuff insertion into the greater tuberosity of the humerus represented degenerative enthesopathy with *secondary calcifications*. These and the secondary calcification of the torn ends of a rotator cuff are irreversible.[84] On the other hand, *"primary" calcification* in the rotator cuff, approximately 1.5 cm away from the tidemark in "Codman's critical area,"[20] occurred in metaplastic fibrocartilage. These deposits were associated with

matrix vesicles and with crystal phagocytosis by macrophages and giant cells. The natural history of such deposits is resorption. Scalloping of the fluffy radiodense deposits on roentgenograms represents the radiologic correlate of cellular resorption of mineral.[64] Others have not found chondroid metaplasia or matrix vesicles in calcific tenosynovitis, but found instead psammoma bodies and calcification within necrotic cells.[40]

Ali has presented electron microscopic evidence for pericellular matrix vesicles in normal articular cartilage, which he regards as a latent growth plate.[2] Vesicles were present at all levels of the cartilage, but were most numerous near the tidemark adjoining the subchondral bone. Microcrystals within mineral nodules (0.6 μm in diameter) were noted in various stages of formation. Both vesicles and mineral were greatly increased in osteoarthritic cartilage; quantitatively, this increase was reflected by a marked increase (up to 30-fold)

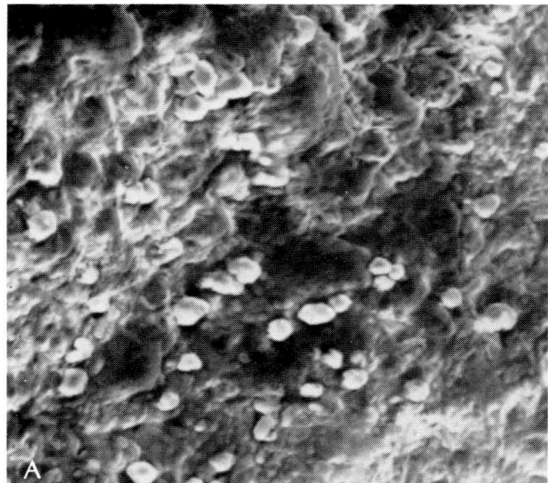

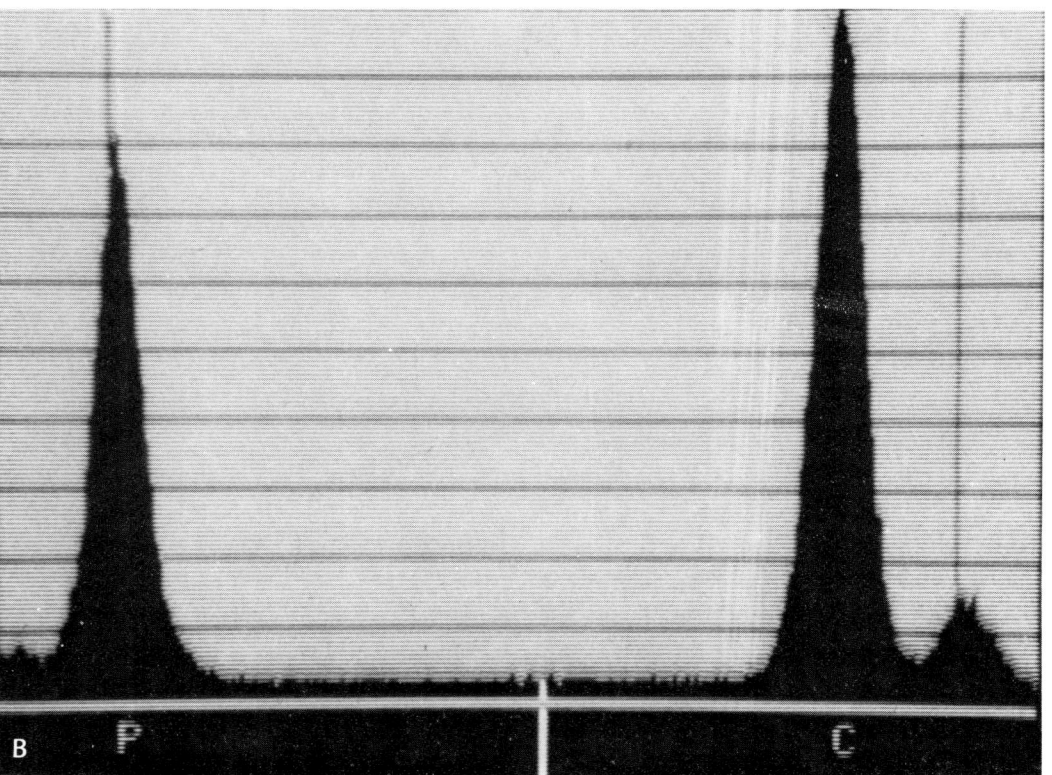

Fig. 95–3. *A*, Scanning electron micrograph of synovial fluid sediment showing typical microspheroidal crystal aggregates (× 525). (From Halverson, P.B., et al.[42]) *B*, Spectrograph from x-ray energy dispersive analysis showing peaks for phosphorus and calcium.

> *Calcific Periarthritis*
> Unifocal[20,72,83,91]
> Multifocal[20,58,75,97]
> Familial[4,11,46,55,88,97]
> *Calcific Tendonitis and Bursitis*[20,35a,64,72,83,92,93]
> *Intra-articular BCP Arthropathies*
> Acute (gout-like) attacks[34,87]
> Milwaukee shoulder/knee syndrome[24,41,57,69,71]
> (Large joint lysis; cuff tear arthropathy)
> Erosive polyarticular disease[86]
> Mixed crystal deposition disease (BCP + CPPD[26,29,41,45])
> *Secondary BCP Crystal Arthropathies/Periarthropathies**
> Chronic renal failure†[9,39,52,65,67]
> ''Collagen'' diseases (calcinosis)[8,78,80]
> Sequel to severe neurologic injury[38,81,96]
> Post local corticosteroid injection[49,56]
> Other (see also Table 66–4)[47,50]
> *Tumoral Calcinosis*
> Hyperphosphatemic[51,54,76]
> Nonhyperphosphatemic[63]

*Mineral deposits may also occur in fibrous tissue remote from joints in these conditions.

†Calcium oxalate[46a] or aluminum salts[70] also may occur in joints in renal failure. Whitlockite ($Ca_3(PO_4)_2$) may deposit in lungs.[21]

in alkaline phosphatase activity in osteoarthritic cartilage. Ali hypothesized that such abnormal mineralization may confer deleterious biomechanical properties to cartilage, and if shed into the synovial fluid, may initiate attacks of joint inflammation. Further studies have shown three distinct types of calcification in osteoarthritic cartilage.[3] In addition to the mineral nodules just discussed, dense cuboidal-shaped crystals resembling Whitlockite morphologically, but with a molar Ca/P of 1.72, were found in pericellular matrix about the surface chondrocytes. Fine needle-shaped crystal clusters were observed on the cartilage surface in the acellular amorphous zone (lamina splendens). These clusters had a molar Ca/P of 1.7, and resembled the crystals found in synovial fluid. Matrix vesicles and crystals were seen in rabbit fibrocartilage that had formed from autologous grafts of synovial tissue implanted into defects produced surgically in hyaline cartilage, but not in sham-operated joints.[90]

A systematic study of articular cartilage from 28 patients with advanced osteoarthritis showed superficial HA-type needle-shaped crystals in 56%; calcified deposits were found in 36% in deeper repair-type fibrocartilage, and calcium pyrophosphate deposition (CPPD) crystals were seen in 11% of cases.[28] Overall, 75% of the cartilages had microcrystalline deposits of some kind. Synovium from the same joints all showed a patchy lining cell hyperplasia and giant cells,

whether or not calcific deposits were present in the area.[28] Calcific deposits were present in 70% of the specimens. All were of the HA type, but four specimens also showed CPPD deposits. The pathologic prevalence of 70 to 75% synovial calcification is in accord with a radiologic survey of osteoarthritic knee joints, wherein 72% showed peri- or intra-articular calcification.[48]

Calcific Periarthritis

Periarticular calcifications are found most commonly around the shoulder, but have been described near many other joints. Calcific scapulohumeral periarthritis was first described in 1870.[83] Roentgenographic demonstration of periarticular shoulder calcifications was first accomplished in 1907,[72] and a classic review of 329 cases of peritendinitis calcarea was presented in 1938.[83] An excellent study disclosed calcium deposits in one or both shoulders of 138 of 5,061 employees of a life insurance company.[7a] More than 70% of patients were under age 40 and many remained asymptomatic, although serial study showed that large deposits usually caused acute painful inflammation eventually. Spontaneous resorption of some deposits, especially the smaller ones, occurred. Nearly half of these subjects had bilateral deposits.

Most cases of acute calcific periarthritis consist of a single attack in a single joint, frequently with localized warmth, erythema, swelling, and pain lasting up to a few weeks. The roentgenographic finding of periarticular calcification is useful as a confirmatory diagnostic aid (see Fig. 85–9).

Recurrent attacks of calcific periarthritis occurring at multiple sites suggest a more generalized condition rather than a chance localized process with resultant calcification.[58,75,97]

Several reports describe familial occurrences of calcific arthritis and periarthritis.[4,11,46,55,88,97] One of three studies that included HLA typing[4,46,55] found a correlation with the haplotype A2, BW35 in patients with two or more deposits.[4]

Episodic attacks of calcific periarthritis have been treated successfully with a variety of nonsteroidal anti-inflammatory drugs and colchicine.[92] Needle aspiration of the paste-like calcific deposits with or without irrigation may be helpful.[7a,20,58] Mechanical disruption and dispersion of the deposits may speed their removal by phagocytosis as outlined by Sarkar and Uhthoff.[84,93] Surgical removal of large calcific deposits usually provides permanent symptomatic relief.[7a] Codman considered this procedure to be essential for symptomatic relief.[20]

BCP Crystal-Related Arthritis

BCP is now recognized as another class of crystals that may be found within joints. Schumacher and associates have described both acute and chronic forms of arthritis.[87] Acute attacks of arthritis in relatively young persons occurred with extreme pain, swelling, and erythema closely resembling gout. Crystals resembling HA were found by transmission electron microscopy in synovial fluid pellets with markedly elevated synovial fluid leukocyte counts and normal joint roentgenograms. The phlogistic potential of HA crystals was also demonstrated by injection into rabbit joints. Individuals with chronic degenerative arthropathy and three patients with erosive arthritis were also described.[86] Recurrent episodes of pain and swelling were associated with gradual erosion and destructive changes in metacarpophalangeal, proximal interphalangeal, and wrist joints. One of the three patients had chronic renal failure. Although all had radiographic evidence of periarticular calcific deposits, no synovial fluid was obtained; therefore, it remains unclear whether or not intrasynovial crystals were present.

In 1976, Dieppe et al. reported that synovial fluid from five patients with clinical evidence of osteoarthritis contained 0.15- to 0.8-µm crystals, which by x-ray energy dispersive analysis were compatible with apatite.[27] Three of these patients had acute inflammatory episodes accompanied by joint effusions, although subsequent analysis of a larger series showed no increase in synovial fluid leukocyte counts of osteoarthritic fluids with apatite crystals as compared to those that had none.[25] These data failed to support the authors' original hypothesis that these crystals were responsible for the intermittent inflammatory episodes of primary generalized osteoarthritis.

Milwaukee Shoulder/Knee Syndrome

Fifteen cases of a peculiar arthropathy, which we named "Milwaukee shoulder/knee syndrome," have been described.[41,57] Salient clinical, radiographic, and synovial fluid findings are listed in Table 95–4.

Clinical Features. The primary findings include female predominance, greater involvement of the dominant arm, glenohumeral joint degeneration, and gross loss of the rotator cuff. Seven patients also had knee involvement with similar synovial fluid findings and a radiographic appearance that differed from ordinary osteoarthritis. Other reports have described patients with similar features.[24,69,71] The average age of these patients was 72.5 years with a range of 54 to 90. Average duration of symptoms was 3.8 years, but the range was variable (1 to 10 years). Symptomatology was also variable. Three patients had asymptomatic shoulders, but most individuals experienced mild to moderate pain, especially after use. One patient

Table 95–4. Features of Milwaukee Shoulder/Knee Syndrome*

Clinical Features
   Elderly, female predominance; M/F = 3/12; mean age 72 years (Range: 54–90)
   Dominant shoulder usually more affected but often bilateral
   Symptoms variable—asymptomatic to severe pain at rest; mostly painful after use and at night. Glenohumeral joint stiffness or instability

Roentgenographic Features
   Glenohumeral joint degeneration, bony destruction of humeral head; small osteophytes
   Soft tissue calcifications (40%)
   Rotator cuff lysis by (1) arthrogram or (2) upward subluxation of the humeral head

Synovial Fluid
   Low leukocyte counts (nearly all)
   Basic calcium phosphate crystal aggregates (nearly all)
   Particulate collagens (all)
   Elevated collagenase (about 50%) and neutral protease activities

had bilateral severe pain at rest. Other symptoms included limitation of motion, stiffness, and pain at night. A history of direct trauma or excessive use of the shoulders was obtained in five. One patient, for example, had severe paraparesis from poliomyelitis and used her shoulders for weight-bearing when standing on crutches or transferring from a wheelchair. Another had a dysplastic left shoulder from birth. Others had fallen on the outstretched hand. All shoulders showed limitation of motion, sometimes with marked joint instability with crepitation and pain when the humerus was grated passively against the glenoid. Two male patients who had previous recurrent shoulder dislocations may have experienced "dislocation arthropathy of the shoulder."[82]

Aspiration of the affected shoulder joints routinely yielded 3 to 40 ml of synovial fluid that was frequently blood-tinged. Occasionally, hydrops of the shoulder yielding 130 ml or more of synovial fluid was encountered (Fig. 95–4). In one man, hydrops was associated with joint rupture and dissection of fluid onto the anterior chest wall.

Neer et al. have described the clinical and pathologic findings in 26 patients encountered over an 8-year period with "cuff-tear arthropathy" for whom they attempted surgical correction by total replacement arthroplasty.[69] Nearly as many cases were encountered where surgery was not performed during the same period. Twenty of these cases were women and all but six involved the dominant shoulder. Their average age was 69 with a range of 50 to 87 years. All but 3 of the 26 patients had some discomfort, with symptoms suggesting subacrom-

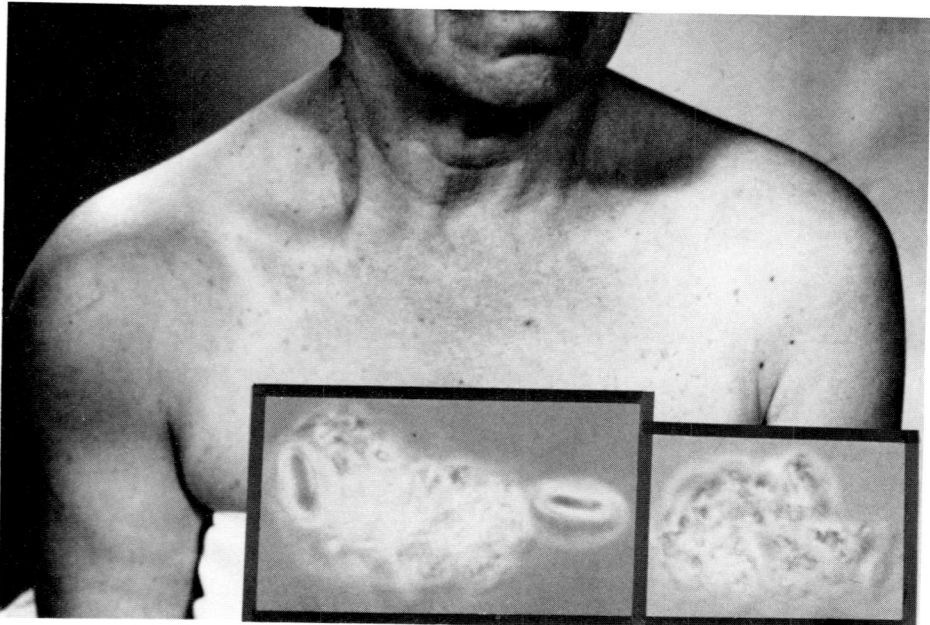

Fig. 95–4. Photograph of a 62-year-old woman with grotesque swelling of the right shoulder. Inserts show two crystal masses found in a wet preparation of fresh joint fluid. Note the erythrocytes for size comparison (phase contrast × 1,000). (From McCarty, D.J., et al.[57])

ial impingement in the contralateral shoulder, but only 5 showed the usual radiologic changes as described subsequently. Only 6 patients had a history of trauma, and none had been active at heavy labor. The symptoms in this group of individuals were nearly identical to those described by our patients. On examination, most patients had swollen shoulders due to synovial fluid accumulation. The fluid was often blood-streaked, and 5 patients had periarticular ecchymoses. The tendon of the long head of the biceps was either ruptured or dislocated in 21 patients, with visible retraction or dislocation of the muscle belly. The incongruity of the glenohumeral joint surfaces resulted in an even greater limitation of motion than usually seen with tears of the rotator cuff per se.

The syndrome of "apatite-associated destructive arthritis," described by Dieppe,[24] also seems identical. Eight of nine patients were female, with a mean age of 74 years (range 68 to 81). Affected joints included 3 shoulders, 6 knees, 6 hips, 2 elbows, and 2 ankles. Radiographic and synovial fluid findings, including the presence of "apatite" crystals, were remarkably similar to those described here.

An isolated case of a patient with shoulder involvement who previously had a total hip replacement for severe arthritis has been recorded.[71]

Roentgenographic Features. Roentgenographic study showed glenohumeral joint degen-

eration in 26 of 27 shoulders examined. Soft tissue calcifications were present in 39% of shoulders, three of which were bilateral. Upward subluxation of the humeral head or arthrographic evidence of rotator cuff defects was evident in 23 of 27 shoulders in our series (Figs. 95–5, 95–6). The distance from the superior rim of the humeral head to the acromion, measured on routine roentgenograms with the patient erect, was reduced to 2 mm or less in all but three patients in the surgical series.[69] Erosion of the coracoid process, of the undersurface of the anterior third of the acromion, and of the acromioclavicular joint was common (Figs. 95–7, 95–8); in many instances a rounding off of the greater tuberosity occurred with loss of the sulcus demarcating the anatomic neck. Erosions, subchondral cysts, and roughening of the bony cortex over the greater tuberosity at the site of the insertion of the rotator cuff were also noted frequently.

Arthrograms or bursagrams were performed in all the patients in the surgical series.[69] Each showed a grossly defective rotator cuff with communication between the glenohumeral and acromioclavicular joints in 10 instances. Arthrograms of the contralateral shoulder were performed in 11 of the 26 patients, and all showed a complete tear of the rotator cuff, although only 5 had typical radiographic changes in the glenohumeral joint. Pseudoarthrosis formation between the humeral head and the acromion and clavicle was common (see

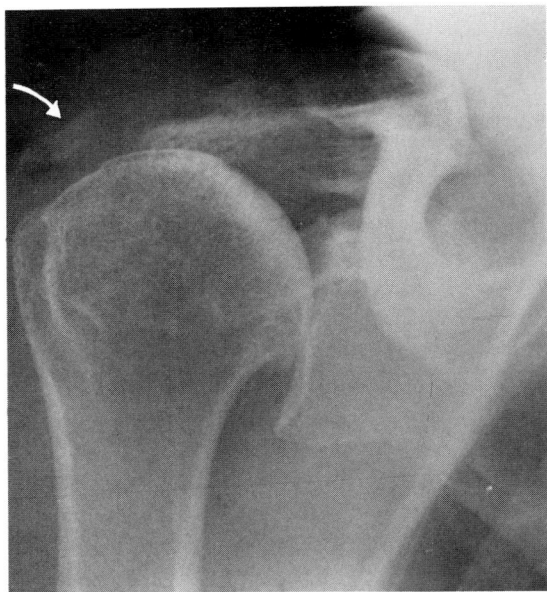

Fig. 95–5. Anteroposterior roentgenogram of the right shoulder showing soft tissue calcifications (arrow) and superior subluxation and sclerosis of the humeral head.

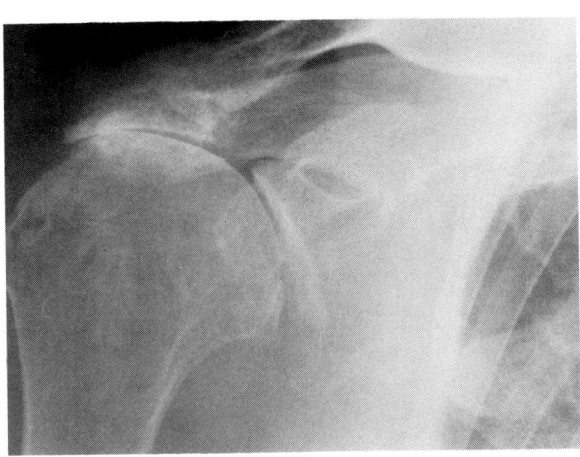

Fig. 95–7. Anteroposterior roentgenogram of the right shoulder in a patient showing more advanced changes. Superior displacement of the humeral head has resulted in a pseudoarticulation with acromion. Sclerosis, cystic changes, and irregularity of the humeral head are also present. (From McCarty, D.J., et al.[57])

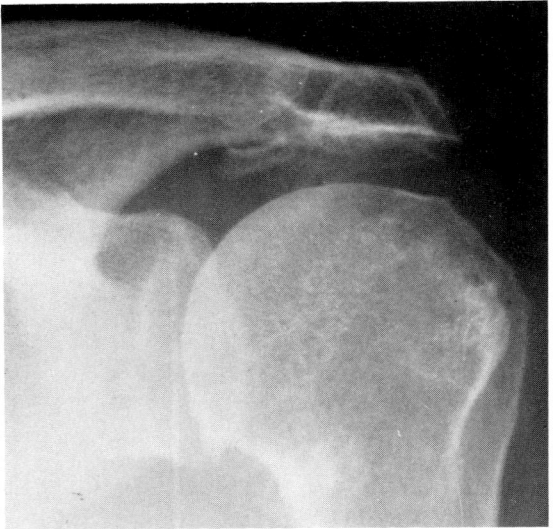

Fig. 95–6. Anteroposterior roentgenogram of an asymptomatic left shoulder in a patient whose dominant right shoulder was severely involved. Calcifications are present in the rotator cuff, and cystic changes are noted at the site of insertion of the rotator cuff on the greater tuberosity of the humerus. An arthrogram showed complete rupture of the rotator cuff. This appearance is characteristic before bony collapse of the articulating surface of the humeral head occurs.

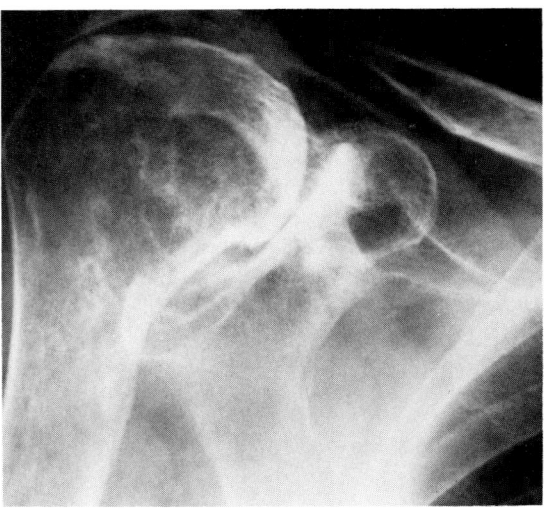

Fig. 95–8. Anteroposterior roentgenogram of the right shoulder of another patient showing superior displacement of the humeral head and pseudoarticulations with the clavicle, acromion, and coracoid process. The humeral head is partly collapsed with eburnation only in its inferomedial articulating surface. Note the absence of osteophytes.

Fig. 95–7). Bony destruction of the humeral head was also common, whereas osteophyte formation was usually modest.[57,69] An area of collapse of the proximal aspect of the humeral articular surface was present in all patients in the series of Neer et al.[69] and was a requirement for the diagnosis of cuff tear arthropathy. We agree with Neer that these changes are not those of osteoarthritis of the shoulder.

Synovial Fluid Features. Synovial fluid leukocyte counts were usually less than 1,000 per cmm (48 of 50 fluids). The fluids were assayed for BCP crystals by (^{14}C) diphosphonate binding as described previously; 47 of 50 fluids showed significant binding.[41] CPPD crystals were also seen in four fluids. Crystal concentrations estimated serially in fluids from two shoulders were remarkably constant for nearly a year, suggesting that they were under homeostatic control. Scanning electron microscopy detected microspheroidal aggregates in 20 of 31 fluids that bound (^{14}C) diphosphonate.

The molar Ca/P of these aggregates ranged from 1.4 to 1.7 by x-ray energy dispersive analysis.[41]

Activated collagenase was found in 16 of 32 fluid samples examined. Although the total protein concentration in these fluids was 3 to 4 g/dl, most was albumin. Low levels of alpha 2 macroglobulin (a natural inhibitor of collagenase) and alpha 1 antitrypsin were found. Synovial fluids also demonstrated type I, II, and III particulate collagens and elevated neutral protease activities.[42] FTIR analyses also showed collagen as a constant feature in these joint fluid pellets.[59]

Knee Involvement. Of our first 15 patients with Milwaukee shoulder syndrome, 7 also had knee involvement, and a patient with isolated knee involvement was included in our initial report.[42] Symptoms included pain during and after ambulation. Medial, or more often lateral, instability was present. CPPD crystal deposition was detected either in synovial fluid or by radiographs in five patients. Roentgenographic study showed degen-

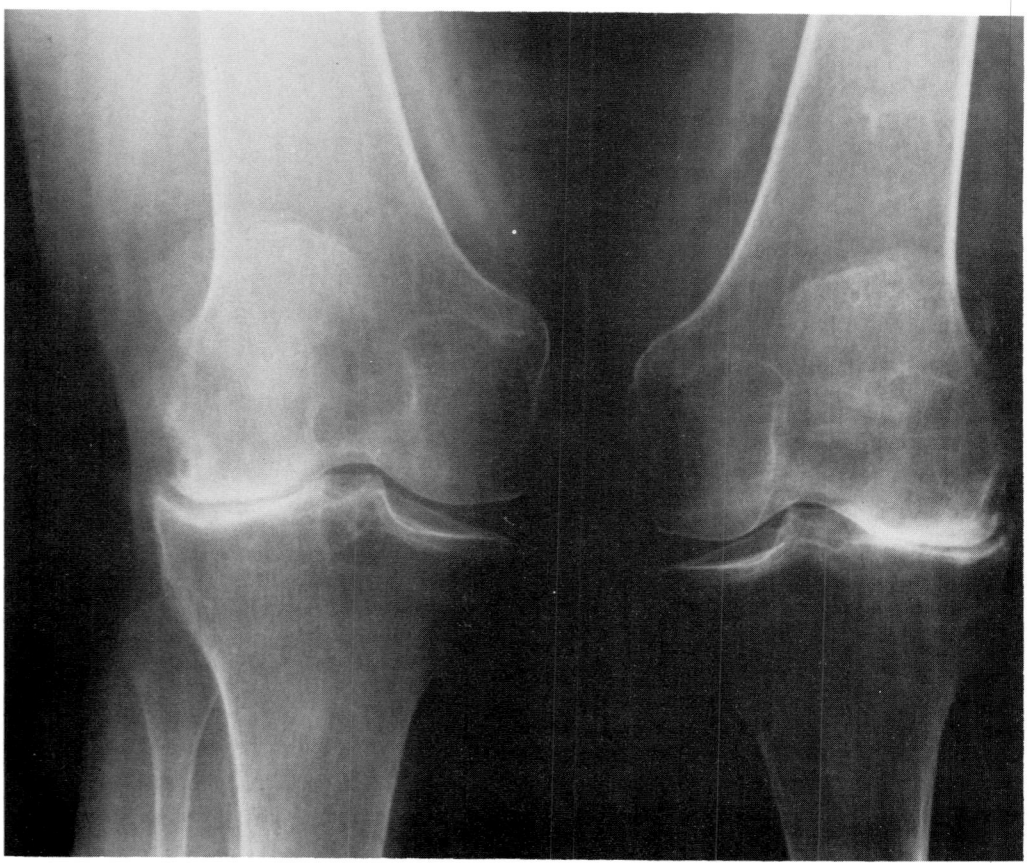

Fig. 95–9. Standing anteroposterior roentgenogram of the knees from a patient with Milwaukee shoulder syndrome showing lateral tibiofemoral compartment narrowing and incongruity with subchondral bony sclerosis, but minimal osteophyte formation.

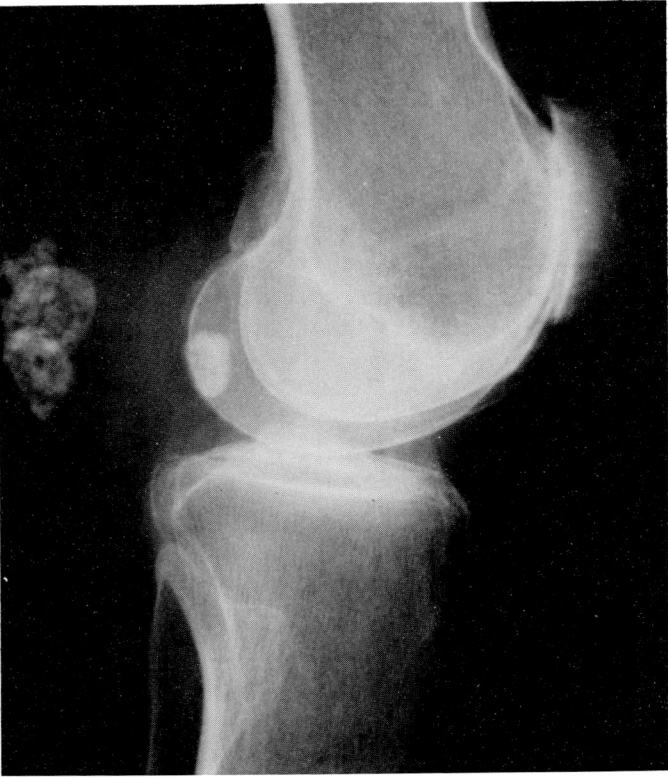

Fig. 95–10. Lateral roentgenogram of the right knee of another patient showing isolated patellofemoral osteoarthritis (patella "wrapped around" the femur), femoral cortical defect, and chondrocalcinosis of the femoral articular cartilage. Osteochondromata can be seen in the posterior joint recess.

erative changes, which again were not typical of primary osteoarthritis. Lateral tibiofemoral and patellofemoral compartmental narrowing (Figs. 95–9, 95–10), such as is seen in CPPD disease (see Chap. 94), was prevalent. One patient each had osteochondromatosis and lateral femoral condylar osteonecrosis, both of which have also been associated with CPPD deposition. The patients with the syndrome of "apatite-associated large joint lysis" described by Dieppe also showed primarily hip and knee involvement.[24]

Other Joint Involvement. Two of our patients had severe degenerative arthritis of the hips, but because they already had prostheses, there was no fluid to study. Whether a similar process was involved in pathogenesis is unclear. We have also studied a man with bilateral elbow joint degeneration and synovial fluid findings consistent with those of "Milwaukee shoulder." As already discussed, the erosive arthropathy of wrists and small hand joints associated with periarticular calcific deposits described by Schumacher et al.[86] may share some of these features, although again, no fluid could be obtained for analysis.

Table 95–5.   Microscopic Features of Synovial Membrane in Milwaukee Shoulder/Knee Syndrome

Villous hyperplasia
Focal synovial lining cell hyperplasia
BCP crystal deposition (extracellular, intracellular)*
Fibrin deposition
Giant cells
Fibrosis
Vascular congestion
No inflammatory cells

*the only specific feature

Pathology. Synovial biopsies obtained at the time of operation from the shoulders of four patients demonstrated increased numbers of villi, focal synovial lining cell hyperplasia, a few giant cells, fibrin, and BCP crystal deposits[44] (Fig. 95–11) (Table 95–5). Electron microscopy showed crystals being engulfed by synovial lining cells and histiocytes (Figs. 95–12, 95–13). Calcific deposits in synovial microvilli appeared to have access to the joint space through areas denuded of synovial lining cells (Fig. 95–14).

In the series of Neer et al., a large, complete

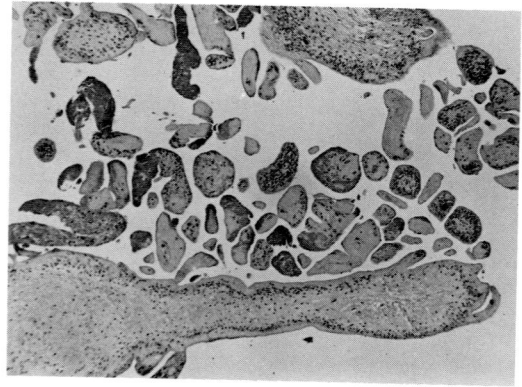

Fig. 95–11. Light micrograph of synovium showing many villi and focal synovial cell hyperplasia. In cross section, the branching villi appear as free bodies. Some villi are partially covered with or contain fibrin in various stages of organization (× 110).

cuff tear was found in each patient at operation.[69] The humeral head could be dislocated passively in 14 instances and was fixed in a dislocated position in the remaining 12 shoulders. The supraspinatus tendon was completely ruptured in all patients and the infraspinatus tendon in all but one instance. The teres minor and subscapularis tendons were usually involved, but some vestiges remained in all patients. The tendon of the long head of the biceps was ruptured, dislocated, or frayed in 18, 3, and 5 patients respectively. The subdeltoid bursa was thickened, forming a large loose pouch about the head of the biceps and contained variable amounts of often sanguineous synovial fluid. The

articular cartilage was pebblestone-like and the collapsed articular surface, the major point of contact with the acromion, was eburnated and denuded of cartilage with small marginal osteophytes. The remainder of the humeral head was covered with degenerated cartilage and fibrous tissue. The subchondral bone could be indented easily with a finger. The anterior acromial epiphysis had failed to fuse in three patients, which may have contributed to subacromial impingement.

Histologically, the atrophic articular cartilage of the humeral head was covered to a variable degree with a fibrous membrane (pannus). In these areas, the adjacent bone was osteoporotic and hypervascularized with attempts at repair at points of bony collapse. At points of contact between the humeral head and scapula, the cartilage was completely denuded and the bone was sclerotic. Fragments of articular cartilage were found in the subsynovium. These fragments resembled those found in neuropathic joints albeit less extensive.

Neer et al. point out that in glenohumeral osteoarthritis, the entire humeral head is sclerotic without large areas of cartilage atrophy and osteoporosis, and that it is enlarged by marginal osteophytes without bone atrophy and collapse.[69] The rotator cuff is nearly always intact.[68]

Overlap with CPPD Crystal Deposition. Several reports of "mixed crystal disease" describe the simultaneous occurrence of BCP and CPPD crystals.[26,29,41,45] No specific clinical syndrome appears to be associated with "mixed crystal disease," but it is intriguing that certain joints can generate both of these different crystal species.

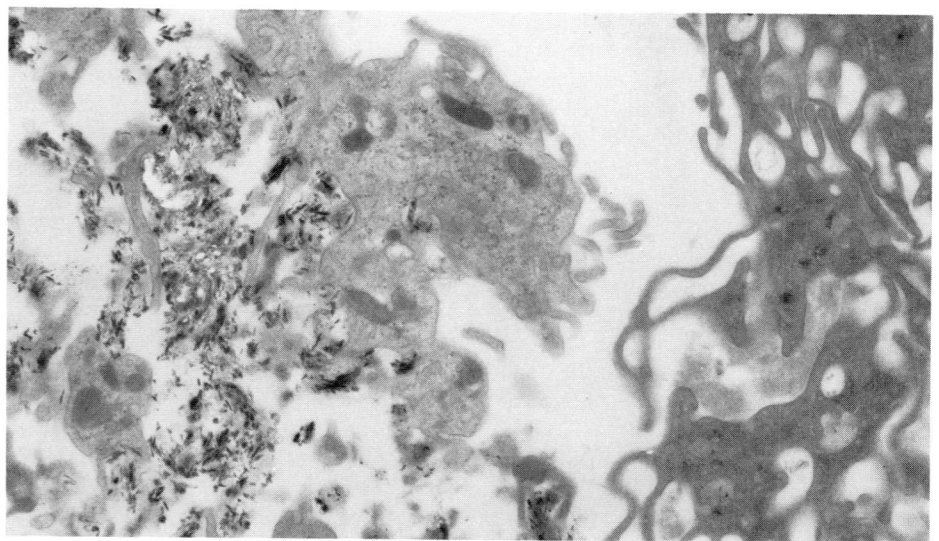

Fig. 95–12. Electron micrograph demonstrating hyperplastic synovial cells engulfing crystals, fibrin, and amorphous material. Extensive cytoplasmic processes form complex interdigitations with processes on adjacent cells (× 14,300).

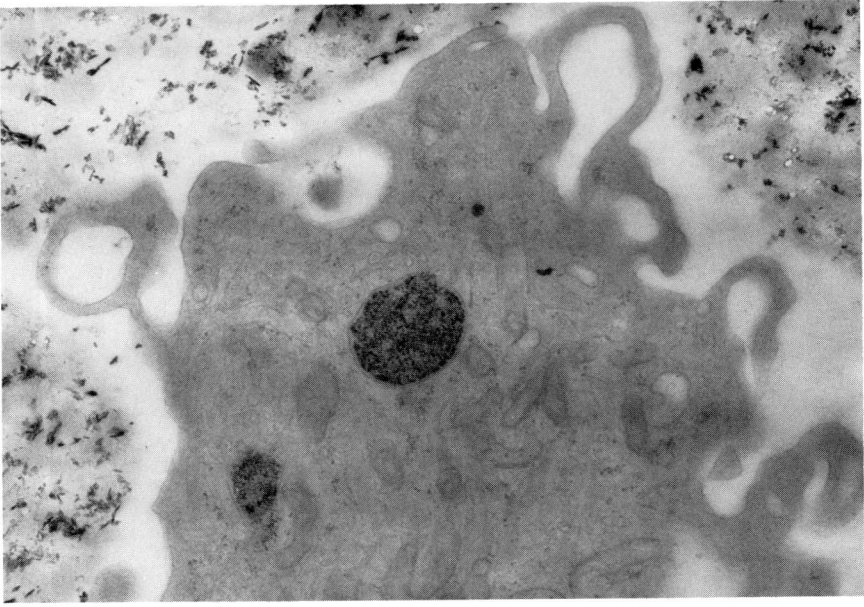

Fig. 95–13. Electron micrograph of a hyperplastic synovial cell. Crystals within phagolysosomes are bounded by distinct limiting membranes. Many extracellular crystals are also present (× 26,400).

Pathogenesis. An hypothesis has been formulated to link the synovial fluid findings to the genesis of this syndrome[42] (Fig. 95–15). BCP crystals, particulate collagens, and low leukocyte counts were associated with activated collagenase and neutral protease activities. Electron microscopy showed crystal aggregates enmeshed in synovial collagenous tissue and within synovial fixed macrophage-like cells. Werb and Reynolds demonstrated that particulates, such as latex beads, added to rabbit synovial cells in culture, are phagocytosed and stimulate increased secretion of proteases, including collagenase.[94] This increased secretion continued relentlessly until the ingested particles were biodegraded, at which time it returned to baseline. Collagen also stimulated collagenase release from cultured human skin fibroblasts,[6] and synovial fluid "wear" particles released neutral proteases from cultured synovial cells.[31]

We postulated that we had discovered the in vivo equivalent of these experiments and that the activated proteases might be instrumental (1) in causing the joint destruction and (2) in releasing additional crystals and particulate collagens into the joint space. Such enzymatic "strip-mining" had

been envisioned previously for sodium urate and CPPD crystal release (see Chap. 93).

This hypothesis was tested by adding natural or synthetic BCP, CPPD, and other crystals to cultured human or canine synovial cells.[13] Neutral protease and collagenase secretion was augmented in a dose-related fashion approximately 5 to 8 times over control cultures incubated without crystals. Chondrocytes in primary culture behaved similarly.[14] As crystals have been described within human chondrocytes,[7,66] it is possible that autolysis of cartilage may occur without crystals first shedding into synovial fluid. Moreover, partially purified mammalian collagenase released BCP crystal microspheroidal aggregates from calcified synovial tissue in vitro.[43] The mean diameter and size ranges of the released aggregates were virtually identical to those observed in synovial fluids obtained from the same patient. Fluid obtained several weeks after synovectomy of the affected shoulder in this patient showed no mineral by (^{14}C) EHDP binding and greatly reduced protease activities.[42] Although degenerating articular cartilage can form mineral as discussed previously, there is little doubt about the synovial origin of the crystals in this patient, who

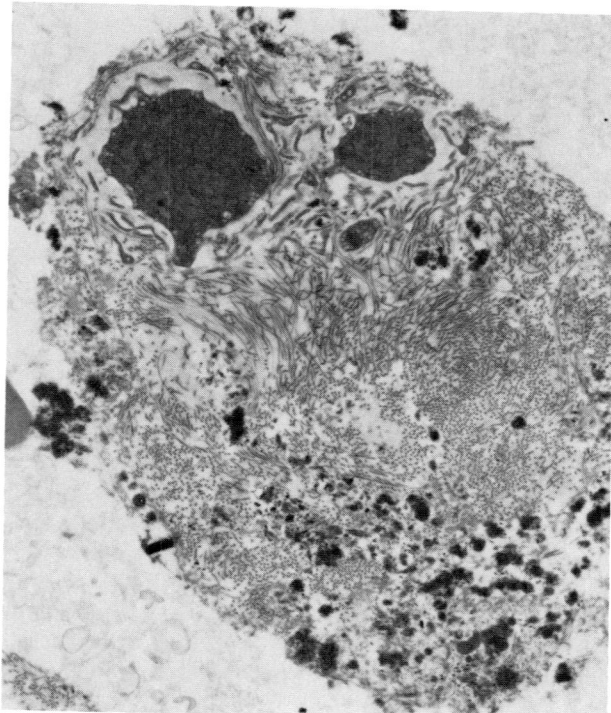

Fig. 95–14. Electron micrograph showing a small villus in cross section. Synovial lining cells are absent. Crystal microaggregates are seen dispersed among collagen fibers, lying free on the surface and in the synovial space. Several fibrocytes are present (× 6,400). (From Garancis, J.C., et al.[36])

PATHOGENESIS OF MILWAUKEE SHOULDER/KNEE SYNDROME

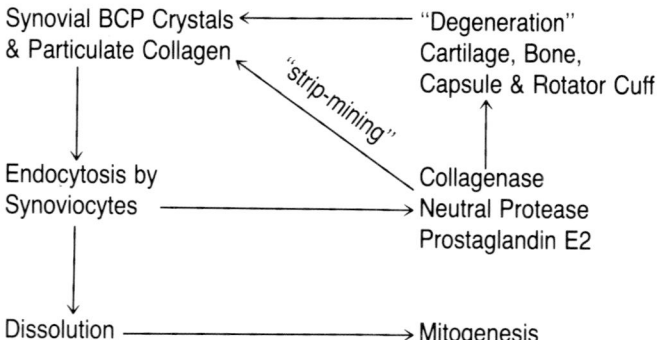

Fig. 95–15. Hypothetical schema relating the various features of Milwaukee shoulder/knee syndrome. Mechanical factors also must contribute to the pathogenesis of joint destruction.

had synovial chondromatosis (chondrometaplasia of subsynovial fibroblasts).

In addition to the stimulation of relentless enzyme secretion, BCP or CPPD crystal endocytosis was associated with a massive genesis of prostaglandins, especially PGE_2.[13,14] All PGE_2 release occurred in the first few hours after crystals were added to the cells. Both PGE_2 release and collagenase release have been found after exposure of macrophages or synovial cells to sodium urate crystals and have been related to the hard tissue destruction in gout as discussed in detail in Chapter 93. CPPD crystal-stimulated prostaglandin and protease release may account for the destructive arthropathies associated with these crystals. PGE_2 was found in joint fluid from our patients,[42] and was isolated from the periarticular calcium phosphate deposits from a patient with phalangeal osteolysis.[10]

This hypothesis is consistent with the concept of "crystal traffic" derived from studies of the fate of radiolabeled CPPD or BCP crystals injected intrasynovially. One-half of a dose of CPPD crystals was cleared from human joints in 30 to 90 days and from rabbit joints in 16 to 20 days.[61,62] Clearance rates were inversely proportional to crystal size. Injected crystals were phagocytosed by synovial cells where virtually all dissolution appeared to take place. This phenomenon was evidenced by localization of all nuclide in synovial tissue, the finding of all crystals inside cells by electron microscopy, the lack of effect on clearance rate of extracellular magnesium depletion by dietary deprivation, the failure of joint lavage to remove significant radionuclide, and reduction of clearance rate by 65% in the presence of synovial cell hemosiderosis induced by injection of autologous blood.[60] Both CPPD crystals and hemosiderin were shown in the same cells by transmission electron microscopy and x-ray energy dispersive analysis. ^{85}Sr-labeled BCP crystals were cleared from rabbit joints with a half-time of about 6 days, about 3 times faster than for CPPD crystals.[73]

The focal cell hyperplasia found in the four synovial membranes we examined[44] was described by Doyle as a constant feature of synovial membranes containing calcium crystals.[28] This finding might be related to their mitogenic properties. BCP, CPPD, calcium urate, calcium diphosphonate, and calcium carbonate, but not crystals or particulates not containing calcium (such as sodium urate, diamond, silicon dioxide, or latex beads) were capable of substituting for serum growth factors in certain cell systems.[15-19] Calcium-containing crystals appear to act as a "competence" factor as they can substitute for growth factors found in serum which are mostly derived from platelets and, like these factors, calcium-containing crystals require a progression factor, such as somatomedin C, for full expression of mitogenic potency.[16] (^{45}Ca) BCP crystals added to cultured synovial cells, skin fibroblasts, or peripheral blood monocytes were phagocytosed and degraded, probably by the ATPase-driven lysosomal proton pump.[32,33] Weak bases, such as chloroquine or $NH_4{}^+$, inhibited BCP crystal solubilization by all three cell types in a dose-dependent fashion.[15] Calcium crystal-induced mitogenesis was also reduced in a parallel dose-dependent fashion by these inhibitors, but mitosis stimulated by serum was unaffected.[17] These data are consistent with the concept that intracellular crystal dissolution is associated with a rise in intracellular calcium, a known stimulus to cell division.

In contrast to these ideas, Neer et al. favor a pathogenesis based on disuse osteoporosis and mechanical instability.[69] The greater severity of the clinical symptoms, radiologic evidence of destruction, the greater joint fluid levels of crystals and enzymes in the shoulder on the dominant side, and the frequent history of increased joint use or trauma support a pathogenetic role of joint movement. But the finding of destructive arthropathies of the knee and possibly other joints in the same patients suggests that other factors are also involved. We agree that biomechanical factors probably play a role in the pathogenetic scheme outlined in Figure 95–15.

Treatment. The treatment of Milwaukee shoulder syndrome is generally unsatisfactory. A conservative approach including prescription of nonsteroidal anti-inflammatory drugs, repeated shoulder aspirations, and decreased shoulder use have sometimes controlled symptoms satisfactorily. Implantation of a subacromial spacer that depresses the humeral head into the glenoid fossa has been performed in two patients resulting in improved motion and decreased pain. Neer et al. suggest a resurfacing total shoulder joint replacement using a nonconstrained prosthesis with rotator cuff reconstruction when the full syndrome is present.[69] They admit that this procedure is difficult and that treatment goals must be limited. They envision three problems: (1) massive rotator cuff loss with instability, (2) painful incongruity of the glenohumeral joint, and (3) painful subacromial impingement. Treatment of the condition at the stage of "precollapse" of the humeral head (radiologic normal bony contour) is by anterior acromioplasty and repair of the rotator cuff. If collapse has occurred, they favor arthroplasty, often using oversized, still experimental, glenoid components for greater stability. Despite residual problems, all but one patient thought that arthroplasty was helpful. Radical acromionectomy had been performed in five patients by other surgeons and had increased the disability in all.

At the time of clinical diagnosis of our patients, advanced destructive changes were usually present, and in three shoulders these changes were asymptomatic. Thus, there is no way to identify persons at risk for this condition. Novel attempts to control the disease with inhibitors of calcification or collagenase inhibitors should probably be directed at the generally less involved nondominant shoulder in patients with established disease on the dominant side.

Secondary BCP Arthropathies. Several disease states, including chronic renal failure, the "collagen" diseases, and neurologic injury, have been associated with calcifications that may occur in almost any tissue. In these conditions, BCP crystals have been found in periarticular soft tissues, in bursae, and within joints and are often associated with rheumatic symptoms. For a more complete listing of conditions associated with calcinosis, see Table 66–4.

Caner and Decker first described periarthritis occurring in hemodialysis patients.[9] Metastatic soft tissue calcifications occur frequently in uremic patients with high calcium × phosphorus products.[52] This phenomenon has been described as a form of calciphylaxis in humans.[37] Several authors have suggested that recurrences of this form of calcific periarthritis could be prevented by control of serum phosphorus levels.[9,65,67] Most of the symptomatic patients appear to have periarthritis or peritendonitis. In cases where synovial fluid was available, leukocytosis was not present. BCP crystals were not specifically sought. Good et al. described three cases of "dialysis shoulder" in which synovial leukocytosis was present and the joints were acutely inflamed.[39] Intra-articular BCP crystals were identified in two instances.

Soft tissue calcifications involving the fibrous tissue in skin or muscle occur in the "collagen" diseases. Rare cases of intra-articular calcification, one with a chalky joint effusion, have been reported in scleroderma.[8,80] Another patient with an "overlap" collagen-vascular disease developed periarticular calcifications in multiple sites.[78]

Heterotopic ossification mimicking arthritis has been described following neurologic catastrophes.[38,81] Such ossification tends to occur in periarticular tissues. The mechanisms are unknown. In some cases of heterotopic ossification, low synovial fluid leukocyte counts and high protein concentrations have been found.[96]

Several miscellaneous causes of BCP crystal deposition have been described. An unusual patient had Laennec's cirrhosis, hypertrophic osteoarthropathy, and synovial calcifications in the knees, which may have been related to vitamin D intoxication.[50] A patient with "draft dodger's knee" developed calcifications about the knee many years after self-injection of olive oil.[47]

The intra-articular injection of triamcinolone hexacetonide has been associated with the formation of periarticular calcifications along the injection tract which may become apparent months after the injection.[49,56] Such calcifications may gradually be resorbed over a period of months to years.

Tumoral Calcinosis. This condition, consisting of massive, expanding calcific deposits in or about one or more large joints, is rare in North America and Europe, but nonhyperphosphatemic cases are relatively common in Africa.[63] Phosphate deprivation constitutes definitive therapy for hyperphosphatemic cases which are often familial.[51,54,76]

Animal Models of BCP Crystal Deposition. Spontaneous periarticular calcinosis has been reported in dogs,[30,95] and may be familial.[95] Reginato et al. successfully calcified articular cartilage or synovium with vitamin D administration to rabbits.[79] These deposits were composed of BCP crystals identical to those found in the synovial fluid of patients.[59]

Novel Treatment. The identification of the calcium-binding amino acid GLA (gamma carboxyglutamic acid) in pathologic soft tissue calcification,[53,53a] provides a rationale for the use of warfarin therapy of these disorders. Synthesis of GLA-containing proteins, such as prothrombin, is vitamin K-dependent. Reports of success, however,[5a] must be viewed in the light of the natural tendency for spontaneous resorption of at least some of these deposits. Probenecid has been used successfully to treat patients with calcinosis, but the same caveat applies in the absence of suitable controls.[89]

UNANSWERED QUESTIONS

Many questions about BCP crystal arthropathies and periarthropathies remain to be answered. Such crystals have been described in the synovial fluids of patients with advanced rheumatoid arthritis.[77] Whether BCP crystals participate in the inflammation of rheumatoid arthritis and other diseases or merely represent an epiphenomenon is unknown.

Perhaps the greatest mystery is the incomplete understanding about mechanisms of pathologic calcification. Codman considered the formation of periarticular calcific deposits in the shoulder to be the result of necrosis,[20] but Uhthoff et al. were unable to detect histologic evidence of necrosis.[93] They hypothesized that hypoxia induces the tendon to transform into fibrocartilage. BCP crystals then form in matrix vesicles generated by metaplastic chondrocytes, subsequently coalescing into larger deposits.[85] Their data suggest that vascular invasion and resorption of the calcific deposits follow, leaving a reconstituted vascularized tendon.

Anderson has presented a unified concept of pathologic calcification encompassing both metastatic and dystrophic forms. Matrix vesicles or mitochondria may serve as repositories for calcium and, upon exposure to sufficient phosphate, mineralization begins.[5] The mechanism responsible for most pathologic calcifications that occur in the absence of hypercalcemia or hyperphosphatemia is unclear. Microcrystalline needles have been found in myelin bodies within degenerating fibrocytes in aging human[50a] and rat[66a] aorta. These crystals were presumed to originate in these cells, but the presence of calcifications on elastin or collagen fibers suggested that the crystals could have formed extracellularly with subsequent phagocytosis.

REFERENCES

1. Alfrey, A.C., et al.: Extraosseous calcification. Evidence for abnormal pyrophosphate metabolism in uremia. J. Clin. Invest., 57:692–699, 1976.
2. Ali, S.Y.: New knowledge of osteoarthritis. J. Clin. Pathol., 31:191–199, 1978.
3. Ali, S.Y., and Griffiths, S.: New types of calcium phosphate crystals in arthritic cartilage. Semin. Arthritis Rheum., 11:124–126, 1981.
4. Amor, B., et al.: Hydroxyapatite rheumatism and HLA markers. J. Rheumatol., 3:101–104, 1977.
5. Anderson, H.C.: Calcific diseases—a concept. Arch. Pathol. Lab. Med., 107:341–348, 1983.
5a. Berger, R.G., and Hadler, N.M.: Treatment of calcinosis universalis secondary to dermatomyositis or scleroderma with low dose warfarin. Arthritis Rheum., 26:S11, 1983.
6. Biswas, C., and Dayer, J.: Stimulation of collagenase production by collagen in mammalian cell cultures. Cell, 18:1035–1041, 1979.
7. Boivin, G., and Lagier, R.: An ultrastructural study of articular chondrocalcinosis in cases of knee osteoarthritis. Virchow's Arch. [A], 400:13–19, 1983.
7a. Bosworth, B.M.: Calcium deposits in the shoulder and subacromial bursitis. J.A.M.A., 116:2477–2482, 1941.
8. Brandt, K.D., and Krey, P.R.: Chalky joint effusion: The result of massive synovial deposition of calcium apatite in progressive systemic sclerosis. Arthritis Rheum., 20:792–796, 1977.
9. Caner, J.E.Z., and Decker, J.L.: Recurrent acute (?gouty) arthritis in chronic renal failure treated with periodic hemodialysis. Am. J. Med., 36:571–582, 1964.
10. Caniggia, A., et al.: Prostaglandin PGE$_2$: A possible mechanism for bone destruction in calcinosis circumscripta. Calif. Tissue Res., 25:53–57, 1978.
11. Cannon, R.B., and Schmid, F.R.: Calcific periarthritis involving multiple sites in identical twins. Arthritis Rheum., 16:393–395, 1973.
12. Cherian, P.V., and Schumacher, H.R.: Diagnostic potential of rapid electron microscopic analysis of joint effusions. Arthritis Rheum., 25:98–100, 1982.
13. Cheung, H.S., et al.: Release of collagenase, neutral protease and prostaglandins from cultured synovial cells by hydroxyapatite and calcium pyrophosphate dihydrate. Arthritis Rheum., 24:1338–1344, 1981.
14. Cheung, H.S., Halverson, P.B., and McCarty, D.J.: Phagocytosis of hydroxyapatite or calcium pyrophosphate dihydrate crystals by rabbit articular chondrocytes stimulates release of collagenase, neutral protease and prostaglandins E$_2$ and F$_2\alpha$. Proc. Soc. Exp. Biol. Med., 173:181–189, 1983.
15. Cheung, H.S., and McCarty, D.J.: Intracellular dissolution is essential for mitogenesis induced by crystals containing calcium (abstract). Arthritis Rheum., 27:549, 1984.
16. Cheung, H.S., and McCarty, D.J.: Biological effects of calcium containing crystals on synoviocytes. In Calcium in Biological Systems. Edited by R.P. Rubin, G. Weiss, and J.W. Putney. New York, Plenum Publishing Co. In press.
17. Cheung, H.S., and McCarty, D.J.: Calcium containing crystals can substitute for platelet derived growth factor (PDGF) in cell cultures. Exp. Cell. Res., in press, 1984.
18. Cheung, H.S., and McCarty, D.J.: Calcium containing crystals can substitute for platelet derived growth factor (PDGF) in cell cultures. Arthritis Rheum., 26:S60, 1983.
19. Cheung, H.S., Story, M.T., and McCarty, D.J.: Mitogenic effects of hydroxyapatite and calcium pyrophosphate on cultured mammalian cells. Arthritis Rheum., 27:668–674, 1984.
20. Codman, E.A.: The Shoulder. Boston, Thomas Todd, 1934.
21. Conger, J.D., et al.: Pulmonary calcification in chronic dialysis patients. Clinical and pathologic studies. Ann. Intern. Med., 83:330–336, 1975.
22. Crocker, P.R.: The identification of particulate matter in biological tissues and fluids. J. Pathol., 121:37–40, 1977.
23. Daculsi, G., Faure, G., and Kerebel, B.: Electron microscopy and microanalysis of a subcutaneous heterotopic calcification. Calcif. Tissue Int., 35:723–727, 1983.
24. Dieppe, P.: Apatite associated destructive arthritis. Brit. J. Rheumatol., 23:84–91, 1984.
25. Dieppe, P.A., et al.: Synovial fluid crystals. Q. J. Med., 192:533–553, 1979.
26. Dieppe, P.A., et al.: Mixed crystal deposition disease and osteoarthritis. Br. Med. J., 1:150, 1977.
27. Dieppe, P.A., et al.: Apatite deposition disease. Lancet, 1:266–269, 1976.
28. Doyle, D.V.: Tissue calcification and inflammation in osteoarthritis. J. Pathol., 136:199–216, 1982.
29. Doyle, D.V., et al.: Mixed crystal deposition in an osteoarthritic joint. J. Pathol., 123:1–5, 1977.
30. Ellison, G.W., and Norrdin, R.W.: Multicentric periarticular calcinosis in a pup. J. Am. Vet. Med. Assoc., 177:542–546, 1980.
31. Evans, C.H., Mears, D.C., and Cosgrove, J.R.: Release of neutral proteinases from mononuclear phagocytes and synovial cells in response to cartilaginous wear particles in vitro. Biochim. Biophys. Acta, 677:287–294, 1981.
32. Evans, R.W., Cheung, H.S., and McCarty, D.J.: Cultured canine synovial cells solubilize ^{45}Ca labeled HA crystals. Arthritis Rheum., 27:829–832, 1984.
33. Evans, R.W., Cheung, H.S., and McCarty, D.J.: Cultured human monocytes and fibroblasts solubilize hydroxyapatite crystals. Calcif. Tissue Int., 36:668–673, 1984.
34. Fam, A.G., et al.: Apatite-associated arthropathy: A clinical study of 14 cases and of 2 patients with calcific bursitis. J. Rheumatol., 6:461–471, 1979.
35. Faure, G., et al.: Apatites in heterotopic calcifications. Scan. Electron Microsc., 4:1624–1634, 1982.
35a. Faure, G., and Daculsi, G.: Calcified tendinitis: A review. Ann. Rheum. Dis., 42:50–53, 1983.
36. Garancis, J.C., et al.: Milwaukee shoulder: Association of microspheroids containing hydroxyapatite crystals, active collagenase and neutral protease with rotator cuff defects. III. Morphologic and biochemical studies of an excised synovium showing chondromatosis. Arthritis Rheum., 24:484–491, 1981.
37. Gipstein, R.M., et al.: Calciphylaxis in man. A syndrome of tissue necrosis and vascular calcification in 11 patients with chronic renal failure. Arch. Intern. Med., 126:1273–1280, 1976.
38. Goldberg, M.A., and Schumacher, H.R.: Heterotopic ossification mimicking acute arthritis after neurologic catastrophes. Arch. Intern. Med., 137:619–621, 1977.
39. Good, A.E., et al.: The dialysis shoulder. Arthritis Rheum., 25:S34, 1982.
40. Gravanis, M.G., and Gaffney, E.F.: Idiopathic calcifying tenosynovitis. Histopathologic features and possible pathogenesis. Am. J. Surg. Pathol., 7:359–361, 1983.

41. Halverson, P.B., et al.: The Milwaukee shoulder syndrome: Eleven additional cases with involvement of the knee in seven. Semin. Arthritis Rheum., *14*:36–44, 1984.

42. Halverson, P.B., et al.: Milwaukee shoulder: Association of microspheroids containing hydroxyapatite crystals, active collagenase and neutral protease with rotator cuff defects. II. Synovial fluid studies. Arthritis Rheum., *24*:474–483, 1981.

43. Halverson, P.B., Cheung, H.S., and McCarty, D.J.: Enzymatic release of microspheroids containing hydroxyapatite crystals from synovium and of calcium pyrophosphate dihydrate crystals from cartilage. Ann. Rheum. Dis., *41*:527–531, 1982.

44. Halverson, P.B., Garancis, J.C., and McCarty, D.J.: Histopathologic and ultrastructural studies of Milwaukee shoulder syndrome—a basic calcium phosphate crystal arthropathy. Ann. Rheum. Dis., *43*:734, 1984.

45. Halverson, P.B., and McCarty, D.J.: Identification of hydroxyapatite crystals in synovial fluid. Arthritis Rheum., *22*:389–395, 1979.

46. Hajirousson, V.J., and Webley, M.: Familial calcific periarthritis. Ann. Rheum. Dis., *42*:469–470, 1983.

46a. Hoffman, G., et al.: Calcium oxalate microcrystalline associated arthritis in end stage renal disease. Ann. Intern. Med., *97*:36–42, 1982.

47. Hood, R.W., and Insall, J.: Draft dodger's knee: Unusual pattern of calcification in the knee secondary to olive oil injection. A case report. Orthopedics, *4*:1241–1244, 1981.

48. Huskisson, E.C., et al.: Another look at osteoarthritis. Ann. Rheum. Dis., *38*:423–428, 1979.

49. Jalava, S., et al.: Periarticular calcification after intra-articular triamcinolone hexacetonide. Scand. J. Rheumatol., *9*:190–192, 1980.

50. Kieff, E.D., and McCarty, D.J.: Hypertrophic osteoarthropathy with arthritis and synovial calcification in a patient with alcoholic cirrhosis. Arthritis Rheum., *12*:261–271, 1969.

50a. Kim, K.M., and Huang, S.N.: Ultrastructural study of calcification of human aortic valve. Lab. Invest., *25*:357–366, 1971.

51. Kirk, T.S., and Simon, M.A.: Tumoral calcinosis: Report of a case with successful medical management. J. Bone Joint Surg., *63A*:1167–1169, 1981.

52. Kuzela, D.C., et al.: Soft tissue calcification in chronic dialysis patients. Am. J. Pathol., *86*:403–424, 1977.

53. Lian, J.B., et al.: Gamma-carboxyglutamate excretion and calcinosis in juvenile dermatomyositis. Arthritis Rheum., *25*:1094–1100, 1982.

53a. Lian, J.B., et al.: The presence of γ-carboxyglutamic acid in the proteins associated with ectopic calcification. Biochim. Biophys. Res. Com., *73*:349–355, 1976.

54. Lufkin, E.G., Kumar, R., and Heath, H.: Hyperphosphatemic tumoral calcinosis: Effects of phosphate depletion on vitamin D metabolism, and of acute hypocalcemia on parathyroid hormone secretion and action. J. Clin. Endocrinol. Metab., *56*:1319–1322, 1983.

55. Marcos, J.C., et al.: Idiopathic familial chondrocalcinosis due to apatite crystal deposition. Am. J. Med., *71*:557–564, 1981.

56. McCarty, D.J.: Treatment of rheumatoid joint inflammation with triamcinolone hexacetonide. Arthritis Rheum., *15*:118–129, 1972.

57. McCarty, D.J., et al.: Milwaukee shoulder: Association of microspheroids containing hydroxyapatite crystals, active collagenase and neutral protease with rotator cuff defects. I. Clinical aspects. Arthritis Rheum., *24*:464–473, 1981.

58. McCarty, D.J., and Gatter, R.A.: Recurrent acute inflammation associated with focal apatite crystal deposition. Arthritis Rheum., *9*:804–819, 1966.

59. McCarty, D.J., Lehr, J.R., and Halverson, P.B.: Crystal populations in human synovial fluid. Identification of apatite, octacalcium phosphate and tricalcium phosphate. Arthritis Rheum., *26*:247–251, 1983.

60. McCarty, D.J., Palmer, D.W., and Garancis, J.C.: Clearance of calcium pyrophosphate dihydrate crystals in vivo. III. Effects of synovial hemosiderosis. Arthritis Rheum., *24*:706–710, 1981.

61. McCarty, D.J., Palmer, D.W., and Halverson, P.B.: Clearance of calcium pyrophosphate dihydrate (CPPD) crystals in vivo. I. Studies using [169]Yb labelled triclinic crystals. Arthritis Rheum., *22*:718–727, 1979.

62. McCarty, D.J., Palmer, D.W., and James, C.: Clearance of calcium pyrophosphate dihydrate (CPPD) crystals in vivo II. Studies using triclinic crystals doubly labelled with [45]Ca and [85]Sr. Arthritis Rheum., *22*:1122–1131, 1979.

63. McKee, P.H., Liomba, N.G., and Hutt, M.S.R.: Tumoral calcinosis: A pathological study of fifty-six cases. Br. J. Dermatol., *107*:669–674, 1982.

64. McKendry, R.J.R., et al.: Calcifying tendinitis of the shoulder: Prognostic value of clinical, histologic and radiologic features in 57 surgically treated cases. J. Rheumatol., *9*:75–80, 1982.

65. Mirahmadi, K.S., Coburn, J.W., and Bluestone, R.: Calcific periarthritis and hemodialysis. J.A.M.A., *223*:548–549, 1973.

66. Mitrovic, D.R.: Pathology of articular deposition of calcium salts and their relationship to osteoarthritis. Ann. Rheum. Dis., *42*:519–526, 1983.

66a. Morgan, A.J.: Mineralized deposits in the thoracic aorta of aged rats: Ultrastructural and electron probe x-ray microanalysis study. J. Gerontol., *15*:563–573, 1980.

67. Moskowitz, R.W., et al.: Crystal induced inflammation associated with chronic renal failure treated with periodic hemodialysis. Am. J. Med., *47*:450–460, 1969.

68. Neer, C.S.: Replacement arthroplasty in glenohumeral osteoarthritis. J. Bone Joint. Surg., *56A*:1–13, 1974.

69. Neer, C.S., Craig, E.V., and Fukuda, H.: Cuff tear arthropathy. J. Bone Joint Surg., *69A*:1232–1244, 1983.

70. Netter, P., et al.: Inflammatory effect of aluminum phosphate. Ann. Rheum. Dis., *42*:114, 1983.

71. Newman, J.H., et al.: Milwaukee shoulder syndrome: A new crystal induced arthritis syndrome associated with hydroxyapatite crystals—a case report. Del. Med. J., *55*:167–169, 1983.

72. Painter, C.F.: Subdeltoid bursitis. Boston Med. Surg. J., *156*:345–349, 1907.

73. Palmer, D.W., and McCarty, D.J.: Clearance of [85]Sr labelled calcium phosphate (CP) crystals from normal rabbit joints. Arthritis Rheum., *27*:427–432, 1984.

74. Paul, H., Reginato, A.J., and Schumacher, H.R.: Alizarin red S staining as a screening test to detect calcium compounds in synovial fluid. Arthritis Rheum., *26*:191–200, 1983.

75. Pinals, R.S., and Short, C.L.: Calcific periarthritis involving multiple sites. Arthritis Rheum., *9*:566–574, 1966.

76. Prince, M.J., et al.: Hyperphosphatemic tumoral calcinosis. Association with elevation of serum 1,25 dihydroxycholecalciferol concentrations. Ann. Intern. Med., *96*:586–591, 1982.

77. Reginato, A.J., Paul, H., and Schumacher, H.R.: Hydroxyapatite (HOA) crystals in rheumatoid arthritis (RA) synovial fluid. Clin. Res., *30*:662A, 1982.

78. Reginato, A.J., and Schumacher, H.R.: Synovial calcification in a patient with collagen-vascular disease: Light and electron microscopic studies. J. Rheumatol., *4*:261–271, 1977.

79. Reginato, A.J., Schumacher, H.R., and Brighton, C.T.: Experimental hydroxyapatite synovial and articular cartilage calcification: Light and electron microscopic studies. Arthritis Rheum., *25*:1239–1249, 1982.

80. Resnick, D., et al.: Intra-articular calcification in scleroderma. Radiology, *124*:685–688, 1977.

81. Rosin, A.J.: Ectopic calcification around joints of paralysed limbs in hemiplegia, diffuse brain damage and other neurological diseases. Ann. Rheum. Dis., *34*:499–505, 1975.

82. Samilson, R.L., and Prieto, V.: Dislocation arthropathy of the shoulder. J. Bone Joint Surg., *65A*:456–460, 1983.

83. Sandstrom, C.: Peritendinitis calcarea: A common disease of middle life; its diagnosis, pathology and treatment. Am. J. Roentgenol., *40*:1–21, 1938.

84. Sarkar, K., and Uhthoff, H.K.: Rotator cuff tendinopathies with calcification. *In* Calcium in Biological Systems. Edited by R.P. Rubin, G. Weiss and J.W. Putney. New York, Plenum Publishing Corp. In press, 1984.

85. Sarkar, K., and Uhthoff, H.K.: Ultrastructural localization

of calcium in calcifying tendonitis. Arch. Pathol. Lab. Med., *102*:266–269, 1978.

86. Schumacher, H.R., et al.: Erosive arthritis associated with apatite crystal deposition. Arthritis Rheum., *24*:31–37, 1981.

87. Schumacher, H.R., et al.: Arthritis associated with apatite crystals. Ann. Intern. Med., *87*:411–416, 1977.

88. Sharp, J.: Heredo-familial vascular and articular calcifications. Ann. Rheum. Dis., *13*:15–26, 1950.

89. Skuterud, E., Sydnes, O.A., and Haavik, T.K.: Calcinosis in dermatomyositis treated with probenecid. Scand. J. Rheumatol., *10*:92–94, 1981.

90. Stein, H., Bab, I.A., and Sela, J.: The occurrence of hydroxyapatite crystals in extracellular matrix vesicles after surgical manipulation of the rabbit knee joint. Cell Tissue Res., *214*:449–454, 1981.

91. Swannell, A.J., Underwood, F.A., and Dixon, A.S.: Peri-

articular calcific deposits mimicking acute arthritis. Ann. Rheum. Dis., *29*:380–385, 1980.

92. Thompson, G.R., et al.: Calcific tendonitis and soft-tissue calcification resembling gout. J.A.M.A., *20*:122–130, 1968.

93. Uhthoff, H.K., Sarkar, K., and Maynard, J.A.: Calcifying tendonitis. Clin. Orthop. Rel. Res., *118*:164–168, 1976.

94. Werb, Z., and Reynolds, J.J.: Stimulation by endocytosis of the secretion of collagenase and neutral protease from rabbit synovial fibroblasts. J. Exp. Med., *140*:1482, 1974.

95. Woodard, J.C. et al.: Calcium phosphate deposition disease in Great Danes. Vet. Pathol., *19*:464–485, 1982.

96. Yue, C.C., Regier, A., and Kushner, I.: The arthritis of heterotopic ossification shows elevated synovial protein concentration without synovial leukocytosis. Clin. Res., *31*:808A, 1983.

97. Zaphiropoulos, G., and Graham, R.: Recurrent calcific periarthritis involving multiple sites. Proc. R. Soc. Med., *66*:351–352, 1973.

Chapter 96

Ochronosis, Hemochromatosis, and Wilson's Disease

H. Ralph Schumacher

ALKAPTONURIA AND OCHRONOSIS

Alkaptonuria is a hereditary disorder characterized by homogentisic acid in the urine, which, when oxidized, imparts a brownish black color to the urine. The term "alkaptonuria," denoting an avidity for oxygen in alkaline solution, was coined by Boedeker in 1859 and is derived from fusion of an Arabic word meaning "alkali" and a Greek word (kaptein), meaning "to suck up avidly." When the freshly passed urine is alkalinized, polymerization of homogentisic acid is accelerated, and the urine turns black. Ochronosis denotes a bluish black pigmentation of connective tissue in patients with alkaptonuria, usually apparent clinically in the cartilage of the ear, in the skin, and in the sclera. This term was originated by Virchow in 1866, who described the microscopic appearance of this pigmentation as "ochre" or dark yellow.

Alkaptonuria itself is a symptomless condition. Clinical signs and symptoms develop when pigment is deposited in cartilage and other connective tissues (ochronosis). The relationship between alkaptonuria and ochronosis was first recognized in 1902 by Albrecht. Table 96–1 lists factors in the diagnosis of these and related conditions.

History

The earliest clinical observation, of a boy who passed dark urine, was made by Scribonius in 1584. Boedeker, in 1859, was the first to isolate homogentisic acid from the urine of a patient with alkaptonuria. Wolkow and Bauman in 1891 established the chemical structure of this compound as 2,5-dihydroxyphenylacetic acid and named it homogentisic acid. A.E. Garrod formulated the concept in 1902 that alkaptonuria was an "inborn error of metabolism" consisting of an inability to oxidize homogentisic acid, an intermediary metabolite of phenylalanine and tyrosine.[6] LaDu and his collaborators in 1958 demonstrated the absence of the enzyme homogentisic acid oxidase in the liver of a patient with alkaptonuria, ochronotic spondylosis, and peripheral arthropathy.[12]

Table 96–1. Diagnostic Features of Alkaptonuria, Ochronosis, Ochronotic Spondylitis, and Peripheral Arthropathy

Alkaptonuria
 Urine turns black:
  On alkalinization
  On standing
  When tested for sugar by Benedict's reagent; in addition, yellow-orange precipitate forms
 Positive family history
Ochronosis
 Pigmentation of cartilage and skin:
  Pinna of ear, ear drum, and cerumen
  Sclera
  Skin over malar area, nose, axilla, groin
 Prostatic calculi
Ochronotic spondylosis
 Calcification and ossification of intervertebral discs
 Disproportionately little osteophytosis
 Sacroiliac joints not fused and no "bamboo" spine
 Loss of lumbar lordosis
 Spine rigid and stooped, knees flexed, stance typical
Ochronotic peripheral arthropathy
 Knees, shoulders, and hips most commonly affected
 Synovial fluid contains small amounts of homogentisic acid and is noninflammatory, except with occasional pseudogout
 Brittle cartilage fragments and pigmented "chards" in the synovium
 Osteochondral joint bodies common
 Small joints of hands and feet not affected

Nature of the Biochemical Lesion

Alkaptonuria is the result of a defect in the metabolic pathway for the aromatic amino acid tyrosine. Normally, the benzene ring of homogentisic acid is broken by the enzyme homogentisic acid oxidase, and maleylacetoacetic acid is formed. LaDu, et al. assayed liver homogenates from ochronotic patients and control subjects and demonstrated that the pattern of enzyme activities of the alkaptonuric liver was essentially the same as in the control liver, except with respect to homogentisic acid oxidase activity, which was completely missing in the alkaptonuric patient.[12] Of interest is the presence of the enzyme maleylacetoacetic acid isomerase in the alkaptonuric liver despite the apparent absence of the substrate maleylacetoacetic acid, which could be derived only from the metabolism of homogentisic acid. The presence of this enzyme in the absence of its substrate demonstrates that the genetic mechanism that controls the synthesis of this enzyme is not regulated by the substrate.

Genetic Factors

Alkaptonuria is felt to be transmitted by a single recessive autosomal gene. The occasional occurrence of this disorder in successive generations of certain families may be the result of consanguineous marriages in which homozygotes mate with heterozygotes. The present concept of the mode of transmission of alkaptonuria, originally advanced by Garrod, and challenged at times, has been substantiated by several careful family studies in which complete pedigrees were available.[11] One family had HLA-B27 in 8 of 10 members with alkaptonuria.[7]

Laboratory Aspects of Alkaptonuria

The freshly passed urine of an alkaptonuric patient is of normal color and does not darken at once unless it is alkaline or contains less than a normal concentration of vitamin C or other reducing agents. On standing, it turns brownish black as the homogentisic acid becomes oxidized. If Benedict's reagent is used in testing the urine for sugar, the yellowish orange precipitate that is formed because homogentisic acid reduces the copper which can be misinterpreted as indicating glucosuria. The color of the supernatant solution in these cases is always brownish black, which is diagnostic for alkaptonuria.

With the the use of copper-reduction tablets (Clinitest), a black supernatant may also be seen in patients with malignant melanoma and after intravenous urography with sodium diatrizoate (Hypaque) and other x-ray contrast media.[14] Specific glucose oxidase tapes (Clinistix) may not detect urine glucose in diabetics with ochronosis because of interference with the peroxidase-indicator chromagen reaction by homogentisic acid.[10] Spuriously increased serum and urinary uric acid determinations have been described in ochronosis when colorimetric methods were used, but values were normal by the uricase spectrophotometric technique.[10] Homogentisic acid in the urine may also falsely elevate creatinine levels when measured by Jaffé's reaction.

Diagnostic Tests for Alkaptonuria

Several presumptive, nonspecific tests for alkaptonuria are available. These tests are color reactions based on the reducing properties of homogentisic acid. Thus, in the Briggs test, molybdate is reduced and a deep blue color is obtained.[2] When a drop of urine is placed on photographic paper, a black spot indicates reduction of silver. When sodium hydroxide is added to the freshly passed urine, homogentisic acid is rapidly oxidized, and the urine promptly darkens in color. A specific enzymatic method for quantitative determination of homogentisic acid in urine and blood has been developed.[27] Thin-layer chromatography can also be used.

Pathologic Features of Ochronosis

The lesions of ochronosis result from the interior intracellular deposition of pigment in many organs or structures. The exact chemical composition of the pigment has not yet been defined, although it is believed to be a polymer derived from homogentisic acid. Benzoquinoneacetic acid may be an intermediate compound that, when bound to connective tissue, may participate in a polymerization process leading to the final pigment formation.[30] Homogentisic acid is concentrated preferentially by connective tissue, but this process is reversible until after polymerization. The typical pathologic findings have been reviewed comprehensively.[16] Granules of insoluble, melanin-like pigment are usually found in the skin and subcutis, the cartilage of joints, the intervertebral discs, including the anulus fibrosus as well as the nucleus pulposus, the tracheal cartilages, the epithelial cells of the renal tubules, and the islets of the pancreas. Pigment granules impregnate the walls of large and medium-sized arteries and arterioles, including the aorta and the pulmonary, coronary, and renal arteries.

Clinical Picture of Ochronosis

Patients with alkaptonuria who live to the fourth decade of life almost invariably develop ochronosis. The cartilage of the ear, especially the concha and anthelix, is frequently involved and takes on a slate blue discoloration while becoming irregularly thickened and inflexible. When the pinna is transilluminated, the opaque pigmented area stands out prominently. The cerumen in the external canal is often black, and the periphery of the tympanic membrane is grayish black. Many patients with long-standing ochronosis have impaired hearing. Pigmentation of the sclera is usually localized to a small area midway between the limbus of the cornea and the inner or outer canthus. The skin over the malar areas, nose, axilla, and groin is often pigmented.

Deposition of pigment in the intervertebral discs and articular cartilages of the large joints leads to spondylosis and peripheral arthropathy.

Loud cardiac murmurs, mostly systolic, have been noted in about 15 to 20% of patients with ochronosis.[22] Pigment deposits in the mitral and aortic valves may be associated with deformity of the leaflets or cusps. Clinically significant aortic stenosis has been successfully treated by aortic valve replacement.[15]

Prostatic calculi occur in a large proportion of men with ochronosis and are readily palpable on rectal examination. Dysuria and frequency of urination may be present, and a prostatic operation may be necessary. Calculi may be passed spontaneously or removed surgically. These calculi have a characteristic black color and contain ochronotic pigment and calcium phosphate salts.

Ochronotic Spondylosis

The majority of patients with ochronosis past the age of 30 develop spondylosis. Symptoms usually consist of stiffness and discomfort in the lower back. In about 10 to 15% of patients with ochronosis, the onset of spondylosis occurs with herniation of a nucleus pulposus.[22] In such instances, the symptoms and signs are indistinguishable from those in typical cases of herniated disc without alkaptonuria. The earliest site of spondylosis is the lumbar spine; years later, the dorsal and finally the cervical spine become involved. Stiffness of the lower back slowly progresses to rigidity and obliteration of normal lumbar lordosis. In many cases, lumbar kyphosis develops. Symptoms may be minimal despite prominent roentgenographic changes.

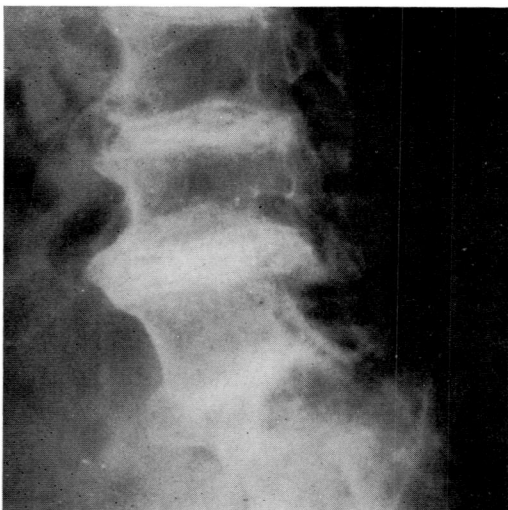

Fig. 96–1. Roentgenogram of the lumbar spine of a 55-year-old man with ochronotic spondylosis. Note the calcification of intervertebral discs. The osteophytes are of only moderate size.

The earliest change apparent in roentgenograms of the spine consists of a wafer of calcification, and actual ossification, in the intervertebral disc of the lumbar spine (Fig. 96–1). Crystallographic study has shown the calcium in these discs to be hydroxyapatite.[3] Radiographic evidence of calcified intervertebral discs in adults is characteristic of ochronosis, but it is not diagnostic in that similar changes can also be seen in pseudogout, in hemochromatosis, in chronic respiratory paralytic poliomyelitis, in spinal fusion of any origin, and occasionally in other disorders or without detectable associated disease.[29] Secondary narrowing of the intervertebral spaces occurs. Osteophytes are usually small. Splits in disc material appear to account for radiolucencies in the discs that have been termed "vacuum discs."[4] In contrast to ankylosing spondylitis, the sacroiliac joints in ochronotic spondylosis are not fused, although they may show degenerative changes, the interfacetal articulations retain a normal radiographic appearance, and anular ossification with a "bamboo" pattern does not appear. The marked narrowing of multiple intervertebral spaces results in a loss of several inches in height. The spinal deformity and forward stoop cause the patient to stand with knees flexed and on a broad base. This posture imparts to the patient with ochronotic spondylosis a stance and gait similar to that of a patient with ankylosing spondylitis (Fig. 96–2).

Ochronotic Peripheral Arthropathy

A degenerative arthritis of the peripheral joints also occurs, although it is less frequent and develops later than spondylosis. The joints most commonly affected are the knees, shoulders, and hips, in descending order of frequency. The knees are involved in the majority of cases of peripheral arthritis. Pain, stiffness, crepitation, flexion contractures, and limitation of motion are the most common features. In the peripheral joints, symptoms often antedate any visible roentgenographic changes. Effusion occurs in about half these cases. Synovial fluid is generally clear, viscous, and yellow, without darkening on exposure to alkali. Although homogentisic acid can be demonstrated, its concentration is much lower than in the urine. Occasionally, black specks of ochronotic cartilage are seen floating in the fluid.[8,23] Leukocyte counts in a large series by Huttl ranged from 112 to 700/mm^3 with predominantly mononuclear cells.[9] Occasional cells have dark inclusions that appear to be phagocytized cartilage containing ochronotic pigment (Fig. 96–3). Synovial effusions or membrane can contain calcium pyrophosphate crystals without inflammation,[13,14,26] or the patient may

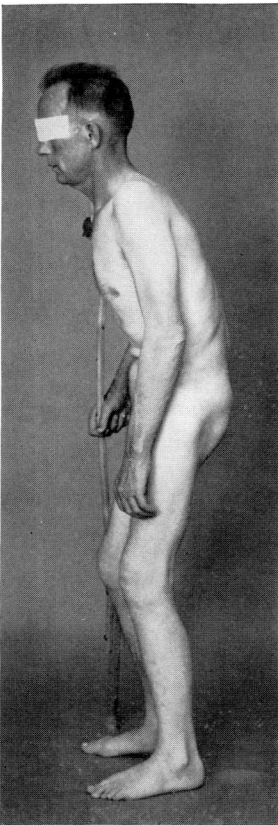

Fig. 96–2. Typical posture and stance of a patient with ochronotic spondylosis: forward stoop, loss of lumbar lordosis, flexed hips and knees, wide-based stance. This 40-year-old man lost 6 inches in height.

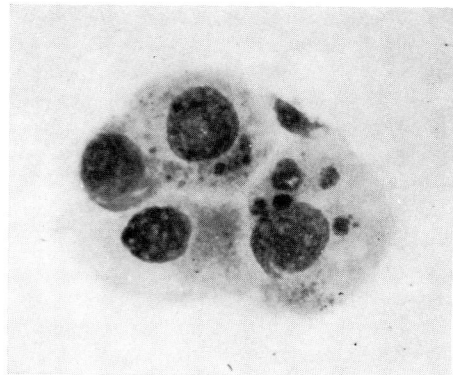

Fig. 96–3. Synovial fluid mononuclear cells in ochronotic arthropathy. The dark cytoplasmic inclusions appear to be phagocytized pigmented debris (Giemsa stain × 1,250). (Courtesy of S. Huttl and Acta Rheum. Baln. Pistiniana.)

have typical acute episodes of pseudogout with increased synovial fluid leukocyte counts.[25]

Pigmentation of the articular cartilage occurs initially in the deeper layers, with relative sparing of the surface. It is seen predominantly in the matrix of the tangential zone, but also in chondrocytes. Necrosis of chondrocytes occurs. Pigment appears by electron microscopy to be associated with the surface of collagen fibers in cartilage, but not in synovium.[20,26] The pigmented articular cartilage is brittle; minute fragments are broken off and are displaced into the synovial tissue (Fig. 96–4). In this location, they sometimes evoke a foreign-body reaction and new formation of bone tissue called osteochondral bodies[21] (Fig. 96–5). These bodies may be several centimeters in diameter and are readily palpable in and around the knee joint. They are often not tender and may be freely movable. Surgical removal may be necessary when the bodies interfere with motion.

The radiographic appearance of the peripheral joints in ochronotic arthritis is not characteristic, in contrast to that of lesions of the spine. The picture is consistent with primary osteoarthritis: narrowing of joint space, small marginal osteophytes, and eburnation.[13] Protrusio acetabuli may be seen.[26] Ossification or calcification of the ligaments and tendons near the joints may be present.[19] Rupture of deeply pigmented ochronotic Achilles tendons has been reported.

In contrast to rheumatoid arthritis (RA) and osteoarthritis, the small joints of hands and feet are rarely affected in ochronosis.

Experimental and Nonalkaptonuric Production of Ochronosis

Rats fed with 8% L-tyrosine for 18 to 24 months develop pigment deposition in joint capsules and cartilages and a degenerative arthritis similar to that of spontaneous human alkaptonuria.[1] The cartilage pigment is melanin-like and includes phenolic bodies as in homogentisic acid or its metabolite benzoquinoneacetic acid.

A grossly bluish black connective tissue pigmentation associated with degenerative arthritis has also been described following prolonged administration of quinacrine in the absence of alkaptonuria.[17] Application of phenol dressings has been reported to produce ochronosis with alkaptonuria and arthropathy. Cartilage pigmentation does not occur in metastatic malignant melanoma.

Treatment

It is not yet feasible to compensate for the enzymatic deficiency of homogentisic acid oxidase. Attempts have been made to treat patients with a diet low in phenylalanine and tyrosine that is, unfortunately, unpalatable. Urinary excretion of

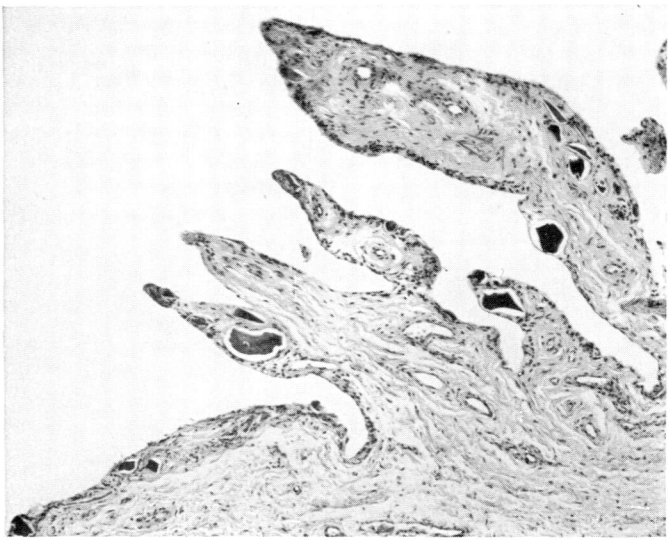

Fig. 96–4. Synovial tissue in ochronotic arthropathy. Minute fragments of darkly pigmented cartilage lie within the superficial portion of the tissue. The sharp edges of the "chards" are characteristic. A foreign-body cell reaction is present at the margins of a few and is accompanied by mild synovial fibrosis. Associated infiltration of lymphocytes and plasma cells may also be present (hematoxylin and eosin stain × 90).

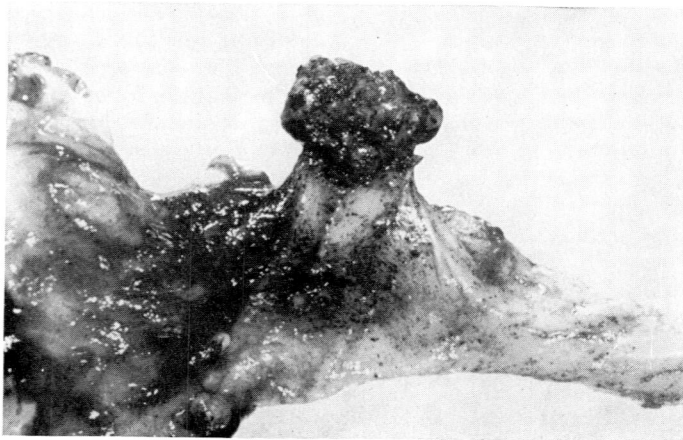

Fig. 96–5. Synovial tissue in ochronotic arthropathy. Numerous pigmented deposits are present. A polypoid nodule has formed in the central portion as an osteochondroid reaction of the displaced cartilage fragments.

homogentisic acid can be decreased, but clinical change was minimal in patients with advanced joint disease. Initiation of this diet at an early age before massive ochronosis develops has not been tried. Reduced protein intake can also decrease urine homogentisic acid levels, but this regimen is impractical for routine treatment. Although high doses of ascorbic acid do not decrease total urine homogentisic acid levels, they have been reported to reduce binding to connective tissue in experimental alkaptonuria of rats.[18] Long-term use of ascorbic acid has not been studied systematically, but it has not been useful in human ochronosis.

Symptomatic measures are of most practical value. Analgesics, braces, program limiting joint overuse, and weight reduction have all provided some help. Adrenal corticosteroids, x-irradiation, tyrosinase, insulin, various vitamins, and phenylbutazone are among the measures tried without benefit. Corrective orthopedic procedures have been helpful in several patients.[5]

HEMOCHROMATOSIS

Hemochromatosis is a chronic disease characterized pathologically by excessive iron deposition and fibrosis in many organs and tissues with ultimate functional impairment in untreated patients. This disorder occurs in about 1 in 7000 people in various populations of European origin. Frequent clinical manifestations are hepatomegaly and cirrhosis, skin pigmentation, mostly from increased melanin, diabetes, other endocrine dysfunction, and heart failure.[40,52] Sicca syndrome has been reported, possibly adding to confusion with other rheumatic diseases.[33] Arthropathy occurs in more than 20% of patients. Hemochromatosis is often idiopathic, with a definite increased familial incidence.[48] It is inherited as an autosomal recessive trait. That patients have an increased frequency of HLA-A3 and HLA-B14 antigens suggests a hemochromatosis locus tightly linked to the HLA region on chromosome 6.[35] Hemochromatosis can also be a late result of alcoholic cirrhosis or occasionally of multiple transfusions, refractory anemia, and long-term excessive oral iron ingestion. In all instances, iron absorption is excessive. Significant overload occurs only after many years, so the onset of symptoms is most common between 40 and 60 years. Hemochromatosis is less frequent in women, presumably because of menstrual blood losses. Tables 96–2 and 96–3 list diagnostic features of hemochromatosis and its related arthropathy.

Pathologic Features and Pathogenesis

Iron as hemosiderin can be identified histologically in all the symptomatically affected tissues, as well as elsewhere. The largest iron deposits are in the liver, and diagnosis is most frequently established by liver biopsy. Large amounts of hemosiderin are seen in parenchymal cells in the liver and in other organs. Iron confined to reticuloendothelial tissues is termed hemosiderosis and does not produce the clinical picture seen in hemochromatosis. Although suspected, the iron has not

Table 96–2.   Diagnostic Features of Hemochromatosis

Cirrhosis with iron deposition, predominantly in parenchymal cells
Iron deposition in other organs causing cardiomyopathy, diabetes, or other endocrine deficiencies
Increased skin pigmentation, largely by melanin
Elevated serum iron concentration and saturated iron-binding capacity

Table 96–3.   Diagnostic Features of Arthropathy of Hemochromatosis

Degenerative arthropathy
Prominent involvement of metacarpophalangeal and proximal and distal interphalangeal joints, hips, and knees.
Chondrocalcinosis
Iron deposition in synovial lining cells

been proved to be the cause of the tissue damage. Organ fibrosis, as in hemochromatosis, has not yet been produced by experimental iron overload alone. Iron may act in an additive fashion with nutritional deficiencies, alcohol, or other, still unidentified, hereditary factors.

Diagnosis

The most important simple diagnostic laboratory test is the determination of serum iron concentration and the percentage of saturation of iron-binding capacity. Both values are elevated in hemochromatosis, but they can also be elevated in hemolytic anemia and other situations. Serum ferritin concentrations are often elevated, but may be normal in precirrhotic disease.[55] Liver biopsy is needed to determine the extent of tissue iron deposition and the degree of tissue damage. One case of hemochromatosis with associated hypoxanthine-guanine phosphoriribosyltransferase deficiency has been recorded where serum iron concentrations and transferrin saturation where normal.[47a]

Osteopenia

Diffuse demineralization of bone can be seen, but its frequency and relationship to the hemochromatosis are difficult to ascertain. A diffuse osteopenia of the hands, without the periarticular demineralization as seen in RA, is most common.[42] The mechanism for osteopenia is not known. Delbarre, who studied this topic extensively, postulated an androgen deficiency secondary to hemochromatosis.[38] Serum calcium, phosphorus, and alkaline phosphatase levels are normal. Biopsy specimens have shown osteoporosis rather than osteomalacia. Because osteopenia is also seen in alcoholic cirrhosis, a direct relation to the defect in iron metabolism is not established.

Degenerative Arthropathy

An arthropathy associated with hemochromatosis was first described in 1964,[50] and since then more than 200 cases have been reported.[37,39,43,44,47] The most frequent joint involvement is degenerative, occurring in 20 to 50% of patients with hemochromatosis.[42] The age of onset varies from 26 to 70, but it is most common in the sixth decade. The onset of arthropathy is usually close in time to the onset of other symptoms of hemochromatosis, but joint symptoms and findings may antedate other clinical manifestations of hemochromatosis and may thus be the first clue to diagnosis.[39,41] Joint symptoms occasionally are first noted many years later, even after completion of phlebotomy therapy.

Hands, knees, and hips are most frequently involved, although other joints can be affected. Characteristic hand findings are a firm, only mildly tender, enlargement of the metacarpophalangeal and the proximal and distal interphalangeal joints. The second and third metacarpophalangeal joints are most often affected (Fig. 96–6). These joints are stiff and have limited motion, but no increased warmth or erythema. Ulnar deviation is not seen. Involvement is generally symmetric. Pain, when present, is accentuated on use. Morning stiffness usually lasts less than half an hour. This arthropathy is gradually progressive. Acute inflammation has occasionally been described, and whether it is always due to associated chondrocalcinosis and crystal-induced synovitis is not certain. Test results for rheumatoid factor are typically negative. Sedimentation rates are only occasionally elevated. Serum uric acid levels are generally normal and occasionally low.[47a,52] Roentgenograms often show the characteristic involvement of the metacarpophalangeal, proximal, and distal interphalangeal joints. Narrowing of the joint space, cystic erosion, joint-space irregularity, subchondral sclerosis, and moderate bony proliferation with frequent hook-like osteophytes are seen[32,50] (Fig. 96–7).

In 30 to 60% of those with arthropathy, especially older patients, chondrocalcinosis is also seen. Roentgenograms of other joints show changes similar to those in the hands and are often indistinguishable from degenerative arthritis and idiopathic chondrocalcinosis. Involvement of the metacarpophalangeal joints 4 and 5 is rare in idiopathic chondrocalcinosis and is most suggestive of underlying hemochromatosis. Synovial fluid is usually noninflammatory, with low leukocyte counts and predominantly mononuclear cells, adequate viscosity, and a pale yellow color. Iron measurements on synovial fluid are comparable to serum levels.[44] Synovial tissue shows a striking deposition of iron, mostly in the synovial lining cells, but also in some deeper cells. On hematoxylin and eosin staining, golden brown hemosiderin granules are seen. The iron can also be stained blue by Prussian blue (Fig. 96–8).

By electron microscopy, the iron is principally seen in type B or synthetic lining cells[49] (Fig. 96–9). This distribution of synovial iron differs from that in hemarthrosis, RA, and other diseases in which iron is presumably derived from gross or microscopic bleeding into the joint. In these conditions, the iron is mostly found in deeper cells and macrophages. In addition to the iron, most synovial membranes in hemochromatosis show only mild lining-cell proliferation, fibrosis, and scattered chronic inflammatory cells. Biopsies of synovium during bouts of acute inflammation have not been reported.

Chondrocalcinosis (see also Chap. 94)

Chondrocalcinosis with hemochromatosis, although usually associated with degenerative arthropathy, can also be an isolated joint finding.[41]

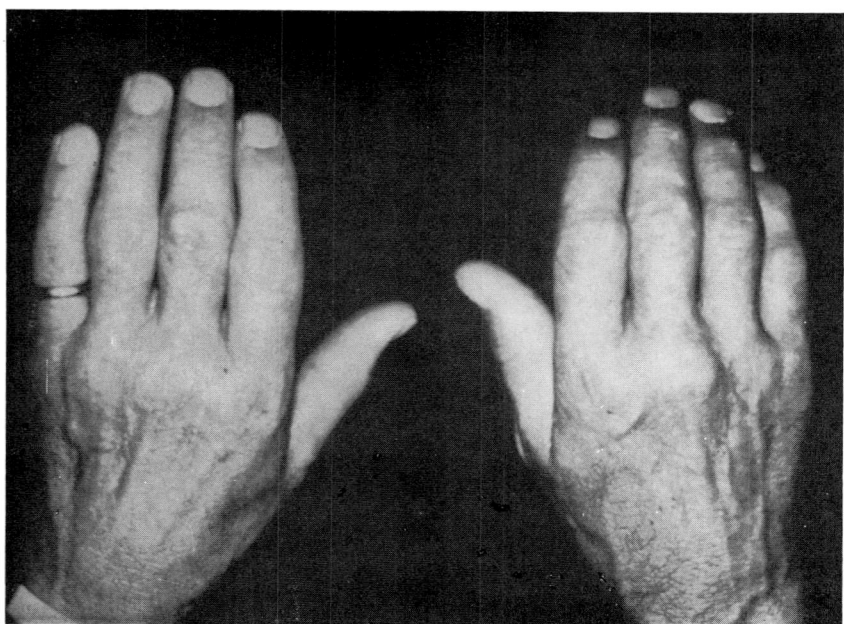

Fig. 96–6. Photograph of the hands of a 45-year-old man with hemochromatosis. Note the knobby enlargement at the metacarpophalangeal, proximal interphalangeal and distal interphalangeal joints. He is unable to extend these joints fully.

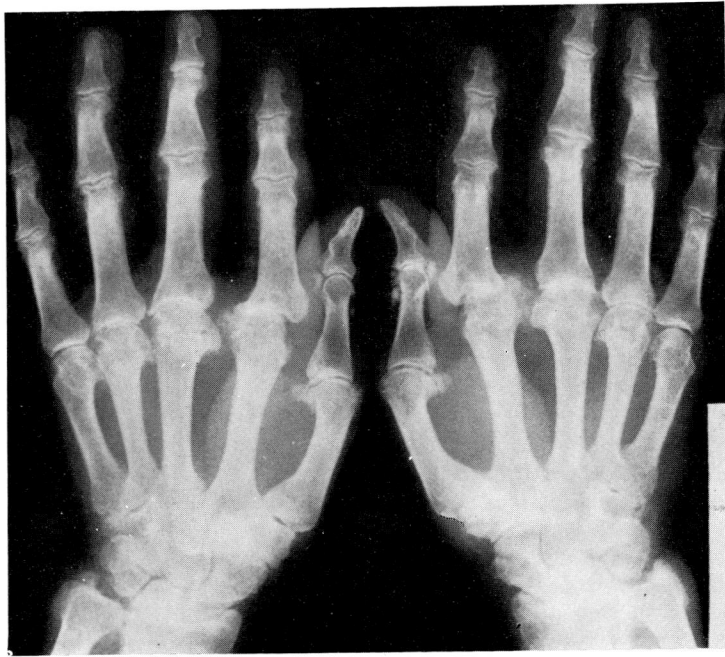

Fig. 96–7. Roentgenogram of hands showing involvement of the metacarpophalangeal and the proximal and distal interphalangeal joints, with characteristic joint-space narrowing, cystic subchondral lesions, joint-space irregularity, subluxation, some osteophytosis, and areas of bony sclerosis. Multiple periarticular calcifications are also present in the interphalangeal joint of the left thumb, and probable chondrocalcinosis is seen at the right ulnocarpal joint. Osteopenia is minimal in these hands.

Calcification is most commonly detected in menisci and articular cartilages at the knee, but it can also be seen at the wrists, fingers, elbows, shoulders, hips, ankles, toes, symphysis pubis, intervertebral discs, and the periarticular soft tissues and bursae. Typical acute pseudogout with calcium pyrophosphate dihydrate crystals can occur. The synovial effusion is inflammatory during such episodes. Menisci and articular cartilages can show grossly evident superficial coating with white crystals. Round intracartilaginous aggregates of positively birefringent calcium pyrophosphate dihydrate crystals identical to those in pseudogout can be seen with compensated polarized light microscopy.

The typical laboratory findings in patients presenting with CPPD crystal deposition are a high serum iron with transferrin saturation in the 60 to 80% range, rather than the nearly complete saturation found in hemochromatosis patients presenting with symptoms due to visceral organ fibrosis.

Iron staining of cartilage has also been noted, but this characteristic is seen in chondrocytes and at the line of ossification, not at the crystal deposits.[48,49] Similarly, x-ray diffraction and chemical studies have shown no iron at the sites of cartilage calcification.[42,48] Periarticular and bursal calcifications have not been studied to determine

the type of calcium salt. Crystals resembling hydroxyapatite have been identified in hemochromatotic synovium and cartilage by electron microscopy.[48,49] Even when no calcification is radiographically visible, cartilage calcium pyrophosphate crystals or apatite are often identifiable by light and electron microscopy.[48]

Possible Mechanisms for Arthropathy

It is attractive to speculate that the iron directly or indirectly causes the osteoarthropathy, but such has not been demonstrated. Arthropathy has only occasionally been reported in patients with transfusion siderosis;[31,51] this finding suggests that factors other than iron deposition are required. Many patients with iron-loading anemias do not survive long enough to develop tissue damage. Aseptic necrosis and osteopenia, but no other arthropathy, have been reported so far in Bantu siderosis.[54] Kashin-Beck disease, an endemic growth disturbance and premature generalized degenerative arthritis seen in Russia and Manchuria, has been attributed by Hiyeda to a high iron content in drinking water.[43] Hiyeda administered iron to vigorously exercised rabbits and believed that this regimen accelerated cartilage deterioration. That experimental iron loading of rabbits produced cartilage degen-

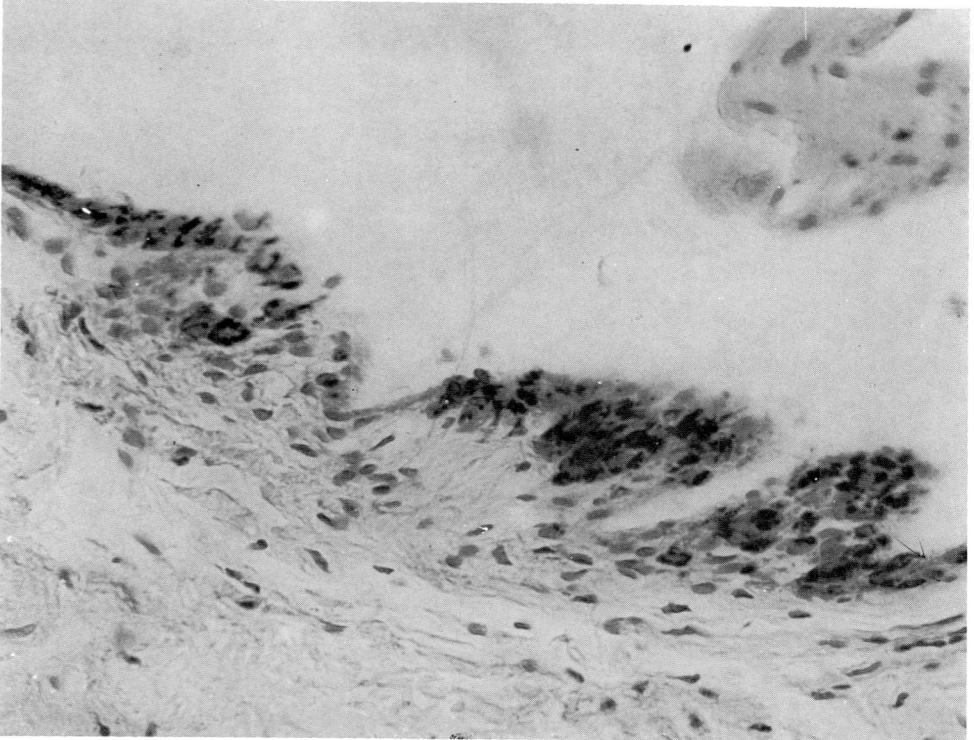

Fig. 96–8.   Synovium in hemochromatosis with dark Prussian blue-stained iron granules in the synovial lining cells (× 400).

eration only when initiated early in life suggests the importance of early initiation of the toxic effect of iron.[34] Localized predominately in synthetic-type cells in cartilage or synovium, iron might cause joint damage by altering the protein polysaccharide or collagen produced by such cells. Iron can injure chondrocytes or other cells by lipid peroxidation of membranes. Ferric ion can irreversibly oxidize ascorbic acid and can impair hydroxylation of proline and thus allow deficient collagen formation.[34] Iron might produce damage by binding to connective tissue protein polysaccharides as it does in vitro in the Hale stain for protein polysaccharide. Some iron is present in lysosomes, and it could increase the release of lysosomal enzymes.

Iron in vitro inhibits pyrophosphatase and might in this manner help to allow the deposition of the calcium pyrophosphate of chondrocalcinosis.[45] Experimental synovial siderosis also inhibited clearance of calcium pyroposphate crystals from rabbit joints.[46] The primary site of joint damage is not established. The cartilage is most suspect in this degenerative process, but subchondral bone or synovial involvement may also be important because cartilage depends on both these areas for nutrition. No correlation has been found between the presence of advanced liver disease, generalized osteopenia, diabetes, or other endocrine disease and the arthropathy. Classic RA has been reported to coexist in several cases, so the arthropathy is not an iron-altered rheumatoid disease.

Treatment

Present therapy of hemochromatosis is directed at removal of the excess iron by phlebotomy, and this approach appears to reverse cardiac failure, to improve liver function, and to ameliorate diabetes. Improvement depends largely on the amount of existing tissue damage. Calcium pyrophosphate dihydrate crystal deposition is not reversed by such therapy. Prevention certainly would be preferable, so serum iron concentrations of relatives should be checked, and prophylactic phlebotomy should be considered. Phlebotomy of 500 ml per week, until the development of mild iron deficiency anemia or demonstrable depletion of liver iron, is usual. Alcohol and excessive vitamin C ingestion can increase iron absorption and should be avoided.[36] Iron chelation with desferrioxamine can also be used. Supportive treatment of the diabetes, liver disease, and heart failure is pursued as needed. Phlebotomy has not had any beneficial effect on the arthritis, and clinical arthritis has even devel-

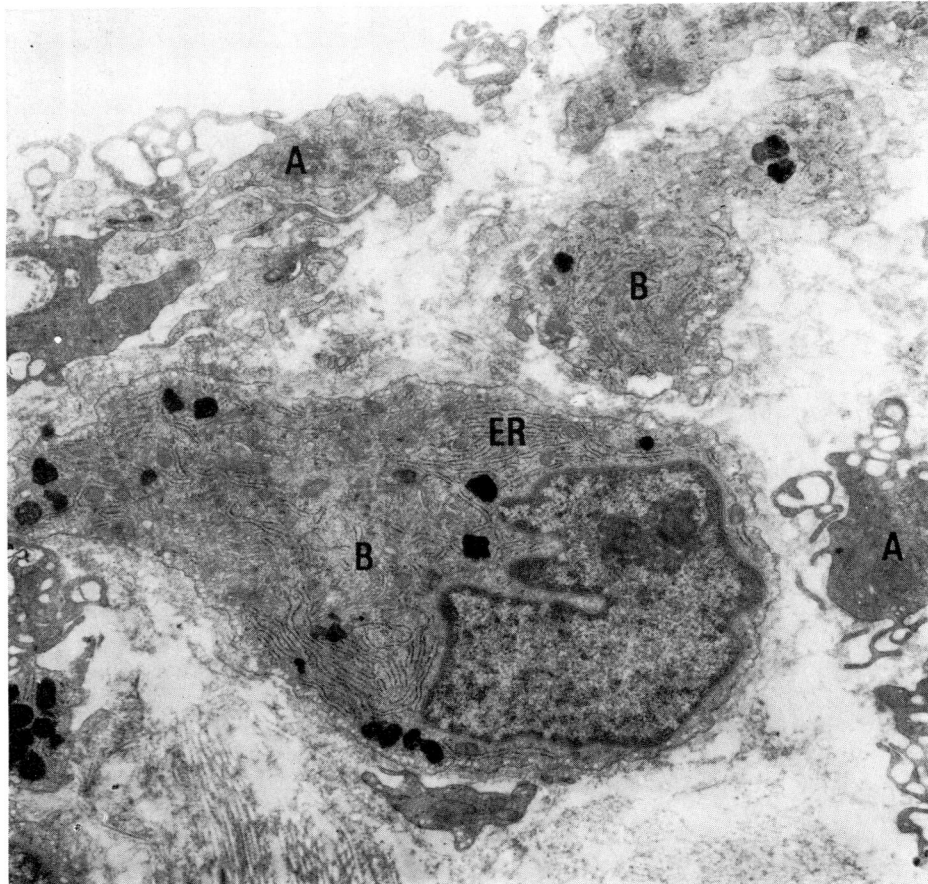

Fig. 96–9. Electron micrograph of electron-dense iron deposits in Type B synovial lining cells (B) in hemochromatosis. Type B cells are primarily synthetic in function and have profuse rough endoplasmic reticulum (ER). The type A cells (A) often have prominent filopodia and vacuoles and are believed to be more active in phagocytosis. Here they contain no identifiable iron (× 13,000).

oped after therapeutic phlebotomy. Irreversible connective tissue and joint change may well become established long before arthritis can be clinically or radiographically detected. Iron is easily demonstrable in the synovium of asymptomatic patients. Treatment of the arthritis is symptomatic; analgesics and systematic range-of-motion exercises are most helpful. Prosthetic hip and knee arthroplasties have been successfully performed in patients with advanced disease, although further breakdown after 18 months has occurred in a knee after prosthetic arthroplasty.

WILSON'S DISEASE

Wilson's disease, or hepatolenticular degeneration,[71] is an uncommon familial disease characterized by a ring of golden brown pigment at the corneal margin, known as the Kayser-Fleischer ring, sometimes visible only on slit-lamp examination, basal ganglion degeneration, and cirrhosis. The condition is inherited as an autosomal recessive trait. Symptoms may first appear between the ages of 4 and 50. Neurologic symptoms are usually earliest and include tremor, rigidity, dysarthria, incoordination, or personality change. Many patients also develop renal tubular disease manifested by aminoaciduria, proteinuria, glucosuria, renal stones, phosphaturia, defective urine acidification, or uricosuria. Uricosuria often results in low serum uric acid levels. Hemolytic anemia can occur. Untreated disease is invariably fatal.[59,67]

Characteristic disorders of copper metabolism are present.[66] Copper concentrations are increased in liver, brain, and other tissues; urine copper excretion is increased; and the serum copper-binding protein, ceruloplasmin, as well as total serum copper are almost always decreased. Measurement of the hepatic copper concentration appears to be the most reliable test. Although the basic underlying defect is not known, increased absorption of copper can be demonstrated. Copper may cause the tissue damage. Mobilization of copper from the body seems to produce an improvement in many patients. Although seen in at least 95% of patients, Kayser-Fleischer rings are not entirely specific and may be seen in other diseases.[70] Table 96–4 lists osseous and articular changes in Wilson's disease.

Osteopenia

Radiographic evidence of demineralization of bone has long been recognized as part of Wilson's disease and is described in 25 to 50% of patients.[61,65] Osteopenia is seen at all ages and usually is asymptomatic. Occasional patients have pathologic fractures. Others have definite rickets,[58] or osteomalacia that can be attributed to the renal tubular disease.

Arthropathy

Boudin, et al. first described articular alterations in Wilson's disease in 1957.[56] Joint changes are rare in childhood, but are seen in up to 50% of adults. Most patients studied have been 20 to 40 years old. Articular involvement ranges from pre-

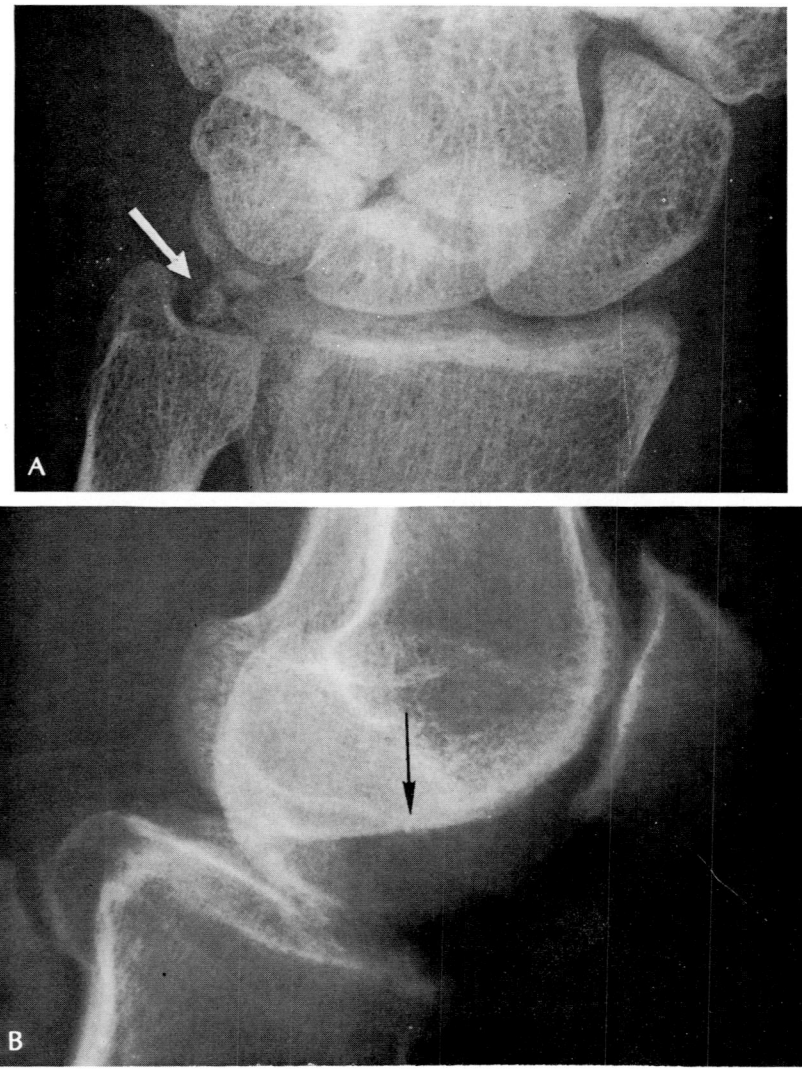

Fig. 96–10. Arthropathy in a 30-year-old woman with Wilson's disease. *A*, Wrist. Note the bony ossicles (arrow) suggested to be a result of cortical fragmentation. Some sclerosis is also present at the distal radius. *B*, Knee. Ossicles are seen near the tibiofibular articulation. Marked chondromalacia patellae with spurs is present on the posterior surface of the patella. The articular cortex of the lateral femoral condyle is irregular, with a suggestion of fragmentation (arrow).

Table 96–4.   Bone and Joint Changes in Wilson's Disease

Bone demineralization
Occasionally, rickets or osteomalacia attributable to renal tubular disease
Premature degenerative arthritis with prominent subchondral bone fragmentation
Prominent involvement of wrists, knees, and, less often, other joints
Periarticular calcifications and bone fragments

mature osteoarthritis with marked symptoms to asymptomatic radiographic findings.[60,61,62,63,65,68] Scattered subchondral bone fragmentations, cortical irregularity, and sclerosis at the margin of wrist, hand, elbow, shoulder, hip, and knee joints are seen (Fig. 96–10). The cartilage space is also often narrowed. Early age of onset and prominent involvement of wrists suggest a difference from the usual osteoarthritis. Tiny periarticular cysts,[65] vertebral wedging and marginal irregularity,[68] osteochondritis dissecans, and chondromalacia patellae[60] have been seen in several patients and may be related to Wilson's disease. Periarticular calcifications are common; many such calcifications occur in ligaments, tendons, and capsule insertions. Other calcifications seem to represent bone fragments or occasional chondrocalcinosis.[60,62] The nature of the calcium crystal deposited in these lesions has not been studied. Joint effusions are usually small, with clear, viscous fluid and 200 to 300 cells/mm³, predominantly mononuclear cells.[60,63] Synovial fluid copper and ceruloplasmin levels have not been studied. Only mild lining-cell hyperplasia and small numbers of chronic inflammatory cells have been noted on synovial biopsies.[63]

No correlation has been found between the severity of the disease, spasticity and tremors, osteopenia, liver or renal disease and the arthropathy. The primary defect may occur in the cartilage or subchondral bone, but no histologic or chemical studies of these tissues have been conducted. Although the joint involvement in Wilson's disease is generally milder, an analogy can be made with that of hemochromatosis. In both diseases, the metal excess is a possible mechanism for direct or indirect production of the arthropathy. Short-term experimental copper loading has not produced arthropathy. McCarty and Pepe have shown in vitro inhibition of inorganic cytosolic pyrophosphatase by cupric as well as by ferrous ions and have suggested this inhibition as a possible mechanism for deposition of calcium pyrophosphate producing chondrocalcinosis in Wilson's diseae and hemochromatosis.[64]

Treatment

Penicillamine, 1 to 4 g/day orally, is the most successful chelating agent for mobilizing copper from the tissue and has produced definite clinical improvement in mental and neurologic changes in many patients. Treatment must be continued for life. Low-copper diets and potassium sulfide may also be used to decrease copper absorption. Symptomatic disease may be preventable by early D-penicillamine treatment of asymptomatic individuals with biochemical abnormalities only.[69] Occasional patients treated with penicillamine still develop arthropathy. Whether early and long-term treatment will decrease the bone and joint disease is not yet known. Occasionally, penicillamine appears to cause polymyositis or lupus-like syndromes. Acute polyarthritis complicated penicillamine therapy in five patients with Wilson's disease.[62] A recent report suggests that zinc may be considered as alternate therapy in patients who cannot tolerate penicillamine.[57]

REFERENCES

Alkaptonuria and Ochronosis

1. Blivaiss, B.B., Rosenberg, E.F., Katuzov, H., and Stoner, R.: Experimental ochronosis: induction in rats by long-term feeding of L-tyrosine. A.M.A. Arch. Pathol., 82:45, 1966.
2. Briggs, A.P.: A colorimetric method for the determination of homogentisic acid in urine. J. Biol Chem., 51:453, 1922.
3. Bywaters, E.G.L., Darling, J., and Sutor, J.: Ochronosis densification. Ann. Rheum. Dis., 29:563, 1970.
4. Deeb, Z., and Frayha, R.: Multiple vacuum disks, an early sign of ochronosis: radiologic findings in 2 biopsies. J. Rheumatol., 3:82, 1976.
5. Detenbeck, L.C., Young, H.H., and Underdahl, L.O.: Ochronotic arthropathy. Arch. Surg., 100:215, 1970.
6. Garrod, A.E.: Inborn Errors of Metabolism. London, Oxford University Press, 1909.
7. Gaucher, A., et al.: HLA antigens and alkaptonuria. J. Rheumatol., 3 (Suppl.):97, 1977.
8. Hunter, T., Gordon, D.A., and Ogryzlo, M.A.: The ground pepper sign of synovial fluid: a new diagnostic feature of ochronosis. J. Rheumatol., 1:45, 1974.
9. Huttl, S.: Synovial effusion. A nosographic and diagnostic study. Part I. Acta Rheum. Baln. Pistiniana, 5:1, 1970.
10. Kelley, W.M., et al.: Significant laboratory artifacts in alkaptonuria. Arthritis Rheum., 12:673, 1969.
11. Knox, W.E.: Sir Archibald Garrod's inborn errors of metabolism. II. Alkaptonuria. Am. J. Hum. Genet., 10:95, 1958.
12. LaDu, B.N., et al.: The nature of the defect in tyrosine metabolism in alcaptonuria. J. Biol. Chem., 230:251, 1958.
13. Lagier, R.: The concept of osteoarthritic remodelling as illustrated by ochronotic arthropathy of the hip: an anatomico-radiological approach. Virchows Arch. (Pathol. Anat.), 385:293, 1981.
14. Lee, S., and Schoen, I.: Black copper reduction reaction simulating alkaptonuria—occurrence after intravenous urography. N. Engl. J. Med., 275:266, 1966.
15. Levine, H.D., et al.: Aortic valve replacement for ochronosis of the aortic valve. Chest, 74:466, 1978.
16. Lichtenstein, L., and Kaplan, L.: Hereditary ochronosis: pathologic changes observed in 2 necropsied cases. Am. J. Pathol., 30:99, 1954.
17. Ludwig, G.D., Toole, J.F., and Wood, J.C.: Ochronosis from quinacrine (Atabrine). Ann. Intern. Med., 59:378, 1963.

18. Lustberg, T.J., Schulman, J.D., and Seegmiller, J.E.: Decreased binding of ^{14}C-homogentisic acid induced by ascorbic acid in connective tissue of rats with experimental alcaptonuria. Nature, 222:770, 1970.
19. MacKenzie, C.R., Major, P., Hunter, T.: Tendon involvement in a case of ochronosis. J. Rheumatol., 9:634, 1982.
20. Mohr, W., Wessinghage, D., Lendschaw, E.: Die Ultrastruktur von Hyalinem Knorpel und Gelenkkapsel-gewebe bei der alkaptonurischen Ochronose. Z. Rheumatol., 39:55, 1980.
21. O'Brien, W.M., Banfield, W.G., and Sokoloff, L.: Studies on the pathogenesis of ochronotic arthropathy. Arthritis Rheum., 4:137, 1961.
22. O'Brien, W.M., LaDu, B.N., and Bunim, J.J.: Biochemistry, pathologic and clinical aspects of alcaptonuria, ochronosis and ochronotic arthropathy. Am. J. Med., 34:813, 1963.
23. Reginato, A.J., Schumacher, H.R., and Martinez, V.A.: Ochronotic arthropathy with calcium pyrophosphate crystal deposition. Arthritis Rheum., 16:705, 1973.
24. Roth, M., and Felgenhaver, W.R.: Recherche de l'excrétion d'acide homogentisique urinaire chez des hétérozygotes pour l'alcaptonurie. Enzymol. Biol. Clin., 9:53, 1968.
25. Rynes, R.J., Sosman, J.L., and Holdsworth, D.E.: Pseudogout in ochronosis: report of a case. Arthritis Rheum., 18:21, 1975.
26. Schumacher, H.R., and Holdsworth, D.E.: Ochronotic arthropathy. 1. Clinicopathologic studies. Semin. Arthritis Rheum., 6:207, 1977.
27. Seegmiller, J.E., et al.: An enzymatic spectrophotometric method for the determination of homogentisic acid in plasma and urine. J. Biol. Chem., 236:774, 1961.
28. Steiger, U., and Lagier, R.: Combined anatomical and radiological study of hip joint in alcaptonuric arthropathy. Ann. Rheum. Dis., 31:369, 1972.
29. Weinberger, A., Myers, A.R.: Intervertebral disc calcification in adults. Semin. Arthritis Rheum., 8:69, 1978.
30. Zannoni, V.G., Malawista, S.E., and LaDu, B.N.: Studies on ochronosis. II. Studies on benzoquinoneacetic acid, a probable intermediate in the connective tissue pigmentation of alcaptonuria. Arthritis Rheum., 5:547, 1962.

Hemochromatosis

31. Abbott, D.F., and Gresham, D.F.: Arthropathy in transfusional hemosiderosis. Br. Med. J., 1:418–419, 1972.
32. Adamson, T.C., et al.: Hand and wrist arthropathies of hemochromatosis and calcium pyrophosphate deposition disease: distinct radiographic features. Radiology, 147:377–381, 1983.
33. Blandford, R.L., et al.: Sicca syndrome associated with idiopathic hemochromatosis. Br. Med. J., 1:1,323, 1979.
34. Brighton, C.T., Bigley, E.C., and Smolenski, B.I.: Iron induced arthritis in immature rabbits. Arthritis Rheum., 13:849–857, 1970.
35. Cartwright, G.E., Edwards, C.Q., and Kravitz, K.: Hereditary hemochromatosis: phenotypic expression of the disease. N. Engl. J. Med., 301:175–179, 1979.
36. Cohen, A., Cohen, I.J., and Schwartz, E.: Scurvy and altered iron stores in thalassemia major. N. Engl. J. Med., 304:158–160, 1981.
37. Delbarre, F.: Les manifestations ostéo-articulaires de l'hémochromatose. Presse Med., 72:2,973–2,978, 1964.
38. Delbarre, F.: L'Ostéoporose des hémochromatoses. Sem. Hop. Paris, 36:3,279–3,294, 1960.
39. Dymock, I.W., et al.: Arthropathy of hemochromatosis. Ann. Rheum. Dis., 29:469–476, 1970.
40. Finch, S.C., and Finch, C.A.: Idiopathic hemochromatosis: an iron storage disease. Medicine, 34:381–340, 1955.
41. Gordon, D.A., Clarke, P.V., and Ogryzlo, M.A.: The chondrocalcific arthropathy of iron overload. Arch. Intern. Med., 134:21–28, 1974.
42. Hamilton, E., et al.: The arthropathy of idiopathic hemochromatosis. Q. J. Med., 145:171–182, 1968.
43. Hiyeda, K.: On cause of endemic diseases prevailing in Manchoukuo (Kaschin-Beck's disease, so called Kokasan

disease endemic goiter). Trans. Soc. Pathol. Jpn., 29:325–331, 1939.
44. Kra, S.J., Hollingsworth, J.W., and Finch, S.C.: Arthritis with synovial iron deposition in a patient with hemochromatosis. N. Engl. J. Med., 272:1,268–1,271, 1965.
45. McCarty, D.J., and Pepe, P.F.: Erythrocyte neutral inorganic pyrophosphatase in pseudogout. J. Lab. Clin. Med., 79:277–284, 1972.
46. McCarty, D.J., Palmer, D.W., and Garancis, J.C.: Clearance of calcium pyrophosphate dihydrate crystals in vivo. III. Effects of synovial hemosiderosis. Arthritis Rheum., 24:706–710, 1981.
47. Mitrovic, D., et al.: Etude histologique et histoclinique des lésion articulaires de la chondrocalcinose survenant au cous d'une hémochromatose. Arch. Anat. Pathol., 14:264–270, 1966.
47a. Rosner, I.A., et al.: Arthropathy, hypouricemic, and normal serum iron studies in hereditary hemochromatosis. Am. J. Med., 70:870–874, 1981.
48. Schumacher, H.R.: Articular cartilage in the degenerative arthropathy of hemochromatosis. Arthritis Rheum., 25:1,460–1,468, 1982.
49. Schumacher, H.R.: Ultrastructural characteristics of the synovial membrane in idiopathic hemochromatosis. Ann. Rheum. Dis., 31:465–473, 1972.
50. Schumacher, H.R.: Hemochromatosis and arthritis. Arthritis Rheum., 7:41–50, 1964.
51. Sella, E.J., and Goodman, A.H.: Arthropathy secondary to transfusion hemochromatosis. J. Bone Joint Surg., 55A:1,077–1,081, 1973.
52. Sheldon, J.H.: Haemochromatosis. London, Oxford University Press, 1935, pp. 1–382.
53. Sinniah, R.: Environmental and genetic factors in idiopathic hemochromatosis. Arch. Intern. Med., 24:455–460, 1969.
54. Solomon, L.: Aseptic necrosis of the femoral head in iron overload osteoporosis. Rev. Rhum. Mal. Osteoartic., 6:457–461, 1974.
55. Wands, J.R., et al.: Normal serum ferritin concentrations in precirrhotic hemochromatosis. N. Engl. J. Med., 294:302–305, 1976.

Wilson's Disease

56. Boudin, G., et al.: Relapsing meningeal tuberculosis, cisternal blocking with symptoms similar to lethargic encephalitis (somnolence, ptosis, extrapyramidial syndromes). Bull. Soc. Med. Hop. Paris, 73:559–561, 1957.
57. Brewer, G.J., et al.: Treatment of Wilson's disease with oral zinc. Clin. Res., 29:758A, 1981.
58. Cavallino, R., and Grossman, H.: Wilson's disease presenting with rickets. Radiology, 90:493–494, 1968.
59. Dobyns, W.B., Goldstein, N.P., and Gordon, H.: Clinical spectrum of Wilson's disease. Mayo Clin. Proc., 54:35–42, 1979.
60. Feller, E., and Schumacher, H.R.: Osteoarticular changes in Wilson's disease. Arthritis Rheum., 15:259–266, 1972.
61. Finby, N., and Bearn, A.G.: Roentgenographic abnormalities of the skeletal system in Wilson's disease (hepatolenticular degeneration). Am. J. Roentgenol., 79:603–611, 1958.
62. Golding, D.N., and Walshe, J.M.: Arthropathy of Wilson's disease: study of clinical and radiological features in 32 patients. Ann. Rheum. Dis., 36:99–111, 1977.
63. Kaklamanis, P., and Spengos, M.: Osteoarticular change and synovial biopsy findings in Wilson's disease. Ann. Rheum. Dis., 32:422–427, 1973.
64. McCarty, D.J., and Pepe, P.F.: Erythrocyte neutral inorganic pyrophosphatase in pseudogout. J. Lab. Clin. Med., 79:277–284, 1972.
65. Mindelzun, R., et al.: Skeletal changes in Wilson's disease: a radiological study. Radiology, 94:127–132, 1970.
66. Perman, J.A., et al.: Laboratory measurements of copper metabolism in the differentiation of chronic active hepatitis and Wilson disease in children. J. Pediatr., 94:564–568, 1979.
67. Roche-Sicot, J., and Benhamou, J.-P.: Acute intravascular hemolysis and acute liver failure associated as a first man-

ifestation of Wilson's disease. Ann. Intern. Med., *86*:301–303, 1977.

68. Rosenoer, V.M., and Michell, R.C.: Skeletal changes in Wilson's disease (hepato-lenticular degeneration). Br. J. Radiol., *32*:805–809, 1959.

69. Sternlieb, I., and Scheinberg, I.H.: Prevention of Wilson's disease in asymptomatic patients. N. Engl. J. Med., *278*:352–359, 1968.

70. Weinberg, L.M., Brasitus, T.A., and Leskowitch, J.H.: Fluctuating Kayser-Fleischer-like rings in a jaundiced patient. Arch. Intern. Med., *142*:246–247, 1981.

71. Wilson, S.A.K.: Progressive lenticular degeneration: a familial nervous disease associated with cirrhosis of the liver. Brain, *34*:295–509, 1912.

Chapter 97

Osteopenic Bone Diseases

Bevra H. Hahn

Diseases of bone constitute a major cause of pain and disability, especially in individuals over the age of 50. Multiple disorders can result in reduced quantities that are inadequate to withstand the stresses of everyday life. Disability results from fractures, from increasing dorsal kyphosis, and from bone pain. The pathophysiologic features of normal bone, and adult osteopenia, with special emphasis on the most common osteopenic diseases in the practice of rheumatology, idiopathic post-menopausal osteoporosis and glucocortoid-induced osteopenia, are the subjects of this chapter.

Confusion surrounds the terms "osteoporosis" and "osteopenia." *Osteopenia* occurs when the total quantity of mineralized bone is less than that expected for a normal individual of the same age, sex, race, and body build. Some authors also use this definition for osteoporosis; others confine the term "osteoporosis" to individuals who have experienced bone fractures as a result of osteopenia. The term "osteopenia" is used here to refer to any disease state involving abnormally reduced quantities of total mineralized bone, and the term "osteoporosis" is used to designate diseases characterized by a high risk of fracture because of low bone mass related to aging or to menopause.

NORMAL BONE

Bone has two major functions in man: (1) it provides a means of support, locomotion, and protection; and (2) it serves as a reservoir of ions necessary for multiple body functions including calcium, phosphorus, magnesium, sodium, and carbonate metabolism. As with other body tissues, continual turnover and remodeling occur; during this process, rates of formation and rates of resorption are normally in equilibrium. The essential role of bone in maintaining normal ion and buffer concentrations in the extracellular fluid takes precedence over the supportive role of bone when formation and resorption rates become uncoupled, however.

Bone is composed of connective tissue that becomes mineralized. Collagen, accounting for approximately 70% of the dry weight of bone, is its major component. Mucopolysaccharides, including chondroitin sulfate, keratin sulfate, and sialic acid are also present, as are other proteins including osteocalcin, a calcium-binding protein, and a glycoprotein called "bone morphogenetic protein" that may signal cells to form bone.

Bone collagen contains two A chains and one B chain; a mature collagen molecule consists of a left-hand helix coil coiled around another axis, which has a right-hand twist (see Chap. 10). Three such coils form tropocollagen, the molecules of which are stacked together in rods with spaces between them. In these spaces mineralization begins. The mineral phase is composed predominantly of hydroxyapatite crystals ($Ca_{10} \times (H_2O)2 \times (PO_4)_6 \times (OH)_2$).

During fetal life and early childhood, bones are formed from cartilaginous growth plates, which form the epiphysis and metaphysis of long bones and most of the mass of short bones such as vertebrae. The cortex of long bones derives from a perichondral area of new bone deposition. Until puberty, bone formation exceeds bone resorption, and bone growth is regulated by mechanical stimuli such as physical activity and weight bearing, which help to shape bone, and by the stimulus of several hormone systems including growth hormone and somatomedins. In adults, bone *modeling* has stopped, as has bone *growth,* and changes in bone thereafter are called *remodeling.*

The two major forms of mature mineralized bone are compact *cortical* bone, which forms the largest portion of long bones of the appendicular skeleton, and transverse interwoven *trabecular* bone, which forms the majority of bone in vertebral bodies and the flat bones of the skull and pelvis. Compact cortical bone is laid down around the Haversian systems in ellipses or circles; the structure is more archlike in trabecular bone. The mechanical relationships of these types of bone and the direction in which they are laid down may be as important in determining skeletal strength as the total quantity of mineralized bone. Consider, for example, the high fracture rate in patients with Paget's disease, in whom the quantity of bone may be great in a given area, but whose structure is mechanically weak.

In both cortical and trabecular bone, the process of remodeling is continual. Remodeling occurs from the three "envelope" areas:[30] (1) from the

Haversian envelope, as shown in Figure 97–1; (2) from the periosteal envelope; and (3) from the endosteal envelope. The Haversian envelope occurs within the structure of cortical bone and consists of tunneling canals in which bone is initially resorbed and then reformed.

The endosteal envelope covers the inner surface of the cortex and the trabecular bone surface, and separates bone from bone marrow. During adult life, the endosteal surface has a higher rate of resorption than formation; the bone marrow cavity consequently expands at the expense of the thickness of cortical and trabecular bone. Frost suggested the concept of bone modeling units, called "basic multicellular units"[29,30] (Figure 97–2). He suggested that two types of such units exist, one in which resorption is the major activity, and one in which bone formation is the major activity. These units occur on each skeletal envelope. In each basic multicellular unit, the following sequence of events occurs: (1) the unit is activated; (2) osteoclasts appear and begin to resorb bone, a process that takes an average of two weeks; (3) osteoblasts that synthesize osteoid, a process that takes approximately six weeks, appear; and (4) finally, mineralization of the new bone occurs. This entire process requires two to six months. In health, a steady state exists between rates of bone formation and resorption in the basic multicellular units. A number of factors can upset this balance, however, including change in the "birth rate" of new multicellular units, an uncoupling of the rates of resorption and formation in multiple units, or failure to mineralize the osteoid that has been formed. Adults have a wider variation in birth rates

of basic multicellular units in the Haversian and endosteal envelopes than in the periosteal; loss of trabecular and cortical bone on the endosteal surface and loss of intracortical bone are more common than losses of subcortical bone. In cortical bone, remodeling caused by basic multicellular units occurs predominantly in the Haversian system; in trabecular bone, remodeling occurs predominantly in Howship's lacunae. In most metabolic bone diseases in adults, the rate of remodeling determines whether total bone formation remains in equilibrium with resorption or whether bone is lost as the rates are uncoupled. The mechanisms by which these rates are controlled are largely unknown; several interesting reviews of this subject are available.[41,70]

Within the basic multicellular units, the origin of functional cells is clearly different. Osteoblasts are probably derived from precursor cells closely related to fibroblasts. They not only synthesize osteoid, but can also produce matrix vesicles, which may be necessary for the initiation of mineralization. Osteoclasts are closely related to macrophages, are probably derived from bone marrow monocytes, and are available in the circulation until they become functionally activated in Haversian canals or Howship's lacunae. The osteocyte is a sessile bone cell, a mature osteoblast, no longer capable of synthesizing either collagen or the ground substance of osteoid.

Hormonal Influences

The movement of calcium and phosphorus ions in and out of the mineral phase of bone is under the control of three major hormones: (1) parathy-

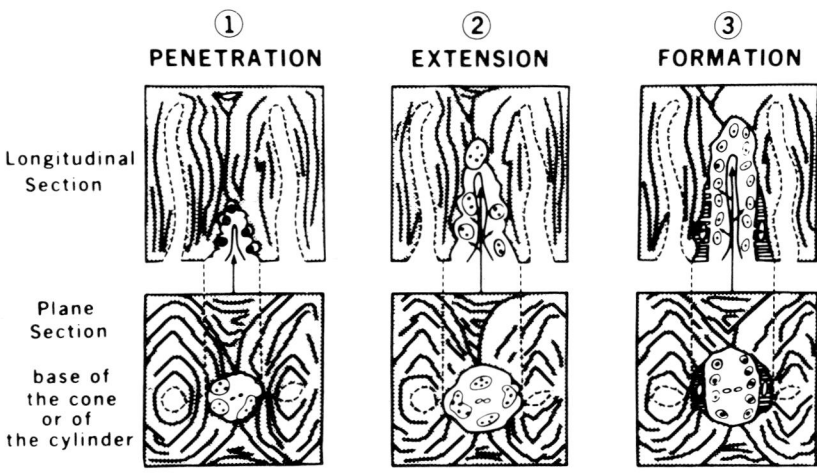

Fig. 97–1. A model of the sequential events in the formation of a new Haversian system in cortical bone. (From Rasmussen, H., and Bordier, P.: The Physiological and Cellular Basis of Metabolic Bone Disease. Baltimore, Williams & Wilkins, 1974.)

roid hormone; (2) the active metabolites of vitamin D; and (3) calcitonin. Parathyroid hormone maintains the level of ionized calcium in the extracellular fluid by: (1) stimulating bone resorption; (2) increasing resorption of calcium in the kidney tubules; and (3) an indirect process involving increased intestinal calcium absorption by stimulating metabolism of vitamin D into its most active form, $1,25(OH)_2D$. Parathyroid hormone is also capable of directly decreasing the synthesis of bone collagen. Vitamin D is formed in the skin from the conversion of 7-dehydrocholesterol to vitamin D_3 (cholecalciferol). Cholecalciferol is hydroxylated to 250H D (calcifediol) in the liver and is further hydroxylated to $1,25(OH)_2D$ (calcitriol) in the kidney. Calcitriol is a potent stimulant of intestinal absorption of calcium and phosphorus. When this process is operating normally, calcitriol promotes bone growth and bone formation by providing adequate levels of mineral. When dietary intake of minerals is low, however, calcitriol is capable of directly resorbing calcium and phosphate from the skeleton. Calcitonin inhibits the resorption of calcium from bone and thus reduces the concentrations of serum calcium. With age, the concentration of parathyroid hormone rises, and the concentrations of $1,25(OH)_2D$ and calcitonin fall.

Several other hormones also act on bone, although their role is less clearly understood than that of the previously described hormones. Thyroid hormone is necessary for normal bone growth and remodeling, and excessive levels of thyroxin can stimulate bone resorption and a rapid birth rate of basic multicellular units. Sex hormones including estrogen, androgens and progestins also affect bone. It has been thought for years that the decline in estrogen levels associated with menopause accounts for rapid loss of bone at that time. As discussed in detail later in this chapter, adrenal glucocorticoids also play an important role in skeletal remodeling. Pharmacologic levels decrease the intestinal absorption of calcium, the conversion of precursor cells to osteoblasts, and the formation of osteoid by osteoblasts. Physiologic levels are probably important in maintaining normal bone formation and resorption rates. Through its effect on somatomedins, growth hormone stimulates collagen synthesis and cell replication in adult bone, as well as growth in children. Insulin stimulates osteoblasts to synthesize collagen.

Other enhancers of bone formation include mechanical stimulation of bone, probably modulated by the generation of small electrical currents, and local factors including prostaglandins, which are produced by bone cells and can stimulate bone resorption as well as formation. Human lymphocytes can be activated to release osteoclast-activating factor (OAF), which stimulates bone resorption. This factor is probably particularly important in the loss of bone characteristic of individuals with multiple myeloma; whether it has a physiologic role is not clear.

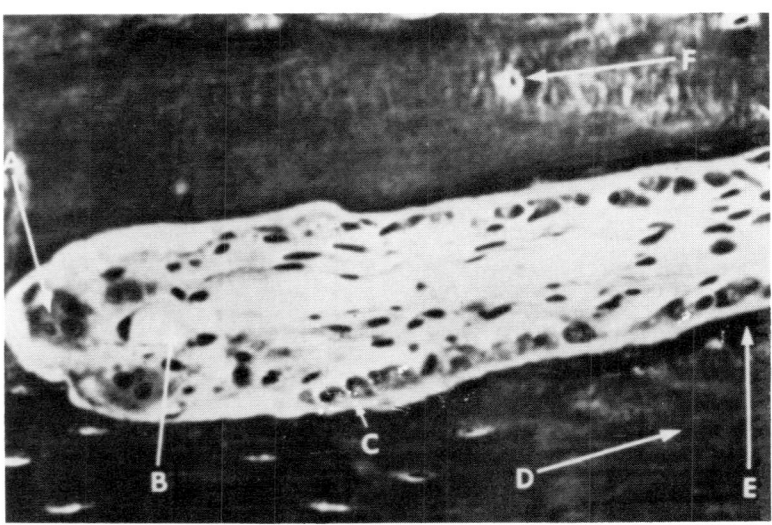

Fig. 97–2.　A basic multicellular unit of bone; longitudinal section through an evolving Haversian system. At the front, the osteoclasts (A) are drilling a tunnel through the bone (D) from right to left, to make a temporary space filled by blood vessels and loose connective tissue (B). Further behind, the osteoblasts (C) lined up along the osteoid seam (E) are refilling the tunnel. (From Parfitt, A.M.: Mineral Electrolyte Metab., *3*:277, 1980. Reprinted with permission of the publisher.)

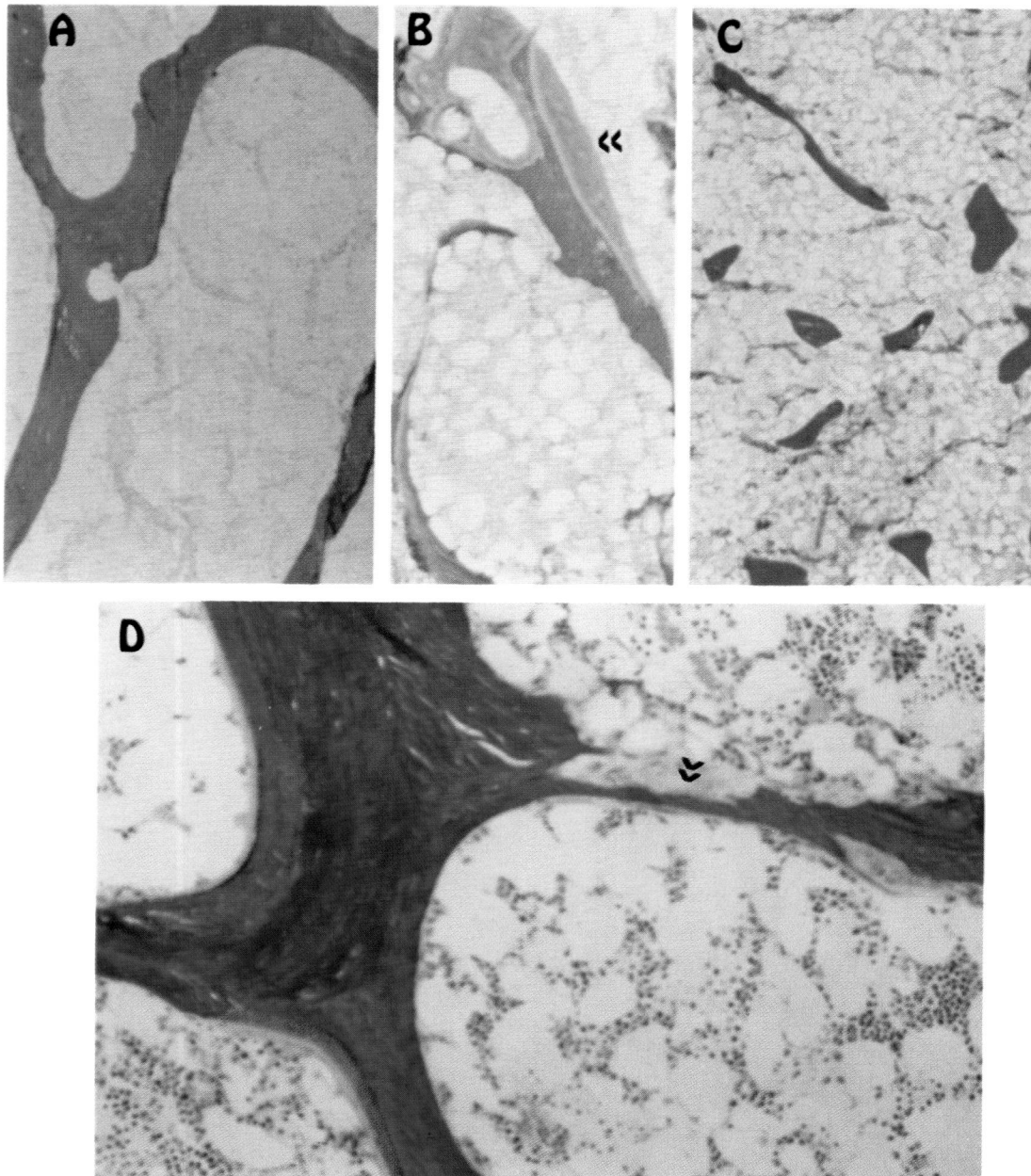

Fig. 97–3. Histologic specimen of bone obtained from iliac crest biopsies. Sections are undemineralized and are stained with the von Kossa stain. Mineralized bone stains blue black; unmineralized osteoid stains pink orange. *A,* Normal bone histologic specimen from a core biopsy of the iliac crest (× 10). *B,* Osteomalacia; note the large quantities of orange-staining undemineralized osteoid (arrows) laid down along all areas of previously mineralized bone (blue) (× 10). *C,* Low-turnover osteoporosis; note the small total quantities of mineralized bone. The absence of areas of osteoid formation and of resorption indicates a low rate of turnover (× 10). *D,* High-turnover osteoporosis; note the large area of resorption of a bone trabecula (arrows) and formation of osteoid (pink). This patient has osteoporosis with a high rate of turnover (× 100). *E,* Osteitis fibrosa of hyperparathyroidism. A line of osteoclasts has resorbed a large area along a trabecula. The space is being replaced by fibrous tissue. At the leading edge of resorption osteoid is being laid down (× 400). *F,* Glucocorticoid-induced osteopenia. Osteoclasts have been activated and have resorbed part of the cortical bone at the endosteal surface (arrows). In contrast to *E,* however, no evidence indicates osteoblast activation; that is, no osteoid is forming (× 100). *G,* Bone biopsy viewed under ultraviolet light after tetracycline labeling; tetracycline deposits at the mineralizing front of new bone. This patient received three days of tetracycline therapy twice, with a two-week interval between doses. The distance between the two fluorescent bands of tetracycline is a measure of the rate of bone formation; the label of the bone indicates osteoid has been formed and mineralized. (Illustrations kindly provided by Steven Teitelbaum, M.D., Professor of Pathology, Washington University/Jewish Hospital of St. Louis.)

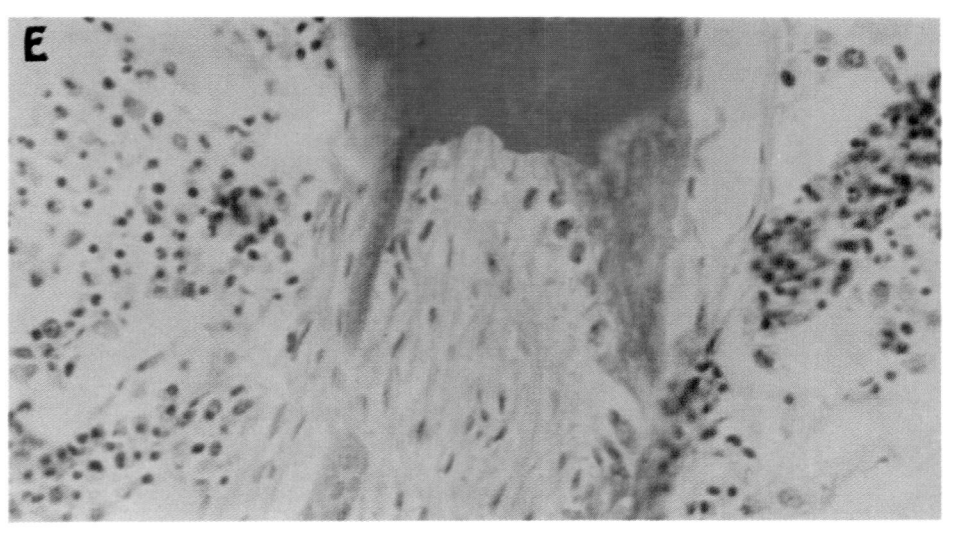

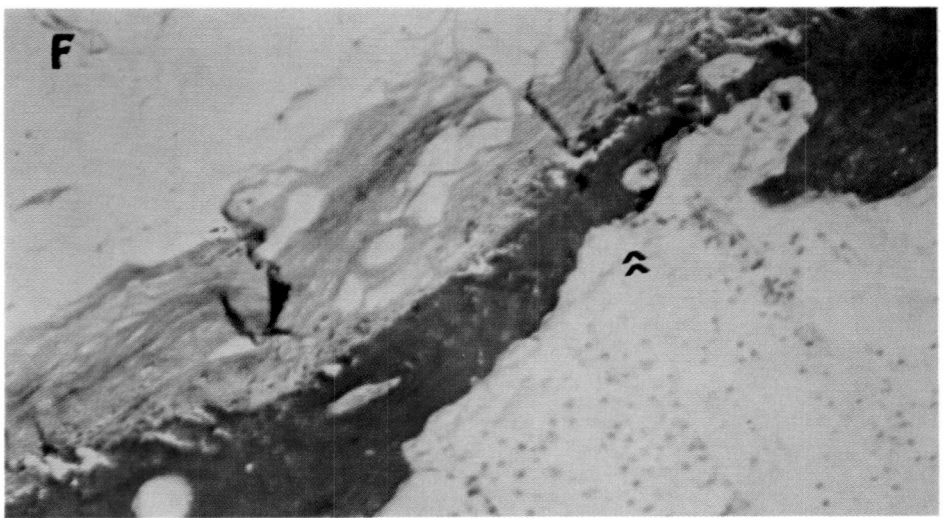

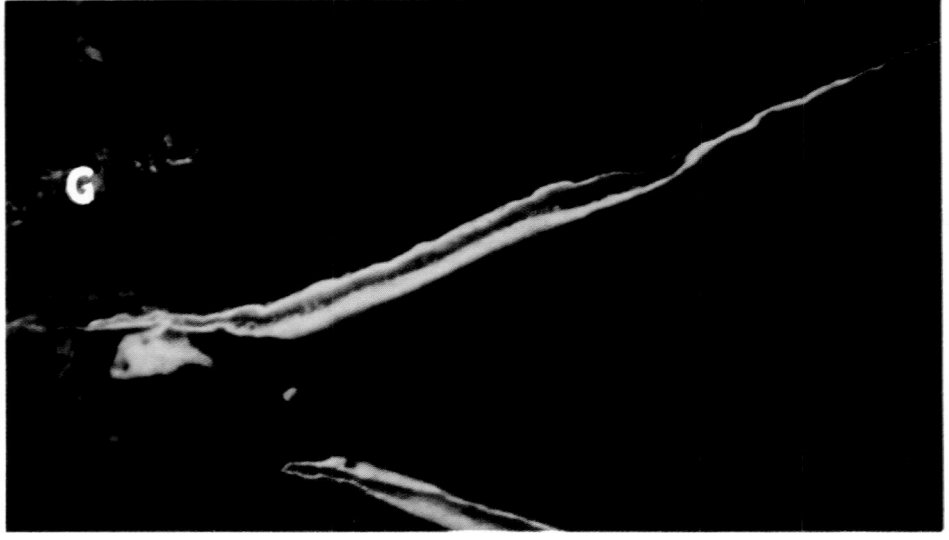

All these hormones affect both osteoblasts and osteoclasts, with the exception of calcitonin, which is a selective inhibitor of osteoclasts. The net result of interaction of these various hormones, mechanical stresses, and the components of the basic multicellular units at all 3 remodeling envelopes is that bone is in a constant dynamic equilibrium. In fact, bone turnover rates in children can be as high as 20% per year; in adults, those rates fall to 3 to 5% annually. To maintain normal bone, an adequate quantity of tropocollagen must be formed, it must be arranged in the correct configuration to permit mineralization, adequate mineral must be available, and mineralization must be mechanically sound to maintain normal tensile strength. When any of these factors or any combination of them becomes abnormal, metabolic bone disease results.

Histologic Features

The morphologic results of the interaction of these multiple factors can be seen histomorphometrically, using the recently developed technique of examining stained, undecalcified bone biopsy sections, usually obtained from the iliac crest. A model of the sequential events in a basic multicellular unit and of the resultant histologic picture is shown in Figure 97–2. Osteoclasts, which can be clearly identified in this figure, form a "cutting cone," that is, a tunnel through cortical bone. Behind the osteoclasts are blood vessels and connective tissue, and farther behind is a line of osteoblasts forming osteoid, which appears as the dark area in Figure 97–2.

In the series of color plates in Figure 97–3, osteoid stains bright orange pink and mineralized bone stains blue black with the von Kossa stain. The osteoblasts and osteoclasts can be differentiated by their morphologic features. From similar bone biopsies, one can measure the quantity of osteoid per unit of bone, the width of the osteoid seam (a wide seam suggests lack of mineralization and osteomalacia), the quantity of trabecular bone, and the numbers of osteoclasts and resorbing surfaces or cavities; all these factors give a picture of the dynamic turnover of bone at the time of biopsy.

The extent of bone formation can be estimated more accurately by the technique of double tetracycline labeling developed by Frost. Before biopsy, 2 short courses of tetracycline are administered 7 to 14 days apart. Tetracycline forms fluorescent bands (Fig. 97–3) after deposition at the mineralization front of bone. The distance between those fluorescent bands divided by the time interval between the midpoints of tetracycline administration is called the "mean mineral apposition rate" and is a measure of osteoblast function, rates of bone formation, and mineralization.

METHODS OF MEASURING BONE MASS

Measurements of bone mass have presented difficulties with regard to sensitivity, accuracy, reproducibility, and general applicability to all parts of the skeleton. (Some areas of the skeleton with a high content of trabecular bone are more metabolically active than others.) Simple radiographic techniques have generally been unsatisfactory. Osteopenia in routine roentgenograms of any bone is defined as: (1) loss of trabeculae; and (2) thinning of cortices. Because these changes are not apparent on standard roentgenograms until 30 to 50% of bone mass is lost, this technique is obviously unsuitable for the detection of early accelerated bone loss and the measurement of increments in bone mass as systemic diseases are controlled or as other therapeutic interventions that affect bone are introduced. Some current techniques are listed in Table 97–1; these methods are reviewed in detail in a recent book.[15]

Several simple radiographic techniques have been tried in the hope of providing greater sensitivity at a low cost. These techniques include metacarpal cortical width, Singh index, and comparison of bone density to an aluminum standard simultaneously irradiated (radiogrammetry). The thickness of several metacarpal bones from the endosteal to the periosteal surface of the cortex at a fixed distance from either the distal or the proximal end of the bone can be used as a sequential measure of bone mass.[60] Although this technique is precise, it is insensitive. When my colleagues and I have employed it in 12- to 18-month studies, during which time bone mass in the appendicular skeleton was shown to change by single-photon osteodensitometry, the metacarpal width did not change. This widely available technique can be used for longitudinal assessment by the practicing physician, however. I have found the Singh index disappointing as a measure of change in bone mass because of its insensitivity, although it is easily reproducible. Radiogrammetry has been largely supplanted by the newer techniques of photon-absorption osteodensitometry, computerized axial tomography (CT scanning), and iliac crest bone biopsy.

In photo-absorption osteodensitometry,[16,58] gamma rays are directed through a selected portion of bone, and a scanning detector measures the degree of interference provided by the minerals contained in bone (Fig. 97–4). This interference correlates directly with bone density and can be converted by computer to a number representing the grams of mineral content per square centimeter of bone scanned. Initially, osteodensitometry was performed using a single low-energy photon beam,

Table 97–1.   **Methods of Measuring Bone Mass**

Technique	Advantages	Disadvantages
Measurement of the cortical width of selected long bones, usually several metacarpals	Simple; inexpensive; accurate for cortical mass; precise in longitudinal studies	Inability to detect loss of trabecular mass or intracortical bone loss; poor correlation with vertebral mass
Singh index, to grade trabecular pattern of the femoral neck	Simple; inexpensive	Better correlation with hip fractures than with vertebral or appendicular bone fractures
Radiogrammetry (density of bone compared to the density of an aluminum standard)	Potential viewing of several bones viewed on one film; bone size and shape and cortical mass measurable simultaneously; accurate correlation with single-photon absorption of appendicular bone and with total body calcium by neutron activation	Precision lessened by uneven film background and large amount of soft tissue; technique largely replaced by single-photon absorptiometry; not good for assessing vertebrae
Single-photon absorptiometry	Inexpensive; low radiation dose; accurate correlation of readings at midradius (diaphyseal mass) or at midmetacarpal with weight of that bone, weight of total skeleton and total body calcium	Poor correlation with mass of vertebrae ($r = .6$); repositioning of arm is a source of error; precision is better at diaphysis than at metaphysis; single low-energy beam not allowing correction for differences in surrounding soft tissues
Dual-photon absorptiometry	Because of second high-energy beam's penetration of soft tissue, potential to measure vertebral mass; correlation with vertebral fractures in osteoporosis more accurate than that of any foregoing techniques	Expensive; time-consuming; repositioning a problem in longitudinal studies; arthritic spurs a possible source of error
Computed tomography of vertebrae	Definition of anatomy of vertebrae and separate measurements of cortical and trabecular bone; correlation with vertebral fractures	Expensive; time-consuming; soft tissue variation around vertebrae a source of error; scanner drifting with time
Neutron activation of restricted area, such as the hand, or of the whole body	Detection of small changes in regional or total body calcium (1–2%) over time	High radiation dose; expensive; time-consuming; unclear correlations with loss of bone mass at specific sites
Histomorphometry, to stain undecalcified iliac crest biopsy specimens	Clearer picture of dynamics of bone metabolism than static measures of bone mass	Poor correlations with vertebral fractures; better for assessing activity of bone formation and resorption than for quantitating mass

which has limited scanning capacity in terms of the thickness of bone and soft tissue it can penetrate. It was applied to readily accessible peripheral bones of the appendicular skeleton; patterns of bone loss in the appendicular and axial skeletons are often dissimilar. Reproducibility is a problem because the peripheral bone must be scanned at exactly the same position at each follow-up visit. Under optimal conditions, the variability of the test is approximately 3% at the midradius and 5% at the distal radius.

In the past few years, dual-photon absorptiometry has come into use.[58] Because two photon sources are available, the density of large amounts of soft tissue can be penetrated, and vertebral mass can thereby be measured. Currently available machines can scan lumbar vertebrae from L1 to L5; their computers can delete the density readings in the soft tissue areas occupied by intervertebral

discs; an average reading for the density of the lumbar vertebrae results. The advantage of this apparatus is that one may directly measure the density of bones with high trabecular content, such as vertebrae. Because vertebral crush fractures and hip fractures are the major disabling consequences of most forms of osteopenia, direct measurement of these areas is desirable. The disadvantages are that the technique is more cumbersome than measurement of the mass of radius or metacarpal bone, it is much more expensive, and the level of radiation exposure is higher.

CT scanning of selected vertebrae has been used at some centers to measure quantities of trabecular and cortical bone in the vertebrae.[33] Defined areas of target vertebrae can be selected for scanning, and the density of bone can be calculated by a computer by comparing energy absorption to that of phantoms containing varying quantities of phos-

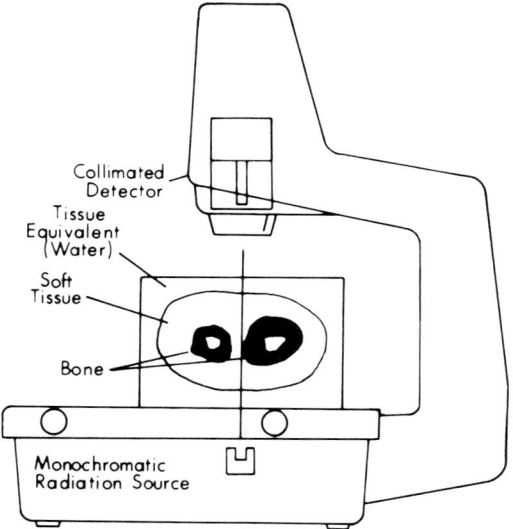

Fig. 97–4. Single-photon absorptiometry. The patient sits beside this absorptiometer, and his arm or hand is placed above the gamma beam and is surrounded with a water-filled cuff. The collimated detector can scan a selected area of the radius or the metacarpal bones.

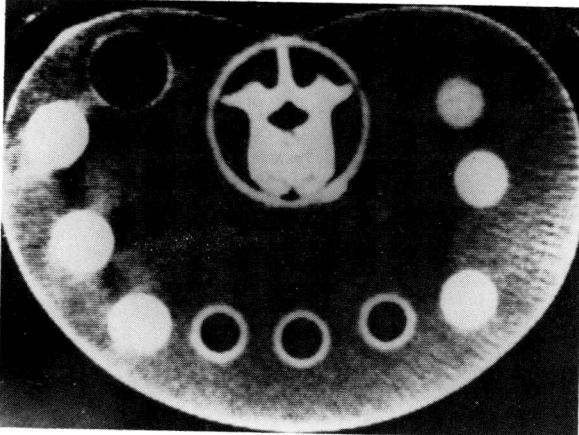

Fig. 97–5. Image of a vertebra analyzed by computerized axial tomography. The patient lies on a plastic board containing tubes (phantoms) filled with varying quantities of phosphates, and scanning is performed. The density of cortical or trabecular portions of vertebrae can be calculated by comparison to density of the phantoms.

phates (Fig. 97–5). The advantages of the technique are its ability to define the anatomic structures of the vertebrae and to obtain separate measurements of trabecular and cortical bone; the correlation with the risk of vertebral fracture is strong. The technique is time consuming and expensive. Differences in the quantities of soft tissue surrounding vertebrae from one subject to another

are a significant source of error, and the scanner drifts with time.

Neutron activation either of restricted areas of the body, such as the hand, or of the total body are available at a small number of centers.[15] Using this technique, the body is bombarded with photons that activate neutrons in the molecules of several different substances, including calcium, to produce ^{46}Ca. The emission of neutrons as the isotope decays can be measured by a detector, and it correlates accurately with the total amount of calcium present in the area bombarded. In population studies in the United States, whole-body neutron activation has been used most frequently to estimate changes in total body calcium as diseases progress or as therapeutic regimens are introduced. The technique is sensitive enough to detect a 1 to 2% change in total body calcium levels. It is assumed that the change in calcium reflects mineralization of bone, and it is unclear how changes in whole-body calcium levels relate to changes in specific areas of the skeleton. The technique requires a high dose of radiation and is expensive.

Histomorphometry can be used to assess total bone volume as well as to quantitate rates of formation and total resorptive surfaces. Bone biopsies are obtained from the iliac crest with a 0.5-cm trocar after tetracycline labeling, and the specimens are stained without prior decalcification using a modified Masson trichrome stain. Fluorescence of the tetracycline label is studied with an ultraviolet microscope. Studies from our center have not shown a strong correlation between total bone volume on biopsy and the number of vertebral compression fractures, the midradius bone density by single-photon absorptiometry, or the metacarpal cortical width.[88] Studies by others have shown an accurate correlation between low total bone volume on biopsy and autopsy diagnosis of osteoporosis, however.[64] Fractional trabecular bone volume is defined as the fraction of a volume of whole trabecular bone tissue, including marrow, occupied by trabecular bone, both mineralized and unmineralized. It does correlate with the weight of iliac bone, but not to a high degree; it also correlates well with the vertebral bone volume. Overall, reduced values for trabecular bone volume have been found in patients with osteoporosis, hyperthyroidism, and secondary hyperparathyroidism from renal disease or glucocorticoids. Nevertheless, the measurements of bone mass by photon absorptiometry or CT scanning are probably more sensitive than those by histomorphometry in regard to loss of bone mass over time; bone biopsy does provide a better understanding of the dynamics of that bone loss. For a detailed review of histomorphometry, the reader is referred to a recent symposium.[62]

DIAGNOSIS AND DIFFERENTIAL DIAGNOSES

Several different symptoms should alert the physician to the possible diagnosis of osteopenia. These symptoms include bone fractures after minor trauma or in the absence of trauma, loss of height, increasing dorsal kyphosis, and bone pain. In addition, some patients with osteomalacia or hyperparathyroidism have muscle symptoms, including stiffness and weakness, that can be confused with inflammatory myopathies. Some patients have no symptoms, but the diagnosis is suspected because of osteopenia seen on roentgenograms obtained for another reason.

The differential diagnosis of generalized osteopenia in adults is shown in Table 97–2. The disorders include osteoporosis, corticosteroid-induced osteopenia, osteomalacia, osteitis fibrosa, and others such as hyperthyroidism, diffuse malignant diseases involving bone, and osteogenesis imperfecta tarda.

A complete evaluation of osteopenia should consist of the following: (1) medical history and physical examination; (2) routine roentgenograms of affected portions of the skeleton; (3) more sensitive measures of bone mass if available (see the preceding discussion of evaluations of bone mass); (4) several measurements of fasting serum calcium, phosphorus, and alkaline phosphatase levels; (5) measurement of the serum parathyroid hormone level; (6) measurement of the serum 25 OH vitamin D level; (7) measurement of 24-hour urine calcium excretion; and (8) iliac crest bone biopsy if available.

Once the radiologic diagnosis of osteopenia is established and a diffuse malignant osteolytic process such as multiple myeloma or a congenital osteopenia such as osteogenesis imperfecta has been excluded, one must establish the basis of the metabolic bone disorder. A good starting point is measurement of fasting serum calcium, phosphorus, and fractionated alkaline phosphatase levels on several occasions. These determinations should be performed on fasting serum because postprandial rises in serum calcium and phosphorus levels can obscure mild decreases in basal levels. Most currently available parathyroid hormone assays can readily

Table 97–2.   Differential Diagnosis of Generalized Osteopenia in Adults

Disorder	Possible Causes, Types, and Characteristics
Osteoporosis (parallel loss of mineral and matrix)	Aging
	Genetic, sex, race, dietary predisposition (osteopenia or senile osteoporosis); fracture, after minor trauma after age 70, especially of hip
	Postmenopausal—fractures of radius, vertebrae
	Idiopathic
	Immobilization or reduced physical activity
	Premature menopause
Glucocorticoid-Induced Osteopenia	Iatrogenic
	Adrenal glucocorticoid overproduction
Osteomalacia (inadequate mineralization)	Vitamin D deficiency
	Inadequate intake and reduced sunlight exposure
	Drug-induced catabolism of vitamin D
	Intestinal malabsorption
	Phosphate-wasting syndromes
	Acquired renal tubular defects with isolated phosphate loss
	Combined tubular defects (Fanconi syndrome)
	Renal tubular acidosis
	Antacid abuse
Osteitis Fibrosa (parathyroid hormone-induced increase in mineral and matrix resorption)	Primary hyperparathyroidism
	Secondary hyperparathyroidism
	Vitamin D deficiency states
	Primary decrease in intestinal calcium absorption with age
	Reduced renal mass
Other Forms of Osteopenia	Hyperthyroidism
	Osteogenesis imperfecta
	Malignant tumors replacing bone

detect the marked increase in serum levels occurring in primary hyperparathyroidism and renal osteodystrophy, but these tests are less likely to detect the usual minor elevations found in states of mild secondary hyperparathyroidism, such as vitamin D deficiency and corticosteroid-induced osteopenia. An elevated serum parathyroid hormone value in combination with other confirmatory data is useful in establishing a diagnosis, however. Serum for parathyroid hormone determinations should also be drawn in the fasting state to increase the likelihood of detecting a minimally elevated basal level. Serum 250H D measurements provide a sensitive means of assessing vitamin D status. The normal ranges for a center in the midwestern United States were 10 to 25 ng/ml in the winter and 15 to 40 ng/ml in the summer. Values at or below normal limits indicate a deficiency state and warrant further evaluation for intestinal malabsorption, drug-induced osteomalacia, and other disorders. The 250H D assays are now available at an increasing number of medical centers and commercial laboratories. Malabsorption syndromes are best defined by determining 72-hour fecal fat excretion and D-xylose absorption.

Determination of 24-hour urinary calcium excretion is a simple and useful, albeit indirect, means of detecting abnormalities in calcium metabolism. With the patient on a 600- to 800-mg calcium diet for several weeks (the average American diet provides that amount), calcium excretions should be between 100 and 200 mg/24 hour. Values below 100 mg on several determinations suggest intestinal calcium malabsorption with a decreased filtered calcium load, and a secondary parathyroid hormone elevation that promotes renal tubular calcium retention, *unless* the patient is taking thiazide drugs, which usually decrease urine calcium excretion to 50 to 60% of basal values. An elevated urine calcium excretion and hyperchloremic acidosis suggests acquired distal renal tubular acidosis. This diagnosis can be confirmed by recording urine pH values for 2 to 3 consecutive days and by failure of urine pH to fall below 5.3 following NH_4Cl loading, in the form of 0.1 mg/kg body weight in 4 divided doses. Other routinely useful tests include determination of urinary hydroxyproline to detect states of increased bone turnover such as osteomalacia, a fasting 4-hour tubular reabsorption of phosphorus test to detect renal phosphate wasting in hyperparathyroidism or renal tubular phosphate "leak" syndromes, and measurement of urinary free cortisol in suspected cases of excessive endogenous glucocorticoid production.

The utility of iliac crest bone biopsy to diagnose

osteomalacia and low or high bone turnover has already been discussed.

OSTEOPOROSIS

The term "osteoporosis" refers to the parallel loss of both mineral and matrix that renders residual quantities of mineralized bone inadequate to withstand minor trauma without fracture. The term is confusing because it has been used to refer to the physiologic loss of bone that occurs with aging, as well as to the syndromes of accelerated or early bone loss that occur with inactivity, in menopausal or early postmenopausal women, and in men in late middle age. Thus, the term "idiopathic osteoporosis," "postmenopausal osteoporosis," "involutional osteoporosis," "senile osteoporosis," "disuse osteoporosis," and "osteopenia" are all in use, with some confusion as to their exact meanings. I agree with the view, expressed by Riggs et al.,[78] that parallel loss of cortical and trabecular bone is physiologic and after many decades results in enough loss of mineralized bone to predispose a person to fractures. This phenomenon should be referred to as "osteopenia" or "senile" or "involutional" osteoporosis. In contrast, a subset of women lose bone mass at a rapid rate after menopause, possibly with a disproportionate loss of trabecular bone, and have a high rate of vertebral fractures in the early postmenopausal period (see Fig. 97–7,A). This disease is properly termed "postmenopausal osteoporosis." Again, the term "osteopenia" can refer to individuals with roentgenographic bone loss, and "osteoporosis" to individuals with bone fractures.

Incidence

Data regarding the rate of bone loss as individuals age have been obtained from weighing bones at autopsy, from the various radiographic techniques discussed earlier, and from histomorphometry. Rates of bone loss vary with age, depending on the particular bone measured and the sex of the individual.

Males have greater bone mass than females. In both sexes, after the age of 40 to 50 years, bone mass is lost from appendicular bone at an average annual rate of 0.5%. In women, however, during the decade following menopause, that rate increases to approximately 1% per year, leveling off to the slower rate after age 60 to 65.[39,70,76] Parallel to this accelerated postmenopausal appendicular bone loss is an increase in the negative calcium balance that occurs after age 40 and almost doubles after menopause.[44] The patterns of bone loss from the midradius in women and in men are shown in Figure 97–6, A,B. Loss of bone from the axial skeleton may occur in a different pattern and at a different rate from that in the appendicular skeleton, however.[76] In vertebrae, bone loss may begin as early as 20 years of age, and it proceeds steadily at a high rate in women, approximately 7% per decade, and at a much slower rate in men, under 2% per decade (Figure 97–6, *C,D*). In contrast to the situation in the midradius, bone loss from vertebrae is not accelerated in the postmenopausal years, nor does the rate of loss decline by age 65; this finding suggests that estrogen responsiveness is lower in the axial than in the appendicular skeleton.[81] Total loss of bone mass in normal women and men over a lifetime, as estimated by the studies of Riggs and colleagues,[76,78] is shown in Table 97–3. If bone loss occurs at different rates in different areas of the skeleton, it is difficult to interpret changes in density or histologic features at a single location as measurements of the impact of therapeutic intervention.

The incidence of vertebral, hip, and distal radial fractures undoubtedly increases with age, hip fractures in the elderly are associated with a mortality rate of 12 to 20% in 6 months,[49] and costs of short- and long-term care for these problems constitute a major expenditure in our society.

Pathogenesis

Although bone turnover rates decrease progressively with age, bone formation is decreased to a slightly greater degree than is resorption, possibly

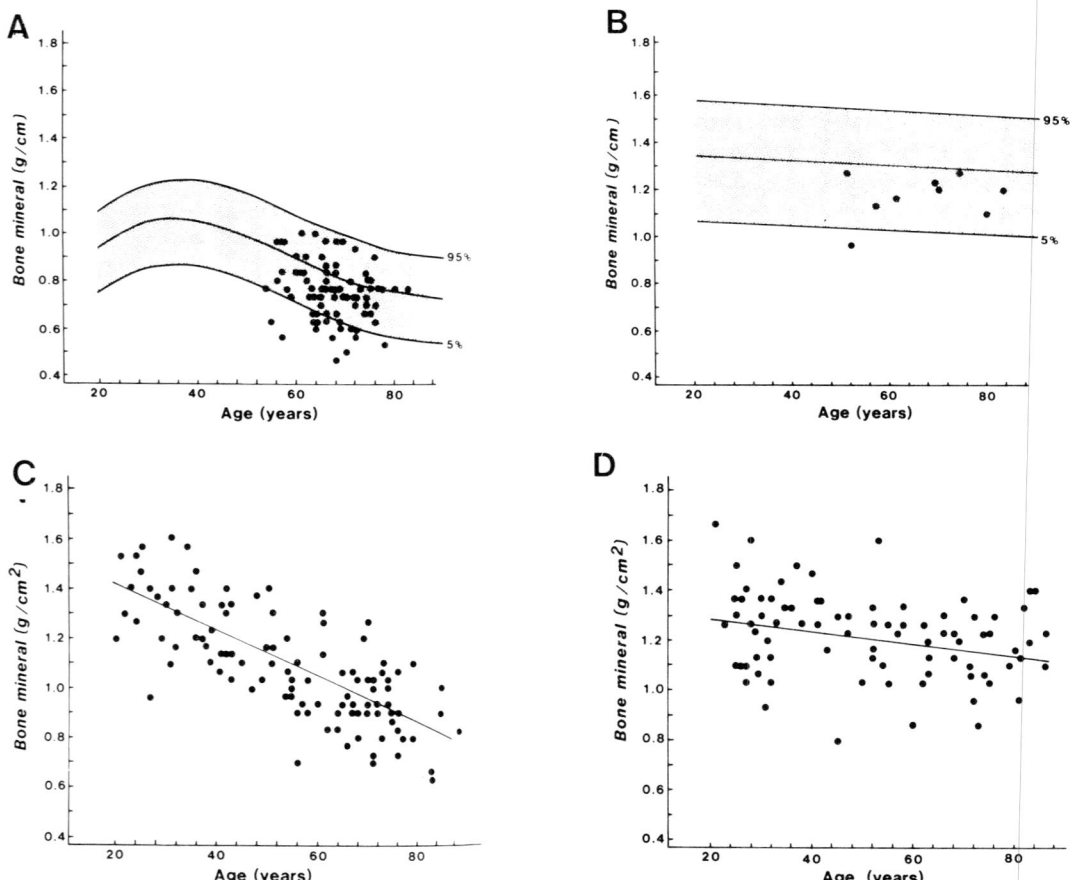

Fig. 97–6. Loss of bone mass with advancing age as determined by single- and dual-photon absorptiometry. *A,* Loss of bone mass from the midradius in normal United States women. Loss begins at age 35 to 40, accelerates around the time of menopause, and slows in rate after age 65. The center line represents the mean density for normal women; the shaded area encloses two standard deviations; dots are the bone mass in women who have osteoporosis and have had one or more vertebral fractures. *B,* Loss of bone mass from the midradius in normal United States men. The rate of loss is slower than in women. *C,* Loss of bone mass from lumbar vertebrae in normal United States women. The pattern is different from the pattern in the midradius. Bone mass begins to fall at age 20 and declines at a rapid rate unchanged by menopause. Dots represent bone mineral content in normal women. *D,* Loss of bone mass from lumbar vertebrae in normal United States men. The rate is much slower than in women. Dots represent values for normal men. (From Riggs, B.L., et al.[78] With permission of the publishers.)

Table 97–3.   Loss of Bone Mass in Normal Individuals

Location	Total Loss in Women (%)	Total Loss in Men (%)
Lumbar vertebrae	42–47	13
Midradius	30	5
Distal radius	39	11
Neck of femur	58	36
Intertrochanteric area of femur	53	35

because resorption rates increase. The result is a gradual net loss of bone. A variety of hypotheses of the nature of this pattern have been suggested, including relative osteoblast failure, calcium and vitamin D deficiencies related to dietary changes, decreased efficiency of intestinal calcium absorption and renal calcium retention, and imbalances among the various hormones that influence bone turnover. Certainly, physiologic osteopenia is a process with many etiologic factors and phenotypic expressions in different individuals. For example, some women with clinically apparent postmenopausal osteopenia actually have osteomalacia on bone biopsy;[50] biopsies showing osteoporosis can contain a spectrum of changes from inactive bone remodeling to high turnover.[88]

Diminished absorption of calcium by the intestine is a physiologic consequence of aging, although the reasons are unknown.[7] In some women, this malabsorption becomes severe enough to add a component of hyperparathyroidism to their osteoporosis. Estrogen loss after menopause probably enhances bone resorption; androgenic hormones and some progestins, levels of which also decline with time, may have positive effects on bone mass. Premature menopause, occurring before the age of 45, is associated with rapid bone loss in some women.[1] Early menopause may be caused by the use of cytotoxic drugs in young women. Diminution in physical activity, in sunlight exposure, in dietary intake of calcium and vitamin D probably play important roles in the osteopenia of aging.

Race and genetic factors are important in predisposing individuals to symptomatic osteoporosis. Black individuals have greater bone mass than white persons, who in turn have greater bone mass than Oriental individuals. Certain populations have a high incidence of osteoporosis, including Eskimos,[59] and Scandinavians. Identical twins have a higher concordance for loss of bone mass than do dizygotic twins.[84] Body build may also be important. Individuals who are "small boned" have low bone mass; osteoporosis is positively correlated with thinness and is negatively correlated with obesity.[20] Total immobilization results in severe

bone loss, as much as 20% over 4 months.[42] Health habits other than nutrition and exercise also play a role in predisposing individuals to osteoporosis. Evidence suggests that alcohol ingestion, smoking, and coffee drinking all have deleterious effects on bone mass.[70] Numerous medications reduce rates of bone turnover and may reduce mass, including prostaglandin inhibitors, glucocorticoids, and methotrexate.[30] The many factors that predispose persons to parallel loss of bone, mineral, and matrix are listed in Table 97–4.

Diagnosis

The clinical diagnosis of idiopathic, postmenopausal, or involutional osteoporosis is essentially one of exclusion. A middle-aged or elderly individual complains of loss of height, increasing dorsal kyphosis, or back pain. Fractures may have occurred (Fig. 97–7,A). In general, patients with hip fractures are a different subset from patients with vertebral and wrist fractures. Radiologic osteopenia, measured either by routine roentgenograms or by one of the more sensitive radiographic techniques discussed previously, is evident. Serum studies show normal levels of calcium, phosphate, alkaline phosphatase, parathyroid hormone, and 250H D. Urine calcium may be low (<100 mg/24 hour), but is usually normal. Other causes of metabolic bone disease should be ruled out, including hyperthyroidism, malignant disorders, hypercortisolism, and alcoholism. Malabsorption, diminished renal function, renal tubular acidosis, or any other factors that might cause osteomalacia or secondary hyperparathyroidism should be excluded. Initial evaluation should include the tests reviewed in the preceding section on diagnosis and differential diagnosis. If special radiographic techniques to measure bone mass are available, baseline studies should be obtained. Similarly, if histomorphometry of bone is available, an iliac crest biopsy can be useful in ruling out an element of osteomalacia or osteitis fibrosa and in establishing the rate of bone turnover, because both high- and low-turnover forms occur, and such information may influence therapy.

Prevention

Because it is difficult to restore clinically significant quantities of bone once that mass is lost in individuals with osteopenia, it is appealing to construct programs that aim to prevent osteopenia or osteoporosis, rather than to treat symptomatic disease. To this end, a number of studies have evaluated the benefits of physical exercise and of dietary and hormonal supplementation in middle-aged, perimenopausal white women. Osteoporosis is a heterogeneous disorder, and measurements of

Table 97–4. Factors Causing Bone Loss and Contributing to Idiopathic or Postmenopausal Osteoporosis

General	Specific
Aging	Reduced intestinal absorption of calcium
	Change in hormone balance
	Senescence of bone multicellular units
Genetics	Race
	Small body build
	Other
Sex	Female (less bone mass and lost more quickly than males)
Premature Menopause	Menopause before age 45
Menopause	Declining levels of estrogen, androgens, progestagens
Drugs	Glucocorticoids, prostaglandin inhibitors, methotrexate
Immobilization	——
Adverse Health Habits	Little physical activity
	Low dietary intake of calcium
	Low dietary intake of vitamin D
	Little sunlight exposure
	Cigarette smoking
	Alcohol abuse
	Coffee drinking

bone mass in a single site or in biopsies at a particular time, or calculations of total body calcium, cannot be considered equivalent to studies of fracture rate. Therefore, studies that actually measure the incidence of fractures determine whether an intervention is efficacious, provided all other variables are well controlled. Detailed discussions of prevention strategies are available elsewhere.[43,70,73]

With regard to exercise, heavy exercise in adolescence leads to a measurable increase in bone mass, and three hours a week of the President's Council on Physical Fitness exercises given to perimenopausal women increase total body calcium levels.[3,68] No firm data show that stimulation of bone formation by longitudinal compression of bone or by exercise against gravity translates into lower fracture rates, however.[42] Thus, moderate, joint sparing exercise programs remain a logical but unproved prevention strategy.

Certain nutritional modifications, on the other hand, have definite positive effects on bone mass. Positive calcium balance correlates directly with increasing calcium intake. The average intake of calcium in the North American diet is 500 to 700 mg daily. To maintain positive calcium balance, most men and premenopausal white females require 1,000 mg elemental calcium a day; postmenopausal women require 1,500 mg daily.[43,45] Therefore, supplements of 500 to 1,000 mg elemental calcium daily may be desirable for many individuals at a high risk for osteoporosis. An 8-ounce glass of milk contains approximately 300 mg calcium; calcium carbonate tablets contain about 40% calcium. Supplementation with calcium alone does reduce the rate of bone loss in postmenopausal women,[45,74] and one study showed much lower hip-fracture rates in a Yugoslavian population with a high calcium intake than in another Yugoslavian group with a low calcium intake.[56] Therefore, calcium supplementation is efficacious in preventing or reducing the rate of bone loss in some individuals and is probably safe. Hypercalcemia occurred in 1% of a population treated with calcium supplements; 1,000 mg supplemental calcium increases urinary calcium by only 70 mg/24 hour.

Strong evidence also indicates that estrogens, and probably low doses of some progestins and androgens, also prevent or slow the rate of bone loss from both appendicular and axial skeleton in perimenopausal women.[54] In individuals who have premature menopause, estrogen replacement clearly slows bone loss, is effective for at least 8 to 10 years, and cannot be discontinued without rapid bone loss. Most authorities recommend that all women with premature menopause be treated with estrogen replacement, in cyclic form, at least 0.625 mg conjugated estrogens (Premarin) 21 days out of 28, unless a specific contraindication exists.

Stabilization of bone mass, without much actual increase, can be achieved by administration of estrogen to women after a natural menopause, especially in those who are within three to five years of cessation of menses. Such replacement therapy is associated with a reduced incidence of hip fractures.[66] Supplemental estrogen administration is associated with an increased risk of endometrial hyperplasia and subsequent malignant disease,[4] however, as well as with exacerbation of hypertension, migraine headaches, and possibly with hypercoagulable states.

If estrogen is to be used to prevent osteoporosis in high-risk individuals, 0.625 mg Premarin daily is a minimal adequate dose to maintain vertebral mass. Recent evidence suggests that the higher the dose of estrogens, the greater the positive effect on bone mass. For example, a minimal daily dose of 15 μg estradiol is required to maintain bone mass; 25 μg or more are required to increase bone mass. The cyclic administration of estrogen, 3 weeks out of 4, is associated with a lower risk of endometrial cancer. The physician may wish to add progesterone, 10 mg daily during days 21 to 28, to minimize endometrial stimulation. New estrogen preparations with little stimulating effect on the endometrium are under study. At a recent National Institutes of Health Consensus Conference on Osteoporosis, the Advisory Panel recommended that cyclic estrogen therapy be considered in all women within 5 years of natural menopause, for the following reasons: (1) many more deaths per year in the United States occur from hip fractures than from endometrial cancer; (2) endometrial carcinoma is not only a rare disease, but also is usually a low-grade, curable malignant disorder; and (3) estrogen is clearly the most effective preventive strategy for maintaining bone mass in women. I agree with all these points, but I believe that data regarding estrogen effects on bone can be applied only to white women with our current state of knowledge, and that the safety of estrogens is sufficiently controversial that replacement therapy should be recommended only for women at a high risk for symptomatic osteoporosis. The use of cyclic estrogen therapy also raises the question of addition of progestagens to prevent withdrawal bleeding; some progestins have adverse effects on lipoproteins, and studies of such combination therapy to prevent osteoporosis have not been completed.

Androgens and some progestagens have similar effects to estrogens on maintaining bone mass in postmenopausal women. Androgens may be useful in men with osteoporosis; estrogens are preferable in women.

Prevention strategies are summarized in Table 97–5.

Therapy

Therapy of symptomatic osteoporosis can be frustrating to both patient and physician because of the uncertainty that any interventions will increase bone mass enough to reduce pain and fractures. Recent data suggest that it is possible to reduce vertebral and hip fracture rates with calcium, fluoride, or estrogens, however.[77]

Calcium has multiple effects on bone. It is required for mineralization, and a positive calcium balance helps to maintain bone mass, as discussed previously. That calcium also suppresses bone turnover may mean that it slows remodeling processes in which the bone-forming unit resorbs more net bone than it produces. Riggs and his colleagues have shown that the rate of recurrence of vertebral fractures can be diminished by approximately 50% if postmenopausal osteoporotic women are treated with calcium carbonate, 1,500 to 2,500 mg daily, for more than a year.[77] This benefit was seen with or without pharmacologic doses of vitamin D.

Vitamin D and its metabolites have been advocated as therapy for osteoporosis, to ensure maximal absorption of dietary calcium and to maintain positive calcium balance. Several recent studies, however, have failed to demonstrate a reduction in fracture rates or an increase in bone mass accompanying vitamin D therapy, without calcium, for osteoporosis. Hypercalciuria, defined as a urine calcium level >300 mg/24 hour, and hypercalcemia are complications of vitamin D therapy occurring in approximately 25% of patients, especially with 25-OH vitamin D and $1,25(OH)_2$ D regimens. Currently, I use supraphysiologic doses of vitamin D or its metabolites only in osteoporotic individuals who have urine calcium levels <100 mg/24 hour. For most patients, vitamin D supplementation greater than 800 U/day is probably undesirable.

Estrogens act primarily as suppressors of bone resorption and thus reduce the rate of remodeling. I have already discussed the evidence that they reduce the loss of bone mass and the hip-fracture rate in postmenopausal women.

In the studies of Recker and colleagues,[74] the combination of calcium and estrogen maintained bone mass in symptomatic postmenopausal women better than did calcium alone. In the studies of Riggs et al.,[77] the combination resulted in vertebral fracture rates much lower than in women receiving calcium alone. Therefore, I prescribe estrogen for women who are continuing to experience fractures in spite of a year or more of therapy with calcium and fluoride. One must judge whether the potential benefit outweighs the risks of endometrial carcinoma, hypertension, and thrombosis. I recommend cyclic therapy, 3 weeks of Premarin out of every 4, to minimize endometrial stimulation. Many patients experience withdrawal bleeding; progesterone, 10 mg daily, during days 21 to 28 prevents this side effect. Many authorities recommend es-

Table 97–5. Prevention of Osteoporosis

Approach	Specifics
Identification of subjects at high risk	Small, white or Oriental women; positive family history; low calcium intake
Prescription of a regular program of physical activity	3 hour/week exercise against gravity; 1–1.5 miles walking daily (suggested regimen)
Ensuring adequate calcium intake	1,000 mg/day elemental calcium in men and premenopausal women; 1,500 mg/day in postmenopausal women
Ensuring adequate vitamin D intake	400 IU/day
Estrogen replacement therapy in women with premature menopause (before age 45)	0.625 mg/day estrogen (Premarin) 3 weeks out of 4 if benefit outweighs risk (some recommend estrogen replacement in all women beginning natural menopause without contraindications; I reserve this therapy for patients at high risk for fractures)

trogen therapy in addition to calcium supplementation early in the treatment of osteoporosis and prefer it to fluoride.

Sodium fluoride has multiple effects on bone. It is the only agent currently available that stimulates formation of osteoid, even in areas that do not contain bone-remodeling units. The danger that the osteoid will not mineralize properly is real, however, so osteomalacia can be induced by fluoride treatment if the dose is high or if inadequate quantities of mineral are available. Therefore, calcium and vitamin D should be given either concomitantly with fluoride or cyclically (see Table 97–6 for recommended regimens). In addition to stimulating bone formation, fluoride incorporated into the hydroxyapatite crystal increases the density of bone. Whether that denser bone is stronger, rather than more brittle, is a point of debate. Therapy of more than a year's duration with fluoride, vitamin D, and calcium has been associated with reduced fracture rates.[77] Undesirable side effects of fluoride therapy are common and include dyspepsia, nausea, diarrhea, anorexia, peptic ulcer, rheumatic symptoms, especially plantar fasciitis, and acne; these side effects occur in 34 to 40% of patients.

In the study of Riggs et al.,[77] the combination of calcium, fluoride, vitamin D, and estrogen was more effective than any two or three of the agents in reducing vertebral fracture rates in osteoporotic women.

Other, less common therapeutic regimens include calcitonin, parathyroid hormone, anabolic hormone, and diphosphanate administration. Their use as single therapeutic agents has not met with consistent success, and the reader is referred to review articles for more information.[5] Each of these agents may be useful in combination therapy. Recent reports also suggest that daily therapy with thiazide prevents loss of bone mass and may reduce fracture rates.

Table 97–6. Treatment of Symptomatic Osteoporosis

1. Measure serum and urine calcium levels
2. If urine calcium <100 mg/24 hour
   a. Give: calcium, 1,000 mg/day
        vitamin D, 50,000 U 2 to 3 times/week*
        or 250H D, 20 µg/day
   b. Monitor urine and serum calcium every 3 to 4 months
3. If urine calcium >100 mg/24 hour
   a. Give: calcium, 1,000 mg/day
        vitamin D, 400 IU/day
   b. If new fractures occur in 6 to 12 months, add:
        sodium fluoride, 20 mg twice/day with meals* (or Luride, 2.2-mg tablets, 6 tablets 3 times/day with meals)
        calcium, 1,000 mg/day
        vitamin D, 50,000 U twice/week or 250H D, 20 µg/day
     Or cycle—6 months sodium fluoride, then discontinue
        6 months of calcium and vitamin D, then discontinue
        Repeat
   c. If new fractures occur after 12 months of therapy with regimen "b," add to the sodium fluoride, calcium, and vitamin D:
        estrogen (Premarin) 0.625 mg/day, 3 weeks out of 4*

*See text for discussion of incidence of undesirable side effects.

Frost has proposed an approach in which one cycle of therapy activates bone-remodeling units; the next cycle inactivates them before a large quantity of bone is resorbed; in the third cycle, no therapy is given, so osteoblasts are free to form bone; the sequence is then repeated.[30] Activators of bone-remodeling units might include parathyroid hormone, growth hormone, thyroxine, or regional electrical stimulation. Suppressors could include diphosphanates, calcitonin, and calcium. A related idea has been offered by Whyte et al.[88] who select therapy according to histologic features. If the patient has low bone turnover with little osteoid and little uptake of tetracycline, one might stimulate osteoid formation with fluoride, in addition to calcium and vitamin D. If the patient has a high rate of bone turnover with multiple areas of osteoid and many resorption sites, remodeling should be suppressed with calcium or estrogen, biopsy should be repeated in six to nine months, and fluoride should be prescribed only if bone turnover has been reduced.

In summary, several available therapeutic approaches to symptomatic osteoporosis, although officially considered experimental, probably reduce fracture rates. They are listed in Table 97–6. Of these, only calcium supplementation is associated with negligible side effects. How aggressive the physician should be with other therapy depends on the degree of disability of the patient and the presence of concomitant disorders.

GLUCOCORTICOID-INDUCED OSTEOPENIA

The bone loss associated with glucocorticoid therapy may be defined as another state in which the rate of bone resorption exceeds the rate of bone formation. The uncoupling of formation and resorption caused by supraphysiologic glucocorticoid levels has two mechanisms; formation is reduced, and resorption is increased. As in many other metabolic bone diseases, especially hyperparathyroid states, bone with a large surface area available for endosteal osteoclastic resorption is lost at a faster rate than compact cortical bone. Therefore, bones with high trabecular content, such as vertebrae and ribs, are at high risk of fracture, a fact recognized for decades in both spontaneous and iatrogenic Cushing's syndrome (Fig. 97–7). Bones of the appendicular skeleton also fracture at a high rate in individuals with rheumatic diseases who are treated on a long-term basis with glucocorticoids (Table 97–7).

Based on the more rapid loss of metabolically active trabecular bone than of compact cortical bone in corticosteroid osteopenia, my colleagues and I have developed a technique for identifying the disease in a population of individuals treated with corticosteroids. As shown in Figure 97–8, the metaphyseal site of the distal human radius has a higher proportion of trabecular bone than does the diaphyseal midradius.[80] In addition, endosteal resorption of cortical bone is more easily measured at metaphyseal than at diaphyseal sites of long bones. Therefore, if a single photon is passed through both diaphyseal and metaphyseal sites of the radius, one can detect differential loss of bone in these two areas. As shown in Figure 97–9, our studies have confirmed this theory; individuals re-

ceiving daily glucocorticoid therapy on a long-term basis had a much greater loss of metaphyseal mass than of diaphyseal mass, whereas individuals with rheumatoid arthritis (RA) who had never received glucocorticoids had a similar loss of metaphyseal and diaphyseal mass.[39,40] The simplest way to express these data is as the ratio of diaphyseal mass to metaphyseal mass. This ratio is constant after puberty and is the same in males and females and in blacks and whites. It does not have to be adjusted for age, sex, or race, as do separate measures of diaphyseal and metaphyseal mass. As discussed previously, the technique of single-photon osteodensitometry has its problems, and measures of appendicular bone mineral content do not correlate as well with vertebral mass as with long bone mass, but the technique is rapid, inexpensive, and useful in screening populations.

Most individuals with rheumatic diseases who receive chronic glucocorticoid therapy develop elevated ratios of diaphyseal to metaphyseal mass because they lose metaphyseal mass at a faster rate than diaphyseal mass. Although patients with primary hyperparathyroidism have a similar pattern of loss (Fig. 97–9), corticosteroid osteopenia can be distinguished easily from primary hyperparathyroidism by the presence of normal serum calcium levels and from other types of secondary hyperparathyroidism by the absence of renal failure, intestinal malabsorption, and hepatic dysfunction.

Although measures of the foregoing ratio have been a useful screening test in our hands, the technique is not widely available to the practicing physician, who must rely on routine roentgenograms to confirm the suspicion that bone mass is declining at a worrisome rate.

The histologic features of iliac crest bone biopsies can be helpful in understanding corticosteroid osteopenia (see Fig. 97–3). Formation rates are usually low, and numbers of resorption sites are increased. Trabecular bone volume is usually low. Sometimes the biopsy shows increased formation or little resorption. None of these histomorphometric findings are specific for corticosteroid osteopenia.

Incidence

Bone fractures of both the axial and the appendicular skeleton in patients receiving glucocorticoid therapy remain a major clinical problem. Such fractures occur in highest frequency in older individuals with long-standing rheumatic disease. Therefore, ''corticosteroid osteopenia'' is usually an insult added to bone loss resulting from age, the postmenopausal state, RA, or inactivity, and it causes enough bone loss to increase fracture rates in a population already at high risk. We have seen

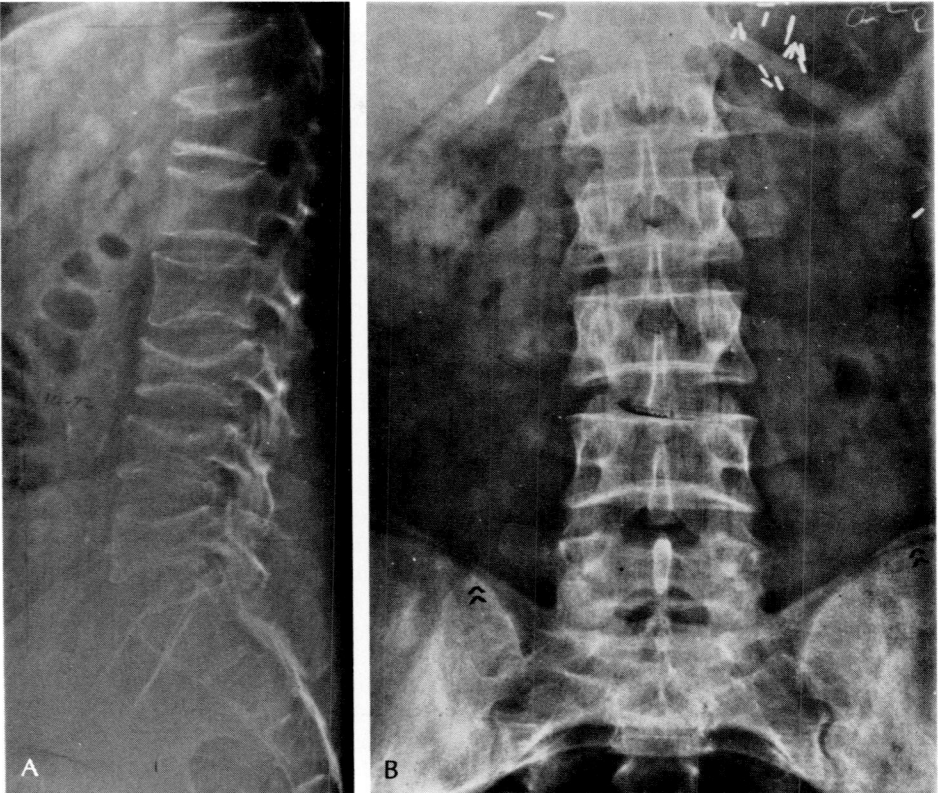

Fig. 97–7. Roentgenograms of patients with glucocorticoid-induced osteopenia. *A*, Multiple vertebral compression fractures in a middle-aged woman with rheumatoid arthritis treated for several years with 10 to 15 mg prednisone daily. Note the anterior wedging of thoracic vertebrae (T12) in contrast to the central collapse of lumbar vertebrae (L1 to L5). Similar radiographic findings occur in idiopathic or postmenopausal or senile osteoporosis. *B*, Lumbar spine and pelvis in a 24-year-old man treated for 10 years with prednisone to suppress glomerulonephritis. Note the mottled appearance of bone in the lumbar vertebrae and ilia indicating bone loss and the failure of the epiphyses of the ilia to close (arrows). (Courtesy of Richard H. Gold, M.D., Professor of Radiology, University of California, Los Angeles.)

Table 97–7. Incidence of Fractures in Rheumatic Disease Patients Receiving Long-term Glucocorticoid Therapy

	Fractures		
	Vertebral (%)	*Extravertebral (%)*	*All (%)*
Patients never receiving systemic glucocorticoid therapy	5–8	6	9
Patients receiving long-term chronic glucocorticoid therapy	12–18	19	30

vertebral fractures as early as three months after the institution of glucocorticoid therapy in older individuals.

The incidence of glucocorticoid osteopenia is not clear because of variations in definition and in populations studied. In studies in which bone mass was measured by direct weight of bones at autopsy, or by calculation of trabecular bone volume from iliac crest biopsies, 85 to 90% of patients treated with corticosteroids had much less bone mass than age-, sex-, and race-matched normal individuals.[63,87] In a cross-sectional study of 161 patients with rheumatic disease treated for more than 6 weeks with various doses of daily or alternate-day prednisone, the incidence of corticosteroid osteopenia, defined as a greater loss of metaphyseal mass than of diaphyseal mass on single-photon absorptiometry of the radius, correlated directly with the cumulative dose of prednisone (Tables 97–7, 97–8, 97–9). More than 80% of individuals who had

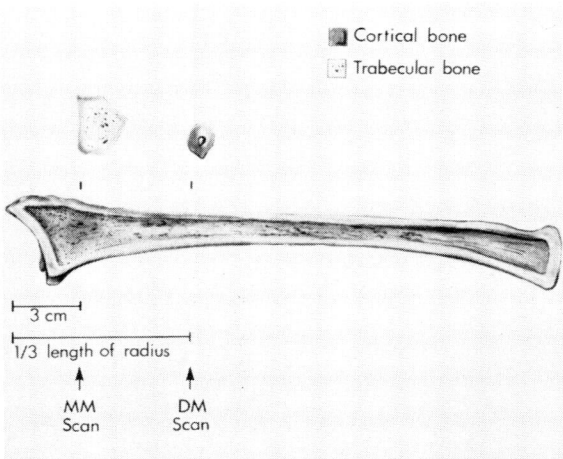

Cortical bone
Trabecular bone

3 cm

1/3 length of radius

MM
Scan

DM
Scan

Fig. 97–8. Sketch of the human radius. The midportion of the radius (diaphyseal mass—DM) contains predominantly compact cortical bone. The distal end (metaphyseal mass—MM) contains a high proportion of trabecular bone.

received >1 g prednisone had corticosteroid osteopenia.[24] *Most individuals receiving glucocorticoid therapy on a long-term basis lose bone to the extent that the risk of fracture is increased.*

Fracture rates in individuals with rheumatic diseases with or without corticosteroid therapy depend on the populations studied. For example, 60% of adults in one series had vertebral or rib fractures;[63] 18% in our study had vertebral collapse.[24] Another study of all ambulatory patients attending a rheumatic disease clinic in Salt Lake City, Utah, used lateral spine roentgenograms. In this all-white population, the incidence of vertebral crush fractures in patients who had never received oral glucocorticoid therapy was 6% in men and 8% in women, whereas in individuals receiving glucocorticoids, it was 12% in men and 16% in women. The mean age of the patients was approximately 50 years; the mean duration of corticosteroid therapy was 60.5 months; the mean daily dose was 9.6 mg prednisone or equivalent. Because my colleagues and I believe that peripheral bone fractures, especially of the shoulder or knee joints, may be as disabling as vertebral fractures, we studied the incidence of fractures in all bones, except the cervical spine and skull. In patients receiving glucocorticoid therapy at a mean daily dose of 15.6 mg prednisone, for a mean duration of 48 months, and at a median age of 50 years, the incidence of fractures in one or more vertebrae was 18%, and in one or more appendicular bones, 19%. The overall incidence of either or both sites in the same individual was 30%. Overall fracture incidence in patients not treated

with glucocorticoids from the same clinic was 9%. In all these studies, the patients receiving glucocorticoids were generally more ill than the group not treated with corticosteroids; it is difficult to control for this variable.

In summary, the available data suggest that patients with rheumatic diseases have a two- to threefold increased incidence of axial or appendicular bone fractures if they are receiving glucocorticoid therapy on a long-term basis (Table 97–8).

Risk Factors

Elderly individuals, especially white women, are the group at highest risk for disabling fractures after the institution of glucocorticoids.[79] This risk is expected because Oriental and white postmenopausal women are also the highest-risk group for fractures related to idiopathic osteoporosis. Children, with their rapidly growing bones, also are at high risk.[9] Factors that may alter this risk include sex, age, race, body build, type of rheumatic disease, duration of disease, glucocorticoid dose, duration of therapy, concomitant therapy, level of activity, nutritional status, especially vitamin D and calcium intake, and amount of exposure to sunlight.

Table 97–8 summarizes factors that increase the risk of elevated ratios of diaphyseal to metaphyseal mass and the risk of fractures.[24] An increasing cumulative glucocorticoid dose gave the strongest positive correlation with a rising ratio of diaphyseal to metaphyseal mass ($p < .05$) (see Table 97–8). Daily prednisone dose and duration of therapy did not correlate with this rising ratio, but both are obviously related to total cumulative doses. Moreover, others have shown that bone mass at the metaphyseal site of the radius falls rapidly with prednisone use, with approximately a 4% loss after 6 months,[75] and a 30% loss after 100 months.[10] Therefore, the duration of glucocorticoid therapy probably correlates inversely with bone mass. With regard to daily dose, my colleagues and I could show no direct effect beyond its relationship to the total cumulative dose. Some have suggested that a low daily dosage level of corticosteroids at which most individuals do not malabsorb calcium may be safe for bones. Klein et al.,[52] who reported that doses of prednisone <10 mg daily do not cause calcium malabsorption, but the level required to reduce the synthesis of osteoid has not been determined. Furthermore, abnormally low intestinal uptake of calcium has been found in several patients with rheumatic disease taking only 5 mg prednisone daily, with an overall fracture rate of 26% in 29 patients receiving ≤5 mg prednisone daily, a rate similar to that of patients taking higher doses.[24] Although it is my opinion that no dose of exogenous glucocorticoids is "safe" in terms of

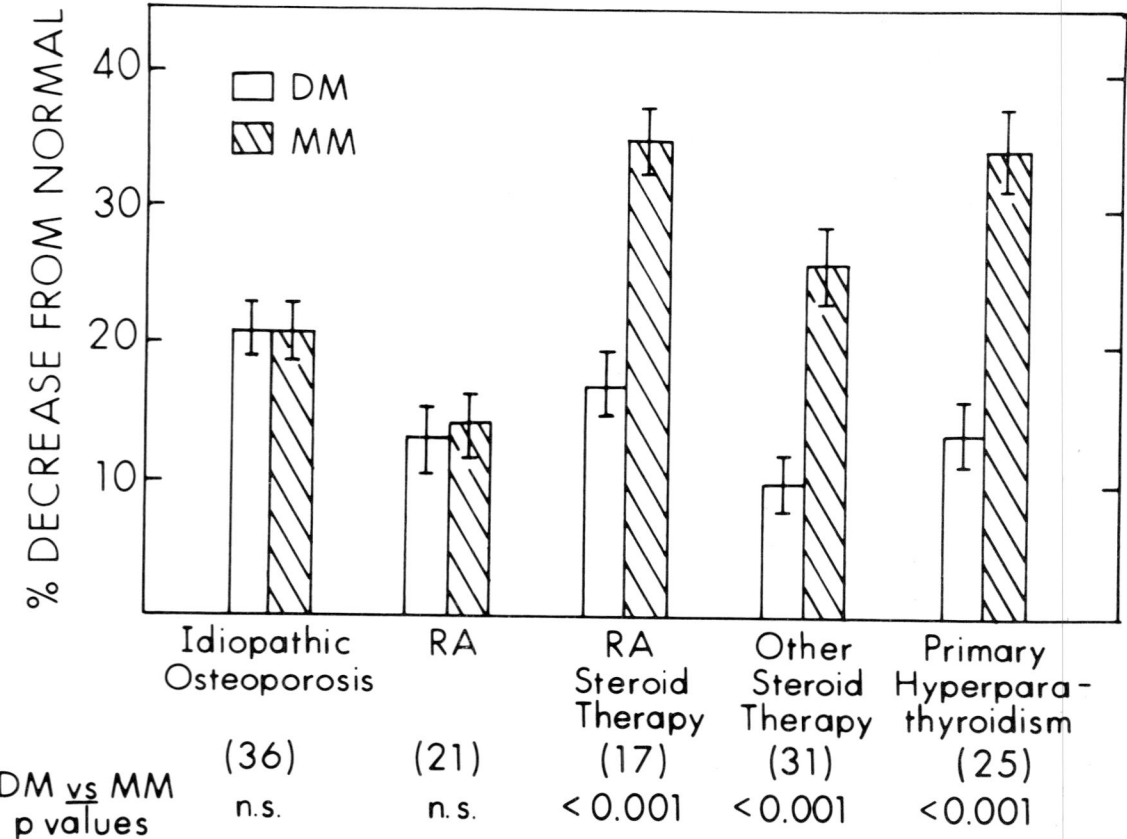

Fig. 97–9. Differential loss of bone mass from the diaphyseal (DM) and metaphyseal (MM) areas of the radius in different disease states. Bone mass is expressed as the percentage of decrease from age- and sex-matched normal individuals living in the same geographic area. In individuals receiving long-term glucocorticoid therapy, more MM is lost than DM; this pattern of bone loss is similar to that seen in primary hyperparathyroidism. RA = Rheumatoid arthritis.

Table 97–8. Daily and Cumulative Effect of Glucocorticoid Doses on Diaphyseal-to-Metaphyseal Mass Ratios (DM/MM) and Fractures

	Elevated DM/MM (%)	p*	Fractures (%)	p*
Daily Dose (mg)				
≤5	11/32 (34)		6/29 (32)	
6–20	42/105 (40)	NS	18/58 (31)	NS
>20	8/24 (33)		4/16 (25)	
Total Dose (g)				
<10	18/77 (23)		10/45 (22)	
10–30	25/61 (40)	p <.002	10/33 (30)	p <.03
>30	18/23 (78)		8/15 (53)	

*Probability by multiple regression analysis; data are based on a cross-sectional survey of 161 patients with various rheumatic diseases attending clinics at Washington University in St. Louis and receiving long-term glucocorticoid therapy. Radiographs were available in 93; the median age was 50 years, the mean prednisone dose was 15.6 mg/day, and the mean duration of therapy was 48 months.

Table 97-9.   Risk Factors for Development of Glucocorticoid-Induced Osteopenia

Definite	Probable	Unlikely
High total cumulative dose of gluco-corticoids	Increasing duration of glucocorticoid therapy	Type of rheumatic disease (when corrected for age of susceptible population)
Increasing age; individuals >50 years old (men or women) at higher risk	High daily doses of glucocorticoids Age <15 years	
Postmenopausal state	Small body size	Sex (after age of 50 years)
	White or Oriental race (may relate to size)	
	Female sex (before menopause or age 50)	

bone loss, it is logical that lower daily doses are desirable. Our data also show that alternate-day glucocorticoid regimens cause bone loss similar to that of daily regimens,[34] again suggesting that the total cumulative dose may be a more powerful risk factor than the daily dose. Others have reported less negative calcium balance in patients receiving alternate-day therapy than in those receiving daily doses,[61] less calcium malabsorption,[52] and better bone growth in animals.[82]

The second strongest risk factor correlating positively with increasing ratios of diaphyseal to metaphyseal mass and fracture rates was increasing age. Individuals over age 50 had a much higher incidence of fractures than did younger patients (p <.05); these findings were similar to those reported by others.[79] Postmenopausal women, including those with premature menopause, had a much higher fracture rate than did premenopausal women. Before age 50, the fracture rate was much lower in men than in women, but thereafter, these rates were essentially the same in both sexes.

Individuals of small body size may be at an increased risk for development of corticosteroid osteopenia. The negative correlation between increasing (precorticosteroid) body surface area and rising ratios of diaphyseal to metaphyseal mass is significant, but no difference in fracture rates has been demonstrated.

Interestingly, no correlations were noted between the type of rheumatic disease and either the ratio of diaphyseal to metaphyseal mass or fracture rates, when data were corrected for age. Clinically, we suspect that older individuals with polymyalgia rheumatica are at unusually high risk for corticosteroid-related fractures, individuals with RA are at high risk, and those with systemic lupus erythematosus are at moderate risk. Data reported by my associates support these perceptions, but show a closer relationship to age than to disease process. This finding is surprising because patients with RA who never received glucocorticoids had much less

bone mass than that found in age-, sex-, and race-matched healthy control subjects.[40]

A significant difference in the ratio of diaphyseal to metaphyseal mass or in fracture rates was not found when black and white patients were compared, but the numbers were small. My colleagues and I did not have enough Oriental or Hispanic individuals in our study group to draw any conclusions regarding race as a risk factor, but we suspect that the racial factors defined for the risk of fracture in idiopathic osteoporosis also apply to corticosteroid-treated patients.

Factors likely to increase the risk of fracture in patients with rheumatic diseases treated with glucocorticoids are listed in Table 97-9.

Mechanisms of Corticosteroid Osteopenia

Several reviews of the pathogenesis of corticosteroid-induced osteopenia have appeared.[10,39,71] The effects resulting in loss of bone are summarized in Table 97-10.

Glucocorticoids undoubtedly inhibit bone formation in vitro and in vivo. In children and in young animals, growth hormone is suppressed;[8] proliferation of epiphyseal cartilage is retarded by pharmacologic levels of glucocorticoids, and complete cessation of longitudinal growth can result (see Fig. 97-7,B).[27] Osteoblasts in culture reduce their synthesis of collagen if glucocorticoids are added to the media.[67] Collagen and noncollagen

Table 97-10.   Mechanisms by which Glucocorticoids Cause Bone Loss

Suppression of Bone Formation
   Reduced conversion of precursor cells to osteoblasts
   Reduced synthesis of osteoid by osteoblasts

Enhancement of Bone Resorption
   Reduced intestinal absorption of calcium
   Stimulation of parathyroid hormone, which activates
     osteoclasts in spite of direct suppression of osteoclast
     function by glucocorticoids

Net Result: Rate of Resorption > Rate of Formation

protein synthesis decline in cultures of fetal rat bone treated with corticosteroids on a long-term basis, and precursor cells do not differentiate into osteoblasts.[21] Decreased bone formation has been found in bone biopsies from humans treated with cortisone or related compounds.[31,51]

The mechanism by which glucocorticoids increase bone resorption is complicated. Many investigators have observed increased numbers of osteoclasts and osteoclast-resorbing surfaces in bone biopsies from patients receiving glucocorticoids.[38,51,64] In culture systems, however, glucocorticoids directly inhibit osteoclast activity.[71,72] Furthermore, short-term administration of these hormones to rats can decrease bone resorption,[89] although in humans receiving long-term glucocorticoid treatment, the indirect effect of those hormones on parathyroid hormone levels predominates. Glucocorticoids decrease the intestinal absorption of calcium and phosphate,[17,38,52] sometimes as early as seven days after the institution of corticosteroid therapy. Malabsorption of calcium stimulates the secretion of parathyroid hormone. In animals, parathyroidectomy abolishes the osteoclastic response to glucocorticoids.[48]

Some studies have shown that levels of circulating parathyroid hormone are higher in patients treated with corticosteroids than in patients with the same diseases but not receiving corticosteroid therapy.[32,38] Other studies have not confirmed that finding.[23,52] In any case, the sensitivity of bone cells to the effects of parathyroid hormone is increased by glucocorticoids. The result is a state of secondary hyperparathyroidism in which the effects of hyperparathyroidism predominate over inhibitory effects on osteoclasts, and osteoclastic resorption of bone is increased. These effects are probably greatest in osseous areas with a large surface for osteoclasts to attack, such as trabecular bone and the endosteal surfaces of cortical bone at the metaphyses of long bones.

Investigators have debated possible alterations in vitamin D metabolism during corticosteroid therapy. Serum levels of $1,25 (OH)_2D$ levels were decreased in corticosteroid-treated children in one study,[12] and these low levels correlated with decreased bone mass. In another study,[52] serum levels of 25OH D correlated inversely with the daily prednisone dose. In studies by my colleagues and myself in adults, differences in the circulating levels of 25OH D or $1,25(OH)_2D$ have not been detected.

In summary, the bone loss of corticosteroid osteopenia is caused by direct suppression of bone formation and increased bone resorption from functional hyperparathyroidism. The results are negative calcium balance[64] and a loss of bone mass that, especially when associated with senile, idiopathic, or disease-related osteoporosis in adults or in rapidly modeling bones in children, contributes to an increased risk of both vertebral and extravertebral fractures.

Diagnosis

As discussed previously, no inexpensive, simple techniques are widely available to confirm a specific diagnosis of glucocorticoid-induced osteopenia. The clinician can only suspect its presence in individuals who have received daily or alternate-day doses of corticosteroids for several months. If routine roentgenograms, especially of vertebrae, show osteopenia, the patient is probably at a high risk for fracture. Simple screening tests should be done to rule out other conditions, including hyperparathyroidism, hyperthyroidism, osteomalacia, and malignant diseases in bone. Generally, a complete blood count, creatinine determination, electrolyte measurement, liver function tests, and determinations of serum levels of calcium, phosphorus, and alkaline phosphatase should suffice. Serum levels of calcium and phosphate are almost always normal in untreated corticosteroid osteopenia. Alkaline phosphatase levels are usually normal, but they may be mildly elevated.

Treatment

The best therapy for corticosteroid-induced osteopenia is complete withdrawal of the glucocorticoids. I have observed exuberant new bone formation in iliac crest bone biopsies obtained from patients with rheumatic disease three to six months after discontinuance of prednisone therapy. Unfortunately, in patients with chronic allergic or inflammatory conditions, it is often undesirable to discontinue glucocorticoids, so other strategies are used, always with the goal of administering the smallest possible dose of this agent.

Two additional strategies might be employed. First, a glucocorticoid less toxic to bone might be formulated. Comparisons of the different types of glucocorticoids currently available in the United States have been made. At equivalent anti-inflammatory doses, they all seem to have similar effects on calcium balance.[10] One new molecule currently designated "Deflazacort," formerly "Oxazacort," in which an oxazoline ring has been added to the prednisolone molecule, has been developed in Europe. In short-term studies in healthy volunteers and in longer-term studies in patients with RA, less calcium wasting was seen with anti-inflammatory doses of Deflazacort than with equivalent doses of prednisone or betamethasone.[11,37] Whether this drug will become available, whether its calcium-sparing effects persist after several months, and whether fracture rates will be diminished remain to be seen.

For the present, only the second strategy, that is, one designed to counteract the adverse effects of glucocorticoids on bone, is practical. This approach is outlined in Table 97–11.

As noted in the discussion of idiopathic osteoporosis, evidence indicates that calcium supplementation alone can diminish the rate of bone loss in postmenopausal women and can reduce the rate of vertebral crush fractures in these individuals. Patients with rheumatic diseases who were receiving long-term glucocorticoid therapy and who had elevated ratios of diaphyseal to metaphyseal mass and intestinal malabsorption of calcium were randomized into 2 groups.[23] The first group received $1,25(OH)_2D$ and 500 mg calcium, as carbonate, daily; the second group received 500 mg calcium, as carbonate, alone. During the subsequent 18 months, most individuals in the calcium-alone group did *not* show a decline of diaphyseal or metaphyseal mass, and the appearance of their iliac crest biopsies did not change; most continued to show increased resorption surfaces. These data suggested that calcium supplementation might be useful to maintain bone mass, at least in the appendicular skeleton.

The use of vitamin D or its metabolites to prevent or to treat corticosteroid-induced osteopenia is more controversial because of the risk of hypercalciuria and hypercalcemia. Treatment with vitamin D, 250H D, or $1,25(OH)_2D$, can partially overcome the intestinal malabsorption of calcium induced by glucocorticoids.[12,18,23,38,39] Such an increase is usually associated with an increase in urinary calcium excretion, so this form of therapy requires regular monitoring of serum and urine calcium levels. Patients with past or present evidence of nephrolithiasis should probably be excluded from such therapy.

Studies by my colleagues and me on rheumatic disease patients with an elevated ratio of diaphyseal to metaphyseal mass while receiving corticosteroids demonstrated a significant increase of 8 to 15% in metaphyseal bone mass after 12 months of therapy with vitamin D, 50,000 U 3 times a week, or 250H D, 20 to 40 μg daily. In the patients receiving 250H D, we also demonstrated increased intestinal absorption of calcium, reduced serum parathyroid hormone levels, and reduced resorption surfaces and osteoclast numbers on iliac crest biopsies. Bone formation rates, judged by tetracycline labeling, were unchanged or increased.[38] In contrast, an 18-month trial of $1,25(OH)_2D$ resulted in improved calcium absorption and reduced parathyroid hormone levels, but metaphyseal mass did not increase. Although resorption surfaces were diminished in iliac crest biopsies, so was the quantity of osteoblastic osteoid.[23] In all these studies, the numbers of patients were inadequate to measure a difference in fracture rates.

In summary, if a vitamin D preparation is to be

Table 97–11. Strategies to Minimize Adverse Effects of Glucocorticoid-Induced Osteopenia

1. Maintain glucocorticoid dose at lowest level possible to control disease
2. Encourage regular exercise (against gravity) when possible to stimulate bone formation
3. Identify high-risk patients and consider prophylactic therapy as follows:
a. Allow glucocorticoid dose to stabilize and hypercalciuric effect of glucocorticoids to diminish (approximately 4 to 12 weeks)
b. Measure serum calcium, phosphate, alkaline phosphate, and 24-hour urine calcium levels

Serum studies normal *Urine calcium >120 mg/24 hour*	*Serum studies normal* *Urine calcium <120 mg/24 hour* *No history of nephrolithiasis*	*Serum studies abnormal*
Add calcium: 500 mg if <50 years old, 1,000 mg if >50 years old	Add calcium: 500 mg if <50 years old, 1,000 mg if >50 years old	Evaluate for additional cause of bone disease
Monitor serum and urine calcium levels every 6 months	Add 250H D, 20 μg/day or vitamin D, 50,000 U three times/week	
	Monitor serum and urine calcium levels every 3 to 4 weeks until stable, then every 3 to 4 months	

4. In patients who develop bone fractures after 12 to 18 months of the foregoing therapy:
   Consider adding fluoride, estrogens, or calcitonin; histologic bone study is helpful at this point; estrogen or calcitonin might be useful (or 250H D if it has not been added) when resorption is occurring at a high rate; fluoride may be useful in patients with little bone formation.
   NOTE: All the regimens listed under 3 and 4 must be considered experimental because none have been proved to reduce fracture rates in glucocorticoid-induced osteopenia.

used, and I recommend it for high-risk patients with 24-hour urine calcium levels <120 mg who are receiving corticosteroids, because they are probably severe malabsorbers of calcium, I prefer 250H D. If vitamin D intoxication occurs, 250H D can be eliminated more quickly than can vitamin D. Vitamin D is largely stored in adipose and muscle tissue,[57] and therefore it has a much longer half-life than 250H D, which has a half-life of 21 days.[85] The most potent metabolite, $1,25(OH)_2D$, may be ineffective in corticosteroid-induced osteopenia. Other investigators could *not* show an increase in bone mass in patients with hematologic and rheumatic diseases treated from the onset of prednisone therapy for 6 months with vitamin D, calcium phosphate, and sodium fluoride.[75] Treatment with either calcium alone or calcium and vitamin-D or its metabolite has not been shown to reduce fracture rates in patients with corticosteroid-induced osteopenia.

In patients who begin or continue to experience bone fractures after 6 to 12 months of therapy with calcium, with or without vitamin D, other, even more experimental, approaches must be considered. The addition of sodium fluoride would probably increase bone formation rates; the addition of estrogens or calcitonin might decrease resorption rates. The use of these regimens is detailed in the section of this chapter on idiopathic osteoporosis. In this situation, I find bone biopsy helpful. If the biopsy shows a large amount of osteoid, which indicates a surprisingly high formation rate, I am reluctant to institute fluoride. If evidence suggests active resorption of bone, then estrogen or calcitonin might be indicated.

Hypercalcemia and hypercalciuria must be sought at regular intervals in patients receiving vitamin D or its metabolites. My colleagues and I do not permit the patient's 24-hour urine calcium excretion to exceed 350 mg; no one knows at what level of urinary calcium the risk of nephrolithiasis increases, so our choice is arbitrary.

In conclusion, glucocorticoid-induced osteopenia is a major problem in terms of high incidence and high association with disability. Although the mechanisms and risk factors are understood and some potential therapies have been studied, none have been shown to lower fracture rates. The need for further investigation is clear.

OSTEOMALACIA

Osteomalacia is a pathologic loss of mineralized bone due to reduction of calcium phosphate levels to below that required for normal mineralization of bone matrix. As a result, the ratio of bone mineral to matrix is reduced, undecalcified matrix (osteoid) accumulates, and bone strength declines. The most common causes of osteomalacia begin-

ning after early childhood are as follows: (1) reduced vitamin D absorption due to biliary, proximal small bowel mucosa, or ileal disease; (2) increased vitamin D catabolism due to drug-induced increases in liver oxidase enzymes; and (3) acquired renal tubular defects with renal phosphate wasting. This third group includes acquired renal tubular phosphate leaks ("adult-onset vitamin D-resistant rickets"), the Fanconi syndrome, and renal tubular acidosis of the variety seen with the chronic dysproteinemias associated with Sjögren's syndrome, systemic lupus erythematosus, monoclonal gammopathies, and heavy metal poisoning. Additionally, an occasional patient with peptic ulcer disease develops phosphate depletion due to magnesium-alumina gel antacid abuse; large amounts of these substances convert dietary phosphate to insoluble complexes in the intestine.

Clinical and Diagnostic Features

Clinically, patients with osteomalacia have many of the symptoms commonly associated with the rheumatic diseases, including generalized aching and fatigability, proximal myopathy, periarticular tenderness, and sensory polyneuropathy.[28,35] When treated, these symptoms all remit rapidly. Radiographs may show only mild generalized demineralization, or they may be more diagnostic and may reveal multiple old rib fractures with poor callus formation or pathognomonic pseudofractures, termed Looser's zones (Fig. 97–10). The presence of nephrocalcinosis suggests renal tubular acidosis.

Characteristic of vitamin D deficiency osteomalacia are a low-normal to decreased calcium

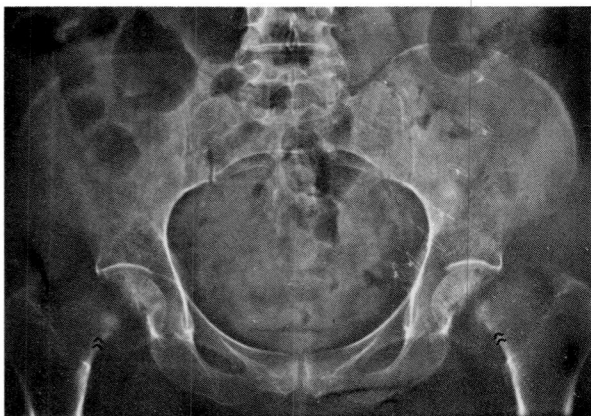

Fig. 97–10. Roentgenogram of the pelvis and hips of a patient with osteomalacia. Note the generalized osteopenia and symmetric pseudofractures in both femoral necks (arrows). (Courtesy of Richard H. Gold, M.D., Professor of Radiology, University of California, Los Angeles.)

level, hypophosphatemia, an elevated bone alkaline phosphatase level, a mild parathyroid hormone elevation, and decreased 250H D levels. In the renal phosphate leak syndromes, levels of serum calcium and 250H D are normal, but serum phosphate levels are low. A mild hyperchloremic acidosis is compatible with severe vitamin D deficiency and secondary hyperparathyroidism leading to proximal tubular bicarbonate wasting. Marked hyperchloremic hypokalemic acidosis suggests renal tubular acidosis, a diagnosis that can be confirmed by inadequate urine acidification after an ammonium chloride load. Vitamin D deficiency decreases urine calcium excretion, sometimes to undetectable levels. In the renal phosphate leak syndromes, urine calcium excretion is generally normal or, in renal tubular acidosis, elevated. In both varieties of osteomalacia, tubular reabsorption of phosphate is inappropriately low for the level of serum phosphate. Bone biopsy in patients with vitamin D deficiency shows changes of both osteomalacia and osteitis fibrosa. In pure phosphate deficiency, osteomalacia predominates.

The differential diagnosis of osteomalacia due to vitamin D deficiency includes severe dietary deprivation, which is rare, intestinal fat malabsorption syndromes, and drug-induced acceleration of hepatic vitamin D catabolism. The diagnosis of dietary deficiency can be established by a careful history, and the patient can be treated rapidly with vitamin D, 50,000 IU 3 times weekly, in addition to calcium supplementation until serum chemistries and urinary calcium excretion return to normal. At that point, an adequate diet with a 400-IU supplement of vitamin D daily is sufficient. Intestinal fat malabsorption may be readily apparent by the patient's medical history, but it is more often occult, as in smoldering ileitis with deficient bile salt reabsorption and consequent deficient solubilization of ingested fats. An adequate evaluation should include appropriate radiologic studies, quantitation of intestinal fat absorption, assessment of mucosal function by D-xylose uptake, and jejunal biopsy, if indicated. Proper treatment involves both control of the primary intestinal disorder and replenishment of body vitamin D and mineral stores. Depending on the severity of the malabsorption syndrome and the degree of vitamin D depletion, one should administer vitamin D, 50,000 IU 3 to 7 times/week, and calcium, 1,000 mg/day. In patients with unusually severe malabsorption, even higher doses may be required.

Therapeutic response can be assessed by following levels of serum calcium, phosphorus, alkaline phosphatase and 250H D, as well as 24-hour urine calcium excretion. A period of several months or longer may be required before these parameters return to normal. At that point, doses can be reduced to maintain normal serum and urine calcium levels. In these disorders especially, it is essential to monitor patients' serum and urine calcium levels frequently because improved intestinal absorption following treatment of the primary disease can lead to vitamin D intoxication if the dose is not adjusted promptly.

Drug-Induced Osteomalacia

The primary basis of this recently recognized disorder appears to be drug induction of hepatic microsomal oxidase enzymes that accelerate the conversion of vitamin D and its active metabolites to polar, inactive compounds that are rapidly excreted.[36] The anticonvulsant drugs, particularly phenobarbital and phenytoin, have been most commonly implicated. All long-acting barbiturates, many sedatives, and a variety of drugs used in rheumatic disease, such as diazepam and phenylbutazone, however, are potent hepatic oxidase inducers that could possibly reduce the levels of vitamin D metabolites. The disorder is most severe in patients with high drug doses, marginal vitamin D intake, and reduced exposure to sunlight. Serum calcium and phosphate levels may be within the normal range in all but the most severe cases; however, serum 250H D levels and urinary calcium excretion are uniformly reduced in patients with clinically significant disease.

Needle bone biopsy is useful to confirm a doubtful diagnosis. It is essential to have a high index of suspicion of this disorder. The diagnosis may be obvious in a patient who experiences seizures and who has been treated with anticonvulsants for a long time; it may be less apparent in an elderly patient with marginal dietary intake who is confined indoors and who has received barbiturate sedatives or phenylbutazone on a long-term basis. Treatment consists of repleting body vitamin D stores with 25,000 to 100,000 IU/week until serum and urine calcium and serum 250H D levels are normal; then one must compensate for the increased hepatic catabolism by supplementing with vitamin D, 1,000 to 2,000 IU/day.

In the renal tubular phosphate leak syndromes, therapy is directed toward reversing the acidosis, if present, compensating for renal phosphate wasting, and maintaining normal calcium absorption with supplemental vitamin D. In the case of an isolated tubular phosphate leak, one should prescribe vitamin D, 50,000 IU 3 times weekly, and phosphate, 1.8 to 2.4 g/day in 2 to 4 divided doses, conveniently given as Fleet's Phospho-soda, 5 ml q.i.d., and Neutra-phos, 2 capsules q.i.d. with meals. In patients with the Fanconi syndrome, it is important to correct the acidosis with bicarbonate of Shol's solution because the acidosis itself impairs bone mineral content. The effect of acidosis appears to be the result of removal of buffering anions and calcium from bone, with resultant renal calcium and phosphate loss. In pure renal tubular acidosis, alkali therapy and calcium supplementation, 500 mg/day, in addition to vitamin D, 2,000 to 5,000 IU/day, are usually sufficient. It is essential to supplement with calcium and vitamin D in renal tubular acidosis because alkali therapy alone may well precipitate tetany in a severely osteomalacic patient. When healing has occurred, vitamin D supplementation should be discontinued; relapse does not usually occur if the acidosis is controlled.

The active metabolites of vitamin D, 25 OH D_3 or $1,25(OH)_2 D_3$, may be substituted for vitamin D_2 in the treatment of osteomalacia. Both metabolites have a shorter half-life than vitamin D; therefore, toxicity can be treated more quickly. Because $1,25(OH)_2 D_3$ is the "final" metabolite, however, it may not be associated with feedback control; hypercalciuria and hypercalcemia are more frequent with $1,25(OH)_2 D_3$ than with vitamin D supplementation. For a more detailed discussion of osteomalacia and its treatment, the reader is referred to recent reviews.[28,35]

OSTEITIS FIBROSA

Osteitis fibrosa is a histological diagnosis based on the findings of increased osteoclast numbers and resorption sites with ultimate replacement of bone by fibrous tissue. The sole basis of these changes is increased secretion of parathyroid hormone, either as a primary process or as a secondary response to a prolonged hypocalcemic stimulus, such as calcium malabsorption due to vitamin D deficiency or decreased intestinal calcium absorption in the aged.

Primary Hyperparathyroidism

The initial manifestations of primary hyperparathyroidism occasionally include generalized osteopenia with vertebral compression or long-bone fractures. Associated clinical findings are a history of weakness and easy fatigability, weight loss, muscular aches and proximal muscle weakness, arthralgias, morning stiffness, or pseudogout, as well as the more classic symptoms of epigastric pain and renal colic.[55,69] Hypertension and proximal myopathy may be observed on physical examination and band keratopathy is an infrequent finding. Radiologic clues include subperiosteal bone resorption, especially in the phalanges (Fig. 97–11,A), occasional brown tumors appearing as smooth, sharply demarcated, cyst-like lesions in any part of the skeleton, and renal calculi. Subperiosteal resorption is the most consistent radiologic finding. Occasionally, erosive and sclerotic

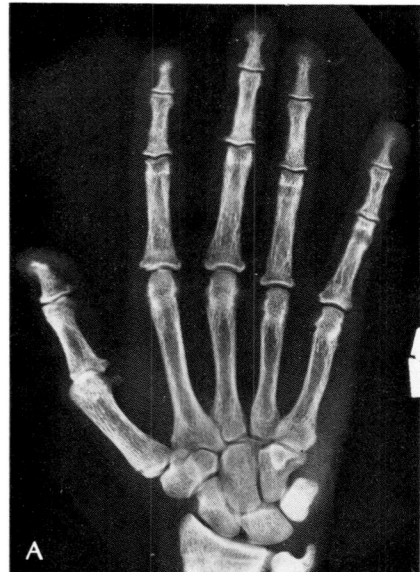

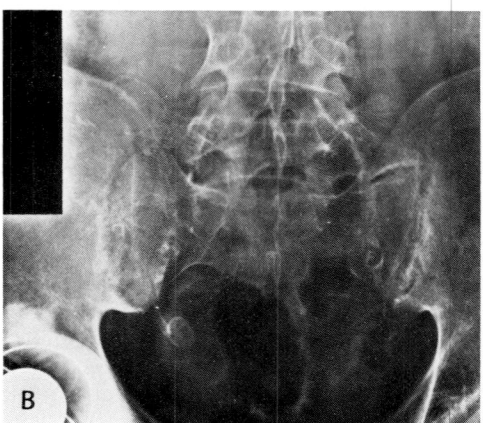

Fig. 97–11. Roentgenograms of patients with hyperparathyroidism. *A,* Hand film from a middle-aged woman with long-standing primary hyperparathyroidism. Note erosions and resorption of digital tufts, subperiosteal resorption of shafts of the proximal and middle phalanges, and bony erosions at the second and fifth metacarpophalangeal joints. *B,* Bilateral erosive changes in the sacroiliac joints in a young man with severe secondary hyperparathyroidism resulting from chronic renal failure. The right femoral head has been replaced because of ischemic necrosis. (Courtesy of Richard H. Gold, M.D., Professor of Radiology, University of California, Los Angeles.)

changes in the sacroiliac joints mimic ankylosing spondylitis (Fig. 97–11,*B*).

The diagnosis can be readily established by demonstrating a consistently elevated serum calcium level, a reduced serum phosphate level, an elevated parathyroid hormone level, and a tubular reabsorption of phosphorus inappropriately low for the level of serum phosphate. In patients with significant bone disease, the bone fraction of serum alkaline phosphatase is likely to be elevated. Hyperuricemia is frequently observed. Whereas urinary calcium excretion may be normal or even low in patients with mild primary hyperparathyroidism because of the renal calcium-retaining effects of parathyroid hormone, patients with significant bone disease usually have an elevated urinary calcium excretion because of the increased filtered load.

The only practical treatment of osteopenia due to primary hyperparathyroidism is parathyroidectomy, following which some return of bone mass is noted.[55,69] In patients who are not operative candidates, serum and urine calcium levels may be reduced by the administration of phosphorus such as Fleet's Phospho-soda, from half to a full teaspoon 3 to 4 times daily. The resultant elevation of urinary phosphate excretion increases the risk of calcium-phosphate stone formation, however, and the increased calcium × phosphate product makes metastatic soft tissue calcification more likely. Moreover, in my experience, no appreciable stabilization of bone mass occurs during phosphate therapy.

Ectopic tumor production of parathyroid hormone accounts for about 15% of cases of hypercalcemic (autonomous) hyperparathyroidism in adult populations,[55] but because of the rapid progression of the underlying malignant process, osteopenia is rarely observed. Approximately 90% of parathyroid hormone-producing tumors occur in the lung, kidney, or urogenital tract; therefore, a normal chest roentgenogram and an intravenous urogram adequately exclude this diagnosis unless definite clinical signs of malignant disease are present elsewhere.

Secondary Hyperparathyroidism

Hyperparathyroidism may be secondary to disorders that decrease intestinal calcium absorption. The commonest of these are vitamin D deficiency states and the idiopathic reduction in intestinal calcium absorption seen occasionally in older individuals. In cases of vitamin D deficiency, fatigability and myopathic symptoms are common. Diagnostic findings include low-normal to mildly reduced serum calcium levels, reduced serum phosphate levels, a mild parathyroid hormone elevation, and much reduced urinary calcium excretion. Treatment consists of restoring intestinal calcium absorption to normal (see the sections of this chapter on osteoporosis and osteomalacia). Although severe secondary hyperparathyroidism is common in chronic renal disease, the radiologic bone picture is generally mixed and can include osteomalacia, osteitis fibrosa, osteoporosis, and even patchy osteosclerosis. The osteitis fibrosa component re-

sponds to therapy with $1,25(OH)_2$ D or 1 alpha OHD, which is metabolized to $1,25(OH)_2$ D, and most patients with bone pain and myopathy benefit. The response of the osteomalacic component to this treatment is variable, however. At least some of the osteomalacia in patients undergoing renal dialysis is due to aluminum toxicity rather than to a deficiency of vitamin D.[22]

In summary, the management of the bone disease associated with renal failure and dialysis is complex and beyond the scope of this chapter, and the reader is referred to detailed reviews of the subject.[6,25]

HYPERTHYROIDISM (HIGH-TURNOVER OSTEOPOROSIS)

The bone disease of hyperthyroidism is high-turnover osteoporosis. Patients may have bone pain and fractures, in addition to other features of hyperthyroidism. Although the disease is usually endogenous, severe osteoporosis can probably be caused by the exogenous administration of thyroid hormones after decades of treatment, possibly in association with postmenopausal osteoporosis.[26] Radiographs usually show diffuse osteopenia; occasionally, abnormal striations of cortical bone are seen. Biochemical parameters usually include slight elevations in serum calcium levels and elevated serum levels of alkaline phosphatase. Urinary studies often show high levels of calcium and hydroxyproline.

The mechanism of this disease is probably direct stimulation of bone resorption by excessive levels of thyroid hormone. This process reduces the levels of serum parathyroid hormone and thereby causes renal retention of phosphate and mild elevations of serum phosphate. Both low parathyroid hormone levels and high serum phosphate levels lead to reduced activity of renal 1-alpha-hydroxylase, with a subsequent decrease in serum levels of $1,25(OH)_2$ D and an increase of $24,25 (OH)_2$ D. In spite of low $1,25(OH)_2$ D levels, bone biopsies rarely show osteomalacia. Typical findings include a high rate of bone turnover, characterized by an increase of osteoclasts and osteoclastic surfaces and increased osteoid formation surfaces, involving cortical as well as trabecular bone; mineralization is normal.[26,47] Increased porosity of cortical bone is typical.

The treatment of this disorder is correction of the hyperthyroid state.

OSTEOGENESIS IMPERFECTA

Occasionally, an adult with multiple fractures, especially on the long bones of the legs, and radiographic osteopenia, a picture typical of idiopathic osteoporosis, actually has osteogenesis imperfecta (see also Chaps. 10 and 75). This group of disorders is characterized by a genetically determined inability to form quantitatively or qualitatively normal collagen; most defects are probably in type I collagen. Most patients develop bone fractures in childhood. One prenatal form is lethal. Some of these individuals are deaf or have blue sclerae, but others have only osseous manifestations. If the disease begins in childhood, bones may grow abnormally. Extremities are short, legs are bowed, and saber shins occur. Pectus excavatum or carinatum can appear, as well as a dome-shaped forehead and lateral widening of the skull. Some individuals have lax joints, are easily bruised, or have small, misshapen, discolored teeth. Fractures usually diminish in frequency at puberty, but they often increase around the time of menopause in women and at a similar age in men.

If none of the phenotypic characteristics of osteogenesis imperfecta are present except for fragile bones, the diagnosis can be difficult. Helpful in establishing the diagnosis are a positive family history and a history of multiple fractures in childhood. Radiographs show thinning of cortical and trabecular areas of bones indistinguishable from that seen in other osteopenias. Platybasia of the skull and bone islands in the cranium also suggest osteogenesis imperfecta. Bone biopsy shows diminished quantities of osteoid with replacement by a blue-staining material. Therapy with sodium fluoride or with sex hormones has been advocated, but it is not clear whether any interventions reduce fracture rates. For a discussion of the different types of this disorder, the reader is referred to recent reviews and to Chapters 10 and 75.[53,83]

REFERENCES

1. Aitken, J.M., et al.: Osteoporosis after oophorectomy for nonmalignant disease in premenopausal women. Br. Med. J., 2:325–328, 1973a.
2. Aitken, J.M., Hart, D.M., and Lindsay, R.: Estrogen replacement therapy for prevention of osteoporosis after oophorectomy. Br. Med. J., 2:515–518, 1973b.
3. Aloia, J.F., et al.: Prevention of involutional bone loss by exercise. Ann. Intern. Med., 89:356–358, 1978.
4. Antunes, C.M.F., et al.: Endometrial cancer and estrogen use. N. Engl. J. Med., 300:9–13, 1979.
5. Avioli, L.V.: Calcitonin therapy for bone disease and hypercalcemia. Arch. Intern. Med., 142:2,076–2,079, 1982.
6. Avioli, L.V.: Renal osteodystrophy. In The Kidney. Edited by B. Brenner and F.C. Rector, Jr. Philadelphia, W.B. Saunders, 1976.
7. Avioli, L.V., McDonald, J.E., and Lee, S.W.: The influence of age on the intestinal absorption of ⁴⁷calcium in women and its relation to ⁴⁷Ca absorption in postmenopausal osteoporosis. J. Clin. Invest., 44:1,960–1,967, 1965.
8. Baxter, J.D.: Mechanisms of glucocorticoid inhibition of growth. Kidney Int., 14:330–333, 1978.
9. Bradley, B.W., and Ansell, B.M.: Fractures in Still's disease. Ann. Rheum. Dis., 19:135–142, 1960.
10. Caniggia, A., et al.: Pathophysiology of the adverse effects of glucoactive corticosteroids on calcium metabolism in man. J. Steroid Biochem., 15:153–161, 1981.
11. Caniggia, A., et al.: Effects of a new glucocorticoid, oxazacort, on some variables connected with bone metabolism in man: a comparison with prednisone. Int. J. Clin. Pharmacol. Biopharm., 15:126–134, 1977.
12. Chesney, R.W., et al.: Reduction of serum 1,25 dihydroxyvitamin D₃ in children receiving glucocorticoids. Lancet, 2:1,123–1,125, 1978.
13. Chesnut, C.H., et al.: Effect of methandrostendone on postmenopausal bone wasting as assessed by changes in total bone mineral mass. Metabolism, 26:267–277, 1977.
14. Clegg, D.O., Egger, M.J., and Ward, J.R.: Osteoporotic vertebral compression fractures. (Abstract.) Arthritis Rheum., 26:547, 1983.
15. Cohn, S.H.: Total body neutron activation. In Noninvasive Bone Measurements of Bone Mass and their Clinical Application. Edited by S.H. Cohn. Boca Raton, CRC Press, 1981, pp. 192–210.
16. Colbert, C., and Bachtell, R.S.: Radiographic absorptiometry (photodensitometry). In Noninvasive Bone Measurements of Bone Mass and their Clinical Application. Edited by S.H. Cohn. Boca Raton, CRC Press, 1981, pp. 52–82.
17. Collins, E.J., Garret, E.R., and Johnston, R.L.: Effects of adrenal steroids on radio-calcium metabolism in dogs. Metabolism, 11:716–726, 1962.
18. Condon, J.R., et al.: Possible prevention and treatment of steroid-induced osteoporosis. Postgrad. Med. J., 54:249–252, 1978.
19. Curtiss, P.H., Clark, W.S., and Herndon, C.H.: Vertebral fractures resulting from prolonged cortisone and corticotrophin therapy. JAMA, 156:467–470, 1954.
20. Dalen, N., Hallberg, D., and Lamke, B.: Bone mass in obese subjects. Acta Med. Scand., 197:353–355, 1975.
21. Dietrich, J.W., et al.: Effects of glucocorticoids on fetal rat bone collagen synthesis in vitro. Endocrinology, 104:715–721, 1979.
22. Drueke, T.: Dialysis osteomalacia and aluminum intoxication. Nephron, 26:207–210, 1980.
23. Dykman, T.R., et al.: Responses of patients with glucocorticoid osteopenia to oral 1,25 dihydroxy vitamin D (OH₂D). Arthritis Rheum., In press.
24. Dykman, T.R., et al.: Steroid osteopenia in rheumatic diseases: incidence and risk factors in rheumatologic patients treated with prednisone. Arthritis Rheum., 26:547, 1983.
25. Editorial: Treatment of renal bone disease. Lancet, 2:1,339–1,340, 1979.
26. Fallon, M.D., et al.: Exogenous hyperthyroidism with osteoporosis. Arch. Intern. Med., 143:442–444, 1983.
27. Follis, R.H.: Effect of cortisone on growing bones of the rat. Proc. Soc. Exp. Biol., 76:722–724, 1954.
28. Frame, B.: Osteomalacia. In Internal Medicine. Edited by J.H. Stein. Boston, Little, Brown, 1983, pp. 1,856–1,860.
29. Frost, H.M.: Clinical management of the symptomatic osteoporotic patient. In Symposium of the Osteoporoses. Edited by H.M. Frost. Orthop. Clin. North Am., 12:671–681, 1981.
30. Frost, H.M.: Coherence treatment of osteoporoses. In Symposium on the Osteoporoses. Edited by H.M. Frost. Orthop. Clin. North Am., 12:649–669, 1981.
31. Frost, H.M., and Villanueva, A.R.: Human osteoblastic activity. III. The effect of cortisone on lamellar osteoblastic activity. Henry Ford Hosp. Med. Bull., 9:97–100, 1961.
32. Fucik, R.F., Kukreja, S.C., and Hargis, G.K.: Effect of glucocorticoids on function of the parathyroid glands in man. J. Clin. Endocrinol. Metab., 40:152–155, 1975.
33. Genant, H., et al.: Computed tomography. In Noninvasive Bone Measurements of Bone Mass and their Clinical Applications. Edited by S.H. Cohn. Boca Raton, CRC Press, 1981, pp. 122–147.
34. Gluck, O.S., et al.: Bone loss in adults receiving alternate day glucocorticoid therapy: a comparison with daily therapy. Arthritis Rheum., 24:892–898, 1981.
35. Goldring, S.R., and Krane, S.M.: Metabolic bone disease: osteoporosis and osteomalacia. DM, 27:1–103, 1981.
36. Hahn, T.J.: Drug-induced disorders of vitamin D and mineral metabolism. Clin. Endocrinol Metab., 9:107–129, 1980.
37. Hahn, T.J., et al.: Comparison of subacute effects of oxazacort and prednisone on mineral metabolism in man. Calcif. Tissue Int., 31:109–115, 1980.
38. Hahn, T.J., et al.: Altered mineral metabolism in glucocorticoid-induced osteopenia: effect of 25-hydroxyvitamin D administration. J. Clin. Invest., 64:655–665, 1979.
39. Hahn, T.J., and Hahn, B.H.: Osteopenia in patients with rheumatic diseases: principles of diagnosis and therapy. Semin. Arthritis Rheum., 6:230–253, 1976.
40. Hahn, T.J., Boisseau, V.C., and Avioli, L.V.: Effect of

chronic corticosteroid administration on diaphyseal and metaphyseal bone mass. J. Clin. Endocrinol. Metab., *39*:274–282, 1974.

41. Harrison, J.E., Murray, T.M., and Bright-Lee, E.: Recent advances in osteoporosis (Symposium). Clin. Invest. Med., *5*:135–201, 1980.

42. Hartman, D.A., et al.: Attempts to prevent disuse osteoporosis by treatment with calcitonin, longitudinal compression, and supplementary calcium and phosphate. J. Clin. Endocrinol. Metab., *36*:845–858, 1973.

43. Heaney, R.P.: Management of osteoporosis: nutritional considerations. Clin. Invest. Med., *5*:185–187, 1982.

44. Heaney, R.P., Recker, R.R., and Saville, P.D.: Menopausal changes in calcium balance performance. J. Lab. Clin. Med., *92*:953–963, 1978.

45. Heaney, R.P., Recker, R.R., and Saville, P.D.: Calcium balance and calcium requirements in middle-aged women. Am. J. Clin. Nutr., *30*:1,603–1,611, 1977.

46. Howland, W.J., Pugh, D.G., and Sprague, R.G.: Roentgenologic changes of the skeletal system in Cushing's syndrome. Radiology, *71*:69–78, 1958.

47. Jastrup, B., et al.: Serum levels of vitamin D metabolites and bone remodeling in hyperthyroidism. Metabolism, *31*:126–132, 1982.

48. Jee, W.S.S., et al.: Corticosteroid and bone. Am. J. Anat., *129*:477–480, 1970.

49. Jensen, J.S., and Tondevold, E.: Mortality after hip fractures. Acta Orthop. Scand., *50*:161–167, 1979.

50. Johnson, K.A., et al.: Osteoid tissue in normal and osteoporotic individuals. J. Clin. Endocrinol. Metab., *33*:745–751, 1971.

51. Jowsey, J., and Riggs, B.L.: Bone formation in hypercortisonism. Acta Endocrinol., *63*:21–31, 1970.

52. Klein, R.G., et al.: Intestinal calcium absorption in exogenous hypercortisonism—role of 25-hydroxyvitamin D and corticosteroid dose. J. Clin. Invest., *60*:253–259, 1977.

53. Krane, S.M.: Osteogenesis imperfecta. *In* Internal Medicine. Edited by J.H. Stein. Boston, Little, Brown, 1983, pp. 1,122–1,123.

54. Lindsay, R., Hart, D.M., and Baird, C.: Prevention of spinal osteoporosis in oophorectemized women. Lancet, *2*:1,151–1,157, 1980.

55. Mallatte, L.E., et al.: Primary hyperparathyroidism: clinical and biochemical features. Medicine, *53*:127, 1974.

56. Matkovic, V., et al.: Fracture rates in two regions of Yugoslavia. Am. J. Clin. Nutr., *32*:540–549, 1979.

57. Mawer, E.B., Blackhouse, J., and Holman, C.: The distribution and storage of vitamin D and its metabolites in man. Clin. Sci., *43*:413–420, 1972.

58. Mazess, R.B.: Photon Absorptiometry. *In* Noninvasive Bone Measurements of Bone Mass and their Clinical Application. Edited by S.H. Cohn. Boca Raton, CRC Press, 1981, pp. 86–93.

59. Mazess, R.B., and Mather, W.E.: Bone mineral content in Canadian Eskimos. Hum. Biol., *47*:45–63, 1975.

60. Meema, H.E., and Meema, S.: Radiogrammetry in noninvasive measurements of bone mass and their clinical application. *In* Noninvasive Bone Measurements of Bone Mass and their Clinical Application. Edited by S.H. Cohn. Boca Raton, CRC Press, 1981, pp. 6–43.

61. Melby, J.C.: Systemic corticosteroid therapy—pharmacology and endocrinologic considerations. Ann. Intern. Med., *81*:505–521, 1974.

62. Melson, F., and Mosekilde, L.: The role of bone biopsy in the diagnosis of metabolic bone disease. Orthop. Clin. North Am., *12*:571–602, 1981.

63. Meunier, P.J., and Bressot, C.: Endocrine influence on bone cells and bone remodeling evaluated by clinical histomorphometry. *In* The Endocrinology of Calcium Metabolism. Edited by J.A. Parson. New York, Raven Press, 1982.

64. Nordin, B.E.C., et al.: The effects of sex steroid and corticosteroid bone hormones on bone. J. Steroid Biochem., *15*:171–174, 1981.

65. Nordin, B.E.C., et al.: Treatment of spinal osteoporosis

in postmenopausal women. Br. Med. J., *280*:451–454, 1980.

66. Paganini-Hill, A., et al.: Menopausal estrogen therapy and hip fractures. Ann. Intern. Med., *95*:28–31, 1981.

67. Peck, W.A., Brandt, J., and Miller, T.: Hydrocortisone-induced inhibition of protein synthesis and uridine incorporation in isolated bone cells in vitro. Proc. Natl. Acad. Sci. U.S.A., *57*:1,599–1,602, 1967.

68. President's Council on Physical Fitness: Adult Physical Fitness: A Program for Men and Women. Washington, D.C., United States Government Printing Office, 1965.

69. Purnell, D.C., et al.: Primary hyperthyroidism: a prospective clinical study. Am. J. Med., *50*:670, 1971.

70. Raisz, L.G.: Osteoporosis. J. Am. Geriatr. Soc., *30*:127–138, 1982.

71. Raisz, L.G.: Effect of corticosteroids on calcium metabolism. Prog. Biochem. Pharmacol., *17*:212–219, 1980.

72. Raisz, L.G., et al.: Effects of glucocorticoids on bone resorption in tissue culture. Endocrinology, *90*:961–967, 1972.

73. Recker, R.R.: Continuous treatment of osteoporosis: current status. *In* Symposium of the Osteoporoses. Edited by H.M. Frost. Orthop. Clin. North Am., *12*:611–627, 1981.

74. Recker, R.R., Saville, P.D., and Heaney, R.P.: Effect of estrogens and calcium carbonate on bone loss in postmenopausal women. Ann. Intern. Med., *87*:649–655, 1977.

75. Rickers, H., et al.: Corticosteroid-induced osteopenia and vitamin D metabolism: effect of vitamin D_2, calcium phosphate and sodium fluoride administration. Clin. Endocrinol., *16*:409–415, 1982.

76. Riggs, B.L., et al.: Changes in the bone mineral density of the proximal femur and spine with aging: difference between the postmenopausal and senile osteoporosis syndromes. J. Clin. Invest., *70*:716–723, 1982.

77. Riggs, B.L., et al.: Effect of the fluoride calcium regimen on vertebral fracture occurrence in postmenopausal osteoporosis: comparison with conventional therapy. N. Engl. J. Med., *306*:446–450, 1982.

78. Riggs, B.L., et al.: Differential changes in bone mineral density of the appendicular and axial skeleton with aging: relationship to spinal osteoporosis. J. Clin. Invest., *67*:328–335, 1981.

79. Saville, P.D., and Karmosh, O.: Osteoporosis of rheumatoid arthritis: influence of age, sex and corticosteroids. Arthritis Rheum., *10*:423–430, 1967.

80. Schlenker, R.A., and von Seggen, W.W.: The distribution of cortical and trabecular bone mass along the lengths of the radius and ulna and the implications for in vivo bone mass measurements. Calcif. Tissue Res., *20*:41–52, 1976.

81. Seeman, E., et al.: Differential effects of endocrine dysfunction on the axial and appendicular skeleton. J. Clin. Invest., *69*:1,302–1,308, 1982.

82. Sheagren, J.N., et al.: Effect on bone growth of daily versus alternate-day corticosteroid administration: an experimental study. J. Lab. Clin. Med., *89*:120–130, 1977.

83. Sillence, D.O., Remoin, D.L., and Danks, D.M.: Clinical variability in osteogenesis imperfecta—variable expressivity or genetic heterogeneity. Birth Defects, *15*:113–129, 1979.

84. Smith, D.M., et al.: Genetic factors in determining bone mass. J. Clin. Invest., *52*:2,800–2,808, 1973.

85. Smith, J.E., and Goodman, D.J.: The turnover and transport of vitamin D and a polar metabolite with the properties of 25-hydroxycholecalciferol in human plasma. J. Clin. Invest., *50*:2,159–2,167, 1971.

86. Soffer, L.J., Iannaccone, A., and Gabrilove, J.L.: Cushing's syndrome: a study of 50 patients. Am. J. Med., *30*:129–138, 1961.

87. Sussman, C.B.: The roentgenologic appearance of the bones in Cushing's syndrome. Radiology, *39*:288–292, 1942.

88. Whyte, M.P., et al.: Postmenopausal osteoporosis. A heterogeneous disorder as assessed by histomorphometric analysis of iliac crest bone from untreated patients. Am. J. Med., *72*:193–201, 1982.

89. Yasumura, S.: Effects of adrenal steroids on resorption in rats. Am. J. Physiol., *230*:90–93, 1976.

Chapter 98

Rheumatic Aspects of Endocrinopathies

Revised by Mary E. Cronin

Hormonal excess or deprivation can lead to a variety of distinctive rheumatologic syndromes. Their recognition is important because they are often treatable. Rheumatic complaints are sometimes the presenting symptom of endocrinopathy, and awareness of these features can suggest the appropriate diagnosis. Such states of altered hormonal balance, including pregnancy, have shed light on the pathogenesis of some rheumatic disorders and promise new insights into their treatment. These relationships are fully described here; standard endocrinology texts are recommeneded for additional information on hormones, diagnosis, and treatment of the endocrinopathies.

ACROMEGALY

Pituitary adenomas may produce excessive quantities of growth hormone, the anabolic effects of which can lead to significant changes in the connective tissues and bony skeleton. Usually, these tumors occur in older individuals, in whom epiphyseal closure has already taken place, and acromegaly results. Excessive growth hormone production before puberty results in gigantism. Although many of the anabolic influences derive from the direct action of this hormone, experimental evidence indicates that stimulation of chondroitin sulfate and collagen synthesis by articular chondrocytes are due to a hepatically derived serum factor called somatomedin or "sulfation factor" induced by growth hormone.[78]

Growth hormone stimulates the proliferation of soft tissues including bursae, joint capsules, synovium, cartilage (Fig. 98–1), and bone. Soft tissue changes of special interest to the rheumatologist include coarse, thickened digits, bursal thickening due to noninflammatory fibrous hyperplasia, particularly of the prepatellar, olecranon, and subacromial bursae, and joint capsular hypertrophy and laxity permitting joint hypermobility. Synovial thickening, villous and usually noninflammatory, is due to increased adipose and fibrous tissue rather than to synovial lining cell hyperplasia. An abnormally thickened heel pad can be found in 35% of acromegalic patients.[79] The contribution of so-

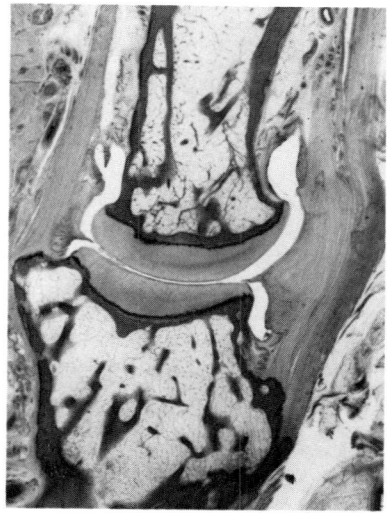

Fig. 98–1. Midsagittal section through the distal toe of a 50-year-old acromegalic man; one sees irregular hypertrophy and hyperplasia of the cartilage and bony overgrowth at the joint margins with sparse, thickened trabeculae (Courtesy of R.T. McCluskey, M.D., Department of Pathology, Massachusetts General Hospital, Boston.)

dium and water retention to the observed soft tissue thickening needs further clarification.

In adults, most endochondral tissues are not as susceptible to growth hormone as they are in the prepubertal state, but some cartilage remains responsive, as in the mandibular condyle, in which the jaw may actually lengthen, and in the costochondral junctions, in which fusiform enlargement may take place leading to a beading pattern and rib lengthening.[90] This process results in an increased anteroposterior diameter of the chest. Cartilaginous overgrowth may even occur in the larynx, interfering with speech and, rarely, with respiratory function. The cartilage space in the joints can be easily quantitated by measuring the second metacarpal phalangeal "joint space" on an anteroposterior radiogram. The normal space in men is less than 3 mm and in women is less than 2 mm. Approximately one-third of acromegalics have increased joint spaces.[1]

Bony thickening results in a thickened calvarium, an enlarged mandible, and *hyperostosis frontalis interna.* Another characteristic finding is widening of the distal ungual tufts, seen in 67% of patients.[1] This widening can lead to a clinical appearance of the hands similar to that of clubbing, but true clubbing is not part of acromegaly. The sesamoid bones are enlarged in approximately half these patients, and even the stapedial footplate of the ear may be affected, causing auditory symptoms.

The rheumatologic manifestations of acromegaly listed in Table 98–1 are found frequently if sought by careful medical history, physical examination, and appropriate laboratory testing. Their presence seems to correlate more with the duration of disease than with absolute levels of growth hormone. With the exception of soft tissue thickening, carpal tunnel symptoms, and paresthesias, many of these rheumatologic consequences of prolonged exposure to growth hormone do not remit with ablative pituitary therapy.

Arthropathy

In general, the usual manifestations of acromegalic arthropathy resemble those of osteoarthritis, with cartilaginous thickening and hypermobility as important distinguishing features. Involvement of large and small peripheral joints has been noted and may occur in as many as 75% of patients.[41] The arthropathy may consist of a noninflammatory proliferation of articular and periarticular structures, with osteophytosis and degenerative changes of the articular cartilage. Kellgren et al. divided the arthropathy into an early form consisting of

hypermobility, recurrent effusions, and widened joint spaces, and an advanced form with bony hypertrophy, loss of motion, and development of deformities.[41] Human necropsy studies and animal experimentation using exogenous growth hormone to produce polyarticular lesions have shed light on the pathogenesis of these changes.[6] The cartilaginous matrix, although massively thickened in acromegaly, is laid down in a random manner, and degenerative changes arise in the middle and basal layers. This process leads to friability, fissuring, and ulceration. Joint hypermobility and laxity due to capsular hypertrophy and redundancy accelerate this degenerative process.

These osteoarthritis-like changes may be monarticular or polyarticular, and they can affect the knees, shoulders, hips, or hands; the elbows and ankles are involved less frequently. Occasionally, patients are afflicted with intermittent painful episodes lasting weeks or months. The exact mechanism responsible for this presentation and the possible role of crystals in its induction remain to be determined. Less commonly, patients complain initially of joint pain and morning stiffness. This presentation, together with the elevated erythrocyte sedimentation rate seen in some patients,[41] can cause confusion with rheumatoid arthritis (RA).

Physical examination often reveals many of the characteristics of osteoarthritis. As mentioned previously, an unusually pronounced degree of joint crepitation, attributed to cartilaginous thickening and joint hypermobility, help to differentiate acromegalic arthropathy from primary osteoarthritis. Palpable dorsal phalangeal ridging just distal to the proximal interphalangeal joints may also be helpful in the diagnosis. Thickened synovium and periarticular tissues may have a swollen appearance, but synovial effusions are rare, and when present are

Table 98–1.   Rheumatologic Manifestations of Acromegaly

Tissue overgrowth	Bursal hyperplasia
	Capsular thickening
	Synovial proliferation and edema
	Cartilage hyperplasia
	Bony proliferation
Arthropathy	Hypermobility of joints
	Cartilage degeneration
	Bony remodeling with osteophytosis and periosteal reaction
	Intermittent (crystal-induced?) synovitis
Muscle abnormalities	Increased muscle mass
	Proximal weakness, fatigue, myalgias, cramps
Neuropathy	Palpable peripheral nerves
	Peripheral neuropathy
	Carpal tunnel syndrome
Others	Back pain and hypermobility
	Kyphosis
	Raynaud's phenomenon

noninflammatory, contain no crystals, and have low leukocyte counts, such as those in synovial fluids in noninflammatory osteoarthritis.

The main radiographic features of acromegaly include widened cartilage spaces, enlarged bones with periosteal remodeling and increased density along the shaft, marginal osteophyte formation, and calcified tendinous and capsular insertions.[6,41] Exostoses at the sites of ligamentous attachments may impart a "squared-off" appearance at bone ends. Although thickening of the trabeculae at the epiphyses occurs, the simultaneous widening may lead to an osteoporotic appearance while the diaphyses remain dense; this phenomenon is especially common at the metacarpal and metatarsal heads (Fig. 98–2). The humeral and femoral heads may develop a mushroom configuration along with the joint-space widening. In the knees, hypertrophic spurring with flaring of the femoral and tibial condyles may be found.

Troublesome symptoms can be treated with nonsteroidal anti-inflammatory agents and other conservative measures, as in osteoarthritis (see Chaps. 28, 44, 90). Aspiration of joint effusions is usually sufficient to promote their resolution. Although intra-articular corticosteroids are reported to be ineffective, a controlled evaluation has not been conducted. Advanced degenerative changes may be treated successfully with surgical intervention, and preoperative corticosteroid administration may be required in a previously treated acromegalic patient who has developed pituitary insufficiency. Owing to the irreversibility of acromegalic arthropathy in spite of pituitary ablation, early diagnosis and treatment of this endocrine disorder prior to the development of significant joint changes are essential.

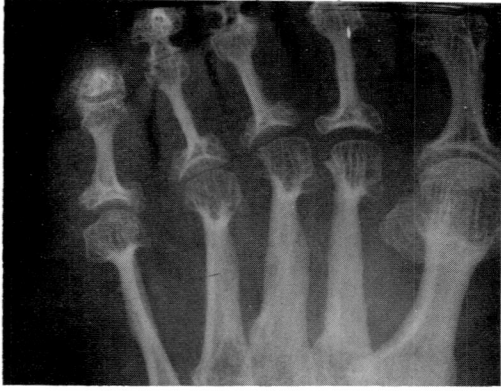

Fig. 98–2. Radiograph of an acromegalic foot showing widened joint spaces, periosteal proliferation, dense diaphyses with pipe-stem configuration, and thickened and widely spaced trabeculae giving a porotic appearance at the metatarsal heads. (From Kellgren, J.H., et al.[41])

Myopathy

Up to 50% of acromegalics with long-standing disease develop a proximal myopathy. Animal experimentation has shown that growth hormone preferentially increases proximal muscle mass, but the muscle is functionally inefficient. Results of examinations of muscle biopsies from patients with acromegaly have been conflicting, but both hypertrophic and atrophic changes have been reported to occur separately or concurrently. Type I fiber hypertrophy, perhaps secondary to peripheral neuropathy, and type IIa and type IIb muscle fiber atrophy predominate. The atrophy is not that of disuse, which primarily affects type I fibers. Disease duration, but not growth hormone levels, correlates with biopsy findings.[52] Ultrastructural findings consist of glycogen and lipofuscin deposits, coiled membranous bodies (probably phospholipid),[69] and pleomorphic mitochondria with abnormal cristae and vacuolization. These abnormalities are consistent with the known influence on glycogen uptake in skeletal muscle by growth hormone and its stimulation of RNA turnover. A definite causal relationship between the mitochondrial disruption noted by electron microscopy and the decreased muscle strength noted clinically has not been established.

The main symptoms are those of proximal weakness and decreased exercise tolerance. Less frequent are myalgias, cramps, and muscle twitching. The muscles may feel flabby, with weakness out of proportion to muscle mass.

The serum creatine phosphokinase and aldolase levels, although usually normal in acromegaly, may be increased as a reflection of patchy necrosis. The electromyogram is abnormal in most acromegalic patients with myopathy, even those without demonstrable weakness, but the findings of low-amplitude, short-duration, and polyphasic potentials are nonspecific myopathic findings.

Return of normal strength after pituitary ablative therapy is gradual and may be incomplete even after two years.[63]

Neuropathy

As noted in Table 98–1, several forms of neuropathy are associated with acromegaly. These neuropathies do not correlate with increased growth hormone levels, may be independent of carpal tunnel syndrome, and may occur without concomitant diabetes mellitus. The pathologic mechanisms are varied and consist of the following: (1) possible metabolic effects on the neuron directly or indirectly related to growth hormone; (2) compression of the spinal cord secondary to bony (foramen magnum, vertebral body) and paraspinal connective tissue overgrowth; and (3) ischemic neuropathy secondary to proliferation of endoneural and perineural tissues. Vague paresthesias involving several peripheral nerves and presumably having a metabolic basis may be the earliest form of neuropathy. These symptoms resolve after treatment of acromegaly. In a series of 11 acromegalic patients, 5 had palpable enlargement of the ulnar or popliteal nerves with paresthesias, decreased or absent deep tendon reflexes, distal wasting, and even footdrop.[47] Sensory loss with decreased vibratory and position sense has also been seen. Microscopic studies of peripheral nerves have revealed a decrease in both myelinated and unmyelinated fibers, with segmental demyelination and remyelination and occasional axonal degeneration. The supporting neural tissues are increased, with marked proliferation, particularly in the hypertrophic form.[47]

Carpal Tunnel Syndrome

A clinically typical carpal tunnel syndrome, usually bilateral, develops in as many as 50% of patients with acromegaly.[6] Although encroachment on the carpal tunnel by enlarging bone and soft tissue is a major part of the pathogenesis of this disorder, local swelling and hypertrophy of the median nerve itself may also contribute. Edema has been observed beneath the transverse carpal ligament at operation. Presumably, the disappearance of this soft tissue swelling after pituitary therapy accounts for the rapid improvement in carpal tunnel symptoms, but the recovery of nerve conduction velocities is more prolonged.

Back Pain

Nearly half of acromegalic patients complain of back pain during the course of their disease. Although most symptoms are in the lumbosacral spine, cervical and thoracic involvement may also occur. In spite of severe pain and sometimes advanced radiographic changes, these patients may have hypermobility of the spine. This striking finding may be a key in distinguishing between this and other spinal disorders and is presumably due to the enlarged intervertebral discs, which retain their resiliency and turgor.[6] Such mobility may be disadvantageous, causing accelerated spinal degeneration and osteophyte formation. On radiographic examination, disc spaces are normal or increased, and occasionally calcified. Hypertrophic spurring develops at the anterior vertebral margin. Posteriorly, the exaggeration of the normal concavity of the vertebral body is probably caused by remodeling or pressure from paraspinal tissues. Kyphosis is frequently observed, possibly secondary to the barrel-chest deformity related to rib elongation.

Raynaud's Phenomenon

This phenomenon has been reported in approximately one-third of acromegalic patients in one series.[41] Although the exact mechanism is uncertain, thickening of the blood vessel walls may contribute to its development.

Gigantism

The accelerated endochondral ossification and lengthening of tubular bone that can occur in the prepubertal patient with a pituitary adenoma is termed gigantism. Because this disorder is rare, the true incidence of rheumatologic manifestations is not known, but the arthropathy, myopathy, and hypertrophic neuropathy noted in acromegaly occur in this entity as well. The incidence of carpal tunnel syndrome may be less frequent. Bony and soft tissue growth occur in tandem, and thus the carpal tunnel may not be compromised.

HYPOTHYROIDISM

In primary hypothyroidism, hyaluronic acid and other mucoproteins deposit in many organs and tissues. Many of the numerous rheumatic syndromes associated with this disorder are probably secondary to such deposits in connective tissues and basement membranes (Table 98–2). The stimulus for the synthesis of the excess hyaluronic acid could be thyroid-stimulating hormone.[5] If this hypothesis is correct, it would account for the apparent paucity of musculoskeletal syndromes in secondary hypothyroidism, in which concentrations of thyroid-stimulating hormone are low. Other reasons for the infrequency of rheumatologic problems include the rarity of this endocrine deficiency and its association with other endocrine disorders, which might mask musculoskeletal problems.

Neuropathy

Neurologic features, although frequent in myxedema, are easily overlooked. Hypothyroid patients have few spontaneous complaints, and the neurologic examination is difficult to perform, owing to the patient's inability to cooperate. Several authors have emphasized the generalized nature of the peripheral neuropathy.[56,68,82] Originally believed to be caused by nerve compression by mucinous deposits, the peripheral neuropathy, in light of more recent evidence, is now thought to be due to a neuronal metabolic dysfunction secondary to the hypothyroid state. Segmental demyelination of nerve fibers has been detected with a proliferation of Schwann cells, together with mucinous infiltration of the endo- and perineurium. This neuropathy is primarily sensory, and slowed sensory conductive velocities have been found in the ulnar, median, and posterior tibial nerves. Abnormalities of

Table 98–2. Possible Rheumatologic Manifestations of Thyroid Disorders

Hypothyroidism	Peripheral neuropathy—carpal tunnel syndrome
	Arthropathy—noninflammatory viscous effusions, chondro-calcinosis (calcium pyrophosphate crystals), Charcot-like destruction, hyperuricemia and gout, flexor tenosynovitis, epiphyseal dysplasia
	Myopathy—aches, pain, stiffness, cramping, weakness, myoedema, hypertrophy
Hyperthyroidism	Thyroid acropachy—clubbing, periosteal proliferation, soft tissue swelling, pretibial myxedema, exophthalmos, LATS (long-acting thyroid stimulator)
	Myopathy—thyrotoxic atrophy, exophthalmic ophthalmoplegia, myasthenia gravis, periodic paralysis
Autoimmune (Hashimoto's) thyroiditis	Fibrositis syndrome
	Chest-wall pains
	Association with connective tissue diseases

conduction in the motor fibers of peripheral nerves have been found, although reports of frequency vary.[68,72]

In a careful review of 25 patients with myxedema, all complained of paresthesias, and 60% had diminished peripheral sensation. The sensory loss primarily involved pain and light touch, whereas decreased vibratory sensations were less common. One of the best recognized neurologic complications of hypothyroidism is *carpal tunnel syndrome*. Approximately 10% of all patients with carpal tunnel syndrome have myxedema.[22] Conversely, median nerve compression can be documented in anywhere from 5 to 80% of those with hypothyroidism.[5,68] Because the severity of the neuropathy often parallels the duration and severity of the hypothyroidism, carpal tunnel syndrome frequently co-exists with other rheumatologic complications of hypothyroidism, such as arthropathy and myopathy. The onset of symptoms of carpal tunnel syndrome can occur before clinical hypothyroidism is apparent. This association is important because treatment by thyroid replacement is followed by complete relief of the neuropathy, and an operation is avoided.

In addition to these effects of hypothyroidism on peripheral nerves, the cerebral cortex, cerebellum, and cranial nerves may also be involved. In hypothyroid patients, the cerebral spinal fluid protein concentration averages 115% above normal, with gamma globulin levels greater than 3 times normal.[56,82] With rare exceptions, all neurologic manifestations of hypothyroidism disappear completely on restoration of the euthyroid state.

Arthropathy

The careful joint evaluations performed by Bland and Frymoyer,[5] and the subsequent clinical pathologic study by Dorwart and Schumacher,[17] have defined a joint disorder distinctive for myxedema.

The characteristic features of this minimally inflammatory arthritis are listed in Table 98–2. The signs and symptoms of joint involvement usually develop concurrently with the onset of hypothyroidism, but occasionally they antedate the development of clinical myxedema. Approximately one-third of hypothyroid patients have symptomatic synovial effusions. Inflammation is neither common nor severe, with minimal pain and tenderness and only slight warmth and erythema. The arthritis of hypothyroidism is usually bilateral and most often affects the knees; the ankles, the metacarpophalangeal joints, and the small joints of the hands and feet are less frequently involved. Periarticular tissues appear thickened, and the increased intra-articular fluid is reflected in a sluggish "bulge" sign. This finding, caused by hyperviscosity, is secondary to an increased concentration of synovial fluid hyaluronic acid.[17] The synovial fluid otherwise is generally noninflammatory, with a white blood cell count of under 1,000/mm³.

Frymoyer and Bland excluded patients with hyaline cartilage calcification from their series, but they did comment that radiograms in 3 cases showed destructive lesions of the tibial plateau and what appeared to be pathologic compression fractures.[22] Because a Charcot-like destructive arthropathy has been associated with chondrocalcinosis (see Chap. 94), it is conceivable that these 3 patients had associated calcium pyrophosphate dihydrate crystal deposition disease. Although controversy still remains, strong evidence suggests an association between calcium pyrophosphate deposition and hypothyroidism. Dorwart and Schumacher found chondrocalcinosis of the knee in 7 of 12 myxedematous patients studied. Nine of the 12 had effusions, with calcium pyrophosphate crystals demonstrable in 6.[17] Conversely, an increased incidence of hypothyroidism (10.5%) has also been reported in a recent study of 105 patients with chondrocalcinosis.[15] Both intraleukocytic and extracellular calcium pyrophosphate and sodium urate crystals were noted, but without an associated inflammatory response.

The frequent failure of patients with myxedema to manifest intense inflammatory joint effusions in response to either sodium urate or calcium pyrophosphate crystals is of considerable interest. Two findings may provide the explanation. Polymorphonuclear leukocyte functions are reduced in hypothyroidism, an abnormality corrected after treatment with thyroxine.[20] Moreover, Brandt has shown that the high intrinsic viscosity and elevated concentration of hyaluronic acid in synovial fluid not only impedes the chemotactic movement of leukocytes, but also diminishes the rate of crystal ingestion by these cells.[8] These experimental findings may explain the blunted response to crystals in hypothyroid patients. On treatment with thyroid hormone, several patients later developed typical crystal-induced inflammatory joint attacks, in contrast to the response to treatment of patients with non-crystal-related joint pain and effusions of hypothyroidism.

Asymptomatic hyperuricemia is seen frequently in hypothyroid men, but not in women.[54] The increased incidence of clinical myxedema in patients with gout is slight but statistically significant.[19] The contributions of obesity to these observations and the influence of thyroid hormone on renal urate excretion remain unclear.

Wrist flexor tenosynovitis, observed in association with hypothyroidism,[17] was reported not to respond to thyroid therapy, but to subside promptly after injections of corticosteroid into the tendon sheaths. Although biopsies were not performed, hyaluronate deposition was believed to be responsible for the thickened, tender, and boggy palmar sheaths.

Ligamentous laxity occurs in approximately one-third of patients with myxedema. The synovial effusions with edematous, lax joint capsules, ligaments, and tendons resemble the changes seen in an animal model of hypothyroidism. These changes in the experimental form were believed to be caused by increased concentrations of hyaluronate in the involved tissues. Myxedematous joint disease has been described only in primary hypothyroidism, in which levels of thyroid-stimulating hormone are increased. This hormone may therefore be the stimulus for increased synovial synthesis of hyaluronate which may result in the changes described.[55]

Both the congenital and the acquired forms of hypothyroidism in children can delay epiphyseal closure and can retard maturation and ossification. This phenomenon, most often seen in the femoral head, may cause slipped capital femoral epiphysis. Helpful diagnostic features in such children include hip pain, limping, and an elevated serum creatine phosphokinase level.[35]

Myopathy

Myopathic features may accompany many different endocrinopathies, but numerically, their occurrence in hypothyroidism is probably the most important. In addition to the slow movements and the delayed muscle contraction and relaxation classically seen in hypothyroidism, about half these patients complain of weakness, and a similar number have muscle cramps, aches and pains, or stiffness.[67] Muscle hypertrophy occurs in about 12% of patients. Pain and stiffness may be present during rest and are exacerbated on exposure to cold, thus resembling primary fibrositis. Several authors have emphasized that muscular symptoms, such as aching and pain, stiffness, or cramps, may be the presenting complaints in many patients who do not have obvious clinical hypothyroidism.[92] Therefore, like other rheumatologic manifestations such as neuropathy and arthropathy, myopathy can antedate the diagnosis of hypothyroidism by several months. These various muscle symptoms of hypothyroidism probably constitute a continuous spectrum, beginning with aches and pains in association with mild disease and progressing to muscle cramping, proximal weakness, and even hypertrophy in association with severe, long-standing hypothyroidism. A case of rhabdomyolysis with hypothyroidism has been reported.[28]

On physical examination, weakness usually is not severe. When present, the proximal muscles are principally affected. Muscle contraction and relaxation are slowed, owing more often to muscle disease than to altered nerve conduction or to defective neuromuscular transmission. Direct percussion of the muscle leads to an interesting sign, termed the "mounding phenomenon" or *myoedema*. This transient focal ridging seen in response to striking or pinching the muscle persists for several seconds and can also be present in patients with hypoalbuminemia. Muscles are usually of normal bulk; atrophy is rare in hypothyroidism. Generalized hypertrophy of muscles, when observed in infants and children, is called the *Kocher-Debre-Semelaigne syndrome*, and in adults, it is called *Hoffman's syndrome*. This unusual finding, producing an athletic or "Herculean" appearance, disappears with therapy. Percussion of these hypertrophic muscles produces prolonged contractions resembling myotonia, although electromyographic studies have shown these muscle responses to be electrically silent.

The activities of most muscle enzymes are increased in the serum of patients with hypothyroidism.[27] Of these enzymes, creatine phosphokinase has been best studied; concentrations correlate well with the severity of hypothyroidism. The exact contribution of cardiac muscle isoenzyme to the serum creatine phosphokinase level in hypothyroidism remains to be resolved. The creatine phosphokinase level returns to normal in one to two months following restoration of the euthyroid state. In the few studies of patients with hypopituitarism and secondary hypothyroidism, myopathy was not a clinically prominent feature, and serum creatine phosphokinase levels were normal. Thus, the possible role of thyroid-stimulating hormone in the pathogenesis of hypothyroid muscle disorders is suggested.

A variety of electromyographic changes are independent of muscle bulk. Approximately half the patients demonstrate increased insertional activity and hyperirritability. An equal number manifest polyphasic motor unit action potentials.[72] Frequently, chains of repetitive discharges are observed after reflex motion.

Light microscopy reveals evidence of degeneration in the muscles of most patients, as well as areas of focal necrosis, regeneration, and basophilia with vacuolization of fibers. Fiber size varies, and the sarcolemmal nuclei are numerous, enlarged, and centrally positioned. Mucoprotein deposits, widespread in multiple organs in hypothyroidism, are found in the muscles of one-third of patients. It appears that these tissue infiltrates in the endo- and perimysium are not the sole cause of hypothyroid myopathy; thyroid hormone deprivation might account for the frequency of some of these muscular signs and symptoms. Histochemical staining has demonstrated a decrease in type II fibers proportional to the severity of the hypothyroidism. This lower percentage of type II fibers correlates with the severity of the disease and with the elevation of creatine phosphokinase levels. With treatment, the ratios of the fiber types return to normal.[49]

Although most cases of thyroid disease and associated connective tissue disease have occurred in patients with autoimmune thyroiditis, a case of hypothyroidism secondary to panhypopituitarism with Raynaud's phenomenon has been reported; all symptoms resolved after thyroid hormone replacement.[75]

HYPERTHYROIDISM

Thyroid Acropachy

This extraordinary rheumatic manifestation of hyperthyroidism usually follows treatment for thyrotoxicosis.[23] Thyroid acropachy, or thickening of

small parts, develops approximately a year after either thyroidectomy or radioablation. The fingers and toes become clubbed, and patients develop periostitis of the digits and distal extremities with swelling of soft tissues. Usually, these patients also have exophthalmos and pretibial myxedema. These features, in addition to the presence in the serum of long-acting thyroid stimulator (LATS), help to differentiate thyroid acropachy from other causes of hypertrophic osteoarthropathy. When this syndrome appears, patients are often clinically hypothyroid. Acropachy, an unusual complication, develops in approximately 1% of patients with past or present hyperthyroidism. Signs of inflammation are not prominent, although the syndrome is painful, especially on palpation over the periosteal new bone. Partial improvement, with incomplete resolution of pains in the extremities and digits and subsidence of the periosteal new bone proliferation, occurs in some patients after treatment with thyroid hormone or prednisone.

Immune factors appear to participate in the pathogenesis of Graves' disease and possibly in extrathyroidal manifestations, including acropachy.[88] Patients with Graves' disease have circulating thyroid-stimulating immunoglobulins, considered to be antibodies to the thyroid-stimulating hormone receptor on thyroid cell membranes. That other thyroid autoantibodies can also be detected suggests a close relationship between Graves' disease and Hashimoto's thyroidits. Evidence indicates cell-mediated immunity in both diseases, with the finding of T-lymphocytes sensitized to a thyroid antigen.[88] Additional evidence linking these two disorders includes the development of acropachy in both, their occurrence in the same families, and their histopathologic co-existence within the same thyroid gland. The finding of the histocompatibility antigen HLA-B8 in great frequency in patients with Graves' disease is evidence of a genetic association. The exact role of the organ-specific autoantibodies and of the sensitized leukocytes in the production of either of these thyroid disorders or of acropachy itself has yet to be studied.

Another rheumatologic association of uncertain pathogenesis is periarthritis of the shoulder. This disorder is said to co-exist with hyperthyroidism and to respond to restoration of the euthyroid state,[25] but controlled populations have not been studied. Marked osteoporosis, also frequently seen in thyrotoxicosis, is due to increased excretion of calcium and phosphorus. This osteoporosis is also reversible when the thyroid disorder is treated.

Thyrotoxic Myopathy

Clinical evidence of weakness can be found in almost all thyrotoxic patients.[67] The myopathy of thyrotoxicosis can be mild, characterized by weakness, fatigability, and minimal atrophy, or it can be extreme, characterized by proximal wasting and severe weakness, resembling polymyositis. Unlike polymyositis, acute inflammatory changes are not evident, and laryngeal and pharyngeal muscles are usually not involved. Atrophy and infiltration by fat cells and lymphocytes occur. "Muscle" enzymes are generally not increased in the serum, although creatinuria is present. Electromyographic abnormalities include short-duration motor unit potentials and an increased percentage of polyphasic potentials. Full recovery of muscle strength occurs as patients become euthyroid.

Less common are three other forms of myopathy seen in thyrotoxicosis. *Exophthalmic ophthalmoplegia* usually parallels the severity of exophthalmos. Associated findings include swelling of the eyelid and conjunctiva and sometimes of the optic nerve head. A second form is the co-existence of Graves' disease in 5% of patients with *myasthenia gravis.* The association of these two disorders has a distinct female sex preponderance. Patients respond to prostigmine, but improvement is incomplete, owing to the thyrotoxicosis. *Hypokalemic periodic paralysis* is the third of the rarer forms of skeletal muscle involvement in thyrotoxicosis. This syndrome has the cardinal features of flaccid paralysis of the extremities, with absent reflexes and diminished electrical excitability. Precipitating factors are thought to be exercise, a high carbohydrate intake, and the administration of insulin or epinephrine. This disorder is rare in the white race and is more common in Oriental males. Serum potassium concentrations are usually low, and the administration of potassium salts can prevent or can abort attacks. Treatment of hyperthyroidism with restoration of the euthyroid state leads to resolution of the paralytic attacks.

AUTOIMMUNE (HASHIMOTO'S) THYROIDITIS

Early in the course of autoimmune thyroiditis, as the thyroid gland gradually enlarges, most patients are euthyroid and some are hyperthyroid. With progressive lymphocytic infiltrations, fibrosis, and obliteration of thyroid follicles, however, approximately 50% of patients develop hypothyroidism. This common cause of diffuse goiter, with a female predilection, is frequently associated with musculoskeletal symptoms. The most common rheumatologic syndrome resembles *fibrositis;* patients complain of stiffness of the joints and muscles. Stiffness is exacerbated by cold or dampness and is worse on arising in the morning or after any period of immobility. This fibrositis syndrome, resembling that seen in hypothyroidism, can be present in autoimmune thyroiditis even in the absence of thyroid deficiency.[3] Another rheumatologic symptom is *unusual chest-wall pains* of intermittent nature. Described in 12% of patients with Hashimoto's disease, these thoracic and shoulder-girdle pains, lasting for several minutes to hours, are relieved by changes of position or by mild exercise.[3] Half the patients with Hashimoto's disease have an *elevated erythrocyte sedimentation rate,* with or without rheumatic symptoms.

Most patients with Hashimoto's disease have high serum titers of thyroid antibodies, both to thyroglobulin and to microsomal antigens. Cellular immunity may also be important in the pathogenesis of the disease.[88] Biologic false-positive tests for syphilis, rheumatoid factors, and antinuclear antibodies are also common. Hashimoto's disease co-exists with other autoimmune disorders, especially pernicious anemia and hemolytic anemia, and possibly with RA, systemic lupus erythematosus, and Sjögren's syndrome.[3,24,58,93] These disorders also appear in family members of patients with autoimmune thyroiditis too often to be coincidental.

The frequency of thyroid disease in patients with rheumatologic disorders has also been examined. Although patients with connective tissue diseases, notably systemic lupus erythematosus and RA, have a high incidence of antibodies to thyroid antigens, the majority are euthyroid and do not have detectable goiters. Despite isolated case reports and uncontrolled series, the co-existence of either hyper- or hypothyroidism with RA, polymyositis, scleroderma, or systemic lupus erythematosus is probably coincidental. Two other associations of rheumatologic disease with thyroid disorders are known, as follows: (1) the administration of antithyroid drugs may be followed by syndromes resembling either RA or systemic lupus erythematosus, especially in children;[11] and (2) falsely low values of serum thyroxine can be seen in patients treated either with salicylates or with corticosteroid hormones.

PARATHYROID DISORDERS

A number of rheumatologic entities are associated with parathyroid hormone excess (Table 98–3). A more detailed discussion of the osseous consequences of increased levels of this hormone, including osteitis fibrosa cystica, may be found in Chapter 97.

The resorptive effects of parathyroid hormone on bone may lead to the characteristic subperiosteal erosive radiographic appearance, particularly at the radial aspect of the middle phalanges, the medial aspect of the proximal femur or tibia, and the inferior aspect of the distal third in the clavicle.

Table 98–3. **Possible Rheumatologic Manifestations of Parathyroid Disorders**

Hyperparathyroidism	Osteitis fibrosa cystica
	Subperiosteal resorption
	Rheumatoid-type erosions
	Joint laxity
	Tendon avulsions
	Back abnormalities
	Degenerative arthritis
	Chondrocalcinosis and pseudogout
	Charcot-like joints
	Hyperuricemia and gout
	Ectopic calcifications
	Neuromyopathy
Hypoparathyroidism and pseudohypoparathyroidism	Subcutaneous calcifications
	Paraspinal ligament calcifications (spondylitis without sacroiliitis)

Erosions may also occur in juxta-articular sites, especially at the interphalangeal, metacarpophalangeal, carpal, and acromioclavicular joints. These lesions can be found in the absence of subperiosteal resorption, can be symmetric, and can be associated with morning stiffness, thus mimicking RA. Several features distinguish parathyroid disorders: (1) the erosions may have a shaggy appearance; (2) they often occur at the distal interphalangeal joints and spare the proximal interphalangeal joints; (3) joint-space narrowing in association with these erosions is uncommon because parathyroid hormone does not directly induce inflammatory synovitis or cartilage dissolution; and (4) the hyperparathyroid patient may have concurrent articular calcification.

Parathyroid hormone increases collagenase activity,[80] and this factor may account for the laxity of capsular and ligamentous structures seen in this disorder. Tendon ruptures and avulsions have been reported.[65] Vertebral subluxation occurs, especially in the cervical spine; dorsal kyphosis is present, with anterior bowing of the sternum; the lumbar spine is hypermobile. Additional back changes include sacroiliac erosions and intervertebral disc calcifications. The laxity leads to joint abuse, which contributes to the back pain, disc protrusion, and degenerative joint changes seen in hyperparathyroidism.

Chondrocalcinosis has been reported in 18 to 25% of patients with hyperparathyroidism[29,66] (see also Chap. 94). Calcium pyrophosphate dihydrate crystal deposition may cause attacks of pseudogout, which can precede the recognition of parathyroid hormone excess and may thus be an initial manifestation of this disease. Pseudogout attacks may flare within two to three days of parathyroidectomy, or they may occur later, often coincident with the postoperative nadir of the serum calcium level.[4] Once chondrocalcinosis is present, it usually persists in spite of parathyroidectomy, and the frequency of episodes of pseudogout continues unabated or even increases. Bywaters and co-workers have described subchondral cyst formation with subsequent destructive joint changes in hyperparathyroidism.[10] More than half their patients had chondrocalcinosis. Because similar joint changes with severe destruction and the development of Charcot-like joints have been described in association with chondrocalcinosis, the relative contributions of calcium pyrophosphate dihydrate and parathyroid hormone to this type of arthropathy remain to be elucidated. The presence of severe degenerative osteoarthritis should alert the physician to search for both parathyroid hormone excess and calcium pyrophosphate dihydrate crystal deposition.

The persistently elevated serum calcium levels in primary hyperparathyroidism may result in nephrocalcinosis and a calcium nephropathy characterized by a tubular defect with an impaired urine-concentrating mechanism. Some hyperparathyroid patients have a decreased uric acid clearance, and this feature may explain the finding of hyperuricemia. The incidence of actual gouty attacks in hyperparathyroidism varies from 3 to 45%.[54] Because the hyperuricemia and gout do not seem to occur without underlying renal changes, they may persist even after parathyroidectomy. Elevated levels of parathyroid hormone have been found in about 70% of patients with calcium pyrophosphate dihydrate crystal deposits and in age- and sex-matched control subjects with osteoarthritis of the knee.[48] Chemical hyperparathyroidism occurred in patients in both groups. Serum levels of parathyroid hormone correlated directly with serum calcium levels, with the severity of osteoarthritis in the female patients, and with bone density. The possible role of parathyroid hormone in the pathogenesis of osteoarthritis needs to be further explored.

In secondary hyperparathyroidism, as well as in

other disorders in which metastatic calcifications are found, deposits of amorphous and crystalline calcium salts, including hydroxyapatite, may occur in periarticular or articular tissues. Their presence can induce a local inflammatory reaction with pain and swelling[51] (see also Chap. 95). Treatment consists of prophylaxis with aluminum hydroxide gels and the use of anti-inflammatory agents or intra-articular corticosteroids during acute episodes.

Fatigue, generalized weakness, and other neuromuscular complaints occur in the majority of patients with primary or secondary hyperparathyroidism. Weakness is usually in the proximal muscles, often only in the lower extremities. This symptom is most commonly secondary to a peripheral neuropathic process.[50,61] Other neurologic findings include abnormalities of the cranial nerves, long-tract signs, and decreased vibratory sensations. Muscle enzyme levels are not elevated, and surprisingly, nerve conduction velocities are reported to be normal despite other electromyographic findings suggesting a neuropathic process. Muscle biopsy reveals neurogenic atrophy of both fiber types, with type II atrophy predominating.[61] Parathyroidectomy usually rapidly reverses these abnormalities. Other causes of neuromuscular symptoms in hyperparathyroid patients are a polymyositis-like myopathy[21] and an ischemic myopathy secondary to intravascular calcifications.[70]

In addition to the bony features of hypoparathyroidism, pseudohypoparathyroidism, and pseudopseudohypoparathyroidism, subcutaneous and ectopic calcifications may be seen. Spondylitis without sacroiliitis, with extensive paraspinal calcifications in hypoparathyroidism and pseudohypoparathyroidism, has been reported.[14] Myopathy, in association with elevated serum levels of creatine phosphokinase and normal muscle biopsy has also been seen in hypoparathyroidism.[42]

DIABETES MELLITUS

The variety of musculoskeletal complications of diabetes mellitus, both articular and periarticular, are listed in Table 98–4. Some of these disorders, such as destructive arthropathy, reflex sympathetic dystrophy, carpal tunnel syndrome, interosseous muscle wasting, and proximal weakness, may be primarily the result of neuropathic changes. Ischemic vascular disease may also contribute to their genesis. Complications that appear to be related to a proliferation of fibrous tissue include the increased incidence of capsulitis of the shoulder, Dupuytren's contractures and flexor tenosynovitis in adults, and flexion contractures in juvenile-onset diabetics. The collagen from skin and tendon samples of young diabetics is stiff and stabilized, similar to samples from normal control subjects 50 to

65 years older.[30] The reason for the excessive fibrosis and accelerated aging of collagen is unclear.

Metabolic consequences of decreased glucose use are also important. Although controversial, some evidence suggests an increased incidence of hyperuricemia and gout in patients with diabetes mellitus.[54] Even less clearly defined are the associations of diabetes mellitus with calcium pyrophosphate dihydrate crystal deposition and the apparent co-existence with ankylosing vertebral hyperostosis[37] (see Chap. 94). Controlled studies have failed to support an association with calcium pyrophosphate dihydrate crystal deposition.

Neuropathy

Diabetic neuropathy may take several forms; (1) a peripheral symmetric sensory or sensorimotor loss; (2) a mononeuropathy multiplex with an increased frequency of cranial nerve involvement; (3) a neuropathy resulting in proximal muscle weakness, termed diabetic amyotrophy; (4) a radiculopathy leading to lancinating pains in a dermatomal distribution; (5) an autonomic neuropathy; and (6) carpal tunnel syndrome. With peripheral neuropathic involvement, patients frequently have a stocking-glove distribution of sensory loss, with decreased vibratory and position sense and decreased or absent deep-tendon reflexes. Wasting of the interosseous muscles of the hands and feet may give a claw-hand or hammer-toe appearance.

Mononeuropathies most commonly affect the third and sixth cranial nerves, and occasionally the fourth and seventh as well. Mononeuropathy involving the motor supply of the proximal hip and leg muscles, and less often of the upper extremities, occurs in a higher incidence in men and often in those with only mild forms of diabetes. This so-called diabetic amyotrophy is usually bilateral but asymmetric. Muscle biopsy shows a predominance of type I fibers, with type II atrophy and no evidence of significant necrosis or inflammation. Muscle enzyme levels are normal, and the electromyogram shows some fibrillation potentials. The weakness may spontaneously remit. Evidence also indicates that control of hyperglycemia contributes to recovery.[46] Diabetic radiculopathy may occur secondary to infarction of a nerve root, with resultant lancinating pains. These pains are sometimes confused with the symptoms of a herniated disc. When proprioceptive loss and ataxia accompany this shooting pain, it is called "diabetic pseudotabes."

Involvement of the autonomic nervous system results in orthostatic hypotension, impotence, dyshidrosis, and diarrhea. Autonomic dysfunction may be related to the unilateral or bilateral reflex dystrophy and to the apparently increased shoulder

Table 98-4.   Possible Rheumatologic Manifestations of Diabetes Mellitus

Neuropathy	Distal sensory and sensorimotor disorders
	Mononeuropathy multiplex
	Carpal tunnel syndrome
	Diabetic amyotrophy
	Radiculopathy
	Autonomic neuropathy and reflex dystrophy
Neuroarthropathy	Osteoporosis and osteolysis
	Charcot joint
	Co-existent osteomyelitis
	Periarthritis of the shoulder
Other Associations	Hyperuricemia and gout
	Ankylosing hyperostosis
	Flexion contractures
	Trigger finger

pain seen in diabetes. Periarthritis (adhesive capsulitis) of the shoulder, often bilateral, has been found in 11% of a large group of diabetic patients.[9] Conversely, in another study, approximately 25% of patients with periarthritis were diabetic.[44] This entity occurs more commonly in women on the nondominant side of the body and produces aching with limitation of shoulder motion. Calcific bursitis and tendinitis may be present. The natural course of the disorder varies, but spontaneous remissions may occur. Physical therapy, anti-inflammatory drugs, and local corticosteroid injections are helpful. Intra-articular corticosteroids are absorbed systemically and, owing to their insulin antagonism, may cause transient problems in controlling blood glucose levels. From 5 to 17% of patients with carpal tunnel syndrome have diabetes, but systematic, controlled observations in diabetic patients have not demonstrated a significant association.[60]

Arthropathy

As a consequence of sensory neuropathy, severe arthropathy with Charcot-like changes develops in approximately 0.1% of long-standing diabetics.[77] The tarsometatarsal and metatarsophalangeal joints are the most common sites of involvement, but changes may also occur in the ankles, knees, and lumbar spine. A combination of microfragmentation from trauma, ischemia from small-blood-vessel disease, and superimposed infection can contribute to the clinical and radiographic changes of neuroarthropathy. In advanced disease, the longitudinal arch of the foot collapses, leading to an unstable gait and a "rocker-sole" appearance. Ulcerations and plantar callosities occur over hypoesthetic pressure points. Actual osteolysis of bone can develop, with periosteal reaction and remodeling, whittling of the metatarsal bones, cupping deformities, and telescoping of the phalanges.[77] Fractures may be the initial lesion in a Charcot

joint or may simply contribute to more extensive joint damage. In all involved joints, the discrepancy between pain, which is minimal or absent, and the destructive radiographic appearance, which is severe, is striking. The mainstay of therapy is rest of the involved area, to prevent further wear and tear, treatment of any concomitant osteomyelitis, and amputation if required (see Chap. 71).

A group of disorders of more obscure pathogenesis has in common excessive proliferation of fibroblastic tissue. *Fibrous palmar nodules* with subsequent Dupuytren's contractures have been reported in as many as 21% of diabetic patients; diabetes is found in 10% of those with Dupuytren's contractures[82] (see Chap. 83). Diabetes has also been described in 10 to 30% of all adult cases of trigger finger or flexor tenosynovitis.[81] In addition, reports exist of interphalangeal flexion deformities in insulin-dependent, juvenile-onset diabetic patients.[26] This progressive stiffness has been seen only in the hands and is not related to Dupuytren's contractures or flexor tenosynovitis. The stiffness and limited mobility appear to be related to a thick, tight, waxy skin. A simple screening test for limited joint mobility consists of asking the patient to place both hands on a table palm down with fingers fanned. The entire palmar surface of the fingers makes contact in normal persons.[26] Rosenbloom et al. showed that, in patients who had had diabetes for 16 years, the presence of stiff joints increased the risk of retinal and renal complications from 25% to 83%.[71]

Several reports exist of insulin-resistant diabetes mellitus secondary to insulin receptor antibodies.[38] This syndrome has been associated with multiple rheumatic complaints suggestive of systemic lupus erythematosus, Sjögren's syndrome, and progressive systemic sclerosis.[31,91] Whenever a patient has extremely insulin-resistant diabetes mellitus, the possibility of circulating antibodies and these associated diseases should be considered.

Finally, caution is required in the use of such drugs as probenecid, aspirin, and phenylbutazone because they may reduce the blood glucose level by augmenting the effect of hypoglycemic agents.

CORTICOSTEROID ADMINISTRATION

Corticosteroid excess due to adrenal hyperproduction or secondary to exogenous administration can profoundly affect the musculoskeletal system. Generalized osteoporosis, avascular necrosis of the humeral and femoral heads, and pathologic fractures are consequences in bone. Changes in the vertebral column can cause severe pain, kyphosis, and loss of height. In children, growth is retarded, and, if not corrected, the result is permanently short stature. A noninflammatory proximal myopathy may progress from the pelvic to the shoulder girdle and, ultimately, to distal musculature. Serum muscle enzyme levels are characteristically normal in states of corticosteroid excess, but urinary creatine excretion is increased. Following correction of hypercortisolism, creatinuria subsides. This dissociation between serum and urine laboratory tests may help to differentiate corticosteroid-related from inflammatory myopathies. The electromyogram in corticosteroid myopathy has yielded confusing results and is not helpful diagnostically. Muscle biopsy reveals a type II atrophy without inflammatory changes in an experimental model.[76] Although some recovery of muscle strength occurs within days after reduction of corticosteroid dose, complete resolution usually takes one to four months.

Adrenal insufficiency after corticosteroid withdrawal may be associated with constitutional symptoms of weakness, fatigue and lassitude, and arthralgias. Corticosteroid withdrawal in patients with RA has been suggested as a causative factor in rheumatoid vasculitis, but this hypothesis needs further substantiation.[74]

CARCINOID ARTHROPATHY

Distinctive rheumatologic findings occur in at least 10% of carcinoid patients. Arthralgias of the wrists and hands, constant stiffness and pain on movement, and marked intensification of pain after a sustained grip are characteristic complaints. Because the arthralgias can be rapidly reversed with parachlorophenylalanine, which blocks serotonin synthesis, serotonin is believed to be responsible for these symptoms. Bradykinin and histamine may also be involved. One may detect juxta-articular demineralization and erosions at the metacarpophalangeal joints and at the proximal and distal interphalangeal joints, with subchondral cystic changes.[64]

ECTOPIC HORMONAL SYNDROMES

Tumor cells can synthesize polypeptide hormones, such as adrenocorticotrophic hormone, growth hormone, thyroid-stimulating hormone, and parathyroid hormone, with structural and functional characteristics similar or identical to those of normal hormones.[57] Because the bony, myopathic, and neuropathic changes associated with endocrinopathies require prolonged hormonal exposure, these syndromes are not seen with ectopic hormone production by malignant tissues. Several cases of hypertrophic pulmonary osteoarthropathy have been reported in patients with acromegalic physical features and increases in growth hormone or similar substances that resolved when the tumor was removed, suggesting a possible relationship.[18] The periosteal proliferation seen in osteoarthropathy may resemble the periosteal remodeling of acromegaly, but further clarification is needed to determine whether any humeral substance mediates this syndrome.

PREGNANCY

The symptoms of RA frequently remit during pregnancy. Since Hench's description in 1938 of the beneficial action of pregnancy,[34] improvement has been reported in numerous other rheumatic disorders as well[62] (Table 98–5). Many of these reports have dealt with a few patients or even a single patient, however, and with rare exception, the observations have been retrospective and anecdotal.

The most complete data have been accumulated on the course of RA during gestation and in the postpartum period.[53] Neely and Persellin collated

Table 98–5. Disorders Reported to be Ameliorated by Pregnancy

Rheumatoid arthritis	Sarcoidosis
Ankylosing spondylitis	Polymyositis
Psoriatic arthropathy (and psoriasis)	Raynaud's phenomenon
	Gout (possibly)
Behçet's syndrome	Cutaneous anaphylaxis
Fibrositis	Angioneurotic edema
Intermittent hydrarthrosis	Bronchial asthma
Periodic diseases	Hay fever
Erythema nodosum	Migraine headache

Experimental Animal Diseases

Experimental vasculitis (dogs)	Carrageenin inflammation (rats)
Adjuvant arthritis (rats)	Allergic thyroiditis (guinea pigs)

Disorders with Variable Course

Systemic lupus erythematosus	Inflammatory bowel diseases
Scleroderma	Necrotizing cutaneous vasculitis
Myasthenia gravis	

the observations in 7 previous publications, including Hench's initial article, together with their own retrospective analysis of 56 pregnancies in patients with RA.[53] As shown in Figure 98–3, improvement was not noted in all these 296 pregnancies described in the literature. Only 219 (74%) had some degree of subsidence of arthritis activity during gestation. The time of onset of clinical improvement is shown in Figure 98–3. Eight percent related improvement in the first month, 17% in the second month, and an additional 25% by the end of the third month of pregnancy. Therefore, 50% of patients with RA had some degree of subsidence of disease activity during the first trimester of pregnancy. Thereafter, an additional 24% experienced relief of symptoms throughout the second and third trimesters, some even waiting until the last month of gestation for improvement. In 26% of published cases, patients failed to note an amelioration of arthritis. Some had more severe symptoms, and others experienced the onset of their disease during pregnancy.

After delivery, the symptoms of RA recurred in more than 90% of patients, although complete data are not available. Information has been published on the postpartum experience of only 128 patients (Fig. 98–4).[53] All related to an exacerbation following parturition; 64% noted a return of symptoms by the eighth week after delivery. Of these patients, 25% had exacerbations during the first month, and an additional 39% had exacerbations in the second month. Thirty-six percent had no joint inflammation until more than 8 weeks post partum. These data indicate that the benefits of pregnancy are temporary, lasting an average of 6 weeks after delivery. The return of symptoms can be abrupt or insidious and is not related either to the resumption of menstruation or to the termination of lactation. A careful quantitation of disease activity has not been performed, but it is generally stated that postpartum RA is at least as severe as prior to gestation.

The other major rheumatic disorder in which a considerable clinical experience during pregnancy has been accumulated is systemic lupus erythematosus.[12] The studies of this relationship have produced controversial and contradictory reports. Most authors have noted a high spontaneous abortion rate in pregnancies occurring before the onset of their first recognizable manifestations of this disease, as well as in pregnancies after the onset of clinical disease. The possibility of heart block in offspring of mothers with systemic lupus erythematosus is now well known[13] and is related to anti-Ro (SSA) antibody. Mothers of babies born with complete heart block should be monitored for signs of lupus because the diagnosis may not be known before delivery. One mother did not develop the disease until 16 years after the birth of the first of 3 children with congenital heart block.[39]

Less certain is the relationship between disease activity and pregnancy, including the progression of renal or other organ dysfunction. As with RA, exacerbations of systemic lupus have been documented frequently in the postpartum period; however, in recent studies in which patients were treated with glucocorticoids and cytotoxic agents, the exacerbation rates varied from 23 to 41%. Because of these uncertainties, a number of investigators have suggested that pregnancies be delayed in these patients until their disease has been inactive for 6 months or more prior to conception.[32] The

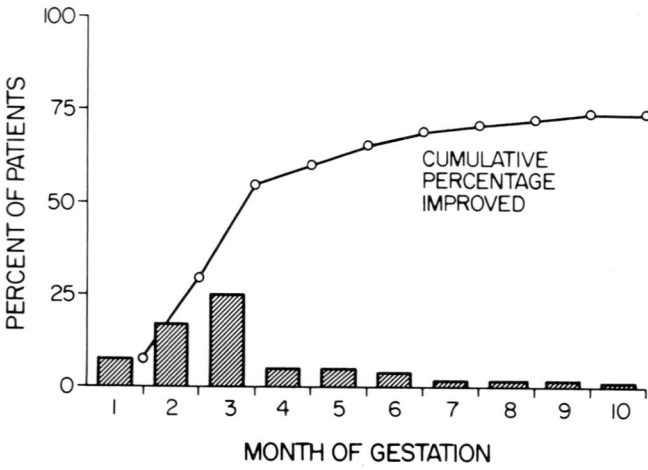

Fig. 98–3. Time of onset of symptomatic improvement in rheumatoid arthritis activity during 296 pregnancies. A total of 50% improved during the first trimester, and an additional 24% improved throughout the remainder of gestation. (From Neely, N.T., and Persellin, R.H.[53])

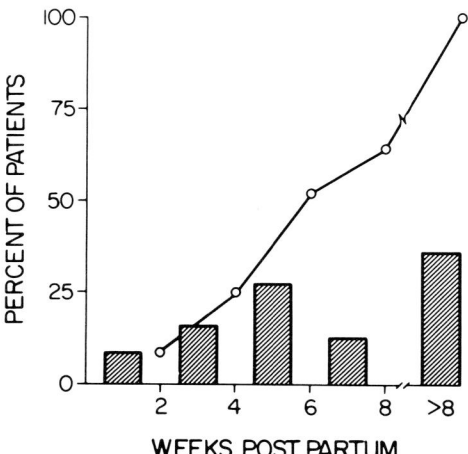

Fig. 98–4. Recurrence of rheumatoid arthritis symptoms in each 2-week period post partum in 128 patients. The cumulative percentage is also presented. (From Neely, N.T., and Persellin, R.H.[53])

same risks during pregnancy have been reported in patients with mixed connective tissue disease.[40]

Factor Responsible for Amelioration

The factor responsible for improvement is not yet known. Robert B. Osgood suggested that "if we could reproduce the biochemical conditions of pregnancy or if we should find that patients who suffer from this disease frequently lack some substance present in the pregnant woman, we might be able to arrest and approach a specific therapy."[59] In considering which factor is reponsible for the subsidence of RA and other inflammatory diseases during pregnancy, one should note both the increased susceptibility of pregnant women to certain infectious diseases and the specific suppression of normal immune responses during pregnancy. During gestation, women are believed to suffer increased morbidity and mortality from certain infectious agents, chiefly viruses and fungi. Included are the agents of infectious hepatitis, poliomyelitis, influenza, and coccidioidomycosis.[62] The virulence of these intracellular micro-organisms may be related to impaired cell-mediated immunity during gestation. Skin-graft rejection is delayed, and in vitro T-lymphocyte responses are depressed, effects believed to be mediated by the serum or plasma of pregnancy.[73] The ameliorating substance is probably responsible for all the clinical alterations associated with gestation.

Hench called attention to the multitude of biochemical alterations in pregnancy.[33] His observations helped to bring about the discovery of cortisone, for which he shared the Nobel Prize in

physiology and medicine in 1950. Because the concentration of blood cortisol increases during pregnancy, it has been related to the suppression of rheumatoid activity. Subsequent studies have shown, however, that the increased corticosteroid concentrations alone were not fully responsible for the observed improvement.[62] Some patients with suppressed RA during pregnancy did not have increased plasma concentrations of corticosteroids, and other patients, who failed to improve or who even experienced exacerbations during pregnancy, had increased cortisol levels. Plasma cortisol levels fall to normal by 48 hours after delivery, and yet RA remains suppressed post partum for more than 6 weeks in 50% of patients. Additional evidence that cortisol is not wholly responsible is that the hormone is mostly transcortin-bound during gestation and is therefore not biologically active. Thus, despite the original enthusiasm for cortisol, other factors responsible for improvement during gestation have been sought.

A variety of other products of pregnancy, including placental extracts, umbilical cord serum, and blood or urine fractions, have been used to treat RA and have been found to be either beneficial or ineffective. No consistently reproducible improvement has been forthcoming. Recently, investigators have focused on nonhormonal constituents of plasma in pregnancy. The concentrations of many plasma proteins are increased during gestation, including: (1) the carrier proteins, such as transcortin, thyroxin-binding globulin, testosterone-binding globulin, estrogen-binding globulin, transferrin, and ceruloplasmin; (2) the coagulation proteins, including fibrinogen and factors VII, VIII, and IX; (3) plasminogen; (4) alpha-2 macroglobulin; (5) C-reactive protein and other so-called "acute phase" proteins; and (5) the pregnancy-associated plasma proteins.[45]

Of these proteins, studies on the biologic activities of the pregnancy zone protein (PZP) have been the most promising. This glycoprotein is found at low concentrations in the serum of women who are not pregnant and increases during gestation in most individuals.[89] Following delivery, the level falls at a slower rate than the other pregnancy-associated plasma proteins. This substance affects a variety of in vitro parameters of inflammation and acts on the membranes of isolated organelles, polymorphonuclear leukocytes, and lymphocytes as well.[62,83] Unlike previous observations using corticosteroid hormones, pregnancy zone protein is effective in vitro in physiologic concentrations. The timing of changes in the concentration of plasma pregnancy zone protein parallels both the remissions and the postpartum exacerbations of RA. Additionally, approximately 25% of women have only minimal elevations of this protein in their plasma during gestation; this finding may explain the failure of this percentage of patients to experience clinical improvements.[62]

The dramatic changes in the metabolism of the sex hormones during pregnancy are well known. Estrogens reduce the metabolic activity of neutrophils, alter delayed skin-test reactivity in experimental animals, and suppress the development and severity of adjuvant arthritis in rats. Progesterone has also been shown in vitro to suppress leukocyte functions. Most of these effects have resulted from large, nonphysiologic amounts of these sex hormones, however.[73] Despite original enthusiasm, the beneficial effects of sex hormones on patients with RA have not been substantiated by clinical trials, but carefully controlled studies have not been performed. Because estrogenic hormones are known to induce a variety of serum protein changes similar to those in pregnancy, their effect on serum concentrations of pregnancy zone protein has been studied. Significant increases in this protein were observed during the administration of either combinations of estrogen and progesterone or of estrogen alone. Serum concentrations of pregnancy zone protein induced by exogenous sex hormone administration reached only one-tenth the levels usually found during pregnancy,[36] however, and this factor may account for the failure of estrogens to produce the clinical response observed during gestation. Thus, sex hormones, corticosteroids, and pregnancy zone protein, the plasma constituents increased during pregnancy, have been demonstrated in vitro and in some animal models to possess anti-inflammatory activity.

SEX HORMONES IN AUTOIMMUNE DISORDERS

Many autoimmune diseases are more common in women than in men. In systemic lupus erythematosus, the best example, the female-to-male ratio can be as high as 15 to 1. The ratio does vary with age. In premenarcheal or postmenopausal women, the ratio falls to 2 to 1. This change in ratio suggests hormonal influence. Oral contraceptive agents either may exacerbate latent systemic lupus erythematosus or may induce the formation of antibodies to nuclear antigens. In a series of 8 patients with antinuclear antibodies believed secondary to oral contraceptives, all had rheumatic complaints of arthralgias, myalgias, and morning stiffness, and 2 had synovitis.[7] A subsequent prospective study by the same investigators confirmed the development of autoantibodies in response to these agents, but other investigators were unable to find either rheumatic symptoms or autoantibodies in large groups of women using oral contraceptives.[85]

Talal et al. have studied the effects of sex steroid hormones on autoimmune disease in murine lupus models. Androgens appear to suppress murine lupus, and estrogens accelerate the disease.[84] Estrogen receptor-like binding has been found in mouse thymus tissue, and estrogens may inhibit the clearance of immune complexes; these findings reflect the probable influence of sex hormones on the immune system by means of thymic epithelium and the reticuloendothelial system. Additionally, that androgens have preserved interleukin-2 (T-cell growth factor) activity in some mice with lupus suggests a relationship between interleukin-2 and sex hormones.[84]

Metabolism of estrogens and androgens in patients with lupus has been investigated by Lahita et al. Patients with systemic lupus erythematosus showed an elevation of 16 hydroxylated metabolites with increased estrogenic activity. First-degree relatives of these patients also had higher levels of 16 hydroxylated metabolites; a genetic predisposition to altered estrogen metabolism is implied.[43]

The results of these and other studies suggest an important role for hormonal modulation of the immune system in autoimmune disorders, in particular systemic lupus erythematosus and may lead to novel therapeutic techniques.

REFERENCES

1. Anton, H.C.: Hand measurements in acromegaly. Clin. Radiol., 23:445–450, 1972.
2. Askari, A., Vignos, P.J., and Moskowitz, R.W.: Steroid myopathy in connective tissue disease. Am. J. Med., 61:485–492, 1976.
3. Becker, K.L., Ferguson, R.H., and McConahey, W.M.: The connective tissue diseases and symptoms associated with Hashimoto's thyroiditis. N. Engl. J. Med., 268:277–280, 1963.
4. Bilezikian, J.P., et al.: Pseudogout after parathyroidectomy. Lancet, 1:445–446, 1973.
5. Bland, J.H., and Frymoyer, J.W.: Rheumatic syndromes of myxedema. N. Engl. J. Med., 282:1,171–1,174, 1970.
6. Bluestone, R., et al.: Acromegalic arthropathy. Ann. Rheum. Dis., 30:243–258, 1971.
7. Bole, G.G., Friedlander, M.H., and Smith, G.K.: Rheumatic symptoms and serological abnormalities induced by oral contraceptives. Lancet, 1:323–326, 1969.
8. Brandt, K.D.: The effect of synovial hyaluronate on the ingestion of monosodium urate crystals by leukocytes. Clin. Chim. Acta, 55:307–315, 1974.
9. Bridgeman, J.E.: Periarthritis of the shoulder and diabetes mellitus. Ann. Rheum. Dis., 31:69–71, 1972.
10. Bywaters, E.G.L., Dixon, A. St. J, and Scott, J.T.: Joint lesions of hyperparathyroidism. Ann. Rheum. Dis., 22:171–184, 1963.
11. Cassorla, F.G., et al.: Vasculitis, pulmonary cavitation and anemia during antithyroid drug therapy. Am. J. Dis. Child., 137:118–122, 1983.
12. Cecere, F.A., and Persellin, R.H.: The interaction of pregnancy and the rheumatic diseases. Clin. Rheum. Dis., 7:747–768, 1981.
13. Chameides, L., et al.: Association of maternal systemic lupus erythematosus with congenital complete heart block. N. Engl. J. Med., 297:1,204–1,207, 1977.
14. Chaykin, L.B., Frame, B., and Sigler, J.W.: Spondylitis:

a clue to hypoparathyroidism. Ann. Intern. Med., 70:995–1,000, 1969.

15. Dieppe, P.A., et al.: Pyrophosphate arthropathy: a clinical and radiological study of 105 cases. Ann. Rheum. Dis., 41:371–376, 1982.

16. Doherty, M.: Pyrophosphate arthropathy—recent clinical advances. Ann. Rheum. Dis., 42:38–44, 1983.

17. Dorwart, B.B., and Schumacher, H.R.: Joint effusions, chondrocalcinosis and other rheumatic manifestations in hypothyroidism. A clinicopathologic study. Am. J. Med., 59:780–790, 1975.

18. DuPont, B., et al.: Plasma growth hormone and hypertrophic osteoarthropathy in carcinoma of the bronchus. Acta Med. Scand., 188:25–30, 1970.

19. Durward, W.F.: Gout and hypothyroidism in males. Arthritis Rheum., 19:123, 1976.

20. Farid, N.R., et al.: Polymorphonuclear leukocyte function in hypothyroidism. Horm. Res., 7:247–253, 1976.

21. Frame, B., et al.: Myopathy in primary hyperparathyroidism: observations in three patients. Ann. Intern. Med., 68:1,023–1,027, 1968.

22. Frymoyer, J.W., and Bland, J.: Carpal-tunnel syndrome in patients with myxedematous arthropathy. J. Bone Joint Surg., 55A:78–82, 1973.

23. Gimlette, T.M.D.: Thyroid acropachy. Lancet, 1:22–24, 1960.

24. Gordon, M.B., et al.: Thyroid disease in progressive systemic sclerosis: increase frequency of glandular fibrosis and hypothyroidism. Ann. Intern. Med., 95:431–435, 1981.

25. Gorman, C.A.: Unusual manifestations of Graves' disease. Mayo Clin. Proc., 47:926–933, 1972.

26. Grgic, A., et al.: Joint contracture—common manifestation of childhood diabetes mellitus. J. Pediatr., 88:584–588, 1976.

27. Griffiths, P.D.: Serum enzymes in diseases of the thyroid gland. J. Clin. Pathol., 18:660–663, 1965.

28. Halverson, P.B., et al.: Rhabdomyolysis and renal failure in hypothyroidism. Ann. Intern. Med., 91:57–58, 1979.

29. Hamilton, E.B.D.: Diseases associated with CPPD deposition disease. Arthritis Rheum., 19:353–357, 1976.

30. Hamlin, C.R., Kohn, R.R., and Luschin, J.H.: Apparent accelerated aging of human collagen in diabetes mellitus. Diabetes, 24:902–904, 1975.

31. Hardin, J.G., and Siegal, A.M.: A connective tissue disease complicated by insulin resistance due to receptor antibodies: report of a case with high titer nuclear ribonucleoprotein antibodies. Arthritis Rheum., 25:458–463, 1982.

32. Hayslett, J.P.: Effect of pregnancy in patients with SLE. Am. J. Kidney Dis., 2:223–228, 1982.

33. Hench, P.S.: Potential reversibility of rheumatoid arthritis. Mayo Clin. Proc., 24:167–178, 1949.

34. Hench, P.S.: The ameliorating effect of pregnancy on chronic atrophic (infectious rheumatoid) arthritis, fibrositis and intermittent hydarthrosis. Mayo Clin. Proc., 13:161–167, 1938.

35. Hirano, T., et al.: Association of primary hypothyroidism and slipped capital femoral epiphysis. J. Pediatr., 93:262–264, 1978.

36. Horne, C.H.W., et al.: Studies on pregnancy associated globulin. Clin. Exp. Immunol., 13:603–611, 1973.

37. Julkunen, H., Heinonen, O.P., Pyörälä, K.: Hyperostosis of the spine in an adult population: its relation to hyperglycaemia and obesity. Ann. Rheum. Dis., 30:605–612, 1971.

38. Kahn, C.R., et al.: The syndromes of insulin resistance and acanthosis nigrans. N. Engl. J. Med., 294:739–745, 1976.

39. Kasinath, S.B., and Katz, A.I.: Delayed maternal lupus after delivery of offspring with congenital heart block. Arch. Intern. Med., 142:2,317, 1982.

40. Kaufman, R.L., and Kitridou, R.C.: Pregnancy in mixed connective tissue disease: comparison with systemic lupus erythematosus. J. Rheumatol., 9:549–555, 1982.

41. Kellgren, J.H., Ball, J., and Tutton, G.K.: The articular and other limb changes in acromegaly. Q. J. Med., 21:405–424, 1952.

42. Kruse, K., et al.: Hypocalcemic myopathy in idiopathic hypoparathyroidism. Eur. J. Pediatr., 138:280–282, 1982.

43. Lahita, R.G., et al.: Abnormal estrogen and androgen metabolism in the human with systemic lupus erythematosus. Am. J. Kidney Dis., 2:206–211, 1982.

44. Lequesne, M., et al.: Increased association of diabetes mellitus with capsulitis of the shoulder and shoulder hand syndrome. Scand. J. Rheumatol., 6:53–56, 1977.

45. Lin, T.M., Halbert, S.P., and Spellacy, W.N.: Measurement of pregnancy-associated plasma proteins during human gestation. J. Clin. Invest., 54:576–582, 1974.

46. Locke, S., Lawrence, D.G., and Legg, M.A.: Diabetic amyotrophy. Am. J. Med., 34:775–785, 1963.

47. Low, P.A., et al.: Peripheral neuropathy in acromegaly. Brain, 97:139–152, 1974.

48. McCarty, D.J., et al.: Diseases associated with calcium pyrophosphate dihydrate crystal deposition: a controlled study. Am. J. Med., 56:704–714, 1974.

49. McKeran, R.O., et al.: Muscle fibre type changes in hypothyroid myopathy. J. Clin. Pathol., 28:659–663, 1975.

50. Mallette, L.E., Patten, B.M., and Engel, W.K.: Neuromuscular disease in secondary hyperparathyroidism. Ann. Intern. Med., 82:474–483, 1975.

51. Mirahmadi, K.S., Coburn, J.W., and Bluestone, R.: Calcific periarthritis and hemodialysis. JAMA, 223:548–549, 1973.

52. Nagulesparen, M., et al.: Muscle changes in acromegaly. Br. Med. J., 2:914–915, 1976.

53. Neely, N.T., and Persellin, R.H.: Activity of rheumatoid arthritis during pregnancy. Tex. Med., 73:59–63, 1977.

54. Newcombe, D.S.: Endocrinopathies and uric acid metabolism. Semin. Arthritis Rheum., 2:281–300, 1972–73.

55. Newcombe, D.S., Ortel, R.W., Levey, G.S.: Activation of synovial membrane adenylate cyclase by thyroid stimulating hormone. Biochem. Biophys. Res. Commun., 48:201–211, 1972.

56. Nickel, S.N., et al.: Myxedema neuropathy and myopathy: a clinical and pathologic study. Neurology, 11:125–137, 1961.

57. Odell, W.D., and Wolfsen, A.R.: Humoral syndromes associated with cancer. Annu. Rev. Med., 29:379–406, 1978.

58. Oren, M.E., and Cohen, M.S.: Immune thrombocytopenia, red cell aplasia, lupus and hyperthyroidism. South. Med. J., 71:1,577–1,578, 1978.

59. Osgood, R.B.: The medical and social approaches to the problem of chronic rheumatism. Am. J. Med. Sci., 200:429–445, 1940.

60. Pastan, R.S., and Cohen, A.S.: The rheumatologic manifestations of diabetes mellitus. Med. Clin. North Am., 62:829–839, 1978.

61. Patten, B.M., et al.: Neuromuscular disease in primary hyperparathyroidism. Ann. Intern. Med., 80:182–193, 1974.

62. Persellin, R.H.: The effect of pregnancy on rheumatoid arthritis. Bull. Rheum. Dis., 27:922–927, 1976–77.

63. Pickett, J.B.E., III, et al.: Neuromuscular complications of acromegaly. Neurology, 25:638–645, 1975.

64. Plonk, J.W., and Feldman, J.M.: Carcinoid arthropathy. Arch. Intern. Med., 134:651–654, 1974.

65. Preston, E.T.: Avulsion of both quadriceps tendons in hyperparathyroidism. JAMA, 221:406–407, 1972.

66. Pritchard, M.H., and Jessop, J.D.: Chondrocalcinosis in primary hyperparathyroidism: influence of age, metabolic bone disease and parathyroidectomy. Ann. Rheum. Dis., 36:146–151, 1977.

67. Ramsey, I.D.: Thyroid Disease and Muscle Dysfunction. London, Whitefriars Press, 1974.

68. Rao, S.N., et al.: Neuromuscular status in hypothyroidism. Acta Neurol. Scand., 61:167–177, 1980.

69. Revel, J.P., Ito, S., and Fawcett, D.W.: Electron micrographs of phospholipids simulating intracellular membranes. J. Biophys. Biocytol., 4:495–498, 1958.

70. Richardson, J.A., et al.: Ischemic ulcerations of skin and necrosis of muscle in azotemic hyperparathyroidism. Ann. Intern. Med., 77:129–138, 1969.

71. Rosenbloom, A.L., et al.: Limited joint mobility in childhood diabetes mellitus indicates increased risk for microvascular disease. N. Engl. J. Med., 305:191–194, 1981.

72. Scarpalezos, S., et al.: Neural and muscular manifestations of hypothyroidism. Arch. Neurol., 29:140–144, 1973.
73. Schiff, R.I., Mercier, D., and Buckley, R.H.: Inability of gestational hormones to account for the inhibitory effects of pregnancy plasmas on lymphocyte responses in vitro. Cell. Immunol., 20:69–80, 1975.
74. Schmid, F.R., et al.: Arteritis in rheumatoid arthritis. Am. J. Med., 30:56–83, 1961.
75. Shagan, B.P., and Friedman, S.A.: Raynaud's phenomenon and thyroid deficiency. Arch. Intern. Med., 140:831–832, 1980.
76. Sheahan, M.G., and Vignos, P.J.: Experimental corticosteroid myopathy. Arthritis Rheum., 12:491–497, 1969.
77. Sinha, S., Munichoodappa, C.S., and Kozak, G.P.: Neuropathy (Charcot joints) in diabetes mellitus. Medicine, 51:191–210, 1972.
78. Sledge, C.: Growth hormone and articular cartilage. Fed. Proc., 32:1,503–1,505, 1973.
79. Steinbach, H.L., and Russell, W.: Measurement of the heel-pad as an aid to diagnosis of acromegaly. Radiology, 82:418–423, 1964.
80. Stern, B.D., et al.: Studies of collagen degradation during bone resorption in tissue culture. Proc. Soc. Exp. Biol. Med., 119:577–583, 1965.
81. Strom, L.: Trigger finger in diabetes. J. Med. Soc. N.J., 74:951–954, 1977.
82. Swanson, J.W., Kelly, J.D., and McConahey, W.M.: Neurologic aspects of thyroid dysfunction. Mayo Clin. Proc., 56:504–512, 1981.
83. Takeuchi, A., and Persellin, R.H.: The inhibitory effect of pregnancy serum on polymorphonuclear leukocyte chemotaxis. J. Clin. Lab. Immunol., 3:121–124, 1980.
84. Talal, N., Dauphinee, M.J., and Wofsy, D.: Interleukin-2 deficiency, genes, and systemic lupus erythematosus. Arthritis Rheum., 25:838–842, 1982.
85. Tarzy, B.J., et al.: Rheumatic disease, abnormal serology and oral contraceptives. Lancet, 2:501–503, 1972.
86. Varshnav, P., and Carasso, B.: Coexistence of polymyositis and carcinoid bronchial adenoma. JAMA, 249:1,266–1,267, 1983.
87. Viljanto, J.A.: Dupuytren's contracture—a review. Semin. Arthritis Rheum., 3:155–176, 1973.
88. Volpé, R.: The role of autoimmunity in hypoendocrine and hyperendocrine function: with special emphasis on autoimmune thyroid disease. Ann. Intern. Med., 87:86–99, 1977.
89. Von Schoultz, B.: A quantitative study of the pregnancy zone protein in the sera of pregnant and puerperal women. Am. J. Obstet. Gynecol., 119:792–797, 1974.
90. Waine, H., Bennett, G.A., and Bauer, W.: Joint disease associated with acromegaly. Am. J. Med. Sci., 209:671–687, 1945.
91. Weinstein, P.S., et al.: Insulin resistance due to receptor antibodies: a complication of progressive systemic sclerosis. Arthritis Rheum., 23:101–105, 1980.
92. Wilke, W.S., Sheeler, L.R., and Makarowski, W.S.: Hypothyroidism with presenting symptoms of fibrositis. J. Rheumatol., 8:626–631, 1981.
93. Withrington, R.H., and Seifert, M.H.: Hypothyroidism associated with mixed connective tissue disease and its response to steroid therapy. Ann. Rheum. Dis., 40:315–316, 1981.

Infectious Arthritis

Chapter 99

Principles of Diagnosis and Treatment of Bone and Joint Infections

Frank R. Schmid

Bone and joint infections are curable if an antimicrobial drug active against the invading micro-organisms is given early and if retained necrotic material is drained. When an infection is eradicated before irreversible tissue damage has occurred, complete restoration of function can be expected. A rational therapeutic program based on these principles should be individually tailored for each patient. A prompt diagnosis is essential for optimal results. A long-range plan such as outlined in Table 99–1 for patients with septic arthritis will avoid errors that can compromise the outcome.

PATHOGENESIS OF BONE AND JOINT INFECTIONS

Septic Arthritis, Bursitis, and Tendinitis

Except in rare cases of direct penetration by instrumentation or trauma,[23,148] invasion of the joint cavity by micro-organisms occurs through the blood and usually reflects the culmination of a series of successive failures of the host's systemic defense mechanisms. A primary focus of infection is first established at a portal of entry, usually remote from the joint. Micro-organisms escaping from this site enter the lymphatic vessels and the circulation,[157,165] where they must resist serum bactericidal activity,[142] as well as elude an active reticuloendothelial system in sufficient numbers and for an adequate time to allow colonization of synovial tissue or juxta-articular bone. Finally, the joint cavity itself must be penetrated from this periarticular location to permit the full-blown expression of acute septic arthritis. In normal circumstances, therefore, the joint is a privileged sanctuary. For each example of overt sepsis, countless instances of failure to infect must occur, considering the low incidence of infectious arthritis in comparison with the much higher incidence of systemic infectious diseases and bacteremia.[25]

Thus, the likelihood of infectious arthritis is greater if host resistance is impaired by prior disease,[53,92,118,165] or by treatment with drugs that interfere with defense mechanisms, such as corticosteroids or immunosuppressive agents.[76,97,158] Although sepsis may develop in normal joints, particularly with gonococcal and staphylococcal infections, previous damage by trauma or by another arthritic disease predisposes a joint to infection.[61,76,88,99,147] The characteristic monarticular presentation of septic arthritis suggests that local factors, even within an apparently "normal" joint, favor its colonization over that of another joint equally exposed to the same blood-borne agent.

As micro-organisms penetrate the joint cavity, a rapid series of events occurs. Although studies of the inflammatory process in septic arthritis are sparse, the process is similar to that produced by other phlogistic stimuli. The synovial microvasculature dilates, subsynovial tissue becomes edematous, and the volume of synovial fluid increases dramatically with a rise in intra-articular pressure.[125,153] Concentrations of macromolecules such as immunoglobulins and complement proteins in joint fluid approach those in plasma.[80] Because hematogenous dissemination usually occurs at least several days after the infection has become established at a primary site, lymphocyte activation and antibody production against the micro-organisms ordinarily will have begun.[1] Thus, immune complexes can form between the antibody and the micro-organism or its antigenic fragments, and these complexes can induce such complement-mediated events in the joint as histamine release, chemotaxis, and phagocytosis.[56,153] Bacterial products alone, even in the absence of antibody, can trigger complement activation through the alternate pathway.[163]

A major difference between a closed-space infection, such as septic arthritis, and one dispersed throughout the fibrillar scaffolding of connective tissue, such as cellulitis, is the slower rate of exchange of its contents with the surrounding vascular and lymphatic spaces. Solutes in synovial fluid must diffuse across the synovial lining, often

Table 99–1. Guidelines for Management of a Patient with Infectious Arthritis

INITIAL EVALUATION

Objective: Develop support for diagnosis of infectious arthritis

1. Historical and physical data
   —Primary site of infection
   —Septicemia: fever, chills, skin rash, polyarthralgia, other metastatic sites of infection
   —Host defense impairment
   —Pre-existing joint damage
2. Initial joint fluid examination
   —Joint fluid analysis: order of priority if amount of joint fluid is limited; smear and culture (or antigen detection); microscopy of wet-mount preparation; glucose and lactate measurement; cell count
3. Joint visualizaiton
   —Radiographs of affected and contralateral joint
   —Radioisotope joint scan, especially for deep-seated joints

INITIAL THERAPEUTIC DECISION

Objective: Selection of antibiotic for the most probable infecting micro-organism

1. Identification of suspected micro-organism
   —Clinical clues: age, geography, environment, primary site of infection
   —Bacteriologic smear of joint fluid
2. Selection of antibiotic(s)
   —Route for administration: intravenous or intramuscular usually
   —Dosage
3. Joint immobilization and support, analgesia

REAPPRAISAL: 24–72 HOURS

Objective: Reassessment of initial antibiotic choice and decision concerning joint drainage

1. Confirmation of antibiotic choice
   —Culture report and sensitivity of invading micro-organism to antibiotic drugs
   —Review of dosage requirements: bacterial assay of synovial fluid if adequacy of drug levels in doubt
2. Institution of joint drainage
   —Needle aspiration and lavage
   —Arthrotomy: reserved initially for such special circumstances as infancy, some deep-seated joint infections, or grossly contaminated wounds
3. Monitoring treatment response
   —Clinical parameters: systemic findings and primary site of infection
   —Infected joint(s): appearance and size; synovial fluid appearance, volume, glucose, lactate, white blood cell count, antigen assay if possible, culture

REAPPRAISAL: 5–8 DAYS

Objective: Assessment of efficacy of joint drainage and antibiotic treatment

1. Assessment of frequency and type of joint drainage
   —Review clinical and laboratory data from monitoring system
   —Criteria for arthrotomy/arthroscopy: micro-organism, treatment response, radiographic changes
2. Problems associated with antibiotic usage
   —Inability to detect an invading micro-organism
   —Hypersensitivity to initial drug choice
   —Decision for duration and dosage: micro-organism, treatment response
   —Postinfectious synovitis
3. Passive or active range-of-motion exercises

REAPPRAISAL: 2–8 WEEKS

Objective: Planning out-patient care

1. Choice of drug for oral use: dosage and duration
2. Joint function
   —Sequential monitoring system to maximal improvement
   —Radiologic comparison with initial films
   —Joint use and weightbearing

REAPPRAISAL: 3–6 MONTHS OR LONGER

Objective: Planning corrective surgical procedure or supportive measures for patients with incomplete restoration of joint function or structure

1. Joint function and structure
   —Evaluation of residual inflammation, motion, and structural integrity of joint
   —Radiologic comparison with previous films
   —Criteria for surgical reconstruction

tamponaded by increased pressure,[120] to reach distant subsynovial vessels, in contrast to the easy access of molecules in interstitial tissues to nearby capillary networks. Diffusion of solutes between joint fluid and blood, although slowed, does reach equilibrium within several hours, however.[116] Proteins leave the joint by lymphatic drainage. Thus, the diminished effectiveness of antibiotics against bacteria in a closed-space infection is not due to suboptimal local concentrations of the drug. Rather, the slowed diffusion from the joint of metabolic by-products of the infection retards bacterial cell growth.[13,37,60,87,150a,168] *Bacteria remain dormant under these conditions and survive in the presence of otherwise bactericidal drug concentrations.* For this reason, the time-honored principle of relief of pressure by drainage of pus is a critical component of an effective therapeutic program.

Other synovial tissues, such as bursae and tendon sheaths, share the same pathogenetic mechanism for infection as described for the joint synovium, except direct penetration of microorganisms from the skin might be a more common means of infection of superficial sacs such as the olecranon and prepatellar bursae.[18,66]

Structures at risk for injury by the infectious process are those lying within the confines of the synovial-lined capsule or sheath, although surrounding soft tissues outside this space are sometimes invaded in rare instances of rupture or sinus formation. Damage to the synovium and capsule of a bursa is reversible, but tendons within synovial sheaths are vulnerable to the effects of the inflammatory process and lose a significant degree of function. Even more vulnerable is articular cartilage. Chondrolysis is readily demonstrated in the presence of pus[29,120,133,170] and destroyed hyaline cartilage cannot be totally or effectively repaired. These anatomic considerations influence the need for drainage, which is obviously even more critical for joints and tendons than for bursae.

Osteomyelitis

Bone becomes infected by the blood or from a site of contiguous infection. Hematogenous osteomyelitis most often involves rapidly growing bone, characteristically the metaphysis of long bones in children and the vertebrae in adults.[42,119,161] Osteomyelitis from an adjacent area of infection may result from trauma, open wounds, compound fractures, or an operative infection.[160,161] In recent years, problems relative to infection of joint prostheses have been of great importance.[38]

The acquisition and spread of such infections are tied closely to differences in the microvascular anatomic structures of growing and of mature bone[161]

(Fig. 99–1). Between the age of one year and puberty, osteomyelitis starts in metaphyseal sinusoidal veins. This site is favored because the afferent loop of the metaphyseal capillary lacks phagocytic lining cells; the efferent loops are frequently multiple, with a broad diameter in which blood flow becomes slow and more turbulent; and the capillary loops adjacent to the epiphyseal growth plate are nonanastomotic, so necrosis can result from obstruction caused by microbial emboli and vascular thrombosis. The metaphyseal infection does not cross the epiphyseal growth plate in children, but spreads laterally, perforating the cortex and lifting the loose periosteum to cause a subperiosteal abscess (Route 4, Fig. 99–1). In some joints, such as the hip and shoulder, the synovial reflection reaches beyond the epiphyseal growth plate, so infection penetrates directly into the joint through cortical bone (Route 1, Fig. 99–1). In the infant less than a year old, capillaries perforate the growth plate, and the infection may thereby spread into the epiphysis and, by further extension, into the joint, with destruction of the epiphyseal growth center (Route 3, Fig. 99–1). An analogous situation can occur in the adult.[5] After resorption of the growth cartilage, anastomoses form between the metaphyseal and the epiphyseal blood vessels and allow the spread of infection from the epiphyseal portion of bone to the joint cavity (Route 2, Fig. 99–1).

Once the infection has started, edema, cellular infiltration, and accumulation of products of inflammation develop in much the same manner as in septic arthritis and contribute to the necrotic breakdown of bone trabeculae and loss of matrix and mineral. The part played by vascular obstruction is even more important in bone infection. Large segments of bone devoid of blood supply can separate to form sequestra. In cross section, the infected bone shows a core of necrosis with fibrin deposits and massive polymorphonuclear cell infiltration surrounded by an area with granulation tissue containing lymphocytes and plasma cells, and finally an outer layer of fibrous tissue in which new bone is formed. When the infection ruptures beneath the periosteum, more common in children than in adults, the periosteum overgrows to form an involucrum. Cortical destruction can predispose such a patient to fractures.[161]

The vertebral body is the most common site of hematogenous osteomyelitis in the adult. This infection spreads readily along the adjacent ligaments by means of freely anastomosing venous channels, thus commonly involving two adjacent vertebral bodies. The disc between each vertebra loses its vascular supply early in life, but it can be infected by direct extension from the vertebral abscess. The

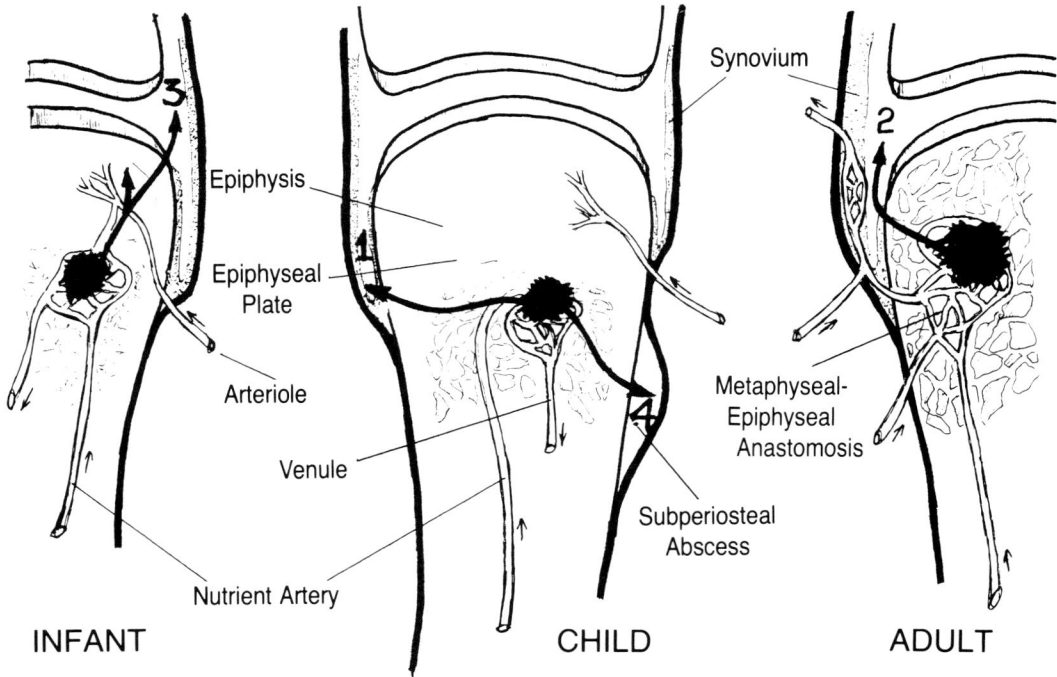

Fig. 99–1. Schematic representation of the vascular supply to the bone and joint in the infant, the child, and the adult. Blood-borne microbial emboli reach the metaphysis where conditions favor their lodgment. The bone abscess that forms can spread in several directions, depending on the age of the patient. In children older than a year of age, the epiphyseal growth plate blocks extension of the infection, so the abscess penetrates laterally to the subperiosteum (route 4) or to the joint, in the case of the shoulder, in which the synovial reflection extends beyond the epiphysis to the metaphysis (route 1). In the infant, small capillaries cross the epiphyseal growth plate and thus permit extension of the infection to the epiphysis and subsequently to the joint (route 3). In the adult, osteomyelitis can spread by the anastomotic metaphyseal-epiphyseal vessels to the subperiosteum and then to the joint (route 2). (Adapted from Waldvogel, F.A., Medoff, G., and Schwartz, M.[161] and from Atcheson, S.G. and Ward, J.R.[5])

infection can also extend centrally into the spinal canal under the dura mater, with resulting spinal cord compression, or externally to paraspinal soft tissues. In the cervical region, osteomyelitis can cause a retropharyngeal abscess or mediastinitis; in the thoracic spine, mediastinitis, empyema, or pericarditis; and in the lumbar spine, peritonitis or an abscess beneath the diaphragm or along fascial planes of the iliopsoas muscle.

An infection anywhere in the body may spread directly to adjacent bone. The source may be exogenous, as in sepsis introduced into a postsurgical or post-traumatic wound, or it may be an already infected neighboring tissue, such as a nasal sinus, tooth, or abdominal organ. The propensity for bone to become infected in these instances appears to be enhanced by concomitant arterial disease. In diabetic feet or in the extremities of patients with rheumatoid vasculitis, an infection in necrotic tissue may involve the underlying bone.[161]

MICRO-ORGANISMS RESPONSIBLE FOR BONE AND JOINT INFECTIONS

Almost any micro-organism can cause infectious arthritis, but most infections are caused by a few common agents (Table 99–2). In children who have a high incidence of pyogenic arthritis,[108] *Staphylococcus aureus* and other cocci are most often found, but gram-negative bacilli and *Haemophilus influenzae* are most frequent in the younger child,[14,42,106] probably as a result of an immature immune system. In those under age two, the absence of antibody has been linked to vulnerability to *H. influenzae*. Even gonococcal arthritis, although rare, occurs in children.[41] In adults, gonococci and staphylococci now cause the majority of joint infections.[2,22,24,46,53,132,145,157,162,165]

Gram-positive cocci are also the most frequent invaders of bone in hematogenous osteomyelitis (Table 99–2). Enterobacteriaceae are next, but

Table 99–2. Estimate of the Incidence of Micro-organisms Commonly Responsible for Acute Pyogenic Arthritis and Osteomyelitis

	Septic Arthritis		Hematogenous Osteomyelitis	
Micro-organism	Adults (%)	Children (%)	Adults (%)	Children (%)
Gram-positive cocci				
Staphylococcus aureus	35	45	65	60
Streptococcus pyogenes, S. pneumoniae, viridans-group streptococci	10	25	10	20
Gram-negative cocci				
Neisseria gonorrhoeae	50	5	—	—
Haeomophilus influenzae*	<1	10	—	—
Gram-negative bacilli				
Escherichia coli, Salmonella sp., Pseudomonas, etc.	5	15	20	15
Mycobacteria, fungi	<1	<1	<5	<5

*H. influenzae are actually coccobacilli, but are listed under "cocci" because they are frequently mistaken on smears for cocci

Neisseria species are rare. In some settings, as in osteomyelitis in heroin addicts, infection with *Pseudomonas aeruginosa* or *Serratia* species stands out;[129] in patients with sickle cell disease, *Salmonella* species are prominent;[113,161] and in the neonate, group B streptococci.[94] Although fungi and mycobacteria are only occasionally the cause of musculoskeletal infections (see Chap. 102), they have a propensity to localize in bone. Diagnosis is especially difficult unless the bone lesion can be aspirated and the material can be cultured. These micro-organisms should always be considered whenever routine cultures are sterile. Occasionally, infection may be caused by several micro-organisms, as, for example, septic arthritis of the hip after perforation of an abdominal organ,[148] or osteomyelitis from a contiguous infection. Both aerobic and anaerobic bacteria may be present together.[33,43]

The micro-organisms that usually infect bone and joint tissues are not the most common causes of clinical septicemia. Gram-negative bacilli, other than *Haemophilus* species are common causes of septicemia, but they invade osseous or synovial tissue usually only when the tissue has suffered previous damage,[52,53] or when the host has become immunocompromised. Bacteria such as the staphylococcus may thus have a special affinity for bone and synovial structures.

MICRO-ORGANISMS ASSOCIATED WITH STERILE JOINT INFLAMMATION

Hematogenous infections of bones and joints almost always occur after the host has had sufficient time to mount an immune response. As part of that response, committed lymphocytes and plasma cells respond to the various products made by the infecting microbial agent or to portions of its structure.[1] Immune complexes that form between these antigens and specific antibody or human cells that are cytolytic for antibody-coated or other target tissues can induce inflammation even in the absence of viable micro-organisms. Furthermore, host tissues that cross-react with microbial antigens may also participate in this response. Thus, a pathogenic spectrum varying from an inflammatory process generated mainly by virulence factors of the actively metabolizing microbe on the one hand to sterile inflammation generated by the host's immune system on the other hand may account to varying degrees for the signs of inflammation seen in different patients infected by the same agent or seen at various times during the course of the disease in a single patient[153] (Fig. 99–2).

Immune-Mediated Forms of Arthritis

Well-known examples of inflammation associated with immune complexes are found in patients with the disseminated gonococcal syndrome[91] (see Chap. 100), with hepatitis[32] and rubella[55] virus infections (see Chap. 103), and most recently, with Lyme disease[58,59] (see Chap. 104). In each instance, viable bacteria, viruses, and spirochetes have been cultured from the inflamed joint, and immune complexes have been detected in the plasma or joint fluid. When both are present at the same time, the relative contribution of either to the inflammation cannot be determined. When cultures of synovial fluid or tissue are sterile, the cause of the inflammation can often be attributed to the host's immune response. Yet even in such patients special culture techniques may be necessary to uncover the presence of a viable agent. For example, spirochetes were recovered from the skin and joints of patients with Lyme disease only after a long search,[150] and rubella virus was "rescued" from the peripheral blood lymphocytes of an arthritic patient who had received live rubella vaccine two

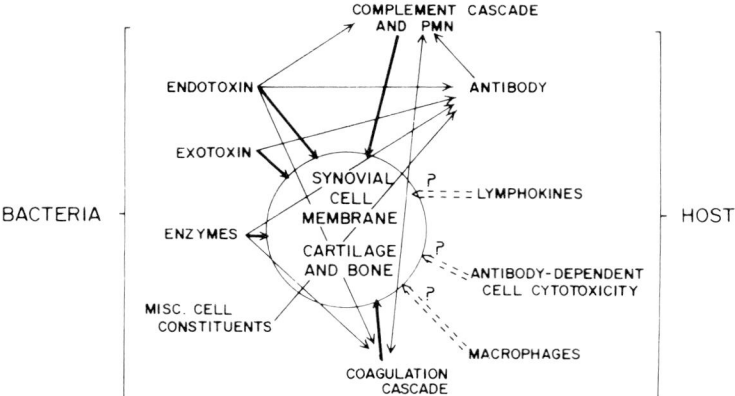

Fig. 99–2. Interaction of bacterial and host factors in the inflammatory process of septic arthritis. A thick arrow indicates a final and direct pathway of tissue damage; a thin arrow represents the interaction of one component with another leading to induction of synovial inflammation; and an interrupted arrow signifies a possible, but insufficiently documented, host effect. PMN = Polymorphonuclear leukocytes. (From Tesar, J.T. and Dietz, F.[153])

years earlier.[21] A unique illustration of the combination of both infectious and noninfectious inflammation in the same patient may be the development of sterile, so-called *"sympathetic"* effusions, in a bursa or joint adjacent to a primary site of septic arthritis or osteomyelitis. No explanation is known for these effusions, and it is assumed that inflammatory mediators are transported to the nearby sac to cause the inflammation. The implications of such observations for antibiotic therapy are discussed later in the section of this chapter on postinfectious synovitis.

A limited number of observations have been made about the immune response in osteomyelitis. Antibodies to a staphylococcal cell-wall constituent, teichoic acid, have been found mainly in the serum of patients with bone infections.[155] Rheumatoid factors develop, but less commonly, in staphylococcal osteomyelitis than in staphylococcal endocarditis.[164] The possible relevance of these serologic findings to the pathogenesis of the bone disease is not known.

Reactive Arthritis

The pathogenesis of sterile inflammation in the joints of patients with infectious diseases at extra-articular sites is even more elusive. Examples are streptococcal pharyngitis in patients with rheumatic fever (see Chap. 68), enteritis due to *Salmonella, Shigella,* or *Yersinia* species, or urethritis due to *Mycoplasma* agents in patients with Reiter's syndrome (see Chap. 54), or bowel lesions related to parasitic infestations,[11] as well as to bacterial residues in patients with Whipple's disease (see Chap. 56). The type of immune or other response responsible for the arthritis in these cases is not known. Pathogenetic immune complexes have not

been found, or if found, do not correlate with the disease process. In some cases, success attends eradication of the triggering infecting agent by administration of appropriate drugs, although most often this approach fails to control the arthritis.

Speculation concerning the mechanism of joint inflammation in such patients can be expanded to the possible contribution of infectious agents to major rheumatic diseases such as rheumatoid arthritis (RA) and systemic lupus erythematosus (see Chap. 27).

CLINICAL PRESENTATIONS

Infectious arthritis may become manifest in a variety of ways, both typical and atypical.

Typical Presentation

Pyogenic arthritis affecting single or, less commonly, two or more joints is usually of acute onset.[3,42,53,165] A migratory polyarthritis may precede this phase, especially in gonococcal and meningococcal arthritis.[15,47,74,75] Large joints, such as the knee and hip, are involved most often, but articular structures of any size or location, including the sacroiliac and spinal joints, may be affected. The infected joint is typically warm, painful, and distended with fluid. Because bacterial entry into a joint is most often hematogenous, the patient may have fever with chills.[132] Signs and symptoms of a primary infection should be sought. Careful examination may reveal pneumonia as a source of pneumococci or a carbuncle as a source of staphylococci. A history of urethritis, pharyngitis, or prostatitis suggesting gonococcal infections might be obtained. In staphylococcal or streptococcal joint disease, and less often in gram-negative bacillary arthritides, a primary site of infection may not be found, however.[53]

Atypical Presentations

Unfortunately, septic arthritis may be atypical. In a joint damaged by prior disease, superimposed infection may not be obvious because the new process may become "lost" among other painful, chronically swollen joints.[33,76,99] Careful questioning usually reveals that the infected joint has become more symptomatic than it was before, however. Elderly patients, or those under treatment with immunosuppressive or corticosteroid drugs, are more vulnerable to superimposed infection and may show less evidence of inflammation than other patients. Some locations may be overlooked, such as a popliteal cyst,[126a] or the sternoclavicular or sternomanubrial joints,[109,129] or the hip joints.[77] Infected bursae are often missed, particularly the superficial prepatellar and olecranon bursae.[18,66]

Infection of the deeply situated axial joints of the body, such as the hip, shoulder, pubic, and sacroiliac joints, can present major difficulties in diagnosis and treatment because evidence of inflammation may be masked or, if present, may be ascribed to noninfectious causes until the process is far advanced.[48,54,77,140,144] This situation is of particular concern in the evaluation of acute shoulder pain. Delay in diagnosis may result in severe joint destruction and loss of motion.[48]

Joint Infections in Children

Septic arthritis in neonates 1 to 28 days of age may induce signs and symptoms of septicemia, such as lethargy, fever, tachycardia, and hypotension. Decreased spontaneous movement of the involved extremity, even in the absence of pain and swelling, helps to locate the infection. Multiple joints may be involved. Although bacteria can gain access into the joint directly by lodging in subsynovial vessels, more commonly they do so from a region of adjacent osteomyelitis (see Route 3, Fig. 99–1). Predisposing factors are a low birth weight and perinatal complications that necessitate instrumentation, such as fetal monitoring or exchange transfusions.[42,94]

In older children, the clinical appearance of septic arthritis more closely parallels that observed in adults.

Diagnostic problems are magnified in children, especially those with an infection of the hip. This joint is affected more often than any other except the knee, particularly in children below the age of six months.[108] Unless treatment is started promptly, irreversible destruction may occur within days.[40,85,152] Distention of the joint can rapidly deprive the femoral head of its blood supply, and

purulent fluids destroy cartilage and bone. Hematogenous dissemination of micro-organisms from a primary portal of entry to the joint or adjacent bone is usual, and prior joint disease or associated illness predisposes the child to infection in the hip just as in other joints.[102] Direct penetration may occur as a complication of femoral venipuncture,[4] or it may result from infection extending from an abdominal abscess into the retroperitoneal space near the iliopsoas muscle.[148]

Symptoms of sepsis in the hip include pain in the groin, lateral upper thigh, or buttocks. Referred pain along the obturator nerve to the knee is common.[44] The thigh is usually held in flexion, adduction, and internal rotation, and pain permits only a few degrees of motion. In adults, external signs of inflammation are rare, but in children, the massive increase in the volume of joint fluid may distend the capsule, obliterating the inguinal crease and causing generalized edema of the thigh. Marked tenderness may be elicited by local pressure.

Infections of Bone

Hematogenous osteomyelitis commonly affects rapidly growing bones in children, frequently the metaphysis of the tibia or the femur. The neonate in particular appears unusually vulnerable to bone infections. In recent years, the prevalence of bone infections in adults has increased, especially in the vertebral bodies.[161]

Most patients have fever, with or without chills, constitutional symptoms such as weight loss and fatigue, and symptoms referable to the local site of bony involvement. Thus, osteomyelitis of the long bones of the lower extremity may be associated with local pain, sometimes accompanied by swelling and erythema, a limp, or in a young child, refusal to walk. Vertebral osteomyelitis may be associated with back pain and local tenderness, spasm of paraspinal or psoas muscles, and limitation of motion. Pelvic osteomyelitis may cause abdominal pain or pain referred to the hip or lower extremities.[101] Findings in patients with spinal or pelvic osteomyelitis may be so subtle that infection in these regions should be considered in any individual who only has systemic signs of inflammation, such as a fever of unknown origin.[10] In such patients, a positive blood culture increases the likelihood of deep-seated osteomyelitis. Sepsis of the sacroiliac joint should be considered in the differential diagnosis of low-back or hip pain, particularly when unilateral sacroiliac disease is noted on a radiograph or scintiphotograph.[27,31]

Infected Joint Prostheses

Infection following a joint implant is a serious complication. Rates of infection initially were greater than 10%, but with extensive experience, they have dropped to less than 1% in most large centers.[38] Although most infections occur during the early postoperative months, they can appear several years later.[70a]

In the postoperative period, systemic signs such as fever may be falsely attributed to other complications such as pneumonia or a urinary tract infection. Persistent joint pain may be the only finding that suggests the real cause of the problem. Its character helps to distinguish mechanical loosening of the prosthesis from infection. With infection, pain is generally dull, is present also at night, is described as deep gnawing, or throbbing, and may diminish after the use of antibiotics. Pain with loosening is related to motion or weight bearing and may be accentuated by sharp movement. If purulent material drains from the wound, and if the infection does not respond to antibiotics, a deep infection around the prosthesis rather than a superficial wound infection should be considered, and exploration of the operative site may be required. *Staphylococcus aureus* or *S. epidermidis* are the most common causes of an infected joint prosthesis; gram-negative bacilli and anaerobic and other bacteria are less common.[12,43,70a,123]

DIAGNOSTIC STUDIES
Differential Diagnosis of Septic Arthritis

Other acute arthritic disorders such as gout, pseudogout, palindromic rheumatism, rheumatic fever, trauma, and the oligoarticular syndromes associated with the spondyloarthropathies or with juvenile RA may be confused with infectious arthritis. Constitutional symptoms such as high fever or chills and marked leukocytosis are uncommon in these conditions. Even when a noninfectious form of arthritis is actually present, an added infectious process must be excluded by bacteriologic examination of synovial fluid. An unusual but distressing example of superimposed infection occurs in crystal-induced synovitis, in which the previous deposition of urate or calcium pyrophosphate crystals in the joint predisposes the patient to sepsis,[57,61,88,147] or more likely, tissue breakdown by septic inflammation releases pre-existing crystal deposits into the joint space, a phenomenon aptly termed "enzymatic strip mining"[86,147] (see Chap. 93). Patients with RA have a high incidence of joint infection, usually due to staphylococci.[76,99] Therefore, suspicion of sepsis should be heightened whenever a primary site of infection or evidence of septicemia is recognized in any arthritic patient.

Differential Diagnosis of Bone Infection

Infections of the vertebral body, disc, or sacroiliac joint may be overlooked because symptoms and signs can mimic other conditions, such as post-traumatic thinning of a disc, congenital absence of a disc, osteochondritis of a disc, metastatic carcinoma, Paget's disease, or Charcot arthropathy.[161] Ankylosing spondylitis or the spondyloarthropathy associated with Reiter's disease, psoriasis, or bowel disease may present problems in the differential diagnosis of sacroiliac joint disease; these conditions usually affect both sacroiliac joints, however, whereas infection is almost always unilateral.[54] Correct diagnosis may require identification or exclusion of an infecting micro-organism by aspiration or surgical exploration.[98]

General Studies

A complete medical history and physical examination are essential, with special attention to the portals of entry for infection: skin, nasal passages including sinuses and the middle ear, lungs, rectum, urethra, and pelvis.

Initial studies in a patient with acute septic arthritis or hematogenous osteomyelitis may reveal leukocytosis with an increased percentage of immature leukocytes, but the absence of leukocytosis does not rule out sepsis, particularly in a debilitated individual. Anemia is not likely to be present early, unless an underlying disease antedates the infectious process. The erythrocyte sedimentation rate and other acute-phase reactants, such as C-reactive protein and the serum precursor of amyloid protein AA (SAA),[140a] are elevated both in infectious arthritis and in noninfectious inflammatory states. That elevated C-reactive protein levels failed to identify infection in patients with systemic lupus erythematosus dashed a hope raised by an earlier study.[68,169] Serum calcium, phosphorus, and alkaline phosphatase levels are usually normal in osteomyelitis. At least two blood cultures for aerobic and anaerobic organisms should be taken within the first several hours in every suspected case of pyogenic arthritis or osteomyelitis. A single positive blood culture may be difficult to interpret because of possible contamination during collection. Two blood cultures containing the same organism virtually rule out contamination. Cultures should also be made of any exudate or secretion at a suspected portal of entry.

Radiologic Examination

Several weeks are usually needed before cartilaginous or bony abnormalities can be detected in previously normal bone or joints (see Chaps. 5–87 through 5–90). In septic arthritis, rarefaction of subchondral bone develops first, followed by erosion of juxta-articular bone and narrowing of the joint space due to destruction of articular cartilage (Fig. 99–3). When superimposed on a diseased

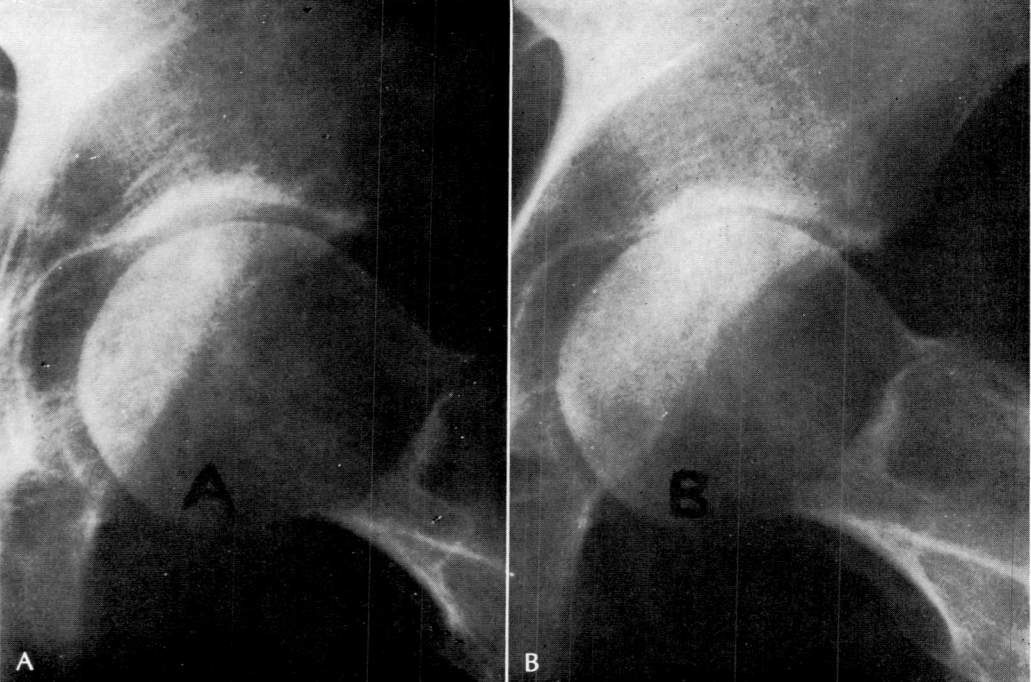

Fig. 99–3.   The hip joint of a patient with septic arthritis due to *Staphyloccus aureus. A,* Radiologic examination within the first week shows no abnormality. *B,* Film repeated three weeks later shows loss of cartilage and beginning bone erosion.

joint, changes caused by infection may be indistinguishable from those already present. The decalcification due to infection is particularly troublesome in children, in whom skeletal immaturity already makes significant bony structures radiolucent.

In osteomyelitis, bone is destroyed locally, but this change does not become visible for 2 to 3 weeks when 30 to 50% of bone mineral has been removed. New bone also forms, but about a month is required for the deposition of mineral to be sufficient to be detected. Thus, areas of lysis and increased bone density appear at about the same time radiographically, although soft tissue swelling and periosteal elevation may be seen earlier. For the same reason, radiologic evidence of healing of osteomyelitis also lags behind clinical improvement and actual bone reconstruction.[161]

Within a few weeks of the onset of vertebral disc or bone infection, thinning of the involved disc and destruction of vertebral bone may occur (see Figs. 5–89 and 5–90). Tomograms may more clearly outline lesions that are obscure on standard films. Lesions may heal by fusion, as illustrated in Figure 99–4. Most infections of the sacroiliac joint are unilateral, in contradistinction to bilateral involvement by the sterile spondylitic syndromes.

In deep-seated joints, such as the hip, soft tissue changes due to joint-space distention may be helpful in diagnosis. The *obturator sign,* a widening and curving of the border of the obturator internus tendon adjacent to the capsule of the hip joint, may be helpful if positive. A radiolucent *air sign* is an unusual finding in lesions produced by some gas-forming micro-organisms. This sign was noted in the disc space of a patient with vertebral osteomyelitis and in joints of patients with septic arthritis due to *Clostridium perfringens,*[117,141] *Streptococcus milleri,* anaerobic bacteria, and gram-negative bacilli.[83]

Although diagnosis of sepsis may not be evident, films taken early document the extent of prior damage and permit an estimate of the degree to which function might ultimately be restored. Comparison with radiographs of the contralateral bone and joint may reveal subtle changes in the involved side. Sequential films are helpful to monitor treatment (see Table 99–1).

Arthrography

In addition to determining placement of structures within the joint, arthrograms may reveal capsular or ligamentous damage. The contrast material does not exacerbate the infectious process, nor does

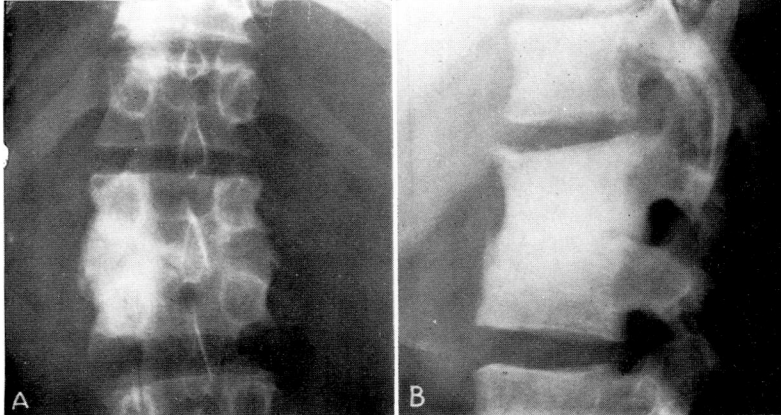

Fig. 99–4. *A* and *B*, specific infectious spondylitis involving lumbar vertebrae 1 and 2. The intervertebral disc has been destroyed, and fusion of the adjacent vertebral bodies is almost complete.

it interfere with antibiotic treatment. Rupture of the rotator cuff, with or without superior subluxation of the humeral head,[48] and delineation of the position and integrity of the femoral head, especially in children,[28,50,143] are often detectable by arthrography. Synovial fluid obtained should be examined for micro-organisms by staining and culture before the contrast dye is injected.

Computed Tomography (CT) Scanning

This procedure is most valuable when the anatomic structures are complex, as in the spine, or when the involved areas are surrounded by bone; it is less valuable in examining peripheral joints and the neck (see Chap. 6).[131] Osteomyelitis in a long bone increases the density of medullary tissues, presumably because of vascular congestion and edema, even before bone destruction becomes apparent. Later, just as on standard radiographs and conventional tomograms, CT scanning can be used to document bone destruction, cavitation, and sequestration.[6] In the spine, this technique permits identification of a soft tissue abscess. Swelling and effusion can be recognized in a deep seated area, such as the sacroiliac joint.[100]

Radioisotope Scanning Techniques

^{99m}Technetium (^{99m}Tc) diphosphonate and ^{67}gallium (^{67}Ga) citrate scintigraphy may detect the presence of infection at an early stage; these techniques are particularly useful in examining deep joints such as the hip, shoulder, and spine.[90,110] Positive results by either isotope are not specific for infection because other inflammatory or even degenerative joint diseases can create the same image.[26] Specificity for bone and joint infection, however, may be enhanced by giving more weight

to a positive ^{67}Ga citrate scan than to a positive ^{99m}Tc scan;[84] for osteomyelitis, one may perform a three-phase study, consisting of the radionuclide angiogram, the immediate postinjection "blood pool" image, and the 2- to 3-hour delayed image, to distinguish bone infection from soft tissue infection and from noninfectious skeletal disease.[93] Using scanning techniques, the pathologic process can be localized to a joint rather than to overlying tissue, as in cellulitis. This feature has been particularly useful in evaluating disease in the sacroiliac joint.[27,36,90]

In acute osteomyelitis, ^{99m}Tc-diphosphonate often fails to demonstrate a lesion in the neonate, in contrast to the expected high yield of abnormal images in the slightly older infant or child.[3] Even in older children, however, fulminant osteomyelitis may escape detection. Instead, a focal decrease in nuclide accumulation occurs, considered to be due to thrombosis in the microcirculation or to intraosseous pressure on the nutrient artery.[105]

The scan should always be interpreted together with findings revealed by the standard radiograph because the detailed anatomic information provided by the radiograph often complements the functional information provided by the newer technique.

Radiology of an Infected Joint Prosthesis

Several weeks or months may elapse before conventional radiographs indicate changes compatible with infection in an endoprosthesis. These changes include the formation of a radiolucent zone at the bone-cement interface, scalloping of the cortical margin, a periosteal reaction resembling lamination, and regions of increased bone density and radiolucency typical of osteomyelitis. Early and minor alterations are not recognizable without a comparison with previous films. Arthrograms are not helpful for the diagnosis of infection itself, but they can demonstrate the extent and location of soft tissue involvement, such as a sinus tract. If a sinus tract has perforated to the exterior, a sinogram can be done. Subtraction technique is essential to verify details when radiopaque cement is present. Bone scanning by ^{99m}Tc-diphosphonate may fail to distinguish mechanical loosening from infection; as mentioned earlier, imaging by ^{67}Ga citrate may be more specific for infection.[81]

Joint Fluid Examination

Aspiration and examination of joint fluid are mandatory whenever infection is considered. These procedures must be done immediately and must not be deferred.

Arthrocentesis requires strict asepsis (see Chap. 34). Inadvertent introduction of infection from skin, blood, or a para-articular focus into a joint cavity represents a hazard of joint aspiration. For this reason, a careful examination of the area is required to define anatomically the exact site of infection. The needle should be introduced into the joint through uninvolved subcutaneous tissue.

An arthrocentesis tray should always contain sterile culture tubes. If indicated, joint fluid should be inoculated into these tubes as well as into tubes for chemical determinations and tubes with heparin or ethylene diamine tetracetate anticoagulant for cell examination. These culture samples should be taken directly to a laboratory by the physician. The synovial fluid should still be warm when inoculated into appropriate bacteriologic media. Some even recommend bedside inoculation of the fluid onto media when infection with fastidious micro-organisms, such as the gonococcus, are anticipated. If only one or two drops of synovial fluid can be obtained, they should be cultured, and any remaining fluid should be smeared onto a slide for Gram staining.

Synovial or Bone Biopsy

Tissue may be required to confirm a diagnosis of sepsis in patients whose synovial fluid has not yielded a positive culture. In some cases, this procedure may prove helpful because the density of bacteria may be greater in tissue,[167] and in other cases, such as in tuberculous and fungal infections,[39] because microbial growth, even on appropriate culture media, is slow and thus may delay diagnosis and appropriate treatment. Tissue can be obtained by a blind synovial biopsy or under direct vision at arthroscopy or arthrotomy. Bone biopsy can be performed with a needle or surgically. The fresh tissue specimen should be transported to the laboratory in a sterile container, in a sterile sponge moistened with saline solution. In addition to the appropriate bacteriologic studies, a portion of the tissue should be fixed and submitted for histologic examination.

Bacteriologic Studies

Blood agar should be used routinely for culturing all synovial fluid or tissue specimens, with chocolate agar used in addition when *Neisseria gonorrhoeae* or *Haemophilus* infection is suspected. The medium designed by Thayer and Martin is suitable for gonococcal isolation, but it contains vancomycin and colistin methanesulfonate because it was designed to isolate gonococci from the mixed flora of the female genital tract.[154] Therefore, many other bacteria such as *Haemophilus* species do not grow on Thayer-Martin media. Media of higher ionic strength have been advocated to culture gonococcal protoplasts. In one patient with gonococcal arthritis, standard cultures were negative, but growth occurred on such hypertonic media.[67] *Haemophilus* species can easily be isolated on peptic digest of blood agar, which is prepared from commercially available products. Placement of about 1 ml synovial fluid in thioglycolate broth allows recovery of many anaerobic and aerobic bacteria. Many microaerophilic bacteria actually grow more rapidly after primary inoculation in thioglycolate broth than on solid media.

Isolation of strict anaerobes may require special anaerobic techniques. Fungal media, such as Sabourand agar, should be inoculated in most instances. If fungal media are not inoculated, fungi may be recovered from the blood agar plates after incubation for as long as two weeks at room temperature. Drying of ordinary blood agar plates can be retarded by sealing the plate with paraffin tape. Culture of *Mycobacterium* species is best done with at least two kinds of media, an egg-glycerol-potato medium, such as A.T.S. medium, and a synthetic medium, such as Middlebrook 7H10 agar. If a large volume of synovial fluid is available, it should be concentrated by centrifugation before inoculating mycobacterial cultures. Because of improvements in culture media, one no longer needs to use guinea pig inoculation as a means of recovering *M. tuberculosis;* results in the guinea pig are rarely positive when mycobacterial cultures are negative.[79] Furthermore, atypical *Mycobacterium* species, which also infect joints, are nonpathogenic for guinea pigs (see also Chap. 102).

After inoculation of joint fluid into all appropriate media, smears are prepared on glass slides, which are air dried, and Gram's stain, Wright's stain, and appropriate stains for acid-fast and fungal organisms are applied. Examination of such slides provides the necessary information to begin treatment.

Certain additional studies of joint fluid are regularly performed (Table 99–3). The total leukocyte count can be determined manually or with an automated cell counter *using physiologic saline solution as a diluent.* The acid diluents used for blood leukocyte counts coagulate the hyaluronate of synovial fluid and trap leukocytes, so counts are falsely low. Although fluids in septic arthritis often appear grossly purulent and have elevated cell counts, predominantly of polymorphonuclear leukocytes, high white blood cell counts containing many polymorphonuclear cells can appear in noninfected fluids obtained from some patients with acute gout, pseudogout, or RA.[130] Therefore, microbiologic stains and cultures provide the only absolute confirmation of sepsis.

The fasting synovial fluid glucose value is usually reduced to less than half the blood glucose value obtained simultaneously.[162] Reductions of this magnitude are unusual in inflammatory joint fluids of nonseptic origin, in infectious arthritis due to viruses, and in gonococcal arthritis. Determinations should be made only on specimens obtained six or more hours after eating or after termination of glucose infusions, to allow equilibration of glucose between blood and synovial fluid. Reduction of glucose concentration in fluid from joints infected with gonoccoci is often less dramatic than in infections with other micro-organisms.[47]

The synovial fluid lactate level is higher in patients with bacterial arthritis than in those with noninfectious inflammatory states such as RA. Lactate values are often just barely elevated, however, in gonococcal arthritis and in partially treated cases of infectious arthritis due to other bacteria.[13,16,103,128] Lactate, along with other metabolites such as succinic acid,[13] may be measured by gas-liquid chromatography, which detects end products of bacterial and host-tissue metabolism, but the method is laborious. A simpler and quicker technique makes use of the enzymatic oxidation of lactate to pyruvate.[9,103] Although the measurement of lactate levels may provide useful information in the diagnosis of joint sepsis, its limitations in patients with gonococcal and, probably, viral disease and in partially treated patients with bacterial sepsis make this test no more informative than the ratio of synovial fluid to serum glucose levels.

Inflammation from any cause increases the vascular permeability of the fenestrated synovial capillaries and augments the influx of serum proteins with a larger proportion of macromolecules, such as the complement proteins. In infectious arthritis, the level of these proteins in synovial fluid does not approach that found in serum because they are consumed intra-articularly in the inflammatory process. Complement proteins of both the classic and the alternate pathways are involved. Therefore, the ratio of C3 to total protein concentration of joint fluid is lower than the ratio of C3 to total serum protein.[17] A similar reduction is well recognized in RA, but not in other inflammatory arthritides such as gout, pseudogout, and seronegative spondyloarthropathy. Thus, decreased joint fluid complement levels are of interest in understanding the pathogenesis of sepsis, but they have a minor role in its diagnosis (see also Chap. 4).

Antigen Detection

Countercurrent immunoelectrophoresis has been used to identify soluble bacterial antigens in various body fluids.[34,95] The method has been particularly helpful to detect the antigens of micro-organisms such as the pneumococcus, meningococcus, and *Haemophilus influenzae* and of viruses such as hepatitis B. Results, available within several hours, provide a quantitative measurement of the amount of antigen within body fluids. In studies

Table 99–3.   Synovial Fluid Findings in Acute Pyogenic Arthritis (see also Chap. 4)

Joint Fluid Examination	Noninflammatory Fluids	Inflammatory Fluids	
		Noninfectious	Infectious
Color	Colorless, pale yellow	Yellow to white	Yellow
Turbidity	Clear, slightly turbid	Turbid	Turbid, purulent
Viscosity	Not reduced	Reduced	Reduced
Mucin clot	Tight clot	Friable	Friable
Cell count (per mm³)	200–1,000	3,000–>10,000	10,000–>100,000
Predominant cell type	Mononuclear	PMN*	PMN*
Synovial fluid/blood glucose ratio	0.8–1.0	0.5–0.8	<0.5
Lactic acid	Same as plasma	Higher than plasma	Often very high
Gram stain for organism	None	None	Positive†
Culture	Negative	Negative	Positive†

*PMN = polymorphonuclear leukocyte
†In some cases, especially in gonococcal infection, no organisms may be demonstrated.

of cerebrospinal and pleural fluids, the quantity of antigen has borne a direct relation to the severity of the infection and to prognosis.[133a]

A reliable test for the diagnosis of active gonococcal disease, using antigens such as pili from the bacterial wall for the detection of specific antibody, is not yet at hand,[126,134] nor have tests for gonococcal antigens in body fluids been developed.

Miscellaneous Tests

Assays using limulus amebocyte lysate to detect endotoxin in body fluids have not been able to distinguish septic arthritis, not even that due to gram-negative organisms, from noninfectious inflammatory arthritis.[149]

Teichoic acid antibodies to staphylococci have been found in the serum of many patients with osteomyelitis, but only infrequently in the serum of patients with septic arthritis due to this organism.[155] The value of this test as a diagnostic procedure seems marginal because staphylococci can be readily cultured from infected fluids and tissues. When the culture is negative or when material for culture is unavailable, the detection of such antibodies may complement the information obtained from the clinical, radiologic, and scanning examinations.

The nitroblue-tetrazolium (NBT) reduction test is useless in confirming the presence of infection in joint fluids. The test depends on the conversion of a soluble, colorless compound into an insoluble, blue granule on phagocytosis by polymorphonuclear or other phagocytic cells. Synovial fluid polymorphonuclear cells usually show a positive reaction, whether they come from infected or noninfected joints. The study of peripheral blood polymorphonuclear cells also does not discriminate between infectious and noninfectious inflammation.[151]

ANTIBIOTIC TREATMENT

Immediate Management

Antibiotics should be given in cases of clear-cut or strongly suspected bone and joint infections, even before an exact identification of the infecting micro-organism is made. When the micro-organism has been identified and its sensitivity to antimicrobial drugs has been assayed, the choice and dose of antibiotic can be reconsidered. If no micro-organism is recovered from the bone or joint, further decisions about drug treatment will depend on the use of other, albeit nonspecific, laboratory tests and on the clinical course.

Antibiotic treatment for septic arthritis should begin within the first few hours after the patient's admission to the hospital. A preliminary estimate of the type of infecting micro-organism can be made on the basis of the findings noted on the Gram-stained smear of synovial fluid, which may show gram-positive cocci, gram-negative cocci or coccobacilli, gram-negative bacilli, or no micro-organisms.

If no organism is detected in an otherwise healthy patient, I treat an adult with penicillin G intravenously (Table 99–4), which is adequate for most infections caused by pneumococci, gonococci, penicillin G-susceptible staphylococci, and a number of less-common bacteria. Gonococcal arthritis in the adult is frequently accompanied by a negative Gram-stained smear, despite clinically convincing evidence of infection.[15,47,74,75] Improvement, often in four to seven days of treatment with large amounts of penicillin G alone, may be dramatic and may suggest the probable cause of the disease. Unlike gonococcal urethritis, only rarely are the gonococci associated with arthritis resistant to penicillin.[127] In an ill patient in whom gram-negative bacillary infection is suspected, I use an aminoglycoside with a penicillinase-resistant penicillin or a cephalosporin. Initial treatment in children, especially in infants under two years of age, should be with chloramphenicol, owing to the likely presence of beta-lactamase-positive *Haemophilus influenzae*. If beta-lactamase-negative micro-organisms are found later on culture, ampicillin is substituted for chloramphenicol.[20] In infants under six months of age, gentamicin and nafcillin are used because of concern for other gram-negative bacilli.

Initial antibiotic treatment for acute hematogenous osteomyelitis is usually a penicillinase-resistant penicillin. If gram-negative sepsis is suspected, an aminoglycoside is added. In nonhematogenous osteomyelitis, which may be due to a polymicrobic infection, dual antibiotic therapy is appropriate, as in the case of gram-negative sepsis.

During the acute phase of the illness, antibiotics should be given parenterally. If the drug is administered intravenously, the daily dose should be divided into fractions, and a fractional dose should be given every 6 to 8 hours over a span of 30 to 60 minutes into a constant infusion. This "piggyback" technique is preferred to continual delivery of the drug by intravenous infusion, to avoid loss due to interruption of flow that might result from subcutaneous infiltration or blockage of the needle or tubing.

When a specific bacterium is seen on the Gram-stained smear, one may attempt a closer approximation to definitive antibiotic therapy. Types and doses of drugs currently recommended for several different kinds of infection are listed in Table 99–4. Infections caused by gram-negative bacilli such as

Table 99–4. Antibiotic Selection Based on Patient's Age and Gram-Stain Findings*

Age (Years)	Gram-Negative Bacilli	Gram-Negative Cocci	Gram-Positive Cocci	No Organism Seen
<½	Gentamicin (*Enterobacteriaceae* or *Pseudomonas aeruginosa*)†	Penicillin G (*Neisseria gonorrhoeae*)	Nafcillin (staphylococci or streptococci)	Nafcillin and gentamicin
½ to 2	Chloramphenicol (*Haemophilus influenzae*)	as above	as above	Chloramphenicol (*Haemophilus influenzae* or streptococci)
2 to 14	Gentamicin (*Enterobocteriaceae* or *Pseudomonas aeruginosa*)	as above	as above	Nafcillin
15 to 39	as above	as above	as above	Penicillin G (*Neisseria gonorrhoeae*)
>40	as above	as above	as above	Nafcillin

*Gentamicin should be added to these regimens for patients with joint trauma, malignant disease, or addiction.
†Presumed identity in parentheses.

Escherichia coli and *Pseudomonas* require a more aggressive approach, usually with two antibiotics.

Transport of Antibiotics into Synovial Fluid

Antibiotics diffuse readily from the circulation into infected and uninfected inflamed joints.[35,63,82,107,114,115,116,139] Early studies of synovial fluid concentrations of penicillin showed inadequate amounts of this drug in the joint, but the dose was much lower than currently recommended.[7,63,112] Effective synovial fluid concentrations of a number of common antibiotics were measured in a study of 75 paired samples of synovial fluid and blood obtained from 29 adult patients with a presumptive diagnosis of infectious arthritis.[115] Parenteral administration of penicillin G, phenoxymethyl penicillin (penicillin V), nafcillin, cloxacillin, cephaloridine, tetracycline, erythromycin, and lincomycin in conventional doses produced bactericidal fluid concentrations within the joint (Fig. 99–5). Similar results have been reported in infants and children for ampicillin, methicillin, penicillin G, and cephalothin.[107] Knowledge of such effective concentrations in infected joints obviates the need for direct instillation of antibiotics into the joint space and thus reduces the risk of introducing a new infectious agent, as well as the risk of producing a "chemical synovitis" from local irritation by excessively high local concentrations of some drugs.[2,63] Protein binding of the antibiotic and the degree of the inflammatory response influence the rate of diffusion of serum constituents into the joint. When the diffusion of nafcillin, which is strongly bound to serum protein, was compared to another penicillin analogue, ampicillin, which shows little pro-

tein binding, comparable, effective joint fluid levels of both drugs were found at four hours, although the rate of entry of ampicillin was initially more rapid than that of nafcillin (Fig. 99–6). Thus, protein binding does not impair the entry into the joint or the efficacy of an antibiotic administered extra-articularly.[116] *The general rule in the use of antibiotics in infectious arthritis is that most drugs reach therapeutic levels in the synovial fluid if adequate amounts are given systemically.*

Amphotericin B may be an exception to this rule because data on this drug are sparse and contradictory.[104,111,121] Information on newly marketed antibiotics may also be unavailable. Therefore, until such data are provided, it is recommended that adequate transport of these drugs be documented by studies in each patient in which they are used. If diffusion of the drug is inadequate, local instillation into the joint might be done once or twice a day, or another antibiotic known to enter the joint more readily can be substituted. Finally, aminoglycoside effectiveness decreases by an order of magnitude at pH 6.5. Thus, effective removal of purulent exudate, which correlates with low pH, is especially important when this antibiotic is used.[86]

Transport of Antibiotics into Bone

Although measurement of antibiotics in bone poses more difficulties than in synovial fluid,[124] most studies indicate that, as in synovial fluid, adequate concentrations of antibiotics are reached when bactericidal doses have been administered systemically. Problems in interpreting drug levels in bone are the use of normal, uninfected bone for the assay, usually from uninfected patients undergoing elective operations, the variations in

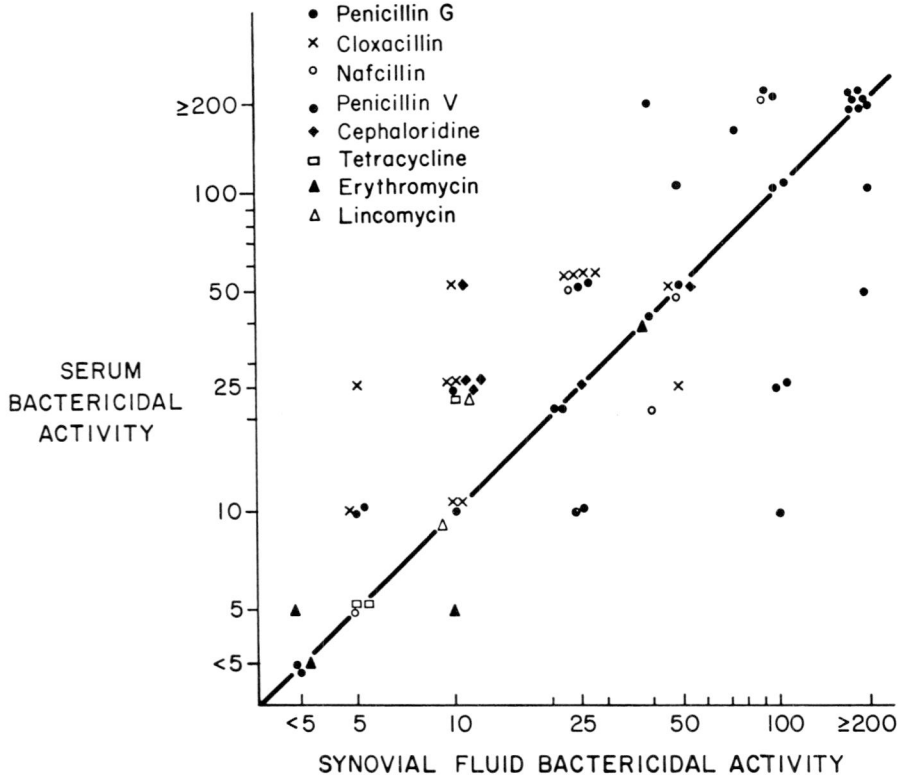

Fig. 99–5. Comparison of the bactericidal activity of 75 paired specimens of serum and synovial fluid obtained from 29 patients during systemic antibiotic therapy. Points on the diagonal line indicate pairs with equal activity. Bactericidal activity is expressed as the reciprocal of the maximum dilution showing this activity. (From Parker, R.H., and Schmid, F.R.[115])

porosity of cancellous and cortical bone, destruction of the test antibiotic by the heat generated by the pulverization process used to grind the bone, and contamination of the specimen by plasma not removed in the washing process. Therefore, only approximate drug levels can be measured. These levels are usually far below those obtained in plasma, yet they are often greater than the concentration needed to achieve bacterial inhibition and killing. Some data are available on most penicillins, cephalosporins, erythromycin, lincomycin, and clindamycin, but few data are available on aminoglycosides.[146]

Definitive Management of Infectious Arthritis

As soon as the exact identity of the micro-organism and its susceptibility to antibiotics are known, definitive therapy can be planned. Details of such management are provided in Chapters 100 through 104. Either the initial antibiotic is continued at the same or modified dose, or a more appropriate antibiotic is selected. Proof that the intravenous antibiotic is actually entering the joint in bactericidal concentrations should be obtained by determining antibacterial activity in paired samples of synovial fluid and serum. A simple tube-dilution technique can be performed in most clinical bacteriologic laboratories, using either the bacterium isolated from the patient or a bacterial species with identical antibiotic susceptibility.[115] Test results indicate the limiting dilution of serum and synovial fluid that still retains bacteriostatic or bactericidal activity. A margin of bactericidal effect ten or more times that found in undiluted synovial fluid provides sufficient antibiotic for antimicrobial action. One should rely on a regimen that produces bactericidal, not just bacteriostatic, activity. If this end has not been achieved, the dose of antibiotic should be increased until adequate bactericidal activity is reached, or else another antibiotic should be substituted. An excellent correlation exists between this simple tube-dilution test and the more quantitative agar-diffusion technique.[115]

Parenteral antibiotic administration should be maintained until clinical signs of active synovitis and inflammatory changes in the joint fluid begin

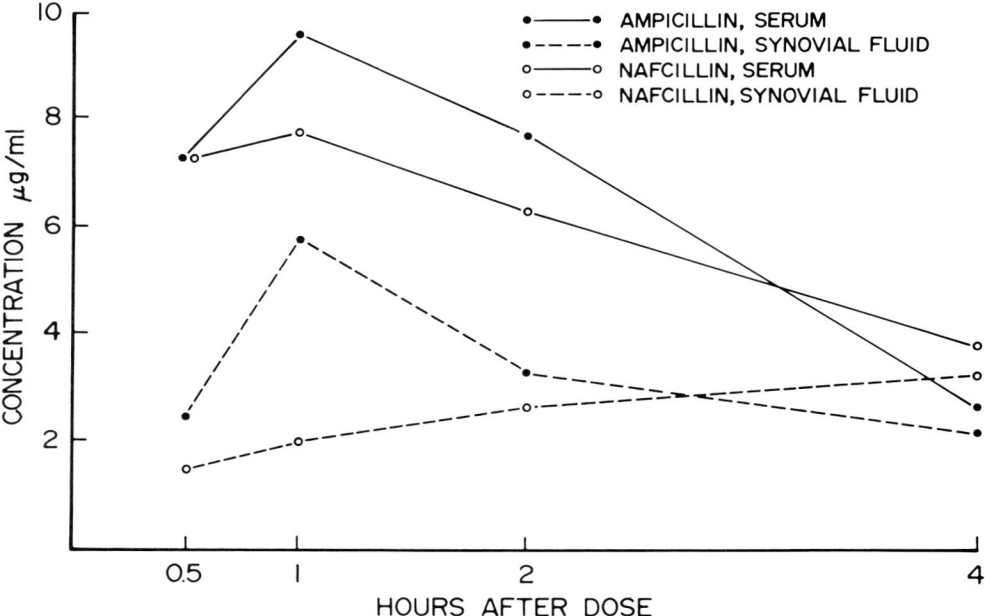

Fig. 99–6. Comparison of serum and synovial fluid concentrations of ampicillin and nafcillin in 6 patients receiving a single dose of each drug, 500 mg intramuscularly, in a cross-over study. (From Parker, R.H., Birbara, C., and Schmid, F.R.[116])

to revert toward normal.[65] Synovial fluid should be recultured repeatedly during the initial stages of therapy to demonstrate sterility. When one is certain that the infection is controlled, the antibiotic may be given orally. The oral route is unreliable in early treatment because patients with sepsis often have nausea, vomiting, and other gastrointestinal disturbances. Sterility and a progressive decline in total joint fluid leukocyte concentration are signs of a good prognosis; conversely, continued bacterial growth and a steady or rising leukocyte level suggest the need to reassess the treatment regimen.[65]

Infections caused by the gonococcus and certain other coccal organisms, such as the pneumococcus and the streptococcus, generally respond rapidly to appropriate antibiotic management. In patients with such infections, the duration of therapy might be expected to be brief, perhaps several weeks or less. Infections caused by staphylococci and gram-negative bacteria respond more slowly to treatment.[14,52,53] No satisfactory explanation for this phenomenon is available, but a change in the drug sensitivity of the micro-organisms present within the joint fluid is not likely to be a factor. In most cases, the strain of organism infecting the joint remains constant and is not replaced by another, drug-resistant variety, unless a contaminating strain is carried into the joint inadvertently during arthrocentesis. This finding contrasts with the

changing bacterial flora noted during the treatment of "open" infections in bone in which a sinus tract has formed or during the open drainage and suction sometimes carried out after arthrotomy. In addition, staphylococci do not usually show spontaneous mutation in their patterns of drug sensitivity. Thus, a strain of *Staphylococcus aureus* sensitive to penicillin G at the outset remains sensitive to this drug during treatment.

Definitive Management of Osteomyelitis

In patients with osteomyelitis, plasma bactericidal levels of antibiotics are an indication of the adequacy of the drug dose. If this information is correlated with the sensitivity of the micro-organism obtained either from blood or an aspirate of the bone lesion, an informed decision can be made. Whether to continue therapy is contingent on an evaluation of the clinical response, which, although less quantitative than the assessment of synovitis and joint fluid changes, provides useful evidence of the effects of treatment.

Suggestions for antibiotic therapy given here provide only general guidelines. Such information quickly becomes outdated as more effective drugs are discovered or as changing patterns of drug resistance emerge in some strains of bacteria. For these reasons, the therapist must have access to current knowledge concerning antibiotics. Knowledge of drug toxicity is also essential. The dosage of antibiotic must be appropriately reduced in a patient with diminished renal function. Blood levels of antibiotic determined by the tube-dilution technique provide the necessary information.

Serum Sickness Arthritis from Antimicrobial Agents

Serum sickness is a well-known but unusual complications of drug therapy. Almost any antibiotic, acting as a hapten, can induce this reaction. When symptoms of fever, rash, and flare of arthritis develop during the course of treatment of infectious arthritis, one must distinguish between a relapse of the primary joint disease and the onset of the polyarthritis of serum sickness (see Chaps. 23 and 63).

Careful examination of the bacterial status of the inflamed joint is mandatory and, if necessary, one must use an unrelated drug. In the interval between stopping the original drug and giving the new antibiotic, the joint fluid should be tested for the presence of micro-organisms by smear and culture, along with cell count and glucose level. Pending the results of these tests, antibiotic treatment can be administered with a drug to which the patient is not known to be sensitive. Only under the most urgent circumstance, such as when no other effective antibiotic is available, is it advisable to challenge the patient with the suspected offending drug. The grave risk of anaphylaxis usually is not warranted.

Postinfectious Synovitis

Tissue injury in septic arthritis is caused directly by toxic factors produced by viable micro-organisms and indirectly by the host's response to microbial antigens. The killing of micro-organisms by the action of antibiotics does not remove microbial products. Such materials may persist within the joint for prolonged periods, either in loculated areas or possibly embedded in articular cartilage. The retention of these substances may thereby contribute to persistence of the inflammatory response.

Such postinfectious synovitis leads to confusion about the adequacy of antibiotic treatment. Because viable micro-organisms may still be present in tissues even after synovial fluid cultures have become sterile, antibiotics are usually not discontinued. Instead, a nonsteroidal anti-inflammatory drug is added, but only after a week or more of antibiotic drug treatment. If the combination of antibiotic and anti-inflammatory therapy controls the inflammatory process, both drugs can be continued until all signs of active disease have diappeared. It is not advisable to initiate nonspecific anti-inflammatory drug use earlier because the patient's initial response to the antibiotic alone provides reassurance

that the infection is under control. A rapid response, particularly in the case of a gonococcal infection, provides added weight for the diagnosis, especially in bacteriologically unproved cases.

ANTIBIOTIC PROPHYLAXIS FOR PATIENTS WITH JOINT PROSTHESES

Infection is the most feared complication of total joint replacement, and removal of the prosthesis is often necessary to eradicate the septic process successfully. Thus, during the perioperative period, ways to avoid infection are emphasized. Attention is also directed to the prevention of a late infection, particularly in situations that might favor bacteremia.

Perioperative Prophylaxis

In addition to the use of scrupulously sterile technique, special operative clothing, avoidance of unnecessary personnel or traffic in the operating room, and sometimes, laminar air-flow systems at the operating table, almost all patients undergoing total joint replacement receive antibiotics prior to and during the procedure and for a number of days postoperatively.[19,62,64] Infections are commonly caused by *Staphylococcus aureus* and *S. epidermidis* and less frequently by such other skin flora as diphtheroids, *Propionibacterium acnes* and coliforms. The rationale for the use of systemic antibiotics is that, despite precautions, most wounds may become contaminated by the end of a long operation. In most centers, the rate of infection has dropped as surgical experience has grown and as the operative time has been shortened. Transient bacteremia with hematogenous seeding of micro-organisms is also a possibility. For this reason, any known focus of infection elsewhere in the body is treated aggressively prior to the operation.

Antibiotic-impregnated cement has also been used; the idea is that a drug reservoir can be maintained at the operative site from which an antibiotic, such as gentamicin, can diffuse throughout the wound.[159] Evidence for its added value to an otherwise exemplary surgical program is not clear; some are concerned that the antibiotic might weaken the mechanical properties of the cement.

Prophylaxis against Late Bacteremia

A few well-placed prostheses become infected months after operation, most likely by hematogenous seeding of bacteria to the implant area.[30] For this reason, antibiotics have been used prophylactically in circumstances in which bacteremia is known to occur. Recommended regimens are as follows: (1) after dental, bronchoscopic, and otorhinolaryngologic procedures, penicillin V, 2.0 g orally an hour before the procedure and 0.5 g every

6 hours for 3 doses for adults; and (2) after urologic procedures, ampicillin, 1.0 g intramuscularly, and streptomycin, 1.0 g intramuscularly before the procedure and again 12 hours later for adults.[78]

DRAINAGE OF INFECTED BONE AND JOINTS

Drainage of Synovial Fluid

Except for infants with septic arthritis of the hip, who require open surgical drainage as soon as the diagnosis is made,[69,102,138] initial drainage can be accomplished by needle aspiration in almost all cases of infectious arthritis. All possible fluid is removed on a regular basis, sometimes daily, or even more frequently if needed. Because some fluid always remains in the joint, some clinicians suggest lavage of the joint cavity with sterile physiologic saline or Ringer's solution. At each aspiration, the volume, cell count, culture, and, at appropriate intervals, the fasting glucose or lactate levels should be determined (see Table 99–1).

In the deep-seated joint of the older child or adult, the decision whether to perform open surgical drainage or needle drainage poses a problem because of the difficulty associated with repeated aspiration. If sepsis is recognized early, and if the organism recovered from the joint is sensitive to antibiotics, particularly if it is a gonococcus or another nonstaphylococcal coccus, then needle drainage is still preferred because it prevents the conversion of a closed-space infection into an open wound. If recognition of sepsis is delayed, however, or if sepsis is due to "difficult" organisms such as staphylococci or gram-negative bacilli, or if the infected joint is the result of extension of infection from a periarticular site such as a contiguous bone or soft tissue, then open drainage may be needed.[8,73] Open drainage is indicated if needle aspiration fails to decompress the joint adequately.

Surgical Drainage

Except for the foregoing circumstances, surgical drainage is withheld unless one sees little or no clinical or laboratory evidence of improvement during the first four to seven days of treatment. This time interval is arbitrary. I would still continue to treat a slowly responding gonococcal infection by needle aspiration for another four to seven days. On the other hand, infections due to staphylococci or to gram-negative bacilli, unrelenting synovitis present a week after treatment is begun calls for arthrotomy or arthroscopy. No adequately controlled study to support this opinion is available, although almost all large series in which this question is examined have failed to demonstrate an advantage of initial open drainage over deferred open drainage.[51,96]

Arthroscopy

This technique offers the prospect of inspecting the joint cavity and the opportunity to lavage its contents and to remove fibrotic or necrotic tissue, some of which might be further examined by culture and histologic study for evidence of persisting infection.[71] Morbidity is much lower from that associated with open drainage. The procedure can be repeated at a later stage if further local debridement is required. Its limitations need to be recognized, however, because current models of arthroscopes are used only for the knee and for a few other large joints such as the shoulder or ankle. Moreover, when adjacent osteomyelitis is extensive, open drainage and debridement may still be needed.

Debridement in Osteomyelitis

For hematogenous osteomyelitis, the prognosis for recovery of function is good with suitable antibiotic therapy. Little or no disability is apt to result, even with spontaneous vertebral fusion, and surgical debridement is not necessary. A diagnostic aspiration of exudate from the body of the vertebra or from the disc space can be done, if necessary, to identify the micro-organisms and its drug sensitivities. If an abscess or spinal cord compression develops, however, surgical drainage and debridement of the infected area are indicated.

GENERAL SUPPORTIVE MEASURES

The affected joint must be kept at rest during the acute phase of the illness. A splint helps to reduce pain and, by immobilization, to control inflammation. A posterior resting splint for the leg or arm is usually sufficient. Patients with infectious spondylitis should stay in bed; if the danger of subluxation exists, they should have the spine immobilized in a plaster shell or brace.

As the process subsides, one should attempt to restore range of motion and to increase muscle strength gradually. Passive exercises, followed by graded active exercises, are begun with the assistance of a physical therapist. Weight bearing should be deferred until signs of acute inflammation have disappeared.[135]

In addition to treatment of the joint, efforts are needed to control the primary infection that led to the arthritis, to supply fluids and nutrition, and to control pain. Anti-inflammatory drugs including aspirin should be withheld for one week or longer until the response of the joint to the antibiotic can be correctly assessed. Codeine or propoxyphene can be used to control pain.

ONGOING EVALUATION OF THE TREATMENT PROGRAM

Acute Stage of Infectious Arthritis

The response of the infection to treatment is assessed by changes in tenderness, heat, swelling, and range of motion of the affected joint. The frequency of aspiration is reduced as the volume and the inflammatory character of the fluid decrease. If one is uncertain whether effective bactericidal levels have been achieved because of a change in the type, dose, or route of administration of an antibiotic drug, a tube-dilution assay of paired serum and synovial fluid should be performed. If joint fluid is no longer obtainable, assay of antibiotic concentrations of blood alone provides an acceptable approximation of the drug concentration in the joint. The results of this continuous monitoring should be charted chronologically, so the effectiveness of the treatment program can be quickly and accurately determined.

Antibiotic therapy is ordinarily continued for at least seven days after all systemic or local findings of inflammation have subsided. In staphylococcal and in some gram-negative bacillary infections, which respond more slowly, this period is extended to four or six weeks. The patient should be observed for another few weeks after cessation of antibiotic therapy for any sign of relapse. If the infection is slow to improve or if it worsens during any phase of the treatment period, one must review all aspects of the program. The following questions should be asked: Was the joint fluid rendered sterile? Were bactericidal levels of antibiotic in the joint fluid achieved? Was needle aspiration successful in decompressing the joint? Answers to these questions dictate the appropriate change in the type or the dosage of antibiotic administered or in the method of drainage. Consultation from the outset with an infectious-disease specialist and with an orthopedic surgeon is invaluable in planning a co-ordinated approach.

Illustrative Case Report

A patient with septic arthritis illustrates the value of continued monitoring of the response to treatment (Fig. 99–7). Gram-positive cocci, subsequently proved to be *Staphylococcus aureus,* were identified in the smear of fluid obtained from the knee. Penicillin G was given intravenously. On the second day of treatment, bactericidal levels of antibiotic against the staphylococcus recovered from the joint were present, but the patient developed an intense allergic response that required the substitution of lincomycin. Again, suitable bactericidal drug concentrations were achieved. As the patient improved, lesser amounts of fluid were obtained by needle aspiration from the joint. For the balance of the treatment schedule, erythromycin was given. Initially, by the intravenous route and later, orally, bactericidal levels of drug were noted. After the patient's discharge from the hospital on the twenty-ninth day, oral medication was continued for another two weeks. Although this patient had developed septic arthritis in a joint already damaged by RA, prompt diagnosis and therapy prevented further loss of joint function.

Late Outcomes of Infectious Arthritis

Any septic joint untreated or inadequately treated for more than one or two weeks may develop some of the pathologic changes of a chronic infection. These manifestations include damage to cartilage and bone, increased fibrosis, and ultimately, destruction of the normal joint mechanism.[69,133] Fortunately, the number of such changes has decreased since the introduction of antibiotic therapy.[108] In one large clinic, the number of cases of bacterial arthritis decreased approximately by half from 1952 to 1957, when compared to two periods extending, respectively, from 1939 to 1945 and from 1946 to 1951. This reduction occurred in the number of patients with chronic, rather than acute, disease.[22]

In patients with chronic disease, a major effort should be directed toward analysis of the factor(s) responsible for the failure of the therapeutic regimen. The bacterial status of the joint should be re-evaluated by a synovial fluid culture obtained several days after withdrawal of all antibiotics and again a week or two later if active synovitis persists.

Open arthrotomy or arthroscopy may be required for adequate drainage and excision of necrotic bone and soft tissue including sinuses.[8,51,71] Tissue should be obtained for culture as well as for histologic examination. Culture of synovial tissue may be positive when the synovial fluid is sterile. Care must be taken to inoculate a wide range of culture media, to facilitate the recovery of fungi or mycobacteria, agents that may have eluded earlier detection. Moreover, during inspection of the joint, a foreign body, such as a plant thorn, that had allowed the inflammatory process to persist may be removed.

Antibiotics, such as the penicillins and cephalosporins, that inhibit bacterial cell-wall synthesis, may induce the formation of cell-wall-free bacteria or protoplasts. Little evidence suggests that these crippled bacteria are pathogenic.[45,67,113] In one case familiar to me, such forms of bacteria, as well as native bacterial forms of *Staphylococcus aureus,* were cultured from the necrotic remnants of a patient's patella after several months of continuous

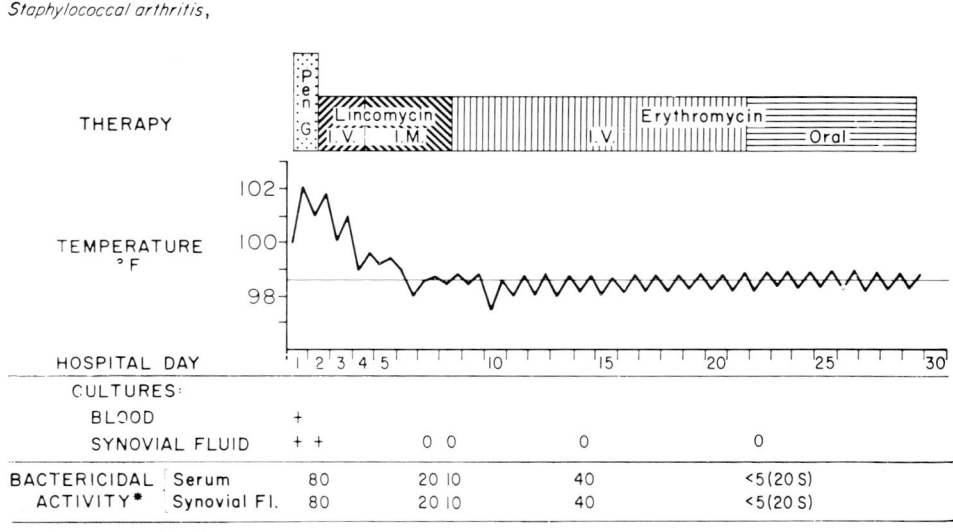

Fig. 99–7. Response of a 56-year-old white male patient with septic arthritis to antibiotic treatment. Comparable bactericidal drug levels were achieved in the joint fluid and blood for each drug. I.V. = Intravenously; I.M. = intramuscularly.

penicillin therapy. In the postoperative period, this patient was treated successfully with erythromycin because this drug influences bacterial metabolism by means other than the inhibition of cell-wall synthesis.

The prognosis for the complete recovery of function in a previously normal joint infected with antibiotic-sensitive bacteria is generally excellent when treatment is begun within a few days of the onset of infection. Delayed diagnosis is directly related to a poorer outcome. The prognosis may be difficult to judge at the outset. In one study, the predictability of good results was not completely ascertained until many months later.[69] Thus, long-term observation is necessary to determine the end result.

Reconstruction of Damaged Joints

If a joint has been damaged, reconstructive procedures may be considered, but the operation should be deferred until all evidence of infection has been absent for several months. Arthroplasty or fusion of a joint may be indicated.[122,156] Prosthetic replacement to restore normal joint function is now widely accepted.[72,89,136,137,166] The possibility of re-exacerbating a dormant infection, however, must always be considered, particularly in patients with tuberculosis. Nevertheless, prosthetic replacement of a damaged hip,[70] knee, and other joint has been undertaken with satisfactory results.

Late Outcomes of Osteomyelitis

The therapeutic program for patients with osteomyelitis needs closer monitoring than that for patients with septic arthritis. Clinical findings at the site of the bone infection and serial radiologic and scintiphotographic examinations are used to determine whether the infection has been eradicated. In hematogenous osteomyelitis of a long bone or a vertebra, antibiotics are given orally for several weeks after initial intravenous use; in chronic osteomyelitis, most often when secondary to continuous infection, long-term oral therapy has been successful.[160] Surgical treatment of osteomyelitis is largely empiric and is based on concepts that have gained wide acceptance, some with and others without scientific documentation. Included are drainage of infected areas, excision of necrotic bone, and removal of sequestra and foreign material, such as cement and prostheses.[160]

The likelihood of only partial eradication of the infection is greater in osteomyelitis than in septic arthritis. Reactivation has been recognized many years after the implantation of the original infection. The late outcome of acute hematogenous osteomyelitis in children between 1947 and 1976 was failure to cure or recurrence in almost 20% of cases, most often in the first year. Half of these patients had more than a single recurrence. With the more effective use of antibiotics, especially in those over age 16, the failure rates were lower.[49]

Treatment of a recurrence requires extended antibiotic administration, usually for months. For staphylococcal osteomyelitis, a penicillinase-resistant penicillin is given orally. At the same time, the involved bone needs to be evaluated by the surgeon for possible osteotomy to remove residual necrotic materials. Persistent treatment almost always eradicates the infection.

REFERENCES

1. Aaskov, J.G., Fraser, J.R.E., and Dalglish, D.A.: Specific and non-specific immunological changes in epidemic polyarthritis patients. Aust. J. Exp. Biol. Med. Sci., 59:599–608, 1981.
2. Argen, R.J., Wilson, C.H., Jr., and Wood, P.: Suppurative arthritis: clinical features of 42 cases. Arch. Intern. Med., 117:661–666, 1966.
3. Ash, J.M., and Gilday, D.L.: The futility of bone scanning in neonatal osteomyelitis. J. Nucl. Med., 21:417–420, 1980.
4. Asnes, R.S., and Arendar, G.M.: Septic arthritis of the hip: a complication of femoral venipuncture. Pediatrics, 38:837–841, 1966.
5. Atcheson, S.G., and Ward, J.R.: Acute hematogenous osteomyelitis progressing to septic synovitis and eventual pyarthrosis: the vascular pathway. Arthritis Rheum., 21:968–971, 1978.
6. Azouz, E.M.: Computed tomography in bone and joint infections. J. Can. Assoc. Radiol., 32:102–106, 1981.
7. Balboni, V.G., Shapiro, I.M., and Kydd, D.M.: The penetration of penicillin into joint fluid following intramuscular administration. Am. J. Med. Sci., 210:588–591, 1945.
8. Ballard, A., et al.: Functional treatment of pyogenic arthritis of the adult knee. J. Bone Joint Surg., 57A:1,119–1,123, 1975.
9. Behn, A.R., Mathews, J.A., and Phillips, I.: Lactate UV-system: a rapid method for diagnosis of septic arthritis. Ann. Rheum., Dis., 40:489–492, 1981.
10. Bernard, T.N., Jr., and Haddad, R.J.: Fever of undetermined etiology masks vertebral osteomyelitis. Orthop. Rev., 9:63–71, 1982.
11. Bocanegra, T.S., et al.: Reactive arthritis induced by parasitic infestation. Ann. Intern. Med., 94:207–209, 1981.
12. Booth, J.E., et al.: Infection of prosthetic arthroplasty by Mycobacterium fortuitum: two case reports. J. Bone Joint Surg., 61A:300–302, 1979.
13. Borenstein, D.G., Gibbs, C.A., and Jacobs, R.P.: Gas-liquid chromatographic analysis of synovial fluid: succinic acid and lactic acid as markers for septic arthritis. Arthritis Rheum., 25:947–953, 1982.
14. Borrela, L., et al.: Septic arthritis in childhood. J. Pediatr., 62:742–747, 1963.
15. Brandt, K.D., Cathcart, E.S., and Cohen, A.S.: Gonococcal arthritis: clinical features correlated with blood, synovial fluid, and genitourinary cultures. Arthritis Rheum., 17:503–510, 1974.
16. Brook, I., et al.: Synovial fluid lactic acid: a diagnostic aid in septic arthritis. Arthritis Rheum., 21:774–779, 1978.
17. Bunch, T.W., et al.: Synovial fluid complement determination as a diagnostic aid in inflammatory joint diseases. Mayo Clin. Proc., 49:715–720, 1974.
18. Canoso, J.J., and Sheckman, P.R.: Septic subcutaneous bursitis: report of sixteen cases. J. Rheumatol., 6:96–102, 1979.
19. Carlsson, A.S., Lidgren, L., and Lindberg, H.: Prophylactic antibiotics against early and late deep infection after total hip replacement. Acta Orthop. Scand., 48:405–410, 1977.
20. Chang, M.J., Contron, G., and Rodriguez, W.J.: Ampicillin-resistant Hemophilus influenzae type B septic arthritis in children. Clin. Pediatr., 20:139–141, 1981.
21. Chantler, J.K., Ford, D.K., and Tingle, A.J.: Rubella-associated arthritis: rescue of rubella virus from peripheral blood lymphocytes two years postvaccination. Infect. Immun., 32:1,274–1,280, 1981.
22. Chartier, Y., Martin, W.J., and Kelly, P.J.: Bacterial arthritis: Experiences in the treatment of 77 patients. Ann. Intern. Med., 50:1,462–1,474, 1959.
23. Chusid, M.J., Jacobs, W.M., and Sty, J.R.: Pseudomonas arthritis following puncture wounds of the foot. J. Pediatr., 94:429–431, 1979.
24. Clarke, J.T.: The antibiotic therapy of septic arthritis. Clin. Rheum. Dis., 4:133–152, 1978.
25. Cluff, L.E., et al.: Staphylococcal bacteremia and altered host resistance. Ann. Intern. Med., 69:859–873, 1968.
26. Coleman, R.E.: Imaging with Tc-99m MDP and Ga-67 citrate in patients with rheumatoid arthritis and suspected septic arthritis. J. Nucl. Med., 23:479–482, 1982.
27. Coy, J.T., III, et al.: Pyogenic arthritis of the sacro-iliac joint: long-term follow-up. J. Bone Joint Surg., 58A:845–849, 1976.
28. Crawford, A.H., and Carothers, T.S.: Hip arthrography in the skeletally immature. Clin. Orthop., 162:54–60, 1982.
29. Curtiss, P.H., and Klein, L.: Destruction of articular cartilage in septic arthritis. J. Bone Joint Surg., 45A:797–806, 1963.
30. D'Ambrosia, R.D., Shoji, H., and Heater, R.: Secondarily infected total joint replacements by hematogenous spread. J. Bone Joint Surg., 58A:450–453, 1976.
31. Delbarre, F., et al.: Pyogenic infection of the sacro-iliac joint: report of thirteen cases. J. Bone Joint Surg., 57A:819–825, 1975.
32. Dienstag, J.L., et al.: Circulating immune complexes in non-A, non-B hepatitis. Lancet, 1:1,265–1,267, 1979.
33. Dodd, M.J.: Pyogenic arthritis due to Bacteroides complicating rheumatoid arthritis. Ann. Rheum. Dis., 41:248–249, 1982.
34. Dorff, G.J., Ziokowski, J.S., and Rytel, M.W.: Detection by counterimmunoelectrophoresis of pneumococcal antigen in synovial fluid from septic arthritis. Arthritis Rheum., 18:613–615, 1975.
35. Drutz, D.J., et al.: The penetration of penicillin and other antimicrobials into joint fluid: three case reports with a reappraisal of the literature. J. Bone Joint Surg., 49A:1,415–1,421, 1967.
36. Dunn, E.J., et al.: Pyogenic infections of the sacro-iliac joint. Clin. Orthop., 118:113–117, 1976.
37. Eagle, H.: Experimental approach to the problem of treatment failure with penicillin. I. Group A streptococcal infection in mice. Am. J. Med., 13:389–399, 1952.
38. Eftekhar, N.S.: Wound infection complicating total hip joint arthroplasty: scope of the problem and its diagnosis. Orthop. Rev., 8:49–64, 1975.
39. Enarson, D.A., et al.: Bone and joint tuberculosis: a continuing problem. Can. Med. Assoc. J., 120:139–145, 1979.
40. Fielding, J.W., and Lieber, W.A.: Septic dislocation of hip joint in infancy: follow-up of fifteen years. N.Y. State J. Med., 61:3,916–3,917, 1961.
41. Fink, C.W.: Gonococcal arthritis in children. JAMA, 194:237–238, 1965.
42. Fink, C.W., et al.: Infections of bones and joints in children. Arthritis Rheum., 20:578–583, 1977.
43. Fitzgerald, R.H., Jr.: Anaerobic septic arthritis. Clin. Orthop., 164:141–148, 1982.
44. Flatman, J.G.: Hip disease with referred pain to the knee. JAMA, 234:967–968, 1975.
45. Garcia-Kutzbach, A., et al.: Identification of Neisseria gonorrhoeae in synovial membrane by electron microscopy. J. Infect. Dis., 130:183–186, 1974.
46. Garcia-Kutzbach, A., and Masi, A.T.: Acute infectious agent arthritis (IAA): a detailed comparison of proved gonococcal and other blood-borne bacterial arthritis. J. Rheumatol., 1:93–101, 1974.
47. Garcia-Kutzbach, A., Dismuke, S.E., and Masi, A.T.: Gonococcal arthritis: clinical features and results of penicillin therapy. J. Rheumatol., 1:210–221, 1974.
48. Gelberman, R.H., et al.: Pyogenic arthritis of the shoulder in adults. J. Bone Joint Surg., 62A:550–553, 1980.

49. Gillespie, W.J.: The management of acute haematogenous osteomyelitis in the antibiotic era: a study of the outcome. J. Bone Joint Surg., *63B*:126–131, 1981.

50. Glassberg, G.B., and Ozonoff, M.B.: Arthrographic findings in septic arthritis of the hip in infants. Radiology, *128*:151–155, 1978.

51. Goldenberg, D.L., et al.: Treatment of septic arthritis: comparison of needle aspiration and surgery as initial modes of joint drainage. Arthritis Rheum., *18*:83–90, 1975.

52. Goldenberg, D.L., et al.: Acute arthritis caused by gram negative bacilli: a clinical characterization. Medicine, *53*:197–208, 1974.

53. Goldenberg, D.L., and Cohen, A.S.: Acute infectious arthritis: a review of patients with nongonococcal joint infections (with emphasis on therapy and prognosis). Am. J. Med., *60*:369–377, 1976.

54. Gordon, G., and Kabins, S.A.: Pyogenic sacroiliitis. Am. J. Med., *69*:50–56, 1980.

55. Grahame, R.: Isolation of rubella virus from synovial fluid in five cases of seronegative arthritis. Lancet, *2*:649–651, 1981.

56. Hadler, N.M.: Phlogistic properties of microbial debris. Semin. Arthritis Rheum., *8*:1–16, 1978.

57. Hamilton, M.E., et al.: Simultaneous gout and pyarthrosis. Arch. Intern. Med., *140*:917–919, 1980.

58. Hardin, J.A., et al.: Circulating immune complexes in Lyme arthritis: detection by the ^{125}I-C1q binding, C1q solid phase, and Raji cell assays. J. Clin. Invest., *63*:468–477, 1979.

59. Hardin, J.A., Steere, A.C., and Malawista, S.E.: Immune complexes and the evolution of Lyme arthritis: dissemination and localization of abnormal C1q-binding activity. N. Engl. J. Med., *301*:1,358–1,363, 1979.

60. Harris, E.D., Jr., and Krane, S.M.: Collagenases. N. Engl. J. Med., *291*:605–609, 1974.

61. Heinicke, M.: Crystal arthropathy as a complication of septic arthritis. J. Rheumatol., *8*:529–531, 1981.

62. Hill, C., et al.: Prophylactic cefazolin versus placebo in total hip replacement. Lancet, *1*:795–797, 1981.

63. Hirsch, H.L., Feffer, H.L., and O'Neil, C.B.: A study of the diffusion of penicillin across the serous membranes of joint cavities. J. Lab. Clin. Med., *31*:535–543, 1946.

64. Hirschmann, J.V., and Inui, T.S.: Antimicrobial prophylaxis: a critique of recent trials. Rev. Infect. Dis., *2*:1–23, 1980.

65. Ho, G., Jr.: Therapy for septic arthritis. JAMA, *247*:797–800, 1982.

66. Ho, G., Jr., and Tice, A.D.: Comparison of nonseptic and septic bursitis: further observations on the treatment of septic bursitis. Arch. Intern. Med., *139*:1,269–1,273, 1979.

67. Holmes, K.K., et al.: Recovery of Neisseria gonorrhoeae from "sterile" synovial fluid in gonococcal arthritis. N. Engl. J. Med., *284*:318–320, 1971.

68. Honig, S., Gorevic, P., and Weissmann, G.: CRP in SLE patients: an aid in diagnosing superimposed infections. Arthritis Rheum., *20*:121, 1977.

69. Howard, J.B., Highgenboten, C.L., and Nelson, J.D.: Residual effects of septic arthritis in infancy and childhood. JAMA, *236*:932–935, 1976.

70. Hunt, D.D., and Larson, C.B.: Treatment of the residua of hip infections by mold arthroplasty: an end-result study of thirty-three hips. J. Bone Joint Surg., *48A*:111–125, 1966.

70a. Inman, R.D., et al.: Clinical and microbiological features of prosthetic joint infection. Am. J. Med., *77*:47–53, 1984.

71. Jarrett, M.P., et al.: The role of arthroscopy in the treatment of septic arthritis. Arthritis Rheum., *24*:737–739, 1981.

72. Jupiter, J.B., et al.: Total hip arthroplasty in the treatment of adult hips with current or quiescent sepsis. J. Bone Joint Surg., *63A*:194–200, 1981.

73. Kawashima, M., et al.: The treatment of pyogenic bone and joint infections by closed irrigation-suction. Clin. Orthop., *148*:240–244, 1980.

74. Keefer, C.S., and Spink, W.W.: Gonococcic arthritis: pathogenesis, mechanism of recovery and treatment. JAMA *109*:1,448–1,453, 1937.

75. Keiser, H., Ruben, F.L., and Wolinsky, E.: Clinical forms of gonococcal arthritis. N. Engl. J. Med., *279*:234–240, 1968.

76. Kellgren, J.H., et al.: Suppurative arthritis complicating rheumatoid arthritis. Br. Med. J., *1*:1,193–1,200, 1958.

77. Kelly, P.J., Martin, W.J., and Coventry, M.B.: Bacterial arthritis of the hip in the adult. J. Bone Joint Surg., *47A*:1,005–1,018, 1965.

78. Keys, T.F.: Antimicrobial prophylaxis for patients with congenital or valvular heart disease. Mayo Clin. Proc., *57*:171–175, 1982.

79. Klein, S.J., Craggs, E., and Konwaler, B.E.: Guinea pig inoculation versus culture for isolation of M. tuberculosis. Am. Rev. Respir. Dis., *87*:451, 1963.

80. Kushner, I., and Somerville, J.A.: Permeability of human synovial membrane to plasma proteins: relationship to molecular size and inflammation. Arthritis Rheum., *14*:560–570, 1971.

81. LaManna, M.M., et al.: An assessment of technetium and gallium scanning in the patient with painful total joint arthroplasty. Orthopedics, *6*:580–582, 1983.

82. Latif, R., et al.: Pharmacokinetic and clinical evaluation of moxalactam in infants and children. Rev. Pharmacol. Ther., *3*:222–231, 1981.

83. Lever, A.M.L., Owen, T., and Forsey, J.: Pneumoarthropathy in septic arthritis caused by Streptococcus milleri. Br. Med. J., *285*:24, 1982.

84. Lisbona, R., and Rosenthall, L.: Observations on the sequential use of ^{99m}Tc-phosphate complex and ^{67}Ga imaging in osteomyelitis, cellulitis, and septic arthritis. Radiology, *123*:123–129, 1977.

85. Lunseth, P.A., and Heiple, K.G.: Prognosis in septic arthritis of the hip in children. Clin. Orthop., *139*:81–85, 1979.

86. McCarty, D.J.: Joint sepsis: a chance for cure. (Editorial.) JAMA, *247*:835, 1982.

87. McCarty, D.J., Jr., Phelps, P., and Pyenson, J.: Crystal-induced inflammation in canine joints. I. An experimental model with quantification of the host response. J. Exp. Med., *124*:99–114, 1966.

88. McConville, J.H., et al.: Septic and crystalline joint disease: a simultaneous occurrence. JAMA, *231*:841–842, 1975.

89. McLaughlin, R.E., and Allen, J.R.: Total hip replacement in the previously infected hip. South. Med. J., *70*:573–575, 1977.

90. Majd, M., and Frankel, R.S.: Radionuclide imaging in skeletal inflammatory and ischemic disease in children. AJR, *126*:832–841, 1976.

91. Manicourt, D.H., and Orloff, S.: Gonococcal arthritis-dermatitis syndrome: study of serum and synovial fluid immune complex levels. Arthritis Rheum., *25*:574–578, 1982.

92. Mathews, M., et al.: Septic arthritis in hemodialyzed patients. Nephron, *25*:87–91, 1980.

93. Maurer, A.H.: Utility of three-phase skeletal scintigraphy in suspected osteomyelitis. J Nucl. Med., *22*:941–949, 1981.

94. Memon, I.A., et al.: Group B streptococcal osteomyelitis and septic arthritis: its occurrence in infants less than two months old. Am. J. Dis. Child., *133*:921–923, 1979.

95. Merritt, K., et al.: Counter immunoelectrophoresis in the diagnosis of septic arthritis caused by Haemophilus influenzae. J. Bone Joint Surg., *58A*:414–415, 1976.

96. Mielants, H.: Long-term functional results of the non-surgical treatment of common bacterial infections of joints. Scand. J. Rheumatol., *11*:101–105, 1982.

97. Mills, L.C., et al.: Septic arthritis as a complication of orally given steroid therapy. JAMA, *164*:1,310–1,314, 1957.

98. Miskew, D.B., Block, R.A., and Witt, P.F.: Aspiration of infected sacro-iliac joints. J. Bone Joint Surg., *61A*:1,071–1,072, 1979.

99. Mitchell, W.S., et al.: Septic arthritis in patients with rheumatoid disease: a still undiagnosed complication. J. Rheumatol., *3*:124–133, 1976.

100. Morgan, G.J., Jr.: Early diagnosis of septic arthritis of the sacroiliac joint by use of computed tomography. J. Rheumatol., 8:979–982, 1981.

101. Morrey, B.F., Bianco, A.J., and Rhodes, K.H.: Hematogenous osteomyelitis at uncommon sites in children. Mayo Clin. Proc., 53:707–713, 1978.

102. Morrey, B.F., Bianco, A.J., and Rhodes, K.H.: Suppurative arthritis of the hip in children. J. Bone Joint Surg., 58A:388–392, 1976.

103. Mossman, S.S.: Synovial fluid lactic acid in septic arthritis. N.Z. Med. J., 93:115–117, 1981.

104. Murray, H.W., Fialk, M.A., and Roberts, R.B.: Candida arthritis: a manifestation of disseminated candidiasis. Am. J. Med., 60:587–595, 1976.

105. Murray, I.P.C.: Photopenia in skeletal scintigraphy of suspected bone and joint infection. Clin. Nucl. Med., 7:13–20, 1982.

106. Nelson, J.D.: The bacterial etiology and antibiotic management of septic arthritis in infants and children. Pediatrics, 50:437–440, 1972.

107. Nelson, J.D.: Antibiotic concentrations in septic joint effusions. N. Engl. J. Med., 284:349–353, 1971.

108. Newman, J.H.: Review of septic arthritis throughout the antibiotic era. Ann. Rheum. Dis., 35:198–205, 1976.

109. Nitsche, J.F.: Septic sternoclavicular arthritis with Pasteurella multocida and Streptococcus sanguis. Arthritis Rheum., 25:467–469, 1982.

110. Norris, S., Ehrlich, M.G., and McKusick, K.: Early diagnosis of disc space infection with ^{67}Ga in an experimental model. Clin. Orthop., 144:293–298, 1979.

111. Noyes, F.R., McCabe, J.D., and Fekety, F.R., Jr.: Acute Candida arthritis: report of a case and use of amphotericin B. J. Bone Joint Surg., 55A:169–176, 1973.

112. Ory, E.M., et al.: Penicillin levels in serum and in some body fluids during systemic and local therapy. J. Lab. Clin. Med., 30:809–820, 1945.

113. Palmer, D.W., and Ellman, M.H.: Septic arthritis and Reiter's syndrome in sickle cell disorders: case reports and implications for management. South. Med. J., 69:902–904, 1976.

114. Pancoast, S.J., and Neu, H.C.: Antibiotic levels in human bone and synovial fluid used in the evaluation of antimicrobial therapy of joint and skeletal infections. Orthop. Rev., 9:49–61, 1980.

115. Parker, R.H., and Schmid, F.R.: Antibacterial activity of synovial fluid during therapy of septic arthritis. Arthritis Rheum., 14:96–104, 1971.

116. Parker, R.H., Birbara, C., and Schmid, F.R.: Passage of nafcillin and ampicillin into synovial fluid. In Staphylococci and Staphylococcal Dieases. Edited by J. Jeljaszewicz. Stuttgart, New York, Gustav Fischer Verlag. 1,151–1,123, 1976.

117. Pate, D., and Katz, A.: Clostridia discitis: a case report. Arthritis Rheum., 22:1,039–1,040, 1979.

118. Petersen, B.H., et al.: Neisseria meningitidis and Neisseria gonorrhoeae bacteremia associated with C6, C7, or C8 deficiency. Ann. Intern. Med., 90:917–920, 1979.

119. Peterson, S.: Acute haematogenous osteomyelitis and septic arthritis in childhood: a 10 year review and follow-up. Acta Orthop. Scand., 51:451–457, 1980.

120. Phemister, D.B.: The effect of pressure on articular surfaces in pyogenic and tuberculous arthritides and its bearing on treatment. Ann. Surg., 80:481–500, 1924.

121. Poplack, D.G., and Jacobs, S.A.: Candida arthritis treated with amphotericin B. J. Pediatr., 87:989–990, 1975.

122. Price, C.T.: Thompson arthrodesis of the hip in children. J. Bone Joint Surg., 62A:1,118–1,123, 1980.

123. Prince, A., and Neu, H.C.: Microbiology of infections of the prosthetic joint. Orthop. Rev., 8:91–96, 1979.

124. Quinlan, W.R., Hall, B.B., and Fitzgerald, R.H., Jr.: Fluid spaces in normal and osteomyelitic canine bone. J. Lab. Clin. Med., 102:78–87, 1983.

125. Reginato, A.J., et al.: Synovitis in secondary syphilis: clinical, light, and electronmicroscopic studies. Arthritis Rheum., 22:170–176, 1979.

126. Reimann, K., Lind, I., and Andersen, K.E.: An indirect haemagglutination test for demonstration of gonococcal antibodies using gonococcal pili as antigen. II. Serological investigation of patients attending a dermatovenereological out-patient clinic in Copenhagen. Acta Pathol. Microbiol. Scand., 88:155–162, 1980.

126a.Richards, A.J.: Ruptured popliteal cyst and pyogenic arthritis. Br. Med. J., 282:1,120–1,121, 1981.

127. Rinaldi, R.Z., Harrison, W.O., and Fan, P.T.: Penicillin-resistant gonococcal arthritis: a report of four cases. Ann. Intern. Med., 97:43–45, 1982.

128. Riordan, T.: Synovial fluid lactic acid measurement in the diagnosis and management of septic arthritis. J. Clin. Pathol., 35:390–394, 1982.

129. Roca, R.P., and Yoshikawa, T.T.: Primary skeletal infections in heroin users: clinical characterization, diagnosis and therapy. Clin. Orthop., 144:238–248, 1979.

130. Ropes, M.W., and Bauer, W.: Synovial Fluid Changes in Joint Disease. Cambridge, Harvard University Press, 1953.

131. Rosenthal, D.I., Mankin, H.J., and Bauman, R.A.: Musculoskeletal applications for computed tomography. Bull. Rheum. Dis., 33:1–4, 1983.

132. Rosenthal, J., Bole, G.G., and Robinson, W.D.: Acute nongonococcal infectious arthritis. Arthritis Rheum., 23:889–897, 1980.

133. Roy, S., and Bhawan, J.: Ultrastructure of articular cartilage in pyogenic arthritis. Arch. Pathol., 99:44–47, 1975.

133a.Rytel, M.W.: Rapid diagnostic methods in infectious diseases. Adv. Intern. Med., 20:37–60, 1975.

134. Salit, I.E., Blake, M., and Gotschlich, E.C.: Intra-strain heterogeneity of gonococcal pili is related to opacity colony variance. J. Exp. Med., 151:716–725, 1980.

135. Salter, R.B.: The protective effect of continuous passive motion on living articular cartilage in acute septic arthritis: an experimental investigation in the rabbit. Clin. Orthop., 159:223–247, 1981.

136. Salvati, E.A.: Total hip replacement in current or recent sepsis. Orthop. Rev., 9:97–102, 1980.

137. Salvati, E.A.: Total hip replacement in presence of subacute or arrested sepsis. Orthop. Rev., 8:103–106, 1979.

138. Samilson, R.L., Bersani, F.A., and Watkins, M.B.: Acute suppurative arthritis in infants and children. The importance of early diagnosis and surgical drainage. Pediatrics, 21:798–803, 1958.

139. Sattar, M.A.: The penetration of metronidazole into synovial fluid. Postgrad. Med. J., 58:20–24, 1982.

140. Schaad, U.B., McCracken, G.H., and Nelson, J.D.: Pyogenic arthritis of the sacroiliac joint in pediatric patients. Pediatrics, 66:375–379, 1980.

140a.Scheinberg, M.A., and Benson, M.D.: SAA amyloid protein levels in amyloid-prone chronic inflammatory disorders: lack of association with amyloid disease. J. Rheumatol., 7:724–726, 1980.

141. Schiller, M., et al.: Clostridium perfringens septic arthritis: Report of a case and review of the literature. Clin. Orthop., 139:92–96, 1979.

142. Schoolnick, G.K., Ochs, H.O., and Buchanan, T.M.: Immunoglobulin class responsible for gonococcal bactericidal activity of normal human sera. J. Immunol., 122:1,771–1,779, 1979.

143. Schwartz, A.M., and Goldberg, M.J.: Medial adductor approach to arthrography of the hip in children. Radiology, 132:483, 1979.

144. Sequeira, W., et al.: Pyogenic infections of the pubic symphysis. Ann. Intern. Med., 96:604–606, 1982.

145. Sharp, J.T., et al.: Infectious arthritis. Arch. Intern. Med., 139:1,125–1,130, 1979.

146. Smith, B.R., et al.: Bone penetration of antibiotics. Orthopedics, 6:187–193, 1983.

147. Smith, J.R., and Phelps, P.: Septic arthritis, gout, pseudogout and osteoarthritis in the knee of a patient with multiple myeloma. Arthritis Rheum., 15:89–96, 1972.

148. Smith, W.S., and Ward, R.M.: Septic arthritis of the hip complicating perforation of abdominal organs. JAMA, 195:1,148–1,150, 1966.

149. Spagna, V.A., and Prior, R.B.: The limulus amebocyte lysate assay. Am. Fam. Physician, 22:125–128, 1980.

150. Steere, A.C., et al.: The spirochetal etiology of Lyme disease. N. Engl. J. Med., 308:733–740, 1983.

150a. Steere, A.C., et al.: Elevated levels of collagenase and prostaglandin E$_2$ from synovium associated with erosion of cartilage and bone in a patient with chronic Lyme arthritis. Arthritis Rheum., *23*:591–599, 1980.

151. Steigbigel, R.T., Johnson, P.K., and Remington, J.S.: The nitroblue tetrazolium reduction test versus conventional hematology in the diagnosis of bacterial infection. N. Engl. J. Med., *290*:235–238, 1974.

152. Stetson, J.W., DePonte, R.J., and Southwick, W.O.: Acute septic arthritis of the hip in children. Clin. Orthop., *56*:105–116, 1968.

153. Tesar, J.T., and Dietz, F.: Mechanisms of inflammation in infectious arthritis. Clin. Rheum. Dis., *4*:51–61, 1978.

154. Thayer, J.D., and Martin, J.E.: Improved medium selective for cultivation of N. gonorrhoeae and N. meningitidis. Public Health Rep., *81*:559–562, 1966.

155. Tuazon, C.U.: Teichoic acid antibodies in osteomyelitis and septic arthritis caused by Staphylococcus aureus. J. Bone Joint Surg., *64A*:762–765, 1982.

156. Tuli, S.M.: Excision arthroplasty for tuberculous and pyogenic arthritis of the hip. J. Bone Joint Surg., *63B*:29–32, 1981.

157. Veal, J.R.: Acute suppurative arthritis. N. Orleans Med. Surg. J., *87*:549–553, 1935.

158. Vincenti, F.: Septic arthritis following renal transplantation. Nephron, *30*:253–256, 1982.

159. Wahlig, H., et al.: The release of gentamicin from polymethylmethacrylate beads. J. Bone Joint Surg., *60B*:270–275, 1978.

160. Waldvogel, F.A., and Vasey, H.: Osteomyelitis: the past decade. N. Engl. J. Med., *303*:360–370, 1980.

161. Waldvogel, F.A., Medoff, G., and Schwartz, M.N.: Osteomyelitis: a review of clinical features, therapeutic considerations and unusual aspects. N. Engl. J. Med., *282*:198–206, 260–266, 316–322, 1970.

162. Ward, J., Cohen, A.S., and Bauer, W.: The diagnosis and therapy of acute suppurative arthritis. Arthritis Rheum., *3*:522–535, 1960.

163. Ward, P.A., et al.: Generation by bacterial proteinases of leukotactic factors from human serum and human C3 and C5. J. Immunol., *111*:1,003–1,006, 1973.

164. Williams, R.C., Jr., and Kunkel, H.G.: Rheumatoid factor, complement and conglutinin aberrations in patients with subacute bacterial endocarditis. J. Clin. Invest., *41*:666–675, 1962.

165. Willkens, R.F., Healey, L.A., and Decker, J.L.: Acute infectious arthritis in the aged and chronically ill. Arch. Intern. Med., *106*:354–364, 1960.

166. Wilson, P.D., Jr., Aglietti, P., and Salvati, E.A.: Subacute sepsis of the hip treated by antibiotics and cemented prosthesis. J. Bone Joint Surg., *56A*:879–898, 1974.

167. Wofsy, D.: Culture-negative septic arthritis and bacterial endocarditis: diagnosis by synovial biopsy. Arthritis Rheum., *23*:605–607, 1980.

168. Yaron, M., et al.: Stimulation of prostaglandin E production by bacterial endotoxins in cultured human synovial fibroblasts. Arthritis Rheum., *23*:921–925, 1980.

169. Zein, N., Ganuza, C., and Kushner, I.: Significance of serum C-reactive protein elevations in patients with systematic lupus erythematosus. Arthritis Rheum., *21*:605, 1978.

170. Ziff, M., Gribetz, H.J., and LoSpalluto, J.: Effect of leukocyte and synovial membrane extracts on cartilage mucoprotein. J. Clin. Invest., *39*:405–412, 1960.

Chapter 100

Gonococcal Arthritis

Don L. Goldenberg

Gonococcal arthritis is now considered to be the most common type of septic arthritis.[2,3,7,12,16] In the past 7 years, 50 patients with culture-proved disseminated gonococcal infection (DGI) were seen at our medical center, and probably twice that many patients had possible DGI without positive cultures.[17] Since the description of *Neisseria gonorrhoeae* in 1879 by Neisser, and since the subsequent recovery of the organism from the joint fluid of a patient with acute arthritis, DGI has been recognized as an important cause of hematogenously acquired septic arthritis. The role of *N. gonorrhoeae* in "reactive" arthritis such as Reiter's disease is still controversial.[7] The frequent absence of positive synovial fluid cultures and the presence of dermatitis and tenosynovitis, not found in other bacterial arthritides, are cited as examples of hypersensitivity or immune mechanisms in DGI. This chapter reviews the microbiologic, serologic, clinical, and therapeutic manifestations of DGI and discusses the possibility that certain of these clinical manifestations may not require the existence of viable organisms.

NEISSERIA GONORRHOEAE

Neisseria gonorrhoeae is a gram-negative diplococcus identified in the laboratory by its growth characteristics and its sugar-fermentation patterns. The gram-stained smear of body secretions reveals the characteristic kidney-bean-shaped pair of organisms, although *Haemophilus* as well as other *Neisseria* species may have a similar appearance. The nutritional requirements of *N. gonorrhoeae* are fastidious, and these bacteria require special care for optimal growth. Genitourinary, anal, and throat secretions should be plated on antibiotic-impregnated media, such as Thayer-Martin or modified New York City plates, to inhibit the growth of other bacteria. All other body fluids should be immediately plated on chocolate agar, prepared by heating red blood cells, and then placed in an atmosphere of increased carbon dioxide tension. Even when optimal culture techniques are followed, the recovery of the organism from body fluids has been disappointing. Growth of the organisms in standard broth cultures can be de-

layed, and blood or joint fluid should be repeatedly checked for bacterial growth for up to seven days.

Currently, one million cases of gonorrhea are reported each year in the United States, and it is estimated that three times as many cases are not reported. Great strides have been made in the past decade in understanding the complicated interactions of *N. gonorrhoeae* with the host and in elucidating the structural and immunologic characteristics of the organism.[5,13,14,19,20,26,27] The cell wall of *N. gonorrhoeae* is a complex structure, which consists of an outer capsule, pili, or protein filaments, an outer membrane that contains protein and lipopolysaccharide, peptidoglycan, and an inner cytoplasmic membrane. Several of these components have identifiable structural or serologic characteristics that vary among specific gonococcal strains. For example, two outer membrane proteins have been identified: (1) protein I, which provides a means for serotyping gonococci; and (2) protein II, responsible for colonial opacity.

At least 60 different pili serologic types have been characterized. The lipopolysaccharide of the outer membrane contains a hydrophobic component, lipid A, and is also characterized serologically into major antigenic determinants, based on variations in carbohydrate structure. One or more of these cell-wall determinants may be important in the virulence of a specific strain.[5,19,20] For example, the nutritional requirements of strains producing DGI are different from those of strains producing uncomplicated local gonococcal infections.[14] My colleagues and I have found that nearly two-thirds of DGI-producing strains possess a nutritional requirement for arginine, hypoxanthine, and uracil, as compared to only 8% of strains from cases of uncomplicated gonorrhea.[17] DGI-producing strains also possess unique principal outer membrane proteins and are resistant to the bactericidal activity of normal human sera, in contrast to many localized strains,[19,20,24] particularly those that cause severe pelvic inflammatory disease in women.[24] Despite this serum resistance, the DGI-producing strains are still uniquely sensitive to antibiotics.[31] Laboratory growth characteristics also distinguish the strains that cause disseminated infections. For example, piliated phenotypes, easily identified on the basis of the growth characteristics of their morphologic colonies, are isolated in primary culture and are probably responsible for DGI.[28] Pili may play a role in the virulence of gonococci by enhancing their attachment to epithelial cells. Transparent colonies are also more common in gonococcal isolates from sites such as the blood or joint, whereas opaque colonies are more often isolated from local sites.[13,17]

INCIDENCE

Most patients with DGI are young and healthy and have no host-defense impairment that might predispose them to bacteremia. It is estimated that 0.1 to 3% of patients with gonococcal urethritis will develop DGI.[12] Although gonococcal arthritis was more common in men than in women prior to the development of antibiotics, in the past 25 years, more women than men developed DGI.[2,5,12,19] The interval from the onset of sexual exposure or genitourinary tract symptoms to DGI varies from a day to many weeks. Patients with DGI do not usually complain of genitourinary symptoms such as pelvic inflammatory disease or prostatitis.[17]

The absence of local symptoms and the female predominance of DGI may be due to failure of a mucosal inflammatory response to block the organism's entrance into the circulation. For example, women are prone to develop DGI during the menses or early in pregnancy. *N. gonorrhoeae* can change its colonial phenotype during menses from opaque to transparent. Thus, the characteristics of the host's mucosa and the adherence traits of the organism, such as the presence of pili, which promotes attachment, are important in the initial gonococcal infection.

The major independent host-defense factor that predisposes individuals to DGI is complement-component deficiency. Patients with congenital complement-component deficiencies, especially those with terminal C5-C8 deficiencies, develop recurrent DGI as well as other recurrent neisserial infections.[18] My colleagues and I have also noted C3 and C4 deficiency in our patients with DGI.[17]

Some of the foregoing interrelated host-microbial factors determine whether a strain of *N. gonorrhoeae* will cause a local infection or whether it will disseminate. Tissue penetration and circulatory invasion seem to depend on specific cell-wall properties that can be altered by genetic mutations.[26] Perhaps the most important factor in dissemination, as well as in the clinical manifestations of DGI is the ability of the various gonococcal strains to resist the bactericidal activity of normal human serum.[19] This activity depends on a natural antibody, which is directed against gonococcal lipopolysaccharide and an uncharacterized unique interaction of gonococci with complement. DGI-producing strains may also effectively bind naturally occurring "blocking antibodies," with a resulting inability of bactericidal antibodies and complement to kill the organism.

CLINICAL MANIFESTATIONS

Most patients with DGI first experience either migratory or additive polyarthralgias (Table 100–1). Fever, chills, and other constitutional symptoms are common; however, genitourinary symptoms are unusual. Only 5 of our 37 patients with positive genitourinary cultures had genitourinary symptoms.[17] Only 1 of 5 patients with positive pharyngeal cultures and none of 10 patients with positive rectal cultures had local symptoms. Tenosynovitis is present in two-thirds of patients with DGI. The tenosynovitis usually involves multiple joints and is especially common over the wrists, fingers, ankles, and toes. Polyarthritis or monoarthritis was present in 42% of our patients with DGI. Although the knees, wrists, and ankles are usually affected, hip, spinal, and temporomandibular joint involvement may occur. In fact, any joint may be affected. When joint effusions can be aspirated, the synovial fluid is usually purulent, with a mean leukocyte count of 50,000 cells/mm³. Occasionally, a small joint effusion that is relatively acellular is present for a few days.

Dermatitis occurs in two-thirds of patients with DGI[2,3,17] (Tables 100–1, 100–2). Skin lesions are usually multiple and are most often found on the extremities or on the trunk, but rarely on the face, palms, or soles (Fig. 100–1). These lesions are often painless, and patients may be unaware of their existence, although some skin lesions are painful. The most common skin lesions are hemorrhagic macules or papules, but pustules, vesicles, bullae, erythema nodosum, or erythema multiforme have also been described. New skin lesions may develop

Table 100–1.   Initial Symptoms and Signs in 49 Patients with Disseminated Gonococcal Infection*

	(%)
Polyarthralgias	70
Tenosynovitis	67
Dermatitis	67
Fever	63
Arthritis†	42
Monoarthritis	32
Polyarthritis	10

*Patients seen from 1975 to 1982 with positive blood or synovial fluid culture or clinical symptoms typical of this infection and positive local cultures

†Documented with synovial fluid aspiration

(Data from O'Brien, Goldenberg, and Rice.[17])

Table 100–2. Clinical and Laboratory Characteristics of Patients with Disseminated Gonococcal Infection with Tenosynovitis and Dermatitis and with Suppurative Arthritis*

	Tenosynovitis and Dermatitis	*Suppurative Arthritis*
Number of patients	30	19
Duration of symptoms prior to hospitalization (median number of days)	4	4
Tenosynovitis	26 (87%)	4 (21%)
Dermatitis	27 (90%)	8 (42%)
Positive blood culture	13 (43%)	0
Positive joint fluid culture	0	9 (47%)
Number of patients with a twofold or greater rise in bactericidal antibody activity	3/18 (17%)	9/13 (69%)
Number of gonococcal strains resistant to all 10 normal sera	18/24 (75%)	9/19 (47%)

*Patients seen at Boston University Medical Center from 1975 to 1982

(Data from O'Brien, Goldenberg, and Rice.[17])

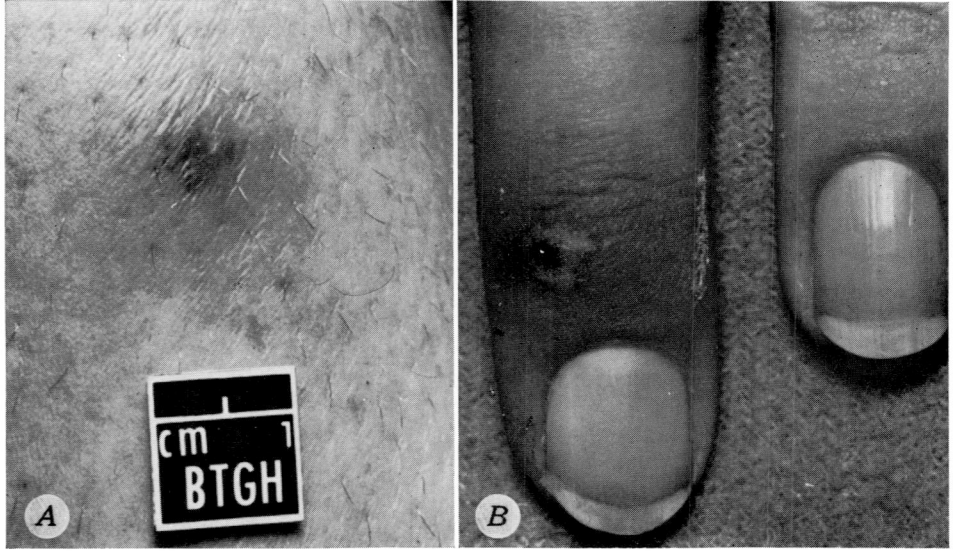

Fig. 100–1.   Skin lesions characteristic of septicemia due to *Neisseria gonorrhoeae, N. meningitidis, Streptobacillus moniliformis,* and *Haemophilus influenzae. A,* Hemorrhagic spot 5 to 6 mm in diameter on the upper arm; the gray area 1 to 2 mm in diameter in the center indicates necrosis. *B,* Pustulovesicular lesion on the finger of the same patient; the necrotic center is evident as a dark gray area.

during the initial 24 to 48 hours of antibiotic therapy.

Most patients are febrile, although the average temperature is usually only moderately elevated. A modest peripheral blood leukocytosis is common. Transiently elevated liver function studies have been described, probably representing subclinical hepatitis during bacteremia.[12,17] Additionally, a perihepatitis, termed the Fitz-Hugh–Curtis syndrome, may occur in women secondary to adhesions between the surfaces of the liver and the peritoneum as a result of intraperitoneal spread of infection. Gonococcal meningitis and endocarditis are rarely reported in the antibiotic era. A presumed immune-mediated glomerulonephritis secondary to DGI has been reported.[4]

Some investigators have proposed that DGI progresses sequentially from a bacteremic phase, characterized by chills, tenosynovitis, and skin lesions, to a joint-localized phase manifested by purulent arthritis.[12] The diagnostic utility of such a classification is suspect, however, because of the significant clinical overlap and the inconsistent temporal sequence of the articular manifestations.[2,3,17] I find that most patients initially have either a predominantly joint-localized disease or tenosynovitis and dermatitis (Table 100–2, Figs. 100–2 and 100–3). No difference is noted in the duration of symptoms prior to the diagnosis of DGI in patients with suppurative arthritis and in those with tenosynovitis. These initial clinical manifestations may be determined by certain microbiologic and serologic features of the strain of *N. gonorrhoeae*.[19] For example, in my experience, the strains of *N. gonorrhoeae* isolated from patients with purulent arthritis are generally phenotypically different from those isolated from patients with dermatitis and tenosynovitis (Table 100–2). In a group studied by my colleagues and myself, 75% of the *N. gonorrhoeae* isolated from patients with tenosynovitis and dermatitis were resistant to the bactericidal activity of normal human sera, whereas only 47% of strains isolated from patients with suppurative arthritis were resistant. Sixty-nine percent of the patients with suppurative arthritis, but only 17% of the patients with tenosynovitis and dermatitis, developed a significant rise in bactericidal antibody activity, as measured in their serum during the acute illness and in convalescence.

PATHOGENESIS

Suppurative arthritis due to *N. gonorrhoeae* is generally considered to be secondary to bacteremic spread of the organisms to the synovium, with replication of bacteria and the subsequent release of proteolytic enzymes from synovial lining cells and polymorphonuclear leukocytes (Table 100–3). Eventually, cartilage is destroyed. This process is the same as in most other types of bacterial arthritis. Gonococcal bacteremia is more likely to cause arthritis or tenosynovitis than infection with pneumococci or other common bacteria. Microscopically, the synovial membrane initially reveals lining-cell hyperplasia and infiltration by polymorphonuclear leukocytes (see Fig. 100–2). Gram-stained smears of the synovial fluid or synovial membrane are often initially positive. If a second synovial membrane specimen is obtained 5 to 7 days after treatment, most of the acute infiltrate will have subsided, but chronic inflammatory cells will be prominent. Synovial fluid and synovial membrane Gram-stained smears and cultures will no longer show *N. gonorrhoeae*. Rarely, a chronic synovitis persists despite appropriate antibiotic therapy.[17] This sterile synovitis may be responsible for persistent pain and joint effusions despite eradication of the acute infection, a phenomenon termed "post-infectious" arthritis.[7]

Although the synovial membrane and fluid characteristics of acute gonococcal arthritis are generally similar to those of arthritis due to other bacteria, DGI rarely destroys cartilage or bone. Even in the preantibiotic era, untreated gonococcal arthritis rarely caused permanent joint destruction.[30] My colleagues and I have also seen patients with DGI undergo complete resolution of arthritis and tenosynovitis without antibiotic treatment.[17]

Clinical and laboratory evidence indicates that the arthralgias, tenosynovitis, dermatitis, and the "sterile" arthritis associated with DGI may be due to immune-mediated mechanisms or hypersensitivity (Table 100–3). The initial presentation of DGI often resembles that of serum sickness, with tenosynovitis and migratory polyarthralgias that are usually transient and often disappear without antimicrobial therapy. Similar musculoskeletal symptoms are common in immune-complex-related infections such as hepatitis, but they are absent in non-neisserial bacterial arthritis. Furthermore, *N. gonorrhoeae* is recovered from fewer than 50% of purulent synovial effusions, in contrast to nongonococcal bacterial arthritis.[8,17] Positive blood cultures are found in fewer than one-third of patients with DGI, and positive blood and synovial fluid cultures are mutually exclusive (see Table 100–2). Investigators have attributed the frequent absence of positive blood and synovial fluid cultures to the fastidious growth requirements of *N. gonorrhoeae*, yet the organisms are easily recovered from the genitourinary tract or other local sites in most cases of DGI. Therefore, some investigators have questioned the role of immune-mediated phenomena or hypersensitivity in the synovitis and dermatitis associated with DGI. Gonococcal urethritis might initiate a "reactive," sterile arthritis. Scandinavian investigators have reported that an aseptic arthritis, clinically similar to Reiter's syndrome, occurs commonly following gonococcal urethritis.[22] Nonviable bacterial antigenic components could also cause a persistent yet sterile synovitis. In some patients with DGI, purulent synovitis does not occur, and circulating or deposited immune complexes may be more important.[7]

The dermatitis associated with DGI is almost always sterile, and the cause of the skin lesions does not seem to be secondary to embolic spread of viable organisms.[1,23,25] Erythema nodosum, erythema multiforme, and vasculitis, which have all been reported in DGI, suggest immune-mediated or hypersensitivity reactions. Although viable *N. gonorrhoeae* are rarely recovered from these skin lesions, immunofluorescent evidence exists of gonococcal cell-wall components, gonococcal antibody, and complement.[5,23,25] Circulating immune complexes have also been detected in patients with DGI.[15,29] These complexes are especially promi-

Fig. 100–2. A 38-year-old man had abrupt onset of pain and swelling in the distal interphalangeal (DIP) joint of the left third finger. One day later, he developed pain and swelling in the right wrist and the dorsum of right hand, and two days later, he had swelling and pain in the right ankle. Ten days after onset, examination confirmed involvement of these areas. No skin lesions or urethral discharge were present. On the eleventh day of illness, the left ankle became swollen and painful. Blood cultures were sterile, and synovial fluid cultures from the right wrist and the left ankle on the fifteenth day of illness showed no growth. Serum uric acid levels, antistreptolysin O titer, and electrocardiograph findings were normal. LE cell preparations and latex fixation for anti-IgG were negative. Nineteen days after onset, the left third DIP and the right wrist joint remained inflamed; the other joints were clear. Fever was present. Diagnostic biopsy was advised by the consultant on the twenty-first day of illness. Tissue from the wrist joint grew *Neisseria gonorrhoeae*. A section of biopsy tissue stained with hematoxylin and eosin is shown in *A* (× 185) and in *B* (× 460). The biopsy shows proliferation of new tissue including prominent neovascularization. Synovial lining cells are not seen on the surface of the section (*A*, right) and are infrequently present throughout the tissue. The inflammatory infiltrate consists of a mixture of cell types. Collections of polymorphonuclear leukocytes are scattered through the section, along with mononuclear cells and lymphocytes. In some areas not shown, plasma cells are prominent.

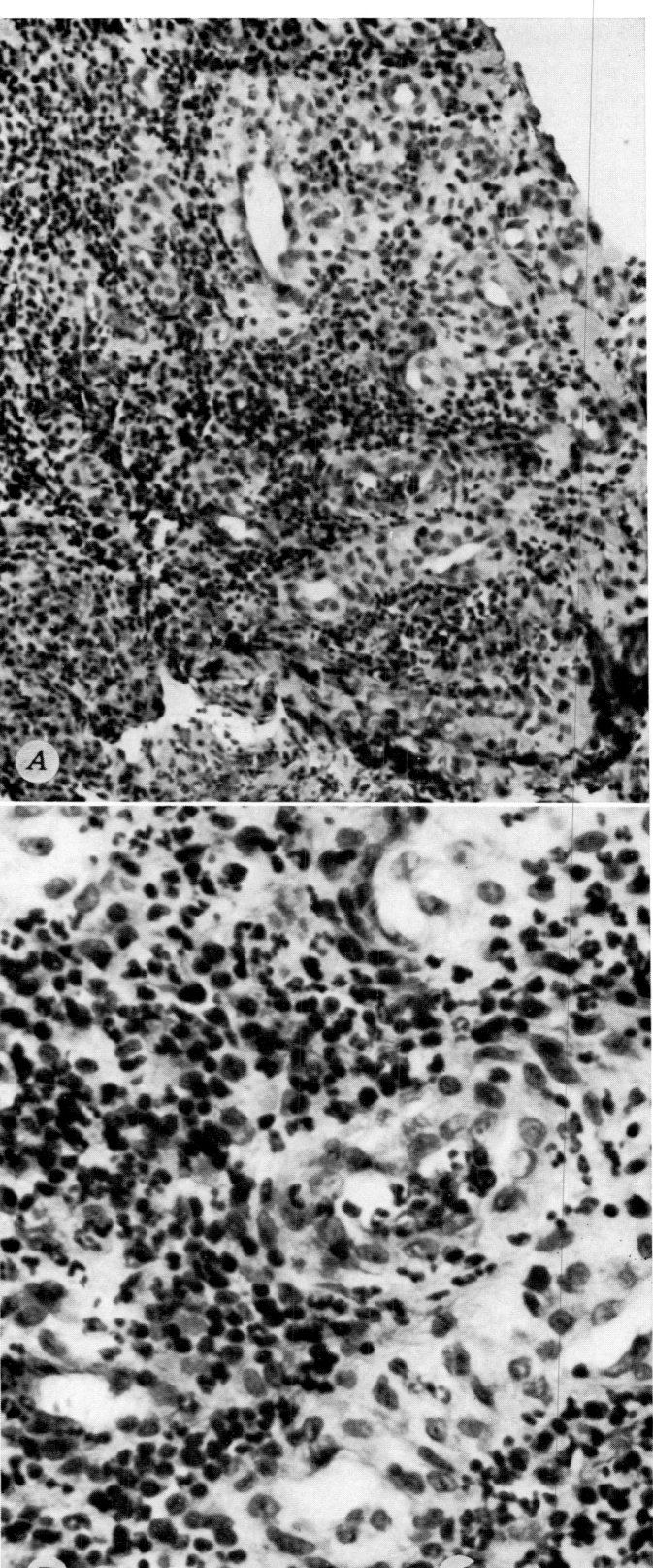

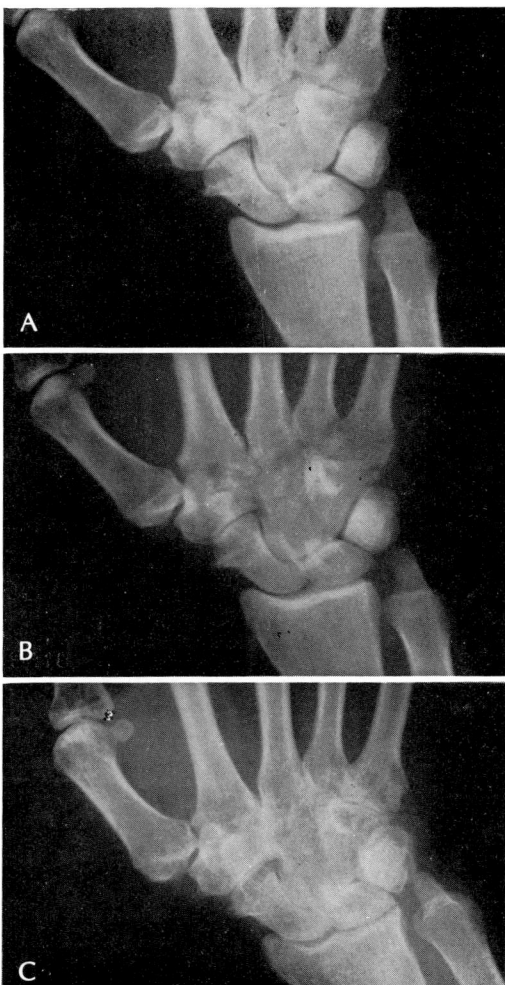

Fig. 100–3. Roentgenograms of the patient whose biopsy specimen is shown in Figure 100–2. *A* was obtained on the eleventh day of illness, 10 days after the onset of pain and swelling in the right wrist; the film is normal. *B* was taken on the nineteenth day of illness; one sees demineralization of the carpal and metacarpal bone, along the carpometacarpal articulations, with a loss of clearly defined trabecular bone markings and a loss of articular cartilage in the same area. *C* was obtained 11 weeks after the onset of arthritis; remineralization has occurred. Joint-space narrowing is present along the carpometacarpal row, the intercarpal articulations, and the radiocarpal joints.

nent early in the clinical course and could cause a sterile synovitis that might promote the later entrance of bacteria into the joint.[15]

My colleagues and I have investigated the role of nonviable bacterial components in DGI using an experimental model of gonococcal arthritis in rabbits.[9] Intra-articular injections of *N. gonorrhoeae* caused an acute arthritis within 24 hours, and at 7 to 10 days, a chronic synovitis developed. Histologically, the changes were identical to those following the intra-articular injection of gram-positive cocci and *Escherichia coli* into rabbits' knees. *N. gonorrhoeae* could not be recovered from the infected joint even 48 hours after injection, however, whereas the gram-positive cocci and the *E. coli* were persistently recovered for days to weeks following their injection. Intra-articular injections of nonviable *N. gonorrhoeae* or gonococcal lipopolysaccharide isolated from the cell wall of *N. gonorrhoeae* also caused an initially acute and then chronic, persistent synovitis. A lipopolysaccharide concentration as low as 5 μg (10^{-6} g dry weight) caused arthritis, whereas much larger concentrations of another gonococcal antigenic component, the outer membrane protein, did not cause synovitis. Therefore, clinical and laboratory evidence indicates that, in some circumstances, the synovitis, tenosynovitis, and dermatitis associated with DGI may not require viable *N. gonorrhoeae*.

DIAGNOSIS

The diagnosis of DGI should be suspected in any young, sexually active patient who has acute arthritis and dermatitis. Although tenosynovitis can occur with other types of arthritis, the presence of tenosynovitis or arthritis in association with a skin rash is sufficient clinical grounds for a presumptive diagnosis of DGI. Most patients are febrile, demonstrate peripheral blood leukocytosis, and have an elevated erythrocyte sedimentation rate. These nonspecific findings are not always present, however. If synovial fluid can be aspirated, the leukocyte count is generally 30,000 to 100,000 cell/mm^3, although the range is wider than in the joint effusions of nongonococcal bacterial arthritis, and some fluids are relatively acellular. A Gram-stained smear of concentrated synovial fluid is positive in fewer than 25% of purulent joint effusions, in contrast to other forms of bacterial arthritis.[8] In most recent series, the genitourinary cultures provided the best yield of *N. gonorrhoeae*, whereas blood and skin cultures were rarely positive[2,4,8,9,10,11,12] (Table 100–4). The urethra should be swabbed to obtain a specimen for culture because most men do not have a urethral discharge. In women, a specimen should be obtained directly from the cervix. Rectal and pharyngeal cultures should be obtained, particularly the latter because pharyngeal gonorrhea may lead to disseminated infection. Investigators are currently using specific polyclonal and monoclonal antisera in attempts to identify gonococcal antigens in sterile joint fluid and blood in patients with DGI. Tests for immunologic detection of gonococcal antigens in cervical specimens are already commercially available.

Table 100–3. **Pathogenesis of Clinical Manifestations of Disseminated Gonococcal Infection**

Mechanism	Evidence
Bacteremic seeding of synovium	Recovery of *Neisseria gonorrhoeae* from synovial fluid
Development of "postinfectious" or "reactive" arthritis	Negative synovial fluid cultures; laboratory models of cell-wall-induced arthritis
Immune mediation	Circulating immune complexes; antibody, complement deposits in skin lesions; clinical resemblance to serum sickness

When Gram-stained smears or cultures of the synovial fluid or blood are negative, a therapeutic response to penicillin or other appropriate antibiotic is so rapidly effective that it may be an important diagnostic clue to DGI. Therefore, it is common to initiate antibiotic therapy in patients with suspected DGI while awaiting the identification of the organisms in the culture specimen. Most patients become afebrile and their clinical manifestations subside within 48 to 72 hours. Some other forms of bacterial arthritis or viral arthritis have initial features similar to those of DGI. Meningococcal arthritis is the most difficult bacterial arthritis to differentiate from DGI, and the musculoskeletal manifestations of the disorders are virtually identical.[32] A chronic purulent monoarthritis may occur in chronic meningococcemia.[6] As in DGI, evidence suggests toxic or immunologic mechanisms because depressed serum complement and deposition of IgG, IgM, complement, and meningococcal antigen have been identified in the synovial membrane and the synovial fluid, and the synovial fluid is usually sterile.

Non-neisserial bacterial arthritides share many clinical features distinct from those of DGI.[8] Gram-positive coccal arthritis or arthritis due to gram-negative bacilli often occurs in the extremely young or in the elderly, it almost always causes monoarthritis, and it often occurs in compromised hosts. These disorders are not associated with tenosynovitis or dermatitis, and they do not usually respond quickly to treatment; repeated needle aspirations or surgical drainage, as well as prolonged parenteral antibiotics, are often required (Table 100–4). Even with optimal treatment, permanent joint destruction is common.

Other major differential diagnostic considerations include hepatitis, Reiter's syndrome, acute rheumatic fever, bacterial endocarditis, other bacteremias, and other connective tissue diseases (Table 100–4). Polyarthritis, tenosynovitis, and a skin rash are common in hepatitis; the rash and arthritis generally occur in the anicteric phase. The skin rash is usually urticarial, and the synovial fluid leukocyte count is usually lower than in DGI. The most helpful diagnostic features are elevated hepatocellular enzymes and the identificaiton of hep-

atitis surface antigen (HB$_s$Ag) in the blood, with negative blood and synovial fluid cultures. Reiter's syndrome may also cause arthritis, tenosynovitis, and urethritis. In classic Reiter's syndrome, the urethritis is not due to *N. gonorrhoeae*, but rather is nongonococcal. Other helpful clinical features include the presence of conjunctivitis, characteristic mucocutaneous lesions, circinate balanitis, and keratoderma blennorrhagicum. Clinical and radiologic evidence of sacroiliitis and the presence of HLA-B27 on lymphocytes are also characteristic of Reiter's syndrome. Acute rheumatic fever may cause polyarthritis in young adults without carditis, chorea, or subcutaneous nodules. Some investigators have termed this disorder poststreptococcal arthritis rather than acute rheumatic fever. If a skin rash is present, it usually is transient (erythema marginatum). The diagnosis relies on evidence of a recent streptococcal throat infection, confirmed by culture or by serologic testing of blood, and a rapid response to salicylates or other anti-inflammatory agents.

Many bacteremias or other systemic infections can cause musculoskeletal and dermatologic manifestations that mimic DGI. Bacterial endocarditis is especially important to differentiate from DGI. Purulent arthritis is not common in bacterial endocarditis unless hematogenous spread to the synovium occurs, such as occasionally seen in endocarditis caused by *Staphylococcus aureus*. Myalgias, arthralgias, tendinitis, and back pain are common musculoskeletal manifestations associated with bacterial endocarditis, particularly subacute disease already present for several weeks. Viral diseases including measles and rubella, as well as various arboviral infections not commonly seen in the United States, can also cause skin lesions and arthritis. Rarely, infections caused by herpes viruses are accompanied by a skin rash and arthralgias.

Lyme disease, caused by a spirochete, is also associated with a skin rash, but the rash is a characteristic enlarging anular lesion (erythema chronicum migrans) and antedates the onset of the arthritis by a few weeks (see Chap. 104). Another disease caused by spirochetes, secondary syphilis, also may cause arthritis and a skin rash.

Table 100–4. Differential Diagnosis of Disseminated Gonococcal Infection

Clinical Diagnosis	Patient	Musculoskeletal Manifestations	Dermatitis	Genitourinary Manifestations	Blood Tests	Therapy
Disseminated gonococcal infection	Young, healthy, more often women	Tenosynovitis (70%); migratory polyarthralgias (70%); monoarthritis, joint fluid culture positive (<25%)	Common (70%), but culture positive in only 5%	Symptoms in <25%, but positive cultures in 80%	Positive cultures in 10 to 30%	Antibiotics (complete and rapid response)
Non-neisserial bacterial arthritis	Often immunocompromised	Monoarthritis with positive joint fluid culture	None	None, unless urinary tract infection is source of bacteremia	Positive cultures in 50 to 70%	Antibiotics, drainage
Hepatitis	Exposed to hepatitis	Tenosynovitis, polyarthritis	Rash, usually urticarial	None	Abnormal liver function tests; HB,Ag	Salicylates or other nonsteroidal anti-inflammatory drugs
Reiter's syndrome	Young, healthy, more often men, with recent history of urethritis, dysentery	Asymmetric arthritis, sacroiliitis	Keratodermia, circinate balanitis	Nongonococcal urethritis	HLA-B27 positive or (+)	Nonsteroidal anti-inflammatory drugs
Acute rheumatic fever	Children, young adults	Migratory arthritis	Erythema marginatum; subcutaneous nodules	None	Serologic evidence of recent streptococcal throat infection	Salicylates
Bacterial endocarditis	Any age	Arthralgias, myalgias, arthritis	Emboli, macules	None	Positive blood culture	Antibiotics
Juvenile rheumatoid arthritis	Children, young adults	Mono- or polyarthritis	Evanescent rash	None	Possibly, striking leukocytosis	Salicylates, other nonsteroidal anti-inflammatory drugs
Lyme disease	Children, young adults; appropriate geographic exposure	Mono- or oligoarthritis	Circular, enlarging lesion 2 weeks before arthritis	None	Antibody to spirochete	Initially antibiotics; later, salicylates, nonsteroidal anti-inflammatory drugs, and (?) antibiotics

Patients with rheumatoid arthritis (RA), systemic lupus erythematosus, or other connective tissue diseases may have initial manifestations similar to those of DGI. Adult-onset juvenile RA is especially confusing, in view of the fever, skin rash, polyarthralgias, and leukocytosis. In addition, patients with underlying connective tissue disease may develop superimposed gonococcal arthritis or other forms of infectious arthritis. Therefore, septic arthritis must always be considered in patients who have an acute exacerbation of an existing joint inflammation.[8]

THERAPY

The principles of therapy of DGI are similar to those of other forms of infectious arthritis, with some notable exceptions. As mentioned, antibiotic therapy is usually so successful that patients are dramatically better within a few days.[16] Patients who predominantly have arthralgias, fever, and dermatitis are often asymptomatic following 24 to 48 hours of antibiotics. These patients do not usually require more than a single needle aspiration of an inflamed joint for diagnostic purposes. Patients with large, purulent joint effusions, however, often require repeated needle aspirations of the joint and longer antimicrobial treatment, such as 7 to 10 days of parenteral antibiotics. In the experience of my colleagues and myself, the average duration of hospitalization of patients with dermatitis and arthralgias was 4 days, whereas the duration of hospitalization in patients with purulent gonococcal arthritis was 8 days.[17] Other investigators also have determined that a large, purulent joint effusion is the single most important determinant of the length of hospitalization in patients with DGI.[11] The response to treatment of patients with DGI and with purulent effusions is more complete and is faster than that of patients with nongonococcal bacterial arthritis. However, even in patients with gonococcal arthritis of the hip, joint drainage is not generally a problem, and only twice in the last 10 years have our patients with gonococcal arthritis required surgical drainage for a recurrent effusion. This finding is in contrast to patients with nongonococcal bacterial arthritis, in whom drainage by needle aspiration is sometimes inadequate, and who often require open drainage, especially when effusions involve the hip or shoulders.[8]

Until recently, the choice of antibiotic in patients with DGI was not difficult because DGI-producing strains were rarely resistant to penicillin. In fact, DGI-producing strains isolated from patients in the United States have been more sensitive to penicillin than strains isolated from patients with local infections.[32] In my experience, the mean inhibitory concentration to penicillin of DGI-producing strains in the past 7 years was 0.0527 μg/ml, as compared to a mean inhibitory concentration of 0.14 μg/ml of strains causing pelvic inflammatory disease and isolated during the same period.[17] None of these DGI-producing strains were penicillinase producing; however, some penicillinase-producing strains causing DGI have been reported,[21] and DGI caused by penicillinase-producing strains is becoming more common in the Far East.

The resistance of certain strains to antibiotics is due to selective mutations that may be promoted by the host-microbial environment. Thus, homosexual males may be infected with organisms that are resistant to the hydrophobic surroundings present in the rectum, and this resistance may also be accompanied by resistance to certain antimicrobial agents. If penicillinase-producing strains become a more common cause of DGI, the choice of antibiotics as well as the utility of a diagnostic trial of antibiotics in DGI will not be nearly as successful. Spectinomycin or some of the newer cephalosporins have been effective in eradicating the penicillin-resistant organisms thus far associated with DGI.[21] At this time, in most patients with DGI, however, penicillin is the antibiotic of choice.

Various treatment regimens have been recommended, and essentially all of them are successful. Large doses of parenteral antibiotics, such as 10 million U penicillin G administered daily for 7 to 10 days, have been recommended by some, but 1.2 million U penicillin intramuscularly or 2 g erythromycin orally have been administered by others[11,16,28] (Table 100–5). At present, no single antibiotic regimen is felt to be superior to others. I generally hospitalize patients with DGI and begin parenteral therapy with 2 to 4 million U penicillin intravenously daily. If the patient responds dramatically or if no large joint effusions are present, I discharge the patient after a few days of parenteral antibiotics and complete a 7-day course of antibiotics with oral drugs. Patients who have significant joint effusions or who are more resistant to therapy receive parenteral antibiotics for 7 days in the hospital or until all signs of joint inflammation have subsided.

In conclusion, DGI has become the most common cause of septic arthritis and is a leading cause of acute arthritis necessitating hospitalization. DGI occurs most often in young, healthy women and generally causes initial polyarthralgias, tenosynovitis, and dermatitis. In contrast to other types of bacterial arthritis, purulent joint effusions are present in fewer than half these patients, and *N. gonorrhoeae* can be recovered from only half the effusions. Other sites of dissemination such as the skin and blood cultures are also usually sterile;

Table 100–5. Treatment of Disseminated Gonococcal Infection*

Patients with arthralgias and tenosynovitis
  24 to 48 hours of moderate-dose penicillin IM or IV, followed by 5 to 7 days of oral ampicillin or other antibiotic
  Outpatient management possible, although with an initial 24 to 48 hours of hospitalization
 	
Patients with large joint effusions
  Hospitalization until signs of sepsis and joint inflammation have disappeared
  Large doses of penicillin (4 to 10 million U/day) IM or IV for 7 to 10 days
  Joint drainage with repeated needle aspirations until purulent effusions fail to reaccumulate
 	
Patients allergic to penicillin
  Same as above, but with spectinomycin, erythromycin, or tetyracyclines
 	
Patients possibly infected with a penicillinase-producing strain
  Same as above, but with spectinomycin or one of the newer cephalosporins and a determination of the sensitivity of the organism

*Always repeat cultures in 3 to 5 days to determine cure
IM = Intramuscularly; IV = intravenously.

therefore, the diagnosis is usually made by a typical clinical picture and by positive genitourinary, pharyngeal, or rectal cultures.

Treatment consists of antibiotic administration and, if necessary, joint drainage with needle aspirations. Response to treatment is rapid, and permanent joint destruction is rare. Antibiotic-resistant strains have only recently been recovered from patients with DGI, and unless these strains become more prevalent, a rapid therapeutic response to penicillin can be used for diagnostic purposes.

The clinical features of DGI that resemble serum sickness and the frequency of negative blood, skin, and joint fluid cultures support the theory that certain of the manifestations of DGI may not require the presence of viable *N. gonorrhoeae*, but rather may relate to toxic or immune-mediated inflammation. The relationship of these mechanisms with certain host and microbial characteristics will require further elucidation.

REFERENCES

1. Barr, J., and Danielson, D.: Septic gonococcal dermatitis. Br. J. Med., *1*:482–485, 1971.
2. Brandt, K.D., Cathcart, E.S., and Cohen, A.S.: Gonococcal arthritis: clinical features correlated with blood, synovial fluid and genito-urinary cultures. Arthritis Rheum., *17*:502–510, 1974.
3. Brogadir, S.P., Schimmer, B.M., and Myers, A.R.: Spectrum of the gonococcal arthritis-dermatitis syndrome. Semin. Arthritis Rheum., *8*:177–183, 1979.
4. Ebright, J.R., and Komorowski, R.: Gonococcal endocarditis associated with immune complex glomerulonephritis. Am. J. Med., *68*:793–796, 1980.
5. Eisenstein, B.I., and Masi, A.T.: Disseminated gonococcal infection (DGI) and gonococcal arthritis (GCA). I. Bacteriology, epidemiology, host factors, pathogen factors, and pathology. Semin. Arthritis Rheum., *10*:155–172, 1981.
6. Fam, A.G., Tenebaum, J., and Stein, J.L.: Clinical forms of meningococcal arthritis: a study of five cases. J. Rheumatol., *6*:567–573, 1979.
7. Goldenberg, D.L.: "Post-infectious" arthritis: a new look at an old concept with particular attention to disseminated gonococcal infection. Am. J. Med., *74*:925–928, 1983.
8. Goldenberg, D.L., and Cohen, A.S.: Acute infectious arthritis. Am. J. Med., *60*:369–377, 1976.
9. Goldenberg, D.L., Chisholm, P.L., and Rice, P.A.: Experimental models of bacterial arthritis: a microbiologic and histopathologic characterization of the arthritis after the intra-articular injection of *Neisseria gonorrhoeae*, *Staphylococcus aureus*, group A streptococci and *Escherichia coli*. J. Rheumatol., *10*:1–7, 1983.
10. Handsfield, H.H.: Clinical aspects of gonococcal infections. *In* The Gonococcus. Edited by R.B. Roberts. New York, John Wiley and Sons, 1977, pp. 57–59.
11. Handsfield, H.H., Wiesner, P.J., and Holmes, K.K.: Treatment of the gonococcal arthritis-dermatitis syndromes. Ann. Intern. Med., *84*:661–667, 1976.
12. Holmes, K.K., Counts, G.W., and Beaty, H.N.: Disseminated gonococcal infection. Ann. Intern. Med., *74*:979–993, 1971.
13. James, J.F., and Swanson, J.: Studies on gonococcus infection. XIII. Occurrence of color/opacity colonial variants in clinical cultures. Infect. Immun., *19*:332–380, 1978.
14. Knapp, J.S., and Holmes, K.K.: Disseminated gonococcal infections caused by *Neisseria gonorrhoeae* with unique nutritional requirements. J. Infect. Dis., *132*:204–208, 1975.
15. Manicourt, D.H., and Orloff, S.: Gonococcal arthritis-dermatitis syndrome. Arthritis Rheum., *25*:574–578, 1982.
16. Masi, A.T., and Eisenstein, B.I.: Disseminated gonococcal infection (DGI) and gonococcal arthritis (GCA). II. Clinical manifestations, diagnosis, complications, treatment, and prevention. Semin. Arthritis Rheum., *10*:173–197, 1981.
17. O'Brien, J.P., Goldenberg, D.L., and Rice, P.A.: Disseminated gonococcal infection: a prospective analysis of 49 patients and a review of the pathophysiology and immune mechanisms. Medicine, *62*:395–406, 1983.
18. Peterson, B.H., et al.: *Neisseria meningitides* and *Neisseria gonorrhoeae* bacteremia associated with C6, C7, or C8 deficiency. Ann. Intern. Med., *90*:917–920, 1979.
19. Rice, P.A., and Goldenberg, D.L.: Clinical manifestations of disseminated infection caused by *Neisseria gonorrhoeae* are linked to differences in bactericidal reactivity of infecting strains. Ann. Intern. Med., *95*:175–178, 1981.
20. Rice, P.A., and Kasper, D.L.: Characterization of serum resistance of gonococci that disseminate: the role of blocking antibody and outer membrane protein. J. Clin. Invest., *70*:157, 1982.
21. Rinaldi, R.Z., Harrison, W.O., and Fan, P.T.: Penicillin-resistant gonococcal arthritis. Ann. Intern. Med., *97*:43–45, 1982.
22. Rosenthal, L., Olhagen, B., and Ek, S.: Aseptic arthritis after gonorrhoeae. Ann. Rheum. Dis., *39*:141–146, 1980.
23. Scherer, R., and Braun-Falco, O.: Alternative pathway complement activation: a possible mechanism inducing skin lesions in benign gonococcal sepsis. Br. J. Dermatol., *95*:303–309, 1976.
24. Schoolnik, G.K., Buchanan, T.M., and Holmes, K.K.: Gonococci causing disseminated gonococcal infection are resistant to the bactericidal action of normal human sera. J. Clin. Invest., *58*:1,163–1,173, 1976.
25. Shapiro, L., Teisch, J.A., and Brownstein, M.H.: Dermatohistopathology of chronic gonococcal sepsis. Arch. Dermatol., *107*:403–406, 1973.
26. Sparling, P.F., Guyman, L., and Biswas, G.: Antibiotic resistance in the gonococcus. *In* Microbiology, 1978. Edited by D. Schlessinger. Washington, D.C., American Society for Microbiology, 1976, pp. 494–500.
27. Swanson, J., Kraus, G.J., and Gotschlich, E.C.: Studies

of gonococcus infection. I. pili and zones of adhesion: their relation to gonococcal growth patterns. J. Exp. Med., *134*:886–906, 1971.

28. Thompson, S.E., et al.: Gonococcal tenosynovitis/dermatitis and septic arthritis: intravenous penicillin vs. oral erythromycin. JAMA, *244*:1,101–1,102, 1980.

29. Walker, L.C., et al.: Circulating immune complexes in disseminated gonorrheal infection. Ann. Intern. Med., *89*:28–33, 1978.

30. Wehrbein, H.L.: Gonococcus arthritis—a study of 610 cases. Surg. Gynecol. Obstet., *49*:105–113, 1929.

31. Wiesner, P.J., Handsfield, H.H., and Holmes, K.K.: Low antibiotic resistance of gonococci causing disseminated infection. N. Engl. J. Med., *288*:1,221–1,222, 1973.

32. Young, E.J., and Morton, G.L.: Meningococcal arthritis simulating gonococcemia. South. Med. J., *68*:636–638, 1975.

Chapter 101

Bacterial Arthritis

Frank R. Schmid

Most bacterial bone and joint infections are caused by cocci; bacilli much less commonly invade these tissues, and when they do, it is often because host resistance is impaired. For this reason, as well as their poorer response to antibiotic drugs, infections with these pathogens are usually prolonged and produce considerable local destruction. Characteristics of the micro-organisms and of the host and the clinical setting in which these bacteria and other microbial agents cause infection are discussed in this chapter. The general principles of infectious arthritis are discussed in Chapter 99. A summary of principles relating to bacterial sepsis is given in Table 101–1. Treatment is given in Table 101–2.

STAPHYLOCOCCAL ARTHRITIS
Characteristics of the Micro-organisms

Staphylococci are distinguished by their hemolytic and biochemical properties. *Staphylococcus epidermidis* differs from *S. aureus* in its lack of hemolysis and of degradation of mannitol and in its inability to coagulate fibrinogen, that is, it is coagulase negative. On the usual media, whitish or yellowish colonies are produced, in contrast to the golden yellow pigment formed by many *S. aureus* strains.[56a] The pathogenicity of *S. epidermidis* is lower than that of *S. aureus,* but *S. aureus* strains have no reliable characteristics by which to predict pathogenicity. Enterotoxin is not produced more often among cocci isolated from cases of chronic osteomyelitis than from other kinds of staphylococcal infections.[230] Some pathogenic strains show hemolysis; others do not. Alpha hemolysis on blood agar medium may parallel virulence. A positive plasma coagulase test and the production of phosphatase are also regarded as signs of pathogenicity. Attempts have been made to identify aggressive strains by lysotrophy or phage typing, but this technique may only provide more exact identification of a given strain and its mammalian species of origin.

The cell wall of various gram-positive cocci is composed of concentric layers of various elements. Next to the plasma membrane of the cell is a coat of peptidoglycans, then teichoic acids with either polyribitol or glycerol phosphate residues, then group- and type-specific polysaccharides, then M protein, and last, a polysaccharide capsule. The cell wall of *S. aureus* has three components: peptidoglycan, teichoic acid, and protein A.

Peptidoglycan appears to be the key cell-wall component in staphylococcal opsonization. Immunoglobulin G (IgG) antibody is the major heat-stable opsonin, and both the classic and alternate pathways of complement participate in opsonization. An effective immune response to peptidoglycan may be related to the development of the natural immunity of most individuals to staphylococci.[188]

In the serum of patients with chronic active osteomyelitis, however, a surprising lack of heat-stable IgG opsonin activity for *S. aureus* has been noted, in contrast to the potent activity found in subacute bacterial endocarditis. The cause for the weak quality of the antibody is not understood, although it is still an effective activator of complement-derived opsonin activity.[266] In these earlier studies, the antigenic specificity of the opsonin antibody was not determined, but it was presumably directed against peptidoglycans.

N-acetylglucosaminyl residues of ribitol teichoic acids comprise as much as 40% by weight of the cell wall. These polymers do not contribute to the opsonization of the bacteria,[188] but serious infections by *S. aureus* do induce the formation of antibodies against teichoic acids. One study reported that antibodies were detected by counterimmunoelectrophoresis and gel-diffusion techniques in 9 of 11 patients with acute and 3 of 7 patients with chronic osteomyelitis and in only 2 of 7 patients with staphylococcal arthritis, but another study noted antibodies in only 4 of 35 patients with acute or chronic osteomyelitis and acute arthritis, detected by gel-diffusion techniques.[159a] None of the 20 patients with chronic osteomyelitis in the second study had positive assays. In contrast, 14 of 23 patients with staphylococcal endocarditis and 6 of 30 with staphylococcal bacteremia had positive tests[159a]; these findings suggest that the presence and the degree of antigenemia are more important than the duration of staphylococcal infection in stimulating the production of teichoic acid anti-

Table 101–1.   Summary of Principles for Diagnosis and Management of Septic Arthritis Due to Bacteria[157]

1. *Suspect* sepsis in a patient: (1) with debilitating disease, especially neoplastic or hepatic disease; (2) who is taking corticosteroids or immunosuppressive agents; (3) who has infection elsewhere, even if receiving antibiotics; or (4) who has pre-existing joint damage due to another type of arthritis.

2. *Diagnose* sepsis by synovial fluid smear and culture, or by counterimmunoelectrophoresis for bacterial antigens. High fluid concentrations of lactate and other organic acids, especially succinate, fluid glucose levels 40 mg/dl or more below plasma glucose levels (after fasting), and poor mucin clot suggest bacterial sepsis. Fluid leukocyte concentrations are usually high; polymorphonuclear leukocytes predominate (>90%).

3. *Splint* affected joint and give analgesic.

4. *Treat* with parenteral antibiotics after obtaining synovial fluid and blood cultures but *before* obtaining the results; time is important. A direct correlation exists between the duration of symptoms before treatment and the time needed to sterilize joint fluid once treatment is begun.[118a] Prescribe empiric antibiotic regimen using clinical clues as to the probable etiologic agent. *Do not* inject antibiotics into the joint because they are irritants and may confuse the clinical picture. Aminoglycoside effectiveness decreases by an order of magnitude at pH 6.5; synovial fluid pH correlates with local leukocyte concentration.[257a] Hence, drainage of exudate is particularly important.

5. *Decompress* joint by daily needle drainage, which gives better results than open drainage, except in infections of long duration and in deeply situated joints, where needle drainage is technically difficult.

6. *Follow* daily joint fluid leukocyte count and cultures for prognosis. Serial fall in leukocyte count and sterile fluid correlates with a good outcome.[118a]

Table 101–2.   Antibiotic Therapy Regimens for Bacterial Arthritis*

Organism	Antibiotic	Alternative	Duration and Comment
Enterobacteriaceae; inludes *Escherichia coli, Salmonella, Klebsiella, Enterobacter,* and *Proteus* species	Gentamicin, 5 mg/kg/day in 3 doses	Tobramycin, 5 mg/kg/day Amikacin, 15 mg/kg/day	2 to 3 weeks; may change to or add ampicillin, carbenicillin, or a cephalosporin when sensitivities are known
Pseudomonas aeruginosa	Tobramycin, 5 mg/kg/day in 3 doses	Gentamicin, 5 mg/kg/day Amikacin, 15 mg/kg/day	2 to 3 weeks; add or change to carbenicillin, 400 mg/kg/day, when confirmed
Haemophilus influenzae	Ampicillin, 50 mg/kg/day in 4 doses	Chloramphenicol, 50/mg/kg/day	2 weeks; if ampicillin resistance is prevalent, chloramphenicol should be added until sensitivities are known
Neisseria gonorrhoeae and *N. meningitidis*	Penicillin G, 10 million U/day in 4 doses	Erythromycin, 2 g/day intravenously in 4 doses for 3 days; cefoxitin, 100 mg/kg/day in 4 doses	After response to penicillin (24 to 72 hours), ampicillin, 2 g/day orally for 1 week; shorter therapy has been effective
Streptococcus	Penicillin G, 250,000 U/kg/day in 2 to 4 doses	Same as for *Staphylococcus aureus*	Enterococci require combined penicillin and aminoglycoside (streptomycin)
Staphylococcus aureus	Nafcillin, 100 mg/kg/day in 4 doses	Cephalothin, 100 mg/kg/day; clindamycin; 30 mg/kg/day; vancomycin, 30 mg/kg/day	Parenteral therapy for a minimum of 3 to 4 weeks; neonatal dose of nafcillin 25 mg/kg/day

*Therapy for a given patient must be individualized to take into account renal and hepatic function. Toxicity may occur with any antibiotic; the patient's status should be monitored to avoid complications.

(Data prepared by Dr. John Clarke, Northwestern University.)

bodies. An ELISA assay, also employed in these studies, was more sensitive, but much less specific.

Most strains of *S. aureus* have cell-wall protein A, a molecule with the unique ability to bind to a site on the Fc region of human IgG-1, IgG-2, and IgG-4, but not IgG-3, and to IgG from many animal species.[142] Aggregation of IgG induced by this property of protein A results in complement attachment and activation much like that caused by

rheumatoid factor.[220] An inflammatory response can be provoked in laboratory animals, but this action has not been correlated with disease in man.[106,226,233] Paradoxically, if the Fc region is completely blocked by excessive amounts of protein A, the inflammatory response will be blunted, presumably by steric interference with C1 binding.[8,62,141,269]

Extracellular matrix proteins such as fibronectin,

laminin, and type IV collagen are exposed when endothelial cells in blood vessels are injured. The gram-positive cocci, staphylococci and streptococci, but not gram-negative bacilli, bind to these matrix proteins. *S. aureus* strains with cell-wall protein A adhere to laminin. *S. aureus* strains with an unknown protein A content also adhere to fibronectin and type IV collagen. In other studies, these three matrix proteins have aggregated fluid suspensions of *S. aureus*. Exposed extracellular matrix proteins, therefore, could attach and assemble blood-borne staphylococci at sites of injury in subsynovial or diaphyseal capillaries, thus leading to tissue colonization and infection. The preferential binding and aggregation of gram-positive cocci also may explain why they, rather than gram-negative bacilli, more often cause bone and joint infections.[253]

Protoplast (cell-wall-free) forms of staphylococci are rarely pathogenic. One patient with osteomyelitis of the femur due to *S. aureus* suffered a relapse two years after an apparently successful course of treatment for six months with methicillin and then oxacillin. At the time of recurrence, only protoplasts of *S. aureus* could be cultured in a high osmotic medium from the surgical specimen. These protoplasts reverted on subculture to the same phage type as the original *S. aureus*.[210]

Penicillin-resistant strains of *S. aureus* are notorious. One center reported 104 patients with septic arthritis over a 30-year period. Between 1944 and 1953, 29% of *S. aureus* strains were resistant to penicillin; the percentage increased to 48% between 1954 and 1963, and to 59% between 1964 and 1973, concomitant with the growing use of various antibiotics, particularly penicillin.[175] Children with suppurative arthritis of the hip due to penicillin-resistant strains of *S. aureus* have less satisfactory outcomes than those infected with penicillin-sensitive strains.[167] Hospital-acquired strains of *S. aureus* are frequently resistant to penicillin. Resistant strains produce penicillinase, which also inactivates penicillin analogs such as ampicillin and carbenicillin. Among penicillin-resistant staphylococci are some strains also resistant to other antibiotics, notably streptomycin, tetracycline, erythromycin, novobiocin, and chloramphenicol.[264] The ability to produce large amounts of penicillinase is also linked with resistance to various antibiotics.[203] Synthetic penicillin analogs not affected by penicillinase are available, such as methicillin, oxacillin, and related compounds, but an increasing number of isolates of methicillin-resistant cocci have appeared in patients seen in hospital practice.[240]

Pathogenesis

Staphylococci are among the most persistent bacteria that parasitize mankind. They reside in the nose and on the skin of almost all individuals.[245,267] They cause infections ranging from small, localized skin pustules to extensive folliculitis to septicemia with widespread metastatic colonization. Nasal carriers and persons with minor skin lesions, with an estimated prevalence of 5 to 9% of the population each year, are important in the spread of staphylococcal disease. Staphylococci are commonly found in open, infected wounds.

Polymorphonuclear leukocytes collect at the point of coccal attack; phagocytosis and killing of bacteria by these cells are critical for control of the infection. Thrombosis in neighboring vessels is followed by local ischemia, necrosis, and abscess formation. Organisms may be carried by the blood to other parts of the body, with deposition occurring preferentially in the long bones and joints, and also in organs such as the kidney, endocardium, meninges, lungs, liver, and spleen. The manner by which staphylococci reach the bone or joint space after implantation either in diaphyseal capillary loops or in the synovial membrane is described in Chapter 99.

In experimental staphylococcal arthritis induced in animals by the intra-articular injection of microorganisms, the synovial membrane showed evidence of an inflammatory reaction within 5 minutes. Within hours, polymorphonuclear leukocytes accumulated in synovial tissues and fluid in large numbers. Synovial membrane necrosis and erosion of the cartilage surface with degeneration and necrosis of chondrocytes began by 24 hours and progressed rapidly.[213] Regeneration occurred from 3 days onward, with the formation of granulation tissue in the subsynovial layer.[19] Loss of glycosaminoglycans and collagen, as measured by the hexosamine and hydroxyproline content in cartilage, accompanied these changes. Collagen loss could be substantially avoided by lavage of the joint on the fourth and seventh days after the inoculation of staphylococci. Preservation of collagen structure assisted in the restoration of cartilage by providing the basis on which newly synthesized proteoglycans could be interpolated[51] (see Chaps. 10 and 11).

The lining synovial cells phagocytize and dispose of invading organisms by their lysosomal enzymes and by the formation of reactive oxygen molecules. The number of lysosomes increases in stimulated synovial cells, an important event for bacterial degradation, but one that forebodes damage to host bone and cartilage.[19,213]

Immune complexes can potentiate and prolong the inflammatory response initiated by the staphylococcus. Microscopic examination of animal articular cartilage by immunofluorescence four weeks after antibiotic cure of an experimental

S. aureus infection still revealed IgG and IgM in both the infected and noninfected knees. Because cartilage damage appeared only in the infected joint, this finding was interpreted as evidence of autoimmunity to cartilage products.[22] The role of staphylococcal antigen or antibody in this model was not studied. Analogous to the situation with antigen-induced synovitis,[44] such antigens and antibodies might have persisted as complexes in cartilage, slowly re-entering the joint space, where they could maintain an inflammatory response long after all viable micro-organisms had vanished. Furthermore, staphylococcal protein A could facilitate this immune aggregation by nonimmune aggregation of both antibody and nonantibody IgG. Evidence for the deposition of immune complexes in the pathogenesis of staphylococcal disease in other tissues has been noted in the development of acute diffuse glomerulonephritis in two patients during the course of acute staphylococcal endocarditis. Improvement of the renal disease was noted after cure of the infection.[246]

In another report, diffuse proliferative glomerulonephritis developed in 11 patients with deep visceral abscesses caused by infection with *S. aureus* or gram-negative bacilli. In many of these patients, blood cultures were consistently sterile. Most had circulating cryoglobulins, and several had soluble immune complexes. Serum complement levels were decreased in approximately a third of these patients. The evolution of the glomerulonephritis, as determined in serial biopsies, generally paralleled the course of the infection. Complete recovery of renal function occurred in 4 patients whose infection was cured, whereas of the 5 patients in whom the infection was not cured, 4 died and 1 developed chronic renal failure. Chronic renal failure developed in 2 patients in whom antibiotic therapy had been delayed.[16] These reports support the concept that autoimmune or antibacterial immune complexes can occur in staphylococcal arthritis and may aggravate or prolong inflammation.

Impairment of Host Defense

Although staphylococci infect bone and joints in normal individuals more easily than many other bacteria, the incidence of septic arthritis and osteomyelitis is even higher in patients with a variety of debilitated states and in patients treated with drugs that impair host resistance. Examples are: (1) the diminished intracellular killing of *S. aureus* within macrophages in virus-infected tissues;[124] and (2) the transient decrease in monocytes and in killing ability of *S. aureus* in normal subjects taking high doses of corticosteroids for as short a time as three days.[205] Critical to the control of staphylo-

coccal infections is an effective polymorphonuclear cell. Impairment of its function is associated with infection, such as impaired phagocytosis in patients with severe infection,[156] diabetes mellitus,[169] rheumatoid arthritis (RA),[170] the Chédiak-Higashi syndrome,[43] and certain types of agammaglobulinemia.[234]

In chronic granulomatous disease, neutrophils are unable to produce adequate free oxygen radicals as superoxide and hydrogen peroxide, which are required to kill catalase-negative bacteria, particularly *S. aureus* and some gram-negative organisms.[48] Correction of this defect was accomplished experimentally by introducing a hydrogen-peroxide-generating system into the phagosome along with the micro-organism.[9] A widespread neutrophilic defect in chemotaxis, phagocytosis, and intracellular killing was described in an adult who developed two episodes of staphylococcal osteomyelitis with suppurative arthritis.[236] Besides their role in phagocytosis and intracellular killing, phagocytic cells must "stick" to endothelial cells prior to extravascular migration. Ethanol, prednisone, and aspirin may inhibit such adherence and may thereby contribute to their anti-inflammatory properties, as well as an impairing resistance to infection.[158] Leukocyte mobilization from noncirculating tissue pools in response to infection is also reduced by glucocorticoid drugs, an effect more pronounced with daily than with alternate-day therapy.[50]

Antibody and complement mediators are necessary agents to control staphylococcal infection. As previously mentioned, a weak IgG opsonic activity, particularly for *S. aureus*, has been found in the serum of many patients with chronic active osteomyelitis.[266] Moreover, teichoic acid antibodies are often absent, although their role in host defense is not established.[163] Many bacteria including staphylococci, pneumococci and gram-negative organisms can elaborate chemotactic factors for neutrophils in the absence of serum.[257] Complement-derived chemotactic factors enhance the host's protection, however. A genetic deficiency of some complement components predisposes individuals to infection; persons without C3 or C3b inactivator are repeatedly infected with pyogenic micro-organisms.[5] Persons affected with a disorder characterized by dysfunction of C5 develop infections with gram-negative bacilli and *S. aureus* during the first 6 to 12 months of life.[5]

Clinical Features

Acute infection with staphylococci involves one or a few joints by metastatic spread in the circulation from a primary site of infection elsewhere. The primary site may not be detected, however.

Staphylococci have a special affinity for localization in bone and joint structures. In comparison, although gram-negative bacilli often cause bacteremia,[81,155,208] they less frequently produce septic arthritis or osteomyelitis.[175,255] The bone or joint infection is accompanied by fever and often a chill. Characteristically, the involved joint is warm, swollen, and painful; the intrasynovial fluid pressure is increased. The knee and hip are most often affected, and hip involvement is more common in children.[94,175] The shoulder, elbow, wrist, and ankle account for almost all the other joints that may become infected. The vertebrae and the sacroiliac joints are involved in fewer than 5% of patients.[91,94,166,175,211]

Hip joint involvement carries an unusually poor prognosis. One series reported poor results in 22 of 59 hips, as compared to only 8 of 43 knees.[175] Children fared the worst; 8 had sequestration and 5 had absorption of the femoral epiphysis, 7 had subluxation or dislocation of the hip, and 3 had coxa magna. Another series confirmed these data.[122] In addition to maldevelopment or avascular necrosis of the femoral head, ankylosis can be another late sequela in children. Ultimate damage to the joint was not recognized in many children at the time of completion of antibiotic treatment. Consequently, long-term observation is necessary to assess correctly the degree to which hip joint function has been restored. The most important cause of a poor prognosis is delay in the initiation of appropriate antibiotic therapy because of a late diagnosis of infection in this deep-seated joint;[84] another cause is the inadequate drainage of pus.[167]

Identification of the staphylococcus in joint fluid by Gram-stained smear and by culture is achieved in over two-thirds of individuals in whom this infection is thought to have occurred. Negative cultures, in the face of convincing clinical evidence of infection, may be due to prior abortive treatment with antibiotics or to the presence of fewer viable micro-organisms in the synovial fluid than in the synovium (see Chap. 4 for other means of diagnosing bacterial joint infection). On the other hand, signs and symptoms of sepsis, including elevated synovial fluid white blood cell counts, predominantly polymorphonuclear cells, and fever may occur in some noninfectious inflammatory arthritides such as pseudogout, gout, and RA. In these instances, however, careful bacteriologic studies need to be carried out before a diagnosis of infection can be correctly excluded.

Hematogenous Osteomyelitis

Osteomyelitis resulting from hematogenous spread has the same general characteristic of infection as pyogenic arthritis. Local findings include bone pain and tenderness, with overlying skin and subcutaneous redness if a peripheral long bone is involved. Vertebral or other deep-seated bone involvement may not be detectable by physical examination.[88,104,115,181,255] Radioactive technetium diphosphonate or gallium scintiphotography may be needed to localize the disorder in these areas. Identification of staphylococci need not be made by biopsy of bone, but it can be inferred from the clinical presentation and the recovery of the bacteria from the blood culture. In patients with recurrent or protracted disease, bone biopsy or debridement often provides the opportunity to obtain tissue for culture.

In the elderly, debilitated, or immunosuppressed patient, the intensity of the inflammatory response in the bone or joint may be muted and may thus be easy to overlook. Such patients, or others under treatment with drugs that reduce host defense mechanisms, are more vulnerable to septic arthritis than others.

In children, osteomyelitis, beginning in the metaphysis, may present as septic arthritis, due to direct extension from bone to joint. Although bacteria can be recovered from the affected joint, prominent tenderness of juxta-articular bone correctly identifies the primary site of infection.

Toxic-Shock Syndrome

Cases have occurred predominantly in menstruating women. The illness is characterized by the sudden onset of fever, diarrhea, shock, a diffuse, macular, erythematous rash followed by desquamation of the palms and soles and hyperemia of conjunctival, oropharyngeal, and vaginal mucous membranes. In addition, the hepatic, renal, muscular, gastrointestinal, cardiopulmonary, and central nervous systems may become involved. S. aureus has been isolated from vaginal cultures in many patients. Mucocutaneous lymph node syndrome, or Kawasaki's disease, is also a multisystemic disease of unknown origin in which vasculitis occurs. It shares many clinical characteristics with toxic shock syndrome. Although the disease is mainly limited to children, a few cases have been described in adults. Therefore, in the differential diagnosis of patients with Kawasaki's disease, one should carefully search for staphylococcal infection, to exclude this specifically treatable entity.[92]

Infection in Rheumatoid Arthritis

Although joints not previously injured can be readily infected by staphylococci, prior joint damage or impairment of host defenses enhances the likelihood of septic involvement. The most striking example of a superimposed infection occurs in patients with RA, as highlighted by Kellgren and co-workers in 1958.[130] Since then, many reports have verified this initial observation.[54,94,105,127,172,204,214,256] In all series, the staphylococcus was by far the most common infecting agent. The course of the illness was severe in most patients, with death and poor restoration of joint function in over one-third. Often, several joints were infected simultaneously. In some infected joints, the clinical signs of sepsis were diminished, so suspicion of infection was not aroused early. Helpful diagnostic findings included: (1) the presence of a primary site of infection, such as an open leg ulcer, perhaps due to vasculitis, or a draining subcutaneous nodule; (2) the development of fever and sometimes a chill; and (3) the appearance of one or more swollen or painful joints in a patient without other evidence of a flare of RA. The complexity of rheumatoid inflammation with its immunologic aberrations, combined with the effects of drug treatment, precludes identification of the precise defect responsible for the increased vulnerability of these patients to sepsis. Adequate polymorphonuclear cell function is a key requirement in the control of staphylococcal infection, however, and such function is often depressed in patients with RA. Prior ingestion of immune complexes by leukocytes in blood or synovial fluid may have diminished their ability to ingest or to kill bacteria.[248]

Infection in Drug Abusers

Septic arthritis and osteomyelitis are well-recognized complications of the habitual use of intravenous heroin. Although gram-negative bacilli, particularly *Pseudomonas* and *Serratia,* are particularly associated with this type of infection, staphylococci constitute an equally common cause of infection.[211] The source of the staphylococcus is usually the skin or nose of the patient; in ten drug abusers with staphylococcal endocarditis, the phage type of the organism carried on the skin or nose matched that of the micro-organism recovered from the blood.[247]

Infection in Prosthetic Joints

Within the past decade, infections at the site of implantation of a joint prosthesis have become a serious problem. *S. epidermidis* and *S. aureus* are recovered most often during the early postoperative period, the result of contamination of the surgical wound. A lesser number of late cases are recognized, some even several years after the operation. Some of these infections are due to reactivation of a latent bacterial nidus that had been introduced into the wound at the time of operation, and others are caused by the hematogenous dissemination of micro-organisms. A full discussion of infection in prosthetic joints is given in Chapter 99.

Treatment

In treating staphylococcal joint infections and osteomyelitis, one must consider the high probability of infection with penicillin-resistant strains, particularly if acquired in a hospital. Initially, a penicillinase-resistant antibiotic should be used intravenously, preferably nafcillin, 100 to 150 mg/kg/day in 4 divided doses. Alternate drugs are indicated in Table 101–2. Treatment can be modified when the sensitivity of the micro-organism becomes known. If the micro-organism proves to be sensitive to penicillin, aqueous penicillin G can be substituted, 20 million U/day, intravenously, in 4 divided doses. Antibiotics other than penicillin are usually reserved for patients infected with staphylococci resistant to penicillin analogs or for those allergic to penicillin. Treatment for 6 weeks or longer may be necessary.

As indicated in Chapter 99, decisions regarding dosage and duration of antibiotic treatment are based on careful monitoring of the response to therapy. Drainage of purulent joint fluid can usually be accomplished successfully by needle aspiration. The response to therapy is assessed at the end of the first week. Persistence of joint swelling and reaccumulation of purulent joint fluid, without evidence of improvement, calls for arthroscopy in selected joints or for arthrotomy. Deep-seated infections of the hip, particularly in young infants, are exceptions to this plan. In these patients, arthrotomy and open drainage should be performed immediately because of the great risk of joint destruction and the difficulty of serial needle aspiration.[94,167,175]

In hematogenous osteomyelitis of long bones or vertebrae due to staphylococci, most authors favor a conservative approach consisting of diminished activity and appropriate long-term antibiotic therapy.[88,104,115] The majority of patients are cured. In vertebral disease, spontaneous fusion may occur. In the face of neurologic complications or extensive bony lesions, surgical intervention may be required. The spinal cord or nerve roots should be decompressed immediately, along with drainage of pus and removal of necrotic bone and soft tissue. A fusion procedure may also be performed to ensure stability of the spine.*

Editor's note: We have been impressed with the results of long-term intravenous antibiotic therapy using a pump and an indwelling Hickman catheter. Antibiotics can be conveniently administered at home for up to six months with this method if oral administration fails.

STREPTOCOCCAL ARTHRITIS

Characteristics of the Micro-organism

Streptococci are classified according to: (1) their hemolytic behavior when grown on blood agar, as alpha-, beta-, or not hemolytic; (2) their growth requirements in various sugars and osmotic media, and (3) their serologic behavior against group- or type-specific antisera. The last reaction depends on specific carbohydrate or protein constituents in their cell walls. Several major groups are recognized, including groups A, B, C, D, F, and G.

Like staphylococci, streptococci also can bind to the Fc region of IgG.[41,140] Isolated membranes and cell walls from group A streptococci and from various other gram-positive micro-organisms are able to activate complement by the alternate pathway. Unlike endotoxin, inulin, or other plant polysaccharides, activation of complement by these cell-wall constituents bypasses properidin.[237] These studies suggest antibody-independent modes of action by which these micro-organisms can contribute to an inflammatory response.

Group A Streptococcal Infection

Almost all strains cause beta hemolysis. More than 50 types have been distinguished by the specific M and T protein in their cell wall. Lipoteichoic acid of group A cell walls mediates adherence of the bacteria to human buccal mucosal cells. Strains stimulated by penicillin to lose their lipoteichoic acid lose this ability; this finding suggests that penicillin may influence bacterial flora by this means as well as by killing sensitive organisms.[2] These bacteria remain sensitive to penicillin. Infection with group A streptococci, usually in the pharynx, precedes and causes rheumatic fever. Arthritis or endocarditis in this disease is not due to colonization of the joint or heart valve by the micro-organism, but rather to a still-undefined toxic or sensitivity-mediated reaction in the host. On other occasions, these pathogens enter the joint from the circulation and cause sepsis.[27,156,184]

Group B Streptococcal Infection

This bacterium is a common cause of neonatal infections, often with a high mortality rate. Bacteremia is followed by focal lesions in the meninges, lung, skin, sinuses, and in the bones and joints. Several distinct serotypes are recognized (Ia, Ib, Ic, II, III), based on the structure of the capsular polysaccharide. Type III appears to be the most virulent. The disease is usually transmitted at the time of delivery from colonized mothers who lack type-specific antibody or from instrumentation such as umbilical catheterization. Infection is not likely to occur if specific antibody is present in umbilical cord blood.[11] S. pneumoniae type 14 cross-reacts with group B streptococci type III, and antisera against the former protect against infection by the latter.[82] These bacteria are penicillin sensitive, although less so than group A streptococci.[3]

During the past decade, osteomyelitis and arthritis due to this bacterium, usually serotype III, have been reported with increased frequency.[163] Symptoms usually first occur several weeks after birth. Because many patients already have radiographically evident osteolytic bony lesions, however, the disease undoubtedly is initiated earlier, probably at or shortly after birth. Most infants have a concomitant arthritis due to the ready route of infection from the bone into the joint space (see Fig. 99–1).

Penicillin G therapy for neonatal osteomyelitis or septic arthritis is generally given for four to six weeks, although shorter regimens have been associated with a cure. Infected bone is decompressed by drilling or by needle aspiration. In contrast to neonatal infections with staphylococci, those due to group B streptococci do not cause a significant functional loss in the early years of life.[163] Some patients develop radiographic changes, such as increased sclerosis, metaphyseal irregularities, or deformity of the articulating angle of a joint. The long-term consequences of these changes remain to be determined.

Group C Streptococcal Infection

These organisms colonize the upper respiratory tract, skin, and vagina in normal persons, but rarely cause disease in man. When they do, they are associated with pharyngitis, pneumonia, peripheral infection, urinary tract infection, meningitis, and endocarditis. One diabetic man with tophaceous gout developed septic arthritis due to group C streptococci in several joints, all of which also contained urate crystals; his infection responded to penicillin.[107]

Group F Streptococcal Infection

These organisms are commonly found in the periodontal area, pharynx, vagina, skin, and gastrointestinal tract. A case of osteomyelitis of a lumbar vertebral body with extension into the epidural space caused by infection with this organism has been reported. The diagnosis was facilitated by a computerized tomogram that outlined the soft tissue lesions and bone destruction.[34]

S. milleri, which possesses group F carbohydrate in its cell wall, is a microaerophilic pathogen particularly associated with abscess formation, notably in the liver. Two patients with monoarthritis due to this micro-organism have been reported, one of whom had RA.[121] The other patient was diabetic, and gas formation in the suprapatellar pouch was recognized radiographically.[150] Gas is seen more often in anaerobic infections, especially those due to clostridia.

Group G Streptococcal Infection

Infectious arthritis due to this pathogen is rare; endocarditis and, less often, other focal infections occur by hematogenous dissemination from the pharynx, skin, vagina, or gastrointestinal tract. The micro-organism is sensitive to penicillin.[87a,214]

Group D and other Streptococcal Infections

In addition to typical enterococci such as *S. faecalis* and *S. faecium*, which are resistant to a variety of antibiotics, group D includes nonenterococcal agents such as *S. bovis* and *S. equinus*, which are sensitive to many antibiotics. Procedures in routine use in clinical laboratories for the isolation and identification of group D streptococci may stop short of separation of these two groups that share the group D antigen. The distinction should be made, however, because therapy for nonenterococci may not require potentially toxic antimicrobial drug combinations.[197]

Streptococcus mutans, some strains of which have produced group E precipitin reactions, are anaerobic inhabitants of the mouth and can be distinguished from group D and alpha-hemolytic (viridans) streptococci by cultural requirements. They are usually sensitive to penicillin.[11]

Alpha-hemolytic streptococci (viridans group) and the strictly anaerobic streptococci lack group-specific carbohydrate in the cell wall. Like the enterococci, *S. bovis* and *S. mutans*, they have a low grade of virulence, but are well-recognized causes of subacute bacterial endocarditis.[56a,110,197]

Diagnosis

The detection of any group of streptococci is usually made by demonstration of gram-positive cocci on the Gram-stained smear and by culture of synovial fluid, bone, or blood. Counterimmunoelectrophoresis has been used to detect group-specific polysaccharide that has been shed into infected fluids or into urine. Additional diagnostic measures are discussed in Chapters 4 and 99.

Treatment

Antibiotic treatment varies according to the drug sensitivity of the streptococcus recovered on culture. Group A streptococci are exquisitely sensitive to penicillin G; enterococci pose formidable problems (see Table 101–2). These resistant organisms may require the use of ampicillin, 12 g daily in divided doses, or the combined use of penicillin

G, 20 million U daily intramuscularly or intravenously, and streptomycin, 0.5 g every 12 hours intramuscularly, or gentamicin, 80 mg every 8 hours intramuscularly or intravenously. Alternatively, vancomycin may be given, 1 g every 12 hours. Duration of treatment is usually 2 to 4 weeks, but as with other infecting micro-organisms, the length of treatment depends on the host's response. Drainage procedures are similar to those outlined for other pyogenic infections.

PNEUMOCOCCAL ARTHRITIS

Although now classified as a member of the *Streptococcus* genus, pathogenetic and clinical features of infections due to this micro-organism are distinctive and merit a separate discussion from those due to the other streptococci.

Characteristics of the Micro-organism

Streptococcus pneumoniae is a normal inhabitant of the human nasopharynx. By agglutination-reaction and capsular-swelling tests using type-specific rabbit antisera, pneumococci can be classified according to their capsular polysaccharides into many types. In the past, types I, II, and III were mainly responsible for lobar pneumonia and its complications in adults, and type XIV most frequently caused the infection in children. Since chemotherapy of pneumococcal infections began, however, typing of pneumococci has become uncommon, so the incidence of the types now responsible for infections is not precisely known. Pneumococci cause bacteremia in 8 to 50% of patients. A higher mortality rate is associated with illness in such patients, especially when infection is due to type III organisms.[31]

The quantity of the same capsular polysaccharide antigen detected in typing can now be accurately measured in body fluids, including synovia. A direct relationship exists between the amount of antigens liberated into the blood or other body fluids and the morbidity and mortality of the infection. Antigen-positive patients have a higher frequency of pleuropericardial effusions,[45] renal impairment,[45] and disseminated intravascular coagulation.[215] The cause of disseminated intravascular coagulation in patients with pneumococcal sepsis is not known. Pneumococci lack the lipopolysaccharide endotoxin in their cell walls responsible for the disseminated intravascular coagulation caused by gram-negative bacilli. A possible explanation is the formation of immune complexes between capsular antigen and antibody, to activate complement and then trigger the coagulation sequence.[215]

Specific antibody to capsular polysaccharide promotes the ingestion of micro-organisms by phagocytic cells. This opsonic requirement may vary among different serotypes.[90] Complement, acting through the classic or the alternate pathway, aids the process. In the presence of complement, one tenth as much IgG is needed to promote phagocytosis as without complement.[198] Membrane receptors for Fc of IgG and for C3b cause particles to adhere to phagocytes and trigger their ingestion. The importance of these events in the resistance to pneumococcal infections is highlighted by the host's increased vulnerability to infection after removal of a major phagocytic organ as the spleen.[25] Decreased clearance of pneumococci from the blood,[262] or depressed antibody response after splenectomy,[212] contributes to the vulnerability of the asplenic individual to pneumococcal infection.

Pneumococcal capsular polysaccharide can also bind to the Fc region of IgG, perhaps only of subclass IgG-1, causing IgG aggregation by a non-immune mechanism. A variety of pneumococcal serotypes are consistently able to react with IgG, whereas others, including types II and III, are not.[235] As with staphylococcal protein A, such reactivity may invoke an inflammatory response in much the same fashion as antigen-antibody complexes, but this hypothesis has not been experimentally proved.

Infection of joints with *Streptococcus pneumoniae* is less frequent than with staphylococci, although suppurative complications such as pericarditis and meningitis are well-recognized complications of infection due to this micro-organism. The low prevalence of pneumococcal arthritis cannot be attributed solely to the emergence of antibiotic therapy because this type of arthritis was also uncommon prior to 1945.[244]

Clinical Presentation and Diagnosis

An antecedent or concomitant pneumococcal infection is frequently present. In addition, the infection may metastasize to other sites, such as the endocardium and meninges. Prior damage to the joint is common;[128] chronic gout is an unusual example of this phenomenon.[68] Underlying conditions disposing patients to pneumococcal infection include chronic alcoholism, asplenia, multiple myeloma, sickle cell disease, and sex-linked agammaglobulinemia.[42,128,134]

Diagnosis is usually confirmed by Gram-stained smear and by culture of joint fluid, although the smear and the culture may be negative when the patient has received antibiotics. Countercurrent immunoelectrophoresis can be used for the specific and rapid detection of pneumococcal capsular antigen in the joint fluid. Multiple type-specific antisera are available.[60]

Treatment

A number of antibiotics are clinically effective against all serotypes of the pneumococcus. Penicillin G is recommended (see Table 101–2). Penicillin-resistant strains, however, have been noted, so drug sensitivities of the micro-organism must now be accurately determined.[123] To reduce the likelihood of the widespread emergence of drug resistance, alternate drugs should ordinarily be reserved for individuals with a penicillin allergy. The duration of therapy is dictated by careful monitoring of the patient's response (see Chap. 99), which may be protracted and associated with juxta-articular osteomyelitis.[42] Usually, however, the treatment regimen is shorter than is needed for staphylococcal infections; two to four weeks of treatment are often sufficient.

MENINGOCOCCAL ARTHRITIS

Characteristics of the Micro-organism

On the basis of serologic reactions against the capsular polysaccharide, *Neisseria meningitidis* can be divided into different groups. Before 1950, most pathogenetic strains belonged to group A; during the next decade, group B became predominant, and since the mid-1960s, it has been group C. Immunization using antigens specific for groups A and C has reduced the risk of infection with these meningococci.[149] As a consequence of this and additional factors, infection with other serotypes is common. Recently, several new groups were identified, of which group Y is the most prominent. As a consequence, joint infections due to group Y,[136,270] as well as to group B,[108,271] have now become more common.

Impairment of Host Immune Systems

N. meningitidis is carried by most individuals in the nasopharynx for prolonged periods with symptoms of only a mild pharyngitis or without any symptoms. Even during an epidemic, most persons remain asymptomatic carriers. Invasive systemic disease is due more to susceptibility of the host rather than to any innate virulence of the infecting micro-organism. Lack of specific antibody and of complement have each been held responsible for the host's vulnerability.

Prevention of disease when large populations are immunized by group-specific polysaccharide antigen supports a major role for antibody.[186] In one study, sera were obtained prospectively from military recruits, and in 51 of 54 patients who later contracted meningococcal disease, predisease sera lacked adequate antibodies to homologous and heterologous strains of pathogenic meningococci. On recovery, these patients showed an antibody response. Their strong antibody response after the illness supports the view that they had not had significant prior exposure to meningococcal antigens.[96]

The complement system also protects against disseminated neisserial infections, both gonococcal and meningococcal. These micro-organisms are especially sensitive to the bactericidal activity provided by the lytic action of the late-acting complement proteins, C6, C7, and C8. Of 24 patients with a complete absence of these proteins (heterozygotes with half-normal values were found not to be at risk), 13 had at least 1 episode and usually 2 or more episodes of either or both of these neisserial infections.[187] Detection of a deficiency of complement proteins is made by a hemolytic assay of serum; the usual serologic test for C3 or C4 does not reveal the defect. Thus, hemolytic complement studies are indicated in patients as well as in family members, particularly siblings, who develop recurrent systemic neisserial infections,[4,229] just as they are for patients with a disease such as systemic lupus erythematosus, which impairs such defense mechanisms as opsonization and immune complex clearing (see also Chap. 100).[219]

Clinical Features

Meningococci enter the blood from the nasopharynx. The meninges, skin, and often the joints are common sites for tissue localization.[117] Protracted meningococcemia is usual, with chills, fever, rash, muscular aches, headaches, nausea, vomiting, and arthritis. Pain in both hips is a common complaint during this phase of the disease. The characteristic rash consists of petechial or purpuric lesions. Sometimes, pustular lesions identical to those seen in gonococcal infections may appear (see Chap. 100).

Overt joint inflammation is seen in a few patients with meningococcal infection. In a postmortem examination of 90 fatal cases, 9 showed purulent synovitis that had been missed clinically. Single or multiple joints as well as tendons and bursae can be involved in patterns that mimic those seen in disseminated gonococcal infections, that is, initial culture-negative polyarthritis followed by culture-positive monoarthritis.[30,69,73,118,144,189,190,218,219,265] These distinct phases are not usually observed during the course of the illness in the same patient, but have been pieced together from observations on different patients. These sequential phases of the same disease process have varying emphasis in different patients.

To account for negative synovial fluid cultures early during septicemia, viable micro-organisms may not have been deposited in sufficient numbers in the tissue or, alternatively, the inflammation may be sterile as a result of immune complex deposition.[69,73,102,144,189] In the later phase, bacterial colonization may have proceeded in one or perhaps two joints to a point that cultures of joint fluid become positive.

On Gram-stain of the joint fluid, the micro-organisms may be identified as gram-negative cocci, many of which may lie within polymorphonuclear cells. Morphologically, these organisms are indistinguishable from *Neisseria gonorrhoeae,* a much more frequent cause of arthritis, or even from *N. catarrhalis,* which has rarely been implicated in arthritis.[49] Joint fluids or tissues should be grown on media identical to that required for the gonococcus or on blood agar. The availability of specific antisera against the major meningococcal groups permits the use of counterimmunoelectrophoresis as a rapid and specific diagnostic aid.[89] White blood cell counts of joint fluids are high; most cells are polymorphonuclear leukocytes. Blood cultures can be positive in patients with chronic meningococcemia who may develop arthritis in the absence of other manifestations of the disease.[189]

Treatment

Penicillin G, 10 to 20 million units daily intravenously, has replaced sulfadiazine as the drug of choice in the treatment of meningococcal infections because of the emergence of sulfadiazine-resistant strains.[145] Nonetheless, one penicillinase-producing strain of a group B meningococcus contained two plasmids, one identical to that from penicillinase-producing gonococci that produce beta-lactamase and another that was a transfer plasmid with the potential for spreading antibiotic-resistant plasmids in meningococci by conjugation.[57] Sensitivity studies against various antibiotics should be performed on organisms recovered on culture. Patients treated with effective amounts of penicillin or other appropriate antibiotic usually enjoy the same rapid and complete recovery as patients with joint infections due to gonococci or streptococci. Resistant cases, which occur at times, can be managed according to procedures discussed in Chapter 99.

GRAM-NEGATIVE BACILLARY BONE AND JOINT INFECTIONS

Gram-negative bacilli encompass a wide range of organisms that share, besides common morphologic features, similar problems in diagnosis, treatment, and prognosis whenever they cause arthritis or osteomyelitis. Although many facets of the bone and joint disease caused by these agents can be discussed together, some practical and theoretic problems associated with infection due to some of these agents are unique, such as the almost exclusive occurrence of *Haemophilus influenzae* arthritis in young children and the strong predilection of *Salmonella* arthritis or osteomyelitis for sickle cell trait or disease. Special attention is therefore devoted to individual micro-organisms and their hosts later in this section of the chapter.

Pathogenesis

Patients with septic arthritis as a result of direct invasion of the joint by gram-negative rods such as *Salmonella*,[52,66,199,251,258] *Shigella*, and *Yersinia*[232] species, and probably others, do not have a known genetic predisposition to their disease. In contrast, HLA-B27-positive individuals who develop a gastrointestinal infection from these same gram-negative bacilli may be predisposed to the noninfectious inflammatory synovitis of Reiter's disease[1,207] (see Chap. 54). The reason for this striking association between the HLA-B27 status of the host and a noninfectious rheumatic disease is unclear, but this risk exists only for the reactive form of arthritis and not for septic arthritis.

Gram-negative rod infections often develop in an immunologically impaired or aged host or in previously damaged or traumatized bones and joints. Occasional patients have no obvious predisposition, however.[14] Factors that contribute to susceptibility for infection include the following: (1) the use of cytotoxic immunosuppressive or corticosteroid drugs that depress host defenses; (2) serious illnesses, such as lymphoma, carcinoma, liver disease, diabetes mellitus, or renal failure; (3) urogenital instrumentation, especially indwelling bladder catheters; and (4) indwelling intravenous catheters or ventriculoatrial shunts used to treat hydrocephalus. Institutionalized, especially bedridden, elderly patients with respiratory disease have a much higher incidence of oropharyngeal colonization by *Klebsiella*, *Escherichia coli*, and *Enterobacter* species, and thus are more likely to develop metastatic infections by these organisms, than independent elderly persons.[250] Any number of host-defense substances and mechanisms may be deficient or compromised in the vulnerable patient, including antibody, complement, phagocytic cell response, and the lymphocyte-machrophage cellular immune system.[14,61,93,94,168,194,263]

Joints that become infected often have sustained prior injury or disease.[93] Even so, the incidence of septic arthritis is lower than that from staphylococcal infection. Serious gram-negative rod bacteremia occurs with a much greater frequency, estimated to be 71,000 cases per year,[268] than does staphylococcal septicemia.

Although acute bacterial infections are often associated with normal or elevated serum hemolytic levels of complement,[65] significant depression of serum complement has been demonstrated in pa-

tients with gram-negative bacteremia in whom shock or death subsequently occurred.[154] Activation was initiated through the alternate pathway by the lipopolysaccharide in gram-negative cell walls in the absence of antibody.[77] In these cases, the normally protective role of complement in controlling infectious agents becomes subverted by the massive, sudden release of biologically active complement products into the circulation.

Clinical Presentation

Gram-negative rods are common pathogens in urinary or gastrointestinal tract infections, from which sites they may enter the blood. Thus, the development of arthritis in a debilitated individual with urinary tract or bowel sepsis suggests a gram-negative bacillary infection. Other sources of bacteria include contaminated intravenous solutions, nebulizers, or human or animal asymptomatic carriers.

The characteristic presentation is usually monoarticular, but occasionally oligoarticular. The onset is acute, with obvious signs of localized heat, swelling, redness, and pain. Sepsis is manifest by chills in some and by fever in most patients, and in patients with severe gram-negative bacteremia, by the development of shock. Serum complement levels in such patients may be depressed, particularly levels of C3 and total hemolytic complement, whereas the values of C4 and of C1 or C2 may be in the normal range. Joint fluid findings are characteristic of septic arthritis, with high white blood cell counts, mostly polymorphonuclear cells, synovial fluid glucose levels low in comparison to serum levels, and high lactate or succinate values (see Chaps. 4 and 99). Micro-organisms may be seen on Gram-stained specimens of joint fluid and are usually cultured from the synovial fluid as well as the blood, although with prior antibiotic therapy, the smear may be negative and the culture sterile.[93]

Treatment

Because patients with arthritis caused by a gram-negative rod often have a major, underlying systemic illness and a joint infection that responds slowly to therapy, treatment must be decisive, vigorous, and prolonged. In addition to an effective antibiotic program, drainage of purulent joint contents must be performed repeatedly. Surgical debridement by arthroscopy or arthrotomy must be prompt if needle aspiration fails. The response of the joint to treatment determines which options to choose (see Chap. 99).

Antibiotic therapy should be initiated even before the specific organism is identified. On suspicion that the bone or joint might be infected by a gram-negative bacillus, initial treatment should consist of parenteral gentamicin, 5 mg/kg/day in 3 divided doses (see Table 101–2).

Amikacin, 15 mg/kg/day, in 2 or 3 divided doses, is an excellent aminoglycoside to which bacteria are less likely to become resistant.[166a] Three mechanisms by which gram-negative bacteria develop resistance to aminoglycosides are known: (1) ribosomal mutation causing decreased binding of the drug; (2) decreased bacterial cell-wall permeability (anaerobic bacteria lack the oxygen-dependent transport system necessary to transport the drug across the cell); and (3) enzyme induction by R-factors (plasmids) found in the cell membrane that inactivate the drug.[205a] The routine use of amikacin does not increase the frequency of resistance.[166a] Rather, the frequency of resistance to tobramycin and to gentamicin decreases.

Carbenicillin, 400 mg/kg/day, may be added particularly if *Pseudomonas aeruginosa* infection is suspected. Sensitivity studies are critical in gram-negative infections because of the likelihood of drug-resistant micro-organisms. Once the sensitivity of the organism is established, more definitive antibiotic treatment can be prescribed. Careful monitoring of the tissue response of the infection is the primary means by which to judge the efficacy of the treatment program. Serial falls in synovial fluid leukocyte concentrations and sterile cultures are encouraging signs;[118a] persistently high cell counts and positive cultures are ominous.

The likelihood that needle aspiration will fail and joint decompression will have to be performed by arthroscopy or arthrotomy may be greater in infections due to gram-negative bacilli than in other types of infection. Such a decision should not be made immediately, however, except in infants with arthritis of the hip. In most other patients, the inflammatory response in the joint can be monitored over the course of the first week, and evidence of improvement, such as a reduction in clinical signs of inflammation, volume of joint fluid, and number of white blood cells in synovial fluid, or a rise in synovial fluid glucose levels, argues for continued needle aspiration. When a patient is not improving, then open drainage by arthrotomy is indicated. At operation, necrotic material and exuberant synovial tissue should be removed for histologic examination and culture.

Infections due to Klebsielleae

A member of the family Enterobacteriaceae is the tribe Klebsielleae, which consists of four genera, *Klebsiella*, *Enterobacter*, *Pectobacterium*, and *Serratia*. All four genera can be identified readily by biochemical means, and complete serotyping of both *Klebsiella* and *Serratia* can be performed.[160]

Klebsiella pneumoniae can be recovered from the urinary tract, often in pure culture in infected patients and from the respiratory tract, wounds, and other infected tissues as part of a mixed flora. Infections with this agent are often hospital acquired.[160] Occasional cases of septic arthritis due to these micro-organisms have been reported,[14,93,224,260,263] often in impaired hosts. Antibiotic response to aminoglycosides, such as gentamicin, often combined with carbenicillin or amikacin, is generally satisfactory, although sometimes complicated by renal disease ototoxicity that is usualy reversible.[160,224]

Serratia marcescens occurs in soil, water, and milk. Until the 1950s, it was generally considered a harmless saprophyte, but in hospitalized patients, drug abusers, and in impaired hosts, it has been implicated as an etiologic agent in almost all kinds of infections, including those in bones and joints.[7,29,36,59,61,132,161,165,179,194,224] A case of septic arthritis of the right hip due to another species, *S. liquefaciens*, occurred in a woman with sickle cell anemia who had had three previous episodes of infections in other joints due to *Klebsiella* and *Enterobacter* species.[109] The predominant mode of spread appears to be hand-to-hand transmission by hospital personnel; point-source outbreaks, from contaminated solutions, disinfectants, and nebulizers account for a minority of cases. A major clinical concern is the resistance to antibiotics of this bacterium. It responds to aminoglycosides such as gentamicin and kanamycin, but resistance mediated by plasmids to these and to other drugs has been reported. Synergistic combinations of drugs as carbenicillin or cefoxitin with aminoglycosides may be successful.[272]

Enterobacter species is rarely reported as a cause of joint infections; a few cases have occurred in children. In one, a premature infant developed joint infections of the hips, knee, and ankle associated with umbilical vein catheterization and intravenous infusions;[99] in another, an older, healthy child incurred monoarthritis of the knee following a penetrating nail wound.[148]

Escherichia coli Infections

This pathogen is a common cause of uncomplicated urinary tract infections and an important cause of sepsis in other tissues. It is the most common agent recovered from the blood of patients with bacteremia due to gram-negative rods. Cases of septic arthritis have been noted in the population at risk, which includes hospitalized, elderly, or impaired hosts of any age.[14,21,93,185,224]

Proteus Infections

These bacilli are widely distributed in nature. In man, they may cause infections similar to those due to *Escherichia coli*. In recent years, *Proteus* species, especially *Proteus mirabilis,* have been isolated with increasing frequency from a variety of tissues. They may be found in pure culture or with other bacteria in urinary infections, abscesses, purulent wounds, burns, peritonitis, and empyema. Patients who develop bone and joint infections usually have pre-existing urinary tract infections and other complicating systemic illnesses.[38,127,168,214,224,241]

Haemophilus influenzae Infections

This micro-organism is an aerobic, pleomorphic, gram-negative coccobacillus that may resemble a coccal bacterium more than a bacillus on Gram-stained smears. Of the 6 typeable strains, A, B, C, D, E, and F, type B is the most virulent; 95% of serious infections of the meninges, respiratory tract, and joints in children are of this type. Osteomyelitis is rare.[75,196] With few exceptions, the remaining 5% are caused by nontypeable strains. In adults, however, the reverse is true; more nontypeable strains cause disease.[171] Exposure to these bacteria, which colonize the upper respiratory tract, usually results in the acquisition of specific immunity. Vaccines using capsular or somatic antigens to induce immunity have proved disappointing so far.[171] Antibodies to type B capsular polysaccharide develop on exposure to cross-reactive antigens of coliform organisms, however, and this finding suggests that some nonpathogenic organisms in the intestine may cause natural immunization.[221] Immunity in early childhood protects against infection, so disease due to this organism is seen mostly in children younger than a few years of age and rarely in older children or adults.[85,100,171] The occasional case of arthritis that occurs in adults may be a consequence of a proved lack of immunity.[37,64,97,119,139,146,147,157a,162,178,183,193,259]

The clinical presentation of this form of arthritis is comparable to that of arthritis due to other micro-organisms. Youngsters experience pain in one or more joints, often the hip or knee. The involved limb may be held immobile. The organism can be cultured from the joint or blood,[174] or antigenic components can be identified by counterimmunoelectrophoresis.[164] Some adults with septic arthritis caused by *H. influenzae* have an associated pustular skin lesion,[139,196] so the differential diagnosis must obviously include infection due to *Neisseria gonorrhoeae* or *N. meningitidis.*

The antibiotic regimen must take into account the recent development of resistance of some strains of *H. influenzae* to ampicillin. Many of the isolates so characterized have been associated with treatment failure.[37,228] Initial therapy should consist of ampicillin, 50 mg/kg/day, and chloramphenicol,

50 mg/kg/day, intravenously. Subsequent drug sensitivity studies indicate which of these two drugs to continue. If the organism is resistant to ampicillin, chloramphenicol alone has proved efficacious.

Salmonella Infections

Salmonella species are classified serologically into a wide variety of subgroups according to their somatic (O) and flagellar (H) antigens. No natural saprophytes exist among them; all are pathogenetic for one or more animal species. Therefore, a sporadic or epidemic infection with salmonellae should always be traced to its source, usually an infected person or animal. So-called healthy carriers are persons or animals who discharge micro-organisms by the fecal route but have no history of symptoms of infection, whereas chronic carriers are hosts who discharge organisms for longer than ten weeks after recovery from an active infection. In septicemia due to these infections, the most common pathogens are *S. typhi* and *S. paratyphi B*; the next most common are *S. paratyphi A* and *S. paratyphi C* and *S. choleraesuis.*[56a]

Salmonellae produce infections that fall into four clinical syndromes: (1) gastroenteritis, which comprises the majority of cases; (2) bacteremia, with or without extraintestinal localization; (3) a typhoid-like illness known as enteric fever; and (4) carrier states. Factors that predispose individuals to hematogenous spread include infection with certain serotypes, loss of gastric acidity, immunosuppression, and sickle cell disease. In occasional patients, no predisposition exists. Focal lesions may appear in almost any organ of the body. Excluding individuals with sickle cell hemoglobinopathies, salmonellae are uncommon causes of osteomyelitis or arthritis.[202,225] When seen, osteomyelitis of the vertebra results from direct implantation of micro-organisms from the blood or by extension from a contiguous abscess. A special instance of this latter type of infection results from an abscess formed at a site in a damaged abdominal aorta seeded by *S. choleraesuis* or *S. typhimurium*. The arteritis or aortitis leads to aneurysmal formation, with extension of infection to the retroperitoneum, the psoas muscle sheath, and the lumbar vertebrae. In 13 cases, the mortality rate was 77%. Successful treatment requires resection of the abdominal aneurysm, debridement of the abscess, and appropriate antimicrobial therapy.[11]

Antibiotic treatment must take into account possible drug resistance, but ampicillin or chloramphenicol are successful in eradicating *Salmonella* infections.

Infection in Sickle Cell Disease

During a crisis, most patients with sickle cell anemia, sickle cell-thalassemia or sickle cell-hemoglobin C disease experience pain in their joints. This short-lived polyarthralgia may be due to blockage of small, subsynovial capillaries by the sickled cells. Gouty arthritis may also occur secondary to the extensive purine production from the erythropoiesis needed to compensate for the hemolysis. Arthritis may be caused by aseptic necrosis or, in rare cases, by hemarthrosis.[70] Bone and joint infections, although not as common as these other arthritides, do occur and, within the differential diagnosis of these other syndromes, represent a critical and difficult problem.

The incidence of infection with *Salmonella* species is increased in patients with the sickle cell gene.[12,251] In an African population with a high incidence of sickle cell disease, no greater frequency of infectious arthritis in general was noted in patients with the gene for S hemoglobin, but all of the three positive cultures for salmonellae were from children with the AS hemoglobin genotype.[135] In several hundred children with infectious arthritis and osteomyelitis observed for almost two decades in a large hospital practice in Texas, two of six children with sickle cell disease had osteomyelitis due to salmonellae.[173] The frequent occurrence of osteomyelitis of this type has also been reported in other patients with sickle cell disease.[120,124] In these and other series,[42] however, patients with sickle cell disease may also have been infected with other bacteria.

When confronted with a patient with sickle cell disease and arthritis, concern for infection must have the highest priority. Joint fluid should be aspirated, and appropriate bacteriologic studies should be undertaken.

Pseudomonas Infection

Pseudomonas species are ubiqitous in the environment. They are contaminants along with the Klebsielleae of many vegetables that are eaten uncooked;[200] they inhabit the gastrointestinal tract and colonize normal skin. Yet, these organisms seldom cause illness in humans with intact defenses. Pathogenicity is related in part to production of a toxin, exotoxin A, that inhibits mammalian protein synthesis. Antibodies against the toxin enhance survival, so the possibility of a vaccine using a modified toxin offers promise to prevent or control the disease.[192] As opposed to earlier experience, in which *P. aeruginosa* was an unusual cause of bone and joint infections, this organism has become the etiologic agent in many such infections in the last two decades.[14] The frequent association of heroin addiction (see the next section of this chapter) with this problem corresponds to the prevalence of this organism in other types of infections in narcotic abusers, especially endocarditis, and to the large number of hospital-acquired infections. The greater incidence of nosocomial disease reflects the increase in the magnitude and number of surgical procedures and instrumentation and the use of immunosuppressive and antibiotic drug therapy,[103] often in patients with severe burns, leukopenia, and debilitating diseases.

The clinical picture of *Pseudomonas aeruginosa* infection is varied. Skin findings include greenish discoloration of nails and indurated black lesions with an erythematous halo and ulcerated center, ecthyma gangrenosum. Local disease can occur in the upper and lower respiratory tracts, the conjunctiva, and the urinary tract. Fever and chills, sometimes with shock, accompany bacteremia. Both joint and bone involvement are reported.[15,103] Arthritis follows the general pattern of infections of joints; osteomyelitis often accompanies joint involvement. The sternoclavicular and sacroiliac joints and the symphysis pubis are often involved in drug abusers.

Another species, *P. pseudomallei*, rarely causes septic arthritis.[24,56] The micro-organism is endemic to Southeast Asia and thus the disease, called melioidosis, may be observed in Vietnam veterans. Manifestations include suppurative skin lesions, septicemia, pneumonia, and liver involvement. The disease may be latent for years.

Treatment is likely to be prolonged. The combined use of an aminoglycoside, such as tobramycin, and carbenicillin is recommended. Surgical debridement is often needed. Although early reports indicated a poor prognosis, the outlook has improved.[14]

Gram-Negative Infections in Drug Abusers

In addition to hepatitis and its vasculitic complication, addicts who inject drugs intravenously may develop infections of their bones and joints. These infections have special characteristics with regard to the type of infecting organism and to the joints that may become involved. Although joint infections in these patients may be caused by all common pathogens including staphylococci, two gram-negative rods have received particular attention, *Pseudomonas* and *Serratia marcescens*.[91,211] Although joints such as the knee may be involved, a greater predisposition is noted for invasion of the sacroiliac joint,[91,211] the symphysis pubis,[222] and the sternoclavicular joint in drug abusers than in the general population.[15,95] Sternoclavicular joint or symphysis pubis involvement is easily confirmed by the appearance of swelling and inflammation, but invasion of the sacroiliac joint is rarely detected on clinical grounds. In some patients, an acute illness associated with pain in the buttocks, fever, or other signs of toxicity appears; in others, symptoms of sepsis are absent or mild.[55] Radioisotope scanning is helpful in patients with low-back pain or stiffness because unilateral involvement is characteristic of infectious sacroiliitis.[47,63] No convincing explanation has been offered for the frequency of gram-negative bacillary infections and for their peculiar localization to certain joints in drug abusers.

In the treatment of drug addicts, the antibiotics initially administered should be effective against gram-negative bacilli, unless evidence of another infecting micro-organism is obtained. Early treatment should result in eradication of the infection and a greater likelihood for restoration of joint function.

Brucellosis

Of the 3 species of the genus *Brucella*,[56a] *B. melitensis* is the most invasive and produces a severe illness in man.[74,111,231] Fewer than 10% of the human cases in the United States are due to *B. melitensis,* but this species is the most common cause of brucellosis in the rest of the world. Another 10 to 20% of the cases of human brucellosis in the United States are due to *B. suis,* for which the natural reservoir is the hog. Suppurative lesions are more common in *B. suis* infections. The most frequent source of brucellosis in the United States is *B. abortus,* which causes about 75% of all cases.[131]

Brucellosis, normally a disease of animals, is rarely transmitted to humans. The organism gains entrance into man through the gastrointestinal tract from contaminated raw milk or through minute abrasions in the skin or mucous membranes after direct contact with cattle or swine or their products. It subsequently localizes in tissues with an abundance of reticuloendothelial cells, such as the bone marrow, lymph nodes, liver, and spleen. Proliferation within macrophages provides protection against the action of antibiotics.[231] The incubation period varies from a few to 21 days, but occasionally, several months elapse between the time of exposure and the first appearance of symptoms.

Generalized aches, backache, and joint pains are the striking clinical manifestations, along with weakness, sweats, chills, headache, and anorexia. Actual joint inflammation, including involvement of the sacroiliac joint, is uncommon,[108a,111,112,143a] reported in under 2% in a certain series.[112] Osteomyelitis involves the vertebrae, discs, pelvis, and long bones.[89,143] Recognition of spinal disease may be delayed for as long as a year after the original infection. The spondylitis of brucellosis resembles tuberculous spondylitis, except recovery is more rapid.

Recognition of brucellosis is often first suggested by the clinical features already noted, especially back pain with fever in individuals exposed to infected animals. Such persons include farmers, livestock producers, veterinarians, and employees in meat packing or rendering plants. Leukopenia with lymphocytosis is often found. Splenomegaly and hepatomegaly may occur, especially in chronic or recurrent cases. The precise diagnosis depends on serologic and cultural evidence. Every attempt should be made to isolate the organism from the blood, bone marrow, excised tissues, or body fluids. Special culture media may be necessary. The serum agglutination test is of considerable diagnostic importance.[28]

An ideal antibiotic program has not been devised, and relapses have occurred after the use of all current available antibiotics. One regimen consists of tetracycline, 2 g, in combination with streptomycin, 1 to 2 g, or another aminoglycoside for at least 3 weeks.[74,116,131] A 20% relapse rate may be expected. Erythromycin has been reported to be effective.[249] Bedrest, back support with casts or braces, and, in rare cases, surgical curettage may be required. Prophylaxis consists of boiling or pasteurizing all milk and destroying or treating infected animals.[101]

Unusual Gram-Negative Bacillary Infections

Haverhill fever, initially recognized as an epidemic in Haverhill, Massachusetts in 1926, was caused by contaminated milk. The contaminant was *Haverhillia multiformis (Streptobacillus moniliformis),* a gram-negative rod that shows extreme polymorphism. The main characteristics of the disease are an abrupt onset of fever and chills, a rubella-like or morbilliform rash, chiefly on the extremities, and joint pains.[191] Mild or marked joint redness and swelling may occur during the first several days of illness and may persist for several days or weeks. The organism can be recovered from the blood and joint fluid of some patients.[114,180] Besides the epidemic, sporadic cases have been reported.[76] Although some cases may follow a rat bite, this disease should not be called rat-bite fever because that term is applied to another disorder.

Rat-bite fever, also called sodoku in Japan, is a disease caused by a short, corkscrew-like rod, *Spirillum minus.* This organism is carried by rats and mice and is transmitted to humans through bites. Joint involvement with arthritis has been noted in a few patients. In two patients from whom the organism was recovered from the blood, a history of swelling about the wrists, elbows, knees, and ankles prior to hospitalization was recorded.[17]

Several types of vibrios are associated with human disease, including: (1) *Vibrio cholerae;* (2) nonagglutinable or noncholera vibrios, called NAG or NCV; (3) *Campylobacter fetus,* which was formerly called *V. fetus;* and (4) halophilic vibrios found in marine life, including *V. parahemolyticus* and *V. alginolyticus.* All four groups are associated with diarrheal diseases; the first two produce a pathogenic enterotoxin that accounts for the symptoms of the disease, and the last two do not always cause diarrhea, but can enter the circulation and may cause septicemia and focal infection. Some halophilic vibrios produce a necrotizing vasculitis and cutaneous ulcers similar to those seen in infections with the unrelated *Pseudomonas aeruginosa* and *Aeromonas hydrophila.*[32]

Of these four types of infection, only *Campylobacter fetus* infection has been linked to septic arthritis, often in an immunocompromised host.[80,83,138] In one report, a reactive arthritis was said to be induced by *C. jejuni.*[18]* Most *Campylobacter* strains are sensitive to erythromycin, tetracycline, aminoglycosides, and chloramphenicol, but are resistant to penicillin and cephalosporin. Many strains produce a beta-lactamase. Erythromycin is the drug of choice.[20]

Pasteurella multocida has recently been shown to cause a variety infections in human beings after contact with cats or dogs. Arthritis may occur after casual exposure, usually with no more contact than a scratch or a lick; osteomyelitis with or without accompanying arthritis is more often associated with animal bites that penetrate the skin and fascia.[13,72,98] Prior joint disease or an impairment of host defenses predisposes individuals to infection. Management follows generally accepted principles. The pathogen is responsive to penicillin.

Moraxella species is a gram-negative coccobacillus that easily can be confused morphologically with *Neisseria* species or *Haemophilus influenzae.* Further, in patients with septic arthritis, the polyarthritis and erythematous macular rash mimics that produced by *H. influenzae.*[88,209] A similar-appearing micro-organism, formerly called *Moraxella kingii,* has been assigned to a new genus, *Kingella.* It has been associated with both arthritis and osteomyelitis.[53,254] The pathogen is sensitive to penicillin.

Yersinia enterocolitica, a well-known intestinal pathogen that has been associated with a reactive arthritis, usually in a HLA-B27-positive host, may also cause an infectious arthritis. In the cases reported, the pattern of illness was characteristic of that seen in septic arthritis. The micro-organism was cultured from the joint.[129,238]

Several other gram-negative rods have been reported as causes of bone or joint infections, usually in compromised hosts. These include *Herrellae* species,[216] *Aeromonas hydrophila,*[40] *Eikenella corrodens,*[33,125] *Arizona hinshawii,*[227] and *Actinobacillus actinomycetemcomitans.*[170a]

BONE AND JOINT INFECTIONS DUE TO MISCELLANEOUS BACTERIA

Gram-Positive Bacillary Infections

Listeria monocytogenes is now appreciated as a rare but important cause of human infection, particularly in the immunosuppressed host. Cellular, rather than humoral, immunity is defective. Smears may reveal coccal forms of this gram-positive rod, so they may be confused with *Streptococcus pneumoniae* or other gram-positive cocci. The micro-organism grows well on blood agar, but it might be dismissed as a diphtheroid contaminant. Two patients, one with diabetes and the other with RA and psoriasis treated with methotrexate, developed septic monoarthritis.[26,176] Joint fluid cultures were positive in both, and blood culture was positive in one. Therapy included ampicillin in one and cephalothin in the other; both patients underwent arthrotomy before the infection was resolved.

Bacillus cereus is an aerobic spore-former recognized as a cause of food-borne disease. Some strains elaborate a toxin similar to that from *Vibrio cholerae.* One patient developed septic arthritis of the knee 36 hours after arthrography. *B. cereus* was cultured from the joint fluid. The infection responded to a penicillin analog. A gas shadow appeared in the radiograph, perhaps because of air entrapped at the time of arthroscopy or because of bacterial metabolism.[206]

Nocardia species are filamentous, aerobic, gram-positive bacteria that fragment into bacillary forms and frequently are acid-fast. *N. asteroides* is responsible for most infections seen in the United States and is associated with cutaneous, localized pulmonary, and disseminated involvement. Most patients are immunosuppressed. Of 25 patients from whom *Nocardia* isolates were obtained, 5 were recovered from the soft tissues or bone. One of these patients had osteomyelitis of the ilium. A combined trimethoprim-sulfamethoxazole regimen is effective.[86] One patient, who had received a kidney transplant and required azathioprine and prednisone for immunosuppression, developed septic monoarthritis due to *N. asteroides.* He responded well to the foregoing antibiotic combination.[195]

Editor's Note: Campylobacter is a common trigger of reactive arthritis in our experience (see Chap. 54).

Rhodococcus, a genus taxonomically related to *Nocardia* and *Mycobacterium*, is a rare pathogen; a young child developed painless enlargement of fingers, a toe, and knees. Radiographs were consistent with osteomyelitis of the phalanges. The knee fluid grew *Rhodococcus*.She was successfully treated with erythromycin and amoxicillin for six months.

An unidentified gram-positive rod adheres to a patient's red blood cells. In one reported case, the patient developed a chronic febrile illness with lymphadenopathy, purpuric nodular lesions in the feet, and arthralgias that responded to cell-wall-active antibiotics and to chloramphenicol.[6] A similar agent has been described in the blood of a patient with systemic lupus erythematosus.[126] Whether these organisms were pathogenic for the associated clinical state is uncertain.

Anaerobic Bacterial Infections

Anaerobes are not always appreciated as pathogens, primarily because of past difficulties in isolation. Now that simplified techniques have been developed, these organisms can be successfully cultivated in most laboratories. Both gram-negative and gram-positive anaerobes are found. *Bacteroides* species, especially *B. fragilis,* are the most common gram-negative anaerobes. *Propionibacterium, Lactobacillus, Clostridium,* and *Peptococcus* are examples of the gram-positive group. The normal microflora on the skin, mouth, large bowel, and vagina consists predominantly of anaerobes, so caution must be exercised in attributing pathogenicity to agents cultured from open areas. Those recovered from closed cavities such as the joint, bone, or blood are more likely to have caused some or all of the pathologic phenomena.[83,151]

Bone and joint infections have been caused by *Bacteroides fragilis* and *B. melaninogenicus,*[39,58,81,83] *Peptococcus,*[83] *Fusobacterium,*[83,87,151] *Propionibacterium,*[83,151,242] and others. *Clostridium perfringens* has been implicated in a handful of cases of septic arthritis.[113,137,153,159,182,223,243] More than half these cases were the result of a puncture wound of the joint. Most patients had monoarthritis; one patient had an infected disc space.[182] This patient and several others had a gas shadow due to bacterial metabolism that could be discerned on the radiograph. These organisms respond to penicillin.

An increasing number of cases of septic arthritis occur in prosthetic joints. Most often, the infection invades the bone and joint space from a contiguous area of infection or directly from the environment. Mixed flora is frequently present, including gram-positive cocci, gram-negative bacilli, as well as anaerobic organisms. In this setting, it is unclear whether one organism is the primary invader or whether several act synergistically to cause infection.

Most anaerobes other than *Bacteroides fragilis* are susceptible to penicillin.[67,151] Parenteral penicillin therefore should be part of the initial antibiotic regimen in patients with suspected or documented anaerobic infection. If the isolated anaerobes are resistant to penicillin, therapy may include parenteral clindamycin, or chloramphenicol may be chosen.

Polymicrobic Infections

Multiple organisms have been recovered from infected bone and joints, mainly those invaded from contiguous abscesses or into which the microorganism was introduced by a penetrating wound.[71,177] In patients who have not had a prior operation, the hip joint may often be involved by rupture of a retroperitoneal or pelvic abscess. *Staphylococcus aureus* and *Escherichia coli* have been isolated, sometimes with gram-negative rods. In patients who have undergone a prior surgical procedure, especially one in which a prosthetic joint is implanted, anaerobes are often recovered, along with streptococci and gram-negative bacilli.[83,151,201] Therapy requires selection of an appropriate spectrum of antibiotics and drainage. Open drainage is preferred because it is necessary to drain the adjacent abscess and to remove necrotic material.[71]

MYCOPLASMAL ARTHRITIS

Mycoplasmas, long recognized as pathogens in animals, are usually associated with respiratory, urogenital, and arthritic diseases. Within the past decade, they have been implicated more strongly in human disease; *Mycoplasma pneumoniae* can cause severe disease not only in the respiratory tract, but also in extrarespiratory site. *Ureaplasma urealyticum,* formerly known as T-strain mycoplasma, produces nongonococcal urethritis in men and is implicated in spontaneous abortion in women and in infertility. *Mycoplasma hominis* causes postpartum fever and probably pelvic inflammatory disease and pyelonephritis.[35]

Recently, all three mycoplasma species known to be pathogenetic in humans have been isolated directly from joints of patients with acute arthritis: *M. hominis* from a young mother who contracted arthritis after delivery, *U. urealyticum* from a patient with Reiter's syndrome, and *U. urealyticum* and *M. pneumoniae* from the joints of hypogammaglobulinemic patients with acute polyarthritis.[35,239,261] Arthritis was associated with proved *M. pneumoniae*-induced respiratory disease in 29 otherwise healthy patients ranging in age from 1 to 64 years. In this form, the arthritis was mild, but lasted up to 18 months. Organisms were not sought from the joints.[35,239] A case similar to this group was reported from another center.[223] *M. pulmonis* was able to induce arthritis in mice; viable organisms were cultured from the joints.[133]

Diagnosis of a mycoplasma infection depends on its isolation from infected secretions or fluids on special media and demonstration of a fourfold rise or fall in specific antibody in a serologic test such as complement fixation. The techniques required for these tests are not unusually difficult, and they are now performed more often in clinical laboratories.[35]

Both *U. urealyticum* and *M. hominis* are susceptible to tetracycline, but some ureaplasma isolates are resistant. *M. pneumoniae* infections are best treated with tetracycline or erythromycin.[35]

Despite these studies and reports, the role of mycoplasmas in human arthritis still remains to be defined. In only rare instances is it likely that these agents cause an infectious arthritis and then probably only in a compromised host. Of great theoretic interest is the long-standing but unanswered concern that mycoplasmas might play a role in acute rheumatic states such as Reiter's syndrome or chronic conditions such as RA.

NONBACTERIAL BONE AND JOINT INFECTIONS

Invasion of the joint or other musculoskeletal tissues such as muscle and bone by pathogens other than various bacteria and selected viruses is rare. More often, systemic effects of illnesses caused by rickettsiae, such as Rocky Mountain spotted fever, Q fever, typhus, and rickettsial pox, produce generalized muscular aches rather than true arthralgia. Moreover, diseases due to chlamydial pathogens, formerly called *Bedsonia*, have not been shown to colonize joint tissue directly, although a possible role as agents triggering reactive arthritis in HLA-B27 positive individuals has been suggested.[217]

Fascinating reports of invasion of bone and joints by parasites have been recorded infrequently along with the better-known examples of invasion of muscle by *Trichinella spiralis* and the larvae of *Taenia solium. Trypanosoma cruzi*, the protozoan that causes Chagas' disease, was found in the muscle of a patient with RA.[46] Two cases of tenosynovitis involving the wrists and ankles were associated with toxoplasmosis. Synovial tissue from one patient was injected into mice, one of whom demonstrated *Toxoplasma gondii* at autopsy.[252] Arthritis of the knee joint in four patients was due to infection by guinea worms. The worms were found at arthrotomy.[197a]

Hydatid disease, a common condition in the Middle East, is caused by the parasite *Echinococ-*

cus granulosus. After ingestion of contaminated meat, this parasite gives rise to lesions in many organs. In a large series of 352 consecutive cases of hydatid disease in man, 21 had bone disease, and 8 others had concurrent soft tissue and bone lesions. Symptoms consisted of bone pain and a progressively enlarging mass in the region of the involved bone. The pelvis, femur, spine, and tibia were affected, in that order. Symptoms had been present for prolonged periods, usually between 5 and 10 years. A few patients had joint as well as bone involvement. The presentation in these latter cases was confused with that of degenerative joint disease because of the chronicity of symptoms.[172a]

Polyarthritis during the course of infestation by the parasites *Strongyloides stercoralis* and *Taenia saginata* was related to evidence of an altered immune response. Immune complexes were found in the serum and synovial fluid, and immunoglobulin deposits were seen in the synovium. The synovitis improved after appropriate antiparasitic treatment.[23]

REFERENCES

1. Aho, K., et al.: HL-A 27 in reactive arthritis: a study of Yersinia arthritis and Reiter's disease. Arthritis Rheum., *17*:521–526, 1974.
2. Alkan, M.L., and Beachey, E.H.: Excretion of lipoteichoic acid by group A streptococci: influence of penicillin on excretion and loss of ability to adhere to human oral mucosal cells. J. Clin. Invest., *61*:671–677, 1978.
3. Allen, J.L., and Sprunt, K.: Discrepancy between minimum inhibitory and minimum bactericidal concentrations of penicillin for group A and group B-beta hemolytic streptococci. J. Pediatr., *93*:69–71, 1978.
4. Alper, C.A., et al.: Homozygous deficiency of C3 in a patient with repeated infections. Lancet, 2:1,179–1,181, 1972.
5. Alper, C.A., Bloch, K.J., and Rosen, F.S.: Increased susceptibility to infection in a patient with Type II essential hypercatabolism of C3. N. Engl. J. Med., *288*:601–606, 1973.
6. Archer, G.L., et al.: Human infection from an unidentified erythrocyte-associated bacterium. N. Engl. J. Med., *301*:897–900, 1979.
7. Atlas, E., and Belding, M.E.: Serratia marcescens arthritis requiring amputation. JAMA, *204*:167–169, 1968.
8. Austin, R.M., and Daniels, C.A.: Inhibition by rheumatoid factor, anti-Fc, and staphylococcal protein A of antibody-dependent cell-mediated cytolysis against herpes simplex virus-infected cells. J. Immunol., *117*:602–607, 1976.
9. Baehner, R.L., Nathan, D.G., and Karnovsky, M.L.: Correction of metabolic deficiencies in the leukocytes of patients with chronic granulomatous disease. J. Clin. Invest., *49*:865–870, 1970.
10. Baird, R.A., Anderson, N.J., and Bloch, J.H.: Salmonella vertebral osteomyelitis: a complication of Salmonella aortitis. Orthop., *4*:1,127–1,133, 1981.
11. Baker, C.J.: Summary of workshop on perinatal infections due to group B streptococcus. J. Infect. Dis., *136*:137–152, 1977.
12. Barrett-Connor, E.: Bacterial infection and sickle cell anemia: an analysis of 250 infections in 166 patients and a review of the literature. Medicine, *50*:97–112, 1971.
13. Barth, W.F., Healey, L.A., and Decker, J.L.: Septic arthritis due to Pasteurella multocida complicating rheumatoid arthritis. Arthritis Rheum., *11*:394–399, 1968.
14. Bayer, A.S., et al.: Gram-negative bacillary septic ar-

thritis: clinical, radiographic, therapeutic, and prognostic features. Semin. Arthritis Rheum., 7:123–132, 1977.

15. Bayer, A.S., et al.: Sternoclavicular pyarthrosis due to gram-negative bacilli. Arch. Intern. Med., 137:1,036–1,040, 1977.

16. Beaufils, M., et al.: Acute renal failure of glomerular origin during visceral abscesses. N. Engl. J. Med., 295:185–189, 1976.

17. Beeson, P.B.: Problem of the etiology of rat bite fever: report of two cases due to Spirillum minus. JAMA, 123:332–334, 1943.

18. Berden, J.H.M., Muyjens, H.L., and van de Putte, L.B.A.: Reactive arthritis associated with Campylobacter jejuni enteritis. Br. Med. J., 1:380–381, 1979.

19. Bhawan, J., Tandon, H.D., and Roy, S.: Ultrastructure of synovial membrane in pyogenic arthritis. Arch. Pathol., 96:155–160, 1973.

20. Blaser, M.J., and Reller, L.B.: Campylobacter enteritis. N. Engl. J. Med., 305:1,444–1,452, 1981.

21. Bliznak, J., and Ramsey, J.: Emphysematous septic arthritis due to Escherichia coli. J. Bone Joint Surg., 58A:138–139, 1976.

22. Bobechko, W.P., and Mandell, L.: Immunology of cartilage in septic arthritis. Clin. Orthop., 108:84–89, 1975.

23. Bocanegra, T.S., et al.: Reactive arthritis induced by parasitic infection. Ann. Intern. Med., 94:207–209, 1981.

24. Borgmeier, P.J., and Kalovidouris, A.E.: Septic arthritis of the sternomanubrial joint due to Pseudomonas pseudomallei. Arthritis Rheum., 23:1,057–1,059, 1980.

25. Bourgault, A.-M., et al.: Severe infection due to Streptococcus pneumoniae in asplenic renal transplant patients. Mayo Clin. Proc., 54:123–126, 1979.

26. Breckenridge, R.L., Jr., et al.: Listeria monocytogenes septic arthritis. Am. J. Clin. Pathol., 73:140–141, 1980.

27. Brosseau, J.D., and Mazza, J.J.: Group A streptococcal sepsis and arthritis: origin from an intrauterine device. JAMA, 238:2,178, 1977.

28. Buchanan, T.M.: Brucellosis in the United States, 1960–1972. Medicine, 53:103, 1974.

29. Burgon, D.S., and Nagel, D.A.: Serratia marcescens infections in orthopedic surgery: a review of the literature and a report of two cases. Clin. Orthop., 89:145–149, 1972.

30. Byeff, P.D., and Suskiewicz, L.: Meningococcal arthritis. JAMA, 235:2,752, 1976.

31. Calder, M.A., McHardy, V.U., and Schonell, M.E.: Importance of pneumococcal typing in pneumonia. Lancet, 1:5–7, 1970.

32. Carpenter, C.C.J.: More pathogenic vibrios. (Editorial.) N. Engl. J. Med., 300:39–40, 1979.

33. Carruthers, M.M., and Sommers, H.M.: Eikenella corrodens osteomyelitis. (Letter.) Ann. Intern. Med., 79:900, 1973.

34. Case records of the Massachusetts General Hospital. N. Engl. J. Med., 306:729–737, 1982.

35. Cassell, G.H. and Cole, B.C.: Mycoplasmas as agents of human disease. N. Engl. J. Med., 305:80–89, 1981.

36. Chan, D.P.K., Kamell, W.M., and Zaky, D.: Multifocal hematogenous Serratia marcescens osteomyelitis in a drug user: case report and review of the literature. Contemp. Orthop., 2:344–347, 1980.

37. Chang, M.J., Controni, G., and Rodriguez, W.J.: Ampicillin resistant Hemophilus influenzae Type B septic arthritis in children. Clin. Pediatr., 20:139–141, 1981.

38. Chartier, Y., Martin, W.J., and Kelly, P.J.: Bacterial arthritis: experiences in the treatment of 77 patients. Ann. Intern. Med., 50:1,462–1,474, 1959.

39. Childers, J.C., Jr.: Pyogenic arthritis due to Bacteroides fragilis infection. Orthop., 3:319–320, 1980.

40. Chmel, J., and Armstrong, D.: Acute arthritis caused by Aeromonas hydrophila. Arthritis Rheum., 19:169–172, 1976.

41. Christensen, P. and Kronvall, G.: Capacity of group A,B,C,D and G streptococci to agglutinate sensitized sheep red cells. Acta Pathol. Microbiol. Scand., 82B:19–24, 1974.

42. Chusid, M.J., and Sty, J.R.: Pneumococcal arthritis and osteomyelitis in children. Clin. Pediatr., 20:105–107, 1981.

43. Clark, R.A., and Kimball, H.R.: Defective granulocyte chemotaxis in the Chediak-Higashi syndrome. J. Clin. Invest., 50:2,645–2,652, 1971.

44. Cooke, T.D., et al.: The pathogenesis of chronic inflammation in experimental antigen-induced arthritis. II. Preferential localization of antigen-antibody complexes to collagenous tissues. J. Exp. Med., 135:323–338, 1972.

45. Coonrod, J.D., and Rytel, M.W.: Detection of type-specific pneumococcal antigens by counterimmunoelectrophoresis. II. Etiologic diagnosis of pneumococcal pneumonia. J. Lab. Clin. Med., 81:778–786, 1973.

46. Cossermelli, W., et al.: Polymositis in Chagas' disease. Ann. Rheum. Dis., 37:277–280, 1978.

47. Coy, J.T., III., et al.: Pyogenic arthritis of the sacro-iliac joint. J. Bone Joint Surg., 58A:845–849, 1976.

48. Curnutte, J.T., Kipnes, R.S., and Babior, B.M.: Defect in pyridine nucleotide dependent superoxide production by a particulate fraction from the granulocytes of patients with chronic granulomatous disease. N. Engl. J. Med., 293:628–632, 1975.

49. Curtis, S.H.: Report of a case of bacteraemia caused by the Micrococcus catarrhalis following tonsillectomy and acute polyarthritis with recovery. N.Y. State J. Med., 32:672, 1932.

50. Dale, D.C., Fauci, A.S., and Wolff, S.M.: Alternate-day prednisone: leukocyte kinetics and susceptibility to infections. New Engl. J. Med., 291:1,154–1,158, 1974.

51. Daniel, D., et al.: Lavage of septic joints in rabbits: effects on chondrolysis. J. Bone Joint Surg., 58A:393–395, 1976.

52. David, J.R., and Black, R.L.: Salmonella arthritis. Medicine, 39:385–403, 1960.

53. Davis, J.M., and Peel, M.M.: Osteomyelitis and septic arthritis caused by Kingella kingii. J. Clin. Pathol., 35:218–222, 1982.

54. De Andrade, J.R., and Tribe, C.R.: Staphylococcal septicaemia with pyoarthrosis in rheumatoid arthritis. Br. Med. J., 1:1,516–1,518, 1962.

55. Delbarre, F., et al.: Pyogenic infection of the sacro-iliac joint: report of thirteen cases. J. Bone Joint Surg., 57A:819–825, 1975.

56. Diamond, H.S., and Pastore, R.: Septic arthritis due to Pseudomonas pseudomallei. Arthritis Rheum., 10:459–466, 1967.

56a. Diem, K., and Lentner, C. (Eds.): Pathogenic Organisms and Infectious Diseases. Basel, Ciba-Geigy, 1971.

57. Dillon, J.R., et al.: Spread of penicillinase-producing and transfer plasmids from the gonococcus to Neisseria meningitidis. Lancet, 1:779, 1983.

58. Dodd, M.J., Griffiths, I.D., and Freeman, R.: Pyogenic arthritis due to Bacteroides complicating rheumatoid arthritis. Ann. Rheum. Dis., 41:248–249, 1982.

59. Donovan, T.L., et al.: Serratia arthritis: report of seven cases. J. Bone Joint Surg., 58A:1,009–1,011, 1976.

60. Dorff, G.J., Ziolkowski, J.S., and Rytel, M.W.: Detection by counterimmunoelectrophoresis of pneumococcal antigen in synovial fluid from septic arthritis. Arthritis Rheum., 18:613–615, 1975.

61. Dorwart, B.B., Abrutyn, E., and Schumacher, H.R.: Serratia arthritis: medical eradication of infection in a patient with rheumatoid arthritis. JAMA, 225:1,642–1,643, 1973.

62. Dossett, J.H., et al.: Antiphagocytic effects of staphylococcal protein A. J. Immunol., 103:1,405–1,410, 1969.

63. Dunn, E.J., et al.: Pyogenic infections of the sacro-iliac joint. Clin. Orthop., 118:113–117, 1976.

64. Dyer, R.F., Romansky, M.J., and Holmes, J.R.: Hemophilus pyarthrosis in an adult. Arch. Intern. Med., 102:580–583, 1958.

65. Ecker, E.E., et al.: Complement in infectious disease in man. J. Clin. Invest., 25:800–808, 1946.

66. Ecker, E.E., Kuehn, A.O., and Recroft, E.W.: Salmonella schottmulleri isolated from sacrolumbar lesion of twenty-four years' duration. JAMA, 118:1,296–1,297, 1942.

67. Edson, R.S., et al.: Recent experience with antimicrobial susceptibility of anaerobic bacteria: increasing resistance to penicillin. Mayo Clin. Proc., 57:737–741, 1982.

68. Edwards, Jr., G.S., and Russell, I.J.: Pneumococcal arthritis complicating gout. J. Rheumatol., 7:907–910, 1980.

69. Eichner, H.L., and Deller, J.J., Jr.: Meningococcal arthritis: report of two cases. Arthritis Rheum., 13:272–275, 1970.

70. Espinoza, L.R., Spilberg, I., and Osterland, K.C.: Joint manifestations of sickle-cell disease. Medicine, 53:295–305, 1974.

71. Esposito, A.L., and Gleckman, R.A.: Acute polymicrobic septic arthritis in the adult: case report and literature review. Am. J. Med. Sci., 267:251–254, 1974.

72. Ewing, R., et al.: Articular and skeletal infections caused by Pasteurella multocida. South Med. J., 73:1,349–1,352, 1980.

73. Fam, A.G., Tenenbaum, J., and Stein, J.L.: Clinical forms of meningococcal arthritis: a study of five cases. J. Rheumatol., 6:567–573, 1979.

74. Farid, Z., and Miale, A., Jr.: Brucella spondylitis: report of the first four cases from Egypt. Trans. Soc. Trop. Med. Hyg., 57:115–118, 1963.

75. Farrand, R.J., Johnstone, J.M.S., and MacCabe, A.F.: Haemophilus osteomyelitis and arthritis. Br. Med. J., 2:334–336, 1968.

76. Farrell, E., Lordi, G.H., and Vogel, J.: Haverhill fever: report of a case with review of the literature. Arch. Intern. Med., 64:1–14, 1939.

77. Fearon, D.T., et al.: Activation of the properdin pathway of complement in patients with gram-negative bacteremia. N. Engl. J. Med., 292:937–940, 1975.

78. Feigin, R.D., et al.: Septic arthritis due to Moraxella osloensis. J. Pediatr., 75:116–117, 1969.

79. Feldman, S.A., and DuClos, T.: Diagnosis of meningococcal arthritis by immunoelectrophoresis of synovial fluid. Appl. Microbiol., 25:1,006–1,007, 1973.

80. Fick, R.B., Jr., Isturiz, R., and Cadman, E.L.: Campylobacter fetus septic arthritis: report of a case. Yale J. Biol. Med., 52:339–344, 1979.

81. Finland, M., Jones, W.F., Jr., and Barnes, M.W.: Occurrence of serious bacterial infections since introduction of antibacterial agents. JAMA, 170:2,188–2,197, 1959.

82. Fischer, G.W., et al.: Demonstration of opsonic activity and in vivo protection against group B streptococci type III by S. pneumoniae type 14 antisera. J. Exp. Med., 148:776–786, 1978.

83. Fitzgerald, R.H., Jr., et al.: Anaerobic septic arthritis. Clin. Orthop., 164:141–148, 1982.

84. Flafman, J.G.: Hip disease with referred pain to the knee. JAMA, 234:967–968, 1975.

85. Fothergill, L.D., and Wright, J.: Influenzal meningitis: the relation of age incidence to the bactericidal power of blood against the causal organism. J. Immunol., 24:273–284, 1933.

86. Frazier, A.R., Rosenow, E.C., III, and Roberts, G.D.: Nocardiosis: a review of 25 cases occurring during 24 months. Mayo Clin. Proc., 50:657–663, 1975.

87. Freedman, H.L., and Cashman, W.F.: Vertebral osteomyelitis caused by Fusobacterium nucleatum: a case report. Orthop., 2:366–369, 1979.

87a. Fujita, N.K., Lam, K., and Bayer, A.S.: Septic arthritis due to Group G streptococci. JAMA, 247:812–813, 1982.

88. Garcia, A., Jr., and Grantham, S.A.: Hematogenous pyogenic vertebral osteomyelitis. J. Bone Joint Surg., 42A:429–436, 1960.

89. Ghormley, R.K.: Pathologic aspects of arthritis. Arch. Phys. Ther., 17:567–571, 1936.

90. Giebink, G.S., et al.: Opsonic requirements for phagocytosis of Streptococcus pneumoniae types VI, XVIII, XXIII and XXV. Infect. Immun., 18:291, 1977.

91. Gifford, D.B., et al.: Septic arthritis due to Pseudomonas in heroin addicts. J. Bone Joint Surg., 57A:631–635, 1975.

92. Glasgow, L.A.: Staphylococcal infection in the toxic-shock syndrome. N. Engl. J. Med., 303:1,473–1,474, 1980.

93. Goldenberg, D.L., et al.: Acute arthritis caused by gram-negative bacilli: a clinical characterization. Medicine, 53:197–208, 1974.

94. Goldenberg, D.L., and Cohen, A.S.: Acute infectious arthritis: a review of patients with nongonococcal joint infections (with emphasis on therapy and prognosis). Am. J. Med., 60:369–377, 1976.

95. Goldin, R.H., et al.: Sternoarticular septic arthritis in heroin users. N. Engl. J. Med., 289:616–618, 1973.

96. Goldschneider, I., Gotschlich, E.C., and Artenstein, M.S.: Human immunity to the meningococcus. I. The role of humoral antibodies. J. Exp. Med., 129:1,307–1,326, 1969.

97. Goldstein, E., and Janoski, A.H.: Hemophilus influenzae pyarthrosis in an adult. Arch. Intern. Med., 114:647–650, 1964.

98. Gomez-Reino, J.J., et al.: Pasteurella multicida arthritis. J. Bone Joint Surg., 62A:1,212–1,213, 1980.

99. Gordon, S.L., Maisels, M.J., and Robbins, W.J.: Multiple joint infections with Enterobacter cloacae. Clin. Orthop., 125:136–138, 1977.

100. Granoff, D.M., and Nankervis, G.A.: Infectious arthritis in the neonate caused by Haemophilus influenzae. Am. J. Dis. Child, 129:730–733, 1975.

101. Green, F.B.: Undulant fever and its relation to public health. Texas State J. Med., 32:549–550, 1936.

102. Greenwood, B.M., Whittle, H.C., and Bryceson, A.D.M.: Allergic complications of meningococcal disease. II. Immunological investigations. Br. Med. J., 2:737–740, 1973.

103. Grieco, M.H.: Pseudomonas arthritis and osteomyelitis. J. Bone Joint Surg., 54A:1,693–1,704, 1972.

104. Griffiths, H.E.D., and Jones, D.M.: Pyogenic infection of the spine: a review of twenty-eight cases. J. Bone Joint Surg., 53B:383–391, 1971.

105. Gristina, A.G., Rovere, G.D., and Shoji, H.: Spontaneous septic arthritis complicating rheumatoid arthritis. J. Bone Joint Surg., 56A:1,180–1,184, 1974.

106. Gustafson, G.T., Sjöquist, J., and Stålenheim, G.: "Protein A" from Staphylococcus aureus. II. Arthus-like reaction produced in rabbits by interaction of protein A and human gammaglobulin. J. Immunol., 98:1,178–1,181, 1967.

107. Hamilton, M.E., and Gibson, R.S.: Group C streptococcal arthritis. N.Y. State J. Med., 80:1,746–1,747, 1980.

108. Hammerschlag, M.R., and Baker, C.J.: Meningococcal osteomyelitis: a report of two cases associated with septic arthritis. J. Pediatr., 88:519–520, 1976.

108a. Handal, G., and LeCompte, M.: Brucellosis: a treatable cause of monarthritis. Clin. Orthop., 168:211–213, 1982.

109. Harden, W.B., et al.: Septic arthritis due to Serratia liquefaciens. Arthritis Rheum., 23:946–948, 1980.

110. Harder, E.J., et al.: Streptococcus mutans endocarditis. Ann. Intern. Med., 80:364–368, 1974.

111. Hardy, A.V.: Arthritis in Brucella melitensis infections. Med. Clin. North Am., 21:1,747–1,749, 1937.

112. Hardy, A.V., et al.: Undulant fever: with special reference to a study of Brucella infection in Iowa. Public Health Rep., 45:2,433–2,476, 1930.

113. Harrington, T.M., et al.: Clostridium perfringens: an unusual cause of septic arthritis. Ann. Emerg. Med., 10:315–317, 1981.

114. Hazard, J.B., and Goodkind, R.: Haverhill fever (erythema arthriticum epidemicum): a case report and bacteriologic study. JAMA, 90:534–538, 1932.

115. Henson, S.W., Jr. and Coventry, M.B.: Osteomyelitis of the vertebrae as the result of infection of the urinary tract. Surg. Gynecol. Obstet., 102:207–214, 1956.

116. Herrell, W.E., and Barber, T.E.: Treatment of brucellosis with Aureomycin or Terramycin combined with dihydrostreptomycin. Postgrad. Med., 11:476–486, 1952.

117. Herrick, W.W.: Meningococcus infections including meningitis. Bull. N.Y. Acad. Med., 7:487–501, 1931.

118. Herrick, W.W., and Parkhurst, G.M.: Meningococcus arthritis. Am. J. Med. Sci., 158:473–481, 1919.

118a. Ho, G., Su, E.Y.: Therapy for septic arthritis. JAMA, 247:797–800, 1982.

119. Hoaglund, F.T., and Lord, G.P.: Hemophilus influenzae: septic arthritis in adults. Arch. Intern. Med., *119*:648–652, 1967.

120. Hook, E.W., et al.: Salmonella osteomyelitis in patients with sickle-cell anemia. N. Engl. J. Med., *257*:403–407, 1957.

121. Houston, B.D., Crouch, M.E., and Finch, R.G.: Streptococcus MG-intermedius septic arthritis in a patient with rheumatoid arthritis. J. Rheumatol., *7*:89, 1980.

122. Howard, J.B., Highgenboten, C.L., and Nelson, J.D.: Residual effects of septic arthritis in infancy and childhood. JAMA, *236*:932–935, 1976.

123. Jacobs, M.R., et al.: Emergence of multiply resistant pneumococci. N. Engl. J. Med., *299*:735–740, 1978.

124. Jakab, G.J., and Green, G.M.: Defect in intracellular killing of Staphylococcus aureus within alveolar macrophages in Sendai virus-infected murine lungs. J. Clin. Invest., *57*:1,533–1,539, 1976.

125. Johnson, S.M., and Pankey, G.A.: Eikenella corrodens osteomyelitis, arthritis, and cellulitis of the hand. South. Med. J., *69*:535–539, 1976.

126. Kallick, C.A., et al.: Systemic lupus erythematosus associated with haemobartonella-like organisms. Nature (New Biol.), *236*:145–146, 1972.

127. Karten, I.: Septic arthritis complicating rheumatoid arthritis. Ann. Intern. Med., *70*:1,147–1,158, 1969.

128. Kauffman, C.A., Watanakunakorn, C., and Phair, J.P.: Pneumococcal arthritis. J. Rheumatol., *3*:409–419, 1976.

129. Keet, E.E.: Yersinia enterocolitica septicemia—source of infection and incubation period identified. N.Y. State J. Med., *74*:2,226–2,230, 1974.

130. Kellgren, J.H., et al.: Suppurative arthritis complicating rheumatoid arthritis. Br. Med. J., *1*:1,193–1,200, 1958.

131. Kelly, P.J., et al.: Brucellosis of the bones and joints: experience with thirty-six patients. JAMA, *174*:347–353, 1960.

132. Kelly, P.J., Wilkowske, C.J., and Washington, J.A., II: Musculoskeletal infections due to Serratia marcescens. Clin. Orthop., *96*:76–83, 1973.

133. Keystone, E.C., et al.: Role of viable mycoplasmas in the pathogenesis of arthritis induced by M. pulmonis. Br. J. Exp. Pathol., *62*:350–356, 1981.

134. Kluge, R., Schmidt, M., and Barth, W.F.: Pneumococcal arthritis. Ann. Rheum. Dis., *32*:21–24, 1973.

135. Kolawole, T.M., and Bohrer, S.P.: Acute septic arthritis in Nigeria: a review of 65 cases involving the hip and shoulder joints. Trop. Geogr. Med., *24*:327–338, 1972.

136. Koppes, G.M., and Arnett, F.C.: Group Y meningococcal arthritis: case report. Milit. Med., *140*:861–862, 1975.

137. Korn, J.A., et al.: Clostridium welchii arthritis. J. Bone Joint Surg., *57A*:555–557, 1975.

138. Kowalek, J.K., Kaminski, Z.C., and Krey, P.R.: Campylobacter arthritis associated with Campylobacter jejuni enteritis. Br. Med. J., *1*:380–381, 1929.

139. Krauss, D.S., et al.: Hemophilus influenzae septic arthritis: a mimicker of gonococcal arthritis. Arthritis Rheum., *17*:267–271, 1974.

140. Kronvall, G.: A surface component in Group A,C and G streptococci with non-immune reactivity for immunoglobulin G. J. Immunol., *111*:1,401–1,406, 1973.

141. Kronvall, G., and Gewurz, H.: Activation and inhibition of IgG mediated complement fixation by staphylococcal protein A. Clin. Exp. Immunol., *7*:211–220, 1970.

142. Kronvall, G., and Williams, R.C., Jr.: Differences in antiprotein A activity among IgG subgroups. J. Immunol., *103*:828–833, 1969.

143. Kulowski, J., and Vinke, T.H.: Undulant (Malta) fever spondylitis: report of a case, due to Brucella melitensis, bovine variety, surgically treated. JAMA, *991*,656–1,659, 1932.

143a.Lam, K., et al.: Disseminated brucellosis initially seen as sternoclavicular arthropathy. Arch. Intern. Med., *142*:1,193–1,194, 1982.

144. Larson, H.E., et al.: Arthritis after meningococcal meningitis. Br. Med. J., *1*:618–619, 1977.

145. Leedom, J.M., et al.: Importance of sulfadiazine resistance in meningococcal disease in civilians. N. Engl. J. Med., *273*:1,395–1,401, 1965.

146. Leek, J.C., and Robbins, D.L.: Infectious arthritis due to Hemophilus influenzae. J. Rheumatol., *6*:432–438, 1979.

147. Lefkovits, A.M., and Noonan, J.R.: Septic arthritis caused by Hemophilus influenzae in an adult: case report. J. Am. Geriatr. Soc., *16*:1,150–1,152, 1968.

148. LeFrock, J.L., et al.: Infectious arthritis resulting from Enterobacter cloacae and Enterobacter hafniae. Clin. Pediatr., *16*:838–839, 1977.

149. Lepow, M.L., and Gold, R.: Further conquest of the meningococcus. N. Engl. J. Med., *297*:721–722, 1977.

150. Lever, A.M.L., Owen, T., and Forsey, J.: Pneumoarthropathy in septic arthritis caused by Streptococcus milleri. Br. Med. J., *285*:24, 1982.

151. Lewis, R.P., Sutter, V.L., and Finegold, S.M.: Bone infections involving anaerobic bacteria. Medicine, *57*:279–305, 1978.

152. This reference has been deleted.

153. Lovell, W.W.: Infection of the knee joint by Clostridium welchii. J. Bone Joint Surg., *28*:398, 1946.

154. McCabe, W.R.: Serum complement levels in bacteremia due to gram-negative organisms. N. Engl. J. Med., *288*:21–23, 1973.

155. McCabe, W.R., and Jackson, G.G.: Gram-negative bacteremia. Arch. Intern. Med., *110*:847–855, 1962.

156. McCall, C.E., and Caves, J.: Dysfunction of human neutrophils during severe bacterial infection. Clin. Res., *18*:444, 1970.

157. McCarty, D.J.: Joint sepsis: a chance for cure. JAMA, *247*:835, 1982.

157a.McClatchey, W.M., and Goldman, J.A.: Pseudopodagra from Hemophilus influenza in an adult. Arthritis Rheum., *22*:681–683, 1979.

158. MacGregor, R.R., Spagnuolo, P.J., and Lentnek, A.L.: Inhibition of granulocyte adherence by ethanol, prednisone, and aspirin, measured with an assay system. N. Engl. J. Med., *291*:642–646, 1974.

159. McNae, J.: An unusual case of Clostridium welchii infection. J. Bone Joint Surg., *48B*:512–513, 1966.

159a.Mackowiak, P.A., and Smith, J.W.: Teichoic acid antibodies in chronic staphylococcal osteomyelitis. Ann. Intern. Med., *89*:494–496, 1978.

160. Martin, W.J., Yu, P.K.W., and Washington, J.A., II: Epidemiologic significance of Klebsiella pneumoniae: 3-month study. Mayo Clin. Proc., *46*:785–793, 1971.

161. Mayer, J.W., DeHoratius, R.J., and Messner, R.P.: Serratia marcescens caused arthritis with negative and positive birefringent crystals. Arch. Intern. Med., *136*:1,323–1,325, 1976.

162. Meligrana, F., Hawks, H., and Marotta, T.: Hemophilus influenzae septicemia with polyarthritis and meningitis in an adult. Can. Med. Assoc. J., *89*:132–134, 1963.

163. Memon, I.A., et al.: Group B streptococcal osteomyelitis and septic arthritis: its occurrence in infants less than 2 months old. Am. J. Dis. Child., *133*:921–923, 1979.

164. Merritt, K., et al.: Counter immunoelectrophoresis in the diagnosis of septic arthritis caused by Hemophilus influenzae. J. Bone Joint Surg., *58A*:414–415, 1976.

165. Mintz, L., and Mollett, G.H.: Serratia vertebral osteomyelitis in narcotic addicts. Ann. Intern. Med., *83*:668–669, 1975.

166. Mitchell, W.S., et al.: Septic arthritis in patients with rheumatoid disease; a still underdiagnosed complication. J. Rheumatol., *3*:124–133, 1976.

166a.Moody, M.M., et al.: Long term amikacin use: effects on aminoglycoside susceptibility patterns of gram negative bacilli. JAMA, *248*:1,199–1,202, 1982.

167. Morrey, B.F., Bianco, A.J., and Rhodes, K.H.: Suppurative arthritis of the hip in children. J. Bone Joint Surg., *58A*:388–392, 1976.

168. Morris, J.L., Zizic, T.M., and Stevens, M.B.: Proteus polyarthritis complicating systemic lupus erythematosus. Johns Hopkins Med. J., *133*:262–269, 1973.

169. Mowat, A.G., and Baum, J.: Chemotaxis of polymorphonuclear leukocytes from patients with diabetes mellitus. New Engl. J. Med., *284*:621–627, 1971.

170. Mowat, A.G., and Baum, J.: Chemotaxis of polymor-

phonuclear leukocytes from patients with rheumatoid arthritis. J. Clin. Invest., *50*:2,541–2,549, 1971.

170a.Muhle, I., Rau, J., and Ruskin, J.: Vertebral osteomyelitis due to Actinobacillus actinomycetemcomitans. JAMA, *241*:1,824–1,825, 1979.

171. Musher, D.M.: Haemophilus influenzae infections. Hosp. Pract., *18*:158–173, 1983.

172. Myers, A.R., Miller, L.M., and Pinals, R.S.: Pyarthrosis complicating rheumatoid arthritis. Lancet, *2*:714–716, 1969.

172a.Nassch, G.A.: Hydatid disease in bone and joint. J. Trop. Med. Hyg., *78*:243–244, 1975.

173. Nelson, J.D.: Sickle cell disease and bacterial bone and joint infection (Letter.) N. Engl. J. Med., *292*:534–535, 1975.

174. Nelson, J.D.: The bacterial etiology and antibiotic management of septic arthritis in infants and children. Pediatrics, *50*:437–440, 1972.

175. Newman, J.H.: Review of septic arthritis throughout the antibiotic era. Ann. Rheum. Dis., *35*:198–205, 1976.

176. Newman, J.H., Waycott, S., and Cooney, L.M., Jr.: Arthritis due to Listeria monocytogenes. Arthritis Rheum., *22*:1,139–1,140, 1979.

177. Nitsche, J.F., et al.: Septic sternoclavicular arthritis with Pasteurella multocida and Streptococcus sanguis. Arthritis Rheum., *25*:467–469, 1982.

178. Norden, C.W., and Sellers, T.F., Jr.: Hemophilus influenza pyarthrosis in an adult. JAMA, *189*:694–695, 1964.

179. Oh, I.: Serratia marcescens arthritis in heroin addicts. Clin. Orthop., *122*:228–230, 1977.

180. Parker, F., Jr., and Hudson, N.P.: The etiology of Haverhill fever (erythema arthriticum). Am. J. Pathol., *2*:357–379, 1926.

181. Partio, E., Hatanpää, S., and Rokkanen, P.: Pyogenic spondylitis. Acta Orthop. Scand., *49*:164–168, 1978.

182. Pate, D., and Katz, A.: Clostridia discitis: a case report. Arthritis Rheum., *22*:1,039–1,040, 1979.

183. Patterson, R.L., Jr., and Levine, D.B.: Hemophilus influenza pyarthrosis in an adult. J. Bone Joint Surg., *47A*:1,250–1,252, 1965.

184. Paul, J.R., Salinger, R., and Zuger, B.: The relation of rheumatic fever to postscarlatinal arthritis and postscarlatinal heart disease—a familial study. J. Clin. Invest., *13*:503–516, 1934.

185. Pearson, R.D., Spiva, D., and Gluckman, J.: Cirrhosis of liver with septic arthritis due to Escherichia coli. N.Y. State J. Med., *78*:1,762–1,763, 1975.

186. Peltola, H., et al.: Clinical efficacy of meningococcus group A capsular polysaccharide vaccine in children three months to five years of age. N. Engl. J. Med., *297*:686–692, 1977.

187. Petersen, B.H., et al.: Neisseria meningitidis and Neisseria gonorrhoeae bacteremia associated with C6, C7, or C8 deficiency. Ann. Intern. Med., *90*:917–920, 1979.

188. Peterson, P.K., et al.: The key role of peptidoglycan in the opsonization of Staphylococcus aureus. J. Clin. Invest., *61*:597–609, 1978.

189. Pinals, R.S.: Meningococcemia presenting as acute polyarthritis. J. Rheumatol., *4*:420–424, 1977.

190. Pinals, R.S., and Ropes, M.W.: Meningococcal arthritis. Arthritis Rheum., *7*:241–258, 1964.

191. Place, E.H., and Sutton, L.E.: Erythema arthriticum epidemicum (Haverhill fever). Arch. Intern. Med., *54*:659–684, 1934.

192. Pollack, M.: Pseudomonas aeruginosa exotoxin A. (Editorial). N. Engl. J. Med., *302*:1,360–1,361, 1980.

193. Raff, M.J., and Dannaher, C.L.: Hemophilus influenzae septic arthritis in adults: report of a case and review of the literature. J. Bone Joint Surg., *56A*:408–412, 1974.

194. Ramsdell, C.M., and Northup, J.D.: Serratia arthritis: report of three cases. South. Med. J., *66*:889–891, 1973.

195. Rao, K.V., O'Brien, T.J., and Andersen, R.C.: Septic arthritis due to Nocardia asteroides after successful kidney transplantation. Arthritis Rheum., *24*:99–101, 1981.

196. Ravn, H.: Acute haematogenous osteomyelitis due to type-B. haemophilus influenzae. Lancet, *1*:517–518, 1966.

197. Ravreby, W.D., Bottone, E.J., and Keusch, G.T.: Group D streptococcal bacteremia with emphasis on the incidence and presentation of infections due to Streptococcus bovis. N. Engl. J. Med., *289*:1,400–1,403, 1973.

197a.Reddy, C.R.R.M., and Sivaramappa, M.: Guinea-worm arthritis of the knee joint. Br. Med. J.,*1*:155–156, 1968.

198. Reed, W.P., Stromquist, D.L., and Williams, R.C., Jr.: Agglutination and phagocytosis of pneumococci by immunoglobulin G antibodies of restricted heterogeneity. J. Lab. Clin. Med., *101*:847–856, 1983.

199. Reeves, B., and Churchill-Davidson, D.: Salmonella infection of the hip. Postgrad. Med. J., *40*:555, 1964.

200. Remington, J.S., and Schimpff, S.C.: Please don't eat the salads. (Editorial.) N. Engl. J. Med., *304*:433–434, 1981.

201. Renne, J.W., Tanowitz, H.B., and Chulay, J.D.: Septic arthritis in an infant due to Clostridium ghoni and Hemophilus parainfluenzae. Pediatrics, *57*:573–574, 1976.

202. Richardson, S.B., Uttley, A.H.C., and Pettingale, K.W.: Acute sacroiliitis due to Salmonella okatie. Br. Med. J., *1*:1,449–1,450, 1977.

203. Richmond, M.H., et al.: High penicillinase production correlated with multiple antibiotic resistance in Staphylococcus aureus. Lancet, *1*:293–300, 1964.

204. Rimoin, D.L., and Wennberg, J.E.: Acute septic arthritis complicating chronic rheumatoid arthritis. JAMA, *196*:617–621, 1966.

205. Rinehart, J.J., et al.: Effects of corticosteroid therapy on human monocyte function. N. Engl. J. Med., *292*:236–241, 1975.

205a.Ristuccia, A.M., and Cunha, B.A.: The aminoglycosides. Med. Clin. North Am., *66*:303–312, 1982.

206. Robinson, S.C.: Bacillus cereus septic arthritis following arthrography. Clin. Orthop., *145*:237–238, 1979.

207. Robitaille, A., et al.: HLA frequencies in less common arthropathies. Ann. Rheum. Dis., *35*:271–273, 1976.

208. Rogers, D.E.: The changing pattern of life-threatening microbial disease. N. Engl. J. Med., *261*:677–683, 1959.

209. Rosenbaum, J., Lieberman, D.H., and Katz, W.A.: Moraxella infectious arthritis: first report in an adult. Ann. Rheum. Dis., *39*:184–185, 1980.

210. Rosner, R.: Isolation of protoplasts of Staphylococcus aureus from a case of recurrent acute osteomyelitis. Am. J. Clin. Pathol., *50*:385–390, 1968.

211. Ross, G.N., Baraff, L.J., and Quismorio, F.P.: Serratia arthritis in heroin users. J. Bone Joint Surg., *57A*:1,158–1,160, 1975.

212. Rowley, D.A.: The formation of circulating antibody in the splenectomized human being following intravenous injection of heterologous erythrocytes. J. Immunol., *65*:515–521, 1950.

213. Roy, S., and Bhawan, J.: Ultrastructure of articular cartilage in pyogenic arthritis. Arch. Pathol., *99*:44–47, 1975.

214. Russell, A.S., and Ansell, B.M.: Septic arthritis. Ann. Rheum. Dis., *331*:40–44, 1972.

215. Rytel, M.W., et al.: Possible pathogenic role of capsular antigens in fulminant pneumococcal disease with disseminated intravascular coagulation (DIC). Am. J. Med., *57*:889–896, 1974.

216. Sampson, C.C., Smith, C.D., and Robinson, H.S.: Isolation of a species of genus Herellea from a patient with acute synovitis. J. Natl. Med. Assoc., *51*:360–362, 1959.

217. Schachter, J.: Chlamydial infections. N. Engl. J. Med., *298*:428–435, 490–495, 540–549, 1978.

218. Schein, A.J.: Articular manifestations of meningococci infections. Arch. Intern. Med., *62*:963–978, 1938.

219. Schenfeld, L., et al.: Bacterial monarthritis due to Neisseria meningitidis in systemic lupus erythematosus. J. Rheumatol., 8:145–148, 1981.

220. Schmid, F.R., Roitt, I.M., and Rocha, M.J.: Complement fixation by a two-component antibody system: immunoglobin G and immunoglobin M anti-globulin (rheumatoid factor) paradoxical effect related to immunoglobulin G concentration. J. Exp. Med., 132:673–693, 1970.

221. Schneerson, R., and Robbins, J.B.: Induction of serum Haemophilus influenzae Type B capsular antibodies in adult volunteers fed cross-reacting Escherichia coli 075:K100:H5. N. Engl. J. Med., 292:1,093–1,096, 1975.

222. Sequeira, W., et al.: Pyogenic infections of the pubis symphysis. Ann. Intern. Med., 96:604–606, 1982.

223. Sequeira, W., Jones, E., and Bronson, D.M.: Mycoplasma pneumoniae infection with arthritis and a varicella-like eruption. JAMA, 246:1,936–1,937, 1981.

224. Schurman, D.J., and Wheeler, R.: Gram negative bone and joint infection: sixty patients treated with amikacin. Clin. Orthop., 134:268–274, 1978.

225. Shiota, K., et al.: Suppurative coxitis due to Salmonella typhimurium in systemic lupus erythematosus. Ann. Rheum. Dis., 40:312–314, 1981.

226. Sjöquist, J., and Stålanheim, G.: Protein A from Staphylococcus aureus. IX. Complement-fixing activity of protein A-IgG complexes. J. Immunol., 103:467–473, 1969.

227. Smilack, J.D., and Goldberg, M.A.: Bone and joint infection with Arizona hinshawii: report of a case and a review of the literature. Am. J. Med. Sci., 270:503–507, 1975.

228. Smith, A.L.: Antibiotics and invasive Haemophilus influenzae. N. Engl. J. Med., 294:1,329–1,331, 1976.

229. Snyderman, R., et al.: Isolated deficiencies of the fifth and eighth components of complement (C) in two families: clinical, genetic and biologic correlations (Abstract.) J. Immunol., 120:1,799, 1978.

230. Sourek, J., et al.: Enterotoxin production by Staphylococcus aureus strains isolated from cases of chronic osteomyelitis. J. Clin. Microbiol., 9:266–268, 1979.

231. Spink, W.W.: What is chronic brucellosis? Ann. Intern. Med., 35:358–374, 1951.

232. Spira, T.J., and Kabins, S.A.: Yersinia enterocolitica septicemia with septic arthritis. Arch. Intern. Med., 136:1,305–1,308, 1976.

233. Stålenheim, G., et al.: Consumption of human complement components by complexes of IgG with protein A of Staphylococcus aureus. Immunochemistry, 10:501–507, 1973.

234. Steerman, R.L., et al.: Intrinsic defect of the polymorphonuclear leucocyte resulting in impaired chemotaxis and phagocytosis. Clin. Exp. Immunol, 9:939–946, 1971.

235. Stephens, C.G., et al.: Reactions between certain strains of pneumococci and Fc of IgG. J. Immunol., 112:1,955–1,960, 1974.

236. Tan, J.S., et al.: Persistent neutrophil dysfunction in an adult: combined defect in chemotaxis, phagocytosis and intracellular killing. Am. J. Med., 57:251–258, 1984.

237. Tauber, J.W., Polley, M.J., and Zabriskie, J.B.: Nonspecific complement activation by streptococcal structures. II. Properdin-independent initiation of the alternate pathway. J. Exp. Med., 143:1,352–1,366, 1976.

238. Taylor, B.G., et al.: Nodular pulmonary infiltrates and septic arthritis associated with Yersinia enterocolitica bacteremia. Am. Rev. Respir. Dis., 116:525–529, 1977.

239. Taylor-Robinson, D.: Mycoplasmal arthritis in man. Isr. J. Med. Sci., 17:616–621, 1981.

240. Thompson, R.L., and Wenzel, R.P.: International recognition of methicillin-resistant strain of Staphylococcus aureus. Ann. Intern. Med., 97:925–926, 1982.

241. Thorpe, M.A., and Buckwalter, J.A.: Hematogenous Proteus mirabilis osteomyelitis. Orthop., 6:865–867, 1983.

242. Tice, A.D., and Oh, W.H.: Anaerobic osteomyelitis due to Propionibacterium acnes. Orthop. Res., 7:67–69, 1978.

243. Torg, J.S., and Lammot, T.R., III: Septic arthritis of the knee due to Clostridium welchii: report of two cases. J. Bone Joint Surg., 50A:1,233–1,236, 1968.

244. Torres, J., Rathbun, H.K., and Greenbough, W.B., III: Pneumococcal arthritis: report of a case and review of the literature. Johns Hopkins Med. J., 132:234–241, 1973.

245. Torrey, J.C., and Reese, M.K.: Initial aerobic flora of newborn infants. Selective tolerance of the upper respiratory tract for bacteria. Am. J. Dis. Child., 69:208–214, 1945.

246. Tu, W.H., Shearn, M.A., and Lee, J.C.: Acute diffuse glomerulonephritis in acute staphylococcal endocarditis. Ann. Intern. Med., 71:335–341, 1969.

247. Tuazon, C.U., and Sheagren, J.N.: Staphylococcal endocarditis in parenteral drug abusers: source of the organism. Ann. Intern. Med., 82:788–790, 1975.

248. Turner, R., Schumacher, H.R., and Myers, A.: Cellular and humoral aspects of neutrophil phagocytosis in rheumatic diseases. Arthritis Rheum., 15:130, 1972.

249. Urtega, O.B., Larrea, P.R., and Calderon, J.M.: Erythromycin in human brucellosis. Antibiot. Med., 1:513–522, 1955.

250. Valenti, W.M., Trudell, R.G., and Bentley, D.W.: Factors predisposing to oropharyngeal colonization with gram-negative bacilli in the aged. N. Engl. J. Med., 298:1,108–1,111, 1978.

251. Vartinen, J., and Hurri, L.: Arthritis due to Salmonella typhimurium: report of 12 cases of migratory arthritis in association with Salmonella typhimurium infection. Acta Med. Scand., 175:771–776, 1964.

252. Vass, M., et al.: Polytenosynovitis caused by Toxoplasma gondii. J. Bone Joint Surg., 59B:229–232, 1977.

253. Vercelloti, G., et al.: Bacterial binding and aggregation to extracellular matrix proteins. Clin. Res., 31:737A, 1983.

254. Vincent, J., et al.: Septic arthritis due to Kingella (Moraxella) kingii. J. Rheumatol., 8:501–503, 1981.

255. Waldvogel, F.A., Medoff, G., and Swartz, M.N.: Osteomyelitis: a review of clinical features, therapeutic considerations and unusual aspects. N. Engl. J. Med., 282:198–206, 1970.

256. Ward, J., Cohen, A.S., and Bauer, W.: The diagnosis and therapy of acute suppurative arthritis. Arthritis Rheum., 3:522–535, 1960.

257. Ward, P.A., Lepow, I.H., and Newman, L.J.: Bacterial factors chemotactic for polymorphonuclear leukocytes. Am. J. Pathol., 52:725–736, 1968.

257a. Ward, T.T., and Steigbigel, R.T.: Acidosis of synovial fluid correlated with synovial fluid leukocytosis. Am. J. Med., 64:933–936, 1978.

258. Warren, C.P.: Arthritis associated with Salmonella infections. Ann. Rheum. Dis., 29:483–487, 1970.

259. Weaver, J.B., and Sherwood, L.: Hematogenous pyarthrosis due to bacillus Haemophilus influenzae and Corynebacterium xerosis. Surgery, 4:908–913, 1938.

260. Weber, R.G., and Ansell, B.F., Jr.: A report of a case of Klebsiella pneumoniae arthritis and a review of extrapulmonary Klebsiella infections. Ann. Intern. Med., 57:281–289, 1962.

261. Webster, A.D.B., et al.: Mycoplasma (ureaplasma) septic arthritis in hypogammaglobinemia. Br. Med. J., 1:478–479, 1981.

262. Whitaker, A.N.: The effect of previous splenectomy on the course of pneumococcal bacteriaemia in mice. J. Pathol. Bacteriol., 95:357–376, 1968.

263. White, A.A., Crelin, E.S., and McIntosh, S.: Septic arthritis of the hip joint secondary to umbilical artery catheterization associated with transient femoral and sciatic neuropathy. Clin. Orthop., 100:190–194, 1974.

264. Whitehead, J.E.M.: Bacterial resistance: changing pat-

terns of some common pathogens. Br. Med. J., 2:224–228, 1973.

265. Williams, D.N., and Geddes, A.M.: Mengococcal meningitis complicated by pericarditis, panophthalmitis, and arthritis. Br. Med. J., 2:93, 1970.

266. Williams, R.C., Jr., Dossett, J.H., and Quie, P.G.: Comparative studies of immunoglobulin opsonins in osteomyelitis and other established infections. Immunology, 17:249–265, 1969.

267. Williams, R.E.O.: Healthy carriage of Staphylococcus aureus: its prevalence and importance. Bacteriol. Rev., 27:56–71, 1963.

268. Wolff, S.M., and Bennett, J.V.: Gram-negative rod bacteremia. (Editorial.) N. Engl. J. Med., 291:733–734, 1974.

269. Wolski, K.P., and Schmid, F.R.: Modulation of immune complex formation by staphylococcal protein A (SPA). Fed. Proc., 34:1,043, 1975.

270. Yee, N.M., Katz, M., and Neu, H.C.: Meningitis, pneumonitis, and arthritis caused by Neisseria meningitidis group Y. JAMA, 232:1,354, 1975.

271. Young, E.J., and Morton, G.L.: Meningococcal arthritis simulating gonococcemia. South. Med. J., 68:636–638, 1975.

272. Yu, V.L.: Serratia marcescens: historical perspective and clinical review. N. Engl. J. Med., 300:887–893, 1979.

Chapter **102**

Arthritis Due to Mycobacteria and Fungi

Ronald P. Messner

Tuberculous and mycotic infections are relatively rare causes of arthritis. They are important because they are potentially curable. Proper diagnosis requires awareness of their clinical presentations together with identification of the organism in synovial fluid or tissue. Certain immunologic tests are helpful but do not replace the need to examine material directly from the involved joints. Constitutional symptoms and radiographic evidence of extra-articular involvement are often absent. These infections should be sought in the evaluation of patients with chronic monoarticular arthritis and should be considered in various other situations, including spondylitis, tendonitis, and erythema nodosum (Table 102–1).

TUBERCULOSIS

The incidence of new cases of tuberculosis of all types has decreased dramatically in the United States in the last 40 years. In 1932 there were 77 new cases per 100,000 population. Since 1972 the attack rate has been stable at 14 to 15 cases per 100,000. The incidence is highest in congested cities. Tuberculosis affects nonwhites six times more frequently than whites, and males twice as often as females. Patients receiving hemodialysis also appear to be at increased risk. Approximately 15% of cases involve extrapulmonary sites,[28] and 1 to 3% of patients have bone and/or joint involvement.[17,21] The rarity of bone and joint tuberculosis has lowered the index of suspicion in the medical community, which often results in unfortunate delays in diagnosis.

In the nonimmune host, primary tuberculosis begins in the lungs. It is characterized by rapid multiplication of tubercle bacilli and dissemination via blood and lymph to all parts of the body. The disease usually resolves coincident with development of delayed hypersensitivity and cellular immunity. In a few patients, it progresses and may result in disseminated tuberculosis or progressive disease limited to one or two organ systems. In contrast, tuberculosis in the immune individual is characterized by a vigorous tissue response with local necrosis but relative containment of the infection.

Dissemination does not occur unless a bronchus or blood vessel is eroded. Tuberculosis of bone can develop in three ways: by hematogenous spread, by lymphatic spread from chronic pleural, renal, or lymph node foci, or by reactivation of latent infection at sites seeded in the primary illness.[47] Involvement of joints may be direct by the hematogenous route or may occur secondary to osseous infection. Articular tuberculosis is often a combination of osteomyelitis and arthritis.[17] An inflammatory reaction in the synovium is followed by formation of granulation tissue, effusion, and production of a pannus. Cartilage destruction begins in the periphery of the joint and proceeds slowly compared to pyogenic infections. Ultimately, the process results in severe destruction of bone, cold abscesses, and sinus tract formation.

Fifty percent of skeletal tuberculosis occurs in the spine. The next most common sites are large weight-bearing joints. The hip and knee are each affected in about 15% of cases and the ankle or wrist in 5 to 10% of cases. Skeletal infection often occurs in the absence of active or even inactive pulmonary disease. The incidence of coexistent active pulmonary infection varies from 10 to 50% in various series.[39,47] Evidence of previous infection has been found in up to 40% of patients and other extrapulmonary disease in about 20% of patients. Multiple skeletal lesions are more common in children but occur in only 5 to 15% of all patients.[39]

Tuberculosis of the Spine. Classic spinal tuberculosis (Pott's disease) is seen in the first and third decades of life. Since 1935, cases in the first decade have almost disappeared.[27] The average patient is now about 25 years old. Typically, the infection starts in the margins of the vertebral bodies and invades the disc space early. The disc space narrows, destruction of bone leads to vertebral collapse with kyphosis or gibbous deformity, and a cold paraspinous abscess forms. The midthoracic to upper lumbar area is usually affected.[2,47] Skip areas with radiographically normal vertebrae in between occur in about 10% of patients. Paraspinous abscesses are common (50 to 96%) and may dissect for long distances up or down the spine or out along

Table 102–1. Typical Clinical Presentations of Arthritis Due to Tuberculosis or Mycoses

Tuberculosis	Spondylitis; monarticular disease of large weight-bearing joints.
Atypical tuberculosis	Tendonitis in hand or wrist.
Leprosy	Polyarthritis with erythema nodosum leprosum; destruction of small bones and joints of hands and feet; neuropathic wrists or ankles.
Coccidioidomycosis	Polyarthritis with erythema nodosum; monarticular arthritis of knee.
Blastomycosis	Monarticular arthritis of large weight-bearing joints associated with lung and skin involvement; spondylitis.
Cryptococcosis	Monarticular arthritis secondary to osseous infection; spondylitis.
Histoplasmosis	Polyarthritis with erythema nodosum.
Sporotrichosis	Monarticular arthritis of knee, wrist, or hand; polyarthritis with disseminated skin lesions.
Candidiasis	Monarticular arthritis of the knee in patient with serious concurrent illness.
Actinomycosis	Spondylitis

the ribs to point in the neck, groin, chest wall, or sternum.[2,47] The most common symptom is back pain.[27] Muscle spasm, local tenderness, kyphosis, and referred pain from root compression complete the typical clinical picture. Neurologic symptoms due to cord compression, Pott's paraplegia, occur in 10 to 25% of patients with spinal tuberculosis.[27,39,42,62] Kyphosis, which is more common in paraplegic patients, is associated with destructive vertebral lesions in the thoracic area more often than in the lumbar area.[2] Altered sensation is present below the level of the lesion. Lower motor neuron weakness due to coexistent root compression is sometimes observed.[27] Cerebral spinal fluid examination reveals a partial or complete block and increased protein with normal cell count and sugar.

Another complication of spinal tuberculosis is a mycotic aneurysm of the aorta, usually created when a paraspinous abscess penetrates the vessel wall. The resulting hematoma walls off to form a false aneurysm. Penetration of the abscess into the arterial blood may lead to secondary hematogenous spread and miliary disease.[23] Other notable frequent sites of tuberculosis of the axial skeleton are the sacroiliac joints and the ribs. Rib lesions are often associated with a local soft tissue mass and pain. They generally occur in patients with other skeletal involvement, particularly in the spine. The sacroiliac joint involvement, usually unilateral, occurs in about 7% of patients with skeletal tuberculosis.

Tuberculosis of Peripheral Joints. Articular tuberculosis presents as chronic monoarticular disease in approximately 85% of patients. It may develop at any age but, similar to spinal tuberculosis, cases in the first decade of life are now rare. The peak incidence is in the fourth and fifth decades. The incidence in males and nonwhites is twice that in females and whites. In the hip, tubercle bacilli may localize in the synovium, acetabulum, or proximal femur. Bony destruction is seen most commonly in the acetabulum. The femoral neck and

capital and trochanteric epiphyses are also frequent sites of involvement.[45] Symptoms include mild to moderate pain in the groin, knee, or thigh, and limitation of motion. A limp is the most common presenting complaint in children. Atrophy of the gluteal muscles and tenderness in the groin are often present. At rest, the hip is held in flexion and abduction. Later severe destruction of the femoral neck and acetabulum occurs with formation of a cold abscess and sinus tract, which usually points to the outer thigh.

In the knee, pain is the first symptom of tuberculosis in 70% of patients. It is insidious in onset and may persist for years before the patient seeks medical attention. About 20% of patients describe swelling, and 10% have stiffness as the initial complaint.[37] Localized heat and muscular wasting are usually present on examination. A limp, synovial swelling and limitation of motion are common. Although pure synovial infection does occur, most patients have involvement of both synovium and bone.[37] Symptoms in other joints are similar to those described in the hip and knee: chronic low-grade pain, swelling, and stiffness with slowly progressive loss of function and eventual abscess formation. Tuberculosis involving tendons in the hand and wrist may cause a carpal tunnel syndrome.[38] Infection of the trochanteric bursa has also been reported. A rare patient with tuberculosis may present with *acute polyarticular arthritis,* a high swinging fever, and evidence of active disease in the chest or lymph nodes (Poncet's disease). In these patients, joints are normal radiographically, and articular symptoms resolve several weeks after initiation of antituberculous drugs.[1]

Radiographic Signs. There are no pathognomonic roentgenographic signs of skeletal tuberculosis. In general, tuberculosis causes destruction of bone without stimulating much reactive new bone formation. Destructive osseous lesions adjacent to joints[47] are often oval with clear margins and no periosteal reaction (Fig. 102–1). As they

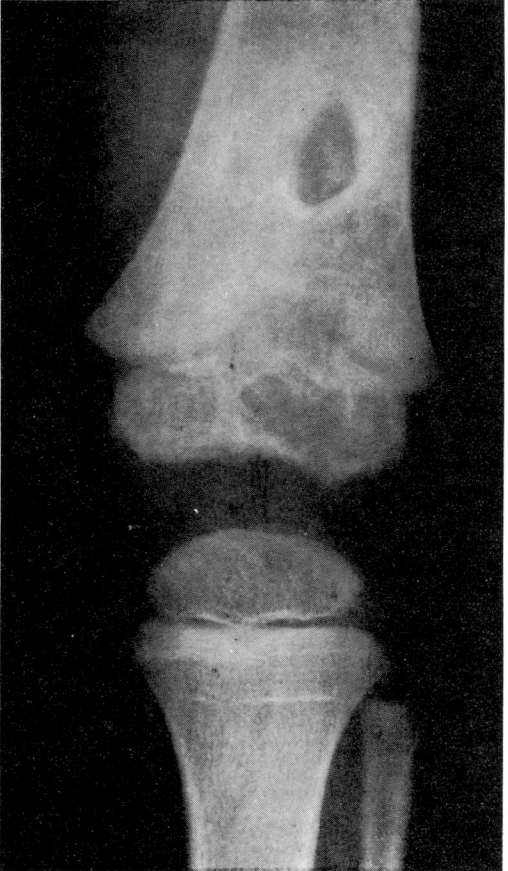

Fig. 102–1. Tuberculosis of the knee and femur in a child.

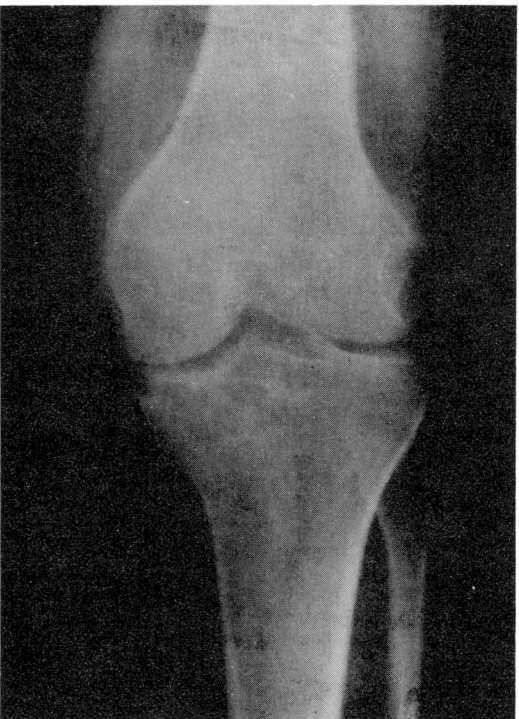

Fig. 102–2. Tuberculosis of the knee in an adult. (Courtesy of Donald Resnick, M.D.)

expand and erode the cortex, some periosteal reaction occurs. Sequestra formation is rare. When the joint itself is involved, local osteopenia and soft tissue swelling are early signs. Later small subchondral erosions appear at the margins of the joint (Fig. 102–2). The cartilage space tends to be preserved until extensive destruction of adjacent cortical bone has occurred (Fig. 102–3). With advanced disease, total destruction of the joint can occur. Destruction is not accompanied by osteophyte formation, but the shadow of a cold abscess may be seen.

In the spine, the classic picture is narrowing of the disc space with vertebral collapse and a paraspinous abscess. Scalloping of the anterior vertebral surface is common.[2] Occasional infection of the central portion of the vertebrae may cause extensive bone destruction without disc space invasion. In about 10% of patients, productive or sclerotic changes, that are difficult to see radiographically, may occur in infected vertebrae.

Diagnostic Tests. Diagnosis of tuberculous arthritis requires an index of suspicion and willingness to obtain material for histologic examination and culture. The quickest and most reliable method of diagnosis is biopsy. A positive diagnosis can be made by either histology or culture of synovial tissue in over 90% of specimens. Synovial fluid culture is positive in approximately 80% and smear in 20% of cases.[9,57] Synovial fluid protein is always elevated, whereas 60% of fluids have low glucose levels. The synovial white blood cell count varies widely, but averages between 10,000 and 20,000/mm³. Polymorphonuclear leukocytes may account for 90% of the total white cell count.[57] The Mantoux test with stabilized purified protein derivative (PPD-S) is positive in most cases of skeletal tuberculosis. In advanced disease or old age, anergy may be present. Anergy may be nonspecific or it may be specific for PPD-S.

Treatment. The keystone of treatment of skeletal tuberculosis is the use of a combination of chemotherapeutic agents. Because skeletal infection is rare compared to pulmonary involvement, the bulk of information on therapy comes from experience with pulmonary disease. The recommended initial combination is isoniazid (5 to 10

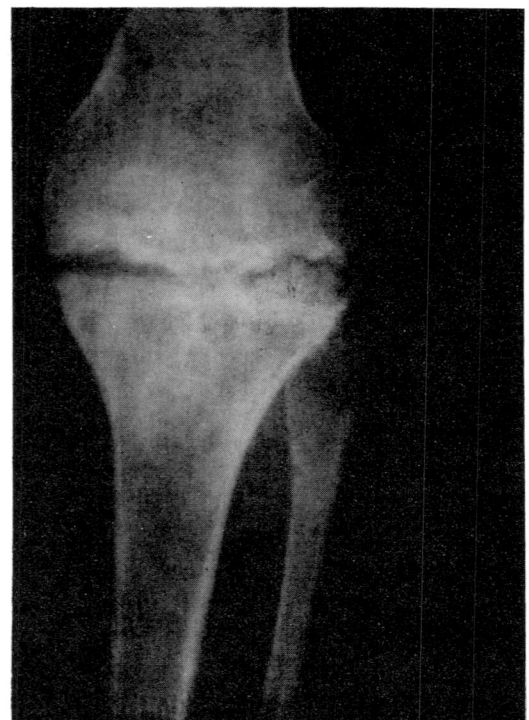

Fig. 102–3. Advanced tuberculosis of the knee. (Courtesy of Donald Resnick, M.D.)

mg/kg, up to 300 mg po daily) and rifampin (10 to 20 mg/kg, up to 600 mg po daily). Ethambutol, 15 mg/kg daily, should be added until drug sensitivity is confirmed if the patient has emigrated from an area with a known high level of initial drug resistance or has a history of previous antituberculosis chemotherapy.[24,28,55] The optimum duration of treatment of skeletal tuberculosis has not been defined. Short-course therapy using isoniazid or rifampin for 9 months has proved equal or superior to other regimens in initial treatment of pulmonary disease. It has been suggested that this form of treatment may also be adequate for extrapulmonary disease,[20] but until its efficacy is proved it seems wise to use the two drugs for at least a year. The major contraindication to the combined use of isoniazid and rifampin is the presence of active liver disease. If alternative drug combinations are used, treatment must be continued for 18 to 24 months.

The role of surgery is more controversial, but some general guidelines can be drawn. In articular disease with absent or minimal bone involvement, drug therapy alone is effective. If bone involvement is more extensive, synovectomy with debridement of foci of bone infection may hasten healing. Synovectomy with curettage may be especially im-

portant in children with hip disease.[45] When destruction is extensive in weight-bearing joints, arthrodesis has been the procedure of choice. In developing countries where sitting cross-legged and squatting are important, Girdlestone excision arthroplasty has been used effectively for hip disease.[54] Experience suggests that total hip replacement may be successful if the active infection is controlled.[34] With respect to spinal tuberculosis, 85% of patients heal in 3 years, with an average 15° increase in kyphosis when given outpatient chemotherapy. No advantage is gained with 6 months of bed rest or spinal immobilization. A similar percentage heals in less time with no increase in kyphosis if surgical fusion is performed.[30] The decision to operate on these patients may be influenced by the availability of surgical facilities and by socioeconomic factors. All patients with paraplegia or paraparesis secondary to Pott's disease should have operative treatment. Many of these individuals show a gratifying recovery of neurologic function.

Atypical Tuberculosis

Atypical mycobacteria are ubiquitous, generally saprophytic organisms that have low pathogenicity for man and do not cause disease in guinea pigs. Surveys with skin tests have shown that up to 48% of healthy young adults have developed delayed hypersensitivity to various members of this group. In addition to producing pulmonary disease resembling typical tuberculosis, these mycobacteria can infect joints, tendons, and bursae. Patients with arthritis rarely have active pulmonary disease. Approximately 50% of patients with articular disease have involvement of tendon sheaths or joints in the hand and wrist, while 20% have infection of the knee.[32,51] Infection in the hip, elbow, ankle, and prepatellar and olecranon bursae as well as in periarticular tissue simulating arthritis have also been described. Several patients with flexor tendonitis at the wrist have had carpal tunnel syndrome. Polyarticular disease has occurred in about 15% of patients. A history of prior trauma or operation has been obtained in 45% of patients, and 36% have had prior intra-articular injection of corticosteroids. About one-quarter of these patients have an underlying illness, most commonly another form of arthritis, such as degenerative joint disease, rheumatoid arthritis, or systemic lupus. The group I photochromogens *Mycobacterium kansasii* and *M. marinum* are the most frequent offenders, followed by the group III nonphotochromogen *M. intracellularis*.

Skin testing with PPDs prepared from atypical mycobacteria correlates well with culture results in children. In adults, cross-reactivity between various PPDs can lead to confusion.[16] Microscopic examination of synovial fluid or biopsy material may reveal granuloma and acid-fast bacilli, but definitive diagnosis of the type of infection requires culture. Although data are not as plentiful on atypical infections, it appears that the yield of positive cultures from biopsies and synovial fluid will be similar to that obtained with *M. tuberculosis.* Treatment should be based on in vitro sensitivity testing because these organisms are often resistant to the standard antituberculosis drug regimen. A combination of four or five drugs and/or synovectomy may be necessary.

LEPROSY

"Those suffering from 'ta feng' have stiff joints, the eyebrows and beard fall off." This quotation from the Chinese medical writings of the "Nei Ching" dates back to approximately 600 B.C. It is believed to be one of the earliest descriptions of leprosy.[11] The "stiff joints" described by these ancient physicians may occur in several ways. The indolent course of leprosy is punctuated by reactions. In *lepromatous leprosy,* these reactions take the form of erythema nodosum leprosum, in which inflamed subcutaneous nodules develop in crops. This condition may be accompanied by fever and arthralgia, or by a frank polyarthritis that involves small joints of the hands, knees, and ankles. Synovial biopsy reveals an acute inflammatory reaction.[35] In most patients, lepra organisms are not detected in the synovium, and the synovial fluid is a transudate.[35,46] It has been postulated that this form of arthritis has an immunologic basis. However, group III fluid, which contains lepra cells with ingested organisms and high synovial fluid complement values, has been found, suggesting that the synovitis in some patients is due to infection.[42] Reactions in *tuberculoid* or borderline leprosy may also be accompanied by joint symptoms which on occasion may simulate rheumatoid arthritis.[46] Another form of arthritis occurs secondary to bone disease. *Direct infection of bone* occurs most commonly in the distal ends of the phalanges. During a reaction, subchondral bone may collapse and cause destruction of the adjacent joint.[35,48]

The most common joint deformities in leprosy occur secondary to disease in the peripheral nerves. Neurotrophic changes lead to absorption of bones, especially in the distal ends of the metatarsals. Sensory loss and repeated trauma are responsible for degenerative changes and aseptic necrosis of bone. These changes, accompanied by infection in soft tissue and bone, are responsible for loss of terminal digits and severe deformities of the hands and feet.[48] The claw hand that occurs secondary to nerve damage can further compound the disability.

Finally, true neuropathic joints with complete disorganization of the weight-bearing surfaces and supporting bone may occur. Charcot joints are most frequently seen at the wrist and ankle.

One of the most puzzling aspects of leprosy is why some patients develop the lepromatous form of diffuse involvement with anergy and large numbers of bacilli present in macrophages, whereas others develop the tuberculoid form of more localized disease with well-organized lymphocyte-rich granulomas containing few viable organisms. Recent data reveal that the T-lymphocytes in lepromatous lesions belong primarily to the OKT8/Leu2a positive suppressor subset, whereas those in the tuberculoid lesions are predominantly OKT4/Leu3a positive helper cells.[56] It has been postulated that the predominance of suppressor cells in the lepromatous form reduces the production of lymphokines, which are critical to effective macrophage killing of the organisms. Whether the different types of reaction to infection relate to genetic factors or to the route of inoculation and whether treatment aimed at reducing T-suppressor activity will prove useful are questions of intense research interest.[49] Fortunately for man but not armadillos, the latter has been found to provide an excellent host for the growth of *Mycobacterium leprae* and now provides a rich source of organisms for research and potentially for development of a vaccine.

The diagnosis of leprosy rests on demonstration of acid-fast bacilli in skin smears and histologic evidence of lepra organisms with involvement of peripheral nerves on skin biopsy. From a clinical standpoint, the cardinal sign is anesthesia of the skin. Typically, thermal and tactile senses are lost before pain and pressure. The ulnar and peroneal nerves frequently are involved early.

Treatment of leprosy requires a coordinated effort that includes attention to the social needs of the patient as well as specialized drug therapy and physical measures to protect the skin and joints and to reduce contractures. In response to the increasing incidence of primary and secondary dapsone resistance, the World Health Organization now recommends the use of three drugs for patients with multibacillary disease: dapsone, rifampin, and clofazimine. Dapsone and rifampin are recommended for those with paucibacillary disease.[49] In the United States, patients with leprosy are entitled to treatment by the U.S. Public Health Service.

COCCIDIOIDOMYCOSIS

Coccidioidomycosis is caused by a fungus found in the soil throughout the lower Sonoran life zone. This zone includes semiarid areas of southern California, Arizona, and New Mexico as well as western Texas. It is characterized by hot summers, moderately wet winters, and infrequent freezes. The fungus multiplies in the soil after the winter rains, resulting in a higher incidence of disease in the summer months.[25] Primary infection occurs 1 to 3 weeks after inhalation of spores. Clinical signs, which are usually self-limited, include fever, malaise, cough, chest pain, and erythema nodosum. A chronic pulmonary infection closely resembling tuberculosis occurs in about 2% of patients, whereas 0.2% develop widely disseminated disease. Dissemination is more common in black and Filipino males. Patients with collagen vascular disease or lymphomas who are taking corticosteroids may be at greater risk, but this association is not as striking as that seen with some other fungal infections.[4]

Arthritis occurs in both the benign primary illness and the chronic disseminated form. In primary disease, it is usually associated with erythema nodosum and clears without residual deformity. In chronic disseminated disease, arthritis may occur alone or secondary to bone infection. Bayer et al. have reviewed 57 cases of coccidioidal arthritis.[5] The most common presentation was a chronic monoarticular arthritis of the knee. The mean age was 36 years, and males outnumbered females by 4 to 1. Patients were otherwise in good health. Only 10% had a major underlying illness. A history of antecedent arthritis or joint injury was rare. Similarly, only 10% had evidence of coccidioidal infection in extra-articular sites. If the organisms seeded directly to synovium, symptoms of an indolent synovitis with effusion, stiffness, and mild pain dominated the early course. If infection began in adjacent bone with later penetration into the joint, the early signs were pain and loss of motion without effusion. In either case, untreated synovial infection gradually progressed to villous hypertrophy and pannus formation, which often led to bony erosive changes later in the course. The indolent nature of this process is reflected in the long interval from onset of symptoms to diagnosis, a mean of 4.5 years. Its destructive nature is clear; fully 42% of patients had radiologically evident destructive changes and/or adjacent osteomyelitis at diagnosis. The knee was involved in 70% of cases, and the wrist, hand, and the ankle were the next most commonly affected sites.

Infection of bone occurs in 10 to 20% of patients with disseminated disease. Sites most often involved are the ends of the long bones, the skull, vertebrae, and ribs. Metacarpals, metatarsals, the tibial tubercle, the malleoli, and the acromial process also appear to be favorite sites of localization.[18] In one series of 72 cases of coccidioidal osteomyelitis, 58% of patients had involvement of a single site, whereas only 17% had infection in three or more sites.[33] Multiple bone lesions are associated with rapid dissemination and a poorer prognosis. In the more indolent forms of disseminated disease, solitary bone lesions are common. The course of these solitary lesions is one of slow destruction of bone that may progress to involve adjacent joints.

Most joint infections have been diagnosed by culture or histologic examination of synovial tissue. Fewer than 5% of synovial fluid cultures have been positive. In purulent material, the characteristic spherules are best seen after digestion with 20% potassium hydroxide. *Coccidioides immitis* can be cultured on Sabouraud's agar. It is important to notify the bacteriology laboratory if coccidioidomycosis is suspected because the spore-forming mycelial cultures are highly infectious. Although most patients with disseminated coccidioidomycosis are anergic, 80% of those with coccidioidal arthritis have a positive skin test to coccidioidin. Serologic tests may also be helpful. The tube precipitation test is useful for detecting early primary disease. It is positive within 1 to 3 weeks of infection in 80% of cases, reverts to negative after 6 months, but becomes positive again with relapse or reinfection. In disseminated disease, complement fixation (CF) and immunodiffusion tests are usually positive. Ninety percent of patients with coccidioidal arthritis have positive CF tests. Circulating immune complexes containing coccidioidin antigen have been found in most patients with active disease. It has been suggested that these complexes or free anticoccidioidin antibodies may play a role in the depressed T-lymphocyte responses that may accompany progressive disease.[62]

If the diagnosis is made prior to bone involvement, the development of villonodular synovitis, or pannus formation, treatment with amphotericin B alone may be effective. If any of these events have occurred, drug treatment should be combined with surgery.[5] Intra-articular amphotericin B has been used with success for a few patients.[61] Ketoconazole, a broad-spectrum fungistatic agent with relatively low toxicity, has been approved recently for use in coccidioidomycosis. It can be given orally and requires gastric acid for absorption. About 80% of patients with osteoarticular disease have shown good initial response. Unfortunately, 40% have relapsed either on the drug or after it has been discontinued.[10,50] It should thus be considered second choice to amphotericin B.

BLASTOMYCOSIS

In the continental United States, blastomycosis occurs primarily in the Ohio and Mississippi river valleys and middle Atlantic States. Peak incidence is in the 20- to 50-year age group. Males are affected 10 times more often than females,[26] presumably owing to their greater exposure through outdoor activities.[52] There is only one documented case of human-to-human transmission. Despite the unique susceptibility of dogs to infection, dog-to-human transmission has been documented in only one instance of a bite from an infected animal. Infection, which begins in the lungs after inhalation of spores, may produce a variety of results ranging from an asymptomatic or acute self-limited illness to acutely or insidiously progressive disease. Extrapulmonary infection spreads from the lungs by lymphatic or hematogenous routes. Skin and bone are the most frequent sites. Skeletal involvement occurs in one-third of patients, and in one large series 3.3% presented with joint pain.[13]

Articular blastomycosis usually presents as an acute monarticular synovitis in a patient who is systemically ill with pulmonary and multifocal extrapulmonary disease. Fully 90% of these patients have active lung infections, and 70% have cutaneous abscesses.[7] The knee is the most frequently involved joint, followed by the ankle and elbow. In approximately 70% of patients joint infection results from hematogenous seeding to synovium; in 30% it is a consequence of extension of an underlying osteomyelitis. Osseous blastomycosis is most common in the vertebrae, ribs, tibia, tarsus, and skull, although involvement of almost every site in bone has been reported. Direct extension into the joint is most often seen at the knee. Spinal infection is associated with destruction of disc spaces, erosion of anterior vertebral bodies, development of paraspinal soft tissue and dissection of the infection beneath the anterior longitudinal ligament. Blastomycosis may also erode into the ribs, where they articulate with the transverse processes.[26] Vertebral infection usually occurs in the thoracic and/or lumbar areas, but is rare in the cervical spine.

Blastomyces dermatitidis organisms may be seen on direct smear of synovial fluid, sputum, or material from abscesses by routine hematoxylin and eosin stain. They are easier to identify after potassium hydroxide digestion or with periodic acid-Schiff reagent.[26] Definitive diagnosis is made on culture. An immunodiffusion test using the A and B antigens of the yeast phase of the organism is specific for *B. dermatitidis* and has a sensitivity of 80%. The drug of choice for treatment of blastomycotic arthritis is amphotericin B. Ketoconazole appears to be moderately effective in disseminated blastomycosis, but should be considered as a second-choice drug on the basis of available information.[18,31] Although the role of operative treatment has not been fully defined, it appears to be of benefit in debridement of devitalized bone or synovium in patients who fail to respond to antifungal drugs.[52]

CRYPTOCOCCOSIS

Infection with *Cryptococcus neoformans* begins in the lungs with inhalation of spores and spreads to other organs, especially the central nervous system. Predisposing factors for susceptibility to this disease include lymphoma, Hodgkin's disease, diabetes mellitus, sarcoidosis, and corticosteroid treatment.[41] The organism is widely distributed in nature. The most dangerous source of infection appears to be pigeon droppings. Rarely, involvement of the joints occurs secondary to infection in adjacent bone, which occurs in only about 10% of patients.[12] Bone infection follows a slowly progressive course. Radiologic changes consist of lytic lesions with sharply scalloped margins and little reaction in adjacent bone or periosteum. These lesions may be found in the metaphyses of long bones, in the flat bones or vertebrae, the ribs, tarsal bones, or carpal bones. Vertebral infection resulting in paraspinal abscess formation can mimic tuberculosis. Only a few detailed reports of cryptococcal arthritis exist in the literature.[3,40] Most involved the knee and were monarticular. About half of these patients had an identifiable underlying illness, including renal transplantation, disseminated histoplasmosis, or possible sarcoidosis. Some synovial fluids were grossly purulent whereas others had a relatively low white count of about 2,000 cells/mm³.

Serologic tests for antibody to cryptococcal antigens are positive in fewer than 50% of proved cases. Cryptococcal antigens in sera or synovial fluid have been detected by agglutination of latex particles coated with rabbit anticryptococcal antibody. Rheumatoid factors can react with rabbit IgG and give a false positive test.[36] Amphotericin B given in combination with 5-fluorocytosine is the recommended treatment.[3] Early reports on the use of ketoconazole are encouraging,[18] but more experience is needed with this fungistatic drug to determine its true efficacy. Although debridement of joints may also be advisable, the data are insufficient to conclude whether medical or combined medical-surgical treatment is more effective.

HISTOPLASMOSIS

Histoplasma capsulatum grows in mycelial form in soil where it produces spores that infect man when inhaled. It thrives in ground contaminated with chicken, bird, or bat excreta. The highest incidence of positive histoplasmin skin tests occurs in individuals from states adjacent to the confluence of the Mississippi and Ohio rivers. In this area, 60 to 90% of young men are positive. Fortunately, both primary infection and reinfection are usually benign self-limited diseases. Symptoms range from a transient pneumonitis to more generalized disease characterized by fever, malaise, chest pain, dyspnea, and weight loss.[29] An acute polyarthritis may occur in association with erythema nodosum,[58] and polyarthritis or an additive polyarthralgia may be the presenting symptom of primary histoplasmosis.[53] Both types of joint involvement clear without residual deformity.

Progressive disease occurs in only 5% of infected individuals. The most common form is a localized pulmonary infection in middle-aged white men. Disseminated histoplasmosis occurs in fewer than 0.1% of infections, usually in older or immune-compromised individuals. Its manifestations are protean, and prognosis is poor. In the chronic form of disease, arthritis is truly an unusual clinical problem. Chronic infection of the knee (both unilateral and bilateral) and of the wrist have been reported.[3] The diagnosis depends upon demonstration of *H. capsulatum* in histologic sections or culture of involved tissues. Immunologic tests play a minor role in diagnosis. In sensitized individuals, the histoplasmin skin test may induce antibodies that will influence serologic tests drawn more than a few days after the skin test. The complement fixation test is positive in 90% of patients, but may also be positive in other fungal diseases. The immunodiffusion test is more specific and should be used together with the complement fixation test. The tube agglutination test, a useful screen in patients with acute primary disease, is often negative in chronic disease.[36]

SPOROTRICHOSIS

Sporotrichosis is a rare form of chronic granulomatous arthritis caused by a ubiquitous fungus that lives on plants or in the soil. Infection with this organism is usually limited to the skin, where it begins as a painful red nodule at the site of a scratch or a thorn prick. Cutaneous sporotrichosis may spread proximally by lymphatics to form multiple necrotic secondary satellite lesions, or it may penetrate directly into adjacent tissues. Only a small percentage of people exposed to the fungus develop the systemic form of infection. In a review of 3,300 cases from South Africa, only 5 systemic infections were reported.

Systemic sporotrichosis occurs primarily in men 40 years of age or older.[43] It has been associated with outdoor occupations or hobbies, alcohol abuse, and diseases or drugs that compromise the immune system. In many patients, however, it develops without history or predisposing factors. Two forms of the disease have been described: unifocal and multifocal.[60] Unifocal systemic sporotrichosis

most commonly affects the lungs as cavitary disease of the upper lobes closely resembling tuberculosis. The other common presentation is as a chronic monarthritis or oligoarthritis. Morning stiffness and fever are absent, but synovial thickening and effusions are found in the involved joints. A history of transient improvement with intra-articular steroids but poor response to oral steroids or aspirin may be obtained. The knee is most often involved, followed in decreasing frequency by the wrist, small joints of the hand, ankle, and elbow. Tenosynovitis may occur in the hand or wrist.[8]

Multifocal systemic sporotrichosis typically involves the skin, joints, and bones. These patients are more likely to have a compromised immune system than those who develop unifocal disease. Skin lesions differ from those in cutaneous sporotrichosis. Dusty red nodules up to several centimeters in diameter develop randomly any place on the body except the palms and soles. The lesions eventually ulcerate and may heal while new ones appear. The skin around joints, on the face, and on the scalp is most often involved.[43] Skin lesions usually precede joint symptoms. In this form of the disease, the arthritis is polyarticular in about two-thirds of patients. As in the unifocal form, tendonitis may be present, and fistulas may develop after surgical procedures on the joints if proper antifungal therapy is not given. Infection of bones spares the vertebrae, ribs, and jaw, but involves long bones near the joints. Joint infection is rarely related to extension of osseous infection. Pulmonary involvement occurs in fewer than 20% of patients with multifocal disease. It differs from unifocal lung disease in that nodules are smaller and do not cavitate.[43] Central nervous system involvement is rare.

Diagnosis of sporotrichosis arthritis rests on culture of *Sporothrix schenckii* from joint fluid or synovial tissue. Both have yielded positive results, but the percentage of positives appears to be higher with cultures of tissue. The best yield occurs with culture of both tissue and fluid. The organisms are difficult to see in tissue sections. The sedimentation rate is elevated, but peripheral white blood counts are normal. Joint fluid shows the pattern of low-grade inflammation with cell counts of 8,000 to 20,000/mm³, a fair to good mucin clot, and decreased glucose concentration.[8,43] Two serologic tests are available for diagnosis. The latex slide test is preferred because it has fewer false positive reactions and comparable sensitivity (94%) to the tube agglutination test. Titers of 1:4 or greater are presumptive evidence of active disease.[36] Soft tissue swelling, osteoporosis, decreased joint space, and erosions similar to those occurring in rheumatoid arthritis may be seen radiographically.

Treatment consists of amphotericin B alone or in combination with surgical debridement of infected joints.[8] In a patient unable to tolerate amphotericin B, iodide therapy plus surgical debridement may be a reasonable alternative. Reports of treatment with ketoconazole have not been encouraging.[18] Results of treatment of unifocal disease are usually excellent. The main cause of poor results is a long delay between onset of disease and diagnosis. The outcome of multifocal sporotrichosis is less certain. In one report, 11 deaths occurred in 37 patients with this form of disease.[43]

CANDIDA ARTHRITIS

Arthritis due to Candida species has been reported with increasing frequency in the past several years. An underlying illness or direct predisposing cause has been present in all patients. Two-thirds of the adults were hospitalized with a serious illness, such as cancer, renal failure, sepsis, or a connective tissue disease. Most were receiving antibiotics, chemotherapy, or immunosuppressive treatment and often had indwelling intravenous catheters.[6,22] The remainder of the adults were ambulatory. In these instances, predisposing causes included osteoarthritis with repeated corticosteroid injections, recent joint surgery, and previous joint infection. Heroin addiction has also been noted as a predisposing cause. A distinctive syndrome of follicular and nodular lesions of the scalp, beard, and pubis with ocular infection or osteoarticular lesions of the intervertebral discs, knee, or chondrocostal junctions has been noted in this group of individuals.[19] Ninety percent of children with candidal arthritis have been less than one year old. All have had a serious underlying illness, and most were critically ill from other causes at the time the arthritis was diagnosed. As in adults, antibiotics, immunosuppression, and catheters were frequently implicated as predisposing causes. Candidal arthritis may occur in as many as 2% of infants receiving hyperalimentation.[63] Only one case has been reported in association with chronic mucocutaneous candidiasis.

In both adults and children, the knee is involved in 75% of cases. The hip and shoulder are the next most frequently involved joints. Small joint involvement is rare. Multiple joint infections occur about twice as often in infants as in adults (35 vs. 15%), and coexistent osteomyelitis is more common in infants. Infection seeds from the blood to the synovium and may follow fungal septicemia by intervals of 2 to 12 weeks. Symptoms include pain, tenderness, synovial thickening, and effusion, but red hot joints are infrequent. Typically,

the synovial fluid contains a mean of 38,000 leukocytes/mm³ with 80% polymorphonuclear leukocytes, but lower counts may be found in patients with leukemia.[22] Synovial fluid glucose has been lower in 70% of reported cases. Culture of synovial fluid is a highly reliable method for identifying Candida species. The Gram's stain is not reliable, however, being negative in 80% of culture-positive samples. *Candida albicans* is the most frequent offender followed by *C. tropicalis*. Serologic tests for serum antibodies to *C. albicans* antigens may show a rising titer with dissemination of infection, but these tests do not clearly differentiate heavy colonization from systemic disease.

The relatively small number of reported cases makes it difficult to draw firm conclusions regarding optimum treatment. Amphotericin B alone has resulted in eradication of the infection in about 60% of cases in which it has been used. The failure rate appears to be somewhat less if it is combined with operation or 5-fluorocytosine. The latter drug alone is not a good choice. Recently, a few reports on the successful use of ketoconazole have appeared.[19] Overall, 60% of adults and 40% of infants have recovered with normal joint function. Twenty percent of patients in both groups have died of Candida sepsis or of the underlying disease. The remainder have survived with significant disability resulting from destruction of the joint.

ACTINOMYCOSIS

Actinomycosis is caused by an anaerobic bacteria-like obligate parasite, *Actinomyces israelii*, which is a normal resident of the human mouth. Infection occurs through the gastrointestinal tract, particularly after dental procedures or injury to the mouth and jaw. It may also follow aspiration into an atelectatic portion of lung. Abscesses form in the neck, jaw, lung, or abdomen. Bone involvement is frequent in the jaw and spine, and is usually secondary to abscesses in adjacent tissues. Infection of the spine typically involves several vertebrae, but not the intervening discs. Adjacent pedicles, transverse processes, and the heads of contiguous ribs may be eroded. In the vertebrae, channels of infection surrounded by sclerotic bone cause a honeycomb or soap bubble radiographic appearance.[14] Long, dense, longitudinal spurs and sclerotic changes in the lateral portions of the vertebrae are sometimes seen when infection spreads from the abdomen to the spine via the psoas muscle. Dense trabeculae and sclerosis make vertebral collapse uncommon.[15] Any level of the spine may be affected. Symptoms vary from mild local pain to severe restriction of motion, radicular pain, or weakness. Extension of the infection into the spinal canal may result in meningitis. Diagnosis is made by identification of "sulfur granules" on Gram's stain of pus from the abscesses and is confirmed by growth of the organism in anaerobic culture. Blood cultures are rarely positive. No serologic test is currently available for actinomycosis. Treatment with tetracycline has been successful, but penicillin is the drug of choice.[59]

MYCETOMA (MADUROMYCOSIS, MADURA FOOT)

Mycetoma is an indolent tumor-like infection found in tropical and semitropical climates. It is caused by a variety of actinomycetes or fungi that gain entrance through the skin. *Petriellidium boydii* is the most common cause in North America, whereas *Nocardia brasiliensis* is the usual cause in Central and South America. Mycetoma commonly involves the foot, where it invades subcutaneous tissue, bone, and ligaments.[44] In long-standing cases, swelling, sinus formation, and clubbing with marked deformity may occur. A similar process may involve the hand. Systemic symptoms and regional lymphadenopathy are uncommon. Effective treatment requires accurate identification of the infecting organism, prolonged high-dose administration of the appropriate antimicrobial agent, and surgical debridement. Prognosis depends to some extent upon the causative organism and is better with actinomycotic than with true fungal mycetoma. In some cases, amputation may be necessary.

REFERENCES

1. Allen, S.C.: A case in favor of Poncet's disease. Br. Med. J., *283*:952, 1981.
2. Bailey, H.L., et al.: Tuberculosis of the spine in children: Operative findings and results in one hundred consecutive patients. J. Bone Joint Surg., *54*:1633–1657, 1972.
3. Bayer, A.S., et al.: Fungal arthritis. V. Cryptococcal and histoplasmal arthritis. Semin. Arthritis Rheum., *9*:218–227, 1980.
4. Bayer, A.S., et al.: Unusual syndromes of coccidioidomycosis: Diagnostic and therapeutic considerations. Medicine, *55*:131–152, 1976.
5. Bayer, A.S., and Guze, L.B.: Fungal arthritis. II. Coccidioidal synovitis: Clinical, diagnostic, therapeutic and prognostic considerations. Semin. Arthritis Rheum., *8*:200–211, 1979.
6. Bayer, A.S., and Guze, L.B.: Fungal arthritis. Part I. Candida arthritis. Semin. Arthritis Rheum., *3*:142–150, 1978.
7. Bayer, A.S., Scott, V.J., and Guze, L.B.: Fungal arthritis. IV. Blastomycotic arthritis. Semin. Arthritis Rheum., *9*:145–151, 1979.
8. Bayer, A.S., Scott, V.J., and Guze, L.B.: Fungal arthritis. III. Sporotrichal arthritis. Semin. Arthritis Rheum., *9*:66–74, 1979.
9. Berney, S., Goldstein, M., and Bishko, F.: Clinical and diagnostic features of tuberculous arthritis. Am. J. Med., *53*:36–42, 1972.
10. Catanzaro, A., et al.: Treatment of coccidioidomycosis with ketoconazole: An evaluation utilizing a new scoring system. Am. J. Med., *74*:64–69, 1983.
11. Cochrane, R.G., and Davey, T.F.: Leprosy in Theory and Practice. Baltimore, Williams & Wilkins, 1964, p. 3.
12. Collins, V.P.: Bone involvement in cryptococcosis (torulosis). Am. J. Roentgenol., *63*:102, 1950.
13. Cooperative Study of the Veterans Administration: Blastomycosis: A review of 198 collected cases in Veterans Administration hospitals. Am. Rev. Respir. Dis., *89*:659–672, 1964.
14. Cope, Z.: Actinomycosis of bone with special reference to infection of the vertebral column. J. Bone Joint Surg., *33*:205–214, 1951.
15. Crank, R.N., Sundaram, M., and Shields, J.B.: Case report 197. Skeletal Radiol., *8*:164–167, 1982.
16. David, H.L., and Selin, M.J.: Immune response to mycobacteria. *In* Manual of Clinical Immunology. Edited by N.R. Rose,and H. Friedmann. Washington, D.C., American Society for Microbiology, 1980, p. 520–525.
17. Davidson, P.T., and Horowitz, I.: Skeletal tuberculosis. Am. J. Med., *48*:77–84, 1970.
18. Dismukes, W.E., et al.: Treatment of systemic mycosis with ketoconazole: Emphasis on toxicity and clinical response in 52 patients. Ann. Intern. Med., *98*:13–20, 1983.
19. Drouhet, E., and Dupont, B.: Laboratory and clinical assessment of ketoconazole in deep seated mycosis. Am. J. Med., *74*:30–47, 1983.
20. Dutt, A.K., and Stead, W.W.: Chemotherapy of tuberculosis for the 1980's. Clin. Chest. Med., *1*:243–252, 1980.
21. Enarsen, D.A., et al.: Bone and joint tuberculosis: A continuing problem. Can. Med. Assoc. J., *120*:139–145, 1979.
22. Fainstein, V., et al.: Septic arthritis due to Candida species in patients with cancer: Report of 5 cases and review of literature. Rev. Infect. Dis., *4*:78–85, 1982.
23. Felson, B., et al.: Mycotic tuberculous aneurysm of the thoracic aorta. J.A.M.A., *237*:1104–1108, 1977.
24. Fox, W.: Whither short-course chemotherapy. Br. J. Dis. Chest., *75*:331–357, 1981.
25. Friese, M.J.: Coccidioidomycosis, Springfield, Illinois, Charles C Thomas, 1958, pp. 53–77.
26. Gehweiler, J.A., Capp, P.M., and Chick, E.W.: Observations on the roentgen patterns in blastomycosis of bone. Am. J. Roent. Rad. Ther. Nucl. Med., *108*:497–510, 1970.
27. Ginsburg, S., et al.: The neurological complications of tuberculous spondylitis. Arch. Neurol., *16*:265–276, 1967.
28. Glassworth, J., Robins, A.G., and Snider, D.E.J.: Tuberculosis in the 1980's. N. Engl. J. Med., *302*:1441–1450, 1980.
29. Goodwin, R.A., Jr., and Des Prez, R.M.: Pathogenesis and clinical spectrum of histoplasmosis. South. Med. J., *66*:13–25, 1973.
30. Griffiths, D.L.: The treatment of tuberculosis in bone and joint. Trans. R. Soc. Trop. Med. Hyg., *72*:559–563, 1978.
31. Hermans, P.E., and Keys, T.F.: Antifungal agents used for deep mycotic infections. Mayo Clin. Proc., *58*:223–231, 1983.
32. Hoffman, G.S., et al.: Septic arthritis associated with mycobacterium avium: A case report and literature review. J. Rheumatol., *5*:199–209, 1978.
33. Iger, M., and Larson, J.: Coccidioidomycosis. Edited by L. Ajello. Tucson, University of Arizona Press, 1967.
34. Jupiter, J.B., et al.: Total hip arthroplasty in the treatment of adult hips with current or quiescent sepsis. J. Bone Joint. Surg., *63A*:194–200, 1981.
35. Karat, A.B.A., et al.: An exudative arthritis in leprosy—Rheumatoid arthritis-like syndrome in association with erythema nodosum leprosum. Br. Med. J., *3*:770–772, 1967.
36. Kaufman, L.: Serodiagnosis of fungal diseases. *In* Manual of Clinical Immunology. Edited by N.R. Rose, and H. Friedman. Washington, D.C., American Society for Microbiology, 1980, pp.553–572.
37. Key, L.A.: Tuberculosis of the knee joint in adults. Br. Med. J., *1*:408, 1940.
38. Klofkorn, R.W., and Steigerwald, J.C.: Carpal tunnel syndrome as the initial manifestation of tuberculosis. Am. J. Med., *60*:583–586, 1976.
39. La Fond, E.M.: An analysis of adult skeletal tuberculosis. J. Bone Joint Surg., *40*:346–364, 1958.
40. Leff, R.D., et al.: Cryptococcal arthritis after renal transplantation. South. Med. J., *74*:1290, 1981.

41. Lewis, J.L., and Rabinovich, S.: Wide spectrum of cryptococcal infections. Am. J. Med., *53*:315–322, 1972.

42. Louie, J.S., and Glovsky, M.: Complement determinations in the synovial fluid and serum of a patient with erythema nodosum leprosum. Int. J. Lepr., *43*:252–255, 1975.

43. Lynch, P.J., Voorhees, J.J., and Harrell, E.R.: Systemic sporotrichosis. Ann. Intern. Med., *73*:23–30, 1970.

44. Mariat, F., Destembes, P., and Segretain, G.: The mycetomas: Clinical features, pathology and epidemiology. Contrib. Microbiol. Immunol., *4*:1–39, 1977.

45. Marmor, L., et al.: Surgical treatment of tuberculosis of the hip in children. Clin. Orthop., *67*:133–142, 1967.

46. Modi, T.H., and Lele, R.D.: Acute joint manifestations in leprosy. J. Assoc. Physicians India, *17*:247–254, 1969.

47. Nathanson, L., and Cohen, W.: A statistical and roentgen analysis of two hundred cases of bone and joint tuberculosis. Radiology, *36*:550–567, 1941.

48. Paterson, D.E., and Job, C.K.: Leprosy in Theory and Practice. Baltimore, Williams & Wilkins, 1964, p. 425.

49. Shepard, C.C.: Leprosy today. N. Engl. J. Med., *307*:1640–1641, 1982.

50. Stevens, D.A., et al.: Experience with ketoconazole in three major manifestations of progressive coccidioidomycosis. Am. J. Med., *74*:58–63, 1983.

51. Sutker, W.L., Laukford, L.L., and Thompsett, R.: Granulomatous synovitis: The role of atypical mycobacteria. Rev. Infect. Dis., *1*:729–735, 1979.

52. Tenenbaum, J.J., Greenspan, J., and Kerkering, T.M.: Blastomycosis. CRC Crit. Rev. Microbiol., *9*:139–163, 1982.

53. Thornberry, D.R., et al.: Histoplasmosis presenting with joint pain and hilar adenopathy. Arthritis Rheum., *25*:1396–1402, 1982.

54. Tulis, M., and Mukherjee, S.K.: Excision arthroplasty for tuberculosis and pyogenic arthritis of the hip. J. Bone Joint. Surg., *63B*:29–32, 1981.

55. Van Scoy, R.E., and Wilkowski, C.T.: Antituberculous agents. Mayo Clin. Proc., *58*:233–240, 1983.

56. Van Vooris, W.C., et al.: Cutaneous infiltrates in leprosy. N. Engl. J. Med., *307*:1593–1597, 1982.

57. Wallace, R., and Cohen, A.S.: Tuberculous arthritis: A report of two cases with review of biopsy and synovial fluid findings. Am. J. Med., *61*:277–282, 1976.

58. Wheat, L.J., et al.: A large urban outbreak of histoplasmosis: Clinical features. Ann. Intern. Med., *94*:331–337, 1981.

59. Wilding, K., and Nade, S.: Actinomycosis of bone. Aust. N. Z. J. Surg., *45*:61–65, 1975.

60. Wilson, D.E., et al.: Clinical features of extracutaneous sporotrichosis. Medicine, *46*:265–279, 1967.

61. Winter, W.G., et al.: Coccidioidal arthritis and its treatment—1975. J. Bone Joint Surg., *57*:1152, 1975.

62. Yoshinoza, S., Cox, R.A., and Pope, R.M.: Circulating immune complexes in coccidioidomycosis. J. Clin. Invest., *66*:655–663, 1980.

63. Yousefzadeh, D.K., and Jackson, J.H.: Neonatal and infantile candidal arthritis with or without osteomyelitis: A clinical and radiographic review of 21 cases. Skeletal Radiol., *5*:77–90, 1980.

Chapter 103

Viral Arthritis

Allen C. Steere
Stephen E. Malawista

Arthritis may be associated with a number of viral infections (Table 103–1). Since the last edition of this textbook, several additional herpes viruses and enteroviruses have been added to the list of arthritogenic agents. Although each agent causes particular syndromes, several generalizations can be made.

Many viral arthritides begin with the nonspecific symptoms often observed with viral infections: malaise and fatigue, chills and fever, headache, stiff neck, sore throat, or nausea and vomiting (Table 103–2). There is often a rash, usually macular or papular, but mild temperature elevation and regional lymphadenopathy may be the only nonarticular physical findings.

No single pattern of joint involvement is characteristic (Table 103–3); in hepatitis B alone, the

Table 103–1   Viral Infections and Arthritis

I. VIRAL INFECTIONS OFTEN ASSOCIATED
   WITH ARTHRITIS
   Hepatitis B
   Rubella (including vaccine-induced)
   Group A arboviruses
      Epidemic polyarthritis of Australia (Ross River
         virus)
      Chikungunya
      O'nyong-nyong
      Sindbis
      Mayaro
   Mumps
   Smallpox (including vaccinia)

II. VIRAL INFECTIONS ASSOCIATED WITH
    ARTHRITIS IN A FEW PATIENTS
    Adenovirus type 7
    Herpes viruses
       Varicella-zoster
       Herpes simplex type 1
       Infectious mononucleosis (Epstein-Barr virus)
       Cytomegalovirus
    Enteroviruses
       Coxsackie viruses
       ECHO viruses types 6 and 9

III. PRESUMED VIRAL INFECTIONS ASSOCIATED
     WITH ARTHRITIS
     Erythema infectiosum
     Transient polyarthritis

arthritis may be symmetric, asymmetric, migratory, or additive and may affect one or many joints. Periarticular structures (tendons and bursae) may also become inflamed. Morning stiffness is usually mentioned only in affected joints. On examination, joints may be red, hot, and swollen, or arthralgia may be the only sign of involvement.

Routine laboratory tests usually show few, if any, abnormalities (Table 103–4). Some patients may be mildly anemic or may have a few atypical lymphocytes. Tests are usually negative for rheumatoid factor (except rubella) and for antinuclear antibodies. Elevated erythrocyte sedimentation rates are the most commonly observed abnormality. Cryoprecipitates and depressed serum complement levels have been found in the serum of patients with hepatitis B. Synovial fluid analyses reflect varying degrees of inflammation, but the findings are nonspecific (Table 103–5). The usual finding, 15,000 to 25,000 cells/mm³ with predominantly polymorphonuclear leukocytes, is also typical for rheumatoid arthritis. However, biopsies generally show less intense signs of synovial inflammation than in rheumatoid arthritis.

Little is known about how viruses induce arthritis, with the exception of hepatitis B, where the evidence suggests an immune-complex-mediated pathogenesis. In rubella, recovery of the virus from the synovial fluid of multiple patients suggests that it may replicate in synovium. Varicella, herpes simplex type 1, and cytomegalovirus have been isolated from joint fluid in only one patient each.

Because many findings are nonspecific, how does one recognize or suspect viral arthritis? Information about exposures can be helpful: a history of drug abuse for hepatitis B, or recent immunization for rubella, or of recent exposure to an endemic area and seasonal onset for arboviruses or enteroviruses. The most characteristic feature of the known viral arthritides, however, is their usual short duration. If inflammatory arthritis disappears in one or two weeks and if the patient has no preceding drug exposures (e.g., penicillin therapy), one thinks of viral arthritis. Indeed, the short duration of arthritis without deforming changes is the

Table 103–2.　**Viral Arthritis: Associated Findings**

Disease	Symptoms	Skin Lesions	Other Signs
I. VIRAL INFECTIONS OFTEN ASSOCIATED WITH ARTHRITIS			
Hepatitis B	Sore throat; nausea, vomiting; myalgias; chills; malaise	Urticarial; macular; papular; petechial	Lymphadenopathy; low-grade fever
Rubella	Coryza; cough; sore throat; headache; myalgia; malaise; fatigue	Morbilliform	Lymphadenopathy; low-grade fever
Rubella vaccine (HPV-77 DK12)	Coryza; cough; sore throat	Morbilliform (often absent)	Lymphadenopathy; low-grade fever; myeloradiculitis
Epidemic polyarthritis of Australia	Headache; rhinorrhea; sore throat; nausea, vomiting	Maculopapular; vesicular; petechial (minor)	Lymphadenopathy; low-grade fever
Chikungunya	Headache and backache; myalgia; malaise; cough; sore throat; mild gastrointestinal complaints	Maculopapular (faint, confluent); petechial (minor)	Conjunctivitis; high fever; lymphadenopathy
O'nyong-nyong	Headache and backache; eye pain; myalgia; cough; coryza; gastrointestinal complaints	Morbilliform; maculopapular	Lymphadenitis; low-grade fever; conjunctivitis
Mumps	Chills; headache; stiff neck; sore throat; vomiting; myalgias		Fever; parotitis; orchitis; pancreatitis
Smallpox	Headache; myalgia; abdominal pain; vomiting	Vesicular	Fever
II. VIRAL INFECTIONS ASSOCIATED WITH ARTHRITIS IN A FEW PATIENTS			
Adenovirus type 7	Sore throat	Maculopapular	Low-grade fever; pericarditis; meningitis
Varicella-zoster	Malaise	Vesicular	Fever
Herpes simplex type 1		Vesicular	
Infectious mononucleosis	Headache; malaise; sore throat	Maculopapular	Lymphadenopathy; sore throat
Cytomegalovirus			Fever
Coxsackie viruses	Sore throat; pleuritis pain	Maculopapular	Fever; myopericarditis
ECHO virus types 6 and 9	Fever; headache; vomiting; sore throat	Macular	Fever; meningitis
III. PRESUMED VIRAL INFECTIONS ASSOCIATED WITH ARTHRITIS			
Erythema infectiosum	Headache; coryza; ocular and abdominal pain	Three stages: red cheeks; maculopapular rash; recurrent lesions	

biggest difference between known types of viral arthritis and established rheumatoid arthritis.

However, observations in the last several years have somewhat blurred this distinction. Hepatitis B arthritis may last for months, and a vasculitis indistinguishable from polyarteritis nodosa may occur. In the latter case, roentgenograms of affected joints may show progressive osteoporosis and a striking loss of articular cartilage. Rubella arthritis associated with HPV-77 DK12 vaccination may recur in the knee for as long as 3 years, although individual attacks remain short. In addition, recent reports suggest that rubella virus may occasionally cause chronic erosive arthritis and that rubella, mumps, and coxsackie viruses may be associated with a condition similar to Still's disease.

When one considers the possible viral etiology of rheumatoid arthritis itself, it becomes even more important to understand the factors leading to chronicity and the effects of chronic inflammation on joints in known viral arthritides.

VIRAL INFECTIONS OFTEN ASSOCIATED WITH ARTHRITIS

Hepatitis B

Although Robert Graves, in 1843, described 8 patients who had transient arthritis followed by jaundice, arthritis associated with liver disease received little attention until the discovery of HB$_s$Ag over a century later. The arthritis typically affects many joints symmetrically, precedes the onset of

Table 103–3.   Viral Arthritis: Musculoskeletal System

Disease	Percentage with Arthritis	Type of Involvement	Duration, Days
I. VIRAL INFECTIONS OFTEN ASSOCIATED WITH ARTHRITIS			
Hepatitis B	10–30%	Symmetric or sometimes asymmetric, migratory, or additive; small, sometimes large joints; tendinitis; bursitis	14 (7–180)
Rubella	15–35% of adult women; uncommon in men, children	Symmetric; knees, wrists; PIPs; carpal tunnel syndrome; tendinitis	5–30
Rubella vaccine (HPV-77 DK12)	1–10% of children; more common in women	Symmetric (PIPs) or monoarticular (knees); carpal tunnel syndrome	7–21; recurrences common
Epidemic polyarthritis of Australia	Majority of adults	Symmetric or sometimes asymmetric or additive; small, sometimes large joints; tendinitis; periarticular swelling	14–21; sometimes months
Chikungunya	Majority	Large (especially knees), sometimes small joints; swelling rare	5–7; may recur for months
O'nyong-nyong	Majority	Large, sometimes small joints; no swelling	~5
Mumps	0.4%	Migratory; large and small joints; tenosynovitis	14 (2–90)
Smallpox	0.25–0.5%	Elbow, other large joints	up to 60
II. VIRAL INFECTIONS ASSOCIATED WITH ARTHRITIS IN A FEW PATIENTS			
Adenovirus type 7	5 patients	Large and small joints	7–35; recurrences possible
Varicella-zoster	8 patients	Knee, other large joints	7
Herpes simplex type 1	3 patients	Knee, other large joints	21 (14–120)
Infectious mononucleosis	4 patients	Large and small joints	68 (7–126)
Cytomegalovirus	1 patient	Knee	7
Coxsackie viruses	9 patients	Large and small joints	unknown
ECHO virus types 6 and 9	2 patients	Large and small joints	9–84
III. PRESUMED VIRAL INFECTIONS ASSOCIATED WITH ARTHRITIS			
Erythema infectiosum	70% of adults; 5% of children	Wrists, knees	5–9

frank hepatitis, and is often associated with a diffuse urticarial, macular, papular, or petechial rash. Both skin and joint lesions usually disappear when the liver disease becomes apparent. There is currently no direct evidence that either hepatitis A or non-A, non-B hepatitis is associated with arthritis.

Pathogenesis. Several observations suggest that circulating immune complexes may play a pathogenetic role in the arthritis and urticaria associated with hepatitis B infection. The complexes appear in the prehepatic period when HB_sAg is in excess and when joints and skin are likely to be clinically active (Fig. 103–1). They contain HB_sAg and anti-HB, other immunoglobulins, and complement components.[17] Their IgG subtypes are primarily 1 and 3, the ones that bind complement,[17] and concomitant serum complement levels, particularly C4 and CH_{50}, may be depressed.[2,3] Immune complexes containing HB_sAg, IgM, and C3 have been found in affected dermal vessels.[4] With the development of antibody excess, the complexes disappear, and the arthritis and rash resolve. This sequence is similar to that in experimental ''one-shot'' serum sickness.[5] The circulating immune complexes may become localized in the synovium or dermal vessels where they elicit an inflammatory response.

Alternatively, hepatitis B virus may invade the synovium directly and replicate there. Particles consistent with HB_sAg, including particles apparently budding from the cell membrane, have been seen in synovial lining cells.[14] Because normal cell structures may resemble viral particles ultrastructurally, however, this finding is not definitive.

Epidemiology. The reported frequency of joint manifestations in patients with hepatitis B infection

Table 103–4. Viral Arthritis: Laboratory Findings in Blood

Disease	Hct	WBC	ESR	RF	ANA	C3	C4	Cryoglobulins	Specific Serology
I. VIRAL INFECTIONS OFTEN ASSOCIATED WITH ARTHRITIS									
Hepatitis B	↔ ↓ *	↔ ↑; rel ↑ cytosis†; atypical lymphs‡	↔ ↑	Negative	Negative	↓ ↔	↓ ↔	Often positive	Yes
Rubella		↔ ↑	↔ ↑	Often positive					Yes
Rubella vaccine (HPV-77 DK12)		↔ ↑	↔ ↑	Rarely positive	Rarely positive				Yes
Epidemic polyarthritis of Australia		↔ ↓; rel ↑ cytosis; atypical lymphs	↔ ↑	Usually negative	Negative	↔	↔ (1 patient)		Yes
Chikungunya	↔	↔ ↑ ↓	↔ ↑						Yes
O'nyong-nyong		↔ ↓; rel ↑ cytosis							Yes
Mumps	↔	↔ ↑	↔ ↑	Rarely positive					Yes
II. VIRAL INFECTIONS ASSOCIATED WITH ARTHRITIS IN A FEW PATIENTS									
Adenovirus type 7		↔ ↑	↔ ↑	Negative	Negative	↓			Yes
Varicella-zoster		↔ ↑	↔ ↑	Negative	Negative			Negative	Yes
Infectious mononucleosis		↔ ↑	↔ ↑	Negative	Usually negative	↑ ↔	↑ ↔	Usually negative	Yes
III. PRESUMED VIRAL INFECTIONS ASSOCIATED WITH ARTHRITIS									
Erythema infectiosum		↔; rel ↑ cytosis							No

*↔ normal, ↓ decreased, ↑ increased
†relative lymphocytosis
‡atypical lymphocytes

Table 103–5. Viral Arthritis: Laboratory Findings in Material from Joints

Disease	Synovial Fluid				Synovium
	WBC × 10⁻³/ mm³	Predominant Cell Type	Total Protein (g/dl)	Virus Cultured	
I. VIRAL INFECTIONS OFTEN ASSOCIATED WITH ARTHRITIS					
Hepatitis B	25 (0.5–90)	PMN or mononuclear cells	4 (2.5–6)	No (HB,Ag detectable)	Limited mononuclear infiltrate
Rubella	30 (15–60) (5 patients)	Mononuclear cells or PMN	2–3.8	Yes	Synovial hyperplasia (2 patients), with ↑ vascularity, mononuclear infiltrate (1 patient)
Epidemic polyarthritis of Australia	10 (1.5–13.8)	Mononuclear cells		No	
Mumps		PMN (1 patient)		No	
Smallpox	Pus	PMN		No (Elementary bodies seen)	
Vaccinia	44 (1 patient)	PMN (1 patient)		Yes	
II. VIRAL INFECTIONS ASSOCIATED WITH ARTHRITIS IN A FEW PATIENTS					
Adenovirus type 7	3–25 (4 patients)	PMN or mononuclear cells		No	
Varicella-zoster	~4 (4 patients)	Mononuclear cells		Yes	
Hepres simplex type 1	~10 (2 patients)	Mononuclear cells		Yes	
Infectious mononucleosis	40 (3 patients)	PMN		No	
Cytomegalovirus	37 (1 patient)	PMN		Yes	
Coxsackie viruses	7–46 (4 patients)	PMN		No	
ECHO viruses types 6 and 9	2.2 (1 patient)	PMN and large mononuclear cells		No	

is variable, but is generally between 10 and 30%.[6,12] Most studies report an age range from the first through the sixth decades (mean, third decade) with males and females affected equally.[1,2,6,15,16]

Clinical Characteristics. The arthritis typically begins with symmetric involvement of many joints.[1,6,9] In some patients, however, the pattern of involvement may be asymmetric,[18] migratory,[10,13] or additive.[6] The small joints of the fingers, particularly the proximal interphalangeal joints, but also the metacarpophalangeal and the distal interphalangeal joints, are most commonly affected, followed by the knee, shoulder, ankle, elbow, and wrist (Fig. 103–2). These joints may be markedly tender and sometimes swollen, red, and hot, or objective signs of inflammation may be absent. Some patients have localized tender areas over the joint, and others have tendinitis.[8,10]

Two patients have been reported with subcutaneous nodules on the extensor surfaces of the forearm.[10,18] The histology of the nodule in one was indistinguishable from that seen in rheumatoid arthritis.[10] The arthritis lasts from several days to 6 months, but usually only for a few weeks.[1,2,10]

The arthritis is often accompanied by a rash that is most commonly urticarial, but may be macular, papular, or petechial.[1,2,6,8,16] All three types of rash may coexist in one patient.[8] In a review of 96 patients, one-half of those with arthritis had an urticarial rash that was often pruritic.[1] The Koebner phenomenon may be noted with respect to urticaria. In another report of 18 patients, 6 had an urticarial eruption and 2 had maculopapular eruptions.[2] The rash is usually on the lower extremities, but it may also involve the upper extremities, trunk, and face.[6] Angioneurotic edema of the soles may

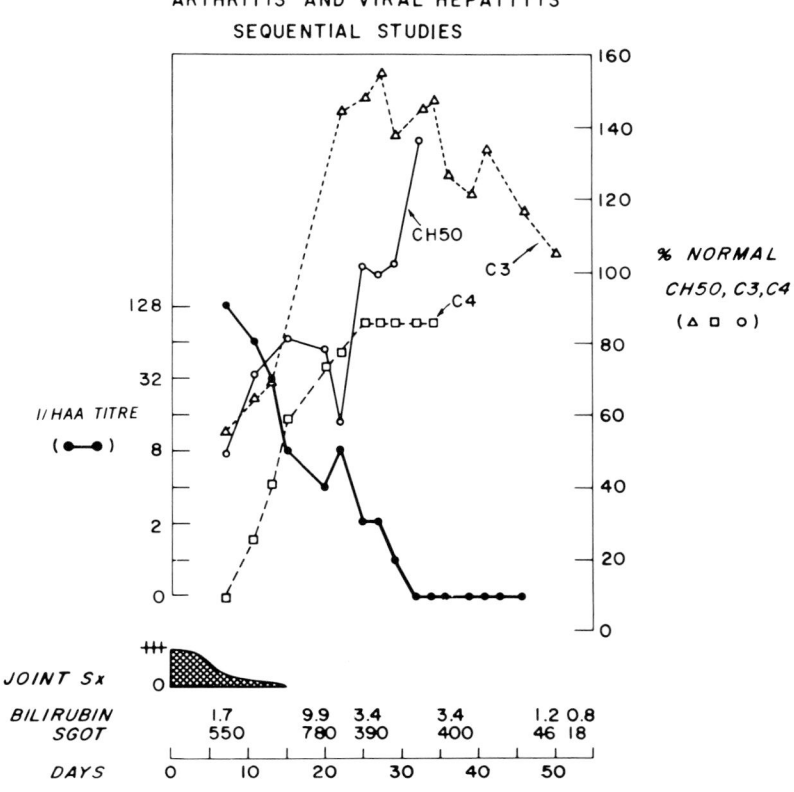

Fig. 103–1. Changes in CH_{50}, C3, and C4 serum concentrations and HB_sAg titers are seen during the course of HB_sAg-associated arthritis followed by hepatitis. HB_sAg is present, and complement components are depressed when the joints are active. With the development of antibody excess (not shown), the arthritis resolves and the hepatitis becomes apparent. (From Alpert, E., et al.[3])

occur.[2] Like the arthritis, the rash lasts from days to weeks.[6]

Patients may experience malaise, sore throat, anorexia, nausea and vomiting, fever and chills, and myalgias.[1,6,13] Fever,[6,10] if present, is low-grade (100 to 102° F). Regional adenopathy may be present.[6,10] These symptoms appear 1 day to 12 weeks before the arthritis.[6]

The joint manifestations usually subside before liver involvement becomes apparent.[1,16] Serum glutamic-oxaloacetic transaminase (SGOT) levels may be elevated while the arthritis is still present; alternatively, some patients never develop abnormal SGOT levels.[6]

Laboratory Findings. When the arthritis is present, HB_sAg is usually recoverable from blood, although it may be necessary to test multiple samples before one obtains a positive result.[6] HB_sAg has been detected in synovial fluid as well as in serum.[6,10,11] As the arthritis improves, HB_sAg usually disappears, and the test for anti-HB becomes positive (see Fig. 103–1). Patients rarely have a positive test for HB_sAg and anti-HB in the serum at the same time.[6]

Cryoprecipitates have been detected in the serum of some patients when the arthritis is present. These precipitates derive from large, circulating immune complexes that may contain HB_sAg, anti-HB, immunoglobulins M, G, and A, and the complement components, Clq, C3, C4, and C5.[17] In addition, putative Dane particles have been seen in the precipitates by electron microscopy.[7]

Complement components may be consumed most quickly when the arthritis is first present (see Fig. 103–1). At such times, C4 and CH_{50} levels are often markedly depressed, C3 levels are low-normal to depressed, and Clq levels are variable.[2,3] Higher concentrations of HB_sAg have been associated with lower levels of C4 and Clq. However, low complement levels are not found in all patients. In one study, only 13 of 29 patients had C3 levels below 120 mg/dl, and only 8 had C4 levels below 20 mg/dl.[6] The complement system apparently may be activated by both the classic and alternative pathways.[17]

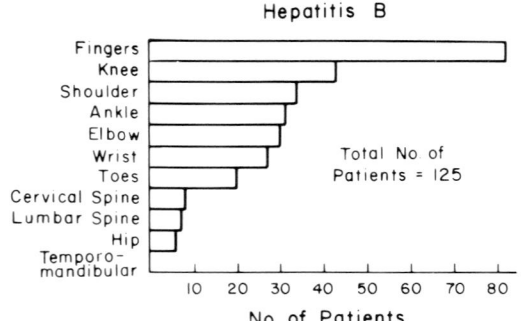

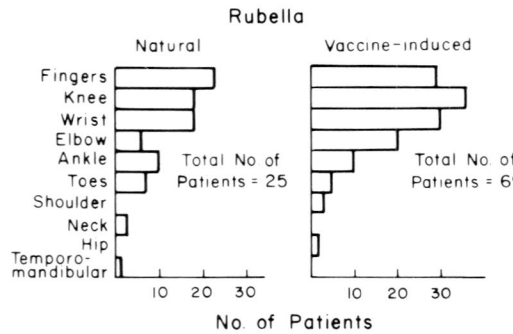

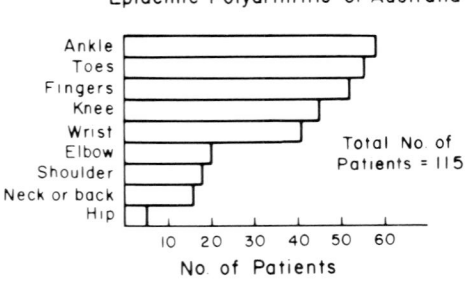

Fig. 103–2. Frequency of joints involved is seen in three viral arthritides. Small joints of the fingers, then knees, are most often affected in hepatitis B[3,8,13,16,17] and rubella.[22,32,41,44,48] Ankles, toes, fingers, and knees are affected most often in epidemic polyarthritis of Australia.[73]

In most patients, the hematocrit and the total white cell count are normal; sometimes a relative lymphocytosis and a few atypical lymphocytes are present.[2] However, hematocrits as low as 31% and total white cell counts as high as 21,500 cells/mm[3] have been noted.[6] The presence of microscopic hematuria and red-cell casts[6] may lead to chronic glomerulonephritis.

The synovial fluid was first thought to be mostly noninflammatory, with a predominance of lymphocytes,[8,10] although counts as high as 5,600

WBC/mm[3] with 56% polymorphs had been recorded. Subsequent observations, however, have shown that white cell counts may be highly variable. In fluid from 6 patients, white counts ranged from 465 to 90,000 cells/mm[3] (mean 24,172), and most were polymorphonuclear leukocytes.[6] The joint fluid total protein and glucose also varied a great deal: protein 2.6 to 6.1 g/dl (mean 4.2) and glucose 62 to 260 mg/dl (mean 114).[6] Joint fluid C3 levels were not low when adjusted for total protein, but CH_{50} was markedly reduced in a fluid with a positive HB_sAg titer.[10]

Synovial biopsies in two patients showed only limited inflammatory changes.[14] Synovial lining cells were 1 to 5 layers thick, some vessels were congested, and occasional scattered lymphocytes were seen. HB_sAg was demonstrated throughout the synovium by direct immunofluorescence, and possible viral particles were observed by electron microscopy in synovial lining cells, blood vessels, and other deep synovial structures.

Treatment. The duration of the arthritis and rash is usually brief regardless of therapy. The rash, which may be quite pruritic, responds poorly to antihistamines or to epinephrine.[6] Some patients have noted dramatic relief of the arthritis with salicylates.[6]

Rubella

Arthritis as a complication of rubella was mentioned in Sir William Osler's textbook. *Principles and Practice of Medicine,* in 1906, and joint symptoms have since been noted in many rubella outbreaks.[31,34,35] Rubella arthritis typically occurs in women[35,48] while the rash is present, or occurs a few days later, often involving the fingers, wrists, and knees symmetrically. Its duration is usually brief.

Epidemiology. Joint involvement occurs in about one-third to one-sixth of women with rubella.[24,35] It is much less common in adult men or in children. In an outbreak in Great Britain in 1953, 16 of 50 patients (32%) developed joint symptoms. All 16 were adults, and 15 were women.[36]

Clinical Characteristics. Patients often have the characteristic morbilliform rash of rubella, posterior cervical lymphadenopathy, low-grade fever, malaise, and fatigue. The onset of arthritis associated with rubella is usually sudden, commonly affecting the fingers, knees, and wrists symmetrically (see Fig. 103–2). Pain on motion and stiffness are often the only symptoms of inflammation. Some patients may also develop carpal tunnel syndrome[32] or tenosynovitis.[20] The arthritis occurs from 6 days before to 6 days after the rash, but usually a few days after its onset.[20] The arthritis may occasionally occur without the rash. The joint symptoms usually do not last longer than one month and are not associated with permanent joint damage.[20,31-33] Aspirin may provide partial relief.[32,47]

Laboratory Findings. Blood counts in most patients are normal; a few patients have mild leukocytosis or an elevated erythrocyte sedimentation rate. In two series, most patients had a positive test for rheumatoid factor;[31,33] in two others, only a few patients did.[32,48] Joint effusions, if present, are usually small (e.g., 20 ml). In fluids aspirated from five patients, synovial fluid white cell counts ranged from 14,600 to 60,000.[20,23a,46] Four patients had predominantly mononuclear cells with no polymorphonuclear leukocytes; the other had 95% polymorphonuclear leukocytes. Rubella antigen was demonstrated in mononuclear cells by immunofluorescence.[23a] The total protein content ranged from 1.9 to 3.8 g/dl. One synovial biopsy showed a nonspecific inflammatory reaction with synovial cell hyperplasia, increased vascularity, a predominantly mononuclear cell infiltrate, and a fibrinopurulent exudate;[48] another showed only mild hyperplasia of synovial lining cells.[23a] Rubella virus has been cultured from the synovial fluid of one infant[29] and three adults[23a] with acute naturally acquired disease.

Chronic Arthritis. Recent articles report the isolation of rubella virus from the synovial fluid of patients with chronic arthritides.[23,27] In some patients, rubella antigen was seen in synovium and synovial fluid mononuclear cells by immunofluorescence, and particles resembling the electron-dense cores of rubella virus were found in synovium by electron microscopy.[27] In another study, the joint fluid mononuclear cells of a patient with unexplained knee arthritis underwent blast transformation when exposed to rubella antigens, but peripheral blood mononuclear cells did not.[23] Rubella virus was subsequently isolated from his joint fluid. These reports suggest that rubella virus may occasionally cause chronic rheumatic disease syndromes, such as rheumatoid arthritis or Still's disease. Alternatively, the virus may simply be present in synovium as an epiphenomenon and may not be the inciting agent.

Rubella Arthritis (Vaccine-Induced)

Because of teratogenic effects of rubella virus on the fetus, rubella vaccines were developed. In 1969, three live attenuated vaccines (HPV-77 DK12, HPV-77 DE5, and Cendehill) became available. It soon became apparent that all three strains, but particularly HPV-77 DK12, could induce arthritis in both children and adults similar to that caused by natural rubella. HPV-77 DK12 has since been withdrawn from the market.

Pathogenesis. The mechanism by which rubella virus induces arthritis is uncertain. The virus was cultured from synovial fluid following vaccination in four reported cases (3 or 4 months after the onset of symptoms in three patients).[37,47] Because of these isolates, it has been postulated that the organism may invade and replicate in synovium. However, the observed sequence of viral isolation from the pharynx or blood, followed by the appearance of the rash and arthritis and the detection of circulating antibody, is compatible with an immune-complex-associated arthritis.[35] Three patients with vaccine-induced rubella arthritis had putative circulating immune complexes, determined by the Clq-binding assay.[46] In other reports, complement levels (Blc and CH_{50}), with one exception,[38] were normal.[42,45]

Epidemiology. Each rubella vaccine, including the newer RA 27/3, has been associated with joint involvement in 5 to 10% of those receiving it.[22,26,30,39,40] These attack rates are somewhat lower than has been found with HPV-77 DK12 vaccine.[42-45] As in natural rubella, the frequency of this complication is greatest in women: 43% of women and 39% of postpubescent, adolescent girls given the HPV-77 DE-5 vaccine developed arthralgias or arthritis, whereas only 3% of children given the same vaccine developed these complications.[19,28,35,47]

In several studies, the mean rubella titers were not significantly different in those who developed arthritis compared to those who did not.[48] In addition, the titers were not significantly different in those with only one attack of arthritis compared to those with recurrent attacks.[42] Arthritis rarely accompanied vaccination if the individual was previously immune due to natural infection.[45]

Clinical Characteristics. The joint symptoms following rubella vaccination are similar to those associated with the natural infection, except that isolated knee involvement and carpal tunnel syndrome are apparently more common (see Fig. 103–2). Of 40 children with arthritis following vaccination with HPV-77 DK12, 50% had predominantly knee complaints, 33% had symptoms that suggested carpal tunnel syndrome, and only 17% had polyarthritis.[45] Pain and stiffness (often mild) are the usual findings in affected joints; swelling, heat, and redness are unusual.[42]

The arthritis usually occurs 2 to 4 weeks after vaccination (range 8 to 55 days); arthralgias typically last a few days and arthritis 1 to 3 weeks (range 1 to 46 days).[19,21,42-45] However, a third to a tenth of those with knee involvement after HPV-77 DK12 vaccination had recurrent attacks for as long as 3 years,[35,42,44] and 3 patients had them for as long as 5 years.[41] Recurrent attacks, usually affecting the same joint, typically last 1 to 5 days with longer intervening periods of complete remission (range 2 weeks to 1 year). Patients tend to have fewer attacks the longer the time from vaccination, but the frequency in an individual patient is unpredictable. One patient experienced synovial hypertrophy in the intercondylar notch 5 years after onset,[41] but permanent joint damage was not reported.[42,44]

As in the natural infection, patients with vaccine-induced arthritis sometimes have the characteristic rash, coryza, cough, sore throat, posterior cervical lymphadenopathy, or low-grade fever.[44,45] However, a rash is less common than in the natural infection; in one study, only 8 of 40 patients developed a rash.[43]

Two distinct neuropathic syndromes have been noted after rubella immunization. One type is characterized by numbness and tingling in the hands and sharp, shooting pains in the arms,[21] and the other by pain mostly in the back of the legs.[25] These children sometimes assume the so-called "catcher's crouch" position, particularly in the morning. In one study of 13 children, 11 had slowing of nerve conduction,[25] a finding also recorded by others.[33]

As in natural rubella, aspirin therapy often provides some symptomatic relief.[45]

Laboratory Findings. Although blood counts are usually normal, white cell counts as high as 11,600 cells/mm^3 and sedimentation rates as high as 46 mm/hour (Westergren) have been seen.[42,43] Tests for rheumatoid factor and for antinuclear antibodies are rarely positive,[44,45] immunoglobulin levels are usually normal,[37] and complement components (Blc and CH$_{50}$), except in one instance,[38] have also been normal.[42,45]

Arboviruses

Joint pain is a common manifestation of many illnesses caused by arboviruses, including dengue. In the following five entities, all caused by group A arboviruses *(alphaviruses),* joint pain is the predominant feature.

Epidemic Polyarthritis of Australia

Epidemic polyarthritis was first described by Nimmo in New South Wales, Australia, in 1928. Outbreaks have been reported subsequently in Australia, New Guinea, the Solomon islands, Fiji, American Samoa, and a number of South Pacific Islands.[78] The illness, caused by a group A arbovirus (the Ross River virus) and transmitted by mosquitoes, usually affects small (and sometimes large) joints, is frequently associated with a diffuse maculopapular rash, and typically lasts for several weeks.

Pathogenesis. The mechanism by which the Ross River virus induces arthritis is unknown. There is no evidence for direct invasion and replication in synovium or for the presence of immune complexes. The virus has been recovered only once, from the blood of an 8-year old boy with headache and fever, but no arthritis.[56] Attempts to isolate the virus from blood, lymphocytes, skin, throat, urine, and synovial fluid specimens of patients with arthritis have been unsuccessful.[49] Unlike classic immune-complex-mediated serum sickness, circulating antibody has always been present when patients are symptomatic rather than appearing as symptoms subside,[50] and levels of complement components (C3 and C4) have been normal in serum and synovial fluid.[51] In one study, patients with epidemic polyarthritis had an increased frequency of the B-cell alloantigen, DR 7.[59]

Epidemiology. Epidemic polyarthritis primarily affects adults of either sex.[50,56,73] Children may show seroconversion against Ross River virus, but they are usually asymptomatic.[50] The illness occurs primarily from December through May (the equivalent of summer and fall in the northern hemisphere).[49,50,53,73] Attack rates in the affected areas may be quite high. During 1979 and 1980, major epidemics of Ross River virus infection occurred in several South Pacific islands; these outbreaks sometimes involved 40 to 50% of the local population.[78] The number of asymptomatic cases may also be high.[54]

The causative agent, the Ross River virus, was first recovered from mosquitoes, *Aëdes vigilex,* in 1959[55] and has been isolated subsequently from other *Aëdes* species and from *Culex* and *Mansonia* mosquitoes.[61,78] The incubation period from the bite to the onset of symptoms is thought to be 2 to 15 days.[49,60] Person-to-person transmission has not been noted.[49,60,73]

Clinical Characteristics. The arthritis, which may begin gradually or suddenly, typically affects two or more joints and may be symmetric, asymmetric, or additive.[57,73,74,76] The ankle and small joints of the toes and fingers are involved most often, followed by knees and wrists (see Fig. 103–2). Although the affected joints are frequently stiff, tender, and painful to move, swelling is rare, and redness and heat are not reported.[76] In addition to arthritis, symptoms that patients may experience include periarticular swelling, tendinitis, and pronounced localized tenderness over one part of a joint capsule or ligament.[57,76] Joint symptoms often persist longer than other manifestations of the illness, typically for 2 to 3 weeks, but sometimes for months.[49,50,57,73] Roentgenograms of affected joints show no abnormality, and no patients have had permanent joint damage.

A fine, nonconfluent, maculopapular rash often accompanies the arthritis,[49,57,73,76] but may precede it by as much as 11 days or follow it by as much as 15 days.[50] The rash may become vesicular, and a few petechiae are sometimes noted. The lesions often begin on the trunk, but in many patients spread quickly to cover the entire body, including the scalp, palms, and soles (lesions on the palms and soles are usually macular).[49,50,57] In a few patients, dark red macules have been noted on the hard and soft palates. The rash, which may be painless or slightly pruritic, typically lasts about 1 week (range 1 to 18 days) and usually fades without desquamation.[49,57,73] It may occur without arthritis, and vice versa.[50]

Constitutional symptoms are often mild. However, some patients experience headache, rhinorrhea, sore throat, nausea and vomiting, myalgia in the legs, malaise, and marked lethargy, particularly at the beginning of the illness.[49,50] Paresthesias with numbness and tingling or soreness of the fingers and toes may be the most distressing symptoms.[50,57,73,76] Temperatures are usually normal or mildly elevated (101°F). Regional or generalized lymphadenopathy may be present, and nodes are sometimes tender.

Aspirin and other analgesic drugs may give partial but not dramatic relief.[59,75]

Laboratory Findings. Complement fixation, hemagglutination inhibition, and neutralization tests are available for serodiagnosis.[74] The white cell count and erythrocyte sedimentation rate are usually normal.[50,76] A few patients have had mild leukopenia, relative lymphocytosis, and a few atypical lymphocytes.[73] In joint fluid from 8 patients, white cell counts ranged from 1,500 to 13,800 cells/mm³ and consisted primarily of monocytes, in which Ross River virus antigen was detected by specific immunofluorescence.[58] In one patient, tests for rheumatoid factor and antinuclear antibodies in serum and synovial fluid were negative, and complement levels (C3 and C4) were normal.[51]

Chikungunya

A large epidemic of a "dengue-like illness" called chikungunya, "that which bends up," was first described in southern Tanganyika (now Tanzania) in 1952.[64,71,72] Epidemics of the same illness have been recognized subsequently in wide areas of Africa, southern India, southeastern Asia, and the Philippine Islands.[67–69,78,79] American servicemen were affected during the Vietnam war.[52] The illness, caused by a group A arbovirus (the chikungunya virus) and transmitted by mosquitoes, is characterized by high fever, severe joint pains, and a maculopapular rash. It usually lasts 5 to 7 days, but residual joint pain may recur for months in some patients.

Epidemiology. Arthritis occurs more often in adults than in children,[67,68,71] and there is no sex predilection. Attack rates during epidemics, which affect primarily rural populations, may be high. During the first outbreak described, 60 to 80% of the inhabitants of affected villages acquired the infection within 2 to 3 weeks.[71] The onset is seasonal, from April through August, during and shortly after periods of unusually heavy rainfall.[52,68]

The virus is usually transmitted by mosquitoes of the species *Aëdes aegypti*,[64,72] although it has also been isolated from *A. africanus* and *A. furcifer*.[78,80] The incubation period from the bite to the onset of symptoms is thought to be 3 to 12 days.[71]

Clinical Characteristics. The illness usually begins abruptly with the onset of high fever and severe, generalized joint pains often associated with prolonged morning stiffness.[63,68,71,72] In some patients, only large joints are involved, particularly the knees.[71] Joint swelling is rare; only 6 of 115 patients experienced it in one epidemic.[71] The arthritis usually lasts from 5 to 7 days, but joint pain and swelling may recur intermittently for more than a year, often in different joints.[63,71] The severity and duration of the joint pain are the primary clinical features distinguishing chikungunya from dengue.[69,71]

The rash is usually a faint, confluent, macular, or maculopapular eruption occurring on the trunk, extremities, or over the entire body,[52,71] and is indistinguishable from the nonhemorrhagic rash of dengue. A few scattered petechiae are sometimes found.[52] Although the rash may precede arthritis, it more often occurs 4 to 5 days after joint symptoms and lasts 2 to 5 days.[71] The rash may also occur without arthritis, and vice versa.

High fever (up to 105°F) is characteristic; it usually lasts for several days, but may be biphasic as in dengue.[52,68,71] Headache, myalgia, backache, and malaise are common. Eye suffusion and conjunctivitis, retro-orbital pain, mild gastrointestinal complaints (vomiting, diarrhea, or constipation), cough, and sore throat occur less often. One patient was described as having paresthesias on the dorsal surface of the arms.[68] Regional lymphadenopathy, particularly of the cervical nodes, is common, and a few patients may have generalized lymphadenopathy and splenomegaly. Mild hemorrhagic phenomena, e.g., a positive tourniquet test, a low normal platelet count, and epistaxis, have been noted in some patients.[69]

Analgesics ranging from aspirin to morphine have been used for relief from the severe joint pain.

Laboratory Findings. Chikungunya virus has

been recovered on numerous occasions from blood specimens of affected patients as long as 3 days after the onset of symptoms.[52,67,68,72] Complement fixation, hemagglutination inhibition, and neutralization tests are available for serodiagnosis.[79] In most instances, the hematocrit is normal, but mild leukopenia or leukocytosis is sometimes found.[52,69,71] The erythrocyte sedimentation rate is sometimes elevated as high as 40/mm hour.[52] In one study, 2 of 20 patients had positive tests for rheumatoid factor.[63] There have been no reports of synovial fluid analyses.

O'nyong-nyong

A large outbreak of a disease similar to chikungunya, called o'nyong-nyong, was first recognized in northern Uganda in 1959.[62,75,81,82] During the subsequent two years, the illness was estimated to have affected about two million inhabitants of Uganda, Kenya, Tanzania, and the Sudan.[81] O'nyong-nyong, caused by a group A arbovirus and transmitted by mosquitoes, is characterized by generalized joint pains, a morbilliform rash, and lymphadenitis. It usually lasts about 5 days, but joint symptoms sometimes persist longer.

Although persons of any age and either sex may be affected, those 10 to 39 years of age are affected most, females more often than males.[75] Attack rates may be high, as many as 78% of the inhabitants of certain villages.[75] Subclinical infections occur in a ratio of 1:6 to overt infections.[82]

The o'nyong-nyong virus has been recovered from both *Anopheles funestes* and *A. gambiae* mosquitoes.[62] The incubation period from the bite to the onset of symptoms is thought to be at least 8 days.[75]

Clinical Characteristics. Onset is sudden with associated fever, rigor, and generalized symmetric joint pain.[75] The knees, elbows, wrists, fingers, and ankles are most frequently involved. The pain in affected joints may range from excruciating to vague weakness and stiffness; swelling, redness, and heat have not been reported. The illness usually lasts about 5 days, but the joint pain may persist longer.

The rash, which is sometimes quite pruritic, is morbilliform, macular, or maculopapular, and cannot be distinguished from that of measles.[75] It generally starts on the face and may descend over the neck, the arms, or the entire body. Punctate erythema of the soft palate is also common. The rash typically erupts on the fourth day of the illness, but may appear at the first sign of symptoms or as long as 7 days later. It lasts approximately 4 to 7 days and then fades without desquamation. About 60 to 70% of individuals with arthritis also have the rash.

Headache, ranging from moderate to severe, is almost universal.[75] Eye pain and suffusion, throbbing postorbital pain, backache, particularly in the lumbar region, dry cough, coryza, colicky abdominal pain, and constipation or diarrhea are also common. About two-thirds of patients have moderate fever (101°F), but high fever is unusual. Lymphadenitis, particularly of the posterior cervical nodes, may be striking and is the principal clinical finding that permits differentiation of this entity from chikungunya.

Laboratory Findings. O'nyong-nyong virus, which is similar to the virus that causes chikungunya has been isolated from the blood of only a few patients.[81] Complement fixation, hemagglutination inhibition, and neutralization tests are available for serodiagnosis.[81,82]

The white cell count is usually normal, but some patients have had neutropenia and a relative lymphocytosis.[75]

Sindbis

Sindbis, a group A arbovirus first isolated from *Culex* and *Mansonia* mosquitoes in 1952,[77] has been reported in Europe, Africa, Asia, Australia, and the Philippines.[78] Its basic maintenance cycle involves mainly *Culex* mosquitoes and wild birds.[78] Although clinical descriptions of the illness are few, it is typically characterized by joint pains, rash, headache, myalgias, and lethargy.[65,66] Arthritis begins suddenly and usually involves small (but sometimes large) joints. Swelling is common, and tendinitis is sometimes present. The rash, which may appear as long as 15 days after the onset of arthritis, is maculopapular, pruritic, and nonconfluent. Vesicles may form on the hands and feet. Red blotches or small ulcers may appear in the pharynx. Headache, stiff neck, periocular pain, myalgias, paresthesias, low-grade fever, and lethargy may accompany the illness. Symptoms usually last 10 to 15 days, but joint involvement has been noted for as long as 10 weeks.

Mayaro

Mayaro, a mosquito-transmitted group A arbovirus, is found in Trinidad, Surinam, Brazil, Colombia, and Bolivia.[78] Forest-dwelling mosquitoes of the genus *Haemagogus* are believed to be the principal vector.[70] The most frequent manifestations of the illness are fever, maculopapular rash, and polyarthralgias; about 20% of the patients develop joint swelling.[70] Associated signs and symptoms include headache, eye pain, myalgia, nausea and vomiting, diarrhea, and lymphadenopathy. The arthritis may persist for more than 2 months.

Mumps

Arthritis as a rare complication of mumps was first mentioned by Rettier in 1850. In the Paris mumps epidemic of 1923 to 1924, it was estimated that 6 of 1,334 patients (0.44%) developed arthritis.

This complication occurs most commonly in men, but may affect either sex at any age.[83] The arthritis, which is often migratory, usually involves large joints, but may also affect small ones. Monarticular involvement, fleeting arthralgias, and tenosynovitis have also been described.[83–87,89] Affected joints may become red, hot, and swollen, or tenderness and pain on motion may be the only signs of inflammation. Although arthritis may precede parotitis by several days, joint symptoms most commonly follow it by 1 to 2 weeks; they usually last only a few weeks, but may linger for months.[84,88] Roentgenograms of affected joints show no signs of permanent damage.

Nonspecific findings may include chills and fever (to 106°F), headache, stiff neck, sore throat, vomiting, and myalgia.[84,86,87] Although patients with mumps arthritis usually experience parotitis, a few cases without parotitis have been recognized by serologic criteria.[88,90] One of these patients had a clinical picture suggestive of adult Still's disease.[88]

Patients often show a leukocytosis (up to 21,000 white cells/mm³) and an elevated erythrocyte sedimentation rate (up to 100 mm/hour).[84,86,87] Several patients have had positive tests for rheumatoid factor.[83,91] Synovial fluid, reported only once, contained many neutrophils; no cell count was given.[83]

Salicylates are completely ineffective, but both phenylbutazone and corticosteroids have been reported to be beneficial.[83,90]

Smallpox (and Vaccinia)

Smallpox, now thought to be extinct, caused arthritis in about 0.25 to 0.5% of patients[92] and usually affected children. The elbow joints were most commonly involved, followed by the wrists, ankles, and knees. In some instances, the arthritis resulted from direct extension of the virus from the metaphysis of bone (osteomyelitis variolosa) to the articular surface. Complete recovery usually occurred within a few months.

Arthritis may also occur as a complication of vaccinia immunization.[93] One such patient developed pain, heat, and swelling of a knee 10 days after vaccination. The joint fluid contained 44,000 white cells/mm³ with 79% polymorphonuclear leukocytes; vaccinia virus was recovered from the fluid. The arthritis resolved completely in 9 days.

VIRAL INFECTIONS ASSOCIATED WITH ARTHRITIS IN A FEW PATIENTS

Adenovirus Type 7

Arthritis related to adenovirus type 7 was first reported in 1974;[94] four additional cases have been noted subsequently.[95,96] Illness begins with pharyngitis and low-grade fever. Within a few days, symmetric arthralgias of large and small joints, myalgias, and a diffuse maculopapular rash develop, and some large joints may become swollen. The arthritis lasts appoximately 1 to 5 weeks, although recurrent attacks are noted in some patients.[95] In addition to arthritis, one patient had aseptic meningitis,[94] and another had pericarditis.[95] Aspirin has been used for symptomatic relief.

The erythrocyte sedimentation rate is usually elevated during attacks. Tests for rheumatoid factor and antinuclear antibodies are negative. Joint fluid white cell counts range from 3,300 to 24,800 cells/mm³, and either polymorphonuclear leukocytes or monocytes may predominate. In one patient, synovial biopsy showed inflammatory synovitis, but attempts to recover the virus from joint fluid were unsuccessful.[94] Complement fixation, hemagglutination inhibition, and neutralization tests are available for serodiagnosis.

Herpes Viruses

All the herpes viruses—varicella-zoster, herpes simplex, Epstein-Barr, and cytomegalovirus—are rare causes of arthritis.

Varicella-Zoster

Arthritis is an unusual complication of chickenpox.[100,103,104,106,110,113] The joint involvement, which typically begins 1 to 5 days after the onset of the rash, most commonly affects the knee, followed by other large joints. In one child, several metatarsophalangeal joints were involved.[110] Some affected joints may become hot and swollen. Complete resolution usually occurs within a week.

The erythrocyte sedimentation rate may be elevated, but tests for rheumatoid factor, antinuclear antibodies, and cryoglobulins are negative. The joint fluid in three patients had 3,600 to 6,000 white cells/mm³, with predominantly mononuclear cells.[103,104,113] In one instance, 90% of the cells were shown to be monocytes.[104] Varicella virus was grown from one knee effusion.[106] Aspirin has been used for treatment.

Arthritis associated with herpes zoster was reported in 1979[98] and again in 1983.[99] One patient experienced involvement of the knees; the other, of a hip. In one instance, varicella antigen was demonstrated in the cytoplasm of joint fluid macrophages by indirect immunofluorescence, but the virus was not recovered from synovial fluid.[98]

Herpes Simplex Type 1

Three patients have had monarticular arthritis in either a knee or an ankle associated with diffuse vesicular rash due to herpes simplex type 1.[101,109] Only one patient had known immunologic impairment. In two cases, the virus was recovered from synovial fluid; in both instances, the joint fluid white cell counts were 10,000 cells/mm³ with predominantly mononuclear cells.[101,109] Joint involvement lasted 2 weeks to 4 months.

Infectious Mononucleosis

Although arthralgias occur in approximately 2% of patients with infectious mononucleosis,[108] frank arthritis is rare.[97] Several case reports, however, suggest that this complication occurs more often than previously thought.[105,111,112] Perhaps the wider availability of serologic tests for Epstein-Barr virus (EBV) has allowed better documentation of unusual cases.

Of the four well-documented cases in the literature, two patients had monarticular or oligoarticular involvement of large joints.[97,105] The other two experienced symmetric polyarthritis.[111,112] The duration of joint involvement ranged from 8 days to 4½ months. Sedimentation rates ranged from 10 to 110 mm/h, and joint fluid leukocyte counts from 18,900 to 80,000 cells/mm³ Antinuclear antibodies were found in low titer in one subject;[112] tests for rheumatoid factor were negative in all four. Three of the four patients lacked heterophil antibody production, but they were diagnosed by a rise in specific EBV antibody titers. In a serologic survey of 9 patients with the acute onset of seronegative polyarthritis, 4 had either acute or continuing active infection with EBV.[107] They did not show other signs and symptoms often associated with infectious mononucleosis.

The pathogenesis of arthritis associated with infectious mononucleosis is not known. Both viral replication within synovium and precipitation of immune complexes have been postulated. However, EB virus is known to replicate only within B lymphocytes, and although one patient had cryoglobulins,[112] another lacked abnormal ¹²⁵I-Clq binding activity.[111]

Cytomegalovirus

Only one patient has been reported with arthritis associated with cytomegalovirus.[101] She developed hip pain, knee pain and swelling, fever, and urinary retention 3 months following renal transplantation. Cytomegalovirus was isolated from the synovial fluid. More recently, the virus has also been recovered from the joint fluid of a patient who had classic seropositive rheumatoid arthritis for 17 years, but who had not been taking corticosteroids

or immunosuppressive agents.[102] The meaning of this isolate is unknown.

Enteroviruses

There are only a few case reports of arthritis induced by either coxsackie or ECHO viruses.[114-117] However, enteroviruses may cause arthritis more commonly than these few case reports might indicate because documentation of these infections is often difficult. There is no single serologic test for enteroviruses; each one must be sought individually.

Coxsackie Viruses

Nine patients are known to have had acute febrile polyarthritis associated with rising or elevated antibody titers against various coxsackie viruses, generally B_2 and B_4.[115,116] In addition to fever and arthritis, symptoms in these patients included rash, sore throat, and pleuritic pain. Three of them also had myopericarditis. Joint fluid white cell counts ranged from 7,000 to 46,000 cells/mm³ with predominantly neutrophils. One of these patients, a 15-year-old boy, had prolonged polyarthritis suggestive of Still's disease.[116]

Echo Viruses Types 6 and 9

Only two patients have been reported with arthritis associated with an ECHO virus infection (types 6 and 9).[114,117] Both patients had polyarthritis of large and small joints, one for 9 days, the other for 3 months. The patient with ECHO virus type 9 infection also experienced the typical clinical manifestations of that infection: fever, myalgias, rash, and meningismus.[114] Her synovial fluid was mildly inflammatory (2,250 leukocytes/mm³).

PRESUMED VIRAL INFECTIONS ASSOCIATED WITH ARTHRITIS

Erythema Infectiosum

Erythema infectiosum, "the fifth disease," a mild exanthematous illness usually of childhood, was first described by Tshamer in 1886 as a variant of rubella and by Escherich in 1896 as a separate clinical entity. It is distinguished by a characteristic, recurrent rash. Joint involvement occurs primarily in adults and affects large joints, usually the knees or wrists. The etiologic agent, presumably a virus, has remained elusive.

The disease occurs in localized epidemics, often during the winter, and usually affects children of school age. It is presumably spread from person-to-person. The incubation period is approximately 4 to 14 days.[118]

Clinical Characteristics. With two exceptions,[120,121] early reports of erythema infectiosum do not mention joint involvement.[119] However, in an outbreak of 364 cases in 1966,[118] 44 of the 57 adults (77%) noted joint pain compared to 24 of the 307 children (8%). Sixty-eight percent of those with joint pain also had joint swelling. The arthritis was confined to large joints, usually the wrists or knees. The symptoms lasted from 5 to 9 days and did not recur.

The illness is defined by a characteristic three-stage rash. The first stage consists of a bright red rash on the face, the so-called "slapped cheek" appearance. Discrete macules may also appear on the forehead, chin, and neck. The rash is warm to the touch and sometimes itches. The second stage begins within 1 to 4 days when a "lace-like" eruption spreads to the extensor surface of the arms and legs and to the buttocks. This stage lasts a few days to several weeks. In the third stage, the lesions may recur for as long as 10 months. Trauma, sunlight, changes in temperature, and emotional stress have been thought to activate the lesions.[119]

Although many patients have no other signs or symptoms, others experience headache, sore eyes, mild coryza, slight sore throat, gastroenteritis, abdominal pain, irritability, depression, or malaise and fatigue. A few patients may have low-grade fever or posterior cervical lymphadenopathy.[118,119] Erythema infectiosum differs from rubella by the usual absence of fever and lymphadenopathy and by the longer duration of the rash. The lack of mucous membrane involvement distinguishes it from measles.

Most patients have a normal white blood cell count, sometimes with a relative lymphocytosis.[120] Animal inoculation and tissue culture studies of blood, throat washing, and stool specimens have failed to yield a causative agent.[118,120]

Transient Polyarthritis

Transient polyarthritis has been described in New Guinea natives,[123] African tribesmen in Nigeria,[122] a Haida Indian family,[125] and other Americans.[124,126] The arthritis in these patients sometimes followed respiratory infections, but the relationship of the two is unclear. Viral etiologies were considered because of the prodromal signs, the short duration of the arthritis, and the lack of permanent joint deformity.

REFERENCES

Hepatitis B

1. Alarcon, G.S., and Townes, A.S.: Arthritis in viral hepatitis: Report of two cases and review of the literature. Johns Hopkins Med. J., 132:1–15, 1973.
2. Alpert, E., Isselbacher, K.J., and Schur, P.H.: The pathogenesis of arthritis associated with viral hepatitis. N. Engl. J. Med., 285:185–189, 1971.
3. Alpert, E., Schur, P.H., and Isselbacher, K.J.: Sequential changes of serum complement in HAA related arthritis. N. Engl. J. Med., 287:103, 1972.
4. Dienstag, J.L., et al.: Urticaria associated with acute viral hepatitis type B: Studies of pathogenesis. Ann. Intern. Med., 89:34–40, 1978.
5. Dixon, F.J., et al.: Pathogenesis of serum sickness. Arch. Pathol., 65:18–28, 1958.
6. Duffy, J., et al.: Polyarthritis, polyarteritis, and hepatitis B. Medicine, 55:19–37, 1976.
7. Farivar, M., et al.: Cryoprotein complexes and peripheral neuropathy in a patient with chronic active hepatitis. Gastroenterology, 71:490–493, 1976.
8. Fernandez, R., and McCarty, D.J.: The arthritis of viral hepatitis. Ann. Intern. Med., 74:207–211, 1971.
9. Inman, R.D.: Rheumatic manifestations of hepatitis B infection. Semin. Arthritis Rheum., 11:406–420, 1982.
10. McCarty, D.J., and Ormiste, V.: Arthritis and HB Ag-positive hepatitis. Arch. Intern. Med., 132:264–268, 1973.
11. McKenna, P.J., et al.: Hepatitis and arthritis with hepatitis-associated antigen in serum and synovial fluid. Lancet, 2:214–215, 1971.
12. Mosley, J., and Galambos, J.: Viral hepatitis. In Diseases of the Liver. Edited by L. Schiff. Philadelphia, J.B. Lippincott Co., 1969.
13. Onion, S.K., Crumpacker, C.S., and Gilliland, B.C.: Arthritis of hepatitis associated with Australia antigen. Ann. Intern. Med., 75:29–33, 1971.
14. Schumacher, H.R., and Gall, E.P.: Arthritis in acute hepatitis and chronic active hepatitis. Am. J. Med., 57:655–664, 1974.
15. Segool, R.A., Lejtenyi, C., and Jaussig, L.M.: Articular and cutaneous prodromal manifestations of viral hepatitis. J. Pediatr., 87:709–712, 1975.
16. Shumaker, J.B., et al.: Arthritis and rash. Arch. Intern. Med., 133:438–485, 1974.
17. Wands, J.R., et al.: The pathogenesis of arthritis associated with acute hepatitis-B surface antigen-positive hepatitis. J. Clin. Invest., 55:930–936, 1975.
18. Wenzel, R.P., et al.: Arthritis and viral hepatitis. Arch. Intern. Med., 130:770–771, 1972.

Rubella (including vaccine-induced)

19. Austin, S.M., et al.: Joint reactions in children vaccinated against rubella. Am. J. Epidemiol., 95:53–58, 1972.
20. Chambers, R.J., and Bywaters, E.G.L.: Rubella synovitis. Ann. Rheum. Dis., 22:263–267, 1963.
21. Cooper, L.Z., et al.: Transient arthritis after rubella vaccination. Am. J. Dis. Child., 118:218–225, 1969.
22. Farquhar, J.D., and Curretjer, J.E.: Clinical experience with Cendehill rubella vaccine in mature women. Am. J. Dis. Child., 118:266–268, 1969.
23. Ford, D.K., et al.: Synovial mononuclear cell responses to rubella antigen in rheumatoid arthritis and unexplained persistent knee arthritis. J. Rheumatol., 9:420–423, 1982.
23a. Fraser, J.R.E., et al.: Rubella arthritis in adults. Isolation of virus, cytology and other aspects of the synovial reaction. Clin. Exp. Rheumatol., 1:287–293, 1983.
24. Geiger, J.C.: Epidemic of German measles in a city adjacent to an army cantonment. J.A.M.A., 70:1818, 1918.
25. Gilmartin, Jr., R.C., Jabbour, J.T., and Duenas, D.A.: Rubella vaccine myeloradiculoneuritis. J. Pediatr., 80:406–412, 1972.
26. Gold, J.A., Prinzie, A., and McKee, J.: Adult women vaccinated with rubella vaccine. Am. J. Dis. Child., 118:264–265, 1969.
27. Grahame, R., et al.: Chronic arthritis associated with the presence of intrasynovial rubella virus. Ann. Rheum. Dis., 42:2–13, 1983.
28. Grand, M.G., et al.: Clinical reactions following rubella vaccination. J.A.M.A., 220:1,569–1,572, 1972.
29. Hildebrandt, H.M., and Maasab, H.F.: Rubella synovitis in a one-year-old-patient. N. Engl. J. Med., 274:1,428–1,429, 1966.
30. Horstmann, D.M., Liebhaber, H., and Kohorn, E.I.: Post-partum vaccination of rubella-susceptible women. Lancet, 2:1003–1006, 1970.

31. Johnson, R.E., and Hall, A.P.: Rubella arthritis. Report of cases studied by latex tests. N. Engl. J. Med., *258*:743–745, 1958.

32. Kantor, T.G., and Tanner, M.: Rubella arthritis and rheumatoid arthritis. Arthritis Rheum., *5*:378–383, 1962.

33. Kilroy, A.W., et al.: Two syndromes following rubella immunization. Clinical observations and epidemiological studies. J.A.M.A., *214*:2287–2292, 1970.

34. Lee, P.R., et al.: Rubella arthritis. A study of twenty cases. California Med., *93*:125–128, 1960.

35. Lerman, S.J., et al.: Immunologic response, virus excretion, and joint reactions with rubella vaccine. Ann. Intern. Med., *74*:67–72, 1971.

36. Loudon, I.S.L.: Polyarthritis in rubella. Br. Med. J., *1*:1388, 1953.

37. Ogra, P.L., and Herd, J.K.: Arthritis associatd with induced rubella infection. J. Immunol., *107*:810–813, 1971.

38. Panush, R.S.: Serum hypocomplementemia with rubella arthritis. Case report. Milit. Med., *140*:117–120, 1975.

39. Plotkin, S.A., Farquhar, J.D., and Ogra, P.L.: Immunologic properties of RA27/3 rubella virus vaccine. J.A.M.A., *225*:585–590, 1973.

40. Rogers, K.D., et al.: Clinical response to immunization with Cendehill strain rubella vaccine. Pediatrics, *47*:7–14, 1971.

41. Spruance, S.L., et al.: Chronic arthropathy associated with rubella vaccination. Arthritis Rheum., *20*:741, 1977.

42. Spruance, S.L., et al.: Recurrent joint symptoms in children vaccinated with HPV-77 DK12 rubella vaccine. J. Pediatr., *80*:413–417, 1972.

43. Spruance, S.L., and Smith, C.B.: Joint complications associated with derivatives of HPV-77 rubella vaccine. Am. J. Dis. Child., *122*:105–111, 1971.

44. Thompson, G.R., et al.: Intermittent arthritis following rubella vaccination. Am. J. Dis. Child., *125*:526–530, 1973.

45. Thompson, G.R., Ferreyra, A., and Brackett, R.G.: Acute arthritis complicating rubella vaccination. Arthritis Rheum., *14*:19–26, 1971.

46. Vergani, D., et al.: Joint symptoms, immune complexes, and rubella (letter). Lancet, *2*:321, 1980.

47. Weibel, R.E., et al.: Rubella vaccination in adult females. N. Engl. J. Med., *280*:682–685, 1969.

48. Yanez, J.E., et al.: Rubella arthritis. Ann. Intern. Med., *64*:772–777, 1966.

Arboviruses

49. Anderson, S.G., and French, E.L.: An epidemic exanthem associated with polyarthritis in the Murray Valley, 1956. Med. J. Aust., *2*:113–117, 1957.

50. Clarke, A.J., Marshall, I.D., and Gard, G.: Annually recurrent epidemic polyarthritis and Ross River virus activity in a coastal area of New South Wales. Am. J. Trop. Med. Hyg., *22*:543–550, 1973.

51. Clarris, B.J., et al.: Epidemic polyarthritis: A cytological, virological, and immunochemical study. Aust. N.Z. J. Med., *5*:450–457, 1975.

52. Deller, J.J., and Russell, P.K.: Chikungunya disease. Am. J. Trop. Med. Hyg., *17*:107–111, 1968.

53. Doherty, R.L., et al.: Epidemic polyarthritis. Occurrence in Eastern Australia 1959–1970. Med. J. Aust., *1*:5–8, 1971.

54. Doherty, R.L., et al.: Studies of arthropod-borne virus infections in Queensland. V. Survey of antibodies to group A arboviruses in man and other animals. Aust. J. Exp. Biol. Med. Sci., *44*:365–377, 1966.

55. Doherty, R.L., et al.: The isolation of a third group A arbovirus in Australia, with preliminary observations on its relationship to epidemic polyarthritis. Aust. J. Sci., *26*:183–189, 1963.

56. Doherty, R.L., Carley, J.G., and Best, J.C.: Isolation of Ross River virus from man. Med. J. Aust., *1*:1,083–1,084, 1972.

57. Dowling, P.G.: Epidemic polyarthritis. Med. J. Aust., *1*:245–246, 1946.

58. Fraser, J.R.E., et al.: Cytology of synovial effusions in epidemic polyarthritis. Aust. N.Z. J. Med., *11*:168, 1981.

59. Fraser, J.R.E., et al.: Possible genetic determinants in epidemic polyarthritis caused by Ross River virus infection. Aust. N.Z. J. Med., *10*:597–603, 1980.

60. Fuller, C.O., and Warner, P.: Some epidemiological and laboratory observations on an epidemic rash and polyarthritis occurring in the upper Murray region of South Australia. Med. J. Aust., *2*:117–120, 1957.

61. Gard, G., Marshall, I.D., and Woodroofe, G.M.: Annually recurrent epidemic polyarthritis and Ross River virus activity in a coastal area of New South Wales. II. Mosquitoes, viruses, and wildlife. Am. J. Trop. Med. Hyg., *22*:551–559, 1973.

62. Haddow, A.J., Davies, C.W., and Walker, A.J.: O'nyong-nyong fever: An epidemic virus disease in East Africa. I. Introduction. Trans. R. Soc. Trop. Med. Hyg., *54*:517–522, 1960.

63. Kennedy, A.C., Fleming, J., and Solomon, L.: Chikungunya viral arthropathy: A clinical description. J. Rheumatol., *7*:231–236, 1980.

64. Lumsden, W.H.R.: An epidemic of virus disease in southern province, Tanganyika territory, in 1952–53. II. General description and epidemiology. Trans. R. Soc. Trop. Med. Hyg., *49*:33–57, 1955.

65. Malherbe, H., Strickland-Cholmley, M., and Jackson, A.L.: Sindbis virus infection in man. Report of a case with recovery of virus from skin lesions. S. Afr. Med. J., *37*:547–552, 1963.

66. McIntosh, M., et al.: Illness caused by Sindbis and west Nile viruses in South Africa. S. Afr. Med. J., *38*:291–294, 1964.

67. Moore, D.L., et al.: Arthropod-borne viral infections of man in Nigeria, 1964–1970. Ann. Trop. Med. Parasitol., *69*:49–64, 1975.

68. Moore, D.L., et al.: An epidemic of chikungunya fever in Ibadan, Nigeria, 1969. Ann. Trop. Med. Parasitol., *68*:59–68, 1974.

69. Nimmannitya, S., et al.: Dengue and chikungunya virus infection in man in Thailand, 1962–1964. I. Observations on hospitalized patients with hemorrhagic fever. Am. J. Trop. Med. Hyg., *18*:954–972, 1969.

70. Pinheiro, F.P., et al.: An outbreak of Mayaro virus disease in Belterra, Brazil. Am. J. Trop. Med. Hyg., *30*:674–681, 1981.

71. Robinson, M.C.: An epidemic of virus disease in southern province, Tanganyika territory, in 1952–53. I. Clinical features. Trans. R. Soc. Trop. Med. Hyg., *49*:28–32, 1955.

72. Ross, R.W.: The Newala epidemic. III. The virus: Isolation, pathogenic properties and relationship to the epidemic. J. Hyg., *54*:177–191, 1956.

73. Seglenieks, Z., and Moore, B.W.: Epidemic polyarthritis in South Australia: Report of an outbreak in 1971. Med. J. Aust., *2*:552–556, 1974.

74. Shope, R.E., and Anderson, S.G.: The virus etiology of epidemic exanthem and polyarthritis. Med. J. Aust., *1*:156–158, 1960.

75. Shore, H.: O'nyong-nyong fever: An epidemic virus disease in East Africa. III. Some clinical and epidemiological observations in the northern province of Uganda. Trans. R. Soc. Trop. Med. Hyg., *55*:361–373, 1961.

76. Sibree, E.W.: Acute polyarthritis in Queensland. Med. J. Aust., *2*:565–567, 1944.

77. Taylor, R.M., et al.: Sindbis virus: A newly recognized arthropod-transmitted virus. Am. J. Trop. Med. Hyg., *4*:844, 1955.

78. Tesh, R.B.: Arthritides caused by mosquito-borne viruses. Ann. Rev. Med., *33*:31–40, 1982.

79. Tesh, R.B., et al.: The distribution and prevalence of group A arbovirus neutralizing antibodies among human populations in southeast Asia and the Pacific Islands. Am. J. Trop. Med. Hyg., *24*:664–675, 1975.

80. Weinbren, M.P., Haddow, A.J., and Williams, M.C.: The occurrence of chikungunya virus in Uganda. Trans. R. Soc. Trop. Med. Hyg., *52*:253–262, 1958.

81. Williams, M.C., Woodhall, J.P., and Gillett, J.D.: O'nyong-nyong fever: An epidemic virus disease in East

Africa. VII. Virus isolations in man and serological studies up to July 1961. Trans. R. Soc. Trop. Med. Hyg., *59*:186–197, 1965.
82. Williams, M.C., Woodhall, J.P., and Portersfield, J.S.: O'nyong-nyong fever: An epidemic virus disease in East Africa. V. Human antibody studies by plaque inhibition and other serological tests. Trans. R. Soc. Trop. Med. Hyg., *56*:166–172, 1962.

Mumps

83. Appelbaum, E., et al.: Mumps arthritis. Arch. Intern. Med., *90*:217–223, 1952.
84. Caranasos, G.J., and Felker, J.R.: Mumps arthritis. Arch. Intern. Med., *119*:394–398, 1967.
85. Filpi, R.G., and Houts, R.L.: Mumps arthritis. J.A.M.A., *205*:216–217, 1968.
86. Ghosh, S.K., and Reddy, T.A.: Arthralgia and myalgia in mumps. Rheumatol. Rehab., *12*:97–99, 1973.
87. Gold, H.E., Boxerbaum, B., and Leslie, Jr., H.J.: Mumps arthritis. Am. J. Dis. Child., *116*:547–548, 1968.
88. Gordon, S.C., and Lauter, C.B.: Mumps arthritis: Unusual presentation as adult Still's disease. Ann. Intern. Med., *97*:45–47, 1982.
89. Lass, R., and Shephard, E.: Mumps arthritis. Br. Med. J., *2*:1613–1614, 1961.
90. Solem, J.H.: Mumps arthritis without parotitis. Scand. J. Infect. Dis., *3*:173–175, 1971.
91. Tracey, J.P., and Riggenbach, R.D.: Mumps arthritis associated with positive latex fixation reaction. South. Med. J., *63*:1,122–1,123, 1970.

Smallpox (including vaccinia)

92. Cockshott, P., and MacGregor, M.: Osteomyelitis variolosa. Q. J. Med., *27*:369–387, 1958.
93. Silby, H.M., et al.: Acute monoarticular arthritis after vaccination. Ann. Intern. Med., *62*:347–350, 1965.

Adenovirus Type 7

94. Panush, R.S.: Adenovirus arthritis. Arthritis Rheum., *17*:534–536, 1974.
95. Rahal, J.J., Millian, S.J., and Noriega, E.R.: Coxsackie and adenovirus infection. J.A.M.A., *235*:2,496–2,501, 1976.
96. Utsinger, P.D.: Immunologic study of arthritis associated with adenovirus infection (abstract). Arthritis Rheum., *20*:138, 1977.

Herpes Viruses

97. Adebonojo, F.O.: Monoarticular arthritis: An unusual manifestation of infectious mononucleosis. Clin. Pediatr., *11*:549–550, 1972.
98. Cunningham, A.L., et al.: A study of synovial fluid and cytology in arthritis associated with herpes zoster. Aust. N.Z. J. Med., *9*:440–443, 1979.
99. Devereaux, M.D., and Hazelton, R.A.: Acute monoarticular arthritis in association with herpes zoster (letter). Arthritis Rheum., *26*:236, 1983.
100. Friedman, A., and Naveh, Y.: Polyarthritis associated with chickenpox. Am. J. Dis. Child., *122*:179–180, 1971.
101. Friedman, H.M., et al.: Acute monoarticular arthritis caused by herpes simplex virus and cytomegalovirus. Am. J. Med., *69*:241–247, 1980.
102. Hamerman, D., Gresser, I., and Smith, C.: Isolation of cytomegalovirus from synovial cells of a patient with rheumatoid arthritis. J. Rheumatol., *9*:658–664, 1982.
103. Mulhern, L.M., Friday, G.A., and Perri, J.A.: Arthritis complicating varicella infection. Pediatrics, *48*:827–829, 1971.

104. Pascual-Gomez, E.: Identification of large mononuclear cells in varicella arthritis (letter). Arthritis Rheum., *23*:519, 1980.
105. Pollack, S., Enat, R., and Barzilai, D.: Monoarthritis with heterophile-negative infectious mononucleosis: Case of an older patient. Arch. Intern. Med., *142*:1,109–1,111, 1980.
106. Priest, J.R., et al.: Varicella arthritis documented by isolation of virus from joint fluid. J. Pediatr., *93*:990, 1978.
107. Ray, C.G., et al.: Acute polyarthritis associated with active Epstein-Barr virus infection. J.A.M.A., *248*:2990–2993, 1982.
108. Schooley, R.T., and Dolin, R.: Epstein-Barr virus (infectious mononucleosis). *In* Principles and Practice of Infectious Diseases. Edited by G.L. Mandell, R.G. Douglas, Jr., and J.E. Bennett. New York, John Wiley & Sons, Inc., 1979.
109. Shelley, W.B.: Herpetic arthritis associated with disseminate herpes simplex in a wrestler. Br. J. Dermatol., *103*:209–212, 1980.
110. Shuper, A., et al.: Varicella arthritis in a child. Arch. Dis. Child., *55*:568–569, 1980.
111. Sigal, L.H., Steere, A.C., and Niederman, J.C.: Symmetric polyarthritis associated with heterophile-negative infectious mononucleosis. Arthritis Rheum., *26*:553–556, 1983.
112. Urman, J.D., and Bobrove, A.M.: Acute polyarthritis and infectious mononucleosis. West. J. Med., *136*:151–153, 1982.
113. Ward, J.R., and Bishop, B.: Varicella arthritis. J.A.M.A., *212*:1954, 1970.

Enteroviruses

114. Blotzer, J.W., and Myers, A.R.: Echovirus-associated polyarthritis. Arthritis Rheum., *21*:978–981, 1978.
115. Hurst, N.P., et al.: Coxsackie B infection and arthritis. Br. Med. J., *286*:605, 1983.
116. Rahal, J.J., Millian, S.J., and Noriega, E.R.: Coxsackie and adenovirus infection. J.A.M.A., *235*:2,496–2,501, 1976.
117. Sanford, J.P., and Sulkin, S.E.: The clinical spectrum of ECHO-virus infection. N. Engl. J. Med., *261*:1,113–1,121, 1959.

Erythema Infectiosum

118. Ager, E.A., Chin, T.D.Y., and Poland, J.D.: Epidemic erythema infectiosum. N. Engl. J. Med., *275*:1,326–1,331, 1966.
119. Auriemma, P.R.: Erythema infectiosum: Report on a familial outbreak. Am. J. Public Health, *44*:1,450–1,454, 1954.
120. Lawton, A.L., and Smith, R.E.: Erythema infectiosum. Arch. Intern. Med., *47*:28–41, 1941.
121. Shaw, H.L.K.: Erythema infectiosum. Am. J. Med. Sci., *129*:16–22, 1905.

Transient Polyarthritis

122. Greenwood, B.M.: Acute tropical polyarthritis. Q. J. Med., *38*:295–306, 1969.
123. Jeremy, R., et al.: Clinical and laboratory studies of a distinctive type of arthritis observed in New Guinea. Med. J. Aust., *1*:1,273–1,279, 1969.
124. Panush, R.S.: Acute arthritis associated with febrile viral-like respiratory syndromes. J. Rheumatol., *1*:299–307, 1974.
125. Price, G.D., et al.: An outbreak of "infectious" polyarthritis in a Haida Indian family. Arthritis Rheum., *66*:633–638, 1963.
126. Schumacher, H.R., and Kitridou, R.C.: Synovitis of recent onset: A clinicopathologic study during the first month of disease. Arthritis Rheum., *15*:465–485, 1972.

Chapter 104

Lyme Disease

Allen C. Steere and Stephen E. Malawista

Lyme disease, originally called Lyme arthritis, was recognized in 1975 because of close geographic clustering in Lyme, Connecticut, of children affected with what was thought to be juvenile rheumatoid arthritis.[35] The illness, now known to be a complex multisystem disorder, usually begins in summer with a characteristic rash called erythema chronicum migrans (ECM) and associated symptoms.[25,34] These manifestations are sometimes followed weeks to months later by cardiac[28] or neurologic abnormalities,[22] and weeks to years later by arthritis.[29,32,34] Lyme disease is caused by a spirochete[4,6,27] that is transmitted by *Ixodes dammini* or related ixodid ticks.[36,39,45] The disorder is associated with characteristic immunologic abnormalities.[14,15,33,37] Patients with severe and prolonged illness often have the B-cell alloantigen, DR2.[31,32] Early in the illness, when ECM is present, oral tetracycline or penicillin therapy shortens the duration of the skin lesion and often prevents the subsequent manifestations.[26,30] The later stages respond to high-dose parenteral penicillin.[35a,40] The known geographic distribution of the disease includes at least 14 states,[9] Europe,[1,13,16,19] and Australia.[41]

PATHOGENESIS

Lyme disease is caused by a newly recognized spirochete that resembles treponemes in its number of flagellae, but its other morphologic features and growth characteristics are like borreliae (Fig. 104–1).[27] The spirochete was first recovered from the tick vector, *I. dammini*, in 1982 in modified Kelly's medium[3,17,42] and subsequently from patient specimens,[4,27] although recovery from patients has been difficult. Of 142 specimens cultured from 56 patients in our study in 1982, three yielded spirochetes: one each from blood, from a skin-biopsy specimen of ECM (the leading edge), and from cerebrospinal fluid.[27] In a study on Long Island, the organism was recovered from the blood of 2 of 36 patients with early Lyme disease.[4] It has not been cultured from joint fluid or synovium.

We believe that the *I. dammini* spirochete either is injected into the skin or blood in tick saliva[36] or is deposited in fecal material on the skin.[6] After an incubation period of 3 to 32 days, the organism probably migrates outward in the skin producing ECM. It is then spread in lymph (regional adenopathy), or is disseminated in blood to organs (e.g., brain and presumably liver or spleen) or to other skin sites (secondary annular lesions). The secondary skin lesions probably do not result from several tick bites because such lesions may be numerous and lack indurated centers. Later in the illness when arthritis is present, therapeutic and immunologic[15] evidence suggests that spirochetes are still alive, and probably in affected joints.

Lyme disease is associated with characteristic immunologic abnormalities.[14,15,33,37] At the beginning of the illness, when ECM is present, many patients have circulating immune complexes.[14,15] At that time, the findings of elevated serum IgM levels and cryoglobulins containing IgM, which correlate directly, predict subsequent nervous system, heart, or joint involvement.[33,37] Serial determinations of serum IgM are often the single most helpful laboratory indicator of disease activity. These abnormalities tend to persist during neurologic or cardiac involvement. Later in the illness, when arthritis is present, serum IgM levels are more often normal, circulating immune complexes and cryoglobulins are usually absent but, as in rheumatoid arthritis, they are found uniformly in joint fluid. Patients who develop neurologic or joint disease have an increased frequency of the B-cell alloantigen, DR2.[31,32]

EPIDEMIOLOGY

Lyme disease seems to occur primarily in three distinct foci in the United States: in the Northeast from Massachusetts to Maryland, in the Midwest in Wisconsin and Minnesota, and in the West in California and Oregon.[9,39] The occurrence of cases correlates closely with the known distribution and frequency of infection of *I. dammini* in the Northeast and Midwest and *I. pacificus* in the West. Cases have also been reported in other states,[9] Germany,[1] Switzerland,[13] France,[16,19] and Australia.[41] Although the overall frequency of Lyme disease is unknown, 444 of the 12,000 residents of the Lyme area are known to have contracted it—a cumulative frequency of 4%[27]—and 858 individuals had participated in Lyme disease studies at Yale University

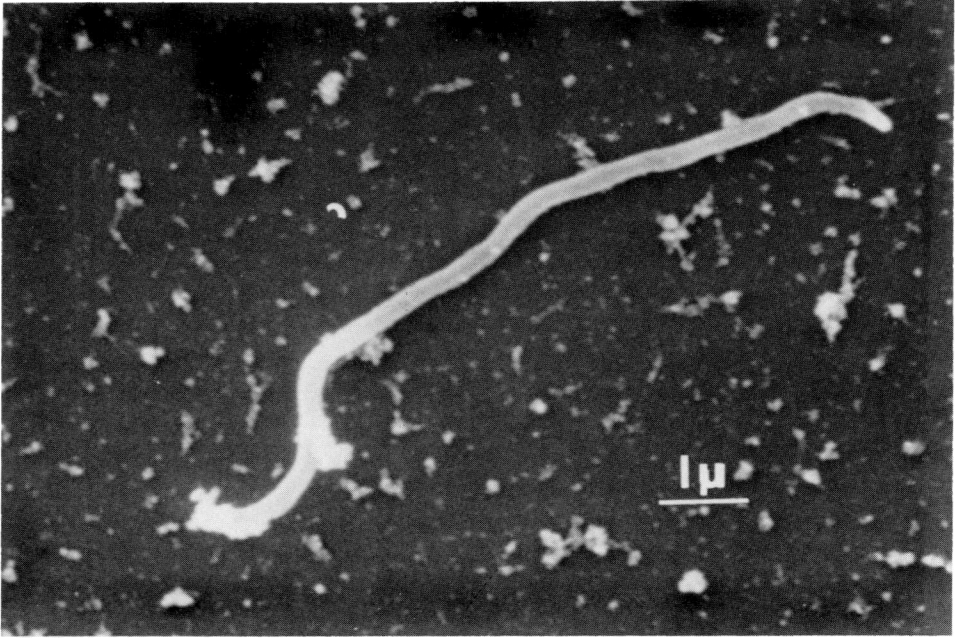

Fig. 104–1. Scanning electron micrograph of the *Ixodes dammini* spirochete. Its length ranges from 4 to 30 μm, and its transverse diameter is about 0.2 μm.

as of 1982. The earliest known cases occurred on Cape Cod in 1962 and in Lyme in 1965.[39] Each year, more individuals have been affected than in the preceding year. In our studies, the ages of patients have ranged from 2 to 88 years (median 28 years), and the sex ratio is nearly one to one.[25] Age-adjusted attack rates show that the risk of acquiring the illness is similar in all age groups through the fourth decade; thereafter, the risk drops, presumably because older residents are less likely to be exposed to tick-infected areas.[38] Onset of the illness is generally between May 1 and November 30 with the majority of cases occurring in June or July.[25]

The vector of Lyme disease is the minute tick, *I. dammini*, or related ixodid ticks.[7,24,36,39,45] Of 314 patients examined from 1976 through 1982, 31% recalled a tick bite at the skin site where ECM developed 3 to 32 days later.[25] Six patients saved the implicated tick, which was identified in all as nymphal *I. dammini*.[39] In addition, the histology of ECM is compatible with that of an arthropod bite.[25,34] The peak questing periods for adult *I. dammini* are spring and fall; for nymphs, May through July; and for larvae, August and September.[8,20] The nymphal stages seems to be primarily responsible for transmission of the disease.[25,39] In concomitant studies of patients and arthropods on both sides of the Connecticut River, the incidence of Lyme disease was almost 30 times as great,[36]

and the number of *I. dammini* on preferred hosts (mice and deer) was over 12 times as great on the east (Lyme) side compared to the west side of the river.[45]

The *I. dammini* spirochete has been recovered from both the vector and animal hosts. In Connecticut, we obtained 21 isolates from 110 nymphal or adult *I. dammini*.[27] In a study on Shelter Island, New York, the prevalence by immunofluorescence was 60%.[6] Spirochetes that are similar, if not identical, to the *I. dammini* agent have been recovered from *I. pacificus* on the West coast[7] and from *I. ricinus* in Europe.[3] The organism has also been isolated from the blood of white-footed mice, a raccoon, and white-tailed deer.[2,5,18] Spirochetal antibody has been found in gray squirrels, chipmunks, opossums, white-footed mice, raccoons, dogs, and deer.[18] Because immature *I. dammini* are aggressive and feed on many animal species, the potential for growth and spread of the organism seems great.

CLINICAL CHARACTERISTICS

As with other spirochetal infections, Lyme disease generally occurs in stages, with remissions and exacerbations and different clinical manifestations at each stage. Although the stages may overlap or occur alone, the illness usually begins with ECM and associated symptoms (stage 1), followed weeks to months later by neurologic or cardiac abnormalities (stage 2), and weeks to years later by arthritis (stage 3). The early symptoms of headache, stiff neck, conjunctivitis, muscle and joint pain, and profound weakness and the neurologic and cardiac abnormalities are reminiscent of other spirochetal infections.[12,23,44] In addition, frank arthritis has been described as a rare feature of leptospirosis,[43] syphilis,[21] and relapsing fever.[23] However, the dermatologic manifestations of Lyme disease, particularly ECM, and the late manifestations, consisting primarily of intermittent or chronic arthritis, seem to be unique.

Early Manifestations

Erythema chronicum migrans, the unique clinical marker for Lyme disease, usually begins as a red macule or papule (Fig. 104–2A, Table 104–1).[25,34] As the area of redness around the center expands (final median diameter, 15 cm; range 3 to 68 cm), most lesions continue to have bright red outer borders (usually flat, but occasionally raised) and partial central clearing (flat) (Fig. 104–2B). The centers of early lesions sometimes become intensely erythematous and indurated, vesicular, or necrotic. In some instances, migrating lesions remain an even intense red, several red rings are found within the outside one, or the central area turns blue before it clears. Although the lesion can be located anywhere, the thigh, groin, and axilla are particularly common sites. The lesion is warm to the touch, but not often painful.

Within several days after onset of the initial skin

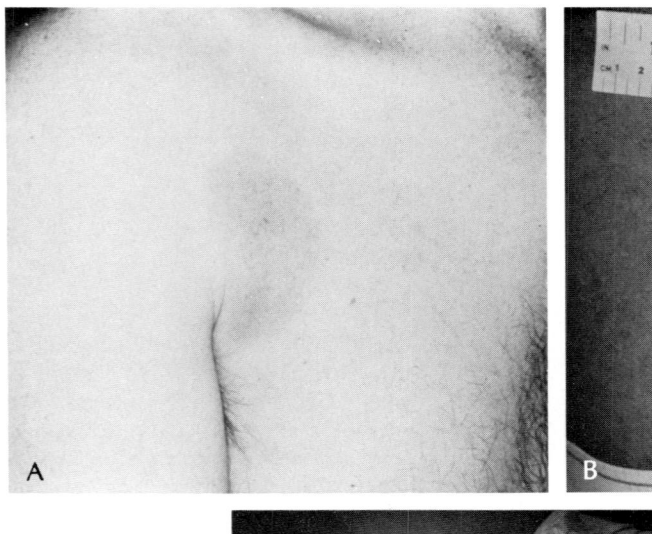
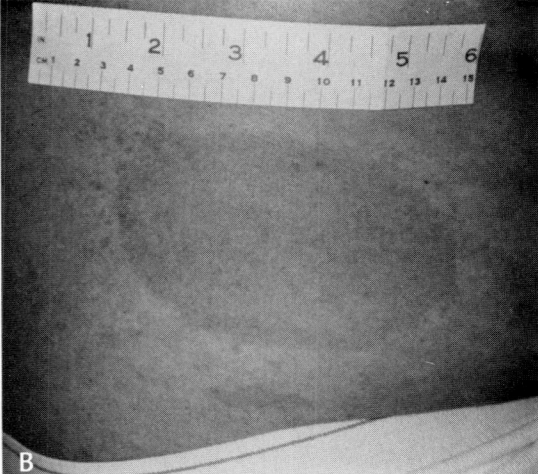
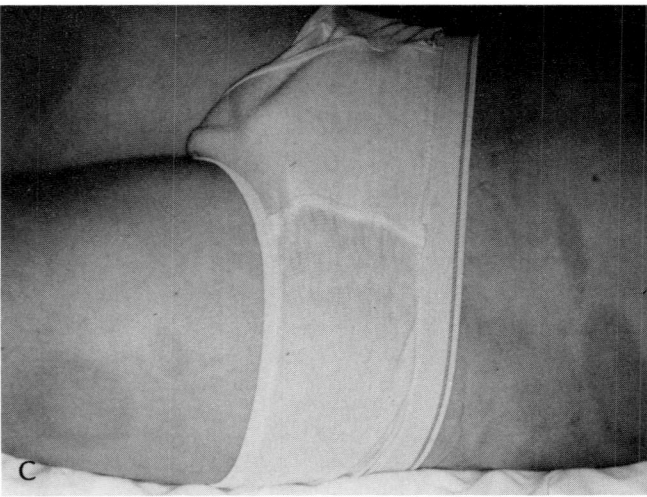

Fig. 104–2. Dermatologic manifestations of Lyme disease. *A*, Erythema chronicum migrans (ECM). An early lesion is seen 4 days after detection. *B*, In a 10-day-old lesion of ECM, the red outer ring has expanded and central clearing is beginning. *C*, Eight days after onset of ECM, similar secondary lesions have appeared, and several of their borders have merged. (From Steere, A.C., et al.[25])

Table 104–1. Early Signs of Lyme Disease

	No. of Patients	
Signs	N = 314	(%)
Erythema chronicum migrans	314	(100)*
Multiple annular lesions	150	(48)
Lymphadenopathy		
Regional	128	(41)
Generalized	63	(20)
Pain on neck flexion	52	(17)
Malar rash	41	(13)
Erythematous throat	38	(12)
Conjunctivitis	35	(11)
Right upper quadrant tenderness	24	(8)
Splenomegaly	18	(6)
Hepatomegaly	16	(5)
Muscle tenderness	12	(4)
Periorbital edema	10	(3)
Evanescent skin lesions	8	(3)
Abdominal tenderness	6	(2)
Testicular swelling	2	(1)

*Erythema chronicum migrans was required for inclusion in this study. (From Steere, A.C., et al.[25])

Table 104–2. Early Symptoms of Lyme Disease

	No. of Patients	
Symptoms	N = 314	(%)
Malaise, fatigue, and lethargy	251	(80)
Headache	200	(64)
Fever and chills	185	(59)
Stiff neck	151	(48)
Arthralgias	150	(48)
Myalgias	135	(43)
Backache	81	(26)
Anorexia	73	(23)
Sore throat	53	(17)
Nausea	53	(17)
Dysesthesia	35	(11)
Vomiting	32	(10)
Abdominal pain	24	(8)
Photophobia	19	(6)
Hand stiffness	16	(5)
Dizziness	15	(5)
Cough	15	(5)
Chest pain	12	(4)
Ear pain	12	(4)
Diarrhea	6	(2)

(From Steere, A.C., et al.[25])

lesion (ECM), almost half of patients develop multiple annular secondary lesions (Fig. 104–2C) (Table 104–1).[25,34] Although their appearance is similar to that of initial lesions, they are generally smaller, migrate less, and lack indurated centers; they are not associated with previous tick bites. Individual lesions sometimes appear and fade at different times, and their borders sometimes merge. During this period, some patients develop malar rash, conjunctivitis, or, rarely, diffuse urticaria. ECM and secondary lesions usually fade within 3 to 4 weeks (range 1 day to 14 months). However, during or soon after their resolution, patients may develop new evanescent lesions (small 2- to 3-cm red circles or blotches) for several more weeks. On a given day, these lesions appear at different sites, but individual lesions do not migrate. Any of the dermatologic manifestations of the illness may recur.

Skin involvement is often accompanied by malaise and fatigue, headache, fever, and chills (Table 104–2).[25,34] In addition, patients sometimes experience meningeal irritation, mild encephalopathy, migratory musculoskeletal pain, hepatitis, generalized lymphadenopathy or splenomegaly, sore throat, nonproductive cough, or testicular swelling. Except for fatigue and lethargy, which are often constant, the early signs and symptoms are typically intermittent and changing. For example, a patient may experience predominantly headache and stiff neck for several days. After a few days of improvement, musculoskeletal pain may begin. Associated symptoms may occur several days before ECM and, conversely, may last for months

(particularly fatigue and lethargy) after the skin lesions have disappeared.

Later Manifestations

Neurologic Findings. Symptoms suggestive of meningeal irritation may occur at the beginning of the illness when ECM is present.[22] Such individuals often have episodic attacks of excruciating headache and neck pain, stiffness, or pressure, typically lasting for hours. During the first 1 or 2 weeks of illness, such symptoms are not associated with spinal fluid pleocytosis or objective neurologic deficit. However, after several weeks to months, about 15% of patients develop frank neurologic abnormalities, including meningitis, encephalitis, chorea, cranial neuritis (including bilateral facial palsy), motor and sensory radiculoneuritis, mononeuritis multiplex, or myelitis, in various combinations. The usual pattern is fluctuating meningoencephalitis with superimposed cranial (particularly facial palsy) and peripheral radiculoneuropathy (Fig. 104–3); facial palsy may occur alone. At this time, patients with meningitic symptoms have a lymphocytic pleocytosis (about 100 cells/mm³) in cerebrospinal fluid and often diffuse slowing on electroencephalograms. Neck stiffness is usually found only on extreme flexion; Kernig and Brudzinski signs are absent. Neurologic abnormalities typically last for months, but usually resolve completely.

Cardiac Findings. Within several weeks after the onset of illness, about 8% of patients develop

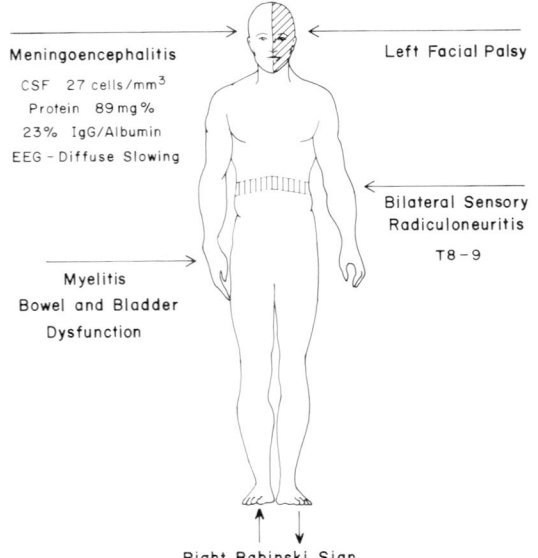

Meningoencephalitis
CSF 27 cells/mm³
Protein 89 mg %
23% IgG/Albumin
EEG - Diffuse Slowing

Left Facial Palsy

Bilateral Sensory
Radiculoneuritis
T 8 - 9

Myelitis
Bowel and Bladder
Dysfunction

Right Babinski Sign

Fig. 104–3. Neurologic abnormalities of Lyme disease that occurred in a 58-year-old man. Three weeks after the onset of erythema chronicum migrans, the patient developed meningoencephalitis, left facial palsy, and bilateral sensory radiculoneuritis. Although long-tract signs are an unusual finding in Lyme disease, this patient had bowel and bladder dysfunction and a right Babinski sign suggestive of myelitis.

cardiac involvement.[28] The most common abnormality is fluctuating degrees of atrioventricular block (first degree, Wenckebach, or complete heart block). Some patients have more diffuse cardiac involvement, including electrocardiographic changes compatible with acute myopericarditis, radionuclide evidence of mild left ventricular dysfunction or, rarely, cardiomegaly. None have had heart murmurs. The duration of cardiac involvement is usually only 3 days to 6 weeks, but it may recur.

Arthritis. Within a few weeks to 2 years after the onset of illness, about 60% of patients develop arthritis.[29,32,34] The typical pattern of early involvement is migratory pain in joints, tendons, bursae, muscle, or bone, often without joint swelling. Pain tends to affect only one or two sites at a time and usually lasts a few hours to several days in a given location.

Frank arthritis with marked joint swelling usually does not begin until months after the onset of the illness. At that time, patients often experience intermittent attacks of swelling and pain in one or two joints, primarily in large joints such as the knee. Affected knees are commonly more swollen than painful. The overlying skin is often warm but rarely red; Baker's cysts may form and rupture

early. However, both large and small joints may be affected, and a few patients have developed symmetrical polyarthritis. Arthritis attacks that generally subside after a few weeks or months typically recur for several years. Fatigue commonly accompanies active joint involvement, but fever and other systemic symptoms are unusual.

Joint fluid white cell counts vary from 500 to 110,000 cells/mm³ with an average of about 25,000 cells/mm³, most of which are polymorphonuclear leukocytes.[34] Total protein ranges from 3 to 8 g/dl. C3 and C4 levels are generally greater than one-third, and fasting glucose levels are usually greater than two-thirds, those of serum.

In about 10% of patients with arthritis, involvement in large joints becomes chronic, with erosion of cartilage and bone (Fig. 104–4A).[10,29,32] Synovial biopsies show surface deposits of fibrin, villous hypertrophy, vascular proliferation, and a heavy infiltration of mononuclear cells, including plasma cells (Fig. 104–4B).[29,32,34] In one patient with chronic Lyme arthritis, synovium grown in tissue culture produced large amounts of collagenase and prostaglandin E_2.[29] Features of Lyme disease resembling RA include joint fluid cell counts; immune reactants, except for rheumatoid factor; synovial histology; and the types and amounts of synovial proteolytic enzymes released. The destruction of cartilage and bone also resembles that of RA. Many agents, including the *I. dammini* spirochete, may be able to trigger a common pathway in the synovium, leading to joint destruction.

LABORATORY TESTS

Culture of the *I. dammini* spirochete from patients permits definitive diagnosis, but has been a low-yield procedure.[27] Similarly, spirochetes are rarely seen by direct examination of blood, plasma, plasma pellets, or skin transudate specimens of ECM.[27] Determination of antibody titers is the most helpful diagnostic test. Specific IgM antibody titers against the *I. dammini* spirochete usually peak between the third and sixth week after disease onset. Specific IgG antibody titers rise slowly and are generally highest months later when arthritis is present (Fig. 104–5).[11,27] Antibody titers are particularly useful in differentiating Lyme disease from other rheumatic syndromes. *I. dammini* spirochetal antibody cross-reacts with other spirochetes, including *Treponema pallidum*, but patients with Lyme disease do not have a positive VDRL test.[11]

The most common nonspecific laboratory abnormalities, particularly early in the illness, are a high erythrocyte sedimentation rate, an elevated serum IgM level, or an increased serum glutamic-oxaloacetic transaminase (SGOT) level (Table

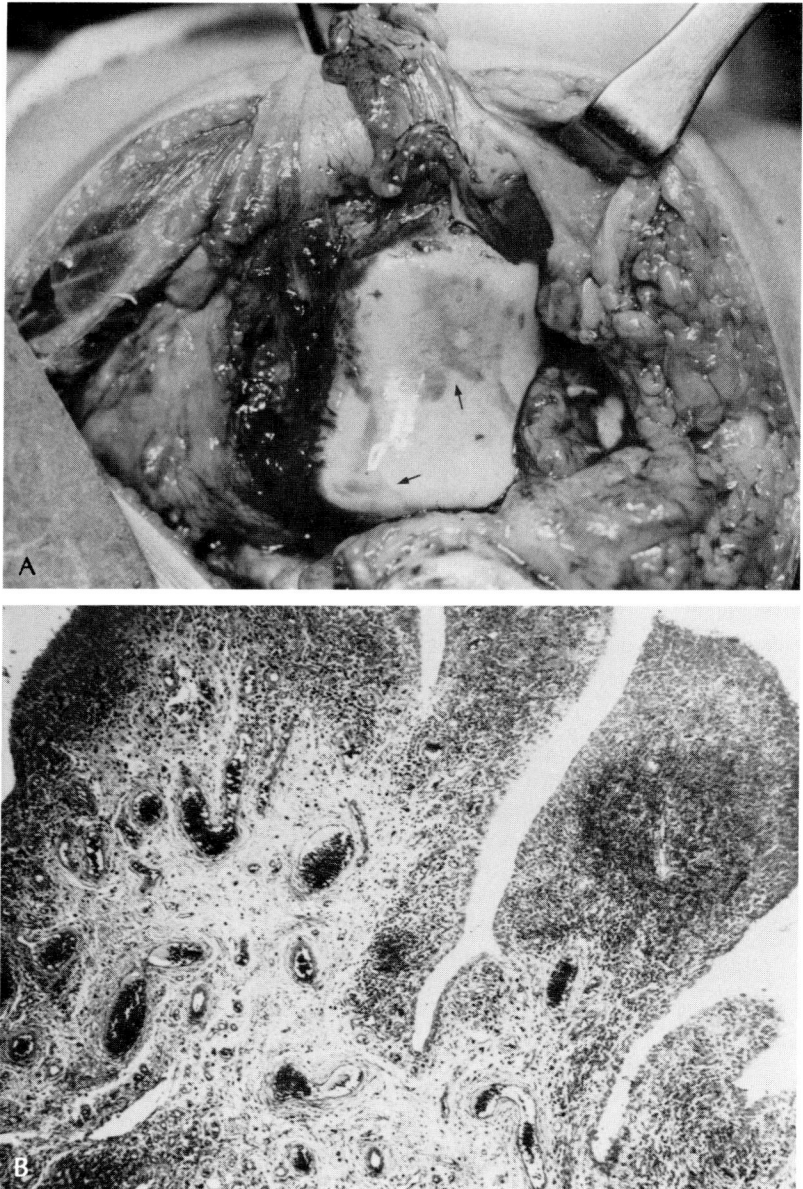

Fig. 104–4. *A,* The knee of a patient with Lyme disease at the time of synovectomy. The patient had typical erythema chronicum migrans in June, 1974 followed by intermittent migratory polyarthritis. Two years later, he developed persistent swelling of the right knee. After 7 months, he underwent a synovectomy. The articular surface of the femur can be seen; the arrows indicate what was the advancing border of pannus, now stripped away from the underlying eroded cartilage. *B,* Tissue structure of affected synovium. Individual polypoid stalks show central edema and vascular proliferation. Surrounding this central core is a rim of predominantly mononuclear cells. In one area an aggregate resembling a lymphoid follicle is seen. (From Steere, A.C., et al.[34])

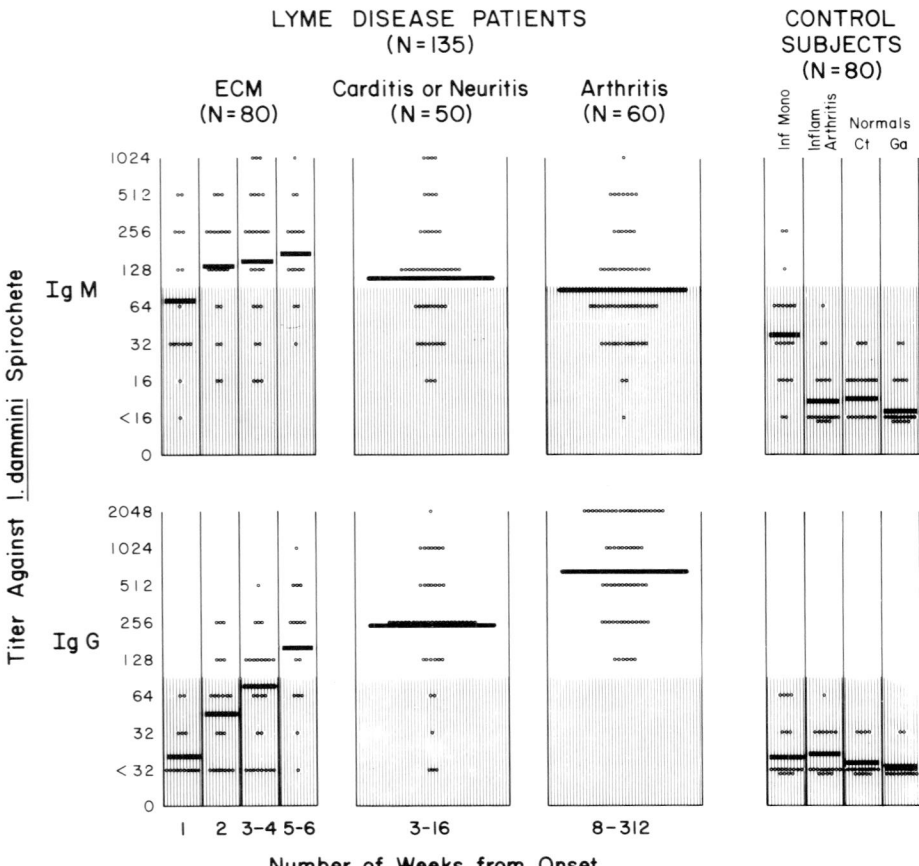

LYME DISEASE PATIENTS
(N=135)

CONTROL
SUBJECTS
(N=80)

Fig. 104–5. Antibody titers against the *Ixodes dammini* spirochete in serum samples from 135 patients with different clinical manifestations of Lyme disease, from 40 control patients with infectious mononucleosis or inflammatory arthritis, and from 40 normal control subjects, determined by indirect immunofluorescence. The heavy bar shows the geometric mean titer for each group; the shaded areas indicate the range of titers generally observed in control subjects. (From Steere, A.C., et al.[27])

104–3).[25,34] Most patients with elevated SGOT levels also have increased levels of serum glutamic-pyruvic transaminase (SGPT) and lactic dehydrogenase (LDH), but no patients have had abnormal creatine phosphokinase (CPK) levels. The enzyme levels generally return to normal within several weeks. Patients may be mildly anemic early in the illness and occasionally have elevated white cell counts with shifts to the left in the differential count. A few patients have microscopic hematuria, sometimes with mild proteinuria. Values for creatinine and blood urea nitrogen (BUN) are normal. Throughout the illness, C3 and C4 levels are generally normal or elevated. Tests for rheumatoid factor or antinuclear antibodies are usually negative.

DIFFERENTIAL DIAGNOSIS

ECM is the unique clinical marker for Lyme disease (see Fig. 104–1). When this lesion is pres-

ent in its classic form, there is little else that might be confused with it. However, in some patients, the lesion expands only slightly, resembling the red papule after an uninfected arthropod bite. In others, the lesion remains an even red as it expands, as in streptococcal cellulitis, or the center becomes vesicular or necrotic, as in tularemia. Patients with secondary lesions might be thought to have erythema multiforme, but we have never noted blistering, mucosal lesions or involvement of the palms and soles. Particularly when multiple lesions are present, a malar rash may occur, as in systemic lupus erythematosus. Rather than typical secondary lesions, a pruritic urticarial rash develops in some patients, similar to the rash in hepatitis B infection or serum sickness. As earlier lesions fade, some patients continue to develop evanescent red blotches and circles. Evanescent lesions may resemble erythema marginatum, but those of Lyme disease do not expand.

Table 104–3.   Laboratory Findings in Early Lyme Disease

Laboratory Test	No. of Patients with Abnormal Values N=314	(%)	Median (Range) of Abnormal Values	
Hematology				
Hematocrit	37	(12)	35	(36–31)
Leukocytes >10 cells × 10³/mm³	24	(8)	12	(11–18)
ESR >20 mm/h	166	(53)	35	(21–68)
Immunoglobulins				
IgM > 250 mg/dl	104	(33)	310	(252– 930)
IgG > 1,500 mg/dl	10	(3)	1580	(1,520–1,760)
IgA > 400 mg/dl	12	(4)	440	(410– 580)
Liver Function				
SGOT > 35 U/ml	59	(19)	71	(36– 251)
SGPT > 32 U/ml*	47	(15)	125	(42– 491)
LDH > 600 U/ml*	49	(16)	775	(608–1,080)
Renal Function				
Microscopic hematuria (red cells/hpf)	18	(6)	15	(10–25)

*Tested only in the 55 patients with abnormal SGOT; CPK was normal in all these patients.
(From Steere, A.C., et al.[25])

The early manifestations of Lyme disease may be confused with viral infections, especially when ECM is absent or overlooked, or is not the first manifestation. The severe headache and stiff neck are reminiscent of aseptic meningitis, abdominal symptoms may suggest hepatitis, and generalized, tender lymphadenopathy and splenomegaly may resemble infectious mononucleosis. As in the last mentioned, profound and persistent fatigue is sometimes a major symptom.

The later manifestations of Lyme disease may mimic several immune-mediated disorders. Sore throat followed by migratory polyarthritis and carditis may suggest rheumatic fever, but we have never seen valvular involvement in Lyme disease. Migratory pain in tendons and joints may also suggest disseminated gonococcal infection. A few patients with neurologic involvement have myelitis, which may be confused with multiple sclerosis, or symmetrical peripheral neuropathy, reminiscent of the Guillain-Barré syndrome. In adults, the large joint effusions, most commonly in knees, resemble those of Reiter's syndrome, and a few patients have had symmetrical polyarthritis, suggestive of RA. In children, arthritis may be identical to the oligoarticular form of juvenile rheumatoid arthritis. However, the duration of attacks is usually shorter, and we have not seen iridocyclitis in Lyme disease.

Treatment

During 1980 and 1981, we compared phenoxymethyl penicillin, erythromycin, and tetracycline in the treatment of early Lyme disease.[26] ECM and its associated symptoms resolved more quickly in patients treated with penicillin or tetracycline than in those given erythromycin (mean duration, 5.4 and 5.7 vs. 9.2 days). More importantly, none of the 39 patients given tetracycline developed major late complications (e.g., myocarditis, meningoencephalitis, or recurrent attacks of arthritis) compared with 3 of 40 patients treated with penicillin (8%) and 4 of 29 given erythromycin (14%) (p = 0.07). In 1982, all 49 adult patients were given tetracycline, again preventing the late disease manifestations. Approximately 10% of patients experienced a Jarisch-Herxheimer-like reaction, consisting of a higher fever, redder rash, or greater pain, during the first 24 hours after the start of therapy.

Thus, early in the illness, tetracycline, 250 mg four times a day, seems to be the drug of choice in adults, followed by phenoxymethyl penicillin, 500 mg four times a day, and erythromycin, 250 mg four times a day. Therapy should be given for at least 10 days, and for up to 20 days if symptoms persist or recur.[26] In children, we recommend phenoxymethyl penicillin 50 mg/kg/day (not less than 1 g/day or more than 2 g/day) in divided doses for the same duration or, in cases of penicillin allergy, erythromycin, 30 mg/kg/day, in divided doses for 15 or 20 days.

Regardless of the antibiotic received, nearly half of patients still experience minor late complications: recurrent episodes of headache or pain in joints, tendons, bursae, or muscles, often accompanied by lethargy.[26] Physical examinations, however, are usually normal. Symptoms are often reminiscent of those experienced at the beginning of the illness, but are generally briefer and less severe. They correlate significantly with the initial severity of the illness. In a given attack, pain usually occurs in one or two sites and lasts from hours to days. With more frequent attacks, pain is often migratory. Some patients may continue to have such attacks for several years. The pathogenesis of these symptoms is unknown.

In patients with frank meningitis, spinal fluid pleocytosis, and cranial or peripheral neuropathies, intravenous penicillin G, 20 million U a day in divided doses for 10 days, is effective.[40] Headache, stiff neck, and radicular pain usually begin to subside by the second day of therapy and are often gone by 7 to 10 days. Patients with motor deficits frequently require 7 to 8 weeks for complete recovery.

Patients with established Lyme arthritis have also been treated successfully with high-dose penicillin.[35a] In a double-blind placebo-controlled trial, 7 of 16 patients given intramuscular benzathine penicillin, 2.4 million units weekly for 3 weeks, were apparently cured (mean follow-up 33 months). All 20 patients given saline continued to have attacks of arthritis. Subsequently, 11 of 20 patients given intravenous penicillin G, 20 million units daily for 10 days, were apparently cured, including two Bicillin failures. Optimal dose, duration, and route of administration are still to be worked out.

REFERENCES

1. Ackermann, R., et al.: Erythema chronicum migrans mit arthritis. Dtsch. Med. Wochenschr., *105*:1779–1781, 1980.
2. Anderson, J.F., et al.: Spirochetes in *Ixodes dammini* and mammals from Connecticut. Am. J. Trop. Med. Hyg., *32*:818–824, 1983.
3. Barbour, A.G., et al.: Isolation of a cultivatable spirochete from *Ixodes ricinus* ticks of Switzerland. Curr. Microbiol., *8*:123–126, 1983.
4. Benach, J.L., et al.: Spirochetes isolated from the blood of two patients with Lyme disease. N. Engl. J. Med., *308*:740–742, 1983.
5. Bosler, E.M., et al.: Natural distribution of the *Ixodes dammini* spirochetes. Science, *220*:321–322, 1983.
6. Burgdorfer, W., et al.: Lyme disease—A tick-borne spirochetosis? Science, *216*:1317–1319, 1982.
7. Burgdorfer, W., and Kierans, J.E.: Ticks and Lyme disease in the United States (editorial). Ann. Intern. Med., *99*:121, 1983.
8. Carey, A.B., Krinsky, W.L., and Main, A.J.: *Ixodes dammini* (Acari: Ixodidae) and associated ixodid ticks in south-central Connecticut, USA. J. Med. Entomol., *17*:89–99, 1980.
9. Centers for Disease Control: Lyme disease. M.M.W.R., *31*:367–368, 1982.
10. Coblyn, J.S., and Taylor, P.: Treatment of chronic Lyme arthritis with hydroxychloroquine. Arthritis Rheum., *24*:1567–1569, 1981.
11. Craft, J.E., Grodzicki, R.L., and Steere, A.C.: The antibody response in Lyme disease: Evaluation of diagnostic tests. J. Infect. Dis., *149*:789–795, 1984.
12. Edwards, G.A., and Domm, B.M.: Human leptospirosis. Medicine, *39*:117–156, 1960.
13. Gerster, J.C., et al.: Lyme arthritis appearing outside the United States: A case report from Switzerland. Br. Med. J., *283*:951–952, 1981.
14. Hardin, J.A., et al.: Circulating immune complexes in Lyme arthritis: Detection by the ^{125}I-Clq binding, Clq solid phase and Raji cell assays. J. Clin. Invest., *63*:468–477, 1979.
15. Hardin, J.A., Steere, A.C., and Malawista, S.E.: Immune complexes and the evolution of Lyme arthritis: Dissemination and localization of abnormal Clq binding activity. N. Engl. J. Med., *301*:1358–1363, 1979.
16. Illouz, G., and Hewitt, J.: A propos de l'arthrite de Lyme: Polyarthrite inflammatoire après un érythème annulaire migrant. Rev. Rhum., *48*:813–815, 1981.
17. Kelly, R.: Cultivation of *Borrelia hermsii*. Science, *173*:443–444, 1971.
18. Magnarelli, L.A., et al.: Parasitism by *Ixodes dammini* (Acari: Ixodidae) and antibodies to spirochetes in mammals in Lyme disease foci of Connecticut, U.S.A. J. Med. Entomol., *21*:52–57, 1984.
19. Mallecourt, J.M., Landurean, M., and Wirth, A.M.: Lyme disease: A clinical case observed in Western France. Nouv. Presse Med., *11*:39, 1982.
20. Piesman, J., and Spielman, A.: Host-associations and seasonal abundance of immature *Ixodes dammini* in southeastern Massachusetts. Ent. Soc. Am., *72*:829–832, 1979.
21. Reginato, A.J., et al.: Synovitis in secondary syphilis: Clinical, light, and electron microscopic studies. Arthritis Rheum., *22*:170–176, 1979.
22. Reik, L., et al.: Neurologic abnormalities of Lyme disease. Medicine, *58*:281–294, 1979.
23. Southern, P.M., Jr., and Sanford, J.P.: Relapsing fever: A clinical and microbiological review. Medicine, *48*:129–149, 1969.
24. Spielman, A., et al.: Human babesiosis on Nantucket Island, USA: Description of the vector, *Ixodes dammini*, N. Sp. (Acarina: Ixodidae). J. Med. Entomol., *15*:218–234, 1979.
25. Steere, A.C., et al.: The early clinical manifestations of Lyme disease. Ann. Intern. Med., *99*:76–82, 1983.
26. Steere, A.C., et al.: Treatment of the early manifestations of Lyme disease. Ann. Intern. Med., *99*:22–26, 1983.
27. Steere, A.C., et al.: The spirochetal etiology of Lyme disease. N. Engl. J. Med., *308*:733–740, 1983.
28. Steere, A.C., et al.: Lyme carditis: Cardiac abnormalities of Lyme disease. Ann. Intern. Med., *93*:8–16, 1980.
29. Steere, A.C., et al.: Elevated levels of collagenase and prostaglandin E$_2$ from synovium associated with erosion of cartilage and bone in a patient with chronic Lyme arthritis. Arthritis Rheum., *23*:591–599, 1980.
30. Steere, A.C., et al.: Antibiotic therapy in Lyme disease. Ann. Intern. Med., *93*:1–8, 1980.
31. Steere, A.C., et al.: Lyme arthritis; Immunologic and immunogenetic markers (abstract). Arthritis Rheum., *22*:662, 1979.
32. Steere, A.C., et al.: Chronic Lyme arthritis: Clinical and immunogenetic differentiation from rheumatoid arthritis. Ann. Intern. Med., *90*:286–291, 1979.
33. Steere, A.C., et al.: Lyme arthritis: Correlation of serum and cryoglobulin IgM with activity and serum IgG with remission. Arthritis Rheum., *22*:471–483, 1979.
34. Steere, A.C., et al.: Erythema chronicum migrans and Lyme arthritis: The enlarging clinical spectrum. Ann. Intern. Med., *86*:685–698, 1977.
35. Steere, A.C., et al.: Lyme arthritis: An epidemic of oligoarticular arthritis in children and adults in three Connecticut communities. Arthritis Rheum., *20*:7–17, 1977.
35a. Steere, A.C., et al.: Curing Lyme arthritis: Successful antibiotic therapy of established joint involvement (abstract). Arthritis Rheum., *27*:S26, 1984.
36. Steere, A.C., Broderick, T.E., and Malawista, S.E.: Erythema chronicum migrans and Lyme arthritis: Epidemiologic evidence for a tick vector. Am. J. Epidemiol., *108*:312–321, 1978.
37. Steere, A.C., Hardin, J.A., and Malawista, S.E.: Erythema chronicum migrans and Lyme arthritis. Cryoimmunoglobulins and clinical activity of skin and joints. Science, *196*:1121–1122, 1977.
38. Steere, A.C., and Malawista, S.E.: The epidemiology of

Lyme disease. *In* Current Topics in Rheumatology: Epidemiology of the Rheumatic Diseases. Proceedings of the Fourth International Conference. Edited by R.C. Lawrence, and L.E. Schulman. New York, Gower Medical Publishing Limited, 1983, pp. 33–42.

39. Steere, A.C., and Malawista, S.E.: Cases of Lyme disease in the United States: Locations correlated with distribution of *Ixodes dammini*. Ann. Intern. Med., *91*:730–733, 1979.

40. Steere, A.C., Pachner, A.R., and Malawista, S.E.: Neurologic abnormalities of Lyme disease: Successful treatment with high-dose intravenous penicillin. Ann. Intern. Med., *99*:767–772, 1983.

41. Stewart, A., et al.: Lyme arthritis in Hunter Valley. Med. J. Aust., *1*:139, 1982.

42. Stoenner, H.G., Dodd, T., and Larsen, C.: Antigenetic variation of *Borrelia hermsii*. J. Exp. Med., *156*:1297–1311, 1982.

43. Sutliff, D.W., Shepard, R., and Dunham, W.B.: Acute *Leptospira pomona* arthritis and myocarditis. Ann. Intern. Med., *39*:134–140, 1953.

44. Tramont, E.C.: *Treponema pallidum*. *In* Principles and Practice of Infectious Diseases. Edited by G.L. Mandel, R.G. Douglas, Jr., and J.E. Bennett. New York, John Wiley & Sons, Inc., 1979, p. 1820.

45. Wallis, R.C., et al.: Erythema chronicum migrans and Lyme arthritis: Field study of ticks. Am. J. Epidemiol., *108*:322–327, 1978.

Index

Page numbers in *italics* indicate illustrations; page numbers followed by "*t*" indicate tables; page numbers followed by "*n*" indicate footnotes.